Effects of Drugs on Clinical Laboratory Tests

FIFTH EDITION

VOLUME TWO
Listing by Drug

Donald S. Young, MD, PhD
Vice-Chair for Laboratory Medicine
Department of Pathology and Laboratory Medicine
University of Pennsylvania
Philadelphia, Pennsylvania, USA

AACC Press
2101 L Street, NW
Suite 202
Washington, DC 20037-1526
www.aacc.org

ISBN 1-890883-24-7

Database design, book assembly, and typography
by Lexi-Comp Inc., Hudson, Ohio, www.lexi.com

INTRODUCTION

This fifth edition of *Effects of Drugs on Clinical Laboratory Tests* contains more than 10,000 additional entries compared with the fourth edition published in 1995. Nonetheless, this number does not reflect the true number of effects of drugs on laboratory tests that have been published in the intervening years. It is impossible for one individual to read all the literature that is published each year concerning the effects on clinical laboratory tests. The primary sources of information of the effects of drugs remain clinical and clinical chemical journals but supplemented by other published information, such as books and manufacturer's product inserts and advertisements.

I have retained the format of the publication from previous editions. The directory is organized in five sections. The first is an index of the tests. Both common and uncommon test names are listed; for those names not used as search terms, the name of the proper search term in indicated. The second section is of drug names. Again, non-search names, often proprietary drug names, are cross-referenced to the actual drugs used in the file. Most of the drugs listed are currently used. Some have been used in the past and some are not used therapeutically. The third section of this publication is a sort of the effects by laboratory test. Within each broad test category there are separate sorts by body fluid, and within these sorts by analytical or physiological effects and whether the effect reported is associated with a decrease, increase, or no effect on the concentration or activity of the analyte. The fourth section is structured similarly, but the sort is by drug. To simplify searches when an analyte is described in either plasma or serum, the fluids are treated as if they were the same unless there are known to be different effects in plasma and serum. For both the third and fourth sections a brief description of the nature of the effect is provided. The final section of the publication lists the references pertinent to the brief descriptions, enabling the reader to get more details of the effects described.

With the expanded number of entries it has become necessary to present the information in two volumes. Each contains the Drug and Test indices. Volume 1 lists the interactions sorted by Test. Volume 2 lists the interactions sorted by Drug. To facilitate easy follow-up of the information listed, the References are included in both volumes.

All the effects described in this publication have been reported in one or more patients. While it is clearly important to describe the magnitude of an effect and the probability of it occurring, much of this important information is not included in the drug effects literature. It is inappropriate to blindly ascribe an effect reported here, e.g., administration of drug A being associated with an increased concentration of analyte X, when confronted with a clinical situation in which a patient is both given drug A and has an increased concentration of analyte X, without considering possible alternative causes of abnormal test results, such as underlying disease or an uncontrolled preanalytical variable. Where the information is contained in an article, I have tried to indicate the possible magnitude of the effect of a drug on a clinical laboratory test. However, many papers do not include such detailed information. In particular, papers published in clinical journals frequently omit details of analytical methods and jump to the conclusion that an effect is an *in vivo* one. It is noteworthy that from edition to edition of this publication the proportion of effects of drugs attributable to interferences with analytical methods has steadily declined. Undoubtedly, this has occurred because of improved methods with greater analytical specificity.

This publication of the *Effects of Drugs on Clinical Laboratory Tests* complements the other publications of the American Association for Clinical Chemistry, of the *Effects of Disease on Clinical Laboratory Tests*, the third edition of which was published in 1997, and the *Effects of Preanalytical Variables on Clinical Laboratory Tests*, the second edition of which also was published in 1997. Together these three publications provide insight into the major causes of alterations of concentrations of a wide range of analytes that are measured in clinical laboratory practice. All three of the publications are oriented more towards unusual conditions than towards the common situation, since the bulk of the contained material is derived from research publications.

In spite of my efforts to minimize the presence and number of errors, it is inevitable that some errors have crept into the files because of the amount of material in the publications of the effects of variables on clinical laboratory tests, and the complexity of the editing process. The errors may be as simple as spelling and grammatical mistakes, but they may also include duplications that I may have overlooked, and conceivably some misinterpretations that I have made of the stated effects. This is why it is very important that no clinician takes any precipitous action with a patient solely on the basis of a report included in the database without very careful consideration of the alleged effect. I would be very grateful if any errors were brought to my attention at donaldyo@mail.med.penn.edu so that I may correct and update the master database.

I am grateful to John Gill of the American Association for Clinical Chemistry for his continued support of the publication of the series of books related to factors affecting the proper interpretation of clinical laboratory test results, to Kenneth Hughes of Lexi-Comp who transforms the single Zip-disk file of Disease, Drug and Preanalytical Variable Effects into the separate hard copies of the series, and to Joyce Dongivin, my secretary, who endlessly downloads the updates of Reference Update (Institute for Scientific Information, Philadelphia, PA) and sends for reprints which provide the bulk of the information included in this and its related publications.

Donald S. Young
October 1999

1 DRUG INDEX

B

C

D

E

F

G

H

I

J

K

L

M

O

P

Q

R

S

T

U

2 LABORATORY TEST INDEX

A

AAP
  see Alanine Aminopeptidase
Abnormal Erythrocytes
Abnormal Leukocytes
Absorbance at 450 nm
ACE
  see Angiotensin-converting Enzyme
Acebutolol
Acecainide
Acenocoumarol
Acetaldehyde
Acetaldehyde Oxidase
Acetaminophen
Acetate
Acetazolamide
Acetoacetate
  see also
    Ketones
Acetoacetate Decarboxylase
Acetoacetic Acid
  see Acetoacetate
Acetone
  see also
    Ketones
Acetyl-N-Ser-Asp-Lys-Pro
Acetylcholine
Acetylcholine Receptor Antibodies
Acetylsalicylic Acid
Acid
α_1-Acid Glycoprotein
Acid Phosphatase
Acid Phosphatase, Prostatic
Acid Phosphatase, Tartrate Resistant
ACP
  see Acid Phosphatase
ACTH
  see Corticotropin
Activated Factor VII
Activated Factor X inhibition
Activated Partial Thromboplastin Time
  see Partial Thromboplastin Time
Activated T Lymphocytes
Acute Phase Reactant
  see C-Reactive Protein
Acyclovir
Acylcarnitine
Acylcarnitine, Long Chain
Acylcarnitine, Short Chain
Acylcholine Acyl Hydrolase
  see Cholinesterase
Adenosine
Adenosine Deaminase Binding Protein
Adenosine Diphosphate
Adenosine Monophosphate
Adenosine Triphosphate
ADH
  see Antidiuretic Hormone
Adipate
Adipic Acid
  see Adipate
Adrenaline
  see Epinephrine
β-Adrenergic Receptors
Adrenocorticotropic Hormone
  see Corticotropin
Adrenocorticotropin
  see Corticotropin
Adriamycin
AFP
  see α-Fetoprotein
Agglutinins
Aggregation Index
AICAR
  see Amino-4-Imidazole-5-Carboxamide Ribotide
ALA
  see δ-Aminolevulinic Acid
Alanine
  see also
    Amino Acids
    Aminoacids
Alanine Aminopeptidase
Alanine Aminotransferase
Albendazole
Albumin
Albumin-corrected Calcium
  see Calcium, Albumin-corrected
Albumin, Glycated
  see Glycated Albumin
Albumin:Globulin Ratio
Alcohol
  see Ethanol
Alcohol Dehydrogenase
Aldehyde Dehydrogenase
Aldolase
Aldosterone
Alendronate
Alfentanil
Alfuzosin
Alkaline DNase
Alkaline Phosphatase
Alkaline Phosphatase, Bone Isoenzyme
Alkaline Phosphatase Isoenzymes
Alkaline Phosphatase, Liver Isoenzyme
Alkaline Phosphatase, Non-bone Isoenzymes
Alkaline Ribonuclease
  see Alkaline RNase
Alkaline RNase
Allopurinol
Allotetrahydrocortisol
Alloxanthine
Alpha$_1$-Acid Glycoprotein
  see α_1-Acid Glycoprotein
Alpha$_1$-Antichymotrypsin
  see α_1-Antichymotrypsin
Alpha$_2$-Antiplasmin
  see α_2-Antiplasmin
Alpidem
Alprazolam
Alprenolol
ALT
  see Alanine Aminotransferase
Aluminum
Amantadine
Amdinocillin
Amikacin
Amino-4-Imidazole-5-Carboxamide Ribotide
Amino Acids
  see also
    α-Amino-N-Butyric Acid
    β-Aminoisobutyric Acid
    Arginine
    Asparagine
    Citrulline
    Glutamine
    Glycine
    Homocystine
    Leucine
    Lysine
    Methylhistidine
    Sarcosine
    Serine
    Threonine
    Tyrosine
    Valine
Amino Nitrogen
  see α-Amino-Nitrogen
α-Amino-Nitrogen
Amino-terminal Peptide of Procollagen III
  see Amino-terminal Propeptide of Type III Procollagen
Amino-terminal Propeptide of Type I Procollagen
Amino-terminal Propeptide of Type III Procollagen
Aminobenzoic Acid
β-Aminobutyric Acid
γ-Aminobutyric Acid
Aminoglycosides
Aminohippurate
Aminohippuric Acid
  see Aminohippurate
Aminolevulinate
  see δ-Aminolevulinic Acid
Aminolevulinic Acid
  see δ-Aminolevulinic Acid
δ-Aminolevulinic Acid
Aminolevulinic Acid Dehydrase
δ-Aminolevulinic Acid Dehydrase
  see Aminolevulinic Acid Dehydrase

B

C

D

E

F

I

K

L

M

N

Q

R

S

T

3 DRUG LISTINGS

Abciximab

Blood *Urine Increase Physiological* Major bleeding at one or more sites observed in 11.1% of 695 patients following bolus injection and minor bleeding in 15.4%. With bolus injection and infusion major bleeding observed in 14.1% and minor bleeding in 16.9% *1707*

Hematocrit *Blood Decrease Physiological* Anemia observed in 1.2% of 678 patients treated with bolus injection and infusion compared with 0.4% after placebo *1707*

Hemoglobin *Blood Decrease Physiological* Anemia observed in 1.2% of 678 patients treated with bolus injection and infusion compared with 0.4% after placebo *1707*

Leukocytes *Blood Increase Physiological* Leukocytosis observed in 1.0% of 678 patients treated with bolus injection and infusion compared with 0.1% after placebo *1707*

Occult Blood *Feces Increase Physiological* Major bleeding at one or more sites observed in 11.1% of 695 patients following bolus injection and minor bleeding in 15.4%. With bolus injection and infusion major bleeding observed in 14.1% and minor bleeding in 16.9% *1707*

Platelets *Blood Decrease Physiological* Thrombocytopenia with platelet count below 50,000 cells/µL observed in 1.6% of 708 patients treated with bolus injection and infusion compared with 0.7% after placebo and to below 100,000 cells/µL in 5.2% of the drug treated group and 3.4% of the placebo-treated group *1707*

Acarbose

1,5-Anhydroglucitol *Serum Increase Physiological* In 16 patients with NIDDM treatment with acarbose (100 mg tds) for one week caused a nonsignificant change in concentration from 18.4 ± 3.2 µmol/L to 19.3 ± 3.1 µmol/L *2730*

Body Mass Index *Patient No Effect Physiological* In 8 individuals treated with 100 mg t.i.d. acarbose for 4 months mean weight changed nonsignificantly from baseline of 32.2 ± 2.3 kg/sq m to 31.7 ± 2.4 kg/sq m *992*

Cholesterol *Serum Decrease Physiological* In 47 patients with NIDDM treated with 300 mg/d for 24 weeks if cholesterol concentration initially low no significant change observed but if high concentration decreased from 273 mg/dL to 251 mg/dL (upper tercile) *3517* In 47 patients with NIDDM treatment with 300 mg/d for 24 weeks caused mean reduction of 40 mg/dL (14%) when initial concentrations above 260 mg/dL *3517*

C-Peptide *Plasma No Effect Physiological* No significant change observed in 47 noninsulin dependent diabetics when treated with 300 mg/d for 24 weeks *2432*

Fatty Acids (FFA), Free *Serum Decrease Physiological* In 16 patients with NIDDM treatment with acarbose (100 mg tds) for one week caused a significant change in concentration from 583 ± 65 µmol/L pretreatment to 403 ± 52 µmol/L following treatment *2730*

Fructosamine *Serum Decrease Physiological* In 16 patients with NIDDM treatment with acarbose (100 mg tds) for one week caused a nonsignificant reduction in concentration from 405 ± 20 µmol/L to 386 ± 15 µmol/L *2730*

Glucose *Serum Decrease Physiological* In 47 NIDDM patients treatment with 300 mg/d for 24 weeks caused significant reduction especially in post-prandial state *3517* In 47 NIDDM patients treatment with 300 mg/d for 24 weeks caused significant reduction, especially in post-prandial state *3517* In 14 type I diabetics 300 mg/d for 6 weeks in addition to insulin caused mean concentration to decrease from 9.7 mmol/L to 8.5 mmol/L *3794* In 8 individuals treated with 100 mg t.i.d. acarbose mean concentration changed significantly following standard breakfast with area under 12-h concentration curve from baseline of 74.3 ± 2.5 $mmol.h^{-1}.L^{-1}$ to 63.6 ± 1.4 $mmol.h^{-1}L^{-1}$ *992* In 47 patients with noninsulin dependent diabetes treatment with 300 mg/d for 24 weeks caused decrease of fasting concentration from mean of 9.8 mmol/L to 8.4 mmol/L but with even greater effect on postprandial glucose concentration *2432* In 20 patients with NIDDM given 300 mg/d caused decrease of fasting blood glucose concentration from baseline of 155 mg/dL to 140 mg/dL after 12 weeks and 143 mg/dL after 24 weeks, and a reduction of post-prandial increase from mean baseline of 83 mg/dL to 55 mg/dL after 12 weeks and 65 mg/dL after 24 weeks *4310*

Serum No Effect Physiological In 8 individuals treated with 100 mg t.i.d. acarbose for 4 months mean concentration changed nonsignificantly from baseline of 5.1 ± 0.2 mmol/L to 5.0 ± 0.2 mmol/L *992*

Urine Decrease Physiological In 16 patients with NIDDM treatment with acarbose (100 mg tds) for one week caused a significant reduction in excretion from 687 ± 172 mmol/d to 298 ± 166 mmol/d *2730*

Glucose Tolerance *Serum Increase Physiological* In 20 patients with NIDDM given 300 mg/d caused increase after 24 weeks in the responders *4310*

HDL-Cholesterol *Serum Increase Physiological* Continuous increase observed in 47 patients with NIDDM treated with 300 mg/d for 24 weeks but change comparable to that observed with placebo *3517*

Serum No Effect Physiological Although concentration steadily increased during treatment of 47 patients with NIDDM when treated with 300 mg/d for 24 weeks similar effect observed with placebo *3517* In 8 individuals treated with 100 mg t.i.d. acarbose for 4 months mean concentration changed nonsignificantly from baseline of 1.13 ± 0.07 mmol/L to 1.10 ± 0.07 mmol/L *992*

Hemoglobin A_{1c} *Blood Decrease Physiological* In 20 patients with NIDDM given 300 mg/d caused decrease from baseline of 6.6% to 6.2% after 12 weeks and 6.4% after 24 weeks *4310* In 47 patients with noninsulin dependent diabetes treatment with 300 mg/d for 24 weeks caused significant decrease (concentration with placebo 9.32%, with acarbose 8.65%) *2432* In 14 type I diabetics 300 mg/d for 3 months in addition to insulin caused decrease from mean of 9.6% to 8.3% *3794* Significant reduction observed in 47 patients with NIDDM treated with 300 mg/d for 24 weeks *3517*

Acarbose *(continued)*

Hemoglobin A_{1c} *(continued)*
Blood No Effect Physiological In 8 individuals treated with 100 mg t.i.d. acarbose for 4 months mean concentration changed nonsignificantly from baseline of 5.9 ± 0.3% to 5.9 ± 0.1% *992*

Insulin *Plasma Decrease Physiological* Postprandial insulin markedly lowered in 47 patients with NIDDM when treated with 300 mg/d for 24 weeks *3517* Significant reduction observed in 47 patients with NIDDM treated with 300 mg/d for 24 weeks especially post-prandially *3517* In 8 individuals treated with 100 mg t.i.d. acarbose mean concentration changed significantly following standard breakfast with area under 12-h concentration curve from baseline of 7.9 ± 0.9 $nmol.h^{-1}.L^{-1}$ to 4.9 ± 0.6 $nmol.h^{-1}L^{-1}$*992*
Plasma No Effect Physiological No significant difference from placebo group in 47 patients with noninsulin dependent diabetes mellitus treated with 300 mg/d for 24 weeks although postprandial insulin increment 30% lower after 24 weeks *2432* In 8 individuals treated with 100 mg t.i.d. acarbose for 4 months mean concentration changed nonsignificantly from baseline of 144 ± 23 pmol/L to 140 ± 30 pmol/L *992*

Triglycerides *Serum Decrease Physiological* In 47 patients with NIDDM treatment with 300 mg/d caused reduction of 19% at 4 weeks, 26% at 8 weeks, 22% at 12 weeks, 24% at 16 weeks, 13% at 20 weeks and 18% at 24 weeks: all greater than reduction observed with placebo *3517* In 8 individuals treated with 100 mg t.i.d. acarbose for 4 months mean concentration changed nonsignificantly from baseline of 2.45 ± 0.65 mmol/L to 1.88 ± 0.36 mmol/L *992*
Serum No Effect Physiological No significant difference in fasting concentration from placebo observed in 47 patients with NIDDM when treated with 300 mg/d for 24 weeks although 1 h post-prandial concentration significantly less with acarbose *3517*

ACE Inhibitors

Bicarbonate *Serum No Effect Physiological* In 194 outpatients using ACE inhibitors mean concentration 27.6 ± 3.2 mmol/L not significantly different compared with 28.2 ± 2.7 mmol/L in 194 controls *4884*

Cholesterol *Serum No Effect Physiological* Treatment of hypertensive patients with normal lipid profiles caused no statistically significant change in concentration *3730*

Creatinine *Serum Increase Physiological* In 194 outpatients using ACE inhibitors mean concentration 120 ± 39 µmol/L compared with 103 ± 25 µmol/L in 194 controls *4884*

Endothelial Leukocyte Adhesion Molecule-1
Serum Increase Physiological In 8 patients receiving angiotensin-convertinginhibitors for 3 months mean concentration increased from 30.1 ± 3.4 ng/mL to 44.1 ± 7.3 ng/mL after 3 months *1496*

Fractional Excretion of Lithium
Urine Increase Physiological In healthy individuals the administration of ACE inhibitors increases urinary fractional excretion of lithium *4399*

Glomerular Filtration Rate *Urine Increase Physiological* In healthy individuals the administration of ACE inhibitors increases GFR *4399*

Glucose *Serum Decrease Physiological* Incidence of 0.8% observed in French Pharmacovigilance database *4106*
Serum No Effect Physiological In 194 outpatients using ACE inhibitors mean concentration 8.8 ± 4.6 mmol/L not significantly different compared with 8.5 ± 3.8 mmol/L in 194 controls *4884*

HDL-Cholesterol *Serum Increase Physiological* Treatment for 12 months of hypertensive patients caused mean 2.6 mg/dL increase in concentration: more marked in patients with hypercholesterolemia *3730*
Serum No Effect Physiological Treatment of hypertensive patients with normal lipid profiles caused no statistically significant change in concentration *3730*

Intercellular Adhesion Molecule-1
Serum No Effect Physiological In 8 patients receiving angiotensin-convertinginhibitors for 3 months mean concentration increased nonsignificantly from 550 ± 63 ng/mL to 564 ± 57 ng/mL after 3 months *1496*

LDL-Cholesterol *Serum Decrease Physiological* Treatment for 12 months of hypertensive patients caused mean 4.2 mg/dL decrease in concentration: more marked in patients with hypercholesterolemia *3730*
Serum No Effect Physiological Treatment of hypertensive patients with normal lipid profiles caused no statistically significant change in concentration *3730*

Potassium *Serum Increase Physiological* In 1818 outpatients using ACE inhibitors 11% developed hyperkalemia *4884*

Sildenafil *Serum No Effect Physiological* CYP2D6 inhibitors such as ACE inhibitors did not affect the pharmacokinetics of sildenafil *4657*

Sodium *Urine Increase Physiological* In healthy individuals the administration of ACE inhibitors increases urinary excretion of sodium *4399*

Triglycerides *Serum Decrease Physiological* Treatment for 12 months of hypertensive patients caused mean 4.2 mg/dL decrease in concentration: more marked in patients with hypercholesterolemia *3730*
Serum No Effect Physiological Treatment of hypertensive patients with normal lipid profiles caused no statistically significant change in concentration *3730*

Tumor Necrosis Factor-α *Serum Increase Physiological* In 8 patients receiving angiotensin-convertinginhibitors for 3 months mean concentration increased from 2.49 ± 0.3 pg/mL to 2.98 ± 0.5 pg/mL after 3 months *1496*

Urea Nitrogen *Serum Increase Physiological* In 194 outpatients using ACE inhibitors mean concentration 8.0 ± 3.7 mmol/L compared with 6.2 ± 2.2 mmol/L in 194 controls *4884*

VLDL-Cholesterol *Serum No Effect Physiological* Treatment of hypertensive patients with normal lipid profiles caused no statistically significant change in concentration *3730*

Acebutolol

Alanine Aminotransferase *Serum Increase Physiological* A small number of cases develop liver function abnormalities with treatment *6569*

Albumin *Serum Decrease Physiological* Significant change in 9 patients with hyperthyroidism within 4 hours of beginning treatment with 200 mg daily but no change observed after one week *3077*

Alkaline Phosphatase *Serum Increase Physiological* A small number of cases develop liver function abnormalities with treatment *6569*

Antinuclear Antibodies *Serum Increase Physiological* Observed in 18.6% diabetics with drug versus 3.8% in normals and 1.3% in diabetics without drug *3456* In 3 of 11 patients treated for 48 weeks: readministration after titer became negative resulted in significant rise *608* In 20% of 35 men and 44% of 23 women in comparison with 10.2% in men and 12.9% women with other antihypertensive drugs *656* Has been associated with the development of antinuclear antibodies with treatment *6569* Developed in 8 of 9 patients treated for 12 to 24 weeks *1072*

Apolipoprotein A-I *Serum No Effect Physiological* Increase by 1 mg/dL in 11 patients given 400 mg daily for 3 mo *4213*

Apolipoprotein B *Serum No Effect Physiological* Decrease by -2 mg/dL in 11 patients given 400 mg daily for 3 mo *4213*

Apolipoprotein C-II *Serum No Effect Physiological* No change in 11 patients given 400 mg daily for 3 mo *4213*

Apolipoprotein C-III *Serum No Effect Physiological* Increase by 1 mg/dL in 11 patients given 400 mg daily for 3 mo *4213*

Apolipoprotein E *Serum No Effect Physiological* Increase by 1 mg/dL in 11 patients given 400 mg daily for 3 mo *4213*

Aspartate Aminotransferase *Serum Increase Physiological* A small number of cases develop liver function abnormalities with treatment *6569*

Bilirubin *Serum Increase Physiological* A small number of cases develop liver function abnormalities with treatment *6569*

Calcium *Serum No Effect Physiological* No significant change in albumin-corrected calcium in 9 patients with hyperthyroidism treated with 200 mg daily for one week *3077*

Cholesterol *Serum Decrease Physiological* Statistically significant reduction in 109 patients with mild essential hypertension treated with 400 mg daily for 2 months *1300* In 132 patients with stage I diastolic hypertension treated with 400 mg/d caused significant reduction from mean baseline of 6.03 ± 1.05 mmol/L by - 0.33 ± 0.06 mmol/L after 12 months and - 0.30 ± 0.06 mmol/L after 48 months *2335*
Serum No Effect Physiological Insignificant change on average in one 6 mo long study *3499* In several studies of about 15 patients treated for 1 to 12 mo *141* In small numbers of patients when treated for 1-12 mo *142* Decrease by -3 mg/dL in 11 patients given 400 mg daily for 3 mo *4213*

Creatinine *Serum Increase Physiological* Significant increase observed over one week in 9 patients with hyperthyroidism treated with 200 mg daily for one week *3077*
Serum No Effect Analytical At 100 mg/L on reversed phase liquid chromatographic procedure of Zhiri et al *6656*

Digoxin *Serum No Effect Physiological* No significant interaction observed *6569*

Fatty Acids (FFA), Free *Serum Decrease Physiological* Significant reduction in 18 patients treated for 6 mo *3501* Significant effect after one month's treatment and then plateaued *3499*

Glucose Tolerance *Serum Decrease Physiological* Increased glucose at 60 and 120 minutes without impaired release of insulin *3501*

HDL-Cholesterol *Serum Decrease Physiological* Slight effect, but no change in ratio of HDL/total cholesterol *3499* Reduction of 11.7% observed in 129 patients with mild essential hypertension after treatment for 2 months with 400 mg daily *1300* But insignificantly in 18 patients treated for 6 mo *3501*
Serum No Effect Physiological In small numbers of patients when treated for 1-12 mo *142* In several studies of about 15 patients treated for 1 to 12 mo *141* In 132 patients with stage I diastolic hypertension treated with 400 mg/d caused insignificant change from mean baseline of 1.14 ± 0.33 mmol/L by - 0.01 ± 0.02 mmol/L after 12 months and - 0.01 ± 0.02 mmol/L after 48 months *2335* Decrease by -2 mg/dL in 11 patients given 400 mg daily for 3 mo *4213* Insignificant change on average in one 6 mo long study *3499*

Hydrochlorothiazide *Serum No Effect Physiological* No significant interaction observed *6569*

17-Ketosteroids *Urine Increase Analytical* Dose dependent increase of concentration when determined by Zimmermann procedure. Same effect produced by acetylated acebutolol *4421*

Lactate Dehydrogenase *Serum Increase Physiological* A small number of cases develop liver function abnormalities with treatment *6569*

LDL-Cholesterol *Serum Decrease Physiological* In 132 patients with stage I diastolic hypertension treated with 400 mg/d caused significant reduction from mean baseline of 4.21 ± 0.92 mmol/L by - 0.26 ± 0.06 mmol/L after 12 months and - 0.30 ± 0.06 mmol/L after 48 months *2335*
Serum No Effect Physiological Insignificant change on average in one 6 mo long study *3499* In several studies of about 15 patients treated for 1 to 12 mo *141* In small numbers of patients when treated for 1-12 mo *142*

LE Cells *Blood Positive Physiological* Observed in several patients treated for 12 to 24 weeks *1072*

Phosphate *Serum Increase Physiological* In 9 patients with hyperthyroidism treated with 200 mg daily for 1 week significant increase within 4 hours and remained high for 1 week *3077*

Potassium *Serum No Effect Physiological* No significant change in 9 patients with hyperthyroidism treated with 200 mg daily for 1 week *3077*

Sodium *Serum No Effect Physiological* No significant change in 9 patients with hyperthyroidism treated with 200 mg daily for one week *3077*

Sulfinpyrazone *Serum No Effect Physiological* No significant interaction observed *6569*

Tirofiban *Serum No Effect Physiological* Coadministration had no significant effect on plasma clearance of tirofiban *3957*

Tolbutamide *Serum No Effect Physiological* No significant interaction observed *6569*

Tramadol *Serum No Effect Physiological* No significant interaction observed *6569*

Triglycerides *Serum No Effect Physiological* Insignificant change on average in one 6 mo long study *3499* No significant effect observed in 109 patients with mild essential hypertension treated with 400 mg daily for 2 months and no change observed after 6 months *1300* In small numbers of patients when treated for 1-12 mo *142* In several studies of about 15 patients treated for 1 to 12 mo *141* Increase by 1 mg/dL in 11 patients given 400 mg daily for 3 mo *4213* In 132 patients with stage I diastolic hypertension treated with 400 mg/d caused change from mean baseline of 1.49 ± 0.77 mmol/L by - 0.11 ± 0.06 mmol/L after 12 months and + 0.01 ± 0.06 mmol/L after 48 months *2335*

Uric Acid *Serum No Effect Analytical* At 100 mg/L on reversed phase liquid chromatographic procedure of Zhiri et al *6656*

VLDL-Cholesterol *Serum No Effect Physiological* In small numbers of patients when treated for 1-12 mo *142* In several studies of about 15 patients treated for 1 to 12 mo *141*

Warfarin *Plasma No Effect Physiological* No significant interaction observed *6569*

Acecarbromal

Bromide *Serum Increase Physiological* Theoretical possibility since drug contains 29% bromide *5116*

Acenocoumarol

Phenytoin *Serum No Effect Physiological* Interactions not been reported (and unlikely to occur due to different routes of elimination) *5966*

Prothrombin Time *Plasma Increase Physiological* Lowers prothrombin of blood: intended action *51*

Tolbutamide *Serum Increase Physiological* Half-life increased in one patient with coadministration probably due to inhibition of liver metabolism *4636*

Uric Acid *Urine No Effect Physiological* No uricosuric action observed *2452*

Acetaminophen

Acid Phosphatase *Serum No Effect Analytical* At concentration of 200 µg/mL (1.3 mmol/L) had no effect on method on Du Pont Dimension *1562*

Alanine Aminotransferase *Serum Increase Analytical* On colorimetric method at 10 times therapeutic concentration *2919*
Serum Increase Physiological In 20 healthy men given acetaminophen 4 g/d in one ALT activity increased to 121 U/L on day 20 *3345* Hepatic necrosis with dose of 10 g reported *678* In 21 patients who had taken accidental overdose peak activity of 2557 ± 3061 U/L and of 1384 ± 2918 U/L in 50 patients with suicidal intent *5344* Manifestation usually of single toxic high dose ingestion in suicide attempt. Liver damage usually of centrizonal hemorrhagic hepatic necrosis *6666*
Serum No Effect Analytical No effect at 300 mg/L on method on Ames Seralyzer *5706* At acute overdose concentration (10 mg/dL) on Technicon SMAC® method *6266* On continuous method at 10 times maximal therapeutic concentration *2919* No effect at 200 mg/L on Boehringer Mannheim Reflotron method *5706* No effect at concentration of 200 µg/mL (1.3 mmol/L) on method on Du Pont Dimension *1563*

Albumin *Serum Decrease Physiological* In severe cases of poisoning (also in some mild) *5824*
Serum No Effect Analytical At 5 times therapeutic concentration on BCG methods on Technicon SMAC® , Ektachem® 400, Hitachi® 705 and KDA *3525* At concentration of 200 mg/L had no effect on Kodak Ektachem® method *5706* At concentration of 1500 mg/L had no effect on BCG method *5704* At acute overdose concentration (10 mg/dL) on Technicon SMAC® method *6266* At concentration of 200 µg/mL (1.3 mmol/L) had no effect on method on Du Pont Dimension *1564* No interference observed at a concentration of 8 mg/L (53 µmol/L) with method used on Du Pont aca *1507*
Urine No Effect Analytical Using a fluorimetric assay with Albumin Blue 580 on a Cobas Fara centrifugal analyzer for the detection of microalbuminuria no significant interference was detected at a concentration of 100 mg/L *3117*

Acetaminophen *(continued)*

Alkaline Phosphatase *Serum Increase Analytical* On continuous method at 10 times maximal therapeutic concentration *2919*
Serum Increase Physiological In severe cases of poisoning (also in some mild) *5824* With overdose and centrolobular hepatic necrosis usually associated with high drug concentration *2894*
Serum No Effect Analytical At concentration of 200 µg/mL (1.3 mmol/L) had no effect on method on Du Pont Dimension *1565* At acute overdose concentration (10 mg/dL) on Technicon SMAC® method *6266*

Alkaline Phosphatase, Bone Isoenzyme
Serum No Effect Analytical At a concentration of 200 mg/L had no effect on Tandem-MP Ostase method *777*

Amino Acids *Urine Increase Analytical* Metabolite reacting with ninhydrin migrates near dihydroxyphenylalanine with 2-dimensional high voltage electrophoresis *5518* False band on high voltage electrophoresis with ninhydrin staining *4717*

Ammonia *Plasma No Effect Analytical* No effect at concentration of 200 µg/mL (1.3 mmol/L) on method on Du Pont Dimension *1566* At concentration of 50 mg/L had no effect on Kodak Ektachem® method *5704*

Ammonium Ions *Urine No Effect Physiological* Without overdose not usually any effect *4777*

Amylase *Serum Increase Physiological* In 26 patients with acetaminophen overdose median activity on admission 50.5 U/L (range 19 - 149 U/L) compared with adult reference range of 0 - 80 U/L. Increase above reference range observed in 31% patients *1340*
Serum No Effect Analytical At 5 times therapeutic concentration on maltotriose method on Du pont aca, maltotetrose method on Roche Cobas-Bio and amylopectin method on Kodak Ektachem® *3525* At concentration of 200 µg/mL (1.3 mmol/L) had no effect on method on Du Pont Dimension *1567* At concentration of 200 mg/L had no effect on method on Boehringer Mannheim Reflotron system *5706*

Amylase, Pancreatic Isoenzyme
Serum Decrease Analytical At toxic concentration of 200 mg/L significant reduction in activity observed with method on Boehringer Mannheim Reflotron *3647*

Apolipoprotein A-I *Serum No Effect Analytical* At a concentration of 86 µmol/L no significant effect observed on automated immunoturbidimetric method on Baxter Paramax analyzer *3005*

Apolipoprotein B *Serum No Effect Analytical* At a concentration of 86 µmol/L no significant effect observed on automated immunoturbidimetric method on Baxter Paramax analyzer *3005*

Aspartate Aminotransferase *Serum Decrease Analytical* On continuous method at 10 times maximal therapeutic concentration *2919*
Serum Increase Analytical At therapeutic concentration may affect Technicon SMA 12/60 method *5576*
Serum Increase Physiological In 21 patients who had taken accidental overdose peak activity of 7430 ± 10309 U/L and of 1501 ± 3555 U/L in 50 patients with suicidal intent *5344* With overdose and centrolobular hepatic necrosis usually associated with high drug concentration *2894* In 20 healthy men given acetaminophen 4 g/d in one AST activity increased to 527 U/L on day 18 *3345* Manifestation usually of single toxic high dose ingestion in suicide attempt. Liver damage usually of centrizonal hemorrhagic hepatic necrosis *6666* Hepatic necrosis with dose of 10 g reported *678*
Serum No Effect Analytical At acute overdose concentration (10 mg/dL) on Technicon SMAC® method *6266* No effect at 200 mg/L on Boehringer Mannheim Reflotron method *5706* At 10 times maximal therapeutic concentration on colorimetric method *2919* No effect at concentration of 1.00 mg/mL (6.62 mmol/L) on method on Du Pont Dimension *1568* No effect at therapeutic concentration on Boehringer Mannheim Reflotron method *3231*

Benzodiazepine Screen *Serum No Effect Analytical* No significant interference observed at a concentration of 1500 µg/mL (9.92 mmol/L) with method on Du Pont aca *1512*

Benzoylecgonine *Urine No Effect Analytical* Negative result observed at a concentration of 1000 µg/mL (6.61 mmol/L) with method on Du Pont aca *1558* No significant interference observed at a concentration of 662 µmol/L with Sung and Neely modification of Syva EMIT procedure *148*

Bicarbonate *Serum No Effect Analytical* At concentration of 1500 mg/L had no effect on method using phenolphthalein *5704*

Bile *Urine Increase Physiological* Hepatic necrosis may occur with dose of 10 g *678*

Bile Acids *Serum Increase Physiological* Manifestation usually of single toxic high dose ingestion in suicide attempt. Liver damage usually of centrizonal hemorrhagic hepatic necrosis *6666* With overdose and centrolobular hepatic necrosis usually associated with high drug concentration *2894*

Bilirubin *Serum Increase Physiological* In 21 patients who had taken accidental overdose peak concentration of 12.0 ± 15.1 mg/dL and of 1.4 ± 2.4 mg/dL in 50 patients with suicidal intent *5344* Manifestation usually of single toxic high dose ingestion in suicide attempt. Liver damage usually of centrizonal hemorrhagic hepatic necrosis *6666* With overdose and centrolobular hepatic necrosis usually associated with high drug concentration *2894* Hepatic damage reported with overdose *5090*
Serum No Effect Analytical At concentration of 200 mg/L had no effect on method on Boehringer Mannheim Reflotron system *5706* No significant effect observed at a concentration of 100 µg/mL (662 µmol/L) with method on Du Pont aca *1548* At 5 times therapeutic concentration on routine methods in use on Technicon SMAC® , Du Pont aca, Roche Cobas-Bio, Kodak Ektachem® , Hitachi® and KDA *3525* At a concentration of 5 mg/dL has no significant effect on method on Kodak Ektachem® systems *2519* At acute overdose concentration (10 mg/dL) on Technicon SMAC® method *6266* No effect at 100 mg/L on Ames Seralyzer method *5706* At concentration of 50 mg/L had no effect on Kodak Ektachem® method *5704* No effect at concentration of 200 µg/mL (1.3 mmol/L) on method on Du Pont Dimension *1589* At concentration of 1500 mg/L had no effect on Jendrassik and Grof method *5704*
Serum No Effect Physiological Insignificant displacement from protein in neonates *6314*

Bilirubin, Conjugated *Serum No Effect Analytical* No effect at concentration of 200 mg/L on method on Kodak Ektachem® *5706* At concentration of 100 µg/mL (662 µmol/L) had no effect on method on Du Pont aca *1517*

Bilirubin, Direct *Serum Increase Physiological* Hepatic necrosis with dose of 10 g reported *678*
Serum No Effect Analytical At concentration of 200 µg/mL (1.3 mmol/L) had no effect on method on Du Pont Dimension *1574*

Bilirubin, Unconjugated *Serum No Effect Analytical* No effect at concentration of 200 mg/L on method on Kodak Ektachem® *5706*

Calcium *Serum No Effect Analytical* At concentration of 1500 mg/L had no effect on cresolphthalein method *5704* No effect at concentration of 200 µg/mL (1.3 mmol/L) on method on Du Pont Dimension *1569* At acute overdose concentration (10 mg/dL) on Technicon SMAC® method *6266* At 5 times therapeutic concentration on o-CPC methods on Technicon SMAC® , Abbott-VP, Du Pont aca, Hitachi® 705 and KDA and arsenazo III method on Ektachem® 400 *3525*

Cannabinoids *Urine No Effect Analytical* No effect on Roche Abuscreen method *5006*

Casts *Urine Increase Physiological* Renal damage due to hemolysis and anuria *2242*

Catecholamines *Plasma No Effect Analytical* No effect on HPLC method of Koller for dopamine, epinephrine, and norepinephrine after extraction with alumina *3230*
Urine Increase Analytical Using reversed phase HPLC-ECD large peak may occur between epinephrine and internal standard (dihydroxybenzylamine) *1257*
Urine No Effect Physiological No effect with short term ingestion of 2.6 g/d *1184*

Cells *Urine Increase Physiological* May be marked increase in renal tubular cells, due to nephrotoxicity *2242* 3 - 6 g for 5 d produces increase in tubular cells but less than with aspirin or phenacetin *4777*

Chloramphenicol *Serum No Effect Analytical* At 100 mg/L has no effect on coupled enzymatic procedure *4122*

Chloride *Serum No Effect Analytical* At concentration of 1500 mg/L had no effect on mercurimetric method *5704* No effect at concentrations up to 50 mg/L with method on Kodak Ektachem® *5706*

Cholesterol *Serum No Effect Analytical* No effect at 100 mg/L on Ames Seralyzer method *5706* No effect at therapeutic concentration on Boehringer Mannheim Reflotron method *3231* At concentration of 1500 mg/L had no effect on Liebermann-Burchard method *5704* At concentration of 200 µg/mL (1.3 mmol/L) had no effect on method on Du Pont Dimension *1570* At concentration of 6 mg/L had no effect on CHOD-PAP method *5704* At 5 times therapeutic concentration on Liebermann-Burchard method on Technicon SMAC® and enzymatic methods on Abbott-VP, Roche Cobas-Bio, Kodak Ektachem® , Hitachi® 705 and KDA *3525* At acute overdose concentration (10 mg/dL) on Technicon SMAC® method *6266* At concentration of 200 mg/L had no effect on method on Boehringer Mannheim Reflotron system *5706*

Cholinesterase *Serum Decrease Physiological* In severe cases of poisoning (also in some mild) *5824*

Serum No Effect Analytical Insignificant increase of 0.30 U/mL at a concentration of 200 µg/mL with method on Du Pont Dimension *3271* Insignificant decrease of 0.10 U/mL at concentration of 200 µg/mL with method on Du Pont aca *3271* No effect observed at concentration of 20 mg/dL with butyrylthiocholine method on Kodak Ektachem® *2504*

Codeine *Serum No Effect Physiological* In 6 healthy individuals coadministration of paracetamol with codeine had no significant effect on area under the concentration curve or clearance *5696*

Color *Urine Increase Analytical* Dark brown urine observed in some patients with overdose, probably due to p-aminophenol *1050*

Cortisol *Plasma No Effect Analytical* At concentration of 200 mg/L no significant effect observed with Boehringer Mannheim CEDIA or Enzymun methods (worst case 96.2% recovery) *1097*

Creatine Kinase *Serum No Effect Analytical* No effect at 100 mg/L on method on Ames Seralyzer *5706* At acute overdose concentration (10 mg/dL) on Technicon SMAC® method *6266* On continuous method at 10 times maximal therapeutic concentration *2919*

Creatine Kinase Isoenzymes *Serum No Effect Analytical* At concentration of 200 µg/mL (1.3 mmol/L) had no effect on CK-MB method on Du Pont Dimension *1571*

Creatinine *Serum Increase Analytical* Mild acute renal failure in two patients following therapeutic ingestion of drug *2001*

Serum Increase Physiological In 21 patients who had taken accidental overdose peak concentration of 2.6 ± 2.6 mg/dL and of 1.0 ± 0.3 mg/dL in 50 patients with suicidal intent *5344* Reversible tubular necrosis reported *678*

Serum No Effect Analytical No effect at 100 mg/L on method on Ames Seralyzer *5706* Although detected by HPLC method of Rosano et al elutes sufficiently later than creatinine so as not to cause interference *5083* At concentration of 50 mg/L had no effect on Kodak Ektachem® method *5704* At 5 times upper limit of therapeutic concentration on routine methods in use on Technicon SMAC® , Abbott-VP, Du Pont aca, Roche Cobas-Bio, Kodak Ektachem® 400, Hitachi® 705, KDA *3525* At concentration of 180 mg/L had no effect on creatinine iminohydrolase method *5704* At 200 mg/L no effect on reversed phase LIquid chrmaographic procedure of Zhiri et al *6656* No effect of concentrations up to 200 mg/L on 2-slide method on Kodak Ektachem® *5706* At concentration of 1500 mg/L had no effect on Technicon AutoAnalyzer® Jaffe method *5704* At acute overdose concentration (10 mg/dL) on Technicon SMAC® method *6266* No effect at concentration of 200 µg/mL (1.3 mmol/L) on method on Du Pont Dimension *1572*

Serum No Effect Physiological Without overdose not usually any effect *4777*

Creatinine Clearance *Urine No Effect Physiological* Without overdose not usually any effect *4777*

Cyclosporine *Blood No Effect Analytical* At concentration of 200 mg/L had no effect on Syva EMIT method *495*

Diflunisal *Serum No Effect Physiological* Concomitant administration of diflunisal with acetaminophen had no significant effect on the diflunisal concentration *3972*

Digoxin *Serum No Effect Analytical* At concentration of 1.00 mg/mL (6.62 mmol/L) had no effect on method on Du Pont Dimension *1573*

Doxazosin *Serum No Effect Physiological* Coadministration with doxazosin had no effect on its pharmacokinetics *4642*

Drugs of Abuse Screen *Urine No Effect Analytical* No effect at concentration of 100 µg/mL on EZ-SCREEN procedure for cannabinoids and cocaine *1739*

Epinephrine *Urine No Effect Physiological* No effect with short term ingestion of 2.6 g/d *1184*

Erythrocytes *Blood Decrease Physiological* May cause hemolytic anemia *3810*

Urine Increase Physiological Renal damage due to hemolysis *2242*

Ethinyl Estradiol *Serum Increase Physiological* When administered in oral contraceptives with acetaminophen: effect probably occurs by reduction of sulfation of ethinyl estradiol in the gastrointestinal tract thereby increasing its absorption: increase only slight *5062*

Felbamate *Serum No Effect Analytical* No significant interference observed with GLC method of Rifai et al *4958*

α-Fetoprotein *Serum Decrease Physiological* After ingestion of 650 mg concentration significantly lower whether measured by radioimmunoassay or enzyme immunoassay (using kits from Amersham and Hybritech) *2230*

Fibrin Degradation Products *Plasma No Effect Analytical* No interference observed at concentrations up to 100 µg/dL (662 µmol/L) with method on Du Pont aca *1525*

F Protein *Serum Increase Physiological* Increased concentration observed in 7 of 9 patients on admission whereas increased ALT observed in only one. Protein concentration reflects extent of centrilobular damage *447*

Glucose *Serum Decrease Analytical* At concentrations of 550 µmol/L and above had significant effect on the method on Medisense Precision QID *904* At concentrations above 25 mg/L (normal therapeutic concentration 20 mg/L) lowered concentration as measured by GOD-PERID method *5704* At concentrations up to 1.30 mmol/L caused nonsignificant reduction of up to 0.08 mmol/L in whole blood glucose concentration as measured by Miles Ames Glucostix analyzer *5904* At concentrations up to 1.30 mmol/L caused nonsignificant reduction of up to 0.13 mmol/L with whole blood glucose concentration as measured by Medisense Satellite G analyzer *5904*

Serum Decrease Physiological Reported effect of metabolite *1258*

Serum Increase Analytical At concentrations of 125 µmol/L and above had significant effect on the methods on Bayer Glucometer Elite and BMC Accu-chek Advantage *904* At concentrations up to 1.30 mmol/L caused significant increase of up to 0.38 mmol/L in whole blood glucose concentration as measured by Medisense Exatech analyzer *5904* In YSI glucose analyzer with potentiometric measurement of hydrogen peroxide produced. Effect can be quite marked *5042* At 1 mmol/L affects Technicon SMA 12/60 method *5576*

Serum No Effect Analytical At 5 times upper limit of therapeutic concentration had no effect on routine methods in use on Technicon SMAC® , Abbott-VP, Du Pont aca, Roche Cobas-Bio, Kodak Ektachem® 400, Hitachi® 705, KDA *3525* At concentrations up to 1.30 mmol/L had no effect on whole blood glucose measurement on Boehringer Mannheim BM 1-44 analyzer *5904* No effect observed with colorimetric glucose oxidase procedure on Technicon AutoAnalyzer® using Boehringer Mannheim kit. No effect on Beckman glucose analyzer with oxygen produced measured by specific electrode *5042* No effect at 10 mmol/L on glucokinase based assay of Scott et al *5414* Unless correcting electrode used as in the Ciba Corning 860 blood gas and critical analyte system at therapeutic concentrations may produce 10 - 20% positive error. In Ciba Corning system therapeutic concentrations produce errors of less than 6 mg/dL and toxic concentrations of less than 10% *1471* At concentration of 200 µg/mL (1.3 mmol/L) has no effect on method on Du Pont Dimension *1575* No effect at therapeutic concentration on Boehringer Mannheim Reflotron method *3231* At concentration of 3 mg/dL had no effect on concentration as measured by enzyme-electrode sensor in Markwell Medical instrument *6132* At concentrations up to 2000 µmol/L had insignificant effect on the methods on Lifescan One Touch Profile, Lifescan SureStep, Radiometer EML 105, J&J Vitros 700 XR, Beckman CX3 and Beckman CX-5 *904* At concentration of 600 mg/L had no effect on hex-

Acetaminophen *(continued)*

Glucose *(continued)*
okinase/G-6-PDH method *5704* At concentration of 57 mg/L had no effect on GOD/POD-PAP method *5704* At acute overdose concentration (10 mg/dL) on Technicon SMAC® method *6266* No effect at 300 mg/L on hexokinase method on Ames Seralyzer *5706* No effect at 10 mmol/L on gluokinase based assay of Scott *5414* At concentrations up to 300 mg/L had no significant effect on whole blood measurement on One Touch II meter *3137* At concentrations up to 200 mg/L no effect on method on Boehringer Mannheim Reflotron system but above this glucose concentration reduced (not clinically important) *5706* No effect at 100 mg/L on glucose oxidase method on Ames Seralyzer *5706*

γ-Glutamyltransferase *Serum Increase Physiological* In severe cases of poisoning (also in some mild) *5824*
Serum No Effect Analytical At concentration of 200 mg/L no effect on method on Boehringer Mannheim Reflotron system *5706* No effect of concentrations up to 50 mg/L on method on Kodak Ektachem® *5706* At concentration of 200 µg/mL (1.3 mmol/L) has no effect on method on Du Pont Dimension *1579* No effect at therapeutic concentration on Boehringer Mannheim Reflotron method *3231*

Glutathione S-Transferase *Serum Increase Physiological* Observed as more sensitive indicator than alanine aminotransferase as marker of hepatic damage (increased activity in 9 patients compared with increased ALT in only one). Increase greater than that of ALT *447*
Serum No Effect Physiological Administration of acetaminophen to a group of healthy individuals caused nonsignificant change from mean baseline of 3.5 ± 3.5 µg/L predose to 3.2 ± 2.5 µg/L postdose *4892*

Glycated Hemoglobin *Blood No Effect Analytical* At a concentration of 300 mg/L had an insignificant 0.0% interference with method on Abbott Vision *1885*

HDL-Cholesterol *Serum No Effect Analytical* No effect of concentrations up to 200 mg/L on method on Kodak Ektachem® *5706* No effect at concentration of 200 µg/mL (1.3 mmol/L) on method on Du Pont Dimension *1576* At a concentration up to 200 mg/L had no significant effect on Reflotron method for whole blood cholesterol *6352*

Hemoglobin *Blood Decrease Physiological* Anemia/pancytopenia may be observed *128*
Blood No Effect Analytical No effect of concentrations up to 50 mg/L on method on Kodak Ektachem® *5706* No effect on method on Boehringer Mannheim Reflotron *5706*

Histamine *Plasma No Effect Analytical* Insignificant inhibition of radio-enzyme assay at concentrations twice physiological *2492*

Hydroxybutyrate Dehydrogenase
Serum No Effect Analytical On continuous method at 10 times maximal therapeutic concentration *2919*

11-Hydroxycorticosteroids *Urine No Effect Physiological* No effect with short term ingestion of 2.6 g/d *1184*

17-Hydroxycorticosteroids *Urine No Effect Physiological* No effect with short term ingestion of 2.6 g/d *1184*

5-Hydroxyindoleacetic Acid *Urine Increase Analytical* May cause false high colorimetric results *1444* Affects nitrosonaphthol procedures *2452*
Urine No Effect Analytical No effect observed with FPIA method on Abbott TDx *695*

Icteric Index *Serum Increase Physiological* May cause hepatic toxicity *3810*

Indomethacin *Serum No Effect Analytical* No effect on HPLC method of Roberts and Smith *4978*

Iron *Serum No Effect Analytical* At concentration of 100 mg/L had no effect on Ferrozine method *5704* At 5 times therapeutic concentration on Ferrozine method on Technicon SMAC® *3525* No effect at concentration of 200 µg/mL (1.3 mmol/L) on method on Du Pont Dimension *1577* No effect of concentrations up to 50 mg/L on method on Kodak Ektachem® *5706* At acute overdose concentration (10 mg/dL) on Technicon SMAC® method *6266* No apparent interference observed in specimens from patients taking acetaminophen when iron measured on Kodak Ektachem® 700 *2590*

Iron-Binding Capacity, Total *Serum No Effect Analytical* No effect at concentration of 200 µg/mL (1.3 mmol/L) on method on Du Pont Dimension *1590*

Ketorolac *Serum No Effect Physiological* At therapeutic concentrations had no effect on ketorolac-protein binding *5035*

17-Ketosteroids *Urine No Effect Physiological* No effect with short term ingestion of 2.6 g/d *1184*

Lactate *Plasma No Effect Analytical* At concentration of 600 mg/L had no effect on enzymatic method *5704*

Lactate Dehydrogenase *Serum Increase Analytical* On colorimetric method at 10 times maximal therapeutic concentration *2919*
Serum No Effect Analytical No effect of concentrations up to 50 mg/L on method on Kodak Ektachem® *5706* No effect at 100 mg/L on method on Ames Seralyzer *5706* At acute overdose concentration (10 mg/dL) on Technicon SMAC® method *6266* On continuous methods using either pyruvate or lactate as substrate at 10 times maximal therapeutic concentration *2919* At concentration of 200 µg/mL (1.3 mmol/L) has no effect on method on Du Pont Dimension *1578*

Leukocytes *Blood Decrease Physiological* May affect bone marrow function/pancytopenia *3624*

Lipase *Serum Increase Physiological* In 26 patients with acetaminophen overdose median activity on admission 87.5 U/L (range 13 - 1550 U/L) compared with adult reference range of 5 - 65 U/L. Increase above reference range observed in 69% patients *1340*
Serum No Effect Analytical No effect observed at a concentration of 20 mg/dL on method on Du Pont aca when colipase incorporated into reaction mixture *4702* No effect at concentration of 200 µg/mL (1.3 mmol/L) with method on Du Pont Dimension *1580* No effect of concentrations up to 500 mg/L on method on Kodak Ektachem® *5706*

Magnesium *Serum No Effect Analytical* No effect of concentrations up to 50 mg/L on method on Kodak Ektachem® *5706* No effect at concentration of 200 µg/mL (1.3 mmol/L) on method on Du Pont Dimension *1581*

Metanephrines, Total *Urine Increase Analytical* Interference with unmodified ion-exchange chromatographic method of Shoup and Kissinger *6493*

Methemoglobin *Blood Increase Physiological* May rarely cause hemolysis *2242*
Urine Increase Physiological Renal damage due to hemolysis *2242*

Morphine *Urine No Effect Analytical* No significant interference observed at concentration of 662 µmol/L with Sung and Neely modification of Syva EMIT procedure *148*

Mycophenolic Acid *Serum No Effect Analytical* No significant interference observed with HPLC method of Shipkova et al *5526*

Mycophenolic Acid Glucuronide
Serum No Effect Analytical No significant interference observed with HPLC method of Shipkova et al *5526*

N-Acetylprocainamide *Serum No Effect Analytical* No significant interference from N-acetyl-p-aminophenol at a concentration of 100 µg/mL (662 µmol/L) with method on Du Pont aca *1536*

Neutrophils *Blood Decrease Physiological* May cause neutropenia/pancytopenia *2242*

Norepinephrine *Urine No Effect Physiological* No effect with short term ingestion of 2.6 g/d *1184*

5'-Nucleotidase *Serum Increase Physiological* In severe cases of poisoning (also in some mild) *5824*

2',5'-Oligoadenylate Synthetase
Neutrophils No Effect Physiological In healthy individuals given a single intramuscular injection of interferon *6519*

Oxaprozin *Serum No Effect Physiological* Coadministration of acetaminophen with oxaprozin caused no significant effect on the pharmacokinetic parameters of oxaprozin in single or multiple dose studies *2065*

p-Aminophenol *Urine No Effect Analytical* With addition of drugs at a concentration of 100 mg/L and of related compounds at 50 mg/L no significant effect observed on colorimetric method of van Bocxlaer on Cobas Mira analyzer which involves reacting free p-aminophenol with resorcinol in the presence of magnesium ions to form an indophenol dye measured at 550 nm *6163*

Phenylalanine *Plasma No Effect Analytical* No interference observed with rapid quantitative whole blood method of Campbell et al using phenylalanine dehydrogenase *867*

Phenytoin *Serum No Effect Analytical* No effect at concentration of 200 µg/mL (1.3 mmol/L) on method on Du Pont Dimension *1583*
Serum No Effect Physiological Insignificant effect in 9 epileptic patients on long-term phenytoin therapy *4260*

Phosphate *Serum No Effect Analytical* At concentration of 1500 mg/L had no effect on phosphomolybdate method *5704* At acute overdose concentration (10 mg/dL) on Technicon SMAC® method *6266* At concentration of 200 µg/mL (1.3 mmol/L) has no effect on method on Du Pont Dimension *1584* No effect of concentrations up to 50 mg/L on method on Kodak Ektachem® *5706* At 5 times therapeutic concentration on molybdate procedures on Technicon SMAC® , Du Pont aca, Hitachi® 705 and KDA *3525*

Platelets *Blood Decrease Physiological* Thrombocytopenia observed in 3.4% of 174 patients with hospital admissions for acute acetaminophen toxicity *1876* Single case of antibodies to SO_4 conjugate of drug *1683*

Potassium *Serum No Effect Analytical* At concentration of 300 mg/L caused nonsignificant 0.4% interference with method on Abbott Vision *681* At concentration of 6 mg/L had no effect on flame-photometric method *5704* No effect of concentrations up to 50 mg/L on method on Kodak Ektachem® *5706* At concentration of 1500 mg/L had no effect on measurement by ISE with predilution *5704*

Procainamide *Serum No Effect Analytical* No significant interference observed at a concentration of 100 µg/mL (662 µmol/L) with method on Du Pont aca *1542*

Protein *Cerebrospinal Fluid Decrease Analytical* Decrease in vitro of 3.2 mg/dL at concentration of 3.0 mg/dL perhaps due to analytical uncertainty of Kodak Ektachem® slide method. Unlikely to have any clinical significance *3654*
Serum No Effect Analytical At 5 times therapeutic concentration on biuret procedures on Technicon SMAC® , Abbott-VP, Kodak Ektachem® 400, Hitachi® 705 and KDA *3525* At acute overdose concentration (10 mg/dL) on Technicon SMAC® method *6266* At concentration of 200 µg/mL (1.3 mmol/L) had negligible effect on method on Du Pont Dimension *1591* At concentration of 1500 mg/L had no effect on biuret method with blank correction *5704*
Urine Increase Physiological Nephrotoxic effect of drug *678*

Prothrombin Time *Plasma Increase Physiological* In 21 patients who had taken accidental overdose peak time of 25.7 ± 18.5 s and of 18.0 ± 12.4 s in 50 patients with suicidal intent *5344* Manifestation usually of single toxic high dose ingestion in suicide attempt. Liver damage usually of centrizonal hemorrhagic hepatic necrosis *6666* In 20 healthy men given acetaminophen 4 g/d in one AST activity increased to 527 U/L on day 18 and ALT activity increased to 121 U/L on day 20, with warfarin 20 mg/d given on days 2 and 16 ptothrombin time increased to 13.3 s on day 18 *3345* Depresses clotting factor synthesis *678* Significant effect in patients receiving warfarin, possibly due to interference with synthesis of factors II, VII, IX, and X *630*
Plasma No Effect Physiological No effect observed in volunteers *5501*

Pyroglutamic Acid *Urine Increase Physiological* Significant increase following drug ingestion although considerably lower than in patients with glutathione synthetase or 5-oxoprolinase deficiency *4717*

SDZ PSC 833 *Blood No Effect Analytical* At a concentration of 164 mg/L had no effect on HPLC method of Scott et al when used to measure PSC with CsD (as internal standard) at a concentration of 5 mg/L *5418*

Sodium *Serum No Effect Analytical* At concentration of 6 mg/L had no effect on flame-photometric method *5704* At concentration of 1500 mg/L had no effect on measurement by ISE with predilution *5704* No interference observed at concentration of 50 mg/dL with Technicon Chromolyte method *969*

Sucrose *Serum No Effect Analytical* Using automated procedure involving sucrose phosphorylase, phosphoglutamase and glucose-6-phosphatase of Vinet et al no significant interference observed at a concentration of 2 mmol/L *6267*
Urine No Effect Analytical Using automated procedure involving sucrose phosphorylase, phosphoglutamase and glucose-6-phosphatase of Vinet et al no significant interference observed at a concentration of 2 mmol/L *6267*

Sulfate *Urine Decrease Physiological* Reduces increased output of rheumatoids *5171*

T3-Uptake *Serum No Effect Analytical* At concentration of 1000 µg/mL (6.62 µmol/L) has no effect on method on Du Pont Dimension *1586* No significant effect observed at a concentration of 1000 µg/mL (6.62 mmol/L) with method on Du Pont aca *1545*

Tacrolimus *Blood No Effect Analytical* No significant effect observed at a concentration of 100 mg/L with MEIA method on Abbott IMx analyzer *1871*
Serum No Effect Analytical At a concentration of 100 mg/L had no significant effect on ELISA method *6329*

Theophylline *Serum No Effect Analytical* At concentration of 250 µg/mL had no effect on method on Ektachem® *6100* At concentration of 200 µg/mL (1.3 mmol/L) had no effect on method on Du Pont Dimension *1585*

Thyroxine (T4) *Serum No Effect Analytical* At concentration of 1000 µg/mL (6.62 mmol/L) has no effect on method on Du Pont Dimension *1587* No significant interference observed at a concentration of 1000 µg/mL (6.62 mmol/L) with method on Du Pont aca *1588 1546*

Ticarcillin *Serum Increase Analytical* Cannot be assayed in presence of acetaminophen with HPLC method used at Mayo Clinic *3858*

Tirofiban *Serum No Effect Physiological* Coadministration had no significant effect on plasma clearance of tirofiban *3957*

Titratable Acidity *Urine No Effect Physiological* Without overdose, not usually any effect *4777*

Tri-iodothyronine, Free (fT3) *Serum No Effect Analytical* At a concentration of 0.5 g/L cross-reactivity of less than 0.1% with free triiodothyronine method on Bayer Technicon Immuno 1® system *425*

Tricyclic Antidepressants Screen
Serum No Effect Analytical No significant interfeerence observed at a concentration of 1500 µg/mL (9.92 mmol/L) with method on Du Pont aca *1550*

Triglycerides *Serum No Effect Analytical* At acute overdose concentration (10 mg/dL) on Technicon SMAC® method *6266* At concentration of 200 µg/mL (1.3 mmol/L) has no effect on method on Du Pont Dimension *1592* No effect at 200 mg/L on Boehringer Mannheim Reflotron method *5706* At 5 times upper limit of therapeutic concentration on routine methods in use on Technicon SMAC® , Abbott-VP, Roche Cobas-Bio, Kodak Ektachem® 400, Hitachi® 705, KDA *3525* At concentration of 1500 mg/L had no effect on lipase/esterase method *5704* No effect at therapeutic concentration on Boehringer Mannheim Reflotron method *3231* At concentration of 300 mg/L had no effect on GPO-PAP method *5704*

Trimantadine *Serum Decrease Physiological* Coadministration of acetaminophen with trimantadine caused reduction of its AUC by approximately 11% *1910*

Troglitazone *Serum No Effect Physiological* Coadministration of acetaminophen with troglitazone had no significant effect on the concentration of either drug *4532*

Urea Nitrogen *Serum Increase Physiological* Mild acute renal failure in two patients following therapeutic ingestion of drug *2001* Reversible tubular necrosis reported *678*
Serum No Effect Analytical At concentration of 200 µg/mL (1.3 mmol/L) had no effect on method on Du Pont Dimension *1593* At acute overdose concentration (10 mg/dL) on Technicon SMAC® method *6266* No effect at 100 mg/L on method on Ames Seralyzer *5706* No effect observed on routine methods in use on Technicon SMAC® , Abbott-VP, Roche Cobas-Bio, Kodak Ektachem® 400, Hitachi® 705, KDA *3525* No effect at 200 mg/L on Boehringer Mannheim Reflotron method *5706* No effect at therapeutic concentration on Boehringer Mannheim Reflotron method *3231* At concentration of 1500 mg/L had no effect on diacetylmonoxime method *5704*
Serum No Effect Physiological Without overdose not usually any effect *4777*

Uric Acid *Serum Increase Analytical* Falsely high values with phosphotungstate methods *2197* At concentrations above 50 mg/L (normal therapeutic concentration 20 mg/L) raised concentration as measured by phosphotungstate reduction method *5704* Reacts as if uric acid with Technicon SMA 12/60 method *5576* 40% increase on Technicon SMAC® at 5 times upper limit of therapeutic concentration on phosphotungstate procedures routinely used. 14% increase on KDA at 5 times upper limit of therapeutic concentration on phosphotungstate procedures routinely used *3525*

Acetaminophen *(continued)*

Uric Acid *(continued)*
Serum *No Effect* *Analytical* No effect at 200 mg/L on Boehringer Mannheim Reflotron method *5706* No effect at therapeutic concentration on Boehringer Mannheim Reflotron method *3231* At 200 mg/L on reversed phase liquid chromatographic procedure of Zhiri et al *6656* At concentration of 810 mg/L had no effect on uricase-PAP method *5704* No effect at concentration of 200 µg/mL (1.3 mmol/L) on method on Du Pont Dimension *1594* At 5 times upper limit of therapeutic concentration on uricase procedures on Abbott-VP, Du Pont aca, Roche Cobas-Bio, Kodak Ektachem® 400, Hitachi® 705 *3525* At acute overdose concentration (10 mg/dL) on Technicon SMAC® method *6266*
Urine *Increase* *Analytical* Falsely high values with phosphotungstate methods *2197*

Vitamin B_{12} *Serum* *No Effect* *Analytical* At concentrations up to 50 mg/dL had no clinically significant cross-reactivity in vitamin B_{12} method on Bayer Technicon Immuno 1® *439*

Volume *Urine* *Decrease* *Physiological* Increases transport of water in diabetes insipidus *2242*

Zidovudine *Serum* *No Effect* *Analytical* No effect on liquid chromatographic method of Hedaya and Sawchuk *2525*
Serum *No Effect* *Physiological* Coadministration of acetaminophen (up to 650 mg/d for 7 days) with 200 mg zidovudine every 4 hours caused slight acceleration of up to 33% in clearance of zidovudine so not likely to potentiate zidovudine toxicity *5289*

Acetanilid

Bilirubin *Serum* *Increase* *Physiological* Hemolysis observed with G-6-PD deficiency *3810*

Bilirubin, Direct *Serum* *Increase* *Physiological* Hemolysis observed with G-6-PD deficiency *3810*

Casts *Urine* *Increase* *Physiological* Due to hemolysis and renal damage *2242*

Color *Blood* *Increase* *Analytical* May cause chocolate colored blood *467*

Erythrocyte Survival *Blood* *Decrease* *Physiological* Due to hemolysis *2242*

Erythrocytes *Blood* *Decrease* *Physiological* Hemolytic anemia/agranulocytosis may occur *4017*
Urine *Increase* *Physiological* Due to hemolysis and renal damage *2242*

Glutathione, Reduced
Red Blood Cells *Decrease* *Physiological* Sharp fall observed before overt hemolysis *3094*

Haptoglobin *Serum* *Decrease* *Physiological* Hemolysis observed with G-6-PD deficiency *3810*

Heinz Body Formation *Blood* *Positive* *Physiological* Occurs initially prior to overt hemolysis *3094*

Hematocrit *Blood* *Decrease* *Physiological* Hemolytic anemia may occur *4013*

Hemoglobin *Blood* *Decrease* *Physiological* Hemolytic anemia may occur *4013*
Plasma *Increase* *Physiological* Occurs with marked hemolysis *3094*
Urine *Increase* *Physiological* Occurs with hemolysis *3094*

Leukocytes *Blood* *Decrease* *Physiological* Leukopenia may occur *3267*

Methemoglobin *Blood* *Increase* *Physiological* Intravascular hemolysis may occur *4013*
Urine *Increase* *Physiological* Due to hemolysis and renal damage *2242*

Occult Blood *Feces* *Increase* *Physiological* Poisoning may cause many gastrointestinal symptoms *467*

Phenylalanine *Plasma* *No Effect* *Analytical* No interference observed with rapid quantitative whole blood method of Campbell et al using phenylalanine dehydrogenase *867*

Protein *Urine* *Increase* *Physiological* Hemolysis may cause renal damage *2242*

Reticulocytes *Blood* *Increase* *Physiological* Occurs during recovery from hemolysis *3094*

Sugar *Urine* *Increase* *Analytical* Acts as reducing substance with Benedict's reagent *4012* Acts as reducing agent with nonspecific tests *2024*

Sulfhemoglobin *Blood* *Increase* *Physiological* Hemolytic anemia in acute poisoning *2242*

Acetazolamide

Albumin *Serum* *No Effect* *Analytical* At concentration of 1,000 mg/L had no effect on BCG method *5704* No effect at 12 mg/dL on Technicon SMA 12/60 method *4390*

Alkaline Phosphatase *Serum* *No Effect* *Analytical* No effect at 12 mg/dL on Technicon SMA 12/60 method *4390*

Ammonia *Plasma* *Increase* *Physiological* ?Diverts NH_3 from kidney to general circulation *2025*
Urine *Decrease* *Physiological* Increased alkalinity *2242*

Amphetamine *Serum* *Increase* *Physiological* Urinary alkalinizing agents increase the nonionized part of the amphetamine molecule, thereby decreasing urinary excretion *5641* Alkalinization of urine increases amount of nonionized amphetamine with increased reabsorption of amphetamine in renal tubules *5126*

Aspartate Aminotransferase *Serum* *No Effect* *Analytical* No effect at 12 mg/dL on Technicon SMA 12/60 method *4390*

Bicarbonate *Serum* *Decrease* *Physiological* Carbonic anhydrase inhibition in renal tubules *1009*
Serum *No Effect* *Analytical* At concentration of 1,000 mg/L had no effect on phenolphthalein method *5704*
Urine *Increase* *Physiological* Inhibition of carbonic anhydrase *2242*

Bilirubin *Serum* *Increase* *Physiological* Single case of cholestatic jaundice reported *3294*
Serum *No Effect* *Analytical* No effect at 12 mg/dL on Technicon SMA 12/60 method *4390* At concentration of 1,000 mg/L had no effect on Jendrassik and Grof method *5704*
Serum *No Effect* *Physiological* At pharmacological concentration probably no significant displacement from protein occurs *6314*

Calcium *Pancreatic Fluid* *Increase* *Physiological* 60 percent increase with infusion in normals *1641*
Serum *Decrease* *Physiological* Defective calcium and PO_4 reabsorption can be induced *1009*
Serum *No Effect* *Analytical* No effect at 12 mg/dL on Technicon SMA 12/60 method *4390* At concentration of 1,000 mg/L had no effect on mercurimetric method *5704*
Urine *Increase* *Physiological* Inhibits tubular reabsorption *4555*

Carbamazepine *Serum* *Increase* *Physiological* Increased plasma concentration observed sometimes with neurotoxicity: presumably due to inhibition of metabolism *3118*

Carbon Dioxide Partial Pressure
Blood *Decrease* *Physiological* Usual effect in bronchitics *3824*

Carbonic Anhydrase
Red Blood Cells *Decrease* *Physiological* Inhibitory effect observed *4821*

Chloride *Pancreatic Fluid* *Increase* *Physiological* 30 percent increase with infusion in normals *1641*
Serum *Increase* *Physiological* Loss of HCO_3 by carbonic anhydrase inhibition *1714*
Urine *Decrease* *Physiological* Significant effect in 5 h after 500 mg orally *1959*

Cholesterol *Serum* *No Effect* *Analytical* No effect at 12 mg/dL on Technicon SMA 12/60 method *4390* At concentration of 1,000 mg/L had no effect on Liebermann-Burchard method *5704*

Citrate *Urine* *Decrease* *Physiological* Alteration of acid base status, diuresis *4555*

Color *Feces* *Increase* *Analytical* Black color reported with acetazolamide ingestion *3388*

Creatinine *Serum* *No Effect* *Analytical* At concentration of 1,000 mg/L had no effect on Tehnicon AutoAnalyzer® Jaffe method *5704* No effect at 12 mg/dL on Technicon SMA 12/60 method *4390*

Crystals *Urine* *Increase* *Physiological* Presence of drug *1714*

Cyclosporine *Serum Increase Physiological* Reported effect although documentation is poor *1069* In one post-transplant patient addition of acetazolamide to therapeutic regime caused increase in previously stable concentration. Mechanism uncertain but possibly due to inhibition of gastric mucosal bicarbonate secretion resulting in increased cyclosporine absorption, inhibition of red cell carbonic anhydrase altering incorporation of cyclosporine into cells, or reduced hepatic metabolism of cyclosporine *6596*

Ephedrine *Serum Increase Physiological* alkalinization of urine increases proportion of nonionized ephedrine with consequent increased tubular reabsorption *6460*

Erythrocytes *Blood Decrease Physiological* May cause pancytopenia/agranulocytosis *3810*
Urine Increase Physiological Occasionally observed adverse reaction *2754*

Erythropoietin *Serum Decrease Physiological* In 6 patients with chronic renal failure administration of 250 mg caused nonsignificant change from mean baseline of 27.5 ± 5.2 mU/mL to 24.0 ± 0.7 mU/mL after 3 h, 39.5 ± 8.6 mU/mL after6 h and 21.2 ± 1.2 mU/mL after 24 h *6134*

Estrogens *Urine Decrease Analytical* Affects hydrolysis of estrogen conjugates *55*
Urine Increase Physiological In pregnant women but mechanism unknown *54*

Glucose *Serum Increase Physiological* In prediabetics and if hypoglycemic agents used *3334*
Serum No Effect Analytical At concentration of 200 mg/L had no effect on GOD/POD-PAP method *5704* No effect at 12 mg/dL on Technicon SMA 12/60 method *4390*
Serum No Effect Physiological Little effect observed in normal individuals *2452*
Urine Increase Physiological Occasionally observed adverse reaction *2754*

Hemoglobin *Blood Decrease Physiological* Anemia may occur due to pancytopenia/agranulocytosis *3810*

Histamine *Plasma No Effect Analytical* Improbable effect on radio-enzyme assay at therapeutic concentrations *2492*

Hydrochloric Acid *Gastric Fluid Decrease Physiological* In large doses reversible effect *1252*

17-Hydroxycorticosteroids *Urine Increase Analytical In vitro* interference with Glenn-Nelson method *1714*

^{131}I Uptake *Serum No Effect Physiological* No effect on test *882*

Inulin Clearance *Urine Decrease Physiological* Infusion at rate of 250 mg/h caused reduction from mean of 128 mL/min to 111 mL/min in 5 healthy young men *632*

Iodide *Urine Decrease Physiological* Significant effect in 5 h after 500 mg orally *1959*

Ketone Body Ratio *Serum No Effect Analytical* When added at a concentration of 8 g/L had no significant effect on AKBR method of Uno et al *6131*

Lactate Dehydrogenase *Serum No Effect Analytical* No effect at 12 mg/dL on Technicon SMA 12/60 method *4390*

LE Cells *Blood Positive Physiological* May produce LE-like syndrome *5869*

Leukocytes *Blood Decrease Physiological* Leukopenia/agranulocytosis may occur *4576*

Lithium *Serum Decrease Physiological* Tubular reabsorption reduced with subsequent reduction in plasma concentration *2986*

Lithium Clearance *Urine Increase Physiological* A single dose of the drug effectively increases lithium clearance *4399*

Magnesium *Pancreatic Fluid Increase Physiological* Approximately 70% increase with infusion in normals *1641*
Urine Decrease Physiological Following acute i.v. administration of 500 mg *5169* Reported effect *6309*
Urine Increase Physiological Reported to cause minor increase in excretion *5169*

Mephentermine *Urine Decrease Physiological* Ingestion of acetazolamide shortly after administration of mephentermine caused decreased excretion of both mephentermine and phentermine in one day *1361*

Methotrexate *Serum Decrease Physiological* 500 mg 6-hourly increased pH above 7.5 in 13 cycles in 10 patients receiving high-dose methotrexate *5470*

Neutrophils *Blood Decrease Physiological* Occasional agranulocytosis reported *6264*

Occult Blood *Feces Increase Physiological* Initial response noted *2754*

Oxalate *Urine No Effect Physiological* Infusion of 250 mg/h in 5 healthy young men had no effect on excretion rate *632*

pH *Blood Decrease Physiological* Due to inhibition of carbonic anhydrase *3810*
Urine Increase Physiological Inhibition of carbonic anhydrase *2242*

Phosphate *Serum Decrease Physiological* Defective calcium and PO_4 reabsorption can be induced *1009*
Serum No Effect Analytical At concentration of 1,000 mg/L had no effect on phosphomolybdate method *5704* No effect at 12 mg/dL on Technicon SMA 12/60 method *4390*
Urine Increase Physiological Inhibits tubular reabsorption *1009*

Platelets *Blood Decrease Physiological* May cause pancytopenia with aplastic anemia *3405*

Potassium *Serum Decrease Physiological* Diuretic action, carbonic anhydrase inhibition *1009*
Serum No Effect Analytical At concentration of 1,000 mg/L had no effect on flame-photometric method *5704*
Urine Increase Physiological Diuretic action *2242*

Procainamide *Serum No Effect Physiological* No effect observed on urinary excretion of procainamide or of N-acetylprocainamide *4903*

Protein *Pancreatic Fluid Increase Physiological* Approximately 40% increase with infusion in normals *1641*
Serum No Effect Analytical No effect at 12 mg/dL on Technicon SMA 12/60 method *4390* At concentration of 1,000 mg/L had no effect on biuret method with blank correction *5704*
Urine Increase Analytical Makes urine highly alkaline, causes false positive *194* When measured by Ponceau S dye method in comparison with sulfosalicylic acid or trichloracetic acid methods *6611*

PSP Excretion *Urine Decrease Physiological* Increased urine flow *1714*

Quinidine *Serum Increase Physiological* Alkalinizes urine, increases reabsorption *2452* Alkalinization of urine increases proportion of nonionized quinidine increasing tubular reabsorption of quinidine. Effect is probable with all agents causing alkalinization of urine especially when it was previously acid *4060*

Quinine *Serum Increase Physiological* Alkalinization of urine reduces the proportion of quinine in unionized form thus enhancing its tubular reabsorption *2388*

Sodium *Serum No Effect Analytical* At concentration of 1,000 mg/L had no effect on flame-photometric method *5704*
Urine Increase Physiological Diuretic action *2242*

Titratable Acidity *Urine Decrease Physiological* Increased alkalinity *2242*

Triglycerides *Serum No Effect Analytical* At concentration of 1,000 mg/L had no effect on lipase/esterase method *5704*

Urea Nitrogen *Serum Increase Physiological* May occur with prolonged treatment *3669*
Serum No Effect Analytical At concentration of 1,000 mg/L had no effect on diacetylmonoxime method *5704*

Uric Acid *Serum Increase Physiological* Decreased urate clearance (?also stimulates synthesis) *1714*
Serum No Effect Analytical At concentration of 1,000 mg/L had no effect on phosphotungstate reduction method *5704* No effect at 12 mg/dL on Technicon SMA 12/60 method *4390*
Urine Decrease Physiological Inhibition of tubular secretion of urate *1714*

Urobilinogen *Urine Increase Physiological* Excretion increased by alkalinization of urine *4060*

Volume *Urine Increase Physiological* Initial response noted *2754*

Acetohexamide

Alanine Aminotransferase *Serum Increase Physiological* May cause intrahepatic cholestatic jaundice *3669*

Alkaline Phosphatase *Serum Increase Physiological* May cause intrahepatic cholestatic jaundice *1009*

Acetohexamide *(continued)*

Aspartate Aminotransferase *Serum Increase Physiological* May cause intrahepatic cholestatic jaundice *3669*

Bile *Urine Increase Physiological* May cause intrahepatic cholestatic jaundice *3810*

Bilirubin *Serum Increase Physiological* May cause intrahepatic cholestatic jaundice *1009*
Urine Increase Physiological May cause intrahepatic cholestatic jaundice *3810*

Bilirubin, Direct *Serum Increase Physiological* May cause hemolytic anemia *1695*

BSP Retention *Serum Increase Physiological* May cause intrahepatic cholestatic jaundice *1009*

Cholesterol *Serum Increase Physiological* May cause intrahepatic cholestatic jaundice *3669*

Creatinine *Serum Increase Analytical* Increase by 63 μmol/L per 1 mol/L acetohexamide with Jaffe procedure on Technicon SMAC® although effect observed much less when patient specimens studied *4976* Increase by 112 μmol/L per 1 mol/L acetohexamide with manual Jaffe method *4976* Increase of 318 μmol/L per 1 mol/L acetohexamide with Jaffe procedure on Roche Cobas-Bio *4976* Increase of 327 μmol/L per 1 mol/L with Jaffe procedure on Beckman Astra® but effect apparently much less in patient specimens *4976* Significant effect on Jaffe methods on Beckman Astra® and Du Pont aca by as much as 2.2 or 3.3 mg/dL respectively at therapeutic concentrations and as little as 0.3 mg/dL on Technicon SMA II *6533* Increase of 536 μmol/L per 1 mol/L acetohexamide with Jaffe procedure on Du Pont aca but effect in patient specimens apparently much less *4976*

Erythrocytes *Blood Decrease Physiological* May cause hemolytic anemia *1695*

Glucose *Serum Decrease Physiological* Sulfonylurea derivative promotes insulin secretion *1009*
Serum No Effect Analytical No effect on Boehringer GOD-PERID method *5480* At concentration of 200 mg/L had no effect on GOD/POD-PAP method *5704* No effect at 4000 mg/L on hexokinase method on Ames Seralyzer *5706*

Haptoglobin *Serum Decrease Physiological* May cause hemolytic anemia *1695*

Hematocrit *Blood Decrease Physiological* May cause anemia and hemolysis if G-6-PD deficiency *1695*

Hemoglobin *Blood Decrease Physiological* May cause anemia and hemolysis if G-6-PD deficiency *1695*

Insulin *Plasma Decrease Physiological* Effect observed after 3 mo therapy *492*
Plasma Increase Physiological Usual effect observed (at 2 mo) *492*

Leukocytes *Blood Decrease Physiological* Leukopenia and aplastic anemia reported *3810*

5'-Nucleotidase *Serum Increase Physiological* Due to cholestasis *2911*

Osmolality *Urine Decrease Physiological* Normal slight diuretic response *4136*

Platelets *Blood Decrease Physiological* Thrombocytopenia and aplastic anemia reported *3810*

Prothrombin Time *Plasma Increase Physiological* Occurs if failure to excrete bile salts *128*

Urea Nitrogen *Serum Increase Analytical* Chemical structure produces reaction with diacetyl *1009*

Uric Acid *Serum Decrease Physiological* Mild uricosuric action *6622*
Urine Increase Physiological Uricosuric action *2378*

Urobilinogen *Feces Decrease Physiological* Theoretical effect if cholestasis occurs *128*
Urine Decrease Physiological Theoretical effect if cholestasis *128*

Water Clearance *Urine Increase Physiological* Normal slight diuretic response *4136*

Acetohydroxamic Acid

Ammonia *Plasma Decrease Physiological* Potent urease inhibitor, effect seen in 1 patient *2452*

Urea Nitrogen *Serum Decrease Physiological* Inhibition of urease (limited *in vivo* effect) *5863*

Acetophenazine

Alanine Aminotransferase *Serum Increase Physiological* Cholestasis with intrahepatic obstruction *3810*

Alkaline Phosphatase *Serum Increase Physiological* Cholestatic hepatitis with obstruction *3810*

Aspartate Aminotransferase *Serum Increase Physiological* Cholestasis with intrahepatic obstruction *3810*

Bile *Urine Increase Physiological* Cholestasis with intrahepatic obstruction *3810*

Bilirubin *Serum Increase Physiological* Cholestasis with intrahepatic obstruction *2024*
Urine Increase Physiological Cholestasis with intrahepatic obstruction *3810*

BSP Retention *Serum Increase Physiological* Cholestasis with intrahepatic obstruction *3810*

Cholesterol *Serum Increase Physiological* Cholestasis with intrahepatic obstruction *4909*

Eosinophils *Blood Increase Physiological* Allergic manifestation *2754*

Erythrocytes *Blood Decrease Physiological* Possible aplastic anemia *3810*

Leukocytes *Blood Decrease Physiological* Transitory leukopenia or agranulocytosis *128*

Platelets *Blood Decrease Physiological* Agranulocytosis or aplastic anemia *128*

Acetophenone

17-Ketogenic Steroids *Urine Increase Analytical* Interferes in measurement by Zimmermann method *5869*

17-Ketosteroids *Urine Increase Analytical* Interferes in measurement by Zimmermann method *5869*

Acetrizoate

Aspartate Aminotransferase *Urine Increase Physiological* Sustained increase due to nephrotoxic action *5935*

Catalase *Urine Increase Physiological* Sustained increase after renal artery injection *5935*

Creatine Kinase *Urine Increase Physiological* Sustained increase after renal artery injection *5935*

Glomerular Filtration Rate *Urine Decrease Physiological* When 70% injected for aortography *116*

^{131}I Uptake *Serum Decrease Physiological* Due to iodine component of material *3669*

Lactate Dehydrogenase *Urine Increase Physiological* Sustained increase due to nephrotoxic action *5935*

PAH Clearance *Urine Decrease Physiological* When 70% acetrizoate injected for aortography *116*

Acetylcysteine

Acetaminophen *Serum No Effect Analytical* No interference observed at a concentration of 2000 μg/mL (1224 μmol/L) with method on Du Pont aca *1506*

Aspartate Aminotransferase *Serum Increase Physiological* In patients who had ingested acetaminophen lower enzyme activity when treated early with N-acetylcysteine than when drug not given, also prognosis better *5612*

Bicarbonate *Serum No Effect Analytical* When used to combat acetaminophen overdose no significant effect observed on method on Beckman CX3 *584*

Chloride *Serum Increase Analytical* In 4 patients in whom Parvolex was taken to combat acetaminophen overdose positive interference observed with method on Beckman Synchron CX3 analyzer. Effect probably due to binding of the thiol group of acetylcysteine with silver ions to form a mercaptide *584*

Cholinesterase *Serum* *No Effect* *Analytical* No effect observed at concentration of 102 mg/dL with butyrylthiocholine method on Kodak Ektachem® *2504*

Creatinine *Serum* *No Effect* *Analytical* When used to combat acetaminophen overdose no significant effect observed on method on Beckman Synchron CX3 *584*

Cysteine *Plasma* *No Effect* *Physiological* No effect of 30 mg/kg on total cysteine concentration in healthy volunteers *813*

Cysteine, Free *Plasma* *Increase* *Physiological* Peak concentration of free cysteine increased, with peak within 45 to 60 minutes by mean increment of 49 nmol/L following dose of 30 mg/kg *813*

Glucose *Serum* *No Effect* *Analytical* When used to combat acetaminophen overdose no significant effect observed on method on Beckman CX3 *584*

Glutathione *Plasma* *No Effect* *Physiological* No effect of 30 mg/kg on concentration of total glutathione in healthy volunteers *813*

Glutathione, Free *Plasma* *No Effect* *Physiological* No effect of 30 mg/kg on concentration in healthy volunteers *813*

Gold *Urine* *Increase* *Physiological* Excretion doubled in response to i.v. drug in patients previously given gold *2199*

Ketones *Serum* *Increase* *Analytical* Strongly positive reaction with aqueous solution containing 5 mmol/L, also observed in one patient receiving intravenous infusion of N-acetylcysteine when blood drawn close to infusion site *6473*

Urine *Increase* *Analytical* Falsely abnormal result produced with Boehringer Mannheim Chemstrip and Miles Multistix in proportion to amount of N-acetylcysteine present *4751* Addition at concentration of 20 mmol/L caused 2+ reaction with Boehringer Mannheim Chemstrip but effect could be eliminated within 2 minutes by the addition of 1 volume 500 g/L iodoacetate to 9 volumes of urine *4749* False positive readings obtained with both Chemstrip and Multistix dipsticks proportional to the amount of N-acetylcysteine *4750* False positive result obtained with this and other compounds containing free sulfhydryl group when Legal method used *1185*

Lipoprotein Lp(a) *Serum* *Decrease* *Physiological* Significant reduction observed in two patients from baselines of 58 and 59 mg/dL to 20 and 18 mg/dL respectively *2057* In 12 patients with high initial concentration (median 87.0 mg/dL) treatment with 1.2 g/d for 6 weeks caused small but significant decrease of 7% *3304*

Serum *No Effect* *Physiological* In 7 patients with a median Lp(a) concentration of 14.3 mg/dL administration of 1.2 g/d for 4 weeks caused no significant effect. Doubling dose to 2.4 g/d for another 2 weeks also had no effect *3304*

Phenylalanine *Plasma* *No Effect* *Analytical* No interference observed with quantitative rapid whole blood method of Campbell et al using phenylalanine dehydrogenase *867*

Phenytoin *Serum* *No Effect* *Analytical* At a concentration of 90 mg/dL had no significant effect on phenytoin concentrations up to 30 µg/mL with method on Johnson and Johnson Ektachem® systems *6356*

Potassium *Serum* *No Effect* *Analytical* When used to combat acetaminophen overdose no interference observed with method on Beckman Synchron CX3 *584*

Sodium *Serum* *No Effect* *Analytical* When administered to combat acetaminophen overdose no interference observed with method on Beckman CX3 *584*

Sulfite *Urine* *Increase* *Analytical* The presence of homocystine had caused significant increase with Merckoquant test for urinary sulfite used to diagnose molybdenum cofactor deficiency *2393*

Urea Nitrogen *Serum* *No Effect* *Analytical* When used to combat acetaminophen overdose no significant effect observed with method on Beckman Synchron CX3 *584*

Acetyldigitoxin

Digoxin *Serum* *Increase* *Analytical* At concentration of 25 ng/mL (30.75 nmol/L) caused 6.0% cross-reactivity with method on Du Pont Dimension *1573* Cross-reactivity of 6.0% observed at concentration of 25 ng/mL (30.75 nmol/L) with method used on Du Pont aca *1522*

Acetyldigoxin

Granulocytes *Blood* *Decrease* *Physiological* Agranulocytosis observed in 30% of patients compared with 11% controls: drug is significantly associated with agranulocytosis *3098*

Acetylglucosamine

Protein *Test Conditions* *Increase* *Analytical* Slight reaction with Folin-Ciocalteu reagent in method of Lowry *2566*

6-Acetylmorphine

Opiates *Urine* *Positive* *Analytical* Significant cross-reactivity observed with Roche Abuscreen method adapted for use with Olympus AU 5121 and 5131 analyzers *214*

Acetylpenicillamine

Copper *Serum* *Decrease* *Physiological* Elimination of heavy metals in cases of mercury poisoning *3043*

Mercury *Serum* *Increase* *Physiological* Mobilization of mercury in case of poisoning *3043*

Urine *Increase* *Physiological* Elimination of heavy metals in cases of mercury poisoning *3043*

Acetylphenylhydrazine

Bilirubin *Serum* *Increase* *Physiological* May cause hemolytic anemia *3810*

Bilirubin, Direct *Serum* *Increase* *Physiological* May cause hemolytic anemia *3810*

Erythrocytes *Blood* *Decrease* *Physiological* May cause hemolytic anemia *3810*

Haptoglobin *Serum* *Decrease* *Physiological* May cause hemolytic anemia *3810*

Hematocrit *Blood* *Decrease* *Physiological* May cause hemolytic anemia *3810*

Hemoglobin *Blood* *Decrease* *Physiological* May cause hemolytic anemia *3810*

Acetylsalicylic Acid

Acetaminophen *Serum* *No Effect* *Analytical* No interference observed at a concentration of 4000 µg/mL (1332 µmol/L) with method on Du Pont aca *1506* At 500 mg/L had no effect on HPLC method *5775*

Alanine Aminotransferase *Serum* *Decrease* *Analytical* At 8300 µmol/L on colorimetric analytical method *2919*

Serum *No Effect* *Analytical* At 5 times upper limit of therapeutic range on methods on Technicon SMAC® , Abbott-VP, Du Pont aca, Roche Cobas-Bio and KDA *3525* At 8300 µmol/L on continuous analytical method *2919* No effect of concentrations up to 1000 mg/L on method on Boehringer Mannheim Reflotron *5706* No effect at therapeutic concentration on Boehringer Mannheim Reflotron method *3231*

Albumin *Serum* *No Effect* *Analytical* At 5 times upper limit of therapeutic range on methods on Technicon SMAC® , Kodak Ektachem® , Hitachi® 705 and KDA *3525* At concentration of 2,000 mg/L had no effect on BCG method *5704* On bromocresol green method on Technicon SMA II at physiological concentration *2922*

Serum *No Effect* *Physiological* No effect seen in patients undergoing treatment *2922*

Urine *No Effect* *Analytical* At concentration of 200 mg/dL had no significant effect on Boehringer Mannheim Tina-quant method *2799* Using a fluorimetric assay with Albumin Blue 580 on a Cobas Fara centrifugal analyzer for the detection of microalbuminuria no significant interference was detected at a concentration of 100 mg/L *3117*

Alkaline Phosphatase *Serum* *No Effect* *Analytical* At 5 times upper limit of therapeutic range on methods on Technicon SMAC® , Abbott-VP, aca, Roche Cobas-Bio, Hitachi® 705 and KDA *3525* At 8300 µmol/L on continuous method *2919*

Acetylsalicylic Acid *(continued)*

Alkaline Phosphatase, Bone Isoenzyme
Serum No Effect Analytical At a concentration of 350 mg/L had no effect on EIA method of Gomez et al *2234*

Ammonia *Plasma No Effect Analytical* At concentration of 300 mg/L had no effect on Kodak Ektachem® method *5704*

Amylase *Serum No Effect Analytical* At concentration of 1000 mg/L had no effect on method on Boehringer Mannheim Reflotron system *5706* At 5 times upper limit of therapeutic range on methods on Du Pont aca, Roche Cobas-Bio, and Kodak Ektachem® *3525*

Amylase, Pancreatic Isoenzyme
Serum No Effect Analytical At toxic concentration of 1000 mg/L had no significant effect on method on Boehringer Mannheim Reflotron *3647*

Angiotensin-converting Enzyme
Serum No Effect Analytical No effect observed even with large amounts *5077*

Antithrombin III *Plasma No Effect Analytical* At concentration of 3 mg/L had no effect on Du Pont aca method *5704*

Antithrombin III Activity *Plasma No Effect Physiological* In 6 healthy volunteers given 6 g/d for 3 days mean activity decreased nonsignificantly from baseline of 96 ± 5% to 94 ± 3% but with return to baseline within 96 hours of treatment being stopped *6522*

Antithrombin III Antigen *Plasma No Effect Physiological* In 6 healthy volunteers treatment with 6 g/d for 3 days caused nonsignificant decrease from mean baseline of 99 ± 5% to 97 ± 4% but with return to baseline within 96 hours of treatment being stopped *6522*

Aspartate Aminotransferase *Serum Increase Analytical* At 5 times upper limit of therapeutic range on method on KDA *3525*
Serum No Effect Analytical At 5 times upper limit of therapeutic range on method on Technicon SMAC®, Abbott-VP, Roche Cobas-Bio, Du Pont aca, and Hitachi® 705 *3525* No effect at 1000 mg/L on Boehringer Mannheim Reflotron method *5706* At 8300 µmol/L on continuous and colorimetric methods *2919* No effect at therapeutic concentration on Boehringer Mannheim Reflotron method *3231*

Benzoylecgonine *Urine No Effect Analytical* Negative result obtained with method on Du Pont aca at a concentration of 1000 µg/mL (3.33 mmol/L) *1558*

Bicarbonate *Serum Decrease Analytical* At concentrations greater than 1,000 mg/L (10 times upper limit of therapeutic range) when using a phenolphthalein indicator method *5704*
Serum Increase Analytical Concentrations above 1030 mg/L increase result as determined by method on Kodak Ektachem® *5706*

Bilirubin *Serum No Effect Analytical* With 8326 µmol/L on Jendrassik - Grof method. With 8326 µmol/L on method using dimethylsulfoxide. With 8326 µmol/L on direct spectrophotometric method *2920* On Jendrassik - Grof, dimethylsulfoxide and spectrophotometric procedures with therapeutic concentrations *2920* At concentration of 300 mg/L had no effect on Kodak Ektachem® method *5704* At concentration of 2,000 mg/L had no effect on Jendrassik and Grof method *5704* No effect at a concentration of 500 mg/L on method on Ames Seralyzer *5706* At a concentration of 1000 mg/L had no effect on method on Boehringer Mannheim Reflotron system *5706* At 5 times upper limit of therapeutic range on methods onTechnicon SMAC®, Du Pont aca, Cobas-Bio, Kodak Ektachem®, Hitachi® 705 and KDA *3525* With 8326 µmol/L on direct spectrophotometric method *2920* On diazo method on Technicon SMA II at physiological concentration *2922*
Serum No Effect Physiological No effect seen in patients undergoing treatment *2922*

Bilirubin, Conjugated *Serum No Effect Analytical* No effect at concentration of 300 mg/L on method on Kodak Ektachem® *5706*

Bilirubin, Unconjugated *Serum No Effect Analytical* No effect at concentration of 300 mg/L on method on Kodak Ektachem® *5706*

Bleeding Time *Patient Increase Physiological* At normal dosage, time enhanced for at least 6 hours after oral ingestion but reduced when very low dosage administered *1482*

Calcium *Serum No Effect Analytical* On cresolphthalein complexone method on Technicon SMA II at physiological concentration *2922* At 5 times upper limit of therapeutic range on method on Technicon SMAC®, Abbott-VP, Du Pont aca, Kodak Ektachem®, Hitachi® 705 and KDA *3525* At concentration of 2,000 mg/L had no effect on cresolphthalein method *5704*
Serum No Effect Physiological No effect seen in patients undergoing treatment *2922*

Cannabinoids *Urine No Effect Analytical* No effect on Roche Abuscreen method *5006* No effect observed at a concentration of 1000 µg/mL (3.33 mmol/L) on method on Du Pont aca *1557*

Catecholamines *Plasma No Effect Analytical* No effect on HPLC method of Koller for dopamine, epinephrine, and norepinephrine *3230*

Chloride *Serum No Effect Analytical* At concentration of 2,000 mg/L had no effect on mercurimetric method *5704* No effect of concentrations up to 300 mg/L with method on Kodak Ektachem® *5706*

Cholesterol *Serum Decrease Analytical* Increase by 9% with 8326 µmol/L on Liebermann-Burchard method *2920*
Serum Increase Physiological Gradual increase during course of treatment with drug *2922*
Serum No Effect Analytical On enzymatic method on Technicon SMA II at physiological concentration *2922* At concentration of 750 mg/L had no effect on method using catalase-Hantzsch reaction *5704* At concentration of 750 mg/L had no effect on catalase-AIDH method *5704* No effect at 500 mg/L on Ames Seralyzer method *5706* At concentration of 2,000 mg/L had no effect on Liebermann - Burchard method *5704* At concentration of 750 mg/L had no effect on CHOD-Iodide method *5704* At concentration of 1000 mg/L no effect on method on Boehringer Mannheim Reflotron system *5706* At concentration of 750 mg/L had no effect on CHOD-PAP method *5704* At 5 times upper limit of therapeutic range on method onTechnicon SMAC®, Abbott-VP, Roche Cobas-Bio, Kodak Ektachem®, Hitachi® 705 and KDA *3525* At therapeutic concentrations on enzymatic and Liebermann - Burchard methods *2920* No effect at therapeutic concentration on Boehringer Mannheim Reflotron method *3231* With 8326 µmol/L on cholesterol esterase/oxidase method *2920*

Cholinesterase *Serum No Effect Analytical* No effect observed at concentration of 30 mg/dL with butyrylthiocholine method on Kodak Ektachem® *2504*

Cortisol *Plasma Increase Analytical* At a concentration of 1000 mg/L caused significant increase with Boehringer Mannheim Enzymun method with 123.2% recovery from female serum and 112.0% recovery with male serum. At therapeutic concentration in plasma of 300 mg/L recovery 111.0% *1097*
Plasma No Effect Analytical At concentration of 1000 mg/L had no significant effect on CEDIA method (worst case 96.3%) *1097*

Cortisol, Free *Urine No Effect Analytical* No significant interference observed with HPLC method of Turpeinen et al *6105*

Creatine Kinase *Serum Decrease Analytical* With 8300 µmol/L on kinetic method *2919*
Serum No Effect Analytical No effect at 500 mg/L on method on Ames Seralyzer *5706* At 5 times upper limit of therapeutic range on methods on Technicon SMAC®, Abbott-VP, Du Pont aca, Roche Cobas-Bio, and Hitachi® 705 *3525*

Creatine Kinase Isoenzymes *Serum No Effect Analytical* No interference observed at a concentration of 500 mg/L (1.67 mmol/L) with CK-MB method on Du Pont aca *1519*

Creatinine *Serum No Effect Analytical* At concentration of 2,000 mg/L had no effect on Technicon AutoAnalyzer® Jaffe method *5704* At 5 times upper limit of therapeutic range on method on Technicon SMAC®, Abbott-VP, Roche Cobas-Bio, Du Pont aca, Kodak Ektachem®, Hitachi® 705 and KDA *3525* No effect observed at a concentration of 4 mg/L with HPLC method of Rosano et al *5083* At concentration of 300 mg/L had no effect on Kodak Ektachem® method *5704* On alkaline picrate method on Technicon SMA II at physiological concentration *2922* With 8326 µmol/L on Technicon AutoAnalyzer® Jaffe method. With 8326 µmol/L on picrate method with deproteinization. With 8326 µmol/L on Slot procedure *2920* On alkaline picrate procedures and Slot method at therapeutic concentrations *2920* At concentration of 600 mg/L had no effect on creatinine iminohydrolase method *5704* At concentration of 600 mg/L had no effect on Jaffe-Fuller's earth method *5704* At concentration of 600 mg/L had no effect on

Jaffe-Fading-Fraction method *5704* At concentration of 500 mg/L had no effect on kinetic Jaffe method on BKA-2 *5704* No effect at 500 mg/L on Ames Seralyzer method *5706* No effect of concentrations up to 300 mg/L on 2-slide method on Kodak Ektachem® *5706* No effect of concentrations up to 300 mg/L on single slide method on Kodak Ektachem® *5706*
Serum No Effect Physiological No effect seen in patients undergoing treatment *2922*

Drugs of Abuse Screen *Urine No Effect Analytical* No effect at concentration of 100 µg/mL on EZ-SCREEN procedure for cannabinoids and cocaine *1739*

Felbamate *Serum No Effect Analytical* No significant interference observed with GLC method of Rifai et al *4958*

Fibrinogen *Plasma No Effect Analytical* At concentration of 500 mg/L had no effect on Du Pont aca method *5704*

Glucose *Serum Decrease Physiological* Enhanced response in healthy volunteers given 3.2 g daily both on basal concentration but also following either arginine orally or intravenously or tolbutamide orally or intravenously *926*
Serum Increase Analytical Increase by 11% with 8326 µmol/L on glucose-peroxidase method with 2,4-Dichlorophenol. Increase by 3% with 8326 µmol/L on glucose-peroxidase method with ABTS *2920*
Serum No Effect Analytical At 5 times upper limit of therapeutic range on method on Technicon SMAC® , Abbott-VP, Roche Cobas-Bio, du Pont aca, Kodak Ektachem® , Hitachi® 705 and KDA *3525* At concentration of 100 mg/L had no effect on Kodak Ektachem® method *5704* At concentration of 1400 mg/L had no effect on hexokinase/G-6-PDH method *5704* At concentration of 500 mg/L had no effect on Ames Seralyzer method *5704* No effect at 1500 mg/L on hexokinase method on Ames Seralyzer *5706* At concentration of 1000 mg/L no effect on glucose oxidase method on Boehringer Mannheim Reflotron system *5706* No effect at 500 mg/L on glucose oxidase method on Ames Seralyzer *5706* At therapeutic concentrations on hexokinase, glucose dehydrogenase 2,4-dichlorophenol, ABTS, and o-toluidine methods *2920* With 8326 µmol/L on hexokinase/G-6-PDH method. With 8326 µmol/L on glucose dehydrogenase method. With 8326 µmol/L on o-toluidine method *2920* No effect at therapeutic concentration on Boehringer Mannheim Reflotron method *3231* On hexokinase method on Technicon SMA II at physiological concentration *2922*
Serum No Effect Physiological No effect seen in patients undergoing treatment *2922*

γ-Glutamyltransferase *Serum No Effect Analytical* At 5 times upper limit of therapeutic range on methods on Technicon SMAC® , Abbott-VP and Hitachi® 705 *3525* At concentration of 1000 mg/L no effect on method on Boehringer Mannheim Reflotron system *5706* No effect at therapeutic concentration on Boehringer Mannheim Reflotron method *3231*

Glycated Hemoglobin *Blood No Effect Analytical* At a concentration of 500 mg/L had an insignificant - 3.7% interference with method on Abbott Vision *1885*

HDL-Cholesterol *Serum No Effect Analytical* At a concentration up to 1000 mg/L had no significant effect on Reflotron method for whole blood cholesterol *6352* No effect of concentrations up to 300 mg/L on method on Kodak Ektachem® *5706*

Hemoglobin *Blood No Effect Analytical* No effect at concentration of 300 mg/L on method on Kodak Ektachem® *5706*

Histamine *Plasma No Effect Analytical* Insignificant inhibition at therapeutic concentration of radio-enzyme assay *2492*

Hydroxybutyrate Dehydrogenase
Serum Decrease Analytical With 8300 µmol/L on kinetic method *2919*

Insulin *Plasma Increase Physiological* In healthy volunteers 3.2 g orally daily enhanced basal secretion and arginine-stimulated secretion following 25 g arginine i.v. over 30 min and tolbutamide-stimulated secretion following either 1 g tolbutamide orally or 0.25 g intravenously in a bolus *926*

Iron *Serum Increase Physiological* Significant effect correlated with duration of treatment (17.95 µmol/L vs 14.98 µmol/L) *2922*
Serum No Effect Analytical On Ferrozine method on Technicon SMA II at physiological concentration *2922* On Ramsay and bathophenanthroline methods at therapeutic concentrations *2920* At a concentration of 1500 mg/L had no effect on Ferrozine method *5704* At 5 times upper limit of therapeutic range on Ferrozine method of Technicon SMAC® *3525* No effect of concentrations up to 300 mg/L on method on Kodak Ektachem® *5706*

11-Keto-thromboxane B_2 *Urine Decrease Physiological* In 9 adults ingestion of a single dose of 500 mg produced a marked reduction the next morning with 5 individuals displaying a decrease of greater than 80% and the other 4 showing decreases of 23 to 49%. In 4 individuals who ingested 30 mg/d for 8 days caused markedly decreased excretion from about 1.0 ng/min to 0.5 ng/min *1446*

Lactate *Plasma No Effect Analytical* At a concentration of 1400 mg/L had no effect on enzyme method *5704*

Lactate Dehydrogenase *Serum Decrease Analytical* With 8300 µmol/L on continuous method with pyruvate substrate *2919* At 5 times upper limit of therapeutic range on method on KDA *3525*
Serum No Effect Analytical At 8300 µmol/L on continuous method with lactate as substrate. At 8300 µmol/L on colorimetric method *2919* No effect at 500 mg/L on method on Ames Seralyzer *5706* At 5 times upper limit of therapeutic range on method on Technicon SMAC® , Abbott-VP, Roche Cobas-Bio, and Hitachi® 705 *3525*

Lipase *Serum No Effect Analytical* No effect of concentrations up to 300 mg/L on method on Kodak Ektachem® *5706* No effect observed at a concentration of 50 mg/dL on revised method on Du Pont aca incorporating colipase *4702*

N-Acetyl-Glucosaminidase *Urine No Effect Analytical* At concentration of 200 mg/dL no significant effect observed on Boehringer Mannheim CPR method *3174*

Occult Blood *Feces Increase Physiological* In 6 healthy volunteers treatment with 1500 mg/d for 5 days caused significant increase from mean baseline of 0.354 ± 0.176 mL/d to 2.018 ± 0.844 mL/d *548*

p-Aminophenol *Urine No Effect Analytical* With addition of drugs at a concentration of 100 mg/L and of related compounds at 50 mg/L no significant effect observed on colorimetric method of van Bocxlaer on Cobas Mira analyzer which involves reacting free p-aminophenol with resorcinol in the presence of magnesium ions to form an indophenol dye measured at 550 nm *6163*

Partial Thromboplastin Time
Plasma Increase Physiological In 6 healthy volunteers given 6 g/d PTT increased nonsignificantly from mean baseline of 36 ± 3 seconds to 41 ± 4 seconds with return to baseline within 96 hours after treatment was stopped although in two of the volunteers the increases were significant *6522*

Phenylalanine *Plasma No Effect Analytical* No interference observed with rapid quantitative whole blood method of Campbell et al using phenylalanine dehyrogenase *867*

Phosphate *Serum No Effect Analytical* At concentration of 2,000 mg/L had no effect on phosphomolybdate method *5704* No effect of concentrations up to 300 mg/L on method on Kodak Ektachem® *5706* At 5 times upper limit of therapeutic range on method on Technicon SMAC® , Du Pont aca, Hitachi® 705, and KDA *3525*

Plasminogen *Plasma No Effect Analytical* At a concentration of 300 mg/L had no effect on Du Pont aca method *5704*

Platelet Aggregation *Blood Increase Physiological* Significant interference with platelet aggregation reported *6557*

Potassium *Serum No Effect Analytical* At concentration of 500 mg/L caused nonsignificant 0.6% interference with method on Abbott Vision *681* At a concentration of 100 mg/L had no effect on flame-photometric method *5704* At a concentration of 3,000 mg/L had no effect on ISE measurement with predilution *5704* At a concentration of 1,000 mg/L had no effect on ISE measurement without predilution *5704* At a concentration of 500 mg/L caused nonsignificant 0.6% interference with method on Abbott Vision *681*

Protein *Cerebrospinal Fluid No Effect Analytical* Insignificant effect when added in vitro and analyzed by Kodak Ektachem® slide method *3654*
Serum Decrease Analytical Increase by 1.5% with 8326 µmol/L on biuret method *2920*
Serum Increase Analytical Increase by 9% with 8326 µmol/L with direct spectrophotometry at 280 nm *2920*
Serum No Effect Analytical At concentration of 2,000 mg/L had no effect on biuret method with blank correction *5704* At therapeutic concentrations on biuret and spectrophotometric methods *2920* On biuret method on Technicon SMA II at

Acetylsalicylic Acid *(continued)*

Protein *(continued)*
physiological concentration *2922* At 5 times upper limit of therapeutic range on methods on Technicon SMAC®, Abbott-VP, Hitachi® 705 and KDA *3525*
Serum No Effect Physiological No effect seen in patients undergoing treatment *2922*

Protein C Activity *Plasma Decrease Physiological* In 6 healthy volunteers given 6 g/d mean activity decreased by 8% after 24 h, 25% after 48 h and 40% after 72 h but with return to almost baseline 96 h after treatment stopped *6522*

Protein C Antigen *Plasma Decrease Physiological* In 6 healthy volunteers treatment with 6 g/d caused mean 5% reduction after 24 h, 15% reduction after 48 h and 25% reduction after 72 h but return to baseline within 96 hours *6522*

Protein Electrophoresis *Serum No Effect Analytical* At a concentration of 1,000 mg/L had no effect on automated Olympus-Hite method *5704*

Prothrombin Time *Plasma Increase Physiological* In 6 healthy volunteers given 6 g/d mean concentration increased nonsignificantly (and still within normal range) from baseline of 14 ± 1 seconds to 15 ± 2 seconds after 72 hours but return to baseline within 96 hours of treatment being stopped *6522*

Sodium *Serum No Effect Analytical* At a concentration of 200 mg/L had no effect on flame-photometric method *5704* At a concentration of 1,000 mg/L had no effect on ISE measurement without predilution *5704* At a concentration of 3,000 mg/L had no effect on ISE measurement with predilution *5704*

Tacrolimus *Serum No Effect Analytical* In HPLC/MS method of Christians et al no significant interference observed with measurement of FK 506 *1010*

Thromboxane B_2 *Plasma Decrease Physiological* Reduction from mean concentration of 95 pg/mL to 10 pg/mL in 22 stroke patients following treatment with 100 mg daily at one month with lower concentrations observed with longer treatment *3478*

Tolbutamide *Serum Decrease Physiological* Insignificant reduction in healthy volunteers pretreated with 3.2 g acetylsalicylic acid following i.v. tolbutamide but percentage of free tolbutamide increased from 5.6% to 8.9% (i.e. increase of 40-50% in free tolbutamide concentration) *926*

Tri-iodothyronine, Free (fT3) *Serum No Effect Analytical* At a concentration of 0.3 g/L cross-reactivity of less than 0.1% with free triiodothyronine method on Bayer Technicon Immuno 1® system *425*

Triglycerides *Serum Decrease Analytical* At concentrations greater than 75 mg/L (within therapeutic range) lowered analyte concentration as measured by GPO-PAP method *5704*
Serum Increase Analytical At 5 times upper limit of therapeutic range on method on KDA *3525*
Serum Increase Physiological Significantly higher in patients receiving drug than in controls (1.69 mmol/L vs 1.47 mmol/L). Also seen in same patients before and after treatment *2922*
Serum No Effect Analytical On enzymatic method on Technicon SMA II at physiological concentration *2922* With 8326 µmol/L on enzymatic procedure with lipase *2920* On enzymatic methods at therapeutic concentrations *2920* At concentration of 2,000 mg/L had no effect on lipase/esterase method *5704* No effect at therapeutic concentration on Boehringer Mannheim Reflotron method *3231* At 5 times upper limit of therapeutic range on method on Technicon SMAC®, Abbott-VP, Kodak Ektachem® and Hitachi® 705 *3525* No effect up to 1000 mg/L on Boehringer Mannheim Reflotron method but above this concentration apparently reduced triglyceride concentration although not of clinical significance *5706*

Urea Nitrogen *Serum No Effect Analytical* At concentration of 50 mg/L had no effect on urease-Berthelot method *5704* At concentration of 100 mg/L had no effect on Kodak Ektachem® method *5704* With 8326 µmol/L on method using glutamate dehydrogenase. With 8326 µmol/L on method using phenol hypochlorite. With 8326 µmol/L on method using diacetyl monoxime *2920* At therapeutic concentrations on glutamate dehydrogenase, phenol-hypochlorite and diacetyl monoxime methods *2920* On diacetyl monoxime method on Technicon SMA II at physiological concentration *2922* No effect at 500 mg/L on method on Ames Seralyzer *5706* No effect at therapeutic concentration on Boehringer Mannheim Reflotron method *3231* At concentration of 2,000 mg/L had no effect on diacetylmonoxime method *5704* At 5 times upper limit of therapeutic range on method onTechnicon SMAC®, Abbott-VP, Roche Cobas-Bio, Kodak Ektachem®, Hitachi® 705 and KDA *3525* No effect at 1000 mg/L on Boehringer Mannheim Reflotron method *5706*
Serum No Effect Physiological No effect seen in patients undergoing treatment *2922*

Uric Acid *Serum Increase Analytical* Increase by 6% with 8326 µmol/L on uricase-catalase method *2920*
Serum No Effect Analytical On phosphotungstate method on Technicon SMA II at physiological concentration *2922* At 5 times upper limit of therapeutic range on method on Technicon SMAC®, Abbott-VP, Roche Cobas-Bio, Du Pont aca, Kodak Ektachem®, Hitachi® 705 and KDA *3525* No effect at 1000 mg/L on method on Boehringer Mannheim Reflotron *5706* At concentration of 900 mg/L had no effect on uricase-PAP method *5704* With 8326 µmol/L on uricase-catalase method with aldehyde dehydrogenase. With 8326 µmol/L on direct UV method with uricase *2920* No effect at therapeutic concentration on Boehringer Mannheim Reflotron method *3231* At therapeutic concentrations on uricase-catalase aldehyde dehydrogenase, direct UV-test and phosphotungstate methods *2920* At concentration of 600 mg/L had no effect on Kageyama-Hantzsch method *5704* With 8326 µmol/L on phosphotungstate reduction method *2920* At concentration of 2,000 mg/L had no effect on phosphotungstate reduction method *5704* At concentration of 600 mg/L had no effect on catalase-AlDH method *5704*
Serum No Effect Physiological No effect seen in patients undergoing treatment *2922*

Vitamin B_{12} *Serum No Effect Analytical* At concentrations up to 12.5 mg/dL had no clinically significant cross-reactivity in vitamin B_{12} method on Bayer Technicon Immuno 1® *439*

Acetylsulfadiazine

Crystals *Urine Increase Physiological* Wheatsheaves eccentric binding (not in alkaline urine) *684*

Acipimox

Apolipoprotein A-I *Serum No Effect Physiological* In 29 patients with NIDDM treatment with acipimox 500 mg twice daily for 12 weeks caused nonsignificant change in mean concentration from 1.2 ± 0.3 g/L to 1.2 ± 0.3 g/L *1284*

Apolipoprotein B *Serum No Effect Physiological* In 29 patients with NIDDM treatment with acipimox 500 mg twice daily for 12 weeks caused nonsignificant change in mean concentration from 1.2 ± 0.2 g/L to 1.0 ± 0.2 g/L *1284*

Cholesterol *Serum Decrease Physiological* In 23 patients with type II hyperlipidemia treatment with 1 g/d for 2 months caused significant reduction from mean baseline of 7.64 ± 0.19 mmol/L to 6.83 ± 0.21 mmol/L (9.4% reduction) *5427* In 82 patients with NIDDM treatment with 750 mg/d for 1 mo caused mean decrease of 0.69 mmol/L and 1.00 mmol/L after 3 mo (14%) *3216*
Serum No Effect Physiological In 29 patients with NIDDM treatment with acipimox 500 mg twice daily for 12 weeks caused nonsignificant change in mean concentration from 5.6 ± 1.3 mmol/L to 5.3 ± 1.3 mmol/L *1284* Insignificant reduction from mean of 216 mg/dL to 206 mg/dL in 11 obese diabetics given 750 mg daily for 1 week *1615*

Fatty Acids (FFA), Free *Serum Decrease Physiological* In 12 patients with NIDDM treatment with 500 mg/d caused significant reduction of both basal and insulin-stimulated concentration *6147* In 82 patients with NIDDM treatment with 750 mg/d caused nonsignificant mean reduction of 0.15 mmol/L after 1 mo and significant reduction of 0.005 mmol/L after 3 mo *3216*
Serum No Effect Physiological In 29 patients with NIDDM treatment with acipimox 500 mg twice daily for 12 weeks caused nonsignificant change in mean concentration from 0.84 ± 0.35 mmol/L to 0.88 ± 0.55 mmol/L *1284*

Fructosamine *Serum No Effect Physiological* In 29 patients with NIDDM treatment with acipimox 500 mg twice daily for 12 weeks caused nonsignificant change in mean concentration from 339 ± 54 mmol/L to 314 ± 47 mmol/L *1284*

Glucose *Serum Decrease Physiological* Significant reduction from mean of 204 mg/dL to 146 mg/dL in 11 obese diabetics given 750 mg daily for 1 week *1615* In 82 patients with NIDDM treatment with 750 mg/d for 1 mo caused nonsignificant decrease of 0.37 mmol/L after 1 mo and 0.70 mmol/L after 3 mo *3216*

Serum No Effect Physiological In 29 patients with NIDDM treatment with acipimox 500 mg twice daily for 12 weeks caused nonsignificant change in mean concentration from 10.8 ± 2.6 mmol/L to 10.1 ± 2.5 mmol/L *1284*

Glucose Tolerance *Serum No Effect Physiological* In 82 patients with NIDDM treatment with 750 mg/d had no significant effect after either 1 or 3 mo *3216*

Glycated Hemoglobin *Blood No Effect Physiological* In 29 patients with NIDDM treatment with acipimox 500 mg twice daily for 12 weeks caused nonsignificant change in mean concentration from 10.9 ± 2.6% to 10.5 ± 2.2% *1284*

HDL-Cholesterol *Serum Increase Physiological* In 82 patients with NIDDM treatment with 750 mg/d for 1 mo caused mean 0.13 mmol/L increase and 0.193 mmol/L after 3 mo (up to 24%) *217* In 31 patients with hypertriglyceridemia concentration significantly increased *6053*

Serum No Effect Physiological In 23 patients with type II hyperlipidemia treatment with 1 g/d for 2 months caused insignificant change from mean baseline of 1.28 ± 0.08 mmol/L to 1.34 ± 0.07 mmol/L *5427* Insignificant reduction from mean of 36 mg/dL to 35 mg/dL in 11 obese diabetics given 750 mg daily for 1 week *1615* In 29 patients with NIDDM treatment with acipimox 500 mg twice daily for 12 weeks caused nonsignificant change in mean concentration from 1.1 ± 0.3 mmol/L to 1.2 ± 0.4 mmol/L *1284*

Hemoglobin A_{1c} *Blood No Effect Physiological* In 82 patients with NIDDM treatment with 750 mg/d had no significant effect after either 1 or 3 mo *3216*

Insulin *Plasma No Effect Physiological* In 29 patients with NIDDM treatment with acipimox 500 mg twice daily for 12 weeks caused nonsignificant change in mean concentration from 14 mIU/L to 14 mIU/L *1284* In 82 patients with NIDDM treatment with 750 mg/d caused no significant change after either 1 or 3 mo *3216*

LDL-Cholesterol *Serum Decrease Physiological* In 23 patients with type II hyperlipidemia treatment with 1 g/d for 2 months caused significant reduction from mean baseline of 5.47 ± 0.16 mmol/L to 4.93 ± 0.19 mmol/L (8.5% reduction) *5427*

Lipoprotein Lp(a) *Serum Decrease Physiological* In 23 patients with type II hyperlipidemia treatment with 1 g/d for 2 months caused significant reduction of antilog of mean log values of 58.1 mg/dL to 52.2 mg/dL *5427*

Serum No Effect Physiological In 29 patients with NIDDM treatment with acipimox 500 mg twice daily for 12 weeks caused nonsignificant change in mean concentration from 116 mg/L to 154 g/L *1284*

Triglycerides *Serum Decrease Physiological* In 82 patients with NIDDM treatment with 750 mg/d for 1 month caused significant mean decrease of 1.06 mmol/L after 1 mo and 1.23 mmol/L after 3 mo (28%) *3216* Reduction from mean concentration of 181 mg/dL to 141 mg/dL in 11 obese diabetics given 750 mg daily for 1 week *1615* In 23 patients with type II hyperlipidemia treatment with 1 g/d for 2 months caused significant reduction from mean baseline of 1.92 ± 0.25 mmol/L to 1.31 ± 0.19 mmol/L (13.2% reduction) *5427*

Serum No Effect Physiological In 29 patients with NIDDM treatment with acipimox 500 mg twice daily for 12 weeks caused nonsignificant change in mean concentration from 2.4 mmol/L to 1.7 mmol/L *1284*

Aconitine

Occult Blood *Feces Increase Physiological* If ingested may cause many gastrointestinal symptoms *467*

Acridine

Chromosomes *Test Conditions Abnormal Physiological* Clastogenic in human diploid fibroblasts *in vitro5484*

Acridine Orange

Chromosomes *Test Conditions Abnormal Physiological* Clastogenic in human diploid fibroblasts *in vitro5484*

Acriflavine

Bile *Urine Increase Analytical* Produces yellow color when urine shaken *703*

Color *Urine Increase Analytical* Greenish fluorescence *4053*

Porphyrin, Total *Urine Increase Analytical* Produce fluorescence *6515*

Urobilin *Urine Increase Analytical* Produces yellow-green fluorescence *2559*

Acrivastine

Histamine *Plasma No Effect Analytical* Improbable inhibition of radio-enzyme assay at physiological concentrations *2492*

Actinomycin

Chromosomes *Test Conditions Abnormal Physiological* Clastogenic in human cells *5484*

Porphobilinogen *Urine Decrease Physiological* Suppressed induction of ALA synthetase in porphyria *1479*

Uroporphyrin *Urine Decrease Physiological* Suppresses induction of ALA synthetase in porphyria *1479*

Activated Charcoal

Acetylsalicylic Acid *Serum Decrease Physiological* Administration of 50 g activated charcoal immediately following 1 g aspirin reduced serum salicylate concentration by 95% *4062*

Urine Decrease Physiological When 50 g activated charcoal administered immediately after 1 g aspirin urinary excretion of salicylic acid and its metabolites reduced by 70% *4062*

Glipizide *Serum Decrease Physiological* In 6 healthy male volunteers concomitant administration of 8 g activated charcoal with single dose of glipizide caused reduction of mean peak plasma concentration from 425 ng/mL to 89 ng/mL *3167*

Nadolol *Serum Decrease Physiological* Concomitant administration reduced area under curve from 2455 ng/h/mL to 1355 ng/h/mL *1601*

Theophylline *Serum Decrease Physiological* Multiple doses rapidly increases the clearance of theophylline at least two-fold by absorption of theophylline secreted into gastrointestinal fluids and reduces its plasma concentration *5999*

Tolbutamide *Serum Decrease Physiological* Following administration of 50 g absorption of 500 mg tolbutamide concentration was reduced by 90% in 6 healthy volunteers *4257*

Valproic Acid *Serum Decrease Physiological* Following ingestion of 50 g activated charcoal by 6 healthy volunteers absorption of 300 mg valproic acid reduced by mean of 65% *4257*

Acyclovir

Alanine Aminotransferase *Serum Increase Physiological* In clinical practice some cases of increased liver function tests *2151*

Alkaline Phosphatase *Serum Decrease Physiological* In clinical practice some cases of leukopenia reported *2151*

Serum Increase Physiological In clinical practice some cases of increased liver function tests *2151*

Aspartate Aminotransferase *Serum Increase Physiological* In clinical practice some cases of increased liver function tests *2151*

Bilirubin *Serum Increase Physiological* Isolated increases reported but not confirmed in large trials *1384* In clinical practice some cases of increased liver function tests *2151*

Acyclovir (continued)

Cholinesterase *Serum No Effect Analytical* No effect observed at concentration of 25 µg/mL on butyrylthiocholine method on Kodak Ektachem® *2504* At a concentration of 25 µg/mL has no significant effect on method on Kodak Ektachem® systems *2519*

Creatinine *Serum Increase Physiological* Observed in 3 of 27 adults with chronic fatigue syndrome treated for 1 month with drug. Renal failure was reversible in all cases *5844* Reversible increase, especially with doses greater than 5 mg/kg i.v. every 8 h. Major adverse effect occurring in as many as 50% patients *1477* Occasional reversible side effect, most often when given as an intravenous bolus: probably due to deposition of crystals in renal tubules *1384* In clinical practice some cases of increased plasma creatinine concentration reported *2151*

Serum No Effect Analytical No effect of concentrations up to 500 mg/L on 2-slide method on Kodak Ektachem® *5706*

Crystals *Urine Increase Physiological* Especially with high-dose bolus infusion and with dehydration and pre-existing renal insufficiency *1477* Crystalluria in 3 of 27 patients with chronic fatigue syndrome in spite of efforts to ensure adequate hydration. In all cases renal failure reversible *5844* Observed in urine of one woman who had received intravenous drug for herpes encephalitis with impairment of renal tubular function: not observed in another 60 patients receiving drug orally or in 20 receiving it intravenously *4635*

Cyclosporine *Blood No Effect Physiological* Coadministration of acyclovir with cyclosporine had no significant effect on cyclosporine concentration but caused some improvement in renal function *859*

Serum No Effect Physiological Coadministration of acyclovir with cyclosporine had no significant effect on cyclosporine concentration but caused some improvement in renal function *859*

Erythrocytes *Blood Decrease Physiological* One case of megaloblastic anemia documented *1477*

Hemoglobin *Blood Decrease Physiological* One case of megaloblastic anemia documented *1477*

Ketone Body Ratio *Serum No Effect Analytical* When added at a concentration of 1.25 g/L had no significant effect on AKBR method of Uno et al *6131*

Lymphocyte response to Pokeweed Mitogen

Blood No Effect Physiological No effect on blastogenic response to mitogens - phytohemagglutin, pokeweed, and concanavilin A *in vitro228*

MCHC *Blood Increase Physiological* Isolated unconfirmed case reported *1384*

MCV *Blood Increase Physiological* Isolated unconfirmed report in one patient *1384*

β_2-Microglobulin *Urine Increase Physiological* Observed in one woman who had acyclovir crystalluria following intravenous infusion for herpes encephalitis: not observed in another 60 patients receiving drug orally or in 20 others receiving it intravenously *4635*

Mycophenolate *Serum No Effect Physiological* Coadministration of mycophenolate mofentil (1 g) with acyclovir (800 mg) in 12 healthy volunteers caused no significant change in mycophenolate AUC or concentration *5017*

Mycophenolate Glucuronide *Serum Increase Physiological* Coadministration of mycophenolate mofentil (1 g) with acyclovir (800 mg) in 12 healthy volunteers caused a 10.6% increase in mycophenolate glucuronide AUC *5017*

Tacrolimus *Serum No Effect Analytical* In HPLC/MS method of Christians et al no significant interference observed with measurement of FK 506 *1010*

Urea Nitrogen *Serum Increase Physiological* Reported reversible effect probably due to deposition of crystals in renal tubules, most often when given as an intravenous bolus *1384* Transient rises reported in some patients *228*

Zalcitabine *Serum No Effect Analytical* At a concentration of 100 mg/L had less than 0.01% cross-reactivity with solid phase extraction and RIA method of Roberts et al *4990*

Zidovudine *Serum No Effect Analytical* No effect on LC method of Hedaya and Sawchuk *2525*

Adenosine

Epinephrine *Plasma Increase Physiological* Increase by 213% after i.v. infusion of 10 to 140 µg/kg/min in 7 normal subjects *544*

Fatty Acids (FFA), Free *Serum No Effect Physiological* In 10 healthy individuals infusion of 100 µg/kg/min had no significant effect on concentration *5903*

Glucose *Serum No Effect Physiological* In 10 healthy individuals infusion of 100 µg/kg/min for 120 minutes had no significant effect on concentration *5903*

Insulin *Plasma No Effect Physiological* In 10 healthy individuals no significant effect of infusion of 100 µg/kg/min for 120 minutes *5903*

Norepinephrine *Plasma Increase Physiological* Increase by 44% after i.v. infusion of 10 to 140 µg/kg/min in 7 normal subjects *544*

Renin Activity *Plasma No Effect Physiological* After i.v. infusion of 10 to 140 µg/kg/min in 7 normal subjects *544*

Adenosine Monophosphate

Cortisol *Plasma Increase Physiological* Hormonal action *1827*

Glucose *Serum Increase Physiological* Hormonal action *1827*

Growth Hormone *Plasma Increase Physiological* Hormonal action *1827*

Insulin *Plasma Increase Physiological* Hormonal action *1827*

β-Adrenergic Drugs

Glucose *Serum Increase Physiological* Masks spurious hypoglycemia from insulin overdose *2024*

Hematocrit *Blood Increase Physiological* But less than expected with change in plasma volume *2988*

Volume *Plasma Decrease Physiological* Decreased by approximately 10% shortly after i.v. injection *2988*

Urine Decrease Physiological Antidiuretic effect mediated centrally *5379*

Aflatoxin

Chromosomes *Test Conditions Abnormal Physiological* Probably clastogenic in human cells *5484*

Ajmaline

Alanine Aminotransferase *Serum Increase Physiological* Intrahepatic cholestasis *453* Hepatotoxicity and intrahepatic cholestasis reported *5395* In 4 patients with centrilobular cholestasis and mild hepatocytic lesions: recovery with drug withdrawal *4514*

Alkaline Phosphatase *Serum Increase Physiological* Intrahepatic cholestasis *453* In 4 patients with centrilobular cholestasis and mild hepatocytic lesions: recovery with drug withdrawal *4514* Hepatotoxicity and intrahepatic cholestasis reported *5395*

Aspartate Aminotransferase *Serum Increase Physiological* In 4 patients with centrilobular cholestasis and mild hepatocytic lesions: recovery with drug withdrawal *4514* Intrahepatic cholestasis *453* Hepatotoxicity and intrahepatic cholestasis reported *5395*

Bile *Urine Increase Physiological* Intrahepatic cholestasis *453*

Bilirubin *Serum Increase Physiological* Hepatotoxicity and intrahepatic cholestasis reported *5395* In 4 patients with centrilobular cholestasis and mild hepatocytic lesions: recovery with drug withdrawal *4514* Intrahepatic cholestasis *453*

Catecholamines *Plasma Increase Physiological* Release of stored norepinephrine *3669*

Creatinine *Serum No Effect Analytical* No interference observed with liquid chromatographic method of Paroni et al *4540*

Digoxin *Serum* *No Effect* *Physiological* No effect on serum concentration reported *558*

Eosinophils *Blood* *Increase* *Physiological* In 4 patients with centrilobular cholestasis and mild hepatocytic lesions: recovery with drug withdrawal *4514*

Glucose *Serum* *No Effect* *Analytical* At concentration of 3.3 mg/L had no effect on GOD/POD-PAP method *5704*

Hydrochloric Acid *Gastric Fluid* *Increase* *Physiological* Strong stimulant action *3669*

4-Hydroxy-3-Methoxy-Phenylglycol
Urine *Increase* *Physiological* Release of stored norepinephrine *3669*

Neutrophils *Blood* *Decrease* *Physiological* Isolated reversible cases of agranulocytosis *5395*

Triglycerides *Serum* *No Effect* *Analytical* At concentration of 3.3 mg/L had no effect on GPO-PAP method *5704*

Uric Acid *Serum* *No Effect* *Analytical* At concentration of 3.3 mg/L had no effect on uricase-PAP method *5704*

Urobilinogen *Feces* *Decrease* *Physiological* Intrahepatic cholestasis *453*
Urine *Decrease* *Physiological* Intrahepatic cholestasis *453*

Vanillylmandelic Acid *Urine* *Increase* *Physiological* Release of stored norepinephrine *3669*

Albendazole

Alanine Aminotransferase *Serum* *Increase* *Physiological* Abnormal liver function tests observed in 15.6% patients with hydatid disease and < 1.0% patients with neurocystercosis *5635* Increase observed in 10 of 12 patients treated with hepatotoxicity occurring in three of them *5793*

Alkaline Phosphatase *Serum* *Increase* *Physiological* Abnormal liver function tests observed in 15.6% patients with hydatid disease and < 1.0% patients with neurocystercosis *5635*

Antipyrine Clearance *Patient* *Decrease* *Physiological* Significant reduction observed in patients with echinococcosis undergoing long term treatment *5793*

Aspartate Aminotransferase *Serum* *Increase* *Physiological* Increase observed in 10 of 12 patients with long term therapy partially due to the drug inhibiting microsomal enzyme function and inducing its own metabolism. Hepatotoxicity observed in 3 of the 12 patients treated *5793* Abnormal liver function tests observed in 15.6% patients with hydatid disease and < 1.0% patients with neurocystercosis *5635*

Bilirubin *Serum* *Increase* *Physiological* Abnormal liver function tests observed in 15.6% patients with hydatid disease and < 1.0% patients with neurocystercosis *5635*

Creatinine *Serum* *Increase* *Physiological* Acute renal failure observed in a few patients receiving albendazole *5635*

Granulocytes *Blood* *Decrease* *Physiological* Granulocytopenia or agranulocytosis or pancytopenia observed in less than 1% treated patients *5635*

Leukocytes *Blood* *Decrease* *Physiological* Reversible reduction of concentration observed in less than 1% treated patients *5635*

Neutrophils *Blood* *Decrease* *Physiological* Neutropenia observed in 3 of 12 patients treated with albendazole over long term *5793*

Platelets *Blood* *Decrease* *Physiological* Incidence of thrombocytopenia of < 1.0% observed in treated patients *5635*

Theophylline *Serum* *No Effect* *Physiological* Pharmacokinetics of theophylline unchanged following a single dose of albendazole *5635*

Urea Nitrogen *Serum* *Increase* *Physiological* Acute renal failure observed in a few patients receiving albendazole *5635*

Albuterol

Adenosine Monophosphate *Plasma* *Increase* *Physiological* Effect mirrored reduction in serum potassium concentration following inhalation of drug *5322*

Aldosterone *Plasma* *Decrease* *Physiological* No significant change in 4 healthy men given i.v. infusion of therapeutic amount *4690*

Calcium *Serum* *Decrease* *Physiological* Significant dose-related effect after i.v. infusion of therapeutic doses in 4 healthy male volunteers *4690*

Catecholamines *Plasma* *No Effect* *Analytical* No effect on HPLC method of Koller for dopamine, epinephrine, and norepinephrine *3230*

Cholesterol *Serum* *Decrease* *Physiological* In 8 healthy males oral administration of 8 mg b.i.d for 14 days caused a significant reduction from mean baseline of 179 ± 9 mg/dL to 162 ± 7 mg/dL *3745*

Cholesterol:HDL-Cholesterol Ratio
Serum *Decrease* *Physiological* In 8 healthy males oral administration of 8 mg b.i.d for 14 days caused a significant reduction from mean baseline of 4.4 ± 0.5 to 3.6 ± 0.4 *3745*

Corticosteroids *Plasma* *Decrease* *Physiological* Significant dose-related effect after i.v. infusion of therapeutic doses in 4 healthy male volunteers *4690*

Cyclosporine *Blood* *No Effect* *Analytical* At concentration of 0.18 mg/L had no effect on Syva EMIT method *495*

Digoxin *Serum* *Decrease* *Physiological* In healthy men coadministration of salbutamol caused significant reduction of digoxin concentration *1661* Coadministration of oral and intravenous albuterol with a single digoxin dose caused reductions of digoxin concentrations of 22% and 16% respectively *5336* During salbutamol infusion area under the concentration curve over 0-6 hours 15% less than during saline infusion due to faster elimination from the central volume of distribution to deeper commpartments *1662*

Eosinophil Cationic Protein *Serum* *No Effect* *Physiological* In 20 asthmatic patients treated with albuterol 400 μg four times daily for two weeks caused insignificant change from mean baseline of 12.8 ± 2.8 μg/L to 13.0 ± 3.1 μg/L *3364*

Estriol *Plasma* *Decrease* *Physiological* Significant reduction when given to women in premature labor *2510*

Glucose *Serum* *Increase* *Physiological* Following 8 mg significant increase by 1.0 mmol/L at 1 h and 0.9 mmol/L at 2 h but falling to baseline at 3 h in 6 healthy volunteers *4064* In patients with hyperkalemia and chronic renal failure intravenous administration of 0.5 mg caused significant increase from mean baseline of 88 ± 4 mg/dL to 101 ± 3 mg/dL after 30 min and to 101 ± 4 mg/dL after 60 min: similar response after inhalation of salbutamol *3600* Significant dose-related effect after i.v. infusion of therapeutic doses in 4 healthy male volunteers *4690*
Serum *No Effect* *Physiological* In 8 healthy males oral administration of 8 mg b.i.d for 14 days caused a nonsignificant change from mean baseline of 92 ± 2 mg/dL to 95 ± 2 mg/dL *3745*

HDL-Cholesterol *Serum* *Increase* *Physiological* In 8 healthy males oral administration of 8 mg b.i.d for 14 days caused a significant increase from mean baseline of 44 ± 4 mg/dL to 48 ± 4 mg/dL *3745* Administration of a dose of 8 mg twice daily for 2 weeks caused mean increase in concentration of 6.9% *975*

Histamine *Plasma* *No Effect* *Analytical* Improbable inhibition of radio-enzyme assay at physiological concentrations *2492*

β-Hydroxybutyrate *Serum* *No Effect* *Physiological* No significant change in 4 healthy men given i.v. infusion of therapeutic amount *4690*

Insulin *Plasma* *Increase* *Physiological* In 15 patients with hyperkalemia and chronic renal failure intravenous injection of 0.5 mg caused significant increase from mean baseline of 28.5 ± 5.7 μU/mL to 45.7 ± 6.7 μU/mL after 30 min and 41.2 ± 6.4 μU/mL after 60 min *3600* Significant dose-related effect after i.v. infusion of therapeutic doses in 4 healthy male volunteers *4690*
Plasma *No Effect* *Physiological* In 8 healthy males oral administration of 8 mg b.i.d for 14 days caused a nonsignificant change from mean baseline of 10.8 ± 1.8 mU/L to 11.0 ± 1.7 mU/L *3745*

Ketones *Serum* *Increase* *Physiological* Significant dose-related effect after i.v. infusion of therapeutic doses in 4 healthy male volunteers *4690*

Lactate *Plasma* *Increase* *Physiological* Significant dose-related effect after i.v. infusion of therapeutic doses in 4 healthy male volunteers *4690*

Albuterol *(continued)*

LDL-Cholesterol *Serum Decrease Physiological* In 8 healthy males oral administration of 8 mg b.i.d for 14 days caused a significant reduction from mean baseline of 115 ± 8 mg/dL to 97 ± 6 mg/dL *3745*

LDL-Cholesterol:HDL-Cholesterol Ratio
Serum Decrease Physiological In 8 healthy males oral administration of 8 mg b.i.d for 14 days caused a significant reduction from mean baseline of 2.9 ± 0.4 to 2.2 ± 0.3 *3745*

Magnesium *Serum Decrease Physiological* In 8 healthy males oral administration of 8 mg b.i.d for 14 days caused a significant change from mean baseline of 1.71 ± 0.04 mEq/L to 1.64 ± 0.05 mEq/L *3745* Significant dose-related effect after i.v. infusion of therapeutic doses in 4 healthy male volunteers *4690*

Norepinephrine *Plasma Increase Physiological* Dose-dependent increase following inhalation of drug *5322*

Phosphate *Serum Decrease Physiological* Significant dose-related effect after i.v. infusion of therapeutic doses in 4 healthy male volunteers *4690*

Platelets *Blood Decrease Physiological* In 5 healthy volunteers given drug i.v.: significant reduction occurred over 6 minutes *3341*

Potassium *Serum Decrease Physiological* Highly significant decrease of 0.6, 0.5, 0.6, and 0.6 mmol/L at 1, 2, 3, and 4 hours respectively after single oral dose of 8 mg in 6 healthy volunteers, but increases observed when propranolol combined with salbutamol (albuterol) *4064* In 15 patients with hyperkalemia and chronic renal failure intravenous administration of 0.5 mg caused significant reduction from mean baseline of 5.53 ± 0.12 mmol/L to 4.64 ± 0.11 mmol/L after 30 min and 4.91 ± 0.11 mmol/L after 1 hour with similar effect after receiving the salbutamol by nebulizer *3600* Significant dose-related effect after i.v. infusion of therapeutic doses in 4 healthy male volunteers *4690* Administration may cause hypokalemia *5336* In 8 healthy males oral administration of 8 mg b.i.d for 14 days caused a significant change from mean baseline of 4.4 ± 0.1 mmol/L to 4.2 ± 0.1 mmol/L *3745* Dose dependent effect in 6 healthy male volunteers with peak effect observed 75 to 90 minutes after first inhalation *5322* At inhaled doses greater than 4.02 mmol/L mean concentration decreased to 3.91 mmol/L *3735*
Serum Increase Physiological Drug may decrease the concentration of potassium *2167*

Renin Activity *Plasma Increase Physiological* Dose-dependent increase following inhalation of drug *5322* Significant dose-related effect after i.v. infusion of therapeutic doses in 4 healthy male volunteers *4690*

Soluble Interleukin-2 Receptor
Serum Increase Physiological In 20 asthmatic patients treated with albuterol 400 μg four times daily for two weeks caused significant change from mean baseline of 505.9 ± 52.1 U/mL to 558.6 ± 47.1 U/mL *3364*

Theophylline *Serum No Effect Analytical* At concentration of 6 mg/L had no effect on methods on Abbott TDx, Kodak DT-60, Abbott Vision with either blood or serum, 3M Diagnostics TheoFAST, Syntex AccμLevel or Ames Seralyzer *1122*
Serum No Effect Physiological Neither systemic or inhaled albuterol had a clinically significant effect on theophylline concentration *5999* Neither systemic or inhaled albuterol has a documented significant interaction with theophylline *6117*

Triglycerides *Serum Decrease Physiological* In 8 healthy males oral administration of 8 mg b.i.d for 14 days caused a nonsignificant reduction from mean baseline of 100 ± 14 mg/dL to 84 ± 18 mg/dL *3745*

Tryptase *Serum No Effect Physiological* In 20 asthmatic patients treated with albuterol 400 μg four times daily for two weeks caused insignificant change from mean baseline of 1.34 ± 0.01 U/L to 1.35 ± 0.01 μg/L *3364*

Uric Acid *Serum Decrease Physiological* In 8 healthy males oral administration of 8 mg b.i.d for 14 days caused a nonsignificant change from mean baseline of 5.98 ± 0.49 mg/dL to 5.95 ± 0.58 mg/dL *3745*

Alclofenac

Tryptophan *Plasma Decrease Physiological* Total measured in rheumatoids on therapy *303*

Tryptophan, Free *Plasma Increase Physiological* In rheumatoids on therapy *303*

Alclometasone

Cortisol *Plasma No Effect Analytical* With twice daily topical application in 39 children over 3 weeks *1168* In 10 volunteers given 30 g over 80% of body surface twice daily *6023*

Cortisol, Free *Urine No Effect Analytical* In 10 volunteers given 30 g over 80% of body surface twice daily *6023*

17-Hydroxycorticosteroids *Urine No Effect Analytical* In 10 volunteers given 30 g over 80% of body surface twice daily *6023*

Alcohols

Occult Blood *Feces Increase Physiological* May cause many gastrointestinal symptoms including bleeding *467*

Alcuronium

Albumin *Serum Decrease Physiological* Negative correlation between sensitivity and albumin concentration *5841*
Serum Increase Physiological Sensitivity to drug associated with albumin concentration *5841*

Histamine *Plasma Decrease Analytical* 50% inhibition of radio-enzyme assay at 1.1 μg/mL (physiological concentration 0.74 - 2.25 μg/mL) *2492*

Aldatense

Alkaline Phosphatase *Serum Decrease Physiological* Increase by 80% in a group of hypertensives compared with controls *2627*

Creatinine *Serum Increase Physiological* Increase by 10-20% in a group of hypertensives compared with controls *2627*

γ-Glutamyltransferase *Serum Decrease Physiological* Increase by 80% in a group of hypertensives compared with controls *2627*

Phosphate *Serum Increase Physiological* Increase by 10-20% in a group of hypertensives compared with controls *2627*

Triglycerides *Serum Increase Physiological* Increase by 30% in a group of hypertensives compared with controls *2627*

Urea Nitrogen *Serum Increase Physiological* Increase by 10-20% in a group of hypertensives compared with controls *2627*

Uric Acid *Serum Increase Physiological* Increase by 10-20% in a group of hypertensives compared with controls *2627*

Aldesleukin

Alanine Aminotransferase *Serum Increase Physiological* Effect observed in 56% of 373 patients with either renal cell cancer or other tumors *997*

Albumin *Serum Decrease Physiological* Effect observed in 8% of 373 patients with either renal cell cancer or other tumors *997*

Alkaline Phosphatase *Serum Increase Physiological* Effect observed in 56% of 373 patients with either renal cell cancer or other tumors *997*

Amylase *Serum No Effect Physiological* Pancreatitis observed in less than 1% of 373 patients with either renal cell cancer or other tumors *997*

Aspartate Aminotransferase *Serum Increase Physiological* Effect observed in 56% of 373 patients with either renal cell cancer or other tumors *997*

Bilirubin *Serum Increase Physiological* Effect observed in 64% of 373 patients with either renal cell cancer or other tumors *997*

Blood *Urine Increase Physiological* Effect observed in 9% of 373 patients with either renal cell cancer or other tumors *997*

Calcium *Serum Decrease Physiological* Effect observed in 15% of 373 patients with either renal cell cancer or other tumors *997*

Serum Increase Physiological Effect observed in 1% of 373 patients with either renal cell cancer or other tumors *997*

Cholesterol *Serum Decrease Physiological* Effect observed in 1% of 373 patients with either renal cell cancer or other tumors *997*

Creatinine *Serum Increase Physiological* Effect observed in 61% of 373 patients with either renal cell cancer or other tumors *997*

Eosinophils *Blood Increase Physiological* Effect observed in 6% of 373 patients with either renal cell cancer or other tumors *997*

Glucose *Serum Decrease Physiological* Effect observed in 2% of 373 patients with either renal cell cancer or other tumors *997*

Serum Increase Physiological Effect observed in 2% of 373 patients with either renal cell cancer or other tumors *997*

Hemoglobin *Blood Decrease Physiological* Effect observed in 77% of 373 patients with either renal cell cancer or other tumors *997*

Leukocytes *Blood Decrease Physiological* Effect observed in 34% of 373 patients with either renal cell cancer or other tumors *997*

Blood Increase Physiological Effect observed in 9% of 373 patients with either renal cell cancer or other tumors *997*

Lipase *Serum No Effect Physiological* Pancreatitis observed in less than 1% of 373 patients with either renal cell cancer or other tumors *997*

Magnesium *Serum Decrease Physiological* Effect observed in 16% of 373 patients with either renal cell cancer or other tumors *997*

pH *Blood Decrease Physiological* Acidosis observed in 16% of 373 patients with either renal cell cancer or other tumors *997*

Blood Increase Physiological Acidosis observed in 4% of 373 patients with either renal cell cancer or other tumors *997*

Phosphate *Serum Decrease Physiological* Effect observed in 11% of 373 patients with either renal cell cancer or other tumors *997*

Serum Increase Physiological Effect observed in 1% of 373 patients with either renal cell cancer or other tumors *997*

Platelets *Blood Decrease Physiological* Effect observed in 64% of 373 patients with either renal cell cancer or other tumors *997*

Potassium *Serum Decrease Physiological* Effect observed in 9% of 373 patients with either renal cell cancer or other tumors *997*

Serum Increase Physiological Effect observed in 4% of 373 patients with either renal cell cancer or other tumors *997*

Protein *Serum Decrease Physiological* Effect observed in 7% of 373 patients with either renal cell cancer or other tumors *997*

Urine Increase Physiological Effect observed in 12% of 373 patients with either renal cell cancer or other tumors *997*

Sodium *Serum Decrease Physiological* Effect observed in 4% of 373 patients with either renal cell cancer or other tumors *997*

Serum Increase Physiological Effect observed in 1% of 373 patients with either renal cell cancer or other tumors *997*

Thyroxine (T4) *Serum No Effect Physiological* Effect observed in less than 1% of 373 patients with either renal cell cancer or other tumors *997*

Urea Nitrogen *Serum Increase Physiological* Effect observed in 63% of 373 patients with either renal cell cancer or other tumors *997*

Uric Acid *Serum Increase Physiological* Effect observed in 9% of 373 patients with either renal cell cancer or other tumors *997*

Aldrin

Cholinesterase *Serum Decrease Analytical In vitro* 6.0% decrease at 1 x 10^{-4} mol/L *2095*

Lactate Dehydrogenase *Serum Decrease Physiological In vitro* 4.5% decrease at 1 x 10^{-4} mol/L *2095*

Alendronate

Alkaline Phosphatase *Serum Decrease Physiological* In osteoporosis treatment with daily oral doses of 10 mg for 6 to 12 months caused activity to decrease by approximately 25 - 30% *3976* In 35 postmenopausal women with osteoporosis median activity of 79.7 ± 4.0 U/L before treatment reduced with treatment to 70.8 ± 4.6 U/L after 3 months and to 64.8 ± 3.5 U/L after 6 months *3349*

Alkaline Phosphatase, Bone Isoenzyme

Serum Decrease Physiological In 35 postmenopausal women with osteoporosis median concentration of 11.0 ± 0.8 µg/L (activity of 21.2 ± 1.4 U/L) before treatment significantly reduced to 8.3 ± 0.6 µg/L (activity of 18.4 ± 1.2 U/L) after 3 months and 7.3 ± 0.5 µg/L (17.1 ± 0.7 U/L) after 6 months *3349* In 477 men and women who had glycocorticoid-induced osteoporosis treatment with 5 or 10 mg alendronate per day for 48 weeks caused 27% reduction in concentration to about 7 ng/mL from 10 ± 5 ng/mL *5175*

Serum No Effect Analytical At a concentration of 50 mg/L had no effect on Tandem-MP Ostase method *777*

Calcium *Serum Decrease Physiological* In long term treatment with alendronate (10 mg/d for 1 month) asymptomatic reduction in concentration of approximately 2% observed but no further change observed for up to 3 years. Transient decreases observed in 18% of treated patients *3976*

Urine Decrease Physiological Daily oral doses of 5, 20, and 40 mg for 6 weeks in postmenopausal women produced dose-independent inhibition of bone reabsorption *3976*

Deoxypyridinoline *Urine Decrease Physiological* Daily oral doses of 5, 20, and 40 mg for 6 weeks in postmenopausal women produced dose-independent inhibition of bone reabsorption with tendency to revert to normal within 3 weeks of ending treatment *3976*

Occult Blood *Feces Increase Physiological* In patients receiving aspirin concomitant treatment with alendronate (more than 10 mg/d) increased the incidence of upper gastrointestinal adverse events *3976*

Osteocalcin *Serum Decrease Physiological* In osteoporosis treatment with daily oral doses of 10 mg for 6 to 12 months caused concentration to decrease by approximately 50% *3976*

Phosphate *Serum Decrease Physiological* In long term treatment with alendronate (10 mg/d for 1 month) asymptomatic reduction in concentration of approximately 4 to 6% observed but no further change observed for up to 3 years. Transient decreases observed in 10% of treated patients *3976*

Type I Collagen Cross-linked N-telopeptide

Urine Decrease Physiological Daily oral doses of 5, 20, and 40 mg for 6 weeks in postmenopausal women produced dose-independent inhibition of bone reabsorption with tendency to revert to normal within 3 weeks of stopping treatment *3976* In 477 men and women who had glycocorticoid-induced osteoporosis treatment with 5 or 10 mg alendronate per day for 48 weeks caused 60% reduction in excretion *5175*

Alfacalcidol

1,25-Dihydroxy Vitamin D *Serum No Effect Physiological* In 46 elderly women with radiological evidence of vertebral osteoporosis treatment with 0.5 µg/d caused nonsignificant change from mean baseline of 62.0 ± 6.5 pmol/L to 60.5 ± 5.5 pmol/L after 3 months and 64.4 ± 4.3 pmol/L after 6 months *1935*

25-Hydroxy Vitamin D *Serum No Effect Physiological* In 46 elderly women with radiological evidence of vertebral osteoporosis treatment with 0.5 µg/d caused nonsignificant change from mean baseline of 51.0 ± 8.3 nmol/L to 47.1 ± 5.1 nmol/L after 3 months and 52.2 ± 7.0 nmol/L after 6 months *1935*

Parathyroid Hormone *Plasma Decrease Physiological* In 46 elderly women with radiological evidence of vertebral osteoporosis treatment with 0.5 µg/d caused significant change from mean baseline of 2.53 ± 0.31 pmol/L to 2.28 ± 0.23 pmol/L after 3 months and 2.10 ± 0.26 pmol/L after 6 months *1935*

Alglucerase

Erythrocytes *Blood* *Increase* *Physiological* In 13 patients with Type I Gaucher disease chronic administration of drug caused concentration to increase *2090*

Hematocrit *Blood* *Increase* *Physiological* In 13 patients with Type I Gaucher disease chronic administration of drug caused hematocrit to increase *2090*

Hemoglobin *Blood* *Increase* *Physiological* In 13 patients with Type I Gaucher disease chronic administration of drug caused concentration to increase, in some cases normalizing after 6 months of treatment *2090*

Platelets *Blood* *Increase* *Physiological* In 13 patients with Type I Gaucher disease chronic administration of drug caused concentration to increase *2090*

Pregnancy Tests *Urine* *Positive* *Analytical* Because drug may contain hCG as it is derived from human placenta administration may cause false positive pregnancy test *2090*

Alimenazine

Tricyclic Antidepressants *Serum* *Increase* *Analytical* May cause false positive reaction in immunoassays for tricyclic antidepressants *3590*

Alkalies

Occult Blood *Feces* *Increase* *Physiological* If ingested may cause many gastrointestinal symptoms *467*

Alkaline Antacids

Calcium *Serum* *Increase* *Physiological* Theoretical possibility with absorption of calcium salts *5620*

Color *Feces* *Decrease* *Analytical* White discoloration or speckling *3810*

Creatinine *Serum* *Increase* *Physiological* May cause milk-alkali syndrome *3669*

Dicyclomine *Serum* *Decrease* *Physiological* May interfere with the absorption of anticholinergic agents *2640*

Digoxin *Serum* *Decrease* *Physiological* By decreasing intestinal digoxin absorption may decrease the digoxin concentration *2161*

Felbamate *Serum* *No Effect* *Physiological* The rate and extent of absorption of felbamate not affected by coadministration of antacids *6324*

Magnesium *Serum* *Increase* *Physiological* Theoretical possibility *5620*

Nalidixic Acid *Urine* *Decrease* *Physiological* May interfere with the absorption of nalidixic acid resulting in lower urine concentrations than desired *5255*

Ofloxacin *Serum* *Decrease* *Physiological* Quinolines form chelates with alkaline earth and transition metal cations resulting in reduced absorption *3914*

Phosphate *Serum* *Decrease* *Physiological* Theoretical possibility *5620*

Urea Nitrogen *Serum* *Increase* *Physiological* Prolonged use may cause nephrotoxicity *3669*

Valproic Acid *Serum* *No Effect* *Physiological* Coadministration of valproate 500 mg with commonly administered antacids (Maalox, Trisogel, Titralac - 160 mEq doses) had no effect on the absorption of valproic acid *17*

Alkoxyglycerols

Leukocytes *Blood* *Increase* *Physiological* Protect against decrease caused by X-rays *743*

Ornithine Carbamoyltransferase
Serum *Decrease* *Physiological* Protects against elevation caused by X-rays *743*

Platelets *Blood* *Increase* *Physiological* Protect against decrease caused by X-rays *743*

Allantoin

Ammonia *Plasma* *No Effect* *Analytical* On indophenol reaction with 5,000 nmoles *2131*

Allopregnanedione

Progesterone *Plasma* *Increase* *Analytical* 2% cross-reactivity observed with method on Abbott IMx *1908*

Allopurinol

Alanine Aminotransferase *Serum* *Increase* *Physiological* In 6 of 73 patients treated for 6 mo *5979* Reversible clinical hepatotoxicity reported *3669*

Albumin *Serum* *No Effect* *Analytical* At concentration of 5 mg/L had no effect on BCG method *5704*

Alkaline Phosphatase *Serum* *Increase* *Physiological* Occasional granulomatous hepatitis as well as massive hepatic necrosis and severe hepatitis *3931* In 1 of 73 patients treated for 6 mo *5979* Reversible clinical hepatotoxicity noted *1009*

Alloxanthine *Serum* *Increase* *Physiological* Accumulates with chronic administration *2242*

Antipyrine *Serum* *Increase* *Physiological* Impairs metabolism *4426*

Ara-Hypoxanthine *Serum* *Increase* *Physiological* Occurs when vidarabine administered as a result of inhibition of xanthine oxidase: ara-hypoxanthine is a metabolite of vidarabine *1384*

Aspartate Aminotransferase
Serum *Decrease* *Physiological* In patients undergoing coronary artery bypass surgery treatment with high dose allopurinol was associated with lower activity than when low dose or no allopurinol given during first 5 days following surgery *5910*
Serum *Increase* *Physiological* Reversible clinical hepatotoxicity reported *3669* Occasional granulomatous hepatitis as well as massive hepatic necrosis and severe hepatitis *3931* In 6 of 73 patients treated for 6 mo *5979*

Atenolol *Serum* *No Effect* *Physiological* 300 mg orally had no effect on bioavailability of atenolol following single oral dose of 100 mg *5309*

Azathioprine *Serum* *Increase* *Physiological* Coadministration of allopurinol with azathioprine inhibits principal pathway for detoxification of azathioprine *2159* Allopurinol inhibits detoxification of azathioprine increasing its plasma concentration *5128* Coadministration of allopurinol with azathioprine to kidney transplant recipients increases systemic availability of azathioprine *3909* Coadministration of allopurinol with azathioprine necessitates a reduction in the azathioprine dose *2152*

Bicarbonate *Serum* *No Effect* *Analytical* At concentration of 5 mg/L had no effect on method using phenolphthalein *5704*

Bile *Urine* *Increase* *Physiological* Hepatotoxic effect *3669*

Bilirubin *Serum* *Increase* *Physiological* Reported in renal failure also in other patients *3564*
Serum *No Effect* *Analytical* At concentration of 136 mg/L had no effect on Jendrassik and Grof method *5704* No effect at 1 mg/L on method on Ames Seralyzer *5706*

Bleomycin *Serum* *No Effect* *Physiological* Coadministration of allopurinol with bleomycin did not affect marrow toxicity of bleomycin *2152*

BSP Retention *Serum* *Increase* *Physiological* Associated with reversible hepatotoxicity *5415*

Calcium *Serum* *No Effect* *Analytical* At concentration of 136 mg/L had no effect on cresolphthalein method *5704*
Serum *No Effect* *Physiological* In 9 patients with stable chroic renal failure treatment with 300 mg/d for 1 week caused nonsignificant increase from mean baseline of 9.3 ± 0.03 mg/dL to 9.5 ± 0.07 mg/dL *6210*

Chloride *Serum* *Decrease* *Analytical* Reduced value obtained with concentration of 20 mg/L with method on Kodak Ektachem® . Probably of no clinical significance since therapeutic concentration is about 2 mg/L *5706*
Serum *No Effect* *Analytical* At concentration of 5 mg/L had no effect on mercurimetric method *5704*

Chlorpropamide *Serum* *Increase* *Physiological* Coadministration of allopurinol with chlorpropamide may prolong its half-life *2152* In several patients receiving drugs concomitantly chlorpropamide concentration increased with prolonged half-life probably due to reduced renal tubular secretion *4636*

Cholesterol *Serum Decrease Analytical* No effect up to 0.5 mg/L on Ames Seralyzer method although at higher concentrations apparently clinically significant reduction of cholesterol concentration since therapeutic concentration is 3.4-19.4 mg/L *5706*

Serum Decrease Physiological Hepatotoxic effect *3669*

Serum No Effect Analytical At concentration of 250 mg/L had no effect on CHOD-Iodide method *5704* At concentration of 250 mg/L had no effect on CHOD-PAP method *5704* At concentration of 250 mg/L had no effect on Liebermann-Burchard method *5704* At concentration of 250 mg/L had no effect on catalase-AIDH method *5704* At concentration of 250 mg/L had no effect on method using catalase-Hantzsch reaction *5704*

Creatine Kinase *Serum No Effect Analytical* No effect at 1 mg/L on method on Ames Seralyzer *5706*

Creatine Kinase Isoenzymes

Serum Decrease Physiological In 30 patients undergoing coronary artery bypass surgery treatment with high dose allopurinol after surgery was associated with lower activity of CK-MB than in those given no or low dose allopurinol *5910*

Creatinine *Serum No Effect Analytical* No effect at 1 mg/L on Ames Seralyzer method *5706* At concentration of 10 mg/L had no effect on kinetic Jaffe method on BKA-2 *5704* At concentration of 60 mg/L had no effect on Technicon AutoAnalyzer® Jaffe method *5704* At concentration of 80 mg/L had no effect on Jaffe-Fading-Fraction method *5704* At concentration of 80 mg/L had no effect on Jaffe-Fuller's earth method *5704* at 200 mg/L on reversed phase liquid chromatographic procedure of Zhiri et al *6656*

Serum No Effect Physiological In 9 patients with stable chronic renal failure treatment with 300 mg/d for 1 week caused nonsignificant reduction from mean baseline of 3.7 mg/dL to 3.5 mg/dL *6210*

Cyclophosphamide *Serum No Effect Physiological* Coadministration of allopurinol with cyclophosphamide did not affect marrow toxicity of cyclophosphamide *2152*

Cyclosporine *Blood Increase Physiological* Coadministration with cyclosporine reported to increase trough cyclosporine concentrations threefold probably due to inhibition of CYP enzymes in liver *859*

Serum Increase Physiological Coadministration with cyclosporine reported to increase trough cyclosporine concentrations threefold probably due to inhibition of CYP enzymes in liver *859* May increase cyclosporine concentration by inhibiting hepatic cytochrome P-450 III A which metabolizes cyclosporine *5236*

Cyclosporine A *Blood Increase Physiological* Rare reports suggest that coadministration of allopurinol with cyclosporine may prolong its half-life *2152*

Dicumarol *Plasma Increase Physiological* Impairs metabolism *4426* Coadministration of allopurinol with dicumarol reported to prolong the half-life of dicumarol *2152* Long term use of drug prolongs half-life *4879*

1,25-Dihydroxy Vitamin D *Serum Increase Physiological* In 9 patients with stable chronic renal failure treatment with 300 mg/d for 1 week caused significant increase from mean baseline of 30.8 ± 2.7 pg/mL to 38.2 ± 4.8 pg/mL *6210*

Doxorubicin *Serum No Effect Physiological* Coadministration of allopurinol with doxorubicin did not affect marrow toxicity of doxorubicin *2152*

Eosinophils *Blood Increase Physiological* Frequently associated with drug-induced hepatitis when it occurs *4844* May cause severe sensitivity reaction *4058*

Erythrocytes *Blood Decrease Physiological* Rare case of anemia may occur *128*

Urine Increase Physiological Associated with severe sensitivity reaction *4058*

Glucose *Serum Decrease Physiological* Hepatotoxic effect *3669*

Serum No Effect Analytical At concentration of 18 mg/L had no effect on Kodak Ektachem® method *5704* At concentration of 100 mg/L had no effect on GOD/POD-PAP method *5704* No effect of concentrations up to 18 mg/L on method on Kodak Ektachem® *5706* No effect at 1 mg/L on glucose oxidase method on Ames Seralyzer *5706*

γ-Glutamyltransferase *Serum Increase Physiological* In 3 of 73 patients treated for 6 mo *5979*

Hematocrit *Blood Decrease Physiological* Rare case of anemia reported *128*

Hemoglobin *Blood Decrease Physiological* Rare case of anemia reported *128*

Histamine *Plasma No Effect Analytical* No inhibition of radio-enzyme assay at therapeutic concentrations *2492*

25-Hydroxy Vitamin D *Serum No Effect Physiological* In 9 patients with stable chronic renal failure treatment with 300 mg/d for 1 week caused nonsignificant increase from mean baseline of 56 ± 4.3 ng/mL to 58 ± 4.3 ng/mL *6210*

Hypoxanthine *Serum Increase Physiological* In 22 patients with gout treatment for 3 to 6 months with 200 or 300 mg/d allopurinol caused significant 2.56-fold increase from mean baseline *6580* Inhibits xanthine oxidase (slight increase only) *128*

Urine Increase Physiological Inhibits xanthine oxidase *128* In 22 patients with gout treatment for 3 to 6 months with 200 or 300 mg/d allopurinol caused significant 4.47-fold increase from mean baseline *6580*

Indomethacin *Serum No Effect Analytical* No effect on HPLC method of Roberts and Smith *4978*

Iron *Serum Decrease Physiological* 40% reduction in 1 week (accumulates in liver) *2740*

Serum No Effect Analytical At therapeutic concentration insignificant reduction of iron concentration on Ferrochem II instrument *4489*

Isocitrate Dehydrogenase *Serum Increase Physiological* Reversible clinical hepatotoxicity reported *3669*

Lactate Dehydrogenase *Serum No Effect Analytical* No effect at 1 mg/L on method on Ames Seralyzer *5706*

Lactate Dehydrogenase Isoenzymes

Serum Decrease Physiological Treatment of 30 patients undergoing coronary artery bypass surgery with high dose allopurinol was associated with lower activities of LD-1 and LD-2 than in those patients receiving no or low dose allopurinol *5910*

Leukocytes *Blood Decrease Physiological* Hypersensitivity reaction (often transient) *3810* In 1 of 73 patients treated for 6 mo *5979* Noted in 3 individuals undergoing therapeutic starvation *5413*

Blood Increase Physiological Hypersensitivity reaction occurs with fever *3810*

Urine Increase Physiological Associated with severe sensitivity reaction *4058*

Lipase *Serum No Effect Analytical* No effect of concentrations up to 1.8 mg/L on method on Kodak Ektachem® *5706*

Mechlorethamine *Serum No Effect Physiological* Coadministration of allopurinol with mechlorethamine did not affect marrow toxicity of mechlorethamine *2152*

Mercaptopurine *Serum Increase Physiological* Coadministration of allopurinol with mercaptopurine necessitates a reduction in the mercaptopurine dose *2152* Administration of allopurinol with 6-mercaptopurine causes significant increase in 6-MP concentration, primarily through influence on gastrointestinal and hepatic xanthine oxidase leading to increased bioavailability of 6-MP *3909*

6-Mercaptopurine *Serum Increase Physiological* Impairs metabolism *4426*

Neutrophils *Blood Decrease Physiological* Occasional agranulocytosis reported *6264* Noted in 3 individuals undergoing therapeutic starvation *5413*

Orotidine *Urine Increase Physiological* In 22 patients with gout treatment for 3 to 6 months with 200 or 300 mg/d allopurinol caused significant change from 0.39 ± 0.17 μmol/m²/d to 5.87 ± 3.27 μmol/m²/d *6580*

Oxypurinol *Serum Increase Physiological* In 14 individuals given 200 mg/d mean maximum concentration of 10.7 μg/mL and mean minimum concentration of 7.2 μg/mL *4164*

Parathyroid Hormone *Plasma No Effect Physiological* In 9 patients with stable chronic renal failure treatment with 300 mg/d for 1 week caused nonsignificant increase from mean baseline of 186 ± 79 pg/mL to 199 ± 85 pg/mL *6210*

Allopurinol *(continued)*

Penciclovir *Serum No Effect Physiological* No significant effect on pharmacokinetics of penciclovir observed following single-dose administatration of 500 mg famciclovir after pre-treatment with multiple doses of allopurinol *5646*

Phenprocoumon *Plasma Increase Physiological* Accumulates for several weeks when drugs coadministered *2886*

Phenylbutazone *Serum No Effect Physiological* No significant effect observed on plasma concentrations *4879*

Phenytoin *Serum Increase Physiological* Possibly capable of increasimg concentration when drugs coadministered *1384*

Phosphate *Serum No Effect Analytical* At concentration of 136 mg/L had no effect on phosphomolybdate reduction method *5704*
Serum No Effect Physiological In 9 patients with stable chronic renal failure treatment with 300 mg/d for 1 week caused nonsignificant increase from mean baseline of 3.1 ± 0.1 mg/dL to 3.4 ± 0.1 mg/dL *6210*

Platelets *Blood Decrease Physiological* In 4 of 73 patients treated for 6 mo *5979* Rare potentially dangerous complication *2222*

Potassium *Serum No Effect Analytical* At concentration of 180 mg/L had no effect on ISE measurement without predilution *5704* At concentration of 5 mg/L had no effect on flame-photometric method *5704*

Prazosin *Serum No Effect Physiological* Coadministration of prazosin with allopurinol had no apparent adverse drug interaction in limited clinical experience *4649*

Procarbazine *Serum No Effect Physiological* Coadministration of allopurinol with procarbazine did not affect marrow toxicity of procarbazine *2152*

Prostate-specific Antigen
Prostatic Fluid Increase Physiological Treatment of 22 patients with prostatitis showed significantly higher expression of 2,603 ± 394 compared with those receiving placebo (1,288 ± 335) *4619*
Serum Increase Physiological Treatment of 22 patients with prostatitis showed significantly higher concentration versus control 1.15 µg/L versus 0.90 µg/L after 30 days, 1.15 µg/L versus 0.75 µg/L at 140 days and 1.35 µg/L versus 0.63 µg/L at 240 days *4619*
Urine Increase Physiological Treatment of 22 patients with prostatitis showed significantly higher excretion versus control of 0.54 ± 0.20 versus 0.17 ± 0.06 after prostate palpation *4619*

Protein *Serum No Effect Analytical* At concentration of 136 mg/L had no effect on biuret method with blank correction *5704*

Protein Electrophoresis *Serum No Effect Analytical* At concentration of 180 mg/L had no effect on automated Olympus-Hite method but with slight displacement of fractions *5704*

Prothrombin Time *Plasma Increase Physiological* Patients on coumarins (unconfirmed clinically) *6244*

Purine Bases *Urine Decrease Physiological* In 22 patients with gout treatment for 3 to 6 months with 200 or 300 mg/d allopurinol caused significant 0.70-fold decrease from mean baseline *6580*

Reticulocytes *Blood Increase Physiological* Mild (may be associated with other drugs) *2152*

Sodium *Serum No Effect Analytical* At concentration of 5 mg/L had no effect on flame-photometric method *5704* At concentration of 180 mg/L had no effect on ISE measurement without predilution *5704*

Theophylline *Serum Increase Physiological* Decreases theophylline clearance at allopurinol doses greater than 600 mg/d and increases serum theophylline concentration by 25% *3125* At a dose of 600 mg/d decreases theophylline clearance, increasing theophylline concentration by about 25% *5999* Large doses of allopurinol reduce theophylline clearance *1384* Up to 25% increase in serum theophylline concentration due to decreased theophylline clearance at allopurinol doses of 600 mg/d or more *6117* Increased half-life and decreased clearance probably due to effect on hepatic metabolizing enzymes *3765*

Triglycerides *Serum No Effect Analytical* At concentration of 5 mg/L had no effect on lipase/esterase method *5704* At concentration of 100 mg/L had no effect on GPO-PAP method *5704*

Urea Nitrogen *Serum Increase Physiological* In 2 of 73 patients treated for 6 mo *5979* Azotemia occurred as sensitivity reaction in 2 cases *4058*
Serum No Effect Analytical At concentration of 136 mg/L had no effect on diacetylmonoxime method *5704* No effect at 1 mg/L on method on Ames Seralyzer *5706* At concentration of 18 mg/L had no effect on Kodak Ektachem® method *5704*

Uric Acid *Serum Decrease Physiological* Therapeutic effect due to inhibition of xanthine oxidase *4847* Inhibition of xanthine oxidase *1714* In 22 patients with gout treatment for 3 to 6 months with 200 or 300 mg/d allopurinol caused significant 0.63-fold decrease from mean baseline *6580* In 3 healthy male volunteers decrease from mean concentration of 5.3 mg/dL to 4.8 mg/dL at 22 hours after administration of 200 mg allopurinol but not affected by coadministration of 80 g ethanol *3026* In 9 patients with stable chronic renal failure treatment with 300 mg/d for 1 week caused significant reduction from mean baseline of 7.3 ± 0.4 mg/dL to 4.0 ± 0.4 mg/dL *6210*
Serum No Effect Analytical At 200 mg/L on reversed phase liquid chromatographic procedure of Zhiri et al *6656* At concentration of 100 mg/L had no effect on uricase method on Du Pont aca *5704* At concentration of 204 mg/L had no effect on uricase-PAP method *5704* At concentration of 250 mg/L had no effect on Kageyama-Hantzsch method *5704* At concentration of 5 mg/L had no effect on phosphotungstate reduction method *5704* At concentration of 80 mg/L had no effect on catalase-AIDH method *5704*
Urine Decrease Physiological In 22 patients with gout treatment for 3 to 6 months with 200 or 300 mg/d allopurinol caused significant 1.26-fold decrease from mean baseline *6580* Inhibition of xanthine oxidase *1714*

Uric Acid Clearance *Urine No Effect Physiological* In 22 patients with gout treatment for 3 to 6 months with 200 or 300 mg/d allopurinol caused nonsignificant change from 7.8 ± 2.4 mL/min to 6.3 ± 1.9 mL/min *6580*

Uridine *Serum Decrease Physiological* In 22 patients with gout treatment for 3 to 6 months with 200 or 300 mg/d allopurinol caused significant decrease from mean baseline of 5.58 ± 1.56 µmol/L to 4.34 ± 1.30 µmol/L *6580*

Urobilin *Urine Increase Physiological* Transient increases reported *4014*

Warfarin *Plasma No Effect Physiological* Overall no change in steady-state plasma concentration although some individual variation *4879*

Xanthine *Serum Increase Physiological* Inhibits xanthine oxidase (slight increase only) *128* In 22 patients with gout treatment for 3 to 6 months with 200 or 300 mg/d allopurinol caused significant 6.60-fold increase from mean baseline *6580*
Urine Increase Physiological In 22 patients with gout treatment for 3 to 6 months with 200 or 300 mg/d allopurinol caused significant 7.46-fold increase from mean baseline *6580* Inhibits xanthine oxidase *128*

Xanthine Calculi *Urine Positive Physiological* Rare side effect *2319*

Alloxan

Acid Phosphatase *White Blood Cells Decrease Analytical* Phenylphosphate enzyme inhibited by 45 mmol/L *298*
White Blood Cells No Effect Analytical Glycerophosphate enzyme no effect with 45 mmol/L *298*

Casts *Urine Increase Physiological* May cause nephrotoxicity *467*

Urea Nitrogen *Serum Increase Physiological* If ingested may cause nephrotoxicity *467*

Allylbarbital

Barbiturate *Urine Increase Analytical* Positive result obtained at a concentration of 3.0 µg/mL (13.4 µmol/L) with method on Du Pont aca *1555*

Allymid

Platelets *Blood Decrease Physiological* Immunologically induced thrombocytopenia *3051*

Aloin

Androstenedione *Plasma Increase Physiological* In 20 premenopausal androgenic women with alopecia mean concentration of 13.9 ± 0.7 nmol/L significantly higher than 5.3 ± 0.7 nmol/L in 10 female controls *3495*

Casts *Urine Increase Physiological* May cause nephrotoxicity *467*

Color *Urine Increase Analytical* Red-brown/yellow pink (alkaline), yellow brown (acid) *3810*

Dehydroepiandrosterone Sulfate
Plasma Increase Physiological In 20 premenopausal androgenic women with alopecia mean concentration of 7.8 ± 0.8 µmol/L significantly higher than 4.5 ± 0.5 nmol/L in 10 female controls *3495*

Testosterone *Serum Increase Physiological* In 20 premenopausal androgenic women with alopecia mean concentration of 2.65 ± 0.1 nmol/L significantly higher than 1.03 ± 0.1 nmol/L in 10 female controls *3495*

Urea Nitrogen *Serum Increase Physiological* May cause nephrotoxicity *467*

Alphacalcidol

Calcium *Serum Increase Physiological* When given intravenously in doses of 1-4 µg/dialysis session over 12 weeks to 51 patients on chronic hemodialysis mean increase of 0.25 mmol/L in calcium concentration observed *3620*

Parathyroid Hormone *Plasma Decrease Physiological* Mean decrease of 60% observed in intact parathyroid hormone concentration observed in 51 patients on chronic hemodialysis when 1-4 µg given intravenously per dialysis session over 12 weeks *3620*

Alprazolam

Alanine Aminotransferase *Serum Increase Physiological* Isolated case, abnormal test value reverted to normal with withdrawal of drug *5138* Administration of alprazolam reported to cause increased hepatic enzyme activity in fewer than 1% of all treated patients *4685*

Albumin *Urine No Effect Analytical* Using a fluorimetric assay with Albumin Blue 580 on a Cobas Fara centrifugal analyzer for the detection of microalbuminuria no significant interference was detected at a concentration of 0.4 mg/L *3117*

Alkaline Phosphatase *Serum Increase Physiological* In a clinical trial involving administration of alprazolam to 1,388 patients mean incidence of high activities of 1.7% compared with 1.8% in 1,231 placebo-treated controls *4685*

Aspartate Aminotransferase *Serum Increase Physiological* Isolated case, abnormal test value reverted to normal with withdrawal of drug *5138* In a clinical trial involving administration of alprazolam to 1,388 patients mean incidence of high activities of 3.2% compared with 1.8% in 1,231 placebo-treated controls *4685*

Benzodiazepine *Urine Positive Analytical* At concentration of 0.1 µg/mL or greater produces positive result with Syva EMIT II assay *1785* With improved Syva EMIT assay detectable limit 0.07 µg/mL with Syva ETS system compared with 0.1 µg/mL with former D.A.U. assay *3370* At concentrations of 0.1 µg/mL or greater produces positive result with Syva EMIT II assay *1785*

Bilirubin *Serum Increase Physiological* In a clinical trial involving administration of alprazolam to 1,388 patients mean incidence of high concentrations of 1.6% compared with less than 1% in 1,231 placebo-treated controls *4685* Administration of alprazolam reported to cause jaundice in fewer than 1% of all treated patients *4685*

Cortisol, Free *Urine No Effect Analytical* No significant interference observed with HPLC method of Turpeinen et al *6105*

Creatinine *Serum Decrease Physiological* In a clinical trial involving administration of alprazolam to 1,388 patients mean incidence of low concentrations of 2.2% compared with 3.5% in 1,231 placebo-treated controls *4685*
Serum Increase Physiological In a clinical trial involving administration of alprazolam to 1,388 patients mean incidence of high concentrations of 1.9% compared with 1.0% in 1,231 placebo-treated controls *4685*

Cyclosporine *Blood No Effect Analytical* At a concentration of 0.37 mg/L had no effect on Syva EMIT method *495*

Desipramine *Serum Increase Physiological* Concomitant administration of alprazolam with imipramine caused an average 20% increase in the steady state concentration of desimipramine *4685*

Digoxin *Serum Increase Physiological* In 12 patients receiving long-term digoxin (0.25 mg/d) administration of 1.0 or 0.5 mg alprazolam for each of 7 days significant increase in area under the curve observed in patients receiving 1 mg/d with increase greater in patients older than 65 years of age (mean trough serum concentration about 1.8 ng/mL) than in those under 65 years (mean trough serum concentration 1.0 ng/mL) *2381* Coadministration with digoxin may increase the digoxin concentration *2161* Observed in one patient when alprazolam coadministered but mechanism not determined *6047*

Eosinophils *Blood Decrease Physiological* In a clinical trial involving administration of alprazolam to 1,388 patients mean incidence of low concentrations of 3.2% compared with 3.3% in 1,231 placebo-treated controls *4685*
Blood Increase Physiological In a clinical trial involving administration of alprazolam to 1,388 patients mean incidence of high concentrations of 9.5% compared with 7.2% in 1,231 placebo-treated controls *4685*

Epinephrine *Plasma Decrease Physiological* In 8 healthy men intravenous administration of 0.014 mg/kg caused significant reduction from mean of about 110 pg/mL to 42 pg/mL 15 minutes after administarion and remained decreased for the next hour *5137*
Plasma No Effect Physiological In 8 healthy individuals administration of 2 mg/d oral alprazolam for 1 week caused nonsignificant decrease from baseline *5137*

Erythrocytes *Urine Increase Physiological* In a clinical trial involving administration of alprazolam to 1,388 patients mean incidence of increased excretion of 3.4% compared with 5.0% in 1,231 placebo-treated controls *4685*

γ-Glutamyltransferase *Serum Increase Physiological* Administration of alprazolam reported to cause increased hepatic enzyme activity in fewer than 1% of all treated patients *4685*

Imipramine *Serum Increase Physiological* Concomitant administration of alprazolam with imipramine caused an average 31% increase in the steady state concentration of imipramine *4685*

Interleukin-1β *Serum Decrease Physiological* In 10 outpatients with panic disorder mean concentration of 38.1 ± 12.4 pg/mL decreased nonsignificantly after treatment with 2 - 2.5 mg/d for one month to 28.8 ± 11.2 pg/mL which was still higher than 13.1 ± 9.1 pg/mL in 10 age-matched controls *688*

Leukocytes *Blood Decrease Physiological* In a clinical trial involving administration of alprazolam to 1,388 patients mean incidence of low concentrations of 1.4% compared with 2.3% in 1,231 placebo-treated controls *4685*
Blood Increase Physiological In a clinical trial involving administration of alprazolam to 1,388 patients mean incidence of high concentrations of 2.3% compared with 2.0% in 1,231 placebo-treated controls *4685*
Urine Increase Physiological In a clinical trial involving administration of alprazolam to 1,388 patients mean incidence of increased excretion of 3.4% compared with 5.0% in 1,231 placebo-treated controls *4685*

Lithium *Serum Increase Physiological* Small but significant increase in area under curve (from 10.3 to 11.1 mEq/h/L) and renal clearance decreased from 31.2 to 22.4 mL/min in 10 normal subjects when lithium coadministered with alprazolam *1770*

Lymphocytes *Blood Decrease Physiological* In a clinical trial involving administration of alprazolam to 1,388 patients mean incidence of low concentrations of 5.5% compared with 5.4% in 1,231 placebo-treated controls *4685*

Monocytes *Blood Decrease Physiological* In a clinical trial involving administration of alprazolam to 1,388 patients mean incidence of low concentrations of 5.3% compared with 6.4% in 1,231 placebo-treated controls *4685*

Alprazolam *(continued)*

Monocytes *(continued)*
Blood Increase Physiological In a clinical trial involving administration of alprazolam to 1,388 patients mean incidence of high concentrations of 2.8% compared with less than 1% in 1,231 placebo-treated controls *4685*

Nefazodone *Serum No Effect Physiological* Administration of 200 mg nefazodone twice daily to individuals dosed with 1 mg alprazolam caused mean concentration of alprazolam to increase approximately twofold but had no effect on the steady state pharmacokinetics of nefazodone or its metabolites *2316*

Neutrophils *Blood Decrease Physiological* In a clinical trial involving administration of alprazolam to 1,388 patients mean incidence of low concentrations of 2.3% compared with 4.2% in 1,231 placebo-treated controls *4685*
Blood Increase Physiological In a clinical trial involving administration of alprazolam to 1,388 patients mean incidence of high concentrations of 3.0% compared with 1.7% in 1,231 placebo-treated controls *4685*

Tricyclic Antidepressants *Serum Increase Physiological* Interacts pharmacokinetically to inhibit metabolism of tricyclic antidepressants *3590*

Alprenolol

Calcium *Serum No Effect Physiological* Concentration remained within normal range in 40 patients with ischemic heart disease treated for 12 months *4611*

ionized Calcium *Serum No Effect Physiological* Concentration remained within normal range in 40 patients with ischemic heart disease treated for 12 months *4611*

17-Ketosteroids *Urine No Effect Analytical* No effect of treatment on concentration as measured by Zimmermann method *4421*

Magnesium *Serum No Effect Physiological* No effect observed on concentration in 40 patients with ischemic heart disease treated for 12 months *4611*

Parathyroid Hormone *Plasma No Effect Physiological* No effect observed in 40 patients with ischemic heart disease treated for 12 months *4611*

Phosphate *Serum No Effect Physiological* Concentration remained within normal range in 40 patients with ischemic heart disease treated for 12 months *4611*

Platelets *Blood Decrease Physiological* In one woman with essential hypertension after 1.5 y treatment: decrease disappeared with withdrawal of drug *931* Marked reduction on two occasions in one patient due to increased destruction *3738*

Potassium *Serum Increase Physiological* Slight increase in patients treated with moderate doses of drug *4739*

T3-Uptake *Serum No Effect Physiological* No significant effect in 9 hyperthyroid patients treated with 100 mg daily for 7 days *4610*

Thyroxine (T4) *Serum No Effect Physiological* No effect observed in 9 hyperthyroid patients treated with 100 mg daily for 7 days *4610*

Tri-iodothyronine, Reverse (rT3)
Serum Increase Physiological Increase from mean of 0.87 nmol/L to 1.05 nmol/L in 9 hyperthyroid patients treated with 100 mg daily for 7 days *4610*

Tri-iodothyronine (T3) *Serum Decrease Physiological* Reduction from mean of 5.3 nmol/L to 4.3 nmol/L in 9 hyperthyroid patients treated with 100 mg daily for 7 days: effect probably due to inhibition of 5'-deiodinase enzyme *4610*

Alprostadil

Blood *Urine Increase Physiological* After intraurethral administration of 1000 μg alprostadil minor urethral bleeding/spotting observed in 5% of 486 patients compared with 1% of 511 given a placebo *6272* Reported to occur as a side effect in fewer than 1% of treated patients *4667*

Creatinine *Serum Increase Physiological* Reported to occur as a side effect in fewer than 1% of treated patients *4667*

Ketone Body Ratio *Serum No Effect Analytical* When added at a concentration of 0.8 mg/L had no significant effect on AKBR method of Uno et al *6131*

Prostaglandin E_1 *Plasma Increase Physiological* Mean maximum concentration in healthy men after intraurethral administration of 1,000 μg alprostadil 11.4 pg/mL but became undetectable after 60 minutes *6272*

Alteplase

α_2-Antiplasmin *Plasma Decrease Physiological* In 10 patients with acute myocardial infarction infusion of 100 mg caused concentration to decrease to 35% of that before infusion *5943*

Blood *Urine Increase Physiological* Bleeding is most common complication of treatment *2081*

Fibrinopeptide A *Plasma Increase Physiological* In 106 patients with acute myocardial infarction significant increase from mean baseline of 21 ng/mL increased significantly to 49, 34, 27, 29 and 30 ng/mL after 0.75, 3, 12, 24 and 36 hours after administration of alteplase with aspirin *4859*

Occult Blood *Feces Increase Physiological* Bleeding is most common complication of treatment *2081*

Plasminogen *Plasma Decrease Physiological* In 10 patients with acute myocardial infarction given 100 mg over 1 hour caused plasminogen to decrease to 70% of value before infusion *5943*

Althesin

Carbon Dioxide Partial Pressure
Blood Increase Physiological Post-induction measurement in arterial blood *5296*

Glucose *Serum Increase Physiological* 30 mg/dL increase observed 1 h after *483*

Oxygen Partial Pressure *Blood Decrease Physiological* Post-induction measurement in arterial blood *5296*

Altretamine

Alkaline Phosphatase *Serum Increase Physiological* Dose related myelosuppression noted with treatment. Increased activity observed in 9% of 78 previously treated ovarian cancer patients receiving single dose drug *6137*

Creatinine *Serum Increase Physiological* Increased concentration of 1.6 - 3.75 mg/dL observed in 7% of 78 previously treated ovarian cancer patients receiving single dose drug *6137*

Hematocrit *Blood Decrease Physiological* Dose related myelosuppression with anemia noted with treatment. Mild anemia observed in 20% and moderate to severe anemia observed in 13% of 78 previously treated ovarian cancer patients receiving single dose drug *6137*

Hemoglobin *Blood Decrease Physiological* Dose related myelosuppression with anemia noted with treatment. Mild anemia observed in 20% and moderate to severe anemia observed in 13% of 78 previously treated ovarian cancer patients receiving single dose drug *6137*

Leukocytes *Blood Decrease Physiological* Moderate effect in half of patients *6497* Dose related myelosuppression noted with treatment. Leukopenia below 3000 cells/μL observed in 15% treated patients. Less than 1% had counts below 1000 cells/μL *6137*

Platelets *Blood Decrease Physiological* Moderate effect in a third of patients *6497* Dose related myelosuppression noted with treatment. Thrombocytopenia below 50,000 cells/μL observed in less than 10% treated patients *6137*

Urea Nitrogen *Serum Increase Physiological* Increased concentration of 25 - 40 mg/dL observed in 5%, of 41 - 60 mg/dL in 3% and of over 60 mg/dL in 1% of 78 previously treated ovarian cancer patients receiving single dose drug *6137*

Aluminum

Magnesium *Serum No Effect Analytical* No effect of concentrations up to 4 μmol/L on Magon dye method on Instrumentation Laboratory Monarch *1263* No effect of concentrations up to 3 mg/L on method on Kodak Ektachem® *5706* At a concentration of 300 µg/dL had no significant effect on method on Kodak Ektachem® systems *2519*

Aluminum Antacids

Alkaline Phosphatase *Serum Decrease Physiological* In 15 men aged from 60 - 80 y taking aluminum containing antacids mean activity of 73.2 ± 17 U/L significantly different from 87.4 ± 22 U/L in healthy age-matched controls *5479*
Serum No Effect Physiological In 10 women older than 50 y taking aluminum antacids mean activity of 93.3 ± 25 U/L not significantly different from 86.2 ± 20 U/L in age-matched controls *5479*

Aluminum *Serum Increase Physiological* In women taking aluminum antacids mean concentration of 9.0 ± 5 µg/L significantly higher than 4.0 ± 2.8 µg/L in 128 women not taking antacids *5479*

Azithromycin *Serum Decrease Physiological* Administration of aluminum- and magnesium-containing antacids reduces peak concentration of azithromycin but not the AUC of azithromycin absorption *4659*

Cefaclor *Serum Decrease Physiological* Absorption reduced if taken within one hour of ingestion of magesium or aluminum hydroxide containing antacids *1627*

Cefdinir *Serum Decrease Physiological* Concomitant administration of aluminum or magnesium-containing antacids with 300 mg cefdinir reduce absorption of cefdinir. Problem can be avoided by giving cefdinir two hours before or after antacid administration *4528*

Ciprofloxacin *Serum Decrease Physiological* Concurrent administration of ciprofloxacin with antacids containing magnesium, aluminum, or calcium may substantially interfere with the absorption of ciprofloxacin and plasma and urine concentrations less than desired *416*
Urine Decrease Physiological Concurrent administration of ciprofloxacin with antacids containing magnesium, aluminum, or calcium may substantially interfere with the absorption of ciprofloxacin and plasma and urine concentrations less than desired *416*

Dicyclomine *Serum Decrease Physiological* May interfere with the absorption of anticholinergic agents *2640*

Digoxin *Serum Decrease Physiological* By decreasing intestinal digoxin absorption may decrease the digoxin concentration *2161*

Enoxacin *Serum Decrease Physiological* Antacids containing aluminum hydroxide and magnesium hydroxide reduce the oral absorption of enoxacin by 75% *4940*

Felbamate *Serum No Effect Physiological* The rate and extent of absorption of felbamate not affected by coadministration of antacids *6324*

Lomerfloxacin *Serum Decrease Physiological* Magnesium and aluminum containing antacids form complexes with lomerfloxacin interfering with its bioavailability with reduction of lomerfloxacin by about 48% when administered together *2068*

Nalidixic Acid *Urine Decrease Physiological* May interfere with the absorption of nalidixic acid resulting in lower urine concentrations than desired *5255*

Ofloxacin *Serum Decrease Physiological* Quinolines form chelates with alkaline earth and transition metal cations resulting in reduced absorption *3914*

Osteocalcin *Serum No Effect Physiological* In 15 men aged from 60 - 80 y taking nonaluminum containing antacids mean concentration of 14.5 ± 6.7 ng/mL not significantly different from 14.4 ± 4 ng/mL in healthy age-matched controls. In 14 women older than 50 y taking nonaluminum antacids mean concentration of 18.7 ± 12.1 µg/mL not significantly different from 14.7 ± 5 ng/mL in age-matched controls *5479*

Procollagen I Peptide *Serum Decrease Physiological* In 13 men aged from 60 - 80 y taking aluminum containing antacids mean concentration of 196 ± 62 (?units) not significantly less than 205 ± 83 (?units) in healthy age-matched controls *5479*
Serum Increase Physiological In 15 women older than 50 y taking aluminum antacids mean concentration of 212 ± 91 (?units) significantly greater than 177 ± 81 (?units) in age-matched controls *5479*

Raloxifene *Serum No Effect Physiological* Reported to have no effect on the systemic exposure of raloxifene *1696*

Sildenafil *Serum No Effect Physiological* Single doses of magnesium hydroxide/aluminum hydroxide did not affect the viability of sildenafil *4657*

Sparfloxacin *Serum Decrease Physiological* Magnesium and aluminum containing antacids form chelation complexes with sparfloxacin and must be given either 2 hours before or after sparfloxacin to avoid reducing its bioavailability *4943*

Tiludronate *Serum Decrease Physiological* Bioavailabilty of tiludronate reduced by 60% when some aluminum or calcium containing antacids are administered one hour before tiludronate *5258*

Trovafloxacin *Serum Decrease Physiological* Coadministration significantly reduces the absorption of trovafloxacin *4663*

Ursodiol *Serum Decrease Physiological* Postulated to cause reduction in absorption of ursodiol from gastrointestinal tract *300*

Valproic Acid *Serum No Effect Physiological* Coadministration of valproate 500 mg with commonly administered antacids (Maalox, Trisogel, Titralac - 160 mEq doses) had no effect on the absorption of valproic acid *17*

Aluminum Hydroxide

Adenosine Monophosphate *Urine No Effect Physiological* Observed in one patient secondary to ingestion of large amounts of compound for long time *2200*

Alkaline Phosphatase *Serum Increase Physiological* Observed in one patient secondary to ingestion of large amounts of compound for long time *2200* Mild effect with drug associated osteomalacia *1769*

Aluminum *Serum Increase Physiological* In 7 nondialyzed patients with chronic renal failure (increase from mean 1.7 to to 3.6 µg/dL) with 15-18 g/d *5924* Very high concentration (3124 µg/L) observed in one individual with renal failure without dialysis but who was receiving oral citrate concurrently with aluminum hydroxide which converted the aluminum to a more soluble form *3158* Moderate increase after ingestion of aluminum hydroxide as antacid *5598*

Calcitonin *Plasma No Effect Physiological* With 15-18 g/d in 7 nondialyzed patients with chronic renal failure *5924*

Calcium *Serum Increase Physiological* Mild effect with osteomalacia due to inhibition of entry into bone *1769* Small increase to 2.37-2.40 mmol/L during administration of 100 mL gel/d for for 28 d *854*
Serum No Effect Physiological Observed in one patient secondary to ingestion of large amounts of compound for long time *2200* With 15-18 g/d in 7 nondialyzed patients with chronic renal failure *5924*
Urine Increase Physiological Observed in one patient secondary to ingestion of large amounts of compound for long time *2200*

Chenodiol *Serum Decrease Physiological* Binds chenodiol in gastrointestinal tract and inhibits its absorption *1384*

Chlorpromazine *Urine Decrease Physiological* Concomitant administration caused reduction in urinary excretion of 10-45% probably through reduced absorption *1917*

Cholesterol *Serum Decrease Physiological* In 28 patients with hypercholesterolemia treatment with 900 mg/d for 2 months caused significant reduction (5.2%) from mean baseline of 6.99 ± 0.17 mmol/L to 6.63 ± 0.17 mmol/L *5744*

Color *Feces Increase Analytical* White discoloration/speckling if taken orally *1957*

Dicumarol *Plasma No Effect Physiological* Although concentration increased with magnesium hydroxide coadministration no effect observed with aluminum hydroxide *136*

Diflunisal *Serum Decrease Physiological* Coadministration reduces extent of absorption of diflunisal *1384*

Digoxin *Serum Decrease Physiological* Gastrointestinal absorption reduced by about 30% *760*

1,25-Dihydroxy Vitamin D_3 *Serum Decrease Physiological* Low compared with normals in 7 patients (nondialyzed) with chronic renal failure. Decreased significantly (19.4 to 11.4 pg/mL) with treatment (15-18 g/d) *5924*

Aluminum Hydroxide *(continued)*

1,25-Dihydroxy Vitamin D_3 *(continued)*
Serum Increase Physiological Observed in one patient secondary to ingestion of large amounts of compound for long time *2200*

Enoxacin *Serum Decrease Physiological* Antacids containing aluminum hydroxide and magnesium hydroxide reduce the oral absorption of enoxacin by 75% *4940*

Fluoride *Feces Increase Physiological* In osteoporotic patients receiving fluoride (50 mg/d) with net decreased absorption of fluoride by 57% when aluminum hydroxide coadministered *5743*
Serum Decrease Physiological When aluminum hydroxide coadministered to osteoporotic patients receiving 50 mg fluoride/d *5743*

HDL-Cholesterol *Serum No Effect Physiological* In 28 hypercholesterolemic patients treatment with 900 mg/d for 2 months caused insignificant change from 1.18 ± 0.06 mmol/L to 1.19 ± 0.05 mmol/L *5744*

HDL-Cholesterol:LDL-Cholesterol Ratio
Serum Increase Physiological In 28 patients with hypercholesterolemia treated with 900 mg/d for 2 months mean ratio increased significantly from 0.23 to 0.26 (13.0%) *5744*

25-Hydroxy Vitamin D_3 *Serum No Effect Physiological* Observed in one patient secondary to ingestion of large amounts of compound for long time *2200*

Isoniazid *Serum Decrease Physiological* Plasma concentration reduced due to inhibition of gastrointestinal absorption *2789*

LDL-Cholesterol *Serum Decrease Physiological* In 28 hypercholesterolemic patients treated with 900 mg/d for 2 months mean concentration decreased from 5.02 ± 0.14 mmol/L to 4.53 ± 0.16 mmmol/L (9.8%) *5744*

Naproxen *Serum Decrease Physiological* Theoretical possibility as rate of absorption is decreased *1384*

Norfloxacin *Urine Decrease Physiological* When aluminum hydroxide coingested with 400 mg norfloxacin urinary excretion of norfloxacin over next 24 hours reduced by 86% due to interference with absorption *865*

Parathyroid Hormone *Plasma Decrease Physiological* Fell approximately 40% in 7 nondialyzed patients with chronic renal failure with 15-18 g/d *5924*

Phosphate *Serum Decrease Physiological* Observed in one patient secondary to ingestion of large amounts of compound for long time *2200* In 7 nondialyzed patients with chronic renal failure: fell from average 6.3 mg/dL to 3.7 mg/dL with 15-18 g/d *5924*
Serum Increase Physiological In 5 normal subjects given 100 mL/d for 28 d (serum phosphate concentration rose to 1.32 mmol/L from 1.18 mmol/L) *854* Mild effect with osteomalacia due to inhibition of entry into bone *1769*

Propranolol *Serum Decrease Physiological* Intestinal absorption greatly reduced *6558*

Pseudoephedrine *Serum Increase Physiological* Increased rate of absorption due to raised gastric pH *6403*

Rifampin *Serum Decrease Physiological* In patients receiving antacid as well as rifampin a statistically greater number had rifampin concentrations less than 6.5 mg/L compared with others not receiving antacid, probably due to delayed gastric emptying due to aluminum ions *657*

Salicylate *Serum Decrease Physiological* Significant reduction from 19.8 mg/dL to 15.8 mg/dL with several days antacid, due to increased alkalinity of urine *2454*
Serum No Effect Analytical No significant effect observed at a concentration of 315 mg/dL with method on Kodak Ektachem® systems *2519*

Tetracycline *Serum Decrease Physiological* Complexes with tetracyclines in gastrointestinal tract and interferes with absorption *1384*

Tolfenamic Acid *Serum Decrease Physiological* Both alone and when combined with magnesium hydroxide retarded absorption of drug and reduced peak plasma concentration *4259*

Triglycerides *Serum No Effect Physiological* In 28 hypercholesterolemic patients treated with 900 mg/d for 2 months mean concentration increased insignificantly (15.2%) from 1.77 ± 0.13 mmol/L to 2.04 ± 0.18 mmol/L *5744*

Valproic Acid *Serum No Effect Physiological* Coadministration of valproate 500 mg with commonly administered antacids (Maalox, Trisogel, Titralac - 160 mEq doses) had no effect on the absorption of valproic acid *17*

Vitamin A *Serum Decrease Physiological* Reduced absorption due to adsorption and oxidation *6403*

VLDL-Cholesterol *Serum No Effect Physiological* In 28 hypercholesterolemic patients treated with 900 mg/d for 2 months no significant effect observed *5744*

VLDL-Triglycerides *Serum No Effect Physiological* In 28 hypercholesterolemic patients treatment with 900 mg/d for 2 months had no significant effect on concentration *5744*

Warfarin *Plasma No Effect Physiological* Coadministration had no effect on plasma concentration *136*

Aluminum Hydroxide: Magnesium Hydroxide

Amoxicillin *Serum Increase Physiological* Increase in concentration from mean of 12.4 mg/L to 15.0 mg/L in 10 healthy volunteers given 10 doses of 10 mL each and 1000 mg amoxicillin *1386*
Serum No Effect Physiological No significant change in 10 healthy volunteers given 10 doses each of 10 mL and 1000 mg amoxicillin concomitantly *1386*

Atorvastatin *Serum Decrease Physiological* Coadministration of Maalox® with atorvastatin plasma concentration of atorvastatin reduced by approximately 35% although reduction of LDL-cholesterol concentration was not affected *4534*

Azithromycin *Serum Decrease Physiological* Administration of aluminum- and magnesium-containing antacids reduces peak concentration of azithromycin but not the AUC of azithromycin absorption *4659*

Capecitabine *Serum Increase Physiological* When antacid administered immediately after capecitabine the AUC and peak plasma concentration of capecitabine by 16% and 35% respectively *5013*

Cephalexin *Serum No Effect Physiological* No significant effect in 10 healthy volunteers given 10 doses of 10 mL concomitantly with 1000 mg cephalexin *1386*

Cerivastatin *Serum No Effect Physiological* Plasma concentrations of cerivastatin not affected by administration of antacid *300*

Ciprofloxacin *Serum Decrease Physiological* Concurrent administration of ciprofloxacin with antacids containing magnesium, aluminum, or calcium may substantially interfere with the absorption of ciprofloxacin and plasma and urine concentrations less than desired *416*
Urine Decrease Physiological Concurrent administration of ciprofloxacin with antacids containing magnesium, aluminum, or calcium may substantially interfere with the absorption of ciprofloxacin and plasma and urine concentrations less than desired *416*

Clavulenic Acid *Serum No Effect Physiological* No significant change in 10 healthy volunteers given 10 doses of 10 mL each and 625 mg amoxicillin and clavulenic acid *1386*

5'-Deoxy-5-fluorocytidine *Serum Increase Physiological* When antacid administered immediately after capecitabine the AUC and peak plasma concentration of 5'-DFCR by 18% and 22% respectively *5013*

Doxycycline *Serum Decrease Physiological* Marked reduction from mean of 2.7 mg/L to 0.45 mg/L in 10 healthy volunteers given 10 doses of 10 mL of antacid and 200 mg doxycycline *1386*

Enoxacin *Serum Decrease Physiological* Antacids containing aluminum hydroxide and magnesium hydroxide reduce the oral absorption of enoxacin by 75% *4940*

Ketoprofen *Serum No Effect Physiological* When coadministered with ketoprofen has no effect on its absorption *6564*

Mycophenolate *Serum Decrease Physiological* Coadministration of mycophenolate mofentil (2 g) with Maalox (10 mL q.i.d.) in 10 patients with rheumatoid arthritis caused a significant decrease in mycophenolate AUC (17%) and concentration (33%) *5017*

Nicardipine *Serum No Effect Physiological* When administered concomitantly Maalox had no effect on nicardipine concentration *5016*

Nitrofurantoin *Serum Decrease Physiological* Antacids containing magnesium trisilicate when administered concomitantly with with nitrofurantoin reduce both the rate and extent of absorption of nitrofurantoin, probably due to adsorption of nitrofurantoin onto the surface of magnesium trisilicate *4800*

Sildenafil *Serum No Effect Physiological* Single doses of magnesium hydroxide/aluminum hydroxide did not affect the viability of sildenafil *4657*

Ursodiol *Serum Decrease Physiological* Postulated to cause reduction in absorption of ursodiol from gastrointestinal tract *300*

Valproic Acid *Serum No Effect Physiological* Coadministration of valproate 500 mg with commonly administered antacids (Maalox, Trisogel, Titralac - 160 mEq doses) had no effect on the absorption of valproic acid *17*

Zalcitabine *Serum Decrease Physiological* Coadministration of Maalox® TC 30 mL and single doses of zalcitabine 1.5 mg to 12 HIV-positive patients decreased mean concentration from 25.2 ng/mL to 18.4 ng/mL and AUC decreased from 75 ng.h/mL to 58 ng.h/mL *5023*

Aluminum Nicotinate

Alanine Aminotransferase *Serum Increase Physiological* Rare hepatotoxic effects *2753*

Aspartate Aminotransferase *Serum Increase Physiological* Rare hepatotoxic effects *2753*

Bilirubin *Serum Increase Physiological* Rare hepatotoxic effects *2753*

Cholesterol *Serum Decrease Physiological* Therapeutic intent through nicotinic acid release *184*

Glucose *Serum Increase Physiological* Produces carbohydrate intolerance over long term *3222*

Glucose Tolerance *Serum Decrease Physiological* Rare hepatotoxic effects *2753*

Uric Acid *Serum Increase Physiological* May increase uric acid to produce gout *184*

Aluminum Nitrate

Potassium *Serum No Effect Analytical* Negligible effect at a concentration of 20 µmol/L on spectrophotometric enzymatic method of Berry et al *523*

Sodium *Serum No Effect Analytical* Negligible effect at a concentration of 20 µmol/L on enzymatic spectrophotometric method of Berry et al *523*

Aluminum Salts

Color *Feces Decrease Analytical* White discoloration or speckling *3810*

Diagnex Blue Excretion *Urine Increase Physiological* Heavy metal displacement of diagnex blue *6515*

Phosphate *Serum Decrease Physiological* Binding of phosphate in gastrointestinal tract *6515*
Urine Decrease Physiological Decreased absorption and excretion *128*

Amantadine

Alkaline Phosphatase *Serum Increase Physiological* Mild transient increase, other liver function tests normal *5388*

Aspartate Aminotransferase *Serum Increase Physiological* Reported effect, no mechanism discussed *3810*

Catecholamines *Plasma No Effect Analytical* No effect on HPLC method of Koller for dopamine, epinephrine, and norepinephrine *3230*

Dopamine *Urine No Effect Physiological* In normals and patients with Parkinson's disease *2966*

Epinephrine *Urine No Effect Physiological* In normals and patients with Parkinson's disease *2966*

Growth Hormone *Plasma No Effect Physiological* No effect observed *3833*

Histamine *Plasma No Effect Analytical* Improbable inhibition of radio-enzyme assay at physiological concentrations *2492*
Urine No Effect Physiological In normals and patients with Parkinson's disease *2966*

Homovanillic Acid *Plasma Increase Physiological* In 30 male schizophrenics treatment with 150 mg/d for 8 weeks caused an increase from the mean baseline of 7.27 ± 1.87 µg/L to 11.34 ± 4.79 µg/L in the 7 responders to treatment *6576*
Urine No Effect Physiological In normals and patients with Parkinson's disease *2966*

5-Hydroxyindoleacetic Acid *Urine No Effect Physiological* In normals but increased in Parkinsonism *2966*

Leukocytes *Blood Decrease Physiological* Leukopenia reported in less than 0.1% treated patients *1600* Occasional leukopenia reported *1384*

1,4-Methylhistamine *Urine No Effect Physiological* In normals but increased in Parkinsonism *2966*

Neutrophils *Blood Decrease Physiological* Neutropenia reported in less than 0.1% treated patients *1600* Occasional neutropenia reported *1384*

Norepinephrine *Urine No Effect Physiological* In normals and patients with Parkinson's disease *2966*

Urea Nitrogen *Serum Increase Physiological* Mild transient elevations reported *5388*

Ambenonium

Cholinesterase *Serum Decrease Physiological* Direct action of drug *1883*

Ambroxol

Lysergic Acid Diethylamide *Urine Increase Analytical* Mucolytics such as ambroxol or pirenzepin cause false positive reaction with Boehringer-Mannheim CEDIA® d.a.u. LSD procedure, not confirmed by HPLC *3658*

Amdinocillin

Glucose *Urine No Effect Analytical* On TesTape® at physiological concentration *305* On Clinitest® at physiological concentration. On Diastix® at physiological concentration *4538*

Amifostine

Calcium *Serum Decrease Physiological* Administration associated with rare hypocalcemia (in fewer than 1% treated patients) *127*

Amikacin

Alanine Aminotransferase *Urine No Effect Physiological* No significant effect in 15 volunteers over 24 hours after receiving 15 mg/kg intravenously *1730*

Albumin *Urine Increase Physiological* Renal function changes may occur that are usually reversible when treatment stopped *270* Increased excretion has been reported as a consequence of treatment, but usually reversible when treatment discontinued *219*

Alkaline Phosphatase *Urine No Effect Physiological* No significant effect in 15 volunteers over 24 hours after receiving 15 mg/kg intravenously *1730*

Amino Acids *Urine Increase Analytical* Peak observed after arginine in same chromatogram and next several chromatograms when short-column postcolumn derivitization used with HPLC. Results likely to be similar regardless of whether o-phthaldehyde or ninhydrin used as detection system *714*

Aspartate Aminotransferase *Urine No Effect Physiological* No significant effect in 15 volunteers over 24 hours after receiving 15 mg/kg intravenously *1730*

Amikacin *(continued)*

Bilirubin *Serum Decrease Analytical* No effect up to 2.5 mg/L on method on Ames Seralyzer but above this concentration apparent reduction of bilirubin concentration. This could be of clinical significance since therapeutic concentration is 15-30 mg/L *5706*

Casts *Urine Increase Physiological* Increased excretion has been reported as a consequence of treatment, but usually reversible when treatment discontinued *219* Renal function changes may occur including excretion of casts. Abnormality usually reversible when treatment stopped *270*

Chloramphenicol *Serum No Effect Analytical* No effect at 100 mg/L on coupled enzymatic method *4122*

Cholesterol *Serum Decrease Analytical* No effect up to 3 mg/L on Ames Seralyzer method although at higher concentrations apparently clinically significant reduction of cholesterol concentration since therapeutic concentration is 15-30 mg/L *5706*

Creatine Kinase *Serum Decrease Analytical* No effect up to 0.08 mg/L on method on Ames Seralyzer although at higher concentrations reduced enzyme activity observed. Effect likely to be of clinical significance since therapeutic concentration 15-30 mg/L *5706*

Creatinine *Serum Decrease Analytical* No effect up to 1 mg/L on Ames Seralyzer method but at higher concentrations apparently clinically significant decreased creatinine concentration *5706*
Serum Increase Physiological Increased concentration has been reported as a consequence of treatment, but usually reversible when treatment discontinued *219* Nephrotoxicity observed in 7 of 54 patients whose drug concentrations were monitored *2050* Renal function changes may occur that are usually reversible when treatment stopped *270*
Serum No Effect Analytical No effect of concentrations up to 15 mg/L on single slide method on Kodak Ektachem® *5706*

Erythrocytes *Urine Increase Physiological* Renal function changes may occur including excretion of red cells. Abnormality usually reversible when treatment stopped *270* Increased excretion has been reported as a consequence of treatment, but usually reversible when treatment discontinued *219*

Gentamicin *Serum No Effect Analytical* No interference observed at concentrations up to 500 µg/mL (858 µmol/L) with method on Du Pont aca *1526* Specimens containing amikacin showed no cross-reactivity when gentamicin measured by method on Bayer Technicon Immuno 1® system *426* No interference observed with Abbott TDx procedure *3858* Has cross-reactivity of less than 0.1% with method on Baxter Stratus *5705*

Glucose *Serum Decrease Analytical* No effect up to 0.2 mg/L on glucose oxidase method on Ames Seralyzer but above this concentration apparently reduced glucose concentration which is of clinical significance since therapeutic concentration is 15-30 mg/L *5706*
Urine No Effect Analytical No effect at up to 2 mg/mL on Clinitest® method and Diastix® and TesTape® procedures *3710*

γ-Glutamyltransferase *Urine No Effect Physiological* No significant effect over 24 hours in 15 volunteers after receiving 15 mg/kg intravenously *1730*

Kanamycin *Serum Increase Analytical* Interferes with Abbott TDx procedure *3858*

Ketone Body Ratio *Serum No Effect Analytical* When added at a concentration of 2.5 g/L had no significant effect on AKBR method of Uno et al *6131*

Lactate Dehydrogenase *Serum Decrease Analytical* No effect up to 0.2 mg/L on method on Ames Seralyzer but at higher concentrations apparently reduced enzyme activity of some clinical significance *5706*
Urine No Effect Physiological No effect in 15 volunteers over 24 hours after receiving 15 mg/kg intravenously *1730*

Leucine Aminopeptidase *Urine Increase Physiological* Significant effect observed in 15 healthy volunteers within 12 hours of receiving 15 mg/kg intravenously indicating involvement of proximal tubule structures *1730*

Leukocytes *Urine Increase Physiological* Renal function changes may occur including excretion of white cells. Abnormality usually reversible when treatment stopped *270* Increased excretion has been reported as a consequence of treatment, but usually reversible when treatment discontinued *219*

Mycophenolic Acid *Serum No Effect Analytical* No significant interference observed with HPLC method of Shipkova et al *5526*

Mycophenolic Acid Glucuronide
Serum No Effect Analytical No significant interference observed with HPLC method of Shipkova et al *5526*

Neomycin *Serum No Effect Analytical* No interference observed with method on Abbott TDx *3858*

Netilmicin *Serum No Effect Analytical* No interference with method on Abbott TDx *3858*

Oligosaccharides *Urine Positive Analytical* When thin-layer chromatography used an abnormal low Rf band observed which reacts like an oligosaccharide *4711*

Phenylalanine *Plasma No Effect Analytical* No interference observed with rapid whole blood quantitative method of Campbell et al using phenylalanine dehydrogenase *867*

Protein *Cerebrospinal Fluid No Effect Analytical* At concentration of 30 mg/L on SDS/Coomassie Blue method of Huang *2745* Insignificant effect when added in vitro when analyzed by Kodak Ektachem® slide method *3654*

SDZ PSC 833 *Blood No Effect Analytical* At a concentration of 29 mg/L had no effect on HPLC method of Scott et al when used to measure PSC with CsD (as internal standard) at a concentration of 5 mg/L *5418*

Streptomycin *Serum No Effect Analytical* No interference observed with method on Abbott TDx *3858*

Tacrolimus *Blood No Effect Analytical* No significant effect observed at a concentration of 30 mg/L with MEIA method on Abbott IMx analyzer *1871*
Serum No Effect Analytical At concentration of 30 mg/L had no significant effect on ELISA method *6329* In HPLC/MS method of Christians et al no significant interference observed with measurement of FK 506 *1010*

Tobramycin *Serum Increase Analytical* Cross-reacts with reagents in method on Du Pont aca *1547* At a concentration of 156 mg/L increased concentration by 25% when measured by method on Baxter Stratus although therapeutic concentration up to 30 mg/L only *5705* About 7.0% cross-reactivity observed with method on Abbott TDx *3858*

Urea Nitrogen *Serum Decrease Analytical* No effect up to 2.5 mg/L on method on Ames Seralyzer but at higher concentrations clinically significant reduction in apparent urea nitrogen concentration which is of clinical importance since normal therapeutic range 15-30 mg/L *5706*
Serum Increase Physiological Azotemia has been reported as a consequence of treatment, but usually reversible when treatment discontinued *219* Renal function changes may occur that are usually reversible when treatment stopped *270*

Vancomycin *Serum No Effect Analytical* No significant interference observed at a concentration of 100 µg/mL (171 µmol/L) with method on Du Pont aca *1561* At concentrations up to 100 µg/mL had no significant cross-reactivity in valproic acid method on Bayer Technicon Immuno 1® *438* No interference observed with method on Abbott TDx *3858*

Volume *Urine Increase Physiological* Renal function changes may occur including oliguria. Abnormality usually reversible when treatment stopped *270* Oliguria has been reported as a consequence of treatment, but usually reversible when treatment discontinued *219*

Amiloride

Aldosterone *Plasma Increase Physiological* In 5 normal subjects given 75 mg daily for 7 d *4037* 3 fold increase observed in 6 healthy subjects given 10 mg/d for 8 d *6304*

Angiotensin-II *Plasma Increase Physiological* Change varies with renin activity *4037*

Bicarbonate *Serum Decrease Physiological* Reduces alkalosis induced by other diuretics *213*
Serum No Effect Physiological No effect seen in 13 men treated for 8 weeks *1014*
Urine Increase Physiological Associated with potassium sparing diuretic action *4329*

Bilirubin *Serum Increase Physiological* Amiloride may cause increased concentration but with a frequency of less than 1% *3983*

Calcium *Serum No Effect Physiological* No effect seen in 13 men treated for 8 weeks *1014*
Urine Increase Physiological Observed in normals if given for 7 d *6309*

Chloride *Serum Decrease Physiological* Amiloride may cause hypochloremia when coadministered with other diuretics *3983*
Serum No Effect Physiological No effect seen in 13 men treated for 8 weeks *1014*
Urine Increase Physiological Diuretic action *2242*

Cholesterol *Serum Decrease Physiological* Significant fall with treatment in 13 men treated with drug: concentration rose when drug discontinued *1014*

Cholinesterase *Serum No Effect Analytical* No effect observed at concentration of 0.1 µg/mL with butyrylthiocholine method on Kodak Ektachem® *2504*

Corticosterone *Plasma No Effect Physiological* In 5 normal subjects given 75 mg daily for 7 d *4037*

Cortisol *Plasma No Effect Physiological* In 5 normal subjects given 75 mg daily for 7 d *4037*

Creatinine *Serum Increase Physiological* May occur with prolonged therapy *6256*
Serum No Effect Physiological No effect seen in 13 men treated for 8 weeks *1014*
Urine No Effect Physiological No effect seen in 13 men treated for 8 weeks *1014*

Deoxycorticosterone *Plasma No Effect Physiological* In 5 normal subjects given 75 mg daily for 7 d *4037*

Digoxin *Serum Decrease Physiological* Mean clearance increased due to increased tubular secretion of digoxin *6304*
Serum Increase Analytical At 50 ng/mL equals 0.6 ng/mL by RIA *6638*
Serum Increase Physiological Reported to increase serum concentration *1384*
Serum No Effect Physiological No apparent effect on serum concentration although renal clearance increased but associated with off-setting reduced nonrenal clearance *6304*

Glucose *Serum No Effect Physiological* No effect seen in 13 men treated for 8 weeks *1014*

Granulocytes *Blood No Effect Physiological* No significant association between use and agranulocytosis *3098*

Hematocrit *Blood No Effect Physiological* No effect seen in 13 men treated for 8 weeks *1014*

Histamine *Plasma No Effect Analytical* Although 50% inhibition at 24 µg/mL unlikely to be of clinical significance since therapeutic concentration about 0.05 µg/mL *2492*

18-Hydroxycorticosterone *Plasma Increase Physiological* In 5 normal subjects given 75 mg daily for 7 d *4037*

18-Hydroxydeoxycorticosterone
Plasma Increase Physiological In 5 normal subjects given 75 mg daily for 7 d *4037*

Inulin Clearance *Urine No Effect Physiological* Unchanged or may be slight increase *6256* No effect on glomerular filtration rate or effective renal plasma flow *1014*

Lithium *Serum Increase Physiological* Amiloride may cause increased concentration because of reduced urinary clearance *3983*

Lithium Clearance *Urine Decrease Physiological* Amiloride may cause increased concentration because of reduced urinary clearance *3983*

Magnesium *Serum Increase Physiological* 20 mg/d produces significant effect sustained for duration of treatment *5169*
Urine Decrease Physiological 5 or 10 mg when administered alone, and also blocked enhanced excretion caused by hydrochlorothiazide *5169*

Occult Blood *Feces Increase Physiological* Amiloride may cause gastrointestinal bleeding but with a frequency of less than 1% *3983*

PAH Clearance *Urine No Effect Physiological* No effect on glomerular filtration rate or effective renal plasma flow *1014*

pH *Urine Increase Physiological* Moderate increase sometimes observed *2242*

Potassium *Serum Increase Physiological* Binds reversibly to luminal membrane, blocking reabsorption of filtered sodium and inhibiting passive potassium and hydrogen ion secretion *4739* Significant rise in 3 patients with creatinines from 0.2 to 0.70 mmol/L when given with hydrochlorothiazide *6430* Increase by 0.9 mmol/L over 7 d in 5 volunteers with 75 mg daily *4037* Also inhibits kaliuresis caused by thiazides *4933* Amiloride may cause hyperkalemia (concentration above 5.5 mmol/L), most often in the absence of a kaliuretic agent. The incidence is higher in patients with renal impairment, diabetes mellitus and in the elderly *3983*
Urine Decrease Physiological May occur even if marked sodium loss *2242* 20 mg/d produces significant effect sustained for duration of treatment *5169* Decreased significantly with start of treatment *4037*
Urine No Effect Physiological No effect seen in 13 men treated for 8 weeks *1014*

Renin Activity *Plasma Increase Physiological* 13.6 fold increase, maximal after 5 d treatment *4037*

Sodium *Serum Decrease Physiological* Increase by 10 mmol/L over 7 d in 5 volunteers with 75 mg daily *4037* In 3 women when drug given with hydrochlorothiazide probably due to direct effect on distal nephrons *5950* Amiloride may cause hyponatremia when coadministered with other diuretics *3983*
Serum Increase Physiological Significant effect in 13 men given drug alone: remained high throughout treatment *1014*
Serum No Effect Physiological No effect seen in 13 men treated for 8 weeks *1014*
Urine Increase Physiological Marked natriuresis observed with start of therapy *4037* Diuretic action of drug *4933*
Urine No Effect Physiological No effect seen in 13 men treated for 8 weeks *1014*

Urea Nitrogen *Serum Increase Physiological* Amiloride may cause increased concentration when coadministered with other diuretics *3983* May occur with excessive saluresis *4014*
Serum No Effect Physiological No effect seen in 13 men treated for 8 weeks *1014*

Uric Acid *Serum Decrease Physiological* Effect observed after 8 weeks in one study *6309*
Serum Increase Physiological Possibly due to decreased clearance *6309* May occur with prolonged therapy particularly if combined with thiazides *6256*
Serum No Effect Physiological No effect observed *2452* No effect seen in 13 men treated for 8 weeks *1014*

Volume *Plasma No Effect Physiological* No effect seen in 13 men treated for 8 weeks *1014*

Amino Acids

Adenosine Triphosphate
Red Blood Cells Decrease Physiological Associated with low serum phosphate *6072*

Albumin *Urine No Effect Analytical* At concentration of 1000 mg/dL had no significant effect on Boehringer Mannheim Tina-quant method *2799*

Amino Acids *Plasma Increase Physiological* Marked increase if amino acids given intravenously, less if intraduodenally *4864*

Bicarbonate *Duodenal Fluid Increase Physiological* With duodenal infusion, no effect if given i.v *4864*

Bilirubin *Duodenal Fluid Increase Physiological* Increase by 800% with duodenal infusion, no effect if given i.v *4864*
Serum Increase Analytical If given i.v. may affect accuracy of estimation *200*

2,3-Diphosphoglycerate
Red Blood Cells Decrease Physiological Associated with low serum phosphate *6072*

Fatty Acids (FFA), Free *Serum Decrease Physiological* More marked if intraduodenal than i.v *4864*

Fructose-6-Phosphate
Red Blood Cells Decrease Physiological Associated with low serum phosphate *6072*

Gastrin *Serum Increase Physiological* Oral feeding produces up to tenfold increase *3250*

Glucose *Serum Decrease Physiological* Significant decrease if i.v. infusion, not if intraduodenal *4864* Fall may occur after intraduodenal infusion *4864*

Amino Acids *(continued)*

Glucose-6-Phosphate
Red Blood Cells Decrease Physiological Associated with low serum phosphate *6072*

Glycerol *Serum Decrease Physiological* More marked if given intraduodenally than i.v *4864*

Growth Hormone *Plasma Increase Physiological* Slight effect, mode of infusion makes no difference *4864*

Hemoglobin *Blood Increase Analytical* If given i.v. reported to affect accuracy of measurement *200*

Histamine *Plasma No Effect Analytical* Apparently no inhibition of radio-enzyme assay at concentration of 100 µg/mL with mixture containing ornithine but excluding glycine *2492* Improbable inhibition of radio-enzyme assay at normal concentrations *2492*

Insulin *Plasma Increase Physiological* Maximum higher if given intraduodenally than if given i.v *4864* ?due to action on beta cells *2909*

N-Acetyl-Glucosaminidase *Urine No Effect Analytical* At concentration of 1000 mg/dL had no significant effect on Boehringer Mannheim CPR method *3174*

Phosphate *Serum Decrease Physiological* If given i.v. hyperalimentation *6072*

Phosphoenolpyruvate
Red Blood Cells Decrease Physiological Associated with low serum phosphate *6072*

2-Phosphoglycerate
Red Blood Cells Decrease Physiological Associated with low serum phosphate *6072*

3-Phosphoglycerate
Red Blood Cells Decrease Physiological Associated with low serum phosphate *6072*

Protein *Serum Increase Analytical* If given i.v. may affect accuracy of measurement *200*

Sodium *Serum Increase Physiological* If Aminosol given i.v. may cause sodium retention *200*

Sugar *Urine Increase Analytical* False positive caused by some amino acids with Benedict's reaction *1714*

Trypsin *Duodenal Fluid Increase Physiological* Increase by 200% with duodenal infusion, no effect if given i.v *4864*

Urea Nitrogen *Serum Increase Analytical* May react with Berthelot if urease not used *4953*
Serum Increase Physiological As result of i.v. infusion *1992*

Volume *Duodenal Fluid Increase Physiological* With duodenal infusion, no effect if given i.v *4864*

Aminoantipyrine

Cholesterol *Serum Decrease Analytical* At concentrations above 400 mg/L lowered concentration as measured by CHOD-PAP method *5704*

p-Aminophenol *Urine No Effect Analytical* With addition of drugs at a concentration of 100 mg/L and of related compounds at 50 mg/L no significant effect observed on colorimetric method of van Bocxlaer on Cobas Mira analyzer which involves reacting free p-aminophenol with resorcinol in the presence of magnesium ions to form an indophenol dye measured at 550 nm *6163*

Aminocaproic Acid

Amino Acids *Urine Increase Analytical* Reacts with ninhydrin, measured as amino acid *6612*

α_1-Antitrypsin *Serum Increase Physiological* Inhibits activation of plasminogen, plasmin and trypsin *3239*

Aspartate Aminotransferase *Serum Increase Physiological* Rare myopathy six weeks after treatment *484*

Bleeding Time *Patient Increase Physiological* Prolongation of the template bleeding time has been observed with continuous intravenous infusion of drug *2815* Effect noted in majority of patients after 24 g/d after 9 d treatment *2304*

Creatine Kinase *Serum Increase Physiological* Increased CK activity with rhabdomyolysis have been observed as complications of drug administration *2815* Rare myopathy 6 weeks after treatment *484*

Granulocytes *Blood Decrease Physiological* Agranulocytosis has been observed as complication of drug administration *2815*

Leucine Aminopeptidase *Urine Decrease Physiological* Due to antifibrinolytic action *4826*

Leukocytes *Blood Decrease Physiological* Leukopenia has been observed as complication of drug administration *2815*

Myoglobin *Urine Increase Physiological* In a few patients inflammatory myopathy observed with myoglobinuria who received doses of 24-38 g/d for more than one month *1384*

Plasmin Activity *Plasma Decrease Physiological* Therapeutic intent *2754*

Platelets *Blood Decrease Physiological* Thrombocytopenia has been observed as complication of drug administration *2815*

Potassium *Serum Increase Physiological* Reported effect especially if renal function impaired *185*

Urea Nitrogen *Serum Increase Physiological* Increased urea nitrogen concentrations and even renal failure have been observed as complications of drug administration *2815*

7-Aminocephalosporanic Acid

Amino Acids *Urine Increase Analytical* Reacts with ninhydrin in paper chromatography, paper electrophoresis and ion-exchange chromatography *4761*

Sugar *Urine Increase Analytical* Reacts positively with Clinitest *4761*

Aminoglutethimide

Alanine Aminotransferase *Serum Increase Physiological* Casual association between drug administration and cholestasis in 2 cases *4608*

Aldosterone *Urine Decrease Physiological* May inhibit aldosterone production *4605*

Alkaline Phosphatase *Serum Increase Physiological* Casual association between drug administration and cholestasis in 2 cases *4608*

Androgens *Plasma Increase Physiological* In 11 postmenopausal women with advanced breast cancer significant increase of plasma androgens observed *3002*

Apolipoprotein A-I *Serum Increase Physiological* In 73 patients with advanced breast cancer receiving 500 mg/d with 40 mg hydrocortisone *653*

Aspartate Aminotransferase *Serum Increase Physiological* Casual association between drug administration and cholestasis in 2 cases *4608*

Bilirubin *Serum Increase Physiological* Casual association between drug administration and cholestasis in 2 cases *4608*

Carcinoembryonic Antigen *Serum No Effect Analytical* At a concentration of up to 398.0 µg/mL caused less than 10% error in the concentration of CEA as measured by the method on Bayer Technicon Immuno 1® *418*

Chloride *Serum Decrease Physiological* With overdose effect observed *1026*

Cholesterol *Serum Increase Physiological* In 73 patients with advanced breast cancer receiving 500 mg/d with 40 mg hydrocortisone *653*

Corticotropin *Plasma No Effect Physiological* In 11 postmenopausal women with advanced breast cancer treated with 500 mg/d for 9 months caused no significant effect *3002*

Cortisol *Plasma Decrease Physiological* Morning concentrations in patients with adrenal carcinomas and ectopic ACTH-producing tumors were reduced on average to about one half of the pretreatment concentrations and in patients with adrenal hyperplasia to about two thirds of the pretreatment concentrations during 1 to 3 months treatment. About 50% reduction observed in patients with adrenal adenomas *1026* In critically ill patients relative hypoadrenalism observed with aminoglutethimide therapy because of its effect on cortisol synthesis *3381*

Plasma *No Effect* *Physiological* In 11 postmenopausal women with advanced breast cancer treatment with 500 mg/d for 9 months had no significant effect on concentration *3002*

Dexamethasone *Serum* *Decrease* *Physiological* Induction of hepatic microsomal enzymes causes reduction of half-life of dexamethasone by up to 50% *5265* Aminoglutethimide accelerates the metabolism of dexamethasone *1026*

Erythrocytes *Blood* *Decrease* *Physiological* Pancytopenia has been reported with drug use *1384*

Estradiol *Plasma* *Decrease* *Physiological* By approximately 50% in women with advanced breast cancer (postmenopausal) *1488*

Estradiol, Free *Plasma* *Decrease* *Physiological* Marked reduction in small number of postmenopausal women with severe breast cancer although no difference in proportion (%) of total estradiol *1488*

Estrogens *Plasma* *Decrease* *Physiological* Significant decrease observed in 11 postmenopausal women with advanced breast cancer treated with 500 mg/d for 9 months *3002*

Glucose *Serum* *Decrease* *Physiological* With overdose effect observed *1026*

γ-Glutamyltransferase *Serum* *Increase* *Physiological* Increased in 26 of 45 patients with breast cancer *4211*

Granulocytes *Blood* *Decrease* *Physiological* Agranulocytosis has been reported with drug use *1384* Single incidence of agranulocytosis in a patient observed in 27 patients with Cushing's syndrome caused by adrenal carcinoma *1026*

HDL-Cholesterol *Serum* *Increase* *Physiological* In 73 patients with advanced breast cancer receiving 500 mg/d with 40 mg hydrocortisone *653*

Hematocrit *Blood* *Decrease* *Physiological* In one patient with adrenal hyperplasia decreased during the course of treatment *1026*

Hemoglobin *Blood* *Decrease* *Physiological* In one patient with adrenal hyperplasia concentration decreased during the course of treatment *1026*

Hydrocortisone *Serum* *No Effect* *Physiological* Although aminoglutethimide accelerates the metabolism of dexamethasone it has no effect on hydrocortisone metabolism *1026*

17-Hydroxycorticosteroids *Urine* *Decrease* *Physiological* Inhibits steroid biosynthesis *2055*

^{131}I Uptake *Serum* *Decrease* *Physiological* Reported effect *3669*

Insulin-like Growth Factor-I *Serum* *Increase* *Physiological* In 15 of 17 postmenopausal women mean concentration increased from 17.0 nmol/L before treatment to 21.1 nmol/L during treatment *3566*

17-Ketosteroids *Urine* *Decrease* *Physiological* Inhibits steroid biosynthesis *2055*

LDL-Cholesterol *Serum* *Increase* *Physiological* In 73 patients with advanced breast cancer receiving 500 mg/d with 40 mg hydrocortisone *653*

Leukocytes *Blood* *Decrease* *Physiological* Single incidence of leukopenia, in a patient also receiving o,p'-DDD, observed in 27 patients with Cushing's syndrome caused by adrenal carcinoma *1026* Leukopenia has been reported with drug use *1384* May cause leukopenia *3810*

Neutrophils *Blood* *Decrease* *Physiological* Single incidence of neutropenia observed in 27 patients with Cushing's syndrome *1026*

Partial Thromboplastin Time
Plasma *Decrease* *Physiological* Aminoglutethimide diminishes the effect of coumarin and warfarin *1026*

Platelets *Blood* *Decrease* *Physiological* Thrombocytopenia has been reported with drug use *1384*

Potassium *Serum* *Increase* *Physiological* With overdose effect observed *1026*

Prothrombin Time *Plasma* *Decrease* *Physiological* Aminoglutethimide diminishes the effect of coumarin and warfarin *1026*

Sodium *Serum* *Decrease* *Physiological* With overdose effect observed *1026*

T3-Uptake *Serum* *Increase* *Physiological* Competes for binding sites *882*

Theophylline *Serum* *Decrease* *Physiological* Up to 25% decrease in serum theophylline concentration due to increased theophylline clearance caused by induction of microsomal enzyme activity *6117* Increases theophylline clearance by induction of microsomal enzyme activity, decreasing theophylline concentration by about 25% *5999* Increases theophylline clearance by induction of microsomal enzyme activity and decreases serum theophylline concentration by 25% *3125*

Thyroid Stimulating Hormone
Serum *Increase* *Physiological* In 9 of 29 patients with prostatic cancer treatment with 1 g/d caused increases above 10 mU/L to mean of 13.1 ± 14.4 mU/L with restoration to normal after administration of levothyroxine *1861* Observed in one patient in whom tested in association with reduced T4 *5295*

Thyroxine (T4) *Serum* *Decrease* *Physiological* On average 1.6 μg/dL decrease in concentration after 3 mo treatment *5295* Hypothyroidism may occur in conjunction with treatment *1026* Competes for T4 binding sites *882*

Warfarin *Plasma* *Decrease* *Physiological* Increases rate of metabolism and may increase warfarin requirement by approximately 100% *1384*

Aminoglycosides

Alanine Aminotransferase *Serum* *No Effect* *Physiological* No change observed in 114 patients observed prospectively before treatment with aminoglycosides *4107*

Alkaline Phosphatase *Serum* *Increase* *Physiological* In prospective study of 114 patients significant increase of alkaline phosphatase activity observed (average increase of 28 U/L on day 6) but no patient had increase above twice the upper limit of normal *4107*

Bilirubin *Serum* *No Effect* *Physiological* No change observed in prospective study of 114 patients *4107*

Clindamycin *Serum* *Positive* *Analytical* Interference observed with bioassay procedure at Mayo Clinic *3858*

Colistin *Serum* *Positive* *Analytical* Interference observed with bioassay procedure at Mayo Clinic *3858*

Erythromycin *Serum* *Increase* *Analytical* Interference observed with bioassay procedure at Mayo Clinic *3858*

Lactate Dehydrogenase *Serum* *No Effect* *Physiological* No change observed in prospective study of 114 patients *4107*

Magnesium *Serum* *Increase* *Physiological* Effect noted in 8 of 32 patients treated by an aminoglycoside alone or with a diuretic *6640*

Metronidazole *Serum* *Increase* *Analytical* Interference observed with bioassay procedure at Mayo Clinic *3858*

Polymyxin *Serum* *Increase* *Analytical* Interference observed with bioassay procedure at Mayo Clinic *3858*

Retinol *Urine* *Increase* *Physiological* In 22 patients with sepsis and pneumonia receiving aminoglycosides significantly higher excretion of 3.06 ± 0.71 μmol/d than 2.34 ± 0.98 μmol/d in 7 patients who did not receive antibiotics *5811*

Tetracycline *Serum* *No Effect* *Analytical* No interference observed with bioassay procedure at Mayo Clinic *3858*

Tobramycin *Serum* *Increase* *Analytical* Cross-react with reagents in method on Du Pont aca *1547*

Trimethoprim *Serum* *No Effect* *Analytical* No interference observed with bioassay procedure at Mayo Clinic *3858*

Aminoguanidine

Histamine *Urine* *No Effect* *Physiological* No effect observed on standard diet *2293*

Imidazoleacetic Acid *Urine* *Decrease* *Physiological* Inhibits diamine oxidase *2292*

Methylhistamine *Urine* *Increase* *Physiological* Methylation increased when diamine oxidase inhibited *2292*

Methylimidazoleacetic Acid *Urine* *Increase* *Physiological* As result of metabolism of increased methyl-histamine *2292*

Aminohippurate

Creatinine *Serum* *Increase* *Analytical* Chromogenicity in color reaction *5869*

Aminohippurate *(continued)*

Creatinine *(continued)*
Serum *No Effect* *Analytical* No inteference observed at a concentration of 10 mg/L with HPLC method of Rosano et al *5083*

Sulfa as Sulfanilamide *Serum* *Increase* *Analytical* Measured as if sulfonamide *4953*

Aminomel LX 6

Amylase *Serum* *No Effect* *Analytical* At concentration of 16 g/L had no effect on maltotetrose method *5704* At concentration of 16 g/L had no effect on p-nitrophenylmaltoheptoside method *5704* At concentration of 16 g/L had no effect on p-nitrophenylmaltopentoside/hexoside method *5704*

Aminomethylcyclohexane

Leucine Aminopeptidase *Urine* *Decrease* *Physiological* Due to antifibrinolytic action *4826*

Aminophenazone

Alanine Aminotransferase *Serum* *Increase* *Analytical* On continuous method at 10 times maximal therapeutic concentration *2919*
Serum *No Effect* *Analytical* On continuous method at 10 times maximal therapeutic concentration *2919*

Alkaline Phosphatase *Serum* *No Effect* *Analytical* On continuous method at 10 times maximal therapeutic concentration *2919*

Aspartate Aminotransferase *Serum* *Decrease* *Analytical* On continuous method at 10 times maximal therapeutic concentration *2919*
Serum *Increase* *Analytical* On continuous method at 10 times maximal therapeutic concentration *2919*

Bilirubin *Serum* *Decrease* *Analytical* With 540 µmol/L on dimethylsulfoxide method *2919*
Serum *No Effect* *Analytical* At therapeutic concentrations no effect on method of Jendrassik and Grof and those using spectrophotometry *2920*

Cholesterol *Serum* *No Effect* *Analytical* No effect at therapeutic concentration on enzymatic and Liebermann-Burchard methods *2920*

Creatine Kinase *Serum* *No Effect* *Analytical* On continuous method at 10 times maximal therapeutic concentration *2919*

Creatinine *Serum* *No Effect* *Analytical* At therapeutic concentrations no effect on alkaline picrate and Slot methods *2920*

Glucose *Serum* *Decrease* *Analytical* Slight reduction at therapeutic concentration on ABTS method *2920* With 540 µmol/L on GOD-PERID/ABTS method *2919*
Serum *No Effect* *Analytical* At therapeutic concentrations no effects on hexokinase, glucose dehydrogenase 2.4-dichlorophenol and o-toluidine methods *2920* With 540 µmol/L on hexokinase method. With 540 µmol/L on glucose dehydrogenase method. With 540 µmol/L on GOD-PERID/2,4-dichlorophenol method. With 540 µmol/L on o-toluidine method *2919*

Hydroxybutyrate Dehydrogenase
Serum *No Effect* *Analytical* On continuous method at 10 times maximal therapeutic concentration *2919*

Iron *Serum* *No Effect* *Analytical* At therapeutic concentration on Ramsay and bathophenanthroline methods *2920*

Lactate Dehydrogenase *Serum* *No Effect* *Analytical* On continuous method with pyruvate as substrate at 10 times maximal therapeutic concentration. On continuous method with lactate as substrate at 10 times maximal therapeutic concentration. On colorimetric method at 10 times maximal therapeutic concentration *2919*

Protein *Serum* *No Effect* *Analytical* No effect on biuret and spectrophotometric methods at therapeutic concentration *2920*

Triglycerides *Serum* *No Effect* *Analytical* At therapeutic concentration on enzymatic methods *2920*

Urea Nitrogen *Serum* *No Effect* *Analytical* At therapeutic concentrations no effects on glutamate dehydrogenase, phenol-hypochlorite, diacetyl monoxime methods *2920* With 540 µmol/L on glutamate dehydrogenase method. With 540 µmol/L on phenol-hypochlorite method. With 540 µmol/L on diacetyl monoxime method *2919*

Uric Acid *Serum* *No Effect* *Analytical* At therapeutic concentrations no effects on methods using uricase-catalase, aldehyde dehydrogenase, direct UV-test phosphotungstate methods *2920*

Aminophylline

Bilirubin *Serum* *No Effect* *Physiological* No significant displacement from protein in neonates *6314*

Catecholamines *Plasma* *Increase* *Physiological* Response to i.v. therapeutic dose *288*

Cholesterol *Serum* *No Effect* *Physiological* No change observed in 9 volunteers after intravenous administration of 0.96 g daily for 3 days *6629*

Clotting Time *Blood* *Decrease* *Physiological* Reported effect *2242*

Color *Feces* *Increase* *Analytical* Black color reported with aminophylline ingestion *3388* Balck color reported with aminophylline ingestion *3388*

Creatinine *Serum* *No Effect* *Analytical* At 400 mg/L on reversed phase liquid chromatographic procedure of Zhiri et al *6656*

Epinephrine *Plasma* *Increase* *Physiological* Increases basal concentration in healthy individuals, also higher during exercise and during recovery *6410*
Urine *Increase* *Physiological* Threefold increase in response to i.v. dose *288* Excretion higher at rest, during and after exercise compared with placebo situation *6410*

Fatty Acids (FFA), Free *Serum* *Increase* *Physiological* After single administration of 0.48 g intravenously in 9 volunteers sharp increase in concentration due to inhibition of phosphodiesterase with increase of intracellular cAMP and hydrolysis of adipose tissue triglycerides *6629*

Ketone Body Ratio *Serum* *No Effect* *Analytical* When added at a concentration of 1.25 g/L had no significant effect on AKBR method of Uno et al *6131*

Lactate *Plasma* *No Effect* *Analytical* No effect at final concentration of 25 µg/mL on method on Kodak Ektachem® *2793*

Leukotriene C_4 *Plasma* *Increase* *Physiological* Treatment of 6 asthmatics with 250 mg aminophylline only intravenously caused increase from mean concentration of 178 ng/L to 213 ng/mL *5529* In 6 asthmatic patients treatment with 250 mg caused increase from mean baseline of 178 pg/mL to 213 pg/mL *5529*

Lipoprotein A-I *Serum* *Decrease* *Physiological* After 3 days treatment with 0.96 g/day intravenously mean reduction of 11% observed in 9 volunteers in parallel with change in lipoprotein lipase *6629*

β-Lipoprotein *Serum* *No Effect* *Analytical* No significant effect of intravenous infusion of 0,96 g/day for 3 days in 9 volunteers *6629*

Lipoproteins, Pre-β *Serum* *No Effect* *Physiological* No significant effect in 9 healthy volunteers with intravenous administration of 0.96 g/day for 3 days *6629*

Lithium Clearance *Urine* *Increase* *Physiological* A single dose of the drug effectively increases lithium clearance *4399*

Midazolam *Serum* *No Effect* *Analytical* On GC-ECD method of Ha et al *2387*

Norepinephrine *Plasma* *Increase* *Physiological* Concentration higher at rest, during and after exercise compared with placebo situation *6410*
Urine *Increase* *Physiological* Concentration higher at rest, during and after exercise compared with placebo situation *6410* Twofold increase in response to i.v. dose *288*

Occult Blood *Feces* *Increase* *Physiological* Hematemesis may occur early with poisoning *4014*

Postheparin Hepatic Triglyceride Lipase
Plasma *No Effect* *Physiological* After 3 days administration of 0.96 g/day intravenously in 9 volunteers no significant change observed following heparin challenge *6629*

Postheparin Lipoprotein Lipase
Plasma Decrease Physiological After 3 days of administration of 0.96 g/day intravenously in 9 volunteers mean decrease of 52% observed following heparin challenge *6629*

Protein *Cerebrospinal Fluid No Effect Analytical* No effect observed at final concentration of 25 μg/mL on method on Kodak Ektachem® *2791*
Urine Increase Physiological Increase in renal disease (occurs early with poisoning) *1714*

Triglycerides *Serum No Effect Physiological* No significant effect observed in 9 volunteers following intravenous administration of 0.96 g/day for 3 days *6629*

Uric Acid *Serum No Effect Analytical* At 400 mg/L on reversed phase liquid chromatographic procedure of Zhiri et al *6656*

Aminopropionitrile

Hydroxyproline *Urine Increase Physiological* Observed in experimental studies *6111*

Aminopterin

Chromosomes *Test Conditions Abnormal Physiological* Clastogenic in human lymphocytes in culture *5484*

Folate *Red Blood Cells Decrease Physiological* Inhibits dihydrofolate reductase by combining irreversibly with it *3383*
Red Blood Cells Increase Analytical High concentrations in samples may have a significant effect on method on Bayer Technicon Immuno 1® *432*
Red Blood Cells No Effect Analytical Cross-reactivity of less than 2% observed at a concentration of 1 μg/mL with method on Bio-Rad Radias *3557*
Serum Decrease Physiological Inhibits dihydrofolate reductase by combining irreversibly with it *3383*
Serum No Effect Analytical At concentration of 5.0 μg/mL no clinically significant effect (0.08%) observed with method on Stratus family of analyzers *4141*

Methotrexate *Serum Increase Analytical* Significant cross-reactivity observed with method on Du Pont aca *1535*

Aminopyrimidine

Bilirubin *Serum No Effect Analytical* At concentration of 57 mg/L had no effect on Kodak Ektachem® method *5704*

Aminopyrine

Alanine Aminotransferase *Serum Increase Physiological* Liver damage up to hepatic necrosis seen *4014*

Albumin *Serum No Effect Analytical* At concentration of 125 mg/L had no effect on BCG method *5704*

δ-Aminolevulinic Acid *Urine Increase Physiological* May precipitate attack of acute porphyria *1687*

Aspartate Aminotransferase *Serum Increase Physiological* Liver damage up to hepatic necrosis seen *4014*

Bilirubin *Serum Increase Physiological* Hemolysis in G-6-PD deficiency *402*
Serum No Effect Analytical At concentration of 125 mg/L had no effect on Jendrassik and Grof method *5704*

Bilirubin, Direct *Serum Increase Physiological* May cause hemolytic anemia *3810*

Calcium *Serum No Effect Analytical* At concentration of 125 mg/L had no effect on cresolphthalein method *5704*

Cannabinoids *Urine No Effect Analytical* No effect on Roche Abuscreen method *5006*

Cholesterol *Serum No Effect Analytical* At concentration of 125 mg/L had no effect on CHOD-PAP method *5704*

Color *Urine Increase Analytical* Red brown *3810*

Creatine *Urine Increase Physiological* Reported effect *3669*

Creatinine *Serum No Effect Analytical* At concentration of 125 mg/L had no effect on Technicon AutoAnalyzer® Jaffe method *5704*

Erythrocytes *Blood Decrease Physiological* Hemolytic anemia in G-6-PD deficient persons *1212*
Urine Increase Physiological Rare nephrotoxicity reported *4014*

γ-Globulin *Serum Increase Physiological* Specific antibodies to drug may develop *3554*

Glucaric Acid *Urine Increase Physiological* Increased excretion occurs as a result of hepatic enzyme induction *3669*

Glucose *Serum No Effect Analytical* No effect of concentrations up to 500 mg/L on method on Kodak Ektachem® *5706* At concentration of 125 mg/L had no effect on hexokinase/G-6-PDH method *5704*

Glutathione, Reduced
Red Blood Cells Decrease Physiological Sharp fall before overt hemolysis *3094*

Haptoglobin *Serum Decrease Physiological* May cause hemolytic anemia *3810*

Heinz Body Formation *Blood Positive Physiological* Occurs initially before overt hemolysis *3094*

Hematocrit *Blood Decrease Physiological* Hemolytic anemia in G-6-PD deficient persons *1212*

Hemoglobin *Blood Decrease Physiological* Hemolytic anemia in G-6-PD deficient persons *1212*
Plasma Increase Physiological May occur with marked hemolysis *3094*
Urine Increase Physiological May occur with marked hemolysis *3094*

Iron *Serum No Effect Analytical* At concentration of 125 mg/L had no effect on Ferrozine method *5704*

Leukocytes *Blood Decrease Physiological* Agranulocytosis occurs within minutes *6654*

Nitrogen *Urine Increase Physiological* Reported effect *3669*

Occult Blood *Feces Increase Physiological* Possibly due to impaired platelet aggregation *915*

Phosphate *Serum No Effect Analytical* At concentration of 125 mg/L had no effect on phosphomolybdate method *5704*
Urine Increase Physiological Reported effect *3669*

Platelet Aggregation *Blood Decrease Physiological* Observed *in vitro*, might cause gastrointestinal bleeding etc *915*

Platelets *Blood Decrease Physiological* May cause hemolytic or aplastic anemia *6654*

Porphyrin, Total *Urine Increase Physiological* Stimulates formation of ALA-synthetase *2242*

Protein *Serum No Effect Analytical* At concentration of 125 mg/L had no effect on biuret method with blank correction *5704*
Urine Increase Physiological Nephrotoxicity reported *4014*

Prothrombin Time *Plasma Increase Physiological* Observed in man and experimental animals *3810*

Reticulocytes *Blood Increase Physiological* May occur during recovery from hemolysis *3094*

Sugar *Urine Increase Analytical* Glucuronide metabolism affects Benedict's, Clinitest® tests *882*

Urea Nitrogen *Serum Increase Physiological* Rare suggestion of nephrotoxic action *4014*
Serum No Effect Analytical No effect of concentrations up to 500 mg/L on method on Kodak Ektachem® *5706* At concentration of 125 mg/L had no effect on diacetylmonoxime method *5704*

Uric Acid *Serum No Effect Analytical* At concentration of 125 mg/L had no effect on phosphotungstate reduction method *5704*

Volume *Plasma Increase Physiological* Fluid retention may occur *4014*

Aminosalicylic Acid

Alanine Aminotransferase *Serum Increase Analytical* At 5 times upper limit of therapeutic range on methods on KDA and Technicon SMAC® *3525*
Serum Increase Physiological In one retrospective study of 7492 patients, drug-induced hepatitis occurred in 38 (0.5%), with the first symptoms usually occurring within 3 months of the start of treatment *2874* Rare side effect *2135* May cause cytotoxic hepatocellular damage *402*

Aminosalicylic Acid *(continued)*

Alanine Aminotransferase *(continued)*
Serum No Effect Analytical At 5 times upper limit of therapeutic range on methods on Abbott-VP, Du Pont aca, and Roche Cobas-Bio *3525*

Albumin *Serum Increase Analytical* Aminosalicylic acid reportedly interferes with dye-binding methods *2874*
Serum No Effect Analytical At 5 times upper limit of therapeutic range on methods on Technicon SMAC® , Kodak Ektachem® , Hitachi® 705 and KDA *3525* No effect at concentration of 1000 mg/L on Kodak Ektachem® method *5706* At concentration of 460 mg/L had no effect on BCG method *5704*

Alkaline Phosphatase *Serum Increase Physiological* In one retrospective study of 7492 patients, drug-induced hepatitis occurred in 38 (0.5%), with the first symptoms usually occurring within 3 months of the start of treatment *2874* Reversible cholestasis may occur *2803*
Serum No Effect Analytical At 5 times upper limit of therapeutic range on methods on Technicon SMAC® , Abbott-VP, Du Pont aca, Roche Cobas-Bio, Hitachi® 705 and KDA *3525*

Amino-4-Imidazole-5-Carboxamide Ribotide
Urine Increase Physiological Occurs with vitamin B_{12} deficiency *6370*

Amylase *Serum Increase Physiological* May cause acute pancreatitis *2242*
Serum No Effect Analytical At 5 times upper limit of therapeutic range on methods on Du Pont aca, Roche Cobas-Bio and Kodak Ektachem® *3525*

Aspartate Aminotransferase *Serum Increase Analytical* Aminosalicylic acid reportedly interferes with azoene dye methods *2874* At 1 mmol/L affects Technicon SMA 12/60 method *5576* With diazonium end point method on Technicon AutoAnalyzer® *2196* At 5 times upper limit of therapeutic range on methods on KDA and Technicon SMAC® *3525*
Serum Increase Physiological Rare side effect *2135* May cause cytotoxic hepatocellular damage *402* In one retrospective study of 7492 patients, drug-induced hepatitis occurred in 38 (0.5%), with the first symptoms usually occurring within 3 months of the start of treatment *2874*
Serum No Effect Analytical At 5 times upper limit of therapeutic range on methods on Abbott-VP, Du Pont aca, Roche Cobas-Bio and Hitachi® 705 *3525*

Bicarbonate *Serum No Effect Analytical* At concentration of 460 mg/L had no effect on method using phenolphthalein *5704* No effect of concentrations up to 230 mg/L on method on Kodak Ektachem® *5706*

Bile *Urine Increase Analytical* Red color with Fouchet procedure *199*
Urine Increase Physiological Hepatotoxicity *3810*

Bilirubin *Serum Increase Analytical* Marked increase at upper limit of therapeutic range on Du Pont aca method. At 5 times upper limit of therapeutic range on Roche Cobas-Bio method *3525*
Serum Increase Physiological In one retrospective study of 7492 patients, drug-induced hepatitis occurred in 38 (0.5%), with the first symptoms usually occurring within 3 months of the start of treatment *2874* Reversible cholestasis caused by drug *464*
Serum No Effect Analytical At concentration of 460 mg/L had no effect on Jendrassik and Grof method *5704* At 5 times upper limit of therapeutic range on methods on Technicon SMAC® , Kodak Ektachem® , Hitachi® 705 and KDA *3525* At concentration of 230 mg/L had no effect on Kodak Ektachem® method *5704*
Serum No Effect Physiological Probable insignificant displacement from protein in neonates *6314*
Urine Increase Analytical Aminosalicylic acid reportedly interferes with qualitative urine test methods *2874*

Bilirubin, Direct *Serum Increase Physiological* Reversible cholestasis caused by drug *464*

BSP Retention *Serum Increase Physiological* Reversible cholestasis caused by drug *4480*

Calcium *Serum No Effect Analytical* At concentration of 460 mg/L had no effect on cresolphthalein method *5704* At 5 times upper limit of therapeutic range on methods on Technicon SMAC® , Abbott-VP, Du Pont aca, Kodak Ektachem® , Hitachi® 705 and KDA *3525*

Chloride *Serum No Effect Analytical* At concentration of 460 mg/L had no effect on mercurimetric method *5704* No effect of concentrations up to 230 mg/L with method on Kodak Ektachem® *5706*

Cholesterol *Serum Decrease Physiological* As effective as neomycin, mechanism obscure *3544*
Serum No Effect Analytical At 5 times upper limit of therapeutic range on methods on Technicon SMAC® , Abbott-VP, Roche Cobas-Bio, Kodak Ektachem® , Hitachi® 705 and KDA *3525* At concentration of 460 mg/L had no effect on Liebermann-Burchard method *5704*

Color *Urine Increase Analytical* Abnormal color (not distinctive) *606*

Coombs' Test *Blood Positive Physiological* Hypersensitivity reactions may be observed after aminosalicylic acid administration including leukopenia, agranulocytosis, and thrombocytopenia, and Coombs' positive hemolytic anemia *2874*

Coombs' Test, Direct *Blood Positive Physiological* Immunological response to drug *2453*

Creatine Kinase *Serum No Effect Analytical* At 5 times upper limit of therapeutic range on methods on Technicon SMAC® , Abbott-VP, Du Pont aca, Roche Cobas-Bio and Hitachi® 705 *3525*

Creatinine *Serum No Effect Analytical* Although p-aminosalicylate elutes at 4.7 min and creatinine at 8.9 min difference is sufficiently great that no interference is observed in HPLC method of Rosano et al *5083* No effect of concentrations up to 1000 mg/L on 2-slide method on Kodak Ektachem® *5706* At concentration of 460 mg/L had no effect on Technicon AutoAnalyzer® method *5704* At 5 times upper limit of therapeutic range on methods onTechnicon SMAC® , Abbott-VP, Du Pont aca, Roche Cobas-Bio, Kodak Ektachem® , Hitachi® 705 and KDA *3525*

Crystals *Urine Increase Physiological* Crystaluria may be prevented after aminosalicylic acid administration by maintenance of a neutral or alkaline urine *2874*

Digoxin *Serum Decrease Physiological* 8 hours after 2 g aminosalicylic acid q.i.d. plasma digoxin concentration was reduced by 40% in two of ten patients although it was unchanged in the others *2874* Slight effect observed in 10 healthy individuals due to reduced absorption *761*

Eosinophils *Blood Increase Physiological* Hypersensitivity reaction *2484* In one retrospective study of 7492 patients, drug-induced hepatitis occurred in 38 (0.5%), with the first symptoms usually occurring within 3 months of the start of treatment. At the time of diagnosis leosnophilia was observed in 55% of the 38 individuals *2874*

Erythrocytes *Blood Decrease Physiological* Hemolytic anemia/megaloblastic anemia *1212*
Urine Increase Physiological Bleeding caused by drug *2024*

Fat *Feces Decrease Physiological* Aminosalicylic acid has been shown to cause a malabsorption syndrome, usually incomplete, with steatorrhea as a consequence *2874*
Feces Increase Physiological Produces steatorrhea possibly because of bile acid chelation *5055*

Ferric Chloride Test *Urine Positive Analytical* Blue-purple color *199*

Fibrinolytic Activity *Plasma No Effect Physiological* No effect of 1.5 g/d or after 250 mg i.v. in 6 patients *6509*

Folate *Serum Decrease Physiological* May occur with protracted therapy *4014*

Glucose *Serum Decrease Physiological* Hypoglycemia may be observed after aminosalicylic acid administration as an uncommon side effect *2874* May cause lowering in diabetics *3669*
Serum Increase Analytical At 1 mmol/L affects Technicon SMA 12/60 method *5576* At concentrations above 100 mg/L raised concentration as measured by Kodak Ektachem® method *5704*
Serum Increase Physiological Hyperglycemia reported with protracted therapy *4133*
Serum No Effect Analytical At 1 g/dL on glucose-oxidase methods. At 1 g/dL on p-HBAH procedure of Lever. At 1 g/dL on o-toluidine procedure *3531* At 5 times upper limit of therapeutic range on methods on Technicon SMAC® , Abbott-VP, Du Pont aca, Roche Cobas-Bio, Kodak Ektachem® , Hitachi® 705 and KDA *3525* No effect on method on Fuji Drichem

1000 at concentration up to 500 mg/L *5706* No effect at 2.5 mmol/L on glucokinase based assay of Scott *5414*
Urine Increase Physiological Glycosuria reported with protracted therapy *4133* Glycosuria reported with long therapy *2452*

γ-Glutamyltransferase *Serum No Effect Analytical* At 5 times upper limit of therapeutic range on methods on Technicon SMAC® , Abbott-VP and Hitachi® 705 *3525*

Granulocytes *Blood Decrease Physiological* Hypersensitivity reactions may be observed after aminosalicylic acid administration including leukopenia, agranulocytosis, and thrombocytopenia, and Coombs' positive hemolytic anemia *2874*

Guanase *Serum Increase Physiological* May cause cytotoxic hepatocellular damage *402*

Haptoglobin *Serum Decrease Physiological* Effect of hemolytic anemia *1212*

HDL-Cholesterol *Serum No Effect Analytical* No effect of concentrations up to 230 mg/L on method on Kodak Ektachem® *5706*

Hematocrit *Blood Decrease Physiological* Hemolytic anemia/megaloblastic anemia *1212* Hypersensitivity reactions may be observed after aminosalicylic acid administration including leukopenia, agranulocytosis, and thrombocytopenia, and Coombs' positive hemolytic anemia *2874*

Hemoglobin *Blood Decrease Physiological* Hypersensitivity reactions may be observed after aminosalicylic acid administration including leukopenia, agranulocytosis, and thrombocytopenia, and Coombs' positive hemolytic anemia *2874* Rare hemolytic anemia *2135* Hemolytic anemia/megaloblastic anemia *1212*
Urine Increase Physiological Actual bleeding caused by drug *1714*

^{131}I Uptake *Serum Decrease Physiological* May cause goitrous hypothyroidism *4691*

Iron *Serum No Effect Analytical* At 5 times upper limit of therapeutic range on Ferrozine method on Technicon SMAC® *3525* No effect of concentrations up to 230 mg/L on method on Kodak Ektachem® *5706*

Isocitrate Dehydrogenase *Serum Increase Physiological* May cause cytotoxic hepatocellular damage *402*

Isoniazid *Serum Decrease Physiological* Aminosalicylic acid at a dose of 12 g has been reported to produce a 20% reduction in the acetylation of isoniazid, especially in rapid acetylators. INH plasma concentration, half-life and excretion is about 50% of those seen in slow acetylators *2874*
Serum Increase Physiological Inhibits acetylation, increases serum concentration *2452* Reduces acetylation of isoniazid *6390*

Ketones *Urine Increase Analytical* Aminosalicylic acid reportedly interferes with qualitative urine test methods *2874*

Lactate Dehydrogenase *Serum No Effect Analytical* At 5 times upper limit of therapeutic range on methods on Technicon SMAC® , Abbott-VP, Roche Cobas-Bio, Hitachi® 705 and KDA *3525*

LE Cells *Blood Positive Physiological* May produce LE-like syndrome *3827*

Leukocytes *Blood Decrease Physiological* Hypersensitivity reactions may be observed after aminosalicylic acid administration including leukopenia, agranulocytosis, and thrombocytopenia, and Coombs' positive hemolytic anemia *2874* Leukopenia but no cases of agranulocytosis *4017*
Blood Increase Physiological In one retrospective study of 7492 patients, drug-induced hepatitis occurred in 38 (0.5%), with the first symptoms usually occurring within 3 months of the start of treatment. At the time of diagnosis leukocytosis was observed in 79% of the 38 individuals *2874* Mainly due to eosinophilia due to hypersensitivity *3810*

Lipase *Serum No Effect Analytical* No effect of concentrations up to 230 mg/L on method on Kodak Ektachem® *5706*

Lymphocytes *Blood Increase Physiological* May produce syndrome like infectious mononucleosis *2242*

MCV *Blood Increase Physiological* If megaloblastic anemia occurs *6370*

Methemoglobin *Blood Increase Physiological* May cause hemolytic anemia *128*

Methylmalonate *Urine Increase Physiological* Occurs with vitamin B_{12} deficiency *6370*

Neutrophils *Blood Decrease Physiological* Occasional case of agranulocytosis reported *6264* If severe megaloblastic anemia occurs *6370*

N-Formiminoglutamic Acid *Urine Increase Physiological* Occurs with vitamin B_{12} deficiency *6370*

Occult Blood *Feces Increase Physiological* Reversible gastritis caused by drug *2242*

Ornithine Carbamoyltransferase
Serum Increase Physiological May cause cytotoxic hepatocellular damage *402*

PAH Clearance *Urine Increase Analytical* Very slight effect, measured as if PAH *4953*

Peripheral Smear *Blood Abnormal Physiological* Atypical lymphocytosis with eosinophilia *4014*

pH *Blood Decrease Physiological* Moderate strong acid, loss of fixed cation leads to acidosis *2242*

Phenylalanine *Plasma No Effect Analytical* No interference observed with rapid quantitative whole blood method of Campbell et al using phenylalanine dehydrogenase *867*

Phenylketones *Urine Positive Analytical* Red-brown with $FeCl_3$, pink to purple Phenistix® *1195*

Phosphate *Serum Increase Analytical* At 5 times upper limit of therapeutic range on methods on Du Pont aca and Hitachi® 705 *3525*
Serum No Effect Analytical At 5 times upper limit of therapeutic range on methods on Technicon SMAC® and KDA *3525* At concentration of 460 mg/L had no effect on phosphomolybdate method *5704*

Platelet Aggregation *Blood No Effect Physiological* No effect on epinephrine or ADP threshold value *6509* No effect on aggregation or fibrinolytic activity in 6 patients with chronic inflammatory bowel disease *6509*

Platelets *Blood Decrease Physiological* Several cases of immune mediated thrombocytopenia reported *4139* Rare reaction *2135* May occur with severe megaloblastic anemia *6370* Hypersensitivity reactions may be observed after aminosalicylic acid administration including leukopenia, agranulocytosis, and thrombocytopenia, and Coombs' positive hemolytic anemia *2874*

Porphobilinogen *Urine Increase Analytical* Aminosalicylic acid reportedly interferes with qualitative urine test methods *2874* Reacts with Ehrlich's reagent *4012*

Potassium *Serum Decrease Physiological* Rare side effect *2135* Due to action on renal tubules or vomiting *3902*
Serum No Effect Analytical At concentration of 460 mg/L had no effect on ISE measurement with predilution *5704*

Protein *Cerebrospinal Fluid Increase Analytical* Reacts as phenol if Folin-Ciocalteu reaction used *5869*
Serum No Effect Analytical At 5 times upper limit of therapeutic range on methods on Technicon SMAC® , Abbott-VP, Kodak Ektachem® , Hitachi® 705 and KDA *3525* At concentration of 460 mg/L had no effect on biuret method with blank correction *5704*
Urine Increase Analytical May cause false positive with sulfosalicylic acid *3044* With sulfosalicylic acid and heat with acetic acid tests *684* Affects acid turbidimetric procedures *882* Reacts with Folin-Ciocalteu of Lowry procedure *2024*
Urine Increase Physiological May occur as result of nephrotoxicity *4134* May cause nephrotoxicity *2024*
Urine No Effect Analytical No effect on Labstix® , heat with acetic acid tests *2452*

Prothrombin Time *Plasma Increase Physiological* Rare side effect *2135* Drug suppresses formation of prothrombin *4860*

Rifampin *Serum Decrease Physiological* May impair gastrointestinal absorption *2452* When rifampin is taken with PAS the rifampin concentration may decrease due to increased hepatic metabolism *2652* Absorption reduced from gastrointestinal tract, possibly due to bentonite present in PAS granules *643* Delayed and reduced absorption due to adsorption to bentonite in PAS granules *6403*
Serum No Effect Physiological Aminosalicylic acid in early reports has been reported to inhibit absorption of rifampin, but later found to be attributable to an excipient in the preparation *2874*

Aminosalicylic Acid *(continued)*

Sodium *Serum No Effect Analytical* At concentration of 460 mg/L had no effect on ISE measurement with predilution *5704*

Sugar *Urine Increase Analytical* Acts as reducing agent with nonspecific methods *2024* Acts as reducing agent with Benedict's reagent *193*

Sulfa as Sulfanilamide *Serum Increase Analytical* Very slight effect, measured as if it were a sulfonamide *4953*

T3-Uptake *Serum Increase Physiological* Resin uptake increase due to impaired synthesis of T4 *3107*

β-Thromboglobulin *Plasma No Effect Physiological* No effect of 1.5 g/d or after 250 mg i.v. in 6 patients *6509*

Thyroxine (T4) *Serum Decrease Physiological* May cause goitrous hypothyroidism *4691* Prolonged administration may lead to hypothyroidism *2135*

Triglycerides *Serum No Effect Analytical* At 5 times upper limit of therapeutic range on methods on Technicon SMAC® , Abbott-VP, Kodak Ektachem® , Hitachi® 705 and KDA *3525* At concentration of 460 mg/L had no effect on lipase/esterase method *5704*

Urea Nitrogen *Serum Increase Analytical* Reacts as urea with dimethylaminobenzaldehyde *5869* At upper limit of therapeutic range on o-phthaldehyde methoxyquinoline method of KDA *3525*

Serum No Effect Analytical At concentration of 460 mg/L had no effect on diacetylmonoxime method *5704* At 5 times upper limit of therapeutic range on methods on Technicon SMAC® , Abbott-VP, Roche Cobas-Bio, Kodak Ektachem® and Hitachi® 705 *3525*

Uric Acid *Serum No Effect Analytical* At concentration of 100 mg/L had no effect on Ames Seralyzer method *5704* At 5 times upper limit of therapeutic range on methods on Technicon SMAC® , Abbott-VP, Du Pont aca, Roche Cobas-Bio, Kodak Ektachem® , Hitachi® 705 and KDA *3525* At concentration of 460 mg/L had no effect on phosphotungstate reduction method *5704* No effect at 100 mg/L on uricase method on Ames Seralyzer *5706*

Urobilinogen *Feces Decrease Physiological* Pale stools may occur if cholestasis *2803*

Urine Increase Analytical Reacts with Ehrlich's reagent (yellow color) *408* Aminosalicylic acid reportedly interferes with qualitative urine test methods *2874*

Vanillylmandelic Acid *Urine Increase Analytical* Reacts with diazo reagent if used *140*

Vitamin B_{12} *Serum Decrease Physiological* Impairs absorption *6370* Aminosalicylic acid at a dose of 5 g has been shown to inhibit vitamin B_{12} absorption by 55% *2874* Reduced absorption noted *6403*

Urine Decrease Physiological Occurs with vitamin B_{12} deficiency *6370*

Xylose *Urine Decrease Physiological* 2 times normal dose produced reversible effect on absorption with reduced excretion *6486*

4-Aminosalicylic Acid

Bilirubin *Serum Increase Analytical* At concentrations above 100 mg/L increases results obtained by method on Kodak Ektachem® . Normal range 30 - 125 mg/L *5706*

Bilirubin, Conjugated *Serum No Effect Analytical* No effect at concentration of 1000 mg/L on method on Kodak Ektachem® *5706*

Bilirubin, Unconjugated *Serum No Effect Analytical* No effect at concentration of 1000 mg/L on method on Kodak Ektachem® *5706*

Aminothiadiazole

Erythrocytes *Blood No Effect Physiological* Hematologic toxicity is unusual *1384*

Leukocytes *Blood No Effect Physiological* Hematologic toxicity is unusual *1384*

Platelets *Blood No Effect Physiological* Hematologic toxicity is unusual *1384*

Uric Acid *Serum Increase Physiological* Drug causes increased synthesis of uric acid whose plasma concentration is usually increased in spite of use of allopurinol *1384*

Aminothiazole

Bilirubin *Serum Increase Physiological* Jaundice with febrile reactions *2242*

Serum No Effect Analytical At concentration of 23 mg/L had no effect on Kodak Ektachem® method *5704*

Amiodarone

Acenocoumarol *Plasma Increase Physiological* Significant potentiation of action so reduced dose of anticoagulant required *9*

Alanine Aminotransferase *Serum Increase Physiological* In 5 of 5 patients with toxic and hypersensitivity liver injury *4960* Effect observed in 5 of 30 patients in one study with effect partially related to serum concentration *4734* Cholestasis, hepatitis and severe hyperbilirubinemia secondary to drug therapy in one patient *4125* Amiodarone administration has been shown to increase liver enzyme activity in 4 to 9% of treated patients *6552* Up to 1.5 to 3 times normal values in 55% patients with hepatitis occurring in 4% *3281* Asymptomatic change in liver function with enzyme activity up to 3 times normal *4108* 1.5 to 4 fold increase in 15 of 100 patients: effect correlated with drug concentration *2479*

Albumin *Serum Decrease Physiological* Reduction observed with 6 months treatment compared with controls *1269* Approximately 10% reduction compared with controls when patients treated for 6 mo: probable direct effect on synthesis or clearance *1938*

Serum No Effect Analytical No effect at up to 10.0 mg/L on bromocresol green method on Technicon SMA II and bromocresol purple on Abbott-VP. Metabolite desethylamiodarone also had no effect *5543*

Alkaline Phosphatase *Serum Increase Physiological* Up to 1.5 to 3 times normal values in 55% patients with hepatitis occurring in 4% *3281* Asymptomatic change in liver function with enzyme activity up to 3 times normal *4108* In 4 of 5 patients with toxic and hypersensitivity liver injury *4960* Rare cases of hepatitis, cholestatic hepatitis or cirrhosis reported with treatment *6552* Cholestasis, hepatitis and severe hyperbilirubinemia secondary to drug therapy in one patient *4125*

Serum No Effect Physiological No effect observed in 100 patients *2479*

δ-Aminolevulinic Acid *Serum Increase Physiological* Increased in all of 10 patients by average of 79% over 18 mo *2479*

Antimicrosomal Antibodies *Serum Increase Physiological* Amiodarone induces thyroid antibodies: in one study almost 50% of 13 patients who received short-term amiodarone developed antimicrosomal antibodies *2468*

Antithyroid Antibodies *Serum Increase Physiological* Increased antithyroid antibodies observed in as many as 40% of patients who became hypothyroid after receiving amiodarone *2468*

Serum No Effect Physiological In one study of 47 patients who received amiodarone no increase in incidence of antithyroid antibodies observed *2468*

Apolipoprotein B *Serum Increase Physiological* Concentration increases as a result of secondary hypothyroidism *3054*

Aprindine *Serum Increase Physiological* Serum concentration increased in two patients when amiodarone was coadministered when patients were previously stabilized but mechanism not established *5731* Concentration increased so dose can be reduced by 50% *6669*

Aspartate Aminotransferase *Serum Increase Physiological* Asymptomatic change in liver function with enzyme activity up to 3 times normal *4108* Effect observed in 5 of 30 patients with some dose dependency observed *4734* Cholestasis, hepatitis and severe hyperbilirubinemia secondary to drug therapy in one patient *4125* In 5 of 5 patients with toxic and hypersensitivity liver injury *4960* Amiodarone administration has been shown to increase liver enzyme activity in 4 to 9% of treated patients *6552* 1.5 to 4 fold increase in 15 of 100 patients:

effect correlated with drug concentration *2479* Up to 1.5 to 3 times normal values in 55% patients with hepatitis occurring in 4% *3281*

Bilirubin *Serum Increase Physiological* Cholestasis, hepatitis and severe hyperbilirubinemia secondary to drug therapy in one patient *4125* Rare cases of hepatitis, cholestatic hepatitis or cirrhosis reported with treatment *6552* Hepatitis occurs in 4% patients *3281*
Serum No Effect Physiological No effect observed in 100 patients *2479* No effect observed in 5 patients with toxic and hypersensitivity liver injury *4960*

Cholesterol *Serum Decrease Physiological* From 214 to 194 mg/dL in 24 patients: continued decrease in female patients but no effect in men after 90 d *5702*
Serum Increase Physiological Concentration increased as a result of secondary hypothyroidism *3054* In 23 patients treatment for 30 months caused significant increase from mean baseline concentration of 5.1 mmol/L to 6.9 mmol/L *6444* 17% increase in concentration observed in 21 patients over one year *4733* Observed effect in 3 individuals but without effect on thyroid function *4730*

Creatinine *Serum Increase Physiological* In 30 consecutive patients receiving amiodarone for up to 12 months mean serum creatinine concentration increased 11% above baseline in 28 patients (correlation coefficient of r = 0.51) *4732* Amiodarone administration has been reported to cause abnormal renal function *6552* Observed effect in some patients *1384*
Serum No Effect Analytical At 50 mg/L on reversed phase liquid chromatographic procedure of Zhiri et al *6656*

Cyclosporine *Blood Increase Physiological* Coadministration with cyclosporine reported to increase trough cyclosporine concentrations by over 30% probably due to inhibtion of CYP enzymes in liver *859*
Serum Increase Physiological Coadministration with cyclosporine reported to increase trough cyclosporine concentrations by over 30% probably due to inhibtion of CYP enzymes in liver *859*

Cyclosporine A *Blood Increase Physiological* Amiodarone administration has been shown to increase cyclosporine concentration with increased creatinine concentration as a consequence *6552*

Digoxin *Serum Increase Physiological* Serum concentration increased 68 to 800% in presence of normal serum creatinine and urea N, possibly due to inhibited tubular secretion of drug *3246* Average increase of 69% with possible toxicity but mechanism not yet established *4631* Amiodarone administration has been shown to increase digoxin concentration *6552* Amiodarone has been reported to reduce both renal and nonrenal elimination of digoxin with effect becoming apparent several days or weeks after drugs first coadministered *5268* Occurs with concomitant administration: mean increase of 280% in four patients, allowing 50% decrease in dosage *2318* Coadministration with digoxin may increase the digoxin concentration *2161* Following treatment with amiodarone for 1 week in 6 volunteers: serum maximum and area under curve increased *3782* Approximate doubling of effect due to inhibition of metabolism *3281* Concentration increased within 24 h of dosing: magnitude of interaction dose related *6669*
Urine Increase Physiological Significant correlation between increases in plasma and urine concentrations. Possible displacement of digoxin from its binding sites *1481*

Disopyramide *Serum Increase Physiological* Increased concentration with possible adverse effects on EKG *3791*

Flecainide *Serum Increase Physiological* When amiodarone coadministered previously stable flecainide concentration shown to increase by about 50% in 8 patients probably by inhibiting metabolism *5487* In healthy individuals receiving amiodarone plasma concentration of flecainide increased twofold or more if flecainide concentration not reduced *3702* Pharmacokinetic interaction with clinical significance *3831*

Glucose *Serum Decrease Physiological* No effect in 10 nondiabetic patients treated with drug over 9 months *3369*
Serum Increase Physiological Significant increase in concentration in parallel with cholesterol in 21 patients followed over one year *4733* Observed effect in 3 individuals but without effect on thyroid function *4730*

Glucose Tolerance *Serum No Effect Physiological* No effect observed in 10 nondiabetic patients treated with drug over 9 months *3369*

γ-Glutamyltransferase *Serum Increase Physiological* But effect minimal in 100 treated patients *2479* Rare cases of hepatitis, cholestatic hepatitis or cirrhosis reported with treatment *6552* Cholestasis, hepatitis and severe hyperbilirubinemia secondary to drug therapy in one patient *4125*

HDL-Cholesterol *Serum No Effect Physiological* In 24 patients given drug for 30-90 d *5702*

Hemoglobin A_{1c} *Blood No Effect Physiological* No effect in 10 nondiabetic patients treated with drug over 9 months *3369*

Indomethacin *Serum No Effect Analytical* No effect on HPLC method of Roberts and Smith *4978*

Interleukin-6 *Serum Increase Physiological* Amiodarone may cause significantly higher concentrations of IL-6 than observed in patients with spontaneous hyperthyroidism *2468* In 27 patients with amiodarone induced thyrotoxicosis mean concentration 573.5 ± 78.7 fmol/L (range 149.4 - 1145.1 fmol/L) compared with 37.8 ± 6.2 fmol/L in healthy controls: in 12 with nodular goiter and/or thyroid autoimmune disease 152.7 ± 46.3 fmol/L concentration also higher than in controls *387*
Serum No Effect Physiological In 10 patients with amiodarone-induced hypothyroidism mean concentration of 43.8 ± 8.4 fmol/L not significantly different from 37.8 ± 6.2 fmol/L in healthy controls *387*

Lactate Dehydrogenase *Serum Increase Physiological* Up to 1.5 to 3 times normal values in 55% patients with hepatitis occurring in 4% *3281* Cholestasis, hepatitis and severe hyperbilirubinemia secondary to drug therapy in one patient *4125*

LDL-Cholesterol *Serum Increase Physiological* Concentration increased as a result of secondary hypothyroidism *3054*

Malate Dehydrogenase *Serum Increase Physiological* In 10-20% of 36 patients *2479*

Mexiletine *Serum Increase Physiological* Increased concentration with possible adverse effects on EKG *3791*

N-Acetylprocainamide *Serum Increase Physiological* Amiodarone administration has been reported to increase N-acetylprocainamide concentration *6552*

Phenytoin *Serum Increase Physiological* Amiodarone administration has been reported to increase procainamide concentration *6552* Possibly capable of increasing plasma concentration when drugs coadministered *1384* Coadministration with phenytoin may increase plasma phenytoin concentration *4522* Concentrations observed to increase by 60-200% above stable baseline before amiodarone coadministered probably by inhibition of phenytoin metabolism *5463* Pharmacokinetic interaction with clinical significance *3831* When amiodarone ingested with fosphenytoin concentration of phenytoin may be increased *4519* Up to 3 fold increase when drugs coadministered, due to inhibition of hepatic metabolism *3898*

Platelets *Blood Decrease Physiological* Thrombocytopenia reported with treatment *6552* Observed in 2 patients with rechallenge probably due to delayed hypersensitivity reaction: occurs early during administration of drug *6385*

Prealbumin *Serum Decrease Physiological* Approximately 20% reduction compared with controls when patients treated for 6 mo: probable direct effect on clearance or synthesis *1938*

Procainamide *Serum Increase Physiological* Administration of amiodarone with procainamide led to plasma procainamide concentrations greater than those with procainamide alone *4530* Amiodarone administration has been reported to increase procainamide concentration *6552* Average 57% in 12 patients allowing 20% reduction in dosage *2318* In 11 of 12 treated patients, probably due to an effect on tissue binding or decrease of clearance *5176* Several documented cases reported but exact mechanisms not discussed *3831* Approximate doubling of effect due to inhibition of metabolism *3281*

Propafenone *Serum Increase Physiological* Increased concentration with probable adverse effects on EKG *3791*

Prothrombin Time *Plasma Increase Physiological* Amiodarone administration has been shown to increase prothrombin time in patients receiving warfarin *6552* Prolongation sufficiently great that 43% reduction in dose of Coumadin® required in 11 patients *2318* Probably by lowering concentrations of vitamin K-dependent coagulation factors *2421* Prolongs prothrombin time when warfarin coadministered through nonselective inhibition of clearance of R and S isomers *2625*

Amiodarone *(continued)*

Prothrombin Time *(continued)*
Metabolism of anticoagulants reduced so patients receiving chronic warfarin or acenocoumarol treatment likely to demonstrate marked increase in prothrombin time when amiodarone coadministered with effect becoming apparent in about one week *3821* May double when warfarin coadministered *3281*
Plasma No Effect Physiological In 0 of 5 patients with toxic and hypersensitivity liver injury *4960*

Quinidine *Serum Increase Physiological* Amiodarone administration has been reported to increase quinidine concentration *6552* Rapid effect possibly due to change in protein or receptor binding *5951* Reported effect but exact mechanism not described *3831* Drug reported to produce 50% increase in concentration *827* Average 32% in 11 patients allowing 37% reduction in dosage *2318*

T3-Uptake *Serum Decrease Physiological* From 0.98 to 0.96 in 13 patients treated for average of 17 mo *659*
Serum Increase Physiological Detectable 24-hour radioiodine uptake observed in 80% of patients with amiodarone-induced hypothyroidism *2468*
Serum No Effect Analytical No significant effect observed at a concentration of 200 µg/mL (293 µmol/L) with method on Du Pont aca *1545*
Serum No Effect Physiological In euthyroid patients treatment for either 1-3 months or longer had no effect on T3 resin uptake *1862*

Thyroglobulin *Serum Increase Physiological* Amiodarone may destroy the thyroid causing increased circulating thyroglobulin in thyrotoxicosis but even higher concentrations of thyroglobulin observed in amiodarone-induced hypothyroidism *2468*

Thyroid Stimulating Hormone
Serum Decrease Physiological In hyperthyroid patients, particularly in areas of iodine deficiency, treatment with amiodarone decreases concentration to low or low-normal level *2412* A mean increase of 44% in serum thyroxine concentration is seen after commencement of amiodarone therapy and before the onset of thyrotoxicosis, which causes a further marked increase in concentration, an increase in T3 concentration and a dramatic 96% decrease in serum TSH concentration *2468* From a survey of lterature amiodarone induces thyrotoxicosis in 1 - 23% of treated patients with a low TSH concentration observed as a result *2468*
Serum Increase Physiological Baseline concentrations are higher in patients who developed hypothyroidism after beginning amiodarone therapy than in those who did not *2468* From a survey of lterature amiodarone induces hypothyroidism in 1 - 32% of treated patients with an increase in TSH concentration as a consequence, but not useful during first 3 months of treatment *2468* In euthyroid patients treatment for1-3 months was associated with transient increase in concentration *1862* Slight increase observed with 6 months treatment although concentrations remained within reference range: effect may be transient and returned to normal within 12 weeks *1269* Median TSH values in individuals treated for 6 mo increased compared with controls but values still within normal range, probable anterior pituitary effect *1938* Initial increase returns to normal in a few months possibly due to inhibition of intracellular binding of T3 to its nuclear receptor by drug *3831* Slight increase to 5-10 mU/L may be observed due to increase of TSH alpha and beta subunit gene expression and increased synthesis of TSH *2412* Slight increase observed in euthyroid patients when treated with amiodarone. More marked increase observed in hypothyroid patients *2412*
Serum No Effect Physiological Slight but insignificant increase at one month in patients with cardiac arrhythmias *4202* Insignificant change in 13 patients treated for average of 17 mo *659* More than 50% of patients receiving long-term amiodarone have abnormal results of thyroid function tests, but most of the patients are euthyroid with serum concentrations of TSH in the normal range *2468* In euthyroid patients treatment for longer than 3 months had no effect on concentration *1862*

Thyroid Stimulating Immunoglobulins
Serum Increase Physiological Baseline concentrations are higher in patients who developed hypothyroidism after beginning amiodarone therapy but only 2 of 32 such patients had higher than normal TSH concentrations *2468*

Thyroxine Binding Globulin *Serum No Effect Physiological* No significant changes after treatment for 2 mo *2203* No effect observed with 6 months treatment *1269*

Thyroxine Binding Prealbumin
Serum Decrease Physiological With six months treatment reduction observed compared with controls *1269*

Thyroxine (T4) *Serum Decrease Physiological* Single case of drug induced myxedema coma and death *3860* Hypothyroidism reported with treatment *6552* From a survey of lterature amiodarone induces hypothyroidism in 1 - 32% of treated patients with a decrease in total thyroxine concentration as a consequence *2468* In patients with hypothyroidism particularly in areas of iodine decifiency concentration when treated with amiodarone reduced to low or low-normal level *2412* Concentration decreased as a result of secondary hypothyroidism *3054*
Serum Increase Analytical Dose-dependent interference by metabolite desethylamiodarone using Syva® EMIT T4 but not with γ-Coat RIA/T4 although concentration in vivo may not be high enough to cause effect *3439*
Serum Increase Physiological In 9 men treated for 28 d caused insignificant increase of 1.4 µg/dL *810* Competes with T4 for cell membrane receptor because of structural similarity and inhibits intracellular type I deiodinase thus reducing breakdown of T4 *2412* From a survey of lterature amiodarone induces thyrotoxicosis in 1 - 23% of treated patients with a further increase in serum thyroxine concentration observed as a result *2468* A mean increase of 44% in serum thyroxine concentration is seen after commencement of amiodarone therapy and before the onset of thyrotoxicosis, which causes a further marked increase in concentration *2468* In euthyroid patients treatment causes slight increase and in hyperthyroidism concentration normal or slightly increased *2412* Significant increase (mean change from 100 to 155 nmol/L, i.e. 55%) after 2 mo probably impaired peripheral conversion of T4 to T3 *2203* In euthyroid patients treatment with amiodarone for 1-3 months caused modest increase with treatment for longer causing concentration to remain increased compared with pretreatment values. Concentrations may be normal or modestly increased *1862* Amiodarone administration has been shown to increase concentration. Hyperthyroidism reported with treatment *6552* Typically increase observed within one week of start of treatment *1269* Significant increase from mean baseline concentration of 105 nmol/L to 165 nmol/L in 23 patients treated for 30 months *6444* After slight decrease in some patients initially in 10 patients over 18 mo *2479* From 7.4 to 9.7 µg/dL in 13 patients treated for average of 17 mo *659* Slight effect in 15 euthyroid volunteers given 400-600 mg/daily for 2 weeks *152* Mean concentration of 131 nmol/L in 38 patients receiving mean 1,420 mg weekly for more than 9 mo *5248* 2 of 92 patients developed hyperthyroidism, whereas 11 developed hypothyroidism in study of up to 4 y *4757* Significant increase from mean of 8 µg/dL to 12 µg/dL after 3 months treatment of patients with cardiac arrhythmias *4202*
Serum No Effect Analytical No significant effect observed at a concentration of 200 µg/mL (293 µmol/L) with method on Du Pont aca *1588 1546*
Serum No Effect Physiological In hyperthyroid patients, particularly those living in iodine deficient areas, treatment with amiodarone was associated with no change in concentration or a slight increase *2412*

Thyroxine (T4), Free *Serum Decrease Physiological* In hypothyroid patients treated with amiodarone concentration low or low-normal *2412* From a survey of lterature amiodarone induces hypothyroidism in 1 - 32% of treated patients with a decrease in free thyroxine concentration as a consequence *2468*
Serum Increase Physiological Change from mean of 22 to 32 pmol/L after 2 mo *2203* Concentration typically increased with inhibition of intracellular type I deiodinase. Amiodarone competes with T4 for cell membrane receptors and transport into cells because of structural similarity *2412* In euthyroid patients slight increase observed with treatment. In patients with hyperthyroidism no effect or slight increase observed *2412* Typically observed within one week of start of treatment *1269* From a survey of lterature amiodarone induces thyrotoxicosis in 1 - 23% of treated patients with a further increase in serum free thyroxine concentration observed as a result *2468* In group treated for 6 mo 9 out of 28 had values above normal range *1938*

Serum No Effect Physiological In 5 healthy subjects given 600 mg daily for 2 weeks *2885* In hyperthyroid patients, particularly those living in iodine deficient areas, treatment with amiodarone associated with no change in concentration or slight increase *2412*

Thyroxine (T4) Index, Free *Serum Decrease Physiological* From a survey of lterature amiodarone induces hypothyroidism in 1 - 32% of treated patients with a decrease in free thyroxine index as a consequence *2468*

Serum Increase Physiological From 7.1 to 9.3 in 13 patients treated for average of 17 mo *659* From a survey of lterature amiodarone induces thyrotoxicosis in 1 - 23% of treated patients with a further increase in serum free thyroxine index observed in some patients as a result *2468*

Serum No Effect Physiological In 5 healthy subjects given 600 mg daily for 2 weeks *2885*

Tri-iodothyronine, Free (fT3)

Serum Decrease Physiological From a survey of lterature amiodarone induces hypothyroidism in 1 - 32% of treated patients with a decrease in free triiodothyronine as a consequence in some patients *2468* Observed effect although not invariable: probably due to partial inhibition of conversion of thyroxine to tri-iodothyronine *3831* In euthyroid patients concentration low or low-normal, as in hypothyroid patients *2412* In both euthyroid and hypothyroid patients concentration low or low-normal *2412* Typically observed within one week of start of treatment *1269* In group treated for 6 mo 10 out of 28 had values below normal range *1938*

Serum Increase Physiological In patients with hyperthyroidism, particularly in areas with iodine deficiency, treatment with amiodarone raises concentration *2412* From a survey of lterature amiodarone induces thyrotoxicosis in 1 - 23% of treated patients with an increase in serum free T3 observed in some patients as a result *2468*

Tri-iodothyronine, Reverse (rT3)

Serum Increase Physiological Amiodarone administration has been shown to increase concentration *6552* Significant increase from mean of 29 ng/dL to 79 ng/dL at 3 months in patients with cardiac arrhythmias *4202* In 9 men treated for 28 d caused increase of 83 ng/dL *810* Typically observed within one week of start of treatment *1269* Significant effect in 15 euthyroid volunteers given 400-600 mg/daily for 2 weeks *152* Mean concentration of 0.85 nmol/L in 38 patients receiving a mean of 1,420 mg weekly for more than 9 mo *5248* Significant increase from mean baseline concentration of 0.33 nmol/L to 0.65 nmol/L in 23 patients treated for 30 months *6444* Concentration increased in euthyroid patients treated for either 1-3 months or for longer *1862* Exceeded normal range after 2 mo in all subjects *2203* Breakdown of rT3 in cells inhibited due to inhibition of type I deiodnase *2412* In euthyroid patients treatment was associated with increase of reverse T3 concentration *2412* Significant rise in mean from 0.59 to 1.47 nmol/L in 5 healthy subjects given 600 mg daily for 2 weeks *2885*

Serum No Effect Physiological In patients with either hypothyroidism or hyperthyroidism when treated with amiodarone no effect observed on concentration *2412*

Tri-iodothyronine (T3) *Serum Decrease Physiological* In patients with hypothyroidism particularly in areas of iodine deficiency concentration low or low-normal when treated with amiodarone *2412* Increases TSH alpha and beta subunit gene expression and reduces inhibiting effect of thyroid hormones on the TSH genes so TSH concentration increased. Amiodarone inhibits intracellular type I iodinase and hence reduces circulating T3 *2412* In euthyroid patients subacute treatment (1-3 months) decreased concentration to lower normal range: chronic treatment for more than 3 months caused concentration to remain slightly decreased but still in normal range *1862* Suggestive decrease in 15 euthyroid volunteers given 400-600 mg/daily for 2 weeks *152* Typically observed within one week of start of treatment *1269* In 9 men treated for 28 d caused mean decrease of 28 ng/dL *810* From a survey of lterature amiodarone induces hypothyroidism in 1 - 32% of treated patients with a decrease in total triiodothyronine as a consequence in some patients *2468* Amiodarone administration has been shown to decrease concentration *6552* Significant decrease from mean baseline concentration of 1.82 nmol/L to 1.55 nmol/L in 23 patients after 30 months treatment *6444* Reduced peripheral conversion from thyroxine in 5% patients *3281* Mean concentration of 1.89 nmol/L in 38 patients receiving mean 1420 mg weekly for more than 9 mo *5248* Significant reduction from mean of 108 ng/dL to 91 ng/dL at 3 months and 98 ng/dL at 18 months in patients with cardiac arrhythmias *4202*

Serum Increase Physiological A mean increase of 44% in serum thyroxine concentration is seen after commencement of amiodarone therapy and before the onset of thyrotoxicosis, which causes a further marked increase in concentration, and an increase in T3 concentration *2468* From 120 to 138 ng/dL in 13 patients treated for average of 17 mo *659* From a survey of lterature amiodarone induces thyrotoxicosis in 1 - 23% of treated patients with an increase in serum T3 observed in some patients as a result *2468* In hyperthyroid patients, particularly in areas of iodine deficiency, treatment with amiodarone increase concentration *2412*

Serum No Effect Physiological Nonsignificant reduction after 2 mo to lower end of normal range *2203* In 5 healthy subjects given 600 mg daily for 2 weeks *2885*

Tri-iodothyronine (T3) Index, Free

Serum Decrease Physiological From a survey of lterature amiodarone induces hypothyroidism in 1 - 32% of treated patients with a decrease in free triiodothyronine index as a consequence in some patients *2468*

Triglycerides *Serum Decrease Physiological* From 140 to 123 mg/dL in 24 patients over 90 d treatment *5702* Treatment of 23 patients for 30 months caused decrease from mean baseline concentration of 1.64 mmol/L to 1.37 mmol/L *6444*

Serum Increase Physiological Significant increase in parallel with increase in cholesterol in 21 patients followed over one year *4733* Observed effect in 3 individuals but without effect on thyroid function *4730*

TSH response to TRH *Serum Decrease Physiological* Observed effect in some patients *1269* In 16 of 44 patients, majority of whom were clinically hyperthyroid: normalized with withdrawal of drug *5779*

Serum Increase Physiological Maximal increment during treatment 32 mU/L compared with 20 mU/L pretreatment *810* Reported effect in some patients *1269*

Serum No Effect Physiological Reported response to treatment *1269* No significant change observed in 23 patients after 30 months treatment *6444*

Urea Nitrogen *Serum Increase Physiological* Amiodarone administration has been reported to cause abnormal renal function *6552*

Uric Acid *Serum No Effect Analytical* At 50 mg/L on reversed phase liquid chromatographic procedure of Zhiri et al *6656*

Warfarin *Plasma Increase Physiological* Effect potentiated and concentration increased as early as third day *6669* Potentiates action of warfarin due to depression of vitamin-K dependent clotting factors *3281* Action prolonged when amiodarone coadministered since warfarin clearance reduced in a concentration related manner. Note effect may persist although amiodarone treatment stopped *3821*

Amitriptyline

Acetaminophen *Serum No Effect Analytical* No interference observed at a concentration of 2000 µg/mL (721 µmol/L) with method on Du Pont aca *1506*

Alanine Aminotransferase *Serum Increase Physiological* Increases of greater than 3 times the upper limit of normal were observed in 2.0% of patients (3 of 181) treated with mirtazepine in short-term clinical trials compared with 0.3% for placebo-treated patients (1 of 328) *4434* Rare cases of transient cholestasis *4113* May rarely cause hepatitis *6645* Occasional case of hypersensitivity associated hepatitis *159*

Serum No Effect Analytical At acute overdose concentration (2.5 mg/dL) on Technicon SMAC® method *6266*

Albumin *Serum No Effect Analytical* At acute overdose concentration (2.5 mg/dL) on Technicon SMAC® method *6266* At concentration of 25 mg/L had no effect on BCG method *5704*

Urine No Effect Analytical Using a fluorimetric assay with Albumin Blue 580 on a Cobas Fara centrifugal analyzer for the detection of microalbuminuria no significant interference was detected at a concentration of 10 mg/L *3117*

Alkaline Phosphatase *Serum Increase Physiological* May rarely cause hepatitis *6645* Occasional case of hypersensitiv-

Amitriptyline *(continued)*

Alkaline Phosphatase *(continued)*
ity associated hepatitis *159* Rare cases of cholestasis (transient) *4113*
Serum No Effect Analytical At acute overdose concentration (2.5 mg/dL) on Technicon SMAC® method *6266*

Antinuclear Antibodies *Serum Increase Physiological* May rarely cause lupus-like syndrome with positive ANA reaction *6645*

Aspartate Aminotransferase *Serum Increase Physiological* Occasional case of hypersensitivity associated hepatitis *159* May rarely cause hepatitis *6645* Rare cases of transient cholestasis *4113*
Serum No Effect Analytical At acute overdose concentration (2.5 mg/dL) on Technicon SMAC® method *6266*

Barbiturate *Serum No Effect Analytical* No significant interference observed at a concentration of 100 µg/mL (0.36 mmol/L) with method on Du Pont aca *1511*

Benzodiazepine Screen *Serum No Effect Analytical* No significant interference observed at a concentration of 100 µg/mL (0.36 mmol/L) with method on Du Pont aca *1512*

Benzoylecgonine *Urine No Effect Analytical* No significant interference observed at a concentration of 360 µmol/L with Sung and Neely modification of Syva EMIT procedure *148* Negative result obtained at a concentration of 100 µg/mL (0.36 mmol/L) with method on Du Pont aca *1558*

Bicarbonate *Serum No Effect Analytical* At concentration of 20 mg/L had no effect on method using phenolphthalein *5704*

Bile *Urine Increase Physiological* Due to transient cholestasis *3810*

Bilirubin *Serum Increase Physiological* May rarely cause hepatitis *6645* Rare cases of transient cholestasis *4113*
Serum No Effect Analytical At acute overdose concentration (2.5 mg/dL) on Technicon SMAC® method *6266* At concentration of 25 mg/L had no effect on Jendrassik and Grof method *5704*
Serum No Effect Physiological Insignificant protein-displacement effect in neonates *6314*

BSP Retention *Serum Increase Physiological* Due to transient cholestasis *3810*

Calcium *Serum No Effect Analytical* At concentration of 25 mg/L had no effect on cresolphthalein method *5704* At acute overdose concentration (2.5 mg/dL) on Technicon SMAC® method *6266*

Cannabinoids *Urine No Effect Analytical* No effect observed at a concentration of 50 µg/mL (0.18 mmol/L) on method on Du Pont aca *1557* No effect on Roche Abuscreen method *5006*

Carbamazepine *Serum Increase Analytical* 9.0% cross-reactivity observed with competitive fluorescence immunoassay used with PB Diagnostics OPUS analyzer *1153*
Serum No Effect Analytical At an amitriptyline concentration of 40 µg/mL had no significant cross-reactivity with carbamazepine at a concentration of 4.0 µg/mL when measured by method on Bayer Technicon Immuno 1® system *417* Cross reactivity of only 0.15% observed with carbamazepine method on Baxter Stratus *5705*

Catecholamines *Plasma No Effect Analytical* No effect on HPLC method of Koller for dopamine, epinephrine, and norepinephrine *3230*

Chloride *Serum No Effect Analytical* At concentration of 20 mg/L had no effect on mercurimetric method *5704*

Cholesterol *Serum No Effect Analytical* At concentration of 0.1 mg/L had no effect on CHOD-PAP method *5704* At acute overdose concentration (2.5 mg/dL) on Technicon SMAC® method *6266* At concentration of 25 mg/L had no effect on Liebermann-Burchard method *5704*
Serum No Effect Physiological Nonfasting increases of up to 20% above normal were observed in 8% of patients treated with mirtazepine compared with 7% for placebo-treated patients *4434*

Cocaethylene *Urine No Effect Analytical* No interference observed with TLC method of Bailey *328*

Color *Urine Increase Analytical* Green urine associated with ingestion of drug *4325* Greenish-blue color *1714*

Creatine Kinase *Serum No Effect Analytical* At acute overdose concentration (2.5 mg/dL) on Technicon SMAC® method *6266*

Creatinine *Serum No Effect Analytical* At concentration of 0.4 mg/L had no effect on creatinine iminohydrolase method *5704* At concentration of 25 mg/L had no effect on Technicon AutoAnalyzer® Jaffe method *5704* At acute overdose concentration (2.5 mg/dL) on Technicon SMAC® method *6266* At 10 mg/L on reversed phase liquid chromatographic procedure of Zhiri et al *6656*

Cyclosporine *Blood No Effect Analytical* At a concentration of 20 mg/L had no effect on Syva EMIT method *495*

Drugs of Abuse Screen *Urine No Effect Analytical* No effect at concentration of 100 µg/mL on EZ-SCREEN procedure for cannabinoids and cocaine *1739*

Eosinophils *Blood Decrease Physiological* May cause bone marrow depression as a side effect with consequent agranulocytosis, leukopenia, thrombocytopenia, purpura and eosinophilia *6645*
Blood Increase Physiological Occasional allergic response *2754* Occasional case of hypersensitivity associated hepatitis *159*

Erythrocytes *Blood Decrease Physiological* Rare transient agranulocytosis *128*

Ethosuximide *Serum No Effect Analytical* Insignificant cross-reactivity observed with method on Du Pont aca *1523*

Glucose *Serum Decrease Physiological* Reported to cause both increases and decreases of blood sugar concentration *6645* Reported observation *2754*
Serum Increase Physiological Reported to cause both increases and decreases of blood sugar concentration *6645* Reported observation *2754*
Serum No Effect Analytical At acute overdose concentration (2.5 mg/dL) on Technicon SMAC® method *6266* At concentration of 6.3 mg/L had no effect on Kodak Ektachem® method *5704* At concentration of 40 mg/L had no effect on hexokinase/G-6-PDH method *5704* No effect of concentrations up to 6.3 mg/L on method on Kodak Ektachem® *5706*

Granulocytes *Blood Decrease Physiological* May cause bone marrow depression as a side effect with consequent agranulocytosis, leukopenia, thrombocytopenia, purpura and eosinophilia *6645*

Growth Hormone *Plasma No Effect Physiological* No effect observed with acute or chronic treatment in depressed patients *2274*

Histamine *Plasma No Effect Analytical* Although 50% inhibition occurs with 19 µg/mL on radio-enzyme assay no clinical effects likely to occur since physiological concentration 0.1 - 0.2 µg/mL *2492*

Imipramine *Serum Increase Analytical* May cause false positive reaction in EMIT immunoassay for imipramine *3590*

Iron *Serum No Effect Analytical* At acute overdose concentration (2.5 mg/dL) on Technicon SMAC® method *6266* At concentration of 25 mg/L had no effect on Ferrozine method *5704*

Lactate Dehydrogenase *Serum No Effect Analytical* At acute overdose concentration (2.5 mg/dL) on Technicon SMAC® method *6266*

Leukocytes *Blood Decrease Physiological* May cause bone marrow depression as a side effect with consequent agranulocytosis, leukopenia, thrombocytopenia, purpura and eosinophilia *6645* Leukopenia/agranulocytosis may occur *301*

Lysergic Acid Diethylamide *Urine Increase Analytical* Minimum concentration that caused a positive result with EMIT method to measure LSD 5 mg/L *4968*

Methadone *Urine No Effect Analytical* Insignificant cross-reactivity of 0.3% observed with Roche Abuscreen ONTRAK method *3279*

Monoamine Oxidase *Platelets Decrease Physiological* Mean decrease of 50% in 8 subjects with primary or secondary depression when given 100 to 300 mg/d *4927*

Mycophenolic Acid *Serum No Effect Analytical* No significant interference observed with HPLC method of Shipkova et al *5526*

Mycophenolic Acid Glucuronide
Serum No Effect Analytical No significant interference observed with HPLC method of Shipkova et al *5526*

Neutrophils *Blood Decrease Physiological* May cause agranulocytosis/neutropenia *4265*

p-Aminophenol *Urine No Effect Analytical* With addition of drugs at a concentration of 100 mg/L and of related compounds at 50 mg/L no significant effect observed on colorimetric method of van Bocxlaer on Cobas Mira analyzer which involves reacting free p-aminophenol with resorcinol in the presence of magnesium ions to form an indophenol dye measured at 550 nm *6163*

Phenobarbital *Serum No Effect Analytical* No interference observed at a concentration of 10 µmol/L with Sung and Neely's modification of the Syva EMIT procedure *148*

Phosphate *Serum No Effect Analytical* At acute overdose concentration (2.5 mg/dL) on Technicon SMAC® method *6266* At concentration of 25 mg/L had no effect on phosphomolybdate method *5704*

Platelets *Blood Decrease Physiological* May cause bone marrow depression as a side effect with consequent agranulocytosis, leukopenia, thrombocytopenia, purpura and eosinophilia *6645* Five cases reported (probably immune response) *4308*

Potassium *Serum No Effect Analytical* At concentration of 20 mg/L had no effect on ISE measurement with predilution *5704* At concentration of 0.1 mg/L had no effect on flame-photometric method *5704*

Prolactin *Plasma Increase Physiological* Marked increase in men and women psychiatric patients treated for up to 4 weeks *6098* In depressive patients: on first day of administration in 6 of 11 patients: nonsignificant decrease after 28 d treatment *2274*

Protein *Serum No Effect Analytical* At acute overdose concentration (2.5 mg/dL) on Technicon SMAC® method *6266* At concentration of 25 mg/L had no effect on biuret method with blank correction *5704*

Rheumatoid Factor *Serum Increase Physiological* May rarely cause lupus-like syndrome with positive reaction *6645*

SDZ PSC 833 *Blood No Effect Analytical* At a concentration of 470 µg/L had no effect on HPLC method of Scott et al when used to measure PSC with CsD (as internal standard) at a concentration of 5 mg/L *5418*

Sodium *Serum No Effect Analytical* At concentration of 0.1 mg/L had no effect on flame-photometric method *5704* At concentration of 20 mg/L had no effect on ISE measurement with predilution *5704*

Thyroid Stimulating Hormone
Serum No Effect Physiological No effect observed with acute or chronic treatment in depressed patients *2274*

Triglycerides *Serum No Effect Analytical* At acute overdose concentration (2.5 mg/dL) on Technicon SMAC® method *6266* At concentration of 25 mg/L had no effect on lipase/esterase method *5704* At concentration of 132 mg/L had no effect on GPO-PAP method *5704*
Serum No Effect Physiological Nonfasting increases of up to 20% above normal were observed in 3% of patients treated with mirtazepine compared with 3% for placebo-treated patients *4434*

Urea Nitrogen *Serum No Effect Analytical* At acute overdose concentration (2.5 mg/dL) on Technicon SMAC® method *6266* At concentration of 6.3 mg/L had no effect on Kodak Ektachem® method *5704* At concentration of 25 mg/L had no effect on diacetylmonoxime method *5704*

Uric Acid *Serum No Effect Analytical* At 10 mg/L on reversed phase liquid chromatographic procedure of Zhiri et al *6656* At acute overdose concentration (2.5 mg/dL) on Technicon SMAC® method *6266* At concentration of 40 mg/L had no effect on uricase-PAP method *5704* At concentration of 25 mg/L had no effect on phosphotungstate reduction method *5704*

Volume *Urine Decrease Physiological* May cause urinary retention *128*

Amlodipine

Alanine Aminotransferase *Serum No Effect Physiological* In post-marketing experience, some patients manifested changes like those of cholestasis, severe to warrant hospitalization *4651*

Alkaline Phosphatase *Serum No Effect Physiological* In post-marketing experience, some patients manifested changes like those of cholestasis, severe to warrant hospitalization *4651*

Aspartate Aminotransferase
Serum No Effect Physiological In post-marketing experience, some patients manifested changes like those of cholestasis, severe to warrant hospitalization *4651*

Bicarbonate *Serum No Effect Physiological* In 10 hypertensive renal transplant patients receiving cyclosporine treatment with up to 10 mg/d for 4 weeks caused nonsignificant change from mean baseline of 26.0 ± 3.6 mmol/L to 26.0 ± 4.3 mmol/L *6062*

Bilirubin *Serum No Effect Physiological* In post-marketing experience, some patients manifested changes like those of cholestasis, severe to warrant hospitalization *4651*

Calcium *Serum Decrease Physiological* In 10 hypertensive renal transplant patients receiving cyclosporine treatment with up to 10 mg/d for 4 weeks caused significant change from mean baseline of 2.37 ± 0.17 mmol/L to 2.29 ± 0.13 mmol/L *6062*

Chloride *Serum No Effect Physiological* In 10 hypertensive renal transplant patients receiving cyclosporine treatment with up to 10 mg/d for 4 weeks caused nonsignificant change from mean baseline of 109.2 ± 3.8 mmol/L to 110.1 ± 4.0 mmol/L *6062*

Cholesterol *Serum Decrease Physiological* In 131 patients with stage I diastolic hypertension treated with 5 mg/d caused change from mean baseline of 5.94 ± 0.99 mmol/L by - 0.03 ± 0.06 mmol/L after 12 months and - 0.15 ± 0.07 mmol/L after 48 months *2335*
Serum No Effect Physiological No clinically significant effect observed in patients receiving amlodipine *4651*

Cortisol, Free *Urine No Effect Analytical* No significant interference observed with HPLC method of Turpeinen et al *6105*

Creatinine *Serum No Effect Physiological* No clinically significant effect observed in patients receiving amlodipine *4651* In 10 hypertensive renal transplant patients receiving cyclosporine treatment with up to 10 mg/d for 4 weeks caused nonsignificant change from mean baseline of 129.2 ± 32.0 µmol/L to 121.8 ± 33.3 µmol/L *6062* In 11 cyclosporine A-treated renal transplant patients coadministration of amlodipine about 5 mg/d caused no significant change from mean baseline of 1.7 ± 0.3 mg/dL to 1.7 ± 0.3 mg/dL during treatment and 1.7 ± 0.4 mg/dL after amlodipine withdrawn *4624*

Cyclosporine A *Blood Increase Physiological* In 11 cyclosporine A-treated renal transplant patients coadministration of amlodipine about 5 mg/d caused a significant 40% increase from mean baseline of 174 ± 34 ng/dL to 244 ± 42 ng/dL during treatment and 174 ± 28 ng/dL after amlodipine withdrawn *4624*
Blood No Effect Physiological In 10 hypertensive renal transplant patients receiving cyclosporine treatment with up to 10 mg/d for 4 weeks caused nonsignificant change from mean baseline of 112.9 ± 24.1 µg/L to 103.3 ± 29.6 µg/L *6062*

Digoxin *Serum No Effect Physiological* No effect observed on serum digoxin concentration or its renal clearance in normal volunteers *4651* No apparent effect observed on digoxin pharmacokinetics in healthy volunteers and patients with congestive heart failure *5345*

Glucose *Serum No Effect Physiological* No clinically significant effect observed in patients receiving amlodipine *4651*

γ-Glutamyltransferase *Serum No Effect Physiological* In post-marketing experience, some patients manifested changes like those of cholestasis, severe to warrant hospitalization *4651*

HDL-Cholesterol *Serum No Effect Physiological* No clinically significant effect observed in patients receiving amlodipine *4651* In 131 patients with stage I diastolic hypertension treated with 5 mg/d caused change from mean baseline of 1.13 ± 0.29 mmol/L by + 0.06 ± 0.02 mmol/L after 12 months and + 0.02 ± 0.02 mmol/L after 48 months *2335*

LDL-Cholesterol *Serum Decrease Physiological* In 131 patients with stage I diastolic hypertension treated with 5 mg/d caused change from mean baseline of 4.13 ± 0.89 mmol/L by - 0.05 ± 0.06 mmol/L after 12 months and - 0.13 ± 0.06 mmol/L after 48 months *2335*

Amlodipine *(continued)*

Phosphate *Serum Decrease Physiological* In 10 hypertensive renal transplant patients receiving cyclosporine treatment with up to 10 mg/d for 4 weeks caused significant change from mean baseline of 1.15 ± 0.27 mmol/L to 1.0 ± 0.28 mmol/L *6062*

Potassium *Serum Decrease Physiological* In 10 hypertensive renal transplant patients receiving cyclosporine treatment with up to 10 mg/d for 4 weeks caused significant change from mean baseline of 4.3 ± 0.3 mmol/L to 4.1 ± 0.3 mmol/L *6062*
Serum No Effect Physiological No clinically significant effect observed in patients receiving amlodipine *4651*

Prothrombin Time *Plasma No Effect Physiological* No effect observed on prothrombin time when amlodipine coadministered with warfarin *4651*

Sildenafil *Serum No Effect Physiological* No interaction observed when amlodipine and sildenafil (100 mg) coadministered to hypertensive patients *4657*

Sodium *Serum No Effect Physiological* In 10 hypertensive renal transplant patients receiving cyclosporine treatment with up to 10 mg/d for 4 weeks caused nonsignificant change from mean baseline of 140.2 ± 2.5 mmol/L to 139.7 ± 1.7 mmol/L *6062*

Tirofiban *Serum No Effect Physiological* Coadministration had no significant effect on plasma clearance of tirofiban *3957*

Triglycerides *Serum Decrease Physiological* In 131 patients with stage I diastolic hypertension treated with 5 mg/d caused change from mean baseline of 1.49 ± 0.90 mmol/L by - 0.19 ± 0.07 mmol/L after 12 months and - 0.08 ± 0.06 mmol/L after 48 months *2335*
Serum No Effect Physiological No clinically significant effect observed in patients receiving amlodipine *4651*

Urea Nitrogen *Serum No Effect Physiological* No clinically significant effect observed in patients receiving amlodipine *4651* In 11 cyclosporine A-treated renal transplant patients coadministration of amlodipine about 5 mg/d caused no significant change from mean baseline of 27 ± 6 mg/dL to 26 ± 5 mg/dL during treatment and 25 ± 6 mg/dL after amlodipine withdrawn *4624*

Uric Acid *Serum Decrease Physiological* In 10 hypertensive renal transplant patients receiving cyclosporine treatment with up to 10 mg/d for 4 weeks caused significant change from mean baseline of 478.3 ± 114.4 µmol/L to 424.6 ± 83.6 µmol/L *6062*
Serum No Effect Physiological No clinically significant effect observed in patients receiving amlodipine *4651*

Ammonium Bromide

Bromide *Serum Increase Physiological* Theoretical possibility since drug contains 80% bromide *5116*

Ammonium Chloride

Aldosterone *Plasma Increase Physiological* In response to metabolic acidosis induced in 12 children by 0.15 g/kg/d for 3 days mean concentration increased from 0.49 ng/mL to 1.52 ng/mL *2386*
Urine Increase Physiological In response to metabolic acidosis induced in 12 children with treatment with 0.15 g/kg/d for 3 days excretion increased from mean of 19.2 µg/d to 71.8 µg/d *2386*

Amphetamine *Serum Decrease Physiological* Urinary acidifying agents by increasing the amount of ionized dextroamphetamine increase the urinary excretion of the drug *5641*

Base Excess *Blood Decrease Physiological* Significant reduction observed in 12 children treated with 0.15 g/kg/d for 3 days *2386*

Bicarbonate *Serum Decrease Physiological* Significant reduction observed in 12 children treated with 0.15 g/kg/d for 3 days *2386*

Bilirubin, Conjugated *Serum No Effect Analytical* No effect at concentration of 0.25 mmol/L on method on Kodak Ektachem® *5706*

Bilirubin, Unconjugated *Serum No Effect Analytical* No effect at concentration of 0.25 mmol/L on method on Kodak Ektachem® *5706*

Calcium *Urine Increase Physiological* During day of administration and following day *3435*

Chloride *Serum Increase Physiological* Added chloride and metabolic acidosis *3810*
Urine Increase Physiological Diuretic action *2242* Marked increase observed in 12 children treated with 0.15 g/kg/d for 3 days *2386*

Chlorpropamide *Serum Increase Physiological* In 6 healthy volunteers prior administration of ammonium chloride increased urinary acidity causing decreased ionization of chlorpropamide and reduced urinary excretion *4258*

Creatinine *Serum Increase Analytical* At ammonia concentrations over 400 µmol/L affects dual-slide method on Kodak Ektachem® systems *2519*
Serum No Effect Analytical No effect of concentrations up to 500 mmol/L on 2-slide method on Kodak Ektachem® *5706* No effect of concentrations up to 1 mmol/L on single slide method on Kodak Ektachem® *5706* At a concentration of 1 mmol/L has no significant effect on single-slide method on Kodak Ektachem® systems *2519*

Epinephrine *Urine No Effect Physiological* No significant effect observed *6065*

Lithium Clearance *Urine No Effect Physiological* A single dose of the compound has no effect on lithium clearance *4399*

Magnesium *Serum No Effect Analytical* At a concentration of 1 mmol/L has no significant effect on method on Kodak Ektachem® systems *2519* No effect of concentrations up to 1 mmol/L on method on Kodak Ektachem® *5706*
Urine Increase Physiological Positive correlation with calcium excretion *3435*

N-Acetyl-Glucosaminidase *Urine No Effect Analytical* No effect at 50 mmol/L on 2 colorimetric analytical methods *2254*

Norepinephrine *Urine No Effect Physiological* No significant effect observed *6065*

pH *Blood Decrease Physiological* significant reduction observed in 12 children following treatment with 0.15 g/kg/d for 3 days *2386* Following administration (metabolic acidosis) *3810*
Urine Decrease Physiological To below 5.3 if acidification normal *1444*

Potassium *Serum Decrease Physiological* Perpetuates potassium deficiency, cation loss *3810*
Serum Increase Physiological Slight but significant increase observed in 12 children treated with 0.15 g/kg/d for 3 days *2386*
Serum No Effect Analytical No effect of concentrations up to 1 mmol/L on method on Kodak Ektachem® *5706* Negligible effect at a concentration of 2.5 mmol/L on spectrophotometric method of Berry et al *523*
Urine Increase Physiological Marked increase observed in 12 children treated with 0.15 g/kg/d for 3 days *2386* Diuretic action and hyperchloremic acidosis *2242*

Procainamide *Serum No Effect Physiological* No effect of acidification of urine on urinary excretion of procainamide or of N-acetylprocainamide *4903*

Renin Activity *Plasma Increase Physiological* Concentration doubled from mean of 4.72 ng/mL/h to 8.13 ng/mL/h in response to metabolic acidosis induced in 12 children by treatment with 0.15 g/kg/d for 3 days *2386*

Sodium *Serum Decrease Physiological* Cation loss as excess chloride excreted *1009*
Serum No Effect Analytical Negligible effect at a concentration of 2.5 mmol/L on spectrophotometric method of Berry et al *523*
Urine Increase Physiological Marked increase in urinary excretion observed in 12 children treated with 0.15 g/kg/d for 3 days *2386* Diuretic action *2242*

Urea Nitrogen *Serum No Effect Analytical* At concentration of 190 µmol/L no effect on urease method on Fuji Drichem 1000 *5706*

Volume *Urine Increase Physiological* Marked increase in urine flow rate observed in 12 children treated with 0.15 g/kg/d for 3 days *2386*

Ammonium Heparin

Alanine Aminotransferase *Serum No Effect Analytical* No effect of concentrations up to 20,000 mg/L on method on Ames Seralyzer *5706*

Creatinine *Serum Decrease Analytical* Concentrations above 600 mg/L decrease result as measured on 2-slide method on Kodak Ektachem® but probably of no clinical significance *5706*
Serum Increase Analytical Ammonium heparin causes interference with dual-slide method on Kodak Ektachem® systems *2519*

Tissue Inhibitor of Metalloproteinase-2
Serum Increase Analytical Mean concentration in heparinized plasma of 142 µg/L significantly increased by 5 to 8-fold compared with that in serum of 26.9 µg/L with concentration in plasma increasing steadily with amount of ammonium heparin added - to 260% with 1.5 IU/mL, 380% with 3.0 IU/mL, 500% with 4.5 IU/mL and to 630% with 7.5 IU/mL *2993*

Ammonium Hydroxide

Creatinine *Urine No Effect Analytical* Causes less than 2% effect with single-slide method with Kodak Ektachem® systems *2519*

Protein *Serum Decrease Analytical* Erroneously low results observed with method on Du Pont aca *1549*

Ammonium Nitrate

Methemoglobin *Blood Increase Physiological* May cause hemolytic anemia *4017*

Amobarbital

Acetaminophen *Serum No Effect Analytical* No interference observed at a concentration of 2000 µg/mL (884 µmol/L) with method on Du Pont aca *1506*

Albumin *Serum No Effect Analytical* At concentration of 150 mg/L had no effect on BCG method *5704*

Amobarbital *Serum Increase Physiological* 600 mg orally produces concentration of 9.6 mg/L *3868*

Antipyrine *Serum Decrease Physiological* Coadministration reduced half-life of antipyrine probably as a result of induction of hepatic microsomal enzymes *5820*

Barbiturate *Urine Increase Analytical* Positive result obtained at a concentration of 2.0 µg/mL (8.8 µmol/L) with method on Du Pont aca *1555*

Bicarbonate *Serum No Effect Analytical* At concentration of 150 mg/L had no effect on method using phenolphthalein *5704*

Bilirubin *Serum No Effect Analytical* At concentration of 150 mg/L had no effect on Jendrassik and Grof method *5704*

BSP Retention *Serum Increase Physiological* Probably nonspecific effect on cells *6238*

Calcium *Serum No Effect Analytical* At concentration of 150 mg/L had no effect on cresolphthalein method *5704*

Cannabinoids *Urine No Effect Analytical* No effect on Roche Abuscreen method *5006*

Carbamazepine *Serum No Effect Analytical* No cross-reactivity observed with method used on Du Pont aca *1513*

Chloride *Serum No Effect Analytical* At concentration of 150 mg/L had no effect on mercurimetric method *5704*

Cholesterol *Serum No Effect Analytical* At concentration of 5 mg/L had no effect on CHOD-PAP method *5704* At concentration of 150 mg/L had no effect on Liebermann-Burchard method *5704*

Creatinine *Serum No Effect Analytical* At concentration of 150 mg/L had no effect on Technicon AutoAnalyzer® Jaffe method *5704*

Glucose *Serum No Effect Analytical* At concentration of 5 mg/L had no effect on GOD/POD-PAP method *5704*

Haloperidol *Serum Decrease Physiological* In chronic schizophrenics treated with 20-70 mg/day haloperidol addition of 200 mg amobarbital per day reduced serum haloperidol concentration by about 50% *469 468*

17-Hydroxycorticosteroids *Urine No Effect Physiological* No significant effect (?small decrease) *5820*

6-β-Hydroxycortisol *Urine Increase Physiological* Significant increase (by approximately 50%) *5820*

^{131}I Uptake *Serum Decrease Physiological* Amytal®, tuinal contain tetraiodofluorescein *4360*

Methionine *Urine Increase Physiological* Contained in large amount in infant formula *2859*

Phenobarbital *Serum Increase Analytical* Significant interference observed at a concentration of 200 µmol/L with Sung and Neely's modification of Syva EMIT method *148*
Serum No Effect Analytical At concentration of 400 µg/mL (1768 µmol/L) has no effect on method on Du Pont Dimension *1582* No significant cross-reactivity observed with method on Du Pont aca *1537* At maximum physiological or pharmacological concentrations no cross-reactivity observed with phenobarbital method on Bayer Technicon Immuno 1® *427*

Phenylbutazone *Serum No Effect Physiological* No significant effect on half-life *5820*

Phenytoin *Serum No Effect Analytical* No significant interference observed at a concentration of 500 µg/mL (2.21 mmol/L) with method on Du Pont aca *1538* No effect at concentration of 500 mg/mL (2209 µmol/L) on method on Du Pont Dimension *1583*

Phosphate *Serum No Effect Analytical* At concentration of 150 mg/L had no effect on phosphomolybdate method *5704*

Potassium *Serum No Effect Analytical* At concentration of 65 mg/L had no effect on ISE measurement with predilution *5704* At concentration of 5 mg/L had no effect on flame-photometric method *5704*

Primidone *Serum No Effect Analytical* No significant cross-reactivity with method on Du Pont aca *1541*

Protein *Serum No Effect Analytical* At concentration of 150 mg/L had no effect on biuret method with blank correction *5704*

Prothrombin Time *Plasma Decrease Physiological* Antagonizes action of coumarins (enzyme induction) *4998*

Sodium *Serum No Effect Analytical* At concentration of 5 mg/L had no effect on flame-photometric method *5704* At concentration of 65 mg/L had no effect on ISE measurement with predilution *5704*

Triglycerides *Serum No Effect Analytical* At concentration of 5 mg/L had no effect on lipase/esterase method *5704*

Urea Nitrogen *Serum No Effect Analytical* At concentration of 150 mg/L had no effect on diacetylmonoxime method *5704*

Uric Acid *Serum No Effect Analytical* At concentration of 150 mg/L had no effect on phosphotungstate reduction method *5704*

Amodiaquine

Alanine Aminotransferase *Serum Increase Physiological* Reported hepatotoxicity *3810* Abnormality usually mild but associated with an immunoallergic hepatotoxicity *3416*

Alkaline Phosphatase *Serum Increase Physiological* Abnormality usually mild but associated with an immunoallergic hepatotoxicity *3416* Reported hepatotoxicity *3810*

Aspartate Aminotransferase *Serum Increase Physiological* Abnormality usually mild but associated with an immunoallergic hepatotoxicity *3416* Reported hepatotoxicity *3810*

Bile *Urine Increase Physiological* Reported hepatotoxicity *3810*

Bilirubin *Serum Increase Physiological* Reported effect *3810* Abnormality usually mild but associated with an immunoallergic hepatotoxicity *3416*

BSP Retention *Serum Increase Physiological* Reported hepatotoxicity *3810*

Erythrocytes *Blood Decrease Physiological* Occasional aplastic anemia reported *6264*

γ-Glutamyltransferase *Serum Increase Physiological* Abnormality usually mild but associated with an immunoallergic hepatotoxicity *3416*

Amodiaquine *(continued)*

Isocitrate Dehydrogenase *Serum Increase Physiological* Reported hepatotoxicity *3810*

Leukocytes *Blood Decrease Physiological* 20 cases associated with agranulocytosis in Switzerland, 12 of which associated with hepatitis *2624* Reported effect (AMA - blood dyscrasia committee) *3810* Occasional aplastic anemia reported *6264*

Neutrophils *Blood Decrease Physiological* Occasional case of agranulocytosis reported *6264* Agranulocytosis observed in 2 patients while receiving prophylactic treatment. Neutrophil IgG antibodies detected in both patients: concentration of antibodies was enhanced by metabolite of amodiaquine *5123*

Platelets *Blood Decrease Physiological* Occasional aplastic anemia reported *6264*

Prothrombin Time *Plasma Increase Physiological* Abnormality usually mild but associated with an immunoallergic hepatotoxicity *3416*

Amoxapine

Alanine Aminotransferase *Serum Increase Physiological* Administration reported to cause possible altered liver function in some patients to whom it was administered *3462*

Alkaline Phosphatase *Serum Increase Physiological* Administration reported to cause possible altered liver function in some patients to whom it was administered *3462*

Amylase *Serum Increase Physiological* Administration reported to cause possible pancreatitis in some patients to whom it was administered *3462*

Aspartate Aminotransferase *Serum Increase Physiological* Administration reported to cause possible altered liver function in some patients to whom it was administered *3462*

Bilirubin *Serum Increase Physiological* Administration reported to cause possible altered liver function with jaundice in some patients to whom it was administered *3462*

Eosinophils *Blood Increase Physiological* Administration reported to cause possible eosinophilia in some patients to whom it was administered *3462*

Glucose *Serum Increase Physiological* Administration reported to cause possible hyperglycemia in some patients to whom it was administered *3462*

Granulocytes *Blood Decrease Physiological* Observed in one 35 year old woman after receiving 18 g over 57 d. Granulocytes reappeared in peripheral blood on 15th day after treatment stopped *5425* Administration reported to cause agranulocytosis in fewer than 1% patients to whom it was administered *3462*

Leukocytes *Blood Decrease Physiological* Administration reported to cause leukopenia in fewer than 1% patients to whom it was administered *3462*

Platelets *Blood Increase Physiological* Observed in one 35 year old woman after receiving 18 g over 57 d. Marked thrombocytosis on 5th day after cessation of treatment. May be early sign of recovery of bone marrow in drug-associated toxic agranulocytosis *5425*

Prolactin *Plasma Increase Physiological* Significant effect in both men and women possibly by blocking dopamine receptors *1126* Administration reported to cause increased concentration in more than 1% patients to whom it was administered *3462*

Tricyclic Antidepressants Screen
Serum Negative Analytical Not detected at concentrations up to 500 µg/mL (1.59 mmol/L) by method on Du Pont aca *1550*

Amoxicillin

Aspartate Aminotransferase *Serum Increase Physiological* Moderate increase observed in a few patients receiving amoxicillin but the significance of this is uncertain *5636*

Bilirubin *Serum No Effect Analytical* No effect at 5000 mg/L on method on Ames Seralyzer *5706*

Chloramphenicol *Serum No Effect Analytical* No effect at 100 mg/L on coupled enzymatic method *4122*

Cholesterol *Serum No Effect Analytical* No effect at 5000 mg/L on Ames Seralyzer method *5706*

Creatine Kinase *Serum No Effect Analytical* No effect up to 500 mg/L but above this reduced enzyme activity observed although clinical significance of this uncertain *5706*

Creatinine *Serum No Effect Analytical* No effect up to 500 mg/L on Ames Seralyzer method but at higher concentrations apparently higher creatinine concentration although of unknown clinical significance *5706*

Doxazosin *Serum No Effect Physiological* Coadministration with doxazosin had no effect on its pharmacokinetics *4642*

Eosinophils *Blood Increase Physiological* Eosinophilia observed in a few patients receiving penicillins, but usually reversible on discontinuation of treatment *5636*

Glucose *Serum No Effect Analytical* No effect at 5000 mg/L on glucose oxidase method on Ames Seralyzer *5706*

Granulocytes *Blood Decrease Physiological* Agranulocytosis observed in a few patients receiving penicillins, but usually reversible on discontinuation of treatment *5636*

Hematocrit *Blood Decrease Physiological* Anemia observed in a few patients receiving penicillins, but usually reversible on discontinuation of treatment *5636*

Lactate Dehydrogenase *Serum No Effect Analytical* No effect at 5000 mg/L on method on Ames Seralyzer *5706*

Leukocytes *Blood Decrease Physiological* Leukopenia observed in a few patients receiving penicillins, but usually reversible on discontinuation of treatment *5636*

Methotrexate *Serum Increase Physiological* In one 16-year old male patient coadministration of 1 g/6 h orally caused significant reduction of methotrexate concentration from mean baseline of about 0.5 uol/L 72 h after infusion to about 5 µmol/L 72 h after infusion when methotrexate infused at a rate of 8 g/sq m over 6 hours: associated with decreased renal clearance probably due to competition at the common tubular secretion system and by methotrexate-induced secondary renal failure *5079*

Midazolam *Serum No Effect Analytical* On GC-ECD method of Ha et al *2387*

Mycophenolic Acid *Serum No Effect Analytical* No significant interference observed with HPLC method of Shipkova et al *5526*

Mycophenolic Acid Glucuronide
Serum No Effect Analytical No significant interference observed with HPLC method of Shipkova et al *5526*

Neutrophils *Blood Decrease Physiological* Absolute count of less than 1500 /µL in 54% of 41 children treated for 10 d *1829*

Phenylalanine *Plasma No Effect Analytical* No interference observed with rapid quantitative whole blood method of Campbell et al using phenylalanine dehydrogenase *867*

Platelets *Blood Decrease Physiological* Thrombocytopenia and thrombocytopenic purpura observed in a few patients receiving penicillins, but usually reversible on discontinuation of treatment *5636*

Theophylline *Serum No Effect Physiological* No documented significant interaction with theophylline reported *6117* No clinically significant effect on theophylline concentration observed when drugs coadministered *5999*

Urea Nitrogen *Serum No Effect Analytical* No effect at 5000 mg/L on method on Ames Seralyzer *5706*

Amphenone B

Aldosterone *Urine Decrease Physiological* May inhibit aldosterone production *4605*

^{131}I Uptake *Serum Decrease Physiological* Reported effect *1279*

Amphepramone

p-Aminophenol *Urine No Effect Analytical* With addition of drugs at a concentration of 100 mg/L and of related compounds at 50 mg/L no significant effect observed on colorimetric method of van Bocxlaer on Cobas Mira analyzer which involves reacting free p-aminophenol with resorcinol in the presence of magnesium ions to form an indophenol dye measured at 550 nm *6163*

Amphetamine

Acetaminophen *Serum No Effect Analytical* No interference observed with 2000 µg/mL (542 µmol/L) amphetamine sulfate with method on Du Pont aca *1506*

Alanine Aminotransferase *Serum No Effect Analytical* No effect at concentrations up to 20 mg/L on Boehringer Mannheim Reflotron method but above this inhibition of enzyme activity but of no clinical significance since normal concentration in serum only up to 0.1 mg/L *5706* At therapeutic concentration on Boehringer Mannheim Reflotron method *3231*

Amino Acids *Urine Increase Analytical* Reacts with ninhydrin; extra spot with TLC, high voltage electrophoresis *4760*

Amphetamine/Methamphetamine
Serum Increase Analytical l-amphetamine at a concentration of 3000 ng/mL caused 61.9% cross-reactivity with method on Abbott AxSYM and 41.9% with method on TDx: dl-amphetamine at a concentration of 1000 ng/mL caused cross-reactivities of 165.0% and 171.8% respectively *6404*

Amylase *Serum No Effect Analytical* At concentration of 10 mg/L had no effect on method on Boehringer Mannheim Reflotron system *5706*

Amylase, Pancreatic Isoenzyme
Serum No Effect Analytical At toxic concentration of 100 mg/L had no significant effect on method on Boehringer Mannheim Reflotron *6203*

Aspartate Aminotransferase *Serum No Effect Analytical* At therapeutic concentration on Boehringer Mannheim Reflotron method *3231* No effect up to 20 mg/L on Boehringer Mannheim Reflotron method but above this decreased enzyme activity. However this is not of clinical significance since therapeutic concentration is up to 0.1 mg/L *5706*

Barbiturate *Urine No Effect Analytical* At concentration of 1000 µg/mL (7.40 mmol/L) with method on Du Pont aca *1555*

Basal Metabolic Rate *Patient Increase Physiological* Metabolic effect of drugs *3669*

Benzodiazepine *Urine No Effect Analytical* Negative result obtained at a concentration of 1000 µg/mL (7.40 mmol/L) with method on Du Pont aca *1556*

Benzodiazepine Screen *Serum No Effect Analytical* No significant interference observed at a concentration of 100 µg/mL (0.74 mmol/L) with method on Du Pont aca *1512*

Benzoylecgonine *Urine No Effect Analytical* No significant interference observed at a concentration of 370 µmol/L with Sung and Neely modification of Syva EMIT procedure *148* Negative result obtained at a concentration of 500 µg/mL (3.70 mmol/L) with method on Du Pont aca *1558*

Bilirubin *Serum No Effect Analytical* At concentration of 10 mg/L had no effect on method on Boehringer Mannheim Reflotron system *5706*

Cannabinoids *Urine No Effect Analytical* No effect on Roche Abuscreen method *5006* No effect observed at a concentration of 100 µg/mL (0.74 mmol/L) on method on Du Pont aca *1557*

Catecholamines *Urine No Effect Analytical* No effect observed *1444*
Urine No Effect Physiological No effect observed *1444*

Cholesterol *Serum No Effect Analytical* At therapeutic concentration on Boehringer Mannheim Reflotron method *3231* No effect of concentrations up to 100 mg/L on method on Boehringer Mannheim Reflotron *5706*

Cocaethylene *Urine No Effect Analytical* No interference observed with TLC method of Baile *328*

Color *Feces Increase Analytical* Black color reported with aminophylline ingestion *3388*

Corticosteroids *Plasma Increase Physiological* Amphetamines may cause a significant increase in concentration, greatest in the evening *5641*

Drugs of Abuse Screen *Urine No Effect Analytical* No effect at concentration of 100 µg/mL on EZ-SCREEN procedure for cannabinoids and cocaine *1739*

Epinephrine *Urine Increase Physiological* 5.8 fold increase noticed with psychosis *2980*

Erythrocytes *Blood Decrease Physiological* Hemolytic anemia (depends on prior sensitivity) *1212*

Ethosuximide *Serum Decrease Physiological* Amphetamines may delay intestinal absorption of ethosuximide *5641*

Fatty Acids (FFA), Free *Serum Increase Physiological* But does not modify carbohydrate utilization *2242*

Glucose *Serum Decrease Physiological* Dextroamphetamine may produce slight effect *2452*
Serum No Effect Analytical At concentrations up to 10 mg/L no effect on method on Boehringer Mannheim Reflotron system but above this concentration reduced (not of clinical importance) *5706* At therapeutic concentration on Boehringer Mannheim Reflotron method *3231*

γ-Glutamyltransferase *Serum No Effect Analytical* At concentration of 100 mg/L no effect on method on Boehringer Mannheim Reflotron system *5706* At therapeutic concentration on Boehringer Mannheim Reflotron method *3231*

Hematocrit *Blood Decrease Physiological* Hemolytic anemia (depends on prior sensitivity) *1212*

Hemoglobin *Blood Decrease Physiological* Hemolytic anemia (depends on prior sensitivity) *1212*

Homovanillic Acid
Cerebrospinal Fluid No Effect Physiological No change in CSF with psychotic dose *2980*

5-Hydroxyindoleacetic Acid
Cerebrospinal Fluid No Effect Physiological No change in CSF with psychotic dose *2980*

Leukocytes *Blood Increase Physiological* Myeloblastic leukemia *522*

Morphine *Urine No Effect Analytical* No significant interference observed at a concentration of 370 µmol/L with Sung and Neely modification of Syva EMIT procedure *148*

Myeloblasts *Blood Increase Physiological* Myeloblastic leukemia *522*

Norepinephrine *Urine Increase Physiological* 2.2 fold increase noted with psychosis *2980*

Occult Blood *Feces Increase Physiological* Reported to cause ulcers of gastrointestinal tract *929*

Opiates *Urine No Effect Analytical* No effect observed at a concentration of 1000 µg/mL (7.4 mmol/L) with method on Du Pont aca *1559*

p-Aminophenol *Urine No Effect Analytical* With addition of drugs at a concentration of 100 mg/L and of related compounds at 50 mg/L no significant effect observed on colorimetric method of van Bocxlaer on Cobas Mira analyzer which involves reacting free p-aminophenol with resorcinol in the presence of magnesium ions to form an indophenol dye measured at 550 nm *6163*

Phenobarbital *Serum Decrease Physiological* Amphetamines may delay intestinal absorption of phenobarbital *5641*

Phenytoin *Serum Decrease Physiological* Amphetamines may delay intestinal absorption of phenobarbital *5641*

Promyeloblasts *Blood Increase Physiological* Myeloblastic leukemia *522*

Thyroxine (T4) Index, Free *Serum Increase Physiological* In 7.5% of patients admitted to a psychiatric hospital with many having ingested amphetamine *4121*

Tri-iodothyronine (T3) *Serum Increase Physiological* In 17% of patients admitted to a psychiatric hospital with many having ingested amphetamine *4121*

Tri-iodothyronine (T3) Index, Free
Serum Increase Physiological In 14% of patients admitted to a psychiatric hospital with many having ingested amphetamine *4121*

Tricyclic Antidepressants *Serum Increase Physiological* Interferes with metabolism of tricyclic antidepressants *1384*

Amphetamine *(continued)*

Tricyclic Antidepressants Screen
Serum No Effect Analytical No significant effect observed at a concentration of 500 µg/mL (3.70 mmol/L) with method on Du Pont aca *1550*

Triglycerides *Serum No Effect Analytical* At therapeutic concentration on Boehringer Mannheim Reflotron method *3231* No effect at 100 mg/L on Boehringer Mannheim Reflotron method *5706*

Urea Nitrogen *Serum No Effect Analytical* At therapeutic concentration on Boehringer Mannheim Reflotron method *3231* No effect at 100 mg/L on Boehringer Mannheim Reflotron method *5706*

Uric Acid *Serum No Effect Analytical* At therapeutic concentration on Boehringer Mannheim Reflotron method *3231* No effect up to 20 mg/L on method on Boehringer Mannheim Reflotron but above this concentration reduced although not of clinical significance since physiological concentration up to 0.1 mg/L only *5706*

Vanillylmandelic Acid *Urine No Effect Analytical* No effect observed *1444*
Urine No Effect Physiological No effect observed *1444*

Amphotericin B

Alanine Aminotransferase *Serum Increase Physiological* Acute liver failure, hepatitis and jaundice have been reported to occur as side effects *222* Acute hepatic failure, hepatitis, jaundice and veno-occlusive liver disease have been reported with amphotericin B administration *5993* Noted in one patient with acute myelogenous leukemia when treated with high dose. Probable idiosyncratic response *4040* Hepatotoxicity reported *3810*

Albumin *Serum No Effect Analytical* At concentration of 20 mg/L had no effect on BCG method *5704*
Serum No Effect Physiological No effect seen in 10 patients with 6 weeks treatment *391*

Alkaline Phosphatase *Serum Increase Physiological* Acute liver failure, hepatitis and jaundice have been reported to occur as side effects *222* Acute hepatic failure, hepatitis, jaundice and veno-occlusive liver disease have been reported with amphotericin B administration *5993* Noted in one patient with acute myelogenous leukemia when treated with high dose. Probable idiosyncratic response *4040* Due to hepatocellular dysfunction *3810*

Amylase *Serum Increase Physiological* Hyperamylasemiahas been reported as a side effect *5993*

Aspartate Aminotransferase *Serum Increase Physiological* Acute liver failure, hepatitis and jaundice have been reported to occur as side effects *222* Acute hepatic failure, hepatitis, jaundice and veno-occlusive liver disease have been reported with amphotericin B administration *5993* Noted in one patient with acute myelogenous leukemia when treated with high dose. Probable idiosyncratic response *4040* Hepatotoxicity reported *3810*

Bicarbonate *Serum No Effect Analytical* At concentration of 20 mg/L had no effect on method using phenolphthalein *5704*

Bile *Urine Increase Physiological* Reported hepatotoxicity *3810*

Bilirubin *Serum Increase Analytical* At concentrations above 96 mg/L (therapeutic concentration about 3.7 mg/L) raised concentration as measured by Jendrassik and Grof method *5704*
Serum Increase Physiological Acute liver failure, hepatitis and jaundice have been reported to occur as side effects *222* Noted in one patient with acute myelogenous leukemia when treated with high dose. Probable idiosyncratic response *4040* In clinical trials with 556 patients treated with amphotericin B 4% had hyperbilirubinemia *5993* May cause hepatocellular dysfunction *2242*

BSP Retention *Serum Increase Physiological* Due to hepatocellular dysfunction *3810*

Calcium *Serum Decrease Physiological* Hypocalcemiahas been reported as a side effect *5993* Hypocalcemia has been reported to occur as a side effect *222*

Serum No Effect Analytical At concentration of 96 mg/L had no effect on cresolphthalein method *5704*

Casts *Urine Increase Physiological* Cylindruria may occur *5985* Granular and hyaline casts with toxicity *128*

Chloride *Serum No Effect Analytical* At concentration of 20 mg/L had no effect on mercurimetric method *5704*

Cholesterol *Serum Increase Analytical* At concentrations above 96 mg/L (therapeutic concentration about 3.7 mg/L) raised concentration as measured by Liebermann-Burchard method *5704*

Color *Feces Increase Analytical* Black color reported with amphotericin B ingestion *3388* Black color reported with amphoteracin B ingestion *3388*

Coombs' Test, Direct *Blood Positive Physiological* Single case reported with hemolytic anemia *2452*

Creatine Kinase *Serum Increase Physiological* Rhabdomyolysis caused by severe hypokalemia *1505*

Creatinine *Serum Increase Physiological* Increased to average of 1.4 mg/dL from 1.0 mg/dL after 2 weeks in 10 patients; further increase with time *391* Nephrotoxic effect *3810* Nephrotoxicity usually develops after a few weeks of treatment, usually reversible unless more than total of 4 g drug given *5985* Azotemia may develop as a side effect with decreased renal function. Renal tubular acidosis and nephrocalcinosis may also occur *222* In clinical trials with 556 patients treated with amphotericin B 11% had serum increased creatinine concentrations *5993* In a study of 22 patients undergoing bone marrow transplantation concurrent administration of cyclosporine A and amphotericin B appeared to increase nephrotoxicity *5993*
Serum No Effect Analytical At concentration of 20 mg/L had no effect on Technicon AutoAnalyzer® Jaffe method *5704* No effect of concentrations up to 15 mg/L on single slide method on Kodak Ektachem® *5706*

Creatinine Clearance *Urine Decrease Physiological* Nephrotoxicity effect (decrease up to 36%) *831* Fell to 69 mL/min from 94 mL/min in 10 patients after 2 weeks. Remained at this value with continued treatment *391*

Cyclosporine *Blood No Effect Analytical* At a concentration of 20 mg/L had no effect on Syva EMIT method *495*

Effective Renal Plasma Flow
Patient Decrease Physiological Occurs in high percentage of patients *128*

Eosinophils *Blood Decrease Physiological* Allergic response *2754*
Blood Increase Physiological Blood dyscrasias have been reported with amphotericin B administration *5993* Eosinophilia has been reported to occur as a side effect *222*

Erythrocytes *Blood Decrease Physiological* Bone marrow depression with hemolytic anemia *6113* Frequently develops after several weeks of therapy due to interference with production of erythrocytes *5985*
Urine Increase Physiological Nephrotoxicity *1714*

Erythropoietin *Serum Decrease Physiological* Response to anemia blunted in individuals receiving amphotericin B *3581*

Flucytosine *Serum No Effect Analytical* No effect at concentrations of up to 25 mg/L on method of Huang et al using creatine iminohydrolase *2747*

Glomerular Filtration Rate *Urine Decrease Physiological* Occurs in high percentage of patients *128*

Glucose *Serum Decrease Physiological* Both hypoglycemia and hyperglycemia have been reported as a side effect *5993*
Serum Increase Physiological Both hypoglycemia and hyperglycemia have been reported as a side effect *5993*

γ-Glutamyltransferase *Serum Increase Physiological* Acute hepatic failure, hepatitis, jaundice and veno-occlusive liver disease have been reported with amphotericin B administration *5993* Acute liver failure, hepatitis and jaundice have been reported to occur as side effects *222*

Granulocytes *Blood Decrease Physiological* Agranulocytosis has been reported to occur as a side effect *222*

Hematocrit *Blood Decrease Physiological* Bone marrow depression with hemolytic anemia *6113*

Hemoglobin *Blood Decrease Physiological* Normochromic normocytic anemia may develop as a side effect *222* Majority of patients receiving drug have fall of 18-35% in concentration

(normocytic normochromic anemia) *3727* Bone marrow depression with hemolytic anemia *6113* In clinical trials with 556 patients treated with amphotericin B 5% had anemia *5993*
Urine Increase Physiological Nephrotoxicity, bleeding actually caused by drug *1714*

Histamine *Plasma No Effect Analytical* Minimal inhibition of radio-enzyme assay at 80 times therapeutic concentration *2492*

Isocitrate Dehydrogenase *Serum Increase Physiological* Due to hepatocellular dysfunction *3810*

Lactate Dehydrogenase *Serum Increase Physiological* Noted in one patient with acute myelogenous leukemia when treated with high dose. Probable idiosyncratic response *4040*

Leukocytes *Blood Decrease Physiological* Leukopenia or agranulocytosis *2754* Occasional complication of treatment *5985* In clinical trials with 556 patients treated with amphotericin B 4% had leukopenia *5993* Both leukopenia and leukocytosis have been reported to occur as side effects *222*
Blood Increase Physiological Both leukopenia and leukocytosis have been reported to occur as side effects *222* Leukocytosis occurs *2754* Blood dyscrasias have been reported with amphotericin B administration *5993*

Magnesium *Serum Decrease Physiological* Significant reduction by 2 weeks from 2.35 mg/dL to 2.0 mg/dL and to 1.6 mg/dL by 4 weeks in 10 patients *391* Hypomagnesemia has been reported to occur as a side effect *222* Occasionally observed, associated with toxic effect of drug *190*
Urine Increase Physiological Following i.v. infusion for 2 h *4014* Significant effect at 4 weeks, but not earlier. Fractional magnesium excretion increased *391*

Methotrexate *Serum Increase Physiological* Administration with methotrexate been demonstrated to increase its elimination half-life and an increase in its AUC *3909*

Mycophenolic Acid *Serum No Effect Analytical* No significant interference observed with HPLC method of Shipkova et al *5526*

Mycophenolic Acid Glucuronide
Serum No Effect Analytical No significant interference observed with HPLC method of Shipkova et al *5526*

Myoglobin *Urine Increase Physiological* Caused by rhabdomyolysis *1505*

Nonprotein Nitrogen *Serum Increase Physiological* Nephrotoxic effect *3810*

Occult Blood *Feces Increase Physiological* Hemorrhagic gastroenteritis and melena have been reported to occur as side effects *222* Melena and hemorrhagic gastroenteritis *128* Melena has been reported with amphotericin B administration *5993*

pH *Blood Decrease Physiological* Acidosis has been reported as a side effect *5993*
Urine Increase Physiological In absence of acid load indicates pending decrease of GFR *812*

Phosphate *Serum No Effect Analytical* At concentration of 96 mg/L had no effect on phosphomolybdate method *5704*

Platelets *Blood Decrease Physiological* Occasional complication of treatment *5985* Bone marrow depression with hemolytic anemia *6113* Thrombocytopenia has been reported to occur as a side effect *222* In clinical trials with 556 patients treated with amphotericin B 5% had thrombocytopenia *5993*

Potassium *Serum Decrease Physiological* In clinical trials with 556 patients treated with amphotericin B 5% had hypokalemia. Hypokalemia is also potentiated with concurrent administration of corticosteroids and corticotropin or potentiate digitalis toxicity *5993* Nephrotoxicity usually develops after a few weeks of treatment, usually reversible unless more than total of 4 g drug given *5985* Hypokalemia may develop as a side effect and may augment the toxicity of coadministered drugs *222* Frequently observed effect, associated with renal damage *190*
Serum Increase Physiological May occur with renal toxicity *831* Hyperkalemia has been reported as a side effect *5993*

Potassium Clearance *Urine Increase Physiological* Dose related inverse relationship to GFR *812*

Protein *Cerebrospinal Fluid No Effect Analytical* At concentration of 1 mg/L on SDS/Coomassie Blue method of Huang *2745*
Serum No Effect Analytical At concentration of 96 mg/L had no effect on biuret method with blank correction *5704*
Serum No Effect Physiological No effect seen in 10 patients with 6 weeks treatment *391*
Urine Increase Physiological Nephrotoxic effect *1714* Nephrotoxicity usually develops after a few weeks of treatment, usually reversible unless more than total of 4 g drug given *5985*

Sodium *Serum Decrease Physiological* Significant effect even in normal subjects *831*

Titratable Acidity *Urine Decrease Physiological* Development of renal tubular acidosis *812*

Triglycerides *Serum No Effect Analytical* At concentration of 20 mg/L had no effect on lipase/esterase method *5704*

Urea Nitrogen *Serum Increase Physiological* Acute renal failure, anuria and oliguria have been reported to occur as side effects *222* In a study of 22 patients undergoing bone marrow transplantation concurrent administration of cyclosporine A and amphotericin B appeared to increase nephrotoxicity *5993* Nephrotoxic effect *3810*
Serum No Effect Analytical At concentration of 96 mg/L had no effect on diacetylmonoxime method *5704*

Uric Acid *Serum No Effect Analytical* At concentration of 96 mg/L had no effect on phosphotungstate reduction method *5704*

Uric Acid Clearance *Urine Increase Physiological* Varies inversely with GFR (consistent change) *812*

Zidovudine *Serum No Effect Analytical* No effect on liquid chromatographic method of Hedaya and Sawchuk *2525*

Ampicillin

Acetate *Feces Increase Physiological* Mild effect when given orally to 6 healthy volunteers for 6 d: normalized after 6 weeks *2734*

Acid Phosphatase *Serum No Effect Analytical* At concentration of 20 µg/mL (57 µmol/L) had no effect on method on Du Pont Dimension *1562*

Alanine Aminotransferase *Serum Increase Physiological* Probable effect of i.m. injection *3199*
Serum No Effect Analytical No effect at concentration of 20 µg/mL (57 µmol/L) on method on Du Pont Dimension *1563* No effect at 1000 mg/L on Boehringer Mannheim Reflotron method *5706* No effect on Boehringer Mannheim Reflotron method at therapeutic concentration *3231*

Albumin *Serum No Effect Analytical* At concentration of 20 µg/mL (57 µmol/L) had no effect on method on Du Pont Dimension *1564* At concentration of 40 mg/L had no effect on BCG method *5704*
Urine No Effect Analytical At concentration of 400 mg/dL no significant effect observed on Boehringer Mannheim Tina-quant method *2799*

Alkaline Phosphatase *Serum No Effect Analytical* At concentration of 20 µg/mL (57 µmol/L) had no effect on method on Du Pont Dimension *1565*

Amino Acids *Urine Increase Analytical* Presence of drug as additional spot *4762* Positive reaction observed with ninhydrin in paper chromatography, paper electrophoresis and ion-exchange chromatography *4761* Produces yellow spots with ninhydrin and thin-layer chromatography *2109*

Ammonia *Plasma No Effect Analytical* No effect at concentration of 20 µg/mL (57 µmol/L) on method on Du Pont Dimension *1566*

Amylase *Serum No Effect Analytical* At concentration of 1000 mg/L had no effect on method on Boehringer Mannheim Reflotron system *5706* At concentration of 20 µg/mL (57 µmol/L) had no effect on method on Du Pont Dimension *1567*

Amylase, Pancreatic Isoenzyme
Serum No Effect Physiological At toxic concentration of 1000 mg/L had no significant effect on method on Boehringer Mannheim Reflotron *3647*

Androstenetriol Sulfate *Urine Decrease Physiological* Increase by 52% after 6 d in pregnant women *6078*

Aspartate Aminotransferase *Serum Increase Physiological* Moderately increased activity has been reported but the significance of this is unknown *6563* Probable effect of i.m. injection (especially in infants) *3199*
Serum No Effect Analytical No effect on Reflotron method at therapeutic concentration *3231* No effect at 1000 mg/L on

Ampicillin *(continued)*

Aspartate Aminotransferase *(continued)* Boehringer Mannheim Reflotron method *5706* No effect at concentration of 20 µg/mL (57 µmol/L) on method on Du Pont Dimension *1568*

Atenolol *Serum Decrease Physiological* Dose related reduction in bioavailability of atenolol, especially above 1 gram. Effect observed in 6 healthy volunteers when studied acutely and over 6 days. Bioavailability reduced from 60 to 36% in acute study and to 24% in longer term study *5309*

Bicarbonate *Serum No Effect Analytical* At concentration of 40 mg/L had no effect on method using phenolphthalein *5704*

Bilirubin *Serum No Effect Analytical* No effect at concentration of 20 µg/mL (70 µmol/L) on method on Du Pont Dimension *1589* At concentration of 40 mg/L had no effect on Jendrassik and Grof method *5704* At concentration of 1000 mg/L had no effect on method on Boehringer Mannheim Reflotron system *5706* No effect at 1250 mg/L on method on Ames Seralyzer *5706*

Serum No Effect Physiological Insignificant displacement from protein in neonates *6314*

Bilirubin, Direct *Serum No Effect Analytical* At concentration of 20 µg/mL (57 µmol/L) had no effect on method on Du Pont Dimension *1574*

Bleeding Time *Patient Increase Physiological* Dose related prolongation of bleeding time in all 5 volunteers studied *756*

Calcium *Serum No Effect Analytical* No effect at concentration of 20 µg/mL (57 µmol/L) on method on Du Pont Dimension *1569* At concentration of 40 mg/L had no effect on cresolphthalein method *5704*

Cannabinoids *Urine No Effect Analytical* No effect on Roche Abuscreen method *5006*

Casts *Urine Increase Physiological* Occurs as result of nephrotoxicity *5942*

Chloramphenicol *Serum No Effect Analytical* At 100 mg/L no effect on coupled enzymatic procedure *4122*

Chloride *Serum No Effect Analytical* At concentration of 40 mg/L had no effect on mercurimetric method *5704*

Cholesterol *Serum Decrease Analytical* At concentrations above 100 mg/L (therapeutic concentration about 320 mg/L) lowered concentration as measured by CHOD-Iodide method *5704*

Serum No Effect Analytical At concentration of 1000 mg/L no effect on method on Boehringer Mannheim Reflotron system *5706* No effect on Boehringer Mannheim Reflotron method at therapeutic concentration *3231* No effect at 1250 mg/L on Ames Seralyzer method *5706* At concentration of 20 µg/mL (57 µmol/L) had no effect on concentration on Du Pont Dimension *1570* At concentration of 900 mg/L had no effect on catalase-Hantzsch method *5704* At concentration of 900 mg/L had no effect on catalase-AIDH method *5704* At concentration of 900 mg/L had no effect on CHOD-PAP method *5704* At concentration of 900 mg/L had no effect on Liebermann-Burchard method *5704*

Cholinesterase *Serum No Effect Analytical* No effect observed at concentration of 5 mg/dL with butyrylthiocholine method on Kodak Ektachem® *2504* Insignificant decrease of 0.02 U/mL at a concentration of 20 µg/mL with method on Du Pont aca *3271* Insignificant increase of 0.27 U/mL at a concentration of 20 µg/mL with method on Du Pont Dimension *3271*

Clot Retraction *Blood No Effect Physiological* In doses as high as 300 mg/kg/d in volunteers *756*

Coombs' Test, Direct *Blood Positive Physiological* Hypersensitivity reaction in 39% of 36 patients receiving drug *3195*

Cortisol *Plasma No Effect Analytical* No effect observed on CEDIA method at concentration of 1000 mg/L (worst case 103.1% recovery) or on Boehringer Mannheim Enzymun method (101.5% recovery) *1097*

Creatine Kinase *Serum Increase Physiological* Probable effect of i.m. injection *3199*

Serum No Effect Analytical No effect at 1250 mg/L on method on Ames Seralyzer *5706*

Creatine Kinase Isoenzymes *Serum No Effect Analytical* No interference observed at a concentration of 500 mg/L (1.43 mmol/L) with CK-MB method on Du Pont aca *1519* At concentration of 20 µg/mL (57 µmol/L) had no effect on method to determine MB isoenzyme on Du Pont Dimension *1571*

Creatinine *Serum No Effect Analytical* At concentration of 12 mg/L had no effect on creatinine iminohydrolase method *5704* At concentration of 1600 mg/L had no effect on kinetic Jaffe method on BKA-2 *5704* At concentration of 40 mg/L had no effect on Technicon AutoAnalyzer® Jaffe method *5704* At concentration of 600 mg/L had no effect on Jaffe-Fading-Fraction method *5704* At concentration of 600 mg/L had no effect on Jaffe-Fuller's earth method *5704* No effect at concentration of 20 µg/mL (57 µmol/L) on method on Du Pont Dimension *1572* No effect of concentrations up to 15 mg/L on single slide method on Kodak Ektachem® *5706* No effect at 1250 mg/L on Ames Seralyzer method *5706*

Crystals *Urine Increase Physiological* Presence of drug maximal at pH 5 *4762*

Dehydroepiandrosterone *Urine Decrease Physiological* Increase by 75% after 6 d administration in pregnant women *6078*

Digitoxin *Serum No Effect Physiological* Insignificant increase in elimination half-life *3672*

Eosinophils *Blood Increase Physiological* Eosinophilia has been reported with ampicillin administration *6563* Allergic reaction *2484* Hypersensitivity reaction in 39% of 36 patients receiving drug *3195*

Erythrocytes *Blood Decrease Physiological* Reversible anemia may occur *2753*

Urine Increase Physiological Necrosis of tubules due to nephrotoxicity *5942*

Estriol *Plasma Decrease Physiological* In pregnant women due to alteration of gut flora *4812* May inhibit synthesis by fetoplacental unit *641*

Urine Decrease Physiological May diminish synthesis by fetoplacental unit *641*

Estrogens *Urine Decrease Physiological* Increase by 46% after 6 d in pregnant women, altered gastrointestinal flora. During luteal phase in normal women. During ovulatory phase in normals *6078*

Estrogens, Conjugated *Urine Decrease Physiological* Increase by 50% after 6 d in pregnant women *6078*

Estrone Sulfate *Plasma Decrease Physiological* Significant reduction in 4 men after taking drug for 5 days, either by reducing bacterial growth in the gastrointestinal tract or by inhibiting estrogen sulfotransferase activity *4890*

Fibrinogen *Plasma No Effect Physiological* In doses as high as 300 mg/kg/d in volunteers *756*

Folate *Serum Decrease Analytical* Inhibits growth of *L. casei5870*

Serum No Effect Analytical Allegedly no effect on autoclave method *2965*

Glucose *Serum No Effect Analytical* At concentration of 1000 mg/L no effect on method on Boehringer Mannheim Reflotron system *5706* No effect at 1250 mg/L on glucose oxidase method on Ames Seralyzer *5706* No effect of concentrations up to 180 mg/L on method on Kodak Ektachem® *5706* No effect on hexokinase, glucose-oxidase methods *4240* At concentration of 1200 mg/L had no effect on hexokinase/G-6-PDH method *5704* At concentration of 20 µg/mL (57 µmol/L) has no effect on method on Du Pont Dimension *1575* At concentration of 180 mg/L had no effect on Kodak Ektachem® method *5704* At concentration of 5 mg/L had no effect on GOD/POD-PAP method *5704* No effect on Boehringer Mannheim Reflotron method at therapeutic concentration *3231*

Urine Decrease Analytical Low with Clinistix® , Diastix® *1826*

Urine Increase Analytical Administration of ampicillin may cause false positive reaction with Benedict's and Fehling's reactions and Clinitest® tablets *6563* At drug concentration of 4 and 10 mg/mL on Clinitest® when no glucose present, but some reduction with 0.5% glucose and higher concentrations *3710*

Urine No Effect Analytical Administration of ampicillin has no effect on enzyme tests such as Clinistix® or TesTape® *6563* No effect at concentration up to 10 mg/mL on Diastix® and TesTape® methods *3710* No effect observed with TesTape® *1826* At concentration of 4,000 mg/L had no effect on Diaburtest *5704*

γ-Glutamyltransferase *Serum No Effect Analytical* At concentration of 1000 mg/L no effect on method on Boehringer Mannheim Reflotron system *5706* At concentration of 20 μg/mL (57 μmol/L) has no effect on method on Du Pont Dimension *1579* No effect on Boehringer Mannheim Reflotron method at therapeutic concentration *3231*

Granulocytes *Blood Decrease Physiological* Agranulocytosis has been reported with ampicillin administration *6563*

HDL-Cholesterol *Serum No Effect Analytical* At a concentration up to 1000 mg/L had no significant effect on Reflotron method for whole blood cholesterol *6352* No effect at concentration of 20 μg/mL (57 μmol/L) on method on Du Pont Dimension *1576*

Hematocrit *Blood Decrease Physiological* Anemia has been reported with ampicillin administration *6563*

Hemoglobin *Blood Decrease Physiological* Reversible hypersensitivity reaction *2754* Anemia has been reported with ampicillin administration *6563*
Urine Increase Physiological Occurs as result of nephrotoxicity *5942*

Histamine *Plasma No Effect Analytical* No effect on radioenzyme assay at therapeutic concentrations *2492*

16-α-Hydroxydehydroepiandrosterone
Urine Decrease Physiological Increase by 72% after 6 d administration in pregnant women *6078*

16-α-Hydroxydehydroepiandrosterone Glucuronide
Urine Decrease Physiological Increase by 45% after 6 d in pregnant women *6078*

6-Hydroxyprogesterone Metabolite
Urine Decrease Physiological Increase by 29% after 6 d in pregnant women *6078*

^{131}I Uptake *Serum Decrease Physiological* Omnipen® contains tetraiodofluorescein *4360*

Iron *Serum No Effect Analytical* No interference observed at concentrations up to 18 mg/mL with method on Kodak Ektachem® 700 *5076* No interference observed with method on Kodak Ektachem® *2792* No effect at concentration on 20 μg/mL (57 μmol/L) on method on Du Pont Dimension *1577*

Iron-Binding Capacity, Total *Serum No Effect Analytical* No effect at concentration of 20 μg/mL (57 μmol/L) on method on Du Pont Dimension *1590*

17-Ketogenic Steroids *Urine Decrease Physiological* Increase by 41% after 7 d administration in pregnant women *6078*
Urine Increase Physiological After 14 d in 1 postmenopausal woman *6078*

Ketone Body Ratio *Serum No Effect Analytical* When added at a concentration of 10 g/L had no significant effect on AKBR method of Uno et al *6131*

17-Ketosteroids *Urine Decrease Physiological* Increase by 42% after 7 d administration in pregnant women *6078*
Urine Increase Physiological After 14 d in 1 postmenopausal woman *6078*

Lactate *Plasma No Effect Analytical* No effect at final concentration of 100 μg/mL on method on Kodak Ektachem® *2793* At concentration of 1200 mg/L had no effect on enzymatic method *5704*

Lactate Dehydrogenase *Serum No Effect Analytical* No effect at 1250 mg/L on method on Ames Seralyzer *5706* At concentration of 20 μg/mL (57 μmol/L) has no effect on method on Du Pont Dimension *1578*

Leukocytes *Blood Decrease Physiological* Leukopenia *2278* Leukopenia has been reported with ampicillin administration *6563*
Blood Increase Physiological Mainly due to eosinophilia of hypersensitivity *3810*

Lipase *Serum No Effect Analytical* No effect at concentration of 20 μg/mL (57 μmol/L) on method on Du Pont Dimension *1580* No effect of concentrations up to 1750 mg/L on method on Kodak Ektachem® *5706*

Magnesium *Serum No Effect Analytical* No effect at concentration of 20 μg/mL (57 μmol/L) on method on Du Pont Dimension *1581*

Monocytes *Blood Increase Physiological* Associated with agranulocytosis *2278*

N-Acetyl-Glucosaminidase *Urine No Effect Analytical* At concentration of 400 mg/dL no significant effect on Boehringer Mannheim CPR method *3174*

Neutrophils *Blood Decrease Physiological* Reported observation *4265*

Partial Thromboplastin Time
Plasma No Effect Physiological In doses as high as 300 mg/kg/d in volunteers *756*

Phenylalanine *Plasma Increase Analytical* When dried blood spot method used similar fluorescent product to phenylalanine produced with ampicillin with procedure of McCaman and Robins. On equal molar basis produced fluorescence 22-45% of that of phenylalanine *1643*
Plasma No Effect Analytical No interference observed with rapid quantitative whole blood method of Campbell et al using phenylalanine dehydrogenase *867*

Phenytoin *Serum No Effect Analytical* No effect at concentration of 20 μg/mL (57 μmol/L) on method on Du Pont Dimension *1583*

Phosphate *Serum No Effect Analytical* At concentration of 40 mg/L had no effect on phosphomolybdate method *5704* No effect of concentrations up to 1750 mg/L on method on Kodak Ektachem® *5706* At concentration of 20 μg/mL (57 μmol/L) has no effect on method on Du Pont Dimension *1584*

Platelet Aggregation *Blood Decrease Physiological* Defective platelet aggregation induced by ADP in 4 of 5 volunteers *756*
Blood No Effect Physiological No effect on collagen or epinephrine induced aggregation *756*

Platelets *Blood Decrease Physiological* Isolated case of platelet-associated IgG and thrombocytopenia *3102* Thrombocytopenia and thrombocytopenic purpura have been reported with ampicillin administration *6563* May be associated with purpura *2754*
Blood No Effect Physiological In doses as high as 300 mg/kg/d in volunteers *756*

Potassium *Serum No Effect Analytical* At concentration of 1800 mg/L had no effect on ISE measurement without predilution *5704* At concentration of 5 mg/L had no effect on flame-photometric method *5704*

Pregnanediol *Urine Decrease Physiological* Increase by 53% after 5 d administration in pregnant women. During luteal phase in normal women *6078*

Pregnenolone *Urine Decrease Physiological* Increase by 44% after 6 d administration in pregnant women *6078*

Progesterone *Plasma Decrease Physiological* Probably decreases synthesis *6078*

Protein *Cerebrospinal Fluid Increase Analytical* At concentration of 10 mg/dL caused 85% increase (generally 1 mg ampicillin gave as much color as 2.5 mg protein) but ampicillin does not diffuse across normal meninges so may be minimal clinical effect when measurements made with Ektachem® slide method *3654*
Cerebrospinal Fluid No Effect Analytical At 20 mg/L on SDS/Coomassie Blue method of Huang *2745*
Serum Increase Analytical At concentrations above 500 mg/L raised concentration as measured by biuret method with blank correction *5704*
Serum No Effect Analytical At concentration of 20 μg/mL (57 μmol/L) had negligible effect on method on Du Pont Dimension *1591*
Urine Increase Physiological Necrosis of tubules due to nephrotoxicity *5942*
Urine No Effect Analytical No effect in patients receiving up to 8 g daily on sulfosalicylic acid, trichloracetic acid or Ponceau S dye methods *6611*

Protein Electrophoresis *Serum No Effect Analytical* At concentration of 1800 mg/L had no effect on automated Olympus-Hite method *5704*

Prothrombin Time *Plasma No Effect Physiological* In doses as high as 300 mg/kg/d in volunteers *756*

Raloxifene *Serum Decrease Physiological* Reported to cause a 28% decrease in peak concentration and of 14% in the overall absorption with coadministration of ampicillin *1696*

Short-Chain Fatty Acids *Feces Decrease Physiological* Mild effect when given orally to 6 healthy volunteers for 6 d: normalized after 6 weeks *2734*

Ampicillin *(continued)*

Sodium *Serum Increase Analytical* At concentrations above 1800 mg/L (therapeutic concentration about 320 mg/L) raised concentration as measured by ISE without predilution *5704*
Serum No Effect Analytical At concentration of 5 mg/L had no effect on flame-photometric method *5704*

Sugar *Urine Increase Analytical* Reacts positively with Clinitest *4761*

T3-Uptake *Serum No Effect Analytical* No significant effect observed at a concentration of 20 µg/mL (57 µmol/L) with method on Du Pont aca *1545* At concentration of 20 µg/mL (57 µmol/L) has no effect on method on Du Pont Dimension *1586*

Tacrolimus *Serum No Effect Analytical* In HPLC/MS method of Christians et al no significant interference observed with measurement of FK 506 *1010*

Theophylline *Serum Increase Analytical* Positive bias of 3.15 mg/L at theophylline concentration of 20 mg/L at ampicillin concentration of 20 mg/L with method used on 3M Diagnostics TheoFAST *1122*
Serum No Effect Analytical No effect at concentration of 10 mg/L on methods used on Kodak DT-60, Abbott TDx, Abbott Vision with either whole blood or serum, Syntex AccµLevel and Ames Seralyzer *1122* At concentration of 20 µg/mL (57 µmol/L) had no effect on method on Du Pont Dimension *1585*
Serum No Effect Physiological No clinically significant effect on theophylline concentration observed when ampicillin with/without sulbactam coadministered *5999* No documented significant interaction with theophylline reported either when administered alone or with sulbactam *6117* No effect observed on half-life *1384*

Thrombin Time *Blood No Effect Physiological* In doses as high as 300 mg/kg/d in volunteers *756*

Thyroxine (T4) *Serum No Effect Analytical* At concentration of 20 µg/mL (57 µmol/L) has no effect on method on Du Pont Dimension *1587* No significant effect observed at a concentration of 20 µg/mL (57 µmol/L) with method on Du Pont aca *1588* *1546*

Triglycerides *Serum No Effect Analytical* No effect at 1000 mg/L on Boehringer Mannheim Reflotron method *5706* At concentration of 20 µg/mL (57 µmol/L) has no effect on method on Du Pont Dimension *1592* At concentration of 11 mg/L had no effect on GPO-PAP method *5704* At concentration of 40 mg/L had no effect on lipase/esterase method *5704* No effect on Boehringer Mannheim Reflotron method at therapeutic concentration *3231*

Urea Nitrogen *Serum No Effect Analytical* No effect at concentration of 20 µg/mL (57 µmol/L) on method on Du Pont Dimension *1593* No effect on Boehringer Mannheim Reflotron method at therapeutic concentration *3231* At concentration of 40 mg/L had no effect on diacetylmonoxime method *5704* No effect at 1000 mg/L on Boehringer Mannheim Reflotron method *5706* No effect at 1250 mg/L on method on Ames Seralyzer *5706* At concentration of 180 mg/L had no effect on Kodak Ektachem® method *5704*

Uric Acid *Serum Increase Analytical* At concentrations above 100 mg/L (therapeutic concentration about 320 mg/L) raised concentration as measured by Ames Seralyzer *5704*
Serum No Effect Analytical No effect at 1000 mg/L on method on Boehringer Mannheim Reflotron *5706* No effect up to 100 mg/L on uricase method on Ames Seralyzer but at higher concentrations disproportionately increased uric acid concentration which may be of clinical significance since therapeutic concentration of drug up to 320 mg/L *5706* At concentration of 300 mg/L had no effect on catalase-AIDH method *5704* At concentration of 40 mg/L had no effect on phosphotungstate reduction method *5704* No effect on Boehringer Mannheim Reflotron method at therapeutic concentration *3231* At concentration of 600 mg/L had no effect on Kageyama-Hantzsch method *5704* No effect at concentration of 20 µg/mL (57 µmol/L) on method on Du Pont Dimension *1594*
Urine Increase Physiological Competes with uric acid for reabsorption and potentiates response to probenecid. Significant uricosuria with ampicillin alone from 0-2 h and 8-24 h after administration *5693*

Urobilin *Urine Increase Physiological* Necrosis of tubules due to nephrotoxicity *5942*

Amrinone

Alanine Aminotransferase *Serum Increase Physiological* Occasional hepatotoxicity reported *1384* Hepatotoxicity has been reported in patients receiving amrinone *5252*

Alkaline Phosphatase *Serum Increase Physiological* Hepatotoxicity has been reported in patients receiving amrinone *5252*

Aspartate Aminotransferase *Serum Increase Physiological* Hepatotoxicity has been reported in patients receiving amrinone *5252* Occasional hepatotoxicity reported *1384*

Bilirubin *Serum Increase Physiological* Hepatotoxicity has been reported in patients receiving amrinone *5252*

Captopril *Serum No Effect Physiological* No untoward clinical observations have been reported in patients receiving amrinone and captopril *5252*

Chlorthalidone *Serum No Effect Physiological* No untoward clinical observations have been reported in patients receiving amrinone and chlorthalidone *5252*

Diazepam *Serum No Effect Physiological* No untoward clinical observations have been reported in patients receiving amrinone and diazepam *5252*

Digoxin *Serum Increase Analytical* Positive interference with Abbott TDx method *4606*
Serum No Effect Analytical No effect on Du Pont aca method *4606* At therapeutic concentration no effect observed on Abbott TDx digoxin II concentration. Note previous report of interference was done at nonphysiological concentration *1063*
Serum No Effect Physiological No untoward clinical observations have been reported in patients receiving amrinone and digoxin *5252*

Ethacrynic Acid *Serum No Effect Physiological* No untoward clinical observations have been reported in patients receiving amrinone and ethacrynic acid *5252*

Furosemide *Serum No Effect Physiological* No untoward clinical observations have been reported in patients receiving amrinone and furosemide *5252*

Heparin *Plasma No Effect Physiological* No untoward clinical observations have been reported in patients receiving amrinone and heparin *5252*

Hydralazine *Serum No Effect Physiological* No untoward clinical observations have been reported in patients receiving amrinone and hydralazine *5252*

Hydrochlorothiazide *Serum No Effect Physiological* No untoward clinical observations have been reported in patients receiving amrinone and hydrochlorothiazde *5252*

Isosorbide *Serum No Effect Physiological* No untoward clinical observations have been reported in patients receiving amrinone and isosorbide *5252*

Lidocaine *Serum No Effect Physiological* No untoward clinical observations have been reported in patients receiving amrinone and lidocaine *5252*

Metoprolol *Serum No Effect Physiological* No untoward clinical observations have been reported in patients receiving amrinone and metoprolol *5252*

Platelets *Blood Decrease Physiological* Dose-dependent, reversible thrombocytopenia reported *1384* Thrombocytopenia has been reported in patients receiving amrinone *5252*

Prazosin *Serum No Effect Physiological* No untoward clinical observations have been reported in patients receiving amrinone and prazosin *5252*

Propranolol *Serum No Effect Physiological* No untoward clinical observations have been reported in patients receiving amrinone and propranolol *5252*

Quinidine *Serum No Effect Physiological* No untoward clinical observations have been reported in patients receiving amrinone and qunidine *5252*

Spironolactone *Serum No Effect Physiological* No untoward clinical observations have been reported in patients receiving amrinone and spironolactone *5252*

Warfarin *Plasma No Effect Physiological* No untoward clinical observations have been reported in patients receiving amrinone and warfarin *5252*

Amsacrine

Leukocytes *Blood Decrease Physiological* Leukopenia develops in almost all patients and is usual dose limiting toxicity. Nadirs occur around day 12 and recovery occurs between days 25 and 28 *1384*

Amygdalin

Sugar *Urine Increase Analytical* Measured as reducing agent with Benedict's reagent *3810*

Amyl Alcohol

Alanine Aminotransferase *Serum Increase Physiological* May cause liver damage if ingested *2183*

Glucose *Urine Increase Physiological* Associated with renal damage *2183*

ionized Calcium *Serum Decrease Analytical* At 0.1 mmol/L to 0.1 mol/L with calcium specific electrode *820*

Methemoglobin *Blood Increase Physiological* May cause hemolysis following ingestion *2183*

Occult Blood *Feces Increase Physiological* May cause gastrointestinal hemorrhage *2183*

Amyl Nitrite

Bilirubin *Serum Increase Physiological* With increased hemolysis *4013*

Casts *Urine Increase Physiological* May cause nephrotoxicity *467*

Erythrocytes *Blood Decrease Physiological* Hemolytic anemia (slight or marked effect) *4013*

Hemoglobin *Plasma Increase Physiological* If intravascular hemolysis occurs *4013*

Methemoglobin *Blood Increase Physiological* Hemolytic anemia *4013*

Reticulocytes *Blood Increase Physiological* Hemolytic anemia (up to 15%) *4013*

Urea Nitrogen *Serum Increase Physiological* May cause nephrotoxicity *467*

Urobilinogen *Feces Increase Physiological* If hemolytic anemia occurs *4013*

Urine Increase Physiological Less reliable index than fecal if hemolysis occurs *4013*

Anabolic Steroids

Alanine Aminotransferase *Serum Increase Physiological* Cholestatic syndrome (intrahepatic cholestasis) *3669*

Alkaline Phosphatase *Serum Increase Physiological* Cholestatic syndrome *2242*

Amylase *Serum Decrease Physiological* Mean decrease from 112 to 89 units in patients with chronic pancreatitis after 3 weeks treatment with combination of anabolic steroids *6067*

Aspartate Aminotransferase *Serum Increase Physiological* Cholestatic syndrome (intrahepatic cholestasis) *3669*

Bile *Urine Increase Physiological* Intrahepatic cholestatic jaundice *2242*

Bilirubin *Serum Increase Physiological* Cholestatic syndrome *1714*

Bilirubin, Direct *Serum Increase Physiological* Cholestatic syndrome *3810*

BSP Retention *Serum Increase Physiological* Cholestatic syndrome *1714*

Calcium *Serum Increase Physiological* Positive effect on calcium retention *129*

Cholesterol *Serum Increase Physiological* Cholestatic phenomenon *3669*

Corticosteroid-Binding Globulin
Serum Increase Physiological Metabolic effect *368*

Cortisol *Plasma No Effect Physiological* No significant change in 7 male power athletes ingesting anabolic steroids for 12 weeks *94*

Creatine *Urine Decrease Physiological* Anabolic effect *2024*

Creatinine *Urine Decrease Physiological* Anabolic effect *2024*

1,25-Dihydroxy Vitamin D_3 *Serum Increase Physiological* Significant effect observed in postmenopausal osteoporotic women following treatment *874*

Erythropoietin *Serum Increase Physiological* Metabolic effect *368*

Estradiol *Plasma Increase Physiological* Insignificant increase from mean of 0.08 nmol/L to 0.12 nmol/L in 7 male power athletes ingesting anabolic steroids for 12 weeks although mean concentration as high as 0.25 nmol/L at 8 weeks *94*

Factor V *Plasma Increase Physiological* Metabolic effect *368*

Factor VII *Plasma Increase Physiological* Metabolic effect *368*

Factor X *Plasma Increase Physiological* Metabolic effect *368*

Fibrinogen *Plasma Decrease Physiological* Metabolic effect *368*

Follicle Stimulating Hormone
Plasma Decrease Physiological In 7 male power athletes ingesting anabolic steroids for 12 weeks: mean fell from 3.2 to 0.9 IU/L *94*

Glucose *Serum Decrease Physiological* Anabolic effect in fasting state *3669*

β-Glucuronidase *Serum Increase Physiological* Metabolic effect *368*

Growth Hormone *Plasma Increase Physiological* Increase from mean of 0.37 µg/L to 4.1 µg/L in 7 male power athletes ingesting anabolic steroids over 12 weeks: change of up to 60-fold increase in some individuals *94*

Guanase *Serum Increase Physiological* Due to cholestatic syndrome *3669*

Haptoglobin *Serum Increase Physiological* Metabolic effect *368*

3-Hydroxyanthranilic Acid *Urine Decrease Physiological* Effect of synthetic androgens given to males *5085*

3-Hydroxykynurenine *Urine Decrease Physiological* Effect of synthetic androgens given to males *5085*

^{131}I Uptake *Serum No Effect Physiological* No effect observed *3107*

Isocitrate Dehydrogenase *Serum Increase Physiological* Due to cholestatic syndrome *3669*

Kynurenine *Urine Decrease Physiological* Effect of synthetic androgens given to males *5085*

Lactate Dehydrogenase *Serum Increase Physiological* May occur as part of cholestatic syndrome *882*

Luteinizing Hormone *Plasma Decrease Physiological* Decreased from mean baseline concentration of 6.8 IU/L to 4.7 IU/L in 7 male power athletes ingesting anabolic steroids for 12 weeks *94*

5'-Nucleotidase *Serum Increase Physiological* Due to cholestasis *2911*

Osteocalcin *Serum Increase Physiological* Significant effect observed in group of postmenopausal osteoporotic women following treatment (note initial concentration low when compared with that of normal females of same age) *874*

Phosphate *Serum Increase Physiological* Augments phosphate retention *1009*

Plasminogen *Plasma Increase Physiological* Metabolic effect *368*

Prealbumin *Serum Increase Physiological* Metabolic effect *368*

Protein *Serum Increase Physiological* Associated with increased protein synthesis *1095*

Prothrombin Time *Plasma Decrease Physiological* Increased prothrombin as metabolic effect *4176*

Anabolic Steroids *(continued)*

Prothrombin Time *(continued)*
Plasma Increase Physiological Exaggerated response to anticoagulants reported *2754* When coadministered with warfarin increases prothrombin time but mechanism of interaction unknown *2625* Increased INR observed in patients receiving warfarin *886*

Sex-Hormone Binding Globulin
Serum Decrease Physiological Significant reduction observed in 7 male power athletes ingesting anabolic steroids for 12 weeks *94*

Sodium *Serum Increase Physiological* Mineralocorticoid effect with retention *3810*

T3-Uptake *Serum Increase Physiological* Decrease level of thyroxine binding globulin *882* Significant increase observed in 7 male power athletes ingesting anabolic steroids for 12 weeks *94*

Testosterone *Serum Increase Physiological* Insignificant increase in 7 male power athletes ingesting anabolic steroids over 12 weeks: actual change was from mean of 21.8 nmol/L to 25.4 nmol/L. Note actual suppression of endogenous secretion since concentration fell markedly once steroid withdrawn *94*

Thyroid Stimulating Hormone
Serum Decrease Physiological Significant decrease observed in 7 male power athletes ingesting anabolic steroids for 12 weeks *94*

Thyroxine Binding Globulin
Serum Decrease Physiological Significant reduction in 7 male power athletes ingesting anabolic steroids for 12 weeks *94* Direct effect of drug *42*

Thyroxine (T4) *Serum Decrease Physiological* Reduction observed due to decreased TBG *2412* Decrease amount of thyroxine binding globulin *882* Significant reduction in 7 male power athletes ingesting anabolic steroids for 12 weeks *94*

Thyroxine (T4), Free *Serum Decrease Physiological* Significant reduction in 7 male power athletes ingesting anabolic steroids for 12 weeks *94*

Thyroxine (T4) (Murphy-Pattee)
Serum Decrease Physiological Decreases circulating thyroxine binding globulin *882*

Tri-iodothyronine (T3) *Serum Decrease Physiological* Significant reduction in 7 male power athletes ingesting anabolic steroids for 12 weeks *94* Concentration reduced due to decreased TBG *2412*

Triglycerides *Serum Decrease Physiological* Concentration reduced in patients receiving anabolic steroids *4989*

Trypsin *Serum Decrease Physiological* Mean decrease from 7.5 to 5.3 mU/dL in patients with chronic pancreatitis after weeks treatment with combination of anabolic steroids *6067*

Trypsin Inhibitor *Serum Increase Physiological* Metabolic effect *368* Mean increase from 401 to 526 mU/dL in patients with chronic pancreatitis after 3 weeks treatment with combination of anabolic steroids *6067*

Urea Nitrogen *Serum Increase Physiological* Improves nitrogen balance *1009*

Uric Acid *Serum Increase Physiological* Improves nitrogen balance *3810*

Xanthurenic Acid *Urine Decrease Physiological* Effect of synthetic androgens given to males *5085*

Anagrelide

Megakaryocytes *Bone Marrow Decrease Physiological* In 5 patients mean number of megakaryocytes in bone marrow fell from 714/250 hpf to 695/250 hpf during anagrelide treatment *5670*

Platelets *Blood Decrease Physiological* 1 to 1.5 mg orally every 6 hours produced decrease in patients with thrombocytosis after 5 days and reaching normal by day 12 but mechanism unknown *5561* In 12 patients with chronic myelogenous leukemia and a high platelet count treatment with anagrelide caused a significant reduction in platelet count from 970,000 to 3,600,000 /μL to less than 600,000 /μL with a median dose of 1.9 mg/d for a period of at least 4 weeks *6070* In 48 patients with essential thrombocytopenia treatment with anagrelide caused a significant reduction in platelet count from 850,000 to 3,100,000 /μL prior to therapy to less than 450,000 /μL in 23 patients and to above 450,000 /μL in the other 19 with a median maintenance dose of 2.5 mg/d for a period of 12 months in complete responders *4639*

Analgesics

Creatine Kinase *Serum Increase Physiological* May cause effect if injected i.m *403*

Methemoglobin *Blood Increase Physiological* May cause intravascular hemolysis *5870*

Anastrozole

Alanine Aminotransferase *Serum Increase Physiological* Increased activity observed in some patients *6642*

Alkaline Phosphatase *Serum Increase Physiological* Increased activity observed in some patients *6642*

Aspartate Aminotransferase *Serum Increase Physiological* Increased activity observed in some patients *6642*

Cholesterol *Serum Increase Physiological* Mean serum concentration increased by 0.5 mmol/L observed in patients receiving anastrozole *6642*

γ-Glutamyltransferase *Serum Increase Physiological* Increased activity observed in some patients *6642*

Hematocrit *Blood Decrease Physiological* Anemia observed in some patients *6642*

Hemoglobin *Blood Decrease Physiological* Anemia observed in some patients *6642*

LDL-Cholesterol *Serum Increase Physiological* Mean serum concentration increased by 0.5 mmol/L observed in patients receiving anastrozole, mainly attributable to LDL-cholesterol *6642*

Thyroid Stimulating Hormone
Serum No Effect Physiological No significant effect observed on TSH concentration *6642*

Ancrod

Fibrinogen *Plasma Decrease Physiological* Converts to fibrin shreds *4715*

Androsterone

Cholesterol *Serum Decrease Physiological* Therapeutic effect *2024*

Anesthetic Agents

Alanine Aminotransferase *Serum Increase Physiological* Occurs without permanent liver damage *6152*

Aspartate Aminotransferase *Serum Increase Physiological* Occurs without permanent liver damage *6152*

Creatine Kinase *Serum Increase Physiological* Occurs if combined with suxamethonium *2823*

Fluoride *Serum Increase Physiological* Slight effect following general anesthetic *1449*

Glucose *Serum Increase Physiological* Presumed response to stress *409*

Isocitrate Dehydrogenase *Serum Increase Physiological* Occurs without permanent liver damage *6152*

Lactate Dehydrogenase *Serum Increase Physiological* Response occurs even with premedication *6152*

Ornithine Carbamoyltransferase
Serum Increase Physiological Occurs without permanent liver damage *6152*

Osmolality *Urine Increase Physiological* Induction of anesthesia produces marked effect *1449*

Osmolar Clearance *Urine Decrease Physiological* Significant effect with general anesthesia *1449*

Phosphate *Serum Decrease Physiological* Observed after anesthesia *2024*

Potassium *Urine Decrease Physiological* Significant effect with general anesthesia *1449*

Prothrombin Time *Plasma Increase Physiological* Observed effect *2754*

Sodium *Urine Decrease Physiological* Significant effect with general anesthesia *1449*

Thyroid Stimulating Hormone
Serum No Effect Physiological No effect observed *4468*

Volume *Urine Decrease Physiological* Induction of anesthesia produces marked effect *1449*

Angiotensin

Aldosterone *Plasma Increase Physiological* Increase of 4 times normal after i.v. for 1 h *1878*
Urine Increase Physiological Approximate doubling in response to i.v. infusion *5313*

Calcium *Urine Decrease Physiological* Hemodynamic effect of drug *3578*

Effective Renal Plasma Flow
Patient Decrease Physiological Marked decrease following administration *4014*

Epinephrine *Plasma Decrease Physiological* Decreased slightly less than norepinephrine increased *6691*

Glomerular Filtration Rate *Urine Decrease Physiological* Vasoconstrictive effect in kidney *2242*

Magnesium *Urine Decrease Physiological* Hemodynamic effect of drug *3578*

Norepinephrine *Plasma Increase Physiological* Of same magnitude as if norepinephrine given *6691*

Prostaglandin E *Urine Increase Physiological* 2.3 fold increase after 3 h in women *1976*

Prostaglandin F *Urine No Effect Physiological* No effect observed after i.v. infusion *1976*

Protein *Serum Increase Physiological* Hemoconcentration effect *2242*

Renin Activity *Plasma Decrease Physiological* Causes decrease in normals when given i.v *1878*

Sodium *Serum Increase Physiological* Due to salt retaining action of aldosterone *2242*
Urine Decrease Physiological Due to effect on renal tubules *2242*

Tetrahydrodeoxycorticosterone
Urine No Effect Physiological No significant effect when infused in normals *5313*

Uric Acid *Serum Increase Physiological* Reduced urate clearance if given i.v *1851*
Urine Decrease Physiological Decreases urate excretion and renal plasma flow *1851*

Uric Acid Clearance *Urine Decrease Physiological* 44% reduction with infusion *1852*

Vanillylmandelic Acid *Urine No Effect Physiological* Epinephrine decrease compensates for norepinephrine increase *6691*

Volume *Plasma Decrease Physiological* Promotes loss of protein-free filtrate to tissues *2242*
Urine Decrease Physiological Vasoconstrictive effect in kidney *2242*

Angiotensin II

Aldosterone *Plasma Increase Physiological* Mean concentration increased from baseline of 7.1 ng/dL to a peak of 43.5 ng/dL 60 minutes after beginning infusion up to 16 ng/kg/min in 7 normal men *1349*

Corticotropin *Plasma Increase Physiological* Concentration increased from mean baseline of 23 pg/mL to a maximum of 65 pg/mL at 150 minutes following intravenous infusion of up to 16 ng/kg/min for 60 minutes in 7 healthy men *1349*

Cortisol *Plasma Increase Physiological* Slight but progressive increase observed at 90 and 120 minutes in 7 healthy men after infusion of up to 16 ng/kg/min for 60 minutes *1349*

Growth Hormone *Plasma Increase Physiological* Increase from mean baseline concentration of 0.8 ng/mL to peak concentration of 6.5 ng/mL in 7 healthy men following intravenous infusion of up to 16 ng/kg/min for 60 minutes with continuing increase at 150 and 180 minutes *1349*

Prolactin *Plasma No Effect Physiological* No change observed in 7 healthy men following intravenous infusion of up to 16 ng/kg/min for 60 minutes *1349*

Renin Activity *Plasma Decrease Physiological* Significant decrease following infusion of 4 ng/kg body weight per minute in 5 normal men *4007*

Renin Substrate *Plasma No Effect Physiological* No change in concentration following infusion of 4 ng/kg body weight per minute in 5 normal men *4007*

Thyroid Stimulating Hormone
Serum No Effect Physiological No effect observed with infusion of up to 16 ng/kg/min for 60 minutes in 7 healthy men *1349*

Anileridine

Vanillylmandelic Acid *Urine Increase Analytical* Interferes with Pisano procedure *1714*

Aniline

Casts *Urine Increase Physiological* Nephrotoxic effect (chronic effect) *467*

Color *Blood Increase Analytical* May produce chocolate color *467*
Urine Increase Analytical May produce red color *1957* Brown color due to intravascular hemolysis *2183*

Erythrocytes *Blood Decrease Physiological* May cause marked hemolytic anemia *467*

Hemoglobin *Blood Decrease Physiological* Hemolysis in glucose-6-phosphate dehydrogenase deficiency or methemoglobin reductase deficiency may be caused by drug *2873* May cause marked hemolytic anemia *467*

Ionized Calcium *Serum Decrease Analytical* At 0.1 mmol/L to 0.1 mol/L with calcium specific electrode *820*

Methemoglobin *Blood Increase Physiological* Occurs as result of intravascular hemolysis *2183*
Urine Increase Physiological Due to intravascular hemolysis *2183*

Sulfa as Sulfanilamide *Serum Increase Analytical* Reacts in Bratton-Marshall procedure *467*

Urea Nitrogen *Serum Increase Physiological* May cause nephrotoxicity (chronic effect) *467*

Aniline Dyes

Color *Urine Increase Analytical* Red from foods and candy *684*

Anisindione

Bilirubin *Serum Increase Physiological* Observed with other indandiones *2754*

Color *Urine Increase Analytical* Orange (alkaline), pink-red-brown (acid) *3810*

Hemoglobin *Urine Increase Physiological* Overdose manifestation *2754*

Leukocytes *Blood Decrease Physiological* Observed with other indandiones *2754*

Occult Blood *Feces Increase Physiological* May indicate toxicity *2754*

Prothrombin Time *Plasma Increase Physiological* Intended effect *2754*

Uric Acid *Urine No Effect Physiological* No uricosuric action observed *2452*

Anistreplase

Blood *Urine Increase Physiological* Administration has been associated with hematuria in 2.4% treated patients compared with < 1% in placebo-treated controls *4979*

Erythrocytes *Urine Increase Physiological* Hematuria observed in 2.4% of 500 patients receiving drug versus < 1% in those receiving placebo *5643*

Fibrinogen *Plasma Decrease Physiological* Marked decrease in concentration following intravenous administration *5643* Intravenous administration causes marked decrease in concentration *4979*

Hematocrit *Blood Decrease Physiological* Administration has been associated with anemia in < 1% treated patients compared with < 1% in placebo-treated controls *4979*

Hemoglobin *Blood Decrease Physiological* Administration has been associated with anemia in < 1% treated patients compared with < 1% in placebo-treated controls *4979*

Urine Increase Physiological Hematuria may occur as side-effect: frequency of 2.4% observed in 500 patients receiving drug versus < 1% in those receiving placebo *5643*

Occult Blood *Feces Increase Physiological* Administration has been associated with gastrointestinal hemorrhage in 2.4% treated patients compared with < 1% in placebo-treated controls *4979* May occur as a result of gastrointestinal bleeding, one of several severe hemorrhagic complications *1384* Frequency of gastrointestinal hemorrhage of 2.0% in patients receiving drug versus 1.4% in those receiving placebo *5643*

Partial Thromboplastin Time
Plasma Increase Physiological Intravenous administration causes increase in time *4979* Marked increase occurs following intravenous administration *5643*

Plasminogen *Plasma Decrease Physiological* Marked decrease occurs after intravenous administration *5643* Intravenous administration causes marked decrease in concentration *4979*

Prothrombin Time *Plasma Increase Physiological* Intravenous administration causes increase in time *4979* Marked prolongation occurs following intravenous administration *5643*

Thrombin Time *Blood Increase Physiological* Marked increase occurs following intravenous administration *5643* Intravenous administration causes increase in time *4979*

Antacids

Acetylsalicylic Acid *Serum Decrease Physiological* Effect observed in both adults and children with large doses of salicylate due to reduced reabsorption in renal tubules because of alkalinization of urine *2454*

Serum Increase Physiological Increased rate of absorption due to faster drug release *6403* Absorption is faster and maximum serum concentration is higher in the presence of antacids although total amount absorbed is not increased *4062*

Atorvastatin *Serum Decrease Physiological* When Maalox TC suspension was coadministered with atorvastatin its plasma concentration was reduced by about 35% *4534*

Azithromycin *Serum Decrease Physiological* In 10 volunteers when 500 mg azithromycin given immediately after 30 mL Maalox mean peak concentration reduced by 24% but area under concentration curve and time to reach peak unchanged. Extent of absorption unaffected by coadministration of antacid *1928* Decreased oral availability *886*

Calcium *Serum Increase Physiological* May occur if calcium containing preparations *4014*

Cefaclor *Serum Decrease Physiological* Absorption reduced if taken within one hour of ingestion of magesium or aluminum hydroxide containing antacids *1627*

Cefdinir *Serum Decrease Physiological* Concomitant administration of aluminum or magnesium-containing antacids with 300 mg cefdinir reduce absorption of cefdinir. Problem can be avoided by giving cefdinir two hours before or after antacid administration *4528*

Cefpodoxime *Serum Decrease Physiological* Administration of sodium bicarbonate and aluminum hydroxide reduced peak plasma concentration by 24% and the extent of absorption by 27% *4684*

Chlorpromazine *Serum Decrease Physiological* Reduced blood concentration observed when antacid containing aluminum hydroxide and magnesium trisilicate coadministered with an oral suspension of chlorpromazine due to effect on gastrointestinal absorption *1795* Absorption decreased by 10 to 45% due to adsorption by antacid *6403*

Chlortetracycline *Serum Decrease Physiological* Absorption of tetracyclines decreased by up to 80% due to adsorption by antacids *6403*

Ciprofloxacin *Serum Decrease Physiological* Antacids containing magnesium, aluminum and to a lesser extent calcium decrease the absorption of oral ciprofloxacin *1384* Concurrent administration of ciprofloxacin with antacids containing magnesium, aluminum, or calcium may substantially interfere with the absorption of ciprofloxacin and plasma and urine concentrations less than desired *416* Decreased oral availability *886*

Urine Decrease Physiological Concurrent administration of ciprofloxacin with antacids containing magnesium, aluminum, or calcium may substantially interfere with the absorption of ciprofloxacin and plasma and urine concentrations less than desired *416*

Diazepam *Serum Decrease Physiological* Delayed absorption due to adsorption *6403*

Dicyclomine *Serum Decrease Physiological* May interfere with the absorption of anticholinergic agents *2640*

Diflunisal *Serum Decrease Physiological* Concomitant administration of diflunisal with antacids decreased the diflunisal concentration significantly *3972* Concomitant administration of antacids with diflunisal may reduce bioavailability of diflunisal but effect is slight with occasional doses of antacids but may be clinically significant during repeated administration *1384*

Digoxin *Serum Decrease Physiological* By decreasing intestinal digoxin absorption may decrease the digoxin concentration *2161* Reduced absorption due to adsorption and faster gastric emptying *6403*

Doxazosin *Serum No Effect Physiological* Coadministration with doxazosin had no effect on its pharmacokinetics *4642*

Doxycycline *Serum Decrease Physiological* Significantly decreased oral availability *886*

Enoxacin *Serum Decrease Physiological* Antacids containing aluminum hydroxide and magnesium hydroxide reduce the oral absorption of enoxacin by 75% *4940*

Etodolac *Serum Decrease Physiological* Administration of antacids with etodolac may cause reduction in peak etodolac concentration by 15 - 20% but have no detectable effect on the time-to-peak concentration *6559*

Felbamate *Serum No Effect Physiological* Addition of antacids to felbamate regime had no significant effect on gastrointestinal absorption and steady state felbamate concentration *6323* The rate and extent of absorption of felbamate not affected by coadministration of antacids *6324*

Fluconazole *Serum No Effect Physiological* Administration of Maalox® (20 mL) to 14 healthy men prior to a single dose of 100 mg fluconazole had no effect on the absorption or elimination of fluconazole *4645*

Folate *Red Blood Cells Decrease Physiological* Associated with malabsorption *5055*

Serum Decrease Physiological Associated with malabsorption *5055*

Gabapentin *Serum Decrease Physiological* Maalox® reduced the bioavailability of gabapentin in 16 patients by 20% when the compounds were coadministered and by 5% when gabapentin administered 2 hours after Maalox® *4526*

Indinavir *Serum Decrease Physiological* Decreased oral availability *886*

Isoniazid *Serum Decrease Physiological* Delayed and reduced absorption due to adsorption and first-pass metabolism *6403* Decreased oral availability *886*

Ketoconazole *Serum Decrease Physiological* Decreased oral availability *886*

Levodopa *Serum Increase Physiological* Increased absorption with faster gastric emptying *6403*

Nalidixic Acid *Urine Decrease Physiological* May interfere with the absorption of nalidixic acid resulting in lower urine concentrations than desired *5255*

Nitrofurantoin *Serum Decrease Physiological* Antacids containing magnesium trisilicate when administered concomitantly with with nitrofurantoin reduce both the rate and extent of absorption of nitrofurantoin, probably due to adsorption of nitrofurantoin onto the surface of magnesium trisilicate *4800*

Nizatidine *Serum No Effect Physiological* No significant effect noted on absorption *1384*

Norfloxacin *Serum Decrease Physiological* Decreased oral availability *886* Administration of antacids within two hours of norfloxacin administration reported to reduce gastrointestinal absorption of norfloxacin with reduction of plasma and urinary concentrations *3987* Multivitamins, or other products containing iron or zinc, may interfere with the absorption of norfloxacin resulting in lower plasma and urine concentrations *4981*

Urine Decrease Physiological Administration of antacids within two hours of norfloxacin administration reported to reduce gastrointestinal absorption of norfloxacin with reduction of plasma and urinary concentrations *3987* Multivitamins, or other products containing iron or zinc, may interfere with the absorption of norfloxacin resulting in lower plasma and urine concentrations *4981*

Ofloxacin *Serum Decrease Physiological* Quinolines form chelates with alkaline earth and transition metal cations resulting in reduced absorption *3914*

Oxaprozin *Serum No Effect Physiological* Coadministration of antacids with oxaprozin caused no significant effect on the pharmacokinetic parameters of oxaprozin in single or multiple dose studies *2065*

Penicillamine *Serum Decrease Physiological* Reduced absorption due to adsorption and chelation *6403*

pH *Blood Increase Physiological* May cause occasional metabolic alkalosis *128*

Piroxicam *Serum Decrease Physiological* When antacids coadministered with piroxicam plasma levels of piroxicam unchanged *4646*

Serum No Effect Physiological No significant effect observed on piroxicam kinetics when antacids (aluminum and magnesium hydroxides) coadministered with 20 mg piroxicam in 15 healthy volunteers (maximum plasma concentration 1.14 to 1.86 µg/mL and maximum concentration reached after mean 7.5 ± 2.1 h) *390*

Pravastatin *Serum No Effect Physiological* Administration one hour prior to pravastatin caused no significant effect on bioavailability of pravastatin *728*

Proquazone *Serum Decrease Physiological* Delayed absorption noted *6403*

Prothrombin Time *Plasma Decrease Physiological* May shorten action of anticoagulants *2753*

Quinine *Serum Decrease Physiological* Antacids containing aluminum may decrease quinine's effectiveness by delaying or decreasing absorption *1384*

Raloxifene *Serum No Effect Physiological* Aluminum and magnesium hydroxide-containing antacids reported to have no effect on the systemic exposure of raloxifene *1696*

Sildenafil *Serum No Effect Physiological* Single doses of magnesium hydroxide/aluminum hydroxide did not affect the viability of sildenafil *4657*

Sparfloxacin *Serum Decrease Physiological* Magnesium and aluminum containing antacids form chelation complexes with sparfloxacin and must be given either 2 hours before or after sparfloxacin to avoid reducing its bioavailability *4943*

Sulfathiazole *Serum Increase Physiological* Due to faster dissolution rate *6403*

Theophylline *Serum No Effect Physiological* In 15 patients with asthma treated stabilized with theophylline addition of 800 mg aluminum hydroxide with 800 mg magnesium hydroxide t.i.d. for 4 days had no significant effect on maximum plasma concentration, time to the maximum concentration, the area under the 24-h time-concentration curve and mean plasma concentration *4154*

Ticlopidine *Serum Decrease Physiological* Administration of ticlopidine after antacids resulted in a 18% decrease in the plasma concentration of ticlopidine *5034*

Serum Increase Physiological Chronic administration of cimetidine reduced the plasma clearance of a single dose of ticlopidine by 50% *5034*

Tiludronate *Serum Decrease Physiological* Bioavailabilty of tiludronate reduced by 60% when some aluminum or calcium containing antacids are administered one hour before tiludronate *5258*

Trovafloxacin *Serum Decrease Physiological* Coadministration significantly reduces the absorption of trovafloxacin *4663*

Valproic Acid *Serum No Effect Physiological* In a study involving the coadministration of a 500 mg dose of valproate with 160 mEq dose of Maalox, Trisogel or Titralac had no effect on the extent of absorption of valproate *15* Coadministration of valproate 500 mg with commonly administered antacids (Maalox, Trisogel, Titralac - 160 mEq doses) had no effect on the absorption of valproic acid *17*

Warfarin *Plasma No Effect Physiological* Neither concentration nor effect affected *2452*

Antazoline

Creatinine *Serum No Effect Analytical* At concentration of 160 mg/L had no effect on Jaffe-Fuller's earth method *5704* At concentration of 160 mg/L had no effect on Jaffe-Fading-Fraction method *5704*

Leukocytes *Blood Decrease Physiological* Leukopenia *6044*

Platelets *Blood Decrease Physiological* Thrombocytopenia (immunologically induced) *6044*

Uric Acid *Serum No Effect Analytical* At concentration of 160 mg/L had no effect on catalase-AIDH method *5704* At concentration of 160 mg/L had no effect on Kageyama-Hantzsch method *5704*

Anthiolimine

LE Cells *Blood Positive Physiological* Observed effect in some cases *1475*

Anthraquinone

Color *Feces Increase Analytical* Brownish staining *3810*

Urine Increase Analytical Pink, red, purple, orange and rust *4012*

PSP Excretion *Urine Increase Analytical* Interference by color of compound *3257*

Antibiotics

Ascorbic Acid *White Blood Cells Decrease Physiological* Observed effect especially in elderly *5964*

Cholesterol *Serum Increase Physiological* Mean concentration rose from baseline of 109 mg/dL to 136 mg/dL following intravenous antibiotics for 2 weeks in 21 patients with cystic fibrosis *982*

Color *Feces Increase Analytical* Black and white speckling reported with ingestion of antibiotics orally *3388*

C-Reactive Protein *Serum Decrease Physiological* In a group of patients with bacterial infections treatment with antibiotics caused decrease from baseline of 134 ± 122 ng/L to 164 ± 107 ng/L after 1 day, 173 ± 48 ng/L after 2 days and 140 ± 110 ng/L after 3 days *4565*

Digoxin *Serum Increase Physiological* In individuals in whom much digoxin is converted to inactive metabolites in the gastrointestinal tract (approximately 10% patients) concurrent administration of oral antibiotics will markedly increase serum concentration *1384*

Granulocyte Colony Stimulating Factor

Serum Decrease Physiological In a group of patients with bacterial infections treatment with antibiotics caused decrease from baseline of 799 ± 1301 ng/L to 466 ± 1432 ng/L after 1 day, 118 ± 79 ng/L after 2 days and 61 ± 35 ng/L after 3 days *4565*

4-Hydroxy-3-Methoxy-Phenylglycol

Urine No Effect Physiological Orally administered has no effect on excretion *660*

Antibiotics *(continued)*

immunoglobulin A *Serum No Effect Physiological* In 13 adult patients with cystic fibrosis and pulmonary infection treatment with an aminoglycoside and ticarcillin or cephtazidime for 14 days caused mean concentration to change nonsignificantly from 2.50 ± 1.89 g/L to 2.41 ± 1.72 g/L *2502*

Immunoglobulin G *Serum Decrease Physiological* In 13 adult patients with cystic fibrosis and pulmonary infection treatment with an aminoglycoside and ticarcillin or cephtazidime for 14 days caused mean concentration to change significantly from 17.21 ± 5.03 g/L to 16.46 ± 5.42 g/L *2502*

Immunoglobulin M *Serum No Effect Physiological* In 13 adult patients with cystic fibrosis and pulmonary infection treatment with an aminoglycoside and ticarcillin or cephtazidime for 14 days caused mean concentration to change nonsignificantly from 2.60 ± 0.88 g/L to 2.69 ± 0.99 g/L *2502*

Interleukin-6 *Serum Decrease Physiological* In a group of patients with bacterial infections treatment with antibiotics caused decrease from baseline of 639 ± 907 ng/L to 248 ± 403 ng/L after 1 day, 89 ± 95 ng/L after 2 days and 201 ± 240 ng/L after 3 days *4565*

Nitroblue Tetrazolium Test *Blood Decrease Physiological* Index drops in 4-6 h if therapy satisfactory *1483*

Potassium *Serum Decrease Physiological* May occur with multiple regime, ?redistribution *5955*
Urine Increase Physiological Some increase often with multiple regimes *5955*

Prothrombin Time *Plasma Increase Physiological* Decreased synthesis of vitamin K by gastrointestinal tract *6515*

Urobilinogen *Feces Decrease Physiological* Inhibit gastrointestinal tract flora *2024*
Urine Decrease Physiological Inhibit gastrointestinal tract flora *2025*

Vanillylmandelic Acid *Urine No Effect Physiological* Sterilization of gut has no effect on excretion *660*

Anticoagulants

Clotting Time *Blood Increase Physiological* Therapeutic intent *3810*

Color *Feces Increase Analytical* Red to black due to internal bleeding *3810*

Creatine Kinase MB-Isoenzyme *Serum Increase Analytical* Specimens from patients receiving anticoagulants with the exception of lithium heparin may yield falsely high results when CK-MB measured by method on Bayer Technicon Immuno 1® system *420*

Digoxin *Serum No Effect Analytical* No significant interference observed with method on Abbott AxSYM *2923*

Osteocalcin *Serum Decrease Physiological* In men aged 25 to 45 years receiving oral anticoagulant therapy mean concentration 3.0 ng/mL compared with 4.2 ng/mL in controls, in those aged 60 to 80 years 2.9 ng/mL compared with 3.6 ng/mL in controls: in women aged 25 to 45 years mean concentration 2.4 ng/mL compared with 3.4 ng/mL in controls and in those aged 60 to 80 years nonsignificant reduction to 2.2 ng/mL compared with 2.6 ng/mL in controls *2937*

Prothrombin Time *Plasma Increase Physiological* Therapeutic intent *3810*

Anticonvulsants

α_1-Acid Glycoprotein *Serum Increase Physiological* In 8 epileptic patients receiving phenobarbital with carbamazepine or phenytoin *4415*

Alanine Aminopeptidase *Serum Increase Physiological* In those individuals in whom anticonvulsants induced activity alanine aminopeptidase activity also increased (by 23%) *5223*

Alanine Aminotransferase *Serum Increase Physiological* Isolated increased activity in 4-19% of 316 patients who had received antiepileptic therapy for at least 6 months: actual frequency depended on which drug taken *1470* In 99 epileptics undergoing treatment mean activity of 22.5 ± 1.6 U/L significantly higher than 15.1 ± 0.8 U/L in 102 healthy controls *998*

Albumin *Serum Decrease Physiological* In 8 epileptic patients receiving phenobarbital with carbamazepine or phenytoin *4415*
Serum Increase Physiological Mean concentration of 39.0 ± 1.0 g/L in 99 epileptics significantly higher than 35.0 ± 1.0 g/L in 102 healthy controls *998*

Alkaline Phosphatase *Serum Increase Physiological* In 99 epileptics receiving anticonvulsants mean concentration 133.0 ± 5.9 U/L significantly higher than 97.6 ± 3.6 U/L in 102 healthy controls *1397* Effect reported in 10% to 60% of patients in various studies with various anticonvulsants *6526* In 8 epileptic patients receiving phenobarbital with carbamazepine or phenytoin *4415* Occurs in 24% children (90% bony origin) *2783* Isolated increase observed in 16-44% of 316 patients who had taken an antiepileptic drug for at least 6 months: frequency depended on which drug taken *1470*

Amino-4-Imidazole-5-Carboxamide Ribotide
Urine Increase Physiological Occurs with megaloblastic anemia *6370*

δ-Aminolevulinic Acid *Serum Increase Physiological* Highly significant increase when multiple drugs given (146 nmol/L versus 99 nmol/L in controls) *2246*
Urine Increase Physiological Reported in one child *4014*

Antinuclear Antibodies *Serum Increase Physiological* Related to number of drugs, higher in women *6411*

α_1-Antitrypsin *Serum No Effect Physiological* In 8 epileptic patients receiving phenobarbital with carbamazepine or phenytoin *4415*

Ascorbic Acid *Serum No Effect Physiological* In 146 epileptics with long-term treatment *3274* No significant difference in either men or women treated for at least 6 months compared with their respective controls *3276*

Aspartate Aminotransferase
Red Blood Cells Decrease Physiological In treated patients compared with controls *4911* Significant increase in male epileptics compared to controls when pyridoxal-5-phosphate added (ratio increase of 1.82 versus 1.76) in men but no significant vitamin B_6 deficiency noted in women *3276*
Serum Increase Physiological Isolated increases reported in 4-13% of 316 patients who had taken an antiepileptic drug for at least 6 months: frequency depended on which drug taken *1470* Observed with chronic administration *5548* In 99 epileptics undergoing treatment mean activity of 29.4 ± 1.7 U/L significantly higher than 24.5 ± 1.2 U/L in 102 healthy controls *998*

Bilirubin *Serum Decrease Physiological* In 99 epileptics receiving anticonvulsants mean concentration of 0.42 ± 0.02 mg/dL significantly less than 0.49 ± 0.03 mg/dL in 102 control individuals *998*

Biotin *Serum Decrease Physiological* Significant reduction in male epileptics treated for at least 6 months from mean of 345 ng/L to mean of 237 ng/L and from mean of 336 ng/L to 223 ng/L in women *3276* Marked effect in 146 epileptics with long-term treatment *3274*

Calcium *Serum Decrease Physiological* Effect reported in 10% to 60% of patients in various studies with various anticonvulsants *6526* Found in 30% children on prolonged therapy *2783*

Carbamazepine *Serum Decrease Physiological* Coadministration of phenobarbital with valproic acid and phenytoin with carbamazepine caused significant decrease in total carbamazepine concentration *4846*

Carbamazepine, Free *Serum Decrease Physiological* Coadministration of phenobarbital, phenytoin and valproic acid with carbamazepine caused significant increase in free carbamazepine concentration *4846*

Carotene *Serum No Effect Physiological* In 146 epileptics with long-term treatment *3274*

β-Carotene *Serum Increase Physiological* Significant increase from mean of 344 µg/L in control women to 419 µg/L in epileptic women treated for at least 6 months whereas nonsignificant reduction observed in epileptic men versus their controls *3276*

Ceruloplasmin *Serum Increase Physiological* In 8 epileptic patients receiving phenobarbital with carbamazepine or phenytoin *4415*

Complement C_3 *Serum* *No Effect* *Physiological* In 8 epileptic patients receiving phenobarbital with carbamazepine or phenytoin *4415*

Complement C_4 *Serum* *No Effect* *Physiological* In 8 epileptic patients receiving phenobarbital with carbamazepine or phenytoin *4415*

Copper *Hair* *Decrease* *Physiological* In 10 treated male epileptics mean concentration 7.54 µg/g significantly reduced compared with 9.97 µg/g in 16 male controls and 8.53 µg/g in 7 treated female epileptics compared with 12.4 µg/g in 12 female controls *5885*
Serum *Increase* *Physiological* In 7 female treated epileptics mean concentration of 186 µg/dL significantly higher than 154 µg/dL in 10 schizophrenics, but no significant difference between 188 µg/dL in 10 male epileptics and 143 µg/dL in 12 male schizophrenics *5885*

Corticosteroid-Binding Globulin
Serum *Increase* *Physiological* 470 nmol/L versus 320 nmol/L in women and 420 nmol/L versus 320 nmol/L in men on long-term therapy *441* In 8 epileptic patients receiving phenobarbitol with carbmazepine or phenytoin *4415*

Cortisol *Plasma* *Increase* *Physiological* 400 nmol/L versus 260 nmol/L in women on long-term treatment *441*
Plasma *No Effect* *Physiological* No difference in concentrations in men on long-term treatment *441*

1,25-Dihydroxy Vitamin D_3 *Serum* *Decrease* *Physiological* Effect reported in 10% to 60% of patients in various studies with various anticonvulsants *6526*

Erythrocyte Sedimentation Rate
Blood *Increase* *Physiological* Observed with SLE-like syndrome *1475*

Estradiol *Plasma* *No Effect* *Physiological* Insignificantly higher in women on long-term therapy *441*

Factor II *Plasma* *Increase* *Physiological* In 8 epileptic patients receiving phenobarbital with carbamazepine or phenytoin *4415*

Factor VII *Plasma* *Increase* *Physiological* In 8 epileptic patients receiving phenobarbital with carbamazepine or phenytoin *4415*

Factor X *Plasma* *Increase* *Physiological* In 8 epileptic patients receiving phenobarbital with carbamazepine or phenytoin *4415*

Ferritin *Serum* *No Effect* *Physiological* In 8 epileptic patients receiving phenobarbital with carbamazepine or phenytoin *4415*

Folate *Cerebrospinal Fluid* *Decrease* *Physiological* Occurs in many long-treated epileptics *4931*
Red Blood Cells *Decrease* *Physiological* In 39% epileptics on chronic therapy *5973*
Serum *Decrease* *Physiological* In pregnant women treated with anticonvulsants mean concentration significantly less than in healthy pregnant women at same stage of pregnancy *3027* Marked effect in 146 epileptics with long-term treatment *3274* Reduced from mean value of 16.2 nmol/L in male controls to mean of 5.3 nmol/L in epileptic men treated for at least 6 months and in women from mean of 7.0 nmol/L in controls to 5.5 nmol/L in epileptics *3276* May cause megaloblastic anemia *5054*

Follicle Stimulating Hormone
Plasma *Decrease* *Physiological* In 33 male epileptics taking at least one drug for long time *5046*

γ-Globulin *Serum* *Increase* *Physiological* Associated with SLE-like syndrome *1475*

Glucaric Acid *Urine* *Increase* *Physiological* Occurs in 94% children (hepatic enzyme induction) *2783*

γ-Glutamyltransferase *Serum* *Increase* *Physiological* In 99 epileptics receiving anticonvulsants mean concentration 155.6 ± 14.9 U/L significantly increased compared with 49.2 ± 2.3 U/L in 102 healthy controls *998* In 8 epileptic patients receiving phenobarbital with carbamazepine or phenytoin *4415* Isolated increase in activity in 9-89% of 316 patients who had taken an antiepileptic drug for at least 6 months: frequency depended on drug taken *1470*
Urine *Increase* *Physiological* In 55 male epileptics receiving anticonvulsants for a mean of 5.2 years mean activity 2550 mU/mmol creatinine. In 42 female epileptics mean activity 2656 mU/mmol creatinine *3396*

Glutathione Reductase
Red Blood Cells *Decrease* *Physiological* Significant increase above ratio of increase due to flavine adenine dinucleotide of 1.11 in control men to 1.15 in male epileptics and from 1.01 in control women to 1.18 in epileptic women, reflecting vitamin B_2 deficiency *3276*

Haptoglobin *Serum* *Increase* *Physiological* In 8 epileptic patients receiving phenobarbital with carbamazepine or phenytoin *4415*

Hematocrit *Blood* *Decrease* *Physiological* May cause megaloblastic/aplastic anemia *5054*

Hemoglobin *Blood* *Decrease* *Physiological* May cause megaloblastic/aplastic anemia *5054*

25-Hydroxy Vitamin D_3 *Serum* *Decrease* *Physiological* Significant reduction from mean of 137 nmol/L in male controls to mean of 95 nmol/L in male epileptics treated for at least 6 months and from 164 nmol/L in control women to 81 nmol/L in treated women *3276* Probably due to increased metabolism of vitamin D *2402* Effect reported in 10% to 60% of patients in various studies with various anticonvulsants *6526* Marked effect in 146 epileptics with long-term treatment *3274*
Serum *No Effect* *Physiological* No significant difference, although slightly less, in men and women on long-term treatment *441*

25-Hydroxy Vitamin D *Serum* *Decrease* *Physiological* Administration of anticonvulsant drugs significantly correlated with hypovitaminosis D ($p = 0.04$) *6008*

Hydroxybutyrate Dehydrogenase
Serum *Increase* *Physiological* In 21% epileptics on chronic therapy *5973* In 4% epileptics on chronic therapy *5973*

5-Hydroxyindoleacetic Acid
Cerebrospinal Fluid *Decrease* *Physiological* Reduction to 18.3 ng/mL from 25.1 ng/mL in lumbar CSF of treated epileptics *6620*

Hydroxyproline *Urine* *Increase* *Physiological* Effect reported in 10% to 60% of patients in various studies with various anticonvulsants *6526*

immunoglobulin A *Serum* *No Effect* *Physiological* In 8 epileptic patients receiving phenobarbital with carbamazepine or phenytoin *4415*

Immunoglobulin G *Serum* *No Effect* *Physiological* In 8 epileptic patients receiving phenobarbital with carbamazepine or phenytoin *4415*

Immunoglobulin M *Serum* *No Effect* *Physiological* In 8 epileptic patients receiving phenobarbital with carbamazepine or phenytoin *4415*

Indocyanine Green *Serum* *Decrease* *Physiological* Mechanism not yet established *3942*

Indoleacetic Acid
Cerebrospinal Fluid *No Effect* *Physiological* Insignificant reduction to 2.60 ng/mL in lumbar CSF from 3.74 ng/mL in untreated epileptics *6620*

Lactate Dehydrogenase
Red Blood Cells *Increase* *Physiological* In 38% epileptics on chronic therapy *5973*
Serum *Decrease* *Physiological* In 99 epileptics undergoing treatment mean activity 144.8 ± 4.6 U/L significantly reduced compared with 161.6 ± 6.0 U/L in 102 healthy controls *998*
Serum *No Effect* *Physiological* No effect of chronic therapy *5973*

LE Cells *Blood* *Positive* *Physiological* May induce lupus-like syndrome in some cases *2575*

Leucine Aminopeptidase Isoenzymes
Serum *Increase* *Physiological* Increase slower running components *5155*

Leukocytes *Blood* *Decrease* *Physiological* May occur with severe megaloblastic anemia *6370*

Lipid Peroxide *Serum* *No Effect* *Physiological* Mean concentrations of 3.9 nmol MDA/mL in both 15 epileptic patients receiving anticonvulsants and in 13 healthy adult controls *3060*

Luteinizing Hormone *Plasma* *Decrease* *Physiological* In 33 male epileptics taking at least one drug for long time *5046*

Magnesium *Hair* *No Effect* *Physiological* In 10 treated epileptic men mean concentration 53 µg/g not significantly less than 80 µg/g in 16 controls but 52 µg/g in 7 treated epileptic women significantly less than 109 µg/g in 12 female controls *5885*

Anticonvulsants *(continued)*

Magnesium *(continued)*
Serum No Effect Physiological In 10 male treated epileptics mean concentration of 2.63 mg/dL not significantly different from 2.60 mg/dL in 12 schizophrenics and mean of 2.47 mg/dL in 7 female treated epileptics not significantly different from 2.50 mg/dL in 10 schizophrenics *5885*

MCV *Blood Increase Physiological* May cause megaloblastic/aplastic anemia *6370*

Neutrophils *Blood Decrease Physiological* May occur without effect on white cell count *2754*

N-Formiminoglutamic Acid *Urine Increase Physiological* Occurs with megaloblastic anemia *6370*

Phosphate *Serum Decrease Physiological* Disturbance of vitamin D metabolism or hepatic enzyme induction *5721*

Platelets *Blood Decrease Physiological* May occur with severe megaloblastic anemia *6370*

Porphobilinogen *Urine Increase Physiological* Drug related effect reported in one child *4014*

Prealbumin *Serum No Effect Physiological* In 8 epileptic patients receiving phenobarbital with carbamazepine or phenytoin *4415*

Prolactin *Plasma Decrease Physiological* In 33 male epileptics taking at least one drug for long time *5046*

Protein *Serum No Effect Physiological* In 99 epileptics mean concentration of 64.0 g/L not significantly different from that in 102 healthy controls *998*

Prothrombin Time *Plasma No Effect Physiological* In 8 epileptic patients receiving phenobarbital with carbamazepine or phenytoin *4415*

Pyridoxal Phosphate *Serum Decrease Physiological* Significant reduction from mean of 5.67 µg/L in male controls to 4.05 µg/L in male epileptics treated for at least 6 months, but no significant reduction observed in women *3276* Increase by 20% at 4 weeks, 60% at 12 weeks *4910*
Serum No Effect Physiological In 146 epileptics with long-term treatment *3274*

Retinol-binding Protein *Serum Increase Physiological* In 8 epileptic patients receiving phenobarbital with carbamazepine or phenytoin *4415*
Serum No Effect Physiological In 146 epileptics with long-term treatment *3274*

Sex-Hormone Binding Globulin
Serum Increase Physiological 83 nmol/L versus 54 nmol/L in women and 32 nmol/L versus 22 nmol/L in men on long-term treatment *441* In 37 male epileptics mean of 49.0 nmol/L versus 23.3 nmol/L in controls receiving chronic therapy *1230*
Serum No Effect Physiological In 8 epileptic patients receiving phenobarbital with carbamazepine or phenytoin *4415*

Taurine *Plasma No Effect Physiological* Concentration quite variable in epileptics compared with controls; no consistent pattern discernible *2241*
Platelets Decrease Physiological Mean concentration significantly lower in epileptics than in control population *2241*

Testosterone *Serum No Effect Physiological* In 33 male epileptics taking at least one drug for long time *5046* No significant difference in men on long-term therapy *441* Insignificant increase in 37 men versus control population on chronic therapy *1230*

Testosterone, Free *Serum Decrease Physiological* 0.35 nmol/L versus 0.55 nmol/L in 37 men on chronic therapy *1230*

Thyroxine Binding Globulin *Serum No Effect Physiological* No difference in men or women on long-term therapy *441* In 8 epileptic patients receiving phenobarbital with carbamazepine or phenytoin *4415*

Thyroxine (T4) *Serum Decrease Physiological* 79 nmol/L versus 99 nmol/L in women and 82 nmol/L versus 100 nmol/L in men on long-term treatment *441* In epileptic pregnant women mean concentration in first and second trimesters about 8 µg/dL compared with 14 µg/dL in healthy pregnant women at same stage of pregnancy and 10.5 µg/dL in third trimester in epileptic women compared with 14 µg/dL in third trimester in healthy pregnant women *3027*

Thyroxine (T4), Free *Serum Decrease Physiological* 16 pmol/L versus 23 pmol/L in women and 16 pmol/L versus 19 pmol/L in men on long-term treatment *441*

Tocopherol *Serum No Effect Physiological* No significant difference between mean concentration of 1.09 mg/dL in 184 adult epileptics receiving anticonvulsants and of 1.12 mg/dL in 22 healthy adult controls *3060*

α-Tocopherol *Serum No Effect Physiological* Nonsignificant reduction in 184 antiepileptic patients (mean concentration 0.92 mg/dL) compared with 1.01 mg/dL in 22 healthy adults *3060*

β-Tocopherol *Serum No Effect Physiological* No significant difference in mean concentration (0.012 mg/dL) in 184 adults receiving anticonvulsants and in 22 healthy adult controls (0.006 mg/dL) *3060*

δ-Tocopherol *Serum No Effect Physiological* No significant difference between concentrations in healthy adults and in those receiving anticonvulsants *3060*

γ-Tocopherol *Serum No Effect Physiological* No significant difference between mean concentrations in 184 patients receiving anticonvulsants (0.15 mg/dL) and in 22 healthy adult controls (0.11 mg/dL) *3060*

Transketolase *Red Blood Cells No Effect Physiological* Minimal reduction in male epileptics from mean of 1.12 units in controls to 1.11 in epileptics. No change observed in women *3276*

Tri-iodothyronine (T3) *Serum Decrease Physiological* 1.6 nmol/L versus 1.9 nmol/L in women and 1.7 nmol/L versus 2.0 nmol/L in men on long-term treatment *441*

Tryptophan *Cerebrospinal Fluid No Effect Physiological* Insignificant reduction to 325 ng/mL from 379 ng/mL in untreated epileptics *6620*

Uroporphyrin *Urine Increase Physiological* Drug related effect reported in one child *4014*

Vitamin A *Serum Decrease Physiological* Significant reduction from mean of 577 µg/L in controls to 527 µg/L in epileptic women treated for at least 6 months but no significant change observed in men *3276*
Serum No Effect Physiological In 146 epileptics with long-term treatment *3274*

Vitamin B_1 *Serum No Effect Physiological* In 146 epileptics with long-term treatment *3274*

Vitamin B_2 *Serum No Effect Physiological* In 146 epileptics with long-term treatment *3274*

Vitamin B_{12} *Cerebrospinal Fluid Decrease Physiological* Significantly lower with long term therapy *1960*
Serum Decrease Physiological Significantly lower than normal controls *4014* Significant reduction in male epileptics treated for at least 6 months from mean of 572 pmol/L to mean of 369 pmol/L but no significant reduction observed in women *3276*
Serum No Effect Physiological In 146 epileptics with long-term treatment *3274*

Vitamin D Binding Globulin *Serum No Effect Physiological* No significant difference in men or women on long-term treatment *441*

Vitamin E *Serum Decrease Physiological* Significant reduction from mean of 13.1 mg/L in control men to 10.1 mg/L in epileptic men treated for at least 6 months but increase observed in women *3276*
Serum Increase Physiological Significant increase from mean of 9.6 mg/L in control women to 10.5 mg/L in epileptic women treated for at least 6 months but reduction observed in men *3276*
Serum No Effect Physiological In 146 epileptics with long-term treatment *3274*

Zinc *Hair Decrease Physiological* In 10 male treated epileptics mean concentration 140 µg/g significantly less than 172 µg/g in 16 male controls and 150 µg/g in 7 treated female epileptics compared with 160 µg/g in 12 control women *5885*
Serum Decrease Physiological In 10 treated male epileptics mean concentration 104 µg/dL significantly reduced compared with 141µg/dL in 12 schizophrenics and insignificant difference of 110 µg/dL in 7 treated female epleptics compared with 115 µg/dL in 10 female schizoprenics *5885*

Antidepressants

Albumin *Serum No Effect Physiological* In 24 patients with major depression treated with antidepressants caused mean serum concentration of 40.1 ± 3.1 g/L to change nonsignificantly to 39.4 ± 4.3 g/L *6189*

Biopterin *Serum No Effect Physiological* Depressant drugs have no significant effect on plasma concentrations *2493*

α_1-Globulin *Serum No Effect Physiological* In 24 patients with major depression treated with antidepressants caused mean serum concentration of 2.39 ± 0.39 g/L to change nonsignificantly to 2.34 ± 0.41 g/L *6189*

α_2-Globulin *Serum No Effect Physiological* In 24 patients with major depression treated with antidepressants caused mean serum concentration of 6.54 ± 1.23 g/L to change nonsignificantly to 6.37 ± 1.25 g/L *6189*

β-Globulin *Serum No Effect Physiological* In 24 patients with major depression treated with antidepressants caused mean serum concentration of 7.84 ± 1.19 g/L to change nonsignificantly to 7.84 ± 1.25 g/L *6189*

γ-Globulin *Serum No Effect Physiological* In 24 patients with major depression treated with antidepressants caused mean serum concentration of 7.07 ± 1.55 g/L to change nonsignificantly to 7.38 ± 1.32 g/L *6189*

5-Hydroxytryptamine *Platelets Decrease Physiological* In 30 drug-free depressed patients treatment with antidepressants caused mean concentration to decrease significantly from mean baseline of 1.405 ng/10^9 platelets to 0.722 ± 0.19 ng/10^9 platelets after one month, 0.452 ± 0.15 ng/10^9 platelets after 2 months and 0.255 ± 0.06 ng/10^9 platelets after 3 months *3041*

Interleukin-6 *Serum No Effect Physiological* In 17 patients with major depression subchronic treatment with fluoxwtine or tricyclic antidepressants caused insignificant change to mean concentration of 3.82 ± 0.58 pg/mL from mean baseline concentration of 4.37 ± 0.83 pg/mL *3734*

Platelets *Blood No Effect Physiological* In 30 drug-free depressed patients mean concentration of treatment with antidepressants caused nonsignificant change from mean baseline of 369000 ± 19000 /μL to 408000 ± 20000 /μL after 1 month, 382000 ± 21000 /μL after 2 months and 353000 ± 17000 /μL after 3 months *3041*

Protein *Serum No Effect Physiological* In 24 patients with major depression treated with antidepressants caused mean serum concentration of 64.0 ± 4.0 g/L to change nonsignificantly to 63.4 ± 5.8 g/L *6189*

Soluble Interleukin-2 Receptor *Serum No Effect Physiological* In 17 patients with major depression subchronic treatment with fluoxwtine or tricyclic antidepressants caused insignificant change to mean concentration of 288 ± 28 U/mL from mean baseline concentration of 291 ± 25 U/mL *3734*

Soluble Interleukin-6 Receptor *Serum No Effect Physiological* In 17 patients with major depression subchronic treatment with fluoxwtine or tricyclic antidepressants caused insignificant change to mean concentration of 91.3 ± 7.7 ng/mL from mean baseline concentration of 86.7 ± 8.0 ng/mL *3734*

Transferrin Receptor *Serum No Effect Physiological* In 17 patients with major depression subchronic treatment with fluoxwtine or tricyclic antidepressants caused insignificant change to mean concentration of 607 ± 41 U/mL from mean baseline concentration of 575 ± 40 U/mL *3734*

Valproic Acid *Serum No Effect Physiological* Inhibition of cytochrome P450 isoenzymes has relatively little effect on the metabolism of valproic acid since P450 microsomal mediated oxidation is a relatively minor secondary pathway *17*

Antifungal Agents

Alanine Aminotransferase *Serum Increase Physiological* Hepatotoxicity may occur *2024*

Alkaline Phosphatase *Serum Increase Physiological* Hepatotoxicity may occur *2024*

Aspartate Aminotransferase *Serum Increase Physiological* Hepatotoxicity may occur *2024*

Bile *Urine Increase Physiological* Hepatotoxicity may occur *2024*

Bilirubin *Serum Increase Physiological* Hepatotoxic effect *2024*

BSP Retention *Serum Increase Physiological* Hepatotoxic effect may impede clearance *2024*

Antihemophiliac Factor (Recombinant)

Antihemophiliac Factor *Plasma Increase Physiological* Administration provides a rapid increase in circulating AHF concentration *935*

Factor VIII Antibodies *Serum Increase Physiological* In a study of previously untreated patients with hemophilia A inhibitor antibodies developed in 17 of 92 patients, 26.7% in patients with severe disease and 11% in patients with moderate disease but 0% in 18 patients with mild disease *937* Administration may provoke development of neutralizing antibodies although true immunogenicity of recombinant AHF not established *937* Prevalence of antibodies in patients receiving plasma derived AHF is 10-20%, typically IgG antibodies *935*

Hemoglobin *Blood Decrease Physiological* In one patient who received 13 infusions out of many receiving a total of 13,394 infusions epistaxis observed associated with each infusion *935*

Antihistamines

Glucose *Serum Decrease Physiological* May occur in susceptible individuals especially children *1334*

^{131}I Uptake *Serum Decrease Physiological* Uncommon reported effect *3669*

Partial Thromboplastin Time *Plasma Decrease Physiological* Reported to partially counteract the anticoagulant action of sodium heparin *6557*

Prothrombin Time *Plasma Decrease Physiological* Accelerate metabolism of anticoagulants *3810*

Antihypertensive Agents

Cholesterol *Serum Increase Physiological* Mean concentration in 1929 medicated individuals 199.1 mg/dL significantly higher than 195.1 mg/dL in 13986 nonmedicated individuals *5847*

HDL-Cholesterol *Serum Decrease Physiological* In 1929 hypertensive individuals receiving antihypertensive medication mean concentration 48.3 mg/dL significantly less than 50.8 mg/dL in 13986 nonmedicated controls *5847*

Homocysteine *Plasma Increase Physiological* In 587 patients with angiographically confirmed coronary artery disease mean concentration 0.7 μmol/L higher in those receiving hypertensive therapy than in those not receiving such therapy *4343*

17-Hydroxycorticosteroids *Urine Increase Analytical* Some may be measured as analytes *467*

17-Ketosteroids *Urine Increase Analytical* Some may be measured as analytes *467*

Antilymphocytic Agents

Platelets *Blood Decrease Physiological* Observed less commonly with other immunosuppressants *5777*

Antimalarials

Bilirubin *Serum Increase Physiological* May cause hemolytic anemia *3094*

Bilirubin, Direct *Serum Increase Physiological* May cause hemolytic anemia *3094*

Erythrocytes *Blood Decrease Physiological* May cause hemolytic anemia *3094*

Glutathione, Reduced *Red Blood Cells Decrease Physiological* Occurs prior to overt hemolysis *3094*

Heinz Body Formation *Blood Positive Physiological* Occurs prior to overt hemolysis *3094*

Antimalarials *(continued)*

Hematocrit *Blood Decrease Physiological* May cause hemolytic anemia *3094*

Hemoglobin *Blood Decrease Physiological* May cause hemolytic anemia *3094*

Plasma Increase Physiological Occurs with marked hemolysis *3094*

Urine Increase Physiological May occur with marked hemolysis *3094*

Methemoglobin *Blood Increase Physiological* May cause hemolytic anemia *3094*

Reticulocytes *Blood Increase Physiological* Occurs during recovery from hemolysis *3094*

Antimicrobial Therapy

α_1-Acid Glycoprotein *Serum Decrease Physiological* In 22 children hospitalized with urinary tract infection mean concentration decreased from 1.96 g/L on admission to 1.62 g/L after 6 days treatment *913*

Amyloid A Protein *Serum Decrease Physiological* In 22 children hospitalized with urinary tract infection mean concentration decreased from 1,084 mg/L at time of admission to 13 mg/L after 6 days treatment *913*

α_1-Antichymotrypsin *Serum Decrease Physiological* In 22 children hospitalized with urinary tract infection mean concentration decreased from 1.11 g/L at time of admission to 0.95 g/L after 6 days treatment *913*

C-Reactive Protein *Serum Decrease Physiological* In 22 children hospitalized with urinary tract infection mean concentration decreased from 122 mg/L on day of admission to 9 mg/L after 6 days treatment *913*

Antineoplastic Agents

Erythrocytes *Blood Decrease Physiological* May cause aplastic anemia *3810*

Hydroxyproline *Urine Decrease Physiological* Catabolic action of cytostatics *6111*

Leukocytes *Blood Decrease Physiological* Often therapeutic intent *3810*

Phenytoin *Serum Decrease Physiological* Decreased plasma condition *886*

Platelets *Blood Decrease Physiological* May cause aplastic anemia *3810*

Uric Acid *Serum Increase Physiological* Destruction of nucleoprotein *189*

Antiplatelet Therapy

α_2-Antiplasmin Inhibitor/Plasmin Complex
Plasma No Effect Physiological In 10 patients with cardioembolic stroke nonsignificant increase from mean baseline of 0.6 ± 0.2 µg/mL to 1.1 ± 0.9 µg/mL observed with treatment *6587*

Antithrombin III *Plasma Increase Physiological* In 10 patients with cardioembolic stroke treatment with antiplatelet therapy caused nonsignificant increase from mean baseline of 93 ± 17% to 106 ± 14% *6587*

D-Dimer *Plasma Increase Physiological* In 10 patients with cardioembolic stroke treatment with antiplatelet agents caused nonsignificant increase from mean baseline of 161 ± 127 ng/mL to 239 ± 316 ng/mL *6587*

Fibrinopeptide A *Plasma Increase Physiological* In 10 patients with cardioembolic stroke treatment caused nonsignificant increase from mean baseline of 5.6 ± 5.3 ng/mL to 9.1 ± 14.0 ng/mL *6587*

Protein C Activity *Plasma No Effect Physiological* In 10 patients with cardioembolic stroke treatment caused nonsignificant change from mean baseline of 124 ± 27% to 122 ± 34% *6587*

Protein C Antigen *Plasma Increase Physiological* In 10 patients with cardioembolic stroke treatment caused nonsignificant increase from mean baseline of 121 ± 32% to 131 ± 32% *6587*

Thrombin/Antithrombin III Complex
Plasma Increase Physiological In 10 patients with cardioembolic stroke treatment with antiplatelet therapy caused nonsignificant increase from 6.1 ± 7.6 ng/mL to 8.9 ± 17.1 ng/mL *6587*

Antipsychotics

Cholesterol *Serum No Effect Physiological* In 14 nonschizophrenic patients treated with antipsychotic drugs mean concentration of 6.3 ± 2.2 µmol/L not significantly different from 6.4 ± 0.9 µmol/L in 14 normal controls *3882*

Homovanillic Acid
Cerebrospinal Fluid Increase Physiological In 14 schizophrenics treatment caused nonsignificant increase from mean baseline of 31.6 ± 17.3 ng/mL to 35.2 ± 21.1 ng/mL *5476*

Lipid Peroxide *Serum No Effect Physiological* In 14 nonschizophrenic patients treated with antipsychotic drugs mean concentration of 0.75 ± 0.39 µmol/L not significantly different from 0.74 ± 0.15 µmol/L in 14 normal controls *3882*

Somatostatin *Cerebrospinal Fluid Increase Physiological* In 14 schizophrenics treatment caused significant increase from mean baseline of 22.7 ± 7.2 to 25.1 ± 8.5 *5476*

Tricyclic Antidepressants *Serum Increase Physiological* Interact pharmacokinetically to inhibit metabolism of tricyclic antidepressants *3590*

Vitamin E *Serum No Effect Physiological* In 14 nonschizophrenic patients treated with antipsychotic drugs mean concentration of 30.2 ± 7.8 µmol/L not significantly different from 29.5 ± 6.3 µmol/L in 14 normal controls *3882*

Vitamin E:Cholesterol Ratio *Serum No Effect Physiological* In 14 nonschizophrenic patients treated with antipsychotic drugs mean ratio of 5.1 ± 0.4 not significantly different from 4.6 ± 0.7 in 14 normal controls *3882*

Antipyretics

Bilirubin *Serum Increase Physiological* Occurs with hemolytic anemia *3094*

Bilirubin, Direct *Serum Increase Physiological* Occurs with hemolytic anemia *3094*

Erythrocytes *Blood Decrease Physiological* May cause hemolytic anemia *3094*

Glutathione, Reduced
Red Blood Cells Decrease Physiological Sharp fall before overt hemolysis *3094*

Heinz Body Formation *Blood Positive Physiological* Occurs prior to overt hemolysis *3094*

Hematocrit *Blood Decrease Physiological* May cause hemolytic anemia *3094*

Hemoglobin *Blood Decrease Physiological* May cause hemolytic anemia *3094*

Plasma Increase Physiological May occur with marked hemolysis *3094*

Urine Increase Physiological Occurs with marked hemolysis *3094*

Porphyrin, Total *Urine Increase Physiological* Reported effect *2024*

Reticulocytes *Blood Increase Physiological* Occurs during recovery from hemolysis *3094*

Antipyrine

Acetoacetate *Urine Increase Analytical* Interferes with ferric chloride test *4012*

Bilirubin *Serum Increase Physiological* Hemolysis in G-6-PD deficiency *402*

Bromide *Serum No Effect Analytical* No effect of antipyrine at concentration of 100 µmol/L when solutions measured by fluorescein or fluorescent excitation methods *692*

Bromine *Serum Decrease Analytical* When total body water or ECF water measured by either gold chloride or rosaniline method inhibitory effect on bromine space corresponded to about 17% for each 100 µmol/L of antipyrine added. With rosaniline method reduction of about 17% for each 100 µmol/L added *692*

Casts *Urine Increase Physiological* May cause nephrotoxicity *467*

Cells *Urine Increase Physiological* Renal action of drug *6447*

Color *Urine Increase Analytical* Red brown (green in reflected light) *3810*

Erythrocytes *Blood Decrease Physiological* Hemolytic anemia in G-6-PD deficient persons *1212*

Ferric Chloride Test *Urine Positive Analytical* May produce red color *684*

Glucaric Acid *Urine Increase Physiological* Reported induction of hepatic enzymes *2782*

Glucose *Serum Increase Physiological* Severe hyperglycemia unresponsive to insulin *4014*
Urine Increase Physiological Renal action of drug *6447*

Heinz Body Formation *Blood Positive Physiological* Occurs initially prior to hemolysis *3094*

Hematocrit *Blood Decrease Physiological* Hemolytic anemia in G-6-PD deficient persons *1212*

Hemoglobin *Blood Decrease Physiological* Hemolytic anemia in G-6-PD deficient persons *1212*
Urine Increase Physiological Occurs with marked hemolysis *3094*

Leukocytes *Blood Decrease Physiological* Leukopenia/agranulocytosis *4014*

Methemalbumin *Serum Increase Physiological* Occurs with intravascular hemolysis *1212*

Methemoglobin *Blood Increase Physiological* Increase seldom occurs *2242*

Neutrophils *Blood Decrease Physiological* Myelotoxic action of drugs *4014*

Phenylketones *Urine Positive Analytical* Red fading with $FeCl_3$, pink to red with Phenistix® *1195*

Platelets *Blood Decrease Physiological* Associated with hemolytic anemia *4014*

Protein *Urine Increase Physiological* Renal action of drug *6447*

Prothrombin Time *Plasma Decrease Physiological* Observed in man and experimental animals *4014*
Plasma Increase Physiological Patients on coumarins *4014*

Reticulocytes *Blood Increase Physiological* Occurs with hemolytic anemia (recovery) *1212*

Sugar *Urine Increase Analytical* Acts as reducing agent *4012*

Urea Nitrogen *Serum Increase Physiological* May cause nephrotoxicity *467*

Urobilinogen *Feces Increase Physiological* Occurs with hemolytic anemia *1212*
Urine Increase Analytical Produces similar color with Ehrlich's reagent *6515*
Urine Increase Physiological Occurs with hemolytic anemia *1212*

Warfarin *Plasma Decrease Physiological* In some patients receiving long-term warfarin treatment plasma concentration decreased and reduced prothrombin time response to warfarin: probably related to hepatic microsomal enzyme induction *6428*

Antithyroid Therapy

Alkaline Phosphatase *Serum Decrease Physiological* Mean activity in 15 women with active Graves' thyrotoxicosis of 2.18 ± 0.2 µkat/L significantly reduced to 1.25 ± 1.0 µkat/L with antithyroid therapy *1418*

Calcium *Serum No Effect Physiological* Mean concentration in 15 women with active Graves' thyrotoxicosis of 2.42 ± 0.04 mmol/L not significantly reduced to 2.35 ± 0.07 mmol/L with antithyroid therapy *1418*

Erythrocytes *Blood Increase Physiological* In 13 hyperthyroid patients treatment with propylthiouracil or thiamazole until the patients were euthyroid caused significant increase from mean baseline of 4.65 ± 0.64 million /µL to 5.14 ± 0.48 million /µL *3312*

Ferritin *Serum Decrease Physiological* In 13 hyperthyroid patients treatment with propylthiouracil or thiamazole until the patients became euthyroid caused significant reduction from mean baseline of 89.5 ± 60.4 µg/L to 24.3 ± 15.8 µg/L *3312*

Hematocrit *Blood Increase Physiological* In 13 hyperthyroid patients treatment with propylthiouracil or thiamazole until the patients became euthyroid caused significant increase from mean baseline of 0.382 ± 0.040 to 0.418 ± 0.042 *3312*

Hemoglobin *Blood Increase Physiological* In 13 hyperthyroid patients treatment with propylthiouracil or thiamazole to produce euthyroid state caused significant increase of mean hemoglobin concentration from 129 ± 16 g/L to 143 ± 15 g/L *3312*

Iron *Serum No Effect Physiological* In 13 hyperthyroid patients treatment with propylthiourcil or thiamazole until they became euthyroid caused nonsignificant change from mean baseline of 19 ± 5 µmol/L to 19 ± 9 µmol/L *3312*

Iron-Binding Capacity, Total *Serum Increase Physiological* In 13 hyperthyroid patients treatment with propylthiouracil or thiamazole until they became euthyroid caused significant increase from mean baseline of 55 ± 11 µmol/L to 71 ± 8 µmol/L *3312*

Iron Saturation *Serum Decrease Physiological* In 13 patients with hyperthyroidism treatment for a mean of 11 ± 6 weeks caused significant reduction from mean baseline of 36.7 ± 10.6% to 26.6 ± 12.9% *3312*

Leukocytes *Blood No Effect Physiological* In 13 hyperthyroid patients treatment with propylthiouracil or thiamazole until the patients became euthyroid caused no significant effect on the leukocyte count *3312*

Osteocalcin *Serum Decrease Physiological* Mean concentration in 15 women with active Graves' thyrotoxicosis of 7.5 ± 0.8 ng/mL significantly reduced to 4.7 ± 0.5 ng/mL with antithyroid therapy *1418*

Platelets *Blood No Effect Physiological* In 13 hyperthyroid patients treatment with propylthiouracil or thiamazole until they became euthyroid caused no significant difference in concentration *3312*

Thyroxine (T4) *Serum Decrease Physiological* Mean concentration in 15 women with active Graves' thyrotoxicosis of 218 ± 12 nmol/L significantly reduced to 97 ± 8 nmol/L with antithyroid therapy *1418*

ANTU

Sugar *Urine Increase Analytical* May reduce Fehling's and Benedict's solutions *467*

Apalcillin

Antithrombin III *Plasma Decrease Physiological* In 21 volunteers with doses up to 225 mg/kg *2089*

Fibrinogen *Plasma No Effect Physiological* In 21 volunteers with doses up to 225 mg/kg *2089*

Partial Thromboplastin Time
Plasma No Effect Physiological In 21 volunteers with doses up to 225 mg/kg *2089*

Prothrombin Time *Plasma No Effect Physiological* In 21 volunteers with doses up to 225 mg/kg *2089*

Thrombin Time *Blood No Effect Physiological* In 21 volunteers with doses up to 225 mg/kg *2089*

Apiol

Alanine Aminotransferase *Serum Increase Physiological* May cause severe liver damage *467*

Aspartate Aminotransferase *Serum Increase Physiological* May cause severe liver damage *467*

Casts *Urine Increase Physiological* May cause nephrotoxicity *467*

Apiol *(continued)*

Urea Nitrogen *Serum Increase Physiological* May cause nephrotoxicity *467*

Apomorphine

Cannabinoids *Urine No Effect Analytical* No effect on Roche Abuscreen method *5006*

Carbon Dioxide Partial Pressure
Blood Increase Physiological May depress respiration *2242*

Growth Hormone *Plasma Increase Physiological* 7 fold increase at 30-45 minutes in 6 children after 12 mg/kg subcutaneously *3834* In control healthy subjects i.v. injection increased mean concentration from 1.8 to 28.3 ng/mL, but weak effect in schizophrenic patients only *5321* Effect greater with 5 μg/kg in 8 depressed individuals than with 1.3 μg/kg of clonidine *1135*

Homovanillic Acid *Plasma No Effect Physiological* No effect when given i.v. to either healthy controls or schizophrenics *5321*

Morphine *Urine No Effect Analytical* Insignificant cross reactivity with RIA procedures *4163*

Prolactin *Plasma Decrease Physiological* In control subjects reduced by 57% when given i.v *5321*

Thyroid Stimulating Hormone
Serum Decrease Physiological In hypothyroidism but can lower basal and TRH-stimulated values *6412*
Serum No Effect Physiological In euthyroids but can lower basal and TRH-stimulated values *6412*

Aprindine

Alanine Aminotransferase *Serum Increase Physiological* Hepatitis is manifestation of chronic toxicity *5395* Hepatitis in 2 patients within 3 weeks of start of therapy resolved with withdrawal of drug *2568*

Alkaline Phosphatase *Serum Increase Physiological* Hepatitis is manifestation of chronic toxicity *5395* Hepatitis in 2 patients within 3 weeks of start of therapy resolved with withdrawal of drug *2568*

Aspartate Aminotransferase *Serum Increase Physiological* Hepatitis is manifestation of chronic toxicity *5395* Hepatitis in 2 patients within 3 weeks of start of therapy resolved with withdrawal of drug *2568*

Bilirubin *Serum Increase Physiological* Hepatitis is manifestation of chronic toxicity *5395* Hepatitis in 2 patients within 3 weeks of start of therapy resolved with withdrawal of drug *2568*

Granulocytes *Blood Decrease Physiological* Agranulocytosis observed in 6.4% of patients versus 0.4% controls: drug identified as being independently associated with agranulocytosis *3098*

Neutrophils *Blood Decrease Physiological* Agranulocytosis may occur between 4th and 16th week of treatment: may be quite severe: usually reversible. Occurs with frequency of 0.1 to 1.0% *5395*

Aprobarbital

Phenobarbital *Serum No Effect Analytical* Cross-reactivity of less than 1.3% with method on Baxter Stratus *5705*

Primidone *Serum No Effect Analytical* At a concentration of more than 1250 mg/L causes 25% increase in concentration as measured by method on Baxter Stratus but clinical concentration only 20 mg/L *5705*

Apronalide

δ-Aminolevulinic Acid *Urine Increase Physiological* May precipitate acute porphyria *2210*

Clot Retraction *Blood Decrease Physiological* Immunological effect *2385*

Coproporphyrin *Feces Increase Physiological* May precipitate acute porphyria *2210*
Urine Increase Physiological May precipitate acute porphyria *2210*

Platelets *Blood Decrease Physiological* Immunological mechanism *4014* Thrombocytopenia (immunologically-induced) *3810*

Porphobilinogen *Urine Increase Analytical* Produces red color with Ehrlich's reagent *2559*
Urine Increase Physiological May precipitate acute porphyria *2210*

Porphyrin, Total *Urine Increase Physiological* May precipitate attack of acute porphyria *4014*

Protoporphyrin *Feces Increase Physiological* May precipitate acute porphyria *2210*

Urobilinogen *Urine Increase Analytical* Produces red color with Ehrlich's reagent *2559*

Arabinose

Glucuronic Acid *Urine Increase Analytical* Large effect on orcinol procedure *612*
Urine No Effect Analytical Minimal effect on carbazole and m-hydroxydiphenyl procedures *612*

Sugar *Urine Increase Analytical* False positive with Benedict's reagent *2559*

Ardeparin

Alanine Aminotransferase *Serum Increase Physiological* Asymptomatic hyperalanine aminotransferasemia of greater than 3 times the upper limit of normal observed in 4 of 16 normal individuals and in 8.7% of patients *6561*

Anti-Factor IIa *Plasma Increase Physiological* After single dose subcutaneous administration of 30 U/kg anti-Xa peak plasma activity barely detectable but peak concentration of 0.07 ± 0.02 U/mL after 100 U/kg, reached in 3.0 ± 1.0 h *6561*

Anti-Factor Xa *Plasma Increase Physiological* After single dose subcutaneous administration of 30 to 100 U/kg anti-Xa peak plasma activity of 0.09 ± 0.03 to 0.32 ± 0.05 U/mL, reached in 2.7 ± 0.6 h *6561*

Aspartate Aminotransferase *Serum Increase Physiological* Asymptomatic hyperaspartate aminotransferasemia of greater than 3 times the upper limit of normal observed in 2 of 16 normal individuals and in 5.5% of patients *6561*

Blood *Urine Increase Physiological* Bleeding can occur from any site as a side effect *6561*

Hematocrit *Blood Decrease Physiological* Bleeding can occur from any site as a side effect *6561*

Occult Blood *Feces Increase Physiological* Bleeding can occur from any site as a side effect *6561*

Platelets *Blood Decrease Physiological* In controlled clinical trials incidence of thrombocytopenia with platelet count of less than 100,000 /μL (2%) comparable to that following aspirin (1%), warfarin (2%) or placebo (0%) *6561*

Triglycerides *Serum Increase Physiological* As with heparin sodium hypertriglyceridemia observed in patients treated with ardeparin *6561*

Argatroban

Factor X *Plasma No Effect Physiological* In patients receiving argatroban as a 350 μg/kg bolus followed by a 5 - 10 μg/kg per minute infusion factor X values were 80 ± 15% *2708*

Arsenicals

Alanine Aminotransferase *Serum Increase Physiological* Hepatotoxic effect (cholestasis/cholangiolitis) *3669*

Alkaline Phosphatase *Serum Decrease Analytical* Arsenates are inhibitors of enzyme in laboratory procedures *6026*
Serum Increase Physiological Hepatotoxic effect (cholestasis/cholangiolitis) *3669*

Aspartate Aminotransferase *Serum Increase Physiological* Hepatotoxic effect (cholestasis/cholangiolitis) *3669*

Bile *Urine Increase Physiological* Hepatotoxicity (cholestasis/cholangiolitis) *3810*

Bilirubin *Serum Increase Physiological* Hepatotoxic effect (cholestasis/cholangiolitis) *3669*

BSP Retention *Serum Increase Physiological* Hepatotoxic effect (cholestasis/cholangiolitis) *3669*

Casts *Urine Increase Physiological* Nephrotoxic effect *3810*

Cholesterol *Serum Increase Physiological* Hepatotoxic effect (may be very high) *3669*

Creatinine *Serum Increase Physiological* Nephrotoxicity (common with therapeutic doses) *2024*

Eosinophils *Blood Increase Physiological* Up to 50% observed in one case, others 10-20% *2434*

Erythrocytes *Blood Decrease Physiological* Megaloblastic anemia/pancytopenia *1212*

Urine Increase Physiological Nephrotoxicity with tubular necrosis *2242*

Folate *Serum Decrease Physiological* Megaloblastic anemia after Fowler's solution *4014*

Glucose *Serum Decrease Physiological* Hepatotoxic effect *3669*

Guanase *Serum Increase Physiological* Hepatotoxic effect *3669*

Heinz Body Formation *Blood Positive Physiological* Some may cause hemolytic anemia *536*

Hematocrit *Blood Decrease Physiological* Pancytopenia *1212*

Hemoglobin *Blood Decrease Physiological* Megaloblastic anemia/pancytopenia *1212*

Urine Increase Physiological May be marked hematuria *2183*

Isocitrate Dehydrogenase *Serum Increase Physiological* Hepatotoxic effect *6461*

Leukocytes *Blood Decrease Physiological* Pancytopenia *1212*

Nonprotein Nitrogen *Serum Increase Physiological* Nephrotoxicity (common with therapeutic doses) *2024*

Occult Blood *Feces Increase Physiological* Observed in several cases with poisoning *2434*

Peripheral Smear *Blood Abnormal Physiological* May produce stippling of red cells *467*

Platelets *Blood Decrease Physiological* Pancytopenia *1212*

Protein *Urine Increase Physiological* Nephrotoxic effect *1714*

Reticulocytes *Blood Increase Physiological* Values observed ranging up to 18% *2434*

Urea Nitrogen *Serum Increase Physiological* Nephrotoxic effect (common with therapeutic doses) *2242*

Xylose *Urine Decrease Physiological* May produce gastrointestinal irritation, impaired absorption and reduced excretion *929*

Arsenobenzenes

Platelets *Blood Decrease Physiological* Thrombocytopenia *3810*

Artesunate

Transforming Growth Factor-α
Serum Decrease Physiological In 37 patients with acute Plasmodium falciparum malaria mean baseline concentration of 172 ± 108 pg/mL reduced to less than 16 pg/mL after treatment with artesunate and mefloquine for 28 days *6407*

Transforming Growth Factor-β
Serum Increase Physiological In 37 patients with acute Plasmodium falciparum malaria mean baseline concentration of 14 ± 11 pg/mL increased to about 58 pg/mL after treatment with artesunate and mefloquine for 28 days *6407*

Transforming Growth Factor Receptor
Serum Decrease Physiological In 37 patients with acute Plasmodium falciparum malaria mean baseline concentration of 22 ± 8.7 pg/mL reduced to 3.7 ± 2.2 pg/mL after treatment with artesunate and mefloquine for 28 days *6407*

Ascorbic Acid

Acetaminophen *Serum No Effect Analytical* At concentrations up to 400 μg/mL no effect observed on enzymic assay of Cambridge Life Sciences, UK *2752*

Urine Decrease Analytical False negative results by screening test of Simpson and Stewart, although corrected by addition of copper sulfate *833*

Acetylsalicylic Acid *Serum No Effect Physiological* No significant effect when compounds coadministered even when ascorbic acid given as much as 3 g daily for several days *2454*

Acid Phosphatase, Prostatic *Serum No Effect Analytical* At a concentration of 2.5 mmol/L had no effect on kinetic method of Osawa et al using 2,6-dichloro-4-acetylphenyl phosphate as substrate *4449*

Alanine *Urine Decrease Physiological* In 10 healthy females given 10 g/d *6080*

Alanine Aminotransferase *Serum No Effect Analytical* No effect at therapeutic concentration on Boehringer Mannheim Reflotron method *3231* No interference observed at concentrations up to 100 mg/L with method on Cobas Ready *5705* No effect of concentrations up to 30 mg/L on method on Kodak Ektachem® *5706* No effect at 300 mg/L on Boehringer Mannheim Reflotron method *5706* No effect at 15 mg/L on method on Ames Seralyzer *5706*

Albumin *Serum No Effect Analytical* No effect at concentration of 30 mg/L on Kodak Ektachem® method *5706* No interference observed at concentrations up to 100 mg/L with method on Cobas Ready *5705* At concentration of 500 mg/L had no effect on BCG method *5704*

Urine No Effect Analytical No interference observed at concentration of 1 g/L with Boehringer Mannheim immunoturbidimetric assay with Hitachi 704 and 717 analyzers, Technicon RA 1000, and Roche Cobas Mira and Fara *2750* At concentration of 1 g/L had no significant effect on Boehringer Mannheim Tina-quant method *2799* Using a fluorimetric assay with Albumin Blue 580 on a Cobas Fara centrifugal analyzer for the detection of microalbuminuria no significant interference was detected at a concentration of 120 mg/L *3117*

Alkaline Phosphatase *Serum No Effect Analytical* No effect at concentration of 30 mg/L on method on Kodak Ektachem® *5706*

Amphetamine *Serum Decrease Physiological* Gastrointestinal acidifying agents lower absorption of amphetamines including dextroamphetamine *5641*

Urine Decrease Analytical At concentration of 10% had slight reduction effect on amphetamine/methamphetamine method on Abbott TDx *5408*

Urine No Effect Analytical No effect observed at a concentration of 100 mg/dL (5.7 mmol/L) with method on Du Pont aca *1554*

Amylase *Serum No Effect Analytical* At concentration of 1,000 mg/L had no effect on maltotetrose method *5704* No interference observed at concentrations up to 50 mg/L with method on Cobas Ready *5705* Up to 1 mmol/L on method of Rauscher et al *4876* At concentration of 30 mg/L had no effect on method on Boehringer Mannheim Reflotron system *5706*

Amylase, Pancreatic Isoenzyme
Serum Increase Analytical At toxic concentration of 300 mg/L significantly increased apparent activity as measured by method on Boehringer Mannheim Reflotron *6203*

Antioxidant Capacity *Serum Increase Physiological* In 4 healthy individuals after consming 1000 mg ascorbic acid mean antioxidant capacity increased significantly from basal 473 ± 57 μmol/L to 576 ± 45 μmol/L after 1 hour and 610 ± 83 μmol/L after 2 hours *6427*

Apolipoprotein A-I *Serum No Effect Analytical* No interference observed with immunoturbidimetric method on Hitachi 717 *2810* At a concentration of 170 μmol/L no significant effect observed on automated immunoturbidimetric method on Baxter Paramax analyzer *3005*

Ascorbic Acid *(continued)*

Apolipoprotein A-II *Serum No Effect Analytical* No interference observed with immunoturbidimetric method on Hitachi 717 *2810*

Apolipoprotein B *Serum No Effect Analytical* At a concentration of 170 µmol/L no significant effect observed on automated immunoturbidimetric method on Baxter Paramax analyzer *3005* No interference observed with immunoturbidimetric method on Hitachi 717 *2810*

Apolipoprotein C-II *Serum No Effect Analytical* No interference observed with immunoturbidimetric method on Hitachi 717 *2810*

Apolipoprotein C-III *Serum No Effect Analytical* No interference observed with immunoturbidimetric method on Hitachi 717 *2810*

Apolipoprotein E *Serum No Effect Analytical* No interference observed with immunoturbidimetric method on Hitachi 717 *2810*

Ascorbic Acid *Serum Increase Physiological* Significant effect in 50 volunteers given 2 g/d for 2 mo *1742* Significant increase with supplement of 200 mg/day in 27 long-stay female elderly patients and even greater increase when supplement increased to 2000 mg/day *246*
Urine Increase Physiological In individuals ingesting 100 mg/d mean excretion 889 µmol/L (range 125 - 3676 µmol/L), with 250 mg/d mean excretion 1765 mol/L (range 153 - 5889 µmol/L), with 500 mg/d mean 3544 µmol/L (range 106 - 12800 µmol/L) and with 1000 mg/d mean excretion 3565 µmol/L (range 123 - 16470 µmol/L) *721* Significant effect in 50 volunteers given 2 g/d for 2 mo *1742*
White Blood Cells Increase Physiological In 178 individuals from rural Swaziland and Zimbabwe administration of 1 - 2 g ascorbic acid daily caused significant increase in concentration from mean baseline of 28.0 ± 16.5 µg/10^8 leukocytes to 33.8 ± 18.4 µg/10^8 leukocytes after 2 days *3131* Significant effect in 50 volunteers given 2 g/d for 2 mo *1742*

Aspartate Aminotransferase *Serum Decrease Analytical* No effect up to 5 mg/L on method on Ames Seralyzer but at higher concentrations apparently reduced enzyme activity observed. Effect likely to be of clinical significance since ascorbic acid concentration may be as high as 18 mg/L *5706*
Serum Increase Analytical At 1 mmol/L affects Technicon SMA 12/60 method *5576*
Serum No Effect Analytical No effect at 300 mg/L on Boehringer Mannheim Reflotron method *5706* No effect of concentration of 30 mg/L on method on Kodak Ektachem® *5706* No effect at therapeutic concentration on Boehringer Mannheim Reflotron method *3231* No interference observed at concentrations up to 100 mg/L with method on Roche Cobas Ready *5705*

Aspartic Acid *Urine Increase Physiological* In 10 healthy females given 10 g/d *6080*

Barbiturate *Urine Decrease Analytical* At concentration of 10% caused slight reduction with barbiturate method on Abbott TDx *5408*
Urine No Effect Analytical No effect at a concentration of 100 mg/dL (5.7 mmol/L) with method on Du Pont aca *1555*

Benzodiazepine *Urine No Effect Analytical* No effect observed at a concentration of 100 mg/dL (5.7 mmol/L) with method on Du Pont aca *1556*

Benzoquinone Acetic Acid *Urine Decrease Physiological* Administration of relatively large amounts to 2 adults was followed by disappearance of compound from urine *6525*

Benzoylecgonine *Urine Decrease Analytical* At a concentration of 10% caused significant reduction when specimen measured on Abbott TDx *5408*
Urine No Effect Analytical No effect observed at a concentration of 100 mg/dL (5.7 mmol/L) with method on Du Pont aca *1558*

Bicarbonate *Serum Decrease Analytical* In one patient given 30 g sodium ascorbate intravenously (reaching concentration of 30 mmol/L) to treat malignant disease mean concentration as measured on Hitachi 747 decreased to 22 mmol/L compared with reference range of 23 - 32 mmol/L *319* At concentration of 20 mmol/L 33% reduction in concentration as measured by Kodak Ektachem® 700 *2828*
Serum No Effect Analytical At concentration of 500 mg/L had no effect on method using phenolphthalein *5704*

Bilirubin *Serum Decrease Analytical* At concentrations above 200 mg/L (normal maximum serum concentration 34 mg/L) lowered concentration as measured by Jendrassik and Grof method *5704*
Serum Increase Analytical In 8 healthy volunteers ingestion of large doses caused mean increase of 14.3% with method on Boehringer Mannheim Hitachi 747-100 but exact mechanism not determined *5383* At therapeutic concentration may affect Technicon SMA 12/60 method *5576*
Serum No Effect Analytical No significant effect observed at a concentration of 15 mg/dL (852 µmol/L) with method on Du Pont aca *1548* On Technicon SMAC® method at therapeutic concentration *6266* No effect at 2000 mg/L on method on Ames Seralyzer *5706* At concentration of 40 mg/L had no effect on Kodak Ektachem® method *5704* No interference observed at concentrations up to 100 mg/dL with method on Roche Cobas Ready *5705* At concentration of 30 mg/L had no effect on method on Boehringer Mannheim Reflotron system *5706*
Urine Decrease Analytical At concentration of 25 mg/dL may cause false negative reaction with Ames Multistix and other reagent test strips *4034*
Urine No Effect Analytical No effect observed with Ames Ictotest reagent tablets *4034*

Bilirubin, Conjugated *Serum No Effect Analytical* No effect at concentration of 40 mg/L on method on Kodak Ektachem® *5706* At concentration of 15 mg/dL (852 µmol/L) had no effect on method on Du Pont aca *1517*

Bilirubin, Direct *Serum No Effect Analytical* No effect observed at concentration up to 200 mg/L with method using bilirubin oxidase and run on Hitachi 7150 *4208*

Bilirubin, Unconjugated *Serum No Effect Analytical* No effect at concentration of 40 mg/L on method on Kodak Ektachem® *5706*

Blood *Urine Decrease Analytical* In 407 of 561 urinary specimens with hematuria by microscopic examination no vitamin C detected by dipstick but 154 had vitamin C present (mean concentration 2173 µmol/L) *3007*
Urine No Effect Analytical No effect observed with occult blood test areas of Ames Multistix and other reagent strip tests and with microscopic examination of urine sediment *4034*

Calcium *Serum No Effect Analytical* No interference observed at concentrations up to 75 mg/L with method on Roche Cobas Ready *5705* At concentration of 2,000 mg/L had no effect on cresolphthalein method *5704*
Urine Increase Physiological In 37 healthy young women 4 hour excretion after ingestion of 1.75 mg increased from mean of 19.8 ± 10.9 mg to 25.7 ± 14.6 mg (105 ± 54 mg/g creatinine to 134 ± 76 mg/g creatinine) *3640*

Cannabinoids *Urine No Effect Analytical* No effect on Roche Abuscreen method *5006* No effect observed at a concentration of 100 mg/dL (5.7 mmol/L) on method on Du Pont aca *1557*

Ceruloplasmin *Serum No Effect Physiological* No effect on protein with 605 mg/d for 3 weeks but up to 21% reduction of oxidase activity *2864*

Chloride *Serum Decrease Analytical* In one patient given 30 g sodium ascorbate intravenously (reaching concentration of 30 mmol/L) to treat malignant disease mean concentration as measured on Hitachi 747 decreased to 93 mmol/L compared with reference range of 96 - 109 mmol/L *319*
Serum No Effect Analytical At concentration of 500 mg/L had no effect on mercurimetric method *5704* At concentration of 40 mg/L had no effect on Kodak Ektachem® method *5704*

Cholesterol *Serum Decrease Analytical* At concentrations of ascorbic acid of 200 µmol/L (just exceeding presumed upper limit of normal) average decrease of ≤ 0.2 mmol/L observed. Correlation of r > 0.97 with ascorbic acid concentration *490* At concentrations above 50 mg/L (maximum serum concentration 34 mg/L) lowered concentration as measured by CHOD-Iodide method *5704* In one patient given 30 g sodium ascorbate intravenously (reaching concentration of 30 mmol/L) to treat malignant disease mean concentration as measured on Hitachi 747 decreased to < 0.1 mmol/L compared with reference range of 0.6 - 5.5 mmol/L *319* At concentrations above 50 mg/L (maximum serum concentration 34 mg/L) lowered con-

centration as measured by CHOD-PAP method *5704* At ascorbic acid concentration of 4 to 5 mmol/L enzymatic method on Olympus Demand completely inhibited and 75% inhibition of method on Abbott TDx. At concentrations that may occur in vivo (0.5 to 1 mmol/L) decrease of 10 to 25% could occur *4577* Increase by 2.1% at 5 mg/dL on enzymatic procedure *103*
Serum Decrease Physiological 16% decrease on average when 1 g/d given to healthy approximately 29 year olds within 2 mo. 14% fall in 58 year olds but required 12 mo. Administration abolished normal rise observed in winter *1453* Tends to fall in people under 25 when 1 g/d given *5753*
Serum Increase Physiological When atherosclerotic, ?mobilization from arteries *5753*
Serum No Effect Analytical At concentrations up to 30 mg/L no effect on method on Boehringer Mannheim Reflotron system, but above this concentration (not likely to occur physiologically) cholesterol concentration decreased *5706* No effect up to 60 mg/L on Ames Seralyzer method although at higher concentrations apparently reduced cholesterol concentration, but not of clinical significance since concentration not at physiological level *5706* No effect at therapeutic concentration on Boehringer Mannheim Reflotron method *3231* No effect at concentrations up to 30 mg/L on method on Kodak Ektachem® *5706* At concentrations up to 25 mg/L no interference observed with method on Roche Cobas Ready *5705* At concentration of 500 mg/L had no effect on Liebermann-Burchard method *5704* No interference reported at a concentration of 3-15 mg/dL (170-852 µmol/L) with method on Du Pont aca *1516* At concentration of 1,000 mg/L had no effect on method using catalase-Hantzsch reaction *5704* At concentration of 400 mg/L had no effect on catalase-AIDH method *5704*
Serum No Effect Physiological No influence on concentration of dietary intake in elderly *2875* No significant effect observed with 1 g/d for 6 weeks in borderline hypertensives and normotensives *4454* No significant effect in 27 elderly female patients with initially low plasma ascorbic acid concentrations when given supplements of either 200 or 2000 mg daily *246*

Cholinesterase *Serum No Effect Analytical* No effect observed at concentration of 3 mg/dL with butyrylthiocholine method on Kodak Ektachem® *2504*

Copper *Serum No Effect Physiological* Not affected by variations in drug intake up to 605 mg/d for 3 weeks *2864*

Cortisol *Plasma No Effect Analytical* At concentration of 300 mg/L no significant effect on CEDIA or Boehringer Mannheim Enzymun methods (worst case 93.6% recovery) *1097*

Creatine Kinase *Serum Decrease Analytical* Recovery of 70% only observed with high doses of ascorbic acid on whole blood method on Boehringer Mannheim Reflotron *2714* Ascorbic acid may lead to apparently reduced concentrations when measured by method on Roche Cobas Ready *5705*
Serum No Effect Analytical No effect at 2000 mg/L on method on Ames Seralyzer *5706*

Creatinine *Serum Decrease Analytical* Marked reduction observed with concentrations as low as 0.6 mmol/L with enzymatic methods of Merck, Wako and PAP and MPA enzymatic methods of Boehringer Mannheim *6375* At concentrations above 1,000 mg/L (maximum serum concentration 34 mg/L) lowered concentration as measured by creatinine amidohydrolase method *5704*
Serum Increase Analytical At concentrations above 25 mg/L (maximum serum concentration 34 mg/L) raised concentration as measured by kinetic Jaffe method *5704* 100 mg/L of ascorbic acid corresponds to 0.01 mg/dL creatinine with method of Heinegard *2539* Chromogenicity in color reaction (as reducing agent) *1714* In one patient given 30 g sodium ascorbate intravenously (reaching concentration of 30 mmol/L) to treat malignant disease mean concentration as measured on Hitachi 747 increased to 0.37 mmol/L compared with reference range of 0.06 - 0.11 mmol/L *319* Marked effect on direct Jaffe methods *4073* At concentrations above 250 mg/L (maximum serum concentration 34 mg/L) raised concentration as measured by Technicon AutoAnalyzer® Jaffe method *5704*
Serum No Effect Analytical No effect at 2000 mg/L on Ames Seralyzer method *5706* On Technicon SMAC® method at therapeutic concentration *6266* At concentration of 400 mg/L had no effect on Jaffe-Fuller's earth method *5704* At 360 mg/dL on ion-exchange method of Mitchell. No effect on Lloyd's procedure *4073* At concentration of 105 mg/L had no effect on creatinine iminohydrolase method *5704* At concentration of 100 mg/L had no effect on Jaffe-Heinegard and Tiderstrom method *5704* Insignificant increase observed with Jaffe methods of Beckman and Merck and apparently no effect observed with manual Fuller's earth method *6375* No effect at concentration of 20 mg/dL (1.1 mmol/L) on method on Du Pont Dimension *1572* No effect of concentrations up to 40 mg/L on 2-slide method on Kodak Ektachem® *5706* No effect of concentrations up to 30 mg/L on single slide method on Kodak Ektachem® *5706* No interference observed at concentrations up to 75 mg/L with method on Roche Cobas Ready *5705* At concentration of 1,000 mg/L had no effect on kinetic Jaffe method on BKA-2 *5704* At concentration of 400 mg/L had no effect on Jaffe-Fading-Fraction method *5704* No interference noted with liquid chromatographic method of Paroni et al *4540* At 500 mg/L on reversed phase liquid chromatographic procedure of Zhiri et al *6656*
Urine Increase Analytical At concentration of 10% 180% increase observed with Abbott TDx REA creatinine method *5408* Acts as reducing agent *189*
Urine No Effect Physiological In 37 healthy young women ingestion of 1.75 g ascorbic acid caused insignificant increase in 4 hour excretion from 189 ± 48 mg to 195 ± 42 mg *3640*

Crystals *Urine Increase Physiological* Acidification may precipitate oxalates, urates, cystine *3384*

C-terminal Telopeptides of Type I Collagen Degradation Products *Serum No Effect Analytical* At a concentration of 100 mg/L had no significant effect when measured by CrossLaps™ procedure *5103*

Cystine *Urine Decrease Physiological* In 10 healthy females given 10 g/d *6080*

Dopamine *Urine Increase Physiological* In 38 healthy young women 4 hour excretion after ingestion of 1.75 g ascorbic acid caused significantly increased excretion from mean of 46.3 ± 14.0 µg to 50.5 ± 13.2 µg (254 ± 68 mg/g creatinine to 270 ± 78 mg/g creatinine) *3640*

Drugs of Abuse Screen *Urine No Effect Analytical* No effect at concentration of 100 µg/mL on EZ-SCREEN procedure for cannabinoids and cocaine *1739*

Epinephrine *Urine No Effect Physiological* In 38 healthy young women ingestion of 1.75 g ascorbic acid caused insignificant decrease in 4 hour excretion from 1.0 ± 0.7 µg to 0.9 ± 0.5 µg (5.6 ± 3.7 mg/g creatinine to 5.0 ± 2.7 mg/g creatinine) *3640*

Erythropoietin *Serum No Effect Analytical* No interference observed at concentrations up to 1.0 g/L with solid phase immunoassay method of Bio-Merieux *4779*

Ethanol *Serum Decrease Physiological* Clearance increased following a single oral dose of 2 g orally before ingestion of 0.5 g/kg body weight by 6 volunteers (33-58%) and following 2 g daily for 2 weeks before alcohol ingestion (25-37%). Plasma alcohol concentration minimally affected *979*
Serum No Effect Analytical No significant interference observed with method on Kodak Ektachem® *1232*

Ethinyl Estradiol *Serum Increase Physiological* In doses of 1 g/d reported to increase plasma concentration *1384*

Ferritin *Serum Decrease Physiological* During 14 week study of varying intakes of drug probably attributable to phlebotomy only *2863*
Serum No Effect Physiological In 178 individuals from rural Swaziland and Zimbabwe administration of 1 - 2 g ascorbic acid daily caused nonsignificant change in concentration from mean baseline of 284 µg/L to 284 µg/L after 2 days *3131*

Fibrinogen *Plasma No Effect Analytical* At concentration of 500 mg/L had no effect on Du Pont aca method *5704*

Fructosamine *Serum Decrease Analytical* Decreases concentration by at least 0.1 mmol/L at concentration of 0.57 mmol/L when method of Baker et al used *2608*
Serum Increase Analytical Interference by more than 0.1 mmol/L but less than 0.3 mmol/L at concentration of 0.57 mmol/L with method of Baker et al *3704*
Serum No Effect Physiological In healthy individuals given 750 or 1500 mg/d for 12 weeks no significant difference from controls observed *6421*

Glucose *Serum Decrease Analytical* At concentrations up to 1.40 mmol/L causes significant reduction of up to 0.63 mmol/L with whole blood measurement by Miles Ames Glucostix analyzer *5904* At concentrations up to 1.40 mmol/L caused nonsignificant 0.1 mmol/L reduction in whole blood glucose concentration as measured by Boehringer Mannheim BM 1-44

Ascorbic Acid *(continued)*

Glucose *(continued)*
analyzer *5904* At concentrations up to 1.40 mmol/L causes nonsignificant reduction of up to 0.22 mmol/L with whole blood method on Medisense Exatech glucose analyzer *5904* At concentrations above 150 mg/L (maximum serum concentration 34 mg/L) lowered concentration as measured by GOD/POD-PAP method *5704* At concentrations above 125 mg/L (maximum serum concentration 34 mg/L) lowered concentration as measured by GOD-PERID method *5704* At concentrations above 100 mg/L (maximum serum concentration 34 mg/L) lowered concentration as measured by Ektachem® method *5704* At concentrations up to 1.40 mmol/L causes significant up to 0.48 mmol/L reduction in whole blood glucose concentration as measured by Medisense Satellite G glucose analyzer *5904* At concentrations above 100 mg/L decreases result as determined by method on Kodak Ektachem® , but of no clinical significance since normal concentration up to 17.5 mg/L only *5706* Slight effect with coupled glucose-oxidase method *2197* At concentrations above 25 mg/L (maximum serum concentration 34 mg/L) lowered concentration as measured by Ames Seralyzer *5704* But reduction insignificant (each 1 mg/dL lowers concentration as measured by 0.65 mg/dL) with glucose oxidase method on Technicon SMAC® *6266*
Serum Decrease Physiological Significant reduction in fasting concentration of diabetics treated for 15 d *5225*
Serum Increase Analytical 17.9% increase in absorbance with 1 mmol/L and 11.4% increase with 0.5 mmol/L on glucokinase based assay of Scott *5414* At 1 mmol/L affects Technicon SMA 12/60 method *5576* Increases sensitivity of o-toluidine procedures: 1 g/dL equivalent to 3.3 mmol/L with alkaline ferricyanide *3531* At concentrations above 60 mg/L (maximum serum concentration 34 mg/L) raised concentration as measured by glucose dehydrogenase method *5704*
Serum No Effect Analytical No interference observed at concentrations of 100 mg/dL with method on Roche Cobas Ready *5705* Insignificant effect at 5 mg/dL on MBTH procedure of Neeley *4241* No effect up to 140 mg/L on hexokinase method on Ames Seralyzer but at higher concentrations disproportionately increased glucose concentration observed but not of clinical significance since test concentration exceeded physiological range *5706* At concentration of 25 mg/dL (1.42 mmol/L) has no effect on method on Du Pont Dimension *1575* No interference observed at a concentration of 2.5-25 mg/dL (132-1420 µmol/L) with method on Du Pont aca *1527* At concentration of 5 mg/dL had no effect on concentration as measured by Markwell Medical instrument *6132* No effect at therapeutic concentration on Boehringer Mannheim Reflotron method *3231* No effect up to 40 mg/L on glucose oxidase method on Ames Seralyzer but above this concentration apparent reduction in glucose concentration although not of clinical significance *5706* No effect at concentration up to 200 mg/L on Boehringer Mannheim Reflotron but decrease with higher concentrations. Note clinical concentrations up to 17.5 mg/L so effect of no clinical relevance *5706* At concentration of 1000 mg/L had no effect on hexokinase/G-6-PDH method *5704* At concentration of 250 mg/L had no effect on hexokinase/G-6-PDH method on Du Pont aca *5704* On p-HBAH procedure of Lever at 1 g/dL *3531*
Serum No Effect Physiological In healthy individuals given 750 or 1500 mg/d for 12 weeks no significant difference from controls observed *6421* In 12 nondiabetic individuals ingestion of 1 g/d for 3 months no significant effect observed *1267*
Urine Decrease Analytical May inhibit TesTape® and Clinistix® *5869* Impaired color develop of chromogen in glucose oxidase method *1714* At concentration of about 100 mg/dL made a urine concentration of 0.1 g/dL react negatively with Chemstrip® 7, Lema-Combistix® and give trace reacftion with Chemstrip® UG *6692* But only very slight effect with BM33071 procedure from Boehringer Mannheim compared with other dipsticks *1210* Significant effect with Redia-test, L-Combur-5-test, Labstix® , Rapignost, Meditest but less effect with BM33071 *497* At concentration of 50 mg/dL may cause false negative results at glucose concentrations of 75-125 mg/dL with Ames Keto-Diastix, Diastix, and Multistix procedures and may cause false negative reaction with Clinistix *4034* At 0.4 g/L interfered with BM33071 in 20% urines containing 1.0 g glucose/L but not with urines containing 5.0 g glucose/L. No effect of ascorbic acid at 0.1 to 0.2 g/L. At 0.4 g/L interfered with Hema-Combistix® in 90% urines containing glucose at 5.0 g/L. No effect of ascorbic acid at 0.1 to 0.2 g/L *5609* At physiological urine amounts, marked reduction of results with especially Ecur-test, Diabur-test 5,000 and Rapignost basis screen but also TesTape® *1211* At concentration of 100 mg/L (normal concentration in urine up to 1290 mg/L) produced false negative result with Diabur-test *5704*
Urine Increase Analytical Effect on Clinitest® causes normal to be read as trace at low concentrations: less effect at high concentrations *1211* At concentration of 250 mg/dL in urine may cause false positive with Ames Clinitest tablets *4034*
Urine No Effect Analytical No effect observed with TesTape® *5869* With DNSA method at usual concentrations *134*

γ-Glutamyltransferase *Serum No Effect Analytical* No effect of concentrations up to 30 mg/L on method on Kodak Ektachem® *5706* At concentration of 2 mg/dL (0.11 mmol/L) had no effect on method on Du Pont aca *1532* *1533* No effect at therapeutic concentration on Boehringer Mannheim Reflotron method *3231* At concentration of 300 mg/L no effect on method on Boehringer Mannheim Reflotron system *5706*

Glutathione *Red Blood Cells Increase Physiological* In 9 healthy individuals administration of 500 mg/d for 2 weeks caused significant increase of 50% from mean baseline (range 8 to 84%). Same change observed after 2000 mg/d for 2 weeks *4194*

Glutathione Peroxidase *Serum Increase Physiological* Significant increase in activity observed when young women given 600 mg daily *4194*

Glycated Albumin *Serum Decrease Physiological* Ingestion of 1 g daily by 12 healthy volunteers caused decrease from mean baseline concentration of 1.56% to 1.04% after 3 months *1266* In 12 nondiabetic healthy individuals mean concentration significantly decreased from mean 1.6% to 1.1% after 1, 2, and 3 months after ingestion of 1 g/d *1267*

Glycated Hemoglobin *Blood Decrease Physiological* In 12 normal individuals, in spite of no change in glucose concentration, ingestion of 1 g ascorbic acid daily caused decrease of mean concentration from baseline of 6.18% to 5.05% after 3 months *1266* In 12 nondiabetic individuals mean concentration decreased by 18% from 6.18 ± 0.48% to 5.05 ± 0.50% after ingesting 1 g/d for 3 months when affinity chromatography used to measure glycosylated hemoglobin *1267*
Blood Increase Analytical Concentration increased in three hemolysates in the presence and absence of glucose in incubates containing either ascorbic acid or dehydroascorbic acid when measurements done by electrophoresis *1265* In 12 nondiabetic individuals ingestion of 1 g/d for 3 months increased in glycosylated hemoglobin as measured by electrophoresis from mean baseline of 6.17 ± 0.61% to 7.16 ± 0.59%. This is a methodological artifact as true glycated Hgb increased *1267* In 12 nondiabetic individuals ingestion of 1 g/d for 3 months increased in glycosylated hemoglobin as measured by electrophoresis from mean baseline of 6.17 ± 0.61% to 7.16 ± 0.59%. This is a methodological artifact as true glycated Hgb increased *1267*
Blood No Effect Analytical Incubation of human hemoglobin with either 1 mmol/L ascorbic acid or dehydroascorbic acid had no effect when measured by affinity chromatography *1265* At a concentration of 100 mg/L had an insignificant + 5.9% interference with method on Abbott Vision *1885*
Blood No Effect Physiological In healthy individuals given 750 or 1500 mg/d for 12 weeks no significant difference from controls observed *6421*

Glycine *Urine Decrease Physiological* In 10 healthy females given 10 g/d *6080*

HDL-Cholesterol *Serum Decrease Analytical* Significant reduction observed at a concentration of 40 mg/L (227 µmol/L) with BMD method on Hitachi 737 probably due to inhibition of oxidation of the indicator dye by hydrogen peroxide *4275* Decreases of from 0.3 to 10% in 6 methods to determine compound with drug concentration of 2.0 mg/dL *4137* Concentrations above 30 mg/L decrease results obtained on Kodak Ektachem® although not of clinical significance because upper limit of normal concentration is 17.5 mg/L *5706*
Serum Decrease Physiological In 256 men for each increment of 0.5 mg/dL in plasma ascorbic acid adjusted concentration did not change but in 221 women decreased by 1.9 mg/dL *2876*
Serum Increase Physiological In 256 men for each increment of 0.5 mg/dL in plasma ascorbic acid adjusted concentration increased by 2.1 mg/dL and in 221 women by 7.4 mg/dL

for ascorbic acid concentrations over 1.05 mg/dL *2876* Significant correlation between drug intake and analyte concentration in elderly *2875*

Serum No Effect Analytical At concentrations up to 50 mg/L no interference observed with method on Roche Cobas Ready *5705* No significant effect observed when added at a concentration of 60 mg/L and measurement made on Boehringer Mannheim Reflotron *4275* At a concentration up to 300 mg/L had no significant effect on Reflotron method for whole blood cholesterol *6352*

Serum No Effect Physiological No significant change in 27 elderly female patients with initially low plasma ascorbic acid concentrations when given supplements of either 200 or 2000 mg/day *246* No significant effect observed in normotensives and borderline hypertensives when treated with 1 g/d for 6 weeks *4454*

Hematocrit *Blood No Effect Physiological* No effect with varying degrees of supplementation over 14 week study period in young men *2863*

Hemoglobin *Blood No Effect Analytical* No effect of concentrations up to 40 mg/L on method on Kodak Ektachem® *5706*

Blood No Effect Physiological No effect with varying degrees of supplementation over 14 week study period in young men *2863*

Urine Decrease Analytical At up to 140 mg/dL made Chemstrip® 7 react negatively to 250 mg/L hemoglobin, also with Hema-Combistix® and some reactions were negative at approximately same concentration with Chemstrip® 9 *6692* In large amounts inhibits guaiac test *1714*

Homogentisic Acid *Urine No Effect Physiological* Administration of relatively large amounts to 2 adults had no effect on excretion but appeared to double excretion in 4 and 5 month old infants presumably through an effect on immature p-hydroxyphenylpyruvic acid oxidase *6525*

Hydrocortisone *Serum Increase Physiological* In adult patients immediately prior to surgery intravenous administration of 1000 mg ascorbic acid on top of 400 mg cimetidine caused significant increase of 15-100% from the second hour to end of study at 3 hours *640*

β-Hydroxybutyrate *Urine Increase Analytical* At concentration of ascorbic acid of 100 mg/dL gave increase of about 1.0 mEq/L with enzymatic procedure of GDS Diagnostics *1824*

17-Hydroxycorticosteroids *Urine Increase Analytical* Interferes with method of Reddy *2451*

Hydroxyproline *Urine Decrease Physiological* Slight effect in osteogenesis imperfecta *6111*

immunoglobulin A *Serum No Effect Analytical* Insignificant effect on method on Du Pont aca at a concentration of 15 mg/dL (0.85 mmol/L) *1528* No significant interference observed with concentrations up to 20 mg/dL with method on Olympus REPLY and AU800 analyzers *3140*

Immunoglobulin G *Serum No Effect Analytical* No significant interference observed with concentrations up to 20 mg/dL with method on Olympus REPLY and AU800 analyzers *3140* No significant interference observed at a concentration of 30 mg/dL (170 mmol/L) with method on Du Pont aca *1529*

Immunoglobulin M *Serum No Effect Analytical* No significant interference observed with concentrations up to 20 mg/dL with method on Olympus REPLY and AU800 analyzers *3140* No significant interference observed at a concentration of 15 mg/dL (0.85 mmol/L) with method on Du Pont aca *1530*

Iodide *Urine Increase Analytical* With an automated method using the ceric-arsenious acid reaction at concentrations less than 5 mmol/L no effect observed but at concentrations as low as 14.2 mmol/L (which can occur physiologically) interfernce definitely does occur *1907*

Iron *Serum No Effect Physiological* In 178 individuals from rural Swaziland and Zimbabwe administration of 1 - 2 g ascorbic acid daily caused nonsignificant change in concentration from mean baseline of 22.2 ± 10.0 μmol/L to 22.2 ± 10.6 μmol/L after 2 days *3131*

Isoleucine *Urine Increase Physiological* In 10 healthy females given 10 g/d *6080*

Ketones *Serum No Effect Analytical* When added at a concentration of 300 mg/L had no significant effect on ketone method of Uno et al *6131*

17-Ketosteroids *Urine Increase Analytical* Due to chemical structure affects Zimmermann procedure *5402*

Lactate *Plasma No Effect Analytical* At concentration of 600 mg/L had no effect on enzymatic method *5704* Interference of less than 0.1 mmol/L at ascorbic acid concentration of 1.2 mg/dL with method on Beckman Synchron CX 4/5 *989*

Lactate Dehydrogenase *Serum Decrease Analytical* At therapeutic concentration may depress Technicon SMA 12/60 value *5576*

Serum No Effect Analytical No effect at 2 mg/L on method on Ames Seralyzer *5706* No effect of concentrations up to 30 mg/L on method on Kodak Ektachem® *5706*

LDL-Cholesterol *Serum Decrease Physiological* In 256 men for each increment of 0.5 mg/dL in plasma ascorbic acid adjusted concentration did not change but in 221 women decreased by 2.1 mg/dL *2876*

Serum No Effect Analytical At concentrations of 150 mg/L had no effect on direct method of Equal Diagnostics performed on a Hitachi 911 analyzer *4959*

Leucine *Urine Increase Physiological* In 10 healthy females given 10 g/d *6080*

Leukocytes *Urine Decrease Analytical* At concentrations above 2,000 mg/L (maximum concentration in urine up to 1290 mg/L) caused false negative result with Cytur-Test *5704*

Lipase *Serum No Effect Analytical* No effect of concentrations up to 120 mg/L on method on Kodak Ektachem® *5706*

Lymphocytes *Blood No Effect Physiological* No effect with megadose supplementation *2245*

Metanephrines, Total *Urine No Effect Analytical* At 5 g/L on modified Pisano procedure *2372*

3-Methylhistidine *Urine Increase Physiological* In 10 healthy females given 10 g/d *6080*

Morphine *Urine No Effect Analytical* At concentration of 10% had no significant effect on method on Abbott TDx *5408*

N-Acetyl-Glucosaminidase *Urine No Effect Analytical* No interference observed with color development of test pad of Boehringer Mannheim dipstick at concentrations tested *3767* No effect at 100 mmol/L on 2 colorimetric analytical methods *2254* At concentration of 100 mg/dL had no significant effect on Boehringer Mannheim CPR method *3174* No significant interference observed with method of Kamiya Biomedical Company at a concentration of 500 mg/dL *3021*

Neutrophils *Blood No Effect Physiological* No effect with megadose supplementation *2245*

Nitrite *Urine Negative Analytical* At concentrations greater than 25 mg/dL may cause false negative results if urine contains nitrite ion in concentrations of 0.06 mg/dL or less with nitrite test area of Ames Multistix and other reagent strip tests *4034*

Norepinephrine *Urine No Effect Physiological* In 38 healthy young women ingestion of 1.75 g ascorbic acid caused insignificant reduction in mean 4 hour norepinephrine excretion from 7.8 ± 3.8 μg to 7.5 ± 3.2 μg (41 ± 15 mg/g creatinine to 39 ± 14 mg/g creatinine) *3640*

Occult Blood *Feces Decrease Analytical* At concentrations above 30 mg/L produced false negative result as measured by Hemoccult® *5704* False reduction at physiological amounts (if taking added vitamin C) on Hemoccult® and other tests with pseudoperoxidase principle, e.g., guaiac, benzidine, or other diamino compound as indicator *2883* Interferes with analytic methods *3810*

Opiates *Urine No Effect Analytical* No effect observed at a concentration of 100 mg/dL (5.7 mmol/L) on method on Du Pont aca *1559*

Oxalate *Urine Decrease Analytical* Reduced concentration observed with methods involving oxalate decarboxylase *5060*

Urine Increase Analytical With Sigma procedure with diluted or undiluted urine, but pretreatment with ferric chloride causes loss of oxalate *2186* Addition of 5.68 mmol/L ascorbate in vitro increased urinary oxalate by 36 μmol/L as measured by HPLC method. Ingestion of 10 g ascorbic acid per day caused 69 μmol/L increase in apparent oxalate excretion but no increase physiologically *6337*

Urine Increase Physiological Normal metabolite excreted *3384*

Urine No Effect Analytical When boric acid used as diluent for low chromatographic measurement procedures *4994* Minimal effect on gas-chromatographic procedure with alkalinization

Ascorbic Acid *(continued)*

Oxalate *(continued)*
of urine *3862* Ingestion of up to 5 g daily caused no effect on automated procedure of Allen et al using modified Boehringer Mannheim kit *109*
Urine No Effect Physiological No effect in 50 volunteers given 2 g/d for 2 mo *1742*

p-Aminophenol *Urine No Effect Analytical* With addition of drugs at a concentration of 100 mg/L and of related compounds at 50 mg/L no significant effect observed on colorimetric method of van Bocxlaer on Cobas Mira analyzer which involves reacting free p-aminophenol with resorcinol in the presence of magnesium ions to form an indophenol dye measured at 550 nm *6163*

pH *Blood No Effect Physiological* Even when 8 $g/m^2/d$ ingested *382*
Urine Decrease Physiological Some effect with ingestion of 3-6 g/d *382* Acidifies urine when ingested in large amounts *3384*

Phencyclidine *Urine No Effect Analytical* At concentration of 10% had insignificant effect on method on Abbott TDx *5408*

Phenylalanine *Plasma Decrease Physiological* Reduces elevated concentration of premature infants *2242*
Plasma No Effect Analytical No interference observed with rapid quantitative whole blood method of Campbell et al using phenylalanine dehydrogenase *867* At a concentration of 300 µmol/L had no significant effect on method of Vilaseca et al using phenylalanine dehydrogenase and adapted to a centrifugal analyzer *6259*
Urine Increase Physiological In 10 healthy females given 10 g/d *6080*

Phosphate *Serum Increase Analytical* In 8 healthy volunteers ingestion of large amounts of ascorbic acid caused significant 9.9% increase as measured by method on Boehringer Mannheim Hitachi 747-100 but exact mechanism not determined *5383*
Serum No Effect Analytical At concentration of 15 mg/dL (0.85 mmol/L) no interference observed with method on Du Pont aca *1539* No effect of concentrations up to 40 mg/L on method on Kodak Ektachem® *5706* At concentration of 150 mg/L had no effect as measured by Du Pont aca method *5704* At concentration of 2,000 mg/L had no effect as measured by phosphomolybdate method *5704*
Urine No Effect Analytical At 20 mg/dL ascorbic acid causes 1% increase with method of Jung/Parekh *2992*
Urine No Effect Physiological In 37 healthy young women 4 hour excretion after ingestion of 1.75 g ascorbic acid changed insignificantly from 84.2 ± 36.3 mg to 91.9 ± 42.6 mg (457 ± 204 mg/g creatinine to 500 ± 320 mg/g creatinine) *3640*

Phosphoethanolamine *Urine Increase Physiological* In 10 healthy females given 10 g/d *6080*

Phosphoserine *Urine Decrease Physiological* In 10 healthy females given 10 g/d *6080*

Porphobilinogen *Urine Decrease Analytical* Inhibition of color development if no prior separation *1839*

Potassium *Serum Increase Analytical* In one patient given 30 g sodium ascorbate intravenously (reaching concentration of 30 mmol/L) to treat malignant disease mean concentration as measured on Hitachi 747 increased to 5.0 mmol/L compared with reference range of 3.5 - 5.0 mmol/L *319*
Serum No Effect Analytical At concentration of 40,000 mg/L had no effect on ISE measurement with predilution *5704* No effect up to 100 mg/L on method on Ames Seralyzer but at higher concentrations apparently higher concentration observed. Since this concentration is above normal clinical concentrations it is of no importance *5706* At concentration of 800 mg/L had no effect on ISE measurement without predilution *5704* No effect of concentrations up to 30 mg/L on method on Kodak Ektachem® *5706* At concentration of 60 mg/L had no effect as measured by flame-photometric method *5704* At concentration of 100 mg/L caused nonsignificant - 0.2% interference with method on Abbott Vision *681*

Protein *Cerebrospinal Fluid No Effect Analytical* No effect on Folin-Ciocalteu procedure *6681* No significant interference observed with benzethonium chloride procedure on Hitachi 704 and 717 analyzers *6549*
Serum No Effect Analytical No interference observed at concentrations up to 100 mg/L with method on Roche Cobas Ready *5705* No effect of concentrations up to 30 mg/L on method on Kodak Ektachem® *5706* At concentration of 2,000 mg/L had no effect as measured by biuret method with blank correction *5704*
Test Conditions Increase Analytical Reacts with Folin-Ciocalteu reagent of Lowry procedure *1102*
Urine Increase Analytical When Kodak Ektachem® slide for CSF protein used to measure protein in urine ascorbic acid reduced both Cu(II) and the dye generating a reduced form of dye which undergoes a hypochromic spectral shift which generates a positive bias. When urine passed over a molecular sieve column to remove low molecular weight compounds results correlated well with Coomassie Blue method *3580*
Urine No Effect Analytical No significant interference observed with benzethonium chloride method on Hitachi 704 and 717 analyzers *6549* No effect observed at a concentration of 100 mg/dL (5.7 mmol/L) on method on Du Pont aca *1553*

Protein Electrophoresis *Serum No Effect Analytical* At concentration of 800 mg/L had no effect on automated Olympus-Hite method but with slight displacement of fractions *5704*

Prothrombin Time *Plasma Decrease Physiological* Case reported when compound given to patient whose time was increased by anticoagulant *382* May shorten action of anticoagulants *2753*
Plasma No Effect Physiological No effect on Thrombotest with dose of 1 g/d *2772* No effect seen in most patients *2452*

Pyridoxine *Urine No Effect Physiological* No effect with varying degrees of supplementation over 14 week study period in young men *2863*

Retinol *Serum No Effect Physiological* No effect with varying degrees of supplementation over 14 week study period in young men *2863*

Sarcosine *Urine Decrease Physiological* In 10 healthy females given 10 g/d *6080*

Selenium *Serum Increase Physiological* Significant increase observed in young women given 600 mg daily *4194*

Serine *Urine Decrease Physiological* In 10 healthy females given 10 g/d *6080*

Sialic Acid *Serum No Effect Analytical* No effect observed at concentrations of more than 200 mg/dL with method of Takahashi et al using N-acetyl-D-mannosamine dehydrogenase *5922*
Urine No Effect Analytical No effect observed at a concentration of 200 mg/dL on method of Takahashi et al using N-acetyl-D-mannosamine dehydrogenase *5922*

Sodium *Serum Increase Analytical* In one patient given 30 g sodium ascorbate intravenously (with ascorbate concentration reaching 30 mmol/L) to treat malignant disease mean concentration as measured on Hitachi 747 increased to 162 mmol/L compared with reference range of 135 - 145 mmol/L *319*
Serum No Effect Analytical No effect of concentrations up to 30 mg/L on method on Kodak Ektachem® *5706* At concentration of 60 mg/L had no effect as measured by flame-photometric method *5704* At concentration of 800 mg/L had no effect on ISE measurement without predilution *5704* At concentration of 40,000 mg/L had no effect on ISE measurement with predilution *5704*

Sorbitol *Red Blood Cells Decrease Physiological* In 9 young adults with IDDM treatment with 100 - 600 mg/d ascorbic acid caused significant reduction from mean baseline of 22.0 ± 3.8 nmol sorbitol/g hemoglobin to 8 nmol sorbitol/g hemoglobin after 30 days and 11 nmol sorbitol/g hemoglobin after 56 days *1197*
Red Blood Cells No Effect Physiological Administration of 100 - 600 mg/d to 11 healthy controls caused nonsignificant decrease from mean baseline of 11.7 nmol sorbitol/g hemoglobin to 9 nmol sorbitol/g hemoglobin after 30 days and 8 nmol sorbitol/g hemoglobin after 58 days *1197*

Sucrose *Serum No Effect Analytical* Using automated procedure involving sucrose phosphorylase, phosphoglutamase and glucose-6-phosphatase of Vinet et al no significant interference observed at a concentration of 5 mmol/L *6267*
Urine No Effect Analytical Using automated procedure involving sucrose phosphorylase, phosphoglutamase and glucose-6-phosphatase of Vinet et al no significant interference observed at a concentration of 5 mmol/L *6267*

Sugar *Urine Increase Analytical* False positive with Benedict's and Clinitest® *1714* Positive with Benedict's, Clinitest® at 50 mg/dL *882*

Tetrahydrocannabinol *Urine No Effect Analytical* At concentration of 10% had no significant effect on method on Abbott TDx *5408*

Theophylline *Serum No Effect Analytical* No effect at 50 mg/L on method on Ames Seralyzer *5706*

Threonine *Urine Increase Physiological* In 10 healthy females given 10 g/d *6080*

α-Tocopherol *Serum No Effect Physiological* No effect with varying degrees of supplementation over 14 week study period in young men *2863*

Transferrin Receptor *Serum Decrease Physiological* In 178 individuals from rural Swaziland and Zimbabwe administration of 1 - 2 g ascorbic acid daily caused significant decrease in concentration from mean baseline of 2.58 ± 1.87 mg/L to 2.26 ± 1.12 mg/L after 2 days *3131*

Triglycerides *Serum Decrease Analytical* At concentrations of ascorbic acid of 200 µmol/L (just exceeding presumed upper limit of normal) average decrease of ≤ 0.2 mmol/L observed. Correlation of r > 0.97 with ascorbic acid concentration *490* In 8 healthy fasting individuals ingestion of large amounts of ascorbic acid caused mean 17% reduction with method on Boehringer Mannheim Hitachi 747-100 although exact mechanism not determined *5383* In one patient given 30 g sodium ascorbate intravenously (reaching concentration of 30 mmol/L) to treat malignant disease mean concentration as measured on Hitachi 747 decreased to < 0.1 mmol/L compared with reference range of 0.6 - 5.5 mmol/L *319* At concentrations above 30 mg/L (maximum serum concentration 34 mg/L) lowered concentration as measured by GPO-PAP method *5704*
Serum Decrease Physiological Effect observed in atherosclerotic patients *5669* In 256 men for each increment of 0.5 mg/dL in plasma ascorbic acid adjusted concentration decreased by 5.2 mg/dL *2876*
Serum Increase Physiological In 221 women for each increment of 0.5 mg/dL in plasma ascorbic acid adjusted concentration increased by 2.0 mg/dL *2876*
Serum No Effect Analytical No effect up to 30 mg/L on method on Boehringer Mannheim Reflotron but above this concentration apparently reduced triglyceride concentration although not of clinical significance *5706* No interference observed at concentrations up to 100 mg/L with method on Roche Cobas Ready *5705* No effect at 200 mg/L on method on Ames Seralyzer *5706* No effect of concentrations up to 30 mg/L on method on Kodak Ektachem® *5706* No significant interference observed at concentration of 3 mg/dL when Beckman reagents used with Synchron CX analyzer *4008* No significant interference observed at concentrations of 0.6-2.0 mg/dL with glycerol blanked method on Hitachi 717, 736, 737 and 747 analyzers *3838* At concentrations up to 3.0 mg/dL interference of less than 5% with new Roche triglycerides method on Roche Cobas Fara and Mira *3540* No effect at therapeutic concentration on Boehringer Mannheim Reflotron method *3231* At concentration of 500 mg/L had no effect as measured by lipase/esterase method *5704*
Serum No Effect Physiological No significant effect in 27 female elderly patients with initially low plasma ascorbic acid concentrations given supplements of either 200 or 2000 mg/day *246* No significant effect observed in normotensives and hypertensives when treated with 1 g/d for 6 weeks *4454*

Tyrosine *Plasma Decrease Physiological* Reduces elevated level in premature infants *2242*

Urea Nitrogen *Serum Decrease Analytical* In 8 healthy fasting volunteers ingestion of large doses caused mean 5.6% reduction in concentration as determined by method on Boehringer Mannheim Hitachi 747-100 but exact mechanism not elucidated *5383* At concentrations above 300 mg/L (maximum serum concentration 34 mg/L) lowered concentration as measured by Ektachem® method *5704* At concentrations above 20 mg/L (maximum serum concentration 34 mg/L) lowered concentration as measured by Ames Seralyzer *5704*
Serum No Effect Analytical No effect at therapeutic concentration on Boehringer Mannheim Reflotron method *3231* No interference observed at concentrations up to 100 mg/L with method on Roche Cobas Ready *5705* No effect at 300 mg/L on Boehringer Mannheim Reflotron method *5706* No effect at 2000 mg/L on method on Ames Seralyzer *5706* At concentration of 2,000 mg/L had no effect on diacetylmonoxime method *5704*

Uric Acid *Serum Decrease Analytical* In one patient given 30 g sodium ascorbate intravenously (reaching concentration of 30 mmol/L) to treat malignant disease mean concentration as measured on Hitachi 747 decreased to 0.05 mmol/L compared with reference range of 0.25 - 0.50 mmol/L *319* At concentrations above 10 mg/L (maximum serum concentration 34 mg/L) lowered concentration as measured by Ames Seralyzer *5704* In 8 healthy volunteers ingestion of large amounts of ascorbic acid caused mean 3.1% reduction in concentration as measured by method on Boehringer Mannheim Hitachi 747-100 but exact mechanism not determined *5383*
Serum Decrease Physiological From 1.2 to 3.1 mg/dL in 3 subjects ingesting 8 g/d due to uricosuria *5798*
Serum Increase Analytical Each 1 mg/dL of drug increases concentration as measured by phosphotungstate method by 0.05 mg/dL *6266* At concentrations above 30 mg/L increases result as determined by method on Kodak Ektachem® but of no clinical significance since this exceeds normal plasma concentration *5706* Measured as reducing substance *1009* At concentrations above 100 mg/L (maximum serum concentration 34 mg/L) raised concentration when measured by phosphotungstate reduction *5704* At 5 mg/dL increases by 3.15 mg/dL method of Klein *3173*
Serum No Effect Analytical At concentration of 250 mg/L had no effect on uricase-PAP method *5704* At concentration of 5,000 mg/L had no effect on catalase-AIDH method *5704* No effect observed at a concentration of 10 mg/dL (0.6 mmol/L) with method on Du Pont aca *1552* No effect at therapeutic concentration on Boehringer Mannheim Reflotron method *3231* At 500 mg/L on reversed phase liquid chromatographic procedure of Zhiri et al *6656* No effect at 20 mg/L on method on Boehringer Mannheim Reflotron but at concentrations above this concentration reduced although apparently not of clinical significance *5706* At concentration of 100 mg/L had no effect on uricase method on Du Pont aca *5704* At 200 mg/L on uricase procedure of Kabasak *2998* At concentration of 1,000 mg/L had no effect on Kageyama-Hantzsch method *5704* No effect on Tripyridyl-s-triazine method of Morin *4117* No effect up to 15 mg/L on method on Ames Seralyzer but at higher concentrations apparently reduced uric acid concentration observed *5706* No interference observed at concentrations up to 20 mg/L with method on Roche Cobas Ready *5705*
Urine Increase Physiological Substantial effect with large amounts of compound: effect inhibited by pyrazinamide *5798*

Valine *Urine Decrease Physiological* In 10 healthy females given 10 g/d *6080*

Vitamin A *Serum No Effect Physiological* No effect with varying degrees of supplementation over 14 week study period in young men *2863*

Vitamin B_{12} *Serum Decrease Physiological* When ingested with food compound causes destruction of substantial amounts of vitamin B_{12}*382*
Serum No Effect Physiological No effect with varying degrees of supplementation over 14 week study period in young men *2863*

Asparaginase

Acetone *Serum No Effect Physiological* In spite of effect on glucose usually no effect observed on serum or urine acetone *3974*
Urine No Effect Physiological In spite of effect on glucose usually no effect observed on serum or urine acetone *3974*

Alanine Aminotransferase *Serum Increase Physiological* Occurs as one of a variety of abnormal liver function tests *3974* Hepatotoxicity *2497* Hepatotoxicity observed in as many as 50-75% treated patients *1384*

Albumin *Serum Decrease Physiological* Occurs as one of a variety of abnormal liver function tests *3974* Hepatotoxicity (observed in 80% patients) *4371* In 71% children and 82% adults reported in various studies *3949* Occurs as result of inhibition of protein synthesis *1384* Depressed in up to 70% of patients treated in different studies: effects usually mild *841*

Alkaline Phosphatase *Serum Increase Physiological* Increased in 30-35% of patients treated in different studies: effects usually mild *841* Occurs as one of a variety of abnor-

Asparaginase *(continued)*

Alkaline Phosphatase *(continued)*
mal liver function tests *3974* May cause hepatotoxicity (frequent) *2497* Hemorrhagic pancreatitis in fewer than 0.5% treated patients *2322* In 31% children and 47% adults reported in various studies *3949*

Ammonia *Plasma Increase Physiological* May be marked, associated with abnormal liver function *2606* Hemorrhagic pancreatitis in fewer than 0.5% treated patients *2322* Concentration may increase during the conversion of asparagine to aspartic acid *3974*

Amylase *Serum Increase Physiological* May cause pancreatic toxicity *2497* Hemorrhagic pancreatitis in fewer than 0.5% treated patients *2322* Pancreatitis may occur as a complication *3974* Reports vary from incidence of 2.5 to 16% cases of acute pancreatitis: usually mild *841*

Antithrombin III *Plasma Decrease Physiological* Mean decrease of 68% (immunological) and 74% (functional assay) in different studies *841* Reported to reduce plasma concentration *3694*

Aspartate Aminotransferase *Serum Increase Physiological* In 46% children and 63% adults reported in various studies *3949* Occurs as one of a variety of abnormal liver function tests *3974* Hemorrhagic pancreatitis in fewer than 0.5% treated patients *2322* Increased in 35-45% of patients treated in different studies: effects usually mild *841* Hepatotoxicity *2497* Hepatotoxicity observed in as many as 50-75% treated patients with fatty metamorphosis of the liver observed *1384*

Aspartic Acid *Plasma Increase Physiological* Azotemia, usually pre-renal, occurs frequently. Acute renal failure and fatal renal insufficiency have been reported during treatment *3974*

Bilirubin *Serum Increase Physiological* Occurs as one of a variety of abnormal liver function tests *3974* Increased in 30-60% of patients treated in different studies: effects usually mild *841* In 29% children and 51% adults reported in various studies *3949* Up to 4 mg/dL (dose related effect) *4371* Hemorrhagic pancreatitis in fewer than 0.5% treated patients *2322*

Bilirubin, Direct *Serum Increase Physiological* Occurs as one of a variety of abnormal liver function tests *3974*

Bilirubin, Indirect *Serum Increase Physiological* Occurs as one of a variety of abnormal liver function tests *3974*

BSP Retention *Serum Increase Physiological* Hepatotoxicity (usually mild) *2497* In 57% children and 84% adults reported in various studies *3949*

Calcium *Serum Decrease Physiological* Observed in 60% (?due to hypoalbuminemia) *4371*
Urine Increase Physiological Atypical response but observed in some *4371*

Ceruloplasmin *Serum Decrease Physiological* Possibly due to inhibition of protein synthesis reported in various studies *3949* Diminished hepatic synthesis *4371*

Cholesterol *Serum Decrease Physiological* Occurs as one of a variety of abnormal liver function tests *3974* Hepatotoxicity (effect marked) *2497* In 82-85% of patients reported in various studies *3949*
Serum Increase Physiological Unusual response in some patients *4371*

Cholesterol Esters *Serum Decrease Physiological* Marked fall maximal at 4 d after single injection *6680* Occurs as one of a variety of abnormal liver function tests *3974*

Cholinesterase *Serum Decrease Physiological* Induces impairment of hepatic synthesis *1190*

Chylomicrons *Serum Increase Physiological* Observed in unusual hyperlipidemic response *4371*

Coombs' Test, Indirect *Blood Positive Physiological* In 4 children who demonstrated hemolytic anemia (direct Coombs' test negative) *841*

Creatinine *Serum Increase Physiological* Azotemia, usually pre-renal, occurs frequently. Acute renal failure and fatal renal insufficiency have been reported during treatment *3974* Prerenal azotemia occurs frequently *1384*

Euglobulin Lysis Time *Blood Decrease Physiological* Occasionally observed with toxicity *4773*

Factor V *Plasma Decrease Physiological* Diminished hepatic synthesis *877* May reduce concentration *3974*

Factor VII *Plasma Decrease Physiological* Diminished hepatic synthesis *877*

Factor VIII *Plasma Decrease Physiological* May variably reduce concentration *3974* Diminished hepatic synthesis *877*

Factor IX *Plasma Decrease Physiological* May variably reduce concentration *3974* In 75 to 100% in different studies *841*

Factor XI *Plasma Decrease Physiological* In 75 to 100% in different studies *841*

Fatty Acids (FFA), Free *Serum Decrease Physiological* Common hepatotoxic response *4773*

Fibrin Degradation Products
Plasma Increase Physiological May infrequently increase concentration as part of a consumption coagulopathy *3974*

Fibrinogen *Plasma Decrease Physiological* Marked effect in almost all patients *4371* In 50 to 100% in different studies *841* Associated with decreased synthesis *1384* Reported to reduce plasma concentration *3694* In 32 of 33 patients reported in various studies *3949* May reduce concentration *3974*

α_2-Globulin *Serum Decrease Physiological* Decreased to 70% of control at 2 weeks *4371*

β-Globulin *Serum Decrease Physiological* Decreased to 70% of control at 2 weeks *4371*

β_1-α-Globulin *Serum Decrease Physiological* Diminished hepatic synthesis *4371*

γ-Globulin *Serum Increase Physiological* Increased continuously to 170% of mean at 4 weeks *4371*

Glucose *Serum Increase Physiological* Reported in 9.7% children, although hypoglycemia reported occasionally *841* Associated with inhibition of insulin synthesis *1384* Hyperglycemia may occur as a complication *3974* Observed in 9.7% children, some within 1 week of start of treatment, observed most commonly in older children *4808* May be hyperosmotic nonketotic hyperglycemia *877*
Urine Increase Physiological Hyperglycemia with glycosuria may occur as a complication *3974*

β_2-Glycoprotein *Serum Decrease Physiological* Diminished hepatic synthesis *4371*

Granulocytes *Blood Decrease Physiological* Slight reduction (not dose dependent) *4371*

Haptoglobin *Serum Decrease Physiological* Possibly due to inhibition of protein synthesis reported in various studies *3949*

Hematocrit *Blood Decrease Physiological* Transient bone marrow depression may occur which is associated with delay in return to normal *3974* May cause anemia *2497*

Hemoglobin *Blood Decrease Physiological* May cause anemia *2497* Transient bone marrow depression may occur which is associated with delay in return of concentration to normal *3974*

immunoglobulin A *Serum Increase Physiological* Increased hepatic synthesis *4371*

Immunoglobulin G *Serum Increase Physiological* Increased hepatic synthesis *4371*

Immunoglobulin M *Serum Increase Physiological* Increased hepatic synthesis *4371*

Insulin *Plasma Decrease Physiological* ?due to decreased production with decreased protein synthesis *877*

Leukocytes *Blood Decrease Physiological* Concentration may decrease to normal or below within a few days of initiation of treatment. Marked leukopenia may occur *3974* Mild effect in up to 25% patients *4371*

Lipase *Serum Increase Physiological* Reports vary from incidence of 2.5 to 16% cases of acute pancreatitis: usually mild *841*

Lipids *Serum Decrease Physiological* Parallel decrease in cholesterol *4371*
Serum Increase Physiological Rare response after initial hypolipidemia *4371*

β-Lipoprotein *Serum Decrease Physiological* Observed in unusual hyperlipidemic response *4371*

Lipoprotein Lipase *Serum Decrease Physiological* Observed in unusual hyperlipidemic response *4371*

Lipoproteins *Serum Decrease Physiological* Possible depressed synthesis *2497*

Lipoproteins, Pre-β *Serum Increase Physiological* Observed in unusual hyperlipidemic response *4371*

Lymphoblasts *Blood Decrease Physiological* Concentration may decrease markedly with initiation of treatment *3974*

Lymphocytes *Blood Decrease Physiological* Slight reduction (not dose dependent) *4371*

Nitrogen *Urine Increase Physiological* Effect greatest in responders to therapy *4371*

5'-Nucleotidase *Serum Increase Physiological* Observed in up to 25% patients *4371* In 15% children and 26% adults reported in various studies *3949*

Partial Thromboplastin Time
Plasma Increase Physiological Observed frequently with toxicity *5611*

Phosphate *Urine Increase Physiological* Response in all treated patients *4371*

Phospholipids *Serum Decrease Physiological* Parallel decrease in cholesterol *4371*
Serum Increase Physiological Rare response after initial hypolipidemia *4371*

Plasminogen *Plasma Decrease Physiological* Mean decrease of 59% (immunological) and 62% (functional assay) in different studies *841* Reported to reduce plasma concentration *3694*

Platelets *Blood Decrease Physiological* May cause bone marrow depression *4371* May infrequently reduce circulating platelet concentration as part of a consumption coagulopathy *3974*

Protein *Urine Increase Physiological* Infrequent transient proteinuria *841* Transient slight effect for few days *4371* Azotemia, usually pre-renal, occurs frequently. Acute renal failure and fatal renal insufficiency have been reported during treatment *3974*

Protein C *Plasma Decrease Physiological* Reported to reduce plasma concentration *3694*

Protein S *Plasma Decrease Physiological* Reported to reduce plasma concentration *3694*

Prothrombin Time *Plasma Increase Physiological* In 18 patients investigated reported in various studies *3949* Diminished synthesis of prothrombin by liver *877*

Thrombin Time *Blood Increase Physiological* Occurs with decreased fibrinogen concentration *4371*

Thyroid Stimulating Hormone
Serum No Effect Physiological No effect during treatment within 3 weeks in 14 children *2534*

Thyroxine Binding Globulin
Serum Decrease Physiological Concentration may decrease significantly within two days of initiation of treatment making interpretation of thyroid function tests difficult, but concentration returns to normal within 4 weeks of the end of treatment *3974* From 29.4 to 8.0 µg/mL within 3 weeks in 14 children *2534*

Thyroxine (T4) *Serum Decrease Physiological* From 10.7 to 2.9 µg/dL within 3 weeks in 14 children *2534* Concentration reduced because L-asparaginase reduces TBG *2412*

Thyroxine (T4), Free *Serum Decrease Physiological* From 1.77 to 0.94 ng/dL within 3 weeks in 14 children *2534*

Transferrin *Serum Decrease Physiological* Reported effect *4371* Possibly due to inhibition of protein synthesis reported in various studies *3949*

Tri-iodothyronine (T3) *Serum Decrease Physiological* From 0.99 to 0.35 ng/mL within 3 weeks in 14 children *2534* Concentration reduced in association with reduction of TBG by L-asparaginase *2412*

Triglycerides *Serum Decrease Physiological* Noted after first week in some patients *4371*
Serum Increase Physiological Rare response after initial hypolipidemia *4371*

Urea Nitrogen *Serum Increase Physiological* Occurs in 50% subjects (prerenal origin) *2497* Increased in from 7.5 to 50% in different studies: usually mild, possibly due to increased availability of ammonia *841*

Uric Acid *Serum Increase Physiological* Concentration of abnormal cells may decrease to normal or below with initiation of treatment with a corresponding increase in the plasma uric acid concentration *3974*
Urine Increase Physiological Marked response if lysis of tissues *4371*

Aspartame

Aspartic Acid *Plasma No Effect Physiological* No significant change in 6 healthy volunteers when given either aspartame sweetened or unsweetened beverage hourly for eight hours *5787* No significant effect on plasma aspartate after 3 successive 12-oz servings of drug-sweetened beverage over 6 hours *5786*

Formate *Serum No Effect Physiological* No effect of ingestion of aspartame-sweetened beverages when ingested over several hours in 6 healthy volunteers *5787*

Methanol *Blood No Effect Physiological* No effect of aspartame-sweetened beverages in 6 healthy volunteers over several hours *5787*

Phenylalanine *Plasma Increase Physiological* Increase by 1.64 to 2.05 µmol/dL 30 to 45 minutes after 12-oz serving of drug-sweetened beverage *5786* Significant increase by 1.41-2.35 µmol/dL above baseline in 6 healthy volunteers given sweetened or unsweetened beverage hourly for 8 hours. Steady state reached after 4-5 servings and did not exceed normal range at any time *5787*

Aspidium

Alanine Aminotransferase *Serum Increase Physiological* May cause hepatic toxicity *3810*

Alkaline Phosphatase *Serum Increase Physiological* May cause hepatic toxicity *3810*

Aspartate Aminotransferase *Serum Increase Physiological* May cause hepatic toxicity *3810*

Bile *Urine Increase Physiological* May cause hepatic toxicity *3810*

Bilirubin *Serum Increase Physiological* May cause hepatic toxicity *1714*

Bilirubin, Direct *Serum Increase Physiological* Probable inhibition of uptake of bilirubin by liver *4014*

BSP Retention *Serum Increase Physiological* Probable inhibition of uptake by liver *4014*

Casts *Urine Increase Physiological* May cause nephrotoxicity *467*

Sugar *Urine Increase Analytical* Acts as reducing agent *1714*

Urea Nitrogen *Serum Increase Physiological* May cause nephrotoxicity *467*

Aspirin

Acetaminophen *Serum Increase Analytical* With Glynn and Kendal technique even with arithmetic corrections, due to metabolites *318* Significant positive effect on unmodified Glynn-Kendal technique *4891*
Serum No Effect Analytical Has no effect on direct acid/ferric reduction method of Liu and Oka *3616*

Acetazolamide *Serum Increase Physiological* Acetazolamide clearance reduced probably as result of competitive inhibition of renal tubular secretion *4062* Acetazolamide displaced from protein-binding sites and excretion inhibited. Clearance reduced by up to 60% *160*

Acetoacetate *Serum Increase Physiological* Due to late metabolic acidosis and renal impairment *2242*
Urine Increase Analytical Reacts with Gerhardt $FeCl_3$ procedure *6515*
Urine Increase Physiological Acidotic response especially in children *2183*

Acetylsalicylic Acid *Serum Increase Physiological* 1 g orally up to 100 mg/L, 12 g = 400 mg/L *3868*

Alanine Aminotransferase *Serum Increase Physiological* Noted in some patients at serum concentrations above 25 mg/dL without signs of hypersensitivity reactions but dose related *6688* Regular administration of doses greater than 50 mg/kg may produce reversible hepatic damage associated with focal hepatocellular necrosis *1384* Reversible, usually mild hepatotoxicity occasionally seen in children with rheumatic disease and in adults with lupus or rheumatoid arthritis usually when serum concentration exceeds 25 mg/dL after 1-4 weeks treatment *1384* Prolonged use may cause hepatic toxicity

Aspirin *(continued)*

Alanine Aminotransferase *(continued)*
1714 Abnormal liver function reported in 0.3% of 1527 patients treated with aspirin in comparison with 0% of 530 patients treated with placebo *5034* In 15% trials of treatment for juvenile rheumatoid arthritis *386*

Albumin *Serum Decrease Analytical* Decreased dye binding capacity *5869*
Serum Decrease Physiological Progressive effect during three days but also noted over longer term study at beginning, eventually reverted towards normal. Effect statistically significant *5122*
Serum No Effect Analytical No significant effect on BCG method at 600 mg/L *4335*

Alkaline Phosphatase *Serum Increase Physiological* Prolonged use may cause hepatic toxicity *3479* Occasional reversible, usually mild, hepatotoxicity observed in patients treated for some time and in whom serum concentration has remained above 25 mg/dL for 1-4 weeks *1384*
Serum No Effect Physiological When approximately 3 g/d ingested for several weeks *5122*
Urine Increase Physiological Due to nephrotoxic effect of drug *4826* Marked increase observed even when as little as 3.5 g aspirin ingested daily *4777*

Alkaline Phosphatase, Bone Isoenzyme
Serum No Effect Analytical At a concentration of 500 mg/L had no effect on Tandem-MP Ostase method *777*

Amino Acids *Urine Increase Physiological* Two fold increase after 1.6 g in normals *1720*

α-Amino-Nitrogen *Urine Increase Physiological* Inhibition of reabsorption, increased protein catabolism *2242*

Amylase *Serum Increase Physiological* Single case reported *6515*
Serum No Effect Physiological When approximately 3 g/d ingested for several weeks *5122*

Ascorbic Acid *Serum Decrease Physiological* Uptake into leukocytes decreased also *3635* In children and adults taking large amount of aspirin since it potentiates excretion of vitamin C *5055*
Urine Increase Physiological Reported effect *1233*
White Blood Cells Decrease Physiological Prolonged administration decreases concentration in buffy coat *1857*

Aspartate Aminotransferase *Serum Increase Physiological* In 15% trials of treatment for juvenile rheumatoid arthritis *386* Occasional hepatotoxicity observed but usually after 1-4 weeks treatment with serum concentration being above 25 mg/dL *1384* Abnormal liver function reported in 0.3% of 1527 patients treated with aspirin in comparison with 0% of 530 patients treated with placebo *5034* Prolonged administration may cause hepatic toxicity *3479* Noted in some patients at serum concentrations above 25 mg/dL without signs of hypersensitivity reactions, but dose related *6688* Rare reversible hepatic damage observed in people receiving doses of more than 50 mg/kg *1384* Probability that a statistically average patient will have an abnormal AST activity (greater than 1.2 times the upper limit of normal) within 12 weeks after beginning treatment 0.02 in patients with osteoarthritis and 0.06 in patients with rheumatoid arthritis compared with 0.02 and 0.01 respectively in patients treated with placebo *1991*
Serum No Effect Physiological When approximately 3 g/d ingested for several weeks *5122*

Aspirin Esterase *Serum Increase Physiological* In all patients except cirrhotics *233*

Atenolol *Serum No Effect Physiological* 300 mg aspirin had no effect on bioavailability of atenolol following single dose of 100 mg atenolol in 6 healthy volunteers *5309*

Barbiturate *Serum No Effect Analytical* No significant interference at a concentration of 1000 µg/mL (5.55 mmol/L) with method on Du Pont aca *1511*

Basal Metabolic Rate *Patient Increase Physiological* Reported metabolic effect *3669*

Benzodiazepine Screen *Serum No Effect Analytical* No significant interference observed at a concentration of 1000 µg/mL (5.55 mmol/L) with method on Du Pont aca *1512*

Bicarbonate *Serum Decrease Physiological* Initial acidosis with excessive doses *1714*
Serum Increase Physiological Later alteration of acid base balance *1009*
Serum No Effect Physiological When approximately 3 g/d ingested for several weeks *5122*
Urine Increase Physiological Response to respiratory alkalosis of early toxicity *2242*

Bile *Urine Increase Analytical* Purple color with Fouchet procedure *199*

Bilirubin *Serum Decrease Physiological* Progressive effect during three days but also noted over longer term study at beginning, eventually reverted towards normal. Effect statistically significant *5122*
Serum Increase Physiological Clinically significant displacement from protein in neonates *6314* Competition for albumin binding *2486* Reversible, usually mild hepatotoxicity observed in patients treated for some time with serum concentration remaining above 25 mg/dL for 1-4 weeks *1384*

Bilirubin, Direct *Serum Increase Physiological* Occurs with hemolytic anemia *5869*

Bleeding Time *Patient Increase Physiological* Significant effect on template bleeding time over 6 d of study *1406* In 6 patients receiving aspirin mean bleeding time increased to 7.4 min compared with 5.0 min in controls without aspirin *1893* Usual analgesic doses increase bleeding time *1384* In 52 healthy volunteers mean bleeding time increased from baseline 5.9 ± 0.4 min before 80 mg aspirin to 7.2 ± 0.6 min 6 h after and 10.6 ± 1.3 min after 14 days. With 325 mg aspirin/d on the same schedule the times were 5.7 ± 0.6 min, 8.0 ± 0.5 min and 10.9 ± 1.1 min respectively. With 325 mg enteric-coated aspirin the times were 6.1 ± 0.5 min, 7.9 ± 1.2 min and 13.8 ± 1.2 min. When the same formulations were given on alternate days the bleeding times were similar *2272* Also inhibits platelet glycolysis *1857* In 25 healthy volunteers treated with 81 mg/d for 1 week mean increased from baseline of 366 ± 17 seconds to 546 ± 44 seconds *6687* In 12 healthy volunteers bleeding time increased from mean baseline of 415 s by 61% to 855 s after treatment with 2250 mg aspirin/d for 5 days *3807* Prolongs bleeding time by itself and when coadministered with warfarin has potential to increase risk of warfarin-associated bleeding *2625* Increase observed in healthy male volunteers regardless of whether aspirin given daily, or in controlled release form or on alternate days *1052* Effect slight in normal subjects, but technical variables such as direction of incision may have influence *4025*

Calcium *Serum Decrease Physiological* Progressive effect during three days but also noted over longer term study at beginning, eventually reverted towards normal. Effect statistically significant *5122*

Carbon Dioxide Partial Pressure
Blood Decrease Physiological In toxicity with increased respiratory rate and pulmonary ventilation *2242*

Casts *Urine Increase Physiological* Occurs with poisoning *2183*

Catecholamines *Urine No Effect Physiological* No effect with short term ingestion 2.6 g/d *1184*

Cells *Urine Increase Physiological* Tubular epithelial cells increased initially, may persist *2242* Tubular cells increased: occur even with therapeutic doses; effect can be quite marked *4777*

Chloride *Serum Increase Analytical* At concentrations substantially above therapeutic, time and concentration dependent increase in concentration with Kone Microlyte potentiometric analyzer. Effect due to salicylate moiety of drug *3548*
Serum Increase Physiological Progressive effect during three days but also noted over longer term study at beginning. Eventually reverted towards normal. Effect statistically significant *5122*

Chlorpropamide *Serum Increase Physiological* Displaces from plasma proteins *2452*

Cholesterol *Serum Decrease Physiological* Doses over 5 g reported to have effect *2242* Progressive effect during three days but also noted over longer term study at beginning, eventually reverted towards normal. Effect statistically significant *5122*
Serum No Effect Physiological In 6 patients with type II hyperlipidemia mean concentration showed no significant effect after treatment with 50 mg/d for 1 week *5585*

Cholinesterase *Serum No Effect Analytical* Insignificant increase of 0.94 U/mL at a concentration of 100 µg/mL with method on Du Pont Dimension *3271* Insignificant decrease of 0.08 U/mL at a concentration of 100 µg/mL with method on Du Pont aca *3271*

Chondrex *Serum No Effect Analytical* Concentrations up to 5 g/L had no significant effect on sandwich-type ELISA procedure of Harvey et al *2491*

Closure Time by PFA-100 *Patient Increase Physiological* In 12 healthy volunteers closing time as measured by PFA-100 increased by 79% from mean baseline of 123 s to 217 s after treatment with 2250 mg aspirin/d for 5 days *3807*

Color *Feces Increase Analytical* Red or black due to gastrointestinal bleeding *3810*

Creatinine *Serum Increase Physiological* Anti-inflammatory doses produced substantial effect in 13 of 23 patients with systemic lupus erythematosus *4777* Average increase of 38% in patients and healthy individuals *824*
Serum No Effect Analytical At 1.0 g/L on reversed phase liquid chromatographic procedure of Zhiri et al *6656* No effect on Jaffe procedure on Technicon AutoAnalyzer® at concentration of 20 mg/dL *4024*
Serum No Effect Physiological When approximately 3 g/d ingested for several weeks *5122*

Creatinine Clearance *Urine Decrease Physiological* Significant effect correlated with plasma salicylate concentration *4195* Observed even with therapeutic doses *4777* As a consequence of increased serum concentrations *824*

Cyclosporine *Blood No Effect Physiological* In individuals taking aspirin while also receiving cyclosporine no significant interactions with pharmacokinetics observed *3264*

D-Dimer *Plasma Decrease Physiological* In 31 patients with chronic atrial fibrillation initial median concentration of 158 ng/mL (interquartile range 81 - 292 ng/mL) changed to 102 ng/mL (interquartile range 77 - 155 ng/mL) after treatment with aspirin for 2 months *2130*

Dehydroepiandrosterone Sulfate
Plasma Decrease Physiological In women with regular use (more than once per week) significant negative correlation of r = - 0.17 *4266*

Diatrizoate Clearance *Urine Decrease Physiological* Observed even with therapeutic doses *4777*

Diclofenac *Serum Decrease Physiological* Coadministration of aspirin with diclofenac reduced the plasma diclofenac concentration by displacing it from its binding sites resulting in lower plasma concentrations, peak plasma concentrations and AUC *1025* Reported to decrease plasma concentration *1384* Coadministration of single doses of each drug reduced area under curve of diclofenac by 52%, similar effect observed when diclofenac given intravenously. Effect probably due to displacement of diclofenac from binding protein sites and increased clearance *4062*

Diflunisal *Serum Decrease Physiological* Concomitant administration of multiple doses of diflunisal and aspirin caused a small decrease in the diflunisal concentration *3972* Small but significant reduction in trough concentration of 17% observed in volunteers but diflunisal did not affect salicylic acid disposition *4062*

Digoxin *Serum No Effect Physiological* Coadministration does not alter elimination of digoxin in healthy volunteers *4062*

2,3-Dinor-6-Keto-Prostaglandin $F_{1\alpha}$
Urine Decrease Physiological Suppression of excretion observed in healthy male volunteers to an extent of about 18% when controlled release aspirin given, 23% when 162.5 mg/d given and 35% when alternate day treatment given *1052* When given for 7 days to patients with mild hypertension not receiving antihypertensive medication for 2 weeks *4065*

2,3-Dinor-Thromboxane B_2 *Urine Decrease Physiological* Reduction observed in mildly hypertensive patients treated for 7 days following two weeks without antihypertensive medication *4065* Single dose aspirin reduced mean excretion from 117 to 33 ng/g creatinine in 8 healthy controls and from 156 to 66 ng/g creatinine in 8 patients with peripheral arteriopathy *4066* Suppression of excretion by 53% in healthy male volunteers given controlled release aspirin, by 80% with daily aspirin and with alternate day aspirin treatment *1052* In 5 healthy adults administration of 2.5 g caused significant decrease from mean baseline of 32.4 nmol/mol creatinine to 3.2 nmol/mol creatinine after administration *1811*

Doxazosin *Serum No Effect Physiological* Coadministration with doxazosin had no effect on its pharmacokinetics *4642*

Drugs of Abuse Screen *Urine Decrease Analytical* Ingestion of aspirin caused decreased rate of change of absorbance with Syva d.a.u. EMIT benzoylecgonone compared with specimens from controls *6292*

EDTA Clearance *Urine No Effect Physiological* Although creatinine clearance apparently affected *824*

Eosinophils *Blood Decrease Physiological* May cause aplastic anemia or pancytopenia *6022*

Epinephrine *Urine No Effect Physiological* No effect with short term ingestion 2.6 g/d *1184*

Erythrocyte Sedimentation Rate
Blood Decrease Physiological If elevated, reduces toward normal value *2242*
Blood Increase Physiological Occurs in some patients (reversible) *2242*

Erythrocyte Survival *Blood Decrease Physiological* Large doses increase destruction *2242*

Erythrocytes *Blood Decrease Physiological* Hemolysis/G-6-PD deficient/gastrointestinal hemorrhage/direct bone marrow depression *5417*
Urine Increase Physiological Initial effect always, may persist *2242* Observed effect with long term low doses for secondary prevention of coronary heart disease *4777*

Ethanol *Serum Increase Physiological* Significant increase in 5 healthy volunteers given 1 g aspirin 1 h before 0.3 g/kg body weight than when no aspirin given. In both situations alcohol ingested 1 h after a standard breakfast. Probably due to inhibition of gastric alcohol dehydrogenase *5065*

Factor VII *Plasma Decrease Physiological* Acts like bishydroxycoumarin *2242*

Fatty Acids (FFA), Free *Serum Decrease Physiological* Increased fatty acid oxidation, decreased lipogenesis *2242* Considerable reduction in concentration in both normals and diabetics and lesser response to oral glucose *4024*

Fenoprofen *Serum Decrease Physiological* Enhances metabolic clearance *1384* Coadministration of aspirin decreases biological half-life of fenoprofen because it increases its metabolic clearance *1439* Area under curve reduced by 19% with single dose and by 33% with multiple dose study but mechanism not determined as yet *4062* Area under curve reduced by both single and multiple doses with probable reduction in half-life but mechanism not established *5141*
Urine Decrease Physiological Coadministration of aspirin decreases biological half-life of fenoprofen because it increases its metabolic clearance and increases the amount of its hydroxylated derivative in the urine *1439*

Ferric Chloride Test *Urine Positive Analytical* Red-purple color may mask true color *882*

α-Fetoprotein *Serum Decrease Physiological* Administration of drug to pregnant women is associated with reduction in concentration in maternal plasma *2229*

Fibrin Degradation Products *Urine Decrease Physiological* Occurs in 2/3 patients with proliferative glomerulonephritis *1053*

Fibrinogen *Plasma Increase Physiological* Associated with increased sedimentation rate *2242*
Plasma No Effect Physiological In 31 patients with chronic atrial fibrillation initial median concentration of 3.78 g/L (interquartile range 3.0 - 4.7 g/L) not significantly changed to 3.83 g/L (interquartile range 2.92 - 4.77 g/L) after treatment with aspirin for 2 months *2130*

Flurbiprofen *Serum Decrease Physiological* Concomitant administration of both drugs reduces plasma concentration of flurbiprofen by 50% *1384* Total clearance increased but elimination half-time unchanged: effect probably due to displacement from plasma protein *4062*

Folate *Serum Decrease Physiological* In 1 study subject brisk, significant but reversible fall in total and bound serum folate. Aspirin *in vitro* also displaced significant amounts of bound serum folate *3441*
Urine No Effect Physiological Small but insignificant rise due to displacement from binding protein in serum *3441*

Fouchet Test *Urine Positive Analytical* Produces purple color *703*

Glomerular Filtration Rate *Urine Decrease Physiological* Nephrotoxicity of drug occurring acutely *451*

Aspirin *(continued)*

Glucagon *Plasma Increase Physiological* Observed in humans and animals but mechanism for this not known *4024*

Glucose *Serum Decrease Physiological* In diabetics and if toxic doses ingested *1714* Also decreased response to oral glucose in normal subjects and diabetics *4024*
Serum Increase Physiological Increased absorption and steroid release inhibits TCA cycle *5869*
Serum No Effect Analytical At 10 mg/dL no effect on glucose oxidase procedure of Gochman. At 10 mg/dL no effect on alkaline ferricyanide procedure *2197* At 1 g/dL on p-HBAH procedure of Lever. At 1 g/dL on o-toluidine procedure *3531*
Urine Decrease Analytical Glucose-oxidase methods inhibited by gentisic acid *1825*
Urine Decrease Physiological May reduce hyperglycemia, glycosuria in diabetes *2242*
Urine Increase Analytical Metabolites may react positively in large doses with Ames Clinitest procedure *4034*
Urine Increase Physiological Inhibits liver and muscle glycogen synthesis due to hyperglycemia *2242*
Urine No Effect Analytical Metabolites have no effect on Ames Keto-Diastix, Diastix, Multistix and Clinistix procedures *4034* With DNSA method at usual concentrations *134*

Glucose Tolerance *Serum No Effect Physiological* No significant effect usually observed *2452*

β-Glucuronidase *Urine Increase Physiological* Marked increase observed even when as little as 3.5 g aspirin ingested daily *4777*

Glutathione, Reduced
Red Blood Cells Decrease Physiological Occurs initially before overt hemolysis *3094*

Guaiacols Spot Test *Urine Positive Analytical* False reaction with screening test of Rogers *5061*

Heinz Body Formation *Blood Positive Physiological* Occur initially but disappear with hemolysis *3094*

Hematocrit *Blood Decrease Physiological* Depresses bone marrow, gastrointestinal bleeding, hemolytic anemia *1212*

Hemoglobin *Blood Decrease Physiological* In 200 individuals aged 70 years or older treatment with 100 mg/d for 1 year caused significant decrease of 0.33 g/dL compared with decrease of 0.11 g/dL in placebo-treated control group *5552* Depresses bone marrow, gastrointestinal bleeding, hemolytic anemia *1212*
Plasma Increase Physiological Occurs with hemolytic anemia *3094*
Urine Increase Physiological Occurs with severe hemolytic anemia *3094*
Urine No Effect Physiological No association observed in over 1000 men aged 60 years and older between aspirin ingestion and dipstick hematuria *732*

Hemoglobin A_{1c} *Blood Increase Analytical* Acetylation of hemoglobin simulates glycosylation when measured by HPLC or electrophoresis but no increase observed with isoelectric focusing and colorimetric techniques *4228*

Heparin-releasable Platelet Factor 4
Plasma Decrease Physiological 5 minutes after intravenous heparin administration significant reduction observed *5182*

Hippuric Acid *Urine Increase Analytical* Salicyluric acid measured by method of Tomokuni *6052*

Homogentisic Acid *Urine Increase Analytical* Interferes with measurement procedure *2025*

Homovanillic Acid *Cerebrospinal Fluid Increase Analytical* Interferes with fluorometric method even if 5 d before *2945*
Urine Increase Analytical May produce interfering fluorescence *882*

11-Hydroxycorticosteroids *Urine No Effect Physiological* No effect with short term ingestion 2.6 g/d *1184*

17-Hydroxycorticosteroids *Plasma Increase Physiological* Large doses stimulate adrenocortical activity *5625*
Urine No Effect Physiological No effect with short term ingestion of 2.6 g/d *1184*

5-Hydroxyindoleacetic Acid *Urine Decrease Analytical* Reported to affect fluorometric method *2452*

Hydroxyproline *Urine Decrease Physiological* At 100 mg/kg in children has significant effect *3556*

^{131}I Uptake *Serum Decrease Physiological* With large doses and chronic administration *2396*

Serum No Effect Physiological No effect observed *3107*

Ibuprofen *Serum Decrease Physiological* Substantial reduction observed when drugs coadministered but mechanism not established *2325* Reduction of up to 60% observed when compared with time prior to administration of aspirin *4062*
Serum No Effect Physiological Single dose studies in normal volunteers of the effect of aspirin on ibuprofen concentrations have shown no effect *3200*

Indomethacin *Serum Decrease Physiological* Substantial reduction observed with coadministration probably due to effect on gastrointestinal absorption *3347* Reported effect with coadministration possibly by interfering with its absorption *1384* Chronic coadministration of 3.6 g/d aspirin with indomethacin in normal volunteers decreased the blood concentration of indomethacin by approximately 20% *3980*
Serum No Effect Analytical No effect on HPLC method of Roberts and Smith *4978*
Serum No Effect Physiological Little or no decrease observed in several studies in which drugs coadministered: maximum reduction of 20% observed after a single oral dose of aspirin but reduction of only 10% with chronic dosing *4062*

Insulin *Plasma Increase Physiological* Increased in response to decreased serum glucose *4024*

Inulin Clearance *Urine Decrease Physiological* Significant effect correlated with plasma salicylate concentration *4195* Observed even with therapeutic doses *4777*

Iron *Serum Decrease Physiological* May be markedly reduced with large doses *2242*

Isoxicam *Serum Decrease Physiological* Area under curve reduced by 23% following a single oral dose of isoxicam when healthy volunteers previously pretreated with aspirin for several days: effect probably related to displacement of isoxicam from plasma protein *4062*

6-Keto-Prostaglandin $F_{1\alpha}$ *Plasma Decrease Physiological* In 52 healthy volunteers administration of 80 mg/d for caused reduction from mean baseline of 4.2 ± 0.6 pg/min to 3.7 ± 0.5 pg/min after 1 day but with return to 4.3 ± 0.7 pg/min on day 14. With 325 mg/d concentration decreased from baseline of 3.6 ± 0.5 pg/min to 3.4 ± 0.7 pg/min after 1 day and 3.3 ± 0.6 pg/min after 14 days. With 325 mg/d enteric aspirin concentration decreased from baseline of 4.6 ± 0.5 pg/min to 2.8 ± 0.4 pg/min after 1 day and 3.0 ± 0.5 pg/min after 14 days. Similar reductions observed when alternate day schedule used *2272* 18% reduction in 34 pregnant women treated with aspirin for 21 days but reduction similar with placebo *5339*
Plasma No Effect Physiological No significant change observed in patients with CAD during aspirin administration *5182* In 8 healthy pregnant women taking 60 to 80 mg aspirin daily from 12 weeks onwards median concentration 626 (326 - 1164) ng/L not significantly different from 862 (471 - 1182) ng/L in 16 pregnant controls *708*
Urine Decrease Physiological Significant reduction observed in mildly hypertensive patients treated for 7 days following two weeks without antihypertensive medication *4065*
Urine No Effect Physiological Insignificant increase in 33 pregnant women treated with 60 mg daily from 12th week until term *481*

Ketone Body Ratio *Serum No Effect Analytical* When added at a concentration of 4 g/L had no significant effect on AKBR method of Uno et al *6131*

Ketones *Serum Decrease Physiological* Increased oxidation of ketone bodies in diabetics *2242*
Serum Increase Physiological Due to induced acidosis *2183*
Urine Decrease Physiological Increased oxidation of ketone bodies in diabetics *2242*
Urine Increase Analytical Reddish color with Gerhardt's test *1714*
Urine Increase Physiological Acidotic response especially in children *2183*
Urine No Effect Analytical No effect of metabolites observed with Ames Multistix and other reagent strip tests and with Ames Acetest reagent tablets *4034*

Ketoprofen *Serum Decrease Physiological* Coadministration decreased protein-binding of ketoprofen and increased its clearance *1384* When coadministered with ketoprofen decreased its protein binding and increased its clearance to 0.07 L/kg/h without aspirin to 0.11 L/kg/h with aspirin *6564*

17-Ketosteroids *Urine No Effect Physiological* No effect with short term ingestion 2.6 g/d *1184*

Lactate *Plasma Increase Physiological* Due to late metabolic acidosis and renal impairment *2242*

Lactate Dehydrogenase *Serum Increase Physiological* Experimental effect seen in rabbits with prolonged use *5159*
Serum No Effect Physiological When approximately 3 g/d ingested for several weeks *5122*
Urine Increase Physiological Renal irritation and desquamation of epithelial cells *4826* Marked increase observed even when as little as 3.5 g aspirin ingested daily *4777*

Leucine Aminopeptidase *Urine Decrease Physiological* Due to antifibrinolytic action *4826*
Urine Increase Physiological Marked increase observed even when as little as 3.5 g aspirin ingested daily *4777*

Leukocytes *Blood Decrease Physiological* Depresses leukocytosis of acute rheumatic fever *6449*
Blood Increase Physiological In 161 individuals aged 70 years or older treatment with 100 mg/d for 1 year caused significant increase of 660 ± 2630 /μL compared with 220 ± 1320 /μL in placebo-treated controls *5552*

Leukotriene E_4 *Urine No Effect Physiological* In 5 healthy adults given 2.5 g aspirin no significant effect observed on urinary excretion changing from mean baseline of 9.34 nmol/mol creatinine to 9.87 nmol/mol creatinine *1811*

Lipoprotein Lp(a) *Serum No Effect Physiological* In 112 individuals receiving aspirin mean and median concentrations of 195 and 93 mg/L respectively not significantly different from 179 and 106 mg/L in 1415 controls *5604*

Lithium *Serum No Effect Physiological* Aspirin administration appears to have no effect on plasma lithium concentration *4399* Administration of 3.9 g/d for 6 days to 7 patients with median age of 61 years did not significantly affect plasma concentration *4831*

Lithium Clearance *Urine No Effect Physiological* Administration of 3.9 g/d for 6 days to 7 patients with median age of 61 years did not significantly affect clearance *4831*

Maclofenamate *Serum Decrease Physiological* When drugs given together concentration of meclofenamate reduced *1384*

Magnesium *Serum Increase Physiological* Prolonged therapy likely to cause elevation *409*

Malondialdehyde *Platelets Decrease Physiological* In 8 healthy pregnant women taking 60 to 80 mg aspirin daily from 12 weeks onwards median concentration of 2.2 (1.9 - 2.7) nmol/10^9 platelets significantly different from 5.2 (4.7 - 5.8) nmol/10^9 platelets in 16 pregnant controls *708*

MCH *Blood Decrease Physiological* In 161 individuals aged 70 years or older treatment with 100 mg/d for 1 year caused significant decrease of 26.8 ± 1.6 pg similar to that observed in placebo-treated controls *5552*

MCV *Blood Increase Physiological* In 161 individuals aged 70 years or older treated with 100 mg/d for 1 year mean increased by 1.62 ± 5.34 fL compared with increase of 1.23 ± 3.08 fL in 162 placebo-treated controls *5552*

Methemoglobin *Blood Increase Physiological* May cause hemolysis with G-6-PD deficiency *6015*

Methotrexate *Serum Increase Physiological* Clearance by kidneys may be halved by large doses of drug *4902* Aspirin reported to reduce methotrexate clearance by 30% and to decrease methotrexate binding to protein by 20-60% *1384* Coadministration in one study reduced renal clearance by 35% with increase in free fraction by 30%: effect probably due to inhibition of active tubular secretion of methotrexate *4062* Displaces from plasma protein binding, if present *2452*

N-Acetyl-Glucosaminidase *Urine Increase Physiological* Marked increase observed even when as little as 3.5 g aspirin ingested daily *4777*

Naproxen *Serum Decrease Physiological* Slight effect noted when drugs coadministered possibly through competition for protein binding sites and increased renal clearance of naproxen *5431* Coadministration reduced area under curve of naproxen by 15%. In another study oral clearance of total naproxen increased by 56% *4062*

Neutrophils *Blood No Effect Physiological* Neutropenia reported in 0.8% of 1527 patients treated with aspirin in comparison with 1.1% of 530 pattients treated with placebo *5034*

Nicotinic Acid *Serum Increase Physiological* Concomitant administration of aspirin with niacin decreases the metabolic clearance of nicotinic acid *3253*

Nitroblue Tetrazolium Test *Blood Decrease Physiological* Mechanism not discussed *1483*

Nitrogen *Urine Increase Physiological* Effect observed in adults *5625*

Nitroglycerin *Serum Increase Physiological* Aspirin may decrease the clearance and enhance the hemodynamic effects of sublingual nitroglycerin *4527*

Norepinephrine *Urine No Effect Physiological* No effect with short term ingestion 2.6 g/d *1184*

5'-Nucleotidase *Serum Increase Physiological* Reversible hepatotoxicity with prolonged administration *5159*

Occult Blood *Feces Increase Physiological* In acute study of 47 healthy volunteers 325 mg enteric-coated aspirin caused excretion to increase to 0.96 ± 0.12 mL/d from baseline of 0.47 ± 0.11 mL/d. With 325 mg plain aspirin excretion increased to 1.82 ± 0.35 mL/d *5298* In 3% of 200 individuals aged 70 years or older treated with 100 mg/d for 1 year clinically evident gastrointestinal bleeding observed *5552* In over 70% patients when more than 3 g/d given *6342* In one drug trial administration of aspirin was associated with a rate of gastrointestinal bleeding of 2.7% *5256* In 1.5% trials of treatment for juvenile rheumatoid arthritis *386*

2',5'-Oligoadenylate Synthetase
Neutrophils No Effect Physiological In healthy individuals given single intramuscular injection of interferon *6519*

PAH Clearance *Urine Decrease Physiological* Observed even with therapeutic doses *4777*
Urine No Effect Physiological Insignificant reduction observed *4195*

pH *Blood Decrease Physiological* Systemic acidosis common in poisoning, more frequent in chronic situation, in patients with severe manifestations and dehydration *2051* May cause acidosis later (respiratory and metabolic) *3810*
Blood Increase Physiological Initial respiratory alkalosis *6201*

Phenylketones *Urine Positive Analytical* Purple with $FeCl_3$, purple with Phenistix® *1714*

Phenytoin *Serum Decrease Physiological* Statistically significant increase of free fraction (0.13 to 0.16) but lower total concentration *1948* With high dose aspirin treatment, total phenytoin concentration decreased from mean of 13.5 mg/L to 10.3 mg/L probably due to displacement form protein-binding sites *4062*
Serum Increase Physiological May displace from plasma protein *2452*

Phosphate *Serum No Effect Physiological* When approximately 3 g/d ingested for several weeks *5122*
Urine Increase Physiological Inhibits tubular reabsorption *2242*
Urine No Effect Analytical No effect with aspirin at a concentration of 20 mg/dL on method of Jung/Parekh *2992*

Phospholipids *Serum Decrease Physiological* Increased fatty acid oxidation, decreased lipogenesis *2242*

Piroxicam *Serum Decrease Physiological* When aspirin 3900 mg/d coadministered plasma levels of piroxicam depressed to 80% of their prior concentrations *4646*

Plasminogen Activator Inhibitor-1
Plasma Decrease Physiological In 34 healthy individuals administration of a single dose of 650 mg caused significant decrease from mean baseline of 100% to 43% after 2 hours but with return to 80% of baseline within 24 hours and 90% within 48 hours *4146*

Plasminogen Activator Inhibitor-1 Activity
Plasma Decrease Physiological In 8 healthy pregnant women taking 60 to 80 mg aspirin daily from 12 weeks onwards median activity 326 (86 - 428) % significantly different from 556 (431 - 829) % in 16 pregnant controls *708*

Plasminogen Activator Inhibitor-1 Antigen
Plasma No Effect Physiological In 8 healthy pregnant women taking 60 to 80 mg aspirin daily from 12 weeks onwards median concentration 101.9 (52.6 - 127.5) ng/mL not significantly different from 101.5 (66.9 - 134) ng/mL in 16 pregnant controls *708*

Aspirin *(continued)*

Plasminogen Activator Inhibitor-2 Antigen
Plasma No Effect Physiological In 8 healthy pregnant women taking 60 to 80 mg aspirin daily from 12 weeks onwards median concentration 168 (146.5 - 209.8) ng/mL not significantly different from 189 (134.4 - 225.8) ng/mL in 16 pregnant controls *708*

Platelet Aggregation *Blood Decrease Physiological* Marked effect observed with treatment *3694* Inhibits collagen induced *5112* In 12 healthy volunteers platelet aggregation in response to arachidonic acid decreased from mean baseline of 337 µmol to undetectable amount at the highest concentration used of 2 mmol/L after treatment with 2250 mg aspirin/d for 5 days *3807* Usual analgesic doses inhibit aggregation *1384* In 34 healthy volunteers after a single dose of 650 mg significant reduction of arachidonic acid induced aggregation with effect lasting for 4 days *4146* Inhibits release of ADP from platelets *2242*
Blood Increase Physiological In 34 healthy volunteers a single dose of 650 mg caused rebound increase of ADP induced platelet aggregation *4146*

Platelets *Blood Decrease Physiological* Decreased platelet survival time, may be purpura *5984* Several cases of immune-mediated thrombocytopenia reported *4139* In 161 individuals aged 70 years or older treatment with 100 mg/d for 1 year caused nonsignificant decrease of 3790 ± 43900 /µL compared with 5610 ± 31120 /µL in placebo-treated controls *5552*
Urine Increase Physiological Loss through damaged glomeruli may occur *5881*

Potassium *Serum Decrease Physiological* Diuretic action, respiratory alkalosis *1009*
Serum No Effect Physiological When approximately 3 g/d ingested for several weeks *5122*
Urine Increase Physiological Direct effect on renal tubules *2242*

Pravastatin *Serum No Effect Physiological* Coadministration with pravastatin caused no significant effect on bioavailability of pravastatin *728*

Prazosin *Serum No Effect Physiological* Coadministration of prazosin with aspirin had no apparent adverse drug interaction in limited clinical experience *4649*

Prolactin response to TRH *Plasma No Effect Physiological* In up to 35 healthy volunteers given 3.6 g daily for 1 week *4841*

Propylthiouracil *Serum Decrease Analytical* Produces negative interference (procedure of Ratliff) *4872*

Prostaglandin E *Plasma Decrease Physiological* In up to 35 healthy volunteers given 3.6 g daily for 1 week *4841*
Urine Decrease Physiological Clearance reduced: increased clearance with sodium restriction *4195*

Prostaglandin F *Plasma Decrease Physiological* In up to 35 healthy volunteers given 3.6 g daily for 1 week *4841*

Protein *Cerebrospinal Fluid Increase Analytical* False positive with Folin-Ciocalteu reagent *6681*
Serum Decrease Physiological Progressive effect during three days but also noted over longer term study at beginning, eventually reverted towards normal. Effect statistically significant *5122*
Urine Increase Analytical Interference with Folin-Ciocalteu reaction *6515*
Urine Increase Physiological Observed effect with long term low doses for secondary prevention of coronary heart disease *4777* May cause nephrotoxicity *2451*

Prothrombin Time *Plasma Decrease Physiological* Small dose effect *3810*
Plasma Increase Physiological Large dose effect (decreased synthesis of clot factors) *1405* Large doses (over 3 g/d) taken for several days may cause hypoprothrobinemia reversible with phytonadione but effect not usually significant except in patients receiving anticoagulants or with severe liver disease *1384*
Plasma No Effect Physiological No effect observed in volunteers *5501*

PSP Excretion *Urine Decrease Physiological* Competes with PSP for excretion *6515*

Pyruvate *Plasma Increase Physiological* Due to late metabolic acidosis and renal impairment *2242*

Renin Activity *Plasma Decrease Physiological* Mean reduction from 2.94 ng/mL/h to 1.41 ng/mL/h when treatment started, but rose following treatment before returning to baseline in 10 weeks *747*
Plasma No Effect Physiological In patients in whom it had been increased with sodium restriction *4195*

Reticulocytes *Blood Increase Physiological* Response during recovery from hemolysis *3094*

Salicylate *Serum Increase Physiological* Due to ingestion of compound *2183* When approximately 3 g/d ingested for several weeks *5122*

Sex-Hormone Binding Globulin
Serum Increase Physiological In women with regular use (more than once per week) significant positive correlation of r = 0.15 *4266*

Sodium *Serum No Effect Physiological* When approximately 3 g/d ingested for several weeks *5122*
Urine Increase Physiological Response to respiratory alkalosis of early toxicity *2242*

Sugar *Urine Increase Analytical* False positive with Clinitest® or Benedict's reagent *1714* Conjugate may react with Benedict's reagent *2559*

T3-Uptake *Serum Increase Physiological* Red cell uptake affected, also affects resin test *1714*
Serum No Effect Physiological When approximately 3 g/d ingested for several weeks *5122*

Taurine *Urine Decrease Physiological* Reduces elevated concentration in rheumatoid patients *5171*

Tenoxicam *Serum Decrease Physiological* Steady-state concentration decreased significantly in the presence of high dose chronic treatment probably due to competitive protein binding interaction *1295*

Thromboxane B_2 *Plasma Decrease Physiological* Although overall no significant reduction in TxB_2 concentration observed after aspirin administration to CAD patients concentration reduced in 7 of 11 patients *5182* In 8 healthy pregnant women taking 60 to 80 mg aspirin daily from 12 weeks onwards median concentration of 37.8 (27.7 - 80) µg/L significantly different from 217 (123 - 326) ng/L in 16 pregnant controls *708* Reduction of concentration to undetectable levels in healthy male volunteers within 2-4 days given aspirin in controlled release, daily or alternate day treatment forms *1052* Significant reduction in 34 pregnant women with treatment for 21 days. Effect slightly less marked in women who developed pregnancy-induced hypertension *5339* In 25 healthy volunteers treatment with 81 mg/d for 1 week caused marked and significant decrease from 381 ± 25 ng/mL to 3.3 ± 0.9 ng/mL *6687* Reduction by about 99% over 24 h, gradually reverted towards normal *3342* In 52 healthy volunteers administration of 80 mg/d caused significant decrease from mean baseline of 2.3 ± 0.2 ng/mL to 1.3 ± 0.2 ng/mL 6 h after first dose and 0.8 ± 03 ng/mL on day 14. With 325 mg day concentration decreased to 1.4 ± 0.6 ng/mL on day 1 and 0.9 ± 0.2 ng/mL on day 14 from mean baseline of 2.6 ± 0.3 ng/mL. Comparable change observed after 325 mg enteric aspirin and only slightly less when alternate day schedule used *2272*
Urine Decrease Physiological In 6 patients with type II hyperlipidemia mean excretion decreased significantly from 79 ± 44 ng/h to 25 ± 13 ng/h after treatment with 50 mg/d for 1 week *5585* Reduced excretion observed in mildly hypertensive patients treated for 7 days following two weeks without antihypertensive medication *4065* About 40% reduction (from 8.6 ng/h to 4.6 ng/h) in 33 pregnant women treated until term with 60 mg daily starting at the 12th week *481*

Thyro-Binding Index *Serum Decrease Physiological* For up to 1 week after treatment *1444*

Thyroid Stimulating Hormone
Serum Decrease Physiological Decreased release after administration *4014*

Thyroxine (T4) *Serum Decrease Physiological* In up to 35 healthy volunteers given 3.6 g daily for 1 week *4841* Progressive effect during three days but also noted over longer term study at beginning, eventually reverted towards normal. Effect statistically significant *5122* Displaces thyroxine from binding sites (thyroxine binding prealbumin) *5869*

Thyroxine (T4), Free *Serum Increase Physiological* Single dose of 4 g may increase concentration 2-3 fold. In long-term treated patients concentrations approximately 20% above pre-

treatment values *1269* Interferes with binding to thyroxine binding globulin and thyroxine binding prealbumin *3421*
Serum No Effect Analytical Toxic concentration caused change of less than 0.01 ng/dL with method on Technicon Immuno-1 *1296*

Thyroxine (T4) Index, Free *Serum Decrease Physiological* Low normal or decreased for 1 week after therapy *1444*

Thyroxine (T4) (Murphy-Pattee)
Serum Decrease Physiological Binds to thyroxine binding prealbumin but not thyroxine binding globulin *882*

Tiludronate *Serum Decrease Physiological* Bioavailabilty of tiludronate reduced by up to 50% when aspirin is administered two hours after tiludronate *5258*

Tirofiban *Serum No Effect Physiological* Coadministration had no significant effect on plasma clearance of tirofiban *3957*

Tissue Plasminogen Activator
Plasma No Effect Physiological In 8 healthy pregnant women taking 60 to 80 mg aspirin daily from 12 weeks onwards median activity 0.8 (0.6 - 1.1) IU/mL not significantly different from 1.0 (0.4 - 1.6) IU/mL in 16 pregnant controls *708*

Tissue Plasminogen Activator Antigen
Plasma No Effect Physiological In 8 healthy pregnant women taking 60 to 80 mg aspirin daily from 12 weeks onwards median concentration 10.8 (6.2 - 12.6) ng/mL not significantly different from 6.5 (4.2 - 16.4) ng/mL in 16 pregnant controls *708*

Tolbutamide *Serum Increase Physiological* Displaces from plasma proteins if present *2452*

Tri-iodothyronine, Free (fT3) *Serum Increase Physiological* Interferes with binding to thyroxine binding globulin *3421* Concentration typically 20% above pretreatment concentration in long-term treated patients *1269*

Tri-iodothyronine (T3) *Serum Decrease Physiological* In up to 35 healthy volunteers given 3.6 g daily for 1 week *4841*

Trimantadine *Serum Decrease Physiological* Coadministration of aspirin with trimantadine caused reduction of its AUC and peak plasma concentration by approximately 10% *1910*

Tryptophan *Plasma Decrease Physiological* Total concentration decreased in rheumatoids on therapy *303*

Tryptophan, Free *Plasma Increase Physiological* In rheumatoids on therapy *303*

TSH response to TRH *Serum Decrease Physiological* In up to 35 healthy volunteers given 3.6 g daily for 1 week *4841*

Urea Nitrogen *Serum Increase Physiological* May have nephrotoxic effect *6191* Anti-inflammatory doses produced substantial effect in 13 of 23 patients with systemic lupus erythematosus. Observed effect with long term low doses for secondary prevention of coronary heart disease *4777*
Serum No Effect Analytical No effect on Berthelot procedure *3033*
Serum No Effect Physiological No effect although creatinine affected *824* When approximately 3 g/d ingested for several weeks *5122*

Uric Acid *Serum Decrease Physiological* Noted in several patients receiving therapeutic amounts of drug *4847* Mild uricosuric action (large dose effect) *1009* Significant effect observed in group of patients with rheumatoid arthritis *1388* Progressive effect during three days but also noted over longer term study at beginning, eventually reverted towards normal. Effect statistically significant *5122*
Serum Increase Analytical Acts as reducing substance with nonspecific methods *2451*
Serum Increase Physiological Low doses reduce renal excretion of uric acid *6515*
Serum No Effect Analytical At 1 g/L on uricase procedure of Kabasak *2998* At 1.0 g/L on reversed phase liquid chromatographic procedure of Zhiri et al *6656* No effect on methods using uricase *4914*
Urine Decrease Physiological Low doses effect *6515*
Urine Increase Analytical Acts as reducing substance with nonspecific methods *2451*
Urine Increase Physiological High dose effect (greater than 3 g daily) *1714*

Urobilin *Urine Increase Physiological* Occurs with poisoning *2183*

Valproic Acid *Serum Increase Physiological* Coadministration of aspirin in doses of 11 - 16 mg/kg with valproic acid to 6 children caused reduced protein binding and inhibition of the metabolism of valproate *17* Coadministration of aspirin, up to 16 mg/kg four times in one day, caused 38% increase in total valproic acid and 51% increase in free concentration in 6 epileptic children receiving valproic acid *6271* In 6 pediatric patients doses of 11 to 16 mg/kg decreased protein binding and an inhibition of metabolism of valproate. Free valproate fraction increased 4-fold in the presence of aspirin compared to valproate alone. The β-oxidation pathway affected so that metabolites produced by it decreased from 25% of total to 8.3% *15* Toxicity has been reported with coadministration probably due to inhibition of β-oxidation of valproic acid through an effect on the CoA-synthetases responsible for the activation of valproic acid *4062*

Valproic Acid, Free *Serum Increase Physiological* Salicylates may displace valproic acid from protein binding sites to cause a sufficiently high free drug concentration to produce toxicity *1384* In 6 pediatric patients doses of 11 to 16 mg/kg decreased protein binding and an inhibition of metabolism of valproate. Free valproate fraction increased 4-fold in the presence of aspirin compared to valproate alone. The β-oxidation pathway affected so that metabolites produced by it decreased from 25% of total to 8.3% *15* Coadministration of aspirin in doses of 11 - 16 mg/kg with valproic acid to 6 children caused reduced protein binding and inhibition of the metabolism of valproate and increased free valproate concentration 4-fold *17*

Volume *Blood Increase Physiological* In 52 healthy volunteers administration of 80 mg/d for 14 days caused increase from mean baseline of 123.4 ± 34.8 mL to 143.6 ± 24.9 mL: with 325 mg/d increase from 120.4 ± 25.1 mL to 168.7 mL and with 325 mg enteric-coated aspirin/d from 111.6 ± 19.8 mL to 135.7 ± 18.2 mL. With an alternate day dose schedule times also showed marked increase *2272*
Plasma Increase Physiological In 52 healthy volunteers ingestion of 80 mg daily for 14 d caused increase from mean baseline of 74.8 ± 19.9 mL to 85.0 ± 14.6 min. Ingestion of 325 mg/d caused increase from mean of 71.5 ± 14.2 mL to 98.1 ± 18.8 mL and ingestion of 325 mg enteric aspirin caused increase from 70.3 ± 12.1 mL to 98.1 ± 10.9 mL. Comparable increases observed when same doses of aspirin given alternate days *2272*
Urine Increase Physiological Decreased renal tubular reabsorption *2242*

von Willebrand Factor *Plasma No Effect Physiological* In 31 patients with chronic atrial fibrillation initial median concentration of 152 IU/dL (interquartile range 108 - 198 IU/dL) not significantly changed to 161 IU/dL (interquartile range 118 - 196 IU/dL) after treatment with aspirin for 2 months *2130*

Xylose *Urine Decrease Physiological* Reduced renal excretion reported with tolerance tests *4777* Affects renal elimination *3105*

Zafirlukast *Serum Increase Physiological* Coadministration of zafirlukast (40 mg/d) at steady state with aspirin (650 mg four times daily) resulted in a mean 45% increase of zafirlukast concentration *6641*

Aspoxicillin

Alanine Aminotransferase *Serum Increase Physiological* In 2 of 5 patients given up to 112 mg/kg intravenously in 3 or 4 divided doses *2488*

Aspartate Aminotransferase *Serum Increase Physiological* In 2 of 5 patients given up to 112 mg/kg intravenously in 3 or 4 divided doses *2488*

Eosinophils *Blood Increase Physiological* In 1 patient given up to 112 mg/kg intravenously in 3 or 4 divided doses *2488*

Astemizole

Histamine *Plasma No Effect Analytical* Improbable inhibition of radio-enzyme assay at physiological concentrations *2492*

Atenolol

Albumin *Serum No Effect Physiological* In 9 patients with essential hypertension treated with atenolol for 6 months baseline value of 42 ± 2 g/L not significantly changed to 43 ± 3 g/L

Atenolol *(continued)*

Albumin *(continued)*
2237 In 14 hypertensive patients with proteinuria treament with up to 100 mg/d for 12 weeks caused nonsignificant increase from mean baseline of 39.0 ± 2.0 g/L to 40.0 ± 3.0 g/L *229*
Urine Decrease Physiological In 12 patients with essential hypertension treatment for 8 weeks caused nonsignificant reduction in excretion of albumin *545*

Aldosterone *Plasma Decrease Physiological* Significant reduction from mean baseline concentration of 73.5 pg/mL to 55.3 pg/mL at 3 days and 43.5 pg/mL at 7 days in 10 patients with uncomplicated essential hypertension treated with 100 mg/d *1086*

Apolipoprotein A *Serum No Effect Physiological* In 18 hypertensive patients treated with 50 mg/d no significant change from mean baseline of 2.6 ± 0.4 g/dL at baseline to 2.5 ± 0.1 g/L after 3 months and 2.6 ± 0.4 g/dL after 12 months *4460*

Apolipoprotein A-I *Serum Decrease Physiological* In 28 hypertensive patients treatment for 6 months caused significant decrease from mean baseline of 106 ± 17 mg/dL to 96 ± 14 mg/dL *3781* 8% reduction from mean baseline of 131 mg/dL to 119 mg/dL in 18 patients with mild to moderate hypertension when treated with up to 150 mg/d for 6 months *966* Reduction by 6% reported from one study *142*
Serum No Effect Physiological In 49 patients with mild to moderate hypertension treatment for 21 weeks little change observed *2733*

Apolipoprotein A-I:Apolipoprotein B Ratio
Serum Decrease Physiological In 28 hypertensive patients treatment for 6 months caused significant decrease in ratio from mean baseline of 0.78 ± 0.2 to 0.70 ± 0.2 *3781*

Apolipoprotein A-II *Serum Decrease Physiological* Nonsignificant decrease from mean baseline of 38 mg/dL to 34 mg/dL in 18 patients with mild to moderate hypertension treated with up to 150 mg/d for 6 months *966*
Serum No Effect Physiological In 49 patients with mild to moderate hypertension little change observed after 21 weeks *2733*

Apolipoprotein B *Serum Increase Physiological* Increase by 3% reported from one study *142* In 28 hypertensive patients treatment for 6 months caused significant increase from mean baseline of 136 ± 16 mg/dL to 142 ± 15 mg/dL *3781* In 49 patients with mild to moderate hypertension treatment for 21 weeks caused nonsignificant increase *2733*
Serum No Effect Physiological Insignificant increase from mean baseline of 126 mg/dL to 130 mg/dL in 18 patients with mild to moderate hypertension treated with up to 150 mg/d for 6 months *966* In 18 hypertensive patients given 50 mg/d no change from baseline of 1.8 ± 0.6 g/dL observed after 3 months and 12 months *4460*

Atrial Natriuretic Peptide *Plasma Increase Physiological* Nonsignificant increase observed in elderly patients with mild essential hypertension both at rest and after exercise *3224* In 10 patients with uncomplicated essential hypertension treated with 100 mg/d significant increase from mean baseline of 49.9 pg/mL to 54.7 pg/mL at 3 days and 73.3 pg/mL at 7 days *1086*

Benazepril *Serum No Effect Physiological* No clinically important pharmacokinetic interactions observed when drugs coadministered *1033*

Bicarbonate *Serum No Effect Physiological* No significant change observed in 18 patients with mild to moderate hypertension when treated with up to 150 mg/d for 6 months *966*

Calcium *Serum No Effect Physiological* No significant effect in 12 healthy volunteers over 24 hours following single dose of 100 mg *3452*
Urine No Effect Physiological No significant effect in 12 healthy volunteers over 24 hours following single oral dose of 100 mg *3452*

Catecholamines *Plasma No Effect Analytical* Not detected when HPLC with electrochemical detection method of Meineke used *3938*
Urine Increase Physiological Significant increase from mean baseline excretion of 39.8 µg/d to 48.5 µg/d at 3 days and 45.0 µg/d at 7 days in 10 patients with uncomplicated essential hypertension treated with 100 mg/d *1086*

Chloride *Serum No Effect Physiological* No significant effect observed in 18 patients with mild to moderate hypertension treated with up to 150 mg/d for 6 months *966* No significant effect in 12 healthy volunteers over 24 hours following single dose of 100 mg *3452*
Urine No Effect Physiological No significant effect in 12 healthy volunteers over 24 hours following single oral dose of 100 mg *3452*

Cholesterol *Serum Decrease Physiological* In 42 patients with mild to moderate hypertension treatment for 6 months caused nonsignificant decrease from mean baseline of 6.69 ± 1.00 mmol/L to 6.38 ± 0.95 mmol/L *2907* Significant reduction observed in hypertensive patients with serum cholesterol concentrations initially greater than 220 mg/dL when treated with 100 mg/d for 1 year *1901*
Serum Increase Physiological In 49 patients with mild to moderate hypertension treatment for 21 weeks caused significant increase *2733* Slight increase (8%) in one 6 mo study *3499* Increase by 49% after 100 mg/d for 5 weeks in 20 hypertensive men *3521* Mean increase of 15 mg/dL in 20 patients with mild to moderate hypertension when treated with mean dose of 76.5 mg for 46 weeks *3571* In 13 hypertensive patients with serum cholesterol concentration greater than 220 mg/dL treatment for 6 months caused nonsignificant increase from mean baseline of 249 ± 13 mg/dL to 258 ± 18 mg/dL and in 15 with serum cholesterol less than 220 mg/dL from 198 ± 11 mg/dL to 202 ± 13 mg/dL *3781*
Serum No Effect Physiological Insignificant increase from mean of 5.62 mmol/L to 5.74 mmol/L in 25 hypertensive patients given mean dose of 67 mg/day for 24 weeks *4736* Insignificant change after 6 mo treatment of 14 hypertensives *1293* In 18 hypertensive men administration of 50 mg/d caused insignificant reduction from mean baseline of 6.7 ± 1.5 mmol/L to 6.5 ± 1.7 mmol/L after 3 months and 6.7 ± 1.6 mmol/L after 12 months *4460* No effect of treatment for either 2 or 6 months with 100 mg daily in 95 patients with mild essential hypertension *1300* In 20 patients with 50 mg/d compared with pre-treatment values after 3 mo *5115* In 9 patients with essential hypertension treated with atenolol for 6 months baseline value of 5.6 ± 0.7 mmol/L not significantly changed to 5.7 ± 0.8 mmol/L *2237* In 15 obese patients with mild to moderate primary hypertension treatment with 50 and 100 mg/d atenolol for 12 weeks caused a nonsignificant increase of 3.9 mg/dL from the mean baseline of 229.4 ± 10.4 mg/dL *671* In 14 patients with essential hypertension treatment with 100 mg/d for 4 weeks caused nonsignificant change from mean baseline of 215 ± 40 mg/dL to 210 ± 46 mg/dL *1305* No significant effect in about 20 hypertensives treated with 100 mg/day for 2 years *1899* Insignificant change in 3 studies of from 1 to 3 mo *3499* In 17 obese, nondiabetic patients with primary hypertension treated with either 50 or 100 mg/d of atenolol for 12 weeks caused a nonsignificant 3.9 mg/dL increase from mean baseline of 229.4 ± 10.4 mg/dL *671* No significant change in 15 hypertensives treated for 8 mo *1713* No change from baseline of 6.3 mmol/L in 18 patients with mild to moderate hypertension treated with up to 150 mg/d for 6 months *966* Typically no significant change from several studies *142*

Clopidogrel *Serum No Effect Physiological* Atenolol administration does not appear to affect the pharmacodynamics of clopidogrel *5256*

Cortisol *Plasma No Effect Analytical* At a concentration of 2 mg/L no significant effect observed on Enzymun method *1097*

C-Peptide *Plasma Decrease Physiological* Reduced activity at 2 and 3 h during glucose tolerance test versus control *3217*

Creatinine *Serum Decrease Physiological* In 9 patients with essential hypertension treated with atenolol for 6 months baseline value of 78 ± 12 µmol/L significantly changed to 70 ± 14 µmol/L *2237*
Serum No Effect Physiological No significant change observed in 18 patients with mild to moderate hypertension treated with up to 150 mg/d for 6 months *966* In 14 hypertensive patients with proteinuria treatment with up to 100 mg/d for 12 weeks caused nonsignificant change from mean baseline of 190 ± 69 µmol/L to 194 ± 77 µmol/L *229* No significant effect in 20 hypertensive patients given up to 100 mg daily for 10 weeks *6495* Nonsignificant increase from mean baseline concentration of 91.6 µmol/L to 93.1 µmol/L in 63 patients with essential hypertension treated with up to 100 mg/d for 8 weeks *454* In 10 hypertensive diabetics treatment with 100 mg/d for

8 months had no significant effect on concentration *1305* No significant effect in 12 healthy volunteers over 24 hours following single dose of 100 mg *3452*
Urine No Effect Physiological No effect in 12 healthy volunteers over 24 hours following single oral dose of 100 mg *3452*

Creatinine Clearance *Urine Decrease Physiological* In 12 patients with essential hypertension treatment for 8 weeks caused nonsignificant decrease from mean baseline of 99.8 ± 2.4 mL/min to 95.1 ± 2.4 mL/min *545*

Cyclosporine *Blood No Effect Analytical* At a concentration of 40 mg/L had no effect on Syva EMIT method *495*

Diazepam *Serum No Effect Physiological* 100 mg daily had no effect on area under concentration curve *2517*

Disopyramide *Serum Increase Physiological* Concurrent administration of both drugs reduced clearance of disopyramide by 20% in one study, but half-life and volume of distribution unchanged *650*

Doxazosin *Serum No Effect Physiological* Coadministration with doxazosin had no effect on its pharmacokinetics *4642*

Effective Renal Plasma Flow
Patient Decrease Physiological In 10 hypertensive diabetics treatment with 100 mg/d for 8 months caused decrease from mean baseline of 582 ± 119 mL/min/1.73 sq m to 562 ± 115 mL/min/1.73 sq m *3481*
Patient No Effect Physiological In 13 hypertensive patients with proteinuria treatment with up to 100 mg/d for 12 weeks caused nonsignificant increase from mean baseline of 164 ± 69 mL/min/1.73 sq m to 170 ± 71 mL/min/1.73 sq m *229*

Erythrocytes *Blood No Effect Physiological* No significant effect observed in 18 patients with mild to moderate hypertension treated with up to 150 mg/d for 6 months *966*

Fatty Acids (FFA), Free *Serum Decrease Physiological* Marked effect with 3 mo treatment given 100 mg/d *1292* In fasting state and after 30 minutes during oral glucose tolerance test *3217* Significant reduction after 3 mo treatment in 14 hypertensives *1293*

Fibrinogen *Plasma Decrease Physiological* In 17 obese, nondiabetic patients with primary hypertension treated with either 50 or 100 mg/d of atenolol for 12 weeks caused a nonsignificant 29 mg/dL decrease from mean baseline of 273 ± 98 mg/dL *671* In 15 obese patients with mild to moderate primary hypertension treatment with 50 and 100 mg/d atenolol for 12 weeks caused a decrease of 29 mg/dL from the mean baseline of 273 ± 98 mg/dL *671* In 25 patients with essential hypertension treatment with 50 mg once daily for 12 weeks caused 9% reduction in concentration *2398*
Plasma No Effect Physiological In 9 patients with essential hypertension treated with atenolol for 6 months baseline value of 2.21 ± 0.69 g/L not significantly changed to 2.19 ± 0.45 g/L *2237*

Filtration Fraction *Urine Decrease Physiological* In 14 hypertensive patients with proteinuria treatment with up to 100 mg/d for 12 weeks caused significant decrease from mean baseline of 26.9 ± 3.8% to 25.0 ± 4.6% *229*

Filtration Rate *Red Blood Cells No Effect Physiological* In 9 patients with essential hypertension treated with atenolol for 6 months baseline value of 62 ± 11 µL/s not significantly changed to 65 ± 11 µL/s *2237*

Geometric Variation in Fibrinolytic Index
Plasma No Effect Physiological In 28 hypertensive patients treatment for 6 months caused nonsignificant change from mean baseline before anoxia of 17.9 ± 1 to 24.4 ± 15 *3781*

GH response to GHRH *Plasma Increase Physiological* In 9 obese children response to GHRH 1-29, 1 µg/kg intravenously significantly less than in 8 age-matched control children except when atenolol given in advance in which case GH response to GHRH same as in control children *3629*

Glomerular Filtration Rate *Urine Decrease Physiological* In 10 hypertensive diabetics treatment with 100 mg/d for 8 months caused decrease from 122 ± 33 mL/min/1.73 sq m to 106 ± 27 mL/min/1.73 sq m *1305*
Urine No Effect Physiological In 14 hypertensive patients with proteinuria treatment with up to 100 mg/d for 12 weeks caused nonsignificant decrease from mean baseline of 43.3 ± 17.8 mL/min/1.73 sq m to 41.6 ± 17.2 mL/min/1.73 sq m *229* In 12 patients with essential hypertension treatment with 100 mg/d for 4 weeks caused nonsignificant increase from mean baseline of 118 ± 33 mL/min to 119 ± 31 mL/min *3481*

Glucagon *Plasma Decrease Physiological* In 18 patients with mild essential hypertension treated with chlorothiazide concomitantly over 4 weeks *1734*
Plasma No Effect Physiological No change in basal concentration or after glucose in 14 hypertensives *1293*

Glucose *Serum Decrease Physiological* Incidence of 0.4% observed in French Pharmacovigilance database *4106*
Serum Increase Physiological In 9 patients with essential hypertension treated with atenolol for 6 months baseline value of 5.7 ± 0.6 mmol/L not significantly changed to 6.6 ± 1.6 mmol/L *2237* In 25 hypertensive patients given mean dose of 67 mg/day for 24 weeks increase from mean concentration of 4.97 mmol/L to 5.19 mmol/L. Plasma glucose concentration also higher at end of i.v. GTT than when placebo ingested *4736* In 42 patients with mild to moderate hypertension treatment for 6 months caused significant increase from mean baseline of 5.53 ± 0.49 mmol/L to 5.73 ± 0.49 mmol/L *2907* In 14 patients with essential hypertension treatment with 100 mg/d for 4 weeks caused significant increase from mean baseline of 116 ± 26 mg/dL to 132 ± 34 mg/dL *3481*
Serum No Effect Physiological In 25 patients with essential hypertension treatment with 50 mg once daily for 12 weeks had no significant effect on concentration *2398* No significant effect in 6 healthy volunteers following single oral dose of 100 mg *4064* In 176 patients with essential years treatment with up to 100 mg/d for 8 weeks caused no significant difference from concentration in those treated with placebo *3841* In 15 obese patients with mild to moderate primary hypertension treatment with 50 and 100 mg/d atenolol for 12 weeks caused a nonsignificant increase of serum glucose of 4.4 mg/dL from mean baseline of 98.4 ± 3.6 mg/dL *671* In 17 obese, nondiabetic patients with primary hypertension treated with either 50 or 100 mg/d of atenolol for 12 weeks caused a nonsignificant 4.4 mg/dL increase from mean baseline of 98.4 ± 3.6 mg/dL *671* No significant effect observed in 18 patients with mild to moderate hypertension treated with up to 150 mg/d for 6 months *966* No significant change after 3 or 6 mo treatment in 14 hypertensives *1293* In 10 hypertensive diabetics treatment with 100 mg/d for 8 months had no significant effect on concentration *1305* In 18 patients with mild essential hypertension treated with chlorothiazide concomitantly over 4 weeks *1734* Compared with controls during oral glucose tolerance test *3217*

Glucose Tolerance *Serum Decrease Physiological* In 15 obese patients with mild to moderate primary hypertension treatment with 50 and 100 mg/d atenolol for 12 weeks caused a significant increase of the area under the serum glucose of 30% *671*
Serum Increase Physiological Significant improvement in 22 patients with primary hypertension and impaired glucose tolerance given 100 mg daily for 3 weeks *1778*
Serum No Effect Physiological In 25 patients with essential hypertension treatment with 50 mg once daily for 12 weeks had no significant effect on OGTT *2398*

γ-Glutamyltransferase *Serum No Effect Physiological* No significant effect observed in 18 patients with mild to moderate hypertension treated with up to 150 mg/d for 6 months *966*

Growth Hormone *Plasma No Effect Physiological* No change in basal concentration or after glucose in 14 hypertensives *1293*

HDL$_2$-Cholesterol *Serum Decrease Physiological* Nonsignificant decrease from mean baseline of 0.59 mmol/L to 0.52 mmol/L in 18 patients with mild to moderate hypertension treated with up to 150 mg/d for 6 months *966*
Serum Increase Physiological In 49 patients with mild to moderate hypertension treated for 21 weeks caused significant increase *2733*

HDL$_3$-Cholesterol *Serum Decrease Physiological* Nonsignificant reduction from mean baseline concentration of 0.73 mmol/L to 0.62 mmol/L in 18 patients with mild to moderate hypertension treated with up to 150 mg/d for 6 months *966*

HDL-Cholesterol *Serum Decrease Physiological* Significant reduction in 22 patients with primary hypertension and impaired or diabetic glucose tolerance given 100 mg daily for 3 weeks *1778* From 1.21 to 1.13 mmol/L with 100 mg drµg/d *3610* Significant effect observed in both normolipemic and moderately hyperlipemic patients with moderate hypertension treated for 6 months *966* Significant decrease from mean baseline of 1.30 mmol/L to 1.12 mmol/L in 18 patients with mild to moderate hypertension treated with up to 150 mg/d for 6

Atenolol *(continued)*

HDL-Cholesterol *(continued)*
months *966* 9.6% reduction in 95 patients with mild essential hypertension treated with 100 mg daily for 2 months, but reversed by 6 months *1300* Slight reduction noted in both normocholesterolemic and hypercholesterolemic hypertensives when treated with 100 mg/d for 6 months *1900* In 41 patients with mild to moderate hypertension treatment for 6 months caused significant decrease from mean baseline of 1.23 ± 0.33 mmol/L to 1.04 ± 0.29 mmol/L *2907* In 17 obese, nondiabetic patients with primary hypertension treated with either 50 or 100 mg/d of atenolol for 12 weeks caused a nonsignificant 23.8 mg/dL decrease from mean baseline of 43.6 ± 4.0 mg/dL *671* Significant reduction observed in hypertensive patients with serum cholesterol concentrations initially greater than 220 mg/dL when treated with 100 mg/d for one year *1901* In about 20 hypertensives treated with 100 mg/day for 2 years reduction from 15-19% observed *1899* In 17 hypertensive patients with serum HDL-cholesterol concentration greater than 40 mg/dL treatment for 6 months caused significant decrease from mean baseline of 50 ± 7 mg/dL to 41 ± 6 mg/dL and in 11 with serum HDL-cholesterol less than 40 mg/dL from 35 ± 6 mg/dL to 30 ± 4 mg/dL *3781* In 15 obese patients with mild to moderate primary hypertension treatment with 50 and 100 mg/d atenolol for 12 weeks caused a significant decrease of 23.8 mg/dL from the mean baseline of 43.6 ± 4.0 mg/dL *671* Reduction by 7 to 12% in 2 studies of 3 to 6 mo *3499* Significant reduction from mean of 1.19 mmol/L to 1.08 mmol/L in 25 patients with hypertension treated with mean dose of 67 mg/day for 24 weeks *4736*
Serum Increase Physiological Insignificant increase from mean baseline of 0.19 mmol/L to 0.23 mmol/L in 18 patients with mild to moderate hypertension treated with up to 150 mg/d for 6 months *966* In 49 patients with mild to moderate hypertension treatent for 21 weeks caused significant increase *2733*
Serum No Effect Physiological In 18 hypertensive men administration of 50 mg/d caused insignificant reduction from mean concentration of 1.21 ± 0.35 mmol/L to 1.18 ± 0.30 mmol/L after 3 months and 1.19 ± 0.30 mmol/L after 12 months *4460* No significant change in 15 hypertensives treated for 8 mo *1713* In 25 patients with essential hypertension treatment with 50 mg once daily for 12 weeks caused nonsignificant reduction of 4% *2398* Typically no significant change but may be slight reduction *142* After 100 mg/d for 5 weeks in 20 hypertensive men *3521* In 9 patients with essential hypertension treated with atenolol for 6 months baseline value of 1.2 ± 0.3 mmol/L not significantly changed to 1.2 ± 0.3 mmol/L *2237* No significant change in one 3 mo long study *3499* In 20 patients with 50 mg/d compared with pre-treatment values after 3 mo *5115*

HDL-Cholesterol:Cholesterol Ratio
Serum No Effect Physiological In 18 hypertensive men administration of 50 mg/d caused no significant change from mean baseline of 0.19 ± 0.07 to 0.20 ± 0.08 at 3 months and 0.19 ± 0.08 after 12 months *4460*

HDL-Triglycerides *Serum Increase Physiological* 34% increase reported from one study *142*
Serum No Effect Physiological In 25 patients with essential hypertension treatment with 50 mg once daily for 12 weeks caused nonsignificant reduction of 4% *2398* In 20 patients with 50 mg/d compared with pre-treatment values after 3 mo *5115* No change in 25 hypertensive patients receiving mean dose of 67 mg/day for 24 weeks *4736*

Hematocrit *Blood No Effect Physiological* In 9 patients with essential hypertension treated with atenolol for 6 months baseline value of 0.42 ± 0.04 not significantly changed to 0.42 ± 0.04 *2237* In 25 patients with essential hypertension treatment with 50 mg once daily for 12 weeks had no significant effect on the hematocrit *2398*

Hemoglobin *Blood No Effect Physiological* In 25 patients with essential hypertension treatment with 50 mg once daily for 12 weeks had no significant effect on the concentration *2398*

Hemoglobin A_{1c} *Blood Increase Physiological* In 25 patients with essential hypertension treatment with 50 mg once daily for 12 weeks increased the concentration by 4% *2398*
Blood No Effect Physiological In 10 hypertensive diabetics treatment with 100 mg/d for 8 months had no significant effect on concentration *1305* In 17 obese, nondiabetic patients with primary hypertension treated with either 50 or 100 mg/d of atenolol for 12 weeks caused a no change from mean baseline of 5.4 ± 0.2% *671*

Histamine *Plasma No Effect Analytical* Probably no effect on radio-enzyme method at clinically relevant concentrations *2492*

Indomethacin *Serum No Effect Analytical* No effect on HPLC method of Roberts and Smith *4978*

Insulin *Plasma No Effect Physiological* In 17 obese, nondiabetic patients with primary hypertension treated with either 50 or 100 mg/d of atenolol for 12 weeks caused a nonsignificant 2.8 mg/dL decrease from mean baseline of 13.7 ± 2.5 mU/L *671* In 25 patients with essential hypertension treatment with 50 mg once daily for 12 weeks had no significant effect on concentration *2398* No change in basal concentration or after glucose in 14 hypertensives *1293* In 18 patients with mild essential hypertension treated with chlorothiazide concomitantly over 4 weeks *1734* Compared with controls during glucose tolerance test *3217*

LDL-Cholesterol *Serum Increase Physiological* Mean increase of 11 mg/dL in 20 patients with mild to moderate hypertension when treated with mean dose of 76.5 mg daily for 46 weeks *3571* Increase by 5.9% after 100 mg/d for 5 weeks in 20 hypertensive men *3521* Slight increase reported from one study *142*
Serum No Effect Physiological No significant effect observed in hypertensive patients with serum cholesterol concentrations initially greater than 220 mg/dL when treated with 100 mg/d for one year *1901* No significant effect in about 20 hypertensives treated with 100 mg/day for 2 years *1899* In 20 patients with 50 mg/d compared with pre-treatment values after 3 mo *5115* No significant change in 4 studies of from 3 to 6 mo *3499* Insignificant increase from mean of 3.99 mmol/L to 4.08 mmol/L in 25 patients treated with average of 67 mg/day for 24 weeks *4736* In 15 obese patients with mild to moderate primary hypertension treatment with 50 and 100 mg/d atenolol for 12 weeks caused a nonsignificant decrease of 0.7 mg/dL from the mean baseline of 152.1 ± 9.2 mg/dL *671* Insignificant change from baseline of 4.42 mmol/L to 4.46 mmol/L in 18 patients with mild to moderate hypertension treated with up to 150 mg/d for 6 months *966* In 18 hypertensive men treated with 50 mg/d nonsignificant reduction to 4.7 ± 1.5 mmol/L observed at 3 and 12 months from mean baseline of 4.7 ± 1.4 mmol/L *4460* In 17 obese, nondiabetic patients with primary hypertension treated with either 50 or 100 mg/d of atenolol for 12 weeks caused a nonsignificant 0.7 mg/dL decrease from mean baseline of 152.1 ± 9.2 mg/dL *671* No effect of treatment with 100 mg/d *3610*

LDL-Triglycerides *Serum Increase Physiological* From 0.46 to 0.51 mmol/L in 15 hypertensives treated for 8 mo *1713* Slight increase reported from one study *142* In 25 patients with essential hypertension treatment with 50 mg once daily for 12 weeks caused significant 8% increase in concentration *2398* Significant increase from mean baseline of 0.67 mmol/L to 1.00 mmol/L in 18 patients with mild to moderate hypertension treated with up to 150 mg/d for 6 months *966* Significant increase from mean of 0.47 mmol/L to 0.52 mmol/L in 25 hypertensive patients receiving average of 67 mg/day for 24 weeks *4736*
Serum No Effect Physiological In 20 patients with 50 mg/d compared with pre-treatment values after 3 mo *5115*

Leukocytes *Blood No Effect Physiological* No significant effect observed in 18 patients with mild to moderate hypertension treated with up to 150 mg/d for 6 months *966*

Magnesium *Muscle No Effect Physiological* No significant effect in 9 volunteers treated with 50 mg daily for 4 weeks *4410*
Serum No Effect Physiological No significant effect in 9 volunteers treated with 50 mg daily for 4 weeks *4410* No significant effect in 12 healthy volunteers over 24 hours following single dose of 100 mg *3452*
Urine No Effect Physiological No significant effect in 12 healthy volunteers over 24 hours following single oral dose of 100 mg *3452*

Melatonin *Urine Decrease Physiological* Nonsignificant reduction observed in 10 hypertensive patients treated with mean dose of 86 mg/day for 4 weeks *724*

Mibefradil *Serum No Effect Physiological* Atenolol coadministration had no significant effect on pharmacokinetics of mibefradil *5009*

Nisoldipine *Serum* *No Effect* *Physiological* Administration of atenolol with nisoldipine caused a variable and insignificant change in the AUC of nisoldipine *6650*

p-Aminophenol *Urine* *No Effect* *Analytical* With addition of drugs at a concentration of 100 mg/L and of related compounds at 50 mg/L no significant effect observed on colorimetric method of van Bocxlaer on Cobas Mira analyzer which involves reacting free p-aminophenol with resorcinol in the presence of magnesium ions to form an indophenol dye measured at 550 nm *6163*

Phosphate *Serum* *No Effect* *Physiological* No significant effect in 12 healthy volunteers over 24 hours following single dose of 100 mg *3452*

Urine *No Effect* *Physiological* No significant effect in 12 healthy volunteers over 24 hours following single oral dose of 100 mg *3452*

Plasminogen Activator Inhibitor-1

Plasma *No Effect* *Physiological* In 28 hypertensive patients treatment for 6 months caused nonsignificant change from mean baseline before anoxia of 18.1 ± 12 U/cm³ to 17.4 ± 14 U/cm³*3781* In 42 patients with mild to moderate hypertension treatment for 6 months caused nonsignificant change from mean baseline of 17.9 ± 13.6 U/mL to 17.4 ± 8.0 U/mL *2907*

Plasminogen Activator Inhibitor Activity

Plasma *Increase* *Physiological* In 25 patients with essential hypertension treatment with 50 mg once daily for 12 weeks caused nonsignificant 17% reduction in concentration *2398*

Potassium *Muscle* *No Effect* *Physiological* No significant effect in 9 volunteers treated with 50 mg daily for 4 weeks *4410*

Serum *Increase* *Physiological* In normal volunteers given exercise training program for 8 weeks postmaximal exercise potassium in individuals given atenolol 100 mg daily rose from 4.95 to 5.16 mmol/L, significantly greater than in placebo control group *1890* Significant increase observed in 6 healthy volunteers of 0.3 and 0.6 mmol/L at 2 and 3 hours respectively after single oral dose of 100 mg *4064*

Serum *No Effect* *Physiological* In 14 hypertensive patients with proteinuria treatment with up to 100 mg/d for 12 weeks caused nonsignificant increase from mean baseline of 4.5 ± 0.4 mmol/L to 4.7 ± 0.3 mmol/L *229* No significant effect in 12 healthy volunteers over 24 hours following single dose of 100 mg *3452* Nonsignificant increase from mean baseline concentration of 4.3 mmol/L to 4.4 mmol/L in 63 patients with essential hypertension treated with up to 100 mg/d for 8 weeks *454* In 10 diabetic hypertensives treatment with 100 mg/d for 8 months had no significant effect on concentration *1305* No significant effect in 9 volunteers treated with 50 mg daily for 4 weeks *4410* No significant effect in 20 hypertensive subjects given up to 100 mg daily for 10 weeks *6495* No significant change observed in 18 patients with mild to moderate hypertension treated with up to 150 mg/d for 6 months *966*

Urine *Increase* *Physiological* Nonsignificant increase observed at 3 and 7 days in 10 patients with uncomplicated essential hypertension treated with 100 mg/d *1086*

Urine *No Effect* *Physiological* No significant effect in 12 healthy volunteers over 24 hours following single oral dose of 100 mg *3452*

Protein *Serum* *No Effect* *Physiological* In 10 diabetic hypertensives treatment with 100 mg/d for 8 months had no significant effect on concentration *1305*

Urine *Decrease* *Physiological* In 10 hypertensive diabetics treatment with 100 mg/d for 8 months caused significant reduction from mean baseline of 3.22 ± 0.23 g/d to 2.56 ± 0.44 g/d *1305* In 14 hypertensive patients with proteinuria treated with up to 100 mg/d for 12 weeks nonsignificant decrease from mean baseline of 2.4 ± 1.9 g/d to 2.1 ± 2.0 g/d observed *229*

Renal Blood Flow *Patient* *No Effect* *Physiological* In 12 patients with essential hypertension treatment with 100 mg/d for 4 weeks caused nonsignificant change from mean baseline of 943 ± 278 mL/min to 947 ± 327 mL/min *3481*

Renal Resistance, Total *Patient* *Decrease* *Physiological* In 10 hypertensive diabetics treatment with 100 mg/d for 8 months caused decrease from mean baseline of 0.23 ± 0.04 mm Hg/mL/min to 0.20 ± 0.04 mm Hg/mL/min *1305*

Renin Activity *Plasma* *Decrease* *Physiological* Significant reduction from mean baseline activity of 2.52 ng/mL/h to 2.19 ng/mL/h at 3 days and 1.58 ng/mL/h at 7 days in 10 patients with uncomplicated essential hypertension treated with 100 mg/d *1086*

Plasma *No Effect* *Physiological* No significant effect on basal activity or after intravenous furosemide in 20 hypertensive patients given up to 100 mg daily for 10 weeks *6495*

Sodium *Serum* *No Effect* *Physiological* No significant change observed in 18 patients with mild to moderate hypertension treated with up to 150 mg/d for 6 months *966* No effect in 20 hypertensive subjects given up to 100 mg daily for 10 weeks *6495* In 14 hypertensive patients with proteinuria treatment with up to 100 mg/d for 12 weeks caused no change from mean baseline of 141.4 ± 1.0 mmol/L *229* No significant effect in 12 healthy volunteers over 24 hours following single dose of 100 mg *3452*

Urine *Increase* *Physiological* Nonsignificant increase observed at 3 and 7 days in 10 patients with uncomplicated essential hypertension treated with 100 mg/d *1086*

Urine *No Effect* *Physiological* In 14 hypertensive patients with proteinuria treatment with up to 100 mg/d caused nonsignificant increase from mean baseline of 110 ± 40 mmol/d to 114 ± 42 mmol/d *229* In 12 patients with essential hypertension treatment for 8 weeks caused nonsignificant change from mean baseline of 135 ± 4.3 mmol/d to 135 ± 3.4 mmol/d *545* No significant effect in 12 healthy volunteers over 24 hours following single oral dose of 100 mg *3452*

T3-Uptake *Serum* *No Effect* *Physiological* Nonsignificant increase from mean baseline of 1.15 arbitrary units to 1.18 arbitrary units after 1 and 3 weeks treatment with 100 mg/d in 8 healthy young normotensive men *3076* No significant effect in 12 hyperthyroid patients treated with 100 mg daily for 7 days *4610*

Tacrolimus *Serum* *No Effect* *Analytical* In HPLC/MS method of Christians et al no significant interference observed with measurement of FK 506 *1010*

Theophylline *Serum* *No Effect* *Physiological* No significant effect observed in 6 male smokers following pretreatment for 7 days with 150 mg/day atenolol *1139* No documented significant interaction with theophylline reported *6117* No clinically significant effect on theophylline concentration observed when drugs coadministered *5999*

Thyroid Stimulating Hormone

Serum *Increase* *Physiological* In 8 healthy young normotensive men treatment with 100 mg/d for 1 week caused increase from mean baseline concentration of 1.76 mU/L to 2.25 mU/L but with gradual decline to baseline concentration with a further 2 weeks treatment *3076*

Serum *No Effect* *Physiological* No significant difference in mean concentration (1.30 mU/L) in 12 atenolol treated patients and in 12 control patients (1.44 mU/L) and no significant difference between within-subject variances *6366*

Thyroxine (T4) *Serum* *Decrease* *Physiological* Nonsignificant decrease observed in 8 normotensive healthy men treated with 100 mg daily with decrease from mean baseline concentration of 94 nmol/L to 89 nmol/L after 1 week and 87 nmol/L after 3 weeks *3076*

Serum *No Effect* *Physiological* No significant effect observed in 23 hyperthyroid patients treated with atenolol for 2-4 weeks in spite of marked clinical improvement *2072* No effect observed in 12 hyperthyroid patients treated with 100 mg daily for 7 days *4610*

Thyroxine (T4), Free *Serum* *No Effect* *Physiological* No significant change from mean baseline concentration of 16.7 pmol/L after either 1 or 3 weeks treatment with 100 mg/d in 8 healthy young normotensive men *3076* Mean concentration 16.03 pmol/L in 12 atenolol treated patients compared with 15.36 pmol/L in 12 control patients but within subject variance greater (4.95 pmol/L) in atenolol treated patients than in controls (2.01 pmol/L) *6366* No significant effect observed in 23 hyperthyroid patients treated for 2-4 weeks in spite of marked clinical improvement *2072*

Thyroxine (T4) Index, Free *Serum* *No Effect* *Physiological* Nonsignificant change from mean baseline of 106 arbitrary units to 103 arbitrary units after 1 week and 108 arbitrary units after 3 weeks treatment with 100 mg/d in 8 healthy young normotensive men *3076*

Tissue Plasminogen Activator

Plasma *Decrease* *Physiological* In 28 hypertensive patients treatment for 6 months caused significant decrease from mean baseline before anoxia of 0.093 ± 0.1 U/cm³ to 0.063 ± 0.3 U/cm³*3781*

Atenolol *(continued)*

Tissue Plasminogen Activator *(continued)*
Plasma No Effect Physiological In 42 patients with mild to moderate hypertension treatment for 6 months caused insignificant change from mean baseline of 0.10 ± 0.26 U/mL to 0.037 ± 0.07 U/mL *2907*

Tissue Plasminogen Activator Activity after Venous Occlusion *Plasma No Effect Physiological* In 42 patients with mild to moderate hypertension treatment for 6 months caused nonsignificant change from mean baseline of 2.19 ± 3.82 U/mL to 1.95 ± 2.94 U/mL *2907*

Tissue Plasminogen Activator Antigen
Plasma No Effect Physiological In 42 patients with mild to moderate hypertension treatment for 6 months caused no significant change from mean baseline of 12.9 ± 6.7 µg/L to 11.8 ± 3.8 µg/L *2907*

Tissue Plasminogen Activator Antigen after Venous Occlusion *Plasma No Effect Physiological* In 42 patients with mild to moderate hypertension treatment for 6 months caused insignificant change from mean baseline of 32.0 ± 18.5 µg/L to 29.5 ± 15.8 µg/L *2907*

Tissue Plasminogen Activator Capacity
Plasma No Effect Physiological In 42 patients with mild to moderate hypertension treatment for 6 months caused nonsignificant change from mean baseline of 2.09 ± 3.71 U/mL to 1.91 ± 2.90 U/mL *2907*

Tissue Plasminogen Activator Release
Plasma No Effect Physiological In 42 patients with mild to moderate hypertension treatment for 6 months caused insignificant change from mean baseline of 19.1 ± 16.6 µg/L to 17.7 ±15.3 µg/L *2907*

Tri-iodothyronine, Free (fT3)
Serum No Effect Physiological No significant difference in concentrations in 12 atenolol treated patients (mean 5.46 pmol/L) and 12 control patients (5.45 pmol/L) but within-subject variance of 0.48 pmol/L significantly greater in atenolol group than in control patients (0.15 pmol/L) *6366* No signifcant effect observed over 2-4 weeks in 23 hyperthyroid patients in spite of marked clinical improvement *2072*

Tri-iodothyronine, Reverse (rT3)
Serum Decrease Physiological Decrease from mean of 0.95 nmol/L to 0.81 nmol/L in 12 hyperthyroid patients treated with 100 mg daily for 7 days: effect probably due to inhibition of 5-deiodinase enzyme *4610*
Serum No Effect Physiological No change from mean baseline concentration of 0.46 nmol/L after either 1 or 3 weeks treatment with 100 mg/d in 8 healthy young normotensive men *3076*

Tri-iodothyronine (T3) *Serum Decrease Physiological* Reduction from mean of 5.0 nmol/L to 4.0 nmol/L in 12 hyperthyroid patients treated with 100 mg daily for 7 days, probably due to inhibition of 5'-deiodinase enzyme *4610*
Serum No Effect Physiological No significant change observed in 23 hyperthyroid patients treated for 2-4 weeks although marked clinical improvement *2072* No significant change observed from mean baseline concentration of 2.3 nmol/L to 2.1 nmol/L after treatment for 1 week with 100 mg/d in 8 healthy young normotensive men with mean concentration of 2.2 nmol/L observed after 3 weeks treatment *3076*

Triglycerides *Serum Increase Physiological* In 49 patients with mild to moderate hypertension treatment for 21 weeks caused nonsignificant increase *2733* In 15 obese patients with mild to moderate primary hypertension treatment with 50 and 100 mg/d atenolol for 12 weeks caused a increase of 21.5 mg/dL from the mean baseline of 212.0 ± 38.0 mg/dL *671* In 25 patients with essential hypertension treatment with 50 mg once daily for 12 weeks caused significant 21% increase in concentration *2398* In about 20 hypertensives treatment with 100 mg/day for 2 years caused increase from 23-30% *1899* In 9 patients with essential hypertension treated with atenolol for 6 months baseline value of 1.9 ± 1.3 mmol/L not significantly changed to 2.7 ± 1.7 mmol/L *2237* In 15 hypertensive patients with serum triglyceride concentration greater than 150 mg/dL treatment for 6 months caused significant increase from mean baseline of 220 ± 18 mg/dL to 244 ± 20 mg/dL and in 13 with serum triglycerides less than 150 mg/dL from 124 ± 19 mg/dL to 136 ± 18 mg/dL *3781* Increase of 6.9% in group of mild to moderate hypertensives treated for 20 weeks *3048* In 17 obese, nondiabetic patients with primary hypertension treated with either 50 or 100 mg/d of atenolol for 12 weeks caused a nonsignificant 21.5 mg/dL increase from mean baseline of 212.0 ± 38.0 mg/dL *671* Significant increase observed in hypertensive patients with serum cholesterol concentrations initially greater than 220 mg/dL when treated with 100 mg/d for one year *1901* Slight effect observed in both normocholesterolemic and hypercholesterolemic hypertensives treated with 100 mg/d for 6 months *1900* Marked effect in 18 patients with mild essential hypertension treated with chlorothiazide concomitantly over 14 weeks *1734* From 1.94 mmol/L to 2.44 mmol/L in 15 hypertensives treated for 8 mo *1713* Mean increase of 15 mg/dL in 20 patients with mild to moderate hypertension treated with mean dose of 76.5 mg daily for 46 weeks *3571* Moderate increase after 6 mo treatment of 14 hypertensives *1293* Up to 60% increase in several studies although no significant chance in some *142* Significant increase from mean baseline concentration of 1.16 mmol/L to 2.3 mmol/L in 18 patients with mild to moderate hypertension treated with up to 150 mg/d for 6 months *966* Increased by 24 to 62% in 4 studies of from 1 to 6 mo *3499* Increase from mean of 1.69 mmol/L to 1.93 mmol/L in 25 hypertensive patients receiving average of 67 mg/day for 24 weeks *4736* In 18 hypertensive men administration of 50 mg/d caused increase from mean baseline of 1.8 ± 1.0 mmol/L to 2.3 ± 1.4 mmol/L at 3 months and at 12 months *4460* Increase by 28% after 100 mg/d for 5 weeks in 20 hypertensive men *3521*
Serum No Effect Physiological In 14 patients with essential hypertension treatment with 100 mg/d for 4 weeks caused nonsignificant increase from mean baseline of 168 ± 105 mg/dL to 155 ± 63 mg/dL *3481* In 42 patients with mild to moderate hypertension treatment for 6 months caused insignificant change from 1.81 ± 0.89 mmol/L to 1.83 ± 0.76 mmol/L *2907* In 20 patients with 50 mg/d compared with pre-treatment values after 3 mo *5115* No significant effect observed in 95 patients with mild essential hypertension treated with 100 mg daily for 2 months, but nonsignificant trend to increase at 6 months *1300*

Urea *Serum Increase Physiological* In 14 hypertensive patients with proteinuria treatment with up to 100 mg/d caused significant increase from mean baseline of 9.0 ± 3.0 mmol/L to 10.5 ± 4.4 mmol/L *229*
Urine Increase Physiological In 14 hypertensive patients with proteinuria treatment with up to 100 mg/d caused significant increase from mean baseline of 271 ± 75 mmol/d to 316 ± 90 mmol/d *229*

Urea Nitrogen *Serum Increase Physiological* In one of 63 patients with essential hypertension treatment with up to 100 mg/d for 8 weeks caused increase from baseline concentration of 8.7 mmol/L to 10.7 mmol/L *454*
Serum No Effect Physiological No significant effect in 12 healthy volunteers over 24 hours following single dose of 100 mg *3452* Nonsignificant increase from mean baseline concentration of 5.1 mmol/L to 5.2 mmol/L in 63 patients with essential hypertension treated with up to 100 mg/d for 8 weeks *454*
Urine No Effect Physiological No significant effect in 12 healthy volunteers over 24 hours following single oral dose of 100 mg *3452*

Uric Acid *Serum Increase Physiological* In 42 patients with mild to moderate hypertension treatment for 6 months caused significant increase from mean baseline of 304 µmol/L to 324 µmol/L *2907* In 25 patients with essential hypertension treatment with 50 mg once daily for 12 weeks increased the concentration by 4% *2398*
Serum No Effect Physiological No significant effect in 12 healthy volunteers over 24 hours following single dose of 100 mg *3452* No significant change observed in 18 patients with mild to moderate hypertension treated with up to 150 mg/d for 6 months *966* After 100 mg/d for 5 weeks in 20 hypertensive men *3521*
Urine No Effect Physiological No significant effect in 12 healthy volunteers over 24 hours following single oral dose of 100 mg *3452*

Verapamil *Serum Increase Physiological* Effect possibly due to inhibitory effect of atenolol on verapamil metabolism. Note atenolol concentration increased by verapamil *3153*
Serum No Effect Physiological No effect observed on plasma concentration when drugs coadministered *6358*

Viscosity *Blood No Effect Physiological* In 9 patients with essential hypertension treated with atenolol for 6 months no significant change over shear rate from 2.25 to 450 /s *2237*
Plasma No Effect Physiological In 9 patients with essential hypertension treated with atenolol for 6 months no significant change over shear rate from 2.25 to 450 /s *2237*

VLDL-Cholesterol *Serum Decrease Physiological* Increase by 5.9% after 100 mg/d for 5 weeks in 20 hypertensive men *3521*
Serum Increase Physiological Increase by 5.9% after 100 mg/d for 5 weeks in 20 hypertensive men *3521* Insignificant increase from mean of 0.45 mmol/L to 0.54 mmol/L in 25 hypertensive patients treated with average dose of 67 mg/day for 24 weeks *4736* From 0.90 to 1.14 mmol/L with 100 mg drμg/d *3610* Significant increase from mean baseline of 0.50 mmol/L to 0.70 mmol/L in the hypertriglyceridemic patients of 18 with mild to moderate hypertension treated with up to 150 mg/d for 6 months *966* From 1.21 to 1.62 mmol/L in 15 hypertensives treated for 8 mo *1713* Significant increase from mean baseline of 0.50 mmol/L to 0.70 mmol/L in 18 hypertriglyceridemic patients with mild to moderate hypertension treated with up to 150 mg/d for 6 months *966* Effect observed in 2 studies, but not significant in one other *142*
Serum No Effect Physiological In 20 patients with 50 mg/d compared with pre-treatment values after 3 mo *5115*

VLDL-Triglycerides *Serum Increase Physiological* 48% effect observed in one study *142* From 1.21 to 1.62 mmol/L in 15 hypertensives treated for 8 mo *1713* Significant increase from mean baseline of 0.70 mmol/L to 1.04 mmol/L observed in the hypertriglyceridemic patients of 18 with mild to moderate hypertension when treated with up to 150 mg/d for 6 months *966* Increase from mean of 1.01 mmol/L to 1.20 mmol/L in 25 hypertensive patients receiving average of 67 mg/day for 24 weeks *4736* In 25 patients with essential hypertension treatment with 50 mg once daily for 12 weeks caused significant 31% increase in concentration *2398* From 0.90 to 1.14 mmol/L with 100 mg drμg/d *3610*
Serum No Effect Physiological In 20 patients with 50 mg/d compared with pre-treatment values after 3 mo *5115*

Volume *Urine Increase Physiological* Nonsignificant increase observed at 3 and 7 days in 10 patients with uncomplicated essential hypertension treated with 100 mg/d *1086*
Urine No Effect Physiological No significant effect in 12 healthy volunteers over 24 hours following single oral dose of 100 mg *3452*

Zinc *Serum No Effect Physiological* No significant effect in 12 healthy volunteers over 24 hours following single dose of 100 mg *3452*
Urine No Effect Physiological No significant effect in 12 healthy volunteers over 24 hours following single oral dose of 100 mg *3452*

Atorvastatin

Alanine Aminotransferase *Serum Increase Physiological* In clinical trials with 2502 patients atorvastatin observed to increase ALT activity in 0.7% *4534* In 6 clinical studies of patients with hyperlipidemias treatment with 5 mg caused mean increases greater than 3 times the upper limit of normal in 1 (8%) of patients *338*

Antipyrine *Serum No Effect Physiological* Atorvastatin had no effect on the pharmacokinetics of antipyrine *4534*

Apolipoprotein B *Serum Decrease Physiological* In one study of 707 hypercholesterolemic patients treatment with 10 mg/d for 16 weeks caused a 28% reduction. In two other studies of 222 and 132 hypercholesterolemic patients 10 mg/d for 16 weeks caused reductions of 27% and 34% respectively *4534* In 6 clinical studies of patients with primary hypercholesterolemia treatment with 5 mg caused mean decreases of 22%, with 10 mg 31%, with 20 mg 31% and with 80 mg 47%. In patients with combined hyperlipidemia treatment with 5 mg. 10 mg, 20 mg and 80 mg caused reductions of 24%, 24%, 31% and 53% respectively. In patients with hypertriglyceridemia treatment with 5 mg. 20 mg and 80 mg caused reductions of 16%, 31% and 40% respectively *338*

Aspartate Aminotransferase *Serum Increase Physiological* In 6 clinical studies of patients with hyperlipidemias treatment with 5 mg caused mean increases greater than 3 times the upper limit of normal in 1 (8%) of patients *338*

Bilirubin *Serum Increase Physiological* In 6 clinical studies of patients with hyperlipidemias treatment caused mean increases greater than 1.5 times the upper limit of normal in 1 (9%) of patients treated with 2.5 mg drug per day, 3 (6%) of those receiving 5 mg/d, 2 (3%) of those receiving 10 mg/d, 1 (2%) of those receiving 20 mg/d, 1 (8%) of those receiving 40 mg/d and 1 (2%) of those receiving 80 mg/d *338*

Cholesterol *Serum Decrease Physiological* In 50 healthy normolipemic volunteers treatment with increasing doses caused at 14 days progressively greater decreases of mean concentration of 6.6% with 0.5 mg/d, 13.3% with 2.5 mg, 21.6% with 10 mg, 29.0% with 20 mg/d, 35.8% with 40 mg/d and 44.8% with 80 mg/d *4759* In 92 patients with primary hypercholesterolemia treatment with upto 80 mg/d for 30 weeks caused significant reduction from mean baseline of 11.0 ± 2.2 mmol/L by 28 ± 9% after 6 weeks, 34 ± 9% after 12 weeks, 38 ± 10% after 18 weeks and 42 ± 10% after 30 weeks *5564* In 6 clinical studies of patients with primary hypercholesterolemia treatment with 5 mg caused mean decreases of 20%, with 10 mg 29%, with 20 mg 29% and with 80 mg 42%. In patients with combined hyperlipidemia treatment with 5 mg. 10 mg, 20 mg and 80 mg caused reductions of 22%, 25%, 30% and 51% respectively. In patients with hypertriglyceridemia treatment with 5 mg. 20 mg and 80 mg caused reductions of 22%, 32% and 42% respectively *338* In one study of 707 hypercholesterolemic patients treatment with 10 mg/d for 16 weeks caused a 27% reduction. In two other studies of 222 and 132 hypercholesterolemic patients 10 mg/d for 16 weeks caused reductions of 25% and 29% respectively *4534*

Creatine Kinase *Serum Increase Physiological* In 6 clinical studies of patients with hyperlipidemias treatment with 10 mg caused mean increases greater than 5 times the upper limit of normal in 1 (2%) of patients *338*

Digoxin *Serum Increase Physiological* Atorvastatin coadministration with digoxin caused a 20% increase in steady state plasma digoxin concentration *4534*

Ethinyl Estradiol *Serum Increase Physiological* When an oral contraceptive was coadministered with atorvastatin the area under the concentration curve of ethinyl estradiol was increased by approximately 20% *4534*

HDL-Cholesterol *Serum Increase Physiological* In clinical trials with 2502 patients atorvastatin observed to increase concentration by 5 - 9% *4534* In one study of 707 hypercholesterolemic patients treatment with 10 mg/d for 16 weeks caused a 7% increase. In two other studies of 222 and 132 hypercholesterolemic patients 10 mg/d for 16 weeks caused increases of 6% and 7% respectively *4534* In 6 clinical studies of patients with primary hypercholesterolemia treatment with 5 mg caused mean increases of 15%, with 10 mg 6%, with 20 mg 18% and with 80 mg 9%. In patients with combined hyperlipidemia treatment with 5 mg. 10 mg, 20 mg and 80 mg caused increases of 12%, 20%, 20% and 9% respectively. In patients with hypertriglyceridemia treatment with 5 mg. 20 mg and 80 mg caused increases of 7%, 11% and 12% respectively *338* In 92 patients with primary hypercholesterolemia treatment with upto 80 mg/d for 30 weeks caused significant increase from mean baseline of 1.1 ± 0.3 mmol/L by 10 ± 12% after 6 weeks, 10 ± 15% after 12 weeks, 10 ± 19% after 18 weeks and 7 ± 15% after 30 weeks *5564*

LDL-Cholesterol *Serum Decrease Physiological* In a group of hypertriglyceridemic patients treatment with 5 mg/d for 4 weeks caused significant 16.7% decrease *5796* In 92 patients with primary hypercholesterolemia treatment with upto 80 mg/d for 30 weeks caused significant reduction from mean baseline of 8.8 ± 2.2 mmol/L by 33 ± 11% after 6 weeks, 40 ± 11% after 12 weeks, 45 ± 12% after 18 weeks and 49 ± 12% after 30 weeks *5564* In 50 healthy normolipemic volunters treatment with increasing doses caused at 14 days progressively greater decreases of mean concentration of 7.9% with 0.5 mg/d, 22.4% with 2.5 mg, 30.5% with 10 mg, 39.2% with 20 mg/d, 46.7% with 40 mg/d and 57.8% with 80 mg/d *4759* In one study of 707 hypercholesterolemic patients treatment with 10 mg/d for 16 weeks caused a 36% reduction. In two other studies of 222 and 132 hypercholesterolemic patients 10 mg/d for 16 weeks caused reductions of 35% and 37% respec-

Atorvastatin *(continued)*

LDL-Cholesterol *(continued)*
tively *4534* In 6 clinical studies of patients with primary hypercholesterolemia treatment with 5 mg caused mean decreases of 27%, with 10 mg 39%, with 20 mg 39% and with 80 mg 57%. In patients with combined hyperlipidemia treatment with 5 mg. 10 mg, 20 mg and 80 mg caused reductions of 27%, 38%, 38% and 64% respectively. In patients with hypertriglyceridemia treatment with 5 mg. 20 mg and 80 mg caused reductions of 12%, 30% and 37% respectively *338* In 55 patients with hypercholesterolemia treatment with 10 mg/d reduced LDLC to below 160 mg/dL in 91% and to 100 mg/dL or below in 27%, with 20 mg/d in 100% and 40% respectively, with 40 mg/d in 100% and 64% respectively and with 80 mg/d in 100% and 82% respectively *1262*

Norethindrone *Serum Increase Physiological* When an oral contraceptive was coadministered with atorvastatin the area under the concentration curve of norethindrone was increased by approximately 30% *4534*

Osmolality *Urine Decrease Physiological* In 50 healthy normolipemic volunteers treatment with increasing doses caused at 14 days progressively greater decreases of mean excretion over placebo over 4 hours of 0 mOsmol/kg with 0.5 µg, 240 mOsmol/kg with 15 µg and 350 mOsmol/kg with 25 µg *4759*

Prothrombin Time *Plasma Increase Physiological* Coadministration of atorvastatin with warfarin had no clinically significant effect on the prothrombin time *4534*

Triglyceride:LDL-Cholesterol Ratio
Serum Decrease Physiological In a group of hypertriglyceridemic patients treatment with 5 mg/d for 4 weeks caused significant 1.6 ratio *5796*

Triglycerides *Serum Decrease Physiological* In a group of hypertriglyceridemic patients treatment with 5 mg/d for 4 weeks caused significant 26.5% decrease *5796* In one study of 707 hypercholesterolemic patients treatment with 10 mg/d for 16 weeks caused a 17% reduction. In two other studies of 222 and 132 hypercholesterolemic patients 10 mg/d for 16 weeks caused reductions of 17% and 23% respectively *4534* In 92 patients with primary hypercholesterolemia treatment with upto 80 mg/d for 30 weeks caused significant reduction from mean baseline of 2.5 ± 1.4 mmol/L by 21 ± 24% after 6 weeks, 28 ± 21% after 12 weeks, 30 ± 20% after 18 weeks and 33 ± 20% after 30 weeks *5564* In 6 clinical studies of patients with primary hypercholesterolemia treatment with 5 mg caused mean decreases of 25%, with 10 mg 17%, with 20 mg 29% and with 80 mg 23%. In patients with combined hyperlipidemia treatment with 5 mg. 10 mg, 20 mg and 80 mg caused reductions of 17%, 27%, 27% and 42% respectively. In patients with hypertriglyceridemia treatment with 5 mg. 20 mg and 80 mg caused reductions of 30%, 34% and 43% respectively *338*

VLDL-Cholesterol *Serum Decrease Physiological* In 6 clinical studies of patients with primary hypercholesterolemia treatment with 5 mg caused mean decreases of 30%, with 10 mg 28%, with 20 mg 33% and with 80 mg 38%. In patients with combined hyperlipidemia treatment with 5 mg. 10 mg, 20 mg and 80 mg caused reductions of 26%, 29%, 34% and 60% respectively. In patients with hypertriglyceridemia treatment with 5 mg. 20 mg and 80 mg caused reductions of 38%, 46% and 53% respectively *338*

Volume *Urine Increase Physiological* In 50 healthy normolipemic volunteers treatment with increasing doses caused at 14 days progressively greater increases of mean excretion over placebo over 4 hours of 20 mL with 0.5 µg, 120 mL with 15 µg and 320 mL with 25 µg *4759*

Water Clearance, Free *Urine Decrease Physiological* In 50 healthy normolipemic volunteers treatment with increasing doses caused at 14 days progressively greater decreases of mean excretion over placebo over 4 hours of - 0.1 mL/min to - 1.6 mL/min with 0.5 µg, 0.8 mL/min to - 0.7 mL/min with 15 µg and - 1.4 mL/min to - 0.1 mL/min with 25 µg *4759*

Atovaquone

Alanine Aminotransferase *Serum Increase Physiological* Increased activity of greater than 5 times the upper limit of normal observed in 6% of patients in an extended trial *2176*

Alkaline Phosphatase *Serum Increase Physiological* Increased activity of greater than 2.5 times the upper limit of normal observed in 8% of patients in an extended trial *2176*

Amylase *Serum Increase Physiological* Increased activity of greater than 1.5 times the upper limit of normal observed in 7% of patients in an extended trial *2176*

Aspartate Aminotransferase *Serum Increase Physiological* Increased activity of greater than 5 times the upper limit of normal observed in 4% of patients in an extended trial *2176*

Creatinine *Serum No Effect Physiological* In an extended trial no cases of increased creatinine concentration in contrast to 5% in patients who received pentamidine *2176*

Hemoglobin *Blood Decrease Physiological* Anemia with hemoglobin concentration of less than 8.0 g/dL observed in 6% of patients in an extended trial *2176*

Neutrophils *Blood Decrease Physiological* Neutropenia of less than 750 cells/µL observed in 3% of patients in an extended trial *2176*

Potassium *Serum No Effect Physiological* In an extended trial no cases of hyperkalemia in contrast to 5% in patients who received pentamidine *2176*

Sodium *Serum Decrease Physiological* Decreased concentration of less than 0.96 times the lower limit of normal observed in 7% of patients in an extended trial *2176*

Zidovudine *Serum Increase Physiological* In 14 HIV-positive volunteers coadministration of 750 mg/12 h atovaquone daily with steady state zidovudine conditions (200 mg/8 h) decreased the zidovudine oral clearance leading to a 35 ± 23% increase in the plasma AUC *2163*

Atracurium

Histamine *Plasma No Effect Analytical* Insignificant effect at physiological concentration on radio-enzyme assay *2492*

Midazolam *Serum No Effect Analytical* On GC-ECD method of Ha et al *2387*

Atropine

Basal Metabolic Rate *Patient Increase Physiological* Temporary effect observed *409*

Cannabinoids *Urine No Effect Analytical* No effect on Roche Abuscreen method *5006*

Cortisol *Plasma Increase Physiological* In 8 patients undergoing abdominal hysterectomy pretreatment with 1.2 mg intramuscularly was unable to stop normal increase from baseline of 387 ± 54 nmol/L to 708 ± 54 nmol/L 60 minutes after start of surgery *1396*

Drugs of Abuse Screen *Urine No Effect Analytical* No effect at concentration of 100 µg/mL on EZ-SCREEN procedure for cannabinoids and cocaine *1739*

Ethanol *Serum Decrease Physiological* Reduced rate of absorption due to delayed gastric emptying *6403*

Gastrin *Serum Decrease Physiological* Significant effect if given i.m *2021*

Glucose *Serum Decrease Physiological* Possible slight fall if given as premedication *3935*
Serum Increase Physiological In 8 patients undergoing abdominal hysterectomy pretreatment with 1.2 mg intramuscularly had no effect on normal increase from mean baseline of 4.6 ± 6.6 mmol/L to 6.6 ± 0.6 mmol/L 60 minutes after start of surgery *1396*

Hematocrit *Blood Increase Physiological* But not to same extent as plasma volume *2988*

Histamine *Plasma Increase Physiological* Associated with dose given associated with anesthesia *3648*
Plasma No Effect Analytical 50% inhibition of radio-enzyme assay at concentration of 40 µg/mL but unlikely to be effect at physiological concentration of less than 0.25 µg/mL *2492*

Hydrochloric Acid *Gastric Fluid Decrease Physiological* Volume also reduced *2242*

Leukocytes *Blood Increase Physiological* May cause leukocytosis (effect in children) *128*

Midazolam *Serum No Effect Analytical* On GC-ECD method of Ha et al *2387*

Pepsin *Gastric Material* *Decrease* *Physiological* Antagonizes cholinergic stimulation *1252*

Prolactin *Plasma* *No Effect* *Physiological* No effect on basal concentration in morning or evening but evening response to hypoglycemia significantly inhibited *4231*

PSP Excretion *Urine* *Decrease* *Physiological* Interferes with secretion by tubules *4953*

Volume *Plasma* *Decrease* *Physiological* Increase by 10-15% after i.v. injection *2988*

Urine *Decrease* *Physiological* Very large doses cause release of ADH *2242*

Auranofin

Alanine Aminotransferase *Serum* *Increase* *Physiological* Increased hepatic enzyme activity reported to occur in more than 1% patients receiving auranofin *5655*

Alkaline Phosphatase *Serum* *Increase* *Physiological* Increased hepatic enzyme activity reported to occur in more than 1% patients receiving auranofin *5655*

Aspartate Aminotransferase *Serum* *Increase* *Physiological* Increased hepatic enzyme activity reported to occur in more than 1% patients receiving auranofin *5655*

Bilirubin *Serum* *Increase* *Physiological* Jaundice reported to occur in fewer than 1% patients receiving auranofin *5655*

Blood *Urine* *Increase* *Physiological* Hematuria reported to occur in more than 1% patients receiving auranofin *5655*

Eosinophils *Blood* *Increase* *Physiological* Eosinophilia reported to occur in more than 1% patients receiving auranofin *5655* Infrequent reversible side effect (occurring in up to 13% patients) *946*

Erythrocytes *Blood* *Decrease* *Physiological* Pure red cell aplasia reported to occur in fewer than 1% patients receiving auranofin *5655* Infrequent reversible side effect (occurring in up to 13% patients) *946*

Granulocytes *Blood* *Decrease* *Physiological* Agranulocytosis reported to occur in fewer than 1% patients receiving auranofin *5655*

Hematocrit *Blood* *Decrease* *Physiological* Infrequent reversible side effect (occurring in up to 13% patients) *946* Anemia reported to occur in more than 1% patients receiving auranofin *5655*

Hemoglobin *Blood* *Decrease* *Physiological* Anemia reported to occur in more than 1% patients receiving auranofin *5655* Infrequent reversible side effect (occurring in up to 13% patients) *946*

Urine *Increase* *Physiological* Occasional drug-associated hematuria: may be partially responsible for anemia *946*

Immunoglobulin G *Serum* *Increase* *Physiological* 26.5% reduction after 12 weeks treatment in patients with rheumatoid arthritis *946*

Serum *No Effect* *Physiological* No effect of 6 mg/d for 1 y *946*

Lactate Dehydrogenase *Serum* *Increase* *Physiological* Increased hepatic enzyme activity reported to occur in more than 1% patients receiving auranofin *5655*

Leukocytes *Blood* *Decrease* *Physiological* Leukopenia reported to occur in more than 1% patients receiving auranofin *5655* Infrequent reversible side effect (occurring in up to 13% patients) *946*

Neutrophils *Blood* *Decrease* *Physiological* Neutropenia reported to occur in 0.1 - 1% patients receiving auranofin *5655*

Occult Blood *Feces* *Increase* *Physiological* Gastrointestinal bleeding reported to occur in 0.1 - 1% patients receiving auranofin *5655*

Phenytoin *Serum* *Increase* *Physiological* Single report that auranofin administration may have increased the plasma concentration of phenytoin *5655*

Platelets *Blood* *Decrease* *Physiological* In one case platelet-reactive IgG antibodies observed in the presence of gold salts *3259* Thrombocytopenia reported to occur in more than 1% patients receiving auranofin *5655*

Blood *Increase* *Physiological* Infrequent reversible side effect (occurring in up to 13% patients) *946*

Protein *Urine* *Increase* *Physiological* In 3% of patients receiving drug, but proteinuria did not persist beyond 12 mo: effect less than when gold given *3066* Proteinuria reported to occur in 3 - 9% patients receiving auranofin *5655*

Testosterone *Serum* *No Effect* *Physiological* In a group of male patients with rheumatoid arthritis taking auranofin mean concentration not significantly different from concentration in untreated male patients *3808*

Zinc *Serum* *Increase* *Physiological* In 10 of 12 patients with initially low concentration *946*

Aurothioglucose

Alanine Aminotransferase *Serum* *Increase* *Physiological* Administration may cause intrahepatic cholestasis, hepatitis with jaundice, toxic hepatitis or acute yellow atrophy *5337*

Alkaline Phosphatase *Serum* *Increase* *Physiological* Administration may cause intrahepatic cholestasis, hepatitis with jaundice, toxic hepatitis or acute yellow atrophy *5337*

Aspartate Aminotransferase *Serum* *Increase* *Physiological* Administration may cause intrahepatic cholestasis, hepatitis with jaundice, toxic hepatitis or acute yellow atrophy *5337*

Bilirubin *Serum* *Increase* *Physiological* Administration may cause intrahepatic cholestasis, hepatitis with jaundice, toxic hepatitis or acute yellow atrophy *5337*

Blood *Urine* *Increase* *Physiological* Administration may cause nephrotic syndrome or glomerulonephritis, which is usually relatively mild and can subside completely if treatment stopped early *5337*

Eosinophils *Blood* *Increase* *Physiological* Administration may rarely cause agranulocytosis or granulocytopenia, thrombocytopenia with or without purpura, leukopenia, or eosinophilia *5337*

γ-Glutamyltransferase *Serum* *Increase* *Physiological* Administration may cause intrahepatic cholestasis, hepatitis with jaundice, toxic hepatitis or acute yellow atrophy *5337*

Granulocytes *Blood* *Decrease* *Physiological* Administration may rarely cause agranulocytosis or granulocytopenia, thrombocytopenia with or without purpura, leukopenia, or eosinophilia *5337*

Hematocrit *Blood* *Decrease* *Physiological* Administration may rarely cause hypoplastic or aplastic anemia *5337*

Hemoglobin *Blood* *Decrease* *Physiological* Administration may rarely cause hypoplastic or aplastic anemia *5337*

immunoglobulin A *Serum* *Decrease* *Physiological* Reduced only at 3 mo in 25 patients with rheumatoid arthritis *6193*

Immunoglobulin G *Serum* *Decrease* *Physiological* Reduced only at 12 mo in 25 patients with rheumatoid arthritis *6193*

Immunoglobulin M *Serum* *Decrease* *Physiological* Substantial reduction at 3 mo in 25 patients with rheumatoid arthritis *6193*

Leukocytes *Blood* *Decrease* *Physiological* Administration may rarely cause agranulocytosis or granulocytopenia, thrombocytopenia with or without purpura, leukopenia, or eosinophilia *5337*

Platelets *Blood* *Decrease* *Physiological* Administration may rarely cause agranulocytosis or granulocytopenia, thrombocytopenia with or without purpura, leukopenia, or eosinophilia *5337*

Protein *Urine* *Increase* *Physiological* Administration may cause nephrotic syndrome or glomerulonephritis, which is usually relatively mild and can subside completely if treatment stopped early *5337*

Aurothiomalate

C-Reactive Protein *Serum* *Decrease* *Physiological* Significant reduction observed in about 200 patients with active rheumatoid arthritis treated for 3-6 months but reduction continued for up to 60 months *5587*

Erythrocyte Sedimentation Rate
Blood *Decrease* *Physiological* Significant reduction observed in about 200 patients with active rheumatoid arthritis treated for 3-6 months but with continued reduction observed for up to 60 months *5587*

Aurothiomalate *(continued)*

Histamine *Plasma No Effect Analytical* Improbable inhibition of radio-enzyme assay at therapeutic concentrations *2492*

Platelets *Blood Decrease Physiological* In patient with rheumatoid arthritis with shortened platelet survival and platelet phagocytosis *3536*

Aza Drugs

BSP Retention *Serum Increase Physiological* May cause hepatotoxicity *2024*

Azacitidine

Alanine Aminotransferase *Serum Increase Physiological* Hepatotoxicity may be observed with treatment *1384*

Aspartate Aminotransferase *Serum Increase Physiological* Hepatotoxicity may occur as an adverse effect *1384*

Erythrocytes *Blood Decrease Physiological* Dose limiting toxicity is effect on bone marrow *1384*

Leukocytes *Blood Decrease Physiological* Dose limiting toxicity is effect on bone marrow *1384*

Platelets *Blood Decrease Physiological* Dose limiting toxicity is effect on bone marrow *1384*

5-Azacytidine

Amino Acids *Urine Increase Physiological* Mean excretion of 16.1 mmol/d in 2 patients with leukemia undergoing chemotherapy not different from 29.1 ± 23.4 mmol/d in 52 patients with acute leukemia and 19.8 ± 10.4 mmol/d in 29 healthy controls of both sexes *6517*

Azapropazone

Alanine Aminotransferase *Serum Increase Physiological* In 9 of 83 patients treated for 6 mo *5979*

Aspartate Aminotransferase *Serum Increase Physiological* In 9 of 83 patients treated for 6 mo *5979*

Chloride *Serum Increase Physiological* In 1 of 83 patients treated for 6 mo *5979*

Cholesterol *Serum No Effect Analytical* At concentration of 250 mg/L had no effect as measured by catalase-AIDH method *5704* At concentration of 250 mg/L had no effect as measured by CHOD-Iodide method *5704* At concentration of 250 mg/L had no effect as measured by CHOD-PAP method *5704* At concentration of 250 mg/L had no effect as measured by catalase-Hantzsch method *5704* At concentration of 250 mg/L had no effect as measured by Liebermann-Burchard method *5704*

Creatinine *Serum Increase Physiological* Initial 10% increase observed in 83 treated patients but thereafter no further increase *5979*

Serum No Effect Analytical At concentration of 360 mg/L had no effect as measured by Jaffe-Fuller's earth method *5704* At concentration of 360 mg/L had no effect as measured by Jaffe-Fading-Fraction method *5704* At concentration of 625 mg/L had no effect as measured by kinetic Jaffe method on BKA-2 *5704*

Eosinophils *Blood Increase Physiological* In 1 of 83 patients treated for 6 mo *5979*

Erythrocytes *Blood Decrease Physiological* In 1 of 83 patients treated for 6 mo *5979*

Glucose *Serum No Effect Analytical* At concentration of 36 mg/L had no effect as measured by Kodak Ektachem® method *5704*

Hemoglobin *Urine Increase Physiological* In 1 of 83 patients treated for 6 mo *5979*

Monocytes *Blood Decrease Physiological* In 1 of 83 patients treated for 6 mo *5979*

Neutrophils *Blood Increase Physiological* In 1 of 83 patients treated for 6 mo *5979*

Phenytoin *Serum Increase Physiological* Probably due to decreased clearance of phenytoin *2071*

Platelets *Blood Decrease Physiological* In 3 of 83 patients treated for 6 mo *5979*

Potassium *Serum No Effect Analytical* At concentration of 360 mg/L had no effect on ISE measurement without predilution *5704*

Protein Electrophoresis *Serum No Effect Analytical* At concentration of 360 mg/L had no effect as measured by automated Olympus-Hite method except for slight displacement of fractions *5704*

Prothrombin Time *Plasma Increase Physiological* Drug has ulcerogenic potential by itself, but enhanced with warfarin *155*

Sodium *Serum No Effect Analytical* At concentration of 360 mg/L had no effect on ISE measurement without predilution *5704*

Thyroxine (T4) *Serum Increase Analytical* Using the Ciba-Corning ACS:180 analyzer mean concentration increased in 6 specimens by 35 to 178% compared with the concentration measured by the Amerlex-M method *5621*

Urea Nitrogen *Serum Increase Physiological* Initial 10% increase observed in 83 treated patients but thereafter no further increase *5979*

Serum No Effect Analytical At concentration of 36 mg/L had no effect as measured by Kodak Ektachem® method *5704*

Uric Acid *Serum Decrease Physiological* Mean fall after 4 d was 31%, and 46% on 2400 mg daily *2598* Therapeutic intent *5979*

Serum No Effect Analytical At concentration of 360 mg/L had no effect as measured by catalase-AIDH method *5704* At concentration of 360 mg/L had no effect as measured by Kageyama-Hantzsch method *5704*

Urine Increase Physiological Potent uricosuric agent (2400 mg daily comparable to 1 g probenecid) *2598*

Azaserine

Alanine Aminotransferase *Serum Increase Physiological* May cause hepatotoxicity *6461*

Aspartate Aminotransferase *Serum Increase Physiological* May cause hepatotoxicity *6461*

Azathioprine

Alanine Aminotransferase *Serum Increase Physiological* Administration of azathioprine may cause hepatotoxicity, primarily in allograft recipients. Hepatotoxicity has been less common (less than 1%) in rheumatoid arthritis patients *2159* Minimal cholestasis and reversible portal fibrosis observed in 8 patients: occasional hepatotoxicity *72* Hepatotoxicity observed in fewer than 1% of 228 patients treated with azathioprine *5240* Canalicular cholestasis and centrilobular ballooning of hepatocytes in one patient *1321* May cause hepatotoxicity *5777* Hepatotoxicity reported as a complication during the course of azathioprine treatment, primarily in allograft recipients, but less than in 1% of rheumatoid arthritis patients *5128*

Albumin *Serum Decrease Physiological* May cause hepatotoxicity *5777*

Alkaline Phosphatase *Serum Decrease Physiological* Improves biliary excretion in biliary cirrhosis *5108*

Serum Increase Physiological Administration of azathioprine may cause hepatotoxicity, primarily in allograft recipients. Hepatotoxicity has been less common (less than 1%) in rheumatoid arthritis patients *2159* Hepatotoxicity reported as a complication during the course of azathioprine treatment, primarily in allograft recipients, but less than in 1% of rheumatoid arthritis patients *5128* Hepatotoxicity observed in fewer than 1% of 228 patients treated with azathioprine *5240* May be very high because of liver damage or biliary stasis *2754* Minimal cholestasis and reversible portal fibrosis observed in 8 patients: occasional hepatotoxicity *72* Canalicular cholestasis and centrilobular ballooning of hepatocytes in one patient *1321*

Serum No Effect Physiological In 58 patients with autoimmune hepatitis treatment with 2 mg azathioprine/kg/d for a median of 67 months caused nonsignificant change from mean baseline of 96 ± 49 U/L to 86 ± 39 U/L *2960*

Amylase *Serum Increase Physiological* 6.2% of 116 patients receiving only drug demonstrated clinical pancreatitis *3758* Administration of azathioprine may cause vomiting with abdominal pain with a hypersensitivity pancreatitis *2159* Unusual side effect but may cause pancreatitis *2754* Pancreatitis reported as a complication during the course of azathioprine treatment *5128*

Apolipoprotein A-I *Serum Decrease Physiological* In patients who had had a renal transplant treatment with azathioprine with prednisone caused significant change from mean baseline of 1477 ± 271 mg/L after 3 months to 1398 ± 285 mg/L after 6 months and 1378 ± 232 mg/L after 12 months *2602*

Apolipoprotein B *Serum No Effect Physiological* In patients who had had a renal transplant treatment with azathioprine with prednisone caused nonsignificant change from mean baseline of 1228 ± 332 mg/L after 3 months to 1257 ± 336 mg/L after 6 months and 1247 ± 338 mg/L after 12 months *2602*

Aspartate Aminotransferase *Serum Increase Physiological* Hepatotoxicity reported as a complication during the course of azathioprine treatment, primarily in allograft recipients, but less than in 1% of rheumatoid arthritis patients *5128* Hepatotoxicity observed in fewer than 1% of 228 patients treated with azathioprine *5240* Minimal cholestasis and reversible portal fibrosis observed in 8 patients: occasional hepatotoxicity *72* Canalicular cholestasis and centrilobular ballooning of hepatocytes in one patient *1321* May cause hepatotoxicity *5777* Administration of azathioprine may cause hepatotoxicity, primarily in allograft recipients. Hepatotoxicity has been less common (less than 1%) in rheumatoid arthritis patients *2159*

Bilirubin *Serum Increase Physiological* Hepatotoxicity observed in fewer than 1% of 228 patients treated with azathioprine *5240* Hepatotoxicity reported as a complication during the course of azathioprine treatment, primarily in allograft recipients, but less than in 1% of rheumatoid arthritis patients *5128* May cause hepatotoxicity (not usually very high) *5777* Administration of azathioprine may cause hepatotoxicity, primarily in allograft recipients. Hepatotoxicity has been less common (less than 1%) in rheumatoid arthritis patients *2159* Canalicular cholestasis and centrilobular ballooning of hepatocytes in one patient *1321* Hypersensitivity reaction without effect on aminotransferases *1277*

Serum No Effect Physiological In 58 patients with autoimmune hepatitis treatment with 2 mg azathioprine/kg/d for a median of 67 months caused nonsignificant change from mean baseline of 0.70 ± 0.35 mg/dL to 0.74 ± 0.57 mg/dL *2960*

Cholesterol *Serum Decrease Physiological* Improves biliary excretion in biliary cirrhosis *5108*

Serum Increase Physiological Administration of 1-2 mg/kg/d or 100-150 mg/d azathioprine to 326 renal transplant patients caused hypercholesterolemia in 11.3% patients *5017*

Serum No Effect Physiological In patients who had had a renal transplant treatment with azathioprine with prednisone caused nonsignificant change from mean baseline of 6.14 ± 1.33 mmol/L after 3 months to 5.85 ± 1.31 mmol/L after 6 months and 5.91 ± 1.43 mmol/L after 12 months *2602*

Cholesterol:HDL-Cholesterol Ratio

Serum Increase Physiological In patients who had had a renal transplant treatment with azathioprine with prednisone caused significant change from mean baseline of 5.11 ± 1.82 after 3 months to 5.69 ± 1.90 after 6 months and 5.73 ± 2.09 after 12 months *2602*

Cholinesterase *Serum No Effect Analytical* No effect observed at concentration of 1 µg/mL with butyrylthiocholine method on Kodak Ektachem® *2504*

Chondrex *Serum No Effect Analytical* Concentrations up to 0.5 g/L had no significant effect on sandwich-type ELISA procedure of Harvey et al *2491*

Chromosomes *Test Conditions Abnormal Physiological* Clastogenic to bone marrow and leukocytes *5484*

Creatinine *Serum Increase Physiological* Reversible increased concentration observed in one patient in association with fever and nasal congestion with same pattern after two rechallenges not associated with renal parenchymal abnormalities: probably due to hypersensitivity *6171* Renal dysfunction observed in 6% of 228 patients treated with azathioprine *5240* Reversible increased concentration observed in one patient in association with fever and nasal congestion with same pattern after two rechallenges not associated with renal parenchymal abnormalities: Probably due to hypersensitivity *6170*

Cyclosporine *Blood No Effect Analytical* At a concentration of 10 mg/L had no effect on Syva EMIT method *495*

Serum No Effect Analytical No interference observed with Incstar RIA procedure *2930*

Diclofenac *Serum No Effect Physiological* Coadministration of azathioprine with diclofenac did not significantly affect the peak concentration or AUC of diclofenac *1025*

Erythrocytes *Blood Decrease Physiological* Bone marrow depression with anemia *128* Principal manifestation of bone marrow depression *72* 18 cases of pancytopenia out of 79 cases with hematological problems out of 328 reports of severe adverse effects *3443*

Fat *Feces Increase Physiological* Administration of azathioprine has been reported to cause steatorrhea with a low frequency *2159* May occasionally cause steatorrhea *2754* Steatorrhea reported as a complication during the course of azathioprine treatment in less than in 1% of patients *5128*

Fractional Excretion of Magnesium

Urine Increase Physiological In 8 renal transplant patients receiving azathioprine and prednisolone mean fractional excretion of 18.0 % significantly greater than 3.5 % in 10 healthy individuals *106*

Glucose *Serum Increase Physiological* Administration of 1-2 mg/kg/d or 100-150 mg/d azathioprine to 326 renal transplant patients caused hyperglycemia in 15.0% patients *5017*

γ-Glutamyltransferase *Serum Decrease Physiological* In 58 patients with autoimmune hepatitis treatment with 2 mg azathioprine/kg/d for a median of 67 months caused significant change from mean baseline of 59 ± 55 U/L to 41 ± 33 U/L *2960*

Serum Increase Physiological Hepatotoxicity observed in fewer than 1% of 228 patients treated with azathioprine *5240*

Urine Increase Physiological In 13 patients following renal transplantation increased excretion observed in about 30% over next 18 months *5953*

HDL-Cholesterol *Serum Decrease Physiological* In patients who had had a renal transplant treatment with azathioprine with prednisone caused significant change from mean baseline of 1.32 ± 0.48 mmol/L after 3 months to 1.13 ± 0.45 mmol/L after 6 months and 1.12 ± 0.37 mmol/L after 12 months *2602*

Hematocrit *Blood Decrease Physiological* Administration of azathioprine may cause macrocytic anemia *2159* Administration of 1-2 mg/kg/d or 100-150 mg/d azathioprine to 326 renal transplant patients caused anemia in 23.6% patients, with hypochromic anemia observed in 9.2% *5017* Macrocytic anemia reported in two patients during the course of azathioprine treatment *5128* In 6 cases of anemia out of 79 cases with hematological problems out of 328 reports of severe adverse effects *3443*

Hemoglobin *Blood Decrease Physiological* Administration of 1-2 mg/kg/d or 100-150 mg/d azathioprine to 326 renal transplant patients caused anemia in 23.6% patients, with hypochromic anemia observed in 9.2% *5017* Macrocytic anemia reported in two patients during the course of azathioprine treatment *5128* Administration of azathioprine may cause macrocytic anemia *2159* Principal manifestation of bone marrow depression *72* In 6 cases of anemia out of 79 cases with hematological problems out of 328 reports of severe adverse effects *3443*

Blood No Effect Physiological In 58 patients with autoimmune hepatitis treatment with 2 mg azathioprine/kg/d for a median of 67 months caused nonsignificant change from mean baseline of 137 ± 13 g/L to 134 ± 14 g/L *2960*

Histamine *Plasma No Effect Analytical* Improbable inhibition of radio-enzyme assay at therapeutic concentrations *2492*

Immunoglobulin M *Serum Decrease Physiological* Reduced when biliary cirrhosis treated *5108*

Ionized Magnesium *Platelets Decrease Physiological* In 8 renal transplant patients receiving azathioprine and prednisolone mean concentration of 1.75 µmol/10^8 significantly lower than 2.84 µmol/10^8 in 10 healthy individuals *106*

Red Blood Cells Decrease Physiological In 8 renal transplant patients receiving azathioprine and prednisolone mean concentration of 2.30 mmol/L significantly lower than 2.56 mmol/L in 10 healthy individuals *106*

Azathioprine *(continued)*

Ionized Magnesium *(continued)*
Serum Decrease Physiological In 8 renal transplant patients receiving azathioprine and prednisolone mean concentration of 0.48 mmol/L significantly lower than 0.58 mmol/L in 10 healthy individuals *106*

LDL-Cholesterol *Serum No Effect Physiological* In patients who had had a renal transplant treatment with azathioprine with prednisone caused nonsignificant change from mean baseline of 3.97 ± 1.08 mmol/L after 3 months to 4.02 ± 1.23 mmol/L after 6 months and 4.04 ± 1.30 mmol/L after 12 months *2602*

Leukocytes *Blood Decrease Analytical* Low count by Coulter S, ?due to fragile cells *3677*
Blood Decrease Physiological Administration of 1-2 mg/kg/d or 100-150 mg/d azathioprine to 326 renal transplant patients caused leukopenia in 24.8% patients *5017* In 58 patients with autoimmune hepatitis treatment with 2 mg azathioprine/kg/d for a median of 67 months caused reduction from mean baseline of 6300 ± 2100 /µL to 5400 ± 1600 /µL *2960* Administration of azathioprine produces dose dependent effect which may occur late in the course of treatment *2159* When azathioprine administered with drugs affecting myelopoesis, such as co-trimoxazole, may exaggerate leukopenia, especially in renal transplant patients. Leukopenia reported in > 50% of renal homograft patients receiving azathioprine and 28% of patients with rheumatoid arthritis receiving azathioprine *5128* In 30 of 79 cases with hematological problem out of 328 reports of severe adverse effects *3443* Principal manifestation of bone marrow depression *72* In 11 patients with Behcet's disease receiving azathioprine low counts observed on 21 occasions but only in 3 patients receiving placebo *6594* Drug related leukopenia (probable effect) *5493*
Blood Increase Physiological Leukopenia observed in 19% of 228 patients treated with azathioprine *5240* Administration of 1-2 mg/kg/d or 100-150 mg/d azathioprine to 326 renal transplant patients caused leukocytosis in 7.4% patients *5017*
Urine Increase Physiological Significant sterile leukocyturia in 62% patients with renal allografts treated with azathioprine and steroid immunotherapy but less than when cyclosporine used *261*

Lipase *Serum Increase Physiological* Administration of azathioprine may cause vomiting with abdominal pain with a hypersensitivity pancreatitis *2159* 6.2% of 116 patients receiving only drug demonstrated clinical pancreatitis *3758* Pancreatitis reported as a complication during the course of azathioprine treatment *5128*

Lipoprotein Lp(a) *Serum No Effect Physiological* In patients who had had a renal transplant treatment with azathioprine with prednisone caused nonsignificant change from mean baseline of 50 (range 25 - 244) mg/L after 3 months to 46 (range 25 - 176) mg/L after 12 months *2602*

Magnesium *Serum Decrease Physiological* In 8 renal transplant patients receiving azathioprine and prednisolone mean concentration of 0.62 mmol/L significantly lower than 0.86 mmol/L in 10 healthy individuals *106*
Urine No Effect Physiological In 13 renal transplant patients receiving azathioprine and prednisolone mean excretion of 3.8 mmol/d not significantly different from 4.4 mmol/d in 10 healthy individuals *106*

MCV *Blood Increase Physiological* Macrocytosis in two-thirds of renal transplant patients *72* Administration of azathioprine may cause macrocytic anemia *2159*

β_2-Microglobulin *Urine Increase Physiological* In 13 patients after renal transplantation increased excretion observed in about 30% over next 18 months *5953*

N-Acetylglucosamine *Urine Increase Physiological* In 11 patients following renal transplantation increased excretion observed in about 30% over next 18 months *5953*

Neutrophils *Blood Decrease Physiological* In 6 of 79 cases with hematological problem out of 328 reports of severe adverse effects *3443* Drug related leukopenia (cured by cessation) *2478*

Nitrogen Balance *Patient Negative Physiological* Administration of azathioprine has been reported to cause negative nitrogen balance with a low frequency *2159* Negative nitrogen balance reported as a complication during the course of azathioprine treatment in less than in 1% of patients *5128*

Phenylalanine *Plasma No Effect Analytical* No interference observed with rapid quantitative whole blood method of Campbell et al using phenylalanine dehydrogenase *867*

Phosphate *Serum Decrease Physiological* Administration of 1-2 mg/kg/d or 100-150 mg/d azathioprine to 326 renal transplant patients caused hypophosphatemia in 11.7% patients *5017*

Platelets *Blood Decrease Physiological* May cause bone marrow depression *5493* Administration of 1-2 mg/kg/d or 100-150 mg/d azathioprine to 326 renal transplant patients caused thrombocytopenia in 13.2% patients *5017* Dose dependent thrombocytopenia reported during the course of azathioprine treatment *5128* Administration of azathioprine produces dose dependent effect which may occur late in the course of treatment *2159* In 13 of 79 cases with hematological problem out of 328 reports of severe adverse effects *3443* Principal manifestation of bone marrow depression *72*
Blood No Effect Physiological In 58 patients with autoimmune hepatitis treatment with 2 mg azathioprine/kg/d for a median of 67 months caused nonsignificant change from mean baseline of 212000 ± 79000 /µL to 213000 ± 84000 /µL *2960*

Potassium *Serum Decrease Physiological* Administration of 1-2 mg/kg/d or 100-150 mg/d azathioprine to 326 renal transplant patients caused hypokalemia in 8.3% patients *5017*
Serum Increase Physiological Administration of 1-2 mg/kg/d or 100-150 mg/d azathioprine to 326 renal transplant patients caused hyperkalemia in 16.9% patients *5017* Observed in only 1 of 13 renal transplant patients after 1 mo treatment also with prednisone *1902*

Protein *Cerebrospinal Fluid No Effect Analytical* No significant effect when added to concentration of 3.0 mg/dL and measured by Ektachem® slide procedure *3654*

Prothrombin Time *Plasma Decrease Physiological* In patients receiving warfarin coadministration of azothioprine caused increased requirement for warfarin to maintain prothrombin time probably due to effect on hepatic microsomal enzymes *5579* May cause hepatotoxicity *5777* Coadministration of azathioprine with warfarin may inhibit warfarin's anticoagulant effect *2159*

Reticulocytes *Blood Decrease Physiological* Gradual reduction observed *3096*

Sperm Count *Semen Decrease Physiological* Not uncommon in males on drug *5106*

Tacrolimus *Blood No Effect Analytical* No significant effect observed at a concentration of 1 mg/L with MEIA method on Abbott IMx analyzer *1871*
Serum No Effect Analytical In HPLC/MS method of Christians et al no significant interference observed with measurement of FK 506 *1010*

Testosterone *Serum No Effect Physiological* In a group of male patients with rheumatoid arthritis taking azathioprine mean concentration not significantly different from concentration in untreated male patients *3808*

Triglycerides *Serum Decrease Physiological* In patients who had had a renal transplant treatment with azathioprine with prednisone caused significant change from mean baseline of 2.03 ± 0.94 mmol/L after 3 months to 1.90 ± 0.99 mmol/L after 6 months and 1.78 ± 0.83 mmol/L after 12 months *2602*

Urea Nitrogen *Serum Increase Physiological* Renal dysfunction observed in 6% of 228 patients treated with azathioprine *5240*

Uric Acid *Serum Decrease Physiological* In patients with gout decreases concentration *5709*
Serum Increase Physiological Rapid destruction of tissues and nucleic acid catabolism *2242*
Urine Decrease Physiological In patients with gout reduces excretion *5709*

Azathymine

Uric Acid *Serum Increase Physiological* Due to tissue destruction *3810*

Azauridine

Crystals *Urine Increase Physiological* May occur due to response to tissue destruction *466*

Orotic Acid *Urine Increase Physiological* Metabolic effect may cause crystalluria *466*

Uric Acid *Serum Increase Physiological* Due to tissue destruction *3810*

Aziridine

Chromosomes *Test Conditions Abnormal Physiological* Clastogenic in human cells *5484*

Azithromycin

Alanine Aminotransferase *Serum Increase Physiological* Administration of azithromycin had a significant effect in 4 - 6% of patients receiving the drug *4659* In one of 39 patients with mycobacterial lung disease treatment with azithromycin was associated with abnormal liver enzyme activity which demonstrated an obstructive or granulomatous pattern *753* In one 69-year old man treatment with 500 mg/d azithromycin for 3 days was associated with acute cholestasis reaching a peak of 156 U/L on day 21 before beginning to subside *3641*

Alkaline Phosphatase *Serum Increase Physiological* In one of 39 patients with mycobacterial lung disease treatment with azithromycin was associated with abnormal liver enzyme activity which demonstrated an obstructive or granulomatous pattern *753* Administration of azithromycin had a significant effect in less than 1% of patients receiving the drug *4659* In one 69-year old man treatment with 500 mg/d azithromycin for 3 days was associated with acute cholestasis reaching a peak of 1200 U/L on day 16 before beginning to subside *3641*

Amylase *Serum Increase Physiological* In one 69-year old man treatment with 500 mg/d azithromycin for 3 days was associated with acute cholestasis reaching a peak of 134 U/L on day 21 before beginning to subside *3641*

Aspartate Aminotransferase *Serum Increase Physiological* Administration of azithromycin had a significant effect in 4 - 6% of patients receiving the drug *4659* In one of 39 patients with mycobacterial lung disease treatment with azithromycin was associated with abnormal liver enzyme activity which demonstrated an obstructive or granulomatous pattern *753* In one 69-year old man treatment with 500 mg/d azithromycin for 3 days was associated with acute cholestasis reaching a peak of 113 U/L on day 16 before beginning to subside *3641*

Astemizole *Serum Increase Physiological* Significantly decreased metabolism resulting in cardiac toxicity or arrhythmias, especially torsade des pointes *886*

Bile Acids *Serum Increase Physiological* In one 69-year old man treatment with 500 mg/d azithromycin for 3 days was associated with acute cholestasis reaching a peak of 15 µmol/L on day 16 before beginning to subside *3641*

Bilirubin *Serum Increase Physiological* In one 69-year old man treatment with 500 mg/d azithromycin for 3 days was associated with acute cholestasis reaching a peak of 16.2 mg/dL on day 16 before beginning to subside *3641* Administration of azithromycin had a significant effect in 1 - 3% of patients receiving the drug *4659*

Bilirubin, Conjugated *Serum Increase Physiological* In one 69-year old man treatment with 500 mg/d azithromycin for 3 days was associated with acute cholestasis reaching a peak of 16.2 mg/dL on day 16 before beginning to subside *3641*

Carbamazepine *Serum Increase Physiological* Significantly decreased metabolism and increased plasma concentration *886* Drugs that inhibit CYP 3A4 inhibit metabolism of carbamazepine producing clinically meaningful effect *1039*
Serum No Effect Physiological No cases of increased concentration reported *4659*

Cetirizine *Serum No Effect Physiological* No clinically significant effect observed *4661*

Creatine Kinase *Serum Increase Physiological* Administration of azithromycin had a significant effect in 1 - 2% of patients receiving the drug *4659*

Creatinine *Serum Increase Physiological* Administration of azithromycin had a significant effect in 4 - 6% of patients receiving the drug *4659*

Cyclosporine *Blood Increase Physiological* In one patient coadministration of azithromycin caused cyclosporine concentration to increase to 149 ng/mL two days after start of azitthromycin *3622*

Cyclosporine A *Blood No Effect Physiological* No cases of increased concentration reported *4659*

Digoxin *Serum No Effect Physiological* No cases of increased concentration reported *4659*

Ergotamine *Serum No Effect Physiological* No cases of increased concentration reported *4659*

Glucose *Serum Increase Physiological* Administration of azithromycin had a significant effect in less than 1% of patients receiving the drug *4659*

γ-Glutamyltransferase *Serum Increase Physiological* Administration of azithromycin had a significant effect in 1 - 2% of patients receiving the drug *4659* In one 69-year old man treatment with 500 mg/d azithromycin for 3 days was associated with acute cholestasis reaching a peak of 230 U/L on day 16 before beginning to subside *3641*

Hexobarbital *Serum No Effect Physiological* No cases of increased concentration reported *4659*

Lactate Dehydrogenase *Serum Increase Physiological* Significant reversible increases observed in clinical trials with a frequency of 1 - 3% *4659*

Leukocytes *Blood Decrease Physiological* Significant reversible decreases observed in clinical trials with a frequency of less than 1% *4659*

Neutrophils *Blood Decrease Physiological* Significant reversible decreases observed in clinical trials with a frequency of less than 1% *4659*

Phenytoin *Serum No Effect Physiological* No cases of increased concentration reported *4659*

Phosphate *Serum Increase Physiological* Administration of azithromycin had a significant effect in less than 1% of patients receiving the drug *4659*

Platelets *Blood Decrease Physiological* Administration of azithromycin had a significant effect in less than 1% of patients receiving the drug *4659*

Potassium *Serum Increase Physiological* Administration of azithromycin had a significant effect in 1 - 2% of patients receiving the drug *4659*

Prothrombin Time *Plasma Increase Physiological* Increased INR observed in patients receiving warfarin *886*
Plasma No Effect Physiological Administration of azithromycin had no effect on the prothrombin time following a single oral dose of warfarin *4659*

Rifabutin *Serum Increase Physiological* Decreased metabolism and increased risk of uveitis *886*

Terfenadine *Serum Increase Physiological* Significantly decreased metabolism resulting in cardiac toxicity or arrhythmias, especially torsade des pointes *886*
Serum No Effect Physiological No cases of increased concentration reported *4659*

Theophylline *Serum Increase Physiological* Decreased metabolism *886*
Serum No Effect Physiological No clinically significant effect on theophylline concentration observed when drugs coadministered *5999* Administration of azithromycin had no effect on plasma concentration or pharmacokinetics of theophylline *4659* No documented significant interaction with theophylline reported *6117*

Triazolam *Serum No Effect Physiological* No cases of increased concentration reported *4659*

Urea Nitrogen *Serum Increase Physiological* Administration of azithromycin had a significant effect in less than 1% of patients receiving the drug *4659*

Zidovudine *Serum Increase Physiological* Azithromycin caused a mean increase of 26% in the AUC when azithromycin coadministered with zidovudine. AUC of phosphorylated zidovudine increased by 75% *4659*

Zidovudine Glucuronide *Serum No Effect Physiological* Azithromycin caused a mean increase of less than 10% in the mean concentration and AUC of zidovudine glucuronide *4659*

Azlocillin

Alanine Aminotransferase *Serum Increase Physiological* Increase observed in 1.7% of 631 patients treated with mean dose of 260 mg/kg/d for mean of 11.1 days: effect mild and reversible *4542*

Albumin *Serum Decrease Physiological* In one patient after intravenous administration of azlocillin sodium concentration decreased from 26 g/L to 21 g/L due to dilutional effect *2368*

Alkaline Phosphatase *Serum No Effect Physiological* No effect observed in 631 patients treated with mean dose of 260 mg/kg/d for mean of 11.1 days *4542*

Aspartate Aminotransferase *Serum Increase Physiological* Mild reversible increase observed in 1.7% of 631 patients treated with mean dose of 260 mg/kg/d for mean of 11.1 days *4542*

Bilirubin *Serum No Effect Analytical* No effect at 10000 mg/L on method on Ames Seralyzer *5706*
Serum No Effect Physiological Probably clinically insignificant displacement from protein in neonates *6314*

Calcium *Serum Decrease Physiological* In one patient following intravenous azlocillin concentration decreased from pretreatment concentration of 1.82 mmol/L to 1.48 mmol/L due to dilution *2368*

Chloride *Serum Decrease Physiological* In one patient after intravenous azlocillin sodium mean concentration decreased from 99 mmol/L to 72 mmol/L due to effect on anion gap *2368*

Cholesterol *Serum No Effect Analytical* No effect at 10,000 mg/L on Ames Seralyzer method *5706*

Creatine Kinase *Serum No Effect Analytical* No effect at 10,000 mg/L on method on Ames Seralyzer *5706*

Creatinine *Serum Increase Analytical* In one patient after intravenous administration of azlocillin sodium concentration increased from 64 µmol/L to 96 µmol/L due to binding to picrate with an absorption peak at 505 nm. Apparent creatinine concentration obtained with 25 g/L azlocillin was 25 µmol/L *2368*
Serum Increase Physiological Observed in 3 of 631 patients treated with mean dose of 260 mg/kg/d for mean of 11.1 days: effect mild and in all cases possible other causes for increase present *4542*
Serum No Effect Analytical No effect at 620 mg/L on Ames Seralyzer method *5706*

Eosinophils *Blood Increase Physiological* Observed in 1.1% of 631 patients treated with mean dose of 260 mg/kg/d for mean of 11.1 days *4542*

Fibrinogen *Plasma Increase Physiological* In one patient following intravenous administration of azlocillin anion gap increased from pretreatment concentration of 11 mmol/L to 65 mmol/L *2368*

Glucose *Serum No Effect Analytical* No effect at 10,000 mg/L on glucose oxidase method on Ames Seralyzer *5706*
Urine Increase Analytical Falsely elevated values with Clinitest® *3446*
Urine No Effect Analytical Concentrations accurately measured by Diastix® . Concentrations accurately measured by TesTape® *3446*

Lactate Dehydrogenase *Serum Increase Physiological* Observed in one of 631 patients treated with mean dose of 260 mg/kg/d for mean 11.1 days: in this patient drug was given intramuscularly and effect might be related to route of administration only *4542*
Serum No Effect Analytical No effect up to 620 mg/L on method on Ames Seralyzer but at higher concentrations apparently reduced enzyme activity *5706*

Leukocytes *Blood Decrease Physiological* Mild transient effect observed in 0.3% of 631 patients treated with mean dose of 260 mg/kg/d for mean of 11.1 days *4542*

Partial Thromboplastin Time
Plasma Increase Physiological Typically mild: observed in some of 631 patients treated with mean dose of 260 mg/kg/d for mean of 11.1 days. Many affected patients also receiving cefamandole and had thrombocytopenia *4542*

Potassium *Serum Decrease Physiological* Observed in 0.5% of 631 patients treated with mean dose of 260 mg/kg/d for mean of 11.1 days *4542*

Protein *Serum Increase Analytical* In one patient following intravenous administration of azlocillin sodium concentration increased from pretreatment value of 38 g/L to 85 g/L due to azlocillin combining with biuret reagent to form a product with absorbance peak at 550 nm. At a concentration of 25 g/L azlocillin produced an apparent concentration of 36 g/L *2368*
Urine Increase Analytical False positive reaction with biuret following precipitation with trichloracetic acid and resuspension *4422*

Prothrombin Time *Plasma Increase Physiological* Typically mild and responds to vitamin K in 631 patients treated with mean dose of 260 mg/kg/d for mean of 11.1 days *4542*

Sodium *Serum Increase Physiological* In one patient after administration of intravenous azlocillin sodium plasma sodium concentration increased from 134 mmol/L to 154 mmol/L *2368*

Tacrolimus *Serum No Effect Analytical* In HPLC/MS method of Christians et al no significant interference observed with measurement of FK 506 *1010*

Urea *Serum Decrease Physiological* In one patient following intravenous administration of azlocillin sodium concentration decreased from 6.2 mmol/L to 1.9 mmol/L probably due to a combination of true fall in concentration with time and dilutional effect of the admixture of azlocillin solution *2368*

Urea Nitrogen *Serum No Effect Analytical* No effect at 10,000 mg/L on method on Ames Seralyzer *5706*

Uric Acid *Serum Decrease Physiological* Fell from average of 6.4 mg/dL to 2.3 mg/dL in 20 hospitalized patients not observed in controls without azlocillin *1755*

Azosemide

Aldosterone *Plasma Increase Physiological* Effect observed in normal male volunteers after 60 mg orally *4373*
Urine Increase Physiological Effect observed in normal male volunteers after 60 mg orally *4373*

Antidiuretic Hormone *Plasma Increase Physiological* Effect observed in normal male volunteers after 60 mg orally *4373*

Calcium *Urine Increase Physiological* Tended to increase but not marked *3343*

Chloride *Serum Decrease Physiological* Slight effect noted in 2 volunteers *3343*
Serum Increase Physiological Delayed effect observed in normal male volunteers after 60 mg orally *4373*
Urine Increase Physiological Effect observed in normal male volunteers after 60 mg orally *4373* Significant effect then gradually decreased *3343*

Creatinine *Urine No Effect Physiological* No clear pattern observed *3343*

Epinephrine *Plasma No Effect Physiological* Effect observed in normal male volunteers after 60 mg orally *4373*

Norepinephrine *Plasma Increase Physiological* Effect observed in normal male volunteers after 60 mg orally *4373*
Urine Increase Physiological Effect observed in normal male volunteers after 60 mg orally *4373*

Osmolality *Serum No Effect Physiological* Effect observed in normal male volunteers after 60 mg orally *4373*

Phosphate *Urine Increase Physiological* Tended to increase but not marked *3343*

Potassium *Serum Decrease Physiological* Slight effect noted in 2 volunteers *3343*
Serum No Effect Physiological Effect observed in normal male volunteers after 60 mg orally *4373*
Urine Increase Physiological Tended to increase but not marked *3343* Slight effect observed in normal male volunteers after 60 mg orally *4373*

Prolactin *Plasma Increase Physiological* Effect observed in normal male volunteers after 60 mg orally *4373*

Protein *Serum Increase Physiological* Slight and delayed effect observed in normal male volunteers after 60 mg orally *4373*

Renin Activity *Plasma Increase Physiological* Effect observed in normal male volunteers after 60 mg orally *4373*

Sodium *Serum Decrease Physiological* Slight effect noted in 2 volunteers *3343*
Serum No Effect Physiological Effect observed in normal male volunteers after 60 mg orally *4373*

Urine *Increase* *Physiological* Effect observed in normal male volunteers after 60 mg orally *4373* Significant effect then gradually decreased *3343*

Urea Nitrogen *Urine* *No Effect* *Physiological* No clear pattern observed *3343*

Uric Acid *Serum* *Increase* *Physiological* Slight effect noted in 2 volunteers *3343*

Urine *Decrease* *Physiological* Slight effect noted on first 2 d *3343*

Volume *Urine* *Increase* *Physiological* Significant effect on first day, but decrease on second *3343*

Urine *No Effect* *Physiological* Effect observed in normal male volunteers after 60 mg orally *4373*

Azosulfamide

PAH Clearance *Urine* *Increase* *Analytical* Slight effect only, measured as if PAH *4953*

Sulfa as Sulfanilamide *Serum* *Increase* *Analytical* Slight effect, measured as if sulfonamide *4953*

Aztreonam

Alanine Aminotransferase *Serum* *Increase* *Physiological* Increase observed in fewer than 1% of individuals to whom drug was administered *713* Mild and reversible increases observed: generally incidence of 4% patients but in some studies up to 36% *1384*

Alkaline Phosphatase *Serum* *Increase* *Physiological* Increased activity observed in fewer than 1% of individuals to whom drug was administered *713*

Aspartate Aminotransferase *Serum* *Increase* *Physiological* Increase observed in less than 1% of individuals to whom drug administered *713* Incidence of 4% observed but in one study up to 36% patients had increased activity but generally increase mild and reversible *1384*

Bilirubin *Serum* *No Effect* *Physiological* Probably clinically insignificant displacement from protein in neonates *6314*

γ-Carboxyglutamic Acid *Urine* *No Effect* *Physiological* No significant change observed in 7 children treated with up to 80 mg/kg daily for up to 14 days *5189*

Cephradine *Serum* *No Effect* *Physiological* In one trial in 48 healthy volunteers no interaction observed between drugs *1384*

Clindamycin *Serum* *No Effect* *Physiological* In one trial in 48 healthy men no interaction observed between drugs *1384*

Serum *Positive* *Analytical* Interference observed with bioassay procedure at Mayo Clinic *3858*

Colistin *Serum* *Positive* *Analytical* Interference observed with bioassay procedure at Mayo Clinic *3858*

Coombs' Test *Blood* *Positive* *Physiological* In rare cases individuals treated with aztreonam demonstrate positive Coombs' test *713*

Creatinine *Serum* *Increase* *Physiological* In rare cases increased concentration observed in individuals receiving aztreonam *713* Single case of deteriorating renal function following treatment with drug for 9 days. Rises reported to occur in 2-4% patients when first treated with drug *4568*

Descarboxyprothrombin *Plasma* *No Effect* *Physiological* Not detected in plasma before treatment begun in 7 children and not detected after up to 80 mg/kg daily for up to 14 days *5189*

Eosinophils *Blood* *Increase* *Physiological* Single case reported of acute renal failure with rash, fever and other features of allergic response to drug administration. Note eosinophilia reported to occur in 1-8% of patients when first treated with drug *4568* In rare cases eosinophilia observed to occur with treatment with aztreonam *713*

Urine *Increase* *Physiological* Marked eosinophiluria in one man treated with drug for 10 days with other evidence of allergic response to drug *4568*

Erythromycin *Serum* *Increase* *Analytical* Interference observed with bioassay procedure at Mayo Clinic *3858*

Gentamicin *Serum* *No Effect* *Physiological* In one trial in 48 healthy men no interaction observed between drugs *1384*

Glucose *Urine* *No Effect* *Analytical* Dark green-black color with Clinitest® , but no effect or slight reduction with glucose concentrations of 1% and up. Concentrations measured accurately by Diastix® . Concentrations measured accurately by TesTape® *3446* Concentrations measured accurately by TesTape® *140*

Immunoglobulin E *Serum* *Increase* *Physiological* Single case reported of markedly increased concentration following treatment for 9 days. Note finding observed in cases of acute interstitial nephritis *4568*

Metronidazole *Serum* *Increase* *Analytical* Interference observed with bioassay procedure at Mayo Clinic *3858*

Serum *No Effect* *Physiological* In one trial in 48 healthy men no interaction observed between drugs *1384*

Nafcillin *Serum* *No Effect* *Physiological* In one trial in 48 healthy men no interaction observed between drugs *1384*

Partial Thromboplastin Time

Plasma *Increase* *Physiological* Occasional increase observed in individuals to whom drug administered *713*

Polymyxin *Serum* *Increase* *Analytical* Interference observed with bioassay procedure at Mayo Clinic *3858*

Prothrombin Time *Plasma* *Increase* *Physiological* Rare instances of prolonged prothrombin time observed in individuals to whom aztreonam administered *713*

Tetracycline *Serum* *Increase* *Analytical* Interference observed with bioassay procedure at Mayo Clinic *3858*

Trimethoprim *Serum* *Increase* *Analytical* Interference observed with bioassay procedure at Mayo Clinic *3858*

Azuresin

Color *Urine* *Increase* *Analytical* Blue or green for a few days after test *2451*

Bacampicillin

Aspartate Aminotransferase *Serum* *Increase* *Physiological* Moderate rise in activity noted in some patients but significance of finding unknown *4654*

Eosinophils *Blood* *Increase* *Physiological* Usually reversible anemia, thrombocytopenia with or without purpura, eosinophilia, leukopenia and agranulocytosis have been reported during treatment with penicillins *4654*

Granulocytes *Blood* *Decrease* *Physiological* Usually reversible anemia, thrombocytopenia with or without purpura, eosinophilia, leukopenia and agranulocytosis have been reported during treatment with penicillins *4654*

Hematocrit *Blood* *Decrease* *Physiological* Usually reversible anemia, thrombocytopenia with or without purpura, eosinophilia, leukopenia and agranulocytosis have been reported during treatment with penicillins *4654*

Hemoglobin *Blood* *Decrease* *Physiological* Usually reversible anemia, thrombocytopenia with or without purpura, eosinophilia, leukopenia and agranulocytosis have been reported during treatment with penicillins *4654*

Leukocytes *Blood* *Decrease* *Physiological* Usually reversible anemia, thrombocytopenia with or without purpura, eosinophilia, leukopenia and agranulocytosis have been reported during treatment with penicillins *4654*

Platelets *Blood* *Decrease* *Physiological* Usually reversible anemia, thrombocytopenia with or without purpura, eosinophilia, leukopenia and agranulocytosis have been reported during treatment with penicillins *4654*

Bacitracin

Casts *Urine* *Increase* *Physiological* Nephrotoxic effect (cylindruria may occur) *3810*

Creatinine *Serum* *No Effect* *Analytical* No effect of concentrations up to 15 mg/L on single slide method on Kodak Ektachem® *5706*

Erythrocytes *Urine* *Increase* *Physiological* Actual bleeding caused by drug *1714*

Hemoglobin *Urine* *Increase* *Physiological* Actual bleeding caused by drug *1714*

Bacitracin *(continued)*

Parathyroid Hormone-related Peptide
Plasma Decrease Analytical When added at a concentration of 50 mg/L only 2% activity retained after storage of specimens at room temperature for 16 hours *4494*

Protein *Urine Increase Physiological* Nephrotoxic effect *1714* May cause nephrotoxicity *2024*

Urea Nitrogen *Serum Increase Physiological* Renal toxicity (especially if given i.v.) *2242*

Baclofen

Alkaline Phosphatase *Serum Increase Physiological* Reported effect *1384*

Aspartate Aminotransferase *Serum Increase Physiological* Reported effect *1384*

Erythrocytes *Urine Increase Physiological* Occasional hematuria may be observed *1031*

Glucose *Serum Increase Physiological* Reported effect *1384*

Occult Blood *Feces Increase Physiological* Positive test for blood in feces may be observed *1031*

Barbital

Alanine Aminotransferase *Serum No Effect Analytical* At acute overdose concentration (20 mg/dL) on Technicon SMAC® method *6266*

Albumin *Serum No Effect Analytical* At acute overdose concentration (20 mg/dL) on Technicon SMAC® method *6266* At concentration of 500 mg/L had no effect as measured by BCG method *5704*

Alkaline Phosphatase *Serum No Effect Analytical* At acute overdose concentration (20 mg/dL) on Technicon SMAC® method *6266*

Aspartate Aminotransferase *Serum No Effect Analytical* At acute overdose concentration (20 mg/dL) on Technicon SMAC® method *6266*

Bicarbonate *Serum No Effect Analytical* At concentration of 500 mg/L had no effect on method using phenolphthalein *5704*

Bilirubin *Serum No Effect Analytical* At concentration of 500 mg/L had no effect as measured by Jendrassik and Grof method *5704* At acute overdose concentration (20 mg/dL) on Technicon SMAC® method *6266*
Serum No Effect Physiological Insignificant protein-displacing effect in neonates *6314*

Calcium *Serum No Effect Analytical* At concentration of 500 mg/L had no effect as measured by cresolphthalein method *5704* At acute overdose concentration (20 mg/dL) on Technicon SMAC® method *6266*

Chloride *Serum No Effect Analytical* At concentration of 500 mg/L had no effect as measured by mercurimetric method *5704*

Cholesterol *Serum No Effect Analytical* At concentration of 500 mg/L had no effect as measured by Liebermann-Burchard method *5704* At acute overdose concentration (20 mg/dL) on Technicon SMAC® method *6266*

Creatine Kinase *Serum No Effect Analytical* At acute overdose concentration (20 mg/dL) on Technicon SMAC® method *6266*

Creatinine *Serum No Effect Analytical* At acute overdose concentration (20 mg/dL) on Technicon SMAC® method *6266* No interference noted with liquid chromatographic method of Paroni et al *4540* At concentration of 500 mg/L had no effect as measured by Technicon AutoAnalyzer® Jaffe method *5704*

Glucose *Serum No Effect Analytical* At acute overdose concentration (20 mg/dL) on Technicon SMAC® method *6266*

Iron *Serum No Effect Analytical* At acute overdose concentration (20 mg/dL) on Technicon SMAC® method *6266* At concentration of 200 mg/L had no effect as measured by Ferrozine method *5704*

Lactate Dehydrogenase *Serum No Effect Analytical* At acute overdose concentration (20 mg/dL) on Technicon SMAC® method *6266*

Phenobarbital *Serum No Effect Analytical* At maximum physiological or pharmacological concentrations no cross-reactivity observed with phenobarbital method on Bayer Technicon Immuno 1® *427* Cross-reactivity of less than 1.3% observed with method on Baxter Stratus *5705*

Phosphate *Serum No Effect Analytical* At concentration of 500 mg/L had no effect as measured by phosphomolybdate method *5704* At acute overdose concentration (20 mg/dL) on Technicon SMAC® method *6266*

Potassium *Serum No Effect Analytical* At concentration of 500 mg/L had no effect on measurement by ISE with predilution *5704*

Primidone *Serum No Effect Analytical* At a concentration of 1250 mg/L causes 25% increase in concentration with method on Baxter Stratus but clinical concentration only up to 10 mg/L *5705*

Protein *Serum No Effect Analytical* At concentration of 500 mg/L had no effect as measured by biuret method with blank correction *5704* At acute overdose concentration (20 mg/dL) on Technicon SMAC® method *6266*

Prothrombin Time *Plasma Decrease Physiological* Antagonizes effect of bishydroxycoumarin *5501*

Sodium *Serum No Effect Analytical* At concentration of 500 mg/L had no effect on measurement by ISE with predilution *5704*

Triglycerides *Serum No Effect Analytical* At acute overdose concentration (20 mg/dL) on Technicon SMAC® method *6266* At concentration of 500 mg/L had no effect as measured by lipase/esterase method *5704*

Urea Nitrogen *Serum No Effect Analytical* At acute overdose concentration (20 mg/dL) on Technicon SMAC® method *6266* At concentration of 500 mg/L had no effect as measured by diacetylmonoxime method *5704*

Uric Acid *Serum No Effect Analytical* At acute overdose concentration (20 mg/dL) on Technicon SMAC® method *6266* At concentration of 500 mg/L had no effect as measured by phosphotungstate reduction method *5704*

Barbiturates

Alanine Aminotransferase *Serum Increase Physiological* Occurs with poisoning, probable muscle origin *6545*

Alkaline Phosphatase *Serum Increase Physiological* Rare case of hepatotoxicity *574*

Amino-4-Imidazole-5-Carboxamide Ribotide
Urine Increase Physiological Occurs if megaloblastic anemia *6370*

δ-Aminolevulinic Acid *Urine Increase Physiological* May precipitate acute porphyria *2210*

Amitriptyline *Serum Decrease Physiological* Stimulates metabolism of tricyclic antidepressants *2452*

Aspartate Aminotransferase *Serum Increase Physiological* Occurs with poisoning, probable muscle origin *6545*

Basal Metabolic Rate *Patient Decrease Physiological* Decreases rate by about 10% *409*

Bilirubin *Serum Decrease Physiological* Induces glucuronyl transferase in newborn infants *2451*
Serum Increase Physiological Rare cases of jaundice following use *574*

BSP Retention *Serum Decrease Physiological* Increase conjugation with glutathione *2242*
Serum Increase Physiological May increase retention if given within 24 h *2240*

Carbon Dioxide Partial Pressure
Blood Increase Physiological Respiratory depressant *2242*

Cholinesterase *Serum Decrease Physiological* May inhibit activity *2754*

Coproporphyrin *Blood Increase Physiological* May precipitate acute cutaneous porphyria *2210*
Feces Increase Physiological May precipitate acute porphyria *2210*
Urine Increase Physiological May precipitate acute porphyria *2210*

Cortisol *Plasma Decrease Physiological* If used preoperatively lower concentration *6141*

Creatine Kinase *Serum Increase Physiological* Occurs with poisoning, probable muscle origin *6545*

Creatinine *Serum Increase Physiological* Shock and renal failure in intoxication *4012*

Dopamine *Urine No Effect Physiological* No effect with addiction or withdrawal *6102*

Doxycycline *Serum Decrease Physiological* Observed to decrease half-life of doxycycline *4357* Decreased plasma concentration because half-life reduced due to increased hepatic metabolism *1384*

Epinephrine *Urine No Effect Physiological* No effect with addiction or withdrawal *6102*

Erythrocytes *Blood Decrease Physiological* Aplastic or megaloblastic anemia *3810*

Estriol *Urine Increase Physiological* Theoretical due to increased hydroxylation *54*

Fludrocortisone *Serum Decrease Physiological* Decreased concentration observed when drugs coadministered due increased metabolic clearance of fludrocortisone because of induction of hepatic enzymes *221*

Folate *Serum Decrease Physiological* May cause megaloblastic anemia (impairs absorption) *6370*

Glucaric Acid *Urine Increase Physiological* As result of hepatic enzyme induction *3669*

Glucose *Serum Decrease Physiological* Reported effect *192*

γ-Glutamyltransferase *Serum Increase Physiological* Possibly due to enzyme induction *6429*

Griseofulvin *Serum Decrease Physiological* Decrease systemic absorption from gastrointestinal tract *1384* Concomitant administration of barbiturates with griseofulvin may depress griseofulvin activity *4447*

Hematocrit *Blood Decrease Physiological* May cause megaloblastic anemia *6370*

Hemoglobin *Blood Decrease Physiological* May cause megaloblastic anemia *6370*

Homovanillic Acid *Urine No Effect Physiological* No effect with addiction or withdrawal *6102*

Hydrochloric Acid *Gastric Fluid Decrease Physiological* Secretion slightly depressed *2242*

17-Hydroxycorticosteroids *Urine Decrease Physiological* With chronic ingestion metabolism diverted to 6-β-hydroxy-cortisol *1184*
Urine No Effect Physiological No effect with short term ingestion *6515*

5-Hydroxyindoleacetic Acid *Urine No Effect Physiological* No effect with addiction or withdrawal *6102*

^{131}I Uptake *Serum Increase Physiological* ?due to enzyme induction *3669*

Imipramine *Serum Decrease Physiological* Plasma concentration of drug may be decreased when hepatic enzyme inducers given concomitantly *1040*

17-Ketosteroids *Urine No Effect Physiological* Short term ingestion produces no effect *1184*

Leukocytes *Blood Decrease Physiological* Leukopenia *6168*

Maprotiline *Serum Decrease Physiological* Concentration may be decreased when hepatic enzyme inducers are coadministered *1034*

MCV *Blood Increase Physiological* May cause megaloblastic anemia *6370*

Myoglobin *Urine Increase Physiological* May be increased in barbiturate poisoning *46*

N-Formiminoglutamic Acid *Urine Increase Physiological* Occurs if megaloblastic anemia *6370*

Norepinephrine *Urine No Effect Physiological* No effect with addiction or withdrawal *6102*

Oxygen Partial Pressure *Blood Decrease Physiological* Slight decrease during sleep with hypnotic dose *2242*

Pepsin *Gastric Material Decrease Physiological* Secretion slightly depressed *2242*

Platelets *Blood Decrease Physiological* Thrombocytopenia *3810*

Porphobilinogen *Urine Increase Physiological* May precipitate acute porphyria *2210*

Porphyrin, Total *Urine Increase Physiological* May precipitate attack of acute porphyria *1687*

Prothrombin Time *Plasma Decrease Physiological* Metabolism of coumarins enhanced (enzyme induction in liver) *2262* Increase metabolic clearance when coadministered with warfarin *2625* Increase metabolic clearance of warfarin when barbiturates coadministered with warfarin *2625*
Plasma Increase Physiological Theoretically if cholestasis occurs *3810*

Protoporphyrin *Blood Increase Physiological* May precipitate acute cutaneous porphyria *2210*
Feces Increase Physiological May precipitate acute porphyria *2210*

T3-Uptake *Serum Increase Physiological* Compete for thyroxine binding prealbumin sites *882*

Testosterone *Serum Increase Physiological* Due to decreased metabolic clearance rate (in women) *3159*

Thyroxine (T4) *Serum Decrease Physiological* Compete with T4 for thyroxine binding prealbumin *882*

Uroporphyrin *Urine Increase Physiological* May precipitate acute porphyria *2210*

Vanillylmandelic Acid *Urine No Effect Physiological* No effect with addiction or withdrawal *6102*

Volume *Urine Decrease Physiological* May produce renal shutdown with oliguria *467*

Barbituric Acid

Felbamate *Serum No Effect Analytical* No significant interference observed with GLC method of Rifai et al *4958*

Barium

Alanine Aminotransferase *Serum Increase Physiological* Severe liver damage if tannic acid in enema *128*

Aspartate Aminotransferase *Serum Increase Physiological* Severe liver damage if tannic acid in enema *128*

Color *Feces Increase Analytical* White discoloration/speckling if taken orally *1957*

Diagnex Blue Excretion *Urine Increase Physiological* Heavy metal displacement of diagnex blue *6515*

^{131}I Uptake *Serum Decrease Physiological* Theoretically if contaminated with I_2*882*

Iron *Serum No Effect Analytical* No significant effect observed at a concentration of 80 μg/dL with method on Kodak Ektachem® systems *2519*

Iron-Binding Capacity, Total *Serum No Effect Analytical* No significant effect observed at a concentration of 80 μg/dL with method on Kodak Ektachem® systems *2519*

Occult Blood *Feces Increase Physiological* May cause severe gastrointestinal tract hemorrhage *2242*

Basiliximab

Albumin *Urine Increase Physiological* Albuminuria reported as side effect in 3 - 10% of patients *3959*

Blood *Urine Increase Physiological* Hematuria reported as side effect in 3 - 10% of patients *3959*

Calcium *Serum Increase Physiological* Hypocalcemia reported as side effect in more than 10% of patients *3959* Hypercalcemia reported as side effect in 3 - 10% of patients *3959*

Cholesterol *Serum Increase Physiological* Hyperlipemia reported as side effect in 3 - 10% of patients *3959* Hypercholesterolemia reported as side effect in more than 10% of patients *3959*

Erythrocytes *Blood Increase Physiological* Polycythemia reported as side effect in 3 - 10% of patients *3959*

Glucose *Serum Decrease Physiological* Hypoglycemia reported as side effect in 3 - 10% of patients *3959*
Serum Increase Physiological Hyperglycemia reported as side effect in more than 10% of patients *3959* Diabetes mellitus reported as side effect in 3 - 10% of patients *3959*

Basiliximab *(continued)*

Hematocrit *Blood Decrease Physiological* Anemia reported as side effect in more than 10% of patients *3959*

Hemoglobin *Blood Decrease Physiological* Anemia reported as side effect in more than 10% of patients *3959*

Magnesium *Serum Decrease Physiological* Hypomagnesemia reported as side effect in 3 - 10% of patients *3959*

Occult Blood *Feces Increase Physiological* Melena reported as side effect in 3 - 10% of patients *3959*

Phosphate *Serum Increase Physiological* Hypophosphatemia reported as side effect in more than 10% of patients *3959*

Platelets *Blood Decrease Physiological* Purpura and thrombocytopenia reported as side effects in 3 - 10% of patients *3959*

Potassium *Serum Decrease Physiological* Both hypokalemia and hyperkalemia reported as side effects in more than 10% of patients *3959*

Serum Increase Physiological Both hypokalemia and hyperkalemia reported as side effects in more than 10% of patients *3959*

Protein *Serum Decrease Physiological* Hypoproteinemia reported as side effect in 3 - 10% of patients *3959*

Uric Acid *Serum Increase Physiological* Hyperuricemia reported as side effect in more than 10% of patients *3959*

BCG Vaccine

Alanine Aminotransferase *Serum Increase Physiological* In 1 of 674 patients with bladder cancer (0.2%) hepatitis occured *4435*

Alkaline Phosphatase *Serum Increase Physiological* In 1 of 674 patients with bladder cancer (0.2%) hepatitis occured *4435*

Aspartate Aminotransferase *Serum Increase Physiological* In 1 of 674 patients with bladder cancer (0.2%) hepatitis occured. *4435*

Bilirubin *Serum Increase Physiological* In 1 of 674 patients with bladder cancer (0.2%) hepatitis occured *4435*

Blood *Urine Increase Physiological* In 175 of 674 patients with bladder cancer (26.0%) hematuria occured *4435*

γ-Globulin *Serum Decrease Physiological* Associated with severe reaction *4014*

Hematocrit *Blood Decrease Physiological* In 9 of 674 patients with bladder cancer (1.3%) anemia occured *4435*

Hemoglobin *Blood Decrease Physiological* In 9 of 674 patients with bladder cancer (1.3%) anemia occured *4435*

Leukocytes *Blood Decrease Physiological* In 2 of 674 patients with bladder cancer (0.3%) leukopenia occured *4435*

Platelets *Blood Decrease Physiological* In 2 of 674 patients with bladder cancer (0.3%) thrombocytopenia occured *4435*

Beclobrate

Alanine Aminotransferase *Serum Increase Physiological* In 1213 cases of hyperlipidemias increase observed in 6 cases *878*

Serum No Effect Physiological No significant effect observed in 15 patients with type IIa hyperlipidemia treated with 100 mg/d for 4 weeks *331*

Alkaline Phosphatase *Serum Decrease Physiological* Significant reduction observed in 15 patients with type IIa hyperlipidemia treated with 100 mg/d for 4 weeks *331* Mean decrease of 15% observed in 16 patients with type II diabetes mellitus and secondary hyperlipidemia treated with beclobrate for about 2 years *3288*

Apolipoprotein A-I *Serum Increase Physiological* Mean increase of 9.1% observed in 10 patients with type IV hyperlipidemia treated with 100 mg/d for 8 weeks *6344* Treatment with 100 mg/d caused average increase of 10% in patients with type IIb hyperlipoproteinemia *878* Increased synthesis. Increased activity of lipoprotein lipase by stimulation of muscle lipoprotein lipase, alteration of capillary endothelial surface and stimulation of apo C-II synthesis *264* Mean increase of 9.1% observed in 10 patients with type IV hyperlipiemia treated with 100 mg/d for 8 weeks *6344*

Apolipoprotein A-II *Serum Increase Physiological* Increased synthesis. Increased activity of lipoprotein lipase by stimulation of muscle lipoprotein lipase synthesis, alteration of capillary endothelial surface and increased synthesis of apo C-II *264*

Apolipoprotein B *Serum Decrease Physiological* Treatment of 10 patients with type IIa hyperlipidemia with 100 mg/d for 8 weeks caused mean reduction of 11.5%. In 10 patients with type IV hyperlipidemia reduction of 10.1% observed *6224 6225* Of fibrates appears to be one of the most effective in decreasing apo B concentrations *5586* In 15 patients with type II hyperlipidemia treatment with 150 mg/d for 2 months caused reduction of 24% *6344* Treatment with 100 mg/d caused average reduction of 13.3% in patients with hyperlipoproteinemia type IIb *878*

Aspartate Aminotransferase *Serum Increase Physiological* In 1213 patients with hyperlipidemias increase observed in 5 cases *878*

Serum No Effect Physiological No significant effect observed in 15 patients with type IIa hyperlipidemia treated with 100 mg/d for 4 weeks *331*

Cholesterol *Serum Decrease Physiological* In type IIa hypercholesterolemia average reduction of 21% observed: in type IIb average reduction of 20% occurred: in hypertriglyceridemia type IV reduction of 4% and in hyperlipoproteinemia type V average reduction of 43% observed *878* Mean reduction of 16% observed in 16 patients with type II diabetes mellitus with secondary hyperlipidemia treated with drug for about 2 years *3288* Reduction of 4.2% observed in 10 patients with type IV hyperlipidemia treated with 100 mg/d for 8 weeks. Reduction of 11.7% observed in 20 patients with type IIb hyperlipidemia treated with 100 mg/d for 8 weeks *6344* Reduction of 4.2% observed in 10 patients with type IV hyperlipidemia treated with 100 mg/d for 8 weeks. Reduction of 11.7% observed in 20 patients with type IIb hyperlipidemia treated with 100 mg/d for 8 weeks *6344*

Creatine Kinase *Serum Increase Physiological* Increase observed in 5 patients of 1213 with hyperlipidemias who were treated with 100 mg/d *878* Isolated but reversible increases observed in 16 patients with type II diabetes mellitus with secondary hyperlipidemia treated for about 2 years *3288*

Serum No Effect Physiological No significant effect observed in 30 patients with types IIa, IIb and IV hyperlipidemias treated with 100 mg/d for 8 weeks *6225 6224* No significant effect observed in 15 patients with type IIa hyperlipidemia treated with 100 mg/d for 4 weeks *331*

Glucose *Serum Decrease Physiological* Nonsignificant decrease from mean concentration of 173 mg/dL to 154 mg/dL in 16 patients with type II diabetes mellitus and secondary hyperlipidemia treated for about 2 years *3288*

HDL-Cholesterol *Serum Increase Physiological* Increase of 23.9% observed in 10 patients with type IV hyperlipidemia treated with 100 mg/d for 8 weeks. 24.6% increase observed in 20 patients with type IIb hyperlipidemia treated with 100 mg/d for 8 weeks. In 15 patients with type II 13% increase seen *6344* Mean increase of 19% observed in 16 patients with type II diabetes mellitus and secondary hyperlipidemia treated with beclobrate for about 2 years *3288* Significant increase of 13% observed in 15 patients with type IIa hyperlipidemia treated with 100 mg/d for 4 weeks *331* Increase of 23.9% observed in 10 patients with type IV hyperlipidemia treated with 100 mg/d for 8 weeks. 24.6% increase observed in 20 patients with type IIb hyperlipidemia treated with 100 mg/d for 8 weeks. In 15 patients with type II 13% increase seen *6344* In patients with type IIa hypercholesterolemia average increase of 33% observed with dose of 100 mg/d: in type IV hypertriglyceridemia average increase of 22% observed *878* Increased synthesis of apo A-I and A-II. Increased activity of lipoprotein lipase by stimulation of muscle lipoprotein lipase, alteration of capillary endothelial surface and increased stimulation of synthesis of apo C-II *264*

Hemoglobin A_{1c} *Blood No Effect Physiological* No significant change observed in 16 patients with type II diabetes mellitus and secondary hyperlipidemia treated for about 2 years with beclobrate *3288*

LDL-Cholesterol *Serum Decrease Physiological* Reduction of 18% observed in 15 patients with type II hyperlipidemia treated with 150 mg/d for 2 months. Reduction of 10.3% observed in 20 patients with type IIb hyperlipidemia treated with 100 mg/d for 8 weeks *6344* Reduction of 18% observed in 15 patients with type II hyperlipidemia treated with 150 mg/d for 2 months. Reduction of 10.3% observed in 20 patients with type IIb hyperlipidemia treated with 100 mg/d for 8 weeks *6344* In 10 type IIa hyperlipidemic patients treatment with 1200 mg/d for 8 weeks caused mean reduction of 25.8% *6225* In hypercholesterolemia type IIa average reduction of 26% observed with dose of 100 mg/d *878* In 10 type IIa hyperlipidemic patients treatment with 1200 mg/d for 8 weeks caused mean reduction of 25.8% *6224* Mean decrease of 28% observed in 15 patients with type IIa hyperlipidemia treated with 100 mg/d for 4 weeks *331* Mean reduction of 15% observed in 16 patients with type II diabetes mellitus and secondary hyperlipidemia not amenable to diet treated for about 2 years *3288*

Platelet Aggregation *Blood Decrease Physiological* Marked effect observed in patients with hyperlipidemias *878*

Platelets *Blood Decrease Physiological* Observed in one patient of 1213 patients with hyperlipidemias treated with 100 mg/d *878*

Quick's Time *Blood Decrease Physiological* Observed in 4 of 1213 patients with hyperlipidemias treated with 100 mg/d *878*

Triglycerides *Serum Decrease Physiological* Treatment of 10 patients with type IV hyperlipidemia with 100 mg/d for 8 weeks caused mean reduction of 58.1% *6225* Reduction observed, but less marked than with gemfibrozil, in 15 patients with type IIa hyperlipidemia when treated with 100 mg/d for 4 weeks *331* Mean decrease of 20% observed in 16 patients with type II diabetes mellitus and secondary hyperlipidemia treated with beclobrate for about 2 years *3288* Mean decrease of 43.3% observed in 20 patients with type IIb hyperlipidemia treated with 100 mg/d for 8 weeks *6344* Treatment of 10 patients with type IV hyperlipidemia with 100 mg/d for 8 weeks caused mean reduction of 58.1% *6224* In patients with type IIa hypercholesterolemia reduction of 34% observed: in patients with mixed hyperlipoproteinemia type IIb average reduction of 45%: in type IV hypertriglyceridemia reduction of 60% and in hyperlipoproteinemia type V reduction of 84% *878*

Urea Nitrogen *Serum Increase Physiological* Increase observed in 2 of 1213 cases of hyperlipidemias when treated with 100 mg/d *878*

VLDL-Cholesterol *Serum Decrease Physiological* Average reduction of 50% observed in patients with hypertriglyceridemia type IV when treated with 100 mg/d *878*

Beclomethasone

Alanine *Plasma No Effect Physiological* No significant effect observed in 9 normal volunteers who inhaled 500 µg twice daily for 4 weeks *3310*

Alkaline Phosphatase *Serum No Effect Physiological* In 13 children with grass pollen hay fever treatment with inhalation of 400 µg/d for 2 months caused nonsignificant decrease from mean baseline of 228.75 ± 89.68 U/L to 219.63 ± 80.07 U/L *3817*

Alkaline Phosphatase, Bone Isoenzyme
Serum No Effect Physiological In 13 children treatment with inhalation of 400 µg/d for 2 months caused nonsignificant decrease from mean baseline of 177.11 ± 77.37 U/L to 135.50 ± 64.56 U/L *3817*

Cholesterol *Serum Increase Physiological* Increase to mean of 4.62 mmol/L from mean of 4.16 mmol/L in 9 normal volunteers following inhalation of 500 µg twice daily for 4 weeks *3310*

Cortisol *Plasma Decrease Physiological* Significant effect observed in asthmatic children given drug by inhalation reflecting compromizing of pituitary-adrenal axis *6216*
Plasma No Effect Physiological No significant effect observed in 9 normal volunteers who inhaled 500 µg twice daily for 4 weeks *3310*
Urine Decrease Physiological Inhalation of compound, up to 800 µg daily, in children with bronchial asthma caused highly significant dose-related suppression of daily output *583*
Urine Increase Physiological Increased excretion in asthmatic children given drug by inhalation although 4 of 31 children had excretions below normal *4586*

Glucose *Serum No Effect Physiological* No significant effect observed in 9 normal volunteers who inhaled 500 µg twice daily for 4 weeks *3310*

Glucose Tolerance *Serum Decrease Physiological* Significant increase at 30 minutes from mean of 6.7 mmol/L to mean of 7.1 mmol/L in 9 normal volunteers following oral ingestion of 75 g glucose after inhaling 500 µg twice daily for 4 weeks *3310*

Glycerol *Serum Decrease Physiological* Significant reduction observed in fasting concentration in 9 normal volunteers who inhaled 500 µg twice daily for 4 weeks *3310*

HDL-Cholesterol *Serum Increase Physiological* Increase to mean of 1.19 mmol/L from mean of 0.97 mmol/L in 9 normal volunteers given 500 µg twice daily for 4 weeks *3310*

Hemoglobin A_{1c} *Blood No Effect Physiological* No significant effect observed in 9 normal volunteers who inhaled 500 µg twice daily for 4 weeks *3310*

β-Hydroxybutyrate *Serum No Effect Physiological* No significant effect observed in 9 normal volunteers who inhaled 500 µg twice daily for 4 weeks *3310*

Insulin *Plasma Increase Physiological* Mean 36% increase in fasting concentration observed in 9 normal volunteers following inhalation of 500 µg twice daily for 4 weeks *3310*

Lactate *Plasma Increase Physiological* Fasting concentrations significantly higher in 9 normal volunteers who inhaled 500 µg twice daily for 4 weeks *3310*

Osteocalcin *Serum Decrease Physiological* In 8 healthy volunteers inhalation of 2000 µg/d for 2 weeks caused mean decrease of 0.73 µg/L observed by day 8 without further change at day 15 *4764*
Serum No Effect Physiological In 39 children with grass pollen hay fever inhalation of 400 µg/d for 2 months caused nonsignificant change from mean baseline of 15.88 ± 4.45 µg/L to 16.03 ± 5.57 µg/L *3817*

Parathyroid Hormone *Plasma No Effect Physiological* In 39 children with grass pollen hay fever inhalation of 400 µg/d for 2 months caused nonsignificant increase from mean baseline of 16.88 ± 4.70 µg/L to 19.25 ± 8.65 µg/L *3817*

Pyruvate *Plasma Increase Physiological* Fasting concentrations significantly higher in 9 normal volunteers who inhaled 500 µg twice daily for 4 weeks *3310*

Type I Collagen Teleopeptide
Serum No Effect Physiological Mean concentration of 13.25 ± 4.06 µg/L in 39 children with grass pollen hay fever treated with 400 µg/d for 2 months by inhalation decreased nonsignificantly to 11.94 ± 4.25 µg/L *3817*

Belladonna

Leukocytes *Blood Increase Physiological* May cause leukocytosis *128*

Benazepril

Acenocoumarol *Plasma No Effect Physiological* No significant effect in 12 healthy male volunteers given 20 mg daily and constant amount of acenocoumarol *6185*

Alanine Aminotransferase *Serum Increase Physiological* Rare clinically important increases observed *1033*

Albumin *Urine No Effect Physiological* Insignificant reduction from mean of 87 µg/min to 79 µg/min in 17 patients with mild to moderate hypertension treated with up to 20 mg daily for 6 weeks *6160*

Aldosterone *Urine Decrease Physiological* Significant reduction from mean concentration of 12 µg/d to 8 µg/d in 17 patients with mild to moderate hypertension treated with up to 20 mg daily for 6 weeks *6160*

Angiotensin-II *Plasma Decrease Physiological* Inhibits ACE resulting in decreased plasma angiotensin II concentration *1033*

Angiotensin-converting Enzyme
Serum Decrease Physiological Inhibits ACE resulting in decreased plasma angiotensin II concentration *1033*

Benazepril *(continued)*

Aspartate Aminotransferase *Serum Increase Physiological* Rare clinically important increases observed *1033*

Atenolol *Serum No Effect Physiological* No clinically important pharmacokinetic interactions observed when drugs coadministered *1033*

Atrial Natriuretic Peptide *Plasma Decrease Physiological* Nonsignificant decrease from mean baseline of 39.98 pg/mL to 27.73 pg/mL in 11 patients with coronary artery disease when treated with 10 mg b.i.d. for 2 weeks *6024*
Plasma No Effect Physiological Concentration unchanged in 11 normotensive men after 2 weeks treatment (mean 28.0 pg/mL versus 26.7 pg/mL with placebo) *6024*

Bilirubin *Serum Increase Physiological* Rare clinically important increases observed *1033*

Chlorthalidone *Serum No Effect Physiological* No clinically important pharmacokinetic interactions observed when drugs coadministered *1033*

Cimetidine *Serum No Effect Physiological* No clinically important pharmacokinetic interactions observed when drugs coadministered *1033*

Creatinine *Serum Increase Physiological* Some hypertensive patients with no apparent preexisting renal vascular disease have developed minor and transient increases in concentration, especially when drug coadministered with a diuretic *1033* During the first 2 months of treatment with benazepril in 300 patients with chronic renal insufficiency serum creatinine concentration increased to a greater extent than in placebo-treated patients but both groups increased from about 2.05 mg/dL to 2.2 mg/dL after 6 months *3826*

Digoxin *Serum No Effect Physiological* No clinically important pharmacokinetic interactions observed when drugs coadministered *1033*

Eosinophils *Blood Increase Physiological* Occasional scattered reports of patients developing eosinophilia *1033*

Erythrocytes *Blood Decrease Physiological* Occasional reports of patients developing thrombocytopenia and hemolytic anemia in patients receiving benazepril *1033*

Furosemide *Serum No Effect Physiological* No clinically important pharmacokinetic interactions observed when drugs coadministered *1033*

Glomerular Filtration Rate *Urine No Effect Physiological* No significant change observed in 17 patients with mild to moderate hypertension treated with up to 20 mg daily for 6 weeks *6160*

Glucose *Serum Decrease Physiological* Incidence of 0.7% observed in French Pharmacovigilance database *4106*
Serum Increase Physiological Rare clinically important increases observed *1033*

Hemoglobin *Blood Decrease Physiological* Occasional reports of patients developing thrombocytopenia and hemolytic anemia in patients receiving benazepril *1033*

Hydrochlorothiazide *Serum No Effect Physiological* No clinically important pharmacokinetic interactions observed when drugs coadministered *1033*

Leukocytes *Blood Decrease Physiological* Occasional scattered reports of patients developing leukopenia *1033*

Lithium *Serum Increase Physiological* Coadministration with lithium caused increased serum lithium concentration with signs of lithium toxicity *1033*

Naproxen *Serum No Effect Physiological* No clinically important pharmacokinetic interactions observed when drugs coadministered *1033*

Platelets *Blood Decrease Physiological* Occasional reports of patients developing thrombocytopenia and hemolytic anemia in patients receiving benazepril *1033*

Potassium *Serum Increase Physiological* Hyperkalemia occurred in approximately 1% of patients receiving drug, in most cases resolving despite continued therapy because benazepril decreases aldosterone secretion *1033* During the first 2 months of treatment with benazepril in 300 patients with chronic renal insufficiency serum potassium increased on an average by 0.5 mmol/L *3826*
Serum No Effect Physiological No significant change observed in 17 patients with mild to moderate hypertension treated with up to 20 mg daily for 6 weeks *6160*
Urine No Effect Physiological No significant change observed in 17 patients with mild to moderate hypertension treated with up to 20 mg daily for 6 weeks *6160*

Propranolol *Serum No Effect Physiological* No clinically important pharmacokinetic interactions observed when drugs coadministered *1033*

Protein *Urine Decrease Physiological* During the first 2 months of treatment with benazepril in 300 patients with chronic renal insufficiency urine protein excretion demonstrated a significant decrease *3826*
Urine Increase Physiological Occasional scattered reports of patients developing proteinuria *1033*

Prothrombin Time *Plasma Decrease Physiological* Significant reduction in 10 healthy males given constant amount of warfarin and 20 mg drug daily for 7 days *6185*
Plasma No Effect Physiological Coadministration with warfarin had no effect on warfarin concentration or prothrombin time *1033* No significant change in 12 healthy male volunteers given 20 mg daily and constant amount of acenocoumarol *6185*

Renal Blood Flow *Patient Increase Physiological* Significant increase from mean of 572 mL/min/1.73 sq m to 770 mL/min/1.73 sq m in 17 patients with mild to moderate hypertension treated with up to 20 mg daily for 6 weeks *6160*

Renal Plasma Flow *Patient Increase Physiological* Significant increase from mean of 317 mL/min/1.73 sq m to 425 mL/min/1.73 sq m in 17 patients with mild to moderate hypertension treated with up 20 mg daily for 6 weeks *6160*

Renin Activity *Plasma Increase Physiological* Significant increase observed in 17 patients with mild to moderate hypertension treated with up to 20 mg daily for 6 weeks (change from baseline of 1.23 ng/mL/h to 5.06 ng/mL/h) *6160* Significant increase observed in 11 patients with coronary artery disease from mean baseline of 1.27 ng/mL/h to 9.62 ng/mL/h when treated with 10 mg b.i.d. for 2 weeks *6024* Dose-related increase observed in mild-to-moderate essential hypertensives treated with benazepril for 4 weeks: mean increases of 0.5, 1.4, 2.0, and 2.4 ng/mL/h observed from baseline with treatment with 2, 5, 10, and 20 mg/d respectively for 4 weeks *4131*

Sodium *Serum Decrease Physiological* Scattered reports of hyponatremia *1033*
Serum No Effect Physiological No significant change observed in 17 patients with mild to moderate hypertension treated with up to 20 mg daily for 6 weeks *6160*
Urine No Effect Physiological No significant change observed in 17 patients with mild to moderate hypertension treated with up to 20 mg daily for 6 weeks *6160*

Thrombotest *Plasma Decrease Physiological* Statistically significant reduction, as for prothrombin time, in 10 healthy male volunteers given constant dose of warfarin and 20 mg benazepril daily for 7 days *6185*
Plasma No Effect Physiological No significant effect in 12 healthy male volunteers given 20 mg daily for 7 days and constant amount of acenocoumarol *6185*

Urea Nitrogen *Serum Increase Physiological* Some hypertensive patients with no apparent preexisting renal vascular disease have developed minor and transient increases in concentration, especially when drug coadministered with a diuretic *1033*

Uric Acid *Serum Increase Physiological* Rare clinically important increases observed *1033*

Warfarin *Plasma No Effect Physiological* No significant effect in 10 healthy male volunteers of 20 mg daily for 7 days when taking constant amount of warfarin *6185* Coadministration with warfarin had no effect on warfarin concentration or prothrombin time *1033*

Bendroflumethiazide

Albumin *Serum No Effect Physiological* No significant difference from control in 6 patients with essential hypertension following oral dose of 5 mg *5573*

Angiotensin-II *Plasma Increase Physiological* Approximately doubled in 5 or 6 hypertensives given 5 mg daily for 6 weeks *6499*

Apolipoprotein A-I *Serum Increase Physiological* In 257 hypertensive patients treatment with 10 mg/d caused significant increase although lower doses had no significant effect on concentration *890*

Apolipoprotein B *Serum Increase Physiological* At a dose of 10 mg/d significant increase observed in 257 patients with hypertension although doses had no significant effect *890*

Bicarbonate *Serum Increase Physiological* Metabolic alkalosis *1856* By 2 mmol/L approximately in 5 or 6 hypertensives given 5 mg daily for 6 weeks *6499* In 7 patients 6 months treatment with bendrofluazide and potassium supplement bicarbonate concentration increased significantly from 24.7 mmol/L to 26.3 mmol/L *5610*

Urine No Effect Physiological Has no effect on carbonic anhydrase and thus has no effect on excretion of bicarbonate *633*

Calcium *Serum Increase Physiological* Due to increased concentration of protein due to temporary Na depletion *4511* In one study of 40 patients with nonmalignant causes of hypercalcemia and low intact PTH concentrations 2 were due to bendrofluazide therapy *3774*

Urine Decrease Physiological Impaired excretion may occur with thiazides *4511*

Urine Increase Physiological Initial diuretic response *174*

Cholesterol *Serum Increase Physiological* 5% increase in 66 subjects when treated for less than 1 y when used as only drug *6249* In 257 hypertensive patients at a dose of 10 mg/d caused significant increase although at lower doses no significant effect observed *890* 5% increase in short term studies *141*

Serum No Effect Physiological No effect with treatment for several years in many patients *141* No significant change in 15 individuals when given as sole treatment for less than 1 y *6450*

Citrate *Urine Decrease Physiological* Up to 30% decrease observed *4014*

Creatinine *Serum No Effect Physiological* No significant difference from control in 6 patients with essential hypertension following oral dose of 5 mg *5573*

Urine No Effect Physiological No significant change compared with controls in 6 patients with essential hypertension following single oral dose of 5 mg *5573*

1,25-Dihydroxy Vitamin D_3 *Serum Decrease Physiological* In 19 healthy early menopausal women given 5 mg/d with calcium supplement due to primary effect on renal tubules and secondary change on vitamin D metabolism *4963*

24,25-Dihydroxy Vitamin D *Serum Increase Physiological* In 19 healthy early menopausal women given 5 mg/d with calcium supplement due to primary effect on renal tubules and secondary change on vitamin D metabolism *4963*

Fructosamine *Serum Increase Physiological* In 257 patients with hypertension treatment with 10 mg/d caused significant increase although lower doses had no significant effect on concentration *890*

Glucose *Serum Increase Physiological* In 257 hypertensive patients treatment with 10 mg/d caused significant increase although lower doses had no significant effect *890* Significant increase after 10 years in middle-aged men treated with bendroflumethiazide and oral potassium to 4.8 mmol/L from baseline of 4.5 mmol/L. Change at 1 and 6 years not significant *167*

Serum No Effect Physiological In 7 outpatients treated with bendrofluazide and potassium supplement for 6 months no significant change observed *5610* After 12 mo treatment of 53 previously untreated hypertensives *507*

Glucose Tolerance *Serum Decrease Physiological* In men and women in 3 y study of patients with mild hypertension *4149*

Serum Increase Physiological Significant decrease in serum glucose at 60 minutes after oral glucose after 1, 6 and 10 years to 8.8 mmol/L, 8.3 mmol/L and 8.1 mmol/L respectively from baseline of 9.6 mmol/L in middle-aged men treated with bendroflumethiazide and oral potassium *167*

HDL-Cholesterol *Serum No Effect Physiological* No significant change in 15 individuals when given as sole treatment for less than 1 y *6450*

Hematocrit *Blood No Effect Physiological* No significant difference from control observed in 6 patients with essential hypertension when treated with 5 mg orally *5573*

Hemoglobin *Blood No Effect Physiological* No significant difference from control observed in 6 patients with essential hypertension treated with 5 mg orally *5573*

25-Hydroxy Vitamin D_3 *Serum No Effect Physiological* In 19 healthy early menopausal women given 5 mg/d with calcium supplement due to primary effect on renal tubules and secondary change on vitamin D metabolism *4963*

Insulin *Plasma No Effect Physiological* After 12 mo treatment of 53 previously untreated hypertensives *507* In 7 outpatients treatment for 6 months with bendrofluazide and potassium supplement caused nonsignificant increase from mean baseline of 7.8 mU/L to 12.3 mU/L *5610*

Lithium *Serum Increase Physiological* Substantial increase in one patient receiving lithium to whose regime bendrofluazide was subsequently added *3112*

Serum No Effect Physiological Short-term administration had no effect on plasma concentration *6017*

Lithium Clearance *Urine No Effect Physiological* Since it lacks effect on carbonic anhydrase does not affect glomerular function *633*

Magnesium *Serum Decrease Physiological* Significant effect noted with prolonged therapy *5490*

Osmolality *Serum Decrease Physiological* Due to hyponatremia *1856*

Parathyroid Hormone *Plasma Decrease Physiological* In one study of 40 patients with nonmalignant causes of low intact PTH concentration and hypercalcemia 2 were attributed to bendrofluazide therapy *3774*

Potassium *Serum Decrease Physiological* From 0.2 to 0.6 mmol/L in 5 or 6 hypertensives given 5 mg daily for 6 weeks *6499* Dose related reduction in concentration observed in 257 patients with hypertension *890* In men and women in 3 y study of patients with mild hypertension *4149* Mean fall from 4.3 to 3.9 mmol/L in 7 essential hypertensives treated for 16 weeks *568* Significant reduction observed in 6 patients with essential hypertension compared with control when treated with 5 mg orally *5573* Marked diuretic response *1856*

Serum No Effect Physiological Nonsignificant reduction from 4.2 mmol/L to 4.0 mmol/L with treatment for 10 years in middle-aged men given potassium supplement *167* After 12 mo treatment of 53 previously untreated hypertensives *507* In 7 patients treated with bendrofluazide for 6 months with potassium supplement although total body potassium decreased plasma concentration unaffected *5610*

Urine Increase Physiological Significant increase observed in 6 patients with essential hypertension in 6 hours following a single oral dose of 5 mg although no significant difference from placebo observed over 24 hours *5573*

Proinsulin *Plasma No Effect Physiological* In 7 outpatients treated with bendrofluazide and potassium supplement for 6 months median baseline concentration of 3.4 pmol/L not significantly changed to 2.9 pmol/L after treatment *5610*

Renin Activity *Plasma Increase Physiological* Significant increase observed at 24 hours observed in 6 patients with essential hypertension compared with controls following oral dose of 5 mg *5573* Mean increase from 3.3 to 5.6 mmol/L in 7 essential hypertensives treated for 16 weeks *568* Approximately doubled in 5 or 6 hypertensives given 5 mg daily for 6 weeks *6499*

Sodium *Serum Decrease Physiological* May cause hyponatremia due to potassium depletion *1856*

Serum No Effect Physiological In 7 essential hypertensives treated for 16 weeks *568* No significant difference from control over 24 hours following 5 mg bendrofluazide *5573*

Urine Increase Physiological Significant increase observed both over first 6 hours and after next 18 hours in 6 patients with essential hypertension following single oral dose of 5 mg *5573*

Triglycerides *Serum Increase Physiological* 20% increase in 66 subjects when treated for less than 1 y when used as only drug *6249* In 257 hypertensive patients treatment with 10 mg/d caused significant increase in concentration although lower doses had no significant effect *890* 20% increase in short term studies *141*

Serum No Effect Physiological No significant change in 15 individuals when given as sole treatment for less than 1 y *6450* After 12 mo treatment of 53 previously untreated hypertensives *507*

Urea Nitrogen *Serum Decrease Physiological* Mean increase from 5.6 to 6.5 mmol/L in 7 essential hypertensives treated for 16 weeks *568*

Bendroflumethiazide *(continued)*

Urea Nitrogen *(continued)*
Serum Increase Physiological In men and women in 3 y study of patients with mild hypertension *4149*
Serum No Effect Physiological No significant difference from control in 6 patients with essential hypertension following 5 mg orally *5573*

Uric Acid *Serum Increase Physiological* In 257 hypertensive patients treatment with as little as 1.25 mg/d caused significant increase in concentration *890* Inhibition of tubular secretion of urate *2378* Increase by 2.7 to 4 mg/dL approximately in 5 or 6 hypertensives given 5 mg daily for 6 weeks *6499* In men and women in 3 y study of patients with mild hypertension *4149*
Serum No Effect Physiological No significant difference from control following dose of 5 mg in 6 patients with essential hypertension *5573* After 12 mo treatment of 53 previously untreated hypertensives *507*

Uric Acid Clearance *Urine No Effect Physiological* Since drug has no effect on carbonic anhydrase has no effect on clearance *633*

Volume *Urine No Effect Physiological* In first 6 hours after 5 mg bendrofluazide no significant difference compared with placebo but significant decrease observed during next 18 hours *5573*

Zinc *Urine Increase Physiological* Increase by 60% in 9 hypertensives treated for 2 weeks *6418*

Benfluorex

Cholesterol *Serum Decrease Physiological* In 7 patients with NIDDM treatment for 6 weeks caused nonsignificant reduction to 216 ± 15 mg/dL compared with 249 ± 26 mg/dL when treated with placebo *930* Increase by 17% in 12 hypertriglyceridemic type 2 diabetic patients given 150 mg tid after 1 mo treatment *5690*

Cortisol *Plasma No Effect Physiological* In 12 middle-aged men treatment with 450 mg/d for 6 weeks caused nonsignificant change from mean baseline of 500 ± 50 nmol/L to 510 ± 60 nmol/L *4251*

Dehydroepiandrosterone Sulfate
Plasma Increase Physiological In 12 middle-aged men treatment with 450 mg/d for 6 weeks caused significant increase from mean baseline of 6.80 ± 0.75 µmol/L to 10.52 ± 1.02 µmol/L *4251*

Dehydroepiandrosterone, Unconjugated
Plasma Increase Physiological In 12 middle-aged men treatment with 450 mg/d for 6 weeks caused significant increase from mean baseline of 13.69 ± 1.95 nmol/L to 22.78 ± 2.90 nmol/L *4251*

Glucose *Serum Decrease Physiological* In 12 middle-aged men treatment with 450 mg/d for 6 weeks caused significant reduction from mean baseline of 5.26 ± 0.10 mmol/L to 4.79 ± 0.08 mmol/L *4251* In 7 patients with NIDDM treated with benfluorex for 6 weeks caused significant reduction of mean to 121.4 ± 5.6 mg/dL compared with 137.0 ± 6.5 mg/dL when treated with placebo *930*

Glucose Tolerance *Serum Increase Physiological* In 12 middle-aged men treatment with 450 mg/d for 6 weeks caused significant improvement in area under the curve from mean baseline of 977 ± 27 mmol/L.min to 814 ± 27 mmol/L.min *4251*

HDL-Cholesterol *Serum No Effect Physiological* In 12 hypertriglyceridemic type 2 diabetic patients given 150 mg tid after 1 mo treatment *5690* In 7 NIDDM patients treated with benfluorex for 6 weeks caused nonsignificant increase to 46 ± 4 mg/dL compared with 42 ± 3 mg/dL during placebo period *930*

Hemoglobin A_{1c} *Blood Decrease Physiological* Significant effect in hypertriglyceridemic type 2 diabetic patients given 150 mg tid after 1 mo treatment *5690* Significant decrease from mean concentration with placebo of 8.3% to 7.7% in 7 mild diet-treated NIDDM patients treated with 450 mg/d for 6 weeks *930*

β-Hydroxybutyrate *Serum Decrease Physiological* Significant decrease from placebo-treated mean concentration of 0.91 mmol/L to 0.60 mmol/L in 7 mild diet-treated NIDDM patients treated with 450 mg/d for 6 weeks *930* In 7 patients with NIDDM treatment with benfluorex for 6 weeks caused significant reduction to 0.66 ± 0.04 mmol/L compared with 0.91 ± 0.06 mmol/L when patients receiving placebo *930*

Insulin *Plasma Decrease Physiological* In 12 middle-aged men treatment with 450 mg/d for 6 weeks caused significant reduction from mean baseline of 174 ± 22 pmol/L to 98 ± 10 pmol/L *4251*
Plasma No Effect Physiological In 7 NIDDM patients treated with benfluorex for 6 weeks mean concentration of fasting insulin nonsignificantly reduced to 11.9 ± 2.9 µU/mL compared with 13.5 ± 2.7 µU/mL in placebo treated controls *930*

Lactate *Plasma Decrease Physiological* In 7 patients with NIDDM treated with 450 mg/d benfluorex for 6 weeks mean fasting concentration significantly reduced to 1.22 ± 0.11 mmol/L compared with 1.82 ± 0.13 mmol/L in placebo treated period *930*

Pyruvate *Plasma Decrease Physiological* In 7 patients with NIDDM treatment with 450 mg/d for 6 weeks caused significant decrease of fasting concentration to 0.095 ± 0.010 mmol/L compared with 0.164 ± 0.011 mmol/L when treated with placebo *930*

Triglycerides *Serum Decrease Physiological* Increase by 33% in 12 hypertriglyceridemic type 2 diabetic patients given 150 mg tid after 1 mo treatment *5690* In 7 patients with NIDDM treatment with benfluorex 450 mg/d for 6 weeks caused nonsignificant reduction to 133 ± 27 mg/dL compared with 210 ± 81 mg/dL during placebo period *930*

VLDL-Cholesterol *Serum Decrease Physiological* Increase by 20% in 12 hypertriglyceridemic type 2 diabetic patients given 150 mg tid after 1 mo treatment *5690*

VLDL-Triglycerides *Serum Decrease Physiological* Increase by 36% in 12 hypertriglyceridemic type 2 diabetic patients given 150 mg tid after 1 mo treatment *5690*

Benserazide

Prolactin *Plasma Increase Physiological* Significant increase in 5 patients with primary hypothyroidism; possibly due to reduction in circulating dopamine *1367*

Thyroid Stimulating Hormone
Serum Increase Physiological In hypothyroidism: is a dopamine antagonist *6412* Significant increase in 5 patients with primary hypothyroidism; possibly due to reduction in circulating dopamine *1367*

Benzaldehyde

ionized Calcium *Serum Decrease Analytical* At 0.1 mmol/L to 0.1 mol/L with calcium specific electrode *820*

Benzamide

Bicarbonate *Serum No Effect Analytical* No effect of concentrations up to 17 mmol/L on method on Kodak Ektachem® *5706* No significant effect observed at a concentration of 20 mmol/L with enzymatic method on Kodak Ektachem® systems *2519*

Benzaprine

Imipramine *Serum Increase Analytical* In liquid-chromatographic method described has similar retention time *5364*

Benzazepine

Hematocrit *Blood Decrease Physiological* Slight effect observed *2845*

Hemoglobin *Blood Decrease Physiological* Slight effect observed *2845*

Leukocytes *Blood Decrease Physiological* Slight effect observed *2845*

Benzbromarone

Cholesterol *Serum No Effect Analytical* At concentration of 60 mg/L had no effect as measured by CHOD-Iodide method *5704* At concentration of 60 mg/L had no effect as measured by catalase-AIDH method *5704* At concentration of 60 mg/L had no effect as measured by CHOD-PAP method *5704* At concentration of 60 mg/L had no effect as measured by Liebermann-Burchard method *5704* At concentration of 60 mg/L had no effect as measured by method using catalase-Hantzsch reaction *5704*
Serum No Effect Analytical At concentration of 20 mg/L had no effect as measured by catalase-AIDH method *5704* At concentration of 20 mg/L had no effect as measured by Kageyama-Hantzsch method *5704*

Creatinine *Serum No Effect Analytical* At concentration of 47 mg/L had no effect as measured by kinetic Jaffe method on BKA-2 *5704* At concentration of 20 mg/L had no effect as measured by Jaffe-Fuller's earth method *5704* At concentration of 20 mg/L had no effect as measured by Jaffe-Fading-Fraction method *5704*

Creatinine Clearance *Urine No Effect Physiological* No significant change observed in 10 healthy men following ingestion of 100 mg *3760*

Glucose *Serum No Effect Analytical* At concentration of 8 mg/L had no effect as measured by Kodak Ektachem® method *5704*

Hypoxanthine *Serum No Effect Physiological* Ingestion of 200 mg had no effect on serum concentration in 5 healthy individuals within 2 hours *6582* In 22 patients with gout treatment for 3 to 6 months with 200 or 300 mg/d benzbromarone caused no significant change from mean baseline of 1.31 ± 0.17 µmol/L to 1.47 ± 0.59 µmol/L *6580*
Urine No Effect Physiological In 22 patients with gout treatment for 3 to 6 months with 200 or 300 mg/d benzbromarone caused nonsignificant change from mean baseline of 42 ± 16 mmol/m²/d to 38 ± 17 mmol/m²/d *6580*

Orotidine *Urine No Effect Physiological* In 22 patients with gout treatment for 3 to 6 months with 200 or 300 mg/d benzbromarone caused nonsignificant change from mean baseline of 0.38 ± 0.11 µmol/m²/d to 0.38 ± 0.11 µmol/m²/d *6580*

Oxypurinol *Serum Decrease Physiological* In 14 adult men coadministration of benzbromarone with allopurinol caused reduction of mean area under the curve of 41% compared to allopurinol administration alone *4164*
Serum No Effect Physiological In 5 healthy men coadministration of benzbromarone with allopurinol had no significant effect on plasma concentration *6581*
Urine Increase Physiological In 5 healthy men coadministration of benzbromarone with allopurinol caused significant increase in ratio of excretion of oxypurinol to creatinine from 0.87 ± 0.14 to 1.67 ± 0.26 *6581*

Potassium *Serum No Effect Analytical* At concentration of 80 mg/L had no effect on ISE measurement without predilution *5704*

Protein Electrophoresis *Serum No Effect Analytical* At concentration of 80 mg/L had no effect as measured by automated Olympus-Hite method *5704*

Purine Bases *Urine Increase Physiological* In 22 patients with gout treatment for 3 to 6 months with 200 or 300 mg/d benzbromarone caused significant change from mean baseline of 2.14 ± 0.51 mmol/m²/d to 2.68 ± 0.47 mmol/m²/d *6580*

Sodium *Serum No Effect Analytical* At concentration of 80 mg/L had no effect on ISE measurement without predilution *5704*

Urea Nitrogen *Serum No Effect Analytical* At concentration of 8 mg/L had no effect as measured by Kodak Ektachem® method *5704*

Uric Acid *Serum Decrease Physiological* Within 2 hours of ingestion of 200 mg significant decrease occurred in 5 healthy individuals *6582* In 22 patients with gout treatment for 3 to 6 months with 200 or 300 mg/d benzbromarone caused significant change from mean baseline of 513 ± 64 µmol/L to 276 ± 60 µmol/L *6580* Potent uricosuric agent: effect enhanced when oxipurinol co-administered *1091* Following ingestion of 100 mg in 3 healthy volunteers decrease from baseline concentration of 6.2 mg/dL to 3.0 mg/dL at 22 hours, not affected by associated ethanol ingestion *3026* At a dose of 100 mg significant reduction observed with a 39% decrease after 6 h and a 53% decrease after 24 h in 10 healthy men associated with increased fractional excretion *3760*
Urine Decrease Physiological Statistically significant reduction in excretion and in clearance versus creatinine clearance in comparison with no treatment *5693*
Urine Increase Physiological In 22 patients with gout treatment for 3 to 6 months with 200 or 300 mg/d benzbromarone caused significant change from mean baseline of 2.07 ± 0.50 mmol/m²/d to 2.61 ± 0.46 mmol/m²/d *6580* Potent uricosuric agent: effect enhanced when oxipurinol co-administered *1091*

Uric Acid Clearance *Urine Increase Physiological* In 22 patients with gout treatment for 3 to 6 months with 200 or 300 mg/d benzbromarone caused significant change from mean baseline of 5.9 ± 1.6 mL/min to 14.3 ± 3.9 mL/min *6580*

Uridine *Serum No Effect Physiological* In 22 patients with gout treatment for 3 to 6 months with 200 or 300 mg/d benzbromarone caused no significant change from mean baseline of 5.22 ± 0.78 µmol/L to 5.00 ± 0.80 µmol/L *6580*

Xanthine *Serum No Effect Physiological* In 22 patients with gout treatment for 3 to 6 months with 200 or 300 mg/d benzbromarone caused nonsignificant change from mean baseline of 0.87 ± 0.17 µmol/L to 1.16 ± 0.31 µmol/L *6580* Ingestion of 200 mg had no effect on serum concentration within 2 hours in 5 healthy individuals *6582*
Urine No Effect Physiological In 22 patients with gout treatment for 3 to 6 months with 200 or 300 mg/d benzbromarone caused nonsignificant change from mean baseline of 36 ± 12 mmol/m²/d to 35 ± 24 mmol/m²/d *6580*

Benzil

Histamine *Plasma No Effect Analytical* Improbable inhibition of radio-enzyme assay at therapeutic concentrations *2492*

Benziodarone

Alanine Aminotransferase *Serum Increase Physiological* May cause hepatic toxicity *3810*

Alkaline Phosphatase *Serum Increase Physiological* May cause hepatic toxicity *3810*

Aspartate Aminotransferase *Serum Increase Physiological* May cause hepatic toxicity *3810*

Bile *Urine Increase Physiological* May cause hepatic toxicity *3810*

Bilirubin *Serum Increase Physiological* May cause hepatic toxicity *3810*

BSP Retention *Serum Increase Physiological* May cause hepatic toxicity *3810*

^{131}I Uptake *Serum Decrease Physiological* Due to iodine component of drug *3669*

Thyroxine (T4) *Serum No Effect Physiological* Relatively constant in 9 normal volunteers receiving 100 mg three times daily for 14 d due to diversion of peripheral metabolism of T4 to rT3 rather than T3 *6575*

Tri-iodothyronine, Reverse (rT3)
Serum Increase Physiological Significant effect in 9 normal volunteers receiving 100 mg three times daily for 14 d due to diversion of peripheral metabolism of T4 to rT3 rather than T3 *6575*

Tri-iodothyronine (T3) *Serum Increase Physiological* Significant effect in 9 normal volunteers receiving 100 mg three times daily for 14 d due to diversion of peripheral metabolism of T4 to rT3 rather than T3 *6575*

Uric Acid *Serum Decrease Physiological* Stimulates secretion of urate *2268*
Urine Increase Physiological Stimulates secretion of urate *2268*

Benzocaine

Cannabinoids *Urine No Effect Analytical* No effect on Roche Abuscreen method *5006*

Benzocaine *(continued)*

Drugs of Abuse Screen *Urine No Effect Analytical* No effect at concentration of 100 μg/mL on EZ-SCREEN procedure for cannabinoids and cocaine *1739*

Erythrocytes *Blood Decrease Physiological* May cause hemolysis *604*

Hematocrit *Blood Decrease Physiological* May cause hemolysis *604*

Hemoglobin *Blood Decrease Physiological* May cause hemolysis *604*

Methemoglobin *Blood Increase Physiological* Hemolysis *604*

Sulfa as Sulfanilamide *Serum Increase Analytical* Diazotizes and interferes *409*

Benzodiazepines

$CD3^+$ Lymphocytes *Blood Decrease Physiological* In 43 benzodiazepine consumers aged less than 45 years mean concentration of 60.4 ± 1.8 significantly less than 68.1 ± 2.4 in age and sex matched controls. In 39 elderly individuals (aged more than 65 y) mean concentration of 51.4 ± 2.1 significantly less than 59.1 ± 1.9 in age and sex matched controls *3457*

$CD4^+$:$CD8^+$ Lymphocyte Ratio *Blood Decrease Physiological* In 43 benzodiazepine consumers aged less than 45 years mean concentration of 1.7 ± 0.2 significantly less than 2.1 ± 0.1 in age and sex matched controls. In 39 elderly individuals (aged more than 65 y) mean concentration of 1.3 ± 0.1 significantly less than 1.7 ± 0.1 in age and sex matched controls *3457*

$CD4^+$ Lymphocytes *Blood Decrease Physiological* In 43 benzodiazepine consumers aged less than 45 years mean concentration of 24.2 ± 1.2 significantly less than 28.5 ± 1.7 in age and sex matched controls. In 39 elderly individuals (aged more than 65 y) mean concentration of 21.9 ± 0.9 significantly less than 24.6 ± 1.6 in age and sex matched controls *3457*

CD11b Lymphocytes *Blood Increase Physiological* In 43 benzodiazepine consumers aged less than 45 years mean concentration of 23.4 ± 2.1 greater than 16.8 ± 4.9 in age and sex matched controls. In 39 elderly individuals (aged more than 65 y) mean concentration of 26.4 ± 3.6 greater than 22.4 ± 1.9 in age and sex matched controls *3457*

$CD16^+$ Lymphocytes *Blood Decrease Physiological* In 43 benzodiazepine consumers aged less than 45 years mean concentration of 4.7 ± 1.3 less than 7.4 ± 1.1 in age and sex matched controls. In 39 elderly individuals (aged more than 65 y) mean concentration of 3.7 ± 0.9 less than 4.8 ± 0.7 in age and sex matched controls *3457*

$CD20^+$ Lymphocytes *Blood No Effect Physiological* In 43 benzodiazepine consumers aged less than 45 years mean concentration of 12.8 ± 0.9 not significantly different from 13.9 ± 3.1 in age and sex matched controls. In 39 elderly individuals (aged more than 65 y) mean concentration of 12.6 ± 1.4 not significantly different from 12.8 ± 2.9 in age and sex matched controls *3457*

$CD57^+$ Lymphocytes *Blood Increase Physiological* In 43 benzodiazepine consumers aged less than 45 years mean concentration of 14.3 ± 1.1 significantly greater than 8.7 ± 0.7 in age and sex matched controls. In 39 elderly individuals (aged more than 65 y) mean concentration of 17.3 ± 1.0 significantly greater than 13.6 ± 0.8 in age and sex matched controls *3457*

Cortisol *Plasma Increase Physiological* In 43 benzodiazepine consumers aged less than 45 years mean concentration of 19.4 ± 2.1 μg/dL significantly greater than 8.9 ± 1.3 μg/dL in age and sex matched controls. In 39 elderly individuals (aged more than 65 y) mean concentration of 29.5 ± 3.3 μg/dL significantly less than 18.6 ± 2.2 μg/dL in age and sex matched controls *3457*

Dopamine *Plasma Decrease Physiological* In 43 benzodiazepine consumers aged less than 45 years mean concentration of 15.2 ± 10 pg/mL less than 17.1 ± 1.2 pg/mL in age and sex matched controls. In 39 elderly individuals (aged more than 65 y) mean concentration of 13.8 ± 2.6 pg/mL less than 14.9 ± 1.6 pg/mL in age and sex matched controls *3457*

Epinephrine *Plasma Increase Physiological* In 43 benzodiazepine consumers aged less than 45 years mean concentration of 41 ± 10 pg/mL significantly greater than 29 ± 3 pg/mL in age and sex matched controls. In 39 elderly individuals (aged more than 65 y) mean concentration of 89 ± 7 pg/mL significantly greater than 67 ± 5 pg/mL in age and sex matched controls *3457*

5-Hydroxytryptamine *Platelets Decrease Physiological* In 43 benzodiazepine consumers aged less than 45 years mean concentration of 152 ± 7 ng/mL less than 196 ± 9 ng/mL in age and sex matched controls. In 39 elderly individuals (aged more than 65 y) mean concentration of 101 ± 13 ng/mL less than 141 ± 6 ng/mL in age and sex matched controls *3457*

5-Hydroxytryptamine, Free *Plasma Increase Physiological* In 43 benzodiazepine consumers aged less than 45 years mean concentration of 4.6 ± 0.9 ng/mL significantly greater than 0.9 ± 0.2 ng/mL in age and sex matched controls. In 39 elderly individuals (aged more than 65 y) mean concentration of 9.4 ± 1.7 ng/mL significantly greater than 3.4 ± 1.1 ng/mL in age and sex matched controls *3457*

Lymphocytes *Blood Decrease Physiological* In 43 benzodiazepine consumers aged less than 45 years mean concentration of 31.4 ± 1.0 significantly less than 37.6 ± 1.2 in age and sex matched controls. In 39 elderly individuals (aged more than 65 y) mean concentration of 24.2 ± 1.3 significantly less than 32.2 ± 1.1 in age and sex matched controls *3457*

Natural Killer Cells *Blood Increase Physiological* In 43 benzodiazepine consumers aged less than 45 years mean cytoxicity against K_{562} target cells of 47.8 ± 1.8 greater than 42.1 ± 2.1 in age and sex matched controls. In 39 elderly individuals (aged more than 65 y) mean cytoxicity against K_{562} target cells of 51.4 ± 2.2 similar to 49.3 ± 2.9 in age and sex matched controls *3457*

Norepinephrine *Plasma Decrease Physiological* In 43 benzodiazepine consumers aged less than 45 years mean concentration of 129 ± 13 pg/mL significantly less than 233 ± 15 pg/mL in age and sex matched controls. In 39 elderly individuals (aged more than 65 y) mean concentration of 89 ± 17 pg/mL significantly less than 292 ± 18 pg/mL in age and sex matched controls *3457*

γ-δ T-Lymphocytes *Blood Increase Physiological* In 57 benzodiazepine consumers mean concentration of 48.2 ± 2.8 greater than 40.1 ± 2.0 in age and sex matched controls *3458*

Tryptophan *Plasma Decrease Physiological* In 43 benzodiazepine consumers aged less than 45 years mean concentration of 10403 ± 23 μg/mL significantly less than 14060 ± 21 μg/mL in age and sex matched controls. In 39 elderly individuals (aged more than 65 y) mean concentration of 6771 ± 34 μg/mL significantly less than 9634 ± 17 μg/mL in age and sex matched controls *3457*

Benzoylecgonine

Amphetamine *Urine No Effect Analytical* Negative result observed with Du Pont aca method at a concentration of 1000 μg/mL (3.46 mmol/L) *1554*

Barbiturate *Urine No Effect Analytical* At a concentration of 1000 μg/mL (3.46 mmol/L) with method on Du Pont aca *1555*

Benzodiazepine *Urine No Effect Analytical* Negative result obtained at a concentration of 1000 μg/mL (3.46 mmol/L) with method on Du Pont aca *1556*

Benzoylecgonine *Urine Increase Analytical* Positive effect observed at a concentration of 0.07 μmol/L with Sung and Neely modification of Syva procedure *148*

Cannabinoids *Urine No Effect Analytical* No effect observed at a concentration of 400 μg/mL (1.38 mmol/L) on method on Du Pont aca *1557* No effect on Roche Abuscreen method *5006*

Morphine *Urine Increase Analytical* Significant interference observed at a concentration of 345 μmol/L with Sung and Neely modification of Syva EMIT method *148*

Opiates *Urine No Effect Analytical* No effect observed at a concentration of 1000 μg/mL (3.46 mmol/L) with method on Du Pont aca *1559*

Benzoylnorecgonine

Benzoylecgonine *Urine No Effect Analytical* No interference observed at concentrations less than 5000 ng/mL with l-benzoylnorecgonine with Roche Abuscreen ONTRAK assay *1106*

Benzphetamine

Lysergic Acid Diethylamide *Urine Increase Analytical* Minimum concentration that caused a positive result with EMIT method to measure LSD < 1000 mg/L *4968*

Benzquinamide

Fatty Acids (FFA), Free *Serum Increase Physiological* 136% increase following single injection i.m. of 300 mg *2675*

Benzthiazide

Amylase *Serum Increase Physiological* Rare, may occur as with other thiazides *2754*

Bilirubin *Serum Increase Physiological* Rare, may occur as with other thiazides *2754*

Chloride *Urine Increase Physiological* Therapeutic diuretic intent *2754*

Erythrocytes *Blood Decrease Physiological* May occur as with other thiazides *2754*

Glucose *Serum Increase Physiological* May occur as with other thiazides *2754*
Urine Increase Physiological Rare, may occur as with other thiazides *2754*

Leukocytes *Blood Decrease Physiological* May occur as with other thiazides *2754*

Platelets *Blood Decrease Physiological* May occur as with other thiazides *2754*

Potassium *Serum Decrease Physiological* May occur as with other thiazides *2754*

Sodium *Urine Increase Physiological* Therapeutic intent (maximum effect 4-6 h) *2754*

Urea Nitrogen *Serum Increase Physiological* May occur as with other thiazides *2754*

Uric Acid *Serum Increase Physiological* May occur as with other thiazides *2754*

Volume *Urine Increase Physiological* Therapeutic diuretic intent *2754*

Benztropine

Histamine *Plasma No Effect Analytical* Improbable inhibition of radio-enzyme assay since concentrations at which enzyme inhibited much greater than physiological *2492*

Prolactin *Plasma No Effect Physiological* No significant response to 1.0 mg given i.m *2352*

Benzyl Alcohol

Bicarbonate *Serum No Effect Analytical* No significant effect observed at a concentration of 20 mmol/L with enzymatic method on Kodak Ektachem® systems *2519*

Glucose *Serum Increase Physiological* Used as saline preservative, effect in mice ?humans *335*

ionized Calcium *Serum Decrease Analytical* At 0.1 mmol/L to 0.1 mol/L with calcium specific electrode *820*

Benzylsulfonic Acid

Bicarbonate *Serum Increase Analytical* Concentrations above 1.5 mmol/L increase result as determined by method on Kodak Ektachem® *5706*

Bepridil

Alanine Aminotransferase *Serum Increase Physiological* In multicenter trials of over 1000 patients clinically significant increases (more than twice the upper limit of normal) observed in approximately treated individuals, with values returning to normal on cessation of treatment *3919*

Aspartate Aminotransferase *Serum Increase Physiological* In multicenter trials of over 1000 patients clinically significant increases (more than twice the upper limit of normal) observed in approximately treated individuals, with values returning to normal on cessation of treatment *3919*

Carbamazepine *Serum Increase Physiological* Concomitant administration of calcium channel blockers with carbamazepine causes marked increase of plasma carbamazepine concentration resulting in toxicity in some cases *282*

Digoxin *Serum Increase Physiological* In two studies of the effect of coadministration of bepridil with digoxin bepridil caused a a modest increase (of about 30%) of the plasma digoxin concentration *3919* Concentration increased by up to 34% in patients in whom two drugs coadministered but effect not observed for one to two weeks after bepridil added to therapeutic regime. However no significant effect reported in another study *474* When coadministered with digoxin increased area under concentration curve, half-life of digoxin, and steady state plasma concentration (34%) of digoxin *5345*
Serum No Effect Physiological In one study of the effect of coadministration of bepridil with digoxin bepridil had no effect on the plasma digoxin concentration *3919*

Leukocytes *Blood Decrease Physiological* In multicenter trials of over 800 patients treated for 5 or more years two cases of marked leukopenia and neutropenia observed *3919*

Neutrophils *Blood Decrease Physiological* In multicenter trials of over 800 patients treated for 5 or more years two cases of marked leukopenia and neutropenia observed *3919*

Potassium *Serum No Effect Physiological* In multicenter trials of over 1000 patients no reports of effects on serum potassium concentration *3919*

Beraprost

Fibrinopeptide A *Plasma Decrease Physiological* In 31 patients with exertional angina 40 µg oral beraprost administered 8-hourly for 1 month caused significant change in concentration following exercise stress test from 4.6 ± 3.2 ng/mL to 2.8 ± 2.1 ng/mL *5190*

Plasminogen Activator Inhibitor-1 Activity
Plasma Decrease Physiological In 31 patients with exertional angina 40 µg oral beraprost administered 8-hourly for 1 month caused significant change in activity following exercise stress test from 5.9 ± 5.8 U/mL to 4.5 ± 4.2 U/mL *5190*

Platelet Factor 4 *Plasma Decrease Physiological* In 31 patients with exertional angina 40 µg oral beraprost administered 8-hourly for 1 month caused significant change in concentration following exercise stress test from 28.7 ± 27.1 ng/mL to 17.6 ± 8.8 ng/mL *5190*

Tissue Plasminogen Activator
Plasma No Effect Physiological In 31 patients with exertional angina 40 µg oral beraprost administered 8-hourly for 1 month caused no significant change in concentration following exercise stress test from 11.1 ± 3.1 ng/mL to 11.1 ± 3.0 ng/mL *5190*

Tissue Plasminogen Activator:Plasminogen Activator Inhibitor-1 Complex *Plasma No Effect Physiological* In 31 patients with exertional angina 40 µg oral beraprost administered 8-hourly for 1 month caused no significant change in concentration following exercise stress test from 16.1 ± 8.0 ng/mL to 13.2 ± 5.0 ng/mL *5190*

Berenil

Histamine *Plasma No Effect Analytical* Improbable inhibition of radio-enzyme assay at therapeutic concentrations *2492*

Beryllium Salts

Alkaline Phosphatase *Serum Decrease Analytical* Inhibitors of enzyme in laboratory procedures *6026*

Protein *Urine Increase Physiological* May cause nephrotoxicity *5377*

Urea Nitrogen *Serum Increase Physiological* May cause nephrotoxicity *5377*

Uric Acid *Serum Increase Physiological* Nephropathy associated with decreased excretion per nephron *3095*
Urine Decrease Physiological Nephropathy associated with decreased excretion per nephron *3095*

Betaine

Histamine *Plasma No Effect Analytical* Improbable inhibition of radio-enzyme assay at therapeutic concentrations *2492*

Betamethasone

Bicarbonate *Serum Increase Physiological* May cause hypokalemic alkalosis *2754*

Cortisol *Plasma Decrease Physiological* Very low values observed in children in whom cream applied topically *1199*

C-Peptide *Plasma Increase Physiological* Progressive and significant increase in 6 healthy volunteers with short-term treatment *4477*

Glucose *Serum Increase Physiological* Progressive and significant increase in 6 healthy volunteers with short-term treatment *4477*

Glucose Tolerance *Serum Decrease Physiological* Marked and significant increase in glucose and insulin peaks during oral glucose tolerance *4477*

17-Hydroxycorticosteroids *Plasma Increase Physiological* Slight effect, absorbed through skin *128*
Urine Increase Physiological Slight increase, may be absorbed through skin *128*

Insulin *Plasma Increase Physiological* Progressive and significant increase in 6 healthy volunteers with short-term treatment *4477*

17-Ketosteroids *Urine Decrease Physiological* Feedback pituitary suppression of ACTH *2025*

Occult Blood *Feces Increase Physiological* May activate peptic ulcer *2754*

Potassium *Serum Decrease Physiological* Occurs infrequently *128*
Urine Increase Physiological Occurs infrequently *293*

Sodium *Serum Increase Physiological* Occurs infrequently with edema *128*

Betaxolol

Alanine Aminotransferase *Serum Increase Physiological* Incidence reported of less than 2% in long-term clinical trials *2067*

Aspartate Aminotransferase *Serum Increase Physiological* Incidence of less than 2% reported in long-term clinical trials *2067*

Cholesterol *Serum Increase Physiological* Incidence of less than 2% reported in long-term clinical trials *2067*

Creatinine *Serum Increase Physiological* Abnormal renal function reported in less than 2% patients in long-term clinical trials *2067*

Glucose *Serum Increase Physiological* Incidence of less than 2% reported in long-term clinical trials *2067*

Growth Hormone *Plasma No Effect Physiological* No significant difference in baseline concentration between controls and hyperthyroid patients with or without drug and no significant difference between groups in effect on concentration during oral glucose tolerance test *3372*

Hematocrit *Blood Decrease Physiological* Anemia reported with frequency of less than 2% in long-term clinical trials *2067*

Hemoglobin *Blood Decrease Physiological* Anemia reported with frequency of less than 2% in long-term clinical trials *2067*

Lactate Dehydrogenase *Serum Increase Physiological* Incidence of less than 2% reported in long-term clinical trials *2067*

Leukocytes *Blood Increase Physiological* Leukocytosis reported with frequency of less than 2% in long-term clinical trials *2067*

pH *Blood Decrease Physiological* Acidosis reported in less than 2% patients in long-term clinical trials *2067*

Platelets *Blood Decrease Physiological* Thrombocytopenia reported with a frequency of less than 2% in long-term clinical trials *2067*

Potassium *Serum Decrease Physiological* Incidence of less than 2% reported in long-term clinical trials *2067*
Serum Increase Physiological Incidence of less than 2% reported in long-term clinical trials *2067*

Protein *Urine Increase Physiological* Incidence of less than 2% reported in long-term clinical trials *2067*

Urea Nitrogen *Serum Increase Physiological* Abnormal renal function reported in less than 2% patients in long-term clinical trials *2067*

Uric Acid *Serum Increase Physiological* Incidence of less than 2% reported in long-term clinical trials *2067*

Betazole

Hydrochloric Acid *Gastric Fluid Increase Physiological* Used to stimulate secretion *128*

Ionized Calcium *Serum Decrease Physiological* Increase by 0.062 mmol/L 1 h after 1.5 mg/kg s.c *2762*

Bethanechol

Albumin *Serum No Effect Analytical* No effect at 0.09 mg/dL on Technicon SMA 12/60 method *4390*

Alkaline Phosphatase *Serum No Effect Analytical* No effect at 0.09 mg/dL on Technicon SMA 12/60 method *4390*

Amylase *Serum Increase Physiological* May cause increased secretion, spasm of sphincter of Oddi *1255*

Aspartate Aminotransferase *Serum Increase Physiological* Impaired excretion due to spasm of sphincter of Oddi *1009*
Serum No Effect Analytical No effect at 0.09 mg/dL on Technicon SMA 12/60 method *4390*

Bilirubin *Serum Increase Physiological* Impaired excretion due to spasm of sphincter of Oddi *1009*
Serum No Effect Analytical No effect at 0.09 mg/dL on Technicon SMA 12/60 method *4390*

BSP Retention *Serum Increase Physiological* Impaired excretion due to spasm of sphincter of Oddi *1009*

Calcium *Serum No Effect Analytical* No effect at 0.09 mg/dL on Technicon SMA 12/60 method *4390*

Cholesterol *Serum No Effect Analytical* No effect at 0.09 mg/dL on Technicon SMA 12/60 method *4390*

Creatinine *Serum No Effect Analytical* No effect at 0.09 mg/dL on Technicon SMA 12/60 method *4390*

Glucose *Serum No Effect Analytical* No effect at 0.09 mg/dL on Technicon SMA 12/60 method *4390*

Lactate Dehydrogenase *Serum No Effect Analytical* No effect at 0.09 mg/dL on Technicon SMA 12/60 method *4390*

Lipase *Serum Increase Physiological* May cause increased secretion, spasm of sphincter of Oddi *1255*

Phosphate *Serum No Effect Analytical* No effect at 0.09 mg/dL on Technicon SMA 12/60 method *4390*

Protein *Serum No Effect Analytical* No effect at 0.09 mg/dL on Technicon SMA 12/60 method *4390*

Uric Acid *Serum No Effect Analytical* No effect at 0.09 mg/dL on Technicon SMA 12/60 method *4390*

Bethanidine

Creatinine *Serum Increase Physiological* Effect reported in one patient *5838*

Norepinephrine *Urine Decrease Physiological* Reported effect *2451*

Platelets *Blood Decrease Physiological* Mild thrombocytopenia reported *6487*

Bezafibrate

Alanine Aminotransferase *Serum No Effect Analytical* No effect at therapeutic concentration on Boehringer Mannheim Reflotron method *3231* No effect at 100 mg/L on Boehringer Mannheim Reflotron method *5706*
Serum No Effect Physiological No significant effect in 20 noninsulin dependent diabetics fed diet and 600 mg bezafibrate daily for 3 months *2970*

Albumin *Urine No Effect Analytical* At concentration of 120 mg/dL had no significant effect on Boehringer Mannheim Tinaquant method *2799*

Alkaline Phosphatase *Serum Decrease Physiological* In 24 individuals with mid to moderate hypertriglyceridemia and low HDL-cholesterol concentration treatment with a triglyceride lowering diet and 400 mg bezafibrate per day for 24 weeks caused significant reduction from mean baseline of 79.6 ± 26.5 U/L to 65.0 ± 25.6 U/L *244* In 10 hyperlipidemic patients treatment resulted in 25% reduction in total activity *1290*

Alkaline Phosphatase, Bone Isoenzyme
Serum No Effect Physiological Treatment of 10 hyperlipidemic patients did not affect bone alkaline phosphatase activity *1290*

Alkaline Phosphatase, Liver Isoenzyme
Serum Decrease Physiological In 10 hyperlipidemic patients treatment caused mean 40% reduction of liver alkaline phosphatase *1290*

Amylase *Serum No Effect Analytical* At concentration of 100 mg/L had no effect on method on Boehringer Mannheim Reflotron system *5706*

Amylase, Pancreatic Isoenzyme
Serum No Effect Analytical No significant effect observed at toxic concentration of 100 mg/L on method on Boehringer Mannheim Reflotron *3647*

Apolipoprotein A-I *Serum Decrease Physiological* In patients with hyperlipoproteinemia type IIb treatment with 400 mg/d for 3 months caused decrease in concentration *644*
Serum Increase Physiological In 25 patients with hyperlipoproteinemia treatment with 400 mg/d bezafibrate for 12 weeks caused significant reduction from mean baseline of 137.8 ± 32.3 mg/dL to 155.6 ± 25.1 mg/dL *2691* Significant effect in 12 individuals with primary hypercholesterolemia when treated with 600 mg daily for 12 weeks *5385* Increased synthesis. Increased activity of lipoprotein lipase by stimulation of muscle lipoprotein lipase synthesis, alteration of the capillary endothelial surface and stimulation of apo C-II synthesis *264* In 12 patients with hypertriglyceridemia treatment with 400 mg/d for 8 weeks caused significant increase (10%) from 120 (SEM 3.1) mg/dL to 132 (SEM 4.6) mg/dL *4573* In 62 hypercholesterolemic patients treatment with up to 1000 mg/d probucol and up to 400 mg/d bezafibrate caused change from mean baseline of 100 ± 2.0 mg/dL to 110 ± 20.6 mg/dL (significant) at 3 months, 111 ± 2.3 mg/dL at 6 months (nonsignificant) and 106 ± 2.1 mg/dL at 12 months (nonsignificant) *5196* In 32 diet-resistant type IIb hyperlipidemic NIDDM patients treatment with 400 mg/d for 1 month caused mean 13% increase *4301* 6 months treatment of 17 patients with type IV hyperlipoproteinemia increased concentration by 29% *3081*
Serum No Effect Physiological In 4 heterogeneous patients with familial LDL-receptor defective hypercholesterolemia treatment with 400 mg/d for 12 weeks caused a nonsignificant change from mean baseline of 156 ± 30 mg/dL to 165 ± 22 mg/dL *2408* In 11 hypertriglyceridemic subjects *5500*

Apolipoprotein A-II *Serum Increase Physiological* In 25 patients with hyperlipoproteinemia treatment with 400 mg/d bezafibrate for 12 weeks caused significant increase from mean baseline of 38.8 ± 7.4 mg/dL to 52.8 ± 8.2 mg/dL *2691* 6 months treatment of 17 patients with type IV hyperlipoproteinemia caused increase of 22% *3081* In 62 hypercholesterolemic patients treatment with up to 1000 mg/d probucol and up to 400 mg/d bezafibrate caused change from mean baseline of 30.4 ± 0.6 mg/dL to 38.0 ± 0.6 mg/dL (significant) at 3 months, 38.8 ± 0.7 mg/dL at 6 months (significant) and 37.7 ± 0.7 mg/dL at 12 months (significant) *5196* Increased synthesis. Increased activity of lipoprotein lipase by stimulation of muscle lipoprotein lipase synthesis, alteration of the capillary endothelial surface and stimulation of apo C-II synthesis *264*
Serum No Effect Physiological In 32 diet-resistant type IIb hyperlipidemic NIDDM patients treatment with 400 mg/d for 1 month caused mean 5% increase *4301* In 11 hypertriglyceridemic subjects *5500* In 4 heterogeneous patients with familial LDL-receptor defective hypercholesterolemia treatment with 40 mg/d for 12 weeks caused a nonsignificant change from mean baseline of 58 ± 5 mg/dL to 57 ± 3 mg/dL *2408* In 12 patients with hypertriglyceridemia treatment with 400 mg/d for 8 weeks caused insignificant change of mean from 26.3 (SEM 0.5) mg/dL to 26.9 (SEM 0.6) mg/dL *4573*

Apolipoprotein B *Serum Decrease Physiological* In 32 diet-resistant type IIb hyperlipidemic NIDDM patients treatment with 400 mg/d for 1 month caused mean 30% decrease *4301* In 12 patients with hypertriglyceridemia treatment with 400 mg/d for 8 weeks caused significant decrease (20%) of mean from 156 (SEM 9.7) mg/dL to 126 (SEM 7.4) mg/dL *4573* 24% reduction in 12 individuals with primary hypercholesterolemia treated with 600 mg daily for 12 weeks *5385* 6 months treatment with 400 mg/day of 17 patients with type IV hyperlipoproteinemia lowered concentration by 26% *3081* In 25 patients with hyperlipoproteinemia treatment with 400 mg/d bezafibrate for 12 weeks caused significant reduction from mean baseline of 128.8 ± 18.8 mg/dL to 106.8 ± 20.6 mg/dL *2691*
Serum No Effect Physiological In 4 heterogeneous patients with familial LDL-receptor defective hypercholesterolemia treatment with 400 mg/d for 12 weeks caused a nonsignificant change from mean baseline of 192 ± 32 mg/dL to 165 ± 26 mg/dL *2408* In 62 hypercholesterolemic patients treatment with up to 1000 mg/d probucol and up to 400 mg/d bezafibrate caused change from mean baseline of 107 ± 1.6 mg/dL to 103 ± 1.7 mg/dL (nonsignificant) at 3 months, 105 ± 1.9 mg/dL at 6 months (nonsignificant) and 99.5 ± 1.8 mg/dL at 12 months (nonsignificant) *5196*

Apolipoprotein C-II *Serum Decrease Physiological* In 25 patients with hyperlipoproteinemia treatment with 400 mg/d bezafibrate for 12 weeks caused significant reduction from mean baseline of 7.5 ± 3.0 mg/dL to 5.5 ± 2.1 mg/dL *2691* 6 months treatment with 400 mg/day of 17 patients with type IV hyperlipoproteinemia caused lowering by 28% *3081*
Serum No Effect Physiological In 32 diet-resistant type IIb hyperlipidemic NIDDM patients treatment with 400 mg/d for 1 month caused mean 4% increase *4301* In 62 hypercholesterolemic patients treatment with up to 1000 mg/d probucol and up to 400 mg/d bezafibrate caused change from mean baseline of 4.4 ± 0.1 mg/dL to 4.3 ± 0.1 mg/dL (nonsignificant) at 3 months, 4.4 ± 0.1 mg/dL at 6 months (nonsignificant) and 4.1 ± 0.1 mg/dL at 12 months (nonsignificant) *5196*

Apolipoprotein C-III *Serum Decrease Physiological* 6 months treatment of 17 patients with type IV hyperlipoproteinemia with 400 mg/day caused lowering by 15% *3081* In 62 hypercholesterolemic patients treatment with up to 1000 mg/d probucol and up to 400 mg/d bezafibrate caused change from mean baseline of 10.6 ± 0.2 mg/dL to 8.4 ± 0.2 mg/dL (significant) at 3 months, 8.2 ± 0.3 mg/dL at 6 months (significant) and 8.0 ± 0.2 mg/dL at 12 months (significant) *5196* In 32 diet-resistant type IIb hyperlipidemic NIDDM patients treatment with 400 mg/d for 1 month caused mean 15% decrease *4301* In 25 patients with hyperlipoproteinemia treatment with 400 mg/d bezafibrate for 12 weeks caused significant reduction from mean baseline of 19.5 ± 8.3 mg/dL to 10.9 ± 4.8 mg/dL *2691*

Apolipoprotein E *Serum Decrease Physiological* In 25 patients with hyperlipoproteinemia treatment with 400 mg/d bezafibrate for 12 weeks caused significant reduction from mean baseline of 8.7 ± 3.5 mg/dL to 5.8 ± 1.9 mg/dL *2691* In 62 hypercholesterolemic patients treatment with up to 1000 mg/d probucol and up to 400 mg/d bezafibrate caused change from mean baseline of 6.9 ± 0.1 mg/dL to 6.2 ± 0.1 mg/dL (significant) at 3 months, 6.3 ± 0.1 mg/dL at 6 months (significant) and 5.7 ± 0.1 mg/dL at 12 months (significant) *5196* 6 months treatment of 17 patients with type IV hyperlipoproteinemia with 400 mg/day caused lowering by 29% *3081* In 32 diet-resistant type IIb hyperlipidemic NIDDM patients treatment with 400 mg/d for 1 month caused mean 14% decrease *4301*

Bezafibrate *(continued)*

Apolipoprotein-LDL *Serum Decrease Physiological* Mean reduction from 171 mg/dL to 137 mg/dL in 9 patients with type IIa hypercholesterolemia treated with 400 mg daily for 12 weeks, but without further significant reduction when cholestyramine added to regime *5449*

Aspartate Aminotransferase *Serum No Effect Analytical* No effect at 100 mg/L on Boehringer Mannheim Reflotron method *5706* No effect at therapeutic concentration on Boehringer Mannheim Reflotron method *3231*
Serum No Effect Physiological No significant effect in 20 noninsulin dependent diabetics fed diet and 600 mg bezafibrate daily for 3 months *2970*

Bicarbonate *Serum No Effect Physiological* No significant effect in 20 noninsulin dependent diabetics fed diet and 600 mg bezafibrate daily for 3 months *2970*

Bilirubin *Serum No Effect Analytical* At concentration of 100 mg/L had no effect on method on Boehringer Mannheim Reflotron system *5706*
Serum No Effect Physiological No significant effect observed in 20 noninsulin dependent diabetics fed diet and 600 mg bezafibrate daily for 3 months *2970*

Chloride *Serum No Effect Physiological* No significant effect in 20 noninsulin dependent diabetics fed diet and 600 mg bezafibrate daily for 3 months *2970*

Cholesterol *Serum Decrease Physiological* In one hyperlipidemic man treatment for 2.5 years was associated with a reduction of total cholesterol from 7.8 mmol/L to 5.7 mmol/L and of HDL-cholesterol from 0.7 mmol/L to 0.1 mmol/L *4404* In the Bezafibrate Coronary Atherosclerosis Intervention Trial of 42 patients treatment with bezafibrate caused mean decrease of 9% *3115* 6 months treatment of 17 patients with type IV hyperlipoproteinemia caused decrease of 16% *3081* In 20 noninsulin dependent diabetics given diet and 600 mg bezafibrate daily reduction from mean baseline of 6.3 mmol/L to 5.6 mmol/L at 1 and 2 months and 5.5 mmol/L at 3 months *2970* In one patient with lipoatrophic diabetes mean concentration changed from mean baseline of 5.8 mmol/L to 4.0 mmol/L after 3 months and 3.8 mmol/L after 6 months treatment with 200 mg t.d.s *4499* Bezafibrate is effective in decreasing cholesterol concentrations *3668* In one patient with familial hypercholesterolemia treated with diet and 400 mg/d bezafibrate for at least 3 months concentration decreased from 8.8 to 6.6 mmol/L *6405* In 25 patients with hyperlipoproteinemia treatment with 400 mg/d bezafibrate for 12 weeks caused significant reduction from mean baseline of 252.0 ± 41.2 mg/dL to 216.2 ± 32.3 mg/dL *2691* In 38 patients with types IIa and IIb primary hypercholesterolemia treatment with 400 mg/d for 12 weeks caused reduction from mean baseline concentration of 363 mg/dL to 325 mg/dL *245* In 4 heterogeneous patients with familial LDL-receptor defective hypercholesterolemia treatment with 400 mg/d for 12 weeks caused a significant decrease from mean baseline of 357 ± 29 mg/dL to 301 ± 14 mg/dL *2408* Mean reduction from 8.10 mmol/L to 6.58 mmol/L in 21 patients with type IIa hypercholesterolemia given 400 mg daily for 12 weeks. Further reduction occurred when cholestyramine also added to regime *5449* In patients with type IIb hyperlipoproteinemia treatment with 400 mg/d for 3 months caused significant decrease in concentration *644* 17% reduction in 12 individuals with primary hypercholesterolemia treated with 600 mg daily for 12 weeks *5385* In patients with hyperlipoproteinemia type IIa concentration reduced by 12% with 42 weeks treatment with 400 mg/d sustained-release drug, and by 18% in hyperlipoproteinemia type IIb *566* In 62 hypercholesterolemic patients treatment with up to 1000 mg/d probucol and up to 400 mg/d bezafibrate caused change from mean baseline of 5.77 ± 0.09 mmol/L to 5.50 ± 0.08 mmol/L (significant) at 3 months, 5.47 ± 0.08 mmol/L at 6 months (significant) and 5.26 ± 0.08 mmol/L at 12 months (significant) *5196* Consistent reduction in 16 hyperlipidemic patients following treatment for 2 months with 400 mg daily *4946* In 20 patients with primary hypercholesterolemia treatment with 400 mg/d of bezafibrate retard caused reduction of 6% at 4 weeks, 8% at 6 weeks, 8% at 10 weeks and 7% at 12 weeks *458* In 12 patients with hypertriglyceridemia treatment with 400 mg/d for 8 weeks caused significant decrease (12%) of mean from 7.1 (SEM 0.3) mmol/L to 6.2 (SEM 0.3) *4573* In 32 diet-resistant type IIb hyperlipidemic NIDDM patients treatment with 400 mg/d for 1 month caused mean reduction of 14% *4301*
Serum No Effect Analytical No effect at therapeutic concentration on Boehringer Mannheim Reflotron method *3231* No effect at concentration of 100 mg/L on method on Boehringer Mannheim Reflotron system *5706*
Serum No Effect Physiological In 10 patients with NIDDM and hyperlipidemia treatment with bezafibrate 400 mg/d for 6 months caused no significant change in concentration from 261 ± 37 mg/dL to 248 ± 32 mg/dL *6607* In 24 individuals with mid to moderate hypertriglyceridemia and low HDL-cholesterol concentration treatment with a triglyceride lowering diet and 400 mg bezafibrate per day for 24 weeks caused nonsignificant change from mean baseline of 5.53 ± 0.76 mmol/L to 5.54 ± 0.93 mmol/L *244*

Cholesterol Ester Transfer Protein
Serum Decrease Physiological In 25 patients with hyperlipoproteinemia treatment with 400 mg/d bezafibrate for 12 weeks caused significant reduction from mean baseline of 110.9 ± 36.2 unit to 89.8 ± 35.6 unit *2691*

Cortisol *Plasma No Effect Analytical* At a concentration of 100 mg/L had no significant effect on CEDIA or Enzymun methods (worst case recovery 96.9%) *1097*

C-Peptide *Plasma Decrease Physiological* In one patient with lipoatrophic diabetes mean concentration changed from mean baseline of 1.5 nmol/L to 1.1 nmol/L after 3 months and 0.9 nmol/L after 6 months treatment with 200 mg t.d.s *4499* Reduction of mean baseline concentration from 0.76 nmol/L to 0.66 nmol/L in 20 noninsulin dependent diabetics fed diet and 600 mg bezafibrate daily for 3 months *2970*

Creatine Kinase *Serum Increase Physiological* In four patients with poor renal function produced myolysis as result of overdose due to renal dysfunction *5154*
Serum No Effect Physiological No significant effect observed in 20 noninsulin dependent diabetics fed diet and 600 mg bezafibrate daily for 3 months *2970*

Creatinine *Serum Increase Physiological* Increase from mean baseline concentration of 82 μmol/L to 93 μmol/L in 20 noninsulin dependent diabetics fed diet and 600 mg bezafibrate daily for 3 months *2970* In four patients with poor renal function produced myolysis as result of overdose due to renal dysfunction *5154*
Serum No Effect Physiological In 10 patients with NIDDM and hyperlipidemia treatment with bezafibrate 400 mg/d for 6 months caused no significant change from 0.8 ± 0.29 mg/dL to 1.0 ± 0.34 mg/dL *6607*

D-Dimer *Plasma No Effect Physiological* In 10 patients with NIDDM and hyperlipidemia treatment with 400 mg/d bezafibrate for 6 months had no effect on increased plasma concentration of D-dimer *6607*

Erythrocytes *Blood No Effect Physiological* No significant change in 20 noninsulin dependent diabetics fed diet and 600 mg bezafibrate daily for 3 months *2970*

Euglobulin Lysis Time *Blood No Effect Physiological* In 12 patients with hypertriglyceridemia treatment with 400 mg/d for 8 weeks caused no significant change either before or after venous occlusion *4573*

Fatty Acids (FFA), Free *Serum Decrease Physiological* In one patient with lipoatrophic diabetes mean concentration changed from mean baseline of 2.3 mmol/L to 1.0 mmol/L after 3 months and 0.7 mmol/L after 6 months treatment with 200 mg t.d.s *4499*

Fibrinogen *Plasma Decrease Physiological* In 12 patients with hypertriglyceridemia treatment with 400 mg/d for 8 weeks caused decrease of mean from 310 mg/dL to 250 mg/dL (21%) *4573* In reported studies bezafibrate reduces mean concentration by 17% (up to -43% in hyperfibrinogenemia) *5585* 15 days treatment with 400 mg daily caused marked reduction in 24 patients with atherosclerotic vasculopathy and hyperfibrinogenemia *4300*
Plasma No Effect Physiological In 10 patients with NIDDM and hyperlipidemia treatment with 400 mg/d bezafibrate for 6 months had no effect on increased plasma concentration of fibrinogen *6607*

Fibrinopeptide A *Plasma Decrease Physiological* significant reduction in group of patients with atherosclerotic vasculopathy and hyperfibrinogenemia treated with 400 mg daily for 15 days *4300*

Glucose *Serum Decrease Physiological* In one patient with lipoatrophic diabetes mean concentration changed from mean baseline of 14.0 mmol/L to 4.8 mmol/L after 3 months and 3.9 mmol/L after 6 months treatment with 200 mg t.d.s *4499*
Serum No Effect Analytical No effect at therapeutic concentration on Boehringer Mannheim Reflotron method *3231* At concentration of 100 mg/L had no effect on method on Boehringer Mannheim Reflotron system *5706*
Serum No Effect Physiological In 10 patients with NIDDM and hyperlipidemia treatment with bezafibrate 400 mg/d for 6 months caused no significant change in fasting concentration from 119 ± 31 mg/dL to 122 ± 35 mg/dL *6607* No effect in 16 hyperlipidemic patients when treated for 2 months with 400 mg daily *4946*

Glucose Tolerance *Serum No Effect Physiological* No effect in 16 hyperlipidemic patients when treated with 400 mg daily for 2 months *4946*

γ-Glutamyltransferase *Serum No Effect Analytical* At concentration of 100 mg/L no effect on method on Boehringer Mannheim Reflotron system *5706* No effect at therapeutic concentration on Boehringer Mannheim Reflotron method *3231*

Glycated Hemoglobin *Blood Decrease Physiological* In one patient with lipoatrophic diabetes mean concentration changed from mean baseline of 8.0% to 7.2% after 3 months and 6.0% after 6 months treatment with 200 mg t.d.s *4499*

HDL_2-Cholesterol *Serum No Effect Physiological* In 62 hypercholesterolemic patients treatment with up to 1000 mg/d probucol and up to 400 mg/d bezafibrate caused change from mean baseline of 0.52 ± 0.016 mg/dL to 0.56 ± 0.017 mg/dL (nonsignificant) at 3 months, 0.55 ± 0.019 mg/dL at 6 months (nonsignificant) and 0.56 ± 0.018 mg/dL at 12 months (nonsignificant) *5196* Insignificant reduction observed in 9 patients with type IIa hypercholesterolemia treated with 400 mg daily for 12 weeks *5449* In 25 patients with hyperlipoproteinemia treatment with 400 mg/d bezafibrate for 12 weeks caused nonsignificant change from mean baseline of 15.4 ± 7.1 mg/dL to 15.8 ± 5.2 mg/dL *2691*

HDL_2-Triglycerides *Serum Decrease Physiological* In 25 patients with hyperlipoproteinemia treatment with 400 mg/d bezafibrate for 12 weeks caused significant reduction from mean baseline of 4.0 ± 2.6 mg/dL to 2.4 ± 1.4 mg/dL *2691*

HDL_{2a}-Cholesterol *Serum No Effect Physiological* In 4 heterogeneous patients with familial LDL-receptor defective hypercholesterolemia treatment with 400 mg/d for 12 weeks caused a nonsignificant change from mean baseline proportion of 12.4 ± 5.0% to 9.6 ± 4.2% *2408*

HDL_{2b}-Cholesterol *Serum No Effect Physiological* In 4 heterogeneous patients with familial LDL-receptor defective hypercholesterolemia treatment with 400 mg/d for 12 weeks caused a nonsignificant change from mean baseline proportion of 8.2 ± 2.4% to 7.6 ± 2.7% *2408*

HDL_3-Cholesterol *Serum Increase Physiological* Mean increase from 190 mg/dL to 312 mg/dL in 9 patients with type IIa hypercholesterolemia treated with 400 mg daily for 12 weeks *5449* In 25 patients with hyperlipoproteinemia treatment with 400 mg/d bezafibrate for 12 weeks caused significant increase from mean baseline of 21.7 ± 4.4 mg/dL to 28.9 ± 5.1 mg/dL *2691*
Serum No Effect Physiological In 62 hypercholesterolemic patients treatment with up to 1000 mg/d probucol and up to 400 mg/d bezafibrate caused change from mean baseline of 0.49 ± 0.010 mg/dL to 0.53 ± 0.011 mg/dL (nonsignificant) at 3 months, 0.54 ± 0.012 mg/dL at 6 months (nonsignificant) and 0.50 ± 0.011 mg/dL at 12 months (nonsignificant) *5196*

HDL_3-Triglycerides *Serum Decrease Physiological* In 25 patients with hyperlipoproteinemia treatment with 400 mg/d bezafibrate for 12 weeks caused significant reduction from mean baseline of 6.1 ± 2.5 mg/dL to 4.6 ± 1.8 mg/dL *2691*

HDL_{3a}-Cholesterol *Serum No Effect Physiological* In 4 heterogeneous patients with familial LDL-receptor defective hypercholesterolemia treatment with 400 mg/d for 12 weeks caused a nonsignificant change from mean baseline proportion of 17.9 ± 5.4% to 17.1 ± 4.1% *2408*

HDL_{3b}-Cholesterol *Serum No Effect Physiological* In 4 heterogeneous patients with familial LDL-receptor defective hypercholesterolemia treatment with 400 mg/d for 12 weeks caused a nonsignificant change from mean baseline proportion of 28.5 ± 5.6% to 30.2 ± 7.2% *2408*

HDL_{3c}-Cholesterol *Serum No Effect Physiological* In 4 heterogeneous patients with familial LDL-receptor defective hypercholesterolemia treatment with 400 mg/d for 12 weeks caused a nonsignificant change from mean baseline proportion of 33.0 ± 11.1% to 35.5 ± 11.8% *2408*

HDL-Cholesterol *Serum Decrease Physiological* In one hyperlipidemic man treatment for 2.5 years was associated with a reduction of total cholesterol from 7.8 mmol/L to 5.7 mmol/L and of HDL-cholesterol from 0.7 mmol/L to 0.1 mmol/L *4404*
Serum Increase Physiological In patients with hyperlipoproteinemia type IIb treatment with 400 mg/d for 3 months increased concentration significantly *644* Increase by 13% in 11 hypertriglyceridemic subjects *5500* In 4 heterogeneous patients with familial LDL-receptor defective hypercholesterolemia treatment with 400 mg/d for 12 weeks caused a nonsignificant increase from mean baseline of 47 ± 8 mg/dL to 61 ± 12 mg/dL *2408* Mean increase from 1.35 mmol/L to 1.65 mmol/L in 21 patients with type IIa hypercholesterolemia when treated for 12 weeks with 400 mg daily. No further reduction when cholestyramine added to regime *5449* Significant effect in 12 individuals with primary hypercholesterolemia when treated with 600 mg daily for 12 weeks *5385* In 12 patients with hypertriglyceridemia treatment with 400 mg/d for 8 weeks caused significant increase (20%) from 1.1 (SEM 0.1) mmol/L to 1.3 (SEM 0.1) mmol/L *4573* Increase by 21% in 7 hypertriglyceridemic type 2 diabetic patients given 200 mg tid after 1 mo treatment *5690* In 32 diet-resistant type IIb hyperlipidemic NIDDM patients treatment with 400 mg/d for 1 month caused mean 19% increase *4301* In the Bezafibrate Coronary Atherosclerosis Intervention Trial of 42 patients treatment with bezafibrate caused mean increase of 9% *3115* Mean increase of 35% observed in 6 patients with hypercholesterolemia treated with 600 mg/d for 12 weeks *4216* In 10 patients with NIDDM and hyperlipidemia treatment with bezafibrate 400 mg/d for 6 months caused no significant change in concentration from 52 ± 14 mg/dL to 62 ± 7 mg/dL *6607* In one patient with lipoatrophic diabetes mean concentration changed from mean baseline of 0.3 mmol/L to 0.5 mmol/L after 3 months and 0.6 mmol/L after 6 months treatment with 200 mg t.d.s *4499* Bezafibrate is more effective than gemfibrozil in increasing HDL-cholesterol concentrations *3668* In 24 individuals with mid to moderate hypertriglyceridemia and low HDL-cholesterol concentration treatment with a triglyceride lowering diet and 400 mg bezafibrate per day for 24 weeks caused significant increase from mean baseline of 0.75 ± 0.11 mmol/L to 0.92 ± 0.18 mmol/L *244* In 38 patients with primary hypercholesterolemia types IIa or IIb treatment with 400 mg/d for 12 weeks caused mean increase of 9% *245* Increased apo A-I and apo A-II synthesis. Increased activity of lipoprotein lipase by stimulation of muscle lipoprotein lipase synthesis, alteration of the capillary endothelial surface and stimulation of apo C-II synthesis *264* In 25 patients with hyperlipoproteinemia treatment with 400 mg/d bezafibrate for 12 weeks caused significant increase from mean baseline of 41.8 ± 12.1 mg/dL to 52.6 ± 12.6 mg/dL *2691* Increase from mean baseline of 1.2 mmol/L in 20 noninsulin dependent diabetics fed diet and 600 mg bezafibrate daily to 1.3 mmol/L at 1, 2 and 3 months *2970* 6 months treatment of 17 patients with type IV hyperlipoproteinemia with 400 mg/day caused increase of 34% *3081* In 20 patients with primary hypercholesterolemia treatment with 400 mg bezafibrate retard daily caused mean increase of 19% at 4 weeks, 14% at 6 weeks, 18% at 10 weeks and 20% at 12 weeks *458*
Serum No Effect Analytical At a concentration up to 100 mg/L had no significant effect on Reflotron method for whole blood cholesterol *6352*
Serum No Effect Physiological In 62 hypercholesterolemic patients treatment with up to 1000 mg/d probucol and up to 400 mg/d bezafibrate caused change from mean baseline of 0.99 ± 0.021 mg/dL to 1.00 ± 0.021 mg/dL (nonsignificant) at 3 months, 1.08 ± 0.024 mg/dL at 6 months (nonsignificant) and 1.05 ± 0.022 mg/dL at 12 months (nonsignificant) *5196*

HDL-Phospholipids *Serum Increase Physiological* In 32 diet-resistant type IIb hyperlipidemic NIDDM patients treatment with 400 mg/d for 1 month caused mean 18% increase *4301* In 62 hypercholesterolemic patients treatment with up to 1000 mg/d probucol and up to 400 mg/d bezafibrate caused change from mean baseline of 1.03 ± 0.021 mg/dL to 1.13 ± 0.022 mg/dL (significant) at 3 months, 1.18 ± 0.024 mg/dL at 6 months (significant) and 1.12 ± 0.023 mg/dL at 12 months

Bezafibrate *(continued)*

HDL-Phospholipids *(continued)*
(nonsignificant) *5196* 6 months treatment of 17 patients with type IV hyperlipoproteinemia with 400 mg/day caused increase of 15% *3081*

HDL-Triglycerides *Serum Decrease Physiological* 6 months treatment of 17 patients with type IV hyperlipoproteinemia caused decrease of 22% *3081* In 62 hypercholesterolemic patients treatment with up to 1000 mg/d probucol and up to 400 mg/d bezafibrate caused change from mean baseline of 0.21 ± 0.005 mg/dL to 0.18 ± 0.005 mg/dL (significant) at 3 months, 0.19 ± 0.006 mg/dL at 6 months (significant) and 0.19 ± 0.005 mg/dL at 12 months (significant) *5196*
Serum Increase Physiological In 32 diet-resistant type IIb hyperlipidemic NIDDM patients treatment with 400 mg/d for 1 month caused mean 49% *4301*

Hemoglobin A_{1c} *Blood No Effect Physiological* In 10 patients with NIDDM and hyperlipidemia treatment with bezafibrate 400 mg/d for 6 months caused no significant change from 6.9 ± 0.93% to 7.1 ± 0.80% *6607* No significant effect observed in 20 noninsulin dependent diabetics fed diet and 600 mg bezafibrate daily for 3 months *2970*

IDL-Cholesterol *Serum Decrease Physiological* In 25 patients with hyperlipoproteinemia treatment with 400 mg/d bezafibrate for 12 weeks caused significant reduction from mean baseline of 15.3 ± 5.9 mg/dL to 9.1 ± 4.7 mg/dL *2691*

IDL-Triglycerides *Serum Decrease Physiological* In 25 patients with hyperlipoproteinemia treatment with 400 mg/d bezafibrate for 12 weeks caused significant reduction from mean baseline of 19.7 ± 9.4 mg/dL to 12.6 ± 7.3 mg/dL *2691*

Insulin *Plasma Decrease Physiological* In 10 patients with NIDDM and hyperlipidemia treatment with bezafibrate 400 mg/d for 6 months caused significant change in concentration from mean of 7.1 µunitsmL to 6.0 µU/mL *6607* In one patient with lipoatrophic diabetes mean concentration changed from mean baseline of 164 pmol/L to 203 pmol/L after 3 months and 125 pmol/L after 6 months treatment with 200 mg t.d.s *4499* Reduction of fasting concentration from mean baseline of 10.1 mU/L to 7.2 mU/L in 20 noninsulin dependent diabetics fed diet and 600 mg bezafibrate daily for 3 months *2970*
Plasma Increase Physiological In one patient with lipoatrophic diabetes mean concentration changed from mean baseline of 164 pmol/L to 203 pmol/L after 3 months and 125 pmol/L after 6 months treatment with 200 mg t.d.s *4499*
Plasma No Effect Physiological No effect in 16 hyperlipidemic patients when treated with 400 mg daily for 2 months *4946*

LDL_1-Cholesterol *Serum No Effect Physiological* In 25 patients with hyperlipoproteinemia treatment with 400 mg/d bezafibrate for 12 weeks caused nonsignificant increase from mean baseline of 78.1 ± 38.5 mg/dL to 89.4 ± 20.9 mg/dL *2691*

LDL_1-Triglycerides *Serum No Effect Physiological* In 25 patients with hyperlipoproteinemia treatment with 400 mg/d bezafibrate for 12 weeks caused nonsignificant increase from mean baseline of 16.2 ± 7.1 mg/dL to 17.2 ± 5.1 mg/dL *2691*

LDL_2-Cholesterol *Serum Decrease Physiological* In 25 patients with hyperlipoproteinemia treatment with 400 mg/d bezafibrate for 12 weeks caused significant reduction from mean baseline of 40.1 ± 13.5 mg/dL to 19.8 ± 8.8 mg/dL *2691*

LDL_2-Triglycerides *Serum Decrease Physiological* In 25 patients with hyperlipoproteinemia treatment with 400 mg/d bezafibrate for 12 weeks caused significant reduction from mean baseline of 6.1 ± 2.6 mg/dL to 2.3 ± 5.4 mg/dL *2691*

LDL-Cholesterol *Serum Decrease Physiological* Treatment of 20 patients with primary hypercholesterolemia with 400 mg bezafibrate retard daily caused mean reduction of 7% at 4 weeks, 8% at 6 weeks, 9% at 10 weeks and 8% at 12 weeks *458* In 32 diet-resistant type IIb hyperlipidemic NIDDM patients treatment with 400 mg/d caused mean 12% reduction *4301* In 12 patients with hypertriglyceridemia treatment with 400 mg/d for 8 weeks caused nonsignificant decrease (7%) from mean of 4.2 (SEM 0.3) mmol/L to 3.9 (SEM 0.3) mmol/L *4573* Mean reduction of 35% in 6 patients with hypercholesterolemia treated with 600 mg/d for 12 weeks *4216* In 38 patients with primary hypercholesterolemia types IIa and IIb the LDL-cholesterol concentration declined to 190 mg/dL or less with 4 wk treatment with 400 mg/d. Treatment for 12 wk caused decrease in all patients from mean of 284 mg/dL to 242 mg/dL *245* In one patient with familial hypercholesterolemia treated with diet and 400 mg/d bezafibrate for at least 3 months concentration decreased from 6.8 to 4.5 mmol/L *6405* 20% reduction in 12 individuals with primary hypercholesterolemia treated with 600 mg daily for 12 weeks *5385* Bezafibrate is more effective than gemfibrozil in decreasing LDL-cholesterol concentrations *3668* Reduction from mean baseline of 4.2 mmol/L in 20 noninsulin dependent diabetics given diet and 600 mg bezafibrate daily to 3.6 mmol/L at 1 month, 3.7 mmol/L at 2 months and 3.5 mmol/L at 3 months *2970* Mean reduction from 5.91 mmol/L to 4.44 mmol/L in 21 patients with type IIa hypercholesterolemia following 12 weeks treatment with 400 mg daily. Further reduction obtained when cholestyramine added to regime *5449* In 4 heterogeneous patients with familial LDL-receptor defective hypercholesterolemia treatment with 400 mg/d for 12 weeks caused a significant decrease from mean baseline of 295 ± 34 mg/dL to 231 ± 18 mg/dL *2408*
Serum Increase Physiological Increase by 16% in 7 hypertriglyceridemic type 2 diabetic patients given 200 mg t.i.d. after 1 mo treatment *5690*
Serum No Effect Physiological In 62 hypercholesterolemic patients treatment with up to 1000 mg/d probucol and up to 400 mg/d bezafibrate caused change from mean baseline of 4.15 ± 0.076 mg/dL to 4.04 ± 0.079 mg/dL (nonsignificant) at 3 months, 4.12 ± 0.088 mg/dL at 6 months (nonsignificant) and 3.94 ± 0.083 mg/dL at 12 months (nonsignificant) *5196* 6 months treatment of 17 patients with type IV hyperlipoproteinemia with 400 mg daily had no effect on concentration *3081* In 10 patients with NIDDM and hyperlipidemia treatment with bezafibrate 400 mg/d for 6 months caused no significant change in concentration from 177 ± 36 mg/dL to 167 ± 32 mg/dL *6607*

LDL-Phospholipids *Serum Increase Physiological* In 32 diet-resistant type IIb hyperlipidemic NIDDM patients treatment with 400 mg/d for 1 month caused mean 25% increase *4301*
Serum No Effect Physiological 6 months treatment of 17 patients with type IV hyperlipoproteinemia with 400 mg daily had no effect on concentration *3081* In 62 hypercholesterolemic patients treatment with up to 1000 mg/d probucol and up to 400 mg/d bezafibrate caused change from mean baseline of 1.34 ± 0.027 mg/dL to 1.39 ± 0.028 mg/dL (nonsignificant) at 3 months, 1.39 ± 0.032 mg/dL at 6 months (nonsignificant) and 1.30 ± 0.030 mg/dL at 12 months (nonsignificant) *5196*

LDL-Triglycerides *Serum Decrease Physiological* 6 months treatment of 17 patients with type IV hyperlipoproteinemia with 400 mg/day caused decrease of 23% *3081*
Serum Increase Physiological In 32 diet-resistant type iib hyperlipidemic NIDDM patients treatment with 400 mg/d for 1 month caused mean 10% increase *4301*
Serum No Effect Physiological In 62 hypercholesterolemic patients treatment with up to 1000 mg/d probucol and up to 400 mg/d bezafibrate caused change from mean baseline of 0.50 ± 0.020 mg/dL to 0.52 ± 0.021 mg/dL (nonsignificant) at 3 months, 0.57 ± 0.023 mg/dL at 6 months (nonsignificant) and 0.55 ± 0.022 mg/dL at 12 months (nonsignificant) *5196*

Lecithin:Cholesterol Acyltransferase
Serum Decrease Physiological In 25 patients with hyperlipoproteinemia treatment with 400 mg/d bezafibrate for 12 weeks caused significant reduction from mean baseline of 120.4 ± 23.9 nmol/mL/h to 93.0 ± 21.6 nmol/mL/h *2691* In 62 hypercholesterolemic patients treatment with up to 1000 mg/d probucol and up to 400 mg/d bezafibrate caused change from mean baseline of 97.0 ± 1.6 nmol/mL/h to 84.1 ± 1.6 nmol/mL/h (significant) at 3 months, 75.7 ± 1.8 nmol/mL/h at 6 months (significant) and 75.7 ± 1.7 nmol/mL/h at 12 months (significant) *5196*

Leukocytes *Blood No Effect Physiological* No significant effect observed in 20 noninsulin dependent diabetics fed diet and 600 mg bezafibrate daily for 3 months *2970*

Lipase, Hepatic *Serum Increase Physiological* In 24 individuals with mid to moderate hypertriglyceridemia and low HDL-cholesterol concentration treatment with a triglyceride lowering diet and 400 mg bezafibrate per day for 24 weeks caused significant increase from mean baseline of 12.99 ± 5.51 U/mL to 15.18 ± 6.8 U/mL *244*

Lipoprotein Lp(a) *Serum Decrease Physiological* In patients with hyperlipoproteinemias and plasma Lp(a) concentration above 30 mg/dL treatment with 400 mg/d sustained-release bezafibrate for 24 weeks caused reduction by 39% *566* In 62 hypercholesterolemic patients treatment with up to 1000 mg/d probucol and up to 400 mg/d bezafibrate caused change from mean baseline of 29 ± 1 mg/dL to 30 ± 1 mg/dL (nonsignificant) at 3 months, 27 ± 1 mg/dL at 6 months (significant) and 25 ± 1 mg/dL at 12 months (significant) *5196*
Serum No Effect Physiological In 12 patients with hypertriglyceridemia treatment with 400 mg/d for 8 weeks caused no significant change from mean baseline of 20.6 (SEM 10.3) mg/dL to 22.8 (SEM 11.5) mg/dL *4573*

Mevalonate *Urine No Effect Physiological* No significant change observed in 20 patients with primary hypercholesterolemia treated with 400 mg bezafibrate retard daily for up to 12 weeks *458*

Myoglobin *Serum Increase Physiological* In four patients with poor renal function produced myolysis as result of overdose due to renal dysfunction *5154*
Urine Increase Physiological In four patients with poor renal function produced myolysis as result of overdose due to renal dysfunction *5154*

N-Acetyl-Glucosaminidase *Urine No Effect Analytical* At concentration of 120 mg/dL had no significant effect on Boehringer Mannheim CPR method *3174*

Phospholipids *Serum Increase Physiological* In 32 diet-resistant type IIb hyperlipidemic NIDDM patients treatment with 400 mg/d for 1 month caused mean 7% increase *4301*
Serum No Effect Physiological In 62 hypercholesterolemic patients treatment with up to 1000 mg/d probucol and up to 400 mg/d bezafibrate caused change from mean baseline of 2.73 ± 0.03 mmol/L to 2.80 ± 0.03 mmol/L (nonsignificant) at 3 months, 2.82 ± 0.04 mmol/L at 6 months (nonsignificant) and 2.72 ± 0.03 mmol/L at 12 months (nonsignificant) *5196*

Plasminogen Activator Inhibitor-1
Plasma No Effect Physiological In 10 patients with NIDDM and hyperlipidemia treatment with 400 mg/d bezafibrate for 6 months had no effect on increased plasma concentration of PAI-1 *6607*

Plasminogen Activator Inhibitor-1 Activity
Plasma No Effect Physiological In 12 patients with hypertriglyceridemia treatment with 400 mg/d for 8 weeks caused insignificant increase from mean 16.7 (SEM 1.6) U/mL to 27.3 (SEM 3.2) U/mL *4573*

Plasminogen Activator Inhibitor-1 Antigen
Plasma No Effect Physiological In 12 patients with hypertriglyceridemia treatment with 400 mg/d for 8 weeks caused insignificant increase from mean of 15.2 (SEM 2.6) ng/mL to 24.0 (SEM 2.6) ng/mL *4573*

Platelet Factor 4 *Plasma Decrease Physiological* Marked reduction with 15 days treatment with 400 mg/day in 23 patients with atherosclerotic vasculopathy and hyperfibrinogenemia *4300*

Platelets *Blood No Effect Physiological* No significant effect in 20 noninsulin dependent diabetics fed diet and 600 mg bezafibrate daily for 3 months *2970*

Postheparin Lipoprotein Lipase
Plasma Increase Physiological In 24 individuals with mid to moderate hypertriglyceridemia and low HDL-cholesterol concentration treatment with a triglyceride lowering diet and 400 mg bezafibrate per day for 24 weeks caused significant increase from mean baseline of 3.39 ± 1.49 U/mL to 5.37 ± 1.81 U/mL *244*

Potassium *Serum No Effect Physiological* No significant effect observed in 20 noninsulin dependent diabetics fed diet and 600 mg bezafibrate daily for 3 months *2970*

Prothrombin Time *Plasma Decrease Physiological* In 10 patients with NIDDM and hyperlipidemia treatment with bezafibrate 400 mg/d for 6 months reduced increased fluorescent prothrombin time to control value *6607*

Sodium *Serum No Effect Physiological* No significant effect observed in 20 noninsulin dependent diabetics fed diet and 600 mg bezafibrate daily for 3 months *2970*

β-Thromboglobulin *Plasma Decrease Physiological* Significant decrease observed with treatment for 15 days with 400 mg/day in group of patients with atherosclerotic vasculopathy and hyperfibrinogenemia *4300*

Tissue Plasminogen Activator Antigen
Plasma No Effect Physiological In 12 patients with hypertriglyceridemia treated with 400 mg/d for 8 weeks caused no change in concentration before venous occlusion and insignificant reduction from 36.5 (SEM 7.7) ng/mL to 26.0 (SEM 2.7) ng/mL after venous occlusion *4573*

Triglycerides *Serum Decrease Physiological* 6 months treatment of 17 patients with type IV hyperlipoproteinemia caused reduction of 43% *3081* Treatment of 20 patients with primary hypercholesterolemia with 400 mg bezafibrate retard daily produced mean decrease of 26% at 4 weeks, 27% at 6 weeks, 30% at 10 weeks and 27% at 12 weeks *458* In 38 patients with types IIa or IIb primary hypercholesterolemia treatment with 40 mg/d for 12 weeks caused decrease from mean baseline concentration of 173 mg/dL to 121 mg/dL *245* In the Bezafibrate Coronary Atherosclerosis Intervention Trial of 42 patients treatment with bezafibrate caused mean decrease of 35% *3115* By average of 58% in 11 hypertriglyceridemic subjects *5500* In 4 heterogeneous patients with familial LDL-receptor defective hypercholesterolemia treatment with 400 mg/d for 12 weeks caused a nonsignificant decrease from mean baseline of 130 ± 70 mg/dL to 87 ± 42 mg/dL *2408* Mean reduction from 2.08 mmol/L to 1.19 mmol/L in 21 patients with type IIa hypercholesterolemia when treated with 400 mg daily for 12 weeks. No further reduction when cholestyramine added to regime *5449* Reduction of mean concentration at baseline of 2.2 mmol/L to 1.7 mmol/L at 1 month, 1.7 mmol/L at 2 months and 1.4 mmol/L at 3 months in 20 noninsulin dependent diabetics given diet and 600 mg bezafibrate daily *2970* 26% reduction in 12 individuals with primary hypercholesterolemia treated with 600 mg daily for 12 weeks *5385* In patients with hyperlipoproteinemia type IIb treatment with 400 mg/d for 3 months caused significant decrease in concentration *644* Mean reduction of 41% observed in 6 patients with hypercholesterolemia treated with 600 mg/d for 12 weeks *4216* In 32 diet-resistant type IIb hyperlipidemic NIDDM patients with 400 mg/d for 1 month caused mean 37% reduction *4301* In 12 patients with hypertriglyceridemia treatment with 400 mg/d for 8 weeks caused significant decrease (45%) of mean from 4.0 (SEM 0.8) mmol/L to 2.2 (SEM 0.4) mmol/L *4573* After 2 months treatment in 16 hyperlipidemic patients with 400 mg daily overall reduction by 46% *4946* In patients with hyperlipoproteinemia type IV plasma triglyceride concentration reduced by 26% with 24 weeks treatment with 400 mg/d sustained-release bezafibrate *566* In 24 individuals with mid to moderate hypertriglyceridemia and low HDL-cholesterol concentration treatment with a triglyceride lowering diet and 400 mg bezafibrate per day for 24 weeks caused significant reduction from mean baseline of 3.56 ± 1.46 mmol/L to 1.84 ± 0.59 mmol/L *244* In 25 patients with hyperlipoproteinemia treatment with 400 mg/d bezafibrate for 12 weeks caused significant reduction from mean baseline of 231.4 ± 130.3 mg/dL to 100.1 ± 49.1 mg/dL *2691* Increase by 54% in 7 hypertriglyceridemic type 2 diabetic patients given 200 mg tid after 1 mo treatment *5690* In 62 hypercholesterolemic patients treatment with up to 1000 mg/d probucol and up to 400 mg/d bezafibrate caused change from mean baseline of 1.49 ± 0.05 mmol/L to 1.13 ± 0.05 mmol/L (significant) at 3 months, 1.21 ± 0.06 mmol/L at 6 months (significant) and 1.15 ± 0.05 mmol/L at 12 months (significant) *5196* Bezafibrate is effective in decreasing triglyceride concentrations *3668* In one patient with lipoatrophic diabetes mean concentration changed from mean baseline of 11.1 mmol/L to 5.1 mmol/L after 3 months and 2.6 mmol/L after 6 months treatment with 200 mg t.d.s *4499* In 10 patients with NIDDM and hyperlipidemia treatment with bezafibrate 400 mg/d for 6 months caused significant change in concentration from 175 ± 144 mg/dL to 96 ± 41 mg/dL *6607*
Serum No Effect Analytical No effect at 100 mg/L on Boehringer Mannheim Reflotron method *5706* No effect at therapeutic concentration on Boehringer Mannheim Reflotron method *3231*
Serum No Effect Physiological In the Bezafibrate Coronary Atherosclerosis Intervention Trial of 42 patients treatment with bezafibrate caused nonsignificant mean decrease of 2% *3115* In one hyperlipidemic man treatment for 2.5 years was associated with a paradoxical reduction of total cholesterol and HDL-cholesterol concentrations but no effect observed on triglyceride concentration *4404*

Bezafibrate *(continued)*

Urea Nitrogen *Serum Increase Physiological* Increase of urea from mean baseline of 5.7 mmol/L to 7.0 mmol/L at 3 months in 20 noninsulin dependent diabetics fed diet and 600 mg bezafibrate daily *2970*
Serum No Effect Analytical No effect at 100 mg/L on Boehringer Mannheim Reflotron method *5706* No effect at therapeutic concentration on Boehringer Mannheim Reflotron method *3231*

Uric Acid *Serum No Effect Analytical* No effect at 100 mg/L on method on Boehringer Mannheim Reflotron *5706* No effect at therapeutic concentration on Boehringer Mannheim Reflotron method *3231*
Serum No Effect Physiological No significant effect in 20 noninsulin dependent diabetics fed diet and 600 mg bezafibrate daily for 3 months *2970*

VLDL-Apolipoprotein B *Serum Decrease Physiological* Residence time in plasma fell from 3.4 to 1.0 h *5500*

VLDL-Cholesterol *Serum Decrease Physiological* In 12 patients with hypertriglyceridemia treatment with 400 mg/d for 8 weeks caused significant decrease (43%) from mean of 1.8 (SEM 0.3) mmol/L to 1.0 (SEM 0.2) mmol/L *4573* In 32 diet-resistant type IIb hyperlipidemic NIDDM patients treatment with 400 mg/d for 1 month caused mean 37% *4301* Consistent reduction in 16 hyperlipidemic patients following 2 months treatment with 400 mg daily *4946* 6 months treatment of 17 patients with type IV hyperlipoproteinemia caused reduction of 54% *3081* In 62 hypercholesterolemic patients treatment with up to 1000 mg/d probucol and up to 400 mg/d bezafibrate caused change from mean baseline of 0.59 ± 0.026 mg/dL to 0.43 ± 0.027 mg/dL (significant) at 3 months, 0.37 ± 0.030 mg/dL at 6 months (significant) and 0.46 ± 0.028 mg/dL at 12 months (significant) *5196* In 25 patients with hyperlipoproteinemia treatment with 400 mg/d bezafibrate for 12 weeks caused significant reduction from mean baseline of 29.7 ± 20.1 mg/dL to 7.3 ± 6.0 mg/dL *2691* Mean reduction from 0.85 mmol/L to 0.50 mmol/L in 21 patients with type IIa hypercholesterolemia following treatment for 12 weeks with 400 mg daily. No further reduction when cholestyramine added to regime *5449* 44% reduction in 12 individuals with primary hypercholesterolemia treated with 600 mg daily for 12 weeks *5385*

VLDL-Phospholipids *Serum Decrease Physiological* 6 months treatment of 17 patients with type IV hyperlipoproteinemia with 400 mg/day caused reduction of 45% *3081* In 62 hypercholesterolemic patients treatment with up to 1000 mg/d probucol and up to 400 mg/d bezafibrate caused change from mean baseline of 0.35 ± 0.018 mg/dL to 0.26 ± 0.019 mg/dL (significant) at 3 months, 0.25 ± 0.021 mg/dL at 6 months (significant) and 0.30 ± 0.020 mg/dL at 12 months (significant) *5196* In 32 diet-resistant type IIb hyperlipidemic NIDDM treatment with 400 mg/d for 1 month caused mean 25% decrease *4301*

VLDL-Remnant Apolipoprotein B
Serum Increase Physiological Metabolism little effect but plasma concentration rose 30% *5500*

VLDL-Triglycerides *Serum Decrease Physiological* In 25 patients with hyperlipoproteinemia treatment with 400 mg/d bezafibrate for 12 weeks caused significant reduction from mean baseline of 133.5 ± 120.8 mg/dL to 33.8 ± 27.1 mg/dL *2691* In 62 hypercholesterolemic patients treatment with up to 1000 mg/d probucol and up to 400 mg/d bezafibrate caused change from mean baseline of 0.81 ± 0.038 mg/dL to 0.51 ± 0.040 mg/dL (significant) at 3 months, 0.56 ± 0.044 mg/dL at 6 months (significant) and 0.55 ± 0.042 mg/dL at 12 months (significant) *5196* Reduction by 50% in 16 hyperlipidemic patients after 2 months treatment with 400 mg daily *4946* 6 months treatment of 17 patients with type IV hyperlipoproteinemia caused reduction of 39%, largely responsible for decrease of plasma total triglycerides *3081* In 32 diet-resistant type IIb hyperlipidemic NIDDM patients treatment with 400 mg/d for 1 month caused mean 56% reduction *4301*

Bicalutamide

Alanine Aminotransferase *Serum Increase Physiological* Increased activity has been reported as an adverse event *6643*

Alkaline Phosphatase *Serum Increase Physiological* Increased activity has been reported as an adverse event *6643*

Aspartate Aminotransferase *Serum Increase Physiological* Increased activity has been reported as an adverse event *6643*

Bilirubin *Serum Increase Physiological* Rarely jaundice has been reported as an adverse event *6643*

Blood *Urine Increase Physiological* Increased concentration has been reported as an adverse event *6643*

Creatinine *Serum Increase Physiological* Increased concentration has been reported as an adverse event *6643*

Glucose *Serum Increase Physiological* Hyperglycemia has been reported as an adverse event in 20 of 401 (5%) of patients treated with bicalutamide with an LHRH analogue *6643*
Urine Increase Physiological Hematuria has been reported as an adverse event in 30 of 401 (7%) of patients treated with bicalutamide with an LHRH analogue *6643*

Hematocrit *Blood Decrease Physiological* Anemia has been reported as an adverse event in 29 of 401 (7%) of patients treated with bicalutamide with an LHRH analogue *6643*

Hemoglobin *Blood Decrease Physiological* Anemia has been reported as an adverse event in 29 of 401 (7%) of patients treated with bicalutamide with an LHRH analogue *6643*

Leukocytes *Blood Decrease Physiological* Leukopenia has been reported as an adverse event *6643*

Occult Blood *Feces Increase Physiological* Rectal bleeding has been reported as an adverse event in 2 to 5% of all treated patients *6643*

Bicarbonate

Acid Phosphatase *Serum No Effect Analytical* No interference observed at a concentration of 40 mmol/L with method on Kodak Ektachem® *2519*

Albumin *Serum No Effect Analytical* No significant effect observed at a concentration of 40 mmol/L with method on Kodak Ektachem® systems *2519* At concentration of 40 mmol/L had no effect on Kodak Ektachem® method *5706*

Bicarbonate *Serum Increase Physiological* Induces metabolic alkalosis *1009*

Bilirubin, Conjugated *Serum No Effect Analytical* At a concentration of 40 mmol/L has no significant effect on method on Kodak Ektachem® systems *2519*

Bilirubin, Unconjugated *Serum No Effect Analytical* No significant effect observed at a concentration of 40 mmol/L with method on Kodak Ektachem® systems *2519*

Calcium *Urine Decrease Physiological* Protects skeleton from reabsorption of PO_4*394*

Chloride *Serum Decrease Analytical* Chloride underestimation on Hitachi 717 = (0.3008 x bicarbonate) - 6.98 mmol/L due to inadequate selectivity for chloride over bicarbonate *1812*
Serum Decrease Physiological Induces metabolic alkalosis *1009*

Cholinesterase *Serum No Effect Analytical* At a concentration of 35 mmol/L has no significant effect on method on Kodak Ektachem® systems *2519* No effect observed at concentrations up to 35 mmol/L with butyrylthiocholine method on Kodak Ektachem® *2504*

Creatinine *Serum No Effect Analytical* At a concentration of 40 mmol/L has no significant effect on either single-slide or dual-slide methods on Kodak Ektachem® systems *2519*

Ethanol *Serum No Effect Analytical* At a concetration of 40 mmol/L had no significant effect on method on Kodak Ektachem® *2519*

γ-Glutamyltransferase *Serum No Effect Analytical* No effect of concentrations up to 40 mmol/L on method on Kodak Ektachem® *5706* At a concentration of 40 mmol/L causes no significant effect on method on Kodak Ektachem® systems *2519*

Iron *Serum No Effect Analytical* No significant effect observed at a concentration of 40 mmol/L with method on Kodak Ektachem® systems *2519* No effect of concentrations up to 38 mmol/L on method on Kodak Ektachem® *5706*

Iron-Binding Capacity, Total *Serum No Effect Analytical* No significant effect observed at a concentration of 40 mmol/L with method on Kodak Ektachem® systems *2519*

Lactate *Plasma Increase Physiological* Intravenous infusion, by altering acid-base balance, may cause increased con-

centration *1531* Small effect after i.v. sodium bicarbonate *2452*
Plasma No Effect Analytical No significant effect observed at a concentration of 40 mmol/L with method on Kodak Ektachem® systems *2519*

Lipase *Serum No Effect Analytical* No significant effect observed at a concentration of 40 mmol/L with method on Kodak Ektachem® systems *2519* No effect of concentrations up to 40 mmol/L on method on Kodak Ektachem® *5706*

Lithium *Serum No Effect Analytical* At a concentration of 40 mmol/L has no effect on method on Kodak Ektachem® systems *2519*

Magnesium *Serum Increase Analytical* In specimens run on the BM/Hitachi 747 analyzer if a bicarbonate specimen was run immediately preceding a magnesium specimen carryover reagent I which contains magnesium acetate caused increase of as much as 20% observed. Problem can be avoided by reconfiguring the chemistries so they do not share the same probe/cuvette *1430*
Serum No Effect Analytical At a concentration of 40 mmol/L had no significant effect on method on Kodak Ektachem® systems *2519* No effect of concentrations up to 40 mmol/L on method on Kodak Ektachem® *5706*

Phosphate *Urine Increase Physiological* Possible competition for same excretory mechanism *1504*

Potassium *Serum Decrease Physiological* Induces metabolic alkalosis *1009*

Protein *Cerebrospinal Fluid No Effect Analytical* No significant observed at a concentration of 40 mmol/L with method on Kodak Ektachem® systems *2519*
Urine Increase Analytical Highly alkaline urine causes false positive *2452*

Pyruvate *Plasma Increase Physiological* By altering acid-base balance intravenous infusion may cause increased concentration *1531*

Salicylate *Serum No Effect Analytical* No significant effect observed at a concentration of 40 mol/L with method on Kodak Ektachem® systems *2519*

Sodium *Serum Decrease Analytical* Concentrations above 30 mmol/L decrease results as determined by method on Kodak Ektachem® *5706*
Serum Decrease Physiological In specimens with high bicarbonate concentrations sodium concentration decreased when measured by direct potentiometry, e.g. concentration by Kone Microlyte 122 mmol/L compared with 133 mmol/L on Baxter Paramax (indirect potentiometry) and 132 mmol/L by flame photometry on Technicon SMA II *4510*
Serum Increase Physiological Induces metabolic alkalosis *1009*

Urea Nitrogen *Serum Increase Analytical* At a concentration of 40 mmol/L causes positive bias of 1.8 mg/dL at urea nitrogen concentration of 27 mg/dL with method on Kodak Ektachem® systems *2519*
Serum No Effect Analytical At concentrations up to 40 mmol/L had no effect on method on Kodak Ektachem® *5706*

Bicine

Protein *Test Conditions Decrease Analytical* Lowry procedure ?non linear absorption *2936*

Bile Acid-binding Resins

LDL-Receptor Activity *Tissue Increase Physiological* Increased activity observed with bile acid binding resin administration *3730*

BIM 23014

GH response to GHRH *Plasma Decrease Physiological* 250 µg subcutaneously significantly reduced GHRH-induced response. Normal response up to 20 µg/L blunted to 8 µg/L *5285*

Glucagon *Plasma No Effect Physiological* During subcutaneous infusion in 8 healthy men no significant changes observed *3319*

Glucose *Serum Increase Physiological* In 8 healthy men administration of 3000 µg/d (also seen with lower doses) by subcutaneous injection caused significant increase after 2 hours *3319*

Growth Hormone *Plasma Decrease Physiological* Continuous subcutaneous administration for 24 hours caused marked reduction to 1.7 ± 0.2 µg/L after 1000 µg, 1.3 ± 0.1 µg/L after 2000 µg and 1.2 ± 0.1 µg/L after 3000 µg *3319* When given subcutaneously to normal men at 8 pm concentration decreased during first part of night but only after 500 µg given *5285* In 8 healthy individuals infusion of BIM 23014 caused peak concentrations during day to be reduced and plasma concentrations were lower than 5 µg/L *3319*

Insulin *Plasma No Effect Physiological* During infusion of 3000 µg/d BIM 23014 in 8 healthy individuals no significant effect observed *3319*

Motilin *Plasma Decrease Physiological* When given subcutaneously to 8 normal young men concentration decreased after doses of 250 and 500 µg but not after lower dose *5285*

Pancreatic Polypeptide *Plasma Decrease Physiological* Concentration decreased in 8 healthy young men after doses of 125 µg or more when given subcutaneously *5285*

Secretin *Plasma Decrease Physiological* When given in dose of up to 500 µg subcutaneously to 8 normal young men had no effect on concentration *5285*

Thyroid Stimulating Hormone
Serum No Effect Physiological Subcutaneous infusion of 2 mg during 12 nighttime hours had no effect on concentration in contrast to effect of placebo which caused increase in all men after 9 p.m *5285*

Biotin

Estradiol *Plasma No Effect Analytical* Negligible interference (less than 15%) observed with method on Boehringer Mannheim ES 300 at a concentration up to 300 ng/dL *2343*

Ferritin *Serum No Effect Analytical* No significant interference observed with BoehringerMannheim ES 300 Enzymun-Test kit method *6402*

Thyroid Stimulating Hormone *Serum No Effect Analytical* No interference observed up to a concentration of 30 ng/mL with Boehringer Mannheim ES 300 method *1937* No significant interference observed at concentrations up to 30 ng/mL with method on Boehringer Mannheim Elecsys analyzer *3268*

Thyroxine (T4), Free *Serum No Effect Analytical* No significant interference observed with method for free T4 on Boehringer Mannheim Elecsys immunoassay system *1652*

Tri-iodothyronine, Free (fT3) *Serum No Effect Analytical* No significant interference observed with method on Boehringer Mannheim Elecsys analyzer *1653*

Tri-iodothyronine (T3) *Serum No Effect Analytical* No significant interference observed with method on Boehringer Mannheim Elecsys analyzer *1653*

Biperiden

Volume *Urine Decrease Physiological* Decreased flow noted in a few patients *2754*

Bisacodyl

Cholesterol *Serum No Effect Analytical* At concentration of 40 mg/L had no effect as measured by catalase-AIDH method *5704* At concentration of 40 mg/L had no effect as measured by CHOD-Iodide method *5704* At concentration of 40 mg/L had no effect as measured by Liebermann-Burchard method *5704* At concentration of 40 mg/L had no effect as measured by method using catalase-Hantzsch reaction *5704* At concentration of 40 mg/L had no effect as measured by CHOD-PAP method *5704*

Creatinine *Serum No Effect Analytical* At concentration of 2 mg/L had no effect as measured by kinetic Jaffe method on BKA-2 *5704* At concentration of 4 mg/L had no effect as measured by Jaffe-Fading-Fraction method *5704* At concentration of 4 mg/L had no effect as measured by Jaffe-Fuller's earth method *5704*

Bisacodyl (continued)

Fat *Feces Increase Physiological* Observed in laxative abusers *5055* May cause steatorrhea if protracted ingestion *6486*

Glucose *Serum No Effect Analytical* At concentration of 4,000 mg/L had no effect as measured by hexokinase/G-6-PDH method *5704* At concentration of 0.2 mg/L had no effect as measured by Kodak Ektachem® method *5704*
Urine Decrease Analytical Low with Clinistix® , Diastix® *1826*
Urine No Effect Analytical No effect observed with Tes-Tape® *1826*

Histamine *Plasma No Effect Analytical* Improbable inhibition of radio-enzyme assay at therapeutic concentrations *2492*

Lactate *Plasma No Effect Analytical* At concentration of 4,000 mg/L had no effect as measured by enzymatic method *5704*

Occult Blood *Feces No Effect Analytical* No effect noted on Hemoquant method *6172*

Potassium *Serum Decrease Physiological* Associated with steatorrhea if used in excess *6486*
Serum No Effect Analytical At concentration of 2 mg/L had no effect on ISE measurement without predilution *5704*

Protein Electrophoresis *Serum No Effect Analytical* At concentration of 2 mg/L had no effect as measured by automated Olympus-Hite method *5704*

Sodium *Serum No Effect Analytical* At concentration of 2 mg/L had no effect on ISE measurement without predilution *5704*

Urea Nitrogen *Serum No Effect Analytical* At concentration of 0.2 mg/L had no effect as measured by Kodak Ektachem® method *5704*

Uric Acid *Serum No Effect Analytical* At concentration of 20 mg/L had no effect as measured by Kageyama-Hantzsch method *5704* At concentration of 4 mg/L had no effect as measured by catalase-AIDH method *5704*

Bismuth

Doxycycline *Serum Decrease Physiological* When given as bismuth subsalicylate decreases bioavailability of doxycycline and must be given two hours after it to avoid effect *1384* Concomitant use of bismuth subsalicylate (Pepto-Bismol) decreased bioavailability of oral deoxycycline *1384*

Salicylate *Serum No Effect Analytical* No significant effect observed at a concentration of 0.3 mol/L with method on Kodak Ektachem® systems *2519*

Bismuth Subnitrate

Methemoglobin *Blood Increase Physiological* May cause hemolytic anemia *4017*

Bismuth Subsalicylate

Alanine Aminotransferase *Serum Increase Physiological* Hepatotoxicity *3810*

Alkaline Phosphatase *Serum Increase Physiological* Hepatotoxicity *3810*

Amino Acids *Plasma Increase Physiological* Toxicity effect *1714*
Urine Increase Physiological Due to proximal tubular dysfunction (Fanconi syndrome) *4851*

Aspartate Aminotransferase *Serum Increase Physiological* Possibly of renal origin due to nephrotoxicity *4851*

Bile *Urine Increase Physiological* Hepatotoxicity *3810*

Bilirubin *Serum Increase Physiological* Hepatotoxicity *3810*

Bismuth *Serum Increase Physiological* Measurable in poisoning *4014*
Urine Increase Physiological Measurable with poisoning *4014*

BSP Retention *Serum Increase Physiological* Hepatotoxicity *3810*

Casts *Urine Increase Physiological* Mainly granular due to nephrotoxicity *4851*

Cells *Urine Increase Physiological* Mainly tubular due to nephrotoxicity *4851*

Color *Feces Increase Analytical* Blackens or discolors stool with 5 g orally *3810*

Enoxacin *Serum Decrease Physiological* Concomitant administration of bismuth subsalicylate, or given 60 minutes later, with enoxacin decreases enoxacin bioavailability by approximately 25% *4940*

Erythrocytes *Blood Decrease Physiological* May cause aplastic anemia *467*
Urine Increase Physiological May cause severe renal damage *4014*

Glucose *Urine Increase Physiological* Due to proximal tubular dysfunction (Fanconi syndrome) *4851*

Hemoglobin *Urine Increase Physiological* May cause severe renal damage *4014*

Lactate Dehydrogenase Isoenzymes
Serum Increase Physiological Especially of LD-1 and LD-2 - probably of renal origin *4851*

Leukocytes *Blood Decrease Physiological* May cause aplastic anemia/agranulocytosis *3810*

Norfloxacin *Urine No Effect Physiological* In 8 healthy men mean excretion after ingestion of 400 mg norfloxacin insignificantly reduced to 137 .4 ± 38.8 mg/d when bismuth subsalicylate coingested with norfloxacin compared with 153.1 ± 34.7 mg/d in control situation *865*

Phosphate *Urine Increase Physiological* Fanconi syndrome with poisoning *4014*

Platelets *Blood Decrease Physiological* May cause aplastic anemia *467*

Protein *Urine Increase Physiological* Nephrotoxic effect *1714* Nephrotoxic effect reported *5377*

Sugar *Urine Increase Analytical* Interferes with Benedict's reaction *1714*

Urea Nitrogen *Serum Increase Physiological* Nephrotoxic effect reported, and even renal failure *5377*

Bisoprolol

Alanine Aminotransferase *Serum Increase Physiological* In clinical trials increased activity of between 1 to 2 times normal was observed in 3.9% patients treated with drug compared with 2.5% when treated with placebo. With long term treatment for 6 to 18 months incidence of increased activity was 6.2% *3471*

Antinuclear Antibodies *Serum Increase Physiological* About 15% of long term treated patients convert to a positive titer *3471*

Apolipoprotein A-I *Serum No Effect Physiological* In 18 patients with mild to moderate hypertension treatment for 3 months caused nonsignificant reduction of 3.2% from mean baseline of 85.6 mmol/L and with 5.0 mg/d nonsignificant reduction of 1.5% *3611*

Apolipoprotein A-II *Serum Decrease Physiological* In 18 patients with mild to moderate hypertension treatment for 3 months with 2.5 mg/d caused significant reduction of 9.1% from mean baseline of 89.7 mmol/L and with 5.0 mg/d significant reduction of 11.1% *3611*

Apolipoprotein B *Serum Decrease Physiological* In 18 patients with mild to moderate hypertension treatment with 2.5 mg/d for 3 months caused significant reduction of 15.9% from mean baseline of 148.7 mmol/L but treatment with 5.0 mg/d caused nonsignificant increase of 4.5% *3611*

Aspartate Aminotransferase *Serum Increase Physiological* In clinical trials increased activity of between 1 to 2 times normal was observed in 3.9% patients treated with drug compared with 2.5% when treated with placebo. With long term treatment for 6 to 18 months incidence of increased activity was 6.2% *3471*

Bisoprolol *Serum Increase Physiological* In 18 patients with mild to moderate hypertension at a dose of 2.5 mg/d mean plasma concentration 3.9 ng/mL and with dose of 5.0 mg/d mean concentration of 6.5 ng/mL *3611*

Cholesterol *Serum Decrease Physiological* In 18 mild to moderate hypertensives treatment for 3 months with 2.5 mg/d caused significant reduction of 0.51 mmol/L from mean baseline of 6.31 mmol/L but only nonsignificant reduction of o.08 mmol/L when 5.0 mg given for same period *3611*
Serum No Effect Physiological Insignificant effect of treatment with 10 mg/day for 2 years in about 20 men with mild to moderate hypertension *1899* In 14 patients with essential hypertension treatment with 10 mg/d for 4 weeks caused nonsignificant increase from mean baseline of 207 ± 51 mg/dL to 210 ± 38 mg/dL *3481*

Creatinine *Serum Increase Physiological* Small increases in concentration reported *3471*

Glomerular Filtration Rate *Urine No Effect Physiological* In 12 patients with essential hypertension treatment with 10 mg/d for 4 weeks caused nonsignificant change from mean baseline of 116 ± 36 mL/min to 117 ± 28 mL/min *3481*

Glucose *Serum Increase Physiological* Small increases in concentration reported *3471*
Serum No Effect Physiological In 14 patents with essential hypertension treatment with 10 mg/d for 4 weeks caused nonsignificant increase from mean baseline of 123 ± 59 mg/dL to 128 ± 54 mg/dL *3481*

HDL-Cholesterol *Serum Decrease Physiological* Slight reduction observed in both normocholesterolemic and hypercholesterolemic hypertensives treated with 10 mg/d for 6 months *1900* In 18 patients with mild to moderate hypertension treatment for 3 months with 2.5 mg/d caused significant reduction of 0.076 mmol/L from mean baseline of 1.27 mmol/L and with 5.0 mg/d caused significant reduction of 0.117 mmol/L *3611* From 1.22 to 1.10 mmol/L with 20 mg drµg/d *3610*
Serum No Effect Physiological Insignificant effect in about 20 mild to moderate hypertensive men treated with 10 mg/day for 2 years *1899*

HDL-Triglycerides *Serum No Effect Physiological* In 18 patients with mild to moderate hypertension treatment for 3 months with 2.5 mg/d caused nonsignificant reduction of 0.025 mmol/L from mean baseline of 0.29 mmol/L and 5.0 mg/d caused nonsignificant reduction of 0.014 mmol/L *3611*

LDL-Cholesterol *Serum Decrease Physiological* In 18 patients with mild to moderate hypertension treatment for 3 months with 2.5 mg/d caused significant reduction of 0.301 mmol/L from mean baseline of 4.42 mmol/L whereas treatment with 5.0 mg/d caused reduction of only 0.248 mmol/L *3611*
Serum No Effect Physiological No effect with 10 or 20 mg/d *3610* Insignificant effect of treatment with 10 mg/day for 2 years in about 20 men with mild to moderate hypertension *1899*

LDL-Triglycerides *Serum No Effect Physiological* In 18 patients with mild to moderate hypertension treatment for 3 months with 2.5 mg/d caused nonsignificant reduction of 0.002 mmol/L from mean baseline of 0.57 mmol/L and with 5.0 mg/d nonsignificant reduction of 0.021 mmol/L *3611*

Leukocytes *Blood Decrease Physiological* Small usually clinically insignificant decreases in concentration reported *3471*

Phosphate *Serum Increase Physiological* Small increases in concentration reported *3471*

Potassium *Serum Increase Physiological* Small increases in concentration reported *3471*

Renal Blood Flow *Patient No Effect Physiological* In 12 patients with essential hypertension treatment with 10 mg/d for 4 weeks caused nonsignificant increase from mean baseline of 955 ± 290 mL/min to 1014 ± 347 mL/min *3481*

Riboflavin *Blood Decrease Physiological* Small usually clinically insignificant decreases in concentration reported *3471*

Triglycerides *Serum Decrease Physiological* In 18 patients with mild to moderate hypertension treatment witn 2.5 mg/d for 3 months caused significant reduction of 0.25 mmol/L from mean baseline of 1.92 mmol/L but 5.0 mg/d for 3 months only caused nonsignificant decrease of 0.05 mmol/L *3611*
Serum Increase Physiological In clinical trials increased plasma triglyceride concentration has been reported as the most common laboratory abnormality with bisoprolol treatment, although this was not a constant finding *3471* In 14 patients with essential hypertension treatment with 10 mg/d for 4 weeks caused significant increase fro mean baseline of 141 ± 63 mg/dL to 192 ± 101 mg/dL *3481* Slight effect noted in both normocholesterolemic and hypercholesterolemic hypertensives treated with 10 mg/d for 6 months *1900* Increase of 20-28% in about 20 mild to moderate hypertensive men treated with 10 mg/day for 2 years *1899*

Urea Nitrogen *Serum Increase Physiological* Small increases in concentration reported *3471*

Uric Acid *Serum Increase Physiological* Gout has been reported as a side effect. Small increases also reported *3471*

VLDL-Cholesterol *Serum Decrease Physiological* In 18 patients with mild to moderate hypertension treatment with 2.5 mg/d for 3 months caused significant reduction of 0.12 mmol/L from mean baseline of 0.60 mmol/L but reduction of 0.02 mmol/L with 5.0 mg/d for 3 months not significant *3611*

VLDL-Triglycerides *Serum Increase Physiological* Significant effect with 10 mg/d (from 1.04 to 1.31 mmol/L) *3610*
Serum No Effect Physiological In 18 patients with mild to moderate hypertension treatment for 3 months with 2.5 mg/d caused nonsignificant reduction of 0.18 mmol/L from mean baseline of 1.03 mmol/L and with 5.0 mg/d nonsignificant reduction of 0.02 mmol/L *3611*

Bisphosphonates

Apolipoprotein A-I *Serum Decrease Physiological* In 9 individuals with plasma Lp(a) concentrations ranging from 6.4 to 17.7 mg/L a single infusion bisphosphonates caused a significant decrease in baseline concentration from 1.68 ± 0.23 g/L to 1.58 ± 0.29 g/L on day 1, 1.52 ± 0.29 g/L on day 2, 1.47 ± 0.25 g/L on day 4 and 1.46 ± 0.22 g/L on day 7 *3603*

Apolipoprotein B *Serum Decrease Physiological* In 9 individuals with plasma Lp(a) concentrations ranging from 6.4 to 17.7 mg/L a single infusion bisphosphonates caused a significant decrease in baseline concentration from 1.22 ± 0.34 g/L to 0.94 ± 0.47 g/L on day 1, 1.1 ± 0.34 g/L on day 2, 1.12 ± 0.34 g/L on day 4 and 1.12 ± 0.35 g/L on day 7 *3603*

Calcium *Serum Decrease Physiological* In 36 patients with hypercalcemia associated with malignant disease mean concentration significantly decreased from 3.22 ± 0.40 mmol/L to 2.32 ± 0.27 mmol/L with treatment *626*
Urine Decrease Physiological In 36 patients with hypercalcemia of malignancy mean excretion decreased significantly from 1.61 ± 0.74 mmol/mmol creatinine to 0.39 ± 0.39 mmol/mmol creatinine with treatment *626*

C-Reactive Protein *Serum Increase Physiological* In 9 individuals with plasma Lp(a) concentrations ranging from 6.4 to 17.7 mg/L a single infusion bisphosphonates caused a significant increase in baseline concentration from 1.3 ± 1.1 mg/L to 1.3 ± 0.6 mg/L on day 1, 8.7 ± 11.2 mg/L on day 2, 5.2 ± 4.4 mg/L on day 4 and 3.5 ± 2.1 mg/L on day 7 *3603*

Deoxypyridinoline *Urine Decrease Physiological* In 36 patients with hypercalcemia of malignancy significant reduction from mean baseline of 20 ± 15 nmol/mmol creatinine to 10 ± 6 nmol/mmol creatinine observed with treatment *626* In 74 patients with Paget's disease mean excretion of 7.8 (range 0.5 - 41.5) nmol/mmol creatinine decreased significantly to 5.6 (range 0.9 - 23.1) nmol/mmol creatinine with treatment with bisphosphonates *4999* In 108 patients with osteoporosis mean excretion of 4.2 (range 2.0 - 7.7) nmol/mmol creatinine decreased significantly to 3.4 (range 1.4 - 6.5) nmol/mmol creatinine with treatment with bisphosphonates *4999*

Erythrocyte Sedimentation Rate
Blood Increase Physiological In 9 individuals with plasma Lp(a) concentrations ranging from 6.4 to 17.7 mg/dL a single infusion bisphosphonates caused a significant increase in baseline rate from 22.0 ± 17.5 mm/h to 24.0 ± 15.1 mm/h on day 1, 28.7 ± 19.9 mm/h on day 2, 32.5 ± 26.1 mm/h on day 4 and 30.0 ± 29.3 mm/h on day 7 *3603*

Hydroxyproline *Urine Decrease Physiological* In 36 patients with hypercalcemia of malignancy treatment caused significant reduction from mean baseline of 71 ± 46 µmol/mmol creatinine to 44 ± 22 µmol/mmol creatinine *626*

ionized Calcium *Serum Decrease Physiological* In 36 patients with hypercalcemia associated with malignant disease mean concentration decreased significantly from mean baseline of 1.66 ± 0.24 mmol/L to 1.20 ± 0.15 mmol/L with treatment *626*

Bisphosphonates *(continued)*

Lipoprotein Lp(a) *Serum Increase Physiological* In 9 individuals with plasma Lp(a) concentrations ranging from 6.4 to 17.7 mg/L a single infusion bisphosphonates caused an increase in baseline concentration from 10.3 mg/dL to 10.6 mg/dL on day 1, 11.3 mg/dL on day 2, 11.2 mg/dL on day 4 and 12.4 mg/dL on day 7 *3603*

Pyridinoline *Urine Decrease Physiological* In 36 patients with hypercalcemia of malignancy significant reduction from mean baseline of 130 ± 62 nmol/mmol creatinine to 90 ± 60 nmol/mmol creatinine *626* In 108 patients with osteoporosis mean excretion of 19.3 (range 9.3 - 30.6) nmol/mmol creatinine decreased significantly to 15.1 (range 7.7 - 33.0) nmol/mmol creatinine with treatment with bisphosphonates *4999* In 74 patients with Paget's disease mean excretion of 29.7 (range 10.9 - 105.5) nmol/mmol creatinine decreased significantly to 21.0 (range 4 - 89.2) nmol/mmol creatinine with treatment with bisphosphonates *4999*

Bitolterol

Alanine Aminotransferase *Serum Increase Physiological* Infrequent effect observed of unknown clinical significance *1628*

Alkaline Phosphatase *Serum Increase Physiological* Infrequent effect observed of unknown clinical significance *1628*

Aspartate Aminotransferase *Serum Increase Physiological* Infrequent effect observed of unknown clinical significance *1628*

Glucose *Serum Increase Physiological* Infrequent effect observed of unknown clinical significance *1628*

Hematocrit *Blood Decrease Physiological* Infrequent effect observed of unknown clinical significance *1628*

Hemoglobin *Blood Decrease Physiological* Infrequent effect observed of unknown clinical significance *1628*

Leukocytes *Blood Increase Physiological* Infrequent effect observed of unknown clinical significance *1628*

Potassium *Serum Decrease Physiological* Infrequent effect observed of unknown clinical significance *1628*

Bleomycin

Alkaline Phosphatase *Serum Increase Physiological* Rare mild abnormality reported: reversible *3949*

Aspartate Aminotransferase *Serum Increase Physiological* Rare mild abnormality reported: reversible *3949*

Bilirubin *Serum Increase Physiological* Rare mild abnormality reported: reversible *3949*

Creatinine *Serum No Effect Analytical* No effect of concentrations of bleomycin sulfate up to 15 mg/L on single slide method on Kodak Ektachem® *5706*

Phenytoin *Serum Decrease Physiological* Decreased plasma condition *886* May reduce plasma concentration when drugs are coadministered *1384*

Platelets *Blood Decrease Physiological* May cause bone marrow aplasia *2385*

Protein *Cerebrospinal Fluid No Effect Analytical* No significant effect when added in vitro on Kodak Ektachem® slide method *3654*

β-blockers

α_2-Antiplasmin *Plasma No Effect Physiological* In 39 hypertensives treated with β-blockers mean concentration of 108 ± 13 %normal not significantly different from 108 ± 11% normal in 346 hypertensives not taking β-blockers and normotensives *2194*

Apolipoprotein A-I *Serum No Effect Physiological* In 39 hypertensives treated with β-blockers mean concentration of 137 ± 29 mg/dL not significantly different from 137 ± 31 mg/dL in 346 hypertensives not taking β-blockers and normotensives *2194*

Apolipoprotein B *Serum No Effect Physiological* In 39 hypertensives treated with β-blockers mean concentration of 135 ± 38 mg/dL not significantly different from 140 ± 41 mg/dL in 346 hypertensives not taking β-blockers and normotensives *2194*

Cholesterol *Serum Increase Physiological* Increased concentration observed with administration of β-blockers *3730*
Serum No Effect Physiological In 39 hypertensives treated with β-blockers mean concentration of 240 ± 48 mg/dL not significantly different from 245 ± 60 mg/dL in 346 hypertensives not taking β-blockers and normotensives *2194*

D-Dimer *Plasma No Effect Physiological* In 39 hypertensives treated with β-blockers mean concentration of 0.10 ± 0.02 µg/mL not significantly different from 0.099 ± 0.03 µg/mL in 346 hypertensives not taking β-blockers and normotensives *2194*

Fibrinogen *Plasma No Effect Physiological* In 39 hypertensives treated with β-blockers mean concentration of 329 ± 59 mg/dL significantly different from 315 ± 67 mg/dL in 346 hypertensives not taking β-blockers and normotensives *2194*

Granulocytes *Blood No Effect Physiological* Agranulocytosis observed in 4.4% of patients taking β-blockers other than propranolol compared with 3.0% of controls (stratified relative risk estimate 1.5) *3098*

HDL-Cholesterol *Serum Decrease Physiological* Decreased concentration observed with administration of β-blockers *3730*
Serum No Effect Physiological In 39 hypertensives treated with β-blockers mean concentration of 42 ± 15 mg/dL not significantly different from 45 ± 15 mg/dL in 346 hypertensives not taking β-blockers and normotensives *2194*

Hemoglobin A_{1c} *Blood Increase Physiological* In 10 patients with NIDDM and hypertension treatment with β-blockers caused mean concentration to increase by 0.50 ± 0.09% after 1 month, 0.99 ± 0.24% after 3 months and 1.12 ± 0.19% after 6 months *5276*

LDL-Cholesterol *Serum Decrease Physiological* In 39 hypertensives treated with β-blockers mean concentration of 139 ± 47 mg/dL significantly different from 156 ± 46 mg/dL in 346 hypertensives not taking β-blockers and normotensives *2194*
Serum Increase Physiological Increased concentration observed with administration of β-blockers *3730*

Lidocaine *Serum Increase Physiological* Reduce clearance and increase plasma concentration *1384*

Lipoprotein Lp(a) *Serum No Effect Physiological* In 94 hypertensives undergoing treatment with β-blockers mean and median concentrations of 216 and 116 mg/L compared with 178 and 104 mg/L respectively in 1433 controls *5604* In 39 hypertensives treated with β-blockers mean concentration of 28 ± 28 mg/dL not significantly different from 29 ± 33 mg/dL in 346 hypertensives not taking β-blockers and normotensives *2194*

Plasminogen *Plasma No Effect Physiological* In 39 hypertensives treated with β-blockers mean concentration of 111 ± 17 %normal not significantly different from 115 ± 20% normal in 346 hypertensives not taking β-blockers and normotensives *2194*

Plasminogen Activator Inhibitor Activity
Plasma Increase Physiological In 39 hypertensives treated with β-blockers mean concentration of 23 ± 16 U/mL significantly different from 18 ± 19 U/mL in 346 hypertensives not taking β-blockers and normotensives *2194*

Plasminogen Activator Inhibitor Antigen
Plasma Increase Physiological In 39 hypertensives treated with β-blockers mean concentration of 40 ± 24 ng/mL significantly different from 32 ± 34 ng/mL in 346 hypertensives not taking β-blockers and normotensives *2194*

Sildenafil *Serum No Effect Physiological* CYP2D6 inhibitors such as nonspecific β-blockers did not affect the pharmacokinetics of sildenafil *4657*

Theophylline *Serum Increase Physiological* May prolong half-life of theophylline *1384*

Tissue Plasminogen Activator
Plasma No Effect Physiological In 39 hypertensives treated with β-blockers mean concentration of 0.58 ± 0.42 IU/mL not significantly different from 0.74 ± 1.19 IU/mL in 346 hypertensives not taking β-blockers and normotensives *2194*

Tissue Plasminogen Activator Antigen
Plasma Increase Physiological In 39 hypertensives treated with β-blockers mean concentration of 9 ± 4 ng/mL significantly different from 8 ± 8 ng/mL in 346 hypertensives not taking β-blockers and normotensives *2194*

Triglycerides *Serum Increase Physiological* Increased concentration observed with administration of β-blockers *3730* In 39 hypertensives treated with β-blockers mean concentration of 311 ± 275 mg/dL significantly different from 254 ± 393 mg/dL in 346 hypertensives not taking β-blockers and normotensives *2194*

Bombesin

Follicle Stimulating Hormone
Plasma Increase Physiological After LHRH after 5 ng/min x 2.5 h in healthy men *4746*

Luteinizing Hormone *Plasma Increase Physiological* After LHRH after 5 ng/min x 2.5 h in healthy men *4746*

Prolactin *Plasma Decrease Physiological* After TRH after 5 ng/min x 2.5 h in healthy men *4746*

Thyroid Stimulating Hormone
Serum Decrease Physiological After TRH after 5 ng/min x 2.5 h in healthy men *4746*

Bopindolol

Chloride *Serum No Effect Physiological* In 10 hypertensive patients treated for either 1 or 21 d *1777*
Urine No Effect Physiological In 10 hypertensive patients treated for either 1 or 21 d *1777*

Cholesterol *Serum No Effect Physiological* In 24 hypertensives treated with drug for 3 mo *6165*

Creatinine *Serum Increase Physiological* Minimal effect observed in large population of hypertensives over 12 weeks study period *6383*
Serum No Effect Physiological In 10 hypertensive patients treated for either 1 or 21 d *1777* No effect observed in hypertensive patients treated with up to 4 mg daily for 4 weeks *5533*

Creatinine Clearance *Urine No Effect Physiological* No effect in hypertensive patients treated with up to 4 mg daily for 4 weeks *5533*

Fractional Excretion of Sodium
Urine No Effect Physiological In 10 hypertensive patients treated for either 1 or 21 d *1777*

HDL-Cholesterol *Serum No Effect Physiological* In 24 hypertensives treated with drug for 3 mo *6165*

Hematocrit *Blood Decrease Physiological* After 1 d but reverted to normal in 10 hypertensives treated for 21 d *1777*

Inulin Clearance *Urine Decrease Physiological* Reduced by 10% in hypertensive patients given up to 4 mg daily for 4 weeks *5533*

LDL-Cholesterol *Serum No Effect Physiological* In 24 hypertensives treated with drug for 3 mo *6165*

Osmolality *Serum No Effect Physiological* In 10 hypertensive patients treated for either 1 or 21 d *1777*
Urine No Effect Physiological In 10 hypertensive patients treated for either 1 or 21 d *1777*

PAH Clearance *Urine No Effect Physiological* No effect in hypertensive patients treated with up to 4 mg daily for 4 weeks *5533*

Potassium *Serum Increase Physiological* Minimal effect observed in large population of hypertensives over 12 weeks study period *6383*
Serum No Effect Physiological In 10 hypertensive patients treated for either 1 or 21 d *1777*
Urine No Effect Physiological In 10 hypertensive patients treated for either 1 or 21 d *1777*

Protein *Serum No Effect Physiological* In 10 hypertensive patients treated for either 1 or 21 d *1777*
Urine No Effect Physiological In 10 hypertensive patients treated for either 1 or 21 d *1777*

Renin Activity *Plasma Decrease Physiological* In 19 patients with essential hypertension reduced mean pretreatment concentration of 2.6 µg/L/h to 1.6 µg/L/h with chronic treatment *2769*

Sodium *Serum No Effect Physiological* In 10 hypertensive patients treated for either 1 or 21 d *1777*
Urine No Effect Physiological In 10 hypertensive patients treated for either 1 or 21 d *1777*

Triglycerides *Serum Increase Physiological* After 4-8 weeks by as much as 41% but disappeared after 12 weeks of therapy in 24 hypertensives *6165*

Urea Nitrogen *Serum No Effect Physiological* No effect observed in hypertensive patients treated with up to 4 mg daily for 4 weeks *5533*

Uric Acid *Serum Increase Physiological* Minimal effect observed in large population of hypertensives over 12 weeks study period *6383*

Volume *Urine No Effect Physiological* In 10 hypertensive patients treated for either 1 or 21 d *1777*

Water Clearance, Free *Urine No Effect Physiological* In 10 hypertensive patients treated for either 1 or 21 d *1777*

Bosentan

Angiotensin-II *Plasma No Effect Physiological* In 293 patients with essential hypertension insignificant changes of - 6.8 ± 5.8 ng/L in those receiving 100 mg/d for 4 weeks, - 2.5 ± 5.0 ng/L in those receiving 500 mg/d, - 0.4 ± 5.8 ng/L in those receiving 1000 mg/d and 2.4 ± 5.1 ng/L in those receiving 2000 mg/d compared with 0.3 ± 6.3 ng/L in placebo treated controls *3307*

Endothelin-1 *Plasma Increase Physiological* In 293 patients with essential hypertension changes of 0.6 ± 0.3 ng/L in those receiving 100 mg/d for 4 weeks, 0.7 ± 0.2 ng/L (significant) in those receiving 500 mg/d, 0.7 ± 0.3 ng/L (significant) in those receiving 1000 mg/d and 1.2 ± 0.2 ng/L (significant) in those receiving 2000 mg/d compared with - 0.3 ± 0.8 ng/L in placebo treated controls *3307*

Endothelin-1, Big *Plasma Increase Physiological* In 293 patients with essential hypertension changes of 2.2 ± 0.9 ng/L (significant) in those receiving 100 mg/d for 4 weeks, 0.9 ± 0.8 ng/L in those receiving 500 mg/d, 2.0 ± 0.9 ng/L (significant) in those receiving 1000 mg/d and 1.2 ± 0.8 ng/L in those receiving 2000 mg/d compared with - 0.3 ± 0.8 ng/L in placebo treated controls *3307*

Norepinephrine *Plasma No Effect Physiological* In 293 patients with essential hypertension nonsignificant changes of 0.4 ± 0.3 ng/L in those receiving 100 mg/d for 4 weeks, 0.5 ± 0.3 ng/L in those receiving 500 mg/d, 0.6 ± 0.3 ng/L in those receiving 1000 mg/d and 0.2 ± 0.3 ng/L in those receiving 2000 mg/d compared with change of 0.3 ± 0.3 ng/L in placebo treated controls *3307*

Renin Activity *Plasma No Effect Physiological* In 293 patients with essential hypertension insignificant changes of 1.4 ± 7.0 mIU/L in those receiving 100 mg/d for 4 weeks, - 4.9 ± 6.2 mIU/L in those receiving 500 mg/d, - 2.7 ± 7.0 mIU/L in those receiving 1000 mg/d and 0.7 ± 6.3 mIU/L in those receiving 2000 mg/d compared with - 2.5 ± 6.6 mIU/L in placebo-treated controls *3307*

Boxidine

Cholesterol *Serum Decrease Physiological* Inhibits transformation of 7-dehydrocholesterol *2003*

7-Dehydrocholesterol *Serum Increase Physiological* Inhibits transformation to cholesterol *2003*

Urea Nitrogen *Serum Increase Physiological* Possible relationship to tumor destruction *2003*

Brodifacoum

Factor II *Plasma Decrease Physiological* Profound reduction for at least 43 days in one subject following intentional ingestion of a large amount of drug *2659*

Factor VII *Plasma Decrease Physiological* Profound reduction in one subject following intentional ingestion of large amount of drug with effect lasting for at least 43 days *2659*

Factor IX *Plasma Decrease Physiological* Profound reduction in one subject following intentional ingestion of large amount of drug with effect lasting for at least 43 days *2659*

Brodifacoum *(continued)*

Factor X *Plasma Decrease Physiological* Profound reduction in one subject following intentional ingestion of large amount of drug with effect lasting for at least 43 days *2659*

Brofaromine

4-Hydroxy-3-Methoxy-Phenylglycol
Urine Decrease Physiological In 6 healthy men 150 mg/day caused 69% reduction from 1.15 mg/g creatinine during first week and 72% reduction during second week *549*

Tryptamine *Urine Increase Physiological* In 6 healthy men 150 mg daily for 2 weeks caused 2.7 fold (from 0.056 to 0.153 mg/g creatinine) increase which normalized by 1 week after treatment stopped *549*

Vanillylmandelic Acid *Urine Decrease Physiological* In 6 healthy men 150 mg/day caused approximately 69% reduction in first week and 72% reduction in second week of treatment *549*

Bromate

Casts *Urine Increase Physiological* Due to renal damage *2183*

Erythrocytes *Blood Decrease Physiological* May cause hemolysis *2242*
Urine Increase Physiological Due to renal damage *2183*

Hemoglobin *Blood Decrease Physiological* May cause hemolysis *2242*

Methemoglobin *Blood Increase Physiological* May cause hemolysis *2242*

Protein *Urine Increase Physiological* Due to renal damage *2183*

Urea Nitrogen *Serum Increase Physiological* Anuria and azotemia may occur within hours *2183*

Bromazepam

Alanine Aminotransferase *Serum No Effect Analytical* At 5 times therapeutic concentration on methods on Technicon SMAC® , Abbott-VP, Du Pont aca, Roche Cobas-Bio and KDA *3525*

Albumin *Serum No Effect Analytical* At 5 times therapeutic concentration on BCG methods on Technicon SMAC® , Kodak Ektachem® 400, Hitachi® 705 and KDA *3525*
Urine No Effect Analytical Using a fluorimetric assay with Albumin Blue 580 on a Cobas Fara centrifugal analyzer for the detection of microalbuminuria no significant interference was detected at a concentration of 4 mg/L *3117*

Alkaline Phosphatase *Serum No Effect Analytical* At 5 times therapeutic concentration on methods on Technicon SMAC® , Abbott-VP, Do Pont aca, Roche Cobas-Bio, Hitachi® 705 and KDA *3525*

Amylase *Serum No Effect Analytical* At 5 times therapeutic concentration on methods on Du Pont aca, Roche Cobas-Bio, Kodak Ektachem® *3525* No effect at concentration of 2 mg/L on method on Kodak Ektachem® *5706*

Aspartate Aminotransferase *Serum No Effect Analytical* At 5 times therapeutic concentration on methods on Technicon SMAC® , Abbott-VP, Du Pont aca, Roche Cobas-Bio, Hitachi® 705 and KDA *3525*

Benzodiazepine *Urine Positive Analytical* Detectable limit 0.3 µg/mL with improved EMIT assay on Syva ETS system compared with 0.5 µg/mL with former d.a.u. assay *3370* At concentration of 0.5 µg/mL or greater produces positive result with Syva EMIT II assay *1785* Reactive with new Syva EMIT assay *3370*

Bilirubin *Serum No Effect Analytical* At 5 times therapeutic concentration on methods on Technicon SMAC® , Du Pont aca, Roche Cobas-Bio, Ektachem® , Hitachi® 705 and KDA *3525*

Bilirubin, Conjugated *Serum No Effect Analytical* No effect at concentration of 2 mg/L on method on Kodak Ektachem® *5706*

Bilirubin, Unconjugated *Serum No Effect Analytical* No effect at concentration of 2 mg/L on method on Kodak Ektachem® *5706*

Bromide *Serum Increase Physiological* In one overdosed patient concentration of bromide determined to be 43 mmol/L *5445*

Calcium *Serum No Effect Analytical* At 5 times therapeutic concentration on methods of Technicon SMAC® , Abbott-VP, Du Pont aca, Kodak Ektachem® 400, Hitachi® 705 and KDA *3525*

Cholesterol *Serum No Effect Analytical* At 5 times therapeutic concentration on methods on Technicon SMAC® , Abbott-VP, Roche Cobas-Bio, Kodak Ektachem® , Hitachi® and KDA *3525*

Creatine Kinase *Serum No Effect Analytical* At 5 times therapeutic concentration on methods on Technicon SMAC® , Abbott-VP, Du Pont aca, Roche Cobas-Bio and and Hitachi® 705 *3525*

Creatinine *Serum No Effect Analytical* At 5 times therapeutic concentration on methods of Technicon SMAC® , Abbott-VP, Du Pont aca, Roche Cobas-Bio, Hitachi® 705 and KDA *3525* No effect of concentrations up to 2 mg/L on 2-slide method on Kodak Ektachem® *5706*

Fibrinogen *Plasma Decrease Analytical* In one overdosed patient serum bromide concentration was measured as 43 mmol/L with measurements on Kodak Ektachem® 1 mole NaBr is equivalent to 5 moles Cl and 3 moles carbon dioxide explaining abnormally low calculated anion gap *5445*

Glucose *Serum No Effect Analytical* At 5 times therapeutic concentration on methods of Technicon SMAC® , Abbott-VP, Du Pont aca, Roche Cobas-Bio, Kodak Ektachem® 400, KDA and Hitachi® 705 *3525*

γ-Glutamyltransferase *Serum No Effect Analytical* At 5 times therapeutic concentration on Technicon SMAC® , Abbott-VP, and Hitachi® 705 *3525*

Iron *Serum No Effect Analytical* At 5 times therapeutic concentration on Ferrozine method on Technicon SMAC® *3525*

Lactate Dehydrogenase *Serum No Effect Analytical* At 5 times therapeutic concentration on Technicon SMAC® , Abbott-VP, Roche Cobas-Bio, Hitachi® , KDA *3525*

Metanephrine *Urine No Effect Analytical* No effect at 2 mg/L on HPLC method *557*

Midazolam *Serum No Effect Analytical* On GC-ECD method of Ha et al *2387*

Normetanephrine *Urine No Effect Analytical* No effect at 2 mg/L on HPLC method *557*

p-Aminophenol *Urine No Effect Analytical* With addition of drugs at a concentration of 100 mg/L and of related compounds at 50 mg/L no significant effect observed on colorimetric method of van Bocxlaer on Cobas Mira analyzer which involves reacting free p-aminophenol with resorcinol in the presence of magnesium ions to form an indophenol dye measured at 550 nm *6163*

Phosphate *Serum No Effect Analytical* At 5 times therapeutic concentration on methods of Technicon SMAC® , Du Pont aca, Hitachi® 705, KDA *3525*

Protein *Serum No Effect Analytical* At 5 times therapeutic concentration on methods of Technicon SMAC® , Abbott-VP, Kodak Ektachem® 400, Hitachi® 705 and KDA *3525*

Tirofiban *Serum No Effect Physiological* Coadministration had no significant effect on plasma clearance of tirofiban *3957*

Triglycerides *Serum No Effect Analytical* At 5 times therapeutic concentration on methods onTechnicon SMAC® , Abbott-VP, Ektachem® 400, Hitachi® 705 and KDA *3525*

Urea Nitrogen *Serum No Effect Analytical* At 5 times therapeutic concentration on methods of Technicon SMAC® , Abbott-VP, Roche Cobas-Bio, Kodak Ektachem® 400, Hitachi® 705 and KDA *3525*

Uric Acid *Serum No Effect Analytical* At 5 times therapeutic concentration on methods of Technicon SMAC® , Abbott-VP, Du Pont aca, Roche Cobas-Bio, Hitachi® 705, Kodak Ektachem® 400 and KDA *3525*

Bromelains

Fibrinogen *Plasma Decrease Physiological* One drug related case reported *2754*

Platelet Aggregation *Blood Decrease Physiological* Reduced sensitivity to ADP induced aggregation *2540*

Prothrombin Time *Plasma Increase Physiological* Effect observed over 4 h period in animals *128*

Bromfenac

Alanine Aminotransferase *Serum Increase Physiological* Activity increased to above 3 times the upper limit of normal occurred at some point during treatment in 2.7% of 926 individuals during clinical trials *6554*

Aspartate Aminotransferase *Serum Increase Physiological* Activity increased to above 3 times the upper limit of normal occurred in 2.7% of 926 individuals during clinical trials *6554*

Creatinine *Serum Increase Physiological* In fewer than 1% treated patients increased creatinine concentration observed *6554*

Glucose *Serum Increase Physiological* In fewer than 1% treated patients hypoglycemia observed *6554*
Urine Increase Physiological In fewer than 1% treated patients glycosuria observed *6554*

Hemoglobin *Blood Decrease Physiological* In fewer than 1% treated patients anemia observed *6554*

Leukocytes *Blood Decrease Physiological* In fewer than 1% treated patients leukopenia observed *6554*

Occult Blood *Feces Increase Physiological* In fewer than 1% treated patients gastrointestinal hemorrhage observed *6554*

Potassium *Serum Increase Physiological* In fewer than 1% treated patients hypokalemia observed *6554*

Sodium *Serum Increase Physiological* In fewer than 1% treated patients hyponatremia observed *6554*

Urea Nitrogen *Serum Increase Physiological* In fewer than 1% treated patients increased serum urea nitrogen observed *6554*

Bromhexine

Ketone Body Ratio *Serum No Effect Analytical* When added at a concentration of 1 mg/L had no significant effect on AKBR method of Uno et al *6131*

p-Aminophenol *Urine No Effect Analytical* With addition of drugs at a concentration of 100 mg/L and of related compounds at 50 mg/L no significant effect observed on colorimetric method of van Bocxlaer on Cobas Mira analyzer which involves reacting free p-aminophenol with resorcinol in the presence of magnesium ions to form an indophenol dye measured at 550 nm *6163*

Bromide

Amylase *Serum No Effect Analytical* At a concentration of 0.5 mmol/L had no significant effect on method on Kodak Ektachem® systems using GEN 11 and above slides *2519* No effect at concentration of 40 mg/L on method on Kodak Ektachem® *5706*

Bicarbonate *Serum Increase Analytical* Increases result with method on Kodak Ektachem® systems *2519* Concentrations above 1 mmol/L increase result as determined by method on Kodak Ektachem® *5706*

Bilirubin, Conjugated *Serum No Effect Analytical* At a concentration of 200 mg/dL had no significant effect on method on Kodak Ektachem® systems *2519*

Bilirubin, Unconjugated *Serum No Effect Analytical* At a concentration of 200 mg/dL had no significant effect on method on Kodak Ektachem® systems *2519*

Bromide *Serum Increase Physiological* Concentration measurable with therapeutic doses *4014*

Chloride *Serum Decrease Physiological* Reversible halide dysequilibration *1009*
Serum Increase Analytical Increased concentration as measured by Kodak Ektachem® at bromide concentrations above 1 mmol/L: probably of clinical significance *5706* Measured concentration on Hitachi® 736-30 increased by 1.5 mmol/L for each 1.0 mmol/L of bromide added. Organic bromine at concentrations up to 10 mmol/L had no effect. No effect of concentration of 2.0 mmol/L on Beckman Synchron CX3 *1728* Measured as Cl by mercurimetric, electrometric methods *2559* Bromide reacts as if it were chloride with method on Kodak Ektachem® systems: positive bias of 3 - 4 mmol/L observed for each mmol/L of bromide *2519* Increases serum chloride by 0.03 mEq/L at a bromide concentration of 20 mEq/L with the method of Fingerhut *1865*
Urine Increase Analytical Bromide measured as chloride *2024*

Cholesterol *Serum Decrease Analytical* Increase by 0.5% at 10 mg/dL (in serum) on enzymatic procedure *103*

Cholinesterase *Serum No Effect Analytical* No effect observed at concentrations up to 1 mEq/L with butyrylthiocholine method on Kodak Ektachem® *2504* At a concentration of 1 mmol/L has no significant effect on method on Kodak Ektachem® systems *2519*

Creatinine *Urine No Effect Analytical* Causes less than 2% effect on single-slide method on Kodak Ektachem® systems *2519*

Glucose *Serum No Effect Analytical* No effect of concentrations up to 65 mg/L on method on Kodak Ektachem® *5706*

Hemoglobin *Urine Increase Analytical* Interferes with guaiac and benzidine tests *6515*

^{131}I Uptake *Serum Decrease Physiological* Theoretically if contaminated with I_2*882*

Occult Blood *Feces Increase Analytical* *In vitro* reaction, ?high enough concentration *in vivo882*

Potassium *Serum No Effect Analytical* Concentration of 10 mmol/L had no effect on ISE method on Hitachi® 736-30 *1728*

Pyruvate Kinase *Red Blood Cells Decrease Analytical* Observed with 0.3 mmol/L PEP in reaction mixture *592*

Salicylate *Serum No Effect Analytical* No significant effect observed at a concentration of 1 mEq/L with method on Kodak Ektachem® systems *2519*

Sodium *Serum No Effect Analytical* At concentration of 10 mmol/L had no effect observed on Hitachi® 736-30 ISE method *1728*

Urea Nitrogen *Serum No Effect Analytical* No effect of concentrations up to 65 mg/L on method on Kodak Ektachem® *5706*

Bromisovalum

Bromide *Serum Increase Physiological* Theoretical possibility since drug contains 36% bromide *5116* Metabolite (concentration may exceed 25 mEq/L) *2242*

Chloride *Serum Increase Analytical* Metabolite may be measured as chloride *2242*

Bromocriptine

Alanine Aminotransferase *Serum Increase Physiological* Asymptomatic increases in activity observed in some patients *1384*

Alkaline Phosphatase *Serum Increase Physiological* In 10 of 45 patients with Parkinson's disease increased by up to 25% without other laboratory abnormalities *3565*

Aspartate Aminotransferase *Serum Increase Physiological* Asymptomatic increases in activity observed in some patients *1384*

Cholinesterase *Serum No Effect Analytical* No effect observed at concentration of 5 ng/mL with butyrylthiocholine method on Kodak Ektachem® *2504*

Corticotropin *Plasma Decrease Physiological* In 6 adult women with Nelson's syndrome administration of 2.5 mg bromocriptine caused mean decrease of 52 ± 8% in the plasma ACTH concentration *3956*

Cyclosporine *Serum Increase Physiological* May increase cyclosporine concentration by inhibiting hepatic cytochrome P-450 III A which metabolizes cyclosporine *5236*

Cyclosporine A *Blood Increase Physiological* Coadministration with cyclosporine A increases its concentration *5240*

Bromocriptine *(continued)*

Follicle Stimulating Hormone
Plasma Increase Physiological Concentration measurable in second postpartum week when treatment with bromocriptine administered although not measurable in first week and initially high FSH/LH ratio observed *3285*

Growth Hormone *Plasma Decrease Physiological* Reduces concentration significantly in patients with acromegaly by 50% or more in approximately half of treated patients *5238*

Histamine *Plasma No Effect Analytical* Concentrations at which inhibition of radio-enzyme occurs greatly exceed physiological concentrations *2492*

Luteinizing Hormone *Plasma Increase Physiological* Concentration undetectable in first postpartum week in 15 women receiving drug but rose in second week although FSH/LH ratio initially high *3285*
Plasma No Effect Physiological No effect observed *2836*

Norepinephrine *Plasma Decrease Physiological* Significant effect of 5 mg/d for 5 d in healthy women but not in hyperprolactinemic women *3762*

Occult Blood *Feces Increase Physiological* In patients with acromegaly may cause intestinal bleding in fewer than 2% treated patients *5238*

Prolactin *Plasma Decrease Physiological* 70% decrease in healthy women and those with prolactin secreting tumors when given 5 mg/d for 5 d *3762* Reduces concentration significantly in patients with physiologically increased plasma prolactin concentrations as well as in patients with hyperprolactinemia *5238*

Tacrolimus *Serum Increase Physiological* By inhibiting cytochrome P-450 IIIA enzyme systems may inhibit the metabolism of tacrolimus *1987*

Tamoxifen *Serum Decrease Physiological* When coadministered with tamoxifen may cause increased steady-state concentrations of tamoxifen and N-desmethyltamoxifen *6648*

Testosterone *Serum Increase Physiological* Causes increase of about 20% *2836*

Thyroxine (T4) *Serum Decrease Physiological* In hypothyroid patients although response to TRH shows no significant change *6412*
Serum No Effect Physiological In euthyroid patients although response to TRH shows no significant change *6412*

Bromodeoxyuridine

Chromosomes *Test Conditions Abnormal Physiological* Clastogenic in human cells *5484*

Bromodiphenhydramine

Bromide *Serum Increase Physiological* Theoretical possibility since drug contains 24% bromide *5116*

Brompheniramine

Amino Acids *Urine Increase Analytical* Orange-brown spot with ninhydrin on thin-layer chromatography *2109*

Amphetamine *Urine Increase Analytical* Metabolites of brompheniramine may cause false positive results with monoclonal Syva EMIT d.a.u. immunoassay *4411*

Bromide *Serum Increase Physiological* Theoretical possibility since brompheniramine maleate contains 25% bromide *5116*

Drugs of Abuse Screen *Urine No Effect Analytical* No effect at concentration of 100 µg/mL on EZ-SCREEN procedure for cannabinoids and cocaine *1739*

Erythrocytes *Blood Decrease Physiological* Occasionally observed with antihistamines *2753*

Felbamate *Serum No Effect Analytical* No significant interference observed with GLC method of Rifai et al even though it is co-extracted *4958*

Hematocrit *Blood Decrease Physiological* Occasionally observed with antihistamines *2753*

Hemoglobin *Blood Decrease Physiological* Occasionally observed with antihistamines *2753*

^{131}I Uptake *Serum Decrease Physiological* Effect observed in some patients *1279*

Leukocytes *Blood Decrease Physiological* Occasional leukopenia/agranulocytosis *2753*

Neutrophils *Blood Decrease Physiological* Occasional case of agranulocytosis reported *6264*

Bromsulfthalein

Bilirubin *Serum No Effect Analytical* At concentration of 150 mg/L had no effect on method on Kodak Ektachem® *5706*

Bilirubin, Conjugated *Serum No Effect Analytical* At concentration of 150 mg/L no effect on method on Kodak Ektachem® *5706*

Bilirubin, Unconjugated *Serum No Effect Analytical* At concentration of 150 mg/L no effect on method on Kodak Ektachem® *5706*

Ketones *Urine Increase Analytical* May cause false positive with Ames Acetest reagent tablets *4034*
Urine No Effect Analytical No effect observed with Ames Multistix and other reagent strip tests *4034*

Lipase *Serum No Effect Analytical* No effect of concentrations up to 1500 mg/L on method on Kodak Ektachem® *5706* At a concentration of 150 mg/dL had no significant effect on method on Kodak Ektachem® systems *2519*

Broxaterol

Bicarbonate *Serum No Effect Physiological* No significant effect observed in 20 patients with reversible obstructive airways disease treated with 1.5 mg/d for up to 12 months *4637*

Carbon Dioxide Partial Pressure
Blood No Effect Physiological No significant effect observed in 20 patients with reversible obstructive airways disease treated with 1.5 mg/d for up to 12 months *4637*

Cholesterol *Serum No Effect Physiological* No significant change observed either up to 3 months or from 3 months to 1 year in 20 patients with reversible obstructive airways disease treated with 1.5 mg/d *4637*

Fatty Acids (FFA), Free *Serum No Effect Physiological* No significant change from mean baseline of 35.1 mg/dL in up to 20 patients treated with 1.5 mg/d for 12 months *4637*

Glucose *Serum No Effect Physiological* No significant change from baseline observed in 20 patients with reversible obstructive airways disease treated for 12 months with 1.5 mg/d *4637*

Glycerol *Serum Increase Physiological* Significant increase from baseline concentration of 9.1 mg/dL to 10.5 mg/dL at 1 month, 11.0 mg/dL at 2 months, 10.1 mg/dL at 3 months but increase at 6 months not significant and normal at 12 months in up to 20 patients given 1.5 mg/d *4637*

HDL-Cholesterol *Serum No Effect Physiological* No significant change observed in up to 20 patients with reversible obstructive airways disease treated with 1.5 mg/d *4637*

Insulin *Plasma Increase Physiological* Significant increase from mean baseline concentration of 8.8 µU/L observed in 20 patients with reversible obstructive airways disease treated with 1.5 mg/d at 1 month (9.8 µU/L), 2 months (9.65 µU/L), and 3 months (9.25 µU/L) but then declined to normal *4637*

LDL-Cholesterol *Serum No Effect Physiological* No significant change observed in up to 20 patients with reversible obstructive airways disease treated with 1.5 mg/d for 12 months *4637*

Oxygen Partial Pressure *Blood No Effect Physiological* Slight but nonsignificant increase observed in 20 patients with reversible obstructive airways disease treated with 1.5 mg/d for up to 12 months *4637*

pH *Blood No Effect Physiological* No significant change observed in 20 patients with reversible obstructive airways disease treated for up to 12 months with 1.5 mg/d *4637*

Potassium *Serum Decrease Physiological* Slight hypokalemia observed during first 3 months treatment with 1.5 mg/d in 20 patients with reversible obstructive airways disease with baseline concentration 4.53 mmol/L and concentrations at 1, 2, and 3 mo respectively of 4.46, 4.25 and 4.25 mmol/L *4637*

Sodium *Serum Increase Physiological* Small but significant increases observed in 20 patients with reversible obstructive airways disease treated with 1.5 mg/d for 12 months *4637*

Triglycerides *Serum No Effect Physiological* No significant change observed in up to 20 patients with reversible airways disease treated for 12 months with 1.5 mg/d *4637*

Bucindolol

Bicarbonate *Serum No Effect Physiological* No effects noted in 8 patients following several weeks on treatment *2117*

Calcium *Serum No Effect Physiological* No effects noted in 8 patients following several weeks on treatment *2117*

Chloride *Serum No Effect Physiological* No effects noted in 8 patients following several weeks on treatment *2117*

Creatine Kinase *Serum Increase Physiological* Effect noted in 3 of 6 patients studied with increased activity originating from skeletal muscle *2117*

Hemoglobin *Blood No Effect Physiological* No effects noted in 8 patients following several weeks on treatment *2117*

Leukocytes *Blood No Effect Physiological* No effects noted in 8 patients following several weeks on treatment *2117*

Norepinephrine *Plasma No Effect Physiological* No effect observed in 15 men with congestive cardiac failure treated with bucindolol for 3 months (mean baseline 403 pg/mL: after treatment 408 pg/mL) *1674*

Platelets *Blood No Effect Physiological* No effects noted in 8 patients following several weeks on treatment *2117*

Potassium *Serum No Effect Physiological* No effects noted in 8 patients following several weeks on treatment *2117*

Renin Activity *Plasma Decrease Physiological* Decrease from mean of 11.6 ng/mL/h to 4.3 ng/mL/h in 15 men with congestive cardiac failure following 3 months treatment *1674*

Sodium *Serum No Effect Physiological* No effects noted in 8 patients following several weeks on treatment *2117*

Urea Nitrogen *Serum No Effect Physiological* No effects noted in 8 patients following several weeks on treatment *2117*

Budesonide

α_1-Acid Glycoprotein *Serum No Effect Physiological* Treatment of 88 patients with Crohn's disease with up to 9 mg/d for 10 weeks caused no change from mean baseline of 1.3 ± 0.4 g/L after 8 weeks *5161*

Alkaline Phosphatase *Serum Increase Physiological* Increase from mean baseline of 2.30 µkat/L in 12 healthy volunteers to 2.43 µkat/L when 0.8 mg/d inhaled, to 2.45 µkat/L with 1.6 µkat/L and 2.43 µkat/L when 3.2 mg/d inhaled *2928*
Serum No Effect Physiological In 15 asthmatic treated with inhaled budesonide caused insignificant reduction from baseline of 532 U/L to 488 U/L after 1 month and 502 U/L after 5 months *5720*

Alkaline Phosphatase, Bone Isoenzyme
Serum No Effect Physiological In 15 asthmatic children treated with inhaled budesonide mean activity decreased insignificantly from mean baseline of 435 U/L to 405 U/L after 1 month and 425 U/L after 5 months *5720*

Amino-terminal Propeptide of Type I Procollagen
Serum Decrease Physiological In 14 prepubertal children with newly detected perennial asthma mean baseline concentration of 13.8 nmol/L treated with 1600 µg/m^2/d for one month and 400 µg/m^2/d for 5 months caused significant reductions to 10.0 nmol/L after 1 month and 9.2 nmol/L after 5 additional months *5719*

Amino-terminal Propeptide of Type III Procollagen
Serum Decrease Physiological In 14 prepubertal children with newly detected perennial asthma mean baseline concentration of 7.8 µg/L treated with 1600 µg/m^2/d for one month and 400 µg/m^2/d for 5 months caused significant reductions to 5.3 µg/L after 1 month and 5.6 µg/L after 5 additional months *5719*

Androstenedione *Plasma Decrease Physiological* Reduction from mean baseline of 6.1 nmol/L to 6.0 nmol/L in 12 healthy volunteers who inhaled 0.8 mg/d, to 5.0 nmol/L when 1.6 mg/d inhaled and to 4.0 nmol/L when 3.2 mg/d inhaled *2928*

Calcium *Serum No Effect Physiological* In 15 asthmatic children mean concentration of 2.43 mmol/L changed insignificantly to 2.45 mmol/L after 1 month inhalation of budesonide and to 2.43 mmol/L after 5 months *5720*

Corticotropin *Plasma No Effect Physiological* In 18 healthy adults a single inhaled dose of budesonide caused an insignificant change from 35.9 ± 27.2 pg/mL to 35.1 ± 33.1 pg/mL and from 28.1 ± 4.8 pg/mL to 27.2 ± 5.6 pg/mL after 2 weeks treatment *4295*

Cortisol *Plasma Decrease Physiological* In 64 patients with Crohn's disease treatment with 15 mg/d caused mean concentration to decrease from 11.5 µg/dL to 3.2 µg/dL after 2 weeks and treatment of 61 patients with 9 mg/d caused mean concentration to decrease from 11.8 µg/dL to 5.0 µg/dL after 2 weeks *2308* Treatment of 88 patients with Crohn's disease with up to 9 mg/d for 10 weeks caused significant change from mean baseline of 15.0 µg/dL to 9.0 µg/dL after 8 weeks *5161* In 18 healthy adults a single inhaled dose of budesonide caused a 40% reduction in the overnight cortisol production and a 37% reduction was observed after 2 weeks *4295* Morning concentration in 76 patients with Crohn's disease who completed 16 weeks of treatment 11.3 ± 7.3 µg/dL with 67% of patients having normal values *6018* Progressively increasing reductions observed with increasing concentration of inhaled drug to about 400 nmol/L with 0.8 mg/d, 360 nmol/L with 1.6 mg/d and 270 nmol/L with 3.2 mg/d in 12 healthy individuals *2928* In a group of asthmatics who received high dose (800 µg/d) budesonide mean fasting morning cortisol decreased from 18.4 ± 2.4 µg/dL to 15.9 ± 2.1 µg/dL after 12 weeks, but were unchanged in a group given low dose budesonide with theophylline, from 13.9 ± 1.2 µg/dL to 13.9 ± 1.3 µg/dL *1767*
Plasma No Effect Physiological In a group of asthmatics who received high dose (800 µg/d) budesonide mean fasting morning cortisol decreased from 18.4 ± 2.4 µg/dL to 15.9 ± 2.1 µg/dL after 12 weeks, but were unchanged in a group given low dose budesonide with theophylline, from 13.9 ± 1.2 µg/dL to 13.9 ± 1.3 µg/dL *1767*
Urine Decrease Physiological Inhalation of compound, up to 800 µg daily, caused highly significant dose-related suppression of output in children with bronchial asthma *583*
Urine Increase Physiological Significant increase in asthmatic children after 6 weeks use of inhaled drug: effect greater than with beclomethasone *4586*

C-Reactive Protein *Serum Decrease Physiological* Treatment of 88 patients with Crohn's disease with up to 9 mg/d for 10 weeks caused nonsignificant reduction from mean baseline of 25 ± 27 mg/L to 20 ± 23 mg/L after 8 weeks *5161*

C-terminal Propeptide of Type I Collagen
Serum Decrease Physiological In 14 prepubertal children with newly detected perennial asthma mean baseline concentration of 3.2 nmol/L treated with 1600 µg/m^2/d for one month and 400 µg/m^2/d for 5 months caused significant reductions to 2.5 nmol/L after 1 month and 2.7 nmol/L after 5 additional months *5719* In 14 children with asthma during daily budesonide inhalations of 800 µg/sq m/d for 1 month and 400 µg/sq m/d for 5 months caused significant decrease from mean baseline of 3.2 nmol/L to 2.5 nmol/L after 1 month and 2.7 nmol/L after 6 months *5719*

C-terminal Propeptide of Type I Procollagen
Serum Decrease Physiological In 15 asthmatic children treated with inhaled budesonide significant reduction from mean baseline of 354 µg/L to 336 µg/L observed after 1 month and to 254 µg/L after 5 months *5720*

Dehydroepiandrosterone Sulfate
Plasma Decrease Physiological Slight increase from mean baseline of 3.9 nmol/L to 4.2 nmol/L in 12 healthy volunteers who inhaled 0.8 mg/d but decrease to 3.0 nmol/L when 1.6 mg/d inhaled and to 2.6 nmol/L when 3.2 mg/d inhaled *2928*

Deoxypyridinoline *Urine Decrease Physiological* In 14 children with asthma during daily budesonide inhalations of 800 µg/sq m/d for 1 month and 400 µg/sq m/d for 5 months caused significant decrease from mean baseline of 18.4 nmol/mmol creatinine to 14.2 nmol/mmol creatinine after 1 month and 14.3 nmol/mmol creatinine after 6 months *5719*

Budesonide *(continued)*

Dipyridinoline *Urine Decrease Physiological* In 14 prepubertal children with newly detected perennial asthma mean baseline concentration of 18.4 nmol/mmol creatinine treated with 1600 μg/m²/d for one month and 400 μg/m²/d for 5 months caused significant reductions to 14.2 nmol/mmol creatinine after 1 month and 14.3 nmol/mmol creatinine after 5 additional months *5719*

Erythrocyte Sedimentation Rate
Blood Decrease Physiological Treatment of 88 patients with Crohn's disease with up to 9 mg/d for 10 weeks caused nonsignificant reduction from mean baseline of 27 ± 18 mm/h to 25 ± 18 mm/h after 8 weeks *5161*

Glucose *Serum Increase Physiological* Treatment of 88 patients with Crohn's disease with up to 9 mg/d for 10 weeks caused significant change from mean baseline of 81 mg/dL to 83 mg/dL after 8 weeks *5161*

Hydroxyproline *Urine Decrease Physiological* After slight increase when 0.8 mg/d inhaled, marked decrease when 1.6 mg/d inhaled and slight increase when 3.2 mg/d inhaled by 12 healthy volunteers *2928*

Insulin-like Growth Factor-I *Serum No Effect Physiological* In 7 asthmatic children treated with inhaled budesonide insignificant increase from mean baseline of 15 nmol/L to 18 nmol/L after 1 month and 17 nmol/L after 5 months *5720*

Ionized Calcium *Serum No Effect Physiological* In 15 asthmatic children treatment with inhaled budesonide for 1 and 5 months caused insignificant increase in concentration from mean baseline of 1.27 mmol/L to 1.29 mmol/L *5720*

Osteocalcin *Serum Decrease Physiological* Reduction from mean baseline of 3.4 μg/L to 3.3 μg/L in 12 healthy volunteers who inhaled 0.8 mg/d, to 3.2 μg/L when 1.6 mg/d inhaled and to 2.7 μg/L when 3.2 mg/d inhaled *2928* In 14 prepubertal children with newly detected perennial asthma mean baseline concentration of 11.5 μg/L treated with 1600 μg/m²/d for one month and 400 μg/m²/d for 5 months caused significant reductions to 9.0 μg/L after 1 month and 7.0 μg/L after 5 additional months *5719*
Serum No Effect Physiological In 15 asthmatic children treated with inhaled budesonide significant reduction from mean baseline of 23.6 μg/L to 21.8 μg/L after 1 month and insignificant reduction to 22.1 μg/L after 5 months *5720*

Phosphate *Serum No Effect Physiological* In 15 asthmatic children treatment with inhaled budesonide caused insignificant reduction from mean baseline of 1.48 mmol/L to 1.39 mmol/L after 1 month and 1.40 mmol/L after 5 months *5720*

Pyridinoline *Urine Decrease Physiological* In 14 prepubertal children with newly detected perennial asthma mean baseline concentration of 150 nmol/mmol creatinine treated with 1600 μg/m²/d for one month and 400 μg/m²/d for 5 months caused significant reductions to 111 nmol/mmol creatinine after 1 month and 106 nmol/mmol creatinine after 5 additional months *5719* In 14 children with asthma during daily budesonide inhalations of 800 μg/sq m/d for 1 month and 400 μg/sq m/d for 5 months caused significant decrease from mean baseline of 150 nmol/mmol creatinine to 111 nmol/mmol creatinine after 1 month and 106 nmol/mmol creatinine after 6 months *5719*

Type I Collagen Cross-linked N-telopeptide
Urine Decrease Physiological In 14 prepubertal children with newly detected perennial asthma mean baseline concentration of 532 nmol/mmol creatinine treated with 1600 μg/m²/d for one month and 400 μg/m²/d for 5 months caused nonsignificant reduction to 473 nmol/mmol creatinine after 1 month and significant reduction to 366 nmol/mmol creatinine after 5 additional months *5719*

Type I Collagen Teleopeptide
Serum Decrease Physiological In 14 children with asthma during daily budesonide inhalations of 800 μg/sq m/d for 1 month and 400 μg/sq m/d for 5 months caused significant decrease from mean baseline of 1.22 nmol/L to 0.85 nmol/L after 1 month and 0.87 nmol/L after 6 months *5719*

Buformin

Cholesterol *Serum Decrease Physiological* Probably inhibits synthesis in liver *1381*

Glucose *Serum Decrease Physiological* Therapeutic intent *4014*

Lactate *Plasma Increase Physiological* Rises but not usually to level of acidosis *4014*

Bufotenine

Volume *Urine Decrease Physiological* 6-7% antidiuretic activity of serotonin *1944*

Bumetanide

Bicarbonate *Serum Increase Physiological* By approximately 1 mEq/L *4405*

Bilirubin *Serum No Effect Physiological* Although displacement observed *in vitro*, insignificant effect likely *in vivo* at pharmacological concentration *6314*

Calcium *Urine Increase Physiological* After 1 mg maximum within 2 h over by 4 h *1268*

Chloride *Serum Decrease Physiological* By approximately 3 mEq/L *4405*
Urine Increase Physiological Marked dose related effect *4405*

Creatinine *Serum No Effect Physiological* No significant effect observed *4405*

Inulin Clearance *Urine No Effect Physiological* Infusion of 0.5 mg/h in 7 healthy young men had no effect on clearance *632*

Leukocytes *Blood Increase Physiological* By up to 6,000 /μL over 3 mo *4405*

Lithium *Serum Increase Physiological* Substantial increase in one patient receiving lithium to whose regime diuretic was subsequently added *3112*

Magnesium *Serum No Effect Physiological* No significant effect observed *4405*
Urine Increase Physiological After 1 mg, maximum within 2 h over by 4 h *1268*

Neutrophils *Blood Decrease Physiological* Occasional case of agranulocytosis reported *6264*

Osmolality *Serum No Effect Physiological* No significant effect observed *4405*

Osmolar Clearance *Urine Increase Physiological* Marked dose related effect *4405*

Oxalate *Urine Increase Physiological* In 7 healthy young men infusion of 0.5 mg/h caused 1.3-1.5 fold increase in specimen collected for 45 min commencing 45 min after start of infusion due to increased tubular secretion or decreased tubular reabsorption *632*

Potassium *Serum Decrease Physiological* By approximately 0.3 mEq/L *4405*
Urine Increase Physiological After 1 mg maximum within 2 h over by 4 h *1268*

Protein *Serum Increase Physiological* By up to 0.6 g/dL over 3 mo *4405*

Sodium *Serum No Effect Physiological* No significant effect observed *4405*
Urine Increase Physiological After 1 mg maximum within 2 h over by 4 h *1613* Marked dose related effect *4405*

Uric Acid *Serum Increase Physiological* Increase by 1 mg/dL over 3 mo *4405*
Urine Decrease Physiological Significantly reduced from 3-6 h *1268*
Urine No Effect Physiological No effect from 0-2 h *1268*

Volume *Urine Increase Physiological* Marked dose related effect *4405* After 1 mg maximum within 2 h over by 4 h *1268*

Water Clearance, Free *Urine Decrease Physiological* Marked dose related effect *4405*

Zinc *Urine Increase Physiological* Increase by 14% in 9 patients with hypertension over 2 weeks *6418*

Bunamiodyl

Bilirubin *Serum Increase Physiological* Competition for hepatic uptake of unconjugated *564*

BSP Retention *Serum Increase Physiological* Competes for hepatocellular protein binding sites *525*

Creatinine Clearance *Urine Decrease Physiological* At dose of 4.5 g; occurred without liver effect *6409*

Protein *Urine Increase Analytical* Affects turbidity tests for up to 3 d *116*

Urine Increase Physiological May cause nephrotoxicity *5377*

Urea Nitrogen *Serum Increase Physiological* May cause nephrotoxicity *5377*

Bunazosin

Cholesterol *Serum No Effect Physiological* In 15 obese patients with mild to moderate primary hypertension treatment with 6 and 12 mg/d bunazosin for 12 weeks caused a nonsignificant decrease of 4.1 mg/dL from the mean baseline of 217.3 ± 9.2 mg/dL *671* In 15 obese, nondiabetic patients with primary hypertension treated with either 6 or 12 mg/d of bunazosin for 12 weeks caused a nonsignificant 4.1 mg/dL reduction from mean baseline of 217.3 ± 9.2 mg/dL *671*

Fibrinogen *Plasma Increase Physiological* In 15 obese patients with mild to moderate primary hypertension treatment with 6 and 12 mg/d bunazosin for 12 weeks caused a increase of 20 mg/dL from the mean baseline of 243 ± 57 mg/dL *671* In 15 obese, nondiabetic patients with primary hypertension treated with either 6 or 12 mg/d of bunazosin for 12 weeks caused a nonsignificant 20 mg/dL increase from mean baseline of 243 ± 57 mg/dL *671*

Glucose *Serum No Effect Physiological* In 15 obese, nondiabetic patients with primary hypertension treated with either 6 or 12 mg/d of bunazosin for 12 weeks caused a nonsignificant 1.3 mg/dL reduction from mean baseline of 105.2 ± 3.0 mg/dL *671* In 15 obese patients with mild to moderate primary hypertension treatment with 6 and 12 mg/d bunazosin for 12 weeks caused a nonsignificant decrease of serum glucose of 1.3 mg/dL from mean baseline of 105.2 ± 3.0 mg/dL *671*

Glucose Tolerance *Serum Increase Physiological* In 15 obese patients with mild to moderate primary hypertension treatment with 6 and 12 mg/d bunazosin for 12 weeks caused a significant decrease in the area under the curve of serum glucose of 30% *671*

HDL-Cholesterol *Serum No Effect Physiological* In 15 obese, nondiabetic patients with primary hypertension treated with either 6 or 12 mg/d of bunazosin for 12 weeks caused a nonsignificant 1.9 mg/dL reduction from mean baseline of 45.8 ± 3.3 mg/dL *671* In 15 obese patients with mild to moderate primary hypertension treatment with 6 and 12 mg/d bunazosin for 12 weeks caused a nonsignificant decrease of 1.9 mg/dL from the mean baseline of 45.8 ± 3.3 mg/dL *671*

Hemoglobin A_{1c} *Blood Decrease Physiological* In 15 obese, nondiabetic patients with primary hypertension treated with either 6 or 12 mg/d of bunazosin for 12 weeks caused a nonsignificant 0.2% reduction from mean baseline of 5.3 ± 0.1% *671*

Blood No Effect Physiological In 15 obese patients with mild to moderate primary hypertension treatment with 6 and 12 mg/d bunazosin for 12 weeks caused a nonsignificant decrease of 0.2% from the mean baseline of 5.3 ± 0.1% *671*

Insulin *Plasma Decrease Physiological* In 15 obese, nondiabetic patients with primary hypertension treated with either 6 or 12 mg/d of bunazosin for 12 weeks caused a nonsignificant 2.3 mU/L reduction from mean baseline of 14.9 ± 1.9 mU/L *671*

Plasma No Effect Physiological In 15 obese patients with mild to moderate primary hypertension treatment with 6 and 12 mg/d bunazosin for 12 weeks caused a nonsignificant decrease of 2.3 mU/L from the mean baseline of 14.9 ± 1.9 mU/L *671*

LDL-Cholesterol *Serum No Effect Physiological* In 15 obese patients with mild to moderate primary hypertension treatment with 6 and 12 mg/d bunazosin for 12 weeks caused a nonsignificant increase of 3.8 mg/dL from the mean baseline of 140.3 ± 8.6 mg/dL *671* In 15 obese, nondiabetic patients with primary hypertension treated with either 6 or 12 mg/d of bunazosin for 12 weeks caused a nonsignificant 3.8 mg/dL increase from mean baseline of 140.3 ± 8.6 mg/dL *671*

Triglycerides *Serum Decrease Physiological* In 15 obese, nondiabetic patients with primary hypertension treated with either 6 or 12 mg/d of bunazosin for 12 weeks caused a nonsignificant 20.2 mg/dL reduction from mean baseline of 118.0 ± 25.4 mg/dL *671* In 15 obese patients with mild to moderate primary hypertension treatment with 6 and 12 mg/d bunazosin for 12 weeks caused a decrease of 20.2 mg/dL from the mean baseline of 118.0 ± 25.4 mg/dL *671*

Bunitrolol

Apolipoprotein A-I *Serum No Effect Physiological* When 30 mg/d given for 12 weeks in normolipidemic patients with mild essential hypertension *5277*

Apolipoprotein A-II *Serum No Effect Physiological* When 30 mg/d given for 12 weeks in normolipidemic patients with mild essential hypertension *5277*

Apolipoprotein B *Serum No Effect Physiological* When 30 mg/d given for 12 weeks in normolipidemic patients with mild essential hypertension *5277*

Apolipoprotein C-II *Serum No Effect Physiological* When 30 mg/d given for 12 weeks in normolipidemic patients with mild essential hypertension *5277*

Apolipoprotein C-III *Serum No Effect Physiological* When 30 mg/d given for 12 weeks in normolipidemic patients with mild essential hypertension *5277*

Apolipoprotein E *Serum No Effect Physiological* When 30 mg/d given for 12 weeks in normolipidemic patients with mild essential hypertension *5277*

Cholesterol *Serum No Effect Physiological* When 30 mg/d given for 12 weeks in normolipidemic patients with mild essential hypertension *5277*

HDL-Cholesterol *Serum Decrease Physiological* When 30 mg/d given for 12 weeks in normolipidemic patients with mild essential hypertension *5277*

LDL-Cholesterol *Serum No Effect Physiological* When 30 mg/d given for 12 weeks in normolipidemic patients with mild essential hypertension *5277*

Triglycerides *Serum No Effect Physiological* When 30 mg/d given for 12 weeks in normolipidemic patients with mild essential hypertension *5277*

VLDL-Cholesterol *Serum No Effect Physiological* When 30 mg/d given for 12 weeks in normolipidemic patients with mild essential hypertension *5277*

Buprenorphine

Histamine *Plasma No Effect Analytical* No inhibition of radio-enzyme assay likely at physiological concentrations *2492*

Bupropion

Alanine Aminotransferase *Serum Increase Physiological* Rare cases of hepatitis observed when drug administered *2168* Infrequently abnormal liver function observed *2171*

Alkaline Phosphatase *Serum Increase Physiological* Rare cases of hepatitis observed when drug administered *2168*

Amphetamine/Methamphetamine *Urine Increase Analytical* False positive results observed from buproprion and its metabolites in urines from patients taking drug when measured by Syva EMIT II procedure *4307*

Aspartate Aminotransferase *Serum Increase Physiological* Infrequently abnormal liver function observed *2171* Rare cases of hepatitis observed when drug administered *2168*

Bilirubin *Serum Increase Physiological* Rare cases of hepatitis observed when drug administered *2168*

Erythrocytes *Blood Decrease Physiological* Rare cases of anemia or pancytopenia observed when drug administered *2168*

Glucose *Urine Increase Physiological* Rare cases of glycosuria observed when drug administered *2168* Infrequently glycosuria observed *2171*

Hematocrit *Blood Decrease Physiological* Rare cases of anemia or pancytopenia observed when drug administered *2168*

Bupropion *(continued)*

Hemoglobin *Blood Decrease Physiological* Infrequently ecchymosis observed and anemia, leukocytosis, leukopenia and pancytopenia *2171* Rare cases of anemia or pancytopenia observed when drug administered *2168*

Homovanillic Acid
Cerebrospinal Fluid No Effect Physiological Insignificant effect in approximately 40 patients with depression or Alzheimer's disease after chronic treatment *4965*

5-Hydroxyindoleacetic Acid
Cerebrospinal Fluid No Effect Physiological Insignificant effect in approximately 40 patients with depression or Alzheimer's disease after chronic treatment *4965*

Leukocytes *Blood Decrease Physiological* Infrequently ecchymosis observed and anemia, leukocytosis, leukopenia and pancytopenia *2171* Rare cases of anemia or pancytopenia observed when drug administered *2168*
Blood Increase Physiological Infrequently ecchymosis observed and anemia, leukocytosis, leukopenia and pancytopenia *2171* Rare cases of leukocytosis observed when drug administered *2168*

Lymphocytes *Blood Decrease Physiological* Rare cases of anemia or pancytopenia observed when drug administered *2168*

Lysergic Acid Diethylamide *Urine Increase Analytical* Minimum concentration that caused a positive result with EMIT method to measure LSD 35 mg/L *4968*

Occult Blood *Feces Increase Physiological* Rare cases of gastrointestinal bleeding observed when drug administered *2168* Rare complication observed with treatment *2171*

Platelets *Blood Decrease Physiological* Rare cases of anemia or pancytopenia observed when drug administered *2168*

Burimamide

Hydrochloric Acid *Gastric Fluid Decrease Physiological* Decrease of up to 60% observed mainly due to decreased volume *6573*

Volume *Gastric Fluid Decrease Physiological* Marked reduction occurs *6573*

Buserelin

Acid Phosphatase, Prostatic
Serum Decrease Physiological When given with nilutamide to men with prostatic cancer steady reduction in concentration from beginning of treatment so that by 2 weeks reduced by 60%. When given with placebo increase above baseline for 2 weeks but 60% reduction occurred by 4 weeks *3320*

Androstanediol Glucuronide
Plasma Decrease Physiological In 8 hirsute women treatment with 200 µg tid as a nasal spray for 6 months caused a decrease from mean baseline of about 13 ng/mL to about 9 ng/mL *528*

Androstenedione *Plasma Decrease Physiological* In 8 hirsute women treatment with 200 µg tid as a nasal spray for 6 months caused a decrease from mean baseline of about 2.6 ng/mL to about 2.0 ng/mL *528*

Cholesterol *Serum No Effect Physiological* When daily administration combined with monthly administration of medroxyprogesterone in patients with endometriosis no significant change in cholesterol concentration noted *3512*

Dehydroepiandrosterone Sulfate
Plasma No Effect Physiological In 8 hirsute women treatment with 200 µg tid as a nasal spray for 6 months caused no significant change from mean baseline *528*

Estradiol *Plasma Decrease Physiological* In women with pelvic endometriosis concentration suppressed to predominantly early follicular phase concentrations *1943* In 13 women entered into an IVF program administration of 0.6 mg/d subcutaneously for 2 weeks caused significant reduction from mean baseline of 36 pg/mL to 20 pg/mL *2448*
Plasma No Effect Physiological In 8 hirsute women treatment with 200 µg tid as a nasal spray for 6 months caused no significant change from mean baseline of about 42 pg/mL *528*

Fibrin Degradation Products
Plasma Decrease Physiological In 13 women entered into an IVF program administration of 0.6 mg/d subcutaneously for 2 weeks caused significant change from mean baseline of 215 ng/mL to 170 ng/mL *2448*

Fibrinogen *Plasma Decrease Physiological* In 13 women entered into an IVF program administration of 0.6 mg/d subcutaneously for 2 weeks caused significant reduction from mean baseline of 2.5 g/dL to 2.0 g/dL *2448*

Fibrinogen Degradation Products
Plasma Decrease Physiological In 13 women entered into an IVF program administration of 0.6 mg/d subcutaneously for 2 weeks caused nonsignificant change from mean baseline of 220 ng/mL to 210 ng/mL *2448*

Follicle Stimulating Hormone
Plasma Decrease Physiological Significant decrease observed in 6 men with prostatic cancer treated with 500 µg s.c. daily for 15 days *6154* In men with prostatic cancer rise from mean of about 7.5 IU/L initially then fall to well below baseline by 4 weeks regardless of whether drug given with nilutamide or by itself *3320*
Plasma No Effect Physiological In 8 hirsute women treatment with 200 µg tid as a nasal spray for 6 months caused no significant change from mean baseline of about 8 mIU/mL to about 8 mIU/mL *528*

Luteinizing Hormone *Plasma Decrease Physiological* With specific IRMA method observed that treatment of 6 men with prostatic cancer with 500 µg s.c. for 15 days caused significant decrease but no change observed with a conventional RIA procedure which cross-reacted with the α-subunit *6154* In 8 hirsute women treatment with 200 µg tid as a nasal spray for 6 months caused a decrease from mean baseline of about 13 mIU/mL to about 8 mIU/mL *528* In men with prostatic cancer rise from mean of about 9.6 IU/L to above 30 - 40 IU/L at 4-5 days then fall to about 3 IU/L at 4 weeks when drug given alone or with nilutamide *3320*
Plasma Increase Physiological In 19 healthy full term infants aged 2 - 4 months a single dose of buserelin caused a significant increase in urinary excretion 4 - 6 h after buserelin administration from 0.6 ± 0.7 mIU/mL to 1.5 ± 1.1 mIU/mL returning to baseline after 24 h *398*

Plasminogen Activator Inhibitor-1
Plasma No Effect Physiological In 13 women entered into an IVF program administration of 0.6 mg/d subcutaneously for 2 weeks caused nonsignificant change from mean baseline of 4.2 ng/mL to 4.3 ng/mL *2448*

Prolactin *Plasma No Effect Physiological* In 8 hirsute women treatment with 200 µg tid as a nasal spray for 6 months caused no significant change from mean baseline *528*

Prostate-specific Antigen *Serum Decrease Physiological* Steady reduction when given with nilutamide to men with prostatic cancer so that reduction of 80% occurred by 2 weeks. In men given drug with placebo reduction did not begin until about 12 days after treatment but 75% reduction observed by 4 weeks *3320*

Sex-Hormone Binding Globulin
Serum No Effect Physiological In 8 hirsute women treatment with 200 µg tid as a nasal spray for 6 months caused no significant change from mean baseline *528*

α-Subunit *Plasma Increase Physiological* Significant increase observed in 6 men with prostatic cancer treated with 500 µg s.c. daily for 15 days *6154*

α-Subunit of Glycoprotein Hormones
Plasma Increase Physiological Significant increase observed in 6 men with prostatic cancer treated with 500 µg s.c. daily for 15 days *6154*

Testosterone *Serum Decrease Physiological* When combined with nilutamide initial rise to mean of 20.7 nmol/L in patients with prostatic cancer then fall with concentration of 0.7 nmol/L being achieved by day 22. When given with placebo rise less marked and concentration of 0.7 nmol/L not reached *3320* In 4 men with prostatic cancer treatment with a slow release form of drug given as 3-month depot injection caused suppression to near castrate range over 21 month duration of study. Same effect observed in 7 previously untreated patients after 7-14 days *6369* In 6 men with prostatic cancer treatment with 500 µg s.c. for 15 days depressed concentration to castration level *6154* In 8 hirsute women treatment with 200 µg tid as a nasal spray for 6 months caused a progressive decrease from mean baseline of about 7.5 ng/mL to about 5 ng/mL *528*

Tissue Plasminogen Activator
Plasma Decrease Physiological In 13 women entered into an IVF program administration of 0.6 mg/d subcutaneously for 2 weeks caused significant reduction from mean baseline of 2.4 ng/mL to 2.0 ng/mL *2448*

Buspirone

Creatinine *Urine No Effect Analytical* In two patients with hypertension administration of 30 mg/d for 2 days caused nonsignificant change from 2142 mg/d to 2285 mg/d in one and from 1306 mg/d to 1350 mg/d in the other when VMA measured by HPLC method with electrochemical detection *1120*

Epinephrine *Urine No Effect Analytical* In two patients with hypertension administration of 30 mg/d for 2 days caused nonsignificant change from 34 µg/d to 40 µg/d in one and from 32 µg/d to 28 µg/d in the other when VMA measured by HPLC method with electrochemical detection *1120*

Growth Hormone *Plasma No Effect Physiological* No significant effect observed in either control patients or those with generalized anxiety following treatment for 4 weeks *6048*

Lysergic Acid Diethylamide *Urine Increase Analytical* Minimum concentration that caused a positive result with EMIT method to measure LSD < 1000 mg/L *4968*

Metanephrine *Urine Increase Analytical* In two patients with hypertension administration of 30 mg/d for 2 days caused significant increase from 47 µg/d to 5913 µg/d in one and from 20 µg/d to 5157 µg/d in the other when VMA measured by HPLC method with electrochemical detection *1120*

Norepinephrine *Urine No Effect Analytical* In two patients with hypertension administration of 30 mg/d for 2 days caused nonsignificant change from 49 µg/d to 78 µg/d in one and from 60 µg/d to 49 µg/d in the other when VMA measured by HPLC method with electrochemical detection *1120*

Normetanephrine *Urine Increase Analytical* In two patients with hypertension administration of 30 mg/d for 2 days caused nonsignificant increase from 377 µg/d to 560 µg/d in one and from 179 µg/d to 204 µg/d in the other when VMA measured by HPLC method with electrochemical detection *1120*

Prolactin *Plasma No Effect Physiological* No significant effect observed in either patients with generalized anxiety or control patients following 4 weeks treatment *6048*

Vanillylmandelic Acid *Urine No Effect Analytical* In two patients with hypertension administration of 30 mg/d for 2 days caused no significant effect when VMA measured by HPLC method with electrochemical detection *1120*

Busulfan

Alanine Aminotransferase *Serum Increase Physiological* Isolated cases of cholestatic jaundice may occur with treatment *2177*

Alkaline Phosphatase *Serum Increase Physiological* Isolated cases of cholestatic jaundice may occur with treatment *2177*

Aspartate Aminotransferase *Serum Increase Physiological* Isolated cases of cholestatic jaundice may occur with treatment *2177*

Bilirubin *Serum Increase Physiological* Occurs with hemolytic anemia *2754* Isolated cases of cholestatic jaundice may occur with treatment *2177*

Erythrocytes *Blood Decrease Physiological* Pancytopenia/hemolytic anemia *2754*

Hematocrit *Blood Decrease Physiological* Pancytopenia/hemolytic anemia *2754* Most serious complication is bone marrow failure with severe pancytopenia *2177*

Hemoglobin *Blood Decrease Physiological* Most serious complication is bone marrow failure with severe pancytopenia *2177* Pancytopenia/hemolytic anemia *2754*

Histamine *Plasma No Effect Analytical* Improbable inhibition of radio-enzyme assay at therapeutic concentrations *2492*

Leukocytes *Blood Decrease Physiological* Most serious complication is bone marrow failure with severe pancytopenia *2177* Pancytopenia/Leukopenia *4014*

Neutrophils *Blood Decrease Physiological* Most serious complication is bone marrow failure with severe pancytopenia *2177*

Platelets *Blood Decrease Physiological* Pancytopenia/thrombocytopenia *2754* Most serious complication is bone marrow failure with severe pancytopenia *2177*

Sperm Count *Semen Decrease Physiological* Aspermia and testicular atrophy may occur *1384*

Urea Nitrogen *Serum Increase Physiological* Renal damage may occur from urate deposition *2242*

Uric Acid *Serum Increase Physiological* As a result of tissue destruction *3810* With cell lysis plasma concentration and urinary excretion may increase *2177*
Urine Increase Physiological With cell lysis plasma concentration and urinary excretion may increase *2177*

Butabarbital

Albumin *Serum No Effect Analytical* At concentration of 100 mg/L had no effect as measured by BCG method *5704*

Barbiturate *Urine Increase Analytical* At a concentration of 1.0 µg/mL (4.7 µmol/L) with method on Du Pont aca *1555*

Bilirubin *Serum No Effect Analytical* At concentration of 100 mg/L had no effect as measured by Jendrassik and Grof method *5704*

Butabarbital *Serum Increase Physiological* 600 mg orally produces concentration of 14 mg/L *3868*

Calcium *Serum No Effect Analytical* At concentration of 100 mg/L had no effect as measured by cresolphthalein method *5704*

Cannabinoids *Urine No Effect Analytical* No effect on Roche Abuscreen method *5006*

Carbamazepine *Serum No Effect Analytical* No cross-reactivity observed with method on Du Pont aca *1513*

Chloride *Serum No Effect Analytical* At concentration of 100 mg/L had no effect as measured by mercurimetric method *5704*

Cholesterol *Serum No Effect Analytical* At concentration of 100 mg/L had no effect as measured by Liebermann-Burchard method *5704*

Creatinine *Serum No Effect Analytical* At concentration of 100 mg/L had no effect as measured by Technicon AutoAnalyzer® Jaffe method *5704*

Drugs of Abuse Screen *Urine No Effect Analytical* No effect at concentration of 100 µg/mL on EZ-SCREEN procedure for cannabinoids and cocaine *1739*

Phenobarbital *Serum Increase Analytical* Significant interference observed at concentration of 200 µmol/L with Sung and Neely's modification of Syva EMIT method *148*
Serum No Effect Analytical No significant cross-reactivity observed with method on Du Pont aca *1537* At maximum physiological or pharmacological concentrations no cross-reactivity observed with phenobarbital method on Bayer Technicon Immuno 1® *427* At concentration of 500 µg/mL (2135 µmol/L) has no effect on method on Du Pont Dimension *1582* Cross-reactivity of less than 1.3% observed with method on Baxter Stratus *5705*

Phenytoin *Serum No Effect Analytical* No significant interference observed at a concentration of 1000 µg/mL (4.27 mmol/L) with method on Du Pont aca *1538* No effect at concentration of 1000 µg/mL (4711 µmol/L) on method on Du Pont Dimension *1583*

Phosphate *Serum No Effect Analytical* At concentration of 100 mg/L had no effect as measured by phosphomolybdate method *5704*

Primidone *Serum No Effect Analytical* No significant cross-reactivity with method on Du Pont aca *1541* At a concentration of 1250 mg/L causes 25% increase in concentration as measured by method on Baxter Stratus but clinical concentration only 15 mg/L *5705*

Protein *Serum No Effect Analytical* At concentration of 100 mg/L had no effect on method using biuret with blank correction *5704*

Butabarbital *(continued)*

Prothrombin Time *Plasma Decrease Physiological* Decreased response to anticoagulants (enzyme induction) *5674*

Triglycerides *Serum No Effect Analytical* At concentration of 100 mg/L had no effect as measured by lipase/esterase method *5704*

Urea Nitrogen *Serum No Effect Analytical* At concentration of 100 mg/L had no effect as measured by diacetylmonoxime method *5704*

Uric Acid *Serum No Effect Analytical* At concentration of 100 mg/L had no effect as measured by phosphotungstate reduction method *5704*

Butalbital

Cannabinoids *Urine No Effect Analytical* No effect on Roche Abuscreen method *5006*

Butanol

ionized Calcium *Serum Decrease Analytical* At 0.1 mmol/L to 0.1 mol/L with calcium specific electrode *820*

Butaperazine

Alanine Aminotransferase *Serum Increase Physiological* Cholestatic hepatitis with obstruction *128*

Aspartate Aminotransferase *Serum Increase Physiological* Cholestatic hepatitis with obstruction *128*

Bilirubin *Serum Increase Physiological* Cholestatic hepatitis with obstruction *128*

Eosinophils *Blood Increase Physiological* Allergic manifestation *2754*

Erythrocytes *Blood Decrease Physiological* Transitory anemia *128*

Hematocrit *Blood Decrease Physiological* Transitory anemia *128*

Hemoglobin *Blood Decrease Physiological* Transitory anemia reported *128*

Leukocytes *Blood Decrease Physiological* Transitory leukopenia *128*

Platelets *Blood Decrease Physiological* Purpura/pancytopenia observed *2754*

Pregnancy Tests *Urine Positive Analytical* May occur with delayed menstruation and ovulation *2754*

Prolactin *Plasma Increase Physiological* Significant response to 5 mg given orally *2352*

Butizide

Cholesterol *Serum No Effect Analytical* At concentration of 440 mg/L had no effect as measured by catalase-AIDH method *5704* At concentration of 440 mg/L had no effect as measured by method using catalase-Hantzsch reaction *5704* At concentration of 440 mg/L had no effect as measured by Liebermann-Burchard method *5704* At concentration of 440 mg/L had no effect as measured by CHOD-PAP method *5704* At concentration of 440 mg/L had no effect as measured by CHOD-Iodide method *5704*

Creatinine *Serum No Effect Analytical* At concentration of 2 mg/L had no effect as measured by kinetic Jaffe method on BKA-2 *5704* At concentration of 2.6 mg/L had no effect as measured by Jaffe-Fuller's earth method *5704* At concentration of 2.6 mg/L had no effect as measured by Jaffe-Fading-Fraction method *5704*

Glucose *Serum No Effect Analytical* At concentration of 0.2 mg/L had no effect as measured by Kodak Ektachem® method *5704*

Potassium *Serum No Effect Analytical* At concentration of 1.98 mg/L had no effect on ISE measurement without predilution *5704*

Protein Electrophoresis *Serum No Effect Analytical* At concentration of 1.98 mg/L had no effect as measured by automated Olympus-Hite method *5704*

Sodium *Serum No Effect Analytical* At concentration of 1.98 mg/L had no effect on ISE measurement without predilution *5704*

Urea Nitrogen *Serum No Effect Analytical* At concentration of 0.2 mg/L had no effect as measured by Kodak Ektachem® method *5704*

Uric Acid *Serum No Effect Analytical* At concentration of 2.6 mg/L had no effect as measured by catalase-AIDH method *5704* At concentration of 260 mg/L had no effect as measured by Kageyama-Hantzsch method *5704*

Butorphanol

Cortisol *Plasma No Effect Physiological* No significant effect in 6 healthy male volunteers given 2 mg i.m *5068*

Follicle Stimulating Hormone *Plasma No Effect Physiological* No significant effect in 6 healthy male volunteers given 2 mg i.m *5068*

Growth Hormone *Plasma No Effect Physiological* No significant effect in 6 healthy male volunteers given 2 mg i.m *5068*

Luteinizing Hormone *Plasma No Effect Physiological* No significant effect in 6 healthy male volunteers given 2 mg i.m *5068*

Prolactin *Plasma Increase Physiological* Significant rise in 6 healthy male volunteers given 2 mg i.m *5068*

Thyroid Stimulating Hormone *Serum No Effect Physiological* No significant effect in 6 healthy male volunteers given 2 mg i.m *5068*

Butylgallate

Catechol-O-Methyltransferase *Test Conditions Decrease Physiological* Observed *in vivo* and *in vitro4856*

Cabergoline

Growth Hormone *Plasma Decrease Physiological* No effect after 0.3 mg in 8 dopamine-responsive acromegalic patients but maximum decrease of 42% after 0.6 mg with effect lasting for up to 3 days *1844*

Prolactin *Plasma Decrease Physiological* Marked fall (49% maximum decrease after 0.3 mg and 63% maximum after 0.6 mg) observed in 8 dopamine-responsive acromegalic individuals lasting for 7 days after 0.3 mg and 14 days after 0.6 mg *1844* In 26 hyperprolactinemic patients treated for 8 weeks with up to 1.2 mg/week caused reduction to normal range in 20 patients (77%) with greater reduction in 4 but only reduction of less than 50% in the other 2 patients *1794* Given to 48 hyperprolactinemic women for 3-18 months at doses from 0.2 to 3 mg/week caused prolactin concentration to decline to normal in 41 women *1843*

Calcipotriol

Albumin *Serum No Effect Physiological* In one 17-year old woman who had treated herself with calcipotriol ointment (50 µg/g) twice daily topically for 26 days had no effect on mean concentration of 43 g/L *2655*

Calcium *Serum Increase Physiological* In one 17-year old woman who had treated herself with calcipotriol ointment (50 µg/g) twice daily topically for 26 days caused mean concentration to increase to 3.55 mmol/L *2655*
Serum No Effect Physiological No significant effect observed when applied topically for psoriasis *5292*

Creatinine *Serum Increase Physiological* In one 17-year old woman who had treated herself with calcipotriol ointment (50 µg/g) twice daily topically for 26 days caused mean concentration to increase to 141 µmol/L *2655*

1,25-Dihydroxy Vitamin D *Serum Increase Analytical* In 5 patients with psoriasis treated with topical calcipotriol mean endogenous calcitriol concentration decreased from baseline of 21.7 pmol/L to 10.0 pmol/L while calciopotriol concentration increased from undetectable to 10.4 pg/L when analyte measured by γ-B-IDS method of Immunodiagnostics System Ltd *2830*

1,25-Dihydroxy Vitamin D_3 *Serum No Effect Physiological* In one 17-year old woman who had treated herself with calcipotriol ointment (50 μg/g) twice daily topically for 26 days had no effect on mean concentration of 74 pmol/L (normal range 24 - 158 pmol/L) *2655*

25-Hydroxy Vitamin D_3 *Serum No Effect Physiological* In one 17-year old woman who had treated herself with calcipotriol ointment (50 μg/g) twice daily topically for 26 days caused decrease in concentration to mean concentration of 9.0 nmol/L (normal range 18.5 - 82 nmol/L) *2655*

Parathyroid Hormone *Plasma Decrease Physiological* In one 17-year old woman who had treated herself with calcipotriol ointment (50 μg/g) twice daily topically for 26 days caused mean concentration of PTH 1-84 to decrease to 10 - 50 ng/L *2655*

Phosphate *Serum No Effect Physiological* In one 17-year old woman who had treated herself with calcipotriol ointment (50 μg/g) twice daily topically for 26 days had no effect on mean concentration of 1.08 mmol/L *2655*

Potassium *Serum No Effect Physiological* In one 17-year old woman who had treated herself with calcipotriol ointment (50 μg/g) twice daily topically for 26 days had no effect on mean concentration of 3.5 mmol/L *2655*

Sodium *Serum No Effect Physiological* In one 17-year old woman who had treated herself with calcipotriol ointment (50 μg/g) twice daily topically for 26 days had no effect on mean concentration of 136 mmol/L *2655*

Calcitonin

Alkaline Phosphatase *Serum Decrease Physiological* Activity may be substantially increased in patients with active Paget's disease due to increased bone formation but calcitonin-salmon, by initially blocking bone absorption decreases activity in 2/3 treated patients *5235*

Alkaline Phosphatase, Bone Isoenzyme
Serum No Effect Analytical Human calcitonin at a concentration of 80 mg/L and salmon calcitonin at a concentration of 80 mg/L had no effect on EIA method of Gomez et al *2234* At a concentration of 1120 IU/L salmon calcitonin had no effect on Tandem-MP Ostase method *777*

Calcitonin *Plasma Increase Physiological* In 19 oophorectomized women given 100 IU intranasal salmon calcitonin daily with 1000 mg oral calcium for 24 months beginning on the seventh day after surgery concentration remained around 1.7 pmol/L for 12 months then increased to 2.4 pmol/L at 18 months *2332*

Calcium *Serum Decrease Physiological* Concentration may be substantially increased in patients with multiple myeloma or hyperparathyroidism but treatment with calcitonin-salmon *5235* Decrease of greater than 0.5 mEq/L observed *2391* 8 of 26 patients with malignant disease associated hypercalcemia achieved normocalcemia with intramuscular injection of drug for 5 days *6353*
Serum No Effect Physiological In 19 oophorectomized women given 100 IU intranasal salmon calcitonin daily with 1000 mg oral calcium for 24 months beginning on the seventh day after surgery concentration remained constant for 24 months *2332* No effect of intravenous injection of bolus of human hormone *3644*
Urine Decrease Physiological In 60 postmenopausal women aged 56 to 82 years dose-dependent reduction in excretion observed when doses of synthetic human calcitonin of 0.25 or 0.125 mg given subcutaneously three times per week for 1 month *3621*
Urine Increase Physiological Acts independently of parathyroid *2391*
Urine No Effect Physiological In 19 oophorectomized women given 100 IU intranasal salmon calcitonin daily with 1000 mg oral calcium for 24 months beginning on the seventh day after surgery excretion remained constant over the 24 months of the study *2332*

Casts *Urine Increase Physiological* Casts containing renal tubular epithelial cells have been reported in young healthy adult volunteers *4935* Possible nephrotoxic effect (increased granular casts) *2455*

Corticotropin *Plasma No Effect Physiological* No effect of nasal administration of 200 IU salmon calcitonin observed in 12 healthy adult men *1932*

Cortisol *Plasma No Effect Physiological* No effect of nasal administration of 200 IU salmon calcitonin observed in 12 healthy adult men *1932*

C-Peptide *Plasma Decrease Physiological* Response to glucose significantly reduced *4547*

Deoxypyridinoline *Urine Decrease Physiological* In 16 healthy volunteers administration of a single dose of salmon calcitonin mean excretion of 118.9 ± 26.0 nmol/d significantly different from 147.2 ± 45.0 nmol/d after placebo *8*

1,25-Dihydroxy Vitamin D_3 *Serum No Effect Physiological* No effect on concentration in group of postmenopausal osteoporotic women following treatment with salmon calcitonin *874*

β-Endorphin *Plasma Increase Physiological* Significant increase from 19.2 ng/L under basal conditions to peak of 27.1 ng/L at 30 minutes after nasal spray administration of 200 IU salmon calcitonin in 12 healthy adult men *1932*

Follicle Stimulating Hormone
Plasma No Effect Physiological No significant effect of 50 IU of synthetic calcitonin in 12 healthy men at rest or following LHRH stimulation *6678*

Glucagon *Plasma Increase Physiological* Inhibitory action of oral glucose on glucagon secretion partially prevented in comparison with control *4547*

Glucose Tolerance *Serum Decrease Physiological* Rise in plasma glucose exaggerated after oral sugar *4547*

Granular Casts *Urine Increase Physiological* Coarse granular casts and casts containing renal tubular epithelial cells have been reported in young healthy adult volunteers *4935* In young healthy adults given salmon calcitonin coarse granular casts and casts containing renal tubular epithelial cells observed which normalized on withdrawal of calcitonin *5235*

Growth Hormone *Plasma No Effect Physiological* No spontaneous surges in concentration observed after intravenous injection of bolus of human calcitonin *3644*

Hydroxyproline *Plasma Decrease Physiological* Excretion may be substantially increased in patients with active Paget's disease due to breakdown of collagen-containing bone matrix but calcitonin-salmon, by decreasing bone turnover decreases activity in 2/3 treated patients *5235*
Urine Decrease Physiological In 19 oophorectomized women given 100 IU intranasal salmon calcitonin daily with 1000 mg oral calcium for 24 months beginning on the seventh day after surgery decreased initially after surgery from baseline of 63 mg/g creatinine to 33 mg/g creatinine at 3 months and 36 mg/g creatinine at 6 and 12 months *2332* Due to anticatabolic action *6111* In 60 postmenopausal women aged 56 to 82 years dose-dependent reduction observed when doses of human synthetic calcitonin of 0.25 mg or 0.125 mg given subcutaneously 3 times per week for 1 month *3621* 400 IU of salmon calcitonin given intranasally for 3 days to 11 women with primary osteoporosis caused significant reduction from placebo level of 24.8 mg/24 hours to 20.1 mg/24 hours. Lower doses produced insignificant reduction *6218*

Insulin *Plasma Decrease Physiological* Response to glucose significantly reduced *4547*

Ionized Calcium *Serum Decrease Physiological* Significant reduction from mean of 4.44 mg/dL to 4.37 mg/dL with 400 IU salmon calcitonin for 3 days in 11 women with primary osteoporosis *6218*

Luteinizing Hormone *Plasma No Effect Physiological* No significant effect of 50 IU synthetic salmon calcitonin in 12 healthy men at rest or after stimulation with LHRH *6678* No effect of intravenous bolus injection of human hormone *3644*

Magnesium *Serum No Effect Physiological* No effect of intravenous injection of bolus of human hormone *3644*
Urine Increase Physiological Acts independently of parathyroid *2391*

Osteocalcin *Serum Decrease Physiological* Within 24 hours continuous infusion caused gradual reduction of increased concentration observed in 14 patients with Paget's

Calcitonin *(continued)*

Osteocalcin *(continued)*
disease *4157* In 60 postmenopausal women aged 56 to 82 years 0.25 mg human synthetic human calcitonin given subcutaneously 3 times per week for 4 months (but not smaller dose or shorter time) caused significant reduction indicating a reduction of bone formation *3621* In 19 oophorectomized women given 100 IU intranasal salmon calcitonin daily with 1000 mg oral calcium for 24 months beginning on the seventh day after surgery decreased initially after surgery but had risen to presurgery baseline after 3 months, but significant increases observed after 18 and 24 months *2332*
Serum Increase Physiological In 19 oophorectomized women given 100 IU intranasal salmon calcitonin daily with 1000 mg oral calcium for 24 months beginning on the seventh day after surgery decreased initially after surgery but had risen to presurgery baseline after 3 months, but significant increases observed after 18 and 24 months *2332*
Serum No Effect Physiological No effect in group of postmenopausal osteoporotic women following treatment with salmon calcitonin *874* In 19 oophorectomized women given 100 IU intranasal salmon calcitonin daily with 1000 mg oral calcium for 24 months beginning on the seventh day after surgery decreased initially after surgery but had risen to presurgery baseline after 3 months, but significant increases observed after 18 and 24 months *2332*

Parathyroid Hormone *Plasma No Effect Physiological* In 19 oophorectomized women given 100 IU intranasal salmon calcitonin daily with 1000 mg oral calcium for 24 months beginning on the seventh day after surgery concentration remained constant for 24 months *2332* No significant effect of treatment with 50 IU synthetic salmon hormone in 12 healthy men *6678*

Phosphate *Serum Decrease Physiological* Due to urinary loss *2242*
Serum No Effect Physiological In 19 oophorectomized women given 100 IU intranasal salmon calcitonin daily with 1000 mg oral calcium for 24 months beginning on the seventh day after surgery concentration remained constant for 24 months *2332*
Urine Increase Physiological Acts independently of parathyroid *2391*

Potassium *Urine Increase Physiological* Acts independently of parathyroid *2391*

Prolactin *Plasma Decrease Physiological* In 9 healthy subjects and 4 patients with hyperprolactinemia after i.v. infusion of salmon preparation *2832*
Plasma Increase Physiological Small but transient rise following intravenous injection of bolus of human hormone. No change in integrated response *3644*

Pyridinoline *Urine No Effect Physiological* In 16 healthy volunteers administration of a single dose of salmon calcitonin mean excretion of 553.5 ± 91.3 nmol/d not significantly different from 592.6 ± 146.3 nmol/d after placebo *8*

Sodium *Urine Increase Physiological* Acts independently of parathyroid *560*

Testosterone *Serum No Effect Physiological* No significant effect of 50 IU synthetic salmon calcitonin in 12 healthy men at rest or after LHRH stimulation *6678*

Thyroid Stimulating Hormone
Serum Increase Physiological Small but transient increase following intravenous injection of bolus of human hormone. No change in integrated response *3644*

Calcitriol

Adenosine Monophosphate *Urine Decrease Physiological* In 6 patients previously treated with cisplatin excretion decreased with calcitriol therapy from mean baseline of 2.86 mmol/d to 2.16 mmol/d *5882*

Alanine Aminotransferase *Serum Increase Physiological* Increased activity is potential complication when calcitriol administered *5031*

Albumin *Urine Increase Physiological* Increased excretion with renal damage is potential complication when calcitriol administered *5031*

Alkaline Phosphatase *Serum Decrease Physiological* Mean reduction from baseline of 261 U/L in 9 patients with secondary hyperparathyroidism undergoing dialysis with treatment with 4 µg twice weekly. Activity reduced to 236 U/L at 4 weeks and 197 U/L at 12 weeks. Reduction at 4 weeks significant *1990* Marked reduction from mean of 489 U/L to 184 U/L with long-term intermittent therapy with intravenous drug in 11 patients on hemodialysis *178*
Serum No Effect Physiological In 16 growth hormone-deficient children treatment with 1.5 µg/d for 4 days caused nonsignificant change from mean baseline of 210 ± 48 U/L to 213 ± 75 U/L *215* Nonsignificant increase in activity observed in 15 healthy men treated with 2 µg/d for 7 days *2286* Insignificant reduction observed in 18 postmenopausal women with osteoporosis treated with up to 2 µg daily for 24 months *2011*

Amylase *Serum Increase Physiological* Pancreatitis is potential complication when calcitriol administered *5031*

Aspartate Aminotransferase *Serum Increase Physiological* Increased activity is potential complication when calcitriol administered *5031*

Bilirubin *Serum No Effect Analytical* At concentration of 80 mg/L had no effect on method on Kodak Ektachem® *5706*

Bilirubin, Conjugated *Serum No Effect Analytical* No effect at concentration of 80 mg/L on method on Kodak Ektachem® *5706*

Bilirubin, Unconjugated *Serum No Effect Analytical* No effect at concentration of 80 mg/L on method on Kodak Ektachem® *5706*

Calcium *Serum Increase Physiological* Significant increase after 1 week treatment in 6 patients with ovarian or testicular cancer and hypomagnesemia induced by cisplatin from mean baseline concentration of 2.37 mmol/L to 2.48 mmol/L at 1 week and 2.59 mmol/L after 4 weeks *5882* Hypercalcemia is potential complication when calcitriol administered with vitamin D and its derivatives *5031* In 18 postmenopausal osteoporotic women treatment with 2 µg daily for 24 months caused increase from mean baseline concentration of 2.36 mmol/L to 2.45 mmol/L *2011* Significant increase after 1 week treatment in 6 patients with hypomagnesemia induced by cisplatin from mean baseline concentration of 2.37 mmol/L to 2.48 mmol/L at 1 weeks and 2.59 mmol/L after 4 weeks *5882* Increase from mean of 2.55 mmol/L to 2.67 mmol/L with long-term intermittent therapy with intravenous calcitriol in 11 patients on hemodialysis *178* In 9 patients with secondary hyperparathyroidism associated with renal failure concentration significantly increased from mean baseline of 2.50 mmol/L to 2.73 mmol/L at 4 weeks at which it remained at 12 weeks following 4 µg calcitriol orally twice weekly *1990*
Serum No Effect Physiological In 16 growth hormone deficient children treatment with 1.5 µg/d for 4 days caused insignificant increase from mean baseline of 9.66 mg/dL to 9.80 ± 0.31 mg/dL *215*
Urine Increase Physiological Nonsignificant increase from baseline of 1.81 mmol/d to 3.63 mmol/d after 1 week and significant increase to 5.72 mmol/d after 4 weeks treatment in 6 patients with ovarian or testicular cancer previously treated with cisplatin *5882* Nonsignificant increase from baseline of 1.81 mmol/d to 3.63 mmol/d after 1 week and significant increase to 5.72 mmol/d after 4 weeks treatment in 6 patients previously treated with cisplatin *5882* Treatment with up to 2 µg daily in 18 postmenopausal osteoporotic women caused increase from mean baseline concentration of 3.6 mmol/d to 8.2 mmol/d at 1 month, 7.6 mmol/d at 3 months, 7.3 mmol/d at 6 months and 6.4 mmol/d at 24 months *2011*

Calcium, Albumin-corrected *Serum No Effect Physiological* In 15 healthy men administration of 2 µg/d for 7 days had no significant effect on albumin-corrected calcium concentration *2286*

Cholesterol *Serum Increase Physiological* Increased concentration is potential complication when calcitriol administered *5031*

Creatinine *Serum No Effect Physiological* No significant change observed in 18 postmenopausal osteoporotic women treated with up to 2 µg daily for 24 months *2011*

Creatinine Clearance *Urine No Effect Physiological* No significant change observed in 18 postmenopausal women with osteoporosis treated with up to 2 µg daily for 24 months *2011*

C-terminal Propeptide of Type I Procollagen
Serum Increase Physiological In 15 healthy men administration of 2 μg/d for 7 days caused mean increase of 15% *2286*

1,25-Dihydroxy Vitamin D *Serum Increase Physiological* Increased in 20 normal subjects when given with vitamin D_2 but fell when vitamin D_2 given alone *2765* Significant increase from mean concentration of 22 pg/mL to 35 pg/mL at 4 hours after last dose in 6 patients with hypomagnesemia induced by cisplatin after 4 weeks treatment *5882*

1,25-Dihydroxy Vitamin D_3 *Serum Increase Physiological* In both placebo-treated and estrogen-treated oophorectomized women calcitriol caused increase from basal concentration to a comparable extent compared with presurgery response (from 24.2% to 34.7% in placebo group, from 34.2% to 26.6% in estrogen group) *2085* Significant effect observed in group of women with postmenopausal osteoporosis following treatment *874* In 15 healthy men aged 28 to 45 years administration of 2 μg/d for 7 days caused significant increase (by about 49%) from mean baseline of 75 pmol/L to 100 pmol/L but concentrations remained within normal range *2286*

Fractional Excretion of Magnesium
Urine Increase Physiological Significant increase from baseline of 9.6% to 14.4% at 2 weeks, 19.3% at 3 weeks and 17.6% at 4 weeks in 6 patients with ovarian or testicular cancer previously treated with cisplatin *5882* Significant increase from baseline of 9.6% to 14.4% at 2 weeks, 19.3% at 3 weeks and 17.6% at 4 weeks in 6 patients previously treated with cisplatin *5882*

Hyaluronan *Serum No Effect Physiological* In 15 healthy men given 2 μg/d for 7 days no significant change observed *2286*

25-Hydroxy Vitamin D *Serum No Effect Physiological* In 15 healthy men treatment with 2 μg/d for 7 days had no significant effect on concentration *2286*

Insulin-like Growth Factor-I *Serum No Effect Physiological* In 16 growth hormone deficient children treatment with 1.5 μg/d for 4 days caused insignificant increase from mean baseline of 61 ± 11 ng/mL to 63 ± 10 ng/mL *215*

Ionized Calcium *Serum Increase Physiological* Significant increase from mean baseline concentration of 1.25 mmol/L to 1.31 mmol/L after one week's treatment with further increase to 1.35 mmol/L after 4 weeks in 6 patients previously treated with cisplatin *5882*

Lipase *Serum Increase Physiological* Pancreatitis is potential complication when calcitriol administered *5031*

Magnesium *Serum Decrease Physiological* Significant decrease from already low baseline concentration in 6 patients previously treated with cisplatin from baseline concentration of 0.44 mmol/L to 0.32 mmol/L after 2 weeks and 0.28 mmol/L after 4 weeks *5882* Significant decrease from already low baseline concentration in 6 patients with ovarian or testicular cancer previously treated with cisplatin from baseline concentration of 0.44 mmol/L to 0.32 mmol/L after 2 weeks and 0.28 mmol/L after 4 weeks *5882*
Serum Increase Physiological Administration of calcitriol with magnesium-containing antacids may be associated with hypermagnesemia *12* Hypermagnesemia is potential complication when calcitriol administered with magnesium-containing antacids in patients on chronic renal dialysis *5031*
Urine No Effect Physiological No significant change observed in 6 patients with ovarian or testicular cancer previously treated with cisplatin after 4 weeks treatment with calcitriol *5882* No significant change observed in 6 patients previously treated with cisplatin after 4 weeks treatment with calcitriol *5882*

N-terminal Propeptide of Type III Procollagen
Serum No Effect Physiological No significant change observed in 15 healthy men aged 28 to 45 years given 2 μg/d for 7 days *2286*

Osteocalcin *Serum Increase Physiological* Significant effect observed in group of postmenopausal women with osteoporosis following treatment *874* In 15 healthy men administration of 2 μg/d for 7 days caused mean increase of 26% *2286* Rose in response to concomitant administration with vitamin D_2 in 20 normal subjects *2765* In 16 growth hormone-deficient prepubertal children treatment with 1.5 μg/d for 4 days caused significant increase in concentration from low pretreatment concentration of 9.39 ± 3.19 ng/mL to 21.32 ± 9.39 ng/mL *215*

Parathyroid Hormone *Plasma Decrease Physiological* In 9 patients with secondary hyperparathyroidism undergoing long-term dialysis 4 μg orally twice weekly caused significant reduction from mean baseline of 108 pmol/L to 67 pmol/L after 4 weeks, and to 44 pmol/L at 12 weeks *1990* Significant reduction observed in 6 patients with ovarian or testicular cancer and hypomagnesemia caused by previous treatment with cisplatin when treated with 0.5-1.0 μg/d calcitriol for 4 weeks *5882* Significant reduction of amino-terminal (from mean of 172 ng/L to 69 ng/L) and nonsignificant reduction of carboxy-terminal concentration from mean of 1486 mL/Eq/L to 1083 mL/Eq/L in 11 patients on hemodialysis following intermittent intravenous therapy *178*

Phosphate *Serum Decrease Physiological* Nonsignificant decrease from mean baseline of 1.90 mmol/L in 9 patients with hyperparathyroidism secondary to renal failure receiving dialysis when treated with 4 μg calcitriol twice weekly to 1.80 mmol/L at 4 weeks and 1.71 mmol/L at 12 weeks *1990*
Serum No Effect Physiological In 16 growth hormone deficient children treatment with 1.5 μg/d for 4 days caused nonsignificant increase from mean baseline of 4.98 ± 0.37 mg/dL to 5.20 ± 0.57 mg/dL *215* No change with long-term intermittent therapy with intravenous drug in 11 patients on hemodialysis *178*

Urea Nitrogen *Serum Increase Physiological* Increased concentration is potential complication when calcitriol administered *5031*

Uric Acid *Serum Increase Physiological* Increased concentration is potential complication when calcitriol administered *5031*

Calcium Bromogalactogluconate

Bromide *Serum Increase Physiological* In patient taking 12 g drug daily for 3 mo serum concentration of 18.7 mmol/L *4778* Theoretical possibility since drug contains 16.7% bromide *5116*

Chloride *Serum Increase Analytical* Relatively small error by coulometric method as used on Beckman Astra® but significant increase at clinical concentrations with thiocyanate methods on Technicon RA-1000 or SMAC® *4778*

Calcium Carbimide

Oxalate *Urine Decrease Analytical* Inhibits enzymatic procedure for measurement *6632*

Calcium Carbonate

Calcium *Serum No Effect Physiological* No rise after 4 g observed *5515*

Ciprofloxacin *Serum Decrease Physiological* Concurrent administration of ciprofloxacin with antacids containing magnesium, aluminum, or calcium may substantially interfere with the absorption of ciprofloxacin and plasma and urine concentrations less than desired *416*
Urine Decrease Physiological Concurrent administration of ciprofloxacin with antacids containing magnesium, aluminum, or calcium may substantially interfere with the absorption of ciprofloxacin and plasma and urine concentrations less than desired *416*

Crystals *Urine Increase Physiological* Small colorless dumbbells/spheres (not in acid urine) *684*

Gastrin *Serum Increase Physiological* 2 fold increase, maximum 30 to 75 minutes after administration *5515*

Raloxifene *Serum No Effect Physiological* Reported to have no effect on the systemic exposure of raloxifene *1696*

Calcium Dobesilate

Albumin *Urine No Effect Analytical* At concentration of 50 mg/dL had no significant effect on Boehringer Mannheim Tinaquant method *2799*

Calcium Dobesilate *(continued)*

Cholesterol *Serum No Effect Analytical* At therapeutic concentrations cholesterol concentration not significantly affected with method on Boehringer Mannheim Hitachi 717 *4179*

Cortisol *Plasma No Effect Analytical* At concentration of 200 mg/L no significant effect on CEDIA or Enzymun methods (worst case 104.0% recovery). At therapeutic concentration of 20 mg/L in plasma no effect observed on recovery with Enzymun method *1097*

Creatine Kinase *Serum Decrease Analytical* Only 85% recovery observed at high drug dose with whole blood method on Boehringer Mannheim Reflotron *2714*

Serum Decrease Physiological Significant reduction observed in drug-treated patients with myocardial infarction compared with untreated controls during first 72 hours *5906*

Creatinine *Serum Decrease Analytical* At therapeutic concentrations concentration of creatinine reduced by 26% with method on Boehringer Mannheim Hitachi 717 *4179*

Glucose *Serum Decrease Analytical* At therapeutic concentrations concentration of glucose reduced by 5.7% with method on Boehringer Mannheim Hitachi 717 *4179*

Glycosaminoglycan *Urine Increase Physiological* Significant increase observed in patients with myocardial infarction when treated with drug than in controls *5906*

HDL-Cholesterol *Serum Increase Analytical* At a concentration of 200 mg/L had a significant effect on Reflotron method for whole blood cholesterol (85% recovery) *6352*

Serum No Effect Analytical At a concentration up to 20 mg/L had no significant effect on Reflotron method for whole blood cholesterol *6352*

Myoglobin *Urine Decrease Physiological* Significant reduction in drug-treated patients during first 72 hours following myocardial infarction compared with controls *5906*

N-Acetyl-Glucosaminidase *Urine No Effect Analytical* At concentration of 50 mg/dL had no significant effect on Boehringer Mannheim CPR method *3174*

Triglycerides *Serum Decrease Analytical* At therapeutic concentrations concentration of triglycerides reduced by 6.1% with method on Boehringer Mannheim Hitachi 717 *4179*

Uric Acid *Serum Decrease Analytical* At therapeutic concentrations concentration of uric acid reduced by 6.2% with method on Boehringer Mannheim Hitachi 717 *4179*

Calcium Gluconate

Calcium *Serum Increase Physiological* Marked effect noted in newborns *2543*

Glucose *Serum Decrease Physiological* Slight effect observed in newborns *2543*

11-Hydroxycorticosteroids *Plasma Increase Physiological* Transient effect maximum at 15 minutes after i.v *2452*

17-Hydroxycorticosteroids *Urine Decrease Physiological* Reduced value reported in a single case *806*

^{131}I Uptake *Serum Decrease Physiological* Wafer of Upjohn contains tetraiodofluorescein *4360*

Insulin *Plasma Increase Physiological* Marked effect noted in newborns *2543*

Ketone Body Ratio *Serum No Effect Analytical* When added at a concentration of 8.5 g/L had no significant effect on AKBR method of Uno et al *6131*

Magnesium *Serum Decrease Analytical* False decrease if measured by titan-yellow *151*

Serum No Effect Physiological No effect on dihydroxyazobenzene method *5867*

Urine Decrease Analytical False decrease if measured by titan-yellow *151*

Calcium Hypochlorite

Cannabinoids *Urine No Effect Analytical* No effect on Roche Abuscreen method *5006*

Calcium Ions

Lipase *Serum Decrease Analytical* At concentrations above 5 mmol/L on method of Tietz *6027*

Serum No Effect Analytical Up to 5 mmol/L on method of Tietz *6027*

Calcium Nitrate

Bilirubin *Serum No Effect Analytical* At concentration of 200 mmol/L had no effect on method on Kodak Ektachem® *5706*

Calomel

Color *Feces Increase Analytical* Green color observed *1957*

Camazepam

Benzodiazepine *Urine Positive Analytical* At concentration of 7.5 µg/mL or greater produces positive result with Syva EMIT II assay *1785*

p-Aminophenol *Urine No Effect Analytical* With addition of drugs at a concentration of 100 mg/L and of related compounds at 50 mg/L no significant effect observed on colorimetric method of van Bocxlaer on Cobas Mira analyzer which involves reacting free p-aminophenol with resorcinol in the presence of magnesium ions to form an indophenol dye measured at 550 nm *6163*

Candesartan Cilexetil

Alanine Aminotransferase *Serum Increase Physiological* In 3260 treated patients small increases observed and severe enough in five to require withdrawal from the trial *269*

Aldosterone *Plasma Decrease Physiological* Once daily administration of 32 mg to hypertensive individuals significantly reduced plasma concentration *269*

Plasma No Effect Physiological Once daily administration of 16 mg to healthy individuals had no effect on plasma concentration *269*

Alkaline Phosphatase *Serum Increase Physiological* In 3260 treated patients small increases observed and severe enough in five to require withdrawal from the trial *269*

Angiotensin-I *Plasma Increase Physiological* Concentrations increased in a dose-dependent manner after single and repeated administration of drug to healthy individuals and hypertensive patients *269*

Angiotensin-II *Plasma Increase Physiological* Concentrations increased in a dose-dependent manner after single and repeated administration of drug to healthy individuals and hypertensive patients *269*

Angiotensin-converting Enzyme
Serum No Effect Physiological Activity unaffected after single and repeated administration of drug to healthy individuals and hypertensive patients *269*

Aspartate Aminotransferase *Serum Increase Physiological* In 3260 treated patients small increases observed and severe enough in five to require withdrawal from the trial *269*

Bilirubin *Serum Increase Physiological* In 3260 treated patients small increases observed and severe enough in five to require withdrawal from the trial *269*

Blood *Urine Increase Physiological* In 3600 treated patients increased concentration observed in more than 0.5% although relationship to administration of candesartan cilexetil not confirmed *269*

Cholesterol *Serum No Effect Physiological* In multiple-dose studies in hypertensive patients no clinically significant change in concentration observed *269*

Creatine Kinase *Serum Increase Physiological* In 3600 treated patients increased creatine kinase activity observed in more than 0.5% although relationship to administration of candesartan cilexetil not confirmed *269*

Creatinine *Serum Increase Physiological* In 3260 treated patients increased concentration observed in 19 (0.6%) although relationship to administration of candesartan cilexetil not confirmed *269*

Glucose *Serum Increase Physiological* In 3600 treated patients increased concentration observed in more than 0.5% although relationship to administration of candesartan cilexetil not confirmed *269*

Serum No Effect Physiological In multiple-dose studies in hypertensive patients no clinically significant change in concentration observed *269*

Hematocrit *Blood Decrease Physiological* In 3260 treated patients decrease of 0.5% observed in some although relationship to administration of candesartan cilexetil not confirmed *269* In a clinical trial anemia caused withdrawal of one patient *269*

Hemoglobin *Blood Decrease Physiological* In a clinical trial anemia caused withdrawal of one patient *269* In 3260 treated patients decrease of 0.2 g/dL observed in some although relationship to administration of candesartan cilexetil not confirmed *269*

Hemoglobin A_{1c} *Blood No Effect Physiological* In a 12 week study of 161 patients with noninsulin-dependent diabetes mellitus no clinically significant change in concentration observed *269*

Leukocytes *Blood Decrease Physiological* In a clinical trial leukopenia caused withdrawal of one patient *269*

Platelets *Blood Decrease Physiological* In a clinical trial thrombocytopenia caused withdrawal of one patient *269* In 3260 treated patients decrease thrombocytopenia caused withdrawal of one patient from clinical trial *269*

Potassium *Serum Decrease Physiological* Once daily administration of 32 mg to hypertensive individuals had no significant effect on plasma potassium concentration although significantly reduced plasma aldosterone concentration *269*

Serum Increase Physiological In 3260 treated patients small increases of about 0.1 mmol/L observed although of no clinical significance *269*

Renin Activity *Plasma Increase Physiological* Concentrations increased in a dose-dependent manner after single and repeated administration of drug to healthy individuals and hypertensive patients *269*

Triglycerides *Serum Increase Physiological* In 3600 treated patients increased concentration observed in more than 0.5% although relationship to administration of candesartan cilexetil not confirmed *269*

Serum No Effect Physiological In multiple-dose studies in hypertensive patients no clinically significant change in concentration observed *269*

Urea Nitrogen *Serum Increase Physiological* In 3260 treated patients increased concentration observed in 19 (0.6%) although relationship to administration of candesartan cilexetil not confirmed *269*

Uric Acid *Serum Increase Physiological* In 3600 treated patients increased concentration observed in 0.6% although relationship to administration of candesartan cilexetil not confirmed *269*

Serum No Effect Physiological In multiple-dose studies in hypertensive patients no clinically significant change in concentration observed *269*

Candoxatril

Atrial Natriuretic Peptide *Plasma Increase Physiological* In patients with essential hypertension concentration increased 2-fold regardless of whether patients were receiving 350 mmol or 10 mmol sodium/d *5572*

N-terminal Pro-atrial Natriuretic Peptide *Serum No Effect Physiological* In patients with essential hypertension concentration increased by high sodium diet (350 mmol/d) but increased concentration not affected by candoxatril *5572*

Renin Activity *Plasma Decrease Physiological* On 10 mmol/d sodium diet concentration suppressed when patient receiving candoxatril but not affected when patients receiving 350 mmol/d sodium *5572*

Sodium *Urine Increase Physiological* With inhibition of endopeptidase 24.11 inhibition by candoxatril urinary excretion increased 3-fold on 10 mmol/d sodium and 6-fold on 350 mmol/d sodium diet *5572*

Cannabis

Catecholamines *Urine No Effect Physiological* Essentially unchanged with moderate dose *2677*

Chloride *Serum Increase Physiological* Reported effect *3669*

Chlorpromazine *Serum Decrease Physiological* In smokers clearance increased by a factor of 1.50 ± 0.28 compared with 1.0 in nonsmokers (191 L/h in cannabis smokers versus 127 L/h in nonsmoking schizophrenics) *987*

Cortisol *Plasma No Effect Physiological* Essentially unchanged with moderate dose *2677*

Creatinine *Serum Decrease Physiological* Reported effect *3669*

Creatinine Clearance *Urine Decrease Physiological* Temporary decrease noted *2677*

Fatty Acids (FFA), Free *Serum No Effect Physiological* No effect observed *2677*

Glucose *Serum Decrease Physiological* Hypoglycemic effect approximately 4 h after use *1437*

Serum Increase Physiological Reported effect *192*

Serum No Effect Physiological No effect observed *2677*

Glucose Tolerance *Serum Decrease Physiological* Increased concentrations noted in some subjects at 1/2 to 1 h *4725*

Insulin *Plasma Increase Physiological* Responsible for hypoglycemia *1437*

Phosphate Clearance *Urine Decrease Physiological* Temporary decrease noted *2677*

Potassium *Serum Increase Physiological* Reported effect *3669*

Sodium *Serum Increase Physiological* Reported effect *3669*

Urea Nitrogen *Serum Increase Physiological* Reported effect *3669*

Uric Acid *Serum Decrease Physiological* Reported effect *3669*

Canola Oil

Alanine Aminotransferase *Serum No Effect Physiological* No significant change observed in 36 hyperlipidemic patients given 30 mL daily for 4 months *555*

Alkaline Phosphatase *Serum No Effect Physiological* No significant effect observed in 36 hyperlipidemic patients given 30 mL daily for 4 months *555*

Aspartate Aminotransferase *Serum Increase Physiological* No significant change observed in 36 hyperlipidemic patients given 30 mL daily for 4 months *555*

Bilirubin *Serum No Effect Physiological* No significant effect observed in 36 hyperlipidemic patients given 30 mL daily for 4 months *555*

Bleeding Time *Patient Increase Physiological* Significant increase from mean baseline of 257 seconds to 400 seconds in 36 hyperlipidemic patients treated with 30 mL daily for 4 months *555*

Calcium *Serum No Effect Physiological* No significant effect observed in 36 hyperlipidemic patients treated with 30 mL daily for 4 months *555*

β-Carotene *Serum Decrease Physiological* Significant reduction from mean baseline concentration of 27.4 μg/dL to 14.9 μg/dL in 36 hypercholesterolemic or hypertriglyceridemic patients given 30 mL daily for 4 months *555*

Cholesterol *Serum No Effect Physiological* Nonsignificant reduction from mean baseline of 254 mg/dL to 248 mg/dL observed in 36 hypercholesterolemic or hypertriglyceridemic patients treated with 30 mL daily for 4 months *555*

Creatinine *Serum No Effect Physiological* No significant effect observed in 36 hyperlipidemic patients given 30 mL daily for 4 months *555*

Canola Oil *(continued)*

Glucose *Serum* *No Effect* *Physiological* No significant effect observed in 36 hyperlipidemic patients treated with 30 mL daily for 4 months *555*

γ-Glutamyltransferase *Serum* *No Effect* *Physiological* No significant change observed in 36 hyperlipidemic patients given 30 mL daily for 4 months *555*

HDL_2-Cholesterol *Serum* *Decrease* *Physiological* Significant decrease from mean baseline concentration of 16.3 mg/dL to 13.1 mg/dL in 24 hypertriglyceridemic or hypercholesterolemic patients treated with 30 mL daily for 4 months *555*

HDL_3-Cholesterol *Serum* *Increase* *Physiological* Significant increase from mean baseline of 33.2 mg/dL to 36.1 mg/dL in 24 hypertriglyceridemic or hypercholesterolemic patients treated with 30 mL daily for 4 months *555*

HDL-Cholesterol *Serum* *No Effect* *Physiological* Nonsignificant increase from mean baseline concentration of 47 mg/dL to 51 mg/dL in 36 hypertriglyceridemic or hypercholesterolemic patients treated with 30 mL daily for 4 months *555*

Iron *Serum* *No Effect* *Physiological* No significant effect observed in 36 hyperlipidemic patients treated with 30 mL daily for 4 months *555*

LDL-Cholesterol *Serum* *Decrease* *Physiological* Significant decrease from mean baseline concentration of 173 mg/dL to 160 mg/dL in 36 hypertriglyceridemic or hypercholesterolemic patients treated with 30 mL daily for 4 months *555*

Phosphate *Serum* *No Effect* *Physiological* No significant change observed in 36 hyperlipidemic patients treated with 30 mL daily for 4 months *555*

Retinol *Serum* *No Effect* *Physiological* Nonsignificant increase from mean baseline concentration of 52.4 µg/d: to 54.3 µg/dL observed in 36 hypertriglyceridemic or hypercholesterolemic patients treated with 30 mL daily for 4 months *555*

α-Tocopherol *Serum* *Decrease* *Physiological* Significant decrease from mean baseline concentration of 1.62 mg/dL to 1.36 mg/dL in 36 hypertriglyceridemic or hypercholesterolemic patients treated with 30 mL daily for 4 months *555*

Triglycerides *Serum* *No Effect* *Physiological* Nonsignificant increase from mean baseline of 214 mg/dL to 226 mg/dL in 36 hypertriglyceridemic or hypercholesterolemic patients treated with 30 mL daily for 4 months *555*

Urea Nitrogen *Serum* *No Effect* *Physiological* No significant effect observed in 36 hyperlipidemic patients given 30 mL daily for 4 months *555*

Uric Acid *Serum* *Decrease* *Physiological* Significant reduction from mean baseline concentration of 6.4 mg/dL to 6.1 mg/dL observed in 36 hyperlipidemic patients treated with 30 mL daily for 4 months *555*

Canrenoate

Digoxin *Serum* *Increase* *Analytical* At normal concentrations in serum if no preincubation *4688*

Canrenone

Digoxin *Serum* *No Effect* *Analytical* At concentrations up to 50 µg/mL no significant effect observed with method on Ciba Corning ACS:180 *1412*

Cantharides

Protein *Urine* *Increase* *Physiological* May cause nephrotoxicity *5377*

Urea Nitrogen *Serum* *Increase* *Physiological* May cause nephrotoxicity *5377*

Volume *Urine* *Decrease* *Physiological* May cause oliguria with renal damage *467*

Canthaxanthine

Carotene *Serum* *Increase* *Analytical* During administration and for 10 d after may affect certain analytical methods *5055*

Color *Serum* *Increase* *Physiological* Constituent of suntan agent imparts strong orange-pink color to plasma *5965*

Vitamin A *Serum* *Increase* *Analytical* During administration and for 10 d after may affect certain analytical methods *5055*

Capecitabine

Alanine Aminotransferase *Serum* *Increase* *Physiological* Capecitabine administration associated with cholestatic hepatitis in 0.2% patients and hepatitis in 0.2% patients *5013*

Alkaline Phosphatase *Serum* *Increase* *Physiological* Capecitabine administration associated with cholestatic hepatitis in 0.2% patients and hepatitis in 0.2% patients *5013*

Aspartate Aminotransferase *Serum* *Increase* *Physiological* Capecitabine administration associated with cholestatic hepatitis in 0.2% patients and hepatitis in 0.2% patients *5013*

Bilirubin *Serum* *Increase* *Physiological* Capecitabine administration associated with cholestatic hepatitis in 0.2% patients and hepatitis in 0.2% patients *5013*

Erythrocytes *Blood* *Decrease* *Physiological* Capecitabine administration associated with pancytopenia in 0.2% patients *5013*

Leukocytes *Blood* *Decrease* *Physiological* Capecitabine administration associated with pancytopenia in 0.2% patients *5013*

Occult Blood *Feces* *Increase* *Physiological* Capecitabine administration associated with rectal bleeding in 0.4% patients and gastrointestinal hemorrhage in 0.4% patients *5013*

Platelets *Blood* *Decrease* *Physiological* Capecitabine administration associated with idiopathic thrombocytopenic purpura in 0.2% patients *5013*

Triglycerides *Serum* *Increase* *Physiological* Capecitabine administration associated with hypertriglyceridemia in 0.2% patients *5013*

Capreomycin

Alanine Aminotransferase *Serum* *No Effect* *Physiological* Decreased BSP excretion observed in patients with preexisting liver disease without effect on liver enzyme activity *1626*

Alkaline Phosphatase *Serum* *Increase* *Physiological* Reported effect on liver *2794*

Aspartate Aminotransferase *Serum* *Increase* *Physiological* Reported effect on liver *2794*
Serum *No Effect* *Physiological* Decreased BSP excretion observed in patients with preexisting liver disease without effect on liver enzyme activity *1626*

BSP Retention *Serum* *Increase* *Physiological* Transient increase in 5% subjects *4014*

Casts *Urine* *Increase* *Physiological* Nephrotoxic effect (usually granular casts) *3810*

Creatinine *Serum* *Increase* *Physiological* Nephrotoxic effect *3810*

Eosinophils *Blood* *Increase* *Physiological* Eosinophilia above 5% observed in the majority of patients treated with daily injections of capreomycin *1626* Allergic reaction (may be up to 35%) *775*

Erythrocytes *Urine* *Increase* *Physiological* May cause nephrotoxicity *2754*

Leukocytes *Blood* *Decrease* *Physiological* May cause leukopenia or leukocytosis *2754* Both leukopenia and leukocytosis observed in patients treated with capreomycin *1626*
Blood *Increase* *Physiological* Both leukopenia and leukocytosis observed in patients treated with capreomycin *1626* Due to eosinophilia of hypersensitivity *3810*

Nonprotein Nitrogen *Serum* *Increase* *Physiological* Nephrotoxic effect *3810*

Phenolsulfonphthalein *Urine* *Decrease* *Physiological* In 36% of 722 patients serum urea nitrogen concentration increased above 30 mg/dL and in many cases depression of PSP excretion observed *1626*

Platelets *Blood* *Decrease* *Physiological* Thrombocytopenia rarely observed in patients treated with capreomycin *1626*

Potassium *Serum* *Decrease* *Physiological* Observed occasionally with therapy *2753*

Protein *Urine Increase Physiological* Nephrotoxic effect (transient) *1714*

PSP Excretion *Urine Decrease Physiological* Observed with other signs of decreased renal function *2754*

Sulfobromophthalein *Serum Increase Physiological* Decreased BSP excretion observed in patients with preexisting liver disease without effect on liver enzyme activity *1626*

Urea Nitrogen *Serum Decrease Physiological* In 36% of 722 patients serum urea nitrogen concentration increased above 30 mg/dL and in many cases depression of PSP excretion observed *1626*

Serum Increase Physiological Nephrotoxic effect (in 6% subjects) *2242*

Uric Acid *Serum Increase Physiological* Nephrotoxic effect associated with hyperuricemia *2548*

Urobilin *Urine Increase Physiological* May cause nephrotoxicity *2754*

Caproxamine

Albumin *Serum Increase Analytical* At 1.5 mg/dL on conventional methods if added to sera *2877*

γ-Globulin *Serum Decrease Analytical* At 1.5 mg/dL on conventional methods when added to sera *2877*

Protein *Serum Decrease Analytical* At 1.5 mg/dL on conventional methods when added to sera *2877*

Urea Nitrogen *Serum Decrease Analytical* At 1.5 mg/dL with conventional methods when added to sera *2877*

Captopril

Albumin *Serum No Effect Physiological* In 17 patients with essential hypertension treatment with up to 40 mg/d quinapril caused caused no significant change in concentration after 12 weeks *4810* In 9 patients with essential hypertension treated with captopril for 6 months baseline value of 43 ± 3 g/L not significantly changed to 43 ± 2 g/L *2237*

Urine Decrease Physiological In 12 patients with sickle cell anemia and persistent microalbuminuria treatment with 25 mg/d caused reduction of 45 mg/d over 6 months *1927* Mean excretion reduced from 78 µg/min to 38 µg/min with 3 months treatment with 0.9 mg/kg/d in 12 insulin-dependent diabetic adolescents including 11 with microalbuminuria *1121* In 19 patients with chronic heart failure treatment with up to 75 mg/d caused significant reduction of mean of 67 µmol/mol creatinine on day 1 to 36 µmol/mol creatinine on day 7, 17 µmol/mol creatinine on day 14 and 11 µmol/mol on day 30 *1717* After 50 mg drug in 24 hours significant reduction after exercise in diabetics with stage II and stage III disease but no effect in normal subjects *5072* In 17 patients with mild to moderate essential hypertension treatment with up to 150 mg/d for 12 weeks caused significant decrease from mean baseline of 59 µg/min to 41 µg/min *4810* In 92 patients with IDDM but no hypertension ingestion of 100 mg/d caused decrease from mean 52 µg/min to 41 µg/min *6254* In 17 patients with essential hypertension treatment with up to 40 mg/d captopril caused decrease in albumin excretion rate from mean baseline of 59 µg/min to 41 µg/min after 12 weeks *4810*

Aldosterone *Plasma Decrease Physiological* Gradual reduction probably due to longer half-life than angiotensin II *287* In 11 patients with resistant heart failure captopril reduced mean concentration from 62 ng/dL to 26 ng/dL *1925* Fell in conjunction with fall of systemic arterial pressure *2811* In 20 normotensive and 7 hypertensive individuals treatment with 25 mg significantly decreased plasma renin activity from a mean of 17.5 ± 1.3 ng/dL to 8.6 ± 1.0 ng/dL in controls *2004* In 24 patients with NIDDM and proteinuria greater than 500 mg/d treatment with captopril (25 - 75 mg/d) for 18 months caused a significant change from mean baseline of 12.31 ± 0.97 ng/mL to 7.24 ± 0.66 ng/mL *3601* Caused reduction in 15 hypertensive patients with advanced liver disease from an increased baseline *5771* From 1.08 nmol/L to 0.22 nmol/L after 3 d treatment in 1 patient with Bartter's syndrome *2553* Parallel decline with sodium in congestive heart failure patients *4282* Nonsignificant reduction observed over 120 minutes in 7 healthy male volunteers following 75 mg orally *4303* With doses up to 800 mg/d for 10 d in 23 hypertensive patients *4739*

Plasma No Effect Physiological Insignificant change observed in 8 normotensive women volunteers and 17 patients with essential hypertension following single oral dose of 25 mg *6082* Treatment of 19 elderly patients with mild to moderate hypertension with up to 75 mg daily for 8 weeks had no significant effect on concentration *3335* In 30 patients with acute myocardial infarction administration of 50 mg twice daily 28 days caused insignificant change from median baseline concentration of 8.3 to 8.0 ng/dL from day 1 to day 3 *798*

Urine Decrease Physiological Fell in conjunction with fall of systemic arterial pressure *2811* Sustained effect: extent related to pretreatment plasma renin activity *287* With doses up to 800 mg/d for 10 d in 23 hypertensive patients *4739*

Alkaline Phosphatase *Serum Increase Physiological* Characteristic pattern of hepatocellular jaundice in one patient. But with secondary cholestatic elements *6204* Isolated case of cholestasis in patient receiving 25 mg t.i.d. for 1 mo *4536*

Angiotensin-II *Plasma Decrease Physiological* Significant reduction observed in 10 patients with stable chronic renal failure with 1 month's treatment *5631* Parallel decline with sodium in congestive heart failure patients *4282* In patients with congestive cardiac failure concentration fell significantly with a single oral dose of 25 mg and during treatment for 2 weeks with 75 mg/d *2271* Prompt and striking reduction following oral administration over 30 minutes *287* Fell in parallel with reduction of blood pressure *2811* Significant effect in 1 h after single dose of 25 mg *292*

Plasma No Effect Physiological In 30 patients with acute myocardial infarction administration of 50 mg twice daily 28 days caused insignificant change from median baseline concentration of 31.6 to 28.2 pg/mL from day 1 to day 3 *798*

Angiotensin-converting Enzyme

Serum Decrease Analytical Marked inhibition of enzyme by drug *5077* 31% inhibition of method using benzyloxycarbonyl-phenylalanyl-histidyl-leucine as substrate *5409*

Serum Decrease Physiological Significant reduction from mean of 12.73 U/L to 5.50 U/L in 8 healthy normotensive volunteers given 50 mg daily for 4 days *3243* Significant decrease observed from 15 minutes after oral administration of 75 mg in 7 healthy male volunteers *4303* May be marked reduction in drug-treated patients *3022*

Anti-DNA Antibodies *Serum Decrease Physiological* In 3 of 78 patients, of IgM class, treated for mean of 11 mo *3013*

Antidiuretic Hormone *Plasma No Effect Physiological* Administration of a single dose of 25 mg drug orally had no effect on plasma concentration in 8 normotensive female volunteers, 17 patients with essential hypertension and 2 patients with primary aldosteronism *6082* No significant effect of drug observed in 15 hypertensives with advanced liver disease *5771*

Urine Decrease Physiological Significant reduction by 57% and 67% respectively in 8 normotensive female volunteers and 17 patients with essential hypertension after 25 mg orally. Magnitude correlated with plasma renin and aldosterone in normotensives but not in hypertensives *6082*

Antinuclear Antibodies *Serum Increase Physiological* In 13 of 78 patients, mainly of IgM class treated for mean of 11 mo *3013*

Apolipoprotein A-I *Serum Decrease Physiological* In 15 patients with essential hypertension treatment with up to 75 mg/d caused nonsignificant reduction from mean baseline of 143.0 ± 5.1 mg/dL to 128.3 ± 7.7 mg/dL after 8 weeks *6145*

Serum Increase Physiological After 12 weeks treatment in 18 patients with mild essential hypertension *5278* Increase from mean concentration of 128 mg/dL to 143 mg/dL in 15 patients with mild essential hypertension treated with 25-100 mg/d for 6 months *1741*

Serum No Effect Physiological Increase by 1 mg/dL in 15 patients given 75 mg daily for 8 weeks *4213* Insignificant increase in 8 men with mild to moderate hypertension treated with up to 150 mg daily for 12 weeks *5931*

Apolipoprotein A-II *Serum Increase Physiological* After 12 weeks treatment in 18 patients with mild essential hypertension *5278*

Apolipoprotein B *Serum Decrease Physiological* In 15 patients with essential hypertension treatment with up to 75 mg/d caused significant decrease from mean baseline of 119.1 ± 5.0 mg/dL to 103.8 ± 5.7 mg/dL after 4 weeks but returned to above baseline at 125.7 ± 4.3 mg/dL after 8 weeks treatment *6145*

Captopril *(continued)*

Apolipoprotein B *(continued)*
Serum No Effect Physiological Insignificant change in 8 men with mild to moderate hypertension treated with up to 150 mg daily for 12 weeks *5931* After 12 weeks treatment in 18 patients with mild essential hypertension *5278* Decrease by -2 mg/dL in 15 patients given 75 mg daily for 8 weeks *4213* No significant effect observed in 15 patients with mild essential hypertension treated with 25-100 mg/d for 6 months *1741*

Apolipoprotein C-II *Serum No Effect Physiological* No change in 15 patients given 75 mg daily for 8 weeks *4213* After 12 weeks treatment in 18 patients with mild essential hypertension *5278*

Apolipoprotein C-III *Serum No Effect Physiological* Increase by 1 mg/dL in 15 patients given 75 mg daily for 8 weeks *4213* After 12 weeks treatment in 18 patients with mild essential hypertension *5278*

Apolipoprotein E *Serum No Effect Physiological* No change in 15 patients given 75 mg daily for 8 weeks *4213* After 12 weeks treatment in 18 patients with mild essential hypertension *5278*

Aspartate Aminotransferase *Serum Increase Physiological* Characteristic pattern of hepatocellular jaundice in one patient. But with secondary cholestatic elements *6204* Isolated case of cholestasis in patient receiving 25 mg tid for 1 mo *4536*

Atrial Natriuretic Peptide *Plasma Increase Physiological* Resting concentration significantly higher in 6 healthy volunteers after 48 hours in those receiving high dose treatment than in those receiving low dose treatment or placebo *6459*

Bilirubin *Serum Increase Physiological* Isolated case of cholestasis in patient receiving 25 mg tid for 1 mo *4536* Characteristic pattern of hepatocellular jaundice in one patient. But with secondary cholestatic elements *6204*

Bilirubin, Direct *Serum Increase Physiological* Characteristic pattern of hepatocellular jaundice in one patient. But with secondary cholestatic elements *6204*

Blood *Urine Decrease Analytical* May cause decreased reactivity with occult blood test areas of Ames Multistix and other reagent strips *4034*
Urine No Effect Analytical Has no effect on occult blood test areas of Ames Multistix and other reagent strips *4034*

Calcium *Serum Increase Physiological* In 17 patients with essential hypertension treatment with up to 40 mg/d quinapril caused insignificant increase in calcium concentration from mean baseline of 0.6 mg/dL after 12 weeks *4810*
Serum No Effect Physiological No significant effect observed in hypertensive patients after 16 weeks treatment *6066*
Urine No Effect Physiological In 17 patients with essential hypertension treatment with up to 40 mg/d captopril caused an insignificant change in calcium excretion from mean baseline of 264 mg/d to 267 mg/d after 12 weeks *4810* In 17 hypertensive patients with mild to moderate renal impairment treatment with up to 150 mg/d for 12 weeks caused nonsignificant change from 264 mg/d to 267 mg/d *4810*

Catecholamines *Plasma Decrease Physiological* Mean decrease from 695 ng/L to 476 ng/L but not significant change in patients with heart failure *1925*

Cholesterol *Serum Decrease Physiological* In 14 patients with normolipidemia but with essential hypertension treatment with 50 mg/d captopril for 5 months caused a nonsignificant 4.8 ± 24.1 mg/dL decrease in concentration *321* In 15 patients with essential hypertension treatment with up to 75 mg/d caused decrease from mean baseline of 240.3 ± 5.9 mg/dL to 218.9 ± 6.6 mg/dL after 24 weeks *6145* Treatment for 6 months of 21 patients with essential hypertension caused mean 18% decrease in concentration *3730* Total cholesterol decreased from mean baseline concentration of 240 mg/dL to 218 mg/dL in 15 patients with mild essential hypertension treated with 25-100 mg/d for 6 months *1741* In 110 mild to moderate hypertensive patients treatment with up to 50 mg/d for 6 months caused significant 10% decrease from mean baseline of 7.3 mmol/L to 6.5 mmol/L *2507* In proteinuric patients treatment with captopril reduced both protein excretion and the increased serum cholesterol concentration *4235*
Serum No Effect Physiological No significant change over 16 weeks in 64 hypertensive patients treated with 37.5 mg daily *4304* After 12 weeks treatment in 18 patients with mild essential hypertension *5278* No significant change in 7,000 hypertensives treated for 3 y *2342* Insignificant change in 8 men with mild to moderate hypertension treated with up to 150 mg daily for 12 weeks *5931* In 40 mild to moderate hypertensives treatment with up to 100 mg/d for 24 weeks had no significant effect *1923* Decrease by -2 mg/dL in 15 patients given 75 mg daily for 8 weeks *4213* In 9 patients with essential hypertension treated with captopril for 6 months baseline value of 5.1 ± 0.8 mmol/L not significantly changed to 5.1 ± 0.9 mmol/L *2237* No significant change in patients in 2 studies treated for 2 and 24 mo *142*

Cholesterol Esters *Serum Decrease Physiological* In 14 patients with normolipidemia but with essential hypertension treatment with 50 mg/d captopril for 5 months caused a nonsignificant 6.7 ± 24.0 mg/dL decrease in concentration *321*

Cholesterol, Free *Serum Increase Physiological* In 14 patients with normolipidemia but with essential hypertension treatment with 50 mg/d captopril for 5 months caused a nonsignificant 2 ± 6.1 mg/dL increase in concentration *321*

Cholesterol:HDL-Cholesterol Ratio
Serum Decrease Physiological In 110 patients with mild to moderate essential hypertension treatment with up to 50 mg/d for 6 months caused significant reduction from mean baseline of 7.8 to 6.3 *2507*

Cortisol *Plasma No Effect Analytical* At a concentration of 50 mg/L had no significant effect on Enzymun method *1097*

Creatinine *Serum Decrease Physiological* In 9 patients with essential hypertension treated with captopril for 6 months baseline value of 88 ± 27 μmol/L significantly changed to 71 ± 18 μmol/L *2237*
Serum Increase Physiological Significant increase in 10 patients with chronic renal failure after 1 month's treatment, which reversed on cessation of the drug *5631* Severe reversible azotemia in a few patients with peripheral vascular disease: in two probably associated with GFR reduction *1013* Eosinophilic interstitial nephritis and membranous glomerulopathy reported. Cases of nephrotic syndrome also reported *1465* Acute reversible renal failure may occur: transient increases common *6257* Occasional reversible azotemia, either due to hypotension or direct renal damage *472*
Serum No Effect Physiological No significant change in 7,000 hypertensives treated for 3 y *2342* No significant change in 8 healthy normotensive volunteers given 50 mg daily for 4 days *3243* In 24 patients with NIDDM and proteinuria greater than 500 mg/d treatment with captopril (25 - 75 mg/d) for 18 months caused a nonsignificant change from mean baseline of 2.2 ± 0.3 mg/dL to 2.1 ± 0.3 mg/dL *3601* Treatment of 40 mild to moderate hypertensives with up to 100 mg/d for 24 weeks caused no significant effect *1923* No significant effect of a single oral dose of 25 mg in 8 normotensive women or in 17 patients with essential hypertension *6082*
Urine Decrease Physiological Significant reduction from mean of 129 mg/2 h to 89 mg/2 h in 8 normotensive women volunteers but no significant change in 17 patients with essential hypertension following single oral dose of 25 mg *6082*

Creatinine Clearance *Urine No Effect Physiological* No significant effect in 10 patients with stable chronic renal failure treated for 1 month *5631* No significant difference observed between patients with mild congestive heart failure when digoxin also ingested *4081*

Cyclosporine *Blood No Effect Analytical* At a concentration of 50 mg/L had no effect on Syva EMIT method *495*

Digoxin *Serum No Effect Physiological* 50 mg captopril daily had no effect on serum concentration in 6 healthy volunteers, nor on gastrointestinal absorption, oral bioavailability or renal clearance of digoxin. However some association between clearances of creatinine and digoxin *5113* No significant difference observed in serum digoxin concentrations between patients with and without captopril *4081*

1,25-Dihydroxy Vitamin D_3 *Serum No Effect Physiological* No significant effect observed in hypertensive patients following 8 or 16 weeks treatment *6066*

2,3-Dinor-6-Keto-Prostaglandin $F_{1\alpha}$
Urine No Effect Physiological In 20 normotensive and 7 hypertensive individuals treatment with 25 mg had no significant effect on excretion *2004*

Dopamine *Urine Decrease Physiological* Insignificant mean reduction in 8 normotensive women and 17 patients with essential hypertension following single oral dose of 25 mg *6082*

Drugs of Abuse Screen *Urine No Effect Analytical* No effect at concentration of 100 µg/mL on EZ-SCREEN procedure for cannabinoids and cocaine *1739*

Effective Renal Plasma Flow
Patient Increase Physiological In 24 patients with NIDDM and proteinuria greater than 500 mg/d treatment with captopril (25 - 75 mg/d) for 18 months caused a significant change from mean baseline of 246 ± 15 mL/min to 276 ± 18 mL/min after 6 months, 278 ± 17 mL/min after 12 months and 258 ± 18 mL/min (nonsignificant) after 18 months *3601* In 13 healthy men administration of a single oral dose of 25 mg caused a mean increase of 23.5 ± 6.1% in the fasting state *639*
Patient No Effect Physiological No significant effect in 10 patients with stable chronic renal failure after 1 month's treatment *5631*

Endothelin *Plasma No Effect Physiological* In 10 patients with congestive cardiac failure treatment with up to 75 mg/d for 16 weeks caused significant change from mean baseline of 8.1 ± 2.9 pg/mL to 8.1 ± 3.8 pg/mL *6064*

Endothelin-1 *Plasma Decrease Physiological* In 16 patients with recent acute myocardial infarction treatment with up to 25 mg every 8 hours caused decrease from 2.31 ± 1.24 fmol/mL to 1.30 ± 0.72 fmol/mL at 24 h, 0.95 ± 0.50 fmol/mL at 48 h and 0.60 ± 0.15 fmol/mL at 72 h significantly less at the same time than in patients treated with placebo *1413* In 11 hypertensives ingestion of 25 mg caused reduction from mean baseline of 1.32 ± 0.63 pg/mL to 1.05 ± 0.66 pg/mL 60 minutes later *6124*
Plasma No Effect Physiological In 9 normotensives ingestion of 25 mg caused insignificant change from mean baseline of 1.39 ± 0.57 pg/mL to 1.33 ± 0.54 pg/mL 60 minutes later *6124* No significant difference observed between captopril-treated and untreated hypertensive nonpregnant women *1896*

Eosinophils *Blood Decrease Physiological* Isolated cases of pancytopenia, usually with pre-existing renal disease *2058*
Blood Increase Physiological Several cases of rash and eosinophilia reported *1465*

Epinephrine *Plasma Decrease Physiological* Treatment of 19 elderly patients with mild to moderate hypertension with up to 75 mg daily for 8 weeks caused mean reduction of 47% at rest *3335* In 30 patients with acute myocardial infarction administration of 50 mg twice daily 28 days caused significant change from median baseline concentration of 56 to 27 pg/mL from day 1 to day 3 *798*
Plasma Increase Physiological Small but significant increase observed in 15 hypertensive patients with advanced liver disease *5771*
Urine No Effect Physiological Insignificant mean reduction in 8 normotensive women volunteers and insignificant mean increase in 17 patients with essential hypertension following single oral dose of 25 mg *6082*

Erythrocytes *Blood Decrease Physiological* Observed in 9 of 12 hypertensive patients on maintenance hemodialysis, maximum effect achieved after about 11 mo *2618* Isolated case of pancytopenia reported *1685*

Factor XI *Plasma Decrease Physiological* High value of essential hypertension significantly reduced *4559*

Factor XII *Plasma Decrease Physiological* High value of essential hypertension significantly reduced *4559*

Fibrinogen *Plasma No Effect Physiological* In 9 patients with essential hypertension treated with captopril for 6 months baseline value of 2.21 ± 0.31 g/L not significantly changed to 2.34 ± 0.50 g/L *2237*

Filtration Fraction *Urine Decrease Physiological* Mean decrease of 23.6% observed in 9 nephrotic patients given 25 mg captopril alone and 14.9% decrease when 800 mg ibuprofen given with 25 mg captopril *114* In 14 healthy uninephrectomized patients admininistration of 25 mg captopril caused significant decrease from mean baseline of 24.6% to 22.1% and in 14 healthy controls 25 mg captopril caused a significant decreas from 24.1% to 22.5% *4285*
Urine Increase Physiological In 24 patients with NIDDM and proteinuria greater than 500 mg/d treatment with captopril (25 - 75 mg/d) for 18 months caused a significant change from mean baseline of 27 ± 1% to 23 ± 1% after 6 months, 22 ± 1% after 12 months and 24 ± 1% (nonsignificant) after 18 months *3601*

Filtration Rate *Red Blood Cells No Effect Physiological* In 9 patients with essential hypertension treated with nicardipine for 6 months baseline value of 65 ± 9 µL/s not significantly changed to 62 ± 14 µL/s *2237*

Fructosamine *Serum Increase Analytical* Positive interference observed with Roche reagents on Roche Cobas Bio at concentration of drug of 1.0 mmol/L, which is well above therapeutic range *5153* When added to serum to a concentration of 1 mmol/L 16% positive interference observed with Roche method on Cobas Fara although this concentration is much higher than therapeutic of about 4 µmol/L *5152*

Glomerular Filtration Rate *Urine Decrease Physiological* Administration of 25 mg caused GFR to decrease nonsignificantly from 80.3 to 74.8 mL/min/kidney/1.73 sq m in 14 healthy uninephrectomized individuals and from 52.9 to 51.2 mL/min/kidney/1.73 sq m in 14 healthy control individuals *4285* In 24 patients with NIDDM and proteinuria greater than 500 mg/d treatment with captopril (25 - 75 mg/d) for 18 months caused a nonsignificant change from mean baseline of 65 ± 5 mL/min to 63 ± 4 mL/min after 6 months, 60 ± 4 mL/min after 12 months and 62 ± 4 mL/min after 18 months *3601*
Urine No Effect Physiological No significant effect in 10 patients with stable chronic renal failure treated for 1 month *5631* In 13 healthy individuals administration of a single oral dose of 25 mg had no significant effect on GFR *639* No significant change observed in 12 adolescent insulin-dependent diabetics treated with 0.9 mg/kg/d for 3 months *1121* Nonsignificant reduction of 4.8% from mean of 60.9 mL/min in 9 nephrotic patients given 25 mg only but 16.5% reduction when also given 800 mg ibuprofen *114*

Glucose *Serum Decrease Physiological* In 15 patients with essential hypertension treatment with up to 75 mg/d caused significant decrease from mean baseline of 102 mg/dL to 86 mg/dL after 24 weeks *6145* In 9 patients with essential hypertension treated with captopril for 6 months baseline value of 5.5 ± 0.5 mmol/L significantly changed to 5.3 ± 0.3 mmol/L *2237* Reduced concentration observed in 12 noninsulin-dependent diabetics possibly through enhanced blood flow to skeletal muscle (effect marginal but beneficial) *3212* Incidence of 0.7% observed in French Pharmacovigilance database *4106*
Serum Increase Physiological In 14 patients with normolipidemia but with essential hypertension treatment with 50 mg/d captopril for 5 months caused a significant 0.08 ± 0.45 mmol/L increase in concentration *321*
Serum No Effect Physiological No significant change in 7,000 hypertensives treated for 3 y *2342* Insignificant reduction in 50 hypertensive patients treated with mean dose of 81 mg/day for 18 weeks *4735* In 188 patients with essential hypertension treated with up to 200 mg/d for 8 weeks no change from placebo concentration *3841*
Urine Increase Physiological Reversible glycosuria reported in one boy with abdominal aortitis and resistant hypertension *1465*

Glucose Tolerance *Serum No Effect Physiological* No significant deterioration with long-term treatment in diabetic hypertensives *5523*

γ-Glutamyltransferase *Serum Increase Physiological* Characteristic pattern of hepatocellular jaundice in one patient. But with secondary cholestatic elements *6204*

HDL_2-Cholesterol *Serum Decrease Physiological* In 14 patients with normolipidemia but with essential hypertension treatment with 50 mg/d captopril for 5 months caused a significant 1.0 ± 1.4 mg/dL decrease in concentration *321*
Serum No Effect Physiological In 14 patients with normolipidemia but with essential hypertension treatment with 50 mg/d captopril for 5 months caused a nonsignificant 1.1 ± 1.4 mg/dL decrease in concentration *321* No change in 8 men with mild to moderate hypertension treated with up to 150 mg daily for 12 weeks *5931*

HDL_2-Cholesterol, Esterified
Serum No Effect Physiological In 14 patients with normolipidemia but with essential hypertension treatment with 50 mg/d captopril for 5 months caused a nonsignificant 0.4 ± 0.8 mg/dL decrease in concentration *321*

HDL_2-Cholesterol, Free *Serum No Effect Physiological* In 14 patients with normolipidemia but with essential hypertension treatment with 50 mg/d captopril for 5 months caused a nonsignificant 0.3 ± 0.6 mg/dL decrease in concentration *321*

Captopril *(continued)*

HDL$_2$-Lecithin *Serum No Effect Physiological* In 14 patients with normolipidemia but with essential hypertension treatment with 50 mg/d captopril for 5 months caused a nonsignificant 0.01 ± 0.01 U/mL decrease in concentration *321*

HDL$_2$-Lysolecithin *Serum No Effect Physiological* In 14 patients with normolipidemia but with essential hypertension treatment with 50 mg/d captopril for 5 months caused a nonsignificant 0.0 ± 0.01 U/mL change in concentration *321*

HDL$_2$-Phosphatidylethanolamine
Serum No Effect Physiological In 14 patients with normolipidemia but with essential hypertension treatment with 50 mg/d captopril for 5 months caused a nonsignificant 0.0 ± 0.0 U/mL change in concentration *321*

HDL$_2$-Phosphatidylinositol *Serum No Effect Physiological* In 14 patients with normolipidemia but with essential hypertension treatment with 50 mg/d captopril for 5 months caused a nonsignificant 0.0 ± 0.0 U/mL change in concentration *321*

HDL$_2$-Sphingomyelin *Serum No Effect Physiological* In 14 patients with normolipidemia but with essential hypertension treatment with 50 mg/d captopril for 5 months caused a nonsignificant 0.0 ± 0.01 U/mL change in concentration *321*

HDL$_2$-Triglycerides *Serum No Effect Physiological* In 14 patients with normolipidemia but with essential hypertension treatment with 50 mg/d captopril for 5 months caused a nonsignificant 0.3 ± 0.9 mg/dL decrease in concentration *321*

HDL$_3$-Cholesterol *Serum Increase Physiological* In 14 patients with normolipidemia but with essential hypertension treatment with 50 mg/d captopril for 5 months caused a nonsignificant 1.5 ± 3.4 mg/dL increase in concentration *321* Increase from mean of 24 mg/dL to 27 mg/dL in 8 men with mild to moderate hypertension treated with up to 150 mg daily for 12 weeks *5931*
Serum No Effect Physiological In 14 patients with normolipidemia but with essential hypertension treatment with 50 mg/d captopril for 5 months caused a nonsignificant 1.5 ± 3.4 mg/dL increase in concentration *321*

HDL$_3$-Cholesterol, Esterified
Serum No Effect Physiological In 14 patients with normolipidemia but with essential hypertension treatment with 50 mg/d captopril for 5 months caused a nonsignificant 0.8 ± 4.9 mg/dL increase in concentration *321*

HDL$_3$-Cholesterol, Free *Serum No Effect Physiological* In 14 patients with normolipidemia but with essential hypertension treatment with 50 mg/d captopril for 5 months caused a nonsignificant 0.5 ± 3.3 mg/dL decrease in concentration *321*

HDL$_3$-Lysolecithin *Serum No Effect Physiological* In 14 patients with normolipidemia but with essential hypertension treatment with 50 mg/d captopril for 5 months caused a nonsignificant 0.01 ± 0.03 U/mL increase in concentration *321* In 14 patients with normolipidemia but with essential hypertension treatment with 50 mg/d captopril for 5 months caused a nonsignificant 0.03 ± 0.07 U/mL decrease in concentration *321*

HDL$_3$-Phosphatidylethanolamine
Serum No Effect Physiological In 14 patients with normolipidemia but with essential hypertension treatment with 50 mg/d captopril for 5 months caused a nonsignificant 0.0 ± 0.01 U/mL change in concentration *321*

HDL$_3$-Phosphatidylinositol *Serum No Effect Physiological* In 14 patients with normolipidemia but with essential hypertension treatment with 50 mg/d captopril for 5 months caused a nonsignificant 0.0 ± 0.01 U/mL change in concentration *321*

HDL$_3$-Sphingomyelin *Serum No Effect Physiological* In 14 patients with normolipidemia but with essential hypertension treatment with 50 mg/d captopril for 5 months caused a nonsignificant 0.0 ± 0.02 U/mL change in concentration *321*

HDL$_3$-Triglycerides *Serum No Effect Physiological* In 14 patients with normolipidemia but with essential hypertension treatment with 50 mg/d captopril for 5 months caused a nonsignificant 0.1 ± 3.0 mg/dL increase in concentration *321*

HDL-Cholesterol *Serum Increase Physiological* Treatment for 6 months of 21 patients with essential hypertension caused mean 27% increase in concentration *3730* In 110 patients with mild to moderate hypertension treatment with up to 50 mg/d for 6 months caused significant 8% increase from mean baseline of 0.93 mmol/L to 1.00 mmol/L *2507* Treatment of 40 mild to moderate hypertensives for 24 weeks with up to 100 mg/d caused mean increase of 6.2% (change from 1.44 mmol/L to 1.53 mmol/L) *1923*
Serum No Effect Physiological In 15 patients with essential hypertension treatment with up to 15 mg/d for 24 weeks caused insignificant change from mean baseline of 51.2 ± 2.2 mg/dL to 52.4 ± 2.3 mg/dL *6145* Insignificant change in 8 men with mild to moderate hypertension treated with up to 150 mg daily for 12 weeks *5931* After 12 weeks treatment in 18 patients with mild essential hypertension *5278* In 9 patients with essential hypertension treated with captopril for 6 months baseline value of 1.3 ± 0.3 mmol/L not significantly changed to 1.4 ± 0.4 mmol/L *2237* No significant effect observed in 15 patients with mild essential hypertension treated with 25-100 mg/d for 6 months *1741* Increase by 1 mg/dL in 15 patients given 75 mg daily for 8 weeks *4213*

HDL-Cholesterol: VLDL + LDL-Cholesterol Ratio
Serum No Effect Physiological Treatment of 40 mild to moderate hypertensives with up to 100 mg/d for 24 weeks caused no significant change *1923*

Hematocrit *Blood Decrease Physiological* Observed in 9 of 12 hypertensive patients on maintenance hemodialysis, maximum effect achieved after about 11 mo *2618*
Blood No Effect Physiological In 9 patients with essential hypertension treated with captopril for 6 months baseline value of 0.43 ± 0.04 not significantly changed to 0.44 ± 0.03 *2237*

Hemoglobin *Blood Decrease Physiological* Observed in 9 of 12 hypertensive patients on maintenance hemodialysis, maximum effect achieved after about 11 mo *2618*

Hemoglobin A$_{1c}$ *Blood No Effect Physiological* In 24 patients with NIDDM and proteinuria greater than 500 mg/d treatment with captopril (25 - 75 mg/d) for 18 months caused a nonsignificant change from mean baseline of 8.2 ± 0.3% to 8.5 ± 0.4% *3601* No significant effect observed in 12 insulin-dependent adolescents treated with 0.9 mg/kg/d for 3 months *1121* No significant effect observed in 50 hypertensive patients treated with mean dose of 81 mg/day for 18 weeks *4735*

Histamine *Plasma No Effect Analytical* Probably no effect at clinically relevant concentrations on radio-enzyme assay *2492*

IgG Clearance:Albumin Clearance Ratio
Urine No Effect Physiological Administration of 25 mg alone to 9 nephrotic patients did not alter ratio but when 800 mg ibuprofen coadministered ratio decreased from mean 23% to 13% suggesting increase in glomerular permselectivity due to direct effect on glomerular capillary wall *114*

immunoglobulin A *Serum Decrease Physiological* Reported reversible or permanent deficiency induced by captopril *2426*

Insulin *Plasma Increase Physiological* In 14 patients with normolipidemia but with essential hypertension treatment with 50 mg/d captopril for 5 months caused a nonsignificant 4.5 ± 5.8 pmol/L increase in concentration *321*
Plasma No Effect Physiological Insignificant reduction in mean fasting concentration from 64 pmol/L to 60 pmol/L in 50 hypertensive patients treated with mean dose of 81 mg/day for 18 weeks. Steady state insulin concentration also unchanged *4735* No decrease during treatment nor effect on glucose tolerance *4830*

ionized Calcium *Serum No Effect Physiological* No significant effect observed in hypertensive patients after 16 weeks treatment *6066*

Iron *Serum No Effect Physiological* In 9 of 12 hypertensive patients although other hematological effects observed *2618*

Iron-Binding Capacity, Total
Serum No Effect Physiological In 9 of 12 hypertensive patients although other hematological effects observed *2618*

6-Keto-Prostaglandin F$_{1\alpha}$ *Urine No Effect Physiological* No significant change in 8 healthy normotensive volunteers given 50 mg daily for 4 days *3243* Nonsignificant increase from mean baseline of 178 ng/d to 192 ng/d in 12 patients with hypertension treated with 25 or 50 mg/d for 4 weeks *851*

Ketones *Urine Increase Analytical* Trace to 3 + reactions in 9 patients with both Diastix® and Chemstrip-6® *6357* At concentration of 2 mmol/L causes ++/+ reaction with Boehringer Mannheim Chemstrip but this can be eliminated within 3 minutes by the addition of 1 volume of 500 g/L iodoacetate to 9 volumes of urine *4749* False positive at concentration of 25 mmol/L on Ames Keto-diastix® , also affected Boehringer Combur Test *2281*

Lactate Dehydrogenase *Serum Increase Physiological* Characteristic pattern of hepatocellular jaundice in one patient. But with secondary cholestatic elements *6204* Isolated case of cholestasis in patient receiving 25 mg tid for 1 mo *4536*

LDL-Cholesterol *Serum Decrease Physiological* In 15 patients with essential hypertension treatment with up to 75 mg/d caused decrease from mean of 152.7 ± 7.1 mg/dL to 135.6 ± .9 mg/dL *6145* In 110 patients with mild to moderate essential hypertension treatment with up to 50 mg/d for 6 months caused significant 12% decrease from mean baseline of 5.0 mmol/L to 4.2 mmol/L *2507*

Serum No Effect Physiological Insignificant change in 8 men with mild to moderate hypertension treated with up to 150 mg daily for 12 weeks *5931* After 12 weeks treatment in 18 patients with mild essential hypertension *5278*

LDL-Cholesterol:HDL-Cholesterol Ratio

Serum Decrease Physiological In 110 patients with mild to moderate essential hypertension treatment with up to 50 mg/d for 6 months caused significant decrease from mean baseline of 5.5 to 4.0 *2507* In 15 patients with essential hypertension and serum cholesterol concentration greater than 240 mg/dL significant reduction observed between 4th and 24th week of treatment *6145*

Lecithin *Serum No Effect Physiological* In 14 patients with normolipidemia but with essential hypertension treatment with 50 mg/d captopril for 5 months caused a nonsignificant 0.02 ± 0.12 U/mL increase in concentration *321*

Leukocytes *Blood Decrease Physiological* Isolated reports of neutropenia and agranulocytosis when first introduced and given in high doses *2881* Isolated cases of pancytopenia, usually with pre-existing renal disease *2058* Isolated case of pancytopenia reported *1685* Agranulocytosis observed in several cases *6257*

Lipoprotein Lp(a) *Serum Decrease Physiological* In 20 patients with acute myocardial infarction treatment with captopril caused a significant reduction from 63 to 46 mg/dL after 30 days compared with an increase from 59 to 72 mg/dL in placebo-treated infarct patients *5668*

Lithium *Serum Increase Physiological* Reported to increase concentration *3590*

Lysolecithin *Serum No Effect Physiological* In 14 patients with normolipidemia but with essential hypertension treatment with 50 mg/d captopril for 5 months caused a nonsignificant 0.01 ± 0.02 U/mL increase in concentration *321*

Magnesium *Serum No Effect Physiological* No significant effect observed in hypertensive patients after 16 weeks treatment *6066*

Malondialdehyde *Serum Decrease Physiological* In 20 patients with acute myocardial infarction treatment with captopril caused a significant reduction from 33 to 26 nmol/mL after 30 days compared with 33 nmol/mL in placebo-treated infarct patients *5668*

MCHC *Blood No Effect Physiological* In 9 of 12 hypertensive patients although other hematological effects observed *2618*

MCV *Blood No Effect Physiological* In 9 of 12 hypertensive patients although other hematological effects observed *2618*

Neutrophils *Blood Decrease Physiological* Isolated cases of pancytopenia, usually with pre-existing renal disease *2058* In approximately 0.3% patients: develops within first 3 to 12 weeks of treatment associated with myeloid hypoplasia of bone marrow *6257* Agranulocytosis reported to occur in 1 of 250 treated patients *6264*

Norepinephrine *Plasma Decrease Physiological* Treatment of 19 elderly patients with mild to moderate essential hypertension with up to 75 mg daily for 8 weeks caused mean reduction of concentration at rest of 17% *3335*

Plasma No Effect Physiological No effect of drug observed in 15 hypertensive patients with advanced liver disease *5771* No effect of drug and concentration responds appropriately to postural changes *6257* In 30 patients with acute myocardial infarction administration of 50 mg twice daily 28 days caused insignificant change from median baseline concentration of 245 to 270 pg/mL from day 1 to day 3 *798*

Urine Decrease Physiological Insignificant reduction from mean of 2.6 µg/2 h to 1.6 µg/2 h in 8 normotensive women volunteers but no change in 17 patients with hypertension following single oral dose of 25 mg *6082*

Osmolality *Serum No Effect Physiological* No significant effect observed in 8 normotensive women and in 17 patients with essential hypertension following single oral dose of 25 mg *6082*

Urine Decrease Physiological Significant reduction from mean of 732 mg/kg to 643 mg/kg in 8 normotensive women volunteers but no significant change in 17 hypertensive patients following single oral dose of 25 mg *6082*

Parathyroid Hormone *Plasma No Effect Physiological* No significant effect observed in hypertensive patients after either 8 or 16 weeks treatment *6066*

Phosphate *Serum No Effect Physiological* No significant effect observed in hypertensive patients after 16 weeks treatment *6066*

Phosphatidylethanolamine *Serum No Effect Physiological* In 14 patients with normolipidemia but with essential hypertension treatment with 50 mg/d captopril for 5 months caused a nonsignificant 0.0 ± 0.01 U/mL change in concentration *321*

Phosphatidylinositol *Serum No Effect Physiological* In 14 patients with normolipidemia but with essential hypertension treatment with 50 mg/d captopril for 5 months caused a nonsignificant 0.0 ± 0.01 U/mL change in concentration *321*

Plasminogen Activator Antigen-1 Activity

Plasma Decrease Physiological In 15 patients with myocardial infarction mean PAI-1 activity in those receiving captopril for 4 weeks 9.0 AU/mL significantly less than 13.2 AU/mL in those treated with placebo *6546*

Plasminogen Activator Antigen-1 Antigen

Plasma Decrease Physiological In 15 patients with myocardial infarction mean PAI-1 concentration in those receiving captopril for 4 weeks 7.8 ng/mL significantly less than 17.3 ng/mL in those treated with placebo *6546*

Platelet Aggregation *Blood No Effect Physiological* No significant effect observed on ADP-induced aggregation in patients with congestive cardiac failure either after a single oral dose of 25 mg or after 75 mg/d for 2 weeks *2271*

Platelets *Blood Decrease Physiological* Isolated case of pancytopenia reported *1685*

Potassium *Serum Decrease Physiological* In 20% of cases treated with captopril hypokalemia observed *1299*

Serum Increase Physiological Rise less than 1.0 mmol/L, but greatest in patients with high baseline renin activity *4739* From 2.9 to 3.3 mmol/L after 1 mo in patient with Bartter's syndrome due to inhibited aldosterone production *2553* In 24 patients with NIDDM and proteinuria greater than 500 mg/d treatment with captopril (25 - 75 mg/d) for 18 months caused a significant change from mean baseline of 4.15 ± 0.11 mmol/L to 4.59 ± 0.11 mmol/L *3601* Resulting from decreased secretion of aldosterone *2811*

Serum No Effect Physiological Treatment of 40 mild to moderate hypertensives with up to 100 mg/d for 24 weeks caused no significant effect *1923* Treatment of 19 elderly patients with mild to moderate hypertension with up to 75 mg daily for 8 weeks had no effect on concentration *3335* No significant change in 7,000 hypertensives treated for 3 y *2342* No significant reduction observed in 8 healthy normotensive volunteers given 50 mg daily for 4 days *3243* No effect observed in either normotensive women or hypertensive patients treated with single oral dose of 25 mg *6082*

Urine No Effect Physiological Insignificant reduction observed in 8 normotensive women volunteers and 17 patients with essential hypertension treated with single oral dose of 25 mg *6082*

Prekallikrein *Plasma Decrease Physiological* Rapid decrease following institution of therapy *4559*

Prolidase *Serum No Effect Physiological* No effect observed in vivo either after single high dose or with chronic treatment although inhibitory activity observed in vitro at concentration much higher than therapeutic *4197*

Prostaglandin E_2 *Plasma No Effect Physiological* No significant change observed in 7 healthy male volunteers following 75 mg orally *4303*

Urine Increase Physiological Significant increase from mean baseline of 349 ng/d to 416 ng/d in 12 patients with hypertension treated with 25 or 50 mg/d for 4 weeks *851*

Captopril *(continued)*

Protein *Serum No Effect Physiological* In 9 of 12 hypertensive patients although other hematological effects observed *2618*

Urine Decrease Physiological In 9 nephrotic individuals administration of 25 mg was followed by a mean reduction of protein excretion of 20% when urine collected from 4 to 8 hours after drug administration. Reduction was 41% when 800 mg ibuprofen combined with captopril *114* In 24 patients with NIDDM and proteinuria greater than 500 mg/d treatment with captopril (25 - 75 mg/d) for 18 months caused a significant change from mean baseline of 2.64 ± 0.47 g/d to 2.01 ± 0.44 g/d after 6 months, 1.76 ± 0.42 g/d after 12 months and 1.93 ± 0.45 g/d after 18 months *3601* Significant reduction in 10 patients with stable chronic renal failure after 1 month's treatment *5631* Significant reduction in patients with advanced diabetic nephropathy *5915*

Urine Increase Physiological Some patients develop heavy proteinuria during use of drug. Reversible with discontinuation *3728* Isolated reports of immune complex glomerulopathy when first introduced and high doses given *2881* In patients with pre-existing renal dysfunction with proteinuria *292* Greater than 1.0 g/d occurs in about 1.2% patients may subside with continuing treatment *6257* Effect observed in small number of patients with excellent control of hypertension *292* Occurs in approximately 1% of 7100 hypertensives most often who had pre-existing renal disease and receiving high doses of drug *2342* Eosinophilic interstitial nephritis and membranous glomerulopathy reported. Cases of nephrotic syndrome also reported *1465*

Renal Blood Flow *Patient Increase Physiological* Mean increase of 11.6% in 9 nephrotic patients given 25 mg captopril alone but no significant change observed when 25 mg captopril given with 800 mg ibuprofen *114*

Renal Plasma Flow *Patient Decrease Physiological* Administration of 25 mg caused RPF to decrease nonsignificantly from mean 334.7 to 329.0 mL/min/kidney/1.73 sq m *1*

Patient Increase Physiological In 20 normotensive and 7 hypertensive individuals treatment with 25 mg significantly increased renal plasma flow *2004* Administration of 25 mg to 14 healthy individuals caused significant increase from mean baseline of 220.8 to 225.1 mL/min/kidney/1.73 sq m *4285*

Patient No Effect Physiological No significant effect observed in 12 adolescent insulin-dependent diabetics treated with 0.9 mg/kg/d for 3 months *1121*

Renin Activity *Plasma Decrease Physiological* In 6 nonazotemic patients with cirrhosis and ascites due to increased renal vasodilatation *4513*

Plasma Increase Physiological Gradually increases over 1 h due to negative feedback on renin activity *287* Significant increase from mean of 1.76 nmol/L/h to 12.54 nmol/L/h in 8 healthy normotensive volunteers given 50 mg daily for 4 days *3243* Oral ingestion of 50 mg by normal volunteers caused approximately 3.5-fold increase *2594* From 10.0 to 34.7 pmol/L/s in one patient with Bartter's syndrome after 1 mo *2553* Significant effect observed in patients with congestive cardiac failure after a single oral dose of 25 mg and after 75 mg/d for 2 weeks *2271* Significant effect in 1 h after single dose of 25 mg *292* Increase from mean of 1.7 ng/mL/h to 12.3 ng/mL/h in 8 normotensive women and from mean of 4.4 ng/mL/h to 33.6 ng/mL/h in 17 patients with essential hypertension following single oral dose of 25 mg *6082* 60 min after ingestion of 25 mg captopril mean concentration increased from 1.40 ± 0.84 ng/mL/h to 3.00 ± 1.89 ng/mL/h in 9 normotensives and from 1.83 ± 1.22 ng/mL/h to 2.58 ± 1.72 ng/mL/h in 11 hypertensives *6124* In 15 patients with advanced liver disease caused further increase from elevated baseline *5771* In 10 patients with stable chronic renal failure 1 month's treatment caused significant increase *5631* Marked effect within 30 minutes on active and total renin with reduction of inactive renin *4559* Significant increase observed in 7 healthy volunteers beginning 45 minutes after both 25 and 75 mg orally *4303* Significant increase in normal subjects following either 25 or 75 mg captopril but response enhanced by prior administration of dexamethasone *4303* Significant increase observed in 12 adolescent insulin-dependent diabetics treated for 3 months with 0.9 mg/kg/d *1121* Significant increase observed in 14 patients with cirrhosis and ascites after 2 days treatment with 12.5 mg/day *786* In 30 patients with acute myocardial infarction administration of 50 mg twice daily 28 days caused significant change from median baseline concentration of 1.8 to 2.9 ng/mL/h from day 1 to day 3 *798* In 69 patients with hypertension after renal transplantation administration of 25 mg captopril caused significant increase from mean baseline of 2.7 ng/mL/h to 5.7 ng/mL/h after 1 hour *3338* In 20 normotensive and 7 hypertensive individuals treatment with 25 mg significantly increased plasma renin activity by a mean of 1.2 ± 0.6 ng angiotensin I/mL/h compared with -0.2 ± 0.2 ng angiotensin I/mL/h in controls *2004* In 24 patients with NIDDM and proteinuria greater than 500 mg/d treatment with captopril (25 - 75 mg/d) for 18 months caused a significant change from mean baseline of 0.76 ± 0.12 ng/mL/h to 3.85 ± 0.21 ng/mL/h *3601*

Plasma No Effect Physiological Treatment of 19 elderly patients with mild to moderate essential hypertension with up to 75 mg/day for 8 weeks had no significant effect *3335*

Renin Concentration *Plasma Increase Physiological* Oral ingestion of 50 mg by normal volunteers caused approximately 4-fold increase in renin concentration *2594*

Renin Substrate *Plasma No Effect Physiological* No significant effect although marked changes in PRA and angiotensin II *292*

Reticulocytes *Blood No Effect Physiological* In 9 of 12 hypertensive patients although other hematological effects observed *2618*

Retinol-binding Protein *Urine No Effect Physiological* In 19 patients with chronic heart failure mean excretion both increased and decreased with treatment with up to 75 mg/d from baseline of 0.64 μmol/mol creatinine to 0.92 μmol/mol after 7 days, 0.41 μmol/mol creatinine on day 14 and 0.59 μmol/mol creatinine on day 30 *1717*

Sodium *Serum Decrease Physiological* In five men with congestive heart failure with fall of sodium by 7 mmol/L on 3rd to 4th day *4282*

Serum No Effect Physiological Insignificant change in either normotensive women or patients with single oral dose of 25 mg *6082* Treatment of 40 mild to moderate hypertensives with up to 100 mg/d caused no significant effect *1923* No effect observed on concentration in 19 elderly patients with mild to moderate hypertension treated with up to 75 mg daily for 8 weeks *3335*

Urine Increase Physiological In 20 normotensive and 7 hypertensive individuals treatment with 25 mg caused a significant increase in urinary excretion to 14.1 ± 1.9 mmol compared with 11.9 ± 1.7 mmol in controls *2004* Significant increase in 14 patients with cirrhosis and ascites following treatment with 12.5 mg/day for 2 days. With withdrawal of treatment sodium excretion rapidly decreased *786*

Urine No Effect Physiological In 24 patients with NIDDM and proteinuria greater than 500 mg/d treatment with captopril (25 - 75 mg/d) for 18 months caused a nonsignificant change from mean baseline of 126 ± 2 mmol/L to 127 ± 2 mmol/L *3601* Insignificant change observed in 8 healthy women volunteers and 17 patients with essential hypertension following single oral dose of 25 mg *6082*

Sphingomyelin *Serum No Effect Physiological* In 14 patients with normolipidemia but with essential hypertension treatment with 50 mg/d captopril for 5 months caused a nonsignificant 0.03 ± 0.04 U/mL increase in concentration *321*

Terazosin *Serum No Effect Physiological* In a study of 6 individuals coadministration of captopril with terazosin had no significant effect on the terazosin concentration *21*

Thromboxane B_2 *Urine No Effect Physiological* Nonsignificant decrease from mean baseline excretion of 191 ng/d to 188 ng/d in 12 hypertensive patients treated with 25 or 50 mg/d for 4 weeks *851*

Tirofiban *Serum No Effect Physiological* Coadministration had no significant effect on plasma clearance of tirofiban *3957*

Tissue Plasminogen Activator Antigen
Plasma Decrease Physiological In 15 patients with myocardial infarction mean t-PA concentration in those receiving captopril for 4 weeks 10.3 ng/mL significantly less than 16.0 ng/mL in those treated with placebo *6546*

Triglycerides *Serum Decrease Physiological* Treatment of 40 mild to moderate hypertensives with up to 100 mg/d for 24 weeks caused mean reduction of 10.6% (change from 1.76 mmol/L to 1.57 mmol/L) *1923* Treatment for 6 months of 21 patients with essential hypertension caused mean 26%

decrease in concentration *3730* In 15 patients with essential hypertension treatment with up to 75 mg/d caused decrease from mean baseline of 181.8 ± 26.4 mg/dL to 154.6 ± 18.8 mg/dL after 24 weeks *6145*
Serum Increase Physiological In 14 patients with normolipidemia but with essential hypertension treatment with 50 mg/d captopril for 5 months caused a nonsignificant 6.3 ± 38.1 mg/dL increase in concentration *321*
Serum No Effect Physiological In 9 patients with essential hypertension treated with captopril for 6 months baseline value of 1.8 ± 0.7 mmol/L not significantly changed to 1.8 ± 1.3 mmol/L *2237* Decrease by -3 mg/dL in 15 patients given 75 mg daily for 8 weeks *4213* No significant change noted in 64 hypertensive patients treated with 37.5 mg daily for 16 weeks *4304* Insignificant change in 8 men with mild to moderate hypertension treated with up to 150 mg daily for 12 weeks *5931* After 12 weeks treatment in 18 patients with mild essential hypertension *5278* No significant effect observed in patients receiving captopril *4989* In 110 patients with mild to moderate essential hypertension treatment with up to 50 mg/d for 6 months caused significant 14% decrease from mean baseline of 2.9 mmol/L to 2.5 mmol/L *2507* No significant change observed in 15 patients with mild essential hypertension treated with 25-100 mg/d for 6 months *1741* No significant change in patients in 2 studies treated for 2 and 24 mo *142*

Urea Nitrogen *Serum Increase Physiological* Severe reversible azotemia in a few patients with peripheral vascular disease two weeks after start of therapy, probably associated with GFR reduction *1013*
Serum No Effect Physiological In 24 patients with NIDDM and proteinuria greater than 500 mg/d treatment with captopril (25 - 75 mg/d) for 18 months caused a nonsignificant decrease from mean baseline of 31 ± 3 mg/dL to 29 ± 2 mg/dL *3601*

Uric Acid *Serum No Effect Physiological* No significant change in 7,000 hypertensives treated for 3 y *2342*

Viscosity *Blood No Effect Physiological* In 9 patients with essential hypertension treated with captopril for 6 months no significant change over shear rate from 2.25 to 450 /s *2237*
Plasma No Effect Physiological In 9 patients with essential hypertension treated with captopril for 6 months no significant change over shear rate from 2.25 to 450 /s *2237*

VLDL + LDL-Cholesterol *Serum Increase Physiological* In 14 patients with normolipidemia but with essential hypertension treatment with 50 mg/d captopril for 5 months caused a nonsignificant 2.9 ± 31.3 mg/dL increase in concentration *321*

VLDL + LDL-Cholesterol Ester
Serum Increase Physiological In 14 patients with normolipidemia but with essential hypertension treatment with 50 mg/d captopril for 5 months caused a nonsignificant 4.1 ± 30.0 mg/dL increase in concentration *321*

VLDL + LDL-Cholesterol, Free
Serum No Effect Physiological In 14 patients with normolipidemia but with essential hypertension treatment with 50 mg/d captopril for 5 months caused a nonsignificant 1.2 ± 7.2 mg/dL decrease in concentration *321*

VLDL + LDL-Lecithin *Serum No Effect Physiological* In 14 patients with normolipidemia but with essential hypertension treatment with 50 mg/d captopril for 5 months caused a nonsignificant 0.02 ± 0.04 U/mL increase in concentration *321*

VLDL + LDL-Lysolecithin *Serum No Effect Physiological* In 14 patients with normolipidemia but with essential hypertension treatment with 50 mg/d captopril for 5 months caused a nonsignificant 0.0 ± 0.01 U/mL change in concentration *321*

VLDL + LDL-Phosphatidylethanolamine
Serum No Effect Physiological In 14 patients with normolipidemia but with essential hypertension treatment with 50 mg/d captopril for 5 months caused a nonsignificant 0.0 ± 0.01 U/mL change in concentration *321*

VLDL + LDL-Phosphatidylinositol
Serum No Effect Physiological In 14 patients with normolipidemia but with essential hypertension treatment with 50 mg/d captopril for 5 months caused a nonsignificant 0.0 ± 0.01 U/mL change in concentration *321*

VLDL + LDL-Sphingomyelin *Serum No Effect Physiological* In 14 patients with normolipidemia but with essential hypertension treatment with 50 mg/d captopril for 5 months caused a nonsignificant 0.02 ± 0.04 U/mL increase in concentration *321*

VLDL + LDL-Triglycerides *Serum Increase Physiological* In 14 patients with normolipidemia but with essential hypertension treatment with 50 mg/d captopril for 5 months caused a nonsignificant 7.9 ± 31.0 mg/dL increase in concentration *321*

VLDL-Cholesterol *Serum No Effect Physiological* After 12 weeks treatment in 18 patients with mild essential hypertension *5278*

Volume *Urine No Effect Physiological* Insignificant increase in 8 normotensive women and 17 patients with essential hypertension following single oral dose of 25 mg *6082*

Caracemide

Erythrocytes *Blood Decrease Physiological* Myelosuppression has been observed with treatment *1384*

Leukocytes *Blood Decrease Physiological* Myelosuppression has been observed with treatment *1384*

Platelets *Blood Decrease Physiological* Myelosuppression has been observed with treatment *1384*

Carbacrylamine Resin

Potassium *Serum Increase Physiological* Part of resin is in form of potassium salt *3810*

Sodium *Serum Decrease Physiological* Cation-exchange with reduced gastrointestinal tract absorption *3810*

Carbamazepine

Acetaminophen *Serum Decrease Physiological* Coadministration with carbamazepine would be expected to decrease concentration of coadministered drug because of induction of hepatic CYP activity *1039*
Serum No Effect Analytical No interference observed at a concentration of 1600 µg/mL (677 µmol/L) with method on Du Pont aca *1506*
Serum No Effect Physiological No significant effect observed when carbamazepine added to therapeutic regime *3118*

Acetylsalicylic Acid *Serum No Effect Physiological* No significant effect on plasma concentration when carbamazepine added to therapeutic regime *3118*

α_1-Acid Glycoprotein *Serum Increase Physiological* Significantly higher in children treated with drug compared with controls *4973* In study of 17 patients mean concentration was 17% higher in those receiving carbamazepine than in controls *6040*
Serum No Effect Physiological In 34 epileptic patients treatment with mean of 10.6 mg/kg/d caused nonsignificant increase to 0.61 g/L from mean baseline of 0.59 g/L in controls *5944*

Alanine Aminotransferase *Serum Increase Physiological* Cholestatic and hepatocellular damage *4845* Abnormalities in liver function tests and cholestatic and hepaocellular jaundice, and hepatitis have been observed as side effects of treatment *1039*
Serum No Effect Physiological No significant change from control activity of 15 U/L compared with activity in 21 men of 14 U/L and 14 U/L in 20 women epileptic patients receiving carbamazepine monotherapy *4394* In 86 epileptic patients of mean age of 31.8 ± 12.2 y mean activity of 16.9 ± 7.8 U/L not significantly different from 13.5 ± 5.5 U/L in 42 healthy controls *6234*

Albumin *Serum Increase Physiological* Concentration higher in epileptic patients receiving carbamazepine only *4347*
Serum No Effect Physiological Osteomalacia observed in 3 of 31 patients given average of 758 mg/d for average of 20.5 mo *4377* In about 20 epileptic patients treated for 2 y *1370*
Urine Increase Physiological Albuminuria may occur as side effect *282* Rare reported side effect *1384*
Urine No Effect Analytical Using a fluorimetric assay with Albumin Blue 580 on a Cobas Fara centrifugal analyzer for the detection of microalbuminuria no significant interference was detected at a concentration of 40 mg/L *3117*

Alkaline Phosphatase *Serum Increase Physiological* Observed effect *3119* Reversible hepatotoxicity with clinical syndrome resembling viral hepatitis in 2 patients *2723* Chole-

Carbamazepine *(continued)*

Alkaline Phosphatase *(continued)*
static and hepatocellular damage *4845* 4 of 21 patients with epilepsy (19%) treated with drug only for average of 40 mo *2664* Abnormalities in liver function tests and cholestatic and hepaocellular jaundice, and hepatitis have been observed as side effects of treatment *1039* In about 20 epileptic patients treated for 2 y *1370* Granulomatous hepatitis observed in small proportion of patients treated for less than 1 mo; resolved within 3 d of cessation of treatment *3547* Serum total alkaline phosphatase activity was increased in 9 of 41 epileptic patients treated with carbamazepine *4393* Osteomalacia observed in 3 of 31 patients given average of 758 mg/d for average of 20.5 mo *4377*
Serum No Effect Physiological Observed 2 times upper limit of normal in none of 36 adult inpatient epileptics (dose and duration of treatment unknown) *1922* No significant difference between mean concentration in 41 treated epileptic patients and controls *4393*

Alkaline Phosphatase, Bone Isoenzyme
Serum Increase Physiological Increased activity observed in 10 of 41 epileptic patients treated with carbamazepine but in 20% of these total alkaline phosphatase activity was normal *4393*

Alkaline Phosphatase, Non-bone Isoenzymes
Serum Increase Physiological Observed in 3 of 41 epileptic patients when treated with carbamazepine *4393*

Alprazolam *Serum Decrease Physiological* Coadministration with carbamazepine would be expected to decrease concentration of coadministered drug because of induction of hepatic CYP activity *1039* Greater than 50% reduction in alprazolam concentration in one patient with atypical bipolar disorder and panic attacks once carbamazepine therapy was instituted *234* Clinical deterioration results when drugs coadministered due to stimulation of hepatic metabolism of alprazolam *3119*

δ-Aminolevulinic Acid *Serum Increase Physiological*
Modest but highly significant statistical increase in drug treated population (132 nmol/L versus 99 nmol/L) *2246*

Aminophylline *Serum Decrease Physiological* Metabolism increased when carbamazepine coadministered *3118*

Ammonia *Plasma No Effect Physiological* No striking effect when given to epileptic patients *6233*

Androgen Index, Free (FAI)
Plasma Decrease Physiological Reduction from mean of 9.8 to 5.9 at 2 and 12 months and to 3.2 in long term treated normally menstruating women with epilepsy *2837* Mean decrease to 68 in 20 male epileptic patients treated for mean of 3.3 years compared with 87 in 17 healthy control subjects *2840* In 11 epileptic patients treatment with carbamazepine caused a significant change in concentration from mean baseline of 98.3 ± 47.4 to 73.0 ± 22.0 after one year and 58.7 ± 16.9 after 5 years *2842*
Plasma No Effect Physiological In 12 epileptic men aged 21 to 40 years treated with carbamazepine mean concentration of 61.5 ± 34.0 not significantly different from normal *2841*

Androstenedione *Plasma Decrease Physiological* Within 7 d of starting 400 mg/d treatment in 6 healthy males probably due to induction of hepatic monooxygenase activity *1109*

Antipyrine Clearance *Patient Increase Physiological* In 12 epileptic men aged 21 to 40 years treated with carbamazepine mean clearance of 112.1 ± 71.4 mL/min significantly different from normal of 23.8 - 51.2 mL/min *2841*

Apolipoprotein A *Serum Increase Physiological* Significantly increased concentration observed in chronically treated epileptics compared with age and sex matched controls *843*

Apolipoprotein A-I *Serum No Effect Physiological* In 23 epileptic children treated with carbamazepine for a mean of 1.58 years mean concentration of 153.33 ± 93.19 mg/dL not significantly different from 111.65 ± 59.75 mg/dL in 57 healthy control children *5727*

Apolipoprotein B *Serum No Effect Physiological* In 23 epileptic children treated with carbamazepine for a mean of 1.58 years mean concentration of 79.47 ± 34.25 mg/dL not significantly different from 75.15 ± 39.67 mg/dL in 57 healthy control children *5727*

Aspartate Aminotransferase *Serum Increase Physiological*
Granulomatous hepatitis observed in small proportion of patients treated for less than 1 mo; resolved within 3 d of cessation of treatment *3547* Cholestatic and hepatocellular damage *4845* Reversible hepatotoxicity with clinical syndrome resembling viral hepatitis in 2 patients *2723* Abnormalities in liver function tests and cholestatic and hepaocellular jaundice, and hepatitis have been observed as side effects of treatment *1039*
Serum No Effect Physiological In 86 epileptic patients of mean age of 31.8 ± 12.2 y mean activity of 31.8 ± 12.2 U/L not significantly different from 15.1 ± 5.6 U/L in 42 healthy controls *6234*

Aspirin Esterase *Serum Increase Physiological* Substantially higher activity in treated epileptics than in controls *4806* Significant increase from mean of 186 μg/mL/h in controls to 366 μg/mL/h in epileptics receiving carbamazepine only *4807*

Bilirubin *Serum Decrease Physiological* Mean reduction of 3.8 μmol/L in 38 epileptic patients treated for several years versus control population *2267* In about 20 epileptic patients treated for 2 y *1370* Significant reduction compared with controls in patients treated for average of 20.5 mo due to hepatic microsomal enzyme induction *4377*
Serum Increase Physiological Abnormalities in liver function tests and cholestatic and hepaocellular jaundice, and hepatitis have been observed as side effects of treatment *1039* Cholestatic and hepatocellular damage *4845* Reversible hepatotoxic damage with clinical syndrome resembling viral hepatitis in 2 patients *2723* Granulomatous hepatitis observed in small proportion of patients treated for less than 1 mo: resolved within 3 d of cessation of treatment *3547*
Serum No Effect Physiological Insignificant displacement from protein in neonates *6314*

Biotin *Serum Decrease Physiological* Dose related effect observed in long term treated epileptic compared with controls *3275*

BSP Retention *Serum Increase Physiological* Cholestatic and hepatocellular damage *2451*

Bupropion *Serum Decrease Physiological* May induce the metabolism of bupropion due to effect on CYP2B6 isoenzyme *2171* Low plasma concentration of bupropion and high plasma concentration of its metabolites when drugs coadministered *3118*

Caffeine *Serum No Effect Physiological* No effect observed on pharmacokinetics of caffeine *3119*

Calcium *Serum Decrease Physiological* Osteomalacia observed in 3 of 31 patients given average of 758 mg/d for average of 20.5 mo *4377* Observed in 3 of 21 (14%) patients whose epilepsy was treated only with drug (mean duration of treatment 40 mo) *2664* In about 20 epileptic patients treated for 2 y *1370* Reported effect *3119* Hypocalcemia has been observed as a side effect of treatment possibly as a consequence of inappropriate secretion of ADH and water retention *1039*

Carbamazepine *Hair Increase Physiological* In 17 patients receiving carbamazepine mean concentration 28.0 μg/g and median 22.1 μg/g as measured by immunoassay on Abbott TDx *6081*
Serum Decrease Physiological Plasma concentration may decrease by 20 to 30% after 2 to 3 weeks of treatment *1815*

Carnitine *Serum No Effect Physiological* In 141 epileptic children treated with carbamazepine mean concentration of 41.5 ± 10.3 nmol/L not significantly less than 57.8 ± 15.4 nmol/mL in 32 healthy control children *2757*

Carnitine, Free *Serum Decrease Physiological* In 141 epileptic children mean concentration of 33.0 ± 8.3 nmol/mL significantly less than 42.5 ± 14.1 nmol/mL in 32 healthy control children *2757*

Ceruloplasmin *Serum Increase Physiological* In 10 epileptic patients receiving carbamazepine as sole therapy higher concentrations of ceruloplasmin observed *4346*

Chloride *Serum Decrease Physiological* Isolated case of dilutional hyponatremia with water intoxication: 7 previous cases reported *3064*
Serum Increase Analytical At 10 times therapeutic concentration caused statistically significant increase with method used on Technicon SRA-2000 *4348*

Serum Increase Physiological Highly significant increase observed in several outpatients treated for several years with carbamazepine alone or in combination with other drugs *4345*

Cholesterol *Serum Increase Physiological* In 23 epileptic children treated with carbamazepine for a mean of 1.58 years mean concentration of 195.61 ± 60.75 mg/dL significantly different from 155.10 ± 35.66 mg/dL in 57 healthy control children *5727* Increased concentration has been reported to occur as a side effect in patients taking anticonvulsants *282* In 27 women and 12 men with bipolar disorder or major depression cholesterol concentrations increased significantly in 77% with mean increase of 25.9 mg/dL after 4 weeks and 26.4 mg/dL after about 12 weeks of therapy *763*

Cholesterol:HDL-Cholesterol Ratio
Serum Increase Physiological In 23 epileptic children treated with carbamazepine for a mean of 1.58 years mean ratio of 4.89 ± 1.99 significantly different from 3.83 ± 10.3 in 57 healthy control children *5727*

Cholinesterase *Serum Increase Physiological* Significant increase from mean of 4.77 U/L in controls to 7.25 U/L in epileptics receiving carbamazepine only *4807*

Cholinesterase (True) *Serum Increase Physiological* Substantially higher activity in treated epileptics than in controls *4806*

Clobazam *Serum Decrease Physiological* Carbamazepine stimulates metabolism causing reduced plasma concentration *3119* Metabolism stimulated *3118*

Clomipramine *Serum Increase Physiological* Coadministration with carbamazepine has been demonstrated to increase concentration of coadministered drug because of induction of hepatic CYP activity *1039*

Clonazepam *Serum Decrease Physiological* Coadministration with carbamazepine would be expected to decrease concentration of coadministered drug because of induction of hepatic CYP activity *1039* Hepatic metabolism stimulated *3118* Carbamazepine increases metabolism so plasma concentration reduced *3119* Increases hepatic metabolism through hepatic enzyme induction *1384*

Clozapine *Serum Decrease Physiological* Coadministration with carbamazepine would be expected to decrease concentration of coadministered drug because of induction of hepatic CYP activity *1039*

Copper *Serum Increase Physiological* In 30 epileptic patients treated for 1 month mean concentration of 99.3 ± 32.9 µg/dL significantly increased compared with 74.7 ± 9.4 µg/dL in 30 healthy controls *3344* As result of increased ceruloplasmin synthesis *2101* In 30 female epileptics treated with a mean of 800 mg/d of phenytoin mean concentration of 99 ± 27 µg/dL not significantly different from 91 ± 27 µg/dL in 35 healthy controls *3614*
Serum No Effect Physiological No significant effect in 26 patients being treated for epilepsy *4710* In 20 epileptic children receiving carbamazepine mean concentration of 1.11 ± 0.33 µg/mL not significantly different from 1.28 ± 0.369 µg/mL in 20 healthy control children *3331*

Copper Zinc Superoxide Dismutase
Serum Increase Physiological In 30 female epileptics treated with a mean of 800 mg/d of phenytoin mean activity of 114 ± 30 U/dL significantly different from 91 ± 24 U/dL in 35 healthy controls *3614*

Cortisol *Plasma Abnormal Physiological* False postivedexamethasone suppression test may occur due to attenuation of dexamethasone induced suppression of both plasma cortisol and urinary free cortisol *3119*
Plasma No Effect Physiological Insignificant variations observed in 10 normally menstruating women with epilepsy treated for up to one year and over long term *2837*

Cortisol, Free *Urine Abnormal Physiological* False postive dexamethasone suppression test may occur due to attenuation of dexamethasone induced suppression of both plasma cortisol and urinary free cortisol *3119*
Urine No Effect Analytical Carbamazepine showed some interference with HPLC method of Turpeinen et al but effect could be reduced by modification of mobile phase *6105*

Creatinine *Serum Increase Physiological* Azotemia and even renal failure have been observed as side effects of treatment *1039*
Serum No Effect Analytical No interference observed at a concentration of 1 mg/L with HPLC method of Rosano et al *5083* At 100 mg/L on reversed phase liquid chromatographic method of Zhiri et al *6656*

Cyclosporine *Blood Decrease Physiological* Coadministration with cyclosporine reported to decrease trough cyclosporine concentrations probably through induction of CYP enzymes in liver *859*
Blood No Effect Analytical At a concentration of 120 mg/L had no effect on Syva EMIT method *495*
Serum Decrease Physiological Increases hepatic metabolism with rate of hydroxylation and elimination *6288* In 3 adult renal transplant patients trough concentrations decreased and increased after carbamazepine discontinued *6595* In a renal transplant patient addition of carbamazepine caused acute decrease in cyclosporine concentration that resolved with discontinuation of carbamazepine and recurred with readministration *3118* Coadministration with cyclosporine reported to decrease trough cyclosporine concentrations probably through induction of CYP enzymes in liver *859* May decrease cyclosporine concentration by inducing hepatic cytochrome P-450 III A which metabolizes cyclosporine *5236* Effect occurs as result of induction of hepatic cytochrome P-450 *1069* Reported to decrease cyclosporine concentration when drugs coadministered *1384*

Cyclosporine A *Blood Decrease Physiological* Coadministration with cyclosporine A decreases its concentration *5240*

Dehydroepiandrosterone *Plasma Decrease Physiological* Significant effect observed in female epileptic patients on carbamazepine *2837*

Dehydroepiandrosterone Sulfate
Plasma Decrease Physiological Significant reduction in 23 treated male epileptic patients compared with untreated patients and controls *2838* In 23 epileptic patients treated with carbamazepine for a median of 14.6 years median concentration in both follicular and luteal phases significantly lower than in controls *4178* Significant reduction in women treated with drug compared with control untreated epileptics. Same effect observed when given in combination with phenytoin *3533* Within 7 d of starting 400 mg/d treatment in 6 healthy males probably due to induction of hepatic monooxygenase activity *1109* Reduction from mean baseline of 6.6 µmol/L to 4.2 µmol/L at 2 months and 3.8 µmol/L at one year and 3.2 µmol/L over long term in normally menstruating women with epilepsy *2837* Reduction to mean of 4.3 µmol/L in 20 male epileptic patients treated for mean of 3.3 years compared with 8.0 µmol/L in healthy control subjects *2840*
Plasma No Effect Physiological In 12 epileptic men aged 21 to 40 years treated with carbamazepine mean concentration of 5.4 ± 1.7 µmol/L not significantly different from normal of 0.8 - 16.0 µmol/L *2841*

Desipramine *Serum Decrease Physiological* Observed in one patient in whom drugs were coadministered *3118*

Dexamethasone *Serum Decrease Physiological* Effect of dexamethasone on suppression of secretion of steroids markedly reduced when carbamazepine coadministered *4791*

Diazepam *Serum Decrease Physiological* Stimulates hepatic metabolism through enzyme induction *1384*

Dicumarol *Plasma Decrease Physiological* Coadministration with carbamazepine would be expected to decrease concentration of coadministered drug because of induction of hepatic CYP activity *1039* Theoretical but undocumented risk that carbamazepine may increase dicoumarol metabolism (since phenytoin does this) *3118*

Digoxin *Serum Decrease Physiological* Coadministration of drugs results in low concentrations of digoxin *3119*

Doxepin *Serum Decrease Physiological* In 17 psychiatric patients in those receiving carbamazepine as well as doxepin concentrations of doxepin decreased to mean 46% of control without carbamazepine and concentration of doxepin and nordoxepin reduced to 45% of control without carbamazepine *3509*

Doxycycline *Serum Decrease Physiological* Hepatic metabolism stimulated by carbamazepine *4599* Observed to decrease half-life of doxycycline *4357* Half-life of drug significantly shortened when drug coadministered with carbamazepine *282* Coadministration with carbamazepine would be expected to decrease concentration of coadministered drug because of induction of hepatic CYP activity *1039* Half-life decreased because of increased hepatic metabolism of drug *1384* Metabolism stimulated by carbamazepine *3118*

Carbamazepine *(continued)*

Eosinophils *Blood Increase Physiological* Isolated hypersensitivity reaction reported. Associated with fever, rash, lymphadenopathy, hepatosplenomegaly and asthma *3550* Eosinophilia, aplastic anemia, pancytopenia and bone marrow depression have been reported as side effects *282* Eosinophilia has been observed as a side effect of treatment *1039* May intensify eosinophilia of filarial infection *2242* Eosinophilia observed occasionally *51*

Erythrocyte Sedimentation Rate
Blood Increase Physiological Associated with rare cases of granulomatous hepatitis *5667*

Erythrocytes *Blood Decrease Physiological* Aplastic anemia, pancytopenia and bone marrow depression have been reported as side effects *282* Aplastic anemia and agranulocytosis have been associated with carbamazepine administration with the risk being 5 to 8 times greater than in an untreated population *1039* Pancytopenia *1464*
Urine Increase Physiological Associated with bleeding tendency *210*

Erythromycin *Serum Increase Physiological* Concomitant administration of carbamazepine with erythromycin may increase its plasma concentration through its effect on cytochrome P450 *20*

Estradiol *Plasma Decrease Physiological* In 23 epileptic patients treated with carbamazepine for a median of 14.6 years median concentration in follicular phase significantly lower than median in 20 age-matched controls *4178*
Plasma Increase Physiological In 23 epileptic patients treated with carbamazepine for a median of 14.6 years median concentration in luteal phase significantly higher than median in 20 age-matched controls *4178* Insignificant increase of mean concentration (0.20 nmol/L) in 20 male epileptic patients compared with 0.15 nmol/L in healthy control subjects *2840*
Plasma No Effect Physiological No change in 10 normally menstruating epileptic women treated with appropriate doses over 1 year. No effect noted either in patients with long term treatment *2837* No difference between concentrations in 23 treated male epileptic patients and untreated patients and controls *2838*

Ethosuximide *Serum Decrease Physiological* Coadministration with carbamazepine would be expected to decrease concentration of coadministered drug because of induction of hepatic CYP activity *1039* Increases hepatic metabolism through enzyme induction *1384* In 2 patients receiving both carbamazepine and ethosuximide mean 48% increase observed between baseline and 4 weeks after withdrawal of carbamazepine *1619* Hepatic metabolism stimulated *3118*
Serum No Effect Analytical Insignificant cross-reactivity with method on Du Pont aca *1523*

Felbamate *Serum Decrease Physiological* Carbamazepine causes an approximate 50% increase in the clearance of felbamate at steady-state, with an approximate 40% decrease in the trough concentration of felbamate *6324*
Serum Increase Physiological Addition of carbamazepine to felbamate regime caused an approximate 40% decrease in steady state felbamate concentration because of 50% increase in its clearance *6323*
Serum No Effect Analytical No significant interference observed with GLC method of Rifai et al *4958*

Felodipine *Serum Decrease Physiological* Marked reduction in concentration when carbamazepine coadministered due to hepatic enzyme induction *876* Coadministration of carbamazepine with felodipine caused a reduction in the maximal plasma concentration of felodipine and a significant reduction to 6% of the area under the time-concentration curve in healthy individuals *266* Reported reduction of area under the curve of 94% when carbamazepine coadministered with felodipine *6623*

Fentanyl *Serum Decrease Physiological* Higher doses of fentanyl required to maintain anesthesia when carbamazepine added to therapeutic regime *3118*

Flecainide *Serum Decrease Physiological* 30% increase in the rate of plasma elimination when drug coadministered with flecainide *3702*

Folate *Red Blood Cells No Effect Physiological* In about 20 epileptic patients treated for 2 y *1370*
Serum No Effect Physiological In about 20 epileptic patients treated for 2 y *1370* Clinically insignificant effects observed on folate absorption and metabolism *3119*

Follicle Stimulating Hormone
Plasma Decrease Physiological Insignificant mean reduction to 4.6 IU/L in 20 male epileptic patients compared with mean of 6.2 IU/L in healthy control volunteers *2840*
Plasma No Effect Physiological In 23 epileptic patients treated with phenobarbital for a median of 14.6 years median concentration of 12.5 mIU/mL in follicular phase and 7.8 mIU/mL in luteal phase not markedly different from medians of 8.1 and 9.4 mIU/mL in 20 age-matched controls *4178* No significant variation in 10 normally menstruating women with epilepsy treated for up to one year or over long term with drug *2837* No difference between 23 treated male epileptic patients and untreated patients and controls *2838* In 12 epileptic men aged 21 to 40 years treated with carbamazepine mean concentration of 5.4 ± 4.0 IU/L not significantly different from normal *2841*

Gabapentin *Serum No Effect Physiological* Administration of 1200 mg/d gabapentin to 12 patients had no effect on steady-state trough plasma concentrations of carbamazepine nor on the pharmacokinetics of gabapentin *4526*

Glucaric Acid *Urine Increase Physiological* Dose dependent correlation: marked effect *4623*

Glucose *Serum No Effect Physiological* No significant effect observed in epileptic patients receiving carbamazepine *4077*
Urine Increase Physiological Single case of glycosuria reported *2451* Glycosuria may occur as side effect *282* Azotemia and even renal failure have been observed as side effects of treatment *1039* Rare reported side effect *1384*

Glutamine *Plasma No Effect Physiological* No striking effect when given to epileptic patients *6233*

γ-Glutamyltransferase *Serum Increase Physiological* In epileptic patients receiving monotherapy with carbamazepine mean increase from controls of 16 U/L to 43 U/L in 21 men and 47 U/L in 20 women *4394* In epileptic patients receiving monotherapy with carbamazepine mean increase from controls of 16 U/L to 43 U/L in 21 men and to 47 U/L in 20 women *4394* Observed 2 times upper limit of normal in 2 of 35 adult inpatient epileptics (dose and duration of treatment unknown) *1922* In 34 epileptic patients treated with mean 10.6 mg/kg/d caused significant mean increase of 60 U/L *5944* Associated with rare cases of granulomatous hepatitis *5667*
Serum No Effect Physiological When administered as sole drug to epileptic patients had no effect on enzyme activity *4078*

Glutathione Peroxidase
Red Blood Cells No Effect Physiological No effect observed in 26 patients being treated for epilepsy *4710*
Serum No Effect Physiological In 20 epileptic children receiving carbamazepine mean activity of 0.65 ± 0.085 U/mL not significantly different from 0.624 ± 0.08 U/mL in 20 healthy control children *3331*

Glutathione, Reduced *Plasma No Effect Physiological* In 30 female epileptics treated with a mean of 800 mg/d of phenytoin mean concentration of 34 ± 7 μmol/L not significantly different from 34 ± 6 μmol/L in 35 healthy controls *3614*

Glycine *Plasma No Effect Physiological* No striking effect when given to epileptic patients *6233*

Granulocytes *Blood Decrease Physiological* May cause agranulocytosis *51* Agranulocytosis has been associated with carbamazepine administration with a risk of it developing in 6 in a million treated patients *1039* Agranulocytosis, aplastic anemia, pancytopenia and bone marrow depression have been reported as side effects *282*

Haloperidol *Serum Decrease Physiological* In one study reductions from mean at 3 weeks of 47 μg/L to 21 μg/L, from 54 μg/L at 4 weeks to 21 μg/L and from 36 μg/L to 21 μg/L at 5 weeks *469 468* Coadministration with carbamazepine would be expected to decrease concentration of coadministered drug because of induction of hepatic CYP activity *1039* Concentration of drug may be significantly reduced when drug coadministered with carbamazepine *282* Mean reduction of 60% of haloperidol concentration in one study when carbamazepine coadministered *235* Carbamazepine can increase metabolism of haloperidol so that a 50% or greater decrease in plasma concentration occurs *3119* Increases hepatic clearance and decreases plasma concentration *1384*

HDL-Cholesterol *Serum Increase Physiological* Increased concentration has been reported to occur as a side effect in

patients taking anticonvulsants *282* Significantly increased concentration observed in chronically treated epileptics compared with age and sex matched controls *843*
Serum No Effect Physiological In 23 epileptic children treated with carbamazepine for a mean of 1.58 years mean concentration of 42.77 ± 11.33 mg/dL not significantly different from 41.31 ± 4.91 mg/dL in 57 healthy control children *5727*

HDL-Cholesterol:LDL-Cholesterol Ratio
Serum Increase Physiological In 23 epileptic children treated with carbamazepine for a mean of 1.58 years mean ratio of 3.33 ± 1.78 significantly different from 2.29 ± 1.04 in 57 healthy control children *5727*

Hematocrit *Blood Decrease Physiological* Pancytopenia *1464*

Hemoglobin *Blood Decrease Physiological* Aplastic anemia and agranulocytosis have been associated with carbamazepine administration with the risk being 5 to 8 times greater than in an untreated population *1039* In about 20 epileptic patients treated for 2 y *1370* Pancytopenia *1464* Aplastic anemia, pancytopenia and bone marrow depression have been reported as side effects *282*
Urine Increase Physiological Associated with bleeding tendency *210*

Histamine *Plasma No Effect Analytical* Improbable inhibition of radio-enzyme assay at physiological concentrations *2492*

Homocysteine *Plasma Increase Physiological* In treated patients concentration increased probably due to interference with folate functions *6123*

25-Hydroxy Vitamin D_3 *Serum Decrease Physiological* Significantly lower (11.1 ng/mL vs 17.6 ng/mL) in 21 patients treated with drug only for average of 40 mo *2664*

25-Hydroxy Vitamin D *Serum Decrease Physiological* Reported effect *3119*
Serum No Effect Physiological Reported effect *3119*

17-Hydroxycorticosteroids *Urine Increase Analytical* Purple color so impossible to quantify with Silber and Porter method at physiological amounts *6657*

6-β-Hydroxycortisol *Urine Increase Physiological* Increase of 193% observed in patients receiving carbamazepine *2016* Marked effect observed when carbamazepine administered due to hepatic enzyme induction *3119*

Imipramine *Serum Decrease Physiological* Significantly lower concentration observed in children receiving both carbamazepine and imipramine than in children receiving only imipramine in spite of receiving larger doses. Concentration of metabolite desipramine also observed *759*

Immunoglobulin A *Serum Decrease Physiological* Significant effect within 1 mo, remained low over next 30 mo *2116*
Serum No Effect Physiological Mean concentration 1.88 ± 0.7 g/L in 39 monotherapy treated epileptics compared with 1.95 ± 0.8 g/L in 40 controls *4475*

Immunoglobulin G *Serum No Effect Physiological* In 39 epileptics treated with monotherapy for at least 2 years mean concentration 10.4 ± 1.7 g/L compared with 10.9 ± 1.4 g/L in 40 healthy controls *4475* No effect regardless of duration of treatment *2116*

Immunoglobulin G_1 *Serum No Effect Physiological* No effect observed with treatment for 6 weeks in 20 epileptic patients *2115*

Immunoglobulin G_2 *Serum Decrease Physiological* Concentration reduced in 13 of 20 epileptic patients treated for 6 weeks. Mean concentration fell from 3.21 to 2.47 g/L. Decrease maintained after 4 and 12 months of treatment *2115*

Immunoglobulin G_3 *Serum No Effect Physiological* No effect observed in 20 epileptic patients after treatment for 6 weeks *2115*

Immunoglobulin G_4 *Serum No Effect Physiological* No effect observed in 20 epileptic patients treated for 6 weeks *2115*

Immunoglobulin M *Serum Decrease Physiological* Significant effect within 1 mo, slight rebound with continuation of treatment for 3 mo *2116*
Serum No Effect Physiological In 39 epileptics treated with carbamazepine for at least 2 years mean concentration 1.53 ± 0.6 g/L not significantly different from 1.42 ± 0.6 g/L in 40 healthy controls *4475*

Indomethacin *Serum No Effect Analytical* No effect on HPLC method of Roberts and Smith *4978*

itraconazole *Serum Decrease Physiological* Itraconazole potently inhibits the cytochrome P450 3A enzyme system thereby affecting the metabolism of drugs by this system: the concentration of itraconazole is substantially reduced with coadministration of carbamazepine *2905*

Lactate *Plasma Increase Physiological* Dose related effect observed in long term treated epileptic compared with controls *3275*
Plasma No Effect Physiological No significant effect observed in epileptic patients receiving carbamazepine *4077*

Lamotrigine *Serum Decrease Physiological* Coadministration of carbamazepine with lamotrigine caused a significant approximately 40% reduction in the plasma concentration of lamotrigine *2160*

LDL-Cholesterol *Serum Increase Physiological* In 23 epileptic children treated with carbamazepine for a mean of 1.58 years mean concentration of 132.23 ± 62.60 mg/dL significantly different from 92.85 ± 38.65 mg/dL in 57 healthy control children *5727*

Leukocytes *Blood Decrease Physiological* Both leukopenia and leukocytosis have been observed as side effects of treatment *1039* Many patients have drop to 3,000 /μL but returns to normal with continued treatment *1815* Pancytopenia (leukopenia in 15% patients) *1464* Leukopenia occurs in approximately 10% treated patients *1384*
Blood Increase Physiological Both leukopenia and leukocytosis have been observed as side effects of treatment *1039* Leukocytosis occasionally observed *51* Often marked leukocytosis maximal on fourth day *2242* Leukocytosis, aplastic anemia, pancytopenia and bone marrow depression have been reported as side effects *282* Granulomatous hepatitis observed in small proportion of patients treated for less than 1 mo; results within 3 d of cessation of treatment *3547*

Lithium *Serum Increase Analytical* May cause positive bias at high concentrations when lithium measured by an ion-specific electrode *3590*
Serum Increase Physiological Coadministration with carbamazepine asociated with increased risk of neurotoxic side effects *1039*

Long-chain Fatty Acid Carnitine Esters
Serum No Effect Physiological In 141 epileptic children treatment with carbamazepine caused nonsignificant reduction to 2.9 ± 1.5 nmol/mL compared with 3.1 ± 2.5 nmol/mL in 32 healthy control children *2757*

Luteinizing Hormone *Plasma Decrease Physiological* Although insignificant reduction at 2 months significant reduction from mean baseline of 9.9 IU/L to 6.6 IU/L at 12 months and 7.6 IU/L in long term treated normally menstruating female patients with epilepsy *2837*
Plasma No Effect Physiological Insignificant mean reduction to 7.8 IU/L in 20 male epileptic patients treated for mean of 3.3 years compared with 8.0 IU/L in healthy volunteers *2840* Insignificant fall in 6 healthy males at 14 d after 400 mg/d treatment *1109* In 23 epileptic patients treated with carbamazepine for a median of 14.6 years median concentration of 10.3 mIU/mL in follicular phase and 8.4 mIU/mL in luteal phase not markedly different from medians of 7.4 and 9.4 mIU/mL in 20 age-matched controls *4178* No difference between 23 treated male epileptics and untreated patients and controls *2838* In 12 epileptic men aged 21 to 40 years treated with carbamazepine mean concentration of 5.0 ± 2.3 IU/L not significantly different from normal *2841*

Luteinizing Hormone:Follicle Stimulating Hormone Ratio
Plasma No Effect Physiological In 23 epileptic patients treated with sodium valproate for a median of 14.6 years median 0.9 in follicular phase and 0.9 in luteal phase not markedly different from medians of 0.9 and 1.0 in 20 age-matched controls *4178*

Magnesium *Cerebrospinal Fluid No Effect Physiological* In 32 patients treated until steady-state concentration achieved nonsignificant change in concentration from mean baseline of 1.13 ± 0.08 mmol/L to 1.12 ± 0.09 mmol/L observed *2091*
Serum No Effect Physiological In 20 epileptic children receiving carbamazepine mean concentration of 23.16 ± 7.16 μg/mL not significantly different from 21.32 ± 5.21 μg/mL in 20 healthy control children *3331*

Carbamazepine *(continued)*

Malondialdehyde *Serum No Effect Physiological* In 30 female epileptics treated with a mean of 800 mg/d of phenytoin mean concentration of 2.1 ± 1.3 µmol/L not significantly different from 1.7 ± 0.8 µmol/L in 35 healthy controls *3614*

Manganese *Serum No Effect Physiological* In 20 epileptic children receiving carbamazepine mean concentration of 42.63 ± 17.25 ng/mL not significantly different from 46.29 ± 15.56 ng/mL in 20 healthy control children *3331*

MCV *Blood Increase Physiological* In about 20 epileptic patients treated for 2 y *1370*

Mebendazole *Serum Decrease Physiological* Increases hepatic clearance and reduces plasma concentration *1384* In one study reduced concentrations observed when carbamazepine administered in comparison with other drugs *3675*

Methadone *Serum Decrease Physiological* During methadone maintenance addition of carbamazepine caused 60% decrease in plasma methadone concentration *3118*

Methsuximide *Serum Decrease Physiological* Coadministration with carbamazepine would be expected to decrease concentration of coadministered drug because of induction of hepatic CYP activity *1039*

Methylprednisolone *Serum Decrease Physiological* Metabolism increased when carbamazepine coadministered *3118*

Mianserin *Serum Decrease Physiological* In 4 psychiatric patients concentration reduced to 30% of concentration when only mianserin given when carbamazepine also administered *3509*

Mycophenolic Acid *Serum No Effect Analytical* No significant interference observed with HPLC method of Shipkova et al *5526*

Mycophenolic Acid Glucuronide
Serum No Effect Analytical No significant interference observed with HPLC method of Shipkova et al *5526*

N-Acetyl-Glucosaminidase *Urine Increase Physiological* In 27 patients with mood disorders treatment with carbamazepine 600 mg/d for median duration of one year caused mean excretion of 53 ± 23 not significantly different from 46 ± 27 in 171 untreated patients. Effect possibly associated with abnormalities of serotonin metabolism *2040*

Natural Killer Cells *Blood Increase Physiological* Increase in natural killer cell activity observed in 39 epileptic patients with epilepsy compared with 40 controls *4475*

Neutrophils *Blood Decrease Physiological* Neutropenia associated with decrease of WBC in small proportion of patients *5158* Occasional case of agranulocytosis reported *6264* Reported to cause neutropenia/agranulocytosis *4265*

Nortriptyline *Serum Decrease Physiological* Low plasma nortriptyline concentrations observed but high hydoxynortriptyline to nortriptyline ratio observed in plasma *3118* Concentration in 8 psychiatric patients receiving carbamazepine in addition to nortriptyline concentration of nortriptyline reduced to 42% of that in patients without carbamazepine and concentration of nortriptyline with amitriptyline reduced to 40% *3509*

5'-Nucleotidase *Serum Increase Physiological* Due to cholestasis *2911*
Serum No Effect Physiological Observed 2 times upper limit of normal in none of 34 adult inpatient epileptics given drug alone (dose and duration of treatment unknown) *1922*

Organic Acids *Urine Increase Physiological* Dose related effect observed in long-term treated epileptics compared with controls *3275*

Ornithine *Plasma No Effect Physiological* No striking effect when given to epileptic patients *6233*

Osmolality *Serum Decrease Physiological* Isolated case of dilutional hyponatremia with water intoxication: 7 previous cases reported *3064* Mean concentration reduced in carbamazepine treated patients, possibly due to stimulation of release of ADH *4621*

p-Aminophenol *Urine No Effect Analytical* With addition of drugs at a concentration of 100 mg/L and of related compounds at 50 mg/L no significant effect observed on colorimetric method of van Bocxlaer on Cobas Mira analyzer which involves reacting free p-aminophenol with resorcinol in the presence of magnesium ions to form an indophenol dye measured at 550 nm *6163*

Phenobarbital *Serum Decrease Physiological* Most commonly slight reduction due to hepatic enzyme induction when drugs coadministered although may occasionally be slight increase *1384*
Serum No Effect Analytical No significant cross-reactivity observed with method on Du Pont aca *1537* At concentration of 500 µg/mL (2117 µmol/L) has no effect on method on Du Pont Dimension *1582* At maximum physiological or pharmacological concentrations no cross-reactivity observed with phenobarbital method on Bayer Technicon Immuno 1® *427*
Serum No Effect Physiological No significant change observed in 23 epileptic patients 4 weeks after withdrawal of carbamazepine *1619*

Phensuximide *Serum Decrease Physiological* Coadministration with carbamazepine would be expected to decrease concentration of coadministered drug because of induction of hepatic CYP activity *1039*

Phenylalanine *Plasma No Effect Analytical* No interference observed with rapid quantitative whole blood method of Campbell et al using phenylalanine dehydrogenase *867*

Phenylbutazone *Serum No Effect Physiological* No significant effect observed when carbamazepine added to therapeutic regime *3118*

Phenytoin *Serum Decrease Physiological* Coadministration with phenytoin may decrease plasma phenytoin concentration *4522* Causes decreased concentration *6350* Half life reduced from 10.6 to 6.4 h *3339* When drugs coadministered typically some reduction of concentration of both drugs due to hepatic anzyme induction but may be slight increase *1384* When carbamazepine ingested with fosphenytoin concentration of phenytoin may be decreased *4519* Half-life of drug significantly shortened when drug coadministered with carbamazepine *282* Coadministration with carbamazepine would be expected to decrease concentration of coadministered drug because of induction of hepatic CYP activity *1039*
Serum Increase Physiological Mean 26% reduction observed in 23 epileptic patients with discontinuation of carbamazepine for 4 weeks *1619* Coadministration with carbamazepine has been demonstrated to increase concentration of coadministered drug because of induction of hepatic CYP activity *1039* Significant increase (36%) after drug added to regime *6659*
Serum No Effect Analytical No effect at concentration of 1000 µg/mL (4230 µmol/L) on method on Du Pont Dimension *1583* No significant interference observed at a concentration of 1000 µg/mL (4.23 mmol/L) with method on Du Pont aca *1538*

Phenytoin, Free *Serum Increase Physiological* Mean 26% reduction in 23 epileptic patients 4 weeks after discontinuation of carbamazepine treatment *1619*

Phosphate *Serum Decrease Physiological* In about 20 epileptic patients treated for 2 y *1370* Hypophosphatemia observed in 1 of 21 patients (5%) treated for average of 40 mo *2664*
Serum No Effect Physiological Osteomalacia observed in 3 of 31 patients given average of 758 mg/d for average of 20.5 mo *4377*

Platelets *Blood Decrease Physiological* Within 2 weeks of commencement of treatment in a single patient. Associated with petechiae *5163* Marked effect in one patient with strongly positive migration inhibition (MIF) test *5531* Thrombocytopenia, aplastic anemia, pancytopenia and bone marrow depression have been reported as side effects *282* In one case drug-dependent IgG antibodies identified *3251* Thrombocytopenia has been observed as a side effect of treatment *1039* Thrombocytopenia may occur after 1 y (immunologic) *1464*

Potassium *Serum Decrease Physiological* Marked reduction observed in several outpatients with epilepsy treated for several years with carbamazepine alone or in combination with other drugs *4345*
Serum No Effect Analytical At concentration of 20 mg/L had no effect on ISE measurement with predilution *5704*
Urine Decrease Physiological Isolated case of dilutional hyponatremia with water intoxication: 7 previous cases reported *3064*

Prealbumin *Serum Increase Physiological* Mean increased above upper reference limit in epileptic patients when treated with carbamazepine alone *4347*

Prednisolone *Serum Decrease Physiological* Concentration reduced when both drugs are given. Prednisolone half-life reduced by 27% and clearance increased by 42% *4408* Metabolism increased when carbamazepine coadministered *3118*

Pregnancy Tests *Urine Negative Analytical* False negative or inconclusive value with Prepurex, Predictor, Gonavislide, Pregnosticon® *3592*

Primidone *Serum Decrease Physiological* Probably occurs as a result of hepatic enzyme induction: concentration of metabolite of phenobarbital increased *3118* Typically slight decrease when drugs coadministered due to hepatic enzyme induction but may be slight increase *1384*
Serum Increase Physiological Coadministration with carbamazepine has been demonstrated to increase concentration of coadministered drug because of induction of hepatic CYP activity *1039*
Serum No Effect Analytical At a concentration of 1250 mg/L causes 25% increase in concentration as measured by method on Baxter Stratus but clinical concentrations up to 12 mg/L only *5705* No significant cross-reactivity observed with method on Du Pont aca *1541*

Progesterone *Plasma Decrease Physiological* Insignificant reduction of mean concentration in 20 male epileptic patients (0.89 nmol/L) compared with 1.01 nmol/L in healthy control subjects *2840* In 23 epileptic patients treated with carbamazepine for a median of 14.6 years median concentration in luteal phase lower than 12.7 nmol/L in 23.0% *4178*
Plasma No Effect Physiological In 23 epileptic patients treated with carbamazepine for a median of 14.6 years median concentration in follicular phase not significantly different from that in controls *4178* No change after 2 months but nonsignificant increase at 12 months in 10 normally menstruating epileptic women and significant reduction to 0.50 nmol/L from typical baseline of 0.93 nmol/L with long term treatment *2837*

Prolactin *Plasma Decrease Physiological* Insignificant reduction to 8.1 µg/L in 20 male epileptic patients treated for mean of 3.3 years compared with 9.5 µg/L in healthy control subjects *2840*
Plasma No Effect Physiological In 12 epileptic men aged 21 to 40 years treated with carbamazepine mean concentration of 11.9 ± 4.5 µg/L not significantly different from normal *2841* In 23 epileptic patients treated with sodium valproate for a median of 14.6 years median concentration of 17.1 ng/mL in follicular phase and 16.1 ng/mL in luteal phase not markedly different from medians of 15.1 and 14.2 ng/mL in 20 age-matched controls *4178* No difference between 23 treated male epileptic patients and untreated patients and controls *2838* Insignificant variation observed in 10 normally menstruating women with epilepsy treated for up to one year and over long term *2837*

Protein *Serum Decrease Physiological* In about 20 epileptic patients treated for 2 y *1370*
Urine Increase Physiological Azotemia and even renal failure have been observed as side effects of treatment *1039* Manifestation of renal damage *51*

Prothrombin Time *Plasma Decrease Physiological* In patients receiving warfarin half-life is reduced and dose must be increased to maintain anticoagulant effect *1384* Increases metabolic clearance of warfarin when it is coadministered *2625* Enhances warfarin metabolism by enzyme induction *2452*

Pyruvate *Plasma No Effect Physiological* No significant effect observed in epileptic patients receiving carbamazepine *4077*

Risperidone *Serum Decrease Physiological* Chronic administration of carbamazepine with risperidone may increase the clearance of risperidone *2904*.

Saquinavir *Serum Decrease Physiological* Coadministration of carbamazepine with saquinavir reduced the latter's concentration by inducing CYP3A4 in the liver *5024*

Selenium *Serum Decrease Physiological* Reduction from mean of 15.9 µg/dL to 13.1 µg/dL in 26 patients being treated with drug for epilepsy *4710*
Serum No Effect Physiological In 20 epileptic children receiving carbamazepine mean concentration of 106.82 ± 16.9 ng/mL not significantly different from 110.72 ± 25.41 ng/mL in 20 healthy control children *3331*

Sex-Hormone Binding Globulin
Serum Increase Physiological Insignificant increase to 37 nmol/L in 20 male epileptic patients treated for mean of 3.3 years compared with 27 nmol/L in healthy control subjects *2840* Within 7 d of starting 400 mg/d treatment in 6 healthy males probably due to induction of hepatic monooxygenase activity *1109* Significant increase in 23 male treated epileptics compared with untreated patients and controls *2838* In 10 normally menstruating epileptic women mean increase from baseline of 42 nmol/L to 59 nmol/L after 2 months treatment and 54 nmol/L with 12 months treatment with drug to control seizures. With long term treatment mean concentration 70 nmol/L *2837* In 11 epileptic patients treatment with carbamazepine caused a significant change in concentration from mean baseline of 28.0 ± 9.3 nmol/L to 32.7 ± 7.0 nmol/L after one year and 47.9 ± 22.2 nmol/L after 5 years *2842* In 12 epileptic men aged 21 to 40 years treated with carbamazepine mean concentration of 50.5 ± 20.6 nmol/L significantly different from normal of 11.2 - 42.0 nmol/L *2841*
Serum No Effect Physiological In 23 epileptic patients treated with carbamazepine for a median of 14.6 years median concentration in both follicular and luteal phases not significantly from that in controls because of wide dispersion of results *4178*

Short-chain Fatty Acid Carnitine Esters
Serum No Effect Physiological In 141 epileptic children treated with carbamazepine mean concentration 8.4 ± 3.9 nmol/mL not significantly less than 15.4 ± 9.1 nmol/mL in 32 healthy control children *2757*

Sodium *Serum Decrease Physiological* Carbamazepine has week antidiuretic effect and low plasma sodium concentrations have been reported in association with carbamazepine administration *3119* Although mean concentration in population of epileptics not affected, significant reduction in 5 of 80 patients *4621* Plasma sodium concentration reported to be decreased when carbamazepine administered alone or in combination with other drugs *282* Hyponatremia has been observed as a side effect of treatment as a consequence of inappropriate secretion of ADH *1039* In 28 of 674 epileptic patients most often when drug combined with barbiturates *3011* Isolated case of dilutional hyponatremia with water intoxication: 7 previous cases reported *3064*
Serum Increase Analytical At 10 times therapeutic concentration caused statistically significant increase with method used on Technicon SRA-2000 *4348*
Serum Increase Physiological In several outpatients receiving drug alone for several years highly increased concentrations observed (also seen with other drugs and when carbamazepine combined with other drugs) *4345*
Serum No Effect Analytical At concentration of 20 mg/L had no effect on ISE measurement with predilution *5704*
Urine Decrease Physiological Isolated case of dilutional hyponatremia with water intoxication: 7 previous cases reported *3064*

Somatostatin *Cerebrospinal Fluid Decrease Physiological* Appears to affect compound whereas other drugs do not *5142*

Superoxide Dismutase
Red Blood Cells No Effect Physiological No significant effect in 26 patients being treated for epilepsy *4710*
Serum No Effect Physiological In 20 epileptic children receiving carbamazepine mean activity of copper:zinc superoxide dismutase of 0.814 ± 0.284 U/mL not significantly different from 0.681 ± 0.298 U/mL in 20 healthy control children *3331*

T3-Uptake *Serum Increase Analytical* At therapeutic concentrations cause interference with CEDIA method *2717*
Serum No Effect Physiological In 32 epileptic patients of mean age of 31.8 ± 12.2 y mean ratio of 0.92 ± 0.1 not significantly different from 0.91 ± 0.1 in 32 healthy controls *6234*

Tacrolimus *Blood No Effect Analytical* No significant effect observed at a concentration of 12 mg/L with MEIA method on Abbott IMx analyzer *1871* No interference observed with radioreceptor assay of Murthy et al *4191*
Serum Decrease Physiological By inducing cytochrome P-450 IIIA enzyme systems may stimulate the metabolism of tacrolimus *1987*
Serum No Effect Analytical At a concentration of 12 mg/L had no significant effect on ELISA method *6329*

Testosterone *Serum Decrease Physiological* Within 7 d of starting 400 mg/d treatment in 6 healthy males probably due to

Carbamazepine *(continued)*

Testosterone *(continued)*
induction of hepatic monooxygenase activity *1109* In 23 epileptic patients treated with carbamazepine for a median of 14.6 years median concentration in follicular phase lower than in controls *4178* In 11 epileptic patients treatment with carbamazepine caused a nonsignificant change in concentration from mean baseline of 24.6 ± 6.6 nmol/L to 23.2 ± 4.9 nmol/L after one year and 25.7 ± 6.6 nmol/L after 5 years *2842*
Serum No Effect Physiological No significant difference between 23 treated male epileptic patients and untreated patients and controls *2838* Usually no effect but may be slight increase *2836* No significant change over one year or with long term treatment in normally menstruating women with epilepsy *2837* No significant difference between 20 male epileptic patients treated for mean of 3.3 years with carbamazepine alone (23.5 pmol/L) and healthy control subjects (23.3 pmol/L) *2840* In 12 epileptic men aged 21 to 40 years treated with carbamazepine mean concentration of 25.8 ± 4.6 nmol/L not significantly different from normal *2841*

Testosterone, Free *Serum Decrease Physiological* Within 7 d of starting 400 mg/d treatment in 6 healthy males probably due to induction of hepatic monooxygenase activity *1109* Observed effect *2836*
Serum No Effect Physiological No significant difference between 20 male epileptic patients treated with carbamazepine alone for mean of 3.3 years (93 pmol/L) and healthy volunteers (91 pmol/L) *2840* Nonsignificant reduction at 2 months, 12 months and over long term in normally menstruating epileptic women *2837* No difference between concentrations in 23 treated male epileptics and untreated patients and controls *2838* In 12 epileptic men aged 21 to 40 years treated with carbamazepine mean concentration of 76.4 ± 20.8 pmol/L not significantly different from normal *2841*

Tetracycline *Serum No Effect Physiological* No effect observed on the metabolism of tetracyclines other than on doxycycline *3118*

Theophylline *Serum Decrease Physiological* Increases theophylline clearance by induction of microsomal enzyme activity, decreasing theophylline concentration by about 30% *5999* Plasma half-life and concentration decreased when carbamazepine coadministered *3118* Coadministration with carbamazepine would be expected to decrease concentration of coadministered drug because of induction of hepatic CYP activity *1039* Increases theophylline clearance by induction of microsomal enzyme activity and decreases serum theophylline concentration by 30% *3125* Half-life of drug significantly shortened when drug coadministered with carbamazepine *282* Half-life reduced from 5.25 h to 2.75 h during treatment probably due to enzyme interaction *5095* Increases hepatic clearance and decreases plasma concentration *1384* Up to 30% decrease in serum theophylline concentration due to increased theophylline clearance caused by induction of microsomal enzyme activity *6117*

Thyroglobulin *Serum No Effect Physiological* No significant effect with 400 mg/d for 21 d *1110*

Thyroid Stimulating Hormone
Serum Decrease Physiological Marked reduction in 26 patients on long-term therapy *3569*
Serum Increase Physiological In 10 patients with chronic epilepsy treatment with carbamazepine with valproic acid caused significant increase to 0 2.5 ± 1.0 mU/L compared with 1.7 ± 0.8 mU/L in 28 healthy controls *2839* Insignificant increase to mean of 1.8 mU/L in 20 male epileptic patients treated for mean of 3.3 years compared with 1.4 mU/L in healthy control subjects *2840*
Serum No Effect Analytical At therapeutic and toxic concentrations on RIA methods *597* No effect observed at both therapeutic and toxic concentrations when added to serum *in vitro597*
Serum No Effect Physiological No change in TSH or in its response to TRH *6412* In 39 patients with depression treatment for about 12 weeks had no significant effect on concentration *763* Therapeutic concentrations of carbamazepine have no effect on plasma TSH concentration *5876* No effect of 400 mg/d on basal or stimulated TSH *1110* In 45 patients with chronic epilepsy treatment with carbamazepine (mean concentration 1.8 mU/L) caused no significant difference from mean concentration of 1.7 ± 0.8 mU/L in 28 healthy controls. In 16 patients treated with carbamazepine with phenytoin mean concentration 2.0 ± 1.0 mU/L *2839* Observed in 9 hypothyroid patients given substitution therapy due to increased extra-thyroidal metabolism of thyroid hormones *2* No significant change in patients on long-term treatment *3568* Basal concentration unchanged in treated patients *1269*

Thyrotropin Releasing Hormone
Cerebrospinal Fluid Increase Physiological In 9 patients with mood disorders mean concentration increased to 4.45 ± 0.35 pg/mL after having taken 950 mg/d carbamazepine for 1 month from 1.50 ± 0.15 pg/mL in medication-free state *3783*

Thyroxine Binding Globulin *Serum Increase Physiological* Observed in 9 hypothyroid patients given substitution therapy due to increased extra-thyroidal metabolism of thyroid hormones *2*
Serum No Effect Analytical At therapeutic and toxic concentrations on Corning radioimmunometric kit method *597* No effect observed at both therapeutic and toxic concentrations when added to serum *in vitro597*

Thyroxine (T4) *Serum Decrease Physiological* Mean concentration of 67 nmol/L in 20 male epileptic patients treated with drug alone for mean of 3.3 years compared with 93 nmol/L in controls *2840* Concentration reduced due to hepatic enzyme induction *2412* Observed in 9 hypothyroid patients given substitution therapy due to increased extra-thyroidal metabolism of thyroid hormones *2* Reduced concentrations observed in treated individuals *1269* Fall from mean of 82 to 75 nmol/L with 400 mg/d carbamazepine after 14 d treatment in 10 healthy males, secondary to hepatic enzyme induction with accelerated nondeiodinative hepatic hormone disposal *1110* In 39 patients with depression treatment for about 12 weeks caused significant decrease from mean baseline of 8.67 ± 1.73 µg/dL to 6.29 ± 1.82 µg/dL *763* In 45 patients with epilepsy treated with long term carbamazepine mean concentration significantly reduced to 66.2 ± 10.7 nmol/L compared with 91.6 ± 12.9 nmol/L in controls. In those treated with carbamazepine with phenytoin mean concentration reduced to 64.5 ± 14.5 nmol/L and in those receiving carbamazepine with valproic acid 59.3 ± 5.7 nmol/L *2839* Decreased thyroid function test values have been reported in patients receiving carbamazepine *1039* Thyroid function tests reported to be decreased when carbamazepine administered alone *282* In 32 epileptic patients of mean age of 31.8 ± 12.2 y mean concentration of 76 ± 14 nmol/L significantly different from 99 ± 19 nmol/L in 32 healthy controls *6234*
Serum Increase Physiological Therapeutic concentrations of carbamazepine displace thyroxine from its binding proteins with increased free T4 but decreased total thyroxine to 74% of untreated concentration *5876*
Serum No Effect Analytical No effect observed at both therapeutic and toxic concentrations when added to serum *in vitro597* At therapeutic and toxic concentrations on an equilibrium dialysis method *597*

Thyroxine (T4), Free *Serum Decrease Physiological* In 45 chronic epileptics treated with long term carbamazepine mean concentration significantly decreased to 13.0 ± 2.4 pmol/L compared with 16.3 ± 2.4 pmol/L in 28 healthy controls. In 16 patients treated with carbamazepine and phenytoin mean concentration 12.3 ± 2.2 pmol/L and in 10 treated with carbamazepine and valproic acid mean concentration 11.7 ± 1.9 pmol/L also significantly less than concentration in healthy controls *2839* Effect observed in treated individuals. In one third patients who took drug for one year concentration below reference range *1269* Fall from mean of 16.0 to 14.2 pmol/L with 400 mg/d in healthy males *1110* Observed in 9 hypothyroid patients given substitution therapy due to increased extra-thyroidal metabolism of thyroid hormones *2* Mean concentration of 13.3 pmol/L in 20 male epileptic patients treated with carbamazepine alone for mean of 3.3 years compared with 16.5 pmol/L in healthy control subjects *2840* As measured by equilibrium dialysis and analog-type radioimmunoassays; not due to displacement from protein *3569*
Serum Increase Analytical Increase observed when FT4 measured by Boehringer Mannheim Enzymun method *2617* As measured by addition of drug to control sera and measured by Analog radioimmunoassay *3569*
Serum No Effect Analytical No effect observed at both therapeutic and toxic concentrations when added to serum *in vitro597* At therapeutic and toxic concentrations on RIA method *597*

Thyroxine (T4), Free Dialyzable
Serum No Effect Physiological Therapeutic concentrations of carbamazepine displace thyroxine from its binding proteins with increased proportion of free T4 but absolute amount of free T4 normal *5876*

Thyroxine (T4) Index, Free *Serum Decrease Physiological* No significant change in patients on long-term treatment *3568*
Serum Increase Physiological In 32 epileptic patients of mean age of 31.8 ± 12.2 y mean concentration of 109.4 ± 12.9 nmol/L significantly different from 106.8 ± 15.4 nmol/L in 32 healthy controls *6234*

Toremifene *Serum Decrease Physiological* Cytochrome P450 3A4 inducers increase the rate of toremifene metabolism thereby reducing its serum concentration *5329*

Tramadol *Serum Decrease Physiological* Coadministration of carbamazepine with tramadol caused a significant increase in the metabolism of tramadol necessitating an increase of perhaps twofold in the tramadol dose *3918*

Transferrin *Serum Increase Physiological* Tendency for higher concentration in epileptics treated only with carbamazepine. Positive correlation observed between carbamazepine and transferrin concentrations *4346*

Tri-iodothyronine, Free (fT3)
Serum Decrease Physiological Observed in 9 hypothyroid patients given substitution therapy due to increased extra-thyroidal metabolism of thyroid hormones *2* As measured by equilibrium dialysis and analog-type radioimmunoassays; not due to displacement from protein *3569*
Serum Increase Analytical As measured by addition of drug to control sera and measured by analog radioimmunoassay *3569*
Serum No Effect Physiological Concentration unchanged or slightly reduced in treated patients *1269* Therapeutic concentrations of carbamazepine displace tri-iodothyronine from its binding proteins with increased proportion of free T3 but absolute amount of free tri-iodothyronine unchanged *5876*

Tri-iodothyronine, Reverse (rT3)
Serum No Effect Physiological No significant change in patients on long-term treatment *3568* No significant effect with 400 mg/d for 21 d *1110*

Tri-iodothyronine (T3) *Serum Decrease Physiological* In 45 chronic epileptics treated with long term carbamazepine mean concentration of 1.5 ± 0.3 nmol/L compared with 1.7 ± 0.2 nmol/L in 28 controls *2839* Observed in 9 hypothyroid patients given substitution therapy due to increased extra-thyroidal metabolism of thyroid hormones *2* Fall from mean of 1.6 to 1.4 nmol/L with 400 mg/d in healthy males *1110* Concentration reduced due to hepatic enzyme induction *2412* Therapeutic concentrations of carbamazepine displace tri-iodothyronine from its binding proteins with increased free T3 but decreased total tri-iodothyronine *5876* In 39 patients with depression treatment for about 12 weeks caused significant decrease from 133.6 ± 26.5 ng/dL to 116.3 ± 28.0 ng/dL *763*
Serum No Effect Analytical No effect observed at both therapeutic and toxic concentrations when added to serum *in vitro597* At therapeutic and toxic concentrations on RIA methods *597*
Serum No Effect Physiological Mean concentration of 1.7 nmol/L in 20 male epileptic patients treated for mean of 3.3 years same as in healthy control volunteers *2840* In 16 chronic epileptics treated with carbamazepine and phenytoin mean concentration 1.7 ± 0.3 nmol/L and in 10 treated with carbamazepine with valproic acid mean concentration 1.6 ± 0.2 nmol/L not significantly different from 1.7 ± 0.2 nmol/L in 28 healthy controls *2839* Concentration unchanged or slightly reduced in treated patients *1269*

Tricyclic Antidepressants *Serum Decrease Physiological* Interacts pharmacokinetically to induce metabolism of tricyclic antidepressants *3590*
Serum Increase Analytical May cause false positive reaction in immunoassays for tricyclic antidepressants *3590*

Tricyclic Antidepressants Screen
Serum No Effect Analytical No significant effect observed at a concentration of 50 µg/mL (0.21 mmol/L) with method on Du Pont aca *1550*

Triglycerides *Serum Increase Physiological* Increased concentration has been reported to occur as a side effect in patients taking anticonvulsants *282*
Serum No Effect Physiological In 23 epileptic children treated with carbamazepine for a mean of 1.58 years mean concentration of 97.57 ± 45.92 mg/dL not significantly different from 98.22 ± 38.83 mg/dL in 57 healthy control children *5727*

TSH response to TRH *Serum Decrease Physiological* Response either decreased or unaffected during the administration of carbamazepine *3119*
Serum No Effect Physiological No change observed typically but in patients treated for affective disorder may be a flat response to TRH *1269*

Urea Nitrogen *Serum Increase Physiological* May cause kidney dysfunction *128* Azotemia and even renal failure have been observed as side effects of treatment *1039* Azotemia may occur as side effect *282*

Uric Acid *Serum Decrease Analytical* At 10 times therapeutic concentration caused statistically significant decrease with method on Technicon SRA-2000 *4348*
Serum No Effect Analytical At 100 mg/L on reversed phase liquid chromatographic method of Zhiri et al *6656*

Valproic Acid *Serum Decrease Physiological* Coadministration with carbamazepine would be expected to decrease concentration of coadministered drug because of induction of hepatic CYP activity *1039* Causes decreased concentration *6350* Concentration of drug may be significantly reduced when drug coadministered with carbamazepine *282* Significant reduction of half-life from 10.9 h to 6.4 h due to enzyme induction *3684* Concentration reduced to about 66% when carbamazepine coadministered *3855* After 2 weeks treatment in 5 healthy adult male volunteers mean serum trough concentrations decreased from 44.0 µg/mL to 27.0 µg/mL *4495* Through induction of hepatic enzymes may increase the plasma clearance of valproate *15* Increases hepatic metabolism through enzyme induction *1384* Concentration in plasma reduced probably due to hepatic enzyme induction *3118* Significant increase by 42% in concentration after 4 weeks withdrawal of carbamazepine in 23 epileptic patients *1619*
Serum No Effect Analytical At concentrations up to 1000 µg/mL had no significant cross-reactivity in valproic acid method on Bayer Technicon Immuno 1® *437* No significant interference observed at a concentration of 1000 µg/mL (4233 µmol/L) with method on Du Pont aca *1560*

VLDL-Cholesterol *Serum No Effect Physiological* In 23 epileptic children treated with carbamazepine for a mean of 1.58 years mean concentration of 24.55 ± 22.37 mg/dL not significantly different from 21.69 ± 19.06 mg/dL in 57 healthy control children *5727*

Volume *Urine Decrease Physiological* Isolated case of dilutional hyponatremia with water intoxication: 7 previous cases reported *3064*

Warfarin *Plasma Decrease Physiological* Coadministration with carbamazepine would be expected to decrease concentration of coadministered drug because of induction of hepatic CYP activity *1039* Decreased plasma concentration observed and decreased prothrombin response to anticoagulant observed in one study when carbamazepine added to therapeutic regime *2442* Increases metabolism to an extent sufficient to interfere with anticoagulant effect *3118* Half-life of drug significantly shortened when drug coadministered with carbamazepine *282* Reported interaction due to alteration of metabolism *3340*

Zinc *Serum Decrease Physiological* Reduction from 670.0 µg/dL to 577.9 µg/dL in 26 patients being treated for epilepsy *4710*
Serum No Effect Physiological In 30 epileptic patients treated with carbamazepine for 1 month insignificant reduction observed to 73.4 ± 11.7 µg/dL from 78.4 ± 12.8 µg/dL in 30 healthy controls *3344* In 20 epileptic children receiving carbamazepine mean concentration of 3.5 ± 0.659 µg/mL not significantly different from 3.44 ± 1.09 µg/mL in 20 healthy control children *3331* In 30 female epileptics treated with a mean of 800 mg/d of phenytoin mean concentration of 85 ± 14 µg/dL not significantly different from 88 ± 13 µg/dL in 35 healthy controls *3614*

Carbamazepine-10,11-epoxide

Carbamazepine *Serum Increase Analytical* 9.8% cross-reactivity observed with competitive fluorescence immunoassay procedure used with PB Diagnostics Systems OPUS analyzer

Carbamazepine-10,11-epoxide *(continued)*

Carbamazepine *(continued)*
1153 Cross reactivity of 18.7% observed with method on Baxter Stratus *5705*
Serum No Effect Analytical Insignificant cross-reactivity observed with method on Johnson and Johnson Ektachem® analyzer *1997* At a concentration of 50 µg/mL had no significant cross-reactivity with carbamazepine at a concentration of 4.0 µg/mL when measured by method on Bayer Technicon Immuno 1® system *417* No interference observed at a concentration of 50 µg/mL with Syva EMIT 2000 assay *4156*

Felbamate *Serum No Effect Analytical* No significant interference observed with GLC method of Rifai et al *4958*

Carbarsone

Alanine Aminotransferase *Serum Increase Physiological* May cause hepatitis/Liver necrosis *128*

Aspartate Aminotransferase *Serum Increase Physiological* May cause hepatitis/Liver necrosis *128*

Bilirubin *Serum Increase Physiological* Cholestasis with cholangiolitis may occur *3171*

BSP Retention *Serum Increase Physiological* Toxic hepatitis may occur *4246*

^{131}I Uptake *Serum Decrease Physiological* Lilly compound contains tetraiodofluorescein *4360*

Protein *Urine Increase Physiological* Nephrotoxic effect *1714*

Carbenicillin

Alanine Aminotransferase *Serum Increase Physiological* In several patients as evidence of drug induced hepatotoxicity *2279* Elevation reported, ?due to hepatotoxicity *2754* In 7 of 27 patients given 270 mg/kg i.v. for 6 d *5475*
Serum No Effect Analytical At 5 times upper limit of therapeutic range on methods on Technicon SMAC® , Abbott-VP, Du Pont aca, Roche Cobas-Bio, and KDA *3525*

Albumin *Serum Decrease Analytical* At concentrations above 5,000 mg/L lowered the concentration as measured by BCG method *5704*
Serum No Effect Analytical At 5 times upper limit of therapeutic range on BCG method on Technicon SMAC® , Kodak Ektachem® 400 Hitachi® 705 and KDA *3525*

Alkaline Phosphatase *Serum Increase Physiological* Transient elevations reported *2242* In 4 of 27 patients given 270 mg/kg i.v. for 6 d *5475*
Serum No Effect Analytical At 5 times upper limit of therapeutic range on methods on Technicon SMAC® , Abbott-VP, Du Pont aca, Roche Cobas-Bio, Hitachi® 705 and KDA *3525*

Amikacin *Serum No Effect Analytical* No interference observed at a concentration of 500 µg/mL (1321 µmol/L) with method used on Du Pont aca *1508*

Amino Acids *Urine Increase Analytical* Unusual ninhydrin positive spot on TLC *2605*

Amylase *Serum No Effect Analytical* At 5 times upper limit of therapeutic range on methods on Du Pont aca, Roche Cobas-Bio and Kodak Ektachem® 400 *3525*

Aspartate Aminotransferase *Serum Increase Physiological* In 6 of 27 patients given 270 mg/kg i.v. for 6 d *5475* Effect of drug ?hepatotoxic *2024* Mild increases in activity may occur infrequently as a side-effect *4647*
Serum No Effect Analytical At 5 times upper limit of therapeutic range on methods on Technicon SMAC® , Abbott-VP, Du Pont aca, Roche Cobas-Bio, Hitachi® 705 and KDA *3525*

Bicarbonate *Serum Increase Physiological* Observed in approximately 8% patients *3170*
Serum No Effect Analytical At concentration of 15,000 mg/L had no effect on method using phenolphthalein *5704*

Bilirubin *Serum Increase Analytical* At 5 times upper limit of therapeutic range on Du Pont aca method *3525*
Serum No Effect Analytical At 5 times upper limit of therapeutic range on methods on Technicon SMAC® , Roche Cobas-Bio, Kodak Ektachem® 400, Hitachi® 705 and KDA *3525* At concentration of 2,000 mg/L had no effect on Jendrassik and Grof method *5704*

Bilirubin, Conjugated *Serum No Effect Analytical* No effect at concentration of 3350 mg/L on method on Kodak Ektachem® *5706*

Bilirubin, Unconjugated *Serum No Effect Analytical* No effect at concentration of 3350 mg/L on method on Kodak Ektachem® *5706*

Bleeding Time *Patient Increase Physiological* Carbenicillin and high doses of other penicillins have the potential for increasing warfarin-associated bleeding *2625* At high concentrations platelet aggregation may be reduced with prolonged bleeding time as result *1384*

Calcium *Serum No Effect Analytical* At 5 times upper limit of therapeutic range on methods on Technicon SMAC® , Abbott-VP, Du Pont aca, Kodak Ektachem® , Hitachi® 705 and KDA *3525* At concentration of 15,000 mg/L had no effect on cresolphthalein method *5704*

Chloride *Serum No Effect Analytical* At concentration of 15,000 mg/L had no effect on mercurimetric method *5704*

Cholesterol *Serum No Effect Analytical* At 5 times upper limit of therapeutic range on methods on Technicon SMAC® , Abbott-VP, Roche Cobas-Bio, Kodak Ektachem® 400, Hitachi® 705 and KDA *3525* At concentration of 15,000 mg/L had no effect on Liebermann-Burchard method *5704*

Clotting Time *Blood Increase Physiological* Reported effect *6299*

Creatine Kinase *Serum Increase Physiological* Probably due to trauma of i.m. injection *3199*
Serum No Effect Analytical At 5 times upper limit of therapeutic range on methods on Technicon SMAC® , Abbott-VP, Du Pont aca, Roche Cobas-Bio and Hitachi® 705 *3525*

Creatine Kinase Isoenzymes *Serum No Effect Analytical* No interference observed at a concentration of 200 mg/L (529 µmol/L) with CK-MB method on Du Pont aca *1519*

Creatinine *Serum No Effect Analytical* No effect of concentrations up to 3350 mg/L on 2-slide method on Kodak Ektachem® *5706* No effect of concentrations up to 15 mg/L on single slide method on Kodak Ektachem® *5706* At 5 times upper limit of therapeutic range on methods on Technicon SMAC® , Abbott-VP, Du Pont aca, Kodak Ektachem® 400, Roche Cobas-Bio, Hitachi® 705 and KDA *3525*

Eosinophils *Blood Increase Physiological* Manifestation of allergic response *2754* In 2 of 27 patients given 270 mg/kg i.v. for 6 d *5475* Eosinophilia may occur infrequently as a side-effect *4647*

Erythrocytes *Blood Decrease Physiological* Hemolytic anemia reported *2754*

Gentamicin *Serum Increase Analytical* At concentrations greater than 750 mg/L (normal clinical concentration up to 500 mg/L) caused concentration (4 mg/L) to increase by approximately 25% *5705*
Serum No Effect Analytical No interference observed at concentrations up to 500 µg/mL (1320 µmol/L) with method on Du Pont aca *1526*

Glucose *Serum No Effect Analytical* At 5 times upper limit of therapeutic range on methods on Technicon SMAC® , Abbott-VP, Du Pont aca, Kodak Ektachem® 400, Roche Cobas-Bio, Hitachi® 705 and KDA *3525*
Urine Increase Analytical At 10 and 20 mg/mL gave false positive with negative urine using Clinitest® but with positive glucose specimens gave falsely low results *3710*
Urine No Effect Analytical No influence of drug at up to 20 mg/mL on Diastix® and TesTape® procedures *3710*

γ-Glutamyltransferase *Serum No Effect Analytical* At 5 times upper limit of therapeutic range on methods on Technicon SMAC® , Abbott-VP, and Hitachi® 705 *3525*

Hematocrit *Blood Decrease Physiological* Anemia may occur infrequently as a side-effect *4647*

Hemoglobin *Blood Decrease Physiological* Hemolytic anemia reported *2754* Anemia may occur infrequently as a side-effect *4647*

Iron *Serum No Effect Analytical* At 5 times upper limit of therapeutic range on Ferrozine method on Technicon SMAC® *3525*
Serum No Effect Physiological No effect although marrow depressed *4928*

Iron-Binding Capacity, Total
Serum No Effect Physiological No effect although marrow depressed *4928*

Lactate Dehydrogenase *Serum Increase Physiological* Transient elevations reported *2242*
Serum No Effect Analytical At 5 times upper limit of therapeutic range on methods on Technicon SMAC® , Abbott-VP, Roche Cobas-Bio, Hitachi® 705 and KDA *3525*

Leukocytes *Blood Decrease Physiological* Leukopenia may occur infrequently as a side-effect *4647* Leukopenia may occur infrequently *2754*

Methotrexate *Serum Increase Physiological* In one patient receiving large doses (30 g daily) increased methotrexate concentration observed *1384*

Monocytes *Blood Increase Physiological* In 1 of 27 patients given 270 mg/kg i.v. for 6 d *5475*

Neutrophils *Blood Decrease Physiological* Neutropenia reported occasionally *2754* Neutropenia may occur infrequently as a side-effect *4647*

Occult Blood *Feces Increase Physiological* Rectal bleeding may occur as a side-effect *4647*

pH *Blood Increase Physiological* High pH observed in most patients *3170*

Phosphate *Serum No Effect Analytical* At 5 times upper limit of therapeutic range on methods on Technicon SMAC® , Du Pont aca, Hitachi® 705 and KDA *3525* At concentration of 15,000 mg/L had no effect on phosphomolybdate method *5704*

Platelet Aggregation *Blood Decrease Physiological* At high concentrations binding to adenosine diphosphate receptors occurs with effect on platelet aggregation *1384*

Platelets *Blood Decrease Physiological* Occasionally thrombocytopenia may occur *2754* Thrombocytopenia may occur infrequently as a side-effect *4647*

Potassium *Serum Decrease Physiological* Observed effect ?redistribution or increased excretion *5955* In one child due to drug having impermeant anion effect on renal tubule *5774* Nonreabsorbable anion increases electrical negativity of lumen of distal nephron with enhanced potassium and hydrogen excretion *984* Hypokalemia may occur because of the large amount of nonreabsorbable anion in the distal tubules *1384*
Urine Increase Physiological Possible increased distal tubular excretion in some patients *5955*

Protein *Serum Increase Analytical* At 5 times upper limit of therapeutic range on methods on Technicon SMAC® , Abbott-VP, Kodak Ektachem® 400 and Hitachi® 705 *3525* Concentrations above 3350 mg/L increase results as determined by method on Kodak Ektachem® but unlikely to be of clinical significance since upper limit of therapeutic concentration is about 14 mg/L *5706*
Serum No Effect Analytical At 5 times upper limit of therapeutic range on biuret method on KDA *3525* At concentrations above 500 mg/L raised the concentration as measured by biuret method with blank correction *5704*

Prothrombin Time *Plasma Increase Physiological* Effect observed especially in uremics *2754*

Tobramycin *Serum No Effect Analytical* At concentrations less than 1000 µg/mL (2.64 mmol/L) had no significant effect on method on Du Pont aca *1547*

Triglycerides *Serum Increase Analytical* At 5 times upper limit of therapeutic range on enzymatic method on Abbott-VP *3525*
Serum No Effect Analytical At 5 times upper limit of therapeutic range on methods on Technicon SMAC® , Kodak Ektachem® 400, Hitachi® 705 and KDA *3525* At concentration of 15,000 mg/L had no effect on lipase/esterase method *5704*

Urea Nitrogen *Serum No Effect Analytical* At 5 times upper limit of therapeutic range on methods on Technicon SMAC® , Abbott-VP, Roche Cobas-Bio, Kodak Ektachem® 400, Hitachi® 705 and KDA *3525* At concentration of 15,000 mg/L had no effect on diacetylmonoxime method *5704*

Uric Acid *Serum No Effect Analytical* At 5 times upper limit of therapeutic range on methods on Technicon SMAC® , Abbott-VP, Du Pont aca, Kodak Ektachem® 400, Roche Cobas-Bio, Hitachi® 705 and KDA *3525* At concentration of 15,000 mg/L had no effect on phosphotungstate reduction method *5704*

Carbenoxolone

Alanine Aminotransferase *Serum Increase Physiological* Associated with myopathy *4071*

Aldolase *Serum Increase Physiological* Due to hypokalemic myopathy *380*

Aldosterone *Plasma Decrease Physiological* In 5 healthy normal volunteers administration of 100 mg carbenoxolone t.i.d. for 14 days (to inhibit both 11βDH and 11βR activities of 11βHSD) caused plasma aldosterone concentration fo decrease from 218.0 pmol/L to 80.0 pmol/L *440*

Allotetrahydrocortisol *Urine Decrease Physiological* In a 7-year old with autosomal recessive pseudohypoaldosteronism given 150 mg/d carbenoxalone caused significant decrease from mean baseline of 904 ± 341 nmol/d to 303 ± 156 nmol/d after 32 days *6127*

Aspartate Aminotransferase *Serum Increase Physiological* Associated with myopathy *4071*

Bicarbonate *Serum Increase Physiological* Hypokalemic alkalosis *4071*

Bilirubin *Serum Increase Physiological* Possible hepatotoxic effect of drug *4071*

BSP Retention *Serum Increase Physiological* Reversible hepatotoxic effect *4071*

Calcium *Serum Decrease Physiological* Aldosterone like effect of drug *4071*

Chloride *Serum Decrease Physiological* Average decrease of 3 mEq/L, associated with alkalosis *1949*

Cortisol, Free *Urine Increase Physiological* In a 7-year old with autosomal recessive pseudohypoaldosteronism given 150 mg/d carbenoxalone caused significant increase from mean baseline of 55 ± 28 nmol/d to 88 ± 28 nmol/d after 32 days *6127*

Cortisone *Urine Decrease Physiological* In a 7-year old with autosomal recessive pseudohypoaldosteronism given 150 mg/d carbenoxalone caused significant decrease from mean baseline of 72 ± 25 nmol/d to 28 ± 11 nmol/d after 32 days *6127*

Creatine Kinase *Serum Increase Physiological* May cause hypokalemic myopathy *1949*

Creatinine Clearance *Urine Decrease Physiological* Due to nephropathy *4071*

Hematocrit *Blood Decrease Physiological* By approximately 4% in adrenalectomized patients *6415*

11-Hydroxycorticosteroids *Plasma Increase Physiological* Transient effect after 100 mg orally *2452*

Magnesium *Serum Decrease Physiological* By approximately 0.1 mEq/L in adrenalectomized patients *6415*

Myoglobin *Urine Increase Physiological* Myopathy following hypokalemia *4071*

5'-Nucleotidase *Serum Increase Physiological* Possible direct hepatotoxicity of drug *4071*

pH *Blood Increase Physiological* Alkalosis occurs in approximately 15% patients *4756*
Urine Increase Physiological Impaired acidification with hypokalemia *4071*

Potassium *Serum Decrease Physiological* In 5 healthy normal volunteers administration of 100 mg carbenoxolone t.i.d. for 14 days (to inhibit both 11βDH and 11βR activities of 11βHSD) caused plasma potassium concentration fo decrease nonsignificantly from 3.9 mmol/L to 3.7 mmol/L *440* Aldosterone like effect *1918* By approximately 0.5 mEq/L in adrenalectomized patients *6415*
Urine Increase Physiological Aldosterone like effect *4071*

Protein *Urine Increase Physiological* Due to myoglobinuria and nephropathy *4071*

Renin Activity *Plasma Decrease Physiological* Significant decrease after adrenalectomy (standing and lying) *6415* In 5 healthy normal volunteers administration of 100 mg carbenoxolone t.i.d. for 14 days (to inhibit both 11βDH and 11βR activities of 11βHSD) caused PRA fo decrease from 1.69 nmol/L/h to 0.38 nmol/L/h *440*

Sodium *Serum Increase Physiological* Significant increase (approximately 5 mEq/L) in adrenalectomized patients *6415*

Specific Gravity *Urine Decrease Physiological* Impaired concentration with hypokalemia Impaired ability to concentrate with low potassium *4071*

Carbenoxolone *(continued)*

Tetrahydrocortisol *Urine Decrease Physiological* In a 7-year old with autosomal recessive pseudohypoaldosteronism given 150 mg/d carbenoxalone caused significant decrease from mean baseline of 1390 ± 491 nmol/d to 437 ± 172 nmol/d after 32 days *6127*

Tetrahydrocortisone *Urine Decrease Physiological* In a 7-year old with autosomal recessive pseudohypoaldosteronism given 150 mg/d carbenoxalone caused significant decrease from mean baseline of 2170 ± 484 nmol/d to 718 ± 374 nmol/d after 32 days *6127*

Urea Nitrogen *Serum Increase Physiological* Due to nephropathy with hypokalemia *380*

Carbidopa

Cortisol *Plasma No Effect Physiological* In 10 normal volunteers given 300 mg daily for 1 week *764*

Dihydroxyphenylalanine *Plasma Increase Physiological* Concentration doubled in 6 men over 5 h after administration, especially if protein also given *6471*

Dopamine *Urine Decrease Physiological* 70% reduction in excretion noted over 5 h *6471*

Epinephrine *Urine No Effect Physiological* No effect over 5 h after ingestion *6471*

Growth Hormone *Plasma No Effect Physiological* In 10 normal volunteers given 300 mg daily for 1 week *764*

Histamine *Plasma No Effect Analytical* Concentrations which inhibit radio-enzyme assay greatly exceed physiological concentrations *2492*

Norepinephrine *Urine No Effect Physiological* No effect over 5 h after ingestion *6471*

Pramipexole *Serum No Effect Physiological* Coadministration of pramipexole with levodopa/carbidopa did not affect the pharmacokinetics of pramipexole *4680*

Prolactin *Plasma Increase Physiological* In 10 normal volunteers given 300 mg daily for 1 week *764*

Tryptamine *Urine Decrease Physiological* Marked effect due to decarboxylase inhibition *764*

Carbimazole

Alanine Aminotransferase *Serum Increase Physiological* Isolated case of jaundice conclusively linked to drug *1434*

Alkaline Phosphatase *Serum Increase Physiological* Isolated case of jaundice conclusively linked to drug *1434* Reversible hypersensitivity response to drug *2926*

Apolipoprotein A-I *Serum No Effect Physiological* From 2.62 to 2.82 g/L in 12 hyperthyroid women patients treated with 10-30 mg daily *1969*

Aspartate Aminotransferase *Serum Increase Physiological* Reversible hypersensitivity response to drug *2926* Isolated case of jaundice conclusively linked to drug *1434*

Bilirubin *Serum Increase Physiological* Isolated case of jaundice conclusively linked to drug *1434*
Serum No Effect Analytical No effect at 1.2 mg/L on Ames Seralyzer method *5706*

Cholesterol *Serum Increase Physiological* From 4.4 to 5.4 mmol/L in 12 hyperthyroid women patients treated with 10-30 mg daily *1969*
Serum No Effect Analytical No effect at 1.2 mg/L on Ames Seralyzer method *5706*

Cortisol *Plasma Increase Analytical* At a concentration of 50 mg/L caused recovery of 136.7% with Enzymun method *1097*
Plasma No Effect Analytical At a concentration of 10 mg/L had no significant effect on Enzymun method (recovery 107.1%) *1097*

Creatine Kinase *Serum No Effect Analytical* No effect at 1.2 mg/L on method on Ames Seralyzer *5706*

Creatinine *Serum No Effect Analytical* No effect at 1.2 mg/L on Ames Seralyzer method *5706*

Erythrocytes *Blood Decrease Physiological* Occasional aplastic anemia reported *6264*

Glucose *Serum No Effect Analytical* No effect at 1.2 mg/L on glucose oxidase method on Ames Seralyzer *5706*

γ-Glutamyltransferase *Serum Increase Physiological* Reversible hypersensitivity response to drug *2926*

Glutathione S-Transferase *Serum Decrease Physiological* Treatment of hyperthyroid patients caused initially high activity to be reduced *448*

HDL-Cholesterol *Serum Increase Physiological* From 1.3 to 1.6 mmol/L in 12 hyperthyroid women patients treated with 10-30 mg daily *1969*

^{131}I Uptake *Serum No Effect Physiological* No effect on uptake by thyroid *3669*

Lactate Dehydrogenase *Serum No Effect Analytical* No effect at 1.2 mg/L on method on Ames Seralyzer *5706*

LDL-Cholesterol *Serum Increase Physiological* From 2.7 to 3.5 mmol/L in 12 hyperthyroid women patients treated with 10-30 mg daily *1969*

Leukocytes *Blood Decrease Physiological* Two case reports with considerable reduction in white cell count and neutrophil count *2424* Occasional aplastic anemia reported *6264* Agranulocytosis *821*

Lymphocyte Autoantibodies *Blood Decrease Physiological* Impaired thyroid microsomal or thyroglobulin antibody secretion due to effect on lymphocytes within thyroid *3907*

Neutrophils *Blood Decrease Physiological* Two case reports with considerable reduction in white cell count and neutrophil count *2424* Occasional case of drug-induced neutropenia *241* May cause agranulocytosis/neutropenia *4265* Occasional agranulocytosis reported *6264*

Platelets *Blood Decrease Physiological* Occasional aplastic anemia reported *6264*

Soluble Interleukin-2 Receptor
Serum Decrease Physiological Increased concentration observed in 18 patients with hyperthyroidism (mean 919 U/mL) fell to 378 U/mL with treatment with dose titration of carbimazole until a euthyroid state was reached (mean duration 3.6 months) *1000*

T3-Uptake *Serum Decrease Physiological* From 1.33 to 0.90 arbitrary units in 12 hyperthyroid women patients treated with 10-30 mg daily *1969*

Thyroxine (T4) *Serum Decrease Physiological* From 184 to 101 nmol/L in 12 hyperthyroid women patients treated with 10-30 mg daily *1969*

Tri-iodothyronine (T3) *Serum Decrease Physiological* From 4.55 to 1.68 nmol/L in 12 hyperthyroid women patients treated with 10-30 mg daily *1969*

Triglycerides *Serum Increase Physiological* From 0.77 to 0.89 mmol/L in 12 hyperthyroid women patients treated with 10-30 mg daily *1969*

Urea Nitrogen *Serum No Effect Analytical* No effect at 1.2 mg/L on method on Ames Seralyzer *5706*

Carbinoxamine

Histamine *Plasma No Effect Analytical* Improbable inhibition of radio-enzyme assay at physiological concentrations, although 50% inhibition observed at 9.2 µg/mL *2492*

Carbochromen

Alanine Aminotransferase *Serum No Effect Analytical* No effect at therapeutic concentration on Boehringer Mannheim Reflotron method *3231*

Amylase, Pancreatic Isoenzyme
Serum No Effect Analytical No significant effect observed at toxic concentration of 30 mg/L on method on Boehringer Mannheim Reflotron *3647*

Aspartate Aminotransferase *Serum No Effect Analytical* No effect at therapeutic concentration on Boehringer Mannheim Reflotron method *3231*

Cholesterol *Serum No Effect Analytical* No effect at therapeutic concentration on Boehringer Mannheim Reflotron method *3231*

Cortisol *Plasma No Effect Analytical* At concentration of 30 mg/L no significant effect (worst case 94.8% recovery) on CEDIA method *1097*

Glucose *Serum No Effect Analytical* No effect at therapeutic concentration on Boehringer Mannheim Reflotron method *3231*

γ-Glutamyltransferase *Serum No Effect Analytical* No effect at therapeutic concentration on Boehringer Mannheim Reflotron method *3231*

HDL-Cholesterol *Serum No Effect Analytical* At a concentration up to 30 mg/L had no significant effect on Reflotron method for whole blood cholesterol *6352*

Triglycerides *Serum No Effect Analytical* No effect at therapeutic concentration on Boehringer Mannheim Reflotron method *3231*

Urea Nitrogen *Serum No Effect Analytical* No effect at therapeutic concentration on Boehringer Mannheim Reflotron method *3231*

Uric Acid *Serum No Effect Analytical* No effect at therapeutic concentration on Boehringer Reflotron method *3231*

Carbohydrate

Aldosterone *Plasma No Effect Physiological* No effect when starved patients refed *2036*

Gastrin *Serum No Effect Physiological* No effect on endogenous secretion if given orally *2021*

Renin Activity *Plasma No Effect Physiological* No effect when starved patients refed *2036*

Sodium *Urine Decrease Physiological* Marked effect when starved patients refed *2036*

Carboplatin

Alkaline Phosphatase *Urine No Effect Physiological* No significant overall increase in excretion of enzyme in patients with solid tumors given several courses of drug *5594*

Creatinine Clearance *Urine No Effect Physiological* No change in patients with solid tumors given several courses of treatment *5594*

Lactate Dehydrogenase *Urine No Effect Physiological* No significant overall increase in excretion of enzyme in patients with solid tumors given several courses of treatment *5594*

β_2-Microglobulin *Urine No Effect Physiological* No change in patients with solid tumors given several courses of treatment *5594*

N-Acetyl-Glucosaminidase *Urine No Effect Physiological* No significant overall increase in excretion in patients with solid tumors given several courses of treatment *5594*

Platinum *Red Blood Cells Increase Physiological* 1 h after bolus injection 2% of drug bound to erythrocytes, stabilizes after 3 h *5492*

Protein *Urine No Effect Physiological* No consistent increase in excretion in patients with solid tumors with several courses of treatment although transient increase observed *5594*

Carboxymethylcysteine

Creatinine *Serum No Effect Analytical* No interference observed with liquid chromatographic method of Paroni *4540*

Carbromal

Alanine Aminotransferase *Serum Increase Physiological* Occurs with poisoning, probable muscle origin *6545*

Aspartate Aminotransferase *Serum Increase Physiological* Occurs with poisoning, probable muscle origin *6545*

Bromide *Serum Increase Physiological* Theoretical possibility since drug contains 34% bromide *5116* Metabolite concentration may exceed 25 mEq/L *2242*

Chloride *Serum Increase Analytical* Bromide as metabolite may be measured as chloride *2242*

Coombs' Test, Direct *Blood Positive Physiological* Unusual cause of hemolytic anemia *3895*

Coombs' Test, Indirect *Blood Positive Physiological* Unusual cause of hemolytic anemia *3895*

Creatine Kinase *Serum Increase Physiological* Occurs with poisoning, probable muscle origin *6545*

Porphyrin, Total *Urine Increase Physiological* May precipitate attack of acute porphyria *3669*

Carbutamide

Alanine Aminotransferase *Serum Increase Physiological* Hepatotoxicity *3810*

Alkaline Phosphatase *Serum Increase Physiological* Hepatotoxicity *3810*

Aspartate Aminotransferase *Serum Increase Physiological* Hepatotoxicity *3810*

Bile *Urine Increase Physiological* Hepatotoxicity *3810*

Bilirubin *Serum Increase Physiological* Hepatotoxicity *3810*

BSP Retention *Serum Increase Physiological* Hepatotoxicity *3810*

Cholesterol *Serum Decrease Physiological* Hepatotoxicity *3810*

Creatinine *Serum Increase Physiological* Nephrotoxic effect *3810*

Fatty Acids (FFA), Free *Serum Increase Physiological* Reported to cause hyperlipemia *3669*

Glucose *Serum Decrease Physiological* Incidence of 4.5% observed in French Pharmacovigilance database *4106* Hepatotoxicity *3810*

^{131}I Uptake *Serum Decrease Physiological* Substantial effect observed in elderly *1279*

Leukocytes *Blood Decrease Physiological* Leukopenia/agranulocytosis *6514*

Nonprotein Nitrogen *Serum Increase Physiological* Nephrotoxic effect *3810*

Platelets *Blood Decrease Physiological* May cause aplastic anemia or thrombocytopenia *6514*

Protein *Urine Increase Physiological* Nephrotoxic effect *6284*

Urea Nitrogen *Serum Increase Physiological* Nephrotoxic effect *3810*

Carfecillin

Chloramphenicol *Serum No Effect Analytical* No effect at 100 mg/L on coupled enzymatic method *4122*

Phenylalanine *Plasma No Effect Analytical* No interference observed with rapid quantitative whole blood method of Campbell et al using phenylanine dehydrogenase *867*

Carinamide

Protein *Urine Increase Analytical* Produces precipitate with acid tests *703*

PSP Excretion *Urine Decrease Physiological* Inhibits secretion *1714*

Sugar *Urine Increase Analytical* False positive with Benedict's reaction *2559*

Carisoprodol

Eosinophils *Blood Increase Physiological* Allergic manifestation *2754*

Leukocytes *Blood Decrease Physiological* Possible consequence/not marked *2754*

Carmine

Color *Feces Increase Analytical* Produces red color *1957*

Carmustine

Alanine Aminotransferase *Serum Increase Physiological* Usually mild and return to normal over few days *3949*

Alkaline Phosphatase *Serum Increase Physiological* Usually mild and return to normal over few days *3949*

Aspartate Aminotransferase *Serum Increase Physiological* Usually mild and return to normal over few days *3949*

Bilirubin *Serum Increase Physiological* Usually mild and return to normal over few days *3949*

Leukocytes *Blood Decrease Physiological* Bone marrow suppression is major dose-limiting toxicity with leukocyte nadirs occurring 5-6 weeks after therapy begins. Leukopenia is usually less severe than thrombocytopenia *1384*

Ondansetron *Serum No Effect Physiological* Coadministration with ondansetron had no effect on its pharmacokinetics *2181*

Platelets *Blood Decrease Physiological* Bone marrow suppression is the usual dose-limiting toxicity with platelet nadirs occurring 4-5 weeks after therapy begins *1384*

Carnitine

HDL-Cholesterol *Serum Increase Physiological* In 7 hemodialyzed children with type IV hyperlipoproteinemia intravenous supplementation over 5 months caused mean increase from baseline of 0.91 mmol/L to 1.13 mmol/L *2187*

Triglycerides *Serum Decrease Physiological* In 7 hemodialyzed children with type IV hyperlipoproteinemia long term intravenous supplementation caused reduction from mean of 3.82 mmol/L to 1.86 mmol/L after 5 months *2187*

Carphenazine

Alanine Aminotransferase *Serum Increase Physiological* Probable cholestatic effect (reversible) *3810*

Aspartate Aminotransferase *Serum Increase Physiological* Probablè cholestatic effect (reversible) *3810*

Bile *Urine Increase Physiological* Probable cholestatic effect (reversible) *3810*

Bilirubin *Serum Increase Physiological* Probable cholestatic effect (reversible) *3810*

BSP Retention *Serum Increase Physiological* Probable cholestatic effect (reversible) *3810*

Carprazidil

Aldosterone *Plasma No Effect Physiological* No consistent effect in 15 men with mild to moderate essential hypertension treated for up to 16 weeks *2093*

Cholesterol *Serum No Effect Physiological* No significant effect in 12 subjects treated for 4 mo *142* In one study involving 12 patients treated for 4 mo *141*

Epinephrine *Plasma No Effect Physiological* No consistent effect in 15 men with mild to moderate essential hypertension treated for up to 16 weeks *2093*

HDL-Cholesterol *Serum Increase Physiological* In 15 men with mild to moderate essential hypertension by 26% over 8 weeks *2093*
Serum No Effect Physiological In one study involving 12 patients treated for 4 mo *141*

LDL-Cholesterol *Serum No Effect Physiological* In one study involving 12 patients treated for 4 mo *141* No consistent effect in 15 men with mild to moderate essential hypertension treated for up to 16 weeks *2093*

α-Lipoproteins *Serum Increase Physiological* In 15 men with mild to moderate essential hypertension by 26% over 8 weeks *2093*

Norepinephrine *Plasma No Effect Physiological* No consistent effect in 15 men with mild to moderate essential hypertension treated for up to 16 weeks *2093*

Renin Activity *Plasma No Effect Physiological* No consistent effect in 15 men with mild to moderate essential hypertension treated for up to 16 weeks *2093*

Triglycerides *Serum No Effect Physiological* In one study involving 12 patients treated for 4 mo *141* No consistent effect in 15 men with mild to moderate essential hypertension treated for up to 16 weeks *2093*

VLDL-Cholesterol *Serum No Effect Physiological* No consistent effect in 15 men with mild to moderate essential hypertension treated for up to 16 weeks *2093* In one study involving 12 patients treated for 4 mo *141*

Carteolol

Aldosterone *Plasma No Effect Physiological* No significant change observed in 10 patients with mild to moderate hypertension treated with 10 mg daily for 6 weeks *312*

Aspartate Aminotransferase
Serum No Effect Physiological No significant effect in 23 hypertensive patients treated with up to 20 mg/day for 50 weeks *5911*

Atrial Natriuretic Peptide *Plasma Increase Physiological* Concentration significantly increased in elderly patients with mild essential hypertension both at rest and after exercise *3224*

Bilirubin *Serum No Effect Physiological* Administration of clarithromycin has been associated with jaundice in fewer than 1% of 1568 patients *13*

Calcium *Serum No Effect Physiological* No significant effect in 23 hypertensive patients treated with up to 23 mg/day for 50 weeks *5911*

Chloride *Serum No Effect Physiological* No significant effect in 23 hypertensive patients treated with up to 20 mg/day for 50 weeks *5911*

Colloid Osmotic Pressure *Serum No Effect Physiological* No significant change observed in 10 patients with mild to moderate hypertension treated with 10 mg daily for 6 weeks *312*

Creatine Kinase *Serum Increase Physiological* Significant effect in 10 of 15 patients with essential hypertension. MM isoenzyme most affected *5275*

Creatinine *Serum No Effect Physiological* No significant effect either of single dose of 10 mg nor of 20 mg/day for 7 days in healthy volunteers or hypertensive patients *5911* No significant change observed in 10 patients with mild to moderate hypertension treated with 10 mg daily for 6 weeks *312*

Creatinine Clearance *Urine No Effect Physiological* Neither single dose of 10 mg nor continuous administration of 20 mg/day for 7 days had any effect in healthy volunteers *5911*

Glomerular Filtration Rate *Urine Decrease Physiological* In 10 patients with mild to moderate hypertension treatment with 10 mg daily for 6 weeks caused mean reduction of 12.3% *312*

Lactate Dehydrogenase *Serum No Effect Physiological* No significant effect in 23 hypertensive patients treated with up to 20 mg/day for 50 weeks *5911*

PAH Clearance *Urine No Effect Physiological* No significant effect of either single dose of 10 mg nor of 20 mg/day for 7 days in healthy volunteers and hypertensive patients *5911*

Potassium *Serum No Effect Physiological* No significant effect in 23 hypertensive patients treated with up to 20 mg/day for 50 weeks *5911*

Protein *Serum No Effect Physiological* No significant change observed in 10 mild to moderate hypertensives treated with 10 mg daily for 6 weeks *312*

Renal Blood Flow *Patient Decrease Physiological* Non-significant reduction of 9.2% observed in 10 patients with mild to moderate hypertension treated with 10 mg daily for 6 weeks *312*

Sodium *Serum No Effect Physiological* No significant effect in 23 hypertensive patients given up to 20 mg/day for 50 weeks *5911*

Urea Nitrogen *Serum No Effect Physiological* No significant effect in 23 hypertensive patients treated for 50 weeks with up to 20 mg/day *5911*

Carvedilol

Alanine Aminotransferase *Serum Decrease Physiological* Significant reduction from mean of 8 U/L to 5 U/L in 9 patients with renal hypertension treated with up to 20 mg daily for up to 4 weeks *3223*

Serum Increase Physiological In 1142 patients with hypertension mild hepatocellular injury was observed in 13 (1.1%) compared with incidence of 0.9% (4 of 462) in those receiving placebo. In patients with congestive cardiac failure abnormal liver function observed in 38 of 765 patients (5.0%) receiving carvedilol compared with 20 of 437 patients (4.6%) receiving placebo *5639* Mild hepatocellular injury observed with treatment. Incidence of abnormalities with carvedilol 1.1% compared with 0.9% in placebo treated controls *1973*

Serum No Effect Physiological No significant effect in 18 patients with essential hypertension given 20 mg daily for 1 week *2595* In 20 patients with mild to moderate hypertension treatment with up to 20 mg/d for 12 weeks caused insignificant change from 41.5 ± 12.5 U/L to 33.4 ± 11.0 U/L *2264* No change in 122 patients with mild to moderate hypertension treated with therapeutic doses for 12 weeks *4374*

Albumin *Urine Increase Physiological* Observed in treated patients with congestive cardiac failure with a frequency of between 1% and 2% *5639*

Aldosterone *Plasma Decrease Physiological* Insignificant reduction in 10 patients with essential hypertension when given a single oral dose of 50 mg but significant reduction from mean of 128 to 104 mg/mL in 10 patients when treated with 50 mg daily for 4 weeks *1624* Significant reduction 30 minutes after single oral dose of 10 mg *2595*

Alkaline Phosphatase *Serum Decrease Physiological* Significant decrease from mean of 191 U/L to 162 U/L in 9 patients with renal hypertension treated with up to 20 mg daily for up to 4 weeks *3223*

Serum Increase Physiological Mild hepatocellular injury observed with treatment. Incidence of abnormalities with carvedilol 1.1% compared with 0.9% in placebo treated controls *1973* Observed in treated patients with congestive cardiac failure with a frequency of between 1% and 2% *5639*

Serum No Effect Physiological No significant change in 83 patients with mild to moderate hypertension treated with therapeutic doses for 12 weeks *4374* No significant effect in 18 patients with essential hypertension treated with 20 mg daily for 1 week *2595* In 16 patients with mild to moderate hypertension treatment with up to 20 mg/d for 12 weeks caused insignificant decrease from 117 ± 21 U/L to 116 ± 21 U/L *2264*

Apolipoprotein A-I *Serum No Effect Physiological* In 25 hypertensive patients treatment for 6 months caused nonsignificant change from mean baseline of 126 ± 16 mg/dL to 124 ± 18 mg/dL *3781* No significant effect observed in 36 patients treated with up to 20 mg daily for 12 weeks *5432* In 14 patients with mild to moderate hypertension treatment with up to 20 mg/d for 12 weeks caused insignificant change from 131.2 ± 6.1 mg/dL to 126.8 ± 4.7 mg/dL *2264*

Apolipoprotein A-I:Apolipoprotein B Ratio

Serum No Effect Physiological In 25 hypertensive patients treatment for 6 months caused nonsignificant change in ratio from mean baseline of 1.0 ± 0.3 to 0.96 ± 0.3 *3781*

Apolipoprotein A-II *Serum No Effect Physiological* In 14 patients with mild to moderate hypertension treatment with up to 20 mg/d for 12 weeks caused insignificant change from 30.7 ± 1.2 mg/dL to 30.2 ± 1.0 mg/dL *2264* No significant effect observed in 36 patients treated with up to 20 mg daily for 12 weeks *5432*

Apolipoprotein B *Serum No Effect Physiological* No significant effect observed in 36 patients treated with up to 20 mg daily for 12 weeks *5432* In 14 patients with mild to moderate hypertension treatment with up to 20 mg/d for up to 12 weeks caused insignificant change from 91.4 ± 4.6 mg/dL to 92.4 ± 5.4 mg/dL *2264* In 25 hypertensive patients treatment for 6 months caused nonsignificant change from mean baseline of 121 ± 8 mg/dL to 128 ± 14 mg/dL *3781*

Apolipoprotein C-II *Serum No Effect Physiological* No significant effect observed in 36 patients treated with up to 20 mg daily for 12 weeks *5432* In 14 patients with mild to moderate hypertension treatment with up to 20 mg/d for 12 weeks caused insignificant change from 3.7 ± 0.4 mg/dL to 3.8 ± 0.4 mg/dL *2264*

Apolipoprotein C-III *Serum No Effect Physiological* No significant effect observed in 36 patients treated with up to 20 mg daily for 12 weeks *5432* In 14 patients with mild to moderate hypertension treatment with up to 20 mg/d for 12 weeks caused insignificant change from 8.5 ± 0.7 mg/dL to 9.0 ± 0.8 mg/dL *2264*

Apolipoprotein E *Serum No Effect Physiological* In 14 patients with mild to moderate hypertension treatment with up to 20 mg/d for 12 weeks caused insignificant change from 4.7 ± 0.4 mg/dL *2264* No significant effect observed in 36 patients treated with up to 20 mg daily for 12 weeks *5432*

Aspartate Aminotransferase *Serum Increase Physiological* In 1142 patients with hypertension mild hepatocellular injury was observed in 13 (1.1%) compared with incidence of 0.9% (4 of 462) in those receiving placebo. In patients with congestive cardiac failure abnormal liver function observed in 38 of 765 patients (5.0%) receiving carvedilol compared with 20 of 437 patients (4.6%) receiving placebo *5639* Mild hepatocellular injury observed with treatment. Incidence of abnormalities with carvedilol 1.1% compared with 0.9% in placebo treated controls *1973*

Serum No Effect Physiological No significant effect in 18 patients with essential hypertension given 20 mg daily for 1 week *2595* No change in 122 patients with mild to moderate hypertension treated with therapeutic doses for 12 weeks *4374* No change in 9 patients with renal hypertension treated with up to 20 mg daily for up to 4 weeks *3223* In 19 patients with mild to moderate hypertension treatment with up to 20 mg/d for 12 weeks caused insignificant change from 30.1 ± 6.7 U/L to 32.2 ± 9.1 U/L *2264*

Atherogenic Index *Serum No Effect Physiological* In 14 patients with mild to moderate hypertension treatment with up to 20 mg/d for 12 weeks caused insignificant change from 3.2 ± 0.3 to 3.3 ± 0.4 *2264*

Atrial Natriuretic Peptide *Plasma No Effect Physiological* No significant change following single oral dose of 10 mg *2595*

Atypical Lymphocytes *Blood Increase Physiological* Observed in treated patients with congestive cardiac failure with a frequency of less than 0.1% *5639*

Bacteriuria *Urine Increase Physiological* Observed in 1.8% of 1142 hypertensive patients receiving carvedilol compared with 0.6% of 462 patients receiving placebo and in 3.1% of 765 patients with congestive heart failure compared with 2.7% of 437 patients receiving placebo *5639*

Bilirubin *Serum Increase Physiological* In 1142 patients with hypertension mild hepatocellular injury was observed in 13 (1.1%) compared with incidence of 0.9% (4 of 462) in those receiving placebo. In patients with congestive cardiac failure abnormal liver function observed in 38 of 765 patients (5.0%) receiving carvedilol compared with 20 of 437 patients (4.6%) receiving placebo *5639* Mild hepatocellular injury observed with treatment. Incidence of abnormalities with carvedilol 1.1% compared with 0.9% in placebo treated controls *1973*

Blood *Urine Increase Physiological* Hematuria observed in 2.9% of 765 patients with congestive failure compared with 2.1% of 437 patients receiving placebo *5639*

Calcium *Serum No Effect Physiological* No significant effect in 9 patients with renal hypertension treated for up to 4 weeks with up to 20 mg daily *3223*

Chloride *Serum Increase Physiological* Significant increase from mean of 104 mmol/L to 105 mmol/L in 118 patients with mild to moderate hypertension treated with therapeutic doses for 12 weeks *4374*

Serum No Effect Physiological No significant effect in 9 patients with renal hypertension treated with up to 20 mg daily for up to 4 weeks *3223* No effect of 20 mg daily for 1 week in 18 patients with essential hypertension *2595* In 20 patients with mild to moderate hypertension treatment with up to 20 mg/d for up to 12 weeks caused insignificant change from mean baseline of 105.5 ± 0.8 mmol/L to 106.6 ± 0.9 mmol/L *2264*

Cholesterol *Serum Decrease Physiological* In 110 patients with mild to moderate hypertension treatment with up to 50 mg/d for 6 months caused significant 11% decrease from mean baseline of 7.4 mmol/L to 6.3 mmol/L *2507* Significant reduction from mean of 198 mg/dL to 173 mg/dL in 9 patients with renal hypertension treated with up to 20 mg daily for up to 4 weeks *3223*

Carvedilol *(continued)*

Cholesterol *(continued)*

Serum Increase Physiological Observed in 4.1% of 765 patients with congestive failure compared with 2.5% of 437 patients receiving placebo *5639*

Serum No Effect Physiological No significant effect observed in 36 patients treated with up to 20 mg daily for 12 weeks *5432* No significant effect in 117 patients with mild to moderate hypertension treated with therapeutic doses for 12 weeks *4374* In a population of hypertensive patients treatment with carvedilol had no significant effect on concentration *5639* In 21 patients with mild to moderate hypertension treatment with up to 20 mg/d for 12 weeks had no significant effect *2264* No significant effect in 32 elderly hypertensive patients treated with 25 mg daily for 12 weeks *5768* No significant effect in 18 patients with essential hypertension treated with 20 mg daily for 1 week *2595* In 9 hypertensive patients with serum cholesterol concentration greater than 220 mg/dL treatment for 6 months caused nonsignificant change from mean baseline of 257 ± 11 mg/dL to 245 ± 27 mg/dL and in 16 with serum cholesterol less than 220 mg/dL from 194 ± 8 mg/dL to 198 ± 14 mg/dL *3781*

Cholesterol:HDL-Cholesterol Ratio

Serum Decrease Physiological In 110 patients with mild to moderate essential hypertension treatment with up to 50 mg/d for 6 months caused significant change in ratio from baseline 7.9 to 6.1 *2507*

Creatine Kinase *Serum No Effect Physiological* No significant change in 81 patients with mild to moderate hypertension treated with therapeutic doses for 12 weeks *4374* In 20 patients with mild to moderate hypertension treatment with up to 20 mg/d for 12 weeks caused insignificant change from 71.4 ± 7.1 U/L to 67.3 ± 7.1 U/L *2264* No significant effect in 18 patients with essential hypertension treated with 20 mg daily for 1 week *2595* No significant effect in 9 patients with renal hypertension treated with up to 20 mg daily for up to 4 weeks *3223*

Creatinine *Serum Increase Physiological* Rare reversible deterioration of renal function, usually in patients with low blood pressure, underlying renal insufficiency, or diffuse vascular disease *1973* Significant increase from 0.8 to 0.9 mg/dL with 20 mg daily for 1 week in 18 patients with essential hypertension *2595*

Serum No Effect Physiological In 12 hypertensive post-renal transplant patients treatment with up to 50 mg/d for 8 weeks caused nonsignificant change from mean baseline of 1.5 ± 0.1 mg/dL to 1.6 mg/dL *3482* No change in 117 patients with mild to moderate hypertension treated with therapeutic doses for 12 weeks *4374* In a population of hypertensive patients treatment with carvedilol had no significant effect on concentration *5639* In 20 patients with mild to moderate hypertension treatment with up to 20 mg/d for 12 weeks caused no change from baseline of 0.9 ± 0.04 mg/dL *2264* No significant effect in 9 patients with renal hypertension treated for up to 4 weeks with 20 mg daily *3223*

Creatinine Clearance *Urine No Effect Physiological* No significant effect in 18 patients with essential hypertension treated with 20 mg daily for 1 week *2595*

Digoxin *Serum Increase Physiological* Mean concentration and area under curve increased when digoxin administered orally. Serum concentration increased from mean of 1.62 µg/L to 2.59 µg/L in 8 individuals when 0.5 mg digoxin given with 25 mg carvedilol. No effect when digoxin given i.v *1319* In 12 hypertensive patients following concomitant doses of 25 mg carvedilol once daily and 0.25 mg digoxin once daily for 14 days steady state AUC and trough concentrations of digoxin were increased by 14% and 16% respectively *5639*

Urine Decrease Physiological Insignificant reduction from mean of 216 ng in 24 hours to 188 ng/24 h when 25 mg carvedilol combined with 0.5 mg digoxin orally in 8 individuals. Effect even less marked when digoxin given intravenously *1319*

Effective Renal Plasma Flow

Patient No Effect Physiological No significant effect observed in 10 patients with essential hypertension following single oral dose of 50 mg. Insignificant reduction in 10 patients when treated with 50 mg daily for 4 weeks *1624*

Erythrocytes *Blood Decrease Physiological* Mean decrease from 3.57 million /µL to 3.24 million /µL in 9 patients with renal hypertension treated with up to 20 mg daily for up tp 4 weeks *3223* Observed in treated patients with congestive cardiac failure with a frequency of between 0.1% and 1% *5639*

Blood No Effect Physiological In 19 patients with mild to moderate hypertension treatment with up to 20 mg/d for 12 weeks caused insignificant change from 4.79 ± 0.12 million /µL to 4.62 ± 0.10 million /µL *2264* Insignificant change in 117 patients with mild to moderate hypertension treated with therapeutic doses for 12 weeks *4374*

Geometric Variation in Fibrinolytic Index

Plasma Increase Physiological In 25 hypertensive patients treatment for 6 months caused significant change from mean baseline before anoxia of 18.2 ± 13 to 28.2 ± 16 *3781*

Glomerular Filtration Rate *Urine Decrease Physiological* Significant reduction observed (from mean of 115 to 106 mL/min per 1.73 sq m) in 10 patients with essential hypertension following single oral dose of 50 mg. Insignificant increase in 10 patients given 50 mg daily for 4 weeks *1624*

Urine No Effect Physiological In 12 hypertensive post-renal transplant patients treatment with up to 50 mg/d for 8 weeks caused no change from mean baseline of 39 ± 3 mL/min *3482*

Glucose *Serum Decrease Physiological* Observed in treated patients with congestive cardiac failure with a frequency of between 1% and 2% *5639*

Serum Increase Physiological Hyperglycemia observed in 12.2% of 765 patients with congestive failure compared with 7.8% of 437 patients receiving placebo *5639*

Serum No Effect Physiological No significant effect in 9 patients with renal hypertension treated with up to 20 mg daily for up to 4 weeks *3223* In a population of hypertensive patients treatment with carvedilol had no significant effect on concentration *5639* No significant effect in 18 patients with essential hypertension treated with 20 mg daily for 1 week *2595* No significant effect on either postprandial or fasting glucose concentration in 25 noninsulin dependent diabetic hypertensives treated with 50 mg daily for 8 weeks *1671* Insignificant change in 59 patients with mild to moderate hypertension treated with therapeutic doses for 12 weeks *4374*

Urine Increase Physiological Observed in treated patients with congestive cardiac failure with a frequency of between 1% and 2% *5639*

Glyburide *Serum No Effect Physiological* In 12 healthy individuals coadministration of drugs had no clinically relevant effect on pharmacokinetics of either compound *5639*

HDL_2-Cholesterol *Serum No Effect Physiological* No significant effect observed in 36 patients with up to 20 mg daily for 12 weeks *5432* In 21 patients with mild to moderate hyperetension treatment with up to 20 mg/d for 12 weeks caused no significant effect on plasma concentration *2264*

HDL_3-Cholesterol *Serum No Effect Physiological* In 21 patients with mild to moderate hypertension treatment with up to 20 mg/d for 12 weeks had no significant effect on plasma concentration *2264* In 21 mild to moderate hypertensives treatment with up to 20 mg/d for 12 weeks had no significant effect on concentration *2264* No significant effect observed in 36 patients treated with up to 20 mg daily for 12 weeks *5432*

HDL-Cholesterol *Serum Decrease Physiological* Observed in treated patients with congestive cardiac failure with a frequency of less than 0.1% *5639*

Serum Increase Physiological In 110 patients with mild to moderate hypertension treatment with up to 50 mg/d for 6 months caused significant 11% increase from mean baseline of 0.93 mmol/L to 1.03 mmol/L *2507*

Serum No Effect Physiological In a population of hypertensive patients treatment with carvedilol had no significant effect on concentration *5639* No significant effect in 18 patients with essential hypertension treated with 20 mg daily for 1 week *2595* No significant effect in 32 elderly hypertensive patients treated with 25 mg daily for 12 weeks *5768* No significant effect observed in 36 patients treated with up to 20 mg daily for 12 weeks *5432* In 16 hypertensive patients with serum HDL-cholesterol concentration greater than 40 mg/dL treatment for 6 months caused significant increase from mean baseline of 49 ± 6 mg/dL to 48 ± 8 mg/dL and in 9 with serum HDL-cholesterol less than 40 mg/dL from 36 ± 4 mg/dL to 37 ± 6 mg/dL *3781* No significant effect in 25 noninsulin dependent diabetic hypertensives treated with 50 mg daily for 8 weeks *1671* In 21 patients with mild to moderate hypertension treatment with up to 20 mg/d had no significant effect on plasma concentration *2264*

Hematocrit *Blood Decrease Physiological* In 19 patients with mild to moderate hypertension treatment with up to 20 mg/d for 12 weeks caused insignificant decrease from 42.9 ± 1.0 % to 41.3 ± 0.9 % *2264* Significant decrease from mean of 32.0 to 29.0% in 9 patients with renal hypertension treated for up to 4 weeks with up to 20 mg daily *3223*
Blood No Effect Physiological No change in 114 patients with mild to moderate hypertension treated with therapeutic doses for 12 weeks *4374*

Hemoglobin *Blood Decrease Physiological* Observed in treated patients with congestive cardiac failure with a frequency of between 0.1% and 1% *5639* Significant reduction from mean of 143 g/L to 141 g/L in 117 patients with mild to moderate hypertension treated with therapeutic doses for 12 weeks *4374* Significant decrease from mean of 10.4 g/dL to 9.5 g/dL in 9 patients with renal hypertension treated with up to 20 mg daily for up to 4 weeks *3223*
Blood No Effect Physiological In 19 patients with mild to moderate hypertension treatment with up to 20 mg/d for 12 weeks caused insignificant change from 14.4 ± 0.4 g/dL to 13.9 ± 0.3 g/dL *2264*

Hemoglobin A_{1c} *Blood No Effect Physiological* No significant effect of treatment with 50 mg daily for 8 weeks in 25 noninsulin dependent diabetics *1671*

Hydrochlorothiazide *Serum No Effect Physiological* In 12 patients with hypertension a single oral dose of 25 mg carvedilol had no clinically relevant effect on the pharmacokinetics of a single oral dose of 25 mg hydrochlorothiazide or vice versa *5639*

Lactate Dehydrogenase *Serum No Effect Physiological* In 20 patients with mild to moderate hypertension treatment with up to 20 mg/d for 12 weeks caused insignificant change from 268 ± U/L to 267 ± 18 U/L *2264* No significant effect in 119 patients with mild to moderate hypertension treated with therapeutic doses for 12 weeks *4374* No significant effect of treatment with up to 20 mg daily for 4 weeks in 9 patients with renal hypertension *3223*

LDL-Cholesterol *Serum Decrease Physiological* In 110 patients with mild to moderate hypertension treatment with up to 50 mg/d for 6 months caused significant 16% reduction from mean baseline of 5.0 mmol/L to 4.0 mmol/L *2507*
Serum No Effect Physiological No significant effect in 32 elderly hypertensive patients treated with 25 mg daily for 12 weeks *5768* No significant effect in 25 noninsulin dependent diabetic hypertensives treated with 50 mg daily for 8 weeks *1671* In 21 mild to moderate hypertensives treatment with up to 20 mg/d for 12 weeks had no significant effect *2264* In 21 patients with mild to moderate hypertension treatment with up to 20 mg/d for 12 weeks had no significant effect on plasma concentration *2264*

LDL-Cholesterol:HDL-Cholesterol Ratio
Serum Decrease Physiological In 110 patients with mild to moderate essential hypertension treatment with up to 50 mg/d for 6 months caused significant change from mean baseline of 5.5 to 3.9 *2507*

Leukocytes *Blood Decrease Physiological* Observed in treated patients with congestive cardiac failure with a frequency of between 0.1% and 1% *5639*
Blood No Effect Physiological In 18 patients with mild to moderate hypertension treatment with up to 20 mg/d for 12 weeks caused insignificant change from 6360 ± 420 /μL to 6390 ± 380 /μL *2264* No effect in 9 patients with renal hypertension treated with up to 20 mg daily for up to 4 weeks *3223* Insignificant change in 117 patients with mild to moderate hypertension treated with therapeutic doses for 12 weeks *4374*

Lipoprotein A *Serum No Effect Physiological* In 13 patients with mild to moderate hypertension treatment with up to 20 mg/d for 12 weeks caused insignificant change from 34.7 ± 1.8 % to 33.9 ± 1.7 % *2264*

β-Lipoprotein *Serum No Effect Physiological* In 13 patients with mild to moderate hypertension treatment with up to 20 mg/d for 12 weeks caused insignificant change from 45.6 ± 1.2 % to 44.3 ± 1.1 % *2264*

Nonprotein Nitrogen *Serum Increase Physiological* Observed in 5.8% of 765 patients with congestive failure compared with 4.6% of 437 patients receiving placebo *5639*

Occult Blood *Feces Increase Physiological* Observed in treated patients with congestive cardiac failure with a frequency of between 1% and 2% *5639*

Plasminogen Activator Inhibitor-1
Plasma No Effect Physiological In 25 hypertensive patients treatment for 6 months caused nonsignificant change from mean baseline before anoxia of 18.05 ± 11 U/cm³ to 18.3 ± 12 U/cm³ *3781*

Platelets *Blood Decrease Physiological* Significant reduction from mean of 240 thousand /μL to 220 thousand /μL in 107 patients with mild to moderate hypertension treated for 12 weeks *4374* Thrombocytopenia observed in 2.0% of 765 patients with congestive failure compared with 0.5% of 437 patients receiving placebo. Observed in 1.1% of 1142 hypertensive patients receiving carvedilol compared with 0.2% of 462 patients receiving placebo *5639*
Blood No Effect Physiological No significant change in 9 patients with renal hypertension treated with up to 20 mg daily for up to 4 weeks *3223* In 16 patients with mild to moderate hypertension treatment with up to 20 mg/d for 12 weeks caused insignificant change from 236 ± 11 thousand /μL to 230 ± 10 thousand /μL *2264*

Potassium *Serum Decrease Physiological* Observed in treated patients with congestive cardiac failure with a frequency of between 0.1% and 1% *5639*
Serum No Effect Physiological In a population of hypertensive patients treatment with carvedilol had no significant effect on concentration *5639* No significant effect in 9 patients with renal hypertension treated with up to 20 mg daily for up to 4 weeks *3223* No significant effect in 118 patients with mild to moderate hypertension treated with therapeutic doses for 12 weeks *4374* No effect of 20 mg daily for 1 week in 18 patients with essential hypertension *2595* In 20 patients with mild to moderate hypertension treatment with up to 20 mg/d for 12 weeks caused no change from mean baseline of 4.3 ± 0.1 mmol/L *2264*

Pre-β-Lipoprotein *Serum No Effect Physiological* In 13 patients with mild to moderate hypertension treatment with up to 20 mg/d for 12 weeks caused insignificant change from 18.8 ± 2.0 % to 20.5 ± 2.1 % *2264*

Protein *Serum Decrease Physiological* In 20 patients with mild to moderate hypertension treatment with up to 20 mg/d for 12 weeks caused significant decrease from men baseline of 7.6 ± 0.1 g/dL to 7.1 ± 0.1 g/dL *2264*
Serum No Effect Physiological No significant change in 9 patients treated with up to 20 mg daily for up to 4 weeks *3223*

Prothrombin Time *Plasma Decrease Physiological* Observed in treated patients with congestive cardiac failure receiving warfarin with a frequency of between 1% and 2% *5639*
Plasma No Effect Physiological In 9 healthy volunteers coadministration of 25 mg/d carvediol with warfarin had no clinically relevant effect on the pharmacokinetics of R(+)- and S(+)-warfarin or on the steady state prothrombin time ratios *5639*

Renal Blood Flow *Patient No Effect Physiological* In 12 hypertensive post-renal transplant patients treatment with up to 50 mg/d for 8 weeks caused nonsignificant change from mean baseline of 311 ± 27 mL/min to 318 ± 14 mL/min *3482*

Renin Activity *Plasma Decrease Physiological* After 10 mg orally concentration decreased 120 minutes later but effect not significant *2595* Insignificant reduction from mean of 2.67 to 2.07 mg/mL/h in 10 patients with essential hypertension given one dose of 50 mg but significant reduction from mean of 2.67 to 1.65 mg/mL/h when 50 mg given daily for 4 weeks *1624*

Sodium *Serum Decrease Physiological* Observed in treated patients with congestive cardiac failure with a frequency of between 1% and 2% *5639*
Serum No Effect Physiological No effect of 20 mg daily for 1 week in 18 patients with essential hypertension *2595* No significant effect in 118 patients with mild to moderate hypertension treated with therapeutic doses for 12 weeks *4374* In 20 patients with mild to moderate hypertension treatment with up to 20 mg/d for 12 weeks caused insignificant change from 143.5 ± 0.6 mmol/L to 143.2 ± 0.6 mmol/L *2264* No significant effect in 9 patients with renal hypertension treated for up to 4 weeks with up to 20 mg daily *3223*
Urine Increase Physiological Insignificant increase from mean of 127 to 141 mmol/24 h in 10 patients with essential hypertension when treated with 50 mg daily for 4 weeks *1624*
Urine No Effect Physiological In 12 hypertensive post-renal transplant patients treatment with up to 50 mg/d caused no change from mean baseline of 80 ± 11 mmol/d *3482*

Carvedilol *(continued)*

Tissue Plasminogen Activator
Plasma No Effect Physiological In 25 hypertensive patients treatment for 6 months caused nonsignificant change from mean baseline before anoxia of 0.084 ± 0.2 U/cm³ to 0.089 ± 0.3 U/cm³ *3781*

Torsemide *Serum No Effect Physiological* In 12 healthy individuals coadministration of 25 mg/d carvedilol and torsemide 5 mg/d for 5 days had no clinically relevant effect on pharmacokinetics of either compound *5639*

Triglycerides *Serum Decrease Physiological* In 110 patients with mild to moderate essential hypertension treatment with up to 50 mg/d for 6 months caused significant decrease from mean baseline of 2.9 mmol/L to 2.5 mmol/L *2507*
Serum Increase Physiological Observed in 1.2% of 1142 hypertensive patients receiving carvedilol compared with 0.2% of 462 patients receiving placebo *5639*
Serum No Effect Physiological No significant effect in 18 patients with essential hypertension treated with 20 mg daily for 1 week *2595* No significant effect in 9 patients with renal hypertension treated for up to 4 weeks with up to 20 mg daily *3223* In 8 hypertensive patients with serum triglyceride concentration greater than 150 mg/dL treatment for 6 months caused significant increase from mean baseline of 236 ± 42 mg/dL to 224 ± 30 mg/dL and in 17 with serum triglycerides less than 150 mg/dL from 121 ± 24 mg/dL to 129 ± 13 mg/dL *3781* No significant effect in 81 patients with mild to moderate hypertension treated with therapeutic doses for 12 weeks *4374* No significant effect observed in 36 patients treated with up to 20 mg daily for 12 weeks *5432* No significant effect in 32 elderly hypertensive patients treated with 25 mg daily for 12 weeks *5768* In a population of hypertensive patients treatment with carvedilol had no significant effect on concentration *5639* No significant effect in 25 noninsulin dependent diabetic hypertensives treated with 50 mg daily for 8 weeks *1671* In 21 mild to moderate hypertensives treatment with up to 20 mg/d for 12 weeks caused no significant effect on concentration *2264*

Urea Nitrogen *Serum Increase Physiological* Rare reversible deterioration of renal function, usually in patients with low blood pressure, underlying renal insufficiency, or diffuse vascular disease *1973* Observed in 6.0% of 765 patients with congestive failure compared with 4.6% of 437 patients receiving placebo *5639*
Serum No Effect Physiological In a population of hypertensive patients treatment with carvedilol had no significant effect on concentration *5639* In 20 patients with mild to moderate hypertension treatment with up to 20 mg/d for 12 weeks caused insignificant change from 15.9 ± 0.6 mg/dL to 15.4 ± 0.7 mg/dL *2264* No change in 123 patients with mild to moderate hypertension treated with therapeutic doses for 12 weeks *4374* No significant effect in 18 patients with essential hypertension given 20 mg daily for 1 week *2595* No significant effect of treatment with up to 20 mg daily for up to 4 weeks in 9 patients with renal hypertension *3223*

Uric Acid *Serum Increase Physiological* Observed in treated patients with congestive cardiac failure with a frequency of between 1% and 2% *5639*
Serum No Effect Physiological No effect in 9 patients with renal hypertension treated with up to 20 mg daily for up to 4 weeks *3223* No effect of 20 mg daily for 1 week in 18 patients with essential hypertension *2595* In 18 patients with mild to moderate hypertension treatment with up to 20 mg/d for 12 weeks caused insignificant change from 5.5 ± 0.3 U/L to 67.3 ± 7.1 U/L *2264* In a population of hypertensive patients treatment with carvedilol had no significant effect on concentration *5639* No significant change in 118 patients with mild to moderate hypertension treated with therapeutic doses for 12 weeks *4374*

Volume *Plasma Increase Physiological* Observed in 2.0% of 765 patients with congestive failure compared with 0.9% of 437 patients receiving placebo *5639*

Warfarin *Plasma No Effect Physiological* In 9 healthy volunteers coadministration of 25 mg/d carvedilol with warfarin had no clinically relevant effect on the pharmacokinetics of R(+)- and S(+)-warfarin or on the steady state prothrombin time ratios *5639*

Cascara

Color *Urine Increase Analytical* Brown (acid), yellow-pink (alkaline), black on standing *1714*

^{131}I Uptake *Serum Decrease Physiological* Lilly compound contains tetraiodofluorescein *4360*

Porphobilinogen *Urine Increase Analytical* Color extractable into chloroform *2559*

PSP Excretion *Urine Increase Physiological* Converted to anthraquinone in the gastrointestinal tract (red color) *1174*

Urobilinogen *Urine Increase Analytical* Reacts with Ehrlich's reagent *2559*

Casodex

Androstenedione *Plasma No Effect Physiological* In 14 patients with benign prostatic hypertrophy receiving 50 mg/d for 24 weeks mean concentration of 3.38 ± 1.88 nmol/L not significantly different from 3.25 ± 2.59 nmol/L in 13 patients with BPH treated with placebo *1745*

Apolipoprotein A-I *Serum No Effect Physiological* In 14 patients with benign prostatic hypertrophy receiving 50 mg/d for 24 weeks mean concentration changed nonsignificantly from baseline of 1.35 ± 0.06 g/L by 0.06 ± 0.04 g/L *1746*

Apolipoprotein B *Serum No Effect Physiological* In 14 patients with benign prostatic hypertrophy receiving 50 mg/d for 24 weeks mean concentration changed nonsignificantly from baseline of 1.56 ± 0.07 g/L by 0.02 ± 0.04 g/L *1746*

Cholesterol *Serum Increase Physiological* In 14 patients with benign prostatic hypertrophy receiving 50 mg/d for 24 weeks mean concentration increased from baseline of 6.31 ± 0.27 mmol/L by 0.11 ± 0.13 mmol/L *1746*

Dehydroepiandrosterone Sulfate
Plasma No Effect Physiological In 14 patients with benign prostatic hypertrophy receiving 50 mg/d for 24 weeks mean concentration of 2.97 ± 1.66 nmol/L not significantly different from 3.42 ± 1.98 nmol/L in 13 patients with BPH treated with placebo *1745*

Dihydrotestosterone *Serum No Effect Physiological* In 14 patients with benign prostatic hypertrophy receiving 50 mg/d for 24 weeks mean concentration of 2.18 ± 1.31 nmol/L not significantly different from 2.20 ± 0.69 nmol/L in 13 patients with BPH treated with placebo *1745*

Estradiol *Plasma No Effect Physiological* In 14 patients with benign prostatic hypertrophy receiving 50 mg/d for 24 weeks mean concentration of 101 ± 20.3 pmol/L not significantly different from 102 ± 27.3 pmol/L in 13 patients with BPH treated with placebo *1745*

Estrone *Plasma No Effect Physiological* In 14 patients with benign prostatic hypertrophy receiving 50 mg/d for 24 weeks mean concentration of 201 ± 41.7 pmol/L not significantly different from 210 ± 76.7 pmol/L in 13 patients with BPH treated with placebo *1745*

Fibrinogen *Plasma Increase Physiological* In 14 patients with benign prostatic hypertrophy receiving 50 mg/d for 24 weeks mean concentration changed significantly from baseline of 3.19 ± 0.21 g/L by 0.34 ± 0.23 g/L *1746*

Follicle Stimulating Hormone
Plasma Increase Physiological In 14 patients with benign prostatic hypertrophy receiving 50 mg/d for 24 weeks mean concentration of 10.7 ± 12.9 IU/L significantly higher than 4.46 ± 2.37 IU/L in 13 patients with BPH treated with placebo *1745*

HDL-Cholesterol *Serum No Effect Physiological* In 14 patients with benign prostatic hypertrophy receiving 50 mg/d for 24 weeks mean concentration changed nonsignificantly from baseline of 1.20 ± 0.08 mmol/L by 0.03 ± 0.09 mmol/L *1746*

Hemoglobin *Blood Decrease Physiological* In 14 patients with benign prostatic hypertrophy receiving 50 mg/d for 24 weeks mean concentration changed significantly from baseline of 152 ± 3 g/L by - 7.6 ± 3.6 g/L *1746*

LDL-Cholesterol *Serum No Effect Physiological* In 14 patients with benign prostatic hypertrophy receiving 50 mg/d for 24 weeks mean concentration changed nonsignificantly from baseline of 4.15 ± 0.29 mmol/L by 0.03 ± 0.18 mmol/L *1746*

Luteinizing Hormone *Plasma Increase Physiological* In 14 patients with benign prostatic hypertrophy receiving 50 mg/d for 24 weeks mean concentration of 7.24 ± 6.89 IU/L significantly higher than 4.33 ± 2.26 IU/L in 13 patients with BPH treated with placebo *1745*

Plasminogen Activator Inhibitor-1 *Plasma Decrease Physiological* In 14 patients with benign prostatic hypertrophy receiving 50 mg/d for 24 weeks mean concentration changed significantly from baseline of 18.9 ± 4.9 U/mL by - 1.8 ± 2.2 U/mL *1746*

Platelets *Blood Decrease Physiological* In 14 patients with benign prostatic hypertrophy receiving 50 mg/d for 24 weeks mean concentration changed significantly from baseline of 230 ± 16 x 10^9/L by - 21 ± 12 x 10^9/L *1746*

Prolactin *Plasma No Effect Physiological* In 14 patients with benign prostatic hypertrophy receiving 50 mg/d for 24 weeks mean concentration of 185 ± 72 mIU/L not significantly different from 189 ± 86 mIU/L in 13 patients with BPH treated with placebo *1745*

Sex-Hormone Binding Globulin *Serum No Effect Physiological* In 14 patients with benign prostatic hypertrophy receiving 50 mg/d for 24 weeks mean concentration of 47.9 ± 34.5 nmol/L not significantly different from 43.3 ± 17.4 nmol/L in 13 patients with BPH treated with placebo *1745*

Testosterone *Serum Increase Physiological* In 14 patients with benign prostatic hypertrophy receiving 50 mg/d for 24 weeks mean concentration of 15.9 ± 8.2 nmol/L not significantly higher than 13.8 ± 4.3 nmol/L in 13 patients with BPH treated with placebo *1745*

Triglycerides *Serum Increase Physiological* In 14 patients with benign prostatic hypertrophy receiving 50 mg/d for 24 weeks mean concentration changed significantly from baseline of 2.14 ± 0.27 mmol/L by 0.42 ± 0.48 mmol/L *1746*

Castor Oil

Cells *Urine Increase Physiological* Multinucleated giant cells in 50% patients *4014*

Protein *Urine Increase Physiological* May cause renal damage *467*

Urea Nitrogen *Serum Increase Physiological* May cause renal damage *467*

Cathartics

Albumin *Serum Decrease Physiological* Rare protein-losing gastroenteropathy *2242*

Potassium *Serum Decrease Physiological* Excessive use may cause hypokalemia *2242*
Urine Increase Physiological Secondary aldosteronism if blood volume reduced *2242*

Protein *Serum Decrease Physiological* Rare protein losing gastroenteropathy *2242*

Prothrombin Time *Plasma Increase Physiological* Accelerated passage and decreased absorption of vitamin K *2452*

Sodium *Serum Decrease Physiological* Excessive use may cause sodium depletion *2242*

Cefaclor

Alanine Aminotransferase *Serum Increase Physiological* Transient hepatitis and cholestatic jaundice has been reported rarely. Slight increases in enzyme activity reported in about one in forty patients *1692*

Alkaline Phosphatase *Serum Increase Physiological* Transient hepatitis and cholestatic jaundice has been reported rarely. Slight increases in enzyme activity reported in about one in forty patients *1692*

Amino Acids *Urine Increase Analytical* Reacts with ninhydrin in paper chromatography, paper electrophoresis and ion-exchange chromatography *4761*

Aspartate Aminotransferase *Serum Increase Physiological* Transient hepatitis and cholestatic jaundice has been reported rarely. Slight increases in enzyme activity reported in about one in forty patients *1692*

Creatinine *Serum Decrease Analytical* At concentration of 1000 mg/L decreased result obtained by enzymatic Boehringer Mannheim creatinine PAP method by 34%, result by Wako creatinine B method by 22% and by Kodak Ektachem® by 15% but no effect observed at therapeutic concentrations *2302*
Serum Increase Analytical Interference of up to 600% observed with certain alkaline picrate methods *2301* At concentration of 1000 mg/L increased result by Jaffe methods on IL Monarch by 156-160%, Technicon SMAC® by 136% and Serono Centrifichem by 516%. However, at therapeutic concentrations only method on Centrifichem produced falsely high result *2302*
Serum Increase Physiological Slight increases in concentration reported in fewer than 1 in 500 treated patients *1692*

Cyclosporine *Blood No Effect Analytical* At a concentration of 230 mg/L had no effect on Syva EMIT method *495*

Eosinophils *Blood Increase Physiological* Eosinophilia has been reported with drug administration in about 1 of 50 treated patients *1692*

Glucose *Urine Increase Analytical* Administration of cefaclor may cause false positive test when Benedict's or Fehling's solutions or Clinitest® tablets used *1627*

Hematocrit *Blood Decrease Physiological* Hemolytic anemia has been rarely reported with drug administration *1692*

Hemoglobin *Blood Decrease Physiological* Hemolytic anemia has been rarely reported with drug administration *1692*

Leukocytes *Blood Decrease Physiological* Leukopenia has been rarely reported with drug administration *1692*

Lymphocytes *Blood Increase Physiological* Transient lymphocytosis has been rarely reported with drug administration *1692*

Neutrophils *Blood Decrease Physiological* Reversible neutropenia has been rarely reported with drug administration *1692*

Platelets *Blood Decrease Physiological* Thrombocytopenia has been rarely reported with drug administration *1692* Rare immune-mediated toxicity *4327*

Protein *Urine Increase Physiological* Abnormal urinalysis reported in fewer than 1 in 200 treated patients *1692*

Prothrombin Time *Plasma Increase Physiological* Rare reports of prolonged prothrombin time with/without clinical bleeding in patients receiving both coumadin and cefaclor *1692* Increased prothrombin time reported with or without bleeding when warfarin coadministered with cefaclor *1627*

Sugar *Urine Increase Analytical* Reacts positively with Clinitest *4761*

Theophylline *Serum No Effect Physiological* No clinically significant effect on theophylline concentration observed when drugs coadministered *5999* No effect on steady state kinetics in healthy young adults *2979* No documented significant interaction with theophylline reported *6117*

Urea Nitrogen *Serum Increase Physiological* Slight increases in concentration reported in fewer than 1 in 500 treated patients *1692*

Cefadroxil

Amino Acids *Urine Increase Analytical* Reacts with ninhydrin in paper chromatography, paper electrophoresis and ion-exchange chromatography *4761*

Sugar *Urine Increase Analytical* Reacts positively with Clinitest *4761*

Cefamandole

Alanine Aminotransferase *Serum Increase Physiological* Occurs in about 4% treated cases *5224* Transient increases in enzyme activity have been reported rarely as a complication of cephalosporin treatment *1702*

Alkaline Phosphatase *Serum Increase Physiological* Fewer than 3 of 53 patients developed reversible hepatotoxicity *1616* Transient increases in enzyme activity have been reported rarely as a complication of cephalosporin treatment *1702*

Aspartate Aminotransferase *Serum Increase Physiological* Occurs in about 4% treated cases *5224* Fewer than 3 of 53

Cefamandole *(continued)*

Aspartate Aminotransferase *(continued)* patients developed reversible hepatotoxicity *1616* Transient increases in enzyme activity have been reported rarely as a complication of cephalosporin treatment *1702*

Bilirubin *Serum No Effect Analytical* At 2.50 mmol/L on method on Eppendorf Epos *2351* No effect at 2000 mg/L on Ames Seralyzer method *5706* At concentration of 533 mg/L had no effect on method on Kodak Ektachem® *5706*

Bilirubin, Conjugated *Serum No Effect Analytical* No effect at concentration of 0.5 mg/L on method on Kodak Ektachem® *5706*

Bilirubin, Unconjugated *Serum No Effect Analytical* No effect at concentration of 0.5 mg/L on method on Kodak Ektachem® *5706*

Cholesterol *Serum No Effect Analytical* At 2.50 mmol/L on method on Eppendorf Epos *2351* No effect at 2000 mg/L on Ames Seralyzer method *5706*

Clindamycin *Serum Positive Analytical* Interferes with bioassays because cannot be inactivated *3858*

Colistin *Serum Positive Analytical* Interferes with bioassays because cannot be inactivated *3858*

Coombs' Test, Direct *Blood Positive Physiological* In about 1% of treated patients (dose related) *5224* Positive direct Coombs' tests have been reported rarely as a complication of cephalosporin treatmen *1702*

Creatine Kinase *Serum No Effect Analytical* No effect at 2000 mg/L on method on Ames Seralyzer *5706*

Creatinine *Serum Decrease Analytical* At 1000 mg/L produced low result by 11% with enzymatic Boehringer Mannheim creatinine PAP method, 14% by Wako creatinine B method and possible increase of less than 10% with method on Kodak Ektachem® . No effects at therapeutic concentrations *2302*
Serum Increase Analytical Slow and slight reaction in Jaffe methods *2351* At concentration of 1000 mg/L caused falsely high results with Jaffe methods on IL Monarch, Technicon SMAC® and Serono Centrifichem, but all by less than 10% and no èffect observed at therapeutic concentrations *2302* No effect up to 60 mg/L on Ames Seralyzer method but at higher concentrations apparently clinically significantly increased creatinine concentration *5706*
Serum Increase Physiological Transient mild increases in concentration have been reported rarely as a complication of cephalosporin treatment, with frequency increased in patients aged over 50 years *1702*
Serum No Effect Analytical At concentration of 1500 mg/L had no effect on kinetic Jaffe method on Du Pont aca *5704* At concentration of 1500 mg/L had no effect on kinetic method on BKA-2 *5704* At concentration of 1500 mg/L had no effect on Technicon AutoAnalyzer® Jaffe method *5704* No significant interference observed at a concentration of 25 mg/dL (4.9 mmol/L) with method on Du Pont aca *1520*

Creatinine Clearance *Urine Decrease Physiological* Decreases in clearance have been reported rarely in patients with prior renal impairment as a complication of cephalosporin treatment *1702*

Eosinophils *Blood Increase Physiological* In 5% cases *5224*

Erythromycin *Serum Increase Analytical* Interferes with bioassays because cannot be inactivated *3858*

Factor VII *Plasma Decrease Physiological* Effect on activity in 30 patients with serious infections. Possibly associated with sulfhydryl group *63*

Fibrinogen *Plasma Decrease Physiological* Effect observed in some cases: associated with vitamin K associated hypoprothrombinemia *5172*

Glucose *Serum No Effect Analytical* No effect at 2000 mg/L on glucose oxidase method on Ames Seralyzer *5706*
Urine Increase Analytical False positive reaction may be given with Fehling's and Benedict's solutions and Clinitest® *1702*
Urine No Effect Analytical No effect observed on Tes-Tape® method *1702*

Hemoglobin *Blood Decrease Physiological* Rare hemolytic anemia *5224*

Lactate Dehydrogenase *Serum No Effect Analytical* No effect up to 650 mg/L on method on Ames Seralyzer but at higher concentrations apparently reduced enzyme activity *5706*

Leukocytes *Blood Decrease Physiological* In 2 patients given 6-9 g daily intravenously *2686*

Lymphocytes *Blood No Effect Physiological* In 2 patients given 6-9 g daily intravenously *2686*

Metronidazole *Serum Increase Analytical* Interferes with bioassays because cannot be inactivated *3858*

Neutrophils *Blood Decrease Physiological* Occasional count below 500 /µL observed *4327* Neutropenia has been reported rarely as a complication of cefamandole treatment, especially with long courses of treatment *1702*

Occult Blood *Feces Increase Physiological* Observed in 3 of 37 patients receiving intravenous nutrition *5224*

Partial Thromboplastin Time
Plasma Increase Physiological In 7 cases developed vitamin K deficient hypoprothrombinemia *5172*

Platelets *Blood Decrease Physiological* Thrombocytopenia has been reported rarely as a complication of cefamandole treatment *1702* Rare immune-mediated toxicity reported *4327*
Blood No Effect Physiological Not known as complication *5224*

Polymyxin *Serum Increase Analytical* Interferes with bioassays because cannot be inactivated *3858*

Protein *Serum No Effect Analytical* At 2.50 mmol/L on method on Eppendorf Epos *2351*
Urine Increase Analytical False positive results may be produced with acid and denatruation-precipitation tests *1702*
Urine No Effect Analytical No effect on sulfosalicylic acid method and Albustix method at concentration of 1 g/L *3927*

Prothrombin *Plasma Decrease Physiological* Hypothrombinemia with/without has been observed rarely but it has been promptly reversed by administration of vitamin K *1702*

Prothrombin Time *Plasma Increase Physiological* Transient plasma appearance of Vitamin K_1 2,3-epoxide in response to 10 mg Vitamin K_1 intravenously *5488* In 3 of 37 patients receiving intravenous nutrition *5224* In 7 cases developed vitamin K deficient hypoprothrombinemia *5172* Occurs due to interference with hepatic vitamin K metabolism by methylthiotetrazole side chain *1384* 4 of 31 patients receiving drug for more than 48 h developed response; reversible but significant bleeding occurred in some *527*

Tetracycline *Serum Increase Analytical* Interferes with bioassays because cannot be inactivated *3858*

Trimethoprim *Serum Increase Analytical* Interferes with bioassays because cannot be inactivated *3858*

Urea Nitrogen *Serum Increase Physiological* Transient increases in concentration have been reported rarely as a complication of cephalosporin treatment, with frequency increased in patients aged over 50 years *1702*
Serum No Effect Analytical At 2.50 mmol/L on method on Eppendorf Epos *2351* No effect up to 1000 mg/L on method on Ames Seralyzer but at higher concentrations apparent reduction in urea nitrogen concentration although not of clinical significance since above therapeutic range *5706*

Uric Acid *Serum No Effect Analytical* At 2.50 mmol/L on method on Eppendorf Epos *2351*

Cefazedone

Bilirubin *Serum No Effect Analytical* On method on Eppendorf Epos at concentration of 2.50 mmol/L *2351*

Cholesterol *Serum No Effect Analytical* On method on Eppendorf Epos at concentration of 2.50 mmol/L *2351*

Creatinine *Serum No Effect Analytical* On Jaffe method at concentration of 2.50 mmol/L *2351*

Protein *Serum No Effect Analytical* On method on Eppendorf Epos at concentration of 2.50 mmol/L *2351*

Urea Nitrogen *Serum No Effect Analytical* On method on Eppendorf Epos at concentration of 2.50 mmol/L *2351*

Uric Acid *Serum No Effect Analytical* On method on Eppendorf Epos at concentration of 2.50 mmol/L *2351*

Cefazolin

Alanine Aminotransferase *Serum Increase Physiological* Transient increase may be observed in response to treatment *5637* Transient increases have rarely been reported in patients receiving cefazolin *1700*

Albumin *Serum No Effect Analytical* At concentration of 117 mg/L had no effect on BCG method *5704*

Alkaline Phosphatase *Serum Increase Physiological* Transient increase may be observed in response to treatment *5637* Transient increases have rarely been reported in patients receiving cefazolin *1700* In 4 of 31 treated cases: transient 2 to 3 fold increase *3744* Reversible hepatotoxicity noted in some patients *1616*

Amino Acids *Urine No Effect Analytical* Negative reaction observed with ninhydrin in paper chromatography, paper electrophoresis and ion-exchange chromatography *4761*

Aspartate Aminotransferase *Serum Increase Physiological* In 4 of 31 treated cases: transient 2 to 3 fold increase *3744* Transient increase may be observed in response to treatment *5637* Reversible hepatotoxicity noted in some patients *1616* Transient increases have rarely been reported in patients receiving cefazolin *1700*

Bicarbonate *Serum No Effect Analytical* At concentration of 110 mg/L had no effect on method using phenolphthalein *5704*

Bilirubin *Serum Increase Physiological* In 4 of 31 treated cases: transient 2 to 3 fold increase *3744*
Serum No Effect Analytical At concentrations up to 1000 mg/L no significant effect observed on DPD method on Hitachi 717 analyzer or method on Kodak Ektachem® analyzers *4695* At concentration of 117 mg/L had no effect on Jendrassik and Grof method *5704* At 2.50 mmol/L on method on Eppendorf Epos *2351*

Calcium *Serum No Effect Analytical* At concentration of 110 mg/L had no effect on cresolphthalein method *5704*

Cefotaxime *Serum Increase Analytical* Cannot be assayed by HPLC method used at Mayo Clinic in presence of cefazolin *3858*

Chloride *Serum No Effect Analytical* At concentration of 110 mg/L had no effect on mercurimetric method *5704*

Cholesterol *Serum No Effect Analytical* At 2.50 mmol/L on method on Eppendorf Epos *2351* At concentration of 110 mg/L had no effect on CHOD-PAP method *5704*

Coombs' Test, Direct *Blood Positive Physiological* Positive tests have been reported: positive reactions have also been observed in the blood of neonates whose mothers received cephalosporins before delivery *1700*

Coombs' Test, Indirect *Blood Positive Physiological* Positive tests have been reported: positive reactions have also been observed in the blood of neonates whose mothers received cephalosporins before delivery *1700* Positive direct and indirect Coomb's tests may be observed and may also occur in neonates whose mothers received cephalosporins before delivery *5637*

Creatinine *Serum Decrease Analytical* At concentration of 1000 mg/L caused increase of less than 10% with Boehringer Mannheim enzymatic creatinine PAP method, and decrease of 10% with Wako creatinine B kit and method on Kodak Ektachem® , but effect not significant at therapeutic concentrations *2302*
Serum Increase Analytical At concentrations above 2,000 mg/L (normal therapeutic concentration 150 mg/L) kinetic Jaffe method on BKA-2 *5704* With Jaffe based procedures concentration increased. 0.13 mg/mL cefazolin equivalent to 0.2 mg/dL with Beckman Synchron CX_5 and CX_3 methods, and 0.2 mg/dL with Hitachi 737 method with effects greater at higher concentrations *2533* With Jaffe based procedures concentration increased. 0.13 mg/mL cefazolin equivalent to 0.2 mg/dL with Beckman Synchron CX5 and CX3 methods, and 0.2 mg/dL with Hitachi 737 method with effects greater at higher concentrations *2533* Increase of 10-20 μmol/L for every 20 mg/L of drug on Ames Seralyzer *4219* Increase of 10-20 μmol/L for every 20 mg/L of drug on Abbott Vision *4219* Slow and slight reaction in Jaffe methods *2351* At concentration of 1000 mg/L caused increases with Jaffe procedures of 42-87% with methods on Instrumentation Laboratory Monarch, 23% with Technicon SMAC® , and 45% with Serono Centrifichem but no effect observed at therapeutic concentrations *2302*
Serum No Effect Analytical At concentration of 2,000 mg/L had no effect on Technicon AutoAnalyzer® Jaffe method *5704* No effect of concentrations up to 500 mg/L on 2-slide method on Kodak Ektachem® *5706* No significant interference observed at a concentration of 50 mg/dL (11.0 mmol/L) with method on Du Pont aca *1520* No effect at up to 250 mg/L on Kodak DT-60 *4219* No effect of concentrations up to 15 mg/L on single slide method on Kodak Ektachem® *5706* At concentration of 2,000 mg/L had no effect on kinetic Jaffe method on Du Pont aca *5704* No significant effect observed with concentrations up to 2.0 mg/mL with Boehringer Mannheim PAP method adapted for use with Beckman Synchron CX5 *2533* No effect at concentration of 50 mg/dL (1.1 mmol/L) on method on Du Pont Dimension *1572* No significant effect observed with concentrations up to 2.0 mg/mL with Boehringer Mannheim PAP method adapted for use with Beckman Synchron CX_5*2533*

Cyclosporine *Blood No Effect Physiological* Coadministration with cyclosporine appeared to have no significant effect on its concentration *859*
Serum No Effect Physiological Coadministration with cyclosporine appeared to have no significant effect on its concentration *859*

Eosinophils *Blood Increase Physiological* Eosinophilia may be observed as an allergic reaction to treatment *5637*

Glucose *Serum No Effect Analytical* At concentration of 110 mg/L had no effect on GOD/POD-PAP method *5704*
Urine Increase Analytical False positive reaction observed with Benedict's, Fehling's and Clinitest® reagents *5637* False positive reaction may be given with Fehling's and Benedict's solutions and Clinitest® *1700*
Urine No Effect Analytical No effect observed with Clinistix® and TesTape® *5637* No effect observed on Tes-Tape® method *1700*

Leukocytes *Blood Decrease Physiological* Leukopenia has been reported in patients receiving cefazolin *1700* Leukopenia may be observed in response to treatment *5637*

Lipase *Serum No Effect Analytical* No effect of concentrations up to 0.35 mg/L on method on Kodak Ektachem® *5706*

Mycophenolic Acid *Serum No Effect Analytical* No significant interference observed with HPLC method of Shipkova et al *5526*

Mycophenolic Acid Glucuronide
Serum No Effect Analytical No significant interference observed with HPLC method of Shipkova et al *5526*

Neutrophils *Blood Decrease Physiological* Neutropenia may be observed in response to treatment *5637* Neutropenia has been reported in patients receiving cefazolin *1700*

Phosphate *Serum No Effect Analytical* At concentration of 110 mg/L had no effect on phosphomolybdate method *5704*

Platelets *Blood Decrease Physiological* Thrombocytopenia may be observed in response to treatment *5637* Rare immune-mediated toxicity reported *4327* Thrombocytopenia has been reported in patients receiving cefazolin *1700*
Blood Increase Physiological Thrombocythemia may be observed in response to treatment *5637*

Potassium *Serum No Effect Analytical* At concentration of 110 mg/L had no effect on flame-photometric method *5704*

Protein *Serum No Effect Analytical* At concentration of 117 mg/L had no effect on biuret method with blank correction *5704* At 2.50 mmol/L on method on Eppendorf Epos *2351*
Urine No Effect Analytical No effect in 9 patients receiving up to 4 g daily on sulfosalicylic acid, trichloracetic acid and Ponceau S dye methods *6611*

Prothrombin Time *Plasma Increase Physiological* Transient plasma appearance of Vitamin K_1 2,3-epoxide after 10 mg intravenously in volunteers as with cephalosporins with N-methylthiotetrazole side chain *5488*

Sodium *Serum No Effect Analytical* At concentration of 110 mg/L had no effect on flame-photometric method *5704*

Sugar *Urine Increase Analytical* Reacts positively with Clinitest *4761*

Theophylline *Serum Increase Analytical* Interference may be observed with some HPLC methods *5999*

Triglycerides *Serum No Effect Analytical* At concentration of 110 mg/L had no effect on lipase/esterase method *5704*

Urea Nitrogen *Serum Increase Physiological* Transient increases have been reported in patients receiving cefazolin,

Cefazolin (continued)

Urea Nitrogen *(continued)*
but without clinical evidence of renal impairment *1700* Transient increase may be observed in response to treatment *5637*
Serum No Effect Analytical At concentration of 117 mg/L had no effect on diacetylmonoxime method *5704* At 2.50 mmol/L on method on Eppendorf Epos *2351*

Uric Acid *Serum No Effect Analytical* At concentration of 117 mg/L had no effect on phosphotungstate reduction method *5704* At 2.50 mmol/L on method on Eppendorf Epos *2351*

Vancomycin *Serum No Effect Analytical* At concentrations up to 500 μg/mL had no significant cross-reactivity in valproic acid method on Bayer Technicon Immuno 1® *438* No significant interference observed at a concentration of 500 μg/mL (1100 μmol/L) with method on Du Pont aca *1561*

Cefdinir

Alanine Aminotransferase *Serum Increase Physiological* During treatment with cefdinir 0.9% patients observed to have increased ALT activity although relationship to cefdinir administration not established exclusively *4528*

Alkaline Phosphatase *Serum Increase Physiological* During treatment with cefdinir 0.2% patients observed to have increased activity although relationship to cefdinir administration not established exclusively *4528*

Aspartate Aminotransferase *Serum Increase Physiological* During treatment with cefdinir 0.4% patients observed to have increased activity although relationship to cefdinir administration not established exclusively *4528*

Bilirubin *Serum Increase Physiological* During treatment with cefdinir 0.2% patients observed to have increased concentration although relationship to cefdinir administration not established exclusively *4528*

Color *Feces Increase Analytical* Concomitant administration of iron with cefdinir caused pink coloration due to formation of a nonabsorbable complex containing iron and cefdinir in the gastrointestinal tract *4528*

Coombs' Test, Direct *Blood Positive Physiological* Cephalosporins may occasionally induce a positive direct Coomb's test *4528*

Eosinophils *Blood Increase Physiological* During treatment with cefdinir 0.6% patients observed to have increased eosinophil concentration although relationship to cefdinir administration not established exclusively *4528*

Erythrocytes *Urine Increase Physiological* During treatment with cefdinir approximately 1% patients observed to have increased red cell excretion although relationship to cefdinir administration not established exclusively *4528*

Glucose *Serum Decrease Physiological* During treatment with cefdinir 0.2% patients observed to have decreased glucose concentration although relationship to cefdinir administration not established exclusively *4528*
Serum Increase Physiological During treatment with cefdinir 0.9% patients observed to have increased glucose concentration although relationship to cefdinir administration not established exclusively *4528*
Urine Increase Analytical False positive reaction may be observed with Benedict's, Fehling's and Clinitest ® *4528*
Urine Increase Physiological During treatment with cefdinir 0.9% patients observed to have increased glucose excretion although relationship to cefdinir administration not established exclusively *4528*
Urine No Effect Analytical Has no effect on Clinistix® or Tes-Tape® *4528*

γ-Glutamyltransferase *Serum Increase Physiological* During treatment with cefdinir approximately 1% patients observed to have increased GGT activity although cefdinir not identified unequivocally as causative agent *4528*

Hemoglobin *Blood Decrease Physiological* During treatment with cefdinir 0.3% patients observed to have decreased concentration although relationship to cefdinir administration not established exclusively *4528*

Ketones *Urine Increase Analytical* False positive test may be observed with tests using nitoprusside *4528*
Urine No Effect Analytical No effect may be observed with tests using nitroferricyanide *4528*

Lactate Dehydrogenase *Serum Increase Physiological* During treatment with cefdinir 0.2% patients observed to have increased activity although relationship to cefdinir administration not established exclusively *4528*

Leukocytes *Blood Decrease Physiological* During treatment with cefdinir 0.7% patients observed to have decreased leukocyte count although relationship to cefdinir administration not established exclusively *4528*
Blood Increase Physiological During treatment with cefdinir 0.8% patients observed to have increased leukocyte count although relationship to cefdinir administration not established exclusively *4528*
Urine Increase Physiological During treatment with cefdinir 0.4% patients observed to have increased excretion although relationship to cefdinir administration not established exclusively *4528*

Lymphocytes *Blood Decrease Physiological* During treatment with cefdinir 0.8% patients observed to have decreased lymphocyte count although relationship to cefdinir administration not established exclusively *4528*
Blood Increase Physiological During treatment with cefdinir 0.2% patients observed to have increased lymphocyte count although relationship to cefdinir administration not established exclusively *4528*

Neutrophils *Blood Decrease Physiological* During treatment with cefdinir 0.2% patients observed to have decreased concentration although relationship to cefdinir administration not established exclusively *4528*

pH *Urine Increase Physiological* During treatment with cefdinir 0.2% patients observed to have increased pH although relationship to cefdinir administration not established exclusively *4528*

Phosphate *Serum Decrease Physiological* During treatment with cefdinir 0.3% patients observed to have decreased phosphate concentration although relationship to cefdinir administration not established exclusively *4528*
Serum Increase Physiological During treatment with cefdinir 0.6% patients observed to have increased phosphate concentration although relationship to cefdinir administration not established exclusively *4528*

Platelets *Blood Increase Physiological* During treatment with cefdinir 0.2% patients observed to have increased concentration although relationship to cefdinir administration not established exclusively *4528*

Potassium *Serum Increase Physiological* During treatment with cefdinir 0.2% patients observed to have increased concentration although relationship to cefdinir administration not established exclusively *4528*

Protein *Urine Increase Physiological* During treatment with cefdinir approximately 1% patients observed to have increased protein excretion although relationship to cefdinir administration not established exclusively *4528*

Specific Gravity *Serum Decrease Physiological* During treatment with cefdinir 0.6% patients observed to have decreased bicarbonate concentration although relationship to cefdinir administration not established exclusively *4528*
Urine Decrease Physiological During treatment with cefdinir 0.8% patients observed to have decreased specific gravity although relationship to cefdinir administration not established exclusively *4528*

Urea Nitrogen *Serum Increase Physiological* During treatment with cefdinir 0.2% patients observed to have increased concentration although relationship to cefdinir administration not established exclusively *4528*

Cefipime

Glucose *Urine Increase Analytical* May give false positive result with Clinitest® *727*
Urine No Effect Analytical Has no effect on Clinistix® or Tes-Tape® methods *727*

Cefixime

Alanine Aminotransferase *Serum Increase Physiological* Transient increases reported in less than 1% treated patients *1384*

Aspartate Aminotransferase *Serum Increase Physiological* Transient increases reported in less than 1% treated patients *1384*

Coombs' Test, Direct *Blood Positive Physiological* False-positive direct Coombs' test has been observed with other cephalosporins *3469*

Creatinine *Serum Increase Analytical* 1 g/L exhibits a positive interference of up to 20% with Jaffe methods involving picrate depending on picrate concentration and reading intervals used. However no effect on enzymatic methods observed *370*

Serum Increase Physiological Transient increases reported in less than 1% treated patients *1384*

Eosinophils *Blood Increase Physiological* Mild and reversible eosinophilia observed in less than 1% treated patients *1384*

Glucose *Urine Increase Analytical* False positive reaction may occur with Clinitest® , Benedict's solution or Fehling solution *3469*

Urine No Effect Analytical No effect observed when measured by methods using glucose oxidase such as Clinistix® or Tes-Tape® *3469*

Interleukin-6 *Serum Decrease Physiological* In 38 children aged 6 months to 14 years with typhoid salmonellosis mean concentration decreased with treatment with intravenous ceftriaxone or oral cefixime from 449 pg/mL to 67 pg/mL after 7 days and 40 pg/mL after 14 days *543*

Ketones *Urine Increase Analytical* False positive reaction may occur with tests using nitroprusside but not with those using ferricyanide *3469*

Urine No Effect Analytical False positive reaction may occur with tests using nitroprusside but not with those using ferricyanide *3469*

Leukocytes *Blood Decrease Physiological* Mild and reversible leukopenia observed in less than 1% treated patients *1384*

Platelets *Blood Decrease Physiological* Mild and reversible thrombocytopenia observed in less than 1% treated patients *1384*

Tumor Necrosis Factor-α *Serum No Effect Physiological* In 38 children aged 6 months to 14 years with typhoid salmonellosis mean concentration changed insignificantly with treatment with intravenous ceftriaxone or oral cefixime from 31 pg/mL to 27 pg/mL after 7 days *543*

Urea Nitrogen *Serum Increase Physiological* Transient increases reported in less than 1% treated patients *1384*

Cefmenoxime

Prothrombin Time *Plasma Increase Physiological* Transient plasma appearance of Vitamin K_1 2,3-epoxide in response to a 10 mg intravenous dose of Vitamin K_1 *5488*

Cefmetazole

Alanine Aminotransferase *Serum Increase Physiological* Transient increases observed *1384*

Aspartate Aminotransferase *Serum Increase Physiological* Transient increases observed *1384*

Bleeding Time *Patient No Effect Physiological* No effect observed in 9 healthy volunteers given 8 g daily intravenously for 6 days *2030*

Eosinophils *Blood Increase Physiological* Transient eosinophilia observed *1384*

Leukocytes *Blood Decrease Physiological* Transient leukopenia observed *1384*

Platelet Aggregation *Blood No Effect Physiological* No effect observed on ADP induced aggregation in 9 healthy volunteers given 8 g intravenously daily for 6 days *4629*

Prothrombin Time *Plasma Increase Physiological* May interfere with hepatic vitamin K metabolism *1384*

Cefodizime

Bilirubin *Serum No Effect Analytical* No effect at 2.50 mmol/L on method on Eppendorf Epos *2351*

Cholesterol *Serum No Effect Analytical* No effect at 2.50 mmol/L on method on Eppendorf Epos *2351*

Creatinine *Serum No Effect Analytical* No effect on Jaffe method at concentration up to 2.50 mmol/L *2351*

Protein *Serum No Effect Analytical* No effect at 2.50 mmol/L on method on Eppendorf Epos *2351*

Urea Nitrogen *Serum No Effect Analytical* No effect at 2.50 mmol/L on method on Eppendorf Epos *2351*

Uric Acid *Serum No Effect Analytical* No effect at 2.50 mmol/L on method on Eppendorf Epos *2351*

Cefonicid

Alanine Aminotransferase *Serum Increase Physiological* Increased activity observed in 1.6% treated patients *5651*

Alkaline Phosphatase *Serum Increase Physiological* Increased activity observed in 1.6% treated patients *5651*

Aspartate Aminotransferase *Serum Increase Physiological* Increased activity observed in 1.6% treated patients *5651*

Coombs' Test *Blood Positive Physiological* Positive Coombs' test observed in less than 1% treated patients *5651*

Creatinine *Serum Increase Physiological* Increased concentration observed in less than 1% treated patients, with rare reports of acute renal failure *5651*

Eosinophils *Blood Increase Physiological* Increased eosinophil count observed in 2.9% treated patients *5651*

γ-Glutamyltransferase *Serum Increase Physiological* Increased activity observed in 1.6% treated patients *5651*

Lactate Dehydrogenase *Serum Increase Physiological* Increased activity observed in 1.6% treated patients *5651*

Leukocytes *Blood Decrease Physiological* Leukopenia observed in less than 1% treated patients *5651*

Neutrophils *Blood Decrease Physiological* Neutropenia observed in less than 1% treated patients *5651*

Platelets *Blood Decrease Physiological* Thrombocytopenia observed in less than 1% treated patients *5651*

Blood Increase Physiological Increased platelet count observed in 1.7% treated patients *5651*

Urea Nitrogen *Serum Increase Physiological* Increased concentration observed in less than 1% treated patients, with rare reports of acute renal failure *5651*

Vanillylmandelic Acid *Serum Increase Physiological* Increased activity observed in 1.6% treated patients *5651*

Cefoperazone

Alanine Aminotransferase *Serum Increase Physiological* Transient increase in 5% of 450 patients *1082* Mild transient increases may occur in 5 - 10% patients *4643*

Alkaline Phosphatase *Serum Increase Physiological* Mild transient increases may occur in 5 - 10% patients *4643*

Aspartate Aminotransferase *Serum Increase Physiological* Mild transient increases may occur in 5 - 10% patients *4643* Transient increase in 5% of 450 patients *1082*

Bilirubin *Serum Increase Physiological* Significant displacement in neonates but possibly only at concentrations above therapeutic *6314* Mild transient increases may occur in 5 - 10% patients *4643*

Serum No Effect Analytical No effect at 2000 mg/L on Ames Seralyzer method *5706* At 2.50 mmol/L on method on Eppendorf Epos *2351*

Cholesterol *Serum No Effect Analytical* No effect at 2000 mg/L on Ames Seralyzer method *5706* At 2.50 mmol/L on method on Eppendorf Epos *2351*

Cholinesterase *Serum No Effect Analytical* No effect observed at concentration of 400 µg/mL with butyrylthiocholine method on Kodak Ektachem® *2504*

Creatine Kinase *Serum No Effect Analytical* No effect at 2000 mg/L on method on Ames Seralyzer *5706*

Creatinine *Serum Increase Analytical* Slow and slight reaction in Jaffe methods *2351*

Cefoperazone *(continued)*

Creatinine *(continued)*
Serum Increase Physiological Transient increases of concentration reported in 1 of 48 treated patients but without significant nephrotoxicity *4643*
Serum No Effect Analytical No effect on Jaffe methods *3299* No effect at 2000 mg/L on Ames Seralyzer method *5706* At up to 1,000 µg/mL on Technicon SMAC® Jaffe method *5729*

Eosinophils *Blood Increase Physiological* Teansient eosinophilia may occur with prolonged administration (1 in 10 patients) *4643* In 8% of 450 patients: effect mild and reversible *1082*

Glucose *Serum No Effect Analytical* No effect at 2000 mg/L on glucose oxidase method on Ames Seralyzer *5706*
Urine Increase Analytical False positive reaction may occur with Benedict's or Fehling's solutions *4643*
Urine No Effect Analytical Dark green-black color with Clinitest® but no effect or slight reduction with glucose concentrations of 1% and up. Concentration measured accurately by Diastix® . Concentrations measured accurately by TesTape® *3446*

Hematocrit *Blood Decrease Physiological* Reversible reductions may occur with prolonged administration (1 in 20 patients) *4643*

Hemoglobin *Blood Decrease Physiological* Reversible reductions may occur with prolonged administration (1 in 20 patients) *4643*

Lactate Dehydrogenase *Serum No Effect Analytical* No effect at 2000 mg/L on method on Ames Seralyzer *5706*

Leukocytes *Blood Decrease Physiological* In 2% of 450 patients: resolved on withdrawal of drug *1082*

Neutrophils *Blood Decrease Physiological* Reversible slight neutropenia may occur with prolonged administration (1 in 50 patients) *4643*

Occult Blood *Feces Increase Physiological* Associated with vitamin K correctable hypoprothrombinemia but mechanism unclear *4451*

Partial Thromboplastin Time
Plasma Increase Physiological Reported in previous study to occur in about 4% treated patients. Mechanism unclear but possibly due to inhibition of prothrombin production. Effect correctable with vitamin K *4451*

Protein *Serum No Effect Analytical* At 2.50 mmol/L on method on Eppendorf Epos *2351*
Urine No Effect Analytical No effect at 1 g/L on sulfosalicylic acid and Albustix methods *3927*

Prothrombin Time *Plasma Increase Physiological* Reported in previous study to occur in about 4% treated patients. Mechanism unclear but possibly due to inhibition of prothrombin production. Effect correctable with vitamin K *4451* Reported effect in some patients with occasional bleeding *4327* In 4% of 450 patients but correctable with vitamin K *1082* May interfere with hepatic vitamin K metabolism *1384* Transient plasma appearance of Vitamin K_1 2,3-epoxide in response to 10 mg Vitamin K_1 intravenously *5488*

Urea Nitrogen *Serum Increase Physiological* Transient increases of concentration reported in 1 of 18 treated patients but without significant nephrotoxicity *4643*
Serum No Effect Analytical No effect at 2000 mg/L on method on Ames Seralyzer *5706* At 2.50 mmol/L on method on Eppendorf Epos *2351*

Uric Acid *Serum No Effect Analytical* At 2.50 mmol/L on method on Eppendorf Epos *2351*

Ceforanide

Creatinine *Serum No Effect Analytical* At up to 1,000 µg/mL on Technicon SMAC® Jaffe method *5729*

Protein *Urine No Effect Analytical* No effect of 1 g/L on sulfosalicylic acid and Albustix methods *3927*

Prothrombin Time *Plasma No Effect Physiological* Not reported to have been associated with hypoprothrombinemia *1384*

Cefotaxime

Alanine Aminotransferase *Serum Increase Physiological* Transient increases in enzyme activity reported to occur with administration in less than 1% cases *2644*

Albumin *Serum Increase Analytical* Slight effect of drug and metabolite on method on American Monitor Parallel *320*

Alkaline Phosphatase *Serum Increase Analytical* Consistent slight increase on American Monitor Parallel method by metabolite *320*
Serum Increase Physiological Transient increases in enzyme activity reported to occur with administration in less than 1% cases *2644*

Amino Acids *Urine No Effect Analytical* Negative reaction observed with ninhydrin in paper chromatography, paper electrophoresis and ion-exchange chromatography *4761*

Ammonia *Plasma Decrease Analytical* Falsely low, even negative, values obtained in several patients receiving cefotaxime in addition to other drugs when concentration measured by Sigma Diagnostics enzymatic kit, but no effect of pure drug or its desacetylcefotaxime metabolite observed *3156*

Amylase *Serum Decrease Analytical* General effect of both drug and metabolite on American Monitor Parallel method *320*

Aspartate Aminotransferase *Serum Increase Physiological* Transient increases in enzyme activity reported to occur with administration in less than 1% cases *2644*

Bilirubin *Serum No Effect Analytical* No effect at 1000 mg/L on Ames Seralyzer method *5706* No effect at 2.50 mmol/L on method on Eppendorf Epos *2351* At concentrations up to 1000 mg/L no significant effect observed on DPD method on Hitachi 717 or method on Kodak Ektachem® analyzers *4695*

Calcium *Serum Increase Analytical* Statistically significant effect of metabolite on American Monitor Parallel method *320*

Ceftriaxone *Serum Increase Analytical* Cannot be assayed in presence of cefotaxime by HPLC method used at Mayo Clinic *3858*

Chloride *Serum Decrease Analytical* Statistically significant effect of metabolite on American Monitor Parallel method *320*
Serum Increase Analytical Statistically significant effect of drug on American Monitor Parallel method *320*

Cholesterol *Serum Increase Analytical* Generally significant increase of drug and metabolite on American Monitor Parallel method *320*
Serum No Effect Analytical No effect at 2.50 mmol/L on method on Eppendorf Epos *2351* No effect at 1000 mg/L on Ames Seralyzer method *5706*

Clindamycin *Serum Positive Analytical* Interferes with bioassays because cannot be inactivated *3858*

Colistin *Serum Positive Analytical* Interferes with bioassays because cannot be inactivated *3858*

Coombs' Test, Direct *Blood Positive Physiological* Some patients reported to develop positive test with administration of cefotaxime, but in less than 1% cases *2644*

Creatine Kinase *Serum Increase Analytical* Statistically significant effect of metabolite on American Monitor Parallel method *320*
Serum No Effect Analytical No effect at 1000 mg/L on method on Ames Seralyzer *5706*

Creatinine *Serum Increase Analytical* Significant increase observed with Jaffe methods of Beckman and Merck at concentrations as low as 0.5 g/L *6375*
Serum Increase Physiological Transient increases in concentration and interstitial nephritis reported to occur with administration in less than 1% cases *2644*
Serum No Effect Analytical No effect on Jaffe methods *3299* No effect at up to 250 mg/L on Kodak DT-60. No effect at up to 250 mg/L on Abbott Vision. No effect at up to 250 mg/L on Ames Seralyzer *4219* No effect at 1000 mg/L on Ames Seralyzer method *5706* No effect of concentrations up to 500 mg/L on 2-slide method on Kodak Ektachem® *5706* At concentration of 500 mg/L had no effect on Jaffe-Fuller's earth method *5704* At concentration of 500 mg/L had no effect on Technicon AutoAnalyzer® Jaffe method *5704* At concentration of 500 mg/L had no effect on kinetic Jaffe method on Du Pont aca *5704* At up to 1,000 µg/mL on Technicon SMAC®

Jaffe method *5729* No significant effect observed with enzymatic methods of Merck, Wako and PAP and MPA methods of Boehringer Mannheim at concentrations up to 4 g/L and at concentration up to 1.0 g/L with manual Fuller's earth method *6375* No effect at 1000 mg/L with Jaffe methods on IL Monarch, Technicon SMAC® , or Serono Centrifichem or enzymatic Boehringer Mannheim creatinine PAP method, Wako creatinine B method or Kodak Ektachem® method *2302* No effect observed on Jaffe procedure at up to 2.50 mmol/L *2351*

Eosinophils *Blood Increase Physiological* Eosinophilia reported to occur with administration in less than 1% cases *2644*

Erythromycin *Serum Increase Analytical* Interferes with bioassays because cannot be inactivated *3858*

Glucose *Cerebrospinal Fluid Decrease Physiological* Mean decrease of 6% observed in 49 children with bacterial meningitis treated with i.v. cefotaxime only for 12 hours *4365*
Cerebrospinal Fluid Increase Physiological Mean increase of 53% after treatment with i.v. cefotaxime for 24 hours in 49 children with bacterial meningitis *4365*
Serum Increase Analytical Statistically significant effect of metabolite on American Monitor Parallel method *320*
Serum No Effect Analytical No effect at 1000 mg/L on glucose oxidase method on Ames Seralyzer *5706*
Urine No Effect Analytical Dark green-black color with Clinitest® but no effect or slight reduction with glucose concentrations of 1% and up. Concentrations measured accurately by Diastix® . Concentrations measured accurately by TesTape® *3446*

γ-Glutamyltransferase *Serum Decrease Analytical* 10% reduction in specimens from patients with liver disease measured on American Monitor Parallel *320*

Granulocytes *Blood Decrease Physiological* Agranulocytosis reported to occur with administration in less than 1% cases *2644*

Iron *Serum Increase Analytical* General effect of both drug and metabolite on American Monitor Parallel method *320*

Iron Saturation *Serum Increase Analytical* Slight but significant increase with both drug and metabolite on method on American Monitor Parallel *320*

Ketone Body Ratio *Serum No Effect Analytical* When added at a concentration of 500 mg/L had no significant effect on AKBR method of Uno et al *6131*

Lactate *Cerebrospinal Fluid Decrease Physiological* Increase of 5% observed at 12 h but decrease of 49% at 24 h in 49 children with bacterial meningitis when treated with i.v. cefotaxime *4365*

Lactate Dehydrogenase *Serum Decrease Analytical* Generally significant decrease of drug and metabolite on American Monitor Parallel method *320*
Serum Increase Physiological Transient increases in enzyme activity reported to occur with administration in less than 1% cases *2644*
Serum No Effect Analytical No effect at 1000 mg/L on method on Ames Seralyzer *5706*

Leukocytes *Blood Decrease Physiological* Observed in 0.5% treated patients *4327* Transient leukopenia reported to occur with administration in less than 1% cases *2644*
Cerebrospinal Fluid Decrease Physiological Mean decrease of 28% observed after 24 hours treatment with i.v. cefotaxime in 49 children with bacterial meningitis *4365*
Cerebrospinal Fluid Increase Physiological Mean 31% increase observed after 12 h in 49 children with bacterial meningitis when treated with i.v. cefotaxime only *4365*

Magnesium *Serum Decrease Analytical* Marked effect of drug and metabolite on specimens containing tobramycin on American Monitor method on Parallel *320*
Serum Increase Analytical Effect of metabolite on method on American Monitor Parallel *320*

Metronidazole *Serum Increase Analytical* Interferes with bioassays because cannot be inactivated *3858*

Neutrophils *Blood Decrease Physiological* Neutropenia reported to occur with administration in less than 1% cases *2644* Occasional count of less than 500 /µL observed *4327*

Occult Blood *Feces Increase Physiological* 21 of 48 children (44%) with bacterial meningitis treated with i.v. cefotaxime observed to have positive guaiac test *4365*

Phenylalanine *Plasma No Effect Analytical* No interference observed with rapid quantitative whole blood method of Campbell et al using phenylalanine dehydrogenase *867*

Phosphate *Serum Decrease Analytical* Effect of drug on most specimens (also of metabolite) on method on American Monitor Parallel *320*
Serum Increase Analytical Marked increase with both drug and metabolite on specimens containing gentamicin and tobramycin on American Monitor Parallel method *320*

Platelet Activating Factor
Cerebrospinal Fluid Decrease Physiological In 49 children with bacterial meningitis treatment with i.v. cefotaxime caused 34% reduction after 12 hours and 57% reduction after 24 hours but reductions less than when i.v. dexamethasone also given *4365*

Platelets *Blood Decrease Physiological* Thrombocytopenia reported to occur with administration in less than 1% cases *2644*

Polymyxin *Serum Increase Analytical* Interferes with bioassays because cannot be inactivated *3858*

Potassium *Serum Increase Analytical* By up to 0.2 mmol/L with both drug and metabolite on method on American Monitor Parallel *320*

Protein *Cerebrospinal Fluid Decrease Physiological* Mean decrease of 36% observed in 49 children with bacterial meningitis treated with i.v. cefotaxime only for 24 hours *4365*
Cerebrospinal Fluid Increase Physiological Mean increase of 13% observed after 12 hours in 49 children with bacterial meningitis treated with i.v. cefotaxime only *4365*
Serum Decrease Analytical Effect of drug and metabolite on specimens containing gentamicin and tobramycin on American Monitor Parallel *320*
Serum No Effect Analytical No effect at 2.50 mmol/L on method on Eppendorf Epos *2351*
Urine No Effect Analytical No effect of 1 g/L on sulfosalicylic acid and Albustix methods *3927*

Prothrombin Time *Plasma No Effect Physiological* In contrast to cephalosporins with N-methylthiotetrazole side chain, no response to intravenous injection of 10 mg Vitamin K_1 *5488*

Salicylate *Serum No Effect Analytical* No interference observed with method on Du Pont aca *6671*

Sodium *Serum Increase Analytical* By up to 5 mmol/L with both drug and metabolite on method on American Monitor Parallel *320*

Sugar *Urine Increase Analytical* Reacts positively with Clinitest *4761*

Tacrolimus *Serum No Effect Analytical* In HPLC/MS method of Christians et al no significant interference observed with measurement of FK 506 *1010*

Tetracycline *Serum Increase Analytical* Interferes with bioassays because cannot be inactivated *3858*

Trimethoprim *Serum Increase Analytical* Interferes with bioassays because cannot be inactivated *3858*

Tumor Necrosis Factor-α
Cerebrospinal Fluid Decrease Physiological Mean decrease of 21% observed in 49 children with bacterial meningitis following i.v. treatment with cefotaxime after 12 hours and decrease of 54% after 24 hours *4365*

Urea Nitrogen *Serum Decrease Analytical* Effect of drug on specimens containing tobramycin on American Monitor Parallel method *320*
Serum Increase Physiological Transient increases in concentration and interstitial nephritis reported to occur with administration in less than 1% cases *2644*
Serum No Effect Analytical No effect at 1000 mg/L on method on Ames Seralyzer *5706* No effect at 2.50 mmol/L on method on Eppendorf Epos *2351*

Uric Acid *Serum Decrease Analytical* Effect of drug on specimens containing tobramycin on American Monitor Parallel method *320*
Serum No Effect Analytical No effect at 2.50 mmol/L on method on Eppendorf Epos *2351*

Vancomycin *Serum No Effect Analytical* No significant interference observed at a concentration of 1000 µg/mL (2195 µmol/L) with method on Du Pont aca *1561* At concentrations up to 1000 µg/mL had no significant cross-reactivity in valproic acid method on Bayer Technicon Immuno 1® *438*

Cefotetan

Alanine Aminotransferase *Serum* *Increase* *Physiological* Increased activity has been reported as an adverse event in 1 in 150 treated patients *6644*

Alkaline Phosphatase *Serum* *Increase* *Physiological* Increased activity has been reported as an adverse event in 1 in 700 treated patients *6644*

Aspartate Aminotransferase *Serum* *Increase* *Physiological* Increased activity has been reported as an adverse event in 1 in 300 treated patients *6644*

Coombs' Test, Direct *Blood* *Positive* *Physiological* Positive direct test has been reported as an adverse event in 1 in 250 treated patients *6644*

Creatinine *Serum* *Increase* *Physiological* Increased concentration has been reported as an adverse event with rare nephrotoxicity *6644*

Eosinophils *Blood* *Increase* *Physiological* Eosinophilia has been reported as an adverse event in 1 in 200 treated patients *6644*

Granulocytes *Blood* *Decrease* *Physiological* Agranulocytosis has been reported as an adverse event *6644*

Hematocrit *Blood* *Decrease* *Physiological* Hemolytic anemia has been reported as an adverse event *6644*

Hemoglobin *Blood* *Decrease* *Physiological* Hemolytic anemia has been reported as an adverse event *6644*

Lactate Dehydrogenase *Serum* *Increase* *Physiological* Increased activity has been reported as an adverse event in 1 in 700 treated patients *6644*

Leukocytes *Blood* *Decrease* *Physiological* Leukopenia has been reported as an adverse event *6644*

Platelets *Blood* *Decrease* *Physiological* Thrombocytopenia has been reported as an adverse event *6644*
Blood *Increase* *Physiological* Thrombocytosis has been reported as an adverse event in 1 in 300 treated patients *6644*

Prothrombin *Plasma* *Increase* *Physiological* Transient plasma appearance of Vitamin K_1 2,3-epoxide in response to 10 mg Vitamin K_1 orally *5488*

Prothrombin Time *Plasma* *Increase* *Physiological* May interfere with hepatic vitamin K metabolism *1384* Prolonged prothrombin time with or without bleeding has been reported as an adverse event *6644* Reported prolongation and occasional bleeding *4327*

Urea Nitrogen *Serum* *Increase* *Physiological* Increased concentration has been reported as an adverse event with rare nephrotoxicity *6644*

Cefotiam

Bilirubin *Serum* *Increase* *Analytical* Significant effect observed at physiological concentrations on method on Kodak Ektachem® analyzer so that at concentration of drug of 31.3 mg/L concentration of bilirubin appeared to be doubled and 125 mg/L increased more than four-fold *4695*
Serum *No Effect* *Analytical* At concentrations as high as 1000 mg/L had no effect on method using 2,5-dichlorodiphenyldiazonium salt (DPD) on Hitachi 717 analyzer *4695* No effect at 5000 mg/L on Ames Seralyzer method *5706* At 2.50 mmol/L on method on Eppendorf Epos *2351*

Bilirubin, δ *Serum* *Increase* *Analytical* At drug concentration of 15.7 mg/L δ-bilirubin concentration increased from 1 mg/L to 5 mg/L, at 31.3 mg/L to 7 mg/L, at 62.5 mg/L to 11 mg/L, at 125 mg/L to 21 mg/L and further increases at higher amounts with method on Kodak Ektachem® analyzer *4695*

Bilirubin Glucuronide *Serum* *No Effect* *Analytical* At drug concentrations up to 250 mg/L no effect observed on method on Kodak Ektachem® analyzer *4695*

Bilirubin, Unconjugated *Serum* *No Effect* *Analytical* At unconjugated bilirubin concentration of 5 mg/L concentrations of drug up to 125 mg/L had no effect but at higher concentrations slight reduction observed *4695*

Cholesterol *Serum* *No Effect* *Analytical* No effect at 5000 mg/L on Ames Seralyzer method *5706* At 2.50 mmol/L on method on Eppendorf Epos *2351*

Creatine Kinase *Serum* *No Effect* *Analytical* No effect at 5000 mg/L on method on Ames Seralyzer *5706*

Creatinine *Serum* *Increase* *Analytical* No effect up to 420 mg/L on Ames Seralyzer method but at higher concentrations apparently increased creatinine concentration of possible clinical significance *5706* Slow and slight reaction in Jaffe methods *2351*

Glucose *Serum* *No Effect* *Analytical* No effect at 5000 mg/L on glucose oxidase method on Ames Seralyzer *5706*

Lactate Dehydrogenase *Serum* *No Effect* *Analytical* No effect up to 1500 mg/L on method on Ames Seralyzer but at higher concentrations inhibition of enzyme activity although of no clinical significance *5706*

Midazolam *Serum* *No Effect* *Analytical* On GC-ECD method of Ha et al *2387*

Protein *Serum* *No Effect* *Analytical* At 2.50 mmol/L on method on Eppendorf Epos *2351*

Urea Nitrogen *Serum* *No Effect* *Analytical* No effect at 5000 mg/L on method on Ames Seralyzer *5706* At 2.50 mmol/L on method on Eppendorf Epos *2351*

Uric Acid *Serum* *No Effect* *Analytical* At 2.50 mmol/L on method on Eppendorf Epos *2351*

Cefotoxine

Lactate Dehydrogenase *Serum* *No Effect* *Analytical* No effect at 2000 mg/L on method on Ames Seralyzer *5706*

Cefoxitin

Alanine Aminotransferase *Serum* *Increase* *Physiological* Transient increases in activity have been reported *3981* Reported incidence of 3% *5224*
Serum *No Effect* *Analytical* At 5 times upper limit of therapeutic range on methods on Technicon SMAC® , Abbott-VP, Du Pont aca, Roche Cobas-Bio and KDA *3525*

Albumin *Serum* *No Effect* *Analytical* At 5 times upper limit of therapeutic range on methods on Technicon SMAC® , Kodak Ektachem® , Hitachi® 705 and KDA *3525*
Urine *No Effect* *Analytical* At concentration of 2400 mg/dL had no significant effect on Boehringer Mannheim Tina-quant method *2799*

Alkaline Phosphatase *Serum* *Increase* *Physiological* Transient 2 to 3-fold increase in 3 of 31 patients following colorectal surgery *3744* Transient increases in activity have been reported *3981*
Serum *No Effect* *Analytical* At 5 times upper limit of therapeutic range on methods on Technicon SMAC® , Abbott-VP, Du Pont aca, Roche Cobas-Bio, Hitachi® 705 and KDA *3525*

Amino Acids *Urine* *No Effect* *Analytical* Negative reaction observed with ninhydrin in paper chromatography, paper electrophoresis and ion-exchange chromatography *4761*

Amylase *Serum* *No Effect* *Analytical* At 5 times upper limit of therapeutic range on methods on Du Pont aca, Roche Cobas-Bio and Kodak Ektachem® *3525*

Aspartate Aminotransferase *Serum* *Increase* *Physiological* Reported incidence of 3% *5224* Transient increases in activity have been reported *3981* Transient 2 to 3-fold increase in 3 of 31 patients following colorectal surgery *3744*
Serum *No Effect* *Analytical* At 5 times upper limit of therapeutic range on methods on Technicon SMAC® , Abbott-VP, Du Pont aca, Roche Cobas-Bio, Hitachi® 705 and KDA *3525*

Bilirubin *Serum* *Increase* *Physiological* Transient 2 to 3-fold increase in 3 of 31 patients following colorectal surgery *3744* Jaundice has been reported as a side effect *3981*
Serum *No Effect* *Analytical* At 5 times upper limit of therapeutic range on methods on Technicon SMAC® , Du Pont aca, Roche Cobas-Bio, Kodak Ektachem® , Hitachi® 705 and KDA *3525* No effect at 2000 mg/L on Ames Seralyzer method *5706* At concentrations up to 1000 mg/L no significant effect observed on DPD method on Hitachi 717 analyzer or method on Kodak Ektachem® analyzer *4695* At concentrations up to 2.50 mmol/L on methods on Eppendorf Epos *2351*

Calcium *Serum* *No Effect* *Analytical* At 5 times upper limit of therapeutic range on methods on Technicon SMAC® , Abbott-VP, Du Pont aca, Kodak Ektachem® , Hitachi® 705 and KDA *3525*

Cefuroxime *Serum Increase Analytical* Cannot be assayed by HPLC method used at Mayo Clinic in presence of cefoxitin *3858*

Cholesterol *Serum No Effect Analytical* At 5 times upper limit of therapeutic range on methods on Technicon SMAC® , Abbott-VP, Roche Cobas-Bio, Kodak Ektachem® , Hitachi® 705, and KDA *3525* No effect at 2000 mg/L on Ames Seralyzer method *5706* At concentrations up to 2.50 mmol/L on methods on Eppendorf Epos *2351*

Clindamycin *Serum Positive Analytical* Interferes with bioassays because cannot be inactivated *3858*

Colistin *Serum Positive Analytical* Interferes with bioassays because cannot be inactivated *3858*

Coombs' Test *Blood Positive Physiological* 6 of 77 patients developed rapidly reversible direct Coombs' test without hemolysis *4327*

Coombs' Test, Direct *Blood Positive Physiological* Positive test may occur in some individuals, especially those with azotemia *3981* In about 2% of treated patients (dose related) *5224*

Creatine Kinase *Serum No Effect Analytical* At 5 times upper limit of therapeutic range on methods on Technicon SMAC® , Abbott-VP, Du Pont aca, Roche Cobas-Bio, and Hitachi® 705 *3525* No effect at 2000 mg/L on method on Ames Seralyzer *5706*

Creatinine *Serum Increase Analytical* At concentrations above 25 mg/L (normal therapeutic concentration 150 mg/L) raised the concentration as measured by kinetic Jaffe method on Du Pont aca *5704* Profound interference with alkaline picrate based reactions *2351* Increased concentrations observed with Jaffe reaction-based procedures. 0.13 mg/mL cefoxitin equivalent to 0.7 mg/dL with Beckman Synchron CX_5, 0.6 mg/dL with Beckman Synchron CX_3 and 0.3 mg/dL with Hitachi 737 *2533* Increase of 50-80 µmol/L for every 100 mg/L of drug on Abbott Vision *4219* Increased concentrations observed with Jaffe reaction-based procedures. 0.13 mg/mL cefoxitin equivalent to 0.7 mg/dL with Beckman Synchron CX5, 0.6 mg/dL with Beckman Synchron CX3 and 0.3 mg/dL with Hitachi 737 *2533* At 5 times upper limit of therapeutic range on methods on Technicon SMAC® , Abbott-VP, Du Pont aca, Roche Cobas-Bio, Hitachi® 705 and KDA *3525* Effect noted on Technicon SMAC® less than with other commercial systems due to lesser dialysis of drug than creatinine *3297* At concentrations above 50 mg/L (normal therapeutic concentration 150 mg/L) raised the concentration as measured by kinetic Jaffe method on BKA-2 *5704* Concentration dependent increase with kinetic Jaffe reaction on Beckman Astra® or Eppendorf system with Merck reagents *5802* At concentrations of cefoxitin greater than 100 µg/mL may interfere with measurements by Jaffe procedure *3981* Increase of 50-80 µmol/L for every 100 mg/L of drug on Ames Seralyzer *4219* At concentrations above 70 mg/L (normal therapeutic concentration 150 mg/L) raised the concentration as measured by kinetic Jaffe method *5704* When used with Jaffe method on Greiner selective analyzer: concentration related effect *110* Linear correlation between drug concentration and that of analyte as measured by Jaffe reaction *2351* At concentration of 1000 mg/L increases results obtained by Jaffe methods on IL Monarch by 262-673%, Technicon SMAC® by 145% and Serono Centrifichem by 813% but significant positive interferences observed at therapeutic concentrations with all methods *2302* At concentrations above 80 mg/L (normal therapeutic concentration 150 mg/L) raised the concentration as measured by Technicon AutoAnalyzer® Jaffe method *5704* Increases concentration by 35-40% as measured by method on Du Pont aca at drug concentration of 5.0 mg/dL (1.2 mmol/L) *1520*
Serum Increase Physiological Increased concentration has been reported as a side effect. Renal failure has been reported rarely *3981*
Serum No Effect Analytical No significant effect at concentrations up to 2.0 mg/mL with Boehringer Mannheim PAP method adapted for use with Beckman Synchron CX_5*2533* In patients at 2 h after 2 g given i.v through interference with Jaffe procedure *1630* At concentration of 1000 mg/L less than 10% interference with enzymatic methods of Boehringer Mannheim creatinine PAP kit, Wako creatinine B kit and Kodak Ektachem® . No interference observed at therapeutic concentrations *2302* No effect of up to 160 mg/L on Boehringer creatinase enzymatic kit *6403* No significant effect at concentrations up to 2.0 mg/mL with Boehringer Mannheim PAP method adapted for use with Beckman Synchron CX5 *2533* At concentration of 500 mg/L had no effect as measured by Jaffe-Fuller's earth method *5704* At concentration of 160 mg/L had no effect on creatinine amidohydrolase method *5704* At concentration of 1 mg/L had no effect on creatinine iminohydrolase method *5704* No effect up to 500 mg/L on Ames Seralyzer method but at higher concentrations apparently higher creatinine concentration although of no clinical significance *5706* No effect of concentrations up to 500 mg/L on 2-slide method on Kodak Ektachem® *5706* No effect at concentration of 5 mg/dL (117 µmol/L) on method on Du Pont Dimension *5706* No effect at up to 250 mg/L on Kodak Ektachem® DT-60 *4219* At 5 times upper limit of therapeutic range on enzymatic method on Kodak Ektachem® 400 *3525*
Urine Increase Analytical When used with Jaffe method on Greiner selective analyzer: concentration related effect *110* Falsely high values with Jaffe methods *1630* At concentrations of cefoxitin greater than 100 µg/mL may interfere with measurements by Jaffe procedure *3981*

Creatinine Clearance *Urine Decrease Analytical* If measured with Jaffe procedure at peak drug concentration, otherwise value will be low, especially near trough concentration *110*
Urine Increase Analytical Artifactually increased for more than 4 h after 2 g drug given i.v *1630*

Eosinophils *Blood Increase Physiological* Reported incidence of 3% *5224* Eosinophilia may occur as a side effect *3981*

Erythromycin *Serum Increase Analytical* Interferes with bioassays because cannot be inactivated *3858*

Gentamicin *Serum Increase Analytical* At concentrations up to 750 mg/L (normal clinical concentration up to 2300 mg/L) caused approximately 25% increase in concentration when added to calibrator containing 4 mg/L with method on Baxter Stratus *5705*

Glucose *Serum No Effect Analytical* At 5 times upper limit of therapeutic range on methods on Technicon SMAC® , Abbott-VP, Du Pont aca, Roche Cobas-Bio, Kodak Ektachem® , Hitachi® 705 and KDA *3525* At concentration of 1,000 mg/L had no effect on GOD/POD-PAP method *5704* No effect at 2000 mg/L on glucose oxidase method on Ames Seralyzer *5706*
Urine Increase Analytical False positive reactions with Clinitest® may be observed *3981*

γ-Glutamyltransferase *Serum No Effect Analytical* At 5 times upper limit of therapeutic range on methods on Technicon SMAC® , Abbott-VP, and Hitachi® 705 *3525*

Glycated Hemoglobin *Blood No Effect Analytical* At a concentration of 25 mg/L had an insignificant - 2.1% interference with method on Abbott Vision *1885*

Granulocytes *Blood Decrease Physiological* Granulocytopenia may occur as a side effect *3981*

Hematocrit *Blood Decrease Physiological* Anemia including hemolytic anemia may occur as a side effect *3981*

Hemoglobin *Blood Decrease Physiological* Rare case of hemolytic anemia reported *5224* Anemia including hemolytic anemia may occur as a side effect *3981*

17-Hydroxycorticosteroids *Urine Increase Analytical* Methodological interference with Porter-Silber reaction not eliminated by sodium bisulfite *1775* High concentrations of cefoxitin in urine may interfere with measurements by Porter-Silber reaction *3981* Increased from 3 to 10-fold in urine from patients when Amberlite XAD-2 Clini-Skreen used for measurement *3298* Substantial effect (up to 3 times actual concentration) when Porter-Silber reaction used on specimen from patients (*in vitro* 5 mg/L reacted as if 14-4 mg/L) *1775*

Iron *Serum No Effect Analytical* At 5 times upper limit of therapeutic range on Ferrozine method on Technicon SMAC® *3525*

Lactate Dehydrogenase *Serum Increase Physiological* Transient increases in activity have been reported *3981*
Serum No Effect Analytical At 5 times upper limit of therapeutic range on methods on Technicon SMAC® , Abbott-VP, Roche Cobas-Bio, Hitachi® 705 and KDA *3525*

Leukocytes *Blood Decrease Physiological* Isolated case of drug-induced leukopenia *2997* Reported in fewer than 0.1% treated patients *4327* Leukopenia may occur as a side effect *3981*

Cefoxitin *(continued)*

Metronidazole *Serum Increase Analytical* Interferes with bioassays because cannot be inactivated *3858*

N-Acetyl-Glucosaminidase *Urine No Effect Analytical* At concentration of 2400 mg/dL had no significant effect on Boehringer Mannheim CPR method *3174* At 2 g/L on 2 colorimetric analytical methods *2254*

Neutrophils *Blood Decrease Physiological* Isolated case of drug-induced leukopenia *2997* Neutropenia may occur as a side effect *3981*

Phosphate *Serum No Effect Analytical* At 5 times upper limit of therapeutic range on methods on Technicon SMAC® , Du Pont aca, Hitachi® 705 and KDA *3525*

Platelets *Blood Decrease Physiological* Rare immune-mediated toxicity reported *4327* Thrombocytopenia, and bone marrow depression, may occur as side effects *3981*

Blood No Effect Physiological No report of thrombocytopenia in response to therapy *5224*

Polymyxin *Serum Increase Analytical* Interferes with bioassays because cannot be inactivated *3858*

Potassium *Serum No Effect Analytical* At concentration of 25 mg/L caused nonsignificant interference of 0% with method on Abbott Vision *681*

Protein *Cerebrospinal Fluid No Effect Analytical* At concentration of 70 mg/L on SDS/Coomassie Blue method of Huang *2745*

Serum No Effect Analytical At 5 times upper limit of therapeutic range on methods on Technicon SMAC® , Abbott-VP, Kodak Ektachem® , Hitachi® 705 and KDA *3525* At concentrations up to 2.50 mmol/L on methods on Eppendorf Epos *2351*

Urine No Effect Analytical No effect in 4 patients receiving up to 8 g daily on trichloracetic acid, sulfosalicylic acid and Ponceau S dye methods *6611* No effect of 1 g/L on sulfosalicylic acid and Albustix methods *3927*

Prothrombin Time *Plasma No Effect Physiological* In contrast to response to intravenous injections of Vitamin K_1 by patients treated with cephalosporins with N-methylthiotetrazole side chain, no effect observed *5488*

Sugar *Urine Increase Analytical* Reacts positively with Clinitest *4761*

Tetracycline *Serum Increase Analytical* Interferes with bioassays because cannot be inactivated *3858*

Theophylline *Serum No Effect Analytical* No effect at concentration of 200 mg/L with methods on Kodak DT60, Abbott TDx, Abbott Vision with either whole blood or serum, 3M Diagnostics TheoFAST, Syntex AccμLevel or Ames Seralyzer *1122*

Triglycerides *Serum No Effect Analytical* At concentration of 1025 mg/L had no effect on GPO-PAP method *5704* At 5 times upper limit of therapeutic range on methods on Technicon SMAC® , Abbott-VP, Kodak Ektachem® , Hitachi® 705 and KDA *3525*

Trimethoprim *Serum Increase Analytical* Interferes with bioassays because cannot be inactivated *3858*

Urea Nitrogen *Serum Increase Physiological* Increased concentration has been reported as a side effect. Renal failure has been reported rarely *3981*

Serum No Effect Analytical At concentrations up to 2.50 mmol/L on methods on Eppendorf Epos *2351* At 5 times upper limit of therapeutic range on methods on Technicon SMAC® , Abbott-VP, Roche Cobas-Bio, Kodak Ektachem® , Hitachi® 705, and KDA *3525* No effect at 2,000 mg/L on method on Ames Seralyzer *5706*

Uric Acid *Serum No Effect Analytical* At concentration of 1,000 mg/L had no effect on uricase-PAP method *5704* At 5 times upper limit of therapeutic range on methods on Technicon SMAC® , Abbott-VP, Du Pont aca, Roche Cobas-Bio, Kodak Ektachem® , Hitachi® 705 and KDA *3525* At concentrations up to 2.50 mmol/L on methods on Eppendorf Epos *2351*

Cefpirome

Bilirubin *Serum No Effect Analytical* At concentration of up to 2.50 mmol/L on methods of Eppendorf Epos *2351*

Cholesterol *Serum No Effect Analytical* At concentration of up to 2.50 mmol/L on methods of Eppendorf Epos *2351*

Creatinine *Serum Increase Analytical* Profound interference with Jaffe reaction *2351* In 14 patients following intravenous administration of cefpirome (1 or 2 g twice daily for 5 to 14 days) when creatinine measured by kinetic Jaffe procedure sharp and significant increase observed with return to baseline in 2 hours compared with little change with other methods *3493* Linear correlation between drug concentration and apparent analyte concentration *2351*

Serum No Effect Analytical Intravenous administration of 1 to 2 g twice daily for 5 to 14 days caused no significant effect on Guy and Legg HPLC method, Kodak Ektachem® two slide method, and Boehringer enzymatic method, with the HPLC method least affected *3493*

Ethanol *Serum No Effect Physiological* In 22 healthy young men administration of 2 g cefpirome intravenously prior to oral ingestion of 0.5 g/kg caused insignificant increase to 229 ± 48 mg/L from 221 ± 56 mg/L. Peak concentrations observed at 0.6 h in both situations. Area under the concentration curve 496 ± 215 mg/L.h compared with 509 ± 183 mg/L *3429*

Protein *Serum No Effect Analytical* At concentration of up to 2.50 mmol/L on methods of Eppendorf Epos *2351*

Urea Nitrogen *Serum No Effect Analytical* At concentration of up to 2.50 mmol/L on methods of Eppendorf Epos *2351*

Uric Acid *Serum No Effect Analytical* At concentration of up to 2.50 mmol/L on methods of Eppendorf Epos *2351*

Cefpodoxime

Alanine Aminotransferase *Serum Increase Physiological* Administration may cause transient increases in activity *4684*

Albumin *Serum Decrease Physiological* Administration may cause decreases in concentration *4684*

Alkaline Phosphatase *Serum Increase Physiological* Administration may cause transient increases in activity *4684*

Aspartate Aminotransferase *Serum Increase Physiological* Administration may cause transient increases in activity *4684*

Basophils *Blood Increase Physiological* Administration may cause transient increases in concentration *4684*

Bilirubin *Serum Increase Physiological* Administration may cause transient increases in concentration *4684*

Coombs' Test, Direct *Blood Positive Physiological* Administration may cause positive direct Coomb's test *4684*

Creatinine *Serum Increase Physiological* Administration may cause transient increases in concentration *4684*

Eosinophils *Blood Increase Physiological* Administration may cause transient increases in concentration *4684*

Glucose *Serum Decrease Physiological* Administration may cause both decreases and increases in concentration *4684*

Serum Increase Physiological Administration may cause both decreases and increases in concentration *4684*

γ-Glutamyltransferase *Serum Increase Physiological* Administration may cause transient increases in activity *4684*

Granulocytes *Blood Increase Physiological* Administration may cause transient increases in concentration *4684*

Hemoglobin *Blood Decrease Physiological* Administration may cause transient decreases in concentration *4684*

Lactate Dehydrogenase *Serum Increase Physiological* Administration may cause transient increases in activity *4684*

Leukocytes *Blood Decrease Physiological* Administration may cause transient decreases in concentration *4684*

Blood Increase Physiological Administration may cause transient increases in concentration *4684*

Lymphocytes *Blood Decrease Physiological* Administration may cause transient decreases in concentration *4684*

Monocytes *Blood Increase Physiological* Administration may cause transient increases in concentration *4684*

Neutrophils *Blood Decrease Physiological* Administration may cause transient decreases in concentration *4684*

Partial Thromboplastin Time
Plasma Increase Physiological Administration may cause prolongation of time *4684*

Platelets *Blood Decrease Physiological* Administration may cause transient decreases in concentration *4684*
Blood Increase Physiological Administration may cause transient increases in concentration *4684*

Protein *Serum Decrease Physiological* Administration may cause decreases in concentration *4684*

Prothrombin Time *Plasma Increase Physiological* Administration may cause prolongation of time *4684*

Urea Nitrogen *Serum Increase Physiological* Administration may cause transient increases in concentration *4684*

Cefsoludine

Bilirubin *Serum No Effect Analytical* At concentrations up to 1000 mg/L no significant effects observed on DPD method on Hitachi or method on Kodak Ektachem® *4695*

Creatinine *Serum Increase Analytical* Significant increase in concentrations with Jaffe methods of Beckman and Merck at concentrations as low as 0.5 g/L *6375*
Serum No Effect Analytical No significant effect observed at a concentration up to 4 g/L with enzymatic methods of Merck, Wako and PAP and MPA methods of Boehringer Mannheim and on manual Fuller's earth method *6375*

Cefsulodin

Creatinine *Serum No Effect Analytical* At up to 1,000 µg/mL on Technicon SMAC® Jaffe method *5729*

Ceftazidime

Alanine Aminopeptidase *Urine Increase Physiological* Significant increase in association with reduced GFR *96*

Alanine Aminotransferase *Serum Increase Physiological* During clinical trials slight increases in activity were observed in 1 in 15 treated patients *5658* Laboratory changes noted during clinical trials are usually mild and transient but increased enzyme activity occurred in 1 of 15 patients *1709* Slight increase in activity observed in 1 of 15 treated patients *2154*

Alkaline Phosphatase *Serum Increase Physiological* Laboratory changes noted during clinical trials are usually mild and transient but increased enzyme activity occurred in 1 of 23 patients *1709* Slight increase in activity observed in 1 of 23 treated patients *2154* During clinical trials slight increases in activity were observed in 1 in 23 treated patients *5658*

Amino Acids *Urine No Effect Analytical* Negative reaction observed with ninhydrin in paper chromatography, paper electrophoresis and ion-exchange chromatography *4761*

Aspartate Aminotransferase *Serum Increase Physiological* During clinical trials slight increases in activity were observed in 1 in 16 treated patients *5658* Slight increase in activity observed in 1 of 16 treated patients *2154* Laboratory changes noted during clinical trials are usually mild and transient but increased enzyme activity occurred in 1 of 16 patients *1709*

Bilirubin *Serum Increase Physiological* Laboratory changes noted during clinical trials are usually mild and transient but increased concentration was observed occasionally *1709*
Serum No Effect Analytical At concentrations up to 1000 mg/L no significant effects observed on DPD method on Hitachi 717 analyzer or on method on Kodak Ektachem® analyzer *4695*

Coombs' Test *Blood Positive Physiological* Laboratory changes noted during clinical trials are usually mild and transient but positive Coombs' test without hemolysis occurred in 1 of 23 patients *1709* During clinical trials positive Coombs' tests without hemolysis were observed in 1 in 23 treated patients *5658* Positive test without hemolysis observed in 1 of 23 treated patients *2154*

Coombs' Test, Direct *Blood Positive Physiological* Acute intravascular hemolysis observed in 1 woman within 5 days of beginning course of ceftazidime. Direct test became strongly positive with both anti-IgG and anticomplement *955*

Creatinine *Serum Increase Physiological* Effect noted in 3 patients given high doses in relation to their renal function *95* During clinical trials transient increases were observed occasionally *5658* Laboratory changes noted during clinical trials are usually mild and transient but increased concentration was observed occasionally *1709* Transient increases in concentration observed in some treated patients *2154*
Serum No Effect Analytical No effect at concentrations up to 250 mg/L on Abbott Vision *4219* No effect on Jaffe methods *3299* No effect at concentrations up to 250 mg/L on Kodak DT-60. No effect at concentrations up to 250 mg/L on Ames Seralyzer *4219* No effect at concentration of 1000 mg/L with Jaffe procedures on IL Monarch, Technicon SMAC® , or Serono Centrifichem or enzymatic Boehringer Mannheim creatinine PAP kit, Wako creatinine B or Kodak Ektachem® methods *2302*
Serum No Effect Physiological Unchanged in most patients with GFR above 30 mL/min *96*

Eosinophils *Blood Increase Physiological* During clinical trials eosinophilia was observed in 1 in 13 treated patients *5658* Laboratory changes noted during clinical trials are usually mild and transient but eosinophilia occurred in 1 of 13 patients *1709* Eosinophilia observed in 1 of 13 treated patients *2154*

Erythrocytes *Blood Decrease Physiological* Rare cases (fewer than 1%) of hemolytic anemia reported *2154*

Factor VII *Plasma No Effect Physiological* In 30 patients with serious infections *63*

Glomerular Filtration Rate *Urine Decrease Physiological* Slight but significant reduction after 3 g daily i.v. in 15 patients for 4 to 9 d *4328* Decreased by mean of 10 mL/min with 4 g drµg/d in 16 patients: initial GFR in patients 30 to 110 mL/min *96*

Glucose *Urine Increase Analytical* May give false positive Clinitest® or positive reaction with Fehling's or Benedict's solutions *2157* *2154* May cause false positive reactions with Fehling's and Benedict's reactions and Clinitest® tablets *5658* False positive tests for glucose by Benedict's, Fehling's or Clinitest methods have been reported with cephalosporins *1709*
Urine No Effect Analytical Does not interfere with tests based on enzymatic glucose oxidase reactions such as Clinistix® or TesTape® *5658* Has no effect on TesTape® or Clinistix® reactions *2157* *2154* Dark green-black color with Clinitest® but no effect or slight reduction with glucose concentrations of 1% and up. Concentrations measured accurately by Diastix® . Concentrations measured accurately by TesTape® *3446*

γ-Glutamyltransferase *Serum Increase Physiological* During clinical trials slight increases in activity were observed in 1 in 19 treated patients *5658* Laboratory changes noted during clinical trials are usually mild and transient but increased enzyme activity occurred in 1 of 19 patients *1709* Slight increase in activity observed in 1 of 19 treated patients *2154*

Granulocytes *Blood Decrease Physiological* During clinical trials transient decreases were observed very rarely *5658* Laboratory changes noted during clinical trials are usually mild and transient but agranulocytosis was observed very rarely *1709*

Hematocrit *Blood Decrease Physiological* Rare cases (fewer than 1%) of hemolytic anemia reported *2154* Laboratory changes noted during clinical trials are usually mild and transient but aplastic anemia, hemolytic anemia and hemorrhage have been reported *1709*

Hemoglobin *Blood Decrease Physiological* Rare cases (fewer than 1%) of hemolytic anemia reported *2154* Laboratory changes noted during clinical trials are usually mild and transient but aplastic anemia, hemolytic anemia and hemorrhage have been reported *1709*

Ketone Body Ratio *Serum No Effect Analytical* When added at a concentration of 450 mg/L had no significant effect on AKBR method of Uno et al *6131*

Lactate Dehydrogenase *Serum Increase Physiological* During clinical trials slight increases in activity were observed in 1 in 18 treated patients *5658* Laboratory changes noted during clinical trials are usually mild and transient but increased enzyme activity occurred in 1 of 18 patients *1709* Slight increase in activity observed in 1 of 18 treated patients *2154*

Leukocytes *Blood Decrease Physiological* During clinical trials transient decreases were observed very rarely *5658* Observed in 0.6% of patients receiving drug *4327* Laboratory changes noted during clinical trials are usually mild and tran-

Ceftazidime *(continued)*

Leukocytes *(continued)*
sient but leukopenia was observed very rarely *1709* Transient decreases in concentration observed very rarely in some treated patients *2154*

Lymphocytes *Blood Increase Physiological* Transient increases in concentration very rarely observed in some treated patients *2154* Laboratory changes noted during clinical trials are usually mild and transient but lymphocytosis was observed very rarely *1709* During clinical trials transient increases were observed very rarely *5658*

β_2-Microglobulin *Serum No Effect Physiological* Unchanged in most patients with GFR above 30 mL/min *96*
Urine No Effect Physiological No effect on proximal tubular function in 15 patients given 3 g daily for 4-9 d *4328* Unchanged in most patients with GFR above 30 mL/min *96*

Neutrophils *Blood Decrease Physiological* During clinical trials transient decreases were observed very rarely *5658* Transient decreases in concentration very rarely observed in some treated patients *2154* Laboratory changes noted during clinical trials are usually mild and transient but neutropenia was observed very rarely *1709*

Platelets *Blood Decrease Physiological* During clinical trials thrombocytopenia was observed in 1 in 45 treated patients *5658* Laboratory changes noted during clinical trials are usually mild and transient but thrombocytopenia occurred in 1 of 45 patients *1709* Thrombocytopenia observed in 1 of 45 treated patients *2154*

Protein *Cerebrospinal Fluid No Effect Analytical* At concentration of 80 mg/L on SDS/Coomassie method of Huang *2745*
Urine No Effect Analytical No effect of 1 g/L on sulfosalicylic acid and Albustix methods *3927*

Prothrombin Time *Plasma Increase Physiological* Laboratory changes noted during clinical trials are usually mild and transient but prolonged prothrombin time has been reported *1709*
Plasma No Effect Physiological In 30 patients with serious infections *63*

Salicylate *Serum No Effect Analytical* No interference observed with method on Du Pont aca *6671*

Sugar *Urine Increase Analytical* Reacts positively with Clinitest *4761*

Tobramycin *Serum No Effect Physiological* No significant effect observed in either normal or anephric patients when ceftazidime coadministered. No effect observed on clearance of tobramycin although 25% in volume of distribution at steady state *249*

Urea Nitrogen *Serum Increase Physiological* Transient increases in concentration observed in some treated patients *2154* During clinical trials transient increases were observed occasionally *5658* Laboratory changes noted during clinical trials are usually mild and transient but increased concentration was observed occasionally *1709*

Ceftibuten

Alanine Aminotransferase *Serum Increase Physiological* May cause increased activity in 1% treated patients *5326*

Alkaline Phosphatase *Serum Increase Physiological* May cause increased activity in fewer than 1% treated patients *5326*

Aspartate Aminotransferase *Serum Increase Physiological* May cause increased activity in fewer than 1% treated patients *5326*

Bilirubin *Serum Increase Physiological* May cause increased concentration in 1% treated patients *5326*

Creatinine *Serum Increase Physiological* May cause increased concentration in fewer than 1% treated patients *5326*

Eosinophils *Blood Increase Physiological* May cause eosinophilia in 3% treated patients *5326*

Hemoglobin *Blood Decrease Physiological* May cause decreased concentration in 2% treated patients *5326*

Leukocytes *Blood Decrease Physiological* May cause decreased concentration in fewer than 1% treated patients *5326*

Platelets *Blood Decrease Physiological* May cause decreased concentration in fewer than 1% treated patients *5326*
Blood Increase Physiological May cause increased concentration in fewer than 1% treated patients *5326*

Urea Nitrogen *Serum Increase Physiological* May cause increased concentration in 4% treated patients *5326*

Ceftizoxime

Alanine Aminotransferase *Serum Increase Physiological* In children 6 months of age or older treatment with ceftizoxime has been associated with transient increases in enzyme activity *1986*

Alkaline Phosphatase *Serum Increase Physiological* Treatment with ceftizoxime has been associated with transient increases in enzyme activity in between 1% and 5% of all patients *1986* In 4 of 110 patients: reversible hepatotoxicity noted *1616* In 3 of 30 patients following colorectal surgery had transient 2 to 3-fold increase *3744*

Aspartate Aminotransferase *Serum Increase Physiological* In 4 of 110 patients: reversible hepatotoxicity noted *1616* In 3 of 30 patients following colorectal surgery had transient 2 to 3-fold Increase *3744* In children 6 months of age or older treatment with ceftizoxime has been associated with transient increases in enzyme activity *1986*

Bilirubin *Serum Increase Physiological* In 3 of 30 patients following colorectal surgery had transient 2 to 3-fold increase *3744* Treatment with ceftizoxime has been associated with rare increases in concentration *1986*
Serum No Effect Analytical At concentrations up to 1000 mg/L no significant effect observed on DPD method on Hitachi 717 analyzer or on method on Kodak Ektachem® analyzer *4695*

Cefotetan *Serum Increase Analytical* Cannot be assayed by HPLC method in use at Mayo Clinic in presence of ceftizoxime *3858*

Coombs' Test *Blood Positive Physiological* Treatment with ceftizoxime has been associated with positive Coombs' test in between 1% and 5% of all patients *1986*

Creatine Kinase *Serum Increase Physiological* In children 6 months of age or older treatment with ceftizoxime has been associated with transient increases in enzyme activity, possibly related to intramuscular administration *1986*

Creatinine *Serum Increase Physiological* Treatment with ceftizoxime has been associated with occasional transient increases in concentration *1986*
Serum No Effect Analytical No effect at concentration of 1000 mg/L on Jaffe methods on IL Monarch, Technicon SMAC® , Serono Centrifichem or enzymatic methods of Boehringer Mannheim creatinine PAP, Wako creatinine B or Kodak Ektachem® *2302*

Eosinophils *Blood Increase Physiological* In children 6 months of age or older treatment with ceftizoxime has been associated with transient eosinophilia. Also observed in between 1% and 5% of treated adults *1986*

Erythrocytes *Blood Decrease Physiological* Treatment with ceftizoxime has been associated with anemia, including hemolytic anemia in less than 1% of all patients *1986*

Glucose *Urine No Effect Analytical* Dark green-black color with Clinitest® but no effect or slight reduction with glucose concentrations of 1% and up. Concentrations measured accurately by Diastix® . Concentrations measured accurately by TesTape® *3446*

Hematocrit *Blood Decrease Physiological* Treatment with ceftizoxime has been associated with anemia, including hemolytic anemia in less than 1% of all patients *1986*

Hemoglobin *Blood Decrease Physiological* Treatment with ceftizoxime has been associated with anemia, including hemolytic anemia in less than 1% of all patients *1986*

Leukocytes *Blood Decrease Physiological* Treatment with ceftizoxime has been associated with leukopenia in less than 1% of all patients *1986*

Neutrophils *Blood Decrease Physiological* Treatment with ceftizoxime has been associated with neutropenia in less than 1% of all patients *1986*

Platelets *Blood Decrease Physiological* Treatment with ceftizoxime has been associated with transient decreases in concentration in between 1% and 5% of all patients *1986*

Protein *Urine No Effect Analytical* No effect of 1 g/L on sulfosalicylic acid and Albustix methods *3927*

Urea Nitrogen *Serum Increase Physiological* Treatment with ceftizoxime has been associated with occasional transient increases in concentration *1986*

Ceftriaxone

Alanine Aminotransferase *Serum Increase Physiological* Ceftriaxone reported to increase ALT activity in 3.3% of patients to whom it is administered *5010*

Alkaline Phosphatase *Serum Increase Physiological* Ceftriaxone reported to increase alkaline phosphatase activity in less than 1% of patients to whom it is administered *5010*

Amino Acids *Urine No Effect Analytical* Negative reaction observed with ninhydrin in paper chromatography, paper electrophoresis and ion-exchange chromatography *4761*

Aspartate Aminotransferase *Serum Increase Physiological* Ceftriaxone reported to increase AST activity in 3.1% of patients to whom it is administered *5010*

Basophils *Blood No Effect Physiological* Ceftriaxone reported to cause basophilia in less than 0.1% of patients to whom it is administered *5010*

Bilirubin *Serum Increase Physiological* Ceftriaxone reported to increase bilirubin concentration in less than 1% of patients to whom it is administered *5010*

Serum No Effect Analytical At concentrations up to 1000 mg/L no significant effect observed on DPD method on Hitachi 717 or method on Kodak Ektachem® analyzers *4695* On method on Eppendorf Epos at concentration of 2.50 mmol/L *2351*

Serum No Effect Physiological In 14 children with sickle cell disease given ceftriaxone (50 mg/kg body weight) intravenously for an average of 3.9 times each no increase in bilirubin concentration observed after 24 hours *6456*

Blood *Urine No Effect Physiological* Ceftriaxone reported to cause hematuria in less than 0.1% of patients to whom it is administered *5010*

Casts *Urine Increase Physiological* Ceftriaxone reported to increase the presence of urinary casts in less than 1% of patients to whom it is administered *5010*

Ceftriaxone *Serum Increase Physiological* In 14 children with sickle cell disease treated over a mean of 3.9 episodes serum concentrations ranged from 96 to 268 mg/L 2 h after administration and 2.7 to 17.5 mg/L 24 h after administration after a single intravenous dose of 50 mg/kg body weight *6456*

Cholesterol *Serum No Effect Analytical* On method on Eppendorf Epos at concentration of 2.50 mmol/L *2351*

Clindamycin *Serum Positive Analytical* Interferes with bioassays because cannot be inactivated *3858*

Colistin *Serum Positive Analytical* Interferes with bioassays because cannot be inactivated *3858*

Creatinine *Serum Increase Physiological* Ceftriaxone reported to increase plasma creatinine concentration in less than 1% of patients to whom it is administered *5010*

Serum No Effect Analytical On Jaffe method at concentration of 2.50 mmol/L *2351*

Eosinophils *Blood Increase Physiological* Ceftriaxone reported to cause eosinophillia in 6% of patients to whom it is administered *5010*

Erythrocytes *Urine No Effect Physiological* Ceftriaxone reported to cause hematuria in less than 0.1% of patients to whom it is administered *5010*

Erythromycin *Serum Increase Analytical* Interferes with bioassays because cannot be inactivated *3858*

Factor VII *Plasma Decrease Physiological* In 30 patients with serious infections possibly due to presence of sulfhydryl group *63*

Glucose *Urine No Effect Analytical* Dark green-black color with Clinitest® but no effect or slight reduction with glucose concentrations of 1% and up. Concentrations measured accurately by Diastix® . Concentrations measured accurately by TesTape® *3446*

Urine No Effect Physiological Ceftriaxone reported to cause glycosuria in less than 0.1% of patients to whom it is administered *5010*

Hematocrit *Blood Decrease Physiological* Ceftriaxone reported to cause anemia or hemolytic anemia in less than 1% of patients to whom it is administered *5010*

Hemoglobin *Blood Decrease Physiological* Ceftriaxone reported to cause anemia or hemolytic anemia in less than 1% of patients to whom it is administered *5010*

Interleukin-6 *Serum Decrease Physiological* In 38 children aged 6 months to 14 years with typhoid salmonellosis mean concentration decreased with treatment with intravenous ceftriaxone or oral cefixime from 449 pg/mL to 67 pg/mL after 7 days and 40 pg/mL after 14 days *543*

Iron *Serum No Effect Analytical* No interference observed with method on Kodak Ektachem® *2792*

Lactate *Plasma No Effect Analytical* No effect at final concentration of 200 µg/mL on method on Kodak Ektachem® *2793*

Leukocytes *Blood Decrease Physiological* Ceftriaxone reported to cause leukopenia in 2.1% of patients to whom it is administered *5010* Reported to occur in fewer than 0.1% patients *4327*

Blood No Effect Physiological Ceftriaxone reported to cause leukocytosis in less than 0.1% of patients to whom it is administered *5010*

Lymphocytes *Blood Decrease Physiological* Ceftriaxone reported to cause lymphopenia in less than 1% of patients to whom it is administered *5010*

Blood No Effect Physiological Ceftriaxone reported to cause lymphocytosis in less than 0.1% of patients to whom it is administered *5010*

Metronidazole *Serum Increase Analytical* Interferes with bioassays because cannot be inactivated *3858*

Monocytes *Blood No Effect Physiological* Ceftriaxone reported to cause monocytosis in less than 0.1% of patients to whom it is administered *5010*

Neutrophils *Blood Decrease Physiological* Ceftriaxone reported to cause neutropenia in less than 1% of patients to whom it is administered *5010*

Phenytoin, Free *Serum Increase Physiological* In one patient, while free phenytoin concentration predicted to be 3.4 µmol/L, measured concentration actually 4.0 µmol/L due to displacement of phenytoin from protein *1242*

Platelets *Blood Decrease Physiological* Ceftriaxone reported to cause thrombocytopenia in less than 1% of patients to whom it is administered *5010*

Blood Increase Physiological Ceftriaxone reported to cause thrombocytosis in 5.1% of patients to whom it is administered *5010*

Polymyxin *Serum Increase Analytical* Interferes with bioassays because cannot be inactivated *3858*

Protein *Cerebrospinal Fluid No Effect Analytical* No effect observed at concentration of 20 µg/mL on method on Kodak Ektachem® *2791* At concentration of 150 mg/L on SDS/Coomassie Blue method of Huang *2745*

Serum No Effect Analytical On method on Eppendorf Epos at concentration of 2.50 mmol/L *2351*

Urine No Effect Analytical No effect at 1 g/L on sulfosalicylic acid and Albustix methods *3927*

Prothrombin Time *Plasma Decrease Physiological* Ceftriaxone reported to decrease prothrombin time in less than 0.1% of patients to whom it is administered *5010*

Plasma Increase Physiological Hypoprothrombinemia is very rare adverse event *1384* In 30 patients with serious infections possibly due to presence of sulfhydryl group *63* Ceftriaxone reported to prolong prothrombin time in less than 1% of patients to whom it is administered. Associated with impaired vitamin K synthesis or low vitamin K stores *5010*

Salicylate *Serum Increase Analytical* On Du Pont aca significant increase observed in one patient with concentration of 76.5 mg/dL observed compared with 2.7 mg/dL on Abbott TDx due to drug forming purple color with ferric nitrate at acidic pH with similar absorbance maximum as salicylate *6671*

Sugar *Urine Increase Analytical* Reacts positively with Clinites *4761*

Tetracycline *Serum Increase Analytical* Interferes with bioassays because cannot be inactivated *3858*

Ceftriaxone *(continued)*

Trimethoprim *Serum Increase Analytical* Interferes with bioassays because cannot be inactivated *3858*

Tumor Necrosis Factor-α *Serum No Effect Physiological* In 38 children aged 6 months to 14 years with typhoid salmonellosis mean concentration changed insignificantly with treatment with intravenous ceftriaxone or oral cefixime from 31 pg/mL to 27 pg/mL after 7 days *543*

Urea Nitrogen *Serum Increase Physiological* Ceftriaxone reported to increase serum urea nitrogen concentration in 1.2% of patients to whom it is administered *5010*
Serum No Effect Analytical On method on Eppendorf Epos at concentration of 2.50 mmol/L *2351*

Uric Acid *Serum No Effect Analytical* On method on Eppendorf Epos at concentration of 2.50 mmol/L *2351*

Valproic Acid, Free *Serum Increase Physiological* At low concentrations of albumin statistically significant increase in concentration of free valproic acid observed at therapeutic concentration of ceftriaxone *1241*

Cefuroxime

Alanine Aminotransferase *Serum Increase Physiological* Transient increases have been reported in 1 of 25 patients *1693* Transient increases reported in 1-2% treated patients *1384* In multiple-dose dosing regimens as part of clinical trials transient increases in activities observed in 1.6% patients *2153* Observed in 24% of 89 patients in one study, but many had pre-existing liver problems *4327*

Alkaline Phosphatase *Serum Increase Physiological* Transient increases have been reported in 1 of 50 patients *1693*

Amino Acids *Urine No Effect Analytical* Negative reaction observed with ninhydrin in paper chromatography, paper electrophoresis and ion-exchange chromatography *4761*

Aspartate Aminotransferase *Serum Increase Physiological* In multiple-dose dosing regimens as part of clinical trials transient increases in activities observed in 2.0% patients *2153* Transient increases observed in 1-2% patients *1384* Transient increases have been reported in 1 of 25 patients *1693* Observed in 24% of 89 patients in one study, but many had pre-existing liver problems *4327*

Bilirubin *Serum Increase Physiological* Transient increases have been reported in 1 of 500 patients *1693*
Serum No Effect Analytical On method on Eppendorf Epos at concentration of 2.50 mmol/L *2351* At concentrations of 1000 mg/L no significant effect observed on DPD method on Hitachi 717 or method on Kodak Ektachem® analyzers *4695*

Blood *Urine Increase Physiological* With single dose of 1 g may cause bleeding and/or pain in urethra in between 0.1% and 1% patients *2153*

Carbenicillin *Serum Increase Analytical* Cannot be assayed by HPLC method used at Mayo Clinic in presence of cefuroxime *3858*

Cholesterol *Serum No Effect Analytical* On method on Eppendorf Epos at concentration of 2.50 mmol/L *2351*

Clindamycin *Serum Positive Analytical* Interferes with bioassays because cannot be inactivated *3858*

Colistin *Serum Positive Analytical* Interferes with bioassays because cannot be inactivated *3858*

Coombs' Test *Blood Positive Physiological* Positive Coombs' test reported in 0.4% treated patients *1384*

Coombs' Test, Direct *Blood Positive Physiological* With multiple doses positive direct Coombs' test may be observed *2153*

Creatinine *Serum Decrease Analytical* At concentration of 1000 mg/L reduced concentration as determined by enzymatic Boehringer Mannheim creatinine PAP method by 11%, Wako creatinine B method by 11% and Kodak Ektachem® method by 10% but no effect demonstrated at therapeutic concentrations *2302*
Serum Increase Analytical At concentration of 1000 mg/L increased results as determined by Jaffe methods on IL Monarch, Technicon SMAC® , and Serono Centrifichem by less than 10% and no effect observed at therapeutic concentrations *2302* Significant increase in concentrations with Jaffe methods of Beckman and Merck at concentrations as low as 0.5 g/L and with manual Fuller's earth method at concentrations above 2.0 g/L *6375* Interference of up to 800% observed with certain alkaline picrate methods *2301*
Serum Increase Physiological Mean change from 112 to 137 µmol/L in 3 patients with chronic osteomyelitis over over 14 d when lysine salt used *6073* Increases have been reported but their relationship to cefuroxime administration is unknown *1693*
Serum No Effect Analytical No analytical interference observed with methods using alkaline picrate *2153* On Jaffe method at concentration of 2.50 mmol/L *2351* Has no effect on methods using alkaline picrate methods *2170* No effect observed on alkaline picrate procedures *1693* No significant effect observed at concentrations up to 4 g/L with enzymatic methods of Merck, Wako, and PAP and MPA methods of Boehringer Mannheim and up to 2.0 g/L with manual Fuller's earth method *6375*
Urine No Effect Analytical No effect observed on alkaline picrate procedures *1693* Has no effect on methods using alkaline picrate methods *2170* No analytical interference observed with methods using alkaline picrate *2153*

Creatinine Clearance *Urine Decrease Physiological* Decreases have been reported but their relationship to cefuroxime administration is unknown *1693*

Eosinophils *Blood Increase Physiological* In multiple-dose dosing regimens as part of clinical trials transient eosinophilia observed in 1.1% patients *2153* Transient eosinophilia observed in 1 of 14 treated patients *1693*

Erythromycin *Serum Increase Analytical* Interferes with bioassays because cannot be inactivated *3858*

Glucose *Serum Decrease Analytical* False negative test may be observed when ferricyanide methods used to measure glucose *2170* False negative reaction may occur with ferricyanide based reactions *2153*
Serum Increase Analytical False positive reaction may be given ferricyanide procedures *1693*
Serum No Effect Analytical No effect observed when hexokinase or glucose oxidase methods used to measure glucose *2170* No analytical interference observed with glucose oxidase or hexokinase based reactions *2153*
Urine Increase Analytical False positive reaction may be given with Fehling's and Benedict's solutions and Clinitest® *1693* False positive reaction may occur with copper reduction methods (Benedict's and Fehling's) or with Clinitest® *2170* False positive reaction may occur with Fehling's solution or Benedict's test or with Clinitest® *2153*
Urine No Effect Analytical No effect observed with enzyme based reactions, e.g. Clinistix® or Tes-Tape® *2153* No effect observed on Tes-Tape® method *1693* No effect observed when TesTape® used to measure glucose *2170*

Granulocytes *Blood Decrease Physiological* Agranulocytosis has been observed, as has hemolysis, aplastic anemia, pancytopenia and thrombocytopenia in treated patients *1693*

Hematocrit *Blood Decrease Physiological* Decrease observed in 1 of 10 treated patients *1693*

Hemoglobin *Blood Decrease Physiological* Decrease observed in 1 of 10 treated patients *1693*

Iron *Serum No Effect Analytical* No interference observed up to a concentration of 300 µg/mL with method on Kodak Ektachem® 700 *2590*

Lactate *Plasma No Effect Analytical* No effect at final concentration of 150 µg/mL on method on Kodak Ektachem® *2793*

Lactate Dehydrogenase *Serum Increase Physiological* In multiple-dose dosing regimens as part of clinical trials transient increases in activities observed in 1.0% patients *2153* Transient increases observed in 1-2% treated patients *1384* Transient increases have been reported in 1 of 75 patients *1693*

Leukocytes *Blood Decrease Physiological* In one case who developed drug-dependent neutrophil antibodies *4183* Transient leukopenia observed in 1 of 750 treated patients *1693*

Metronidazole *Serum Increase Analytical* Interferes with bioassays because cannot be inactivated *3858*

β_2-Microglobulin *Serum Increase Physiological* Mean change from 4,000 to 6,000 µg/L in 3 patients with chronic osteomyelitis over 14 d when lysine salt used *6073*

Neutrophils *Blood Decrease Physiological* Transient neutropenia observed in 1 of 100 treated patients *1693* In one case who developed drug-dependent neutrophil antibodies *4183*

Platelets *Blood Decrease Physiological* Agranulocytosis has been observed, as has hemolysis, aplastic anemia, pancytopenia and thrombocytopenia in treated patients *1693*

Polymyxin *Serum Increase Analytical* Interferes with bioassays because cannot be inactivated *3858*

Protein *Cerebrospinal Fluid No Effect Analytical* At concentration of 40 mg/L on SDS/Coomassie Blue method of Huang *2745* No effect observed at final concentration of 10 µg/mL with method on Kodak Ektachem® *2791*

Serum No Effect Analytical On method on Eppendorf Epos at concentration of 2.50 mmol/L *2351*

Prothrombin Time *Plasma Increase Physiological* Prolonged prothrombin time has been reported in some patients *1693*

Salicylate *Serum No Effect Analytical* No interference observed with method on Du Pont aca *6671*

Sugar *Urine Increase Analytical* Reacts positively with Clinitest *4761*

Tetracycline *Serum Increase Analytical* Interferes with bioassays because cannot be inactivated *3858*

Trimethoprim *Serum Increase Analytical* Intereferes with bioassays because cannot be inactivated *3858*

Urea Nitrogen *Serum Increase Physiological* Increases have been reported but their relationship to cefuroxime administration is unknown *1693*

Serum No Effect Analytical On method on Eppendorf Epos at concentration of 2.50 mmol/L *2351*

Uric Acid *Serum No Effect Analytical* On method on Eppendorf Epos at concentration of 2.50 mmol/L *2351*

Cefuzonam

Ketone Body Ratio *Serum No Effect Analytical* When added at a concentration of 300 mg/L had no significant effect on AKBR method of Uno et al *6131*

Celiprolol

Cholesterol *Serum Decrease Physiological* Significant reduction observed in hypertensive patients with serum cholesterol concentrations initially greater than 220 mg/dL when treated with 400 mg/d for 1 year *1901* Slight reduction of concentration over 6 weeks in over 15000 patients with essential hypertension *2576*

Serum No Effect Physiological Insignificant effect in about 20 mild to moderately hypertensive men treated with 400 mg/day for 2 years *1899* In patients with hyperlipoproteinemia types IIa, IIb or IV with 300 mg drug for 4 weeks *4789*

Effective Renal Plasma Flow

Patient Increase Physiological In 13 healthy men administration of a single oral dose of 200 mg caused a mean increase of 11.0 ± 5.3% in the fasting state *639*

Glomerular Filtration Rate *Urine Increase Physiological* In 13 healthy men administration of a single oral dose of 200 mg caused a nonsignificant mean increase of 3.9 ± 4.2% in the fasting state *639*

HDL-Cholesterol *Serum Increase Physiological* Significant increase observed in hypertensive patients with serum cholesterol concentrations initially greater than 220 mg/dL when treated with 400 mg/d for one year *1901* From 42 to 54 mg/dL in patients with hyperlipoproteinemia types IIa, IIb or IV with 300 mg drug for 4 weeks *4789* Increase by 8-14% in about 20 mild to moderate hypertensively men treated with 400 mg/day for 2 years *1899*

LDL-Cholesterol *Serum Decrease Physiological* Progressive reduction with time observed in hypertensive patients with serum cholesterol concentrations initially greater than 220 mg/dL when treated with 400 mg/d for one year *1901*

Serum Increase Physiological Effect slight in patients with hyperlipoproteinemia types IIa, IIb, or IV with 300 mg drug for 4 weeks *4789*

Serum No Effect Physiological Insignificant effect of treatment with 400 mg/day for 2 years in about 20 mild to moderately hypertensive men *1899*

Platelet Aggregation *Blood Decrease Physiological* In 21 patients with non-treated essential hypertension treatment with 300 mg/d for 1 week significant reduction in epinephrine-induced aggregation (from 19 to 13%) and ADP-induced aggregation (15 to 13%) observed *4395*

β-Thromboglobulin *Plasma Decrease Physiological* Non-significant reduction from mean baseline of 180 µg/L to 166 µg/L observed in 21 hospitalized patients with untreated essential hypertension treated with 300 mg/d for 1 week *4395*

Triglycerides *Serum Decrease Physiological* Slight reduction over 6 weeks in over 15000 patients with essential hypertension *2576* Reduction by 14-21% in about 20 mild to moderately hypertensive men treated with 400 mg/day for 2 years *1899* Significant reduction observed in hypertensive patients with serum cholesterol concentrations initially greater than 220 mg/dL when treated with 400 mg/d for one year *1901* In patients with hyperlipoproteinemia types IIa, IIb or IV with 300 mg drug for 4 weeks *4789*

Cellulose

Cholesterol *Serum Decrease Physiological* Observed in young girls with 100 g/d *2523*

Cellulose Phosphate

Calcium *Serum Increase Physiological* Without changing calcium balance *4483*

Urine Decrease Physiological By impairing absorption decreases output *4483* As result of decreased gastrointestinal absorption *4482*

Citrate *Urine Decrease Physiological* Observed in 3 of 5 cases *4482*

Copper *Serum No Effect Physiological* No significant effect observed *4482*

Urine No Effect Physiological No significant effect observed *4482*

Creatinine Clearance *Urine No Effect Physiological* No significant effect observed *4482*

Parathyroid Hormone *Plasma No Effect Physiological* In patients with absorptive hypercalciuria *4483*

Phosphate *Urine Increase Physiological* With decrease of activity product ratio *4482*

Potassium *Serum No Effect Physiological* No significant effect observed *4482*

Sodium *Serum No Effect Physiological* With decrease of activity product ratio *4482*

Zinc *Serum No Effect Physiological* With decrease of activity product ratio *4482*

Urine No Effect Physiological No significant effect observed *4482*

Cephalexin

Alanine Aminotransferase *Serum Increase Physiological* Transient hepatitis and cholestatic jaundice reported as a complication *1438 1699*

Alkaline Phosphatase *Serum Increase Physiological* Transient hepatitis and cholestatic jaundice reported as a complication *1699*

Amino Acids *Urine Increase Analytical* Reacts with ninhydrin in paper chromatography, paper electrophoresis and ion-exchange chromatography *4761* Reacts with ninhydrin; extra spot with TLC, high voltage electrophoresis *4760* Yellow spot with ninhydrin on thin-layer chromatography *2109*

Aspartate Aminotransferase *Serum Increase Physiological* Transient hepatitis and cholestatic jaundice reported as a complication *1699 1438*

Bicarbonate *Serum Increase Physiological* If given with gentamicin to leukemics *6614*

Cephalexin *(continued)*

Coombs' Test, Direct *Blood Positive Physiological* Incidence low *1772* Positive tests have been reported during administration of cephalosporins *1699 1438*

Creatinine *Serum Increase Analytical* At concentration of 1000 mg/L caused increase of 48-54% with Jaffe methods on Instrumentation Laboratory Monarch, 71% with method on Technicon SMAC® and 32% with method on Serono Centrifichem. Changes not significant at therapeutic concentration *2302* At concentration of 1000 mg/L caused increase of 48-54% with Jaffe methods on Instrumentation Laboratory Monarch, 71% with method on Technicon SMAC® and 32% with method on Serono Centrifichem. Changes not significant at therapeutic concentration *2302*
Serum Increase Physiological Increased serum concentration reported as complication of treatment *1699*
Serum No Effect Analytical No effect of concentrations up to 15 mg/L on single slide method on Kodak Ektachem® *5706* No effect at concentration of 25 mg/dL (720 µmol/L) on method on Du Pont Dimension *1572* No interference observed at a concentration of 25 mg/dL (7.2 mmol/L) with method on Du Pont aca *1520* At 1000 mg/L interference of less than 10% with enzymatic Boehringer Mannheim creatinine PAP method and Wako creatinine B methods, negative interference of 10% with method on Kodak Ektachem® but no effect on any method at therapeutic concentrations *2302* No effect of concentrations up to 500 mg/L on 2-slide method on Kodak Ektachem® *5706*

Eosinophils *Blood Increase Physiological* Occasional eosinophilia reported *1438* In 16% of 74 patients all children given 25-150 mg/kg/d for 5 to 15 d *4142* Allergic response *4691* Occasional eosinophilia reported *1699*

Glucose *Urine Increase Analytical* Positive tests with Benedict's and Fehling's solutions and Clinitest® have been reported during administration of cephalosporins *1699* Positive tests with Benedict's and Fehling's solutions have been reported during administration of cephalosporins *1438*
Urine No Effect Analytical No effect on TesTape® *2794* At concentration of 10,000 mg/L had no effect on Diabur-test *5704* No false positive reactions with Tes-Tape® have been reported during administration of cephalosporins *1699 1438*

Histamine *Plasma No Effect Analytical* No effect at therapeutic concentrations on radio-enzyme assay *2492*

Leukocytes *Blood Decrease Physiological* Leukopenia reported as a complication *1699* In 12% of 74 patients all children given 25-150 mg/kg/d for 5 to 15 d *4142*
Urine Decrease Analytical May cause decreased test results with leukocyte test area of Ames Multistix and other reagent test strips *4034*

Neutrophils *Blood Decrease Physiological* Occasional neutropenia reported as a complication *1699* Agranulocytosis reported to occur occasionally *6264* Occasional neutropenia reported as a complication *1438*
Blood No Effect Physiological In 74 patients all children given 25-150 mg/kg/d for 5 to 15 d *4142*

Platelets *Blood Decrease Physiological* Occasional thrombocytopenia reported as a complication *1438 1699*

Potassium *Serum Decrease Physiological* If given with gentamicin to leukemics *6614*

Prothrombin Time *Plasma Increase Physiological* Increased prothrombin time reported as a complication *1699*

Sugar *Urine Increase Analytical* False positive with Benedict's, Fehlings, Clinitest® *2794* Reacts positively with Clinitest *4761*

Theophylline *Serum No Effect Physiological* No effect observed on half-life *1384*

Urea Nitrogen *Serum Increase Physiological* Increased serum concentration reported as complication of treatment *1699*

Cephaloglycin

Alanine Aminotransferase *Serum Increase Physiological* Slight elevation reported *2754*

Aspartate Aminotransferase *Serum Increase Physiological* Slight elevation reported *2754*

Coombs' Test *Blood Positive Physiological* Rare observed side effect *198*

Creatinine *Serum No Effect Analytical* No effect of concentrations up to 15 mg/L on single slide method on Kodak Ektachem® *5706*

Eosinophils *Blood Increase Physiological* Allergic response *2754*

Glucose *Urine No Effect Analytical* No effect on TesTape® *2754*

Neutrophils *Blood Decrease Physiological* Neutropenia reported *2754*

Protein *Urine Increase Physiological* Of cephalosporins one of most likely to cause nephrotoxicity *4327*

Sugar *Urine Increase Analytical* Affects Benedict's, Fehlings, Clinitest® *2754*

Cephaloridine

Alanine Aminotransferase *Serum Increase Physiological* Transient slight rise ?hepatotoxicity *1695*

Alkaline Phosphatase *Serum Increase Physiological* Mechanism not listed *2451*

Aspartate Aminotransferase *Serum Increase Physiological* Transient slight rise ?hepatotoxicity *1695*

Bilirubin *Serum No Effect Analytical* At 2.50 mmol/L on method on Eppendorf Epos *2351*

Casts *Urine Increase Physiological* Nephrotoxicity (hyaline and granular) *1695*

Cholesterol *Serum No Effect Analytical* At 2.50 mmol/L on method on Eppendorf Epos *2351*

Coombs' Test, Direct *Blood Positive Physiological* No immunological response (complex binds to cell in 8% cases) *2453*

Creatinine *Serum Increase Analytical* Pronounced interference with alkaline picrate based reactions *2351* Linear correlation between drug concentration and analyte concentration as measured by Jaffe method *2351*
Serum Increase Physiological Nephrotoxic especially if combined with diuretic *4691*
Serum No Effect Analytical No significant interference observed at a concentration of 25 mg/dL (6.0 mmol/L) with method on Du Pont aca *1520* No effect of concentrations up to 15 mg/L on single slide method on Kodak Ektachem® *5706* No effect of concentrations up to 500 mg/L on 2-slide method on Kodak Ektachem® *5706* No effect at concentration of 25 mg/dL (602 µmol/L) on method on Du Pont Dimension *1572*

Eosinophils *Blood Increase Physiological* May be up to 10% in 1% people *1695*

Erythrocytes *Blood Decrease Physiological* May cause anemia *128*

Glucose *Urine No Effect Analytical* No effect observed with TesTape® *1695*

Hematocrit *Blood Decrease Physiological* May cause anemia *128*

Hemoglobin *Blood Decrease Physiological* May cause anemia *128*

17-Ketogenic Steroids *Urine Increase Analytical* On day of administration - method of Wilson and Lipsett *2913*

17-Ketosteroids *Urine Increase Analytical* On day of administration with Zimmermann reaction *2913*

Leukocytes *Blood Decrease Physiological* May cause neutropenia/Leukopenia *1695*

Nonprotein Nitrogen *Serum Increase Physiological* Nephrotoxic especially if combined with diuretic *4691*

Potassium *Serum Increase Physiological* May occur with nephrotoxicity *3810*

Protein *Serum No Effect Analytical* At 2.50 mmol/L on method on Eppendorf Epos *2351*
Urine Increase Analytical Affects acid turbidimetric procedures *882* Precipitate occurs with sulfosalicylic acid. Weak positive with Albustix at high concentrations *3546*
Urine Increase Physiological Of cephalosporins one of most likely to produce nephrotoxicity *4327* May be result of nephrotoxicity *2614*

Prothrombin Time *Plasma Increase Physiological* Reported effect *128*

Sugar *Urine Increase Analytical* Abnormal dark color with Benedict's and Clinitest® *1825*

Urea Nitrogen *Serum Increase Physiological* High doses, nephrotoxicity reported *139*
Serum No Effect Analytical At 2.50 mmol/L on method on Eppendorf Epos *2351*

Uric Acid *Serum No Effect Analytical* At 2.50 mmol/L on method on Eppendorf Epos *2351*

Volume *Urine Decrease Physiological* Suggestive of nephrotoxicity *1695*

Cephalosporin C

Histamine *Plasma No Effect Analytical* No inhibition of radio-enzyme assay at therapeutic concentrations *2492*

Cephalosporins

Alanine Aminotransferase *Serum Increase Physiological* Observed with all cephalosporins at frequency of from 1 to 7% *4327*

Alkaline Phosphatase *Serum Increase Physiological* Observed with all cephalosporins at frequency of from 1 to 7% *4327*

Antithrombin III *Plasma No Effect Analytical* At concentration of 30 mg/L had no effect on Du Pont aca method *5704*

Aspartate Aminotransferase *Serum Increase Physiological* Observed with all cephalosporins at frequency of from 1 to 7% *4327*

Clindamycin *Serum No Effect Analytical* If inactivated most cephalosporins do not interfere with bioassay procedure *3858*

Colistin *Serum No Effect Analytical* If inactivated most cephalosporins do not interfere with bioassay procedures *3858*

Coombs' Test, Direct *Blood Positive Physiological* Approximately 3% incidence, immunologic effect *2452*

Eosinophils *Blood Increase Physiological* In about 4% patients treated with drugs *4327*

Erythromycin *Serum No Effect Analytical* If inactivated most cephalosporins do not intefere with bioassay procedures *3858*

Glucose *Urine Increase Analytical* May cause false positive or atypical reaction with Ames Clinitest tablet procedure *4034*
Urine No Effect Analytical Have no effect on Ames Keto-Diastix, Diastix, Multistix and Clinistix methods *4034*

Metronidazole *Serum No Effect Analytical* If inactivated most cephalosporins do not interfere with bioassay procedures *3858*

Plasminogen *Plasma No Effect Analytical* At concentration of 30 mg/L had no effect on Du Pont aca method *5704*

Polymyxin *Serum No Effect Analytical* If inactivated most cephalosporins do not intefere with bioassay procedures *3858*

Potassium *Serum No Effect Analytical* At concentration of 100 mg/L had no effect on ISE measurement with predilution *5704*

Pramipexole *Serum No Effect Physiological* Coadministration of cephalosporins with pramipexole presumed to have no effect on the oral clearance of pramipexole *4680*

Prothrombin Time *Plasma Increase Physiological* Second and third generation cephalosporins increase prothrombin time when coadministered with warfarin through inhibition of cyclic interconversion of vitamin K *2625*

Sodium *Serum No Effect Analytical* At concentration of 100 mg/L had no effect on ISE measurement with predilution *5704*

Tetracycline *Serum No Effect Analytical* If inactivated most cephalosporins do not interfere with bioassay procedures *3858*

Trimethoprim *Serum No Effect Analytical* If inactivated most cephalosporins do not interfere with bioassay procedures *3858*

Cephalothin

Alanine Aminotransferase *Serum Increase Physiological* Single case reported *4014*
Serum No Effect Analytical At 5 times upper limit of therapeutic range on methods on Technicon SMAC® , Abbott-VP, aca, Roche Cobas-Bio and KDA *3525*

Albumin *Serum No Effect Analytical* At concentration of 1,000 mg/L had no effect on BCG method *5704* At 5 times upper limit of therapeutic range on methods on Technicon SMAC® , Kodak Ektachem® , Hitachi® 705 and KDA *3525*

Alkaline Phosphatase *Serum No Effect Analytical* At 5 times upper limit of therapeutic range on methods on Technicon SMAC® , Abbott-VP, Du pont aca, Roche Cobas-Bio, Hitachi® 705 and KDA *3525*

Amikacin *Serum No Effect Analytical* No interference observed at a concentration of 500 µg/mL (1261 µmol/L) with method on Du Pont aca *1508*

Amylase *Serum No Effect Analytical* At 5 times upper limit of therapeutic range on methods on Du Pont aca, Roche Cobas-Bio and Kodak Ektachem® *3525*

Aspartate Aminotransferase *Serum Increase Physiological* Transient rise reported *2754*
Serum No Effect Analytical At 5 times upper limit of therapeutic range on methods on Technicon SMAC® , Abbott-VP, Du Pont aca, Roche Cobas-Bio, Hitachi® 705 and KDA *3525*

Azlocillin *Serum Increase Analytical* Cannot be assayed by HPLC method used at Mayo Clinic in presence of cephalothin *3858*

Bicarbonate *Serum No Effect Analytical* At concentration of 1,000 mg/L had no effect on method using phenolphthalein *5704*

Bilirubin *Serum Increase Physiological* May cause hemolytic anemia *2284*
Serum No Effect Analytical No effect a 2.50 mmol/L on method on Eppendorf Epos *2351* At concentration of 1,000 mg/L had no effect on Jendrassik and Grof method *5704* At 5 times upper limit of therapeutic range on methods on Technicon SMAC® , Du Pont aca, Roche Cobas-Bio, Kodak Ektachem® , Hitachi® 705 and KDA *3525*
Serum No Effect Physiological Clinically insignificant displacement from protein in neonates *6314*

Bilirubin, Conjugated *Serum No Effect Analytical* No effect at concentration of 500 mg/L on method on Kodak Ektachem® *5706*

Bilirubin, Direct *Serum Increase Physiological* May cause hemolytic anemia *2284*

Bilirubin, Unconjugated *Serum No Effect Analytical* No effect at concentration of 500 mg/L on method on Kodak Ektachem® *5706*

Calcium *Serum No Effect Analytical* At 5 times upper limit of therapeutic range on methods on Technicon SMAC® , Abbott-VP, Du Pont aca, Kodak Ektachem® , Hitachi® 705 and KDA *3525* At concentration of 1,000 mg/L had no effect on cresolphthalein method *5704* No effect of concentrations up to 500 mg/L with method on Kodak Ektachem® *5706*

Cefamandole *Serum Increase Analytical* Cannot be assayed by HPLC method used at Mayo Clinic in presence of cephalothin *3858*

Cefoperazone *Serum Increase Analytical* Cannot be assayed by HPLC method used at Mayo Clinic in presence of cephalothin *3858*

Cephalexin *Serum Increase Analytical* Cannot be assayed by HPLC method used at Mayo Clinic in presence of cephalothin *3858*

Chloride *Serum No Effect Analytical* At concentration of 1,000 mg/L had no effect on mercurimetric method *5704*

Cholesterol *Serum No Effect Analytical* At 5 times upper limit of therapeutic range on methods on Technicon SMAC® , Abbott-VP, Roche Cobas-Bio, Kodak Ektachem® , Hitachi® 705 and KDA *3525* No effect at concentrations up to 500 mg/L on method on Kodak Ektachem® *5706* At concentration of 1,000 mg/L had no effect on CHOD-PAP method *5704* No effect a 2.50 mmol/L on method on Eppendorf Epos *2351*

Coombs' Test, Direct *Blood Positive Physiological* Nonimmunologic phenomenon, complex binds to cell *2453*

Cortisol *Plasma No Effect Physiological* No physiological effect *2913*

Cephalothin *(continued)*

Creatine Kinase *Serum No Effect Analytical* At 5 times upper limit of therapeutic range on methods on Technicon SMAC® , Abbott-VP, Du Pont aca, Roche Cobas-Bio and Hitachi® 705 *3525*

Creatine Kinase Isoenzymes *Serum No Effect Analytical* No interference observed at a concentration of 1000 mg/L (2.52 mmol/L) with CK-MB method on Du Pont aca *1519*

Creatinine *Serum Decrease Analytical* At concentration of 1000 mg/L caused 14% reduction with Boehringer Mannheim enzymatic creatinine PAP method, 14% with enzymatic Wako creatinine B method and 12% with Kodak Ektachem® method. No interference observed at therapeutic concentrations *2302* At concentration of 100 mg/dL (25.2 mmol/L) decreases concentration by 20-25% with method used on Du Pont aca *1520* Positive interference with kinetic Jaffe reactions in first 45 s, thereafter negative effect with reduced concentration *3300* As measured by Du Pont aca due to decrease of absorbance of product with picrate with time *3300*

Serum Increase Analytical Dose related interference with Jaffe procedure on Greiner selective analyzer *110* Pronounced interference with alkaline picrate based reactions *2351* Concentration related increase when Jaffe method used *2351* Marked effect at therapeutic concentrations on Jaffe type procedures but substantially greater on Beckman Astra® 8 (by 162 µmol/L) than on Technicon SMAC® II because of earlier reaction reading time. Discrepancy not observed with other cephalosporins *2589* At concentrations above 100 mg/L (normal therapeutic concentration 17 mg/L) raised concentration as measured by kinetic Jaffe method on BKA-2 *5704* Interference of up to 200% observed with certain alkaline picrate methods *2301* At concentration of 1000 mg/L caused 131-220% increase with Jaffe methods on IL Monarch, 28% increase with Technicon SMAC® , and 80% increase with method on a Serono Centrifichem. Significant interference also observed at therapeutic concentration *2302* At concentrations above 500 mg/L (normal therapeutic concentration 17 mg/L) raised concentration as measured by Technicon AutoAnalyzer® Jaffe method *5704* Significant increase in concentrations as measured by Jaffe methods of Beckman and Merck at concentrations as low as 0.5 g/L and with manual Fuller's earth method at concentrations above 1.0 g/L *6375* At 5 times upper limit of therapeutic range on methods on Technicon SMAC® , Abbott-VP, Roche Cobas-Bio and Hitachi® 705 *3525*

Serum Increase Physiological High rate of nephrotoxicity observed with combined with aminoglycosides, more than when other drugs given with aminoglycosides *6287*

Serum No Effect Analytical At concentration of 1,000 mg/L had no effect on kinetic Jaffe method on Du Pont aca *5704* No effect at concentration of 100 mg/dL (2.5 mmol/L) on method on Du Pont Dimension *1572* No effect of concentrations up to 1200 mg/L on 2-slide method on Kodak Ektachem® *5706* No effect of concentrations up to 15 mg/L on single slide method on Kodak Ektachem® *5706* At 5 times upper limit of therapeutic range on methods on Du Pont aca, Kodak Ektachem® and KDA *3525* No significant effect observed at concentrations up to 4 g/L with enzymatic methods of Merck, Wako and PAP and MPA methods of Boehringer Mannheim and up to 1.0 g/L with manual Fuller's earth method *6375* No interference observed at a concentration of 10 mg/L with HPLC method of Rosano et al *5083*

Urine Increase Analytical Dose related interference with Jaffe procedure on Greiner selective analyzer *110*

Creatinine Clearance *Urine Decrease Analytical* If Jaffe procedure used and plasma concentration of drug is near peak; values low if drug concentration low *110*

Eosinophils *Blood Increase Physiological* Modest increase with prolonged high dose i.v. administration *5222* Allergic response *4001*

Erythrocyte Sedimentation Rate
Blood Increase Physiological With high doses and prolonged i.v. administration *5222*

Erythrocytes *Blood Decrease Physiological* Hemolytic anemia *2285*

Gentamicin *Serum No Effect Analytical* No interference observed at concentrations up to 500 µg/mL (1261 µmol/L) with method on Du Pont aca *1526*

Glucose *Serum No Effect Analytical* At 5 times upper limit of therapeutic range on methods on Technicon SMAC® , Abbott-VP, Du pont aca, Roche Cobas-Bio, Kodak Ektachem® , Hitachi® 705 and KDA *3525* At concentration of 1,000 mg/L had no effect on GOD/POD-PAP method *5704* At concentration of 1046 mg/L had no effect on glucose dehydrogenase method *5704*

γ-Glutamyltransferase *Serum No Effect Analytical* At 5 times upper limit of therapeutic range on methods on Technicon SMAC® , Abbott-VP, and Hitachi® 705 *3525*

Hematocrit *Blood Decrease Physiological* Hemolytic anemia *2285*

Hemoglobin *Blood Decrease Physiological* Coombs' positive hemolytic anemia *2285*

Histamine *Plasma No Effect Analytical* No inhibition of radio-enzyme assay at therapeutic concentrations *2492*

17-Hydroxycorticosteroids *Urine Increase Analytical* 5 mg/L reacted as if 7.2 mg/L: effect eliminated if Allen correction used *1775*

Iron *Serum No Effect Analytical* At 5 times upper limit of therapeutic range on methods on Ferrozine method on Technicon SMAC® *3525*

17-Ketogenic Steroids *Urine Increase Analytical* Non specificity of method of Wilson and Lipsett *2913*

17-Ketosteroids *Plasma Increase Analytical* Marked effect on Zimmermann procedure with 6 g dose *3141*

Urine Increase Analytical Non specificity of Zimmermann reaction on day of administration *2913* Marked effect on Zimmermann procedure with 6 g dose *3141*

Lactate Dehydrogenase *Serum No Effect Analytical* At 5 times upper limit of therapeutic range on methods on Technicon SMAC® , Abbott-VP, Roche Cobas-Bio, Hitachi® 705 and KDA *3525*

Leukocytes *Blood Decrease Physiological* Marked decrease in one case after prolonged high i.v. doses *5222* In 2 patients given 12 g daily intravenously *2686* Rare response to therapy *3810*

Blood Increase Physiological Due to eosinophilia of hypersensitivity *3810*

Urine Decrease Analytical May cause decreased test results with leukocyte test area of Ames Multistix and other reagent strip tests *4034*

Lymphocytes *Blood No Effect Physiological* In 2 patients given 12 g daily intravenously *2686*

Neutrophils *Blood Decrease Physiological* Neutropenia or leukopenia rare *129* Occasional count below 500 /µL observed *4327*

Phosphate *Serum No Effect Analytical* At 5 times upper limit of therapeutic range on methods on Technicon SMAC® , Du Pont aca, Hitachi® 705 and KDA *3525* At concentration of 1,000 mg/L had no effect on phosphomolybdate method *5704*

Platelets *Blood Decrease Physiological* Increased resistance to osmotic fragility *4013*

Potassium *Serum No Effect Analytical* At concentration of 1,000 mg/L had no effect on flame-photometric method *5704*

Protein *Serum Increase Analytical* At concentrations above 500 mg/L (normal therapeutic concentration 17 mg/L) raised concentration as measured by biuret method with blank correction *5704*

Serum No Effect Analytical At 5 times upper limit of therapeutic range on methods on Technicon SMAC® , Abbott-VP, Kodak Ektachem® , Hitachi® 705 and KDA *3525* No effect at 2.50 mmol/L on method on Eppendorf Epos *2351*

Urine Increase Analytical Precipitate occurs with sulfosalicylic acid. Weak positive with Albustix at high concentrations *3546* Affects acid turbidimetric procedures *882*

Urine Increase Physiological Rare effect following i.v. infusion *4014*

Urine No Effect Analytical No effect of 1 g/L on sulfosalicylic acid and Albustix methods *3927*

Sodium *Serum No Effect Analytical* At concentration of 1,000 mg/L had no effect on flame-photometric method *5704*

Sugar *Urine Increase Analytical* Brown-black color with Clinitest® (false positive) *193* False positive with copper reduction procedures *5869*

Theophylline *Serum Increase Analytical* Interference may be observed with some HPLC methods *5999*

Tobramycin *Serum No Effect Analytical* At concentrations less than 1000 μg/mL (2.52 mmol/L) no significant effect observed on method on Du Pont aca *1547*

Triglycerides *Serum No Effect Analytical* At concentration of 1,000 mg/L had no effect on lipase/esterase method *5704* At 5 times upper limit of therapeutic range on methods on Technicon SMAC® , Abbott-VP, Kodak Ektachem® , Hitachi® 705 and KDA *3525*

Urea Nitrogen *Serum Increase Physiological* Rare elevation noted (possible nephrotoxicity) *1695* When given in large doses has caused tubular necrosis or when patients have had preexisting renal impairment *1384*
Serum No Effect Analytical At 5 times upper limit of therapeutic range on methods on Technicon SMAC® , Abbott-VP, Roche Cobas-Bio, Kodak Ektachem® , Hitachi® 705 and KDA *3525* No effect at 2.50 mmol/L on method on Eppendorf Epos *2351* At concentration of 1,000 mg/L had no effect on diacetylmonoxime method *5704*

Uric Acid *Serum No Effect Analytical* At 5 times upper limit of therapeutic range on methods on Technicon SMAC® , Abbott-VP, Du pont aca, Roche Cobas-Bio, Kodak Ektachem® , Hitachi® 705 and KDA *3525* At concentration of 1,000 mg/L had no effect on phosphotungstate reduction method *5704* No effect a 2.50 mmol/L on method on Eppendorf Epos *2351*

Cephapirin

Ampicillin *Serum Positive Analytical* Cannot be assayed by HPLC method used at Mayo Clinic in presence of cephapirin *3858*

Cefaclor *Serum Increase Analytical* Cannot be assayed by HPLC method used at Mayo Clinic in presence of cephapirin *3858*

Cefazolin *Serum Increase Analytical* Cannot be assayed by HPLC method used at Mayo Clinic in presence of cephapirin *3858*

Cephradine *Serum Increase Analytical* Cannot be assayed by HPLC method used at Mayo Clinic in presence of cephrapirin *3858*

Creatinine *Serum No Effect Analytical* At concentration of 1,000 mg/L had no effect on kinetic Jaffe method on Du Pont aca *5704* No significant interference observed at a concentration of 25 mg/dL (5.6 mmol/L) with method on Du Pont aca *1520* No effect at concentration of 25 mg/dL (562 μmol/L) on method on Du Pont Dimension *1572* At concentration of 100 mg/L had no effect on kinetic Jaff'e method on BKA-2 *5704* At concentration of 1,000 mg/L had no effect on Technicon AutoAnalyzer® Jaffe method *5704* No effect of concentrations up to 500 mg/L on 2-slide method on Kodak Ektachem® *5706*

Eosinophils *Blood Increase Physiological* Modest increase with prolonged high dose i.v. administration *5222*

Erythrocyte Sedimentation Rate
Blood Increase Physiological With high doses and prolonged i.v. administration *5222*

Leukocytes *Blood Decrease Physiological* Marked decrease in one case with prolonged high i.v. doses *5222*

Neutrophils *Blood Decrease Physiological* Occasional count of below 500 /μL reported *4327*

Cephradine

Amino Acids *Urine Increase Analytical* Reacts with ninhydrin in paper chromatography, paper electrophoresis and ion-exchange chromatography *4761*

Chloramphenicol *Serum No Effect Analytical* No effect at 100 mg/L on coupled enzymatic method *4122*

Creatinine *Serum Decrease Analytical* At concentration of 1000 mg/L reduced concentrations as determined by enzymatic Boehringer Mannheim creatinine PAP method by 16%, Wako creatinine B method by 10% and Kodak Ektachem® by 12% but no effect at therapeutic concentrations *2302*
Serum Increase Analytical Increased concentrations observed when cephradine at a concentration of 0.13 mg/mL added to serum when concentrations measured by Jaffe reaction. Effect of order of 0.3 mg/dL with Beckman CX_5, 0.2 mg/dL with Synchron CX_3 and 0.3 mg/dL with Hitachi 737 *2533* Significant increase in concentrations as measured by Jaffe methods of Beckman and Merck at concentrations as low as 0.5 g/L and on manual Fuller's earth method at 0.5 g/L and above *6375* At concentration of 1000 mg/L increased results obtained by Jaffe methods on IL Monarch by 52-73%, on Technicon SMAC® by 60% and by Serono Centrifichem by 38% but no effect at therapeutic concentrations *2302* Increased concentrations observed when cephradine at a concentration of 0.13 mg/mL added to serum when concentrations measured by Jaffe reaction. Effect of order of 0.3 mg/dL with Beckman CX5, 0.2 mg/dL with Synchron CX3 and 0.3 mg/dL with Hitachi 737 *2533*
Serum No Effect Analytical No significant interference observed at concentrations up to 2.0 mg/mL when Boehringer Mannheim PAP adapted for use with Beckman Synchron CX_5*2533* No significant interference observed at concentrations up to 2.0 mg/mL when Boehringer Mannheim PAP adapted for use with Beckman Synchron CX5 *2533* No significant interference observed at a concentration of 25 mg/dL (7.1 mmol/L) with method on Du Pont aca *1520* No effect of concentrations up to 15 mg/L on single slide method on Kodak Ektachem® *5706* No significant effect observed at concentrations up to 4 g/L with enzymatic methods of Merck, Wako and PAP and MPA methods of Boehringer Mannheim and with manual Fuller's earth method at concentrations up to 0.5 g/L *6375* No effect at concentration of 25 mg/dL (769 μmol/L) on method on Du Pont Dimension *1572*

Eosinophils *Blood Increase Physiological* In 28% of 86 children given 25-110 mg/kg daily orally for 5 to 15 d *4142*

Leukoagglutinins *Serum Positive Physiological* In a single patient either due to a toxic effect on bone marrow or immune mediated mechanism, probably immune basis *3442*

Leukocytes *Blood Decrease Physiological* In 12% of 86 children given 25-110 mg/kg daily orally for 5 to 15 d *4142*

Lysergic Acid Diethylamide *Urine Increase Analytical* Minimum concentration that caused a positive result with EMIT method to measure LSD 580 mg/L *4968*

Neutrophils *Blood Decrease Physiological* In a single patient either due to toxic effect on bone marrow or immune-mediated *3442* In 1 of 86 children given 25-110 mg/kg daily orally for 5 to 15 d *4142*

Phenylalanine *Plasma No Effect Analytical* No interference observed with rapid quantitative whole blood method of Campbell et al using phenylalanine dehydrogenase *867*

Sugar *Urine Increase Analytical* Reacts positively with Clinitest *4761*

Cerivastatin

Alanine Aminotransferase *Serum Increase Physiological* In less than 1% of treated patients increased activity of greater than 3 times the upper limit of normal reported on two or more occasions *300*

Alkaline Phosphatase *Serum Increase Physiological* Activity increased with cholestatic jaundice, hepatitis (including chronic active hepatitis) or fatty change in the liver when cerivastatin administered *300*

Amylase *Serum Increase Physiological* Activity increased occasionally when pancreatitis develops when cerivastatin administered *300*

Aspartate Aminotransferase *Serum Increase Physiological* In less than 1% of treated patients increased activity of greater than 3 times the upper limit of normal reported on two or more occasions *300*

Bilirubin *Serum Increase Physiological* Bilirubin increased occasionally when hepatitis develops when cerivastatin administered *300*

Cortisol *Plasma No Effect Physiological* Plasma cortisol concentration not affected when cerivastatin administered *300*

Creatine Kinase *Serum Increase Physiological* Treatment with 0.3 mg/d cerivastatin caused rhabdomyolysis occasionally *300*

Digoxin *Serum No Effect Physiological* Plasma concentrations of digoxin not affected by coadministration of cerivastatin *300*

Cerivastatin *(continued)*

Factor VII *Plasma No Effect Physiological* Clotting factor VII concentration not affected when cerivastatin coadministered with warfarin *300*

HDL-Cholesterol *Serum Increase Physiological* Treatment with 0.3 mg/d in two studies of over 300 patients in each for 12 and 24 weeks caused mean 10% increase in concentration *300*

LDL-Cholesterol *Serum Decrease Physiological* Treatment with 0.3 mg/d in two studies of over 300 patients in each for 12 and 24 weeks caused mean 30% reduction in concentration *300*

Lipase *Serum Increase Physiological* Activity increased occasionally when pancreatitis develops when cerivastatin administered *300*

Prothrombin Time *Plasma No Effect Physiological* Prothrombin time not affected when cerivastatin coadministered with warfarin *300*

Sperm Count *Semen No Effect Physiological* Concentration not affected when cerivastatin administered *300*

Thyroid Stimulating Hormone
Serum No Effect Physiological Concentration not affected when cerivastatin administered *300*

Triglycerides *Serum Decrease Physiological* Treatment with 0.3 mg/d in two studies of over 300 patients in each for 12 and 24 weeks caused mean 11.5% reduction in concentration with baseline concentration of ≤200 mg/dL and of 21% with baseline > 200 mg/dL *300*

Warfarin *Plasma No Effect Physiological* Neither plasma concentrations of (R) and (S) isomers of warfarin affected by coadministration of cerivastatin *300*

Cetirizine

Alanine Aminotransferase *Serum Increase Physiological* Abnormal hepatic function, hepatitis and cholestasis reported as adverse events *4661*

Alkaline Phosphatase *Serum Increase Physiological* Abnormal hepatic function, hepatitis and cholestasis reported as adverse events *4661*

Aspartate Aminotransferase *Serum Increase Physiological* Abnormal hepatic function, hepatitis and cholestasis reported as adverse events *4661*

Azithromycin *Serum No Effect Physiological* No clinically significant interaction observed *4661*

Bilirubin *Serum Increase Physiological* Abnormal hepatic function, hepatitis and cholestasis reported as adverse events *4661*

Creatinine *Serum Increase Physiological* In foreign post-marketing studies glomerulonepritis reported as an adverse event *4661*

Erythromycin *Serum No Effect Physiological* No clinically significant interaction observed *4661*

γ-Glutamyltransferase *Serum Increase Physiological* Abnormal hepatic function, hepatitis and cholestasis reported as adverse events *4661*

Hematocrit *Blood Decrease Physiological* In foreign post-marketing studies hemolytic anemia reported as an adverse event *4661*

Hemoglobin *Blood Decrease Physiological* In foreign post-marketing studies hemolytic anemia reported as an adverse event *4661*

Ketoconazole *Serum No Effect Physiological* No clinically significant interaction observed *4661*

Occult Blood *Feces Increase Physiological* Rectal hemorrhage and hemorrhoids reported as adverse events *4661*

Platelets *Blood Decrease Physiological* In foreign post-marketing studies thrombocytopenia reported as an adverse event *4661*

Pseudoephedrine *Serum No Effect Physiological* No clinically significant interaction observed *4661*

Theophylline *Serum No Effect Physiological* No clinically significant interaction observed *4661*

Urea Nitrogen *Serum Increase Physiological* In foreign post-marketing studies glomerulonepritis reported as an adverse event *4661*

Cetrorelix

Estradiol *Plasma Decrease Physiological* Administration of 3 mg/d for 7 days beginning on cycle day 8 to 5 normal cycling women caused mean decrease to 17.9 ± 0.4% of baseline during entire period of application with nadir on cycle day 15 *5691*

Follicle Stimulating Hormone
Plasma Decrease Physiological Administration of 3 mg/d for 7 days beginning on cycle day 8 to 5 normal cycling women caused mean decrease to 58.7 ± 1.3% of baseline during entire period of application with nadir on cycle day 15 *5691*

Luteinizing Hormone *Plasma Decrease Physiological* Administration of 3 mg/d for 7 days beginning on cycle day 8 to 5 normal cycling women caused mean decrease to 16.1 ± 0.7% of baseline during entire period of application with nadir on cycle day 15 *5691*

CGS 16617

Angiotensin-converting Enzyme
Serum Decrease Physiological 50 mg daily to 8 normal volunteers caused persistent marked decrease to 5.58 nmol/L/min at 15 days and 5.38 nmol/L/min at 29 days (8 hours after drug ingestion) in 8 normal volunteers *6290* Peak inhibition between 2 and 12 h after drug intake. Reduction from 96 to 14.9 nmol/L/min with 20 mg after 12 h. After 50 mg lowest activity 4.8 nmol/L/min and after 100 mg 5.0 nmol/L/min in 9 normal volunteers. Activity still low after 3 days *6290*

Renin Activity *Plasma Increase Physiological* Significant increase in normal volunteers when treated with 50 mg daily for 29 days. On day 15 activity approximately 13 ng/mL/h 8 hours after drug ingestion and about 14 ng/mL/h 8 hours after drug on day 29 compared with about 1 ng/mL/h in control *6290*

Sodium *Urine No Effect Physiological* Excretion unchanged in 8 normal volunteers given 50 mg daily for 29 days *6290*

CGS 16949A

Aldosterone *Plasma Decrease Physiological* In 16 postmenopausal women receiving 16 mg/day for 2 weeks significant reduction in basal and ACTH-stimulated production observed. Basal concentration reduced from about 310 pmol/L to 100 pmol/L with 16 mg/day and to 180 pmol/L with 8 mg/day/for 2 weeks *1377*

Potassium *Serum No Effect Physiological* No significant change observed in 16 postmenopausal women treated with up to 16 mg daily for 12 weeks *1377*
Urine No Effect Physiological No significant effect observed in 16 women treated with up to 16 mg daily for 12 weeks *1377*

Renin Activity *Plasma Increase Physiological* Nonsignificant increase observed in 16 postmenopausal women receiving 16 mg/day for 2 weeks (mean baseline 1.13 ng/mL/h, final concentration 2.56 ng/mL/h) *1377*

Sodium *Serum No Effect Physiological* No significant change observed in 16 postmenopausal women treated with increasing doses up to 16 mg/day for 12 weeks *1377*
Urine No Effect Physiological No significant change observed in 16 postmenopausal women treated with up to 16 mg daily for 12 weeks *1377*

Charcoal

Acetylsalicylic Acid *Serum Decrease Physiological* Reduced absorption due to adsorption *6403*

Carbamazepine *Serum Decrease Physiological* Reduced absorption due to adsorption *6403*

Color *Feces Increase Analytical* Black due to ingested material *1957*

Digoxin *Serum Decrease Physiological* Reduced absorption due to adsorption *6403*

Flecainide *Serum Decrease Physiological* Effective in reducing absorption from gastrointestinal tract *1384*

Phenobarbital *Serum Decrease Physiological* In one neonate administration of activated charcoal caused marked reduction of serum concentration *6217* Reduced absorption and increased elimination rate with adsorption reducing availability *6403*

Phenylbutazone *Serum Decrease Physiological* Reduced absorption and increased elimination rate with adsorption reducing availability *6403*

Phenytoin *Serum Decrease Physiological* Reduced absorption due to adsorption *6403*

Chemotherapy

Acetyl-N-Ser-Asp-Lys-Pro *Serum Decrease Physiological* In 20 patients with acute myeloid leukemia treatment caused reduction from mean baseline of 6.79 ± 1.33 pmol/mL to 4.26 ± 1.22 pmol/mL during aplasia and 5.77 ± 1.89 pmol/mL during recovery *3602*

Alkaline Phosphatase *Serum Decrease Physiological* In 4 patients with gynecologic malignancies activity declined in two with 1,25-dihydroxy vitamin D_3 concentration after one or two courses of chemotherapy *2023*

α_2-Antiplasmin *Plasma Decrease Physiological* In 28 adult patients with AML mean concentration of 96% with chemotherapy changed to 88% after 7 days, 62% after 17 days and 93% after 31 days *945*

Antithrombin III *Plasma Decrease Physiological* In 28 adult patients with AML mean concentration of 89% with chemotherapy changed to 89% after 7 days, 67% after 17 days and 79% after 31 days *945*

Aspartic Acid *Urine Increase Physiological* In 17 patients with acute leukemia mean excretion during chemotherapy 3.38 ± 3.32 mmol/d significantly higher than 1.45 ± 1.20 mmol/d when off chemotherapy *6517*

c-erb-B_2 *Serum Decrease Physiological* In 10 patients with metastatic breast cancer who were c-erbB_2 positive, two demonstrated increases in c-erbB_2 concentration in response to treatment and eight demonstrated decreases *4924*

Serum Increase Physiological In 10 patients with metastatic breast cancer who were c-erbB_2 positive, two demonstrated increases in c-erbB_2 concentration in response to treatment and eight demonstrated decreases *4924*

CA 125 *Serum Decrease Physiological* In 25 women with ovarian carcinoma treatment with 3 courses of chemotherapy caused significant decrease *3763*

Calcitonin Gene-related Peptide

Serum Decrease Physiological In 30 patients with small cell lung carcinoma treatment with chemotherapy caused a decrease in 18 although they remained increased compared with normal controls *5342*

Calcium *Serum No Effect Physiological* In 4 patients with gynecologic malignancies concentration not appreciably changed after one or two courses of chemotherapy *2023*

Cholesterol *Serum No Effect Physiological* In 12 patients with stage I to IV non-Hodgkin's lymphoma treatment with with one cycle of intravenous cyclophosphamide, adriamycin and vincristine and prednisolone caused nonsignificant change from mean baseline of 6.1 ± 0.4 mmol/L to 6.2 ± 0.5 mmol/L *2444*

C-Reactive Protein *Serum Increase Physiological* In 28 adult patients with AML mean concentration of 6 mg/L with chemotherapy changed significantly to 16 mg/L after 7 days, 63 mg/L after 17 days and 28 mg/L after 31 days *945*

Serum No Effect Physiological In 20 patients with primary lung cancer treatment with chemotherapy for 24 days caused no significant change in concentration *1988*

Creatinine *Serum No Effect Physiological* In 4 patients with gynecologic malignancies no significant change in concentration observed after one or two courses of chemotherapy *2023*

Creatinine Clearance *Urine Decrease Physiological* In 4 patients with gynecologic malignancies gradual decrease observed in three evaluated patients after one or two courses of chemotherapy *2023*

Cystine *Plasma No Effect Physiological* In 12 patients mean concentration of 109.6 ± 30.7 μmol/L changed insignificantly to 111.2 μmol/L 6 to 10 days after treatment *1395*

24,25-Dihydroxy Vitamin D_3 *Serum Decrease Physiological* In 4 patients with gynecologic malignancies concentration fluctuated irregularly in two patients, increased in one and decreased in one *2023*

Serum Increase Physiological In 4 patients with gynecologic malignancies concentration fluctuated irregularly in two patients, increased in one and decreased in one *2023*

Serum No Effect Physiological In 4 patients with gynecologic malignancies concentration fluctuated irregularly in two patients, increased in one and decreased in one *2023*

Elastase-α_1-Proteinase Inhibitor Complex

Serum Decrease Physiological In 15 patients with chronic myelogenous leukemia anti-leukemic treatment was associated with a significant reduction in concentration *4118*

Serum Increase Physiological In 20 patients with primary lung cancer mean concentration decreased from about 200 ng/mL to about 80 ng/mL after 8 days treatment returning to about 1800 ng/mL after24 days of treatment *1988*

Eosinophils *Blood Decrease Physiological* In one patient with non-Hodgkin's lymphoma receiving chemotherapy caused significant decrease from mean baseline of about 1400 u/L to close to 0 /u/L after 2 days treatment after initial increase to about 2400 /μL on the first day of treatment *6578*

Estradiol *Plasma Decrease Physiological* Significant reduction observed in 25 women with ovarian carcinoma following 3 courses of treatment *3763*

Fibrinogen *Plasma Increase Physiological* In 28 adult patients with AML mean concentration of 2.5 g/L with chemotherapy changed significantly to 3.5 g/L after 7 days, 6.8 g/L after 17 days and 3.8 g/L after 31 days *945*

Fibrinopeptide A *Plasma Decrease Physiological* In 28 adult patients with AML mean concentration of 4.8 ng/mL with chemotherapy changed to 3.1 ng/mL after 7 days, 7.5 ng/mL after 17 days and 3.3 ng/mL after 31 days *945*

Plasma Increase Physiological In 28 adult patients with AML mean concentration of 4.8 ng/mL with chemotherapy changed to 3.1 ng/mL after 7 days, 7.5 ng/mL after 17 days and 3.3 ng/mL after 31 days *945*

Glutamic Acid *Urine Increase Physiological* In 17 patients with acute leukemia mean excretion during chemotherapy 4.52 ± 2.80 mmol/d not significantly higher than 2.96 ± 2.45 mmol/d when off chemotherapy *6517*

Glycine *Urine Increase Physiological* In 17 patients with acute leukemia mean excretion during chemotherapy 17.6 ± 11.4 mmol/d significantly higher than 10.8 ± 6.45 mmol/d when off chemotherapy *6517*

HDL-Cholesterol *Serum No Effect Physiological* In 12 patients with stage I to IV non-Hodgkin's lymphoma treatment with with one cycle of intravenous cyclophosphamide, adriamycin and vincristine and prednisolone caused nonsignificant change from mean baseline of 1.3 ± 0.2 mmol/L to 1.5 ± 0.1 mmol/L *2444*

Hemoglobin *Blood Decrease Physiological* Chemotherapy of patients with small cell carcinoma of lung produced immediate decrease in hemoglobin concentration *4059*

25-Hydroxy Vitamin D_3 *Serum Decrease Physiological* In 4 patients with gynecologic malignancies concentration fluctuated irregularly in two patients, increased in one and decreased in one *2023*

Serum Increase Physiological In 4 patients with gynecologic malignancies concentration fluctuated irregularly in two patients, increased in one and decreased in one *2023*

Serum No Effect Physiological In 4 patients with gynecologic malignancies concentration fluctuated irregularly in two patients, increased in one and decreased in one *2023*

Iron *Serum Increase Physiological* Chemotherapy of patients with small cell carcinoma of lung produced significant increase in concentration *4059*

LDL-Cholesterol *Serum No Effect Physiological* In 12 patients with stage I to IV non-Hodgkin's lymphoma treatment with with one cycle of intravenous cyclophosphamide, adriamycin and vincristine and prednisolone caused nonsignificant change from mean baseline of 4.4 ± 0.3 mmol/L to 4.3 ± 0.4 mmol/L *2444*

Leucine *Urine Increase Physiological* In 17 patients with acute leukemia mean excretion during chemotherapy 2.25 ± 4.89 mmol/d not significantly higher than 0.625 ± 0.891 mmol/d when off chemotherapy *6517*

Chemotherapy *(continued)*

Leukocytes *Blood Decrease Physiological* In 20 patients with primary lung cancer mean concentration decreased from about 6000 /μL to about 1000 /μL after 15 days *1988*
Blood Increase Physiological In 20 patients with primary lung cancer treatment treatment caused increase from nadir of about 1000 /μL reached at 15 days after treatment begun to about 5000 /μL after 24 days *1988*

Lipoprotein Lp(a) *Serum No Effect Physiological* In 12 patients with stage I to IV non-Hodgkin's lymphoma treatment with with one cycle of intravenous cyclophosphamide, adriamycin and vincristine and prednisolone caused nonsignificant change from mean baseline of 190 mg/L to 196 mg/L *2444*

Methionine *Plasma No Effect Physiological* In 12 patients after 6 to 10 days treatment mean concentration changed insignificantly from 18.5 ± 4.8 μmol/L to 24.0 ± 14.5 μmol/L *1395*
Urine Increase Physiological In 17 patients with acute leukemia mean excretion during chemotherapy 2.90 mmol/d not significantly higher than 2.07 mmol/d when off chemotherapy *6517*

Myelin Basic Protein *Serum Decrease Physiological* In one patient with non-Hodgkin's lymphoma receiving chemotherapy caused significant decrease from mean baseline of about 180 ng/mL to close to 0 ng/mL after 7 days treatment *6578*

Neuron-specific Enolase *Serum Decrease Physiological* Serum neuron specific enolase activity increased in 88% of 120 patients with SCLC but activity reduced in response to treatment. Successful outcomes were associated with lower NSE activity *1882*

Parathyroid Hormone *Plasma Increase Physiological* In 2 patients with gynecologic malignancies concentration concentration increased from baselines of 11 and 16 pg/mL to 2- or 3-times after one or two courses of chemotherapy *2023*

Phosphate *Serum No Effect Physiological* In 4 patients with gynecologic malignancies concentration not appreciably changed after one or two courses of chemotherapy *2023*

Plasminogen *Plasma Decrease Physiological* In 28 adult patients with AML mean concentration of 101% with chemotherapy changed to 89% after 7 days, 58% after 17 days and 76% after 31 days *945*

Plasminogen Activator Inhibitor
Plasma Increase Physiological In 28 adult patients with AML mean concentration of 9.3 U/mL with chemotherapy changed to 7.3 U/mL after 7 days, 18.3 U/mL after 17 days and 10.2 U/mL after 31 days *945*

Platelets *Blood Decrease Physiological* In 28 adult patients with AML mean concentration of 86 x 10^9/L with chemotherapy changed significantly to 68 x 10^9/L after 7 days, 22 x 10^9/L after 17 days and 21 x 10^9/L after 31 days *945*

Protein C *Plasma No Effect Physiological* In 28 adult patients with AML mean concentration of 94% with chemotherapy changed nonsignificantly to 81% after 7 days, 96% after 17 days and 86% after 31 days *945*

Serine *Urine Increase Physiological* In 17 patients with acute leukemia mean excretion during chemotherapy 1.56 ± 1.83 mmol/d significantly higher than 0.642 ± 0.650 mmol/d when off chemotherapy *6517*

Taurine *Plasma Decrease Physiological* In 12 patients 6 to 10 days after completing intensive cytotoxic treatment mean concentration decreased from 37.2 ± 11.6 μmol/L to 24.3 ± 6.0 μmol/L *1395*
Urine Increase Physiological In 6 patients following cytotoxic therapy mean excretion increased from 0.6 ± 0.5 μmol/mg creatinine to 1.9 ± 2.3 μmol/mg creatinine after treatment but with concentration returning to low value 2 weeks after completion of therapy *1395*

Threonine *Urine Increase Physiological* In 17 patients with acute leukemia mean excretion during chemotherapy 2.95 ± 3.25 mmol/d significantly higher than 1.06 ± 1.08 mmol/d when off chemotherapy *6517*

Thrombomodulin *Plasma Decrease Physiological* In 15 patients with chronic myelogenous leukemia significant decrease observed with anti-leukemic therapy *4118*

Tissue Plasminogen Activator Antigen
Plasma No Effect Physiological In 28 adult patients with AML mean concentration of 3.2 ng/mL with chemotherapy changed nonsignificantly to 8.1 ng/mL after 7 days, 9.3 ng/mL after 17 days and 7.8 ng/mL after 31 days *945*

Transferrin Saturation *Serum Increase Physiological* Chemotherapy of patients with small cell carcinoma of lung produced significant increase in saturation *4059*

Triglycerides *Serum No Effect Physiological* In 12 patients with stage I to IV non-Hodgkin's lymphoma treatment with with one cycle of intravenous cyclophosphamide, adriamycin and vincristine and prednisolone caused nonsignificant change from mean baseline of 2.1 ± 0.3 mmol/L to 1.9 ± 0.3 mmol/L *2444*

Urea Nitrogen *Serum Increase Physiological* In 4 patients with gynecologic malignancies gradual increases in concentration occurred in two after one or two courses of chemotherapy *2023*

Chenodiol

Alanine Aminotransferase *Serum Increase Physiological* Mild elevation usually less than 3 times normal in up to 30% patients receiving 750 mg/d *5369* Slight transient increases may be observed: clinically significant hepatic injury in 3% *5368*

Alkaline Phosphatase *Serum Increase Physiological* Mild transient elevation observed *1237* In 7.2% of 916 patients given up to 750 mg/d for 2 y *5369*
Serum No Effect Physiological After 3 mo in patients with gallstones *462*

Apolipoprotein A-I *Serum No Effect Physiological* No significant effect of 12 mo treatment in 252 patients *90*

Apolipoprotein A-II *Serum No Effect Physiological* No significant effect of 12 mo treatment in 252 patients *90*

Apolipoprotein B *Serum No Effect Physiological* No significant effect of 12 mo treatment in 252 patients *90*

Aspartate Aminotransferase *Serum Increase Physiological* Mild transient elevation observed *1237* Mild elevation usually less than 3 times normal in up to 30% patients receiving 750 mg/d *5369* Slight transient increases may be observed: clinically significant hepatic injury in 3% *5368*
Serum No Effect Physiological After 3 mo in patients with gallstones *462*

Bile Salts *Bile No Effect Physiological* No change in patients with gallstones *462*

Bilirubin *Serum Increase Physiological* In 4.9% in 916 patients given up to 750 mg/d for 2 y *5369*

BSP Retention *Serum No Effect Physiological* No effect noticed even if ICD increased *462*

Cholestanol *Serum Decrease Physiological* In one 36 year old man with cerebrotendinous xanthomatosis treatment with 0.6 g/d for 2 years caused reduction from 3.12 mg/dL to 1.96 mg/dL. When pravastatin (10 mg/d) added to regime concentration decreased to 0.92 mg/dL after 1 year *4215*

Cholesterol *Bile Decrease Physiological* In patients with gallstones, not in normals *462*
Serum Increase Physiological Increase by 10% or more in 82% of 916 patients given up to 750 mg/d for 2 y *5369* Elevation of about 10 mg/dL attributable to drug *5368* Mean increase of 20 mg/dL in 252 individuals treated for 12 mo *90*
Serum No Effect Physiological No significant change over 3 mo with treatment of gallstones *462* No significant change with 150 mg four times daily in patients with endogenous hypertriglyceridemias *905*

Creatinine *Serum No Effect Physiological* No significant effect with up to 750 mg/d in 916 patients treated for 2 y *5369*

Erythrocytes *Blood No Effect Physiological* No significant effect with up to 750 mg/d over 2 y in 916 patients *5369*
Urine No Effect Physiological No significant effect with up to 750 mg/d in 916 patients treated for 2 y *5369*

Glucose *Urine No Effect Physiological* No significant effect with up to 750 mg/d in 916 patients treated for 2 y *5369*

HDL-Cholesterol *Serum Decrease Physiological* Increase by 46% in 8 normolipemic patients receiving 16 g drug daily *3510*
Serum Increase Physiological Significant effect with 150 mg four times daily in patients with endogenous hypertriglyceridemias *905*

Serum *No Effect* *Physiological* No significant effect of 12 mo treatment in 252 patients *90*

HDL-Triglycerides *Serum* *Decrease* *Physiological* In 8 normolipemic patients receiving 1 g drug daily *3510*

Hematocrit *Blood* *No Effect* *Physiological* No significant effect with up to 750 mg/d over 2 y in 916 patients *5369*

Hemoglobin *Blood* *No Effect* *Physiological* No significant effect with up to 750 mg/d over 2 y in 916 patients *5369*
Urine *No Effect* *Physiological* No significant effect with up to 750 mg/d in 916 patients treated for 2 y *5369*

Isocitrate Dehydrogenase *Serum* *Increase* *Physiological* Slight effect in almost 30% cases *462*

LDL-Cholesterol *Serum* *Increase* *Physiological* Increase by 12.2 mg/dL in 916 patients given up to 750 mg/d for 2 y *5369*
Serum *No Effect* *Physiological* By 26% in 8 normolipemic patients receiving 16 g drug daily *3510*

LDL-Triglycerides *Serum* *Decrease* *Physiological* In 8 normolipemic patients receiving 1 g drug daily *3510*

Leukocytes *Blood* *No Effect* *Physiological* No significant effect with up to 750 mg/d over 2 y in 916 patients *5369*
Urine *No Effect* *Physiological* No significant effect with up to 750 mg/d in 916 patients treated for 2 y *5369*

β-Lipoprotein *Serum* *No Effect* *Physiological* No effect observed during treatment of gallstones *1237*

Phospholipids *Bile* *No Effect* *Physiological* No significant effect in patients with gallstones *462*

Platelets *Blood* *No Effect* *Physiological* No significant effect with up to 750 mg/d in 916 patients treated for 2 y *5369*

Protein *Urine* *No Effect* *Physiological* No significant effect with up to 750 mg/d in 916 patients treated for 2 y *5369*

Reticulocytes *Blood* *No Effect* *Physiological* No significant effect with up to 750 mg/d over 2 y in 916 patients *5369*

Triglycerides *Serum* *Decrease* *Physiological* Significant effect with 150 mg four times daily in patients with endogenous hypertriglyceridemias *905* By up to 20% in patients given 10 to 25 mg/kg body weight for 6 mo. Increase by 18.6% in 916 patients given up to 750 mg/d for 2 y *5369* Mean fall by 20 mg/dL over 3 mo *462* By 26% in 8 normolipemic patients receiving 16 g drug daily *3510*

VLDL-Cholesterol *Serum* *No Effect* *Physiological* By 26% in 8 normolipemic patients receiving 16 g drug daily *3510*

VLDL-Triglycerides *Serum* *No Effect* *Physiological* In 8 normolipemic patients receiving 1 g drug daily *3510*

Chiniofon

Alanine Aminotransferase *Serum* *Increase* *Physiological* Large doses may occasionally cause hepatic damage *2242*

Chloral Hydrate

Alanine Aminotransferase *Serum* *Increase* *Physiological* May cause liver damage *467*

Aspartate Aminotransferase *Serum* *Increase* *Physiological* May cause liver damage *467*

Bilirubin *Serum* *Increase* *Physiological* Probably nonspecific effect on cells *2467*

BSP Retention *Serum* *Increase* *Physiological* Probably nonspecific effect on cells *2467*

Catecholamines *Urine* *Increase* *Analytical* Interferes with fluorometric procedures *2451*

Chloral Hydrate *Blood* *No Effect* *Physiological* Not detectable after 1 g orally *3868*

Ethanol *Serum* *Increase* *Physiological* Coadministration increases both concentration of ethanol and trichloroethanol, the major metabolite of chloral hydrate. This metabolite inhibits ethanol metabolism *5441*

Glucose *Urine* *Decrease* *Analytical* Low with Clinistix® , Diastix® *1826*
Urine *No Effect* *Analytical* Has no effect on Ames Keto-Diastix, Diastix, Multistix, Clinistix and Clinitest procedures *4034* No effect observed with TesTape® *1826*

17-Hydroxycorticosteroids *Urine* *Increase* *Analytical* Interferes with Porter-Silber reaction *5869*

Methylmalonate *Urine* *No Effect* *Analytical* Drug has no effect on GC/MS assay which can be used to assess vitamin B_{12} deficiency *4326*

Porphyrin, Total *Urine* *Increase* *Physiological* May precipitate attack of acute porphyria *3669*

Potassium *Serum* *No Effect* *Analytical* At concentration of 200 mg/L had no effect on measurement by ISE with predilution *5704*

Prolactin *Plasma* *No Effect* *Physiological* No significant effect in response to up to 9 g/d *2352*

Protein *Urine* *Increase* *Physiological* Renal damage with high concentration: Parenchymatous renal injury in chronic intoxication *2242*

Prothrombin Time *Plasma* *Decrease* *Physiological* Accelerates rate of inactivation of coumarins *3810*
Plasma *Increase* *Physiological* Displaces anticoagulants from albumin *5674*
Plasma *No Effect* *Physiological* No significant effect noted in 10 patients on warfarin when receiving 0.5 g daily *6118*

Sodium *Serum* *No Effect* *Analytical* At concentration of 200 mg/L had no effect on measurement by ISE with predilution *5704*

Sugar *Urine* *Increase* *Analytical* Excreted as glucuronide false positive with Benedict's reagent *1714*

Trichlorethanol *Blood* *Increase* *Physiological* 1 g orally produces concentration of 1.5 mg/L *3868*

Urea Nitrogen *Serum* *Increase* *Analytical* Reacts with Nessler reagent *5869*

Uric Acid *Serum* *Increase* *Analytical* Affects phosphotungstate reduction methods *3669*

Vitamin B_{12} *Serum* *Increase* *Analytical* Falsely high values obtained with a radioimmunoassay even at very low drug concentrations *4326* Significant increase on Dual Count (Diagnostic Products) methods, both boil and no-boil *3337*
Serum *No Effect* *Analytical* No effect found on Magic (Ciba-Corning) and Combostat II (Micromedics) assays *3337*

Warfarin *Plasma* *Increase* *Physiological* TCA displaces from protein (temporary effect) *2452*

Chlorambucil

Alanine Aminotransferase *Serum* *Increase* *Physiological* Occasional hepatotoxicity reported *2242* Hepatotoxicity and jaundice with drug fever may occur as a complication of treatment *2175*

Albumin *Serum* *Increase* *Physiological* In 17 patients with severe membranous glomerulonephritis and proteinuria of more than 10 g/d treatment with prednisolone and chlorambucil on alternate months for 6 months caused significant change from mean baseline of 22.6 ± 1.5 g/L to 24.7 ± 1.8 g/L (nonsignificant) after 3 months and 29.0 ± 2.5 g/L after 6 months *785*

Aspartate Aminotransferase *Serum* *Increase* *Physiological* Hepatotoxicity and jaundice with drug fever may occur as a complication of treatment *2175* Hepatotoxicity with centrolobular necrosis *3171*

Bilirubin *Serum* *Increase* *Physiological* Hepatotoxicity with centrolobular necrosis *3171* Hepatotoxicity and jaundice with drug fever may occur as a complication of treatment *2175*

Cholesterol *Serum* *Decrease* *Physiological* In 17 patients with severe membranous glomerulonephritis and proteinuria of more than 10 g/d treatment with prednisolone and chlorambucil on alternate months for 6 months caused significant change from mean baseline of 14.2 ± 1.2 mmol/L to 12.7 ± 1.2 mmol/L after 3 months and 13.0 ± 1.5 mmol/L after 6 months *785*

Chromosomes *Test Conditions* *Abnormal* *Physiological* In lymphocytes with chronic lympholeukemia *3440*

Creatinine *Serum* *Decrease* *Physiological* In 17 patients with severe membranous glomerulonephritis and proteinuria of more than 10 g/d treatment with prednisolone and chlorambucil on alternate months for 6 months caused significant change from mean baseline of 162 ± 27 μmol/L to 138 ± 20 μmol/L after 3 months and 134 ± 18 μmol/L after 6 months *785*

Erythrocytes *Blood* *Decrease* *Physiological* Dose dependent bone marrow depression *128*

Histamine *Plasma* *No Effect* *Analytical* Improbable inhibition of radio-enzyme assay at therapeutic concentrations *2492*

Chlorambucil *(continued)*

Leukocytes *Blood Decrease Physiological* Leukopenia develops after the third week of treatment and continues for up to 10 days after the last dose but subsequently the leukocyte count usually returns to normal *1384* Neutropenia (dose related) *822*

Lymphocyte response to Phytohemagglutinin *Blood Decrease Physiological* Significant reduction with chemotherapy observed *685*

Lymphocytes *Blood Decrease Physiological* Many patients develop a slowly progressive lymphopenia during treatment *2175* Marked decrease may occur *2754*
Blood Increase Physiological Persistent lymphocytosis suggests bone marrow infiltration *2175*

Neutrophils *Blood Decrease Physiological* Severe neutropenia may be produced *2754* Many patients have some neutropenia after the third week of treatment and this may continue for up to 10 days after the last dose. Subsequently the neutrophil count usually rapidly returns to normal *2175*

Platelets *Blood Decrease Physiological* Dose dependent bone marrow depression *128* A persistently low platelet count may occur and suggests bone marrow infiltration *2175*

Protein *Serum Increase Physiological* In 17 patients with severe membranous glomerulonephritis and proteinuria of more than 10 g/d treatment with prednisolone and chlorambucil on alternate months for 6 months caused nonsignificant change from mean baseline of 44.4 ± 1.5 g/L to 46.6 ± 1.7 g/L (nonsignificant) after 3 months and 52.1 ± 2.7 g/L after 6 months *785*
Urine Decrease Physiological In 17 patients with severe membranous glomerulonephritis and proteinuria of more than 10 g/d treatment with prednisolone and chlorambucil on alternate months for 6 months caused significant change from mean baseline of 16.9 ± 2.0 g/d to 9.7 ± 1.1 g/d after 3 months and 7.8 ± 1.4 g/d after 6 months *785*

Sperm Count *Semen Decrease Physiological* Azoospermia may be observed in adult men *1384*

Triglycerides *Serum No Effect Physiological* In 17 patients with severe membranous glomerulonephritis and proteinuria of more than 10 g/d treatment with prednisolone and chlorambucil on alternate months for 6 months caused nonsignificant change from mean baseline of 4.9 ± 0.6 mmol/L to 5.1 ± 0.6 mmol/L after 3 months and 5.0 ± 0.7 mmol/L after 6 months *785*

Uric Acid *Serum Increase Physiological* Increased concentration may be observed with successful destruction of malignant cells *1384*

Chloramine

Chromosomes *Test Conditions Abnormal Physiological* Clastogenic in human lymphocyte cultures *5484*

Chloramphenicol

Acetaminophen *Serum No Effect Analytical* No effect at therapeutic concentration on o-cresol reaction based method *949*

Alanine Aminotransferase *Serum Increase Physiological* Hepatotoxic-cholestatic effect *3669*
Serum No Effect Analytical No effect at therapeutic concentration on Boehringer Mannheim Reflotron method *3231* No effect at 200 mg/L on Boehringer Mannheim Reflotron method *5706*

Alkaline Phosphatase *Serum Increase Physiological* ?Hepatotoxic-cholestatic effect *3669*

Amikacin *Serum No Effect Analytical* No interference observed at a concentration of 500 µg/mL (1547 µmol/L) with method on Du Pont aca *1508*

Amylase *Serum No Effect Analytical* At concentration of 200 mg/L had no effect on method on Boehringer Mannheim Reflotron system *5706*

Amylase, Pancreatic Isoenzyme *Serum No Effect Analytical* No significant effect observed at toxic concentration of 200 mg/L with method on Boehringer Mannheim Reflotron *3647*

Antithrombin III *Plasma No Effect Analytical* At concentration of 25 mg/L had no effect on Du Pont aca method *5704*

Aspartate Aminotransferase *Serum Increase Physiological* Hepatotoxic-cholestatic effect *3669* Isolated case of hepatitis and pancytopenia reported which resolved with discontinuation of drug *907*
Serum No Effect Analytical No effect at therapeutic concentration on Boehringer Mannheim Reflotron method *3231* No effect at 200 mg/L on Boehringer Mannheim Reflotron method *5706*

Bile *Urine Increase Physiological* Hepatotoxicity *3810*

Bilirubin *Serum Increase Physiological* Hepatotoxic-cholestatic effect *3669*
Serum No Effect Analytical At concentration of 200 mg/L had no effect on method on Boehringer Mannheim Reflotron system *5706* No effect at 50 mg/L on Ames Seralyzer method *5706*
Serum No Effect Physiological Clinically insignificant displacement from protein in neonates *6314*

BSP Retention *Serum Increase Physiological* Hepatotoxicity *3669*

Chlorpropamide *Serum Increase Physiological* Half-life of chlorpropamide prolonged to 100 hours in one patient in whom drugs coadministered *4636* Drugs that are highly protein-bound compete with chlorpropamide for binding sites and may potentiate hypoglycemic action of sulfonylurea *4644* Inhibits hepatic microsomal metabolizing enzymes thus prolonging half-life *6498*

Cholesterol *Serum No Effect Analytical* At concentration of 600 mg/L had no effect on catalase-AIDH method *5704* No effect at therapeutic concentration on Boehringer Mannheim Reflotron method *3231* At concentration of 600 mg/L had no effect on method using catalase-Hantzsch reaction *5704* At concentration of 600 mg/L had no effect on Liebermann-Burchard method *5704* At concentration of 600 mg/L had no effect on CHOD-Iodide method *5704* At concentration of 600 mg/L had no effect on CHOD-PAP method *5704* At concentration of 200 mg/L no effect on method on Boehringer Mannheim Reflotron system *5706* No effect at 50 mg/L on Ames Seralyzer method *5706*
Serum No Effect Physiological No effect seen even when administration orally *2452*

Cholinesterase *Serum No Effect Analytical* No effect observed at concentration of 25 mg/dL with butyrylthiocholine method on Kodak Ektachem® *2504*

Chromosomes *Test Conditions No Effect Physiological* Not clastogenic in human cells *5484*

Clindamycin *Serum Positive Analytical* Interferes with bioassays *3858*

Cloxacillin *Serum Increase Analytical* Cannot be assayed by HPLC method in use at Mayo Clinic in presence of chloramphenicol *3858*

Colistin *Serum Positive Analytical* Interferes with bioassays *3858*

Color *Feces Increase Analytical* Blue color reported with chloramphenicol ingestion *3388*

Cortisol *Plasma No Effect Analytical* At a concentration of 200 mg/L no significant effect observed on CEDIA method *1097*

Creatine Kinase *Serum No Effect Analytical* No effect at 50 mg/L on method on Ames Seralyzer *5706*

Creatinine *Serum No Effect Analytical* At concentration of 20 mg/L had no effect on creatinine iminohydrolase method *5704* At concentration of 600 mg/L had no effect on Jaffe-Fading-Fraction method *5704* At concentration of 100 mg/L had no effect on kinetic Jaffe method on BKA-2 *5704* No effect at 50 mg/L on Ames Seralyzer method *5706*

Cyclosporine *Blood No Effect Analytical* At a concentration of 250 mg/L had no effect on Syva EMIT method *495*

Dicumarol *Plasma Increase Physiological* Inhibits hepatic microsomal metabolizing enzymes thus prolonging half-life *6498* Half-life increased 2-4 times in four patients treated with dicumarol in one study, possibly by inhibiting hepatic microsomal enzymes although effect could also be related to decreased gut flora producing less vitamin K *1005*

Eosinophils *Blood Increase Physiological* Occasional hypersensitivity reaction occurs *6498* Allergic reaction *2484*

Erythrocytes *Blood Decrease Physiological* Occurs either as dose-related or idiosyncratic bone marrow suppression: dose- related usually occurs 5-7 d after start of therapy: idiosyncratic reaction is rare occurring 1 case per 40,000 courses of therapy *6498* Aplastic anemia reported to occur in from 1 to 10,000 or 40,000 cases *6264* Dose related response usual/aplastic anemia *1429* Most severe complications, sometimes fatal, are aplastic anemia, hypoplastic anemia, thrombocytopenia and granulocytopenia *4520*

Erythromycin *Serum Increase Analytical* Interferes with bioassays *3858*

Folate *Serum Decrease Analytical* Inhibits growth of *L. casei5870*

Gentamicin *Serum No Effect Analytical* No interference observed at concentrations up to 500 µg/mL (1547 µmol/L) with method on Du Pont aca *1526*

Glucose *Serum Decrease Physiological* Reported effect *192*
Serum No Effect Analytical No effect at therapeutic concentration on Boehringer Mannheim Reflotron method *3231* At concentration of 400 mg/L had no effect on hexokinase/G-6-PDH method *5704* At concentration of 100 mg/L had no effect on Kodak Ektachem® method *5704* No effect at 50 mg/L on glucose oxidase method on Ames Seralyzer *5706* At concentration of 3,000 mg/L had no effect on GOD/POD-PAP method *5704* At concentration of 200 mg/L no effect on method on Boehringer Mannheim Reflotron system *5706*
Urine No Effect Analytical At concentration of 400 mg/L had no effect on Diabur-test *5704*

γ-Glutamyltransferase *Serum Increase Physiological* Isolated case of hepatitis and pancytopenia reported, which resolved with discontinuation of drug *907*
Serum No Effect Analytical At concentration of 200 mg/L no effect on method on Boehringer Mannheim Reflotron system *5706* No effect at therapeutic concentration on Boehringer Mannheim Reflotron method *3231*

Granulocytes *Blood Decrease Physiological* Most severe complications, sometimes fatal, are aplastic anemia, hypoplastic anemia, thrombocytopenia and granulocytopenia *4520*

HDL-Cholesterol *Serum No Effect Analytical* At a concentration up to 200 mg/L had no significant effect on Reflotron method for whole blood cholesterol *6352*

Hematocrit *Blood Decrease Physiological* Normally slight response: may be pancytopenia *1429* Most severe complications, sometimes fatal, are aplastic anemia, hypoplastic anemia, thrombocytopenia and granulocytopenia *4520*

Hemoglobin *Blood Decrease Physiological* Normally slight response: may be pancytopenia *1429* Isolated cases of hepatitis and pancytopenia reported which resolved with discontinuation of drug *907* Most severe complications, sometimes fatal, are aplastic anemia, hypoplastic anemia, thrombocytopenia and granulocytopenia *4520*

Histamine *Plasma No Effect Analytical* No inhibition of radio-enzyme assay at therapeutic concentrations *2492*

17-Hydroxycorticosteroids *Urine No Effect Analytical* No effect on modified Reddy procedure *2452*

Iron *Serum Increase Physiological* Occurs either as dose-related or idiosyncratic bone marrow suppression: dose-related usually occurs 5-7 d after start of therapy: idiosyncratic reaction is rare occurring 1 case per 40,000 courses of therapy *6498* Reversible toxic reaction *4691*
Serum No Effect Analytical At concentration of 5,000 mg/L had no effect on Ferrozine method *5704* No interference observed with method on Kodak Ektachem® *2792*

Iron-Binding Capacity, Total
Serum Decrease Physiological Decreased uptake by erythroid tissue *3669*

17-Ketosteroids *Urine Increase Analytical* Affects some methods but not modified Reddy method *2451*

Lactate *Plasma No Effect Analytical* No effect at final concentration of 20 µg/mL on method on Kodak Ektachem® *2793* At concentration of 400 mg/L had no effect on enzymatic method *5704*

Lactate Dehydrogenase *Serum Increase Physiological* Isolated case of hepatitis and pancytopenia reported which resolved with discontinuation of drug *907*
Serum No Effect Analytical No effect at 50 mg/L on method on Ames Seralyzer *5706*

Leukocytes *Blood Decrease Physiological* Isolated case of hepatitis and pancytopenia reported which resolved with discontinuation of drug *907* Pancytopenia/aplastic anemia *1429* Occurs either as dose-related or idiosyncratic bone marrow suppression: dose- related usually occurs 5-7 d after start of therapy: idiosyncratic reaction is rare occurring in one case per 40,000 courses of therapy *6498* Aplastic anemia reported to occur in from 1 to 10,000 or 40,000 cases *6264* Most severe complications, sometimes fatal, are aplastic anemia, hypoplastic anemia, thrombocytopenia and granulocytopenia *4520*
Blood Increase Physiological Leukemia may occur as sequel to marrow depression *128*

Methemoglobin *Blood Increase Physiological* May cause hemolysis in G-6-PD deficiency *6015*

Methotrexate *Serum Decrease Physiological* Concomitant administration of chloramphenicol may decrease absorption of methotrexate *2818*

Metronidazole *Serum Increase Analytical* Interferes with bioassays *3858*

Mexiletine *Serum Increase Physiological* Decreases clearance of drug and prolongs half-life *3281*

Mycophenolic Acid *Serum No Effect Analytical* No significant interference observed with HPLC method of Shipkova et al *5526*

Mycophenolic Acid Glucuronide
Serum No Effect Analytical No significant interference observed with HPLC method of Shipkova et al *5526*

Neutrophils *Blood Decrease Physiological* Occurs either as dose-related or idiosyncratic bone marrow suppression: dose- related usually occurs 5-7 d after start of therapy: idiosyncratic reaction is rare occurring in one case per 40,000 courses of therapy *6498* Agranulocytosis reported to occur occasionally *6264* Most severe complications, sometimes fatal, are aplastic anemia, hypoplastic anemia, thrombocytopenia and granulocytopenia *4520* Common toxic reaction: aplastic anemia *4014*

5'-Nucleotidase *Serum Increase Physiological* Due to cholestasis *3669*

Occult Blood *Feces Increase Physiological* Occasional case of pseudomembranous colitis reported with mucus or bloody diarrhea *689* May be gastrointestinal hemorrhage, with low prothrombin *128*

Phenylalanine *Plasma No Effect Analytical* No interference observed with rapid quantitative whole blood method of Campbell et al using phenylalanine dehydrogenase *867*

Phenytoin *Serum Increase Physiological* Inhibits hepatic microsomal metabolizing enzymes thus prolonging half-life *6498* When chloramphenicol ingested with fosphenytoin concentration of phenytoin may be increased *4519* May increase from 2.5 to 9 µg/mL (at 2 g/d) *3339* Coadministration with phenytoin may increase plasma phenytoin concentration *4522* Inhibition of metabolism *3340* Significant increases in concentration when drugs coadministered *1384* Concentration observed to be increased in several studies due to inhibition of hepatic microsomal enzyme activity *1005*

Plasminogen *Plasma No Effect Analytical* At concentration of 25 mg/L had no effect on Du Pont aca method *5704*

Platelets *Blood Decrease Physiological* Isolated case of hepatitis and pancytopenia reported which resolved with discontinuation of drug *907* Most severe complications, sometimes fatal, are aplastic anemia, hypoplastic anemia, thrombocytopenia and granulocytopenia *4520* Aplastic anemia reported to occur in from 1 to 10,000 or 40,000 cases *6264* Pancytopenia/aplastic anemia *1429* Occurs either as dose-related or idiosyncratic bone marrow suppression: dose- related usually occurs 5-7 d after start of therapy: idiosyncratic reaction is rare occurring in one case per 40,000 courses of therapy *6498*

Polymyxin *Serum Increase Analytical* Interferes with bioassays *3858*

Potassium *Serum No Effect Analytical* At concentration of 6,000 mg/L had no effect on measurement by ISE without predilution *5704*

Protein *Cerebrospinal Fluid Increase Analytical* Slight effect on Folin-Ciocalteu procedure *6681*

Chloramphenicol *(continued)*

Protein *(continued)*
Cerebrospinal Fluid *No Effect* *Analytical* At concentration of 20 mg/L on SDS/Coomassie Blue method of Huang *2745* No effect observed at final concentration of 10 µg/mL with method on Kodak Ektachem® *2791*
Serum *Increase* *Analytical* At concentrations above 500 mg/L (normal therapeutic concentration 10 mg/L) raised concentration as measured by biuret method with blank correction *5704*

Protein Electrophoresis *Serum* *No Effect* *Analytical* At concentration of 6,000 mg/L had no effect on automated Olympus-Hite method but with slight displacement of fractions *5704*

Prothrombin Time *Plasma* *Increase* *Physiological* May cause lowered prothrombin and hemorrhage *1405*

Reticulocytes *Blood* *Decrease* *Physiological* Reversible toxic reaction or pancytopenia *4013*

SDZ PSC 833 *Blood* *No Effect* *Analytical* At a concentration of 55 mg/L had no effect on HPLC method of Scott et al when used to measure PSC (with CsD as internal standard) at a concentration of 5 mg/L *5418*

Sodium *Serum* *No Effect* *Analytical* At concentration of 6,000 mg/L had no effect on measurement by ISE without predilution *5704*

Sugar *Urine* *Increase* *Analytical* False positive with copper reduction procedures *5869*

Tetracycline *Serum* *Increase* *Analytical* Interferes with bioassays *3858*

Tobramycin *Serum* *No Effect* *Analytical* At concentrations less than 1000 µg/mL (3.09 µmol/L) no significant effect observed on method on Du Pont aca *1547*

Tolbutamide *Serum* *Increase* *Physiological* May cause 3 fold increase in half life *2452* Threefold increase in half-life of tolbutamide reported in one study due to inhibition of hepatic metabolism *1005* Inhibits hepatic microsomal metabolizing enzymes thus prolonging half-life *6498*

Triglycerides *Serum* *No Effect* *Analytical* No effect at therapeutic concentration on Boehringer Mannheim Reflotron method *3231* No effect at 200 mg/L on Boehringer Mannheim Reflotron method *5706* At concentration of 3,000 mg/L had no effect on GPO-PAP method *5704*

Trimethoprim *Serum* *Increase* *Analytical* Interferes with bioassays *3858*

Urea Nitrogen *Serum* *Decrease* *Analytical* Inhibits Berthelot reaction *5869*
Serum *Increase* *Analytical* Reacts with Nessler reagent *5869*
Serum *No Effect* *Analytical* At concentration of 2500 mg/L had no effect on urease/Berthelot method *5704* No effect at therapeutic concentration on ehringer Mannheim Reflotron method *3231* No effect at 50 mg/L on method on Ames Seralyzer *5706* No effect at 200 mg/L on Boehringer Mannheim Reflotron method *5706* At concentration of 600 mg/L had no effect on Kodak Ektachem® method *5704*

Uric Acid *Serum* *Decrease* *Analytical* At concentrations greater than 600 mg/L (normal therapeutic concentration 10 mg/L) lowered concentration as measured by Kageyama-Hantzsch method *5704*
Serum *No Effect* *Analytical* No effect at 200 mg/L on method on Boehringer Mannheim Reflotron *5706* At concentration of 600 mg/L had no effect on catalase-AIDH method *5704* At concentration of 3,000 mg/L had no effect on uricase-PAP method *5704* No effect at therapeutic concentration on Boehringer Mannheim Reflotron method *3231*

Urobilinogen *Feces* *Decrease* *Physiological* Reduction of flora in gastrointestinal tract *2451*
Urine *Decrease* *Physiological* Reduction of flora in gastrointestinal tract *2451*

Vancomycin *Serum* *No Effect* *Analytical* No significant interference observed at a concentration of 100 µg/mL (309 µmol/L) with method on Du Pont aca *1561* At concentrations up to 100 µg/mL had no significant cross-reactivity in valproic acid method on Bayer Technicon Immuno 1® *438*

Chlordane

Alanine Aminotransferase *Serum* *Increase* *Physiological* Due to hepatotoxicity *2183*

Bilirubin *Serum* *Increase* *Physiological* Due to hepatotoxicity *2183*

Creatine Kinase *Serum* *Increase* *Physiological* Activity increased in pest-control operators compared with nonexposed individuals *4372*

Erythrocytes *Blood* *Decrease* *Physiological* Pancytopenia (AMA Blood dyscrasias) *4017*

Lactate Dehydrogenase *Serum* *Increase* *Physiological* Activity increased in pest-control operators compared with nonexposed individuals *4372*

Leukocytes *Blood* *Decrease* *Physiological* Pancytopenia (AMA Blood dyscrasias) *4017*

Platelets *Blood* *Decrease* *Physiological* Pancytopenia (AMA Blood dyscrasias) *4017*

Prothrombin Time *Plasma* *Decrease* *Physiological* Induces hepatic metabolism of anticoagulants *2242*

Triglycerides *Serum* *Increase* *Physiological* Concentration increased compared with controls in pest-control operators than in nonexposed individuals *4372*

Chlordiazepoxide

Alanine Aminotransferase *Serum* *Increase* *Analytical* At 5 times upper limit of therapeutic range on kinetic methods on KDA *3525*
Serum *Increase* *Physiological* Rare cases of jaundice and hepatic dysfunction reported with treatment *5040* May produce hepatotoxic effect *30*
Serum *No Effect* *Analytical* No effect at therapeutic concentration on Boehringer Mannheim Reflotron method *3231* At 5 times upper limit of therapeutic range on methods on Technicon SMAC® , Abbott-VP, Du Pont aca, and Roche Cobas-Bio *3525* At acute overdose concentration (5 mg/dL) on Technicon SMAC® method *6266* No effect at 30 mg/L on Boehringer Mannheim Reflotron method *5706*

Albumin *Serum* *No Effect* *Analytical* At concentration of 50 mg/L had no effect on BCG method *5704* At acute overdose concentration (5 mg/dL) on Technicon SMAC® method *6266* At 5 times upper limit of therapeutic range on methods on Technicon SMAC® , Kodak Ektachem® , Hitachi® 705 and KDA *3525*
Urine *No Effect* *Analytical* Using a fluorimetric assay with Albumin Blue 580 on a Cobas Fara centrifugal analyzer for the detection of microalbuminuria no significant interference was detected at a concentration of 4 mg/L *3117*

Alkaline Phosphatase *Serum* *Increase* *Physiological* Infrequent cholestatic effect *3669* Rare cases of jaundice and hepatic dysfunction reported with treatment *5040*
Serum *No Effect* *Analytical* At 5 times upper limit of therapeutic range on methods onTechnicon SMAC® , Abbott-VP, Du Pont aca, Roche Cobas-Bio, Hitachi® 705 and KDA *3525* At acute overdose concentration (5 mg/dL) on Technicon SMAC® method *6266*

δ-Aminolevulinic Acid *Urine* *Increase* *Physiological* May precipitate acute porphyria *2210*

Amitriptyline *Serum* *No Effect* *Physiological* No effect on serum concentration if given together *5559*

Amylase *Serum* *No Effect* *Analytical* At 5 times upper limit of therapeutic range on methods on Du Pont aca, Roche Cobas-Bio and Kodak Ektachem® *3525* At concentration of 30 mg/L had no effect on method on Boehringer Mannheim Reflotron system *5706*

Aspartate Aminotransferase *Serum* *Increase* *Analytical* At 5 times upper limit of therapeutic range on kinetic methods on KDA *3525*
Serum *Increase* *Physiological* May produce hepatotoxic effect *30* Rare cases of jaundice and hepatic dysfunction reported with treatment *5040*
Serum *No Effect* *Analytical* No effect at 30 mg/L on Boehringer Mannheim Reflotron method *5706* At acute overdose concentration (5 mg/dL) on Technicon SMAC® method *1419* At 5 times upper limit of therapeutic range on methods on Technicon SMAC® , Abbott-VP, Du Pont aca, Roche Cobas-

Bio and Hitachi® 705 *3525* No effect at therapeutic concentration on Boehringer Mannheim Reflotron method *3231*

Benzodiazepine *Urine Positive Analytical* Positive result observed at a concentration of 3.0 µg/mL (10.01 µmol/L) with method on Du Pont aca *1556*

Bicarbonate *Serum No Effect Analytical* At concentration of 5 mg/L had no effect on method using phenolphthalein *5704*

Bile *Urine Increase Physiological* Hepatotoxic effect *3810*

Bilirubin *Serum Increase Physiological* Infrequent cholestatic effect *1714* Rare cases of jaundice and hepatic dysfunction reported with treatment *5040*

Serum No Effect Analytical No effect at 1.7 mg/L on Ames Seralyzer method *5706* At concentration of 50 mg/L had no effect on Jendrassik and Grof method *5704* At 5 times upper limit of therapeutic range on methods on Technicon SMAC® , Du Pont aca, Roche Cobas-Bio, Kodak Ektachem® , Hitachi® 705 and KDA *3525* At acute overdose concentration (5 mg/dL) on Technicon SMAC® method *6266* At concentration of 30 mg/L had no effect on method on Boehringer Mannheim Reflotron system *5706*

Serum No Effect Physiological Insignificant protein displacement effect in neonates *6314*

Bilirubin, Conjugated *Serum No Effect Analytical* No effect at concentration of 25 mg/L on method on Kodak Ektachem® *5706*

Bilirubin, Unconjugated *Serum No Effect Analytical* No effect at concentration of 25 mg/L on method on Kodak Ektachem® *5706*

BSP Retention *Serum Increase Physiological* Infrequent cholestatic effect *2803*

Bufotenin *Urine No Effect Physiological* Ingestion of low doses (10 mg/d for 7 days) had no significant effect on urinary excretion in one man *3046*

Calcium *Serum No Effect Analytical* At concentration of 50 mg/L had no effect on cresolphthalein method *5704* At acute overdose concentration (5 mg/dL) on Technicon SMAC® method *6266* At 5 times upper limit of therapeutic range on methods on Technicon SMAC® , Abbott-VP, Du Pont aca, Kodak Ektachem® , Hitachi® 705 and KDA *3525*

Cannabinoids *Urine No Effect Analytical* No effect on Roche Abuscreen method *5006*

Catecholamines *Urine No Effect Physiological* No effect of short term ingestion of 30 mg/d *1184*

Chlordiazepoxide *Serum Increase Physiological* 150 mg orally produces concentration of 10 mg/L, 600 mg/d produces a concentration of 40 mg/L *3868*

Chloride *Serum No Effect Analytical* At concentration of 5 mg/L had no effect on mercurimetric method *5704*

Cholesterol *Serum No Effect Analytical* At concentration of 30 mg/L no effect on method on Boehringer Mannheim Reflotron system *5706* At concentration of 160 mg/L had no effect on CHOD-PAP method *5704* At concentration of 160 mg/L had no effect on method using catalase-Hantzsch reaction *5704* No effect at 1.7 mg/L on Ames Seralyzer method *5706* At 5 times upper limit of therapeutic range on methods on Technicon SMAC® , Abbott-VP, Roche Cobas-Bio, Kodak Ektachem® , Hitachi® 705 and KDA *3525* At acute overdose concentration (5 mg/dL) on Technicon SMAC® method *6266* At concentration of 160 mg/L had no effect on CHOD-Iodide method *5704* At concentration of 160 mg/L had no effect on catalase-AIDH method *5704* At concentration of 160 mg/L had no effect on Liebermann-Burchard method *5704* No effect at therapeutic concentration on Boehringer Mannheim Reflotron method *3231*

Copper *Urine No Effect Physiological* No significant effect observed *6283*

Coproporphyrin *Feces Increase Physiological* May precipitate acute porphyria *2210*

Urine Increase Physiological May precipitate acute porphyria *2210*

Cortisol *Plasma No Effect Analytical* At a concentration of 30 mg/L no significant effect observed on CEDIA method *1097*

Creatine Kinase *Serum No Effect Analytical* At acute overdose concentration (5 mg/dL) on Technicon SMAC® method *6266* At 5 times upper limit of therapeutic range on methods on Technicon SMAC® , Abbott-VP, Du Pont aca, Roche Cobas-Bio and Hitachi® 705 *3525* No effect at 1.7 mg/L on method on Ames Seralyzer *5706*

Creatinine *Serum No Effect Analytical* At acute overdose concentration (5 mg/dL) on Technicon SMAC® method *6266* At concentration of 20 mg/L had no effect on Jaffe-Fading-Fraction method *5704* At concentration of 20 mg/L had no effect on kinetic Jaffe method on BKA-2 *5704* At concentration of 20 mg/L had no effect on creatinine iminohydrolase method *5704* No effect of concentrations up to 25 mg/L on 2-slide method on Kodak Ektachem® *5706* At 5 times upper limit of therapeutic range on methods on Technicon SMAC® , Abbott-VP, Du Pont aca *3525* At 16 mg/L on reversed phase liquid chromatographic procedure of Zhiri et al *6656* At concentration of 50 mg/L had no effect on Technicon AutoAnalyzer® Jaffe method *5704* No effect at 1.7 mg/L on Ames Seralyzer method *5706* At concentration of 20 mg/L had no effect on Jaffe-Fuller's earth method *5704*

Epinephrine *Urine No Effect Physiological* No effect of short term ingestion of 30 mg/d *1184*

Erythrocytes *Blood Decrease Physiological* Aplastic anemia occasionally occurs *6264*

Glucose *Serum No Effect Analytical* At acute overdose concentration (5 mg/dL) on Technicon SMAC® method *6266* At concentration of 30 mg/L no effect on method on Boehringer Mannheim Reflotron system *5706* At concentration of 50 mg/L had no effect on GOD/POD-PAP method *5704* No effect at therapeutic concentration on Boehringer Mannheim Reflotron method *3231* At concentration of 1.8 mg/L had no effect on Kodak Ektachem® method *5704* At 5 times upper limit of therapeutic range on methods on Technicon SMAC® , Abbott-VP, Du Pont aca, Roche Cobas-Bio, Kodak Ektachem® , Hitachi® 705 and KDA *3525* No effect at 1.7 mg/L on glucose oxidase method on Ames Seralyzer *5706* At concentration of 6 mg/L had no effect on hexokinase/G-6-PDH method *5704*

γ-Glutamyltransferase *Serum No Effect Analytical* At concentration of 30 mg/L no effect on method on Boehringer Mannheim Reflotron system *5706* No effect at therapeutic concentration on Boehringer Mannheim Reflotron method *3231* At 5 times upper limit of therapeutic range on methods on Technicon SMAC® , Abbott-VP, and Hitachi® 705 *3525*

Granulocytes *Blood Decrease Physiological* Rare cases of agranulocytosis reported with treatment *5040*

11-Hydroxycorticosteroids *Urine No Effect Physiological* No effect of short term ingestion of 30 mg/d *1184*

17-Hydroxycorticosteroids *Urine No Effect Physiological* No effect of short term ingestion of 30 mg/d *1184*

6-β-Hydroxycortisol *Urine Increase Physiological* Observed in 2 out of 5 patients *4436*

5-Hydroxyindoleacetic Acid *Urine Increase Analytical* Slight effect observed *in vitro* in method of Udenfriend *1051*

^{131}I Uptake *Serum Decrease Physiological* ?Antithyroid effect *383*

Iron *Serum No Effect Analytical* At 5 times upper limit of therapeutic range on Ferrozine method of Technicon SMAC® *3525* At acute overdose concentration (5 mg/dL) on Technicon SMAC® method *6266* At concentration of 50 mg/L had no effect on Ferrozine method *5704*

Isocitrate Dehydrogenase *Serum Increase Physiological* Infrequent cholestatic effect *3810*

17-Ketogenic Steroids *Urine Decrease Analytical* Interferes with Zimmermann reaction *5869*

Urine Increase Analytical Interferes with Zimmermann reaction *4245*

17-Ketosteroids *Urine No Effect Physiological* No effect of short term ingestion of 30 mg/d *1184*

Lactate *Plasma No Effect Analytical* At concentration of 6 mg/L had no effect on enzymatic method *5704*

Lactate Dehydrogenase *Serum No Effect Analytical* No effect at 1.7 mg/L on method on Ames Seralyzer *5706* At 5 times upper limit of therapeutic range on methods on Technicon SMAC® , Abbott-VP, Roche Cobas-Bio, Hitachi® 705 and KDA *3525* At acute overdose concentration (5 mg/dL) on Technicon SMAC® method *6266*

Leukocytes *Blood Decrease Physiological* Aplastic anemia occasionally occurs *6264* Agranulocytosis reported (leukopenia more common) *3810*

Neutrophils *Blood Decrease Physiological* Occasional case of agranulocytosis reported *6264*

Chlordiazepoxide *(continued)*

Norepinephrine *Urine No Effect Physiological* No effect of short term ingestion of 30 mg/d *1184*

Nortriptyline *Serum No Effect Physiological* No effect on serum concentration if given together *5559*

p-Aminophenol *Urine No Effect Analytical* With addition of drugs at a concentration of 100 mg/L and of related compounds at 50 mg/L no significant effect observed on colorimetric method of van Bocxlaer on Cobas Mira analyzer which involves reacting free p-aminophenol with resorcinol in the presence of magnesium ions to form an indophenol dye measured at 550 nm *6163*

Phenobarbital *Serum No Effect Analytical* No significant cross-reactivity observed with method on Du Pont aca *1537* At concentration of 1.00 mg/mL (3.34 mmol/L) has no effect on method on Du Pont Dimension *1582*

Phenytoin *Serum Increase. Physiological* When chlordiazepoxide ingested with fosphenytoin concentration of phenytoin may be increased *4519* Coadministration with phenytoin may increase plasma phenytoin concentration *4522* Inhibition of metabolism (by 60%) *3340*

Serum No Effect Analytical No significant interference observed at a concentration of 100 µg/mL (334 µmol/L) with method on Du Pont aca *1538* No effect at concentration of 100 µg/mL (334 µmol/L) on method on Du Pont Dimension *1583*

Phosphate *Serum No Effect Analytical* At 5 times upper limit of therapeutic range on methods on Technicon SMAC®, Du Pont aca, Hitachi® 705 and KDA *3525* At concentration of 50 mg/L had no effect on phosphomolybdate method *5704* At acute overdose concentration (5 mg/dL) on Technicon SMAC® method *6266*

Platelets *Blood Decrease Physiological* Aplastic anemia occasionally occurs *6264* May rarely cause bone marrow depression *2385*

Porphobilinogen *Urine Increase Physiological* May precipitate acute porphyria *2210*

Porphyrin, Total *Urine Increase Physiological* May precipitate attack of acute porphyria *3669*

Potassium *Serum No Effect Analytical* At concentration of 18 mg/L had no effect on measurement by ISE without predilution *5704* At concentration of 20 mg/L had no effect on measurement by ISE with predilution *5704* At concentration of 5 mg/L had no effect on flame-photometric method *5704*

Prazosin *Serum No Effect Physiological* Coadministration of prazosin with chlordiazepoxide had no apparent adverse drug interaction in limited clinical experience *4649*

Pregnancy Tests *Urine No Effect Analytical* No effect on UCG test *2452*

Urine Positive Analytical False positive with Gravindex™ *2452*

Protein *Serum No Effect Analytical* At concentration of 50 mg/L had no effect on biuret method with blank correction *5704* At 5 times upper limit of therapeutic range on methods on Technicon SMAC®, Abbott-VP, Kodak Ektachem®, Hitachi® 705 and KDA *3525* At acute overdose concentration (5 mg/dL) on Technicon SMAC® method *6266*

Protein Electrophoresis *Serum No Effect Analytical* At concentration of 18 mg/L had no effect on automated Olympus-Hite method except for slight displacement of fractions *5704*

Prothrombin Time *Plasma Decrease Physiological* May shorten action of anticoagulants *2753*

Plasma Increase Physiological Associated with failure of excretion of bile salts *2803*

Plasma No Effect Physiological. Does not affect action of administered coumarins *4998*

Protoporphyrin *Feces Increase Physiological* May precipitate acute porphyria *2210*

Sodium *Serum No Effect Analytical* At concentration of 18 mg/L had no effect on measurement by ISE without predilution *5704* At concentration of 5 mg/L had no effect on flame-photometric method *5704* At concentration of 20 mg/L had no effect on measurement by ISE with predilution *5704*

T3-Uptake *Serum Decrease Physiological* ?Antithyroid effect (resin test affected) *383*

Triglycerides *Serum No Effect Analytical* At 5 times upper limit of therapeutic range on methods on Technicon SMAC®, Abbott-VP, Kodak Ektachem®, Hitachi® 705 and KDA *3525* No effect at 30 mg/L on Boehringer Mannheim Reflotron method *5706* At acute overdose concentration (5 mg/dL) on Technicon SMAC® method *6266* At concentration of 51 mg/L had no effect on GPO-PAP method *5704* At concentration of 50 mg/L had no effect on lipase/esterase method *5704* No effect at therapeutic concentration on Boehringer Mannheim Reflotron method *3231*

Urea Nitrogen *Serum No Effect Analytical* At concentration of 50 mg/L had no effect on diacetylmonoxime method *5704* No effect at 30 mg/L on Boehringer Mannheim Reflotron method *5706* At 5 times upper limit of therapeutic range on methods on Technicon SMAC®, Abbott-VP, Roche Cobas-Bio, Kodak Ektachem®, Hitachi® 705 and KDA *3525* At concentration of 1.8 mg/L had no effect on Kodak Ektachem® method *5704* At acute overdose concentration (5 mg/dL) on Technicon SMAC® method *6266* No effect at 1.7 mg/L on method on Ames Seralyzer *5706* No effect at therapeutic concentration on Boehringer Mannheim Reflotron method *3231*

Uric Acid *Serum No Effect Analytical* No effect at therapeutic concentration on Boehringer Mannheim Reflotron method *3231* At acute overdose concentration (5 mg/dL) on Technicon SMAC® method *6266* At 16 mg/L on reversed phase liquid chromatographic procedure of Zhiri et al *6656* No effect of concentrations up to 25 mg/L on method on Kodak Ektachem® *5706* At concentration of 50 mg/L had no effect on phosphotungstate reduction method *5704* At concentration of 20 mg/L had no effect on Kageyama-Hantzsch method *5704* At concentration of 20 mg/L had no effect on catalase-AIDH method *5704* At concentration of 50 mg/L had no effect on uricase-PAP method *5704* At 5 times upper limit of therapeutic range on methods on Technicon SMAC®, Abbott-VP, Du Pont aca *3525* No effect at 30 mg/L on method on Boehringer Mannheim Reflotron *5706*

Urobilinogen *Feces Decrease Physiological* Infrequent cholestatic effect *2803*

Urine Decrease Physiological Infrequent cholestatic effect *2803*

Warfarin *Plasma Increase Analytical* Spectrophotometric method shows interference *4998*

Chlorhexidine

Bilirubin *Urine Decrease Analytical* Large quantities may cause false negative with Ames Multistix and other reagent strip tests *4034*

Urine No Effect Analytical No effect observed with Ames Ictotest reagent tablets *4034*

Protein *Urine Increase Analytical* False positive with Stix alkalinization *199* May cause false positive with protein test areas on Ames Multistix and other reagent test strips *4034*

Urine No Effect Analytical Has no effect on Sulfosalicylic Acid and Exton's reagent tests *4034*

Specific Gravity *Urine Increase Analytical* Large quantities may increase result as measured by Ames Multistix and other reagent strip tests as may also be observed with T.S. meter (refractometer) *4034*

Urine No Effect Analytical No effect observed hen S.G. measured by urinometer (hydrometer) *4034*

Chloride Salts

Amylase *Serum Increase Analytical* Chloride enhances enzyme activity *5504*

Chloride *Serum Increase Physiological* Increased absorption with increased serum levels *1009*

Orthophosphate *Test Conditions Decrease Analytical* 85% inhibition at 0.4 mol/L on method of Horder *2713*

Protein *Test Conditions Increase Analytical* If glyoxylic acid used to measure tryptophan *154*

Pyruvate Kinase *Red Blood Cells Decrease Analytical* Observed with 0.3 mmol/L PEP in reaction mixture *592*

Sugar *Urine Increase Analytical* If anthrone method used *154*

Zinc *Serum No Effect Analytical* At 6,000 to 1 with flameless atomic absorption *3333*
Urine No Effect Analytical At 6,000 to 1 with flameless atomic absorption *3333*

Chlorine

Uric Acid *Serum Decrease Analytical* If in water affects phosphotungstate procedure *882*

Chlormadinone

Cholesterol *Serum No Effect Physiological* No significant effect observed *2193*

Factor VIII *Plasma Increase Physiological* Significant effect observed by 3 mo *4063*

Factor IX *Plasma Increase . Physiological* Significant effect observed by 3 mo *4063*

Factor X *Plasma Decrease Physiological* Significant effect observed by 3 mo *4063*

Luteinizing Hormone *Urine Decrease Physiological* Usual effect in normal women *5817*

Prothrombin Time *Plasma Increase Physiological* Significant effect observed by 3 mo *1226*

Thyroxine Binding Globulin *Serum Increase Physiological* Therapeutic effect *3810*

Triglycerides *Serum No Effect Physiological* No significant effect observed *2193*

Chlormerodrin

Protein *Urine Increase Physiological* May produce nephrotic syndrome *1958*

Urea Nitrogen *Serum Increase Physiological* May produce nephrotic syndrome *1958*

Chlormethiazole

Indomethacin *Serum No Effect Analytical* No effect on HPLC method of Roberts and Smith *4978*

Chlormethine

Chromosomes *Test Conditions Abnormal Physiological* Clastogenic in human cells *5484*

Chlormezanone

Alanine Aminotransferase *Serum Increase Physiological* Reversible cholestatic jaundice occurs rarely *5260* Occasional reversible cholestasis *3810*

Albumin *Serum No Effect Analytical* At concentration of 100 mg/L had no effect on BCG method *5704*

Alkaline Phosphatase *Serum Increase Physiological* Occasional reversible cholestasis *3810* Reversible cholestatic jaundice occurs rarely *5260*

Aspartate Aminotransferase *Serum Increase Physiological* Occasional reversible cholestasis *3810* Reversible cholestatic jaundice occurs rarely *5260*

Bicarbonate *Serum No Effect Analytical* At concentration of 100 mg/L had no effect on method using phenolphthalein *5704*

Bile *Urine Increase Physiological* Occasional reversible cholestasis *3810*

Bilirubin *Serum Increase Physiological* Reversible cholestatic jaundice occurs rarely *5260* Occasional reversible cholestasis *3810*
Serum No Effect Analytical At concentration of 100 mg/L had no effect on Jendrassik and Grof method *5704*

Calcium *Serum No Effect Analytical* At concentration of 100 mg/L had no effect on cresolphthalein method *5704*

Chloride *Serum No Effect Analytical* At concentration of 100 mg/L had no effect on mercurimetric method *5704*

Cholesterol *Serum No Effect Analytical* At concentration of 100 mg/L had no effect on Liebermann-Burchard method *5704*

Creatinine *Serum No Effect Analytical* At concentration of 100 mg/L had no effect on Technicon AutoAnalyzer® Jaffe method *5704*

γ-Glutamyltransferase *Serum Increase Physiological* Reversible cholestatic jaundice occurs rarely *5260*

Phenylalanine *Plasma No Effect Analytical* No interference observed with rapid quantitative whole blood method of Campbell et al using phenylalanine dehydrogenase *867*

Phosphate *Serum No Effect Analytical* At concentration of 100 mg/L had no effect on phosphotungstate reduction method *5704*

Potassium *Serum No Effect Analytical* At concentration of 100 mg/L had no effect on measurement by ISE with predilution *5704*

Protein *Serum No Effect Analytical* At concentration of 100 mg/L had no effect on biuret method with blank correction *5704*

Sodium *Serum No Effect Analytical* At concentration of 100 mg/L had no effect on measurement by ISE with predilution *5704*

Triglycerides *Serum No Effect Analytical* At concentration of 100 mg/L had no effect on lipase/esterase method *5704*

Urea Nitrogen *Serum No Effect Analytical* At concentration of 100 mg/L had no effect on diacetylmonoxime method *5704*

Uric Acid *Serum No Effect Analytical* At concentration of 100 mg/L had no effect on phosphotungstate reduction method *5704*

Chloroform

Alanine Aminotransferase *Serum Increase Physiological* Hepatotoxic effect with necrosis *3810*

Alkaline Phosphatase *Serum Increase Physiological* Hepatotoxic effect with necrosis *3810*

Aspartate Aminotransferase *Serum Increase Physiological* Hepatotoxic effect with necrosis *3810*

Bile *Urine No Effect Analytical* As preservative has no effect on Stix tests *3805*

Bilirubin *Serum Increase Physiological* Hepatotoxic effect with necrosis *3810*

BSP Retention *Serum Increase Physiological* Hepatotoxic effect with necrosis *3810*

Cholesterol *Serum Decrease Physiological* Hepatotoxic effect with necrosis *3810*

Glucose *Serum Decrease Physiological* Hepatotoxic effect with necrosis *3810*
Urine No Effect Analytical As preservative has no effect on Stix tests *3805*

Hemoglobin *Urine No Effect Analytical* As preservative has no effect on Stix tests *3805*

Ketones *Urine No Effect Analytical* As preservative has no effect on Stix tests *3805*

Leukocytes *Blood Increase Physiological* Normal response to anesthesia *409*

Ornithine Carbamoyltransferase
Serum Increase Physiological Hepatotoxic effect with necrosis *6461*

pH *Urine No Effect Analytical* As preservative has no effect on Stix tests *3805*

Phosphate *Serum Decrease Physiological* Follows most forms of anesthesia *467*

Protein *Urine Increase Physiological* May cause renal damage *467*
Urine No Effect Analytical As preservative has no effect on Stix tests *3805*

Sugar *Urine Increase Analytical* Positive with Benedict's, Fehling's solutions *6515*

Urea Nitrogen *Serum Increase Physiological* May cause renal damage *467*

Uric Acid *Serum Increase Physiological* May occur with marked tissue destruction *467*

Chloroguanide

Casts *Urine Increase Physiological* Nephrotoxic effect *3810*

Cells *Urine Increase Physiological* May cause transient appearance of epithelial cells *2242*

Erythrocytes *Urine Increase Physiological* Drug produces actual bleeding *1714*

Folate *Serum Decrease Physiological* Antagonizes folic acid *128*

Hemoglobin *Urine Increase Physiological* Drug produces actual bleeding *1714*

Myelocytes *Blood Increase Physiological* Up to 10% in patients with overt malaria *2242*

Chlorophenothane

Alanine Aminotransferase *Serum Increase Physiological* May cause liver damage *467*

Aldosterone *Urine Decrease Physiological* May inhibit synthesis of hormone *4605*

Aspartate Aminotransferase *Serum Increase Physiological* May cause liver damage *467*

Bilirubin *Serum Decrease Physiological* Effect on congenital non-hemolytic hyperbilirubinemia *5869*

Cortisol *Plasma No Effect Physiological* Occupational exposure no effect *1059*

Dexamethasone Suppression
Patient No Effect Physiological Normal in subjects with occupational exposure *1059*

Erythrocytes *Blood Decrease Physiological* Pancytopenia (AMA blood dyscrasias) *4017*

Leukocytes *Blood Decrease Physiological* Pancytopenia (AMA blood dyscrasias) *4017*

Occult Blood *Feces Increase Physiological* May cause gastrointestinal tract bleeding and other symptoms *467*

Phenobarbital *Serum Decrease Physiological* Reported interaction due to alteration of metabolism *3340*

Phenytoin *Serum Decrease Physiological* Decrease from 9 to 1 parts per billion (with dose of 300-400 mg) *3339*

Platelets *Blood Decrease Physiological* Pancytopenia (AMA blood dyscrasias) *4017*

Chlorophenylalanine

Eosinophils *Blood Increase Physiological* Observed in isolated case *6200*

Homovanillic Acid
Cerebrospinal Fluid No Effect Physiological After 1 g/d for 4 d or after single dose *5591*

5-Hydroxyindoleacetic Acid
Cerebrospinal Fluid No Effect Physiological After 1 g/d for 4 d or after single dose *5591*
Urine Decrease Physiological Inhibits biosynthesis of serotonin *1167*

Chlorophenylpiperazine

Cortisol *Plasma Increase Physiological* In 10 patients with seasonal affective disorder treatment with m-chlorophenylpiperazine in winter caused mean concentration to increase from 8.73 ± 1.28 μg/mL to 9.58 ± 1.44 μg/mL *2027*

Homovanillic Acid *Plasma No Effect Physiological* In 10 healthy men administration of 0.35 mg/kg had no significant effect on concentration with concentration decreasing with time (over 210 minutes) from mean baseline concentration of 10.3 ng/mL to 8.0 ng/mL *3004*

Prolactin *Plasma Increase Physiological* In 10 healthy men administration of 0.35 mg/kg orally caused significant increase from mean baseline of 6.0 ng/mL to 10.5 ng/mL at 120 minutes and 10.0 ng/mL at 210 minutes *3004*
Plasma No Effect Physiological In 10 patients with seasonal affective disorder treatment with m-chlorophenylpiperazine in winter caused mean concentration to change nonsignificantly from 7.35 ± 0.67 μg/mL to 7.31 ± 0.69 μg/mL *2027*

Chloroquine

Aspartate Aminotransferase *Serum Increase Physiological* Reported effect: no mechanism cited *3810*

Bilirubin *Serum Increase Physiological* Hemolytic anemia in G-6-PD deficiency *2754*

Calcium *Serum Decrease Physiological* Reduction in one patient with sarcoidosis from 3.54 mmol/L to normal concentration after 18 days treatment with 500 mg daily *47*
Urine Decrease Physiological In 2 patients with sarcoidosis given 500 mg daily while receiving corticosteroid at same time *4402*

Cannabinoids *Urine No Effect Analytical* No effect on Roche Abuscreen method *5006*

Cholesterol *Serum No Effect Analytical* At concentration of 60 mg/L had no effect on Liebermann-Burchard method *5704* At concentration of 60 mg/L had no effect on CHOD-Iodide method *5704* At concentration of 60 mg/L had no effect on method using catalase-Hantzsch reaction *5704* At concentration of 60 mg/L had no effect on catalase-AIDH method *5704* At concentration of 200 mg/L had no effect on CHOD-PAP method *5704*

Color *Urine Increase Analytical* Brown color *1714*

Creatinine *Serum No Effect Analytical* At concentration of 100 mg/L had no effect on Jaffe-Fading-Fraction method *5704* At concentration of 100 mg/L had no effect on Jaffe-Fuller's earth method *5704* At concentration of 0.5 mg/L had no effect on creatinine iminohydrolase method *5704* At concentration of 50 mg/L had no effect on kinetic Jaffe method on BKA-2 *5704*

Diclofenac *Serum No Effect Physiological* Coadministration of chloroquine with diclofenac did not significantly affect the peak concentration or AUC of diclofenac *1025*

1,25-Dihydroxy Vitamin D_3 *Serum Decrease Physiological* Reduction of inappropriately high concentration began within 3 days in one patient with sarcoidosis due to reduced synthesis of analyte. Concentration fell by 37% by fifth day and 67% by seventh day *47* In 2 patients with sarcoidosis given 500 mg daily while receiving corticosteroid at same time *4402*

Erythrocytes *Blood Decrease Physiological* Aplastic anemia reported to occur occasionally *6264* Hemolytic anemia in G-6-PD deficient persons *5899*

Glucose *Serum Decrease Physiological* In 20 patients with noninsulin-dependent diabetes mellitus controlled by diet with 1.0 g for 3 days mean fasting concentration reduced from 200 mg/dL to 166 mg/dL *4770*
Serum No Effect Analytical At concentration of 5 mg/L had no effect on Kodak Ektachem® method *5704* At concentration of 250 mg/L had no effect on GOD/POD-PAP method *5704*

Hematocrit *Blood Decrease Physiological* G-6-PD hemolytic anemia/pancytopenia *5899*

Hemoglobin *Blood Decrease Physiological* Hemolytic anemia in G-6-PD deficient persons *5899*

Histamine *Plasma No Effect Analytical* 50% inhibition of radio-enzyme assay at 3 times therapeutic concentration *2492*

25-Hydroxy Vitamin D_3 *Serum No Effect Physiological* Possibly inhibits conversion of 25-hydroxyvitamin D to 1,25-dihydroxyvitamin D *4402*

Leukocytes *Blood Decrease Physiological* Aplastic anemia reported to occur occasionally *6264* Agranulocytosis/pancytopenia *5899*

Opiates *Urine No Effect Analytical* No effect observed at a concentration of 250 μg/mL (0.78 mmol/L) with method on Du Pont aca *1559*

Platelets *Blood Decrease Physiological* Pancytopenia *5899* Aplastic anemia reported to occur occasionally *6264*

Potassium *Serum Decrease Physiological* Marked prolonged reduction in two cases of acute massive intoxication *3632*
Serum No Effect Analytical At concentration of 50 mg/L had no effect on measurement by ISE without predilution *5704*

Protein Electrophoresis *Serum No Effect Analytical* At concentration of 50 mg/L had no effect on automated Olympus-Hite method *5704*

Sodium *Serum No Effect Analytical* At concentration of 50 mg/L had no effect on measurement by ISE without predilution *5704*

Spermidine Oxidase *Serum No Effect Analytical* At concentration of 0.2 mmol/L had no effect on method of Tabor and Kellogg *1884*

Triglycerides *Serum No Effect Analytical* At concentration of 250 mg/L had no effect on GPO-PAP method *5704*

Urea Nitrogen *Serum No Effect Analytical* No effect of concentrations up to 5 mg/L on method on Kodak Ektachem® *5706*

Uric Acid *Serum No Effect Analytical* At concentration of 100 mg/L had no effect on catalase-AIDH method *5704* At concentration of 250 mg/L had no effect on uricase-PAP method *5704* At concentration of 100 mg/L had no effect on Kageyama-Hantzsch method *5704* No effect at 50 mg/L on uricase method on Ames Seralyzer *5706*

Urobilinogen *Urine Increase Physiological* Hemolytic anemia in G-6-PD deficiency *2754*

Uroporphyrin *Urine Increase Physiological* Transient increase may occur with cutaneous porphyria *2210*

8-Chlorotheophylline

Theophylline *Serum Increase Analytical* Cross-reactivity of 6% observed with whole blood Theophylline II assay used with Abbott Vision *5707* Approximately 25% cross-reactivity on a molar basis independent of theophylline concentration when measured on Abbott TDx. Effect of 2 Dramamine® tablets (1000 mg) would increase measured theophylline concentration by about 7 µmol/L *302* Cross-reactivity of 6.8% observed with method on Baxter Stratus *5705* At a concentration of 100 µg/mL increases concentration as measured by Kodak Ektachem® systems by 3.14 µg/mL *2519*
Serum No Effect Analytical No significant interference observed awith Syva EMIT 2000 assay *413* No significant interference observed at a concentration of 50 µg/mL (233 µmol/L) with method on Du Pont aca *1544* No effect up to 3 mg/L on method on Ames Seralyzer but at higher concentrations clinically significant increase due to presence of compound *5706* No effect at concentration of 50 µg/mL (233 µmol/L) on method on Du Pont Dimension *1585* No effect of concentrations up to 50 mg/L on method on Kodak Ektachem® *5706*

Chlorothiazide

Alanine Aminotransferase *Serum Increase Physiological* May cause cholestatic jaundice *3810* Thiazides may rarely cause intrahepatic cholestasis *3971*

Alkaline Phosphatase *Serum Increase Physiological* Thiazides may rarely cause intrahepatic cholestasis *3971* May cause cholestatic jaundice *3810*

Ammonia *Plasma Increase Physiological* Decreased potassium and alkalosis *2025*

Amylase *Serum Increase Physiological* 10 of 20 patients developed 50 to 100% increase in serum amylase shortly after beginning treatment *3758* Thiazides may rarely cause pancreatitis *3971* Infrequent consequence of therapy *581*

Aspartate Aminotransferase *Serum Increase Physiological* Thiazides may rarely cause intrahepatic cholestasis *3971* May cause cholestatic jaundice *3810*

Bicarbonate *Serum No Effect Analytical* No effect of concentrations up to 30 mg/L on method on Kodak Ektachem® *5706*
Urine Increase Physiological Increased excretion probably due to suppression of proximal tubular reabsorption through carbonic anhydrase inhibition *633*

Bile *Urine Increase Physiological* May cause cholestatic jaundice *3810*

Bilirubin *Serum Increase Physiological* Reported to cause cholestatic jaundice *4555* Thiazides may rarely cause intrahepatic cholestasis *3971*
Serum No Effect Physiological Displacement from protein observed *in vitro*, but unlikely at pharmacological concentrations *in vivo6314*

Blood *Urine Increase Physiological* Thiazides may rarely cause renal failure, renal dysfunction or interstitial nephritis with hematuria occurring after intravenous use *3971*

BSP Retention *Serum Increase Physiological* May cause cholestatic jaundice *3810*

Calcium *Feces Decrease Physiological* Accentuates positive calcium balance *4014*
Lymphocytes No Effect Physiological No significant effect on lymphocyte calcium in 6 patients with hypertension treated with 500 mg daily for at least 12 months *37*
Red Blood Cells No Effect Physiological No significant effect in 6 patients with hypertension given 500 mg daily for at least 12 months *37*
Serum Decrease Physiological Initial response to administration *174*
Serum Increase Physiological Impaired excretion with chronic administration *5869* Due to increased tubular reabsorption but usually associated with mild primary hyperparathyroidism *3089* Thiazides may decrease urinary excretion of calcium which may cause intermittent and slight increases of serum calcium in the absence of known disorders of calcium metabolism. Marked hypercalcemia may be evidence of hidden hyperparathyroidism *3971*
Serum No Effect Analytical No effect of concentrations up to 30 mg/L with method on Kodak Ektachem® *5706*
Serum No Effect Physiological No effect in 6 patients with hypertension given 500 mg drug daily for at least 12 months *37*
Urine Decrease Physiological Impaired excretion with chronic administration *5869* Thiazides may decrease urinary excretion of calcium *3971*
Urine Increase Physiological Initial diuretic response *174*

Catecholamines *Urine No Effect Physiological* No effect observed *1444*

Chloride *Serum Increase Physiological* With prolonged therapy hyperchloremic alkalosis *3669*

Cholesterol *Serum Increase Physiological* Thiazides may cause increased concentration *3971*
Serum No Effect Analytical No effect at concentrations up to 30 mg/L on method on Kodak Ektachem® *5706*

Citrate *Urine Decrease Physiological* Up to 30% decrease observed *4014*

Creatine Kinase Isoenzymes *Serum No Effect Analytical* No interference observed at a concentration of 12.5 mg/L (42.3 µmol/L) with CK-MB method on Du Pont aca *1519*

Creatinine *Serum Increase Physiological* Thiazides may rarely cause renal failure, renal dysfunction or interstitial nephritis *3971*

Creatinine Clearance *Urine Decrease Physiological* Reported effect *3669*

Erythrocytes *Blood Decrease Physiological* Aplastic anemia reported to occur occasionally *6264* Pancytopenia/aplastic anemia *132*
Urine Increase Physiological occurred in one case after i.v. administration *2754*

Estriol *Urine No Effect Analytical* No interference with hydrolysis observed *5105*

Glomerular Filtration Rate *Urine Decrease Physiological* Increased glomerular-tubular feedback activity in association with carbonic anhydrase inhibition and suppression of proximal tubular reabsorption *633*

Glucose *Serum Increase Physiological* Diabetogenic properties of drug affect glucose tolerance test *5869* Hyperglycemia may occur in certain patients receiving thiazides *3971*
Serum No Effect Analytical No effect of concentrations up to 30 mg/L on method on Kodak Ektachem® *5706*
Urine Increase Physiological Diabetogenic-like action of drug affects glucose tolerance test *5869* Thiazides may cause hyperglycemia and glycosuria *3971*

Glucose Tolerance *Serum Decrease Physiological* Diabetogenic-like action of drug *4555*

Granulocytes *Blood Decrease Physiological* Thiazides may rarely cause agranulocytosis *3971*

HDL-Cholesterol *Serum No Effect Analytical* No effect of concentrations up to 30 mg/L on method on Kodak Ektachem® *5706*

Hematocrit *Blood Decrease Physiological* Pancytopenia *132* Thiazides may rarely cause aplastic or hemolytic anemia *3971*

Hemoglobin *Blood Decrease Physiological* Thiazides may rarely cause aplastic or hemolytic anemia *3971* Pancytopenia *132*

Chlorothiazide *(continued)*

17-Hydroxycorticosteroids *Urine Increase Analytical* Interferes with Porter-Silber reaction *in vitro6515*

17-Ketogenic Steroids *Urine No Effect Analytical* Probably minimal interference with Zimmermann reaction *5869*

LE Cells *Blood Positive Physiological* May produce LE-like syndrome *5870*

Leukocytes *Blood Decrease Physiological* Leukopenia/pancytopenia *132* Aplastic anemia reported to occur occasionally *6264* Thiazides may rarely cause leukopenia *3971*

Lipase *Serum Increase Physiological* Thiazides may rarely cause pancreatitis *3971*
Serum No Effect Analytical No effect of concentrations up to 30 mg/L on method on Kodak Ektachem® *5706*

Lithium *Serum Increase Physiological* Thiazides may decrease lithium clearance resulting in higher serum concentrations *3971*

Lithium Clearance *Urine Decrease Physiological* Thiazides may decrease lithium clearance resulting in higher serum concentrations *3971*
Urine Increase Physiological Acute administration increased clearance by about 25% in sodium-restricted healthy adults *633*

Magnesium *Red Blood Cells No Effect Physiological* No significant effect in 6 patients with hypertension given 500 mg daily for at least 12 months *37*
Serum Decrease Physiological Hypermagnesuria may occur in certain patients receiving thiazides which may result in hypomagnesemia *3971*
Serum No Effect Physiological No effect in 6 patients with hypertension given 500 mg drug daily for at least 12 months *37*
Urine Increase Physiological 1.5 g/d for 2 d produces 33% increase *2452* Hypermagnesuria may occur in certain patients receiving thiazides which may result in hypomagnesemia *3971*

Neutrophils *Blood Decrease Physiological* Occasionally observed *4014* Occasional case of agranulocytosis reported *6264*

5'-Nucleotidase *Serum Increase Physiological* May cause cholestatic jaundice *3810*

PAH Clearance *Urine Decrease Physiological* Competitive inhibition of secretion *2378*

Phosphate *Serum No Effect Analytical* No effect of concentrations up to 30 mg/L on method on Kodak Ektachem® *5706*

Platelets *Blood Decrease Physiological* Aplastic anemia reported to occur occasionally *6264* Pancytopenia due to aplastic anemia may occur *289* Thiazides may rarely cause thrombocytopenia *3971*

Potassium *Red Blood Cells No Effect Physiological* No significant effect in 6 patients with hypertension treated with 500 mg daily for at least 12 months *37*
Serum Decrease Physiological Hypokalemia may develop with brisk diuresis *3971* Significant reduction observed in 6 patients with hypertension given 500 mg daily for at least 12 months *37* Diuretic action *5869*
White Blood Cells Decrease Physiological Significant reduction in lymphocyte potassium in 6 patients with hypertension treated with 500 mg daily for at least 12 months *37*

Prothrombin Time *Plasma No Effect Physiological* Does not affect action of administered coumarins *4998*

Quinidine *Serum Increase Physiological* Drugs that alkalinize the urine reduce the renal elimination of quinidine *5996* Alkalinizes urine, increases reabsorption *2452*

Sodium *Serum Decrease Physiological* May cause hyponatremia *3669* Dilutional hyponatremia may occur in edematous patients *3971*
Urine Increase Physiological Diuretic action *3669*

Theophylline *Serum Increase Analytical* Slight effect, 0.11 mg/dL, at 100 mg/L and 0.23 mg/dL at 1000 mg/L, on method on Kodak Ektachem® 700 *586*

Triglycerides *Serum Increase Physiological* Thiazides may cause increased concentration *3971*
Serum No Effect Analytical No effect of concentrations up to 30 mg/L on method on Kodak Ektachem® *5706*

Urea Nitrogen *Serum Increase Physiological* Thiazides may rarely cause renal failure, renal dysfunction or interstitial nephritis *3971*

Uric Acid *Serum Decrease Physiological* If given i.v. in large doses has uricosuric effect *2378*
Serum Increase Physiological Decreased urate clearance *5869* Diuretic induced gout observed in one patient with hypertension *5416* Hyperuricemia may occur or acute gout may be precipitated in certain patients receiving thiazides *3971*
Serum No Effect Analytical No effect of concentrations up to 30 mg/L on method on Kodak Ektachem® *5706*
Urine Decrease Physiological Impaired clearance *3669*
Urine Increase Physiological If given i.v. in large doses has uricosuric effect *2378*

Uric Acid Clearance *Urine Increase Physiological* Concomitant increase with increase in lithium clearance with acute administration of diuretic *633*

Vanillylmandelic Acid *Urine No Effect Physiological* No effect observed *1444*

Volume *Urine Increase Physiological* Increase in maximum urine flow in association with administration of diuretic *633*

Warfarin *Plasma No Effect Physiological* No effect of 1 g/d for 21 d *2452*

Chlorphenesin

Albumin *Serum No Effect Analytical* At concentration of 150 mg/L had no effect on BCG method *5704*

Bicarbonate *Serum No Effect Analytical* At concentration of 150 mg/L had no effect on method using phenolphthalein *5704*

Bilirubin *Serum No Effect Analytical* At concentration of 150 mg/L had no effect on Jendrassik and Grof method *5704*

Calcium *Serum No Effect Analytical* At concentration of 150 mg/L had no effect on cresolphthalein method *5704*

Chloride *Serum No Effect Analytical* At concentration of 150 mg/L had no effect on mercurimetric method *5704*

Cholesterol *Serum No Effect Analytical* At concentration of 150 mg/L had no effect on Liebermann-Burchard method *5704*

Creatinine *Serum No Effect Analytical* At concentration of 150 mg/L had no effect on Technicon AutoAnalyzer® Jaffe method *5704*

Leukocytes *Blood Decrease Physiological* Rare leukopenia/agranulocytosis/pancytopenia *2754*

Occult Blood *Feces Increase Physiological* Two cases of gastrointestinal bleeding reported *2754*

Phosphate *Serum No Effect Analytical* At concentration of 150 mg/L had no effect on phosphomolybdate method *5704*

Platelets *Blood Decrease Physiological* Rare thrombocytopenia/pancytopenia *2754*

Potassium *Serum No Effect Analytical* At concentration of 150 mg/L had no effect on measurement by ISE with predilution *5704*

Protein *Serum No Effect Analytical* At concentration of 150 mg/L had no effect on biuret method with blank correction *5704*

Sodium *Serum No Effect Analytical* At concentration of 150 mg/L had no effect on measurement by ISE with predilution *5704*

Triglycerides *Serum No Effect Analytical* At concentration of 150 mg/L had no effect on lipase/esterase method *5704*

Urea Nitrogen *Serum No Effect Analytical* At concentration of 150 mg/L had no effect on diacetylmonoxime method *5704*

Uric Acid *Serum No Effect Analytical* At concentration of 150 mg/L had no effect on phosphotungstate reduction method *5704*

Chlorpheniramine

Alanine Aminotransferase *Serum Increase Physiological* May cause liver damage *467*
Serum No Effect Analytical At acute overdose concentration (20 mg/dL) on Technicon SMAC® method *6266*

Albumin *Serum No Effect Analytical* At concentration of 3 mg/L had no effect on BCG method *5704* At acute overdose concentration (20 mg/dL) on Technicon SMAC® method *6266*

Alkaline Phosphatase *Serum No Effect Analytical* At acute overdose concentration (20 mg/dL) on Technicon SMAC® method *6266*

Aspartate Aminotransferase *Serum Increase Physiological* May cause liver damage *467*
Serum No Effect Analytical At acute overdose concentration (20 mg/dL) on Technicon SMAC® method *6266*

Bicarbonate *Serum No Effect Analytical* At concentration of 200 mg/L had no effect on method using phenolphthalein *5704*

Bilirubin *Serum No Effect Analytical* At acute overdose concentration (20 mg/dL) on Technicon SMAC® method *6266* At concentration of 200 mg/L had no effect on Jendrassik and Grof method *5704*

Calcium *Serum No Effect Analytical* At acute overdose concentration (20 mg/dL) on Technicon SMAC® method *6266* At concentration of 200 mg/L had no effect on cresolphthalein method *5704*

Cannabinoids *Urine No Effect Analytical* No effect on Roche Abuscreen method *5006*

Chloride *Serum No Effect Analytical* At concentration of 2 mg/L had no effect on mercurimetric method *5704*

Cholesterol *Serum No Effect Analytical* At acute overdose concentration (20 mg/dL) on Technicon SMAC® method *6266* At concentration of 200 mg/L had no effect on Liebermann-Burchard method *5704*

Color *Blood Increase Analytical* May cause chocolate color *467*

Creatine Kinase *Serum No Effect Analytical* At acute overdose concentration (20 mg/dL) on Technicon SMAC® method *6266*

Creatinine *Serum No Effect Analytical* At concentration of 200 mg/L had no effect on Technicon AutoAnalyzer® Jaffe method *5704* At acute overdose concentration (20 mg/dL) on Technicon SMAC® method *6266*

Doxazosin *Serum No Effect Physiological* Coadministration with doxazosin had no effect on its pharmacokinetics *4642*

Drugs of Abuse Screen *Urine No Effect Analytical* No effect at concentration of 100 µg/mL on EZ-SCREEN procedure for cannabinoids and cocaine *1739*

Erythrocytes *Blood Decrease Physiological* Reported to cause hemolytic anemia *2753* Destroys cells on absorption *2242*

Felbamate *Serum No Effect Analytical* No significant interference observed with GLC method of Rifai et al *4958*

Glucose *Serum No Effect Analytical* At acute overdose concentration (20 mg/dL) on Technicon SMAC® method *6266*

Haptoglobin *Serum Decrease Physiological* May cause hemolytic anemia *467*

Hematocrit *Blood Decrease Physiological* Case of aplastic anemia after 10 y of low dose treatment *3030*

Hemoglobin *Blood Decrease Physiological* Case of aplastic anemia after 10 y of low dose treatment *3030* Reported to cause hemolytic anemia *2753* Causes hemolysis *2242* One case of aplastic anemia after 1 mo therapy, reversible with discontinuation of drug discontinuation of drug *1390*

Histamine *Plasma No Effect Analytical* Improbable inhibition of radio-enzyme assay at physiological concentrations although 50% inhibition at 3.2 µg/mL *2492*

^{131}I Uptake *Serum Decrease Physiological* Ornade®, Teldrin contain tetraiodofluorescein *4360*
Serum No Effect Physiological 16 mg/d reduced uptake by 48% *882*

Iron *Serum No Effect Analytical* At acute overdose concentration (20 mg/dL) on Technicon SMAC® method *6266*

Lactate Dehydrogenase *Serum No Effect Analytical* At acute overdose concentration (20 mg/dL) on Technicon SMAC® method *6266*

Leukocytes *Blood Decrease Physiological* Leukopenia (AMA Blood dyscrasias) *4017* One case of aplastic anemia after 1 mo therapy, reversible with discontinuation of drug *1390* Case of aplastic anemia after 10 y of low dose treatment *3030*

Methadone *Urine No Effect Analytical* Insignificant cross-reactivity of 0.3% observed with Roche Abuscreen ONTRAK method *3279*

Methemoglobin *Blood Increase Physiological* May cause hemolysis *2242*

p-Aminophenol *Urine No Effect Analytical* With addition of drugs at a concentration of 100 mg/L and of related compounds at 50 mg/L no significant effect observed on colorimetric method of van Bocxlaer on Cobas Mira analyzer which involves reacting free p-aminophenol with resorcinol in the presence of magnesium ions to form an indophenol dye measured at 550 nm *6163*

Phenytoin *Serum Increase Physiological* Possibly capable of increasing plasma concentration when drugs coadministered *1384*

Phosphate *Serum No Effect Analytical* At concentration of 200 mg/L had no effect on phosphomolybdate method *5704* At acute overdose concentration (20 mg/dL) on Technicon SMAC® method *6266*

Platelets *Blood Decrease Physiological* One case of aplastic anemia after 1 mo therapy, reversible with discontinuation of drug *1390* Case of aplastic anemia after 10 y of low dose treatment *3030* Thrombocytopenia reported *2754*

Protein *Serum No Effect Analytical* At concentration of 200 mg/L had no effect on biuret method with blank correction *5704* At acute overdose concentration (20 mg/dL) on Technicon SMAC® method *6266*
Urine Increase Physiological May cause renal damage *467*

Theophylline *Serum No Effect Analytical* No effect on method on Kodak Ektachem® 700 *1716*

Triglycerides *Serum No Effect Analytical* At concentration of 200 mg/L had no effect on lipase/esterase method *5704* At acute overdose concentration (20 mg/dL) on Technicon SMAC® method *6266*

Urea Nitrogen *Serum Increase Physiological* May cause renal damage *467*
Serum No Effect Analytical At concentration of 200 mg/L had no effect on diacetylmonoxime method *5704* At acute overdose concentration (20 mg/dL) on Technicon SMAC® method *6266*

Uric Acid *Serum No Effect Analytical* At acute overdose concentration (20 mg/dL) on Technicon SMAC® method *6266* At concentration of 200 mg/L had no effect on phosphotungstate reduction method *5704*

Volume *Urine Decrease Physiological* May cause oliguria with renal damage *467*

Chlorphentermine

Amobarbital *Urine No Effect Analytical* No interference using TLC with ethyl acetate: methanol: water: ammonium hydroxide and modified Dragendorff's reagent for detection *6502*

Amphetamine *Urine No Effect Analytical* No interference using TLC with ethyl acetate: methanol: water: ammonium hydroxide and modified Dragendorff's reagent for detection *6502*

Hydromorphone *Urine No Effect Analytical* No interference using TLC with ethyl acetate: methanol: water: ammonium hydroxide and modified Dragendorff's reagent for detection *6502*

Mescaline *Urine No Effect Analytical* No interference using TLC with ethyl acetate: methanol: water: ammonium hydroxide and modified Dragendorff's reagent for detection *6502*

Methamphetamine *Urine No Effect Analytical* No interference using TLC with ethyl acetate: methanol: water: ammonium hydroxide and modified Dragendorff's reagent for detection *6502*

Morphine *Urine No Effect Analytical* No interference using TLC with ethyl acetate: methanol: water: ammonium hydroxide and modified Dragendorff's reagent for detection *6502*

Pentobarbital *Urine No Effect Analytical* No interference using TLC with ethyl acetate: methanol: water: ammonium hydroxide and modified Dragendorff's reagent for detection *6502*

Phenmetrazine *Urine Positive Analytical* Similar R_f and color reaction on TLC using ethyl acetate: methanol: water: ammonium hydroxide and modified Dragendorff's reagent *6502*

Chlorphentermine *(continued)*

Phenobarbital *Urine No Effect Analytical* No interference using TLC with ethyl acetate: methanol: water: ammonium hydroxide and modified Dragendorff's reagent for detection *6502*

Phentermine *Urine Positive Analytical* Similar R_f and color reaction on TLC using ethyl acetate: methanol: water: ammonium hydroxide and modified Dragendorff's reagent *6502*

Phenylpropanolamine *Urine No Effect Analytical* No interference using TLC with ethyl acetate: methanol: water: ammonium hydroxide and modified Dragendorff's reagent for detection *6502*

Quinine *Urine Increase Analytical* Similar R_f and color reaction on TLC using ethyl acetate: methanol: water: ammonium hydroxide and modified Dragendorff's reagent *6502*

Secobarbital *Urine No Effect Analytical* No interference using TLC with ethyl acetate: methanol: water: ammonium hydroxide and modified Dragendorff's reagent for detection *6502*

Chlorpromazine

Alanine Aminotransferase *Serum Increase Physiological* Low incidence of jaundice observed with treatment, probably as a result of a sensitivity reaction, usually occurring between the second and fourth weeks of therapy, usually reversible on withdrawal of treatment *5659* May be damage of biliary canaliculi *6461* Of phenothiazines has greatest propensity to cause cholestatic jaundice *1384*

Albumin *Serum No Effect Analytical* No interference observed at a concentration of 20 mg/L (63 µmol/L) with method used on Du Pont aca *1507* At concentration of 3 mg/L had no effect on BCG method *5704*

Alkaline Phosphatase *Serum Increase Physiological* Low incidence of jaundice observed with treatment, probably as a result of a sensitivity reaction, usually occurring between the second and fourth weeks of therapy and usually reversible on withdrawal of medication *5659* Of phenothiazines has greatest propensity to cause cholestatic jaundice *1384* Hepatic sensitivity to drug (in up to 2% patients) *5485* In one patient who developed cholestasis with fever and leukopenia after 260 mg drug *4745*

Amitriptyline *Serum No Effect Analytical* Cross-reactivity less than 5% with Abbott TDx procedure *2487*

Amphetamine *Urine Increase Analytical* False positive results observed in 13 of 13 assays using Syva EMIT amphatamine method using a monoclonal antibody *1160* Metabolites of chlorpromazine may cause false positive urinary amphetamine results with Syva EMIT monoclonal d.a.u. immunoassay *4411*
Urine No Effect Analytical Observed reaction with method on Du Pont aca method at a concentration of 12 µg/L (37.6 µmol/L) *1554* No false positive results observed in 13 assays using Syva EMIT amphatamine method using a polyclonal antibody *1160*

Amphetamine/Methamphetamine *Urine Positive Analytical* False positive result observed in some patients taking chlorpromazine with/without chlorprothixene and promethazine when measured by Syva EMIT II procedure *5634*

Angiotensin-converting Enzyme
Cerebrospinal Fluid Increase Physiological In 14 schizophrenics treated for 254 ± 158 months with approximately 1000 mg chlorpromazine equivalents daily mean activity of 0.99 ± 0.10 U/L significantly higher than 0.75 ± 0.10 U/L in 9 controls *6296*
Serum No Effect Physiological In 14 schizophrenics treated with approximately 1000 mg chlorpromazine equivalents daily for 154 ± 158 months mean concentration of 29.1 ± 9.0 U/L not significantly different from 25.0 ± 7.2 U/L in 9 controls *6296*

Anti-ds DNA Antibodies *Serum Increase Physiological* In 40% to native-DNA of schizophrenic patients given long-term treatment *6633*

Anticardiolipin Antibodies *Serum Increase Physiological* Observed in 31 of 96 psychiatric patients treated chronically with chlorpromazine. 54 of the patients had IgM-lupus anticoagulant. Anticardiolipin antibodies observed in 31 of these, but only observed in 5 patients without lupus anticoagulant *873*

Anticardiolipin-specific IgM Antibodies
Serum Increase Physiological In 23 of 97 treated psychiatric patients increased anticardiolipin-specific IgM antibodies observed *3576*

Antidiuretic Hormone *Plasma Decrease Physiological* Mean concentration in 37 chlorpromazine treated schizophrenics was 0.95 pg/mL versus 2.74 pg/mL in 23 untreated controls *5271*
Plasma No Effect Physiological In 14 schizophrenics treated for 154 ± 158 months with approximately 1000 mg chlorpromazine equivalents daily mean concentration 3.93 ± 2.94 ng/L not significantly different from 4.08 ± 2.68 ng/L in 9 controls *6296* No effect of intramuscular injection of drug *4866*

Antinuclear Antibodies *Serum Increase Physiological* In patients treated for a long time with chlorpromazine high prevalence of antinuclear antibodies observed *0* In 63% of schizophrenic patients given long-term treatment *6633* Single case reported associated with rash and fever *1609*

Antinucleoprotein Antibodies
Serum Positive Physiological In 58% of schizophrenic patients given long-term treatment *6633*

Antithrombin III *Plasma No Effect Analytical* At concentration of 3 mg/L had no effect on Du Pont aca method *5704*

Aspartate Aminotransferase *Serum Increase Physiological* Hepatic sensitivity to drug (in up to 2% patients) *5485* In one patient who developed cholestasis with fever and leukopenia after 260 mg drug *4745* Low incidence of jaundice observed with treatment, probably as a result of a sensitivity reaction, usually occurring between the second and fourth weeks of therapy and usually reversible on withdrawal of treatment *5659* Of phenothiazines has greatest propensity to cause cholestatic jaundice *1384*

Barbiturate *Urine No Effect Analytical* Negative result obtained at a concentration of 12 µg/mL (38 µmol/L) with method on Du Pont aca *1555*

Benzodiazepine *Urine No Effect Analytical* Negative result obtained at a concentration of 12 µg/mL (38 µmol/L) with method on Du Pont aca *1556*

Benzoylecgonine *Urine No Effect Analytical* No significant interference observed at a concentration of 38 µmol/L with Sung and Neely modification of Syva EMIT procedure *148* Negative result obtained at a concentration of 12 µg/mL (38 µmol/L) with method on Du Pont aca *1558*

Bicarbonate *Serum No Effect Analytical* At concentration of 3 mg/L had no effect on method using phenolphthalein *5704*

Bile *Urine Increase Analytical* Alleged interference with BiliLabstix® *2451*

Bilirubin *Serum Increase Physiological* Sensitivity reaction (may cause jaundice in infant) *5485* In one patient who developed cholestasis with fever and leukopenia after 260 mg drug *4745* Low incidence of jaundice observed with treatment, probably as a result of a sensitivity reaction, usually occurring between the second and fourth weeks of therapy and usually reversible on withdrawal of treatment *5659* Has greatest propensity of phenothiazines to cause cholestatic jaundice *1384*
Serum No Effect Analytical At concentration of 3 mg/L had no effect on Jendrassik and Grof method *5704*
Urine Increase Analytical Metabolites may cause false positive in large quantities with Ames Ictotest reagent tablets *4034*
Urine No Effect Analytical No effect of metabolites observed with Ames Multistix and other reagent strip tests *4034*

Bilirubin, Direct *Serum Increase Physiological* In one patient who developed cholestasis with fever and Leukopenia after 260 mg drug *4745* Sensitivity reaction to drug (in up to 2% patients) *5485*

BSP Retention *Serum Increase Physiological* Induces transient cholestatic hepatitis (1 case) *1421*

Calcium *Serum No Effect Analytical* At concentration of 3 mg/L had no effect on cresolphthalein method *5704*

Cannabinoids *Urine No Effect Analytical* No effect on Roche Abuscreen method *5006* No effect observed at a concentration of 12 µg/mL (38 µmol/L) on method on Du Pont aca *1557*

Carbamazepine *Serum No Effect Analytical* At a concentration of 40 µg/mL had no significant cross-reactivity with carbamazepine at a concentration of 4.0 µg/mL when measured by method on Bayer Technicon Immuno 1® system *417* No cross-reactivity observed with method on Du Pont aca *1513*

Catecholamines *Plasma Increase Physiological* Increased metabolism, decreased organ uptake of norepinephrine *2024*
Plasma No Effect Analytical No effect on HPLC method of Koller for dopamine, epinephrine, and norepinephrine *3230*

Chloride *Serum No Effect Analytical* At concentration of 3 mg/L had no effect on mercurimetric method *5704*

Cholesterol *Serum Increase Analytical* 50 µg in reaction mixture produces color *882*
Serum Increase Physiological Associated with hepatocanalicular cholestatic jaundice *402*
Serum No Effect Analytical At concentration of 3 mg/L had no effect on CHOD-PAP method *5704*

Chromosomes *Test Conditions Abnormal Physiological* Clastogenic in human lymphocytes *in vitro5484*

Coombs' Test *Blood Positive Physiological* Immunological response to drug *2453*

Creatine Kinase *Serum Increase Physiological* May be due to injection only (occurs in 20%) *3946*

Creatinine *Serum No Effect Analytical* At concentration of 3 mg/L had no effect on Technicon AutoAnalyzer® Jaffe method *5704*

Drugs of Abuse Screen *Urine No Effect Analytical* No effect at concentration of 100 µg/mL on EZ-SCREEN procedure for cannabinoids and cocaine *1739*

Effective Renal Plasma Flow
Patient Increase Physiological Slight increase in renal blood flow *2242*

Eosinophils *Blood Increase Physiological* Eosinophilia rarely observed with treatment *5659* Often precursor of jaundice *4014*

Erythrocytes *Blood Decrease Physiological* Hemolytic anemia *1127* Occasional aplastic anemia reported *6264*

Estrogens *Urine Increase Physiological* Blocks ovulation, maintains decidual reaction *2242*

Ethosuximide *Serum No Effect Analytical* Insignificant cross-reactivity with method on Du Pont aca *1523*

Fatty Acids (FFA), Free *Serum Increase Physiological* 51% increase following single i.m. injection of 50 mg *2675*

Ferric Chloride Test *Urine Positive Analytical* Purple color *199*

Glucose *Serum Decrease Physiological* Hypoglycemia has been observed with treatment *5659*
Serum Increase Physiological Abnormally high with repeated doses *2604* Hyperglycemia has been observed with treatment *5659*
Serum No Effect Analytical At concentration of 0.1 mg/L had no effect on Kodak Ektachem® method *5704* At concentration of 3 mg/L had no effect on GOD/POD-PAP method *5704*
Urine Increase Physiological Due to hyperglycemia *2754* Glycosuria has been observed with treatment *5659*

Glucose Tolerance *Serum Decrease Physiological* Acute high dose effect in normal subjects *1751* Abnormal curves in 40% patients *4014*
Serum No Effect Physiological Low dose effect in normal subjects *4978*

β-Glucuronidase *Serum Increase Physiological* Result of toxic hepatitis *6461*

γ-Glutamyltransferase *Serum Increase Physiological* Low incidence of jaundice observed with treatment, probably as a result of a sensitivity reaction, usually occurring between the second and fourth weeks of therapy and reversible on withdrawal of medication *5659*

Gonadotropins *Urine Decrease Physiological* Blocks ovulation, maintains decidual reaction *2242*

Granulocytes *Blood Decrease Physiological* Of phenothiazines has greatest propensity to produce agranulocytosis *1384* Agranulocytosis rarely observed with treatment *5659*

Growth Hormone *Plasma Decrease Physiological* Probably inhibits secretion of pituitary growth hormone *5506*
Plasma No Effect Physiological No significant difference in patients receiving drug on continuing basis versus controls *6491*

Guaiacols Spot Test *Urine Positive Analytical* False reaction with screening test of Rogers *5061*

Haptoglobin *Serum Decrease Physiological* Hemolytic anemia *3810*

Hematocrit *Blood Decrease Physiological* Hemolytic or aplastic anemia rarely observed with treatment *5659* Hemolytic anemia *1127*

Hemoglobin *Blood Decrease Physiological* Hemolytic anemia *1127* Hemolytic or aplastic anemia rarely observed with treatment *5659*

Histamine *Plasma No Effect Analytical* Although 50% inhibition of radio-enzyme assay occurs at 25 µg/mL no clinical effect likely to occur since physiological concentration is 0.002-0.122 µg/mL *2492*

17-Hydroxycorticosteroids *Urine Decrease Physiological* Inhibition of hypothalamus and decreased ACTH secretion *2055*

5-Hydroxyindoleacetic Acid *Urine Decrease Analytical* Interferes with method of Goldenberg *2219* Inhibits color development *1444*
Urine No Effect Analytical No effect on FPIA method on Abbott TDx *695*

^{131}I Uptake *Serum Increase Physiological* With procyclidine decreased renal clearance (45 to 27 mL/min) *882*

Imipramine *Serum No Effect Analytical* Cross-reactivity less than 5% with Abbott TDx procedure *2473*

Immunoglobulin M *Serum Increase Physiological* Significant correlation with dose and duration of treatment in schizophrenic patients *6633* After continuous treatment for 5 years with chlorpromazine 6 of 29 schizophrenic patients had progressive increase of serum IgM and one developed an IgM monoclonal gammopathy and a lymphocyte immunoglobulin heavy and kappa light chain rearrangement *0*

Isocitrate Dehydrogenase *Serum Increase Physiological* May be hypersensitive reaction *6461*

17-Ketogenic Steroids *Urine Increase Analytical* Interferes with Zimmermann reaction *5869*

17-Ketosteroids *Urine Decrease Physiological* Inhibition of hypothalamus and decreased ACTH secretion *2055*
Urine Increase Analytical Interferes with Zimmermann reaction *5869*
Urine Increase Physiological Alters steroid metabolism *661*

Lactate Dehydrogenase *Serum Increase Physiological* In one patient who developed cholestasis with fever and leukopenia after 260 mg drug *4745*

LE Cells *Blood Positive Physiological* Single case reported associated with rash and fever *1609*

Leukocytes *Blood Decrease Physiological* In one patient who developed cholestasis with fever and leukopenia after 260 mg drug *4745* Occasional aplastic anemia reported *6264* Isolated case of agranulocytosis reported in elderly woman (general incidence of 1 in 1300 in psychiatric population dose related) *3792* Agranulocytosis/Leukopenia/granulocytopenia *3693* Leukopenia rarely observed with treatment *5659*

Lipids *Serum Increase Physiological* Xanthomatous biliary cirrhosis may occur *3221*

Lupus Anticoagulant *Plasma Increase Physiological* IgM-lupus anticoagulant observed in 54 of 96 chronically treated psychiatric patients *873*

Lymphocyte T-Cells *Blood Decrease Physiological* In 13 of 41 patients with schizophrenia with long term treatment *6633*

Lysergic Acid Diethylamide *Urine Increase Analytical* Minimum concentration that caused a positive result with EMIT method to measure LSD < 4 mg/L *4968*

Malondialdehyde *Blood No Effect Physiological* Following treatment in schizophrenic patients significantly lower values *567*

Metanephrines, Total *Urine No Effect Analytical* At 15 mg/L on modified Pisano procedure *2372*

Metyrapone Test *Patient No Effect Physiological* May interfere with response to test *1444*

Monocytes *Blood Increase Physiological* Occasionally before agranulocytosis *3693*

Morphine *Urine No Effect Analytical* No significant interference observed at a concentration of 38 µmol/L with Sung and Neely modification of Syva EMIT procedure *148*

Neutrophils *Blood Decrease Physiological* Isolated case of agranulocytosis reported in elderly woman (general incidence of 1 in 1300 in psychiatric population dose related) *3792* Reported to cause agranulocytosis/neutropenia *4265* Occasional case of agranulocytosis reported *6264*

Chlorpromazine *(continued)*

Norepinephrine *Plasma Increase Physiological* Increases metabolism, decreases organ uptake *2242*

Nortriptyline *Serum No Effect Analytical* Cross-reactivity less than 5% with Abbott TDx procedure *2487*

Opiates *Urine No Effect Analytical* No effect observed at a concentration of 12 mg/dL (38 μmol/L) with method on Du Pont aca *1559*

Osmolality *Serum Decrease Physiological* Mean osmolarity 287 mosmol/L in 35 treated schizophrenic patients versus 295 mosmol/L in 23 controls *5271*
Serum No Effect Physiological In 14 schizophrenics treated for 154 ± 158 months with approximately 1000 chlorpromazine equivalents daily mean concentration 292 .8 ± 10.0 mOsm/kg compared with 294.1 ± 4.2 mOsm/kg in 9 controls *6296*
Urine No Effect Physiological In 14 schizophrenics treated for 154 ± 158 months with approximately 1000 mg chlorpromazine equivalents daily mean concentration of 554.6 ± 162.0 mOsm/kg compared with 685.0 ± 211.9 mOsm/kg in 9 controls *6296*

p-Aminophenol *Urine No Effect Analytical* With addition of drugs at a concentration of 100 mg/L and of related compounds at 50 mg/L no significant effect observed on colorimetric method of van Bocxlaer on Cobas Mira analyzer which involves reacting free p-aminophenol with resorcinol in the presence of magnesium ions to form an indophenol dye measured at 550 nm *6163*

Partial Thromboplastin Time
Plasma Increase Physiological Caused by circulating inhibitor resembling that seen in systemic lupus in schizophrenic patients *6633* In 97 psychiatric patients treated with chlorpromazine time prolonged in 5 patients with the use of an insensitive APTT reagent and in 14 patients with a lower phosopholipid content *3576*

Phenobarbital *Serum No Effect Analytical* No effect observed at a concentration of 52 μmol/L with Sung and Neely modification of Syva EMIT procedure *148* At concentration of 1.00 mg/mL (3.136 mmol/L) has no effect on method on Du Pont Dimension *1582* No significant cross-reactivity observed with method on Du Pont aca *1537*

Phenylketones *Urine Positive Analytical* Light purple with $FeCl_3$, same with Phenistix® *1195*

Phenytoin *Serum Increase Physiological* Reported impairment of metabolism *3340*
Serum No Effect Analytical No significant interference observed at a concentration of 1000 μg/mL (3.14 mmol/L) with method on Du Pont aca *1538* No effect at concentration of 1000 μg/mL (3136 μmol/L) on method on Du Pont Dimension *1583*

Phosphate *Serum No Effect Analytical* At concentration of 3 mg/L had no effect on phosphomolybdate method *5704* No effect of concentrations up to 50 mg/L on method on Kodak Ektachem® *5706*

Phospholipids *Serum Increase Physiological* May cause xanthomatous biliary cirrhosis *2377*

Plasminogen *Plasma No Effect Analytical* At concentration of 5 mg/L had no effect on Du Pont aca method *5704*

Platelets *Blood Decrease Physiological* Occasional aplastic anemia reported *6264* Thrombocytopenic purpura rarely observed with treatment *5659* Significant reduction, although still in normal range in 17 psychiatric patients treated for more than 1 y *2684* Associated with purpura and pancytopenia *128*

Porphobilinogen *Urine Increase Analytical* Reacts with Ehrlich's aldehyde reagent *6515*

Potassium *Serum No Effect Analytical* At concentration of 3 mg/L had no effect on flame-photometric method *5704* At concentration of 3 mg/L had no effect on measurement by ISE with predilution *5704*
Serum No Effect Physiological In 14 schizophrenics treated for 154 ± 159 months with approximately 1000 mg equivalents daily mean concentration 4.25 ± 0.21 mmol/L compared with 4.08 ± 0.20 mmol/L in 9 controls *6296*

Pregnancy Tests *Urine Positive Analytical* False positive pregnancy tests observed with treatment, although these are less common with serum tests *5659*

Primidone *Serum No Effect Analytical* No significant cross-reactivity with method on Du Pont aca *1541*

Progestins *Urine Decrease Physiological* Blocks ovulation, maintains decidual reaction *2242*

Prolactin *Plasma Increase Physiological* Significant increase within 5 minutes of ingestion of 50 mg orally and 3 to 27 times baseline at 2 h. Functions as potent dopamine antagonist in the tuberoinfundibular system. Effect dose related *5179* In 28 male schizophrenics treatment with neuroleptics for 3 weeks caused increase from mean baseline of 7.87 ± 4.9 μg/L to 39.65 ± 27.91 μg/L and in 20 schizophrenic women from 13.42 ± 10.31 μg/L to 102.54 ± 66.03 μg/L *3332* Neuroleptic drugs increase plasma prolactin concentrations with the increasing persisting throughout chronic treatment *5659* In 41 patients receiving mean dose of 1901 ± 1760 ng/d average plasma prolactin concentration 30.5 ± 17.3 ng/mL compared with 5 ± 3 ng/mL in normal male volunteers *6639* Marked increase in male and female psychiatric patients treated for up to 4 weeks *6098* Marked increase in normals in 2 h *6097* Normal response to intravenous TRH *891*

Propranolol *Serum Increase Physiological* Plasma concentration of both drugs increased when they are coadministered *6558* Coadministration of chlorpromazine with propranolol caused significant increase in propranolol concentration due to inhibition of metabolism and enhanced bioavailability *6245* Concomitant administration increases the concentrations of both drugs *5659*

Protein *Cerebrospinal Fluid Increase Analytical* Reacts as if phenol with Folin-Ciocalteu reagent *5869*
Serum No Effect Analytical At concentration of 3 mg/L had no effect on biuret method with blank correction *5704*
Urine Increase Analytical Affects turbidity tests for up to 3 d *116* In 2 patients receiving therapeutic doses on Ponceau S dye method in comparison with sulfosalicylic acid and trichloracetic acid methods *6611*

Prothrombin Time *Plasma Increase Physiological* Associated with failure of excretion of bile salts *2803*

Salicylate *Serum Increase Analytical* At 100 mg/L had significant positive interference on colorimetric methods of Heller (and modified version) and Trinder *2910*

Sodium *Serum No Effect Analytical* At concentration of 3 mg/L had no effect on flame-photometric method *5704* At concentration of 3 mg/L had no effect on measurement by ISE with predilution *5704*
Serum No Effect Physiological In 14 schizophrenics receiving approximately 1000 mg chlorpromazine equivalents daily for 154 ± 159 months mean concentration 140.7 ± 3.9 mmol/L compared with 141.8 ± 2.0 mmol/L in 9 controls *6296*

Specific Gravity *Urine No Effect Physiological* In 14 schizophrenics treated for 154 ± 158 months with approximately 1000 mg chlorpromazine equivalents daily mean SG 1.016 ± 0.004 compared with 1.020 ± 0.005 in 9 controls *6296*

Thyroid Stimulating Hormone
Serum Increase Physiological In hypothyroidism although no change in euthyroidism, increases TRH-induced TSH response *6412*

Thyroxine (T4) *Serum Decrease Physiological* Increased metabolism by hepatic microsomes *5869*

Tricyclic Antidepressants *Serum Increase Analytical* May cause false positive reaction in immunoassays for tricyclic antidepressants *3590*

Tricyclic Antidepressants Screen
Serum No Effect Analytical No significant effect observed at a concentration of 200 ng/mL (0.62 μmol/L) with method on Du Pont aca *1550*
Serum Positive Analytical High therapeutic concentrations may cause a positive response with method on Du Pont aca *1550*

Triglycerides *Serum No Effect Analytical* At concentration of 3 mg/L had no effect on lipase/esterase method *5704*

Urea Nitrogen *Serum No Effect Analytical* At concentration of 0.1 mg/L had no effect on Kodak Ektachem® method *5704* At concentration of 3 mg/L had no effect on diacetylmonoxime method *5704*
Test Conditions Increase Analytical Produces turbidity with Berthelot's reagent *3144*

Uric Acid *Serum Decrease Physiological* Uricosuric action within 2-3 d *5869*
Serum No Effect Analytical At concentration of 3 mg/L had no effect on phosphotungstate reduction method *5704*

Urine *Increase* *Physiological* Uricosuric action reported *3669*

Urobilinogen *Feces* *Decrease* *Physiological* Pale stools, due to cholestasis *2803*
Urine *Decrease* *Physiological* May be cholestasis *2803*
Urine *Increase* *Analytical* Reacts with Erhlich's aldehyde reagent *6515*

Valproic Acid *Serum* *Increase* *Physiological* In a study involving the coadministration of a 100 to 300 mg/d doses of chlorpromazine to schizophrenics with 400 mg/d dose of valproate resulted in a 15% increase in trough plasma concentrations of valproate *15* Administration of 100 - 300 mg/d of chlorpromazine to schizophrenic patients already receiving 200 mg b.i.d. revealed a 15% increase in trough valproic acid concentration *17*

Vanillylmandelic Acid *Urine* *Increase* *Physiological* Increased metabolism and decreased organ uptake of norepinephrine *6515*
Urine *No Effect* *Analytical* No effect on Gitlow method *2452*

Vitamin B_{12} *Serum* *Decrease* *Analytical* Possible inhibition effect on some strains *E. gracilis4014*

Volume *Urine* *Increase* *Physiological* ?depresses ADH secretion or water reabsorption *2242*

Chlorpropamide

Alanine Aminotransferase *Serum* *Increase* *Physiological* Cholestatic jaundice may occur rarely *4644* May cause cytotoxic liver damage *402*

Albumin *Serum* *Decrease* *Physiological* In isolated case with diabetes who developed proliferative glomerulonephritis indicating immunologically mediated reaction *226*
Serum *No Effect* *Analytical* At concentration of 150 mg/L had no effect on BCG method *5704*

Alkaline Phosphatase *Serum* *Increase* *Physiological* Infrequent intrahepatic cholestasis *2803* Cholestatic jaundice observed in one patient in association with red cell aplasia (prevalence of jaundice as high as 0.5%) *2118* Cholestatic jaundice may occur rarely *4644*

δ-Aminolevulinic Acid *Urine* *Increase* *Physiological* May precipitate cutaneous porphyria *2210*

Antidiuretic Hormone *Urine* *Increase* *Physiological* Stimulates release from neurohypophysis *2026*

Apolipoprotein A-I *Serum* *No Effect* *Analytical* At a concentration of 2710 μmol/L no significant effect observed on automated immunoturbidimetric method on Baxter Paramax analyzer *3005*

Apolipoprotein B *Serum* *No Effect* *Analytical* At a concentration of 2710 μmol/L no significant effect observed on automated immunoturbidimetric method on Baxter Paramax analyzer *3005*

Aspartate Aminotransferase *Serum* *Increase* *Physiological* May cause cytotoxic liver damage *402* Cholestatic jaundice observed in one patient in association with red cell aplasia (prevalence of jaundice as high as 0.5%) *2118* Cholestatic jaundice may occur rarely *4644* In isolated case of hypersensitivity reaction producing hepatic granulomas also in bone marrow *4961*

Bicarbonate *Serum* *No Effect* *Analytical* At concentration of 150 mg/L had no effect on method using phenolphthalein *5704*

Bile *Urine* *Increase* *Physiological* Cholestatic jaundice *139*

Bilirubin *Serum* *Increase* *Physiological* Cholestatic jaundice observed in one patient in association with red cell aplasia (prevalence of jaundice as high as 0.5%) *2118* Cholestatic jaundice of allergic nature may occur *2451* Cholestatic jaundice may occur rarely *4644* Isolated case of drug-induced hemolytic anemia *5183*
Serum *No Effect* *Analytical* At concentration of 150 mg/L had no effect on Jendrassik and Grof method *5704*

BSP Retention *Serum* *Increase* *Physiological* Infrequent cholestatic effect *2803*

Calcium *Serum* *Increase* *Analytical* At concentrations above 7.5 mg/L (normal therapeutic concentration 150 mg/L) raised concentration as measured by cresolphthalein method *5704*

Chloride *Serum* *Decrease* *Physiological* Drug-induced syndrome of inappropriate ADH secretion *4302*
Serum *No Effect* *Analytical* At concentration of 150 mg/L had no effect on mercurimetric method *5704*

Cholesterol *Serum* *Decrease* *Physiological* With 8 weeks treatment of 8 C-peptide negative insulin dependent diabetics *5456* May inhibit hepatic synthesis (?also absorption) *3669*
Serum *Increase* *Physiological* Infrequent cholestatic effect *2803*
Serum *No Effect* *Analytical* At concentration of 150 mg/L had no effect on CHOD-PAP method *5704*

Color *Feces* *Increase* *Analytical* Black color reported with chlorpropamide ingestion *3388*

Complement C_1q *Serum* *Increase* *Physiological* In isolated case with diabetes who developed proliferative glomerulonephritis indicating immunologically mediated reaction *226*

Complement CH50 *Serum* *Increase* *Physiological* In isolated case with diabetes who developed proliferative glomerulonephritis indicating immunologically mediated reaction *226*

Coombs' Test *Blood* *Positive* *Physiological* Immunological response to drug *2453*

Coombs' Test, Direct *Blood* *Positive* *Physiological* Single case with hemolytic anemia *2452* Isolated case of drug-induced hemolytic anemia *5183*

Coproporphyrin *Blood* *Increase* *Physiological* May precipitate cutaneous porphyria *2210*
Feces *Increase* *Physiological* May precipitate cutaneous porphyria *2210*

Creatinine *Serum* *Increase* *Physiological* In isolated case with diabetes who developed proliferative glomerulonephritis indicating immunologically mediated reaction *226*
Serum *No Effect* *Analytical* At 5 times therapeutic concentration on Technicon SMAC® , Beckman Astra® and Du Pont aca or Roche Cobas Bio methods or manual Jaffe method *4976* At concentration of 150 mg/L had no effect on Technicon AutoAnalyzer® Jaffe method *5704* No effect on liquid chromatographic method of Paroni *4540*

Creatinine Clearance *Urine* *Decrease* *Physiological* In isolated case with diabetes who developed proliferative glomerulonephritis indicating immunologically mediated reaction *226*

Eosinophils *Blood* *Increase* *Physiological* Allergic response *2484* Eosinophilia has been reported as an adverse reaction *4644* In isolated case with diabetes who developed proliferative glomerulonephritis indicating immunologically mediated reaction *226*

Erythrocytes *Blood* *Decrease* *Physiological* Occasional aplastic anemia reported *6264* Isolated case of pure red blood cell aplasia *4720* Mild anemia, rare aplastic or hemolytic anemia or pancytopenia *4644*

Glucagon *Plasma* *No Effect* *Physiological* No effect i.v. if given rapidly or slowly *4590*

Glucose *Serum* *Decrease* *Analytical* At concentrations above 500 mg/L (normal therapeutic concentration 150 mg/L) lowered concentration as measured by GOD-PERID method *5704*
Serum *Decrease* *Physiological* Sulfonylurea derivative promotes insulin secretion *4644* Incidence of 10.0% observed in French Pharmacovigilance database *4106*
Serum *No Effect* *Analytical* No effect at 10 mmol/L on glucokinase based assay of Scott *5414* No effect on glucose oxidase (GOD-PERID) method of Boehringer *5480* No effect at 5000 mg/L on hexokinase method on Ames Seralyzer *5706* At concentration of 1,000 mg/L had no effect on GOD/POD-PAP method *5704*

γ-Glutamyltransferase *Serum* *Increase* *Physiological* Cholestatic jaundice may occur rarely *4644* Cholestatic jaundice observed in one patient in association with red cell aplasia (prevalence of jaundice as high as 0.5%) *2118*

Glycated Hemoglobin *Blood* *No Effect* *Analytical* At a concentration of 750 mg/L had an insignificant - 6.1% interference with method on Abbott Vision *1885*

Granulocytes *Blood* *Decrease* *Physiological* Agranulocytosis has been reported as an adverse reaction: may even be pancytopenia *4644*

Guanase *Serum* *Increase* *Physiological* May cause cytotoxic liver damage *402*

Chlorpropamide *(continued)*

HDL_3-Cholesterol *Serum Decrease Physiological* With 8 weeks treatment of 8 C-peptide negative insulin dependent diabetics *5456*

HDL-Cholesterol *Serum Decrease Physiological* With 8 weeks treatment of 8 C-peptide negative insulin dependent diabetics *5456*

Hematocrit *Blood Decrease Physiological* Isolated case of drug-induced hemolytic anemia *5183* Mild anemia, rare aplastic anemia *4644*

Hemoglobin *Blood Decrease Physiological* Mild anemia, rare aplastic anemia *4644* Isolated case of drug-induced hemolytic anemia *5183*
Urine Increase Physiological Isolated case of drug-induced hemolytic anemia *5183*

Insulin *Plasma Decrease Physiological* Observed when initial level high *492*
Plasma Increase Physiological Effect observed during tolerance test *3687* Observed in most patients (especially if low initially) *492*

Lactate Dehydrogenase *Serum Increase Physiological* Isolated case of drug-induced hemolytic anemia *5183* In isolated case of hypersensitivity reaction producing hepatic granulomas: also in bone marrow *4961*

LDL-Cholesterol *Serum Decrease Physiological* With 8 weeks treatment of 8 C-peptide negative insulin dependent diabetics *5456*

Leukocytes *Blood Decrease Physiological* Leukopenia has been reported as an adverse reaction: may even be pancytopenia *4644* Occasional aplastic anemia reported *6264* Isolated case of agranulocytosis observed *6087* Agranulocytosis *6423*
Blood Increase Physiological Due to eosinophilia of hypersensitivity *3810*

Lovastatin *Serum No Effect Physiological* In patients with hypercholesterolemia and noninsulin-dependent diabetes mellitus coadministration of lovastatin and oral hypoglycemics had no interactions *3982*

Lymphocytes *Blood Increase Physiological* Mild, of no clinical significance *2754*

Neutrophils *Blood Decrease Physiological* Isolated case of agranulocytosis observed *6087* Occasional aplastic anemia reported *6264*

5'-Nucleotidase *Serum Increase Physiological* Due to cholestasis *2911*

Occult Blood *Feces Increase Physiological* Associated with severe diarrhea and bleeding *4644*

Ornithine Carbamoyltransferase
Serum Increase Physiological May cause cytotoxic liver damage *402*

Osmolality *Serum Decrease Physiological* May rarely cause syndrome of inappropriate ADH secretion *4644*
Urine Increase Physiological Normal diuretic response also if diabetes insipidus *4136* May rarely cause syndrome of inappropriate ADH secretion *4644*

Phosphate *Serum No Effect Analytical* At concentration of 150 mg/L had no effect on phosphomolybdate method *5704*

Platelets *Blood Decrease Physiological* Thrombocytopenia has been reported as an adverse reaction: may even be pancytopenia *4644* Occasional aplastic anemia reported *6264* Thrombocytopenia or aplastic anemia may occur *132*

Porphobilinogen *Urine Increase Physiological* May aggravate cutaneous porphyria *2210*

Porphyrin, Total *Urine Increase Physiological* May precipitate attack of acute porphyria *1687*

Potassium *Serum No Effect Analytical* At concentration of 150 mg/L had no effect on flame-photometric method *5704*

Pramipexole *Serum No Effect Physiological* Coadministration of chlorpropamide with pramipexole presumed to have no effect on the oral clearance of pramipexole *4680*

Prazosin *Serum No Effect Physiological* Coadministration of prazosin with chlorpropamide had no apparent adverse drug interaction in limited clinical experience *4649*

Protein *Serum No Effect Analytical* At concentration of 150 mg/L had no effect on biuret method with blank correction *5704*
Urine Increase Physiological Nephrotoxic effect *6284* In isolated case with diabetes who developed proliferative glomerulonephritis indicating immunologically mediated reaction *226* Isolated case of drug-induced hemolytic anemia *5183*

Prothrombin Time *Plasma Increase Physiological* Associated with failure of excretion of bile salts *2803*

Protoporphyrin *Blood Increase Physiological* May precipitate cutaneous porphyria *2210*
Feces Increase Physiological May precipitate cutaneous porphyria *2210*
Urine Increase Physiological May precipitate cutaneous porphyria *2210*

Reticulocytes *Blood Decrease Physiological* Isolated case of pure red blood cell aplasia *4720*

Sodium *Serum Decrease Physiological* Induces inappropriate ADH secretion *6399* May rarely cause syndrome of inappropriate ADH secretion *4644* Drug-induced syndrome of inappropriate ADH secretion *4302*
Serum No Effect Analytical At concentration of 150 mg/L had no effect on flame-photometric method *5704*

T3-Uptake *Serum Increase Physiological* Competes for thyroxine binding globulin sites *882*

Thyroxine (T4) *Serum Decrease Physiological* Displaces thyroxine from thyroxine binding globulin *5869*

Thyroxine (T4) (Murphy-Pattee)
Serum Decrease Physiological May be competition for thyroxine binding globulin *882*

Triglycerides *Serum No Effect Analytical* At concentration of 150 mg/L had no effect on lipase/esterase method *5704*

Urea Nitrogen *Serum No Effect Analytical* At concentration of 150 mg/L had no effect on diacetylmonoxime method *5704*

Uric Acid *Serum No Effect Analytical* At concentration of 150 mg/L had no effect on phosphotungstate reduction method *5704*

Urobilinogen *Feces Decrease Physiological* Pale stools due to cholestasis (infrequent) *2803*
Urine Decrease Physiological Cholestasis may occur infrequently *2803*

Uroporphyrin *Urine Increase Physiological* May precipitate cutaneous porphyria *2210*

Volume *Urine Decrease Physiological* In patients with diabetes insipidus *5394*

Water Clearance, Free *Urine Decrease Physiological* Normal antidiuretic response in normals *4136*

Chlorprothixene

Alanine Aminotransferase *Serum Increase Physiological* May cause hepatotoxicity (reversible) *3810*

Albumin *Serum No Effect Analytical* At concentration of 1 mg/L had no effect on BCG method *5704*
Urine No Effect Analytical Using a fluorimetric assay with Albumin Blue 580 on a Cobas Fara centrifugal analyzer for the detection of microalbuminuria no significant interference was detected at a concentration of 10 mg/L *3117*

Alkaline Phosphatase *Serum Increase Physiological* Hepatotoxicity (reversible) cholestatic effect *3810*

Amphetamine/Methamphetamine
Urine No Effect Analytical No false positive results observed in 9 urines from 9 patients taking drug when measured by Syva EMIT II procedure *5634*

Aspartate Aminotransferase *Serum Increase Physiological* May cause hepatotoxicity (reversible) *3810*

Bicarbonate *Serum No Effect Analytical* At concentration of 1 mg/L had no effect on method using phenolphthalein *5704*

Bile *Urine Increase Physiological* May cause hepatotoxicity (reversible) *2024*

Bilirubin *Serum Increase Physiological* Hepatotoxicity (reversible) cholestatic effect *3810*
Serum No Effect Analytical At concentration of 1 mg/L had no effect on Jendrassik and Grof method *5704*
Urine Increase Physiological May cause hepatotoxicity (reversible) *3810*

BSP Retention *Serum Increase Physiological* May cause hepatotoxicity (reversible) *3810*

Calcium *Serum* *No Effect* *Analytical* At concentration of 1 mg/L had no effect on cresolphthalein method *5704*

Catecholamines *Plasma* *No Effect* *Analytical* No effect on HPLC method of Koller for dopamine, epinephrine, and norepinephrine *3230*

Chloride *Serum* *No Effect* *Analytical* At concentration of 1 mg/L had no effect on mercurimetric method *5704*

Cholesterol *Serum* *No Effect* *Analytical* At concentration of 1 mg/L had no effect on Liebermann-Burchard method *5704*

Creatinine *Serum* *No Effect* *Physiological* Constant concentration regardless of dose of drug co-administered and duration *5467*

Eosinophils *Blood* *Increase* *Physiological* Allergic manifestation *2754*

Glucose *Serum* *Increase* *Physiological* Due to altered endocrine function *2754*
Urine *Increase* *Physiological* Due to altered endocrine function *2754*

Histamine *Plasma* *No Effect* *Analytical* Although 50% inhibition of radio-enzyme assay occurs at 50 µg/mL unlikely to be of clinical significance since physiological concentration about 0.01 µg/mL *2492*

LE Cells *Blood* *Positive* *Physiological* May produce LE-like syndrome *5870*

Leukocytes *Blood* *Decrease* *Physiological* Possible hematological disorder *2242*

Phosphate *Serum* *No Effect* *Analytical* At concentration of 1 mg/L had no effect on phosphomolybdate method *5704*

Platelets *Blood* *Decrease* *Physiological* Purpura or pancytopenia may occur *2754*

Pregnancy Tests *Urine* *Positive* *Analytical* Endocrine abnormality *2754*

Protein *Serum* *No Effect* *Analytical* At concentration of 1 mg/L had no effect on biuret method with blank correction *5704*

Triglycerides *Serum* *No Effect* *Analytical* At concentration of 1 mg/L had no effect on lipase/esterase method *5704*

Urea Nitrogen *Serum* *No Effect* *Analytical* At concentration of 1 mg/L had no effect on diacetylmonoxime method *5704*
Serum *No Effect* *Physiological* Constant concentration regardless of dose of drug co-administered and duration *5467*

Uric Acid *Serum* *Decrease* *Physiological* Reduction of from 8 to 69% in 30 psychiatric patients *5467* Uricosuric effect within 2-3 d of start of drug *5869*
Serum *No Effect* *Analytical* At concentration of 1 mg/L had no effect on phosphotungstate reduction method *5704*
Urine *Increase* *Physiological* Significant increase during treatment *5467* Uricosuric action *2521*

Chlortetracycline

Alanine Aminotransferase *Serum* *Increase* *Physiological* Hepatotoxic effect with centrolobular necrosis *2024*

Alkaline Phosphatase *Serum* *Increase* *Physiological* Hepatotoxic effect with centrolobular necrosis *2024*

Aspartate Aminotransferase *Serum* *Increase* *Physiological* Hepatotoxic effect with centrolobular necrosis *2024*

Bile *Urine* *Increase* *Physiological* Hepatotoxic effect with centrolobular necrosis *2024*

Bilirubin *Serum* *Increase* *Physiological* Hepatotoxic effect with centrolobular necrosis *2024*
Serum *No Effect* *Physiological* Critically insignificant displacement from protein in neonates *6314*

BSP Retention *Serum* *Increase* *Physiological* Hepatotoxic effect with centrolobular necrosis *4012*

Catecholamines *Urine* *Increase* *Analytical* Interference with fluorometric methods *4243*

Cholesterol *Serum* *Decrease* *Physiological* Hepatotoxic effect with centrolobular necrosis *2024* Not as effective as neomycin reacts with bile acids *2452*

Eosinophils *Blood* *Increase* *Physiological* Probably allergic response *2754*

Erythrocytes *Blood* *Decrease* *Physiological* Pancytopenia (AMA Blood dyscrasias) *4017*

Folate *Urine* *Increase* *Physiological* With dose of 3 g/d *2242*

Hemoglobin *Blood* *Decrease* *Physiological* Hemolytic anemia may occur *2754*

Leukocytes *Blood* *Decrease* *Physiological* Pancytopenia (AMA Blood dyscrasias) *4017*

Nitrogen *Urine* *Increase* *Physiological* Effect observed in malnourished *2242*

N-Methylnicotinamide *Urine* *Increase* *Physiological* With dose of 3 g/d *2242*

Nonprotein Nitrogen *Serum* *Increase* *Physiological* Effect observed in malnourished *2242*

Occult Blood *Feces* *Increase* *Physiological* Occasional case of pseudomembranous colitis reported with mucus and bloody diarrhea *689*

Platelets *Blood* *Decrease* *Physiological* Pancytopenia (AMA Blood dyscrasias) *4017*

Prothrombin Time *Plasma* *Increase* *Physiological* Reported effect due to action in gastrointestinal tract *51*

Riboflavin *Urine* *Increase* *Physiological* With dose of 3 g/d *2242*

Sugar *Urine* *Increase* *Analytical* Acts as reducing substance *2025*

Urea Nitrogen *Serum* *Increase* *Physiological* Dose related antianabolic action *2754*

Chlorthalidone

Alanine Aminotransferase *Serum* *Increase* *Physiological* Single case of severe reversible myopathy noted *2929*

Aldosterone *Plasma* *Increase* *Physiological* At 3 d but not after 3 mo in 8 patients with mild hypertension given 50 mg/d *5081* At least 50% increase in pre- and post-menopausal women given 100 mg/d for 6 weeks *628*
Urine *Increase* *Physiological* Single case of severe reversible myopathy noted *2929*

Ammonia *Plasma* *Increase* *Physiological* Partially due to decreased potassium and alkalosis *179*

Amylase *Serum* *Increase* *Physiological* May precipitate acute pancreatitis *2972*

Antidiuretic Hormone *Plasma* *Increase* *Physiological* Secreted in response to hyponatremia *1856*

Apolipoprotein A-I *Serum* *No Effect* *Physiological* During diuretic therapy for 6 weeks in 23 subjects *2191* No effect of monotherapy for 6 weeks *141* In 22 premenopausal and 18 postmenopausal women given 100 mg/d for 6 weeks *628* Decrease by -1 mg/dL in 10 patients given 100 mg daily for 1 mo *4213*

Apolipoprotein A-II *Serum* *No Effect* *Physiological* No effect of monotherapy for 6 weeks *141* In 22 premenopausal and 18 postmenopausal women given 100 mg/d for 6 weeks *628* During diuretic therapy for 6 weeks in 23 subjects *2191*

Apolipoprotein B *Serum* *Increase* *Physiological* Increase by 11 mg/dL in 10 patients given 100 mg daily for 1 mo *4213* Increase by 16% in 18 postmenopausal women given 100 mg/d for 6 weeks *628*
Serum *No Effect* *Physiological* In 22 premenopausal women given 100 mg/d for 6 weeks *628* No effect of monotherapy for 6 weeks *141* During diuretic therapy for 6 weeks in 23 subjects *2191*

Apolipoprotein C-II *Serum* *No Effect* *Physiological* Increase by 1 mg/dL in 10 patients given 100 mg daily for 1 mo *4213*

Apolipoprotein C-III *Serum* *No Effect* *Physiological* Increase by 2 mg/dL in 10 patients given 100 mg daily for 1 mo *4213*

Aspartate Aminotransferase *Serum* *Increase* *Physiological* Single case of severe reversible myopathy noted *2929*

Atrial Natriuretic Peptide *Plasma* *Decrease* *Physiological* In 19 hypertensive patients treated with an average of 25 mg/d for 6 weeks caused nonsignificant increase to 19.8 ± 3.3 pg/mL from mean baseline of 19.1 ± 2.2 pg/mL but with further treatment for a total of 3 months mean concentration decreased nonsignificantly to 16.7 ± 3.4 pg/mL *553*

Benazepril *Serum* *No Effect* *Physiological* No clinically important pharmacokinetic interactions observed when drugs coadministered *1033*

Chlorthalidone *(continued)*

Betaxolol *Serum No Effect Physiological* Coadministration had no effect on pharmacokinetics of betaxolol *2067*

Bicarbonate *Serum Increase Physiological* From 2 to 3 mmol/L at doses from 25 to 200 mg/d in 37 patients over 8 weeks *6110* Metabolic alkalosis in severe cases *1856*

Calcium *Serum Increase Physiological* Occurs in normal and hyperparathyroid *3511*
Urine Decrease Physiological Decreased in normals and hyperparathyroid *3511*

Casts *Urine No Effect Physiological* Normally but augments effects of acidifying agents *2814*

Chloride *Serum Decrease Physiological* Hypochloremic alkalosis is common in patients receiving chlorthalidone *2726* Progressive effect with dose: from 3 mmol/L with 25 mg/d to 6 mmol/L at 200 mg/d in 37 patients treated for 8 weeks *6110* Single case of severe reversible myopathy noted *2929*
Urine Increase Physiological May produce marked diuresis *4014*

Cholesterol *Serum Decrease Physiological* Statistically significant decrease of 3 mg/dL in 12 men receiving drug in conjunction with diet to reduce cholesterol *145*
Serum Increase Physiological 5% change during monotherapy in 302 subjects for 1 y *2224* 5% in long term, 9% in short term in several studies with monotherapy *141* Increase by 10 mg/dL in 1,000 men and women with mild hypertension treated for 1 y *2224* In short term studies administration of chlorthalidone increased concentration of cholesterol by 10 to 20% within a year *3730* 9% change in 39 subjects treated with drug only for less than 1 y *2337* Increase by 26 mg/dL in 10 patients given 100 mg daily for 1 mo *4213* Increase by 13% in 18 postmenopausal women given 100 mg/d for 6 weeks *628*
Serum No Effect Physiological In 22 premenopausal women given 100 mg/d for 6 weeks *628* In 136 patients with stage I diastolic hypertension treated with 15 mg/d caused change from mean baseline of 5.94 ± 0.99 mmol/L by + 0.03 ± 0.06 mmol/L after 12 months and - 0.15 ± 0.07 mmol/L after 48 months *2335*

Creatine Kinase *Serum Increase Physiological* Single case of severe reversible myopathy noted *2929*

Creatinine *Serum Increase Physiological* Nephrotoxic effect *3669* Increased in hypertensives; most marked in those individuals whose initial values were lower *4841* Effect observed at dose of 100 mg/d and upwards in 37 patients treated for 8 weeks *6110*

Creatinine Clearance *Urine Decrease Physiological* Significantly reduced in 10 hypertensive patients given 25 mg daily for 16 weeks *2015*

Dopamine β-Hydroxylase *Serum Decrease Physiological* In 76 patients with mild hypertension treatment with chlorthalidone 50 mg/d was associated with an insignificant change in the plasma enzyme activity (- 13.0 U/L) in 20 in whom there was a significant reduction in blood pressure *2295*

Epinephrine *Plasma No Effect Physiological* In 22 premenopausal and 18 postmenopausal women given 100 mg/d for 6 weeks *628*

Erythrocytes *Blood Decrease Physiological* Leukopenia, agranulocytosis, thrombocytopenia and aplastic anemia have been observed in patients receiving chlorthalidone *2726* Aplastic anemia may occur *2754*

Estradiol *Plasma No Effect Physiological* In 22 premenopausal and 18 postmenopausal women given 100 mg/d for 6 weeks *628*

Fatty Acids (FFA), Free *Serum No Effect Physiological* In 22 premenopausal and 18 postmenopausal women given 100 mg/d for 6 weeks *628*

Glucose *Serum Increase Physiological* Increase by 15 mg/dL in 39 mildly hypertensives treated for 6 weeks *2337* Hyperglycemia may occur or latent diabetes mellitus may become manifest in patients receiving chlorthalidone *2726* Diabetogenic-like action affects pre- or diabetic *164* Progressive effect with dose: by 5 mg/dL with 25 mg/d to 14 mg/dL with 200 mg/d in 37 patients treated for 8 weeks *6110* In 28 hypertensive men treatment with 50 mg/d for 2 months caused significant increase of fasting concentration from mean baseline of 4.6 mmol/L to 5.3 mmol/L *5544*
Serum No Effect Physiological In 22 premenopausal and 18 postmenopausal women given 100 mg/d for 6 weeks *628*
Urine Increase Physiological Diabetogenic-like action of drug affects glucose tolerance test *5870* *5869* Hyperglycemia may occur or latent diabetes mellitus may become manifest in patients receiving chlorthalidone *2726*

Glucose Tolerance *Serum Decrease Physiological* In 21 essential hypertensives glucose and insulin concentrations increased to a greater extent after chlorthalidone administration than after administration of a placebo *4722* Diabetogenic-like action of drug *4555* Significant reduction in 10 hypertensive patients given 25 mg daily for 16 weeks *2015*

Granulocytes *Blood Decrease Physiological* Leukopenia, agranulocytosis, thrombocytopenia and aplastic anemia have been observed in patients receiving chlorthalidone *2726*

HDL-Cholesterol *Serum No Effect Physiological* In long or short term in several studies with monotherapy *141* In 136 patients with stage I diastolic hypertension treated with 15 mg/d caused change from mean baseline of 1.13 ± 0.29 mmol/L by + 0.06 ± 0.02 mmol/L after 12 months and + 0.02 ± 0.02 mmol/L after 48 months *2335* In 1,000 men and women with mild hypertension treated for 1 y *2224* Nonsignificant change during monotherapy in 302 subjects for 1 y *2224* Nonsignificant change in 39 subjects treated with drug only for less than 1 y *2337* In 22 premenopausal and 18 postmenopausal women given 100 mg/d for 6 weeks *628* In 19 hypertensives treated with mean dose of 25 mg/d for 3 months mean concentration nonsignificantly reduced from mean baseline of 43 ± 2 mg/dL to 41 ± 2 mg/dL but when combined with metoprolol mean concentration significantly reduced to 37 ± 1 mg/dL *553* In 22 premenopausal women without decrease in blood pressure treated for less than 1 y *628* Increase by 1 mg/dL in 10 patients given 100 mg daily for 1 mo *4213*

HDL-Triglycerides *Serum No Effect Physiological* In 22 premenopausal and 18 postmenopausal women given 100 mg/d for 6 weeks *628*

Hematocrit *Blood Decrease Physiological* Leukopenia, agranulocytosis, thrombocytopenia and aplastic anemia have been observed in patients receiving chlorthalidone *2726*
Blood Increase Physiological Increase by 1.4% in 39 mildly hypertensives treated for 6 weeks *2337*

Hemoglobin *Blood Decrease Physiological* Leukopenia, agranulocytosis, thrombocytopenia and aplastic anemia have been observed in patients receiving chlorthalidone *2726*

17-Hydroxycorticosteroids *Urine Increase Physiological* Reported effect *3669*

Insulin *Plasma Increase Physiological* In 28 hypertensive men treatment with 50 mg/d for 2 months caused significant increase of fasting concentration from mean baseline of 80.4 pmol/L to 144.9 pmol/L *5544*
Plasma No Effect Physiological In 22 premenopausal and 18 postmenopausal women given 100 mg/d for 6 weeks *628*

17-Ketosteroids *Urine Increase Physiological* Alleged increased excretion *2451*

Lactate Dehydrogenase *Serum Increase Physiological* Single case of severe reversible myopathy noted *2929*

LDL-Apolipoprotein B *Serum No Effect Physiological* In 19 hypertensives treated with an average of 25 mg/d for 3 months caused nonsignificant change from mean baseline of 109 ± 5 mg/dL to 110 ± 5 mg/dL but when metoprolol (in Logotron) added to regime concentration decreased nonsignificantly to 102 ± 7 mg/dL *553*

LDL-Cholesterol *Serum Increase Physiological* 10% change in 39 subjects treated with drug only for less than 1 y *2337* Increase by 13 mg/dL in 1,000 men and women with mild hypertension treated for 1 y *2224* Increase by 21% in 18 postmenopausal women given 100 mg/d for 6 weeks *628* 10% change during monotherapy in 302 subjects for 1 y *2224* 10% in long term, 10% in short term in several studies with monotherapy *141* In short term studies administration of chlorthalidone increased concentration of LDL-cholesterol by 10 to 20% within a year *3730*
Serum No Effect Physiological In 136 patients with stage I diastolic hypertension treated with 15 mg/d caused change from mean baseline of 4.13 ± 0.89 mmol/L by + 0.05 ± 0.06 mmol/L after 12 months and - 0.13 ± 0.06 mmol/L after 48 months *2335* In 22 premenopausal women without decrease in blood pressure treated for less than 1 y *628* In 22 premenopausal and 18 postmenopausal women given 100 mg/d for 6

weeks *628* In 19 hypertensives treated with mean dose of 25 mg/d for 3 months caused nonsignificant increase from mean baseline of 127 ± 7 mg/dL to 131 ± 8 mg/dL: when combined with metoprolol mean concentration reduced to 124 ± 8 mg/dL *553*

LDL-Triglycerides *Serum No Effect Physiological* In 22 premenopausal and 18 postmenopausal women given 100 mg/d for 6 weeks *628*

Leukocytes *Blood Decrease Physiological* Agranulocytosis *3176* Leukopenia, agranulocytosis, thrombocytopenia and aplastic anemia have been observed in patients receiving chlorthalidone *2726*

Lithium *Serum Increase Physiological* Lithium clearance may be reduced in patients receiving chlorthalidone, thus increasing serum lithium concentration *2726*

Lithium Clearance *Urine Decrease Physiological* Lithium clearance may be reduced in patients receiving chlorthalidone, thus increasing serum lithium concentration *2726*

Magnesium *Serum Decrease Physiological* Significant effect with prolonged treatment *5490*

Myoglobin *Urine Increase Physiological* Single case of severe reversible myopathy noted *2929*

Neutrophils *Blood Decrease Physiological* Occasional case of agranulocytosis reported *6264* Few cases reported *4014*

Norepinephrine *Plasma No Effect Physiological* In 22 premenopausal and 18 postmenopausal women given 100 mg/d for 6 weeks *628*

Urine Decrease Physiological In 76 patients with mild hypertension treatment with chlorthalidone 50 mg/d was associated with an insignificant change in the urine norepinephrine excretion (- 1.0 µg/g creatinine) in 20 in whom there was a significant reduction in blood pressure *2295*

Urine Increase Physiological After 3 d and 3 mo in 8 patients with mild hypertension given 50 mg/d *5081*

Osmolality *Serum Decrease Physiological* With ADH secretion in response to diuresis *1856*

Parathyroid Hormone *Plasma No Effect Physiological* But probable enhancement of peripheral action *3511*

pH *Blood Increase Physiological* Hypochloremic alkalosis is common in patients receiving chlorthalidone *2726*

Phospholipids *Serum No Effect Physiological* In 22 premenopausal and 18 postmenopausal women given 100 mg/d for 6 weeks *628*

Platelets *Blood Decrease Physiological* Leukopenia, agranulocytosis, thrombocytopenia and aplastic anemia have been observed in patients receiving chlorthalidone *2726* Associated with rare agranulocytosis *4014*

Potassium *Red Blood Cells Decrease Physiological* Not significant but tendency to fall in 10 hypertensive patients given 25 mg for 16 weeks *5588*

Serum Decrease Physiological Significant effect in pre- and postmenopausal women given 100 mg/d for 6 weeks *628* Progressive effect with dose: from 0.4 mmol/L with 25 mg/d to 1.0 mmol/L at 200 mg/d in 37 patients treated for 8 weeks *6110* In majority of children during course of treatment *313* 43% patients with hypokalemia given long term 25-100 mg/d *506* Hypokalemia is common in patients receiving chlorthalidone *2726* Diuretic induced depletion *2024* In 21 essential and 9 diabetic hypertensive patients during OGTT hypokalemia developed in 7 of the essential hypertensives whereas only one of diabetics developed hypokalemia below 3.5 mmol/L *4722* 0.5 mmol/L reduction in drug-treated versus placebo-treated patients *5632* Significant decrease observed in 19 hypertensive patients treated with 50 mg/d for 4 weeks *799* Hyperaldosteronism major causal factor in diuretic induced hypokalemia *2390* Significant fall from 8 weeks in 10 hypertensive patients given 25 mg daily for for 16 weeks *2015*

Urine Increase Physiological May produce marked diuresis *4014*

Protein *Urine Increase Physiological* Nephrotoxic effect *2024*

Prothrombin Time *Plasma Increase Physiological* Patients on coumarins *4013*

Renin Activity *Plasma Increase Physiological* In 19 hypertensive patients treatment with an average of 25 mg/d caused significant increase from mean baseline of 0.63 ± 0.10 ng/mL/h to 1.18 ± 0.20 ng/mL/h after 6 weeks and to 1.17 ± 0.19 ng/mL/h after 12 weeks *553* At 3 d and after 3 mo in 8 patients with mild hypertension given 50 mg/d *5081* At least 3 fold increase in pre- and post-menopausal women given 100 mg/d for 6 weeks *628*

Plasma No Effect Physiological Insignificant change in 10 hypertensives patients given 25 mg daily for 16 weeks *2015*

Sodium *Serum Decrease Physiological* Hyponatremia is common in patients receiving chlorthalidone *2726* Severe hyponatremia with potassium depletion *1856*

Serum Increase Physiological Single case of severe reversible myopathy noted *2929*

Serum No Effect Physiological No significant change in 10 hypertensive patients given 25 mg daily for 16 weeks *2015*

Urine Increase Physiological May produce marked diuresis *4014*

Urine No Effect Physiological After 3 d and 3 mo in 8 patients with mild hypertension given 50 mg/d *5081*

Testosterone *Serum No Effect Physiological* No significant effect observed although higher incidence of sexual dysfunction than in control population *2074*

Triglycerides *Serum Decrease Physiological* Statistically significant decrease of 10 mg/dL in 12 men receiving drug in conjunction with diet to reduce cholesterol *145*

Serum Increase Physiological 15% in short term, no effect in long term in several studies with monotherapy *141* But insignificant change in 10 hypertensive patients given 25 mg daily for 16 weeks *2015* 15% change in 39 subjects treated with drug only for less than 1 y *2337* In short term studies administration of chlorthalidone increased concentration of triglycerides by as much as 50% within a year *3730* Increase by 10 mg/dL in 1,000 men and women with mild hypertension treated for 1 y *2224*

Serum No Effect Physiological Nonsignificant change during monotherapy in 302 subjects for 1 y *2224* Increase by 6 mg/dL in 10 patients given 100 mg daily for 1 mo *4213* In 22 premenopausal and 18 postmenopausal women given 100 mg/d for 6 weeks *628* In 136 patients with stage I diastolic hypertension treated with 15 mg/d caused change from mean baseline of 1.49 ± 0.90 mmol/L by - 0.19 ± 0.07 mmol/L after 12 months and - 0.08 ± 0.06 mmol/L after 48 months *2335*

Urea Nitrogen *Serum Increase Physiological* Nephrotoxic effect *129*

Uric Acid *Serum Increase Physiological* Hyperuricemia may occur or frank gout may be precipitated in patients receiving chlorthalidone *2726* Slight and insignificant in 10 hypertensive patients given 25 mg daily for 16 weeks *2015* From 1.2 to 1.8 mg/dL at doses from 25 to 200 mg/d in 37 patients over 8 weeks *6110* Significantly different in post-menopausal women but still increased in premenopausal given drug 100 mg/d for 6 weeks *628* Significant increase observed in 19 hypertensive patients treated with 50 mg/d for 4 weeks *799* By 1.7 mg/dL in 39 mg/dL mildly hypertensives treated for 6 weeks *2337* 0.9 mg/dL in drug-treated versus placebo-treated patients *5632* Decreases urate clearance *790* Increased in hypertensives; most marked in those individuals whose initial values were lower *4841* Diuretic induced gout observed in two patients with hypertension *5416*

Urine Decrease Physiological Decreased clearance *3669*

Vanillylmandelic Acid *Urine No Effect Physiological* In 22 premenopausal and 18 postmenopausal women given 100 mg/d for 6 weeks *628*

VLDL-Apolipoprotein B *Serum No Effect Physiological* In 19 hypertensive patients treatment with an average of 25 mg/d caused insignificant increase from mean baseline of 18 ± 3 mg/dL to 21 ± 4 mg/dL but when metoprolol added to regime concentration increased significantly to 22 ± 3 mg/dL *553*

VLDL-Cholesterol *Serum Increase Physiological* 7% in short term in several studies with monotherapy *141* 7% change in 39 subjects treated with drug only for less than 1 y *2337* In short term studies administration of chlorthalidone increased concentration of VLDL-cholesterol by as much as 50% within a year *3730*

Serum No Effect Physiological In 19 hypertensives treated with an average of 25 mg/d for 3 months nonsignificant increase from 29 ± 3 mg/dL to 33 ± 4 mg/dL observed and further nonsignificant increase to 35 ± 3 mg/dL when metoprolol added to regime *553* In 22 premenopausal and 18 postmenopausal women given 100 mg/d for 6 weeks *628*

Chlorthalidone *(continued)*

VLDL-Triglycerides *Serum* *No Effect* *Physiological* In 22 premenopausal and 18 postmenopausal women given 100 mg/d for 6 weeks *628*

Volume *Blood* *Decrease* *Physiological* At 3 d but not after 3 mo in 8 patients with mild hypertension given 50 mg/d *5081*
Plasma *Decrease* *Physiological* At 3 d but not after 3 mo in 8 patients with mild hypertension given 50 mg/d *5081*
Plasma *No Effect* *Physiological* In 22 premenopausal and 18 postmenopausal women given 100 mg/d for 6 weeks *628*
Urine *Increase* *Physiological* May produce marked diuresis *4014*

Zinc *Serum* *Increase* *Physiological* In hypertensive males taking drug for at least 6 mo: probably due to release from tissues but also possibly due to contracted blood volume *2074*
Urine *Increase* *Physiological* Increase by 65% in 9 hypertensives treated for 2 weeks *6418*

Chlorzoxazone

Alanine Aminotransferase *Serum* *Increase* *Physiological* May cause hepatotoxicity *3810*

Alkaline Phosphatase *Serum* *Increase* *Physiological* May cause hepatotoxicity *3810*

Aspartate Aminotransferase *Serum* *Increase* *Physiological* May cause hepatotoxicity *3810*

Bile *Urine* *Increase* *Physiological* May cause hepatotoxicity *1714*

Bilirubin *Serum* *Increase* *Physiological* May cause hepatotoxicity *3810*

BSP Retention *Serum* *Increase* *Physiological* May cause hepatotoxicity *3810*

Color *Urine* *Increase* *Analytical* Orange to purple-red *1714*

Cholecalciferol

Alkaline Phosphatase *Serum* *No Effect* *Physiological* In 29 free living elderly individuals treatment with 20 μg/d for 4 weeks caused nonsignificant change from 1.15 ± 0.57 μkat/L to 1.20 ± 0.72 μkat/L *1953*

Calcium *Serum* *No Effect* *Physiological* In 29 free living elderly adults treatment with 20 μg/d for 4 weeks caused nonsignificant change from 2.37 ± 0.10 mmol/L to 2.35 ± 0.11 mmol/L *1953*

Creatinine *Serum* *No Effect* *Physiological* In 29 free living elderly individuals treatment with 20 μg/d for 4 weeks caused nonsignificant change from 89 ± 35 μmol/L to 95 ± 34 μmol/L *1953*

C-terminal Propeptide of Type I Procollagen
Serum *Decrease* *Physiological* In 5 elderly patients largely confined to bed for 12 months mean concentration after treatment with calcium and cholecalciferol for 40 weeks caused significant reduction from mean baseline of 104 ± 24 μg/L to 83 ± 18 μg/L *5717*

1,25-Dihydroxy Vitamin D *Serum* *Increase* *Physiological* In 5 elderly patients largely confined to bed treatment with calcium and cholecalciferol (vitamin D_3) for 40 weeks nonsignificant change from mean baseline of 89 pmol/L to 139 pmol/L observed *5717*

25-Hydroxy Vitamin D *Serum* *Increase* *Physiological* In 5 elderly patients largely confined to bed treatment with calcium and cholecalciferol (vitamin D_3) for 40 weeks significant change from mean baseline of 12.6 nmol/L to 57.2 nmol/L observed *5717* In 29 free living elderly individuals treatment with 20 μg/d for 4 weeks caused significant increase from 13 ± 12 nmol/L to 25 ± 14 nmol/L *1953*

Insulin-like Growth Factor-I *Serum* *No Effect* *Physiological* In 5 elderly patients largely confined to bed for 12 months mean concentration of 12.1 ± 3.0 nmol/L after treatment with cholecalciferol and calcium for 40 weeks not significantly different from baseline of 14.4 ± 3.7 nmol/L *5717*

Ionized Calcium *Serum* *No Effect* *Physiological* In 5 elderly patients largely confined to bed treatment with calcium and cholecalciferol (vitamin D_3) for 40 weeks nonsignificant change from mean baseline of 1.25 mmol/L to 1.23 mmol/L observed *5717*

LDL-Cholesterol *Serum* *Increase* *Physiological* In 102 postmenopausal women treatment with 300 IU/d cholecalciferol caused significant change from mean baseline of 4.02 ± 0.11 mmol/L to 4.26 ± 0.12 mmol/L after 6 months and 4.27 ± 0.11 mmol/L after 12 months *6096*
Serum *No Effect* *Physiological* In 101 postmenopausal women treatment with 2 mg/d estradiol valerate, 1 mg/d cyptoterone acetate sequentially and 300 IU/d cholecalciferol caused nonsignificant change from mean baseline of 3.87 ± 0.12 mmol/L to 3.82 ± 0.10 mmol/L after 6 months and 3.79 ± 0.10 mmol/L after 12 months *6096*

Parathyroid Hormone *Plasma* *No Effect* *Physiological* In 5 elderly patients largely confined to bed treatment with calcium and cholecalciferol (vitamin D_3) for 40 weeks nonsignificant change from mean baseline of 38 ng/L to 32 ng/L observed *5717* In 29 free living elderly individiuals treatment with 20 μg/d for 4 weeks caused nonsignificant reduction from 6.3 ± 2.8 pmol/L to 5.8 ± 2.3 pmol/L *1953*

pH *Blood* *Increase* *Physiological* In 5 elderly patients largely confined to bed treatment with calcium and cholecalciferol (vitamin D_3) for 40 weeks significant change from mean baseline of 7.372 to 7.440 observed *5717*

Phosphate *Serum* *No Effect* *Physiological* In 29 free living elderly individuals treatment with 20 μg/d for 4 weeks caused nonsignificant change from 1.17 ± 0.26 mmol/L to 1.19 ± 0.20 mmol/L *1953* In 5 elderly patients largely confined to bed treatment with calcium and cholecalciferol (vitamin D_3) for 40 weeks nonsignificant change from mean baseline of 1.07 mmol/L to 1.05 mmol/L observed *5717*

Pyridinoline Crosslinked Telopeptide of Type I Collagen
Serum *No Effect* *Physiological* In 5 elderly patients largely confined to bed for 12 months mean concentration of 7.9 ± 5.6 μg/L after treatment with calcium and cholecalciferol for 40 weeks not significantly different from baseline of 7.3 ± 3.6 μg/L *5717*

Cholecystokinin

Glucagon *Plasma* *No Effect* *Physiological* No effect with intravenous infusion on effect produced by intravenous infusion of amino acids alone or in combination with glucose *5347*

Hydrochloric Acid *Gastric Fluid* *No Effect* *Physiological* May occasionally cause increase *3348*

Insulin *Plasma* *No Effect* *Physiological* In healthy volunteers low-dose cholecystokinin infusion in increasing doses of 5, 10, and 20 pmol/kg/h had no effect on basal, glucose-, or amino acid stimulated insulin release *5347*

Pancreatic Polypeptide *Plasma* *Increase* *Physiological* Intravenous infusion caused increase in dose-related manner. Effect enhanced with infusion of some amino acids but effect abolished by infusion of glucose *5347*

Choleretics

BSP Retention *Serum* *Increase* *Physiological* Reported effect (?competition for excretion) *1714*

Cholesterol-lowering Drugs

Fatty Acids (FFA), Free *Serum* *No Effect* *Physiological* In 20 patients with hypercholesterolemia treated with diet and a cholesterol-lowering drug for at least one month mean concentration 0.72 ± 0.41 mmol/L not significantly different when compared with 0.74 ± 0.80 mmol/L in 20 controls *1375*

Fractional Excretion of Potassium
Urine *Decrease* *Physiological* In 20 patients with hypercholesterolemia treated with diet and a cholesterol-lowering drug for at least one month mean concentration 5.92 ± 1.40 mmol/L compared with 5.05 ± 0.39 mmol/L in 20 controls *1375*

HDL-Cholesterol *Serum* *No Effect* *Physiological* In 20 patients with hypercholesterolemia treated with diet and a cholesterol-lowering drug for at least one month mean concentration 1.17 ± 0.49 mmol/L not significantly different when compared with 1.14 ± 0.29 mmol/L in 20 controls *1375*

5-Hydroxytryptophan *Platelets No Effect Physiological* In 20 patients with hypercholesterolemia treated with diet and a cholesterol-lowering drug for at least one month mean concentration 3.90 ± 1.12 nmol/10^9 platelets not significantly different when compared with 3.44 ± 1.15 nmol/10^9 in 20 controls *1375*

LDL-Cholesterol *Serum No Effect Physiological* In 20 patients with hypercholesterolemia treated with diet and a cholesterol-lowering drug for at least one month mean concentration 3.88 ± 1.40 mmol/L not significantly different when compared with 3.28 ± 0.92 mmol/L in 20 controls *1375*

Triglycerides *Serum Increase Physiological* In 20 patients with hypercholesterolemia treated with diet and a cholesterol-lowering drug for at least one month mean concentration 2.10 ± 1.30 mmol/L not significantly different when compared with 1.33 ± 0.62 mmol/L in 20 controls *1375*

Tryptophan *Plasma No Effect Physiological* In 20 patients with hypercholesterolemia treated with diet and a cholesterol-lowering drug for at least one month mean concentration 11.67 ± 3.27 µg/mL not significantly different when compared with 11.37 ± 2.82 µg/mL in 20 controls *1375*

Tryptophan, Free *Plasma No Effect Physiological* In 20 patients with hypercholesterolemia treated with diet and a cholesterol-lowering drug for at least one month mean concentration 0.77 ± 0.20 µg/mL not significantly different when compared with 0.83 ± 0.24 µg/mL in 20 controls *1375*

Cholestyramine

Acetaminophen *Serum Decrease Physiological* Decreased oral bioavailability *886* Plasma concentrations reduced because of reduced gastrointestinal absorption *1473*

Acetylsalicylic Acid *Serum Decrease Physiological* Coadministration of cholestyramine with aspirin appears to delay the time to reach peak plasma concentration but does not reduce total amount absorbed *4062*

Alanine Aminotransferase *Serum Increase Physiological* Few cases reported, probably not hepatotoxicity *2754* In 358 hypercholesterolemic patients under age 65 years treatment for 48 weeks caused mean 15% increase *3945*
Serum No Effect Physiological No effect noted in 5 patients with hyperlipoproteinemia treated with up to 12 g b.i.d. for 12 weeks *6621* Treatment of 50 hypercholesterolemic patients aged over 65 y nonsignificant 6% increase observed *3945*

Amiodarone *Serum Decrease Physiological* Concurrent administration with amiodarone has been reported to reduce concentration of amiodarone by increasing its enterohepatic elimination *6552* Serum concentration reduced when amiodarone coadministered probably due to increased elimination through reduced enterohepatic circulation *4305*

Androstenedione *Plasma No Effect Physiological* In a group of patients with heterozygous familial hypercholesterolemia treatment for 12 weeks had no significant effect on concentration *2912*

Apolipoprotein A-I *Serum Increase Physiological* Increased synthesis of intestinal apo A-I *264* Slight effect observed with treatment with 16 g/d for 12 weeks *372*
Serum No Effect Analytical At a concentration of 6.0 mg/L no significant effect observed on automated immunoturbidimetric method on Baxter Paramax analyzer *3005*
Serum No Effect Physiological In 40 patients with primary hypercholesterolemia treated with up to 24 g/d for 12 weeks no significant change observed from mean baseline of 1.5 ± 0.3 g/L *1651*

Apolipoprotein A-II *Serum Decrease Physiological* Slight effect observed with treatment with 16 g/d for 12 weeks *372*
Serum No Effect Physiological No significant effect observed *264*

Apolipoprotein B *Serum Decrease Physiological* Reduction of 21.7-30.5% observed with treatment with 16 g/d for 4 to 12 weeks *372* In 40 patients with primary hypercholesterolemia treated with up to 24 g/d significant reduction of 23.3% observed from mean baseline of 1.7 ± 0.4 g/L to 1.3 ± 0.3 g/L *1651*
Serum No Effect Analytical At a concentration of 6.0 mg/L no significant effect observed on automated immunoturbidimetric method on Baxter Paramax analyzer *3005*

Apolipoprotein C-III *Serum No Effect Physiological* No significant effect observed with treatment with 16 g/d for 12 weeks *372*

Apolipoprotein E *Serum No Effect Physiological* No significant effect observed with treatment with 16 g/d for up to 12 weeks *372*

Aspartate Aminotransferase *Serum Increase Physiological* In 358 hypercholesterolemic patients under 65 years of age treatment for 48 weeks caused mean 18% increase and in 50 patients over 65 years of age caused 24% increase *3945* Few cases reported, probably not hepatotoxicity *2754*

Bicarbonate *Serum Decrease Physiological* In 8 patients aged 5 weeks to 70 years treated with cholestyramine plasma bicarbonate concentrations reduced to 5.4 to 14 mmol/L *5318*

Bile Acids *Feces Increase Physiological* When treatment is initiated with cholestyramine excretion is increased to about 2 - 3 g/d from normal 1 g/d *5586* Due to increased binding in gastrointestinal tract *2754*
Serum Decrease Physiological Binds acids in gastrointestinal tract *2754* In 15 patients with hyperlipidemia and pruritus of primary biliary cirrhosis receiving 8 - 16 g/d for 2 months significant reduction induced *6675*

Bilirubin, Conjugated *Serum Increase Physiological* In 19 patients suffering from intrahepatic cholestasis of pregnancy *2536*

BSP Retention *Serum Increase Physiological* Few cases reported, probably not hepatotoxicity *2754*

Calcium *Urine Increase Physiological* Binds heavy metals *1714*

Cephalexin *Serum Decrease Physiological* Reduced absorption due to adsorption or steatorrhea *6403*

Cerivastatin *Serum Decrease Physiological* AUC and plasma concentrations of cerivastatin reduced by 22% and 40% respectively when cerivastatin coadministered with cholestyramine *300*

Chenodeoxycholic Acid *Serum Decrease Physiological* In 19 patients suffering from intrahepatic cholestasis of pregnancy *2536*

Chenodiol *Serum Decrease Physiological* Binds chenodiol and inhibits its absorption *1384*

Chloride *Serum Increase Physiological* In 8 patients aged 5 weeks to 70 years treatment with cholestyramine caused hyperchloremic metabolic acidosis with plasma chloride concentrations ranging from 112 to 130 mmol/L *5318* Severe hyperchloremia up to 128 mmol/L in 2 pediatric patients receiving drug for some weeks *4787* Is chloride salt of basic anion exchange resin *6515*

Cholesterol *Serum Decrease Physiological* Therapeutic goal (?increased binding of bile salts in gut) *2738* In 7 hyperlipidemic men treatment with 24 g/d for 48 weeks caused a 8.3% decrease from mean baseline of 272 mg/dL to 250 mg/dL *1450* In the Lipid Research Clinic Coronary Primary Prevention Trial of 3.806 asymptomatic middle aged men with primary hypercholesterolemia treatment with cholestyramine for an average of 7.4 years caused mean decrease of 8.5% *3115* In 21 patients with NIDDM well controlled with glyburide or insulin treatment with cholestyramine with 16 g/d for 6 weeks caused significant change from mean baseline of 6.02 mmol/L to 4.85 mmol/L *2032* Concentration reduced in plasma associated with increased fecal loss of bile acids with normal loss being increased from 1 g/d to 2-3 g/d with reduction of body pools of cholesterol *5586* Significant reduction observed in 15 patients with pruritus of primary biliary cirrhosis when treated with 8-16 g/d for 2 months *6675* In 5 patients with hyperlipoproteinemia type II treated with up to 12 g b.i.d. for 12 weeks reduction from mean of 10.4 mmol/L to 7.6 mmol/L observed *6621* Mean reduction of 16% observed in 9 women with xanthomatous familial hypercholesterolemia treated with 12 g/d and of 31% when cholestyramine combined with ketoconazole *2384* Treatment with resin for 48 weeks caused 16% reduction in nonelderly and 18% reduction in elderly in about 400 patients with hypercholesterolemia *3945* In 88 patients with hypercholesterolemia treatment with 24 g/d for 12 weeks caused a mean decrease of 17% *3982* Treatment of a population of patients with primary hypercholesterolemia for 12 weeks caused significant 19.7% reduction in concentration

Cholestyramine *(continued)*

Cholesterol *(continued)*

4349 In 8 patients with primary hypercholesterolemia treatment with diet and cholestyramine caused significant reduction from mean baseline of 7.4 ± 0.36 mmol/L to 5.7 ± 0.41 mmol/L after 6 months, 6.2 ± 0.45 mmol/L after 12 months and 5.8 ± 0.19 mmol/L after 24 months *4153* In 14 patients with familial hypercholesterolemia treatment with 12 g/d for 3 months caused decrease from mean baseline of 440 mg/dL to 367 mg/dL *1209* In 40 patients with primary hypercholesterolemia treated with up to 24 g/d for 12 weeks significant reduction of 24.3% observed from mean baseline of 10.0 ± 2.1 mmol/L to 7.5 ± 1.9 mmol/L *1651* Significant decrease from mean concentration of 319 mg/dL to 266 mg/dL in 101 patients taking 24 g daily *3035*

Cholesterol:HDL-Cholesterol Ratio
Serum Decrease Physiological In 88 patients with hypercholesterolemia treatment with 24 g/d for 12 weeks caused a mean decrease of 21% *3982*

Cholic Acid *Serum No Effect Physiological* In 19 patients suffering from intrahepatic cholestasis of pregnancy *2536*

Clofibrate *Serum Decrease Physiological* Cholestyramine can decrease the rate of absorption of clofibrate and reducing its plasma concentration, although clinical significance not established *3668*

Corticosteroids *Plasma Decrease Physiological* Decreased oral bioavailability *886*

Cortisol response to Tetracosactrin
Plasma No Effect Physiological In 11 patients with heterozygous familial hypercholesterolemia treatment for 12 weeks caused no significant difference from response in controls *2912*

Creatine Kinase *Serum Increase Physiological* About 9% patients have demonstrated increased activity on one or more occasions *3982*
Serum No Effect Physiological In 408 patients with hypercholesterolemia treatment for 48 weeks caused insignificant 2% increase *3945*

Creatine Kinase MM-Isoenzyme
Serum Increase Physiological About 9% patients have demonstrated increased activity on one or more occasions, attributable to the CK-MM fraction *3982*

Creatinine *Serum No Effect Physiological* In 408 patients with hypercholesterolemia treatment for 48 weeks caused nonsignificant change *3945*

Cyclosporine *Blood Decrease Physiological* No consistent effect observed on cyclosporine concentration when cholestyramine coadministered but decreases of as much as 23% observed in cyclosporine concentration *859*
Blood Increase Physiological No consistent effect observed on cyclosporine concentration when cholestyramine coadministered but increases of as much as 55% observed in cyclosporine concentration *859*
Serum Decrease Physiological No consistent effect observed on cyclosporine concentration when cholestyramine coadministered but decreases of as much as 23% observed in cyclosporine concentration *859*
Serum Increase Physiological No consistent effect observed on cyclosporine concentration when cholestyramine coadministered but increases of as much as 55% observed in cyclosporine concentration *859*

Dehydroepiandrosterone Sulfate
Plasma No Effect Physiological In a group of patients with heterozygous familial hypercholesterolemia treatment for 12 weeks had no significant effect on concentration *2912*

Digitoxin *Serum Decrease Physiological* Digitoxin bound in gastrointestinal tract causing reduction in its absorption *4700* Increased elimination rate with interrupted enterohepatic circulation *6403* Reduces bioavailability in gastrointestinal tract due to binding of drug *4631*

Digoxin *Serum Decrease Physiological* By decreasing intestinal digoxin absorption may decrease the digoxin concentration *2161* Reduces bioavailability in gastrointestinal tract due to binding of drug *4631* After 8 g daily 32% reduction in area under concentration curve observed *762*

Dolichol *Serum No Effect Physiological* No significant change observed in 6 patients with heterozygous familial hypercholesterolemia treated with cholestyramine for 12 weeks *1725*

Estradiol *Plasma No Effect Physiological* In a group of patients with heterozygous familial hypercholesterolemia treatment for 12 weeks had no significant effect on concentration *2912*

Fat *Feces Increase Physiological* Dose-dependent: forms nonabsorbable complexes with bile salts which are lost in feces *5055* Occurs with doses over 15 g/d *2754*

Fluvastatin *Serum Decrease Physiological* Administration of cholestyramine with, or up to 4 hours after, fluvastatin was associated with a 50% decrease in the AUC and 50-80% decrease in maximum concentration of fluvastatin *5232*

Folate *Serum Decrease Physiological* Reduction of concentration reported with long-term administration *1384*

Glipizide *Serum Decrease Physiological* Concomitant administration of 8 g cholestyramine with a single dose of glipizide caused 29% reduction in absorption of glipizide in six healthy male volunteers with reduction of mean peak plasma concentration from 425 ng/mL to 285 ng/mL *3167*

Glucose *Serum Decrease Physiological* In 21 patients with NIDDM well controlled with glyburide or insulin treatment with cholestyramine with 16 g/d for 6 weeks caused significant change from mean baseline of 7.3 mmol/L to 6.5 mmol/L *2032*
Serum Increase Physiological In 358 patients younger than 65 years with hypercholesterolemia treatment for 48 weeks caused significant 1% increase of concentration *3945*
Serum No Effect Physiological In 50 hypercholesterolemic patients aged more than 65 years treatment for 48 weeks had nonsignificant 2.5% reduction effect on plasma glucose concentration *3945*
Urine Decrease Physiological In 21 patients with NIDDM well controlled with glyburide or insulin treatment with cholestyramine with 16 g/d for 6 weeks caused significant change from mean baseline of 1.227 g/d to 0.177 g/d *2032*

Glycated Hemoglobin *Blood Decrease Physiological* In 21 patients with NIDDM well controlled with glyburide or insulin treatment with cholestyramine with 16 g/d for 6 weeks caused significant change from mean baseline of 9.2% to 8.3% *2032*

HDL-Cholesterol *Serum Increase Physiological* In 7 hyperlipidemic men treatment with 24 g/d for 48 weeks caused a 10.7% increase from mean baseline of 43.5 mg/dL to 48.1 mg/dL *1450* In 88 patients with hypercholesterolemia treatment with 24 g/d for 12 weeks caused a mean increase of 8% *3982* After 12 weeks treatment with up to 12 g b.i.d. 5 patients with hyperlipoproteinemia had mean nonsignificant increase of 9% *6621* In a population of patients with primary hypercholesterolemia treatment for 12 weeks caused nonsignificant 6.4% increase in concentration *4349* In about 400 hypercholesterolemic patients treatment for 48 weeks caused 2% increase in nonelderly and 12% increase in elderly *3945* Concentration slightly increased with treatment with 16 g/d for 12 weeks *372* Treatment of 14 patients with familial hypercholesterolemia with 12 g/d for 3 months caused increase from mean baseline of 43 mg/dL to 44 mg/dL *1209* Increased synthesis of intestinal apo A-I *264*
Serum No Effect Physiological Insignificant increase from 45 mg/dL to 48 mg/dL in 101 patients taking 24 g daily *3035* In 8 patients with primary hypercholesterolemia treatment with diet and cholestyramine caused nonsignificant change from mean baseline of 1.34 ± 0.29 mmol/L to 1.52 ± 0.41 mmol/L after 6 months, 1.37 ± 0.04 mmol/L after 12 months and 1.34 ± 0.26 mmol/L after 24 months *4153* No significant change observed in 15 patients with primary biliary cirrhosis treated with 8-16 g/d for 2 months *6675* In 21 patients with NIDDM well controlled with glyburide or insulin treatment with cholestyramine with 16 g/d for 6 weeks caused nonsignificant change from mean baseline of 1.04 mmol/L to 1.07 mmol/L *2032* In 40 patients with familial hypercholesterolemia nonsignificant increase of 7.7% from mean baseline of 1.33 ± 0.43 mmol/L to 1.39 ± 0.41 mmol/L *1651* No significant change observed in 9 women with xanthomatous familial hypercholesterolemia when given 12 g/d *2384*

Hemoglobin *Blood Decrease Physiological* Impairs absorption of iron *3197*

Hydrochlorothiazide *Serum Decrease Physiological* A single dose of cholestyramine reduces the absorption of hydrochlorothiazide by 85% *1028* Effect probably occurs through cholestyramine binding thiazide in gastrointestinal tract with reduced absorption of diuretic as a consequence *2778*

Hydrocortisone *Serum Decrease Physiological* Area under time-concentration curve reduced by 35% when drugs coadministered due to binding of hydrocortisone in gastrointestinal tract *2946*

7α-Hydroxycholesterol *Serum Increase Physiological* In hypercholesterolemic patients treatment for 3-5 days caused significant increase in concentration from mean baseline of 0.04 mg/L to 1 mg/L but when treatment stopped concentration decreased rapidly with a half-life analogous to that of LDLs (also seen in normocholesterolemic individuals) *396*

17-Hydroxyprogesterone *Plasma No Effect Physiological* In a group of patients with heterozygous familial hypercholesterolemia treatment for 12 weeks had no significant effect on concentration of 17α-progesterone *2912*

Iron *Serum Decrease Physiological* Impairs absorption of iron *3197*

Ketoprofen *Serum Increase Physiological* Administration of 8 g to 6 healthy men caused significant effect on concentration of ketoprofen 1.5 hours after intramuscular injection of 50 mg (with 24% reduction in area under concentration curve) *1726*

Lathosterol *Serum Increase Physiological* Treatment of 6 patients with heterozygous familial hypercholesterolemia with cholestyramine for 12 weeks caused mean increase in concentration of 125% *1725*

LDL-Cholesterol *Serum Decrease Physiological* Treatment of about 400 hypercholesterolemic patients with resin caused 27% reduction in nonelderly and 30% reduction in elderly *3945* Increase in LDL receptors in liver together with increased HMG-CoA reductase occurs in response to treatment with cholestyramine with enhanced uptake of LDL from plasma and reduction of LDL-cholesterol *5586* In 8 patients with primary hypercholesterolemia treatment with diet and cholestyramine caused significant change from mean baseline of 5.2 ± 0.30 mmol/L to 3.7 ± 0.36 mmol/L after 6 months, 4.2 ± 0.39 mmol/L after 12 months and 3.8 ± 0.41 mmol/L after 24 months *4153* In 7 hyperlipidemic men treatment with 24 g/d for 48 weeks caused a 22.9% decrease from mean baseline of 202 mg/dL to 155 mg/dL *1450* After 12 weeks receiving up to 12 g b.i.d. 5 patients with hyperlipoproteinemia type II had mean reduction of 33% *6621* In 88 patients with hypercholesterolemia treatment with 24 g/d for 12 weeks caused a mean decrease of 23% *3982* In the Lipid Research Clinic Coronary Primary Prevention Trial of 3.806 asymptomatic middle aged men with primary hypercholesterolemia treatment with cholestyramine for an average of 7.4 years caused mean decrease of 12.6% *3115* In 21 patients with NIDDM well controlled with glyburide or insulin treatment with cholestyramine with 16 g/d for 6 weeks caused significant change from mean baseline of 4.19 mmol/L to 2.98 mmol/L *2032* Treatment with 12 g/d for 3 months caused reduction from mean baseline of 366 mg/dL to 290 mg/dL in 14 patients with familial hypercholesterolemia *1209* In 40 patients with primary hypercholesterolemia treatment with up to 24 g/d for 12 weeks caused significant 32.1% decrease from mean of 7.8 ± 2.2 mmol/L to 5.2 ± 1.9 mmol/L *1651* Decrease of 25.1-35.0% observed over 4-12 weeks with treatment with 16 g/d *372* Significant decrease from mean concentration of 242 mg/dL to 179 mg/dL in 101 patients taking 24 g daily *3035* Significant decrease from mean concentration of 242 mg/dL to 1.79 mg/dL in 101 patients taking 24 g daily *3035* Mean reduction of 21% observed in 9 women with xanthomatous familial hypercholesterolemia when given 12 g/d and of 41% when cholestyramine combined with ketoconazole *2384* In 6 patients with heterozygous familial hypercholesterolemia decreased concentration by 32% with 12 weeks treatment *1725* In a population of patients with primary hypercholesterolemia treatment for 12 weeks caused significant 31.8% reduction in concentration *4349*

LDL-Cholesterol:HDL-Cholesterol Ratio
Serum Decrease Physiological In 40 patients with familial hypercholesterolemia treatment with up to 24 g/d caused significant reduction of 35.5% from mean baseline of 6.5 ± 2.8 to 4.0 ± 1.6 *1651* In a population of patients with primary hypercholesterolemia treatment for 12 weeks caused significant 33.6% reduction in ratio *4349* In 88 patients with hypercholesterolemia treatment with 24 g/d for 12 weeks caused a mean decrease of 27% *3982*

Leukocytes *Blood Decrease Physiological* Possible relationship to drug administration *2754*

Lipids *Serum Decrease Physiological* Lowers bile acids by ionic binding *3810*

β-Lipoprotein *Serum Decrease Physiological* But does not affect very low density lipoproteins *2242*

Lipoprotein Lp(a) *Serum No Effect Physiological* In 7 hyperlipidemic men treatment with 40 mg/d for 48 weeks caused caused no significant change from mean baseline of 7.5 mg/dL *1450*

Lithium *Serum Increase Physiological* Hydrochlorothiazide reduces lithium clearance thereby increasing serum lithium concentration *1028*

Lithium Clearance *Urine Decrease Physiological* Hydrochlorothiazide reduces lithium clearance thereby increasing serum lithium concentration *1028*

Methylmalonate *Urine Increase Physiological* Increase by 28% in patients with heterozygous familial hypercholesterolemia when treated with 16 g/day *4506*

Mycophenolate *Serum Decrease Physiological* Administration of mycophenolate mofentil (1.5 g) to 12 healthy volunteers pretreated with cholestyramine 4 g t.i.d. for 4 days caused a significant 40% decrease in mycophenolate AUC, probably due to interruption of enterohepatic recirculation *5017*

Occult Blood *Feces No Effect Analytical* No effect noted on Hemoquant procedure *6172*

pH *Blood Decrease Physiological* In 6 patients aged 5 weeks to 70 years treated with cholestyramine blood pH reduced to 6.83 to 7.34 *5318*
Urine Decrease Physiological In 5 patients aged 5 weeks to 70 years treated with cholestyramine urinary pH ranged from 5.0 to 6.0 *5318*

Phenytoin *Serum No Effect Physiological* In 6 healthy men pretreatment with 5 g cholestyramine appeared to have no effect on absorption of 100 mg phenytoin over 72 hours *847*

Phospholipids *Serum Decrease Physiological* Therapeutic effect *3669*

Pravastatin *Serum Decrease Physiological* Concomitant administration of cholestyramine and colestipol with pravastatin caused an approximately 40 - 50% decrease of AUC of pravastatin *728*
Serum No Effect Physiological Administration of cholestyramine four hours before or one hour after pravastatin caused no effect on concentration of pravastatin *728*

Propranolol *Serum Decrease Physiological* Significant reduction of peak plasma concentration and area under curve due to binding in gastrointestinal tract *2587*
Serum No Effect Physiological Coadministration of the two drugs had no effect on propranolol concentration *5392*

Prothrombin Time *Plasma Decrease Physiological* May shorten action of anticoagulants *2753* When coadministered with warfarin reduces its absorption *2625*
Plasma Increase Physiological Combines with bile acids (vitamin K not absorbed) *1405*

Raloxifene *Serum Decrease Physiological* Reported to cause a 60% decrease in the absorption and enterohepatic cycling of raloxifene *1696*

Retinol *Serum No Effect Physiological* In 35 patients with primary hypercholesterolemia treatment with diet and cholestyramine caused nonsignificant increase from mean baseline of 3.20 ± 0.66 mmol/L to 3.99 ± 0.73 mmol/L after 24 months *4153*

Sex-Hormone Binding Globulin
Serum No Effect Physiological In a group of patients with heterozygous familial hypercholesterolemia treatment for 12 weeks had no significant effect on concentration *2912*

Sodium *Serum Increase Physiological* Severe hypernatremia (sodium 175 mmol/L) in 2 pediatric patients receiving drug for some weeks *4787*

Sulfamethoxazole *Serum Decrease Physiological* Reduced absorption due to adsorption or steatorrhea *6403*

Teicoplanin *Serum Decrease Physiological* Bound and inactivated in the gastrointestinal tract by cholestyramine *1384*

Testosterone *Serum No Effect Physiological* In a group of patients with heterozygous familial hypercholesterolemia treatment for 12 weeks had no significant effect on concentration *2912*

Thyroxine (T4) *Serum Decrease Physiological* Concentration reduced due to fecal loss *2412* Decreased intestinal

Cholestyramine *(continued)*

Thyroxine (T4) *(continued)*
absorption of thyroxine *5869* Reduced absorption from gastrointestinal tract due to adsorption *6403*

α-Tocopherol *Serum Decrease Physiological* ?inhibits synthesis of carrier lipoprotein *6395*

Tri-iodothyronine (T3) *Serum Decrease Physiological* Concentration reduced due to increased fecal excretion *2412*

Triglycerides *Serum Decrease Physiological* In 5 patients with hyperlipoproteinemia type II treated with up to 12 g b.i.d. nonsignificant mean reduction of 14% observed *6621* In a population of patients with primary hypercholesterolemia treatment for 12 weeks caused significant 37.5% reduction in concentration *4349* Significant decrease from mean concentration of 157 mg/dL to 129 mg/dL in 101 patients taking 24 g daily *3035* Therapeutic effect *3669*
Serum Increase Physiological Mechanism obscure (may occur in diabetics) *2976* Slight increase observed with treatment for 12 weeks with 16 g/d *372* In 7 hyperlipidemic men treatment with 24 g/d for 48 weeks caused a 43.3% increase from mean baseline of 118 mg/dL to 168 mg/dL *1450* In 40 patients with familial hypercholesterolemia treatment with up to 24 g/d for 12 weeks significant increase (3.7%) from mean baseline of 1.9 ± 0.7 mmol/L *1651* In about 400 hypercholesterolemic patients treatment for 48 weeks caused 15% increase in nonelderly and 30% increase in elderly *3945* In 88 patients with hypercholesterolemia treatment with 24 g/d for 12 weeks caused a mean increase of 11% *3982* In 21 patients with NIDDM well controlled with glyburide or insulin treatment with cholestyramine with 16 g/d for 6 weeks caused change from mean baseline of 1.93 mmol/L to 2.13 mmol/L *2032* Treatment of 14 patients with familial hypercholesterolemia with 12 g/d for 3 months caused increase from mean baseline of 158 mg/dL to 171 mg/dL *1209*
Serum No Effect Physiological In 8 patients with primary hypercholesterolemia treatment with diet and cholestyramine caused nonsignificant change from mean baseline of 1.75 ± 0.60 mmol/L to 1.18 ± 0.48 mmol/L after 6 months, 1.15 ± 0.11 mmol/L after 12 months and 1.45 ± 0.45 mmol/L after 24 months *4153* No significant change observed in 9 women with xanthomatous familial hypercholesterolemia when treated with 12 g/d *2384*

Trimethoprim *Serum Decrease Physiological* Delayed absorption due to adsorption *6403*

Troglitazone *Serum Decrease Physiological* Coadministration of cholestyramine with troglitazone caused decreased absorption of troglitazone by approximately 70% *4532* In 12 healthy volunteers administration of 12 g cholestyramine 1 hour after 400 mg orally caused AUC of troglitazone to decrease from 17.9 µg/mL/h to 5.2 µg/mL/h *6615*

Ubiquinone *Serum No Effect Physiological* No significant change observed in 6 patients with heterozygous familial hypercholesterolemia treated with cholestyramine for 12 weeks *1725*

Ubiquinone Q_{10} *Serum Increase Physiological* Increase from mean pretreatment concentration of 0.85 µg/mL to 0.94 µg/mL in 101 patients treated with 24 g daily *3035*
Serum No Effect Physiological No significant change observed in 6 patients with heterozygous familial hypercholesterolemia treated with cholestyramine for 12 weeks *1725*

Ursodiol *Serum Decrease Physiological* May cause reduction in absorption of ursodiol from gastrointestinal tract *300* Administration has been shown to decrease absorption of ursodiol *1020*

Vancomycin *Serum Decrease Physiological* When vancomycin given orally with cholestyramine it is bound and inactivated in the gastrointestinal tract *1384*

Vitamin A *Serum Decrease Physiological* Due to bile acid sequestration, but values still remain within normal range *5055*
Serum No Effect Physiological Absorption not significantly impaired *4014*

Vitamin B_{12} *Serum Decrease Physiological* Reported to cause ileal malabsorption *5055*

Vitamin E *Serum Decrease Physiological* Decreased but values still in normal range over 1-2 y in children with familial hypercholesterolemia *5055*

VLDL-Cholesterol *Serum Decrease Physiological* Concentration reduced over 12 weeks with treatment with 16 g/d *372*
Serum No Effect Physiological In 21 patients with NIDDM well controlled with glyburide or insulin treatment with cholestyramine with 16 g/d for 6 weeks caused no change from mean baseline of 0.79 mmol/L to 0.79 mmol/L *2032* In 88 patients with hypercholesterolemia treatment with 24 g/d for 12 weeks caused a mean increase of 2% *3982* No significant change observed in 9 women with xanthomatous familial hypercholesterolemia when treated with 12 g/d *2384*

Warfarin *Plasma Decrease Physiological* Decreased oral bioavailability *886* Reduced absorption from gastrointestinal tract due to adsorption *6403*

Choline Magnesium Trisalicylate

Alanine Aminotransferase *Serum Increase Physiological* Increased activity and hepatitis reported occasionally *5998*

Aspartate Aminotransferase *Serum Increase Physiological* Two cases reported with increased activity at week one *5998*

Salicylate *Serum Increase Physiological* Concentration increased when salicylate preparations are coadministered with choline magnesium trisalicylate *5998*

Cholinergics

Amylase *Serum Increase Physiological* Cause spasm of sphincter of Oddi *189*

Aspartate Aminotransferase *Serum Increase Physiological* Impaired excretion due to spasm of sphincter of Oddi *1009*

Bilirubin *Serum Increase Physiological* Impaired excretion due to spasm of sphincter of Oddi *1009*

BSP Retention *Serum Increase Physiological* Impaired excretion due to spasm of sphincter of Oddi *1009*

Lipase *Serum Increase Physiological* Impaired excretion spasm of sphincter of Oddi *2242*

Chromium

Nickel *Test Conditions Increase Analytical* Possible interference with atomic absorption procedures *5866*

Chromonar Hydrochloride

Alanine Aminotransferase *Serum No Effect Analytical* No effect at 30 mg/L on Boehringer Mannheim Reflotron method *5706*

Amylase *Serum No Effect Analytical* At concentration of 30 mg/L had no effect on method on Boehringer Mannheim Reflotron system *5706*

Aspartate Aminotransferase *Serum No Effect Analytical* No effect at 30 mg/L on Boehringer Mannheim Reflotron method *5706*

Bilirubin *Serum No Effect Analytical* At concentration of 30 mg/L had no effect on method on Boehringer Mannheim Reflotron system *5706* No effect at 9.5 mg/L on Ames Seralyzer method *5706*

Cholesterol *Serum No Effect Analytical* At concentration of 900 mg/L had no effect on CHOD-Iodide method *5704* At concentration of 900 mg/L had no effect on catalase-AIDH method *5704* At concentration of 900 mg/L had no effect on method using catalase-Hantzsch reaction *5704* At concentration of 30 mg/L no effect on method on Boehringer Mannheim Reflotron system *5706* At concentration of 900 mg/L had no effect on Liebermann-Burchard method *5704* At concentration of 900 mg/L had no effect on CHOD-PAP method *5704* No effect at 9.5 mg/L on Ames Seralyzer method *5706*

Creatine Kinase *Serum No Effect Analytical* No effect at 9.5 mg/L on method on Ames Seralyzer *5706*

Creatinine *Serum No Effect Analytical* At concentration of 180 mg/L had no effect on kinetic Jaffe method on BKA-2 *5704* At concentration of 90 mg/L had no effect on Jaffe-Fuller's earth method *5704* No effect at 9.5 mg/L on Ames Seralyzer method *5706* At concentration of 90 mg/L had no effect on Jaffe-Fading-Fraction method *5704*

Glucose *Serum No Effect Analytical* At concentration of 180 mg/L had no effect on hexokinase/G-6-PDH method *5704* At concentration of 30 mg/L no effect on method on Boehringer Mannheim Reflotron system *5706* No effect of concentrations up to 18 mg/L on method on Kodak Ektachem® *5706* No effect at 9.5 mg/L on glucose oxidase method on Ames Seralyzer *5706*

γ-Glutamyltransferase *Serum No Effect Analytical* At concentration of 30 mg/L no effect on method on Boehringer Mannheim Reflotron system *5706*

Lactate *Plasma No Effect Analytical* At concentration of 180 mg/L had no effect on enzymatic method *5704*

Lactate Dehydrogenase *Serum No Effect Analytical* No effect at 9.5 mg/L on method on Ames Seralyzer *5706*

Potassium *Serum No Effect Analytical* At concentration of 180 mg/L had no effect on ISE measurement without predilution *5704*

Protein Electrophoresis *Serum No Effect Analytical* At concentration of 180 mg/L had no effect on automated Olympus-Hite method *5704*

Sodium *Serum No Effect Analytical* At concentration of 180 mg/L had no effect on ISE measurement without predilution *5704*

Triglycerides *Serum No Effect Analytical* No effect at 30 mg/L on Boehringer Mannheim Reflotron method *5706*

Urea Nitrogen *Serum No Effect Analytical* At concentration of 18 mg/L had no effect on Kodak Ektachem® method *5704* No effect at 9.5 mg/L on method on Ames Seralyzer *5706* No effect at 30 mg/L on Boehringer Mannheim Reflotron method *5706*

Uric Acid *Serum No Effect Analytical* At concentration of 90 mg/L had no effect on catalase-AlDH method *5704* At concentration of 200 mg/L had no effect on Kageyama-Hantzsch method *5704* No effect at 30 mg/L on method on Boehringer Mannheim Reflotron *5706*

Chronic Back Pain

Substance P *Cerebrospinal Fluid Decrease Physiological* Concentration reduced in patients with chronic low back pain compared with healthy individuals *4541*

Plasma Decrease Physiological Concentration reduced in patients with chronic low back pain syndrome compared with healthy human volunteers *4541*

Saliva Decrease Physiological Concentration reduced in patients with chronic low back pain compared with healthy individuals *4541*

Chrysarobin

Color *Urine Increase Analytical* Oxidation product colors alkaline urine red *2242*

Protein *Urine Increase Physiological* Kidney irritation by metabolite *128*

Chymotrypsin

Albumin *Urine No Effect Analytical* Using a fluorimetric assay with Albumin Blue 580 on a Cobas Fara centrifugal analyzer for the detection of microalbuminuria no significant interference was detected at a concentration of 100 mg/L *3117*

Prothrombin Time *Plasma Increase Physiological* May prolong action of anticoagulants *2753*

CI-924

Apolipoprotein A-I *Serum Increase Physiological* Significant increase at 8 weeks only in type IV hyperlipoproteinemic patients with doses from 300 to 1200 mg daily, but no effect in type IV patients over 12 weeks *1133*

Apolipoprotein A-II *Serum No Effect Physiological* No effect observed over 12 weeks in patients with type II hyperlipoproteinemia given daily doses from 300 to 1200 mg but in patients with type IV hyperlipoproteinemia increased following treatment for 8 to 12 weeks with 600 mg/day *1133*

Apolipoprotein E *Serum No Effect Physiological* No effect observed in patients with type II hyperlipoproteinemia treated with 300 to 1200 mg daily for 12 weeks; similar lack of response observed in patients with type IV hyperlipoproteinemia *1133*

Cholesterol *Serum Decrease Physiological* With 4 to 8 weeks therapy with 600 mg daily in 3 patients with type II hyperlipoproteinemia but unaffected both by higher and lower doses and with 600 mg daily at 12 weeks: no effect observed in patients with type IV hyperlipoproteinemia *1133*

HDL-Cholesterol *Serum Increase Physiological* Significant increase in patients with type II hyperlipoproteinemia at 4 weeks with daily doses of 300 or 600 mg although 1200 mg daily had no effect. In patients with type IV hyperlipoproteinemia HDL increased at 4 and 8 weeks with 600 and 1200 mg daily *1133*

LDL-Apolipoprotein B *Serum Decrease Physiological* Significant reduction in patients with type II hyperlipoproteinemia treated with 600 mg daily for 4 weeks and by 300 mg daily for 12 weeks. No effect observed in type IV patients *1133*

LDL-Cholesterol *Serum Increase Physiological* In type IV hyperlipoproteinemic patients significant increase at 12 weeks with treatment with 1200 mg daily but not significant with lower amounts. In type IV patients significant increase at 8 weeks with either 600 or 1200 mg daily *1133*

Triglycerides *Serum Decrease Physiological* 600 mg daily caused significant reduction at 4 weeks in 3 patients with type II hyperlipoproteinemia and with 300 mg/day at 12 weeks; average reduction of 53% at 12 weeks. In 5 type IV patients significant reduction with 600 mg daily at 4 weeks *1133*

VLDL-Cholesterol *Serum Decrease Physiological* Significant reduction from 4 weeks in patients with type II hyperlipoproteinemia treated with daily doses from 300 mg daily and upwards; in patients with type IV hyperlipoproteinemia significant reduction from 4 weeks with doses of 300 mg and above *1133*

Cibenzoline

Glucose *Serum Decrease Physiological* Marked hypoglycemia observed in one 84-year old woman in the presence of normal plasma insulin concentration *2731* Incidence of 24.6% observed in French Pharmacovigilance database *4106*

Protein *Urine Increase Analytical* Positive reaction in 23 of 53 patients when bromphenol reagent strips used to measure protein *3263*

Urine No Effect Analytical Negative reaction in 23 of 53 patients when sulfosalicylic acid or acetic acid/sodium acetate heat coagulation used to measure protein *3263*

Cicletanine

Albumin *Serum No Effect Physiological* No significant difference from control in 6 patients with essential hypertension following either 50 or 100 mg *5573*

Antidiuretic Hormone *Plasma No Effect Physiological* No significant difference in 9 healthy male volunteers in comparison with placebo following ingestion of a single oral dose of 150 mg *514*

Atrial Natriuretic Peptide *Plasma No Effect Physiological* No significant change observed at rest or after exercise compared with placebo in 9 normotensive healthy male volunteers following a single oral dose of 150 mg *514*

Bicarbonate *Serum No Effect Physiological* No significant difference observed between ingestion of 150 mg and placebo in 9 healthy male volunteers *514*

Chloride *Serum No Effect Physiological* No significant difference observed in 9 healthy male volunteers between ingestion of 150 mg cicletanine and placebo *514*

Cicletanine *(continued)*

Creatinine *Serum No Effect Physiological* No significant difference from control in 6 patients with essential hypertension following either 50 or 100 mg *5573*

Urine No Effect Physiological No significant change observed in 6 patients with essential hypertension compared with controls following single oral doses of either 50 or 100 mg *5573*

Glucose *Serum No Effect Physiological* No significant effect of treatment with 50 mg/day for 3 months in 10 patients with mild to moderate hypertension *1058*

Glucose Tolerance *Serum No Effect Physiological* No significant effect in 10 mild to moderate hypertensives treated with 50 mg/day for 3 months *1058*

Guanosine Monophosphate

Plasma No Effect Physiological No significant difference observed in 9 healthy male normotensive male volunteers following single oral dose of 150 mg compared with placebo *514*

Urine No Effect Physiological No significant difference observed in 9 healthy male volunteers following ingestion of a single oral dose of 150 mg compared with placebo *514*

Hematocrit *Blood No Effect Physiological* No significant difference from control observed in 6 patients with essential hypertension treated with either 50 or 100 mg *5573*

Hemoglobin *Blood No Effect Physiological* No significant difference from control observed in 6 patients with essential hypertension given either 50 or 100 mg *5573*

Insulin *Plasma No Effect Physiological* No significant effect on plasma concentration in 10 mild to moderate hypertensives treated with 50 mg daily for 3 months *1058*

6-Keto-Prostaglandin $F_{1\alpha}$ *Plasma Increase Physiological* Mean concentration in 9 hypertensive patients increased significantly from baseline of 3.21 ± 1.25 pg/mL to 3.79 ± 1.41 pg/mL after 1 h, 3.88 ± 1.44 pg/mL 3 h after and 3.43 ± 0.86 pg/mL 24 h after a single dose of 100 mg *6591*

Urine Increase Physiological Excretion increased by 45% in 12 hypertensive patients from initially low concentrations with dose of 150 mg *2721*

Potassium *Serum No Effect Physiological* No significant difference from control in 6 patients with essential hypertension when treated with 50 or 100 mg *5573* No significant difference observed in 9 healthy male volunteers following ingestion of a single oral dose of 150 mg compared with placebo *514*

Urine Increase Physiological Significant increase observed in 6 patients with essential hypertension in 6 hours following single oral dose of 100 mg although no change observed after 50 mg and total excretion over 24 hours no different from placebo *5573*

Urine No Effect Physiological No significant difference observed in 9 healthy male volunteers after ingestion of a single oral dose of 150 mg compared with placebo *514*

Prostaglandin E_2 *Plasma Increase Physiological* Mean concentration in 9 hypertensive patients increased from baseline of 1.41 ± 1.09 pg/mL to 1.81 ± 1.98 pg/mL after 1 h (nonsignificant), 2.45 ± 1.45 pg/mL (significant) 3 h after and 1.59 ± 0.82 pg/mL 24 h (nonsignificant) after a single dose of 100 mg *6591*

Urine Increase Physiological With 150 mg increase in urinary excretion by 59% from initially low concentration in 12 hypertensive patients *2721*

Renin Activity *Plasma Increase Physiological* Mean concentration in 9 hypertensive patients increased from baseline of 1.04 ± 0.69 ng/mL/h to 1.58 ± 1.68 ng/mL/h after 1 h (nonsignificant), 1.32 ± 1.26 ng/mL/h (nonsignificant) 3 h after and 2.36 ± 2.86 ng/mL/h 24 h (significant) after a single dose of 100 mg *6591*

Plasma No Effect Physiological No significant effect observed at 24 hours in 6 patients with essential hypertension when treated with either 50 or 100 mg compared with controls *5573*

Sodium *Serum No Effect Physiological* No significant difference from control over 24 hours following either 50 or 100 mg *5573* No significant difference observed in 9 healthy male volunteers following ingestion of a single oral dose of 150 mg compared with placebo *514*

Urine Increase Physiological In 2 hours following ingestion of 150 mg orally by 9 healthy male volunteers increase from 15.3 mmol/L with placebo to 31.8 mmol/L and from 20 mmol/L during second hour to 33.3 mmol/L *514*

Urine No Effect Physiological Not significantly different from placebo in 24 hours following doses of 50 or 100 mg in 6 patients with uncomplicated essential hypertension *5573*

Urea Nitrogen *Serum No Effect Physiological* No significant difference from control in 6 patients with essential hypertension following either 50 or 100 mg *5573*

Uric Acid *Serum No Effect Physiological* No significant difference from control following either 50 or 100 mg *5573*

Volume *Urine No Effect Physiological* No significant difference observed in 9 healthy male volunteers between ingestion of 150 mg orally and placebo *514* No significant difference observed in 6 patients following oral doses of 50 or 100 mg compared with placebo over 24 hours *5573*

Cidofovir

Alanine Aminotransferase *Serum Increase Physiological* In one patient (< 1%) serious metabolic acidosis occurred with liver failure, panreatitis, mucormycosis, aspergillus, disseminated mycobacterial infection and progression to death *2114*

Alkaline Phosphatase *Serum Increase Physiological* In one patient (< 1%) serious metabolic acidosis occurred with liver failure, panreatitis, mucormycosis, aspergillus, disseminated mycobacterial infection and progression to death *2114*

Amylase *Serum Increase Physiological* In one patient (< 1%) serious metabolic acidosis occurred with liver failure, panreatitis, mucormycosis, aspergillus, disseminated mycobacterial infection and progression to death *2114*

Aspartate Aminotransferase *Serum Increase Physiological* In one patient (< 1%) serious metabolic acidosis occurred with liver failure, panreatitis, mucormycosis, aspergillus, disseminated mycobacterial infection and progression to death *2114*

Bicarbonate *Serum Decrease Physiological* Dose-dependent nephrotoxicity may be observed as side effect of cidofovir administration. Continued administration may lead to additional proximal tubular damage and Fanconi's syndrome in 2% patients. At a maintenance dose of 5 mg/kg every other week reductions of bicarbonate concentration below 16 mmol/L occurred in 9% patients *2114*

Bilirubin *Serum Increase Physiological* In one patient (< 1%) serious metabolic acidosis occurred with liver failure, panreatitis, mucormycosis, aspergillus, disseminated mycobacterial infection and progression to death *2114*

Blood *Urine Increase Physiological* Dose-dependent nephrotoxicity may be observed as side effect of cidofovir administration *2114*

Calcium *Serum Decrease Physiological* Hypocalcemia observed as a rare side effect *2114*

Creatinine *Serum Increase Physiological* Dose-dependent nephrotoxicity may be observed as side effect of cidofovir administration *2114*

Creatinine Clearance *Urine Decrease Physiological* Dose-dependent nephrotoxicity may be observed as side effect of cidofovir administration. Reduced clearance observed in 47 of 80 patients (53%) receiving a maintenance dose of 5 mg/kg every other week *2114*

Glucose *Serum Increase Physiological* Hyperglycemia observed as a rare side effect *2114*

Urine Increase Physiological Dose-dependent nephrotoxicity may be observed as side effect of cidofovir administration. Continued administration may lead to additional proximal tubular damage and Fanconi's syndrome *2114*

Lipase *Serum Increase Physiological* In one patient (< 1%) serious metabolic acidosis occurred with liver failure, panreatitis, mucormycosis, aspergillus, disseminated mycobacterial infection and progression to death *2114*

Myoglobin *Urine Increase Physiological* Rhabdomyolysis may occur with possible myoglobinuric acute renal failure *2154*

Neutrophils *Blood Decrease Physiological* Dose-dependent neutropenia may be observed as side effect of cidofovir administration] Reduction below 500 cells/µL occurred in 20% of patients at a maintenance dose of 5 mg/kg *2114*

Occult Blood *Feces Increase Physiological* Melena observed in clinical trials as possible side effect of drug *2114*

pH *Blood Decrease Physiological* In one patient (< 1%) serious metabolic acidosis occurred with liver failure, panreatitis, mucormycosis, aspergillus, disseminated mycobacterial infection and progression to death *2114*

Phosphate *Serum Decrease Physiological* Dose-dependent nephrotoxicity may be observed as side effect of cidofovir administration. Continued administration may lead to additional proximal tubular damage and Fanconi's syndrome *2114*

Platelets *Blood Increase Physiological* In 13 patients with Type I Gaucher disease chronic administration of drug caused concentration to increase *2114*

Potassium *Serum Decrease Physiological* Hypokalemia observed as a rare side effect *2114*
Serum Increase Physiological Hyperkalemia may occur as an adverse reaction *2154*

Protein *Urine Increase Physiological* Dose-dependent nephrotoxicity may be observed as side effect of cidofovir administration *2114*

Uric Acid *Serum Decrease Physiological* Dose-dependent nephrotoxicity may be observed as side effect of cidofovir administration. Continued administration may lead to additional proximal tubular damage and Fanconi's syndrome *2114*

Zidovudine *Serum No Effect Physiological* Intravenous cidofovir has no effect on pharmacokinetics of zidovudine *2114*

Cilastatin

Bilirubin *Serum No Effect Analytical* At concentrations up to 1000 mg/L mixture of cilastatin with imipenem had no significant effect on DPD method on Hitachi 717 or method on Kodak Ektachem® analyzer *4695*

Cyclosporine *Serum Decrease Physiological* Reported to decrease concentration when drugs coadministered *1384*

Tacrolimus *Serum No Effect Analytical* In HPLC/MS method of Christians et al no significant interference observed with measurement of FK 506 *1010*

Cilazapril

Alanine Aminotransferase *Serum No Effect Physiological* Treatment with up to 5.0 mg daily for 1 month had no effect in 11 patients with renal disease and hypertension *5893*

Albumin *Urine Decrease Physiological* Nonsignificant reduction in 11 patients with renal disease and hypertension when treated with up to 5.0 mg daily for 1 month *5893*

Aldosterone *Plasma Decrease Physiological* Significant decrease observed in 11 patients with renal disease and hypertension when treated with up to 5.0 mg daily for 1 month *5893* Significant reduction observed in 6 healthy volunteers following single doses ranging from 1.25 to 10.0 mg *3179*
Urine Decrease Physiological Significant decrease observed in 11 patients with renal disease and hypertension when treated with up to 5.0 mg daily for 1 month *5893*

Angiotensin-I *Plasma Increase Physiological* Concentration increased in parallel with renin activity in 6 healthy male volunteers given 2.5 mg drug with peak after 2 hours *473* Significant effect observed in 6 healthy volunteers following doses ranging from 1.25 mg to 10.0 mg *3179*

Angiotensin-II *Plasma Decrease Physiological* Significant reduction in 6 healthy volunteers following single dose of from 1.25 to 10.0 mg in 6 healthy volunteers *3179*
Plasma No Effect Physiological Insignificant reduction in 6 healthy male volunteers given 2.5 mg drug *473* No significant change observed in 11 patients with renal disease and hypertension when treated with up to 5.0 mg daily for 1 month *5893*

Angiotensin-converting Enzyme
Serum Decrease Physiological Reversible potent selective inhibition of enzyme activity in 6 healthy volunteers from 1 to 8 hours after doses ranging from 1.25 to 10.0 mg with up to 100% inhibition observed *3179* In 13 hypertensives treated with up to 5 mg/d for up to 82 weeks significantly reduced from mean of about 15 U/L in wash out period to less than 2 U/L in treatment period *706* Almost complete inhibition of activity in 6 healthy male volunteers 2 hours following 2.5 mg drug, with 60% inhibition after 24 hours *473*

Antidiuretic Hormone *Plasma No Effect Physiological* Treatment with up to 5.0 mg daily for 1 month caused no significant change in 11 patients with renal disease and hypertension *5893*

Apolipoprotein A-I *Serum Increase Physiological* Mean increase of 6 mg/dL in 7 hypertensive patients with normal glucose tolerance and of 1 mg/dL in 12 patients with abnormal glucose tolerance when treated for mean of 6.4 months *5524*

Apolipoprotein B *Serum Decrease Physiological* Mean decrease of 4 mg/dL in 7 hypertensive patients with normal glucose tolerance and of 14 mg/dL in 12 hypertensive patients with abnormal glucose tolerance *5524*

Aspartate Aminotransferase
Serum No Effect Physiological Treatment with up to 5.0 mg daily for 1 month had no effect in 11 patients with renal disease and hypertension *5893*

Atrial Natriuretic Peptide *Plasma No Effect Physiological* No significant effect in 6 healthy volunteers following single doses of from 1.25 mg to 10.0 mg *3179*

Bilirubin *Serum No Effect Physiological* Treatment with up to 5.0 mg daily for 1 month had no effect in 11 patients with renal disease and hypertension *5893*

Chloride *Urine Increase Physiological* Slight increase or no change in 6 healthy volunteers given single doses of from 1.25 mg to 10.0 mg due to decreased aldosterone concentration *3179*

Cholesterol *Serum Decrease Physiological* Mean reduction of 24 mg/dL in 7 hypertensive patients with normal glucose tolerance and of 11 mg/dL (nonsignificant) in 12 hypertensive patients with abnormal glucose tolerance when treated for mean of 6.4 months *5524*
Serum No Effect Physiological Nonsignificant reduction observed in 84 patients with hypertension treated with 2.5 or 5.0 mg daily for 8 weeks *4115*

Cortisol *Plasma No Effect Physiological* Treatment of 11 patients with renal disease and hypertension with up to 5.0 mg daily for 1 month had no effect *5893*

Creatinine Clearance *Urine No Effect Physiological* No significant change in 11 patients with renal disease and hypertension treated with up to 5.0 mg daily for 1 month *5893*

Effective Renal Plasma Flow
Patient Increase Physiological In 6 healthy volunteers doses of from 1.25 mg to 10.0 mg increased ERPF by 10 to 20% as measured by hippuran clearance *3179*
Patient No Effect Physiological When 10 mg daily combined with 12.5 to 25 mg hydrochlorothiazide in 38 patients with severe hypertension had no effect on measurement *5218* No significant change in 11 patients with renal disease and hypertension treated with up to 5.0 mg daily for 1 month *5893*

Erythrocytes *Blood No Effect Physiological* Nonsignificant increase in 84 patients with hypertension treated with 2.5 or 5.0 mg daily for 8 weeks *4115*

Glomerular Filtration Rate *Urine No Effect Physiological* When 10 mg daily combined with 12.5 to 25 mg hydrochlorothiazide in 38 severely hypertensive patients had no effect on measurement *5218* No significant effect observed in 6 healthy volunteers given single doses from 1.25 mg to 10.0 mg as determined by inulin clearance *3179* No significant change in 11 patients with renal disease and hypertension treated with up to 5.0 mg daily for 1 month *5893*

Glucose *Serum No Effect Physiological* Treatment of 11 patients with renal disease and hypertension with up to 5.0 mg daily for 1 month had no effect *5893* Nonsignificant reduction in 84 patients with hypertension treated with 2.5 or 5.0 mg daily for 8 weeks *4115*

γ-Glutamyltransferase *Serum No Effect Physiological* Nonsignificant increase in 84 patients with hypertension treated with 2.5 or 5.0 mg daily for 8 weeks *4115*

HDL-Cholesterol *Serum Increase Physiological* Insignificant mean increase of 6.9 mg/dL in 7 hypertensive patients with normal glucose tolerance and of 3.0 mg/dL in 12 hypertensive patients with abnormal glucose tolerance following treatment for mean of 6.4 months *5524*

Hematocrit *Blood No Effect Physiological* Nonsignificant increase in 84 patients treated with 2.5 or 5.0 mg daily for 8 weeks *4115*

Cilazapril *(continued)*

Hemoglobin *Blood No Effect Physiological* No significant effect in 15 healthy male volunteers when measured 4 hours after first dose of 2.5 mg and last dose after 14 days treatment *1754* Treatment for 1 month with up to 5.0 mg daily had no effect in 11 patients with renal disease and hypertension *5893*

Hemoglobin A_{1c} *Blood Decrease Physiological* Decrease from mean of 8.67% to 7.75% in 12 hypertensive patients with abnormal glucose tolerance when treated for mean of 6.4 months but no change observed in 7 hypertensive patients with normal glucose tolerance *5524*

LDL-Cholesterol *Serum Decrease Physiological* Mean decrease of 22 mg/dL in 7 hypertensive patients with normal glucose tolerance and of 6 mg/dL in 12 patients with abnormal glucose tolerance *5524*

Leukocytes *Blood No Effect Physiological* Treatment with up to 5.0 mg daily for 1 month had no effect in 11 patients with renal disease and hypertension *5893*

Lithium Clearance *Urine Decrease Physiological* Lithium clearance reduced with antihypertensive therapy *5562*

Magnesium *Muscle No Effect Physiological* No significant effect of treatment with 2.5 mg daily for 4 weeks in 9 volunteers *4410*

Serum No Effect Physiological No significant effect of treatment with 2.5 mg daily for 4 weeks in 9 volunteers *4410*

N-Acetyl-Glucosaminidase *Urine Decrease Physiological* Increased concentration associated with hypertension reduced with treatment *5562*

Platelets *Blood No Effect Physiological* Treatment with up to 5.0 mg daily for 1 month had no effect in 11 patients with renal disease and hypertension *5893*

Potassium *Muscle No Effect Physiological* No significant effect of treatment with 2.5 mg daily for 4 weeks in 9 volunteers *4410*

Serum Increase Physiological Significant increase in 11 patients with renal disease and hypertension when treated with up to 5.0 mg daily for 1 month *5893*

Serum No Effect Physiological No change observed in 84 patients with hypertension treated with 2.5 or 5.0 mg daily for 8 weeks *4115* No significant effect of treatment with 2.5 mg daily for 4 weeks in 9 volunteers *4410*

Urine Decrease Physiological Slight decrease or no change in 6 healthy volunteers given single doses of from 1.25 mg to 10.0 mg due to decrease of aldosterone concentration *3179*

Urine No Effect Physiological No significant change in excretion in 11 patients with renal disease and hypertension when treated with up to 5.0 mg daily for 1 month *5893*

Renin Activity *Plasma Increase Physiological* Significant increase from initial normal value in 11 patients with renal disease and hypertension when treated with up to 5.0 mg daily for 1 month *5893* Significant increase observed in 13 hypertensives treated with up to 5 mg/d for up to 82 weeks from about 0.8 ng/mL/h in wash out period to about 2.3 ng/mL/h in treatment period *706* Ten-fold increase in concentration at 2 hours postdose with only a very weak effect at 24 hours in 6 healthy male volunteers given 2.5 mg drug *473*

Sodium *Urine Increase Physiological* Slight increase or no change in 6 healthy volunteers given single doses of from 1.25 mg to 10.0 mg due to decreased aldosterone concentration *3179*

Urine No Effect Physiological No significant change in 11 patients with renal disease and hypertension when treated with up to 5.0 mg daily for 1 month *5893*

Triglycerides *Serum Decrease Physiological* Reduction by average of 23 mg/dL in 84 patients with hypertension treated with 2.5 or 5.0 mg daily for 8 weeks *4115* Mean reduction of 48 mg/dL in 7 hypertensive patients with normal glucose tolerance and of 37 mg/dL in 12 hypertensive patients with abnormal glucose tolerance treated for mean of 6.4 months *5524*

Urea Nitrogen *Serum No Effect Physiological* Nonsignificant increase in 84 patients with hypertension treated with 2.5 or 5.0 mg daily for 8 weeks *4115*

Uric Acid *Serum No Effect Physiological* Nonsignificant reduction in 84 patients with hypertension treated with 2.5 or 5.0 mg daily for 8 weeks *4115*

Viscosity *Blood No Effect Physiological* No significant change observed when measurement made 4 hours after first dose of 2.5 mg and 4 hours after last dose after treatment with 2.5 mg daily for 14 days in 15 healthy male volunteers *1754*

Plasma No Effect Physiological No effect observed 4 hours after first and last dose when 2.5 mg given daily for 14 days to 15 healthy male volunteers *1754*

Cilostazol

Albumin *Urine Decrease Physiological* In 13 patients with NIDDM administration of 100 mg/d for 3 months caused decrease in excretion from mean baseline of 25.0 ± 7.7 µg/mg creatinine to 19.4 ± 7.4 µg/mg creatinine *6360*

Antithrombin III *Plasma Decrease Physiological* In 159 patients treatment caused significant change from mean baseline of 27.7 ± 10.3 mg/dL to 26.8 ± 6.1 mg/dL *186*

Bleeding Time *Patient Increase Physiological* Mean increase from 135 to 177 seconds in 10 patients with cerebral thrombosis when treated with 100 mg daily for 4 weeks *6121*

Patient No Effect Physiological In 100 patients treatment caused nonsignificant change from mean baseline of 146.0 ± 67.8 s to 146.4 ± 61.2 s *186*

Fibrin Degradation Products

Plasma No Effect Physiological In 290 patients treatment caused nonsignificant change from mean baseline of 8.4 ± 14.2 µg/mL to 8.4 ± 12.1 µg/mL *186*

Fibrinogen *Plasma No Effect Physiological* In 452 patients treatment caused nonsignificant change from mean baseline of 298.9 ± 85.2 mg/dL to 304.8 ± 86.9 mg/dL *186*

Glucose *Serum No Effect Physiological* In 13 patients with NIDDM administration of 100 mg/d for 3 months caused nonsignificant decrease from mean baseline of 6.6 ± 0.3 mmol/L to 6.5 ± 0.3 mmol/L *6360*

Hemoglobin A_{1c} *Blood No Effect Physiological* In 13 patients with NIDDM treatment with 100 mg/d for 3 months caused no significant change from baseline of 6.8 ± 0.3% *6360*

6-Keto-Prostaglandin $F_{1\alpha}$ *Urine Decrease Physiological* In 13 patients with NIDDM treatment with 100 mg/d for 3 months caused nonsignificant decrease from mean baseline of 797.2 ± 79.4 pg/mL to 563.9 ± 66.9 pg/mL *6360*

β_2-Microglobulin *Urine Decrease Physiological* In 13 patients with NIDDM treatment with 100 mg/d for 3 months caused nonsignificant decrease from mean baseline of 164.4 ± 46.2 µg/L to 148.8 ± 23.2 µg/L *6360*

N-Acetyl-Glucosaminidase *Urine No Effect Physiological* In 13 patients with NIDDM treatment with 100 mg/d for 3 months caused nonsignificant increase from mean baseline of 7.1 ± 0.7 U/L to 7.4 ± 1.2 U/L *6360*

Partial Thromboplastin Time

Plasma No Effect Physiological In 409 patients treatment caused nonsignificant change from mean baseline of 31.8 ± 7.2 s to 32.0 ± 7.6 s *186*

Plasminogen *Plasma No Effect Physiological* In 96 patients treatment caused nonsignificant change from mean baseline of 12.5 ± 3.5 mg/dL to 12.7 ± 3.7 mg/dL *186*

Platelet Aggregation *Blood Decrease Physiological* Epinephrine-induced aggregation reduced from mean of 57 to 44 with 1.0 µg/mL *6121* ADP-induced aggregation reduced from mean of 46 to 27 with 3 µmol/L and 25 to 12 with 1.5 µmol/L ADP *6121* Arachidonic acid induced aggregation reduced from mean of 67 to 51 with 200 µg/mL *6121* Collagen-induced aggregation reduced from mean of 63 to 56 with 2.5 µg/mL *6121*

Platelet Factor 4 *Plasma Decrease Physiological* Reduction from mean value of 46.1 to 36.6 in 10 patients with cerebral thrombosis treated with 100 mg/day for 4 weeks *6121*

Prostaglandin E_2 *Urine Decrease Physiological* In 13 patients with NIDDM administration of 100 mg/d for 3 months caused nonsignificant decrease from mean baseline of 370.4 ± 59.1 pg/mL to 349.9 ± 54.1 pg/mL *6360*

Prothrombin Time *Plasma No Effect Physiological* In 395 patients treatment caused nonsignificant change from mean baseline of 12.2 ± 4.7 s to 12.1 ± 1.7 s *186*

β-Thromboglobulin *Platelets Decrease Physiological* Reduction from mean of 87.5 to 49.5 in 10 patients with cerebral thrombosis when treated with 100 mg daily for 4 weeks *6121*

Thromboxane B_2 *Urine Decrease Physiological* Administration of 100 mg/d for 3 months caused significant decrease from mean baseline of 547.1 ± 66.0 ng/g creatinine to 354.8 ± 49.9 ng/g creatinine *6360*

Triglycerides *Serum No Effect Physiological* In 13 patients with NIDDM treatment with 100 mg/d for 3 months caused nonsignificant increase from mean baseline of 5.38 ± 0.20 mmol/L to 5.65 ± 0.20 mmol/L *6360*

Cimetidine

Acecainide *Serum Increase Physiological* Reported to reduce renal clearance *1384*

Acenocoumarol *Plasma Increase Physiological* In 9 healthy volunteers plasma concentration remained consistently higher when a 10 mg dose of acenocoumarol was given with cimetidine when volunteers followed for 36 h. Clearance of acenocoumarol decreased by 25% *3305*

Acetaminophen *Serum No Effect Physiological* Coadministration of cimetidine had no effect on plasma concentration and fractional clearances through renal and metabolic routes were not altered *5599*

Acetylsalicylic Acid *Serum Increase Physiological* Plasma clearance reduced by about 20% in healthy volunteers treated with 1 g/day for 4 days: half-life prolonged but no change in unbound fraction observed: effect probably due to inhibition of metabolism *4062* Absorption rate of aspirin probably increased when two compounds coadministered *4558*
Serum No Effect Physiological Prior administration of 1 g/day for 4 days had no significant effect on plasma concentration or the time to reach it *4062*

α_1-Acid Glycoprotein *Serum No Effect Physiological* No significant effect observed in 6 healthy male volunteers after 1.2 g for 2 days *4515*

Adenosine Monophosphate
Platelets Decrease Physiological Probable activation of endogenous cyclic AMP phosphodiesterase involved in favoring action of platelet aggregating agents *6635*

Alanine Aminotransferase *Serum Increase Physiological* Dose-related increases in activity have been reported with the administration of cimetidine, with rare reports of cholestatic or mixed cholestatic-hepatocellular effects that are usually reversible *5657* In isolated case treated for 7 mo with 400 mg/d progressed to bridging hepatic necrosis *5149*

Albendazole *Bile Increase Physiological* Concentration increased by about twofold in bile and cystic fluid when cimetidine administered with 20 mg/kg/d albendazole *5635*
Cyst Fluid Increase Physiological Concentration increased by about twofold in bile and cystic fluid when cimetidine administered with 20 mg/kg/d albendazole *5635*
Serum No Effect Physiological Concentration unchanged four hours later when cimetidine administered with 20 mg/kg/d albendazole *5635*

Albumin *Serum No Effect Analytical* At concentration of 1 mg/L had no effect on BCG method *5704*
Urine No Effect Physiological No change observed during treatment of 13 ulcer patients *1002*

Alfentanil *Serum Increase Physiological* Concomitant administration of cimetidine with alfentanil significantly inhibits its clearance, thereby increasing its plasma concentration *2899*

Alfuzosin *Serum No Effect Physiological* Mean concentration in 10 healthy volunteers not significantly affected by coadministration of cimetidine *1392*

Alkaline Phosphatase *Serum Increase Physiological* Mild increase in reversible cholestatic jaundice in a few children *3577* Rare reports of cholestatic or mixed cholestatic-hepatocellular effects that are usually reversible *5657* In isolated case treated for 7 mo with 400 mg/d progressed to bridging hepatic necrosis *5149*

Alpidem *Serum No Effect Physiological* No apparent effect observed of cimetidine on plasma pharmacokinetics of a single oral dose of 50 mg alpidem *1394*

Alprazolam *Serum Increase Physiological* By inhibiting CYP 3A cimetidine increased the alprazolam concentration by 86%, decreasing its plasma clearance by 42% and increasing its half-life by 16% *4685*

δ-Aminolevulinic Acid *Urine Decrease Physiological* Marked effect in patient with acute intermittent porphyria possibly due to inhibition of hepatic δ-aminolevulinic acid synthetase *2715*

Amiodarone *Serum Increase Physiological* Concurrent administration with amiodarone has been reported to increase concentration of amiodarone *6552*

Amitriptyline *Serum Increase Physiological* When coadministered, by inhibiting cytochrome P450 2D6, may increase the concentration of amitriptyline *6645*

Amlodipine *Serum No Effect Physiological* Coadministration of cimetidine with amlodipine had no effect on its pharmacokinetics *4651*

Amylase *Serum Increase Physiological* Rare reports of pancreatitis that cleared on withdrawal of the drug *5657*

Anti-Smooth Muscle Antibodies
Serum No Effect Physiological No effect noted in 12 patients treated for acid-peptic disease *3900*

Antimitochondrial Antibodies
Serum No Effect Physiological No effect noted in 12 patients treated for acid-peptic disease *3900*

Antinuclear Antibodies *Serum No Effect Physiological* No effect noted in 12 patients treated for acid-peptic disease *3900*

Antipyrine *Serum Increase Physiological* Clearance reduced: probably by inhibition of drug metabolism with increased half-life *5450* Plasma clearance reduced from 54 mL/min to 48 mL/min in 7 healthy subjects given 1 g/d *4988*

Aspartate Aminotransferase *Serum Increase Physiological* Dose-related increases in activity have been reported with the administration of cimetidine, with rare reports of cholestatic or mixed cholestatic-hepatocellular effects that are usually reversible *5657* Reversible cholestatic jaundice in a few children *3577* In isolated case treated for 7 mo with 400 mg/d progressed to bridging hepatic necrosis *5149*

Atorvastatin *Serum No Effect Physiological* Cimetidine coadministration had no effect on the atorvastatin concentration or its reduction of plasma LDL-cholesterol concentration *4534*

Azelastine *Serum Increase Physiological* Coadministration of cimetidine (600 mg b.i.d.) with azelastine (4 mg b.i.d.) increased the mean maximum concentration and AUC of azelastine by approximately 65% *6320*

Azithromycin *Serum No Effect Physiological* Administration of cimetidine 2 hours before azithromycin in 8 healthy volunteers had no effect on serum concentration of azithromycin *1928* Administration of 800 mg cimetidine 2 hours before azithromycin had no effect on azithromycin absorption *4659*

Benazepril *Serum No Effect Physiological* No clinically important pharmacokinetic interactions observed when drugs coadministered *1033*

Betaxolol *Serum No Effect Physiological* Coadministration with betaxolol had no effect on pharmacokinetics of betaxolol *2067*

Bicarbonate *Serum No Effect Analytical* At concentration of 1 mg/L had no effect on method using phenolphthalein *5704*

Bile Acids *Serum Increase Physiological* 8 to 9 fold increase reversible cholestatic jaundice in a few children *3577*

Bile Salts *Feces Decrease Physiological* By about 30%; in 17 patients with cystic fibrosis receiving constant concomitant therapy with pancreatic enzymes *952*

Bilirubin *Serum Increase Physiological* Reversible cholestatic jaundice in a few children *3577* Rare reports of cholestatic or mixed cholestatic-hepatocellular effects that are usually reversible *5657* In isolated case treated for 7 mo with 400 mg/d progressed to bridging hepatic necrosis *5149*
Serum No Effect Analytical At concentration of 1 mg/L had no effect on Jendrassik and Grof method *5704*

Bupropion *Serum Increase Physiological* May inhibit the metabolism of bupropion due to effect on CYP2B6 isoenzyme *2171*

Calcium *Serum No Effect Analytical* At concentration of 1 mg/L had no effect on cresolphthalein method *5704*

Carbamazepine *Serum Increase Physiological* Increased concentration observed due to effect on hepatic metabolism.

Cimetidine *(continued)*

Carbamazepine *(continued)*
Effect is transient *1384* Increased concentration when co-administered, as elimination affected, although urinary excretion increased *1228* Concentration increased since carbamazepine metabolism is inhibited by cimetidine but at steady state effect is minimal *3119* Drugs that inhibit CYP 3A4 inhibit metabolism of carbamazepine producing clinically meaningful effect *1039* Concomitant administration with carbamazepine causes marked increase of plasma carbamazepine concentration resulting in toxicity in some cases *282* Significant increase observed when cimetidine first coadministered with carbamazepine although concentration tends to revert to normal subsequently *5977*
Serum No Effect Physiological No significant effect on carbamazepine concentration when co-administered *3541*

Carvedilol *Serum Increase Physiological* In 10 healthy men coadministration of 1000 mg/d cimetidine with carvedilol increased the AUC of carvedilol by 30% without change in its maximum concentration *5639*
Serum No Effect Physiological In 10 healthy men coadministration of 1000 mg/d cimetidine with carvedilol increased the AUC of carvedilol by 30% without change in its maximum concentration *5639*

CD2+ Lymphocytes *Blood Increase Physiological* Increase from mean of 1.4 cells /nL to 2.0 cells /nL and from 69.5% to 77.8% in 12 healthy volunteers given 1600 mg/day for 21 days *734*

CD3+ Lymphocytes *Blood No Effect Physiological* Insignificant increase in both absolute number and percentage of total cells in 12 healthy volunteers given 1600 mg/day for 21 days *734*

CD4+ Lymphocytes *Blood Increase Physiological* Significant increase in absolute numbers from mean of 0.8600 /nL to 1.2103 /nL and percentage from mean of 41.5% to 56.3% in 12 healthy volunteers given 1600 mg/day for 21 days *734*

CD8+ Lymphocytes *Blood No Effect Physiological* Insignificant increase in absolute count and percentage of cells in 12 healthy volunteers given 1600 mg/day for 21 days *734*

Cefaclor *Serum No Effect Physiological* When coadministered with cefaclor reported to have no effect on its rate or extent of absorption *1627*

Cefpodoxime *Serum Decrease Physiological* Administration of H_2-blockers reduced peak plasma concentration by 42% and the extent of absorption by 32% *4684*

Cerivastatin *Serum No Effect Physiological* Plasma concentrations of cerivastatin not affected by administration of cimetidine *300*

Chlordiazepoxide *Serum Increase Physiological* Due to impaired clearance and impairment of hydroxylation of desmethyl derivative *5148*

Chloride *Serum No Effect Analytical* At concentration of 1 mg/L had no effect on mercurimetric method *5704*

Chloroquine *Serum Increase Physiological* Significant reduction in oral clearance from 0.49 L/d/kg to 0.23 L/d/kg and elimination half-life increased from 3.11 d to 4.62 d in test group *1766*

Chlorpromazine *Serum Decrease Physiological* Coadministration of cimetidine with chlorpromazine reduced chlorpromazine plasma concentration probably through effect on gastrointestinal absorption *2739*

Cholecystokinin *Plasma Increase Physiological* In 12 healthy volunteers administration of cimetidine plasma concentration of CCK increased with a peak after 30 min and a smaller one 120 min after cimetidine *5829*

Cholesterol *Serum No Effect Analytical* At concentration of 1 mg/L had no effect on CHOD-PAP method *5704*
Serum No Effect Physiological No significant change in 9 healthy men given 1600 mg/day for 14 days *2006* In 25 patients pretreatment 174 mg/dL, after 181 mg/dL over 5 weeks *5986* In healthy individuals and in subjects with high serum glucose concentration *2703*

Cifenline *Serum Increase Physiological* Coadministration of cimetidine 300 mg four times daily with a sing,e dose of 160 mg cifenline caused maximum serum concentration to increase by 27%, area under concentration curve to increase by 44% and prolonged half-life by 30% *3836* Coadministration of cimetidine 300 mg four times daily with a single dose of 160 mg cifenline caused maximum serum concentration to increase by 27%, area under concentration curve to increase by 44% and prolong half-life by 30% *3836*

Cisapride *Serum Increase Physiological* Coadministration of cimetidine with cisapride leads to an increase in the peak concentration and AUC of cisapride *2903* Mean peak plasma concentration increased from 58 ng/mL to 84 ng/mL when two drugs coadministered in 8 healthy volunteers due to inhibition of metabolism *3148*

Clonazepam *Serum Increase Physiological* Reported to increase plasma concentration *1384*

Clopidogrel *Serum No Effect Physiological* Cimetidine administration does not appear to affect the pharmacodynamics of clopidogrel *5256*

Clorazepate *Serum Increase Physiological* Probable effect as a result of inhibition of hepatic microsomal drug metabolising enzymes *1384*

Clozapine *Serum Increase Physiological* Cimetidine administration with clozapine may increase the plasma concentration of clozapine enhancing its side effects *5229*

Cocaethylene *Urine No Effect Analytical* No interference observed with TLC method of Bailey *328*

Complement C_3 *Serum Increase Physiological* Significant increase from mean of 0.986 g/L to 1.187 g/L in 12 healthy volunteers given 1600 mg/day for 21 days *734*

Complement C_4 *Serum No Effect Physiological* No change in 12 healthy volunteers given 1600 mg/day for 21 days *734*

Complement, Total *Serum No Effect Physiological* Insignificant increase in 12 healthy volunteers given 1600 mg/day for 21 days *734*

Coproporphyrin *Urine No Effect Physiological* No measurable change in one patient with acute intermittent porphyria *2715*

Creatine *Urine Increase Physiological* Significant effect at 3 weeks in 9 patients given 1.6 g daily *1634*

Creatine Kinase *Serum No Effect Physiological* No significant effect observed in 9 patients given 1.6 g daily *1634*

Creatinine *Serum Increase Physiological* Rises because of competitive inhibition of creatinine secretion following i.v. bolus of 300 mg *811* In 13 ulcer patients average increase of 22% which fell on cessation on therapy *1002* Small but detectable increases compared with placebo, but rarely exceeding 2 mg/dL *3900* Small, possibly dose related increases in plasma creatinine have been reported, presumably due to competition for renal tubular secretion, are not uncommon. Rare cases of interstitial nephritis that cleared on withdrawal of the drug have been reported *5657* Single case of reversible renal failure probably attributable to drug *5434* Significant effect from first day of treatment and at 3 weeks but not after 12 weeks *1634*
Serum No Effect Analytical At concentration of 4 mg/L had no effect on creatinine iminohydrolase method *5704* At 300 mg/L on reversed phase liquid chromatographic procedure of Zhiri et al *6656* At concentration of 1 mg/L had no effect on Technicon AutoAnalyzer® Jaffe method *5704* No effect of concentrations up to 500 mg/L on 2-slide method on Kodak Ektachem® *5706*
Serum No Effect Physiological No effect in volunteers receiving 1.2 g daily for 12 d *491*
Urine No Effect Physiological No significant effect observed in 9 patients given 1.6 g daily *1634*

Creatinine Clearance *Urine Decrease Physiological* In 13 ulcer patients average fall of 28 mL/min (26%) *1002* Administration of 1200 mg/d gabapentin to 12 patients had caused a 14% decrease in the mean apparent oral clearance of gabapentin but a decrease of creatinine clearance of 10% *4526* Significant effect within 6 h, normalized after several weeks *1634* By at least 20% in patients with renal failure maximal after 2 to 3 d *3424*

Cyclosporine *Blood Increase Physiological* With coadministration of cimetidine absorption of cyclosporine is delayed and dosage:concentration ratio decreased leading to increased cyclosporine concentration *859*
Blood No Effect Analytical At a concentration of 100 mg/L had no effect on Syva EMIT method *495*

Serum Increase Physiological Reports have been made that concomitant administration of drugs both does and does not have an effect on cyclosporine concentration. Has been reported that cimetidine reduces cyclosporine clearance but also that it does not affect its pharmacokinetics *1069* With coadministration of cimetidine absorption of cyclosporine is delayed and dosage:concentration ratio decreased leading to increased cyclosporine concentration *859* Increased concentration presumably due to effect on liver metabolism *1075*

Serum No Effect Physiological Coadministration of cimetidine with cyclosporine had no effect on plasma concentration *6596* No significant difference in trough concentration, area under curve, and clearance in 2 renal transplant patients before and during treatment *2908*

Cyclosporine A *Blood Increase Physiological* Concomitant administration of cyclosporine with lomerfloxacin probably increases its half-life and AUC as occurs with other quinolones *2068*

Diazepam *Serum Increase Physiological* 40-50% increase due to reduction of total body clearance *3194* Mean decrease of clearance of 38% and increased half-life of 39% in 8 healthy men when 0.1 mg/kg administered intravenously following treatment with 400 mg cimetidine b.d. for 1 week *170* Impaired clearance, increasing half-life by 40% *5148*

Digitoxin *Serum Increase Physiological* Reported to increase concentration, although effect on metabolism uncertain *827*

Diltiazem *Serum Increase Physiological* Administration of diltiazem concurrently with cimetidine in six normal volunteers resulted in a 58% increase in the diltiazem concentration and a 53% increase in the area under the curve after one week, possibly due to cimetidine's inhibition of hepatic cytochrome P450 *4937* Diltiazem clearance may be reduced when drugs are coadministered *1384* Significant increase in area under curve and peak concentration observed when drugs coadministered; similar effect noted on metabolites *6505* Administration of a single dose of 60 mg diltiazem concomitantly with 1200 mg/d cimetidine to 6 healthy volunteers caused a 58% increase in diltiazem concentration and 53% increase in area under the curve after one week's treatment *1911* Coadministration of 1200 mg/d cimetidine for 1 week with a single 60 mg dose of diltiazem to 6 healthy volunteers caused a 58% increase in peak diltiazem concentration and 53% increase in its AUC *2643*

Donepezil *Serum No Effect Physiological* Cimetidine reported to have no effect on the metabolism of donepezil *4662*

Doxazosin *Serum Increase Physiological* In a placebo-controlled clinical trial in normal volunteers a single 1 mg dose of doxazosin together with 4 days of oral cimetidine (400 mg b.i.d.) resulted in a 10% increase in mean AUC of doxazosin and a slight but not statistically significant increase in the maximum concentration of doxazosin *4642*

Doxepin *Serum Increase Physiological* Concentration approximately doubled when cimetidine coadministered in 6 healthy men: effect probably due to action on liver enzymes *5880*

EDTA Clearance *Urine Decrease Physiological* Significant effect within 6 h, normalized after several weeks *1634*

Encainide *Serum Increase Physiological* Increases concentration of encainide and its metabolites by more than 30% possibly due to inhibition of its metabolism or excretion *4820* Concomitant administration increases drug concentration by 30 to 40% *3281*

Erythrocytes *Blood Decrease Physiological* Isolated case of pancytopenia reported possibly due to cimetidine *6143*

Estradiol *Plasma Decrease Physiological* Significantly reduced only in midproliferative phase of cycle *460*

Plasma Increase Physiological Significant increase from mean of 142.8 pmol/L to 171.1 pmol/L in 9 healthy men given 1600 mg/day for 14 days *2006* After 4 weeks treatment with up to 2400 mg/d for 1 month in 5 postmenopausal women concentration increased significantly from mean baseline of 30.0 pg/mL to 59.8 pg/mL *4022*

Plasma No Effect Physiological In 3 premenopausal women smokers administration of 1600 mg daily for 1 month serum concentration unaltered when measured during follicular phase (similar to response in nonsmokers) *4022* No significant effect of treatment with 800 mg/day for 2 weeks in healthy male volunteers on estradiol-17β concentration *1092* In 25 men treated for duodenal ulcer or duodenitis *3900*

Urine No Effect Physiological No significant change in 9 healthy men given 1600 mg/day for 14 days *2006*

Estriol *Urine No Effect Physiological* No significant change in 9 healthy men given 1600 mg/day for 14 days *2006*

Estrogens *Urine Decrease Physiological* Reduction in excretion of total estrogens from mean of 10.7 nmol/nmol creatinine to 9.9 nmol/nmol creatinine in 9 healthy men given 1600 mg/day for 14 days *2006*

Estrone *Plasma No Effect Physiological* Insignificant change from mean of 146.4 pmol/L to 140.5 pmol/L in 9 healthy men given 1600 mg/day for 14 days *2006*

Urine Decrease Physiological Reduction from mean of 3.80 nmol/nmol creatinine to 3.32 nmol/nmol creatinine in 9 healthy men given 1600 mg/day for 14 days *2006*

Ethanol *Serum Increase Physiological* Prior administration of drug caused increased concentration probably due to enhanced absorption rather than effect on metabolism *5437* Coadministration of cimetidine with alcohol increased the concentration of the latter *5064* In 6 men after ingestion of 0.3 g/kg body weight with ingestion of 1000 mg/d cimetidine for 1 week area under curve increased from 6.5 ± 0.6 mmol/L/h to 12.6 ± 2.1 mmol/L/h and peak concentration increased from 6.4 ± 0.9 mmol/L to 12.4 ± 1.5 mmol/L *1436* Peak ethanol concentration and area under time-concentration curve increased due to either inhibition of ethanol metabolism or increased gastrointestinal absorption *1822*

Serum No Effect Physiological Ingestion of alcohol in patients receiving cimetidine for several days prior to alcohol was not associated with any change in the integrated postprandial blood alcohol concentration *1947*

Fat *Feces Decrease Physiological* By about 30%; in 17 patients with cystic fibrosis receiving constant concomitant therapy with pancreatic enzymes *952*

Felodipine *Serum Increase Physiological* Coadministration of cimetidine with felodipine caused a 50% increase in the area under the curve and its maximum plasma concentration *266*

Flecainide *Serum Increase Physiological* Increases elimination half-life and decreases clearance by 13 to 27% *3281* In healthy individuals receiving cimetidine 1 g/d for one week plasma concentration of flecainide increased by about 30% and half-life increased by about 10% *3702* Plasma concentration increased in 8 healthy volunteers with area under curve increased by 28% and time to reach peak plasma concentration increased from 1.8 to 3.6 hours. Effect due to inhibition of hepatic metabolism *6041*

Fluconazole *Serum Decrease Physiological* When cimetidine ingested as a single dose of 400 mg by 6 healthy men and 100 mg fluconazole ingested 2 h later there was a mean decrease of fluconazole AUC of 13 ± 11% and maximum concentration of 19 ± 14% *4645*

Flurbiprofen *Serum Increase Physiological* Although peak concentration not increased area under curve increased *5860*

Fluvastatin *Serum Increase Physiological* Administration of cimetidine with fluvastatin to patients with hypercholesterolemia caused a significant increase of 43% in the AUC of fluvastatin and 24 - 33% in its maximum concentration and 18 - 23% decrease in its plasma clearance *5232*

Follicle Stimulating Hormone

Plasma Increase Physiological With 1.2 g/d caused significant increase in periovulatory period *460* In 11 male subjects with chronic duodenal ulcer given drug 1 g/d for 3 mo *6338*

Plasma No Effect Physiological In 6 patients treated for 1 mo with 1 g/d *5853* In 3 studied men with duodenal ulcer or duodenitis *3900*

Fosfomycin *Serum No Effect Physiological* When coadministered with fosfomycin has no effect on the pharmacokinetics of fosfomycin *1912*

Furosemide *Serum No Effect Physiological* In 10 patients with hepatic cirrhosis mean serum furosemide concentration had same concentration decay curve in the presence or absence of prior furosemide *1061*

Gabapentin *Serum Increase Physiological* Administration of 1200 mg/d gabapentin to 12 patients had caused a 14% decrease in the mean apparent oral clearance of gabapentin *4526*

Cimetidine *(continued)*

Gastrin *Serum Increase Physiological* Increase higher in people ingesting drug in response to food *3900*
Serum No Effect Physiological No effect noted after short-term treatment and no effect on nocturnal serum concentration *3900* In 12 healthy volunteers administration of cimetidine had no effect on basal concentration of gastrin *5829* No effect reported in spite of long-term treatment *2736* No significant effect observed in healthy male volunteers treated with 800 mg/day for 2 weeks *1092*

Glimepiride *Serum No Effect Physiological* When cimetidine at a dose of 800 mg/d coadministered with a single oral dose of 4 mg glimepiride no effect on absorption and disposition of glimepiride noted *2639*

Glipizide *Serum Increase Physiological* Inhibition of metabolism observed with increase in serum concentration *1820*

Glucose *Serum Decrease Physiological* After 100 mg/h for 4 h caused decrease of 15% at 150 minutes in normal subjects. Mean value fell from 5.4 to 4.8 mmol/L on average in 6 patients given 1 g/d for 1 mo *5853*
Serum No Effect Analytical At concentration of 4 mg/L had no effect on GOD/POD-PAP method *5704*
Serum No Effect Physiological Oral drug for 48 h had little effect in normal subjects *5853*

γ-Glutamyltransferase *Serum Increase Physiological* In isolated case treated for 7 mo with 400 mg/d progressed to bridging hepatic necrosis *5149* Rare reports of cholestatic or mixed cholestatic-hepatocellular effects that are usually reversible *5657*

Glyburide *Serum Increase Physiological* Effect observed in normal volunteers due to inhibition of metabolism of glyburide *3311*

Glycated Hemoglobin *Blood No Effect Analytical* At a concentration of 75 mg/L had an insignificant 7.5% interference with method on Abbott Vision *1885*

Granulocytes *Blood Decrease Physiological* Administration of cimetidine reported to cause agranulocytosis in approximately 3 per million patients *5657*
Blood No Effect Physiological No decrease in bone marrow granulocyte reserves *5801*

Growth Hormone *Plasma No Effect Physiological* In 6 patients treated for 1 mo with 1 g/d *5853*

HDL_2-Cholesterol *Serum Increase Physiological* In 8 individuals with peptic ulcer given 1 g/d for 1 mo *6490*

HDL_3-Cholesterol *Serum No Effect Physiological* In 8 individuals with peptic ulcer given 1 g/d for 1 mo *6490*

HDL-Cholesterol *Serum Increase Physiological* Increased proportion of HDL-cholesterol when 600 mg given b.i.d. to 6 males for 1 week *4420* Significant increase in 25 patients over 5 weeks from 37 mg/dL to 42 mg/dL *5986*
Serum No Effect Physiological In healthy individuals and in subjects with high serum glucose concentration *2703* Insignificant increase from mean of 1.15 mmol/L to 1.22 mmol/L in 9 healthy men given 1600 mg/day for 14 days *2006*

Hematocrit *Blood Decrease Physiological* Administration of cimetidine reported to cause immune hemolytic anemia extremely rarely *5657*

Hemoglobin *Blood Decrease Physiological* Administration of cimetidine reported to cause immune hemolytic anemia extremely rarely *5657* Reported in one case in which drug given intravenously *2893*

Hippuran Clearance *Urine Decrease Physiological* Significant effect within 6 h, normalized after several weeks *5369*

Histamine *Plasma No Effect Analytical* Improbable inhibition of radio-enzyme assay at therapeutic concentration of 0.5-1.5 µg/mL although 50% inhibition at 24 µg/mL *2492*

Hydrocortisone *Serum Decrease Physiological* In 7 of 8 adult patients when 400 mg cimetidine given immediately prior to surgery concentration reduced by 0-60% due to blocking of cytochrome P-450 by cimetidine *640*

2-Hydroxyestrone *Urine Decrease Physiological* Significant reduction from mean of 1.71 nmol/nmol creatinine to 1.27 nmol/nmol creatinine in 9 healthy men given 1600 mg/day for 14 days *2006*

16α-Hydroxyestrone *Urine No Effect Physiological* No significant change in 9 healthy men given 1600 mg/day for 14 days *2006*

Hydroxynefazodone *Serum No Effect Physiological* When cimetidine coadministered with nefazodone no significant effect observed on the concentrations of nefazodone or its principal metabolite hydroxynefazodone *363*

Ibuprofen *Serum No Effect Physiological* Coadministration of cimetidine with ibuprofen had no effect on the ibuprofen serum concentration *3913* Cimetidine has been shown to have no effect on ibuprofen concentrations *3200*

Imipramine *Serum Increase Physiological* Marked increase in concentration observed in one patient when cimetidine coadministered: effect probably due to impairment of hepatic metabolism *4043* Plasma concentration of drug may be increased when hepatic enzyme inhibitors given concomitantly *1040* Although peak concentration not different, clearance significantly reduced so higher concentration overall *2550*

immunoglobulin A *Serum Increase Physiological* Significant increase from mean of 1.7 g/L to 2.0 g/L in 12 healthy volunteers given 1600 mg/day for 21 days *734*

Immunoglobulin G *Serum Increase Physiological* Significant increase from mean of 11.0 g/L to 13.0 g/L in 12 healthy volunteers given 1600 mg/day for 21 days *734*

Immunoglobulin M *Serum No Effect Physiological* Insignificant increase in 12 healthy volunteers given 1600 mg/day for 21 days *734*

Indinavir *Serum No Effect Physiological* Administration of a single dose of indinavir (800 mg) after 6 days of cimetidine 600 mg every 12 hours resulted in no change in indinavir AUC *3966*

Insulin *Plasma Decrease Physiological* After 100 mg/h for 4 h caused decrease of 34% at 150 minutes in normal subjects *5853*

Intrinsic Factor *Gastric Material Decrease Physiological* Marked effect on basal and stimulated concentrations *5803*

itraconazole *Serum Decrease Physiological* Itraaconazole inhibits the cytochrome P450 3A enzyme system thereby affecting the metabolism of drugs by this system: cimetidine reduces the plasma concentration of itraconazole *2905* Decreased oral bioavailability *886*

6-Keto-Prostaglandin $F_{1\alpha}$ *Plasma Decrease Physiological* Probable activation of endogenous cyclic AMP phosphodiesterase involved in favoring action of platelet aggregating agents *6635*

Ketoconazole *Serum Decrease Physiological* Effect probably related to reduced gastrointestinal absorption due to increased pH *6177* Decreased oral bioavailability *886* Absorption reduced by about one half when administered with cimetidine *1384*

Labetalol *Serum Increase Physiological* Cimetidine has been shown to increase the bioavailability of labetalol but it is unknown whether this is through enhanced absorption or by alteration of its hepatic metabolism *5335*

Lactate Dehydrogenase *Serum Increase Physiological* In isolated case treated for 7 mo with 400 mg/d progressed to bridging hepatic necrosis *5149* In isolated case of drug associated bridging hepatic necrosis *1355*

LDL-Cholesterol *Serum No Effect Physiological* Insignificant decrease from mean of 2.93 mmol/L to 2.67 mmol/L in 9 healthy men given 1600 mg/day for 14 days *2006* In healthy individuals and in subjects with high serum glucose concentration *2703*

Leu Cells *Blood No Effect Physiological* Insignificant increase in absolute number and percentage of cells in 12 healthy volunteers given 1600 mg/day for 21 days *734*

Leukocyte Migration Inhibition
Blood No Effect Physiological No effect noted in 12 patients treated for acid-peptic disease *3900*

Leukocytes *Blood Decrease Physiological* Significant reduction observed in one patient *1093* Proved case of drug induced agranulocytopenia *888* Administration of cimetidine reported to cause decreased white blood cell count in approximately 1 per 100,000 patients *5657* Reported in one case in which drug given intravenously *2893* Isolated case of pancytopenia reported possibly due to cimetidine *6143*

Blood No Effect Physiological In Medicaid patients from 6 States neither a dose-response relationship nor a duration-response relationship could be established between cell count and cimetidine treatment *5850* No significant change in 12 healthy volunteers given 1600 mg/day for 21 days *734*

Levofloxacin *Serum Increase Physiological* Concurrent administration of cimetidine with levofloxacin increased AUC and and half-life of levofloxacin by 27-38% and 30% respectively *3916* No significant effect observed of cimetidine on the rate and extent of levofloxacin absorption but AUC and half-life of levofloxacin increased by 27 - 38% and 30% respectively *3916*

Serum No Effect Physiological The AUC of levofloxacin was increased 30% in healthy volunteers but not enough to require alteration of dosage *4448*

Lidocaine *Serum Increase Physiological* Reported to reduce clearance and increase its half-life *1384* Slight increase in plasma concentration observed in several studies probably related to decreased metabolism but possibly also due to reduced hepatic blood flow and altered protein binding *410*

Lipase *Serum Increase Physiological* Rare reports of pancreatitis that cleared on withdrawal of the drug *5657*

Lomerfloxacin *Serum Increase Physiological* Concomitant administration of cimetidine with lomerfloxacin probably increases its half-life and AUC as occurs with other quinolones *2068*

Loratadine *Serum Increase Physiological* With coadministration increased plasma concentrations (24 hour AUC) of loratidine (103%) and descarboethoxyloratidine (6%) observed in normal volunteers but without clinical effects *5327*

Lorazepam *Serum No Effect Physiological* No effect observed on concentration since almost entirely metabolized through glucuronidation *1384* Not subject to N-dealkylation or hydroxylation by cytochrome P-450 so not affected by drug *5148*

Losartan *Serum Increase Physiological* Coadministration of cimetidine with losartan caused an increase of about 18% in the AUC of losartan but did not affect the pharmacokinetics of its active metabolite *3965* Coadministration caused an 18% increase in the AUC of losartan but had no effect on on the pharmacokinetics of its active metabolite *3979*

Serum No Effect Physiological Coadministration of losartan with cimetidine had no significant effect on the concentration of either drug *1596*

Luteinizing Hormone *Plasma No Effect Physiological* In 3 studied men with duodenal ulcer or duodenitis *3900* No significant effect of drug during menstrual cycle *460* In 6 patients treated for 1 mo with 1 g/d *5853* In 11 male subjects with chronic duodenal ulcer given drug 1 g/d for 3 mo *6338*

Lymphocyte B-Cells *Blood Increase Physiological* Increase from mean of 0.26 /nL to 0.34 /nL in 12 healthy volunteers given 1600 mg/day for 21 days *734*

Lymphocyte response to Concanavalin A
Blood Increase Physiological Threefold increase in cpm with 1 µg/mL and fourfold increase with 2 µg/mL in 12 healthy volunteers given 1600 mg/day for 21 days *734*

Lymphocyte response to Phytohemagglutinin
Blood Increase Physiological 2.5 fold increase in cpm with both 1 µg/mL and 2 µg/mL in 12 healthy volunteers given 1600 mg/day for 21 days *734*

Lymphocyte response to Pokeweed Mitogen
Blood Increase Physiological Threefold increase in cpm with both 1 µg/mL and 2 µg/mL in 12 healthy volunteers given 1600 mg/day for 21 days *734*

Lymphocyte Transformation *Blood Increase Physiological* Serum from patients treated with drug enhanced lymphocyte response to phytohemagglutinin *3900*

Lymphocytes *Blood No Effect Physiological* No significant change in percentage of total white cells or absolute number of lymphocytes in 12 healthy volunteers given 1600 mg/day for 21 days *734*

Maprotiline *Serum Increase Physiological* Concentration may be raised when hepatic enzyme inhibitors are coadministered *1034*

Mebendazole *Serum Increase Physiological* Cimetidine inhibits mebendazole metabolism thereby increasing its plasma concentration *2906*

Metformin *Serum Increase Physiological* In both single and multiple dose studies during which cimetidine and metformin were coadministered cimetidine increased the maximum concentration and AUC of metformin by 60% and 40% respectively by competing for common renal tubular transport systems *726*

Metoprolol *Serum Increase Physiological* Substantial increase reported with coadministration due to inhibition of hepatic microsomal enzymes *4196* In 12 volunteers given 200 mg metoprolol daily with 800 mg cimetidine daily area under metoprolol's curve increased by 60% due to inhibition of metabolizing enzymes *6054*

Metronidazole *Serum Increase Physiological* By decreasing microsomal hepatic enzyme activity may prolong the half-life of metronidazole and decrease its plasma clearance, thus increasing its plasma concentration *5420* Administration of drugs that induce microsomal liver enzymes may prolong the half-life and decrease the plasma clearance of metronidazole *4446* Clearance prolonged and toxic blood concentrations may occur, probably by inhibiting hepatic metabolizing enzymes *1384* In 6 healthy volunteers half-life increased to mean of 7.9 hours from 6.2 hours and clearance of intravenous dose reduced by 29% *2360* When drugs that decrease hepatic microsomal enzyme activity are coadministered the half-life of metronidazole may be prolonged and the elimination of metronidazole may be decreased *2066*

Mexiletine *Serum Increase Physiological* Decreases clearance of drug and prolongs half-life *3281*

Serum No Effect Physiological Administration of cimetidine with on-going mexiletine treatment had no effect on steady-state peak and trough mexiletine concentrations in 11 patients *3172* No effect on distribution or elimination or its overall kinetics or excretion of its metabolites *733*

Mibefradil *Serum No Effect Physiological* Cimetidine coadministration had no significant effect on pharmacokinetics of mibefradil *5009*

β₂-Microglobulin *Urine No Effect Physiological* No change observed during treatment of 13 ulcer patients *1002*

Microscopy *Urine No Effect Physiological* Unchanged although there may be slight increases in creatinine, not progressive; decreases with continued treatment *3900*

Midazolam *Serum Increase Physiological* By inhibiting cytochrome P450 3A4 may reduce plasma clearance of midazolam when drugs coadministered. Coadministration caused an increase in steady-state concentration from 57 to 71 ng/mL *5037*

Moclobemide *Serum Increase Physiological* After a single oral dose of 100 mg moclobemide following 2 weeks of administration of 1000 mg cimetidine daily mean concentration in 8 healthy individuals increased from 575 ng/mL to 787 ng/mL *5371*

Moricizine *Serum Increase Physiological* Concomitant oral administration of cimetidine, 1200 mg/d, decreases clearance of moricizine by 48%, increases its mean plasma elimination half-life by 35% and increases its plasma concentration by 40% *1062* In healthy individuals concomitant administration decreases moricizine clearance by 49% and increased plasma concentrations 1.4 fold *1384*

Mycophenolic Acid *Serum No Effect Analytical* No significant interference observed with HPLC method of Shipkova et al *5526*

Mycophenolic Acid Glucuronide
Serum No Effect Analytical No significant interference observed with HPLC method of Shipkova et al *5526*

Nefazodone *Serum No Effect Physiological* When cimetidine coadministered with nefazodone no significant effect observed on the concentrations of nefazodone or its principal metabolite hydroxynefazodone *363* Coadministration of nefazodone 200 mg b.i.d. with 300 mg q.i.d. cimetadine for 1 week had no effect on the concentration of either drug *729*

Neutrophils *Blood Decrease Physiological* Occasional case of agranulocytosis reported *6264* Proved case of drug induced agranulocytopenia *888*

Blood No Effect Physiological In Medicaid patients from 6 States neither a dose-response relationship nor a duration-response relationship could e established between cell count and cimetidine treatment *5850*

Nicardipine *Serum Increase Physiological* Cimetidine administration has been shown to increase nicardipine concen-

Cimetidine *(continued)*

Nicardipine *(continued)*
tration *6551* When administered concomitantly increases nicardipine concentration *5016*

Nicoumalone *Serum Increase Physiological* Coadministration causes statistically significant increase in serum concentration of the R(+) but not the S(-) enantiomer because of reduced clearance of the former: rate, but not extent, of absorption of both enantiomers increased by cimetidine *2119*

Nifedipine *Serum Increase Physiological* Impairs disposition and increases plasma concentration *1384* Coadministration of cimetidine with nifedipine in 6 healthy volunteers caused a significant 80% increase in peak plasma nifedipine concentration and 74% increase in its AUC after a 1 week course of cimetidine 1000 mg/d and nifedipine 40 mg/d *4652* In 18 healthy men coadministration of cimetidine with nifedipine caused mean peak concentration to increase to 76 ± 40 μg/L compared with 33 ± 14 μg/L after placebo. Area under curve increased significantly to 211 ± 64 μg/L/h compared with 105 ± 40 μg/L/h after placebo *3127* In 11 healthy subjects 1.2 g daily increased area under curve by approximately 80% when they were also ingesting 60 mg daily for 1 week. Clearance of nifedipine reduced by up to 50%. Effects probably due to inhibition of P-450 cytochrome by cimetidine *5397* With coadministration significant increase in area under the curve possibly attributable to increase in gastric pH. Plasma concentration also increased by about 80% *5629* Metabolism inhibited to a greater extent than occurs with ranitidine *1384* Peak plasma concentration and AUC of nifedipine may increase following administration of cimetidine, possibly mediated by inhibition of cytochrome P-450 *415*

Nisoldipine *Serum Increase Physiological* Plasma concentration increased because of inhibition of hepatic mono-oxygenases *3147* Administration of cimetidine 400 mg twice daily with nisoldipine caused a 30 - 45% increase in the AUC and plasma concentration of nisoldipine *6650*

Nitrendipine *Serum Increase Physiological* Plasma concentration increased with coadministration due to inhibition of hepatic mono-oxygenases *6184*

Nitrogen *Feces Decrease Physiological* By about 30%; in 17 patients with cystic fibrosis receiving constant concomitant therapy with pancreatic enzymes *952*

Nortriptyline *Serum Increase Physiological* Effect observed with coadministration in one patient: effect probably related to impairment of hepatic metabolism *4044* Area under curve increased, most noticeably for its 10-hydroxy metabolite *2550*

o-Desmethylvenlafaxine *Serum No Effect Physiological* Concomitant administration of cimetidine and venlafaxine to 18 healthy men reduced had no effect on the pharmacokinetics of o-desmethylvenlafaxine *6555*

Occult Blood *Feces Increase Analytical* At concentrations above 1500 mg/L on Hemoccult® method *5704* When added to Hemoccult® test paper as pure chemical applied at pH of gastric juice *2512*
Feces No Effect Analytical No effect noted on Hemoquant method *6172*

Oxaprozin *Serum Increase Physiological* Coadministration of cimetidine with oxaprozin caused a 20% decrease in its total body clearance *2065*

Oxazepam *Serum No Effect Physiological* No effect on concentration since eliminated by glucuronidation *1384* Not subject to N-dealkylation or hydroxylation by cytochrome P-450 so not affected by drug *5148*

Parathyroid Hormone *Plasma Decrease Physiological* Affect C-terminal component only: observed in normals and patients with renal failure: slight increase of N-terminal component *1868*

Paroxetine *Serum Increase Physiological* When paroxetine (30 mg q.i.d.) was given orally for 4 weeks with cimetidine 300 mg (t.i.d.) for the final week caused an increase of 50% in the plasma concentration of paroxetine *5654*

Penciclovir *Serum No Effect Physiological* No significant effect on pharmacokinetics of penciclovir observed following single-dose administatration of 500 mg famciclovir after pretreatment with multiple doses of cimetidine *5646*

Pepsin *Gastric Material Decrease Physiological* Marked effect on basal and stimulated concentrations *5803*

pH *Gastric Material Increase Physiological* Effectively reduces gastric acidity both before and after meals *3876*
Urine Increase Physiological Mean increase of 0.4 in healthy volunteers *3407*

Phenytoin *Serum Increase Physiological* Significant increases in concentration observed when drugs coadministered *1384* Significant increase due to inhibition of metabolism probably by reversibly binding to hepatic microsomal cytochrome P-450 *3541* When cimetidine ingested with fosphenytoin concentration of phenytoin may be increased *4519* Causes increase in concentration when drugs coadministered through enzyme inhibition *6350* Significant increases when coadministered, due to effect on hepatic metabolism *5201*

Phosphate *Serum No Effect Analytical* At concentration of 1 mg/L had no effect on phosphomolybdate method *5704*

Platelets *Blood Decrease Physiological* Observed in one patient with cancer in absence of leukopenia: fell again with rechallenge by drug *3768* Administration of cimetidine reported to cause thrombocytopenia in approximately 3 per million patients *5657* Significant reduction observed in one patient *1093* Isolated case of drug effect together with psoriasis *6592* Reported in one case in which drug given intravenously *2893* Isolated case of pancytopenia reported possibly due to cimetidine *6143* Isolated case of platelet-associated IgG and thrombocytopenia *3102*

Porphobilinogen *Urine Decrease Physiological* Slight decrease in patient with acute intermittent porphyria *2715*

Porphyrin, Total *Feces No Effect Physiological* No measurable change in one patient with acute intermittent porphyria *2715*

Potassium *Serum No Effect Analytical* At concentration of 1 mg/L had no effect on flame-photometric method *5704* At concentration of 75 mg/L caused nonsignificant 2.6% interference with method on Abbott Vision *681*

Pramipexole *Serum Increase Physiological* Coadministration of pramipexole with cimetidine caused a 50% increase in pramipexole AUC and a 40% increase in its half-life *4680*

Pravastatin *Serum No Effect Physiological* Coadministration with pravastatin caused no significant effect on bioavailability of pravastatin *728*

Prazepam *Serum Increase Physiological* Probable effect as a result of inhibition of drug metabolizing hepatic microsomal enzymes *1384*

Procainamide *Serum Increase Physiological* Administration of cimetidine decreases renal clearance of procainamide leading to clinically significant increases in plasma procainamide concentration *4530* Reduces renal clearance of both procainamide and its active metabolite *1384* NAPA metabolite also increased not due to effect on hepatic blood flow or liver cytochrome enzymes; interaction occurs at renal tubular excretion level *2597* Renal clearance of procainamide reduced by 43% and clearance of N-acetylprocainamide reduced by 24% in healthy volunteers. Area under curve increased by 44%. Effects due to reduced renal tubular secretion *5697* Area under curve increased by 43%, renal clearance decreased 36% and decreased ratio of clearance to bioavailability *5053*

Progesterone *Plasma No Effect Physiological* No significant effect of drug during menstrual cycle *460*

Prolactin *Plasma Increase Physiological* Significant increase in basal values observed *4609* Sustained effect throughout luteal phase of menstrual cycle *460* In 5 of 11 male subjects with chronic duodenal ulcer given drug 1 g/d for 3 mo *6338* Following either i.v. or oral drug, may be associated with larger doses of drug, possible effect on dopamine receptors in anterior pituitary, or on inhibition of uptake in peripheral tissues *3900*
Plasma No Effect Physiological In 2 studied men with duodenal ulcer or duodenitis *3900* No significant effect with 800 mg/day for 2 weeks in healthy male volunteers *1092* In 6 patients treated for 1 mo with 1 g/d *5853*

Propafenone *Serum Increase Physiological* Concomitant administration of propafenone with cimetidine in 12 healthy individuals resulted in a 20% increase in the propafenone concentration *3204*

Propranolol *Serum Increase Physiological* Coadministration of cimetidine with propranolol caused 50-100% increase of both peak and steady-state concentrations of propranolol due to inhibition of hepatic microsomal enzymes *1821* Reduces oral clearance by as much as 50% *4905* Cimetidine administration decreases the hepatic metabolism of propranolol delaying its elimination and increasing its blood concentration *6558* In 12 volunteers given 1.2 g daily area under curve increased by 47% and 17% increase in propranolol's elimination half-life with reduction of 4-hydroxypropranolol to propranolol ratio due to decreased metabolism *1467*

Protein *Serum No Effect Analytical* At concentration of 1 mg/L had no effect on biuret method with blank correction *5704*
Urine No Effect Physiological Although drug cleared principally by glomerular filtration and partial reabsorption in proximal renal tubules *3900*

Prothrombin Time *Plasma Increase Physiological* In 6 patients mean prolongation of time by 12.6 s in patients receiving warfarin, nicoumalone and phenindone *5450*
Plasma No Effect Physiological Causes minimal prolongation of stereoselective inhibition of clearance of R isomer of warfarin when it is coadministered *2625*

Quinapril *Serum No Effect Physiological* Coadministration of cimetidine with quinapril had no effect on the pharmacokinetics of a single dose of quinapril *4516*

Quinidine *Serum Increase Physiological* Drug probably competes with quinidine for secretion of basic compounds by the proximal renal tubules *2459* By mechanisms not understood concentration of quinidine increased when cimetidine coadministered *5996* In 6 normal individuals, administration of 1.2 g/day for 7 days increased quinidine half-life by 55% and reduced quinidine clearance from mean of 26 L/h to 16 L/h *2460* Increased area under curve and prolonged half-life and decreased total body clearance *3229*

Rimantadine *Serum Increase Physiological* Coadministration in normal volunteers caused increase in area under concentration-time curve, reduced apparent total clearance (by 18%) and elimination rate constant *2668*

Salicylate *Serum Increase Physiological* Influence on serum concentration in drug treated group compared with enteric-coated drug administered group (180 µg/mL vs 161 µg/mL) *6477*

Sertraline *Serum Increase Physiological* On second day of administration of cimetidine (800 mg/d) for 8 days and 100 mg of sertraline mean AUC of sertraline increased by 50% and maximum concentration increased by 24% with increase of half life of 26% *4660*

Sex-Hormone Binding Globulin
Serum Decrease Physiological Reduction of about 30% observed in 3 smoking premenopausal women given 1600 mg/d for 1 month *4022*
Serum No Effect Physiological No significant effect observed in 5 postmenopausal women treated with up to 2400 mg/d for 1 month *4022* No significant change in 9 healthy men given 1600 mg/day for 14 days *2006*

Sibutramine *Serum Increase Physiological* Concomitant administration of 400 mg cimetidine b.i.d. with 20 mg sibutramine per day for 7 days to 12 healthy individuals caused increases of AUC metabolites M_1 and M_2 of 3.4% and of combined concentration of 7.3% *3203*

Sildenafil *Serum Increase Physiological* Following treatment with cimetidine (800 mg) concentration of sildenafil increases 56% after a single 50 mg dose *4657*

Sodium *Serum No Effect Analytical* At concentration of 1 mg/L had no effect on flame-photometric method *5704*
Urine No Effect Physiological Although drug cleared principally by glomerular filtration and partial reabsorption in proximal renal tubules *3900*

Sparfloxacin *Serum No Effect Physiological* Cimetidine has no effect on the pharmacokinetics of sparfloxacin *4943*

Sperm Count *Semen Decrease Physiological* In 7 patients treated for 9 weeks with 1200 mg/d compared with their pretreatment values *3900* In 11 male subjects with chronic duodenal ulcer given drug 1 g/d for 3 mo *6338*

Sperm Morphology *Semen No Effect Physiological* In 11 male subjects with chronic duodenal ulcer given drug 1 g/d for 3 mo *6338*

Sperm Motility *Semen No Effect Physiological* In 11 male subjects with chronic duodenal ulcer given drug 1 g/d for 3 mo *6338*

Tacrine *Serum Increase Physiological* Coadministration of cimetidine with tacrine increased the maximum concentration and AUC of tacrine by 54% and 64% respectively *4521*

Tacrolimus *Serum Increase Physiological* By inhibiting cytochrome P-450 IIIA enzyme systems may inhibit the metabolism of tacrolimus *1987*
Serum No Effect Analytical In HPLC/MS method of Christians et al no significant interference observed with measurement of FK 506 *1010*

Temazepam *Serum No Effect Physiological* Pharmacokinetic properties of temazepam not affected by administration of cimetidine *5239*

Tenidap *Serum No Effect Physiological* In 24 healthy volunteers coadministration of 800 mg of cimetidine on one day when individuals ingesting 120 mg tenidap daily caused no significant clinical change in the plasma concentration of tenidap although area under the curve increased by 4% and maximum concentration changed from placebo concentration of 26.8 µg/mL to 25.8 µg/L with cimetidine *6480*

Tenoxicam *Serum No Effect Physiological* In 6 healthy volunteers mean peak plasma concentration of 3.76 ± 1.19 µg/mL after pretreatment with 1 g/d cimetidine for 7 days not significantly different from 3.48 ± 0.64 µg/mL when 20 mg tenoxicam given alone *1294*

Terbinafine *Serum Increase Physiological* Cimetidine decreased the clearance of terbinafine by 33%, a CyP450 enzyme inhibitor *5231*

Testosterone *Serum Decrease Physiological* Observed in one 66 y old man, together with increased serum gonadotropin possibly due to reversible defect in 17-β-hydroxysteroid dehydrogenase *3412*
Serum Increase Physiological In 11 male subjects with chronic duodenal ulcer given drug 1 g/d for 3 mo *6338* Up to 20% increase on chronic administration and displaces DHT from its binding sites at pituitary and hypothalamic level *2836*
Serum No Effect Physiological In 6 patients treated for 1 mo with 1 g/d *5853* No significant change in 9 healthy men given 1600 mg/day for 14 days *2006* No significant effect of treatment with 800 mg/day for 2 weeks in healthy male volunteers *1092* In 25 men treated for duodenal ulcer or duodenitis *3900*

Theophylline *Serum Increase Physiological* In 17 patients with COPD given theophylline for 42 days coadministration of cimetidine caused 32% increase in mean AUC_{0-12} from 113.95 mg/h/L to 151.03 mg/h/L and mean maximum concentration from 9.5 mg/L to 12.6 mg/L *316* In group of young adults and elderly with increased area under curve, increased half-life and reduced clearance *1078* In 6 young male nonsmokers administration of 400 mg p. o. every 12 h for 7 days caused decrease of theophylline clearance by 25% *3638* Plasma concentration following aminophylline infusion higher in cimetidine treated volunteers than in placebo treated volunteers *6606* Decreases theophylline clearance by inhibiting cytochrome P450 1A2 and increases serum theophylline concentration by 70% *3125* Decreases theophylline clearance by inhibiting cytochrome P450 1A2, increasing theophylline concentration by about 25% *5999* Plasma clearance reduced from 71 mL/min to 56 mL/min in 7 healthy subjects given 1 g/d *4988* Half-life increased by 60% with coadministration *6387* Up to 70% increase in serum theophylline concentration due to decreased theophylline clearance caused by inhibition of cytochrome P450 1A2 *6117* Average increase of 32% when 800 mg cimetidine given daily for one week to 15 patients with chronic obstructive airway disease. Two patients had concentrations that exceeded 20 mg/L *627* Single case reported in which serum concentration doubled: effect reversible: effect possibly due to direct inhibition of hepatic metabolism *862*

Thromboxane B_2 *Plasma Increase Physiological* Probable activation of endogenous cyclic AMP phosphodiesterase involved in favoring action of platelet aggregating agents *6635*

Thyroid Stimulating Hormone
Serum No Effect Physiological No significant changes caused by drug *4609* In 6 patients treated for 1 mo with 1 g/d *5853* No change after 1 g daily for 28 d, although different findings by other group *6412*

Thyroxine (T4) *Serum No Effect Physiological* In 6 patients treated for 1 mo with 1 g/d *5853* No significant difference in drug treated healthy volunteers: no difference in response to TRH *2763*

Cimetidine *(continued)*

Titratable Acidity *Urine No Effect Physiological* Although drug cleared principally by glomerular filtration and partial reabsorption in proximal renal tubules *3900*

Tocainide *Serum No Effect Physiological* No clinically significant interaction observed *268*

Tolbutamide *Serum Increase Physiological* When coadministered with tolbutamide, cimetidine caused increase in half-life of 17% and area under curve of 20% in 12 healthy volunteers due to inhibition of metabolism *922*

Tramadol *Serum Decrease Physiological* Coadministration of cimetidine with tramadol had no significant effect on the pharmacokinetics of tramadol *3918*

Trandolapril *Serum Increase Physiological* Coadministration of cimetidine with trandolapril led to a 44% increase in the maximum plasma concentration of trandopril *3202*

Tri-iodothyronine, Reverse (rT3)
Serum Increase Physiological Basal concentration increased by treatment due to drug effect on hepatic metabolism *4609*
Serum No Effect Physiological No significant difference in drug treated healthy volunteers: no difference in response to TRH *2763*

Tri-iodothyronine (T3) *Serum Decrease Physiological* From average of 1.49 to 1.25 nmol/L after 1.2 g for 5 d in 8 healthy male volunteers reduces response to TRH *2763*
Serum No Effect Physiological No significant changes caused by drug *4609* In 6 patients treated for 1 mo with 1 g/d *5853*

Triazolam *Serum Increase Physiological* Coadministration may approximately double elimination half-life and plasma concentration of triazolam *4677*

Tricyclic Antidepressants *Serum Increase Physiological* Interacts pharmacokinetically to inhibit cytochrome P450 enzymes thereby inhibiting metabolism of tricyclic antidepressants and increasing their plasma concentration by up to 2-fold *3590*

Triglycerides *Serum No Effect Analytical* At concentration of 1 mg/L had no effect on lipase/esterase method *5704* At concentration of 4 mg/L had no effect on GPO-PAP method *5704*
Serum No Effect Physiological In healthy individuals and in subjects with high serum glucose concentration *2703* In 25 patients pretreatment 139 mg/dL, after 146 mg/dL over 5 weeks *5986*

Trimantadine *Serum Increase Physiological* Coadministration of cimetidine with trimantadine in normal volunteers caused reduction of its clearance by 18% compared to the apparent clearance in the absence of cimetidine *1910*

Trovafloxacin *Serum No Effect Physiological* No significant interaction observed *4663*

Urea Nitrogen *Serum Increase Physiological* Rare cases of interstitial nephritis that cleared on withdrawal of the drug have been reported *5657* Single case of reversible renal failure probably attributable to drug *5434*
Serum No Effect Analytical At concentration of 1 mg/L had no effect on diacetylmonoxime method *5704*
Serum No Effect Physiological Unchanged although there may be slight increases in creatinine, not progressive: decreases with continued treatment *3900* No significant effect observed in 9 patients given 1.6 g daily *1634*

Uric Acid *Serum Increase Physiological* Slight increase in patients with renal failure *3424*
Serum No Effect Analytical At concentration of 1 mg/L had no effect on phosphotungstate reduction method *5704* At concentration of 4 mg/L had no effect on uricase-PAP method *5704* At 300 mg/L on reversed phase liquid chromatographic procedure of Zhiri et al *6656*
Serum No Effect Physiological No effect in volunteers receiving 1.2 g daily for 12 d *491* Unchanged although there may be slight increases in creatinine, not progressive: decreases with continued treatment *3900*
Urine No Effect Physiological No effect in volunteers receiving 1.2 g daily for 12 d *491* Although drug cleared principally by glomerular filtration and partial reabsorption in proximal renal tubules *3900*

Uroporphyrin *Urine No Effect Physiological* No measurable change in one patient with acute intermittent porphyria *2715*

Valproic Acid *Serum No Effect Physiological* In a study involving the coadministration of cimetidine with valproate resulted in no significant effect on the trough plasma concentrations of valproate *15* Coadministration with valproic acid did not affect its clearance *17*

Venlafaxine *Serum Increase Physiological* Concomitant administration of cimetidine and venlafaxine to 18 healthy men reduced the oral clearance of venlafaxine by about 43% *6555*

Verapamil *Serum Increase Physiological* Clearance reduced in most patients but not constant since in some serum concentration actually reduced *3639* Coadministration led to significant increase of area under concentration versus time curve. Increase significantly greater for S-verapamil than for R-verapamil. Effects due to stereoselective inhibition of hepatic and renal elimination of verapamil *4031* Variable effects of cimetidine on verapamil clearance have been reported with clearance of verapamil either reduced or unchanged *3470* Coadministration of cimetidine with verapamil may decrease verapamil clearance or have no effect on its clearance *3201* Cimetidine reportedly reduces verapamil clearance *1384*
Serum No Effect Physiological Variable effects of cimetidine on verapamil clearance have been reported with clearance of verapamil either reduced or unchanged *3470* Coadministration of cimetidine with verapamil may decrease verapamil clearance or have no effect on its clearance *3201*

Vitamin B_{12} *Urine Decrease Physiological* Excretion reduced because of markedly reduced absorption *5206*

VLDL-Cholesterol *Serum No Effect Physiological* In healthy individuals and in subjects with high serum glucose concentration *2703*

VLDL-Triglycerides *Serum No Effect Physiological* In healthy individuals and in subjects with high serum glucose concentration *2703*

Volume *Urine No Effect Physiological* Although drug cleared principally by glomerular filtration and partial reabsorption in proximal renal tubules *3900*

Warfarin *Plasma Increase Physiological* Clearance reduced: probably by inhibition of drug metabolism with increased half-life *5450*

Zalcitabine *Serum Increase Physiological* When single doses of zalcitabine 1.5 mg and cimetidine 800 mg to 12 HIV-positive patients, mean renal clearance of zalcitabine decreased from 224 mL/min to 171 mL/min and AUC increased from 75 ng.h/mL to 102 ng.h/mL *5023*

Zolmitriptan *Serum Increase Physiological* Coadministration of cimetidine with zolmitriptan caused a doubling of the AUC and half-life of zolmitriptan *6653*

Zolpidem *Serum No Effect Physiological* Coadministration of cimetidine with zolpidem had no effect on the pharmacokinetics or pharmacodynamics of zolpidem *2062*

Cinchophen

Alanine Aminotransferase *Serum Increase Physiological* May cause hepatotoxicity (viral-hepatitis like) *3810*

Alkaline Phosphatase *Serum Increase Physiological* May cause intrahepatic cholestasis *3810*

Aspartate Aminotransferase *Serum Increase Physiological* May cause hepatotoxicity (viral-hepatitis like) *3810*

Bile *Urine Increase Physiological* May cause hepatotoxicity (viral-hepatitis like) *3810*

Bilirubin *Serum Increase Physiological* May cause hypersensitive cholestasis *3810*

BSP Retention *Serum Increase Physiological* May cause hepatotoxicity (viral-hepatitis like) *3810*

Cholesterol *Serum Increase Physiological* May cause intrahepatic cholestasis *2377*

Color *Urine Increase Analytical* Red brown *3810*

Leukocytes *Blood Decrease Physiological* Leukopenia or agranulocytosis may occur *4017*

Occult Blood *Feces Increase Physiological* May cause severe ulceration of gastrointestinal tract *929*

Prothrombin Time *Plasma Increase Physiological* May prolong action of anticoagulants *2753*

Sugar *Urine Increase Analytical* Acts as a reducing substance *4012*

Uric Acid *Serum Decrease Physiological* Uricosuric action *3810*

Cinepazide

Granulocytes *Blood Decrease Physiological* Increased risk of agranulocytosis observed in small study population in Spain *3098* Risk of agranulocytosis reported to be between 0.07% and 1.1% depending on duration of treatment in data reported to Spanish Centre for Drug Monitoring *3410*

Leukocytes *Blood Decrease Physiological* Risk of agranulocytosis presumed to be between 0.07% and 1.1% depending on duration of treatment *3410*

Cinoxacin

Alanine Aminotransferase *Serum Increase Physiological* Reported effect in some patients *1384*

Alkaline Phosphatase *Serum Increase Physiological* Reported effect observed in some patients *1384*

Aspartate Aminotransferase *Serum Increase Physiological* Reported effect in some patients *1384*

Creatinine *Serum Increase Physiological* Reported effect in some patients *1384*

Eosinophils *Blood Increase Physiological* Reported effect in some patients *1384*

Hemoglobin *Blood Decrease Physiological* Anemia reported to occur in some patients *1384*

Urea Nitrogen *Serum Increase Physiological* Reported effect in some patients *1384*

Ciprofibrate

Apolipoprotein A-I *Serum Decrease Physiological* In one 41 year old women treatment with 100 mg/d for 2 weeks caused significant decrease of concentration *1178*
Serum Increase Physiological Treatment of 127 patients with primary hyperlipidemia types IIa, IIb and IV with 100 mg/d for 12 weeks caused a significant reduction in concentration *928* Increased synthesis. Increased activity of lipoprotein lipase by stimulation of muscle lipoprotein lipase synthesis, alteration of the capillary endothelial surface and stimulation of apo C-II synthesis *264*

Apolipoprotein A-II *Serum Increase Physiological* Increased synthesis. Increased activity of lipoprotein lipase by stimulation of muscle lipoprotein lipase synthesis, alteration of capillary endothelial surface and stimulation of apo C-II synthesis *264*

Apolipoprotein B *Serum Decrease Physiological* Treatment of 104 patients with primary hyperlipidemia (types IIa, and IIb) for 12 weeks with 100 mg/d caused significant reduction *928*
Serum No Effect Physiological No significant change observed in 23 patients with type IV hyperlipidemia treated with 100 mg/d for 12 weeks *928*

Cholesterol *Serum Decrease Physiological* In 127 diet resistant primary hyperlipidemic patients (types IIa, IIb and IV) treatment with 100 mg/d for 12 weeks caused significant reduction *928* Ciprofibrate is effective in decreasing cholesterol concentrations *3668*

C-Reactive Protein *Serum No Effect Physiological* In 48 hypercholesterolemic patients (cholesterol concentration greater than 6.5 mmol/L) treatment with 100 mg/d ciprofibrate caused an insignificant change from mean baseline concentration of 1.28 mg/L to 1.32g/L *1317*

Fibrinogen *Plasma Decrease Physiological* In 48 hypercholesterolemic patients (cholesterol concentration greater than 6.5 mmol/L) treatment with 100 mg/d ciprofibrate caused significant reduction from mean baseline concentration of 3.38 g/L to 2.42 g/L *1317* In reported studies ciprofibrate reduces mean concentration by up to -18% *5585*

γ-Glutamyltransferase *Serum Decrease Physiological* In one 41 year old women treatment with 100 mg/d for 2 weeks caused significant decrease of activity from 227 to 65 U/L *1178*

HDL-Cholesterol *Serum Decrease Physiological* In one 41 year old women treatment with 100 mg/d for 2 weeks caused significant decrease of plasma HDL-cholesterol concentration from 1.05 mmol/L to 0.12 mmol/L but with fluctuations up to 0.8 mmol/L over next 3 months with continued treatment *1178*
Serum Increase Physiological Increased apo A-I and A-II synthesis. Increased activity of lipoprotein lipase by stimulation of muscle lipoprotein lipase synthesis, alteration of the capillary endothelial surface and stimulation of apo C-II synthesis *264* Ciprofibrate has been reported to be more effective than other fibrates in increasing HDL-cholesterol concentrations *3668* Treatment of 127 patients with primary hyperlipidemia (types IIa, IIb and IV) for 12 weeks with 100 mg/d caused significant reduction *928*

Triglycerides *Serum Decrease Physiological* Treatment of 127 patients with diet resistant primary hyperlipidemia (types IIa, IIb and IV) for 12 weeks with 100 mg/d caused significant reduction *928* Ciprofibrate is effective in decreasing triglyceride concentrations *3668*

VLDL-Cholesterol *Serum Decrease Physiological* Treatment of 127 patients with diet resistant hyperlipidemia (types IIa, IIb and IV) with 100 mg/d for 12 weeks caused significant reduction *928*

Ciprofloxacin

Alanine Aminotransferase *Serum Increase Physiological* Rare cases reported during clinical trials *237*

Alkaline Phosphatase *Serum Increase Physiological* Rare cases reported during clinical trials *237*

Aspartate Aminotransferase *Serum Increase Physiological* Rare cases reported during clinical trials *237*

Bilirubin *Serum No Effect Physiological* Clinically insignificant displacement from protein in neonates *6314*

Caffeine *Serum Increase Physiological* Reported to reduce clearance *1384* Concurrent administration of ciprofloxacin with caffeine may cause reduced clearanceof caffeine and prolongation of its half-life *416* Clearance inhibited to some extent *2704*

Clindamycin *Serum Increase Analytical* Interferes with bioassays *3858*

Colistin *Serum Increase Analytical* Interferes with bioassays *3858*

Coproporphyrin I *Urine Increase Analytical* In urine to which ciprofloxacin added to a concentration of 0.25 mmol/L and coproporphyrin I measured by HPLC with fluorescence 3% increase in peak area observed *5366*

Coproporphyrin III *Urine Increase Analytical* In urine to which ciprofloxacin added to a concentration of 0.25 mmol/L peak area increased by 3% when measured by HPLC method with fluorescence detection *5366*

Cortisol *Plasma No Effect Physiological* No significant effect noted in 8 healthy men given 500 mg orally every 12 hours for 4 days *6300*

Creatinine *Serum Increase Physiological* Acute renal failure developed in one patient following administration of ciprofloxacin for 7 days: caused by allergic tubulointerstitial nephritis *4869* Concurrent administration of ciprofloxacin with cyclosporine has been associated with transient increases of creatinine concentration *416* Mild and transient cases reported although 1 case each of acute renal failure, interstitial nephritis and nonspecific nephritis reported in population of 2829 patients *237*

Crystals *Urine Increase Physiological* Observed in 4 of 2829 patients without change in renal function *237* Crystals of ciprofloxacin have been observed rarely in the urine of humans but more commonly in animals *416*

Cyclosporine *Blood Increase Physiological* Coadministration of 500 to 1500 mg/d ciprofloxacin with cyclosporine caused a 156% increase in whole blood cyclosporine concentration with 37.5% increase in serum creatinine concentration *859*
Blood No Effect Analytical At a concentration of 43 mg/L had no effect on Syva EMIT method *495*
Blood No Effect Physiological Coadministration of 500 mg ciprofloxacin twice daily with cyclosporine to bone marrow transplant patients had no significant effect on cyclosporine trough concentration or AUC *859*

Ciprofloxacin *(continued)*

Cyclosporine *(continued)*
Serum Increase Physiological Coadministration of 500 to 1500 mg/d ciprofloxacin with cyclosporine caused a 156% increase in whole blood cyclosporine concentration with 37.5% increase in serum creatinine concentration *859*
Serum No Effect Physiological In 10 bone marrow transplant no clinically or statistically significant changes observed in plasma trough concentration when 500 mg ciprofloxacin given every 12 hours for 4 days *3287* Pharmacokinetics unaffected by coadministration *2704* Coadministration of 500 mg ciprofloxacin twice daily with cyclosporine to bone marrow transplant patients had no significant effect on cyclosporine trough concentration or AUC *859* In one study of transplant patients addition of ciprofloxacin to therapeutic regime had no significant effect on concentration of cyclosporine *6596*

Diazepam *Serum Increase Physiological* In 12 healthy individuals pretreatment with ciprofloxacin significantly reduced diazepam clearance after 5 mg intravenously from 19.5 mL/h/kg to 12.3 mL/h/kg with increase of diazepam half-life *3018*

Eosinophils *Blood Increase Physiological* In one case following administration of ciprofloxacin allergic tubulointerstitial nephritis developed with rapid onset of azotemia, peripheral blood eosinophilia and eosinophiluria. Blood eosinophil count rose to almost 4000/µL *4869* Observed in 16 of 2829 patients and not serious *237*
Urine Increase Physiological Marked eosinophiluria observed in one patient who developed ciprofloxacin-associated allergic tubulointerstitial nephritis. More than 5% of leukocytes in urine were eosinophils *4869*

Erythromycin *Serum Increase Analytical* Interferes with bioassays *3858*

Glucose *Serum Decrease Physiological* Concurrent administration of ciprofloxacin with glyburide has, on rare occasions, been associated with severe hypoglycemia *416*

Lactate Dehydrogenase *Serum Increase Physiological* Rare cases reported during clinical trials *237*

Leukocytes *Blood Decrease Physiological* Seen in 7 of 2829 patients: in all cases mild and not clearly drug related *237*

Metronidazole *Serum Increase Analytical* Interferes with bioassays *3858*

Neutrophils *Blood Decrease Physiological* Reversible rare effect, often in association with administration of other drugs *304*

Norfloxacin *Serum Increase Analytical* Cannot be assayed by HPLC method used at Mayo Clinic in presence of ciprofloxacin *3858*

Phenytoin *Serum Decrease Physiological* Concurrent administration of ciprofloxacin with diphenylhydantoin has been associated with both increased and decreased plasma concentrations of phenytoin *416*
Serum Increase Physiological Concurrent administration of ciprofloxacin with diphenylhydantoin has been associated with both increased and decreased plasma concentrations of phenytoin *416*

Polymyxin *Serum Increase Analytical* Interferes with bioassays *3858*

Porphyrin, Total *Urine Increase Analytical* In urine to which ciprofloxacin added to a concentration of 0.25 mmol/L peak area as obtained by HPLC with fluorescence detection increased by 3% *5366* In one patient treated with ciprofloxacin 2-fold increase in apparent concentration observed with screening method of Porphyrin Products *5366*

Prostate-specific Antigen, Free *Serum No Effect Analytical* Ciprofloxacin hydrochloride at a concentration of 46 mg/L had no significant effect on the Hybritech Tandem® -R free PSA immunoassay *4286*

Prothrombin Time *Plasma Increase Physiological* Increased INR in patients receiving warfarin *886* Concurrent administration of ciprofloxacin with warfarin has been associated with an enhanced effect of warfarin *416*

Quinidine *Serum No Effect Physiological* Ciprofloxacin has no effect on the pharmacokinetics of quinidine *5996*

Tacrolimus *Serum Increase Analytical* In HPLC/MS method of Christians et al interference observed with measurement of metabolites of FK 506 because of similar retention time *1010*

Testosterone *Serum No Effect Physiological* No effect observed in 8 healthy men given 500 mg orally every 12 hours for 4 days *6300*

Tetracycline *Serum Increase Analytical* Interferes with bioassays *3858*

Theophylline *Serum Increase Physiological* In 6 healthy young nonsmoking men administration of 500 mg p. o. every 12 h for 7 days caused 32% decrease of theophyllne clearance due to inhibition of N-demethylation pathway *3638* Coadministration in 8 healthy volunteers reduced clearance by 18% or more due to inhibition of demethylation *4306* Approximate doubling of concentration in 33 hospitalized patients with respiratory tract infections. In 20 patients increase into toxic range. Effect probably due to inhibition of hepatic microsomal enzymes by ciprofloxacin *4857* In 9 male volunteers ciprofloxacin 500 mg 12 hourly for 7 days together with theophylline 125 mg 8 hourly caused reduction of theophylline clearance by 27% due to decreased clearance via 1,3-demethylation and 8-hydroxylation *5003* In one case clearance fell from 2.3 L/h to 0.8 L/h when drug added to treatment regime *6019* Concurrent administration of ciprofloxacin with theophylline causes an increase in its plasma concentration and prolongation of its half-life *416* Decreased metabolism and increased plasma concentration *886* Decreases theophylline clearance by inhibiting cytochrome P450 1A2 and increases serum theophylline concentration by 40% *3125* Decreases theophylline clearance by inhibiting cytochrome P450 1A2, increasing theophylline concentration by about 40% *5999* Up to 40% increase in serum theophylline concentration due to decreased theophylline clearance caused by inhibition of cytochrome P450 1A2 *6117* Significant effect observed probably due to interference with hepatic metabolism *1384* Clearance inhibited to some extent *2704* Coadministration of 3.4 mg/kg theophylline before and after 60 h of ciprofloxacin at a dose of 500 mg twice daily was associated with mean reduction of clearance of theophylline of 19% *405*

Trimethoprim *Serum Increase Analytical* Interferes with bioassays *3858*

Urea Nitrogen *Serum Increase Physiological* Mild and transient cases reported although 1 case each of acute renal failure, interstitial nephritis and nonspecific nephritis reported in population of 2829 patients *237*

Uroporphyrin *Urine Increase Analytical* In urine to which ciprofloxacin added to a concentration of 0.25 mmol/L and uroporphyrin measured by HPLC with fluorescence 3% increase in peak area observed *5366*

Cisapride

Cimetidine *Serum Increase Physiological* Peak plasma concentration increased and occurred earlier when two drugs coadministered because of enhanced gastrointestinal absorption *3148*
Serum No Effect Physiological In patients receiving cimetidine together with cisapride no effect reported on gastrointestinal absorption of cimetidine *2903*

Cyclosporine *Blood Increase Physiological* With coadministration of drugs increase of maximum concentration of 24% and decrease of 38% in half-life *859*
Serum Increase Physiological With coadministration of drugs increase of maximum concentration of 24% and decrease of 38% in half-life *859*

Prothrombin Time *Plasma Increase Physiological* In patients receiving oral anticoagulants together with cisapride coagulation times reported to be prolonged *2903*

Ranitidine *Serum No Effect Physiological* In patients receiving ranitidine together with cisapride no effect reported on gastrointestinal absorption of ranitidine *2903*

Cisplatin

Adenosine Deaminase Binding Protein
Urine Increase Physiological Fivefold increase 12 children given drug 100 mg/m^2 for 6 h. Changes observed before alteration in serum creatinine *2255*

Alanine Aminopeptidase *Urine Increase Physiological* In 8 women with malignant diseases treatment caused significant increase from mean baseline of 15.1 µmol/s/mol creatinine to 57.6 µmol/s/mol creatinine after 3 days and 35.4 µmol/s/mol creatinine after 5 days *6237* Fivefold increase 12 children given drug 100 mg/m^2 for 6 h. Changes observed before alteration in serum creatinine *2255*

Alanine Aminotransferase *Serum Increase Physiological* Slight and transient increases in 45 patients receiving drug *6235*

Albumin *Urine Increase Physiological* In 8 women with cancer treatment caused significant increase from mean baseline of 0.63 mg/mol creatinine to 3.30 mg/mol creatinine after 3 days and 6.43 mg/mol creatinine after 5 days *6237* In 5 men aged 30 -39 y with testicular cancer treatment with cisplatin with doses up to 100 mg/d/sq m for up to 15 days caused significant increase to 90.5 ± 34.19 mg/g during treatment from mean baseline of 5.21 ± 2.18 mg/g with subsequent change to 9.81 ± 3.26 mg/g 2 weeks after treatment completed *5927*

Amino Acids *Urine Increase Physiological* Significant effect with each cycle of treatment in 30 patients with germ-cell tumors: all neutral amino acids except phenylalanine and tyrosine affected but lysine only basic and glutamic acid only acidic amino acid affected in all 3 treatment cycles *1249*

Amylase *Serum Increase Physiological* 10 cycles in 4 patients associated with increased activity: increase mild and transient up to 2 times normal limit *6235*

Antidiuretic Hormone *Plasma Increase Physiological* Significant increase in 30 patients with germ-cell tumors with first cycle of treatment but did not change with subsequent cycles of treatment *1249*

Aspartate Aminotransferase *Serum Increase Physiological* Slight and transient increases in 45 patients receiving drug *6235*

CA549 *Serum No Effect Analytical* No statistically significant effect observed over a concentration range of 4.4 to 66.7 mg/L with BRESMARQ assay *958* No interference observed at concentrations from 4.4 - 66.7 mg/L with immunoradiometric BRESMARQ procedure *958*

Calcium *Serum Decrease Physiological* Marked effect in 15 patients treated with drug *6689* In 3rd and 4th week of treatment of one girl with malignant ovarian germ cell tumor probably related to renal tubular dysfunction *3385* One patient with head and neck cancer after second course of treatment developed marked hyponatremia, hypophosphatemia, hypokalemia and hypocalcemia and increased urinary sodium excretion *1686* Calcium regulation impaired by magnesium deficit *591* Observed in 5.8% of 17 patients receiving drug, associated with low serum magnesium increased urine excretion and decreased intestinal absorption of Mg *5821*
Serum No Effect Physiological No effect noted in 11 children treated for 0.1 to 3.8 y *5492* Concentration remained within normal range in 17 patients with germ cell tumors of the testis following single course of chemotherapy with bleomycin, etoposide and cisplatin *2423*

Carbamazepine *Serum Decrease Physiological* Significant reduction in one patient when two drugs co-administered together with adriamycin *4239* Drugs that induce CYP 3A4 enhance metabolism of carbamazepine producing clinically meaningful effect *1039*

Coombs' Test, Direct *Blood Positive Physiological* Observed in 2 individuals receiving drug *2096*

Copper *Serum No Effect Physiological* Insignificant change in 15 patients treated with drug *6689*
Urine Increase Physiological Marked effect in 15 patients treated with drug *6689*

Creatinine *Serum Increase Physiological* In 8 women with various forms of cancer daily treatments caused significant increases from mean baseline of 68 µmol/L to 83 µmol/L after 3 days and 88 µmol/L after 5 days *6237* Nephrotoxicity evidenced by increase in 12 children receiving chemotherapy *2255* Significant increases concentration: typically observed when used in patients with hypertension, diabetes, a single functioning kidney or abdominal irradiation but not significant change typically seen with cardiac insufficiency or pelvic tumors *1308* In 5% of 96 cancer patients given drug for 5 d repeated at 4-6 week intervals *5200* Observed in one patient, but major side effect renal toxicity *1963*
Serum No Effect Physiological No significant change in 17 patients with germ cell tumors of the testis following single course of bleomycin, etoposide and cisplatin chemotherapy *2423*

Creatinine Clearance *Urine Decrease Physiological* Observed in one patient, but major side effect renal toxicity *1963*

EDTA Clearance *Urine Decrease Physiological* From 108 to 90 mL/min/1.73 m^2; irreversible *5711*

Endothelin *Urine Increase Physiological* Urinary excretion in individuals with cisplatin nephrotoxicity reported to be significantly higher than in healthy individuals *6*

Endothelin-1 *Urine Increase Physiological* In 8 patients with testicular cancer administration of 75 mg/sq m/d together with 100 mg/sq m/d for 5 days caused significant increase in excretion to 130.2 ± 48.8 pg/mg creatinine during treatment from mean baseline of 48.3 ± 29.8 pg/mg creatinine with decline from peak to 121.0 ± 50.8 pg/mg one week after treatment *5926* In 5 men aged 30 -39 y with testicular cancer treatment with cisplatin with doses up to 100 mg/d/sq m for up to 15 days caused significant increase to 134.4 ± 50.2 pg/mg during treatment from mean baseline of 51.5 ± 33.2 pg/mg with subsequent change to 94.8 ± 32.3 pg/mg 2 weeks after treatment completed *5927*

Erythropoietin *Serum Decrease Physiological* In 25 patients with head or neck cancer cisplatin chemotherapy was associated with inappropriately low serum concentrations of erythropoietin *5616*
Serum No Effect Physiological In 25 patients with cancer undergoing cisplatin-based chemotherapy 21 had concentrations appropriate for their degree of anemia *5616*

Etoposide *Serum No Effect Physiological* Cisplatin administration has no effect on etoposide binding to plasma proteins *2270*

β-Galactosidase *Urine Increase Physiological* In 8 women with malignant disease treatment caused significant increase from mean baseline of 5.96 µmol/s/mol creatnine to 14.6 µmol/s/mol creatinine after 3 days and 11.8 µmol/s/mol creatinine after 5 days *6237*

Glomerular Filtration Rate *Urine Decrease Physiological* Significant reduction observed with initiation of intravenous treatment in 30 patients with germ-cell tumors *1249* Decrease from mean of 132 mL/min to 103 mL/min in 17 patients with germ cell tumors of the testis 8 to 60 months following treatment with bleomycin, etoposide and cisplatin *2423*

γ-Glutamyltransferase *Serum Increase Physiological* Slight and transient increases in 45 patients receiving drug *6235*

Hemoglobin *Blood Decrease Physiological* In 23% of 74 evaluable cancer patients given drug for 5 d repeated at 4-6 weeks intervals *5200* By more than 2 g/dL in 2 of 20 patients *2296* Observed in 2 individuals receiving drug *2096*

5-Hydroxyindoleacetic Acid *Urine Increase Physiological* Mean excretion increased from 49 µg/h to 1242 µg/h in 4 to 6 hours post-infusion in 28 patients with cancer *1187*

Ionized Calcium *Serum No Effect Physiological* No effect noted in 11 children treated for 0.1 to 3.8 y *5492*

Iron *Serum Increase Physiological* Mean increase from 67 to 128 µmol/L observed in 14 of 20 patients. Normalized few months after therapy *2296* Both towards beginning and during treatment marked increase in concentration observed *5273* Increase noted in 9 children with malignancies (mean increase from 76 µg/dL to 162 µg/dL) with first treatment course *4232*

Iron-Binding Capacity, Unsaturated
Serum Decrease Physiological Decrease with first course of treatment in 9 children with malignancies from mean of 182 µg/dL to 86 µg/dL *3184*

Leukocytes *Blood Decrease Physiological* Leukopenia is most frequent dose limiting adverse effect. White cell nadirs occur between 8 and 14 days and recovery usually occurs by days 16-21 *1384*

Cisplatin *(continued)*

Magnesium *Red Blood Cells No Effect Physiological* In 11 children given drug for 0.1-3.8 y although serum concentration reduced *5492*

Serum Decrease Physiological Typical response largely avoided by prophylactic magnesium *3708* In 76% of 50 patients receiving low dose cisplatin in combination with 4 other drugs every 4 weeks. Lower incidence when chemotherapy less frequently *795* Marked effect in 15 patients treated with drug *6689* Incidence and severity dose-dependent in patients receiving multiple drugs: extent of effect may be related to interaction with another drug *795* Significant reduction with increased urinary clearance in all 3 treatment cycles in 30 patients with germ-cell tumors *1249* In 13 patients with ovarian cancer previously treated with cisplatin 69% were found to be hypomagnesemic with a mean interval of 19 months since previous treatment *3798* In 3rd and 4th week of treatment of one girl with malignant ovarian germ cell tumor probably related to renal tubular dysfunction *3385* In 41 of 69 gynecologic oncology patients *259* Two cases of renal loss described, with observation that hypokalemia could not be corrected until magnesium had been replaced *5050* Observed in 5 of 6 patients who developed orthostatic hypotension when treated with drug for several months *2797* As result of renal tubular defect induced by drug may be severe enough to cause tetany and grand mal fits *3708* In 22 of 29 of patients with tumors of testis *5343* Cisplatin causes decreased renal absorption of magnesium *5882* In 4 % of 140 cycles in 96 cancer patients given drug for 5 d repeated at 4-6 weeks intervals *5200*

Serum No Effect Physiological Concentration remained within normal range in 17 patients with germ cell tumors of the testis following treatment with a course of bleomycin, etoposide and cisplatin *2423*

Urine Increase Physiological Urine wasting common manifestation *591* Renal loss of magnesium responsible for low serum concentration *5821* Marked effect in 15 patients treated with drug *6689*

Urine No Effect Physiological In 11 children given drug for 0.1-3.8 y although serum concentration reduced *5492*

Methotrexate *Serum Increase Physiological* Administration with methotrexate been demonstrated to increase its elimination half-life and an increase in its AUC *3909*

β_2-Microglobulin *Serum No Effect Physiological* Concentration remained within normal range in 17 patients with germ cell tumors of the testis following single course of chemotherapy with bleomycin, etoposide and cisplatin *2423*

Urine Increase Physiological In 5 men aged 30 -39 y with testicular cancer treatment with cisplatin with doses up to 100 mg/d/sq m for up to 15 days caused significant increase to 6.21 ± 3.28 mg/g during treatment from mean baseline of 0.4 ± 0.14 mg/g with subsequent change to 0.50 ± 0.19 mg/g 2 weeks after treatment completed *5927* In 16 patients with malignant disease treatment for 35 cycles with 100 mg/sq m cisplatin caused significant increase from mean baseline of 0.1 ± 0.05 µg/mg creatinine to 1.7 ± 1.6 µg/mg creatinine *609* Significant increase with each cycle of treatment in 30 patients with germ-cell tumors *1249* Transient 2 to 5-fold increase during treatment *5711* In 8 patients with testicular cancer administration of 75 mg/sq m/d together with 100 mg/sq m/d for 5 days caused significant increase in excretion to 6.56 ± 3.23 mg/g creatinine during treatment from mean baseline of 0.5 ± 0.16 mg/g creatinine with decline from peak to 0.92 ± 0.41 mg/g one week after treatment *5926*

N-Acetyl-Glucosaminidase *Urine Increase Physiological* In 8 patients with testicular cancer administration of 75 mg/sq m/d together with 100 mg/sq m/d for 5 days caused significant increase in excretion to 43.52 ± 12.18 U/g creatinine during treatment from mean baseline of 3.21 ± 1.26 U/g creatinine with decline from peak to 20.48 ± 7.01 U/g one week after treatment *5926* In 16 patients with malignant disease treatment for 35 cycles with 100 mg/sq m cisplatin caused significant increase from mean baseline of 1.1 ± 0.2 mU/mg creatinine to 5.0 ± 1.5 mU/mg creatinine *609* Commonly observed increased excretion as a result of nephrotoxicity *2254* In 5 men aged 30 -39 y with testicular cancer treatment with cisplatin with doses up to 100 mg/d/sq m for up to 15 days caused significant increase to 39.28 ± 11.56 U/g during treatment from mean baseline of 2.90 ± 1.28 U/g with subsequent change to 5.41 ± 3.34 U/g 2 weeks after treatment completed *5927* In 8 women with cancer treatment caused significant increase from mean baseline of 13.4 µmol/s/mol creatinine to 38.5 µmol/s/mol creatinine after 3 days and 35.7 µmol/s/mol creatinine after 5 days *6237* Significant effect observed in 30 patients with germ-cell tumors with each cycle of treatment *1249* Fivefold increase in 12 children given drug 100 mg/m^2 for 6 h. Changes observed before alteration in serum creatinine *2255*

Urine No Effect Analytical At 1 mg/L had no effect on 2 colorimetric analytical methods *2254*

Ondansetron *Serum No Effect Physiological* Coadministration with ondansetron had no effect on its pharmacokinetics *2181*

Phenytoin *Serum Decrease Physiological* Reduction to 37% of original concentration in one patient when two drugs co-administered together with adriamycin *4239* Possible reduction of plasma concentration when drugs are coadministered *1384*

Phosphate *Serum Decrease Physiological* One patient with head and neck cancer after second course of treatment developed marked hyponatremia, hypophosphatemia, hypokalemia and hypocalcemia and increased urinary sodium excretion *1686*

Serum No Effect Physiological No effect noted in 11 children treated for 0.1 to 3.8 y *5492*

Platinum *Serum Increase Physiological* Marked effect in 15 patients treated with drug *6689*

Urine Increase Physiological Marked effect in 15 patients treated with drug *6689*

Potassium *Serum Decrease Physiological* One patient with head and neck cancer after second course of treatment developed marked hyponatremia, hypophosphatemia, hypokalemia and hypocalcemia and increased urinary sodium excretion *1686* Significant reduction in all 3 treatment cycles in 30 patients with germ-cell tumors but without significantly increased urinary clearance *1249* Associated with magnesium deficiency *591* Marked effect in 15 patients treated with drug *6689* Two cases of hypokalemia with hypomagnesemia described due to renal loss with observation that hypokalemia could not be corrected until magnesium replaced *5050*

Protein *Urine Increase Physiological* Significant increase with each cycle of treatment in 30 patients with germ-cell tumors *1249* In 8 women with various forms of cancer treatment caused significant increase fro mean baseline of 7.26 mg/mol creatinine to 16.1 mg/mol creatinine after 3 days and 18.6 mg/mol creatinine after 5 days *6237*

Retinol-binding Protein *Urine Increase Physiological* In 8 women with cancer treatment caused significant increase from mean baseline of 12.3 µg/mol creatinine to 72.9 µg/mol creatinine after 3 days and 39.1 µg/mol creatinine after 5 days *6237*

Sodium *Serum Decrease Physiological* One patient with head and neck cancer after second course of treatment developed marked hyponatremia, hypophosphatemia, hypokalemia and hypocalcemia and increased urinary sodium excretion *1686* In 3rd and 4th week of treatment of one girl with malignant ovarian germ cell tumor probably related to renal tubular dysfunction *3385*

Urine Increase Physiological Excretion increased in all of 6 patients who developed orthostatic hypotension following several months treatment with drug *2797* One patient with head and neck cancer after second course of treatment developed marked hyponatremia, hypophosphatemia, hypokalemia and hypocalcemia and increased urinary sodium excretion *1686* In single case in 3rd and 4th treatment course, identified with renal tubular dysfunction *3385*

Thromboxane B_2 *Urine Increase Physiological* In 16 patients with malignant disease treatment for 35 cycles with 100 mg/sq m cisplatin caused significant increase from mean baseline of 45.5 ± 4.9 ng/h to 142.7 ± 62.0 ng/h (3.1-fold increase) *609*

Urea Nitrogen *Serum Increase Physiological* In 11 of 18 cases with doses of less than 50 mg/m^2 surface area: extent of change equivalent to 50% reduction in renal function *591* Observed in one patient, but major side effect renal toxicity *1963*

Uric Acid *Serum Increase Physiological* Probable consequence of drug-induced nephrotoxicity *4218*

Valproic Acid *Serum Decrease Physiological* Significant reduction in concentration when two drugs co-administered together with adriamycin *4239*

Zinc *Serum No Effect Physiological* Insignificant change in 15 patients treated with drug *6689*

Urine Increase Physiological Marked effect in 15 patients treated with drug *6689*

Citalopram

Albumin *Urine No Effect Analytical* Using a fluorimetric assay with Albumin Blue 580 on a Cobas Fara centrifugal analyzer for the detection of microalbuminuria no significant interference was detected at a concentration of 4 mg/L *3117*

Cortisol *Plasma Increase Physiological* In 8 healthy men infusion of 20 mg citalopram over 30 minutes caused a significant increase from mean baseline of about 100 ng/mL to a peak of 156.9 ± 62.3 ng/mL at about 60 minutes after the start of the infusion *5435*

Growth Hormone *Plasma Increase Physiological* In 8 healthy men infusion of 20 mg citalopram over 30 minutes caused an increase from mean baseline of about 1.41 ± 1.68 ng/mL but significantly less than 6.63 ± 5.41 ng/mL in patients who received an infusion of saline *5435*

Imipramine *Serum No Effect Physiological* In healthy volunteers coadministration of citalopram caused a significant (about 50%) increase in the area under the desipramine curve and a corresponding decrease in the concentration of 2-hydroxydesipramine. Desipramine elimination half-life was significantly increased. Nevertheless niether the imipramine area under the curve nor half-life were affected by citalopram administration *2288*

Levomepromazine *Serum No Effect Physiological* In healthy volunteers no significant effect observed on levomepromazine kinetics *2288*

Lithium *Serum No Effect Physiological* Coadministration of citalopram with lithium had no significant effect on lithium kinetics *2288*

Prolactin *Plasma Increase Physiological* In 8 healthy men infusion of 20 mg citalopram over 30 minutes caused a significant increase from mean baseline of 8.81 ± 3.53 ng/mL to a peak of 17.80 ± 4.65 ng/mL at 80 minutes after the start of the infusion *5435*

Citalopramin

Cortisol, Free *Urine No Effect Analytical* No significant interference observed with HPLC method of Turpeinen et al *6105*

Citruplexina

Urea Nitrogen *Serum Increase Analytical* Absorbance relative to urea = 1.5 with diacetyl procedure *882*

CL 277082

Apolipoprotein A-I *Serum No Effect Physiological* No significant effect in 8 healthy men treated with 750 mg daily for 20 days (127 mg/dL with placebo, 129 mg/dL with treatment) *2480*

Apolipoprotein B *Serum No Effect Physiological* No significant change in 8 healthy men treated with 750 mg daily for 20 days (68 mg/dL with placebo, 71 mg/dL with treatment) *2480*

Cholesterol *Serum No Effect Physiological* No significant change observed in 8 healthy men given 750 mg daily for 20 days (placebo 169 mg/dL; treatment 175 mg/dL) *2480*

HDL-Cholesterol *Serum No Effect Physiological* No significant change in 8 healthy men given 750 mg daily for 20 days (47 mg/dL with placebo, 44 mg/dL with treatment) *2480*

LDL-Cholesterol *Serum No Effect Physiological* No significant change in 8 healthy men given 750 mg/day for 20 days (placebo 112 mg/dL; treatment 117 mg/dL) *2480*

Triglycerides *Serum No Effect Physiological* No significant change in 8 healthy men treated with 750 mg daily for 20 days (68 mg/dL with placebo, 82 mg/dL with treatment) *2480*

VLDL-Cholesterol *Serum No Effect Physiological* No significant change in 8 healthy men given 750 mg/day for 20 days (placebo 10 mg/dL; treatment 14 mg/dL) *2480*

Cladribine

Alanine Aminotransferase *Serum Increase Physiological* Reversible, generally mild, increases observed *4441*

Aspartate Aminotransferase *Serum Increase Physiological* Reversible, generally mild, increases observed *4441*

Bilirubin *Serum Increase Physiological* Reversible, generally mild, increases observed *4441*

CD4+ Lymphocytes *Blood Decrease Physiological* Treatment with cladribine is associated with prolonged depression of CD4 counts. Mean nadir, occurring 4 to 6 months after treatment was 272 /μL compared with 766 /μL prior to treatment *4441*

CD8+ Lymphocytes *Blood Decrease Physiological* Treatment with cladribine is associated with prolonged depression of CD8 counts. Mean nadir, occurred 4 to 6 months after treatment but increasing counts were observed after 9 months *4441*

Hematocrit *Blood Decrease Physiological* Severe bone marrow suppression, including neutropenia, anemia and thrombocytopenia has been commonly observed, especially at high doses *4441*

Hemoglobin *Blood Decrease Physiological* Severe bone marrow suppression, including neutropenia, anemia and thrombocytopenia has been commonly observed, especially at high doses *4441*

Neutrophils *Blood Decrease Physiological* Severe bone marrow suppression, including neutropenia, anemia and thrombocytopenia has been commonly observed, especially at high doses *4441*

Platelets *Blood Decrease Physiological* Severe bone marrow suppression, including neutropenia, anemia and thrombocytopenia has been commonly observed, especially at high doses *4441*

Clarithromycin

Alanine Aminotransferase *Serum Increase Physiological* Administration of clarithromycin has been associated with increased activity above 5-times upper limit of normal in 3% of all patients receiving drug compared with 2% in placebo-treated controls *11*

Serum No Effect Physiological Administration of clarithromycin has been associated with increased activity in fewer than 1% of all patients receiving drug *11*

Alkaline Phosphatase *Serum No Effect Physiological* Administration of clarithromycin has been associated with increased activity in fewer than 1% of all patients receiving drug *11*

Aspartate Aminotransferase *Serum Increase Physiological* Administration of clarithromycin has been associated with increased activity above 5-times upper limit of normal in 4% of all patients receiving drug compared with 2% in placebo-treated controls *11*

Serum No Effect Physiological Administration of clarithromycin has been associated with increased activity in fewer than 1% of all patients receiving drug *11*

Astemizole *Serum Increase Physiological* Significantly decreased metabolism resulting in cardiac toxicity or arrhythmias, especially torsade des pointes *886*

Bilirubin *Serum No Effect Physiological* Administration of clarithromycin has been associated with increased concentration in fewer than 1% of all patients receiving drug *11*

Carbamazepine *Serum Increase Physiological* Significantly decreased metabolism and increased plasma concentration *886* Drugs that inhibit CYP 3A4 inhibit metabolism of carbamazepine producing clinically meaningful effect *1039* Coadministration of clarithromycin with carbamazepine has caused a significant increase in the carbamazepine concentration *11*

Clarithromycin *(continued)*

Cisapride *Serum Increase Physiological* By inhibiting cytochrome P450 3A4 inhibits metabolism of cisapride and increases its plasma concentration *2903*

Creatinine *Serum Increase Physiological* Administration of clarithromycin has been associated with increased concentration in less than 1% of all patients receiving drug *11*

Cyclosporine *Blood Increase Physiological* Coadministration of clarithromycin with cyclosporine reported to cause a 60-200% increase in cyclosporine concentration probably due to competitive inhibition of cyclosporine metabolism *859*
Serum Increase Physiological May increase cyclosporine concentration by inhibiting hepatic cytochrome P-450 III A which metabolizes cyclosporine *5236* Coadministration of clarithromycin with cyclosporine reported to cause a 60-200% increase in cyclosporine concentration probably due to competitive inhibition of cyclosporine metabolism *859*

Digoxin *Serum Increase Physiological* Coadministration with digoxin may increase the digoxin concentration *2161*

γ-Glutamyltransferase *Serum No Effect Physiological* Administration of clarithromycin has been associated with increased activity in fewer than 1% of all patients receiving drug *11*

Hemoglobin *Blood No Effect Physiological* Administration of clarithromycin has been associated with a reduction of concentration below 8 g/dL in 3% treated patients compared with 5% in placebo treated group *11*

Indinavir *Serum Increase Physiological* Causes a 29% increase in area under the concentration curve when clarithromycin coadministered *1891* Administration of indinavir 800 mg every 8 hours with clarithromycin 500 mg every 12 hours for 1 week resulted in a 29 ± 42% increase in indinavir AUC and a 53 ± 36% increase in clarithromycin AUC *3966*

Lactate Dehydrogenase *Serum No Effect Physiological* Administration of clarithromycin has been associated with increased activity in fewer than 1% of all patients receiving drug *11*

Leukocytes *Blood Decrease Physiological* Administration of clarithromycin has been associated with a reduction of concentration below 1000/µL in 4% treated patients compared with 5% in placebo treated group *11*
Blood No Effect Physiological Administration of clarithromycin has been associated with decreased concentration in fewer than 1% of all patients receiving drug *11*

Platelets *Blood No Effect Physiological* Administration of clarithromycin has been associated with a reduction of concentration below 50,000/µL in 4% treated patients compared with 5% in placebo treated group *11*

Prothrombin Time *Plasma Increase Physiological* Increased INR observed in patients receiving warfarin *886*
Plasma No Effect Physiological Administration of clarithromycin has been associated with prolonged time in 1% of all patients receiving drug *11*

Rifabutin *Serum Increase Physiological* Decreased metabolism and increased risk of uveitis *886*

Ritonavir *Serum Increase Physiological* Increases area under the concentration curve by 12% when clarithromycin coadministered *1891*

Tacrolimus *Serum Increase Physiological* By inhibiting cytochrome P-450 IIIA enzyme systems may inhibit the metabolism of tacrolimus *1987*

Terfenadine *Serum Increase Physiological* Significantly decreased metabolism resulting in cardiac toxicity or arrhythmias, especially torsade des pointes *886* Decreases the clearance of terfenadine but effect on plasma concentration uncertain *2653* Coadministration of clarithromycin with terfenadine has caused a significant threefold increase in the active acid terfenadine metabolites concentration *11*

Theophylline *Serum Increase Physiological* Coadministration of clarithromycin with theophylline has caused a significant (20%) increase in the theophylline concentration and AUC *11* Decreased metabolism *886* Metabolite decreases theophylline clearance by inhibiting cytochrome P450 3A3, increasing theophylline concentration by about 25% *5999* Up to 35% increase in serum theophylline concentration due to decreased theophylline clearance caused by inhibition of cytochrome P450 3A3 by an erythromycin metabolite *6117* Decreases theophylline clearance by inhibiting cytochrome P450 1A2 and increases serum theophylline concentration by 25% *3125*

Urea Nitrogen *Serum Increase Physiological* Administration of clarithromycin has been associated with increased concentration in 4% of all patients receiving drug *11*

Clavulinic Acid

Amino Acids *Urine No Effect Analytical* No reaction observed with ninhydrin in paper chromatography, paper electrophoresis and ion-exchange chromatography *4761*

Sugar *Urine Increase Analytical* Reacts positively with Clinitest *4761*

Clazolam

LE Cells *Blood Positive Physiological* SLE may occur, usually normalized when stopped *5102*

Clemastine

Granulocytes *Blood Decrease Physiological* Agranulocytosis may occur as a complication *5243*

Hematocrit *Blood Decrease Physiological* Hemolytic anemia may occur as a complication *5243*

Hemoglobin *Blood Decrease Physiological* Hemolytic anemia may occur as a complication *5243*

Mycophenolic Acid *Serum No Effect Analytical* No significant interference observed with HPLC method of Shipkova et al *5526*

Mycophenolic Acid Glucuronide
Serum No Effect Analytical No significant interference observed with HPLC method of Shipkova et al *5526*

Platelets *Blood Decrease Physiological* Thrombocytopenia may occur as a complication *5243*

Theophylline *Serum No Effect Analytical* No effect on Kodak Ektachem® 700 slide method *1716*

Clindamycin

Acetate *Feces Increase Physiological* Marked proportional increase in 6 healthy individuals fed orally for 6 d *2734*

Alanine Aminotransferase *Serum Increase Physiological* Jaundice and other abnormal liver function tests have been observed during clindamycin therapy *4668* Mild transient rises seen *4689* Uncommon side effect *6498*

Alkaline Phosphatase *Serum Increase Physiological* Transient abnormality noted *4668* Uncommon side effect *6498*

Amikacin *Serum No Effect Analytical* No interference observed at a concentration of 500 µg/mL (1177 µmol/L) with method on Du Pont aca *1508*

Aspartate Aminotransferase *Serum Increase Physiological* Uncommon side effect *6498* Transient abnormality noted *4668*

Bilirubin *Serum Increase Physiological* Jaundice and other abnormal liver function tests have been observed during clindamycin therapy *4668* Occurs especially if pre-existing liver disease *4689* Uncommon side effect *6498*

BSP Retention *Serum Increase Physiological* Probable hepatotoxic effect *1809*

Chloramphenicol *Serum No Effect Analytical* No effect at 100 mg/L on coupled enzymatic method *4122*

Colistin *Serum Increase Analytical* Interferes with bioassays *3858*
Serum Positive Analytical Interferes with bioassays *3858*

Color *Feces Increase Analytical* Black color reported with clindamycin ingestion *3388*

Creatine Kinase *Serum Increase Physiological* Probably due to muscle damage (common with i.m.) *1311*

Creatinine *Serum Increase Physiological* Possible associated azotemia has been observed during clindamycin therapy *4668*

Serum No Effect Analytical No effect of concentrations up to 15 mg/L on single slide method on Kodak Ektachem® *5706*

Eosinophils *Blood Increase Physiological* Transient eosinophilia has been observed during clindamycin therapy *4668* Common hypersensitivity reaction *6498* Occasional allergic response *4689*

Erythromycin *Serum Increase Analytical* Interferes with bioassays *3858*

Gentamicin *Serum No Effect Analytical* No interference observed at concentrations up to 500 µg/mL (1183 µmol/L) with method on Du Pont aca *1526*

Granulocytes *Blood Decrease Physiological* Reports of agranulocytosis during clindamycin therapy have been made *4668*

Isocitrate Dehydrogenase *Serum Increase Physiological* Mild transient increase *1809*

Ketone Body Ratio *Serum No Effect Analytical* When added at a concentration of 1 g/L had no significant effect on AKBR method of Uno et al *6131*

Lactate Dehydrogenase *Serum Increase Physiological* ?hepatic or muscle origin (transient) *1809*

Leukocytes *Blood Decrease Physiological* May cause agranulocytosis *4691* Transient leukopenia and neutropenia have been observed during clindamycin therapy *4668*

Metronidazole *Serum Increase Analytical* Interferes with bioassays *3858*

Neutrophils *Blood Decrease Physiological* Transient leukopenia and neutropenia have been observed during clindamycin therapy *4668* Transient neutropenia may occur *2753*

Blood Increase Physiological Uncommon side effect *6498*

Occult Blood *Feces Increase Physiological* Occasionally bloody mucus, especially in elderly *2753* Reported frequency of 1 case of pseudomembranous colitis in 10 treated cases associated with mucus or bloody diarrhea *689*

Ornithine Carbamoyltransferase
Serum Increase Physiological Mild increase noted (transient) *1809*

Phenylalanine *Plasma No Effect Analytical* No interference observed with rapid quantitative whole blood method of Campbell et al using phenylalanine dehydrogenase *867*

Platelets *Blood Decrease Physiological* Reports of thrombocytopenia during clindamycin therapy have been made *4668* Some cases reported *187*

Blood Increase Physiological Uncommon side effect *6498*

Polymyxin *Serum Increase Analytical* Interferes with bioassays *3858*

Potassium *Serum No Effect Analytical* At concentration of 150 mg/L had no effect on measurement by ISE with predilution *5704*

Protein *Urine Increase Physiological* Possible associated proteinuria has been observed during clindamycin therapy *4668*

Short-Chain Fatty Acids *Feces Decrease Physiological* Marked effect in 6 healthy individuals fed orally for 6 d *2734*

Sodium *Serum No Effect Analytical* At concentration of 150 mg/L had no effect on measurement by ISE with predilution *5704*

Tetracycline *Serum Increase Analytical* Interferes with bioassays *3858*

Theophylline *Serum Increase Analytical* At clindamycin concentration of 20 mg/L produced false positive bias of 3.30 mg/L at theophylline concentration of 20 mg/L with method on Syntex AccµLevel *1122*

Serum No Effect Analytical No effect at concentration of 20 mg/L on methods on Kodak DT-60, Abbott TDx, Abbott Vision with either whole blood or serum, 3M Diagnostics TheoFAST and Ames Seralyzer *1122*

Tobramycin *Serum No Effect Analytical* At concentrations less than 1000 µg/mL (2.35 mmol/L) no significant effect observed on method on Du Pont aca *1547*

Trimethoprim *Serum Increase Analytical* Interferes with bioassays *3858*

Urea Nitrogen *Serum Increase Physiological* Possible associated azotemia has been observed during clindamycin therapy *4668*

Clinofibrate

Cholesterol *Serum No Effect Physiological* No significant effect in 10 patients with diabetes mellitus treated with 600 mg/kg for 4 weeks *4389*

HDL_2-Cholesterol *Serum Increase Physiological* Significant effect in insulin-dependent diabetics treated with 600 mg/kg for 4 weeks *4389*

HDL_3-Cholesterol *Serum No Effect Physiological* No significant effect in 10 patients with diabetes mellitus treated with 600 mg/kg for 4 weeks *4389*

HDL-Cholesterol *Serum Increase Physiological* Significant effect in 10 patients with diabetes mellitus, both insulin-dependent and noninsulin-dependent, treated with 600 mg/kg for 4 weeks *4389*

Lecithin:Cholesterol Acyltransferase
Serum Increase Physiological Significant effect in 10 patients with diabetes mellitus treated with 600 mg/kg for 4 weeks *4389*

Triglycerides *Serum No Effect Physiological* No significant effect in 10 patients with diabetes mellitus treated with 600 mg/kg for 4 weeks *4389*

Clobazam

Albumin *Urine No Effect Analytical* Using a fluorimetric assay with Albumin Blue 580 on a Cobas Fara centrifugal analyzer for the detection of microalbuminuria no significant interference was detected at a concentration of 4 mg/L *3117*

Benzodiazepine *Urine Positive Analytical* At concentrations of 0.3 µg/mL or greater produces positive result with Syva EMIT II assay *1785*

Carbamazepine *Serum No Effect Physiological* No apparent effect of coadministration of clobazam on total carbamazepine concentration in epileptic patients *4173*

Carbamazepine-10,11-Epoxide
Serum Increase Physiological Although total carbamazepine concentration not apparently affected by coadministration of drugs in epileptics increased concentrations of epoxide metabolites observed *4173*

Clodronate

Albumin *Serum No Effect Physiological* In 8 patients with various malignant diseases treatment with clodronate 1500 mg intravenously for 4 h caused nonsignificant change from mean baseline of 43.7 ± 0.8 g/L to 42.8 ± 1.4 g/L when measured after 24 h and 42.6 ± 1.2 g/L at 48 h *5294*

Alkaline Phosphatase *Serum Decrease Physiological* In 20 patients with increased bone resorption mean activity decreased from 387 ± 40 U/L to 262 ± 25 U/L after 1 week's treatment with intravenous infusions of 300 mg/d *1933*

Calcium *Serum Decrease Physiological* In patients with hypercalcemia of malignancy doses of up to 6 mg/kg given intravenously daily for 3-5 days caused normalization of concentration *562* In 10 normocalcemic patients with multiple osteolytic bone metastases 300 mg/d intravenous sodium clodronate for 20 days caused significant decrease in serum calcium after 10 and 20 days *1324* In 20 patients with increased bone resorption significant decrease in mean concentration observed from 10.6 ± 0.1 mg/dL to 9.1 ± 0.1 mg/dL following infusion of 300 mg over 1 hour for 7 days *1933*

Urine Decrease Physiological In 10 normocalcemic patients with multiple osteolytic bone metastases intravenous infusion of 300 mg/d for 20 days of sodium clodronate caused significant reduction in excretion after 10 and 20 days *1324*

Calcium, Albumin-corrected *Serum No Effect Physiological* In 8 patients with various malignant diseases treatment with clodronate 1500 mg intravenously for 4 h caused nonsignificant change from mean baseline of 2.31 ± 0.03 mmol/L to 2.22 ± 0.05 mmol/L when measured after 48 h *5294*

Clodronate *(continued)*

1,25-Dihydroxy Vitamin D *Serum Increase Physiological* In 20 women with normocalcemic women with breast cancer and bone metastases 12 were treated with 300 mg intravenously over 5 days and later 1600 mg orally for 6 months mean concentration increased from 67 ± 21 pmol/L to 91 ± 46 pmol/L after 2 months, 96 ± 46 pmol/L after 4 months but had reverted to 67 ± 33 pmol/L after 6 months *3820*

β-Endorphin *Plasma No Effect Physiological* In 20 patients with increased bone resorption daily intravenous infusion of 300 mg over 1 hour for 7 days had no effect on concentration 2 hours after infusions *1933*

Histamine *Plasma No Effect Analytical* Improbable inhibition of radio-enzyme assay at therapeutic concentrations *2492*

25-Hydroxy Vitamin D *Serum Decrease Physiological* In 20 women with normocalcemic women with breast cancer and bone metastases 12 were treated with 300 mg intravenously over 5 days and later 1600 mg orally for 6 months mean concentration decreased from 46 ± 19 nmol/L to 38 ± 24 nmol/L after 2 months, 24 ± 14 nmol/L after 4 months and 22 ± 19 nmol/L after 6 months *3820*

Hydroxyproline *Urine Decrease Physiological* In 20 patients with increased bone resorption mean excretion decreased from 32.9 ± 1.8 mg/24 h/sq m to 18.9 ± 1.4 mg/24 h/sq m after daily hourly intravenous infusions of 300 mg for 7 days *1933* In 10 normocalcemic patients with multiple osteolytic bone mestastes treatment with 300 mg/d intravenously for 20 days caused significant reduction in excretion after 10 and 20 days *1324*

Interleukin-6 *Serum No Effect Physiological* In 8 patients with various malignant diseases treatment with clodronate 60 mg intravenously for 4 h caused nonsignificant change from mean baseline of 10 pg/mL to 5 pg/mL when measured after 24 h and 6 pg/mL at 48 h *5294*

ionized Calcium *Serum Decrease Physiological* In 20 women with normocalcemic women with breast cancer and bone metastases 12 were treated with 300 mg intravenously over 5 days and later 1600 mg orally for 6 months mean concentration decreased from 1.25 ± 0.04 mmol/L to 1.22 ± 0.06 mmol/L *3820*

Leukocytes *Blood No Effect Physiological* In 8 patients with various malignant diseases treatment with clodronate 1500 mg intravenously for 4 h caused nonsignificant change from mean baseline of 4,350 ± 475 /μL to 4,540 ± 626 /μL when measured after 24 h and 4,726 ± 696 /μL at 48 h *5294*

Lymphocytes *Blood Increase Physiological* In 8 patients with various malignant diseases treatment with clodronate 1500 mg intravenously for 4 h caused significant change from mean baseline of 923 ± 131 /μL to 1211 ± 196 /μL when measured after 24 h and nonsigificant change to 1033 ± 156 /μL at 48 h *5294*

Monocytes *Blood No Effect Physiological* In 8 patients with various malignant diseases treatment with clodronate 1500 mg intravenously for 4 h caused nonsignificant change from mean baseline of 166 ± 20 /μL to 202 ± 38 /μL when measured after 24 h and 162 ± 29 /μL at 48 h *5294*

Osteocalcin *Serum Increase Physiological* In 10 normocalcemic patients with multiple bone metastases treatment with 300 mg/d intravenously for 20 days caused significant increase after 20 days treatment but not after 10 days *1324*

Parathyroid Hormone *Plasma Increase Physiological* Significant increase in midmolecule hormone observed in 10 normocalcemic patients with multiple bone metastases after first treatment with 300 mg intravenous sodium clodronate and more markedly after 10 days of daily intravenous infusions *1324* In 20 women with normocalcemic women with breast cancer and bone metastases 12 were treated with 300 mg intravenously over 5 days and later 1600 mg orally for 6 months mean concentration increased from 4 ± 2 pmol/L to 5 ± 2 pmol/L *3820*

Platelets *Blood No Effect Physiological* In 8 patients with various malignant diseases treatment with clodronate 1500 mg intravenously for 4 h caused significant change from mean baseline of 219,000 ± 33,000 /μL to 215,000 ± 30,000 /μL when measured after 24 h and nonsigificant change to 218,000 ± 30,000 /μL at 48 h *5294*

Tumor Necrosis Factor-α *Serum No Effect Physiological* In 8 patients with various malignant diseases treatment with clodronate 60 mg intravenously for 4 h caused nonsignificant change from mean baseline of 12 pg/mL to 10 pg/mL when measured after 24 h and 8 pg/mL at 48 h *5294*

Clofazimine

Alanine Aminotransferase *Serum Increase Physiological* Hepatitis may occur as a side effect in less than 1% of treated patients *1030*

Albumin *Serum Increase Physiological* Increased concentration may occur occasionally *1030*

Aspartate Aminotransferase *Serum Increase Physiological* Hepatitis may occur as a side effect in less than 1% of treated patients *1030*

Bilirubin *Serum Increase Physiological* Hepatitis may occur as a side effect in less than 1% of treated patients *1030*

Color *Feces Increase Physiological* May cause discoloration of skin from red to brownish black and also discolor body fluids *1030*

Sputum Increase Physiological May cause discoloration of skin from red to brownish black and also discolor body fluids *1030*

Sweat Increase Physiological May cause discoloration of skin from red to brownish black and also discolor body fluids *1030*

Tears Increase Physiological May cause discoloration of skin from red to brownish black and also discolor body fluids *1030*

Urine Increase Physiological May cause discoloration of skin from red to brownish black and also discolor body fluids *1030*

Eosinophils *Blood Increase Physiological* Eosinophilia may occur occasionally *1030*

Occult Blood *Feces Increase Physiological* Gastrointestinal bleeding may occur in less than 1% patients *1030*

Potassium *Serum Increase Physiological* Hypokalemia may occur occasionally *1030*

Clofibrate

Acid Phosphatase *Serum Increase Physiological* Reported effect (?mechanism) *1714*

Alanine Aminotransferase *Serum Increase Physiological* Single case of granulomatous hepatitis associated with drug administration *4697* Hepatotoxic effect *3810*

Aldosterone *Plasma No Effect Physiological* No significant change in 6 men with hyperlipidemia treated for average of 26 days with 2 g daily *2582*

Alkaline Phosphatase *Serum Decrease Physiological* Continuous reduction from 82 U/L to 52 U/L in 26 type IIa hyperlipoproteinemic patients: same response seen in type IV patients *5307* Reduction of bone isoenzyme when activity increased in patients on chronic hemodialysis *3136* Significant reduction in 27 patients, half of whom had hypertriglyceridemia, after 1 week *1845*

Serum Increase Physiological Hepatotoxic effect *3810* Single case of granulomatous hepatitis associated with drug administration *4697*

Apolipoprotein A-I *Serum Increase Physiological* Increased apo A-I and apo A-II synthesis. Increased activity of lipoprotein lipase by stimulation of muscle lipoprotein lipase synthesis, alteration of the capillary endothelial surface and stimulation of apo C-II synthesis *264* Increase by 10 to 20% in 10 hyperlipidemic patients *4249*

Apolipoprotein A-II *Serum Increase Physiological* Increased synthesis. Increased activity of lipoprotein lipase by stimulation of muscle lipoprotein lipase synthesis, alteration of the capillary endothelial surface, stimulation of apolipoprotein A-II synthesis *264*

Aspartate Aminotransferase *Serum Increase Physiological* Abnormal liver function tests have been reported as adverse events *6550* Transiently elevated during early therapy *512*

Bile *Urine Increase Physiological* Hepatotoxic effect *3810*

Bile Acids *Feces Decrease Physiological* After 2 weeks treatment significant fall *4075*

Bilirubin *Serum Increase Physiological* Single case of granulomatous hepatitis associated with drug administration *4697* Hepatotoxic effect *3810*

Bilirubin, Direct *Serum Increase Physiological* Single case of granulomatous hepatitis associated with drug administration *4697*

Blood *Urine Increase Physiological* Hematuria has been reported as adverse event *6550*

BSP Retention *Serum Increase Physiological* Intrahepatic cholestasis reported *1714*

Carnitine *Serum Increase Physiological* In patients receiving carnitine (2 g/d) with probucol (1 g/d) basal concentrations abnormally high *4254*

Carotenoids *Serum No Effect Physiological* Insignificant change in about 26 subjects given 2 g daily *4794*

Cholesterol *Serum Decrease Physiological* By 40% in first year became normal after this in patients with hyperlipoproteinemia and impaired glucose tolerance given diet plus 2 g drµg/d. 14 patients monitored for 5 y *4874* Marked reduction within 6 weeks in 10 hyperlipidemic patients *4249* Reduction from mean of 253 mg/dL to 201 mg/dL in 6 hyperlipidemic men treated with 2 g daily for average of 26 days *2582* Significant reduction in 27 patients, half of whom had hypertriglyceridemia, after 1 week *1845* Therapeutic goal (probably diminished synthesis) *701* In both normals with hypertriglyceridemia and diabetics *1842* Effect mediated through reduction of VLDL and LDL *878* By 40% in first year but normalized later in 14 patients with primary hyperlipoproteinemia given 2.0 g daily over 5 y *4874* In the Stockholm Ischemic Heart Study of 555 myocardial infarction patients treatment with clofibrate and nicotinic acid caused mean decrease of 13% *3115*
Serum Increase Physiological Paradoxical effect in patients with biliary cirrhosis *4765*
Serum No Effect Analytical At concentration of 1,000 mg/L had no effect on CHOD-PAP method *5704* At concentration of 1400 mg/L had no effect on method using catalase-Hantzsch reaction *5704*

Corticosterone *Plasma Increase Physiological* Increase to mean of 9.4 ng/mL from 3.4 ng/mL in 6 men with hyperlipidemia treated with 2 g daily for average of 26 days *2582*

Cortisol *Plasma No Effect Physiological* No effect of drug after 1 week in healthy individuals with hypertriglyceridemia *1842* No significant effect in 6 men with hyperlipidemia treated with 2 g daily for average of 26 days *2582*

Creatine Kinase *Serum Increase Physiological* Originates from skeletal muscle (in up to 15%) *5869* Increased activity has been reported as adverse event *6550*

Creatinine *Serum Increase Physiological* Possibly derived from muscle damage (in 15%) *3669*
Serum No Effect Analytical At concentration of 400 mg/L had no effect on Jaffe-Fading-Fraction method *5704* At concentration of 500 mg/L had no effect on creatinine iminohydrolase method *5704* At concentration of 400 mg/L had no effect on Jaffe-Fuller's earth method *5704*

Dehydroepiandrosterone *Plasma No Effect Physiological* No significant effect in 6 men with hyperlipidemia treated with 2 g daily for average of 26 days *2582*

Dehydroepiandrosterone Sulfate
Plasma No Effect Physiological No significant effect in 6 men with hyperlipidemia treated with 2 g daily for average of 26 days *2582*

11-Deoxycortisol *Plasma No Effect Physiological* No change in 6 men with hyperlipidemia treated with 2 g daily for average of 26 days *2582*

Eosinophils *Blood Increase Physiological* Eosinophilia has been reported as adverse event *6550*

Euglobulin Lysis Time *Blood Decrease Physiological* Reported observation *4014*

Fatty Acids (FFA), Free *Serum Decrease Physiological* Displacement from albumin *2242* Reduction observed in diabetics after 1 week treatment *1842*

Fibrinogen *Plasma Decrease Physiological* Reported observation in some cases *948* In reported studies clofibrate reduces mean concentration by 13% (up to -30%) *5585*

Glucose *Serum Decrease Physiological* If previously abnormal *2452* Clofibrate can enhance the hypoglycemic effect of intravenous tolbutamide administered at the same time through displacing tolbutamide from albumin binding sites and increasing the amount of free drug. Similar effect observed with biguanides such as metformin *3668* After 1 week in both normals and diabetics but more marked in latter *1842*
Serum No Effect Analytical At concentration of 500 mg/L had no effect on GOD/POD-PAP method *5704*

Glucose Tolerance *Serum Decrease Physiological* After 1 week in both normals and diabetics but more marked in latter *1842*
Serum Increase Physiological In diabetic patients receiving clofibrate reportedly improved glucose tolerance *3668* Improved in most patients in 14 patients with primary hyperlipoproteinemia given 2.0 g daily over 5 y *4874* Improvement relative to degree of abnormal triglycerides *512*

γ-Glutamyltransferase *Serum Decrease Physiological* Significant reduction in 27 patients, half of whom had hypertriglyceridemia, after 1 week *1845*

Granulocytes *Blood Decrease Physiological* Agranulocytosis has been reported as adverse event *6550*

Growth Hormone *Plasma No Effect Physiological* No effect of drug after 1 week in healthy individuals with hypertriglyceridemia *1842*

HDL-Cholesterol *Serum Decrease Physiological* In patients receiving clofibrate (2 g/d) and probucol (1 g/d) mean concentration reduced *4254* When probucol administered with clofibrate reduction of HDL-cholesterol concentration may be enhanced *3668*
Serum Increase Physiological Possible effect due to decreased apo A-I synthesis with expression of apo E and activation of cholesterol ester transfer protein *264* Increase by 10 to 20% in 10 hyperlipidemic patients *4249*

Hematocrit *Blood Decrease Physiological* Anemia has been reported as adverse event *6550*

Hemoglobin *Blood Decrease Physiological* Anemia has been reported as adverse event *6550*

Histamine *Plasma No Effect Analytical* No inhibition of radio-enzyme assay at therapeutic concentrations *2492*

17-Hydroxyprogesterone *Plasma No Effect Physiological* No change in 6 men with hyperlipidemia treated with 2 g daily for average of 26 days *2582*

^{131}I Uptake *Serum Decrease Physiological* Up to 2.5 g/d produces effect for up to 4 mo *882*

Insulin *Plasma Decrease Physiological* After 1 week in both normals and diabetics but more marked in latter *1842*

Lactate Dehydrogenase *Serum Decrease Physiological* Possibly derived from muscle damage *3669*
Serum Increase Physiological May cause muscle fiber atrophy in many patients *3065*

LDL-Cholesterol *Serum Decrease Physiological* Effect due to decreased synthesis and increased catabolism *878*

LDL-Triglycerides *Serum Decrease Physiological* Effect due to decreased synthesis and increased catabolism *878*

Leukocytes *Blood Decrease Physiological* Leukopenia has been reported as adverse event *6550* May cause leukopenia *4995*

Lipids *Serum Decrease Physiological* Normal response (may increase in diabetics) *4014*

β-Lipoprotein *Serum Decrease Physiological* Therapeutic effect (mechanism disputed) *128*

Lipoproteins, Pre-β *Serum Decrease Physiological* Therapeutic intent *254*

Neutral Steroids *Feces Decrease Physiological* After 2 weeks treatment fall observed *4075*

Occult Blood *Feces Increase Physiological* Gastrointestinal hemorrhage has been reported as probable adverse event *6550*

Phenytoin *Serum Increase Physiological* Potentiates action so amount of phenytoin should be reduced *1384*

Phospholipids *Serum Decrease Physiological* Effect less marked than with triglycerides *701*

Platelets *Blood Decrease Physiological* Thrombocytopenic purpura has been reported as probable adverse event *6550*

Clofibrate *(continued)*

Potassium *Serum Increase Physiological* Hyperkalemia has been reported as adverse event in association with renal insufficiency and continuous ambulatory peritoneal dialysis *6550*
Serum No Effect Physiological No effect of treatment of 6 men with hyperlipidemia with 2 g daily for average of 26 days *2582*
Urine No Effect Physiological No effect of treatment of 6 men with hyperlipidemia with 2 g daily for average of 26 days *2582*

Progesterone *Plasma No Effect Physiological* No significant effect in 6 men with hyperlipidemia treated for average of 26 days with 2 g daily *2582*

Protein *Serum Increase Physiological* Reported effect, mechanism not discussed *4174*
Urine Increase Physiological Proteinuria has been reported as adverse event *6550*

Prothrombin Time *Plasma Decrease Physiological* Prothrombin time may be increased by 50% in patients taking anticoagulants *6550*
Plasma Increase Physiological Displaces anticoagulants from binding protein *4406* Observed when coadministered with warfarin *2625* In patients receiving warfarin prothrombin time likely to be prolonged when clofibrate added to regime *3668*

Renin Activity *Plasma No Effect Physiological* No effect of treatment with 2 g daily in 6 men with hyperlipidemia for average of 26 days *2582*

Sodium *Serum No Effect Physiological* No effect of treatment with 2 g daily for average of 26 days in 6 men with hyperlipidemia *2582*
Urine Increase Physiological Clofibrate can enhance the diuretic effect of furosemide administered at the same time through displacing furosemide from albumin binding sites and increasing the amount of free drug *3668*
Urine No Effect Physiological No effect of treatment of 6 hyperlipidemic men with 2 g daily for average of 26 days *2582*

Sulfobromophthalein *Serum Increase Physiological* Abnormal liver function tests have been reported as adverse events as evidenced by increased BSP retention *6550*

T3-Uptake *Serum Decrease Physiological* Due to increased thyroxine binding globulin *4766*

Thyroid Stimulating Hormone
Serum Decrease Physiological In hypothyroidism but no change in euthyroid patients presumed to have direct action at hypothalamic or pituitary level *6412*

Thyroxine Binding Globulin *Serum Increase Physiological* Increases concentration (small dose effect) *5869*

Thyroxine (T4) *Serum Decrease Physiological* Due to increased binding capacity of drug *4766*
Serum Increase Physiological Insignificant increase due to increased binding capacity (augmentation of transport proteins) *6412* Increase observed due to increased thyroxine-binding globulin *2412*

Thyroxine (T4), Free *Serum Decrease Physiological* Percentage of free decreased (large doses) *4766*

α-Tocopherol *Serum Decrease Physiological* ?inhibits synthesis of carrier lipoprotein *6395*

Tolbutamide *Serum Increase Physiological* Potntiates action of tolbutamide so dose should be reduced *1384*

Tri-iodothyronine (T3) *Serum Increase Physiological* Increase observed due to increased throxine-binding globulin *2412*

Triglycerides *Serum Decrease Physiological* Marked reduction within 6 weeks in 10 hyperlipidemic patients *4249* Increase by 80% in first year in patients with hyperlipoproteinemia and impaired glucose tolerance given diet plus 2 g drμg/d monitored for 5 y *4874* In the Stockholm Ischemic Heart Study of 555 myocardial infarction patients treatment with clofibrate and nicotinic acid caused mean decrease of 19% *3115* In both normals with hypertriglyceridemia and diabetics *1842* Effect mediated through reduction of VLDL and LDL *878* Inhibits transfer from liver to plasma *701* Reduction from mean of 232 mg/dL to 138 mg/dL in 6 hyperlipidemic men treated with 2 g daily for average of 26 days *2582* Significant reduction in 27 patients, half of whom had hypertriglyceridemia, after 1 week *1845*
Serum No Effect Analytical At concentration of 500 mg/L had no effect on GPO-PAP method *5704*

Uric Acid *Serum Decrease Physiological* Occurs in about 10% (may occasionally cause gout) *92* Reduction observed in diabetics after 1 week treatment *1842*
Serum No Effect Analytical At concentration of 400 mg/L had no effect on Kageyama-Hantzsch method *5704* At concentration of 400 mg/L had no effect on catalase-AIDH method *5704* At concentration of 500 mg/L had no effect on uricase-PAP method *5704*
Urine Increase Physiological Weak transient uricosuric effect *128*

Vitamin A *Serum No Effect Physiological* Insignificant change in about 26 subjects given 2 g daily *4794*

VLDL-Cholesterol *Serum Decrease Physiological* Effect due to increased catabolism, decreased synthesis and increased uptake of VLDL *878*

VLDL-Triglycerides *Serum Decrease Physiological* Effect due to decreased synthesis and increased catabolism and hepatic uptake of VLDL *878*

Clometacin

Lithium *Serum Increase Physiological* Administration of 450 mg/d to 6 women increased serum concentration from an average of 0.64 mEq/L to 1.01 mEq/L within 6 days but concentration had reverted to normal within 7 days of discontinuation of clometacin *4831*

Lithium Clearance *Urine Decrease Physiological* With increase of serum concentration corresponding reduction of lithium clearance observed together with increased tubular lithium reabsorption *4831*

Clomiphene

Alanine Aminotransferase *Serum Increase Physiological* Post-marketing reports suggest hepatitis or transient increases of enzyne activity may occur *2645*

Androstenedione *Plasma Increase Physiological* Liberates LH, anti-steroid hormone effect of drug *924*

Aspartate Aminotransferase *Serum Increase Physiological* Post-marketing reports suggest hepatitis or transient increases of enzyne activity may occur *2645*

BSP Retention *Serum Increase Physiological* May cause hepatotoxicity *2024*

Cholesterol *Serum Decrease Physiological* Possible interference with synthesis *128*
Serum No Effect Physiological No significant effect observed with treatment *5451*

Dehydroepiandrosterone *Plasma Increase Physiological* Liberates LH, anti-steroid hormone effect of drug *924*

Dehydroepiandrosterone Sulfate
Plasma Increase Physiological Liberates LH, anti-steroid hormone effect of drug *924*

Desmosterol *Serum Increase Physiological* Patients on prolonged treatment may show increased concentrations, most likely due to direct interference with cholesterol synthesis *2645*

Estradiol *Plasma Increase Physiological* Increase in both follicular and luteal phases over normal *4991* Maximum with induced ovulation *2139*
Plasma No Effect Analytical Clomiphene citrate at a concentration of 100 ng/mL had less than 0.1% cross-reactivity with method on Bayer Technicon Immuno 1® *422*

Estrogens *Urine Increase Physiological* Due to action on hypothalamic-pituitary axis *4269*

Follicle Stimulating Hormone
Plasma Increase Physiological Maximum increase of 350% of control in males *5264*
Urine Increase Physiological Due to action on hypothalamic-pituitary axis *4269*

Histamine *Plasma No Effect Analytical* Improbable inhibition of radio-enzyme assay at therapeutic concentrations *2492*

Leukocytes *Blood Increase Physiological* Post-marketing reports suggest leukocytosis may occur with use of the drug *2645*

Luteinizing Hormone *Plasma Increase Physiological* Maximum with induced ovulation *2139* Up to 700% in normal males for first 21 d *5264*
Urine Increase Physiological Due to action on hypothalamic-pituitary axis *4269*

Progesterone *Plasma Increase Physiological* Increased over normal in luteal phase *4991*

Sperm Count *Semen Increase Physiological* In men with oligozoospermia but pregnancy rate unchanged *1499*

Sulfobromophthalein *Serum Increase Physiological* Greater than 5% retention observed in from 10 - 20% treated patients. Effect greatest with chronic treatment or with unrelated liver disease *5451*

T3-Uptake *Serum No Effect Physiological* 100 mg/d no effect on test *882*

Testosterone *Serum Increase Physiological* Liberates LH, anti-steroid hormone effect of drug *924*
Urine Increase Physiological Liberates LH, anti-steroid hormone effect of drug *374*

Thyroid Stimulating Hormone
Serum Increase Physiological Small but significant effect with basal and TRH-stimulated value: hypophyseal effect *6412*

Thyroxine (T4) *Serum No Effect Physiological* Probably direct thyroid inhibition *6412*

Thyroxine (T4) Index, Free *Serum Decrease Physiological* Probably direct thyroid inhibition *6412*

Tri-iodothyronine (T3) *Serum Decrease Physiological* Probably direct thyroid inhibition *6412*

Clomipramine

Alanine Aminotransferase *Serum Decrease Physiological* Administration has been occasionally shown to increase activity (to above 3 times the upper limit of normal) in approximately 3% patients *1021*
Serum Increase Physiological Reversible increase in activity observed but not usually of much significance *1384*
Serum No Effect Physiological No significant effect observed in 13 patients treated with a mean daily dose of 84 mg for 4 weeks *4289*

Albumin *Urine No Effect Analytical* Using a fluorimetric assay with Albumin Blue 580 on a Cobas Fara centrifugal analyzer for the detection of microalbuminuria no significant interference was detected at a concentration of 10 mg/L *3117*

Alkaline Phosphatase *Serum No Effect Physiological* No significant effect observed in 13 patients treated with a mean daily dose of 84 mg for 4 weeks *4289*

Antidiuretic Hormone
Cerebrospinal Fluid Decrease Physiological In 17 children and adolescents with obsessive-compulsive disorders and long-term administration of clomipramine mean concentration decreased from 1.30 ± 0.57 pmol/L to 0.86 ± 0.54 pmol/L *123*

Aspartate Aminotransferase
Serum Decrease Physiological Administration has been occasionally shown to increase activity (to above 3 times the upper limit of normal) in approximately 1% patients *1021*
Serum Increase Physiological Reversible increase of enzyme activity observed but not usually of much significance *1384*
Serum No Effect Physiological No significant effect observed in 13 patients treated with a mean daily dose of 84 mg for 4 weeks *4289*

Bilirubin *Serum No Effect Physiological* No significant effect observed in 13 patients treated with a mean daily dose of 84 mg for 4 weeks *4289*

Cholesterol *Serum No Effect Physiological* No significant effect observed in 13 patients treated with a mean daily dose of 84 mg for 4 weeks *4289*

Corticotropin *Plasma Increase Physiological* Insignificant increase following i.v. infusion of 10 mg, but significant effect with 20 mg in 10 healthy volunteers *2218*

Corticotropin-releasing Hormone
Cerebrospinal Fluid Decrease Physiological In 17 children and adolescents with obsessive-compulsive disorder and long-term administration of clomipramine mean concentration decreased from 175 ± 32 pmol/L to 152 ± 25 pmol/L *123*

Cortisol *Plasma Increase Physiological* Significant effect in 10 healthy volunteers following i.v. infusion of 10 mg *2218*

Creatinine *Serum No Effect Physiological* No significant effect observed in 13 patients treated with a mean daily dose of 84 mg for 4 weeks *4289*

Erythrocytes *Blood Decrease Physiological* In postmarketing reports administration has been occasionally shown to cause anemia and pancytopenia *1021*
Blood No Effect Physiological No significant effect observed in 13 patients treated for 4 weeks with a mean daily dose of 84 mg *4289*

Glucose *Serum No Effect Physiological* No significant effect noted in 13 patients treated with a mean daily dose of 84 mg for 4 weeks *4289*

γ-Glutamyltransferase *Serum Increase Physiological* Moderate increase observed in 2 of 13 patients treated with a mean dose of 84 mg daily for 4 weeks *4289*

Granulocytes *Blood Decrease Physiological* In postmarketing reports administration has been occasionally shown to cause agranulocytosis and pancytopenia *1021*

Growth Hormone *Plasma Increase Physiological* In depressive patients: increase in 5 of 8 patients with acute treatment: no effect observed after 28 d *2274*
Plasma No Effect Physiological No significant effect in 10 healthy adult volunteers following i.v. infusion of either 10 or 20 mg *2218*

Hematocrit *Blood No Effect Physiological* No significant effect observed in 13 patients treated with a mean daily dose of 84 mg for 4 weeks *4289*

Hemoglobin *Blood Decrease Physiological* In postmarketing reports administration has been occasionally shown to cause anemia *1021*
Blood No Effect Physiological No significant effect observed in 13 patients treated with a mean daily dose of 84 mg for 4 weeks *4289*

Homovanillic Acid
Cerebrospinal Fluid Decrease Physiological In 17 children and adolescents with obsessive compulsive disorder and long-term administration of clomipramine mean concentration decreased from 273 ± 111 pmol/mL to 237 ± 101 pmol/mL *123*

4-Hydroxy-3-Methoxy-Phenylglycol
Cerebrospinal Fluid Decrease Physiological In 17 children and adolescents with obsessive-compulsive disorder and long-term administration of clomipramine mean concentration decreased from 42.4 ± 10.2 pmol/L to 36.1 ± 4.8 pmol/mL *123*

5-Hydroxyindoleacetic Acid
Cerebrospinal Fluid Decrease Physiological In 17 children and adolescents with obsessive-compulsive disorder and long-term administration of clomipramine mean concentration decreased from 109 ± 31 pmol/mL to 77 ± 23 pmol/mL *123*

5-Hydroxytryptamine *Plasma Increase Physiological* In 27 patients with major depression treatment with clomipramine intravenously caused a nonsignificant increase from 32.5 ± 10.9 nmol/L to 62.2 ± 19.4 nmol/L from 0800 to 1130 on day 1 in those treated intravenously and significantly from 20.4 ± 6.7 nmol/L to 41.9 ± 16.7 nmol/L in those treated orally *5758*
Platelets No Effect Physiological In 27 patients with major depression treatment with clomipramine intravenously caused a nonsignificant change from 693 ± 74 nmol/L to 743 ± 77 nmol/L from 0800 to 1130 on day 1 in those treated intravenously and from 646 ± 107 nmol/L to 696 ± 104 nmol/L in those treated orally *5758*

Leukocytes *Blood Decrease Physiological* In postmarketing reports administration has been occasionally shown to cause leukopenia and pancytopenia *1021*
Blood No Effect Physiological No significant effect observed in 13 patients treated with a mean dose of 84 mg/d for 4 weeks *4289*

Melatonin *Plasma No Effect Physiological* No significant effect in 10 healthy adults following i.v. infusion of either 10 or 20 mg *2218*

Neutrophils *Blood Decrease Physiological* Occasional case of agranulocytosis reported *6264*

Norepinephrine *Plasma No Effect Physiological* No significant difference between either 10 or 20 mg of drug by i.v. infusion and effect of placebo *2218*

Clomipramine (continued)

Oxytocin *Cerebrospinal Fluid Increase Physiological* In 17 children and adolescents with obsessive-compulsive disorder and long-term administration of clomipramine mean concentration increased from 6.05 ± 1.60 pmol/L to 6.70 ± 1.44 pmol/L *123*

Phenobarbital *Serum Increase Physiological* Coadministration with clomipramine has been reported to increase the plasma concentration of phenobarbital *1021*

Platelets *Blood Decrease Physiological* In postmarketing reports administration has been occasionally shown to cause thrombocytopenia and pancytopenia *1021*
Blood No Effect Physiological No significant effect observed in 13 patients treated with a mean daily dose of 84 mg for 4 weeks *4289*

Potassium *Serum No Effect Physiological* No significant effect observed in 13 patients treated with a mean daily dose of 84 mg for 4 weeks *4289*

Prolactin *Plasma Increase Physiological* In 10 normal volunteers mean increase from 3.1 µg/L to 4.8 µg/L 30 min following start of i.v. infusion of 10 mg *2218* In depressive patients: temporary increase during first day with lag after drug peak in 6 out of 11 patients. Significant effect after 28 d *2274*

Sodium *Serum No Effect Physiological* No significant effect observed in 13 patients treated with a mean daily dose of 84 mg for 4 weeks *4289*

Somatostatin *Cerebrospinal Fluid Decrease Physiological* In 17 children and adolescents with obsessive-compulsive disorder and long-term administration of clomipramine mean concentration decreased from 21.3 ± 8.5 pmol/L to 15.3 ± 9.8 pmol/L *123*

Thyroid Stimulating Hormone
Serum No Effect Physiological No effect with acute or chronic treatment in depressive patients *2274*

Tri-iodothyronine (T3) *Serum Decrease Physiological* Observed effect *2412*

Tricyclic Antidepressants *Serum Increase Analytical* May cause false positive reaction in immunoassays for tricyclic antidepressants *3590*

Triglycerides *Serum No Effect Physiological* No significant effect observed in 13 patients treated with a mean daily dose of 84 mg for 4 weeks *4289*

Urea Nitrogen *Serum No Effect Physiological* No significant effect observed in 13 patients treated with a mean daily dose of 84 mg for 4 weeks *4289*

Uric Acid *Serum No Effect Physiological* No significant effect observed in 13 patients treated with a mean daily dose of 84 mg for 4 weeks *4289*

Clonazepam

Albumin *Urine No Effect Analytical* Using a fluorimetric assay with Albumin Blue 580 on a Cobas Fara centrifugal analyzer for the detection of microalbuminuria no significant interference was detected at a concentration of 2 mg/L *3117*

Benzodiazepine *Urine Positive Analytical* Positive result observed at a concentration of 2.0 µg/mL (6.33 µmol/L) with method on Du Pont aca *1556*

Bilirubin *Serum No Effect Physiological* Insignificant displacement from protein in neonates *6314*

Carbamazepine *Serum No Effect Physiological* No significant effect on concentrations observed *2942* No consistent effect on plasma concentration *1384*

Eosinophils *Blood Increase Physiological* Occasional cases of eosinophilia reported *1384* Administration of clonazepamhas been associated with anemia, leukopenia, eosinophilia and thrombocytopenia *5025*

Erythrocytes *Blood Decrease Physiological* Minor cases of anemia reported *1384*

Felbamate *Serum No Effect Analytical* No significant interference observed with GLC method of Rifai et al *4958*

Hematocrit *Blood Decrease Physiological* Administration of clonazepam has been associated with anemia, leukopenia, eosinophilia and thrombocytopenia *5025*

Hemoglobin *Blood Decrease Physiological* Administration of clonazepam has been associated with anemia, leukopenia, eosinophilia and thrombocytopenia *5025* Occasional cases of anemia reported *1384*

Leukocytes *Blood Decrease Physiological* Occasional cases of leukopenia reported *1384*

Mycophenolic Acid *Serum No Effect Analytical* No significant interference observed with HPLC method of Shipkova et al *5526*

Mycophenolic Acid Glucuronide
Serum No Effect Analytical No significant interference observed with HPLC method of Shipkova et al *5526*

Phenobarbital *Serum No Effect Physiological* No consistent effect on plasma concentration *1384* No effect observed when both drugs coadministered *2942*

Phenytoin *Serum No Effect Physiological* No consistent effect observed on plasma concentration *1384* No effect on plasma concentration observed when drugs coadministered *2942*

Platelets *Blood Decrease Physiological* Occasional cases of thrombocytopenia reported *1384* Administration of clonazepam has been associated with anemia, leukopenia, eosinophilia and thrombocytopenia *5025*

Primidone *Serum No Effect Physiological* No consistent effect observed on plasma concentration *1384*

Valproic Acid *Serum No Effect Analytical* At concentrations up to 100 µg/mL had no significant cross-reactivity in valproic acid method on Bayer Technicon Immuno 1® *437* No significant interference observed at a concentration of 100 µg/mL (317 µmol/L) with method on Du Pont aca *1560*

Clonidine

Alanine Aminotransferase *Serum Increase Physiological* Single probable case of toxic hepatitis *2108*

Aldosterone *Plasma Decrease Physiological* General tendency to decrease observed in 11 hypertensive patients given 150 µg/d for 4 days but effect not significant *4079* Premedication with 300 µg clonidine prior to neurosurgery in 9 patients was associated with significant reduction of plasma aldosterone concentration *2053*
Plasma No Effect Physiological No significant change observed in 8 normal volunteers treated with 150 µg daily for 1 week *6381*
Urine Decrease Physiological Secondary to effect on renin *2666*

Alkaline Phosphatase *Serum Increase Physiological* Single probable case of toxic hepatitis *2108*

Angiotensin-II *Plasma Increase Physiological* General tendency to increase observed in 11 hypertensive patients given 150 µg/d for 4 days but effect not significant *4079*

Antidiuretic Hormone *Plasma Decrease Physiological* Significant reduction observed in 13 patients given intravenous infusion of 7 µg/kg over 2 hours when compared with response following placebo in control group of 16 patients *4824*
Plasma No Effect Physiological No significant effect observed in 11 hypertensive patients given 150 µg/d for 4 days *4079*

Aspartate Aminotransferase *Serum Increase Physiological* Single probable case of toxic hepatitis *2108*

Atrial Natriuretic Peptide *Plasma Decrease Physiological* Reduction of 65% observed in basal concentration in 8 normal volunteers given 150 µg daily for 1 week with 15% increase following acute infusion of 2 liters of saline *6381*
Plasma No Effect Physiological No significant change observed in 11 hypertensive patients given 150 µg/d for 4 days *4079*

Bilirubin *Serum Increase Physiological* Toxic hepatitis reported *2108*

BSP Retention *Serum Increase Physiological* Single probable case of toxic hepatitis *2108*

Catecholamines *Plasma Increase Physiological* Increase observed in response to exercise but overall response blunted *6611*
Plasma No Effect Analytical No effect on HPLC method of Koller for dopamine, epinephrine, and norepinephrine *3230*
Plasma No Effect Physiological In a group of patients prior to neurosurgery 300 µg clonidine had the same effect as placebo *2053*

Urine *Decrease* *Physiological* Dose related effect (primary action of drug) *2666*

Cholesterol *Serum* *Decrease* *Physiological* In 16 patients treated for 2 mo (by 8%) *142*

Serum *Increase* *Physiological* Increase by 6% in 59 patients with primary hypertension given up to 300 mg daily for 6 mo *3047*

Coombs' Test, Indirect *Blood* *Positive* *Physiological* Mechanism not discussed *6616*

Corticotropin *Plasma* *Decrease* *Physiological* Significant reduction with 0.45 mg daily for 3 days in normal individuals as well as hypertensive and obese subjects *5602* Reduced in response to single oral dose in all of 6 healthy adults studied *3398*

Cortisol *Plasma* *Decrease* *Physiological* In 9 neurosurgical patients premedication with 300 µg for surgery with clonidine caused significant reduction in concentration *2053* In 10 postoperative patients following 150 µg extradurally but to a lesser extent than with 4·mg morphine *3682* Lower level in growth hormone deficient children: did not change with 0.1 mg/m^2 daily for 60 d *4709* Significant reduction with 0.45 mg daily for 3 days in normal subjects as well hypertensive and obese subjects *5602* Overall decrease in mean concentration in melancholic and control subjects after intravenous administration *150* In normal subjects reduced by 50% with 0.15 mg/d but no effect in opiate addicts *2110*

Plasma *No Effect* *Physiological* No change greater than with normal diurnal variation *1723*

Creatine Kinase *Serum* *Increase* *Physiological* Temporary effect of unknown significance *2108*

Creatinine *Serum* *Increase* *Physiological* Approximately 0.1 mg/dL *6616*

Serum *No Effect* *Analytical* At 10 mg/L on reversed phase liquid chromatographic procedure of Zhiri et al *6656*

Dopamine β-Hydroxylase

Cerebrospinal Fluid *No Effect* *Physiological* In 5 patients with essential hypertension treatment with clonidine for 6 weeks caused nonsignificant change from mean baseline of 25.7 ± 3.8 ng/mL to 28.8 ± 3.8 ng/mL of dopamine β-hydroxylase *4358*

Serum *Increase* *Physiological* In 6 patients with essential hypertension treatment for 6 weeks mean concentration of dopamine β-hydroxylase increased nonsignificantly from 13.7 ± 3.8 µg/mL to 16.8 ± 7.2 µg/mL *4358* In 5 patients with essential hypertension treatment for 6 weeks caused nonsignificant increase in activity of dopamine β-hydroxylase from mean baseline of 31.1 ± 8.1 U/L to 39.3 ± 10.2 U/L *4358*

Drugs of Abuse Screen *Urine* *No Effect* *Analytical* No effect at concentration of 100 µg/mL on EZ-SCREEN procedure for cannabinoids and cocaine *1739*

Effective Renal Plasma Flow

Patient *Increase* *Physiological* Sustained rise after initial drop with i.v. injection *735*

β-Endorphin *Plasma* *Decrease* *Physiological* Significant reduction in normal individuals with 0.45 mg daily for 3 days but in obese individuals basal value was high and did not change in response to treatment. In hypertensives, both obese and normal, significant increase noted *5602*

Plasma *No Effect* *Physiological* In normal subjects with 0.15 mg/d but raised to normal values in opiate addicts *2110*

Epinephrine *Plasma* *Decrease* *Physiological* Depressed concentration noted on average, although not significant, in 8 normal volunteers treated with 150 µg daily for 1 week *6381* In 5 patients with essential hypertension treatment for 6 weeks caused significant reduction from mean baseline of 29 ± 5 pg/mL to 21 ± 4 pg/mL *4358* Significant reduction observed in 13 patients given intravenous infusion of 7 µg/kg over 2 hours compared with placebo *4824* In 9 volunteers administration of 150 µg orally caused significant reduction from 286 ± 64 pmol/L to 190 ± 43 pmol/L in one study, 197 ± 62 pmol/L to 138 ± 30 pmol/L in a second and 307 ± 44 pmol/L to 186 ± 34 pmol/L in a third *4818* After 0.3 mg orally mean decrease of 0.06 ± 0.04 nmol/L (from 0.21 ± 0.03 nmol/L to 0.14 ± 0.03 nmol/L) in 10 normotensive men and 0.09 ± 0.02 nmol/L (from 0.14 ± 0.03 nmol/L to 0.05 ± 0.01 nmol/L) in 21 normotensive women over next 140 minutes *1357*

Plasma *No Effect* *Physiological* No significant change observed in 11 hypertensive patients given 150 µg/d for 4 days *4079*

Urine *Decrease* *Physiological* Primary action of drug *2666*

Fatty Acids (FFA), Free *Serum* *Increase* *Physiological* In 10 healthy volunteers administration of 0.2 mg caused significant increase from mean baseline of 445 µEq/mL to 500 µEq/mL after 1 hour and 525 µEq/mL after 4 hours *5903*

Follicle Stimulating Hormone

Plasma *No Effect* *Physiological* No effect seen in 12 healthy adults after single oral dose *3398*

Glomerular Filtration Rate *Urine* *Decrease* *Physiological* Nonsignificant reduction by 1.1 mL/min in 5 patients with idiopathic membranous nephropathy treated with mean dose of 0.3 mg/d for 3 weeks: reduction increased to 2.1 mL/min with later rechallenge *5293*

Urine *Increase* *Physiological* Sustained rise after initial fall with i.v. injection *735*

Glucagon *Plasma* *No Effect* *Physiological* No effect observed on normal response to moderate or heavy exercise *2940* No effect when given i.v. to 6 healthy volunteers *3371*

Glucose *Serum* *Increase* *Physiological* In 9 preoperative patients premedicated with 300 µg clonidine concentration increased but were lower in the clonidine-treated patients than placebo-treated patients *2053* Increase observed in response to exercise but overall response blunted *6611* In 10 healthy volunteers administration of 0.2 mg caused transient but significant increase from mean baseline of 90.8 ± 14.8 mg/dL to 96.5 ± 7.5 mg/dL after1 hour and 96.7 ± 12.6 mg/dL after 2 hours *5903* When given i.v. over 10 minutes increase of about 15 mg/dL preceded other changes in normal volunteers *3371* Significant increase in 10 postoperative patients following 150 µg extradurally *3682*

Serum *No Effect* *Physiological* In children with growth hormone deficiency 0.1 mg/m^2 daily for 60 d *4709*

Gonadotropins *Plasma* *No Effect* *Physiological* In children with growth hormone deficiency 0.1 mg/m^2 daily for 60 d *4709*

Growth Hormone *Plasma* *Increase* *Physiological* In children who are growth hormone responders significantly greater increase in hormone concentration following dose of about 0.15 ng/sq meter than in nonresponders given same dose *2660* In 10 patients with panic disorder and 14 control individuals given mean intravenous dose of 124 µg concentration increased from mean baseline of 1.3 µg/L to 10.6 µg/L after 45 minutes in control individuals and to 3.9 µg/L from mean baseline of 0.8 µg/L in patients with panic disorder (not significant) *33* In children with growth hormone deficiency 0.1 mg/m^2 daily for 60 d *4709* In 13 healthy short stature children oral clonidine (0.15 mg/sq m) caused mean increase of 0.9 nmol/L *2111* Peak of 6.4 to 30 ng/mL when given i.v. to 6 healthy normals *3371*

Plasma *No Effect* *Physiological* No effect observed on normal response to moderate or heavy exercise *2940*

Urine *No Effect* *Physiological* In 11 prepubertal children treatment with 0.15 mg/sq m daily caused insignificant change from mean baseline of 10.0 ± 5.3 ng/d (22.4 ± 11.4 ng/g creatinine) to 14.1 ± 7.9 ng/d (28.2 ± 13.7 ng/g creatinine) at 6 months and 14.2 ± 9.5 ng/d (28.0 ± 16.1 ng/g creatinine) at 12 months *5247*

Growth Hormone Releasing Hormone

Plasma *Increase* *Physiological* Maximal mean increment of 6.82 pmol/L observed in 13 healthy short stature children given oral clonidine (0.15 mg/sq m) *2111*

Guanosine Monophosphate

Plasma *No Effect* *Physiological* No effect noted on basal concentration in 8 volunteers treated with 150 µg daily for 1 week but 40% increase with acute infusion of 2 liters of saline *6381*

Urine *No Effect* *Physiological* No change in basal excretion in 8 volunteers given 150 µg daily for 1 week compared with placebo-treated controls but 60% increase following acute infusion of 2 liters of saline *6381*

HDL-Cholesterol *Serum* *No Effect* *Physiological* In 59 patients with primary hypertension given up to 300 mg daily for 6 mo *3047*

Histamine *Plasma* *No Effect* *Analytical* Although 50% inhibition of radio-enzyme assay at 27 µg/mL unlikely to be of clinical significance since therapeutic concentration 0.0003-0.0018 µg/mL *2492*

4-Hydroxy-3-Methoxy-Phenylglycol

Cerebrospinal Fluid *Decrease* *Physiological* In 5 patients with essential hypertension treatment for 6 weeks treatment for 6 weeks caused nonsignificant reduction from mean baseline of 6.74 ± 2.09 ng/mL to 4.89 ± 1.33 ng/mL *4358*

Clonidine *(continued)*

4-Hydroxy-3-Methoxy-Phenylglycol *(continued)*
Plasma Decrease Physiological In 10 patients with panic disorder and 14 age and sex matched controls reduction of concentrations observed from 4.0 µg/L to 3.5 µg/L at 45 minutes in patients with panic disorder and from 3.3 µg/L to 3.2 µg/L at 45 minutes in control patients following intravenous administration of mean dose of 124 µg *33*

Insulin *Plasma No Effect Physiological* No effect observed on normal response to moderate or heavy exercise *2940* In 10 healthy individuals no significant difference observed between ingestion of 0.2 mg and after placebo *5903*

Insulin-like Growth Factor-I *Serum Increase Physiological* In children with growth hormone deficiency 0.1 mg/m² daily for 60 d *4709*
Urine No Effect Physiological In 11 prepubertal children treatment with 0.15 mg/sq m daily caused insignificant change from mean baseline of 0.69 ± 0.29 U/mL to 0.83 ± 0.26 U/mL at 6 months and 0.70 ± 20 U/mL at 12 months *5247*

LDL-Cholesterol *Serum No Effect Physiological* In 59 patients with primary hypertension given up to 300 mg daily for 6 mo *3047*

LDL-Triglycerides *Serum Decrease Physiological* Small effect in 59 patients with primary hypertension given up to 300 mg daily for 6 mo *3047*

Luteinizing Hormone *Plasma No Effect Physiological* No effect seen in 12 healthy adults after single oral dose *3398*

Neuropeptide Y *Plasma No Effect Physiological* In 3 studies of 9 volunteers administration of 150 µg orally caused reduction from 3.5 ± 0.4 pmol/L to 2.8 ± 0.4 pmol/L in one study, but no significant change from 2.7 ± 0.7 pmol/L to 2.8 ± 0.5 pmol/L in a second study and from 3.6 ± 0.6 pmol/L to 3.6 ± 0.5 pmol/L in another study *4818*

Norepinephrine *Cerebrospinal Fluid Decrease Physiological* In 5 patients with essential hypertension treatment for 6 weeks caused a significant decrease from mean baseline of 310 ± 111 pg/mL to 147 ± 26 pg/mL *4358*
Plasma Decrease Physiological After 0.3 mg administered orally mean concentration decreased by 0.63 ± 0.07 nmol/L (from 0.87 ± 0.07 nmol/L to 0.24 ± 0.03 nmol/L) in 21 normotensive women and by 0.3 ± 0.1 nmol/L (from 1.16 ± 0.26 nmol/L to 0.85 ± 0.32 nmol/L) in 10 normotensive men *1357* In 5 patients with essential hypertension treatment for 6 weeks caused nonsignificant decrease from mean baseline of 199 ± 36 pg/mL to 164 ± 24 pg/mL *4358* Decrease of 159 pg/mL in 11 hypertensive patients given 150 µg/d for 4 days *4079* In 9 volunteers administration of 150 µg orally caused significant reduction from 2187 ± 326 pmol/L to 1769 ± 346 pmol/L in one study, 2101 ± 236 pmol/L to 1838 ± 272 pmol/L in another and 2030 ± 380 pmol/L to 1945 ± 493 pmol/L in a third *4818* Significant reduction observed compared with placebo treated group when 7 µg/kg infused over 2 hours *4824* Depressed concentration, although not significant, noted in 8 normal volunteers treated with 150 µg daily for 1 week *6381*
Urine Decrease Physiological Dose related effect (primary action of drug) *2666*

PAH Clearance *Urine Increase Physiological* Nonsignificant effect in hypertensives *620*

Potassium *Saliva Increase Physiological* Mechanism not discussed *620*

Prolactin *Plasma No Effect Physiological* No effect seen in 12 healthy adults after single oral dose *3398* In children with growth hormone deficiency given 0.1 mg/m² daily for 60 d *4709* No effect observed on normal response to moderate or heavy exercise *2940*

Protein *Urine Decrease Physiological* In 5 patients with idiopathic membranous nephropathy excretion slightly reduced by 0.3 g/day when treated with mean dose of 0.3 mg/day over 3 weeks (but no different from situation observed with natural history of disease) *5293*

Quinidine *Serum No Effect Analytical* Clonidine at a concentration of 100 µg/mL had no significant cross-reactivity with quinidine at a concentration of 2.0 µg/mL in method on Bayer Technicon Immuno 1® *431* No significant interference observed at a concentration of 100 µg/mL (435 µmol/L) with method on Du Pont aca *1543*

Renin Activity *Plasma Decrease Physiological* Significant reduction observed in 13 patients when compared against placebo following intravenous infusion of 7 µg/kg over 2 hours *4824* Dose related effect (secondary to action of catecholamines) *2666* Significant decrease of 0.81 ng/mL/h observed in 11 hypertensive patients given 150 µg/d for 4 days *4079*
Plasma No Effect Physiological No effect observed in 8 normal subjects treated with 150 µg daily for 1 week *6381*

Sodium *Serum Increase Physiological* Probable direct action on renal tubules *2242*

Tacrolimus *Serum No Effect Analytical* In HPLC/MS method of Christians et al no significant interference observed with measurement of FK 506 *1010*

Thyroid Stimulating Hormone
Serum No Effect Physiological In children with growth hormone deficiency 0.1 mg/m² daily for 60 d *4709*

Triglycerides *Serum No Effect Physiological* No significant effect observed in 10 healthy subjects following 0.2 mg clonidine *5903*

Urea Nitrogen *Serum Increase Physiological* Associated with decreased GFR at start of therapy *4922*

Uric Acid *Serum No Effect Analytical* At 10 mg/L on reversed phase liquid chromatographic procedure of Zhiri et al *6656*

Vanillylmandelic Acid *Urine Decrease Physiological* Dose related effect *2666*

Vasopressin *Plasma Decrease Physiological* Significant reduction observed in 13 patients given intravenous infusion of 7 µg/kg over 2 hours when compared with response following placebo in control group of 16 patients *4824*

VLDL-Cholesterol *Serum No Effect Physiological* In 59 patients with primary hypertension given up to 300 mg daily for 6 mo *3047*

Volume *Saliva Decrease Physiological* Mechanism not discussed *620*
Urine No Effect Physiological No change compared with placebo treated controls in 8 normal volunteers treated with 150 µg daily for 1 week *6381*

Clopamide

Alanine Aminotransferase *Serum Increase Physiological* Single case of diuretic associated myopathy *2929*

Aldolase *Serum Increase Physiological* Single case of diuretic associated myopathy *2929*

Ammonia *Plasma No Effect Physiological* No significant effects observed *2452*

Apolipoprotein A-I *Serum Increase Physiological* No significant change in 17 individuals treated for less than 1 y when used as sole treatment *5341*

Apolipoprotein A-II *Serum No Effect Physiological* No significant change in 17 individuals treated for less than 1 y when used as sole treatment *5341*

Apolipoprotein B *Serum No Effect Physiological* No significant change in 17 individuals treated for less than 1 y when used as sole treatment *5341*

Aspartate Aminotransferase *Serum Increase Physiological* Single case of diuretic associated myopathy *2929*

Catecholamines *Urine No Effect Physiological* Single case of diuretic associated myopathy *2929*

Chloride *Serum Decrease Physiological* Single case of diuretic associated myopathy *2929*
Urine Increase Physiological Diuretic action *4829*

Cholesterol *Serum No Effect Physiological* No significant change in 17 individuals treated for less than 1 y when used as sole treatment *5341*

Creatine Kinase *Serum Increase Physiological* Single case of diuretic associated myopathy *2929*

Glucose *Serum Increase Physiological* Mild effect ?due to induced hypokalemia *2452*

Glucose Tolerance *Serum Decrease Physiological* Possible effect of hypokalemia *6516*

Granulocytes *Blood No Effect Physiological* No significant association between use and agranulocytosis *3098*

HDL-Cholesterol *Serum No Effect Physiological* No significant change in 17 individuals treated for less than 1 y when used as sole treatment *5341*

17-Hydroxycorticosteroids *Urine No Effect Physiological* Single case of diuretic associated myopathy *2929*

17-Ketosteroids *Urine No Effect Physiological* Single case of diuretic associated myopathy *2929*

Lactate Dehydrogenase *Serum Increase Physiological* Single case of diuretic associated myopathy *2929*

LDL-Cholesterol *Serum Increase Physiological* 13% change in 17 individuals treated for less than 1 y when used as sole treatment *5341*

Myoglobin *Urine Increase Physiological* Single case of diuretic associated myopathy *2929*

Potassium *Serum Decrease Physiological* Result of diuretic action *6516* Single case of diuretic associated myopathy *2929*
Urine Increase Physiological Diuretic action *4829*

Sodium *Serum Increase Physiological* Single case of diuretic associated myopathy *2929*
Urine Increase Physiological Diuretic action (rapid effect) *4829*

Triglycerides *Serum No Effect Physiological* No significant change in 17 individuals treated for less than 1 y when used as sole treatment *5341*

Vanillylmandelic Acid *Urine No Effect Physiological* Single case of diuretic associated myopathy *2929*

VLDL-Cholesterol *Serum No Effect Physiological* No significant change in 17 individuals treated for less than 1 y when used as sole treatment *5341*

Volume *Urine Increase Physiological* Diuretic action *4829*

Clopenthixol

Glucose *Serum Increase Physiological* Hyperglycemic effect reported *4014*

Clopidogrel

Alanine Aminotransferase *Serum Increase Physiological* Administration of clopidogrel was associated with increased hepatic enzyme activity in 1.0 to 2.5% treated patients *5256*

Aspartate Aminotransferase *Serum Increase Physiological* Administration of clopidogrel was associated with increased hepatic enzyme activity in 1.0 to 2.5% treated patients *5256*

Atenolol *Serum No Effect Physiological* Clopidogrel administration does not appear to affect the pharmacokinetics of atenolol *5256*

Bilirubin *Serum Increase Physiological* Administration of clopidogrel was associated with hyperbilirubinemia in less than 1.0% of 9599 treated patients *5256*

Bleeding Time *Patient Increase Physiological* Administration of clopidogrel prolongs bleding time *5256*

Blood *Urine Increase Physiological* Administration of clopidogrel was associated with hematuria in less than 1.0% of 9599 treated patients *5256*

Cholesterol *Serum Increase Physiological* Administration of clopidogrel was associated with hypercholesterolemia in 4.0% of 9599 treated patients *5256*

Digoxin *Serum No Effect Physiological* Coadministration of clopidogrel does not affect the pharmacokinetics of digoxin *5256*

Hematocrit *Blood Decrease Physiological* Administration of clopidogrel was associated with anemia in 1.0 to 2.5% treated patients *5256*

Hemoglobin *Blood Decrease Physiological* Administration of clopidogrel was associated with anemia in 1.0 to 2.5% treated patients *5256*

Heparin *Plasma No Effect Physiological* In healthy volunteers clopidogrel administration does not appear to modify the heparin effect on coagulation *5256*

Leukocytes *Blood Decrease Physiological* Administration of clopidogrel was associated with leukopenia in less than 1.0% treated patients *5256*

Neutrophils *Blood Decrease Physiological* Administration of clopidogrel was associated with severe neutropenia in 4 of 9599 patients in a clinical trial of the drug *5256*

Nifedipine *Serum No Effect Physiological* Clopidogrel administration does not appear to affect the pharmacodynamics of nifedipine *5256*

Nonprotein Nitrogen *Serum Increase Physiological* Administration of clopidogrel was associated with increased plasma nonprotein nitrogen concentration in 1.0 to 2.5% patients *5256*

Occult Blood *Feces Increase Physiological* Administration of clopidogrel was associated with a rate of gastrointestinal bleeding of 2.0% *5256*

Platelet Aggregation response to ADP
Blood Decrease Physiological Inhibits ADP-induced platelet aggregation *5256*

Platelets *Blood Decrease Physiological* Administration of clopidogrel was associated with decreased platelet concentration in 1.0 to 2.5% treated patients *5256*

Theophylline *Serum No Effect Physiological* Coadministration of clopidogrel does not affect the pharmacokinetics of theophylline *5256*

Uric Acid *Serum Increase Physiological* Administration of clopidogrel was associated with gout and increased plasma uric acid concentration in 1.0 to 2.5% patients *5256*

Clorazepate

Alanine Aminotransferase *Serum Increase Physiological* Administration associated with rare abnormal liver function tests *28*

Aspartate Aminotransferase *Serum Increase Physiological* Administration associated with rare abnormal liver function tests *28*

Benzodiazepine *Urine Positive Analytical* At concentration of 1.0 µg/mL or greater produces positive result with Syva EMIT II assay *1785*

Creatinine *Serum Increase Physiological* Administration associated with rare abnormal renal function *28*

Urea Nitrogen *Serum Increase Physiological* Mild elevation in 10% patients reported *3053*

Clorexolone

Glucose *Serum Increase Physiological* Diabetogenic action *3810*

Potassium *Serum Decrease Physiological* Diuretic action *4014*

Uric Acid *Serum Increase Physiological* Occurs as with thiazide drugs *4014*

Clorgiline

Homovanillic Acid
Cerebrospinal Fluid Decrease Physiological Significant reduction in 43 patients with depression or Alzheimer's disease chronically treated with drug *4965*

5-Hydroxyindoleacetic Acid
Cerebrospinal Fluid Decrease Physiological Significant reduction in 43 patients with depression or Alzheimer's disease chronically treated with drug *4965*

Clotermine

Amobarbital *Urine No Effect Analytical* No interference on TLC using ethyl acetate: methanol: water: ammonium hydroxide and modified Dragendorff's reagent for detection *6502*

Amphetamine *Urine No Effect Analytical* No interference on TLC using ethyl acetate: methanol: water: ammonium hydroxide and modified Dragendorff's reagent for detection *6502*

Fenfluramine *Urine Positive Analytical* Similar R_fs and color reaction on TLC using ethyl acetate: methanol: water: ammonium hydroxide and modified Dragendorff's reagent *6502*

Clotermine *(continued)*

Hydromorphone *Urine* *No Effect* *Analytical* No interference on TLC using ethyl acetate: methanol: water: ammonium hydroxide and modified Dragendorff's reagent for detection *6502*

Mescaline *Urine* *No Effect* *Analytical* No interference on TLC using ethylacetate: methanol: water: ammonium hydroxide and modified Dragendorff's reagent for detection *6502*

Methamphetamine *Urine* *No Effect* *Analytical* No interference on TLC using ethyl acetate: methanol: water: ammonium hydroxide and modified Dragendorff's reagent for detection *6502*

Morphine *Urine* *No Effect* *Analytical* No interference on TLC using ethyl acetate: methanol: water: ammonium hydroxide and modified Dragendorff's reagent for detection *6502*

Nicotine *Urine* *Positive* *Analytical* Similar R_fs and color reaction on TLC using ethyl acetate: methanol: water: ammonium hydroxide and modified Dragendorff's reagent *6502*

Pentobarbital *Urine* *No Effect* *Analytical* No interference on TLC using ethyl acetate: methanol: water: ammonium hydroxide and modified Dragendorff's reagent for detection *6502*

Phenobarbital *Urine* *No Effect* *Analytical* No interference on TLC using ethyl acetate: methanol: water: ammonium hydroxide and modified Dragendorff's reagent for detection *6502*

Phenylpropanolamine *Urine* *No Effect* *Analytical* No interference on TLC using ethylacetate: methanol: water: ammonium hydroxide and modified Dragendorff's reagent for detection *6502*

Secobarbital *Urine* *No Effect* *Analytical* No interference on TLC using ethyl acetate: methanol: water: ammonium hydroxide and modified Dragendorff's reagent for detection *6502*

Clothiapine

Aspartate Aminotransferase *Serum* *Decrease* *Analytical* At 9 mg/L when added to serum and conventional method *2877*
Serum *No Effect* *Analytical* No effect of concentrations up to 9 mg/L on method on Kodak Ektachem® *5706*

Creatine Kinase *Serum* *Decrease* *Analytical* At 9 mg/L when added to serum and conventional method *2877*

γ-Globulin *Serum* *Decrease* *Analytical* At 9 mg/L when added to serum and conventional method *2877*

Clotiazepam

Alanine Aminotransferase *Serum* *Increase* *Physiological* In single case acute hepatitis with extensive hepatocellular necrosis observed 7 months after onset of administration of drug *2394*

Aspartate Aminotransferase *Serum* *Increase* *Physiological* 7 months after start of administration of drug in a single case acute hepatitis observed with extensive hepatocellular necrosis *2394*

Benzodiazepine *Urine* *Positive* *Analytical* At concentrations of 1.0 µg/mL or greater produces positive result with Syva EMIT II method *1785*

Bilirubin *Serum* *Increase* *Physiological* 7 months after start of treatment acute hepatitis observed with extensive hepatocellular necrosis *2394*

γ-Glutamyltransferase *Serum* *Increase* *Physiological* 7 months after onset of treatment acute hepatitis with extensive hepatic necrosis observed in a single patient *2394*

Clotrimazole

Aspartate Aminotransferase *Serum* *Increase* *Physiological* Reversible increased activity observed in up to 15% patients who had received troches *1384*

Tacrolimus *Serum* *Increase* *Physiological* By inhibiting cytochrome P-450 IIIA enzyme systems may inhibit the metabolism of tacrolimus *1987*

Cloxacillin

Alanine Aminotransferase *Serum* *Increase* *Physiological* Increases linked to drug administration observed in some hemodialysis patients *500*

Albumin *Serum* *No Effect* *Analytical* At concentration of 5 mg/L had no effect on BCG method *5704*

Amino Acids *Urine* *Increase* *Analytical* 2 orange colored spots with ninhydrin on paper or thin-layer chromatography, not present following peroxide oxidation of specimen but new spot appeared *2605*

Aspartate Aminotransferase *Serum* *Increase* *Physiological* Few cases reported, ?due to i.m. injection *128*

Bicarbonate *Serum* *No Effect* *Analytical* At concentration of 5 mg/L had no effect on method using phenolphthalein *5704*

Bilirubin *Serum* *No Effect* *Analytical* At concentration of 5 mg/L had no effect on Jendrassik and Grof method *5704*

Calcium *Serum* *No Effect* *Analytical* At concentration of 5 mg/L had no effect on cresolphthalein method *5704*

Chloride *Serum* *No Effect* *Analytical* At concentration of 5 mg/L had no effect on mercurimetric method *5704*

Cholesterol *Serum* *No Effect* *Analytical* At concentration of 5 mg/L had no effect on CHOD-PAP method *5704*

Creatinine *Serum* *No Effect* *Analytical* No effect of concentrations up to 15 mg/L on single slide method on Kodak Ektachem® *5706* At concentration of 5 mg/L had no effect on Technicon AutoAnalyzer® Jaffe method *5704*

Eosinophils *Blood* *Increase* *Physiological* Hypersensitivity response *2484*

Glucose *Serum* *No Effect* *Analytical* At concentration of 5 mg/L had no effect on GOD/POD-PAP method *5704*

17-Ketosteroids *Urine* *Increase* *Analytical* Interferes with Zimmermann reaction *5869*

Leukocytes *Blood* *Decrease* *Physiological* May cause leukopenia *3810*
Blood *Increase* *Physiological* Due to eosinophilia of hypersensitivity *3810*

Oxacillin *Serum* *Increase* *Analytical* Cannot be assayed by HPLC method used at Mayo Clinic in presence of cloxacillin *3858*

Phosphate *Serum* *No Effect* *Analytical* At concentration of 5 mg/L had no effect on phosphomolybdate method *5704*

Potassium *Serum* *No Effect* *Analytical* At concentration of 5 mg/L had no effect on flame-photometric method *5704*

Protein *Serum* *No Effect* *Analytical* At concentration of 5 mg/L had no effect on biuret method with blank correction *5704*

Sodium *Serum* *No Effect* *Analytical* At concentration of 5 mg/L had no effect on flame-photometric method *5704*

Triglycerides *Serum* *No Effect* *Analytical* At concentration of 5 mg/L had no effect on lipase/esterase method *5704*

Urea Nitrogen *Serum* *No Effect* *Analytical* At concentration of 5 mg/L had no effect on diacetylmonoxime method *5704*

Uric Acid *Serum* *No Effect* *Analytical* At concentration of 5 mg/L had no effect on phosphotungstate reduction method *5704*

Clozapine

Alanine Aminotransferase *Serum* *Increase* *Physiological* In a clinical trial involving 842 patients liver function abnormalities were observed in 1% of treated patients *5229* In 167 patients treated with clozapine 66.9% had activity greater than the upper limit of normal *2773*

Alkaline Phosphatase *Serum* *Increase* *Physiological* In a clinical trial involving 842 patients liver function abnormalities were observed in 1% of treated patients *5229* In 167 patients treated with clozapine 40.6% had activity greater than the upper limit of normal *2773*

Amylase *Serum* *Increase* *Physiological* Acute pancreatitis observed in some patients during post-marketing observations *5229*

Aspartate Aminotransferase *Serum* *Increase* *Physiological* In a clinical trial involving 842 patients liver function abnormalities were observed in 1% of treated patients *5229* In 167 patients treated with clozapine 46.6% had activity greater than the upper limit of normal *2773*

Bilirubin *Serum Increase Physiological* In a clinical trial involving 842 patients liver function abnormalities were observed in 1% of treated patients *5229* In 167 patients treated with clozapine 6.3% had a concentration greater than the upper limit of normal *2773*

Clara Cell Protein *Serum Increase Physiological* In 14 patients with schizophrenia treatment with a mean of 353 ± 163 mg/d clozapine for a median of 12 days caused mean concentration of 40 ± 17 ng/mL to change significantly to 48 ± 18 ng/mL *3731*

Creatine Kinase *Serum Increase Physiological* In 17 acutely psychotic patients treatment with clozapine (1 - 9 determinations per patient) was associated with 2 marked elevations (in 11.8% of the patients) *3947* Increased activity observed in some patients during post-marketing observations *5229*

Digitoxin *Serum Increase Physiological* Because both drugs are highly protein-bound administration of clozapine may increase the plasma concentration of digitoxin *5229*

Eosinophils *Blood Decrease Physiological* Eosinophilia occurred in 1% of 842 treated patients during clinical trials *5229*

Erythrocyte Sedimentation Rate
Blood Increase Physiological Increase observed in some patients during post-marketing observations *5229*

Glucose *Serum Increase Physiological* Increased concentration observed in some patients during post-marketing observations *5229*

γ-Glutamyltransferase *Serum Increase Physiological* In 167 patients treated with clozapine 45.9% had activity greater than the upper limit of normal *2773* In a clinical trial involving 842 patients liver function abnormalities were observed in 1% of treated patients *5229*

Granulocytes *Blood Decrease Physiological* Mechanism of clozapine-induced agranulocytosis unknown, but occurred in 1% of 1700 treated patients during clinical trials *5229* Risk of developing agranulocytosis about 1-2% in treated patients, possibly highest in Jews of Eastern European background. Most commonly condition develops between the 6th and 18th week *1384* In 205 patients with refractory schizophrenia treated for one year neutropenia of less than 1500 granulocytes/µL observed in 8 patients with agranulocytosis developing in 3 of them *5100*

Hematocrit *Blood Decrease Physiological* Anemia occurred in less than 1% of 842 treated patients during clinical trials *5229*
Blood Increase Physiological Hemoconcentration observed in some patients during post-marketing observations *5229*

Hemoglobin *Blood Decrease Physiological* Anemia occurred in less than 1% of 842 treated patients during clinical trials *5229*
Blood Increase Physiological Increased concentration observed in some patients during post-marketing observations *5229*

Interleukin-1 Receptor Antagonist
Serum Increase Physiological In 14 patients with schizophrenia treatment with a mean of 353 ± 163 mg/d clozapine for a median of 12 days caused mean concentration of 0.31 ± 0.37 ng/mL to change significantly to 0.39 ± 0.46 ng/mL *3731*

Interleukin-6 *Serum Increase Physiological* In 14 patients with schizophrenia treatment with a mean of 353 ± 163 mg/d clozapine for a median of 12 days caused 25th to 75th quartiles of 3.7 to 9.9 pg/mL to increase significantly to 7.2 to 14.8 pg/mL *3731*

Leukocytes *Blood Decrease Physiological* Incidence of agranulocytosis of 0.6% reported in patients treated in United States *344* Leukopenia occurred in 3% of 842 treated patients during clinical trials *5229* Agranulocytosis developed in 73 patients out of 11555 who received the drug. Episodes of agranulocytosis occurred in 61 patients within 3 months of after they began treatment. Risk of agranulocytosis increased with age and was greater in women *126* In 205 patients with refractory schizophrenia treated for one year leukopenia of less than 3000 leukocytes/µL observed in 4 patients *5100*
Blood Increase Physiological Leukocytosis occurred in less than 1% of 842 treated patients during clinical trials *5229*

Lipase *Serum Increase Physiological* Acute pancreatitis observed in some patients during post-marketing observations *5229*

Neutrophils *Blood Decrease Physiological* Leukopenia or neutropenia occurred in 3% of 842 treated patients during clinical trials *5229* Occasional case of agranulocytosis reported *6264*

Occult Blood *Feces Increase Physiological* Rectal bleeding or hematemesis occurred in less than 1% of 842 treated patients during clinical trials *5229*

Peptides, Low-molecular Weight
Urine Decrease Physiological In one schizophrenic patient treatment with 400 mg/d for 5 weeks caused significant reduction from 44.1 µmol/d to 16.1 µmol/d *4901*

Platelets *Blood Increase Physiological* Thrombocytosis observed in some patients during post-marketing observations *5229*

Prolactin *Plasma No Effect Physiological* No response to 12.5 mg given orally *2352*

Risperidone *Serum Increase Physiological* Chronic administration of clozapine with risperidone may increase the clearance of risperidone *2904*

Sodium *Serum Decrease Physiological* Decreased concentration observed in some patients during post-marketing observations *5229*

Soluble CD8+ *Serum Increase Physiological* In 14 patients with schizophrenia treatment with clozapine mean 353 ± 163 mg/d for a median of 12 days caused mean concentration at baseline of 489 ± 185 U/mL to increase to 604 ± 236 U/mL *3731*

Soluble Interleukin-6 Receptor
Serum No Effect Physiological In 14 patients with schizophrenia treatment with a mean of 353 ± 163 mg/d clozapine for a median of 12 days caused mean concentration of 179 ± 67 pg/mL to change nonsignificantly to 178 ± 67 pg/mL *3731*

Transferrin Receptor *Serum No Effect Physiological* In 14 patients with schizophrenia treatment with a mean of 353 ± 163 mg/d clozapine for a median of 12 days caused mean concentration of 567 ± 169 U/mL to change nonsignificantly to 616 ± 218 U/mL *3731*

Uric Acid *Serum Increase Physiological* Increased concentration observed in some patients during post-marketing observations *5229*

Warfarin *Plasma Increase Physiological* Because both drugs are highly protein-bound administration of clozapine may increase the plasma concentration of warfarin *5229*

Co-dergocrine

Aldosterone *Plasma No Effect Physiological* Treatment of patients with essential hypertension with 4 mg daily for 3 weeks had no effect on concentration *6122*

Angiotensin-II *Plasma No Effect Physiological* Treatment of patients with essential hypertension with 4 mg daily for 3 weeks had no effect on concentration *6122*

Cholesterol *Serum Decrease Physiological* Concentration reduced by 6% in patients with essential hypertension following treatment with 4 mg daily for 3 weeks *6122*

Epinephrine *Plasma No Effect Physiological* Treatment of patients with essential hypertension with 4 mg daily for 3 weeks had no effect on concentration *6122*

HDL-Triglycerides *Serum Decrease Physiological* Treatment of patients with essential hypertension with 4 mg daily for 3 weeks caused reduction of concentration by 6% *6122*

Norepinephrine *Plasma Decrease Physiological* Reduced concentration of both upright and supine concentrations by 24% in patients with essential hypertension following treatment with 4 mg daily for 3 weeks *6122*

Renin Activity *Plasma No Effect Physiological* Treatment of patients with essential hypertension with 4 mg daily for 3 weeks had no effect *6122*

Volume *Blood No Effect Physiological* Treatment of patients with essential hypertension with 4 mg daily for 3 weeks had no effect *6122*
Plasma No Effect Physiological Treatment of patients with essential hypertension with 4 mg daily for 3 weeks had no effect *6122*

Co-trimoxazole

Chloramphenicol *Serum No Effect Analytical* No effect at 100 mg/L on coupled enzymatic method *4122*

Chlorpropamide *Serum Increase Physiological* Effects of compound may be potentiated *1071*

Creatinine *Serum Increase Physiological* Usually reversible effect (in many patients) *3016* By 0.2 mg/dL in 21 patients: probably due to competitive inhibition of tubular secretion of trimethoprim *505* Change of 0.12 mg/dL in 5 volunteers after 7 days *5136*

Creatinine Clearance *Urine Decrease Physiological* Usually reversible effect (in many patients) *3016*

Crystals *Urine Increase Physiological* Single case reported *3016* May occur with high doses of drug, particularly in patients with severe renal insufficiency *1071*

Hematocrit *Blood Increase Physiological* May cause megaloblastic anemia *1156*

Hemoglobin *Blood Decrease Physiological* May cause hemolysis if G-6-PD deficiency *4466*

Leukocytes *Blood Decrease Physiological* Isolated cases reported *1046* May cause leukopenia *1156*

Methemoglobin *Blood Increase Physiological* Possible effect of drug or sulfonamides *2753*

Neutrophils *Blood Decrease Physiological* Also reduced survival of transfused platelets due to drug associated antibodies *1046*

Nifedipine *Serum No Effect Physiological* In 9 healthy volunteers no effect on maximum plasma concentration, elimination half-life or area under plasma concentration curve of nifedipine or its primary oxidized metabolite after a single oral dose of 20 mg with/without co-trimoxazole pretreatment *1665*

Phenylalanine *Plasma Increase Physiological* 4 h after 0.1 g/kg orally *1735*
Plasma No Effect Analytical No interference observed with rapid quantitative whole blood method of Campbell et al using phenylalanine dehydrogenase *867*

Phenytoin *Serum Increase Physiological* Effects of compound may be potentiated *1071*

Platelets *Blood Decrease Physiological* Highly significant effect in warfarin treated patients but no effect on warfarin half-life *1046* May cause thrombocytopenia *1156* Effects of compound may be potentiated *3102*

Protein *Urine No Effect Analytical* No effect of up to 4 tablets daily in 4 patients on sulfosalicylic acid, trichloroacetic acid and Ponceau S Dye Methods *6611*

Prothrombin Time *Plasma Increase Physiological* Several cases of platelet-associated IgG and thrombocytopenia *4430*

Theophylline *Serum No Effect Physiological* No documented significant interaction with theophylline reported *6117* No clinically significant effect on theophylline concentration observed when drugs coadministered *5999*

Thyroid Stimulating Hormone
Serum No Effect Physiological In men or women with treatment for 10 days *1077*

Thyroxine (T4) *Serum Decrease Physiological* Marked decrease possibly due to intrathyroidal inhibition of conversion of iodine to organic form *6412* From 97.1 to 83.0 nmol/L in men and 92.6 to 87.2 nmol/L in women with 10 days treatment *1077*

Thyroxine (T4) Index, Free *Serum Decrease Physiological* Marked decrease possibly due to intrathyroidal inhibition of conversion of iodine to organic form *6412* From 95.2 to 82.6 in men and 90.1 to 86.4 in women with 10 days treatment *1077*

Tolbutamide *Serum Increase Physiological* Effects of compound may be potentiated *1071*

Tri-iodothyronine (T3) *Serum Decrease Physiological* From 2.33 to 1.96 nmol/L in men and 1.76 to 1.53 nmol/L in women after 10 days treatment *1077* Marked decrease possibly due to intrathyroidal inhibition of conversion of iodine to organic form *3297*

Urea Nitrogen *Serum Increase Analytical* In patients receiving high oral doses or intravenously concentration significantly increased when urea measured by o-phthaldehyde although no effect observed on urease procedure *3545*
Serum Increase Physiological Uremia occurs if anemia, urine infection G-6-PD deficiency *4466* Usually reversible effect (in many patients) *3016*

Warfarin *Plasma Increase Physiological* Effects of compound may be potentiated *1071*

Cobalamin

Albumin *Urine No Effect Analytical* Using a fluorimetric assay with Albumin Blue 580 on a Cobas Fara centrifugal analyzer for the detection of microalbuminuria no significant interference was detected at a concentration of 0.006 mg/L *3117*

Methylmalonate *Serum Decrease Physiological* High concentration in cobalamin deficient individuals reduced with intramuscular administration of cobalamin *4867*

Cobalt

Erythrocytes *Blood Increase Physiological* Reported to cause increased red cell production *3661*

Hematocrit *Blood Increase Physiological* Polycythemia observed with poisoning *3661*

^{131}I Uptake *Serum Decrease Physiological* Reported effect *3669* Due to impaired synthesis of thyroxine *3107*

Lipids *Serum Increase Physiological* Profound hyperlipemia, xanthomatosis in one case *3661*

Nickel *Test Conditions Increase Analytical* Possible interference with atomic absorption *5866*

T3-Uptake *Serum Increase Physiological* Resin uptake increased with impaired synthesis of T4 *3107*

Thyroxine (T4) *Serum Decrease Physiological* Impaired synthesis from tyrosine *3107*

Cobinamide

Vitamin B_{12} *Serum No Effect Analytical* Cross-reactivity of about 0.75% observed over a wide range of concentrations in vitamin B_{12} method on Bayer Technicon Immuno 1® *439*

Cod-Liver Oil

Albumin *Urine No Effect Physiological* Insignificant reduction with 8 weeks treatment of 18 patients with insulin-dependent diabetes mellitus and albuminuria *2931*

Glomerular Filtration Rate *Urine No Effect Physiological* No effect of 8 weeks dietary supplementation in 18 patients with insulin-dependent diabetes mellitus and albuminuria *2931*

Glucose *Serum No Effect Physiological* Insignificant increase in 18 patients with diabetes mellitus and albuminuria with 8 weeks therapy *2931*

Hemoglobin A_{1c} *Blood No Effect Physiological* No change in 18 patients with insulin-dependent diabetes mellitus given dietary supplement for 8 weeks *2931*

Volume *Plasma No Effect Physiological* No significant effect of 8 weeks dietary supplementation in 18 patients with insulin-dependent diabetes mellitus and albuminuria *2931*

Codeine

Acetaminophen *Serum No Effect Analytical* At concentration of 10 mg/L had no effect on HPLC method *5775* No interference at a concentration of 2000 µg/mL (668 µmol/L) with method on Du Pont aca *1506*

Alanine Aminotransferase *Serum Increase Physiological* Rise in intrabiliary pressure especially if liver disease *5869*
Serum No Effect Analytical At acute overdose concentration (2.0 mg/dL) on Technicon SMAC® method *6266*

Albumin *Serum No Effect Analytical* At concentration of 20 mg/L had no effect on BCG method *5704* At acute overdose concentration (2.0 mg/dL) on Technicon SMAC® method *6266*

Alkaline Phosphatase *Serum No Effect Analytical* At acute overdose concentration (2.0 mg/dL) on Technicon SMAC® method *6266*

Amylase *Serum Increase Physiological* May cause spasm of sphincter of Oddi *2242*

Aspartate Aminotransferase *Serum Increase Physiological* May cause rise in intrabiliary pressure *5869*
Serum No Effect Analytical At acute overdose concentration (2.0 mg/dL) on Technicon SMAC® method *6266*

Benzoylecgonine *Urine No Effect Analytical* Negative result obtained at a concentration of 500 µg/mL (1.60 mmol/L) with method on Du Pont aca *1558* No interference observed at a concentration of 167 µmol/L with Sung and Neely modification of Syva EMIT procedure *148*

Bicarbonate *Serum No Effect Analytical* At concentration of 1 mg/L had no effect on method using phenolphthalein *5704*

Bilirubin *Serum No Effect Analytical* At concentration of 20 mg/L had no effect on Jendrassik and Grof method *5704* At acute overdose concentration (2.0 mg/dL) on Technicon SMAC® method *6266*

Calcium *Serum No Effect Analytical* At acute overdose concentration (2.0 mg/dL) on Technicon SMAC® method *6266* At concentration of 20 mg/L had no effect on cresolphthalein method *5704*

Cannabinoids *Urine No Effect Analytical* No effect on Roche Abuscreen method *5006*

Carbon Dioxide Partial Pressure
Blood Increase Physiological May cause respiratory depression *2242*

Chloride *Serum No Effect Analytical* At concentration of 1 mg/L had no effect on mercurimetric method *5704*

Cholesterol *Serum No Effect Analytical* At acute overdose concentration (2.0 mg/dL) on Technicon SMAC® method *6266* At concentration of 20 mg/L had no effect on Liebermann-Burchard method *5704* At concentration of 0.1 mg/L had no effect on CHOD-PAP method *5704*

Cholinesterase *Serum No Effect Analytical* No effect observed at concentration of 25 mg/dL with butyrylthiocholine method on Kodak Ektachem® *2504*

Cocaethylene *Urine No Effect Analytical* No interference observed with TLC method of Bailey *328*

Codeine *Cerebrospinal Fluid Increase Physiological* In 8 patients given 125 mg codeine median concentration 2 h later 387 nmol/L *5571*
Serum Increase Physiological In 8 patients given 125 mg codeine median concentration 2 h later 485 nmol/L *5571*

Creatine Kinase *Serum No Effect Analytical* At acute overdose concentration (2.0 mg/dL) on Technicon SMAC® method *6266*

Creatinine *Serum No Effect Analytical* At acute overdose concentration (2 mg/dL) on Technicon SMAC® method *6266* At concentration of 20 mg/L had no effect on Technicon AutoAnalyzer® Jaffe method *5704*

Doxazosin *Serum No Effect Physiological* Coadministration with doxazosin had no effect on its pharmacokinetics *4642*

Drugs of Abuse Screen *Urine No Effect Analytical* No effect at concentration of 100 µg/mL on EZ-SCREEN procedure for cannabinoids and cocaine *1739*

Glucose *Serum No Effect Analytical* At acute overdose concentration (2.0 mg/dL) on Technicon SMAC® method *6266* At concentration of 0.1 mg/L had no effect on GOD/POD-PAP method *5704*

Histamine *Plasma No Effect Analytical* Improbable inhibition of radio-enzyme assay at therapeutic concentrations *2492*

Iron *Serum No Effect Analytical* At acute overdose concentration (2.0 mg/dL) on Technicon SMAC® method *6266* At concentration of 20 mg/L had no effect on Ferrozine method *5704*

Lactate Dehydrogenase *Serum Increase Physiological* May cause rise in intrabiliary pressure *5869*
Serum No Effect Analytical At acute overdose concentration (2.0 mg/dL) on Technicon SMAC® method *6266*

Lipase *Serum Increase Physiological* Causes spasm of sphincter of Oddi *6377*

Morphine *Serum Increase Physiological* In 8 patients given 125 mg codeine median concentration 2 h later 9.86 nmol/L *5571*
Urine Increase Analytical Significant interference observed at a concentration of 3.3 µmol/L with Sung and Neely modification of Syva EMIT method *148* Cross reacts equally (or more) with RIA procedures. Greater reaction than morphine with EMIT procedure. Substantial cross reaction hemagglutination inhibition procedure *4163*

Opiates *Urine Positive Analytical* At concentration of 1.0 µg/mL (3.33 µmol/L) with method on Du Pont aca *1559* Significant cross-reactivity observed with Roche Abuscreen method adapted for use with Olympus AU 5121 and 5131 analyzers *214* Cross-reactivity of over 50% observed with Roche Abuscreen Online procedure when adapted for use with Roche Cobas Fara II analyzer *5547*

p-Aminophenol *Urine No Effect Analytical* With addition of drugs at a concentration of 100 mg/L and of related compounds at 50 mg/L no significant effect observed on colorimetric method of van Bocxlaer on Cobas Mira analyzer which involves reacting free p-aminophenol with resorcinol in the presence of magnesium ions to form an indophenol dye measured at 550 nm *6163*

Phenylalanine *Plasma No Effect Analytical* No interference observed from codeine phosphate with rapid quantitative whole blood method of Campbell et al using phenylalanine dehydrogenase *867*

Phosphate *Serum No Effect Analytical* At acute overdose concentration (2.0 mg/dL) on Technicon SMAC® method *6266* At concentration of 20 mg/L had no effect on phosphomolybdate method *5704*

Platelets *Blood Decrease Physiological* Thrombocytopenia reported to occur *2385*

Potassium *Serum No Effect Analytical* At concentration of 0.1 mg/L had no effect on flame-photometric method *5704*

Protein *Serum No Effect Analytical* At acute overdose concentration (2.0 mg/dL) on Technicon SMAC® method *6266* At concentration of 20 mg/L had no effect on biuret method with blank correction *5704*
Urine Increase Physiological May cause nephropathy *4265*

Sodium *Serum No Effect Analytical* At concentration of 0.1 mg/L had no effect on flame-photometric method *5704*

Theophylline *Serum No Effect Analytical* No effect on Kodak Ektachem® 700 method *1716*

Triglycerides *Serum No Effect Analytical* At concentration of 20 mg/L had no effect on lipase/esterase method *5704* At acute overdose concentration (2.0 mg/dL) on Technicon SMAC® method *6266*

Urea Nitrogen *Serum Increase Physiological* May cause nephropathy *4265*
Serum No Effect Analytical At acute overdose concentration (2.0 mg/dL) on Technicon SMAC® method *6266* At concentration of 20 mg/L had no effect on diacetylmonoxime method *5704*

Uric Acid *Serum No Effect Analytical* At acute overdose concentration (2.0 mg/dL) on Technicon SMAC® method *6266* At concentration of 20 mg/L had no effect on phosphotungstate reduction method *5704*

Coenzyme Q10

Aldosterone *Urine No Effect Physiological* In 10 patients with essential hypertension treated with 100 mg/d for 10 weeks no significant effect observed *1427*

Cholesterol *Serum Decrease Physiological* In 10 patients with essential hypertension treated with 100 mg/d for 10 weeks mean concentration decreased from 227 ± 24 mg/dL to 204 ± 21 mg/dL *1427*

Coenzyme Q_{10} *Serum Increase Physiological* In 10 patients with essential hypertension treated with 100 mg/d for 10 weeks concentration of CoQ10 increased from 0.69 ± 0.1 µg/mL to 1.95 ± 0.3 µg/mL *1427*

HDL-Cholesterol *Serum Increase Physiological* In 10 patients with essential hypertension treatment with 100 mg/d for 10 weeks caused increase from 42 ± 3 mg/dL to 46 ± 3 mg/dL *1427*

Potassium *Serum No Effect Physiological* In 10 patients with essential hypertension treatment with 100 mg/d for 10 weeks had no significant effect on concentration *1427*
Urine No Effect Physiological In 10 patients with essential hypertension treatment with 100 mg/d for 10 weeks had no significant effect on excretion *1427*

Coenzyme Q10 *(continued)*

Renin Activity *Plasma No Effect Physiological* In 10 patients with essential hypertension treated with 100 mg/d for 10 weeks no significant change in concentration observed *1427*

Sodium *Serum No Effect Physiological* In 10 patients with essential hypertension treatment with 100 mg/d for 10 weeks had no significant effect *1427*

Urine No Effect Physiological In 10 patients with essential hypertension treatment with 100 mg/d for 10 weeks had no significant effect on excretion *1427*

Colchicine

Alanine Aminotransferase *Serum Increase Physiological* Possible hepatotoxic effect *3669*

Serum No Effect Physiological Treatment of 44 patients with primary sclerosing cholangitis 1 mg/d for up to 3 years had no significant effect on test values *4414*

Albumin *Serum No Effect Physiological* Treatment of 44 patients with primary sclerosing cholangitis 1 mg/d for up to 3 years had no significant effect on test values *4414*

Alkaline Phosphatase *Serum Decrease Physiological* In 24 patients with primary biliary cirrhosis treatment with 1 mg/d for 2 years caused nonsignificant change of 351 ± 68 U/L from mean baseline *4026*

Serum Increase Physiological Possible hepatotoxic effect *3669*

Serum No Effect Physiological Treatment of 44 patients with primary sclerosing cholangitis 1 mg/d for up to 3 years had no significant effect on test values *4414*

Amino-4-Imidazole-5-Carboxamide Ribotide

Urine Increase Physiological Megaloblastic anemia with B_{12} deficiency *6370*

α_1-Antitrypsin *Serum No Effect Physiological* Treatment of 44 patients with primary sclerosing cholangitis 1 mg/d for up to 3 years had no significant effect on test values *4414*

Aspartate Aminotransferase *Serum Increase Physiological* Possible hepatotoxic effect *3669*

Serum No Effect Physiological Treatment of 44 patients with primary sclerosing cholangitis 1 mg/d for up to 3 years had no significant effect on test values *4414*

Bile *Urine Increase Physiological* May cause hepatotoxicity *3810*

Bilirubin *Serum Increase Physiological* May cause hepatic toxicity *3810*

Serum No Effect Physiological In 24 patients with primary biliary cirrhosis treatment with 1 mg/d for 2 years caused nonsignificant change of 0.0 ± 2.5 μmol/L from mean baseline *4026* Treatment of 44 patients with primary sclerosing cholangitis 1 mg/d for up to 3 years had no significant effect on test values *4414*

BSP Retention *Serum Increase Physiological* May cause hepatic toxicity *3810*

Campesterol *Serum Increase Physiological* In 24 patients with primary biliary cirrhosis treatment with 1 mg/d for 2 years caused nonsignificant change of + 59 ± 33 x 10 mmol/mol cholesterol from mean baseline of 291 ± 40 x 10 mmol/mol cholesterol *4026*

Ceruloplasmin *Serum No Effect Physiological* Treatment of 44 patients with primary sclerosing cholangitis 1 mg/d for up to 3 years had no significant effect on test values *4414*

Cholestanol *Serum Decrease Physiological* In 24 patients with primary biliary cirrhosis treatment with 1 mg/d for 2 years caused significant change of - 19 ± 10 x 10 mmol/mol cholesterol from mean baseline of 320 ± 44 x 10 mmol/mol cholesterol *4026*

δ^8-Cholestanol *Serum Increase Physiological* In 24 patients with primary biliary cirrhosis treatment with 1 mg/d for 2 years caused significant change of + 3.8 ± 1.6 x 10 mmol/mol cholesterol from mean baseline of 11.0 ± 1.1 x 10 mmol/mol cholesterol *4026*

Cholesterol *Serum Decrease Physiological* In 24 patients with primary biliary cirrhosis treatment with 1 mg/d for 2 years caused significant change of - 0.72 ± 0.31 mmol/L from mean baseline of 6.45 ± 0.40 mmol/L *4026* May have hepatotoxic effect *5145* In 24 patients with primary biliary cirrhosis treatment with 1 mg/d for 2 years caused nonsignificant change of - 1.00 ± 0.64 mmol/L from mean baseline of 7.08 ± 0.98 mmol/L *4026*

Cholesterol, Esterified *Serum Decrease Physiological* In 24 patients with primary biliary cirrhosis treatment with 1 mg/d for 2 years caused nonsignificant change of - 0.33 ± 0.26 mmol/L from mean baseline of 4.40 ± 0.26 mmol/L *4026*

Cholesterol, Free *Serum Decrease Physiological* In 24 patients with primary biliary cirrhosis treatment with 1 mg/d for 2 years caused nonsignificant change of - 0.68 ± 0.41 mmol/L from mean baseline of 2.68 ± 0.75 mmol/L *4026*

Cholinesterase *Serum No Effect Analytical* No effect observed at concentration of 35 ng/dL with butyrylthiocholine method on Kodak Ektachem® *2504*

Chromosomes *Test Conditions Abnormal Physiological* Inhibits mitosis at metaphase in human cells *5484*

Cyclosporine *Blood Increase Physiological* Coadministration of colchicine with cyclosporine to a single renal transplant recipient caused a significant increase in the cyclosporine concentration and was associated with renal impairment *859* Observed in one renal transplant recipient within 2 days of receiving 4 mg oral colchicine, associated with renal impairment *3955*

Serum Increase Physiological Coadministration of colchicine with cyclosporine to a single renal transplant recipient caused a significant increase in the cyclosporine concentration and was associated with renal impairment *859* In one renal transplant patient 4 mg colchicine caused increased cyclosporine and creatinine concentrations within two days *6596*

Desmosterol *Serum Increase Physiological* In 24 patients with primary biliary cirrhosis treatment with 1 mg/d for 2 years caused nonsignificant change of + 4 ± 3 x 10 mmol/mol cholesterol from mean baseline of 63 ± 6 x 10 mmol/mol cholesterol *4026*

Erythrocytes *Blood Decrease Physiological* Megaloblastic anemia (impaired absorption of vitamin B_{12}) *6370*

Urine Increase Physiological May cause bleeding *3810*

Fat *Feces Increase Physiological* May cause villus damage and impaired regeneration of the epithelial cells of small intestine *5055*

HDL-Cholesterol *Serum Decrease Physiological* In 24 patients with primary biliary cirrhosis treatment with 1 mg/d for 2 years caused nonsignificant change of - 0.01 ± 0.25 mmol/L from mean baseline of 1.65 ± 0.22 mmol/L *4026*

HDL-Cholesterol, Esterified *Serum Increase Physiological* In 24 patients with primary biliary cirrhosis treatment with 1 mg/d for 2 years caused nonsignificant change of + 0.07 ± 0.17 mmol/L from mean baseline of 1.14 ± 0.18 mmol/L *4026*

HDL-Cholesterol, Free *Serum Decrease Physiological* In 24 patients with primary biliary cirrhosis treatment with 1 mg/d for 2 years caused nonsignificant change of - 0.08 ± 0.09 mmol/L from mean baseline of 0.51 ± 0.07 mmol/L *4026*

HDL-Phospholipids *Serum Decrease Physiological* In 24 patients with primary biliary cirrhosis treatment with 1 mg/d for 2 years caused nonsignificant change of - 0.17 ± 0.15 mmol/L from mean baseline of 1.72 ± 0.16 mmol/L *4026*

HDL-Triglycerides *Serum Decrease Physiological* In 24 patients with primary biliary cirrhosis treatment with 1 mg/d for 2 years caused nonsignificant change of - 0.03 ± 0.03 mmol/L from mean baseline of 0.22 ± 0.03 mmol/L *4026*

Hematocrit *Blood Decrease Physiological* Megaloblastic anemia (impaired absorption of vitamin B_{12}) *6370*

Hemoglobin *Blood Decrease Physiological* Megaloblastic anemia (impaired absorption of vitamin B_{12}) *6370*

Urine Increase Physiological May cause bleeding *3810*

17-Hydroxycorticosteroids *Urine Increase Analytical* Interferes with Porter-Silber reaction *5869*

IDL-Cholesterol *Serum Increase Physiological* In 24 patients with primary biliary cirrhosis treatment with 1 mg/d for 2 years caused nonsignificant change of + 0.03 ± 0.03 mmol/L from mean baseline of 0.26 ± 0.05 mmol/L *4026*

IDL-Cholesterol, Esterified *Serum Increase Physiological* In 24 patients with primary biliary cirrhosis treatment with 1 mg/d for 2 years caused significant change of + 0.04 ± 0.02 mmol/L from mean baseline of 0.15 ± 0.03 mmol/L *4026*

IDL-Cholesterol, Free *Serum Decrease Physiological* In 24 patients with primary biliary cirrhosis treatment with 1 mg/d for 2 years caused nonsignificant change of - 0.01 ± 0.01 mmol/L from mean baseline of 0.11 ± 0.19 mmol/L *4026*

IDL-Phospholipids *Serum Increase Physiological* In 24 patients with primary biliary cirrhosis treatment with 1 mg/d for 2 years caused nonsignificant change of + 0.01 ± 0.01 mmol/L from mean baseline of 0.12 ± 0.03 mmol/L *4026*

IDL-Triglycerides *Serum Increase Physiological* In 24 patients with primary biliary cirrhosis treatment with 1 mg/d for 2 years caused nonsignificant change of + 0.01 ± 0.02 mmol/L from mean baseline of 0.11 ± 0.03 mmol/L *4026*

Immunoglobulin A *Serum No Effect Physiological* Treatment of 44 patients with primary sclerosing cholangitis 1 mg/d for up to 3 years had no significant effect on test values *4414*

Immunoglobulin G *Serum No Effect Physiological* Treatment of 44 patients with primary sclerosing cholangitis 1 mg/d for up to 3 years had no significant effect on test values *4414*

Immunoglobulin M *Serum No Effect Physiological* Treatment of 44 patients with primary sclerosing cholangitis 1 mg/d for up to 3 years had no significant effect on test values *4414*

Interleukin-2 *Serum Decrease Physiological* In 28 patients with primary biliary cirrhosis mean concentration decreased with treatment from 57 ± 24 pg/mL to 40 ± 22 pg/mL *4047*

Lathosterol *Serum Increase Physiological* In 24 patients with primary biliary cirrhosis treatment with 1 mg/d for 2 years caused significant change of + 27 ± 13 x 10 mmol/mol cholesterol from mean baseline of 119 ± 11 x 10 mmol/mol cholesterol *4026*

LDL-Cholesterol *Serum Decrease Physiological* In 24 patients with primary biliary cirrhosis treatment with 1 mg/d for 2 years caused nonsignificant change of - 0.96 ± 0.57 mmol/L from mean baseline of 4.14 ± 0.94 mmol/L *4026*

LDL-Cholesterol, Esterified *Serum Decrease Physiological* In 24 patients with primary biliary cirrhosis treatment with 1 mg/d for 2 years caused nonsignificant change of - 0.41 ± 0.25 mmol/L from mean baseline of 2.43 ± 0.31 mmol/L *4026*

LDL-Cholesterol, Free *Serum Decrease Physiological* In 24 patients with primary biliary cirrhosis treatment with 1 mg/d for 2 years caused nonsignificant change of - 0.55 ± 0.34 mmol/L from mean baseline of 1.71 ± 0.66 mmol/L *4026*

LDL-Phospholipids *Serum Decrease Physiological* In 24 patients with primary biliary cirrhosis treatment with 1 mg/d for 2 years caused nonsignificant change of - 0.67 ± 0.55 mmol/L from mean baseline of 2.10 ± 0.91 mmol/L *4026*

LDL-Triglycerides *Serum Decrease Physiological* In 24 patients with primary biliary cirrhosis treatment with 1 mg/d for 2 years caused nonsignificant change of - 0.08 ± 0.16 mmol/L from mean baseline of 0.39 ± 0.17 mmol/L *4026*

Leukocytes *Blood Decrease Physiological* Leukopenia *4013*

Blood Increase Physiological Leukocytosis follows initial leukopenia *2242*

MCV *Blood Increase Physiological* Megaloblastic anemia with B_{12} deficiency *6370*

Methylmalonate *Urine Increase Physiological* Occurs with impaired absorption of B_{12}*6370*

Neutrophils *Blood Decrease Physiological* Occasional case of agranulocytosis reported *6264*

N-Formiminoglutamic Acid *Urine Increase Physiological* Megaloblastic anemia with B_{12} deficiency *6370*

Occult Blood *Feces Increase Physiological* Toxicity effect *3810*

Phospholipids *Serum Decrease Physiological* In 24 patients with primary biliary cirrhosis treatment with 1 mg/d for 2 years caused nonsignificant change of - 0.69 ± 0.34 mmol/L from mean baseline of 4.48 ± 0.79 mmol/L *4026*

Platelets *Blood Decrease Physiological* Selective thrombocytopenia or aplastic anemia *4013*

Prazosin *Serum No Effect Physiological* Coadministration of prazosin with colchicine had no apparent adverse drug interaction in limited clinical experience *4649*

Prothrombin *Plasma No Effect Physiological* Treatment of 44 patients with primary sclerosing cholangitis 1 mg/d for up to 3 years had no significant effect on test values *4414*

Prothrombin Time *Plasma Decrease Physiological* Patients on coumarins *4013*

Sitosterol *Serum Increase Physiological* In 24 patients with primary biliary cirrhosis treatment with 1 mg/d for 2 years caused nonsignificant change of + 13 ± 19 x 10 mmol/mol cholesterol from mean baseline of 222 ± 31 x 10 mmol/mol cholesterol *4026*

Sperm Count *Semen Decrease Physiological* Potent antispermatogenic action observed *4726*

Squalene *Serum Increase Physiological* In 24 patients with primary biliary cirrhosis treatment with 1 mg/d for 2 years caused nonsignificant change of + 4.8 ± 3.5 x 10 mmol/mol cholesterol from mean baseline of 35.3 ± 2.7 x 10 mmol/mol cholesterol *4026*

Triglycerides *Serum Increase Physiological* In 24 patients with primary biliary cirrhosis treatment with 1 mg/d for 2 years caused significant change of + 0.18 ± 0.22 mmol/L from mean baseline of 1.37 ± 0.27 mmol/L *4026*

Tumor Necrosis Factor-α *Serum Decrease Physiological* In 28 patients with primary biliary cirrhosis treatment with colchicine caused decrease from mean of 586 ± 295 pg/mL to 445 ± 295 pg/mL *4047*

Uric Acid *Serum No Effect Analytical* No effect at 3000 mg/L on uricase method on Ames Seralyzer *5706*

Vitamin B_{12} *Serum Decrease Physiological* Reduced absorption due to ileal blockade *6403* Impairs absorption *6370*

Urine Decrease Physiological Occurs with impaired absorption of B_{12}*6370*

VLDL-Cholesterol *Serum Increase Physiological* In 24 patients with primary biliary cirrhosis treatment with 1 mg/d for 2 years caused significant change of + 0.14 ± 0.11 mmol/L from mean baseline of 0.41 ± 0.10 mmol/L *4026*

VLDL-Cholesterol, Esterified *Serum Increase Physiological* In 24 patients with primary biliary cirrhosis treatment with 1 mg/d for 2 years caused significant change of + 0.12 ± 0.08 mmol/L from mean baseline of 0.22 ± 0.06 mmol/L *4026*

VLDL-Cholesterol, Free *Serum Increase Physiological* In 24 patients with primary biliary cirrhosis treatment with 1 mg/d for 2 years caused significant change of + 0.02 ± 0.04 mmol/L from mean baseline of 0.19 ± 0.04 mmol/L *4026*

VLDL-Phospholipids *Serum Increase Physiological* In 24 patients with primary biliary cirrhosis treatment with 1 mg/d for 2 years caused significant change of + 0.08 ± 0.04 mmol/L from mean baseline of 0.26 ± 0.05 mmol/L *4026*

VLDL-Triglycerides *Serum Increase Physiological* In 24 patients with primary biliary cirrhosis treatment with 1 mg/d for 2 years caused significant change of + 0.28 ± 0.15 mmol/L from mean baseline of 0.56 ± 0.15 mmol/L *4026*

Xylose *Urine Decrease Physiological* Decreased absorption from gut, disturbs epithelial cell function and causes reduced excretion *4828*

Colestipol

Alanine Aminotransferase *Serum Increase Physiological* Transient increases in activity have rarely in patients treated with colestipol *4669*

Alkaline Phosphatase *Serum Increase Physiological* Transient increases in activity have rarely in patients treated with colestipol *4669*

Apolipoprotein A-I *Serum Increase Physiological* Increased intestinal apo A-I synthesis *264*

Apolipoprotein A-II *Serum No Effect Physiological* No significant effect observed *264*

Apolipoprotein B *Serum Decrease Physiological* In 18 patients with familial hypercholesterolemia 8 weeks treatment with 15 g/d caused mean reduction of 8.6% *6400*

Aspartate Aminotransferase *Serum Increase Physiological* Transient increases in activity have rarely in patients treated with colestipol *4669*

Atorvastatin *Serum Decrease Physiological* When colestipol was coadministered with atorvastatin the latter's plasma concentration was reduced by about 25% although LDL-cholesterol concentration was reduced to a greater extent *4534*

Bile Acids *Feces Increase Physiological* Binds bile acids in intestine and increases fecal loss from normal 1 g/d to about 2 - 3 g/d *5586*

Colestipol *(continued)*

Carotenoids *Serum Decrease Physiological* Increase by 30% with 30 g daily of drug *4794*

Chenodiol *Serum Decrease Physiological* Binds chenodiol in gastrointestinal tract and inhibits its absorption *1384*

Chlorophenoxyisobutyric acid
Serum Decrease Physiological Cholestyramine can decrease the rate of absorption of clofibrate and reduce its plasma concentration, although clinical significance not established *3668*

Chlorothiazide *Serum Decrease Physiological* Effect probably occurs through colestipol inhibiting absorption of diuretic in gastrointestinal tract *2778* Reduced absorption due to binding *6403*
Urine Decrease Physiological Absorption from gastrointestinal tract markedly reduced when administered one hour before colestipol: urinary excretion rather than serum concentration of chlorothiazide used as marker of overall absorption *4669*

Cholesterol *Serum Decrease Physiological* Therapeutic intent *1480* In 98 patients with moderate hypercholesterolemia treatment with 10 g/d for 12 weeks caused significant 12% reduction in concentration *3698* Concentration reduced because of loss of bile acids in gastrointestinal tract and reduction of body pools of cholesterol *5586*

Clindamycin *Serum No Effect Physiological* Absorption from gastrointestinal tract apparently unaffected when drug administered simultaneously with colestipol *4669*

Clofibrate *Serum No Effect Physiological* Absorption from gastrointestinal tract apparently unaffected when drug administered simultaneously with colestipol *4669*

Digitoxin *Serum Decrease Physiological* Reduced bioavailability due to binding in gastrointestinal tract *4631* Absorption from gastrointestinal tract may be affected when drug administered simultaneously with colestipol *4669*

Digoxin *Serum Decrease Physiological* In one patient drug given for 2 d reduced half-life of digoxin by approximately 50% (from 4 to 2 d) *827* Absorption from gastrointestinal tract may be affected when drug administered simultaneously with colestipol *4669*

Fat *Feces Increase Physiological* Bile acid sequestrant may cause steatorrhea with conventional dosage schedules *5055*

Furosemide *Serum Decrease Physiological* Absorption from gastrointestinal tract markedly reduced when administered simultaneously with colestipol *4669*

Gemfibrozil *Serum Decrease Physiological* Colestipol may inhibit the absorption of gemfibrozil when drugs are coadministered, probably due to binding of gemfibrozil to colestipol in the gastrointestinal tract *3668* Absorption from gastrointestinal tract markedly reduced when administered simultaneously with colestipol *4669*

HDL-Cholesterol *Serum Increase Physiological* Increased intestinal apo A-I synthesis *264* In 98 patients with moderate hypercholesterolemia treatment with 10 g/d for 12 weeks caused significant 7% increase in concentration *3698*

Homocysteine *Plasma Increase Physiological* Concentration increased when colestipol administered with niacin possibly through interference with folate absorption *6123*

Hydrochlorothiazide *Serum Decrease Physiological* Absorption from gastrointestinal tract markedly reduced when administered simultaneously with colestipol *4669* A single dose of colestipol reduces the absorption of hydrochlorothiazide by 43% *1028*

Hydroflumethiazide *Serum Decrease Physiological* May inhibit gastrointestinal absorption unless colestipol given one hour before or 4 after hydroflumethiazide administration *6553*

Ketoprofen *Serum No Effect Physiological* Administration of 10 g to 6 healthy men had no significant effect on concentration of ketoprofen after intramuscular injection of 50 mg *1726*

LDL-Cholesterol *Serum Decrease Physiological* Treatment caused disproportionate decrease relative to that of LDL Apo B *6619* In 98 patients with moderate hypercholesterolemia treatment with 10 g/d for 12 weeks caused significant 19% reduction *3698* Compensatory increase of LDL-receptors in liver observed in response to loss of bile acids in gastrointestinal tract and reduction of cholesterol pool leading to increased uptake of LDL from plasma and reduction of LDL-cholesterol *5586* In 18 patients with familial hypercholesterolemia 8 weeks treatment with 15 g/d caused mean reduction of 18.4% *6400*

Methyldopa *Serum No Effect Physiological* Absorption from gastrointestinal tract apparently unaffected when drug administered simultaneously with colestipol *4669*

Nicotinic Acid *Serum No Effect Physiological* Absorption from gastrointestinal tract apparently unaffected when drug administered simultaneously with colestipol *4669*

Penicillin G *Serum Decrease Physiological* Absorption from gastrointestinal tract markedly reduced when administered simultaneously with colestipol *4669*

Phenytoin *Serum No Effect Physiological* Absorption from gastrointestinal tract apparently unaffected when drug administered simultaneously with colestipol *4669* Pretreatment with 10 g appeared to have no effect on absorption of 100 mg phenytoin over 72 hours in 6 healthy men *847*

Pravastatin *Serum Decrease Physiological* Concomitant administration of cholestyramine and colestipol with pravastatin caused an approximately 40 - 50% decrease of AUC of pravastatin *728*
Serum No Effect Physiological Administration of colestipol one hour after pravastatin caused no effect on concentration of pravastatin *728*

Propranolol *Serum Decrease Physiological* Repeated doses of colestipol given before a single dose of propranolol reported to reduce its absorption *4669* Significant reduction of peak concentration and area under curve due to binding in gastrointestinal tract *2587*

Salicylate *Serum No Effect Physiological* Absorption from gastrointestinal tract apparently unaffected when aspirin administered simultaneously with colestipol *4669*

T3-Uptake *Serum Increase Physiological* Observed in euthyroid patients when drug given together with niacin *912*

Tetracycline *Serum Decrease Physiological* Absorption from gastrointestinal tract markedly reduced when administered simultaneously with colestipol *4669*

Thyroxine Binding Globulin
Serum Decrease Physiological Observed in euthyroid patients when drug given together with niacin *912*

Thyroxine (T4) *Serum Decrease Physiological* Observed in euthyroid patients when drug given together with niacin *912* Concentration reduced because of increased fecal excretion *2412*
Serum No Effect Physiological Reduced reabsorption of thyroid hormones from gastrointestinal tract *6412*

Tolbutamide *Serum No Effect Physiological* Absorption from gastrointestinal tract apparently unaffected when drug administered simultaneously with colestipol *4669*

Tri-iodothyronine (T3) *Serum Decrease Physiological* Concentration reduced due to increased fecal loss *2412* Reduced reabsorption of thyroid hormones from gastrointestinal tract *6412*

Triglycerides *Serum Decrease Physiological* Therapeutic intent *1480*
Serum Increase Physiological Increase of 7% noted *4793* In 98 patients with moderate hypercholesterolemia treatment with 10 g/d for 12 weeks caused nonsignificant 8.9% increase in concentration *3698*

Ursodiol *Serum Decrease Physiological* Administration has been shown to decrease absorption of ursodiol *1020*

Vitamin A *Serum Decrease Physiological* With prolonged treatment due to bile acid sequestration but values still in normal range *5055*
Serum No Effect Physiological No effect with 30 g daily of drug *4794*

VLDL-Cholesterol *Serum Increase Physiological* Significant increase in 18 patients with familial hypercholesterolemia treated with 15 g/d for 8 weeks *6400*

Warfarin *Plasma No Effect Physiological* Absorption from gastrointestinal tract apparently unaffected when drug administered simultaneously with colestipol *4669*

Colistimethate

Casts *Urine Increase Physiological* Nephrotoxic effect *3810*

Creatinine *Serum Increase Physiological* Nephrotoxic effect (usually reversible) *4691*

Erythrocytes *Urine Increase Physiological* Common nephrotoxic effect *4691*

Hemoglobin *Urine Increase Physiological* Common nephrotoxic effect *4691*

Leukocytes *Blood Decrease Physiological* Neutropenia/Leukopenia/granulocytopenia *128*

Nonprotein Nitrogen *Serum Increase Physiological* Nephrotoxic effect (usually reversible) *4691*

Protein *Urine Increase Physiological* Nephrotoxic effect *3810* Common nephrotoxic effect *4691*

Urea Nitrogen *Serum Increase Physiological* Nephrotoxic effect (usually reversible) *3810*

Colistin

Amino Acids *Urine Increase Analytical* Reacts with ninhydrin; extra spot with TLC, high voltage electrophoresis *4760*

Casts *Urine Increase Physiological* Cylindruria may occur with nephrotoxicity *1618*

Chloramphenicol *Serum No Effect Analytical* No effect at 100 mg/L on coupled enzymatic method *4122*

Creatinine *Serum Increase Physiological* Nephrotoxic effect (reversible renal damage) *3810*
Serum No Effect Analytical No effect of concentrations up to 15 mg/L on single slide method on Kodak Ektachem® *5706*

Erythrocytes *Urine Increase Physiological* Hematuria may occur with nephrotoxicity *1618*

Leucine Aminopeptidase *Urine Increase Physiological* Probably associated with proximal renal tubular injury *135*

Leukocytes *Blood Decrease Physiological* May cause leukopenia/granulocytopenia *3810*

Nonprotein Nitrogen *Serum Increase Physiological* Nephrotoxic effect (reversible renal damage) *3810*

Phenylalanine *Plasma No Effect Analytical* No interference observed with rapid quantitative whole blood method of Campbell et al using phenylalanine dehydrogenase *867*

Potassium *Serum No Effect Analytical* At concentration of 150 mg/L had no effect on measurement by ISE with predilution *5704*

Protein *Urine Increase Physiological* Nephrotoxic effect (reversible renal damage) *4133*

Sodium *Serum No Effect Analytical* At concentration of 150 mg/L had no effect on measurement by ISE with predilution *5704*

Specific Gravity *Urine Decrease Physiological* Concentrating ability may be impaired *1618*

Urea Nitrogen *Serum Increase Physiological* Nephrotoxic effect/may occur after large doses *3810*

Collidine

ionized Calcium *Serum Increase Analytical* At concentrations > 0.1 mmol/L on calcium specific electrode *820*

Congo Red

Color *Urine Increase Analytical* Dye not taken up by amyloid *128*

Conjugated Estrogens

α_1-Acid Glycoprotein *Serum Decrease Physiological* In postmenopausal women treatment for 14 days caused mean decrease to 65% of baseline *2494*

Alanine Aminotransferase *Serum Increase Physiological* May cause cholestatic jaundice *6566*

Albumin *Serum No Effect Physiological* No significant effect observed in 23 postmenopausal women treated for 21 days *2494*

Alkaline Phosphatase *Serum Increase Physiological* May cause cholestatic jaundice *6566*

Amylase *Serum Increase Physiological* In patients with familial hyperlipoproteinemia administration may cause massive increases in plasma triglyceride concentration, possibly leading to pancreatitis *6566*

Amyloid P *Serum Decrease Physiological* Treatment of postmenopausal women for 14 days caused decrease to mean 85% of pretreatment concentration *2494*

Angiotensinogen *Plasma Increase Physiological* In 23 healthy postmenopausal women treatment with conjugated estrogens 0.625 mg and 5 mg medroxyprogesterone acetate in 21-day sequences over 12 cycles caused significant change in concentration from 1889 ± 80 ng/mL to 4341 ± 271 ng/mL *588*

Antithrombin III *Plasma Decrease Physiological* In postmenopausal women treatment for 14 days caused decrease to 78% of pretreatment concentrations *2494* In 21 healthy postmenopausal women treatment with conjugated estrogens 0.625 mg and 5 mg medroxyprogesterone acetate in 21-day sequences over 12 cycles caused significant change in concentration from 1.11 ± 0.024 mg/L to 1.05 ± 0.024 mg/L *588*

α_1-Antitrypsin *Serum Increase Physiological* In 23 postmenopausal women treatment for 14 days caused increase to mean 144% of baseline *2494*

α_2-AP-Glycoprotein *Serum Increase Physiological* Increase to mean of 337% of baseline observed in 23 postmenopausal women 21 days after start of conjugated estrogen treatment *2494*

Apolipoprotein A-I *Serum Increase Physiological* In most studies of effect of conjugated estrogens in postmenopausal women concentration observed to increase (effect about 17% when women treated for at least 3 months with 0.625 mg/d) *3628*
Serum No Effect Physiological Nonsignificant mean increase of 0.20 g/L in 15 postmenopausal women treated with about 0.625 mg/day for an average of 8 months *1668* In 18 post-menopausal women treatment for 28 days had no significant effect on concentration *1888* In 43 postmenopausal women treatment with 0.6 mg CEE and 5 mg medrogesterone for 3 months caused nonsignificant change from mean baseline of 1.54 ± 0.26 g/L to 1.62 ± 0.32 g/L *2989* In 390 healthy postmenopausal women randomized to treatment with 0.625 mg/d conjugated equine estrogen and 2.5 mg/d medroxyprogesterone acetate caused median insignificant decrease of 4 ± 1% at both 3 and 6 months *6332*

Apolipoprotein A-II *Serum No Effect Physiological* Nonsignificant mean increase of 0.06 g/L in 15 postmenopausal women treated with about 0.625 mg/day for an average of 8 months *1668* In 18 post-menopausal women treatment for 28 days had no significant effect on concentration *1888*

Apolipoprotein B *Serum Decrease Physiological* Observed to decrease in most studies of postmenopausal women treated with 0.625 mg/d (effect about 12% when treated for at least 3 months) *3628*
Serum Increase Physiological In 390 healthy postmenopausal women randomized to treatment with 0.625 mg/d conjugated equine estrogen and 2.5 mg/d medroxyprogesterone acetate caused median significant increase of 12 ± 1% at both 3 and 6 months *6332*
Serum No Effect Physiological In 43 postmenopausal women treatment with 0.6 mg CEE and 5 mg medrogesterone for 3 months caused nonsignificant change from mean baseline of 1.08 ± 0.23 g/L to 1.08 ± 0.22 g/L *2989* Nonsignificant mean increase of 0.19 g/L in 15 postmenopausal women treated with about 0.625 mg/day for an average of 8 months *1668* In 18 post-menopausal women treatment for 28 days had no significant effect on plasma concentration *1888*

Aspartate Aminotransferase *Serum Increase Physiological* May cause cholestatic jaundice *6566*

Bilirubin *Serum Increase Physiological* May cause cholestatic jaundice *6566*

Bleeding Time *Patient Decrease Physiological* In four patients with renal failure, prolonged bleeding time and clinical bleeding, administration of 50 mg conjugated estrogens daily normalized bleeding time in two and reduced time to less than 50% of pretreatment in other two: mechanism unknown *5494*

CA549 *Serum No Effect Analytical* No statistically significant effect observed over a concentration range of 0.4 to 6.7

Conjugated Estrogens *(continued)*

CA549 *(continued)*
mg/L with BRESMARQ assay *958* No interference observed at concentrations of premarin from 0.4 - 6.7 mg/L with immunoradiometric BRESMARQ procedure *958*

Ceruloplasmin *Serum Increase Physiological* In 23 postmenopausal women treatment for 21 days caused mean to increase to 156% of baseline *2494*

Cholesterol *Serum Decrease Physiological* In 18 postmenopausal women treatment for 28 days caused significant decrease after 2 weeks *1888* Significant decrease of 4% in 31 healthy postmenopausal women from mean baseline of 5.71 mmol/L (220 mg/dL) given 0.625 mg I.M. twice for 3 months and of 6% when given 1.25 mg I.M. twice for 3 months *6333* In postmenopausal women treated with 0.625 mg/d for 1 year mean concentration decreased by 6% *3628* In 45 postmenopausal women treatment with conjugated equine estrogens and L-norgestrel causedsignificant decrease from mean of 7.09 ± 1.31 mmol/L to 6.43 ± 0.99 mmol/L *4853* In 31 healthy normolipidemic postmenopausal women treatment with 0.625 mg/d for 3 mo caused mean decrease of 0.23 mg/dL from mean baseline of 5.7 ± 0.9 mg/dL and 0.34 mg/dL with 1.25 mg/d *5181*

Serum Increase Physiological Mean concentration in postmenopausal women 191 mg/dL decreased to 175 mg/dL after treatment for 14 days *2494* In 43 postmenopausal women treatment with 0.6 mg CEE and 5 mg medrogesterone for 3 months caused significant increase from mean baseline of 5.78 ± 0.66 mmol/L to 5.40 ± 0.58 mmol/L *2989*

Serum No Effect Physiological In 140 postmenopausal women treatment with 0.625 mg conjugated equine estrogens daily for 25 days per month caused a nonsignificant change from mean baseline of 5.29 ± 0.91 mmol/L to 5.03 ± 0.82 mmol/L after 2 months, 5.13 ± 0.81 mmol/L after 6 months and 5.30 ± 0.85 mmol/L after 12 months *3138* In 25 healthy postmenopausal women treatment with 0.625 mg/d (three weeks out of four) for 2 months caused a nonsignificant change from mean value with placebo of 212 ± 31 mg/dL to 204 ± 28 mg/dL *2359* In 20 healthy postmenopausal women treatment with conjugated estrogens 0.625 mg and 5 mg medroxyprogesterone acetate in 21-day sequences over 12 cycles caused nonsignificant change in concentration from 5.00 ± 0.17 mmol/L to 5.07 ± 0.16 mmol/L in estrogenic phase and 4.90 ± 0.13 mmol/L in progestogenic phase *588* Nonsignificant mean increase of 0.42 mmol/L in 15 postmenopausal women treated with about 0.625 mg/day for about 8 months *1668*

Cholesterol Ester Transfer Protein
Serum No Effect Physiological In 31 healthy normolipidemic postmenopausal women treatment with 0.625 mg/d for 3 mo caused mean 0.01 mg/dL decrease from mean baseline of 2.26 ± 0.54 mg/dL and 0.00 mg/dL with 1.25 mg/d *5181*

Chylomicron Triglycerides *Serum No Effect Physiological* In 43 postmenopausal women treatment with 0.6 mg CEE and 5 mg medrogesterone for 3 months caused nonsignificant increase from mean baseline of 0.02 ± 0.08 mmol/L to 0.03 ± 0.07 mmol/L *2989*

Complement C_1s-Inactivator
Serum Decrease Physiological In postmenopausal women treatment for 14 days caused decrease to mean of 68% of pretreatment concentrations *2494*

Complement C_3 *Serum No Effect Physiological* No significant effect observed in 23 postmenopausal women treated for 21 days *2494*

Complement C_3-Proactivator
Serum No Effect Physiological No significant effect observed in 23 postmenopausal women treated for 21 days *2494*

Complement C_5 *Serum No Effect Physiological* No significant effect observed in 23 postmenopausal women treated for 21 days *2494*

Complement C_9 *Serum No Effect Physiological* No significant effect observed in 23 postmenopausal women treated for 21 days *2494*

C-terminal Telopeptide of Type I Collagen
Urine Decrease Physiological In 33 postmenopausal women treated with 0.625 mg/d conjugated equine estrogens and 2.5 mg/d medroxyprogesterone acetate for 12 months caused significant change from mean baseline of 280 µg/mmol creatinine to 120 µg/mmol creatinine after 6 momths and 70 µg/mmol creatinine after one year *5912*

D-Dimer *Plasma Increase Physiological* In 30 healthy postmenopausal women aged 55 ± 5 years treatment with 0.625 mg oral conjugated estrogen daily for one month caused nonsignificant increase from mean baseline of 441 ± 501 ng/mL to 551 ± 579 ng/mL *3219*

Dehydroepiandrosterone Sulfate
Plasma Decrease Physiological In 23 healthy postmenopausal women treatment with conjugated estrogens 0.625 mg and 5 mg medroxyprogesterone acetate in 21-day sequences over 12 cycles caused nonsignificant decrease in concentration from 3.17 ± 0.43 µmol/L to 2.82 ± 0.75 µmol/L *588*

Deoxypyridinoline *Urine Decrease Physiological* In 33 postmenopausal women treated with 0.625 mg/d conjugated equine estrogens and 2.5 mg/d medroxyprogesterone acetate for 12 months caused significant change from mean baseline of 6.7 pmol/µmol creatinine to 4.2 pmol/µmol creatinine after 6 momths and 3.6 pmol/µmol creatinine after one year *5912*

1,25-Dihydroxy Vitamin D_3 *Serum Increase Physiological* In 7 postoophorectomy women 0.625 mg/day for 6 months caused a mean increase of 10.3% whereas a detectable but not significant decrease occurred in the absence of estrogen therapy *2085*

Estradiol *Plasma Increase Physiological* In 5 hospitalized postmenopausal women administration of 0.625 mg/d at 08:00 h for 21 days caused significant increase from mean of 23 ± 20 pg/mL to 78 ± 36 pg/mL *1055* In 28 healthy postmenopausal women treatment with conjugated estrogens 0.625 mg and 5 mg medroxyprogesterone acetate in 21-day sequences over 12 cycles caused significant increase in concentration from 62 ± 17 pmol/L to 313 ± 40 pmol/L *588* In 23 postmenopausal women treatment for 14 days with conjugated estrogens caused increase from mean baseline of 10.4 pg/mL to 66.2 pg/mL *2494* In postmenopausal women treatment with 0.3 mg caused mean concentration of 18 pg/mL, 0.625 mg caused 39 pg/mL and 1.25 mg caused 60 pg/mL *3628*

17β-Estradiol *Plasma Increase Physiological* In 25 healthy postmenopausal women treatment with 0.625 mg/d (three weeks out of four) for 2 months caused a significant change from mean value with placebo of 22 ± 28 pg/mL to 75 ± 52 pg/mL *2359* In 30 healthy postmenopausal women aged 55 ± 5 years treatment with 0.625 mg oral conjugated estrogen daily for one month caused significant increase from mean baseline of 20 ± 13 pg/mL to 75 ± 30 pg/mL *3219*

Estrone *Plasma Decrease Physiological* In 20 healthy postmenopausal women treatment with conjugated estrogens 0.625 mg and 5 mg medroxyprogesterone acetate in 21-day sequences over 12 cycles caused significant decrease in concentration from 2361 ± 17 pmol/L to 729 ± 64 pmol/L *588*

Plasma Increase Physiological In 30 healthy postmenopausal women aged 55 ± 5 years treatment with 0.625 mg oral conjugated estrogen daily for one month caused significant increase from mean baseline of 24 ± 12 pg/mL to 130 ± 76 pg/mL *3219* In postmenopausal women treatment with 0.3 mg caused mean concentration of 76 pg/mL. with 0.625 mg caused concentration of 153 pg/mL and with 1.25 mg caused 220 pg/mL *3628*

Fibrinogen *Plasma Decrease Physiological* In 23 healthy postmenopausal women treatment with conjugated estrogens 0.625 mg and 5 mg medroxyprogesterone acetate in 21-day sequences over 12 cycles caused significant change in concentration from 3.01 ± 0.11 g/L to 2.82 ± 0.08 g/L *588*

Plasma No Effect Physiological In 390 healthy postmenopausal women randomized to treatment with 0.625 mg/d conjugated equine estrogen and 2.5 mg/d medroxyprogesterone acetate caused median insignificant decrease of 3 ± 3% at both 3 and 6 months *6332*

Fibrinopeptide A *Plasma No Effect Physiological* In 390 healthy postmenopausal women randomized to treatment with 0.625 mg/d conjugated equine estrogen and 2.5 mg/d medroxyprogesterone acetate caused median insignificant increase of 16 ± 7% at both 3 and 6 months *6332*

Follicle Stimulating Hormone
Plasma Decrease Physiological In 5 postmenopausal women administration of 0.625 mg/d at 08:00 h caused significant decrease from mean of 33.6 ± 6.7 mIU/L to 28.9 ± 9.2 mIU/L *1055* In 31 healthy normolipidemic postmenopausal women treatment with 0.625 mg/d for 3 mo caused 30% decrease from mean baseline of 81 ± 12 IU/L and 57% with 1.25 mg/d *5181* Reduction observed in patients receiving drug *5703* In 29 healthy postmenopausal women treatment with conjugated estrogens 0.625 mg and 5 mg medroxyprogesterone acetate in 21-day sequences over 12 cycles caused significant decrease in concentration from 70.3 ± 6.8 IU/L to 22.8 ± 2.2 IU/L *588*

Gc-Globulin *Serum Increase Physiological* In 23 postmenopausal women treatment for 14 days caused increase to mean 128% of pretreatment concentrations *2494*

Glucose *Serum No Effect Physiological* No change observed in fasting concentration and insignifcant increase in 2-hour post glucose concentration in 15 postmenopausal women treated with an average of 0.625 mg daily for about 8 months *1668*

Glucose Tolerance *Serum Decrease Physiological* May reduce carbohydrate tolerance *6566*

γ-Glutamyltransferase *Serum Decrease Physiological* Activity reduced in patients receiving drug *5703*

β_2-Glycoprotein I *Serum Decrease Physiological* In postmenopausal women treatment for 14 days caused decrease to mean 84% of baseline *2494*

β_2-Glycoprotein III *Serum Increase Physiological* In 23 postmenopausal women treatment for 14 days caused mean increase to 119% of baseline *2494*

α_1-Glycoprotein B *Serum No Effect Physiological* No significant effect observed in 23 postmenopausal women treated for 21 days *2494*

Haptoglobin *Serum Decrease Physiological* In postmenopausal women treatment for 14 days caused decrease to 65% of mean baseline concentration *2494*

HDL_2-Apolipoprotein A-I *Serum Increase Physiological* Mean increase of 46% from mean baseline of 9.28 µmol/L (26 mg/dL) in 31 healthy postmenopausal women given 0.625 mg I.M. twice for 3 months and of 39% when given 1.25 mg twice for 3 months *6333*

HDL_2-Apolipoprotein A-II *Serum Decrease Physiological* Nonsignificant decrease of 6% in 31 healthy postmenopausal women given 0.625 mg I.M. twice for 3 months and of 3% when given 1.25 mg I.M. twice for 3 months *6333*

HDL_2-Cholesterol *Serum Increase Physiological* Largely responsible for increase in HDL-cholesterol observed when conjugated equine estrogens given to postmenopausal women (approximate 27% increase with 0.625 mg/d for at least 3 months) *3628* Mean increase of 50% from mean baseline of 0.36 mmol/L (14 mg/dL) in 31 healthy postmenopausal women given 0.625 mg I.M. twice for 3 months and of 59% when given 1.25 mg I.M. twice for 3 months *6333* In 390 healthy postmenopausal women randomized to treatment with 0.625 mg/d conjugated equine estrogen and 2.5 mg/d medroxyprogesterone acetate caused median significant increase of 33 ± 4% at both 3 and 6 months *6332*
Serum No Effect Physiological In 43 postmenopausal women treatment with 0.6 mg CEE and 5 mg medrogesterone for 3 months caused nonsignificant change from mean baseline of 0.22 ± 0.15 mmol/L to 0.21 ± 0.12 mmol/L *2989* In 18 postmenopausal women treatment for 4 weeks had no significant effect on concentration *1888*

HDL_3-Apolipoprotein A-I *Serum Increase Physiological* Significant increase of mean concentration by 14% from mean baseline of 54.6 µmol/L (153 mg/dL) in 31 healthy postmenopausal women given 0.625 mg I.M. twice for 3 months and of 22% when given 1.25 mg I.M. twice for 3 months *6333*

HDL_3-Apolipoprotein A-II *Serum Increase Physiological* Significant mean increase of 10% from mean baseline concentration of 17.8 µmol/L (31 mg/dL) in 31 healthy postmenopausal women treated with 0.625 mg I.M. twice for 3 months and of 10% when given 1.25 mg I.M. twice for 3 months *6333*

HDL_3-Cholesterol *Serum Increase Physiological* Significant increase of mean concentration by 6% from mean baseline of 1.34 mmol/L (52 mg/dL) in 31 healthy postmenopausal women given 0.625 mg I.M. and of 6% when given 1.25 mg I.M. twice for 3 months *6333*
Serum No Effect Physiological In 18 post-menopausal women treatment for 28 days had no significant effect on concentration *1888* In 43 postmenopausal women treatment with 0.6 mg CEE and 5 mg medrogesterone for 3 months caused nonsignificant change from mean baseline of 1.30 ± 0.28 mmol/L to 1.29 ± 0.26 mmol/L *2989*

HDL-Apolipoprotein A *Serum Increase Physiological* In 31 healthy normolipidemic postmenopausal women treatment with 0.625 mg/d for 3 mo caused mean increase of 27 mg/dL from mean baseline of 180 ± 25 mg/dL and 27 mg/dL with 1.25 mg/d *5181*

HDL-Cholesterol *Serum Increase Physiological* In 25 healthy postmenopausal women treatment with 0.625 mg/d (three weeks out of four) for 2 months caused a significant change from mean value with placebo of 58 ± 18 mg/dL to 64 ± 20 mg/dL *2359* In 390 healthy postmenopausal women randomized to treatment with 0.625 mg/d conjugated equine estrogen and 2.5 mg/d medroxyprogesterone acetate caused median significant increase of 11 ± 2% at both 3 and 6 months *6332* In 30 healthy postmenopausal women aged 55 ± 5 years treatment with 0.625 mg oral conjugated estrogen daily for one month caused significant increase from mean baseline of 58 ± 15 mg/dL to 69 ± 17 mg/dL *3219* In 140 postmenopausal women treatment with 0.625 mg conjugated equine estrogens daily for 25 days per month caused a significant change from mean baseline of 1.75 ± 0.55 mmol/L to 1.87 ± 0.46 mmol/L after 2 months, 2.05 ± 0.51 mmol/L after 6 months and 2.06 ± 0.46 mmol/L after 12 months *3138* Mean increase of 16% observed from mean baseline of 1.67 mmol/L (66 mg/dL) in 31 healthy postmenopausal women given 0.625 mg twice for 3 months and of 18% when given 1.25 mg twice for 3 months *6333* In 31 healthy normolipidemic postmenopausal women treatment with 0.625 mg/d for 3 mo caused mean increase of 0.26 mg/dL from mean baseline of 1.7 ± 0.3 mg/dL and 0.28 mg/dL with 1.25 mg/d *5181* In 45 postmenopausal women treatment with conjugated equine estrogens and L-norgestrel significant increase from baseline of 1.94 ± 0.54 mmol/L to 2.15 ± 0.53 mmol/L *4853* In the Postmenopausal Estrogen/Progestin Intervention Trial of 875 healthy postmenopausal women with primary hypercholesterolemia treatment with estrogen/progestin or estrogen alone caused mean increase of 4 - 8% *3115* In postmenopausal women treated with 0.625 mg daily for 1 year increased concentration by mean of 13.5% *3628*
Serum No Effect Physiological In 20 healthy postmenopausal women treatment with conjugated estrogens 0.625 mg and 5 mg medroxyprogesterone acetate in 21-day sequences over 12 cycles caused nonsignificant change in concentration from 1.60 ± 0.08 mmol/L to 1.62 ± 0.07 mmol/L in estrogenic phase and 1.57 ± 0.07 mmol/L in progestogenic phase *588* Nonsignificant mean increase of 0.11 mmol/L in 15 postmenopausal women treated with about 0.625 mg/day for an average of 8 months *1668* In 18 post-menopausal women treatment for 28 days had no significant effect on concentration *1888* In 43 postmenopausal women treatment with 0.6 mg CEE and 5 mg medrogesterone for 3 months caused nonsignificant change from mean baseline of 1.52 ± 0.33 mmol/L to 1.50 ± 0.31 mmol/L *2989*

HDL-Triglycerides *Serum Increase Physiological* In 31 healthy normolipidemic postmenopausal women treatment with 0.625 mg/d for 3 mo caused mean increase of 0.07 mg/dL from mean baseline of 0.2 ± 0.1 mg/dL and 0.09 mg/dL with 1.25 mg/d *5181* Mean increase of 32% observed from mean baseline of 0.21 mmol/L (19 mg/dL) in 31 healthy postmenopausal women given 0.625 mg twice for 3 months and of 43% when 1.25 mg given twice for 3 months *6333*

Hemopexin *Serum Decrease Physiological* In postmenopausal women treatment for 14 days caused decrease to mean of 77% of pretreatment concentrations *2494*

α_2-HS Glycoprotein *Serum Increase Physiological* In 23 postmenopausal women treatment for 14 days caused increase from mean baseline of 123% *2494*

Hydroxyproline *Urine Decrease Physiological* In 33 postmenopausal women treated with 0.625 mg/d conjugated equine estrogens and 2.5 mg/d medroxyprogesterone acetate for 12 months caused significant change from mean baseline of 20 mg/g creatinine to 13 mg/g creatinine after 6 momths and 12 mg/g creatinine after one year *5912*

Conjugated Estrogens *(continued)*

Immunoglobulin G *Serum No Effect Physiological* No significant effect observed in 23 postmenopausal women treated for 21 days *2494*

Immunoglobulin M *Serum No Effect Physiological* No significant effect observed in 23 postmenopausal women treated for 21 days *2494*

Insulin *Plasma Decrease Physiological* In 30 healthy postmenopausal women aged 55 ± 5 years treatment with 0.625 mg oral conjugated estrogen daily for one month caused nonsignificant decrease from mean baseline of 10.4 ± 9.6 μU/mL to 8.1 ± 4.6 μU/mL *3219*
Plasma No Effect Physiological Nonsignificant increase of 1.40 mU/L in basal concentration and 18.40 mU/L in 2-hour post-glucose concentration in 15 postmenopausal women treated with an average of 0.625 mg/day for about 8 months *1668*

LDL-Apolipoprotein B *Serum Decrease Physiological* In 31 healthy normolipidemic postmenopausal women treatment with 0.625 mg/d for 3 mo caused mean decrease of 8.9 mg/dL from mean baseline of 0.24 ± 0.05 mg/dL and 7.7 mg/dL with 1.25 mg/d *5181* Mean decrease of 10% from mean baseline of 1560 nmol/L (86 mg/dL) observed in 31 healthy postmenopausal women given 0.625 mg twice for 3 months and of 9% when 1.25 mg twice for 3 months *6333*

LDL-Cholesterol *Serum Decrease Physiological* In 18 post-menopausal women treatment with conjugated estrogens for 28 days caused significant decrease after 2 weeks *1888* In 30 healthy postmenopausal women aged 55 ± 5 years treatment with 0.625 mg oral conjugated estrogen daily for one month caused significant decrease from mean baseline of 152 ± 31 mg/dL to 131 ± 27 mg/dL *3219* In 31 healthy normolipidemic postmenopausal women treatment with 0.625 mg/d for 3 mo caused mean decrease of 0.54 mg/dL from mean baseline of 3.6 ± 0.7 mg/dL and 0.70 mg/dL with 1.25 mg/d *5181* In 140 postmenopausal women treatment with 0.625 mg conjugated equine estrogens daily for 25 days per month caused a nonsignificant change from mean baseline of 3.30 ± 0.75 mmol/L to 2.81 ± 0.60 mmol/L after 2 months, 2.78 ± 0.62 mmol/L after 6 months and 2.91 ± 0.60 mmol/L after 12 months *3138* Mean decrease of 15% from baseline of 3.6 mmol/L (139 mg/dL) observed in 31 healthy postmenopausal women given 0.625 mg twice for 3 months and of 19% when given 1.25 mg twice for 3 months *6333* In 390 healthy postmenopausal women randomized to treatment with 0.625 mg/d conjugated equine estrogen and 2.5 mg/d medroxyprogesterone acetate caused median significant decrease of 13 ± 1% at both 3 and 6 months *6332* In the Postmenopausal Estrogen/Progestin Intervention Trial of 875 healthy postmenopausal women with primary hypercholesterolemia treatment with estrogen/progestin or estrogen alone caused mean decrease of 10 - 12% *3115* In postmenopausal women treated with 0.625 mg/d for 1 year concentration decreased by mean of 16% *3628* In 25 healthy postmenopausal women treatment with 0.625 mg/d (three weeks out of four) for 2 months caused a significant change from mean value with placebo of 134 ± 29 mg/dL to 115 ± 31 mg/dL *2359*
Serum Increase Physiological In 43 postmenopausal women treatment with 0.6 mg CEE and 5 mg medrogesterone for 3 months caused significant increase from mean baseline of 3.46 ± 0.71 mmol/L to 3.11 ± 0.51 mmol/L *2989*
Serum No Effect Physiological In 20 healthy postmenopausal women treatment with conjugated estrogens 0.625 mg and 5 mg medroxyprogesterone acetate in 21-day sequences over 12 cycles caused nonsignificant change in concentration from 2.84 ± 0.17 mmol/L to 2.87 ± 0.15 mmol/L in estrogenic phase and 2.88 ± 0.15 mmol/L in progestogenic phase *588* Nonsignificant mean increase of 0.12 mmol/L in 15 postmenopausal women treated with about 0.625 mg/day for an average of 8 months *1668*

LDL-Cholesterol:HDL-Cholesterol Ratio
Serum Decrease Physiological In 18 post-menopausal women treatment with conjugated estrogens caused significant reduction after 1 week *1888*

LDL-Triglycerides *Serum Increase Physiological* Mean increase of 20% from mean baseline of 0.24 mmol/L (21 mg/dL) observed in 31 healthy postmenopausal women given 0.625 mg twice for 3 months and of 30% when 1.25 mg given twice for 3 months *6333* In 31 healthy normolipidemic postmenopausal women treatment with 0.625 mg/d for 3 mo caused mean increase of 0.05 mg/dL from mean baseline of 0.24 ± 0.11 mg/dL and 0.07 mg/dL with 1.25 mg/d *5181*

Lipase *Serum Increase Physiological* In patients with familial hyperlipoproteinemia administration may cause massive increases in plasma triglyceride concentration, possibly leading to pancreatitis *6566*

Lipoprotein A-I *Serum Increase Physiological* Treatment of 23 postmenopausal women for 14 days caused increase to 122% of mean baseline *2494*

β-Lipoprotein *Serum Decrease Physiological* Concentration in postmenopausal women decreased to 80% of concentration prior to treatment for 14 days *2494*

Lipoprotein Lp(a) *Serum Decrease Physiological* In postmenopausal women with initial lipoprotein Lp(a) concentration greater than 10 mg/dL treatment with 0.6 mg CEE and 5 mg medrogesterone for 3 months caused significant decrease from mean baseline by 10% *2989* In 140 postmenopausal women treatment with 0.625 mg conjugated equine estrogens daily for 25 days per month caused significant reduction from mean baseline of 22.6 ± 21.6 mg/dL to 15.0 ± 16.2 mg/dL after 2 months, 13.7 ± 14.6 mg/dL after 6 months and 13.3 ± 15.6 mg/dL after 12 months *3138* In 390 healthy postmenopausal women randomized to treatment with 0.625 mg/d conjugated equine estrogen and 2.5 mg/d medroxyprogesterone acetate caused median significant decrease of 16 ± 3% at both 3 and 6 months *6332* In 31 healthy normolipidemic postmenopausal women treatment with 0.625 mg/d for 3 mo caused 14% decrease from mean baseline of 20.4 ± 14.6 mg/dL and 16% with 1.25 mg/d *5181*
Serum No Effect Physiological In 30 healthy postmenopausal women aged 55 ± 5 years treatment with 0.625 mg oral conjugated estrogen daily for one month caused nonsignificant decrease from mean baseline of 29.9 ± 22.5 mg/dL to 26.7 ± 20.2 mg/dL *3219*

Luteinizing Hormone *Plasma Decrease Physiological* Concentration reduced in patients taking conjugated estrogens *5703* In 29 healthy postmenopausal women treatment with conjugated estrogens 0.625 mg and 5 mg medroxyprogesterone acetate in 21-day sequences over 12 cycles caused significant decrease in concentration from 58.6 ± 8.0 IU/L to 34.0 ± 3.1 IU/L *588*
Plasma No Effect Physiological In 5 hospitalized postmenopausal women administration of 0.625 mg/d at 08:00 h for 21 days caused nonsignificant decrease from mean of 41.3 ± 6.9 mIU/L to 40.5 ± 7.5 mIU/L *1055*

α_2-Macroglobulin *Serum No Effect Physiological* No significant effect observed in 23 postmenopausal women treated for 21 days *2494*

Oxaprozin *Serum No Effect Physiological* Coadministration of conjugated estrogens with oxaprozin caused no significant effect on the pharmacokinetic parameters of oxaprozin in single or multiple dose studies *2065*

Partial Thromboplastin Time
Plasma No Effect Physiological In 21 healthy postmenopausal women treatment with conjugated estrogens 0.625 mg and 5 mg medroxyprogesterone acetate in 21-day sequences over 12 cycles caused nonsignificant change in concentration from 90.7 ± 2.4% to 89.4 ± 2.5% *588*

Plasminogen *Plasma No Effect Physiological* No significant effect observed in 23 postmenopausal women treated for 21 days *2494*

Plasminogen Activator Inhibitor-1
Plasma Decrease Physiological In 30 healthy postmenopausal women aged 55 ± 5 years treatment with 0.625 mg oral conjugated estrogen daily for one month caused significant decrease from mean baseline of 32 ± 34 ng/mL to 14 ± 10 ng/mL *3219* In 390 healthy postmenopausal women randomized to treatment with 0.625 mg/d conjugated equine estrogen and 2.5 mg/d medroxyprogesterone acetate caused median significant decrease of 29 ± 3% at both 3 and 6 months *6332*

Prealbumin *Serum Decrease Physiological* Decrease to mean of 78% of pretreatment concentration in postmenopausal women after 14 days *2494*

Progesterone *Plasma No Effect Physiological* In 5 hospitalized postmenopausal women administration of 0.625 mg/d at 08:00 h for 21 days caused nonsignificant increase from mean of 1.04 ± 0.4 ng/mL to 1.2 ± 0.3 ng/mL *1055*

Prolactin *Plasma Decrease Physiological* Concentration reduced in patients taking conjugated estrogens *5703*

Protein *Serum Decrease Physiological* Slight decrease from mean of 64.6 g/L to 63.3 g/L observed in postmenopausal women after 14 days treatment *2494*

Prothrombin Fragment 1.2 *Plasma No Effect Physiological* In 390 healthy postmenopausal women randomized to treatment with 0.625 mg/d conjugated equine estrogen and 2.5 mg/d medroxyprogesterone acetate caused median insignificant increase of 16 ± 7% at both 3 and 6 months *6332*

Prothrombin Time *Plasma No Effect Physiological* In 22 healthy postmenopausal women treatment with conjugated estrogens 0.625 mg and 5 mg medroxyprogesterone acetate in 21-day sequences over 12 cycles caused nonsignificant change in concentration from 96.8 ± 0.7% to 96.9 ± 0.9% *588*

Pyridinoline *Urine Decrease Physiological* In 33 postmenopausal women treated with 0.625 mg/d conjugated equine estrogens and 2.5 mg/d medroxyprogesterone acetate for 12 months caused significant change from mean baseline of 30 pmol/µmol creatinine to 22 pmol/µmol creatinine after 6 momths and 20 pmol/µmol creatinine after one year *5912*

Renin Activity *Plasma No Effect Physiological* In 23 healthy postmenopausal women treatment with conjugated estrogens 0.625 mg and 5 mg medroxyprogesterone acetate in 21-day sequences over 12 cycles caused nonsignificant change in concentration from 4.1 ± 0.53 ng/mL/h to 3.9 ± 0.66 ng/mL/h *588*

Retinol-binding Protein *Serum Decrease Physiological* In postmenopausal women treatment for 14 days caused decrease to mean of 84% of baseline *2494*

Sex-Hormone Binding Globulin
Serum Increase Physiological In 21 healthy postmenopausal women treatment with conjugated estrogens 0.625 mg and 5 mg medroxyprogesterone acetate in 21-day sequences over 12 cycles caused significant increase in concentration from 50.6 ± 4.2 nmol/L to 117.2 ± 9.9 nmol/L *588*

T3-Uptake *Serum No Effect Physiological* In 25 healthy postmenopausal women treatment with conjugated estrogens 0.625 mg and 5 mg medroxyprogesterone acetate in 21-day sequences over 12 cycles caused nonsignificant change in concentration from 0.53 ± 0.10 to 0.48 ± 0.09 *588*

Testosterone *Serum Decrease Physiological* In 17 healthy postmenopausal women treatment with conjugated estrogens 0.625 mg and 5 mg medroxyprogesterone acetate in 21-day sequences over 12 cycles caused nonsignificant decrease in concentration from 1.39 ± 0.15 nmol/L to 1.27 ± 0.13 nmol/L *588*

Thyroid Stimulating Hormone
Serum Increase Physiological In 28 healthy postmenopausal women treatment with conjugated estrogens 0.625 mg and 5 mg medroxyprogesterone acetate in 21-day sequences over 12 cycles caused nonsignificant increase in concentration from 2.11 ± 0.52 mIU/L to 2.82 ± 0.75 mIU/L *588*

Thyroxine (T4) *Serum Increase Physiological* In 29 healthy postmenopausal women treatment with conjugated estrogens 0.625 mg and 5 mg medroxyprogesterone acetate in 21-day sequences over 12 cycles caused significant increase in concentration from 101.5 ± 5.6 mmol/L to 132.8 ± 3.7 mmol/L *588*

Triglycerides *Serum Decrease Physiological* In 30 healthy postmenopausal women aged 55 ± 5 years treatment with 0.625 mg oral conjugated estrogen daily for one month caused significant decrease from mean baseline of 231 ± 36 mg/dL to 224 ± 32 mg/dL *3219*
Serum Increase Physiological Concentration observed to increase in postmenopausal women treated with 0.625 mg/d for 1 year (approximately 14% increase when treated for at least 3 months. Effect may be dose-dependent but probably not significantly different *3628* In postmenopausal women mean concentration of 96 mg/dL increased to 128 mg/dL after 14 days treatment *2494* In 43 postmenopausal women treatment with 0.6 mg CEE and 5 mg medrogesterone for 3 months caused significant increase from mean baseline of 0.90 ± 0.36 mmol/L to 1.04 ± 0.36 mmol/L *2989* In 25 healthy postmenopausal women treatment with 0.625 mg/d (three weeks out of four) for 2 months caused a nonsignificant change from mean value with placebo of 103 ± 71 mg/dL to 121 ± 67 mg/dL *2359* In patients with familial hyperlipoproteinemia administration may cause massive increases in plasma triglyceride concentration, possibly leading to pancreatitis *6566* In 30 healthy postmenopausal women aged 55 ± 5 years treatment with 0.625 mg oral conjugated estrogen daily for one month caused significant increase from mean baseline of 103 ± 59 mg/dL to 120 ± 63 mg/dL *3219* Significant mean increase of 24% in 31 healthy postmenopausal women given 0.625 mg I.M. twice for 3 months and of 38% when given 1.25 mg I.M. twice for 3 months *6333* In 20 healthy postmenopausal women treatment with conjugated estrogens 0.625 mg and 5 mg medroxyprogesterone acetate in 21-day sequences over 12 cycles caused significant change in concentration from 0.98 ± 0.09 mmol/L to 1.45 ± 0.17 mmol/L in estrogenic phase and 1.18 ± 0.11 mmol/L in progestogenic phase *588* In 390 healthy postmenopausal women randomized to treatment with 0.625 mg/d conjugated equine estrogen and 2.5 mg/d medroxyprogesterone acetate caused median significant increase of 20 ± 5% at both 3 and 6 months *6332* In 31 healthy normolipidemic postmenopausal women treatment with 0.625 mg/d for 3 mo caused mean increase of 0.24 mg/dL from mean baseline of 0.95 ± 0.07 mg/dL and 0.36 mg/dL with 1.25 mg/d *5181* In the Postmenopausal Estrogen/Progestin Intervention Trial of 875 healthy postmenopausal women with primary hypercholesterolemia treatment with estrogen/progestin or estrogen alone caused mean increase of 15 - 20% *3115*
Serum No Effect Physiological In 18 post-menopausal women treatment for 28 days had no significant effect *1888* In 140 postmenopausal women treatment with 0.625 mg conjugated equine estrogens daily for 25 days per month caused a nonsignificant change from mean baseline of 1.35± 0.56 mmol/L to 1.63 ± 0.90 mmol/L after 2 months, 1.55 ± 0.71 mmol/L after 6 months and 1.52 ± 0.70 mmol/L after 12 months *3138* Nonsignificant mean increase of 0.44 mmol/L in 15 postmenopausal women treated with about 0.625 mg/day for an average of 8 months *1668* In 45 postmenopausal women treatment with conjugated equine estrogens and L-norgestrel caused nonsignificant increase from mean baseline of 1.20 ± 0.60 mmol/L to 1.33 ± 0.62 mmol/L *4853*

Type I Collagen Cross-linked N-telopeptide
Urine Decrease Physiological In 33 postmenopausal women treated with 0.625 mg/d conjugated equine estrogens and 2.5 mg/d medroxyprogesterone acetate for 12 months caused significant change from mean baseline of 54 nMBCE/mmol creatinine to 33 nMBCE/mmol creatinine after 6 momths and 24 nMBCE/mmol creatinine after one year *5912*

VLDL-Apolipoprotein B *Serum Increase Physiological* Mean increase of 29% observed from mean baseline of 38 nmol/L (2.1 mg/dL) in 31 healthy postmenopausal women given 0.625 mg twice for 3 months and increase of 22% when 1.25 mg given twice for 3 months *6333*
Serum No Effect Physiological In 31 healthy normolipidemic postmenopausal women treatment with 0.625 mg/d for 3 mo caused mean 0.6 mg/dL increase from mean baseline of 2.1 ± 1.7 mg/dL and 0.5 mg/dL with 1.25 mg/d *5181*

VLDL-Cholesterol *Serum Increase Physiological* In most studies of postmenopausal women concentration of VLDL observed to increase (effect about 14% in women treated with 0.625 mg/d for at least 3 months) *3628* Mean increase of 16% from mean baseline of 0.24 mmol/L (9.3 mg/dL) in 31 healthy postmenopausal women given 2 doses of 0.625 mg for 3 months and increase of 30% in those given 1.25 mg twice for 3 months *6333*
Serum No Effect Physiological In 43 postmenopausal women treatment with 0.6 mg CEE and 5 mg medrogesterone for 3 months caused nonsignificant change from mean baseline of 0.38 ± 0.20 mmol/L to 0.41 ± 0.21 mmol/L *2989* In 140 postmenopausal women treatment with 0.625 mg conjugated equine estrogens daily for 25 days per month caused a nonsignificant change from mean baseline of 0.28 ± 0.17 mmol/L to 0.34 ± 0.25 mmol/L after 2 months, 0.30 ± 0.22 mmol/L after 6 months and 0.33 ± 0.24 mmol/L after 12 months *3138* In 18 post-menopausal women treatment for 28 days had no significant effect on concentration *1888* In 20 healthy postmenopausal women treatment with conjugated estrogens 0.625 mg and 5 mg medroxyprogesterone acetate in 21-day sequences over 12 cycles caused nonsignificant change in concentration from 0.56 ± 0.06 mmol/L to 0.58 ± 0.07 mmol/L in estrogenic phase and 0.46 ± 0.05 mmol/L in progestogenic phase *588* In 31 healthy normolipidemic postmenopausal women treatment with 0.625 mg/d for 3 mo caused mean 0.04 mg/dL nonsignificant increase from mean baseline of 0.24 ± 0.05 mg/dL and 0.07 mg/dL with 1.25 mg/d *5181*

Conjugated Estrogens *(continued)*

VLDL-Triglycerides *Serum Increase Physiological* In 31 healthy normolipidemic postmenopausal women treatment with 0.625 mg/d for 3 mo caused mean increase of 0.11 mg/dL from mean baseline of 0.24 ± 0.05 mg/dL and 0.20 mg/dL with 1.25 mg/d *5181* Mean increase from mean baseline of 0.49 mmol/L (43 mg/dL) of 24% observed in 31 healthy postmenopausal women given 0.625 mg twice for 3 months and increase of 42% when given 1.25 mg twice for 3 months *6333*
Serum No Effect Physiological In 43 postmenopausal women treatment with 0.6 mg CEE and 5 mg medrogesterone for 3 months caused nonsignificant increase from mean baseline of 0.50 ± 0.28 mmol/L to 0.53 ± 0.27 mmol/L *2989*

Zinc-α_2-Glycoprotein *Serum Decrease Physiological* Decrease to mean of 88% of pretreatment concentrations in postmenopausal women after 14 days treatment *2494*

Corbadrin

Cholesterol *Serum No Effect Analytical* At concentration of 200 mg/L had no effect on Kageyama-Hantzsch method *5704* At concentration of 200 mg/L had no effect on CHOD-PAP method *5704* At concentration of 200 mg/L had no effect on method using catalase-Hantzsch reaction *5704*

Corn Oil

Arachidonic Acid *Serum No Effect Physiological* No change from basal concentration of 110 mg/L in 78 hypertensive patients treated with 6.0 g daily for 10 weeks *646*

Cholesterol *Serum No Effect Physiological* No significant effect observed in 78 hypertensive patients treated with dietary supplement of 6.0 g corn oil daily for 10 weeks *646*

Docosahexaenoic Acid *Serum Decrease Physiological* Reduction from mean basal concentration of 113 mg/L to 106 mg/L in 78 hypertensive patients treated with dietary supplement of 6.0 g daily for 10 weeks *646*

Eicosapentaenoic Acid *Serum Decrease Physiological* Reduction from mean baseline concentration of 45 mg/L to 34 mg/L in 78 hypertensive patients treated with dietary supplement of 6.0 g daily for 10 weeks *646*

HDL-Cholesterol *Serum Increase Physiological* Increase from mean baseline of 1.33 mmol/L to 1.40 mmol/L in 78 hypertensive patients treated with dietary supplement of 6.0 g corn oil daily for 10 weeks *646*

Linoleic Acid *Serum Increase Physiological* Increase from mean concentration of 269 mg/L to 295 mg/L in 78 hypertensive patients treated with dietary supplement of 6.0 g daily for 10 weeks *646*

Triglycerides *Serum No Effect Physiological* No significant change observed in 78 hypertensive patients treated with dietary supplement of 6.0 g corn oil daily for 10 weeks *646*

Corticosteroids

Amylase *Serum Increase Physiological* Condition like acute idiopathic pancreatitis *5864*

Calcium *Serum Decrease Physiological* Antagonizes action of vitamin D and parathyroid *128*
Urine Increase Physiological Metabolic effect *3669*

Chloride *Serum Decrease Physiological* Metabolic alkalosis with reduced chloride reabsorption *4053*
Serum Increase Physiological May cause retention *3810*
Urine Decrease Physiological Promotes retention (mineralocorticoid effect) *128*

Cholesterol *Serum Increase Analytical* Many steroids react with $FeCl_3$ reagent *2559*
Serum Increase Physiological Effect of prolonged hormone action *1095*

Color *Feces Increase Analytical* Black color reported with corticosteroid ingestion *3388*

Cortisol *Plasma Decrease Physiological* In critically ill patients relative hypoadrenalism observed with previously unknown corticosteroid therapy *3381*

Creatinine *Urine Increase Physiological* Associated with negative nitrogen balance *3810*

D. farinae-specific IgE Antibodies
Serum No Effect Physiological In 39 patients with perennial allergic rhinitis treatment with corticosteroids for up to 8 weeks caused a nonsignificant reduction from mean baseline of 78.2 ± 150.3 ARU/mL to 43.4 ± 42.2 ARU/mL (0.6 ± 57.9%) *4381*

Doxazosin *Serum No Effect Physiological* Coadministration with doxazosin had no effect on its pharmacokinetics *4642*

Erythrocytes *Blood Decrease Physiological* May cause gastrointestinal bleeding with low iron stores *536*

Glucose *Serum Increase Physiological* Tends to be high (as in Cushing's syndrome) *2242*
Urine Increase Physiological As result of hyperglycemia *3810*

Growth Hormone *Plasma Decrease Physiological* Suppresses secretion of hormone *4014*

Hematocrit *Blood Decrease Physiological* May cause gastrointestinal bleeding with low iron stores *536*

Hemoglobin *Blood Decrease Physiological* May cause gastrointestinal bleeding with low iron stores *536*

25-Hydroxy Vitamin D_3 *Serum Decrease Physiological* Observed effect in some children *5055*

17-Hydroxycorticosteroids *Urine Decrease Physiological* If given orally, inhaled or topically *2452*

Hydroxyproline *Urine Decrease Physiological* Alleged normal metabolic effect *6111*
Urine Increase Physiological Stimulate growth in children *4014*

^{131}I Uptake *Serum Decrease Physiological* Observed effect may last 8 d *2452*
Serum No Effect Physiological No effect observed *3107*

Interleukin-4 *Serum No Effect Physiological* In 39 patients with perennial allergic rhinitis treatment with corticosteroids for up to 8 weeks caused a nonsignificant change of 2.0 ± 38.9% from mean baseline of 13.6 ± 13.2 pg/mL *4381*

Isoniazid *Serum Decrease Physiological* Decreased plasma condition *886*

17-Ketosteroids *Urine Decrease Physiological* If given orally, inhaled or topically *2452*

LE Cells *Blood Positive Physiological* Implicated as activators of SLE *1608*

Leukocytes *Blood Decrease Physiological* May cause leukopenia *3810*

Occult Blood *Feces Increase Physiological* May increase incidence of gastric ulcers *536*

Osmolality *Serum Increase Physiological* Associated with sodium and chloride retention *2242*

Osteocalcin *Serum Decrease Physiological* In patients treated with long term corticosteroids significant reduction to 4.3 ± 0.5 ng/mL compared with 6.2 ± 0.2 ng/mL in normal individuals *1372*

Phosphate *Urine Increase Physiological* Metabolic effect *3669*

Potassium *Serum Decrease Physiological* Mineralocorticoid effect with increase renal excretion *129*
Urine Increase Physiological Promotes excretion (mineralocorticoid effect) *128*

Protein *Serum Increase Physiological* Physiological doses promote protein synthesis *1095*
Urine Increase Physiological Nephrotoxic especially in children with chronic disease *2452*

Prothrombin Time *Plasma Decrease Physiological* Accelerate metabolism of anticoagulants *3810*
Plasma Increase Physiological Alleged potentiation of effect of anticoagulants *2754*

Salicylate *Serum Decrease Physiological* Levels did not rise above 150 µg/mL in patients given corticosteroids and 4.8 g aspirin/d *2280* Increases glomerular filtration, decreases tubular reabsorption *2452* Concomitant administration causes accelerated metabolism, most marked in males *2985*

Sodium *Serum Increase Physiological* May cause retention *3810*
Urine Decrease Physiological Promotes retention (mineralocorticoid effect) *128*

T3-Uptake *Serum Increase Physiological* Resin uptake increased due to decreased thyroxine binding globulin *3107*

Thyro-Binding Index *Serum Decrease Physiological* May occur for up to 1 week after therapy *1444*

Thyroid Stimulating Hormone
Serum Decrease Physiological Effect observed in patients with Hashimoto's thyroiditis as autoimmune process is suppressed *1269* Usual response in patients on steroids *3669*

Thyroxine Binding Globulin
Serum Decrease Physiological Large dose response *3107* Decreased concentration observed with corticosteroid treatment *277* Observed effect with corticosteroid treatment *1269*

Thyroxine Binding Prealbumin
Serum Increase Physiological Reciprocal increase observed in response to reduction of TBG *1269*

Thyroxine (T4) *Serum Decrease Physiological* Minor effect observed with systemic therapy. Concentrations usually remain within reference range *1269* May occur for up to 1 week after therapy *1444* Decreased concentration observed with corticosteroid treatment which reduces TBG concentration *277*
Serum Increase Physiological In patients with Hashimoto's thyroiditis concentration may increase as autoimmune process is suppressed *1269*

Thyroxine (T4), Free *Serum Decrease Physiological* Minor effect observed with systemic therapy. Concentrations usually remain within reference range *1269*

Thyroxine (T4) Index, Free *Serum Decrease Physiological* Low normal or slight decrease for 1 week after treatment *1444*

Tri-iodothyronine, Free (fT3)
Serum Decrease Physiological Minor effect observed with systemic therapy. Concentrations usually remain within reference range *1269*

Tri-iodothyronine, Reverse (rT3)
Serum Increase Physiological Increase observed with systemic therapy although concentrations rarely outside reference range *1269*

Tri-iodothyronine (T3) *Serum Decrease Physiological* Minor effect observed with systemic therapy. Concentrations usually remain within reference range *1269*

Tri-iodotyrosine, Reverse *Serum Increase Physiological* Increase observed with systemic therapy although concentrations rarely outside reference range *1269*

Uric Acid *Serum Decrease Physiological* Produces negative nitrogen balance *3810*

Uropepsinogen *Urine Increase Physiological* Increase renal clearance *1252*

Volume *Plasma Increase Physiological* Expansion of extracellular fluid due to water retention *2242*

Zinc *Serum Decrease Physiological* Rapid sustained drop in burn and surgical patients *1898*

Corticosterone

Cortisol *Plasma No Effect Analytical* At concerntrations 40 times that usually present in plasma 1.0% cross reactivty observed with method on Baxter Stratus *5705*

Cortisol, Free *Urine No Effect Analytical* No significant interference observed with HPLC method of Turpeinen et al *6105*

Digitoxin *Serum No Effect Analytical* At concentration of 1.4 mg/L no cross reactivity observed with method on Baxter Stratus *5705*

Digoxin *Serum No Effect Analytical* Cross reactivity of less than 10% observed with method on Baxter Stratus *5705*

Progesterone *Plasma No Effect Analytical* Corticosterone at a concentration of up to 1000 ng/mL had a cross-reactivity of only 0.3% in progesterone method on Bayer Technicon Immuno 1® *429* Cross-reactivity of 0.2% observed with method on Ciba Corning ACS:180 *1113* 1% or less cross reactivity with RIA *858*

Corticotropin

Aldolase *Serum Increase Physiological* Probably due to muscle damage at site of injection *463*

Aldosterone *Plasma Increase Physiological* In 7 healthy individuals intravenous administration of ACTH 1-24 caused significant increases from 1545 ± 441 pmol/L to 3606 ± 860 pmol/L after 0.1 µg, from 1062 ± 241 pmol/L to 3859 ± 499 pmol/L after 1 µg and from 1379 ± 391 pmol/L to 4572 ± 1140 pmol/L after 250 µg *1216*
Urine Increase Physiological Effect less marked than on tetrahydro-DOC *5313*

Amino Acids *Urine Increase Physiological* Catabolism of body tissues *6515*

α-Amino-Nitrogen *Plasma Increase Physiological* Tissue and protein catabolism *2024*
Urine Increase Physiological Catabolism of body tissues *6515*

Amylase *Serum Increase Physiological* Increase may be marked (both short and long term) *950*

Androstenedione *Plasma Increase Physiological* Increase from baseline mean of 4.8 to 6.1 nmol/L at 30 min following intravenous administration of 100 units ACTH in 22 normal women and comparable increases in women with hirsutism from a variety of causes *5545*

Androsterone *Plasma Increase Physiological* Hormonal effect *4028*
Urine Increase Physiological Normal response to 2 d ACTH test *2425*

Ascorbic Acid *Urine Increase Physiological* Mobilizes vitamin stored in adrenal cortex *655*

Basal Metabolic Rate *Patient Decrease Physiological* Metabolic action of hormone *3669*

Calcium *Urine Increase Physiological* Average or large doses promote excretion *2754*

Chloride *Serum Decrease Physiological* May cause hypochloremic alkalosis *3809*

Cholesterol *Serum Decrease Physiological* Ester concentration reduced by stimulation of adrenal *1009*
Serum Increase Physiological Effect of hormone action after initial fall *3669*

Cholesterol Esters *Serum Increase Physiological* Initial fall then rise about 10% *3809*

Corticosteroids *Plasma Increase Physiological* Maximum response seen after 4 h *258*

Corticosterone *Urine No Effect Physiological* No effect observed in normals *3228*

Cortisol *Plasma Increase Physiological* Therapeutic intent *2754* Increase from mean of 367 nmol/L to 620 nmol/L in 22 normal women at 30 min following intravenous administration of 100 units ACTH and comparable increases in women with hirsutism from a variety of causes *5545* In 7 healthy individuals intravenous administration of ACTH 1-24 caused significant increases from 232 ± 28 nmol/L to 497 ± 72 nmol/L after 0.1 µg, from 235 ± 22 nmol/L to 761 ± 25 nmol/L after 1 µg and from 190 ± 25 nmol/L to 670 ± 36 nmol/L after 250 µg *1216*
Urine Increase Physiological Progressive increase with repeated injection *3228*

Cortisone *Plasma Increase Physiological* In one individual continuous infusion of β_1-24 ACTH for 2.5 h caused 60 nmol/L increase with magnitude of increase linearly related to the duration of infusion *1854*

Dehydroepiandrosterone *Plasma Increase Physiological* Increase in 22 normal women from mean of 18.7 to 34.6 nmol/L at 30 min and in women with hirsutism following intravenous administration of 100 units ACTH *5545* In 7 healthy individuals intravenous administration of ACTH 1-24 caused significant increases from 11.1 ± 1.4 nmol/L to 15.9 ± 1.4 nmol/L after 0.1 µg, from 10.4 ± 1.0 nmol/L to 25.0 ± 2.1 nmol/L after 1 µg and from 9.7 ± 1.0 nmol/L to 29.1 ± 3.5 nmol/L after 250 µg *1216* Hormonal effect *4028*
Urine Increase Physiological Normal response to 2 d ACTH test *2425*

Dehydroepiandrosterone Sulfate
Plasma Increase Physiological Increase from mean of 4921 to 5029 nmol/L in 22 normal women at 30 min following intravenous administration of 100 units ACTH but reduction in women with hirsutism from most causes *5545*

Corticotropin *(continued)*

11-Deoxycortisol *Plasma Increase Physiological* Increase from mean of 1.2 to 3.6 nmol/L in 22 normal women at 30 min following intravenous administration of 100 units and comparable increases in women with hirsutism from a variety of causes *5545*
Urine Increase Physiological Progressive increase with repeated injection *3228*

21-Deoxycortisol *Plasma Increase Physiological* In 25 normal women mean concentration rose from 0.173 nmol/L to 1.09 nmol/L post-ACTH, in 18 normal men from 0.23 nmol/L to 1.09 nmol/L, in 8 normal children from 0.20 nmol/L to 1.03 nmol/L. In 27 late onset congenital adrenal hyperplasia patients mean concentration increased from 6.00 nmol/L to 29.72 nmol/L after ACTH, from 0.77 to 4.24 nmol/L in 18 heterozygotes for late onset congenital adrenal hyperplasia and from 0.69 to 5.28 nmol/L after ACTH in 30 heterozygotes for classical congenital adrenal hyperplasia *1860*

Eosinophils *Blood Decrease Physiological* Striking response in normals *2242*

Epinephrine *Urine No Effect Physiological* No effect observed in normals or rheumatoids *467*

Erythrocyte Sedimentation Rate
Blood Decrease Physiological Particularly in rheumatoid patients *409*

Erythrocytes *Blood Increase Physiological* Especially marked if given to anemics *2242*

Estriol *Urine Increase Physiological* In pregnant increased production of adrenal precursors *54*

Estrogens *Urine Increase Physiological* Hormonal effect in men and women *3646*

Etiocholanolone *Urine Increase Physiological* Normal response to 2 d ACTH test *2425*

Glucose *Serum Increase Physiological* Gluconeogenesis, insulin antagonism *6515*
Urine Increase Physiological Increased blood glucose, reduced TMG *6515*

Glucose Tolerance *Serum Decrease Physiological* Corticosteroid impairment of insulin secretion *322*

Growth Hormone *Plasma Decrease Physiological* Reduces maximum of hormone during sleep *2150*
Plasma Increase Physiological Up to 1 mg i.v. has marked effect *3090* Increase in 50%, moderate effect only *3584*

Hematocrit *Blood Increase Physiological* Especially in anemics *463*

Hydrochloric Acid *Gastric Fluid Increase Physiological* Effect of protracted therapy *2754*

11-Hydroxyandrosterone *Urine Increase Physiological* Normal response to 2 d ACTH test *2425*

11-Hydroxycorticosteroids *Plasma Increase Analytical* Increased cholesterol with nonspecific fluorescent procedure *2277*

17-Hydroxycorticosteroids *Urine Decrease Physiological* Reduction even if given orally or topically *687*
Urine Increase Physiological Marked response to i.v. infusion *578*

11-Hydroxyetiocholanolone *Urine Increase Physiological* Normal response to 2 d ACTH test *2425*

5-Hydroxyindoleacetic Acid *Urine Decrease Physiological* Mechanism not described *2451*

17-Hydroxypregnenolone *Plasma Increase Physiological* Increase at 30 min in 13 women with decreased activity of 3β-hydroxy-δ5-steroid dehydrogenase following 100 units ACTH intravenously compared with 22 normal women (increase from 5.6 to 24.0 nmol/L) and those with other causes of hirsutism *5545*

17-Hydroxyprogesterone *Plasma Increase Physiological* Increase at 30 min in 5 hirsute women with decreased acivity of 21-hydroxylase following 100 units ACTH intravenously compared with response in 22 normal women (increase from mean of 1.9 to 4.3 nmol/L) and in those with other causes of hirsutism *5545*

^{131}I Uptake *Serum Decrease Physiological* ?effect on TSH: lasts up to 8 d *2396*

Iron *Serum Decrease Physiological* Decrease in iron binding globulin *6515*

Iron-Binding Capacity, Total
Serum Decrease Physiological Decrease in iron binding globulin *6515*

Iron-Binding Capacity, Unsaturated
Serum Decrease Physiological Decrease in iron binding globulin *6515*

11-Ketoetiocholanolone *Urine Increase Physiological* Normal response to 2 d ACTH test *2425*

17-Ketosteroids *Urine Decrease Physiological* Reduction even if orally or topically given *687*
Urine Increase Physiological Stimulation of adrenal *2451*

Leukocytes *Blood Increase Physiological* Significant neutrophilic granulocytosis *4014*

Lymphocytes *Blood Decrease Physiological* Marked drop occurs within 2 h *2242*

Norepinephrine *Urine Decrease Physiological* Observed effect in normals and rheumatoids *467*

pH *Urine Decrease Physiological* Metabolic effect *2658*

Potassium *Serum Decrease Physiological* Increased urinary excretion (mineralocorticoid effect) *6515*
Urine Increase Physiological Mobilization of potassium from tissues *2242*

Pregnanediol *Urine Increase Physiological* Hormonal effect *3646*

Progesterone *Plasma Increase Physiological* Significant increase at 30 min in 5 hirsute women with decreased 21-hydroxylase activity following 100 units of ACTH intravenously compared with 22 normal women or those with hirsutism from other causes. In normal increased from mean of 0.9 to 2.1 nmol/L *5545*

Protein *Serum Increase Physiological* Physiological doses promote protein synthesis *1095*
Urine Increase Physiological May be nephrotoxic in chronic disease *2586*

Prothrombin Time *Plasma Decrease Physiological* Patients on coumarins (may induce enzymes) *4013*
Plasma Increase Physiological Prolongs action of anticoagulants *3810*

Reticulocytes *Blood Increase Physiological* Especially if given to anemics *2242*

Sodium *Serum Increase Physiological* Causes retention with edema *128*

Testosterone *Urine Increase Physiological* Moderate effect in men *5107*

Tetrahydrodeoxycorticosterone
Urine Increase Physiological Fivefold increase in response to infusion in normals *5313*

Thyro-Binding Index *Serum Decrease Physiological* Occurs for up to 1 week after treatment *1444*

Thyroxine Binding Globulin
Serum Decrease Physiological Reduced synthesis *6515*

Thyroxine (T4) *Serum Decrease Physiological* Decreased thyro-binding globulin (occurs for up to 1 week) *6515*

Thyroxine (T4) Index, Free *Serum Decrease Physiological* Low normal or slight decrease 1 week after therapy *1444*

Uric Acid *Serum Decrease Physiological* Uricosuric action *2378*
Urine Increase Physiological Uricosuric action *2378*

Volume *Plasma Increase Physiological* Moderate doses can cause salt and water retention *2754*

Zinc *Serum Increase Physiological* Occurs in most subjects (decreased in others) *5962*

Corticotropin-Releasing Hormone

Cortisol *Plasma Increase Physiological* Significant increase observed in all phases of menstrual cycle following 100 μg intravenously *362*

Follicle Stimulating Hormone
Plasma Decrease Physiological Significant reduction with 100 μg intravenously during midluteal phase of menstrual cycle although not during other phases of cycle *362*

Luteinizing Hormone *Plasma Decrease Physiological* 100 µg intravenously caused 50% decrease during late follicular phase of menstrual cycle, 52% decrease during midluteal phase but had no effect during midfollicular phase. Hormone concentration decreased within 4 h of injection, normalized within 5 h *362*

Cortisone

Alanine Aminotransferase *Serum Increase Physiological* May contribute to long duration of hepatitis *3669*

α-Amino-Nitrogen *Urine Increase Physiological* Increased tissue catabolism *6515*

Aspartate Aminotransferase *Serum Increase Physiological* May contribute to long duration of hepatitis *3669*

Calcium *Serum Decrease Physiological* If elevated due to sarcoidosis or vitamin D *128*

Cells *Urine Increase Physiological* Increased number observed with long-term treatment *4014*

Chloride *Serum Decrease Physiological* May cause hypochloremic alkalosis *6686*
Urine Decrease Physiological Causes retention *128*

Cholesterol *Serum Increase Physiological* Increase about 20% with vigorous treatment *6686*

Cholesterol Esters *Serum Increase Physiological* Increase about 20% with vigorous treatment *6686*

Cortisol *Plasma Increase Physiological* Effect lasts for 24 h at least *2895*
Plasma No Effect Analytical Cortisone caused an insignificant cross-reactivity of 3.0% with method on Bayer Technicon Immuno 1® *419* At concentrations 40 times greater than in plasma 2.1% cross reactivity observed with method on Baxter Stratus *5705*

Cortisol, Free *Urine No Effect Analytical* No significant interference observed with HPLC method of Turpeinen et al *6105*

Digoxin *Serum No Effect Analytical* At concentrations up to 40 µg/mL no significant effect observed on method on Ciba Corning ACS:180 *1412*

Eosinophils *Blood Decrease Physiological* Normal physiological response to injection *3671*

Epinephrine *Urine Decrease Physiological* Decreased output with 200 mg/d *467*

Erythrocyte Sedimentation Rate
Blood Decrease Physiological Particularly in rheumatoid patients *409*

Estradiol *Plasma No Effect Analytical* At a concentration of 4000 ng/mL had less than 0.01% cross-reactivity with method on Bayer Technicon Immuno 1® *422*

Glomerular Filtration Rate *Urine Decrease Physiological* Probably does this by decreased secretion of creatinine *1444*

Glucose *Serum Increase Physiological* Gluconeogenesis *3669*

Glucose Tolerance *Serum Decrease Physiological* Gluconeogenesis and anti-insulin effects *3669*

17-Hydroxycorticosteroids *Urine Increase Physiological* Measuring excretory products of cortisone *6515*

^{131}I Uptake *Serum Decrease Physiological* Probably diminishes TSH secretion *4014*

Iron *Serum Decrease Physiological* Reduced synthesis of transferrin *6515*

Iron-Binding Capacity, Total
Serum Decrease Physiological Reduced synthesis of transferrin *6515*

17-Ketogenic Steroids *Urine Increase Physiological* Metabolic products *3669*

17-Ketosteroids *Urine Decrease Physiological* Pituitary suppression of ACTH *6515*

Neutrophils *Blood Increase Physiological* Significant granulocytosis observed *2242*

Occult Blood *Feces Increase Physiological* May cause hemorrhage or ulceration of gastrointestinal tract *929*

Potassium *Serum Decrease Physiological* Mineralocorticoid effect *6515*
Urine Increase Physiological Promotes excretion *128*

Prothrombin Time *Plasma Decrease Physiological* Patients on coumarins *3950*

Sodium *Serum Increase Physiological* Mineralocorticoid effect *6515*
Urine Decrease Physiological Causes retention *128*

Thyroxine Binding Globulin
Serum Decrease Physiological Reduced synthesis *6515*

Thyroxine (T4) *Serum Decrease Physiological* Decreased synthesis *5869*

Transferrin *Serum Decrease Physiological* Reduced synthesis *6515*

Uric Acid *Serum Decrease Physiological* Observed in normals after 200 mg daily *5353*
Urine Increase Physiological Observed in normals after 200 mg daily *5353*

Cotrifamole

Thyroid Stimulating Hormone
Serum No Effect Physiological No change in men or women over 10 d *1077*

Thyroxine (T4) *Serum No Effect Physiological* Possible intrathyroidal inhibition of conversion of iodine to organic form *6412* No change in men or women over 10 d *1077*

Thyroxine (T4) Index, Free *Serum No Effect Physiological* No change in men or women over 10 d *1077*

Tri-iodothyronine (T3) *Serum Decrease Physiological* Possible intrathyroidal inhibition of conversion of iodine to organic form *6412* From 2.50 to 2.17 nmol/L in men and 1.90 to 1.65 nmol/L in women when treated for 10 d *1077*

Cotrimoxazole

Cyclosporine *Blood No Effect Physiological* Coadministration with cyclosporine appears to have no effect on the cyclosporine concentration *859*
Serum No Effect Physiological Coadministration with cyclosporine appears to have no effect on the cyclosporine concentration *859*

Coumaric Acid

5-Hydroxyindoleacetic Acid *Urine Increase Analytical* May interfere with colorimetric methods *1444*

Coumarin

Alanine Aminotransferase *Serum Increase Physiological* Infrequent occurences of hepatitis or cholestatic hepatic injury reported *1595* May cause hepatic toxicity *6461*

Alkaline Phosphatase *Serum Increase Physiological* Infrequent occurences of hepatitis or cholestatic hepatic injury reported *1595* May cause hepatotoxicity *6461*

Aspartate Aminotransferase *Serum Increase Physiological* Infrequent occurences of hepatitis or cholestatic hepatic injury reported *1595* May cause hepatic toxicity *6461*

Bile *Urine Increase Physiological* May cause hepatotoxicity *6461*

Bilirubin *Serum Increase Physiological* Infrequent occurences of hepatitis or cholestatic hepatic injury reported *1595* May cause hepatotoxicity *6461*

BSP Retention *Serum Increase Physiological* May cause hepatotoxicity *6461*

Chlorpropamide *Serum Decrease Physiological* Coadministration of coumarin may cause drug to accumulate as a result of interference with either metabolism or excretion *1595*
Serum Increase Physiological Drugs that are highly protein-bound compete with chlorpropamide for binding sites and may potentiate hypoglycemic action of sulfonylurea *4644*

Cyclosporine *Serum Increase Physiological* Poorly documented effect reported *1069*

Erythrocytes *Urine Increase Physiological* Actual bleeding may occur with high doses *1714*

Coumarin *(continued)*

Hemoglobin *Urine Increase Physiological* Actual bleeding may occur with high doses *2024*

Heparin *Plasma Increase Analytical* In patients receiving both heparin and coumarin Heptest results exceeded true heparin concentrations by more than 0.2 int U/mL, sometimes up to 0.4 int U/mL. Effect due to coumarin-induced decrease of plasma prothrombin *1875*

Phenobarbital *Serum Decrease Physiological* Coadministration of coumarin may cause drug to accumulate as a result of interference with either metabolism or excretion *1595*

Phenytoin *Serum Decrease Physiological* Coadministration of coumarin may cause drug to accumulate as a result of interference with either metabolism or excretion *1595*

T3-Uptake *Serum Increase Physiological* Competes with T3 for thyroxine binding albumin sites *882*

Tolbutamide *Serum Decrease Physiological* Coadministration of coumarin may cause drug to accumulate as a result of interference with either metabolism or excretion *1595*

Uric Acid *Serum Decrease Physiological* Uricosuric effect *2024*
Urine Increase Physiological Uricosuric effect *2024*

Cremomycin

^{131}I Uptake *Serum Decrease Physiological* Merck compound contains tetraiodofluorescein *4360*

Prothrombin Time *Plasma Increase Physiological* May cause hypoprothrombinemia *128*

Urea Nitrogen *Serum Increase Physiological* Dehydration may simulate renal disease *128*

Cromakalim

Aldosterone *Plasma Increase Physiological* Insignificant increase from mean of 16.5 ng/dL to 18.2 ng/dL in 12 healthy volunteers treated with up to 1 mg daily for 1 week *3573*
Plasma No Effect Physiological Insignificant reduction in 8 healthy men given 1 mg daily for 5 days *1850*
Urine No Effect Physiological Insignificant increase from mean of 14.3 µg/24 h to mean of 15.4 µg/24 h in 12 healthy volunteers treated with up to 1 mg daily for 1 week *3573*

Angiotensin-II *Plasma Increase Physiological* Doubling of concentration to 10.5 pg/mL in 8 healthy men given 1 mg daily for 5 days *1850* Insignificant increase from mean of 42.8 pg/mL to mean of 62.2 pg/mL in 12 healthy volunteers after 1 week treatment with up to 1 mg daily *3573*

Atrial Natriuretic Peptide *Plasma No Effect Physiological* Insignificant effect in 8 healthy men given 1 mg daily for 5 days *1850* Insignificant increase from mean of 18.1 pg/mL to 19.0 pg/mL in 12 healthy volunteers treated for i week with up to 1 mg daily *3573*

Calcium *Serum No Effect Physiological* No effect observed in 8 healthy men given 1 mg daily for 5 days *1850*

Creatinine *Serum No Effect Physiological* No effect observed in 8 healthy men given 1 mg daily for 5 days *1850*

Creatinine Clearance *Urine No Effect Physiological* Insignificant reduction in 8 healthy men given 1 mg daily for 5 days *1850*

Dopamine *Plasma No Effect Physiological* Insignificant increase in 8 healthy men given 1 mg daily for 5 days *1850*

Epinephrine *Plasma Increase Physiological* Insignificant increase from mean of 0.22 ng/mL to 0.29 ng/mL in 12 healthy volunteers treated with up to 1 mg daily for 1 week *3573* Insignificant increase from 2.47 to 3.23 ng/dL in 8 healthy men given 1 mg daily for 5 days *1850*

Kallikrein *Urine No Effect Physiological* Insignificant increase from mean of 0.575 U/24 h to 0.773 U/24 h in 12 healthy volunteers treated with up to 1 mg daily for 1 week *3573*

Norepinephrine *Plasma Increase Physiological* Significant increase (61%) from mean of 11.5 to 18.5 ng/dL in 8 healthy men given 1 mg daily for 5 days *1850* Insignificant increase from mean of 0.24 pg/mL to 0.38 pg/mL in 12 healthy volunteers treated with up to 1 mg daily for 1 week *3573*

Potassium *Serum No Effect Physiological* No effect observed in 8 healthy men given 1 mg daily for 5 days *1850*
Urine No Effect Physiological Insignificant reduction observed in 8 healthy men given 1 mg daily for 5 days *1850*

Renin Activity *Plasma Increase Physiological* Significant increase from mean of 0.76 ng/mL/h to 1.41 ng/mL/h in 12 healthy volunteers treated for 1 week with up to 1 mg daily *3573* Doubling of concentration of Angiotensin-I to 3.87 ng/mL/h following treatment with 1 mg daily for 5 days *1850*

Sodium *Serum No Effect Physiological* No change observed in 8 healthy men given 1 mg daily for 5 days *1850*
Urine No Effect Physiological Insignificant reduction observed in 8 healthy men given 1 mg daily for 5 days *1850*

Cromolyn

Alanine Aminotransferase *Serum No Effect Physiological* No clinical significant change observed *744*

Aspartate Aminotransferase
Serum No Effect Physiological No clinical significant change observed *744*

Eosinophils *Blood No Effect Physiological* No clinical significant change observed *744*

Erythrocyte Sedimentation Rate
Blood No Effect Physiological No clinical significant change observed *744*

Ethanol *Serum No Effect Physiological* No significant effect on ethanol concentration observed *1165*

Hemoglobin *Blood No Effect Physiological* No clinically significant change observed *744*
Urine No Effect Physiological No clinical significant change observed *744*

Histamine *Plasma No Effect Analytical* No inhibition of radio-enzyme assay even at concentrations much greater than physiological *2492*

17-Hydroxycorticosteroids *Plasma Decrease Physiological* Significant effect observed if given prior to exercise *2681*
Urine No Effect Physiological No proportional increase in relation to blood change *2681*

Leukocytes *Blood No Effect Physiological* No clinical significant change observed *744*

Protein *Urine No Effect Physiological* No clinical significant change observed *744*

Theophylline *Serum No Effect Analytical* No effect on method on Kodak Ektachem® 700 *1716* At concentration of 15 mg/L produced no interference with methods used on Kodak DT60, Abbott TDx, Abbott Vision with both whole blood and serum, 3M Diagnostics TheoFAST, Syntex AccµLevel, and Ames Seralyzer *1122*

Urea Nitrogen *Serum No Effect Physiological* No clinical significant change observed *744*

Urobilin *Urine No Effect Physiological* No clinical significant change observed *744*

Croton Oil

Agglutinins *Blood Positive Physiological* May induce formation *467*

Cyclacillin

Glucose *Urine Increase Analytical* Falsely elevated value of 0.25% approximately at physiological concentration *4538*
Urine No Effect Analytical No effect on Diastix® at physiological concentration. No effect on TesTape® at physiological concentration *4538*

Cyclamate

Amphetamine *Urine Positive Analytical* False positive measurement observed with Abbott TDx system due to metabolite cyclohexylamine *3822*

Chromosomes *Test Conditions Abnormal Physiological* Potent clastogen in human cells *5484*

Lincomycin *Serum Decrease Physiological* Inhibits gastro-intestinal absorption *2452*

Cyclazocine

Morphine *Urine No Effect Analytical* Insignificant cross reactivity with RIA procedures. Insignificant cross reactivity with EMIT procedure for opiates *4163*

Cyclobenzaprine

Alanine Aminotransferase *Serum Increase Physiological* In less than 1% of treated patients abnormal liver function has been reported with rare reports of hepatitis, jaundice and cholestasis *3975*

Alkaline Phosphatase *Serum Increase Physiological* In less than 1% of treated patients abnormal liver function has been reported with rare reports of hepatitis, jaundice and cholestasis *3975*

Amitriptyline *Serum Increase Analytical* Reported interference with EMIT, TLC, GC, LC and GC/MS procedures: may also interfere with other antidepressants *4815*

Aspartate Aminotransferase *Serum Increase Physiological* In less than 1% of treated patients abnormal liver function has been reported with rare reports of hepatitis, jaundice and cholestasis *3975*

Bilirubin *Serum Increase Physiological* In less than 1% of treated patients abnormal liver function has been reported with rare reports of hepatitis, jaundice and cholestasis *3975*

Desipramine *Serum Increase Analytical* May cause false positive reaction for desipramine when measured by HPLC *3590*

Eosinophils *Blood Increase Physiological* Bone marrow depression and eosinophilia have been reported rarely *3975*

Glucose *Serum Increase Physiological* Both hyperglycemia and hypoglycemia have been reported rarely as complications *3975*

Leukocytes *Blood Decrease Physiological* Bone marrow depression and leukopenia have been reported rarely *3975*

Platelets *Blood Decrease Physiological* Purpura, bone marrow depression and thrombocytopenia have been reported rarely *3975*

Tricyclic Antidepressants *Serum Increase Analytical* May cause false positive reaction in immunoassays for tricyclic antidepressants *3590*

Tricyclic Antidepressants Screen *Serum No Effect Analytical* No significant interference observed at a concentration of 200 ng/mL (0.73 µmol/L) with method on Du Pont aca *1550*

Cyclofenil

Alanine Aminotransferase *Serum Increase Physiological* In 1 case, but total of 30 cases reported up to 1980; Considered to be metabolic idiosyncrasy and reversible in all cases *4416* Slightly and transiently increased in 6 of 19 patients over 4 mo of treatment, especially with high doses *4618*

Alkaline Phosphatase *Serum Increase Physiological* In 1 case, but total of 30 cases reported up to 1980; Considered to be metabolic idiosyncrasy and reversible in all cases *4416*

Apolipoprotein A-I *Serum Increase Physiological* Increase by 15% after 2 and 4 mo after therapy in 19 patients given 600 mg daily for 4 mo *4618*

Aspartate Aminotransferase *Serum Increase Physiological* Slightly and transiently increased in 6 of 19 patients over 4 mo of treatment, especially with high doses *4618* In 1 case, but total of 30 cases reported up to 1980; Considered to be metabolic idiosyncrasy and reversible in all cases *4416*

Bilirubin *Serum Increase Physiological* In 1 case, but total of 30 cases reported up to 1980; Considered to be metabolic idiosyncrasy and reversible in all cases *4416*

Cholesterol *Serum Increase Physiological* Slight effect in 19 patients given 600 mg daily for 4 mo *4618*

Estradiol *Urine No Effect Physiological* Normal amounts observed with GC/MS *54*

HDL-Cholesterol *Serum Increase Physiological* By approximately 15% with 2 and 4 mo of therapy in 19 patients given 600 mg daily for 4 mo *4618*

LDL-Cholesterol *Serum No Effect Physiological* Non-significant tendency to increase in 19 patients given 600 mg daily for 4 mo *4618*

Triglycerides *Serum Increase Physiological* Slight increase over 4 mo in 19 patients given 600 mg daily for therapy *4618*

Cycloheximide

Leukocytes *Blood Decrease Physiological* Leukopenia (AMA Blood dyscrasias) *4017*

Cycloleucine

Arginine *Urine Increase Physiological* Reversible marked aminoaciduria *770*

Cystine *Urine Increase Physiological* Reversible marked aminoaciduria *770*

Lysine *Urine Increase Physiological* Reversible marked aminoaciduria *770*

Cyclopenthiazide

Cholesterol *Serum No Effect Physiological* No significant effect in 53 mild hypertensives treated with 50 to 500 µg daily for 8 weeks *3925*

Coombs' Test *Blood Positive Physiological* Reported observation *4265*

Glucose *Serum No Effect Physiological* No significant effect in 53 patients with mild hypertension given from 50 to 500 µg daily for 8 weeks *3925*

Neutrophils *Blood Decrease Physiological* Reported to cause neutropenia/agranulocytosis *4265*

Platelets *Blood Decrease Physiological* Thrombocytopenia reported *4265*

Uric Acid *Serum Increase Physiological* Diuretic induced gout observed in 4 patients with either hypertension or myocardial ischemia *5416*

Cyclopentobarbital

Cannabinoids *Urine No Effect Analytical* No effect on Roche Abuscreen method *5006*

Cyclophosphamide

Alanine Aminotransferase *Serum Increase Physiological* May cause hepatotoxicity *5777*
Serum No Effect Physiological No significant perturbation in 41 patients *3949*

Albumin *Serum Decrease Physiological* May cause hepatotoxicity *5777*

Alkaline Phosphatase *Serum Increase Physiological* May cause hepatotoxicity *3810*
Serum No Effect Physiological No significant perturbation in 41 patients *3949*

Anti-DNA Antibodies *Serum Decrease Physiological* In 9 patients with SLE given monthly i.v. infusions of drug for 6 months *3885*

Aspartate Aminotransferase *Serum Increase Physiological* May cause hepatotoxicity *5777*
Serum No Effect Physiological No significant perturbation in 41 patients *3949*

Bile *Urine Increase Physiological* May cause hepatotoxicity *3810*

Bilirubin *Serum Increase Physiological* May cause hepatotoxicity *3810*
Serum No Effect Physiological No significant perturbation in 41 patients *3949*

BSP Retention *Serum Increase Physiological* May cause hepatotoxicity *3810*

Cyclophosphamide *(continued)*

CA549 *Serum No Effect Analytical* No statistically significant effect observed over a concentration range of 22 to 330 mg/L with BRESMARQ assay *958* No interference observed at concentrations up to 330 mg/L with immunoradiometric BRESMARQ procedure *958*

Cholesterol *Serum Increase Physiological* Single case of drug induced myxedema *1073*
Serum No Effect Analytical At concentration of 240 mg/L had no effect on Liebermann-Burchard method *5704* At concentration of 240 mg/L had no effect on CHOD-PAP method *5704* At concentration of 240 mg/L had no effect on CHOD-Iodide method *5704* At concentration of 240 mg/L had no effect on method using catalase-Hantzsch reaction *5704* At concentration of 240 mg/L had no effect on catalase-AIDH method *5704*

Cholinesterase *Serum Decrease Physiological* Causes inhibition of activity *6684*

Chromosomes *Test Conditions Abnormal Physiological* Clastogenic in human cells *5484*

Color *Feces Increase Analytical* Black color reported with cyclophosphamide ingestion *3388*

Complement C_3 *Serum Increase Physiological* In 9 patients with SLE given i.v. infusions of drug monthly for 6 months *3885*

Complement C_4 *Serum Increase Physiological* In 9 patients with SLE given i.v. infusions of drug monthly for 6 months *3885*

Complement CH50 *Serum Increase Physiological* In 9 patients with SLE given i.v. infusions of drug monthly for 6 months *3885*

Coombs' Test, Direct *Blood Positive Physiological* May cause hemolytic anemia *3895*

Creatinine *Serum No Effect Analytical* At concentration of 40 mg/L had no effect on Jaffe-Fuller's earth method *5704* At concentration of 452 mg/L had no effect on kinetic Jaffe method on BKA-2 *5704* At concentration of 40 mg/L had no effect on Jaffe-Fading-Fraction method *5704*

Creatinine Clearance *Urine Increase Physiological* In 9 patients with SLE given i.v. drug infusions monthly for 6 months *3885*
Urine No Effect Physiological In majority of patients although decreased urine volume. With decreased sodium excretion in one patient *1343*

Cyclosporine *Blood No Effect Analytical* At a concentration of 250 mg/L had no effect on Syva EMIT method *495*

Erythrocyte Sedimentation Rate
Blood Decrease Physiological In 9 patients with SLE given i.v. infusions of drug monthly for 6 months *3885*

Erythrocytes *Blood Decrease Physiological* May cause anemia, usually reversible *2754*
Urine Increase Physiological Actual bleeding may be caused by drug *1714*

Glomerular Filtration Rate *Urine No Effect Physiological* In majority of patients although decreased urine volume *1343*

Glucose *Serum No Effect Analytical* At concentration of 40 mg/L had no effect on GOD/POD-PAP method *5704* At concentration of 8 mg/L had no effect on Kodak Ektachem® method *5704*

Hemoglobin *Blood Decrease Physiological* May cause megaloblastic anemia *4265*
Urine Increase Physiological Actual bleeding caused by drug *1714*

Histamine *Plasma No Effect Analytical* Improbable inhibition of radio-enzyme assay at therapeutic concentrations *2492*

^{131}I Uptake *Serum Decrease Physiological* Single case of drug induced myxedema *1073*

Kininogen *Plasma Decrease Physiological* Maximum effect with onset of leukopenia *1200*

Leukocytes *Blood Decrease Physiological* Bone marrow depression (reversible leukopenia) *133*

Lymphocyte response to Phytohemagglutinin
Blood Decrease Physiological Significant reduction with chemotherapy observed *685*

Methotrexate *Serum No Effect Analytical* No significant interference observed at a concentration of 10 µmol/L with method on Du Pont aca *1535*

Neutrophils *Blood Decrease Physiological* Reported observation *4265*

Occult Blood *Feces Increase Physiological* Hemorrhagic colitis reported *4014*

Osmolality *Serum Decrease Physiological* Average of 15 mosm/kg for 1 d (due to metabolites) *1344*
Urine Increase Physiological Impaired water excretion 500 mosm/kg increase *1344*

Platelets *Blood Decrease Physiological* May cause bone marrow depression *133*

Potassium *Serum No Effect Analytical* At concentration of 80 mg/L had no effect on measurement by ISE without predilution *5704*

Prostate-specific Antigen *Serum No Effect Analytical* Cyclophosphamide at a concentration of up to 700 µg/mL caused less than 0.1% cross-reactivity with method on PSA method on Bayer Technicon Immuno 1® *430*

Prostate-specific Antigen, Free *Serum No Effect Analytical* Cyclophosphamide at a concentration of 330 mg/L had no significant effect on the Hybritech Tandem® -R free PSA immunoassay *4286*

Protein *Urine Decrease Physiological* In 9 patients with SLE given monthly i.v. infusions of drug for 6 months *3885* In 10 patients with active lupus lupus nephritis administration of intravenous cyclophosphamide over 18 months caused reduction or disappearance of protein in 6 *3818*

Protein Electrophoresis *Serum No Effect Analytical* At concentration of 80 mg/L had no effect on automated Olympus-Hite method *5704*

Prothrombin Time *Plasma Increase Physiological* May cause hypoprothrombinemia *5777*

Sodium *Serum Decrease Physiological* Average 8.5 mEq/L (H_2O retention by metabolites) *1344*
Serum No Effect Analytical At concentration of 80 mg/L had no effect on measurement by ISE without predilution *5704*

Testosterone *Serum Decrease Physiological* Due to induced testicular atrophy *2836*

Triglycerides *Serum No Effect Analytical* At concentration of 40 mg/L had no effect on GPO-PAP method *5704*

Urea Nitrogen *Serum No Effect Analytical* At concentration of 8 mg/L had no effect on Kodak Ektachem® method *5704*

Uric Acid *Serum No Effect Analytical* At concentration of 40 mg/L had no effect on catalase-AIDH method *5704* At concentration of 40 mg/L had no effect on uricase-PAP method *5704* At concentration of 60 mg/L had no effect on Kageyama-Hantzsch method *5704*

Volume *Plasma Increase Physiological* Water retention due to metabolites *1343*
Urine Decrease Physiological To 60 mL/h from 160 mL/h for d (4-12 h after drug) *1344*

Cyclopropane

Alanine Aminotransferase *Serum Increase Physiological* May cause hepatotoxicity (lasts several days) *3810*

Alkaline Phosphatase *Serum Increase Physiological* May cause hepatotoxicity (lasts several days) *3810*

Aspartate Aminotransferase *Serum Increase Physiological* May cause hepatotoxicity (lasts several days) *3810*

Bile *Urine Increase Physiological* May cause hepatotoxicity (lasts several days) *3810*

Bilirubin *Serum Increase Physiological* May cause hepatotoxicity (lasts several days) *3810*

Bleeding Time *Patient No Effect Physiological* Anesthesia has no effect *2242*

BSP Retention *Serum Increase Physiological* May cause hepatotoxicity (lasts several days) *3810*

Capillary Fragility *Patient No Effect Physiological* Anesthesia has no effect *2242*

Catecholamines *Plasma Decrease Analytical* Falsely low with ethylene diamine method *3766*

Plasma Increase Physiological Significant increase, may reduce blood to kidneys etc *128*

Clotting Time *Blood No Effect Physiological* Anesthesia has no effect *2242*

Fibrinogen *Plasma No Effect Physiological* Anesthesia has no effect *2242*

Glucose *Serum Increase Physiological* Moderate with depletion of liver glycogen *128*

Hematocrit *Blood Increase Physiological* Possible effect due to decreased plasma volume *2242*

Indocyanine Green *Serum Increase Physiological* Hepatic extraction impaired after injection *2242*

pH *Blood Decrease Physiological* May cause metabolic acidosis *2242*

Platelets *Blood No Effect Physiological* Anesthesia has no effect *2242*

Prothrombin Time *Plasma No Effect Physiological* Anesthesia has no effect *2242*

Thrombin Time *Blood No Effect Physiological* Anesthesia has no effect *2242*

Cycloserine

Alanine Aminotransferase *Serum Increase Physiological* May cause hepatotoxicity *3810*

Alkaline Phosphatase *Serum Increase Physiological* May cause hepatotoxicity *3810*

Amino-4-Imidazole-5-Carboxamide Ribotide
Urine Increase Physiological Occurs with folic acid deficiency *6370*

Aspartate Aminotransferase *Serum Increase Physiological* May cause hepatotoxicity *3810*

Bile *Urine Increase Physiological* May cause hepatotoxicity *3810*

Bilirubin *Serum Increase Physiological* May cause hepatotoxicity *3810*

BSP Retention *Serum Increase Physiological* May cause hepatotoxicity *3810*

Creatinine *Serum No Effect Analytical* No effect of concentrations up to 15 mg/L on single slide method on Kodak Ektachem® *5706*

Erythrocytes *Blood Decrease Physiological* May cause megaloblastic anemia *6370*

Folate *Serum Decrease Physiological* May cause megaloblastic anemia *6370* Low serum folate in half patients treated with cycloserine plus isoniazid in contrast to 2 of 55 treated with isoniazid alone, but mechanism unknown *3383*

Hematocrit *Blood Decrease Physiological* May cause megaloblastic anemia *6370*

Hemoglobin *Blood Decrease Physiological* May cause megaloblastic anemia *6370*

Histamine *Plasma No Effect Analytical* Improbable inhibition of radio-enzyme assay at therapeutic concentrations *2492*

Homocysteine *Plasma Increase Physiological* As a vitamin B_6 antagonist causes increased concentration *6123*

^{131}I Uptake *Serum Decrease Physiological* Seromycin® contains tetraiodofluorescein *4360*

Leukocytes *Blood Decrease Physiological* May occur with megaloblastic anemia *6370*

MCV *Blood Increase Physiological* May cause megaloblastic anemia *6370*

N-Formiminoglutamic Acid *Urine Increase Physiological* Occurs with folic acid deficiency *6370*

Platelets *Blood Decrease Physiological* May occur with megaloblastic anemia *6370*

Cyclosporine

Alanine Aminotransferase *Serum Decrease Physiological* Mean reduction of 38 U/L in 19 patients with primary biliary cirrhosis when treated with cyclosporine for one year *6445* In 85 patients with severe psoriasis treated for 8 weeks mean decrease of 23% seen when given 3 mg/kg daily, 29% decrease when given 5 mg/kg daily and 22% in patients given 7.5 mg/kg daily compared with increase of 4% in patients given vehicle only *1722*
Serum Increase Physiological Occcasional abnormality observed in 58% of 59 patients with endogenous uveitis treated with 2-10 mg/kg/d for 6-36 months who developed abnormal liver function tests *3057* Hepatotoxicity associated with cyclosporine use has been observed in 4% renal transplant cases, 7% of cardiac transplant cases and 4% of liver transplant cases *5236* Mean increase of 132% observed in 21 post-transplant children receiving cyclosporine for at least 3 months *2829*

Albumin *Serum Increase Physiological* Mean increase of 3.2 g/L in 19 patients with primary biliary cirrhosis treated with cyclosporine for one year *6445*

Alkaline Phosphatase *Serum Decrease Physiological* Mean reduction of 438 U/L in 19 patients with primary biliary cirrhosis when treated with cyclosporine for one year *6445*
Serum Increase Physiological Mild transient increase of activity observed as most common abnormality of liver function in 59 patients with endogenous uveitis treated with 2-10 mg/kg/d for 6-36 months, 58% of whom developed at least one abnormality of liver function *3057* Hepatotoxicity associated with cyclosporine use has been observed in 4% renal transplant cases, 7% of cardiac transplant cases and 4% of liver transplant cases *5236*
Serum No Effect Physiological No significant effect observed in 21 post-transplant children following treatment for at least 3 months *2829*

Antimitochondrial Antibodies
Serum Decrease Physiological Decrease of mean titer by 273 (reciprocal of titer) in 19 patients with primary biliary cirrhosis when treated with cyclosporine for one year *6445*

Apolipoprotein A-I *Serum No Effect Physiological* No significant effect noted in 21 post-transplant children receiving treatment for at least 3 months *2829*

Apolipoprotein A-II *Serum No Effect Physiological* No significant effect observed in 21 post-transplant children receiving treatment for at least 3 months *2829*

Apolipoprotein B *Serum Increase Physiological* Mean increase of 33% in 21 post-transplant children receiving cyclosporine for at least 3 months *2829*

Aspartate Aminotransferase
Serum Decrease Physiological Mean decrease of 16% in patients with severe psoriasis when treated with 3 mg/kg daily for 8 weeks, 10% decrease with 5 mg/kg daily and 11% decrease with 7.5 mg/kg daily compared with increase of 12% in patients given vehicle only *1722*
Serum Increase Physiological Occasional abnormality observed in 58% of 59 patients with endogenous uveitis who developed abnormal liver function in response to treatment with 2-10 mg/kg/d for 6-36 months *3057* Hepatotoxicity associated with cyclosporine use has been observed in 4% renal transplant cases, 7% of cardiac transplant cases and 4% of liver transplant cases *5236*

Atrial Natriuretic Peptide *Plasma Increase Physiological* In 9 patients with uveitis treated with cyclosporine no change in concentration observed over first 7 days (mean of 44 pg/mL versus 40 pg/mL in control state) but increase to 76 pg/mL at 30 days and 62 pg/mL at 60 days with return to normal by 6 months *1333*

Bilirubin *Serum Decrease Physiological* In 19 patients with primary biliary cirrhosis decrease of mean concentration from baseline of 3.4 µmol/L after treatment for one year *6445*
Serum Increase Physiological Mean increase of 41% in 21 post-transplant children receiving cyclosporine for at least 3 months *2829* Occasional increase observed in 58% of patients with endogenous uveitis who developed an abnormality of liver function in response to 6-36 months treatment with 2-10 mg/kg/d *3057* Hepatotoxicity associated with cyclosporine use has been observed in 4% renal transplant cases, 7% of cardiac transplant cases and 4% of liver transplant cases *5236*

Bilirubin, Direct *Serum Increase Physiological* In 85 patients with severe psoriasis treated for 8 weeks mean increase of 50% with 3 mg/kg daily, 75% with 5 mg/kg daily and 124% with 7.5 mg/kg daily *1722*

Cyclosporine *(continued)*

Bilirubin, Indirect *Serum Increase Physiological* In 85 patients with severe psoriasis treated for 8 weeks mean increase of 18% with 3 mg/kg daily, 35% with 5 mg/kg daily and 58% with 7.5 mg/kg daily *1722*

Chloride *Serum Increase Physiological* Significant hyperkalemia, sometimes associated with hyperchloremic metabolic acidosis, and hyperuricemia has been seen in individual patients receiving cyclosporine A *5236*

Cholesterol *Serum Increase Physiological* In 85 patients with severe psoriasis treated for 8 weeks with 3 mg/kg daily mean increase of 3% observed, 7% with 5 mg/kg daily and 12% with 7.5 mg/kg daily compared with increase of 1% only when vehicle administered *1722* Mean increase of 52% observed in 21 post-transplant children receiving cyclosporine for at least 3 months *2829*

Cholinesterase *Serum No Effect Analytical* No effect observed at concentration of 3.5 µg/mL with butyrylthiocholine method on Kodak Ektachem® *2504*

Creatinine *Serum Increase Physiological* In 21 post-transplant children mean increase of 159% observed after at least 3 months treatment *2829* Increase observed at 8 weeks in 85 patients with severe psoriasis: 5% with 3 mg/kg daily, 10% with 5 mg/kg daily and 22% with 7.5 mg/kg daily *1722* Gradual rise in serum creatinine concentration of < 0.15 mg/dL/d is often sign of nephrotoxicity *5236* After 24 weeks of treatment in patients with rheumatoid arthritis, at which time the dose was 3.9 mg/kg/d, the mean serum creatinine increased to 1.04 mg/dL (32% above baseline) *6388* Observed in 9 patients with uveitis treated with cyclosporine with increase from mean of 70 µmol/L to 87 µmol/L after 2 months *1333* In 266 patients mean concentration increased from baseline of 1.0 ± 0.4 mg/dL (88 ± 35 µmol/L) to 1.5 ± 0.5 mg/dL (133 ± 44 µmol/L) 1 year after liver transplant with cyclosporine used as immunosuppressant *6000*

Creatinine Clearance *Urine Decrease Physiological* In 9 renal allograft transplant patients with normal renal function at least 6 months after surgery treated with cyclosporine, azathioprine and prednisone (66 mL/min) compared with 10 patients treated with only azathioprine and prednisone (69 mL/min) *3427* In 85 patients with severe psoriasis treated for 8 weeks mean decrease of 3% with 3 mg/kg daily, 7% with 5 mg/kg daily and 14% with 7.5 mg/kg daily *1722* Reduction from mean of 121 mL/min to 107 mL/min in 9 patients with uveitis after 2 months of treatment *1333*

Digoxin *Serum Increase Physiological* Reduced clearance observed when digoxin coadministered with cyclosporine *5236*

2,3-Dinor-Thromboxane B_2 *Urine Increase Physiological* Significant increase observed after 2 weeks treatment with 4 mg/kg/d in patients with rheumatoid arthritis *6388*

Endothelin *Urine Increase Physiological* Urinary excretion in individuals with cyclosporine nephrotoxicity reported to be significantly higher than in healthy individuals *6*

Endothelin-1 *Plasma No Effect Physiological* In 21 patients treated with cyclosporine mean concentration increased to 3.2 ± 0.3 pg/mL, 0.8-fold normal values *404*

FSH response to GnRH *Plasma Decrease Physiological* FSH response to GnRH reduced in patients who had received heart transplants and under treatment with cyclosporine *4843*

γ-Globulin *Serum Decrease Physiological* Mean decrease of 5.0 g/L in 19 patients with primary biliary cirrhosis treated with cyclosporine for one year *6445*

Glomerular Filtration Rate *Urine Decrease Physiological* Significant effect observed in 9 patients with normal renal allograft function at least 6 months after surgery treated with cyclosporine, azathioprine and prednisone (64 mL/min) compared with 10 treated only with azathioprine and prednisone (75 mL/min) *3427* In 266 patients mean GFR decreased from baseline of 93.0 ± 35.0 mL/min to 62.6 ± 28.4 mL/min 1 year after liver transplant with cyclosporine used as immunosuppressant *6000* In 34 patients with severe psoriasis given mean dose of 5.2 mg/kg daily for 8 weeks median decrease of 16% observed *1722* In patients with rheumatoid arthritis treatment for 24 weeks caused mean decrease of 16% when patients treated with 3.9 mg/kg/d *6388*

Glucose *Serum Increase Physiological* In 266 patients hyperglycemia observed in 38 (14%) 1 year after liver transplant with cyclosporine used as immunosuppressant *6000*

γ-Glutamyltransferase *Serum Increase Physiological* Hepatotoxicity associated with cyclosporine use has been observed in 4% renal transplant cases, 7% of cardiac transplant cases and 4% of liver transplant cases *5236*

HDL-Cholesterol *Serum No Effect Physiological* No significant effect observed in 21 post-transplant children following treatment for at least 3 months *2829*

Immunoglobulin G *Serum Decrease Physiological* Mean decrease of 2.70 g/L in 19 patients with primary biliary cirrhosis treated with cyclosporine for one year *6445*

Immunoglobulin M *Serum Decrease Physiological* Mean decrease of 3.24 g/L in 19 patients with primary biliary cirrhosis when treated with cyclosporine for one year *6445*

Inulin Clearance *Urine Decrease Physiological* In 25 patients with renal transplants mean inulin clearance 73.3 mL/min/1.73 sq m 3 months after transplantation compared with 89.6 mL/min/1.73 sq m in patients receiving azothioprine but not cyclosporine in whom transplant performed earlier *2531*

LH response to GnRH *Plasma Decrease Physiological* Blunted response observed in patients who had received heart transplant and under treatment with cyclosporine *4843*

Lovastatin *Serum Increase Physiological* Reduced clearance observed when digoxin coadministered with cyclosporine *5236*

Magnesium *Serum Decrease Physiological* In 85 patients with severe psoriasis treated for 8 weeks mean decrease of 11% with 3 mg/kg daily, 14% with 5 mg/kg daily and 14% with 7.5 mg/kg daily compared with no change when vehicle only administered *1722* Hypomagnesemia has been reported in some, but not all, patients exhibiting convulsions while on cyclosporine therapy *5236*

N-Acetyl-Glucosaminidase *Urine No Effect Physiological* Only in one of 23 patients receiving immunosuppression following corneal grafting was excretion increased *3134*

PAH Clearance *Urine Decrease Physiological* In 35 patients 3 months after renal transplant mean clearance 263 mL/min/1.73 sq m compared with 338.7 mL/min/1.73 sq m in 15 patients transplanted earlier but who were being treated with azothioprine and not cyclosporine *2531*

pH *Blood Decrease Physiological* Significant hyperkalemia, sometimes associated with hyperchloremic metabolic acidosis, and hyperuricemia has been seen in individual patients receiving cyclosporine A *5236*

Potassium *Serum Increase Physiological* Significant hyperkalemia, sometimes associated with hyperchloremic metabolic acidosis, and hyperuricemia has been seen in individual patients receiving cyclosporine A *5236* In 266 patients hyperkalemia observed in 26 (10%) 1 year after liver transplant with cyclosporine used as immunosuppressant *6000*

Prednisolone *Serum Increase Physiological* Reduced clearance observed when prednisolone coadministered with cyclosporine *5236*

Prolactin *Plasma Decrease Physiological* In heart and renal transplant patients receiving cyclosporine prolactin concentration reduced *4843*

Prolactin response to TRH *Plasma Decrease Physiological* Response blunted in patients with renal or heart transplants *4843*

Protein *Urine Increase Physiological* In 4 of 8 patients treated with cyclosporine showed evidence of glomerular damage and 4 showed evidence of both glomerular and tubular damage *2728* In 704 renal transplant recipients receiving long-term cyclosporine immunosuppression, 71 patients had proteinuria greater than 1 g/d beyond the first month post-transplant *6213*

Renal Blood Flow *Patient Decrease Physiological* In patients with rheumatoid arthritis treatment for 24 weeks, at which the daily dose was 3.9 mg/kg/d, renal blood flow decreased by 21% *6388*

Sodium *Urine Decrease Physiological* Slight but not significant decrease in 9 patients with uveitis treated for two months with cyclosporine together with unrestricted sodium diet *1333*

Tacrolimus *Blood No Effect Analytical* No significant effect observed at a concentration of 1.50 mg/L with MEIA method on Abbott IMx analyzer *1871*

Serum Increase Analytical In HPLC/MS method of Christians et al interference observed from metabolites AM1A and AM1 with measurement of FK 506 because of similar retention time *1010*

Triglycerides *Serum Increase Physiological* In 85 patients with severe psoriasis treated for 8 weeks mean increase of 16% with 3 mg/kg daily, 23% with 5 mg/kg daily and 41% with 7.5 mg/kg daily compared with increase of 17% when vehicle only administered *1722*

TSH response to TRH *Serum Decrease Physiological* Response blunted in patients who had received kidney or heart transplants *4843*

Tubular Cells *Urine Increase Physiological* Excretion of tubular cells with vacuolization and granularization is suggestive of nephrotoxicity in patients receiving cyclosporine A *5236*

Urea Clearance *Urine Decrease Physiological* In 9 renal allograft patients with normal renal function at least 6 months after surgery treated with cyclosporine, azathioprine and prednisone (32 mg/mL/min) compared with 10 patients treated with only azathioprine and prednisone (37 mg/mL/min) *3427*

Urea Nitrogen *Serum Increase Physiological* In 9 renal allograft transplant patients with normal renal function 6 months after surgery and treated with cyclosporine, azathioprine and prednisone (22 mg/dL) compared with 10 patients treated with only azathioprine and prednisone (18 mg/dL) *3427* Serum creatinine:Urea nitrogen ratio of ≥ 20 is suggestive of nephrotoxicity in patients receiving cyclosporine A *5236* Increase observed in 85 patients with severe psoriasis when treated over 8 weeks: increase of 25% with 3 mg/kg daily, 44% with 5 mg/kg daily and 42% with 7.5 mg/kg daily *1722* In 21 post-transplant children receiving cyclosporine for at least 3 months 250% mean increase in uren nitrogen observed *2829*

Uric Acid *Serum Increase Physiological* In 85 patients with severe psoriasis treated for 8 weeks mean decrease of 1% with 3 mg/kg daily, increase of 5% with 5 mg/kg daily and 13% with 7.5 mg/kg daily *1722* Significant hyperkalemia, sometimes associated with hyperchloremic metabolic acidosis, and hyperuricemia has been seen in individual patients receiving cyclosporine A *5236* Mean increase of 51% in 21 post-transplant children receiving cyclosporine for at least 3 months *2829*

Volume *Urine Decrease Physiological* In 9 renal allograft transplant patients with normal renal function at least 6 months after surgery treated with cyclosporine, azathioprine and prednisone (87 mL/min) compared with 10 patients treated with only azathioprine and prednisone (97 mL/min) *3427*

Cyclosporine A

α_1-Acid Glycoprotein *Serum Decrease Physiological* Reduction from mean of 37 µmol/L to 29 µmol/L at 2 weeks at which concentration it remained for 3 months duration of study in 37 patients with chronic Crohn's disease *791*

Alanine Aminotransferase *Serum Decrease Physiological* In 85 patients with severe psoriasis treated for 8 weeks mean decrease of 23% seen when given 3 mg/kg daily, 29% decrease when given 5 mg/kg daily and 22% in patients given 7.5 mg/kg daily compared with increase of 4% in patients given vehicle only *1722* Mean reduction of 38 U/L in 19 patients with primary biliary cirrhosis when treated with cyclosporine for one year *6445*

Serum Increase Physiological Increase to 109 U/L on average as manifestation of hepatotoxicity in 18 bone-marrow transplant recipients *284* Occcasional abnormality observed in 58% of 59 patients with endogenous uveitis treated with 2-10 mg/kg/d for 6-36 months who developed abnormal liver function tests *3056* Both early and late toxicity observed but effects mild in comparison with nephrotoxicity in renal transplant patients *3189* Mean increase of 132% observed in 21 post-transplant children receiving cyclosporine for at least 3 months *2829* Hepatotoxicity observed in < 1% patients treated with cyclosporine A *5240*

Serum No Effect Analytical At concentration of 41.5 mmol/L (50 µg/L) on methods on Technicon SMAC® II and Hitachi® 705 *1848*

Serum No Effect Physiological No effect observed in 23 patients with inflammatory ocular disease treated for 6 mo *4487*

Albumin *Serum Increase Physiological* Mean increase of 3.2 g/L in 19 patients with primary biliary cirrhosis treated with cyclosporine for one year *6445* Significant increase after treatment for 4 weeks with 5 mg/kg/day in group of patients with IgA nephropathy *3366*

Serum No Effect Analytical At concentration of 41.5 mmol/L (50 µg/L) on methods on Technicon SMAC® II and Hitachi® 705 *1848*

Aldosterone *Plasma Decrease Physiological* Inappropriately low in several patients receiving drug possibly due to concomitant β-blockers *4739*

Plasma No Effect Physiological No significant effect of infusion of 4 mg/kg over 6 hours in 8 healthy women *6392*

Alkaline Phosphatase *Serum Decrease Physiological* Mean reduction of 438 U/L in 19 patients with primary biliary cirrhosis when treated with cyclosporine for one year *6445*

Serum Increase Physiological Mild transient increase of activity observed as most common abnormality of liver function in 59 patients with endogenous uveitis treated with 2-10 mg/kg/d for 6-36 months, 58% of whom developed at least one abnormality of liver function *3056* Increase to 124 U/L on average as manifestation of hepatotoxicity in 18 bone-marrow transplant recipients *284* Slight increase or normal in association with hepatotoxicity in renal transplant patients *3189* Persistent increase observed in some renal transplant patients: speculation that it is due to increased sensitivity of bone to action of parathyroid hormone *3631* Persistent increase reported in some renal transplant patients occurring within short time of start of treatment, possibly due to cholestasis *1075* Hepatotoxicity observed in < 1% patients treated with cyclosporine A *5240*

Serum No Effect Analytical At concentration of 41.5 mmol/L (50 µg/L) on methods on Technicon SMAC® II and Hitachi® 705 *1848*

Serum No Effect Physiological No significant effect observed in 21 post-transplant children following treatment for at least 3 months *2829*

Amylase *Serum Increase Physiological* Pancreatitis observed rarely in patients treated with cyclosporine A *5240*

Serum No Effect Analytical At concentration of 41.5 mmol/L (50 µg/L) on methods on Technicon SMAC® II and Hitachi® 705 *1848*

Androstenedione *Plasma No Effect Physiological* In 16 patients who developed hypertrichosis but also given added cortisone *5352*

Angiotensin-II *Plasma No Effect Physiological* No significant effect of infusion of 4 mg/kg over 6 hours in 8 healthy women *6392* No signifcant increase observed in 8 patients with Alport's syndrome during treatment for 8 months *848*

Antimitochondrial Antibodies

Serum Decrease Physiological Decrease of mean titer by 273 (reciprocal of titer) in 19 patients with primary biliary cirrhosis when treated with cyclosporine for one year *6445*

Apolipoprotein A-I *Serum Decrease Physiological* In patients who had had a renal transplant treatment with cyclosporine alone caused significant change from mean baseline of 1538 ± 325 mg/L after 3 months to 1350 ± 328 mg/L after 6 months and 1426 ± 326 mg/L after 12 months *2602*

Serum No Effect Physiological In 50 patients who had undergone renal transplantation treatment with cyclosporine A for a mean of 36 months had no significant effect on concentration of 98.8 ± 24.3 mg/dL compared with 105.3 ± 25.2 mg/dL in those patients treated with azothioprine and prednisolone *766* No significant effect noted in 21 post-transplant children receiving treatment for at least 3 months *2829*

Apolipoprotein A-II *Serum No Effect Physiological* No significant effect observed in 21 post-transplant children receiving treatment for at least 3 months *2829*

Apolipoprotein B *Serum Increase Physiological* Mean increase of 33% in 21 post-transplant children receiving cyclosporine for at least 3 months *2829* Increase of 12 % on average in 36 men with amyotrophic lateral sclerosis after 2 months treatment *353* In patients who had had a renal transplant treatment with cyclosporine alone caused significant change from mean baseline of 1295 ± 399 mg/L after 3 months to 1314 ± 347 mg/L after 6 months and 1386 ± 409 mg/L after 12 months *2602*

Cyclosporine A *(continued)*

Apolipoprotein B *(continued)*
Serum No Effect Physiological In 50 patients who had undergone renal transplantation treatment with cyclosporine A for a mean of 36 months had no significant effect on concentration of 105.3 ± 29.2 mg/dL compared with 109.7 ± 29.8 mg/dL in those patients treated with azothioprine and prednisolone *766*

Aspartate Aminotransferase
Serum Decrease Physiological Mean decrease of 16% in patients with severe psoriasis when treated with 3 mg/kg daily for 8 weeks, 10% decrease with 5 mg/kg daily and 11% decrease with 7.5 mg/kg daily compared with increase of 12% in patients given vehicle only *1722*
Serum Increase Physiological Hepatotoxicity observed in < 1% patients treated with cyclosporine A *5240* Both early and late toxicity observed but effects mild in comparison with nephrotoxicity in renal transplant patients *3189* Occasional abnormality observed in 58% of 59 patients with endogenous uveitis who developed abnormal liver function in response to treatment with 2-10 mg/kg/d for 6-36 months *3056*
Serum No Effect Analytical At concentration of 41.5 mmol/L (50 µg/L) on methods on Technicon SMAC® II and Hitachi® 705 *1848*
Serum No Effect Physiological No effect observed in 23 patients with inflammatory ocular disease treated for 6 mo *4487*

Atrial Natriuretic Peptide *Plasma Increase Physiological* In 9 patients with uveitis treated with cyclosporine no change in concentration observed over first 7 days (mean of 44 pg/mL versus 40 pg/mL in control state) but increase to 76 pg/mL at 30 days and 62 pg/mL at 60 days with return to normal by 6 months *1333*

Bicarbonate *Serum No Effect Analytical* No effect of concentrations up to 20 mg/L on method on Kodak Ektachem® *5706*

Bilirubin *Serum Decrease Physiological* In 19 patients with primary biliary cirrhosis decrease of mean concentration from baseline of 3.4 µmol/L after treatment for one year *6445*
Serum Increase Physiological In 18 of 21 patients after bone marrow transplantation *284* Both early and late toxicity observed but effects mild in comparison with nephrotoxicity in renal transplant patients *3189* Mean increase of 41% in 21 post-transplant children receiving cyclosporine for at least 3 months *2829* Occasional increase observed in 58% of patients with endogenous uveitis who developed an abnormality of liver function in response to 6-36 months treatment with 2-10 mg/kg/d *3056* In 15 patients with chronic plaque psoriasis treatment with low-dose cyclosporine for 3 months caused significant change from mean baseline of 10.1 ± 6.1 µmol/L to 14.8 ± 9.0 µmol/L *1664* Association in 4 cadaveric renal transplant patients with cyclosporine trough concentration (reversible) *3433* Observed in 1 of 23 patients with inflammatory ocular disease treated for 6 mo *4487* Transient increase observed in 20% of renal transplant patients *1075* Hepatotoxicity observed in < 1% patients treated with cyclosporine A *5240*
Serum No Effect Analytical At concentration of 238 mg/L had no effect on method on Kodak Ektachem® *5706* At concentration of 41.5 mmol/L (50 µg/L) on methods on Technicon SMAC® II and Hitachi® 705 *1848*

Bilirubin, Conjugated *Serum No Effect Analytical* No effect at concentration of 238 mg/L on method on Kodak Ektachem® *5706*

Bilirubin, Direct *Serum Increase Physiological* In 85 patients with severe psoriasis treated for 8 weeks mean increase of 50% with 3 mg/kg daily, 75% with 5 mg/kg daily and 124% with 7.5 mg/kg daily *1722*
Serum No Effect Analytical At concentration of 41.5 mmol/L (50 µg/L) on methods on Technicon SMAC® II and Hitachi® 705 *1848*

Bilirubin, Indirect *Serum Increase Physiological* In 85 patients with severe psoriasis treated for 8 weeks mean increase of 18% with 3 mg/kg daily, 35% with 5 mg/kg daily and 58% with 7.5 mg/kg daily *1722*

Bilirubin, Unconjugated *Serum No Effect Analytical* No effect at concentration of 238 mg/L on method on Kodak Ektachem® *5706*

Calcium *Serum No Effect Analytical* No effect of concentrations up to 20 mg/L with method on Kodak Ektachem® *5706* At concentration of 41.5 mmol/L (50 µg/L) on methods on Technicon SMAC® II and Hitachi® 705 *1848*

Casts *Urine Increase Physiological* Usually cellular or granular characteristic feature of nephrotoxicity in most common form of renal damage to drug *285*

Chloride *Serum Increase Physiological* Hyperchloremic metabolic acidosis out of proportion to reduction in GFR *4739* Hyperchloremic acidosis in 7 of 43 renal allograft patients *59*
Serum No Effect Analytical At concentration of 41.5 mmol/L (50 µg/L) on methods on Technicon SMAC® II and Hitachi® 705 *1848*

Cholesterol *Serum Increase Physiological* In 85 patients with severe psoriasis treated for 8 weeks with 3 mg/kg daily mean increase of 3% observed, 7% with 5 mg/kg daily and 12% with 7.5 mg/kg daily compared with increase of 1% only when vehicle administered *1722* Significant increase by 90 days in patients with renal transplants when receiving only cyclosporine or with prednisolone. Effect persisted for at least 2 years and unrelated to renal function *4836* Mean increase of 52% observed in 21 post-transplant children receiving cyclosporine for at least 3 months *2829* In 500 cyclosporine treated renal transplant patients 37.6% incidence of hypercholesterolemia which occurred within 6 months post-transplant in 82% of patients but strong correlation between coadministered prednisone dose and cholesterol concentration *6214* In 15 patients with chronic plaque psoriasis treatment with low-dose cyclosporine for 3 months caused significant change from mean baseline of 5.4 ± 0.9 mmol/L to 6.6 ± 1.9 mmol/L *1664* Increase of 21% after 2 months treatment in 36 men with amyotrophic lateral sclerosis *353*
Serum No Effect Analytical At concentration of 41.5 mmol/L (50 µg/L) on methods on Technicon SMAC® II and Hitachi® 705 *1848* No effect observed when added in vitro to a concentration of 2500 µg/L and enzymatic cholesterol measurements made *5459*
Serum No Effect Physiological In 50 patients who had undergone renal transplantation treatment with cyclosporine A for a mean of 36 months caused a nonsignificant reduction of concentration to 6.66 ± 1.58 mmol/L compared with 6.77 ± 1.43 mmol/L in those patients treated with azothioprine and prednisolone *766* In patients who had had a renal transplant treatment with cyclosporine alone caused nonsignificant change from mean baseline of 6.31 ± 1.63 mmol/L after 3 months to 6.19 ± 1.40 mmol/L after 6 months and 6.28 ± 1.86 mmol/L after 12 months *2602* When coadministered with prednisolone to patients following kidney transplantation no significant effect on concentration observed *6068*

Cholesterol:HDL-Cholesterol Ratio
Serum Increase Physiological In patients who had had a renal transplant treatment with cyclosporine alone caused significant change from mean baseline of 5.23 ± 2.05 after 3 months to 6.82 ± 2.78 after 6 months and 6.72 ± 3.33 after 12 months *2602*

Cholinesterase *Serum No Effect Analytical* No effect observed at concentration of 3.5 µg/mL with butyrylthiocholine method on Kodak Ektachem® *2504*

Cortisol *Plasma No Effect Analytical* At a concentration of 20 mg/L no significant effect observed on CEDIA or Enzymun methods *1097*
Plasma No Effect Physiological In 16 patients who developed hypertrichosis but also given added cortisone *5352*

Creatine Kinase *Serum No Effect Analytical* At concentration of 41.5 mmol/L (50 µg/L) on methods on Technicon SMAC® II and Hitachi® 705 *1848*

Creatine Kinase Isoenzymes *Serum No Effect Analytical* At concentration of 41.5 mmol/L (50 µg/L) on methods on Technicon SMAC® II and Hitachi® 705 *1848*

Creatinine *Serum Increase Physiological* In patients with rheumatoid arthritis: significant effect unrelated to initial *1428* In 8 of 23 patients with ocular inflammatory disease treated for 1 mo (mean change from 1.0 to 1.5 mg/dL) *4487* In 21 post-transplant children mean increase of 159% observed after at least 3 months treatment *2829* Observed in 9 patients with uveitis treated with cyclosporine with increase from mean of 70 µmol/L to 87 µmol/L after 2 months *1333* Median concentration increased from 80 µmol/L to 89 µmol/L after 3 months treatment in 37 patients with chronic Crohn's disease *791* In over 70 patients with rheumatoid arthritis treatment with 2.5 mg/kg for 6 months caused mean 15.6 µmol/L increase in concentration *6088* Mean change from 1.0 to 1.5 mg/dL in 8 of 23 patients with 2 to 6 mo treatment (patients with inflammatory ocular disease). 30% increase in more than half patients *4487* Increase observed at 8 weeks in 85 patients with severe psoriasis: 5% with 3 mg/kg daily, 10% with 5 mg/kg daily and 22% with 7.5 mg/kg daily *1722* In 62 renal allograft recipients from 28 to 90 d after transplant: effect greater than with azathioprine and prednisolone: reversible *968* In 347 patients with cyclosporine treated renal transplantation concentration significantly increased compared with 64 patients who had a minimum of 55 months of graft function and no cyclosporine coverage *117* In 4 patients with primary biliary cirrhosis in whom creatinine and drug concentration rose as bleeding occurred *5004* Significant increase in group of patients with IgA nephropathy within 2 weeks of starting 5 mg/kg/day *3366* Renal dysfunction observed in 32% patients treated with cyclosporine A *5240* After 24 weeks of treatment in patients with rheumatoid arthritis, at which time the dose was 3.9 mg/kg/d, the mean serum creatinine increased to 1.04 mg/dL (32% above baseline) *6388* Characteristic feature of nephrotoxicity in most common form of renal damage to drug *285*

Serum *No Effect* *Analytical* At concentration of 41.5 mmol/L (50 µg/L) on methods on Technicon SMAC® II and Hitachi® 705 *1848*

Serum *No Effect* *Physiological* No significant effect in 8 healthy women with intravenous infusion of 4 mg/kg over 6 hours *6392*

Creatinine Clearance *Urine* *Decrease* *Physiological* In 85 patients with severe psoriasis treated for 8 weeks mean decrease of 3% with 3 mg/kg daily, 7% with 5 mg/kg daily and 14% with 7.5 mg/kg daily *1722* After 6 weeks of treatment with 5 mg/kg/day in group of patients with IgA nephropathy *3366* Reduction from mean of 121 mL/min to 107 mL/min in 9 patients with uveitis after 2 months of treatment *1333* In 9 renal allograft transplant patients with normal renal function at least 6 months after surgery treated with cyclosporine, azathioprine and prednisone (66 mL/min) compared with 10 patients treated with only azathioprine and prednisone (69 mL/min) *3427*

Urine *No Effect* *Physiological* In 8 patients with Alport's syndrome treatment for 8 months caused no permanent decrease *848*

Dehydroepiandrosterone Sulfate

Plasma *No Effect* *Physiological* In 16 patients who developed hypertrichosis but also given added cortisone *5352*

Digoxin *Serum* *Increase* *Physiological* Higher concentration after digoxin administered for 4 d possibly due to diminished renal clearance *6288* Coadministration with cyclosporine A reduces its clearance and increases its concentration *5240* Coadministration of cyclosporine with digoxin has been reported to cause severe digitalis toxicity *859*

2,3-Dinor-Thromboxane B_2 *Urine* *Increase* *Physiological* Significant increase observed after 2 weeks treatment with 4 mg/kg/d in patients with rheumatoid arthritis *6388*

Doxorubicinol *Serum* *Increase* *Physiological* Coadministration of cyclosporine with daunorubicin caused a twofold increase in the concentration of doxorubicinol its primary metabolite and reduction of its plasma clearance by 37% *859*

Effective Renal Plasma Flow

Patient *Decrease* *Physiological* In 25 recently liver-transplanted patients total loss 53% *5958*

Patient *No Effect* *Physiological* No significant effect observed in 8 healthy female volunteers being 480 mL/min before infusion with 4 mg/kg over 6 hours and 463 mL/min during infusion *6392*

Endothelin-1 *Plasma* *Increase* *Physiological* In two studies increases observed, 0.8-fold in one and 3.5-fold in the other *404*

Erythrocyte Sedimentation Rate

Blood *Increase* *Physiological* Mean increase from 35 to 52 mm/1h in 16 patients with inflammatory ocular disease with 3 to 6 mo treatment *4487*

Erythrocytes *Blood* *Decrease* *Physiological* In 6 of 23 patients normochromic normocytic anemia in first 6 mo treatment (patients with inflammatory ocular disease) *4487*

Urine *No Effect* *Physiological* No effect observed in 23 patients with inflammatory ocular disease treated for 6 mo *4487*

Erythromycin *Serum* *Increase* *Physiological* Concomitant administration of cyclosporine with erythromycin may increase its plasma concentration through its effect on cytochrome P450 *20*

Estradiol *Plasma* *No Effect* *Physiological* In 16 patients who developed hypertrichosis but also given added cortisone *5352*

Etopside *Serum* *Increase* *Physiological* Coadministration of cyclosporine with etopside caused a 60% increase in its AUC and a 35% reduction of its plasma clearance *859*

Euglobulin Lysis Time *Blood* *Increase* *Physiological* In 26 renal transplanted patients treated with cyclosporine A and prednisolone mean time 7.80 ± 0.25 h significantly increased compared with 6.90 ± 0.15 h in 20 patients treated with azathioprine and prednisolone *6120*

Folate *Serum* *No Effect* *Physiological* No significant effect observed in 23 patients with inflammatory ocular disease treated for 6 mo *4487*

Fractional Excretion of Magnesium

Urine *Increase* *Physiological* In 8 renal transplant patients receiving cyclosporine, azathioprine and prednisolone mean fractional excretion of 12.8 % significantly greater than 3.5 % in 10 healthy individuals *106*

FSH response to GnRH *Plasma* *Decrease* *Physiological* FSH response to GnRH reduced in patients who had received heart transplants and under treatment with cyclosporine *4843*

γ-Globulin *Serum* *Decrease* *Physiological* Mean decrease of 5.0 g/L in 19 patients with primary biliary cirrhosis treated with cyclosporine for one year *6445*

Glomerular Filtration Rate *Urine* *Decrease* *Physiological* In 15 patients with chronic plaque psoriasis treatment with low-dose cyclosporine for 3 months caused significant change from mean baseline of 101 ± 23 mL/min/1.73 m² to 86 ± 19 mL/min/1.73 m² *1664* 51 versus 93 mL/min in 17 cardiac transplant recipients compared with those on azathioprine *4199* Significant effect observed in 9 patients with normal renal allograft function at least 6 months after surgery treated with cyclosporine, azathioprine and prednisone (64 mL/min) compared with 10 treated only with azathioprine and prednisone (75 mL/min) *3427* Acute reduction, on average, by 13% in patients with renal allografts immediately following administration of a dose of cyclosporine *3132* In 34 patients with severe psoriasis given mean dose of 5.2 mg/kg daily for 8 weeks median decrease of 16% observed *1722* In 25 recently liver-transplanted patients mean total loss 25% *5958* In 27 patients with psoriasis treatment with low dose cyclosporine A (< 5 mg/kg/d) for 6 months caused reduction by about 10% from mean baseline of 119 ± mL/min/1.73 m². With treatment for 12 months reduction was about 12% *4004* In patients with rheumatoid arthritis treatment for 24 weeks caused mean decrease of 16% when patients treated with 3.9 mg/kg/d *6388* Reduction from mean of 109 mL/min to 91 mL/min in 8 healthy women after infusion of 4 mg/kg over 6 hours *6392* In type I diabetics with disease of recent origin 25% decrease observed after 3 months on 6.3 mg/kg/d *5045*

Glucose *Serum* *No Effect* *Analytical* At concentration of 41.5 mmol/L (50 µg/L) on methods on Technicon SMAC® II and Hitachi® 705 *1848*

γ-Glutamyltransferase *Serum* *Increase* *Physiological* Hepatotoxicity observed in < 1% patients treated with cyclosporine A *5240*

Serum *No Effect* *Analytical* At concentration of 41.5 mmol/L (50 µg/L) on methods on Technicon SMAC® II and Hitachi® 705 *1848*

Urine *Increase* *Physiological* In 13 patients following renal transplantation 30 to 40% had increased excretion over next 2 weeks *5953*

HDL_2-Cholesterol *Serum* *Decrease* *Physiological* In 50 patients who had undergone renal transplantation treatment with cyclosporine A for a mean of 36 months caused a significant reduction in concentration to 0.63 ± 0.34 mmol/L compared with 0.86 ± 0.38 mmol/L in those patients treated with azothioprine and prednisolone *766*

Serum *No Effect* *Physiological* In 15 patients with chronic plaque psoriasis treatment with low-dose cyclosporine for 3 months caused nonsignificant change from mean baseline of 0.64 ± 0.12 mmol/L to 0.66 ± 0.20 mmol/L *1664*

Cyclosporine A *(continued)*

HDL_3-Cholesterol *Serum No Effect Physiological* In 50 patients who had undergone renal transplantation treatment with cyclosporine A for a mean of 36 months had no significant effect on concentration of 0.59 ± 0.15 mmol/L compared with 0.56 ± 0.13 mmol/L in those patients treated with azothioprine and prednisolone *766* In 15 patients with chronic plaque psoriasis treatment with low-dose cyclosporine for 3 months caused nonsignificant change from mean baseline of 0.80 ± 0.35 mmol/L to 0.97 ± 0.58 mmol/L *1664*

HDL-Cholesterol *Serum Decrease Physiological* In patients who had had a renal transplant treatment with cyclosporine alone caused significant change from mean baseline of 1.31 ± 0.38 mmol/L after 3 months to 1.01 ± 0.34 mmol/L after 6 months and 1.06 ± 0.38 mmol/L after 12 months *2602* In 50 patients who had undergone renal transplantation treatment with cyclosporine A for a mean of 36 months caused a significant reduction in concentration to 1.24 ± 0.39 mmol/L compared with 1.41 ± 0.40 mmol/L in those patients treated with azothioprine and prednisolone *766*

Serum No Effect Analytical No effect when added in vitro to concentration of 2500 µg/L and β-lipoprotein precipitation methods used followed by enzymatic cholesterol measurements *5459*

Serum No Effect Physiological In 15 patients with chronic plaque psoriasis treatment with low-dose cyclosporine for 3 months caused nonsignificant change from mean baseline of 1.45 ± 0.45 mmol/L to 1.52 ± 0.60 mmol/L *1664* No significant effect observed in 21 post-transplant children following treatment for at least 3 months *2829*

Hematocrit *Blood Decrease Physiological* Reduction from median of 0.37 to 0.35 in 37 patients with chronic Crohn's disease treated for 3 months *791*

Hemoglobin *Blood Decrease Physiological* Reduction of 2- 4 g/dL over 6 mo treatment in 6 of 23 patients with inflammatory ocular disease *4487* In 4 patients with primary biliary cirrhosis in whom creatinine and drug concentration rose as bleeding occurred *5004*

Blood No Effect Analytical No effect of concentrations up to 20 mg/L on method on Kodak Ektachem® *5706*

Urine Increase Physiological In approximately 5% patients given drug versus 8% given azathioprine in over 200 renal transplant patients *870*

β-Hydroxy-Simvastatin *Serum Increase Physiological* Coadministration of cyclosporine with simvastatin caused a higher mean concentration of β-hydroxy-simvastatin the major metabolite of simvastatin *859*

5-Hydroxyindoleacetic Acid *Plasma Increase Physiological* In 26 renal transplanted patients treated with cyclosporine A and prednisolone mean concentration 0.61 ± 0.25 ng/mL significantly increased compared with 0.42 ± 0.12 ng/mL in 20 patients treated with azathioprine and prednisolone *6120*

17-Hydroxyprogesterone *Plasma No Effect Physiological* In 16 patients who developed hypertrichosis but also given added cortisone *5352*

Hydroxyproline *Urine Increase Physiological* In 18 patients with biliary cirrhosis receiving cyclosporine A median hydroxyproline:creatinine ratio of 0.097 significantly higher than 0.031 in 20 patients with biliary cirrhosis receiving placebo *2356*

5-Hydroxytryptamine *Blood Increase Physiological* In 26 renal transplanted patients treated with cyclosporine A and prednisolone mean concentration 203.53 ± 82.61 ng/mL increased compared with 156.32 ± 36.98 ng/mL in 20 patients treated with azathioprine and prednisolone *6120*

Plasma Increase Physiological In 26 renal transplanted patients treated with cyclosporine A and prednisolone mean concentration 13.43 ± 3.56 ng/mL significantly increased compared with 10.48 ± 1.56 ng/mL in 20 patients treated with azathioprine and prednisolone *6120*

Immunoglobulin A *Serum Decrease Physiological* Concentration fell in 7 of 9 patients with IgA nephropathy treated for 12 weeks with 5 mg/kg/day *3366*

Immunoglobulin G *Serum Decrease Physiological* Mean decrease of 2.70 g/L in 19 patients with primary biliary cirrhosis treated with cyclosporine for one year *6445*

Immunoglobulin M *Serum Decrease Physiological* Mean decrease of 3.24 g/L in 19 patients with primary biliary cirrhosis when treated with cyclosporine for one year *6445*

Insulin *Plasma No Effect Physiological* No significant effect observed in post-renal transplant patients with regard to basal insulin concentration, peak insulin response to glucose and area under the insulin curve *1761*

Interferon-γ *Serum Decrease Physiological* In 8 patients with psoriasis treatment with 10 mg/kg/d for 8 weeks caused initially high concentration to decrease to mean baseline (less than 0.02 U/mL) after 4 weeks *5521*

Interleukin-1α *Serum No Effect Physiological* In 8 patients with psoriasis treated with 10 mg/kg/d for 8 weeks no significant difference from mean baseline despite clinical improvement *5521*

Inulin Clearance *Urine Decrease Physiological* In 25 patients with renal transplants mean inulin clearance 73.3 mL/min/1.73 m^2 3 months after transplantation compared with 89.6 mL/min/1.73 m^2 in patients receiving azothioprine but not cyclosporine in whom transplant performed earlier *2531*

Ionized Magnesium *Serum Decrease Physiological* In 8 renal transplant patients receiving cyclosporine, azathioprine and prednisolone mean concentration of 0.43 mmol/L significantly less than 0.58 mmol/L in 10 healthy individuals *106*

Iron *Serum No Effect Analytical* At concentration of 41.5 mmol/L (50 µg/L) on methods on Technicon SMAC® II and Hitachi® 705 *1848*

Serum No Effect Physiological No significant effect observed in 23 patients with inflammatory ocular disease treated for 6 mo *4487*

Kallikrein *Urine Decrease Physiological* After 3 and 6 months therapy of 6 to 8 mg/kg/day in 10 patients with rheumatoid arthritis excretion had fallen to 44% and 46% respectively of baseline (98 µg/24h) *5756*

6-Keto-Prostaglandin $F_{1\alpha}$ *Urine No Effect Physiological* No difference in excretion between azathioprine and cyclosporine renal- transplant patients *360* No significant change in 8 healthy women following intravenous infusion of 4 mg/kg over 6 hours *6392*

Ketone Body Ratio *Serum No Effect Analytical* When added at a concentration of 200 mg/L had no significant effect on AKBR method of Uno et al *6131*

Lactate Dehydrogenase *Serum No Effect Analytical* At concentration of 41.5 mmol/L (50 µg/L) on methods on Technicon SMAC® II and Hitachi® 705 *1848*

LDL-Cholesterol *Serum Increase Physiological* Increased by 45% in patients given cyclosporine only following renal transplantation and by 28% when prednisolone also given. Increase persisted for at least 2 years following transplant and change unrelated to renal function *4836* In 15 patients with chronic plaque psoriasis treatment with low-dose cyclosporine for 3 months caused significant change from mean baseline of 3.1 ± 1.3 mmol/L to 4.2 ± 1.5 mmol/L *1664* Increase of 31% on average after 2 months treatment in 36 men with amyotrophic lateral sclerosis *353*

Serum No Effect Physiological In 50 patients who had undergone renal transplantation treatment with cyclosporine A for a mean of 36 months caused a nonsignificant change of concentration to 4.39 ± 1.21 mmol/L compared with 4.33 ± 1.22 mmol/L in those patients treated with azothioprine and prednisolone *766* In patients who had had a renal transplant treatment with cyclosporine alone caused nonsignificant change from mean baseline of 4.23 ± 1.51 mmol/L after 3 months to 4.12 ± 1.16 mmol/L after 6 months and 4.22 ± 1.67 mmol/L after 12 months *2602*

Leukocytes *Blood Decrease Physiological* In approximately 1% patients given drug versus 12% given azathioprine in over 200 renal transplant patients *870*

Blood Increase Physiological Leukopenia observed in 2% of 227 patients treated with cyclosporine A *5240*

Urine Increase Physiological Significantly greater excretion of white cells in renal allograft patients treated with cyclosporine and steroid immunotherapy than in those treated with azathioprine and steroid immunotherapy (93% versus 62%) *261*

Urine No Effect Physiological No effect observed in 23 patients with inflammatory ocular disease treated for 6 mo *4487*

Levofloxacin *Serum Increase Physiological* Cyclosporine A slightly lowered the maximum plasma concentration of levofloxacin and slightly increased its half-life *3916*

Serum No Effect Physiological Concurrent administration of levofloxacin with cyclosporine A caused a slight reduction in the peak plasma concentration with longer half life of levofloxacin although not clinically significant *3916*

LH response to GnRH *Plasma Decrease Physiological* Blunted response observed in patients who had received heart transplant and under treatment with cyclosporine *4843*

Lipase *Serum Increase Physiological* Pancreatitis observed rarely in patients treated with cyclosporine A *5240*

Lipoprotein Lp(a) *Serum Decrease Physiological* In patients with chronic renal failure 6 months to one year after renal transplantation treated with cyclosporine A and prednisone mean concentration after transplantation decreased by 42% *308*
Serum Increase Physiological In patients who had had a renal transplant treatment with cyclosporine alone caused significant change from mean baseline of 61 (range 25 - 168) mg/L after 3 months to 105 (42 - 340) mg/L after 12 months *2602* In 50 patients who had undergone renal transplantation treatment with cyclosporine A for a mean of 36 months had a significant effect on mean concentration of 32.0 mg/dL compared with 18.3 mg/dL in those patients treated with azothioprine and prednisolone *766*
Serum No Effect Physiological In 15 patients with chronic plaque psoriasis treatment with low-dose cyclosporine for 3 months caused nonsignificant change from mean baseline of 6.9 (1.7 - 163.0) mg/dL to 7.8 (1.7 - 129.0) mg/dL *1664*

Lovastatin *Serum Increase Physiological* Coadministration with cyclosporine A reduces its clearance and increases its concentration *5240* Increased frequency of myopathy observed when lovastatin given with cyclosporine and lovastatin concentration or that of its metabolites observed to be increased *1069*

Lymphocyte T-Cells *Blood Decrease Physiological* In renal transplant patients with normal graft function compared with normal controls, higher values seen in individuals with acute cyclosporine nephrotoxicity *5496*

Lymphocytes *Blood Decrease Physiological* In renal transplant patients with normal graft function compared with normal controls, higher values seen in individuals with acute cyclosporine nephrotoxicity *5496*

Magnesium *Platelets Decrease Physiological* In 8 renal transplant patients receiving cyclosporine, azathioprine and prednisolone mean concentration of 1.75 µmol/10^8 significantly less than 2.84 µmol/10^8 in 10 healthy individuals *106*
Red Blood Cells Decrease Physiological In 8 renal transplant patients receiving cyclosporine, azathioprine and prednisolone mean concentration of 2.18 mmol/L significantly less than 2.56 mmol/L in 10 healthy individuals *106*
Serum Decrease Physiological In 85 patients with severe psoriasis treated for 8 weeks mean decrease of 11% with 3 mg/kg daily, 14% with 5 mg/kg daily and 14% with 7.5 mg/kg daily compared with no change when vehicle only administered *1722* Hypomagnesemia has been reported in some, but not all patients exhibiting convulsions, while being treated with cyclosporine A *5240* Observed in 5 of 9 patients treated with drug *6640* In 8 renal transplant patients receiving cyclosporine, azathioprine and prednisolone mean concentration of 0.61 mmol/L significantly less than 0.86 mmol/L in 10 healthy individuals *106* Mean of 1.06 mEq/L versus 1.33 mEq/L in methotrexate treated patients after 3 mo treatment of patients with bone marrow transplant *2990*
Serum No Effect Analytical No effect of concentrations up to 0.15 mg/L on method on Kodak Ektachem® *5706*
Urine Increase Physiological Renal loss due to nephrotoxicity observed in many patients with bone marrow transplantation *2990*
Urine No Effect Physiological In 8 renal transplant patients receiving cyclosporine, azathioprine and prednisolone mean excretion of 4.4 mmol/d the same as 4.4 mmol/d in 10 healthy individuals *106*

β_2-Microglobulin *Serum Increase Physiological* Nephrotoxicity observed after bone marrow transplantation *1629*
Urine Increase Physiological In 13 patients following renal transplantation 30 to 40% had increased excretion over next 18 months *5953*

Mycophenolic Acid *Serum No Effect Analytical* No significant interference observed with HPLC method of Shipkova et al *5526*

Mycophenolic Acid Glucuronide
Serum No Effect Analytical No significant interference observed with HPLC method of Shipkova et al *5526*

N-Acetyl-Glucosaminidase *Urine No Effect Physiological* Only in one of 23 patients receiving immunosuppression following corneal grafting was excretion increased *3134*

N-Acetylglucosamine *Urine Increase Physiological* 30 to 40% of 13 patients following renal transplantation receiving cyclosporine had increased excretion over 18 months *5953*

Neutrophils *Blood No Effect Physiological* No significant effect observed in 23 patients with inflammatory ocular disease treated for 6 mo *4487*

Occult Blood *Feces Increase Physiological* In approximately 3% patients given drug versus 6% given azathioprine in over 200 renal transplant patients *870* Upper gastrointestinal tract bleeding observed rarely in patients treated with cyclosporine A *5240*

Osteocalcin *Serum Increase Physiological* In 18 patients with biliary cirrhosis receiving cyclosporine A median concentration of 7.8 ng/mL significantly higher than 5.4 ng/mL in 20 patients with biliary cirrhosis receiving placebo *2356*

PAH Clearance *Urine Decrease Physiological* In 35 patients 3 months after renal transplant mean clearance 263 mL/min/1.73 sq m compared with 338.7 mL/min/1.73 sq m in 15 patients transplanted earlier but who were being treated with azothioprine and not cyclosporine *2531*

Parathyroid Hormone *Plasma Increase Physiological* In 18 patients with biliary cirrhosis receiving cyclosporine A median concentration of 4.3 pmol/L significantly higher than 3.1 pmol/L in 20 patients with biliary cirrhosis receiving placebo *2356*

Phenylalanine *Plasma No Effect Analytical* No interference observed with rapid quantitative whole blood method of Campbell et al using phenylalanine dehydrogenase *867*

Plasminogen Activator Inhibitor Antigen
Plasma Increase Physiological In 26 renal transplanted patients treated with cyclosporine A and prednisolone mean concentration 24.50 ± 7.40 ng/mL significantly increased compared with 19.30 ± 5.80 ng/mL in 20 patients treated with azathioprine and prednisolone *6120*

Platelets *Blood No Effect Physiological* No significant effect observed in 23 patients with inflammatory ocular disease treated for 6 mo *4487*

Potassium *Serum Increase Physiological* Observed in 13 of 50 renal transplant patients after 1 mo *1902* Reported in 7 of 43 patients with good renal function following kidney transplantation: single case reported here which responded to fludrocortisone *4632* Sustained hyperkalemia (6.0 to 7.1 mmol/L) inappropriate for renal function in in 7 of 43 renal allograft patients *59* Median concentration increased from 4.1 mmol/L to 4.2 mmol/L in 37 patients with chronic Crohn's disease treated for 3 months *791* Probably occurs as manifestation of nephrotoxicity with tubular dysfunction *1075* Hyperkalemia out of proportion to reduction in GFR *4739*
Serum No Effect Analytical At concentration of 41.5 mmol/L (50 µg/L) on methods on Technicon SMAC® II and Hitachi® 705 *1848* No effect of concentrations up to 20 mg/L on method on Kodak Ektachem® *5706*
Urine Decrease Physiological Reduction from mean of 63 mmol/day to 22 mmol/day on day of infusion of 4 mg/kg over 6 hours in 8 healthy women *6392*

Pravastatin *Serum Increase Physiological* Coadministration of cyclosporine with pravastatin caused a significantly higher mean AUC of pravastatin, 1304 ± 783 µg.h/L compared with control of 57 ± 40 µg.h/L. Cyclosporine probably inhibits hepatic metabolism of pravastatin *859* In one single dose study in cardiac transplant patients administration of cyclosporine with pravastatin caused an increase in pravastatin concentrations *728*

Prednisolone *Serum Increase Physiological* Increase of area under curve and half-life with reduction of body clearance by 22% *6288* Coadministration with cyclosporine A reduces its clearance and increases its concentration *5240* Clearance reduced with coadministration although for short period of time following transplant metabolism of prednisolone is normal *1069*

Prolactin *Plasma Decrease Physiological* Decreased concentrations observed in both kidney and heart recipients *4843* In heart and renal transplant patients receiving cyclosporine prolactin concentration reduced *4843*

Cyclosporine A *(continued)*

Prolactin *(continued)*
Plasma No Effect Physiological In 16 patients who developed hypertrichosis but also given added cortisone *5352*

Prolactin response to TRH *Plasma Decrease Physiological* Response blunted in patients with renal or heart transplants *4843*

Prostaglandin E *Urine No Effect Physiological* No significant effect of infusion of 4 mg/kg over 6 hours in 8 healthy women *6392*

Prostaglandins *Urine No Effect Physiological* No difference in excretion between azathioprine and cyclosporine treated renal- transplant patients *360*

Protein *Serum No Effect Analytical* At concentration of 41.5 mmol/L (50 µg/L) on methods on Technicon SMAC® II and Hitachi® 705 *1848*
Urine Decrease Physiological Proteinuria reduced in 11 of 15 patients with nephrotic syndrome in response to conventional therapy *6662* In 8 patients with Alport's syndrome treatment for 8 months proteinuria abated in 5 patients and decreased from mean of 183.3 ± 29.7 mg/sq m/h to 32.5 mg/sq m/h *848* In 9 patients with IgA nephropathy given 5 mg/kg/day for 12 weeks with significant reduction observed by one week *3366*
Urine Increase Physiological In 704 renal transplant recipients receiving long-term cyclosporine immunosuppression, 71 patients had proteinuria greater than 1 g/d beyond the first month post-transplant *6213* Characteristic feature of nephrotoxicity in most common form of renal damage to drug *285*
Urine No Effect Physiological No effect observed in 23 patients with inflammatory ocular disease treated for for 6 mo *4487*

Renal Blood Flow *Patient Decrease Physiological* 320 mL/min versus 480 mL/min in 17 cardiac transplant recipients compared with those on azathioprine *4199* In patients with rheumatoid arthritis treatment for 24 weeks, at which the daily dose was 3.9 mg/kg/d, renal blood flow decreased by 21% *6388*

Renin Activity *Plasma Decrease Physiological* Significantly lower than in azathioprine treated patients or in those with renal insufficiency, possibly due to expansion of extracellular fluid *360* Inappropriately low in several patients receiving drug possibly due to concomitant β-blockers concentration *4739*
Plasma No Effect Physiological No significant effect of a dose of cyclosporine in renal allograft recipients immediately following a dose of drug. Predose mean 0.6 ng/L/s, postdose 0.4 ng/L/s *3132* No significant effect of infusion of 4 mg/kg over 6 hours in 8 healthy women *6392*

SDZ PSC 833 *Blood No Effect Analytical* At a concentration of 360 µg/L had no effect on HPLC method of Scott et al when used to measure PSC (with CsD as internal standard) at a concentration of 5 mg/L *5418*

Sex-Hormone Binding Globulin
Serum No Effect Physiological In 16 patients who developed hypertrichosis but also given added cortisone *5352*

Sodium *Serum No Effect Analytical* At concentration of 41.5 mmol/L (50 µg/L) on methods on Technicon SMAC® II and Hitachi® 705 *1848*
Urine Decrease Physiological Reduction from mean excretion of 88 mmol/day to 58 mmol/day in 8 healthy women on day of infusion of 4 mg/kg over 6 hours *6392* Slight but not significant decrease in 9 patients with uveitis treated for two months with cyclosporine together with unrestricted sodium diet *1333*

Tacrolimus *Blood No Effect Analytical* No interference observed with radioreceptor method of Murthy et al *4191*
Serum Increase Physiological By inhibiting cytochrome P-450 IIIA enzyme systems may inhibit the metabolism of tacrolimus *1987*
Serum No Effect Analytical At concentrations up to 1500 µg/L had no significant effect on ELISA method *6329*

Terbinafine *Serum No Effect Physiological* Cyclosporine had no effect on the clearance of terbinafine *5231*

Testosterone *Serum No Effect Physiological* In 16 patients who developed hypertrichosis but also given added cortisone *5352*

Thromboxane B_2 *Urine Increase Physiological* Marked increase from 40 ng/h in control period in 8 healthy women to 86 ng/h after intravenous infusion of 4 mg/kg over 6 hours *6392*

Tissue Plasminogen Activator Antigen
Plasma Decrease Physiological In 26 renal transplanted patients treated with cyclosporine A and prednisolone mean concentration 5.95 ± 2.74 ng/mL significantly decreased compared with 7.1 ± 1.99 ng/mL in 20 patients treated with azathioprine and prednisolone *6120*

Triglycerides *Serum Increase Physiological* In 7 of 8 patients with psoriasis treament with 2.0-7.5 mg/kg/d cyclosporine caused significant increase in triglycerde concentration *2350* In 85 patients with severe psoriasis treated for 8 weeks mean increase of 16% with 3 mg/kg daily, 23% with 5 mg/kg daily and 41% with 7.5 mg/kg daily compared with increase of 17% when vehicle only administered *1722* In patients who had had a renal transplant treatment with cyclosporine alone caused significant change from mean baseline of 1.91 ± 0.97 mmol/L after 3 months to 2.53 ± 1.42 mmol/L after 6 months and 2.37 ± 1.99 mmol/L after 12 months *2602* Present in 14.7% of 500 postrenal transplant patients but more severe in cyclosporine/prednisone than in azathioprine/prednisone treated patients. Hypertriglyceridemia occurred later than hypercholesterolemia. Correlated with increased creatinine *6214*
Serum No Effect Physiological No change observed in renal transplant recipients when coadministered with prednisolone *6068* In 15 patients with chronic plaque psoriasis treatment with low-dose cyclosporine for 3 months caused nonsignificant change from mean baseline of 1.33 (0.61 - 4.99) mmol/L to 1.78 (0.69 - 5.55) mmol/L *1664* In 50 patients who had undergone renal transplantation treatment with cyclosporine A for a mean of 36 months caused a nonsignificant change in concentration to 1.84 mmol/L compared with 1.79 mmol/L in those patients treated with azothioprine and prednisolone *766*

Trovafloxacin *Serum No Effect Physiological* No significant interaction observed *4663*

TSH response to TRH *Serum Decrease Physiological* Response blunted in patients who had received kidney or heart transplants *4843*

Urea Clearance *Urine Decrease Physiological* In 9 renal allograft patients with normal renal function at least 6 months after surgery treated with cyclosporine, azathioprine and prednisone (32 mg/mL/min) compared with 10 patients treated with only azathioprine and prednisone (37 mg/mL/min) *3427*

Urea Nitrogen *Serum Increase Physiological* In 9 renal allograft transplant patients with normal renal function 6 months after surgery and treated with cyclosporine, azathioprine and prednisone (22 mg/dL) compared with 10 patients treated with only azathioprine and prednisone (18 mg/dL) *3427* Mean change from 13 to 27 mg/dL in 8 of 23 patients with 2 to 6 mo treatment (patients with inflammatory ocular disease) *4487* Increase observed in 85 patients with severe psoriasis when treated over 8 weeks: increase of 25% with 3 mg/kg daily, 44% with 5 mg/kg daily and 42% with 7.5 mg/kg daily *1722* In 21 post-transplant children receiving cyclosporine for at least 3 months 250% mean increase in uren nitrogen observed *2829* Renal dysfunction observed in 32% patients treated with cyclosporine A *5240* Characteristic feature of nephrotoxicity in most common form of renal damage to drug *285*
Serum No Effect Analytical At concentration of 41.5 mmol/L (50 µg/L) on methods on Technicon SMAC® II and Hitachi® 705 *1848*

Uric Acid *Serum Increase Physiological* In 72% of male heart-transplant patients and in 81% of female patients treated with cyclosporine hyperuricemia developed *805* Mean increase of 51% in 21 post-transplant children receiving cyclosporine for at least 3 months *2829* In 85 patients with severe psoriasis treated for 8 weeks mean decrease of 1% with 3 mg/kg daily, increase of 5% with 5 mg/kg daily and 13% with 7.5 mg/kg daily *1722* Hyperuricemia occurred in 84% of renal-transplant recipients receiving cyclosporine and prednisone versus 30% in patients receiving azathioprine and prednisone. Gout developed in 7% of cyclosporine treated versus none in the azathioprine treated group *3582* In 62 renal allograft recipients from 28 to 90 d after transplant: effect greater than with

azathioprine and prednisolone: reversible *968* Mean increase from 5.7 to 7.0 mg/dL in 26 patients with inflammatory ocular disease after 3 to 6 mo treatment. 9 patients had increase greater than 2.0 mg/dL *4487*
Serum No Effect Analytical At concentration of 41.5 mmol/L (50 µg/L) on methods on Technicon SMAC® II and Hitachi® 705 *1848*

Vitamin B_{12} *Serum No Effect Physiological* No significant effect observed in 23 patients with inflammatory ocular disease treated for 6 mo *4487*

VLDL-Cholesterol *Serum No Effect Physiological* In 50 patients who had undergone renal transplantation treatment with cyclosporine A for a mean of 36 months caused a non-significant change in concentration to 0.58 mmol/L compared with 0.58 mmol/L in those patients treated with azothioprine and prednisolone *766* In 15 patients with chronic plaque psoriasis treatment with low-dose cyclosporine for 3 months caused nonsignificant change from mean baseline of 0.38 (1.03 - 2.54) mmol/L to 0.54 (0.77 - 2.71) mmol/L *1664*

Volume *Urine Decrease Physiological* In 9 renal allograft transplant patients with normal renal function at least 6 months after surgery treated with cyclosporine, azathioprine and prednisone (87 mL/min) compared with 10 patients treated with only azathioprine and prednisone (97 mL/min) *3427*

Cyclothiazide

Alanine Aminotransferase *Serum Increase Physiological* Occasional intrahepatic cholestatic jaundice *2754*

Amylase *Serum Increase Physiological* Occasional case of pancreatitis observed *2754*

Aspartate Aminotransferase *Serum Increase Physiological* Occasional intrahepatic cholestatic jaundice *2754*

Bilirubin *Serum Increase Physiological* Occasional intrahepatic cholestatic jaundice *2754*

Chloride *Urine Increase Physiological* Intended diuretic action *2754*

Erythrocytes *Blood Decrease Physiological* Occasional response to thiazides *2754*

Glucose *Urine Increase Physiological* Diabetogenic action of thiazides *2754*

^{131}I Uptake *Serum Decrease Physiological* Anhydron contains tetraiodofluorescein *4360*

Leukocytes *Blood Decrease Physiological* Occasional response to thiazides *2754*

Osmolality *Serum Decrease Physiological* Syndrome of inappropriate ADH secretion seen *2722*

Platelets *Blood Decrease Physiological* Occasional response to thiazides *2754*

Potassium *Serum Decrease Physiological* Same degree of hypokalemia as hydrochlorothiazide *1351*

Sodium *Serum Decrease Physiological* Syndrome of inappropriate ADH secretion seen *2722*
Urine Increase Physiological Intended diuretic action *2754*

Urea Nitrogen *Serum Increase Physiological* May occur with decreased renal flow *2754*

Uric Acid *Serum Increase Physiological* Inhibition of tubular secretion of urate *2378*

Volume *Urine Increase Physiological* Potent diuretic, same as hydrochlorothiazide *1351*

Cyproheptadine

Alanine Aminotransferase *Serum Increase Physiological* Isolated case of jaundice due to cholestasis: reversed on withdrawal of drug *2557*

Alkaline Phosphatase *Serum Increase Physiological* Isolated case of jaundice due to cholestasis: reversed on withdrawal of drug *2557*

Amylase *Serum Increase Physiological* Mechanism not listed *2451*

Aspartate Aminotransferase *Serum Increase Physiological* Isolated case of jaundice due to cholestasis: reversed on withdrawal of drug *2557*

Bilirubin *Serum Increase Physiological* Jaundice has been reported as an adverse reaction *3989* Isolated case of jaundice due to cholestasis: reversed on withdrawal of drug *2557*

Corticotropin *Plasma Decrease Physiological* In 6 adult women with Nelson's syndrome administration of 8 mg cyproheptadine caused mean decrease of 17 ± 15% in the plasma ACTH concentration *3956*

Glucose *Serum Decrease Physiological* Small decrease (10%), often no change *2451*
Serum No Effect Physiological Reported to have no effect *2452*

Glucose Tolerance *Serum No Effect Physiological* Reported to have no effect *2452*

Granulocytes *Blood Decrease Physiological* Agranulocytosis has been reported as an adverse reaction *3989*

Growth Hormone *Plasma No Effect Physiological* No effect observed in 9 of 10 acromegalics treated with 4 mg 6-hourly for 21 days either in basal state or after glucose *1244*

Hematocrit *Blood Decrease Physiological* Hemolytic anemia has been reported as an adverse reaction *3989*

Hemoglobin *Blood Decrease Physiological* Hemolytic anemia has been reported as an adverse reaction *3989*

Histamine *Plasma No Effect Analytical* 50% inhibition of radio-enzyme assay at 1000 times therapeutic concentration *2492*

Leukocytes *Blood Decrease Physiological* Leukopenia has been reported as an adverse reaction *3989*

Platelets *Blood Decrease Physiological* Thrombocytopenia has been reported as an adverse reaction *3989*

Prolactin *Plasma No Effect Physiological* No effect on basal concentration or response to hypoglycemia in morning or evening *4231*

Tricyclic Antidepressants *Urine Increase Analytical* As measured by Syva d.a.u. assay false positive in urine specimen observed at a concentration above that obtained with concentrations above therapeutic *6434*

Cyproterone

Alkaline Phosphatase, Bone Isoenzyme
Serum Decrease Physiological In 16 healthy postmenopausal women treatment with 2 mg/d estradiol valerate and 1 mg/d cyproterone acetate for 12 months caused a significant decrease in activity from mean baseline of 78.0 ± 7.4 U/L to 57.9 ± 5.7 U/L at 6 months and 52.8 ± 4.7 U/L at 12 months *2535*

Androstenedione *Plasma Decrease Physiological* Reduction from mean of 2.1 ng/mL in 8 hirsute women to 1.6 ng/mL at 2 months, 1.7 ng/mL at 4 months and 1.3 ng/mL at 6 months when treated with 300 mg intramuscularly monthly for 6 months *3788*
Plasma Increase Physiological By up to 450% if acetate derivative used *5708*
Plasma No Effect Physiological In 27 women treated for total of 194 cycles with 50 µg ethinyl estradiol and 2.0 mg cyproterone acetate *3757*

Angiotensinogen *Plasma Increase Physiological* In 16 healthy postmenopausal women treatment with estradiol valerate 2 mg and 1 mg cyproterone acetate in 21-day sequences over 12 cycles caused significant change in concentration from 2029 ± 120 ng/mL to 4151 ± 497 ng/mL *588*

Cholesterol *Serum Decrease Physiological* In oophorectomized women (slight effect) when given alone *3586* In 16 healthy postmenopausal women treatment with estradiol valerate 2 mg and 1 mg cyproterone acetate in 21-day sequences over 12 cycles caused significant change in concentration from 5.60 ± 0.13 mmol/L to 5.25 ± 0.13 mmol/L in estrogenic phase and 5.39 ± 0.15 mmol/L in progestogenic phase *588* In 94 postmenopausal women treatment with 2 mg/d estradiol valerate and 1 mg/d cyptoterone acetate sequentially caused significant reduction from mean baseline of 6.47 mmol/L by 4.8% after 6 months and 6.2% after 12 months *6096*
Serum Increase Physiological When given in combination with ethinyl estradiol *3586*

Cholesterol, Free *Serum Decrease Physiological* In oophorectomized women when given alone *3586*

Cyproterone (continued)

Cholesterol, Free *(continued)*
Serum *No Effect* *Physiological* When given in combination with ethinyl estradiol *3586*

C-Peptide *Plasma* *No Effect* *Physiological* Unchanged following oral glucose when given with ethinyl estradiol combination causes insulin resistance *5426*

C-terminal Telopeptide of Type I Collagen
Serum *Decrease* *Physiological* In 16 healthy postmenopausal women treatment with 2 mg/d estradiol valerate and 1 mg/d cyproterone acetate for 12 months caused a significant decrease in concentration from mean baseline of 3.57 ± 0.22 µg/L to 2.78 ± 0.12 µg/L at 6 months and 2.84 ± 0.17 µg/L at 12 months *2535*

Dehydroepiandrosterone *Plasma* *No Effect* *Physiological* In 27 women treated for total of 194 cycles with 50 µg ethinyl estradiol and 2.0 mg cyproterone acetate *3757*

Dehydroepiandrosterone Sulfate
Plasma *Decrease* *Physiological* In 27 women treated for total of 194 cycles with 50 µg ethinyl estradiol and 2.0 mg cyproterone acetate *3757* In 29 healthy postmenopausal women treatment with estradiol valerate 2 mg and 1 mg cyproterone acetate in 21-day sequences over 12 cycles caused significant change in concentration from 3.99 ± 0.36 µmol/L to 2.13 ± 0.31 µmol/L *588*
Plasma *No Effect* *Physiological* Insignificant reduction observed in 8 hirsute women treated with 300 mg intramuscularly monthly for 6 months *3788*

Estradiol *Plasma* *Decrease* *Physiological* In 27 women treated for total of 194 cycles with 50 µg ethinyl estradiol and 2.0 mg cyproterone acetate *3757* Reduction from mean concentration of 35 pg/mL in 8 hirsute women to 22 pg/mL at 2 months, 25 pg/mL at 4 months and 21 pg/mL at 6 months when treated with 300 mg intramuscularly monthly for 6 months *3788*
Plasma *Increase* *Physiological* In 25 healthy postmenopausal women treatment with estradiol valerate 2 mg and 1 mg cyproterone acetate in 21-day sequences over 12 cycles caused significant increase in concentration from 86 ± 21 pmol/L to 742 ± 160 pmol/L *588*

Estrone *Plasma* *Decrease* *Physiological* In 27 women treated for total of 194 cycles with 50 µg ethinyl estradiol and 2.0 mg cyproterone acetate *3757*
Plasma *Increase* *Physiological* In 19 healthy postmenopausal women treatment with estradiol valerate 2 mg and 1 mg cyproterone acetate in 21-day sequences over 12 cycles caused significant increase in concentration from 276 ± 24 pmol/L to 1561 ± 220 pmol/L *588*

Fibrinogen *Plasma* *No Effect* *Physiological* In 16 healthy postmenopausal women treatment with estradiol valerate 2 mg and 1 mg cyproterone acetate in 21-day sequences over 12 cycles caused nonsignificant change in concentration from 2.95 ± 0.10 g/L to 2.95 ± 0.11 g/L *588*

Follicle Stimulating Hormone
Plasma *Decrease* *Physiological* In 29 healthy postmenopausal women treatment with estradiol valerate 2 mg and 1 mg cyproterone acetate in 21-day sequences over 12 cycles caused significant change in concentration from 70.3 ± 6.8 IU/L to 22.8 ± 2.2 IU/L *588*
Plasma *No Effect* *Physiological* No significant effect in 8 hirsute women treated with 300 mg intramuscularly monthly for 6 months *3788* No change following oral administration *5708*

Glucose *Serum* *Decrease* *Physiological* When given with ethinyl estradiol: combination causes insulin resistance *5426*

Glucose Tolerance *Serum* *Decrease* *Physiological* When given with ethinyl estradiol: combination causes insulin resistance *5426*

HDL-Cholesterol *Serum* *No Effect* *Physiological* In 16 healthy postmenopausal women treatment with estradiol valerate 2 mg and 1 mg cyproterone acetate in 21-day sequences over 12 cycles caused nonsignificant change in concentration from 1.68 ± 0.09 mmol/L to 1.69 ± 0.09 mmol/L in estrogenic phase and 1.69 ± 0.10 mmol/L in progestogenic phase *588*

Insulin *Plasma* *Increase* *Physiological* Fasting concentration when given with ethinyl estradiol: combination causes insulin resistance *5426*

LDL-Cholesterol *Serum* *Decrease* *Physiological* In 94 postmenopausal women treatment with 2 mg/d estradiol valerate and 1 mg/d cyptoterone acetate sequentially caused significant reduction from mean baseline of 4.26 ± 0.93 mmol/L to 3.97 ± 0.09 mmol/L after 6 months and 3.94 ± 0.09 mmol/L after 12 months *6096* In 16 healthy postmenopausal women treatment with estradiol valerate 2 mg and 1 mg cyproterone acetate in 21-day sequences over 12 cycles caused significant change in concentration from 3.41 ± 0.13 mmol/L to 2.98 ± 0.17 mmol/L in estrogenic phase and 3.12 ± 0.17 mmol/L in progestogenic phase *588*
Serum *No Effect* *Physiological* In 101 postmenopausal women treatment with 2 mg/d estradiol valerate, 1 mg/d cyptoterone acetate sequentially and 300 IU/d cholecalciferol caused nonsignificant change from mean baseline of 3.87 ± 0.12 mmol/L to 3.82 ± 0.10 mmol/L after 6 months and 3.79 ± 0.10 mmol/L after 12 months *6096*

Luteinizing Hormone *Plasma* *Decrease* *Physiological* In 29 healthy postmenopausal women treatment with estradiol valerate 2 mg and 1 mg cyproterone acetate in 21-day sequences over 12 cycles caused significant change in concentration from 52.6 ± 5.1 IU/L to 26.3 ± 2.6 IU/L *588* Slight but significant decrease observed from 2 months onwards in 8 hirsute women treated with 300 mg intramuscularly monthly for 6 months *3788*
Plasma *No Effect* *Physiological* No change following oral administration *5708*

Osteocalcin *Serum* *Decrease* *Physiological* In 16 healthy postmenopausal women treatment with 2 mg/d estradiol valerate and 1 mg/d cyproterone acetate for 12 months caused significant 29.2% decrease in concentration from mean baseline of 3.12 ± 0.59 ng/mL to 2.77 ± 0.50 ng/mL at 6 months and 2.46 ± 0.44 ng/mL at 12 months *2535*

Partial Thromboplastin Time
Plasma *No Effect* *Physiological* In 16 healthy postmenopausal women treatment with estradiol valerate 2 mg and 1 mg cyproterone acetate in 21-day sequences over 12 cycles caused nonsignificant change in concentration from 90.8 ± 2.7% to 94.3 ± 2.9% *588*

Phospholipids *Serum* *Decrease* *Physiological* In oophorectomized women (slight effect) when given alone *3586*
Serum *Increase* *Physiological* When given in combination with ethinyl estradiol *3586*

Progesterone *Plasma* *Decrease* *Physiological* In 27 women treated for total of 194 cycles with 50 µg ethinyl estradiol and 2.0 mg cyproterone acetate *3757*

Prolactin *Plasma* *No Effect* *Physiological* In 27 women treated for total of 194 cycles with 50 µg ethinyl estradiol and 2.0 mg cyproterone acetate 2.0 mg cyproterone acetate *3757*

Prothrombin Time *Plasma* *No Effect* *Physiological* In 16 healthy postmenopausal women treatment with estradiol valerate 2 mg and 1 mg cyproterone acetate in 21-day sequences over 12 cycles caused nonsignificant change in concentration from 1.09 ± 0.030 mg/L to 1.08 ± 0.041 mg/L *588*

Renin Activity *Plasma* *No Effect* *Physiological* In 16 healthy postmenopausal women treatment with estradiol valerate 2 mg and 1 mg cyproterone acetate in 21-day sequences over 12 cycles caused nonsignificant change in activity from 2.7 ± 0.33 ng/mL/h to 2.7 ± 0.53 ng/mL/h *588*

Sex-Hormone Binding Globulin
Serum *Decrease* *Physiological* Significant reduction in SHBG binding capacity at 2 and 6 months in 8 hirsute women treated with 300 mg intramuscularly monthly for 6 months *3788*
Serum *Increase* *Physiological* In 20 healthy postmenopausal women treatment with estradiol valerate 2 mg and 1 mg cyproterone acetate in 21-day sequences over 12 cycles caused significant increase in concentration from 43.6 ± 5.2 nmol/L to 79.2 ± 7.1 nmol/L *588*

Sperm Count *Semen* *Decrease* *Physiological* May completely inhibit spermatogenesis with high doses *1499*

T3-Uptake *Serum* *Decrease* *Physiological* In 25 healthy postmenopausal women treatment with estradiol valerate 2 mg and 1 mg cyproterone acetate in 21-day sequences over 12 cycles caused nonsignificant change in concentration from 0.63 ± 0.13 to 0.56 ± 0.12 *588*

Testosterone *Serum* *Decrease* *Physiological* Increase by 20-40% (antiandrogenic effect) *5708* Decreases hormone in adult men but does not affect concentration in children with precocious puberty. Decreases concentration in hirsute women

2836 In 15 healthy postmenopausal women treatment with estradiol valerate 2 mg and 1 mg cyproterone acetate in 21-day sequences over 12 cycles caused significant change in concentration from 1.52 ± 0.17 nmol/L to 1.05 ± 0.14 nmol/L *588*
Serum No Effect Physiological In 27 women treated for total of 194 cycles with 50 µg ethinyl estradiol and 2.0 mg cyproterone acetate *3757* No significant effect over 6 months on the high initial concentration in 8 hirsute women treated with 300 mg intramuscularly monthly *3788* No significant effect observed over 6 months in a population receiving monophasic cyproterone acetate as oral contraceptive agent even though free testosterone concentration reduced *6179*

Testosterone, Free *Serum Decrease Physiological* In 27 women treated for total of 194 cycles with 50 µg ethinyl estradiol and 2.0 mg cyproterone *3757*

Thyroid Stimulating Hormone
Serum Decrease Physiological In 29 healthy postmenopausal women treatment with estradiol valerate 2 mg and 1 mg cyproterone acetate in 21-day sequences over 12 cycles caused nonsignificant change in concentration from 2.67 ± 0.76 mIU/L to 2.13 ± 0.31 mIU/L *588*

Thyroxine (T4) *Serum Increase Physiological* In 25 healthy postmenopausal women treatment with estradiol valerate 2 mg and 1 mg cyproterone acetate in 21-day sequences over 12 cycles caused nonsignificant change in concentration from 105.2 ± 4.0 nmol/L to 126.8 ± 2.6 nmol/L *588*

Triglycerides *Serum Increase Physiological* In 16 healthy postmenopausal women treatment with estradiol valerate 2 mg and 1 mg cyproterone acetate in 21-day sequences over 12 cycles caused nonsignificant change in concentration from 1.07 ± 0.13 mmol/L to 1.37 ± 0.14 mmol/L in estrogenic phase and 1.29 ± 0.25 mmol/L in progestogenic phase *588* When given in combination with ethinyl estradiol *3586*
Serum No Effect Physiological In oophorectomized women when given alone *3586*

VLDL-Cholesterol *Serum No Effect Physiological* In 16 healthy postmenopausal women treatment with estradiol valerate 2 mg and 1 mg cyproterone acetate in 21-day sequences over 12 cycles caused nonsignificant change in concentration from 0.51 ± 0.06 mmol/L to 0.57 ± 0.06 mmol/L in estrogenic phase and 0.57 ± 0.10 mmol/L in progestogenic phase *588*

Cytarabine

Alanine Aminotransferase *Serum Increase Physiological* Hepatic dysfunction may occur with cytarabine administration *4670* Hepatotoxic effect *2242*

Alkaline Phosphatase *Serum Increase Physiological* At 3 g/m² every 12 h for 6 d, some mild and reversible abnormalities in about 75% of 12 cases *2580* In two cases with acute leukemia: unlikely to have been due to other drugs co-administered: effects slight *4719* Slight effect and returned to normal while still under treatment *3949* Hepatic dysfunction may occur with cytarabine administration *4670*

Amino Acids *Urine Increase Physiological* Mean excretion of 20.3 mmol/d in 3 patients with leukemia undergoing chemotherapy not different from 29.1 ± 23.4 mmol/d in 52 patients with acute leukemia and 19.8 ± 10.4 mmol/d in 29 healthy controls of both sexes *6517*

Amylase *Serum Increase Physiological* Acute pancreatitis reported in patients who had prior treatment with asparaginase *1384*

Aspartate Aminotransferase *Serum Increase Physiological* Slight effect and returned to normal while still under treatment *3949* In two cases with acute leukemia: unlikely to have been due to other drugs co-administered: effect slight *4719* Hepatic dysfunction may occur with cytarabine administration *4670* At 3 g/m² every 12 h for 6 d, some mild and reversible abnormalities of AST activity observed in about 75% of 12 cases *2580*

Bilirubin *Serum Increase Physiological* Hepatic dysfunction may occur with cytarabine administration *4670* At 3 g/m² every 12 h for 6 d, some mild and reversible abnormalities in about 75% of 12 cases *2580* Significant elevation in 7 of 42 patients with previously normal liver function *3949*

Bilirubin, Direct *Serum Increase Physiological* In two cases with acute leukemia: unlikely to have been due to other drugs co-administered: effects slight *4719*

Chromosomes *Test Conditions Abnormal Physiological* Clastogenic in human cells *5484*

Color *Feces Increase Analytical* Black color reported with cytarabine ingestion *3388*

Digitoxin *Serum No Effect Physiological* No effect on concentration reported when drug coadministered with cytarabine *4670*

Digoxin *Serum Decrease Physiological* Reversible decrease reported in some patients receiving multiple chemotherapeutic agents both with and without cytarabine *4670*
Urine Decrease Physiological Reversible decrease reported in some patients receiving multiple chemotherapeutic agents both with and without cytarabine *4670*

Erythrocytes *Blood Decrease Physiological* Megaloblastic anemia (relatively infrequent) *3810* Aplasia of bone marrow developed in nearly all of 57 leukemics *2580*

Hematocrit *Blood Decrease Physiological* Anticipated response with cytarabine administration *4670*

Hemoglobin *Blood Decrease Physiological* May cause anemia *3810* Anticipated response with cytarabine administration *4670* In 20 patients with HIV infection and progressive multifocal leukoencephalopathy antiretroviral treatment for 24 weeks with intravenous cytarabine caused reduction of hemoglobin concentration to below 6.5 g/dL in 3 (15%) *2411*

Histamine *Plasma No Effect Analytical* No inhibition of radio-enzyme assay at 100 µg/mL *2492*

Leukocytes *Blood Decrease Physiological* Anticipated response with cytarabine administration *4670* Aplasia of bone marrow developed in nearly all of 57 leukemics *2580* Agranulocytosis/Leukopenia *3810*

Neutrophils *Blood Decrease Physiological* In 20 patients with HIV infection and progressive multifocal leukoencephalopathy antiretroviral treatment for 24 weeks with intravenous cytarabine caused reduction of absolute neutrophil count to below 749 /µL in 4 (20%): in 19 given intrathecal cytarabine with antiretroviral therapy neutrophil count reduced to below 749 /µL in 3 (16%): in 17 given antiretroviral therapy only count reduced below 749/µL in 5 (29%) *2411*

Occult Blood *Feces Increase Physiological* Gastrointestinal hemorrhage in fewer than 2% *2754*

Platelets *Blood Decrease Physiological* Anticipated response with cytarabine administration *4670* Due to bone marrow depression *3810* In 20 patients with HIV infection and progressive multifocal leukoencephalopathy antiretroviral treatment for 24 weeks with intravenous cytarabine caused reduction of platelet count to below 49,999 /µL in 8 (40%): in 19 given intrathecal cytarabine with antiretroviral therapy platelet count reduced to below 49,000 /µL in 3 (16%) *2411* Aplasia of bone marrow developed in nearly all of 57 leukemics *2580*

Protein *Cerebrospinal Fluid Decrease Analytical* False low value with Folin-Ciocalteu reagent. False low with turbidimetric method on standing *6693*

Reticulocytes *Blood Decrease Physiological* In fewer than 2% *2754* Anticipated response with cytarabine administration *4670*

Uric Acid *Serum Increase Physiological* Secondary to rapid lysis of neoplastic cells *2754*

Zalcitabine *Serum No Effect Analytical* At a concentration of 100 mg/L had less than 0.01% cross-reactivity with solid phase extraction and RIA method of Roberts et al *4990*

Cytostatic Therapy

Protein *Serum Decrease Physiological* In 27 patients with various malignancies treatment caused significant reduction from mean of 75.5 g/L to 74.2 g/L *1445*

Thyroglobulin *Serum No Effect Physiological* Insignificant increase from mean concentration of 31 µg/L to 35 µg/L in 27 patients with various malignancies *1445*

Thyroid Stimulating Hormone
Serum Decrease Physiological Treatment of 27 patients with various malignancies caused nonsignificant decrease from mean of 5.68 mIU/L to 4.96 mIU/L *1445*

Thyroxine Binding Globulin
Serum Decrease Physiological Treatment of 27 patients with various malignancies caused significant reduction from mean concentration of 14.89 mg/L to 12.68 mg/L *1445*

Cytostatic Therapy *(continued)*

Thyroxine (T4) *Serum Decrease Physiological* Treatment of 27 patients with various malignancies caused significant decrease from mean concentration of 71 nmol/L to 64 nmol/L *1445*

Tri-iodothyronine (T3) *Serum No Effect Physiological* In 27 patients with various malignancies treatment caused non-significant increase from mean of 1.65 nmol/L to 1.73 nmol/L *1445*

Cytotoxic Drugs

Digoxin *Serum Decrease Physiological* May reduce bioavailability *1384*

Lactoferrin *Plasma Decrease Physiological* Mean concentration in 8 patients with chronic myeloid leukemia treated with cytotoxic agents had subnormal concentrations (0.01 - 0.54 µg/mL) compared with concentrations in normal women (1.62 µg/mL) and in healthy men (1.62 µg/mL) *487*

Dacarbazine

Leukocytes *Blood Decrease Physiological* Myelosuppression is usually dose limiting: platelets and leukocytes most affected *1384*

Platelets *Blood Decrease Physiological* Myelosuppression is usually dose limiting: Platelets and leukocytes most affected *1384*

Daclizumab

Lymphocytes *Blood No Effect Physiological* No change observed in count before renal transplant and 6 months after in daclizumab treated patients *6265*

Dactinomycin

Alanine Aminotransferase *Serum Increase Physiological* Dactinomycin may cause liver toxicity including ascites, hepatomegaly, hepatitis and liver function test abnormalities *3964*

Alkaline Phosphatase *Serum Increase Physiological* Dactinomycin may cause liver toxicity including ascites, hepatomegaly, hepatitis and liver function test abnormalities *3964*

Aspartate Aminotransferase *Serum Increase Physiological* Dactinomycin may cause liver toxicity including ascites, hepatomegaly, hepatitis and liver function test abnormalities *3964*

Bilirubin *Serum Increase Physiological* Dactinomycin may cause liver toxicity including ascites, hepatomegaly, hepatitis and liver function test abnormalities *3964*

Erythrocytes *Blood Decrease Physiological* Anemia/pancytopenia *128*

γ-Glutamyltransferase *Serum Increase Physiological* Dactinomycin may cause liver toxicity including ascites, hepatomegaly, hepatitis and liver function test abnormalities *3964*

Granulocytes *Blood Decrease Physiological* Dactinomycin may cause agranulocytosis and even aplastic anemia *3964*

Hematocrit *Blood Decrease Physiological* Dactinomycin may cause anemia, even to the point of aplastic anemia *3964*

Hemoglobin *Blood Decrease Physiological* May cause anemia *128* Dactinomycin may cause anemia, even to the point of aplastic anemia *3964*

Histamine *Plasma No Effect Analytical* Improbable inhibition of radio-enzyme assay at therapeutic concentrations *2492*

Leukocytes *Blood Decrease Physiological* Leukopenia/pancytopenia *128* Dactinomycin may cause leukopenia and even aplastic anemia *3964*

Occult Blood *Feces Increase Physiological* Dactinomycin may cause gastrointestinal ulceration *3964*

Platelets *Blood Decrease Physiological* Thrombocytopenia/pancytopenia *128* Dactinomycin may cause thrombocytopenia and even aplastic anemia *3964*

Reticulocytes *Blood Decrease Physiological* Dactinomycin may cause reticulocytopenia and even aplastic anemia *3964* Reticulocytopenia/pancytopenia *128*

Dalteparin

Alanine Aminotransferase *Serum Increase Physiological* Mean asymptomatic increases more than 3 times the upper limit of normal observed in 4.3% treated patients *4674*

Anti-Factor Xa *Plasma Increase Physiological* Mean increases in activity of 0.19 ± 0.04 IU/mL, 0.41 ± 0.07 IU/mL and 0.82 ± 0.10 IU/mL observed about 4 hours after single subcutaneous doses of 2,500, 5,000 and 10,000 IU respectively in normal volunteers *4674*

Aspartate Aminotransferase *Serum Increase Physiological* Mean asymptomatic increases more than 3 times the upper limit of normal observed in 1.7% treated patients *4674*

Platelets *Blood Decrease Physiological* In trials in patients for thromboprophylaxis thrombocytopenia with a count below 50,000 cells/µL observed in less than 1% of treated patients and of less than 100,000 cells/µL observed in less than 1% treated patients *4674*

Danazol

α_1-Acid Glycoprotein *Serum No Effect Physiological* No significant change over 8 weeks in 7 women with endometriosis treated with 600 mg daily *3434*

Alanine Aminotransferase *Serum Increase Physiological* Significantly increased mean activity in women with endometriosis treated for 6 months *2562* Significant effect at 4,8, 12 and 16 weeks after 600 mg daily in 18 women with endometriosis *892* Hepatic dysfunction has been reported in patients receiving 400 mg danazol or more on a daily basis *5251*

Albumin *Serum No Effect Physiological* No effect in 7 women with endometriosis over 8 weeks when treated with 600 mg daily *3434* No change during treatment of women with endometriosis *4297* No change in 18 women with endometriosis given 600 mg/d for 6 mo *892*

Alkaline Phosphatase *Serum Decrease Physiological* Mean 6.9% decrease in almost 100 patients with endometriosis treated with 400 mg daily for 6 months *5069*
Serum Increase Physiological Hepatic dysfunction has been reported in patients receiving 400 mg danazol or more on a daily basis *5251*
Serum No Effect Physiological No abnormalities observed in patients taking drug *6574*

Alkaline Phosphatase, Bone Isoenzyme
Serum Increase Physiological Mean increase of 30-40% observed in 6 women with confirmed endometriosis treated with 600 mg/day orally for 6 months *6600*

Aminoterminal Propeptide of Type III Collagen
Serum No Effect Physiological No significant change observed in 6 women with confirmed endometriosis treated with 600 mg/day orally for 6 months *6600*

Androstenedione *Plasma Decrease Physiological* Significant reduction in 6 women with endometriosis treated with 600 mg daily with reduction from mean of 7.2 nmol/L at baseline to 5.5 nmol/L at 3 months and 5.0 nmol/L at 6 months *6157*
Plasma Increase Analytical May interfere with some analytical methods *5251*
Plasma Increase Physiological Increase by 70% in 7 normal subjects given drug 800 mg daily *3674*
Plasma No Effect Physiological Nonsignificant reduction from mean of 5.8 nmol/L to 4.5 nmol/L in 6 nonobese women with minimal endometriosis treated with 400 mg daily for 6 weeks *2233*

α_1-Antichymotrypsin *Serum No Effect Physiological* Insignificant change over 8 weeks in 7 women with endometriosis treated with 600 mg daily *3434*

α_2-Antiplasmin *Plasma No Effect Physiological* Insignificant increase in 7 women with endometriosis treated with 600 mg daily for 8 weeks *3434*

Antithrombin III *Plasma Increase Physiological* Approximately 41% increase in 7 women with endometriosis treated with 600 mg daily for 8 weeks *3434*

α_1-Antitrypsin *Serum No Effect Physiological* Insignificant reduction in 7 women with endometriosis treated with 600 mg daily for 8 weeks *3434*

Apolipoprotein A-I *Serum Decrease Physiological* Reduction by 35% in 6 women with endometriosis at 3 months when treated with 600 mg daily *6157*

Apolipoprotein A-II *Serum No Effect Physiological* No change observed in 6 women with endometriosis treated with 600 mg daily for 6 months *6157*

Aspartate Aminotransferase *Serum Increase Physiological* Significant increase in women with endometriosis treated for 6 months *2562* Hepatic dysfunction has been reported in patients receiving 400 mg danazol or more on a daily basis *5251* In 1 of 4 men and 0 in 7 women *6574* In study of almost 100 women with endometriosis treated with 400 mg daily for 6 months increase of aspartate aminotransferase twice as much as for those patients treated with nafarelin *5069*

Bilirubin *Serum Increase Physiological* Abnormal liver function tests and jaundice occasionally reported *1384* Hepatic dysfunction has been reported in patients receiving 400 mg danazol or more on a daily basis *5251*

Blood *Urine Increase Physiological* Hematuria has been reported in patients receiving danazol *5251*

BSP Retention *Serum Increase Physiological* Develops in over one third of patients taking drug *6574*

C_1-Esterase Inhibitor *Serum Increase Physiological* Approximately 54% increase in 7 women with endometriosis treated with 600 mg daily for 8 weeks *3434*

C_1-Inhibitor *Serum Increase Physiological* Approximate doubling in 5 patients with hereditary angioneurotic edema treated for up to 10 mo *5406*

CA 125 *Serum Decrease Physiological* Concentration decreased significantly in 40 patients with stage III or IV endometriosis to < 20 U/mL at 8 weeks but after 12 weeks in those patients who were poor responders significant increase (to 20.8 U/mL) compared with good responders (8.5 U/mL) *5921* Elevated concentration in patients with moderate or severe endometriosis (mean in excess of 30 U/mL) fell to within normal range during treatment but rose again following cessation of treatment. Some correlation between high value and recurrence *40*

Calcitonin *Plasma No Effect Physiological* In 6 women with endometriosis treatment with 800 mg/d oral danazol over 24 weeks had no effect on the plasma calcitonin concentration *1286* No significant effect observed in 6 women with confirmed endometriosis treated with 600 mg/day orally for 6 months *6600*

Calcium *Serum No Effect Physiological* No significant effect observed in 6 women with confirmed endometriosis treated with 600 mg/day orally for 6 months *6600*
Urine No Effect Physiological Insignificant change in excretion observed in 6 women with confirmed endometriosis treated with 600 mg/day orally for 6 months *6600*

Carbamazepine *Serum Increase Physiological* Due to effect on hepatic metabolism *1384* Increased concentrations and neurotoxicity reported with coadministration of drugs *3119* Coadministration of 600 mg/day caused steady-state plasma concentrations of carbamazepine to increase by 50-100%. Effect due to inhibition of hepatic oxidative metabolism *3270* Drugs that inhibit CYP 3A4 inhibit metabolism of carbamazepine producing clinically meaningful effect *1039* Concentration increased almost 2 fold when drug added for treatment of fibrocystic breast disease *6660* May increase carbamazepine concentration in patients receiving both drugs *5251*

Ceruloplasmin *Serum No Effect Physiological* Insignificant reduction in 7 women with endometriosis treated with 600 mg daily for 8 weeks *3434*

Cholesterol *Serum Increase Physiological* During clinical trials of patients who had cholesterol concentrations initially below 250 mg/dL 2% demonstrated increased cholesterol concentration after treatment *2070* During clinical trials of patients who had cholesterol concentrations initially below 250 mg/dL 18% demonstrated increased cholesterol concentration after treatment *2070* Increase in almost 100 patients with endometriosis treated with 400 mg daily for 6 months *5069*
Serum No Effect Physiological No significant effect in 6 women with endometriosis treated with 600 mg daily for 6 months *6157* No significant change over 24 weeks in 12 women with endometriosis given 600 mg daily for 24 weeks *1782* No effect after 6 mo of 600 mg/d *6574* Inconsistent changes observed in 62 patients with endometriosis treated with 600 mg daily for up to 24 weeks *5410* Insignificant change in 9 women with endometriosis treated for 6 mo *108*

Cholinesterase *Serum Decrease Physiological* Approximately 19% reduction in 7 women with endometriosis treated with 600 mg daily for 8 weeks *3434*

Complement C_3 *Serum Decrease Physiological* Approximately 22% reduction over 8 weeks in 7 women with endometriosis treated with 600 mg daily *3434*

Complement C_4 *Serum Increase Physiological* Up to 8 fold increase in 5 patients with hereditary angioneurotic edema treated for up to 10 mo *5406*
Serum No Effect Physiological No significant change in 7 women with endometriosis treated with 600 mg daily for 8 weeks *3434*

Corticosteroid-Binding Globulin
Serum No Effect Physiological No significant change in 5 patients with hereditary angioneurotic edema treated for up to 10 mo *5406* No significant change in 7 women with endometriosis treated with 600 mg daily for 8 weeks *3434*

Cortisol *Plasma Decrease Analytical* Concentrations low: in case of cortisol and testosterone displacement from plasma proteins occurs and protein binding assays are probably invalid *2435*
Plasma Decrease Physiological Affect binding in women treated with drug so that proportion of free drug high *2435*
Plasma Increase Analytical Probably invalid results because of high cross-reactivity with protein in competitive binding assays *2435*
Plasma No Effect Analytical At concentrations up to 160 mg/L no significant effect observed on Enzymun method *1097*

Cortisol, Free *Plasma Increase Physiological* Proportion high due to displacement of hormone from protein *2435*

C-Peptide *Plasma No Effect Physiological* Nonsignificant increase in fasting concentration from 410 pmol/L to 750 pmol/L in 6 nonobese women with minimal endometriosis treated with 400 mg daily for 6 weeks: but significant increase from 11.42 nmol/L to 20.09 nmol/L in summed OGTT concentration *2233*

C-Reactive Protein *Serum No Effect Physiological* No significant effect of treatment with 600 mg daily for 8 weeks in 7 women with endometriosis *3434*

Creatine Kinase *Serum Increase Physiological* Significant increase in women with endometriosis treated for 6 months *2562* Increased activity has been reported in patients receiving danazol *5251*

Creatinine *Serum Increase Physiological* Slight effect in 18 women with endometriosis given 600 mg/d for 6 mo *892*

Cyclosporine *Blood Increase Physiological* Coadministration of danazol with cyclosporine caused 2- to 4-fold increase in cyclosporine concentration possibly due to increased intestinal absorption or decreased metabolism *859*
Serum Increase Physiological May increase cyclosporine concentration by inhibiting hepatic cytochrome P-450 III A which metabolizes cyclosporine *5236* Increased concentrations observed when drugs coadministered *1384* Observed effect presumed to be due to inhibition of hepatic microsomal enzymes *1069* Coadministration of danazol with cyclosporine caused 2- to 4-fold increase in cyclosporine concentration possibly due to increased intestinal absorption or decreased metabolism *859* 2-fold increase observed in one 15-year old renal transplant patient within days of beginning danazol treatment *6596*

Cyclosporine A *Blood Increase Physiological* Coadministration with cyclosporine A increases its concentration *5240*

Dehydroepiandrosterone *Plasma Decrease Physiological* Significant effect at 8,12 weeks after 600 mg daily in 18 women with endometriosis *892*
Plasma Increase Analytical May interfere with some analytical methods *5251*

Dehydroepiandrosterone Sulfate
Plasma Increase Physiological Significant effect at 2, 4 and 8 weeks after 600 mg daily in 18 women with endometriosis *892* Increase by 40% in 7 normal subjects given drug 800 mg daily *3674*
Plasma No Effect Physiological Nonsignificant mean increase from 3.8 µmol/L to 4.6 µmol/L in 6 nonobese women with minimal endometriosis treated with 400 mg daily for 6

Danazol (continued)

Dehydroepiandrosterone Sulfate *(continued)*
weeks *2233* No consistent change noted in patients with prostatic cancer *1088*

Eosinophils *Blood Increase Physiological* Eosinophilia has been reported in patients receiving danazol *5251*

Erythrocytes *Blood Increase Physiological* Reversible increased erythrocyte count has been reported in patients receiving danazol *5251*

Estradiol *Plasma Decrease Physiological* But normal mid-follicular values during treatment in 62 patients with endometriosis treated with 600 mg daily for up to 24 weeks *5410* In 10 infertile patients with endometriosis mean concentration of 126.1 ± 11.1 pg/mL decreased to 111.1 ± 5.0 pg/mL during treatment with 600 mg/d danazol for 6 months *4496* In 6 patients with confirmed endometriosis 600 mg orally reduced concentration below 21.6 pg/mL after 3 months *6600* Mean decrease from early follicular phase baseline of about 55% in almost 100 women with endometriosis treated with 400 mg daily for 6 months *5069* In 6 women with endometriosis treatment with 800 mg oral danazol daily concentration decreased from mean baseline of about 60 pg/mL to > 47 pg/mL after about 8 weeks *1286* Mean concentration reduced in women with endometriosis following administration of 800 mg/day *6093* Significant reduction in 6 women with endometriosis treated with 600 mg daily with reduction from mean baseline concentration of 0.49 nmol/L to 0.11 nmol/L at 3 months and 0.07 nmol/L at 6 months *6157* In patients with stage III or IV endometriosis who responded well significant reduction (from baseline of 30 pg/mL to 11 pg/mL at 4 weeks) although it reverted to prior level at 12 weeks. In poor responders no change in estradiol concentration *5921*
Plasma No Effect Physiological No change from baseline, 170 pmol/L, observed in 6 patients with minimal endometriosis when treated with 600 mg/d for 2 months *3779* In 7 normal women given 800 mg daily for 2 mo amenorrheic state induced drug *3674* No effect observed in 9 nondiabetics with pelvic endometriosis with 6 weeks of treatment *6215* No consistent change noted in patients with prostatic cancer *1088*

Estrone *Plasma No Effect Physiological* In 7 normal women given 800 mg daily for 2 mo amenorrheic state induced by drug *3674*

Factor VIII *Plasma No Effect Physiological* In 21 hemophiliacs given drug for 2 weeks *4339*

Factor IX *Plasma No Effect Physiological* In 21 hemophiliacs given drug for 2 weeks *4339*

Fc-γ Receptors *Monocytes Decrease Physiological* In 22 patients with myelodysplastic syndrome treatment with 600 - 800 mg/d for 3 - 12 months caused significant reduction in numbers *5764*

Fibrinogen *Plasma Decrease Physiological* Significant effect in 21 hemophiliacs given drug for 2 weeks *4339*

Follicle Stimulating Hormone
Plasma Decrease Physiological Mean 20% decrease observed in 6 women with minmal endometriosis treated with 600 mg/d for 2 months but nonsignificant increase in FSH pulse amplitude and in pulse frequency *3779* Effect noted in 6 orchidectomized patients with prostatic cancer *1088*
Plasma Increase Physiological In 10 infertile patients with endometriosis mean concentration of 6.9 ± 1.2 mIU/mL increased nonsignificantly to 7.6 ± 0.8 mIU/mL during treatment with 600 mg/d danazol for 6 months *4496*
Plasma No Effect Physiological No significant effect of treatment observed in women with endometriosis *3780* In 7 normal women given 800 mg daily for 2 mo amenorrheic state induced by drug *3674* No significant change observed in 6 nonobese women with minimal endometriosis treated with 400 mg daily for 6 weeks *2233*

Gc-Globulin *Serum No Effect Physiological* 25% reduction in 7 women with endometriosis treated with 600 mg daily for 8 weeks *3434*

Glucagon *Plasma Increase Physiological* Significant reduction in one woman with systemic lupus erythematosus on withdrawal of drug *1254* Concentration above 50 pmol/L observed in 7 women treated with up to 600 mg/d for up to 24 weeks: slight fall with glucose tolerance test *6466* Significant increase from mean baseline of 17 pmol/L to 59 pmol/L in 6 nonobese women with minimal endometriosis treated with 400 mg daily for 6 weeks and from 94 pmol/L to 238 pmol/L in summed concentration following oral glucose tolerance test *2233*

Glucose *Serum No Effect Physiological* No significant change in fasting concentration in 6 nonobese women with minimal endometriosis: likewise no significant change in summed concentration in response to oral glucose tolerance test following treatment with 400 mg daily for 6 weeks *2233*

Glucose Tolerance *Serum Decrease Physiological* In patients receiving drug, although baseline concentration normal *6466* Abnormal response has been reported in patients receiving danazol *5251* Mild deterioration observed in 9 women with pelvic endometriosis 6 weeks after starting treatment. At same time marked increase in insulin response to glucose loading *6215* In response to oral and i.v. glucose tolerance associated with insulin resistance *6574*

Haptoglobin *Serum Increase Physiological* Approximately 77% increase over 8 weeks in 7 women with endometriosis treated with 600 mg daily *3434*

HDL_2-Cholesterol *Serum Decrease Physiological* Increase by 73% after 2 weeks in 12 women with endometriosis given 600 mg daily for 24 weeks *1782* After 1 month treatment with 600 mg daily in 6 women with endometriosis mean concentration decreased by 58% *6157*

HDL_2-Phospholipids *Serum Decrease Physiological* After 1 month treatment of 6 women with endometriosis with 600 mg daily mean concentration decreased by 79% *6157*

HDL_2-Triglycerides *Serum Decrease Physiological* After 1 month treatment of 6 women with endometriosis with 600 mg daily mean concentration decreased by 65% *6157*

HDL_3-Cholesterol *Serum Decrease Physiological* Increase by 29% after 2 weeks in 12 women with endometriosis given 600 mg daily for 24 weeks *1782*
Serum No Effect Physiological Insignificant change in 6 women with endometriosis treated with 600 mg daily for 6 months *6157*

HDL_3-Phospholipids *Serum No Effect Physiological* Insignificant change in 6 women with endometriosis treated with 600 mg daily for 6 months *6157*

HDL_3-Triglycerides *Serum No Effect Physiological* Insignificant change in 6 women with endometriosis treated with 600 mg daily for 6 months although slight reduction post-treatment *6157*

HDL-Cholesterol *Serum Decrease Physiological* Mean reduction at 3 months of 45% in 6 women with endometriosis treated with 600 mg daily but reverted to normal within 3 months after treatment stopped *6157* In 9 subjects studied for 6 mo significant reduction: returned to normal at end of therapy *108* In 12 women with pelvic endometriosis treated with 600 mg/d danazol for 24 weeks mean concentration decreased by 49% after 2 weeks and by 59% after 6 weeks. Eight weeks after cessation of treatment concentrations had reverted to baseline *1782* Significant effect in women with endometriosis treated for 6 months *2562* Increase by 50% in 6 patients with endometriosis given 600 mg daily for 3 to 6 mo *3754* During clinical trials of patients 43% had abnormal concentrations below 30 mg/dL at the end of treatment *2070* Reduction observed in almost 100 women with endometriosis treated with 400 mg daily for 6 months *5069* By about 45% during first 2 mo in 62 patients with endometriosis treated with 600 mg daily for up to 24 weeks *5410*

Hematocrit *Blood Increase Physiological* In 16 patients with SLE and corticosteroid refractory autoimmune throbocytopenia treatent with up to 1200 mg/d caused increase to above 39% within 2 months of starting treatment *943* During clinical trials of patients danazol treatment was associated with an increase at the end of treatment *2070*

Hemoglobin *Blood Increase Physiological* In one patient with systemic lupus erythematosus who had failed to respond to conventional therapy treatment with 600 mg/d caused increase in blood hemoglobin and a reduction in RBC transfusion requirement *957*

Hemopexin *Serum Increase Physiological* Approximately 19% increase over 8 weeks in 7 women with endometriosis treated with 600 mg daily *3434*

Hydroxyproline *Urine Increase Physiological* Oral administration of 600 mg/day for 6 months caused approximate 50% increase in excretion in 6 women with confirmed endometriosis *6600*

Insulin *Plasma No Effect Physiological* No significant change observed in fasting concentration in 6 nonobese women with minimal endometriosis treated with 400 mg daily for 6 weeks but summed concentration from oral glucose tolerance test increased from 1.08 nmol/L to 3.00 nmol/L *2233* But rose to higher extent than in controls when given oral glucose tolerance test *6466*

17-Ketosteroids *Urine Increase Physiological* 80% increase in 7 women given 800 mg daily for 2 mo *3674*

LDL-Cholesterol *Serum Increase Physiological* Increase by 51% in 6 patients with endometriosis given 600 mg daily for 3 to 6 mo *3754* Increase observed in almost 100 women with endometriosis treated with 400 mg daily for 6 months *5069* Constant but significant effect in 62 patients with endometriosis treated with 600 mg daily for up to 24 weeks *5410* Nonsignificant increase of 41% in 6 women with endometriosis treated with 600 mg daily for 6 months *6157* In 12 women with pelvic endometriosis mean concentration increased by 14% after 2 weeks and by 34% after 8 weeks when treated with 600 mg/d. Eight weeks after cessation of 24 weeks treatment concentration had reverted to baseline *1782* During clinical trials of patients 15% had abnormal concentrations above 190 mg/dL at the end of treatment *2070* Significant effect in women with endometriosis treated for 6 months *2562*

LDL-Cholesterol:HDL-Cholesterol Ratio
Serum Increase Physiological During clinical trials of patients the ratio was increased approximately twofold at the end of treatment *2070*

LDL-Phospholipids *Serum Increase Physiological* Mean increase of 23% (not significant) in 6 women with endometriosis treated with 600 mg daily for 6 months *6157*

LDL-Triglycerides *Serum Increase Physiological* Mean increase of 24% (not significant) in 6 women with endometriosis treated with 600 mg daily for 6 months *6157*

Leukocytes *Blood Decrease Physiological* Leukopenia has been reported in patients receiving danazol *5251*
Blood Increase Physiological Reversible leukocytosis has been reported in patients receiving danazol *5251* In 5 patients with paroxysmal nocturnal hemoglobinuria unresponsive to other therapies treatment with 400 - 800 mg/d caused changes from 6.2 to 7.7, 3.0 to 5.0, 4.0 to 4.9, 4.9 to 5.7 and 8.4 to 10.5 x 1000 /µL in the different patients *2475* During clinical trials of patients danazol treatment was associated with an increase at the end of treatment *2070*

Lipoprotein A *Serum Decrease Physiological* Approximately 15% reduction in 7 women with endometriosis treated with 600 mg daily for 8 weeks *3434*

Luteinizing Hormone *Plasma Decrease Physiological* Mean 22% decrease observed in 6 women with minimal endometriosis given 600 mg/d for 2 months but 16% increase in mean pulse amplitude with 20% decrease in pulse frequency *3779* Effect noted in 6 orchidectomized patients with prostatic cancer *1088*
Plasma Increase Physiological In 10 infertile patients with endometriosis mean concentration of 6.3 ± 0.9 mIU/mL increased nonsignificantly to 8.7 ± 1.7 mIU/mL during treatment with 600 mg/d danazol for 6 months *4496*
Plasma No Effect Physiological In 7 normal women given 800 mg daily for 2 mo amenorrheic state induced by drug *3674* No significant change in 5 patients with hereditary angioneurotic edema treated for up to 10 mo *5406* No significant change observed in 6 nonobese women with minimal endometriosis treated with 400 mg daily for 6 weeks *2233* No significant effect of treatment observed in women with endometriosis *3780*

α_2-Macroglobulin *Serum Decrease Physiological* Approximately 44% reduction in 7 women with endometriosis treated with 600 mg daily for 8 weeks *3434*

Osteocalcin *Serum Increase Physiological* Mean increase of 80-120% observed in 6 women with confirmed endometriosis treated with 600 mg/day orally for 6 months: still increased 3 months after end of treatment *6600*

Parathyroid Hormone *Plasma No Effect Physiological* No significant change observed in 6 women with confirmed endometriosis treated with 600 mg/day orally for 6 months *6600*

Plasminogen *Plasma Increase Physiological* Approximately 60% increase in 7 women with endometriosis treated with 600 mg daily for 8 weeks *3434* Significant effect in 21 hemophiliacs given drug for 2 weeks *4339*

Platelet-associated IgG *Serum No Effect Physiological* No significant effect observed on increased concentration observed in 22 patients with myelodysplastic syndrome when treated with 600 - 800 mg/d for 3 - 12 months *5764*

Platelets *Blood Decrease Physiological* Thrombocytopenia has been reported in patients receiving danazol *5251*
Blood Increase Physiological In 22 patients with myelodysplasia treatment with oral danazol 600-800 mg/d for 3-12 months caused significant increase *5764* Probable increase observed in one patient with cyclic thrombocytopenia although possibly due to spontaneous remission. Following 2 months treatment platelet counts at nadirs were considerably higher than previously *5005* In 16 patients with SLE and corticosteroid refractory autoimmune throbocytopenia treatent with up to 1200 mg/d caused increase to above 100,000 /µL within 2 months of starting treatment *943* Probable increase observed in one patient with cyclic thrombocytopenia although possibly due to spontaneous remission. Following 2 months treatment platelet counts at nadirs were considerably higher than previously *5005* In 5 patients with paroxysmal nocturnal hemoglobinuria unresponsive to other therapies treatment with 400 - 800 mg/d caused changes from 340 to 414, 61 to 100, 18 to 133, 60 to 274 and 267 to 476 x 1000 /µL in the different patients *2475*

Potassium *Serum Increase Physiological* Slight effect in 18 women with endometriosis given 600 mg/d for 6 mo *892*

Prealbumin *Serum Increase Physiological* Approximately 52% increase in 7 women with endometriosis over 8 weeks when treated with 600 mg daily *3434*

Pregnancy Zone Protein *Serum Decrease Physiological* 70% reduction over 8 weeks in 7 women with endometriosis treated with 600 mg daily *3434*

Progesterone *Plasma Decrease Physiological* Often to nondetectable level in 62 patients with endometriosis treated with 600 mg daily for up to 24 weeks *5410* Mean concentration reduced in women with endometriosis following administration of 800 mg/day *6093*
Plasma No Effect Analytical Danazol at a concentration of up to 1000 ng/mL had a cross-reactivity of less than 0.01% in progesterone method on Bayer Technicon Immuno 1® *429*

Prolactin *Plasma Increase Physiological* Effect noted in 6 orchidectomized patients with prostatic cancer *1088*
Plasma No Effect Physiological In patients with endometriosis treatment with danazol had no effect on mean plasma concentration *4497*

Prolactin response to Insulin
Plasma No Effect Physiological In patients with endometriosis treatment with danazol caused no significant ly different effect compared with healthy controls *4497*

Prolactin response to TRH *Plasma No Effect Physiological* In patients with endometriosis treatment with danazol had no significant effect on mean concentration compared with controls *4497*

Prothrombin *Plasma Increase Physiological* Approximately 67% increase in 7 women with endometriosis treated with 600 mg daily for 8 weeks *3434*

Prothrombin Time *Plasma Increase Physiological* May prolong prothrombin time in patients receiving warfarin *5251*

Reticulocytes *Blood Decrease Physiological* In 5 patients with paroxysmal nocturnal hemoglobinuria unresponsive to other therapies treatment with 400 - 800 mg/d caused changes from 15 to 20%, 10 to 12%, 6.1 to 3.5%, 4.5 to 5.7% and 8 to 6% in the different patients *2475*
Blood Increase Physiological In 5 patients with paroxysmal nocturnal hemoglobinuria unresponsive to other therapies treatment with 400 - 800 mg/d caused changes from 15 to 20%, 10 to 12%, 6.1 to 3.5%, 4.5 to 5.7% and 8 to 6% in the different patients *2475*

Danazol *(continued)*

Sex-Hormone Binding Globulin
Serum Decrease Physiological In 6 women with endometriosis treatment with 600 mg daily for 6 months caused reduction from mean of 69.7 nmol/L to 8.4 nmol/L with reduction to 8.1 nmol/L apparent at 3 months *6157* Reduced up to 5 fold in 5 patients with hereditary angioneurotic edema treated for up to 10 mo *5406* Reduction of 80% in 9 nondiabetic women within 6 weeks of starting treatment for pelvic endometriosis *6215* When used for treatment of endometriosis can cause increase of up to 20% *2836* Marked reduction in women over 3 mo *6574* Reduction from mean of 65 nmol/L to 9 nmol/L on 6 nonobese women with minmal endometriosis treated with 400 mg daily for 6 weeks *2233* Reduction of binding capacity by 80% during treatment of women with endometriosis *4297* 90% reduction over 8 weeks in 7 women with endometriosis treated with 600 mg daily *3434*

Sodium *Serum No Effect Physiological* No change in 18 women with endometriosis given 600 mg/d for 6 mo *892*

Tacrolimus *Serum Increase Physiological* By inhibiting cytochrome P-450 IIIA enzyme systems may inhibit the metabolism of tacrolimus *1987*

Testosterone *Serum Decrease Analytical* Concentrations low: in case of cortisol and testosterone displacement from plasma proteins occurs and protein binding assays are probably invalid *2435*
Serum Decrease Physiological Marked reduction in some patients in 5 patients with hereditary angioneurotic edema treated for up to 10 mo *5406* Affect binding in women treated with drug so that proportion of free drug high *2435* Throughout treatment period after 600 mg daily in 18 women with endometriosis *892*
Serum Increase Analytical Nonspecificity in RIA kits produced by Diagnostic Products Corporation, Farmos Diagnostica and Bio-RIA *5477* May interfere with some analytical methods *5251* Probably invalid results because of high cross-reactivity with protein in competitive binding assays *2435* May be cross-reactivity in certain radioimmunoassays *1088*
Serum Increase Physiological Increase by 70% in 7 normal subjects given drug 800 mg daily for 2 mo *3674*
Serum No Effect Analytical No detectable cross-reactivity observed with in testosterone method on Bayer Technicon Immuno 1® *433*
Serum No Effect Physiological No effect observed on total concentration in 9 nondiabetic women with pelvic endometriosis within 6 weeks of starting treatment *6215* No significant change observed in 6 nonobese women with minimal endometriosis treated with 400 mg daily for 6 weeks *2233* No change during treatment of women with endometriosis *4297* No consistent change noted in patients with prostatic cancer *1088*

Testosterone, Free *Serum Increase Physiological* Marked rise observed in women with endometriosis. Due to displacement from sex hormone binding globulin *4297* Proportion high due to displacement of hormone from protein *2435* Causes displacement of hormone from SHBG and may result in increase of up to 90% *2836*

Testosterone Index, Free *Serum Increase Physiological* Increase from mean of 3.3 to 13.3 in 6 nonobese women with minimal endometriosis treated with 400 mg daily for 6 weeks *2233*

Thyroid Stimulating Hormone
Serum Decrease Physiological Not initially, but after 4 weeks in 12 healthy female post-menopausal volunteers given up to 800 mg daily *1642*
Serum No Effect Physiological No effect after 2 weeks with 800 mg/d but slight decrease after 4 weeks *1642*

Thyroxine Binding Globulin
Serum Decrease Physiological Approximately halved in 5 patients with hereditary angioneurotic edema treated for up to 10 mo *5406* In healthy postmenopausal women after 2 weeks treatment with 400 to 800 mg daily through direct effect on thyroxine binding globulin production at cellular level *1642* 60% reduction in 7 women with endometriosis treated with 600 mg daily for 8 weeks *3434* Mean fall of 19% in 10 people due to competition for binding sites or androgen-like effect *4498*

Thyroxine (T4) *Serum Decrease Analytical* Concentrations low: in case of cortisol and testosterone displacement from plasma proteins occurs and protein binding assays are probably invalid *2435*
Serum Decrease Physiological In healthy postmenopausal women after 2 weeks treatment with 400 to 800 mg daily through direct effect on thyroxine binding globulin production at cellular level *1642* Fell by 26% in 9 individuals due to competition for binding sites or androgen-like effect *4498* Affect binding in women treated with drug so that proportion of free drug high *2435*

Thyroxine (T4), Free *Serum Increase Physiological* Slight effect after 4 weeks in 12 healthy female post-menopausal volunteers *1642* Proportion high due to displacement of hormone from protein *2435*
Serum No Effect Physiological No effect after 2 weeks with 800 mg/d but slight increase after 4 weeks *1642*

Thyroxine (T4) Index, Free *Serum No Effect Physiological* No consistent change due to competition for binding sites or androgen-like effect *4498*

Transferrin *Serum Increase Physiological* 55% increase in 7 women with endometriosis treated with 600 mg daily for 8 weeks *3434*

Tri-iodothyronine (T3) *Serum Decrease Physiological* In 12 healthy postmenopausal women after 2 weeks treatment with 400 to 800 mg daily through direct effect on thyroxine binding globulin production at cellular level *1642*

Triglycerides *Serum Decrease Physiological* Reduction of 33% in 6 women with endometriosis treated for 1 month with 600 mg daily. Effect persisted with prolonged treatment and for 3 months after treatment stopped *6157*
Serum Increase Physiological In 12 women with pelvic endometriosis mean concentration increased by 20% after treatment with 600 mg/d for 2 weeks. Eight weeks after cessation of 24 weeks treatment concentration had reverted to baseline *1782* During clinical trials of patients who had triglycerides concentrations measured 7% demonstrated increased concentration after treatment *2070*
Serum No Effect Physiological No effect after 6 mo of 600 mg/d *6574* No significant effect in 9 women with endometriosis treated for 6 mo *108* Inconsistent changes observed in 62 patients with endometriosis treated with 600 mg daily for up to 24 weeks *5410*

VLDL-Cholesterol *Serum No Effect Physiological* Non-significant reduction observed in 6 women with endometriosis treated with 600 mg daily for 6 months *6157*

VLDL-Phospholipids *Serum No Effect Physiological* Non-significant reduction observed in 6 women with endometriosis treated with 600 mg daily for 6 months *6157*

VLDL-Triglycerides *Serum Decrease Physiological* Concentration fell in parallel with total triglyceride concentration in 6 women with endometriosis treated with 600 mg daily *6157*

Dantrolene

Alanine Aminotransferase *Serum Increase Physiological* In 1.8% of 1044 patients, hepatocellular damage with acute or subacute hepatic disease or chronic active hepatitis *6140* Increase observed temporarily in about 10% treated patients regardless of dose *1384* Dantrolene hepatotoxicity may occur *4797* Chronic active hepatitis reported in a few patients *3725*

Albumin *Serum Decrease Physiological* Single observation, ?significance *1017*

Aldolase *Serum No Effect Physiological* No significant effect observed in patients with Duchenne muscular dystrophy *529*

Alkaline Phosphatase *Serum Increase Physiological* Dantrolene hepatotoxicity may occur *4797* Acute hepatitis as result of drug ingestion in 4 patients returned to normal after drug stopped *6462* In 1.8% of 1044 patients, hepatocellular damage with acute or subacute hepatic disease or chronic active hepatitis *6140* Observed effect, cause uncertain *1017*

Aspartate Aminotransferase *Serum Increase Physiological* Chronic active hepatitis reported in a few patients *3725* Observed effect, cause uncertain *1017* In 1.8% of 1044 patients, hepatocellular damage with acute or subacute hepatic disease or chronic active hepatitis *6140* Increase observed in about 10% treated patients regardless of dose *1384* Dantrolene hepatotoxicity may occur *4797* Acute hepatitis as result of drug ingestion in 4 patients returned to normal after drug stopped *6462*

Bilirubin *Serum Increase Physiological* Acute hepatitis as result of drug ingestion in 4 patients returned to normal after drug stopped *6462* In 1.8% of 1044 patients, hepatocellular damage with acute or subacute hepatic disease or chronic active hepatitis *6140* Dantrolene hepatotoxicity may occur *4797* Isolated observation in one individual *1017*

Cholesterol *Serum Increase Physiological* Isolated observation in one individual *1017*

Creatine Kinase *Serum Decrease Physiological* Significant reduction observed in patients with Duchenne muscular dystrophy *529*
Serum Increase Physiological Isolated observation, uncertain relevance *1017*

Crystals *Urine Increase Physiological* Crystalluria may occur as a toxic side effect *4797*

Eosinophils *Blood Increase Physiological* Isolated instance reported *1017*

γ-Glutamyltransferase *Serum Increase Physiological* Dantrolene hepatotoxicity may occur *4797*

Hematocrit *Blood Decrease Physiological* Aplastic anemia may occur as a toxic side effect *4797* Rare effect of no consequence *1017*

Hemoglobin *Blood Decrease Physiological* Aplastic anemia may occur as a toxic side effect *4797* Rare effect of no consequence *1017*

Leukocytes *Blood Decrease Physiological* Leukopenia may occur as a toxic side effect *4797*
Urine Increase Physiological Possible effect, perhaps urinary infection *1017*

Occult Blood *Feces Increase Physiological* Gastrointestinal bledding has been reported as a side effect *4797*

Protein *Serum Decrease Physiological* Single observation, ?significance *1017*
Urine Increase Physiological Possible effect, perhaps urinary infection *1017*

Prothrombin Time *Plasma Increase Physiological* Acute hepatitis as result of drug ingestion in 4 patients returned to normal after drug stopped *6462*

Uric Acid *Serum Increase Physiological* Isolated observation in one individual *1017*

Dapsone

Alanine Aminotransferase *Serum Increase Physiological* Sulfone syndrome in one 16 year old girl given 50 mg daily short-term administration *6049* Toxic hepatitis and cholestatic jaundice have been reported early in therapy. Hyperbilirubinemia may occur more often in G6PD deficient patients *2873*

Albumin *Serum Decrease Physiological* To below 2.0 g/dL in one woman with dermatitis herpetiformis: possibly associated with increased intravascular catabolism of albumin *1149* Significant effect after 32 mo treatment in 1 woman with dermatitis herpetiformis *1924* Sulfone syndrome in one 16 year old girl given 50 mg daily short-term administration *6049* In 2 patients given long-term treatment *3143*

Alkaline Phosphatase *Serum Increase Physiological* In 3 individuals treated for 3 to 36 weeks *5835* Sulfone syndrome in one 16 year old girl given 50 mg daily short-term administration *6049* Toxic hepatitis and cholestatic jaundice have been reported early in therapy. Hyperbilirubinemia may occur more often in G6PD deficient patients *2873* Associated with hemolytic anemia when occurs as main side effect *5763*

Aspartate Aminotransferase *Serum Increase Physiological* Sulfone syndrome in one 16 year old girl given 50 mg daily short-term administration *6049* Toxic hepatitis and cholestatic jaundice have been reported early in therapy. Hyperbilirubinemia may occur more often in G6PD deficient patients *2873* Components of typical sulfone or dapsone syndrome *3301*

Bilirubin *Serum Increase Physiological* Sulfone syndrome in one 16 year old girl given 50 mg daily short-term administration *6049* Toxic hepatitis and cholestatic jaundice have been reported early in therapy. Hyperbilirubinemia may occur more often in G6PD deficient patients *2873* In 3 individuals treated for 3 to 36 weeks *5835* Associated with hemolytic anemia when occurs as main side effect *5763*
Urine Increase Physiological Associated with hemolytic anemia in sulfone syndrome *6049*

Bilirubin, Direct *Serum Increase Physiological* Sulfone syndrome in one 16 year old girl given 50 mg daily short-term administration *6049*

Chloride *Serum Decrease Physiological* Sulfone syndrome in one 16 year old girl given 50 mg daily short-term administration *6049*

Cholesterol *Serum Increase Physiological* In 3 individuals treated for 3 to 36 weeks *5835*

Eosinophils *Blood Increase Physiological* Components of typical sulfone or dapsone syndrome *3301* Observed in 66% (2 of 3 patients) treated with drug who had rheumatoid arthritis *5617*

Erythrocyte Lifespan *Blood Decrease Physiological* Almost all treated patients, regardless of whether they are G6PD deficient or not, show a loss of 1 - 2 g/dL hemoglobin and an interrelated 2 - 12% increase in reticulocyte count and shortened erythrocyte life span and an increase in methemoglobin concentration *2873*

Erythrocytes *Blood Decrease Physiological* May cause hemolytic anemia *2629*

Haptoglobin *Serum Decrease Physiological* Associated with hemolytic anemia when occurs as main side effect *5763*

Heinz Body Formation *Blood Positive Physiological* Early stage of hemolytic anemia *536* Hemolysis and Heinz body formation may be exaggerated in individuals with a glucose-6-phosphate dehydrogenase deficiency or methemoglobin reductase deficiency, or hemoglobin M, often dose-related response *2873*

Hematocrit *Blood Decrease Physiological* Hemolysis (hemolytic anemia) *2629*

Hemoglobin *Blood Decrease Physiological* Hemolysis and Heinz body formation may be exaggerated in individuals with a glucose-6-phosphate dehydrogenase deficiency or methemoglobin reductase deficiency, or hemoglobin M, often dose-related response. Almost all patients show a loss of 1 - 2 g/dL hemoglobin *2873* Associated with hemolytic anemia when occurs as main side effect *5763* May cause hemolytic anemia *2629* Anemia developed in 61% of 51 patients with leprosy *3953*

Lactate Dehydrogenase *Serum Increase Physiological* Sulfone syndrome in one 16 year old girl given 50 mg daily short-term administration *6049* Associated with hemolytic anemia when occurs as main side effect *5763* In 3 individuals treated for 3 to 36 weeks *5835*

Leukocytes *Blood Decrease Physiological* After 7-9 weeks of treatment with drug plus pyrimethamine in 7 patients taking drug as prophylaxis against malaria *1970* Agranulocytosis *2629*

Methemoglobin *Blood Increase Physiological* May cause hemolytic anemia *2629* Almost all treated patients, regardless of whether they are G6PD deficient or not, show a loss of 1 - 2 g/dL hemoglobin and an interrelated 2 - 12% increase in reticulocyte count and shortened erythrocyte life span and an increase in methemoglobin concentration *2873*

Neutrophils *Blood Decrease Physiological* Isolated case of agranulocytoisis reported *1872* After 7-9 weeks of treatment with drug plus pyrimethamine in 7 patients taking drug as prophylaxis against malaria *1970* Occasional case of agranulocytosis reported *6264*

Osmotic Fragility *Red Blood Cells Increase Physiological* In 20 of 51 patients with leprosy, most of whom were receiving 51 to 100 mg drug daily *3953*

Platelets *Blood No Effect Physiological* After 7-9 weeks of treatment with drug plus pyrimethamine in 7 patients taking drug as prophylaxis against malaria *1970*

Protein *Serum Decrease Physiological* Sulfone syndrome in one 16 year old girl given 50 mg daily short-term administration *6049*

Reticulocytes *Blood Increase Physiological* Almost all treated patients, regardless of whether they are G6PD deficient or not, show a loss of 1 - 2 g/dL hemoglobin and a 2 - 12% increase in reticulocyte count *2873*

Sodium *Serum Decrease Physiological* To 117 mmol/L in one woman with dermatitis herpetiformis: possibly associated

Dapsone *(continued)*

Sodium *(continued)*
increased intravascular catabolism of albumin *1149* Sulfone syndrome in one 16 year old girl given 50 mg daily short-term administration *6049*

Trimethoprim *Serum Decrease Physiological* Decreased metabolism and increased risk of marrow toxicity *886*
Serum Increase Physiological Increased concentration observed in patients with AIDS when drugs coadministered *1384* When coadministered with dapsone (100 mg/d) trimethoprim (3 mg/kg/q6 h) on day 7 dapsone concentration averaged 2.1 ± 1.0 µg/mL compared with 1.5 ± 0.5 µg/mL when dapsone given alone and trimethoprim concentration averaged 18.4 ± 5.2 µg/mL compared with 12.4 ± 4.5 µg/mL when given alone *2873*

Urobilinogen *Urine Increase Physiological* Associated with hemolytic anemia when occurs as main side effect *5763*

Daunorubicin

Chromosomes *Test Conditions Abnormal Physiological* Clastogenic in human cells *5484*

Color *Urine Increase Analytical* Red color observed following ingestion of daunorubacin *3388*

Erythropoietin *Serum Increase Physiological* Observed in 6 patients with acute leukemia in response to first treatment with daunorubicin when combined with different chemotherapeutic agents including ARA-C and vincristine with subsequent reduction to below initial value *4712*

Hemoglobin *Blood No Effect Physiological* Although inappropriate increase in erythropoietin concentration in 6 leukemics treated with daunorubicin and other chemotherapeutic agents no effect on blood hemoglobin noted *4712*

Debrisoquin

Homovanillic Acid *Plasma Decrease Physiological* In 5 healthy volunteers administration of 10 mg caused significant reduction from mean baseline of 8.5 ng/mL to 5.3 ng/mL after 6 hours *5091*

Vanillylmandelic Acid *Urine Decrease Physiological* Mechanism not discussed *199*

Decaborane

Catecholamines *Urine Decrease Physiological* Markedly decreases output *6277*

Deferiprone

Alanine Aminotransferase *Serum Increase Physiological* In 44% of 84 treated patients transient liver enzyme abnormalities observed *4409*

Alkaline Phosphatase *Serum Increase Physiological* In 44% of 84 treated patients transient liver enzyme abnormalities observed *4409*

Anti-DNA Antibodies *Serum No Effect Physiological* No significant effect observed in one study over several years *4409*

Anti-Histone Antibodies *Serum No Effect Physiological* No significant effect observed in one study over several years *4409*

Antinuclear Antibodies *Serum No Effect Physiological* No significant effect observed in one study over several years *4409*

Aspartate Aminotransferase *Serum Increase Physiological* In 44% of 84 treated patients transient liver enzyme abnormalities observed *4409*

Ferritin *Serum Decrease Physiological* In 29 patients with thalassemia treatment with 70 mg/kg/d for a mean of 21.8 months caused significant reduction in concentration from mean baseline of 3748 ng/mL to 2550 ng/mL *3861* In two studies sustained decreased ferritin concentration during 12 - 22 months treatment *4409*
Serum No Effect Physiological In two early studies no reports of sustained decreased ferritin concentration during 1 - 15 months treatment *4409*

Granulocytes *Blood Decrease Physiological* Agranulocytosis observed as toxic effect in patients as early as 6 weeks and up to 21 months after instigation of treatment *4409*

Iron *Liver Increase Physiological* In 29 patients with thalassemia treatment with 70 mg/kg/d for a mean of 21.8 months caused significant change in concentration from mean baseline of 16.09 mg/g to 20.99 mg/g *3861*
Urine Increase Physiological Effective in patients with thalassemia in removing iron *4409* In 29 patients with thalassemia treatment with 70 mg/kg/d for a mean of 21.8 months caused significant change in concentration from mean baseline of 17.25 mg/dL to 20.98 mg/dL *3861*

Neutrophils *Blood Decrease Physiological* Neutropenia observed as toxic effect in 8 treated patients *4409*

Non-transferrin-bound Iron *Serum Decrease Physiological* Mean non-transferrin-bound iron concentration measured 12 hours after administration of deferiprone significantly less than at the start of therapy *4409*

Rheumatoid Factor *Serum No Effect Physiological* No significant effect observed in one study over several years *4409*

Transferrin Saturation *Serum Decrease Physiological* Lowest saturation in 16 patients with iron overload decreased to 54.5 ± 17.2% occurring 72.5 ± 50.0 minutes after deferiprone administration compared with baseline saturation of 16.4 ± 3.0% in 10 normal volunteers *121*

Zinc *Serum Decrease Physiological* 14% incidence of zinc deficiency observed in treated patients *4409*

Deferoxamine

Alkaline Phosphatase *Serum Decrease Physiological* In a 59-year old woman with impaired renal function, severe osteomalacia and aluminum intoxication infusions of desferrioxamine caused slight decrease from initial activity of 1700 U/L *1264*

Aluminum *Serum Decrease Physiological* Significant reduction observed in patients with aluminum-associated encephalopathy especially during hemodialysis during which part of the deferoxamine-aluminum complex is removed in the dialysate *1384*
Serum Increase Physiological In one 59-year old woman with impaired renal function, severe osteomalacia and aluminum intoxication infusion of 2 g desferrioxamine caused plasma aluminum concentration to increase to 730 µg/L (27.0 µmol/L) 24 hours later from preinfusion concentration of 160 µg/L (5.9 µmol/L) *1264*
Urine Increase Physiological In one 59-year old women with impaired renal function, severe osteomalacia and aluminum intoxication a single infusion of 2 g desferrioxamine caused excretion to increase from 312 - 531 µg/d to 652 µg/d (24.4 µmol/d) *1264*

Color *Urine Increase Analytical* Forms iron chelate with reddish color *2451*

C-Peptide *Plasma Increase Physiological* In 9 patients with NIDDM treatment with 10 mg/kg intravenously for a minimum of 6 weeks caused significant increase from mean of 0.74 ± 0.12 nmol/L to 1.13 ± 0.18 nmol/L *4888*

Ferritin *Serum Decrease Physiological* In 9 patients with NIDDM and increased serum ferritin concentration treatment with 10 mg/kg intravenously twice weekly for a minimum of 6 weeks caused significant reduction from mean of 478 ± 65 µg/L to 313 ± 54 µg/L *4888*

Glucose *Serum No Effect Physiological* In 9 patients with NIDDM treatment with 10 mg/kg intravenously twice per week for a minimum of 6 weeks caused nonsignificant change from mean of 11.6 ± 1.2 mmol/L to 11.3 ± 1.5 mmol/L *4888*

Hemoglobin A_{1c} *Blood Decrease Physiological* In 9 patients with NIDDM treatment with 10 mg/kg intravenously twice weekly for a minimum of 6 weeks caused significant reduction from mean of 9.3 ± 0.7% to 8.8 ± 0.7% *4888*

Insulin *Plasma Increase Physiological* In 5 patients with NIDDM treatment with 10 mg/kg intravenously twice weekly for a minimum of 6 weeks caused a nonsignificant increase of fasting concentration from 125 pmol/L to 175 ± 73 pmol/L *4888*

Iron *Serum Decrease Analytical* Because it chelates iron makes iron unavailable to react with most chromogens thereby

giving falsely low iron concentration *1384* At concentrations above 140 mg/L lowered concentration as measured by Ferrozine method *5704*
Serum Decrease Physiological Chelates iron and reduces serum concentration *1384* Therapeutic intent *5323*
Serum No Effect Analytical No effect on method on Du Pont aca when thioglycolic acid added to test packs with both normal and toxic iron concentrations measured in presence of chelating agent at a concentration of 130 mg/L *6435*
Urine Increase Physiological Deferoxamine can promote iron excretion in patients with secondary iron overload *1027* In healthy individuals urinary excretion is less than 1 µmol/d but increased up to 10-fold following deferoxamine administration *5510* Primary affinity for trivalent iron *128*

Osteocalcin *Serum Increase Physiological* In one 59-year old woman with impaired renal function, severe osteomalacia and aluminum intoxication concentration 1 month after starting 1,25-dihydroxyvitamin D_3 mean concentration of 72 ng/mL (12.6 nmol/L) but increased to 456 ng/mL (81.4 nmol/L) after 3 infusions of 0.5 g desferrioxamine and rose to 580 ng/mL (101.5 nmol/L) after several additional infusions. Three weeks after cessation of desferrioxamine concentration fell to 130 ng/mL (12.0 nmol/L) *1264*

Procollagen I Peptide *Urine No Effect Physiological* In one 59-year old woman with impaired renal function, severe osteomalacia and aluminum intoxication a series of infusions of desferrioxamine had little effect on initial concentration of 254 ng/mL *1264*

Deferoxamine B

Aluminum *Urine Increase Physiological* Administration of 2 g to a man with bizarre neuropsychiatric symptoms caused increase from baseline of 20.0 ± 1.0 µg/L to 32 µg/48 h after administration of drug *5078*

Calcium *Urine No Effect Physiological* In one man with bizarre psychiatric neuropsychiatric symptoms administration of 2 g caused no significant change over 48 h from predrug excretion of 504 ± 10 mg/L *5078*

Iron *Urine Increase Physiological* In one man with bizarre neuropsychiatric symptoms administration of 2 g caused increase from baseline of 6.2 ± 3.0 µg/L to 1765 µg/48 h after drug *5078*

Lead *Red Blood Cells No Effect Physiological* In one man with bizarre neuropsychiatric symptoms administration of 2 g caused insignificant change from 188 ± 8 µg/L to 189 ± 5 µg/L *5078*
Urine Increase Physiological In one man with bizarre neuropsychiatric symptoms administration of 2 g caused significant increase from 3.1 ± 0.3 µg/L to remove 52 µg lead over 48 h *5078*

Magnesium *Urine No Effect Physiological* Administration of 2 g to a man with bizarre neuropsychiatric symptoms caused no significant change from predrug excretion of 114 ± 12 mg/L *5078*

Defibrotide

Fibrinogen *Plasma No Effect Physiological* In 22 patients treated with 800 mg/d mean concentration changed insignificantly from 270 ± 43.4 mg/dL to 271 ± 55.9 mg/dL after 30 days *6269*

6-Keto-Prostaglandin $F_{1\alpha}$ *Plasma Increase Physiological* Marked and prolonged elevation with infusion of 1200 mg *1068*

Partial Thromboplastin Time
Plasma No Effect Physiological In 22 patients treated with 800 mg/d APTT ratio changed insignificantly from mean of 0.99 ± 0.09 to 1.03 ± 0.07 after 30 days treatment *6269*

Plasminogen Activator Antigen-1 Antigen
Plasma Decrease Physiological In 22 patients treated with 800 mg/d for 30 days mean concentration decreased from 17 ng/mL to 11 ng/mL *6269*

Plasminogen Activator Inhibitor-1 Activity
Plasma Decrease Physiological In 22 patients treated with 800 mg/d for 30 days mean activity decreased significantly from 22 U/mL to 12 U/mL *6269*

Prothrombin Time *Plasma No Effect Physiological* In 22 patients treated with 800 mg/d INR changed insignificantly from 1.07 ± 0.1 to 1.03 ± 0.07 after 30 days treatment *6269*

Tissue Plasminogen Activator
Plasma Increase Physiological In 22 patients treatment with 800 mg/d for 30 days caused significant increase of activity before stasis from mean of 2.18 ± 1.0 U/mL to 3.38 ± 1.77 U/mL and of activity after stasis from 8.81 ± 4.99 U/mL to 14.3 ± 6.62 U/mL *6269*

Tissue Plasminogen Activator Antigen
Plasma No Effect Physiological In 22 patients treated with 800 mg/d for 30 days nonsignificant increase in TPA antigen concentration before stasis from 4.5 ± 2.52 ng/mL to 4.62 ± 2.73 ng/mL and from 14.0 ± 8.39 ng/mL to 14.7 ± 8.4 ng/mL after stasis *6269*

Uric Acid *Serum Increase Physiological* Slight but significant increase following i.v. infusion of 1200 mg *1068*

Deflazacort

Adenosine Monophosphate *Urine No Effect Physiological* In 7 patients who needed high-dose corticosteroid therapy concentration changed nonsignificantly from mean baseline of 464 ± 79 nmol/mmol creatinine to 471 ± 45 nmol/mmol creatinine after 15 days treatment with 34.3 mg/d *3625*

Alkaline Phosphatase *Serum Decrease Physiological* In 7 patients who needed high-dose corticosteroid therapy concentration changed significantly from mean baseline of 89.2 ± 37 U/L to 71.8 ± 28 U/L after 15 days treatment with 34.3 mg/d *3625*

Calcium *Serum No Effect Physiological* In 7 patients who needed high-dose corticosteroid therapy concentration changed nonsignificantly from mean baseline of 2.42 ± 0.07 mmol/L to 2.34 ± 0.08 mmol/L after 15 days treatment with 34.3 mg/d *3625*
Urine No Effect Physiological In 7 patients who needed high-dose corticosteroid therapy concentration changed nonsignificantly from mean baseline of 0.33 ± 0.16 mmol/mmol creatinine to 0.33 ± 0.16 mmol/mmol creatinine after 15 days treatment with 34.3 mg/d *3625*

Glucose *Serum No Effect Physiological* No modification of basal concentration observed in 6 healthy volunteers after short-term administration *4477*

Glucose Tolerance *Serum Decrease Physiological* Increased peak glucose, C-peptide and insulin concentrations in 6 healthy volunteers although to lesser extent than when following short term betamethasone *4477*

Hydroxyproline *Urine No Effect Physiological* In 7 patients who needed high-dose corticosteroid therapy concentration changed nonsignificantly from mean baseline of 1.82 ± 0.86 mmol/mmol creatinine to 1.88 ± 1.21 mmol/mmol creatinine after 15 days treatment with 34.3 mg/d *3625*

Parathyroid Hormone *Plasma No Effect Physiological* In 7 patients who needed high-dose corticosteroid therapy concentration changed nonsignificantly from mean baseline of 44.6 ± 17.3 pmol/L to 46.7 ± 17.6 pmol/L after 15 days treatment with 34.3 mg/d *3625*

Phosphate *Serum No Effect Physiological* In 7 patients who needed high-dose corticosteroid therapy concentration changed nonsignificantly from mean baseline of 1.22 ± 0.14 mmol/L to 1.45 ± 0.45 mmol/L after 15 days treatment with 34.3 mg/d *3625*

Dehydrobenzperidole

β-Endorphin *Plasma No Effect Physiological* No reduction of increased values induced by stress when given alone but significant decrease when given with fentanyl also *3408*

Dehydrocholic Acid

BSP Retention *Serum Increase Physiological* Hepatic uptake or biliary excretion impaired *2451*

Hemoglobin *Blood Decrease Physiological* Mild hemolytic action if injected *128*

Dehydrocholic Acid *(continued)*

Volume *Urine Increase Physiological* Mild diuretic action *128*

Dehydroemetine

Aspartate Aminotransferase *Serum Increase Physiological* Possibly due to generalized myositis *4014*

Delalande 69276

Thyroxine (T4) *Serum Increase Analytical* At 37.5 mg/dL with usual methods when added to serum *2877*

Thyroxine (T4) Index, Free *Serum Increase Analytical* At 37.5 mg/dL with usual methods when added to serum *2877*

Delavirdine

Indinavir *Serum Increase Physiological* Causes a 72% increase in area under the concentration curve when delavirdine coadministered *1891*

Ritonavir *Serum Increase Physiological* Increases area under the concentration curve by 2% when delavirdine coadministered *1891*

Saquinavir *Serum Increase Physiological* The area under the concentration curve increased by 520% when delavirdine coadministered *1891*

Demecarium

Cholinesterase *Serum Decrease Physiological* Therapeutic intent *128*

Demeclocycline

Alanine Aminotransferase *Serum Increase Physiological* Increased liver enzyme activity and hepatic toxicity have been reported as rare side effects *3463*

Alkaline Phosphatase *Serum Increase Physiological* Increased liver enzyme activity and hepatic toxicity have been reported as rare side effects *3463*

Amylase *Serum Increase Physiological* Pancreatitis reported as a rare side effect *3463*

Aspartate Aminotransferase *Serum Increase Physiological* Increased liver enzyme activity and hepatic toxicity have been reported as rare side effects *3463*

Catecholamines *Urine Increase Analytical* Produces interfering fluorescence with analysis *3192*

Chloramphenicol *Serum No Effect Analytical* No effect at 100 mg/L on coupled enzymatic method *4122*

Creatinine *Serum Increase Physiological* Dose related nephrotoxicity *3463*

Serum No Effect Analytical No effect of concentrations up to 15 mg/L on single slide method on Kodak Ektachem® *5706*

Eosinophils *Blood Increase Physiological* Eosinophilia has been reported as a rare side effect *3463* Rare, but reported to occur *2754*

Erythrocytes *Blood Decrease Physiological* Rare, but reported to occur *2754*

Hematocrit *Blood Decrease Physiological* Hemolytic anemia has been reported as a rare side effect *3463*

Hemoglobin *Blood Decrease Physiological* Hemolytic anemia has been reported as a rare side effect *3463*

^{131}I Uptake *Serum Decrease Physiological* Declomycin® contains tetraiodofluorescein *4360*

LE Cells *Blood Positive Physiological* Rare exacerbation may occur *2754*

Lipase *Serum Increase Physiological* Pancreatitis reported as a rare side effect *3463*

Neutrophils *Blood Decrease Physiological* Neutropenia has been reported as a rare side effect *3463* Rare, but reported to occur *2754*

Osmolality *Urine Decrease Physiological* Maximum osmolality in response to dehydration *5574*

Phenylalanine *Plasma No Effect Analytical* No interference observed with rapid quantitative whole blood method of Campbell et al using phenylalanine dehydrogenase *867*

Platelets *Blood Decrease Physiological* Thrombocytopenia has been reported as a rare side effect *3463* Rare, but reported to occur *2754*

Protein *Urine Increase Physiological* Nephrotoxic effect *3463*

Prothrombin Time *Plasma Decrease Physiological* Reported to depress prothrombin time so dose of anticoagulants may need to be reduced *3463*

Plasma Increase Physiological Depresses plasma prothrombin activity *2754*

Sperm Count *Semen Decrease Physiological* Potent antispermatogenic action observed *4726*

Urea Nitrogen *Serum Increase Physiological* Dose related nephrotoxicity *3463*

Volume *Urine Increase Physiological* Rare induction of reversible nephrogenic diabetes *2754* Reversible nephrogenic diabetes insipidus may occur *5574*

Demoxepam

Benzodiazepine *Urine Positive Analytical* Positive result observed at a concentration of 2.0 µg/mL (7.00 µmol/L) with method on Du Pont aca *1556* Detectable limit 0.7 µg/mL with improved assay with Syva ETS system compared with 1.0 µg/mL of former d.a.u. assay *3370*

Deoxyglucose

Glucose *Serum Decrease Analytical* At 4.0 mmol/L if hexokinase from Leuconostoc Mesent *649*

2-Deoxyglucose

Glucose *Serum No Effect Analytical* No effect at 2.5 mmol/L on glucokinase based assay of Scott *5414*

Deoxypyridoxine

3-Hydroxyanthranilic Acid *Urine Increase Physiological* After 2 g tryptophan load *5089*

3-Hydroxykynurenine *Urine Increase Physiological* After 2 g tryptophan load *3340*

Quinolinic Acid *Urine Increase Physiological* After 2 g tryptophan load *5089*

Xanthurenic Acid *Urine Increase Physiological* After 2 g tryptophan load *5089*

Desalkylflurazepam

Benzodiazepine *Urine Positive Analytical* Positive result observed at a concentration of 2.0 µg/mL (6.92 µmol/L) with method on Du Pont aca *1556*

Deserpidine

Platelets *Blood Decrease Physiological* Possible effect as related compounds cause this *2754*

Desiccated Thyroid

Thyroxine (T4) *Serum Increase Physiological* Increases by 1-2 µg/dL/d per grain given *572*

Desipramine

Alanine Aminotransferase *Serum Increase Physiological* Rare transient cholestasis *3810* Hepatitis, jaundice (simulating obstructive), altered liver function may occur as complications of treatment *2650*
Serum No Effect Physiological In 42 children or adolescents treated for up to 24 mo *2662*

Albumin *Serum No Effect Analytical* At concentration of 8 mg/L had no effect on BCG method *5704*

Alkaline Phosphatase *Serum Increase Physiological* Hepatitis, jaundice (simulating obstructive), altered liver function may occur as complications of treatment *2650* Transient cholestasis (rare) *3810* Significant effect in 46 patients but values did not rise above reference range *4785*
Serum No Effect Physiological In 42 children and adolescents treated for up to 24 mo *2662*

γ-Aminobutyric Acid *Plasma No Effect Physiological* In 5 patients with major depression treatment with doses to maintain plasma desipramine concentration between 115 and 250 ng/mL caused nonsignificant decrease or no change in concentration *4641*

Amylase *Serum Increase Physiological* Increased pancreatic enzyme activity may occur as a complication of treatment *2650*

Aspartate Aminotransferase *Serum Increase Physiological* Hepatitis, jaundice (simulating obstructive), altered liver function may occur as complications of treatment *2650* Idiosyncratic response observed in 4 of 46 patients *4785* Rare transient cholestasis *3810*
Serum No Effect Physiological Increase observed in 4 of 46 patients but previously increased value decreased in 5 others so probably not dose-dependent toxic effect *4785* In 42 children and adolescents treated for up to 24 mo *2662*

Basophils *Blood Increase Physiological* Mild effect noted in some patients *4014*

Bicarbonate *Serum No Effect Analytical* At concentration of 8 mg/L had no effect on method using phenolphthalein *5704*

Bile *Urine Increase Physiological* Rare transient cholestasis *3810*

Bilirubin *Serum Increase Physiological* Hepatitis, jaundice (simulating obstructive), altered liver function may occur as complications of treatment *2650* Rare transient cholestasis *2451*
Serum No Effect Analytical At concentration of 8 mg/L had no effect on Jendrassik and Grof method *5704*
Serum No Effect Physiological No effect observed in 46 treated patients *4785* In 42 children and adolescents treated for up to 24 mo *2662* Insignificant protein-displacement effect in neonates *6314*

Bilirubin, Direct *Serum Decrease Physiological* Slight effect observed in 46 treated patients *4785*

BSP Retention *Serum Increase Physiological* Rare transient cholestasis *3810*

Butaperazine *Serum Increase Physiological* When large doses of desipramine given to 6 patients concentration of butaperazine increased probably as a result of inhibited metabolism *1727*

Calcium *Serum No Effect Analytical* At concentration of 8 mg/L had no effect on cresolphthalein method *5704*

Carbamazepine *Serum Increase Physiological* In one patient coadministration of both drugs caused increase in plasma concentration of carbamazepine 6 days after desipramine added to therapeutic regime *3118*

Chloride *Serum No Effect Analytical* At concentration of 8 mg/L had no effect on mercurimetric method *5704*

Cholesterol *Serum No Effect Analytical* At concentration of 8 mg/L had no effect on Liebermann-Burchard method *5704*

Cocaethylene *Urine No Effect Analytical* No interference observed with TLC method of Bailey *328*

Cortisol *Plasma No Effect Physiological* In group of depressed patients *846*

Creatinine *Serum No Effect Analytical* At concentration of 8 mg/L had no effect on Technicon AutoAnalyzer® Jaffe method *5704*

Eosinophils *Blood Decrease Physiological* Agranulocytosis *1158*
Blood Increase Physiological Bone marrow depression may occur with agranulocytosis, eosinophilia, thrombocytopenia and purpura *2650* In 4 of 46 patients as manifestation of idiosyncratic response but no value exceeded 10% of total white cell count: uncorrelated with drug plasma concentration *4785* Allergic reaction *6488*

Epinephrine *Plasma No Effect Physiological* Observed with long term, high or low dose, treatment under experimental conditions *5110*

Erythrocytes *Blood Decrease Physiological* Transient agranulocytosis (up to 25% reported) *128*

Fatty Acids (FFA), Free *Serum Increase Physiological* 41% increase following single injection i.m. of 50 mg *2675*

Glucose *Serum Decrease Physiological* Mechanism not understood *2754* Both increased and decreased concentrations may occur as complications of treatment *2650*
Serum Increase Physiological Both increased and decreased concentrations may occur as complications of treatment *2650* Mechanism not understood *2754*

Granulocytes *Blood Decrease Physiological* Bone marrow depression may occur with agranulocytosis, eosinophilia, thrombocytopenia and purpura *2650*

Growth Hormone *Plasma Increase Physiological* Substantial effect in some patients in group of depressed patients *846*

Homovanillic Acid
Cerebrospinal Fluid No Effect Physiological In 43 patients with depression or Alzheimer's disease chronically treated with drug *4965*

5-Hydroxyindoleacetic Acid
Cerebrospinal Fluid Decrease Physiological In 43 patients with depression or Alzheimer's disease chronically treated with drug *4965*

Leukocytes *Blood Decrease Physiological* May cause agranulocytosis *3810*
Blood Increase Physiological Due to eosinophilia of hypersensitivity *3810*

Lipase *Serum Increase Physiological* Increased pancreatic enzyme activity may occur as a complication of treatment *2650*

Luteinizing Hormone *Plasma No Effect Physiological* In group of depressed patients *846*

Lysergic Acid Diethylamide *Urine Increase Analytical* Minimum concentration that caused a positive result with EMIT method to measure LSD 75 mg/L *4968*

Mycophenolic Acid *Serum No Effect Analytical* No significant interference observed with HPLC method of Shipkova et al *5526*

Mycophenolic Acid Glucuronide
Serum No Effect Analytical No significant interference observed with HPLC method of Shipkova et al *5526*

Neutrophils *Blood Decrease Physiological* Occasional case of agranulocytosis reported *6264*

Norepinephrine *Plasma Increase Physiological* Observed with long term, high or low dose, treatment under experimental conditions *5110*

Nortriptyline *Serum Increase Analytical* May cause false positive reaction in EMIT immunoassay for nortriptyline *3590*

p-Aminophenol *Urine No Effect Analytical* With addition of drugs at a concentration of 100 mg/L and of related compounds at 50 mg/L no significant effect observed on colorimetric method of van Bocxlaer on Cobas Mira analyzer which involves reacting free p-aminophenol with resorcinol in the presence of magnesium ions to form an indophenol dye measured at 550 nm *6163*

Phenylbutazone *Serum Decrease Physiological* Inhibits gastrointestinal absorption *2452*

Phosphate *Serum No Effect Analytical* At concentration of 8 mg/L had no effect on phosphomolybdate method *5704*

Platelets *Blood Decrease Physiological* Bone marrow depression may occur with agranulocytosis, eosinophilia, thrombocytopenia and purpura *2650* Immune response after some weeks *2385*

Prolactin *Plasma Increase Physiological* Acute response in group of depressed patients *846*
Plasma No Effect Physiological No significant effect with 50 mg orally *2352*

Protein *Serum No Effect Analytical* At concentration of 8 mg/L had no effect on biuret method with blank correction *5704*

Desipramine *(continued)*

Triglycerides *Serum No Effect Analytical* At concentration of 8 mg/L had no effect on lipase/esterase method *5704*

Urea Nitrogen *Serum No Effect Analytical* At concentration of 8 mg/L had no effect on diacetylmonoxime method *5704*

Uric Acid *Serum No Effect Analytical* At concentration of 8 mg/L had no effect on phosphotungstate reduction method *5704*

Volume *Urine Decrease Physiological* Temporary due to anticholinergic action *2754*

Deslanoside

Albumin *Serum No Effect Analytical* No effect on Technicon SMA 12/60 method at 0.06 mg/dL *4390*

Alkaline Phosphatase *Serum No Effect Analytical* No effect on Technicon SMA 12/60 method at 0.06 mg/dL *4390*

Aspartate Aminotransferase *Serum No Effect Analytical* No effect on Technicon SMA 12/60 method at 0.06 mg/dL *4390*

Bilirubin *Serum No Effect Analytical* No effect on Technicon SMA 12/60 method at 0.06 mg/dL *4390*

Calcium *Serum No Effect Analytical* No effect on Technicon SMA 12/60 method at 0.06 mg/dL *4390*

Cholesterol *Serum No Effect Analytical* No effect on Technicon SMA 12/60 method at 0.06 mg/dL *4390*

Creatinine *Serum No Effect Analytical* No effect on Technicon SMA 12/60 method at 0.06 mg/dL *4390*

Digitoxin *Serum No Effect Analytical* No cross reactivity observed at concentrations up to 0.01 mg/L with method on Baxter Stratus *5705*

Glucose *Serum No Effect Analytical* No effect on Technicon SMA 12/60 method at 0.06 mg/dL *4390*

Lactate Dehydrogenase *Serum No Effect Analytical* No effect on Technicon SMA 12/60 method at 0.06 mg/dL *4390*

Phosphate *Serum No Effect Analytical* No effect on Technicon SMA 12/60 method at 0.06 mg/dL *4390*

Protein *Serum No Effect Analytical* No effect on Technicon SMA 12/60 method at 0.06 mg/dL *4390*

Uric Acid *Serum No Effect Analytical* No effect on Technicon SMA 12/60 method at 0.06 mg/dL *4390*

Desmethylchlorpromazine

Amitriptyline *Serum No Effect Analytical* Cross-reactivity less than 5% with Abbott TDx procedure *2487*

Imipramine *Serum No Effect Analytical* Cross-reactivity less than 5% with Abbott TDx procedure *2473*

Nortriptyline *Serum No Effect Analytical* Cross-reactivity less than 5% with Abbott TDx procedure *2487*

Desmethylquinidine

Quinidine *Serum No Effect Analytical* No significant interference observed with o-desmethylquinidine at a concentration of 0.6 µg/mL (1.94 µmol/L) with method on Du Pont aca *1543*

6-Desmethylquinidine

Quinidine *Serum Increase Analytical* At concentrations of 1.5 mg/L causes 30% increase with method on Baxter Stratus but not ascertained whether this is clinically significant *5705*

Desmethylthioridazine

Amitriptyline *Serum No Effect Analytical* Cross-reactivity less than 5% with Abbott TDx procedure *2487*

Imipramine *Serum No Effect Analytical* Cross-reactivity less than 5% with Abbott TDx procedure *2473*

Nortriptyline *Serum No Effect Analytical* Cross-reactivity less than 5% with Abbott TDx procedure *2487*

Desmopressin

Adenosine Monophosphate *Plasma Increase Physiological* In normal individuals administration causes increase but in 7 males with nephrogenic diabetes no effect observed *546*

α_1-Antitrypsin *Serum No Effect Physiological* In 7 healthy individuals infusion of 0.3 µg/kg concentration decreased non-significantly from mean baseline of 223.9 ± 10.6 mg/dL to 215.1 ± 11.7 mg/dL after 30 min and 218.0 ± 10.9 mg/dL after 120 min. Similar effect observed in uremics *81*

Aquaporin-2 *Urine Increase Physiological* In 5 healthy individuals who received a 20 minute infusion of desmopressin excretion increased from mean baseline of 0.8 ± 0.3 pmol/mg creatinine to 11.2 ± 1.6 pmol/mg creatinine *3029*

Aspartate Aminotransferase *Serum Increase Physiological* Transient increases in activity, but no higher than 1.5 times the upper limit of normal,have been observed but return to normal with continuing treatment *4936*

Bleeding Time *Patient Decrease Physiological* Following intravenous infusion of 0.4 µg/kg in 11 uremic patients observed within 1 hour of infusion *1758* In patients taking 1 g aspirin per day for 5 days administration of 2 doses of DDAVP of 0.3 µg/kg caused reduction of previously prolonged bleeding time to a value within normal range *1893*

Factor VIII *Plasma Increase Physiological* In one patient with von Willebrand's disease treatment with 0.3 µg/kg desmopressin caused increase in factor VIII activity from baseline of 66 U/dL to 305 U/dL *2775* Up to 4-fold increase following i.v. administration and 3.1-fold increase when given s.c *3220*

Factor VIII Coagulant *Plasma Increase Physiological* In normal individuals administration stimulates release but no effect observed in 7 male subjects with nephrogenic diabetes insipidus *546* Statistically significant increase in 11 uremic patients 1 hour after intravenous infusion of 0.4 µg/kg *1758* In 4 healthy volunteers 0.3 µg/kg intravenously alone and with dextran caused increased concentration *1894*

Leukocytes *Blood Increase Physiological* 1.4- to 1.6-fold increase 4 h after i.v. and s.c. administration *3220*

Norepinephrine *Plasma Increase Physiological* Statistically significant increase observed in 11 uremic patients 1 hour following intravenous infusion of 0.4 µg/kg *1758*

Plasminogen Activator Inhibitor-1 *Plasma Decrease Physiological* Significant decrease observed in 4 healthy volunteers given 0.3 µg/kg intravenously either alone or with dextran *1894*

Plasminogen Activator Inhibitor-3 *Plasma No Effect Physiological* In 7 healthy individuals infusion of 0.3 µg/kg caused nonsignificant reduction from mean baseline of 85.3 ± 11.7% to 77.0 ± 6.8% after 30 min, and 74.1 ± 14.3% after 120 min. Similar response seen in uremics *81*

Protein C *Plasma Increase Physiological* Significant increase observed in 4 healthy volunteers given 0.3 µg/kg intravenously either alone or with dextran *1894*

Protein C Activity *Plasma Decrease Physiological* In 7 healthy controls after 0.3 µg/kg body weight activity declined from mean baseline of 110.8 ± 12.1% to 78.9 ± 12.5% after 30 min and 74.3 ± 13.3% after 120 min. Similar change observed in uremic individuals *81*

Protein C Antigen *Plasma No Effect Physiological* In 7 healthy controls infusion of 0.3 µg/kg caused nonsignificant reduction from mean baseline of 116.6 ± 9.5% to 109.7 ± 8.0% after 30 min and 114.6 ± 2.3% after 120 min. Similar results seen in uremics *81*

Renin Activity *Plasma Increase Physiological* In normal individuals increase observed but no effect observed with administration in 7 cases of nephrogenic diabetes insipidus *546*

Ristocetin Cofactor Activity *Plasma Increase Physiological* In one patient with von Willebrand's disease treatment caused significant increase from mean baseline of 13 U/dL to 177 U/dL, towards the upper limit of the normal range of 47 - 196 U/dL *2775*

Sodium *Serum Decrease Physiological* In 6 children receiving the drug intranasally (in 4 only once) concentrations ranged from 118 to 125 mmol/L *5387* In one adult with von Willebrand's disease after 3 intravenous doses of 18 µg; 0.3 µg/kg caused decrease of plasma concentration to 121 mmol/L *2775*

Tissue Plasminogen Activator
Plasma Increase Physiological Significant increase observed in 4 healthy volunteers given 0.3 µg/kg intravenously either alone or with dextran *1894* Highly significant increase observed after intravenous infusion of 0.4 µg/kg in 15 minutes in patient group with proven coronary artery disease *1625*

Tissue Plasminogen Activator Antigen
Plasma Increase Physiological Up to 1.9-fold increase above basal value following i.v. administration and 2.2-fold increase following s.c. administration *3220* Highly significant increase observed in patients with proven coronary artery disease following intravenous infusion of 0.4 µg/kg over 15 minutes *1625*

von Willebrand Factor *Plasma Increase Physiological* Statistically significant increase in 11 uremic patients 1 hour following intravenous infusion of 0.4 µg/kg *1758* In normal individuals administration stimulates release but in 7 males with nephrogenic diabetes insipidus no effect observed *546*

von Willebrand Factor Antigen
Plasma Increase Physiological In 4 healthy volunteers administration of 0.3 µg/kg intravenously either alone or with dextran caused significant increase *1894*

Desogestrel

Apolipoprotein A-I *Serum Increase Physiological* Increase by 20% when 150 µg desogestrel given with 30 µg ethinyl estradiol for 3 mo. Results normal within 2 mo after treatment stopped *504*

Apolipoprotein B *Serum No Effect Physiological* (ratio apo B: apo A-I decreased by 17%) when 150 µg desogestrel given with 30 µg ethinyl estradiol for 3 mo. Results normal within 2 mo after treatment stopped *504*

Ceruloplasmin *Serum No Effect Physiological* With daily dose of 0.125 mg in 30 healthy female volunteers when given alone. Normal values 30 d after treatment stopped *5157*

Cholesterol *Serum No Effect Physiological* When 150 µg desogestrel given with 30 µg ethinyl estradiol for 3 mo. Results normal within 2 mo after treatment stopped *504*

Corticosteroid-Binding Globulin
Serum Increase Physiological In 30 women given a combination of 150 µg desogestrel and 30 µg ethinyl estradiol mean concentration rose from 700 ± 122 nmol/L on day 1 of first cycle to 1350 ± 259 nmol/L on day 1, 1882 ± 383 nmol/L on day 10 and 2064 ± 415 nmol/L on day 21 of third cycle *2428*
Serum No Effect Physiological With daily dose of 0.125 mg in 30 healthy female volunteers when given alone. Normal values 30 d after treatment stopped *5157*

Cortisol *Urine Decrease Physiological* In 30 women given a combination of 150 µg desogestrel and 30 µg ethinyl estradiol mean excretion declined from 76.5 ± 32.8 µg/d on day 1 of first cycle to 54.4 ± 23.9 µg/d on day 1, 51.1 ± 22.7 µg/d on day 10 and 51.0 ± 31.7 µg/d on day 21 of third cycle *2428*

Glycated Protein *Serum No Effect Physiological* When 150 µg desogestrel given with 30 µg ethinyl estradiol for 3 mo. Results normal within 2 mo after treatment stopped *504*

HDL-Cholesterol *Serum Decrease Physiological* With daily dose of 0.125 mg in 30 healthy female volunteers when given alone. Normal values 30 d after treatment stopped *5157*
Serum Increase Physiological Increase by 12% (% HDL-cholesterol increased by 15%) when 150 µg desogestrel given with 30 µg ethinyl estradiol for 3 mo. Results normal within 2 mo after treatment stopped *504*

6-β-Hydroxycortisol *Urine Decrease Physiological* In 30 women given a combination of 150 µg desogestrel and 30 µg ethinyl estradiol mean concentration declined from 278 ± 142 µg/d on day 1 of first cycle to 224 ± 109 µg/d on day 1, 236 ± 129 µg/d on day 10 and 238 ± 120 µg/d on day 21 of third cycle *2428*

Sex-Hormone Binding Globulin
Serum Decrease Physiological With daily dose of 0.125 mg in 30 healthy female volunteers when given alone. Normal values 30 d after treatment stopped *5157*

Triglycerides *Serum Increase Physiological* Increase by 35% when 150 µg desogestrel given with 30 µg ethinyl estradiol for 3 mo. Results normal within 2 mo after treatment stopped *504*

Desoximetasone

Cortisol *Plasma Decrease Physiological* Rapid and sustained suppression in 5 patients with psoriasis and topical application of glucocorticoid *2029*

Glucose Tolerance *Serum Decrease Physiological* In 2 of 5 patients with psoriasis and topical application of glucocorticoid *2029*

Insulin *Plasma Increase Physiological* 2 to 3 fold increase in 5 patients with psoriasis and topical application of glucocorticoid *2029*

Leukocytes *Blood Increase Physiological* 2 to 3 fold increase in 5 patients with psoriasis and topical application of glucocorticoid *2029*

Dexamethasone

Absorbance at 450 nm *Amniotic Fluid Decrease Analytical* Time-dependent decrease when added to bilirubin containing amniotic fluid *in vitro4061*

Adenosine Monophosphate
Plasma No Effect Physiological Antenatal administration of one or two courses of dexamethasone (mean total dose 42.8 ± 26.3 mg) with last dose given within 7 d of delivery caused no significant change in concentration, mean with treatment 113 nmol/L compared with 105 nmol/L in untreated group, within 12 h after birth in infants *3014*

Albendazole *Serum Increase Physiological* Steady state trough concentration about 56% higher when 8 mg dexamethasone coadministered with each dose of albendazole *5635*

Aldosterone *Plasma Decrease Physiological* Reduction from mean baseline concentration of 175 pmol/L to 122 pmol/L at 60 minutes, 115 pmol/L at 90 minutes and 114 pmol/L at 120 minutes after 1 mg orally *4303*
Plasma No Effect Physiological In 28 healthy volunteers administration of 2 mg in one day had no significant effect on mean concentration *3487* No significant effect in 6 volunteers with acute mountain sickness given 4 mg/6 hours for 48 hours compared with placebo treated controls *3538*

Amino Acids *Plasma Increase Physiological* In preterm infants with bronchopulmonary dysplasia treatment with dexamethasone caused increased concentrations of plasma amino acids *2552*

Amylase *Serum Increase Physiological* May cause pancreatitis as side effect *2754*

Androstanediol Glucuronide
Plasma Decrease Physiological In some women with hirsutism dexamethasone administration caused a reduction in plasma 3α-androstanediol glucuronide concentration *1416*

Androstenedione *Plasma No Effect Physiological* No effect of treatment on initially high concentrations in hirsute women *1198*

Androsterone *Urine Decrease Physiological* Suppression of ACTH *4006*

Bicarbonate *Serum Increase Physiological* May cause hypokalemic alkalosis *2754*

Bilirubin *Serum No Effect Analytical* No effect at 0.2 mg/L on Ames Seralyzer method *5706*

Calcium *Urine Increase Physiological* Metabolic effect *2754*

CD3+ Lymphocytes *Blood Decrease Physiological* In 25 patients with acute rheumatoid arthritis pulse therapy of 200 mg dexamethasone given within one hour on 3 successive alternate days in conjunction with a disease modifying antirheumatic drug caused a significant decrease from mean baseline of 60.7 ± 9.5% positive cells to 50.9 ± 15.0% after one day and 57.3 ± 11.1% (nonsignificant) after 4 weeks *6173*

CD4+:CD8+ Lymphocyte Ratio
Blood No Effect Physiological In 25 patients with acute rheumatoid arthritis pulse therapy of 200 mg dexamethasone given within one hour on 3 successive alternate days in conjunction with a disease modifying antirheumatic drug caused a nonsignificant change from mean baseline ratio of 1.9 to 1.9 after one day and 1.7 after 4 weeks *6173*

Dexamethasone *(continued)*

$CD4^+$ Lymphocytes *Blood Decrease Physiological* In 25 patients with acute rheumatoid arthritis pulse therapy of 200 mg dexamethasone given within one hour on 3 successive alternate days in conjunction with a disease modifying antirheumatic drug caused a nonsignificant decrease from mean baseline of 45.6 ± 7.6% positive cells to 38.1 ± 9.7% after one day and 44.2 ± 5.9% after 4 weeks *6173*

$CD8^+$ Lymphocytes *Blood Decrease Physiological* In 25 patients with acute rheumatoid arthritis pulse therapy of 200 mg dexamethasone given within one hour on 3 successive alternate days in conjunction with a disease modifying antirheumatic drug caused a significant decrease from mean baseline of 24.6 ± 8.4% positive cells to 20.2 ± 5.1% after one day and 26.1 ± 8.0% (nonsignificant increase) after 4 weeks *6173*

$CD16^+$ Lymphocytes *Blood No Effect Physiological* In 25 patients with acute rheumatoid arthritis pulse therapy of 200 mg dexamethasone given within one hour on 3 successive alternate days in conjunction with a disease modifying antirheumatic drug caused a nonsignificant change from mean baseline of 16.4 ± 10% of positive cells to 13.4 ± 10.7% after one day and 18.8 ± 11.6% after 4 weeks *6173*

Cholesterol *Serum No Effect Analytical* No effect at 0.2 mg/L on Ames Seralyzer method *5706*

Chondrex *Serum No Effect Analytical* Concentrations up to 1 g/L had no significant effect on sandwich-type ELISA procedure of Harvey et al *2491*

Corticosteroids *Plasma Decrease Physiological* Effect seen following morning if given in evening *5301*

Corticotropin *Plasma Decrease Physiological* In 28 healthy volunteers treatment with 2 mg dexamethasone caused significant reduction from mean baseline of 7.06 ± 0.64 pmol/L to 0.47 ± 0.05 pmol/L *3487* In 9 healthy individuals mean concentration decreased from 4.6 ± 2.1 pmol/L to less than 1.0 pmol/L 12 hours after ingestion 1.0 mg dexamethasone when measured by IRMA kit of Nichols *5478* Effect measured after 9 h *258*

Cortisol *Plasma Decrease Physiological* Following 7 days treatment of 27 preterm infants with bronchopulmonary dysplasia significant decrease observed. Peak concentration in response to ACTH also reduced *6485* In 28 healthy volunteers treatment with 2 mg in one day caused significant reduction from mean baseline of 420.9 ± 19.7 nmol/L to 12.45 ± 2.31 nmol/L *3487* Marked effect for 4 d after i.v. injection *1208* Significant reduction in 6 volunteers with acute mountain sickness given 4 mg/6 hours for 48 hours compared with controls *3538* Normal response not always observed in psychiatric patients *3948* Effect observed in hospitalized depressed patients maximal in those whose spontaneous afternoon cortisol was lowest *1006* In 25 patients with acute rheumatoid arthritis pulse therapy of 200 mg dexamethasone given within one hour on 3 successive alternate days in conjunction with a disease modifying antirheumatic drug caused a significant decrease from mean baseline of 0.4 ± 0.2 μmol/L to 0.07 ± 0.1 μmol/L after one day and 0.32 ± 0.2 μmol/L (nonsignificant) after 4 weeks *6173* In 5 healthy men administration of 3.0 mg/day for 7 days caused decrease of mean from 540 ± 109 nmol/L to less than 80 nmol/L *6223* In 7 healthy male volunteers significant reduction from mean baseline concentration of 245 nmol/L to 173 nmol/L at 60 minutes, 151 nmol/L at 90 minutes and 132 nmol/L at 120 minutes after 1 mg orally *4303* In 9 healthy individuals plasma concentration decreased from baseline of 382 ± 222 nmol/L to 63 ± 30 nmol/L 12 hours after ingestion of 1.0 mg dexamethasone *5478*

Plasma No Effect Analytical Reactivity of less than 1% possible with RIA *1803* At concentration up to the upper limit of usual concentration only had 0.1% cross reactivity with method on Baxter Stratus *5705*

Urine Decrease Physiological In 9 healthy individuals ingestion of 1.0 mg dexamethasone caused excretion to decrease from mean baseline of 161 ± 58 nmol/d to less than 20 nmol/d *5478*

Cortisol, Free *Urine No Effect Analytical* No significant interference observed with HPLC method of Turpeinen et al *6105*

C-Reactive Protein *Serum Decrease Physiological* In 25 patients with acute rheumatoid arthritis pulse therapy of 200 mg dexamethasone given within one hour on 3 successive alternate days in conjunction with a disease modifying antirheumatic drug caused a significant decrease from mean baseline of 75 μg/dL to 6 ± 6 μg/dL after one day and 32 ± 29 μg/dL after 4 weeks *6173*

Creatine Kinase *Serum No Effect Analytical* No effect at 0.2 mg/L on method on Ames Seralyzer *5706*

Creatinine *Serum No Effect Analytical* No effect at 0.2 mg/L on Ames Seralyzer method *5706*

Dehydroepiandrosterone *Plasma Decrease Physiological* In 25 patients with acute rheumatoid arthritis pulse therapy of 200 mg dexamethasone given within one hour on 3 successive alternate days in conjunction with a disease modifying antirheumatic drug caused a significant decrease from mean baseline of 5.2 ± 8.0 ng/mL to 2.0 ± 2.0 ng/mL after one day and 4.8 ± 5.2 ng/mL (nonsignificant) after 4 weeks *6173*

Urine Decrease Physiological Suppression of ACTH *4006*

Dehydroepiandrosterone Sulfate

Plasma Decrease Physiological Suppressed by treatment in hirsute women from mean of 8.6 to 3.4 μmol/L *1198* In 25 patients with acute rheumatoid arthritis pulse therapy of 200 mg dexamethasone given within one hour on 3 successive alternate days in conjunction with a disease modifying antirheumatic drug caused a significant decrease from mean baseline of 3.2 ± 2.3 μg/mL to 0.98 ± 0.6 μg/mL after one day and 2.58 ± 1.8 μg/mL after 4 weeks *6173* In 5 healthy men administration of 3.0 mg daily for 7 days caused decrease of mean from 6.0 ± 1.6 μmol/L to 1.7 ± 0.3 μmol/L *6223*

21-Deoxycortisol *Plasma Decrease Physiological* In 5 normal women post-dexamethasone concentrations were undetectable *3948*

Dexamethasone *Serum Increase Physiological* Following overnight administration of 1 mg dexamethasone to individuals without Cushing's syndrome concentration at 8:00 a.m. varied from 3.3 to 19.6 nmol/L *6538* In 9 healthy individuals ingestion of 1.0 mg at bedtime caused a plasma concentration of 9.2 ± 2.4 nmol/L *5478*

3,4-Dihydroxyphenylglycol *Plasma No Effect Physiological* Antenatal administration of one or two courses of dexamethasone (mean total dose 42.8 ± 26.3 mg) with last dose given within 7 d of delivery caused no significant change in concentration, mean with treatment 30 nmol/L compared with 26 nmol/L in untreated group, within 12 h after birth in infants *3014*

β-Endorphin *Plasma Decrease Physiological* Postoperative induced secretion of compound reduced by all amounts of drug given but amount of pain increased *2464*

Epidermal Growth Factor *Urine Increase Physiological* In preterm infants excretion of EGF increased from 17 ± 1 μmol/μmol creatinine to peak of 150 ± 46 μmol/μmol creatinine in 10 responders and from 15 ± 5 μmol/μu]mol creatinine to 75 ± 30 μmol/μmol creatinine in 10 nonresponders when treated with dexamethasone for chronic lung disease or presumed airway edema *5419*

Epinephrine *Plasma Decrease Physiological* Antenatal administration of one or two courses of dexamethasone (mean total dose 42.8 ± 26.3 mg) with last dose given within 7 d of delivery caused significant reduction in concentration, mean with treatment 6.42 nmol/L compared with 7.02 nmol/L in untreated group, within 12 h after birth in infants *3014*

Urine No Effect Physiological No effect on increased concentration caused by simulated high altitude in 6 volunteers given 4 mg/6 hours for 48 hours *3538*

Erythrocyte Sedimentation Rate

Blood Decrease Physiological In 25 patients with acute rheumatoid arthritis pulse therapy of 200 mg dexamethasone given within one hour on 3 successive alternate days in conjunction with a disease modifying antirheumatic drug caused a significant decrease from mean baseline of 80 ± 38 mm/h to 41 ± 24 mm/h after one day and 57 ± 34 mm/h after 4 weeks *6173*

Blood Increase Physiological Slight dose related effect observed in 6 normal volunteers 24 hours after oral administration of 4-8 mg/square meter surface area *4067*

Erythrocytes *Blood No Effect Physiological* No significant effect over 8 hours in 6 healthy volunteers following oral or intravenous administration of 4-8 mg/square meter surface area *4067*

Estradiol *Plasma Decrease Physiological* In 5 men administration of 3.0 mg daily for 1 week caused decrease of mean from 144 ± 18 pmol/L to 99 ± 18 pmol/L *6223*
Plasma No Effect Physiological No effect of treatment on initially high concentrations in hirsute women *1198*

Estriol *Plasma No Effect Physiological* No effect of treatment on initially high concentrations in hirsute women *1198*

Estrogens *Urine Decrease Physiological* Decreased conversion of neutral steroids *54*

Etiocholanolone *Urine Decrease Physiological* Suppression of ACTH *4006*

Glucose *Cerebrospinal Fluid Increase Physiological* Increase of 86% observed after 12 hours and 115% after 24 hours in 52 children with bacterial meningitis treated with i.v. dexamethasone in addition to the i.v. cefotaxime with which controls only treated *4365*
Serum Increase Physiological Significant increase to 7.3 mmol/L in 6 dexamethasone (4 mg/6 hourly for 48 hours) treated volunteers with simulated acute mountain sickness compared with 4.8 mmol/L in placebo treated controls *3538* Hormonal action *4174*
Serum No Effect Analytical No effect at 0.2 mg/L on glucose oxidase method on Ames Seralyzer *5706*
Urine Increase Physiological Associated with hyperglycemia *2754*

Glucose Tolerance *Serum Decrease Physiological* May impair carbohydrate tolerance *2754* Observed in normal subjects and associated with enhanced insulin, C-peptide and glucagon responses to a test meal and blunted gastric inhibitory polypeptide response *2347*

Granulocyte Colony Stimulating Factor
Serum Increase Physiological In 9 healthy men infusion of of 0.04 mg/kg dexamethasone caused mean baseline concentration of 15.5 ng/L to increase by 240% at 24 h and a dose of 1.0 mg/kg caused a 871% increase from the baseline of 12.3 ng/L *2938*

Growth Hormone *Plasma Increase Physiological* In 5 healthy men administration of 3.0 mg/day for 7 days caused increase from mean baseline of 1.2 ± 0.90 µg/L to 4.2 ± 1.5 µg/L *6223* Significant increase observed after intravenous administration *908*

Hematocrit *Blood No Effect Physiological* No significant effect over 8 hours in 6 healthy volunteers following oral or intravenous administration of 4-8 mg/square meter surface area *4067*

Hemoglobin *Blood Increase Physiological* In 25 patients with acute rheumatoid arthritis pulse therapy of 200 mg dexamethasone given within one hour on 3 successive alternate days in conjunction with a disease modifying antirheumatic drug caused a significant increase from mean baseline of 7.1 ± 1.1 g/dL to 7.5 ± 1.0 g/dL after one day and 7.4 ± 1.0 g/dL (nonsignificant) after 4 weeks *6173*

17-Hydroxycorticosteroids *Urine Decrease Physiological* Pituitary feedback with suppression of ACTH *3563*
Urine Increase Analytical Measured as endogenous steroids by Reddy method *4006*

Insulin-like Growth Factor-I *Serum Increase Physiological* In 5 healthy men administration of 3.0 mg daily for 7 days caused increase from mean baseline of 0.74 ± 0.08 U/mL to 2.0 ± 0.35 U/mL *6223*

Interleukin-6 *Serum Decrease Physiological* In 25 patients with acute rheumatoid arthritis pulse therapy of 200 mg dexamethasone given within one hour on 3 successive alternate days in conjunction with a disease modifying antirheumatic drug caused a significant decrease from mean baseline of 17 ± 4 pg/mL to 4 ± 2 pg/mL after one day and 9 ± 3.2 pg/mL after 4 weeks *6173*

Interleukin-8 *Serum Decrease Physiological* In 25 patients with acute rheumatoid arthritis pulse therapy of 200 mg dexamethasone given within one hour on 3 successive alternate days in conjunction with a disease modifying antirheumatic drug caused a significant decrease from mean baseline of 48 ± 10 pg/mL to 15 ± 4 pg/mL after one day and 18 ± 5.3 pg/mL after 4 weeks *6173*

17-Ketogenic Steroids *Urine Decrease Physiological* Suppression of ACTH *4006*

17-Ketosteroids *Urine Increase Analytical* Affects method of Reddy *2766*

Lactate *Cerebrospinal Fluid Decrease Physiological* In 52 children with bacterial meningitis given i.v. dexamethasone in addition to i.v. cefotaxime mean reduction of 27% after 12 hours and 62% after 24 hours *4365*

Lactate Dehydrogenase *Serum No Effect Analytical* No effect at 0.2 mg/L on method on Ames Seralyzer *5706*

Leukocytes *Blood Increase Physiological* In 25 patients with acute rheumatoid arthritis pulse therapy of 200 mg dexamethasone given within one hour on 3 successive alternate days in conjunction with a disease modifying antirheumatic drug caused a significant increase from mean baseline of 7100 ± 2000 /µL to 13400 ± 4500 /µL after one day and nonsignificant change to 7000 ± 2500 /µL after 4 weeks *6173*
Cerebrospinal Fluid Decrease Physiological Mean reduction of 43% after 12 hours and 69% after 24 hours in 52 children with bacterial meningitis given i.v. dexamethasone in addition to the i.v. cefotaxime only given to controls *4365*

Luteinizing Hormone *Plasma No Effect Physiological* In 5 healthy men administration of 3.0 mg daily for 7 days insignificant reduction from mean baseline of 5.3 ± 1.2 IU/L to 4.2 ± 0.61 IU/L *6223*

Lymphocyte Interleukin-2 Receptor
Blood No Effect Physiological In 25 patients with acute rheumatoid arthritis pulse therapy of 200 mg dexamethasone given within one hour on 3 successive alternate days in conjunction with a disease modifying antirheumatic drug caused a nonsignificant change from mean baseline of 17.8 ± 2.3% positive cells to 16.4 ± 8.7% after one day and 19.4 ± 7.9% after 4 weeks *6173*

Lymphocytes *Blood Decrease Physiological* As neutrophil count increases following oral or intravenous administration lymphocyte count decreases *4067*
Blood Increase Physiological Peak observed at 24 hours after oral administration of 4-8 mg/square meter surface area *4067*

MCH *Blood No Effect Physiological* No significant effect over 8 hours in 6 healthy volunteers given 4-8 mg/square meter surface area either orally or intravenously *4067*

MCHC *Blood No Effect Physiological* No significant effect observed in 6 healthy volunteers over 8 hours when given 4-8 mg/square meter surface area either orally or intravenously *4067*

MCV *Blood No Effect Physiological* No significant effect over 8 hours in 6 healthy volunteers given 4-8 mg/square meter surface area either orally or intravenously *4067*

3-Methylhistidine *Urine Increase Physiological* In preterm infants treatment with dexamethasone caused increased excretion of 3-methylhistidine in association with endogenous protein catabolism *2552*

Neutrophils *Blood Increase Physiological* Maximum effect observed in 6 healthy volunteers at 4-6 hours following either oral or intravenous injection of 4-8 mg/square meter surface area. Direct correlation between plasma concentration of drug and blood neutrophils after i.v. drug but not oral *4067* Second peak observed 24 hours after oral administration of 4-8 mg/square meter surface area *4067*

Nitrogen Balance *Patient Negative Physiological* Due to protein catabolism *2754* Administration has been reported to increase protein catabolism thus reducing nitrogen balance *3969*

Norepinephrine *Plasma Decrease Physiological* Antenatal administration of one or two courses of dexamethasone (mean total dose 42.8 ± 26.3 mg) with last dose given within 7 d of delivery caused significant reduction in concentration, mean with treatment 1.20 nmol/L compared with 1.92 nmol/L in untreated group, within 12 h after birth in infants *3014*
Urine No Effect Physiological No effect in 6 volunteers exposed to simulated high altitude given 4 mg/6 hours for 48 hours *3538*

Occult Blood *Feces Increase Physiological* Observed in 12 of 51 (24%) children with bacterial meningitis treated with i.v. dexamethasone in addition to cefotaxime *4365* May aggravate peptic ulcer and cause bleeding *2754*

Dexamethasone *(continued)*

Platelet Activating Factor
Cerebrospinal Fluid Decrease Physiological In 52 children with bacterial meningitis treatment with i.v. dexamethasonewith cefotaxime caused mean reduction of 70% after 12 h compared with increase of 34% in control group (cefotaxime only) and decreases of 92% and 57% respectively at 24 h *4365*

Potassium *Serum Decrease Physiological* May promote increased urinary loss *2754* Administration has been reported to cause potassium loss *3969*
Serum Increase Physiological Significant increase observed in healthy volunteers following treatment with 1 mg orally 2 hours previously *4303*
Serum No Effect Analytical At concentration of 1.4 mg/L had no effect on measurement by ISE with predilution *5704*
Serum No Effect Physiological No significant change observed in 7 healthy men for 2 hours following 1 mg orally *4303*
Urine Increase Physiological Metabolic effect *2754* Significant increase observed in 6 healthy volunteers given 4-8 mg/square meter surface area over subsequent 24 hours *4067*

Prolactin *Plasma Decrease Physiological* Normal response not always observed in psychiatric patients *3948*

Prostaglandin E_2 *Plasma No Effect Physiological* No significant change over 2 hours in 7 healthy male volunteers following 1 mg orally *4303*

Protein *Cerebrospinal Fluid Decrease Physiological* Mean reduction of 22% observed at 12 hours and 58% observed at 24 hours in 52 children with bacterial meningitis treated with i.v. dexamethasone in addition to i.v. cefotaxime with which controls only treated *4365*
Cerebrospinal Fluid No Effect Analytical No significant effect when added to concentration of 10.0 mg/dL on Ektachem® slide method *3654*

Rheumatoid Factor (IgM) *Serum Decrease Physiological* In 25 patients with acute rheumatoid arthritis pulse therapy of 200 mg dexamethasone given within one hour on 3 successive alternate days in conjunction with a disease modifying antirheumatic drug caused a nonsignificant decrease from mean baseline of 1094 ± 1853 µg/L to 1115 ± 1853 µg/L after one day and significant decrease to 655 ± 1403 µg/L after 4 weeks *6173*

Saquinavir *Serum Decrease Physiological* Coadministration of dexamethasone with saquinavir reduced the latter's concentration by inducing CYP3A4 in the liver *5024*

Sex-Hormone Binding Globulin
Serum Decrease Physiological In 25 patients with acute rheumatoid arthritis pulse therapy of 200 mg dexamethasone given within one hour on 3 successive alternate days in conjunction with a disease modifying antirheumatic drug caused a significant decrease from mean baseline of 46 ± 22 nmol/L to 38 ± 26 nmol/L after one day and 50 ± 23 nmol/L (nonsignificant) after 4 weeks *6173*
Serum Increase Physiological Mean increase from 35.2 to 47.7 nmol/L in 14 women hirsute women *1198*

Sodium *Serum No Effect Analytical* At concentration of 1.4 mg/L had no effect on measurement by ISE with predilution *5704*
Serum No Effect Physiological No significant change observed in 7 healthy men over 2 hours following 1 mg orally *4303* No effect observed in 6 healthy volunteers over 8 hours following oral or intravenous administration of 4-8 mg/square meter surface area *4067*
Urine Increase Physiological Mild diuresis with sodium loss may occur initially *128*
Urine No Effect Physiological No effect observed over 24 hours in 6 healthy volunteers given 4-8 mg/square meter surface area either orally or intravenously *4067*

Soluble Interleukin-2 Receptor
Serum Decrease Physiological In 25 patients with acute rheumatoid arthritis pulse therapy of 200 mg dexamethasone given within one hour on 3 successive alternate days in conjunction with a disease modifying antirheumatic drug caused a significant decrease from mean baseline of 1523 ± 186 U/mL to 1170 ± 170 U/mL after one day and 1158 ± 158 U/mL after 4 weeks *6173*

Tacrolimus *Serum No Effect Analytical* In HPLC/MS method of Christians et al no significant interference observed with measurement of FK 506 *1010*

Testosterone *Serum Decrease Physiological* Decreased metabolic clearance and binding in women *3159*
Serum No Effect Physiological No effect of treatment on initially high concentrations in hirsute women *1198*
Urine Decrease Physiological Slight effect in men *5107*

Testosterone, Free *Serum Decrease Physiological* In 5 healthy men administration of 3.0 mg daily for 7 days caused decrease of mean from 105 ± 10 pmol/L to 87 ± 10 pmol/L *6223*

Thromboxane *Plasma No Effect Physiological* No effect of up to 100 µmol/L on formation during clotting *4817*

Thyroxine (T4) *Serum Decrease Physiological* 8 mg/d for 2 d reduced concentration in normal individuals due to altered secretion and peripheral metabolism *1352*

Tri-iodothyronine (T3) *Serum Decrease Physiological* 8 mg/d for 2 d reduced concentration in normal and hypothyroid patients *1352*

Tumor Necrosis Factor-α
Cerebrospinal Fluid Decrease Physiological In 52 children with bacterial meningitis i.v. drug caused reduction of 84% after 12 h compared with 21% in controls and of 93% in treatment group and of 54% in controls after 24 h when i.v. dexamethasone given in addition to the cefotaxime in controls *4365*

Urea Nitrogen *Serum Increase Physiological* Highly significant increase in concentration of nearly 5.0 mmol/L in preterm infants undergoing treatment for chronic lung disease. Dxamethasone therapy significantly increases the rate of endogenous protein catabolism in very low birth weight infants *2552*
Serum No Effect Analytical No effect at 0.2 mg/L on method on Ames Seralyzer *5706*

Volume *Urine Increase Physiological* Significant increase over 24 hours following intravenous administration of 4-8 mg/square meter surface area in 6 healthy volunteers *4067*

Dexbrompheniramine

Bromide *Serum Increase Physiological* Theoretical possibility since drug contains 25% bromide *5116*

Dexfenfluramine

Alanine Aminotransferase *Serum Increase Physiological* Infrequently hepatitis and melena may occur with treatment *6568*
Serum No Effect Physiological No significant effect observed in 17 premenopausal obese normotensive women treated with 30 mg/d for 4 days *165*

Alkaline Phosphatase *Serum Increase Physiological* Hepatic failure, jaundice and liver damage have been reported to occur with treatment *6568*
Serum No Effect Physiological No significant effect observed in 17 premenopausal obese normotensive women treated with 30 mg/d for 4 days *165*

Amphetamine *Urine Positive Analytical* Reported false positive effect with ELISA methods *6568*

Amylase *Serum Increase Physiological* Rarely pancreatitis may occur with treatment *6568*

Aspartate Aminotransferase *Serum Increase Physiological* Infrequently hepatitis and melena may occur with treatment *6568*
Serum No Effect Physiological No significant effect observed in 17 normotensive obese premenopausal women treated with 30 mg/d for 4 days *165*

Bilirubin *Serum Increase Physiological* Hepatic failure, jaundice and liver damage have been reported to occur with treatment *6568*
Serum No Effect Physiological No significant effect observed in 17 normotensive obese premenopausal women treated with 30 mg/d for 4 days *165*

Cholesterol *Serum Decrease Physiological* In 10 healthy nondiabetic obese individuals treated with 15 mg/d for 8 days concentration significantly reduced from mean baseline of 6.07 ± 0.41 mmol/L to 5.48 ± 0.38 mmol/L *158*

Serum *No Effect* *Physiological* No significant change observed in 17 normotensive obese premenopausal women treated with 30 mg/d for 4 days *165*

Corticotropin *Plasma* *Increase* *Physiological* In 9 obese men treated with 30 mg/d for 8 days caused nonsignificant increase in fasting concentration from mean baseline of 11.09 pg/mL compared with 3.2 pg/mL in controls *1442*

Cortisol *Plasma* *No Effect* *Physiological* No significant effect observed in 17 premenopausal obese normotensive women treated with 30 mg/d for 4 days *165*

C-Peptide *Plasma* *Decrease* *Physiological* In 10 healthy nondiabetic obese individuals treatment with 15 mg/d for 8 days caused significant derease from mean baseline of 0.68 ± 0.03 nmol/L to 0.58 ± 0.02 nmol/L *158*

Plasma *No Effect* *Physiological* No significant effect observed in 17 normotensive obese premenopausal women treated with 30 mg/d for 4 days *165*

β-Endorphin *Plasma* *Decrease* *Physiological* Significant reduction compared with placebo treated controls (33.4 ng/mL versus 40.9 ng/mL) in 17 premenopausal obese normotensive women when treated with 30 mg/d for 4 days *165*

Erythrocytes *Blood* *Increase* *Physiological* Rarely polycythemia may occur with treatment *6568*

Fatty Acids (FFA), Free *Serum* *No Effect* *Physiological* In 10 healthy nondiabetic obese individuals treatment with 15 mg/d for 8 days caused nonsignificant reduction from mean baseline of 0.765 ± 0.091 mmol/L to 0.794 ± 0.051 mmol/L *158* In 9 obese men treated with 30 mg/d for 8 days caused nonsignificant decrease in fasting concentration from mean baseline of 0.07 mmol/L compared with increase of 0.10 mmol/L in controls *1442*

Glucose *Serum* *Decrease* *Physiological* Infrequently hypoglycemia may occur with treatment *6568* In 10 healthy nondiabetic obese individuals treatment with 15 mg/d for 8 days caused significant decrease from mean baseline of 6.2 ± 0.2 mmol/L to 5.7 ± 0.2 mmol/L *158*

Serum *Increase* *Physiological* Rarely hyperglycemia may occur with treatment *6568*

Serum *No Effect* *Physiological* In 9 obese men treated with 30 mg/d for 8 days caused nonsignificant decrease in fasting concentration from mean baseline of 3 mg/dL compared with decrease of 2 mg/dL in controls *1442* No significant effect observed in 17 normotensive obese premenopausal women treated with 30 mg/d for 4 days *165*

Glucose Tolerance *Serum* *No Effect* *Physiological* treatment of 10 healthy nondiabetic individuals with 15 mg/d for 8 days had no effect on oral glucose tolerance curve *158*

γ-Glutamyltransferase *Serum* *Increase* *Physiological* Hepatic failure, jaundice and liver damage have been reported to occur with treatment *6568*

Granulocytes *Blood* *Decrease* *Physiological* Agranulocytosis may occur with treatment *6568*

Growth Hormone *Plasma* *No Effect* *Physiological* In 9 obese men treated with 30 mg/d for 8 days caused nonsignificant increase in fasting concentration from mean baseline of 0.3 ng/mL compared with increase of 0.21 ng/mL in controls *1442*

HDL-Cholesterol *Serum* *No Effect* *Physiological* In 10 healthy nondiabetic obese individuals treatment with 15 mg/d for 8 days caused nonsignificant change from mean baseline of 1.07 ± 0.08 mmol/L *158*

Hematocrit *Blood* *Decrease* *Physiological* Infrequently anemia may occur with treatment *6568*

Hemoglobin *Blood* *Decrease* *Physiological* Infrequently anemia may occur with treatment *6568*

Insulin *Plasma* *Decrease* *Physiological* In 10 healthy nondiabetic obese individuals treatment with 15 mg/d for 8 days caused significant decrease from mean baseline of 168.0 ± 14.5 pmol/L to 138.9 ± 7.9 pmol/L *158* In 9 obese men treatment with 30 mg/d for 8 days caused significant reduction of 22 μU/mL in 08:00 concentration of about 45 μU/mL *1442*

Plasma *No Effect* *Physiological* No significant change observed in 17 obese normotensive premenopausal women treated with 30 mg/d for 4 days *165*

LDL-Cholesterol *Serum* *Decrease* *Physiological* In 10 healthy nondiabetic obese individuals treatment with 15 mg/d for 8 days caused significant reduction from mean baseline of 3.99 ± 0.40 mmol/L to 3.64 ± 0.37 mmol/L *158*

Lipase *Serum* *Increase* *Physiological* Rarely pancreatitis may occur with treatment *6568*

Lipids *Serum* *Increase* *Physiological* Rarely hyperlipemia may occur with treatment *6568*

Norepinephrine *Plasma* *Decrease* *Physiological* In 9 obese men treated with 30 mg/d for 8 days caused significant decrease in fasting concentration from mean baseline of 165 ng/mL compared with increase of 8 ng/mL in controls *1442* Significant reduction observed from mean placebo concentration of 0.28 ng/mL to 0.15 ng/mL in 17 normotensive obese premenopausal women treated with 30 mg/d for 4 days *165*

Occult Blood *Feces* *Increase* *Physiological* Infrequently gastrointestinal hemorrhage and melena may occur with treatment *6568*

Platelets *Blood* *Increase* *Physiological* Rarely thrombocythemia may occur with treatment *6568*

Potassium *Serum* *Decrease* *Physiological* Infrequently hypokalemia may occur with treatment *6568*

Serum *Increase* *Physiological* Rarely hyperkalemia may occur with treatment *6568*

Prolactin *Plasma* *Increase* *Physiological* Hyperprolactinemia may occur with treatment *6568*

Renin Activity *Plasma* *Decrease* *Physiological* Significant reduction in 17 obese normotensive premenopausal women treated with 30 mg/d for 4 days from baseline of 1.09 ng angiotensin I/mL/h to 0.76 ng angiotensin I/mL/h *165*

Sex-Hormone Binding Globulin

Serum *No Effect* *Physiological* No significant effect observed in 17 normotensive obese premenopausal women treated with 30 mg/d for 4 days *165*

Testosterone *Serum* *No Effect* *Physiological* No significant effect observed in 17 normotensive obese normotensive premenopausal women treated with 30 mg/d for 4 days *165*

Thyroid Stimulating Hormone

Serum *No Effect* *Physiological* No significant effect observed in 17 obese normotensive premenopausal women treated with 30 mg/d for 4 days *165*

Thyroxine (T4) *Serum* *Increase* *Physiological* Rarely hypothyroidism may occur with treatment *6568*

Serum *No Effect* *Physiological* No significant effect observed in 17 premenopausal obese normotensive women treated with 30 mg/d for 4 days *165*

Tri-iodothyronine, Reverse (rT3)

Serum *No Effect* *Physiological* No significant effect observed in 17 premenopausal obese normotensive women treated with 30 mg/d for 4 days *165*

Tri-iodothyronine (T3) *Serum* *No Effect* *Physiological* No significant effect observed in 17 premenopausal obese normotensive women treated with 30 mg/d for 4 days *165*

Triglycerides *Serum* *Decrease* *Physiological* In 10 healthy nondiabetic obese individuals treatment with 15 mg/d for 8 days caused significant reduction from mean baseline of 2.25 ± 0.45 mmol/L to 1.70 ± 0.21 mmol/L *158*

Serum *No Effect* *Physiological* No significant change observed in 17 premenopausal obese normotensive women treated with 30 mg/d for 4 days *165*

Uric Acid *Serum* *Increase* *Physiological* Infrequently gout may occur with treatment *6568*

Serum *No Effect* *Physiological* No significant effect observed in 17 obese premenopausal normotensive women treated with 30 mg/d for 4 days *165*

Dexrazoxane

Alanine Aminotransferase *Serum* *Increase* *Physiological* Coadministration of dexrazoxane with fluorouracil, doxorubicin and cyclophosphamide (FAC) was associated with similar toxicity as when FAC alone was administered *4687*

Alkaline Phosphatase *Serum* *Increase* *Physiological* Coadministration of dexrazoxane with fluorouracil, doxorubicin and cyclophosphamide (FAC) was associated with similar toxicity as when FAC alone was administered *4687*

Aspartate Aminotransferase *Serum* *Increase* *Physiological* Coadministration of dexrazoxane with fluorouracil, doxorubicin and cyclophosphamide (FAC) was associated with similar toxicity as when FAC alone was administered *4687*

Dexrazoxane *(continued)*

Creatinine *Serum Increase Physiological* Coadministration of dexrazoxane with fluorouracil, doxorubicin and cyclophosphamide (FAC) was associated with similar toxicity as when FAC alone was administered *4687*

Doxorubicin *Serum No Effect Physiological* Coadministration of dexrazoxane with doxorubicin had no effect on its pharmacokinetics and its principal metabolite, doxorubicinol *4687*

Granulocytes *Blood Decrease Physiological* Coadministration of dexrazoxane with fluorouracil, doxorubicin and cyclophosphamide (FAC) was associated with greater toxicity when FAC alone was administered *4687*

Leukocytes *Blood Decrease Physiological* Coadministration of dexrazoxane with fluorouracil, doxorubicin and cyclophosphamide (FAC) was associated with greater toxicity when FAC alone was administered *4687*

Platelets *Blood Decrease Physiological* Coadministration of dexrazoxane with fluorouracil, doxorubicin and cyclophosphamide (FAC) was associated with greater toxicity when FAC alone was administered *4687*

Urea Nitrogen *Serum Increase Physiological* Coadministration of dexrazoxane with fluorouracil, doxorubicin and cyclophosphamide (FAC) was associated with similar toxicity as when FAC alone was administered *4687*

Dextran

Albumin *Serum Decrease Physiological* 30% after Macrodex® , no effect after Rheomacrodex® *5596*
Serum No Effect Analytical No effect at concentration of 10,000 mg/L on Kodak Ektachem® method *5706* At concentration of 30,000 mg/L had no effect on BCG method *5704*

Ammonia *Plasma No Effect Analytical* At concentration of 10,000 mg/L had no effect on Kodak Ektachem® method *5704*

α_1-Antitrypsin *Serum Increase Physiological* Possibly associated with underlying disease *5596*

Aspartate Aminotransferase *Serum No Effect Analytical* No significant interference observed with IFCC method on Baxter Paramax Analytical system *5622*

Bilirubin *Serum Increase Analytical* Causes turbidity with methanol in Evelyn-Malloy method *5869*
Serum No Effect Analytical At concentration of 10,000 mg/L had no effect on Kodak Ektachem® method *5704*

Bilirubin, Conjugated *Serum No Effect Analytical* No effect at concentration of 10,000 mg/L on method on Kodak Ektachem® *5706*

Bilirubin, Direct *Serum Increase Analytical* Turbidity develops with Evelyn-Malloy method *1009*

Bilirubin, Unconjugated *Serum No Effect Analytical* No effect at concentration of 10,000 mg/L on method on Kodak Ektachem® *5706*

Bleeding Time *Patient Increase Physiological* Interference with platelet function observed especially when higher molecular weight products used *1384* After infusion reported to prolong bleeding time *3694* Observed effect but explanation uncertain *3810*

Calcium *Serum No Effect Analytical* No effect of concentrations up to 10,000 mg/L with method on Kodak Ektachem® *5706*

Chloride *Serum No Effect Analytical* No effect of concentrations up to 10,000 mg/L with method on Kodak Ektachem® *5706*

Cholesterol *Serum Increase Analytical* At concentrations above 10,000 mg/L on method on Kodak Ektachem® causes increase that may be of clinical significance since therapeutic range is between 8,000-14,500 mg/L *5706*

Cholinesterase *Serum No Effect Analytical* No effect observed at concentration of 3000 mg/dL with butyrylthiocholine method on Kodak Ektachem® *2504*

Complement C_4 *Serum Decrease Physiological* Complex formation or increased consumption *5596*

Creatine *Serum No Effect Analytical* No effect on method of Heinegard and Tiderstrom *2539*

Creatinine *Serum Increase Physiological* Blocks tubules causing renal failure *995*
Serum No Effect Analytical No effect of concentrations up to 10,000 mg/L on 2-slide method on Kodak Ektachem® *5706* No effect of concentrations up to 10,000 mg/L on single slide method on Kodak Ektachem® *5706*

Erythrocyte Sedimentation Rate
Blood Increase Physiological Due to cell aggregating properties *3810*

Euglobulin Lysis Time *Blood Decrease Physiological* Marked decrease noted *515*

Factor V *Plasma Decrease Physiological* Slight effect (more than hemodilution) *4014*

Factor VII *Plasma Decrease Physiological* Decrease by 50% in normals *4014*

Factor VIII *Plasma Decrease Physiological* Marked decrease noted in single case *515*

Factor IX *Plasma Decrease Physiological* Slight effect (more than hemodilution) *4014*

Factor XI *Plasma Decrease Physiological* Marked reduction in one case *515*

Fibrinogen *Plasma Decrease Physiological* Complex formation or increased consumption *5596*

β_1-α-Globulin *Serum Decrease Physiological* Complex formation or increased consumption *5596*

Glucose *Serum Increase Analytical* 10 g/dL equivalent to 0.3 mmol/L in alkaline ferricyanide. 10 g/dL equivalent to 0.7 mmol/L in p-HBAH procedure *3531* 10 g/dL equivalent to 6.7 mmol/L with o-toluidine procedure. 10 g/dL equivalent to 0.3 mmol/L with glucose oxidase procedures *3531*
Serum No Effect Analytical No effect on hexokinase, glucose oxidase methods *4240* At 1 g/dL on MBTH procedure of Neeley *4241* No effect at 500 mg/L on glucose oxidase method on Ames Seralyzer *5706* No effect at concentrations up to 30,000 mg/L with method on Fuji Drichem 1000 but at concentrations above 30,000 mg/L caused increase. Since clinical concentrations are up to 14,500 mg/L this is of no significance *5706* At concentration of 500 mg/L had no effect on Ames Seralyzer method *5704*

Haptoglobin *Serum Decrease Physiological* Complex formation or increased consumption *5596*

HDL-Cholesterol *Serum No Effect Analytical* No effect of concentrations up to 10,000 mg/L on method on Kodak Ektachem® *5706*

Hematocrit *Blood Decrease Physiological* Macrodex® increases blood volume, no effect of Rheomacrodex® *5596*

Hemoglobin *Blood No Effect Analytical* No effect of concentrations up to 10,000 mg/L on method on Kodak Ektachem® *5706*

immunoglobulin A *Serum Decrease Physiological* Complex formation or increased consumption *5596*

Immunoglobulin G *Serum Decrease Physiological* Complex formation or increased consumption *5596*

Immunoglobulin M *Serum Decrease Physiological* Complex formation or increased consumption *5596*

Inulin Clearance *Urine Increase Analytical* Interferes with analytical procedure *4014*

Iron *Serum No Effect Analytical* At concentration of 10,000 mg/L had no effect on Ferrozine method *5704*

α_2-Macroglobulin *Serum Decrease Physiological* Complex formation or increased consumption *5596*

Midazolam *Serum No Effect Analytical* On GC-ECD method of Ha et al *2387*

Partial Thromboplastin Time
Plasma Increase Physiological 15% increase noted in one case *515*

Phosphate *Serum No Effect Analytical* No effect of concentrations up to 10,000 mg/L on method on Kodak Ektachem® systems *5706*

Plasminogen *Plasma Decrease Physiological* Marked reduction *515*

Platelet Adhesiveness *Blood Decrease Physiological* After infusion reported to reduce platelet adhesion and aggregation *3694*

Platelet Aggregation *Blood Decrease Physiological* After infusion reported to reduce platelet adhesion and aggregation *3694*

Blood *Increase* *Physiological* Significant interference with platelet aggregation reported *6557*

Potassium *Serum* *No Effect* *Analytical* At concentration of 30,000 mg/L had no effect on Ektachem® ISE method *5704*

Protein *Serum* *Decrease* *Analytical* Reported effect with method on Du Pont aca *1549* Reported effect on methods such as that used on Du Pont Dimension *1591*
Serum *Decrease* *Physiological* 30% after Macrodex® , no effect after Rheomacrodex® *5596*
Serum *Increase* *Analytical* At concentrations greater than 5,000 mg/L (normal therapeutic concentration 14,500 mg/L) raised concentration as measured by biuret method with blank correction *5704* Turbidity effect with biuret reaction *5869* Concentrations above 30,000 mg/L increase results as determined by method on Kodak Ektachem® but unlikely to be of clinical significance *5706*
Serum *No Effect* *Analytical* No effect on modified biuret method of Moore *4105* If dextranase used to remove protein *4237*

Prothrombin Time *Plasma* *Increase* *Physiological* May prolong action of anticoagulants *2753*

Reptilase ® Time *Plasma* *Decrease* *Physiological* After infusion reported to reduce reptilase time *3694*

Sodium *Serum* *No Effect* *Analytical* No effect of concentrations up to 10,000 mg/L on method on Kodak Ektachem® *5706*

Specific Gravity *Urine* *Increase* *Analytical* High molecular weight *1714*

Thrombin Time *Blood* *Decrease* *Physiological* After infusion reported to reduce thrombin time *3694* Slight reduction noted in one case *515*

Transferrin *Serum* *Decrease* *Physiological* 30% after Macrodex® , no effect after Rheomacrodex® *5596*

Triglycerides *Serum* *No Effect* *Analytical* No effect of concentrations up to 10,000 mg/L on method on Kodak Ektachem® *5706*

Urea Nitrogen *Serum* *Increase* *Analytical* Reacts as if urea with dimethylaminobenzaldehyde *5869*
Serum *Increase* *Physiological* Blocks tubules causing renal failure *995*

Uric Acid *Serum* *Increase* *Analytical* Reduces phosphotungstate *3669*
Serum *No Effect* *Analytical* No effect of concentrations up to 10,000 mg/L on method on Kodak Ektachem® *5706*

Volume *Plasma* *Increase* *Physiological* Hemodynamic effect, also increases urine flow *2242* Effect of Macrodex® , not observed with Rheomacrodex® *5596*
Urine *Increase* *Physiological* Hemodynamic effect *2242*

Dextran 40

Albumin *Urine* *No Effect* *Analytical* At concentration of 1000 mg/dL had no significant effect on Boehringer Mannheim Tina-quant method *2799*

Amylase *Serum* *No Effect* *Analytical* At concentration of 80,000 mg/L had no effect on maltotetrose method *5704* At concentration of 80,000 mg/L had no effect on p-nitrophenylmaltoheptoside method *5704* At concentration of 80,000 mg/L had no effect on p-nitrophenylmaltopentoside/-hexoside method *5704*

Glucose *Serum* *Increase* *Analytical* At concentrations above 10,000 mg/L raised concentration as measured by Kodak Ektachem® method *5704*
Serum *No Effect* *Analytical* At concentration of 25 g/L has no effect on method on Du Pont Dimension *1575* At concentration of 2,500 mg/L had no effect on hexokinase/G-6-PDH method on Du Pont aca *5704* No interference observed at a concentration of 5-25 g/L with method on Du Pont aca *1527*

N-Acetyl-Glucosaminidase *Urine* *No Effect* *Analytical* At concentration of 1000 mg/dL had no significant effect on Boehringer Mannheim CPR method *3174*

Oncotic Pressure *Plasma* *Increase* *Physiological* Increase to 34 mm Hg in one patient (normal 19.7 to 24.7) who had received daily infusions of 500 mL of 10% Dextran 40 (to a total of 350 g) *1502*

Potassium *Serum* *No Effect* *Analytical* At concentration of 9,100 mg/L had no effect on measurement by ISE with predilution *5704*

Protein *Serum* *Decrease* *Analytical* At concentrations above 30 g/L causes falsely low results with Du Pont aca, although results could be corrected if ethylene glycol previously injected into packs *379*
Serum *No Effect* *Analytical* At concentrations up to 30 g/L no effect on Roche Cobas-Bio, Kodak Ektachem® 400 and Beckman Astra® 8 *379* Since 1987 no interference up to 120 g/L on American Monitor Parallel method *4356*

Sodium *Serum* *No Effect* *Analytical* At concentration of 9,100 mg/L had no effect on measurement by ISE with predilution *5704*

Urea Nitrogen *Serum* *No Effect* *Analytical* At concentration of 10,000 mg/L had no effect on Kodak Ektachem® method *5704*

Dextran 60

Albumin *Serum* *Decrease* *Physiological* In postoperative patients even on eighth day after surgery when dextran given concentration only 77-83% of preoperative concentration *508*

Cholesterol *Serum* *No Effect* *Analytical* At concentration of 6,000 mg/L had no effect on CHOD-PAP method *5704* At concentration of 6,000 mg/L had no effect on CHOD-Iodide method *5704* At concentration of 6,000 mg/L had no effect on method using catalase-Hantzsch reaction *5704* At concentration of 6,000 mg/L had no effect on catalase-AIDH method *5704* At concentration of 6,000 mg/L had no effect on Liebermann-Burchard method *5704*

Creatinine *Serum* *No Effect* *Analytical* At concentration of 6,000 mg/L had no effect on Jaffe-Fuller's earth method *5704* At concentration of 6,000 mg/L had no effect on Jaffe-Fading-Fraction method *5704* At concentration of 81250 mg/L had no effect on kinetic Jaffe method on BKA-2 *5704*

Glucose *Serum* *No Effect* *Analytical* At concentration of 6,000 mg/L had no effect on hexokinase/G-6-PDH method *5704* At concentration of 1,800 mg/L had no effect on Kodak Ektachem® method *5704*

Immunoglobulin G *Serum* *Decrease* *Physiological* In a group of postoperative surgical patients even with dextran infusion concentration was still below preoperative level on day 8. Preoperative concentration about 11 g/L, postoperative on day 8 about 7.5 g/L *508*

Immunoglobulin M *Serum* *Increase* *Physiological* Postoperatively in patients receiving dextran concentration returned to normal from decrease immediately following surgery *508*

Lactate *Plasma* *No Effect* *Analytical* At concentration of 6,000 mg/L had no effect on enzymatic method *5704*

Potassium *Serum* *No Effect* *Analytical* At concentration of 18,000 mg/L had no effect on measurement by ISE without predilution *5704*

Protein Electrophoresis *Serum* *No Effect* *Analytical* At concentration of 18,000 mg/L had no effect on automated Olympus-Hite method except for slight displacement of fractions *5704*

Sodium *Serum* *No Effect* *Analytical* At concentration of 18,000 mg/L had no effect on measurement by ISE without predilution *5704*

Urea Nitrogen *Serum* *No Effect* *Analytical* At concentration of 1800 mg/L had no effect on Kodak Ektachem® method *5704*

Uric Acid *Serum* *No Effect* *Analytical* At concentration of 6,000 mg/L had no effect on catalase-AIDH method *5704* At concentration of 6,000 mg/L had no effect on Kageyama-Hantzsch method *5704*

Dextran 70

Antithrombin III *Plasma* *Increase* *Physiological* Slight increase observed in 4 healthy volunteers following 30 g intravenously *1894*
Plasma *No Effect* *Analytical* At concentration of 1500 mg/L had no effect on Du Pont aca method *5704*

Factor VIII Coagulant *Plasma* *Decrease* *Physiological* Moderate decrease observed in 4 healthy volunteers following 30 g intravenously *1894*

Fibrinogen *Plasma* *No Effect* *Analytical* At concentration of 1500 mg/L had no effect on Du Pont aca method *5704*

Dextran 70 *(continued)*

Glucose *Serum No Effect Analytical* At concentration of 1,000 mg/L had no effect on Kodak Ektachem® method *5704*

Plasminogen *Plasma No Effect Analytical* At concentration of 1500 mg/L had no effect on Du Pont aca method *5704*

Potassium *Serum No Effect Analytical* At concentration of 5400 mg/L had no effect on measurement by ISE with predilution *5704*

Protein *Serum Increase Analytical* Progressive increase in concentration as dextran concentrations increased from 6 to 36 g/L when measurements made by refractometer *1605* When added to serum 13% increase in concentration when measured by biuret reaction at dextran concentrations of 12 g/L and 65% at dextran concentrations of 24 g/L but in vivo at "therapeutic" concentration of dextran no effect observed *1605*
Serum No Effect Analytical No effect observed even at concentrations as high as 36 g/L when measurements made by Bio-Rad dye binding method and Pierce bincinchoninic acid (BCA) color reagent *1605*

Sodium *Serum No Effect Analytical* At concentration of 5400 mg/L had no effect on measurement by ISE with predilution *5704*

Uric Acid *Serum No Effect Analytical* At concentration of 1,000 mg/L had no effect on Kodak Ektachem® method *5704*

von Willebrand Factor Antigen
Plasma Decrease Physiological Moderate decrease observed in 4 healthy volunteers following 30 g intravenously *1894*

Dextran 75

Apolipoprotein A-I *Serum No Effect Analytical* At a concentration of 25 g/L no significant effect observed on automated immunoturbidimetric method on Baxter Paramax analyzer *3005*

Apolipoprotein B *Serum No Effect Analytical* At a concentration of 25 g/L no significant effect observed on automated immunoturbidimetric method on Baxter Paramax analyzer *3005*

Fibrinogen *Plasma No Effect Analytical* No interference observed at a concentration of 15 g/L with method on Du Pont aca *1524*

Glucose *Serum No Effect Analytical* No interference observed at a concentration of 3-15 g/L with method on Du Pont aca *1527* At concentration of 15 g/L has no effect on method on Du Pont Dimension *1575* At concentration of 1500 mg/L had no effect on hexokinase/G-6-PDH method *5704*

Lipase *Serum No Effect Analytical* No effect observed at a concentration of 2.5 g/dL with revised method incorporating colipase on Du Pont aca *4702*

Dextroamphetamine

Amphetamine *Serum No Effect Physiological* Not detected after 30 mg/d *3868*
Urine Positive Analytical At concentration of 0.7 µg/mL (5.18 µmol/L) produced positive result with method on Du Pont aca *1554*

Corticosteroids *Plasma Increase Physiological* Effect most marked in evenings *532*

Cortisol *Plasma Decrease Physiological* Mean reduction of 60.7 nmol/L between 9.00 am and 10.30 am in 12 depressed patients given up to 20 mg drug compared with increase of 30.3 nmol/L when given placebo *4198*

Dopamine *Urine No Effect Physiological* In children with attention deficit disorder and hyperactivity treatment with dextroamphetamine had no effect on excretion *6628*

Epinephrine *Urine Increase Physiological* For 3 h after administration *2452*

Glucose *Serum Decrease Physiological* Reported to produce decrease of fasting glucose *2452*
Serum Increase Physiological Metabolic effect *3810*
Urine Increase Physiological Will occur if hyperglycemia *3810*

4-Hydroxy-3-Methoxy-Phenylglycol
Urine Decrease Physiological In children with attention deficit disorder and hyperactivity treatment with dextroamphetamine caused significant reduction in MHPG excretion *6628*

17-Hydroxycorticosteroids *Urine No Effect Analytical* No effect on modified Glenn-Nelson procedure *2452*

17-Ketosteroids *Urine No Effect Analytical* No effect on modified Holtorff-Koch procedure *2452*

Methamphetamine *Urine No Effect Analytical* Less than 0.5% cross-reactivity with Hycor accuPINCH method *162*

Norepinephrine *Urine No Effect Physiological* In children with attention deficit disorder and hyperactivity treatment had no significant effect on excretion *6628* No effect observed *2452*

Normetanephrine *Urine No Effect Physiological* In children with attention deficit disorder and hyperactivity treatment with dextroamphetamine had no significant effect on excretion *6628*

Phenylalanine *Plasma No Effect Analytical* No interference observed from dexamphetamine sulfate with rapid quantitative whole blood method of Campbell et al using phenylalanine dehydrogenase *867*

Phenylethylamine *Urine Increase Physiological* In children with attention deficit disorder and hyperactivity treatment with dextroamphetamine caused 1600% increase in excretion *6628*

Platelets *Blood Decrease Physiological* Thrombocytopenia reported to occur *2385*

Vanillylmandelic Acid *Urine No Effect Analytical* Apparently no method interference *2452*
Urine No Effect Physiological No physiological effect *2452*

Dextromethorphan

Amphetamine *Urine No Effect Analytical* Observed result with Du Pont aca at a concentration of 1000 µg/L (3.68 mmol/L) *1554*

Benzodiazepine *Urine No Effect Analytical* Negative result observed at a concentration of 1000 µg/mL (3.68 mmol/L) with method on Du Pont aca *1556*

Benzoylecgonine *Urine No Effect Analytical* Negative result obtained at a concentration of 175 µg/mL (0.64 mmol/L) with method on Du Pont aca *1558*

Bromide *Serum Increase Physiological* Theoretical possibility if hydrobromide salt is administered since drug contains 43% bromide *5116*

Cannabinoids *Urine No Effect Analytical* No effect on Roche Abuscreen method *5006*

Carbon Dioxide Partial Pressure
Blood Increase Physiological High doses may produce respiratory depression *2242*

Drugs of Abuse Screen *Urine No Effect Analytical* No effect at concentration of 100 µg/mL on EZ-SCREEN procedure for cannabinoids and cocaine *1739*

Histamine *Plasma No Effect Analytical* Although 50% inhibition of radio-enzyme assay at 8.5 µg/mL unlikely to be of clinical significance since therapeutic concentration about 0.08 µg/mL *2492*

Morphine *Urine No Effect Analytical* Insignificant cross reactivity with RIA procedures Insignificant cross react with hemagglutination inhibition. Insignificant cross reactivity with EMIT procedure for opiates *4163*

Opiates *Urine No Effect Analytical* No effect observed at a concentration of 175 µg/mL (0.64 mmol/L) with method on Du Pont aca *1559*

Phencyclidine *Urine No Effect Analytical* Cross-reactivity of only 0.01% observed with Roche Abuscreen method adapted for use with the Roche Cobas Mira *909*

Platelets *Blood Decrease Physiological* Thrombocytopenia (AMA Blood dyscrasias) *4017*

Theophylline *Serum No Effect Analytical* No effect on Kodak Ektachem® 700 method *1716*

Tricyclic Antidepressants Screen
Serum No Effect Analytical No significant efffect observed at a concentration of 1000 µg/mL (2.84 mmol/L) with method on Du Pont aca *1550*

Dextromoramide

Epinephrine *Plasma Decrease Physiological* Mechanism obscure *2854*

Norepinephrine *Plasma Decrease Physiological* Mechanism obscure *2854*

Dextropropoxyphene

p-Aminophenol *Urine No Effect Analytical* With addition of drugs at a concentration of 100 mg/L and of related compounds at 50 mg/L no significant effect observed on colorimetric method of van Bocxlaer on Cobas Mira analyzer which involves reacting free p-aminophenol with resorcinol in the presence of magnesium ions to form an indophenol dye measured at 550 nm *6163*

Dextrose

Bicarbonate *Serum No Effect Analytical* At concentration of 10.0 mg/mL (55.5 mmol/L) had no effect on method on Du Pont aca *1514*

Dextrothyroxine

Basal Metabolic Rate *Patient No Effect Physiological* No significant effect noted in normal subjects *51*

Bilirubin *Serum Increase Physiological* One case of possible cholestasis reported *51*

Cholesterol *Serum Decrease Physiological* Therapeutic intent (enhances excretion) *2451* Concentration reduced by more than 20% in hypercholesterolemic patients due to stimulated liver LDL receptor synthesis *5586*
Serum No Effect Analytical No effect at concentrations up to 0.75 mg/L on method on Kodak Ektachem® *5706*

Factor VII *Plasma Decrease Physiological* Reported effect *51*

Factor VIII *Plasma Decrease Physiological* Reported effect *51*

Factor IX *Plasma Decrease Physiological* Reported effect *51*

Glucose *Serum Increase Physiological* Increase observed probably related to metabolic effect when administered with antidiabetic drugs *206* Effect seen in diabetics *2451*
Urine Increase Physiological Occurs due to hyperglycemia *2451*

HDL-Cholesterol *Serum Decrease Physiological* Increased catabolism *264*

^{131}I Uptake *Serum Decrease Physiological* Marked effect observed even in normals *51*
Serum No Effect Physiological No effect reported *3669*

LDL-Cholesterol *Serum Decrease Physiological* Concentration reduced by more than 20% in hypercholesterolemic patients due to stimulation of LDL receptor synthesis *5586*

Lipids *Serum Decrease Physiological* Therapeutic effect *51*

β-Lipoprotein *Serum Decrease Physiological* Therapeutic effect *128*

Phospholipids *Serum Decrease Physiological* Therapeutic effect *128*

Prothrombin Time *Plasma Increase Physiological* Increases receptor site affinity for anticoagulants *5676*

T3-Uptake *Serum Increase Physiological* Binds to usual T4 sites, decreases thyroxine binding globulin *882*

Thyroxine (T4) *Serum Increase Analytical* Cross-reactivity of 58.0% observed with method on Baxter Stratus *5705*
Serum Increase Physiological Mechanism not discussed *2451*

Thyroxine (T4), Free *Serum No Effect Analytical* Has cross-reactivity of 62.8% with method on Baxter Stratus *5705*

Thyroxine (T4) (Murphy-Pattee) *Serum Increase Analytical* Reacts as if levo compound *882*

Tri-iodothyronine (T3) *Serum No Effect Analytical* Cross-reactivity of 0.2% observed with method on Baxter Stratus *5705*

Triglycerides *Serum Decrease Physiological* Therapeutic effect *128*

Dezocine

Alkaline Phosphatase *Serum Increase Physiological* Increased activity reported to occur in less than 1% of 2192 treated patients *272*

Aspartate Aminotransferase *Serum Increase Physiological* Increased activity reported to occur in less than 1% of 2192 treated patients *272*

Diallylbarbituric Acid

Cannabinoids *Urine No Effect Analytical* No effect on Roche Abuscreen method *5006*

1,2-Diaminopropane

Creatinine Clearance *Urine Decrease Physiological* In 11 patients who showed glomerular injury including minimal change nephrotic syndrome with a membranous pattern of immune complex deposition as well as other patterns of deposition *1934*

Leukocytes *Blood Decrease Physiological* In 3% of 90 patients with rheumatoid arthritis *2413*

Platelets *Blood Decrease Physiological* In 3% of 90 patients with rheumatoid arthritis *2413*

Protein *Urine Increase Physiological* Good correlation between amount of protein and duration of proteinuria moderate doses not preclude reinstitution of therapy once protein has cleared *4270* In 16% of 90 patients with rheumatoid arthritis *2413* HLA DRB positive patients had 11 times risk of this side effect than those antigen *2289*

Pyruvate Kinase *Red Blood Cells Decrease Analytical* Most marked with larger side chain *592*

Diapamide

Chloride *Urine Increase Physiological* Diuretic action *3717*

Glucose *Serum Increase Physiological* Alters glucose tolerance *3717*
Urine Increase Physiological Result of marked hyperglycemia *3717*

Glucose Tolerance *Serum Decrease Physiological* Modification of glucose tolerance *3717*

Potassium *Serum Decrease Physiological* Diuretic action *3717*
Urine Increase Physiological Diuretic action *3717*

Sodium *Urine Increase Physiological* Diuretic action *3717*

Uric Acid *Serum Increase Physiological* Impaired excretion *3717*

Volume *Urine Increase Physiological* Diuretic action *3717*

Diaprim

Leukocytes *Blood Decrease Physiological* Leukopenia *4013*

Diazepam

Acetaminophen *Serum No Effect Analytical* No interference observed at a concentration of 2000 µg/mL (700 µmol/L) with method on Du Pont aca *1506* At concentration of 2 mg/L had no effect on HPLC method *5775*

Acid Phosphatase *Serum No Effect Analytical* At concentration of 20 µg/dL (70 µmol/L) had no effect on method on Du Pont Dimension *1562*

Alanine Aminotransferase *Serum Increase Physiological* Isolated case of drug induced hepatitis *5975*
Serum No Effect Analytical At 5 times upper limit of therapeutic range on methods on Technicon SMAC® , Abbott-VP,

Diazepam *(continued)*

Alanine Aminotransferase *(continued)*
Du Pont aca, Roche Cobas-Bio, and KDA *3525* No effect at concentration of 20 µg/mL (70 µmol/L) on method on Du Pont Dimension *1563* At acute overdose concentration (2.5 mg/dL) on Technicon SMAC® method *6266*

Albumin *Serum No Effect Analytical* At concentration of 25 mg/L had no effect on BCG method *5704* At acute overdose concentration (2.5 mg/dL) on Technicon SMAC® method *6266* No effect observed at a concentration of 0.8 mg/L (2.8 µmol/L) with method on Du Pont aca *1507* At concentration of 20 µg/dL (70 µmol/L) had no effect on method on Du Pont Dimension *1564* At 5 times upper limit of therapeutic range on methods on Technicon SMAC®, Kodak Ektachem®, Hitachi® 705 and KDA *3525*
Urine No Effect Analytical Using a fluorimetric assay with Albumin Blue 580 on a Cobas Fara centrifugal analyzer for the detection of microalbuminuria no significant interference was detected at a concentration of 4 mg/L *3117*

Alkaline Phosphatase *Serum Increase Physiological* Mild effect reported in one patient *3053* Isolated case of drug induced hepatitis *5975*
Serum No Effect Analytical At 5 times upper limit of therapeutic range on methods on Technicon SMAC®, Abbott-VP, Du Pont aca, Roche Cobas-Bio, Hitachi® 705 and KDA *3525* At acute overdose concentration (2.5 mg/dL) on Technicon SMAC® method *6266* At concentration of 20 µg/dL (70 µmol/L) had no effect on method on Du Pont Dimension *1565*

δ-Aminolevulinic Acid *Urine Increase Physiological* May precipitate attack of acute porphyria *1687*

Amitriptyline *Serum No Effect Physiological* No effect on serum concentration if given together *5559*

Ammonia *Plasma No Effect Analytical* No effect at concentration of 20 µg/mL (70 µmol/L) on method on Du Pont Dimension *1566*

Amylase *Serum No Effect Analytical* At concentration of 20 µg/mL (70 µmol/L) had no effect on method on Du Pont Dimension *1567* At 5 times upper limit of therapeutic range on methods on Du Pont aca, Roche Cobas-Bio, and Kodak Ektachem® *3525*

Aspartate Aminotransferase *Serum Increase Physiological* Isolated case of drug induced hepatitis *5975*
Serum No Effect Analytical At 5 times upper limit of therapeutic range on methods on Technicon SMAC®, Abbott-VP, Du Pont aca, Roche Cobas-Bio, Hitachi® 705 and KDA *3525* At acute overdose concentration (2.5 mg/dL) on Technicon SMAC® method *6266* No effect at concentration of 20 µg/dL (70 µmol/L) on method on Du Pont Dimension *1568*

Barbiturate *Serum No Effect Analytical* No significant interference observed at a concentration of 100 µg/mL (0.35 mmol/L) with method on Du Pont aca *1511*

Benzodiazepine *Urine Positive Analytical* Positive result observed at a concentration of 2.0 µg/mL (7.01 µmol/L) with method on Du Pont aca *1556* Detectable limit 0.06 µg/mL with improved assay and Syva ETS system compared with 0.2 µg/mL with former d.a.u. assay *3370*

Bicarbonate *Serum No Effect Analytical* At concentration of 1.5 mg/L had no effect on method using phenolphthalein *5704*

Bilirubin *Serum Increase Physiological* Presumed hepatic toxic effect *6515*
Serum No Effect Analytical At acute overdose concentration (2.5 mg/dL) on Technicon SMAC® method *6266* At concentration of 25 mg/L had no effect on Jendrassik and Grof method *5704* No effect at concentration of 20 µg/mL (70 µmol/L) on method on Du Pont Dimension *1589* At 5 times upper limit of therapeutic range on methods on Technicon SMAC®, Du Pont aca, Roche Cobas-Bio, Kodak Ektachem®, Hitachi® 705 and KDA *3525*
Serum No Effect Physiological Insignificant displacement from protein in neonates *6314*

Bilirubin, Conjugated *Serum No Effect Analytical* No effect at concentration of 10 mg/L on method on Kodak Ektachem® *5706*

Bilirubin, Direct *Serum No Effect Analytical* At concentration of 20 µg/mL (70 µmol/L) had no effect on method on Du Pont Dimension *1574*

Bilirubin, Unconjugated *Serum No Effect Analytical* No effect at concentration of 10 mg/L on method on Kodak Ektachem® *5706*

Busulphan *Serum No Effect Physiological* In 8 patients prior to bone-marrow transplantation concentration of 453 ± 118 ng/mL after pretreatment with diazepam not significantly different from mean concentration of 481 ± 98 ng/mL in the absence of diazepam: no effect observed on pharmacokinetics *2503*

Calcium *Serum No Effect Analytical* At concentration of 25 mg/L had no effect on cresolphthalein method *5704* At 5 times upper limit of therapeutic range on methods on Technicon SMAC®, Abbott-VP, Du Pont aca, Kodak Ektachem®, Hitachi® 705 and KDA *3525* At acute overdose concentration (2.5 mg/dL) on Technicon SMAC® method *6266* No effect at concentration of 20 µg/dL (70 µmol/L) on method on Du Pont Dimension *1569*
Serum No Effect Physiological No effect when given in normal therapeutic amounts to elderly *6618*

Cannabinoids *Urine No Effect Analytical* No effect on Roche Abuscreen method *5006*

Carbamazepine *Serum No Effect Analytical* No cross-reactivity observed with method on Du Pont aca *1513*

Carbon Dioxide Partial Pressure
Blood Increase Physiological In healthy volunteers but change of short duration *1748*

Catecholamines *Plasma No Effect Analytical* No effect on HPLC method of Koller for dopamine, epinephrine, and norepinephrine *3230*
Urine No Effect Physiological No effect with short term ingestion of 15 mg/d *1184*

Chloride *Serum No Effect Analytical* At concentration of 1.5 mg/L had no effect on mercurimetric method *5704*

Cholesterol *Serum No Effect Analytical* At concentration of 1.5 mg/L had no effect on CHOD-PAP method *5704* At concentration of 20 µg/mL (70 µmol/L) had no effect on method on Du Pont Dimension *1570* At acute overdose concentration (2.5 mg/dL) on Technicon SMAC® method *6266* At 5 times upper limit of therapeutic range on methods on Technicon SMAC®, Abbott-VP, Roche Cobas-Bio, Kodak Ektachem®, Hitachi® 705 and KDA *3525* At concentration of 25 mg/L had no effect on Liebermann-Burchard method *5704*

Cholinesterase *Serum No Effect Analytical* Insignificant decrease of 0.05 U/mL at a concentration of 20 µg/mL with method on Du Pont aca *3271* Insignificant increase of 0.07 U/mL at a concentration of 20 µg/mL with method on Du Pont Dimension *3271*

Creatine Kinase *Serum No Effect Analytical* At acute overdose concentration (2.5 mg/dL) on Technicon SMAC® method *6266* At 5 times upper limit of therapeutic range on methods on Technicon SMAC®, Abbott-VP, Du Pont aca, Roche Cobas-Bio, and Hitachi® 705 *3525*

Creatine Kinase Isoenzymes *Serum No Effect Analytical* At concentration of 20 µg/mL (20 µmol/L) had no effect on method for CK-MB on Du Pont Dimension *1571*

Creatinine *Serum No Effect Analytical* At 5 times upper limit of therapeutic range on methods on Technicon SMAC®, Abbott-VP, Du Pont aca, Roche Cobas-Bio, Kodak Ektachem®, Hitachi® 705 and KDA *3525* No effect of concentrations up to 10 mg/L on 2-slide method on Kodak Ektachem® *5706* At concentration of 25 mg/L had no effect on Technicon AutoAnalyzer® Jaffe method *5704* At acute overdose concentration (2.5 mg/dL) on Technicon SMAC® method *6266* At 50 mg/L on reversed phase liquid chromatographic procedure of Zhiri et al *6656* No effect at concentration of 20 µg/mL (70 µmol/L) on method on Du Pont Dimension *1572*

Digoxin *Serum Increase Physiological* Half-life increased and reduced urinary excretion observed but mechanism not yet established *918*

Disopyramide *Serum No Effect Physiological* When drugs coadministered no significant effect observed on the pharmacokinetics of either drug *2069*

Doxazosin *Serum No Effect Physiological* Coadministration with doxazosin had no effect on its pharmacokinetics *4642*

Drugs of Abuse Screen *Urine No Effect Analytical* No effect at concentration of 100 µg/mL on EZ-SCREEN procedure for cannabinoids and cocaine *1739*

Epinephrine *Urine No Effect Physiological* No effect with short term ingestion of 15 mg/d *1184*

Estradiol *Plasma Increase Physiological* Observed in 5 of 5 men with gynecomastia *509*

Ethosuximide *Serum No Effect Analytical* Insignificant cross-reactivity observed with method on Du Pont aca *1523*

Fosphenytoin *Serum No Effect Physiological* Diazepam had no effect on the protein binding or pharmacokinetics of fosphenytoin when coadministered *4519*

Glucose *Serum Decrease Physiological* Incidence of 0.4% observed in French Pharmacovigilance database *4106*
Serum No Effect Analytical At 5 times upper limit of therapeutic range on methods on Technicon SMAC® , Abbott-VP, Du Pont aca, Roche Cobas-Bio, Kodak Ektachem® , Hitachi® 705 and KDA *3525* At concentration of 4 mg/L had no effect on Kodak Ektachem® method *5704* At concentration of 20 µg/mL (70 µmol/L) has no effect on method on Du Pont Dimension *1575* At concentration of 1.5 mg/L had no effect on GOD/POD-PAP method *5704* At acute overdose concentration (2.5 mg/dL) on Technicon SMAC® method *6266*
Urine Decrease Analytical Low with Clinistix® and Diastix® test strips *1826*
Urine No Effect Analytical No effect observed on TesTape® *1826*

γ-Glutamyltransferase *Serum No Effect Analytical* At 5 times upper limit of therapeutic range on methods on Technicon SMAC® , Abbott-VP, and Hitachi® 705 *3525* At concentration of 20 µg/mL (70 µmol/L) has no effect on method on Du Pont Dimension *1579*

Growth Hormone *Plasma Increase Physiological* Response to diazepam much less in both treated and untreated patients with epilepsy than in controls *2008*

HDL-Cholesterol *Serum No Effect Analytical* No effect at concentration of 20 µg/mL (70 µmol/L) has no effect on method on Du Pont Dimension *1576*

Histamine *Plasma No Effect Analytical* Improbable inhibition of radio-enzyme assay likely at physiological concentrations *2492*

Homovanillic Acid
Cerebrospinal Fluid Decrease Physiological Probably due to decreased turnover of dopamine *4505*

Hydrochloric Acid *Gastric Fluid Decrease Physiological* Presumed central action lasts for 5 h after 10 mg *580*

11-Hydroxycorticosteroids *Urine No Effect Physiological* No effect with short term ingestion of 15 mg/d *1184*

17-Hydroxycorticosteroids *Urine No Effect Physiological* No effect with short term ingestion of 15 mg/d *1184*

5-Hydroxyindoleacetic Acid *Urine Increase Analytical* With method of Udenfriend et al Due to reaction of nitrosonaphthol on the reactive fused benzene ring of the benzodiazepine nucleus. Effect unlikely to produce clinical misinterpretation. Effect also seen with N-desmethyldiazepam *1051*

^{131}I Uptake *Serum Decrease Physiological* Conflicting reports. ?no effect *2024*
Serum No Effect Physiological No effect after i.v. administration *882*

Iron *Serum No Effect Analytical* At acute overdose concentration (2.5 mg/dL) on Technicon SMAC® method *6266* At concentration of 25 mg/L had no effect on Ferrozine method *5704* At 5 times upper limit of therapeutic range on Ferrozine method on Technicon SMAC® *3525* No effect at concentration of 20 µg/mL (70 µmol/L) on method on Du Pont Dimension *1577*

Iron-Binding Capacity, Total *Serum No Effect Analytical* No effect at concentration of 20 µg/mL (70 µmol/L) on method on Du Pont Dimension *1590*

17-Ketosteroids *Urine No Effect Physiological* No effect with short term ingestion of 15 mg/d *1184*

Lactate Dehydrogenase *Serum No Effect Analytical* At 5 times upper limit of therapeutic range on methods on Technicon SMAC® , Abbott-VP, Roche Cobas-Bio, Hitachi® 705 and KDA *3525* At concentration of 20 µg/dL (70 µmol/L) has no effect on method on Du Pont Dimension *1578* At acute overdose concentration (2.5 mg/dL) on Technicon SMAC® method *6266*

Leukocytes *Blood Decrease Physiological* Leukopenia *5012*

Lipase *Serum No Effect Analytical* No effect at concentration of 20 µg/mL (70 µmol/L) on method on Du Pont Dimension *1580*

Magnesium *Serum No Effect Analytical* No effect at concentration of 20 µg/mL (70 µmol/L) on method on Du Pont Dimension *1581*

Midazolam *Serum No Effect Analytical* On GC-ECD method of Ha et al *2387*

Mitrazepine *Serum No Effect Physiological* Concomitant administration of diazepam (15 mg) had minimal effect on the plasma concentration of mitrazepine (after 15 mg) in 12 healthy men *4434*

Mycophenolic Acid *Serum No Effect Analytical* No significant interference observed with HPLC method of Shipkova et al *5526*

Mycophenolic Acid Glucuronide
Serum No Effect Analytical No significant interference observed with HPLC method of Shipkova et al *5526*

Neutrophils *Blood Decrease Physiological* Occasional case of agranulocytosis reported *6264* Transitory neutropenia reported *128*

Norepinephrine *Urine No Effect Physiological* No effect with short term ingestion of 15 mg/d *1184*

Nortriptyline *Serum No Effect Physiological* No effect on serum concentration if given together *5559*

o-Desmethylvenlafaxine *Serum No Effect Physiological* When a single 10 mg dose of diazepam was administered to 18 healthy men no effect observed on steady state pharmacokinetics of venlafaxine or o-desmethylvenlafaxine when venlafaxine administered 50 mg every 8 hours *6555*

Oxygen Partial Pressure *Blood Decrease Physiological* In healthy volunteers but changes of short duration *1748*
Blood Increase Physiological In healthy volunteers but changes of short duration *1748*

p-Aminophenol *Urine No Effect Analytical* With addition of drugs at a concentration of 100 mg/L and of related compounds at 50 mg/L no significant effect observed on colorimetric method of van Bocxlaer on Cobas Mira analyzer which involves reacting free p-aminophenol with resorcinol in the presence of magnesium ions to form an indophenol dye measured at 550 nm *6163*

Paroxetine *Serum No Effect Physiological* No significant effect on the pharmacokinetics of paroxetine observed when the drugs coadministered *5654*

Phenobarbital *Serum No Effect Analytical* No significant cross-reactivity observed with method on Du Pont aca *1537* At concentration of 1.00 mg/mL (3.51 mmol/L) has no effect on method on Du Pont Dimension *1582*

Phenylalanine *Plasma No Effect Analytical* No interference observed with rapid quantitative whole blood method of Campbell et al using phenylalanine dehydrogenase *867*

Phenytoin *Serum Increase Physiological* Coadministration with phenytoin may increase plasma phenytoin concentration *4522* From 20 to 40 µg/mL (unknown dose) inhibits metabolism *4011*
Serum No Effect Analytical No significant interference observed at a concentration of 100 µg/mL (351 µmol/L) with method on Du Pont aca *1538*
Serum No Effect Physiological Diazepam had no effect on the protein binding or pharmacokinetics of phenytoin when coadministered *4519*

Phosphate *Serum No Effect Analytical* At concentration of 25 mg/L had no effect on phosphomolybdate method *5704* At 5 times upper limit of therapeutic range on methods on Technicon SMAC® , Du Pont aca, Hitachi® 705 and KDA *3525* At concentration of 20 µg/mL (70 µmol/L) has no effect on method on Du Pont Dimension *1584* At acute overdose concentration (2.5 mg/dL) on Technicon SMAC® method *6266*

Porphyrin, Total *Urine Increase Physiological* May precipitate attack of acute porphyria *1687*

Potassium *Serum No Effect Analytical* At concentration of 10 mg/L had no effect on measurement by ISE with predilution *5704* At concentration of 1.5 mg/L had no effect on flamephotometric method *5704*

Prazosin *Serum No Effect Physiological* Coadministration of prazosin with diazepam had no apparent adverse drug interaction in limited clinical experience *4649*

Diazepam *(continued)*

Primidone *Serum No Effect Analytical* No significant cross-reactivity with method on Du Pont aca *1541*

Prolactin *Plasma No Effect Physiological* No effect with 20 mg given i.m *2352*

Protein *Serum No Effect Analytical* At concentration of 25 mg/L had no effect on biuret method with blank correction *5704* At acute overdose concentration (2.5 mg/dL) on Technicon SMAC® method *6266* At 5 times upper limit of therapeutic range on methods on Technicon SMAC® , Abbott-VP, Kodak Ektachem® , Hitachi® 705 and KDA *3525*

Prothrombin Time *Plasma No Effect Physiological* No effect when given 15 mg/d *4436*

Sodium *Serum No Effect Analytical* At concentration of 1.5 mg/L had no effect on flame-photometric method *5704* At concentration of 10 mg/L had no effect on measurement by ISE with predilution *5704*

T3-Uptake *Serum Decrease Physiological* Resin test affected *3669*

Serum No Effect Analytical No significant effect observed at a concentration of 20 µg/mL (70 µmol/L) with method on Du Pont aca *1545* At concentration of 20 µg/mL (70 µmol/L) has no effect on method on Du Pont Dimension *1586*

Serum No Effect Physiological No effect after i.v. administration *882*

Tacrolimus *Serum No Effect Analytical* In HPLC/MS method of Christians et al no significant interference observed with measurement of FK 506 *1010*

Theophylline *Serum No Effect Analytical* At concentration of 20 µg/mL (70 µmol/L) had negligible effect on method on Du Pont Dimension *1591*

Thyroxine (T4) *Serum Decrease Physiological* Due to competition for transport proteins *6412*

Serum No Effect Analytical No significant effect observed at a concentration of 20 µg/dL (70 µmol/L) with method on Du Pont aca *1546* At concentration of 20 µg/mL (70 µmol/L) has no effect on method on Du Pont Dimension *1587* No significant effect observed at a concentration of 20 µg/dL (70 µmol/L) with method on Du Pont aca *1588*

Serum No Effect Physiological Conflicting reports. ?no effect *2451*

Tirofiban *Serum No Effect Physiological* Coadministration had no significant effect on plasma clearance of tirofiban *3957*

Tricyclic Antidepressants Screen

Serum No Effect Analytical No significant effect observed at a concentration of 500 µg/mL (1.76 mmol/L) with method on Du Pont aca *1550*

Triglycerides *Serum No Effect Analytical* At concentration of 20 µg/mL (70 µmol/L) has no effect on method on Du Pont Dimension *1592* At 5 times upper limit of therapeutic range on methods on Technicon SMAC® , Abbott-VP, Kodak Ektachem® , Hitachi® 705 and KDA *3525* At concentration of 25 mg/L had no effect on lipase/esterase method *5704* At acute overdose concentration (2.5 mg/dL) on Technicon SMAC® method *6266*

Urea Nitrogen *Serum Increase Physiological* Slight elevation in one hypertensive *3053*

Serum No Effect Analytical At concentration of 25 mg/L had no effect on diacetylmonoxime method *5704* At concentration of 4 mg/L had no effect on Kodak Ektachem® method *5704* At acute overdose concentration (2.5 mg/dL) on Technicon SMAC® method *6266* No effect at concentration of 20 µg/dL (70 µmol/L) on method on Du Pont Dimension *1593* At 5 times upper limit of therapeutic range on methods on chnicon SMAC® , Abbott-VP, Roche Cobas-Bio, Kodak Ektachem® , Hitachi® 705 and KDA *3525*

Uric Acid *Serum No Effect Analytical* No effect at concentration of 20 µg/mL (70 µmol/L) on method on Du Pont Dimension *1594* At acute overdose concentration (2.5 mg/dL) on Technicon SMAC® method *6266* At 50 mg/L on reversed phase liquid chromatographic procedure of Zhiri et al *6656* At concentration of 25 mg/L had no effect on phosphotungstate reduction method *5704* At 5 times upper limit of therapeutic range on methods on Technicon SMAC® , Abbott-VP, Du Pont aca, Roche Cobas-Bio, Kodak Ektachem® , Hitachi® 705 and KDA *3525*

Valproic Acid *Serum No Effect Analytical* No significant interference observed at a concentration of 100 µg/mL (351 µmol/L) with method on Du Pont aca *1560* At concentrations up to 100 µg/mL had no significant cross-reactivity in valproic acid method on Bayer Technicon Immuno 1® *437*

Venlafaxine *Serum No Effect Physiological* When a single 10 mg dose of diazepam was administered to 18 healthy men no effect observed on steady state pharmacokinetics of venlafaxine or o-desmethylvenlafaxine when venlafaxine administered 50 mg every 8 hours *6555*

Volume *Gastric Fluid Decrease Physiological* Presumed central action lasts for 5 h after 10 mg *580*

Diaziquone

Alanine Aminotransferase *Serum Increase Physiological* Mild increases occasionally observed *1384*

Aspartate Aminotransferase *Serum Increase Physiological* Mild increases occasionally observed *1384*

Erythrocytes *Blood Decrease Physiological* Myelosuppression is dose-limiting toxicity *1384*

Leukocytes *Blood Decrease Physiological* Myelosuppression is dose-limiting toxicity *1384*

Platelets *Blood Decrease Physiological* Myelosuppression is dose-limiting toxicity *1384*

Diazo Dyes

T3-Uptake *Serum Increase Physiological* Compete for binding sites *882*

Thyroxine (T4) *Serum Decrease Physiological* Compete for binding sites *882*

Diazoxide

Albumin *Urine Increase Physiological* Albuminuria reported to occur as a frequent side effect *337*

Alkaline Phosphatase *Serum Increase Physiological* Increased activity reported to occur as a frequent side effect *337*

Amylase *Serum Increase Physiological* May cause acute pancreatitis rarely *5332* Acute pancreatitis or pancreatic necrosis reported to occur as a frequent side effect *337*

Androstenedione *Plasma No Effect Physiological* 300 mg daily for 10 days caused no effect on concentration in 5 obese women with polycystic ovary disease *4250*

Aspartate Aminotransferase *Serum Increase Physiological* Increased activity reported to occur as a frequent side effect *337*

Bicarbonate *Urine Decrease Physiological* Effect not as marked as on sodium excretion *188*

Catecholamines *Plasma Increase Physiological* Increased release from tissue *208*

Chloride *Serum Increase Physiological* May cause salt retention *2242*

Urine Decrease Physiological Decreased excretion observed as a side effect *337* Effect over 2 h of 4 mg/kg given i.v. or orally *2951*

Cortisol *Plasma Decrease Physiological* Decreased secretion reported to occur following drug administration *337*

Plasma Increase Physiological May cause decreased secretion *5332*

Creatinine Clearance *Urine Decrease Physiological* Decreased clearance reported to occur as a frequent side effect *337* Effect over 2 h of 4 mg/kg given i.v *2951*

Dehydroepiandrosterone Sulfate

Plasma No Effect Physiological 300 mg daily for 10 days had no effect on concentration in 5 obese women with polycystic ovary disease *4250*

Effective Renal Plasma Flow

Patient Decrease Physiological After i.v. injection immediate reduction noted *188*

Eosinophils *Blood Increase Physiological* Eosinophilia may occur *337*

Erythrocytes *Urine Increase Physiological* Hematuria reported to occur as a frequent side effect *337*

Estradiol *Plasma No Effect Physiological* 300 mg daily for 10 days had no effect on concentration in 5 obese women with polycystic ovary disease *4250*

Estrone *Plasma No Effect Physiological* 300 mg daily for 10 days had no effect on concentration in 5 obese women with polycystic ovary disease *4250*

Fatty Acids (FFA), Free *Serum Increase Physiological* Significant rise observed after oral or i.v. administration *188* Increased plasma concentration observed as a side effect *337*

Follicle Stimulating Hormone
Plasma No Effect Physiological 300 mg daily for 10 days administered to 5 obese women with polycystic ovary disease had no effect on serum concentration or LH to FSH ratio *4250*

Glomerular Filtration Rate *Urine Decrease Physiological* Effect over 2 h of 4 mg/kg given i.v *2951*
Urine No Effect Physiological Decreased PAH clearance observed without appreciable effect on glomerular filtration rate *337*

Glucose *Serum Increase Physiological* Predictable effect due to direct inhibition of insulin secretion *697* 300 mg daily for 10 days in 5 obese women with polycystic ovary disease caused increase in fasting concentration from mean of 4.91 mmol/L to 6.64 mmol/L *4250* Inhibits insulin release, peripheral glucose utilization *973* May cause hyperglycemia, especially in diabetics after repeated injections of diazoxide *5332* Oral administration produces a prompt dose-related increase in blood glucose concentration, due primarily to inhibition of insulin release from the pancreas as well as to an extrapancreatic effect. Response begins within 1 h and lasts no more than 8 hours in the presence of normal renal function. Hyperglycemia is reversible with insulin or tolbutamide *337*
Urine Increase Physiological If hyperglycemia occurs *973* Oral administration produces a prompt dose-related increase in blood glucose concentration with resulting increased urinary excretion *337*

Glucose Tolerance *Serum Decrease Physiological* 300 mg daily administered to 5 obese women with polycystic ovary disease caused increased concentration and prolonged rise with no reduction in concentration at 3 hours *4250*

Hematocrit *Blood Decrease Physiological* Decreased hemoglobin and hematocrit may occur with excessive bleeding *337*

Hemoglobin *Blood Decrease Physiological* Decreased hemoglobin and hematocrit may occur with excessive bleeding *337*
Urine Increase Physiological Hematuria reported to occur as a frequent side effect *337*

Immunoglobulin G *Serum Decrease Physiological* Decreased concentration reported to occur as a frequent side effect *337* Effect may be persistent. ?mechanism *188*
Serum Increase Physiological May cause increased concentration *5332* Increased concentration reported to occur following drug administration *337*

Insulin *Plasma Decrease Physiological* After 300 mg daily for 10 days fasting concentration in 5 obese women with polycystic ovary syndrome decreased from mean of 177 pmol/L to 123 pmol/L *4250*

Insulin response to Glucagon
Plasma Decrease Physiological May cause false negative insulin response to glucagon *5332*

Inulin Clearance *Urine Decrease Physiological* Effect over 2 h of 4 mg/kg given i.v *2951*

Ketones *Serum Increase Physiological* Infrequently diabetic ketoacidosis and hyperosmolar nonketotic coma may develop rapidly *337*

Leukocytes *Blood Decrease Physiological* May cause leukopenia *6306*

Lipase *Serum Increase Physiological* Acute pancreatitis or pancreatic necrosis reported to occur as a frequent side effect *337* May cause acute pancreatitis rarely *5332*

Luteinizing Hormone *Plasma No Effect Physiological* 300 mg daily for 10 days had no effect on serum concentration, pulse frequency and amplitude, and LH to FSH ratio in 5 obese women with polycystic ovary disease. Integrated response to stimulation by GnRH also unaffected *4250*

Neutrophils *Blood Decrease Physiological* Occasional case of agranulocytosis reported *6264* Transient neutropenia may occur but is not associated with increased susceptibility to infection and ordinarily does not require discontinuation of the drug *337*

Osmolar Clearance *Urine Decrease Physiological* Effect over 2 h of 4 mg/kg given i.v *2951*

PAH Clearance *Urine Decrease Physiological* Effect over 2 h of 4 mg/kg given i.v *2951* Decreased clearance observed without appreciable effect on glomerular filtration rate *337*

pH *Urine Decrease Physiological* Due to decreased bicarbonate excretion *188*

Phenytoin *Serum Decrease Physiological* Greatly reduced serum concentration observed in children with increased urinary excretion suggesting enhanced metabolism *5058*

Platelets *Blood Decrease Physiological* Thrombocytopenia may occur with or without purpura and may require discontinuation of the drug *337* Immunologic response occurs from days to months *6306*

Potassium *Urine Decrease Physiological* Effect over 2 h of 4 mg/kg given i.v *2951*

Progesterone *Plasma No Effect Physiological* 300 mg daily for 10 days had no effect on concentration in 5 obese women with polycystic ovary disease *4250*

Prothrombin Time *Plasma Increase Physiological* Displaces anticoagulants from albumin *5440*

Renin Activity *Plasma Increase Physiological* May cause increased renin secretion *5332* Increased renin secretion reported to occur following drug administration *337* Effect observed in some hypertensives *2242*

Sex-Hormone Binding Globulin
Serum Increase Physiological Nonsignificant increase from mean concentration of 70 nmol/L to 80 nmol/L in 5 normal nonobese women given 300 mg daily for 10 days *4252* Slight but insignificant increase in 5 obese women with polycystic ovary disease given 300 mg daily for 10 days *4250*

Sodium *Serum Increase Physiological* May cause salt retention *2242*
Urine Decrease Physiological Decreased excretion of sodium and water observed as side effects with possibly clinically significant fluid retention *337* Effect over 2 h of 4 mg/kg given i.v *2951*

Testosterone *Serum Decrease Physiological* After 300 mg/day for 10 days concentration in 5 obese women with polycystic ovary syndrome fell from mean of 2.5 nmol/L to 2.1 nmol/L *4250*
Serum No Effect Physiological In 5 nonobese normal women administration of 300 mg daily for 10 days caused increase of total testosterone from 0.69 nmol/L to 0.73 nmol/L although increase not significant *4252*

Urea Nitrogen *Serum Increase Physiological* Azotemia reported to occur as a frequent side effect *337*

Uric Acid *Serum Increase Physiological* Increased plasma concentration occurs because of decreased urinary excretion *337* Inhibition of tubular uric acid excretion *2951* May cause hyperuricemia *5332*
Urine Decrease Physiological Effect over 2 h of 4 mg/kg given i.v *2951* Decreased excretion occurs as a side effect *337*

Uric Acid Clearance *Urine Decrease Physiological* Effect over 2 h of 4 mg/kg given i.v *2951*

Volume *Plasma Increase Physiological* Causes salt and water retention *2242*
Urine Decrease Physiological Effect over 2 h of 4 mg/kg given i.v *2951* Decreased urinary output reported to occur as a frequent side effect *337*

Dibekacin

Amikacin *Serum Increase Analytical* About 7.3% cross-reactivity observed with method on Abbott TDx *3858*

Gentamicin *Serum No Effect Analytical* No interference observed with method on Abbott TDx *3858*

Kanamycin *Serum Increase Analytical* Interferes with method on Abbott TDx *3858*

Neomycin *Serum No Effect Analytical* No interference observed with method on Abbott TDx *3858*

Dibekacin *(continued)*

Netilmicin *Serum No Effect Analytical* No interference observed with method on Abbott TDx *3858*

Streptomycin *Serum No Effect Analytical* No interference observed with method on Abbott TDx *3858*

Tobramycin *Serum Increase Analytical* Interferes with method on Abbott TDx *3858*

Vancomycin *Serum No Effect Analytical* No interference observed with method on Abbott TDx *3858*

Dibenzepine

Catecholamines *Plasma No Effect Analytical* No effect on HPLC method of Koller for dopamine, epinephrine, and norepinephrine *3230*

Dichloralphenazone

δ-Aminolevulinic Acid *Urine Increase Physiological* May precipitate acute porphyria *2210*

Coproporphyrin *Feces Increase Physiological* May precipitate acute porphyria *6537*

Urine Increase Physiological May precipitate acute porphyria *2210*

Porphobilinogen *Urine Increase Physiological* May precipitate acute porphyria *2210*

Porphyrin, Total *Urine Increase Physiological* May precipitate attack of acute porphyria *1687*

Prothrombin Time *Plasma Decrease Physiological* Antagonizes action of administered coumarins *4998*

Protoporphyrin *Feces Increase Physiological* May precipitate acute porphyria *2210*

Dichlorobenzene

Protein *Urine Increase Physiological* May cause renal damage *467*

Urea Nitrogen *Serum Increase Physiological* May cause renal damage *467*

Dichlorphenamide

Chloride *Serum Increase Physiological* Administration increases the excretion of potassium and may cause hypokalemia and hyperchloremia *3968*

Granulocytes *Blood Decrease Physiological* Administration has been reported to cause agranulocytosis *3968*

Leukocytes *Blood Decrease Physiological* Administration has been reported to cause leukopenia *3968* May cause leukopenia *3810*

Platelets *Blood Decrease Physiological* Administration has been reported to cause thrombocytopenia *3968* Probable effect (like acetazolamide) *128*

Potassium *Serum Decrease Physiological* Administration increases the excretion of potassium and may cause hypokalemia *3968* Diuretic action (inhibits carbonic anhydrase) *3810*

Urine Increase Physiological Administration increases the excretion of potassium *3968*

Sodium *Serum Decrease Physiological* Cation loss as excess chloride is excreted *1009*

Uric Acid *Serum Increase Physiological* Administration may cause hyperuricemia *3968*

Diclofenac

Alanine Aminotransferase *Serum Increase Physiological* Meaningful increased activity of more than 3 times the upper limit of normal reported in about 2% of treated patients during first two weeks of treatment *1025* Incidence of acute liver injury of 3.6 per 100,000 treated patients with reported in United Kingdom. Liver damage among all cases primarily hepatocellular in some and primarily cholestatic in others *5049* Occasional cholestatic jaundice observed, most often in women and after several months treatment *1384* Liver disease observed in 7 patients treated with diclofenac for several weeks but resolved several weeks after withdrawal of drug although one fatality occurred *2546* In one patient treated with diclofenac for 13 days for arthritis attributed to gout the patient developed erythema multiforme followed by muscular weakness and an increase in CK from 101 to 83,770 U/L as a result of rhabdomyolysis with ALT activity of 131 U/L (reference range 0 - 55 U/L), rising over 17 days to 322 U/L *1374*

Serum No Effect Analytical On continuous method at 10 times maximal therapeutic concentration. On colorimetric method at 10 times maximal therapeutic concentration *2919*

Albumin *Serum Decrease Physiological* In one patient treated with diclofenac for 13 days for arthritis attributed to gout the patient developed erythema multiforme followed by muscular weakness and an increase in CK from 101 to 83,770 U/L as a result of rhabdomyolysis with a decrease in albumin concentration to 24 g/L (reference range 32 - 55 g/L) *1374* Low or low normal concentration observed in 5 patients who developed acute hepatitis within 3 months of starting drug. Effect reversible when treatment stopped *2851*

Serum No Effect Analytical On bromocresol green method on Technicon SMA II at physiological concentration *2922*

Serum No Effect Physiological No effect seen in patients undergoing treatment *2922*

Urine No Effect Analytical Using a fluorimetric assay with Albumin Blue 580 on a Cobas Fara centrifugal analyzer for the detection of microalbuminuria no significant interference was detected at a concentration of 20 mg/L *3117*

Aldolase *Serum Increase Physiological* In one patient treated with diclofenac for 13 days for arthritis attributed to gout the patient developed erythema multiforme followed by muscular weakness and an increase in CK from 101 to 83,770 U/L as a result of rhabdomyolysis with aldolase activity of 160 U/L (reference range 0 - 6 U/L) over 17 days after cessation of drug *1374*

Alkaline Phosphatase *Serum Increase Physiological* Occasional cholestatic jaundice observed, most often in women and after several months treatment *1384* Liver disease developed in 7 patients treated with diclofenac for several weeks but resolved with withdrawal of treatment although one fatality occurred *2546* Acute drug-induced hepatitis observed in 5 patients but activity reverted to normal with withdrawal of drug *2851*

Serum No Effect Analytical On continuous method at 10 times maximal therapeutic concentration *2919*

Aspartate Aminotransferase *Serum Increase Analytical* On continuous method at 10 times maximal therapeutic concentration *2919*

Serum Increase Physiological Meaningful increased activity of more than 3 times the upper limit of normal reported in about 2% of treated patients during first two months of treatment *1025* Sharp increase observed in 5 patients who developed drug-induced acute hepatitis but activity reverted to normal with withdrawal of drug *2851* Liver disease developed in 7 patients several weeks after initiation of treatment with diclofenac but resolved several weeks after withdrawal although one fatality occurred *2546* Occasional cholestatic jaundice observed, most often in women and after several months treatment *1384* In one patient treated with diclofenac for 13 days for arthritis attributed to gout the patient developed erythema multiforme followed by muscular weakness and an increase in CK from 101 to 83,770 U/L as a result of rhabdomyolysis with AST activity of 389 U/L (reference range 0 - 50 U/L), rising over 17 days to 1,505 U/L *1374* Incidence of acute liver injury of 3.6 per 100,000 treated patients with reported in United Kingdom. Liver damage among all cases primarily hepatocellular in some and primarily cholestatic in others *5049* Probability that a statistically average patient will have an AST activity greater than 1.2 times upper limit of normal within 12 weeks after beginning treatment 0.12 in osteoarthritis patients and 0.07 in rheumatoid arthritis patients compared with 0.02 and 0.01 respectively in patients treated with placebo *1991*

Serum No Effect Analytical On colorimetric method at 10 times maximal therapeutic concentration *2919*

Bilirubin *Serum Increase Physiological* Rare cases of jaundice observed in a few extreme cases liver necrosis and fulminant fatal hepatitis with or without jaundice *1025* Occasional cholestatic jaundice observed, most often in women and after several months treatment *1384* Liver disease developed several weeks after treatment initiated in 7 patients with resolution several weeks after drug withdrawn. One fatality occurred *2546* 3 of 5 patients who developed hepatitis demonstrated jaundice. Overall picture of acute hepatitis with inflammation and hepatocyte damage. Toxicity developed within 3 months of starting drug. Liver function normalized with withdrawal of drug in 4 of 5 *2851*

Serum No Effect Analytical No effect at therapeutic concentrations on methods of Jendrassik-Grof and those using spectrophotometry *2920* On diazo method on Technicon SMA II at physiological concentration *2922*

Serum No Effect Physiological No effect seen in patients undergoing treatment *2922*

Bleeding Time *Patient No Effect Physiological* Diclofenac does not affect bleeding time *1025*

Calcium *Serum No Effect Analytical* On cresolphthalein complex one method on Technicon SMA II at physiological concentration *2922* At concentration of 23 mg/L had no effect on cresolphthalein method *5704*

Serum No Effect Physiological No effect seen in patients undergoing treatment *2922*

Cholesterol *Serum Increase Physiological* Significantly higher (5.16 vs 4.60 mmol/L) than in controls *2922*

Serum No Effect Analytical On enzymatic method on Technicon SMA II at physiological concentration *2922* At concentration of 23 mg/L had no effect on CHOD-PAP method *5704* No effect at therapeutic concentrations on enzymatic and Liebermann-Burchard methods *2920*

Chondrex *Serum No Effect Analytical* Concentrations up to 5 g/L had no significant effect on sandwich-type ELISA procedure of Harvey et al *2491*

Clotting Time *Blood No Effect Physiological* Diclofenac does not affect plasma thrombin clotting time *1025*

Cortisol *Plasma Increase Analytical* At a concentration of 20 mg/L recovery of 112.5% with female serum and 107.9% with male serum with Enzymun methods *1097*

Plasma No Effect Analytical At therapeutic concentration of 4 mg/L in plasma recovery 99.2% *1097*

Creatine Kinase *Serum Increase Physiological* In one patient treated with diclofenac for 13 days for arthritis attributed to gout the patient developed erythema multiforme followed by muscular weakness and an increase in CK from 101 to 83,770 U/L *1374*

Serum No Effect Analytical On continuous method at 10 times maximal therapeutic concentration *2919*

Creatinine *Serum Increase Physiological* In one patient treated with diclofenac for 13 days for arthritis attributed to gout the patient developed erythema multiforme followed by muscular weakness and an increase in CK from 101 to 83,770 U/L, and creatinine from 1.0 to 2.1 mg/dL *1374* In a study of over 4000 patients 11 (0.3%) experienced serum urea concentrations of more than 2.0 mg/dL *1025*

Serum No Effect Analytical At concentration of 23 mg/L had no effect on Technicon AutoAnalyzer® Jaffe method *5704* No effect at therapeutic concentrations on alkaline picrate and Slot methods *2920* On alkaline picrate method on Technicon SMA II at physiological concentration *2922*

Serum No Effect Physiological No effect seen in patients undergoing treatment *2922*

Cyclosporine *Serum Increase Physiological* May increase toxicity particularly in patients with impaired renal function *1384*

Digitoxin *Serum No Effect Physiological* No effect observed on toxicity even in patients with impaired renal function *1384*

Digoxin *Serum Increase Physiological* Toxicity may be increased with coadministration particularly in patients with impaired renal function *1384* Coadministration of diclofenac with digoxin may increase its plasma concentration *1025*

Eosinophils *Blood Increase Physiological* Diclofenac associated with eosinophilia in less than 1% of treated patients *1025*

Factor VII *Plasma No Effect Physiological* Diclofenac does not affect plasma factors VII through XII *1025*

Factor VII Activity *Plasma No Effect Physiological* Diclofenac does not affect plasma factors VII through XII *1025*

Factor VIII *Plasma No Effect Physiological* Diclofenac does not affect plasma factors VII through XII *1025*

Factor VIII Activity *Plasma No Effect Physiological* Diclofenac does not affect plasma factors VII through XII *1025*

Factor IX *Plasma No Effect Physiological* Diclofenac does not affect plasma factors VII through XII *1025*

Factor X *Plasma No Effect Physiological* Diclofenac does not affect plasma factors VII through XII *1025*

Factor XI *Plasma No Effect Physiological* Diclofenac does not affect plasma factors VII through XII *1025*

Factor XII *Plasma No Effect Physiological* Diclofenac does not affect plasma factors VII through XII *1025*

Fibrinogen *Plasma No Effect Physiological* Diclofenac does not affect plasma fibrinogen concentration *1025*

Glucose *Serum Increase Analytical* Increase at therapeutic concentration with glucose oxidase/peroxidase method with ABTS *2920*

Serum No Effect Analytical On hexokinase method on Technicon SMA II at physiological concentration *2922* At concentration of 23 mg/L had no effect on hexokinase/G-6-PDH method *5704* No effect a therapeutic concentrations on hexokinase, glucose dehydrogenase, 2,4-dichloro, and o-toluidine methods *2920*

Serum No Effect Physiological No effect seen in patients undergoing treatment *2922* Diclofenac has no effect on glucose metabolism in healthy individuals *1025*

γ-Glutamyltransferase *Serum Increase Physiological* Acute drug-induced hepatitis developed in 5 patients within 3 months of start of treatment but activity normalized with withdrawal of drug *2851*

Granulocytes *Blood Decrease Physiological* Diclofenac associated with agranulocytosis in less than 1% of treated patients *1025*

Hemoglobin *Blood Decrease Physiological* Rare cases of anemia sometimes seen with treatment as with other NSAIDs *1025*

Hydroxybutyrate Dehydrogenase

Serum No Effect Analytical On continuous method at 10 times maximal therapeutic concentration *2919*

Iron *Serum No Effect Analytical* No effect at therapeutic concentrations on Ramsay and bathophenanthroline methods *2920* At concentration of 23 mg/L had no effect on Ferrozine method *5704* On Ferrozine method on Technicon SMA II at physiological concentration *2922*

Serum No Effect Physiological No effect seen in patients undergoing treatment *2922*

Isradipine *Serum Increase Physiological* In 18 healthy men coadministration of diclofenac with isradipine maximum isradipine concentration increased by 19.6% (from 5.06 ng/mL to 6.05 ng/mL) although total body clearance and steady state area under the concentration curve remained unchanged *5692*

Lactate Dehydrogenase *Serum Increase Physiological* In one patient treated with diclofenac for 13 days for arthritis attributed to gout the patient developed erythema multiforme followed by muscular weakness and an increase in CK from 101 to 83,770 U/L as a result of rhabdomyolysis with a LD activity of 566 U/L (reference range 0 - 250 U/L), rising over 17 days to 2,351 U/L *1374*

Serum No Effect Analytical On continuous method with lactate or pyruvate as substrate at 10 times maximal therapeutic concentration. On colorimetric method at 10 times maximal therapeutic concentration *2919*

Leukocytes *Blood Decrease Physiological* Diclofenac associated with leukopenia in less than 1% of treated patients *1025*

Lithium *Serum Increase Physiological* Coadministration of diclofenac with lithium reduces its renal clearance and increases its plasma concentration *1025* Lithium toxicity reported with the concomitant administration of diclofenac *4399* In 5 normal women administration of 250 mg/day for 7-10 days with previously steady state plasma concentration increased concentration by 26% *4831* Decreased renal clearance and increased plasma concentration by 26% in 5 normal women *4906*

Lithium Clearance *Urine Decrease Physiological* Lithium toxicity reported with the concomitant administration of diclofenac *4399* In 5 normal women administration of 250 mg diclofenac per day for 7-10 days reduced lithium clearance by 23%. Concentrations normalized with withdrawal of diclofenac

Diclofenac *(continued)*

Lithium Clearance *(continued)*
4831 Coadministration of diclofenac with lithium reduces its renal clearance and increases its plasma concentration *1025*

Methotrexate *Serum Increase Physiological* Coadministration of diclofenac with methotrexate may increase its plasma concentration *1025* Toxicity may be increased with coadministration particularly in patients with impaired renal function *1384*

Midazolam *Serum No Effect Analytical* On GC-ECD method of Ha et al *2387*

Myoglobin *Serum Increase Physiological* In one patient treated with diclofenac for 13 days for arthritis attributed to gout the patient developed erythema multiforme followed by muscular weakness and an increase in CK from 101 to 83,770 U/L, and urinary myoglobin to 1,190 µg/dL *1374*

Occult Blood *Feces Increase Physiological* Diclofenac reported to cause peptic ulcer or gastrointestinal bleeding in 0.6% of patients in a clinical trial of approximately 1800 patients *1025*

p-Aminophenol *Urine No Effect Analytical* With addition of drugs at a concentration of 100 mg/L and of related compounds at 50 mg/L no significant effect observed on colorimetric method of van Bocxlaer on Cobas Mira analyzer which involves reacting free p-aminophenol with resorcinol in the presence of magnesium ions to form an indophenol dye measured at 550 nm *6163*

Partial Thromboplastin Time
Plasma Increase Physiological Diclofenac causes statistically but not clinically significant mean increase in time, of less than 1 second *1025*

Phenobarbital *Serum Increase Physiological* Coadministration of diclofenac was associated with phenobarbital toxicity in one patient on chronic phenobarbital treatment *1025*

Phosphate *Serum No Effect Physiological* No effect seen in patients undergoing treatment *2922*

Platelet Aggregation *Blood Decrease Physiological* Effect less marked that observed with treatment with aspirin *3694*
Blood Increase Physiological Diclofenac increases platelet aggregation time *1025*
Blood No Effect Physiological Administration had no effect on aggregation response to adenosine diphosphate, collagen or epinephrine *5692*

Platelets *Blood Decrease Physiological* Diclofenac associated with thrombocytopenia in less than 1% of treated patients *1025*

Protein *Serum No Effect Analytical* On biuret method on Technicon SMA II at physiological concentration *2922* No effect at therapeutic concentrations on biuret and spectrophotometric methods *2920* At concentration of 23 mg/L had no effect on biuret method with blank correction *5704*
Serum No Effect Physiological No effect seen in patients undergoing treatment *2922*

Prothrombin Time *Plasma Increase Physiological* Diclofenac causes statistically but not clinically significant mean increase in time, of less than 1 second *1025*

Thyroid Stimulating Hormone
Serum No Effect Physiological In 8 individuals treated with a mean dose of 141 mg/d for at least 3 weeks mean concentration of 1.3 ± 0.2 mU/L not significantly different from 1.5 ± 0.2 mU/L in 22 controls *585*

Thyroxine (T4) *Serum No Effect Analytical* Using the Ciba-Corning ACS:180 analyzer mean concentration not significantly changed in 3 specimens where concentrations varied by -5 to +2% compared with the concentration measured by the Amerlex-M method *5621*
Serum No Effect Physiological In 8 individuals who had received a mean dose of 141 mg/d for at least 3 weeks mean concentration of 85 ± 6 nmol/L not significantly different from 94 ± 4 nmol/L in 22 controls *585*

Thyroxine (T4) Index, Free *Serum No Effect Physiological* In 8 individuals treated with a mean dose of 141 mg/d for at least 3 weeks mean FTI 89 ± 6 not significantly different from 93 ± 4 in 22 controls *585*

Tiludronate *Serum No Effect Physiological* Bioavailabilty of tiludronate not significantly altered when diclofenac coadministered *5258*

Tri-iodothyronine (T3) *Serum Decrease Physiological* In 8 individuals treated with a mean dose of 141 mg/d for at least 3 weeks mean concentration of 1.5 ± 0.1 nmol/L significantly less than 2.0 ± 0.1 nmol/L in 22 controls *585*

Triglycerides *Serum No Effect Analytical* No effect on enzymatic methods at therapeutic concentrations *2920* On enzymatic method on Technicon SMA II at physiological concentration *2922*
Serum No Effect Physiological No effect seen in patients undergoing treatment *2922*

Urea Nitrogen *Serum Increase Physiological* Significantly higher in treated patients (6.87 mmol/L vs 5.32 mmol/L) than in controls *2922* In a study of over 4000 patients 11 (0.3%) experienced serum urea concentrations of more than 40 mg/dL *1025* In one patient treated with diclofenac for 13 days for arthritis attributed to gout the patient developed erythema multiforme followed by muscular weakness and an increase in CK from 101 to 83,770 U/L, and urea nitrogen from 15 to 87 mg/dL *1374*
Serum No Effect Analytical On diacetyl monoxime complexone method on Technicon SMA II at physiological concentration *2922* No effect at therapeutic concentrations with glutamate dehydrogenase, phenol hypochlorite and diacetyl monoxime procedures *2920*

Uric Acid *Serum Increase Physiological* In one patient treated with diclofenac for 13 days for arthritis attributed to gout the patient developed erythema multiforme followed by muscular weakness and an increase in CK from 101 to 83,770 U/L as a result of rhabdomyolysis with an increase in uric acid concentration to 7.8 mg/dL (reference range 4.0 - 8.5 mg/dL) *1374*
Serum No Effect Analytical No effect at therapeutic concentrations on uricase-catalase, aldehyde dehydrogenase, direct UV-test and phosphotungstate methods *2920* At concentration of 23 mg/L had no effect on phosphotungstate reduction method *5704* On phosphotungstate method on Technicon SMA II at physiological concentration *2922*
Serum No Effect Physiological No effect seen in patients undergoing treatment *2922*

Dicloxacillin

Aspartate Aminotransferase *Serum Increase Physiological* Mild hepatic dysfunction observed *195*

Bilirubin *Serum Increase Physiological* Possible displacement from protein especially in critically ill neonates *6314*

Creatinine *Serum No Effect Analytical* No effect of concentrations up to 15 mg/L on single slide method on Kodak Ektachem® *5706*

Eosinophils *Blood Increase Physiological* Mild allergic response *195*

Nafcillin *Serum Increase Analytical* Cannot be assayed by HPLC method used at Mayo Clinic in presence of dicloxacillin *3858*

Dicumarol

Alanine Aminotransferase *Serum Increase Physiological* May be high enough to simulate myocardial infarction *402*

Aspartate Aminotransferase *Serum Increase Physiological* May simulate myocardial infarction (greater than ALT) *402*

Chlorpropamide *Serum Increase Physiological* In three diabetic patients concentration increased with coadministration due to inhibition of hepatic metabolism *3292* Increases half life, augments hypoglycemia *2452*

Clotting Time *Blood Increase Physiological* Slight effect in glass, greater in silicone *2242*

Erythrocyte Sedimentation Rate
Blood No Effect Physiological Unaltered by coumarins *2242*

Erythrocytes *Blood Decrease Physiological* May cause anemia (AMA Blood dyscrasias committee) *4017*

Factor VII *Plasma Decrease Physiological* Dose related effect *2242*

Factor IX *Plasma Decrease Physiological* Dose related effect *2242*

Factor X *Plasma Decrease Physiological* Dose related effect *2242*

Glucose *Serum Decrease Physiological* Reported effect *192*

Lactate Dehydrogenase *Serum Increase Physiological* May be high enough to simulate myocardial infarction *402*

Leukocytes *Blood Decrease Physiological* Reported effect (AMA Blood dyscrasias committee) *4017*

Mexiletine *Serum Increase Physiological* Decreases clearance and prolongs half-life *3281*

Midazolam *Serum No Effect Analytical* On GC-ECD method of Ha et al *2387*

Occult Blood *Feces Increase Physiological* May cause intramural hemorrhage even if no ulcer *5864*

Phenytoin *Serum Increase Physiological* Coadministration with phenytoin may increase plasma phenytoin concentration *4522* Increase by 38 to 250% in six volunteers probably due to inhibition of para-hydroxylation in liver *5966* May increase concentration 5 to 15 µg/mL (at dose for prothrombin time = 30%) *3339* When dicumarol ingested with fosphenytoin concentration of phenytoin may be increased *4519* Significant increases in concentration when drugs coadministered *1384* Causes increase in concentration when drugs coadministered through enzyme inhibition *6350*

Platelet Adhesiveness *Blood Decrease Physiological* Related to dose *2242*

Platelet Aggregation *Blood Increase Physiological* In response to ADP *2242*

Prothrombin Time *Plasma Increase Physiological* Dose related effect *2242*

Recalcification Time *Plasma Increase Physiological* Effect on citrated plasma *2242*

T3-Uptake *Serum Increase Physiological* Red cell uptake affected *881*

Tolbutamide *Serum Increase Physiological* Half-life substantially prolonged in healthy individuals when drugs coadministered probably due to inhibition of hepatic metabolism of tolbutamide *5677* Increases half life, augments hypoglycemia *2452*

Uric Acid *Serum Decrease Physiological* Uricosuric action *194*
Urine Increase Physiological Uricosuric action *2378*

Dicyclomine

Digoxin *Serum Increase Physiological* May increase gastrointestinal absorption thereby increasing plasma concentration *2640*

Didanosine

Alanine Aminotransferase *Serum Increase Physiological* At recommended dose in ACTG 1168/117 and 116A trials of almost 500 adult patients caused ALT activity of more than 5 times ULN in 9 and 6% patients respectively, and of greater than 10 times ULN in 5% of 281 children *730* In 281 children with AIDS treatment with didanosine for a median of 20 months 14% had serum alanine aminotransferase activity exceeding 10 times the upper limit of normal *1736*

Alkaline Phosphatase *Serum Increase Physiological* At recommended dose in ACTG 1168/117 and 116A trials of almost 500 adult patients caused alkaline phosphatase activity of more than 5 times ULN in 4 and 1% patients respectively, and of greater than 2 times ULN in 6% of 281 children *730*

Amylase *Serum Increase Physiological* Pancreatitis ranging from mild abdominal pain and increased serum amylase activity to fatal disease occurs in 5 to 10% patients being treated for HIV-1 infection especially in those with renal disease or previous pancreatitis *2623* At recommended dose in ACTG 1168/117 and 116A trials of almost 500 adult patients caused amylase activity of more than 1.4 times ULN in 17 and 15% patients respectively, and of greater than 3.1 ULN in 5% children *730* In 281 children with AIDS treatment with dianosine for a median of 20 months 14% had serum amylase activity exceeding 3 times the upper limit of normal *1736* In 230 patients in one trial intolerant or resistant to zidovudine treatment with 250 mg q12 h 3.9% demonstrated increased activity *5023*

Aspartate Aminotransferase *Serum Increase Physiological* In 230 patients in one trial intolerant or resistant to zidovudine treatment with 250 mg q12 h 5.7% demonstrated increased activity *5023* At recommended dose in ACTG 1168/117 and 116A trials of almost 500 adult patients caused AST activity of more than 5 times ULN in 9 and 7% patients respectively, and in 14% of 281 children *730*

Bilirubin *Serum Increase Physiological* In 281 children with AIDS treatment with didanosine for a median of 20 months 9% had serum total bilirubin concentration exceeding 2.6 times the upper limit of normal *1736* In 230 patients in one trial intolerant or resistant to zidovudine treatment with 250 mg q12 h 0.8% demonstrated hyperbilirubinemia *5023* At recommended dose in ACTG 1168/117 and 116A trials in almost 500 adult patients caused an increase in bilirubin concentration to more than 2.6 times ULN in 1 and 1% patients respectively, and in 6% of 281 children *730*

CD4+ Lymphocytes *Blood Increase Physiological* In patients with HIV-1 infection treatment with didanosine caused increased concentrations in Phase I trials *2623*

Ciprofloxacin *Serum Decrease Physiological* Decreased oral availability *886*

Creatine Kinase *Serum Increase Physiological* At recommended dose in ACTG 152 trial of 281patients caused creatine kinase activity of more than 5.1 times ULN in 6% patients. Increased creatine kinase activity also observed in adults in association with rhabdomyolysis *730*
Serum No Effect Physiological None of 230 patients in one trial intolerant or resistant to zidovudine treatment with 250 mg q12 h demonstrated increased activity *5023*

Dapsone *Serum Decrease Physiological* Decreased oral availability *886*

Doxycycline *Serum Decrease Physiological* Decreased oral availability *886*

Ganciclovir *Serum Decrease Physiological* At an oral dose of 1000 mg ganciclovir every 8 h and didanosine 200 mg every 12 h the steady state AUC of ganciclovir decreased 21 ± 17% when didanosine administered 2 h before ganciclovir but AUC of ganciclovir not affected when drugs administered simultaneously *5018*
Serum No Effect Physiological At an oral dose of 1000 mg ganciclovir every 8 h and didanosine 200 mg every 12 h the steady state AUC of ganciclovir decreased 21 ± 17% when didanosine administered 2 h before ganciclovir but AUC of ganciclovir not affected when drugs administered simultaneously *5018*

Glucose *Serum Increase Physiological* In 230 patients in one trial intolerant or resistant to zidovudine treatment with 250 mg q12 h 3.9% demonstrated hyperglycemia *5023*

Granulocytes *Blood Decrease Physiological* At recommended dose in ACTG 1168/117 and 116A trials of almost 500 adult patients caused granulocyte concentrations of less than 750/µL in 6 and 8% patients respectively, and 11% in 281 children *730*

Hematocrit *Blood Decrease Physiological* In 230 patients in one trial intolerant or resistant to zidovudine treatment with 250 mg q12 h 7.4% demonstrated anemia *5023*

Hemoglobin *Blood Decrease Physiological* In 281 children with AIDS treatment with didanosine for a median of 20 months 11% had hemoglobin concentration of less than 7.5 g/dL *1736* At recommended dose in ACTG 1168/117 and 116A trials of almost 500 adult patients caused hemoglobin concentrations of less than 80 g/L in 6 and 3% patients respectively, and hemoglobin of less than 75 g/L in 5% of 281 children *730*

HIV p24 Antigen *Serum Decrease Physiological* Decreased concentration observed in adults with treatment during Phase I trials *2623*

Indinavir *Serum Decrease Physiological* Decreased oral availability *886*

Isoniazid *Serum Decrease Physiological* Decreased oral availability *886*

itraconazole *Serum Decrease Physiological* Decreased oral availability *886*

Ketoconazole *Serum Decrease Physiological* Decreased oral availability *886*
Serum No Effect Physiological No significant effect observed on the concentration of either drug when two drugs coadministered *730*

Didanosine *(continued)*

Leukocytes *Blood Decrease Physiological* In 230 patients in one trial intolerant or resistant to zidovudine treatment with 250 mg q12 h 9.6% demonstrated leukopenia *5023* At recommended dose in ACTG 1168/117 and 116A trials of almost 500 adult patients caused leukocyte concentrations of less than 2000/μL in 13 and 16% patients respectively, but less than 1% in 281 children *730*
Blood Increase Physiological In 230 patients in one trial intolerant or resistant to zidovudine treatment with 250 mg q12 h 1.7% demonstrated eosinophilia *5023*

Lipase *Serum Increase Physiological* Pancreatitis occurs in 5-10% patients being treated with drug *2623*

Loperamide *Serum No Effect Physiological* No significant effect observed on the concentration of either drug when two drugs coadministered *730*

Metoclopramide *Serum No Effect Physiological* No significant effect observed on the concentration of either drug when two drugs coadministered *730*

Nelfinavir *Serum No Effect Physiological* Has no significant effect on area under the concentration curve when didanosine coadministered *1891*

Neutrophils *Blood Decrease Physiological* In 281 children with AIDS treatment with didanosine for a median of 20 months 28% had absolute neutrophil count of less than 500 cells/μL *1736* In 230 patients in one trial intolerant or resistant to zidovudine treatment with 250 mg q12 h 11.7% demonstrated neutropenia *5023*

Norfloxacin *Serum Decrease Physiological* Decreased oral availability *886*

Platelets *Blood Decrease Physiological* In 230 patients in one trial intolerant or resistant to zidovudine treatment with 250 mg q12 h 4.5% demonstrated thrombocytopenia *5023* At recommended dose in ACTG 1168/117 and 116A trials of about 500 adult patients caused platelet concentrations of less than 50,000/μL in 2 and 2% patients respectively, and 6% in 281 children *730*

Ranitidine *Serum No Effect Physiological* No significant effect observed on the concentration of either drug when two drugs coadministered *730*

Rifabutin *Serum No Effect Physiological* No significant effect observed on the concentration of either drug when two drugs coadministered *730*

Ritonavir *Serum No Effect Physiological* Has no effect on the area under the concentration curve when didanosine coadministered *1891*

Triglycerides *Serum Increase Physiological* In one man with AIDS mean concentration increased from 155 mg/dL at start of didanosine treatment (600 mg/d) to 1630 mg/dL 2 weeks after treatment begun with gradual decline after didanosine withdrawn. Increase recurred after didanosine reinstituted *5932*

Uric Acid *Serum Increase Physiological* In some patients with HIV-1 infection treatment increased plasma uric acid concentrations observed *2623* At recommended dose in ACTG 1168/117 and 116A trials caused increased uric acid concentration to more than 12 mg/dL in 3 and 2% patients respectively, and to above 3.5 times ULN in less than 1% of 281 children *730*

Didemnim B

Alanine Aminotransferase *Serum Increase Physiological* Hepatic dysfunction may occur *1384*

Aspartate Aminotransferase *Serum Increase Physiological* Hepatic dysfunction may occur *1384*

Dideoxycytidine

Amylase *Serum Increase Physiological* In 163 (149 men, 14 women) consecutive asymptomatic HIV-infected outpatients of whom only 6 were receiving dideoxyinosine, known to cause pancreatitis, 39 (24%) had increased serum amylase activity. In all of the 6 patients receiving ddi amylase activity was increased, in four it was due to pancreatic isoamylasse and in the other two to macroamylase *1905*

Amylase, Pancreatic Isoenzyme
Serum Increase Physiological In 163 (149 men, 14 women) consecutive asymptomatic HIV-infected outpatients of whom only 6 were receiving dideoxyinosine, known to cause pancreatitis, 39 (24%) had increased serum amylase activity. In all of the 6 patients receiving ddi amylase activity was increased, in four it was due to pancreatic isoamylasse and in the other two to macroamylase *1905*

CD4+ Lymphocytes *Blood Increase Physiological* Most patients with AIDS receiving 0.06 to 0.54 mg daily had increased count within 2 weeks *6590*

HIV p24 Antigen *Serum Decrease Physiological* In most patients with AIDS receiving from 0.06 to 0.54 mg per kilogram daily *6590*

Macroamylase *Serum Increase Physiological* In 163 (149 men, 14 women) consecutive asymptomatic HIV-infected outpatients of whom only 6 were receiving dideoxyinosine, known to cause pancreatitis, 39 (24%) had increased serum amylase activity. In all of the 6 patients receiving ddi amylase activity was increased, in four it was due to pancreatic isoamylasse and in the other two to macroamylase *1905*

Dideoxyinosine

Alanine Aminotransferase *Serum Decrease Physiological* In 7 of 14 children with enzyme activity more than 3 times at start of treatment reduction of more than 50% observed with treatment of up to 540 mg/sq m daily for 24 weeks *830*
Serum Increase Physiological Observed in 13 of 37 patients with AIDS or AIDS related complex when treated with up to 12 mg/kg/d. In 6 increased to above 5 times normal *3378* Observed in 13 of 37 patients with AIDS or AIDS related complex when treated with up to 12 mg/kg/d. In 6 patients increased to above 5 times normal *3378* Observed in 5 of 34 patients with AIDS or AIDS related complex following treatment with doses from 4.0 to 30.4 mg/kg/d *1090*

Amylase *Serum Increase Physiological* Pancreatitis developed in 5 of 37 patients with AIDS or AIDS related complex when treated with drug for up to 20 weeks, resolved when drug withdrawn *3378* Pancreatitis developed in 2 of 34 patients with AIDS or AIDS related complex after 10 to 12 weeks treatment with 30.4 mg/kg/d *1090* In 4 of 32 children with HIV infection who initially had normal serum amylase treatment with up to 540 mg/sq m daily for 24 weeks caused increases to more than twice normal activities. Asymptomatic hyperamylasemia observed in 35% of patients at some time *830*

Aspartate Aminotransferase
Serum Decrease Physiological Reduction of more than 50% observed in 7 of 14 children with HIV infection and initial enzyme activity more than three times normal treated with up to 540 mg/sq m daily for 24 weeks *830*
Serum Increase Physiological Observed in 13 of 37 patients with AIDS or AIDS related complex when treated with up to 12 mg/kg/d. In 6 activity increased to above times normal *3378* Observed in 5 of 34 patients with AIDS or AIDS related complex when treated with doses from 4.0 to 30.4 mg/kg/d *1090*

CD4+ Lymphocytes *Blood Increase Physiological* Increase observed from mean baseline concentration of 125 /μL to 313 /μL after 24 weeks in 33 patients with AIDS or AIDS related complex treated with 24 weeks of drug treatment *1090* Significant increase from mean of 0.218 to 0.327/μL in 38 children with HIV infection treated with up to 540 mg/sq m daily for 24 weeks. Effect most marked in children with initially high count *830* Mean count increased in 35 patients with AIDS or AIDS related complex when examined after 2, 6, 10 and 20 weeks treatment *3378*

CD8+ Lymphocytes *Blood Increase Physiological* Significantly higher counts observed at 2 and 6 weeks of treatment with trend towards higher count at 10 weeks in 36 patients with AIDS or AIDS related complex *3378* Increase from mean baseline concentration of 557 /μL to 829 /μL after 24 weeks in 33 patients with AIDS or AIDS related complex following treatment with drug first intravenously then orally *1090*

Creatine Kinase *Serum Increase Physiological* Observed in 3 patients being treated with the drug together with muscle weakness. Drug appears to be toxic to muscle mitochondria *1220* Observed in one of 34 patients with AIDS or AIDS related complex treated with drug for up to 24 weeks: originated from skeletal muscle *1090*

Creatinine *Serum Increase Physiological* In 5 of 43 children with HIV infection treatment with up to 540 mg/sq m daily for 24 weeks caused mild and transient increase *830*

Granulocytes *Blood Increase Physiological* Nonsignificant increase observed in 33 patients with AIDS or AIDS related complex when treated with drug for up to 24 weeks. Mean baseline concentration 2400 /μL, 2600 /μL at 2 to 12 weeks and 3100 /μL after 24 weeks treatment *1090*

Hematocrit *Blood Increase Physiological* From mean baseline of 0.38 increased to 0.42 at 12 weeks and 0.45 at 24 weeks in 17 patients with AIDS or AIDS related complex when treated with drug *1090*

Hemoglobin *Blood Decrease Physiological* 27 of 43 children with HIV infection had hemoglobin concentration of less than 95 g/L on at least one occasion during 24 week study with up to 540 mg/sq m body surface area daily. Effect possibly related to frequency of phlebotomy only *830*
Blood Increase Physiological Significant increase from mean baseline concentration of 129 g/L to 141 g/L observed in 17 patients with AIDS or AIDS related complex following treatment for 12 weeks, with further increase to 150 g/L at 24 weeks *1090* In 35 patients with AIDS or AIDS related complex increase from mean baseline concentration of 127 g/L to 139 g/L after 10 weeks treatment *3378*

HIV-1 p24 Antigen *Serum Decrease Physiological* Significant response observed in majority of 34 patients with AIDS or AIDS related complex treated with drug for up to 24 weeks *1090* In 35 children with HIV infection treatment with up to 540 mg/sq m daily for 24 weeks caused significant reduction in mean concentration *830* Statistically significant decrease of concentration in 17 patients with AIDS and 20 patients with AIDS related complex with treatment up to 12 mg/kg/d *3378*

HIV p24 Antigen *Serum Decrease Physiological* Significant response observed in majority of 34 patients with AIDS or AIDS related complex treated with drug for up to 24 weeks *1090* Statistically significant decrease of concentration in 17 patients with AIDS and 20 patients with AIDS related complex with treatment up to 12 mg/kg/d *3378* In 35 children with HIV infection treatment with up to 540 mg/sq m daily for 24 weeks caused significant reduction in mean concentration *830*

Immunoglobulin G *Serum Decrease Physiological* 80% children with HIV infection had initially high concentration but in 25% treatment with up to 540 mg/sq m daily for 24 weeks caused decrease of more than 10% *830*

Leukocytes *Blood Increase Physiological* Increase from mean baseline of 3700 /μL to 4300 /μL at 2 weeks and sustained for further 22 weeks during treatment with drug in 33 patients with AIDS or AIDS related complex *1090* In 35 patients with AIDS or AIDS related complex during 10 weeks of administration increase from mean baseline of 3500 /μL to 4100 /μL *3378*

Lipase *Serum Increase Physiological* Pancreatitis observed in 5 of 36 patients with AIDS or AIDS related complex when treated with drug for up to 20 weeks but activity reverted to normal when drug withdrawn *3378* Pancreatitis observed in 2 of 34 patients with AIDS or AIDS related complex between 10 and 12 weeks treatment with 30.4 mg/kg/d *1090* Increased activity observed in 3 of 16 children with HIV infection treated with up to 540 mg/sq m daily for 24 weeks *830*

Lymphocytes *Blood Increase Physiological* In 35 patients with AIDS or AIDS related complex increase from mean baseline of 1000/ μL to 1300/ μL after 10 weeks treatment *3378* Increase observed as early as two weeks after start of treatment in 33 patients with AIDS or AIDS related complex when treated with drug. Mean concentration at baseline 800 /μL, 1200 /μL after 2 weeks and 1300 /μL after 24 weeks *1090* In 35 patients with AIDS or AIDS related complex increase from mean baseline of 1000 /μL to 1300 /μL after 10 weeks treatment *3378*

Neutrophils *Blood Increase Physiological* Significant increase from mean baseline concentration of 1900 /μL in 35 patients with AIDS or AIDS related complex to 2500 /μL after 10 weeks treatment *3378*

Platelets *Blood Decrease Physiological* Eight of 43 children with HIV infection had thrombocytopenia at some time during 24 week study when treated with up to 540 mg/sq m daily. Five of these patients had history of thrombocytopenia *830*
Blood Increase Physiological In 35 patients with AIDS or AIDS related complex treatment for 10 weeks increased concentration from mean baseline of 175,000 /μL to 203,000 /μL *3378* Nonsignificant increase from mean baseline concentration of 190,000 /μL to 201,000 /μL at 12 weeks and 208,000 /μL at 24 weeks in 17 patients with AIDS or AIDS related complex when treated with drug *1090*

Triglycerides *Serum Increase Physiological* Probable increase observed in 13 of 18 children with HIV infection treated with doses of up to 540 mg/sq m daily for 24 weeks *830*

Urea Nitrogen *Serum Increase Physiological* In 11 children with HIV infection treatment with up to 540 mg/sq m daily for 24 weeks caused increase, often mild and transient *830*

Uric Acid *Serum Increase Physiological* Asymptomatic hyperuricemia observed in 19 of 34 patients with AIDS or AIDS related complex when treated for up to 24 weeks: dose related effect apparent *1090* Dose-related increase observed in 37 patients with AIDS or AIDS related complex with uric acid concentrations ranging from 0.56 to 0.83 mmol/L in 10 patients who had received more than 30 mg/kg/d *3378* Ten of 42 children with HIV infection had asymptomatic increase in concentration to between 473 and 811 μmol/L at some time during treatment with up to 540 mg/sq m daily for 24 weeks *830*

Dieldrin

Cholinesterase *Serum Decrease Analytical In vitro* 7.2% decrease at 1 x 10^{-4} mol/L *2095*

Lactate Dehydrogenase *Serum Decrease Physiological In vitro* 8.0% decrease at 1 x 10^{-4} mol/L *2095*

Leukocytes *Blood Increase Physiological* May occur in acute response *2183*

Dienestrol

Alanine Aminotransferase *Serum Increase Physiological* Reported to cause cholestasis *2754*

Aspartate Aminotransferase *Serum Increase Physiological* Reported to cause cholestasis *2754*

Bilirubin *Serum Increase Physiological* May cause cholestasis *2754*

Calcium *Serum Increase Physiological* May occur with extended high dosage *2754*

Volume *Plasma Increase Physiological* Fluid retention with large dose estrogens *2754*

Diethazine

Leukocytes *Blood Decrease Physiological* May cause leukopenia *3810*

Diethylaminoethanol

Albumin *Serum No Effect Analytical* At concentration of 30 mg/L had no effect on BCG method *5704*

Bicarbonate *Serum No Effect Analytical* At concentration of 30 mg/L had no effect on method using phenolphthalein *5704*

Bilirubin *Serum No Effect Analytical* At concentration of 30 mg/L had no effect on Jendrassik and Grof method *5704*

Calcium *Serum No Effect Analytical* At concentration of 30 mg/L had no effect on cresolphthalein method *5704*

Chloride *Serum No Effect Analytical* At concentration of 30 mg/L had no effect on mercurimetric method *5704*

Cholesterol *Serum No Effect Analytical* At concentration of 30 mg/L had no effect on Liebermann-Burchard method *5704*

Creatinine *Serum No Effect Analytical* At concentration of 30 mg/L had no effect on Technicon AutoAnalyzer® method *5704*

Phosphate *Serum No Effect Analytical* At concentration of 30 mg/L had no effect on phosphomolybdate method *5704*

Protein *Serum No Effect Analytical* At concentration of 30 mg/L had no effect on biuret method with blank correction *5704*

Diethylaminoethanol *(continued)*

Triglycerides *Serum* *No Effect* *Analytical* At concentration of 30 mg/L had no effect on lipase/esterase method *5704*

Urea Nitrogen *Serum* *No Effect* *Analytical* At concentration of 30 mg/L had no effect on diacetylmonoxime method *5704*

Uric Acid *Serum* *No Effect* *Analytical* At concentration of 30 mg/L had no effect on phosphotungstate reduction method *5704*

Diethylaminoethyl-Dextran

Bile Acids *Serum* *Decrease* *Physiological* Significant reduction observed in 15 patients with primary biliary cirrhosis when treated with 4 - 6 g/d for 2 months *6675*

Cholesterol *Serum* *Decrease* *Physiological* Significant reduction observed in 15 patients with primary biliary cirrhosis treated with 4-6 g/d for 2 months *6675*

HDL-Cholesterol *Serum* *No Effect* *Physiological* No significant change observed in 15 patients with primary cirrhosis treated with 4-6 g/d for 2 months *6675*

Diethylpropion

Alanine Aminotransferase *Serum* *No Effect* *Analytical* At acute overdose concentration (10 mg/dL) on Technicon SMAC® method *6266*

Albumin *Serum* *No Effect* *Analytical* At acute overdose concentration (10 mg/dL) on Technicon SMAC® method *6266* At concentration of 100 mg/L had no effect on BCG method *5704*

Alkaline Phosphatase *Serum* *No Effect* *Analytical* At acute overdose concentration (10 mg/dL) on Technicon SMAC® method *6266*

Amobarbital *Urine* *No Effect* *Analytical* No interference with TLC using ethyl acetate: methanol: water: ammonium hydroxide and modified Dragendorff's reagent for detection *6502*

Amphetamine *Urine* *No Effect* *Analytical* Negative result observed with Du Pont aca at a concentration of 50 µg/L (0.24 mmol/L) *1554* No interference with TLC using ethyl acetate: methanol: water: ammonium hydroxide and modified Dragendorff's reagent for detection *6502*

Aspartate Aminotransferase *Serum* *No Effect* *Analytical* At acute overdose concentration (10 mg/dL) on Technicon SMAC® method *6266*

Bilirubin *Serum* *No Effect* *Analytical* At acute overdose concentration (10 mg/dL) on Technicon SMAC® method *6266* At concentration of 100 mg/L had no effect on Jendrassik and Grof method *5704*

Calcium *Serum* *No Effect* *Analytical* At acute overdose concentration (10 mg/dL) on Technicon SMAC® method *6266* At concentration of 100 mg/L had no effect on cresolphthalein method *5704*

Cholesterol *Serum* *No Effect* *Analytical* At acute overdose concentration (10 mg/dL) on Technicon SMAC® method *6266* At concentration of 100 mg/L had no effect on Liebermann-Burchard method *5704*

Cocaine *Urine* *Increase* *Analytical* Similar R_f and color reaction on TLC using ethyl acetate: methanol: water: ammonium hydroxide and modified Dragendorff's reagent *6502*

Creatine Kinase *Serum* *No Effect* *Analytical* At acute overdose concentration (10 mg/dL) on Technicon SMAC® method *6266*

Creatinine *Serum* *No Effect* *Analytical* At acute overdose concentration (10 mg/dL) on Technicon SMAC® method *6266* At concentration of 100 mg/L had no effect on Technicon AutoAnalyzer® Jaffe method *5704*

Diazepam *Urine* *Positive* *Analytical* Similar R_f and color reaction on TLC using ethyl acetate: methanol: water: ammonium hydroxide and modified Dragendorff's reagent *6502*

Erythrocytes *Blood* *Decrease* *Physiological* May cause bone marrow depression *183*

Glucose *Serum* *No Effect* *Analytical* At acute overdose concentration (10 mg/dL) on Technicon SMAC® method *6266*

Hydromorphone *Urine* *No Effect* *Analytical* No interference with TLC using ethyl acetate: methanol: water: ammonium hydroxide and modified Dragendorff's reagent for detection *6502*

Iron *Serum* *No Effect* *Analytical* At concentration of 100 mg/L had no effect on Ferrozine method *5704* At acute overdose concentration (10 mg/dL) on Technicon SMAC® method *6266*

Lactate Dehydrogenase *Serum* *No Effect* *Analytical* At acute overdose concentration (10 mg/dL) on Technicon SMAC® method *6266*

Leukocytes *Blood* *Decrease* *Physiological* Marrow depression with leukopenia/agranulocytosis *4000*

Mescaline *Urine* *No Effect* *Analytical* No interference with TLC using ethyl acetate: methanol: water: ammonium hydroxide and modified Dragendorff's reagent for detection *6502*

Methamphetamine *Urine* *No Effect* *Analytical* No interference with TLC using ethyl acetate: methanol: water: ammonium hydroxide and modified Dragendorff's reagent for detection *6502*

Methaqualone *Urine* *Positive* *Analytical* Similar R_f and color reaction on TLC using ethyl acetate: methanol: water: ammonium hydroxide and modified Dragendorff's reagent *6502*

Morphine *Urine* *No Effect* *Analytical* No interference with TLC using ethyl acetate: methanol: water: ammonium hydroxide and modified Dragendorff's reagent for detection *6502*

Pentobarbital *Urine* *No Effect* *Analytical* No interference with TLC using ethyl acetate: methanol: water: ammonium hydroxide and modified Dragendorff's reagent for detection *6502*

Phencyclidine *Urine* *Increase* *Analytical* Similar R_f and color reaction on TLC using ethyl acetate: methanol: water: ammonium hydroxide and modified Dragendorff's reagent *6502*

Phenobarbital *Urine* *No Effect* *Analytical* No interference with TLC using ethyl acetate: methanol: water: ammonium hydroxide and modified Dragendorff's reagent for detection *6502*

Phenylpropanolamine *Urine* *No Effect* *Analytical* No interference with TLC using ethyl acetate: methanol: water: ammonium hydroxide and modified Dragendorff's reagent for detection *6502*

Phosphate *Serum* *No Effect* *Analytical* At concentration of 100 mg/L had no effect on phosphomolybdate method *5704* At acute overdose concentration (10 mg/dL) on Technicon SMAC® method *6266*

Platelets *Blood* *Decrease* *Physiological* Isolated cases of bone marrow depression *2753*

Protein *Serum* *No Effect* *Analytical* At acute overdose concentration (10 mg/dL) on Technicon SMAC® method *6266* At concentration of 100 mg/L had no effect on biuret method with blank correction *5704*

Secobarbital *Urine* *No Effect* *Analytical* No interference with TLC using ethyl acetate: methanol: water: ammonium hydroxide and modified Dragendorff's reagent for detection *6502*

Triglycerides *Serum* *No Effect* *Analytical* At acute overdose concentration (10 mg/dL) on Technicon SMAC® method *6266* At concentration of 100 mg/L had no effect on lipase/esterase method *5704*

Urea Nitrogen *Serum* *No Effect* *Analytical* At concentration of 100 mg/L had no effect on diacetylmonoxime method *5704* At acute overdose concentration (10 mg/dL) on Technicon SMAC® method *6266*

Uric Acid *Serum* *No Effect* *Analytical* At concentration of 100 mg/L had no effect on phosphotungstate reduction method *5704* At acute overdose concentration (10 mg/dL) on Technicon SMAC® method *6266*

Diethylstilbestrol

Acid Phosphatase *Prostatic Fluid* *Decrease* *Physiological* Markedly lower in benign hypertrophy *3109*

Alanine Aminotransferase *Serum* *Increase* *Physiological* Hepatotoxicity with centrolobular necrosis *3171*

Albumin *Serum Decrease Physiological* In women in third trimester of pregnancy mean concentration 32.5 ± 1.6 g/L compared with mean of 1.2 g/L in healthy controls *262*

Amino Acids *Plasma Decrease Physiological* Specific amino acids affected in men *1154*

Antithrombin III *Plasma Decrease Physiological* Administration of estrogens to women is likely to decrease antithrombin III *1694* In 22 patients with metastatic prostatic cancer treatment significant decrease observed. Effect noticed within one month of commencement of treatment *1731*

Aspartate Aminotransferase *Serum Increase Physiological* Five cases of increased bilirubin alone but additional cases of increased bilirubin concentration together with increased activity of LDH and/or AST observed in 93 patients receiving treatment *4673* Hepatotoxicity with centrolobular necrosis *3171*

Bilirubin *Serum Increase Physiological* Five cases of increased bilirubin alone but additional cases of increased bilirubin concentration together with increased activity of LDH and/or AST observed in 93 patients receiving treatment *4673* Hepatotoxicity with centrolobular necrosis *3171*

Blood *Urine Increase Physiological* Hematuria observed in 4 of 101 treated patients *5945*

Calcium *Serum Increase Physiological* One case of transiently increased calcium concentration observed in 93 patients receiving treatment *4673* Rapid increase in 24 h in patients with breast cancer *5896* Administration of estrogens to women with breast cancer may produce marked hypercalcemia *1694*

Carcinoembryonic Antigen *Serum No Effect Analytical* At a concentration of up to 5.0 µg/mL caused less than 10% error in the concentration of CEA as measured by the method on Bayer Technicon Immuno 1® *418*

Coproporphyrin *Feces Increase Physiological* May induce porphyria cutanea tarda *6364*
Urine Increase Physiological May induce porphyria cutanea tarda *6364*

Corticosteroid-Binding Globulin
Serum Increase Physiological Can be doubled in males with treatment *5992*

Factor VII *Plasma Increase Physiological* Administration of estrogens to women is likely to increase factor VII *1694*

Factor VIII *Plasma Increase Physiological* Administration of estrogens to women is likely to increase factor VIII *1694*

Factor IX *Plasma Increase Physiological* Administration of estrogens to women is likely to increase factor IX *1694*

Factor X *Plasma Increase Physiological* Administration of estrogens to women is likely to increase factor IX *1694*

Folate *Serum Decrease Physiological* Administration of estrogens to women is likely to reduce serum folate concentration *1694*

Follicle Stimulating Hormone
Plasma Decrease Physiological At doses affecting pituitary-gonadal axis *3109*

Glucose Tolerance *Serum Decrease Physiological* May provoke mild to moderate deterioration *3012* Presumed decrease as is common in individuals receiving estrogen-containing oral contraceptives *1694*

Hematocrit *Blood Decrease Physiological* Anemia observed in 5 of 101 treated patients *5945*

Hemoglobin *Blood Decrease Physiological* Anemia observed in 5 of 101 treated patients *5945*

17-Hydroxycorticosteroids *Urine Increase Physiological* Can be doubled in males with treatment *5992*

6-β-Hydroxycortisol *Urine Increase Physiological* Increased conversion of cortisol produced *55*

Leukocytes *Blood Decrease Physiological* Two cases of leukopenia observed in 93 patients receiving treatment *4673*

Luteinizing Hormone *Plasma Decrease Physiological* At doses affecting pituitary-gonadal axis *3109*

Metyrapone Test *Patient Decrease Physiological* Administration of estrogens to women is likely to reduce response to metyrapone *1694*

Occult Blood *Feces No Effect Physiological* No cases of gastrointestinal bleeding observed in 93 patients receiving treatment *4673*

Phospholipids *Serum Increase Physiological* Administration of estrogens to women is likely to increase serum phospholipid concentration *1694*

Platelet Aggregation response to Epinephrine
Blood Increase Physiological Administration of estrogens to women is likely to increase norepinephrine-induced platelet aggregability *1694*

Platelets *Blood Decrease Physiological* Thrombocytopenia (AMA Blood dyscrasias) *4017* Two cases of thrombocytopenia observed in 93 patients receiving treatment *4673*

Prealbumin *Serum Decrease Physiological* Mean concentration in patients undergoing stilbestrol treatment 200 ± 12 mg/L compared with mean of 263 mg/L in healthy normal controls *262*

Pregnanediol *Urine Decrease Physiological* Administration of estrogens to women is likely to reduce excretion of pregnanediol *1694*

Prolactin *Plasma Increase Physiological* Over 1 week in normal males *6597*

Prostate-specific Antigen *Serum No Effect Analytical* Diethylstilbestrol at a concentration of up to 5 µg/mL caused less than 0.1% cross-reactivity with method on PSA method on Bayer Technicon Immuno 1® *430*

Prostate-specific Antigen, Free *Serum No Effect Analytical* Diethylstilbestrol at a concentration of 1 mg/L had no significant effect on the Hybritech Tandem® -R free PSA immunoassay *4286*

Prothrombin *Plasma Increase Physiological* Administration of estrogens to women is likely to increase prothrombin *1694*

Protoporphyrin *Feces Increase Physiological* May induce porphyria cutanea tarda *6364*

Sex-Hormone Binding Globulin
Serum Increase Physiological Observed when given to men with androgen-dependent prostatic cancer *2836*

Sulfobromophthalein *Serum Increase Physiological* Administration of estrogens to women is likely to cause BSP retention *1694*

Testosterone *Serum Decrease Physiological* At doses affecting pituitary-gonadal axis *3109* When given to men with androgen-dependent prostatic cancer reduced concentration to normal female range *2836*

Testosterone, Free *Serum Decrease Physiological* In men with androgen-dependent prostatic cancer and reduction of total hormone concentration with SHBG *2836*

Thyroxine Binding Globulin *Serum Increase Physiological* Administration of estrogens to women is likely to increase concentration of TBG *1694* Mean concentration in patients undergoing stilbestrol therapy 27.5 ± 4.8 g/L compared with mean of 10.2 g/L in healthy controls *262* Direct effect of drug *42*

Thyroxine (T4) *Serum Increase Physiological* Mean concentration 158.3 ± 4.6 nmol/L in patients receiving stilbestrol therapy compared with mean of 102.5 nmol/L in healthy controls *262*

Thyroxine (T4), Free *Serum No Effect Physiological* Administration of estrogens to women is likely to increase concentration of TBG and thus total T4 concentration but free T4 concentration is unaffected *1694*

Triglycerides *Serum Increase Physiological* Administration of estrogens to women is likely to increase serum triglyceride concentration *1694*

Tyrosine *Plasma Decrease Physiological* Observed with 5 mg daily for 5 d *1313*

Uric Acid *Serum Decrease Physiological* In men on therapy (hormonal effect) *4280*
Urine Increase Physiological In men on therapy (hormonal effect) *4280*

Uric Acid Clearance *Urine Increase Physiological* In men on therapy (hormonal effect) *4280*

Uroporphyrin *Feces Increase Physiological* May induce porphyria cutanea tarda *6364*
Urine Increase Physiological May induce porphyria cutanea tarda *6364*

Vitamin A *Serum Decrease Physiological* Hormonal effect when given to lactating women *2005*

Diflunisal

Acetaminophen *Serum Increase Physiological* Increases plasma concentration *1384* Concomitant administration of diflunisal with acetaminophen increased the acetaminophen concentration by approximately 50% *3972*

Alanine Aminotransferase *Serum Increase Physiological* Diflunisal has been reported to cause increases in activity of over three times the upper limit of normal in less than 1% of patients *3972* Significant increase, three times upper limit of normal. occurred in less than 1% of patients but borderline increases may occur in as many as 15% *1384*

Aspartate Aminotransferase *Serum Increase Physiological* Significant increase observed in less than 1% of all patients but borderline increases observed in as many as 15% *1384* Diflunisal has been reported to cause increases in activity of over three times the upper limit of normal in less than 1% of patients *3972*

Bilirubin *Serum Increase Physiological* Diflunisal has been reported to cause increases in bilirubin with occasional severe reactions *3972*
Serum No Effect Physiological At pharmacological concentrations has little or no protein displacement effect *6314*

Bleeding Time *Patient Increase Physiological* Moderate but not significant increase at 1,000 mg b.i.d. whereas 250 mg and 500 mg had no effect. Effect reverted to normal in 24 h *2303*

Cortisol *Plasma No Effect Analytical* No effect on FETI methods of Syva® Advance® *2768*

Cyclosporine *Serum Increase Physiological* Concomitant administration of NSAIDs with cyclosporine increased its concentration by reducing its tubular secretion possibly due to decreased synthesis of renal prostaglandin *3972*

Digoxin *Serum No Effect Analytical* No effect on FETI methods of Syva® Advance® *2768*

Hydrochlorothiazide *Serum Increase Physiological* Concomitant administration of both drugs caused increase in hydrochlorothiazide concentration and decreased hyperuricemic effect of the diuretic *1384* Significantly increases plasma concentration *1384* Concomitant administration of diflunisal with hydrochlorothiazide increased the hydrochlorothiazide concentration significantly *3972*

Indomethacin *Serum Increase Physiological* Renal clearance decreased and plasma concentration increased *1384* Maximum plasma concentration increased by 40% with renal clearance reduced by 21.9 to 1.8 mL/min when indomethacin administered rectally and 1000 mg diflunisal given orally each day *1750* Steady-state plasma concentration and area under curve increased 2- to 3-fold during treatment with diflunisal. Clearance and volume of distribution significantly decreased. Due to selective inhibition of glucuronidation of indomethacin by diflunisal *6187* Diflunisal administration decreased the renal clearance and significantly increased the plasma concentration of indomethacin *3980* Concomitant administration of diflunisal with indomethacin increased its concentration by decreasing its renal clearance thereby significantly increasing its plasma concentration *3972*

Malondialdehyde *Blood Decrease Physiological* Production reduced with 1,000 mg b.i.d. whereas no effect observed at lesser amounts. Effects observed only for 24 h after administration for 1 d *2303*

Methotrexate *Serum Increase Physiological* Concomitant administration of diflunisal with methotrexate increased the methotrexate concentration by reducing its tubular secretion *3972*

Naproxen *Serum No Effect Physiological* No effect noted on plasma concentration but significantly decreased urinary excretion of naproxen and its glucuronide metabolite *1384* Concomitant administration of diflunisal with naproxen had no effect on the plasma concentration of naproxen but significantly decreased its urinary excretion *3972*
Urine Decrease Physiological Concomitant administration of diflunisal with naproxen had no effect on the plasma concentration of naproxen but significantly decreased its urinary excretion *3972*

Naproxen Glucuronide *Urine Decrease Physiological* Concomitant administration of diflunisal with naproxen had no effect on the plasma concentration of naproxen but significantly decreased its urinary excretion and that of its glucuronide metabolite *3972*

Occult Blood *Feces Increase Physiological* When administered with indomethacin has been associated with fatal gastrointestinal hemorrhage *1384* Significant increase when 1,000 mg given b.i.d. whereas no effect with 250 mg or 500 mg b.i.d *2303* Two reported cases of hematemesis attributable to drug, although other drugs also ingested *3829* Diflunisal has been reported to cause gastrointestinal tract ulceration with bleeding *3972*

Prothrombin Time *Plasma Increase Physiological* Displaces oral anticoagulants from plasma protein binding sites *1384* Concomitant administration of diflunisal with warfarin, acencoumarol or phenprocoumon has been reported to prolong the prothrombin time *3972*

Renal Blood Flow *Patient Decrease Physiological* Diflunisal has been reported to cause a form of renal toxicity associated with decreased renal blood flow or blood volume *3972*

Salicylate *Serum Increase Analytical* Concomitant administration of diflunisal with salicylate may cause falsely increased concentrations of salicylate with some assay methods *3972* At 100 mg/L on colorimetric methods of Keller (and modified version) and Trinder: effect approximately half of that of salicylate *2910* Half to two thirds concentration of salicylate when measured by Trinder and Du Pont aca methods *1227* 2 to 3 times higher concentration than salicylate measured by Abbott TDx method *1227*

Sulindac *Serum Decrease Physiological* Concomitant administration of diflunisal with sulindac decreased the plasma concentration of the active sulindac sulfide metabolite by approximately one-third *3972*
Serum No Effect Physiological Coadministration of diflunisal with sulindac had no effect on plasma concentration of active sulfide metabolite of sulindac *1384*

T3-Uptake *Serum Decrease Analytical* Same interference as with thyroxine but to lesser extent *2768*

Thyroid Stimulating Hormone
Serum No Effect Physiological In 9 individuals given a mean dose of 833 mg/d for at least 3 weeks mean concentration 1.4 ± 0.2 mU/L not significantly different from 1.5 ± 0.2 mU/L in 22 controls *585*

Thyroxine (T4) *Serum Decrease Analytical* Using FETI in Syva® Advance® system in a patient receiving 250 mg drug twice per day although mechanism not clear *2768*
Serum No Effect Physiological In 9 individuals treated with a mean dose of 833 mg/d for at least 3 weeks 94 ± 8 nmol/L not significantly different from 94 ± 4 nmol/L in 22 controls *585*

Thyroxine (T4) Index, Free *Serum No Effect Physiological* In 9 individuals treated with a mean dose of 833 mg/d for at least 3 weeks mean FTI 91 ± 6 not significantly different from 93 ± 4 in 22 controls *585*

Tolbutamide *Serum No Effect Physiological* Concomitant administration of diflunisal with tolbutamide had no effect on tolbutamide concentrations or the plasma glucose concentration *3972* No significant effect observed on plasma concentration when drugs coadministered *1384*

Tri-iodothyronine (T3) *Serum No Effect Physiological* In 9 individuals treated with a mean dose of 833 mg/d for at least 3 weeks mean concentration 1.9 ± 0.1 nmol/L not significantly different from 2.0 ± 0.1 nmol/L in 22 controls *585*

Uric Acid *Serum Decrease Physiological* Dose-dependent effect: at dose of 1 g/d concentration was 30% lower than at baseline, maximum effect within 2 weeks *3932*

Volume *Blood Decrease Physiological* Diflunisal has been reported to cause a form of renal toxicity associated with decreased renal blood flow or blood volume *3972*

Digitalis

Carbamazepine *Serum Increase Physiological* In one old man addition of carbamazepine to therapeutic regime resulted in high concentration of carbamazepine *3119*

Chloride *Urine Increase Physiological* Diuretic action in cardiac failure *2242*

Color *Feces Increase Analytical* Black color reported with digitalis ingestion *3388*

Eosinophils *Blood Increase Physiological* Allergic response may be large with toxicity *2484*

Erythrocytes *Blood Decrease Physiological* Aplastic anemia/pancytopenia *3810*

Glomerular Filtration Rate *Urine Increase Physiological* Improvement with relief of edema *2242*

^{131}I Uptake *Serum Decrease Physiological* Lilly product contains tetraiodofluorescein *4360*

LE Cells *Blood Positive Physiological* SLE may occur, usually normalizes when stopped *5102*

Leukocytes *Blood Decrease Physiological* Agranulocytosis/Leukopenia *3810*
Blood Increase Physiological Rare leukocytosis *3810*

Occult Blood *Feces Increase Physiological* May occasionally cause gastrointestinal hemorrhagic necrosis *1016*

Partial Thromboplastin Time
Plasma Decrease Physiological Reported to partially counteract the anticoagulant action of sodium heparin *6557*

Platelets *Blood Decrease Physiological* Rare pancytopenia/thrombocytopenia may occur *6617*

Potassium *Serum Increase Physiological* But only with doses 20 to 40 times therapeutic *4739*

Prazosin *Serum No Effect Physiological* Coadministration of prazosin with digitalis had no apparent adverse drug interaction in limited clinical experience *4649*

Protein *Serum Increase Physiological* Improved hepatic function and decreased hypovolemia *2242*

Sodium *Urine Increase Physiological* Diuretic action in cardiac failure *2242*

Volume *Urine Increase Physiological* Diuretic action in cardiac failure *2242*

Xylose *Urine Decrease Physiological* May produce gastrointestinal intolerance, impaired absorption with consequent reduced excretion *929*

Digitonin

Cholesterol *Serum Increase Analytical* Affects Liebermann-Burchard and Zlatkis-Zak procedure *2991*

Digitoxigenin

Digitoxin *Serum Increase Analytical* Cross-reacts by 190% at concetration of 10 ng/mL with method on Du Pont aca *1521*

Digoxin *Serum No Effect Analytical* Less than 10% cross reactivity observed with method on Baxter Stratus *5705*

Digitoxigenin bis-Digitoxoside

Digitoxin *Serum Increase Analytical* Cross-reactivity of 113% observed with method on Du Pont aca *1521*

Digitoxigenin mono-Digitoxoside

Digitoxin *Serum Increase Analytical* Cross-reactivity of 129% at a concentration of 10 ng/mL with method on Du Pont aca *1521*

Digitoxin

Albumin *Serum No Effect Analytical* At concentration of 6 mg/L had no effect on BCG method *5704* No effect at 21 mg/dL on Technicon SMA 12/60 method *4390*

Alkaline Phosphatase *Serum No Effect Analytical* No effect at 21 mg/dL on Technicon SMA 12/60 method *4390*

Antithrombin III *Plasma No Effect Analytical* At concentration of 20 mg/L had no effect on Du Pont aca method *5704*

Aspartate Aminotransferase *Serum No Effect Analytical* No effect at 21 mg/dL on Technicon SMA 12/60 method *4390*

Bicarbonate *Serum No Effect Analytical* At concentration of 6 mg/L had no effect on method using phenolphthalein *5704*

Bilirubin *Serum No Effect Analytical* No effect at 21 mg/dL on Technicon SMA 12/60 method *4390* At concentration of 6 mg/L had no effect on Jendrassik and Grof method *5704*

Calcium *Serum No Effect Analytical* At concentration of 6 mg/L had no effect on cresolphthalein method *5704* No effect at 21 mg/dL on Technicon SMA 12/60 method *4390*

Chloride *Serum No Effect Analytical* At concentration of 6 mg/L had no effect on mercurimetric method *5704*

Cholesterol *Serum No Effect Analytical* No effect at 21 mg/dL on Technicon SMA 12/60 method *4390* At concentration of 6 mg/L had no effect on Liebermann-Burchard method *5704*

Creatinine *Serum No Effect Analytical* At concentration of 6 mg/L had no effect on Technicon AutoAnalyzer® Jaffe method *5704* No effect at 21 mg/dL on Technicon SMA 12/60 method *4390*

Diclofenac *Serum No Effect Physiological* Coadministration of digitoxin with diclofenac did not significantly affect the peak concentration or AUC of diclofenac *1025*

Digoxin *Serum Increase Analytical* At normal concentrations in serum if no preincubation (RIA) *4688* Cross-reactivity of 6.1% at concentration of 25 ng/mL (32.75 nmol/L) with method on Du Pont aca *1522* At concentration of 25 ng/mL (32.75 nmol/L) caused 6.1% cross-reactivity with method on Du Pont Dimension *1573* Due to cross-reactivity (RIA) if given i.m. recently *3323*
Serum No Effect Analytical Less tha 1% cross-reactivity observed with CEDIA method adapted for use with Hitachi 717 *1144* Digitoxin had no detectable cross-reactivity with method on Bayer Technicon Immuno 1® *421* Less than 10% cross reactivity observed with method on Baxter Stratus *5705*

Glucose *Serum No Effect Analytical* No effect at 21 mg/dL on Technicon SMA 12/60 method *4390*

17-Hydroxycorticosteroids *Urine Increase Analytical* Moderate effect with *in vitro* test *2451*

^{131}I Uptake *Serum Decrease Physiological* Purodigin, Crystodigin® contain tetraiodofluorescein *4360*
Serum No Effect Physiological With 0.01 mg/kg/week orally no effect *882*

Lactate Dehydrogenase *Serum No Effect Analytical* No effect at 21 mg/dL on Technicon SMA 12/60 method *4390*

Phosphate *Serum No Effect Analytical* No effect at 21 mg/dL on Technicon SMA 12/60 method *4390* At concentration of 6 mg/L had no effect on phosphomolybdate method *5704*

Plasminogen *Plasma No Effect Analytical* At concentration of 20 mg/L had no effect on Du Pont aca method *5704*

Platelets *Blood Decrease Physiological* Several cases of immune-mediated thrombocytopenia reported *4139* Rare thrombocytopenia (due to immune mechanism) *6617*

Potassium *Serum No Effect Analytical* At concentration of 6 mg/L had no effect on measurement by ISE with predilution *5704*

Protein *Serum No Effect Analytical* No effect at 21 mg/dL on Technicon SMA 12/60 method *4390* At concentration of 6 mg/L had no effect on biuret method with blank correction *5704*

Quinidine *Serum No Effect Analytical* No significant interference observed at a concentration of 0.1 μg/mL (0.131 μmol/L) with method on Du Pont aca *1543* At concentrations exceeding 0.25 mg/L concentration as measured by method on Baxter Stratus increased by 30% but physiological concentrations are up to 0.02 mg/L only *5705*

Sodium *Serum No Effect Analytical* At concentration of 6 mg/L had no effect on measurement by ISE with predilution *5704*

Tacrolimus *Blood No Effect Analytical* No significant effect observed at a concentration of 0.04 mg/L with MEIA method on Abbott IMx analyzer *1871*
Serum No Effect Analytical At a concentration of 40 μg/L had no significant effect on ELISA method *6329*

Triglycerides *Serum No Effect Analytical* At concentration of 6 mg/L had no effect on lipase/esterase method *5704*

Urea Nitrogen *Serum No Effect Analytical* At concentration of 6 mg/L had no effect on diacetylmonoxime method *5704*

Digitoxin *(continued)*

Uric Acid *Serum* *No Effect* *Analytical* No effect at 21 mg/dL on Technicon SMA 12/60 method *4390* At concentration of 6 mg/L had no effect on phosphotungstate reduction method *5704*

Digoxigenin

Digitoxin *Serum* *Increase* *Analytical* Cross-reactivity of 359% observed at a concentration of 10 ng/mL with method on Du Pont aca *1521*
Serum *No Effect* *Analytical* At concentration of 0.01 mg/L had no effect on method on Baxter Stratus *5705*

Digoxin *Serum* *Increase* *Analytical* At concentration of 2ng/mL (5.12 nmol/L) caused 156.3% cross-reactivity with method on Du Pont Dimension *1573* Cross-reactivity of 156.3% observed with method on Du Pont aca at concentration of 2 ng/mL (5.12 nmol/L) *1522* At concentration of 5 ng/mL 6% cross-reactivity observed with CDC proposed RIA reference method *4238*
Serum *No Effect* *Analytical* Digoxigenin had an insignificant cross-reactivity of 6% with method on Bayer Technicon Immuno 1® *421*

Digoxigenin bis-Digitoxoside

Digitoxin *Serum* *Increase* *Analytical* Cross-reactivity of 153% observed at a concentration of 10 ng/L with method on Du Pont aca *1521*

Digoxin *Serum* *Increase* *Analytical* At concentration of 5 ng/mL 104% cross-reactivity with proposed CDC RIA reference method *4238* Digoxigenin bisdigitoxoside had a significant cross-reactivity of 82% with method on Bayer Technicon Immuno 1® *421*

Digoxigenin mono-Digitoxoside

Digitoxin *Serum* *Increase* *Analytical* Cross-reactivity of 200% at concentration of 10 ng/mL with method on Du Pont aca *1521*

Digoxin *Serum* *Increase* *Analytical* At concentration of 5 ng/mL 69% cross-reactivity observed with CDC proposed RIA reference method *4238* Digoxigenin monodigitoxoside had a significant cross-reactivity of 12% with method on Bayer Technicon Immuno 1® *421*

Digoxin

Acid Phosphatase *Serum* *No Effect* *Analytical* At concentration of 20 ng/mL (26 nmol/L) had no effect on method on Du Pont Dimension *1562*

Alanine Aminotransferase *Serum* *No Effect* *Analytical* No effect at concentration of 20 ng/mL (26 nmol/L) on method on Du Pont Dimension *1563*

Albumin *Serum* *No Effect* *Analytical* At concentration of 20 ng/mL (26 nmol/L) had no effect on method on Du Pont Dimension *1564* At concentration of 9 mg/L had no effect on BCG method *5704* No effect at 0.04 mg/dL on Technicon SMA 12/60 method *4390*

Alkaline Phosphatase *Serum* *No Effect* *Analytical* No effect at 0.04 mg/dL on Technicon SMA 12/60 method *4390* At concentration of 20 ng/mL (26 nmol/L) had no effect on method on Du Pont Dimension *1565*

Ammonia *Plasma* *No Effect* *Analytical* No effect at concentration of 20 ng/mL (26 nmol/L) on method on Du Pont Dimension *1566*

Amylase *Serum* *No Effect* *Analytical* At concentration of 20 ng/mL (26 nmol/L) had no effect on method on Du Pont Dimension *1567*

Androstenedione *Plasma* *No Effect* *Physiological* No significant effect with long-term administration *4248*

Antithrombin III *Plasma* *No Effect* *Analytical* At concentration of 10 mg/L had no effect on Du Pont aca method *5704*

Aspartate Aminotransferase *Serum* *No Effect* *Analytical* No effect at concentration of 20 ng/mL (26 nmol/L) on method on Du Pont Dimension *1568* No effect at 0.04 mg/dL on Technicon SMA 12/60 method *4390*

Benazepril *Serum* *No Effect* *Physiological* No clinically important pharmacokinetic interactions observed when drugs coadministered *1033*

Bicarbonate *Serum* *No Effect* *Analytical* At concentration of 9 mg/L had no effect on method using phenolphthalein *5704*

Bilirubin *Serum* *No Effect* *Analytical* No effect at concentration of 20 ng/mL (26 nmol/L) on method on Du Pont Dimension *1589* No effect at 0.04 mg/dL on Technicon SMA 12/60 method *4390* At concentration of 9 mg/L had no effect on Jendrassik and Grof method *5704*

Bilirubin, Direct *Serum* *No Effect* *Analytical* At concentration of 20 ng/mL (26 nmol/L) had no effect on method on Du Pont Dimension *1574*

Calcium *Serum* *No Effect* *Analytical* At concentration of 9 mg/L had no effect on cresolphthalein method *5704* No effect at concentration of 20 ng/mL (26 nmol/L) on method on Du Pont Dimension *1569* No effect at 0.04 mg/dL on Technicon SMA 12/60 method *4390*

Catecholamines *Urine* *No Effect* *Analytical* No effect observed *1444*

Cerivastatin *Serum* *No Effect* *Physiological* Plasma concentrations of cerivastatin not affected by coadministration of digoxin *300*

Chloride *Serum* *No Effect* *Analytical* At concentration of 9 mg/L had no effect on mercurimetric method *5704*

Cholesterol *Serum* *No Effect* *Analytical* No effect at 0.04 mg/dL on Technicon SMA 12/60 method *4390* At concentration of 9 mg/L had no effect on Liebermann-Burchard method *5704* At concentration of 100 mg/L had no effect on method using catalase-Hantzsch reaction *5704* At concentration of 100 mg/L had no effect on CHOD-PAP method *5704* At concentration of 20 ng/mL (26 nmol/L) had no effect on concentration on Du Pont Dimension *1570*

Cholinesterase *Serum* *No Effect* *Analytical* Insignificant increase of 0.16 U/mL at a concentration of 0.02 µg/mL with method on Du Pont Dimension *3271* Insignificant decrease of 0.04 U/mL at a concentration of 0.02 µg/mL with method on Du Pont aca *3271*

Cortisol, Free *Urine* *No Effect* *Analytical* Digoxin showed some interference with HPLC method of Turpeinen et al but effect could be reduced by modification of mobile phase *6105*

C-Reactive Protein *Serum* *No Effect* *Analytical* At concentration of 2.5 µg/L (3.2 nmol/L) had no effect on Du Pont aca method *5403* No significant interference of concentrations up to 2.5 ng/mL (3.2 nmol/L) with method on Du Pont aca *1518*

Creatine Kinase *Serum* *Increase* *Physiological* 15 to 17 x increase after i.m. injection (increase for 8 d) *2312*

Creatine Kinase Isoenzymes *Serum* *No Effect* *Analytical* At concentration of 20 ng/mL (26 nmol/L) had no effect on method for CK-MB on Du Pont Dimension *1571* No interference observed at a concentration of 7.5 µg/L (9.6 nmol/L) with CK-MB method on Du Pont aca *1519*

Creatinine *Serum* *No Effect* *Analytical* No effect at concentration of 20 ng/mL (26 nmol/L) on method on Du Pont Dimension *1572* No effect at 0.04 mg/dL on Technicon SMA 12/60 method *4390* At 10 mg/L on reversed phase liquid chromatographic procedure of Zhiri et al *6656* At concentration of 9 mg/L had no effect on Technicon AutoAnalyzer® Jaffe method *5704* At concentration of 0.15 mg/L had no effect on Jaffe-Fading-Fraction method *5704* No interference observed at a concentration of 1 mg/L with HPLC method of Rosano et al *5083* At concentration of 0.15 mg/L had no effect on Jaffe-Fuller's earth method *5704* At concentration of 0.15 mg/L had no effect on kinetic Jaffe method on BKA-2 *5704*

Cyclosporine *Blood* *No Effect* *Analytical* At a concentration of 0.02 mg/L had no effect on Syva EMIT method *495*

Dehydroepiandrosterone *Plasma* *No Effect* *Physiological* No significant effect with long-term administration *4248*

Digitoxin *Serum* *Increase* *Analytical* Cross-reactivity of 159% observed at a concentration of 5 ng/mL with method on Du Pont aca *1521*
Serum *No Effect* *Analytical* No cross reactivity observed at concentrations up to 0.01 mg/L with method on Baxter Stratus *5705*

Donepezil *Serum No Effect Physiological* Digoxin reported to have no effect on the metabolism of donepezil *4662*

Drugs of Abuse Screen *Urine No Effect Analytical* No effect at concentration of 100 µg/mL on EZ-SCREEN procedure for cannabinoids and cocaine *1739*

Estrogens *Plasma Increase Physiological* 2-fold in men, 1.5-fold in postmenopausal women with chronic administration *5832*

Estrone *Plasma Increase Physiological* Major estrogen with chronic administration *5832*

Glucose *Serum No Effect Analytical* At concentration of 0.25 mg/L had no effect on GOD/POD-PAP method *5704* At concentration of 20 ng/mL (26 nmol/L) has no effect on method on Du Pont Dimension *1575* No effect at 0.04 mg/dL on Technicon SMA 12/60 method *4390* At concentration of 0.015 mg/L had no effect on Kodak Ektachem® method *5704*
Urine Decrease Analytical Low values observed with Clinistix® , Diastix® dipsticks *1826*
Urine No Effect Analytical No effect observed with Tes-Tape® *1826*

γ-Glutamyltransferase *Serum No Effect Analytical* At concentration of 20 ng/mL (26 nmol/L) has no effect on method on Du Pont Dimension *1579*

Granulocytes *Blood Decrease Physiological* Agranulocytosis observed in 7.4% patients compared with 4.2% in controls: drug significantly associated with agranulocytosis *3098*

HDL-Cholesterol *Serum No Effect Analytical* No effect at concentration of 20 ng/mL (26 nmol/L) on method on Du Pont Dimension *1576*

Histamine *Plasma No Effect Analytical* No effect on radioenzyme assay at therapeutic concentrations *2492*

17-Hydroxycorticosteroids *Urine Increase Analytical* Moderate effect with *in vitro* test *2451*

Indomethacin *Serum No Effect Analytical* No effect on HPLC method of Roberts and Smith *4978*

Iron *Serum No Effect Analytical* No effect at concentration of 20 ng/mL (26 nmol/L) on method on Du Pont Dimension *1577*

Iron-Binding Capacity, Total *Serum No Effect Analytical* No effect at concentration of 20 ng/mL (26 nmol/L) on method on Du Pont Dimension *1590*

Ketorolac *Serum No Effect Physiological* At therapeutic concentrations had no effect on ketorolac-protein binding *5035*

Lactate Dehydrogenase *Serum No Effect Analytical* At concentration of 20 ng/mL (26 nmol/L) has no effect on method on Du Pont Dimension *1578* No effect at 0.04 mg/dL on Technicon SMA 12/60 method *4390*

Levofloxacin *Serum No Effect Physiological* Concurrent administration of levofloxacin with digoxin had no significant effect on the absorption and disposition of levofloxacin in healthy volunteers *3916*

Lidocaine *Serum No Effect Analytical* No significant interference observed at a concentration of 0.1 µg/mL (0.128 µmol/L) with method on Du Pont aca *1534* At a concentration of 1250 mg/L (normal therapeutic concentration 0.001 mg/L) had an effect of less than 10% when measured by method on Baxter Stratus *5705*

Lipase *Serum No Effect Analytical* No effect at concentration of 20 ng/mL (26 nmol/L) on method on Du Pont Dimension *1580*

Losartan *Serum No Effect Physiological* Coadministration of losartan with digoxin had no significant effect on the concentration of either drug *1596*

Luteinizing Hormone *Plasma Decrease Physiological* 50% in men, 40% decrease in postmenopausal women *5832*

Magnesium *Serum Decrease Physiological* Important factor in digitalis toxicity, possibly associated with prior diuretic use *1892*
Serum No Effect Analytical No effect at concentration of 20 ng/mL (26 nmol/L) on method on Du Pont Dimension *1581*

Midazolam *Serum No Effect Analytical* On GC-ECD method of Ha et al *2387*

Mycophenolic Acid *Serum No Effect Analytical* No significant interference observed with HPLC method of Shipkova et al *5526*

Mycophenolic Acid Glucuronide
Serum No Effect Analytical No significant interference observed with HPLC method of Shipkova et al *5526*

N-Acetylprocainamide *Serum No Effect Analytical* No significant interference at a concentration of 0.1 µg/mL (0.128 µmol/L) with method on Du Pont aca *1536*

Nefazodone *Serum No Effect Physiological* In 18 healthy male volunteers phenotyped as P450IID6 extensive metabolizers coadministration of nefazodone 200 mg b.i.d. with 0.2 mg q.i.d. digoxin for 9 days had no effect on the concentration of nefazodone *729*

Neutrophils *Blood Decrease Physiological* Reported observation *4265*

Nisoldipine *Serum No Effect Physiological* No significant interaction observed between nisoldipine and digoxin *6650*

Paroxetine *Serum No Effect Physiological* No significant effect on the pharmacokinetics of either lithium carbonate or paroxetine observed when the drugs coadministered *5654*

Phenytoin *Serum No Effect Analytical* No effect at concentration of 20 ng/mL (26 nmol/L) on method on Du Pont Dimension *1583*

Phosphate *Serum No Effect Analytical* No effect at 0.04 mg/dL on Technicon SMA 12/60 method *4390* At concentration of 9 mg/L had no effect on phosphomolybdate method *5704* At concentration of 20 ng/mL (26 nmol/L) has no effect on method on Du Pont Dimension *1584*

Plasminogen *Plasma No Effect Analytical* At concentration of 2 mg/L had no effect on Du Pont aca method *5704*

Potassium *Red Blood Cells Decrease Physiological* 6% drop within 2 d, affects membrane ATP-ase *3120*
Serum Increase Physiological In 10 healthy individuals who had received digoxin for 10 days serum potassium concentration increased from mean baseline of 4.24 ± 0.27 mmol/L to 4.43 ± 0.30 mmol/L after 2 hours supine rest whereas in those who did not have potassium no significant change was observed. Effect probably related to digitalis-induced depression of Na-K-ATPase activity *1663*
Serum No Effect Analytical At concentration of 0.15 mg/L had no effect on measurement by ISE without predilution *5704* At concentration of 0.002 mg/L had no effect on flame-photometric method *5704* At concentration of 9 mg/L had no effect on measurement by ISE with predilution *5704*

Pravastatin *Serum No Effect Physiological* Concurrent administration of digoxin with pravastatin to 18 healthy men caused no significant effect on the bioavailability of pravastatin plus its metabolites SQ 31,906 and SQ 31,945 *728*

Prazosin *Serum No Effect Physiological* Coadministration of prazosin with digoxin had no apparent adverse drug interaction in limited clinical experience *4649*

Procainamide *Serum No Effect Analytical* No significant interference observed at a concentration of 0.1 µg/mL (0.13 µmol/L) with method on Du Pont aca *1542*

Protein *Serum No Effect Analytical* No effect at 0.04 mg/dL on Technicon SMA 12/60 method *4390* At concentration of 9 mg/L had no effect on biuret method with blank correction *5704* At concentration of 20 ng/mL (26 nmol/L) had negligible effect on method on Du Pont Dimension *1591*

Protein Electrophoresis *Serum No Effect Analytical* At concentration of 0.15 mg/L had no effect on automated Olympus-Hite method *5704*

Quinidine *Serum No Effect Analytical* No significant interference observed at a concentration of 0.1 µg/mL (0.128 µmol/L) with method on Du Pont aca *1543* Digoxin at a concentration of 100 µg/mL had no significant cross-reactivity with quinidine at a concentration of 2.0 µg/mL in method on Bayer Technicon Immuno 1® *431* At concentrations greater than 0.25 mg/L causes 30% increase in concentration as measured by method on Baxter Stratus but physiological concentrations are only up to 0.002 mg/L *5705*
Serum No Effect Physiological Digoxin has no effect on the pharmacokinetics of quinidine *5996*

Riluzole *Serum No Effect Physiological* No effect on riluzole binding observed *4941*

SDZ PSC 833 *Blood No Effect Analytical* At a concentration of 2.3 µg/L had no effect on HPLC method of Scott et al when used to measure PSC (with CsD as internal standard) at a concentration of 5 mg/L *5418*

Digoxin *(continued)*

Sodium *Red Blood Cells Increase Physiological* 16% increase, due to effect on membrane ATP-ase *3120*
Serum No Effect Analytical At concentration of 0.002 mg/L had no effect on flame-photometric method *5704* At concentration of 9 mg/L had no effect on measurement by ISE with predilution *5704* At concentration of 0.15 mg/L had no effect on measurement by ISE without predilution *5704*

T3-Uptake *Serum No Effect Analytical* No significant effect observed at a concentration of 20 ng/mL (26 nmol/L) with method on Du Pont aca *1545* At concentration of 20 ng/mL (26 nmol/L) has no effect on method on Du Pont Dimension *1586*

Tacrolimus *Blood No Effect Analytical* No interference observed with radioreceptor assay of Murthy et al *4191* No significant effect observed at a concentration of 0.003 mg/L with MEIA method on Abbott IMx analyzer *1871*
Serum No Effect Analytical At a concentration of 3 µg/L had no significant effect on ELISA method *6329*

Testosterone *Serum Decrease Physiological* 30% decrease in men with chronic administration *5832*

Theophylline *Serum No Effect Analytical* At concentration of 20 ng/mL (26 nmol/L) had no effect on method on Du Pont Dimension *1585* No effect at 2.2 µg/L on method on Ames Seralyzer *5706* At concentration of 0.005 mg/L produced no interference with methods used on Kodak DT60, Abbott TDx, Abbott Vision with either whole blood or serum, 3M Diagnostics TheoFAST, Syntex AccµLevel or Ames Seralyzer *1122*

Thyroxine (T4) *Serum No Effect Analytical* At concentration of 20 ng/mL (26 nmol/L) has no effect on method on Du Pont Dimension *1587* No significant effect observed at a concentration of 20 ng/mL (26 nmol/L) with method on Du Pont aca *1546 1588*

Tirofiban *Serum No Effect Physiological* Coadministration had no significant effect on plasma clearance of tirofiban *3957*

Tocainide *Serum No Effect Physiological* No clinically significant interaction observed *268*

Triglycerides *Serum No Effect Analytical* At concentration of 20 ng/mL (26 nmol/L) has no effect on method on Du Pont Dimension *1592* At concentration of 9 mg/L had no effect on lipase/esterase method *5704* At concentration of 0.25 mg/L had no effect on GPO-PAP method *5704*

Trovafloxacin *Serum No Effect Physiological* No significant interaction observed *4663*

Urea Nitrogen *Serum No Effect Analytical* At concentration of 9 mg/L had no effect on diacetylmonoxime method *5704* At concentration of 0.015 mg/L had no effect on Kodak Ektachem® method *5704* No effect at concentration of 20 ng/mL (26 nmol/L) on method on Du Pont Dimension *1593*

Uric Acid *Serum No Effect Analytical* No effect at concentration of 20 ng/mL (26 nmol/L) on method on Du Pont Dimension *1594* At concentration of 9 mg/L had no effect on phosphotungstate reduction method *5704* At concentration of 0.15 mg/L had no effect on catalase-AIDH method *5704* At concentration of 0.15 mg/L had no effect on Kageyama-Hantzsch method *5704* No effect at 0.04 mg/dL on Technicon SMA 12/60 method *4390* At concentration of 0.25 mg/L had no effect on uricase-PAP method *5704* At 10 mg/L on reversed phase liquid chromatographic procedure of Zhiri et al *6656*

Valaciclovir *Serum No Effect Physiological* Coadministration of valaciclovir with digoxin had no effect on the pharmacokinetics of either drug *5725*

Vanillylmandelic Acid *Urine No Effect Analytical* No effect observed *1444*
Urine No Effect Physiological No effect observed *1444*

Water *Red Blood Cells Increase Physiological* Slight effect only due to action on membrane *3120*

Digoxin Immune Fab

Digoxin *Serum Decrease Physiological* Used to remove drug in overdose situations *2786*
Serum Increase Analytical Specimens containing Digibind may cause falsely high results when digoxin measured by method on Bayer Technicon Immuno 1® system *421* Assays that are interfered with by antidigoxin Fab fragments include Abbott PEG, Becton Dickinson solid phase, Bio RAD, Corning MAGIC, Clinical Assays, Diagnostic Products, Du Pont NEN, Kallsted, Medical & Scientific Designs, Ventrex, Micromedic Systems *2438*
Serum Increase Physiological Total serum concentration may rise precipitously following Digoxin Immune Fab administration but almost entirely due to Fab-bound digoxin *2155*
Serum No Effect Analytical Assays unaffected by presence of antibodies used to treat digoxin toxicity include Abbott PEG and TDx, Baxter Healthcare STRATUS, Becton Dickinson ARIA II, Du Pont aca, Leeco Diagnostics and Nuclear Medical Laboratories *2438*

Potassium *Serum Decrease Physiological* Hypokalemia may develop rapidly and require correction *1384* Concentration may devekop rapidly with digoxin immune Fab administration as potassium shifts back into cells *2155*

Digoxin-like Immunoreactive Factors

Digoxin *Serum Increase Analytical* In serum from 40 newborns not receiving digoxin mean concentration < 0.3 µg/L when measured by Johnson and Johnson Vitros method and 0.5 ± 0.1 µg/L when measured by Abbott Digoxin II method *6371*
Serum No Effect Analytical In serum from 40 newborns not receiving digoxin mean concentration 0.0 ± 0.0 µg/L when measured by Roche OnLine method *6371*

Dihydralazine

Aldosterone *Plasma No Effect Physiological* No significant change in basal values in 8 normal subjects treated with 50 mg daily for 1 week *6381*

Epinephrine *Plasma Increase Physiological* In general increase observed in 8 normal volunteers treated with 50 mg daily for 1 week *6381*

Guanosine Monophosphate *Plasma Increase Physiological* Increase of 30% observed in basal values in 8 volunteers treated with 50 mg daily for 1 week but significant increase following acute infusion of 2 liters of saline *6381*
Urine Increase Physiological Basal excretion increased by 90% in 8 volunteers given 50 mg daily for 1 week compared with placebo or clonidine treated individuals but with no change induced by volume loading *6381*

Norepinephrine *Plasma Increase Physiological* In general increase observed in 8 normal volunteers treated with 150 µg daily for 1 week *6381*

Renin Activity *Plasma Increase Physiological* Approximately 100% increase in 8 normal volunteers treated with 50 mg daily for 1 week *6381*

Volume *Urine No Effect Physiological* No change noted in normal volunteers treated with 50 mg daily for 1 week compared with placebo treated controls *6381*

Dihydrocodeine

Albumin *Urine No Effect Analytical* Using a fluorimetric assay with Albumin Blue 580 on a Cobas Fara centrifugal analyzer for the detection of microalbuminuria no significant interference was detected at a concentration of 14 mg/L *3117*

Cannabinoids *Urine No Effect Analytical* No effect on Roche Abuscreen method *5006*

Opiates *Urine Positive Analytical* Significant cross-reactivity observed with Roche Abuscreen method adapted for use with Olympus AU 5121 and 5131 analyzers *214* Cross-reactivity of over 50% observed with Roche Abuscreen Online procedure when adapted for use with Roche Cobas Fara II analyzer *5547*

p-Aminophenol *Urine No Effect Analytical* With addition of drugs at a concentration of 100 mg/L and of related compounds at 50 mg/L no significant effect observed on colorimetric method of van Bocxlaer on Cobas Mira analyzer which involves reacting free p-aminophenol with resorcinol in the presence of magnesium ions to form an indophenol dye measured at 550 nm *6163*

Phenylalanine *Plasma* *No Effect* *Analytical* No interference observed with rapid quantitative whole blood method of Campbell et al using phenylalanine dehydrogenase *867*

Dihydrodigitoxin

Digitoxin *Serum* *Increase* *Analytical* At a concentration of 10 ng/mL cross-reacts to an extent of 16% with method on Du Pont aca *1521*
Serum *No Effect* *Analytical* No cross reactivity observed at concentration of 0.01 mg/L with method on Baxter Stratus *5705*

Dihydrodigoxigenin

Digitoxin *Serum* *Increase* *Analytical* At a concentration of 10 ng/mL cross-reacts to an extent of 120% with method used on Du Pont aca *1521*

Digoxin *Serum* *No Effect* *Analytical* At concentration of 5 ng/mL no cross-reactivity observed in CDC proposed RIA reference method *4238*

Dihydrodigoxin

Digitoxin *Serum* *Increase* *Analytical* Cross-reactivity of 68.5% observed at a concentration of 10 ng/mL with method on Du Pont aca *1521*
Serum *No Effect* *Analytical* At concentration of 0.05 mg/L caused no significant cross reactivity with method on Baxter Stratus *5705*

Digoxin *Serum* *Increase* *Analytical* Cross-reactivity of 10.0% observed with method on Du Pont aca at a concentration of 25 ng/mL (30.50 nmol/L) *1522* At concentration of 25 ng/mL (30.50 nmol/L) caused 10.0% cross-reactivity with method on Du Pont Dimension *1573* Dihydrodigoxin had a significant cross-reactivity of 55% with method on Bayer Technicon Immuno 1® *421*
Serum *No Effect* *Analytical* Cross reactivity less than 10% observed with method on Baxter Stratus *5705*

Dihydroergotamine

p-Aminophenol *Urine* *No Effect* *Analytical* With addition of drugs at a concentration of 100 mg/L and of related compounds at 50 mg/L no significant effect observed on colorimetric method of van Bocxlaer on Cobas Mira analyzer which involves reacting free p-aminophenol with resorcinol in the presence of magnesium ions to form an indophenol dye measured at 550 nm *6163*

Dihydroergotoxine

Aldosterone *Plasma* *Decrease* *Physiological* Eight of 13 men with chronic heart failure showed marked suppression 30 minutes after oral administration although no effect observed in other 5 patients *4069*

Epinephrine *Plasma* *No Effect* *Physiological* Although effect observed on norepinephrine concentration, no effect of 9 mg orally observed on epinephrine concentration over next 4 hours in 8 elderly mild hypertensives *4101*

Norepinephrine *Plasma* *Decrease* *Physiological* After 9 mg orally over next 4 hours concentration decreased to 115 pg/mL from 154 pg/mL and remained significantly reduced for some time longer in 8 mildly hypertensive 60 year-olds *4101*
Urine *Decrease* *Physiological* Marked reduction in excretion over 4 hours following oral ingestion of 9 mg orally in 8 mildly hypertensive 60 year-olds *4101*

Renin Activity *Plasma* *Decrease* *Physiological* Nonsignificant reduction at 30 minutes from mean baseline of 3.08 ng/mL/h to 2.31 ng/mL/h in 13 men with chronic cardiac failure given i.v. bolus dose of 6 µg/kg *4069*

Dihydrofolic Acid

Methotrexate *Serum* *No Effect* *Analytical* At concentration of 10 µmol/L no significant interference observed with method on Du Pont aca *1535*

Dihydroquinidine

Quinidine *Serum* *Increase* *Analytical* At concentrations of 1 mg/L cause increase of 30% with method on Baxter Stratus but significance of this is unknown since physiological concentration is unknown *5705*
Serum *No Effect* *Analytical* No significant interference observed at a concentration of 0.6 µg/mL (1.84 µmol/L) with method on Du Pont aca *1543*

Dihydrospirorenone

Aldosterone *Plasma* *Increase* *Physiological* Significant increase observed in 6 healthy women receiving 2 mg/d during days 8-13 of their menstrual cycle compared with 6 controls *2060*
Urine *Increase* *Physiological* Significant increase observed in 6 women who took 2 mg/d during days 8-13 of their menstrual cycle compared with 6 control women *2060*

Potassium *Urine* *No Effect* *Physiological* No significant effect observed in 6 women who took 2 mg/d during days 8-13 of their menstrual cycle compared with 6 control women *2060*

Renin Activity *Plasma* *Increase* *Physiological* Significant increase observed in 6 women who took 2 mg/d during days 8-13 of their menstrual cycle compared with 6 control women *2060*

Sodium *Urine* *Increase* *Physiological* In 6 healthy women given 2 mg/d on days 8-13 of their menstrual cycle excreted mean of 98.5 mmol/d compared with 79 mmol/d in control women *2060*

Dihydrostreptomycin

Bilirubin *Serum* *No Effect* *Physiological* Clinically insignificant displacement from protein in neonates *6314*

Dihydrotachysterol

Calcium *Serum* *Increase* *Physiological* Delayed elimination of drug from plasma in hypothyroid state *3375* Weak antirachitic activity *3810* Increases plasma calcium concentration by stimulating calcium absorption and mobilizing bone calcium in the absence of parathyroid hormone and functioning renal tissue *5129*
Urine *Increase* *Physiological* Hypercalciuric effect *1714*

Hemoglobin *Blood* *Decrease* *Physiological* Adverse effect with severe hypercalcemia *2754*

Phosphate *Urine* *Increase* *Physiological* Increases renal phosphate excretion *5129* Diuresis almost as great as with vitamin D_3 *128*

Protein *Urine* *Increase* *Analytical* Increased glomerular permeability *1714*
Urine *Increase* *Physiological* May induce increased glomerular permeability *1714*

24,25-Dihydroxy-Vitamin D_3

Calcium *Serum* *No Effect* *Physiological* No significant change observed in 20 patients receiving chronic ambulatory peritoneal dialysis when given 24,25-Dihydroxy-Vitamin D_3 with calcium, remaining within normal range although occasional hypercalcemic episodes *478*

Parathyroid Hormone *Plasma* *Decrease* *Physiological* In 20 patients with chronic ambulatory peritoneal dialysis significant decrease of concentration of intact molecule PTH from 382 pg/mL to 245 pg/mL in 9 patients whose initial concentration was high *478*

Dihydroxyacetone

Lactate *Plasma No Effect Analytical* No significant effect observed at a concentration of 30 mg/dL with method on Kodak Ektachem® systems *2519*

Triglycerides *Serum Increase Analytical* Measured as glycerol with enzymatic methods *4953*

Dihydroxycholecalciferol

Calcium *Serum No Effect Physiological* No effect observed *719*

Urine Increase Physiological 30-100% increase within 2 d up to 2.7 µg/d *719*

Phosphate *Serum No Effect Physiological* No effect observed *719*

Urine No Effect Physiological No effect observed *719*

20-α-Dihydroxyprogesterone

16-α-Hydroxyprogesterone *Plasma Increase Analytical* Up to 25% cross reactivity *38*

Dilevalol

Aldosterone *Plasma Decrease Physiological* Concentration lower over 4 hours of recumbency following single dose of 200 mg than when placebo ingested *6433*

Plasma No Effect Physiological No significant change observed in 10 patients with mild to moderate hypertension treated with 100 mg daily for 6 weeks *3846 312*

Colloid Osmotic Pressure *Serum No Effect Physiological* No change observed in 10 patients with mild to moderate hypertension treated with 100 mg daily for 6 weeks *312*

Creatinine *Serum No Effect Physiological* No significant change observed in 10 mild to moderate hypertensives treated with 100 mg daily for 6 weeks *312*

Glomerular Filtration Rate *Urine No Effect Physiological* No change observed in 10 patients with mild to moderate hypertension treated with 100 mg daily for 6 weeks *312*

Norepinephrine *Plasma Increase Physiological* At 100 watts exercise level mean concentration increased from 5.1 nmol/L to 7.6 nmol/L *1497*

Protein *Serum No Effect Physiological* No significant change observed in 10 patients with mild to moderate hypertension treated with 100 mg daily for 6 weeks *312*

Renal Blood Flow *Patient Decrease Physiological* Non-significant decrease of 4.6% observed in 10 mild to moderate hypertensives treated with 100 mg daily for 6 weeks *312*

Renin Activity *Plasma Decrease Physiological* Activity reduced in 10 patients with mild to moderate hypertension to a greater extent when receiving 100 mg dilevalol daily for 6 weeks than when receiving 10 mg carteolol daily for 6 weeks *312* Concentration lower in 6 normal men receiving 200 mg drug after 4 hours recumbency than after placebo *6433*

Renin Concentration *Plasma No Effect Physiological* No effect of 200 mg on total renin concentration in 6 normal men when compared against effect of placebo *6433*

Diltiazem

Alanine Aminotransferase *Serum Increase Physiological* In rare instances significantly increased activity observed but reversible with withdrawal of drug therapy. Mild increases may occur with/without concomitant increases of bilirubin and alkaline phosphatase: usually transient and often resolved even with continued treatment *2643* Administration of diltiazem reported to cause mild increases in enzyme activity *1911* Mild increases in activity have been observed with/without concomitant increases in alkaline phosphatase activity and observed but return to normal with continuing treatment. Increases usually transient. Rarely significant increases occur with acute hepatic injury *4937*

Alkaline Phosphatase *Serum Increase Physiological* Administration of diltiazem reported to cause mild increases in enzyme activity *1911* In rare instances significantly increased activity observed but reversible with withdrawal of drug therapy *2643* Mild increases in activity have been observed with/without concomitant increases in alkaline phosphatase activity and observed but return to normal with continuing treatment. Increases usually transient. Rarely significant increases occur with acute hepatic injury *4937*

Antipyrine *Serum Increase Physiological* Administration of 30 mg q.i.d. caused significant increase in concentration probably due to inhibition of oxidative metabolism in the liver *411*

Aspartate Aminotransferase *Serum Increase Physiological* Administration of diltiazem reported to cause mild increases in enzyme activity *1911* In rare instances significantly increased activity observed but reversible with withdrawal of drug therapy. Mild increases may occur with/without concomitant increases of alkaline phosphatase and bilirubin: usually transient and often resolved even with continued treatment *2643* Mild increases in activity have been observed with/without concomitant increases in alkaline phosphatase activity and observed but return to normal with continuing treatment. Increases usually transient. Rarely significant increases occur with acute hepatic injury *4937*

Bilirubin *Serum Increase Physiological* Mild increases in activity have been observed with/without concomitant increases in alkaline phosphatase activity and observed but return to normal with continuing treatment. Increases usually transient. Rarely significant increases occur with acute hepatic injury *4937* May occur with acute hepatic injury *2643*

Bleeding Time *Patient Increase Physiological* Post-marketing reports suggest that administration of diltiazem (orally) may cause increased bleeding times *2643* Administration of diltiazem reported to prolong bleeding time in postmarketing studies *1911*

Patient No Effect Physiological In 25 healthy volunteers treated with up to 360 mg/d for 1 week mean concentration changed insignificantly from baseline of 366 ± 17 seconds to 387 ± 21 seconds *6687*

Buspirone *Serum Increase Physiological* In 9 healthy volunteers coadministration of diltiazem with buspirone caused increase in AUC of buspirone by 5.5-fold with a 4.1-fold increase in peak plasma concentration *3376*

Calcium *Serum No Effect Physiological* No significant effect observed after 16 weeks treatment in hypertensive patients *6066*

Urine Increase Physiological Change from mean of 3.4 mmol/24 h to 4.3 mmol/24 h in 15 normo- or hypertensive individuals given 240 mg/day for 3 days. Reduction observed in 100% subjects *5429*

Carbamazepine *Serum Increase Physiological* Coadministration of diltiazem with carbamazepine has been reported to cause a 40 to 72% increase in plasma carbamazepine concentration *2643* Concentration increased during coadministration due to probable inhibition of hepatic oxidative metabolism *3119* Presumed reduction in elimination of drug: drug dose reduced by 60% to reduce toxicity *1677* Due to effect on hepatic metabolism *1384* Coadministration of diltiazem 60 mg t.i.d. caused 40% increase in carbamazepine concentration after 3 days in several patients *739* Rarely significant increases may occur when drugs coadministered resulting in toxicity in some cases *4937* Drugs that inhibit CYP 3A4 inhibit metabolism of carbamazepine producing clinically meaningful effect *1039* Administration of diltiazem concomitantly with carbamazepine caused a 40 to 72% increase in carbamazepine concentration *1911* Single cases of 40% and 50% increase observed when diltiazem coadministered with carbamazepine with concentrations reverting to normal with withdrawal of diltiazem. Marked reduction in carbamazepine dose required to maintain therapeutic concentration *5411* Concomitant administration of calcium channel blockers with carbamazepine causes marked increase of plasma carbamazepine concentration resulting in toxicity in some cases *282*

Cholesterol *Serum Decrease Physiological* Decrease from mean of 5.76 mmol/L to 5.54 mmol/L in 26 hypertensive patients given average of 329 mg/day for 24 weeks *4736*

Serum No Effect Physiological Treatment of 96 patients over 8 weeks had no statistically significant effect on concentration *3730* No significant change in 31 subjects treated for 6 mo *142*

Creatine Kinase *Serum Increase Physiological* Administration of diltiazem (orally) reported to cause increased enzyme activity *2643* Administration of diltiazem reported to increase creatine kinase activity in less than 1% of all patients to whom drug was administered *1911*

Creatinine *Serum No Effect Physiological* No change in 15 normo- or hypertensive individuals given 240 mg daily for 3 days *5429* No significant effect observed in 8 non-insulin dependent hypertensive diabetics treated with mean dose of 196 mg daily for 6 weeks *339*

Creatinine Clearance *Urine No Effect Physiological* No significant effect observed in 14 noninsulin-dependent diabetics treated with mean dose of 214 mg/d long-acting diltiazem for 6 weeks *1376* No significant effect in 8 non-insulin dependent hypertensive diabetics treated with mean dose of 196 mg daily for 6 weeks *339*

Cyclosporine *Blood Increase Physiological* Coadministration with cyclosporine reported to increase trough cyclosporine concentrations from 245 to 822 μg/L in a renal transplant recipient after addition of oral diltiazem to therapeutic regime probably due to inhibtion of CYP enzymes in liver. The concentration of metabolite M17 increased significantly *859*
Serum Increase Physiological Increased concentrations observed when drugs coadministered *1384* May increase cyclosporine concentration by inhibiting hepatic cytochrome P-450 III A which metabolizes cyclosporine *5236* Administration of diltiazem concomitantly with cyclosporine necessitated a 15 to 48% reduction in cyclosporine dose to maintain its serum concentration constant *1911* Coadministration with cyclosporine reported to increase trough cyclosporine concentrations from 245 to 822 μg/L in a renal transplant recipient after addition of oral diltiazem to therapeutic regime probably due to inhibtion of CYP enzymes in liver. The concentration of metabolite M17 increased significantly *859* Significant increase observed when drugs are coadministered with marked reduction in clearance noted: effect due to inhibition of cytochrome P-450 system. Dose reduction of about 40% required *2338* In 126 renal transplant patients in whom 26 received diltiazem cyclosporine concentrations increased by 17 to 400% first observed 3 to 4 days after diltiazem started *6596* Probable interference with demethylation and binding to cytochrome P-450 *6288* Concomitant administration of diltiazem with cyclosporine necessitated 30% reduction in cyclosporine dose to maintain blood cyclosporine concentrations comparable to those in control group *5411*

Cyclosporine A *Blood Increase Physiological* Coadministration with cyclosporine A increases its concentration *5240* Coadministration of diltiazem with cyclosporine necessitated a 15 - 48% reduction of cyclosporine A trough dose in renal and cardiac transplant patients *2643*

Digitoxin *Serum Increase Physiological* Serum concentration increased by up to 21% when two drugs coadministered due to effect on nonrenal elimination *3318* In 10 patients receiving concomitant diltiazem 180 mg/d and digitoxin plasma digitoxin increased by a mean of 7% but in only five did an increase occur. In the others there was a mean increase of 21% (range 6 to 31%) *5345*

Digoxin *Serum Increase Physiological* Increase of up to 20% observed in patients when two drugs coadministered although effect not constant among patients. Half-life prolonged by about 0.5 h. Renal and total clearance reduced *4840* When coadministered with digoxin increased its area under the concentration curve, its half-life and minimum plasma concentration (39% and 50% in two different stidies) *5345* Increased plasma concentration after single oral dose, or for 1 week in 6 healthy subjects. Renal clearance decreased *6603* Increased mean trough concentration from 1.11 ng/mL to 1.54 ng/mL after 3 d coadministration in 11 patients with congestive cardiac failure *176* Administration of diltiazem concurrently with digoxin in 24 normal volunteers resulted in an approximate 20% increase in the digoxin concentration *4937* Administration of diltiazem concomitantly with digoxin to 24 healthy male volunteers caused a 20% increase in digoxin concentration *1911* Coadministration of diltiazem with digoxin reported to have no effect in 12 patients with coronary artery disease but another study of 24 healthy male volunteers demonstrated a 20% increase in the plasma digoxin concentration *2643*
Serum No Effect Physiological Coadministration of diltiazem with digoxin reported to have no effect in 12 patients with coronary artery disease but another study of 24 healthy male volunteers demonstrated a 20% increase in the plasma digoxin concentration *2643* Probably does not cause clinically important increase *1384* Administration of diltiazem concurrently with digoxin in 12 patients with coronary artery disease had no significant effect on the digoxin concentration *4937*

1,25-Dihydroxy Vitamin D_3 *Serum No Effect Physiological* No significant effect observed in hypertensive patients after either 8 or 16 weeks treatment *6066*

Encainide *Serum Increase Physiological* Coadministration in one poor metabolizer caused area under the encainide concentration curve to increase by 33% and half-life of encainide to increase from 8 to 12.3 h. In extensive metabolizers encainide area under the curve increased by 60% *5345*

Glucose *Serum Decrease Physiological* Incidence of 0.8% observed in French Pharmacovigilance database *4106*
Serum Increase Physiological Administration of diltiazem reported to cause effect *1911* Mean increase from 98 to 105 mg/dL after 16 weeks in approximately 120 hypertensives *3837* In nondiabetic hypertensives significant increase observed although concentrations remained within normal range *2528*
Serum No Effect Physiological No effect on basal glucose concentration in 26 hypertensive patients given mean dose of 329 mg daily for 24 weeks *4736* Treatment of 96 patients over 8 weeks had no statistically significant effect on concentration *3730*

HDL-Cholesterol *Serum Increase Physiological* Increase by 15% in 31 subjects treated for 6 mo *142*
Serum No Effect Physiological No change in 26 hypertensive patients treated with average of 329 mg/day for 24 weeks *4736*

Hematocrit *Blood Decrease Physiological* Administration of diltiazem reported to cause hemolytic anemia *1911*
Blood Increase Physiological Post-marketing reports suggest that administration of diltiazem (orally) may cause hemolytic anemia *2643*

Hemoglobin *Blood Decrease Physiological* Administration of diltiazem reported to cause hemolytic anemia *1911*
Blood Increase Physiological Post-marketing reports suggest that administration of diltiazem (orally) may cause hemolytic anemia *2643*

Hemoglobin A_{1c} *Blood Decrease Physiological* In 5 patients with NIDDM and hypertension treatment with β-blockers caused mean concentration to decrease nonsignificantly by 0.07 ± 0.15% after 1 month, 0.24 ± 0.15% after 3 months and 0.13 ± 0.07% after 6 months *5276*

Histamine *Plasma No Effect Analytical* 50% inhibition of radio-enzyme assay at 100 μg/L but therapeutic concentration 0.05-0.2 μg/mL so unlikely to be clinical effect *2492*

Indocyanine Green Clearance
Serum Increase Physiological In 18 patients administration of 90 mg every 8 h for 4 d caused modest increase from 0.484 ± 0.087 L/h/kg to 0.550 ± 0.081 L/h/kg (14% increase) *5345*

Insulin *Plasma Decrease Physiological* Significant decrease in peak insulin value and nonsignificant decrease in value at end of intravenous GTT but insignificant change in baseline value in 26 hypertensive patients given mean dose of 329 mg/day for 24 weeks *4736*

Inulin Clearance *Urine No Effect Physiological* No change in 15 normo- or hypertensive individuals given 240 mg daily for 3 days *5429*

ionized Calcium *Serum Increase Physiological* Slight but insignificant change in 15 normo- or hypertensive individuals given 240 mg/day for 3 days. Increase from mean of 1.12 mmol/L to 1.20 mmol/L *5429*
Serum No Effect Physiological No significant effect observed with 16 weeks treatment in hypertensive patients *4065*

Ketone Body Ratio *Serum No Effect Analytical* When added at a concentration of 5 mg/L had no significant effect on AKBR method of Uno et al *6131*

Lactate Dehydrogenase *Serum Increase Physiological* Administration of diltiazem reported to cause mild increases in enzyme activity *1911* In rare instances significantly increased activity observed but reversible with withdrawal of drug therapy *2643* Rarely significant increases occur with acute hepatic injury *4937*

LDL-Cholesterol *Serum Decrease Physiological* Treatment of 40 patients over 8 weeks caused a statistically significant decrease in concentration *3730*

Diltiazem *(continued)*

LDL-Cholesterol *(continued)*

Serum No Effect Physiological No change in concentration in 26 patients with hypertension treated with average of 329 mg/day for 24 weeks *4736* No significant change in 31 subjects treated for 6 mo *142*

LDL-Triglycerides *Serum No Effect Physiological* No change over 24 weeks in 26 hypertensive patients receiving average of 329 mg/day *4736*

Leukocytes *Blood Decrease Physiological* Administration of diltiazem reported to cause leukopenia *1911*

Blood Increase Physiological Post-marketing reports suggest that administration of diltiazem (orally) may cause leukopenia *2643*

Lithium *Serum Increase Physiological* In some patients diltiazem might have been responsible for inducing lithium toxicity but patients also receiving other drugs at the same time *5345*

Lysergic Acid Diethylamide *Urine Increase Analytical* Minimum concentration that caused a positive result with EMIT method to measure LSD 900 mg/L *4968*

Magnesium *Serum No Effect Physiological* No change in 15 normo- or hypertensive subjects given 240 mg daily for 3 days *5429* No significant effect observed with 16 weeks treatment in hypertensive patients *6066*

Urine Decrease Physiological Insignificant reduction from mean of 5.6 mmol/24 h to 4.9 mmol/24 h in 15 normo- or hypertensive individuals given 240 mg daily for 3 days *5429*

Midazolam *Serum Increase Physiological* By inhibiting cytochrome P450 3A4 may reduce plasma clearance of midazolam when drugs coadministered. Half-life of midazolam increased from 5 to 7 hours *5037*

Serum No Effect Analytical On GC-ECD method of Ha et al *2387*

Nifedipine *Serum Increase Physiological* In 6 healthy volunteers 180 mg diltiazem orally for 3 days produced marked increase in area under curve when 20 mg nifedipine taken orally. Mean increase of 140% observed with reduced clearance and increase in biological half life *4379*

Norepinephrine *Plasma No Effect Physiological* No significant effect observed in hypertensive patients with chronic administration *2528*

PAH Clearance *Urine No Effect Physiological* No change in 15 normo- or hypertensive individuals given 240 mg daily for 3 days *5429*

Parathyroid Hormone *Plasma Decrease Physiological* In 15 normo- or hypertensive individuals given 240 mg daily for 3 days reduction of midmolecule PTH from 1.07 to 0.87 pg/L. Reduction observed in 87% subjects *5429*

Plasma No Effect Physiological No significant effect at either 8 or 16 weeks with treatment in hypertensive patients *6066*

Phosphate *Serum No Effect Physiological* No significant effect of 16 weeks treatment in hypertensive patients with 16 weeks treatment *4065* No change in 15 normo- or hypertensive individuals given 240 mg daily for 3 days *5429*

Urine Decrease Physiological Significant reduction from mean of 32 mmol/24 h to 29 mmol/24 h in 15 normo- or hypertensive individuals given 240 mg/day for 3 days. Reduction observed in 84% subjects *5429*

Platelet Aggregation *Blood Decrease Physiological* Initial platelet aggregation significantly reduced by 50% in 15 patients with essential hypertension after treatment with 180 mg/d for 1 week *4589*

Blood No Effect Physiological In 15 patients with essential hypertension treatment with 180 mg/d for 1 week had no significant effect on epinephrine- and ADP-induced platelet aggregation *1804*

Platelets *Blood Decrease Physiological* Administration of diltiazem reported to cause thrombocytopenia and purpura *1911*

Blood Increase Physiological Post-marketing reports suggest that administration of diltiazem (orally) may cause thrombocytopenia and purpura *2643*

Pramipexole *Serum Increase Physiological* Coadministration of diltiazem with pramipexole presumed to decrease the oral clearance of pramipexole by about 20% *4680*

Propranolol *Serum Increase Physiological* Administration of diltiazem concurrently with propranolol in five normal volunteers resulted in increased concentration in all individuals and a 50% increase in the bioavailability of propranolol *4937* Administration of 180 mg daily diltiazem for 5 days reduced clearance of propranolol by 40% *1431* With coadministration increase observed in d-propranolol maximal concentration of 43% and in area under concentration curve of 37%: maximal plasma concentration of l-propranolol increased by 40% and area under concentration curve increased by 31%. Half-lifes of both enantiommers were unchanged *5411* Administration of diltiazem concomitantly with propranolol to 5 healthy volunteers caused increased bioavailability of propranolol by approximately 50% and increased serum concentration *1911* Coadministration of diltiazem with propranolol to 5 healthy volunteers caused increased propranolol concentrations and its bioavailability was increased approximately 50% *2643*

Prostaglandins *Plasma Increase Physiological* Increase by 63 pg/mL in 20 patients with essential hypertension with 14 weeks treatment *5898*

Protein *Urine Decrease Physiological* Reduction from mean excretion of 4.0 g/d to 2.8 g/d in 8 non-insulin dependent diabetics with hypertension treated with mean dose of 196 mg/d for 6 weeks *339* Decrease from mean baseline excretion of 2.7 g/d to 1.3 g/d in 14 noninsulin-dependent diabetics treated with men 214 mg/d long-acting diltiazem for 6 weeks *1376*

Quinidine *Serum No Effect Physiological* No reported interactions between diltiazem and quinidine *5345* Diltiazem has no effect on the pharmacokinetics of quinidine *5996* No effect of diltiazem on quinidine concentration reported *3839*

Renin Activity *Plasma Increase Physiological* Increase by 0.8 ng/mL/h in 20 patients with essential hypertension with 14 weeks treatment *5898*

Sodium *Urine No Effect Physiological* No significant effect observed in 8 non-insulin dependent hypertensive diabetics treated with mean dose of 196 mg daily for 6 weeks *339*

Tacrolimus *Blood No Effect Analytical* No significant effect observed at a concentration of 1 mg/L with MEIA method on Abbott IMx analyzer *1871*

Serum Increase Physiological By inhibiting cytochrome P-450 IIIA enzyme systems may inhibit the metabolism of tacrolimus *1987*

Serum No Effect Analytical In HPLC/MS method of Christians et al no significant interference observed with measurement of FK 506 *1010*

Theophylline *Serum Increase Physiological* After theophylline 5 mg/kg was administered as a single dose in healthy nonsmokers after 7 days pretreatment with diltiazem mean area under concentration curve increased by 14.6% and mean oral theophylline clearance decreased by 12% with prolongation of half-life *5345*

Serum No Effect Physiological No clinically significant effect on theophylline concentration observed when drugs coadministered *5999* No documented significant interaction with theophylline reported *6117* Coadministration of theophylline with diltiazem had no effect on theophylline metabolism *657*

β-Thromboglobulin *Plasma No Effect Physiological* In 15 patients with essential hypertension treatment with 180 mg/d for 1 week had no significant effect on plasma concentration *4589*

Thromboxane B_2 *Plasma No Effect Physiological* In 25 healthy volunteers treatment with up to 360 mg/d for 1 week caused nonsignificant increase from mean baseline of 381 ± 25 ng/mL to 398 ± 21 ng/mL *6687*

Tirofiban *Serum No Effect Physiological* Coadministration had no significant effect on plasma clearance of tirofiban *3957*

Triglycerides *Serum Decrease Physiological* Reduction from mean of 1.49 mmol/L to 1.29 mmol/L in 26 hypertensive patients receiving average of 329 mg/day for 24 weeks *4736*

Serum No Effect Physiological No significant change in 31 subjects treated for 6 mo *142* No significant effect observed in patients receiving diltiazem *4989* Treatment of 96 patients over 8 weeks had no statistically significant effect on concentration *3730*

Uric Acid *Serum Increase Physiological* Administration of diltiazem reported to cause effect *1911* Administration of diltiazem may cause gout as a side effect *4937*

VLDL-Cholesterol *Serum* *No Effect* *Physiological* No significant change in 31 subjects treated for 6 mo *142* Insignificant reduction from mean of 0.40 mmol/L to 0.35 mmol/L in 26 patients with hypertension given mean dose of 329 mg/day for 24 weeks *4736*

VLDL-Triglycerides *Serum* *Decrease* *Physiological* Reduction from mean of 0.85 mmol/L to 0.69 mmol/L in 26 hypertensive patients receiving average of 329 mg/day for 24 weeks *4788* *4736*

Dimenhydrinate

Theophylline *Serum* *Increase* *Analytical* When Clinical Assays RIA kit used: almost 3 fold increase observed *2401*

Dimercaprol

Arsenic *Urine* *Increase* *Physiological* If poisoning due to arsenic *128*

Bicarbonate *Serum* *Decrease* *Physiological* Associated with metabolic acidosis *1714*

Bilirubin *Serum* *Increase* *Physiological* May cause hemolysis with G-6-PD deficiency *402*

Calcium *Urine* *Increase* *Physiological* Effective but less good than edetic acid *128*

Copper *Urine* *Increase* *Physiological* If cause of poisoning (penicillamine better) *128*

Erythrocytes *Blood* *Decrease* *Physiological* Hemolytic anemia in G-6-PD deficient persons *1212* May induce hemolytic anemia in patients with glucose-6-phosphate dehydrogenase deficiency *1384*

Glucose *Serum* *Decrease* *Physiological* After initial increase *3810*
Serum *Increase* *Physiological* Initial response to toxic doses *3810*

Gold *Urine* *Increase* *Physiological* If poisoning due to gold *128*

Haptoglobin *Serum* *Decrease* *Physiological* May cause hemolysis *402*

Hematocrit *Blood* *Decrease* *Physiological* Hemolytic anemia in G-6-PD deficient persons *1212*

Hemoglobin *Blood* *Decrease* *Physiological* May induce hemolysis in patients with glucose-6-phosphate dehydrogenase deficiency *1384* Hemolytic anemia in G-6-PD deficient persons *1212*
Plasma *Increase* *Physiological* Occurs with intravascular hemolysis *1212*

^{131}I Uptake *Serum* *Decrease* *Physiological* Elemental iodine trapped in thyroid *3810*

Ketones *Urine* *Increase* *Analytical* False positive result obtained with this and other compounds containing free sulfhydryl group when Legal method used *1185*

Lactate *Plasma* *Increase* *Physiological* May induce metabolic acidosis with associated increased blood lactate concentration *1384* Associated with metabolic acidosis *128*

Lead *Urine* *Increase* *Physiological* If poisoning due to lead *128*

Mercury *Urine* *Increase* *Physiological* If poisoning due to mercury *128*

Methemalbumin *Serum* *Increase* *Physiological* Occurs with intravascular hemolysis *1212*

Methemoglobin *Blood* *Increase* *Physiological* May cause hemolysis in G-6-PD deficiency *6015*

Odor *Breath* *Positive* *Physiological* Unpleasant odor present in breath of patients receiving drug *1384*

pH *Blood* *Decrease* *Physiological* May induce metabolic acidosis *128*

Reticulocytes *Blood* *Increase* *Physiological* Hemolytic anemia in G-6-PD deficient persons *1212*

Dimercaptoethane

N-Acetyl-Glucosaminidase *Urine* *No Effect* *Analytical* At 60 mmol/L on 2 colorimetric analytical methods *2254*

Dimercaptopropanol

Salicylate *Serum* *No Effect* *Analytical* No significant effect observed at a concentration of 5 mg/dL with method on Kodak Ektachem® systems *2519*

Dimethadione

Albumin *Serum* *No Effect* *Analytical* At concentration of 2,000 mg/L had no effect on BCG method *5704*

Bicarbonate *Serum* *Decrease* *Physiological* Displacement of bicarbonate by dimethadione *6518*
Serum *No Effect* *Analytical* At concentration of 2,000 mg/L had no effect on method using phenolphthalein *5704*

Bilirubin *Serum* *No Effect* *Analytical* At concentration of 2,000 mg/L had no effect on Jendrassik and Grof method *5704*

Calcium *Serum* *No Effect* *Analytical* At concentration of 2,000 mg/L had no effect on cresolphthalein method *5704*

Chloride *Serum* *No Effect* *Analytical* At concentration of 2,000 mg/L had no effect on mercurimetric method *5704*

Cholesterol *Serum* *No Effect* *Analytical* At concentration of 2,000 mg/L had no effect on Liebermann-Burchard method *5704*

pH *Blood* *Decrease* *Physiological* Extracellular acidosis induced *6518*

Phosphate *Serum* *No Effect* *Analytical* At concentration of 2,000 mg/L had no effect on phosphomolybdate method *5704*

Protein *Serum* *No Effect* *Analytical* At concentration of 2,000 mg/L had no effect on biuret method with blank correction *5704*

Urea Nitrogen *Serum* *No Effect* *Analytical* At concentration of 2,000 mg/L had no effect on diacetylmonoxime method *5704*

Uric Acid *Serum* *No Effect* *Analytical* At concentration of 2,000 mg/L had no effect on phosphotungstate reduction method *5704*

Dimethindene

Erythrocytes *Blood* *Decrease* *Physiological* Rare hemolytic anemia with antihistamines *2753*

Hemoglobin *Blood* *Decrease* *Physiological* Rare hemolytic anemia with antihistamines *2753*

Leukocytes *Blood* *Decrease* *Physiological* Rare reported effect of antihistamines *2754*

Dimpylate

Cholinesterase *Serum* *Decrease* *Analytical* *In vitro* 8.2% decrease at 1 x 10^{-4} mol/L *2095*

Dinitrophenol

Alanine Aminotransferase *Serum* *Increase* *Physiological* Hepatotoxicity with centrolobular necrosis *2242*

Aspartate Aminotransferase *Serum* *Increase* *Physiological* Hepatotoxicity with centrolobular necrosis *2242*

Bile *Urine* *Increase* *Physiological* Due to hepatotoxicity *2183*

Bilirubin *Serum* *Increase* *Physiological* Due to toxic hepatitis *2183*

Casts *Urine* *Increase* *Physiological* Due to toxic nephritis *2183*

Color *Urine* *Increase* *Analytical* Red brown due to hematuria *3810*

Erythrocytes *Blood* *Decrease* *Physiological* May cause anemia/aplastic anemia *2242*
Urine *Increase* *Physiological* Due to toxic nephritis *2183*

Hemoglobin *Blood* *Decrease* *Physiological* May cause anemia/aplastic anemia *2242*

Leukocytes *Blood* *Decrease* *Physiological* May cause agranulocytosis/aplastic anemia *2242*

Methemoglobin *Blood* *Increase* *Physiological* May cause hemolysis/aplastic anemia *4017*

Dinitrophenol *(continued)*

Protein *Urine Increase Physiological* Due to nephrotoxicity *2183*

T3-Uptake *Serum Increase Physiological* Competes for sites on thyroxine binding prealbumin *882*

Thyroxine (T4) *Serum Decrease Physiological* Displaced from binding sites on thyroxine binding globulin *5869*

Thyroxine (T4) (Murphy-Pattee)
Serum Decrease Physiological Competes with T4 for thyroxine binding globulin *882*

Urea Nitrogen *Serum Increase Physiological* Reported to cause renal damage *2242*

Dinoprost

Ketone Body Ratio *Serum No Effect Analytical* When added at a concentration of 2 mg/L had no significant effect on AKBR method of Uno et al *6131*

Dioxane

Protein *Urine Increase Physiological* May cause renal damage *467*

Urea Nitrogen *Serum Increase Physiological* May cause renal damage *467*

Diphenhydramine

Alanine Aminotransferase *Serum No Effect Analytical* At acute overdose concentration (20 mg/dL) on Technicon SMAC® method *6266*

Albumin *Serum No Effect Analytical* At concentration of 200 mg/L had no effect on BCG method *5704* At acute overdose concentration (20 mg/dL) on Technicon SMAC® method *6266*

Alkaline Phosphatase *Serum No Effect Analytical* At acute overdose concentration (20 mg/dL) on Technicon SMAC® method *6266*

Aminosalicylic Acid *Serum Decrease Physiological* Delayed absorption due to delayed gastric emptying *6403* Gastrointestinal absorption reduced probably due to effect on gastrointestinal motility *3438*

Ammonia *Plasma Decrease Physiological* Reported effect in exogenous NH_3 toxicity *3160*

Antipyrine *Serum No Effect Physiological* No significant effect on half-life *5820*

Aspartate Aminotransferase *Serum No Effect Analytical* At acute overdose concentration (20 mg/dL) on Technicon SMAC® method *6266*

Bicarbonate *Serum No Effect Analytical* At concentration of 10 mg/L had no effect on method using phenolphthalein *5704*

Bilirubin *Serum Increase Physiological* May occur with hemolytic anemia *6044*
Serum No Effect Analytical At acute overdose concentration (20 mg/dL) on Technicon SMAC® method *6266* At concentration of 200 mg/L had no effect on Jendrassik and Grof method *5704*

Calcium *Serum No Effect Analytical* At concentration of 200 mg/L had no effect on cresolphthalein method *5704* At acute overdose concentration (20 mg/dL) on Technicon SMAC® method *6266*

Catecholamines *Urine No Effect Physiological* No effect with short term ingestion of 150 mg/d *1184*

Chloride *Serum No Effect Analytical* At concentration of 10 mg/L had no effect on mercurimetric method *5704*

Cholesterol *Serum No Effect Analytical* At acute overdose concentration (20 mg/dL) on Technicon SMAC® method *6266* At concentration of 200 mg/L had no effect on Liebermann-Burchard method *5704*

Cholinesterase *Serum No Effect Analytical* No effect observed at concentration of 0.20 µg/mL with butyrylthiocholine method on Kodak Ektachem® *2504*

Cocaethylene *Urine Increase Analytical* Possible interference with TLC method of Bailey *328*

Creatine Kinase *Serum No Effect Analytical* At acute overdose concentration (20 mg/dL) on Technicon SMAC® method *6266*

Creatinine *Serum No Effect Analytical* At acute overdose concentration (20 mg/dL) on Technicon SMAC® method *6266* At concentration of 200 mg/L had no effect on Technicon AutoAnalyzer® Jaffe method *5704*

Drugs of Abuse Screen *Urine No Effect Analytical* No effect at concentration of 100 µg/mL on EZ-SCREEN procedure for cannabinoids and cocaine *1739*

Epinephrine *Urine No Effect Physiological* No effect with short term ingestion of 150 mg/d *1184*

Erythrocytes *Blood Decrease Physiological* Hemolytic anemia *6044*

Glucose *Serum No Effect Analytical* At acute overdose concentration (20 mg/dL) on Technicon SMAC® method *6266*

Granulocytes *Blood Decrease Physiological* Agranulocytosis has been reported with treatment *4517*

Haptoglobin *Serum Decrease Physiological* Consequence of hemolytic anemia *6044*

Hematocrit *Blood Decrease Physiological* Hemolytic anemia has been reported with treatment *4517* Hemolytic anemia *6044*

Hemoglobin *Blood Decrease Physiological* Hemolytic anemia *6044* Hemolytic anemia has been reported with treatment *4517*

Histamine *Plasma No Effect Analytical* Improbable inhibition of radio-enzyme assay at physiological concentrations of 0.1-1.0 µg/mL although 50% inhibition observed at 26 µg/mL *2492*

11-Hydroxycorticosteroids *Urine No Effect Physiological* No effect with short term ingestion of 150 mg/d *1184*

17-Hydroxycorticosteroids *Urine No Effect Physiological* No effect with short term ingestion of 150 mg/d *1184*

^{131}I Uptake *Serum Decrease Physiological* Benadryl® contains tetraiodofluorescein *4360*

Iron *Serum No Effect Analytical* At acute overdose concentration (20 mg/dL) on Technicon SMAC® method *6266* At concentration of 200 mg/L had no effect on Ferrozine method *5704*

17-Ketosteroids *Urine No Effect Physiological* No effect with short term ingestion of 150 mg/d *1184*

Lactate Dehydrogenase *Serum No Effect Analytical* At acute overdose concentration (20 mg/dL) on Technicon SMAC® method *6266*

Methadone *Urine Increase Analytical* At concentrations above 100 mg/L positive results obtained with Syva® EMIT-ASSAY for drugs of abuse *79*
Urine No Effect Analytical Insignificant cross-reactivity of 0.33% observed with Roche Abuscreen ONTRAK method *3279*

Norepinephrine *Urine No Effect Physiological* No effect with short term ingestion of 150 mg/d *1184*

p-Aminophenol *Urine No Effect Analytical* With addition of drugs at a concentration of 100 mg/L and of related compounds at 50 mg/L no significant effect observed on colorimetric method of van Bocxlaer on Cobas Mira analyzer which involves reacting free p-aminophenol with resorcinol in the presence of magnesium ions to form an indophenol dye measured at 550 nm *6163*

Phenylbutazone *Serum No Effect Physiological* No significant effect on half-life *5820*

Phosphate *Serum No Effect Analytical* At concentration of 200 mg/L had no effect on phosphomolybdate method *5704* At acute overdose concentration (20 mg/dL) on Technicon SMAC® method *6266*

Platelets *Blood Decrease Physiological* Thrombocytopenia has been reported with treatment *4517*

Potassium *Serum No Effect Analytical* At concentration of 23 mg/L had no effect on measurement by ISE with predilution *5704*

Prolactin *Plasma No Effect Physiological* No significant effect with 50 mg given i.m *2352*

Protein *Serum No Effect Analytical* At acute overdose concentration (20 mg/dL) on Technicon SMAC® method *6266* At concentration of 200 mg/L had no effect on biuret method with blank correction *5704*

Prothrombin Time *Plasma No Effect Physiological* Probably no effect on response to anticoagulant *2452*

Sodium *Serum No Effect Analytical* At concentration of 23 mg/L had no effect on measurement by ISE with predilution *5704*

Theophylline *Serum No Effect Analytical* No effect on Kodak Ektachem® 700 method *1716*

Tri-iodothyronine (T3) *Serum No Effect Analytical* At acute overdose concentration (20 mg/dL) on Technicon SMAC® method *6266*

Tricyclic Antidepressants *Serum Increase Analytical* May cause false positive reaction in immunoassays for tricyclic antidepressants *3590* False positive observed with EMIT-ST test for tricyclic antidepressants *5713*
Urine Increase Analytical Large proportion of false positive tricyclic antidepressant results due to cross-reactivity from diphenhydramine with method on Abbott ADx *4535*

Triglycerides *Serum No Effect Analytical* At concentration of 200 mg/L had no effect on lipase/esterase method *5704* At acute overdose concentration (20 mg/dL) on Technicon SMAC® method *6266*

Urea Nitrogen *Serum No Effect Analytical* At concentration of 200 mg/L had no effect on diacetylmonoxime method *5704* At acute overdose concentration (20 mg/dL) on Technicon SMAC® method *6266*

Uric Acid *Serum No Effect Analytical* At acute overdose concentration (20 mg/dL) on Technicon SMAC® method *6266* At concentration of 200 mg/L had no effect on phosphotungstate reduction method *5704*

Diphenoxylate

Digoxin *Serum Increase Physiological* By decreasing gut motility may increase digoxin absorption thus coadministration with digoxin may increase the digoxin concentration *2161*

Diphenylhydantoin

γ-Glutamyltransferase *Serum Increase Physiological* In 10 epileptic patients treated with mean 5.5 mg/kg/d caused mean activity to increase by 60 U/L *5944*

Tri-iodothyronine (T3) *Serum No Effect Analytical* No cross-reactivity observed with method on Baxter Stratus *5705*

Diphosphonate

Hydroxyproline *Urine Decrease Physiological* Normal response in Paget's disease *6111*

Diprafenone

Digoxin *Serum Increase Physiological* When diprafenone administered 3 x 100 mg/d coadministered with digoxin 0.5 mg/d clinically significant increase of digoxin trough concentration from 1.4 ± 0.2 ng/mL to 1.6 ± 0.3 ng/mL observed with maximum concentration increased from 3.9 ± 0.6 ng/mL to 5.5 ± 0.9 ng/mL and AUC increased from 41 ± 7 ng/h/mL to 48 ± 9 ng/h/mL *3265*

Dipyridamole

Acetylsalicylic Acid *Serum Increase Physiological* Coadministration in one study caused increase of peak plasma concentration by 32% and area under curve by 37% probably through inhibition of aspirin esterase *4062*

Adenosine *Serum Increase Physiological* Coadministration with adenosine potentiates its effects *1985*

Adenosine Monophosphate *Urine No Effect Physiological* In 64 patients with low renal phosphate threshold infusion with 1 mg/kg body weight dipyridamole for 30 min had no significant effect on mean excretion changing it only from 348.9 ± 20.6 nmol/mmol to 347.3 ± 20.7 nmol/mmoL *4782*

Albumin *Urine Decrease Physiological* 150 mg/day orally to 15 patients with diabetes but without clinically discernible nephropathy caused decrease in ratio of urinary albumin to creatinine after 9 months from 9.8 to 5.6. In hospitalized patients decreased from 68.0 to 21.9 after 10 days *77*
Urine No Effect Physiological No difference observed in 42 children with insulin-dependent diabetes treated with 5 mg/kg/day compared with placebo-treated controls at 1 year *2105*

Atrial Natriuretic Peptide *Plasma Increase Physiological* In 6 adults who experienced chest pain during dipyramidole test significant increase from mean baseline of 42 ± pmol/L to 55 ± 12 pmol/L *914*

Cortisol *Plasma No Effect Analytical* At concentration of 20 mg/L no significant effect on CEDIA or Enzymun methods (worst case 93.5% recovery) *1097*

Creatinine *Serum No Effect Physiological* No significant change observed in 48 patients with diabetes mellitus without clinically discernible nephropathy when treated with dipyridamole for variable periods of time up to several months *77*

Cyclosporine *Blood No Effect Analytical* At a concentration of 25 mg/L had no effect on Syva EMIT method *495*

Endothelin *Plasma No Effect Physiological* In 6 patients who experienced chest pain during dipyramidole test no significant change from mean baseline of 4.3 ± 0.6 pmol/L observed *914*

Glomerular Filtration Rate *Urine No Effect Physiological* No difference observed in 42 children with insulin-dependent diabetes given 5 mg/kg/day compared with placebo treated controls at 12 months *2105*

Glucose *Serum No Effect Analytical* At concentration of 40 mg/L had no effect on hexokinase/G-6-PDH method *5704*
Serum No Effect Physiological No significant effect on glycemia control in 48 patients with diabetes mellitus without clinically discernible nephropathy when treated for variable periods of time up to several months *77*

Granulocytes *Blood Decrease Physiological* Significant reduction observed in patients (3.0%) versus 1.1% in controls (multivariate relative risk estimate 2.7%) *3098*

HDL-Cholesterol *Serum No Effect Analytical* At a concentration up to 100 mg/L had no significant effect on Reflotron method for whole blood cholesterol *6352*

Histamine *Plasma No Effect Analytical* Since minimal inhibition of radio-enzyme assay at 100 μg/mL unlikely to be any effect at therapeutic concentration of 0.1-4 μg/mL *2492*

Ionized Calcium *Serum No Effect Physiological* In 64 patients with low renal phosphate threshold treatment with 300 mg/d dipyridamole for 2 years had no significant effect on mean concentration which changed from 1.20 ± 0.01 mmol/L to 1.21 ± 0.01 mmol/L over one year *4782*

Lactate *Plasma No Effect Analytical* At concentration of 40 mg/L had no effect on enzymatic method *5704*

β_2-Microglobulin *Urine No Effect Physiological* No change observed in 48 patients with diabetes mellitus without clinically discernible nephropathy when treated with 150 mg dipyridamole daily for variable periods of time up to several months *77*

N-Acetyl-Glucosaminidase *Urine No Effect Physiological* No difference in 42 insulin-dependent diabetic children treated with 5 mg/kg/day compared with placebo-treated controls at 12 months *2105*

Nicardipine *Serum No Effect Physiological* Had no effect on plasma protein binding in vitro and presumed to have no effect on nicardipine concentration in vivo *5016*

Parathyroid Hormone *Plasma No Effect Physiological* In 64 patients with low renal phosphate threshold treatment with 300 mg/d dipyridamole for 2 years had no significant effect on mean concentration which changed from 36.9 ± 1.6 pg/mL to 36.8 ± 3.1 pg/mL over one year *4782*

Dipyridamole *(continued)*

Phosphate *Serum Increase Physiological* In 64 patients with low renal phosphate threshold treatment with 300 mg/d dipyridamole for 2 years caused significant increase in mean concentration from 0.77 ± 0.01 mmol/L to 0.93 ± 0.05 mmol/L *4782*

Platelet Aggregation *Blood Decrease Physiological* Weak inhibition of adenosine deaminase *1857*
Blood Increase Physiological Significant interference with platelet aggregation reported *6557*

Platelets *Blood Increase Physiological* Possibly due to alteration of turnover *1857*

Retinol-binding Protein *Urine No Effect Physiological* No significant difference in 42 insulin-dependent diabetic children given 5 mg/kg/day for 12 months compared with controls *2105*

Tubular Maximum for Phosphate
Urine Increase Physiological In 64 patients with low renal phosphate threshold treatment with 300 mg/d dipyridamole for 2 years caused significant increase in mean $TmPO_4$/GFR from 0.56 ± 0.04 mmol/L to 0.67 ± 0.02 mmol/L *4782*

Dipyridoglutethimide

Aldosterone *Plasma No Effect Physiological* In 9 postmenopausal women with breast cancer treatment with up to 2400 mg/d for 2 weeks had no significant effect on concentration *1486*

Androstenedione *Plasma Decrease Physiological* In 9 postmenopausal women with breast cancer treatment appeared to cause dose-related reduction so that decrease of about 1 nmol/L observed with dose of 1600 mg/d after 2 weeks *1486*

Cortisol *Plasma No Effect Physiological* In 9 postmenopausal women with breast cancer treatment with up to 2400 mg/d caused nonsignificant increase of concentration *1486*

Dehydroepiandrosterone *Plasma Decrease Physiological* In 9 postmenopausal women with breast cancer treatment showed dose related reduction so that decrease of about 1.6 nmol/L observed with 2400 mg/d for 2 weeks *1486*

Dehydroepiandrosterone Sulfate
Plasma Decrease Physiological In 9 postmenopausal women with breast cancer treatment was associated with dose-related reduction so that with 2400 mg/d for 2 weeks concentration reduced by 1.2 µmol/L *1486*

17-Hydroxyprogesterone *Plasma Increase Physiological* In 9 postmenopausal women with breast cancer dose related increase in concentration observed from mean baseline of 1.0 ± 0.1 nmol/L by 0.1 nmol/L after 2 weeks with 800 mg/d, 0.3 nmol/L after 2 weeks with 1600 mg/d and 0.6 nmol/L after 2 weeks with 2400 mg/d *1486*

Testosterone *Serum Decrease Physiological* in 9 postmenopausal women with breast cancer mean concentration decreased in a dose-related manner so that decrease observed of about 0.3 nmol/L after 2 weeks treatment with 1600 mg/d *1486*

Dipyrone

Alanine Aminotransferase *Serum Decrease Analytical* In vitro interference observed at concentration of 89 µmol/L with methods on Kodak Ektachem® and Hitachi 747 *2043*

Aspartate Aminotransferase *Serum Decrease Analytical* Interference observed in vitro at concentration of 89 µmol/L with methods on Kodak Ektachem® and Hitachi 747 analyzers *2043*

Bilirubin *Serum Increase Physiological* May cause hemolytic anemia *3895*

Bilirubin, Direct *Serum Increase Physiological* May cause hemolytic anemia *3895*

Calcium *Serum No Effect Analytical* No interference observed at any concentrations tested with methods on Kodak Ektachem® and Hitachi 747 *2043*

Carcinoembryonic Antigen *Serum Decrease Analytical* At a concentration of 44 µmol/L and higher caused significant decrease with Amerlite method on Kodak Amerlite analyzer *2044*

Chloride *Serum No Effect Analytical* No interference observed at any concentration tested in vitro with methods on Kodak Ektachem® and Hitachi 747 *2043*

Cholesterol *Serum Decrease Analytical* In vitro interference observed at concentration of 44 µmol/L with methods on Kodak Ektachem® and Hitachi 747 analyzers. After 2 g intravenously at 2 min 18% reduction and 6% reduction at 60 min with method on Kodak Ektachem® and 11% reduction at 2 min and 5% reduction at 60 min with method on Hitachi 747 *2043*

β-Chorionic Gonadotropin *Plasma Decrease Analytical* At a concentration of 89 µmol/L and higher caused significant decrease with Amerlite method on Kodak Amerlite analyzer *2044*
Plasma Increase Analytical At a concentration of 44 µmol/L caused significant increase with Amerlite method on Kodak Amerlite analyzer *2044*

Coombs' Test *Blood Positive Physiological* May produce immune hemolytic anemia *575*

Cortisol *Plasma Increase Analytical* At a concentration of 712 µmol/L and higher caused significant increase with Amerlite method on Kodak Amerlite analyzer *2044*

Creatine Kinase *Serum Decrease Analytical* In vitro interference interference observed at concentration of 44 µmol/L with methods on Kodak Ektachem® and Hitachi 747 analyzers. After 2 g intravenously reduction of 16% observed after 2 min and 8% after 180 min with method on Kodak Ektachem® and 10% after 2 min and 8% after 180 min with method on Hitachi 747 *2043*

Creatinine *Serum Decrease Analytical* At concentration of 22 µmolL interference observed with method on Kodak Ektachem® analyzer but no interference observed with method on Boehringer Mannheim Hitachi 747 analyzer. After 2 g intravenously concentration reduced by 54% at 2 min and 26% at 180 min with method on Kodak Ektachem® but with no effect on method on Hitachi 747 *2043* Main metabolite of methyl-amino-antipyrine caused 25 - 75% reduction with enzymatic methods on Kodak Ektachem® analyzers and in Boehringer Mannheim kit used with Roche Cobas Mira *325*
Serum No Effect Analytical No interference observed in vitro at any concentration tested with method on Boehringer Mannheim Hitachi 747 *2043*

Cyclosporine *Serum Decrease Physiological* Reported in three well documented cases *1069*

Erythrocytes *Blood Decrease Physiological* Hemolytic anemia *3444*

Estradiol *Plasma Increase Analytical* At a concentration of 2846 µmol/L and higher caused significant increase with Amerlite method on Kodak Amerlite analyzer *2044*

α-Fetoprotein *Serum Decrease Analytical* At a concentration of 44 µmol/L and higher caused significant decrease with Amerlite method on Kodak Amerlite analyzer *2044*

Glucose *Urine Decrease Analytical* May cause false negative with enzyme tests *2559*

γ-Glutamyltransferase *Serum No Effect Analytical* No interference observed at any concentration tested with methods on Kodak Ektachem® and Hitachi 747 *2043*

Haptoglobin *Serum Decrease Physiological* May cause hemolytic anemia *3895*

Hematocrit *Blood Decrease Physiological* Hemolytic anemia *3444*

Hemoglobin *Blood Decrease Physiological* Hemolytic anemia *3444*

Histamine *Plasma No Effect Analytical* Improbable inhibition of radio-enzyme assay at physiological concentrations *2492*

Lactate Dehydrogenase *Serum Decrease Analytical* Interference observed in vitro at a concentration of 44 µmol/L with methods on Kodak Ektachem® and Hitachi 747. After 2 g intravenously 16% reduction of activity at 2 min and 5% reduction at 60 min with method on Kodak Ektachem® and 11% reduction at 2 min and 8% reduction at 60 min with method on Hitachi 747 *2043*

Leukocytes *Blood Decrease Physiological* Leukopenia or agranulocytosis *2764*

Methemalbumin *Serum Increase Physiological* Occurs with hemolytic anemia *3444*

Neutrophils *Blood Decrease Physiological* Rate of agranulocytosis 23.7 times higher than in nonusers *1830*

Occult Blood *Feces Increase Physiological* May cause gastrointestinal bleeding *128*

Phenylalanine *Plasma No Effect Analytical* No interference observed with rapid quantitative whole blood method of Campbell et al using phenylalanine dehydrogenase *867*

Phosphate *Serum No Effect Analytical* No interference observed at any concentration tested in vitro with methods on Kodak Ektachem® and Hitachi 747 *1459*

Platelets *Blood Decrease Physiological* Thrombocytopenic purpura reported *2754*

Potassium *Serum No Effect Analytical* No interference observed at any concentration tested in vitro with methods on Kodak Ektachem® and Hitachi 747 *2043*

Progesterone *Plasma Increase Analytical* At a concentration of 14230 µmol/L and higher caused significant increase with Amerlite method on Kodak Amerlite analyzer *2044*

Protein *Serum No Effect Analytical* No interference observed at any concentration tested in vitro with methods on Kodak Ektachem® and Hitachi 747 *2043*

Prothrombin Time *Plasma Increase Physiological* May aggravate prothrombin deficiency *2754*

Sodium *Serum No Effect Analytical* No interference observed at any concentration tested in vitro with methods on Kodak Ektachem® and Hitachi 747 *2043*

Tri-iodothyronine, Free (fT3) *Serum Increase Analytical* At a concentration of 712 µmol/L and higher caused significant increase with Amerlite method on Kodak Amerlite analyzer *2044*

Triglycerides *Serum Decrease Analytical* In vitro interference observed at a concentration of 44 µmol/L with methods on Kodak Ektachem® analyzer and Hitachi 747. After 2 g intravenously 15% reduction observed at 2 min and 6% at 60 min with method on Kodak Ektachem® and 21% at 2 min and 4% at 60 min with method on Hitachi 747 *2043*

Urea Nitrogen *Serum Decrease Analytical* In vitro interference observed at a concentration of 1,423 µmol/L with methods on Kodak Ektachem® and Hitachi 747 *2043*
Serum Increase Physiological Reported to cause anuria *128*

Uric Acid *Serum Decrease Analytical* Interference observed in vitro at 44 µmol/L with method on Kodak Ektachem® analyzer and at 22 µmol/L with method on Hitachi 747. After 2 g intravenously at 2 min 9% reduction and 3% reduction at 60 min with method on Kodak Ektachem® but 54% reduction at 2 min and 13% reduction at 180 min with method on Hitachi 747 *2043*

Dirithromycin

Theophylline *Serum Decrease Physiological* Mean steady state concentration unchanged before, during and after dirithromycin administration but mean average steady state plasma concentration declined by 18% during treatment and mean peak plasma concentration declined by 26%. Clearance increased *314*
Serum No Effect Physiological No clinically significant effect on theophylline concentration observed when drugs coadministered *5999* No documented significant interaction with theophylline reported *6117*

Disopyramide

Alanine Aminotransferase *Serum Increase Physiological* Increased activity observed in fewer than 1% of treated patients *2069* Occasional case of cholestatic jaundice reported *5395*

Albumin *Serum No Effect Analytical* At concentration of 4 mg/L had no effect on BCG method *5704*

Alkaline Phosphatase *Serum Increase Physiological* Occasional case of cholestatic jaundice reported *5395* Increased activity observed in fewer than 1% of treated patients *2069*

Aspartate Aminotransferase *Serum Increase Physiological* Increased activity observed in fewer than 1% of treated patients *2069* Occasional case of cholestatic jaundice reported *5395*

Bicarbonate *Serum No Effect Analytical* At concentration of 4 mg/L had no effect on method using phenolphthalein *5704*

Bilirubin *Serum Increase Physiological* Occasional case of cholestatic jaundice reported *5395* Cholestatic jaundice reported as side effect infrequently *2069*
Serum No Effect Analytical At concentration of 4 mg/L had no effect on Jendrassik and Grof method *5704*

Calcium *Serum No Effect Analytical* At concentration of 4 mg/L had no effect on cresolphthalein method *5704*

Chloride *Serum No Effect Analytical* At concentration of 4 mg/L had no effect on mercurimetric method *5704*

Cholesterol *Serum No Effect Analytical* At concentration of 4 mg/L had no effect on CHOD-PAP method *5704*

Creatinine *Serum Increase Physiological* Increased concentration observed in fewer than 1% of treated patients *2069*
Serum No Effect Analytical At 200 mg/L on reversed phase liquid chromatographic procedure of Zhiri et al *6656* At concentration of 4 mg/L had no effect on Technicon AutoAnalyzer® Jaffe method *5704*

Creatinine Clearance *Urine No Effect Physiological* No effect when drug given to total of 300 or 600 mg daily *4967*

Cyclosporine *Blood No Effect Analytical* At a concentration of 30 mg/L had no effect on Syva EMIT method *495*

Diazepam *Serum No Effect Physiological* When drugs coadministered no significant effect observed on the pharmacokinetics of either drug *2069*

Digoxin *Serum Increase Physiological* Mean change for 1.3 to 1.5 nmol/L but clinically unimportant: disopyramide concentrations above therapeutic range when this effect noted *3775*
Serum No Effect Physiological Although disopyramide may cause reduction in volume of distribution and half-life of digoxin serum concentration is unchanged since drug clearance is unaffected. No significant effect after 3 doses of 100 mg per day. Slight effect noted when daily dose doubled *4967* When drugs coadministered no effect observed on plasma digoxin concentration *2069* No significant effect on concentration observed *1384*

Digoxin Clearance *Urine No Effect Physiological* No effect when drug given to total of 300 or 600 mg daily *4967*

Glucose *Serum Decrease Physiological* Incidence of 12.0% observed in French Pharmacovigilance database *4106* Case report together with discussion of 13 other cases reported. Risk factors appear to be pre-existing chronic renal failure, advanced age, and malnutrition *837* Severe hypoglycemia reported in one patient but mechanism not determined *2211* Hypoglycemia reported as side effect in rare instances *2069* To below 10 mg/dL observed in 2 patients both receiving other drugs and occurring with hypotension *4221*
Serum No Effect Analytical At concentration of 4 mg/L had no effect on GOD/POD-PAP method *5704*

γ-Glutamyltransferase *Serum Increase Physiological* Increased activity observed in fewer than 1% of treated patients *2069*

Granulocytes *Blood Decrease Physiological* Reversible agranulocytosis reported as side effect rarely *2069*

Hematocrit *Blood Decrease Physiological* Decreased value observed in fewer than 1% of treated patients *2069*

Hemoglobin *Blood Decrease Physiological* Decreased value observed in fewer than 1% of treated patients *2069*

Histamine *Plasma No Effect Analytical* Although 50% inhibition of radio-enzyme assay at 45 µg/mL, unlikely to be of clinical significance since therapeutic concentration 2-5 µg/mL *2492*

Lactate *Plasma Increase Physiological* Marked effect observed in 2 patients both receiving other drugs and occurring with hypotension *4221*

Lidocaine *Serum No Effect Analytical* At a concentration of 1250 mg/L (normal therapeutic up to 6 mg/L) had an effect of less than 10% on method on Baxter Stratus *5705*

Midazolam *Serum No Effect Analytical* On GC-ECD method of Ha et al *2387*

Mycophenolic Acid *Serum No Effect Analytical* No significant interference observed with HPLC method of Shipkova et al *5526*

Disopyramide *(continued)*

Mycophenolic Acid Glucuronide
Serum No Effect Analytical No significant interference observed with HPLC method of Shipkova et al *5526*

N-Acetylprocainamide *Serum No Effect Analytical* No significant interference observed at a concentration of 100 μg/mL (295 μmol/L) with method on Du Pont aca *1536*

Neutrophils *Blood Decrease Physiological* Occasional case of agranulocytosis reported *6264* Isolated case of agranulocytosis reported *5395*

p-Aminophenol *Urine No Effect Analytical* With addition of drugs at a concentration of 100 mg/L and of related compounds at 50 mg/L no significant effect observed on colorimetric method of van Bocxlaer on Cobas Mira analyzer which involves reacting free p-aminophenol with resorcinol in the presence of magnesium ions to form an indophenol dye measured at 550 nm *6163*

Phosphate *Serum No Effect Analytical* At concentration of 4 mg/L had no effect on phosphomolybdate method *5704*

Platelets *Blood Decrease Physiological* Thrombocytopenia reported as side effect rarely *2069*

Potassium *Serum No Effect Analytical* At concentration of 4 mg/L had no effect on flame photometric method *5704*

Procainamide *Serum No Effect Analytical* No significant cross-reactivity observed with method on Du Pont aca at a concentration of 100 μg/mL (295 μmol/L) with method on Du Pont aca *1542*

Propranolol *Serum No Effect Physiological* When drugs coadministered no significant effect observed on the pharmacokinetics of either drug *2069*

Protein *Serum No Effect Analytical* At concentration of 4 mg/L had no effect on biuret method with blank correction *5704*

Quinidine *Serum Decrease Physiological* When drugs coadministered slight increase in plasma disopyramide concentration observed together with a slight decrease in the plasma quinidine concentration *2069* Small effect noted, but elimination half-life not significantly affected *332*
Serum Increase Physiological Small increases in concentration observed but mechanism not determined *3042*
Serum No Effect Analytical No significant interference observed at a concentration of 100 μg/mL (295 μmol/L) with method on Du Pont aca *1543* Disopyramide at a concentration of 100 μg/mL had no significant cross-reactivity with quinidine at a concentration of 2.0 μg/mL in method on Bayer Technicon Immuno 1® *431* At concentrations greater than 10,000 mg/L cause 30% increase with method on Baxter Stratus but physiological concentration only up to 6 mg/L *5705*

SDZ PSC 833 *Blood No Effect Analytical* At a concentration of 5.2 mg/L had no effect on HPLC method of Scott et al when used to measure PSC (with CsD as internal standard) at a concentration of 5 mg/L *5418*

Sodium *Serum No Effect Analytical* At concentration of 4 mg/L had no effect on flame photometric method *5704*

Tacrolimus *Blood No Effect Analytical* No significant effect observed at a concentration of 4 mg/L with MEIA method on Abbott IMx analyzer *1871*
Serum No Effect Analytical At a concentration of 4 mg/L had no significant effect on ELISA method *6329*

Triglycerides *Serum No Effect Analytical* At concentration of 4 mg/L had no effect on lipase/esterase method *5704*

Urea Nitrogen *Serum Increase Physiological* Increased concentration observed in fewer than 1% of treated patients *2069*
Serum No Effect Analytical At concentration of 4 mg/L had no effect on diacetylmonoxime method *5704*

Uric Acid *Serum No Effect Analytical* At concentration of 4 mg/L had no effect on phosphotungstate reduction method *5704* At 200 mg/L on reversed phase liquid chromatographic procedure of Zhiri et al *6656*

Disulfiram

Acetaldehyde *Blood Increase Physiological* Ethanol metabolism diverted (10 times normal concentration) *2242*

Acetaldehyde Oxidase *Test Conditions Decrease Analytical* Inhibitory effect observed *4821*

Acetoacetate *Serum Increase Physiological* In 1 of 6 volunteers rapid and short lasting effect *5842*

Acetone *Serum Increase Physiological* In all of 6 volunteers rapid and short lasting effect *5842*

Alanine Aminotransferase *Serum Increase Physiological* In 6 patients: proved to be drug associated in one by challenge test *4852* One case of questionable cholestasis reported *2754* Case reported of disulfiram induced hepatitis in 38-year old alcoholic woman probably due to allergic or hypersensitivity reaction *3832* Reversible toxic liver damage in one nonalcoholic woman *3293*

Albumin *Serum No Effect Analytical* At concentration of 120 mg/L had no effect on BCG method *5704*

Alcohol Dehydrogenase *Serum Increase Physiological* In 40 chronic non-cirrhotic alcoholics treatment with disulfiram caused significant change from mean baseline of 0.82 ± 0.28 kU/L to 2.17 ± 0.88 kU/L *814*

Aldehyde Dehydrogenase
Red Blood Cells Decrease Physiological Maximal inhibition (90%) attained after 3-6 days treatment with 200-400 mg/day: remained 90% inhibited for 1 week after treatment stopped *2544*
White Blood Cells Decrease Physiological Maximally inhibited within 2-3 days of initial treatment with 200 or 400 mg orally: remained inhibited at same level for 2 days after treatment stopped then reverted to normal about 6-7 days after treatment stopped *2544*

Alkaline Phosphatase *Serum Increase Physiological* In 6 patients: proved to be drug associated in one by challenge test *4852* One possible case of cholestasis reported *2754* Reversible toxic liver damage in one nonalcoholic woman *3293*

Antipyrine *Serum Increase Physiological* Inhibits hydroxylation, prolongs action *4426*

Aspartate Aminotransferase *Serum Increase Physiological* Reversible toxic liver damage in one nonalcoholic woman *3293* Observed in one patient and similar results followed challenge test *4124* Case reported of drug related hepatitis in 38-year old alcoholic woman which resolved with withdrawal of drug *3832*

Bicarbonate *Serum No Effect Analytical* At concentration of 120 mg/L had no effect on method using phenolphthalein *5704*

Bilirubin *Serum Increase Physiological* One possible case of cholestasis reported *2754* In 6 patients: proved to be drug associated in one by challenge test *4852* Case reported in a 38-year old alcoholic woman in whom acute hepatitis occurred but resolved with withdrawal of drug probably due to allergic or hypersensitivity response *3832*
Serum No Effect Analytical At concentration of 120 mg/L had no effect on Jendrassik and Grof method *5704*

Calcium *Serum No Effect Analytical* At concentration of 120 mg/L had no effect on cresolphthalein method *5704*

Carbamazepine *Serum No Effect Physiological* No significant changes observed in carbamazepine or carbamazepine epoxide concentrations when drugs are coadministered *3119*

Carbon Disulfide *Blood Increase Physiological* In 4 abstinent alcoholics dose response relationship observed following oral administration of 100 to 400 mg doses with peak concentrations observed at 12 h for free carbon disulfide although bound carbon disulfide concentration continued to increase to 23 h (free concentration approximately one fifth of total at 12 h) *895*

Chlordiazepoxide *Serum Increase Physiological* Toxic concentrations may occur when disulfiram coadministered *1384* Clearance reduced and half-life prolonged when drugs coadministered probably as a result of inhibition of hepatic metabolism of chlordiazepoxide *3720*

Chloride *Serum No Effect Analytical* At concentration of 120 mg/L had no effect on mercurimetric method *5704*

Chlorzoxazone *Serum Increase Physiological* In 6 healthy volunteers administration of 750 mg orally pretreatment with 500 mg oral disulfiram causedmarkedly decreased chlorzoxazone elimination clearance to 15% of control values and caused a 2-fold increase in peak plasma concentration from 20.6 ± 9.9 μg/mL to 38.7 ± 10.3 μg/mL *3129*

Cholesterol *Serum Increase Physiological* 500 mg/d raised mean concentration from 193 mg/dL to 227 mg/dL after 3 weeks and 264 mg/dL after 6 weeks in alcoholic subjects. No fall in cholesterol with abstinence *3743*
Serum No Effect Analytical At concentration of 120 mg/L had no effect on Liebermann-Burchard method *5704*

Clonazepam *Serum Increase Physiological* Reported to increase plasma concentration *1384*

Clorazepate *Serum Increase Physiological* Toxic concentrations may occur when disulfiram coadministered *1384*

Creatinine *Serum No Effect Analytical* At concentration of 120 mg/L had no effect on Technicon AutoAnalyzer® Jaffe method *5704*

Diazepam *Serum Increase Physiological* Toxic concentrations may occur with coadministration of disulfiram *1384* Clearance reduced and half-life prolonged as a result of inhibition of hepatic metabolizing enzymes *3720*

Dopamine β-Hydroxylase *Serum No Effect Physiological* In abstinent alcoholics neither administration of a single oral dose of 100 to 400 mg or daily administration of 200 mg for one month had a significant effect on activity of dopamine β-hydroylase, causing a mean 6.4% decrease only from baseline of 18.0 ± 14.0 µmol/min/L in the latter situation in 20 individuals *895*

Epinephrine *Plasma No Effect Physiological* No effect observed after 1 week *3008*

Flurazepam *Serum Increase Physiological* Toxic concentrations may occur when disulfiram coadministered *1384*

γ-Glutamyltransferase *Serum Increase Physiological* Reversible toxic liver damage in nonalcoholic woman *3293*

Halazepam *Serum Increase Physiological* Toxic concentrations may occur when disulfiram coadministered *1384*

Histamine *Plasma No Effect Analytical* Improbable inhibition of radio-enzyme assay at therapeutic concentrations *2492*

Homovanillic Acid *Urine Increase Physiological* Probably due to inhibition of dopamine hydroxylase *6243*

4-Hydroxy-3-Methoxy-Phenylglycol
Urine Increase Physiological Inhibition of aldehyde dehydrogenase *3669*

β-Hydroxybutyrate *Serum Increase Physiological* In 1 of 6 volunteers rapid and short lasting effect *5842*

^{131}I Uptake *Serum Decrease Physiological* Uncommon reported effect *3669*

Isoniazid *Serum Increase Physiological* Toxic concentrations may occur with coadministration of disulfiram *1384*

Mexiletine *Serum Increase Physiological* Decreases clearance and prolongs half-life *3281*

Norepinephrine *Plasma Decrease Physiological* Significant decrease after 1 week therapy *3008*

p-Aminophenol *Urine No Effect Analytical* With addition of drugs at a concentration of 100 mg/L and of related compounds at 50 mg/L no significant effect observed on colorimetric method of van Bocxlaer on Cobas Mira analyzer which involves reacting free p-aminophenol with resorcinol in the presence of magnesium ions to form an indophenol dye measured at 550 nm *6163*

Phenytoin *Serum Increase Physiological* Toxic concentrations may occur with coadministration of disulfiram *1384* May increase from 7/15 to 25/39 µg/mL (at 400-800 mg/d) *3339* Inhibits hydroxylation, prolongs action *4426* Marked increase observed with concomitant administration of disulfiram; effect due to inhibition of hepatic metabolism of phenytoin *5887* Causes increase in concentration when drugs coadministered through enzyme inhibition *6350* When disulfiram ingested with fosphenytoin concentration of phenytoin may be increased *4519* Coadministration with phenytoin may increase plasma phenytoin concentration *4522* Metabolism inhibited, with half-life increased and decrease in mean metabolic clearance rate *5967*

Phosphate *Serum No Effect Analytical* At concentration of 120 mg/L had no effect on phosphomolybdate method *5704*

Prazepam *Serum Increase Physiological* Toxic concentrations may occur when disulfiram coadministered *1384*

Protein *Serum No Effect Analytical* At concentration of 120 mg/L had no effect on biuret method with blank correction *5704*

Prothrombin Time *Plasma Increase Physiological* Inhibits metabolism of coumarins *5117* Causes stereoselective inhibition of clearance of S isomer of warfarin *2625* Augmented S-warfarin hypoprothrombinemia but not that of R- warfarin *4425*

Rifampin *Serum Increase Physiological* Toxic concentrations may occur with coadministration of disulfiram *1384*

Theophylline *Serum Increase Physiological* Dose dependent reduction in clearance decreasing from mean of 106 mL/kg/h to 83 mL/kg/h with 250 mg and from mean of 94 mL/kg/h to 65 mL/kg/h in 500 mg group. Cytochrome P-450 isoenzymes inhibited. Hydroxylation more affected than demethylation pathway *3636* Decreases theophylline clearance by inhibiting hydroxylation and demethylation and increases serum theophylline concentration by 50% *3125* Decreases theophylline clearance by inhibiting hydroxylation and demethylation, increasing theophylline concentration by about 50% *5999* Up to 50% increase in serum theophylline concentration due to decreased theophylline clearance caused by inhibition of hydroxylation and demethylation *6117* Toxic concentrations may occur with coadministration of disulfiram *1384*

Triglycerides *Serum No Effect Analytical* At concentration of 120 mg/L had no effect on lipase/esterase method *5704*

Urea Nitrogen *Serum No Effect Analytical* At concentration of 120 mg/L had no effect on diacetylmonoxime method *5704*

Uric Acid *Serum No Effect Analytical* At concentration of 120 mg/L had no effect on phosphotungstate reduction method *5704*

Vanillylmandelic Acid *Urine Decrease Physiological* Probably due to inhibition of dopamine hydroxylase *6243* Although HMPG excretion increased *660*
Urine Increase Analytical ?Interference from acetaldehyde from ethanol *2451*

Warfarin *Plasma Increase Physiological* Toxic concentrations may occur with coadministration of disulfiram *1384* If administered together *4426*
Plasma No Effect Physiological No effect on plasma concentrations of either R- or S- warfarin *4425*

Dithiazanine

Color *Feces Increase Analytical* Green to blue *3810*
Urine Increase Analytical Blue *3810*

^{131}I Uptake *Serum Decrease Physiological* Due to iodine component of drug *3669*

Protein *Urine Increase Analytical* Reacts with Folin-Ciocalteu of Lowry procedure *4012*
Urine Increase Physiological Transient proteinuria may occur *4014*

Dithionite

Ethanol *Serum No Effect Analytical* Over 16 weeks at 20 °C at concentration of 0.5% w/v on blood ethanol concentration *5608*

Dithiothreitol

Protein *Test Conditions Increase Analytical* Reacts with Folin-Ciocalteu of Lowry procedure *1102*

Dithranol

Histamine *Plasma No Effect Analytical* Improbable inhibition of radio-enzyme assay at therapeutic concentrations *2492*

Diuretics

Albumin *Urine Decrease Physiological* In 12 patients with essential hypertension and proteinuria treatment for 8 weeks caused nonsignificant reduction in albumin excretion *545*

Calcium *Serum Decrease Physiological* Excretion enhanced by most diuretics *174*
Urine Increase Physiological Excretion enhanced by most diuretics *174*

Cell Water *White Blood Cells No Effect Physiological* No change observed in normal individuals *1660*

Diuretics *(continued)*

Chloride *Serum Decrease Physiological* Diuretic action if excessive *3810*

Creatine Kinase *Serum Increase Physiological* May occur as result of i.m. injections *403*

Creatinine *Serum Increase Physiological* May be associated with acute sodium depletion *174*

Creatinine Clearance *Urine Increase Physiological* In 12 patients with essential hypertension treatment for 8 weeks caused nonsignificant increase from mean baseline of 98.2 ± 2.1 mL/min to 102.2 ± 4.8 mL/min *545*

Epinephrine *Urine No Effect Physiological* No significant effect during diuresis *6065*

Glomerular Filtration Rate *Urine Decrease Physiological* Effect on clearances *4555*

Glucose *Serum Decrease Physiological* Incidence of 0.4% observed in French Pharmacovigilance database *4106*

Lipoprotein Lp(a) *Serum Increase Physiological* In 50 diuretic users (in whom 43 were being treated for hypertension) mean and median concentrations 288 and 176 mg/L compared with 176 and 103 mg/L respectively in 1477 non-diuretic using controls but 23 of these were postmenopausal women and sex and systolic blood pressure predicted the Lp(a) concentration whereas use of diuretics did not reach statistical significance *5604*

Norepinephrine *Urine No Effect Physiological* No significant effect during diuresis *6065*

Potassium *Serum Decrease Physiological* Loss in urine *3810*
Urine Increase Physiological Diuretic action *3810*
White Blood Cells No Effect Physiological No change observed in normal individuals *1660*

Prothrombin Time *Plasma Decrease Physiological* In patients receiving anticoagulants *3810*
Plasma Increase Physiological May prolong action of anticoagulants *2753*

PSP Excretion *Urine Decrease Physiological* Blocking of secretory mechanism *1714*

Quinidine *Serum Increase Physiological* If administration concomitantly and alkalinize urine *2452*

Sodium *Serum Decrease Physiological* Diuretic action *4555*
Serum No Effect Physiological May appear normal if hypovolemia occurs *174*
Urine Decrease Physiological In 12 patients with essential hypertension treatment with diuretics for 8 weeks caused nonsignificant decrease from mean baseline of 142 ± 4.0 mmol/d to 138 ± 3.5 mmol/d *545*
White Blood Cells No Effect Physiological No change observed in normal individuals *1660*

Urea Clearance *Urine Increase Physiological* May be observed after use of diuretics *703*

Urea Nitrogen *Serum Increase Physiological* Reduced clearance *4555*

Uric Acid *Serum Increase Physiological* Reduced clearance *189*

Volume *Plasma Decrease Physiological* May occur if rapid diuretic action *2242*

Zinc *Urine Decrease Physiological* Although other cations increased *5782*

Dixyrazine

Albumin *Urine No Effect Analytical* Using a fluorimetric assay with Albumin Blue 580 on a Cobas Fara centrifugal analyzer for the detection of microalbuminuria no significant interference was detected at a concentration of 10 mg/L *3117*

Doans® Pills

Color *Urine Increase Analytical* Greenish blue *3810*

Dobutamine

Aldosterone *Plasma Increase Physiological* In 8 normal individuals infusion of a mean of 4.92 ± 0.40 µg/kg/min over 2 hours caused significant increase from mean baseline of 328 ± 50 pmol/L to 457 ± 86 pmol/L *4412*

Antidiuretic Hormone *Plasma No Effect Physiological* In 10 patients with congestive cardiac failure *6135*

Cholesterol *Serum Decrease Analytical* Concentrations significantly changed with increasing concentrations of dopamine up to 200 mg/L with method on BMC/Hitachi 747 analyzer: concentration at baseline of 1070 mg/L reduced to 990 mg/L at 25 mg/L, 920 mg/L at 50 mg/L and 590 mg/L at a dobutamine concentration of 200 mg/L dobutamine *3050*

Creatinine *Serum Decrease Analytical* Concentrations significantly changed with increasing concentrations of dopamine up to 200 mg/L with method on J&J Vitros 750 analyzer: concentration at baseline of 52 mg/L reduced to 36 mg/L at 25 mg/L, 24 mg/L at 50 mg/L and < 1 mg/L at a dobutamine concentration of 200 mg/L dobutamine *3050*
Serum No Effect Analytical Concentrations not significantly changed with increasing concentrations of dopamine up to 200 mg/L with method on BMC/Hitachi 747 analyzer *3050*

Effective Renal Plasma Flow
Patient No Effect Physiological In 8 normal individuals infusion of 4.92 ± 0.40 µg/kg/min over 2 hours caused no significant change *4412*

Fractional Excretion of Lithium
Urine No Effect Physiological In 8 normal individuals infusion of a mean of 4.92 ± 0.40 µg/kg/min over 2 hours caused nonsignificant increase from mean baseline of 28% to 29% *4412*

Glomerular Filtration Rate *Urine No Effect Physiological* In 8 normal individuals infusion of a mean 4.92 ± 0.40 µg/kg/min over 2 h caused no significant change in GFR *4412*

Ketone Body Ratio *Serum No Effect Analytical* When added at a concentration of 9.5 mg/L had no significant effect on AKBR method of Uno et al *6131*

Lithium Clearance *Urine No Effect Physiological* In 8 normal individuals infusion of a mean of 4.92 ± 0.40 µg/kg/min caused nonsignificant increase from mean baseline of 30 mL/min/1.73 sq m to 33 mL/min/1.73 sq m *4412*

Midazolam *Serum No Effect Analytical* On GC-ECD method of Ha et al *2387*

Myosin *Serum Increase Physiological* All patients receiving intravenous infusion demonstrated increase of cardiac-specific myosin light-chains up to 42 ng/mL *981*

Norepinephrine *Plasma Decrease Physiological* In 10 patients with congestive cardiac failure *6135* Significant reduction from mean of 771 to 524 pg/mL in 13 patients with cardiomyopathy given infusion of 10 µg/kg/min *2221*

Potassium *Serum Decrease Physiological* Mean decrease from 4.6 to 4.2 mmol/L in 13 patients with various forms of cardiomyopathy following infusion of 10 µg/kg/min at peak of infusion with decrease continuing for at least 45 min after infusion *2221*

Renin Activity *Plasma Increase Physiological* In 10 patients with congestive cardiac failure from 11.3 to 17.8 ng/mL/h on average *6135* In 8 normal individuals infusion of a mean of 4.92 ± 0.40 µg/kg/min over 2 hours caused nonsignificant increase from mean baseline of 23 ± 3 mIU/L to 38 ± 6 mIU/L *4412*

Thyroid Stimulating Hormone
Serum Decrease Physiological Infusion of 5-20 µg/kg/min from 8 pm to midnight in normal volunteers initially caused small but significant fall but towards end of infusion rose to same concentration seen with placebo *625*

Triglycerides *Serum Decrease Analytical* Concentrations significantly changed with increasing concentrations of dopamine up to 200 mg/L with method on BMC/Hitachi 747 analyzer: concentration at baseline of 1020 mg/L reduced to 850 mg/L at 25 mg/L, 730 mg/L at 50 mg/L and 270 mg/L at a dobutamine concentration of 200 mg/L dobutamine *3050*

Uric Acid *Serum Decrease Analytical* Concentrations significantly changed with increasing concentrations of dopamine up to 200 mg/L with method on BMC/Hitachi 747 analyzer: concentration at baseline of 64 mg/L reduced to 37 mg/L at 25 mg/L, 24 mg/L at 50 mg/L and 4 mg/L at a dobutamine concentration of 200 mg/L dobutamine: with J&J Vitros 750 analyzer uric acid concentrations at the same concentration of dobutamine were baseline 68 mg/L and 51, 40 and 10 mg/L respectively *3050*

Docetaxel

Alanine Aminotransferase *Serum Increase Physiological* In over 1400 patients treated with 100 mg/m^2 and normal LFTs at baseline 18.1% patients had activities more than 1.5 times the upper limit of normal *4942*

Alkaline Phosphatase *Serum Increase Physiological* In over 1400 patients treated with 100 mg/m^2 and normal LFTs at baseline 7.6% patients had activities more than 2.5 times the upper limit of normal *4942*

Aspartate Aminotransferase *Serum Increase Physiological* In over 1400 patients treated with 100 mg/m^2 and normal LFTs at baseline 18.1% patients had activities more than 1.5 times the upper limit of normal *4942*

Bilirubin *Serum Increase Physiological* In over 1400 patients treated with 100 mg/m^2 and normal LFTs at baseline 8.9% patients had concentrations above the upper limit of normal *4942*

Hemoglobin *Blood Decrease Physiological* In 55 breast cancer patients treated with 75 mg/m^2 89.1% patients had concentrations below 11 g/dL *4942*

Neutrophils *Blood Decrease Physiological* In 55 breast cancer patients treated with 75 mg/m^2 98.1% patients had cell counts below 2000 /µL and 80.0% had counts below 500 /µL *4942*

Occult Blood *Feces Increase Physiological* In some patients treated with docetaxel gastrointestinal hemorrhage has been reported as a complication *4942*

Platelets *Blood Decrease Physiological* In 55 breast cancer patients treated with 75 mg/m^2 5.5% patients had cell counts below 100,000 /µL but none had counts below 20,000 /µL *4942*

Docusate

Tirofiban *Serum No Effect Physiological* Coadministration had no significant effect on plasma clearance of tirofiban *3957*

Domperidone

Aldosterone *Plasma No Effect Physiological* No effect observed 15 minutes after 1 mg/kg intravenously in healthy volunteers *5765* After 10 mg intravenously in 8 healthy males *5732*

Corticotropin *Plasma No Effect Physiological* No effect 15 minutes after 1 mg/kg intravenously in healthy volunteers *5765*

Cortisol *Plasma No Effect Physiological* After 10 mg intravenously in 8 healthy males *5732* No effect 15 minutes after 1 mg/kg intravenously in healthy volunteers *5765*

Growth Hormone *Plasma No Effect Physiological* No significant change in concentration after 0.17 mg/kg bolus i.v. in 10 children *3834*

18-Hydroxycorticosterone *Plasma No Effect Physiological* After 10 mg intravenously in 8 healthy males *5732*

p-Aminophenol *Urine No Effect Analytical* With addition of drugs at a concentration of 100 mg/L and of related compounds at 50 mg/L no significant effect observed on colorimetric method of van Bocxlaer on Cobas Mira analyzer which involves reacting free p-aminophenol with resorcinol in the presence of magnesium ions to form an indophenol dye measured at 550 nm *6163*

Prolactin *Plasma Increase Physiological* After 10 mg intravenously in 8 healthy males *5732* Quick and marked effect when given i.m. to 12 normal subjects and to a group of patients with subclinical hypothyroidism *1366*

Renin Activity *Plasma No Effect Physiological* After 10 mg intravenously in 8 healthy males *5732*

Thyroid Stimulating Hormone
Serum Increase Physiological Small but significant effect when given i.m. to 12 normal subjects and to a group of patients with subclinical hypothyroidism *1366* In euthyroid and hypothyroid patients: drug is a dopamine antagonist *6412* After 10 mg intravenously in 8 healthy males *5732*
Serum No Effect Physiological No effect on basal or TRH-stimulated TSH observed during treatment of 18 euthyroid patients with 60 mg daily for 6 months *1203*

Donepezil

Amylase *Serum Increase Physiological* Post-marketing studies have shown that donepezil causes pancreatitis infrequently *4662*

Blood *Urine Increase Physiological* Donepezil causes hematuria infrequently *4662*

Cimetidine *Serum No Effect Physiological* Donepezil had no significant effect on pharmacokinetics of cimetidine *1008*

Creatine Kinase *Serum Increase Physiological* Donepezil causes increased activity infrequently *4662*

Digoxin *Serum No Effect Physiological* Donepezil had no significant effect on pharmacokinetics of digoxin *4662 1008*

Eosinophils *Blood Increase Physiological* Donepezil causes eosinophilia infrequently *4662*

Erythrocytes *Blood Decrease Physiological* Donepezil causes erythrocytopenia infrequently *4662*

Glucose *Serum Increase Physiological* Donepezil causes infrequent diabetes mellitus *4662*

Hematocrit *Blood Decrease Physiological* Donepezil causes anemia infrequently *4662*

Hemoglobin *Blood Decrease Physiological* Donepezil causes anemia infrequently *4662*

Hydrochloric Acid *Gastric Fluid Increase Physiological* Donepezil expected to increase gastric acid secretion through increased cholinergic activity *4662*

Lactate Dehydrogenase *Serum Increase Physiological* Donepezil causes increased activity infrequently *4662*

Lipase *Serum Increase Physiological* Post-marketing studies have shown that donepezil causes pancreatitis infrequently *4662*

Occult Blood *Feces Increase Physiological* Donepezil causes frequent gastrointestinal bleeding *4662*

Platelets *Blood Decrease Physiological* Donepezil causes thrombocytopenia infrequently *4662*
Blood Increase Physiological Donepezil causes thrombocythemia infrequently *4662*

Potassium *Serum Decrease Physiological* Donepezil causes hypokalemia infrequently *4662*

Theophylline *Serum No Effect Physiological* Donepezil had no significant effect on pharmacokinetics of theophylline *4662*

Uric Acid *Serum Increase Physiological* Donepezil causes gout infrequently *4662*

Warfarin *Plasma No Effect Physiological* Donepezil had no significant effect on pharmacokinetics of warfarin *4662*

Dopexamine

Aldosterone *Plasma Decrease Physiological* In 8 normal individuals infusion of a mean of 1.00 ± 0.02 µg/kg/min over 2 hours caused nonsignificant decrease from mean baseline of 345 ± 105 pmol/L to 198 ± 42 pmol/L *4412*

Amyloid A *Serum Decrease Physiological* In 44 patients receiving 0.5, 1.0 or 2 µg/kg/min preoperatively, during cardiopulmonary bypass surgery and postoperatively increases of serum amyloid A were less in those receiving dopexamine than in those receiving placebo *494*

C-Reactive Protein *Serum Decrease Physiological* In 44 patients receiving 0.5, 1.0 or 2 µg/kg/min preoperatively, during cardiopulmonary bypass surgery and postoperatively increases of C-reactive protein were less in those receiving dopexamine than in those receiving placebo *494*

Dopexamine (continued)

Creatinine Clearance *Urine Increase Physiological* In 44 patients receiving 0.5, 1.0 or 2 µg/kg/min preoperatively, during cardiopulmonary bypass surgery and postoperatively increases of creatinine clearance were observed in those receiving dopexamine with the increases greatest in those receiving lower doses *494*

Effective Renal Plasma Flow
Patient Increase Physiological In 8 normal individuals infusion of 1.00 ± 0.02 µg/kg/min over 2 h caused significant 10% increase *4412*

Fractional Excretion of Lithium
Urine Increase Physiological In 8 normal individuals infusion of a mean of 1.00 ± 0.02 µgkg/min over 2 hours caused significant increase from mean baseline of 28% to 33% *4412*

Glomerular Filtration Rate *Urine Increase Physiological* In 8 normal individuals infusion of 1.00 ± 0.02 µg/kg/min over 2 h caused significant increase from mean baseline of 121 mL/min/1.73 sq m to 130 mL/min/1.73 sq m *4412*

Interleukin-6 *Serum Decrease Physiological* In 44 patients receiving 0.5, 1.0 or 2 µg/kg/min preoperatively, during cardiopulmonary bypass surgery and postoperatively increases of IL-6 were least in those receiving 2.0 µg/kg/min *494*

Lithium Clearance *Urine Increase Physiological* In 8 normal individuals infusion of a mean of 1.00 ± 0.02 µg/kg/min over 2 hours caused significant increase from mean baseline of 33 mL/min/1.73 sq m to 42 mL/min/1 73 sq m *4412*

Renin Activity *Plasma No Effect Physiological* In 8 normal individuals infusion of a mean of 1.00 ± 0.02 µg/kg/min over 2 hours had no effect on mean baseline of 26 ± 5 mIU/L *4412*

Thyroid Stimulating Hormone
Serum Decrease Physiological Infusion of 1.0 to 4.0 µg/kg/min from 8 pm to midnight in normal volunteers initially caused small but significant decrease but by end of infusion concentration had risen to same level as with placebo *625*

Dorzolamide

Bicarbonate *Serum No Effect Physiological* In 12 healthy volunteers topical administration of 7.7 µg/d for 14 days caused nonsignificant decrease of 0.1% *571*
Urine No Effect Physiological In 12 healthy volunteers topical administration of 7.7 µg/d for 14 days caused significant increase of 17.7% *571*

Carbon Dioxide Partial Pressure
Blood No Effect Physiological In 12 healthy volunteers topical administration of 7.7 µg/d for 14 days caused nonsignificant increase of 2.1% *571*

Chloride *Serum No Effect Physiological* In 12 healthy volunteers topical administration of 7.7 µg/d for 14 days caused nonsignificant decrease of 0.3% *571*
Urine No Effect Physiological In 12 healthy volunteers topical administration of 7.7 µg/d for 14 days caused nonsignificant increase of 8.8% *571*

Citrate *Urine No Effect Physiological* In 12 healthy volunteers topical administration of 7.7 µg/d for 14 days caused nonsignificant increase of 3.2% *571*

Creatinine *Serum No Effect Physiological* In 12 healthy volunteers topical administration of 7.7 µg/d for 14 days caused nonsignificant decrease of 0.4% *571*
Urine No Effect Physiological In 12 healthy volunteers topical administration of 7.7 µg/d for 14 days caused nonsignificant increase of 6.3% *571*

Osmolality *Serum No Effect Physiological* In 12 healthy volunteers topical administration of 7.7 µg/d for 14 days caused nonsignificant increase of 0.3% *571*
Urine No Effect Physiological In 12 healthy volunteers topical administration of 7.7 µg/d for 14 days caused significant increase of 3.1% *571*

pH *Blood No Effect Physiological* In 12 healthy volunteers topical administration of 7.7 µg/d for 14 days caused nonsignificant decrease of 1.8% *571*

Phosphate *Serum No Effect Physiological* In 12 healthy volunteers topical administration of 7.7 µg/d for 14 days caused nonsignificant decrease of 3.8% *571*
Urine No Effect Physiological In 12 healthy volunteers topical administration of 7.7 µg/d for 14 days caused nonsignificant increase of 11.4% *571*

Potassium *Urine No Effect Physiological* In 12 healthy volunteers topical administration of 7.7 µg/d for 14 days caused nonsignificant increase of 2.6% *571*

Protein *Serum No Effect Physiological* In 12 healthy volunteers topical administration of 7.7 µg/d for 14 days caused nonsignificant increase of 1.2% *571*

Sodium *Serum No Effect Physiological* In 12 healthy volunteers topical administration of 7.7 µg/d for 14 days caused nonsignificant decrease of 0.7% *571* In 12 healthy volunteers topical administration of 7.7 µg/d for 14 days caused nonsignificant increase of 0.1% *571*
Urine No Effect Physiological In 12 healthy volunteers topical administration of 7.7 µg/d for 14 days caused nonsignificant increase of 12.6% *571*

Urea Nitrogen *Serum No Effect Physiological* In 12 healthy volunteers topical administration of 7.7 µg/d for 14 days caused nonsignificant increase of 0.6% *571*
Urine No Effect Physiological In 12 healthy volunteers topical administration of 7.7 µg/d for 14 days caused nonsignificant increase of 8.5% *571*

Uric Acid *Serum No Effect Physiological* In 12 healthy volunteers topical administration of 7.7 µg/d for 14 days caused nonsignificant decrease of 1.0% *571*
Urine No Effect Physiological In 12 healthy volunteers topical administration of 7.7 µg/d for 14 days caused nonsignificant increase of 5.1% *571*

Volume *Urine No Effect Physiological* In 12 healthy volunteers topical administration of 7.7 µg/d for 14 days caused significant increase of 3.1% *571*

Dosulepin

Albumin *Urine No Effect Analytical* Using a fluorimetric assay with Albumin Blue 580 on a Cobas Fara centrifugal analyzer for the detection of microalbuminuria no significant interference was detected at a concentration of 4 mg/L *3117*

Doxapram

Erythrocytes *Blood Decrease Physiological* Noted postoperatively in a few patients *3810*

Hematocrit *Blood Decrease Physiological* Noted postoperatively in a few patients *68*

Hemoglobin *Blood Decrease Physiological* Noted postoperatively in a few patients *68*

Leukocytes *Blood Decrease Physiological* Further decrease noted in patient with leukopenia *68*

Protein *Urine Increase Physiological* May have nephrotoxic effect *1714*

Urea Nitrogen *Serum Increase Physiological* ?nephrotoxic effect *1714*

Doxazosin

Acetaminophen *Serum No Effect Physiological* In clinical trials with doxazosin in some patients were taking other drugs no significant interactions were observed *4642*

Acetylsalicylic Acid *Serum No Effect Physiological* In clinical trials with doxazosin in some patients were taking other drugs no significant interactions were observed *4642*

Alanine Aminotransferase *Serum No Effect Physiological* In clinical trials of 3960 patients no clinically adverse reactions reported *4642*

Aldosterone *Plasma No Effect Physiological* No significant effect observed in 17 patients with mild to moderate uncomplicated essential hypertension treated with mean dose up to 4.4 mg/d for 12 weeks *4407*

Alkaline Phosphatase *Serum No Effect Physiological* In clinical trials of 3960 patients no clinically adverse reactions reported *4642*

Amoxicillin *Serum No Effect Physiological* In clinical trials with doxazosin in some patients were taking other drugs no significant interactions were observed *4642*

Apolipoprotein A *Serum No Effect Physiological* No significant effect in 14 mildly hypertensive patients treated with up to 16 mg/day for 10 weeks *144*

Apolipoprotein A-I *Serum Increase Physiological* In 25 hypertensive patients treatment for 6 months caused significant increase from mean baseline of 102 ± 17 mg/dL to 117 ± 16 mg/dL *3781*
Serum No Effect Physiological In 17 hypertensive nondiabetics treatment with up to 16 mg/d for 12 weeks caused non significant change from mean baseline of 138 ± 8 mg/dL to 137 ± 5 mg/dL and in 13 hypertensives with NIDDM caused nonsignificant change from mean baseline of 135 ±10 mg/dL *3741*

Apolipoprotein A-I:Apolipoprotein B Ratio
Serum Increase Physiological In 25 hypertensive patients treatment for 6 months caused significant increase in ratio from mean baseline of 0.74 ± 0.1 to 0.94 ± 0.2 *3781*

Apolipoprotein B *Serum Decrease Physiological* In 25 hypertensive patients treatment for 6 months caused significant decrease from mean baseline of 137 ± 18 mg/dL to 124 ± 14 mg/dL *3781*
Serum No Effect Physiological In 17 hypertensive nondiabetics treatment with up to 16 mg/d for 12 weeks caused non significant change from mean baseline of 114 ± 7 mg/dL to 101 ± 7 mg/dL and in 13 hypertensives with NIDDM caused nonsignificant change from mean baseline of 94 ±9 mg/dL to 86 ± 7 mg/dL *3741* No significant effect observed in 14 mildly hypertensive patients treated for 10 weeks with up to 16 mg/day *144*

Aspartate Aminotransferase
Serum No Effect Physiological In clinical trials of 3960 patients no clinically adverse reactions reported *4642*

Atenolol *Serum No Effect Physiological* In clinical trials with doxazosin in some patients were taking other drugs no significant interactions were observed *4642*

Bilirubin *Serum No Effect Physiological* In clinical trials of 3960 patients no clinically adverse reactions reported *4642*

Chlorpheniramine *Serum No Effect Physiological* In clinical trials with doxazosin in some patients were taking other drugs no significant interactions were observed *4642*

Cholesterol *Serum Decrease Physiological* In 17 hypertensive nondiabetics treatment with up to 16 mg/d for 12 weeks caused significant decrease from mean baseline of 5.50 ± 0.23 mmol/L to 4.97 ± 0.22 mmol/L *3741* Significant mean reduction of 6.6% observed after 14 weeks treatment in 153 patients with mild to moderate hypertension *3776* In 134 patients with stage I diastolic hypertension treated with 2 mg/d caused change from mean baseline of 5.92 ± 0.98 mmol/L by - 0.33 ± 0.06 mmol/L after 12 months and - 0.42 ± 0.07 mmol/L after 48 months *2335* Concentration reduced with treatment in hypertensive patients *3502* Nonsignificant mean reduction of 3.1% in 96 hypertensive adults treated for 12 weeks with mean dose up to 3.4 mg daily *652* Nonsignificant decrease of 2.66% observed in 53 patients with mild to moderate hypertension treated with up to 8 mg daily for 12 weeks *2470* Significant reduction (3.64%) from mean of 5.73 mmol/L to 5.53 mmol/L follwing treatment with up to 8 mg/d for 6 weeks in 25 patients with mild to moderate essential hypertension *3863* Significant reduction observed in hypertensive patients after treatment for 26 weeks *3498* Decrease from baseline mean of 7.31 mmol/L to 6.96 mmol/L in 77 patients with mild essential hypertension treated with up to 16 mg daily for 26 weeks *3502* Nonsignificant trend to decrease in 32 patients with hypertension treated with up to 16 mg/d for 28 weeks *5970* Mean reduction of 25 mg/dL in 20 patients treated with mean dose of 9.2 mg daily for 46 weeks *3571* In 38 treated hypertensives given 1 to 16 mg/d over 10 weeks *4226*
Serum No Effect Physiological No significant change in 44 patients treated for 3 mo *142* No effect in 14 mildly hypertensive patients treated with up to 16 mg/day for 10 weeks *144* In 13 hypertensive patients with NIDDM treatment with up to 16 mg/d for 12 weeks caused nonsignificant change from mean baseline of 4.80 ± 0.36 mmol/L to 4.84 ± 0.42 mmol/L *3741* In 10 hypertensive patients with serum cholesterol concentration greater than 220 mg/dL treatment for 6 months caused nonsignificant change from mean baseline of 250 ± 24 mg/dL to 246 ± 30 mg/dL and in 15 with serum cholesterol less than 220 mg/dL from 197 ± 14 mg/dL to 190 ± 12 mg/dL *3781* In 42 patients with mild to moderate hypertension treatment for 6 months caused insignificant change from mean baseline of 6.66 ± 0.86 mmol/L to 6.37 ± 1.27 mmol/L *2907* Compared with controls over 10-12 weeks, although 9% increase in HDL/total cholesterol ratio *4747*

Codeine *Serum No Effect Physiological* In clinical trials with doxazosin in some patients were taking other drugs no significant interactions were observed *4642*

Creatinine *Serum No Effect Physiological* In clinical trials of 3960 patients no clinically adverse reactions reported *4642* No significant effect observed on renal function in 17 patients with mild to moderate uncomplicated essential hypertension treated with mean dose up to 4.4 mg/d for 12 weeks *4407*

Creatinine Clearance *Urine No Effect Physiological* No effect on clearance or on renal blood flow in 24 patients with 6 weeks treatment *6482*

Diazepam *Serum No Effect Physiological* In clinical trials with doxazosin in some patients were taking other drugs no significant interactions were observed *4642*

Erythromycin *Serum No Effect Physiological* In clinical trials with doxazosin in some patients were taking other drugs no significant interactions were observed *4642*

Geometric Variation in Fibrinolytic Index
Plasma Increase Physiological In 25 hypertensive patients treatment for 6 months caused significant change from mean baseline before anoxia of 18.8 ± 12 to 36.1 ± 16 *3781*

Glucose *Serum Decrease Physiological* Reduction from baseline mean of 4.54 mmol/L to 4.33 mmol/L in 77 mild essential hypertensives treated with up to 16 mg daily for 26 weeks *3502* In hypertensive individuals treatment for 26 weeks caused significant decrease in plasma concentration. Effect also observed at 4 weeks *3413*
Serum No Effect Physiological In 42 patients with mild to moderate hypertension treatment for 6 months caused nonsignificant change from mean baseline of 5.36 ± 0.57 mmol/L to 5.49 ± 0.44 mmol/L *2907* In clinical trials of 3960 patients no clinically adverse reactions reported *4642*

HDL_2-Cholesterol *Serum No Effect Physiological* No significant effect observed in 14 mildly hypertensive patients treated with up to 16 mg/day for 10 weeks *144*

HDL_3-Cholesterol *Serum No Effect Physiological* No significant effect observed in 14 mildly hypertensive patients treated with up to 16 mg/day for 10 weeks *144*

HDL-Cholesterol *Serum Increase Physiological* Nonstatistical increase in concentration observed in group of individuals with mild to moderate hypertension treated for 20 weeks *3048* Nonsignificant tendency to increase observed in 32 hypertensive patients for up to 28 weeks with doses up to 16 mg/d *5970* Significantly increased concentration observed with administration of $alpha_1$-inhibitors such as doxazosin in short and long term studies *3730* In 16 hypertensive patients with serum HDL-cholesterol concentration greater than 40 mg/dL treatment for 6 months caused significant increase from mean baseline of 48 ± 7 mg/dL to 54 ± 5 mg/dL and in 9 with serum HDL-cholesterol less than 40 mg/dL from 37 ± 6 mg/dL to 40 ± 4 mg/dL *3781*
Serum No Effect Physiological In 42 patients with mild to moderate hypertension treatment for 6 months caused insignificant change from mean baseline of 1.25 ± 0.34 mmol/L to 1.27 ± 0.36 mmol/L *2907* In 17 hypertensive nondiabetics treatment with up to 16 mg/d for 12 weeks caused non significant change from mean baseline of 1.23 ± 0.08 mmol/L to 1.26 ± 0.08 mmol/L and in 13 hypertensives with NIDDM caused nonsignificant change from mean baseline of 1.08 ± 0.06 mmol/L to 1.16 ± 0.07 mmol/L *3741* No significant change in 14 mildly hypertensive patients treated with up to 16 mg/day for 10 weeks *144* No significant effect observed in hypertensive patients treated for 26 weeks *3498* No significant change over 26 weeks in 77 mild essential hypertensives treated with up to 16 mg daily *3502* In 134 patients with stage I diastolic hypertension treated with 2 mg/d caused change from mean baseline of 1.16 ± 0.28 mmol/L by + 0.06 ± 0.02 mmol/L after 12 months and + 0.02 ± 0.02 mmol/L after 48 months *2335* Compared with controls over 10-12 weeks, although 9% increase in HDL/total cholesterol ratio *4747*

Doxazosin *(continued)*

HDL-Triglycerides *Serum Decrease Physiological* In 17 hypertensive nondiabetics treatment with up to 16 mg/d for 12 weeks caused significant decrease from mean baseline of 0.13 ± 0.01 mmol/L to 0.12 ± 0.01 mmol/L *3741*
Serum No Effect Physiological In 13 hypertensive patients with NIDDM treatment with up to 16 mg/d for 12 weeks caused nonsignificant change from mean baseline of 0.15 ± 0.01 mmol/L to 0.16 ± 0.02 mmol/L *3741*

Hydrochlorothiazide *Serum No Effect Physiological* In clinical trials with doxazosin in some patients were taking other drugs no significant interactions were observed *4642*

Ibuprofen *Serum No Effect Physiological* In clinical trials with doxazosin in some patients were taking other drugs no significant interactions were observed *4642*

IDL-Cholesterol *Serum No Effect Physiological* In 17 hypertensive nondiabetics treatment with up to 16 mg/d for 12 weeks caused no change from mean baseline of 0.29 ± 0.05 mmol/L and in 13 hypertensives with NIDDM caused nonsignificant change from mean baseline of 0.19 ± 0.04 mmol/L to 0.23 ± 0.4 mmol/L *3741*

IDL-Triglycerides *Serum No Effect Physiological* In 17 hypertensive nondiabetics treatment with up to 16 mg/d for 12 weeks caused non significant change from mean baseline of 0.14 ± 0.01 mmol/L to 0.13 ± 0.01 mmol/L and in 13 hypertensives with NIDDM caused nonsignificant change from mean baseline of 0.13 ± 0.02 mmol/L *3741*

Indomethacin *Serum No Effect Physiological* In clinical trials with doxazosin in some patients were taking other drugs no significant interactions were observed *4642*

Insulin *Plasma Decrease Physiological* Reduction from baseline mean of 11.36 mU/L to 9.41 mU/L in 77 mild essential hypertensives treated for 26 weeks with up to 16 mg daily *3502* Significant effect observed after 4 weeks treatment in hypertensives and even more marked effect observed after 26 weeks treatment *3498*

Kallikrein *Urine Increase Physiological* Urinary excretion augmented 2.47 fold in 17 patients with uncomplicated mild to moderate essential hypertension treated with mean dose up to 4.4 mg/d for 12 weeks *4407*

LDL-Cholesterol *Serum Decrease Physiological* Reduction from baseline mean of 5.13 mmol/L to 4.78 mmol/L in 77 mild essential hypertensives treated with up to 16 mg daily for 26 weeks *3502* Mean reduction of 32 mg/dL in 20 patients with mild to moderate hypertension when treated with mean daily dose of 9.2 mg daily for 46 weeks *3571* Significant reduction observed in hypertensive patients with treatment for 26 weeks *3498* In 134 patients with stage I diastolic hypertension treated with 2 mg/d caused change from mean baseline of 4.09 ± 0.91 mmol/L by - 0.21 ± 0.06 mmol/L after 12 months and - 0.34 ± 0.06 mmol/L after 48 months *2335* Significantly decreased concentration observed with administration of $alpha_1$-inhibitors such as doxazosin in short and long term studies *3730*
Serum No Effect Physiological In 17 hypertensive nondiabetics treatment with up to 16 mg/d for 12 weeks caused non significant change from mean baseline of 2.84 ± 0.20 mmol/L to 2.68 ± 0.18 mmol/L and in 13 hypertensives with NIDDM caused nonsignificant change from mean baseline of 2.37 ± 0.18 mmol/L to 2.30 ± 0.15 mmol/L *3741* No significant effect in 14 mildly hypertensive patients treated with up to 16 mg/day for 10 weeks *144*

LDL-Triglycerides *Serum Decrease Physiological* In 17 hypertensive nondiabetics treatment with up to 16 mg/d for 12 weeks caused significant decrease from mean baseline of 0.21 ± 0.02 mmol/L to 0.19 ± 0.02 mmol/L *3741*
Serum No Effect Physiological In 13 hypertensive patients with NIDDM treatment with up to 16 mg/d for 12 weeks caused nonsignificant change from mean baseline of 0.24 ± 0.02 mmol/L to 0.23 ± 0.02 mmol/L *3741*

Leukocytes *Blood Decrease Physiological* In clinical trials with 474 hypertensive patients treated with doxazosin 2.4% had leukopenia *4642*

Neutrophils *Blood Decrease Physiological* In clinical trials with 474 hypertensive patients treated with doxazosin 1.0% had neutropenia *4642*

Norepinephrine *Plasma Increase Physiological* After 6 weeks in 24 patients treated for 6 weeks *6482*

Plasminogen Activator Inhibitor-1
Plasma No Effect Physiological In 25 hypertensive patients treatment for 6 months caused nonsignificant change from mean baseline before anoxia of 17.3 ± 13 U/cm³ to 18.4 ± 15 U/cm³*3781* In 42 patients with mild to moderate hypertension treatment for 6 months caused nonsignificant change from mean baseline of 17.7 ± 14.2 U/mL to 18.0 ± 11.5 U/mL *2907*

Platelet Aggregation *Blood Decrease Physiological* Concentration related inhibition in response to collagen, epinephrine and adenosine diphosphate in both normotensives and hypertensives *2572*

Potassium *Serum Decrease Physiological* In clinical trials of 3960 patients hypokalemia reported in less than 0.5% of patients *4642*
Serum No Effect Physiological In clinical trials involving 3,960 patients no clinically adverse reactions reported *4642* No significant change over 26 weeks in 77 mild essential hypertensives treated with up to 16 mg daily *3502*
Urine No Effect Physiological No significant effect observed in 17 patients with mild to moderate uncomplicated essential hypertension treated with mean dose of up to 4.4 mg/d for 12 weeks *4407*

Propranolol *Serum No Effect Physiological* In clinical trials with doxazosin in some patients were taking other drugs no significant interactions were observed *4642*

Prostate-specific Antigen *Serum No Effect Physiological* In clinical trials with doxazosin patients treated for 3 years failed to show a change in concentration *4642*

Renin Activity *Plasma Increase Physiological* Acute increase in 24 patients treated for 6 weeks *6482*
Plasma No Effect Physiological No significant effect observed in 17 patients with mild to moderate uncomplicated essential hypertension when treated with mean dose of up to 4.4 mg/d for 12 weeks *4407*

Sodium *Urine No Effect Physiological* No significant effect observed in 17 patients with mild to moderate uncomplicated essential hypertension treated for 12 weeks with mean dose up to 4.4 mg/d *4407*

Sulfamethoxazole *Serum No Effect Physiological* In clinical trials with doxazosin in some patients were taking other drugs no significant interactions were observed *4642*

Tissue Plasminogen Activator
Plasma Increase Physiological In 25 hypertensive patients treatment for 6 months caused significant increase from mean baseline before anoxia of 0.056 ± 0.6 U/cm³ to 0.083 ± 0.6 U/cm³*3781*
Plasma No Effect Physiological In 42 patients with mild to moderate hypertension treatment for 6 months caused nonsignificant change from mean baseline of 0.036 ± 0.08 U/mL to 0.068 ± 0.149 U/mL *2907*

Tissue Plasminogen Activator Activity after Venous Occlusion *Plasma Increase Physiological* In 42 patients with mild to moderate hypertension treatment for 6 months caused significant increase from mean baseline of 1.02 ± 1.30 U/mL to 2.10 ± 2.81 U/mL *2907*

Tissue Plasminogen Activator Antigen
Plasma No Effect Physiological In 42 patients with mild to moderate hypertension treatment for 6 months caused nonsignificant change from mean baseline of 9.5 ± 4.4 µg/L to 8.3 ± 3.9 µg/L *2907*

Tissue Plasminogen Activator Antigen after Venous Occlusion *Plasma No Effect Physiological* In 42 patients with mild to moderate hypertension treatment for 6 months caused nonsignificant change from mean baseline of 26.0 ± 11.9 µg/L to 24.2 ± 11.9 µg/L *2907*

Tissue Plasminogen Activator Capacity
Plasma Increase Physiological In 42 patients with mild to moderate hypertension treatment for 6 months caused significant increase from mean baseline of 0.98 ± 1.29 U/mL to 2.03 ± 2.75 U/mL *2907*

Tissue Plasminogen Activator Release
Plasma No Effect Physiological In 42 patients with mild to moderate hypertension treatment for 6 months caused nonsignificant change from mean baseline of 16.5 ± 11.2 µg/L to 15.9 ± 11.2 µg/L *2907*

Triglycerides *Serum Decrease Physiological* Nonsignificant reduction from 1.54 mmol/L to 1.34 mmol/L in 25 patients with mild to moderate essential hypertension following treatment with up to 8 mg/d for 6 weeks *3863* Significant reduction observed in 32 patients with hypertension treated for 28 weeks with up to 16 mg/d *5970* In 38 treated hypertensives given 1 to 16 mg/d over 10 weeks *4226* Nonsignificant mean reduction of 3.8% observed in 96 hypertensive adults treated for 12 weeks with dose up to mean of 3.4 mg/d *652* In 42 patients with mild to moderate hypertension treatment for 6 months caused significant decrease from mean baseline of 1.55 ± 0.98 mmol/L to 1.38 ± 1.02 mmol/L *2907* Reduction of 24.4% observed in mild to moderate hypertensive patients treated for 20 weeks *3048* Mean decrease of 54 mg/dL observed in approximately 20 patients with mild to moderate hypertension when treated with mean daily dose of 9.2 mg daily for 46 weeks *3571* In 17 hypertensive nondiabetics treatment with up to 16 mg/d for 12 weeks caused significant decrease from mean baseline of 2.03 ± 0.34 mmol/L to 1.71 ± 0.24 mmol/L *3741* Nonsignificant reduction of 8.8% observed in 53 patients with mild to moderate hypertension treated for 12 weeks with up to 8 mg/d *2470* In 8 hypertensive patients with serum triglyceride concentration greater than 150 mg/dL treatment for 6 months caused significant increase from mean baseline of 224 ± 23 mg/dL to 202 ± 19 mg/dL and in 17 with serum triglycerides less than 150 mg/dL from 131 ± 21 mg/dL to 122 ± 19 mg/dL *3781* In 134 patients with stage I diastolic hypertension treated with 2 mg/d caused change from mean baseline of 1.47 ± 0.74 mmol/L by - 0.38 ± 0.05 mmol/L after 12 months and - 0.23 ± 0.06 mmol/L after 48 months *2335* Increase by 13% in 44 patients treated for 3 mo *142*

Serum No Effect Physiological In 13 hypertensive patients with NIDDM treatment with up to 16 mg/d for 12 weeks caused nonsignificant change from mean baseline of 2.38 ± 0.52 mmol/L to 2.51 ± 0.56 mmol/L *3741* No significant effect observed in hypertensive patients treated for 26 weeks *3498* No significant change compared with controls *4747* No significant change observed in 77 mild essential hypertensives treated with up to 16 mg daily for 26 weeks *3502* No effect of treatment for 10 weeks with up to 16 mg/day in 14 mildly hypertensive patients *144*

Trimethoprim *Serum No Effect Physiological* In clinical trials with doxazosin in some patients were taking other drugs no significant interactions were observed *4642*

Urea Nitrogen *Serum No Effect Physiological* In clinical trials of 3960 patients no clinically adverse reactions reported *4642*

Uric Acid *Serum Decrease Physiological* Slight reduction from baseline mean of 362 µmol/L to 351 µmol/L in 77 mild essential hypertensives treated with up to 16 mg daily for 26 weeks *3502*

Serum Increase Physiological In clinical trials of 3960 patients gout reported in less than 0.5% of patients *4642* In 42 patients with mild to moderate hypertension treatment for 6 months caused change from mean baseline of 279 ± 53.2 µmol/L to 291 ± 68.9 µmol/L *2907*

Serum No Effect Physiological In clinical trials of 3960 patients no clinically adverse reactions reported *4642*

VLDL-Cholesterol *Serum Decrease Physiological* In 17 hypertensive nondiabetics treatment with up to 16 mg/d for 12 weeks caused significant decrease from mean baseline of 1.10 ± 0.20 mmol/L to 0.72 ± 0.14 mmol/L *3741* Significantly decreased concentration observed with administration of alpha$_1$-inhibitors such as doxazosin in short and long term studies *3730* In 38 treated hypertensives given 1 to 16 mg/d over 10 weeks *4226*

Serum No Effect Physiological No significant change in 14 mildly hypertensive patients treated with up to 16 mg/day for 10 weeks *144* In 13 hypertensive patients with NIDDM treatment with up to 16 mg/d for 12 weeks caused nonsignificant change from mean baseline of 1.15 ± 0.32 mmol/L to 1.16 ± 0.30 mmol/L *3741* No significant effect observed in hypertensive patients treated for 26 weeks *3498*

VLDL-Triglycerides *Serum Decrease Physiological* In 17 hypertensive nondiabetics treatment with up to 16 mg/d for 12 weeks caused significant decrease from mean baseline of 1.55 ± 0.32 mmol/L to 1.27 ± 0.22 mmol/L *3741*

Serum No Effect Physiological In 13 hypertensive patients with NIDDM treatment with up to 16 mg/d for 12 weeks caused nonsignificant change from mean baseline of 1.87 ± 0.51 mmol/L to 1.99 ± 0.55 mmol/L *3741*

Doxepin

Bile *Urine Increase Physiological* Theoretical possibility due to class of compound *128*

Bilirubin *Serum Increase Physiological* Theoretical possibility due to class of compound *128* Rare cases of jaundice reported in patients taking doxepin *4653*

Catecholamines *Plasma No Effect Analytical* No effect on HPLC method of Koller for dopamine, epinephrine, and norepinephrine *3230*

Cholesterol *Serum No Effect Analytical* At concentration of 150 mg/L had no effect on method using catalase-Hantzsch reaction *5704* At concentration of 150 mg/L had no effect on CHOD-PAP method *5704* At concentration of 150 mg/L had no effect on catalase-AIDH method *5704* At concentration of 150 mg/L had no effect on CHOD-Iodide method *5704* At concentration of 150 mg/L had no effect on Liebermann-Burchard method *5704*

Cocaethylene *Urine Increase Analytical* Possible interference observed with TLC method of Bailey *328*

Creatinine *Serum No Effect Analytical* At 1.2 g/L on reversed phase liquid chromatographic procedure of Zhiri et al *6656* At concentration of 30 mg/L had no effect on Jaffe-Fading-Fraction method *5704* At concentration of 10 mg/L had no effect on kinetic Jaffe method on BKA-2 *5704* At concentration of 0.3 mg/L had no effect on creatinine iminohydrolase method *5704* At concentration of 30 mg/L had no effect on Jaffe-Fuller's earth method *5704*

Eosinophils *Blood Increase Physiological* Eosinophilia has been reported as a side effect in a few patients *3656* Eosinophilia has been reported in a few patients *4653*

Glucose *Serum Decrease Physiological* In one patient with type II diabetes maintained on tolazamide 1 g/d severe hypoglycemia occurred 11 days after the addition of doxepin 75 mg/d *4653* Occasional reports of both hypoglycemia and hyperglycemia *3656*

Serum Increase Physiological Both increased and decreased blood glucose concentrations reported in patients taking doxepin *4653* Occasional reports of both hypoglycemia and hyperglycemia *3656*

Serum No Effect Analytical At concentration of 6 mg/L had no effect on Kodak Ektachem® method *5704*

Granulocytes *Blood Decrease Physiological* Occasional reports of bone marrow depression manifesting as agranulocytosis, leukopenia, thrombocytopenia, and purpura *4653* Occasional reports of bone marrow depression, including leukopenia, thrombocytopenia, purpura and agranulocytosis *3656*

Histamine *Plasma No Effect Analytical* Although 50% inhibition of radio-enzyme assay occurs at 4.8 µg/mL no clinical effects likely since physiological concentration 0.02-0.15 µg/mL *2492*

Leukocytes *Blood Decrease Physiological* Occasional reports of bone marrow depression, including leukopenia, thrombocytopenia, purpura and agranulocytosis *3656* Occasional reports of bone marrow depression manifesting as agranulocytosis, leukopenia, thrombocytopenia, and purpura *4653* Theoretical possibility due to class of compound *128*

Lysergic Acid Diethylamide *Urine Increase Analytical* Minimum concentration that caused a positive result with EMIT method to measure LSD 11 mg/L *4968*

Osmolality *Serum Decrease Physiological* Syndrome of inappropriate ADH secretion reported in patients taking doxepin *4653*

Urine Increase Physiological Syndrome of inappropriate ADH secretion reported in patients taking doxepin *4653*

p-Aminophenol *Urine No Effect Analytical* With addition of drugs at a concentration of 100 mg/L and of related compounds at 50 mg/L no significant effect observed on colorimetric method of van Bocxlaer on Cobas Mira analyzer which involves reacting free p-aminophenol with resorcinol in the presence of magnesium ions to form an indophenol dye measured at 550 nm *6163*

Platelets *Blood Decrease Physiological* Occasional reports of bone marrow depression, including leukopenia, thrombocytopenia, purpura and agranulocytosis *3656* Occasional reports of bone marrow depression manifesting as agranulocytosis, leukopenia, thrombocytopenia, and purpura *4653* Single case observed (probably immune response) *4308*

Doxepin *(continued)*

Potassium *Serum No Effect Analytical* At concentration of 60 mg/L had no effect on measurement by ISE without predilution *5704*

Protein Electrophoresis *Serum No Effect Analytical* At concentration of 60 mg/L had no effect on automated Olympus-Hite method *5704*

Sodium *Serum Decrease Physiological* Occasional reports of syndrome of inappropriate ADH secretion with tricyclic antidepressants *3656* Syndrome of inappropriate ADH secretion reported in patients taking doxepin *4653*
Serum No Effect Analytical At concentration of 60 mg/L had no effect on measurement by ISE without predilution *5704*
Urine Increase Physiological Occasional reports of syndrome of inappropriate ADH secretion with tricyclic antidepressants *3656*

Tricyclic Antidepressants *Serum Increase Analytical* May cause false positive reaction in immunoassays for tricyclic antidepressants *3590*

Urea Nitrogen *Serum No Effect Analytical* At concentration of 6 mg/L had no effect on Kodak Ektachem® method *5704*

Uric Acid *Serum No Effect Analytical* At concentration of 30 mg/L had no effect on Kageyama-Hantzsch method *5704* At 1.2 g/L on reversed phase liquid chromatographic procedure of Zhiri et al *6656* At concentration of 30 mg/L had no effect on catalase-AIDH method *5704*

Doxorubicin

Adenosine Deaminase Binding Protein
Urine No Effect Physiological No effect in 12 children given drug for 3 d *2255*

Alanine Aminotransferase *Serum Increase Physiological* May produce idiosyncratic hepatic dysfunction, as observed in 6 patients *299* Increased activity observed in 1 to 5% of 753 patients with AIDS Kaposi syndrome *5448*

Albumin *Urine Increase Physiological* Increased excretion observed in 1 to 5% of 753 patients with AIDS Kaposi syndrome *5448*

Alkaline Phosphatase *Serum Increase Physiological* Cholestatic jaundice observed in less than 1% of 753 treated patients *5448* May produce idiosyncratic hepatic dysfunction, as observed in 6 patients *299*

Amino Acids *Urine Increase Physiological* Mean excretion of 40.0 mmol/d in 8 patients with leukemia undergoing chemotherapy different from 29.1 ± 23.4 mmol/d in 52 patients with acute leukemia and 19.8 ± 10.4 mmol/d in 29 healthy controls of both sexes *6517*

Amylase *Serum Increase Physiological* Pancreatitis observed in less than 1% of 753 treated patients *5448*

Aspartate Aminotransferase *Serum Increase Physiological* May produce idiosyncratic hepatic dysfunction, as observed in 6 patients *299* Cholestatic jaundice observed in less than 1% of 753 treated patients *5448*

Atrial Natriuretic Peptide *Plasma Increase Physiological* In 16 patients aged 5 to 19 years treatment with 45 mg/sq m for various malignancies 6 had increased concentrations of ANP after 3 weeks (5 of whom had received high cumulative doses and 2 of whom entered cardiac failure) *406*

Bilirubin *Serum Increase Physiological* Increased concentration observed in 1 to 5% of 753 patients with AIDS Kaposi syndrome. Cholestatic jaundice observed in less than 1% treated patients *5448*

Bilirubin, Direct *Serum Increase Physiological* May produce idiosyncratic hepatic dysfunction, as observed in 6 patients *299*

Blood *Urine Increase Physiological* Hematuria observed in less than 1% of 753 patients with AIDS Kaposi syndrome *5448*

CA549 *Serum No Effect Analytical* No statistically significant effect observed over a concentration range of 0.4 to 6.6 mg/L with BRESMARQ assay *958* No interference observed at concentrations up to 6.6 mg/L with immunoradiometric BRESMARQ method *958*

Calcium *Serum Decrease Physiological* Decreased concentration observed in 1 to 5% of 753 patients with AIDS Kaposi syndrome *5448*
Serum Increase Physiological Increased concentration observed in less than 1% of 753 treated patients *5448*

Carbamazepine *Serum Decrease Physiological* Significant reduction in concentration when two drugs co-administered together with cisplatin in one patient *4239* Drugs that induce CYP 3A4 enhance metabolism of carbamazepine producing clinically meaningful effect *1039*

Carcinoembryonic Antigen *Serum No Effect Analytical* At a concentration of up to 51.80 µg/mL caused less than 10% error in the concentration of CEA as measured by the method on Bayer Technicon Immuno 1® *418*

Cholinesterase *Serum No Effect Analytical* No effect observed at concentration of 0.55 µg/mL with butyrylthiocholine method on Kodak Ektachem® *2504*

Color *Urine Increase Analytical* Red color observed following ingestion of doxorubicin *3388*

Creatine Kinase Isoenzymes
Serum No Effect Physiological In 17 children receiving anthracycline chemotherapy no significant change in mass concentration observed for 72 hours after start of treatment *2086*

Creatinine *Serum Increase Physiological* Increased concentration observed in less than 1% of 753 treated patients *5448*

Eosinophils *Blood Increase Physiological* Eosinophilia observed in less than 1% of 753 treated patients *5448*

Erythrocytes *Blood Decrease Physiological* Impaired but not as marked as WBC decrease *611*

Glucose *Serum Decrease Physiological* Decreased concentration observed in less than 1% of 753 treated patients *5448*
Serum Increase Physiological Increased concentration observed in 1 to 5% of 753 patients with AIDS Kaposi syndrome *5448*
Urine Increase Physiological Increased excretion observed in less than 1% of 753 patients with AIDS Kaposi syndrome *5448*

γ-Glutamyltransferase *Serum Increase Physiological* Cholestatic jaundice observed in less than 1% of 753 treated patients *5448*

Hematocrit *Blood Decrease Physiological* Anemia observed in about 20% of patients with AIDS Kaposi syndrome *5448*

Hemoglobin *Blood Decrease Physiological* Anemia observed in about 20% of patients with AIDS Kaposi syndrome *5448*

Lactate Dehydrogenase *Serum Increase Physiological* Increased activity observed in less than 1% of 753 treated patients *5448*

Leukocytes *Blood Decrease Physiological* In 70% patients with 60 mg/sq m for 21 d *611* Leukopenia observed in about 60% of patients with AIDS Kaposi syndrome *5448*

Lipase *Serum Increase Physiological* Pancreatitis observed in less than 1% of 753 treated patients *5448*

Lipids *Serum Decrease Physiological* Decreased concentration observed in less than 1% of 753 treated patients *5448*
Serum Increase Physiological Hyperlipemia observed in less than 1% of 753 treated patients *5448*

Magnesium *Serum Decrease Physiological* Decreased concentration observed in less than 1% of 753 treated patients *5448*

Methotrexate *Serum No Effect Analytical* No significant interference at a concentration of 50 µmol/L with method on Du Pont aca *1535*

N-Acetyl-Glucosaminidase *Urine No Effect Analytical* At 50 mg/L on 2 colorimetric analytical methods *2254*

Neutrophils *Blood Decrease Physiological* Neutropenia (< 1000 neutrophils/µL) observed in 49% of 753 patients with AIDS Kaposi syndrome, 13% patients having at least one episode with a count of less than 500 cells/µL *5448*

Occult Blood *Feces Increase Physiological* Ulceration and bleeding of the colon may occur, especially the cecum, leading to bleeding or severe infections which can be fatal *4664* Gastrointestinal hemorrhage observed in less than 1% of 753 treated patients *5448*

Phenytoin *Serum Decrease Physiological* Coadministration may cause decreased concentration of phenytoin *273*

Reduced to 37% of original value in a patient when drugs co-administered together with cisplatin. Effect possibly due to increased metabolism or increased volume of distribution *4239*

Phosphate *Serum Decrease Physiological* Decreased concentration observed in less than 1% of 753 treated patients *5448*

Platelets *Blood Decrease Physiological* Thrombocytopenia observed in about 10% of patients with AIDS Kaposi syndrome *5448* Impaired but not as marked as WBC decrease, possible bone marrow aplasia *611*

Potassium *Serum Decrease Physiological* Decreased concentration observed in less than 1% of 753 treated patients *5448*
Serum Increase Physiological Increased concentration observed in less than 1% of 753 treated patients *5448*

Prostate-specific Antigen *Serum No Effect Analytical* Doxorubicin hydrochloride at a concentration of up to 51.8 µg/mL caused less than 0.1% cross-reactivity with method on PSA method on Bayer Technicon Immuno 1® *430*

Prostate-specific Antigen, Free *Serum No Effect Analytical* Doxorubicin hydrochloride at a concentration of 6.6 mg/L had no significant effect on the Hybritech Tandem® -R free PSA immunoassay *4286*

Protein *Serum Decrease Physiological* Decreased concentration observed in less than 1% of 753 treated patients *5448*
Serum Increase Analytical Significant positive interference observed with 2,2'-bicinchoninic acid (BCA) method of Smith PK et al whether assayed in the presence or absence of a bovine serum albumin protein calibrator, although at therapeutic concentrations interference is unlikely to be significant *3001*

Prothrombin Time *Plasma Increase Physiological* Increased prothrombin time observed in 1 to 5% of 753 patients with AIDS Kaposi syndrome *5448*

Sodium *Serum Decrease Physiological* Decreased concentration observed in less than 1% of 753 treated patients *5448*
Serum Increase Physiological Increased concentration observed in less than 1% of 753 treated patients *5448*

Thromboplastin Generation *Blood Decrease Physiological* Decreased thromboplastin observed in less than 1% of 753 treated patients *5448*

Troponin T *Serum No Effect Physiological* In 17 children treated with anthracycline chemotherapy for 72 hours no significant change in concentration observed *2086*

Urea Nitrogen *Serum Increase Physiological* Increased concentration observed in less than 1% of 753 treated patients *5448*

Uric Acid *Serum Increase Physiological* Increased concentration observed in less than 1% of 753 treated patients *5448* Administration may cause tumor lysis and hyperuricemia in patients with rapidly growing tumors *273*

Valproic Acid *Serum Decrease Physiological* Significant reduction in one patient when drugs co-administered together with cisplatin *4239*

Doxycycline

Alanine Aminotransferase *Serum Increase Physiological* Hepatotoxicity has been reported rarely *4658*

Alkaline Phosphatase *Serum Increase Physiological* Hepatotoxicity has been reported rarely *4658*

Aspartate Aminotransferase *Serum Increase Physiological* Hepatotoxicity has been reported rarely *4658* Reported effect (?hepatic origin) *128*

Bilirubin *Serum Increase Physiological* Hepatotoxicity has been reported rarely *4658*
Serum No Effect Analytical At concentration of 9 mg/L had no effect on method on Kodak Ektachem® *5706*

Bilirubin, Conjugated *Serum No Effect Analytical* No effect at concentration of 9 mg/L on method on Kodak Ektachem® *5706*

Bilirubin, Unconjugated *Serum No Effect Analytical* No effect at concentration of 9 mg/L on method on Kodak Ektachem® *5706*

Catecholamines *Urine Increase Analytical* False increase may occur due to interference with fluorescence *4357*

Chloramphenicol *Serum No Effect Analytical* No effect at 100 mg/L on coupled enzymatic method *4122*

Creatinine *Serum Increase Physiological* Nephrotoxic effect *4658*
Serum No Effect Analytical No effect of concentrations up to 15 mg/L on single slide method on Kodak Ektachem® *5706*

Cyclosporine *Serum Increase Physiological* Single documented but substantiated case reported with coadministration of both drugs *1069*

Diclofenac *Serum No Effect Physiological* Coadministration of doxycycline with diclofenac did not significantly affect the peak concentration or AUC of diclofenac *1025*

Eosinophils *Blood Increase Physiological* Hemolytic anemia, thrombocytopenia, neutropenia, and eosinophilia have been reported with tetracycline *4357* Reported as an adverse event *4523* Allergic response reported *4658*

γ-Glutamyltransferase *Serum Increase Physiological* Hepatotoxicity has been reported rarely *4658*

Hematocrit *Blood Decrease Physiological* Hemolytic anemia reported as an adverse event *4523* Hemolytic anemia has been reported as an adverse event *4658* Hemolytic anemia, thrombocytopenia, neutropenia, and eosinophilia have been reported with tetracycline *4357*

Hemoglobin *Blood Decrease Physiological* Hemolytic anemia has been reported as an adverse event *4658* Hemolytic anemia, thrombocytopenia, neutropenia, and eosinophilia have been reported with tetracycline *4357* Observed with other tetracyclines *2754* Hemolytic anemia reported as an adverse event *4523*

Histamine *Plasma No Effect Analytical* No inhibition of radio-enzyme assay at about 40 times therapeutic concentration *2492*

LE Cells *Blood Positive Physiological* May produce exacerbation of SLE *2754*

Leukocytes *Blood Decrease Physiological* Neutropenia reported *4658*

L-Lactate *Plasma Increase Physiological* In one patient receiving doxycycline on admission to hospital L-lactate concentration 2.1 mmol/L compared with reference range of 0.6 - 1.7 mmol/L *1137*

Neutrophils *Blood Decrease Physiological* Observed with other tetracyclines *2754* Neutropenia reported *4658* Reported as an adverse event *4523* Hemolytic anemia, thrombocytopenia, neutropenia, and eosinophilia have been reported with tetracycline *4357* Occasional case of agranulocytosis reported *6264*

p-Aminophenol *Urine No Effect Analytical* With addition of drugs at a concentration of 100 mg/L and of related compounds at 50 mg/L no significant effect observed on colorimetric method of van Bocxlaer on Cobas Mira analyzer which involves reacting free p-aminophenol with resorcinol in the presence of magnesium ions to form an indophenol dye measured at 550 nm *6163*

pH *Blood Decrease Physiological* In one patient receiving doxycycline on admission to hospital L-lactate concentration 2.1 mmol/L and pH of 7.32 associated with lactate acidosis *1137*

Phenylalanine *Plasma No Effect Analytical* No interference observed with rapid quantitative whole blood method of Campbell et al using phenylalanine dehydrogenase *867*

Platelets *Blood Decrease Physiological* Reported as an adverse event *4523* Thrombocytopenia reported *4658* Hemolytic anemia, thrombocytopenia, neutropenia, and eosinophilia have been reported with tetracycline *4357*

Protein *Urine Increase Physiological* Nephrotoxic effect *4658*

Prothrombin Time *Plasma Decrease Physiological* Tetracyclines have been shown to depress plasma prothrombin activity *4658* Reported to decrease prothrombin activity *4523*
Plasma Increase Physiological Depresses prothrombin activity *2754*

T3-Uptake *Serum No Effect Physiological* Although discoloration of thyoid glands reported no apparent effect on thyroid function tests reported *4523* When given over a prolonged time tetracyclines have been reported to produce brown-black microscopic discoloration of thyroid glands but without effect on thyroid function tests *4658*

Doxycycline *(continued)*

Thyroid Stimulating Hormone
Serum *No Effect* *Physiological* Although discoloration of thyoid glands reported no apparent effect on thyroid function tests reported *4523* When given over a prolonged time tetracyclines have been reported to produce brown-black microscopic discoloration of thyroid glands but without effect on thyroid function tests *4658*

Thyroxine (T4) *Serum* *No Effect* *Physiological* Although discoloration of thyoid glands reported no apparent effect on thyroid function tests reported *4523* When given over a prolonged time tetracyclines have been reported to produce brown-black microscopic discoloration of thyroid glands but without effect on thyroid function tests *4658*

Urea Nitrogen *Serum* *Increase* *Physiological* Nephrotoxic effect *4658* Dose-related increase in concentration reported *4523*

Doxylamine

Methadone *Urine* *No Effect* *Analytical* Insignificant cross-reactivity of 0.2% observed with Roche Abuscreen ONTRAK method *3279*

Opiates *Urine* *No Effect* *Analytical* No effect observed at a concentration of 500 µg/mL (1.85 mmol/L) on method on Du Pont aca *1559*

Dromostanolone

Calcium *Serum* *Decrease* *Physiological* May occur with regression *128*
Serum *Increase* *Physiological* Usually if osteolytic metastases *128*

Erythrocytes *Blood* *Increase* *Physiological* Response to androgens *128*

Hematocrit *Blood* *Increase* *Physiological* Response to androgens *128*

Hemoglobin *Blood* *Increase* *Physiological* Response to androgens *128*

Dronabinol

Alanine Aminotransferase *Serum* *Increase* *Physiological* Incidence of increased hepatic liver enzyme activity observed in less than 1% of treated patients but causal relationship not established *5131*

Aspartate Aminotransferase *Serum* *Increase* *Physiological* Incidence of increased hepatic liver enzyme activity observed in less than 1% of treated patients but causal relationship not established *5131*

Droperidol

Histamine *Plasma* *No Effect* *Analytical* 50% inhibition of radio-enzyme assay observed at 4.5 µg/mL although clinical significance of this unknown *2492*

D-Thyroxine

T3-Uptake *Serum* *Increase* *Analytical* 104% recovery observed when D-thyroxine added at a concentration of 3.0 µg/dL (38.7 nmol/L) with method on Du Pont aca *1545*

Thyroxine (T4) *Serum* *Increase* *Analytical* 161% recovery when D-thyroxine at concentration of 3.0 µg/dL (38.7 nmol/L) added with method on Du Pont aca *1546* *1588*

Thyroxine (T4), Free *Serum* *Increase* *Analytical* D-thyroxine at a concentration of 5.0 µg/dL was recovered as 0.87 ng/dL of FT4 with method on Bayer Technicon Immuno 1® *424* Tetraiodoacetic acid at a concentration of 5.0 µg/dL was recovered as 0.19 ng/dL of FT4 with method on Bayer Technicon Immuno 1® *424*

Tri-iodothyronine, Free (fT3) *Serum* *No Effect* *Analytical* At a concentration of 5.0 x 10^{-5} g/L cross-reactivity of less than 0.1% with free triiodothyronine method on Bayer Technicon Immuno 1® system *425* No significant cross-reactivity observed with either D- or L-thyroxine with method on Organon Teknika AuraFlex random access immunoassay analyzer *885*

DTNB

Cholesterol *Serum* *Decrease* *Analytical* Falsely reduced plasma cholesterol determinations when made by enzymatic method of Allain et al when 50 µL of a DTNB solution containing 15.8 mg/mL used *2481*

Triglycerides *Serum* *Increase* *Physiological* Falsely increased result when determined by method of Bucolo and David when 50 µL of a DTNB solution (15.8 mg/mL) added in vitro but effect largely abolished by use of glycerol blanking *2481*

D-Trp-6

Prolactin *Plasma* *Decrease* *Physiological* Long acting capsules of this chorionic gonadotropic-releasing hormone analog caused reduction of concentration of prolactin in a young hyperprolactinemic woman but had no effect in individuals with normal prolactin concentrations *2207*

D-Trp-6-LHRH

Androstenedione *Plasma* *No Effect* *Physiological* In 21 men with prostatic cancer treatment with 3.75 mg 4-weekly intramuscularly had no significant effect over 6 months *1336*

Dehydroepiandrosterone *Plasma* *No Effect* *Physiological* In 21 men with prostatic cancer treatment with 3.75 mg 4-weekly for 6 months had no significant effect on concentration *1336*

Dehydroepiandrosterone Sulfate
Plasma *No Effect* *Physiological* In 21 men with prostatic cancer treatment with 3.75 mg 4-weekly intramuscularly for up to 6 months had no significant effect *1336*

Estradiol *Plasma* *Decrease* *Physiological* In 21 men with prostatic cancer treatment with 3.75 mg 4-weekly intramuscularly for 6 months caused significant decrease from mean baseline of 32.3 ± 2.5 pg/mL to 18.6 ± 1.8 pg/mL *1336*

Follicle Stimulating Hormone
Plasma *Decrease* *Physiological* In 21 men with prostatic cancer treatment with 3.75 mg 4-weekly intramuscularly for 6 months caused significant decrease from mean baseline of 21.3 ± 3.5 mIU/mL to 14.3 ± 1.6 mIU/mL *1336*

Luteinizing Hormone *Plasma* *Decrease* *Physiological* In 21 men with prostatic cancer treatment with 3.75 mg 4-weekly intramuscularly for 6 months caused significant decrease from mean baseline of 18.0 ± 2.9 mIU/mL to 9.4 ± 0.9 mIU/mL *1336*

Prolactin *Plasma* *Decrease* *Physiological* In 21 men with prostatic cancer treatment with 3.75 mg 4-weekly intramuscularly for 6 months caused significant decrease from mean baseline of 12.4 ± 1.9 ng/mL to 9.0 ± 1.1 ng/mL *1336*

Testosterone *Serum* *Decrease* *Physiological* In 21 men with prostatic cancer treatment with 3.75 mg intramuscularly for 4-weekly caused significant decrease from mean baseline of 5.0 ± 0.4 ng/mL to 0.1 ± 0.1 ng/mL *1336*

DuP 128

Apolipoprotein A-I *Serum* *Decrease* *Physiological* In 28 healthy individuals treated with up to 3600 mg QD mean concentration changed significantly from mean baseline of 150 ± 21 mg/dL to 142 ± 17 mg/dL after 13 days *2409*
Serum *No Effect* *Physiological* In 28 healthy individuals treated with up to 3600 mg QD mean concentration changed significantly from mean baseline of 150 ± 21 mg/dL to 147 ± 21 mg/dL after 42 days *2409*

Apolipoprotein B *Serum* *Decrease* *Physiological* In 28 healthy individuals treated with up to 3600 mg QD mean concentration changed nonsignificantly from mean baseline of 124 ± 23 mg/dL to 115 ± 22 mg/dL after 42 days *2409*

Serum *Increase* *Physiological* In 28 healthy individuals treated with up to 3600 mg QD mean concentration changed significantly from mean baseline of 124 ± 23 mg/dL to 131 ± 22 mg/dL after 13 days *2409*

Cholesterol *Serum* *No Effect* *Physiological* In 28 healthy individuals treated with up to 3600 mg QD mean concentration changed nonsignificantly from mean baseline of 212 ± 28 mg/dL to 215 ± 32 mg/dL after 13 days and 200 ± 32 mg/dL after 42 days *2409*

HDL-Cholesterol *Serum* *Decrease* *Physiological* In 28 healthy individuals treated with up to 3600 mg QD mean concentration changed nonsignificantly from mean baseline of 43 ± 11 mg/dL to 40 ± 19 mg/dL after 13 days and to 43 ± 11 mg/dL after 42 days *2409*

LDL-Cholesterol *Serum* *Decrease* *Physiological* In 28 healthy individuals treated with up to 3600 mg QD mean concentration changed nonsignificantly from mean baseline of 149 ± 30 mg/dL to 149 ± 31 mg/dL after 13 days and significantly to 140 ± 29 mg/dL after 42 days *2409*

Triglycerides *Serum* *Decrease* *Physiological* In 28 healthy individuals treated with up to 3600 mg QD mean concentration changed significantly from mean baseline of 167 ± 77 mg/dL to 120 ± 60 mg/dL after 13 days *2409*

Serum *Increase* *Physiological* In 28 healthy individuals treated with up to 3600 mg QD mean concentration changed nonsignificantly from mean baseline of 167 ± 77 mg/dL to 180 ± 84 mg/dL after 13 days *2409*

Dydrogesterone

Leukocytes *Blood* *Increase* *Physiological* Mild leukocytosis reported *128*

Dyphylline

Albumin *Urine* *Increase* *Physiological* Albuminuria has been reported as adverse event *6325*

Blood *Urine* *Increase* *Physiological* Gross and microscopic hematuria have been reported as adverse events *6325*

Glucose *Serum* *Increase* *Physiological* Hyperglycemia has been reported as adverse event *6325*

Occult Blood *Feces* *Increase* *Physiological* Hematemesis has been reported as adverse event *6325*

Theophylline *Serum* *No Effect* *Analytical* No significant interference with Syva EMIT 2000 assay *413* No effect observed on immunoassay measurement systems *5999*

Ecgonine Methyl Ester

Ecgonine *Urine* *No Effect* *Analytical* No interference observed with l-ecgonine methyl ester at a concentration of 5000 ng/mL with Roche Abuscreen ONTRAK assay *1106*

Echinomycin

Alanine Aminotransferase *Serum* *Increase* *Physiological* Transient increases may be observed *1384*

Aspartate Aminotransferase *Serum* *Increase* *Physiological* Transient increases may occur *1384*

Creatinine *Serum* *Increase* *Physiological* Prerenal azotemia may occur *1384*

Platelets *Blood* *Decrease* *Physiological* Mild thrombocytopenia may occur *1384*

Urea Nitrogen *Serum* *Increase* *Physiological* Prerenal azotemia may occur *1384*

Echothiophate

Cholinesterase *Red Blood Cells* *Decrease* *Physiological* Direct effect of drug (specific inhibitor of enzyme) *5900*

Serum *Decrease* *Physiological* After few weeks of eyedrop therapy *2753*

Ectylurea

Alanine Aminotransferase *Serum* *Increase* *Physiological* May cause cholestasis with cholangiolitis *3810*

Alkaline Phosphatase *Serum* *Increase* *Physiological* May cause cholestasis with cholangiolitis *3810*

Aspartate Aminotransferase *Serum* *Increase* *Physiological* May cause cholestasis with cholangiolitis *3810*

Bile *Urine* *Increase* *Physiological* May cause cholestasis with cholangiolitis *3810*

Bilirubin *Serum* *Increase* *Physiological* May cause cholestasis with cholangiolitis *3810*

BSP Retention *Serum* *Increase* *Physiological* May cause cholestasis with cholangiolitis *3810*

Edrophonium

Cholinesterase *Serum* *Decrease* *Physiological* Direct action of drug *1883*

Cholinesterase (True)

Red Blood Cells *No Effect* *Physiological* Administration of 1.43 mg/kg to healthy individuals had no significant efffect over 60 minutes *5197*

Growth Hormone *Plasma* *No Effect* *Physiological* No difference in response in patients with Alzheimer's disease from that in healthy elderly subjects *1259*

Eflornithine

Erythrocytes *Blood* *Decrease* *Physiological* Due to myelosuppression *1384*

Hemoglobin *Blood* *Decrease* *Physiological* Anemia occasionally reported *1384*

Leukocytes *Blood* *Decrease* *Physiological* Due to myelosuppression *1384* Leukopenia occasionally reported *1384*

Platelets *Blood* *Decrease* *Physiological* Due to effect on bone marrow: may be pronounced reduction: is usually dose limiting adverse effect *1384*

Eicosapentaenoic Acid

HDL_2-Cholesterol *Serum* *No Effect* *Physiological* In patients treated with 2.7 g/d for 12 weeks no significant change in concentration observed *2690*

HDL_2-Phospholipids *Serum* *No Effect* *Physiological* In patients treated with 2.7 g/d for 12 weeks no significant change in concentration observed *2690*

HDL_2-Triglycerides *Serum* *No Effect* *Physiological* In patients treated with 2.7 g/d for 12 weeks no significant change in concentration observed *2690*

HDL_3-Apolipoprotein A-I *Serum* *No Effect* *Physiological* Treatment with 2.7 g/d for 12 weeks had no significant effect on concentration *2690*

HDL_3-Cholesterol *Serum* *No Effect* *Physiological* Treatment with 2.7 g/d for 12 weeks had no significant effect on concentration *2690*

HDL_3-Phospholipids *Serum* *No Effect* *Physiological* In patients treatment with 2.7 g/d for 12 weeks had no significant effect on concentration *2690*

HDL_3-Triglycerides *Serum* *Decrease* *Physiological* Treatment with 2.7 g/d for 12 weeks caused significant decrease in concentration *2690*

HDL-Apolipoprotein A-I *Serum* *No Effect* *Physiological* In patients treated with 2.7 g/d for 12 weeks no significant change in concentration observed *2690*

IDL-Apolipoprotein B *Serum* *No Effect* *Physiological* Treatment with 2.7 g/d for 12 weeks had no significant effect on concentration *2690*

IDL-Cholesterol *Serum* *No Effect* *Physiological* Treatment with 2.7 g/d for 12 weeks had no significant effect *2690*

IDL-Phospholipids *Serum* *No Effect* *Physiological* Treatment with 2.7 g/d for 12 weeks had no significant effect on concentration *2690*

Eicosapentaenoic Acid *(continued)*

IDL-Triglycerides *Serum No Effect Physiological* Treatment with 2.7 g/d for 12 weeks had no significant effect on concentration *2690* In patients treated with 2.7 g/d for 12 weeks mean concentration unaffected *691*

LDL_1-Apolipoprotein B *Serum Decrease Physiological* In patients treated with 2.7 g/d for 12 weeks mean concentration decreased by 23.5% *2690*

LDL_1-Cholesterol *Serum Decrease Physiological* In patients treated with 2.7 g/d for 12 weeks mean concentration decreased by 18.7% *2690*

LDL_2-Apolipoprotein B *Serum No Effect Physiological* In patients treated with 2.7 g/d for 12 weeks no significant change in concentration observed *2690*

LDL_2-Phospholipids *Serum No Effect Physiological* In patients treated with 2.7 g/d for 12 weeks no significant effect observed on concentration *2690*

LDL_2-Triglycerides *Serum Increase Physiological* In patients treated with 2.7 g/d for 12 weeks mean concentration increased by 25.7% *2690*
Serum No Effect Physiological In patents treated with 2.7 g/d for 12 weeks no significant change in concentration observed *2690*

LDL-Phospholipids *Serum Decrease Physiological* In patients treated with 2.7 g/d for 12 weeks mean concentration decreased by 19.1% *2690*

Lecithin:Cholesterol Acyltransferase
Serum No Effect Physiological In patients treated with 2.7 g/d for 12 weeks no significant effect observed on activity *2690*

Lipid Transfer Protein *Serum Increase Physiological* In patients treated with 2.7 g/d concentration increased by 24.8% after 4 weeks and by 32.1% after 12 weeks *2690*

VLDL-Apolipoprotein B *Serum Decrease Physiological* Treatment with 2.7 g/d for 12 weeks caused mean 32.5% decrease *2690*

VLDL-Apolipoprotein C-II *Serum Decrease Physiological* In patients treated with 2.7 g/d for 12 weeks mean 34.7% decrease observed *2690*

VLDL-Apolipoprotein C-III *Serum Decrease Physiological* In patients treated with 2.7 g/d for 12 weeks mean concentration decreased by 34.1% *2690*

VLDL-Cholesterol *Serum Decrease Physiological* Administration of 2.7 g/d for 12 weeks caused mean decrease of 32.8% *2690*

VLDL-Phospholipids *Serum Decrease Physiological* Treatment with 2.7 g/d for 12 weeks caused mean 31.5% decrease *2690*

VLDL-Triglycerides *Serum Decrease Physiological* Administration of 2.7 g/d for 12 weeks caused mean 31.2% decrease *2690*

Emepronium

Histamine *Plasma No Effect Analytical* 50% inhibition of radio-enzyme assay at 34 µg/mL but unlikely to be effect at physiological concentrations *2492*

Midazolam *Serum No Effect Analytical* On GC-ECD method of Ha et al *2387*

Enalapril

Alanine Aminotransferase *Serum Increase Physiological* Enalapril may cause hepatic failure rarely or cholestatic jaundice *3997*
Serum No Effect Physiological In 427 patients with essential hypertension treatment for 6 months caused nonsignificant change from mean baseline of 22 ± 11 U/L to 21 ± 12 U/L *3559*

Albumin *Serum Increase Physiological* In 13 hypertensive patients with proteinuria treatment with up to 40 mg/d caused significant increase from mean baseline of 39.8 ± 2.0 g/L to 41.6 ± 3.8 g/L *229*
Serum No Effect Physiological Nonsignificant increase from mean baseline of 623 µmol/L to 625 µmol/L in 27 patients with hypertension treated with 2.5 mg/d and upwards for 90 days *3023*
Urine Decrease Physiological In 12 patients with essential hypertension and proteinuria treatment caused significant reduction from mean baseline of about 50 µg/min to 26 µg/min after 4 and 8 weeks *545* Microalbuminuria, non-nephrotic and nephrotic range proteinurias all reduced with enalapril treatment. Microalbuminuria in type I diabetics observed with both short and long-term studies. Cited reductions were from 51 to 12 mg/d and from 33 to 23 mg/d *5627* Microalbuminuria, non-nephrotic and nephrotic range proteinurias all reduced with enalapril treatment. Microalbuminuria in type I diabetics observed with both short and long-term studies. Cited reductions were from 51 to 12 mg/d and from 33 to 23 mg/d *5627* In 6 hypertensive type 1 diabetics treatment with 10-20 mg/d caused reduction of 55% after 3 weeks and 35% after 6 months. In 6 normotensive diabetics the same treatment caused reduction of 65% at 3 weeks and 61% at 6 months *5146*
Urine No Effect Physiological No significant change from mean baseline of 188 µg/mg creatinine observed in 12 hypertensive diabetics with excretion of 112 µg/mg observed at 10 weeks, 70 µg/mg at 20 weeks and 163 µg/mg at 30 weeks *1849* In 9 patients with essential hypertension treatment with a mean dose of 11.3 ± 1.3 mg/d for 3 months caused nonsignificant change from mean baseline of 18 ± 8 µg/min to 11 ± 5 µg/min over 24 h and from 32 ± 9 µg/min to 17 ± 4 µg/min during clearances *4945*

Aldosterone *Plasma Decrease Physiological* In 10 nonazotemic cirrhotics treatment with enalapril caused 66% and 68% decrease in concentration after 2 and 8 days respectively from mean baseline of 240.9 ± 67 pg/mL *4384* Gradual reduction following effect on angiotensin II due to longer half-life *287* Significant effect observed in 15 patients with essential hypertension treated with 40 mg once daily for 2 months *3068* Increase by 1 mo as part of long-term response in 6 responders of 10 treated hypertensives *1926* Treatment of 24 patients with congestive heart failure with 5 mg/d enalapril for 16 weeks caused a mean decrease of 0.05 pg/mL *1326*
Plasma No Effect Physiological No significant effect in patients receiving drug *2636* In 9 patients with essential hypertension treatment with a mean dose of 11.3 ± 1.3 mg/d for 3 months caused nonsignificant change from mean baseline of 16.7 ± 3.4 ng/dL to 12.6 ± 2.2 ng/dL *4945*
Urine Decrease Physiological Sustained effect: extent related to pretreatment plasma renin activity *287*

Alkaline Phosphatase *Serum Increase Physiological* Enalapril may cause hepatic failure rarely or cholestatic jaundice *3997*

Amylase *Serum Increase Physiological* Apparent case of pancreatitis in one patient within 1 day of starting treatment with drug *6034* Enalapril may cause pancreatitis rarely *3997*

Angiotensin-I *Plasma Increase Physiological* Increases as angiotensin II falls after first dose *2636* Increase from mean baseline concentration of 30.2 pg/mL to 118 pg/mL at 6 hours with fall off to 55 pg/mL at 8 hours and similar concentration for next 16 hours in 8 healthy volunteers *3075*

Angiotensin-II *Plasma Decrease Physiological* Reduction observed in 15 patients with essential hypertension treated with 40 mg once daily for 2 months *3068* Significant reduction from mean baseline concentration of 7.29 pg/mL to 2.89 pg/mL at 4 hours, 2.59 pg/mL at 8 hours in 8 healthy volunteers after single oral dose of 10 mg but returned to 9.69 pg/mL at 24 hours *3075* Prompt and striking reduction following i.v. administration over 30 min: more gradual reduction when given orally *287* Significant fall after first dose, subsequently remains depressed *2636*
Plasma No Effect Physiological In 50 patients with essential hypertension nonsignificant change of - 2.8 ± 6.5 ng/L in those receiving 20 mg/d for 4 weeks, compared with 0.3 ± 6.3 ng/L in placebo-treated controls *3307*

Angiotensin-converting Enzyme
Serum Decrease Physiological Significant reduction from mean of 12.20 U/L to 2.30 U/L in 8 healthy normotensive volunteers given 20 mg daily for 4 days *3243* Almost complete inhibition observed in group of volunteers given 20 mg previous day and another 20 mg 2 hours before measurement *4007* Significant reduction from mean baseline activity of 13.3 mU/mL to 5.06 mU/mL at 2 hours, 2.55 mU/mL at 6 hours but returned to 11.4 mU/mL at 24 hours in 8 healthy volunteers given single oral dose of 10 mg *3075* Good correlation between serum concentration of drug and inhibition of enzyme

in both acute and chronic studies *2857* In 10 non-azotemic cirrhotics treatment with enalapril caused 61% and 53% decrease after 2 and 8 days respectively from mean baseline of 25.8 ± 1.8 U/L *4384* Significant fall even on first day of treatment *2636* Significant reduction observed in 6 normotensive and 6 hypertensive diabetics after 3 weeks and 6 months treatment with 10-20 mg/d *5146* Treatment for 4 weeks in 18 normotensive, normoalbuminuric Type 1 insulin-dependent diabetic children caused marked and significant inhibition *1503* Marked effect in 4 d as part of long-term response in 6 responders of 10 treated hypertensives *1926*

Angiotensinogen *Plasma No Effect Physiological* No significant change from mean baseline concentration of 1.38 µg/mL over 24 hours following a single oral dose of 10 mg in 8 healthy volunteers *3075*

Apolipoprotein A-I *Serum No Effect Physiological* Insignificant change observed in 12 patients with mild uncomplicated essential hypertension treated for 24 weeks with 30 mg daily *964* In 50 patients with NIDDM and hypertension treatment with up to 40 mg/d for 12 weeks caused nonsignificant increase of 3.8 mg/dL *960*

Apolipoprotein B *Serum No Effect Physiological* Insignificant change observed in 12 patients with mild uncomplicated hypertension treated for 24 weeks with 30 mg daily *964* In 50 patients with NIDDM and hypertension treatment with up to 40 mg/d for 12 weeks caused nonsignificant decrease of 8.2 mg/dL *960*

Aspartate Aminotransferase *Serum Increase Physiological* Enalapril may cause hepatic failure rarely or cholestatic jaundice *3997*

Serum No Effect Physiological In 427 patients with essential hypertension treatment for 6 months caused no change from mean baseline of 21 ± 9 U/L *3559*

Bilirubin *Serum Increase Physiological* Enalapril may cause hepatic failure rarely or cholestatic jaundice *3997*

Cholesterol *Serum Decrease Physiological* In proteinuric patients treatment with enalapril reduced both protein excretion and the increased serum cholesterol concentration *4235* In 427 patients with essential hypertension treatment with enalapril for 6 months caused significant decrease from mean baseline of 5.61 ± 1.08 mmol/L to 5.40 ± 0.91 mmol/L *3559* In 135 patients with stage I diastolic hypertension treated with 5 mg/d caused change from mean baseline of 5.84 ± 0.94 mmol/L by - 0.21 ± 0.06 mmol/L after 12 months and - 0.29 ± 0.06 mmol/L after 48 months *2335*

Serum Increase Physiological In 10 middle-aged patients with essential hypertension treatment with up to 40 mg/d for up to 12 weeks caused increase of 0.21 ± 0.26 mmol/L from mean baseline of 5.00 ± 0.24 mmol/L *4397*

Serum No Effect Physiological In nonobese patients with essential hypertension treatment with 10 mg/d for 6 months caused nonsignificant increase from mean 5.2 ± 0.7 mmol/L to 5.5 ± 0.9 mmol/L *311* Insignificant change observed in 12 patients with mild uncomplicated hypertension given 30 mg daily for 24 weeks *964* In 12 normotensive patients with NIDDM treatment with 5 mg/d for 48 months caused nonsignificant change from mean baseline of 5.53 ± 0.41 mmol/L to 5.46 ± 0.41 mmol/L *5250* In 10 patients with essential hypertension treatment with up to 40 mg/d for 8 - 12 weeks caused nonsignificant increase in concentration of 0.21 ± 0.26 mmol/L from mean baseline of 5.00 ± 0.24 mmol/L *4397* No effect observed in patients with essential hypertension when given as monotherapy *6470* In 50 patients with NIDDM and hypertension treatment with up to 40 mg/d for 12 weeks caused nonsignificant decrease of 0.26 mmol/L *960* In 53 patients given up to 160 mg daily or when combined with hydrochlorothiazide *3752*

Cortisol, Free *Urine No Effect Analytical* No significant interference observed with HPLC method of Turpeinen et al *6105*

Creatinine *Serum Increase Physiological* Observed in patients with both initially normal and initially increased concentrations. In 12 patients with mean concentration of 1.3 mg/dL increased to 3.0 mg/dL and in 7 with initial concentration of 1.8 mg/dL increased to 2.6 mg/dL over 2 years *5627* Reversible renal insufficiency reported in some patients without evidence of renal artery stenosis *1465* Nonsignificant increase from mean baseline concentration of 375 µmol/L to 418 µmol/L in 27 hypertensive patients treated with 2.5 mg/d and upwards for 90 days *3023* In 2111 patients with asymptomatic left ventricular failure treated with enalapril 20 mg/d for an average of 37.4 months was associated with slight but significant increase in concentration of 3.5 µmol/L *5686* Associated with selective glomerular efferent arteriolar dilatation and possible interference with autoregulatory capacity of kidney in response to severe renovascular hypertension *475* Enalapril inhibits the renin-angiotensin-aldosterone system and changes in renal function may be anticipated in susceptible individuals *3997*

Serum No Effect Physiological No change in 8 healthy normotensive volunteers given 20 mg daily for 4 days *3243* No significant effect in 20 hypertensive patients given up to 20 mg daily for 10 weeks *6495* In 10 hypertensive diabetics treatment with 20 mg/d for 8 months had no significant effect on concentration *1305* In 13 hypertensive patients with proteinuria treatment with up to 40 mg/d caused nonsignificant increase from mean baseline of 199 ± 77 µmol/L to 209 ± 91 µmol/L *229*

Creatinine Clearance *Urine Increase Physiological* In 10 non-azotemic cirrhotics treatment with enalapril caused significant increases of 24% and 34% from mean baseline of 7.4 ± 4.3 mL/min after 6 and 8 days treatment respectively *4384*

Urine No Effect Physiological In 12 normotensive patients with NIDDM treatment with 5 mg/d for 48 months caused nonsignificant increase from mean baseline of 89.6 ± 10.5 mL/min to 94.1 ± 13.4 mL/min *5250* In 12 patients with essential hypertension treatment for 8 weeks caused nonsignificant reduction from mean baseline of 99.5 ± 2.4 mL/min to 95.4 ± 2.2 mL/min *545* In 53 patients given up to 160 mg daily or when combined with hydrochlorothiazide *3752*

Effective Renal Plasma Flow

Patient Decrease Physiological Associated with selective glomerular efferent arteriolar dilatation and possible interference with autoregulatory capacity of kidney in response to severe renovascular hypertension *475*

Patient Increase Physiological In 13 hypertensive patients with proteinuria treatment with up to 40 mg/d for 12 weeks caused significant increase from mean baseline of 179 ± 93 mL/min/1.73 sq m to 191 ± 99 mL/min/1.73 sq m *229* In majority of studies enalapril observed to cause increase regardless of whether patients had previously normal or reduced ERPF *5627* Slight but not significant increase observed with 4 weeks treatment in 18 normotensive, normoalbuminuric Type 1 diabetic children without change in filtration fraction *1503* In 10 hypertensive diabetics treated with 20 mg/d for 8 months caused significant increase from mean baseline of 500 ± 130 mL/min/1.73 sq m to 560 ± 165 mL/min/1.73 sq m *1305* In 6 normotensive type 1 diabetics treatment with 10-20 mg/d for 6 months showed increase at 3 weeks and 6 months but in 6 hypertensive type 1 diabetics no effect observed on renal plasma flow when given the same treatment *5146*

Patient No Effect Physiological In 9 patients with essential hypertension treatment with a mean dose of 11.3 ± 1.3 mg/d for 3 months caused nonsignificant change from mean baseline of 493 ± 44 mL/min/1.73 sq m to 530 ± 55 mL/min/1.73 sq m *4945*

Endothelin-1 *Plasma No Effect Physiological* In 50 patients with essential hypertension nonsignificant change of - 0.1 ± 0.2 ng/L in those receiving 20 mg/d for 4 weeks, compared with - 0.1 ± 0.3 ng/L in placebo-treated controls *3307*

Endothelin-1, Big *Plasma Increase Physiological* In 50 patients with essential hypertension significant change of 2.3 ± 0.8 ng/L in those receiving 20 mg/d for 4 weeks, compared with - 0.3 ± 0.8 ng/L in placebo-treated controls *3307*

Eosinophils *Blood Increase Physiological* Reversible and associated with rash in one patient *1465*

Erythrocytes *Blood No Effect Physiological* In 53 patients given up to 160 mg daily or when combined with hydrochlorothiazide *3752*

Erythropoietin *Serum Decrease Physiological* Increased concentration present in 18 patients with dilated cardiomyopathy (mean 37 pmol/L) normalized during 48 weeks treatment (mean concentration 17.5 pmol/L) when enalapril added to regime of digoxin and diuretic therapy *1996* Significant reduction observed from mean baseline concentration of 32 U/L to 24 U/L in 27 hypertensive patients treated with 2.5 mg/d and upwards for 90 days *3023*

Enalapril *(continued)*

Erythropoietin *(continued)*
Serum No Effect Physiological In 7 patients with chronic renal failure administration of 5 mg caused nonsignificant change from mean baseline of 28.0 ± 8.4 mU/mL to 31.4 ± 4.3 mU/mL after 6 h and 26.8 ± 6.0 mU/mL after 24 h *6134*

Filtration Fraction *Urine Decrease Physiological* In 6 normotensive type 1 diabetics treatment with 10-20 mg/d decreased after 3 weeks *5146* In 10 hypertensive diabetics treated with 20 mg/d for 8 months caused decrease from mean baseline of 0.23 ± 0.05 to 0.21 ± 0.05 *1305* In 13 hypertensive patients with proteinuria treatment with up to 40 mg/d for 12 weeks caused significant decrease from mean baseline of 25.1 ± 4.6% to 21.4 ± 4.0% *229*
Urine No Effect Physiological In 9 patients with essential hypertension treatment with a mean dose of 11.3 ± 1.3 mg/d for 3 months caused nonsignificant change from mean baseline of 0.23 ± 0.01 to 0.22 ± 0.01 *4945*

Glomerular Filtration Rate *Urine Decrease Physiological* Nonsignificant reduction by 1.9 mL/min in 5 patients with idiopathic membranous nephropathy treated with 0.15 mg/kg/d over 3 weeks: reduction increased to 3.2 mL/min with later rechallenge *5293* Associated with selective glomerular efferent arteriolar dilatation and possible interference with autoregulatory capacity of kidney in response to severe renovascular hypertension *475* Nonsignificant reduction from mean baseline of 15 mL/min/1.73 sq m to 13 mL/min/1.73 sq m following treatment with 2.5 mg/d and upwards for 90 days in 27 patients with hypertension *3023* In 26 chronic hypertensives on treatment and in 5 untreated normotensives following a single mean dose of 9 mg GFR fell from median 14 mL/min/173 sq m to 12 mL/min/1.73 sq m after 24 hours *3024* In 13 hypertensive patients with proteinuria treatment with up to 40 mg/d for 12 weeks caused significant decrease from mean baseline of 43.6 ± 20.0 mL/min/1.73 sq m to 39.6 ± 19.7 mL/min/1.73 sq m *229*
Urine Increase Physiological When baseline glomerular filtration rate is below normal dose dependent increase observed. In one study increase from mean of 103 to 110 mL/min. In another, 10% increase when baseline less than 100 mL/min *5627* Slight but not significant increase observed in 18 normotensive, normoalbuminuric Type 1 diabetic children treated for 4 weeks without change in filtration fraction *1503* In 10 hypertensive diabetics treatment with 20 mg/d for 8 months caused significant increase from mean baseline of 119 ± 14 mL/min/1.73 sq m to 135 ± 11 mL/min/1.73 sq m *1305* When baseline glomerular filtration rate is below normal dose dependent increase observed. In one study increase from mean of 103 to 110 mL/min. In another, 10% increase when baseline less than 100 mL/min *5627*
Urine No Effect Physiological No significant change observed in 15 patients with essential hypertension treated with 40 mg daily for 2 months *3068* In 9 patients with essential hypertension treatment with a mean dose of 11.3 ± 1.3 mg/d for 3 months caused nonsignificant change from mean baseline of 110 ± 9 mL/min/1.73 sq m to 111 ± 6 mL/min/1.73 sq m *4945* Mean GFR remained unchanged in 6 hypertensive and 6 normotensive type 1 diabetics treated with 10 - 20 mg/d for 6 months *5146*

Glucose *Serum Decrease Physiological* Incidence of 1.0% observed in French Pharmacovigilance database *4106* In 427 patients with essential hypertension treatment for 6 months caused significant reduction from mean baseline of 5.4 ± 1.0 mmol/L to 5.3 ± 0.8 mmol/L *3559* In 10 middle-aged patients with essential hypertension treatment with up to 40 mg/d for up to 12 weeks caused reduction of 0.2 ± 0.2 mmol/L from mean baseline of 6.2 ± 0.3 mmol/L *4397*
Serum No Effect Physiological No significant effect observed in either diabetics or normal subjects in response to acute ingestion of drug *3851* Nonsignificant decrease from mean baseline of 9.0 mmol/L to 8.7 mmol/L in 12 hypertensive diabetic patients treated for 30 weeks *1849* In 53 patients given up to 160 mg daily or when combined with hydrochlorothiazide *3752* In 10 hypertensive diabetics treatment with 20 mg/d for 8 months had no significant effect on concentration *1305* In 50 patients with NIDDM and hypertension treatment with up to 40 mg/d for 12 weeks caused significant decrease of 0.24 mmol/L *960* In 10 patients with essential hypertension treatment with up to 40 mg/d for 8 - 12 weeks caused nonsignificant decrease of 0.2 ± 0.2 mmol/L of fasting glucose concentration from mean baseline of 6.2 ± 0.3 mmol/L *4397* No significant effect observed at 3 weeks and 6 months when 6 normotensive and 6 hypertensive type 1 diabetics were treated with 10-20 mg/d *5146*
Urine Increase Physiological Reported in one patient with mild uncomplicated essential hypertension *1465*

Glucose Tolerance *Serum No Effect Physiological* Treatment of patients with essential hypertension treatment for 8 - 12 weeks had no significant effect *4397* Concomitant administration of enalapril had no effect on glucose tolerance in response to IVGTT in 8 nonobese hypertensive patients *311*

γ-Glutamyltransferase *Serum Increase Physiological* Enalapril may cause hepatic failure rarely or cholestatic jaundice *3997*
Urine No Effect Physiological In 53 patients given up to 160 mg daily or when combined with hydrochlorothiazide *3752*

HDL-Cholesterol *Serum Decrease Physiological* In 10 patients with essential hypertension treatment with up to 40 mg/d for 8 - 12 weeks caused nonsignificant decrease of 0.21 ± 0.1 mmol/L from mean baseline of 1.07 ± 0.07 mmol/L *4397*
Serum Increase Physiological In 427 patients with essential hypertension treatment with enalapril for 6 months caused nonsignificant increase from mean baseline of 1.19 ± 0.36 mmol/L to 1.22 ± 0.28 mmol/L *3559*
Serum No Effect Physiological Insignificant change observed in 12 patients with mild uncomplicated essential hypertension given 30 mg daily for 24 weeks *964* In 8 nonobese patients with essential hypertension treatment with 10 mg/d for 6 months caused nonsignificant increase from mean baseline of 1.3 ± 0.2 mmol/L to 1.4 ± 0.2 mmol/L *311* In 50 patients with NIDDM and hypertension treatment with up to 40 mg/d for 12 weeks caused nonsignificant decrease of 0.03 mmol/L *960* In 135 patients with stage I diastolic hypertension treated with 5 mg/d caused change from mean baseline of 1.13 ± 0.32 mmol/L by + 0.07 ± 0.01 mmol/L after 12 months and + 0.02 ± 0.02 mmol/L after 48 months *2335* No effect observed in patients with essential hypertension when given as monotherapy *6470*

Hematocrit *Blood Decrease Physiological* Enalapril may cause neutropenia, thrombocytopenia or bone marrow depression rarely. Hematocrit reduced by 1.0% regularly *3997*
Blood No Effect Physiological In 53 patients given up to 160 mg daily or when combined with hydrochlorothiazide *3752*

Hemoglobin *Blood Decrease Physiological* Significant reduction from mean baseline concentration of 7.6 mmol/L to 6.7 mmol/L after 90 days treatment of 27 patients with hypertension with 2.5 mg/d and upwards *3023* Enalapril may cause neutropenia, thrombocytopenia or bone marrow depression rarely. Hemoglobin decreased by 0.3 g/dL regularly *3997*

Hemoglobin A_{1c} *Blood Decrease Physiological* In 50 patients with NIDDM and hypertension treatment with up to 40 mg/d for 12 weeks caused significant decrease of 0.49% *960*
Blood No Effect Physiological No significant effect observed in 6 hypertensive and 6 normotensive type 1 diabetics treated with 10-20 mg/d for 6 months *5146* In 11 patients with NIDDM and hypertension treatment with β-blockers caused mean concentration to change nonsignificantly by -0.27 ± 0.12% after 1 month, +0.18 ± 0.15% after 3 months and +0.39 ± 0.24% after 6 months *5276* No significant effect observed in diabetics after 3 months of treatment *3851* In 10 hypertensive diabetics treatment with 20 mg/d for 8 months had no significant effect on concentration *1305* Nonsignificant increase from mean baseline of 6.9% to 7.1% in 12 hypertensive diabetic patients treated for 30 weeks *1849* In 8 nonobese patients with essential hypertension treatment with 10 mg/d for 6 months had no effect on blood concentration *311*

Indocyanine Green Clearance
Serum Decrease Physiological 35% reduction in clearance observed in 9 healthy volunteers 4 hours following 40 mg orally. Apparent 23% decrease in volume of distribution of ICG. Half-life not significantly affected. Effect probably due to pooling of blood in hepatosplanchnic area *2084*

Insulin *Plasma Decrease Physiological* In 10 hypertensive patients treated with up to 40 mg/d treated for 8 - 12 weeks caused significant decrease of fasting insulin concentration of 5.3 ± 1.7 μU/mL from mean baseline of 8.2 ± 1.2 μU/mL *4397*

Insulin response to Glucose
Plasma No Effect Physiological In 8 nonobese hypertensive patients concomitant administration of enalapril had no effect on plasma insulin concentration during IVGTT *311*

Kallikrein *Urine Increase Physiological* In 10 patients with non-azotemic cirrhosis treatment with enalapril caused significant increase from mean baseline of 103.1 ± 28.9 µg/d to 165.0 ± 46.9 µg/d after 2 days (64%) with no further increase thereafter *4384*

Urine No Effect Physiological In 9 patients with essential hypertension treatment with a mean dose of 11.3 ± 1.3 mg/d for 3 months caused nonsignificant change from mean baseline of 7.7 ± 1.7 nkat/d to 9.5 ± 1.6 nkat/d and from 9.1 ± 1.8 nkat/d to 9.9 ± 2.1 nkat/d during clearances *4945*

6-Keto-Prostaglandin $F_{1\alpha}$ *Urine Increase Physiological* In 10 non-azotemic cirrhotics treatment with enalapril caused significant increases of 101% and 53% on days 8 and 6 respectively from mean baseline of 350.7 ± 64.0 ng/d *4384* Significant increase from baseline excretion of 167 ng/d to 231 ng/d in 12 patients with hypertension treated with 10 or 20 mg/d for 4 weeks *851*

Urine No Effect Physiological Insignificant increase in 8 healthy normotensive volunteers given 20 mg daily for 4 days *3243*

Lactate Dehydrogenase *Serum Decrease Physiological* Significant reduction from mean baseline of 333 U/L to 287 U/L in 27 patients with hypertension treated with 2.5 mg/d and upwards for 90 days *3023*

LDL-Cholesterol *Serum Decrease Physiological* In 135 patients with stage I diastolic hypertension treated with 5 mg/d caused change from mean baseline of 3.97 ± 0.87 mmol/L by - 0.11 ± 0.05 mmol/L after 12 months and - 0.25 ± 0.06 mmol/L after 48 months *2335* In 427 patients with essential hypertension treatment with enalapril for 6 months caused significant decrease from mean baseline of 3.59 ± 1.08 mmol/L to 3.41 ± 1.06 mmol/L *3559*

Serum No Effect Physiological In 50 patients with NIDDM and hypertension treatment with up to 40 mg/d for 12 weeks caused nonsignificant decrease of 0.18 mmol/L *960* In 8 nonobese patients with essential hypertension treatment with 10 mg/d for 6 months caused nonsignificant increase from mean baseline of 3.2 ± 0.7 mmol/L to 3.5 ± 0.8 mmol/L *311* Insignificant change observed in 12 patients with mild uncomplicated hypertension given 30 mg daily for 24 weeks *964* No effect observed in patients with essential hypertension when given as monotherapy *6470*

Leukocytes *Blood Decrease Physiological* Nonsignificant reduction from mean baseline concentration of 5500 /µL to 5300 /µL in 27 hypertensive patients treated with 2.5 mg/d and upwards for 90 days *3023*

Blood No Effect Physiological In 53 patients given up to 160 mg daily or when combined with hydrochlorothiazide *3752*

Lipase *Serum Increase Physiological* Enalapril may cause pancreatitis rarely *3997*

Lysozyme *Urine No Effect Physiological* In 53 patients given up to 160 mg daily or when combined with hydrochlorothiazide *3752*

Mibefradil *Serum No Effect Physiological* Enalapril coadministration had no significant effect on pharmacokinetics of mibefradil *5009*

β_2-Microglobulin *Urine No Effect Physiological* In 12 normotensive patients with NIDDM treatment with 5 mg/d for 48 months caused nonsignificant reduction from mean baseline of 12.3 ± 3.0 nmol/L to 10.8 ± 3.0 nmol/L *5250*

Na/K-ATPase *Red Blood Cells Increase Physiological* Effect of drug on erythrocyte membrane so intracellular sodium reduced and potassium increased *3752*

N-Acetyl-Glucosaminidase *Urine No Effect Physiological* In 12 normotensive patients with NIDDM treatment with 5 mg/d for 48 months caused nonsignificant change from mean baseline of 4.0 ± 0.7 U/L to 4.1 ± 0.9 U/L *5250*

Neutrophils *Blood Decrease Physiological* Enalapril may cause neutropenia, thrombocytopenia or bone marrow depression rarely *3997*

Norepinephrine *Plasma Decrease Physiological* Treatment of 24 patients with congestive heart failure with 5 mg/d enalapril for 16 weeks caused a mean decrease of 131 pg/mL *1326*

Plasma No Effect Physiological In 15 patients treated for 2 months with 40 mg once daily no significant effect observed on mean concentration (0.92 nmol/L versus 1.33 nmol/L on placebo) *3068* Nonsignificant increase as part of long-term response in 6 responders of 10 treated hypertensives *1926* In 50 patients with essential hypertension nonsignificant change of 0.3 ± 0.3 ng/L in those receiving 20 mg/d for 4 weeks, compared with 0.3 ± 0.3 ng/L in placebo-treated controls *3307*

Occult Blood *Feces Increase Physiological* Enalapril may cause melena rarely *3997*

Platelets *Blood Decrease Physiological* Enalapril may cause neutropenia, thrombocytopenia or bone marrow depression rarely *3997* Nonsignificant reduction from 248,000 /µL to 226,000 /µL in 27 patients with hypertension treated with 2.5 mg/d and upwards for 90 days *3023*

Blood No Effect Physiological In 53 patients given up to 160 mg daily or when combined with hydrochlorothiazide *3752*

Potassium *Serum Decrease Physiological* In 20% of treated cases hypokalemia observed *1299*

Serum Increase Physiological Enalapril may cause hyperkalemia (more than 5.7 mmol/L) in approximately 1% treated patients *3997* In 9 patients with essential hypertension treatment with a mean dose of 11.3 ± 1.3 mg/d for 3 months caused significant change from mean baseline of 3.6 ± 0.1 mmol/L to 3.9 ± 0.1 mmol/L *4945* In 427 patients with essential hypertension treatment for 6 months caused significant increase from mean baseline of 4.2 ± 0.4 mmol/L to 4.3 mmol/L *3559* Produces mild potassium retention and hyperkalemia *4739* In 2111 patients with asymptomatic left ventricular failure treated with enalapril 20 mg/d for an average of 37.4 months was associated with slight but significant increase in concentration of 0.1 mmol/L *5686* In 13 hypertensive patients with proteinuria treatment with up to 40 mg/d for 12 weeks caused significant increase from mean baseline of 4.4 ± 0.5 mmol/L to 5.0 ± 0.5 mmol/L *229*

Serum No Effect Physiological In 10 hypertensive diabetics treatment with 20 mg/d for 8 months had no significant effect on concentration *1305* No significant effect in 20 hypertensive patients given up to 20 mg daily for 10 weeks *6495* Insignificant increase in 8 healthy normotensive volunteers given 20 mg daily for 4 days *3243*

Urine No Effect Physiological In 9 patients with essential hypertension treatment with a mean dose of 11.3 ± 1.3 mg/d for 3 months caused nonsignificant change from mean baseline of 77 ± 8 mmol/d to 73 ± 9 mmol/d *4945*

Prolactin *Plasma Increase Physiological* In 30 patients (22 women and 8 men) with mild to moderate hypertension treatment with 20 mg/d for 6 weeks caused significant increase from mean baseline of 5.28 ± 0.7 ng/mL to 6.93 ± 1.02 ng/mL *2520*

Prolidase *Serum No Effect Analytical* Slight inhibitory effect observed in vitro but at much higher concentration than therapeutic *4197*

Prostaglandin E_2 *Urine Increase Physiological* Significant increase from mean baseline of 337 ng/d to 425 ng/d in 12 patients treated with 10 or 20 mg/d for 4 weeks *851* In 10 non-azotemic cirrhotics treatment with enalapril caused significant increase from mean baseline of 500.7 ± 140.5 ng/d by 101% and 53% on days 8 and 6 respectively *4384*

Protein *Serum No Effect Physiological* In 10 hypertensive diabetics treatment with 20 mg/d for 8 months had no significant effect on concentration *1305*

Urine Decrease Physiological In 17 patients with nondiabetic essential hypertension treated with 40 mg enalapril daily proteinuria decreased from 133 to 72 mg/day. In patients with renal insufficiency caused mean reductions of 1.9 g/d and 2.9 g/d *5627* Often reduction and rarely increased during treatment *3894* Treatment of 10 hypertensive diabetic patients for 8 months with 20 mg/d caused significant reduction from mean 3.38 ± 0.29 g/d to 2.72 ± 0.49 g/d *1305* In 13 hypertensive patients with proteinuria treated with up to 40 mg/d for 12 weeks significant decrease observed from mean baseline of 2.2 ± 1.8 g/d to 1.0 ± 1.3 g/d *229*

Urine Increase Physiological Mean increase of 3.9 g/24 h in 5 patients with idiopathic membranous nephropathy when treated with 0.15 mg/kg/d during first 3 weeks of treatment: subsequently excretion reduced to below initial level *5293*

Renal Blood Flow *Patient Increase Physiological* May increase without increase in GFR in patients with normal renal function, but GFR may increase if initial GFR below 80 $mL/min/m^2$ *1270*

Patient No Effect Physiological No significant effect observed in 15 patients with essential hypertension treated with 40 mg daily for 2 months *3068*

Enalapril *(continued)*

Renal Resistance, Total *Patient Decrease Physiological* In 10 hypertensive diabetics treatment with 20 mg/d for 8 months caused decrease from 0.27 ± 0.08 mm Hg/mL/min to 0.22 ± 0.07 mm Hg/mL/min *1305*

Renin Activity *Plasma Increase Physiological* Treatment of 24 patients with congestive heart failure with 5 mg/d enalapril for 16 weeks caused a significant mean increase of 3.2 pmol/mL/h *1326* In 9 patients with essential hypertension treatment with a mean dose of 11.3 ± 1.3 mg/d for 3 months caused significant change from mean baseline of 1.52 ± 0.54 ng/mL/h to 6.16 ± 2.50 ng/mL/h *4945* In 10 non-azotemic cirrhotics treatment caused significant increase from mean baseline of 4.1 ± 1.0 ng/mL/h to 9.2 ± 2.5 ng/mL/h on day 2 and 11.3 ± 2.7 ng/mL/h on day 8 *4384* Treatment of 18 normotensive, normoalbuminuric insulin-dependent Type 1 diabetic children caused significant increase over 4 weeks *1503* In 50 patients with essential hypertension significant changes of 44.1 ± 6.5 mIU/L in those receiving 20 mg/d for 4 weeks, compared with - 2.5 ± 6.6 mIU/L in placebo-treated controls *3307* Within 4 d as part of long-term response in 6 responders of 10 treated hypertensives *1926* Significant increase from mean of 1.46 nmol/L/h to 13.39 nmol/L/h in 8 healthy normotensive volunteers given 20 mg daily for 4 days *3243* Significant increase from mean baseline concentration of 2.00 ng/mL/h to 9.37 ng/mL/h at 6 hours with gradual decline to 4.07 ng/mL/h at 24 hours in 8 healthy volunteers given single oral dose of 10 mg *3075* Significant change observed in 15 patients with essential hypertension treated with 40 mg once daily for 2 months *3068* Significant increase in basal activity and following intravenous furosemide in 20 hypertensive patients given up to 20 mg daily *6495* Steady increase from administration of first dose *2636* Gradually increases over 1 h (due to negative feedback on renin secretion) *287*

Sodium *Serum No Effect Physiological* In 427 patients with essential hypertension treated for 6 months mean concentration was unchanged from baseline of 141 ± 4 mmol/L *3559* In 9 patients with essential hypertension treatment with a mean dose of 11.3 ± 1.3 mg/d for 3 months caused nonsignificant change from mean baseline of 140 ± 1 mmol/L to 140 ± 1 mmol/L *4945* In 13 hypertensive patients with proteinuria treatment with up to 40 mg/d for 12 weeks caused nonsignificant change from 141.4 ± 1.7 mmol/L to 140.7 ± 2.0 mmol/L *229*

Urine Decrease Physiological In 12 patients with essential hypertension treatment for 8 weeks caused nonsignificant reduction from mean baseline of 147 ± 7.1 mmol/d to 133 ± 3.0 mmol/d *545*

Urine Increase Physiological In 10 non-azotemic cirrhotics treatment caused increases of 40% and 54% after 6 and 8 days treatment respectively *4384*

Urine No Effect Physiological In 13 hypertensive patients with proteinuria treated with up to 40 mg/d for 12 weeks nonsignificant decrease observed from mean baseline of 124 ± 40 mmol/d to 116 ± 47 mmol/d *229* In 9 patients with essential hypertension treatment with a mean dose of 11.3 ± 1.3 mg/d for 3 months caused nonsignificant change from mean baseline of 164 ± 18 mmol/d to 143 ± 17 mmol/d *4945*

Thromboxane B_2 *Urine No Effect Physiological* Insignificant increase from mean baseline of 196 ng/d to 197 ng/d in 12 hypertensive patients treated with 10 or 20 mg/d for 4 weeks *851*

Tirofiban *Serum No Effect Physiological* Coadministration had no significant effect on plasma clearance of tirofiban *3957*

Triglycerides *Serum Decrease Physiological* In 135 patients with stage I diastolic hypertension treated with 5 mg/d caused change from mean baseline of 1.60 ± 1.16 mmol/L by - 0.36 ± 0.06 mmol/L after 12 months and - 0.14 ± 0.08 mmol/L after 48 months *2335* In 427 patients with essential hypertension treatment with enalapril for 6 months caused significant decrease from mean baseline of 1.74 ± 1.04 mmol/L to 1.63 ± 0.54 mmol/L *3559* Downward trend in 12 patients with mild uncomplicated hypertension given up to 30 mg daily for 24 weeks *964*

Serum Increase Physiological In 10 patients with essential hypertension treatment with up to 40 mg/d for 8 - 12 weeks caused significant increase of 0.26 ± 0.19 mmol/L from mean baseline of 1.54 ± 0.15 mmol/L *4397*

Serum No Effect Physiological No effect observed in patients with essential hypertension when given as monotherapy *6470* In 8 nonobese patients with essential hypertension treatment with 10 mg/d for 6 months caused nonsignificant increase from baseline of 1.4 ± 0.3 mmol/L to 1.5 ± 0.2 mmol/L *311* In 50 patients with NIDDM and hypertension treatment with up to 40 mg/d for 12 weeks caused significant decrease of 0.36 mmol/L *960* In 12 normotensive patients with NIDDM treatment with 5 mg/d for 48 months caused nonsignificant change from mean baseline of 1.83 ± 0.39 mmol/L to 1.85 ± 0.29 mmol/L *5250* No significant effect observed in patients receiving enalapril *4989* In 53 patients given up to 160 mg daily or when combined with hydrochlorothiazide *3752*

Urea *Serum Increase Physiological* In 13 hypertensive patients with proteinuria treatment with up to 40 mg/d for 12 weeks caused significant increase from mean baseline of 8.2 ± 3.1 mmol/L to 11.4 ± 3.4 mmol/L *229*

Serum No Effect Physiological In 427 patients with essential hypertension treatment for 6 months caused nonsignificant reduction from mean baseline of 13.2 ± 3.9 mmol/L to 12.8 ± 3.2 mmol/L *3559*

Urine Increase Physiological In 13 hypertensive patients with proteinuria treatment with up to 40 mg/d caused significant increase from mean baseline of 272 ± 97 mmol/d to 311 ± 74 mmol/d *229*

Urine No Effect Physiological In 9 patients with essential hypertension treatment with a mean dose of 11.3 ± 1.3 mg/d for 3 months caused nonsignificant change from mean baseline of 425 ± 42 mmol/d to 453 ± 38 mmol/d *4945*

Urea Nitrogen *Serum Increase Physiological* Enalapril inhibits the renin-angiotensin-aldosterone system and changes in renal function may be anticipated in susceptible individuals *3997*

Uric Acid *Serum Decrease Physiological* In 427 patients with essential hypertension treatment for 6 months caused significant reduction from mean baseline of 309 ± 77 µmol/L to 297 ± 65 µmol/L *3559* After enalapril alone (up to 160 mg/daily) but may be increased when combined with hydrochlorothiazide *3752*

VLDL-Cholesterol *Serum No Effect Physiological* Insignificant change observed in 12 patients with mild uncomplicated essential hypertension treated with 30 mg daily for 24 weeks *964*

Volume *Blood No Effect Physiological* As part of long-term response in 6 responders of 10 treated hypertensives *1926*

Urine Increase Physiological In 10 non-azotemic cirrhotics treatment with enalapril caused 12% and 25% increases on days 6 and 8 of treatment *4384*

Encainide

Cyclosporine *Blood No Effect Analytical* At a concentration of 1050 mg/L had no effect on Syva EMIT method *495*

Glucose *Serum Increase Physiological* Five episodes of marked hyperglycemia observed in 4 patients previously not requiring treatment for hyperglycemia out of 23 patients studied. Mean glucose concentration rose from 190 mg/L pretreatment to 397 mg/dL 1 month after start in hyperglycemics *5203*

β-Endorphin

Cortisol *Plasma No Effect Physiological* No effect with i.v. infusion in depressed patients or methadone treated addicts *925*

Growth Hormone *Plasma No Effect Physiological* No effect with i.v. infusion in depressed patients or methadone treated addicts *925*

Prolactin *Plasma Increase Physiological* Prompt 2-4 fold increase in 4 depressed psychiatric patients with i.v. infusion *925*

Endralazine

Aldosterone *Plasma Increase Physiological* A single oral dose of 93% caused a mean increase of 93% in 7 hypertensive patients *6380*

Glomerular Filtration Rate *Urine Decrease Physiological* In 7 hypertensive patients a single oral dose of 10 - 15 mg caused a mean reduction of 33% *6380*

Urine *Increase* *Physiological* Treatment with 15 - 90 mg daily for 8 - 17 days in 7 hypertensive patients caused a mean increase of 27% *6380*

PAH Clearance *Urine* *Decrease* *Physiological* A single oral dose of 10-15 mg in 7 hypertensive patients caused a mean reduction of 5% *6380*

Urine *Increase* *Physiological* Treatment of 7 hypertensive patients with 15-90 mg daily for 8-17 days caused a mean increase of 46% *6380*

Potassium Clearance *Urine* *Decrease* *Physiological* A single oral dose of 10-15 mg caused a mean reduction of 12% in 7 hypertensive patients *6380*

Renin Activity *Plasma* *Decrease* *Physiological* Treatment of 7 hypertensive patients with 15-90 mg daily for 8-17 days caused a mean decrease of 33% *6380*

Plasma *Increase* *Physiological* Significant effect in 20 hypertensive patients (WHO phase I and II) *2508* A single oral dose of 10-15 mg caused a mean increase of 40% in 7 hypertensive patients *6380*

Sodium Clearance *Urine* *Decrease* *Physiological* A single oral dose of 10-15 mg caused a mean decrease of 32% in 7 hypertensive patients *6380*

Urea Clearance *Urine* *Decrease* *Physiological* A single oral dose of 10-15 mg caused a mean reduction of 53% in 7 hypertensive patients *6380*

Uric Acid Clearance *Urine* *Decrease* *Physiological* A single oral dose of 54% caused a mean reduction of 54% in 7 hypertensive patients *6380*

Volume *Urine* *Decrease* *Physiological* A single oral dose of 10-15 mg caused a mean reduction of 37% in 7 hypertensive patients *6380*

Urine *Increase* *Physiological* Treatment of 7 hypertensive patients with 15-90 mg daily for 8-17 days caused a mean increase of 65% although this increase was not constant and not significant *6380*

Enflurane

Alanine Aminotransferase *Serum* *Increase* *Physiological* Evidence of hepatocellular damage; characteristically centrilobular necrosis: mechanism of injury most probably metabolic idiosyncrasy *3551* In up to 10 % patients given 2 to 3 administrations of anesthetic agent *1818*

Alkaline Phosphatase *Serum* *Increase* *Physiological* Evidence of hepatocellular damage; characteristically centrilobular necrosis: mechanism of injury most probably metabolic idiosyncrasy *3551*

Aspartate Aminotransferase *Serum* *Increase* *Physiological* Evidence of hepatocellular damage; characteristically centrilobular necrosis: mechanism of injury most probably metabolic idiosyncrasy *3551* Slight effect but decreased in others *1670*

Serum *No Effect* *Physiological* In all patients given 2 to 3 administrations of anesthetic agent *1818*

Bicarbonate *Serum* *Increase* *Physiological* Postoperatively moderately high but still normal *1670*

Bilirubin *Serum* *Increase* *Physiological* Evidence of hepatocellular damage; characteristically centrilobular necrosis: mechanism of injury most probably metabolic idiosyncrasy *3551*

Calcium *Serum* *Decrease* *Physiological* Slight decrease noted postoperatively *1670*

Cortisol *Plasma* *No Effect* *Physiological* No difference between pre-induction and values during anesthesia *5808*

Creatinine *Serum* *Increase* *Physiological* In one patient with initially normal renal function following comparatively long exposure to anesthetic. Normal renal function eventually returned *1675*

Erythrocytes *Urine* *Increase* *Physiological* In one patient with initially normal renal function following comparatively long exposures to anesthetic. Normal renal function eventually returned *1675*

Fatty Acids (FFA), Free *Serum* *Decrease* *Physiological* Fall during anesthesia, but increases in recovery *4470*

Glucose *Serum* *Increase* *Physiological* Effect of anesthesia and surgery *1670*

γ-Glutamyltransferase *Serum* *Increase* *Physiological* In about 10% patients given 2 to 3 administrations of anesthetic agent *1818*

Growth Hormone *Plasma* *No Effect* *Physiological* No effect of anesthesia alone *4470* No effect unless given with propranolol *3833*

Insulin *Plasma* *No Effect* *Physiological* No effect during anesthesia, slight increase after *4470*

Lactate Dehydrogenase *Serum* *Increase* *Physiological* In about 10% patients given 2 to 3 administrations of anesthetic agent *1818*

Leukocytes *Blood* *Increase* *Physiological* May also partly reflect surgery *1670*

Midazolam *Serum* *No Effect* *Analytical* On GC-ECD method of Ha et al *2387*

Potassium *Serum* *Decrease* *Physiological* Slight decrease noted postoperatively *1670*

Prolactin *Plasma* *Increase* *Physiological* In both men and women when used to induce anesthesia with peak at 30 minutes *5808*

Protein *Serum* *No Effect* *Physiological* No effect observed *1670*

Urine *Increase* *Physiological* In one patient with initially normal renal function following comparatively long exposure to anesthetic. Normal renal function eventually returned *1675*

Theophylline *Serum* *No Effect* *Physiological* No clinically significant effect on theophylline concentration observed when drugs coadministered *5999* No documented significant interaction with theophylline reported *6117*

Urea Nitrogen *Serum* *Decrease* *Physiological* Partly due to surgery possibly *1670*

Serum *Increase* *Physiological* In one patient with initially normal renal function following comparatively long exposure to anesthetic. Normal renal function eventually returned *1675*

Enoxacin

Alanine Aminotransferase *Serum* *Increase* *Physiological* Increased activity observed in more than 1% patients receiving multiple doses of enoxacin *4940*

Aspartate Aminotransferase *Serum* *Increase* *Physiological* Increased activity observed in more than 1% patients receiving multiple doses of enoxacin *4940*

Bilirubin *Serum* *No Effect* *Physiological* Clinically insignificant displacement from protein in neonates *6314*

Caffeine *Serum* *Increase* *Physiological* Clearance inhibited *2704* Reported to reduce clearance *1384* Enoxacin is a potent inhibitor of cytochrome P450. In a multiple dose study, enoxacin caused a dose-related increase in the mean elimination half-life of caffeine, decreasing its clearance by up to 80%, and leading to a five-fold increase in the AUC and half-life of caffeine *4940*

Clotting Time *Blood* *No Effect* *Physiological* Enoxacin has no effect on the clearance of the active S-isomer of warfarin and no effect on the clotting time has been observed when the drugs are co-administered *4940*

Cyclosporine A *Blood* *Increase* *Physiological* Increased concentration of cyclosporine have been reported with concomitant use of other members of the quinolone class of drugs *4940*

Digoxin *Serum* *Increase* *Physiological* Increased concentration of digoxin has been reported when enoxacin co-administered *4940*

Theophylline *Serum* *Increase* *Physiological* Up to 300% increase in serum theophylline concentration due to decreased theophylline clearance caused by inhibition of cytochrome P450 1A2 *6117* Probably caused by interference with hepatic metabolism *1384* Clearance inhibited *2704* 400 mg twice daily added to a regime of 150 mg twice daily caused increase in mean theophylline concentration from 3.17 mg/L to 8.23 mg/L with reduction in concentration of theophylline metabolites, with increase of metabolites as soon as theophylline withdrawn *5063* Since enoxacin is a potent inhibitor of cytochrome P450 it interferes with the metabolism of theophylline resulting in a 42% to 74% dose-related theophylline clearance and a subsequent 260% to 350% increase in plasma theophyl-

Enoxacin *(continued)*

Theophylline *(continued)*
line concentration *4940* Decreases theophylline clearance by inhibiting cytochrome P450 1A2, increasing theophylline concentration by about 300% *5999* Decreases theophylline clearance by inhibiting cytochrome P450 1A2 and increases serum theophylline concentration by 300% *3125* 50% reduction in dose necessary to maintain established therapeutic effect *3262* Plasma concentration increased and reduced theophylline clearance by 40-63% with chronic administration due to inhibited demethylation *6448*

Warfarin *Plasma No Effect Physiological* Enoxacin has no effect on the clearance of the active S-isomer of warfarin *4940*

Enoxaparin

Alanine Aminotransferase *Serum Increase Physiological* Asymptomatic increases in activity above 3 times the upper limit of normal observed in 2 of 10 normal individuals and in up to 4% of treated patients *4938*

Aspartate Aminotransferase *Serum Increase Physiological* Asymptomatic increases in activity above 3 times the upper limit of normal observed in 2 of 10 normal individuals and in up to 4% of treated patients *4938*

Bilirubin *Serum Increase Physiological* Asymptomatic increases in aminotransferase activity above 3 times the upper limit of normal observed in 2 of 10 normal individuals and in up to 4% of treated patients, rarely associated with increases in bilirubin concentration *4938*

Fatty Acids (FFA), Free *Serum Increase Physiological* Specimens collected three hours after enoxapirin injection and analyzed within 9 hours had increased concentration of FFA, 0.45 ± 0.07 mmol/L versus 0.12 ± 0.01 mmol/L preheparin *5819*
Serum No Effect Physiological Specimens collected three hours after enoxapirin injection and analyzed within 9 hours had increased concentration of FFA, 0.45 ± 0.07 mmol/L versus 0.12 ± 0.01 mmol/L preheparin but after 24 hours concentration was similar to baseline at 0.14 ± 0.03 mmol/L *5819*

Hematocrit *Blood Decrease Physiological* Severe hypochromic anemia observed in fewer than 1%of 1080 treated patients but hypochromic anemia of any kind observed in 2% *4938*

Hemoglobin *Blood Decrease Physiological* Severe hypochromic anemia observed in fewer than 1%of 1080 treated patients but hypochromic anemia of any kind observed in 2% *4938*

Platelets *Blood Decrease Physiological* Administration of enoxaparin may be associated with thrombocytopenia: counts between 50,000 and 100,000 /µL occurred in 1.9% treated patients compared with 2.0% of patients given heparin and 1.7% given placebo: platelet counts of less than 50,000 /µL occurred in 0.1% patients given enoxaparin and 0.5% patients given heparin *4938*

Thyroid Stimulating Hormone
Serum No Effect Physiological Specimens collected three hours after enoxapirin injection and analyzed within 9 hours had ino significant change in concentration, 1.64 ± 0.43 mIU/L versus 1.59 ± 0.41 mIU/L preheparin *5819*

Thyroxine (T4), Free *Serum Increase Physiological* In 10 cardiac patients receiving multiple doses of enoxapirin specimens FT4 concentration increased by up to 171% *5819*
Serum No Effect Physiological Specimens collected three hours after enoxapirin injection and analyzed within 9 hours had ino significant change in concentration, 12.2 ± 0.5 pmol/L versus 12.4 ± 0.49 pmol/L preheparin *5819*

Triglycerides *Serum No Effect Physiological* Specimens collected three hours after enoxapirin injection and analyzed within 9 hours had ino significant change in concentration, 1.60 ± 0.31 mmol/L versus 1.76 ± 0.38 mmol/L preheparin. 24 hours after enoxapirin concentration remained unchanged at 1.54 ±0.30 mIU/L *5819*

Enoxaprin

Hematocrit *Blood Decrease Physiological* In 2 of 153 patients treated with enoxaprin and compression stockings anemia occurred *64*

Hemoglobin *Blood Decrease Physiological* In 2 of 153 patients treated with enoxaprin and compression stockings anemia occurred *64*

Occult Blood *Feces Increase Physiological* In 2 of 153 patients treated with enoxaprin and compression stockings anemia occurred with melena *64*

Enoximone

Antidiuretic Hormone *Plasma No Effect Physiological* In 10 patients with congestive cardiac failure *6135*

Effective Renal Plasma Flow
Patient Decrease Physiological Significant reduction in 14 patients following intravenous administration but change following oral administration *1060*

Glomerular Filtration Rate *Urine Decrease Physiological* Mean reduction of about 20% following intravenous administration in 14 patients but no significant change following oral administration *1060*

Norepinephrine *Plasma No Effect Physiological* In 10 patients with congestive cardiac failure *6135*

Renin Activity *Plasma Increase Physiological* In 10 patients with congestive cardiac failure from 13.6 to 16.6 ng/mL/h on average *6135*

Volume *Plasma Decrease Physiological* In 8 patients following oral administration 14% reduction observed although this was not significant. When combined with furosemide reduction of 31% observed in 10 patients which was significant *1060*

Enprostil

Apolipoprotein A-I *Serum No Effect Physiological* In 8 normocholesterolemic individuals 9 days of treatment with 70 µg/day failed to alter concentration *5398*

Apolipoprotein B *Serum Decrease Physiological* In 8 normocholesterolemic subjects 9 days of treatment with 70 µg/day caused reduction of concentration by 16% *5398*

Cholesterol *Serum Decrease Physiological* 10% or more reduction in concentration in 64%, 64%, and 67% respectively of hypercholesterolemic subjects receiving 140, 70, or 14 µg drug daily. Median reductions were respectively 17%, 13%, and 11%. 8 normal subjects had reduction of 16% after 9 days *5398*

C-Peptide *Plasma Decrease Physiological* Suppression of peak concentration by 16% in 8 healthy male volunteers after test meal given 70 µg/day when compared with controls *5399*

Fatty Acids (FFA), Free *Serum No Effect Physiological* No effect of treatment with 70 µg/day in 8 healthy male subjects *5399*

Gastrin *Serum Decrease Physiological* Significant reduced response after meals following 35 µg. Significant reduction in overall nocturnal secretion following 35 µg twice daily (from mean of 9450 pmol/min/L to 4393 pmol/min/L from 8.30 pm to 8.00 am in 9 healthy volunteers) *1895*

Glucose *Serum Decrease Physiological* Significant reduction in peak concentration after glucose ingestion in 8 normal men given 70 µg/day with delayed peak when compared with controls *5399*

Glucose-dependent Insulinotropic Peptide
Plasma Decrease Physiological Suppression of peak concentration by 60% in 8 healthy males following test meal compared with controls when test subjects given 70 µg/day *5399*

HDL-Cholesterol *Serum No Effect Physiological* In 8 normocholesterolemic individuals 9 days of treatment with 70 µg/day failed to alter concentration *5398*

Insulin *Plasma Decrease Physiological* Suppression of peak concentration by 36% following ingestion of test meal in 8 normal volunteers given 70 µg/day when compared with controls *5399*

LDL-Cholesterol *Serum Decrease Physiological* In 8 normocholesterolemic subjects 9 days of treatment with 70 µg/day caused reduction of concentration by 22% from baseline *5398*

Propranolol *Serum No Effect Physiological* No effect on propranolol elimination or hepatic metabolism *4905*

Triglycerides *Serum No Effect Physiological* In 8 normocholesterolemic individuals 9 days of treatment with 70 µg/day failed to alter concentration *5398*

Eosin

Vancomycin *Serum Decrease Analytical* Topical application of eosin to burns caused significant bakground interference that increased linearly with increasing amounts of eosin when specimens measured by Abbott TDx system, thereby reducing apparent concentration of vancomycin. Effect can be lessened by ultrafiltration of specimen *3450*

Epalrestat

Fructose-3-Phosphate
Red Blood Cells Decrease Physiological Administration of 150 mg/d of epalrestat for at least one month to 3 NIDDM patients caused significant reduction from mean baseline of 8.3 ± 1.7 µmol/L erythrocytes to 3.0 ± 2.2 µmol/L erythrocytes *2419*

Glucose *Serum No Effect Physiological* Administration of 150 mg/d of epalrestat for at least one month to 3 NIDDM patients caused nonsignificant change from mean baseline of 9.1 ± 2.9 mmol/L to 7.8 ± 1.8 mmol/L *2419*

Hemoglobin A_{1c} *Blood No Effect Physiological* Administration of 150 mg/d of epalrestat for at least one month to 3 NIDDM patients caused nonsignificant change from mean baseline of 8.0 ± 0.2% to 8.0 ± 0.1% *2419*

Sorbitol-3-Phosphate
Red Blood Cells Decrease Physiological Administration of 150 mg/d of epalrestat for at least one month to 3 NIDDM patients caused significant reduction from mean baseline of 24.7 ± 1.9 µmol/L erythrocytes to 16.2 ± 0.7 µmol/L erythrocytes *2419*

Epanolol

Cholesterol *Serum No Effect Physiological* In 10 patients with chronic stable angina mean concentration changed nonsignificantly with 6 months treatment from mean baseline of 6.7 ± 1.0 mmol/L to 7.1 ± 0.6 mmol/L *6547*

Digoxin *Serum No Effect Physiological* In 10 healthy men 200 mg epanolol daily for 7 days had no effect on either trough or peak plasma concentration of digoxin *3489*

Glucose *Serum No Effect Physiological* In 10 patients with chronic stable angina mean fasting concentration changed nonsignificantly with 6 months treatment from mean baseline of 5.1 ± 0.3 mmol/L to 5.3 ± 0.4 mmol/L *6547*

HDL-Cholesterol *Serum No Effect Physiological* In 10 patients with chronic stable angina mean concentration changed nonsignificantly with 6 months treatment from mean baseline of 1.1 ± 0.2 mmol/L to 1.2 ± 0.2 mmol/L *6547*

Insulin *Plasma No Effect Physiological* In 10 patients with chronic stable angina mean fasting concentration changed nonsignificantly with 6 months treatment from mean baseline of 16.6 ± 8.6 mU/L to 14.4 ± 7.8 mU/L *6547*

Plasminogen Activator Inhibitor-1
Plasma No Effect Physiological In 10 patients with chronic stable angina mean concentration did not change significantly with 6 months treatment from mean baseline of 101 ng/mL *6547*

Tissue Plasminogen Activator Antigen
Plasma No Effect Physiological In 10 patients with chronic stable angina mean concentration did not change significantly with 6 months treatment from mean baseline of 6.1 ng/mL *6547*

Triglycerides *Serum No Effect Physiological* In 10 patients with chronic stable angina mean concentration changed nonsignificantly with 6 months treatment from mean baseline of 2.0 ± 1.0 mmol/L to 2.8 ± 1.8 mmol/L *6547*

Ephedrine

Amino Acids *Urine Increase Analytical* Reacts with ninhydrin; extra spot TLC, high voltage electrophoresis *4760*

Amphetamine *Urine No Effect Analytical* Less than 1% cross-reactivity with Roche Abuscreen method when adapted for use with Roche Cobas Mira analyzer *5120*
Urine Positive Analytical At concentrations of D,L-ephedrine greater than 1.0 µg/mL (6.06 µmol/L) with method on Du Pont aca *1554*

Amphetamine/Methamphetamine
Serum No Effect Analytical At a concentration of 3000 mg/mL caused no detectable cross-reactivity with methods on Abbott AxSYM and TDx *6404*

Catecholamines *Plasma No Effect Analytical* No effect on HPLC method of Koller for dopamine, epinephrine, and norepinephrine *3230*
Urine No Effect Analytical No effect observed *1444*
Urine No Effect Physiological No effect observed *1444*

Cortisol *Plasma Decrease Physiological* Accelerated steroid clearance due to increased hepatic blood flow and induction of enzymes in liver *2985*

Dexamethasone *Serum Decrease Physiological* Metabolic clearance enhanced and conjugated fraction in urine increased *2985* May enhance metabolic clearance resulting in decreased plasma concentrations and lessened physiologic effects *3969* Decrease of 36% in half-life of dexamethasone reported when drugs coadministered: clearance of dexamethasone increased by 42% *748*

Epinephrine *Urine Increase Physiological* For 3 h after administration (slight) *2452*

Glucose *Serum Increase Physiological* Less effective than epinephrine *2242*
Urine Increase Physiological May cause glycosuria *1714*

Histamine *Plasma No Effect Analytical* No significant effect on radio-enzyme assay observed at physiological concentration *2492*

5-Hydroxyindoleacetic Acid *Urine Increase Analytical* May cause false increase in color *1444*

^{131}I Uptake *Serum Decrease Physiological* Lilly, P-D products contain tetraiodofluorescein *4360*

Lidocaine *Serum No Effect Analytical* At a concentration of 1250 mg/L (normal therapeutic concentration 0.1 mg/L) had less than 10% effect on method on Baxter Stratus *5705* No significant interference observed at a concentration of 100 µg/mL (605 µmol/L) with method on Du Pont aca *1534*

Metanephrines, Total *Urine No Effect Analytical* At 5 mg/L on modified Pisano procedure *2372*

Methamphetamine *Urine No Effect Analytical* Less than 1% cross-reactivity with Roche Abuscreen Online assay as performed on Roche Cobas Mira *6347* Less than 0.5% cross-reactivity with Hycor accuPINCH method *162*

Norepinephrine *Urine No Effect Physiological* No effect observed *2452*

p-Aminophenol *Urine No Effect Analytical* With addition of drugs at a concentration of 100 mg/L and of related compounds at 50 mg/L no significant effect observed on colorimetric method of van Bocxlaer on Cobas Mira analyzer which involves reacting free p-aminophenol with resorcinol in the presence of magnesium ions to form an indophenol dye measured at 550 nm *6163*

Quinidine *Serum No Effect Analytical* No significant interference observed at a concentration of 100 µg/mL (605 µmol/L) with method on Du Pont aca *1543*

Theophylline *Serum No Effect Analytical* At concentration of 40 mg/L produced no interference with methods used on Kodak DT-60, Abbott TDx, Abbott Vision with either whole blood or serum, 3M Diagnostics TheoFAST, Syntex AccµLevel or Ames Seralyzer *1122* No effect on Kodak Ektachem® 700 method *1716*

Vanillylmandelic Acid *Urine No Effect Physiological* No effect observed *1444*

Epicillin

Eosinophils *Blood Increase Physiological* Marked increase up to 18% in some cases *120*

Epoetin Alfa

Bleeding Time *Patient Decrease Physiological* Prolonged bleeding time characteristic of chronic renal failure decreases towards normal after correction of anemia *146*

Creatinine *Serum Increase Physiological* During clinical trials in patients on dialysis modest increases in concentration observed *146*

Hematocrit *Blood Increase Physiological* Increased hematocrit reflects successful treatment *146* In chronic renal failure patients treatment with starting dose of 50 U/kg caused increase of 0.11%/d and 1.5%/2 wk, with 100 U/kg 0.18%/d and 2.5%/2 wk and with 150 U/kg increase of 0.25%/d and 3.5%/2 wk. Similar increases in patients with cancer undergoing chemotherapy *4445*

Leukocytes *Blood Increase Physiological* During clinical trials modest statistically significant increases in counts observed *146*

Blood No Effect Physiological Treatment with erythropoietin had no effect on concentration *4445* Typically no change in concentration observed with treatment *146*

Phosphate *Serum Increase Physiological* During clinical trials in patients on dialysis modest increases in concentration observed, also in some patients with chronic renal failure not on dialysis *146*

Platelets *Blood Increase Physiological* During clinical trials modest statistically significant increases in counts observed *146*

Blood No Effect Physiological Typically no change in concentration observed with treatment *146* Treatment with erythropoietin had no effect on concentration *4445*

Potassium *Serum Increase Physiological* During clinical trials in patients on dialysis modest increases in concentration observed *146*

Urea Nitrogen *Serum Increase Physiological* During clinical trials in patients on dialysis modest increases in concentration observed *146*

Uric Acid *Serum Increase Physiological* During clinical trials in some patients with chronic renal failure not on dialysis modest statistically significant increases in concentration observed *146*

Epoprostenol

Platelets *Blood Decrease Physiological* Thrombocytopenia reported in patients participating in uncontrolled clinical trials *2156*

Potassium *Serum Decrease Physiological* Hypokalemia observed in 6 of 52 patients compared with 4% in patients receiving standard treatment *2156*

Epostane

β-Chorionic Gonadotropin *Plasma Decrease Physiological* In women who aborted following ingestion of 800 mg daily for 7 days decreased from baseline of 73 kIU/L to 18 kIU/L at 7 days and 9 kIU/L at day 14 *1172*

Cortisol *Plasma Increase Physiological* In pregnant women taking 800 mg/day for 7 days in those who did not abort concentration increased to mean of 412 nmol/L on day 7 from baseline of 268 nmol/L whereas no significant change observed in those who did abort *1172*

Estradiol *Plasma Decrease Physiological* Mean area under curve in 10 women with normal ovulatory cycles but with endometriosis receiving 600 mg/day was lower than during control cycles *4854* In 4 pregnant women who aborted following ingestion of 800 mg/day for 7 days concentration of estradiol-17β decreased from baseline value at 0 day of 959 pmol/L to 222 pmol/L at day 14 *1172*

Plasma Increase Physiological Mean area under curve in 10 women with regular menstrual cycles receiving 150 mg/day somewhat higher than during control cycles despite apparently lower preovulatory estradiol surges. During medication highest estradiol occurred during luteal phase *4854*

17-Hydroxyprogesterone *Plasma Decrease Physiological* Mean area under curve of 17α-hydroxyprogesterone concentration markedly reduced in 10 women with regular ovulatory cycles but with endometriosis who received 600 mg/day compared with individuals receiving smaller doses and against control cycles *4854* Mean area under curve in 10 women with normal ovulatory cycles receiving 150 mg/day reduced during luteal surge in 17α-hydroxyprogesterone concentration by approximately 45% *4854* In pregnant women receiving 800 mg/day for 7 days reduction of17α-hydroxyprogesterone concentration from baseline of 13-18 nmol/L to 4 nmol/L at day 14 in those who aborted but no change (13 nmol/L at day 14) in those who did not, although concentration declined in both groups from day 0 to 14 *1172*

Progesterone *Plasma Decrease Physiological* In pregnant women who aborted following 800 mg/day for 7 days mean decrease from 76 nmol/L to 16 nmol/L by day 7 and 10 nmol/L by day 14. In those who did not abort progesterone decreased slightly to 52 nmol/L at day 7 and rose to 81 nmol/L at day 14 *1172* Mean area under curve in 10 women with normal ovulatory cycles receiving 150 mg/day reduced during luteal surge by approximately 45% *4854*

Eptastatin

Apolipoprotein A-I *Serum Increase Physiological* Effect noted in type IIb but not type IIa hypercholesterolemics when treated for 3 months with 10 or 20 mg/day *6608*

Apolipoprotein A-II *Serum Increase Physiological* Effect noted in type IIb but not type IIa hypercholesterolemics when treated for 3 months with 10 or 20 mg/day *6608*

Apolipoprotein B *Serum Decrease Physiological* Treatment with 10 or 20 mg daily for 3 months caused reduction in concentration in 47 individuals with hypercholesterolemia *6608*

Apolipoprotein C-II *Serum Decrease Physiological* Effect noted in type IIb hypercholesterolemics but not type IIa individuals when treated for 3 months with 10 or 20 mg daily *6608*

Cholesterol *Serum Decrease Physiological* Concentration reduced with 10 or 20 mg daily for 3 months in 47 patients with hypercholesterolemia *6608*

HDL-Cholesterol *Serum Increase Physiological* Effect noted in type IIb but not type IIa hypercholesterolemics when treated for 3 months with 10 or 20 mg/day *6608*

LDL-Cholesterol *Serum Decrease Physiological* Treatment for 3 months with 10 or 20 mg/day caused reduction in concentration in 47 individuals with hypercholesterolemia *6608*

LDL-Phospholipids *Serum Decrease Physiological* Treatment with 10 or 20 mg daily for 3 months caused reduction in concentration in 47 individuals with hypercholesterolemia *6608*

LDL-Triglycerides *Serum Decrease Physiological* In 47 patients with hypercholesterolemia treatment for 3 months with 10 or 20 mg/day caused reduction in concentration *6608*

Phospholipids *Serum Decrease Physiological* 10 or 20 mg given daily for 3 months to 47 patients with hypercholesterolemia caused significant reduction in concentration *6608*

Triglycerides *Serum Decrease Physiological* Effect noted only in patients with type IIb hypercholesterolemia, not with type IIa, when treated for 3 months with 10 or 20 mg/day *6608*

VLDL-Triglycerides *Serum Decrease Physiological* Effect noted in type IIb but not type IIa hypercholesterolemics when treated for 3 months with 10 or 20 mg/day *6608*

Ergocalciferol

Calcium *Serum Increase Physiological* Slight but significant increase in 20 normal subjects given vitamin D_2 alone or with 1,25-dihydroxyvitamin D_3*2765* Enhances absorption from gastrointestinal tract *1009*

Urine Increase Physiological As result of increased absorption *1009*

Cholecalciferol *Serum No Effect Physiological* Daily administration of 400 IU for 1 week to 8 healthy individuals caused insignificant change in concentration *3847*

1,25-Dihydroxy Vitamin D_2 *Serum Increase Physiological* Minimal increase observed after single dose of 4000 IU over that obtained over baseline which was very small after daily doses of 400 IU for 1 week *3847*

24,25-Dihydroxy Vitamin D_2 *Serum* *No Effect* *Physiological* No compound detected in serum of 8 healthy volunteers given 400 IU daily for 1 week. A single dose of 4000 IU caused only slightly higher concentration *3847*

Ergocalciferol *Serum* *No Effect* *Physiological* No compound detected in serum of 8 healthy volunteers given 400 IU daily for 1 week. A single oral dose of 4000 IU caused only slightly higher concentration than when repeated doses given *3847*

25-Hydroxy Vitamin D_2 *Serum* *Increase* *Physiological* Rose in 20 normal subjects regardless of whether they also received 1,25-dihydroxyvitamin D_3*2765* Daily administration of 400 IU to 8 healthy volunteers caused slight increase in concentration *3847*

Parathyroid Hormone *Plasma* *No Effect* *Physiological* No significant effect in 20 normal subjects when given alone or with 1,25-dihydroxyvitamin D_3*2765*

Phosphate *Serum* *Increase* *Physiological* Better absorption and utilization *1009*
Serum *No Effect* *Physiological* No significant effect when given alone but fell between 5th and 8th day when 1,25-dihydroxyvitamin D_3 also given *2765*

Ergoloid Mesylate

Creatinine *Serum* *No Effect* *Analytical* At 10 mg/L on reversed phase liquid chromatographic procedure of Zhiri et al *6656*

Homovanillic Acid
Cerebrospinal Fluid *Decrease* *Physiological* In 10 of 12 patients with Alzheimer's dementia treatment for two weeks caused decrease in concentration *5428*

4-Hydroxy-3-Methoxy-Phenylglycol
Cerebrospinal Fluid *No Effect* *Physiological* In none of 12 patients with Alzheimer's dementia was a significant change observed over two weeks *5428*

5-Hydroxyindoleacetic Acid
Cerebrospinal Fluid *No Effect* *Physiological* In none of 12 patients with Alzheimer's dementia treated for two weeks no significant change observed *5428*

Uric Acid *Serum* *No Effect* *Analytical* At 10 mg/L on reversed phase liquid chromatographic procedure of Zhiri et al *6656*

Ergot Preparations

δ-Aminolevulinic Acid *Urine* *Increase* *Physiological* May precipitate attack of acute porphyria *1687*

Occult Blood *Feces* *Increase* *Physiological* May cause gastrointestinal bleeding with overdose *467*

Porphyrin, Total *Urine* *Increase* *Physiological* May precipitate attack of acute porphyria *1687*

Protein *Urine* *Increase* *Physiological* May cause renal damage with poisoning *467*

Urea Nitrogen *Serum* *Increase* *Physiological* May cause renal damage with poisoning *467*

Ergotamine

Histamine *Plasma* *No Effect* *Analytical* Improbable inhibition of radio-enzyme assay at therapeutic concentrations *2492*

Erythromycin

Alanine Aminotransferase *Serum* *Increase* *Physiological* Estolate produces mild hepatotoxicity in about 15% treated individuals. Jaundice in 2% patients on drug for more than 2 weeks *4627* Observed to some extent in some patients with different erythromycin salts: usually cholestatic hepatitis *3088* May cause hepatic toxicity *1874*
Serum *No Effect* *Analytical* No effect at 100 mg/L on method on Ames Seralyzer *5706*

Albumin *Urine* *No Effect* *Analytical* At concentration of 200 mg/dL had no significant effect on Boehringer Mannheim Tina-quant method *2799*

Alfentanil *Serum* *Increase* *Physiological* Concomitant administration of erythromycin with alfentanil significantly inhibits its clearance, thereby increasing its plasma concentration *2899*

Alkaline Phosphatase *Serum* *Increase* *Physiological* May cause intrahepatic cholestasis (reversible) *1874* Moderate increase with hepatitis mixed in type with both cholestasis and mild necrosis. Ethylsuccinate and propionate derivatives produce similar jaundice *4627* Observed to some extent in some patients with different erythromycin salts: usually cholestatic hepatitis *3088*

Amikacin *Serum* *No Effect* *Analytical* No interference observed at a concentration of 500 μg/mL (661 μmol/L) with method on Du Pont aca *1508*

Amino Acids *Urine* *Increase* *Analytical* Yellow spot with ninhydrin on thin-layer chromatography *2109*

Aspartate Aminotransferase *Serum* *Increase* *Analytical* Colorimetric assay if DNPH or diazonium salt used *5869*
Serum *Increase* *Physiological* Estolate produces mild hepatotoxicity in about 15% treated individuals. Jaundice in 2% patients on drug for more than 2 weeks *4627* Observed to some extent in some patients with different erythromycin salts: usually cholestatic hepatitis *3088* Causes hepatic toxicity in some cases *1874*

Astemizole *Serum* *Increase* *Physiological* Coadministration of erythromycin with astemizole caused significant increase in terfenadine concentration due to inhibition of cytochrome P450IIIA4 in the liver *729* Concomitant administration of erythromycin with astemizole causes increased astemizole concentration because erythromycin inhibits cytochrome P450 which metabolizes astemizole *2901* Significantly decreased metabolism resulting in cardiac toxicity or arhythmias, especially torsade des pointes *886*

Atorvastatin *Serum* *Increase* *Physiological* When erythromycin was coadministered with atorvastatin the latter's plasma concentration was increased by about 40% due to inhibition of cytochrome P450 *20* Erythromycin coadministration with atorvastatin to healthy individuals caused approximately 40% increase in plasma atorvastatin concentration due to inhibition of cytochrome P450 3A4 *4534*

Azelastine *Serum* *No Effect* *Physiological* Coadministration of erythromycin (500 mg t.i.d. for 7 days) with azelastine had no effect on the pharmacokinetics of azelastine *6320*

Bile *Urine* *Increase* *Physiological* Intrahepatic cholestatic jaundice *139*

Bilirubin *Serum* *Increase* *Physiological* Causes cholestasis in approximately 15% patients *1874* Observed to some extent in some patients with different erythromycin salts: usually cholestatic hepatitis *3088* Estolate produces mild hepatotoxicity in about 15% treated individuals. Jaundice in 2% patients on drug for more than 2 weeks *4627*
Serum *No Effect* *Analytical* At concentration of 73 mg/L had no effect on Jendrassik and Grof method *5704*

Bilirubin, Direct *Serum* *Increase* *Physiological* Reported effect *3810*

BSP Retention *Serum* *Increase* *Physiological* Intrahepatic cholestatic jaundice *139*

Calcium *Serum* *No Effect* *Analytical* At concentration of 73 mg/L had no effect on cresolphthalein method *5704*

Cannabinoids *Urine* *No Effect* *Analytical* No effect on Roche Abuscreen method *5006*

Carbamazepine *Serum* *Increase* *Physiological* Due to effect on hepatic metabolism *1384* Carbamazepine half-life significantly increased as well as 24 hour postdose concentration with decrease of oral clearance following addition of erythromycin to regime of daily carbamazepine in healthy volunteers *4035* Interferes with liver microsomal metabolism of drug *2529* Concomitant administration with carbamazepine causes marked increase of plasma carbamazepine concentration resulting in toxicity in some cases *282* Drugs that inhibit CYP 3A4 inhibit metabolism of carbamazepine producing clinically meaningful effect *1039* Clearance reduced from 0.36 to 0.29 L/kg/d with 1 g/d for 5 d, probably due to effect on metabolism *6535* Metabolism of carbamazepine inhibited, possibly by forming complexes with cytochrome P-450 *3118* Significantly decreased metabolism and increased plasma concentration *886*

Erythromycin *(continued)*

Cerivastatin *Serum* *Increase* *Physiological* Plasma concentration and AUC of cerivastatin increased by approximately 50% and 24% respectively after coadministration of erythromycin for 10 days *300*

Cetirizine *Serum* *No Effect* *Physiological* No clinically significant effect observed *4661*

Chloramphenicol *Serum* *No Effect* *Analytical* No effect at 100 mg/L on coupled enzymatic method *4122*

Cholesterol *Serum* *Decrease* *Physiological* Hepatotoxic effect *3669*

Cholinesterase *Serum* *No Effect* *Analytical* No effect observed at concentration of 20 mg/dL with butyrylthiocholine method on Kodak Ektachem® *2504*

Cisapride *Serum* *Increase* *Physiological* By inhibiting cytochrome P450 3A4 inhibits metabolism of cisapride and increases its plasma concentration *2903* Coadministration of erythromycin with cisapride caused significant increase in terfenadine concentration due to inhibition of cytochrome P450IIIA4 in the liver *729*

Clindamycin *Serum* *Positive* *Analytical* Interferes with bioassays *3858*

Colistin *Serum* *Positive* *Analytical* Interferes with bioassays *3858*

Cyclosporine *Blood* *Increase* *Physiological* Coadministration of daily doses as low as 500 mg have been associated with a five-fold increase in cyclosporine trough concentration probably due to enhanced cyclosporine absorption (but mechanism unclear) and impaired metabolism of cyclosporine *859* With coadministration of drugs absorption of oral cyclosporine increased from 36 ± 12% to 60 ± 20% but mechanism unclear *859*

Blood *No Effect* *Analytical* At a concentration of 200 mg/L had no effect on Syva EMIT method *495*

Serum *Increase* *Physiological* Concentration increased when cyclosporine coadministered with erythromycin probably due to induction of 1 or more P-450 enzymes that convert erythromycin to a nitrosalkane metabolite that then binds and inhibits subsequent metabolism by the enzyme. Effect observed in many renal transplant patients becoming apparent 2-14 days after erythromycin started *6595* Because of competition for protein binding sites in serum *6498* One case reported in which marked increase in serum concentration occurred after administration of erythromycin possibly due to inhibition of hepatic clearance *4805* Coadministration of daily doses as low as 500 mg have been associated with a five-fold increase in cyclosporine trough concentration probably due to enhanced cyclosporine absorption (but mechanism unclear) and impaired metabolism of cyclosporine *859* Peak concentration increased from about 0.9 µg/mL to about 2.5 µg/mL in six patients following coadministration. Area under curve also increased. Concentration of metabolite 17 increased. No changes after i.v. cyclosporine suggesting increased absorption *2373* With coadministration of drugs absorption of oral cyclosporine increased from 36 ± 12% to 60 ± 20% but mechanism unclear *859* May increase cyclosporine concentration by inhibiting hepatic cytochrome P-450 III A which metabolizes cyclosporine *5236*

Cyclosporine A *Blood* *Increase* *Physiological* Coadministration with cyclosporine A increases its concentration *5240*

Digoxin *Serum* *Increase* *Physiological* Two fold increase noted in some individuals when antibiotic given orally. In 10% patients but bacteria convert digoxin to cardioinactive reduced metabolites *3589* Coadministration with digoxin may increase the digoxin concentration *2161* Concomitant administration of erythromycin with digoxin may increase its plasma concentration *20*

Dihydroergotamine *Serum* *Increase* *Physiological* Concomitant administration of erythromycin with dihydroergotamine may increase its plasma concentration and cause acute ergot toxicity *20*

Disopyramide *Serum* *Increase* *Physiological* In two patients plasma concentration increased when erythromycin added to therapeutic regime *1384*

Doxazosin *Serum* *No Effect* *Physiological* Coadministration with doxazosin had no effect on its pharmacokinetics *4642*

Drugs of Abuse Screen *Urine* *No Effect* *Analytical* No effect at concentration of 100 µg/mL on EZ-SCREEN procedure for cannabinoids and cocaine *1739*

Eosinophils *Blood* *Increase* *Physiological* Associated with hypersensitivity reaction *3828* Hypersensitivity reaction in 45% individuals *4627*

Ergotamine *Serum* *Increase* *Physiological* Concomitant administration of erythromycin with ergotamine may increase its plasma concentration and cause acute ergot toxicity *20*

Felbamate *Serum* *No Effect* *Physiological* Coadministration of 1000 mg/d erythromycin for 10 days did not alter the concentration, AUC or t_{max} of felbamate when either 3000 or 3600 mg/d was given to 10 healthy volunteers *6324*

Fexofenadine *Serum* *Increase* *Physiological* Coadministration of erythromycin 500 mg every 8 hours (twice normal dose) with 7 days of fexofenadine 120 mg every 12 hours (twice recommended dose) caused an 82% increase in concentration and 109% increase in area under time-concentration curve *2637*

Folate *Serum* *Decrease* *Analytical* Inhibits growth of *L. casei5870*

Gentamicin *Serum* *No Effect* *Analytical* No interference observed at concentrations up to 500 µg/mL (680 µmol/L) with method on Du Pont aca *1526*

Glucose *Serum* *Decrease* *Physiological* Hepatotoxic effect *3669*

Histamine *Plasma* *No Effect* *Analytical* Improbable inhibition of radio-enzyme assay by estolate salt at therapeutic concentrations *2492*

17-Hydroxycorticosteroids *Urine* *Increase* *Analytical* Reported interference with measuring procedure *2451*

^{131}I Uptake *Serum* *Decrease* *Physiological* Tetraiodofluorescein is included in pedimycin *4360*

Indomethacin *Serum* *No Effect* *Analytical* No effect on HPLC method of Roberts and Smith *4978*

17-Ketosteroids *Urine* *Increase* *Analytical* Interference with measuring procedure *2451*

Leukocytes *Blood* *Decrease* *Physiological* Leukopenia or neutropenia may occur *3828*

Blood *Increase* *Physiological* Leukocytosis observed *3828*

Loratadine *Serum* *Increase* *Physiological* With coadministration increased plasma concentrations (24 hour AUC) of loratidine (40%) and descarboethoxyloratidine (46%) observed in normal volunteers but without clinical effects *5327*

Methylprednisolone *Serum* *Increase* *Physiological* Hepatic drug metabolism inhibited by erythromycin *1384*

Metronidazole *Serum* *Increase* *Analytical* Interferes with bioassays *3858*

Midazolam *Serum* *Increase* *Physiological* By inhibiting cytochrome P450 3A4 may reduce plasma clearance of midazolam when drugs coadministered. After 500 mg erythromycin t.i.d. for 1 week in 6 individuals the half-life of midazolam approximately doubled *5037*

N-Acetyl-Glucosaminidase *Urine* *No Effect* *Analytical* At concentration of 200 mg/dL no significant effect observed on Boehringer Mannheim CPR method *3174*

Nadolol *Serum* *Increase* *Physiological* Administration of erythromycin together with neomycin orally caused doubling (from 146 to 397 ng/mL) of nadolol concentration following a single oral dose. Effect probably related to increased bioavailability *1601*

Phenylalanine *Plasma* *No Effect* *Analytical* No interference observed with rapid quantitative whole blood method of Campbell et al using phenylalanine dehydrogenase *867*

Phosphate *Serum* *No Effect* *Analytical* At concentration of 73 mg/L had no effect on phosphomolybdate method *5704*

Platelets *Blood* *Decrease* *Physiological* Thrombocytopenia reported to occur *2754*

Polymyxin *Serum* *Increase* *Analytical* Interferes with bioassays *3858*

Potassium *Serum* *No Effect* *Analytical* At concentration of 10 mg/L had no effect on measurement by ISE with predilution *5704*

Protein *Cerebrospinal Fluid* *No Effect* *Analytical* No effect on Folin-Ciocalteu procedure *6681*

Serum *No Effect* *Analytical* At concentration of 73 mg/L had no effect on biuret method with blank correction *5704*

Prothrombin Time *Plasma* *Increase* *Physiological* Increase by 40% in a patient within 3 d of adding drug to a regime stabilized with warfarin: possible effect on metabolism *2795* Convincing interaction with warfarin when drugs coadministered but mechanism unknown *2625* Increased INR observed in patients receiving warfarin *886* Associated with impaired availability of bile salts *3669*

Rifabutin *Serum* *Increase* *Physiological* Decreased metabolism and increased risk of uveitis *886*

Sibutramine *Serum* *Increase* *Physiological* Concomitant administration of 500 mg erythromycin t.d.s. with 20 mg sibutramine 50 mg/d for 7 days to 12 obese but otherwise healthy individuals caused increases of AUCs of metabolites M_1 and M_2 of less than 14% and a dcrease of the concentration of M_1 of 11% but increase in concentration of M_2 of 10% *3203*

Sildenafil *Serum* *Increase* *Physiological* Following treatment with erythromycin (1000 mg for 5 days) area under concentration curve of sildenafil increased by 182% due to CYP3A4 inhibition *4657*

Sodium *Serum* *No Effect* *Analytical* At concentration of 10 mg/L had no effect on measurement by ISE with predilution *5704*

Tacrolimus *Blood* *No Effect* *Analytical* No significant effect observed at a concentration of 5 mg/L with MEIA method on Abbott IMx analyzer *1871*

Serum *Increase* *Physiological* By inhibiting cytochrome P-450 IIIA enzyme systems may inhibit the metabolism of tacrolimus *1987*

Serum *No Effect* *Analytical* In HPLC/MS method of Christians et al no significant interference observed with measurement of FK 506 *1010*

Terfenadine *Serum* *Increase* *Physiological* Significantly decreased metabolism resulting in cardiac toxicity or arrhythmias, especially torsade des pointes *886* Coadministration of erythromycin with terfenadine caused significant increase in terfenadine concentration due to inhibition of cytochrome P450IIIA4 in the liver *729* Decreases the clearance of terfenadine but effect on plasma concentration uncertain *2653*

Tetracycline *Serum* *Increase* *Analytical* Interferes with bioassays *3858*

Theophylline *Serum* *Increase* *Physiological* 40% increase in concentration due to 26% reduction in clearance after 1 week therapy *3363* Clearance reduced after several days treatment due to inhibition of metabolism *4546* Clearance significantly reduced. Plasma concentration increased by 28% in 12 patients *4913* Decreased metabolism *886* Up to 35% increase in serum theophylline concentration due to decreased theophylline clearance caused by inhibition of cytochrome P450 3A3 by an erythromycin metabolite *6117* Has steroid sparing action and also prolongs theophylline half-life by reducing its clearance *1384* In patients receiving high doses of theophylline may further increase its concentration *20* Erythromycin metabolite decreases theophylline clearance by inhibiting cytochrome P450 3A3 and increases serum theophylline concentration by 35% *3125* Metabolite decreases theophylline clearance by inhibiting cytochrome P450 3A3, increasing theophylline concentration by about 35% *5999*

Tobramycin *Serum* *No Effect* *Analytical* At concentrations less than 1000 µg/mL (1.36 mmol/L) no significant effect observed on method on Du Pont aca *1547*

Triazolam *Serum* *Decrease* *Physiological* Coadministration may approximately double elimination half-life and plasma concentration of triazolam *4677*

Serum *Increase* *Physiological* In normal volunteers reduced clearance and increased plasma concentration *1384* Concomitant administration of erythromycin with triazolam may increase its plasma concentration by reducing its plasma clearance *20*

Tricyclic Antidepressants *Serum* *No Effect* *Physiological* Concomitant administration appeared to have no effect on either hepatic or gastrointestinal tract metabolism *149*

Trimethoprim *Serum* *Increase* *Analytical* Interferes with bioassays *3858*

Urea Nitrogen *Serum* *No Effect* *Analytical* At concentration of 73 mg/L had no effect on diacetylmonoxime method *5704*

Uric Acid *Serum* *No Effect* *Analytical* At concentration of 73 mg/L had no effect on phosphotungstate reduction method *5704*

Urobilinogen *Feces* *Decrease* *Physiological* May cause cholestasis (reversible) *2803*

Urine *Decrease* *Physiological* May occur with cholestasis *2803*

Valproic Acid *Serum* *Increase* *Physiological* Causes increase in concentration when drugs coadministered *6350*

Warfarin *Plasma* *Increase* *Physiological* Clearance decreased by 14% in 12 individuals given 1 g/d for 8 d *315*

Zafirlukast *Serum* *Decrease* *Physiological* In 11 asthmatic patients coadministration of a single dose of zafirlukast (40 mg) with erythromycin (1500 mg/d) for 5 days to steady state caused a significant decrease of 40% in the mean plasma concentration of zafirlukast due to a decrease in its bioavailability *6641*

Erythromycin Acistrate

Alanine Aminotransferase *Serum* *Increase* *Physiological* In 1549 patients treated for 7-10 days moderate increase observed in 9.9% with clear increase observed in 0.6% *3507*

Serum *No Effect* *Physiological* In 1549 patients treated for 7-10 days moderate increase observed in 9.9%, clearly increased in 0.6%, and normalized in 3.5% *3507*

Alkaline Phosphatase *Serum* *No Effect* *Physiological* In 1549 patients treated for 7-10 days moderate increase observed in 1.0%, with normalization in 1.3% *3507*

Aspartate Aminotransferase

Serum *No Effect* *Physiological* In 1549 patients treated for 7-10 days moderate increase observed in 2.4%, clear increase observed in 0.3% and decrease observed in 2.0% *3507*

γ-Glutamyltransferase *Serum* *Increase* *Physiological* In 1549 patients treated for 7-10 days moderate increase observed in 3.5%, clear increase in 0.3%, and decreased to normal in 3.3% *3507*

Erythropoietin

Alanine *Plasma* *No Effect* *Physiological* Treatment with 150 - 250 U/kg/wk in 10 patients with chronic renal failure undergoing regular hemodialysis caused nonsignificant change from mean baseline of 278 ± 24 µmol/L to 270 ± 21 µmol/L after 3 months, 268 ± 23 µmol/L after 6 months, 274 ± 29 µmol/L after 9 months and 284 ± 35 µmol/L after 12 months *2034*

Albumin *Serum* *No Effect* *Physiological* Treatment with recombinant erythropoietin for 6 months caused In 11 patients on chronic hemodialysis in whom hematocrit increased by more than 5% a nonsignificant change in concentration from mean baseline of 4.4 ± 0.2 g/dL to 4.5 ± 0.1 g/dL and in 11 in whom hematocrit increased by less than 5% changed nonsignificantly from 4.2 ± 0.1 g/dL to 4.3 ± 0.1 g/dL *6051*

Aluminum *Serum* *No Effect* *Physiological* Treatment with recombinant erythropoietin for 6 months caused In 11 patients on chronic hemodialysis in whom hematocrit increased by more than 5% no significant change in concentration from mean baseline of 34.9 ± 4.3 µg/L and in 11 in whom hematocrit increased by less than 5% a nonsignificant change from 26.1 ± 4.2 µg/L *6051*

Aminolevulinic Acid Dehydrase

Serum *Increase* *Physiological* Greater than 3-fold increase observed in 17 chronic uremic patients treated with erythropoietin for 3 weeks (change from mean of 4.8 U/mL to 15.5 U/mL) *3273*

Antithrombin III *Plasma* *No Effect* *Physiological* In 20 patients receiving chronic hemodialysis administration of recombinant human erythropoietin 40 IU/kg body weight 3 times weekly intravenously after each dialysis mean time changed insignificantly from baseline of 93 ± 20% to 95 ± 21% after 4 weeks, 90 ± 14% after 8 weeks and 96 ± 19% after 12 weeks *3852*

Erythropoietin *(continued)*

Arginine *Plasma No Effect Physiological* Treatment with 150 - 250 U/kg/wk in 10 patients with chronic renal failure undergoing regular hemodialysis caused nonsignificant change from mean baseline of 73 ± 7 µmol/L to 64 ± 5 µmol/L after 3 months, 63 ± 5 µmol/L after 6 months, 62 ± 5 µmol/L after 9 months and 66 ± 6 µmol/L after 12 months *2034*

Aspartic Acid *Plasma No Effect Physiological* Treatment with 150 - 250 U/kg/wk in 10 patients with chronic renal failure undergoing regular hemodialysis caused nonsignificant change from mean baseline of 38 ± 3 µmol/L to 34 ± 3 µmol/L after 3 months, 43 ± 5 µmol/L after 6 months, 42 ± 5 µmol/L after 9 months and 40 ± 5 µmol/L after 12 months *2034*

Atrial Natriuretic Peptide *Plasma Decrease Physiological* Significant reduction observed in 15 patients undergoing long-term hemodialysis when given recombinant erythropoietin for 6 weeks *5288*

Bleeding Time *Patient .Decrease Physiological* In 20 patients receiving chronic hemodialysis administration of recombinant human erythropoietin 40 IU/kg body weight 3 times weekly intravenously after each dialysis mean time changed significantly from baseline of 21 ± 4.3 min to 14 ± 4.3 min after 4 weeks, 12 ± 6.4 min after 8 weeks and 10 ± 4.9 min after 12 weeks *3852*

Calcium *Serum Decrease Physiological* In 43 pateints receiving maintenance hemodialysis for 2-16 years when given intravenous erythropoietin following each session for one year mean predialysis serum concentration decreased from 2.45 mmol/L to 2.36 mmol/L *4148*

Citrulline *Plasma No Effect Physiological* Treatment with 150 - 250 U/kg/wk in 10 patients with chronic renal failure undergoing regular hemodialysis caused nonsignificant change from mean baseline of 85 ± 4 µmol/L to 87 ± 7 µmol/L after 3 months, 84 ± 8 µmol/L after 6 months, 85 ± 8 µmol/L after 9 months and 94 ± 9 µmol/L after 12 months *2034*

Corticotropin *Plasma Increase Physiological* In 7 patients with chronic end stage renal disease mean concentration significantly increased with initiation of treatment with erythropoietin *6363*

Creatinine *Serum Decrease Physiological* Treatment with recombinant erythropoietin for 6 months caused In 11 patients on chronic hemodialysis in whom hematocrit increased by less than 5% a nonsignificant decrease in concentration from mean baseline of 13.2 ± 1.3 mg/dL to 12.7 ± 1.0 mg/dL *6051*

Serum Increase Physiological During treatment with recombinant erythropoietin following each dialysis throughout one year pretreatment serum creatinine concentrations were increased *4148*

Serum No Effect Physiological Treatment with recombinant erythropoietin for 6 months caused In 11 patients on chronic hemodialysis in whom hematocrit increased by more than 5% a nonsignificant increase in concentration from mean baseline of 13.6 ± 0.7 mg/dL to 14.1 ± 0.9 mg/dL *6051*

Cysteine *Plasma No Effect Physiological* Treatment with 150 - 250 U/kg/wk in 10 patients with chronic renal failure undergoing regular hemodialysis caused nonsignificant change from mean baseline of 110 ± 12 µmol/L to 108 ± 12 µmol/L after 3 months, 102 ± 11 µmol/L after 6 months, 102 ± 12 µmol/L after 9 months and 90 ± 11 µmol/L after 12 months *2034*

Erythrocytes *Blood Increase Physiological* Increase observed in 85% of 13 patients with anemia associated with myeloma with median time to response of 5 weeks *3676* In 17 chronic uremic patients treated with erythropoietin for 3 weeks mean increase of 11.4% observed *3273*

Erythropoietin *Serum Increase Physiological* In 32 patients who gave 2 units of blood treatment with 500 U rhEPO/kg body weight twice weekly for 3 weeks caused significant increase at peak to about 40 U/L compared with about 11 U/L in 30 patients who gave two units but did not receive EPO *556*

Fibrinogen *Plasma No Effect Physiological* In 20 patients receiving chronic hemodialysis administration of recombinant human erythropoietin 40 IU/kg body weight 3 times weekly intravenously after each dialysis mean time changed insignificantly from baseline of 415 ± 120 mg/dL to 400 ± 119 mg/dL after 4 weeks, 411 ± 118 mg/dL after 8 weeks and 399 ± 115 mg/dL after 12 weeks *3852*

Follicle Stimulating Hormone

Plasma Increase Physiological In 7 patients with end stage renal disease already high FSH concentration further increased by erythropoietin administration *6363*

Glycine *Plasma No Effect Physiological* Treatment with 150 - 250 U/kg/wk in 10 patients with chronic renal failure undergoing regular hemodialysis caused nonsignificant change from mean baseline of 281 ± 14 µmol/L to 303 ± 14 µmol/L after 3 months, 305 ± 16 µmol/L after 6 months, 291 ± 18 µmol/L after 9 months and 288 ± 14 µmol/L after 12 months *2034*

Hematocrit *Blood Increase Physiological* In 43 patients on maintenance hemodialysis for 2 to 16 years treatment with recombinant erythropoietin intravenously following each dialysis for 1 year corrected anemia with effects becoming apparent in about 4 weeks *4148* Increase from to 20.0% to 33.0% observed in 15 patients undergoing long-term hemodialysis after 6 weeks of recombinant erythropoietin therapy *5288* In 20 patients receiving chronic hemodialysis administration of recombinant human erythropoietin 40 IU/kg body weight 3 times weekly intravenously after each dialysis mean concentration increased from baseline of 22.1 ± 1.8% to 24.8 ± 1.8% after 4 weeks, 26.3 ± 2.0% after 8 weeks and 26.7 ± 2.9% after 12 weeks *3852* Significant increase observed in 10 patients with hemoglobin less than 8 g/dL receiving CAPD when treated for 16 weeks *3713* Significant increase observed in 85% of 13 patients with anemia associated with myeloma with median time to response of 5 weeks *3676*

Hemoglobin *Blood Increase Physiological* Treatment with 150 - 250 U/kg/wk in 10 patients with chronic renal failure undergoing regular hemodialysis caused significant increase of blood hemoglobin from mean baseline of 7.0 ± 0.3 g/dL to 10.1 ± 0.3 g/dL after 3 months thereafter remaining steady *2034* In 32 patients who gave 2 units of blood treatment with 500 U rhEPO/kg body weight twice weekly for 3 weeks caused significant increase at peak to 13.7 ± 1.3 g/dL compared with 11.9 ± 1.3 g/dL in 30 patients who gave two units but did not receive EPO *556* In 10 severely anemic patients receiving chronic ambulatory peritoneal dialysis mean hemoglobin concentration increased from less than 8 g/dL to more than 10 g/dL within 16 weeks. In 5 individuals low or no response observed *3713* Increase of greater than 20 g/L observed in majority of patients (85%) with anemia associated with myeloma with median response time of 5 weeks *3676* In 6 children with end-stage renal disease and anemia receiving hemodialysis thrice weekly intravenous bolus doses of 100-150 U/kg of human recombinant erythropoietin thrice weekly produced response within 9-13 weeks *4962* In 17 chronic uremic patients treated with erythropoietin for 3 weeks mean increase of 10.3% observed *3273*

Plasma Increase Physiological In 20 patients receiving chronic hemodialysis administration of recombinant human erythropoietin 40 IU/kg body weight 3 times weekly intravenously after each dialysis mean concentration increased from baseline of 0.164 ± 0.053 mg/dL to 0.190 ± 0.071 mg/dL after 4 weeks, 0.210 ± 0.057 mg/dL after 8 weeks and 0.222 ± 0.086 mg/dL after 12 weeks *3852*

Histidine *Plasma No Effect Physiological* Treatment with 150 - 250 U/kg/wk in 10 patients with chronic renal failure undergoing regular hemodialysis caused nonsignificant change from mean baseline of 87 ± 3 µmol/L to 90 ± 3 µmol/L after 3 months, 87 ± 3 µmol/L after 6 months, 87 ± 3 µmol/L after 9 months and 94 ± 5 µmol/L after 12 months *2034*

Interleukin-1β *Serum No Effect Physiological* In 4 patients with myelodysplastic syndrome who responded to treatment with recombinant erythropietin mean concentration 30 ± 24.8 pg/mL not significantly different from 36.1 ± 21.7 pg/mL in 42 healthy controls *4193*

Isoleucine *Plasma No Effect Physiological* Treatment with 150 - 250 U/kg/wk in 10 patients with chronic renal failure undergoing regular hemodialysis caused nonsignificant change from mean baseline of 41 ± 2 µmol/L to 40 ± 2 µmol/L after 3 months, 41 ± 2 µmol/L after 6 months, 42 ± 2 µmol/L after 9 months and 39 ± 3 µmol/L after 12 months *2034*

Lactate Dehydrogenase *Serum No Effect Physiological* In 20 patients receiving chronic hemodialysis administration of recombinant human erythropoietin 40 IU/kg body weight 3 times weekly intravenously after each dialysis mean activity changed insignificantly from baseline of 130 ± 21 U/L to 134 ± 26 U/L after 4 weeks, 136 ± 27 U/L after 8 weeks and 136 ± 14 U/L after 12 weeks *3852*

Leucine *Plasma No Effect Physiological* Treatment with 150 - 250 U/kg/wk in 10 patients with chronic renal failure undergoing regular hemodialysis caused nonsignificant change from mean baseline of 76 ± 4 µmol/L to 71 ± 3 µmol/L after 3 months, 72 ± 3 µmol/L after 6 months, 74 ± 3 µmol/L after 9 months and 72 ± 4 µmol/L after 12 months *2034*

Leukocytes *Blood Increase Physiological* In 43 patients on maintenance hemodialysis for 2-16 years treatment with recombinant human erythropoietin intravenously following each dialysis caused mean increase from 5880/µL to 6600/µL *4148*

Blood No Effect Physiological No consistent pattern of change observed in patients with anemia of myeloma when treated with recombinant erythropoietin at same time as given chemotherapy *3676*

Lysine *Plasma No Effect Physiological* Treatment with 150 - 250 U/kg/wk in 10 patients with chronic renal failure undergoing regular hemodialysis caused nonsignificant change from mean baseline of 148 ± 10 µmol/L to 149 ± 11 µmol/L after 3 months, 153 ± 11 µmol/L after 6 months, 154 ± 9 µmol/L after 9 months and 151 ± 14 µmol/L after 12 months *2034*

MCV *Blood Decrease Physiological* In patients with chronic renal failure 2 months treatment with recombinant erythropoietin caused decrease from mean baseline of 88.0 86.9 fL, 4 to 5 months treatment from 89.3 to 86.1 fL and 7 to 8 months treatment from 89.2 to 88.8 fL *5391*

Blood Increase Physiological In 32 patients who gave 2 units of blood treatment with 500 U rhEPO/kg body weight twice weekly for 3 weeks caused significant increase from 91.8 ± 3.6 fL to 97.0 ± 6.0 fL at peak compared with change from 90.9 ± 5.2 fL to 92.2 ± 6.5 fL in 30 patients who gave two units but did not receive EPO *556*

Ornithine *Plasma No Effect Physiological* Treatment with 150 - 250 U/kg/wk in 10 patients with chronic renal failure undergoing regular hemodialysis caused nonsignificant change from mean baseline of 68 ± 4 µmol/L to 69 ± 5 µmol/L after 3 months, 71 ± 7 µmol/L after 6 months, 70 ± 8 µmol/L after 9 months and 70 ± 7 µmol/L after 12 months *2034*

Parathyroid Hormone *Plasma No Effect Physiological* Treatment with recombinant erythropoietin for 6 months caused In 11 patients on chronic hemodialysis in whom hematocrit increased by more than 5% no significant change in concentration from mean baseline of 1.71 ± 0.46 ng/mL and in 11 in whom hematocrit increased by less than 5% a nonsignificant change from 2.14 ± 0.39 ng/mL *6051*

Phenylalanine *Plasma No Effect Physiological* Treatment with 150 - 250 U/kg/wk in 10 patients with chronic renal failure undergoing regular hemodialysis caused nonsignificant change from mean baseline of 43 ± 1 µmol/L to 43 ± 3 µmol/L after 3 months, 43 ± 3 µmol/L after 6 months, 43 ± 3 µmol/L after 9 months and 43 ± 3 µmol/L after 12 months *2034*

Phosphate *Serum Increase Physiological* In 43 patients on maintenance hemodialysis for 2-16 years who received intravenous recombinant erythropoietin following each session over one year mean predialysis concentration increased *4148*

Platelets *Blood Increase Physiological* In 20 patients receiving chronic hemodialysis administration of recombinant human erythropoietin 40 IU/kg body weight 3 times weekly intravenously after each dialysis mean concentration increased from baseline of 210 ± 62 x 10^9/L to 246 ± 104 x 10^9/L after 4 weeks, 244 ± 76 x 10^9/L after 8 weeks and 258 ± 84 x 10^9/L after 12 weeks *3852*

Blood No Effect Physiological No consistent pattern observed in 13 patients with anemia associated with myeloma when treated with recombinant erythropoietin simultaneously with chemotherapy *3676*

Potassium *Serum Increase Physiological* In 43 patients on maintenance hemodialysis for 2-16 years treatment with recombinant erythropoietin intravenously following each session for one year caused increase in mean pretreatment serum concentration *4148*

Proline *Plasma No Effect Physiological* Treatment with 150 - 250 U/kg/wk in 10 patients with chronic renal failure undergoing regular hemodialysis caused nonsignificant change from mean baseline of 346 ± 49 µmol/L to 308 ± 32 µmol/L after 3 months, 304 ± 39 µmol/L after 6 months, 307 ± 41 µmol/L after 9 months and 312 ± 39 µmol/L after 12 months *2034*

Protein C *Plasma No Effect Physiological* In 20 patients receiving chronic hemodialysis administration of recombinant human erythropoietin 40 IU/kg body weight 3 times weekly intravenously after each dialysis mean time changed insignificantly from baseline of 90 ± 9% to 93 ± 8% after 4 weeks, 91 ± 12% after 8 weeks and 87 ± 11% after 12 weeks *3852*

Protein S *Plasma No Effect Physiological* In 20 patients receiving chronic hemodialysis administration of recombinant human erythropoietin 40 IU/kg body weight 3 times weekly intravenously after each dialysis mean time changed insignificantly from baseline of 92 ± 13% to 90 ± 15% after 4 weeks, 94 ± 12% after 8 weeks and 93 ± 8% after 12 weeks *3852*

Prothrombin Time *Plasma No Effect Physiological* In 20 patients receiving chronic hemodialysis administration of recombinant human erythropoietin 40 IU/kg body weight 3 times weekly intravenously after each dialysis mean time changed insignificantly from baseline of 14.5 ± 1.3 s to 14.3 ± 1.1 s after 4 weeks, 14.0 ± 1.5 s after 8 weeks and 13.8 ± 0.8 s after 12 weeks *6406*

Protoporphyrin, Free

Red Blood Cells Increase Physiological In 32 patients who gave 2 units of blood treatment with 500 U rhEPO/kg body weight twice weekly for 3 weeks caused significant increase at peak to 520 µmol/L RBC compared with 305 µmol/L RBC in 30 patients who gave two units but did not receive EPO *556*

Red Cell Distribution Width *Blood Increase Physiological* In 32 patients who gave 2 units of blood treatment with 500 U rhEPO /kg body weight twice weekly for 3 weeks caused significant increase from 28.2 ± 1.8 fL to 36.5 ± 5.2 fL at peak compared with change from 27.8 ± 2.0 fL to 29.8 ± 2.7 fL in 30 patients who gave two units but did not receive EPO *556*

Reticulocytes *Blood Increase Physiological* In 6 children with end-stage renal failure with anemia receiving thrice weekly hemodialysis given intravenous bolus of 100-150 U/kg recombinat human erythropoietin thrice weekly with response from 9-13 weeks *4962* In 32 patients who gave 2 units of blood treatment with 500 U rhEPO/kg body weight twice weekly for 3 weeks caused significant increase at peak to 230 /µL compared with 110 /µL in 30 patients who gave two units but did not receive EPO *556* Significant increase above baseline observed in 85% of 13 patients with anemia associated with myeloma with median change of 370% and maximum individual increase up to 10-fold *3676*

Serine *Plasma No Effect Physiological* Treatment with 150 - 250 U/kg/wk in 10 patients with chronic renal failure undergoing regular hemodialysis caused nonsignificant change from mean baseline of 66 ± 2 µmol/L to 64 ± 2 µmol/L after 3 months, 70 ± 4 µmol/L after 6 months, 77 ± 5 µmol/L (significant increase) after 9 months and 75 ± 6 µmol/L after 12 months *2034*

Threonine *Plasma No Effect Physiological* Treatment with 150 - 250 U/kg/wk in 10 patients with chronic renal failure undergoing regular hemodialysis caused nonsignificant change from mean baseline of 86 ± 6 µmol/L to 89 ± 4 µmol/L after 3 months, 85 ± 7 µmol/L after 6 months, 87 ± 8 µmol/L after 9 months and 91 ± 8 µmol/L after 12 months *2034*

Thrombin Time *Blood No Effect Physiological* In patients on chronic hemodialysis administration for 16 weeks had no effect on thrombin time *2785*

Thyroid Stimulating Hormone

Serum No Effect Physiological Treatment with recombinant erythropoietin for 6 months caused in 11 patients on chronic hemodialysis in whom hematocrit increased by more than 5% a nonsignificant change in concentration from mean baseline of 3.6 ± 0.6 /µU/mL to 3.5 ± 0.6 /µU/mL and in 11 in whom hematocrit increased by less than 5% no change from 5.6 ± 0.9 /µU/mL to 5.6 ± 1.0 /µU/mL *6051*

Erythropoietin *(continued)*

Thyroxine Binding Globulin *Serum Increase Physiological* Treatment with recombinant erythropoietin for 6 months caused in 11 patients on chronic hemodialysis in whom hematocrit increased by more than 5% a nonsignificant increase in concentration from mean baseline of 18.7 ± 1.8 µg/mL to 21.2 ± 1.6 µg/mL and in 11 in whom hematocrit increased by less than 5% a nonsignificant change from 15.3 ± 1.4 µg/mL to 16.6 ± 1.5 µg/mL *6051*

Thyroxine (T4) *Serum Increase Physiological* Treatment with recombinant erythropoietin for 6 months caused in 11 patients on chronic hemodialysis in whom hematocrit increased by more than 5% a significant increase in concentration from mean baseline of 6.7 ± 0.5 µg/dL to 8.5 ± 0.6 µg/dL and in 11 in whom hematocrit increased by less than 5% a nonsignificant increase from 5.3 ± 0.5 µg/dL to 6.3 ± 0.5 µg/dL *6051*

Thyroxine (T4), Free *Serum Increase Physiological* Treatment with recombinant erythropoietin for 6 months caused in 11 patients on chronic hemodialysis in whom hematocrit increased by more than 5% a significant increase in concentration from mean baseline of 0.79 ± 0.07 ng/dL to 0.98 ± 0.08 ng/dL and in 11 in whom hematocrit increased by less than 5% a nonsignificant change from 0.67 ± 0.03 ng/dL to 0.71 ± 0.05 ng/dL *6051*

Transferrin Receptor *Serum Increase Physiological* In 32 patients who gave 2 units of blood treatment with 500 U rhEPO/kg body weight twice weekly for 3 weeks caused significant increase at peak to 16 µg/mL compared with 5 µg/mL in 30 patients who gave two units but did not receive EPO *556*

Tri-iodothyronine, Free (fT3)
Serum Decrease Physiological Treatment with recombinant erythropoietin for 6 months caused in 11 patients on chronic hemodialysis in whom hematocrit increased by less than 5% a nonsignificant decrease in concentration from mean baseline of 1.9 ± 0.1 to 1.7 ± 0.2 pg/mL *6051*
Serum Increase Physiological Treatment with recombinant erythropoietin for 6 months caused in 11 patients on chronic hemodialysis in whom hematocrit increased by more than 5% a significant increase in concentration from mean baseline of 1.7 ± 0.2 pg/mL to 2.4 ± 0.1 pg/mL *6051*

Tri-iodothyronine (T3) *Serum Increase Physiological* Treatment with recombinant erythropoietin for 6 months caused in 11 patients on chronic hemodialysis in whom hematocrit increased by more than 5% a nonsignificant increase in concentration from mean baseline of 77.0 ± 4.9 ng/dL to 96.5 ± 6.8 ng/dL and in 11 in whom hematocrit increased by less than 5% a nonsignificant change from 74.4 ± 4.2 ng/dL to 77.6 ± 5.3 ng/dL *6051*

Tumor Necrosis Factor-α *Serum No Effect Physiological* In 4 patients with myelodysplastic syndrome who responded to treatment with recombinant erythropoietin mean concentration 8.2 ± 9.6 pg/mL not significantly different from 4.2 ± 7.9 pg/mL in 42 healthy controls *4193*

Tyrosine *Plasma No Effect Physiological* Treatment with 150 - 250 U/kg/wk in 10 patients with chronic renal failure undergoing regular hemodialysis caused nonsignificant change from mean baseline of 39 ± 2 µmol/L to 39 ± 3 µmol/L after 3 months, 40 ± 3 µmol/L after 6 months, 42 ± 2 µmol/L after 9 months and 39 ± 3 µmol/L after 12 months *2034*

Urea Nitrogen *Serum No Effect Physiological* Treatment with recombinant erythropoietin for 6 months caused in 11 patients on chronic hemodialysis in whom hematocrit increased by more than 5% no significant change in concentration from mean baseline of 84.9 ± 3.6 mg/dL to 85.0 ± 3.4 mg/dL and in 11 in whom hematocrit increased by less than 5% a nonsignificant change from 82.3 ± 5.0 mg/dL to 82.8 ± 3.7 mg/dL *6051*

Valine *Plasma No Effect Physiological* Treatment with 150 - 250 U/kg/wk in 10 patients with chronic renal failure undergoing regular hemodialysis caused nonsignificant change from mean baseline of 137 ± 9 µmol/L to 133 ± 6 µmol/L after 3 months, 133 ± 6 µmol/L after 6 months, 135 ± 6 µmol/L after 9 months and 133 ± 7 µmol/L after 12 months *2034*

Viscosity *Blood Increase Physiological* Progressive increase observed in patients with renal anemia during first 4 months of treatment in association with rise in hemoglobin concentration *1393*

Volume *Blood No Effect Physiological* No change observed in 15 patients undergoing long-term hemodialysis following 6 weeks treatment with recombinant erythropoietin *5288*
Plasma Decrease Physiological Significant decrease observed in 10 patients undergoing CAPD with hemoglobin less than 8 g/dL treated with subcutaneous erythropoietin for 16 weeks *3713*

Erythrosine

Iodide *Serum Increase Physiological* Significant dose related increases in 30 men receiving 20 to 200 mg/d for 15 d *2031*
Urine Increase Physiological Significant effect of daily doses of 60 mg and higher in 30 men treated for 15 d *2031*

T3-Uptake *Serum No Effect Physiological* In 30 men receiving up to 200 mg daily for 15 d *2031*

Thyroid Stimulating Hormone
Serum Increase Physiological Significant increase from 1.7 to 2.2 µU/mL after 15 d on up to 200 mg/d in 30 men *2031*

Thyroxine (T4) *Serum No Effect Physiological* In 30 men receiving up to 200 mg daily for 15 d *2031*

Tri-iodothyronine, Reverse (rT3)
Serum No Effect Physiological In 30 men receiving up to 200 mg daily for 15 d *2031*

Tri-iodothyronine (T3) *Serum No Effect Physiological* In 30 men receiving up to 200 mg daily for 15 d *2031*

TSH response to TRH *Serum Increase Physiological* Increase from peak increment of 6.3 to 10.5 µU/mL after 15 d on 200 mg/d in 30 men but no significant effect at lower doses *2031*

Estazolam

Aspartate Aminotransferase *Serum Increase Physiological* Administration associated with rare increase in activity *27*

Erythrocytes *Urine Increase Physiological* Administration associated with rare hematuria *27*

Granulocytes *Blood Decrease Physiological* Administration associated with rare granulocytosis *27*

Leukocytes *Blood Decrease Physiological* Administration associated with rare leukopenia *27*

Esterified Estrogens

Alanine Aminotransferase *Serum Increase Physiological* Cholestatic jaundice observed in some treated patients *5650* May cause cholestatic jaundice *5684*

Alkaline Phosphatase *Serum Increase Physiological* Cholestatic jaundice observed in some treated patients *5650* May cause cholestatic jaundice *5684*

Aspartate Aminotransferase *Serum Increase Physiological* May cause cholestatic jaundice *5684* Cholestatic jaundice observed in some treated patients *5650*

Bilirubin *Serum Increase Physiological* Cholestatic jaundice observed in some treated patients *5650* May cause cholestatic jaundice *5684*

Cholesterol *Serum Decrease Physiological* In 406 postmenopausal women given 1000 mg/d calcium and 0.3, 0.625 or 1.25 mg/d esterified estrogens for 24 months caused change from baseline of -0.15 ± 0.08 mmol/L with 0.3 mg/d, 0.03 ± 0.09 with 0.625 mg/d and -0.35 ± 0.12 mmol/L after 24 months *2078*

γ-Glutamyltransferase *Serum Increase Physiological* Cholestatic jaundice observed in some treated patients *5650* May cause cholestatic jaundice *5684*

HDL-Cholesterol *Serum Increase Physiological* In 406 postmenopausal women given 1000 mg/d calcium and 0.3, 0.625 or 1.25 mg/d esterified estrogens for 24 months caused change from baseline of 0.07 ± 0.03 mmol/L with 0.3 mg/d, 0.14 ± 0.03 with 0.625 mg/d and 0.15 ± 0.04 mmol/L after 24 months *2078*

LDL-Cholesterol *Serum Decrease Physiological* In 406 postmenopausal women given 1000 mg/d calcium and 0.3, 0.625 or 1.25 mg/d esterified estrogens for 24 months caused change from baseline of -0.23 ± 0.08 mmol/L with 0.3 mg/d, -0.18 ± 0.08 with 0.625 mg/d and -0.63 ± 0.11 mmol/L after 24 months *2078*

Triglycerides *Serum Increase Physiological* In 406 postmenopausal women given 1000 mg/d calcium and 0.3, 0.625 or 1.25 mg/d esterified estrogens for 24 months caused change from baseline of 0.05 ± 0.06 mmol/L with 0.3 mg/d, 0.04 ± 0.06 with 0.625 mg/d and 0.29 ± 0.10 mmol/L after 24 months *2078*

17β-Estradiol

Alkaline Phosphatase *Serum Decrease Physiological* In post-menopausal women given different amounts of drug *1011*

β-Aminobutyric Acid *Plasma No Effect Physiological* In 22 healthy men aged over 65 years administration of 0.5 to 2.0 mg/d 17β-estradiol for 9 weeks caused insignificant change from mean baseline of 15.8 ± 3.6 mmol/L to 13.8 ± 2.5 mmol/L *2134*

Antithrombin III *Plasma No Effect Physiological* In 22 healthy men aged over 65 years administration of 0.5 to 2.0 mg/d 17β-estradiol for 9 weeks caused insignificant change from mean baseline of 96 ± 30% to 95 ± 33% *2134*

Apolipoprotein A-I *Serum Increase Physiological* In 20 postmenopausal women patients with type II diabetes mellitus treatment with 2 mg/d micronized 17β-estradiol for 6 weeks caused a 14% increase in concentration compared with that in placebo-treated contols *787* In 6 normolipidemic postmenopausal healthy women treatment with 2 mg/d micronized 17β-micronized estradiol for 6 weeks caused significant change from mean baseline of 1.46 ± 0.23 g/L to 1.59 ± 0.36 g/L *6419*
Serum No Effect Physiological In 22 healthy men aged over 65 years administration of 0.5 to 2.0 mg/d 17β-estradiol for 9 weeks caused insignificant increase from mean baseline of 157 ± 20 mg/dL to 158 ± 28 mg/dL *2134*

Apolipoprotein B *Serum Decrease Physiological* In 20 postmenopausal women patients with type II diabetes mellitus treatment with 2 mg/d micronized 17β-estradiol for 6 weeks caused a 11% decrease in concentration compared with that in placebo-treated contols *787* In 22 healthy men aged over 65 years administration of 0.5 to 2.0 mg/d 17β-estradiol for 9 weeks caused significant decrease from mean baseline of 103 ± 23 mg/dL to 94 ± 21 mg/dL *2134*
Serum No Effect Physiological In 6 normolipidemic postmenopausal healthy women treatment with 2 mg/d micronized 17β-micronized estradiol for 6 weeks caused nonsignificant change from mean baseline of 0.59 ± 0.14 g/L to 0.55 ± 0.14 g/L *6419*

Apolipoprotein Lp(a) *Serum No Effect Physiological* In 22 healthy men aged over 65 years administration of 0.5 to 2.0 mg/d 17β-estradiol for 9 weeks caused insignificant change from mean baseline of 6.5 ± 6.9 mg/dL to 6.6 ± 6.3 mg/dL *2134*

CA 19-9 *Serum Increase Physiological* Sensitivity of 67% (n = 6) *2563*

Cholesterol *Serum Decrease Physiological* In 20 postmenopausal women patients with type II diabetes mellitus treatment with 2 mg/d micronized 17β-estradiol for 6 weeks caused a 6% reduction in concentration compared with that in placebo-treated controls *787* Almost 10% reduction in 38 healthy postmenopausal women given 2-4 mg orally or 3 mg cutaneously over 6 mo *1783*
Serum No Effect Physiological In 22 healthy men aged over 65 years administration of 0.5 to 2.0 mg/d 17β-estradiol for 9 weeks caused insignificant decrease from mean baseline of 211 ± 34 mg/dL to 205 ± 33 mg/dL *2134* In 20 healthy postmenopausal women treatment with 17β-estradiol 0.1 mg/d or 17β-estradiol 0.1 mg/d with 2.5 mg/d oral medroxyprogesterone acetate for 1 month caused nonsignificant change in concentration from 235 ± 30 mg/dL to 220 ± 28 mg/dL *3218* In 6 normolipidemic postmenopausal healthy women treatment with 2 mg/d micronized 17β-micronized estradiol for 6 weeks caused nonsignificant change from mean baseline of 5.63 ± 0.83 mmol/L to 5.48 ± 0.39 mmol/L *6419*

Cholesterol:HDL-Cholesterol Ratio
Serum Decrease Physiological In 22 healthy men aged over 65 years administration of 0.5 to 2.0 mg/d 17β-estradiol for 9 weeks caused significant change from mean baseline of 4.61 ± 0.96 to 3.98 ± 0.93 *2134*

C-Peptide *Plasma No Effect Physiological* In 20 postmenopausal women patients with type II diabetes mellitus treatment with 2 mg/d micronized 17β-estradiol for 6 weeks caused no sgnificant change in concentration compared with that in placebo-treated contols *787*

Cystathionine *Plasma No Effect Physiological* In 22 healthy men aged over 65 years administration of 0.5 to 2.0 mg/d 17β-estradiol for 9 weeks caused insignificant change from mean baseline of 165 ± 56 nmol/L to 152 ± 39 nmol/L *2134*

Cysteine *Plasma No Effect Physiological* In 22 healthy men aged over 65 years administration of 0.5 to 2.0 mg/d 17β-estradiol for 9 weeks caused insignificant change from mean baseline of 355 ± 27 mmol/L to 335 ± 26 mmol/L *2134*

D-Dimer *Plasma No Effect Physiological* In 22 healthy men aged over 65 years administration of 0.5 to 2.0 mg/d 17β-estradiol for 9 weeks caused insignificant change from mean baseline of 15.4 ± 20.5 ng/mL to 17.4 ± 26.4 ng/mL *2134*

Digoxin *Serum No Effect Analytical* Cross reactivity of less than 10% observed with method on Baxter Stratus *5705*

Dimethylglycine *Plasma No Effect Physiological* In 22 healthy men aged over 65 years administration of 0.5 to 2.0 mg/d 17β-estradiol for 9 weeks caused insignificant change from mean baseline of 3.4 ± 0.8 mmol/L to 3.5 ± 0.7 mmol/L *2134*

Estradiol *Plasma Increase Physiological* In 6 normolipidemic postmenopausal healthy women treatment with 2 mg/d micronized 17β-micronized estradiol for 6 weeks caused significant change from mean baseline of 50 ± 31 pmol/L to 336 ± 124 pmol/L *6419*

17β-Estradiol *Plasma Increase Physiological* In 20 healthy postmenopausal women treatment with 17β-estradiol 0.1 mg/d or 17β-estradiol 0.1 mg/d with 2.5 mg/d oral medroxyprogesterone acetate for 1 month caused significant increase in concentration from 16 ± 8 pg/mL to 122 ± 50 pg/mL *3218*

Estrone *Plasma Increase Physiological* In 6 normolipidemic postmenopausal healthy women treatment with 2 mg/d micronized 17β-micronized estradiol for 6 weeks caused significant change from mean baseline of 123 ± 39 pmol/L to 1925 ± 667 pmol/L *6419*

Fatty Acids (FFA), Free *Serum No Effect Physiological* In 20 postmenopausal women patients with type II diabetes mellitus treatment with 2 mg/d micronized 17β-estradiol for 6 weeks caused no sgnificant change in concentration compared with that in placebo-treated contols *787*

Fibrinogen *Plasma Decrease Physiological* In 22 healthy men aged over 65 years administration of 0.5 to 2.0 mg/d 17β-estradiol for 9 weeks caused significant change from mean baseline of 297 ± 57 g/L to 260 ± 35 g/L *2134*

Follicle Stimulating Hormone
Plasma Decrease Physiological In 6 normolipidemic postmenopausal healthy women treatment with 2 mg/d micronized 17β-micronized estradiol for 6 weeks caused significant change from mean baseline of 89 ± 36 IU/L to 39 ± 15 IU/L *6419*

Glutathione S-Transferase *Serum Increase Physiological* Treatment of 64 postmenopausal women with 17β-estradiol for one cycle caused nonsignificant increase to 2.25 µg/L from mean baseline of 1.94 µg/L *4162*

Glycated Hemoglobin *Blood Decrease Physiological* In 20 postmenopausal women patients with type II diabetes mellitus treatment with 2 mg/d micronized 17β-estradiol for 6 weeks caused a 3% decrease in concentration compared with that in placebo-treated contols *787*

Glycine *Plasma No Effect Physiological* In 22 healthy men aged over 65 years administration of 0.5 to 2.0 mg/d 17β-estradiol for 9 weeks caused insignificant change from mean baseline of 301 ± 34 mmol/L to 300 ± 44 mmol/L *2134*

HDL_2-Cholesterol *Serum Increase Physiological* In 20 postmenopausal women patients with type II diabetes mellitus treatment with 2 mg/d micronized 17β-estradiol for 6 weeks caused a 49% increase in concentration compared with that in placebo-treated contols *787*

HDL_3-Cholesterol *Serum Increase Physiological* In 20 postmenopausal women patients with type II diabetes mellitus treatment with 2 mg/d micronized 17β-estradiol for 6 weeks caused a 5% increase in concentration compared with that in placebo-treated contols *787*

17β-Estradiol *(continued)*

HDL-Cholesterol *Serum Increase Physiological* In 14 oophorectomized women over 6 mo when 50 mg drug given as implant *1801* By up to 20% in 38 healthy post-menopausal women given 2-4 mg orally or 3 mg cutaneously over 6 mo *1783* In 20 postmenopausal women patients with type II diabetes mellitus treatment with 2 mg/d micronized 17β-estradiol for 6 weeks caused a 20% increase in concentration compared with that in placebo-treated contols *787* In 22 healthy men aged over 65 years administration of 0.5 to 2.0 mg/d 17β-estradiol for 9 weeks caused significant increase from mean baseline of 47 ± 9 mg/dL to 53 ± 10 mg/dL *2134*
Serum No Effect Physiological In 20 healthy postmenopausal women treatment with 17β-estradiol 0.1 mg/d or 17β-estradiol 0.1 mg/d with 2.5 mg/d oral medroxyprogesterone acetate for 1 month caused nonsignificant change in concentration from 63 ± 15 mg/dL to 61 ± 13 mg/dL *3218* In 6 normolipidemic postmenopausal healthy women treatment with 2 mg/d micronized 17β-micronized estradiol for 6 weeks caused nonsignificant change from mean baseline of 1.61 ± 0.41 mmol/L to 1.69 ± 0.32 mmol/L *6419*

HDL-Phospholipids *Serum Increase Physiological* By about 10% in 38 healthy postmenopausal women given 2-4 mg orally or 3 mg subcutaneously over 6 mo *1783*

HDL Size *Serum Increase Physiological* In 22 healthy men aged over 65 years administration of 0.5 to 2.0 mg/d 17β-estradiol for 9 weeks caused significant change from mean baseline of 9.1 ± 0.4 nm to 9.3 ± 0.4 nm *2134*

HDL-Triglycerides *Serum No Effect Physiological* In 6 normolipidemic postmenopausal healthy women treatment with 2 mg/d micronized 17β-micronized estradiol for 6 weeks caused nonsignificant change from mean baseline of 0.27 ± 0.08 mmol/L to 0.37 ± 0.06 mmol/L *6419*

Homocysteine *Plasma Decrease Physiological* In 22 healthy men aged over 65 years administration of 0.5 to 2.0 mg/d 17β-estradiol for 9 weeks caused significant decrease from mean baseline of 8.7 ± 3.0 μmol/L to 7.7 ± 2.6 μmol/L *2134*

IDL-Cholesterol *Serum Decrease Physiological* In 6 normolipidemic postmenopausal healthy women treatment with 2 mg/d micronized 17β-micronized estradiol for 6 weeks caused significant change from mean baseline of 0.62 ± 0.36 mmol/L to 0.47 ± 0.27 mmol/L *6419*

IDL-Triglycerides *Serum No Effect Physiological* In 6 normolipidemic postmenopausal healthy women treatment with 2 mg/d micronized 17β-micronized estradiol for 6 weeks caused nonsignificant change from mean baseline of 0.15 ± 0.08 mmol/L to 0.17 ± 0.06 mmol/L *6419*

Insulin-like Growth Factor-I *Serum Decrease Physiological* In 6 normolipidemic postmenopausal healthy women treatment with 2 mg/d micronized 17β-micronized estradiol for 6 weeks caused significant change from mean baseline of 130.5 ± 71.9 ng/mL to 91.7 ± 30.3 ng/mL *6419*

Intercellular Adhesion Molecule-1
Serum Decrease Physiological In 20 healthy postmenopausal women treatment with 17β-estradiol 0.1 mg/d or 17β-estradiol 0.1 mg/d with 2.5 mg/d oral medroxyprogesterone acetate for 1 month caused significant change in concentration from mean 280 ± 16.3 ng/mL to 254 ± 17.6 ng/mL *3218*

Kynurenic Acid *Serum No Effect Physiological* In 22 healthy men aged over 65 years administration of 0.5 to 2.0 mg/d 17β-estradiol for 9 weeks caused insignificant change from mean baseline of 33.1 ± 4.5 nmol/L to 31.4 ± 7.4 nmol/L *2134*

LDL-Cholesterol *Serum Decrease Physiological* In 14 oophorectomized women over 6 mo when 50 mg drug given as implant *1801* In 20 postmenopausal women patients with type II diabetes mellitus treatment with 2 mg/d micronized 17β-estradiol for 6 weeks caused a 16% reduction in concentration compared with that in placebo-treated contols *787* Marked reduction in 38 healthy post-menopausal women given 2-4 mg orally or 3 mg cutaneously over 6 mo *1783* In 22 healthy men aged over 65 years administration of 0.5 to 2.0 mg/d 17β-estradiol for 9 weeks caused significant decrease from mean baseline of 141 ± 28 mg/dL to 137 ± 30 mg/dL *2134*
Serum No Effect Physiological In 6 normolipidemic postmenopausal healthy women treatment with 2 mg/d micronized 17β-micronized estradiol for 6 weeks caused nonsignificant change from mean baseline of 3.10 ± 0.77 mmol/L to 2.91 ± 0.67 mmol/L *6419* In 20 healthy postmenopausal women treatment with 17β-estradiol 0.1 mg/d or 17β-estradiol 0.1 mg/d with 2.5 mg/d oral medroxyprogesterone acetate for 1 month caused nonsignificant change in concentration from 152 ± 26 mg/dL to 139 ± 23 mg/dL *3218*

LDL Particles *Serum Decrease Physiological* In 22 healthy men aged over 65 years administration of 0.5 to 2.0 mg/d 17β-estradiol for 9 weeks caused significant change from mean baseline of 1665 ± 483 nmol/L to 1513 ± 479 nmol/L *2134*

LDL-Phospholipids *Serum Decrease Physiological* By about 12% in 38 healthy postmenopausal women given 2-4 mg orally or 3 mg subcutaneously over 6 mo *1783*

LDL Size *Serum Increase Physiological* In 22 healthy men aged over 65 years administration of 0.5 to 2.0 mg/d 17β-estradiol for 9 weeks caused significant change from mean baseline of 20.7 ± 0.6 nm to 20.9 ± 0.6 nm *2134*

LDL-Triglycerides *Serum No Effect Physiological* In 6 normolipidemic postmenopausal healthy women treatment with 2 mg/d micronized 17β-micronized estradiol for 6 weeks caused nonsignificant change from mean baseline of 0.29 ± 0.16 mmol/L to 0.25 ± 0.04 mmol/L *6419*

Lipase, Hepatic *Serum Decrease Physiological* In 6 normolipidemic postmenopausal healthy women treatment with 2 mg/d micronized 17β-micronized estradiol for 6 weeks caused significant change from mean baseline of 417 ± 84 U/L to 284 ± 71 U/L *6419*

Lipoprotein Lipase *Serum No Effect Physiological* In 6 normolipidemic postmenopausal healthy women treatment with 2 mg/d micronized 17β-micronized estradiol for 6 weeks caused nonsignificant change from mean baseline of 136 ± 38 U/L to 123 ± 30 U/L *6419*

Methionine *Plasma No Effect Physiological* In 22 healthy men aged over 65 years administration of 0.5 to 2.0 mg/d 17β-estradiol for 9 weeks caused insignificant change from mean baseline of 23.1 ± 2.8 mmol/L to 23.8 ± 4.3 mmol/L *2134*

Methylcitrate Acid *Serum No Effect Physiological* In 22 healthy men aged over 65 years administration of 0.5 to 2.0 mg/d 17β-estradiol for 9 weeks caused insignificant change from mean baseline of 131 ± 38 mmol/L to 119 ± 31 mmol/L *2134*

Methylglycine *Plasma No Effect Physiological* In 22 healthy men aged over 65 years administration of 0.5 to 2.0 mg/d 17β-estradiol for 9 weeks caused insignificant change from mean baseline of 1.5 ± 0.3 mmol/L to 1.4 ± 0.3 mmol/L *2134*

Methylmalonate *Serum No Effect Physiological* In 22 healthy men aged over 65 years administration of 0.5 to 2.0 mg/d 17β-estradiol for 9 weeks caused insignificant change from mean baseline of 242 ± 261 mmol/L to 219 ± 168 mmol/L *2134*

Phospholipids *Serum No Effect Physiological* Insignificant change in 38 healthy post-menopausal women given 2 - 4 mg orally or 3 mg cutaneously over 6 mo *1783*

Plasminogen Activator Inhibitor-1
Plasma Decrease Physiological In 22 healthy men aged over 65 years administration of 0.5 to 2.0 mg/d 17β-estradiol for 9 weeks caused significant change from mean baseline of 21.8 ± 10.7 ng/mL to 17.2 ± 9.5 ng/mL *2134*

Protein C *Plasma No Effect Physiological* In 22 healthy men aged over 65 years administration of 0.5 to 2.0 mg/d 17β-estradiol for 9 weeks caused insignificant change from mean baseline of 106 ± 17% to 109 ± 20% *2134*

Protein S *Plasma No Effect Physiological* In 22 healthy men aged over 65 years administration of 0.5 to 2.0 mg/d 17β-estradiol for 9 weeks caused insignificant change from mean baseline of 120 ± 21% to 116 ± 19% *2134*

Prothrombin Fragment 1.2 *Plasma No Effect Physiological* In 22 healthy men aged over 65 years administration of 0.5 to 2.0 mg/d 17β-estradiol for 9 weeks caused insignificant change from mean baseline of 3.6 ± 1.4 ng/mL to 3.8 ± 1.4 ng/mL *2134*

Quinolinic Acid *Serum No Effect Physiological* In 22 healthy men aged over 65 years administration of 0.5 to 2.0 mg/d 17β-estradiol for 9 weeks caused insignificant change from mean baseline of 425 ± 236 nmol/L to 359 ± 67 nmol/L *2134*

Serine *Plasma No Effect Physiological* In 22 healthy men aged over 65 years administration of 0.5 to 2.0 mg/d 17β-estradiol for 9 weeks caused insignificant change from mean baseline of 108 ± 16 mmol/L to 101 ± 19 mmol/L *2134*

Sf > 1000 Cholesterol *Serum No Effect Physiological* In 6 normolipidemic postmenopausal healthy women treatment with 2 mg/d micronized 17β-micronized estradiol for 6 weeks caused nonsignificant change from mean baseline of 0.11 ± 0.029 mmol/L to 0.1 ± 0.07 mmol/L *6419*

Sf > 1000 Triglycerides *Serum No Effect Physiological* In 6 normolipidemic postmenopausal healthy women treatment with 2 mg/d micronized 17β-micronized estradiol for 6 weeks caused nonsignificant change from mean baseline of 0.08 ± 0.05 mmol/L to 0.09 ± 0.05 mmol/L *6419*

Sf < 1000 Cholesterol *Serum No Effect Physiological* In 6 normolipidemic postmenopausal healthy women treatment with 2 mg/d micronized 17β-micronized estradiol for 6 weeks caused nonsignificant change from mean baseline of 5.33 ± 1.11 mmol/L to 5.39 ± 0.28 mmol/L *6419*

Sf < 1000 Triglycerides *Serum No Effect Physiological* In 6 normolipidemic postmenopausal healthy women treatment with 2 mg/d micronized 17β-micronized estradiol for 6 weeks caused nonsignificant change from mean baseline of 1.8 ± 1.4 mmol/L to 1.4 ± 0.47 mmol/L *6419*

Soluble E-selectin *Serum No Effect Physiological* In 20 healthy postmenopausal women treatment with 17β-estradiol 0.1 mg/d or 17β-estradiol 0.1 mg/d with 2.5 mg/d oral medroxyprogesterone acetate for 1 month caused nonsignificant change in concentration from 54.2 ± 16.3 ng/mL to 50.4 ± 17.6 ng/mL *3218*

Soluble Vascular Cell Adhesion Molecule-1
Serum Decrease Physiological In 20 healthy postmenopausal women treatment with 17β-estradiol 0.1 mg/d or 17β-estradiol 0.1 mg/d with 2.5 mg/d oral medroxyprogesterone acetate for 1 month caused nonsignificant change in concentration from mean 572 ± 123 ng/mL to 547 ± 110 ng/mL *3218*

Thrombin Precursor Protein
Plasma No Effect Physiological In 22 healthy men aged over 65 years administration of 0.5 to 2.0 mg/d 17β-estradiol for 9 weeks caused insignificant change from mean baseline of 0.08 ± 0.16 μg/mL to 0.00 ± 0.00 μg/mL *2134*

Thrombin/Antithrombin III Complex
Plasma No Effect Physiological In 22 healthy men aged over 65 years administration of 0.5 to 2.0 mg/d 17β-estradiol for 9 weeks caused insignificant change from mean baseline of 5.4 ± 3.9 ng/mL to 6.4 ± 5.6 ng/mL *2134*

Tissue Plasminogen Activator Inhibitor
Plasma No Effect Physiological In 22 healthy men aged over 65 years administration of 0.5 to 2.0 mg/d 17β-estradiol for 9 weeks caused insignificant change from mean baseline of 11.1 ± 2.4 ng/mL to 12.1 ± 3.0 ng/mL *2134*

Triglycerides *Serum Decrease Physiological* In 22 healthy men aged over 65 years administration of 0.5 to 2.0 mg/d 17β-estradiol for 9 weeks caused significant decrease from mean baseline of 113 ± 52 mg/dL to 98 ± 37 mg/dL *2134*
Serum Increase Physiological Slight increase in 38 healthy post-menopausal women given 2-4 mg orally or 3 mg cutaneously over 6 mo *1783*
Serum No Effect Physiological In 20 postmenopausal women patients with type II diabetes mellitus treatment with 2 mg/d micronized 17β-estradiol for 6 weeks caused no sgnificant change in concentration compared with that in placebo-treated contols *787* In 20 healthy postmenopausal women treatment with 17β-estradiol 0.1 mg/d or 17β-estradiol 0.1 mg/d with 2.5 mg/d oral medroxyprogesterone acetate for 1 month caused nonsignificant change in concentration from 102 ± 52 mg/dL to 98 ± 50 mg/dL *3218* In 6 normolipidemic postmenopausal healthy women treatment with 2 mg/d micronized 17β-micronized estradiol for 6 weeks caused nonsignificant change from mean baseline of 1.47 ± 0.69 mmol/L to 1.62 ± 0.59 mmol/L *6419*

VLDL-Cholesterol *Serum No Effect Physiological* In 20 postmenopausal women patients with type II diabetes mellitus treatment with 2 mg/d micronized 17β-estradiol for 6 weeks caused no sgnificant change in concentration compared with that in placebo-treated contols *787* In 6 normolipidemic postmenopausal healthy women treatment with 2 mg/d micronized 17β-micronized estradiol for 6 weeks caused nonsignificant change from mean baseline of 0.39 ± 0.27 mmol/L to 0.36 ± 0.20 mmol/L *6419* Insignificant change in 38 healthy postmenopausal women given 2-4 mg orally or 3 mg cutaneously over 6 mo *1783*

VLDL Size *Serum No Effect Physiological* In 22 healthy men aged over 65 years administration of 0.5 to 2.0 mg/d 17β-estradiol for 9 weeks caused insignificant change from mean baseline of 46.5 ± 5.7 nm to 46.6 ± 6.3 nm *2134*

VLDL-Triglycerides *Serum No Effect Physiological* Insignificant change in 38 healthy postmenopausal women given 2-4 mg orally or 3 mg cutaneously over 6 mo *1783* In 6 normolipidemic postmenopausal healthy women treatment with 2 mg/d micronized 17β-micronized estradiol for 6 weeks caused nonsignificant change from mean baseline of 0.77 ± 0.46 mmol/L to 0.81 ± 0.36 mmol/L *6419*

von Willebrand Factor *Plasma No Effect Physiological* In 22 healthy men aged over 65 years administration of 0.5 to 2.0 mg/d 17β-estradiol for 9 weeks caused insignificant change from mean baseline of 140 ± 48% to 147 ± 49% *2134*

Xanthurenic Acid *Serum No Effect Physiological* In 22 healthy men aged over 65 years administration of 0.5 to 2.0 mg/d 17β-estradiol for 9 weeks caused insignificant change from mean baseline of 10.4 ± 3.6 nmol/L to 10.7 ± 5.5 nmol/L *2134*

Estradiol Valerate

Alkaline Phosphatase, Bone Isoenzyme
Serum Decrease Physiological In 16 healthy postmenopausal women treatment with 2 mg/d estradiol valerate and 1 mg/d cyproterone acetate for 12 months caused a significant decrease in activity from mean baseline of 78.0 ± 7.4 U/L to 57.9 ± 5.7 U/L at 6 months and 52.8 ± 4.7 U/L at 12 months *2535*

Angiotensinogen *Plasma Increase Physiological* In 16 healthy postmenopausal women treatment with estradiol valerate 2 mg and 1 mg cyproterone acetate in 21-day sequences over 12 cycles caused significant change in concentration from 2029 ± 120 ng/mL to 4151 ± 497 ng/mL *588*

Apolipoprotein A-I *Serum Increase Physiological* In 12 women with surgically induced menopause treatment with 2 mg/d estradiol valerate for 16 weeks caused significant change to 1.82 ± 0.26 g/L from mean baseline of 1.60 ± 0.16 g/L *2328*

Apolipoprotein B *Serum No Effect Physiological* In 12 women with surgically induced menopause treatment with 2 mg/d estradiol valerate for 16 weeks caused nonsignificant change to 0.68 ± 0.18 g/L from mean baseline of 0.71 ± 0.18 g/L *2328*

Cholesterol *Serum Decrease Physiological* In 16 healthy postmenopausal women treatment with estradiol valerate 2 mg and 1 mg cyproterone acetate in 21-day sequences over 12 cycles caused significant change in concentration from 5.60 ± 0.13 mmol/L to 5.25 ± 0.13 mmol/L in estrogenic phase and 5.39 ± 0.15 mmol/L in progestogenic phase *588*
Serum No Effect Physiological In 12 women with surgically induced menopause treatment with 2 mg/d estradiol valerate for 16 weeks caused nonsignificant change to 5.52 ± 1.16 mmol/L from mean baseline of 5.59 ± 1.30 mmol/L *2328*

C-terminal Telopeptide of Type I Collagen
Serum Decrease Physiological In 16 healthy postmenopausal women treatment with 2 mg/d estradiol valerate and 1 mg/d cyproterone acetate for 12 months caused a significant decrease in concentration from mean baseline of 3.57 ± 0.22 μg/L to 2.78 ± 0.12 μg/L at 6 months and 2.84 ± 0.17 μg/L at 12 months *2535*

Dehydroepiandrosterone Sulfate
Plasma Decrease Physiological In 29 healthy postmenopausal women treatment with estradiol valerate 2 mg and 1 mg cyproterone acetate in 21-day sequences over 12 cycles caused significant change in concentration from 3.99 ± 0.36 μmol/L to 2.13 ± 0.31 μmol/L *588*

Estradiol *Plasma Increase Physiological* In 25 healthy postmenopausal women treatment with estradiol valerate 2 mg and 1 mg cyproterone acetate in 21-day sequences over 12 cycles caused significant increase in concentration from 86 ± 21 pmol/L to 742 ± 160 pmol/L *588*

Estradiol Valerate *(continued)*

Estrone *Plasma Increase Physiological* In 19 healthy postmenopausal women treatment with estradiol valerate 2 mg and 1 mg cyproterone acetate in 21-day sequences over 12 cycles caused significant increase in concentration from 276 ± 24 pmol/L to 1561 ± 220 pmol/L *588*

Fibrinogen *Plasma No Effect Physiological* In 16 healthy postmenopausal women treatment with estradiol valerate 2 mg and 1 mg cyproterone acetate in 21-day sequences over 12 cycles caused nonsignificant change in concentration from 2.95 ± 0.10 g/L to 2.95 ± 0.11 g/L *588*

Follicle Stimulating Hormone
Plasma Decrease Physiological In 29 healthy postmenopausal women treatment with estradiol valerate 2 mg and 1 mg cyproterone acetate in 21-day sequences over 12 cycles caused significant change in concentration from 70.3 ± 6.8 IU/L to 22.8 ± 2.2 IU/L *588*

HDL_2-Cholesterol *Serum Increase Physiological* In 12 women with surgically induced menopause treatment with 2 mg/d estradiol valerate for 16 weeks caused significant change to 0.62 ± 0.19 mmol/L from mean baseline of 0.50 ± 0.17 mmol/L *2328*

HDL_3-Cholesterol *Serum No Effect Physiological* In 12 women with surgically induced menopause treatment with 2 mg/d estradiol valerate for 16 weeks caused nonsignificant change to 1.09 ± 0.19 mmol/L from mean baseline of 1.10 ± 0.26 mmol/L *2328*

HDL-Cholesterol *Serum Increase Physiological* In 12 women with surgically induced menopause treatment with 2 mg/d estradiol valerate for 16 weeks caused significant change to 1.84 ± 0.41 mmol/L from mean baseline of 1.65 ± 0.30 mmol/L *2328*
Serum No Effect Physiological In 16 healthy postmenopausal women treatment with estradiol valerate 2 mg and 1 mg cyproterone acetate in 21-day sequences over 12 cycles caused nonsignificant change in concentration from 1.68 ± 0.09 mmol/L to 1.69 ± 0.09 mmol/L in estrogenic phase and 1.69 ± 0.10 mmol/L in progestogenic phase *588*

LDL-Cholesterol *Serum Decrease Physiological* In 16 healthy postmenopausal women treatment with estradiol valerate 2 mg and 1 mg cyproterone acetate in 21-day sequences over 12 cycles caused significant change in concentration from 3.41 ± 0.13 mmol/L to 2.98 ± 0.17 mmol/L in estrogenic phase and 3.12 ± 0.17 mmol/L in progestogenic phase *588*
Serum No Effect Physiological In 12 women with surgically induced menopause treatment with 2 mg/d estradiol valerate for 16 weeks caused nonsignificant change to 3.21 ± 1.01 mmol/L from mean baseline of 3.52 ± 1.24 mmol/L *2328*

Luteinizing Hormone *Plasma Decrease Physiological* In 29 healthy postmenopausal women treatment with estradiol valerate 2 mg and 1 mg cyproterone acetate in 21-day sequences over 12 cycles caused significant change in concentration from 52.6 ± 5.1 IU/L to 26.3 ± 2.6 IU/L *588*

Osteocalcin *Serum Decrease Physiological* In 16 healthy postmenopausal women treatment with 2 mg/d estradiol valerate and 1 mg/d cyproterone acetate for 12 months caused significant 29.2% decrease in concentration from mean baseline of 3.12 ± 0.59 ng/mL to 2.77 ± 0.50 ng/mL at 6 months and 2.46 ± 0.44 ng/mL at 12 months *2535*

Prothrombin Time *Plasma No Effect Physiological* In 16 healthy postmenopausal women treatment with estradiol valerate 2 mg and 1 mg cyproterone acetate in 21-day sequences over 12 cycles caused nonsignificant change in concentration from 1.09 ± 0.030 mg/L to 1.08 ± 0.041 mg/L *588*

Renin Activity *Plasma No Effect Physiological* In 16 healthy postmenopausal women treatment with estradiol valerate 2 mg and 1 mg cyproterone acetate in 21-day sequences over 12 cycles caused nonsignificant change in activity from 2.7 ± 0.33 ng/mL/h to 2.7 ± 0.53 ng/mL/h *588*

Sex-Hormone Binding Globulin
Serum Increase Physiological In 20 healthy postmenopausal women treatment with estradiol valerate 2 mg and 1 mg cyproterone acetate in 21-day sequences over 12 cycles caused significant increase in concentration from 43.6 ± 5.2 nmol/L to 79.2 ± 7.1 nmol/L *588*

Testosterone *Serum Decrease Physiological* In 15 healthy postmenopausal women treatment with estradiol valerate 2 mg and 1 mg cyproterone acetate in 21-day sequences over 12 cycles caused significant change in concentration from 1.52 ± 0.17 nmol/L to 1.05 ± 0.14 nmol/L *588*

Thyroid Stimulating Hormone
Serum Decrease Physiological In 29 healthy postmenopausal women treatment with estradiol valerate 2 mg and 1 mg cyproterone acetate in 21-day sequences over 12 cycles caused nonsignificant change in concentration from 2.67 ± 0.76 mIU/L to 2.13 ± 0.31 mIU/L *588*

Thyroxine (T4) *Serum Increase Physiological* In 27 healthy postmenopausal women treatment with estradiol valerate 2 mg and 1 mg cyproterone acetate in 21-day sequences over 12 cycles caused nonsignificant change in concentration from 105.2 ± 4.0 nmol/L to 126.8 ± 2.6 nmol/L *588*

Triglycerides *Serum Increase Physiological* In 16 healthy postmenopausal women treatment with estradiol valerate 2 mg and 1 mg cyproterone acetate in 21-day sequences over 12 cycles caused nonsignificant change in concentration from 1.07 ± 0.13 mmol/L to 1.37 ± 0.14 mmol/L in estrogenic phase and 1.29 ± 0.25 mmol/L in progestogenic phase *588*
Serum No Effect Physiological In 12 women with surgically induced menopause treatment with 2 mg/d estradiol valerate for 16 weeks caused nonsignificant change to 1.33 ± 1.03 mmol/L from mean baseline of 1.21 ± 0.58 mmol/L *2328*

VLDL-Cholesterol *Serum No Effect Physiological* In 12 women with surgically induced menopause treatment with 2 mg/d estradiol valerate for 16 weeks caused nonsignificant change to 0.48 ± 0.40 mmol/L from mean baseline of 0.43 ± 0.25 mmol/L *2328* In 16 healthy postmenopausal women treatment with estradiol valerate 2 mg and 1 mg cyproterone acetate in 21-day sequences over 12 cycles caused nonsignificant change in concentration from 0.51 ± 0.06 mmol/L to 0.57 ± 0.06 mmol/L in estrogenic phase and 0.57 ± 0.10 mmol/L in progestogenic phase *588*

Estramustine

Aspartate Aminotransferase *Serum Increase Physiological* One case of increased bilirubin alone but additional cases of increased bilirubin concentration together with increased activity of LDH and/or AST observed in 93 patients receiving treatment *4673* Altered liver function tests are common with treatment *1384*

Bilirubin *Serum Increase Physiological* One case of increased bilirubin alone but additional cases of increased bilirubin concentration together with increased activity of LDH and/or AST observed in 93 patients receiving treatment *4673*

Calcium *Serum Increase Physiological* Although uncommon adverse side effect is serious *1384*

Lactate Dehydrogenase *Serum Increase Physiological* Altered liver function tests are common *1384* Five cases of increased bilirubin alone but additional cases of increased bilirubin concentration together with increased activity of LDH and/or AST observed in 93 patients receiving treatment *4673* One case of increased bilirubin alone but additional cases of increased bilirubin concentration together with increased activity of LDH and/or AST observed in 93 patients receiving treatment *4673*

Leukocytes *Blood Decrease Physiological* Four cases of leukopenia observed in 93 patients receiving treatment *4673*

Occult Blood *Feces Increase Physiological* One case of gastrointestinal bleeding observed in 93 patients receiving treatment *4673*

Platelets *Blood Decrease Physiological* One case of thrombocytopenia observed in 93 patients receiving treatment *4673*

Prostate-specific Antigen, Free *Serum No Effect Analytical* Estramustine at a concentration of 81.7 mg/L had no significant effect on the Hybritech Tandem® -R free PSA immunoassay *4286*

Estrogen Therapy

Ceruloplasmin *Serum No Effect Physiological* In 4 women aged 50-59 years receiving estrogen therapy mean concentration 593 (480-700) mg/L versus 516 (410-723) mg/L in 13 controls when measured enzymatically and 384 (300-460) mg/L versus 370 (250-490) when measured by RID *3519*

Cholesterol *Serum Decrease Physiological* In 15 postmenopausal women treatment with 17β-estradiol for 6 months and a 10 day course of methoxyprogesterone every 3 months caused significant decrease in concentration from mean baseline of 5.63 ± 0.90 mmol/L to 5.00 ± 1.11 mmol/L *534*

Clopidogrel *Serum No Effect Physiological* Estrogen administration does not appear to affect the pharmacodynamics of clopidogrel *5256*

Copper *Serum Increase Physiological* In 4 women aged 50 to 59 years mean concentration 19.2 (16.5-20.8) µmol/L not significantly greater than mean of 17.0 (12.7-23.6) µmol/L in 13 healthy control women of same age *3519*

Endothelin-1 *Plasma Decrease Physiological* In 15 postmenopausal women treatment with 17β-estradiol for 6 months and a 10 day course of methoxyprogesterone every 3 months caused significant decrease in concentration from mean baseline of 16.4 ± 7.9 pg/mL to 12.5 ± 5.7 pg/mL *534*

Estradiol *Plasma Increase Physiological* In 15 postmenopausal women treatment with 17β-estradiol for 6 months and a 10 day course of methoxyprogesterone every 3 months caused significant increase in concentration from mean baseline of 63.9 ± 18.6 pmol/L to 278.5 ± 163.5 pmol/L *534*

HDL-Cholesterol *Serum Increase Physiological* In 15 postmenopausal women treatment with 17β-estradiol for 6 months and a 10 day course of methoxyprogesterone every 3 months caused significant increase in concentration from mean baseline of 1.05 ± 0.35 mmol/L to 1.23 ± 0.48 mmol/L *534*

Iron-Binding Capacity, Total *Serum Increase Physiological* May increase TIBC to 90 µmol/L from typical reference range of 50 - 70 µmol/L *5510*

LDL-Cholesterol *Serum Decrease Physiological* In 15 postmenopausal women treatment with 17β-estradiol for 6 months and a 10 day course of methoxyprogesterone every 3 months caused significant decrease in concentration from mean baseline of 3.79 ± 0.71 mmol/L to 2.92 ± 0.77 mmol/L *534*

Nitric Acid Products *Serum Increase Physiological* In 15 postmenopausal women treatment with 17β-estradiol for 6 months and a 10 day course of methoxyprogesterone every 3 months caused significant increase in concentration from mean baseline of 27.5 ± 13.1 nmol/mL to 34.7 ± 18.2 nmol/mL *534*

Nitric Acid:Endothelin-1 Ratio
Plasma Increase Physiological In 15 postmenopausal women treatment with 17β-estradiol for 6 months and a 10 day course of methoxyprogesterone every 3 months caused significant increase in ratio from mean baseline of 2.0 ± 1.3 to 3.2 ± 1.9 *534*

Superoxide Dismutase
Red Blood Cells No Effect Physiological In 4 women aged 50-59 y mean activity 2840 U/g hemoglobin not significantly different from 3327 U/g hemoglobin in healthy control women of same age *3519*

Thyroxine (T4), Free *Serum Decrease Physiological* In patients with non-functioning thyroid glands receiving levothyroxine free T4 may be decreased: if the patient's thyroid gland is functioning the decreased free thyroxine will result in a compensatory increase in thyroxine output by the thyroid *277*

Triglycerides *Serum Decrease Physiological* In 15 postmenopausal women treatment with 17β-estradiol for 6 months and a 10 day course of methoxyprogesterone every 3 months caused nonsignificant decrease in concentration from mean baseline of 1.93 ± 1.22 mmol/L to 1.84 ± 1.14 mmol/L *534*

Estrogen/Progestin Therapy

Albumin *Serum Decrease Physiological* In 300 postmenopausal women treatment with hormone replacement therapy caused significant reduction from mean baseline of 42.8 g/L to 42.1 g/L *1977*

Alkaline Phosphatase *Serum No Effect Physiological* In 17 postmenopausal women treatment for 25 days had no effect on baseline activity of 29.7 ± 1.45 U/L *119*

Alkaline Phosphatase, Bone Isoenzyme
Serum Decrease Physiological In 17 postmenopausal women treatment for 25 days caused insignificant reduction from mean baseline of 14.9 ± 0.81 U/L to 13.0 ± 1.39 U/L *119*

Apolipoprotein A-I *Serum Decrease Physiological* In postmenopausal women treated with 0.625 mg conjugated estrogens with progestogens decreases observed as follows: medroxyprogesterone 5 mg 5% and 10 mg 11%, norethindrone 1 mg 11%, and with norgestrel at either 0.15 or 0.25 mg 15% *3628*
Serum No Effect Physiological Nonsignificant mean increase of 0.19 g/L in 39 postmenopausal women treated with combination therapy for an average of 16 months *1668*

Apolipoprotein A-II *Serum No Effect Physiological* Nonsignificant mean increase of 0.02 g/L in 39 postmenopausal women treated with combination therapy for an average of 16 months *1668*

Apolipoprotein B *Serum Increase Physiological* In postmenopausal women treatment with 0.625 mg conjugated estrogens with progestogens caused increases as follows: 10 mg medroxyprogesterone 3%, 1 mg norethindrone 10%, 0.15 mg norgestrel 8% and 0.25 mg norethindrone 10% *3628*
Serum No Effect Physiological Nonsignificant mean increase of 0.14 g/L in 39 postmenopausal women treated with combination therapy for an average of 16 months *1668*

Calcitonin *Plasma Increase Physiological* In 17 postmenopausal women treatment for 25 days caused significant increase from mean baseline of 30.2 ± 6.3 pg/mL to 39.7 ± 6.5 pg/mL *119*

Calcium *Serum Decrease Physiological* In 17 postmenopausal women treatment for 25 days caused significant reduction from mean baseline of 9.06 ± 0.09 mg/dL to 8.80 ± 0.09 mg/dL *119*

Cholesterol *Serum Decrease Physiological* In 58 postmenopausal women with fasting serum cholesterol concentrations greater than 250 mg/dL treatment with up to 1.25 mg conjugated equine estrogens daily with 5 mg medroxyprogesterone acetate daily for 8 weeks caused significant change from mean baseline of 305 ± 41 mg/dL to 255 ± 32 mg/dL *1239*
Serum No Effect Physiological Nonsignificant mean increase of 0.23 mmol/L in 39 postmenopausal women treated for an average of 16 months with combination therapy *1668*

C-terminal Telopeptides of Type I Collagen Degradation Products *Serum Decrease Physiological* Mean concentration of a group of postmenopausal women actively treated with hormone replacement therapy decreased by 75% over 12 months *5103*

1,25-Dihydroxy Vitamin D *Serum Increase Physiological* In 17 postmenopausal women treatment for 25 days caused significant increase from mean baseline of 29.9 ± 1.66 pg/mL to 34.2 ± 1.95 pg/mL *119*

1,25-Dihydroxy Vitamin D, Free
Serum Increase Physiological In 17 postmenopausal women treated for 25 days mean concentration increased nonsignificantly from baseline of 69.4 ± 5.37 pg/mL to 83.6 ± 6.38 pg/mL *119*

Estradiol *Plasma Increase Physiological* In 17 postmenopausal women treated for 25 days caused significant increase from mean baseline of 14.2 ± 3.36 pg/mL to 85.2 ± 7.15 pg/mL *119*

Fibrinogen *Plasma Decrease Physiological* In 300 postmenopausal women treatment with hormone replacement therapy caused significant reduction from mean baseline of 2.68 g/L to 2.21 g/L *1977*

Follicle Stimulating Hormone
Plasma Decrease Physiological In 17 postmenopausal women treatment for 25 days caused significant decrease from mean baseline of 72.6 ± 0.51 mIU/mL to 44.3 ± 7.01 mIU/mL *119*

Glucose *Serum No Effect Physiological* Nonsignificant decrease of 0.39 mmol/L in fasting concentration and 0.09 mmol/L in 2-hour post-glucose concentration in 39 postmenopausal women treated with combination therapy for about 16 months *1668*

Estrogen/Progestin Therapy *(continued)*

HDL_2-Cholesterol *Serum Decrease Physiological* In postmenopausal women 0.625 mg conjugated estrogens with progestogens caused decreases as follows: medroxyprogesterone 5 mg 11%, 10 mg 19%, norethindrone 1 mg 27%, norgestrel 0.15 mg 23% and 0.25 mg 25% *3628*
Serum Increase Physiological Although estrogen effect is lessened during combined therapy in postmenopausal women, even with doses of 5 mg medroxyprogesterone acetate or 1 mg norethindrone, HDL-concentration remains increased and increases further with withdrawal of the progestin *3628*

HDL_3-Cholesterol *Serum Decrease Physiological* Slight effect observed in postmenopausal women treated with 0.625 mg conjugated estrogens and progestogens as follows: 2% decrease with 10 mg medroxyprogesterone, 1% with 1 mg norethindrone and 8% with 0.25 mg norgestrel but no effect with lower doses *3628*

HDL-Cholesterol *Serum Decrease Physiological* In postmenopausal women 0.625 mg conjugated estrogens with 200 mg micronized progesterone caused 2% decrease, with 5 or 10 mg medroxyprogesterone 6% decrease, with 1 mg norethindrone 10% decrease: with 0.15 and 0.25 mg norgestrel 14 and 18% decrease *3628*
Serum Increase Physiological In the Postmenopausal Estrogen/Progestin Intervention Trial of 875 healthy postmenopausal women with primary hypercholesterolemia treatment with estrogen/progestin or estrogen alone caused mean increase of 4 - 8% *3115*
Serum No Effect Physiological Nonsignificant mean increase of 0.02 mmol/L in 39 postmenopausal women treated with combination therapy for an average of 16 months *1668* In 58 postmenopausal women with fasting serum cholesterol concentrations greater than 250 mg/dL treatment with up to 1.25 mg conjugated equine estrogens daily with 5 mg medroxyprogesterone acetate daily for 8 weeks caused nonsignificant change from mean baseline of 63 ± 17 mg/dL to 67 ± 16 mg/dL *1239*

25-Hydroxy Vitamin D *Serum Increase Physiological* In 17 postmenopausal women treatment for 25 days caused nonsignificant increase from mean baseline of 25.4 ± 1.66 ng/mL to 27.3 ± 2.44 ng/mL *119*

25-Hydroxy Vitamin D, Free *Serum Increase Physiological* In 17 postmenopausal women treatment for 25 days caused nonsignificant increase from mean baseline of 7.21 ± 0.42 pg/mL to 9.29 ± 1.1 pg/mL *119*

Hydroxyproline *Urine Decrease Physiological* In 17 postmenopausal women treatment for 25 days caused significant reduction from mean baseline of 23.5 ± 1.4 mg/g creatinine to 18.0 ± 1.7 mg/g creatinine *119*

Insulin *Plasma No Effect Physiological* Nonsignificant increase of 2.80 mU/L in fasting concentration and 3.20 mU/L in 2-hour post-glucose concentration in 39 postmenopausal women treated with combination therapy for about 16 months *1668*

LDL-Cholesterol *Serum Decrease Physiological* In 58 postmenopausal women with fasting serum cholesterol concentrations greater than 250 mg/dL treatment with up to 1.25 mg conjugated equine estrogens daily with 5 mg medroxyprogesterone acetate daily for 8 weeks caused significant change from mean baseline of 212 ± 40 mg/dL to 154 ± 29 mg/dL *1239* In the Postmenopausal Estrogen/Progestin Intervention Trial of 875 healthy postmenopausal women with primary hypercholesterolemia treatment with estrogen/progestin or estrogen alone caused mean decrease of 10 - 12% *3115*
Serum Increase Physiological In postmenopausal women treatment with 0.625 mg conjugated estrogens with progestogens caused increases as follows: 3% with 5 mg and 7% with 10 mg medroxyprogesterone, 10% with 1 mg norethindrone, 6% with 0.15 mg and 1% with 0.25 mg norgestrel *3628*
Serum No Effect Physiological Nonsignificant mean increase of 0.05 mmol/L in 39 postmenopausal women treated with combination therapy for an average of 16 months *1668*

Lipoprotein Lp(a) *Serum Decrease Physiological* In 58 postmenopausal women with fasting serum cholesterol concentrations greater than 250 mg/dL treatment with up to 1.25 mg conjugated equine estrogens daily with 5 mg medroxyprogesterone acetate daily for 8 weeks caused significant change from mean baseline of 34.5 ± 38.6 mg/dL to 23.8 ± 25.3 mg/dL *1239*

Luteinizing Hormone *Plasma Decrease Physiological* In 17 postmenopausal women treatment for 25 days caused significant decrease from mean baseline of 27.9 ± 2.01 mIU/mL to 19.4 ± 2.30 mIU/mL *119*

Osteocalcin *Serum Decrease Physiological* In 17 postmenopausal women treatment for 25 days caused significant decrease from mean baseline of 3.52 ± 0.31 ng/mL to 2.65 ± 0.21 ng/mL *119*

Parathyroid Hormone *Plasma Increase Physiological* In 17 postmenopausal women treatment for 25 days caused significant increase from mean baseline of 30.0 ± 2.54 pg/mL to 34.9 ± 3.46 pg/mL *119*

Phosphate *Serum No Effect Physiological* In 17 postmenopausal women treatment for 25 days caused no significant change from mean baseline of 3.39 ± 0.09 mg/dL to 3.40 ± 0.13 mg/dL *119*

Testosterone *Serum Increase Physiological* Observed in 9 postmenopausal women with signs and symptoms of androgen excess following long-term use of an injectable androgen-estrogen combination. Concentrations increased in 8 of 9 women (5.7-14.9 nmol/L, compared with normal up to 2.43 nmol/L) *6136*

Triglycerides *Serum Increase Physiological* In 58 postmenopausal women with fasting serum cholesterol concentrations greater than 250 mg/dL treatment with up to 1.25 mg conjugated equine estrogens daily with 5 mg medroxyprogesterone acetate daily for 8 weeks caused significant change from mean baseline of 151 ± 60 mg/dL to 172 ± 59 mg/dL *1239* In the Postmenopausal Estrogen/Progestin Intervention Trial of 875 healthy postmenopausal women with primary hypercholesterolemia treatment with estrogen/progestin or estrogen alone caused mean increase of 15 - 20% *3115*
Serum No Effect Physiological Increase caused by estrogens may be eliminated with progestins during treatment of postmenopausal women *3628* Nonsignificant mean increase of 0.36 mmol/L in 39 postmenopausal women treated with combination therapy for an average of 16 months *1668*

Viscosity *Plasma Decrease Physiological* In 300 postmenopausal women treatment with hormone replacement therapy caused reduction from mean baseline of 1.176 mPa/s to 1.147 mPa/s *1977*

Estrogens

Alkaline DNase *Serum Decrease Physiological* Activity reduced in old women given estrogens compared with those not given estrogens *294*

Alkaline Phosphatase *Serum Decrease Physiological* Reported effect in postmenopausal women with estrogen replacement therapy *3679*

Alkaline Phosphatase, Bone Isoenzyme
Serum No Effect Analytical At a concentration of 0.4 mg/L had no effect on Tandem-MP Ostase method *777* At a concentration of 100 mg/L had no effect on EIA method of Gomez et al *2234*

Apolipoprotein A-I *Serum Increase Physiological* Significant increase observed in postmenopausal women treated with estrogens *868* In postmenopausal women administration of 0.625 mg/d for one year caused mean increase of 18% *3628* Concentrations significantly higher in postmenopausal women taking estrogens regardless of type of menopause *869*

Apolipoprotein B *Serum Decrease Physiological* In postmenopausal women administration of 0.625 mg/d for one year caused mean decrease of about 12% *3628*

Calcitonin *Plasma Decrease Physiological* Significant decrease observed in 13 postmenopausal women studied over 8 weeks of hormone replacement therapy *1889*

Ceruloplasmin *Serum No Effect Physiological* In 4 healthy women aged 50 - 59 years taking estrogens mean concentration of 593 ± 100 mg/L (enzymatic) and 383 ± 72 (by RID) not significantly increased compared with 517 ± 85 mg/L (enzymatic) and 370 ± 77 mg/L (by RID) in 12 healthy women aged 50 - 59 years not taking estrogens *2959*

Cholesterol *Serum Decrease Physiological* Significantly reduced in women taking estrogens following natural menopause compared with those not taking estrogens *869* In postmenopausal women administration of 0.625 mg/d for one year caused mean decrease of 6% *3628*

Copper *Serum No Effect Physiological* In 4 healthy women aged 50 - 59 years taking estrogens mean concentration of 19.7 ± 2.0 μmol/L not significantly increased compared with 17.2 ± 2.8 μmol/L in 12 healthy women aged 50 - 59 years not taking estrogens *2959*

Corticosteroid-Binding Globulin
Serum Increase Physiological False positive results for dexamethasone suppression test may be observed due to increased corticosteroid binding globulin concentration in the circulation *6538*

Cortisol *Plasma Increase Analytical* Estrogens, as in oral contraceptives, may cause a clinically significant effect with method on Bayer Technicon Immuno 1® *419*

Cytochrome c Oxidase *Monocytes No Effect Physiological* In 3 healthy women aged 50 - 59 years taking estrogens mean concentration of 0.318 ± 0.077 U/mg protein not significantly different from 0.384 ± 0.083 U/mg protein in 6 healthy women aged 50 - 59 years not taking estrogens *2959*
Platelets No Effect Physiological In 3 healthy women aged 50 - 59 years taking estrogens mean concentration of 3.54 ± 1.55 U/10^6 platelets not significantly different from 3.93 ± 0.97 U/10^6 platelets in 11 healthy women aged 50 - 59 years not taking estrogens *2959*

Dexamethasone Suppression
Patient Abnormal Physiological False positive results for dexamethasone suppression test may be observed due to increased corticosteroid binding globulin concentration in the circulation *6538*

Estradiol *Plasma Increase Physiological* In postmenopausal women administration of 0.625 mg/d for at least 2 weeks caused increase of mean concentration to 39 pg/mL *3628*

Estrone *Plasma Increase Physiological* In postmenopausal women administration of 0.625 mg/d for at least 2 weeks caused increase of mean to 153 pg/mL *3628*

Fibrinogen *Plasma Decrease Physiological* In 300 postmenopausal women treatment with hormone replacement therapy caused significant reduction from mean baseline of 2.68 g/L to 2.38 g/L *1977*

Fludrocortisone *Serum Increase Physiological* Estrogens increase corticosteroid-binding globulin concentration increasing bound fraction of steroid, although may be offset partially by decreased metabolism *221*

Glucose *Serum Decrease Physiological* Concentration significantly lower in postmenopausal women taking estrogens regardless of type of menopause *869*

HDL_2-Cholesterol *Serum Increase Physiological* In postmenopausal women administration of 0.625 mg/d for one year caused mean increase of 28% *3628*

HDL-Cholesterol *Serum Increase Physiological* In 18 postmenopausal women receiving replacement estrogen therapy mean concentration mean concentration of 63 ± 6 mg/dL significantly higher than in 72 who did not (48 ± 2 mg/dL) *2697* Increases of both 0-6% and 25% observed in postmenopausal women treated with either subdermal or transdermal estrogens but effect only observed when serum estradiol concentration increased above 60 pg/mL and treatment for at least 3 months *3628* In postmenopausal women concentration significantly higher in those taking estrogens following oophorectomy: also higher in those with natural menopause but not significantly so *869*

Insulin-like Growth Factor-I *Serum Decrease Physiological* In about 10 healthy postmenopausal women treatment with 0.625 mg/d premarin caused significant decrease from mean baseline of 18.89 ± 1.10 nmol/L to 13.97 ± 1.54 nmol/L after 4 weeks, 13.25 ± 1.47 nmol/L after 8 weeks and 14.20 ± 1.21 nmol/L after 12 weeks *5512*

Insulin-like Growth Factor Binding Protein-3
Serum No Effect Physiological In about 10 healthy postmenopausal women treatment with 0.625 mg/d premarin caused nonsignificant change from mean baseline of 3.64 ± 0.13 mg/mL to 3.70 ± 0.26 mg/mL after 4 weeks, 3.51 ± 0.26 mg/mL after 8 weeks and 3.29 ± 0.19 mg/mL after 12 weeks *5512*

LDL-Cholesterol *Serum Decrease Physiological* Significantly lower in women with natural menopause taking estrogens than in those not taking estrogens *869* In postmenopausal women administration of 0.625 mg/d for one year caused mean decrease of 16.5% *3628*

Lipoprotein Lp(a) *Serum Decrease Physiological* In about 10 healthy postmenopausal women treatment with 0.625 mg/d premarin caused decrease from mean baseline of 19.4 ± 1.3 mg/dL to 14.4 ± 1.4 mg/dL after 4 weeks (significant), 15.4 ± 1.4 mg/dL after 8 weeks (significant) and 15.7 ± 1.4 mg/dL (nonsignificant) after 12 weeks *5512* Oral estrogen may decrease concentration in some postmenopausal women *3628*

Metyrapone Test *Patient Decrease Physiological* Subnormal response may be observed in patients taking estrogens *1035*

Osteocalcin *Serum Decrease Physiological* In postmenopausal women during prophylactic treatment for osteoporosis concentration reduced *5948* In 20 postmenopausal women undergoing hormonal replacement therapy mean midregion osteocalcin concentration decreased by 39% *5104*

Phenytoin *Serum Increase Physiological* Coadministration with phenytoin may increase plasma phenytoin concentration *4522* When estrogens ingested with fosphenytoin concentration of phenytoin may be increased *4519*

Platelets *Blood No Effect Physiological* In 4 healthy women aged 50 - 59 years taking estrogens mean concentration of 239 ± 58 x 10^6/L not significantly different from 278 ± 51 x 10^6/L in 12 healthy women aged 50 - 59 years not taking estrogens *2959*

Sex-Hormone Binding Globulin
Serum Increase Physiological Plasma concentrations increased by estrogens possibly by regulating hepatic synthesis *5439*

Superoxide Dismutase
Red Blood Cells No Effect Physiological In 3 healthy women aged 50 - 59 years taking estrogens mean concentration of 2839 ± 225 U/g hemoglobin not significantly different from 3360 ± 823 U/g hemoglobin in 12 healthy women aged 50 - 59 years not taking estrogens *2959*

Theophylline *Serum Increase Physiological* Up to 30% increase in serum theophylline concentration in a dose-related manner *6117* Estrogens decrease theophylline clearance in a dose-dependent manner and increases serum theophylline concentration by 30% *3125*

Thyroxine Binding Globulin *Serum Increase Physiological* Increased concentration observed as a physiological response *277*

Thyroxine (T4) *Serum Increase Physiological* Increased concentration observed as a response to physiological increase of TBG *277*

Triglycerides *Serum Increase Physiological* In postmenopausal women administration of 0.625 mg/d for one year caused a significant increase (about 14%) *3628*

VLDL-Cholesterol *Serum Decrease Physiological* Significantly lower in women with natural menopause taking estrogens than in those not taking estrogens *869*

VLDL-Triglycerides *Serum Increase Physiological* General effect of oral treatment on VLDL, but not observed in all cases of treatment of postmenopausal women *3628*

Estropipate

Alanine Aminotransferase *Serum Increase Physiological* Administration of estrogens may cause cholestatic jaundice *4443*

Alkaline Phosphatase *Serum Increase Physiological* Administration of estrogens may cause cholestatic jaundice *4443*

Amylase *Serum Increase Physiological* Administration may lead to massive increases in concentration in patients with familial hyperlipoproteinemia with pancreatitis as a complication *4682* Administration of estrogens may lead to massive increases in concentration in patients with familial defects of lipoprotein metabolism leading to pancreatitis and other complications *4443*

Angiotensinogen *Serum Increase Physiological* Administration of estrogens increases concentration *4443*

Anti-Factor Xa *Plasma Decrease Physiological* Administration of estrogens may lead to decreased concentration *4443* Administration may decrease concentration *4682*

Estropipate *(continued)*

Antithrombin *Plasma Increase Physiological* Administration may lead to dose- and duration-related hypercoagulability, primarily related to decreased antithrombin activity *4682*

Antithrombin III *Plasma Decrease Physiological* Administration of estrogens may lead to decreased concentration *4443* Administration may decrease concentration *4682*

Antithrombin III Activity *Plasma Decrease Physiological* Administration of estrogens may lead to hypercoagulability primarily related to decreased antithrombin activity *4443* Administration may decrease concentration *4682*

α_1-Antitrypsin *Serum Increase Physiological* Administration of estrogens increases concentration *4443*

Aspartate Aminotransferase *Serum Increase Physiological* Administration of estrogens may cause cholestatic jaundice *4443*

Bilirubin *Serum Increase Physiological* Administration of estrogens may cause cholestatic jaundice *4443*

Calcium *Serum Decrease Physiological* Administration of estrogens may lead to severe hypercalcemia in patients with breast cancer and bone metastases *4443*
Serum Increase Physiological Administration may lead to severe hypercalcemia in patients with breast cancer and bone metastases *4682*

Ceruloplasmin *Serum Increase Physiological* Administration of estrogens increases concentration *4443*

Cholesterol *Serum No Effect Physiological* Insignificant reduction from mean baseline of 232 mg/dL to 216 mg/dL in 6 postmenopausal women treated with 1.25 mg/d for 6 months *323*

Cholesterol, Free *Serum Decrease Physiological* Significant reduction observed from mean baseline of 73.4 mg/dL to 53.7 mg/dL in 6 postmenopausal women treated with 1.25 mg/d for 6 months *323*

Corticosteroid-Binding Globulin
Serum Increase Physiological Administration of estrogens increases concentration *4443*

Factor II *Plasma Increase Physiological* Administration of estrogens may lead to increased concentration *4443* Administration may increase concentration *4682*

Factor II-Factor VII-Factor X Complex
Plasma Increase Physiological Administration of estrogens may lead to increased concentration *4443* Administration may increase concentration *4682*

Factor VII Antigen *Plasma Increase Physiological* Administration of estrogens may lead to increased concentration *4443* Administration may increase concentration *4682*

Factor VII-Factor X Complex
Plasma Increase Physiological Administration of estrogens may lead to increased concentration *4443* Administration may increase concentration *4682*

Factor VIII Antigen *Plasma Increase Physiological* Administration of estrogens may lead to increased concentration *4443* Administration may increase concentration *4682*

Factor VIII Coagulant *Plasma Increase Physiological* Administration of estrogens may lead to increased concentration *4443* Administration may increase concentration *4682*

Factor IX *Plasma Increase Physiological* Administration of estrogens may lead to increased concentration *4443* Administration may increase concentration *4682*

Factor X *Plasma Increase Physiological* Administration may increase concentration *4682* Administration of estrogens may lead to increased concentration *4443*

Factor XII *Plasma Increase Physiological* Administration may increase concentration *4682* Administration of estrogens may lead to increased concentration *4443*

Fibrinogen *Plasma Increase Physiological* Administration of estrogens may lead to increased concentration *4443* Administration may increase concentration *4682*

Fibrinogen Activity *Plasma Increase Physiological* Administration may increase concentration *4682* Administration of estrogens may lead to increased activity *4443*

Folate *Serum Decrease Physiological* Administration of estrogens decreases concentration *4443* Administration of estrogens may decrease concentration *4682*

Glucose Tolerance *Serum Decrease Physiological* Administration of estrogens may decrease glucose tolerance *4682* Administration of estrogens decreases glucose tolerance *4443*

γ-Glutamyltransferase *Serum Increase Physiological* Administration of estrogens may cause cholestatic jaundice *4443*

HDL_2-Cholesterol *Serum Increase Physiological* Administration of estrogens may increase concentration *4682* Administration of estrogens increases concentration *4443*

HDL-Cholesterol *Serum Increase Physiological* Administration of estrogens increases concentration *4443* Administration of estrogens may increase concentration *4682*
Serum No Effect Physiological Insignificant decrease from mean baseline of 57.8 mg/dL to 55.6 mg/dL in 6 postmenopausal women treated with 1.25 mg/d for 6 months *323*

LDL-Cholesterol *Serum Decrease Physiological* Administration of estrogens may decrease concentration *4682* Administration of estrogens decreases concentration *4443*

Lecithin *Serum Increase Physiological* Significant increase from mean baseline of 2.12 mg/dL to 2.47 mg/dL in 6 postmenopausal women treated with 1.25 mg/d for 6 months *323*

Lipase *Serum Increase Physiological* Administration of estrogens may lead to massive increases in concentration in patients with familial defects of lipoprotein metabolism leading to pancreatitis and other complications *4443* Administration may lead to massive increases in concentration in patients with familial hyperlipoproteinemia with pancreatitis as a complication *4682*

Metyrapone Test *Patient Decrease Physiological* Administration of estrogens decreases response to metyrapone test *4443*

Partial Thromboplastin Time
Plasma Decrease Physiological Administration of estrogens may lead to accelerated partial thromboplastin time *4443* Administration may accelerate time *4682*

Plasminogen Activity *Plasma Increase Physiological* Administration of estrogens may lead to increased activity *4443* Administration may increase concentration *4682*

Plasminogen Antigen *Plasma Increase Physiological* Administration may increase concentration *4682* Administration of estrogens may lead to increased concentration *4443*

Platelet Aggregation *Blood Decrease Physiological* Administration of estrogens may lead to accelerated platelet aggregation *4443*
Blood Increase Physiological Administration may accelerate platelet aggregation time *4682*

Platelets *Blood Increase Physiological* Administration of estrogens may lead to increased platelet count *4443* Administration may increase platelet count *4682*

Prothrombin Time *Plasma Decrease Physiological* Administration of estrogens may lead to accelerated prothrombin time *4443* Administration may accelerate time *4682*

Sex-Hormone Binding Globulin
Serum Increase Physiological Administration of estrogens increases concentration *4443*

T3-Uptake *Serum Decrease Physiological* Administration of estrogens may lead to reduced uptake due to increased TBG concentration *4443* Administration of estrogens may increase concentration of TBG and reduce T3-uptake *4682*

β-Thromboglobulin *Plasma Increase Physiological* Administration may increase concentration *4682* Administration of estrogens may lead to increased concentration *4443*

Thyroxine Binding Globulin *Serum Increase Physiological* Administration of estrogens may increase concentration *4682* Administration of estrogens may lead to increased concentration *4443*

Thyroxine (T4) *Serum Increase Physiological* Administration of estrogens may lead to increased concentration due to increased TBG concentration *4443* Administration of estrogens may increase concentration of TBG and that of total thyroxine *4682*

Thyroxine (T4), Free *Serum No Effect Physiological* Administration of estrogens may increase concentration of TBG and reduce total T4concentration, but has no effect on free T4 *4682* Administration of estrogens has no effect on free hormone concentration although total concentration is increased because of increased TBG concentration *4443*

Tri-iodothyronine, Free (fT3)
Serum No Effect Physiological Administration of estrogens may increase concentration of TBG and reduce total T3concentration, but has no effect on free T3 *4682* Administration of estrogens has no effect on free hormone concentration although total concentration is increased because of increased TBG concentration *4443*

Tri-iodothyronine (T3) *Serum Increase Physiological* Administration of estrogens may increase concentration of TBG and that of triiodothyronine *4682*

Triglycerides *Serum Increase Physiological* Administration may lead to massive increases in concentration in patients with familial hyperlipoproteinemia *4682* Administration of estrogens may lead to massive increases in concentration in patients with familial defects of lipoprotein metabolism *4443* Administration of estrogens increases concentration *4443*
Serum No Effect Physiological Insignificant increase from mean baseline concentration of 135 mg/dL to 143 mg/dL observed in 6 postmenopausal women treated with 1.25 mg/d for 6 months *323*

Ethacrynic Acid

Alanine Aminotransferase *Serum Increase Physiological* Administration of ethacrynic acid has rarely caused jaundice and abnormal liver function in a few seriously ill patients receiving multiple drugs *3973* Cholestasis with hepatocellular damage *1246*

Albumin *Serum No Effect Analytical* At 2.5 mg/dL no effect on Technicon SMA 12/60 method *4390*

Alkaline Phosphatase *Serum Increase Physiological* Administration of ethacrynic acid has rarely caused jaundice and abnormal liver function in a few seriously ill patients receiving multiple drugs *3973*
Serum No Effect Analytical At 2.5 mg/dL no effect on Technicon SMA 12/60 method *4390*

Ammonia *Plasma Increase Physiological* ?Due to hypokalemia and alkalosis *2451*

Amylase *Serum Increase Physiological* Isolated case of acute pancreatitis *2451*

Aspartate Aminotransferase *Serum Increase Physiological* Cholestasis with hepatocellular damage *1246* Administration of ethacrynic acid has rarely caused jaundice and abnormal liver function in a few seriously ill patients receiving multiple drugs *3973*
Serum No Effect Analytical At 2.5 mg/dL no effect on Technicon SMA 12/60 method *4390*

Bicarbonate *Serum Increase Physiological* Associated with hypochloremic alkalosis *5394*

Bilirubin *Serum Increase Physiological* Administration of ethacrynic acid has rarely caused jaundice and abnormal liver function in some seriously ill patients receiving multiple drugs including ethacrynic acid *3973* Cholestasis or hepatocellular damage *5394*
Serum No Effect Analytical At 2.5 mg/dL no effect on Technicon SMA 12/60 method *4390*
Serum No Effect Physiological Although *in vitro* effect observed no significant effect at pharmacological concentrations *6314*

Calcium *Serum No Effect Analytical* At 2.5 mg/dL no effect on Technicon SMA 12/60 method *4390*
Urine Increase Physiological Impaired reabsorption *4555*

Casts *Urine Increase Physiological* Hyaline casts without proteinuria (orosomucoid) *2814*

Chloride *Serum Decrease Physiological* Diuretic action (inhibits tubular reabsorption) *4555* Administration of ethacrynic acid may cause hyponatremia, hypokalemia and/or hypochloremic alkalosis *3973*
Urine Increase Physiological Present as major anion *2242*

Cholesterol *Serum No Effect Analytical* At 2.5 mg/dL no effect on Technicon SMA 12/60 method *4390*

Color *Feces Increase Analytical* Black color reported with ethacrynic acid ingestion *3388*

Cortisol *Plasma No Effect Physiological* No effect observed with therapy *4014*
Urine Decrease Physiological ?due to changed secretion or renal handling *2451*

Creatinine *Serum No Effect Analytical* At 2.5 mg/dL no effect on Technicon SMA 12/60 method *4390*

Erythrocytes *Urine Increase Physiological* Rare case of hematuria reported *2754*

Glomerular Filtration Rate *Urine No Effect Physiological* Administration of ethacrynic acid has little or no effect on the GFR unless the plasma volume has been substantially reduced *3973*

Glucose *Serum Decrease Physiological* Administration of ethacrynic acid caused acute symptomatic hypoglycemia with convulsions in two uremic patients *3973* Symptomatic hypoglycemia reported *5394*
Serum Increase Physiological Diabetogenic properties *5869* Administration of ethacrynic acid has caused hyperglycemia *3973*
Serum No Effect Analytical At 2.5 mg/dL no effect on Technicon SMA 12/60 method *4390*
Urine Increase Physiological Diabetogenic properties *5869*

Glucose Tolerance *Serum Decrease Physiological* Diabetogenic-like action of drug *4555*

Granulocytes *Blood Decrease Physiological* Administration of ethacrynic acid has rarely caused agranulocytosis or severe neutropenia in a few seriously ill patients receiving multiple drugs including ethacrynic acid *3973*

Histamine *Plasma No Effect Analytical* Improbable inhibition of radio-enzyme assay at therapeutic concentrations *2492*

Insulin *Plasma Decrease Physiological* Reduction in fasting state noted *4014*

Lactate Dehydrogenase *Serum No Effect Analytical* At 2.5 mg/dL no effect on Technicon SMA 12/60 method *4390*

Leukocytes *Blood Decrease Physiological* Agranulocytosis *6313*

Lithium *Serum Increase Physiological* Administration of ethacrynic acid may reduce lithium clearance thereby increasing the plasma lithium concentration *3973*

Lithium Clearance *Urine Decrease Physiological* Administration of ethacrynic acid may reduce lithium clearance thereby increasing the plasma lithium concentration *3973*
Urine No Effect Physiological A single dose of the drug has no effect on lithium clearance *4399*

Magnesium *Serum Decrease Physiological* Administration of ethacrynic acid may cause increased excretion of magnesium with resultant decreased plasma concentration *3973*
Urine Increase Physiological Increase up to seven times reported *2451* Administration of ethacrynic acid may cause increased excretion of magnesium with resultant decreased plasma concentration *3973*

Neutrophils *Blood Decrease Physiological* Occasional case of agranulocytosis reported *6264* Occasional neutropenia or agranulocytosis *4014* Administration of ethacrynic acid has rarely caused agranulocytosis or severe neutropenia in a few seriously ill patients receiving multiple drugs including ethacrynic acid *3973*

Occult Blood *Feces Increase Physiological* One case reported (26% if given i.v. possibly) *581*

pH *Blood Increase Physiological* Administration of ethacrynic acid may cause hyponatremia, hypokalemia and/or hypochloremic alkalosis *3973* Hypochloremic alkalosis may occur *5394*

Phosphate *Serum No Effect Analytical* At 2.5 mg/dL no effect on Technicon SMA 12/60 method *4390*
Urine No Effect Physiological No effect observed on excretion *6309*

Platelets *Blood Decrease Physiological* Thrombocytopenia reported *4555* Administration of ethacrynic acid has rarely caused thrombocytopenia. Henoch-Schölein purpura has been reported rarely in patients with rheumatic heart disease *3973*

Potassium *Serum Decrease Physiological* Diuretic action *5869* Administration of ethacrynic acid may cause hyponatremia, hypokalemia and/or hypochloremic alkalosis *3973*
Urine Increase Physiological Marked diuretic response may occur *2451*

Protein *Serum No Effect Analytical* At 2.5 mg/dL no effect on Technicon SMA 12/60 method *4390*

Ethacrynic Acid *(continued)*

Prothrombin Time *Plasma Increase Physiological* Displaces coumarins from albumin *5440* Administration of ethacrynic acid may cause displacement of warfarin from plasma protein thereby increasing the plasma PT *3973*

Renal Blood Flow *Patient No Effect Physiological* Administration of ethacrynic acid has little or no effect on the RBF unless the plasma volume has been substantially reduced *3973*

Sodium *Serum Decrease Physiological* Administration of ethacrynic acid may cause hyponatremia, hypokalemia and/or hypochloremic alkalosis *3973* Diuretic action *3810*
Urine Increase Physiological Therapeutic intent *5394*

Urea Nitrogen *Serum Increase Physiological* Administration of ethacrynic acid may cause transient increases in concentration, usually reversible when the drug is discontinued *3973* May cause deterioration if renal function impaired *139*

Uric Acid *Serum Decrease Physiological* If given i.v. in large doses has uricosuric effect *5783*
Serum Increase Physiological Administration of ethacrynic acid may cause reversible hyperuricemia and gout *3973* Decreased urate clearance with low doses *5869*
Serum No Effect Analytical At 2.5 mg/dL no effect on Technicon SMA 12/60 method *4390*
Urine Decrease Physiological Decreased urate clearance *1714*
Urine Increase Physiological If given i.v. in large doses has uricosuric effect *5783*

Volume *Plasma Decrease Physiological* Initial diuretic response may cause hypovolemia *174*
Urine Increase Physiological Therapeutic intent *5394*

Zinc *Urine Increase Physiological* When given i.v. brief effect only *5782*

Ethambutol

Alanine Aminotransferase *Serum Increase Physiological* In 72 patients with tuberculosis all receiving isoniazid and rifampin and, in addition, pyrazinamide in 72.2%, ethambutol in 80% and streptomycin in 16.7% drug-induced hepatitis observed with AST activity reaching mean of 330.2 ± 425.5 U/L *5577* Transient impairment of liver function has been reported as a side effect *3466* Decreased liver function reported *128*

Alkaline Phosphatase *Serum Increase Physiological* Transient impairment of liver function has been reported as a side effect *3466*

Aspartate Aminotransferase *Serum Increase Physiological* Transient impairment of liver function has been reported as a side effect *3466* In 72 patients with tuberculosis all receiving isoniazid and rifampin and, in addition, pyrazinamide in 72.2%, ethambutol in 80% and streptomycin in 16.7% drug-induced hepatitis observed with AST activity reaching mean of 428.4 ± 666.0 U/L *5577* Decreased liver function reported *128*

Bilirubin *Serum Increase Physiological* In 72 patients with tuberculosis all receiving isoniazid and rifampin and, in addition, pyrazinamide in 72.2%, ethambutol in 80% and streptomycin in 16.7% drug-induced hepatitis observed with bilirubin concentration reaching mean of 5.34 ± 4.68 mg/dL *5577* Transient impairment of liver function has been reported as a side effect *3466*

BSP Retention *Serum Increase Physiological* Few cases reported *4014*

Creatinine *Serum Increase Physiological* Rare case of renal damage reported *198*
Serum No Effect Analytical No effect of concentrations up to 15 mg/L on single slide method on Kodak Ektachem® *5706*

Creatinine Clearance *Urine Decrease Physiological* Rare case of renal damage reported *198*

Diazepam *Serum No Effect Physiological* No significant effect observed on clearance in normal volunteers *4354*

Histamine *Plasma No Effect Analytical* Minimal inhibition of radio-enzyme assay at concentration 20 times therapeutic *2492*

Iron *Serum No Effect Analytical* At a concentration of 50 µg/mL had no significant effect on Ferrochem II method (mean concentration 9.90 µmol/L versus 9.91 µmol/L in controls) and 11.58 µmol/L by atomic absorption versus 11.40 µmol/L in controls *5217*

Phentolamine Test *Patient Increase Physiological* False positive, mechanism unknown *1999*

Urea Nitrogen *Serum Increase Physiological* Rare renal damage reported *198*

Uric Acid *Serum Increase Physiological* Due to decreased renal clearance, usually occurs by third week of treatment *4758* In 66% patients with tuberculosis when combined with streptomycin and isoniazid not seen when same drugs given with thioacetazone, during first 60-90 d of treatment. Reverted to normal when ethambutol withdrawn *3128* Increased uric acid and precipitation of gout have been reported as side effects *3466* May occur within 24 h, by decreasing clearance *4758*
Urine Decrease Physiological Decreases clearance but mechanism not known *4758*

Ethamivan

Carbon Dioxide Partial Pressure
Blood Decrease Physiological Increased depth of respiration and improved pulmonary ventilation *128*

Ethamsylate

Creatinine *Serum Decrease Analytical* In patients in whom ethamsylate ingested peroxidase-coupled enzymatic method (Ono Pharmaceutical Co.) gave falsely low value (by about 11-23%) compared with kinetic Jaffe method *1994* In one patient with renal dysfunction taking ethamsylate to to stabilize capillary vessels mean concentration observed to be 22 mg/L by an automated POD-coupled method compared with 83 mg/L as measured by Jaffe reaction-rate method on Beckman Astra® 8, 79 mg/L by a deproteinized Jaffe method, and 85 mg/L by a coupled-enzyme ultraviolet absorbance method (Boehringer Mannheim Co) *3740*

Phenytoin *Serum No Effect Analytical* At a concentration of 3 mg/dL had no significant effect on phenytoin concentrations up to 30 µg/mL with method on Johnson and Johnson Ektachem® systems *6356*

Ethanediol

Ionized Calcium *Serum Decrease Analytical* At 0.1-1.0 mol/L with calcium specific electrode *820*

Ethaverine

Alanine Aminotransferase *Serum No Effect Analytical* No effect at therapeutic concentration on Boehringer Mannheim Reflotron method *3231* No effect at 2 mg/L on Boehringer Mannheim Reflotron method *5706*

Amylase *Serum No Effect Analytical* At concentration of 2 mg/L had no effect on method on Boehringer Mannheim Reflotron system *5706*

Amylase, Pancreatic Isoenzyme
Serum No Effect Analytical No significant effect observed at toxic concentration of 2 mg/L on method on Boehringer Mannheim Reflotron *3647*

Aspartate Aminotransferase *Serum No Effect Analytical* No effect at therapeutic concentration on Boehringer Mannheim Reflotron method *3231* No effect at 2 mg/L on Boehringer Mannheim Reflotron method *5706*

Bilirubin *Serum No Effect Analytical* At concentration of 2 mg/L had no effect on method on Boehringer Mannheim Reflotron system *5706*

Cholesterol *Serum No Effect Analytical* At concentration of 2 mg/L no effect on method on Boehringer Mannheim Reflotron system *5706* No effect at therapeutic concentration on Boehringer Mannheim Reflotron method *3231*

Glucose *Serum No Effect Analytical* At concentration of 2 mg/L no effect on method on Boehringer Mannheim Reflotron system *5706* No effect at therapeutic concentration on Boehringer Mannheim Reflotron method *3231* At concentration of 400 mg/L had no effect on hexokinase/G-6-PDH method *5704*

γ-Glutamyltransferase *Serum No Effect Analytical* At concentration of 2 mg/L no effect on method on Boehringer Mannheim Reflotron system *5706* No effect at therapeutic concentration on Boehringer Mannheim Reflotron method *3231*

Lactate *Plasma No Effect Analytical* At concentration of 400 mg/L had no effect on enzymatic method *5704*

Triglycerides *Serum No Effect Analytical* No effect at therapeutic concentration on Boehringer Mannheim Reflotron method *3231* No effect at 2 mg/L on Boehringer Mannheim Reflotron method *5706*

Urea Nitrogen *Serum No Effect Analytical* No effect at therapeutic concentration on ehringer Mannheim Reflotron method *3231* No effect at 2 mg/L on Boehringer Mannheim Reflotron method *5706*

Uric Acid *Serum No Effect Analytical* No effect at 2 mg/L on method on Boehringer Mannheim Reflotron *5706* No effect at therapeutic concentration on Boehringer Mannheim Reflotron method *3231*

Ethchlorvynol

Alanine Aminotransferase *Serum Increase Physiological* Occurs with poisoning, probable muscle origin *6545*
Serum No Effect Analytical At acute overdose concentration (20 mg/dL) on Technicon method *6266*

Albumin *Serum No Effect Analytical* At concentration of 400 mg/L had no effect on BCG method *5704* At acute overdose concentration (20 mg/dL) on Technicon method *6266*

Alkaline Phosphatase *Serum No Effect Analytical* At acute overdose concentration (20 mg/dL) on Technicon method *6266*

Aspartate Aminotransferase *Serum Increase Physiological* Occurs with poisoning, probable muscle origin *6545*
Serum No Effect Analytical At acute overdose concentration (20 mg/dL) on Technicon method *6266*

Benzodiazepine Screen *Serum No Effect Analytical* No significant interference observed at a concentration of 300 µg/mL (2.07 mmol/L) with method on Du Pont aca *1512*

Bicarbonate *Serum No Effect Analytical* At concentration of 400 mg/L had no effect on method using phenolphthalein *5704*

Bilirubin *Serum No Effect Analytical* At acute overdose concentration (20 mg/dL) on Technicon method *6266* At concentration of 400 mg/L had no effect on Jendrassik and Grof method *5704*

Calcium *Serum No Effect Analytical* At acute overdose concentration (20 mg/dL) on Technicon method *6266* At concentration of 400 mg/L had no effect on cresolphthalein method *5704*

Chloride *Serum No Effect Analytical* At concentration of 400 mg/L had no effect on mercurimetric method *5704*

Cholesterol *Serum No Effect Analytical* At acute overdose concentration (20 mg/dL) on Technicon method *6266* At concentration of 400 mg/L had no effect on Liebermann-Burchard method *5704*

Creatine Kinase *Serum Increase Physiological* Occurs with poisoning, probable muscle origin *6545*
Serum No Effect Analytical At acute overdose concentration (20 mg/dL) on Technicon method *6266*

Creatinine *Serum No Effect Analytical* At acute overdose concentration (20 mg/dL) on Technicon method *6266* At concentration of 400 mg/L had no effect on Technicon AutoAnalyzer® Jaffe method *5704*

Ethchlorvynol *Serum Increase Physiological* 200 mg orally may produce concentration of 2 mg/L in blood *3868*
Urine Increase Physiological 200 mg orally may produce concentration of 1 mg/L *3868*

Glucose *Serum No Effect Analytical* At acute overdose concentration (20 mg/dL) on Technicon method *6266*

Iron *Serum No Effect Analytical* At acute overdose concentration (20 mg/dL) on Technicon method *6266* At concentration of 400 mg/L had no effect on Ferrozine method *5704*

Lactate Dehydrogenase *Serum No Effect Analytical* At acute overdose concentration (20 mg/dL) on Technicon SMAC® method *6266*

Phosphate *Serum No Effect Analytical* At acute overdose concentration (20 mg/dL) on Technicon method *6266* At concentration of 400 mg/L had no effect on phosphomolybdate method *5704*

Platelets *Blood Decrease Physiological* Administration associated with fatal immune thrombocytopenia in one patient *26* One case of fatal immune thrombocytopenia described *1384*

Potassium *Serum No Effect Analytical* At concentration of 400 mg/L had no effect on measurement by ISE with predilution *5704*

Protein *Serum No Effect Analytical* At concentration of 400 mg/L had no effect on biuret method with blank correction *5704* At acute overdose concentration (20 mg/dL) on Technicon method *6266*

Prothrombin Time *Plasma Decrease Physiological* Administration with coumarin anticoagulants may decrease prothrombin time *26* Decreased potency of coumarin anticoagulants (enzyme induction) *2949*

Sodium *Serum No Effect Analytical* At concentration of 400 mg/L had no effect on measurement by ISE with predilution *5704*

Tricyclic Antidepressants Screen
Serum No Effect Analytical No significnat effect observed at a concentration of 500 µg/mL (3.46 mmol/L) with method on Du Pont aca *1550*

Triglycerides *Serum No Effect Analytical* At concentration of 400 mg/L had no effect on lipase/esterase method *5704* At acute overdose concentration (20 mg/dL) on Technicon method *6266*

Urea Nitrogen *Serum No Effect Analytical* At acute overdose concentration (20 mg/dL) on Technicon method *6266* At concentration of 400 mg/L had no effect on diacetylmonoxime method *5704*

Uric Acid *Serum No Effect Analytical* At concentration of 400 mg/L had no effect on phosphotungstate reduction method *5704* At acute overdose concentration (20 mg/dL) on Technicon method *6266*

Ether

Alanine Aminotransferase *Serum Increase Physiological* Hepatic disturbance (transient) *3810*

Alkaline Phosphatase *Serum Increase Physiological* Hepatic disturbance (transient) *5401*

Antidiuretic Hormone *Plasma Increase Physiological* Effect in moderate to deep anesthesia *2242*

Aspartate Aminotransferase *Serum Increase Physiological* Hepatic disturbance (transient) *5401*

Bile *Urine Increase Physiological* Hepatic disturbance (transient) *3810*

Bilirubin *Serum Increase Physiological* Hepatic disturbance (transient) *5401*

Bleeding Time *Patient No Effect Physiological* Anesthesia has no effect *2242*

Bogen Test *Urine Positive Analytical* Reacts as if ethanol *2183*

BSP Retention *Serum Increase Physiological* Hepatic disturbance (transient) *3810*

Capillary Fragility *Patient No Effect Physiological* Anes`thesia has no effect *2242*

Carbon Dioxide Partial Pressure
Blood Decrease Physiological May be slight effect during anesthesia *2242*

Catecholamines *Plasma Decrease Analytical* Falsely low with ethylenediamine method *3766*
Plasma Increase Physiological Response to stress *4784*

Cholesterol *Serum Increase Physiological* Reportedly may cause hypercholesterolemia *2452*

Clotting Time *Blood No Effect Physiological* No effect of anesthesia *2242*

Cortisol *Plasma Increase Physiological* Effect observed in moderate to deep anesthesia *2242*

Ether *(continued)*

Effective Renal Plasma Flow
Patient Decrease Physiological Probably due to renal vasoconstriction *2242*

Epinephrine *Plasma Increase Physiological* Response to stress *4784*

Glomerular Filtration Rate *Urine Decrease Physiological* Due to renal vasoconstriction *2242*

Glucose *Serum Increase Physiological* Metabolic effect (transient effect) *6605*
Urine Increase Physiological Due to hyperglycemia *3810*

Insulin *Plasma Decrease Physiological* Due to release of epinephrine causing inhibition *6605*

Ketones *Urine Increase Physiological* May follow anesthesia *2452*

Lactate *Plasma Increase Physiological* Metabolic effect *6605*

Leukocytes *Blood Increase Physiological* Normal response to anesthesia *409*

Norepinephrine *Plasma Increase Physiological* Response to stress *4784*

pH *Blood Decrease Physiological* Metabolic acidosis especially in children *128*

Phosphate *Serum Decrease Physiological* Observed after most types of anesthesia *2242*

Platelets *Blood No Effect Physiological* Anesthesia has no effect *2242*

Protein *Urine Increase Physiological* May cause nephrotoxicity *5377*

Prothrombin Time *Plasma No Effect Physiological* Anesthesia has no effect *2242*

Pyruvate *Plasma Increase Physiological* Metabolic effect *6605*

Sugar *Urine Increase Analytical* May cause positive Benedict's and Fehling's tests *467*

Thyroxine (T4) *Serum Increase Physiological* Effect observed in moderate to deep anesthesia *2242*

Urea Nitrogen *Serum Increase Physiological* May cause nephrotoxicity *5377*

Volume *Urine Decrease Physiological* Due to vasoconstriction *128*

Ethinamate

Alanine Aminotransferase *Serum No Effect Analytical* At acute overdose concentration (20 mg/dL) on Technicon SMAC® method *6266*

Albumin *Serum No Effect Analytical* At acute overdose concentration (20 mg/dL) on Technicon SMAC® method *6266* At concentration of 200 mg/L had no effect on BCG method *5704*

Alkaline Phosphatase *Serum No Effect Analytical* At acute overdose concentration (20 mg/dL) on Technicon SMAC® method *6266*

Aspartate Aminotransferase *Serum No Effect Analytical* At acute overdose concentration (20 mg/dL) on Technicon SMAC® method *6266*

Bilirubin *Serum No Effect Analytical* At concentration of 200 mg/L had no effect on Jendrassik and Grof method *5704* At acute overdose concentration (20 mg/dL) on Technicon SMAC® method *6266*

Calcium *Serum No Effect Analytical* At acute overdose concentration (20 mg/dL) on Technicon SMAC® method *6266* At concentration of 200 mg/L had no effect on cresolphthalein method *5704*

Cholesterol *Serum No Effect Analytical* At concentration of 200 mg/L had no effect on Liebermann-Burchard method *5704* At acute overdose concentration (20 mg/dL) on Technicon SMAC® method *6266*

Creatine Kinase *Serum No Effect Analytical* At acute overdose concentration (20 mg/dL) on Technicon SMAC® method *6266*

Creatinine *Serum No Effect Analytical* At concentration of 200 mg/L had no effect on Technicon AutoAnalyzer® Jaffe method *5704* At acute overdose concentration (20 mg/dL) on Technicon SMAC® method *6266*

Glucose *Serum No Effect Analytical* At acute overdose concentration (20 mg/dL) on Technicon SMAC® method *6266*

17-Hydroxycorticosteroids *Urine Increase Analytical* Minimum effect with Glenn-Nelson method *2451*

Iron *Serum No Effect Analytical* At acute overdose concentration (20 mg/dL) on Technicon SMAC® method *6266* At concentration of 200 mg/L had no effect on Ferrozine method *5704*

Lactate Dehydrogenase *Serum No Effect Analytical* At acute overdose concentration (20 mg/dL) on Technicon SMAC® method *6266*

Phosphate *Serum No Effect Analytical* At concentration of 200 mg/L had no effect on phosphomolybdate method *5704* At acute overdose concentration (20 mg/dL) on Technicon SMAC® method *6266*

Platelets *Blood Decrease Physiological* Throbocytopenic purpura and fever have been reported occasionally *1384* Thrombocytopenia (AMA Blood dyscrasias) *4017*

Protein *Serum No Effect Analytical* At acute overdose concentration (20 mg/dL) on Technicon SMAC® method *6266* At concentration of 200 mg/L had no effect on biuret method with blank correction *5704*

Sugar *Urine Increase Analytical* Theoretical effect as excreted as glucuronide *2242*

Triglycerides *Serum No Effect Analytical* At concentration of 200 mg/L had no effect on lipase/esterase method *5704* At acute overdose concentration (20 mg/dL) on Technicon SMAC® method *6266*

Urea Nitrogen *Serum No Effect Analytical* At concentration of 200 mg/L had no effect on diacetylmonoxime method *5704* At acute overdose concentration (20 mg/dL) on Technicon SMAC® method *6266*

Uric Acid *Serum No Effect Analytical* At concentration of 200 mg/L had no effect on phosphotungstate reduction method *5704* At acute overdose concentration (20 mg/dL) on Technicon SMAC® method *6266*

Ethinyl Estradiol

Cortisol *Plasma Increase Physiological* In 7 girls aged 13 years treatment with 0.5 mg/d caused increase from mean baseline of 145 ± 90 µg/L to 510 ± 40 µg/L *1104*

Estradiol *Plasma Decrease Physiological* In 7 girls aged 13 years treatment with 0.5 mg/d caused reduction from mean baseline of 36 ± 2.0 pg/mL to 17 ± 1.6 pg/mL *1104*
Plasma No Effect Analytical At a concentration of 20 ng/mL had less than 1.0% cross-reactivity with method on Bayer Technicon Immuno 1® *422*

Follicle Stimulating Hormone
Plasma Decrease Physiological Administration of 20 µg/d for 3 months to 7 postmenopausal women caused decrease from mean of 36 ± 2 mIU/mL to 15 ± 3 mIU/mL *2632* In 7 girls aged 13 years treatment with 0.5 mg/d caused reduction from mean baseline of 1.2 ± 0.04 µg/L to < 0.6 µg/L *1104*

Growth Hormone *Plasma Increase Physiological* In 7 postmenopausal women mean concentration increased to 7.0 ± 0.6 U/mL from 2.0 ± 0.4 U/mL when 20 µg/d administered. Significant increase in mean nadir concentration observed and rise in GH concentration characterized by increased pulse amplitude *2632* Oral administration to postmenopausal women significantly increased mean concentration from 2.0 ± 0.4 mIU/mL to 7.0 ± 2.5 mIU/mL but transdermal administration did not affect 24-hour growth hormone secretion *6397*

Insulin-like Growth Factor-I *Serum Decrease Physiological* Oral administration to postmenopausal women significantly reduced circulating concentration from 0.70 ± 0.09 U/mL to 0.47 ± 0.04 U/mL *6397* In 7 postmenopausal women administration of 20 µg/d caused decrease from mean of 0.70 ± 0.09 U/mL to 0.47 ± 0.04 U/mL *2632*
Serum Increase Physiological Transdermal administration significantly increased concentration in postmenopausal women from mean of 0.96 ± 0.15 U/mL to 1.10 ± 0.14 U/mL, comparable to concentrations observed in premenopausal women *6397*

Luteinizing Hormone *Plasma Decrease Physiological* In 7 postmenopausal women administration of 20 μg/d caused decrease from mean of 44 ± 4 mIU/mL to 18 ± 5 mIU/mL *2632* In 7 girls aged 13 years treatment with 0.5 mg/d caused reduction from mean baseline of 2.0 ± 0.2 μg/L to < 1.1 μg/L *1104*

Melatonin *Plasma Decrease Physiological* In 7 girls aged 13 years treatment with 0.5 mg/d caused reduction from mean maximum baseline of about 88 ng/L to about 70 ng/mL *1104*

Ethionamide

Alanine Aminotransferase *Serum Increase Physiological* Intrahepatic bile duct damage, toxic hepatitis *3324*

Alkaline Phosphatase *Serum Increase Physiological* Hepatotoxic effect *3810*
Urine Decrease Analytical Interference with determination procedure *4826*

Aspartate Aminotransferase *Serum Increase Physiological* Intrahepatic cholestatic jaundice *2242*

Bile *Urine Increase Physiological* Hepatotoxic effect *3810*

Bilirubin *Serum Increase Physiological* Hepatotoxicity in about 2% cases *2451*

BSP Retention *Serum Increase Physiological* Hepatotoxic effect *3810*

Glucose *Serum Increase Physiological* Hyperglycemia reported *3669*
Urine Increase Physiological Due to hyperglycemia *3669*

Lactate Dehydrogenase *Urine Decrease Analytical* Interference with determination procedure *4826*

Thyroxine (T4) *Serum Decrease Physiological* Antithyroid effect after several weeks *2451*

Xylose *Urine Decrease Physiological* May cause gastrointestinal irritation, impaired absorption and subsequent reduced excretion *929*

Ethoheptazine

Phenylalanine *Plasma No Effect Analytical* No interference observed with rapid quantitative whole blood method of Campbell et al using phenylalanine dehydrogenase *867*

Ethosuximide

Albumin *Serum No Effect Analytical* At concentration of 390 mg/L had no effect on BCG method *5704*

Antinuclear Antibodies *Serum Increase Physiological* Related to number of drugs, higher in women *6411*

Aspartate Aminotransferase *Serum Increase Physiological* Increased in one third cases *4014*

Bicarbonate *Serum No Effect Analytical* At concentration of 390 mg/L had no effect on method using phenolphthalein *5704*

Bilirubin *Serum Increase Physiological* Rare idiosyncratic hepatitis reported *128*
Serum No Effect Analytical At concentration of 390 mg/L had no effect on Jendrassik and Grof method *5704*
Serum No Effect Physiological Insignificant displacement of protein in neonates *6314*

Blood *Urine Increase Physiological* Reported to cause microscopic hematuria as side effect *4533*

Calcium *Serum No Effect Analytical* At concentration of 390 mg/L had no effect on cresolphthalein method *5704*

Carbamazepine *Serum No Effect Analytical* Cross reactivity of about 0.05% observed with method on Baxter Stratus *5705* No cross-reactivity observed with method on Du Pont aca *1513* At a concentration of 500 μg/mL had no significant cross-reactivity with carbamazepine at a concentration of 4.0 μg/mL when measured by method on Bayer Technicon Immuno 1® system *417*

Chloride *Serum No Effect Analytical* At concentration of 390 mg/L had no effect on mercurimetric method *5704*

Cholesterol *Serum No Effect Analytical* At concentration of 390 mg/L had no effect on Liebermann-Burchard method *5704*

Coombs' Test *Blood Positive Physiological* Mechanism obscure *2453*

Coombs' Test, Direct *Blood Positive Physiological* 3 cases reported with SLE and anemia *2452*

Creatinine *Serum No Effect Analytical* At concentration of 390 mg/L had no effect on Technicon AutoAnalyzer® Jaffe method *5704*

Eosinophils *Blood Decrease Physiological* Reported to cause as side effects leukopenia, agranulocytosis, pancytopenia, with or without bone marrow suppression, and eosinophilia *4533*
Blood Increase Physiological Rare eosinophilia reported *128*

Erythrocytes *Blood Decrease Physiological* Aplastic anemia/pancytopenia *3810* Reported to cause as side effects leukopenia, agranulocytosis, pancytopenia, with or without bone marrow suppression, and eosinophilia *4533*

Felbamate *Serum No Effect Analytical* No significant interference observed with GLC method of Rifai et al *4958*

Glucaric Acid *Urine Increase Physiological* Induces hepatic enzymes *2782*

Granulocytes *Blood Decrease Physiological* Reported to cause as side effects leukopenia, agranulocytosis, pancytopenia, with or without bone marrow suppression, and eosinophilia *4533*

Hematocrit *Blood Decrease Physiological* Aplastic anemia *128*

Hemoglobin *Blood Decrease Physiological* Aplastic anemia *128*
Urine Increase Physiological Rare side effect observed *3340*

Histamine *Plasma No Effect Analytical* No inhibition of radio-enzyme assay at physiological concentrations *2492*

Indomethacin *Serum No Effect Analytical* No effect on HPLC method of Roberts and Smith *4978*

LE Cells *Blood Positive Physiological* Rare immune response reported *793*

Leukocytes *Blood Decrease Physiological* Reported to cause as side effects leukopenia, agranulocytosis, pancytopenia, with or without bone marrow suppression, and eosinophilia *4533* Aplastic anemia/pancytopenia/Leukopenia in 10% *128*

Mycophenolic Acid *Serum No Effect Analytical* No significant interference observed with HPLC method of Shipkova et al *5526*

Mycophenolic Acid Glucuronide
Serum No Effect Analytical No significant interference observed with HPLC method of Shipkova et al *5526*

Neutrophils *Blood Decrease Physiological* Reported to cause as side effects leukopenia, agranulocytosis, pancytopenia, with or without bone marrow suppression, and eosinophilia *4533* Occasional case of agranulocytosis reported *6264*

Phenobarbital *Serum No Effect Analytical* At concentration of 500 μg/mL (3542 μmol/L) has no effect on method on Du Pont Dimension *1582* No significant cross-reactivity observed with method on Du Pont aca *1537*

Phenylalanine *Plasma No Effect Analytical* No interference observed with rapid quantitative whole blood method of Campbell et al using phenylalanine dehydrogenase *867*

Phenytoin *Serum Increase Physiological* When ethosuximide ingested with fosphenytoin concentration of phenytoin may be increased *4519* May be increased plasma levels (impaired metabolism) *4011*
Serum No Effect Analytical No significant interference observed at a concentration of 1000 μg/mL (7.08 mmol/L) with method on Du Pont aca *1538* No effect at concentration of 1000 μg/mL (7.08 mmol/L) on method on Du Pont Dimension *1583*

Phosphate *Serum No Effect Analytical* At concentration of 390 mg/L had no effect on phosphotungstate reduction method *5704*

Platelets *Blood Decrease Physiological* Aplastic anemia/thrombocytopenia/pancytopenia *128*

Potassium *Serum No Effect Analytical* At concentration of 390 mg/L had no effect on measurement by ISE with predilution *5704*

Ethosuximide *(continued)*

Primidone *Serum* *No Effect* *Analytical* At concentrations exceeding 1250 mg/L causes 25% increase in concentration as measured by method on Baxter Stratus but physiological concentrations up to 100 mg/L only *5705* No significant cross-reactivity with method on Du Pont aca *1541*

Protein *Serum* *No Effect* *Analytical* At concentration of 390 mg/L had no effect on biuret method with blank correction *5704*
Urine *Increase* *Physiological* Possible reversible nephropathy *1714*

SDZ PSC 833 *Blood* *No Effect* *Analytical* At a concentration of 108 mg/L had no effect on HPLC method of Scott et al when used to measure PSC (with CsD as internal standard) at a concentration of 5 mg/L *5418*

Sodium *Serum* *No Effect* *Analytical* At concentration of 390 mg/L had no effect on measurement by ISE with predilution *5704*

Tacrolimus *Blood* *No Effect* *Analytical* No significant effect observed at a concentration of 100 mg/L with MEIA method on Abbott IMx analyzer *1871*
Serum *No Effect* *Analytical* At a concentration of 100 mg/L had no significant effect on ELISA method *6329*

Triglycerides *Serum* *No Effect* *Analytical* At concentration of 390 mg/L had no effect on lipase/esterase method *5704*

Urea Nitrogen *Serum* *Increase* *Physiological* Possible reversible nephropathy *128*
Serum *No Effect* *Analytical* At concentration of 390 mg/L had no effect on diacetylmonoxime method *5704*

Uric Acid *Serum* *No Effect* *Analytical* At concentration of 390 mg/L had no effect on phosphotungstate reduction method *5704*

Valproic Acid *Serum* *No Effect* *Analytical* At concentrations up to 1000 µg/mL had no significant cross-reactivity in valproic acid method on Bayer Technicon Immuno 1® *437*

Ethotoin

Alanine Aminotransferase *Serum* *Increase* *Physiological* Hepatotoxicity *3810*

Alkaline Phosphatase *Serum* *Increase* *Physiological* Probable idiosyncratic hepatitis *3810*

Aspartate Aminotransferase *Serum* *Increase* *Physiological* Hepatotoxicity *3810*

Bile *Urine* *Increase* *Physiological* Hepatotoxicity *3810*

Bilirubin *Serum* *Increase* *Physiological* Probable idiosyncratic hepatitis *3810*

BSP Retention *Serum* *Increase* *Physiological* Probable idiosyncratic hepatitis *3810*

Erythrocytes *Blood* *Decrease* *Physiological* May cause marrow depression or megaloblastic anemia *128*

Leukocytes *Blood* *Decrease* *Physiological* Possible bone marrow depression *128*

MCV *Blood* *Increase* *Physiological* Theoretical effect on folic acid metabolism *2754*

Phenobarbital *Serum* *No Effect* *Analytical* No significant cross-reactivity observed with method on Du Pont aca *1537* At concentration of 1.00 mg/mL (4.90 mmol/L) has no effect on method on Du Pont Dimension *1582*

Phenytoin *Serum* *No Effect* *Analytical* No detectable influence at 40 µg/mL *6029*

Ethoxazene

Alanine Aminotransferase *Serum* *Increase* *Physiological* Hepatotoxic effect *3810*

Alkaline Phosphatase *Serum* *Increase* *Physiological* Hepatotoxic effect *3810*

Aspartate Aminotransferase *Serum* *Increase* *Physiological* Hepatotoxic effect *3810*

Bile *Urine* *Increase* *Analytical* Atypical red color with Bili-Labstix® and Ictotest® *2451*
Urine *Increase* *Physiological* Hepatotoxic effect *3810*

Bilirubin *Serum* *Increase* *Analytical* Postulated production of color with Ehrlich's diazo reaction *139*
Serum *Increase* *Physiological* Hepatotoxic effect *1714*
Urine *Increase* *Physiological* Hepatotoxic effect *1714*

BSP Retention *Serum* *Increase* *Analytical* Increases absorbancy in test, falsely high result *2451*
Serum *Increase* *Physiological* Hepatotoxic effect *4012*

Color *Urine* *Increase* *Analytical* red, pink, orange and rust colors *4012*

Porphyrin, Total *Urine* *Increase* *Analytical* False positive with fluorescent methods *6515*
Urine *Increase* *Physiological* Hepatotoxic effect *1714*

PSP Excretion *Urine* *Increase* *Analytical* Produces interfering background color *1714*

Ethoxycaffeine

Chromosomes *Test Conditions* *Abnormal* *Physiological* Clastogenic in human cells *5484*

Ethoxyethanol

Protein *Urine* *Increase* *Physiological* May cause nephrotoxicity *5377*

Urea Nitrogen *Serum* *Increase* *Physiological* May cause nephrotoxicity *5377*

Ethoxzolamide

Leukocytes *Blood* *Decrease* *Physiological* Leukopenia *3810*

pH *Blood* *Decrease* *Physiological* May cause metabolic acidosis *3669*

Platelets *Blood* *Decrease* *Physiological* Thrombocytopenia *4013*

Potassium *Serum* *Decrease* *Physiological* Probable effect (like acetazolamide) *128*

Uric Acid *Serum* *Increase* *Physiological* Decreases urate clearance *3669*
Urine *Decrease* *Physiological* Decreases urate clearance *3669*

2-Ethyl-2-phenylmalondiamide

Ethosuximide *Serum* *No Effect* *Analytical* Insignificant cross-reactivity observed with method on Du Pont aca *1523*

Phenobarbital *Serum* *No Effect* *Analytical* At concentration of 1.00 mg/mL has no effect on method on Du Pont Dimension *1582* No significant cross-reactivity observed with method on Du Pont aca *1537*

5-Ethyl-5-phenylhydantoin

Phenytoin *Serum* *No Effect* *Analytical* No effect at concentration of 1000 µg/mL (4.897 mmol/L) on method on Du Pont Dimension *1583* No significant interference observed at a concentration of 1000 µg/mL (4.90 mmol/L) with method on Du Pont aca *1538*

Ethyl Biscoumacetate

Platelet Aggregation *Blood* *Decrease* *Physiological* Inhibits if due to ATP, collagen, epinephrine, thrombin *941*

Uric Acid *Serum* *Decrease* *Physiological* Uricosuric action *2378*
Urine *Increase* *Physiological* Uricosuric action *2378*

Ethyl Chloride

Alanine Aminotransferase *Serum* *Increase* *Physiological* May cause liver damage *128*

Aspartate Aminotransferase *Serum* *Increase* *Physiological* May cause liver damage *128*

Bilirubin *Serum Increase Physiological* May cause liver damage *128*

Ethyl Morphine

Opiates *Urine Positive Analytical* Significant cross-reactivity observed with Roche Abuscreen method adapted for use with Olympus AU 5121 and 5131 analyzers *214* Cross-reactivity of over 50% observed with Roche Abuscreen Online procedure when adapted for use with Roche Cobas Fara II analyzer *5547*

Ethylamine

Pyruvate Kinase *Red Blood Cells Decrease Analytical* Most marked with larger side chain *592*

Ethylene

Glucose *Serum Increase Physiological* After prolonged use may be moderate increase *128*

Phosphate *Serum Decrease Physiological* Observed after most forms of anesthesia *467*

Ethylenediamine

Amino Acids *Urine Increase Analytical* Reacts with ninhydrin; extra spot TLC, high voltage electrophoresis *4760*

Ethylestrenol

Haptoglobin *Serum Increase Physiological* Metabolic effect *368*

Plasminogen *Plasma Increase Physiological* Metabolic effect *368*

Sialic Acid *Serum Increase Physiological* Metabolic effect *368*

Ethylphenacemide

Alkaline Phosphatase *Serum Increase Physiological* Frequently occurs *2242*

Glucaric Acid *Urine Increase Physiological* Induces hepatic enzymes (more potent than phenobarbital) *2782*

Leukocytes *Blood Decrease Physiological* Leukopenia reported *2242*

Ethynodiol

Glucose *Serum No Effect Physiological* With doses of 0.25, 0.35, 0.5 mg/d *2225*

Insulin *Plasma No Effect Physiological* With doses of either 0.25, 0.35 or 0.5 mg/d *2225*

Triglycerides *Serum Increase Physiological* Decreased removal from circulation *5869*

Etidocaine

Creatine Kinase *Serum Increase Physiological* Intramuscular injection of drug may cause release of enzyme *274*

Etidronate

Acid Phosphatase, Tartrate Resistant
Serum No Effect Physiological In 14 patients with Paget's disease treatment with etidronate for 6 months caused non-significant mean 7% reduction in concentration *613*

Adenosine Monophosphate *Urine No Effect Physiological* No effect of drug alone *4886*

Alkaline Phosphatase *Serum Decrease Physiological* Steady decline from mean activity of 80 U/L to 69 U/L in 105 postmenopausal women with osteoporosis treated with 400 mg daily for 2 weeks *6367* In 4 children aged 9 to 14 years with cherubism initial normal activity decreased with treatment with diphosphonate etidronate over 9 months *5730* Significant decrease observed observed at 30, 60, 120 and 150 weeks of treatment with 400 mg daily in 33 postmenopausal women with osteoporosis *5837*
Serum No Effect Physiological In 14 patients with Paget's disease treatment with etidronate for 6 months caused non-significant mean 41% reduction in concentration *613*

Alkaline Phosphatase, Bone Isoenzyme
Serum No Effect Analytical At a concentration of 1050 mg/L had no effect on Tandem-MP Ostase method *777* At a concentration of 350 mg/L had no effect on EIA method of Gomez et al *2234*

Calcium *Serum Decrease Physiological* Therapeutic intent when drug administered for hypercalcemia of malignancy. 88% of patients had reductions of 1.0 mg/dL or more. Total serum calcium returned to normal in 63% of patients within 7 days *4015* In majority of patients with hypercalcemia of malignancy when drug given i.v. for 3-5 d *2499* In 12 patients with cancer-associated hypercalcemia treatment with 7.5 mg/kg intravenously daily for 7 days caused significant decrease from mean of 12.5 mg/dL to 9.4 mg/dL *562*
Serum No Effect Physiological In 33 women with postmenopausal osteoporosis administration of 400 mg/d over 150 weeks had no effect on serum calcium *5837* No significant effect observed in 105 postmenopausal women with osteoporosis treated with 400 mg daily for 2 weeks *6367*
Urine Decrease Physiological In 12 patients with cancer-associated hypercalcemia treatment with 7.5 mg/kg intravenously daily for 7 days caused significant reduction from mean baseline of 1200 mg/g creatinine to 400 mg/g creatinine *562* In 4 children aged 9 to 14 years with cherubism initial high concentration decreased with treatment with diphosphonate etidronate over 9 months *5730* Therapeutic intent when drug administered for hypercalcemia of malignancy. Reduced urine calcium becomes apparent after 24 hours *4015*
Urine No Effect Physiological No significant effect on calcium:creatinine ratio in 105 postmenopausal women with osteoporosis treated with 400 mg daily for 2 weeks *6367*

Creatinine *Serum Increase Physiological* Transient mild effect in patients with hypercalcemia of malignancy given drug i.v. for 3-5 d *2499* Occasional mild to moderate increases observed with intravenous infusion for hypercalcemia of malignancy *4015*
Serum No Effect Physiological No significant change observed in 105 postmenopausal women with osteoporosis treated with 400 mg daily for 2 weeks *6367*

Creatinine Clearance *Urine No Effect Physiological* No effect of drug alone *4886*

Deoxypyridinoline *Urine Decrease Physiological* In 4 children aged 9 to 14 years with cherubism initial high concentration decreased with treatment with diphosphonate etidronate over 9 months *5730* In 14 patients with Paget's disease treatment with etidronate for 6 months caused mean 59% reduction in excretion *613*

Deoxypyridinoline, Free *Serum Decrease Physiological* In 14 patients with Paget's disease treatment with etidronate for 6 months caused mean 42% reduction in concentration as measured by Metra Biosystems method *613*

Erythrocytes *Blood Decrease Physiological* Rare reports of pancytopenia in conjunction wth etidronate administration *4798*

Granulocytes *Blood Decrease Physiological* Rare reports of agranulocytosis in conjunction wth etidronate administration *4798*

Hematocrit *Blood Decrease Physiological* Rare reports of pancytopenia in conjunction wth etidronate administration *4798*

Hemoglobin *Blood Decrease Physiological* Rare reports of pancytopenia in conjunction wth etidronate administration *4798*

Hydroxyproline *Urine Decrease Physiological* In 14 patients with Paget's disease treatment with etidronate for 6 months caused mean 45% reduction in excretion *613* In 12 patients with hypercalcemia associated with malignancy treatment with 7.5 mg/kg intravenously daily for 7 days caused significant reduction from mean baseline of 160 mg/g creatinine to

Etidronate *(continued)*

Hydroxyproline *(continued)*
100 mg/g creatinine *562* In 4 children aged 9 to 14 years with cherubism initial high concentration decreased with treatment with diphosphonate etidronate over 9 months *5730*
Urine No Effect Physiological No significant effect on hydroxyproline:creatinine ratio in 105 postmenopausal women with osteoporosis treated with 400 mg daily for 2 weeks *6367*

Leukocytes *Blood Decrease Physiological* Rare reports of pancytopenia in conjunction wth etidronate administration *4798*

N-terminal Telopeptide of Type I Collagen
Serum Decrease Physiological In 14 patients with Paget's disease treatment with etidronate for 6 months caused mean 76% reduction in concentration *613*

Phosphate *Serum Increase Physiological* Significant effect of treatment with etidronate over 150 weeks in 33 postmenopausal women. Effect probably due to increased reabsorption of phosphate in renal tubules *5837* Increases tubular reabsorption, no effect on PTH action *4886* Effect observed when 10-20 mg/kg/d given presumably because of increased renal absorption. Increased concentrations usually revert to normal 2-4 weeks after therapy stopped *1384* Often observed with oral administration at doses of 10 - 20 mg/kg/d occurs less frequently with intravenous medication of patients with hypercalcemia of malignancy, due to increased tubular reabsorption of phosphate in the kidney. Serum concentration usually reverts to normal 2 - 4 weeks after therapy is discontinued *4015*
Serum No Effect Physiological No significant effect observed in 105 postmenopausal women with osteoporosis treated with 400 mg daily for 2 weeks *6367* In 12 patients with hypercalcemia associated with malignancy treatment with 7.5 mg/d intravenously daily for 7 days caused insignificant change from mean baseline of 2.8 mg/dL to 2.6 mg/dL *562*
Urine No Effect Physiological Increases tubular reabsorption, no effect on PTH action *4886*

Phosphate Clearance *Urine Decrease Physiological* Increases tubular reabsorption, no effect on PTH action *4886*

Phosphate, Diffusible *Serum Increase Physiological* Increases tubular reabsorption, no effect on PTH action *4886*

Platelets *Blood Decrease Physiological* Rare reports of pancytopenia in conjunction wth etidronate administration *4798*

Prothrombin Time *Plasma Increase Physiological* Isolated reports of increased prothrombin time when drug coadministered with warfarin *4798*

Pyridinoline *Urine Decrease Physiological* In 14 patients with Paget's disease treatment with etidronate for 6 months caused mean 48% reduction in excretion *613* In 4 children aged 9 to 14 years with cherubism initial high concentration decreased with treatment with diphosphonate etidronate over 9 months *5730*

Pyridinoline Crosslinked Telopeptide of Type I Collagen
Serum Decrease Physiological In 14 patients with Paget's disease treatment with etidronate for 6 months caused mean 14% reduction in concentration *613*
Urine Decrease Physiological In 14 patients with Paget's disease treatment with etidronate for 6 months caused mean 73% reduction in excretion *613*

Pyridinoline, Free *Serum Decrease Physiological* In 14 patients with Paget's disease treatment with etidronate for 6 months caused mean 38% reduction in concentration as measured by Metra Biosystems method *613*

Urea Nitrogen *Serum Increase Physiological* Occasional mild to moderate increases observed with intravenous infusion for hypercalcemia of malignancy *4015*

Etilefrine

Histamine *Plasma No Effect Analytical* Improbable inhibition of radio-enzyme assay at therapeutic concentrations *2492*

Etintidine

Propranolol *Serum Increase Physiological* Significantly increased area under curve and prolonged elimination half-life: also protracted elimination of 4-hydroxypropranolol, an active metabolite *2749*

Etiocholanolone

BSP Retention *Serum Increase Physiological* In almost 50% patients with induced fever *598*

Leukocytes *Blood Increase Physiological* Pyrogen increases number of granulocytes *4014*

Etodolac

Alanine Aminotransferase *Serum Increase Physiological* Administration of etodolac caused borderline increases in about 15% of treated patients. Increases to above 3 times the upper limit of normal observed in about 1% patients *6559*

Aspartate Aminotransferase *Serum Increase Physiological* Administration of etodolac caused borderline increases in about 15% of treated patients. Increases to above 3 times the upper limit of normal observed in approximately 1% of all patients *6559*

Bilirubin *Urine Increase Analytical* Metabolites may cause false positive or atypical result with Ames Multistix and other reagent strip tests and with Ames Ictotest reagent tablets *4034*

Chloride *Urine Decrease Physiological* Both in normal subjects but also to greater extent in individuals with renal insufficiency *699*

Chondrex *Serum No Effect Analytical* Concentrations up to 10 g/L had no significant effect on sandwich-type ELISA procedure of Harvey et al *2491*

Creatinine *Serum No Effect Physiological* No cumulative effect observed over 24 h in individuals with normal renal function or with renal insufficiency when given 500 mg b.i.d. for 4 d *699*

Creatinine Clearance *Urine No Effect Physiological* No cumulative effect observed over 24 h in individuals with normal renal function or with renal insufficiency when given 500 mg b.i.d. for 4 d *699*

Cyclosporine *Serum Increase Physiological* Coadministration of etodolac with cyclosporine caused increased concentration due to an effect on renal prostaglandins *6559*

Digoxin *Serum Increase Physiological* Coadministration of etodolac with digoxin caused increased concentration due to an effect on renal prostaglandins *6559*

Hematocrit *Blood Decrease Physiological* Administration of etodolac may cause anemia due to fluid retention or gastrointestinal blood loss or an incompletely described effect on erythropoietin *6559*

Hemoglobin *Blood Decrease Physiological* Administration of etodolac may cause anemia due to fluid retention or gastrointestinal blood loss or an incompletely described effect on erythropoietin *6559*

Interleukin-6 *Serum Decrease Physiological* In 18 patients with osteoarthritis treatment with 1200 mg/d caused a significant decrease in mean concentration from 398 ± 113 pg/mL to 280 ± 121 pg/mL *5386*

Inulin Clearance *Urine No Effect Physiological* No effect with acute or chronic treatment in individuals with normal renal function but transient reduction in people with renal insufficiency *699*

6-Keto-Prostaglandin $F_{1\alpha}$ *Urine Decrease Physiological* 6-keto- less than 30% in people with normal renal function but about 60% in individuals with renal insufficiency *699*

Ketones *Urine Increase Analytical* Administration of etodolac may cause false positive measurement with dip-stick tests *6559*

Leukocytes *Blood Decrease Physiological* In 18 patients with osteoarthritis treatment with 1200 mg/d caused a significant decrease in mean concentration from 239 /µL to 138 /µL *5386*

Lithium *Serum Increase Physiological* Coadministration of etodolac with lithium caused increased concentration due to an effect on renal prostaglandins *6559*

Methotrexate *Serum Increase Physiological* Coadministration of etodolac with methotrexate caused increased concentration due to an effect on renal prostaglandins *6559*

PAH Clearance *Urine No Effect Physiological* No effect with acute or chronic treatment in individuals with normal renal function but transient reduction in people with renal insufficiency *699*

Potassium *Serum No Effect Physiological* No cumulative effect observed over 24 h in individuals with normal renal function or with renal insufficiency when given 500 mg b.i.d. for 4 d *699*

Prostaglandin E_2 *Plasma Decrease Physiological* In 18 patients with osteoarthritis treatment with 1200 mg/d caused a significant decrease in mean concentration from 4.2 ± 0.3 pg/mL to 3.3 ± 0.4 ng/mL *5386*

Prostaglandins *Urine Decrease Physiological* About 40% reduction in people with normal renal function but 70% in people with renal insufficiency *699*

Prothrombin Time *Plasma No Effect Physiological* Administration of etodolac with warfarin caused reduced protein binding of warfarin but there was no change in the clearance of free warfarin or of the pharmacodynamic effects of warfarin as judged by no effect on the prothrombin time *6559*

Sodium *Urine Decrease Physiological* Both in normal subjects but also to greater extent in individuals with renal insufficiency *699*
Urine No Effect Physiological No cumulative effect observed over 24 h in individuals with normal renal function or with renal insufficiency when given 500 mg b.i.d. for 4 d *699*

Thyroxine (T4) *Serum No Effect Analytical* Using the Ciba-Corning ACS:180 analyzer mean concentration not significantly changed in 1 specimen whose concentration differed by +4% compared with the concentration measured by the Amerlex-M method *5621*

Tumor Necrosis Factor-α *Serum Increase Physiological* In 18 patients with osteoarthritis treatment with 1200 mg/d caused a significant increase in mean concentration from 69 ± 32 pg/mL to 382 ± 142 pg/mL *5386*
Synovial Fluid Increase Physiological In 18 patients with osteoarthritis obese women with polycystic ovary syndrome showed a significant change from 17.37 ± 1.83 nmol/L to 77.99 ± 22.70 nmol/L and in 11 healthy obese women from 20.94 ± 2.17 nmol/L to 59.08 ± 11.99 nmol/L *5386*

Urea Nitrogen *Serum No Effect Physiological* Fewer than 2% patients showed pattern of deviant renal function tests *5471*

Uric Acid *Serum Decrease Physiological* Administration of etodolac may cause slight decreases in concentration (mean decreases of 1 to 2 mg/dL) after 4 weeks of therapy *6559*

Urobilin *Urine Increase Analytical* Administration of etodolac may cause false positive measurement of urobilin due to the presence of interfering phenolic metabolites *6559*

Etofibrate

Apolipoprotein A-I *Serum Increase Physiological* Increased synthesis. Increased activity of lipoprotein lipase by stimulation of muscle lipoprotein lipase synthesis, alteration of capillary endothelial surface and stimulation of apolipoprotein C-II synthesis *264*

Apolipoprotein A-II *Serum Increase Physiological* Increased synthesis. Increased activity of lipoprotein lipase by stimulation of muscle lipoprotein lipase, alteration of capillary endothelial surface and stimulation of apo C-II synthesis *264*

HDL-Cholesterol *Serum Increase Physiological* Increased synthesis of apo A-I and A-II. Increased activity of lipoprotein lipase by stimulation of muscle lipoprotein lipase synthesis, alteration of capillary endothelial surface and stimulation of apo C-II synthesis *264*

Etomidate

Aldosterone *Plasma Decrease Physiological* Clear suppression when induction compared with induction by thiopentone *113*

Corticosterone *Plasma Decrease Physiological* Clear suppression when induction compared with induction by thiopentone *113*

Corticotropin *Plasma Increase Physiological* Nonsignificant increase vs thiopentone-treated controls in 7 men *113* Apparently direct suppressive effect on adrenal cortical function *976*

Cortisol *Plasma Decrease Physiological* Apparently direct suppressive effect on adrenal cortical function *976* Attributable to direct antisteroidogenic effects on adrenal gland *1111* Clear suppression when induction compared with induction by thiopentone *113* Similar effect to that of thiopental but reduction with induction of anesthesia *5423* Subnormal increase observed following surgery during which etomidate was administered to optimize respiratory assistance, despite increases in corticotropin and deoxycortisol secretion, because of selective of adrenal 11β-hydroxylase *3381*

11-Deoxycortisol *Plasma Increase Physiological* Clear effect 3.5 h after induction demonstrating inhibition of 11β-hydroxylation of glucocorticoid and mineralocorticoid intermediates *113*

17-Hydroxyprogesterone *Plasma No Effect Physiological* No significant difference in 7 men given drug in induction dose versus thiopentone *113*

Midazolam *Serum No Effect Analytical* On GC-ECD method of Ha et al *2387*

Progesterone *Plasma No Effect Physiological* No significant difference in 7 men given drug in induction dose versus thiopentone *113*

Etoposide

Adenosine Deaminase Binding Protein
Urine No Effect Physiological No effect in 12 children given drug for 2 d *2255*

Alanine Aminotransferase *Serum Increase Physiological* Hepatic toxicity may occur, especially in patients receiving higher doses of the drug than recommended *275* Hepatic toxicity reported in 3% treated patients *191*

Albumin *Serum Decrease Physiological* In 28 patients with solid tumors treatment with etoposide and cisplatin on 3 alternate days was associated with mean concentration of 3.5 ± 0.4 g/dL, remaining at lower end of normal range *5822*

Alkaline Phosphatase *Serum Increase Physiological* Hepatic toxicity may occur, especially in patients receiving higher doses of the drug than recommended *275* Hepatic toxicity reported in 3% treated patients *191*

Aspartate Aminotransferase *Serum Increase Physiological* Hepatic toxicity reported in 3% treated patients *191* Hepatic toxicity may occur, especially in patients receiving higher doses of the drug than recommended *275* In 28 patients with solid tumors treatment with etoposide and cisplatin on 3 alternate days for one week was associated with increased activity to mean of 109 ± 200 U/L although increased activity present in some before treatment *5822*

Bilirubin *Serum Increase Physiological* Hepatic toxicity reported in 3% treated patients *191* In 28 patients with solid tumors treatment with cisplatin and etoposide on 3 alternate days during one week was associated with significantly increased concentration of 2.5 ± 5.4 mg/dL although several had increases prior to treatment *5822* Hepatic toxicity may occur, especially in patients receiving higher doses of the drug than recommended *275*

Carcinoembryonic Antigen *Serum No Effect Analytical* At a concentration of up to 415.2 µg/mL caused less than 10% error in the concentration of CEA as measured by the method on Bayer Technicon Immuno 1® *418* At a concentration of up to 48.0 µg/mL caused less than 10% error in the concentration of CEA as measured by the method on Bayer Technicon Immuno 1® *418*

Creatinine *Serum No Effect Physiological* In 28 patients with solid tumors who received treatment with cisplatin and etoposide for 3 alternate days for one week concentration of 0.86 ± 0.18 mg/dL remained within normal range *5822*

Creatinine Clearance *Urine Decrease Physiological* In 24 patients with solid tumors treatment with etoposide and cisplatin on 3 alternate days caused mean concentration to remain at lower end of normal range, 82.8 ± 27.8 mL/min/1.73 sq m *5822*

Etoposide *(continued)*

Erythrocytes *Blood Decrease Physiological* Myelosuppression is dose related and dose limiting with platelet nadirs occurring 9 to 16 days after drug administration. Anemia observed in 0 - 30% treated patients *275*

γ-Glutamyltransferase *Serum Increase Physiological* Hepatic toxicity may occur, especially in patients receiving higher doses of the drug than recommended *275*

Granulocytes *Blood Decrease Physiological* Myelosuppression is dose related and dose limiting with granulocyte nadirs occurring 7 to 14 days after drug administration *275*

Leukocytes *Blood Decrease Physiological* Dose-limiting noncumulative leukopenia in 60-90% patients *191* In 28 patients with solid tumors treatment with etoposide and cisplatin on 3 alternate days during one week was associated with significant decrease from mean baseline of 8764 ± 4840 /µL to 3157 ± 2137 /µL *5822* Occurs 7-10 d after therapy started: recovery occurs by day 20 to 24 *5581* 12 of 37 patients had transient leukopenia for 3-4 d *6532* Myelosuppression is dose related and dose limiting with platelet nadirs occurring 9 to 16 days after drug administration. Leukopenia of less than 1000 /µL observed in 3 - 17% treated patients and less than 4,000 /µL in 60 - 91% patients *275*

Neutrophils *Blood Decrease Physiological* Nadir at 7 to 14 d after administration *191*

Ondansetron *Serum No Effect Physiological* Coadministration with ondansetron had no effect on its pharmacokinetics *2181*

Platelets *Blood Decrease Physiological* In 28 patients with solid tumors treatment on 3 alternate days within cisplatin and etoposide was associated with significant decrease from mean baseline of 318,600 /µL ± 124,000 /µL to 175,400 ± 97,900 /µL *5822* Occurs 9-13 d after therapy started *5581* Myelosuppression is dose related and dose limiting with platelet nadirs occurring 9 to 16 days after drug administration. Thrombocytopenia of less than 50,000 /µL observed 1 - 30% treated patients and less than 100,000 /µL in 22 - 41% patients *275* Nadir at 9 to 16 d after administration *191*

Blood No Effect Physiological In all of 37 patients given drug orally *6532*

Uric Acid *Serum Increase Analytical* Values of more than 3 times uricase values with direct phosphotungstate method *3842*

Serum No Effect Analytical No effect on uricase method on Du Pont aca at therapeutic concentration *3842*

Etozoline

Alanine Aminotransferase *Serum No Effect Physiological* No effect in 17 hypertensive patients treated for 6 months with 200 mg daily *809*

Apolipoprotein A-I *Serum No Effect Physiological* Non-significant increase over 6 months with treatment with 200 mg daily in 17 hypertensive patients *809*

Apolipoprotein B *Serum No Effect Physiological* No effect of treatment for 6 months with 200 mg daily in 17 hypertensive patients *809*

Aspartate Aminotransferase
Serum No Effect Physiological No effect of treatment of 17 hypertensive patients with 200 mg daily for 6 months *809*

Cholesterol *Serum No Effect Physiological* No significant effect of treatment with 200 mg daily for 6 months in 17 hypertensive patients *809*

Creatinine *Serum No Effect Physiological* No effect of treatment with 200 mg daily for 4 months in 17 hypertensive patients *809*

Creatinine Clearance *Urine No Effect Physiological* No significant effect of treatment with 200 mg daily over 6 months in 17 hypertensive patients *809*

Glucose *Serum No Effect Physiological* No effect of 200 mg daily for 6 months in 17 hypertensive patients *809*

HDL_2-Cholesterol *Serum Increase Physiological* Significant increase from 20.5 mg/dL to 26.4 mg/dL in 17 hypertensive patients treated with 200 mg daily for 6 months *809*

HDL-Cholesterol *Serum No Effect Physiological* No significant effect in 17 hypertensive patients treated with 200 mg daily for 6 months although general trend towards increase *809*

HDL-Triglycerides *Serum No Effect Physiological* No significant effect of treatment of 17 hypertensive patients with 200 mg daily for 6 months *809*

LDL-Cholesterol *Serum No Effect Physiological* No significant effect in 17 hypertensive patients treated with 200 mg daily for 6 months although a general trend towards reduction *809*

LDL-Triglycerides *Serum No Effect Physiological* No significant effect in 17 hypertensive patients treated for 6 months with 200 mg daily *809*

Potassium *Serum No Effect Physiological* No effect of 200 mg daily for 6 months in 17 hypertensive patients *809*

Sodium *Serum No Effect Physiological* No effect of treatment for 6 months with 200 mg daily in 17 hypertensive patients *809*

Triglycerides *Serum No Effect Physiological* No significant effect of treatment for 6 months with 200 mg daily in 17 hypertensive patients *809*

Urea Nitrogen *Serum No Effect Physiological* No effect of 200 mg daily for 6 months in 17 hypertensive patients *809*

Uric Acid *Serum No Effect Physiological* No effect of 200 mg daily for 6 months in 17 hypertensive patients *809*

VLDL-Cholesterol *Serum No Effect Physiological* No significant effect in 17 hypertensive patients treated with 200 mg daily for 6 months *809*

VLDL-Triglycerides *Serum No Effect Physiological* No significant effect in 17 hypertensive patients treated with 200 mg daily for 6 months *809*

Etretinate

Acetone *Urine Increase Physiological* Acetonuria observed in 1 to 10% of treated patients *5033*

Alanine Aminotransferase *Serum Increase Physiological* Increased activity observed in 10 to 25% of treated patients *5033* In 2 of 20 patients treated for 1 y *3037* In one 74-year old woman treated for severe psoriasis: normalized with withdrawal of therapy and recurred when reinstituted *6396* Reversible increase reported in 15-25% patients *1384*

Albumin *Serum Decrease Physiological* Increased or decreased concentration observed in 1 to 10% of treated patients *5033*

Serum Increase Physiological Increased or decreased concentration observed in 1 to 10% of treated patients *5033*

Alkaline Phosphatase *Serum Increase Physiological* Hepatitis observed in from 1 to 10% of treated patients *5033* In one 74-year old woman treated for severe psoriasis: normalized with withdrawal of therapy and recurred when reinstituted *6396* Increased activity observed in 10 to 25% of treated patients *5033*

Apolipoprotein A-I *Serum No Effect Physiological* In 13 patients with hyperkeratotic disorders given 50 mg daily for 2 mo *6150*

Apolipoprotein A-II *Serum No Effect Physiological* In 13 patients with hyperkeratotic disorders given 50 mg daily for 2 mo *6150*

Apolipoprotein B *Serum Increase Physiological* From 133 to 147% in 13 patients with hyperkeratotic disorders given 50 mg daily for 2 mo *6150*

Aspartate Aminotransferase *Serum Increase Physiological* Reversible increase reported in 15-25% patients *1384* Increased activity observed in 10 to 25% of treated patients *5033* In 2 of 20 patients treated for 1 y *3037* In one 74-year old woman treated for severe psoriasis: normalized with withdrawal of therapy and recurred when reinstituted *6396*

Bicarbonate *Serum Decrease Physiological* Increased or decreased concentration observed in 10 to 25% of treated patients *5033*

Serum Increase Physiological Increased or decreased concentration observed in 10 to 25% of treated patients *5033*

Bilirubin *Serum Increase Physiological* No marked effect seen but slight change noted *6500* Increased concentration observed in 1 to 10% of treated patients *5033* Hepatitis observed in from 1 to 10% of treated patients *5033*

Serum *No Effect* *Analytical* At concentration of 1.2 mg/L had no effect on method on Kodak Ektachem® *5706*
Serum *No Effect* *Physiological* In 2 of 20 patients treated for 1 y *3037*

Bilirubin, Conjugated *Serum* *No Effect* *Analytical* No effect at concentration of 1.2 mg/L on method on Kodak Ektachem® *5706*

Bilirubin, Unconjugated *Serum* *No Effect* *Analytical* No effect at concentration of 1.2 mg/L on method on Kodak Ektachem® *5706*

Blood *Urine* *Increase* *Physiological* Microscopic hematuria observed in 1 to 10% of treated patients *5033*

Calcium *Serum* *Decrease* *Physiological* Increased or decreased concentration observed in 25 to 50% of treated patients *5033*
Serum *Increase* *Physiological* Increased or decreased concentration observed in 25 to 50% of treated patients *5033*

Casts *Urine* *Increase* *Physiological* Increased excretion observed in 1 to 10% of treated patients *5033*

Chloride *Serum* *Decrease* *Physiological* Increased or decreased concentration observed in 10 to 25% of treated patients *5033*
Serum *Increase* *Physiological* Increased or decreased concentration observed in 10 to 25% of treated patients *5033*

Cholesterol *Serum* *Increase* *Physiological* From 5.75 to 6.05 mmol/L in 13 patients with hyperkeratotic disorders given 50 mg daily for 2 mo *6150* In 4 of 11 patients who showed hypertriglyceridemia: effect slight but measured over 1 y therapy *3037* Increased concentration observed in 10 to 25% of treated patients *5033*

Creatine Kinase *Serum* *Increase* *Physiological* Increased activity observed in 10 to 25% of treated patients *5033*

Creatinine *Serum* *Increase* *Physiological* Increased concentration observed in 1 to 10% of treated patients *5033*

Eosinophils *Blood* *Increase* *Physiological* In one 74-year old woman treated for severe psoriasis: normalized with withdrawal of therapy and recurred when reinstituted *6396*

Erythrocyte Sedimentation Rate
Blood *Increase* *Physiological* Increased rate observed in 25 to 50% of treated patients *5033*

Erythrocytes *Blood* *Decrease* *Physiological* No marked effect seen but slight change noted *6500*
Blood *Increase* *Physiological* Increased concentration observed in 1 to 10% of treated patients *5033*

Globulin *Serum* *Increase* *Physiological* Increased concentration observed in 10 to 25% of treated patients *5033*

Glucose *Serum* *Decrease* *Physiological* Increased or decreased concentration observed in 10 to 25% of treated patients *5033*
Serum *Increase* *Physiological* Increased or decreased concentration observed in 10 to 25% of treated patients *5033*
Urine *Increase* *Physiological* Increased excreion observed in 1 to 10% of treated patients *5033*

γ-Glutamyltransferase *Serum* *Increase* *Physiological* In 2 of 20 patients treated for 1 y *3037* Increased activity observed in 10 to 25% of treated patients *5033*

HDL-Cholesterol *Serum* *Decrease* *Physiological* Decrease observed in about half treated patients *1384* Decreased concentration observed in 37% of 652 patients with keratosis or a disorder of keratinization treated in clinical trials *5033*
Serum *No Effect* *Physiological* In 13 patients with hyperkeratotic disorders given 50 mg daily for 2 mo *6150*

HDL-Triglycerides *Serum* *No Effect* *Physiological* In 13 patients with hyperkeratotic disorders given 50 mg daily for 2 mo *6150*

Hematocrit *Blood* *Decrease* *Physiological* Decrease observed in 10 to 25% of treated patients *5033*

Hemoglobin *Blood* *Decrease* *Physiological* Decrease observed in 10 to 25% of treated patients *5033*
Blood *Increase* *Physiological* Increased concentration observed in 1 to 10% of treated patients *5033* Increase observed in 1 to 10% of treated patients *5033*
Urine *Increase* *Physiological* Hemoglobinuria observed in 1 to 10% of treated patients *5033*

High Density Lipoproteins *Serum* *Decrease* *Physiological* Decrease observed in about half treated patients *1384*

Interferon-γ *Serum* *Decrease* *Physiological* In 8 patients with psoriasis treated with 1.6 mg/kg/d for 12 weeks caused increased concentration at beginning of treatment to return to mean baseline (less than 0.02 U/mL) within the first 2 weeks of therapy *5521*

Interleukin-1α *Serum* *No Effect* *Physiological* In 8 patients with psoriasis treatment with 1.6 mg/kg/d for 12 weeks caused no significant change from mean baseline in spite of clnical improvement *5521*

Lactate Dehydrogenase *Serum* *Increase* *Physiological* Reversible increase reported in 15-25% patients *1384* In one 74-year old woman treated for severe psoriasis: normalized with withdrawal of therapy and recurred when reinstituted *6396*

LDL-Cholesterol *Serum* *Increase* *Physiological* From 3.82 to 4.16 mmol/L in 13 patients with hyperkeratotic disorders given 50 mg daily for 2 mo *6150*

Leukocytes *Blood* *Decrease* *Physiological* Increased or decreased concentration of leukocytes and components observed in 10 to 25% of treated patients *5033*
Blood *Increase* *Physiological* Increased or decreased concentration of leukocytes and components observed in 10 to 25% of treated patients *5033*
Urine *Increase* *Physiological* Increased excreion observed in 10 to 25% of treated patients *5033*

MCH *Blood* *Decrease* *Physiological* Decreased concentration observed in 1 to 10% of treated patients *5033*
Blood *Increase* *Physiological* Increased concentration observed in 25 to 50% of treated patients *5033*

MCHC *Blood* *Decrease* *Physiological* Decreased concentration observed in 1 to 10% of treated patients *5033*
Blood *Increase* *Physiological* Increased concentration observed in 60% of treated patients *5033*

MCV *Blood* *Decrease* *Physiological* Decrease observed in 10 to 25% of treated patients *5033*

Methotrexate *Serum* *Increase* *Physiological* In 6 patients with psoriasis concomitant treatment with etretinate increased mean maximum methotrexate concentration from 721 nmol/L to 992 nmol/L after intramuscular administration of 0.2 mg/kg body weight of methotrexate *3418*

Occult Blood *Feces* *Increase* *Physiological* Melena observed in less than 1% of treated patients *5033*

Partial Thromboplastin Time
Plasma *Decrease* *Physiological* Decreased time observed in 1 to 10% of treated patients *5033*
Plasma *Increase* *Physiological* Increased time observed in 25 to 50% of treated patients *5033*

Phosphate *Serum* *Decrease* *Physiological* Increased or decreased concentration observed in 25 to 50% of treated patients *5033*
Serum *Increase* *Physiological* Increased or decreased concentration observed in 25 to 50% of treated patients *5033*

Platelets *Blood* *Decrease* *Physiological* Decreased time observed in 1 to 10% of treated patients *5033*
Blood *Increase* *Physiological* Increased concentration observed in 10 to 25% of treated patients *5033*

Potassium *Serum* *Decrease* *Physiological* Increased or decreased concentration observed in 25 to 50% of treated patients *5033*
Serum *Increase* *Physiological* Increased or decreased concentration observed in 25 to 50% of treated patients *5033*

Protein *Serum* *Decrease* *Physiological* Increased or decreased concentration observed in 1 to 10% of treated patients *5033*
Serum *Increase* *Physiological* Increased or decreased concentration observed in 1 to 10% of treated patients *5033*
Urine *Increase* *Physiological* Increased excreion observed in 1 to 10% of treated patients *5033*

Prothrombin Time *Plasma* *Decrease* *Physiological* Increased or decreased time observed in 10 to 25% of treated patients *5033*
Plasma *Increase* *Physiological* Increased or decreased time observed in 10 to 25% of treated patients *5033*

Reticulocytes *Blood* *Increase* *Physiological* Increased concentration observed in 25 to 50% of treated patients *5033*

Sodium *Serum* *Decrease* *Physiological* Increased or decreased concentration observed in 10 to 25% of treated patients *5033*

Etretinate *(continued)*

Sodium *(continued)*
Serum Increase Physiological Increased or decreased concentration observed in 10 to 25% of treated patients *5033*

Triglycerides *Serum Increase Physiological* Observed in about half the treated patients *1384* In 11 of 20 patients but not to more than 2 times normal over 1 y *3037* Increased concentration observed in 25 to 50% of treated patients *5033*
Serum No Effect Physiological In 13 patients with hyperkeratotic disorders given 50 mg daily for 2 mo *6150*

Tumor Necrosis Factor-α *Serum Decrease Physiological* In 8 patients with psoriasis treatment with 1.6 mg/kg/d for 12 weeks caused gradual decrease of concentration concurrent with clinical improvement *5521*

Urea Nitrogen *Serum Increase Physiological* Increased concentration observed in 1 to 10% of treated patients *5033*

VLDL-Cholesterol *Serum No Effect Physiological* In 13 patients with hyperkeratotic disorders given 50 mg daily for 2 mo *6150*

VLDL-Triglycerides *Serum No Effect Physiological* In 13 patients with hyperkeratotic disorders given 50 mg daily for 2 mo *6150*

Evans Blue

Color *Urine Increase Analytical* Blue color due to presence of dye *703*

Thyroxine (T4) *Serum Decrease Physiological* Compete for binding sites *882*

Exemestane

Dehydroepiandrosterone Sulfate
Plasma Decrease Physiological In 56 postmenopausal women with advanced breast cancer administration of 12.5, 5 and 2.5 mg/day caused significant reductions from mean baselines of 886, 979 and 1076 ng/mL to 726, 804 and 1061 ng/mL respectively after 14 days *6663*
Plasma Increase Physiological In 56 postmenopausal women with advanced breast cancer administration of 25 mg/day caused increase from mean baseline of 869 ng/mL to 7964 ng/mL after 14 days *6663*

Estradiol *Plasma Decrease Physiological* In 56 postmenopausal women with advanced breast cancer administration of 25, 12.5, 5 and 2.5 mg/day caused significant reductions from mean baselines of 15.3, 18.9, 20.6 and 12.6 pmol/L to 5.3, 5.8, 5.7 and 6.0 pmol/L respectively after 14 days *6663*

Estrone *Plasma Decrease Physiological* In 56 postmenopausal women with advanced breast cancer administration of 25, 12.5, 5 and 2.5 mg/day caused significant reductions from mean baselines of 71.0, 91.9, 98.4 and 75.2 pmol/L to 34.4, 30.9, 30.6 and 33.1 pmol/L respectively after 14 days *6663*

Estrone Sulfate *Plasma Decrease Physiological* In 56 postmenopausal women with advanced breast cancer administration of 25 mg/day caused significant change from mean baseline of 606 pmol/L to 159, 164, 150 and 190 pmol/L respectively after 7, 14, 28 and 56 days *6663*

Follicle Stimulating Hormone
Plasma Increase Physiological In 56 postmenopausal women with advanced breast cancer administration of 2.5 to 25 mg/day caused slight increase from mean baseline *6663*

17-Hydroxycorticosteroids *Urine No Effect Physiological* In 56 postmenopausal women with advanced breast cancer administration of 12.5, 5 and 2.5 mg/day caused no significant change from mean baselines of 5.1, 6.8, 5.8 and 6.3 ng/mL to 5.7, 6.8, 5.7 and 5.4 μmol/12 h respectively after 14 days *6663*

Luteinizing Hormone *Plasma Increase Physiological* In 56 postmenopausal women with advanced breast cancer administration of 2.5 to 25 mg/day caused slight increase from mean baseline *6663*

Sex-Hormone Binding Globulin
Serum Decrease Physiological In 56 postmenopausal women with advanced breast cancer administration of 25, 12.5, 5 and 2.5 mg/day caused significant reductions from mean baselines of 60.7, 64.0, 78.1 and 54.1 nmol/L to 48.5, 53.4, 76.9 and 47.9 nmol/L respectively after 14 days *6663*

Factor VIII Concentrate

Haptoglobin *Serum Decrease Physiological* Of factor VIII-deficient hemophiliacs 19 (39%) had reduced haptoglobin concentration. 46% of patients receiving only monoclonally purified factor VIII products had reduced concentration. Hypohaptoglobulinemia may be due to dissolution of hematomas etc *792*

Factor IX Complex, Human

Alkaline Phosphatase *Serum Increase Physiological* 62% of cases developed hepatitis after use *4392*

Aspartate Aminotransferase *Serum Increase Physiological* 62% cases developed hepatitis after use *4392*

Bilirubin *Serum Increase Physiological* 62% cases developed hepatitis after use *4392*

Factor VIIa

Antithrombin III *Plasma Decrease Physiological* In 10 cirrhotics mean concentration unchanged after doses of 5 μg/kg, 20 μg/kg and 80 μg/kg *519*

D-Dimer *Plasma Decrease Physiological* In 2 of 10 cirrhotics with extremely high mean concentrations administration of factor VIIa decreased after doses of 20 μg/kg and 80 μg/kg *519*
Plasma Increase Physiological In 8 of 10 cirrhotics administration of factor VIIa increased concentration at 6 h after doses of 80 μg/kg *519*

Fibrinogen *Plasma Decrease Physiological* In 10 cirrhotics mean concentration unchanged after doses of 5 μg/kg, 20 μg/kg and 80 μg/kg *519*

Fibrinopeptide A *Plasma Increase Physiological* In 10 cirrhotics administration of factor VIIa increased concentration at 6 h after doses of 80 μg/kg *519*

Partial Thromboplastin Time
Plasma Decrease Physiological In 10 cirrhotics mean time normalized after doses of 20 μg/kg and 80 μg/kg *519*
Plasma No Effect Physiological In 10 cirrhotics mean time of about 40 s unaffected after a dose of 5 μg/kg *519*

Platelets *Blood Decrease Physiological* In 10 cirrhotics mean number unchanged after doses of 5 μg/kg, 20 μg/kg and 80 μg/kg *519*

Prothrombin Fragment 1.2 *Plasma Increase Physiological* In 10 cirrhotics administration of factor VIIa had no effect on concentration after doses of 5 or 20 μg/kg *519* In 10 cirrhotics administration of factor VIIa increased concentration at 2 and 4 h after doses of 80 μg/kg *519*

Prothrombin Time *Plasma Decrease Physiological* In 10 cirrhotics mean time at least 2 s greater than the upper limit of normal but after a dose of 5 μg/kg mean PT normalized for 2 h, after 20 μg/kg normalized for 6 h and after 80 μg/kg normalized for 12 h *519*

Fadrozole

Aldosterone *Plasma Decrease Physiological* In 8 healthy men administration of 4 mg/d for 13 days caused significant reduction from mean basal concentration of 102.9 ± 16.6 pmol/Lto 59.1 ± 13.9 pmol/L *6077* In 16 postmenopausal women receiving 16 mg/day for 2 weeks significant reduction in basal and ACTH-stimulated production observed. Basal concentration reduced from about 310 pmol/L to 100 pmol/L with 16 mg/day and to 180 pmol/L with 8 mg/day/for 2 weeks *1377*
Plasma No Effect Physiological At a dose of 1-2 mg/d CGS 16949A inhibits aromatase but does not alter aldosterone production *1377* In 54 postmenopausal women treatment with up to 4.0 mg/d for 12 weeks caused nonsignificant reduction (of the order of 10%) *5263*

Androstenedione *Plasma Increase Physiological* In 26 postmenopausal women with advanced metastatic breast cancer treatment with fadrozole (CGS 169 49A) caused increase from mean baseline of 2.1 nmol/L to 3.0 nmol/L after 1 month, but change not significant over next 11 months *5891* In 54 postmenopausal women with breast cancer treatment for 12 weeks caused significant increase to about 165% of baseline with 1.8 mg/d, to 160% of baseline with 2.0 mg/d and 150% of baseline with 4.0 mg/d *5263*

Cortisol *Plasma No Effect Physiological* In 8 healthy men administration of 4 mg/d for 13 days caused no significant difference from mean baseline of 302.4 ± 41.4 nmol/L to 306.2 ± 50.0 nmol/L *6077* In 54 postmenopausal women with breast cancer treatment with up to 4.0 mg/d for 12 weeks had no significant effect on concentration (reduction of about 6% observed) *5263*

Urine Decrease Physiological In 54 postmenopausal women with breast cancertreatment with 1.8 mg/d for 12 weeks caused approximately 20% reduction although reduction with higher doses less *5263*

Urine No Effect Physiological No significant difference observed between excretions of 174 ± 29.0 nmol/d before treatment and 178.8 ± 33.9 nmol/d after 13 days treatment with mg/d for 13 days *6077*

Cortisol response to ACTH

Plasma Decrease Physiological At a dose of 16 mg/d in postmenopausal women with metastatic breast cancer cortisol response to ACTH significantly blunted *1377*

Estradiol *Plasma Decrease Physiological* In 54 postmenopausal women treatment with 4.0 mg/d caused significant reduction from mean baseline of 48 pmol/L to 22 pmol/L after 2 weeks (decrease of 67-78% from mean baseline observed with different doses) *5263* In 8 healthy men administration of 4 mg/d for 13 days caused significant decrease from mean baseline of 84.4 ± 13.2 pmol/L at 08:00 h to 68.2 ± 10.3 pmol/L *6077*

Urine Decrease Physiological In 54 postmenopausal women with breast cancer treatment with 4.0 mg/d caused significant reduction from baseline of 4.5 nmol/d to 1.5 nmol/d after 2 weeks (decrease of 47-53% observed with different doses) *5263*

Estrone *Plasma Decrease Physiological* In 8 healthy men treatment with 4 mg/d for 13 days caused significant decrease of 08:00 h concentration from mean 109.1 ± 10.7 pmol/L to mean of 52.9 ± 8.5 pmol/L *6077* In 54 postmenopausal women with breast cancer treatment with 4.0 mg/d caused signifcant decrease from mean baseline of 155 pmol/L to 55 pmol/L after 2 weeks (decrease of 42-51% from basal concentration observed with different doses) *5263* In 26 postmenopausal women with advanced metastatic breast cancer treatment with fadrozole (CGS 169 49A) caused decrease from mean baseline of 120 pmol/L to 68 pmol/L after 1 month, 70 pmol/L after 6 months and 60 pmol/L after 12 months *5891*

Urine Decrease Physiological In 54 postmenopausal women with breast cancer treatment with up to 4.0 mg/d caused significant reduction from 12.0 nmol/d to 2.0 nmol/d after 2 weeks (decrease of 33-39% observed with different doses) *5263*

Estrone Sulfate *Plasma Decrease Physiological* In 26 postmenopausal women with advanced metastatic breast cancer treatment with fadrozole (CGS 169 49A) caused decrease from mean baseline of 1300 pmol/L to 800 pmol/L after 1 month, 700 pmol/L after 6 months and 800 pmol/L after 12 months *5891* In 54 postmenopausal women with breast cancer treatment with 4.0 mg/d caused significant reduction from mean baseline of 1150 pmol/L to 400 pmol/L after 2 weeks (decrease of 40-50% from baseline observed with different doses) *5263*

17-Hydroxyprogesterone *Plasma Increase Physiological* In 54 postmenopausal women with breast cancer treatment for 12 weeks with 1.8 mg/d caused increase to 115% of baseline, with 2.0 mg/d to 122% and with 4.0 mg/d to 145% of baseline *5263*

Potassium *Serum No Effect Physiological* No significant change observed in 16 postmenopausal women treated with up to 16 mg daily for 12 weeks *1377* In 54 postmenopausal women with breast cancer treatment with up to 4.0 mg/d caused no significant effect *5263* In 8 healthy men treatment with 4 mg/d caused no significant effect on concentration *6077*

Renin Activity *Plasma Increase Physiological* In 8 healthy men administration of 4 mg/d for 13 days caused significant increase from mean 09:00 h baseline concentration of 0.28 ± 0.03 ng/L/s to 0.47 ± 0.08 ng/L/s *6077* Nonsignificant increase observed in 16 postmenopausal women receiving 16 mg/day for 2 weeks (mean baseline 1.13 ng/mL/h, final concentration 2.56 ng/mL/h) *1377*

Renin Concentration *Plasma Increase Physiological* In 54 postmenopausal women with breast cancer treatment for 12 weeks with 1.8 mg/d caused increase from 1.72 ± 0.84 ng/mL to 3.00 ± 0.76 ng/mL, from 1.09 ± 0.35 ng/mL to 6.4 ± 3.5 ng/mL with 2 mg/d and from 1.35 ± 0.42 ng/mL to 3.38 ± 0.61 ng/mL with 4 mg/d *5263*

Sex-Hormone Binding Globulin

Serum Decrease Physiological In 26 postmenopausal women with advanced metastatic breast cancer treatment with fadrozole (CGS 169 49A) caused decrease from mean baseline of 90 nmol/L to 78 nmol/L after 1 month, 60 nmol/L after 6 months and 50 nmol/L after 12 months *5891*

Sodium *Serum Decrease Physiological* In 8 healthy men administration of 4 mg/d for 13 days caused significant decrease from mean baseline of 143 ± 0.4 mmol/L to 141 ± 0.5 mmol/L *6077*

Serum No Effect Physiological No significant change observed in 16 postmenopausal women treated with increasing doses up to 16 mg/day for 12 weeks *1377*

Urine No Effect Physiological No significant change observed in 16 postmenopausal women treated with up to 16 mg daily for 12 weeks *1377*

Tetrahydroaldosterone *Urine Decrease Physiological* In 8 healthy men treated with 4 mg/d for 13 days mean excretion decreased insignificantly from 93.0 ± 10.4 nmol/d to 62.8 ± 9.9 nmol/d *6077*

Thyroid Stimulating Hormone

Serum No Effect Physiological In 54 postmenopausal women with breast cancer treatment with up to 4.0 mg/d for 12 weeks had no consistent effect *5263*

Thyroxine (T4) *Serum No Effect Physiological* In 54 postmenopausal women with breast cancer treatment with up to 4.0 mg/d for 12 weeks had no consistent effect *5263*

Thyroxine (T4), Free *Serum No Effect Physiological* In 54 postmenopausal women with breast cancer treatment with up to 4.0 mg/d for 12 weeks had no consistent effect on concentration *5263*

Famotidine

Alanine Aminotransferase *Serum Increase Physiological* Cholestatic jaundice has been reported infrequently *3988*

Serum No Effect Physiological In 9 patients with Zollinger-Ellison syndrome when followed for 33 weeks *2736*

Alkaline Phosphatase *Serum Increase Physiological* Cholestatic jaundice has been reported infrequently *3988*

Aminopyrine *Serum No Effect Physiological* Administration of famotidine with aminopyrine had no effect on its concentration or that of others metabolized by the cytochrome P450 system *3988*

Antipyrine *Serum No Effect Physiological* Administration of famotidine with antipyrine had no effect on its concentration or that of others metabolized by the cytochrome P450 system *3988*

Aspartate Aminotransferase *Serum Increase Physiological* Cholestatic jaundice has been reported infrequently *3988*

Serum No Effect Physiological In 9 patients with Zollinger-Ellison syndrome when followed for 33 weeks *2736*

Bilirubin *Serum Increase Physiological* Cholestatic jaundice has been reported infrequently *3988*

Creatinine *Serum No Effect Physiological* No significant change from pretreatment values in 9 patients with Zollinger-Ellison syndrome over 33 weeks *2736*

Cyclosporine *Blood Increase Physiological* With coadministration of famotidine absorption of cyclosporine is delayed and dosage:concentration ratio decreased leading to increased cyclosporine concentration *859*

Blood No Effect Physiological In 10 renal transplant patients treatment with 40 mg/d famotidine for 7 days caused nonsignificant increase in area under the curve from 2776 ng/mL to 3128 ng/mL *4111*

Famotidine *(continued)*

Cyclosporine *(continued)*
Serum Increase Physiological With coadministration of famotidine absorption of cyclosporine is delayed and dosage:concentration ratio decreased leading to increased cyclosporine concentration *859*

Diazepam *Serum No Effect Physiological* No interference observed with hepatic oxidative metabolism *1384* Administration of famotidine with diazepam had no effect on its concentration or that of others metabolized by the cytochrome P450 system *3988*

Estradiol *Plasma No Effect Physiological* No effect of short-term or long-term treatment in male patients with duodenal ulcers *1134*

Ethanol *Serum No Effect Physiological* In 6 healthy men given alcohol 0.3 g/kg body weight when also given 40 mg/d famotidine for 1 week mean area under the curve 8.0 ± 1.3 mmol/L/h compared with 8.9 ± 1.6 mmol/L/h in controls and peak blood concentration 6.5 ± 1.2 mmol/L compared with 6.1 ± 1.1 mmol/L in controls *1436* Ingestion of famotidine for several days prior to ingestion of alcohol had no effect on integrated postprandial ethanol concentration *1947*

Follicle Stimulating Hormone
Plasma No Effect Physiological No effect of short-term or long-term treatment in male patients with duodenal ulcers *1134*

Gastrin *Serum No Effect Physiological* No effect in 9 patients with Zollinger-Ellison syndrome treated for 33 weeks *2736*

γ-Glutamyltransferase *Serum Increase Physiological* Cholestatic jaundice has been reported infrequently *3988*

Granulocytes *Blood Decrease Physiological* Rare cases of pancytopenia with agranulocytosis reported *3988*

Hydrochloric Acid *Gastric Fluid Increase Physiological* Therapeutic effect as drug is long-acting histamine H_2-receptor antagonist *2736*

Indocyanine Green *Serum No Effect Physiological* Administration of famotidine with indocyanine green had no effect on its concentration or that of others metabolized by the cytochrome P450 system *3988*

itraconazole *Serum Decrease Physiological* Decreased oral bioavailability *886*

Ketoconazole *Serum Decrease Physiological* Decreased oral bioavailability *886*

Ketone Body Ratio *Serum No Effect Analytical* When added at a concentration of 50 mg/L had no significant effect on AKBR method of Uno et al *6131*

Leukocytes *Blood Decrease Physiological* Rare cases of pancytopenia with leukopenia reported *3988*
Blood No Effect Physiological No significant change from pretreatment values in 9 patients with Zollinger-Ellison syndrome over 33 weeks *2736*

Luteinizing Hormone *Plasma No Effect Physiological* No effect of short-term or long-term treatment in male patients with duodenal ulcers *1134*

Parathyroid Hormone *Plasma Decrease Physiological* 20 mg daily for 6 months caused significant, but not definitive, reduction in concentration in 10 hemodialysis patients with end-stage renal disease *2008*

pH *Gastric Material Increase Physiological* Significant increase observed in 8 patients given 2 daily doses of 40 mg but no significant effect compared with control with placebo when only single dose of 40 mg given (mean pH increased to 6.2 after evening and morning dose) *1607*

Phenytoin *Serum No Effect Physiological* Administration of famotidine with phenytoin had no effect on its concentration or that of others metabolized by the cytochrome P450 system *3988* No interference observed with hepatic oxidative metabolism *1384*

Platelets *Blood Decrease Physiological* Rare cases of pancytopenia with thrombocytopenia reported *3988*

Procainamide *Serum No Effect Physiological* Concomitant administration did not appear to affect the plasma concentration or metabolism of procainamide *3193*

Progesterone *Plasma No Effect Physiological* No effect of short-term or long-term treatment in male patients with duodenal ulcers *1134*

Prothrombin Time *Plasma No Effect Physiological* No significant effect observed in 8 healthy male volunteers (mean increase from 16.62 seconds to 16.98 seconds) when 40 mg famotidine added daily to therapeutic regime of 4.0 mg warfarin daily *1316*

Testosterone *Serum No Effect Physiological* No effect of short-term or long-term treatment in male patients with duodenal ulcers *1134*

Theophylline *Serum Increase Physiological* In 7 patients with chronic pulmonary obstructive disease treatment with 40 mg/d for 8 days caused substantial and statistically significant slowing of theophylline elimination with area under plasma concentration curve increasing from 3081 ± 337 mg/L/min to 4792 ± 403 mg/L/min *1219*
Serum No Effect Physiological No interference with hepatic oxidative metabolism observed *1384* No clinically significant effect on theophylline concentration observed when drugs coadministered *5999* Administration of famotidine with theophylline had no effect on its concentration or that of others metabolized by the cytochrome P450 system *3988* No documented significant interaction with theophylline reported *6117*

Thrombotest *Plasma No Effect Physiological* No significant effect observed when 40 mg/day famotidine added to therapeutic regime involving 4.0 mg warfarin daily as maintenance dose in 8 healthy male volunteers *1316*

Thyroid Stimulating Hormone
Serum No Effect Physiological No effect of short-term or long-term treatment in male patients with duodenal ulcers *1134*

Thyroxine (T4) *Serum No Effect Physiological* No effect of short-term or long-term treatment in male patients with duodenal ulcers *1134*

Tri-iodothyronine (T3) *Serum No Effect Physiological* No effect of short-term or long-term treatment in male patients with duodenal ulcers *1134*

Volume *Gastric Fluid Decrease Physiological* Significant reduction to mean of 7.8 mL in 8 outpatients treated with evening and morning doses, each of 40 mg, compared with 19.9 mL in 15 placebo treated controls with no significant change observed with single evening dose of 40 mg *1607*

Warfarin *Plasma No Effect Physiological* No interference observed with hepatic oxidative metabolism *1384* No significant effect observed when 40 mg famotidine added daily to maintenance therapeutic regime of 4.0 mg warfarin daily in 8 healthy male volunteers *1316* Administration of famotidine with warfarin had no effect on its concentration or that of others metabolized by the cytochrome P450 system *3988*

Felbamate

Alanine Aminotransferase *Serum Increase Physiological* Increased activity observed in 5.2% of 58 patients *6323* Hepatitis and hepatic failure have been reported as adverse events *6323*

Alkaline Phosphatase *Serum Increase Physiological* Hepatitis and hepatic failure have been reported as adverse events *6323* Increased activity observed infrequently with treatment *6323*

Ammonia *Plasma Increase Physiological* Hyperammonemia has been reported as an adverse event *6323*

Amylase *Serum Increase Physiological* Pancreatitis has been reported as an adverse event *6323*

Antinuclear Factor *Serum Increase Physiological* Positive antinuclear factor test observed rarely with treatment *6323*

Aspartate Aminotransferase *Serum Increase Physiological* Hepatitis and hepatic failure have been reported as adverse events *6323*

Bilirubin *Serum Increase Physiological* Hepatitis and hepatic failure have been reported as adverse events *6323*

Calcium *Serum Decrease Physiological* Hypocalcemia has been reported as adverse event *6323*

Carbamazepine *Serum Decrease Physiological* In 9 healthy individuals steady state trough concentration decreased 31% to 5 ± 1 µg/mL when 3000 mg/d felbamate coadministered with carbamazepine from baseline of 8 ± 2 µg/mL *6323* In 26 epileptic patients coadministration of felbamate with carbamazepine caused significant decrease from ean baseline concentration of 7.48 ± 1.83 µg/mL or when placebo administered

(7.51 ± 1.75 µg/mL) *6294* Mean reduction of 25% observed in 22 patients treated with carbamazepine and 4 weeks treatment with felbamate with dose of carbamazepine held constant *87* Drugs that induce CYP 3A4 enhance metabolism of carbamazepine producing clinically meaningful effect *1039* Coadministration of 300 mg/d felbamate with carbamazepine caused the steady-state plasma concentration of carbamazepine to decrease from 8 ± 2 µg/mL to 5 ± 1 µg/mL *6324*

Carbamazepine-10,11-Epoxide
Serum Increase Physiological Coadministration of 300 mg/d felbamate with carbamazepine caused the steady-state plasma concentration of carbamazepine-10,11-epoxide to increase from 1.0 ± 0.3 µg/mL to 1.6 ± 0.4 µg/mL *6324* In 26 epileptic patients coadministration of felbamate with carbamazepine caused mean increase from 1.8 µg/mL during placebo to 2.4 µg/mL *6294* In 9 healthy individuals steady state trough concentration increased 57% to 1.6 ± 0.4 µg/mL when 3000 mg/d felbamate coadministered with carbamazepine from baseline of 1.0 ± 0.3 µg/mL *6323* Drugs that induce CYP 3A4 enhance metabolism of carbamazepine producing clinically meaningful effect. Carbamazepine concentration decreased and carbamazepine-10,11-epoxide concentration increased *1039* Ratio of CBZ-E to CBZ increased from 0.20 to 0.43 following addition of felbamate to a steady dose carbamazepine regime in 4 patients with carbamazepine concentration decreasing from 10.30 µg/mL to 7.30 µg/mL and CBZ-E increased from 2.12 to 3.09 µg/mL *87*

Carbamazepine-trans-10,11-diol
Serum No Effect Physiological In 26 patients coadministration of felbamate with carbamazepine no significant difference in concentration observed compared with placebo *6294*

Creatine Kinase *Serum Increase Physiological* Increased activity observed rarely with treatment *6323*

Eosinophils *Blood Increase Physiological* Eosinophilia has been reported as adverse event *6323*

Ethinyl Estradiol *Serum No Effect Physiological* In 24 healthy nonsmoking women coadministration of 2400 mg/d felbamatefor 3 months with oral contraceptives containing 30 µg ethinyl estradiol and 75 µg gestodene had no significant effect on the pharmacokinetic parameters of ethinyl estradiol *6324*

Gestodene *Serum Decrease Physiological* In 24 healthy nonsmoking women coadministration of 2400 mg/d felbamatefor 3 months with oral contraceptives containing 30 µg ethinyl estradiol and 75 µg gestodene resulted in a 42% decrease in the AUC of gestodene *6324*

Glucose *Serum Decrease Physiological* Hypoglycemia has been reported as adverse event *6323*
Serum Increase Physiological Hyperglycemia has been reported as adverse event *6323*

γ-Glutamyltransferase *Serum Increase Physiological* Increased activity observed rarely with treatment *6323*

Granulocytes *Blood Decrease Physiological* Granulocytopenia observed infrequently with treatment *6323*
Blood Increase Physiological Granulocytosis observed rarely with treatment *6323*

Hematocrit *Blood Decrease Physiological* Anemia, hypochromic anemia, aplastic anemia, hemolytic anemia and pancytopenia have been reported as adverse events *6323*

Hemoglobin *Blood Decrease Physiological* Anemia, hypochromic anemia, aplastic anemia, hemolytic anemia and pancytopenia have been reported as adverse events *6323*

Lactate Dehydrogenase *Serum Increase Physiological* Increased activity observed infrequently with treatment *6323*

Lamotrigine *Serum Increase Physiological* In 21 healthy men given 100 mg every 12 hours addition of 1,200 mg felbamate every 12 hours caused an increase in the maximum plasma concentration of felbamate of 13% and increased its AUC by 14% *1100*
Urine No Effect Physiological In 21 healthy men given 100 mg every 12 hours addition of 1,200 mg felbamate every 12 hours caused an increase in the maximum plasma concentration of felbamate of 13% but had no effect on its urinary excretion *1100*

Leukocytes *Blood Decrease Physiological* Leukopenia observed in 6.5% of 31 patients *6323*
Blood Increase Physiological Leukocytosis observed infrequently with treatment *6323*

Lipase *Serum Increase Physiological* Pancreatitis has been reported as an adverse event *6323*

Magnesium *Serum Decrease Physiological* Hypomagnesemia has been reported as adverse event *6323*

MCV *Blood Increase Physiological* Increased mean corpuscular volume has been reported as adverse event *6323*

Occult Blood *Feces Increase Physiological* Gastrointestinal hemorrhage has been reported as an adverse event *6323*

Phenobarbital *Serum Increase Physiological* In 12 healthy men coadministration of 2400 mg/d felbamate with valproic acid caused the mean steady-state plasma concentration of phenobarbital to increase from 14.2 µg/mL to 17.8 µg/mL *6324*

Phenytoin *Serum Increase Physiological* Coadministration of 1200 mg/d felbamate with phenytoin in 10 healthy volunteers caused the steady-state plasma concentration of phenytoin to increase from 17 ± 5 µg/mL to 21 ± 5 µg/mL. Increasing felbamate to 1800 mg/d caused the steady-state phenytoin concentration to increase to 25 ± 7 µg/mL *6324* In 10 healthy individuals steady state trough concentration increased to 21 ± 5 µg/mL when 1200 mg/d felbamate coadministered with phenytoin from baseline of 17 ± 5 µg/mL. When 1500 mg/d felbamate administered phenytoin concentration increased to 25 ± 7 µg/mL *6323*

Phosphate *Serum Decrease Physiological* Hypophosphatemia observed in 3.4% of 58 patients *6323* Hypophosphatemia observed infrequently with treatment *6323*

Platelets *Blood Decrease Physiological* In one 26-year old man given felbamate for 3 days platelet count decreased from 0.320 million/µL to 0.023 million /µL while other hematological indices remained normal: platelet count returned to normal after felbamate withdrawn *4271* Thrombocytopenia observed infrequently with treatment *6323*

Potassium *Serum Decrease Physiological* Hypokalemia observed infrequently with treatment *6323*

Prothrombin Time *Plasma Decrease Physiological* Increased and decreased prothrombin times have been reported as adverse events *6323*
Plasma Increase Physiological Increased and decreased prothrombin times have been reported as adverse events *6323*

Sodium *Serum Decrease Physiological* Hyponatremia observed infrequently with treatment *6323*
Serum Increase Physiological Hypernatremia has been reported as adverse event *6323*

Valproic Acid *Serum Increase Physiological* In 4 individuals with epilepsy steady state trough concentration increased to 78 ± 14 µg/mL when 1200 mg/d felbamate coadministered with valproic acid from baseline of 63 ± 16 µg/mL. When 2400 mg/d felbamate administered valproic acid concentration to 96 ± 25 µg/mL *6323* In 10 patients with epilepsy who also received 1200 mg/d felbamate mean valproate concentration increased by 35% from 86 µg/mL to 115 µg/mL. Increasing the felbamate concentration to 2400 mg/d caused a further 16% increase in the valproate concentration *15* In 18 healthy volunteers who received 400 mg/day valproic acid for 21 days coadministration of felbamate from 1200 to 3600 mg/d from day 8 to day 21 caused increase from mean baseline of 32 - 42 µg/mL to 55 - 64 µg/mL *2706* Coadministration of felbamate in doses of 1200 mg/d with valproic acid to 10 patients with epilepsy caused a mean increase of 35% from 86 to 115 µg/mL in the valproic acid concentration *17* In 4 epileptics coadministration of 1200 mg/d felbamate with valproic acid caused the steady-state plasma concentration of valproate to increase from 63 ± 16 µg/mL to 78 ± 14 µg/mL. When 2400 mg/d felbamate give the valproate concentration increased to 96 ± 25 µg/mL *6324*

Valproic Acid, Free *Serum Increase Physiological* In 4 epileptics coadministration of 1200 mg/d felbamate with valproic acid caused the steady-state plasma concentration of free valproic acid to increase from 7 ± 3 µg/mL to 8 ± 4 µg/mL. When 2400 mg/d felbamate give the valproate concentration increased to 11 ± 6 µg/mL *6324*

Felodipine

Alanine Aminotransferase *Serum No Effect Physiological* No significant change observed in 16 hypertensive patients with hyperlipoproteinemia treated with 10 mg/d for 2 years *5363*

Felodipine *(continued)*

Albumin *Serum Increase Physiological* In 11 healthy volunteers administration of 825 μg intravenously over 150 minutes caused significant increase from mean baseline of 44 ± 1 g/L to 46 ± 1 g/L *3415*

Aldosterone *Plasma No Effect Physiological* In 11 healthy volunteers administration of 825 μg intravenously over 150 minutes caused nonsignificant change from mean baseline of 6.1 ± 1.1 ng/dL to 6.9 ± 1.1 ng/dL *3415* Treatment of 28 mild to moderate hypertensive patients with 10 mg/d felodipine-ER for 2 weeks had generally no effect on concentration *3213*
Urine Increase Physiological With 20 mg daily in 10 men with essential hypertension over 8 weeks *3069*

Alkaline Phosphatase *Serum Increase Physiological* Nonsignificant increase from mean baseline of 88 U/L to 108 U/L at 1 year and 129 U/L at 2 years in 16 hypertensive patients with hyperlipoproteinemia when treated with 10 mg/d *5363*

Angiotensin-II *Plasma No Effect Physiological* With 20 mg daily in 10 men with essential hypertension over 8 weeks *3069*

Antidiuretic Hormone *Plasma No Effect Physiological* In 11 healthy volunteers administration of 825 μg intravenously over 150 minutes caused change from mean baseline of 7.88 ± 1.00 pg/mL to 9.30 ± 0.50 pg/mL not significantly different from response following placebo *3415*

Apolipoprotein A-I *Serum No Effect Physiological* Nonsignificant increase from mean baseline of 140 mg/dL to 159 mg/dL at 1 year and 146 mg/dL at 2 years in 16 hypertensives with hyperlipoproteinemia when treated with 10 mg/d *5363*

Apolipoprotein B *Serum No Effect Physiological* Nonsignificant decrease from mean baseline of 119 mg/dL to 106 mg/dL at 1 year and 103 mg/dL at 2 years in 16 hypertensive patients with hyperlipoproteinemia when treated with 10 mg/d *5363*

Aspartate Aminotransferase
Serum No Effect Physiological No significant effect observed in 16 hypertensive patients with hyperlipoproteinemia when treated with 10 mg/d for 2 years *5363*

Atrial Natriuretic Peptide *Plasma No Effect Physiological* In 11 healthy volunteers administration of 825 μg intravenously over 150 min caused nonsignificant changes of concentration of C-terminal ANF from 10.5 ± 1.7 pmol/L to 9.1 ± 0.5 pmol/L and of N-terminal ANF from 461 ± 43 pmol/L to 452 ± 62 pmol/L *3415*

Bicarbonate *Serum No Effect Physiological* No significant effect observed on concentration with either short or long-term administration of felodipine *266*

Calcium *Serum No Effect Physiological* No significant change observed in 16 hypertensive patients with hyperlipoproteinemia treated with 10 mg/d for 2 years *5363*

Carbamazepine *Serum Increase Physiological* Concomitant administration of calcium channel blockers with carbamazepine causes marked increase of plasma carbamazepine concentration resulting in toxicity in some cases *282*

Chloride *Serum No Effect Physiological* No significant effect observed on concentration with either short or long-term administration of felodipine *266*

Cholesterol *Serum No Effect Physiological* Nonsignificant reduction from mean baseline of 275 mg/dL to 258 mg/dL at 1 year and 250 mg/dL at 2 years in 16 hypertensives with hyperlipoproteinemia when treated with 10 mg/d for 2 years *5363*

Creatinine *Serum No Effect Physiological* In 11 healthy volunteers administration of 825 μg intravenously over 150 minutes caused nonsignificant change from baseline of 78 ± 4 μmol/L to 75 ± 4 μmol/L *3415*

Digoxin *Serum Increase Physiological* At steady state caused an increase of 11% in digoxin concentration but mechanism not described *3149* Nonsignificant increase observed in patients with congestive heart failure when drugs coadministered and instant release formulation of felodipine used, but no effect with sustained release formulation *1623*
Serum No Effect Physiological Coadministration of felodipine with digoxin had no significant on the area under the curve or its maximum plasma concentration *266* No apparent effect observed with coadministration on digoxin pharmacokinetics in healthy volunteers and patients with congestive heart failure *5345*

Endothelin-1 *Plasma No Effect Physiological* Drug administration had no significant effect when administeed before microvascular surgery: concentration prior to surgery 4.6 - 7.7 pg/mL *6061*

Epinephrine *Plasma No Effect Physiological* No effect in 14 healthy male volunteers given 10 mg/day for 14 days *5446* In 28 mild to moderate hypertensive patients treatment with 10 mg felodipine-ER for 2 weeks generally had no effect on plasma concentration *3213*
Urine No Effect Physiological With 20 mg daily in 10 men with essential hypertension over 8 weeks *3069*

Erythrocyte Aggregation *Blood No Effect Physiological* In 28 mild to moderate hypertensives treatment with 10 mg/d felodipine ER for 2 weeks caused nonsignificant change from mean baseline of 10.3 ± 0.34 units to 10.4 ± 0.31 units *3215*

Erythrocytes *Blood No Effect Physiological* No significant effect observed in 16 patients with hypertension and hyperlipoproteinemia when treated with 10 mg/d for 2 years *5363*

Euglobulin Lysis Time *Blood No Effect Physiological* No significant effect in 14 healthy male volunteers given 10 mg/day for 14 days *5446*

Glomerular Filtration Rate *Urine Decrease Physiological* In 11 healthy volunteers administration of 825 μg intravenously over 150 minutes caused significant reduction from mean baseline of 100 ± 4 mL/min to 91 ± 4 mL/min *3415*

Glucose *Serum No Effect Physiological* No significant change observed in fasting and maximal glucose concentrations in 18 type II male diabetics treated with up to 20 mg/d for 4 weeks *3169* No significant effect observed on concentration with either short or long-term administration of felodipine *266* No significant change observed in 16 hypertensive patients with hyperlipoproteinemia when treated with 10 mg/d for 2 years *5363*

Glucose Tolerance *Serum Decrease Physiological* Small (4%) but statistically significant increase in area under the glucose concentration versus time curve in 18 type II male diabetics treated with up to 20 mg/g for 4 weeks. Effect probably not clinically significant *3169*

γ-Glutamyltransferase *Serum No Effect Physiological* No significant change observed in 16 hypertensives with hyperlipoproteinemia treated with 10 mg/d for 2 years *5363*

Guanosine Monophosphate
Plasma No Effect Physiological In 11 healthy volunteers administration of 825 μg intravenously over 150 minutes caused nonsignificant change in comparison with placebo from 5.36 ± 0.27 pmol/L to 4.40 ± 0.27 pmol/L *3415*
Urine No Effect Physiological In 11 healthy volunteers administration of 825 μg intravenously over 150 minutes caused nonsignificant decrease in comparison with placebo from mean baseline of 0.53 ± 0.10 nmol/min to 0.41 ± 0.04 nmol/min *3415*

HDL-Cholesterol *Serum No Effect Physiological* No significant change observed in 16 hypertensives with hyperlipoproteinemia when treated with 10 mg/d for 2 years *5363*

Hematocrit *Blood No Effect Physiological* No significant effect observed in 16 patients with hypertension and hyperlipoproteinemia when treated with 10 mg/d for 2 years *5363* In 11 healthy volunteers administration of 825 μg intravenously over 150 minutes caused nonsignificant change from 0.42 ± 0.01 to 0.43 ± 0.01 *3415* In 8 mild to moderate hypertensives treated with 10 mg felodipine ER per day for 2 weeks nonsignificant change from mean baseline of 45.1 ± 0.83% to 45.50 ± 0.34% observed *3215*

Hemoglobin *Blood No Effect Physiological* In 11 healthy volunteers administration of 825 μg intravenously over 150 minutes caused nonsignificant change from 146 ± 3 g/L to 152 ± 3 g/L *3415* No significant effect observed in 16 hypertensive patients with hyperlipoproteinemia when treated with 10 mg/d for 2 years *5363*

Hemoglobin A_{1c} *Blood No Effect Physiological* No change observed in 18 male type II diabetics treated with up to 20 mg/d for 4 weeks *3169*

Indomethacin *Serum No Effect Physiological* No significant effect observed on either felodipine or indomethacin concentrations when drugs coadministered *266*

Insulin *Plasma No Effect Physiological* No change in fastimg plasma insulin concentration in 18 type II male diabetics during treatment with up to 20 mg/d for 4 weeks *3169*

Inulin Clearance *Urine No Effect Physiological* No significant effect in 9 volunteers given 0.075 mg/kg orally over next 2.5 hours *2925*

Kallikrein *Urine No Effect Physiological* No change in urinary excretion rate in 9 volunteers after having been given 0.075 mg/kg orally *2925*

6-Keto-Prostaglandin $F_{1\alpha}$ *Urine No Effect Physiological* No significant effect on excretion in 9 volunteers given 0.075 mg/kg orally *2925*

Lactate Dehydrogenase *Serum No Effect Physiological* No significant change observed in 16 hypertensives with hyperlipoproteinemia when treated with 10 mg/d for 2 years *5363*

LDL-Cholesterol *Serum No Effect Physiological* Nonsignificant reduction from mean baseline of 169 mg/dL to 154 mg/dL at 1 year and 164 mg/dL at 2 years in 16 hypertensive patients with hyperlipoproteinemia when treated with 10 mg/d *5363*

Leukocytes *Blood No Effect Physiological* No significant effect in 14 healthy male volunteers given 10 mg/day for 14 days *5446* No significant effect observed in 16 patients with hypertension and hyperlipoproteinemia when treated with 10 mg/d for 2 years *5363*

Magnesium *Serum Increase Physiological* Significant increase from mean baseline of 0.74 mmol/L to 0.80 mmol/L at 24 and 52 weeks and 0.79 mmol/L at 1.5 and 2 years in 16 hypertensive patients with hyperlipoproteinemia when treated with 10 mg/d *5363*

Metoprolol *Serum Increase Physiological* In healthy volunteers coadministration for 5 days caused increase in area under concentration curve of metoprolol of about 31% and increased maximum plasma concentration *5630* Coadministration of felodipine with metoprolol caused s 31% increase in the area under the curve and a 38% increase in its maximum plasma concentration *266* In healthy volunteers receiving metoprolol 100 mg twice daily mean maximum concentration and area under the curve increased by 38% and 31% respecively compared with placebo when felodipine 10 mg twice daily was coadministered, although effect not likely to be of clinical significance, since intersubject variations were large *5411*

Norepinephrine *Plasma Increase Physiological* When infused in 10 healthy normotensive volunteers *5603* In 28 mild to moderate hypertensive patients treatment with 10 mg felodipine-ER for 2 weeks significantly increased plasma norepinephrine concentration *3213* Significant increase due to increased sympathetic tone *2528*

Plasma No Effect Physiological Insignificant increase in 14 healthy male volunteers given 10 mg/day for 14 days *5446*

Urine Increase Physiological With 20 mg daily in 10 men with essential hypertension over 8 weeks *3069*

Osmolar Clearance *Urine Increase Physiological* In 11 healthy volunteers administration of 825 µg intravenously over 150 minutes caused significant increase from mean baseline of 3.4 ± 0.4 mL/min to 5.8 ± 0.5 mL/min *3415*

PAH Clearance *Urine No Effect Physiological* No significant effect in 9 male volunteers given 0.075 mg/kg orally, over next 2.5 hours *2925*

Platelet Aggregation *Blood No Effect Physiological* No significant effect in 14 healthy male volunteers given 10 mg/day for 14 days on ADP induced aggregation *5446* No significant effect in 14 healthy male volunteers given 10 mg/day for 14 days on epinephrine-induced aggregation *5446*

Platelet Factor 4 *Plasma Decrease Physiological* With 14 days treatment of 14 healthy male volunteers with 10 mg/day reduction from mean of 18.8 ng/mL to 12.6 ng/mL observed *5446*

Platelets *Blood No Effect Physiological* No significant effect in 14 healthy male volunteers given 10 mg/day for 14 days *5446* No significant effect observed in 16 hypertensive patients with hyperlipoproteinemia when treated with 10 mg/d for 2 years *5363*

Potassium *Serum Increase Physiological* Significant increase from mean baseline of 4.67 mmol/L in 16 hypertensives with hyperlipoproteinemia treated with 10 mg/d for 24 weeks but with nonsignificant increase thereafter for 2 years *5363*

Serum No Effect Physiological No significant effect observed on concentration with either short or long-term administration of felodipine *266*

Urine Decrease Physiological In 11 healthy volunteers administration of 825 µg intravenously over 150 minutes caused significant decrease from mean baseline of 103 ± 10 µmol/min to 67 ± 5 µmol/min *3415*

Urine No Effect Physiological No significant change in 9 volunteers given 0.075 mg/kg orally although higher in individuals when pretreated with indomethacin *2925* Mild diuresis, natriuresis or kaliuresis may occur with administration of felodipine diring the first week of therapy *266*

Prostaglandin E_2 *Urine Increase Physiological* Transient increase in 9 male volunteers at 90 minutes after having been given 0.075 mg/kg orally *2925*

Prostaglandin $F_{2\alpha}$ *Plasma No Effect Physiological* No significant effect in 14 healthy male volunteers given 10 mg/day for 14 days *5446*

Quinidine *Serum No Effect Physiological* Felodipine has no effect on the pharmacokinetics of quinidine *5996* Insignificant increase of maximum plasma concentration from mean baseline of 747 ± 52 ng/mL to 855 ± 66 ng/mL when felodipine coadministered with quinidine *327*

Red Cell Transit Time *Blood No Effect Physiological* In 28 mild to moderate hypertensives treatment with 10 mg/d felodipine ER for 2 weeks caused nonsignificant change from 15.2 ± 0.61 units to 16.3 ± 0.72 units *3215*

Relative Filtration Rate *Blood No Effect Physiological* In 28 mild to moderate hypertensives treatment with 10 mg/d felodipine ER for 2 weeks caused nonsignificant change from mean baseline of 0.24 ± 0.009 units to 0.23 ± 0.007 units *3215*

Renal Blood Flow *Patient No Effect Physiological* In 11 healthy volunteers administration of 825 µg intravenously over 150 minutes caused nonsignificant increase from mean baseline of 987 ± 107 mL/min to 1052 ± 54 mL/min *3415*

Renal Plasma Flow *Patient No Effect Physiological* In 11 healthy volunteers administration of 825 µg intravenously over 150 minutes caused nonsignificant change from mean baseline of 571 ± 58 mL/min to 584 ± 35 mL/min *3415*

Renin Activity *Plasma Increase Physiological* In 11 healthy volunteers administration of 825 µg intravenously over 150 minutes caused significant increase from mean baseline of 0.57 ± 0.2 ng/mL/h to 1.20 ± 0.30 ng/mL/h *3415* When infused into 10 healthy normotensive volunteers *5603* With 20 mg daily in 10 men with essential hypertension over 8 weeks *3069*

Plasma No Effect Physiological No significant change in 9 male volunteers given 0.075 mg/kg orally *2925* In 28 mild to moderate hypertensive patients treatment with 10 mg felodipine-ER for 2 weeks generally had no effect on activity *3213*

Sodium *Serum No Effect Physiological* No significant effect observed on concentration with either short or long-term administration of felodipine *266* No significant change observed in 16 hypertensives with hyperlipoproteinemia treated with 10 mg/d for 2 years *5363*

Urine Increase Physiological In 11 healthy volunteers administration of 825 µg intravenously over 150 minutes caused significant increase from mean baseline of 277 ± 39 µmol/min to 546 ± 69 µmol/min *3415* Significant effect in 9 male volunteers given 0.075 mg/kg, which was not affected by indomethacin pretreatment *2925*

Urine No Effect Physiological Mild diuresis, natriuresis or kaliuresis may occur with administration of felodipine during the first week of therapy *266*

Spironolactone *Serum No Effect Physiological* No significant effect observed on either felodipine or spironolactone concentrations when drugs coadministered *266*

Theophylline *Serum Decrease Physiological* In healthy volunteers administration of 5 mg every 8 h for 4 days decreased area under theophylline concentration curve was decreased by 18.3% with concomitant reduction of plasma minimal and maximal concentrations of theophylline *5345* Coadministration in 10 healthy male volunteers caused reduction of area under theophylline curve of 18.3% with metabolic and renal clearances unchanged. Effect probably due to interference with absorption of theophylline *778*

Serum No Effect Physiological No documented significant interaction with theophylline reported *6117* No clinically significant effect on theophylline concentration observed when drugs coadministered *5999*

Felodipine *(continued)*

β-Thromboglobulin *Plasma Decrease Physiological* In 14 healthy male volunteers treatment with 10 mg/day caused reduction from mean of 73.8 ng/mL to 47.7 ng/mL at rest *5446*

Thromboxane B_2 *Plasma No Effect Physiological* No significant effect in 14 healthy male volunteers given 10 mg/day for 14 days *5446*

Triglycerides *Serum No Effect Physiological* Nonsignificant reduction from mean baseline of 422 mg/dL to 388 mg/dL at 1 year and 383 mg/dL at 2 years in 16 hypertensives with hyperlipoproteinemia when treated with 10 mg/d *5363*

Urea Nitrogen *Serum No Effect Physiological* Nonsignificant increase observed in 16 hypertensive patients with hyperlipoproteinemia when treated with 10 mg/d for 2 years *5363*

Uric Acid *Serum No Effect Physiological* No significant effect observed in 16 hypertensive patients with hyperlipoproteinemia when treated with 10 mg/d for 2 years *5363*

Viscosity *Plasma No Effect Physiological* In 28 mild to moderate hypertensives treatment with 10 mg/d felodipine ER for 2 weeks caused nonsignificant change from mean baseline of 1.29 ± 0.02 mPa/s to 1.30 ± 0.01 mPa/s *3215*

VLDL-Cholesterol *Serum No Effect Physiological* Nonsignificant reduction from mean baseline of 69 mg/dL to 63 mg/dL at 1 year and 46 mg/dL at 2 years in 16 hypertensive patients with hyperlipoproteinemia when treated with 10 mg/d *5363*

Volume *Urine Decrease Physiological* In 11 healthy volunteers administration of 825 μg intravenously over 150 minutes caused significant decrease from mean baseline of 10.1 ± 1.3 mL/min to 8.9 ± 0.6 mL/min *3415* 65% decrease in urinary volume maximal at 1 hour following 0.075 mg/kg in 9 male volunteers, but effect delayed if subjects pretreated with indomethacin *2925*

Urine No Effect Physiological Mild diuresis, natriuresis or kaliuresis may occur with administration of felodipine during the first week of therapy *266*

Water Clearance *Urine Decrease Physiological* In 11 healthy volunteers administration of 825 μg intravenously over 150 minutes caused significant decrease from mean baseline of 6.8 ± 0.9 mL/min to 3.0 ± 0.3 mL/min *3415*

Fenbufen

Alanine Aminotransferase *Serum Increase Physiological* Incidence of acute liver injury of 11.9 per 100,000 treated patients with reported in United Kingdom. Liver damage among all cases primarily hepatocellular in some and primarily cholestatic in others *5049*

Aspartate Aminotransferase *Serum Increase Physiological* Incidence of acute liver injury of 11.9 per 100,000 treated patients with reported in United Kingdom. Liver damage among all cases primarily hepatocellular in some and primarily cholestatic in others *5049*

Thyroxine (T4) *Serum No Effect Analytical* Using the Ciba-Corning ACS:180 analyzer mean concentration not significantly changed in 1 specimen whose concentration differed by -7% compared with the concentration measured by the Amerlex-M method *5621*

Fenclofenac

Thyroid Stimulating Hormone
Serum No Effect Physiological May be short-term reduction (beginning of therapy) at hypophyseal level *6412* None of 8 patients receiving 1.2 g/d had altered values *4944* No effect observed in patients treated for long term and they remain euthyroid clinically *1269*

Thyroxine Binding Globulin *Serum No Effect Physiological* In 7 out of 8 patients receiving 1.2 g/d no change observed *4944*

Thyroxine (T4) *Serum Decrease Physiological* From 173 nmol/L to 70 nmol/L in 4 women with thyrotoxicosis given 1.2 g/d for 7 d *4575* In 7 out of 8 individuals receiving 1.2 g/d values below normal range. T4 displaced from binding protein *4944* In therapeutic doses reduction of plasma concentration by approximately one third after two weeks of treatment *1269*

Thyroxine (T4), Free *Serum Decrease Physiological* Significant decrease but not to normal in 4 women with thyrotoxicosis given 1.2 g/d for 7 d *4575* Nonsignificant decrease reported in several studies *6412* Circulating concentration reduced but remaining within reference range with long-term treatment *1269*

Thyroxine (T4) Index, Free *Serum Decrease Physiological* In 7 out of 8 individuals receiving 1.2 g/d values below normal range. Thyroxine displaced from binding protein *4944*

Tri-iodothyronine, Free (fT3)
Serum No Effect Physiological Values at lower end of normal range in individuals receiving 1.2 g/d *4944*

Tri-iodothyronine, Reverse (rT3)
Serum Decrease Physiological From 0.63 nmol/L to 0.52 nmol/L in 4 women with thyrotoxicosis given 1.2 g/d for 7 d *4575*

Tri-iodothyronine (T3) *Serum Decrease Physiological* In 7 out of 8 individuals receiving 1.2 g/d values below normal range. Thyroxine displaced from binding protein *4944* From 6.2 nmol/L to 3.8 nmol/L in 4 women with thyrotoxicosis given 1.2 g/d for 7 d *4575*

Tri-iodothyronine (T3) Index, Free
Serum Decrease Physiological In 7 out of 8 individuals receiving 1.2 g/d values below normal range. Thyroxine displaced from binding protein *4944*

TSH response to TRH *Serum Decrease Physiological* During long-term treatment suppressed response observed: also observed at beginning of treatment *1269*

Fendiline

Digoxin *Serum No Effect Physiological* No significant interaction reported from one study with chronic combination therapy *1304*

Fenfluramine

Amobarbital *Urine No Effect Analytical* No interference on TLC using ethyl acetate: methanol: water: ammonium hydroxide and Dragendorff's reagent for detection *6502*

Amphetamine *Urine No Effect Analytical* No interference on TLC using ethyl acetate, methanol, water, ammonium hydroxide and modified Dragendorff's reagent for detection *6502*

Amylase *Serum No Effect Physiological* In 15 female patients with bulimia nervosa treated with 45 mg/d mean activity changed nonsignificantly from 4.57 ± 2.1 μkat/L at baseline to 3.88 ± 1.8 μkat/L after 8 weeks *3303*

Amylase, Salivary Isoenzyme
Serum No Effect Physiological In 15 female patients with bulimia nervosa treated with 45 mg/d mean activity changed nonsignificantly from 3.14 ± 1.6 μkat/L at baseline to 2.60 ± 1.6 μkat/L after 8 weeks *3303*

Clotermine *Urine Positive Analytical* Similar R_f and color reaction on TLC using ethyl acetate: methanol: water: ammonium hydroxide and modified Dragendorff's reagent *6502*

Corticotropin *Plasma No Effect Physiological* No significant effect in 40 depressed patients at 2 and 4 hours after oral administration of 60 mg D,L-fenfluramine *3733*

Cortisol *Plasma Increase Analytical* Fluoresces with sulfuric acid *199*

Plasma Increase Physiological Baseline concentration increased in depressed patients but further increased in response to 60 mg orally. Increase somewhat greater in normals but from a lower baseline *4072*

Plasma No Effect Physiological No significant effect observed in 40 depressed patients at 2 and 4 hours after administration of 60 mg D,L-fenfluramine orally *3733*

Drugs of Abuse Screen *Urine Increase Analytical* False positive produced with Abbott ADx method for amphetamine/methamphetamine *4279*

β-Endorphin *Plasma No Effect Physiological* No significant effect observed in 40 depressed patients at 2 and 4 hours after oral administration of 60 mg D,L-fenfluramine *3733*

Erythrocytes *Blood No Effect Physiological* No adverse reaction reported *818*

Glucose *Serum Decrease Physiological* Direct effect, increased glucose uptake by muscle *6106*

Glucose Tolerance *Serum Increase Physiological* Significant improvement (mean decrease of 25 mg/dL) *603*

Growth Hormone *Plasma Increase Physiological* Action on brain stimulating release *3553*

Hematocrit *Blood No Effect Physiological* No adverse reaction reported *818*

Hydromorphone *Urine No Effect Analytical* No interference on TLC using ethyl acetate: methanol: water: ammonium hydroxide and modified Dragendorff's reagent for detection *6502*

Insulin *Plasma No Effect Physiological* Variable response (some increased, some decreased) *603*

Ketones *Serum Increase Physiological* Average increase of 57% observed *4566*

β-Lipoprotein *Serum Decrease Physiological* Small but significant reduction *603*

Melatonin *Plasma No Effect Physiological* In 8 healthy volunteers administration of 30 mg d-fenfluramine at 20:00 h caused no significant effect on nocturnal plasma melatonin concentration *4230*

Mescaline *Urine No Effect Analytical* No interference on TLC using ethyl acetate: methanol: water: ammonium hydroxide and modified Dragendorff's reagent for detection *6502*

Methamphetamine *Urine No Effect Analytical* No interference on TLC using ethyl acetate: methanol: water: ammonium hydroxide and modified Dragendorff's reagent for detection *6502*

Morphine *Urine No Effect Analytical* No interference on TLC using ethyl acetate: methanol: water: ammonium hydroxide and modified Dragendorff's reagent for detection *6502*

Nicotine *Urine Positive Analytical* Similar R_f and color reaction on TLC using ethyl acetate: methanol: water: ammonium hydroxide and modified Dragendorff's reagent *6502*

Pentobarbital *Urine No Effect Analytical* No interference on TLC using ethyl acetate: methanol: water: ammonium hydroxide and modified Dragendorff's reagent for detection *6502*

Phenobarbital *Urine No Effect Analytical* No interference on TLC using ethyl acetate: methanol: water: ammonium hydroxide and modified Dragendorff's reagent for detection *6502*

Phenylpropanolamine *Urine No Effect Analytical* No interference on TLC using ethyl acetate: methanol: water: ammonium hydroxide and modified Dragendorff's reagent for detection *6502*

Prolactin *Plasma Increase Physiological* Following 60 mg orally in depressed patients increased concentration of prolactin observed but not to same extent as in healthy controls but difference not significant *4072* Significant increase observed in 40 depressed patients 2 and 4 hours after oral administration of 60 mg D,L-fenfluramine but only in major and not in minor depressives *3733*

Secobarbital *Urine No Effect Analytical* No interference on TLC using ethyl acetate: methanol: water: ammonium hydroxide and modified Dragendorff's reagent for detection *6502*

Triglycerides *Serum Decrease Physiological* Not constant finding *5869*

Fengabine

Alanine Aminotransferase *Serum No Effect Physiological* No significant effect observed in 11 patients treated with a mean daily dose of 1070 mg for 4 weeks *4289*

Alkaline Phosphatase *Serum No Effect Physiological* No significant effect observed in 11 patients treated with a mean daily dose of 1070 mg for 4 weeks *4289*

Aspartate Aminotransferase *Serum No Effect Physiological* No significant effect observed in 11 patients treated with a mean daily dose of 1070 mg for 4 weeks *4289*

Bilirubin *Serum No Effect Physiological* No significant effect noted in 11 patients treated with a mean dose of 1070 mg daily for 4 weeks *4289*

Cholesterol *Serum No Effect Physiological* No significant effect observed in 11 patients treated with a mean daily dose of 1070 mg for 4 weeks *4289*

Creatinine *Serum No Effect Physiological* No significant effect noted in 11 patients treated with mean daily dose of 1070 mg for 4 weeks *4289*

Erythrocytes *Blood No Effect Physiological* No significant effect observed in 11 patients treated with mean daily dose of 1070 mg for 4 weeks *4289*

Glucose *Serum No Effect Physiological* No significant effect observed in 11 patients treated with a mean daily dose of 1070 mg for 4 weeks *4289*

γ-Glutamyltransferase *Serum Increase Physiological* Moderate increase observed in one of 11 patients treated with mean dose of 1070 mg/d for 4 weeks *4289*

Hematocrit *Blood No Effect Physiological* No significant effect observed in 11 patients treated with mean daily dose of 1070 mg for 4 weeks *4289*

Hemoglobin *Blood No Effect Physiological* No significant effect observed in 11 patients treated with mean daily dose of 1070 mg for 4 weeks *4289*

Leukocytes *Blood No Effect Physiological* No significant effect noted in 11 patients treated with mean dose of 1070 mg daily for 4 weeks *4289*

Platelets *Blood No Effect Physiological* No significant effect noted in 11 patients treated with mean dose of 1070 mg daily for 4 weeks *4289*

Potassium *Serum No Effect Physiological* No significant effect observed in 11 patients treated for 4 weeks with a mean daily dose of 1070 mg *4289*

Sodium *Serum No Effect Physiological* No significant effect observed in 11 patients treated with a mean daily dose of 1070 mg for 4 weeks *4289*

Triglycerides *Serum No Effect Physiological* No significant effect observed in 11 patients treated with a mean daily dose of 1070 mg for 4 weeks *4289*

Urea Nitrogen *Serum No Effect Physiological* No significant effect noted in 11 patients treated with mean daily dose of 1070 mg for 4 weeks *4289*

Uric Acid *Serum No Effect Physiological* No significant effect observed in 11 patients treated with a mean daily dose of 1070 mg for 4 weeks *4289*

Fenofibrate

Alanine Aminotransferase *Serum Increase Physiological* Transient increases occur commonly in hypertriglyceridemic or hypercholesterolemic patients when treated with doses of 200 to 400 mg daily *349*

Apolipoprotein A-I *Serum Decrease Physiological* In patients with type IIb hyperlipoproteiemia treatment with 300 mg/d for 3 months caused significant decrease in concentration *644*

Serum Increase Physiological Significant effect in 18 patients with familial hypercholesterolemia given 0.25 g/d for 8 weeks *6400* Increased synthesis. Increased activity of lipoprotein lipase by stimulation of muscle lipoprotein lipase synthesis, alteration of the capillary endothelial surface and stimulation of apolipoprotein C-II synthesis *264*

Serum No Effect Physiological In 15 patients with type IIa hyperlipidemia treatment with 200 mg/d for 3 months caused nonsignificant reduction from mean baseline of 152 ± 27 mg/dL to 144 ± 28 mg/dL and in 11 with type IIb hyperlipidemia from 147 ± 30 mg/dL to 141 ± 38 mg/dL *1805*

Apolipoprotein B *Serum Decrease Physiological* Of fibrates appears to be one of the most effective in reducing apo B concentration *5586* In 18 patients with familial hypercholesterolemia 8 weeks treatment with 0.25 g/d caused mean reduction of 10.6% *6400* In 15 patients with type IIa hyperlipidemia treatment with 200 mg/d for 3 months caused marked reduction from mean baseline of 154 ± 22 mg/dL to 110 ± 20 mg/dL and in 11 with type IIb hyperlipidemia from 175 ± 21 mg/dL to 124 ± 23 mg/dL *1805*

Aspartate Aminotransferase *Serum Increase Physiological* Transient increases commonly occur in hypertriglyceridemic or hypercholesterolemic patients when treated with 200 to 400 mg daily *349*

Fenofibrate *(continued)*

Cholesterol *Serum Decrease Physiological* Drug is effective in reducing plasma cholesterol concentration. In one study of 92 type IIa patients in the United States reduced concentration by 18% *3668* In 15 patients with type IIa hyperlipidemia treatment with 200 mg/d for 3 months caused significant decrease from mean baseline of 8.30 ± 1.41 mmol/L to 6.03 ± 1.31 mmol/L and in 11 with type IIb from 7.80 ± 1.08 mmol/L to 6.04 ± 1.05 mmol/L *1805* Increase by 18% over 24 weeks in 92 type IIa given 100 mg 3 times per day with similar responses in type IIb patients when compared with baseline values *773* In patients with type IIb hyperlipoproteinemia treatment with 300 mg/d for 3 months caused significant reduction *644* In 10 postmenopausal women and 13 age-matched men with hypercholesterolemia treatment with fenofibrate 250 mg/d for 96 weeks caused significant reduction from mean baseline of 299 ± 40 mg/dL to 234 ± 21 mg/dL in the women and in the men from 265 ± 11 mg/dL to 233 ± 22 mg/dL *5857* At daily doses of 200 to 400 mg produces substantial reduction in cholesterol concentration in hypercholesterolemic patients *349* In 27 patients with severe hypertriglyceridemia treatment with 250 mg/d for 6 weeks caused significant reduction from median baseline of 11.6 ± 3.49 mmol/L to 9.20 ± 3.62 mmol/L *3086* In 41 patients with combined hyperlipidemia treatment with fenofibrate 300 mg/d for 2 years caused significant reduction of 9.0% *1718*

Cholesterol:HDL-Cholesterol Ratio
Serum Decrease Physiological In 39 patients with combined hyperlipidemia treatment with fenofibrate 300 mg/d for 2 years caused significant decrease from 8.62 pretreatment to 5.48 *1718*

Creatine Kinase *Serum Increase Physiological* Transient increases commonly occur in hypertriglyceridemic or hypercholesterolemic patients when treated with 200 to 400 mg daily *349*

Fibrinogen *Plasma Decrease Physiological* Decreased concentration associated with decreased platelet aggregation *349*

Glucose *Serum Decrease Physiological* Fenofibrate has a tendency to reduce serum glucose concentrations *3668*

HDL-Cholesterol *Serum Increase Physiological* Increase by 11% over 24 weeks in 92 type IIa given 100 mg 3 times per day with similar responses in type IIb patients when compared with baseline values *773* In 11 patients with type IIb hyperlipidemia treatment with 200 mg/d for 3 months caused increase from mean baseline of 1.06 ± 0.36 mmol/L to 1.32 ± 0.41 mmol/L *1805* In 41 patients with combined hyperlipidemia treatment with fenofibrate 300 mg/d for 2 years caused significant increase of 14.1% *1718* Increased apo A-I and apo A-II synthesis. Increased activity of lipoprotein lipase by stimulation of muscle lipoprotein lipase synthesis, alteration of the capillary endothelial surface and stimulation of apo C-II synthesis *264* Drug is effective in increasing plasma HDL-cholesterol concentration *3668* In 27 patients with severe hypertriglyceridemia treatment with 250 mg/d for 6 weeks caused significant increase from median baseline of 0.71 ± 0.22 mmol/L to 0.93 ± 0.32 mmol/L *3086* Generally increased in both hypertriglyceridemic and hypercholesterolemic patients when treated with 200 to 400 mg daily when initial concentration low *349* Significant effect in 18 patients with familial hypercholesterolemia given 0.25 g/d for 8 weeks *6400* In patients with type IIb hyperlipoproteinemia treatment with 300 mg/d for 3 months was associated with slight increase in concentration *644* Increase by 16% in 9 hypertriglyceridemic type 2 diabetic patients given 100 mg tid after 1 mo treatment *5690* In 10 postmenopausal women and 13 age-matched men with hypercholesterolemia treatment with fenofibrate 250 mg/d for 96 weeks caused significant increase from mean baseline of 53 ± 16 mg/dL to 63 ± 12 mg/dL in the women and in the men from 45 ± 10 mg/dL to 50 ± 10 mg/dL *5857*
Serum No Effect Physiological In 15 patients with type IIa hyperlipidemia treatment with 200 mg/d for 3 months caused nonsignificant change from mean baseline of 1.50 ± 0.42 mmol/L to 1.52 ± 0.33 mmol/L *1805*

HDL-Cholesterol:LDL-Cholesterol Ratio
Serum Decrease Physiological In 10 postmenopausal women and 13 age-matched men with hypercholesterolemia treatment with fenofibrate 250 mg/d for 96 weeks caused significant reduction from mean baseline of 4.3 ± 1.2 to 2.5 ± 0.8 in the women and in the men from 4.4 ± 1.0 to 3.4 ± 0.8 *5857*

LDL-Cholesterol *Serum Decrease Physiological* In 15 patients with type IIa hyperlipidemia treatment with 200 mg/d for 3 months caused significant decrease from mean baseline of 6.36 ± 1.35 mmol/L to 4.23 ± 1.17 mmol/L and in 11 with type IIb hyperlipidemia from mean baseline of 5.55 ± 1.04 mmol/L to 4.15 ± 0.89 mmol/L *1805* In 10 postmenopausal women and 13 age-matched men with hypercholesterolemia treatment with fenofibrate 250 mg/d for 96 weeks caused significant reduction from mean baseline of 210 ± 30 mg/dL to 151 ± 24 mg/dL in the women and in the men from 192 ± 11 mg/dL to 160 ± 20 mg/dL *5857* Increase by 20% over 24 weeks in 92 type IIa given 100 mg 3 times per day with similar responses in type IIb patients when compared with baseline values *773* In 18 patients with familial hypercholesterolemia 8 weeks treatment with 0.25 g/d caused mean reduction of 17.4% *6400* Drug is more effective than other fibrates in reducing plasma LDL-cholesterol concentration. In one study of 92 type IIa patients in the United States reduced the concentration by 20% *3668*
Serum Increase Physiological Increase by 22% in 9 hypertriglyceridemic type 2 diabetic patients given 100 mg t.i.d. after 1 mo treatment *5690*
Serum No Effect Physiological In 41 patients with combined hyperlipidemia treatment with fenofibrate 300 mg/d for 2 years caused nonsignificant increase of 0.1% *1718*

LDL-Cholesterol:HDL-Cholesterol Ratio
Serum Decrease Physiological In 41 patients with combined hyperlipidemia treatment with fenofibrate 300 mg/d for 2 years caused significant change from 5.30 to 4.28 *1718*

Lipoprotein Lp(a) *Serum No Effect Physiological* In 15 patients with type IIa hyperlipidemia treatment with 200 mg/d fenofibrate for 3 months caused nonsignificant change from mean baseline of 25.4 ± 18.5 mg/dL to 23.5 ± 19.4 mg/dL and in 11 with type IIb hyperlipidemia from 36.0 ± 39.5 mg/dL to 29.3 ± 31.9 mg/dL *1805*

Plasminogen Activator Inhibitor-1 Activity
Plasma No Effect Physiological In 27 patients with severe hypertriglyceridemia treatment with 250 mg/d for 6 weeks caused nonsignificant reduction from median baseline of 36.5 IU/mL to 34.2 IU/mL *3086*

Plasminogen Activator Inhibitor-1 Antigen
Plasma Decrease Physiological In 27 patients with severe hypertriglyceridemia treatment with 250 mg/d for 6 weeks caused nonsignificant reduction from median baseline of 48.3 ng/mL to 37.6 ng/mL *3086*

Platelet Aggregation *Blood Decrease Physiological* Decreased aggregation observed with treatment *349*

Postheparin Lipase *Plasma Increase Physiological* In 18 patients with familial hypercholesterolemia 8 weeks treatment with 0.25 g/d caused mean stimulation of enzyme by 16.1% *6400*

Prothrombin Time *Plasma Increase Physiological* Fenofibrate reported to prolong the prothrombin time when coadministered with an oral anticoagulant *3668*

Tissue Plasminogen Activator
Plasma Decrease Physiological In 27 patients with severe hypertriglyceridemia treatment with 250 mg/d for 6 weeks caused significant reduction from median baseline of 1.06 IU/mL to 0.94 IU/mL *3086*

Tissue Plasminogen Activator Antigen
Plasma Decrease Physiological In 27 patients with severe hypertriglyceridemia treatment with 250 mg/d for 6 weeks caused significant reduction from median baseline of 14.5 ng/mL to 11.9 ng/mL *3086*

Triglycerides *Serum Decrease Physiological* At dose of 200 to 400 mg daily substantial reduction observed in hypertriglyceridemic patients *349* In 27 patients with severe hypertriglyceridemia treatment with 250 mg/d for 6 weeks caused significant reduction from median baseline of 17.0 ± 10.9 mmol/L to 10.4 ± 11.9 mmol/L *3086* Increase by 38% over 24 weeks in 92 type IIa given 100 mg 3 times per day with similar responses in type IIb patients when compared with baseline values *773* Increase by 50% in 9 hypertriglyceridemic type 2 diabetic patients given 100 mg tid after 1 mo treatment *5690* In 10 postmenopausal women and 13 age-matched men with hypercholesterolemia treatment with fenofibrate 250 mg/d for 96 weeks caused significant reduction from mean baseline of 182 ± 97 mg/dL to 98 ± 34 mg/dL in the women and in the men from 147 ± 67 mg/dL to 113 ± 49 mg/dL *5857* In 15 patients with type IIa hyperlipidemia treatment with 200 mg/d for 3 months caused significant decrease from mean baseline of 0.97 ± 0.34 mmol/L to 0.62 ± 0.42 mmol/L and in 11 with type IIb hyperlipidemia from 2.63 ± 1.04 mmol/L to 1.23 ± 0.46 mmol/L *1805* In 41 patients with combined hyperlipidemia treatment with fenofibrate 300 mg/d for 2 years caused significant reduction of 40.7% *1718* Drug is effective in reducing plasma triglyceride concentration *3668* In patients with type IIb hyperlipoproteinemia treatment with 300 mg/d for 3 months caused significant decrease in concentration *644*

Uric Acid *Serum Decrease Physiological* Fenofibrate has been reported to increase clearance of uric acid reducing its serum concentration *3668* Drug has uricosuric effect *349*

VLDL-Cholesterol *Serum Decrease Physiological* Drug is more effective than other fibrates in reducing plasma VLDL-cholesterol concentration. In one study of 92 type IIa patients in the United States reduced the concentration by 38% *3668* Significant reduction in 18 patients with familial hypercholesterolemia given 0.25 g/d for 8 weeks *6400* Increase by 38% over 24 weeks in 92 type IIa given 100 mg 3 times per day with similar responses in type IIb patients when compared with baseline values *773*

VLDL-Triglycerides *Serum Decrease Physiological* Increase by 60% in 9 hypertriglyceridemic type 2 diabetic patients given 100 mg tid after 1 mo treatment *5690*

Fenoldopam

Aldosterone *Plasma Increase Physiological* In 10 healthy volunteers infusion of drug caused significant increase from mean baseline of 0.51 nmol/L to 0.70 nmol/L *2133* In 10 patients with chronic heart failure treatment with either 50, 100 or 200 mg/d for 4 days caused significant increase with the greatest effect observed after 200 mg/d *2133*

Calcium *Serum No Effect Physiological* Infusion of 0.5 µg/kg/min in 7 healthy volunteers had no effect on concentration at 25 minutes *341*
Urine Increase Physiological Infusion of 0.05-0.50 µg/kg/min for 1 hour caused significant increase in 10 healthy volunteers *2133*

Creatinine Clearance *Urine Increase Physiological* In 9 severely hypertensive patients with impaired renal function intravenous infusion until diastolic blood pressure declined to 100 to 110 mm Hg caused increase in clearance from 39 ± 7 mL/min to 75 ± 16 mL/min *5542*
Urine No Effect Physiological No significant change observed in 5-6 patients with severe hypertension in whom a mean of 0.32 µg/kg/min was infused for 2 hours *2133*

Dopamine *Plasma No Effect Physiological* No significant effect observed in 10 healthy volunteers with intravenous infusion *2133*
Urine Increase Physiological Infusion of fenoldopam intravenously in 10 healthy volunteers caused significant increase from mean baseline of 96.2 µmol/mol creatinine to 143 µmol/mol creatinine *2133*

Effective Renal Plasma Flow
Patient Increase Physiological Increase observed in 10 healthy volunteers with infusion of doses ranging from 0.05-0.50 µg/kg/min for 1 hour *2133*

Follicle Stimulating Hormone
Plasma No Effect Physiological Similar effects in drug infused and control situation in 9 volunteers *635*

Glomerular Filtration Rate *Urine No Effect Physiological* No significant effect observed in 10 healthy volunteers following infusion of doses ranging from 0.05 - 0.50 µg/kg/min for 1 hour *2133*

Growth Hormone *Plasma No Effect Physiological* Similar effects on basal concentrations in drug infused and control situations in 9 volunteers *635*

Luteinizing Hormone *Plasma No Effect Physiological* Similar effects observed in drug infused and control situation in 9 volunteers *635*

Norepinephrine *Plasma Increase Physiological* Significant increase observed in 10 patients with chronic heart failure treated with either 50, 100 or 200 mg/d for 4 days but no further increase observed when norepinephrine concentration already increased *2133*

Parathyroid Hormone *Plasma No Effect Physiological* Infusion of 0.5 µg/kg/min for 25 minutes in 7 normal volunteers had no effect on concentration *341*

Potassium *Urine Increase Physiological* In 9 hypertensive patients with impaired renal function intravenous infusion of fenoldopam until diastolic blood pressure fell to 100 to 110 mm Hg caused significant increase from mean baseline of 25.4 µEq/min to 68.5 ± 20.9 µEq/min *5542*

Prolactin *Plasma Increase Physiological* Mean 128% increase versus decline to 85% in control situation in volunteers given intravenous infusion *635*

Renal Plasma Flow *Patient Increase Physiological* In healthy volunteers fenoldopam increases increases renal plasma flow which, however, was attenuated by metoclopramide according to one report but not according to another *2133*

Renin Activity *Plasma Increase Physiological* In 10 patients with chronic heart failure treatment for 4 days with either 50, 100 or 200 mg/d caused significant increase with 200 mg/d causing the greatest effect *2133* Effect observed due to lack of DA_2- and α_2-agonist action *2846* Effect due to its lack of DA_2- and α_2-agonist action *2846* Significant increased observed in 10 healthy volunteers with intravenous infusion increasing with increasing dose *2133*

Sodium *Urine Increase Physiological* Infusion of doses ranging from 0.05-0.50 µg/kg/min for 1 hour caused significant increase *2133* In 9 hypertensive patients with impaired renal function intravenous infusion of fenoldopam until blood pressure decreased to 100 to 110 mm Hg caused significant increase from mean baseline of 75 ± 22 µEq/min to 227 ± 60 µEq/min *5542* Infusion of a mean of 0.32 µg/kg/min for 2 hours in 5-6 patients with severe hypertension caused increased sodium excretion *2133*

T3-Uptake *Serum No Effect Physiological* No effect of drug infusion in 9 volunteers *635*

Testosterone *Serum Decrease Physiological* Reduction by 26% in 9 volunteers given drug infusion compared with controls, affecting both basal and GnRH/TRH stimulated concentrations *635*

Thyroid Stimulating Hormone
Serum Decrease Physiological Significant decrease in basal concentration to 71% during drug infusion compared with 82% in control infusion in 9 volunteers *635*

Thyroxine (T4) *Serum No Effect Physiological* No effect of infusion of drug on basal concentration in 9 volunteers *635*

Tri-iodothyronine (T3) *Serum No Effect Physiological* No effect of infusion on basal concentration in 9 volunteers *635*

Volume *Urine Increase Physiological* In 5-6 patients with severe hypertension intravenous infusion of a mean of 0.32 µg/kg/min for 2 hours caused increased urine flow rate *2133* In 9 hypertensive patients with impaired renal function intravenous infusions until diastolic blood pressure fell to 100 to 110 mm Hg caused significant increase from mean baseline of 119 ± 37 mL/h to 275 ± 84 mL/h *5542*

Fenoprofen

Alanine Aminotransferase *Serum Increase Physiological* Occasional cholestatic jaundice observed, especially in women, after several months treatment *1384* With administration cholestatic hepatitis may occur in less than 1% patients *1439*
Serum No Effect Physiological In 49 patients with juvenile rheumatoid arthritis when some abnormal results in patients with same therapeutic outcome given aspirin *712*

Alkaline Phosphatase *Serum Increase Physiological* Occasional cholestatic jaundice observed, most often in women and after several months treatment *1384* With administration cholestatic hepatitis may occur in less than 1% patients *1439*

Aspartate Aminotransferase *Serum Increase Physiological* With administration cholestatic hepatitis may occur in less than 1% patients *1439* Occasional cholestatic jaundice observed, most often in women, after several months treatment *1384*
Serum No Effect Physiological In 49 patients with juvenile rheumatoid arthritis when some abnormal results in patients with same therapeutic outcome given aspirin *712*

Barbiturate *Urine Increase Analytical* At concentration occurring in urine following ingestion positive result obtained with Abbott TDx procedure *3420*

Fenoprofen *(continued)*

Benzodiazepine *Urine No Effect Analytical* No significant interference observed with new Syva EMIT assay in urines of patients taking fenoprofen *3370*
Urine Positive Analytical At concentration occurring in urine following ingestion positive result obtained with Abbott TDx *3420*

Bilirubin *Serum Increase Physiological* Occasional cholestatic jaundice observed, most often in women and after several months treatment *1384* With administration cholestatic hepatitis may occur in less than 1% patients *1439*
Serum No Effect Physiological At pharmacological concentrations has little or no protein displacement effect *6314*

Blood *Urine Increase Physiological* Renal damage with hematuria may occur in less than 1% patients *1439*

Chondrex *Serum No Effect Analytical* Concentrations up to 5 g/L had no significant effect on sandwich-type ELISA procedure of Harvey et al *2491*

Cortisol *Plasma Increase Analytical* At a concentration of 480 mg/L increased recovery to 146.3% with Enzymun method *1097*
Plasma No Effect Analytical At a concentration of 96 mg/L had no significant effect on Enzymun method (105.7% recovery) *1097*

Creatinine *Serum Increase Physiological* Renal failure with azotemia may occur in less than 1% patients *1439* In 2 isolated cases of patients with arthritis in the absence of hypertension *715*

Creatinine Clearance *Urine Decrease Physiological* Rare case of acute tubulointerstitial nephritis with acute renal failure (probable association with drug administration) *6016*

11-Deoxycorticosterone *Plasma Increase Analytical* False positive results reported with Amerlex-M kit procedure as result of chemical cross-reaction that directly interferes with the assay *1439*

Erythrocytes *Blood Decrease Physiological* Hemolytic or aplastic anemia may occur in less than 1% patients *1439* In 6.5% of patients treated for juvenile rheumatoid arthritis *386*
Urine Increase Physiological Rare case of acute tubulointerstitial nephritis with acute renal failure (probable association with drug administration) *6016*

Granulocytes *Blood Decrease Physiological* Agranulocytosis or pancytopenia may occur in less than 1% patients *1439*

Hemoglobin *Blood Decrease Physiological* Hemolytic or aplastic anemia or pancytopenia may occur in less than 1% patients *1439*
Urine Increase Physiological In 6.5% of patients treated for juvenile rheumatoid arthritis *386* Rare case of acute tubulointerstitial nephritis with acute renal failure (probable association with drug administration) *6016*

Lactate Dehydrogenase *Serum Increase Physiological* With administration cholestatic hepatitis may occur in less than 1% patients *1439*

Leukocytes *Blood Decrease Physiological* Hemolytic or aplastic anemia or pancytopenia may occur in less than 1% patients *1439*
Urine Increase Physiological Rare case of acute tubulointerstitial nephritis with acute renal failure (probable association with drug administration) *6016*

Meprobamate *Serum Increase Physiological* In clinical trials some patients demonstrated increased activity *1439*

Neutrophils *Blood Decrease Physiological* Occasional case of agranulocytosis reported *6264*

Occult Blood *Feces Increase Physiological* Significant effect but less than with aspirin *4955* Occasional case of gastrointestinal bleeding reported but much less frequent than with aspirin *1384* With administration gastrointestinal hemorrhage may occur in less than 1% patients *1439* In 9% in patients treated for juvenile rheumatoid arthritis *386*
Feces No Effect Physiological In 49 patients with juvenile rheumatoid arthritis when some abnormal results in patients with same therapeutic outcome given aspirin *712*

Platelets *Blood Decrease Physiological* Purpura with/without thrombocytopenia may occur in less than 1% patients *1439* Single case with approximately 1 g/d for 6 to 8 weeks, although patient also taking niacin *5568*

Protein *Urine Increase Physiological* Renal damage with interstitial nephritis, nephrosis or papillary necrosis may occur in less than 1% patients *1439* In 4% in patients treated for juvenile rheumatoid arthritis *386* In 2 isolated cases of patients with arthritis in the absence of hypertension *715*

Thyroid Stimulating Hormone *Serum No Effect Analytical* No effect observed on analytical procedures *1439*
Serum No Effect Physiological No effect noted physiologically or on methods *6035*

Thyroxine (T4) *Serum No Effect Analytical* No effect observed on analytical procedures *1439*
Serum No Effect Physiological No effect noted physiologically or on methods *6035*

Tri-iodothyronine, Free (fT3) *Serum Increase Analytical* Tripled in 2 volunteers over 2 weeks as also observed in some patients due to metabolite cross-reacting with antisera from Amersham and to lesser extent with that from Corning *6035*
Serum No Effect Analytical At a concentration of 0.6 g/L cross-reactivity of less than 0.1% observed with free triiodothyronine method on Bayer Technicon Immuno 1® system *425*

Tri-iodothyronine (T3) *Serum Increase Analytical* Doubled in 2 volunteers over 2 weeks as also observed in some patients due to metabolite cross-reacting with antisera from Amersham and to lesser extent with that from Corning *6035*

Triolein ^{131}I Test *Serum Increase Analytical* False positive results reported with Amerlex-M kit procedure as result of chemical cross-reaction that directly interferes with assay *1439*

Urea Nitrogen *Serum Increase Physiological* Renal failure with azotemia may occur in less than 1% patients *1439*

Fenoterol

Adenosine Monophosphate *Plasma Increase Physiological* Effect mirrored reduction in serum potassium concentration following inhalation of drug *5322*

Erythropoietin *Serum Increase Physiological* In patients given 2 µg/min caused significant increase from mean baseline of 7 mU/L to 14 mU/L after 24 h *2185*

Norepinephrine *Plasma Increase Physiological* Dose-dependent increase following inhalation of drug *5322*

Placental Lactogen *Plasma No Effect Physiological* In patients given 2 µg/min caused insignificant change from mean baseline of 5.3 µg/mL over 50 h *2185*

Potassium *Serum Decrease Physiological* Dose dependent reduction observed in 6 healthy male volunteers with peak effect 75 to 90 minutes after first inhalation. At same concentration effect considerably greater than when salbutamol given *5322* In patients given 2 µg/min caused insignificant change from mean baseline of 3.8 mmol/L over 50 h after initial significant decrease to 3.0 mmol/L after 1 h *2185* Reduction of up to 0.9 mmol/L in normal subjects with inhalation of drug *2389*
Serum No Effect Physiological In patients given 2 µg/min caused insignificant change from mean baseline of 3.8 mmol/L over 50 h after initial significant decrease to 3.0 mmol/L after 1 h *2185*

Renin Activity *Plasma Increase Physiological* Dose-dependent increase observed following inhalation of drug *5322*

Fenquizone

Creatinine *Serum No Effect Analytical* No interference observed with liquid chromatographic method of Paroni *4540*

Fentanyl

Amylase *Serum Increase Physiological* May cause spasm of sphincter of Oddi *128*

Epinephrine *Plasma Increase Physiological* Mechanism obscure *2854*

Hemoglobin *Plasma Increase Physiological* In a single patient with low haptoglobin following high dose administration dose related effect *2813*
Urine Increase Physiological In a single patient with low haptoglobin following high dose administration. dose related effect *2813*

Histamine *Plasma No Effect Analytical* Improbable inhibition of radio-enzyme assay at physiological concentrations *2492*

Lysergic Acid Diethylamide *Urine Increase Analytical* Minimum concentration that caused a positive result with EMIT method to measure LSD 0.1 mg/L *4968*

Midazolam *Serum No Effect Analytical* On GC-ECD method of Ha et al *2387*

Norepinephrine *Plasma Decrease Physiological* Mechanism obscure *2854*

p-Aminophenol *Urine No Effect Analytical* With addition of drugs at a concentration of 100 mg/L and of related compounds at 50 mg/L no significant effect observed on colorimetric method of van Bocxlaer on Cobas Mira analyzer which involves reacting free p-aminophenol with resorcinol in the presence of magnesium ions to form an indophenol dye measured at 550 nm *6163*

Ferric Polymaltose

Ferritin *Serum Increase Physiological* Significant increase in iron-deficient blood donors who received 200 mg elemental iron for 56 days *3719*

Hemoglobin *Blood Increase Physiological* Significant increase in blood donors following treatment with 200 mg elemental iron for 56 days when initial hemoglobin was low *3719*

Ferrous Ascorbate

Glucose Tolerance *Serum Decrease Physiological* Mechanism not reported *2451*

Ferrous Gluconate

Ciprofloxacin *Serum Decrease Physiological* When administered with 600 mg ferrous gluconate peak serum concentration reduced by 1.3 mg/L and area under curve reduced by 4.1 mg/Lh probably due to oxidation of ferrous iron to ferric iron and binding of ferric iron by ciprofloxacin *3038*

Occult Blood *Feces Increase Analytical* 50% false positive with Hemoccult® ; 65% false positive with Hematest® in 10 male volunteers taking 300 mg 3 times per day for 1 week *3570*

Ferrous Sulfate

Cefdinir *Serum Decrease Physiological* Concomitant administration of 60 mg elemental iron as ferrous sulfate or vitamins supplemented with 10 mg of elemental iron with cefdinir reduced its absorption by 80% and 31% respectively *4528*

Ciprofloxacin *Serum Decrease Physiological* Bioavailability reduced with both peak concentration and area under concentration-time curve markedly reduced *1384* Simultaneous administration of ferrous sulfate with ciprofloxacin caused reduction of area under the curve (mean 5.4 µg/h/mL versus 14.5 µg/h/mL in cotrols) in 12 healthy adult male volunteers *4731* In 8 healthy volunteers coadministration of ferrous sulfate with 500 mg ciprofloxacin caused significant reduction from control baseline of 2.15 ± 0.37 µg/mL to 0.95 ± 0.32 µg/mL *3497* When ferrous sulfate and 500 mg ciprofloxacin coadministered AUC of ciprofloxacin reduced by 57% and peak plasma concentration reduced by 54% *3497* When administered with 300 mg ferrous sulfate peak serum concentration reduced from 3.0 to 2.0 mg/L and area under curve from 12.3 mg/Lh to 6.7 mg/Lh probably due to oxidation of ferrous iron to ferric iron and its binding by ciprofloxacin *3038*

Color *Urine Increase Analytical* Black, brown or dark color observed following ingestion of ferrous sulfate *3388*

Cortisol *Plasma No Effect Physiological* No significant change observed on basal cortisol concentration in 11 anemic patients given ferrous sulfate for 7 days *5174*

Cortisol, Free *Urine No Effect Analytical* No significant interference observed with HPLC method of Turpeinen et al *6105*

Cortisol response to ACTH
Plasma Decrease Physiological No significant difference from situation before administration of ferrous sulfate for 7 days in 11 anemic patients compared with healthy controls i.e. significantly reduced response observed *5174*

Doxycycline *Serum Decrease Physiological* Reduced absorption due to chelation which also affects elimination *6403* Greatly reduced gastrointestinal absorption observed with reduced serum concentration when drugs coadministered *4255*

Ferritin *Serum Increase Physiological* In 107 apparently healthy female nurse students admnistration of 105 mg ferrous sulfate for 30 days caused significant change from mean baseline of 29.2 ± 24.4 µg/L to 46.4 ± 30.3 µg/L *2565*

Glucose *Urine Decrease Analytical* Low measurements obtained with Clinistix® , Diastix® *1826*
Urine No Effect Analytical No effect observed with Tes-Tape® *1826*

Hemoglobin *Blood Increase Physiological* In 107 apparently healthy female nurse students admnistration of 105 mg ferrous sulfate for 30 days caused significant change from mean baseline of 13.4 ± 0.9 g/dL to 13.9 ± 0.8 g/dL *2565*

Iron *Serum Increase Physiological* In 107 apparently healthy female nurse students admnistration of 105 mg ferrous sulfate for 30 days caused nonsignificant change from mean baseline of 19.8 ± 7.7 µmol/L to 22.1 ± 8.0 µmol/L *2565*

Iron-Binding Capacity, Total
Serum Decrease Physiological In 107 apparently healthy female nurse students admnistration of 105 mg ferrous sulfate for 30 days caused significant change from mean baseline of 78.1 ± 13.2 µmol/L to 73.0 ± 12.5 µmol/L *2565*

Levodopa *Serum Decrease Physiological* Ingestion of 325 mg ferrous sulfate together with 250 mg levodopa caused a 55% reduction in peak levodopa concentration due to oxidation of ferrous to ferric iron which binds strongly to levodopa. Clinical significance of this chelation is unknown *6682*

Methacycline *Serum Decrease Physiological* Reduced absorption due to chelation which also affects elimination *6403* Concomitant administration of ferrous sulfate with antibiotic caused reduced gastrointestinal absorption and reduced serum concentration *4255*

Norfloxacin *Serum Decrease Physiological* In 8 healthy volunteers coadministration of ferrous sulfate with 400 mg norfloxacin caused decrease of 75% from mean control baseline of 0.84 ± 0.37 µg/mL to 0.19 ± 0.08 µg/mL *3497*
Urine Decrease Physiological In 8 healthy men after ingestion of 400 mg norfloxacin excretion significantly reduced by 55% when ferrous sulfate coingested due to interference with absorption *865*

Occult Blood *Feces Increase Analytical* 65% false positive with Hemoccult® ; 25% false positive with Hematest® in 10 male volunteers taking 300 mg 3 times per day for 1 week *3570*

Ofloxacin *Serum Decrease Physiological* In 8 healthy volunteers coadministration of ferrous sulfate with 400 mg ofloxacin caused mean concentration to decrease from control baseline of 3.02 ± 0.47 µg/mL to 1.89 ± 0.39 µg/mL *3497*

Oxytetracycline *Serum Decrease Physiological* Reduced absorption due to chelation which also affects elimination *6403* Concomitant administration of 200 mg ferrous sulfate caused reduced absorption and serum concentration of antibiotic *4255*

Penicillamine *Serum Decrease Physiological* Reduced absorption due to chelation which also affects elimination *6403* Marked reduction (by about 35%) in 6 healthy men when 300 mg ferrous sulfate given orally due to effect on absorption *4455*

T3-Uptake *Serum No Effect Physiological* Coadministration of ferrous sulfate with thyroxine to 14 patients with primary hypothyroidism for 12 weeks had no effect on serum T3 resin uptake assay *864*

Tetracycline *Serum Decrease Physiological* Reduced absorption due to chelation which also affects elimination *6403* Absorption of all tetracyclines reduced due to ferrous ion chelation *1384* Concomitant administration of 200 mg ferrous sulfate caused reduction of absorption of antibiotic and reduced serum concentration *4255*

Ferrous Sulfate *(continued)*

Thyroid Stimulating Hormone
Serum Increase Physiological In 11 of 14 patients with established primary hypothyroidism coadministration of ferrous sulfate with thyroxine caused mean plasma TSH concentration to increase to 2.7 ± 0.6 mU/L from mean baseline of 1.6 ± 0.5 mU/L *864*

Thyroxine (T4) *Serum No Effect Physiological* Nonsignificant reduction from mean baseline of 135 ± 22 nmol/L to 127 ± 28 nmol/L when ferrous sulfate coadministered with thyroxine to patients with primary hypothyroidism *864*

Thyroxine (T4) Index, Free *Serum Decrease Physiological* In 10 of 14 patients with primary hypothyroidism coadministration of ferrous sulfate with thyroxine was associated with a reduction of FTI after 12 weeks *864*

Fexofenadine

Pseudoephedrine *Serum No Effect Physiological* Coadministration of drugs has no effect on the pharmacokinetics of each other *2637*

Fibrates

Cholesterol *Serum Increase Physiological* Effect not always clear cut but hypercholesterolemia reduced particularly with relatively marked increases (familial type IIA) and normal triglyceridemia *5586*

Fibrinogen *Plasma Decrease Physiological* Prolonged administration observed to reduce plasma concentration *3186* Some fibrates possess potent plasma fibrinogen reducing activity *5586*

HDL-Cholesterol *Serum Increase Physiological* By activating VLDL catabolism concentration of HDL-cholesterol increased in most patients *5586*

Platelet Aggregation *Blood Decrease Physiological* Some reports of reduced sensitivity to different aggregants in fibrate-treated patients *5586*

VLDL-Triglycerides *Serum Decrease Physiological* In about 80% of patients with increased plasma triglycerides activation of lipoprotein catabolism by fibrates can bring concentration close to normal *5586*

Fibrin Hydrolysate

Ammonia *Plasma Increase Physiological* Due to high ammonia content of solution *6311*

Hemoglobin *Blood Decrease Physiological* ?due to septicemia or hypophosphatemia *6311*

Phosphate *Serum Decrease Physiological* Intracellular transfer *6311*

Fibrinolysin

Aspartate Aminotransferase *Serum Increase Physiological* Hepatitis as late complication of administration *128*

Urea Nitrogen *Serum Increase Physiological* Renal failure reported (rare complication) *128*

Finasteride

Aldosterone *Plasma Decrease Physiological* In 48 patients with benign prostatic hyperplasia treatment with 5 mg/d caused a nonsignificant decrease from mean baseline of 140.9 ± 57.5 pg/mL to 150.6 ± 54.6 µg/mL after 3 months and 122.9 ± 55.9 pg/mL after 6 months *6142*

Androstanediol Glucuronide
Plasma Decrease Physiological Significant reduction observed in male volunteers receiving doses of 0.04 mg, 0.12 mg, 0.2 mg or 1.0 mg daily for 14 days but no difference between groups *2256*

Androstenedione *Plasma Increase Physiological* In 12 young women with idiopathic hirsutism treatment with 5 mg/d caused mean concentration to change significantly from 10.9 ± 1.1 nmol/L to 12.6 ± 1.3 nmol/L after one month and 15.8 ± 1.0 nmol/L after 6 months *4087* Nonsignificant increase from mean of 5.9 to 6.7 nmol/L in 10 male volunteers given 25 mg/day for 11 days, but significant increase from 5.8 to 7.5 nmol/L with 50 mg/day and from 5.6 to 9.1 nmol/L with 100 mg/day *2256*
Plasma No Effect Physiological In 9 hirsute patients treatment with 7.5 mg/d orally caused change from mean baseline of 1.84 ± 0.12 ng/mL to 1.32 ± 0.08 ng/mL at 3 months (nonsignificant), 1.89 ± 0.09 ng/mL at 6 months (nonsignificant) and 1.83 ± 0.11 ng/mL at 9 months (nonsignificant) *1045*

Androsterone Glucuronide *Plasma Decrease Physiological* Significant reduction in male volunteers receiving daily doses from 0.04 mg, 0.12 mg, 0.4 mg or 1.0 mg daily for 14 days but no significant difference between groups *2256*

Antipyrine *Serum No Effect Physiological* In 12 patients receiving 19 mg/d finasteride no effect observed on pharmacokinetics of antipyrine or its metabolite *3991*

Blood *Urine Decrease Physiological* In 18 patients with BPH and gross hematuria treatment with finasteride for a mean follow-up of 31 months caused marked reduction in hematuria *4051*

Cholesterol *Serum No Effect Physiological* No significant change observed in 10 male volunteers given doses up to 100 mg/day for 11 days *2256*

Cortisol *Plasma No Effect Physiological* No significant change observed in morning concentration in 10 male volunteers given doses up to 100 mg daily for 11 days *2256*

Dehydroepiandrosterone *Plasma Decrease Physiological* In 48 patients with benign prostatic hyperplasia treatment with 5 mg/d caused a nonsignificant decrease from mean baseline of 3.2 ± 1.8 ng/mL to 3.0 ± 1.5 ng/mL after 3 months and 2.9 ± 1.6 ng/mL after 6 months *6142* In 48 patients with benign prostatic hyperplasia treatment with 5 mg/d caused a nonsignificant decrease from mean baseline of 20.0 ± 9.2 µg/mL to 19.5 ± 9.8 µg/mL after 3 months and 18.4 ± 8.4 µg/mL after 6 months *6142*

Dehydroepiandrosterone Sulfate
Plasma Decrease Physiological In 9 hirsute patients treatment with 7.5 mg/d orally caused change from mean baseline of 2.0 µg/mL to 1.9 µg/mL at 3 months (nonsignificant), 1.8 µg/mL at 6 months (significant) and 1.9 µg/mL at 9 months (nonsignificant) *1045*
Plasma No Effect Physiological In 12 young women with idiopathic hirsutism treatment with 5 mg/d caused mean concentration to change nonsignificantly from 6.6 ± 1.1 µmol/L to 6.4 ± 0.3 µmol/L after one month and 7.4 ± 0.5 µmol/L after 6 months *4087*

Digoxin *Serum No Effect Physiological* In 17 normal volunteers receiving 5 mg/d finasteride for 10 days no effect observed on plasma concentration of digoxin after a single dose *3991*

Dihydrotestosterone *Serum Decrease Physiological* In 21 men aged 58 - 79 years with benign prostatic hypertrophy treatment with 5 mg/d for 12 months caused significant decrease from mean baseline of 2.86 ± 0.924 nmol/L to 0.59 ± 0.186 nmol/L *2879* In 9 healthy men aged 52.1 ± 7.2 y treated with finasteride 5 mg/d caused 69% and 72% reduction after 4 and 12 weeks respectively from baseline of 1.16 ± 0.27 nmol/L *1196* Significant reduction from baseline in 10 male volunteers given 25 mg/day for 11 days from mean of 2.20 to 0.63 nmol/L, in 10 given 50 mg/day from mean of 1.98 to 0.63 nmol/L and in 10 given 100 mg/day from mean of 2.02 to 0.44 nmol/L *2256* In 69 men with benign prostatic hypertrophy mean baseline concentration of 1.37 ± 0.13 nmol/L in placebo treated population reduced to 0.50 ± 0.04, 0.50 ± 0.05, 0.4 ± 0.06, 0.2 ± 0.03 and 0.3 ± 0.05 nmol/L respectively when treated with 1, 5, 10, 50 and 100 mg/d for 8 days *3878* In 48 patients with benign prostatic hyperplasia treatment with 5 mg/d caused significant decrease from mean baseline of 43.2 ± 8.7 ng/dL to 26.8 ± 5.2 ng/dL after 3 months and 10.8 ± 2.8 ng/dL after 6 months *6142* In normal men treatment with doses from 5 to 400 mg caused 60 to 80% reduction in concentration. In men given 0.4 to 100 mg daily for 11 to 14 days concentration decreased by 63 to 78% *4970*

Serum Increase Physiological In men treated with long term drug mean concentration increased by about 10% *4970* In 9 hirsute patients treatment with 7.5 mg/d orally caused change from mean baseline of 340 pg/mL to 210 pg/mL at 3 months (significant), 180 pg/mL at 6 months (significant) and 160 pg/mL at 9 months (significant) *1045*

Estradiol *Plasma No Effect Physiological* In 9 hirsute patients treatment with 7.5 mg/d orally caused change from mean baseline of 52.6 ± 4.4 pg/mL to 57.4 ± 4.7 pg/mL at 3 months (nonsignificant), 58.7 ± 4.5 pg/mL at 6 months (nonsignificant) and 57.9 ± 3.7 pg/mL at 9 months (nonsignificant) *1045* In 12 young women with idiopathic hirsutism treatment with 5 mg/d caused mean concentration to change nonsignificantly from 90 ± 10 pmol/L to 92 ± 6 pmol/L after one month and 116 ± 14 pmol/L after 6 months *4087* No significant deviation from baseline in 10 male volunteers given doses up to 100 mg daily for 11 days *2256*

17β-Estradiol *Plasma Decrease Physiological* In 21 men aged 58 - 79 years with benign prostatic hypertrophy treatment with 5 mg/d for 12 months caused nonsignificant decrease from mean baseline of 62.5 ± 17.6 pmol/L to 55.7 ± 12.8 pmol/L *2879*

Follicle Stimulating Hormone

Plasma Decrease Physiological In 48 patients with benign prostatic hyperplasia treatment with 5 mg/d caused a significant decrease from mean baseline of 9.7 ± 6.2 mIU/mL to 7.5 ± 5.2 mIU/mL after 3 months and 5.8 ± 2.6 mIU/mL after 6 months *6142*

Plasma Increase Physiological In 12 young women with idiopathic hirsutism treatment with 5 mg/d caused mean concentration to change significantly from 4.7 ± 0.4 IU/L to 5.6 ± 0.6 IU/L after one month and 5.1 ± 0.4 IU/L after 6 months *4087*

Plasma No Effect Physiological In young men receiving 5 mg/d for 28 days no significant effect observed on concentration *4970* No significant change observed in mean concentrations in 10 male volunteers given doses of either 25 mg/day, 50 mg/day or 100 mg/day for 11 days *2256* In 9 hirsute patients treatment with 7.5 mg/d orally caused change from mean baseline of 3.6 mIU/mL to 3.4 mIU/mL at 3 months (nonsignificant), 3.7 mIU/mL at 6 months (nonsignificant) and 3.4 mIU/mL at 9 months (nonsignificant) *1045*

HDL-Cholesterol *Serum No Effect Physiological* No significant change observed in 10 male volunteers given doses up to 100 mg daily for 11 days *2256*

17-Hydroxyprogesterone *Plasma No Effect Physiological* In 12 young women with idiopathic hirsutism treatment with 5 mg/d caused mean concentration to change nonsignificantly from 2.2 ± 0.2 nmol/L to 2.6 ± 0.4 nmol/L after one month and 2.0 ± 0.3 nmol/L after 6 months *4087*

17α-Hydroxyprogesterone *Plasma No Effect Physiological* In 9 hirsute patients treatment with 7.5 mg/d orally caused change from mean baseline of 408.9 ± 23.9 µg/mL to 381.1 ± 16.7 µg/mL at 3 months (nonsignificant), 403.3 ± 11.2 µg/mL at 6 months (nonsignificant) and 405.5 ± 20.6 µg/mL at 9 months (nonsignificant) *1045*

LDL-Cholesterol *Serum No Effect Physiological* No significant change observed in 10 male volunteers given doses up to 100 mg daily for 11 days *2256*

Luteinizing Hormone *Plasma Decrease Physiological* In 48 patients with benign prostatic hyperplasia treatment with 5 mg/d caused a significant decrease from mean baseline of 9.1 ± 4.4 mIU/mL to 7.7 ± 3.7 mIU/mL after 3 months and 6.8 ± 3.5 mIU/mL after 6 months *6142*

Plasma Increase Physiological In 12 young women with idiopathic hirsutism treatment with 5 mg/d caused mean concentration to change significantly from 3.6 ± 0.6 IU/L to 5.6 ± 0.5 IU/L after one month and 5.4 ± 0.8 IU/L after 6 months *4087* In 250 men who received 5 mg daily for 12 months mean concentration increased from 6.6 IU/L to 7.6 IU/L, unlikely to be of clinical significance *4970*

Plasma No Effect Physiological In healthy young men treatment with 5 mg daily for 28 days had no effect on concentration *4970* No significant change observed in mean concentrations in 10 male volunteers given doses of either 25 mg/day, 50 mg/day or 100 mg/day for 11 days *2256* In 9 hirsute patients treatment with 7.5 mg/d orally caused change from mean baseline of 5.7 mIU/mL to 5.8 mIU/mL at 3 months (nonsignificant), 6.0 mIU/mL at 6 months (nonsignificant) and 6.0 mIU/mL at 9 months (nonsignificant) *1045*

Prolactin *Plasma Decrease Physiological* In 48 patients with benign prostatic hyperplasia treatment with 5 mg/d caused a nonsignificant decrease from mean baseline of 10.4 ± 7.4 ng/mL to 8.2 ± 3.6 ng/mL after 3 months and 7.6 ± 3.9 ng/mL after 6 months *6142*

Propranolol *Serum No Effect Physiological* In 19 normal volunteers receiving 5 mg/d finasteride for 10 days no effect observed on plasma concentration of propranolol after a single dose *3991*

Prostate-specific Antigen *Serum Decrease Physiological* In men with benign prostatic hypertrophy treatment for 3 months caused mean reduction of 50% *4970* In 10 men in phase 3 trial serum PSA decreased by 26% and in 13 concentration decreased by 15% after 6 weeks without evidence of tumor regression *4970*

Prostate-specific Antigen, Free *Serum No Effect Analytical* Finasteride at a concentration of 370 µg/L had no significant effect on the Hybritech Tandem® -R free PSA immunoassay *4286*

Prothrombin Time *Plasma No Effect Physiological* In 12 patients chronically treated with warfarin the prothrombin time and plasma concentration of warfarin were not altered after treatment with finasteride 5 mg/d for 14 days *3991*

Sex-Hormone Binding Globulin

Serum Decrease Physiological In 9 hirsute patients treatment with 7.5 mg/d orally caused change from mean baseline of 2.17 ± 0.13 µg/mL to 2.08 ± 0.07 µg/mL at 3 months (nonsignificant), 1.89 ± 0.12 µg/mL at 6 months (nonsignificant) and 1.87 ± 0.08 µg/mL at 9 months (nonsignificant) *1045*

Serum No Effect Physiological In 21 men aged 58 - 79 years with benign prostatic hypertrophy treatment with 5 mg/d for 12 months caused nonsignificant change from mean baseline of 44.1 ± 4.5 nmol/L to 45.2 ± 5.7 nmol/L *2879*

Testosterone *Serum Decrease Physiological* In 12 young women with idiopathic hirsutism treatment with 5 mg/d caused mean concentration to change significantly from 1.7 ± 0.1 nmol/L to 2.3 ± 0.3 nmol/L after one month and 2.4 ± 0.2 nmol/L after 6 months *4087*

Serum Increase Physiological No significant change in 10 male volunteers given 25 mg daily for 11 days (mean baseline 21.6 nmol/L increased to 23.8 nmol/L) but significant increase from mean of 21.3 to 26.5 nmol/L with 50 mg daily and from 21.6 to 26.9 nmol/L with 100 mg daily *2256* In 9 hirsute patients treatment with 7.5 mg/d orally caused change from mean baseline of 0.52 ng/mL to 0.58 ng/mL at 3 months (nonsignificant), 0.71 ng/mL at 6 months (significant) and 0.74 ng/mL at 9 months (significant) *1045* In 48 patients with benign prostatic hyperplasia treatment with 5 mg/d caused significant increase from mean baseline of 3.82 ± 1.24 ng/mL to 4.44 ± 1.40 ng/mL after 3 months and 4.82 ± 1.38 ng/mL after 6 months *6142* In 21 men aged 58 - 79 years with benign prostatic hypertrophy treatment with 5 mg/d for 12 months caused significant increase from mean baseline of 16.38 ± 1.66 nmol/L to 19.4 ± 1.67 nmol/L *2879*

Serum No Effect Physiological In 69 men with benign prostatic hypertrophy mean baseline concentration of 16.0 ± 1.4 nmol/L not significantly reduced to 15.7 ± 1.9 nmol/L when treated with 100 mg/d for 8 days *3878* In 9 healthy men aged 52.1 ± 7.2 y treated with finasteride 5 mg/d caused no significant change after 4 and 12 weeks respectively from baseline of 16.54 ± 2.64 nmol/L *1196* No significant effect observed in male volunteers given doses of 0.04 mg, 0.12 mg, or 0.2 mg daily for 14 days but initial slight reduction observed when daily dose of 1.0 mg used although concentration remained within normal range *2256*

Testosterone, Bioavailable *Serum Increase Physiological* In 21 men aged 58 - 79 years with benign prostatic hypertrophy treatment with 5 mg/d for 12 months caused nonsignificant increase from mean baseline of 3.12 ± 0.38 nmol/L to 3.467 ± 0.30 nmol/L *2879*

Testosterone, Free *Serum No Effect Physiological* In 12 young women with idiopathic hirsutism treatment with 5 mg/d caused mean concentration to change nonsignificantly from 8.2 ± 0.6 pmol/L to 10.1 ± 1.5 pmol/L after one month and 10.6 ± 1.2 pmol/L after 6 months *4087* In 9 hirsute patients treatment with 7.5 mg/d orally caused change from mean baseline of 2.86 ± 0.11 pg/mL to 2.97 ± 0.13 pg/mL at 3 months (nonsignificant), 2.97 ± 0.11 pg/mL at 6 months (nonsignificant) and 3.04 ± 0.08 pg/mL at 9 months (nonsignificant) *1045*

Finasteride *(continued)*

Theophylline *Serum Decrease Physiological* In 12 normal volunteers receiving 5 mg/d finasteride for 8 days significantly increased the plasma clearance of theophylline by 7% and decreased its half-life by 10% after intravenous administration of aminophylline, although the changes were not clearly significant *3991*
Serum No Effect Physiological No clinically significant effect on theophylline concentration observed when drugs coadministered *5999* No documented significant interaction with theophylline reported *6117*

Triglycerides *Serum No Effect Physiological* No significant change observed in 10 male volunteers given up to 100 mg daily for 11 days *2256*

Flavaspidic Acid

Bilirubin *Serum Increase Physiological* Inhibits UDP-glucuronyl transferase *4332*

Bilirubin, Direct *Serum Increase Physiological* Inhibits uptake of bilirubin by liver cells *563*

BSP Retention *Serum Increase Physiological* Competition for hepatocellular binding sites *4332*

Flavoxate

Eosinophils *Blood Increase Physiological* Single reversible case reported *2754* Rare case observed as a side effect *1384*

Leukocytes *Blood Decrease Physiological* Reversible leukopenia observed in one patient *1384* Reversible leukopenia reported *5662* Single reversible case reported *2754*

Flax Seed Oil

Apolipoprotein A-I *Serum No Effect Physiological* No significant effect noted in 10 healthy men in whom 6% of carbohydrate in diet was replaced by flax seed oil for 55 days *3662*

Apolipoprotein B *Serum No Effect Physiological* No effect observed in 10 healthy men in whom 6% carbohydrate was replaced by flax seed oil for 55 days *3662*

Cholesterol *Serum No Effect Physiological* No significant effect observed in 10 healthy men in whom 6% of total carbohydrate in diet was replaced by flax seed oil for 55 days *3662*

HDL-Cholesterol *Serum No Effect Physiological* No significant effect observed in 13 healthy men in whom 6% of carbohydrate in diet was replaced with flax seed oil for 55 days *3662*

LDL-Cholesterol *Serum No Effect Physiological* No significant effect noted in 10 healthy men in whom 6% of carbohydrate was replaced by flax seed oil for 55 days *3662*

Triglycerides *Serum Decrease Physiological* In 10 healthy men replacement of 6% dietary carbohydrate with n-3 fatty acids in the form of flax seed oil caused mean reduction of triglyceride concentration by 29.6% after 55 days *3662*

Flecainide

Alanine Aminotransferase *Serum Increase Physiological* Rare reports of isolated increases of enzyme activity *3702*

Alkaline Phosphatase *Serum Increase Physiological* Rare reports of isolated increases of enzyme activity *3702* Mild increases in activity reported *3281*

Amitriptyline *Serum Increase Physiological* When coadministered, by inhibiting cytochrome P450 2D6, may increase the concentration of amitriptyline *6645*

Aspartate Aminotransferase *Serum Increase Physiological* Rare reports of isolated increases of enzyme activity *3702*

Digoxin *Serum Increase Physiological* Small increases in plasma concentration (13 - 19%) are observed at 6 h post-dose when digoxin coadministered with flecainide *3702* Increases serum concentration *3281* Trough concentrations increased by 24% in 15 healthy volunteers when drugs coadministered but mechanism not determined *6378*

Granulocytes *Blood Decrease Physiological* Rare reports in less than 1% of treated patients *3702*

Leukocytes *Blood Decrease Physiological* Rare reports in less than 1% of treated patients *3702*

Platelets *Blood Decrease Physiological* Rare reports in less than 1% of treated patients *3702*

Propranolol *Serum Increase Physiological* Small increases in plasma concentration are observed (30%) when propranolol coadministered with flecainide *3702* Increases hypotensive and negative inotropic effects as well as concentration *3281*

Tacrolimus *Blood No Effect Analytical* No significant effect observed at a concentration of 1 mg/L with MEIA method on Abbott IMx analyzer *1871*
Serum No Effect Analytical At a concentration of 1 mg/L no significant effect observed on ELISA method *6329*

Verapamil *Serum No Effect Physiological* Coadministration of had no effect on pharmacokinetics of verapamil *5345*

Fleroxicin

Theophylline *Serum No Effect Physiological* No significant change with either a single dose or multiple doses of fleroxicin. Significant changes in urinary excretion of unchanged theophylline and its metabolites after a single dose of fleroxicin but no changes after multiple doses *4509*

Flomoxef

Antithrombin III *Plasma No Effect Physiological* In 10 volunteers treatment for 5 days caused no change from baseline of 104.7 ± 7.8% *932*

Fibrinogen *Plasma No Effect Physiological* In 10 volunteers treatment for 5 days caused insignificant decrease from 368 ± 116 mg/dL to 350 ± 116 mg/dL *932*

Hepato Quick *Plasma No Effect Physiological* In 10 volunteers treatment for 5 days caused insignificant change in Hepato Quick (a measure of factors II, VIII and X) from 88.1 ± 24.4% to 91.9 ± 23.2 *932*

Partial Thromboplastin Time
Plasma No Effect Physiological In 10 volunteers treatment for 5 days caused insignificant change of PTT ratio from 1.015 ± 0.097 to 1.011 ± 0.091 *932*

Protein C *Plasma No Effect Physiological* In 10 volunteers treatment for 5 days caused insignificant change from 102.6 ± 20.0% to 102.0 ± 18.6% although when broken out by gender significant increase observed in men and decrease in women *932*

Protein S *Plasma No Effect Physiological* In 10 volunteers treatment for 5 days caused insignificant change from 92.3 ± 12.9% to 99.1 ± 10.1% although when broken out by gender significant increase observed in men and nonsignificant decrease in women *932*

Prothrombin Time *Plasma No Effect Physiological* In 10 volunteers caused insignificant change of prothrombin ratio from 1.047 ± 0.092 to 1.039 ± 0.078 after 5 days treatment *932*

Florantyrone

Alanine Aminotransferase *Serum Increase Physiological* Hepatotoxic effect *3810*

Alkaline Phosphatase *Serum Increase Physiological* Hepatotoxic effect *3810*

Aspartate Aminotransferase *Serum Increase Physiological* Hepatotoxic effect *3810*

Bile *Urine Increase Physiological* Hepatotoxic effect *3810*

BSP Retention *Serum Increase Physiological* Hepatotoxic effect *1714*

Eosinophils *Blood Increase Physiological* In patients with pre-existing liver disease *3810*

Leukocytes *Blood Increase Physiological* In patients with pre-existing liver disease *3810*

Floxuridine

Alanine Aminotransferase *Serum Increase Physiological* Manifestation of toxicity *2754* Increased activity probably associated with drug administration observed in some treated patients *5020*

Alkaline Phosphatase *Serum Increase Physiological* Hepatotoxic manifestation *2754* Increased activity probably associated with drug administration observed in some treated patients *5020*

Aspartate Aminotransferase *Serum Increase Physiological* Manifestation of toxicity *2754* Increased activity probably associated with drug administration observed in some treated patients *5020*

Bilirubin *Serum Increase Physiological* Hepatotoxic manifestation *2754* Increased concentration probably associated with drug administration observed in some treated patients *5020*

BSP Retention *Serum Increase Physiological* Manifestation of toxicity *2754*

Chromosomes *Test Conditions Abnormal Physiological* Clastogenic in human cells *5484*

Erythrocyte Sedimentation Rate
Blood Increase Physiological Increased ESR probably associated with drug administration observed in some treated patients *5020* Manifestation of toxicity *2754*

Erythrocytes *Blood Decrease Physiological* Bone marrow depression *2754*

Hematocrit *Blood Decrease Physiological* Bone marrow depression *2754* Anemia probably associated with drug administration observed in some treated patients *5020*

Hemoglobin *Blood Decrease Physiological* Bone marrow depression *2754* Anemia probably associated with drug administration observed in some treated patients *5020*

Lactate Dehydrogenase *Serum Increase Physiological* Manifestation of toxicity *2754* Increased activity probably associated with drug administration observed in some treated patients *5020*

Leukocytes *Blood Decrease Physiological* Early indication of toxicity on bone marrow *2754* Leukopenia probably associated with drug administration observed in some treated patients *5020*

Occult Blood *Feces Increase Physiological* Gastrointestinal bleeding probably associated with drug administration observed in some treated patients *5020* May cause gastrointestinal bleeding *6479*

Platelets *Blood Decrease Physiological* Thrombocytopenia probably associated with drug administration observed in some treated patients *5020* Toxic effect on bone marrow *6479*

Protein *Serum Decrease Physiological* Decreased protein probably associated with drug administration observed in some treated patients *5020* Manifestation of toxicity *2754*

Prothrombin Time *Plasma Increase Physiological* Manifestation of toxicity *2754* Decreased prothrombin probably associated with drug administration observed in some treated patients *5020*

Sulfobromophthalein *Serum Increase Physiological* BSP retention increased probably associated with drug administration in some treated patients *5020*

Flucloxacillin

Alanine Aminotransferase *Serum Increase Physiological* In a single patient on hemodialysis: abnormal results only mild *3627*

Alkaline Phosphatase *Serum Increase Physiological* In a single patient on hemodialysis: abnormal results only mild *3627*

Aspartate Aminotransferase *Serum Increase Physiological* In a single patient on hemodialysis: abnormal results only mild *3627*

Bilirubin *Serum No Effect Physiological* In a single patient on hemodialysis: abnormal results only mild *3627*

Chloramphenicol *Serum No Effect Analytical* No effect at 100 mg/L on coupled enzymatic method *4122*

Lactate Dehydrogenase *Serum No Effect Physiological* In a single patient on hemodialysis: abnormal results only mild *3627*

Midazolam *Serum No Effect Analytical* On GC-ECD method of Ha et al *2387*

Phenylalanine *Plasma No Effect Analytical* No interference observed with rapid quantitative whole blood method of Campbell et al using phenylalanine dehydrogenase *867*

Protein *Urine No Effect Analytical* At concentration of 8 g/L had no effect on benzethonium chloride method *1171*

Tacrolimus *Serum No Effect Analytical* In HPLC/MS method of Christians et al no significant interference observed with measurement of FK 506 *1010*

Fluconazole

Alanine Aminotransferase *Serum Increase Physiological* Rare cases of serious hepatic reactions to drug including clinical hepatitis, cholestasis and fulminant hepatic failure including hepatitis *4645* Observed in about 5% treated patients but increase reversible *1384*

Alkaline Phosphatase *Serum Increase Physiological* Rare cases of serious hepatic reactions to drug including clinical hepatitis, cholestasis and fulminant hepatic failure including hepatitis *4645*

Aspartate Aminotransferase *Serum Increase Physiological* Fluconazole reported to significantly increase AST activity from 30 to 41 U/L in one large study and from 34 to 66 U/L in a second study. Rare cases of serious hepatic reactions to drug including clinical hepatitis, cholestasis and fulminant hepatic failure including hepatitis *4645* Observed in about 5% patients but increase is reversible *1384*

Astemizole *Serum Increase Physiological* Coadministration of fluconazole with astemizole presumed from preliminary evidence to cause increase in astemizole concentration since it is metabolized by P450 enzyme system *4645* Decreased metabolism, increased risk of cardiac toxicity or arrhythmia *886*

Benzoylecgonine *Urine Decrease Analytical* Presence of fluconazole caused false negative result with TMS-derivatised benzoylecgonine by GC/MS *161*

Bilirubin *Serum Increase Physiological* Rare cases of serious hepatic reactions to drug including clinical hepatitis, cholestasis and fulminant hepatic failure including hepatitis *4645*

Cefotaxime *Serum Increase Physiological* Hypercholesterolemia reported as adverse reaction *4645*

Cisapride *Serum Increase Physiological* Coadministration of fluconazole with cisapride presumed from preliminary evidence to cause increase in cisapride concentration since it is metabolized by P450 enzyme system *4645* By inhibiting cytochrome P450 3A4 inhibits metabolism of cisapride and increases its plasma concentration *2903*

Cyclosporine *Blood Increase Physiological* Coadministration may cause two-fold increase in cyclosporine concentration but severe nephrotoxicity is rare *859*
Blood No Effect Analytical At a concentration of 81 mg/L had no effect on Syva EMIT method *495*
Serum Increase Physiological May increase cyclosporine concentration by inhibiting hepatic cytochrome P-450 III A which metabolizes cyclosporine *5236* Coadministration may cause two-fold increase in cyclosporine concentration but severe nephrotoxicity is rare *859* Doubling in concentration observed in some patients when drugs coadministered 6 days after both drugs given *6595* Occasional increase noted with coadministration in renal transplant patients with or without renal impairment. In 8 renal transplant patients treated with cyclosporine A for at least 6 months and on a stable dose for at least 6 weeks the administration of fluconazole 200 mg/d for 14 days caused AUC to increase by 92 ± 43%, and maximum and minimum concentrations to increase by 60 ± 48% and 157 ± 96% respectively *4645*
Serum No Effect Physiological No effect on concentration either following single dose of 100 mg or after 100 mg daily for 14 days *3306*

Cyclosporine A *Blood Increase Physiological* Coadministration with cyclosporine A increases its concentration *5240*

Eprosartan *Serum No Effect Physiological* When fluconazole administered with eposartan no effect observed on its AUC or maximum concentration *3078*

Fluconazole *(continued)*

Ethinyl Estradiol *Serum Increase Physiological* Mean concentrations of ethinyl estradiol were significantly increased after 150 mg fluconazole in patients taking either Ortho-Novum 7/7/7 (from 148 to 185 pg/mL) or Triphasil (from 102 pg/mL to 127 pg/mL) *5583*
Serum No Effect Physiological When oral contraceptives ingested as a single dose before and after the oral administration of fluconazole 50 mg/d for 10 days in 10 healthy women no significant effect observed on ethinyl estradiol AUC (+6%) *4645*

Fluconazole *Serum No Effect Physiological* In 12 people with HIV infection treatment with fluconazole 200 mg/d for 2 weeks together with 300 mg/d rifabutin caused an insignficant decrease to 197 ± 45 µg.h/mL from 201 ± 36 µg.h/mL in the absence of rifabutin *6069*

Glipizide *Serum Increase Physiological* Coadministration of 100 mg/d fluconazole for 7 days with glipizide caused a mean increase of 56.9% in the AUC of glipizide *4648* Fluconazole observed to reduce the metabolism of sulfonylureas and related drugs and increases the concentration of these drugs leading to hypoglycemia. AUC of glipizide increased by 49 ± 13% and peak plasma concentration increased by 19 ± 23% *4645*

γ-Glutamyltransferase *Serum Increase Physiological* Rare cases of serious hepatic reactions to drug including clinical hepatitis, cholestasis and fulminant hepatic failure including hepatitis *4645*

Glyburide *Serum Increase Physiological* Fluconazole observed to reduce the metabolism of sulfonylureas and related drugs and increases the concentration of these drugs leading to hypoglycemia. AUC of glyburide increased by 44 ± 29% and peak plasma concentration increased by 19 ±19% *4645*

Granulocytes *Blood Decrease Physiological* Leukopenia, including neutropenia and agranulocytosis reported as adverse reactions *4645*

Indinavir *Serum Decrease Physiological* Causes a 19% decrease in area under the concentration curve when fluconazole coadministered *1891* Administration of indinavir 1000 mg every 6 hours with fluconazole 400 mg/d for 1 week resulted in a 19 ± 33% decrease in indinavir AUC *3966*

Ketone Body Ratio *Serum No Effect Analytical* When added at a concentration of 100 mg/L had no significant effect on AKBR method of Uno et al *6131*

Leukocytes *Blood Decrease Physiological* Leukopenia, including neutropenia and agranulocytosis reported as adverse reactions *4645*

Levonorgestrel *Serum No Effect Physiological* When oral contraceptives ingested as a single dose before and after the oral administration of fluconazole 50 mg/d for 10 days in 10 healthy women no significant effect observed on ethinyl estradiol AUC (+17%) *4645*

LM565 *Serum Increase Physiological* In 12 people with HIV infection treatment with fluconazole 200 mg/d for 2 weeks together with 300 mg/d rifabutin caused a significant 82% increase in the rifabutin area under the concentration curve from 3025 ± 1117 ng.h/mL to 5442 ± 2404 ng.h/mL with 216% increase in area under curve of LM565 over the 24-hour dosing interval *6069*

Losartan *Serum Increase Physiological* When fluconazole administered with losartan its AUC was increased by 66% and its maximum concentration by 30% *3078*

Methadone *Serum Increase Physiological* Coadministration of 200 mg/d fluconazole with methadone caused an average 35% increase in AUC of methadone with an increase in mean peak and trough concentrations of 27% and 48%, respectively *1065*

Neutrophils *Blood Decrease Physiological* Leukopenia, including neutropenia and agranulocytosis reported as adverse reactions *4645*

Phenytoin *Serum Increase Physiological* Decreased metabolism and increased risk of phenytoin toxicity *886* Fluconazole observed to reduce the metabolism of phenytoin and increases its plasma concentration. Phenytoin AUC increased by 88 ± 68% after 4 days of 200 mg/d phenytoin for 3 days followed by 200 mg fluconazole for 16 days in 10 normal male volunteers *4645*

Platelets *Blood Decrease Physiological* Rare reversible thrombocytopenia reported *1384* Thrombocytopenia reported as adverse reaction *4645*

Potassium *Serum Decrease Physiological* Hypokalemia reported as adverse reaction *4645*

Prothrombin Time *Plasma Increase Physiological* In 7 men who were receiving low dose warfarin therapy addition of low dose fluconazole (100 mg/d) for 7 days caused increase from mean baseline of 15.8 ± 1 seconds to 18.9 ± 1.9 seconds on day 5 and 21.9 ± 2.2 seconds on day 8 *1183* Fluconazole observed to reduce the metabolism of coumarin-type drugs thereby increasing prothrombin time when these are administered. In 13 normal male volunteers after a single oral 15 mg dose of warfarin the AUC prothrombin time increased by 7 ± 4% *4645* Increased INR in patients taking warfarin *886* Probable interaction with warfarin when drugs coadministered *2625*

Rifabutin *Serum Increase Physiological* In 12 people with HIV infection treatment with fluconazole 200 mg/d for 2 weeks together with 300 mg/d rifabutin caused a significant 82% increase in the rifabutin area under the concentration curve from 3025 ± 1117 ng.h/mL to 5442 ± 2404 ng.h/mL with 216% increase in area under curve of LM565 over the 24-hour dosing interval *6069* Increased plasma concentration *886*
Urine Decrease Physiological In 12 people with HIV infection treatment with fluconazole 200 mg/d for 2 weeks together with 300 mg/d rifabutin caused a significant reduction of rifabutin excretion from 6.2 ± 2.0% to 2.5 ± 1.5% of administered dose although renal clearance of rifabutin unchanged *6069*

Ritonavir *Serum Increase Physiological* Increases area under the concentration curve by 12% when fluconazole coadministered *1891*

Tacrolimus *Serum Increase Physiological* By inhibiting cytochrome P-450 IIIA enzyme systems may inhibit the metabolism of tacrolimus *1987*

Terfenadine *Serum Increase Physiological* Decreased metabolism, increased risk of cardiac toxicity or arrhythmia *886* Because of similar chemical structure to ketoconazole and itraconazole which markedly inhibit the metabolism of terfenadine, probably has similar effect *2653*
Serum No Effect Physiological Fluconazole has no significant effect on the plasma concentration of terfenadine *4645*

Testosterone *Serum No Effect Physiological* At doses up to 50 mg/day for 28 days had no effect on concentration in 10 male volunteers *2433*

Theophylline *Serum Increase Physiological* Fluconazole 200 mg/d for 14 days increased the plasma concentration of theophylline (after a single IV dose of 6 mg/kg aminophylline) in 10 normal male volunteers by 13 ± 17%, AUC by 21 ± 16% and increased theophylline half-life from 6.6 ± 1.7 h to 7.9 ± 1.5 h *4645*

Tolbutamide *Serum Increase Physiological* Fluconazole observed to reduce the metabolism of sulfonylureas and related drugs and increases the concentration of these drugs leading to hypoglycemia. Increase of tolbutamide AUC of 26 ± 9% and peak plasma concentration increased by 11 ± 9% *4645*

Triglycerides *Serum Increase Physiological* Hypertriglyceridemia reported as adverse reaction *4645*

Zidovudine *Serum Increase Physiological* In 12 HIV-positive volunteers coadministration of 400 mg fluconazole daily with steady state zidovudine conditions (200 mg/8 h) increased the zidovudine AUC by a mean of 74% and the zidovudine half life by 128% *2163* Administration of 200 mg fluconazole for 15 days 13 volunteers with AIDS or ARC on a stable dose of zidovudine for 2 weeks caused a significant 20 ± 32% increase in the zidovudine AUC *4645*

Flucytosine

Alanine Aminotransferase *Serum Increase Physiological* May cause hepatic dysfunction and jaundice *5015* Reversible hepatotoxicity in 10% *5784*

Alkaline Phosphatase *Serum Increase Physiological* Occurs in about 25% treated patients: usually mild but necessitates discontinuation of therapy *5985* Reversible hepatotoxicity in 10% *5784* May cause hepatic dysfunction and jaundice *5015*

Aspartate Aminotransferase *Serum Increase Physiological* Occurs in about 25% treated patients: usually mild but necessitates discontinuation of therapy *5985* May cause hepatic dysfunction and jaundice *5015* Reversible hepatotoxicity in 10% *5784*

Bilirubin *Serum Increase Physiological* Reversible hepatotoxicity in 10% *5784* May cause hepatic dysfunction and jaundice *5015*

Clindamycin *Serum No Effect Analytical* Has no effect on bioassay procedure at Mayo Clinic *3858*

Colistin *Serum No Effect Analytical* Has no effect on bioassay procedure at Mayo Clinic *3858*

Creatinine *Serum Increase Analytical* At 10 μg/mL and above on Ektachem® 700 2 slide procedure: change in proportion to concentration *5728* Interferes with enzymatic method on Johson and Johnson Vitros *5015* At concentrations above 5 mg/L on 2-slide method on Kodak Ektachem® significantly increase concentration: effect of clinical importance *5706*

Serum Increase Physiological May have nephrotoxic effect *2753* May cause azotemia and renal failure *5015*

Serum No Effect Analytical At 100 μg/mL on Jaffe methods on Technicon SMAC® and Du Pont aca *5728* Has no effect on methods using Jaffe reaction *5015* No effect of concentrations up to 50 mg/L on single slide method on Kodak Ektachem® *5706*

Crystals *Urine Increase Physiological* May cause crystalluria *5015*

Eosinophils *Blood Increase Physiological* May cause eosinophilia and other hematological abnormalities *5015*

Erythrocytes *Blood Decrease Physiological* May depress bone marrow function *2753* Usually mild, occurs in 8 to 13% patients: occasionally pancytopenia occurs *5985*

Erythromycin *Serum No Effect Analytical* Has no effect on bioassay procedure at Mayo Clinic *3858*

Glucose *Serum Decrease Physiological* May cause hypoglycemia *5015*

γ-Glutamyltransferase *Serum Increase Physiological* May cause hepatic dysfunction and jaundice *5015*

Granulocytes *Blood Decrease Physiological* May cause agranulocytosis or pancytopenia *5015*

Hematocrit *Blood Decrease Physiological* May cause anemia, aplastic anemia or pancytopenia *5015*

Hemoglobin *Blood Decrease Physiological* May depress bone marrow function *2753* May cause anemia, aplastic anemia or pancytopenia *5015*

Leukocytes *Blood Decrease Physiological* Usually mild, occurs in 8 to 13% patients: occasionally pancytopenia occurs *5985* Reported effect (with agranulocytosis) *5784* May cause leukopenia or pancytopenia *5015*

Metronidazole *Serum No Effect Analytical* Has no effect on bioassay procedure at Mayo Clinic *3858*

Neutrophils *Blood Decrease Physiological* Occasional case of agranulocytosis reported *6264*

Occult Blood *Feces Increase Physiological* May cause gastrointestinal hemorrhage *5015*

pH *Gastric Material Decrease Physiological* Effect on both basal and submaximal pentagastrin simulated gastric acid secretion. Effect dose related *844*

Platelets *Blood Decrease Physiological* Occasional thrombocytopenia observed *2753* Usually mild, occurs in 8 to 13% patients: occasionally pancytopenia occurs *5985* May cause thrombocytopenia or pancytopenia *5015*

Polymyxin *Serum No Effect Analytical* Has no effect on bioassay procedure at Mayo Clinic *3858*

Potassium *Serum Decrease Physiological* May cause hypokalemia *5015*

Protein *Cerebrospinal Fluid No Effect Analytical* At concentration of 100 mg/L on SDS/Coomassie Blue method of Huang *2745*

Tetracycline *Serum No Effect Analytical* Has no effect on bioassay procedure at Mayo Clinic *3858*

Trimethoprim *Serum No Effect Analytical* Has no effect on bioassay procedure at Mayo Clinic *3858*

Urea Nitrogen *Serum Increase Physiological* May have nephrotoxic effect *2753* May cause azotemia and renal failure *5015*

Volume *Gastric Fluid Decrease Physiological* Effect on both basal and submaximal pentagastrin-stimulated gastric acid secretion. Effect dose related *844*

Zidovudine *Serum No Effect Analytical* No effect on liquid chromatographic method of Hedaya and Sawchuk *2525*

Fludarabine

Creatinine *Serum Increase Physiological* Renal insufficiency has been reported as an adverse reaction *1384* In one patient with stage C chronic lymphatic leukemia treatment with fludarabine 25 mg/m^2 caused significant increase to 416 μmol/L with further increase to 424 μmol/L during hospitalization *3447*

Erythrocytes *Blood Decrease Physiological* Myelosuppression is dose-limiting toxicity *1384*

Hemoglobin *Blood Decrease Physiological* In one patient with stage C chronic lymphatic leukemia treatment with fludarabine 25 mg/m^2 caused significant reduction from mean baseline of 11.3 g/dL to 9.9 g/dL *3447*

Blood Increase Physiological In 35 previously treated patients with advanced and progressed B-cell chronic lymphocytic leukemia and 6 previously untreated patients treated with 25 mg/sq m/d for 5 days for 6 courses caused significant reduction from mean baseline of 10.5 g/dL to 11.5 g/dL *6668*

Leukocytes *Blood Decrease Physiological* Myelosuppression is dose limiting with leukocytes most affected *1384* In one patient with stage C chronic lymphatic leukemia treatment with fludarabine 25 mg/m^2 caused significant reduction from mean baseline of 105 x 10^9/L to 4.2 x 10^9/L 3 days after completion of therapy *3447*

Lymphocytes *Blood Decrease Physiological* In one patient with stage C chronic lymphatic leukemia treatment with fludarabine 25 mg/m^2 caused significant reduction from mean baseline of 100 x 10^9/L *3447* In 35 previously treated patients with advanced and progressed B-cell chronic lymphocytic leukemia and 6 previously untreated patients treated with 25 mg/sq m/d for 5 days for 6 courses caused significant reduction from mean baseline of 100000 /μL to about 10000 /μL *6668*

Neutrophils *Blood Decrease Physiological* In 41 patients with advanced and progressed B-cell chronic lymphocytic leukemia and 6 previously untreated patients treated with 25 mg/sq m/d for 5 days for 6 courses caused significant reduction from mean baseline in 41 (27%) patients: 10 patients had grade 1, 15 had grade 2 and 2 had grade 4 neutropenia *6668* In 35 previously treated patients with advanced and progressed B-cell chronic lymphocytic leukemia and 6 previously untreated patients treated with 25 mg/sq m/d for 5 days for 6 courses caused significant reduction from mean baseline of 200 /μL to 1400 /μL *6668*

Platelets *Blood Decrease Physiological* Myelosuppression is dose-limiting toxicity *1384* In one patient with stage C chronic lymphatic leukemia treatment with fludarabine 25 mg/m^2 caused significant reduction from mean baseline of 82 x 10^9/L to 55 x 10^9/L *3447* In 41 previously treated patients with advanced and progressed B-cell chronic lymphocytic leukemia and 6 previously untreated patients treated with 25 mg/sq m/d for 5 days for 6 courses significant reduction from mean baseline concentration observed in 4 patients: 2 with grade 1 and 2 with grade 2 reduction *6668*

Blood Increase Physiological In 35 previously treated patients with advanced and progressed B-cell chronic lymphocytic leukemia and 6 previously untreated patients treated with 25 mg/sq m/d for 5 days for 6 courses caused significant increase from mean baseline of 87000 /μL to 120000 /μL *6668*

Urea Nitrogen *Serum Increase Physiological* Renal insufficiency has been reported as adverse reaction *1384*

Uric Acid *Serum Increase Physiological* In one patient with stage C chronic lymphatic leukemia treatment with fludarabine 25 mg/m^2 caused significant increase to 1780 μmol/L changing to 1761 μmol/L with supportive therapy during hospitalization *3447*

Fludrocortisone

Aldosterone *Urine Decrease Physiological* Marked reduction following administration *5313*

Amylase *Serum Increase Physiological* May cause hemorrhagic pancreatitis *2754*

Bicarbonate *Serum Increase Physiological* May cause hypokalemic alkalosis *2754*

Glucose *Serum Increase Physiological* May occur as a metabolic effect *221* Endocrine response *2754*
Urine Increase Physiological Endocrine response *2754* May occur as a metabolic effect *221*

Glucose Tolerance *Serum Decrease Physiological* Endocrine response *2754*

Nitroblue Tetrazolium Test *Blood Decrease Analytical* Corticosteroids may cause false negative reactions *221*

Nitrogen Balance *Patient Negative Physiological* Due to protein catabolism *2754* Negative nitrogen balance may occur as a metabolic effect *221*

Occult Blood *Feces Increase Physiological* May activate peptic ulcer *2754*

Potassium *Serum Decrease Physiological* May cause increased urinary excretion *128*
Urine Increase Physiological Increases urinary elimination *128*

Prothrombin Time *Plasma Decrease Physiological* Decreased prothrombin time response reported when fludrocortisone coadministered with warfarin *221*

Sodium *Serum Increase Physiological* May cause sodium retention and edema *128*

Tetrahydrodeoxycorticosterone
Urine Decrease Physiological Slight effect following administration *5313*

Volume *Blood Increase Physiological* May cause fluid retention and increase blood volume *1384*

Flufenamic Acid

Alanine Aminotransferase *Serum Increase Physiological* Transient elevation reported *4014*

Albumin *Urine No Effect Analytical* Using a fluorimetric assay with Albumin Blue 580 on a Cobas Fara centrifugal analyzer for the detection of microalbuminuria no significant interference was detected at a concentration of 12 mg/L *3117*

Aspartate Aminotransferase *Serum Increase Physiological* Transient elevation reported *4014*

Bile *Urine Increase Analytical* Probably due to interfering metabolite *2451*

Uric Acid *Serum Decrease Physiological* Uricosuric action of drug *5002*

Flumazenil

Corticotropin *Plasma No Effect Physiological* Administration of 0.5 mg intravenously to 9 normal volunteers had no significant effect on the area under the concentration curve (-36.5 ± 63.5 pmol/L/x min) compared with -53.5 ± 31.8 pmol/L/x min after placebo *6056*

Cortisol *Plasma No Effect Physiological* Administration of 0.5 mg intravenously to 9 normal volunteers had no significant effect on the area under the concentration curve (-2.4 ± 2.4 nmol/L/minx10-3) compared with -0.56 ± 1.4 nmol/L/minx10-3 after placebo *6056*

Flumecinolone

Bilirubin *Serum Decrease Physiological* Inhibits hyperbilirubinemia of term or premature newborns due to enzyme induction *3799*

Flumethiazide

Uric Acid *Serum Increase Physiological* Inhibition of tubular secretion of urate *2378*

Flunarizine

Follicle Stimulating Hormone
Plasma No Effect Physiological After 90 d in 8 women *3736*

Luteinizing Hormone *Plasma No Effect Physiological* After 90 d in 8 women *3736*

Lymphocyte response to Phytohemagglutinin
Blood Increase Physiological Enhanced response suggesting differential sensitivity of lymphocytes to calcium-entry blockers *742*

Prolactin *Plasma Increase Physiological* Significant increase of baseline value in men and women *3736* Significant increase observed in patients with migraine with chronic treatment *1916*

Thyroid Stimulating Hormone
Serum Increase Physiological Significant increase in men noted *3736*
Serum No Effect Physiological Basal concentration not affected but increase of domperidone blunted in women *3736*

Flunisolide

Cortisol *Plasma No Effect Physiological* No effect observed when high doses are inhaled by children with asthma *2129*

Cortisol, Free *Urine No Effect Physiological* No effect observed when high doses are inhaled by children with asthma *2129*

Flunitrazepam

Albumin *Urine No Effect Analytical* Using a fluorimetric assay with Albumin Blue 580 on a Cobas Fara centrifugal analyzer for the detection of microalbuminuria no significant interference was detected at a concentration of 0.4 mg/L *3117*

Benzodiazepine *Urine Positive Analytical* Detectable limit 0.1 µg/mL with improved Syva EMIT assay with Syva ETS system compared with 0.5 µg/mL with former d.a.u. assay *3370* At concentrations of 0.2 µg/mL or greater produces positive result with Syva EMIT II assay *1785* Reactive with new Syva EMIT assay *3370* Positive result observed at a concentration of 2.0 µg/mL (6.38 µmol/L) with method on Du Pont aca *1556*

Midazolam *Serum No Effect Analytical* On GC-ECD method of Ha et al *2387*

Fluocinolone

Corticotropin *Plasma Decrease Physiological* About 23% reduced when 30 g/d drug applied as topical ointment over large area *124*

Cortisol *Plasma Decrease Physiological* About 43% suppression in 4 d when 30 g/d drug applied as topical ointment over large area *124*

α-Melanocyte Stimulating Hormone
Plasma No Effect Physiological When 30 g/d drug applied as topical ointment over large area *124*

Fluoromethylhistidine

Histamine *Plasma No Effect Analytical* Improbable inhibition of radio-enzyme assay at physiological concentrations *2492*

5-Fluoronicotinic Acid

Fatty Acids (FFA), Free *Serum Decrease Physiological* Max effect of 50% at 2 h, starts in 15 minutes *5124*

Glucose *Serum No Effect Physiological* No effect seen in normals *5124*

Fluorophenylalanine

Chromosomes *Test Conditions Abnormal Physiological* Clastogenic in human lymphocyte cultures *5484*

Fluoroquinolones

Prothrombin Time *Plasma Increase Physiological* Increased INR in patients receiving warfarin *886*

Theophylline *Serum Increase Physiological* Decreased metabolism and increased plasma concentration *886*

Fluorouracil

Alanine Aminotransferase *Serum Increase Physiological* Observed in 3 of more than 600 patients treated with levamisole alone or with fluorouracil following resection of colon carcinoma. Activity normalized with withdrawal of therapy *4085*

Alkaline Phosphatase *Serum Increase Physiological* In over 600 cases following resection of colon carcinoma treated with levamisole alone or with fluorouracil increased activity observed in 7 patients and activity subsided when therapy withdrawn *4085*

Bilirubin *Serum Increase Physiological* In 9 of over 600 patients treated with fluorouracil and levamisole or levamisole alone following resection of colon carcinoma with in all cases improvement after therapy withdrawn *4085* Single case reported *2451*
Serum No Effect Analytical At concentration of 130 mg/L had no effect on Jendrassik and Grof method *5704*

Bilirubin, Conjugated *Serum No Effect Analytical* At concentration of 38.6 µg/mL (300 µmol/L) had no effect on method on Du Pont aca *1517*

CA549 *Serum No Effect Analytical* No interference observed at concentrations from 21 - 280 mg/L with immunoradiometric BRESMARQ procedure *958*

Calcium *Serum No Effect Analytical* At concentration of 130 mg/L had no effect on cresolphthalein method *5704*

Color *Feces Increase Analytical* Black color reported with fluorouracil ingestion *3388*

Creatinine *Serum No Effect Analytical* No interference observed with liquid chromatographic method of Paroni *4540*

Eosinophils *Blood Increase Physiological* Eosinophilia probably associated with drug administration observed in some treated patients *5019*

Erythrocytes *Blood Decrease Physiological* May cause bone marrow depression *128*

Flucytosine *Serum No Effect Analytical* No effect at concentration of up to 150 mg/L on enzymatic method of Huang et al using creatine iminohydrolase *2747*

Glucose-6-Phosphate Dehydrogenase
Red Blood Cells Increase Physiological In 14 patients with gastric or colorectal adenocarcinomas treated with intravenous 5-fluorouracil for up to 120 min with 300 to 500 mg/m² caused significant change from 10.5 ± 0.7 µmol/min/g hemoglobin to 15.1 ± 4.4 µmol/min/g hemoglobin *6301*

Glutathione *Red Blood Cells Decrease Physiological* In 14 patients with gastric or colorectal adenocarcinomas treated with intravenous 5-fluorouracil for up to 120 min with 300 to 500 mg/m² caused significant change from 5.1 ± 1.5 µmol/g hemoglobin to 3.5 ± 1.4 µmol/g hemoglobin *6301*

Glutathione Peroxidase
Red Blood Cells Increase Physiological In 14 patients with gastric or colorectal adenocarcinomas treated with intravenous 5-fluorouracil for up to 120 min with 300 to 500 mg/m² caused significant change from 21.5 ± 7.1 µmol/min/g hemoglobin to 28.6 ± 10 µmol/min/g hemoglobin *6301*

Glutathione Reductase
Red Blood Cells Decrease Physiological In 14 patients with gastric or colorectal adenocarcinomas treated with intravenous 5-fluorouracil for up to 120 min with 300 to 500 mg/m² caused significant change from 8.2 ± 3.2 µmol/min/g hemoglobin to 5.2 ± 1.9 µmol/min/g hemoglobin *6301*

Glutathione S-Transferase
Red Blood Cells Increase Physiological In 14 patients with gastric or colorectal adenocarcinomas treated with intravenous 5-fluorouracil for up to 120 min with 300 to 500 mg/m² caused significant change from 1.5 ± 0.7 µmol/min/g hemoglobin to 2.8 ± 1.6 µmol/min/g hemoglobin *6301*

Hematocrit *Blood Decrease Physiological* Anemia probably associated with drug administration observed in some treated patients *5019*

Hemoglobin *Blood Decrease Physiological* Anemia probably associated with drug administration observed in some treated patients *5019*

5-Hydroxyindoleacetic Acid *Urine Increase Physiological* In patients with carcinoid, due to cell destruction *2451*

Kininogen *Plasma Decrease Physiological* Maximum effect with onset of leukopenia *1200*

Leukocytes *Blood Decrease Physiological* Rare and not usually severe side effect in patients given levamisole and fluorouracil following resection of colon carcinoma *4085* May cause bone marrow depression *128*

Lipase *Serum No Effect Analytical* No effect of concentrations up to 3 mg/L on method on Kodak Ektachem® *5706*

Methotrexate *Serum No Effect Analytical* No significant interference at a concentration of 50 µmol/L with method on Du Pont aca *1535*

Occult Blood *Feces Increase Physiological* Gastrointestinal ulceration and bleeding probably associated with drug administration observed in some treated patients *5019* Manifestation of toxicity *2754*

Phosphate *Serum No Effect Analytical* At concentration of 130 mg/L had no effect on phosphomolybdate method *5704*

6-Phosphogluconate Dehydrogenase
Red Blood Cells Increase Physiological In 14 patients with gastric or colorectal adenocarcinomas treated with intravenous 5-fluorouracil for up to 120 min with 300 to 500 mg/m² caused nonsignificant change from 10.7 ± 4.1 µmol/min/g hemoglobin to 12.1 ± 3.2 µmol/min/g hemoglobin *6301*

Platelets *Blood Decrease Physiological* Thrombocytopenia probably associated with drug administration observed in some treated patients *5019* May cause bone marrow depression *128*

Protein *Cerebrospinal Fluid No Effect Analytical* No significant effect when added in vitro to concentration of 10.0 mg/dL on Kodak Ektachem® slide method *3654*
Serum No Effect Analytical At concentration of 130 mg/L had no effect on biuret method with blank correction *5704*

Thyroxine (T4) *Serum Increase Physiological* Increased binding capacity (augmentation of transport proteins) *6412* Increase observed due to increased thyroxine-binding globulin *2412*

Tri-iodothyronine (T3) *Serum Increase Physiological* Increase observed due to increased thyroxine-binding globulin *2412* Increased binding capacity (augmentation of transport proteins) *6412*

Urea Nitrogen *Serum No Effect Analytical* At concentration of 130 mg/L had no effect on diacetylmonoxime method *5704*

Uric Acid *Serum No Effect Analytical* At concentration of 130 mg/L had no effect on phosphotungstate reduction method *5704*

Zalcitabine *Serum No Effect Analytical* At a 5-fluorouracil concentration of 100 mg/L had less than 0.01% cross-reactivity with solid phase extraction and RIA method of Roberts et al *4990*

5-Fluorouracil

Bleeding Time *Patient Increase Physiological* Administration of 5-fluorouracil with warfarin been demonstrated to increase bleeding time *3909*

CA549 *Serum No Effect Analytical* No statistically significant effect observed over a concentration range of 21 to 280 mg/L with BRESMARQ assay *958*

Carcinoembryonic Antigen *Serum No Effect Analytical* At a concentration of up to 346.0 µg/mL caused less than 10% error in the concentration of CEA as measured by the method on Bayer Technicon Immuno 1® *418*

Creatine Kinase *Serum Increase Physiological* In one man with stage B2 colon cancer activity began to increase dramatically 4 weeks after initiation of combined therapy with levamisole and 5-fluorouracil: increased activity due to CK-MM *942*

Creatine Kinase MM-Isoenzyme
Serum Increase Physiological In one man with stage B2 colon cancer activity began to increase dramatically 4 weeks after initiation of combined therapy with levamisole and 5-fluorouracil: increased activity due to CK-MM *942*

5-Fluorouracil *(continued)*

Fibrinogen *Plasma Decrease Physiological* In 11 patients treatment with 5-fluorouracil caused decrease from 4.31 ± 1.69 g/L on day 1 to 3.49 ± 1.93 g/L on day 4 *1205*

Glucose-6-Phosphate Dehydrogenase
Red Blood Cells Increase Physiological In 14 patients with gastrointestinal malignancies treatment with intravenous infusion of up to 500 mg/m^2 weekly caused significant increase from mean baseline of 10.5 ± 0.7 µmol/min/g hemoglobin to 15.1 ± 4.4 µmol/min/g hemoglobin *6301*

Glutathione *Red Blood Cells Decrease Physiological* In 14 patients with gastrointestinal malignancies treatment with intravenous infusion of up to 500 mg/m^2 weekly caused significant reduction from mean baseline of 5.1 ± 1.5 µmol/g hemoglobin to 3.5 ± 1.4 µmol/g hemoglobin *6301*

Glutathione Peroxidase
Red Blood Cells Increase Physiological In 14 patients with gastrointestinal malignancies treatment with intravenous infusion of up to 500 mg/m^2 weekly caused significant increase from mean baseline of 21.5 ± 7.1 µmol/min/g hemoglobin to 28.6 ± 10 µmol/min/g hemoglobin *6301*

Glutathione Reductase
Red Blood Cells Decrease Physiological In 14 patients with gastrointestinal malignancies treatment with intravenous infusion of up to 500 mg/m^2 weekly caused significant reduction from mean baseline of 8.2 ± 3.2 µmol/min/g hemoglobin to 5.2 ± 1.9 µmol/min/g hemoglobin *6301*

Glutathione S-Transferase
Red Blood Cells Increase Physiological In 14 patients with gastrointestinal malignancies treatment with intravenous infusion of up to 500 mg/m^2 weekly caused significant increase from mean baseline of 1.5 ± 0.7 µmol/min/g hemoglobin to 2.8 ± 1.6 µmol/min/g hemoglobin *6301*

Hematocrit *Blood Decrease Physiological* In 11 patients treatment with 5-fluorouracil caused decrease from 42.1 ± 2.7% on day 1 to 40.0 ± 3.1% on day 4 *1205*

Partial Thromboplastin Time
Plasma Increase Physiological Administration of 5-fluorouracil with warfarin been demonstrated to increase PTT *3909*

6-Phosphogluconate Dehydrogenase
Red Blood Cells No Effect Physiological In 14 patients with gastrointestinal malignancies treatment with intravenous infusion of up to 500 mg/m^2 weekly caused nonsignificant increase from mean baseline of 10.7 ± 4.1 µmol/min/g hemoglobin to 12.1 ± 3.2 µmol/min/g hemoglobin *6301*

Viscosity *Plasma Decrease Physiological* In 11 patients treatment with 5-fluorouracil caused decrease from 1.86 ± 0.15 (relative to water) to 1.75 ± 0.18 on day 4 *1205*

Fluosol-DA

Alanine Aminotransferase *Serum Decrease Analytical* Decrease by 86% on Du Pont aca III at concentration of 50% *4167*
Serum No Effect Analytical On Technicon SMA IIC at concentration of 50% *4167*

Albumin *Serum Decrease Analytical* Albumin results very variable with Kodak Ektachem® due to poor spreading accounting for imprecise results *4167*
Serum Increase Analytical Albumin results very variable with Kodak Ektachem® due to poor spreading accounting for imprecise results *4167*
Serum No Effect Analytical On Technicon SMA IIC at a concentration of 50%. On Du Pont aca III at a concentration of 50% *4167* Albumin results very variable with Kodak Ektachem® due to poor spreading accounting for imprecise results *4167*

Alkaline Phosphatase *Serum No Effect Analytical* On Technicon SMA IIC at concentration of 50%. On Du Pont aca III at concentration of 50% *4167*

Aspartate Aminotransferase *Serum Decrease Analytical* Decrease by 100% on Du Pont aca III at concentration of 50% *4167*
Serum No Effect Analytical On Technicon SMA IIC at concentration of 50% *4167*

Bicarbonate *Serum Decrease Analytical* Reduction from 9.6 mmol/L to 9.3 mmol/L with method on Beckman Astra® 400 at concentration of 50% *4167*
Serum No Effect Analytical On Technicon SMA IIC at concentration of 50% *4167*

Bilirubin *Serum Increase Analytical* Increase by 500% on Du Pont aca III at concentration of 50% *4167*
Serum No Effect Analytical On Technicon SMA IIC at concentration of 50% *4167*

Calcium *Serum No Effect Analytical* On Technicon SMA IIC at concentration of 50% or on Kodak Ektachem® 400 at concentration of 50% *4167* On Du Pont aca III at concentration of 50% *4167*

Carbamazepine *Serum No Effect Analytical* As measured on Du Pont aca III at concentration up to 50% *4167*

Chloride *Serum Decrease Analytical* Unpredictable variation in concentrations as measured on Technicon SMA® IIC, Beckman Astra® 8 and Kodak Ektachem® 400 *4167*
Serum Increase Analytical Unpredictable variation in concentrations as measured on Technicon SMA® IIC, Beckman Astra® 8 and Kodak Ektachem® 400 *4167*
Serum No Effect Analytical Unpredictable variation in concentrations as measured on Technicon SMA® IIC, Beckman Astra® 8 and Kodak Ektachem® 400 *4167*

Cholesterol *Serum Increase Analytical* Increase by 20% on Technicon SMA IIC at concentration of 50% *4167*
Serum No Effect Analytical No significant effect on Du Pont aca III at concentration of 50% *4167*

Creatine Kinase Isoenzymes *Serum No Effect Analytical* No effect on electrophoresis although added fluorescent band *4167*

Creatinine *Serum No Effect Analytical* No significant effect on Technicon SMA® IIC and Beckman Astra® at concentration of 50% *4167*

Digoxin *Serum No Effect Analytical* As measured by Abbott TD_x at concentration up to 50% *4167*

Glucose *Serum Increase Analytical* Increase by 14% with Du Pont aca III at concentration of 50% *4167*
Serum No Effect Analytical On Technicon SMA IIC at concentration of 50% *4167* No significant effect on methods on Kodak Ektachem® 400 and Beckman Astra® at concentration of 50% *4167*

Lactate Dehydrogenase *Serum Increase Analytical* Increase by 37% on Technicon SMA IIC at concentration of 50%. Increase by 18% on Du Pont aca III at concentration of 50% *4167*

Lipoprotein Electrophoresis *Serum No Effect Analytical* Not affected by presence of compound in specimen *4167*

Magnesium *Serum No Effect Analytical* No effect at 50% on atomic absorption measurement *4167*

Phenobarbital *Serum No Effect Analytical* As measured on Du Pont aca III at concentration up to 50% *4167*

Phenytoin *Serum No Effect Analytical* As measured on Du Pont aca III at concentration up to 50% *4167*

Phosphate *Serum Increase Analytical* Increase by 16% on Technicon SMA IIC at concentration of 50%. Increase by 82% on Du Pont aca III at concentration of 50% *4167*

Potassium *Serum Decrease Analytical* Possible 5% decrease with method on Kodak Ektachem® 400 at concentration of 50% *4167*
Serum Increase Analytical Increase from 2.2 mmol/L to 2.7 mmol/L with method on Beckman Astra® 400 at concentration of 50% *4167* Increase by 33% with method on Technicon SMA IIC at concentration of 50% *4167*

Protein *Serum Decrease Analytical* Decrease by 20% on Du Pont aca III at concentration of 50% *4167*
Serum Increase Analytical By 18% on Kodak Ektachem® 400 at concentration of 50% *4167*
Serum No Effect Analytical On Technicon SMA IIC at concentration of 50% *4167*

Protein Electrophoresis *Serum No Effect Analytical* Not affected by presence of compound in specimen *4167*

Sodium *Serum Decrease Analytical* Unpredictable variation in concentrations as measured on Technicon SMA® IIC, Beckman Astra® 8 and Kodak Ektachem® 400 *4167*
Serum Increase Analytical Unpredictable variation in concentrations as measured on Technicon SMA® IIC, Beckman Astra® 8 and Kodak Ektachem® 400 *4167*

Serum *No Effect* *Analytical* Unpredictable variation in concentrations as measured on Technicon SMA® IIC, Beckman Astra® 8 and Kodak Ektachem® 400 *4167*

Theophylline *Serum* *No Effect* *Analytical* As measured by Syva® EMIT at concentration up to 50% on Roche Cobas-Bio centrifugal analyzer *4167*

Triglycerides *Serum* *Increase* *Analytical* Directly proportional to Fluosinal concentration with methods on Beckman Astra®, Technicon SMA® IIC, Du Pont aca and Kodak Ektachem®, since emulsion contains glycerol *4167*

Urea Nitrogen *Serum* *No Effect* *Analytical* On Technicon SMA IIC at concentration of 50% *4167* Insignificant effect on Kodak Ektachem® 400 and Beckman Astra® at a concentration of 50% *4167*

Uric Acid *Serum* *No Effect* *Analytical* On Technicon SMA IIC at concentration of 50%. On Du Pont aca III at concentration of 50% *4167*

Fluoxetine

Albumin *Serum* *No Effect* *Physiological* No significant change observed in 44 depressed patients treated for 6 weeks *4615*

Urine *No Effect* *Analytical* Using a fluorimetric assay with Albumin Blue 580 on a Cobas Fara centrifugal analyzer for the detection of microalbuminuria no significant interference was detected at a concentration of 8 mg/L *3117*

Alprazolam *Serum* *Increase* *Physiological* In 11 healthy men administration of fluoxetine together with alprazolam caused significantly greater area under the curve and reduced clearance although degree of impairment not significantly associated with plasma fluoxetine or norfluoxetine concentrations *2314* Concomitant administration of fluoxetine with alprazolam caused an average 46% increase in the steady state concentration of alprazolam, decreased its plasma clearance by 31% and increased its half-life by 17% *4685* Concurrent administration of fluoxetine with alprazolam caused increased concentration of alprazolam *1440*

Amitriptyline *Serum* *Increase* *Physiological* When coadministered, by inhibiting cytochrome P450 2D6, may increase the concentration of amitriptyline *6645*

Bleeding Time *Patient* *Increase* *Physiological* Time prolonged to 11.5 minutes in one 44 year old postmenopausal woman treated with 20 mg on alternate days for 2 years but returned to normal within 2 weeks of withdrawal of drug *2776*

Patient *No Effect* *Physiological* In 10 normal volunteers receiving 60 mg daily for 4 or 6 weeks time remained within normal range *357*

Calcium *Serum* *No Effect* *Physiological* No significant change observed in 44 depressed patients treated for 6 weeks *4615*

Carbamazepine *Serum* *Increase* *Physiological* Increased concentration with toxicity observed in 2 patients when drugs coadministered *3118* Drugs that inhibit CYP 3A4 inhibit metabolism of carbamazepine producing clinically meaningful effect *1039* Concurrent administration of fluoxetine with carbamazepine caused increased plasma concentration probably due to effect on P450IIIA4 in liver *1440* Insignificant increase in concentration of drug and ratio of serum concentration to dose when fluoxetine coadministered possibly due to impaired hepatic metabolism *236* In 7 patients with epilepsy coadministration of fluoxetine with carbamazepine caused tendency for plasma clearance to be reduced from mean baseline with carbamazepine alone of 5.9 ± 2.4 L/h to 4.2 ± 2.2 L/h *2107*

Serum *No Effect* *Physiological* In 8 epileptics receiving chronic carbamazepine treatment administration of 20 mg/d for 3 weeks had no significant effect on plasma concentration (mean baseline 28.5 ± 5.7 µmol/L and 27.8 ± 5.7 µmol/L during treatment) *5749*

Carbamazepine-10,11-Epoxide
Serum *No Effect* *Physiological* In 8 epileptic patients receiving chronic carbamazepine therapy treatment with 20 mg/d fluoxetine for 3 weeks had no significant effect on concentration (mean baseline 6.1 ± 2.3 µmol/L and 6.0 ± 2.6 µmol/L during treatment) *5749*

Cholesterol *Serum* *No Effect* *Physiological* No significant change observed in 44 depressed patients treated for 6 weeks *4615*

Clonazepam *Serum* *No Effect* *Physiological* In 11 healthy men no significant interaction observed between fluoxetine and clonazepam administration *2314*

Clozapine *Serum* *Increase* *Physiological* Concurrent administration of fluoxetine with clozapine caused increased concentration of clozapine *1440* Coadministration of the drugs in 6 patients caused significant increase of clozapine metabolites *938*

Cortisol, Free *Urine* *No Effect* *Analytical* No significant interference observed with HPLC method of Turpeinen et al *6105*

Desipramine *Serum* *Increase* *Physiological* Possible doubling of concentration when fluoxetine coadministered perhaps due to impaired hepatic metabolism *236* Concurrent administration of fluoxetine with desipramine has caused a 2 - 10 fold increase in previously stable concentration *1440*

Diazepam *Serum* *Increase* *Physiological* Concurrent administration of fluoxetine with diazepam caused increased half-life of diazepam *1440*

Digoxin *Serum* *Increase* *Physiological* In a 93-year old woman treatment with fluoxetine caused serum digoxin concentration to increase from mean baseline of 1.4 nmol/L to 2.0 nmol/L after 2 days and to 2.8 nmol/L after 4 days *3508*

Erythrocytes *Blood* *No Effect* *Physiological* No significant change observed in RBC count in 44 depressed patients treated for 6 weeks *4615*

Haloperidol *Serum* *Increase* *Physiological* 7-10 days treatment with 20 mg/d was added to stable dose regime of haloperidol in 8 psychotic patients and caused mean increase of haloperidol concentration of 20% *2205* Concurrent administration of fluoxetine with haloperidol caused increased concentration of haloperidol *1440*

Hematocrit *Blood* *No Effect* *Physiological* No significant change observed in 44 depressed patients treated for 6 weeks *4615*

Hemoglobin *Blood* *No Effect* *Physiological* No significant change observed in 44 depressed patients treated for 6 weeks *4615*

Homovanillic Acid
Cerebrospinal Fluid *Decrease* *Physiological* In 9 patients with major depression treatment with 20 mg/d for at least 4 weeks caused nonsignificant decrease from mean of 182.9 ± 49.7 pmol/L to 167.6 ± 57.0 pmol/mL *1301*

4-Hydroxy-3-Methoxy-Phenylglycol
Cerebrospinal Fluid *Decrease* *Physiological* In 9 patients with major depression treatment with 20 mg/d for at least 4 weeks caused significant decrease from mean concentration of 46.7 ± 14.2 pmol/mL to 42.6 ± 11.6 pmol/mL *1301*

5-Hydroxyindoleacetic Acid
Cerebrospinal Fluid *Decrease* *Physiological* In 9 patients with major depression administration of 20 mg/d for at least 4 weeks caused significant decrease of mean concentration from 95.9 ± 24.6 pmol/L to 64.2 ± 26.1 pmol/L *1301*

Imipramine *Serum* *Increase* *Physiological* Concurrent administration of fluoxetine with imipramine has caused a 2 - 10 fold increase in previously stable concentration *1440* Plasma concentration of drug may be increased when hepatic enzyme inhibitors given concomitantly *1040* Marked increase in one patient when fluoxetine coadministered (486% increase in ratio of drug concentration to dose) possibly due to impaired hepatic metabolism *236* Several days after drug added to regime markedly increased concentration of imipramine and desipramine observed in serum *1816*

Lithium *Serum* *Decrease* *Physiological* Concurrent administration of fluoxetine with lithium has been associated with increased lithium concentration with toxicity and decreased concentration of lithium *1440*

Serum *Increase* *Physiological* Concurrent administration of fluoxetine with lithium has been associated with increased lithium concentration with toxicity and decreased concentration of lithium *1440*

Lysergic Acid Diethylamide *Urine* *Increase* *Analytical* Minimum concentration that caused a positive result with EMIT method to measure LSD 6 mg/L *4968*

Maprotiline *Serum* *Increase* *Physiological* Concentration may be raised when hepatic enzyme inhibitors are coadministered *1034*

Fluoxetine *(continued)*

Melatonin *Plasma No Effect Physiological* Short-term treatment had no effect on nighttime plasma melatonin concentration in healthy individuals *4102* In 10 patients with seasonal affective disorder treatment with 20 mg/d fluoxetine for 6 weeks caused significant reduction in concentration *994*

Nortriptyline *Serum Increase Physiological* Marked increase in concentration when fluoxetine coadministered possibly due to decreased hepatic metabolism *236*

Osmolality *Serum Decrease Physiological* In two elderly patients being treated with fluoxetine sodium concentrations changed to 404 mOsm/kg and 230 mOsm/kg after being normal previously *5980*
Serum Increase Physiological In two elderly patients being treated with fluoxetine sodium concentrations changed to 404 mOsm/kg and 230 mOsm/kg after being normal previously *5980*
Urine Decrease Physiological In two elderly patients being treated with fluoxetine sodium concentrations fell to 209 mOsm/kg and 247 mOsm/kg after being normal previously *5980*

Phenytoin *Serum Increase Physiological* When fluoxetine ingested with fosphenytoin concentration of phenytoin may be increased *4519* Concurrent administration of fluoxetine with phenytoin caused increased plasma concentration probably due to effect on P450IIIA4 in liver *1440*

Platelet Aggregation *Blood No Effect Physiological* Response to collagen or arachidonic acid in 10 normal volunteers receiving 60 mg daily for either 4 or 6 weeks remained within normal limits *357*

Ritonavir *Serum Increase Physiological* Increases area under the concentration curve by 19% when fluoxetine coadministered *1891*

Sodium *Serum Decrease Physiological* Hyponatremia reported, especially in older patients and those taking diuretics who were otherwise volume depleted *1384* In two elderly patients being treated with fluoxetine sodium concentrations fell to 103 mmol/L and 110 mmol/L after being normal previously *5980*
Urine Decrease Physiological In two elderly patients being treated with fluoxetine sodium concentrations fell to 30 mmol/L and 61 mmol/L after being normal previously *5980*

Trazodone *Serum Increase Physiological* 30% increase in ratio of drug concentration to dose when fluoxetine coadministered possibly due to impaired hepatic metabolism *236*

Tricyclic Antidepressants *Serum Increase Physiological* Previously stable plasma concentrations reported to be doubled with exacerbation of their adverse reactions *1384* Interacts pharmacokinetically to inhibit metabolism of tricyclic antidepressants *3590*

Warfarin *Plasma Increase Physiological* Concurrent administration of fluoxetine with warfarin has been associated with altered anticoagulation effects including increased bleeding *1440*

Fluoxymesterone

Alanine Aminotransferase *Serum Increase Physiological* Cholestatic hepatitis and jaundice may occur with 17α-alkyl-androgens. These drugs have also been associated with development of hepatic adenomas, hepatocellular carcinomas and peliosis hepatitis *4678* Intrahepatic cholestatic jaundice *2242*

Alkaline Phosphatase *Serum Increase Physiological* Cholestatic hepatitis and jaundice may occur with 17α-alkyl-androgens. These drugs have also been associated with development of hepatic adenomas, hepatocellular carcinomas and peliosis hepatitis *4678* Intrahepatic cholestatic jaundice *2242*

Aspartate Aminotransferase *Serum Increase Physiological* Cholestatic hepatitis and jaundice may occur with 17α-alkyl-androgens. These drugs have also been associated with development of hepatic adenomas, hepatocellular carcinomas and peliosis hepatitis *4678* Intrahepatic cholestatic effect *51*

Bile *Urine Increase Physiological* Intrahepatic cholestatic jaundice *2242*

Bilirubin *Serum Increase Physiological* Intrahepatic cholestatic jaundice *2242* Cholestatic hepatitis and jaundice may occur with 17α-alkyl-androgens. These drugs have also been associated with development of hepatic adenomas, hepatocellular carcinomas and peliosis hepatitis *4678*

BSP Retention *Serum Increase Physiological* ?hepatotoxic, cholestatic effect *2024*

Calcium *Serum Increase Physiological* Hypercalcemia may occur in immobilized patients and in those with breast cancer *4678* May occur in immobilized patients or if cancer *2753*

Cefotaxime *Serum Increase Physiological* Serum cholesterol concentration may increase during androgen treatment *4678*

Cholesterol *Serum Decrease Physiological* Observed effect *2754*
Serum Increase Physiological Observed effect *2754*

Creatine *Urine Increase Physiological* For up to 2 weeks when treatment stopped *2754*

Creatinine *Urine Increase Physiological* For up to 2 weeks when treatment stopped *2754*

Erythropoietin *Serum Increase Physiological* Observed if anemia of renal failure *1757*

Factor II *Plasma Increase Physiological* Metabolic effect *51*

Factor V *Plasma Increase Physiological* Metabolic effect *51*

Factor VII *Plasma Increase Physiological* Metabolic effect *51*

Factor X *Plasma Increase Physiological* Metabolic effect *51*

Glucose *Serum Decrease Physiological* Metabolic action *51* Serum glucose concentration in diabetics may decrease during androgen treatment *4678*
Serum Increase Physiological Endocrine response *2754*

Glucose Tolerance *Serum Increase Physiological* Metabolic effect *51*

β-Glucuronidase *Serum Increase Physiological* Metabolic effect *368*

γ-Glutamyltransferase *Serum Increase Physiological* Cholestatic hepatitis and jaundice may occur with 17α-alkyl-androgens. These drugs have also been associated with developments of hepatic adenomas, hepatocellular carcinoma and peliosis hepatitis *4678*

Haptoglobin *Serum Increase Physiological* Metabolic effect *368*

Hematocrit *Blood Increase Physiological* Polycythemia may occur with long term treatment with 17α-alkyl-androgens *4678* Observed if anemia of renal failure *1757*

Hemoglobin *Blood Increase Physiological* Polycythemia may occur with long term treatment with 17α-alkyl-androgens *4678*

^{131}I Uptake *Serum Decrease Physiological* Metabolic effect *51*

17-Ketosteroids *Urine Decrease Physiological* Endogenous hormone suppression *2754*

Leukocytes *Blood Decrease Physiological* Leukopenia may occur *51*

Metyrapone Test *Patient Positive Physiological* At concentration of 23 mg/L had no effect when Kodak Ektachem® method used for measurement of cortisol *51*

Oxyphenbutazone *Serum Increase Physiological* Serum oxyphenbutazone concentration may increase during concomitant androgen treatment *4678*

Plasminogen *Plasma Increase Physiological* Metabolic effect *368*

Prothrombin Time *Plasma Increase Physiological* Increased sensitivity to anticoagulant reported *51*

Sperm Count *Semen Decrease Physiological* After prolonged administration or excess dosage *2753*

T3-Uptake *Serum Decrease Physiological* Serum concentration of TBG may decrease during androgen treatment with a reduction in T3-uptake *4678*
Serum Increase Physiological Affects RBC and resin uptake *51*

Thyroxine Binding Globulin *Serum Decrease Physiological* Metabolic effect *2754* Serum concentration of TBG, and thus thyroxine, may decrease during androgen treatment *4678*

Thyroxine (T4), Free *Serum No Effect Physiological* No change observed *51* Although serum concentration of TBG, and thus total thyroxine, may decrease during androgen treatment, the concentration of free thyroxine is unaffected *4678*

Volume *Plasma Increase Physiological* With retention of water and electrolytes *2754*

Flupenthixole

Albumin *Urine No Effect Analytical* Using a fluorimetric assay with Albumin Blue 580 on a Cobas Fara centrifugal analyzer for the detection of microalbuminuria no significant interference was detected at a concentration of 0.4 mg/L *3117*

Amphetamine/Methamphetamine *Urine No Effect Analytical* No false positive results observed in 9 urines from 4 patients taking drug when measured by Syva EMIT II procedure *5634*

p-Aminophenol *Urine No Effect Analytical* With addition of drugs at a concentration of 100 mg/L and of related compounds at 50 mg/L no significant effect observed on colorimetric method of van Bocxlaer on Cobas Mira analyzer which involves reacting free p-aminophenol with resorcinol in the presence of magnesium ions to form an indophenol dye measured at 550 nm *6163*

Fluphenazine

Alanine Aminotransferase *Serum Increase Physiological* Isolated case of hepatotoxicity with centrilobular cholestasis *5665* Hypersensitivity response *3810* Liver damage as manifested by cholestatic jaundice may occur particularly during the first month of treatment *224*

Alkaline Phosphatase *Serum Increase Physiological* Liver damage as manifested by cholestatic jaundice may occur particularly during the first month of treatment *224* Hypersensitivity response *3810* Isolated case of hepatotoxicity with centrilobular cholestasis *5665*

Aspartate Aminotransferase *Serum Increase Physiological* Hypersensitivity response *3810* Isolated case of hepatotoxicity with centrilobular cholestasis *5665* Liver damage as manifested by cholestatic jaundice may occur particularly during the first month of treatment *224*

Bile *Urine Increase Physiological* Hypersensitivity response *3810*

Bilirubin *Serum Increase Physiological* Liver damage as manifested by cholestatic jaundice may occur particularly during the first month of treatment *224* Hypersensitivity response *3810* Rare jaundice observed but not reported after use of depot preparation *1384*
Urine Increase Physiological Hypersensitivity response *3810*

Bilirubin, Direct *Serum Increase Physiological* Relatively high compared with total *2242*

BSP Retention *Serum Increase Physiological* Hypersensitivity response *3810*

Eosinophils *Blood Increase Physiological* Allergic response with phenothiazines *2753* Blood dyscrasias may occur including eosinophilia *224*

Erythrocytes *Blood Decrease Physiological* Rare pancytopenia with phenothiazines *2753*

Granulocytes *Blood Decrease Physiological* Blood dyscrasias may occur including agranulocytosis *224*

Lactate Dehydrogenase *Serum Increase Physiological* Isolated case of hepatotoxicity with centrilobular cholestasis *5665*

Leukocytes *Blood Decrease Physiological* Agranulocytosis/Leukopenia rarely *2753* Blood dyscrasias may occur including leukopenia *224*

Neutrophils *Blood Decrease Physiological* Occasional case of agranulocytosis reported *6264*

Platelets *Blood Decrease Physiological* Rare thrombocytopenia with/without purpura *2753* Significant reduction observed in 18 psychiatric patients treated for at least 1 y although mean value still in normal range *2684* Blood dyscrasias may occur including thrombocytopenia or nonthrombocytopenic purpura *224*

Pregnancy Tests *Urine Positive Analytical* False positive results may occur *224* False reactions may occur with phenothiazines *2753*

Prolactin *Plasma Increase Physiological* Marked increase in male and female psychiatric patients treated for up to 4 weeks *6098* In schizophrenics treated with fluphenazine by injection all patients exhibited an increase in prolactin concentration *6454* Typical dose-related response to i.m. administered drug due to antidopaminergic action *3402* Neuroleptics increase plasma prolactin concentrations, the increase persisting with chronic administration *224*

Flurazepam

Alanine Aminotransferase *Serum Increase Physiological* Rare cases of increased activity reported with treatment *5039* May cause hepatic toxicity *5007*
Serum No Effect Analytical At acute overdose concentration (2.5 mg/dL) on Technicon SMAC® method *6266* At 5 times upper limit of therapeutic range on methods on Technicon SMAC® , Abbott-VP, Du Pont aca, Roche Cobas-Bio, and KDA *3525*

Albumin *Serum No Effect Analytical* At acute overdose concentration (2.5 mg/dL) on Technicon SMAC® method *6266* At 5 times upper limit of therapeutic range on methods on Technicon SMAC® , Kodak Ektachem® , Hitachi® 705 and KDA *3525* At concentration of 25 mg/L had no effect on BCG method *5704*

Alkaline Phosphatase *Serum Increase Physiological* May cause hepatic toxicity *5007* Rare cases of increased activity reported with treatment *5039*
Serum No Effect Analytical At acute overdose concentration (2.5 mg/dL) on Technicon SMAC® method *6266* At 5 times upper limit of therapeutic range on methods on Technicon SMAC® , Abbott-VP, Roche Cobas-Bio, Du Pont aca, Hitachi® 705 and KDA *3525*

Amylase *Serum No Effect Analytical* At 5 times upper limit of therapeutic range on methods on Du Pont aca, Roche Cobas-Bio, and Kodak Ektachem® *3525*

Aspartate Aminotransferase *Serum Increase Physiological* May cause hepatic toxicity *5007* Rare cases of increased activity reported with treatment *5039*
Serum No Effect Analytical At acute overdose concentration (2.5 mg/dL) on Technicon SMAC® method *6266* At 5 times upper limit of therapeutic range on methods on Technicon SMAC® , Abbott-VP, Roche Cobas-Bio, Du Pont aca, Hitachi® 705 and KDA *3525*

Benzodiazepine *Urine Positive Analytical* At concentration of 0.2 µg/mL produces positive result with Syva EMIT II assay *1785* Positive result observed at a concentration of 2.0 µg/mL (5.15 µmol/L) with method on Du Pont aca *1556*

Bicarbonate *Serum No Effect Analytical* At concentration of 0.1 mg/L had no effect on method using phenolphthalein *5704*

Bile *Urine Increase Physiological* May cause hepatotoxicity *5007*

Bilirubin *Serum Increase Physiological* May cause hepatic toxicity *5007* Rare cases of increased concentration reported with treatment *5039*
Serum No Effect Analytical At concentration of 25 mg/L had no effect on Jendrassik and Grof method *5704* At 5 times upper limit of therapeutic range on methods on Technicon SMAC® , Roche Cobas-Bio, Du Pont aca, Kodak Ektachem® , Hitachi® 705 and KDA *3525* At acute overdose concentration (2.5 mg/dL) on Technicon SMAC® method *6266*

Bilirubin, Conjugated *Serum No Effect Analytical* No effect at concentration of 2 mg/L on method on Kodak Ektachem® *5706*

Bilirubin, Direct *Serum Increase Physiological* May cause hepatic toxicity *5007* Rare cases of increased concentration reported with treatment *5039*

Bilirubin, Unconjugated *Serum No Effect Analytical* No effect at concentration of 2 mg/L on method on Kodak Ektachem® *5706*

Flurazepam *(continued)*

BSP Retention *Serum Increase Physiological* May cause hepatotoxicity *5007*

Calcium *Serum No Effect Analytical* At 5 times upper limit of therapeutic range on methods on Technicon SMAC®, Abbott-VP, Du Pont aca, Kodak Ektachem®, Hitachi® 705 and KDA *3525* At concentration of 25 mg/L had no effect on cresolphthalein method *5704* At acute overdose concentration (2.5 mg/dL) on Technicon SMAC® method *6266*

Catecholamines *Plasma No Effect Analytical* No effect on HPLC method of Koller for dopamine, epinephrine, and norepinephrine *3230*

Chloride *Serum No Effect Analytical* At concentration of 0.1 mg/L had no effect on mercurimetric method *5704*

Cholesterol *Serum No Effect Analytical* At 5 times upper limit of therapeutic range on methods on Technicon SMAC®, Abbott-VP, Roche Cobas-Bio, Kodak Ektachem®, Hitachi® 705 and KDA *3525* At concentration of 0.1 mg/L had no effect on CHOD-PAP method *5704* At concentration of 25 mg/L had no effect on Liebermann-Burchard method *5704* At acute overdose concentration (2.5 mg/dL) on Technicon SMAC® method *6266*

Creatine Kinase *Serum No Effect Analytical* At 5 times upper limit of therapeutic range on methods on Technicon SMAC®, Abbott-VP, Du Pont aca, Roche Cobas-Bio, and Hitachi® 705 *3525* At acute overdose concentration (2.5 mg/dL) on Technicon SMAC® method *6266*

Creatinine *Serum No Effect Analytical* No effect of concentrations up to 2 mg/L on 2-slide method on Kodak Ektachem® *5706* At concentration of 25 mg/L had no effect on Technicon AutoAnalyzer® Jaffe method *5704* At acute overdose concentration (2.5 mg/dL) on Technicon SMAC® method *6266* At 5 times upper limit of therapeutic range on methods on Technicon SMAC®, Abbott-VP, Du Pont aca, Roche Cobas-Bio, Kodak Ektachem®, Hitachi® 705, and KDA *3525*

Glucose *Serum No Effect Analytical* At 5 times upper limit of therapeutic range on methods on Technicon SMAC®, Abbott-VP, Du Pont aca, Roche Cobas-Bio, Kodak Ektachem®, Hitachi® 705, and KDA *3525* At concentration of 0.1 mg/L had no effect on GOD/POD-PAP method *5704* At acute overdose concentration (2.5 mg/dL) on Technicon SMAC® method *6266*

Urine Decrease Analytical Lowered result with Clinistix®, Diastix® *1826*

Urine No Effect Analytical No effect observed with Tes-Tape® *1826*

γ-Glutamyltransferase *Serum No Effect Analytical* At 5 times upper limit of therapeutic range on methods on Technicon SMAC®, Abbott-VP, and Hitachi® 705 *3525*

Granulocytes *Blood Decrease Physiological* Rare cases of granulocytopenia reported with treatment *5039*

5-Hydroxyindoleacetic Acid *Urine Increase Analytical* Slight effect when added *in vitro* in method of Udenfriend *1051*

Iron *Serum No Effect Analytical* At concentration of 25 mg/L had no effect on Ferrozine method *5704* At 5 times upper limit of therapeutic range on Ferrozine method on Technicon SMAC® *3525* At acute overdose concentration (2.5 mg/dL) on Technicon SMAC® method *6266*

Lactate Dehydrogenase *Serum No Effect Analytical* At acute overdose concentration (2.5 mg/dL) on Technicon SMAC® method *6266* At 5 times upper limit of therapeutic range on methods on Technicon SMAC®, Abbott-VP, Du Pont aca, Roche Cobas-Bio, Hitachi® 705 and KDA *3525*

Leukocytes *Blood Decrease Physiological* Rare cases of leukopenia reported with treatment *5039*

Phosphate *Serum No Effect Analytical* At concentration of 25 mg/L had no effect on phosphomolybdate method *5704* At 5 times upper limit of therapeutic range on methods on Technicon SMAC®, Du Pont aca, Hitachi® 705 and KDA *3525* At acute overdose concentration (2.5 mg/dL) on Technicon SMAC® method *6266*

Potassium *Serum No Effect Analytical* At concentration of 0.1 mg/L had no effect on flame-photometric method *5704*

Protein *Serum No Effect Analytical* At acute overdose concentration (2.5 mg/dL) on Technicon SMAC® method *6266* At concentration of 25 mg/L had no effect on biuret method with blank correction *5704* At 5 times upper limit of therapeutic range on methods on Technicon SMAC®, Abbott-VP, Kodak Ektachem®, Hitachi® 705 and KDA *3525*

Sodium *Serum No Effect Analytical* At concentration of 0.1 mg/L had no effect on flame-photometric method *5704*

Sugar *Urine Increase Analytical* Excreted as glucuronide, sulfate: affect Benedict's reaction *5400*

Triglycerides *Serum No Effect Analytical* At concentration of 25 mg/L had no effect on lipase/esterase method *5704* At acute overdose concentration (2.5 mg/dL) on Technicon SMAC® method *6266* At 5 times upper limit of therapeutic range on methods on Technicon SMAC®, Abbott-VP, Kodak Ektachem®, Hitachi® 705 and KDA *3525*

Urea Nitrogen *Serum No Effect Analytical* At acute overdose concentration (2.5 mg/dL) on Technicon SMAC® method *6266* At concentration of 25 mg/L had no effect on diacetylmonoxime method *5704* At 5 times upper limit of therapeutic range on methods on Technicon SMAC®, Abbott-VP, Roche Cobas-Bio, Kodak Ektachem®, Hitachi® 705 and KDA *3525*

Uric Acid *Serum No Effect Analytical* At 5 times upper limit of therapeutic range on methods on Technicon SMAC®, Abbott-VP, Du Pont aca, Roche Cobas-Bio, Kodak Ektachem®, Hitachi® 705, and KDA *3525* At acute overdose concentration (2.5 mg/dL) on Technicon SMAC® method *6266* At concentration of 25 mg/L had no effect on phosphomolybdate reduction method *5704*

Volume *Saliva Increase Physiological* Excessive salivation may occur *2753*

Warfarin *Plasma No Effect Physiological* No effect on plasma concentrations noted in one study of eight healthy volunteers *4997*

Flurbiprofen

Bilirubin *Serum No Effect Physiological* At pharmacological concentrations has little or no effect on displacement from protein *6314*

Bleeding Time *Patient Increase Physiological* Prolongs bleeding time with associated bleeding complications *1384*

Chondrex *Serum No Effect Analytical* Concentrations up to 0.05 g/L had no significant effect on sandwich-type ELISA procedure of Harvey et al *2491*

Cortisol *Plasma Increase Analytical* At a concentration of 60 mg/L caused increase in recovery to 118.0% with Enzymun method *1097*

Plasma No Effect Analytical At a concentration of 12 mg/L had no significant effect on Enzymun method *1097*

Phenprocoumon *Plasma No Effect Physiological* In one study no effect observed on plasma concentrations with coadministration of drugs *3784*

Platelet Aggregation *Blood Decrease Physiological* Inhibits platelet aggregation *1384*

Flurithromycin

Carbamazepine *Serum Increase Physiological* Inhibits metabolism and increases plasma concentration *3118*

Fluroxene

Alanine Aminotransferase *Serum Increase Physiological* Potentially hepatotoxic *128*

Aspartate Aminotransferase *Serum Increase Physiological* Potentially hepatotoxic *128*

Bilirubin *Serum Increase Physiological* Potentially hepatotoxic *128*

Bleeding Time *Patient Increase Physiological* Prolonged during anesthesia, normal in 24 h *128*

BSP Retention *Serum Increase Physiological* Potentially hepatotoxic *128*

Factor V *Plasma No Effect Physiological* No significant effect noted *2964*

Fibrinogen *Plasma Decrease Physiological* From 283 mg/dL to 257 mg/dL postoperatively *2964*

Hemoglobin *Urine No Effect Physiological* No significant effect noted *2964*

Leukocytes *Blood Increase Physiological* Normal response to anesthesia *5818*

Occult Blood *Feces Increase Physiological* In 1 of 8 patients (slight only) *2964*

Partial Thromboplastin Time
Plasma No Effect Physiological No significant effect noted *2964*

Platelets *Blood Increase Physiological* Slight from 217,000 /μL to 251,000 /μL postoperatively *2964*

Prothrombin Time *Plasma No Effect Physiological* No significant effect noted *2964*

Thrombin Time *Blood No Effect Physiological* No significant effect noted *2964*

Fluspirilene

Alkaline Phosphatase *Serum Decrease Physiological* Slight but observable trend *358*

Amphetamine *Urine Increase Analytical* 5 false positive results observed in 5 assays using Syva EMIT amphatamine method using a monoclonal antibody *1160*
Urine No Effect Analytical No false positive results observed in 5 assays using Syva EMIT amphatamine method using a polyclonal antibody *1160*

Aspartate Aminotransferase
Serum Decrease Physiological Slight but observable trend *358*

Catecholamines *Plasma No Effect Analytical* No effect on HPLC method of Koller for dopamine, epinephrine, and norepinephrine *3230*

Granulocytes *Blood Decrease Physiological* Decreased values noted (not marked) *358*

Leukocytes *Blood Increase Physiological* Initial effect observed *358*

Flutamide

Alanine Aminotransferase *Serum Increase Physiological* Hepatitis and jaundice occurred in fewer than 1% of treated patients *5328* Transient increases observed in up to 33% patients with severe toxic hepatitis occurring in some *1384* In 4 of 1091 patients with stage C or D prostatic cancer more than fourfold increase observed but only two developed clinical manifestations of liver disease *2235*

Alkaline Phosphatase *Serum Increase Physiological* Hepatitis and jaundice occurred in fewer than 1% of treated patients *5328* In one of 1091 patients with stage C or D prostatic cancer xignificant increase to 640 U/L observed *2235*

Androstanediol Glucuronide
Plasma No Effect Physiological In 9 women with hirsutism no significant effect observed with treatment with 750 mg/d for 3 months *3789*

Androstenedione *Plasma No Effect Physiological* No effect of treatment with 750 mg daily for 10 days in 6 men with untreated advanced prostatic cancer *355*

Aspartate Aminotransferase *Serum Increase Physiological* In 4 of 1091 patients with stage C or D prostatic cancer increase of at least fourfold observed over course of treatment but only developed clinical manifestations of liver disease *2235* Hepatitis and jaundice occurred in fewer than 1% of treated patients *5328*

Bilirubin *Serum Increase Physiological* Hepatitis and jaundice occurred in fewer than 1% of treated patients *5328* In one of 1091 patients with stage C or D prostatic cancer concentration increased significantly to 126 mmol/L *2235* Transient increases observed in up to 33% treated patients with toxic hepatitis occuring in some *1384*

Dehydroepiandrosterone *Plasma No Effect Physiological* No effect of treatment with 750 mg daily for 10 days in 6 men with untreated advanced prostatic cancer *355*

Dehydroepiandrosterone Sulfate
Plasma No Effect Physiological No effect of treatment with 750 mg daily for 10 days in 6 men with untreated advanced prostatic cancer *355*

FSH response to GnRH *Plasma No Effect Physiological* In 9 women with hirsutism no observed in response observed after GnRH *3789*

γ-Glutamyltransferase *Serum Increase Physiological* Hepatitis and jaundice occurred in fewer than 1% of treated patients *5328*

Hematocrit *Blood Decrease Physiological* Anemia occurred in 6% of treated patients *5328*

Hemoglobin *Blood Decrease Physiological* Anemia occurred in 6% of treated patients *5328*

17-Hydroxypregnenolone *Plasma No Effect Physiological* No effect of 750 mg/day for 10 days in 6 men with untreated advanced prostatic cancer *355*

17-Hydroxyprogesterone *Plasma No Effect Physiological* No effect of 750 mg daily for 10 days in 6 men with untreated advanced prostatic cancer *355*

Leukocytes *Blood Decrease Physiological* Leukopenia occurred in 3% of treated patients *5328*

LH response to GnRH *Plasma No Effect Physiological* In 9 women with hirsutism response to GnRH unchanged *3789*

Prostate-specific Antigen *Serum Decrease Physiological* In 11 men with benign prostatic hypertrophy treatment with 750 mg/d for 6 months caused decrease from mean of 10.7 ng/mL (range 1.9 to 42 ng/mL) to 3.8 ng/mL (range 0.5 to 16) *5834*
Serum No Effect Analytical Flutamide at a concentration of up to 10 μg/mL caused less than 0.1% cross-reactivity with method on PSA method on Bayer Technicon Immuno 1® *430*

Prostate-specific Antigen, Free *Serum No Effect Analytical* Flutamide at a concentration of 78 μg/L had no significant effect on the Hybritech Tandem® -R free PSA immunoassay *4286*

Riboflavin *Blood Decrease Physiological* Thrombocytopenia occurred in 1% of treated patients *5328*

Sex-Hormone Binding Globulin
Serum No Effect Physiological In 9 women with hirsutism treated with 750 mg/d for 3 months no significant effect observed on concentration *3789*

Testosterone *Serum Increase Physiological* Significant increase in mean concentration in 6 men with untreated advanced prostatic cancer given 750 mg daily for 10 days *355* In 11 men with benign prostatic hypertrophy treatment with 750 mg/d for 6 months caused increase from mean baseline of 336 ng/dL (range 250 to 597) to 518 ng/dL (range 400 to 732) with increased concentration returning to baseline 6 weeks after end of treatment *5834*
Serum No Effect Physiological In 9 women with hirsutism treated with 750 mg/d for 3 months no significant effect observed on plasma concentration *3789*

Testosterone, Bound *Serum No Effect Physiological* In 9 women with hirsutism treated with 750 mg/d for 3 months no significant effect observed on concentration *3789*

Testosterone, Free *Serum No Effect Physiological* In 9 women with hirsutism treatment with 750 mg/d for 3 months had no significant effect on concentration *3789*

Fluvastatin

Alanine Aminotransferase *Serum Increase Physiological* Administration of fluvastatin caused an increase to over 3 times the upper limit of normal in 1.1% (25) of 2969 patients in multiple trials *5232*
Serum No Effect Physiological In 42 hypercholesterolemic patients receiving cyclosporine after renal transplantation treatment with 20 mg/d for 12 weeks caused no significant change from mean baseline of 25 ± 2 U/L to 24 ± 2 U/L and to 21 ± 2 U/L at week 20 after 40 mg/d *2669*

Alkaline Phosphatase *Serum Increase Physiological* Administration of statins rarely causes a hepatitis including chronic active hepatitis, cholestatic jaundice, fatty changes in the liver and even more rarely cirrhosis, fulminant hepatic necrosis and hepatoma *5232*

Amylase *Serum Increase Physiological* Administration of statins rarely causes pancreatitis *5232*

Antinuclear Antibodies *Serum Increase Physiological* Administration of fluvastatin rarely causes a hypersensitivity reaction with positive ANA titer *5232*

Fluvastatin *(continued)*

Antipyrine *Serum* *No Effect* *Physiological* Administration of fluvastatin to patients with hypercholesterolemia together with antipyrine had no effect on its metabolism and excretion *5232*

Apolipoprotein A *Serum* *No Effect* *Physiological* In 31 patients with primary hypercholesterolemia treatment with 40 mg/d caused nonsignificant change to 13.4 g/L (6%) from mean baseline of 12.7 ± 0.5 g/L *5614* In 24 patients with a history of angina pectoris (randomized from 27 men and 21 women) with mean age 59 years treatment with 40 mg/d fluvastatin caused no significant change from mean baseline of 118.6 ± 17.4 mg/dL to 119.5 ± 16.8 mg/dL after 20 weeks *537*

Apolipoprotein A-I *Serum* *Increase* *Physiological* In 337 hypercholesterolemic patients treatment with up to 30 mg/d for 12 weeks caused nonsignificant 3.3% increase from mean baseline of 136.5 ± 1.4 mg/dL *5982*

Serum *No Effect* *Physiological* In 4 heterogeneous patients with familial LDL-receptor defective hypercholesterolemia treatment with 40 mg/d for 12 weeks caused a nonsignificant change from mean baseline of 168 ± 26 mg/dL to 174 ± 27 mg/dL *2408* In 24 patients with familial hypercholesterolemia treatment with up to 60 mg/d for 2 years caused nonsignificant change from mean baseline of 115.4 mg/dL to 112.8 mg/dL *3227*

Apolipoprotein A-II *Serum* *No Effect* *Physiological* In 4 heterogeneous patients with familial LDL-receptor defective hypercholesterolemia treatment with 40 mg/d for 12 weeks caused a nonsignificant change from mean baseline of 59 ± 7 mg/dL to 57 ± 4 mg/dL *2408*

Apolipoprotein B *Serum* *Decrease* *Physiological* In 24 patients with familial hypercholesterolemia treatment with up to 60 mg/d for 2 years caused significant change from mean baseline of 142.0 mg/dL to 111.1 mg/dL *3227* In 4 heterogeneous patients with familial LDL-receptor defective hypercholesterolemia treatment with 40 mg/d for 12 weeks caused a significant change from mean baseline of 174 ± 20 mg/dL to 141 ± 27 mg/dL *2408* In 337 hypercholesterolemic patients treatment with up to 30 mg/d for 12 weeks caused significant 16.8% decrease from mean baseline of 132.6 ± 1.5 mg/dL *5982* In 31 patients with primary hypercholesterolemia treatment with 40 mg/d caused significant change to 7.0 g/L (17%) from mean baseline of 8.5 ± 0.5 g/L *5614* In 86 hypercholesterolemic patients treated with 10 mg/d for 6 weeks significant reduction from mean baseline of 189 ± 58 mg/dL to 173 ± 51 mg/dL observed. With 80 mg/d for 6 weeks significant reduction from 185 ± 63 mg/dL to 148 ± 56 mg/dL observed *1225* Administration of fluvastatin to patients with hypercholesterolemia reduced the serum apolipoprotein B concentration *5232*

Serum *No Effect* *Physiological* In 24 patients with a history of angina pectoris (randomized from 27 men and 21 women) with mean age 59 years treatment with 40 mg/d fluvastatin caused no significant change from mean baseline of 109.5 ± 27.5 mg/dL to 100.0 ± 24.0 mg/dL after 20 weeks *537*

Apolipoprotein E *Serum* *Decrease* *Physiological* In 337 hypercholesterolemic patients treatment with up to 30 mg/d for 12 weeks caused significant 14.5% decrease from mean baseline of 7.8 ± 0.2 mg/dL *5982*

Aspartate Aminotransferase *Serum* *Increase* *Physiological* Administration of fluvastatin caused an increase to over 3 times the upper limit of normal in 1.1% (25) of 2969 patients in multiple trials *5232*

Serum *No Effect* *Physiological* In 42 hypercholesterolemic patients receiving cyclosporine after renal transplantation treatment with 20 mg/d for 12 weeks caused no significant change from mean baseline of 24 ± 1 U/L to 26 ± 2 U/L and to 25 ± 2 U/L at week 20 after 40 mg/d *2669*

Bilirubin *Serum* *Increase* *Physiological* Administration of statins rarely causes a hepatitis including chronic active hepatitis, cholestatic jaundice, fatty changes in the liver and even more rarely cirrhosis, fulminant hepatic necrosis and hepatoma *5232*

Chenodeoxycholic Acid *Bile* *No Effect* *Physiological* In 19 patients with hypercholesterolemia types IIa or IIb treatment with 30 mg/d for 12 weeks caused caused nonsignificant change from mean baseline proportion of 42.75 ± 2.61% to 44.88 ± 2.20% *5972*

Cholesterol *Serum* *Decrease* *Physiological* In 918 patients with primary hypercholesterolemia treatment with 20 mg/d fluvastatin caused significant reduction of 16.5% from mean baseline after 9 weeks treatment *6636* In 337 hypercholesterolemic patients treatment with up to 30 mg/d for 12 weeks caused significant 17.0% reduction from mean baseline of 288.7 ± 3.0 mg/dL *5982* In 4 heterogeneous patients with familial LDL-receptor defective hypercholesterolemia treatment with 40 mg/d for 12 weeks caused a significant decrease from mean baseline of 376 ± 60 mg/dL to 284 ± 19 mg/dL *2408* In 19 patients with hypercholesterolemia types IIa or IIb treatment with 30 mg/d for 4 weeks caused caused significant 24% reduction from mean baseline of 280 mg/dL after 4 weeks but with slight increase thereafter with continuing treatment with concentration remaining significantly reduced *5972* In 31 patients with primary hypercholesterolemia treatment with 40 mg/d caused reduction to 6.38 mmol/L (22%) from mean baseline of 8.18 ± 0.40 mmol/L *5614* Administration of fluvastatin to patients with hypercholesterolemia reduced the total serum cholesterol concentration *5232* In 24 patients with familial hypercholesterolemia treatment with up to 60 mg/d for 2 years caused significant decrease from mean baseline of 318.0 mg/dL to 232.3 mg/dL *3227* In 20 patients with type IIa hypercholesterolemia treatment with 40 mg/d for 4 weeks caused mean 27% decrease from mean baseline of 293 ± 23 mg/dL *4033* In 42 hypercholesterolemic patients receiving cyclosporine after renal transplantation treatment with 20 mg/d for 12 weeks caused significant reduction from mean baseline of 313 ± 12 mg/dL to 262 ± 12 mg/dL and to 228 ± 12 mg/dL at week 20 after 40 mg/d *2669* In 19 renal transplant recipients with hypercholesterolemia treatment with 20 mg/d caused mean reductions of 16.1% after 6 weeks and 16.3% after 14 weeks from mean baseline of 313 ± 44 mg/dL *2216* In 44 individuals with LDL-cholesterol concentration greater than 4.0 mmol/L after 8 weeks of dietary therapy treated with 40 mg/d for 12 weeks caused decrease of 21 ± 8.5% but with magnitude associated with alleles of LPL *953* In 46 men with LDL-cholesterol concentrations greater than 160 mg/dL treatment with 20 mg/d fluvastatin for 27 weeks caused mean decrease of 46.4 ± 22.6 mg/dL versus increase of 13.2 ± 27.8 mg/dL in placebo-treated controls *5874* In 24 patients with a history of angina pectoris (randomized from 27 men and 21 women) with mean age 59 years treatment with 40 mg/d fluvastatin caused significant reduction from mean baseline of 246.1 ± 47.5 mg/dL to 216.0 ± 44.0 mg/dL after 20 weeks *537*

Cholesterol:HDL-Cholesterol Ratio
Serum *Decrease* *Physiological* In 20 patients with type IIa hypercholesterolemia treatment with 40 mg/d for 4 weeks caused mean decrease of 50% *4033*

Cholic Acid *Bile* *No Effect* *Physiological* In 19 patients with hypercholesterolemia types IIa or IIb treatment with 30 mg/d for 12 weeks caused caused nonsignificant change from mean baseline proportion of 28.01 ± 3.18% to 28.57 ± 2.26% *5972*

Cortisol *Plasma* *No Effect* *Physiological* Administration of fluvastatin had no effect on unstimulated cortisol concentration *5232*

Creatine Kinase *Serum* *Increase* *Physiological* Administration of fluvastatin rarely causes rhabdomyolysis with creatine kinase activity above 10 times the upper limit of normal with renal failure due to myoglobinuria *5232*

Serum *No Effect* *Physiological* In 42 hypercholesterolemic patients receiving cyclosporine after renal transplantation treatment with 20 mg/d for 12 weeks caused no significant change from mean baseline of 101 ± 11 U/L to 114 ± 13 U/L and to 116 ± 13 U/L at week 20 after 40 mg/d *2669*

Creatinine *Serum* *No Effect* *Physiological* In 42 hypercholesterolemic patients receiving cyclosporine after renal transplantation treatment with 20 mg/d for 12 weeks caused no significant change from mean baseline of 174 ± 15 μg/L to 181 ± 18 μg/L and to 180 ± 16 μg/L at week 20 after 40 mg/d *2669*

Cyclosporine *Serum* *No Effect* *Physiological* In 42 hypercholesterolemic patients receiving cyclosporine after renal transplantation treatment with 20 mg/d for 12 weeks caused no significant change from mean baseline of 115 ± 15 μg/L to 146 ± 8 μg/L and to 142 ± 14 μg/L at week 20 after 40 mg/d *2669*

Deoxycholic Acid *Bile No Effect Physiological* In 19 patients with hypercholesterolemia types IIa or IIb treatment with 30 mg/d for 12 weeks caused caused nonsignificant change from mean baseline proportion of 25.20 ± 3.40% to 21.98 ± 3.54% *5972*

Digoxin *Serum Increase Physiological* In 18 patients chronically receiving digoxin administration of a single oral 40 mg dose of fluvastatin had no effect on the digoxin AUC but caused a 11% increase in the digoxin concentration and small increase in urinary clearance *5232*

Urine Increase Physiological In 18 patients chronically receiving digoxin administration of a single oral 40 mg dose of fluvastatin had no effect on the digoxin AUC but caused a 11% increase in the digoxin concentration and small increase in urinary clearance *5232*

Eosinophils *Blood Increase Physiological* Administration of fluvastatin rarely causes a hypersensitivity reaction with eosinophilia *5232*

Erythrocyte Sedimentation Rate

Blood Increase Physiological Administration of fluvastatin rarely causes a hypersensitivity reaction with increased ESR *5232*

Erythrocytes *Blood Decrease Physiological* Administration of fluvastatin rarely causes a hypersensitivity reaction with hemolytic anemia *5232*

Erythromycin *Serum No Effect Physiological* Administration of fluvastatin to patients with hypercholesterolemia together with erythromycin had no effect on its metabolism and excretion *5232*

Fibrinogen *Plasma Increase Physiological* Administration of fluvastatin to patients with hypercholesterolemia had no consistent effect on concentration *5232*

Gemfibrozil *Serum No Effect Physiological* Administration of fluvastatin to patients with hypercholesterolemia together with gemfibrozil had no effect on its metabolism and excretion *5232*

γ-Glutamyltransferase *Serum Increase Physiological* Administration of statins rarely causes a hepatitis including chronic active hepatitis, cholestatic jaundice, fatty changes in the liver and even more rarely cirrhosis, fulminant hepatic necrosis and hepatoma *5232*

Glyburide *Serum Increase Physiological* In 16 healthy individuals coadministration of 40 mg fluvastatin in single dose caused 16% increase and in multiple doses caused 31% increase in maximum glyburide concentration relative to placebo-treated controls *227*

HDL_{2a}-Cholesterol *Serum No Effect Physiological* In 4 heterogeneous patients with familial LDL-receptor defective hypercholesterolemia treatment with 40 mg/d for 12 weeks caused a nonsignificant change from mean baseline of 13.8 ± 6.4% to 11.1 ± 6.3% *2408*

HDL_{2b}-Cholesterol *Serum No Effect Physiological* In 4 heterogeneous patients with familial LDL-receptor defective hypercholesterolemia treatment with 40 mg/d for 12 weeks caused a nonsignificant change from mean baseline of 9.1 ± 3.1% to 7.4 ± 3.9% *2408*

HDL_{3a}-Cholesterol *Serum No Effect Physiological* In 4 heterogeneous patients with familial LDL-receptor defective hypercholesterolemia treatment with 40 mg/d for 12 weeks caused a nonsignificant change from mean baseline of 14.3 ± 4.1% to 13.4 ± 3.3% *2408*

HDL_{3c}-Cholesterol *Serum No Effect Physiological* In 4 heterogeneous patients with familial LDL-receptor defective hypercholesterolemia treatment with 40 mg/d for 12 weeks caused a nonsignificant change from mean baseline of 39.2 ± 15.5% to 42.1 ± 16.8% *2408*

HDL-Cholesterol *Serum Increase Physiological* Administration of fluvastatin to patients with hypercholesterolemia increased the serum HDL-cholesterol concentration to a variable extent *5232* In 24 patients with a history of angina pectoris (randomized from 27 men and 21 women) with mean age 59 years treatment with 40 mg/d fluvastatin caused significant increase from mean baseline of 47.6 ± 13.5 mg/dL to 57.0 ± 13.9 mg/dL after 20 weeks *537* In 622 patients with heterozygous familial hypercholesterolemia treatment with 40 mg/d for 19.4 ± 15.5 weeks caused a change of + 4.5% from mean baseline in those with serum cholesterol concentrations greater than 240 mg/dL and + 4.5% in those with serum cholesterol less than 240 mg/dL *4630* In 19 patients with hypercholesterolemia types IIa or IIb treatment with 30 mg/d for 12 weeks caused caused significant increase to 50 mg/dL from mean baseline of 47 mg/dL *5972* In 337 hypercholesterolemic patients treatment with up to 30 mg/d for 12 weeks caused significant 6.0% increase from mean baseline of 53.0 ± 0.8 mg/dL to 56.2 ± 0.6 mg/dL *5982* In 24 patients with familial hypercholesterolemia treatment with up to 60 mg/d for 76 weeks caused significant increase from mean baseline of 45.5 mg/dL by 11.0 ± 3.3% and nonsignificant increase to 46.8 mg/dL after two years *3227* In 19 renal transplant recipients with hypercholesterolemia treatment with 20 mg/d caused mean nonsignificant increases of 4.7% after 6 weeks and 6.9% after 14 weeks from mean baseline of 54 ± 12 mg/dL *2216*

Serum No Effect Physiological In 31 patients with primary hypercholesterolemia treatment with 40 mg/d caused nonsignificant reduction to 1.17 mmol/L (3%) from mean baseline of 1.22 ± 0.08 mmol/L *5614* In 918 patients with primary hypercholesterolemia treatment with 20 mg/d fluvastatin caused nonsignificant increase of 2.2% from mean baseline after 9 weeks treatment *6636* In 42 hypercholesterolemic patients receiving cyclosporine after renal transplantation treatment with 20 mg/d for 12 weeks caused no change from mean baseline of 58 ± 4 mg/dL to 58 ± 4 mg/dL and to 58 ± 4 mg/dL at week 20 after 40 mg/d *2669* In 46 men with LDL-cholesterol concentrations greater than 160 mg/dL treatment with 20 mg/d fluvastatin for 27 weeks caused mean increase of 1.3 ± 7.3 mg/dL versus increase of 1.2 ± 7.3 mg/dL in placebo-treated controls *5874* In 4 heterogeneous patients with familial LDL-receptor defective hypercholesterolemia treatment with 40 mg/d for 12 weeks caused a nonsignificant change from mean baseline of 47 ± 5 mg/dL to 47 ± 8 mg/dL *2408*

Hemoglobin *Blood Decrease Physiological* Administration of fluvastatin rarely causes a hypersensitivity reaction with hemolytic anemia *5232*

LDL-Cholesterol *Serum Decrease Physiological* In 19 renal transplant recipients with hypercholesterolemia treatment with 20 mg/d caused mean reductions of 24.0% after 6 weeks and 25.3% after 14 weeks from mean baseline of 211 ± 42 mg/dL *2216* In 24 patients with familial hypercholesterolemia treatment with up to 60 mg/d for 2 years caused significant decrease from mean baseline of 245.9 mg/dL to 163.8 mg/dL *3227* In 20 patients with type IIa hypercholesterolemia treatment with 40 mg/d for 4 weeks caused mean 33% decrease from mean baseline of 213 ± 47 mg/dL *4033* Administration of fluvastatin caused a 20 to 30% decrease according to 18 published, controlled trials *5232* In 42 hypercholesterolemic patients receiving cyclosporine after renal transplantation treatment with 20 mg/d for 12 weeks caused significant reduction from mean baseline of 212 ± 12 mg/dL to 166 ± 12 mg/dL and to 131 ± 12 mg/dL at week 20 after 40 mg/d *2669* In 622 patients with heterozygous familial hypercholesterolemia treatment with 40 mg/d for 19.4 ± 15.5 weeks caused a significant change of 25 - 26% from mean baseline *4630* In 4 heterogeneous patients with familial LDL-receptor defective hypercholesterolemia treatment with 40 mg/d for 12 weeks caused a significant change from mean baseline of 304 ± 58 mg/dL to 214 ± 23 mg/dL *2408* In 85 hypercholesterolemic patients treated with 10 mg/d for 6 weeks significant reduction from mean baseline of 261 ± 75 mg/dL to 236 ± 70 mg/dL observed. With 80 mg/d for 6 weeks significant reduction from 243 ± 60 mg/dL to 195 ± 51 mg/dL observed *1225* In 918 patients with primary hypercholesterolemia treatment with up to 40 mg/d fluvastatin caused significant reduction from mean baseline of 227 mg/dL by 30.7% after one year and 30.6% after 2 years *6636* In 44 individuals with LDL-cholesterol concentration greater than 4.0 mmol/L after 8 weeks of dietary therapy treated with 40 mg/d for 12 weeks caused decrease of 28 ± 8.5% but with magnitude nonsignificantly associated with alleles of LPL *953* In 46 men with LDL-cholesterol concentrations greater than 160 mg/dL treatment with 20 mg/d fluvastatin for 27 weeks caused mean decrease of 42.4 ± 16.7 mg/dL versus increase of 9.7 ± 30.3 mg/dL in placebo-treated controls *5874* In 337 hypercholesterolemic patients treatment with up to 30 mg/d for 12 weeks caused significant 23.8% reduction from mean baseline of 204.3 ± 2.8 mg/dL to 154.8 ± 2.5 mg/dL *5982* In 19 patients with hypercholesterolemia types IIa or IIb treatment with 30 mg/d for 12 weeks caused caused significant 33% reduction from mean baseline of 205 mg/dL after 4 weeks

Fluvastatin *(continued)*

LDL-Cholesterol *(continued)*
but increased thereafter *5972* In 24 patients with a history of angina pectoris (randomized from 27 men and 21 women) with mean age 59 years treatment with 40 mg/d fluvastatin caused significant reduction from mean baseline of 172.8 ± 39.9 mg/dL to 134.4 ± 43.8 mg/dL after 20 weeks *537* In 31 patients with primary hypercholesterolemia treatment with 40 mg/d caused significant reduction to 4.52 mmol/L (28%) from mean baseline of 6.20 ± 0.42 mmol/L *5614*

LDL-Cholesterol:HDL-Cholesterol Ratio
Serum Decrease Physiological In 918 patients with primary hypercholesterolemia treatment with 20 mg/d fluvastatin caused significant decrease of ratio of 23.2% *6636*
Serum Increase Physiological In 19 renal transplant recipients with hypercholesterolemia treatment with 20 mg/d caused mean significant increases of 29.2% after 14 weeks *2216*

Leukocytes *Blood Decrease Physiological* Administration of fluvastatin rarely causes a hypersensitivity reaction with leukocytopenia *5232*

Lipase *Serum Increase Physiological* Administration of statins rarely causes pancreatitis *5232*

Lipoprotein C-III:Lipoprotein B Ratio
Serum Decrease Physiological In 86 hypercholesterolemic patients treated with 10 mg/d for 6 weeks nonsignificant reduction from mean baseline of 20.5 ± 17 mg/dL to 19.0 ± 15 mg/dL observed. With 80 mg/d for 6 weeks significant reduction from 19.5 ± 15 mg/dL to 17.5 ± 13 mg/dL observed *1225*

Lipoprotein E:Lipoprotein B Ratio
Serum Decrease Physiological In 86 hypercholesterolemic patients treated with 10 mg/d for 6 weeks significant reduction from mean baseline of 44.0 ± 39 mg/dL to 33.0 ± 30 mg/dL observed *1225*
Serum No Effect Physiological In 86 hypercholesterolemic patients treated with 10 mg/d for 6 weeks nonsignificant reduction from mean baseline of 43.5 ± 38 mg/dL to 40.5 ± 41 mg/dL observed *1225*

Lipoprotein Lp(a) *Serum Decrease Physiological* In 83 hypercholesterolemic patients treated with 80 mg/d for 6 weeks nonsignificant change from mean baseline of 38.0 ± 34 mg/dL to 34.0 ± 32 mg/dL observed *1225*
Serum Increase Physiological Administration of fluvastatin to patients with hypercholesterolemia had no consistent effect on concentration *5232*
Serum No Effect Physiological In 24 patients with a history of angina pectoris (randomized from 27 men and 21 women) with mean age 59 years treatment with 40 mg/d fluvastatin caused no significant change from mean baseline of 57.3 ± 14.8 mg/dL to 56.2 ± 17.9 mg/dL after 20 weeks *537* In 80 hypercholesterolemic patients treated with 10 mg/d for 6 weeks nonsignificant change from mean baseline of 15.0 ± 33 mg/dL to 15.0 ± 32 mg/dL observed *1225*

Lithocholic Acid *Bile No Effect Physiological* In 19 patients with hypercholesterolemia types IIa or IIb treatment with 30 mg/d for 12 weeks caused caused nonsignificant change from mean baseline proportion of 1.53 ± 0.29% to 1.52 ± 0.42% *5972*

Low Density Lipoprotein Diameter
Serum No Effect Physiological In 46 men with LDL-cholesterol concentrations greater than 160 mg/dL treatment with 20 mg/d fluvastatin for 27 weeks caused mean decrease of 2.3 ± 5.1 angstroms versus decrease of 0.6 ± 6.2 angstroms in placebo-treated controls *5874*

Luteinizing Hormone *Plasma No Effect Physiological* Administration of fluvastatin caused a slight reduction in testosterone concentration without any change in luteinizing hormone concentration *5232*

Myoglobin *Urine Increase Physiological* Administration of fluvastatin rarely causes rhabdomyolysis with creatine kinase activity above 10 times the upper limit of normal with renal failure due to myoglobinuria *5232*

Nicotinic Acid *Serum No Effect Physiological* Administration of fluvastatin to patients with hypercholesterolemia together with niacin had no effect on the metabolism and excretion of nicotinic acid *5232*

Plasminogen Activator Inhibitor-1 Activity
Plasma Increase Physiological In 24 patients with a history of angina pectoris (randomized from 27 men and 21 women) with mean age 59 years treatment with 40 mg/d fluvastatin caused nonsignificant change from mean baseline of 3.1 AU/mL to 8.9 AU/mL after 20 weeks *537*

Plasminogen Activator Inhibitor-1 Antigen
Plasma Increase Physiological In 24 patients with a history of angina pectoris (randomized from 27 men and 21 women) with mean age 59 years treatment with 40 mg/d fluvastatin caused nonsignificant change from mean baseline of 17.9 ± 11.0 ng/mL to 26.0 ± 10.4 ng/mL after 20 weeks *537*

Platelets *Blood Decrease Physiological* Administration of fluvastatin rarely causes a hypersensitivity reaction with purpura and/on thrombocytopenia *5232*

Testosterone *Serum Decrease Physiological* Administration of fluvastatin caused a slight reduction in testosterone concentration without any change in luteinizing hormone concentration *5232*

Tissue Plasminogen Activator
Plasma Decrease Physiological In 24 patients with a history of angina pectoris (randomized from 27 men and 21 women) with mean age 59 years treatment with 40 mg/d fluvastatin caused significant change from mean baseline of 6.5 ± 2.0 ng/mL to 4.7 ± 2.1 ng/mL after 20 weeks *537*

Tolbutamide *Serum No Effect Physiological* In 16 healthy individuals coadministration of 40 mg fluvastatin in either single or multiple doses had no significant effect on maximum tolbutamide concentration *227*

Triglycerides *Serum Decrease Physiological* In 622 patients with heterozygous familial hypercholesterolemia treatment with 40 mg/d for 19.4 ± 15.5 weeks caused a significant change of - 7.7% from mean baseline in those with serum cholesterol concentrations greater than 240 mg/dL and - 6.8% in those with serum cholesterol less than 240 mg/dL *4630* Administration of fluvastatin to patients with hypercholesterolemia moderately reduced the serum triglycerides concentration *5232* In 24 patients with familial hypercholesterolemia treatment with up to 60 mg/d for 2 years caused significant decrease from mean baseline of 133 mg/dL to 108.8 mg/dL *3227* In 46 men with LDL-cholesterol concentrations greater than 160 mg/dL treatment with 20 mg/d fluvastatin for 27 weeks caused mean decrease of 2.5 ± 41.1 mg/dL versus increase of 11.1 ± 54.2 mg/dL in placebo-treated controls *5874* In 20 patients with type IIa hypercholesterolemia treatment with 40 mg/d for 4 weeks caused mean 30% decrease from mean baseline of 186 ± 119 mg/dL *4033* In 42 hypercholesterolemic patients receiving cyclosporine after renal transplantation treatment with 20 mg/d for 12 weeks caused significant reduction from mean baseline of 230 ± 37 mg/dL to 186 ± 27 mg/dL and to 177 ± 18 mg/dL at week 20 after 40 mg/d *2669* In 918 patients with primary hypercholesterolemia treatment with 20 mg/d fluvastatin caused significant reduction of 7.4% from mean baseline after 9 weeks treatment *6636* In 19 patients with hypercholesterolemia types IIa or IIb treatment with 30 mg/d for 4 weeks caused caused nonsignificant reduction from mean baseline of 145 mg/dL and a slight increase after treatment was stopped *5972* In 19 renal transplant recipients with hypercholesterolemia treatment with 20 mg/d caused mean nonsignificant decreases of about 3% after 6 weeks and 9% after 14 weeks from mean baseline of 250 ± 111 mg/dL *2216*
Serum Increase Physiological In 24 patients with a history of angina pectoris (randomized from 27 men and 21 women) with mean age 59 years treatment with 40 mg/d fluvastatin caused significant increase from mean baseline of 116.7 ± 42.0 mg/dL to 123.7 ± 64.7 mg/dL after 20 weeks *537*
Serum No Effect Physiological In 31 patients with primary hypercholesterolemia treatment with 40 mg/d caused nonsignificant change to 1.55 mmol/L (4%) from mean baseline of 1.68 ± 0.17 mmol/L *5614* In 4 heterogeneous patients with familial LDL-receptor defective hypercholesterolemia treatment with 40 mg/d for 12 weeks caused a nonsignificant change from mean baseline of 156 ± 52 mg/dL to 160 ± 45 mg/dL *2408* In 337 hypercholesterolemic patients treatment with up to 30 mg/d for 12 weeks caused nonsignificant 0.2% reduction from mean baseline of 165.9 ± 6.4 mg/dL *5982*

Ursodeoxycholic Acid *Bile No Effect Physiological* In 19 patients with hypercholesterolemia types IIa or IIb treatment with 30 mg/d for 12 weeks caused caused nonsignificant change from mean baseline proportion of 2.51 ± 0.97% to 3.03 ± 0.97% *5972*

Warfarin *Plasma No Effect Physiological* Concomitant administration of a single dose of 30 mg of warfarin with 40 mg/d fluvastatin for 8 days to young healthy males had no effect on racemic warfarin concentration *5232*

Fluvoxamine

Alanine Aminotransferase *Serum Increase Physiological* Fluvoxamine administration reported to cause increased activity frequently *5684* In 12 of 250 (4%) cases of overdose altered liver function observed *2558*

Alprazolam *Serum Increase Physiological* By inhibiting CYP 3A fluvoxamine may cause an approximate two-fold increase in alprazolam concentration, decreasing its plasma clearance by 49% and increasing its half-life by 71% *4685* Fluvoxamine increases concentration presumably by inhibiting metabolism of alprazolam by cytochrome P450IIIA4. When drugs coadministered AUC, maximum concentration and half-life of alprazolam approximately doubled *5684*

Aminophylline *Serum Increase Physiological* Fluvoxamine (50 mg b.i.d) coadministered with a single dose of 375 mg theophylline or 442 mg aminophylline in 12 healthy male volunteers increased concentration by reducing clearance by approximately 3-fold *5684*

Amitriptyline *Serum Increase Physiological* Fluvoxamine co-administration reported to increase significantly the concentration of amitriptyline *5684*

Aspartate Aminotransferase *Serum Increase Physiological* In 12 of 250 (4%) reported overdose cases abnormal liver function observed *2558* Fluvoxamine administration reported to cause increased activity frequently *5684*

Atenolol *Serum No Effect Physiological* Coadministration of fluvoxamine (100 mg/d) and atenolol (100 mg/d) in 6 healthy volunteers did not affect the plasma concentration of atenolol *5684*

Bilirubin *Serum Increase Physiological* Administration of fluvoxamine rarely associated with jaundice *5684*

Carbamazepine *Serum Increase Physiological* Fluvoxamine co-administration reported to increase significantly the concentration of carbamazepine *5684* Coadministration of fluvoxamine with carbamazepine increased concentration of carbamazepine and caused symptoms of toxicity *0*
Serum No Effect Physiological In 7 epileptic patients receiving chronic carbamazepine therapy treatment with 100 mg/d for 3 weeks had no significant effect on concentration (mean baseline 27.2 ± 4.8 µmol/L and 28.3 ± 4.0 µmol/L during treatment) *5749*

Carbamazepine-10,11-Epoxide
Serum No Effect Physiological In 7 epileptics receiving chronic carbamazepine treatment administration of 100 mg/d fluvoxamine for 3 weeks had no significant effect on plasma concentration (mean baseline 6.1 ± 2.4 µmol/L and 6.1 ± 2.3 µmol/L during treatment) *5749*

Cholesterol *Serum Increase Physiological* Fluvoxamine administration reported to cause hypercholesterolemia infrequently *5684* Administration of fluvoxamine infrequently associated with hypercholesterolemia *5684*

Clomipramine *Serum Increase Physiological* Coadministration of fluvoxamine with tricyclic antidepressants increased concentration of these *5684* Fluvoxamine co-administration reported to increase significantly the concentration of clomipramine *5684*

Clozapine *Serum Increase Physiological* In a female patient coadministration of fluvoxamine caused serum clozapine concentration to increase from 267 ng/mL to 2166 ng/mL after 4 days and 3151 ng/mL on day 8 *2593* Fluvoxamine administration reported to increase clozapine concentration *5684*

Clozapine N-Oxide *Serum Increase Physiological* In a female patient coadministration of fluvoxamine caused serum clozapine N-oxide concentration to decrease from 199 ng/mL to 70 ng/mL after 4 days and 151 ng/mL on day 8 *2593*

Desipramine *Serum No Effect Physiological* In 12 healthy volunteers given 100 mg/d for 10 days no significant observed on kinetics ofdesipramine after a single dose of 100 mg *5751*

Diazepam *Serum Increase Physiological* Fluvoxamine increases concentration presumably by inhibiting metabolism by cytochrome P450IIIA4 reducing clearance of diazepam (65%) and its major metabolite, N-desmethyldiazepam *5684*

Digoxin *Serum No Effect Physiological* Coadministration of fluvoxamine (100 mg/d for 18 days) with a single intravenous 1.25 mg dose of digoxin had no significant effect on the pharmacokinetics of digoxin *5684*

Diltiazem *Serum Increase Physiological* Coadministration of fluvoxamine (100 mg/d for 18 days) with diltiazem caused bradycardia, presumably because of an increased diltiazem concentration *5684*

Glucose *Serum Decrease Physiological* Fluvoxamine administration reported to cause hypoglycemia rarely *5684*
Serum Increase Physiological Administration of fluvoxamine rarely associated with hyperglycemia *5684*

Hematocrit *Blood Decrease Physiological* Fluvoxamine administration reported to cause anemia infrequently *5684*

Hemoglobin *Blood Decrease Physiological* Administration of fluvoxamine infrequently associated with anemia *5684*

Homovanillic Acid *Urine No Effect Physiological* In 15 depressed outpatients treatment with up to 223 ± 60 mg/d for 6 weeks caused nonsignificant reduction from mean baseline of 28.1 ± 7.1 µmol/d to 27.3 ± 7.1 µmol/d *2958*

4-Hydroxy-3-Methoxy-Phenylglycol
Urine Decrease Physiological In 15 depressed outpatients treatment with up to 223 ± 60 mg/d for 6 weeks caused non-significant decrease from mean baseline of 10.7 ± 3.0 µmol/d to 9.9 ± 3.0 µmol/d *2958*

Imipramine *Serum Increase Physiological* Coadministration of fluvoxamine with tricyclic antidepressants increased concentration of these *5684* Fluvoxamine co-administration reported to increase significantly the concentration of imipramine *5684* In 12 healthy controls given 100 mg/d fluvoxamine for 10 days imipramine half-life increased from 22.8 ± 6.4 h to 40.5 ± 5.0 h and decrease in apparent oral clearance from 1.02 ± 0.19 L/h/kg to 0.28 ± 0.06 L/h/kg *5751*

Lactate Dehydrogenase *Serum Increase Physiological* Fluvoxamine administration reported to cause increased activity rarely *5684* Administration of fluvoxamine rarely associated with increased enzyme activity *5684*

Leukocytes *Blood Decrease Physiological* Administration of fluvoxamine rarely associated with leukopenia *5684*
Blood Increase Physiological Administration of fluvoxamine infrequently associated with leukocytosis *5684*

Lipids *Serum Increase Physiological* Administration of fluvoxamine rarely associated with hyperlipidemia *5684*

Lorazepam *Serum No Effect Physiological* Because it is metabolized through glucuronidation lorazepam concentration unaffected unlike those drugs that are metabolized by cytochrome P450IIIA4 *5684*

Metanephrine *Urine Decrease Physiological* In 15 depressed outpatients treatment with up to 223 mg/d for 6 weeks caused nonsignificant reduction from mean baseline of 0.68 ± 0.38 µmol/d to 0.61 ± 0.29 µmol/d *2958*

Methadone *Serum Increase Physiological* Fluvoxamine co-administration reported to increase significantly the concentration of methadone *5684* Coadministration of fluvoxamine with methadone increased concentration of methadone with symptoms of opiod intoxication in one patient *5684*

Metoprolol *Serum Increase Physiological* Two cases of hypotension observed with coadministration of fluvoxamine and metoprolol presumably due to decreased metabolism of metoprolol *5684*

Midazolam *Serum Increase Physiological* Through probable inhibition of cytochrome P450IIIA4, fluvoxamine blocks the metabolism of midazolam leading to a higher plasma concentration *5684*

N-Desmethylclozapine *Serum Increase Physiological* In a female patient coadministration of fluvoxamine caused serum N-desmethylclozapine concentration to increase from 206 ng/mL to 615 ng/mL after 4 days and 855 ng/mL on day 8 *2593*

Fluvoxamine *(continued)*

N-Desmethyldiazepam *Serum Increase Physiological* Fluvoxamine reduces the clearance of both diazepam and N-desmethyldiazepam *5684*

Norepinephrine *Plasma No Effect Physiological* In 15 depressed outpatients treatment with up to 223 ± 14 mg/d for 6 weeks caused increase from mean baseline of 2.73 ± 1.42 pmol/mL to 1.94 ± 0.90 pmol/L, similar to change in placebo-treated group *2958*

Normetanephrine *Urine Decrease Physiological* In 15 depressed outpatients treatment with up to 223 ± 60 mg/d for 6 weeks caused nonsignificant reduction from mean baseline of 1.50 ± 0.56 μmol/d to 1.35 ± 0.66 μmol/d *2958*

Occult Blood *Feces Increase Physiological* Fluvoxamine administration reported to cause gastrointestinal hemorrhage infrequently with melena *5684*

Oxazepam *Serum No Effect Physiological* Because it is metabolized through glucuronidation oxazepam concentration unaffected unlike those drugs that are metabolized by cytochrome P450IIIA4 *5684*

Platelets *Blood Decrease Physiological* Fluvoxamine administration reported to cause thrombocytopenia infrequently and purpura rarely *5684*

Potassium *Serum Decrease Physiological* Administration of fluvoxamine rarely associated with hypokalemia *5684* Hypokalemia observed in 25 (8%) of overdose cases *2558*

Prolactin *Plasma Increase Physiological* In 8 healthy men mean concentration increased significantly from baseline of 8.4 ± 4.3 μg/L to 13.7 ± 9.9 μg/L after 4 weeks with increasing weekly doses of up to 200 mg/d *5746*

Propranolol *Serum Increase Physiological* Coadministration of fluvoxamine (100 mg/d) with propranolol (160 mg/d) caused a mean 5-fold increase in the minimum plasma concentration of propranolol in healthy volunteers *5684*

Prothrombin Time *Plasma Increase Physiological* Fluvoxamine (50 mg t.i.d) coadministered with warfarin for two weeks increased plasma concentration by 98% with increase of prothrombin times *5684*

Sodium *Serum Decrease Physiological* In 8 healthy men mean concentration decreased nonsignificantly from baseline of 141.5 ± 2.2 mmol/L to 140.1 ± 1.6 mmol/L after 4 weeks with increasing weekly doses of up to 200 mg/d *5746*

Temazepam *Serum No Effect Physiological* Because it is metabolized through glucuronidation temazepam concentration unaffected unlike those drugs that are metabolized by cytochrome P450IIIA4 *5684*

Theophylline *Serum Increase Physiological* Decreases theophylline clearance by inhibiting cytochrome P450 1A2 and increases serum theophylline concentration by 70% *3125* Up to 70% increase in serum theophylline concentration due to decreased theophylline clearance caused by inhibition of cytochrome P450 1A2 *6117* Decreases theophylline clearance by inhibiting cytochrome P450 1A2, increasing theophylline concentration by about 25% *5999* Fluvoxamine (50 mg b.i.d) coadministered with a single dose of 375 mg theophylline or 442 mg aminophylline in 12 healthy male volunteers increased concentration by reducing clearance by approximately 3-fold *5684*

Thyroxine (T4) *Serum Decrease Physiological* Administration of fluvoxamine infrequently associated with hypothyroidism and rarely associated with goiter *5684*

Triazolam *Serum Increase Physiological* Through probable inhibition of cytochrome P450IIIA4, fluvoxamine blocks the metabolism of triazolam leading to a higher plasma concentration *5684*

Tricyclic Antidepressants *Serum Increase Physiological* Interacts pharmacokinetically to inhibit demethylation of tricyclic antidepressants especially tertiary amines *3590*

Vanillylmandelic Acid *Urine Decrease Physiological* In 15 depressed outpatients treatment with up to 223 ± 60 mg/d for 6 weeks caused nonsignificant reduction from 19.7 ± 5.9 μmol/d to 18.3 ± 7.5 μmol/d *2958*

Warfarin *Plasma Increase Physiological* When fluvoxamine (50 mg t.i.d.) was administered concomitantly with warfarin for two weeks warfarin concentration increased by 98% with prolongation of prothrombin time *5684*

Folic Acid

Folate *Serum Increase Analytical* Increase by 20% if chloramphenicol method of O'Broin used *4352*
Serum Increase Physiological In a group of patients given 30 g cereal fortified with 127 μg folic acid folate concentration increasd by 30.8%, in those receiving cereal fortified with 499 or 665 μg of folic acid per 30 g of cereal increased homocysteine concentrations by 64.8% and 105.7% respectively *3753*

Homocysteine *Plasma Decrease Physiological* In 31 of 33 patients with AMI treatment with either 2.5 mg or 10 mg folic acid/d caused mean decrease of 4.4 μmol/L (27%) after 6 weeks *3393* In a group of patients given 30 g cereal fortified with 127 μg folic acid homocysteine concentration reduced by 3.7%, in those receiving cereal fortified with 499 or 665 μg of folic acid per 30 g of cereal reduced homocysteine concentrations by 11.0% and 14.0% respectively *3753*
Plasma Increase Physiological High doses of folate (5 mg daily) cause variable increases in patients with renal failure and in healthy individuals without overt deficiency *6123*

^{131}I Uptake *Serum Decrease Physiological* Filibon, Iberet® contain tetraiodofluorescein *4360*

Lymphocytes *Blood Decrease Physiological* Significant effect with megadose supplementation *2245*

Methotrexate *Serum No Effect Analytical* No significant interference observed at a concentration of 10 μmol/L with method on Du Pont aca *1535*

N-Acetyl-Glucosaminidase *Urine No Effect Analytical* At 50 mmol/L no effect on 2 colorimetric analytical methods *2254*

Neutrophils *Blood No Effect Physiological* No effect with megadose supplementation *2245*

Phenobarbital *Serum Decrease Physiological* Occurs with pharmacologic doses; lowers plasma concentration *5056*

Phenytoin *Serum Decrease Physiological* In 3 of 4 healthy individuals administration of folic acid caused significant decrease in serum phenytoin concentration probably due to enhanced metabolism *2182* Occurs with pharmacologic doses; lowers plasma concentration *5056* Possibly capable of decreasing concentration when drugs coadministered *1384* Increase by 8 to 48% in 4 male patients associated with increase in drug oxidative metabolism *499* If patients folate deficient, stimulate metabolism *2452*

Vitamin B_{12} *Red Blood Cells Increase Physiological* During treatment of folate deficient anemia *2482*

Follicle Stimulating Hormone, Recombinant

Androstenedione *Plasma No Effect Physiological* In 9 men with isolated gonadotropin deficiency or panhypopituitarism treatment with recombinant FSH up 225 IU/d for 21 days caused an insignificant change from mean baseline of 14 ng/dL to 12 ng/dL after 3 weeks *3769*

Estradiol *Plasma No Effect Physiological* In 9 men with isolated gonadotropin deficiency or panhypopituitarism treatment with recombinant FSH up 225 IU/d for 21 days caused an insignificant change from mean baseline of 14 pg/dL to 14 pg/dL after 3 weeks *3769*

Follicle Stimulating Hormone
Plasma Increase Physiological In 9 men with isolated gonadotropin deficiency or panhypopituitarism treatment with recombinant FSH up 225 IU/d for 21 days caused a significant increase from mean baseline of 0.5 mIU/mL to 13.6 mIU/mL after 3 weeks *3769*

Inhibin *Plasma Increase Physiological* In 9 men with isolated gonadotropin deficiency or panhypopituitarism treatment with recombinant FSH up 225 IU/d for 21 days caused a significant increase from mean baseline of 116 IU/L to 350 IU/L after 3 weeks *3769*

Luteinizing Hormone *Plasma No Effect Physiological* In 9 men with isolated gonadotropin deficiency or panhypopituitarism treatment with recombinant FSH up 225 IU/d for 21 days caused an insignificant change from mean baseline of 0.2 mIU/mL to 0.1 mIU/mL after 3 weeks *3769*

Testosterone *Serum Decrease Physiological* In 9 men with isolated gonadotropin deficiency or panhypopituitarism treatment with recombinant FSH up 225 IU/d for 21 days caused an significant change from mean baseline of 58 ng/dL to 17 ng/dL after 3 weeks *3769*

Food Ingestion

Homocysteine *Plasma No Effect Physiological* No influence of food intake observed in healthy adults *1838*

Formestane

Aldosterone *Plasma No Effect Physiological* In 43 postmenopausal women treated with up to 500 mg/d for 4 wk followed by 250 mg/d for 4 wk caused no consistent change in concentration *1487*

Cortisol *Plasma No Effect Physiological* In 43 postmenopausal women with breast cancer treatment with up to 500 mg/d for 4 wk followed by 250 mg/d for 4 wk caused no consistent change in concentration *1487*

Estradiol *Plasma Decrease Physiological* In 43 postmenopausal women with breast cancer treatment with up to 500 mg/d for 4 weeks followed by 250 mg/d for 4 weeks caused suppression of estradiol concentration *1487*

Estrone *Plasma Decrease Physiological* In 43 postmenopausal women with breast cancer treatment with up to 500 mg/d for 4 weeks followed by 250 mg/d for 4 weeks caused suppression of secretion *1487*

17-Hydroxyprogesterone *Plasma No Effect Physiological* In 43 postmenopausal women with breast cancer treatment with up to 500 mg/d for 4 wk followed by 250 mg/d for 4 wk caused no consistent change in concentration *1487*

Formoterol

Potassium *Serum Decrease Physiological* At inhaled doses of more than 36 µg decrease from mean concentration of 4.16 to 3.83 mmol/L *3735*

Foscarnet

Alanine Aminotransferase *Serum Increase Physiological* Increase in ALT or AST activity of more than fivefold observed in 1 of 24 patients with AIDS treated with intravenous drug for 10-42 days *5184* Increased enzyme activity observed in 1% to 5% treated patients *276*

Alkaline Phosphatase *Serum Increase Physiological* Greater than 2.6 fold increase observed in 2 of 24 patients with AIDS treated with drug intravenously daily for 10-42 days *5184* Increased enzyme activity observed in 1% to 5% treated patients *276*

Amylase *Serum Increase Physiological* Increased enzyme activity observed in less than 1% treated patients *276*

Aspartate Aminotransferase *Serum Increase Physiological* Greater than 5-fold increase of ALT or AST activity observed in 1 of 24 patients with AIDS treated with drug intravenously daily for 10-42 days *5184* Increased enzyme activity observed in 1% to 5% treated patients *276*

Calcium *Serum Decrease Physiological* Coadministration with intravenous pentamidine may cause hypocalcemia. Hypocalcemia, independent of other drugs, observed in 15 - 30% treated patients *276* Observed in 5 of 24 patients with AIDS treated with intravenous drug for 10-42 days *5184*
Serum No Effect Physiological In 2 patients with AIDS 2-hour infusion had no effect on concentration *1979* In 5 HIV positive patients daily infusion of 120 mg/kg body weight caused no significant change from mean baseline of 2.25 ± 0.25 mmol/L to 2.14 ± 0.25 mmol/L *5180*

Chloride *Serum Decrease Physiological* Hypochloremia observed in less than 1% treated patients *276*

Creatine Kinase *Serum Increase Physiological* Increased enzyme activity observed in less than 1% treated patients *276*

Creatinine *Serum Increase Physiological* Approximately 33% of 189 patients with AIDS and CMV retinitis who received foscarnet 60 mg/kg t.i.d. without adequate hydration developed significant impairment of renal function (serum creatinine ≥2.0 mg/dL) *276* Concentration increased above 1.1 times upper limit of normal in 3 of 24 AIDS patients treated with intravenous drug for 10-42 days *5184*

Creatinine Clearance *Urine Decrease Physiological* Decreased creatinine clearance observed in 27% of 189 patients with AIDS who received foscarnet *276*

Erythrocytes *Urine Increase Physiological* Hematuria and glomerulonephritis observed in less than 1% treated patients *276*

Ganciclovir *Serum No Effect Physiological* Coadministration has no effect on the pharmacokinetics of either drug *276*

Glucose *Serum Decrease Physiological* Observed in 1 of 24 patients with AIDS treated with intravenous drug for 10-42 days *5184*
Serum Increase Physiological Observed in 1 of 24 patients with AIDS treated with drug intravenously for 10-42 days *5184* Hyperglycemia observed in less than 1% treated patients *276*
Urine Increase Physiological Glycosuria observed in less than 1% treated patients *276*

Glucose Tolerance *Serum Decrease Physiological* Glucose tolerance impaired in less than 1% treated patients *276*

Granulocytes *Blood Decrease Physiological* Observed in less than 1% treated patients (1 in 189 patients) *276*

Hemoglobin *Blood Decrease Physiological* Anemia observed in more than 33% treated patients in controlled studies *276* Decreased below 79 g/L in 3 of 24 patients with AIDS treated with drug intravenously for 10-42 days *5184*
Urine Increase Physiological Hematuria and glomerulonephritis observed in less than 1% treated patients *276*

Ionized Calcium *Serum Decrease Physiological* In 5 HIV positive patients receiving a daily infusion of 120 mg/kg body weight mean concentration decreased from 1.25 ± 0.05 mmol/L to 0.98 ± 0.03 mmol/L at the end of an infusion *5180* Administration may cause decreased concentrations of ionized calcium *276* In 2 patients with AIDS 2-hour infusion caused acute reduction to below lower limit of normal and remained suppressed *1979* Administration of 120 mg/kg caused mean 0.25 mmol/L *2872*

Ionized Magnesium *Serum Decrease Physiological* In 5 HIV positive patients receiving daily infusions of 120 mg/kg body weight mean concentration decreased from 0.55 ± 0.05 mmol/L to 0.34 ± 0.05 mmol/L after an infusion *5180*

Lactate Dehydrogenase *Serum Increase Physiological* Increased enzyme activity observed in 1% to 5% treated patients *276*

Leukocytes *Blood Decrease Physiological* Leukopenia observed in more than 5% treated patients *276*

Magnesium *Serum Decrease Physiological* Hypomagnesemia observed in 15 - 30% treated patients *276*
Serum No Effect Physiological In 5 HIV positive patients daily infusion of 120 mg/kg body weight caused no significant change from mean baseline of 0.79 ± 0.07 mmol/L to 0.80 ± 0.07 mmol/L *5180*

Neutrophils *Blood Decrease Physiological* Decrease below 5000 /µL observed in 1 of 24 patients with AIDS treated with intravenous drug for 10-42 days *5184* Decrease below 5000/µL observed in 1 of 24 patients with AIDS treated with intravenous drug for 10-42 days *5184*

Occult Blood *Feces Increase Physiological* Melena observed in 1% to 5% treated patients *276*

Parathyroid Hormone *Plasma Increase Physiological* In 2 patients with AIDS 2-hour infusion of foscarnet caused 3-fold increase in PTH concentration and in spite of low ionized calcium concentration remained within normal range *1979* In 5 HIV positive patients daily infusion of 120 mg/kg caused significant increase from mean baseline of 29.4 ± 9.3 pg/mL to 54 ± 17 pg/mL *5180*

Phosphate *Serum Decrease Physiological* Hypophosphatemia observed in 8 - 26% treated patients *276* In 2 patients with AIDS 2-hour infusion caused small decrease *1979* Observed in 3 of 24 patients with AIDS treated with intravenous drug for 10-42 days *5184*
Serum Increase Physiological Observed in 6 of 24 patients with AIDS treated with intravenous drug for 10-42 days *5184* Hyperphosphatemia observed in 6% treated patients *276*

Potassium *Serum Decrease Physiological* Hypokalemia observed in 16 - 48% treated patients *276* Observed in 5 of 24 patients with AIDS treated with intravenous drug for 10-42 days *5184*

Protein *Serum Decrease Physiological* Hypoproteinemia observed in less than 1% treated patients *276*
Urine Increase Physiological Observed in 7 of 24 patients with AIDS treated with drug intravenously for 10-42 days *5184*

Foscarnet *(continued)*

Sodium *Serum Decrease Physiological* Observed in 4 of 24 patients with AIDS treated with intravenous drug for 10-42 days *5184*

Urea Nitrogen *Serum Increase Physiological* Increased concentration observed in 1% to 5% treated patients *276*

Volume *Blood Increase Physiological* Hypervolemia observed in less than 1% treated patients *276*

Fosfomycin

Ketone Body Ratio *Serum No Effect Analytical* When added at a concentration of 0.75 g/L had no significant effect on AKBR method of Uno et al *6131*

Fosinopril

Alanine Aminotransferase *Serum No Effect Physiological* In 8 patients with mild to moderate hypertension treatment with up to 10 mg/d for 8 weeks caused no significant effect on concentration *1919*

Albumin *Serum No Effect Physiological* In 15 patients with mild to moderate proteinuria treatment with 10 mg/d for 15 weeks caused nonsignificant mean reduction of 0.1 g/L from mean baseline of 37.1 ± 1.2 g/L *3092*

Urine Decrease Physiological In 13 hypertensives with mild to moderate renal impairment treatment for 12 weeks caused significant reduction from mean baseline of 3,800 mg/24 h to 2,750 mg/24 h *5346* In 17 patients with mild to moderate proteinuria treatment with 10 mg/d for 8 weeks caused significant mean reduction of 0.89 g/d from mean baseline of 3.69 ± 0.42 g/d *3092*

Aldosterone *Plasma Decrease Physiological* Significant decrease observed in 5 patients on chronic ambulatory peritoneal dialysis following single oral dose of 10 mg *2073* During first 8 hours after administration of single doses of 10 mg upwards significant decrease observed although it reverted to normal with almost all doses within 24 hours *1611*

Plasma Increase Physiological In 8 patients with mild to moderate hypertension treatment with up to 10 mg/d for 8 weeks caused nonsignificant increase from mean baseline of 259 ± 188 pmol/L to 286 ± 255 pmol/L *6030*

Plasma No Effect Physiological No effect observed in 11 moderately hypertensive men treated for 8 weeks with up to 40 mg/day *5861*

Angiotensin-converting Enzyme

Serum Decrease Physiological In 17 patients with mild to moderate proteinuria treatment with 10 mg/d for 8 weeks caused mean reduction of 4.6 µU/mL/min from mean baseline of 15.9 ± 1.5 µU/mL/min *3092* Activity significantly reduced (94% after 24 hours, and 71% after 48 hours) in 5 patients on chronic ambulatory peritoneal dialysis after oral administration of 10 mg *2073* In 13 hypertensives with mild to moderate renal impairment treatment for 12 weeks caused significant decrease from mean baseline of 15 µU/mL/min to 6 µU/mL/min *5346* Almost immediate complete inhibition observed in volunteers given either 40 mg or 80 mg b.i.d. but activity increased to 40% of baseline 36 hours after last dose and 82% after 60 hours after last dose *1611*

Apolipoprotein Lp(a) *Serum Decrease Physiological* In those proteinuric patients in whom treatment with fosinopril reduced protein excretion the serum lipoprotein Lp(a) concentration was also reduced *4235*

Aspartate Aminotransferase

Serum No Effect Physiological In 8 patients with mild to moderate hypertension treatment with up to 10 mg/d for 10 weeks caused no significant effect *1919*

Atrial Natriuretic Peptide *Plasma No Effect Physiological* In 8 patients with mild to moderate hypertension treatment with up to 10 mg/d for 8 weeks caused nonsignificant increase from mean baseline of 18 ± 22 pg/mL to 19 ± 24 pg/mL *1919*

Bilirubin *Serum No Effect Physiological* In 8 patients with mild to moderate hypertension treatment with up to 10 mg/d for 8 weeks had no significant effect on concentration *2907*

Cholesterol *Serum Decrease Physiological* In 13 patients with hypertension and mild to moderate renal impairment treatment with fosinopril for 12 weeks caused reduction from 255 mg/dL to 225 mg/dL *5346* In proteinuric patients treatment with fosinopril reduced both protein excretion and the increased serum cholesterol concentration *4235* In 15 patients with mild to moderate proteinuria treatment with 10 mg/d for 8 weeks caused a decrease from a mean of 6.39 mmol/L to 5.82 mmol/L *3092*

Serum Increase Physiological In 8 patients with mild to moderate hypertension treatment with up to 10 mg/d for 8 weeks caused nonsignificant increase to 5.91 ± 1.4 mmol/L from mean baseline of 5.51 ± 0.9 mmol/L *1919*

Creatinine *Serum No Effect Physiological* In 8 patients with mild to moderate hypertension treatment with up to 50 mg/d for 8 weeks caused nonsignificant change from mean baseline of 85.1 ± 14.4 µmol/L to 84.9 ± 12.6 µmol/L *1919*

Creatinine Clearance *Urine No Effect Physiological* In 17 patients with mild to moderate proteinuria treatment for 8 weeks with 10 mg/d caused nonsignificant increase of 0.04 mL/s from mean baseline of 0.92 ± 0.14 mL/s *3092*

Glucose *Serum Decrease Physiological* In 8 patients with mild to moderate hypertension treatment for 8 weeks with up to 10 mg/d caused significant increase from 5.4 ± 0.38 mmol/L to 5.1 ± 0.33 mmol/L *1919*

Hemoglobin *Blood No Effect Physiological* In 8 patients with mild to moderate hypertension treatment with up to 10 mg/d for 8 weeks caused insignificant change from mean baseline of 132 ± 12.8 g/L to 133 ± 9.90 g/L *1919*

LDL-Cholesterol *Serum Decrease Physiological* In 13 hypertensives with mild to moderate renal impairment treatment for 12 weeks caused significant reduction from mean baseline of 175 mg/dL to 150 mg/dL *5346*

Leukocytes *Blood No Effect Physiological* In 8 patients with mild to moderate hypertension treatment with up to 10 mg/d for 8 weeks caused no change from mean baseline of 4,900 ± 1,100 /µL *1919*

Lipoprotein Lp(a) *Serum Decrease Physiological* In 17 patients with mild to moderate renal impairment treatment with fosinopril for 12 weeks reduced mean concentration from about 4.5 mg/dL to 3.5 mg/dL *5346* In 17 patients with mild to moderate proteinuria treatment with 10 mg/d for 12 weeks caused reduction from mean baseline of 3.94 mg/dL to 3.33 mg/dL *3092* In 26 hypertensive patients with mild to moderate renal impairment treatment for 12 weeks caused significant reduction in concentration *4923*

Potassium *Serum Decrease Physiological* In 11 moderately hypertensive men treated for 8 weeks with up to 40 mg/day with reduction from mean of 4.25 mmol/L to 3.98 mmol/L in resting state *5861*

Serum No Effect Physiological In 8 patients with mild to moderate hypertension treatment with up to 10 mg/d for 8 weeks caused nonsignificant change from 4.1 ± 0.3 mmol/L to 4.2 ± 0.1 mmol/L *1919*

Protein *Urine Decrease Physiological* In 17 patients with mild to moderate renal impairment and proteinuria treatment with to 10 mg/d for 8 weeks caused significant decrease from 5.56 g/d to 4.28 g/d *3092* In 26 hypertensive patients with mild to moderate renal impairment treatment for 12 weeks caused significant reduction in excretion *5346*

Renin Activity *Plasma Increase Physiological* Significant increase observed in 5 patients on chronic ambulatory peritoneal dialysis following single oral dose of 10 mg *2073* In 11 moderately hypertensive men given up to 40 mg/day for 8 weeks with increase from mean of 0.99 ng/mL/h to 4.80 ng/mL/h in resting state *5861*

Plasma No Effect Physiological In 8 patients with mild to moderate hypertension treatment with up to 10 mg/d for 8 weeks caused nonsignificant increase from mean baseline of 1.77 ± 0.42 ng/mL to 1.87 ± 0.92 ng/mL *1919*

Sodium *Serum No Effect Physiological* In 8 patients with mild to moderate hypertension treatment with up to 10 mg/d for 8 weeks had no significant effect on concentration *1919*

Triglycerides *Serum Decrease Physiological* In 8 patients with mild to moderate hypertension treatment with up to 10 mg/d for 8 weeks caused nonsignificant reduction from mean baseline of 1.22 ± 0.57 mmol/L to 1.05 ± 0.37 mmol/L *1919*

Urea Nitrogen *Urine No Effect Physiological* In 17 patients with mild to moderate proteinuria treatment with 10 mg/d for 8 weeks caused insignificant increase of 20 mmol/d from mean baseline of 378 ± 36 mmol/d *3092*

Uric Acid *Serum No Effect Physiological* In 8 patients with mild to moderate hypertension treatment with up to 10 mg/d for 8 weeks caused no change from mean baseline of 250 ± 64 µmol/L *1919*

Fosphenytoin

Alanine Aminotransferase *Serum Increase Physiological* Fosphenytoin is infrequently associated with abnormal liver function tests *4519*

Alkaline Phosphatase *Serum Increase Physiological* Fosphenytoin is infrequently associated with abnormal liver function tests *4519*

Aspartate Aminotransferase *Serum Increase Physiological* Fosphenytoin is infrequently associated with abnormal liver function tests *4519*

Bilirubin *Serum Increase Physiological* Fosphenytoin is infrequently associated with abnormal liver function tests *4519*

Diazepam *Serum No Effect Physiological* Fosphenytoin had no effect on the protein binding or pharmacokinetics of diazepam when coadministered *4519*

Glucose *Serum Increase Physiological* Fosphenytoin is frequently associated with hyperglycemia *4519*

γ-Glutamyltransferase *Serum Increase Physiological* Fosphenytoin is infrequently associated with abnormal liver function tests *4519*

Hematocrit *Blood Decrease Physiological* Fosphenytoin is infrequently associated with hypochromic anemia *4519*

Hemoglobin *Blood Decrease Physiological* Fosphenytoin is infrequently associated with hypochromic anemia *4519*

Ketones *Serum Increase Physiological* Fosphenytoin is infrequently associated with ketosis *4519*
Urine Increase Physiological Fosphenytoin is infrequently associated with ketosis *4519*

Leukocytes *Blood Decrease Physiological* Fosphenytoin is infrequently associated with leukopenia *4519*
Blood Increase Physiological Fosphenytoin is infrequently associated with leukocytosis *4519*

Occult Blood *Feces Increase Physiological* Fosphenytoin is infrequently associated with gastrointestinal hemorrhage *4519*

pH *Blood Decrease Physiological* Fosphenytoin is infrequently associated with acidosis or alkalosis *4519*
Blood Increase Physiological Fosphenytoin is infrequently associated with acidosis or alkalosis *4519*

Phosphate *Serum Decrease Physiological* Fosphenytoin is frequently associated with hypophosphatemia *4519*

Platelets *Blood Decrease Physiological* Fosphenytoin is infrequently associated with thrombocytopenia *4519*

Potassium *Serum Decrease Physiological* Fosphenytoin is frequently associated with hypokalemia *4519*
Serum Increase Physiological Fosphenytoin is infrequently associated with hyperkalemia *4519*

Fotemustine

Effective Renal Plasma Flow
Patient No Effect Physiological No significant change from mean baseline of 418 mL/min in 7 patients with advanced malignancies after infusion of 100 mg/sq meter with decrease to 394 mL/min on one occasion and 392 mL/min on a second *1389*

Glomerular Filtration Rate *Urine No Effect Physiological* In 7 patients with advanced malignancies infusion of 100 ng/sq meter caused insignificant change from mean baseline of 108 mL/min to 117 mL/min on one occasion and to 124 mL/min on a second *1389*

β_2-Microglobulin *Urine No Effect Physiological* After infusion of 100 mg/sq meter in 7 patients with advanced malignancies on two occasions excretion showed slight reduction within normal range *1389*

N-Acetyl-Glucosaminidase *Urine No Effect Physiological* Insignificant increase from mean baseline excretion of 208 nmol/h to 220 nmol/h on one occasion after infusion of 100 mg/sq meter and to 240 nmol/h on a second in 7 patients with advanced malignancies *1389*

Fumagillin

Leukocytes *Blood Decrease Physiological* Leukopenia (AMA Blood dyscrasias) *4017*

Furadaltone

Bilirubin *Serum Increase Physiological* May cause hemolysis with G-6-PD deficiency *402*

Erythrocytes *Blood Decrease Physiological* May cause hemolysis with G-6-PD deficiency *402*

Haptoglobin *Serum Decrease Physiological* Due to hemolysis *402*

Heinz Body Formation *Blood Positive Physiological* Early stage of hemolytic anemia *536*

Hematocrit *Blood Decrease Physiological* May cause hemolysis with G-6-PD deficiency *402*

Hemoglobin *Blood Decrease Physiological* May cause hemolysis with G-6-PD deficiency *402*

Methemalbumin *Serum Increase Physiological* May occur with hemolysis *402*

Reticulocytes *Blood Increase Physiological* Occurs with hemolysis *402*

Furapromidium

Ammonia *Plasma Increase Physiological* Occasional increase observed *4014*

Furazolidone

Alanine Aminotransferase *Serum Increase Physiological* Frequency of hepatic dysfunction 0.01% reported in 10,443 patients *122*

Amphetamine *Serum Increase Physiological* A metabolite of furazolidone slows metabolism of amphetamines increasing their effect on the release of norepinehrine and other monoamines from adrenergic nerve endings *5641*

Aspartate Aminotransferase *Serum Increase Physiological* Frequency of hepatic dysfunction reported to be 0.01% in 10,443 treated patients *122*

Bilirubin *Serum Increase Physiological* May cause hemolysis with G-6-PD deficiency *402* Frequency of 0.05% reported in 10,443 treated patients *122*

Color *Urine Increase Analytical* Metabolites may produce brown color *2451*

Creatinine *Serum No Effect Analytical* No effect of concentrations up to 15 mg/L on single slide method on Kodak Ektachem® *5706*

Eosinophils *Blood Increase Physiological* Frequency of 0.06% reported in 10,443 treated patients *122*

Erythrocytes *Blood Decrease Physiological* May cause hemolysis with G-6-PD deficiency *402*

Glucose *Urine Increase Analytical* Due to presence of glucose in vaginal powder *2024*

Haptoglobin *Serum Decrease Physiological* Due to hemolysis *402*

Heinz Body Formation *Blood Positive Physiological* Early stage of hemolytic anemia *536*

Hematocrit *Blood Decrease Physiological* May cause hemolysis with G-6-PD deficiency *402*

Hemoglobin *Blood Decrease Physiological* Frequency of 0.09% reported in 10,443 treated patients *122* May cause hemolysis with G-6-PD deficiency *402*

Leukocytes *Blood Decrease Physiological* Frequency of 0.15% reported in 10,443 treated patients *122*
Blood Increase Physiological Frequency of 0.01% reported in 10,443 treated patients *122*

Methemalbumin *Serum Increase Physiological* May occur with hemolysis *402*

Methemoglobin *Blood Increase Physiological* May cause hemolysis with G-6-PD deficiency *6015*

Reticulocytes *Blood Increase Physiological* Occurs with hemolysis *402*

Furazolidone *(continued)*

Sugar *Urine Increase Analytical* Metabolites may give false positive with Benedict's reagent *2451*

Furazolium

Color *Urine Increase Analytical* Red, pink, purple, orange and rust colors *2024*

Furosemide

Adenosine Monophosphate
Plasma No Effect Physiological In 8 normal subjects associated with secondary hyperparathyroidism *1989*
Urine Increase Physiological In 8 normal subjects associated with secondary hyperparathyroidism *1989*

Alanine Aminotransferase *Serum Increase Physiological* Effect observed in 7 patients with systematic decrease in systolic blood pressure for less than 6 hours following short parenteral infusion *3399*
Serum No Effect Analytical No effect at therapeutic concentration on Boehringer Mannheim Reflotron method *3231* No effect at 1750 mg/L on Boehringer Mannheim Reflotron method *5706*

Albumin *Serum Increase Physiological* In 14 healthy young men ingestion of 40 mg caused significant 14.0 ± 3.6% increase in albumin concentration 3 hours later *866*
Serum No Effect Analytical No effect at 1.4 mg/dL on Technicon SMA 12/60 method *4390* At concentration of 4 mg/L had no effect on BCG method *5704*
Urine Decrease Physiological In 6 Albustix negative diabetics addition of furosemide to therapeutic regime caused reduction of daytime albumin excretion from 12.38 µg/min to 7.22 ± 6.44 µg/min and nighttime excretion from 4.50 ± 1.12 µg/min to 3.82 ± 1.69 µg/min *1128*
Urine No Effect Physiological In 10 healthy men ingestion of 40 mg had no significant effect on excretion *2890*

Aldosterone *Plasma Decrease Physiological* May be marked reduction in patients with congestive cardiac failure when given drug i.v. if initial concentration high, otherwise usually slight increase *4158*
Plasma Increase Physiological Slower response than angiotensin to i.v. injection *3892*
Urine Increase Physiological Significant increase in 6 volunteers given 80 mg/day for 3 days *1813* Effect observed after 40 mg orally in normal male volunteers *4373*

Alkaline Phosphatase *Serum No Effect Analytical* No effect at 1.4 mg/dL on Technicon SMA 12/60 method *4390*
Serum No Effect Physiological No effect observed despite effect on other enzymes following short parenteral infusion which was associated with decrease in systolic blood pressure for less than 6 hours *3399*

Ammonia *Plasma Increase Physiological* Acts like thiazides causes hypokalemia and alkalosis *2451*

Amylase *Serum Increase Physiological* Isolated case of acute hemorrhagic pancreatitis *2973* Not significant increase in total amylase in 12 hypertensives Increase by 16% on average in 12 hypertensives *3290* May induce mild pancreatitis *5869*
Serum No Effect Analytical At a concentration of 1,750 mg/L had no effect on method on Boehringer Mannheim Reflotron system *5706*

Amylase, Pancreatic Isoenzyme
Serum Increase Physiological Increase by 17% on average in 12 hypertensives *3290*
Serum No Effect Analytical No significant effect at toxic concentration of 100 mg/L on method on Boehringer Mannheim Reflotron *3647*

Angiotensin-II *Plasma Increase Physiological* Rapid response to i.v. injection *1633*

Antidiuretic Hormone *Plasma Increase Physiological* Effect observed after 40 mg orally in normal male volunteers *4373*
Urine No Effect Physiological No significant effect observed in 6 volunteers given 80 mg/day for 3 days *1813*

Apolipoprotein A *Serum Increase Physiological* In 14 healthy young men ingestion of 40 mg furosemide caused 9.6 ± 4.1% increase in apolipoprotein A concentration 3 hours later *866*

Apolipoprotein A-I *Serum No Effect Analytical* At a concentration of 60 µmol/L no significant effect observed on automated immunoturbidimetric method on Baxter Paramax analyzer *3005*
Serum No Effect Physiological Decrease by -2 mg/dL in 12 patients given 40 to 80 mg daily for 3 mo *4213*

Apolipoprotein B *Serum Increase Physiological* In 14 healthy young men ingestion of 40 mg caused significant 12.3 ± 5.8% increase 3 hours later *866*
Serum No Effect Analytical At a concentration of 60 µmol/L no significant effect observed on automated immunoturbidimetric method on Baxter Paramax analyzer *3005*
Serum No Effect Physiological Increase by 2 mg/dL in 12 patients given 40 to 80 mg daily for 3 mo *4213*

Apolipoprotein C-II *Serum No Effect Physiological* Increase by 1 mg/dL in 12 patients given 40 to 80 mg daily for 3 mo *4213*

Apolipoprotein C-III *Serum No Effect Physiological* Increase of 4 mg/dL in 12 patients given 40 to 80 mg daily for 3 mo *4213*

Aspartate Aminotransferase *Serum Increase Physiological* Effect observed in 7 patients following short parenteral infusion with systematic drop in systolic blood pressure for less than 6 hours *3399*
Serum No Effect Analytical No effect at therapeutic concentration on Boehringer Mannheim Reflotron method *3231* No effect at 1.4 mg/dL on Technicon SMA 12/60 method *4390* No effect at 1750 mg/L on Boehringer Mannheim Reflotron method *5706*

Atenolol *Serum No Effect Physiological* Concomitant administration had no effect on renal clearance of atenolol *3152*

Benazepril *Serum No Effect Physiological* No clinically important pharmacokinetic interactions observed when drugs coadministered *1033*

Bicarbonate *Serum Increase Physiological* In 24% in 204 hospitalized patients receiving the drug *5752*
Serum No Effect Analytical At concentration of 4 mg/L had no effect on method using phenolphthalein *5704*

Bilirubin *Serum Increase Physiological* Mild increase observed in 7 patients who had decrease of systolic blood pressure for less than 6 hours following short parenteral infusion *3399*
Serum No Effect Analytical At concentration of 1750 mg/L had no effect on method on Boehringer Mannheim Reflotron system *5706* No effect at 20 mg/L on Ames Seralyzer method *5706* At concentration of 4 mg/L had no effect on Jendrassik and Grof method *5704* No effect at 1.4 mg/dL on Technicon SMA 12/60 method *4390*
Serum No Effect Physiological Although *in vitro* effect observed at pharmacological concentrations no significant effect *6314*

Calcium *Lymphocytes No Effect Physiological* No significant effect in lymphocyte calcium in 9 patients with congestive cardiac failure treated with drug alone for at least 6 months, and in 12 others treated with drug with Slow K for same time *37*
Red Blood Cells No Effect Physiological No significant effect in 9 patients with congestive cardiac failure treated with drug alone for at least 6 months and in 12 others given drug with Slow K for same time *37*
Serum Decrease Physiological Diuretic action (different effect hydrochlorothiazide) *718* If increase due to dihyrotachysterol, also if normal *4907* Hypocalcemia may occur with treatmen *2647*
Serum No Effect Analytical At concentration of 4 mg/L had no effect on cresolphthalein method *5704* No effect at 1.4 mg/dL on Technicon SMA 12/60 method *4390*
Serum No Effect Physiological No effect observed in 9 patients with congestive cardiac failure given drug alone for at least 6 months and 12 given drug with Slow K for the same time *37* In 8 normal subjects associated with secondary hyperparathyroidism *1989*
Urine Increase Physiological In 7 healthy individuals treatment with a single dose of 80 mg caused increase in mean calcium/creatinine ratio from 0.20 to 0.46 due to increased

excretion of calcium *4900* In 8 normal subjects associated with secondary hyperparathyroidism *1989* Impaired reabsorption (initial effect only) *4555* Slight increase with administration *3343*

Casts *Urine Increase Physiological* Hyaline casts without proteinuria (orosomucoid) *2814*

Catecholamines *Plasma No Effect Analytical* No effect on HPLC method of Koller for dopamine, epinephrine, and norepinephrine *3230*
Plasma No Effect Physiological In 7 healthy individuals treated with a single oral dose of 80 mg had no significant effect on concentration *4900*

Cephaloridine *Serum Increase Physiological* Increased plasma concentration (by 100% in first hour) in healthy volunteers due to reduced renal clearance *6037*

Chloride *Serum Decrease Physiological* Reduced often in association with hyponatremia *2311* In 36% of 204 hospitalized patients receiving the drug *5752* Diuretic action (inhibits tubular reabsorption) *129* Hypochloremic alkalosis may occur *2647* Observed after drug administration *3343*
Serum No Effect Analytical At concentration of 4 mg/L had no effect on mercurimetric method *5704*
Urine Increase Physiological Marked effect: decreased sharply when administration stopped *3343* Diuretic action *2647*

Cholesterol *Serum Increase Physiological* In 14 healthy young men ingestion of 40 mg furosemide caused 10.9 ± 5.1% increase in cholesterol concentration after 3 hours *866* 5% change in 12 normotensive men when treated with drug alone for less than 1 y *2981* 6% change in 16 subjects treated for less than 1 y with drug only *2190*
Serum No Effect Analytical No effect at 1.4 mg/dL on Technicon SMA 12/60 method *4390* No effect at therapeutic concentration on Boehringer Mannheim Reflotron method *3231* At concentration of 60 mg/L had no effect on method using catalase-Hantzsch reaction *5704* No effect at 20 mg/L on Ames Seralyzer method *5706* At concentration of 60 mg/L had no effect on catalase-AIDH method *5704* At concentration of 60 mg/L had no effect on Liebermann-Burchard method *5704* At concentration of 60 mg/L had no effect on CHOD-Iodide method *5704* At concentration of 1750 mg/L no effect on method on Boehringer Mannheim Reflotron system *5706* At concentration of 60 mg/L had no effect on CHOD-PAP method *5704*
Serum No Effect Physiological Increase by 2 mg/dL in 12 patients given 40 to 80 mg daily for 3 mo *4213*

Cholinesterase *Serum No Effect Analytical* No effect observed at concentration of 2 mg/dL with butyrylthiocholine method on Kodak Ektachem® *2504*

Cortisol *Plasma Increase Analytical* At a concentration of 100 mg/L had a recovery of 118.1% with female serum with Enzymun method. At therapeutic concentration in plasma of 10 mg/L caused 113.6% recovery with Enzymun method *1097*
Plasma No Effect Analytical At concentration of 100 mg/L no significant effect on CEDIA method (worst case 102.2% recovery): no significant effect with male serum with Enzymun method in which case recovery 102.9% *1097*

Cortisol, Free *Urine No Effect Analytical* No significant interference observed with HPLC method of Turpeinen et al *6105*

Creatine Kinase *Serum No Effect Analytical* No effect at 20 mg/L on method on Ames Seralyzer *5706*

Creatine Kinase Isoenzymes *Serum No Effect Analytical* No interference observed at a concentration of 15 mg/L (45.3 µmol/L) with CK-MB method on Du Pont aca *1519*

Creatinine *Serum Increase Physiological* Treatment of 8 healthy male volunteers with 80 mg/d for 8 days caused mean increase from baseline of 73.6 mmol/L to 98.8 mmol/L *5469*
Serum No Effect Analytical At concentration of 30 mg/L had no effect on kinetic Jaffe method on BKA-2 *5704* At concentration of 20 mg/L had no effect on Jaffe-Fading-Fraction method *5704* No effect at 20 mg/L on Ames Seralyzer method *5706* At concentration of 20 mg/L had no effect on Jaffe-Fuller's earth method *5704* No interference observed with liquid chromatographic method of Paroni *4540* At concentration of 4 mg/L had no effect on Technicon AutoAnalyzer® Jaffe method *5704* At concentration of 5 mg/L had no effect on creatinine iminohydrolase method *5704* No effect at 1.4 mg/dL on Technicon SMA 12/60 method *4390*
Serum No Effect Physiological Ingestion of 40 mg orally by 10 healthy men had no effect on concentration *2890* In 8 normal subjects associated with secondary hyperparathyroidism *1989*
Urine No Effect Physiological No clear pattern observed with drug administration *3343*

Creatinine Clearance *Urine Decrease Physiological* In 8 healthy male volunteers 8 days treatment with 80 mg/d caused mean 21% decrease *5469*
Urine Increase Physiological In 10 healthy men after ingestion of 40 mg orally mean clearance increased from 123 ± 19 mL/min to 133 ± 28 mL/min over next 4 hours *2890* If given intravenously especially *4707*
Urine No Effect Physiological No significant effect observed in 6 volunteers given 80 mg/day for 3 days *1813*

Cyclosporine *Blood No Effect Analytical* At a concentration of 20 mg/L had no effect on Syva EMIT method *495*

Digoxin *Serum No Effect Analytical* Furosemide had no detectable cross-reactivity with method on Bayer Technicon Immuno 1® *421*
Serum No Effect Physiological No effect observed on renal clearance in 27 healthy volunteers *6037*

1,25-Dihydroxy Vitamin D *Serum No Effect Physiological* In 7 healthy individuals treatment with a single oral dose of 80 mg had no significant effect on plasma concentration *4900*

Dopamine *Urine Increase Physiological* Significant effect in 15 minutes following 30 mg intravenously *2918*

Epinephrine *Plasma No Effect Physiological* Effect observed after 40 mg orally in normal male volunteers *4373*

Erythrocytes *Blood Decrease Physiological* May cause anemia *2647*

Erythropoietin *Serum Decrease Physiological* In 6 patients with chronic renal failure administration of 500 mg caused significant change from mean baseline of 51.6 ± 11.6 mU/mL to 31.4 ± 4.3 mU/mL after 6 h and 26.8 ± 6.0 mU/mL after 24 h *6134*

Gentamicin *Serum Increase Physiological* Clearance reduced with increase in plasma concentration of 70% in one hour in healthy volunteers *6037*

Glomerular Filtration Rate *Urine Decrease Physiological* Excessive diuresis may cause effect *4014*

Glucose *Serum Decrease Physiological* Incidence of 0.8% observed in French Pharmacovigilance database *4106*
Serum Increase Physiological Diabetogenic-like action of drug affects glucose tolerance test *5869* In 6% in 204 hospitalized patients receiving the drug *5752* Hyperglycemia and alterations in glucose tolerance may occur with treatment *2647*
Serum No Effect Analytical At concentration of 1750 mg/L no effect on method on Boehringer Mannheim Reflotron system *5706* At concentration of 5 mg/L had no effect on GOD/POD-PAP method *5704* At concentration of 40 mg/L had no effect on Kodak Ektachem® method *5704* At concentration of 100 mg/L had no effect on hexokinase/G-6-PDH method *5704* No effect at 1.4 mg/dL on Technicon SMA 12/60 method *4390* No effect at 20 mg/L on glucose oxidase method on Ames Seralyzer *5706* No effect at therapeutic concentration on Boehringer Mannheim Reflotron method *3231*
Urine Decrease Analytical Lowered result with Clinistix® , Diastix® *1826*
Urine Increase Physiological Observed in 0.2% of 2580 medical inpatients *3666* Hyperglycemia and glycosuria and alterations in glucose tolerance may occur with treatment *2647* Diabetogenic-like action of drug *5869*
Urine No Effect Analytical No effect observed with Tes-Tape® *1826*

Glucose Tolerance *Serum Decrease Physiological* Diabetogenic-like action of drug *4555* Hyperglycemia and alterations in glucose tolerance may occur with treatment *2647*

γ-Glutamyltransferase *Serum No Effect Analytical* No effect at therapeutic concentration on Boehringer Mannheim Reflotron method *3231* At concentration of 1750 mg/L no effect on method on Boehringer Mannheim Reflotron system *5706*
Serum No Effect Physiological No effect observed in 7 patients who had decrease in systolic blood pressure for less than 6 hours following short parenteral infusion *3399*

Granulocytes *Blood No Effect Physiological* No significant association between ingestion and agranulocytosis *3098*

Furosemide (continued)

HDL-Cholesterol *Serum Increase Physiological* In 14 healthy young men ingestion of 40 mg furosemide caused significant 12.7 ± 5.2% increase after 3 hours *866*
Serum No Effect Analytical At a concentration up to 1750 mg/L had no significant effect on Reflotron method for whole blood cholesterol *6352*
Serum No Effect Physiological Reduced by -4 mg/dL in 12 patients given 40 to 80 mg daily for 3 mo *4213* Not significant change in 12 normotensive men when treated with drug alone for less than 1 y *2981* No significant change in 16 subjects treated for less than 1 y with drug only *2190*

Hematocrit *Blood Decrease Physiological* Risk of aplastic anemia increased to 1.7 per million (3-fold increase) *3098* May cause anemia *2647*

Hemoglobin *Blood Decrease Physiological* In 14 healthy young men ingestion of 40 mg caused significant 6.3 ± 2.4% increase in blood hemoglobin concentration 3 hours later *866* May cause anemia *2647* Risk of aplastic anemia increased to 1.7 per million (3-fold increase) *3098*

Histamine *Plasma No Effect Analytical* Improbable inhibition of radio-enzyme assay at therapeutic concentrations *2492*

Indomethacin *Serum No Effect Analytical* No effect on HPLC method of Roberts and Smith *4978*

Insulin *Plasma Decrease Physiological* Intravenous injection effect, little effect on blood sugar *4014*

Inulin Clearance *Urine Decrease Physiological* In one study clearance observed to be reduced in 20 of 27 healthy volunteers *6037*

Ionized Calcium *Serum No Effect Physiological* In 7 healthy individuals treatment with a single oral dose of 80 mg had no effect on plasma concentration *4900* In 8 normal subjects associated with secondary hyperparathyroidism *1989*

6-Keto-Prostaglandin $F_{1\alpha}$ *Urine No Effect Physiological* No significant difference between older and younger individuals in response to intravenous infusion of 0.5 mg/kg *6496*

Lactate *Plasma No Effect Analytical* At concentration of 100 mg/L had no effect on enzymatic method *5704*

Lactate Dehydrogenase *Serum Increase Physiological* Effect observed in 7 patients with systematic decrease in systolic blood pressure for less than 6 hours following short parenteral infusion *3399*
Serum No Effect Analytical No effect at 1.4 mg/dL on Technicon SMA 12/60 method *4390* No effect at 20 mg/L on method on Ames Seralyzer *5706*

LDL-Cholesterol *Serum Increase Physiological* In 14 healthy young men ingestion of 40 mg furosemide caused significant 10.4 ± 6.8% increase 3 hours later *866* 15% change in 16 subjects treated for less than 1 y with drug only *2190*
Serum No Effect Physiological Not significant change in 12 normotensive men when treated with drugs alone for less than 1 y *2981*

Leukocytes *Blood Decrease Physiological* Frequency of aplastic anemia observed to be about 1.7 per million (risk of aplastic anemia increased 3-fold) *3098* May cause leukopenia or aplastic anemia *3810*

Lidocaine *Serum No Effect Analytical* At a concentration of 1250 mg/L (normal therapeutic concentration up to 50 mg/L) had less than 10% effect on method on Baxter Stratus *5705* No significant interference observed at a concentration of 100 µg/mL (302 µmol/L) with method on Du Pont aca *1534*

Lipase *Serum Increase Physiological* Isolated case of acute hemorrhagic pancreatitis *2973*
Serum No Effect Analytical No effect of concentrations up to 16 mg/L on method on Kodak Ektachem® *5706*

Lithium *Serum Increase Physiological* In patients receiving lithium diuretics may reduce lithium clearance increasing the risk of lithium toxicity *2647*
Serum No Effect Physiological No effect observed in normal volunteers given drug over 2 weeks (40 mg/d) *2916*

Lithium Clearance *Urine Decrease Physiological* In patients receiving lithium diuretics may reduce lithium clearance increasing the risk of lithium toxicity *2647*
Urine No Effect Physiological A single dose of the drug has no effect on lithium clearance *4399* Nonsignificant decrease from mean baseline of 29.8 mL/min to 28.4 mL/min in 8 healthy volunteers given 80 mg/d furosemide for 8 days and single dose of 24 mmol lithium *5469*

Lymphocytes *Blood Decrease Physiological* Significantly reduced concentration in congestive heart failure patients treated with drug *5169*

Magnesium *Lymphocytes Decrease Physiological* Significantly reduced concentration in congestive heart failure patients treated with drug *5169*
Red Blood Cells No Effect Physiological No significant effect in 9 patients with congestive cardiac failure treated with drug for at least 6 months and in 12 others given drug with Slow K for same time *37*
Serum Decrease Physiological Hypomagnesemia may occur with treatment *2647* Observed in several patients on long term therapy or with short term vigorous treatment *5490*
Serum No Effect Physiological In 7 healthy individuals treatment with a single oral dose of 80 mg caused no significant effect on concentration *4900* No effect observed in 9 patients with congestive cardiac failure treated for at least 6 months with drug alone and 12 treated with drug plus Slow K for 6 months *37*
Urine Increase Physiological Renal wasting of magnesium reported with loop-blocking diuretics *5169* Diuretic action on divalent cations *6309*

Metformin *Serum Increase Physiological* In a single dose study during which furosemide and metformin were coadministered furosemide increased the maximum concentration and AUC of metformin by 22% and 15% respectively *726*

β_2-Microglobulin *Serum No Effect Physiological* In 10 healthy men ingestion of 40 mg had no significant effect on concentration *2890*
Urine Increase Physiological In 10 healthy men ingestion of 40 mg caused increase from mean baseline of 133 ± 34 µg/d to 289 ± 97 µg/d over next 4 hours *2890*

N-Acetyl-Glucosaminidase *Urine Increase Physiological* In 10 healthy men ingestion of 40 mg caused significant increase from mean baseline of 2.4 ± 0.8 nmol/h/µmol creatinine to 3.4 ± 0.9 nmol/h/µmol creatinine over next 4 hours *2890* In 10 healthy men after ingestion of 40 mg mean excretion increased from mean baseline of 0.20 ± 0.04 U/mmol creatinine to 0.42 ± 0.21 U/mmol creatinine over next 4 hours *2890* Excretion increased by drug induced diuresis *2458*

N-Acetylprocainamide *Serum No Effect Analytical* No significant interference at a concentration of 100 µg/mL (302 µmol/L) with method on Du Pont aca *1536*

Neutrophils *Blood Decrease Physiological* Reported to cause neutropenia *4265*

Nicardipine *Serum No Effect Physiological* Had no effect on plasma protein binding in vitro and presumed to have no effect on nicardipine concentration in vivo *5016*

Norepinephrine *Plasma Increase Physiological* Effect observed after 40 mg orally in normal male volunteers *4373*
Urine Increase Physiological Effect observed after 40 mg orally in normal male volunteers *4373*

Osmolality *Urine Increase Physiological* In 10 healthy men administration of 40 mg orally caused significant increase in excretion from 2.6 ± 0.4 mL/min to 7.1 ± 1.4 mL/min over next 4 hours *2890*

p-Aminophenol *Urine No Effect Analytical* With addition of drugs at a concentration of 100 mg/L and of related compounds at 50 mg/L no significant effect observed on colorimetric method of van Bocxlaer on Cobas Mira analyzer which involves reacting free p-aminophenol with resorcinol in the presence of magnesium ions to form an indophenol dye measured at 550 nm *6163*

Parathyroid Hormone *Plasma Increase Physiological* In patients with chronic renal failure rate of increase with progression of renal failure greater in patients receiving furosemide than in others. In 7 normal individuals given 80 mg concentration higher 3 hours after drug than on a control day (3.9 pmol/L versus 1.8 pmol/L) and 6 hours after drug (4.0 pmol/L versus 2.6 pmol/L) *4900* Small but significant increase in 5 patients with primary hyperparathyroidism treated with 40 mg daily for up to 29 weeks *4640* 10% increase in normal individuals after 8 d administration *1989*

pH *Blood Increase Physiological* Hypochloremic alkalosis may occur with treatment *2647*

Phenprocoumon *Plasma No Effect Physiological* In 17 healthy volunteers 40 mg b.i.d. for 7 days did not interact with phenprocoumon to a significant extent *4095*

Phosphate *Serum Increase Physiological* Temporary increase when fluid losses continuously replaced *4907*
Serum No Effect Analytical At concentration of 4 mg/L had no effect on phosphomolybdate method *5704* No effect at 1.4 mg/dL on Technicon SMA 12/60 method *4390*
Urine Increase Physiological Slight increase with administration *3343*

Platelet Aggregation *Blood Decrease Physiological* Inhibits primary ADP-induced agglutination. Effect seen *in vitro* but not *in vivo5111*

Platelets *Blood Decrease Physiological* Observed in 0.2% of 2580 medical inpatients *3666* Risk of aplastic anemia about 1.7 per million (3-fold increase in risk) *3098* May be associated with purpura *2647*

Potassium *Red Blood Cells No Effect Physiological* No significant effect in 9 patients with congestive cardiac failure treated with drug alone for at least 6 months and in 12 others given drug with Slow K for same time *37*
Serum Decrease Physiological Slight decrease with 80 mg/day for 3 days in 6 volunteers *1813* 12% patients with hypokalemia given 40-80 mg/d over long term *506* In 25% of 204 hospitalized patients receiving the drug *5752* Diuretic action *5869* Observed after drug administration *3343* In 8 healthy male volunteers treatment with 80 mg/d for 8 days caused mean decrease of 0.58 mmol/L *5469* Clinically important in about 3.6% patients *2311* In 12% patients with hypokalemia given 40-80 mg/d over long term *506*
Serum Increase Physiological Diuretic action: hypokalemia occurs especially with brisk diuresis, inadequate electrolyte intake, when cirrhosis is present, or during concomitant use of corticosteroids or ACTH *2647*
Serum No Effect Analytical At concentration of 4 mg/L had no effect on flame-photometric method *5704* At concentration of 6,000 mg/L had no effect on measurement by ISE with predilution *5704* At concentration of 400 mg/L had no effect on measurement by ISE without predilution *5704*
Serum No Effect Physiological No effect observed in 9 patients with congestive cardiac failure treated for at least 6 months: also no effect observed in 12 patients treated for at least 6 months with furosemide and Slow K *37*
Urine Increase Physiological Slight increase with administration *3343* Diuretic action: hypokalemia occurs especially with brisk diuresis, inadequate electrolyte intake, when cirrhosis is present, or during concomitant use of corticosteroids or ACTH *2647* Significant increase from mean baseline of 74 mmol/d to 103 mmol/d in 8 healthy male volunteers given 80 mg/d for 8 days *5469*
White Blood Cells Decrease Physiological Significant reduction in lymphocyte potassium in 9 patients with congestive cardiac failure treated with drug alone for at least 6 months, and in 12 others given drug with Slow K *37*

Practolol *Serum Increase Physiological* One study showed that renal clearance of practolol reduced by furosemide *6037*

Procainamide *Serum No Effect Analytical* No significant interference observed at a concentration of 100 µg/mL (302 µmol/L) with method on Du Pont aca *1542*

Prolactin *Plasma Increase Physiological* Effect observed after 40 mg orally in normal male volunteers *4373*

Propranolol *Serum Increase Physiological* Although mechanism not established, coadministration of 25 mg furosemide with 40 mg propranolol in 10 volunteers caused substantial increase in propranolol concentration *991*

Prostaglandin $F_{2\alpha}$ *Urine No Effect Physiological* No significant effect observed in 6 volunteers given 80 mg daily for 3 days *1813*

Prostaglandins *Urine No Effect Physiological* No effect observed in 6 volunteers given 80 mg daily for 3 days *1813*

Protein *Serum Increase Physiological* In 14 healthy young men ingestion of 40 mg caused significant 11.4 ± 4.1% increase in total protein concentration 3 hours later *866*
Serum No Effect Analytical At concentration of 4 mg/L had no effect on biuret method with blank correction *5704* No effect at 1.4 mg/dL on Technicon SMA 12/60 method *4390*
Urine Increase Physiological If pre-existing proteinuria *4707*
Urine No Effect Analytical At concentration of 250 mg/L had no effect on concentration as measured by benzethonium chloride method *1171*

Protein Electrophoresis *Serum No Effect Analytical* At concentration of 400 mg/L had no effect on automated Olympus-Hite method *5704*

Quinidine *Serum No Effect Analytical* Furosemide at a concentration of 100 µg/mL had no significant cross-reactivity with quinidine at a concentration of 2.0 µg/mL in method on Bayer Technicon Immuno 1® *431* No significant interference observed at a concentration of 100 µg/mL (302 µmol/L) with method on Du Pont aca *1543*

Renin Activity *Plasma Increase Physiological* Effect observed after 40 mg orally in normal male volunteers *4373* Most often slight increase in patients with chronic congestive heart failure in response to i.v. drug but not consistent pattern of response *4158* Injection of 40 mg into normal volunteers followed by standing for 1 hour caused significant increase (2.5 fold increase) *2594* Significant increase observed in 6 volunteers given 80 mg/day for 3 days *1813* Increment in response to infusion of 0.5 mg/kg intravenously much less in individuals older than 50 years than in those aged 18 to 30 years *6496*

Renin Concentration *Plasma Increase Physiological* In normal volunteers injection of 40 mg followed by 1 hour in upright position caused significant increase in renin concentration (approximately 3.5 fold increase) *2594*

Rifampin *Serum Increase Physiological* Effect observed after 40 mg orally in normal male volunteers *4373*

Salicylate *Serum Increase Physiological* If given concomitantly, competes for excretion *2753* In patients receiving salicylates competitive renal excretion may increase salicylate concentration *2647*

Sodium *Serum Decrease Physiological* In 8 healthy male volunteers treatment with 80 mg daily for 8 days caused mean decrease of 8.4 mmol/L *5469* Diuretic action with sodium depletion *129* In 25% of 204 hospitalized patients receiving the drug *5752* Observed after drug administration *3343*
Serum No Effect Analytical At concentration of 6,000 mg/L had no effect on measurement by ISE with predilution *5704* At concentration of 4 mg/L had no effect on flame-photometric method *5704* At concentration of 400 mg/L had no effect on measurement by ISE without predilution *5704*
Serum No Effect Physiological No effect of 80 mg/day for 3 days in 6 volunteers *1813*
Urine Increase Physiological Excretion 48% higher in older (above age 50 years) men and 26% higher in older women compared with 18 to 30 year olds in response to infusion of 0.5 mg/kg *6496* In 10 healthy men ingestion of 40 mg caused increase from mean baseline of 178 ± 48 mmol/L to 989 ± 227 mmol/L over next 4 hours *2890* In 8 patients with congestive cardiac failure intravenous bolus infusion of furosemide caused significantly increased urinary volume approximately 4 times and sodium excretion approximately 5 times compared to the output during first 4 hours of continuous infusion *5* Marked effect: decreased sharply when administration stopped *3343* Therapeutic intent of drug administration *1989* Diuretic action *2647*
Urine No Effect Physiological Nonsignificant increase from mean baseline of 144 mmol/d to 155 mmol/d in 8 healthy volunteers given 80 mg/d for 8 days *5469*

T3-Uptake *Serum Increase Analytical* At therapeutic concentrations caused interference with CEDIA method *2717*
Serum Increase Physiological Diminished protein binding at time of peak drug concentration *5830* Transient significant effect seen 2-5 h after ingestion of various amounts of drug chronically in 34 patients with congestive cardiac failure *4268*

Theophylline *Serum Decrease Physiological* Significantly lower when coadministered with drug *896*
Serum Increase Physiological May prolong half-life of theophylline *1384*
Serum No Effect Analytical At concentration of 20 mg/L produced no interference with methods on Kodak DT60, Abbott TDx, Abbott Vision with either whole blood or serum, 3M Diagnostics TheoFAST, Syntex AccµLevel or Ames Seralyzer *1122*

Thromboxane B_2 *Urine Increase Physiological* Significant increase in older individuals (above 50 years) compared with 18 to 30 year olds: in men 58 vs 30 ng/4 h and in women 48 vs 29 ng/4 h in response to intravenous infusion of 0.5 mg/kg *6496*

Furosemide *(continued)*

Thyroid Stimulating Hormone
Serum Increase Physiological Increased after drug treatment stopped *5830*
Serum No Effect Physiological No effect typically observed in spite of changes in concentration of peripheral hormones *4268*

Thyroxine Binding Globulin *Serum No Effect Physiological* At same time as thyroxine concentration reduced *5830*

Thyroxine (T4) *Serum Decrease Physiological* Transient significant effect seen 2-5 h after ingestion of various amounts of drug chronically in 34 patients with congestive cardiac failure *4268* In 4 patients high concentrations of drug inhibit T4 binding in plasma *5830* Probably due to enhanced clearance due to displacement from serum protein binding sites *4268*

Thyroxine (T4), Free *Serum Decrease Physiological* At same time as thyroxine concentration reduced *5830*
Serum Increase Analytical Increase observed when FT4 concentration measured by Boehringer Mannheim Enzymun method *2617* Significant increase observed at concentrations above 9,5 µmol/L with methods on Abbott AxSYM, Chiron ACS 180 and Ortho Vitros *2516*
Serum Increase Physiological Effect similar to that of fT4 index with analog tracer assay *4268* Transient significant effect seen 2-5 h after ingestion of various amounts of drug chronically in 34 patients with congestive cardiac failure *4268*

Thyroxine (T4) Index, Free *Serum Increase Physiological* occurring 2-5 h after single morning dose of 80 to 250 mg *4268* Transient significant effect seen 2-5 h after ingestion of various amounts of drug chronically in 34 patients with congestive cardiac failure *4268*

Tirofiban *Serum No Effect Physiological* Coadministration had no significant effect on plasma clearance of tirofiban *3957*

Trandolapril *Serum No Effect Physiological* Coadministration of furosemide with trandolapril led to a 25% increase in the renal clearance of trandoprilat but had no effect on the pharmacokinetics of furosemide *3202*

Tri-iodothyronine (T3) *Serum Decrease Physiological* At same time as thyroxine concentration reduced *5830*

Triglycerides *Serum Increase Physiological* Increase by 29 mg/dL in 12 patients given 40 to 80 mg daily for 3 mo *4213* In 14 healthy young mean ingestion of 40 mg furosemide caused significant 14.4 ± 8.2% increase 3 hours later *866* 37% change in 12 normotensive men when treated with drug alone for less than 1 year *2981*
Serum No Effect Analytical No effect at therapeutic concentration on Boehringer Mannheim Reflotron method *3231* At concentration of 5 mg/L had no effect on GPO-PAP method *5704* At concentration of 4 mg/L had no effect on lipase/esterase method *5704* No effect at 1750 mg/L on Boehringer Mannheim Reflotron method *5706*
Serum No Effect Physiological No significant change in 16 subjects treated for less than 1 y with drug only *2190*

Urea Nitrogen *Serum Increase Physiological* In patients with chronic renal failure: associated with decreased renal clearance and increased tubular reabsorption of urea *1218* Reversible increases in concentration may occur with treatment and are associated with dehydration *2647* In 9 patients with chronic failure when treated for 6 d average plasma urea rose from 18.7 mmol/L to 28.8 mmol/L secondary to reduced urea excretion which occurred in spite of increased urea filtration *1218* In 8% of 204 hospitalized patients receiving the drug *5752* ?Nephrotoxic effect (reversible) usually dehydration *139* Largely as consequence of volume depletion: effect most marked in patients receiving additional diuretics *2311*
Serum No Effect Analytical No effect at 20 mg/L on method on Ames Seralyzer *5706* At concentration of 4 mg/L had no effect on diacetylmonoxime method *5704* At concentration of 40 mg/L had no effect on Kodak Ektachem® method *5704* No effect at 1750 mg/L on Boehringer Mannheim Reflotron method *5706* No effect at therapeutic concentration on Boehringer Mannheim Reflotron method *3231*
Urine Decrease Physiological Occurs when diuretic given to patients with chronic failure, due to increased tubular reabsorption of urea, presumably in distal part of nephron, secondary to extracellular fluid volume depletion *1218*
Urine No Effect Physiological No clear pattern observed with drug administration *3343*

Uric Acid *Serum Increase Physiological* In 5 patients with hypertension , heart failure or myocardial ischemia diuretic induced gout observed *3666* Observed after drug administration *3343* Asymptomatic hyperuricemia can occur and gout may rarely be precipitated with treatment *2647* In 10% of 204 hospitalized patients receiving the drug *5752* In about 0.4% of patients receiving drug *2311* Decreased urate clearance *5869*
Serum No Effect Analytical No effect at 1750 mg/L on method on Boehringer Mannheim Reflotron *5706* At concentration of 20 mg/L had no effect on Kageyama-Hantzsch method *5704* No effect at 1.4 mg/dL on Technicon SMA 12/60 method *4390* At concentration of 4 mg/L had no effect on phosphotungstate reduction method *5704* At concentration of 20 mg/L had no effect on catalase-AIDH method *5704* At concentration of 5 mg/L had no effect on uricase-PAP method *5704* No effect at therapeutic concentration on Boehringer Mannheim Reflotron method *3231*
Urine Decrease Physiological Slight effect observed on first and second day *3343*

VLDL-Cholesterol *Serum Increase Physiological* 56% change in 12 normotensive men when treated with drug alone for less than 1 y *2981* 6% change in 16 subjects treated for less than 1 y with drug only *2190*
Serum No Effect Physiological No significant change in 16 subjects treated for less than 1 y with drug only *2190*

VLDL-Triglycerides *Serum Increase Physiological* 56% change in 12 normotensive men when treated with drug alone for less than 1 y *2981* 6% change in 16 subjects treated for less than 1 y with drug only *2190*

Volume *Blood Decrease Physiological* Diuretic action may cause dehydration, particularly in elderly patients *2647*
Plasma Decrease Physiological Excess diuresis may cause reduction in blood volume *51*
Urine Increase Physiological In 8 patients with congestive cardiac failure intravenous bolus infusion of furosemide caused significantly increased urinary volume approximately 4 times and sodium excretion approximately 5 times compared to the output during first 4 hours of continuous infusion *5* In 10 healthy volunteers given 40 mg orally mean excretion increased by 782% in next 4 hours, but returned to normal within 24 hours *2890* Significant effect, peak between 1 and 3 h after single 40 mg dose *4373* Diuretic action *2647* Significant increase on first day but decrease on second *3343*
Urine No Effect Physiological Nonsignificant increase from mean baseline of 3.6 L/d to 3.8 L/d in 8 healthy volunteers given 80 mg/d for 8 days *5469*

Zinc *Urine Increase Physiological* Increase by 12% in 9 hypertensive patients treated for 2 weeks *6418* When given i.v. brief effect only *5782*
Urine No Effect Physiological No effect observed on excretion *4484*

Fusaric Acid

Dopamine *Urine Increase Physiological* Significant increase in 6 men with pheochromocytoma treated with 300-600 mg daily for several days *4207*

Dopamine β-Hydroxylase *Serum Decrease Physiological* Administration of 300-600 mg/d to 6 patients with pheochromocytoma caused significant reduction in dopamine β-hydroxylase *4207* Total inhibitor *in vivo* possible for up to 122 h after 300 mg *4209* Most effective if given with levodopa *4856*

Epinephrine *Urine Decrease Physiological* Initial reduction followed by increase in 6 men with pheochromocytoma treated with 300-600 mg daily for several days *4207*

Metanephrine *Urine No Effect Physiological* No significant effect in 6 men with pheochromocytoma treated with 300 - 600 mg daily for several days *4207*

Norepinephrine *Urine Decrease Physiological* Significant reduction in 6 men with pheochromocytoma then rise following treatment with 300-600 mg daily for several days *4207*
Urine Increase Physiological May cause increase release early, later increased metabolism *4471*

Normetanephrine *Urine No Effect Physiological* No significant effect in 6 men with pheochromocytoma treated with 300-600 mg daily for several days *4207*

Thyroid Stimulating Hormone
Serum Decrease Physiological Inhibition of dopamine degradation in hypothyroidism *6412*

Vanillylmandelic Acid *Urine No Effect Physiological* No significant effect in 6 men with pheochromocytoma treated with 300-600 mg daily for several days *4207*

Fuscin

Color *Urine Increase Analytical* Red from foods and candy *684*

Fusidic Acid

Alanine Aminotransferase *Serum Increase Physiological* Reported in 6 patients in UK, although causal relationship could not be established with certainty *5933*

Alkaline Phosphatase *Serum Increase Physiological* Reported in 6 patients in UK, although causal relationship could not be established with certainty *5933* Jaundice developed in 34% of 112 patients given drug, highest when drug given intravenously. Jaundice resolved when drug withdrawn *2771*

Aspartate Aminotransferase *Serum Increase Physiological* Jaundice developed in 34% of 112 patients given drug, highest when drug given intravenously. Jaundice resolved when drug withdrawn *2771* Reported in 6 patients in UK, although causal relationship could not be established with certainty *5933*

Bile Acids *Serum Increase Analytical* In methods using 3-α-hydroxysteroid dehydrogenase for which drug functions as substrate *2450*

Bilirubin *Serum Increase Physiological* Jaundice developed in 34% of 112 patients given drug, highest when drug given intravenously. Jaundice resolved when drug withdrawn *2771* Clinically significant displacement from protein in neonates *6314* Reported in 6 patients in UK, although causal relationship could not be established with certainty *5933*

Phenylalanine *Plasma No Effect Analytical* No interference observed with rapid quantitative whole blood method of Campbell et al using phenylalanine dehydrogenase *867*

Vancomycin *Serum No Effect Analytical* No significant interference observed at a concentration of 500 µg/mL (968 µmol/L) with method on Du Pont aca *1561*

Gabapentin

Bleeding Time *Patient Increase Physiological* Rarely increase of bleeding time increase reported with gabapentin administration *4526*

Blood *Urine Increase Physiological* Rarely hematuria reported with gabapentin administration *4526*

Carbamazepine *Serum No Effect Physiological* Administration of 1200 mg/d gabapentin to 12 patients had no effect on steady-state trough plasma concentrations of carbamazepine and carbamazepine10,11 epoxide *4526*

Carbamazepine-10,11-Epoxide
Serum No Effect Physiological Administration of 1200 mg/d gabapentin to 12 patients had no effect on steady-state trough plasma concentrations of carbamazepine and carbamazepine10,11 epoxide *4526*

Cortisol, Free *Urine No Effect Analytical* No significant interference observed with HPLC method of Turpeinen et al *6105*

Creatinine *Serum Increase Physiological* Rarely acute renal failure reported with gabapentin administration *4526*

Ethinyl Estradiol *Serum No Effect Physiological* The half-life and AUC of norethindrone and ethinyl estradiol administered as an oral contraceptive were not affected by the coadministration of 1200 mg/d gabapentin to 13 patients *4526*

Glucose *Urine Increase Physiological* Rarely glycosuria reported with gabapentin administration *4526*

Hematocrit *Blood Decrease Physiological* Infrequently anemia reported with gabapentin administration *4526*

Hemoglobin *Blood Decrease Physiological* Infrequently anemia reported with gabapentin administration *4526*

5-Hydroxytryptamine *Blood Increase Physiological* Significant increase in concentration observed in 6 volunteers in parallel with serum concentration of drug *4855*

Leukocytes *Blood Increase Physiological* Rarely leukocytosis reported with gabapentin administration *4526*

Lymphocytes *Blood Increase Physiological* Rarely lymphocytosis reported with gabapentin administration *4526*

Melatonin *Plasma No Effect Physiological* No effect observed in 6 healthy volunteers given doses that affected concentration of blood serotonin *4855*

Norethindrone *Serum Increase Physiological* The half-life and AUC of norethindrone and ethinyl estradiol administered as an oral contraceptive were not affected by the coadministration of 1200 mg/d gabapentin to 13 patients although the maximum concentration of norethindrone was increased by 13% *4526*

Occult Blood *Feces Increase Physiological* Gabapentin administration leads infrequently to bloody stools *4526*

Phenobarbital *Serum No Effect Physiological* Coadministration of phenobarbital with gabapentin to 12 patients had no effect on the pharmacokinetics of phenobarbital *4526*

Phenytoin *Serum No Effect Physiological* Administration of 1200 mg/d gabapentin to 8 epileptic patients maintained on phenytoin monotherapy for at least 2 months had no effect on phenytoin concentration *4526*

Platelets *Blood Decrease Physiological* Infrequently thrombocytopenia reported with gabapentin administration *4526*

Protein *Urine Increase Analytical* Gabapentin appears to react positively with urinary protein component of Ames N-Multistix SG® dipsticks *4526*
Urine No Effect Analytical Gabapentin appears to react positively with urinary protein component of Ames N-Multistix SG® dipsticks but has no effect on sulfosalicylic acid precipitation procedures *4526*

Thyroxine (T4) *Serum Decrease Physiological* Rare hyperthyroidism or hypothyroidism and goiter reported with gabapentin administration *4526*
Serum Increase Physiological Rare hyperthyroidism or hypothyroidism and goiter reported with gabapentin administration *4526*

Urea Nitrogen *Serum Increase Physiological* Rarely acute renal failure reported with gabapentin administration *4526*

Valproic Acid *Serum No Effect Physiological* Administration of 1200 mg/d gabapentin to 17 epileptic patients had no effect on steady-state trough plasma concentration *4526*

Gabexate

Ketone Body Ratio *Serum No Effect Analytical* When added at a concentration of 25 mg/L had no significant effect on AKBR method of Uno et al *6131*

Gallamine

Albumin *Serum Increase Physiological* Sensitivity to drug correlated with concentration *5841*

Histamine *Plasma Increase Physiological* Observed with injection for anesthesia *3648*

^{131}I Uptake *Serum Decrease Physiological* Due to iodine component of drug *3669*

Gallium Nitrate

Bicarbonate *Serum Decrease Physiological* Decreased concentration, possibly secondary to mild respiratory alkalosis reported in 40 - 50% treated patients with cancer *5679*

Calcium *Serum Decrease Physiological* In two patients with hypercalcemia due to parathyroid carcinoma *6354* 18 of 24 patients with malignant disease associated hypercalcemia achieved normocalcemia following intravenous drug for 5 days *6353* In patients with hypercalcemia of malignancy mean concentration reduced to normal more frequently (75%) than with calcitonin (31%) and for a longer period (6 days versus 1 day) *562* Hypocalcemia may occur after treatment *5679*
Urine Decrease Physiological In patients with hypercalcemia of malignancy excretion reduced as a result of its inhibition of bone resorption *562* In two patients with hypercalcemia due to parathyroid carcinoma *6354*

Gallium Nitrate *(continued)*

Creatinine *Serum Increase Physiological* Increasing concentration reported in 12.5% treated patients, with acute renal failure reported in some patients *5679*

Creatinine Clearance *Urine No Effect Physiological* In two patients with hypercalcemia due to parathyroid carcinoma *6354*

Hematocrit *Blood Decrease Physiological* With high doses, up to 1400 mg/sq m, anemia may occur *5679*

Hemoglobin *Blood Decrease Physiological* With high doses, up to 1400 mg/sq m, anemia may occur *5679*

Hydroxyproline *Urine Decrease Physiological* In two patients with hypercalcemia due to parathyroid carcinoma *6354* Excretion in patients with hypercalcemia of malignancy reduced due to inhibitory action on bone resorption *562*

Ionized Calcium *Serum Decrease Physiological* Change paralleled that of total calcium in two patients with hypercalcemia due to parathyroid carcinoma *6354*

Leukocytes *Blood Decrease Physiological* Leukopenia may occur with treatment *5679*

Parathyroid Hormone *Plasma Decrease Physiological* In two patients with hypercalcemia due to parathyroid carcinoma *6354*

Phosphate *Serum Decrease Physiological* Hypophosphatemia of mild to moderate degree may occur in up to 79% of hypercalcemic treated patients. In one trial 33% of patients had at least one measurement between 1.5 - 2.4 mg/dL and 46% had at least one measurement below 1.5 mg/dL *5679*

Urea Nitrogen *Serum Increase Physiological* Increasing concentration reported in 12.5% treated patients, with acute renal failure reported in some patients *5679*

Gallopamil

Digoxin *Serum Increase Physiological* 16% increase when concomitantly administered with drug *472*
Serum No Effect Physiological Coadministration generally did not affect serum concentrations although in individual patients increase observed *472*

Platelet Aggregation *Blood Decrease Physiological* In 12 healthy volunteers after platelet rich plasma incubated with 250 µmol gallopamil significant reduction of ADP- and collagen-induced platelet aggregation observed *3232*

Ganciclovir

Alanine Aminotransferase *Serum Increase Physiological* Abnormal liver function tests observed in 2% treated patients *5018*

Alkaline Phosphatase *Serum Increase Physiological* Abnormal liver function tests observed in 2% treated patients *5018*

Aspartate Aminotransferase *Serum Increase Physiological* Abnormal liver function tests observed in 2% treated patients *5018*

Bilirubin *Serum Increase Physiological* Abnormal liver function tests observed in 2% treated patients *5018*

Blood *Urine Increase Physiological* Hematuria observed in some treated patients *5018*

Clindamycin *Serum No Effect Analytical* No interference observed with bioassays *3858*

Colistin *Serum No Effect Analytical* No interference observed with bioassays *3858*

Creatine Kinase *Serum Increase Physiological* Increased activity observed in some treated patients *5018*

Creatinine *Serum Increase Physiological* In transplant patients coadministration of ganciclovir with cyclosporine A or amphoteracin B observed to increase serum creatinine concentrations. Maximum concentration of greater than 2.5 mg/dL observed in 1% patients and between 1.5 and 2.5 mg/dL in 12% in 320 patients with CMV retinitis receiving 3000 mg/d ganciclovir *5018* In 20 bone marrow transplant recipients 20% had increases in plasma concentrations to above 2.5 mg/dL during a 120 day course of intravenous ganciclovir. The values decreased after treatment was discontinued *1182* In 4 of 20 patients with positive CMV culture following bone marrow transplantation treated with prophylactic ganciclovir serum creatinine concentration increased above 221 µmol/L as compared with no increases in controls *5351*

Creatinine Clearance *Urine Decrease Physiological* Decreased clearance observed in some treated patients *5018*

Cyclosporine A *Blood No Effect Physiological* In 93 liver transplant patients coadministration of ganciclovir (infusion of 5 mg/kg over 1 h every 12 h) with therapeutic doses of cyclosporine A had no effect on cyclosporine A concentrations *5018*

Didanosine *Serum Increase Physiological* Increased plasma concentration *886* At an oral dose of 1000 mg ganciclovir every 8 h and didanosine 200 mg every 12 h the steady state AUC of didanosine increased 111 ± 114% *5018*

Eosinophils *Blood Increase Physiological* Eosinophilia observed in some treated patients *5018*

Erythromycin *Serum No Effect Analytical* No interference observed with bioassays *3858*

Glucose *Serum Decrease Physiological* Hypoglycemia observed in some treated patients *5018*
Serum Increase Physiological Increased concentration observed in some treated patients *5018*

Hemoglobin *Blood Decrease Physiological* In 320 patients with CMV retinitis administration of ganciclovir 3000 mg/d caused anemia with hemoglobin concentration of less than 65 g/L in 2% patients, between 65 and 80 g/L in 10% and between 80 and 95 g/L in 25% *5018*

Ketone Body Ratio *Serum No Effect Analytical* When added at a concentration of 1.0 g/L had no significant effect on AKBR method of Uno et al *6131*

Lactate Dehydrogenase *Serum Increase Physiological* Increased concentration observed in some treated patients *5018*

Metronidazole *Serum No Effect Analytical* No interference observed with bioassays *3858*

Mycophenolate *Serum No Effect Physiological* Coadministration of single doses of mycophenolate mofentil with ganciclovir (1.5 mg/d) in 12 stable renal transplant patients had no significant effect on AUC and concentration of mycophenolate *5017*

Neutrophils *Blood Decrease Physiological* In patients with CMV retinitis treatment with intravenous ganciclovir followed by maintenance therapy for 3 months, approximately 40% had granulocytopenia with neutrophil count less than 1000 /µL. With oral treatment the incidence was less *1182* In 320 patients with CMV retinitis administration of ganciclovir 3000 mg/d caused neutropenia of less than 500 cells/µL in 18% patients, between 500 and 749 cells/µL in 17% and between 750 and 1000 cells/µL in 19% *5018*

Occult Blood *Feces Increase Physiological* Gastrointestinal hemorrhage or melena observed in 2% treated patients *5018*

Platelets *Blood Decrease Physiological* In 76 patients with heart allografts administration of ganciclovir caused thrombocytopenia of less than 50,000 cells/µL in 8% patients *5018* In patients with CMV retinitis treatment with intravenous ganciclovir followed by maintenance therapy for 3 months, approximately 40% had thrombocytopenia with platelet count less than 50,000 /µL. With oral treatment the incidence was less. Problem can be avoided with concomitant administration of G-CSF or GM-CSF *1182*

Polymyxin *Serum No Effect Analytical* No interference observed with bioassays *3858*

Potassium *Serum Decrease Physiological* Decreased concentration observed in some treated patients *5018*

Tacrolimus *Serum No Effect Analytical* In HPLC/MS method of Christians et al no significant interference observed with measurement of FK 506 *1010*

Tetracycline *Serum No Effect Analytical* No interference observed with bioassays *3858*

Trimethoprim *Serum No Effect Analytical* No interference observed with bioassays *3858*

Urea Nitrogen *Serum Increase Physiological* Increased concentration observed in some treated patients *5018*

Zalcitabine *Serum No Effect Analytical* At a concentration of 100 mg/L had less than 0.01% cross-reactivity with solid phase extraction and RIA method of Roberts et al *4990*

Zidovudine *Serum Increase Physiological* At an oral dose of 1000 mg ganciclovir every 8 h mean steady-state AUC of zidovudine increased 19 ± 27% in the presence of zidovudine 100 mg every 4 h *5018*
Serum No Effect Analytical No effect on liquid chromatographic method of Hedaya and Sawchuk *2525*

Ganglionic Blocking Agents

Effective Renal Plasma Flow
Patient Decrease Physiological Returns to normal usually within 2 h *2242*

Glomerular Filtration Rate *Urine Decrease Physiological* Returns to normal usually within 2 h *2242*

Hydrochloric Acid *Gastric Fluid Decrease Physiological* Volume and acidity generally reduced *2242*

Ganirelix

Estradiol *Plasma Decrease Physiological* In a group of healthy women intranasal administration of single doses up to 6 mg caused reduction of plasma estradiol from mean baseline of 51.4 ± 11.4 pg/mL to 34.4 ± 8.3 pg/mL 12 h after dosing, with smaller reduction after 3 mg *1982*

Luteinizing Hormone *Plasma Decrease Physiological* In a group of healthy women intranasal administration of single doses up to 6 mg caused reduction of plasma luteinizing hormone by ≥ 35% relative to baseline from 2 to 12 hours after dosing. Mean maximal decrease was 62% at 8 hours after dosing in the group receiving 3 mg and 74% at 6 h in the group receiving 6 mg *1982*

Gemcitabine

Alanine Aminotransferase *Serum Increase Physiological* In patients with pancreatic cancer increased activity was observed in 68% patients *1697*

Alkaline Phosphatase *Serum Increase Physiological* In patients with pancreatic cancer increased activity was observed in 55% patients *1697*

Aspartate Aminotransferase *Serum Increase Physiological* In patients with pancreatic cancer increased activity was observed in 67% patients *1697*

Bilirubin *Serum Increase Physiological* In patients with pancreatic cancer increased concentration was observed in 13% patients *1697*

Blood *Urine Increase Physiological* In patients with pancreatic cancer increased concentration was observed in 35% patients *1697*

Creatinine *Serum Increase Physiological* In patients with pacreatic cancer increased concentration was observed in 8% patients *1697*

Hematocrit *Blood Decrease Physiological* In patients with pancreatic cancer anemia was observed in 68% patients *1697*

Leukocytes *Blood Decrease Physiological* In patients with pancreatic cancer leukopenia was observed in 62% patients *1697*

Neutrophils *Blood Decrease Physiological* In patients with pancreatic cancer neutropenia was observed in 63% patients *1697*

Platelets *Blood Decrease Physiological* In patients with pancreatic cancer thrombocytopenia was observed in 24% patients *1697*

Protein *Urine Increase Physiological* In patients with pancreatic cancer increased concentration was observed in 45% patients *1697*

Urea Nitrogen *Serum Increase Physiological* In patients with pancreatic cancer increased concentration was observed in 16% patients *1697*

Gemfibrozil

Alanine Aminotransferase *Serum Increase Physiological* May occur as a side effect *4524*
Serum No Effect Physiological No significant effect observed in 25 patients with type IIa hyperlipidemia treated with 900 mg/d for 4 weeks *331*

Alkaline Phosphatase *Serum Increase Physiological* May occur as a side effect *4524*
Serum No Effect Physiological No significant effect observed in 25 patients with type IIa hyperlipidemia treated with 900 mg/d for 4 weeks *331*

Androstanediol Glucuronide
Plasma Increase Physiological In 90 dyslipidemic men (serum cholesterol greater than or equal to 5.2 mmol/L) treatment with gemfirozil for one year caused significant change from mean baseline of 8.4 ± 3.1 nmol/L to 18.3 ± 8.2 nmol/L *2513*

Androstenedione *Plasma Increase Physiological* In 90 dyslipidemic men (serum cholesterol greater than or equal to 5.2 mmol/L) treatment with gemfirozil for one year caused nonsignificant change from mean baseline of 5.1 ± 1.3 nmol/L to 5.7 ± 2.1 nmol/L *2513*

Antinuclear Antibodies *Serum Increase Physiological* Positive ANA reported as a possible side effect *4524*

Antithrombin III *Plasma Increase Physiological* Mean increase of 19% observed in 27 hyperlipidemic patients treated with 1200 mg daily for 12 weeks *5849*
Plasma No Effect Physiological In 20 patients with primary hypertriglyceridemia treatment with 1200 mg/d caused nonsignificant change from mean baseline of 91.43 ± 10.35 to 93.25 ± 22.15 *295*

Apolipoprotein A *Serum Increase Physiological* Significant increase in 20 hyperlipidemic out patients treated with 1200 mg daily for 90 days *5177*

Apolipoprotein A-I *Serum Increase Physiological* Nonsignificant increase from mean baseline of 1.44 g/L to 1.51 g/L in 18 patients with familial combined hyperlipidemia treated with 1200 mg/d for 6 weeks *4367* Significant increase (7%) observed in 10 patients with type IV hyperlipoproteinemia treated with 1200 mg/d for 3 months but increase not significant in 10 patients with type IIb hyperlipoproteinemia *4919* Increase by 29% in 6 patients with primary familial endogenous hypertriglyceridemia from baseline values. Synthetic rates of apo A-I and apo A-II increased by 27% and 34% respectively *5193* Of fibrates gemfibrozil appears to be most effective in increasing concentration *5586* In 10 patients with noninsulin-dependent diabetes mellitus treatment for 3 months caused nonsignificant increase from mean baseline of 12.6% *3006* Significant increase from mean of 104 mg/dL to 132 mg/dL in 10 patients with hyperglyceridemia and abnormal glucose tolerance but no significant increase in hypertriglyceridemic patients with normal glucose tolerance *5990* In 63-69 patients with hypercholesterolemia treatment for 12 weeks caused increase from mean baseline of 1.41 ± 0.03 g/L to 1.49 ± 0.04 g/L (5.1%) *6463* In 8 patients with familial dysbetalipoproteinemia treatment with 1200 mg/d for 1 month caused significant increase from mean baseline of 158 mg/dL to 176 mg/dL *6655* In 109 patients with dyslipidemia treatment with 1200 mg/d for 12 months caused increase from mean baseline of about 120 mg/dL to about 135 mg/dL *3254* Mean concentration of 106.1 ± 10.4 mg/dL in 20 patients with primary hypertriglyceridemia treatment with 1200 mg/d for 12 weeks caused significant increase to 122.4 ± 12.7 mg/dL *295* In 20 patients with hypertriglyceridemia treatment with 1200 mg/d caused significant increase from mean baseline of 107.4 ± 12.3 mg/dL to 115.4 ± 10.3 mg/dL after 4 weeks and 126.9 ± 12.1 mg/dL after 12 weeks *296* Treatment of 48 patients with primary hyperlipidemia with 900 mg/d for 16 weeks caused mean increase of 9.7% whereas treatment with 600 mg b.i.d. caused mean increase of 13.5% *297* Increased synthesis. Increased activity of lipoprotein lipase by stimulation of muscle lipoprotein lipase synthesis, alteration of the capillary endothelial surface and stimulation of apo C-II synthesis *264*
Serum No Effect Physiological In 12 type IIa hyperlipidemic patients treatment with gemfibrozil for 12 weeks caused nonsignificant change from mean baseline of 184.6 ± 42.9 mg/dL to 176.1 ± 30.3 mg/dL *1929* No significant change observed in 14 hypertriglyceridemic patients treated with 1200 mg daily

Gemfibrozil *(continued)*

Apolipoprotein A-I *(continued)*
for 24 weeks *4564* In 30 patients with familial defective apolipoprotein B-100 treatment with 1200 mg/d for 8 weeks caused an insignificant change from mean baseline of 1.08 ± 0.02 g/L to 1.11 ± 0.03 g/L *2445* No significant effect observed in 9 patients with familial hypercholesterolemia after treatment with 1200 mg daily for 16 weeks *1930* In 21 men with combined hyperlipidemia treatment with 1200 mg/d for a mean 11.0 weeks caused caused an insignificant change from mean baseline of 1.25 ± 0.03 g/L to 1.28 ± 0.05 g/L *752* In 14 men with low HDL-cholesterol concentration treatment with gemfibrozil for 3 months had no significant effect on plasma concentration (no change from 1.23 ± 0.03 g/L) *4049* In 17 male patients with established atherosclerosis and high triglycerides and low high-density lipoprotein cholesterol treated 1200 mg/d for 12 weeks nonsignificant change from mean baseline of 1.11 g/L to 1.13 g/L observed *3198*

Apolipoprotein A-I:Apolipoprotein B Ratio
Serum Increase Physiological In 109 patients with dyslipidemia treatment with 1200 mg/d for 12 months caused increase from mean baseline of 0.68 ± 0.19 to 0.90 ± 0.29 *3254*

Apolipoprotein A-II *Serum Increase Physiological* In 109 patients with dyslipidemia treatment with 1200 mg/d for 12 months caused increase from mean baseline of about 33 mg/dL to 40 mg/dL *3254* Slight but significant increase observed after 24 weeks treatment with 1200 mg daily in 14 hypertriglyceridemic patients *4564* In 12 type IIa hyperlipidemic patients treatment with gemfibrozil for 12 weeks caused significant change from mean baseline of 44.7 ± 6.5 mg/dL to 49.3 ± 5.7 mg/dL *1929* In 8 patients with familial dysbetalipoproteinemia treatment with 1200 mg/d for 1 month caused significant increase from mean baseline of 50 mg/dL to 64 mg/dL *4148* Significant increase from mean of 24.0 mg/dL to 28.6 mg/dL in 9 patients with familial hypercholesterolemia treated with 1200 mg daily for 16 weeks *1930* Small but significant increase observed in 27 hyperlipidemic patients treated with 1200 mg daily for 12 weeks *5849* Increased synthesis. Increased activity of lipoprotein lipase by stimulation of muscle lipoprotein lipase synthesis, alteration of the capillary surface and stimulation of apo C-II synthesis *264* In 10 patients with noninsulin-dependent diabetes mellitus treatment for 3 months caused significant increase from mean baseline of 28% *3006* Increase by 38% in 6 patients with primary familial endogenous hypertriglyceridemia from from baseline values. Synthetic rates of apo A-I and apo A-II increased by 27% and 34% respectively *5193* In 14 men with low total HDL-cholesterol concentration treatment for 3 months caused slight increase in concentration (change from 0.23 ± 0.09 g/L to 0.25 ± 0.13 g/L) *4049*

Apolipoprotein B *Serum Decrease Physiological* Significant reduction of 16.4% in 8 patients with hypercholesterolemia treated with 1.2 g/day for 6 weeks and of 24.4% in 19 patients with serum cholesterols above 7.8 mmol/L treated with 1.2 g/day for 6 weeks *4387* In patients with type IIb hyperlipoproteinemia drug alone reduced concentration by 18% *1644* Significant reduction from mean baseline of 2.08 g/L to 1.59 g/L in 18 patients with familial combined hyperlipidemia treated with 1200 mg/d for 6 weeks *4367* Significant reduction from mean of 260 mg/dL to 202 mg/dL in 9 patients with familial hypercholesterolemia after treatment with 1200 mg daily for 16 weeks *1930* In 12 type IIa hyperlipidemic patients with gemfibrozil for 12 weeks caused significant reduction from mean baseline of 216.3 ± 24.0 mg/dL to 177.9 ± 24.3 mg/dL *1929* In 109 patients with dyslipidemia treatment with 1200 mg/d for 12 months caused reduction from about 180 mg/dL to about 155 mg/dL *3254* Treatment of 10 patients with type IIa hyperlipidemia with 1200 mg/d for 8 weeks caused mean reduction of 5.4%. In 10 patients with type IV hyperlipidemia reduction of 5.4% also observed *6224* In 20 patients with primary hypertriglyceridemia treatment with 1200 mg/d caused significant reduction from mean baseline of 165.8 ± 18.1 mg/dL to 153.4 ± 14.3 mg/dL after 4 weeks and 128.7 ± 12.8 mg/dL after 12 weeks *296* Treatment of 10 patients with type IIa hyperlipidemia with 1200 mg/d for 8 weeks caused mean reduction of 5.4%. In 10 patients with type IV hyperlipidemia reduction of 5.4% also observed *6225* In 20 patients with primary hypertriglyceridemia treatment with 1200 mg/d for 12 weeks caused significant decrease from mean baseline of 169.5 ± 14.9 mg/dL to 124.7 ± 11.3 mg/dL *295* Treatment of 48 patients with primary hyperlipidemia with 900 mg/d for 16 weeks caused mean decrease of 16.5% whereas treatment with 600 mg b.i.d. caused mean decrease of 19.4% *297* Significant reduction from mean of 118 mg/dL to 101 mg/dL in 10 patients with hypertriglyceridemia with normal glucose tolerance and from 115 mg/dL to 96 mg/dL in 10 with abnormal glucose tolerance after treatment with 1200 mg daily for 1 month *5990* In 10 patients with type IIb apolipoproteinemia 1200 mg/d for 3 months caused mean decrease of 20% and in 10 type IV hyperlipoproteinemia patients a mean decrease of 6% *4919* In 30 patients with familial defective apolipoprotein B-100 treatment with 1200 mg/d for 8 weeks caused a significant change from mean baseline of 1.52 ± 0.06 g/L to 1.41 ± 0.06 g/L *2445* In 21 men with combined hyperlipidemia treatment with 1200 mg/d for a mean 11.0 weeks caused caused an insignificant decrease from mean baseline of 1.79 ± 0.16 g/L to 1.43 ± 0.09 g/L *752* In 63-69 patients with hypercholesterolemia treatment for 12 weeks caused significant decrease from mean baseline of 1.62 ± 0.05 g/L to 1.37 ± 0.04 g/L (15.3%) *6463*
Serum Increase Physiological Slight but not significant increase observed after 24 weeks treatment with 1200 mg daily in 14 patients with hypertriglyceridemia *4564*
Serum No Effect Physiological In 5 patients with hypertriglyceridemia treatment with 1200 mg/d for 8 weeks caused insignificant decrease to 103 ± 27 mg/dL compared with 105 ± 35 mg/dL in those receiving placebo and in 5 patients with combined hyperlipidemia concentration decreased to 114 ± 32 mg/dL versus 116 ± 25 mg/dL in those receiving placebo *6589* In 17 male patients with established atherosclerosis and high triglycerides and low high-density lipoprotein cholesterol treated 1200 mg/d for 12 weeks nonsignificant change from mean baseline of 1.59 g/L to 1.67 g/L observed *3198* In 14 men with low HDL-cholesterol concentration treatment with gemfibrozil for 3 months had no significant effect on plasma concentration (no change from 1.10 ± 0.04 g/L) *4049*

Apolipoprotein C-II *Serum No Effect Physiological* No significant change observed in 14 patients with hypertriglyceridemia treated with 1200 mg daily for 14 weeks *4564*

Apolipoprotein C-III *Serum Decrease Physiological* Significant decrease from mean baseline concentration of about 23 mg/dL to 13 mg/dL in 14 patients with hypertriglyceridemia treated with 1200 mg daily for 24 weeks *4564*

Apolipoprotein E *Serum Decrease Physiological* In 5 patients with hypertriglyceridemia treatment with 1200 mg/d for 8 weeks caused significant decrease to 4.4 ± 0.9 mg/dL compared with 9.4 ± 3.8 mg/dL in those receiving placebo and in 5 patients with combined hyperlipidemia concentration decreased to 4.4 ± 7.2 mg/dL versus 7.2 ± 3.2 mg/dL in those receiving placebo *6589* Significant reduction from mean baseline concentration of about 16 mg/dL to about 8 mg/dL after 12 weeks treatment with 1200 mg daily in 14 hypertriglyceridemic patients and nonsignificant reduction to 10 mg/dL at 24 weeks *4564*

Apolipoprotein E:Apolipoprotein B Ratio
Serum Decrease Physiological In 5 patients with hypertriglyceridemia treatment with 1200 mg/d for 8 weeks caused significant decrease in ratio to 0.7 ± 0.3 compared with 1.5 ± 0.7 in those receiving placebo *6589*
Serum Increase Physiological In 5 patients with combined hyperlipidemia treatment with 1200 mg/d gemfibrozil for 8 weeks increased ratio to 1.0 ± 0.3 versus 0.6 ± 0.2 in those receiving placebo *6589*

Apolipoprotein Lp(a) *Serum Increase Physiological* In 30 patients with familial defective apolipoprotein B-100 treatment with 40 mg/d for 8 weeks caused an insignificant change from mean baseline of 9.19 mg/dL to 10.31 mg/dL *2445*

Aspartate Aminotransferase *Serum Increase Physiological* May occur as a side effect *4524*
Serum No Effect Physiological No significant effect observed in 25 patients with type IIa hyperlipidemia treated with 900 mg/d for 4 weeks *331*

Bilirubin *Serum Increase Physiological* May occur as a side effect *4524*

Bleeding Time *Patient No Effect Physiological* No significant difference between survivors of myocardial infarction who received 1200 mg daily for 8 weeks and controls *157*

Carbamazepine *Serum Increase Physiological* Plasma concentrations of carbamazepine may be increased with coadministration of drugs *3119*

Cholesterol *Serum Decrease Physiological* In the Helsinki Heart Study of 4,081 asymptomatic middle-aged male patients with primary dyslipidemia treatment with 1200 mg/d caused mean decrease of 11% *3115* Mean decrease of 10% in dyslipidemic men treated over 5 years, most marked in Fredrickson type IIa *3773* In 24 patients with hypertriglyceridemia greater than 5.67 mmol/L treatment with 1200 mg/d gemfibrozil caused significant reduction in concentration from 8.02 ± 3.60 mmol/L to 6.44 ± 2.68 mmol/L *5800* In 17 patients with mean basal concentration of 6.53 ± 0.44 mmol/L 6 weeks treatment with 1200 mg/d for caused significant reduction *3905* Gemfibrozil decreases plasma cholesterol concentration *3668* In 35 patients with primary hypercholesterolemia treatment with diet and gemfibrozil caused significant reduction from mean baseline of 7.9 ± 0.28 mmol/L to 6.8 ± 0.17 mmol/L after 6 months, 6.7 ± 0.19 mmol/L after 12 months and 6.3 ± 0.14 mmol/L after 24 months *4153* In 63 male patients with coronary heart disease treated with gemfibrozil for 2 months mean concentration decreased by 12% (9 to 15%) during treatment *6457* Significant reduction from mean baseline concentration of 8.0 mmol/L to 6.8 mmol/L in 18 patients with familial combined hyperlipidemia treated with 1200 mg/d for 6 weeks. Addition of cholestyramine caused further 9% decrease *4367* In 5 patients with hypertriglyceridemia treatment with 1200 mg/d for 8 weeks caused significant decrease to 231 ± 45 mg/dL compared with 272 ± 68 mg/dL in those receiving placebo *6589* In 30 patients with familial defective apolipoprotein B-100 treatment with 1200 mg/d for 8 weeks caused a significant change from mean baseline of 8.22 ± 0.27 mmol/L to 7.78 ± 0.24 mmol/L *2445* In 21 men with combined hyperlipidemia treatment with 1200 mg/d for a mean 11.0 weeks caused caused a significant decrease from mean baseline of 7.8 ± 0.3 mmol/L to 6.5 ± 0.3 mmol/L *752* In 8 patients with familial dyslipoproteinemia treatment with 1200 mg/d for 4 weeks caused concentration to decrease by 45% from mean baseline of 11.87 mmol/L to 6.51 mmol/L. After 3 months the concentration had decreased to 5.95 mmol/L and after 10 months to 6.19 mmol/L *6655* In 63-69 patients with hypercholesterolemia treatment for 12 weeks caused significant reduction from mean baseline of 7.32 ± 0.14 mmol/L to 6.20 ± 0.12 mmol/L (15.2%) *6463* Mean reduction of 15% observed in 18 patients with familial combined hypercholesterolemia when treated with 1200 mg/d for 6 weeks. Addition of cholestyramine caused further decrease of 9% *4367* Insignificant decrease from mean baseline concentration of 6.4 mmol/L to 6.0 mmol/L after 24 weeks treatment 1200 mg daily in 14 hypertriglyceridemic patients *4564* Treatment with 1200 mg daily for 8 weeks caused reduction from mean of 10.88 mmol/L to 5.62 mmol/L in 13 patients with type V hyperlipidemia *3448* In 8 patients with hypercholesterolemia insignificant reduction of 3.7% at 6 weeks with 1.2 g/day but in 19 patients with serum cholesterol concentrations above 7.8 mmol/L given 1.2 g/day significant reduction of 13.2% after 6 weeks *4387* In 38 renal allograft patients who had persistent hyperlipidemia and stable renal function treatment with up to 1200 mg/d caused significant change from mean baseline of 297.6 ± 41.0 mg/dL (7.69 ± 1.06 mmol/L) to 249.2 ± 43.7 mg/dL(6.44 ± 1.13 mmol/L) *962* In 295 patients with NIDDM treatment with 1200 mg/d caused significant decrease from mean baseline of about 233 mg/dL to 221 mg/dL after 4 weeks, 224 mg/dL after 12 weeks and 222 mg/dL after 20 weeks *6268* In 12 healthy men treatment for 10 days with 600 mg/d caused decrease from baseline of 166.9 ± 25.6 mg/dL to 157.3 ± 17.2 mg/dL and for 10 days with 1200 mg/d for 10 days 145.6 ± 18.8 mg/dL *2724* In 48 patients with hyperlipidemia treatment with 900 mg/d caused mean reduction of 19.8% over 16 weeks. Treatment with 600 mg b.i.d. caused mean decrease of 15.6% *297* In 20 patients with primary triglyceridemia treatment with 1200 mg/d for 12 weeks caused significant decrease from mean baseline of 248.5 ± 50.5 mg/dL to 219.7 ± 50.2 mg/dL *295* Mean reduction of 15 % in 75 patients with primary hypercholesterolemia treated with mean dose of 1200 mg/day for 12 weeks *6031* In 27 patients with severe hypertriglyceridemia treatment with 1200 mg/d for 6 weeks caused significant reduction from median baseline of 11.6 ± 3.49 mmol/L to 8.65 ± 2.85 mmol/L *3086* In 90 dyslipidemic men (serum cholesterol greater than or equal to 5.2 mmol/L) treatment with gemfirozil for one year caused significant reduction from 7.62 ± 0.91 mmol/L to 6.42 ± 1.14 mmol/L *2513* In 10 patients with type IIb hyperlipoproteinemia 1200 mg/d gemfibrozil caused mean decrease of 18% after 3 months and 14% reduction in 10 patients with type IV hyperlipoproteinemia *4919* In 55 middle-aged ambulatory men treatment with 1200 mg/d for 3 months caused significant decrease of 8% from mean baseline of 6.18 ± 0.85 mmol/L to 5.61 ± 0.90 mmol/L *5143* Mean reduction of 6.8% in 51 noninsulin dependent diabetics with primary hypercholesterolemia treated with 1200 mg daily for 24 weeks *2215* Significant reduction observed in 15 patients with familial type IV hyperlipoproteinemia when given 1200 mg daily *1103* Significant effect of 1200 mg daily for 90 days in 20 out patients with hyperlipidemia *5177* Mean reduction of 11.3% observed in 27 hyperlipidemic patients given 1200 mg daily for 12 weeks *5849* In 109 patients with dyslipidemia treatment with 1200 mg/d for 12 months caused reduction from mean baseline of 7.42 ± 1.00 mmol/L to 6.82 ± 1.02 mmol/L *3254* 17% reduction observed in 22 survivors of a myocardial infarction when given 1200 mg daily for 8 weeks but not statistically different from control group *157* In patients with type IIb hyperlipoproteinemia reduced concentration by 11% *1644* Significant reduction from mean of 390 mg/dL to 319 mg/dL in 9 patients with familial hypercholesterolemia after treatment with 1200 mg daily for 16 weeks *1930* Significant reduction from mean of 297 mg/dL to 238 mg/dL in 10 patients with hypertriglyceridemia and normal glucose tolerance and from 259 mg/dL to 206 mg/dL in 10 with abnormal glucose tolerance treated with 1200 mg daily for 1 month *5990* In 12 type IIa hyperlipidemic patients treatment with gemfibrozil for 12 weeks caused significant reduction from mean baseline of 313.9 ± 40.6 mg/dL to 260.4 ± 26.9 mg/dL *1929* In 20 patients with primary hypertriglyceridemia treatment with 1200 mg/d caused decrease from mean baseline of 244.2 ± 27.3 mg/dL to 225.9 ± 18.5 mg/dL after 4 weeks and 210.5 ± 22.4 mg/dL after 12 weeks *296* Increase by 11% in extensive 5 year double-blinded trial with 2,000 men receiving 600 mg drug twice daily *1962*

Serum No Effect Physiological In 17 male patients with established atherosclerosis and high triglycerides and low high-density lipoprotein cholesterol treated 1200 mg/d for 12 weeks nonsignificant reduction from mean baseline of 7.15 mmol/L to 6.76 mmol/L observed *3198* In 5 patients with combined hyperlipidemia treatment with 1200 mg/d for 8 weeks caused insignificant change to 245 ± 40 mg/dL compared with 249 ± 31 mg/dL in those receiving placebo *6589* In 14 men with low total cholesterol concentration treatment for 3 months caused insigniicant reduction from mean of 147.2 ± 3.8 mg/dL to 145.5 ± 4.3 mg/dL *4049*

Cholesterol Ester Transfer Protein

Serum Increase Physiological In 10 patients with noninsulin-dependent diabetes mellitus treatment for 3 months caused significant increase from mean baseline of 56 ± 15.1 nmol/mL/h *3006*

Cholesterol:HDL-Cholesterol Ratio

Serum Decrease Physiological In 20 patients with primary hypertriglyceridemia treatment with 1200 mg/d for 12 weeks caused significant decrease from mean baseline of 7.7 ± 2.4 to 5.7 ± 1.2 *295* In 17 patients treatment with 1200 mg/d for 6 weeks caused reduction from mean baseline ratio of 7.50 ± 0.76 to 5.57 ± 0.93 *3905* Treatment of 48 patients with primary hyperlipidemia with 900 mg/d for 16 weeks caused mean decrease of 30.4% whereas treatment with 600 mg b.i.d. caused mean decrease of 31% *297*

Chylomicrons *Serum Decrease Physiological* Virtual disappearance observed in 13 patients with type V hyperlipidemia treated with 1200 mg daily for 8 weeks *3448*

Cortisol *Plasma Increase Physiological* In 90 dyslipidemic men (serum cholesterol greater than or equal to 5.2 mmol/L) treatment with gemfibrozil for one year caused significant change from mean baseline of 358 ± 110 nmol/L to 426 ± 140 nmol/L *2513*

Coumarin *Plasma Increase Physiological* By displacing oral anticoagulants from their plasma protein binding sites gemfibrozil increases their plasma concentration and may cause bleeding problems *3668*

C-Peptide *Plasma No Effect Physiological* No effect on fasting or post oral glucose tolerance test concentrations in 10 hypertriglyceridemic patients with normal glucose tolerance and 10 with abnormal glucose tolerance following treatment with 1200 mg daily for 1 month *5990*

Gemfibrozil *(continued)*

C-Reactive Protein *Serum Decrease Physiological* In 51 hypercholesterolemic patients (cholesterol concentration greater than 6.5 mmol/L) treatment with 1200 mg/d gemfibrozil caused significant reduction from mean baseline concentration of 0.93 mg/L to 0.51 mg/L after 6 weeks *1317*
Serum No Effect Physiological In 51 hypercholesterolemic patients (cholesterol concentration greater than 6.5 mmol/L) treatment with 1200 mg/d gemfibrozil caused an insignificant change from mean baseline concentration of 0.93 mg/L to 1.25 mg/L after 12 weeks *1317*

Creatine Kinase *Serum Increase Physiological* Significant increase to above 1000 U/L observed in 2 of 52 noninsulin dependent diabetics with primary hypercholesterolemia treated with 1200 mg daily for 24 weeks. Activity returned to normal in spite of continued treatment. No myopathy observed *2215* May occur as a side effect, particularly when administered with lovastain *4524* Significant increase observed in 30 patients with types IIa, IIb and IV hyperlipidemia treated with 1200 mg/d for 8 weeks *6225 6224*
Serum No Effect Physiological No significant effect observed in 25 patients with type IIa hyperlipidemia when treated with 900 mg/d for 4 weeks *331*

Creatinine *Serum Increase Physiological* Increased concentration may occur in patients in whom initial concentration was increased (greater than 2.0 mg/dL) *4524*

D-Dimer Agglutination *Blood Increase Physiological* Increase from 3 to 5 in DDAVP stimulated D-dimer agglutination in 22 postmyocardial infarction survivors following treatment with 1200 mg daily for 8 weeks similar to change observed in placebo control group *157*

11-Dehydro-thromboxane B_2 *Urine Increase Physiological* In 21 men with combined hyperlipidemia treatment with 1200 mg/d for a mean 11.0 weeks caused caused a significant 54% change in excretion to 670 ng/mmol creatinine at night and 505 ng/mmol creatinine during the day *752*

Dehydroepiandrosterone *Plasma Increase Physiological* In 90 dyslipidemic men (serum cholesterol greater than or equal to 5.2 mmol/L) treatment with gemfirozil for one year caused nonsignificant change from mean baseline of 8.0 ± 4.2 nmol/L to 10.2 ± 7.3 nmol/L *2513*

Dehydroepiandrosterone Sulfate
Plasma Increase Physiological In 90 dyslipidemic men (serum cholesterol greater than or equal to 5.2 mmol/L) treatment with gemfirozil for one year caused significant increase from mean baseline of 5.8 ± 2.8 μmol/L to 8.0 ± 5.0 μmol/L *2513*

Eosinophils *Blood Increase Physiological* Eosinophilia may occur as a side effect *4524*

Epinephrine *Plasma No Effect Physiological* In 21 men with combined hyperlipidemia treatment with 1200 mg/d for a mean 11.0 weeks caused caused a nonsignificant change from mean baseline of 0.13 ± 0.02 nmol/L to 0.14 ± 0.02 nmol/L *752*
Urine Decrease Physiological In 21 men with combined hyperlipidemia treatment with 1200 mg/d for a mean 11.0 weeks caused caused a significant change from mean baseline of 3.4 ± 0.9 nmol/mmol creatinine to 2.5 ± 0.8 nmol/mmol creatinine *752*

Euglobulin Lysis Time *Blood Decrease Physiological* Insignificant reduction from mean of 37 min to 33.5 min in 22 survivors of a myocardial infarction who had received 1200 mg daily for 8 weeks but reduction in placebo group even greater (from 38 to 29 minutes) *157*

Factor VII *Plasma Decrease Physiological* In 20 patients with primary hypertriglyceridemia treatment with 1200 mg/d caused significant decrease from mean baseline of 132.0 ± 19.5% to 115.8 ± 16.8% after 4 weeks and 106.8 ± 15.6% after 12 weeks *296* In 20 patients with primary hypertriglyceridemia treatment with 1200 mg/d for 12 weeks caused significant decrease from mean baseline of 128.30 ± 20.17% to 107.10 ± 17.87% *295*

Factor VII Activity *Plasma Decrease Physiological* Significant reduction observed in 27 hyperlipidemic patients treated with 1200 mg daily for 12 weeks *5849*
Plasma No Effect Physiological In 63 men with coronary heart disease mean activity unaffected by disease *6457*

Factor VII Antigen *Plasma No Effect Physiological* In men with coronary heart disease no significant effect observed on concentration *6457*

Factor VII Coagulant *Plasma Decrease Physiological* Significant reduction observed in 27 hyperlipidemic patients treated with 1200 mg daily for 12 weeks *5849*

Factor VII Phospholipid Complex
Plasma Decrease Physiological In a reported study of patients with myocardial infarction gemfibrozil decreased mean concentration significantly from 47.5% to 19.0% after 8 weeks treatment *5585* Reduction (60%) from mean of 47.5% to 19.0% in 22 survivors of myocardial infarction treated with 1200 mg daily for 8 weeks compared with 18% reduction in placebo group *157*

Fibrinogen *Plasma Decrease Physiological* In 20 patients with primary hypertriglyceridemia treatment with 1200 mg/d caused significant decrease from mean baseline of 625.7 ± 133.6 mg/dL to 512.1 ± 119.6 mg/dL after 4 weeks and 472.5 ± 99.5 mg/dL after 12 weeks *296* In 51 hypercholesterolemic patients (cholesterol concentration greater than 6.5 mmol/L) treatment with 1200 mg/d gemfibrozil caused significant reduction from mean baseline concentration of 3.44 g/L to 3.01 g/L *1317* In 24 patients with hypertriglyceridemia greater than 5.67 mmol/L treatment with 1200 mg/d gemfibrozil caused an insignificant reduction in concentration from 3.76 ± 1.20 g/L to 3.41 ± 0.81 g/L *5800* In 20 patients with primary hypertriglyceridemia treatment with 1200 mg/d for 12 weeks caused significant reduction from mean baseline of 642.30 ± 125.85 mg/dL to 431.71 ± 93.21 mg/dL *295*
Plasma Increase Physiological Mean increase of 17.6% observed in 27 hyperlipidemic patients treated with 1200 mg daily for 12 weeks *5849* In a reported study of patients with myocardial infarction gemfibrozil increased mean concentration nonsignificantly from 2.35 g/L to 2.95 g/L after 8 weeks treatment *5585* In 63 men with coronary heart disease mean concentration determined gravimetrically increased by 5 (2 to 9)% *6457* Increase from mean of 2.35 g/L to 2.95 g/L in 22 survivors of myocardial infarction who received 1200 mg daily for 8 weeks but not significantly different from those who did not receive drug *157*
Plasma No Effect Physiological Gemfibrozil has no effect on the plasma fibrinogen concentration *3668* In reported studies gemfibrozil had no significant effect on concentration *5585*

Fibrinopeptide A *Plasma Decrease Physiological* In 20 patients with primary hypertriglyceridemia treatment with 1200 mg/d for 12 weeks caused significant decrease from mean baseline of 7.64 ± 3.10 ng/mL to 3.55 ± 1.83 ng/mL *295*
Plasma No Effect Physiological No significant effect observed with treatment in 63 men with coronary heart disease *6457*

Glucose *Serum Decrease Physiological* Significant reduction in basal glucose concentration in 10 patients with hypertriglyceridemia and abnormal glucose tolerance but no change observed in 10 with normal glucose tolerance following one month treatment with 1200 mg daily *5990* By enhancing action of glyburide gemfibrozil may cause clinical hypoglycemia *3668*
Serum Increase Physiological Mean increase of 11.5% in 52 noninsulin dependent diabetics with primary hypercholesterolemia treated with 20 mg daily for 24 weeks *2215*
Serum No Effect Physiological In 20 patients with primary hypertriglyceridemia treatment with 1200 mg/d caused no significant change over 12 weeks *296*

HDL_2-Cholesterol *Serum No Effect Physiological* In 14 men with low HDL-cholesterol concentrations treatment with gemfibrozil for 3 months had no significant effect on plasma concentration (change from 8.4 ± 1.6 mg/dL to 8.1 ± 1.4 mg/dL) *4049* No significant change in 9 patients with familial hypercholesterolemia treated with 1200 mg daily for 16 weeks *1930* In 10 patients with noninsulin-dependent diabetes mellitus treatment for 3 months caused nonsignificant change from mean baseline of 0.60 ± 0.16 mmol/L to 0.61 ± 0.12 mmol/L *3006* In 12 healthy men treatment with 600 mg/d for 10 days caused nonsignificant change from mean baseline of 15.7 ± 5.6 mg/dL to 16.8 ± 5.9 mg/dL and to 15.9 ± 4.9 mg/dL after 1200 mg/d for 10 days *2724*

HDL_2-Phospholipids *Serum No Effect Physiological* In 10 patients with noninsulin-dependent diabetes mellitus treatment for 3 months caused nonsignificant change from mean baseline of 35.5 ± 11.4 mg/dL to 35.3 ± 13.1 mg/dL *3006*

HDL_2-Triglycerides *Serum No Effect Physiological* In 10 patients with noninsulin-dependent diabetes mellitus treatment for 3 months caused nonsignificant change from mean baseline of 0.14 ± 0.03 mmol/L to 0.12 ± 0.05 mmol/L *3006*

HDL_3-Cholesterol *Serum Increase Physiological* In 14 men with low total HDL-cholesterol concentration treatment with gemfibrozil for 3 months as associated with slight increase in concentration (increase from 22.1 ± 1.1 mg/dL to 24.9 ± 1.2 mg/dL) *4049* Main HDL subfraction affected in study of 60 participants in Helsinki heart study *3777* Significant increase from mean baseline concentration of 0.52 mmol/L to 0.65 mmol/L in 14 hypertriglyceridemic patients after treatment with 1200 mg daily for 24 weeks *4564* In 10 patients with noninsulin-dependent diabetes mellitus treatment for 3 months caused significant change from mean baseline of 0.55 ± 0.12 mmol/L to 0.64 ± 0.13 mmol/L *3006*

Serum No Effect Physiological No significant change in 9 patients with familial hypercholesterolemia treated with 1200 mg daily for 16 weeks *1930* In 12 healthy men treatment with up to 1200 mg/d for 10 days caused nonsignificant change from mean baseline of 27.6 ± 4.1 mg/dL *2724*

HDL_3-Phospholipids *Serum Increase Physiological* In 10 patients with noninsulin-dependent diabetes mellitus treatment for 3 months caused significant change from mean baseline of 35.9 mg/dL to 43.1 ± 7.8 mg/dL *3006*

HDL_3-Triglycerides *Serum No Effect Physiological* In 10 patients with noninsulin-dependent diabetes mellitus treatment for 3 months caused no change from mean baseline of 0.11 ± 0.07 mmol/L *3006*

HDL-Apolipoprotein A-I *Serum Increase Physiological* Significant increase of 8% observed in 10 patients with type IV hyperlipoproteinemia when treated with 1200 mg/d for 3 months *4919*

Serum No Effect Physiological Nonsignificant increase of 7% observed in 10 patients with type IIb hyperlipoproteinemia when treated with 1200 mg/d for 3 months *4919*

HDL-Cholesterol *Serum Decrease Physiological* In the Helsinki Heart Study of 4,081 asymptomatic middle-aged male patients with primary dyslipidemia treatment with 1200 mg/d caused mean decrease of 14% *3115*

Serum Increase Physiological Significant increase from mean of 40 mg/dL to 50 mg/dL in 10 patients with hypertriglyceridemia and normal glucose tolerance and from 37 mg/dL to 44 mg/dL in 10 with abnormal glucose tolerance when treated with 1200 mg daily for 1 month *5990* 12% increase observed in 22 survivors of a myocardial infarction after treatment with 1200 mg daily for 8 weeks but not statistically different from control population *157* Significant increase observed in 8 type III hyperlipoproteinemic patients treated for up to 28 months *3330* Gemfibrozil increases plasma HDL-cholesterol concentration *3668* Small but significant mean increase observed in 27 hyperlipidemic patients treated with 1200 mg daily for 12 weeks *5849* Of fibrates gemfibrozil appears to be most effective in increasing HDL concentration *5586* Raised concentration by 26% in patients with type IIb hyperlipoproteinemia *1644* Increase by 36% in 6 patients with primary familial endogenous hypertriglyceridemia from baseline values. Synthetic rates of apo A-I and apo A-II increased by 27% and 34% respectively *5193* Significant increase in 20 hyperlipidemic out patients treated with 1200 mg daily for 90 days *5177* In 55 ambulatory middle-aged men treatment with 1200 mg/d for 3 months caused significant 11% increase from mean baseline of 0.90 ± 0.13 mmol/L to 1.01 ± 0.18 mmol/L *5143* Significant increase (27%) observed in 10 patients with type IV hyperlipoproteinemia when treated with 1200 mg/d for 3 months. 11% increase observed in 10 patients with type IIb hyperlipoproteinemia *4919* Significant increase from mean baseline concentration from about 0.6 mmol/L to about 0.8 mmol/L in 14 patients with hypertriglyceridemia treated with 1200 mg daily for 24 weeks *4564* Increase by 50% in 18 patients with chronic renal failure treated with 1200 mg/d for 28 weeks. Simultaneous activation of postheparin plasma lipoprotein and hepatic lipases. Effects reversed when drug discontinued *4550* Significant increase of 11.0% in 8 hypercholesterolemic patients treated with 1.2 g/day for 6 weeks and of 23.3% in 19 patients with serum cholesterols above 7.8 mmol/L treated with 1.2 g/day for 6 weeks *4387* Slight increase from mean of 51.0 mg/dL to 54.2 mg/dL in 9 patients with familial hypercholesterolemia after treatment with 1200 mg daily for 16 weeks *1930* By more than 10% in extensive 5 year double-blinded trial with 2,000 men receiving 600 mg drug twice daily *1962* Mean increase of 21.3% in 51 noninsulin dependent diabetics with primary hypercholesterolemia treated with 1200 mg daily for 24 weeks *2215* In 24 patients with hypertriglyceridemia greater than 5.67 mmol/L treatment with 1200 mg/d gemfibrozil caused significant increase in concentration from 0.66 ± 0.24 mmol/L to 0.80 ± 0.23 mmol/L *5800* Increased apo A-I and apo Apo A-II synthesis. Increased activity of lipoprotein lipase by stimulation of muscle lipoprotein lipase synthesis, alteration of the capillary surface and stimulation of apo C-II synthesis *264* In 109 patients with dyslipidemia treatment with 1200 mg/d for 12 months caused increase from mean baseline of 1.24 ± 0.37 mmol/L to 1.45 ± 0.42 mmol/L *3254* In 17 male patients with established atherosclerosis and high triglycerides and low high-density lipoprotein cholesterol treated 1200 mg/d for 12 weeks significant change from mean baseline of 0.82 mmol/L to 0.99 mmol/L observed *3198* Increased by lovastatin in patients with hyperlipidemia type IIb both with serum cholesterol below and above 7.8 mmol/L but gemfibrozil 600 mg b.i.d. more effective than 20 mg/d lovastatin for patients with lower cholesterol and 40 mg/d for higher *4387* In 21 men with combined hyperlipidemia treatment with 1200 mg/d for a mean 11.0 weeks caused caused a significant increase from mean baseline of 0.78 ± 0.04 mmol/L to 0.93 ± 0.04 mmol/L *752* In 27 patients with severe hypertriglyceridemia treatment with 1200 mg/d for 6 weeks caused significant increase from median baseline of 0.71 ± 0.22 mmol/L to 0.89 ± 0.33 mmol/L *3086* In 10 patients with noninsulin-dependent diabetes mellitus treatment for 3 months caused significant change from mean baseline of 1.15 ± 0.19 mmol/L to 1.25 ± 0.21 mmol/L *3006* In 90 dyslipidemic men (serum cholesterol greater than or equal to 5.2 mmol/L) treatment with gemfirozil for one year caused significant increase from 1.25 ± 0.31 mmol/L to 1.39 ± 0.34 mmol/L *2513* Significant increase from mean baseline concentration of 1.1 mmol/L to 1.3 mmol/L in 18 patients with familial combined hyperlipidemia treated with 1200 mg/d for 6 weeks *4367* Mean increase of 16% in 75 patients with primary hypercholesterolemia treated with mean dose of 1200 mg/day for 12 weeks *6031* Mean increase of 18% observed in 18 patients with familial hypercholesterolemia when treated with 1200 mg/d for 6 weeks. Addition of 4 g cholestyramine/d to regime had no further effect *4367* In 73 patients with type IIa hyperlipoproteinemia treatment with 1200 mg/d for 12 weeks caused mean increase of about 6% *6033* Mean increase of 18% from 1.1 mmol/L to 1.3 mmol/L observed in 18 patients with familial hypercholesterolemia when treated with 1200 mg/d for 6 weeks. Addition of 4 g cholestyramine/d to regime had no further effect *4367* In 8 type IIb hyperlipoproteinemic patients with moderately increased total cholesterol treatment with 1200 mg/d for 6 weeks caused mean increase of 11%: treatment of 19 patients with high cholesterol caused mean increase of 23% *6033* In 20 patients with primary hypertriglyceridemia treatment with 1200 mg/d caused significant increase from mean baseline of 33.3 ± 8.9 mg/dL to 38.9 ± 5.4 mg/dL after 4 weeks and to 39.5 ± 4.0 mg/dL after 12 weeks *296* In 8 type IIb hyperlipoprtoeinemic patients with moderately increased total cholesterol treatment with 1200 mg/d for 6 weeks caused mean increase of 11%: treatment of 19 patients with high cholesterol caused mean increase of 23% *6033* In 14 men with low HDL-cholesterol concentrations treated with gemfibrozil for 3 months total HDL-cholesterol concentration significantly increased by 9.2% (from 31.6 ± 0.9 mg/dL to 34.5 ± 1.1 mg/dL) *4049* In 61 middle-aged men with low HDL concentration treatment increased mean HDL-cholesterol concentration by 10% *6219* In 17 patients treatment with 1200 mg/d caused concentration to increase from mean baseline of 0.88 ± 0.09 mmol/L to 1.04 ± 0.13 mmol/L *3905* In 295 patients with NIDDM treatment with 1200 mg/d caused significant increase from mean baseline of 37 mg/dL of 8.4% after 4 weeks and by 12.2% after 12 weeks *6268* Concentration observed to be increased in 60 patients in Helsinki heart study *3777* In 63-69 patients with hypercholesterolemia treatment for 12 weeks caused significant increase from mean baseline of 1.20 ± 0.05 mmol/L to 1.39 ± 0.04 mmol/L (15.2%) *6463* Mean increase of 11% in dyslipidemic men treated over 5 years *3773* In 13 patients with type V hyperlipidemia treatment with 1200 mg daily for 8 weeks caused increase from mean of 0.62 mmol/L (with placebo) to 0.85 mmol/L (without placebo) *3448* In 8 patients with familial dysbetalipoproteinemia treatment with 1200 mg/d for 1 month caused significant increase from mean baseline of 0.95 mmol/L to 1.22

Gemfibrozil *(continued)*

HDL-Cholesterol *(continued)*

mmol/L *6655* In 30 patients with familial defective apolipoprotein B-100 treatment with 1200 mg/d for 8 weeks caused a significant change from mean baseline of 1.30 ± 0.07 mmol/L to 1.42 ± 0.08 mmol/L *2445* In 5 patients with hypertriglyceridemia treatment with 1200 mg/d for 8 weeks caused nonsignificant increase to 31 ± 10 mg/dL compared with 24 ± 5 mg/dL in those receiving placebo and in 5 patients with combined hyperlipidemia concentration increased to 38 ± 11 mg/dL versus 33 ± 10 mg/dL in those receiving placebo *6589* Mean concentration of 32.2 ± 13.2 mg/dL in 20 patients with primary hypertriglyceridemia treated with 1200 mg/d for 12 weeks caused significant increase to 38.2 ± 5.7 mg/dL *295* Treatment of 48 patients with primary hypercholesterolemia with 900 mg/d for 16 weeks caused mean increase of 15% whereas treatment with 600 mg b.i.d. caused mean decrease of 18.7% *297*

Serum No Effect Physiological In 12 healthy men treatment with 600 mg/d for 10 days caused non significant reduction from mean baseline of 46.8 ± 8.2 mg/dL to 44.5 ± 7.5 mg/dL and to 44.9 ± 5 mg/dL after 1200 mg/d for 10 days *2724* In 38 patients with primary hypercholesterolemia treatment with diet and gemfibrozil caused nonsignificant change from mean baseline of 1.31 ± 0.04 mmol/L to 1.37 ± 0.05 mmol/L after 6 months, 1.42 ± 0.05 mmol/L after 12 months and 1.32 ± 0.05 mmol/L after 24 months *4153* No significant effect observed in 25 patients with type IIa hyperlipidemia treated with 900 mg/d for 4 weeks *331* In 38 renal allograft patients who had persistent hyperlipidemia and stable renal function treatment with up to 1200 mg/d caused nonsignificant change from mean baseline of 48.8 ± 12.0 mg/dL (1.26 ± 0.31 mmol/L) to 51.9 ± 17.0 mg/dL(1.34 ± 0.44 mmol/L) *962* In 12 type IIa hyperlipidemic patients treatment with gemfibrozil for 12 weeks caused nonsignificant change from mean baseline of 65.1 ± 17.8 mg/dL to 65.8 ± 15.7 mg/dL *1929*

HDL-Cholesterol:LDL-Cholesterol Ratio

Serum Increase Physiological Insignificant increase of 12.7% in 8 hypercholesterolemic patients treated with 20 mg daily for 6 weeks but significant increase of 43.5% in 19 patients with serum cholesterols initially above 7.8 mmol/L treated with 1.2 g/day for 6 weeks *4387*

HDL-Phospholipids *Serum Increase Physiological* In 10 patients with noninsulin-dependent diabetes mellitus treatment for 3 months caused nonsignificant change from mean baseline of 71.5 ± 15.0 mg/dL to 78.4 ± 18.9 mg/dL *3006*

HDL-Triglycerides *Serum Decrease Physiological* In 21 men with combined hyperlipidemia treatment with 1200 mg/d for a mean 11.0 weeks caused caused a significant decrease from mean baseline of 0.34 ± 0.03 mmol/L to 0.22 ± 0.03 mmol/L *752*

Serum No Effect Physiological In 10 patients with noninsulin-dependent diabetes mellitus treatment for 3 months caused nonsignificant change from mean baseline of 0.25 ± 0.08 mmol/L to 0.23 ± 0.06 mmol/L *3006* In 8 patients with familiail dysbetalipoproteinemia treatment with 1200 mg/d for 1 month caused nonsignificant change from mean baseline of 0.31 mmol/L to 0.27 mmol/L *6655*

Hematocrit *Blood Decrease Physiological* Anemia may occur as a side effect *4524*

Hemoglobin *Blood Decrease Physiological* Anemia may occur as a side effect *4524*

Hemoglobin A_{1c} *Blood Increase Physiological* In 295 patients with NIDDM treatment with 1200 mg/d caused nonsignificant increase from mean baseline of 6.8% to 7.31% (8.6%) *6268* Nonsignificant mean increase of 4.3% in 49 noninsulin dependent diabetics with primary hypercholesterolemia treated with 1200 mg daily for 24 weeks *2215*

High Density Lipoproteins *Serum Increase Physiological* Significant increase in 20 hyperlipidemic outpatients treated with 1200 mg daily for 90 days *5177*

HMW β-Thromboglobulin *Plasma No Effect Physiological* In 21 men with combined hyperlipidemia treatment with 1200 mg/d for a mean 11.0 weeks caused caused a nonsignificant change in concentration *752*

Urine Increase Physiological In 21 men with combined hyperlipidemia treatment with 1200 mg/d for a mean 11.0 weeks caused caused a nonsignificant change in excretion from 2.4 and 2.5 ng/mmol creatinine during the night and day respectively with placebo and 3.8 and 2.7 ng/mmol creatinine at night and during the day with gemfibrozil *752*

IDL-Cholesterol *Serum Decrease Physiological* In 8 patients with familial dysbetalipoproteinemia treatment with 1200 mg/d for 1 month caused significant decrease from mean baseline of 2.47 mmol/L to 1.62 mmol/L *6655* Nonsignificant reduction from mean baseline concentration of 0.34 mmol/L to 0.23 mmol/L after treatment for 24 weeks with 1200 mg daily in 14 hypertriglyceridemic patients *4564*

IDL-Triglycerides *Serum Decrease Physiological* Significant reduction from mean baseline concentration of 0.11 mmol/L to 0.07 mmol/L in 14 hypertriglyceridemic patients treated with 1200 mg daily for 24 weeks *4564* In 8 patients with familial dysbetalipoproteinemia treatment with 1200 mg/d for 1 month caused significant decrease from mean baseline of 0.70 mmol/L to 0.34 mmol/L *6655*

Insulin *Plasma No Effect Physiological* No effect observed on fasting and post oral glucose tolerance test concentrations in 10 hypertriglyceridemic patients with normal glucose tolerance and 10 with abnormal glucose tolerance after 1 month treatment with 1200 mg daily *5990*

LDL-Apolipoprotein B *Serum Decrease Physiological* Significant reduction of 19% observed in 10 patients with type IIb hyperlipoproteinemia when treated with 1200 mg/d for 3 months *4919*

Serum No Effect Physiological In 8 patients with familial dysbetalipoproteinemia treatment with 1200 mg/d for 1 month caused nonsignificant change from mean baseline of 55 mg/dL to 56 mg/dL *6655* Insignificant increase of 1% observed in 10 patients with type IV hyperlipoproteinemia when treated with 1200 mg/d for 3 months *4919*

LDL-Cholesterol *Serum Decrease Physiological* Mean decrease of 11% over 5 years in dyslipidemic men, most marked in Fredrickson type IIa and least in type IV *3773* During treatment for 28 months significant reduction observed in 8 patients with type III hyperlipoproteinemia *3330* Observed reduction dependent on triglyceride concentration in cohort of 60 people in Helsinki heart study *3777* In 109 patients with dyslipidemia treatment with 1200 mg/d for 12 months caused reduction from mean baseline of 5.47 ± 1.01 mmol/L to 4.32 ± 0.97 mmol/L *3254* In 17 patients treated with 1200 mg/d for 6 weeks concentration significantly reduced from mean baseline of 4.67 ± 0.36 mmol/L to 4.23 ± 0.59 mmol/L *3905* Mean reduction of 28% observed in 25 patients with type IIa hyperlipidemia treated with 900 mg/d for 4 weeks *331* In 38 patients with primary hypercholesterolemia treatment with diet and gemfibrozil caused significant change from mean baseline of 5.8 ± 0.27 mmol/L to 4.9 ± 0.17 mmol/L after 6 months, 4.7 ± 0.19 mmol/L after 12 months and 4.4 ± 0.16 mmol/L after 24 months *4153* In 18 patients with familial combined hypercholesterolemia addition of 4 g cholestyramine/d to a regime of 1200 mg gemfibrozil/d for 6 weeks caused further reduction of 9% to already reduced concentration *4367* Nonsignificant reduction from mean baseline concentration of 5.4 mmol/L to 4.7 mmol/L in 18 patients with familial combined hyperlipidemia treated with 1200 mg/d for 6 weeks *4367* In 8 patients with type IIb hyperlipidemia and serum cholesterol 6.2-7.8 mmol/L treatment with 1200 mg/d for 6 weeks caused increase of 1% but treatment of 19 patients with serum cholesterol above 7.9 mmol/L caused mean decrease of 12% *4387* In 12 healthy men treatment for 10 days with 600 mg/d caused nonsignificant decrease from mean baseline of 105.1 ± 19.8 mg/dL to 103.4 ± 14.7 mg/dL and to 91.6 ± 15.1 mg/dL after 1200 mg/d for 10 days *2724* Significant reduction from mean of 324 mg/dL to 255 mg/dL in 9 patients with familial hypercholesterolemia after treatment with 1200 mg daily for 16 weeks *1930* Significant reduction of 16% observed in 10 patients with type IIb hyperlipoproteinemia when treated with 1200 mg/d for 3 months *4919* Treatment of 48 patients with primary hyperlipidemia with 900 mg/d for 16 weeks caused mean decrease of 19.9% whereas treatment with 600 mg b.i.d. caused mean decrease of 17.6% *297* In 90 dyslipidemic men (serum cholesterol greater than or equal to 5.2 mmol/L) treatment with gemfirozil for one year caused significant reduction from 5.39 ± 0.90 mmol/L to 4.55 ± 1.12 mmol/L *2513* In 55 middle-aged ambulatory men treatment with 1200 mg/d for 3 months caused reduction from mean baseline of 4.19 ± 0.85

mmol/L to 4.03 ± 0.83 mmol/L *5143* Significant reduction in 20 hyperlipidemic out patients with 1200 mg daily for 90 days *5177* Mean reduction of 19.9% observed in 27 hyperlipidemic patients treated with 1200 mg daily for 12 weeks *5849* Mean reduction of 17% in 75 patients with primary hypercholesterolemia treated with mean dose of 1200 mg/day for 12 weeks *6031* In 73 type IIa hyperlipoproteinemic patients with serum cholesterol greater than 7.8 mmol/L treatment with 1200 mg/d for 12 weeks caused mean reduction of about 18% *6033* In 8 type IIb hyperlipidemic patients with moderately increased serum cholesterol treatment with 1200 mg/d for 6 weeks had no significant effect but in 19 patients with high cholesterol caused mean reduction of 12% *6033* Slight reduction observed with treatment in 61 middle-aged men with low HDL *6219* In 10 patients with type IIa treatment with 1200 mg/d for 8 weeks caused mean reduction of 15.5% *6225* *6224* In 38 renal allograft patients who had persistent hyperlipidemia and stable renal function treatment with up to 1200 mg/d caused significant change from mean baseline of 203.8 ± 37.4 mg/dL (5.28 ± 0.97 mmol/L) to 174.5 ± 42.5 mg/dL(4.52 ± 1.10 mmol/L) *962* In 63-69 patients with hypercholesterolemia treatment for 12 weeks caused significant reduction from mean baseline of 5.18 ± 0.13 mmol/L to 4.29 ± 0.11 mmol/L (16.8%) *6463* Increase by 10% in extensive 5 year double-blinded trial with 2,000 men receiving 600 mg drug twice daily *1962* In 30 patients with familial defective apolipoprotein B-100 treatment with 1200 mg/d for 8 weeks caused a significant change from mean baseline of 6.16 ± 0.25 mmol/L to 5.83 ± 0.23 mmol/L *2445* In 12 type IIa hyperlipidemic patients treated with gemfibrozil for 12 weeks caused significant reduction from mean baseline of 197.6 ± 36.6 mg/dL to 154.2 ± 22.9 mg/dL *1929* In the Helsinki Heart Study of 4,081 asymptomatic middle-aged male patients with primary dyslipidemia treatment with 1200 mg/d caused mean decrease of 10% *3115* Gemfibrozil has a variable effect on plasma LDL-cholesterol concentration *3668*

Serum Increase Physiological Gemfibrozil has a variable effect on plasma LDL-cholesterol concentration *3668* In 21 men with combined hyperlipidemia treatment with 1200 mg/d for a mean 11.0 weeks caused caused an insignificant increase from mean baseline of 4.2 ± 0.4 mmol/L to 4.6 ± 0.3 mmol/L *752* In 295 patients with NIDDM treatment with 1200 mg/d caused significant increase from mean baseline of 145 mg/dL to 146 mg/dL after 12 and 20 weeks although no change observed after 4 weeks *6268* Significant increase observed in 15 patients with familial type IV hyperlipoproteinemia in response to ingestion of 1200 mg daily *1103* Nonsignificant increase observed from mean baseline concentration of about 3.2 mmol/L to 4.3 mmol/L at 12 weeks and 3.6 mmol/L at 24 weeks after treatment with 1200 mg daily in 14 patients with hypertriglyceridemia *4564* In 13 patients with type V hyperlipidemia treatment with 1200 mg daily for 8 weeks caused increase from mean of 1.84 mmol/L (with placebo) to 3.08 mmol/L with gemfibrozil *3448*

Serum No Effect Physiological Had no effect on concentration in patients with type IIb hyperlipoproteinemia *1644* In 17 male patients with established atherosclerosis and high triglycerides and low high-density lipoprotein cholesterol treated 1200 mg/d for 12 weeks nonsignificant change from mean baseline of 4.92 mmol/L to 4.95 mmol/L observed *3198* Gemfibrozil has a variable effect on plasma LDL-cholesterol concentration *3668* In 8 patients with familial dysbetalipoproteinemia treatment with 1200 mg/d for 1 month caused nonsignificant change from mean baseline of 1.87 mmol/L to 1.86 mmol/L *6655* Insignificant reduction of 1.1% in 38 patients with noninsulin dependent diabetes and primary hypercholesterolemia after treatment for 24 weeks with 1200 mg daily *2215* In 14 men with low HDL-cholesterol concentrations treatment with gemfibrozil for 3 months had no significant effect on concentration (change from 94.8 ± 3.7 mg/dL to 98.1 ± 4.3 mg/dL) *4049* Insignificant increase of 2% observed in 10 patients with type IV hyperlipoproteinemia when treated with 1200 mg/d for 3 months *4919* Insignificant increase of 1.1% in 8 patients with hypercholesterolemia treated with 1.2 g/day for 6 weeks but significant decrease of 12.3% in 19 patients with higher serum cholesterols treated with 40 mg/day for 6 weeks *4387*

LDL-Cholesterol:HDL-Cholesterol Ratio

Serum Decrease Physiological In 17 patients treatment with 1200 mg/d for 6 weeks caused mean ratio to decrease from 5.36 ± 0.58 to 4.14 ± 0.84 *3905*

LDL-Triglycerides *Serum Decrease Physiological* Significant reduction of 23% observed in 10 patients with type IIb hyperlipoproteinemia when treated with 1200 mg/d for 3 months *4919* In 8 patients with familial dysbetalipoproteinemia treatment with 1200 mg/d for 1 month caused significant decrease from mean baseline of 0.41 mmol/L to 0.21 mmol/L *6655* In 21 men with combined hyperlipidemia treatment with 1200 mg/d for a mean 11.0 weeks caused caused a significant decrease from mean baseline of 0.51 ± 0.04 mmol/L to 0.37 ± 0.03 mmol/L *752*

Serum No Effect Physiological Insignificant increase of 2% observed in 10 patients with type IV hyperproteinemia when treated with 1200 mg/d for 3 months *4919*

Lecithin:Cholesterol Acyltransferase

Serum No Effect Physiological In 9 patients with primary hypertriglyceridemia treatment for 8 weeks had no significant effect *541*

Leukocytes *Blood Decrease Physiological* In 63 men with coronary heart disease mean concentration decreased by 6 (2 to 10)% with treatment for 2 months *6457* Leukopenia may occur as a side effect *4524* In 21 men with combined hyperlipidemia treatment with 1200 mg/d for a mean 11.0 weeks caused caused a nonsignificant decrease from mean baseline of 7.0 ± 0.5 x 10^9/L to 6.4 ± 0.4 x 10^9/L *752*

Lipase, Hepatic *Serum Increase Physiological* In 10 patients with noninsulin-dependent diabetes mellitus treatment for 3 months caused significant increase from mean baseline of 36.2 ± 20.4 μmol FFA/mL/min by 18.8% *3006* In 12 healthy men treatment with up to 1200 mg/d for 10 days caused significant increase to about 210 mU/mL from mean baseline of 140 mU/mL *2724*

Lipid Peroxide *Serum Decrease Physiological* Significant reduction observed in 27 hyperlipidemic patients treated with 1200 mg daily for 12 weeks *5849*

Lipoprotein Lipase *Serum Increase Physiological* In 12 healthy men treatment with up to 1200 mg/d for 10 days caused significant increase from mean baseline of 520 mU/mL to 675 mU/mL *2724*

Lipoprotein Lp(a) *Serum Increase Physiological* In 5 patients with hypertriglyceridemia treatment with 1200 mg/d for 8 weeks caused significant increase to 19.2 ± 29.3 mg/dL compared with 7.6 ± 8.0 mg/dL in those receiving placebo *6589* In 21 men with combined hyperlipidemia treatment with 1200 mg/d for a mean 11.0 weeks caused caused an insignificant change from mean baseline of 88 mg/L to 112 mg/L *752*

Serum No Effect Physiological In 12 type IIa hyperlipidemic patients treatment with gemfibrozil for 12 weeks caused nonsignificant change from mean baseline of 78.2 mg/dL to 76.2 mg/dL *1929* In 17 male patients with established atherosclerosis and high triglycerides and low high-density lipoprotein cholesterol treated 1200 mg/d for 12 weeks nonsignificant change from mean baseline of 26.13 g/L to 21.56 g/L observed *3198* In 5 patients with combined hyperlipidemia treatment with 1200 mg/d for 8 weeks caused insignificant change to 8.2 ± 2.8 mg/dL compared with 7.5 ± 2.0 mg/dL in those receiving placebo *6589* In 14 men with low plasma HDL-cholesterol concentration treatment with gemfibrozil for 3 months had no significant on plasma concentration (insignificant change from 0.09 ± 0.03 g/L to 0.11 ± 0.02 g/L) *4049*

Myoglobin *Urine Increase Physiological* May occur as a side effect, particularly when administered with lovastain *4524*

Norepinephrine *Plasma No Effect Physiological* In 21 men with combined hyperlipidemia treatment with 1200 mg/d for a mean 11.0 weeks caused caused a nonsignificant change from mean baseline of 1.68 ± 0.21 nmol/L to 1.72 ± 0.17 nmol/L *752*

Urine Increase Physiological In 21 men with combined hyperlipidemia treatment with 1200 mg/d for a mean 11.0 weeks caused caused a nonsignificant change from mean baseline of 34.8 ± 4.3 nmol/mmol creatinine to 42.6 ± 6.7 nmol/mmol creatinine *752*

Partial Thromboplastin Time

Plasma Increase Physiological By inhibiting p-hydroxylation of warfarin increases its plasma concentration, with a further decrease in the synthesis of clotting factors, and may cause bleeding problems *3668*

Plasminogen *Plasma Decrease Physiological* In 20 patients with primary hypertriglyceridemia treatment with 1200 mg/d caused significant decrease from mean baseline of 14.5 ± 2.3 mg/dL to 12.8 ± 2.1 mg/dL after 4 weeks and 11.5 ± 1.8 mg/dL after 12 weeks *296*

Gemfibrozil *(continued)*

Plasminogen *(continued)*
Plasma No Effect Physiological In 20 patients with primary hypertriglyceridemia treatment with 1200 mg/d for 12 weeks caused significant decrease from mean baseline of 14.7 ± 2.1 mg/dL to 11.1 ± 2.1 mg/dL *295*

Plasminogen Activator Inhibitor
Plasma Decrease Physiological In 20 patients with primary hypertriglyceridemia treatment with 1200 mg/d for 12 weeks caused significant decrease from mean baseline of 8.6 ± 2.1 U/mL to 4.2 ± 2.6 U/mL *295* In 20 patients with primary hypertriglyceridemia treatment with 1200 mg/d caused significant decrease from mean baseline of 8.9 ± 1.9 U/mL to 5.6 ± 2.1 U/mL after 4 weeks and 5.0 ± 1.9 U/mL after 12 weeks *296*

Plasminogen Activator Inhibitor-1 Activity
Plasma No Effect Physiological In 27 patients with severe hypertriglyceridemia treatment with 1200 mg/d for 6 weeks caused nonsignificant reduction from median baseline of 36.5 IU/mL to 36.3 IU/mL *3086*

Plasminogen Activator Inhibitor-1 Antigen
Plasma Decrease Physiological In 27 patients with severe hypertriglyceridemia treatment with 1200 mg/d for 6 weeks caused nonsignificant reduction from median baseline of 48.3 ng/mL to 40.3 ng/mL *3086*

Plasminogen Activator Inhibitor Antigen
Plasma Decrease Physiological In a reported study of patients with myocardial infarction gemfibrozil decreased mean concentration significantly from 47 ng/mL to 38 ng/mL after 8 weeks treatment *5585*

Platelet Volume *Blood No Effect Physiological* In 21 men with combined hyperlipidemia treatment with 1200 mg/d for a mean 11.0 weeks caused caused no significant change from in median platelet volume mean baseline of 9.1 0.1 fL to 9.0 ± 0.1 fL *752*

Platelets *Blood Decrease Physiological* Thrombocytopenia reported as a possible side effect *4524*
Blood Increase Physiological In 21 men with combined hyperlipidemia treatment with 1200 mg/d for a mean 11.0 weeks caused caused a significant increase from mean baseline of 212 ± 10 x 10^9/L to 248 ± 13 x 10^9/L *752* In 63 male coronary heart disease patients treated for 2 months mean concentration increased by 11% (8 to 13%) *6457*
Blood No Effect Physiological No significant difference between survivors of myocardial infarction who received 1200 mg daily for 8 weeks and those who did not *157*

Postheparin Lipoprotein Lipase
Plasma Increase Physiological In 10 patients with noninsulin-dependent diabetes mellitus treatment for 3 months caused significant increase from mean baseline of 20.2 ± 5.9 µmol FFA/mL/min by 14.7% *3006*

Pravastatin *Urine Increase Physiological* In one single dose study in 20 healthy men administration of cyclosporine with pravastatin caused a significant increase in excretion of pravastatin *728*

Protein *Serum No Effect Physiological* In 24 patients with hypertriglyceridemia greater than 5.67 mmol/L treatment with 1200 mg/d gemfibrozil caused an significant change in concentration from 0.74 ± 0.06 g/L to 0.75 ± 0.05 g/L *5800*

Protein C *Plasma No Effect Physiological* In 20 patients with primary hypertriglyceridemia treatment with 1200 mg/d for 12 weeks caused nonsignificant change from mean baseline of 120.76 ± 23.15% to 123.22 ± 20.47% *295*

Prothrombin Fragment 1.2 *Plasma Decrease Physiological* In 63 male patients with coronary heart disease treatment with gemfibrozil for 2 months mean concentration decreased by 25% (12 to 37%) *6457*

Prothrombin Time *Plasma Increase Physiological* By displacing oral anticoagulants from their plasma protein binding sites gemfibrozil increases their plasma concentration and may cause bleeding problems *3668*

Retinol *Serum No Effect Physiological* In 35 patients with primary hypercholesterolemia treatment with diet and gemfibrozil caused nonsignificant increase from mean baseline of 3.57 ± 0.12 mmol/L to 3.73 ± 0.10 mmol/L after 24 months *4153*

Sex-Hormone Binding Globulin
Serum Decrease Physiological In 90 dyslipidemic men (serum cholesterol greater than or equal to 5.2 mmol/L) treatment with gemfirozil for one year caused nonsignificant change from mean baseline of 46.4 ± 18.7 nmol/L to 41.7 ± 14.6 nmol/L *2513*

SQ 31,906 *Serum Increase Physiological* In one single dose study in 20 healthy men administration of cyclosporine with pravastatin caused a significant increase in the AUC and peak concentration of the pravastatin metabolite SQ 31,906 *728*

Testosterone *Serum Decrease Physiological* In 90 dyslipidemic men (serum cholesterol greater than or equal to 5.2 mmol/L) treatment with gemfirozil for one year caused nonsignificant change from mean baseline of 18.8 ± 6.4 nmol/L to 17.7 ± 5.4 nmol/L *2513*

Tissue Plasminogen Activator
Plasma Decrease Physiological In 20 patients with primary hypertriglyceridemia treatment with 1200 mg/d caused significant reduction from mean baseline of 7.5 ± 2.2 ng/dL to 5.0 ± 1.7 ng/dL *295* In 20 patients with primary hypertriglycetridemia treatment with 1200 mg/d caused significant decrease from mean baseline of 7.7 ± 1.9 ng/dL to 6.4 ± 1.6 ng/dL after 4 weeks and 5.2 ± 1.7 ng/dL after 12 weeks *296*
Plasma Increase Physiological In 22 postmyocardial infarction survivors given 1200 mg daily for 8 weeks increased from mean of 4.9 IU/mL to 5.8 IU/mL but less than in placebo-treated control group (change from 5.0 to 8.6 IU/mL) *157*
Plasma No Effect Physiological In 27 patients with severe hypertriglyceridemia treatment with 1200 mg/d for 6 weeks caused nonsignificant reduction from median baseline of 1.06 IU/mL to 1.01 IU/mL *3086*

Tissue Plasminogen Activator Antigen
Plasma Decrease Physiological In 27 patients with severe hypertriglyceridemia treatment with 1200 mg/d for 6 weeks caused significant reduction from median baseline of 14.5 ng/mL to 12.5 ng/mL *3086*
Plasma No Effect Physiological Insignificant increase from mean of 35.0 µg/L to 37.2 µg/L in 22 postmyocardial infarction survivors treated with 1200 mg daily for 8 weeks compared with change from 44.8 µg/L to 43.8 µg/L in placebo-treated controls *157*

Tissue Plasminogen Activator Inhibitor
Plasma Increase Physiological In a reported study of patients with myocardial infarction gemfibrozil increased mean concentration significantly from 35.0 ng/mL to 37.2 ng/mL after 8 weeks treatment *5585*
Plasma No Effect Physiological Insignificant increase from mean of 25 IU/mL to 27 IU/mL in 22 postmyocardial infarction survivors treated with 1200 mg daily for 8 weeks compared with decrease from 28 to 24 IU/mL in placebo-treated controls *157*

Tissue Plasminogen Activator Inhibitor Antigen
Plasma Decrease Physiological Significant reduction in 22 postmyocardial infarction survivors from mean of 47 µg/L to 38 µg/L following treatment with 1200 mg daily for 8 weeks compared with reduction from 63 to 60 µg/L in placebo-treated controls *157*

Triglycerides *Serum Decrease Physiological* In 61 middle-aged men with low HDL concentration treatment effectively lowered plasma triglyceride concentration *6219* Marked decrease (about 33%) observed in 73 type IIa hyperlipoproteinemic patients treated with 1200 mg/d for 12 weeks *6033* In 8 type IIb hyperlipoproteinemic patients with moderately increased serum cholesterol treatment with 1200 mg/d for 6 weeks caused mean decrease of 34%: treatment of 19 patients with high serum cholesterol caused mean decrease of 49% *6033* Mean reduction of 32% in 75 patients with primary hypercholesterolemia treated with mean dose of 1200 mg/day for 12 weeks *6031* Significant reduction from mean of 277 mg/dL to 129 mg/dL in 10 hypertriglyceridemic patients with normal glucose tolerance and from 269 mg/dL to 152 mg/dL in 10 with abnormal glucose tolerance following 1200 mg gemfibrozil for one month *5990* In 6 patients with hypertriglyceridemia treatment with 1200 mg/d for 6 weeks caused significant reduction from mean baseline of 776 ± 573 mg/dL to 226 ± 82 mg/dL *5959* Mean reduction of 42.3% observed in 27 hyperlipidemic patients treated with 1200 mg daily for 12 weeks *5849* Increase by 54% in 6 patients with primary familial endogenous hypertriglyceridemia from baseline values. Synthetic rates of apo A-I and apo A-II increased by 27% and 34% respectively *5193* Significant reduction with 1200 mg daily for 90 days in 20 hyperlipidemic out patients *5177* In 55 ambulatory middle-aged men treated with 1200 mg/d for 3 months significant 41% decrease observed from mean baseline of 2.41 ± 1.30 mmol/L to 1.33 ± 0.84 mmol/L *5143* In 9 patients with primary hypertriglyceridemia treatment for 8 weeks caused significant reduction from mean of 6.05 mmol/L (2.48-10.99 mmol/L) to 1.76 mmol/L (1.16-11.90 mmol/L) *541* Mean reduction of 54% observed in 10 patients with type IIb hyperlipoproteinemia given 1200 mg/d for 3 months and of 60% in 10 type IV hyperlipoproteinemia patients *4919* Decrease from mean baseline concentration of 4.54 mmol/L to 2.02 mmol/L in 14 hypertriglyceridemic patients treated wuth 1200 mg daily for 24 weeks *4564* Decrease from mean baseline concentration of 4.54 mmol/L to 2.02 mmol/L in 14 hypertriglyceridemic patients treated with 1200 mg daily for 24 weeks *4564* Significant reduction of 34.1% in 8 hypercholesterolemic patients treated with 1.2 g/day for 6 weeks and 49.3% reduction in 19 hypercholesterolemic patients (cholesterol above 7.8 mmol/L) treated with 1.2 g/day for 6 weeks *4387* Significant reduction from mean baseline concentration of 3.4 mmol/L to 1.8 mmol/L (47%) in 18 patients with familial combined hyperlipidemia treated with 1200 mg/d for 6 weeks. Addition of 4 g/d cholestyramine to regime had no further effect *4367* Mean decrease of 47% observed in 18 patients with familial combined hypercholesterolemia when treated with 1200 mg/d for 6 weeks. Addition of 4 g cholestyramine/d to regime had no further effect *4367* In 38 patients with primary hypercholesterolemia treatment with diet and gemfibrozil caused significant change from mean baseline of 1.69 ± 0.12 mmol/L to 1.22 ± 0.11 mmol/L after 6 months, 1.23 ± 0.13 mmol/L after 12 months and 1.42 ± 0.15 mmol/L after 24 months *4153* In 14 men with low HDL-cholesterol concentrations treatment with gemfibrozil for 3 months caused significant decrease of plasma triglyceride concentration by 38% (from 102.0 mg/dL to 63.6 ± 3.3 mg/dL) *4049* In 17 patients treatment with 1200 mg/d for 6 weeks caused significant reduction from mean baseline of 2.02 ± 0.77 mmol/L to 0.98 ± 0.64 mmol/L *3905* Mean decrease of 35% in dyslipidemic men treated over 5 years *3773* In 13 patients with type V hyperlipidemia treatment for 8 weeks with 1200 mg daily caused reduction from mean of 21.03 mmol/L to 5.50 mmol/L *3448* In 20 patients with primary hypertriglyceridemia treatment with 1200 mg/d weeks caused significant decrease from mean baseline of 388.6 ± 103.4 mg/dL to 237.1 ± 88.2 mg/dL after 4 weeks and 205.7 ± 67.8 mg/dL after 12 weeks *296* Reduction observed in 25 patients with type IIa hyperlipidemia treated with 900 mg/d for 4 weeks *331* In 12 healthy men treatment with 600 mg/d for 10 days caused significant decrease from mean baseline of 75.3 ± 41.0 mg/dL to 47.1 ± 22.9 mg/dL and to 45.3 ± 19.7 mg/dL after 1200 mg/d for 10 days *2724* In 295 patients with NIDDM treatment with 1200 mg/d caused significant reduction from mean baseline of 273 mg/dL to 177 mg/dL after 20 weeks. Decrease of 31.6% observed after 4 weeks *6268* In 63 male patients with coronary heart disease treated with gemfibrozil for 2 months mean nonfasting concentration decreased by 43% (34 to 51%) during active treatment *6457* In 63-69 patients with hypercholesterolemia treatment for 12 weeks caused significant decrease from mean baseline of 1.80 ± 0.08 mmol/L to 1.03 ± 0.05 mmol/L (42.2%) *6463* Mean reduction of 41.1% observed in 10 patients with type IV hyperlipidemia treated with 1200 mg/d for 8 weeks *6225* *6224* In 109 patients with dyslipidemia treatment with 1200 mg/d for 12 months caused reduction from mean baseline of 2.21 ± 1.06 mmol/L to 1.36 ± 0.87 mmol/L *3254* In 8 patients with familial dysbetalipoproteinemia treatment with 1200 mg/d for 4 weeks caused significant decrease of 63% from mean baseline of 6.08 mmol/L to 2.23 mmol/L. After 3 months the concentration had decreased to 2.06 mmol/L and after 10 months to 2.27 mmol/L *6655* In 5 patients with hypertriglyceridemia treatment with 1200 mg/d for 8 weeks caused significant decrease to 293 ± 88 mg/dL compared with 1175 ± 112 mg/dL in those receiving placebo and in 5 patients with combined hyperlipidemia concentration decreased to 213 ± 163 mg/dL versus 449 ± 202 mg/dL in those receiving placebo *6589* In 21 men with combined hyperlipidemia treatment with 1200 mg/d for a mean 11.0 weeks caused caused a significant decrease from mean baseline of 5.3 ± 0.7 mmol/L to 2.1 ± 0.2 mmol/L *752* In the Helsinki Heart Study of 4,081 asymptomatic middle-aged male patients with primary dyslipidemia treatment with 1200 mg/d for caused mean decrease of 43% *3115* In 24 patients with hypertriglyceridemia greater than 5.67 mmol/L treatment with 1200 mg/d gemfibrozil caused significant reduction in concentration from 5.75 to 77.75 mmol/L to 0.58 - 16.65 mmol/L *5800* Gemfibrozil decreases triglyceride concentration by decreasing VLDL-cholesterol production in the liver and increases lipoprotein lipase activity *3668* Treatment of 48 patients with primary hyperlipidemia with 900 mg/d for 16 weeks caused mean decrease of 44.8% whereas treatment with 600 mg b.i.d. caused mean decrease of 41% *297* In 90 dyslipidemic men (serum cholesterol greater than or equal to 5.2 mmol/L) treatment with gemfirozil for one year caused significant reduction from 2.28 ± 2.09 mmol/L to 1.08 ± 0.64 mmol/L *2513* Mean reduction of 36.0% in 51 noninsulin dependent diabetics with primary hypercholesterolemia treated with 1200 mg daily for 24 weeks *2215* Increase by 43% in extensive 5 year double-blinded trial with 2,000 men receiving 600 mg drug twice daily *1962* In 12 type IIa hyperlipidemic patients treatment with gemfibrozil for 12 weeks caused significant reduction from mean baseline of 109.8 ± 33.4 mg/dL to 64.4 ± 19.1 mg/dL *1929* In 38 renal allograft patients who had persistent hyperlipidemia and stable renal function treatment with up to 1200 mg/d caused significant change from mean baseline of 231.9 ± 116.8 mg/dL (2.62 ± 1.32 mmol/L) to 125.7 ± 58.4 mg/dL(1.42 ± 0.66 mmol/L) *962* Significant reduction from mean of 130 mg/dL to 66 mg/dL in 9 patients with familial hypercholesterolemia after treatment with 1200 mg daily for 16 weeks *1930* In 30 patients with familial defective apolipoprotein B-100 treatment with 1200 mg/d for 8 weeks caused a significant change from mean baseline of 1.35 mmol/L to 1.01 mmol/L *2445* 44% reduction observed in 22 individuals who had survived a myocardial infarction when given 1200 mg daily for 8 weeks *157* Significant decrease observed in 15 patients with familial type IV hyperlipoproteinemia when 1200 mg ingested daily *1103* In 20 patients with primary hypertriglyceridemia treatment with 1200 mg/d for 12 weeks caused significant decrease from mean baseline of 414.1 ± 138.2 mg/dL to 210.2 ± 72.1 mg/dL *295* In 27 patients with severe hypertriglyceridemia treatment with 1200 mg/d for 6 weeks caused significant reduction from median baseline of 17.0 ± 10.9 mmol/L to 8.76 ± 8.71 mmol/L *3086* In 17 male patients with established atherosclerosis and high triglycerides and low high-density lipoprotein cholesterol treated 1200 mg/d for 12 weeks significant change from mean baseline of 3.65 mmol/L to 1.82 mmol/L observed *3198*

Viscosity *Plasma Decrease Physiological* In 24 patients with hypertriglyceridemia greater than 5.67 mmol/L treatment with 1200 mg/d gemfibrozil caused a significant reduction in viscosity from 1.340 - 2.383 mPa/s to 1.290 - 1.851 mPa/s *5800*

Serum Decrease Physiological In 24 patients with hypertriglyceridemia greater than 5.67 mmol/L treatment with 1200 mg/d gemfibrozil caused a significant reduction in viscosity from 1.422 ± 0.155 mPa/s to 1.336 ± 0.091 mPa/s *5800*

VLDL$_1$-Cholesterol *Serum Decrease Physiological* In 8 patients with familial dysbetalipoproteinemia treatment for one month with 1200 mg/d caused significant decrease from mean baseline of 1.63 mmol/L to 0.47 mmol/L *6655*

VLDL$_1$-Triglycerides *Serum Decrease Physiological* In 8 patients with familial dysbetalipoproteinemia treatment with 1200 mg/d for 1 month caused significant decrease from mean baseline of 1.88 mmol/L to 0.57 mmol/L *6655*

VLDL$_2$-Cholesterol *Serum No Effect Physiological* In 8 patients with familial dysbetalipoproteinemia treatment with 1200 mg/d for 1 month caused significant decrease from mean baseline of 4.94 mmol/L to 1.34 mmol/L *6655*

VLDL$_2$-Triglycerides *Serum Decrease Physiological* In 8 patients with familial dysbetalipoproteinemia treatment with 1200 mg/d for 1 month caused significant decrease from mean baseline of 2.78 mmol/L to 0.84 mmol/L *6655*

VLDL-Apolipoprotein B *Serum Decrease Physiological* Significant reduction of 34% observed in 10 patients with type IIb hyperlipoproteinemia and of 40% in 10 patients with type IV hyperlipoproteinemia when treated with 1200 mg/d for 3 months *4919*

VLDL-Cholesterol *Serum Decrease Physiological* Significant reduction from mean of 23 mg/dL to 9 mg/dL in 9 patients with familial hypercholesterolemia after treatment with 1200 mg

Gemfibrozil *(continued)*

VLDL-Cholesterol *(continued)*
daily for 16 weeks *1930* Mean reduction of 41.1% in 38 noninsulin dependent diabetics with primary hypercholesterolemia treated with 1200 mg daily for 24 weeks *2215* In 5 patients with hypertriglyceridemia treatment with 1200 mg/d for 8 weeks caused significant decrease to 1.6 ± 0.8 U/dL compared with 8.9 ± 1.6 U/dL in those receiving placebo *6589* In 63-69 patients with hypercholesterolemia treatment for 12 weeks caused significant decrease from mean baseline of 0.64 ± 0.05 mmol/L to 0.32 ± 0.02 mmol/L (49.1%) *6463* In 21 men with combined hyperlipidemia treatment with 1200 mg/d for a mean 11.0 weeks caused caused a significant decrease from mean baseline of 2.9 ± 0.4 mmol/L to 1.0 ± 0.1 mmol/L *752* Reduction largely responsible for reduction in total cholesterol in 15 patients with familial type IV hyperlipoproteinemia when treated with 1200 mg daily *1103* Significant decrease from mean baseline concentration of about 2.2 mmol/L to 0.8 mmol/L after 24 weeks treatment with 1200 mg daily in 14 patients with hypertriglyceridemia *4564* Significant reduction of 44% observed in 10 patients with type IIb hyperlipoproteinemia when treated with 1200 mg/d for 3 months and of 40% in 10 type IV hyperlipoproteinemic patients *4919* Significant reduction from mean baseline of 1.6 mmol/L to 0.9 mmol/L in 18 patients with familial combined hyperlipidemia treated with 1200 mg/d for 6 weeks *4367* Increase by 50% in 18 patients with chronic renal failure treated with 1200 mg/d for 28 weeks. Simultaneous activation of plasma postheparin lipoprotein and hepatic lipases. Effects reversed when drug discontinued *4550* In 17 patients treatment with 1200 mg/d for 6 weeks caused significant reduction from mean baseline of 0.93 ± 0.35 mmol/L to 0.45 ± 0.16 mmol/L *3905* In 13 patients with type V hyperlipidemia treatment with 1200 mg daily for 8 weeks caused reduction from mean of 6.66 mmol/L to 2.15 mmol/L *3448* Significant reduction observed in 8 type III hyperlipoproteinemic patients treated for 28 months *3330*
Serum No Effect Physiological In 5 patients with combined hyperlipidemia treatment with 1200 mg/d for 8 weeks caused insignificant change to 1.0 ± 0.8 U/dL compared with 2.6 ± 1.5 U/dL in those receiving placebo *6589*

VLDL-Triglycerides *Serum Decrease Physiological* In 21 men with combined hyperlipidemia treatment with 1200 mg/d for a mean 11.0 weeks caused caused a significant decrease from mean baseline of 4.5 ± 0.7 mmol/L to 1.5 ± 0.2 mmol/L *752* Reduction largely responsible for reduction in total triglycerides in 15 patients with familial type IV hyperlipoproteinemia when treated with 1200 mg daily *1103* Significant reduction of 66% observed in 10 patients with type IIb hyperlipoproteinemia and of 67% in 10 type IV hyperlipoproteinemic patients when treated with 1200 mg/d for 3 months *4919* Significant reduction observed in 8 type III hyperlipoproteinemic patients treated for up to 28 months *3330* Treatment of 13 type V hyperlipidemics with 1200 mg daily for 8 weeks caused reduction from mean of 14.40 mmol/L to 4.59 mmol/L *3448* Significant reduction from mean baseline concentration of 2.4 mmol/L to 1.2 mmol/L in 18 patients with familial combined hyperlipidemia treated with 1200 mg/d for 6 weeks *4367* Significant decrease from mean baseline concentration of about 4.0 mmol/L to 1.3 mmol/L in 14 patients with hypertriglyceridemia treated with 1200 mg daily for 24 weeks *4564* Increase by 50% in 18 patients with chronic renal failure treated with 1200 mg/d for 28 weeks. Simultaneous activation of postheparin plasma lipoprotein and hepatic lipases. Effects reversed when drug discontinued *4550*

Warfarin *Plasma Increase Physiological* By inhibiting p-hydroxylation of warfarin increases its plasma concentration, with a further decrease in the synthesis of clotting factors, and may cause bleeding problems *3668*

Gentamicin

Acid Phosphatase *Serum No Effect Analytical* At concentration of 16 µg/mL (29 µmol/L) had no effect on method on Du Pont Dimension *1562*

Alanine Aminopeptidase *Urine Increase Physiological* In 24 patients with carefully monitored plasma concentration significant infradian rhythms observed with periods between 2.2 and 8.1 days and in 10 of these patients (42%) a circaseptan period was detected *354* Marked effect especially with treatment for more than 12 d *4283*

Alanine Aminotransferase *Serum Increase Physiological* Observed in some patients treated with gentamicin *5331* May cause hepatotoxicity *3669*
Serum No Effect Analytical No effect at concentration of 16 µg/mL (29 µmol/L) on method on Du Pont Dimension *1563*
Urine No Effect Physiological No significant effect in 15 volunteers up to 24 hours after receiving 1 mg/kg intravenously *1730*

Albumin *Serum No Effect Analytical* No interference observed at a concentration of 8 mg/L with method on Du Pont aca *1507* At concentration of 16 µg/mL (29 µmol/L) had no effect on method on Du Pont Dimension *1564* At concentration of 150 mg/L had no effect on BCG method *5704*
Urine Increase Physiological In 31 patients treatment caused increased excretion after 3 and 7 days of treatment *6045*
Urine No Effect Analytical At concentration of 80 mg/dL of gentamicin sulfate had no significant effect on Boehringer Mannheim Tina-quant method *2799*

Aldosterone *Plasma No Effect Physiological* Effect observed in 2 patients following larger doses of gentamicin. Associated with massive urinary loss of magnesium and potassium *361*

Alkaline Phosphatase *Serum Increase Physiological* Hepatotoxic effect *2242*
Serum No Effect Analytical At concentration of 16 µg/mL (29 µmol/L) had no effect on method on Du Pont Dimension *1565*
Urine Increase Physiological Significant effect 12 to 24 hours after 15 volunteers received 1 mg/kg intravenously indicating brush border involvement *1730*

Amikacin *Serum No Effect Analytical* Error of less than 5% observed when added at a concentration of 100 mg/L to a specimen containing 15 mg/L amikacin and measured on Baxter Stratus *5705* No interference observed with method on Abbott TDx *3858* No interference observed at a concentration of 100 µg/mL (216 µmol/L) with method on Du Pont aca *1508*

Amino Acids *Urine Increase Analytical* Reacts with ninhydrin; extra spot TLC, high voltage electrophoresis *4760*

Ammonia *Plasma No Effect Analytical* No effect at concentration of 16 µg/mL (29 µmol/L) on method on Du Pont Dimension *1566*

Amylase *Serum No Effect Analytical* At concentration of 16 µg/mL (29 µmol/L) had no effect on method on Du Pont Dimension *1567*

Aspartate Aminotransferase *Serum Increase Analytical* False elevation with Babson procedure *5178*
Serum Increase Physiological May cause hepatotoxicity (or due to i.m. injection) *3669* Observed in some patients treated with gentamicin *5331*
Serum No Effect Analytical No effect at concentration of 16 µg/mL (29 µmol/L) on method on Du Pont Dimension *1568*
Urine No Effect Physiological No significant effect in 15 volunteers up to 24 hours after receiving 1 mg/kg intravenously *1730*

Bicarbonate *Serum Increase Physiological* If given with cephalexin to leukemics *6614*
Serum No Effect Analytical At concentration of 150 mg/L had no effect on method using phenolphthalein *5704*

Bilirubin *Serum Increase Physiological* Observed in some patients treated with gentamicin *5331* Affects liver function *128*
Serum No Effect Analytical At concentration of 150 mg/L had no effect on Jendrassik and Grof method *5704* At concentration of 5 mg/L had no effect on method on Kodak Ektachem® *5706* No effect at concentration of 16 µg/mL (29 µmol/L) on method on Du Pont Dimension *1589*
Serum No Effect Physiological Clinically insignificant displacement from protein in neonates *6314*

Bilirubin, Conjugated *Serum No Effect Analytical* No effect at concentration of 5 mg/L on method on Kodak Ektachem® *5706* At concentration of 15.8 µg/mL (34.1 µmol/L) had no effect on method on Du Pont aca *1517*

Bilirubin, Direct *Serum No Effect Analytical* At concentration of 16 µmol/L (29 µmol/L) had no effect on method on Du Pont Dimension *1574*

Bilirubin, Unconjugated *Serum No Effect Analytical* No effect at concentration of 5 mg/L on method on Kodak Ektachem® *5706*

Calcium *Serum Decrease Physiological* Observed in some patients treated with gentamicin *5331* Effect observed in 2 patients following larger doses of gentamicin. Associated with massive urinary loss of magnesium and potassium *361*
Serum No Effect Analytical At concentration of 150 mg/L had no effect on cresolphthalein method *5704* No effect at concentration of 16 µg/mL (29 µmol/L) on method on Du Pont Dimension *1569*

Casts *Urine Increase Physiological* Observed in association with drug associated nephrotoxicity *5325* Nephrotoxicity occurred rarely in treated patients, most often in patients with a history of renal impairment and in patients treated for longer periods or with larger doses than recommended *5331*

Cells *Urine Increase Physiological* Nephrotoxicity occurred rarely in treated patients, most often in patients with a history of renal impairment and in patients treated for longer periods or with larger doses than recommended *5331*

Chloramphenicol *Serum No Effect Analytical* No effect at 100 mg/L on coupled enzymatic method *4122*

Chloride *Serum No Effect Analytical* At concentration of 150 mg/L had no effect on mercurimetric method *5704*

Cholesterol *Serum No Effect Analytical* At concentration of 6 mg/L had no effect on CHOD-PAP method *5704* At concentration of 16 µg/mL (29 µmol/L) had no effect on method on Du Pont Dimension *1570* At concentration of 150 mg/L had no effect on Liebermann-Burchard method *5704*

Cholinesterase *Serum No Effect Analytical* Insignificant decrease of 0.04 U/mL at a concentration of 16 µg/mL with method on Du Pont Dimension *3271* Insignificant reduction of 0.07 U/mL at a concentration of 16 µg/mL with method on Du Pont aca *3271*

C-Reactive Protein *Serum No Effect Analytical* At concentration of 15 mg/L (32.4 µmol/L) had no effect on method on Du Pont aca *5403* No interference observed at concentrations up to 15 µg/mL (32.4 µmol/L) with method on Du Pont aca *1518*

Creatine Kinase Isoenzymes *Serum No Effect Analytical* At concentration of 16 µg/mL (29 µmol/L) had no effect on method to measure MB isoenzyme on Du Pont Dimension *1571* No interference observed at a concentration of 20 mg/L (36.8 µmol/L) with CK-MB method on Du Pont aca *1519*

Creatinine *Serum Increase Physiological* 24% incidence of nephrotoxicity but unrelated to initial renal function or prior use of drug, drug concentration, amount given, duration of treatment or concurrent treatment with other drugs *5325* 10.2% incidence in 49 patients given drug by McHenry method versus 8% in 50 patients given drug by Sawchuk/Zaske method *3850* Nephrotoxicity observed in 26% patients treated with drug for sepsis. Mean increase for all population studied 0.4 mg/dL *5615* Nephrotoxic effect *3669* Nephrotoxicity occurred rarely in treated patients, most often in patients with a history of renal impairment and in patients treated for longer periods or with larger doses than recommended *5331*
Serum No Effect Analytical At concentration of 6 mg/L had no effect on Jaffe-Fading-Fraction method *5704* At concentration of 6 mg/L had no effect on Jaffe-Fuller's earth method *5704* At concentration of 150 mg/L had no effect on Technicon AutoAnalyzer® Jaffe method *5704* No effect at concentration of 16 µg/mL (29 µmol/L) on method on Du Pont Dimension *1572* No effect of concentrations up to 15 mg/L on single slide method on Kodak Ektachem® *5706* No effect at therapeutic concentration on method on Kodak Ektachem® 700 *586*
Serum No Effect Physiological No effect observed in 18 neonates although tubular damage observed during treatment *263*

Creatinine Clearance *Urine No Effect Physiological* No effect observed in 18 neonates although renal tubular damage observed *263*

Cyclosporine *Blood No Effect Analytical* At a concentration of 120 mg/L had no effect on Syva EMIT method *495*

Eosinophils *Blood Increase Physiological* Observed in some patients treated with gentamicin *5331*

Erythrocytes *Blood Decrease Physiological* May cause anemia *128*

Fibrin Degradation Products *Plasma No Effect Analytical* No interference observed at concentrations up to 50 µg/mL (92 mmol/L) with method on Du Pont aca *1525*

Glomerular Filtration Rate *Urine Decrease Physiological* Using chromium labeled EDTA even with subnormal amounts of drug. Noticeable before effect on serum creatinine *6074*

Glucose *Serum No Effect Analytical* At concentration of 10 mg/L had no effect on GOD/POD-PAP method *5704* At concentration of 16 µg/mL (29 µmol/L) has no effect on method on Du Pont Dimension *1575*
Urine No Effect Analytical At concentration of 200 mg/L had no effect on Diabur-test *5704* At up to 250 µg/mL had no effect on measured glucose concentrations using Clinitest®, Diastix® and TesTape® *3710*

γ-Glutamyltransferase *Serum No Effect Analytical* At concentration of 16 µg/mL (29 µmol/L) has no effect on method on Du Pont Dimension *1579*
Urine No Effect Physiological No significant effect in 15 volunteers up to 24 hours after receiving 1 mg/kg intravenously *1730*

Granulocytes *Blood Decrease Physiological* Observed in some patients treated with gentamicin *5331*

HDL-Cholesterol *Serum No Effect Analytical* No effect at concentration of 16 µg/mL (29 µmol/L) on method on Du Pont Dimension *1576*

Hematocrit *Blood Decrease Physiological* Observed in some patients treated with gentamicin *5331*

Hemoglobin *Blood Decrease Physiological* Observed in some patients treated with gentamicin *5331*

Heparin Sulfate *Urine Increase Physiological* Reacts with heparin to form precipitate *1414*

Histamine *Plasma No Effect Analytical* No inhibition of radio-enzyme assay at concentration 10 times therapeutic *2492*

Immunoglobulin G *Urine Increase Physiological* Increased excretion observed in 31 patients with 3 days of treatment but excretion normalized by 7 days even with continuing treatment *6045*

Immunoglobulin Light Chains
Urine Increase Physiological Marked effect especially with treatment for more than 12 d *4283*

Iron *Serum No Effect Analytical* No effect at concentration of 16 µg/mL (29 µmol/L) on method on Du Pont Dimension *1577*

Iron-Binding Capacity, Total *Serum No Effect Analytical* No effect at concentration of 16 µg/mL (29 µmol/L) on method on Du Pont Dimension *1590*

Kanamycin *Serum No Effect Analytical* No interference observed with method on Abbott TDx *3858*

17-Ketosteroids *Urine No Effect Analytical* With normal dose on Zimmermann procedure *3141*

Lactate Dehydrogenase *Serum Increase Physiological* Observed in some patients treated with gentamicin *5331*
Serum No Effect Analytical At concentration of 16 µg/mL (29 µmol/L) has no effect on method on Du Pont Dimension *1578*
Urine Increase Physiological Significant effect in 15 volunteers 12 to 24 hours after receiving 1 mg/kg intravenously indicating cytoplasmic damage *1730*

Leucine Aminopeptidase *Urine Increase Physiological* Significant effect between 12 and 24 hours in 15 volunteers after receiving 1 mg/kg intravenously indicating involvement of proximal tubule structures *1730*

Leukocytes *Blood Decrease Physiological* Observed in some patients treated with gentamicin *5331*

Lipase *Serum No Effect Analytical* No effect at concentration of 16 µg/mL (29 µmol/L) on method on Du Pont Dimension *1580*

Lysozyme *Serum No Effect Physiological* Remained in normal range in 26 patients given course of treatment *4283*
Urine Increase Physiological Marked effect especially with treatment for more than 12 d *4283*

Magnesium *Serum Decrease Physiological* Observed in some patients treated with gentamicin *5331* Effect observed in 2 patients following larger doses of gentamicin. Associated with massive urinary loss of magnesium and potassium *361* In 2 patients, one of whom was also receiving furosemide, con-

Gentamicin *(continued)*

Magnesium *(continued)*
centrations of less than 12 mg/L observed *6640* Decreased concentration observed due to increased renal excretion in some patients *3113*
Serum No Effect Analytical No effect at therapeutic concentration on method on Kodak Ektachem® 700 *586* No effect at concentration of 16 µg/mL (29 µmol/L) on method on Du Pont Dimension *1581*
Urine Increase Physiological Effect observed in 2 patients following larger doses of gentamicin. Associated with massive urinary loss of magnesium and potassium *361* Increased excretion observed in some patients *3113*

β₂-Microglobulin *Serum Increase Physiological* Significant effect observed in the absence of change in the serum creatinine *6074*
Serum No Effect Physiological No difference during or following treatment in 26 patients given drug *4283*
Urine Increase Physiological Effect observed, and used as measure of tubular damage, in 18 neonates treated with drug *263* Marked effect especially with treatment for more than 12 d *4283* Competitively inhibits reabsorption of compound when drug excretion rates exceed 150 mg/min *6305* Significant effect observed in the absence of change in the serum creatinine *6074* Increased excretion observed in 31 patients after 3 days but excretion normalized by 7 days even with continuing treatment *6045*

Mycophenolic Acid *Serum No Effect Analytical* No significant interference observed with HPLC method of Shipkova et al *5526*

Mycophenolic Acid Glucuronide
Serum No Effect Analytical No significant interference observed with HPLC method of Shipkova et al *5526*

N-Acetyl-Glucosaminidase *Urine Increase Physiological* Marked effect especially with treatment for more than 12 d *4283*
Urine No Effect Analytical No effect at 50 g/L on 2 colorimetric analytical methods *2254* At concentration of 80 mg/dL no significant effect observed on Boehringer Mannheim CPR method *3174*

Netilmicin *Serum Increase Analytical* Interferes with method on Abbott TDx *3858*

Neutrophils *Blood Decrease Physiological* Occasional case of agranulocytosis reported *6264*

Nonprotein Nitrogen *Serum Increase Physiological* Nephrotoxicity occurred rarely in treated patients, most often in patients with a history of renal impairment and in patients treated for longer periods or with larger doses than recommended *5331*

Parathyroid Hormone *Plasma Decrease Physiological* Effect observed in 2 patients following larger doses of gentamicin. Associated with massive urinary loss of magnesium and potassium *361*

Phenylalanine *Plasma No Effect Analytical* No interference observed with rapid quantitative whole blood method of Campbell et al using phenylalanine dehydrogenase *867*

Phenytoin *Serum No Effect Analytical* No effect at concentration of 16 µg/mL (29 µmol/L) on method on Du Pont Dimension *1583*

Phosphate *Serum No Effect Analytical* At concentration of 150 mg/L had no effect on phosphomolybdate method *5704* At concentration of 16 µg/mL (29 µmol/L) has no effect on method on Du Pont Dimension *1584*

Platelets *Blood Decrease Physiological* Observed in some patients treated with gentamicin *5331*

Potassium *Serum Decrease Physiological* Effect observed in 2 patients following larger doses of gentamicin. Associated with massive urinary loss of magnesium and potassium *361* If given with cephalexin to leukemics *6614* Observed in some patients treated with gentamicin *5331*
Serum No Effect Analytical At concentration of 14 mg/L had no effect on measurement by ISE with predilution *5704* At concentration of 6 mg/L had no effect on flame-photometric method *5704*
Urine Increase Physiological Effect observed in 2 patients following larger doses of gentamicin. Associated with massive urinary loss of magnesium and potassium *361*

Protein *Cerebrospinal Fluid No Effect Analytical* No significant effect when added in vitro to concentration of 100.0 mg/dL on Ektachem® slide method *3654* At concentration of 7.5 mg/L on SDS/Coomassie Blue method of Huang *2745*
Serum No Effect Analytical At concentration of 150 mg/L had no effect on biuret method with blank correction *5704* At concentration of 16 µg/mL (29 µmol/L) had negligible effect on method on Du Pont Dimension *1591*
Urine Increase Analytical On Ponceau S dye method in comparison with sulfosalicylic acid method in 7 patients receiving therapeutic doses *6341*
Urine Increase Physiological Nephrotoxicity occurred rarely in treated patients, most often in patients with a history of renal impairment and in patients treated for longer periods or with larger doses than recommended *5331* Manifestation of drug-induced nephrotoxicity *5325* Nephrotoxic effect *1714*
Urine No Effect Analytical No difference between sulfosalicylic acid and trichloracetic acid methods in patients receiving therapeutic doses *6341* At concentration of 160 mg/L had no effect on concentration as measured by benzethonium chloride method *1171*

Renin Activity *Plasma No Effect Physiological* Effect observed in 2 patients following larger doses of gentamicin. Associated with massive urinary loss of magnesium and potassium *361*

Reticulocytes *Blood Decrease Physiological* Observed in some patients treated with gentamicin *5331*
Blood Increase Physiological Observed in some patients treated with gentamicin *5331*

Retinol-binding Protein *Serum No Effect Physiological* No difference during or following treatment in 26 patients given drug *4283*
Urine Increase Physiological Marked effect especially with treatment for more than 12 d *4283*

SDZ PSC 833 *Blood No Effect Analytical* At a concentration of 6 mg/L had no effect on HPLC method of Scott et al when used to measure PSC (with CsD as internal standard) at a concentration of 5 mg/L *5418*

Sodium *Serum Decrease Physiological* Observed in some patients treated with gentamicin *5331*
Serum No Effect Analytical At concentration of 6 mg/L had no effect on flame-photometric method *5704* At concentration of 14 mg/L had no effect on measurement by ISE with predilution *5704*

Streptomycin *Serum No Effect Analytical* No interference observed with method on Abbott TDx *3858*

T3-Uptake *Serum No Effect Analytical* At concentration of 16 µg/mL (29 µmol/L) has no effect on method on Du Pont Dimension *1586* No significant effect observed at a concentration of 16 µg/mL (29 µmol/L) with method on Du Pont aca *1545*

Tacrolimus *Blood No Effect Analytical* No significant effect observed at a concentration of 10 mg/L with MEIA method on Abbott IMx analyzer *1871*
Serum No Effect Analytical In HPLC/MS method of Christians et al no significant interference observed with measurement of FK 506 *1010* At concentration of 10 mg/L no significant effect on ELISA procedure observed *6329*

Theophylline *Serum No Effect Analytical* At concentration of 20 mg/L produced no interference with methods used on Kodak DT60, Abbott TDx, Abbott Vision with either whole blood or serum, 3M Diagnostics TheoFAST, Syntex AccµLevel or Ames Seralyzer *1122* At concentration of 16 µg/mL (29 µmol/L) had no effect on method on Du Pont Dimension *1585*

Thyroxine (T4) *Serum No Effect Analytical* At concentration of 16 µg/mL (29 µmol/L) has no effect on method on Du Pont Dimension *1587* No significant effect observed at a concentration of 16 µg/mL (29 µmol/L) with method on Du Pont aca *1546 1588*

Tobramycin *Serum No Effect Analytical* No interference observed with method on Abbott TDx *3858* At concentrations less than 100 µg/mL (216 µmol/L) no significant effect observed on method on Du Pont aca *1547* No detectable cross-reactivity of observed with tobramycin method on Bayer Technicon Immuno 1® *435* At a concentration of 1250 mg/L produces 15% increase in concentration when measured by method on Baxter Stratus but therapeutic concentration only up to 10 mg/L *5705*

Transferrin *Urine Increase Physiological* Significant increase observed in 31 patients after 3 days of treatment but normalized by 7 days even with continuing treatment *6045*
Urine No Effect Physiological No effect observed in 26 patients given drug *4283*

Triglycerides *Serum No Effect Analytical* At concentration of 10 mg/L had no effect on GPO-PAP method *5704* At concentration of 150 mg/L had no effect on lipase/esterase method *5704* At concentration of 16 μg/mL (29 μmol/L) has no effect on method on Du Pont Dimension *1592*

Urea Nitrogen *Serum Increase Physiological* Nephrotoxicity occurred rarely in treated patients, most often in patients with a history of renal impairment and in patients treated for longer periods or with larger doses than recommended *5331* Nephrotoxic effect with large doses *3669*
Serum No Effect Analytical At concentration of 150 mg/L had no effect on diacetylmonoxime method *5704* No effect at concentration of 16 μg/mL (29 μmol/L) on method on Du Pont Dimension *1593*

Uric Acid *Serum Increase Physiological* Reported effect of i.m. injection *4727*
Serum No Effect Analytical At concentration of 6 mg/L had no effect on catalase-AIDH method *5704* At concentration of 6 mg/L had no effect on Kageyama-Hantzsch method *5704* At concentration of 10 mg/L had no effect on uricase-PAP method *5704* At concentration of 150 mg/L had no effect on phosphotungstate reduction method *5704*

Vancomycin *Serum No Effect Analytical* Mo interference observed with method on Abbott TDx *3858* No significant interference observed at a concentration of 500 μg/mL (1079 μmol/L) with method on Du Pont aca *1561*

Gepirone

Cortisol *Plasma Increase Physiological* In 14 patients with major depression administration of 10 mg drug orally concentration increased at 90 minutes to mean of 19.6 μg/dL versus 14.2 μg/dL in placebo treated controls. Insignificant difference from control observed with chronic administration *4875*

Growth Hormone *Plasma Increase Physiological* In 14 patients with major depression mean concentration 90 minutes after oral ingestion of 10 mg caused increase to 2.1 μg/L compared with 1.1 μg/L in placebo treated controls. Little difference from controls observed with chronic treatment *4875*

Prolactin *Plasma No Effect Physiological* Little change compared with placebo following oral ingestion of 10 mg in 14 patients with major depression *4875*

Gestodene

Corticosteroid-Binding Globulin
Serum Increase Physiological In 30 women given a combination of 75 μg gestodene and 30 μg ethinyl estradiol mean concentration rose from 772 ± 189 nmol/L on day 1 of first cycle to 1401 ± 374 nmol/L on day 1, 1958 ± 479 nmol/L on day 10 and 2136 ± 514 nmol/L on day 21 of third cycle *2428*

Cortisol *Urine Decrease Physiological* In 30 women given a combination of 75 μg gestodene and 30 μg ethinyl estradiol mean excretion declined from 82.5 ± 42.5 μg/d on day 1 of first cycle to 70.5 ± 44.8 μg/d on day 1, 50.0 ± 25.9 μg/d on day 10 and 57.1 ± 39.2 μg/d on day 21 of third cycle *2428*

6-β-Hydroxycortisol *Urine No Effect Physiological* In 30 women given a combination of 75 μg gestodene and 30 μg ethinyl estradiol mean concentration changed insignificantly from 312 ± 169 μg/d on day 1 of first cycle to 311 ± 266 μg/d on day 1, 244 ± 166 μg/d on day 10 and 261 ± 141 μg/d on day 21 of third cycle *2428*

Gestrinone

Cholesterol *Serum Decrease Physiological* In 16 women with pelvic endometriosis treatment with 2.5 mg twice weekly over 24 weeks caused a significant reduction in concentration *1285*

Estradiol *Plasma Decrease Physiological* In 16 women with pelvic endometriosis treatment with up to 2.5 mg twice weekly over 24 weeks caused a ≥30% decrease to 50 to 100 pg/mL although it was not significant *1285*

Follicle Stimulating Hormone
Plasma Increase Physiological In 16 women with pelvic endometriosis treatment with up to 2.5 mg twice weekly over 24 weeks caused a slight increase in plasma FSH concentration although it was not significant *1285*

HDL-Cholesterol *Serum Decrease Physiological* In 16 women with pelvic endometriosis treatment with 2.5 mg twice weekly over 24 weeks caused a significant reduction in concentration *1285*

LDL-Cholesterol *Serum Decrease Physiological* In 16 women with pelvic endometriosis treatment with 2.5 mg twice weekly over 24 weeks caused a significant reduction in concentration *1285*

Luteinizing Hormone *Plasma Increase Physiological* In 16 women with pelvic endometriosis treatment with up to 2.5 mg twice weekly over 24 weeks caused a slight increase in plasma LH concentration although it was not significant *1285*

Progesterone *Plasma Decrease Physiological* In 16 women with pelvic endometriosis treatment with up to 2.5 mg twice weekly over 24 weeks caused a decrease to 0.08 to 0.47 ng/mL *1285*

Sex-Hormone Binding Globulin
Serum Decrease Physiological In 16 women with pelvic endometriosis treatment with up to 2.5 mg twice weekly over 24 weeks caused a decrease from about 5 μg/mL to about 1 μg/mL *1285*

Testosterone, Free *Serum No Effect Physiological* In 16 women with pelvic endometriosis treatment with up to 2.5 mg twice weekly over 24 weeks caused no significant effect on concentration *1285*

Thyroxine (T4), Free *Serum No Effect Physiological* In 16 women with pelvic endometriosis treatment with up to 2.5 mg twice weekly over 24 weeks caused no significant effect on concentration *1285*

Triglycerides *Serum Decrease Physiological* In 16 women with pelvic endometriosis treatment with 1.25 mg twice weekly over 24 weeks caused a significant reduction in concentration, not seen with a dose of 2.5 mg *1285*

Gitoxin

Digoxin *Serum Increase Analytical* Cross-reactivity of 2.8% observed with method on Du Pont aca at concentration of 25 ng/mL (32.02 nmol/L) *1522* At concentration of 25 ng/mL (32.02 nmol/L) caused 2.8% cross-reactivity with method on Du Pont Dimension *1573*

Glaucarubin

Leukocytes *Blood Decrease Physiological* Leukopenia *3810*

Glibenclamide

Albumin *Urine No Effect Analytical* Using a fluorimetric assay with Albumin Blue 580 on a Cobas Fara centrifugal analyzer for the detection of microalbuminuria no significant interference was detected at a concentration of 2 mg/L *3117*

Cholesterol *Serum No Effect Physiological* In 417 type 2 diabetics treatment for 12 months caused no significant change in concentration *1490*

C-Peptide *Plasma Increase Physiological* In 417 type 2 diabetics treatment with glibenclamide over 12 months caused significant increase in fasting C-peptide concentration from mean baseline of 1.98 ng/mL to 2.43 ng/mL *1490*

Glucose *Serum Decrease Physiological* Incidence of 12.3% observed in French Pharmacovigilance database *4106*
Serum Increase Physiological In 453 type 2 diabetics treatment with glibenclamide over 12 months caused nonsignificant increase in fasting glucose concentration from mean baseline of 8.8 mmol/L to 9.3 mmol/L *1490*

Glibenclamide *(continued)*

HDL-Cholesterol *Serum No Effect Physiological* In 417 type 2 diabetics treatment for 12 months caused no significant change in concentration *1490*

Hemoglobin A_{1c} *Blood Increase Physiological* In 451 type 2 diabetics treatment with glibenclamide over 12 months caused increase from mean baseline of 7.80% to 8.32% *1490*

Insulin *Plasma Increase Physiological* In 425 type 2 diabetics treatment with glibenclamide over 12 months caused significant increase in fasting insulin concentration from mean baseline of 15.62 µU/mL to 17.77 µU/mL *1490*

LDL-Cholesterol *Serum No Effect Physiological* In 417 type 2 diabetics treatment for 12 months caused no significant change in concentration *1490*

Triglycerides *Serum No Effect Physiological* In 417 type 2 diabetics treatment for 12 months caused no significant change in concentration *1490*

Glibonuride

Cholesterol *Serum No Effect Physiological* No significant effect observed after 4 weeks *492*

Fatty Acids (FFA), Free *Serum Decrease Physiological* Small immediate rise then fall to 25% at 90 minutes *2511*

Glucose *Serum Decrease Physiological* Therapeutic intent *2511*

Glucose Tolerance *Serum Increase Physiological* Reported but not universal effect *492*

Glycerol *Serum Decrease Physiological* Response similar to that of free fatty acids *2511*

Insulin *Plasma Increase Physiological* Immediate sharp increase, lasting for 20 minutes *2511*

Lipoproteins *Serum No Effect Physiological* No significant effect observed after 4 weeks *492*

Phenprocoumon *Plasma No Effect Physiological* No effect noted on half-life or plasma concentration with coadministration *2538*

Triglycerides *Serum No Effect Physiological* No significant effect observed after 4 weeks *492*

Glibornuride

Glucose *Serum Decrease Physiological* Incidence of 4.6% observed in French Pharmacovigilance database *4106*

Gliclazide

Albumin *Urine No Effect Analytical* Using a fluorimetric assay with Albumin Blue 580 on a Cobas Fara centrifugal analyzer for the detection of microalbuminuria no significant interference was detected at a concentration of 4 mg/L *3117*

CA 19-9 *Serum Increase Physiological* In one diabetic patient with Lewis(a-,b-) blood phenotype administration of gliclazide was associated with an increase of CA 19-9 to about 1200 U/mL from baseline of about 200 U/mL on different occasions during which drug was administered *6609*

C-Peptide *Plasma No Effect Physiological* No significant difference from baseline observed in maximum concentration or in concentration 2 hours post-meal in 10 noninsulin dependent diabetics regardless of when drug given, before, during or after the meal *399*

Glucose *Serum Decrease Physiological* Incidence of 11.2% observed in French Pharmacovigilance database *4106* In 10 noninsulin dependent diabetics decrease from mean baseline of 15.5 mmol/L to 14.7 mmol/L when drug given 30 minutes before a meal but no significant reduction when drug given with meal or 30 minutes after. No differences observed 2 hours after meal *399*

Insulin *Plasma No Effect Physiological* No significant effect observed in maximum concentration or in concentration 2 hours after the meal in 10 noninsulin dependent diabetics when drug given, either before, during or after a meal *399*

Plasminogen Activator Inhibitor-1 Antigen *Plasma Decrease Physiological* In 23 male nonobese male type I diabetics administration of 160 mg or 240 mg glicazide/d for 6 months caused considerable variation but no significant change in concentration over 6 months *2287*

Span-1 *Serum Increase Physiological* In one diabetic patient with Lewis(a-,b-) blood phenotype administration of gliclazide was associated with an increase of CA 19-9 to about 300 U/mL from baseline on one occasion during which drug was administered *6609*

Glimepiride

Alanine Aminotransferase *Serum Increase Physiological* Cholestatic jaundice reported to occur rarely with sulfonylureas *2639*

Alkaline Phosphatase *Serum Increase Physiological* Cholestatic jaundice reported to occur rarely with sulfonylureas *2639*

Aspartate Aminotransferase *Serum Increase Physiological* Cholestatic jaundice reported to occur rarely with sulfonylureas *2639*

Bilirubin *Serum Increase Physiological* Cholestatic jaundice reported to occur rarely with sulfonylureas *2639*

Cholesterol *Serum No Effect Physiological* In 455 type 2 diabetics treatment for 12 months caused no significant change in concentration *1490*

C-Peptide *Plasma Increase Physiological* In 429 type 2 diabetics treatment with glimepiride over 12 months caused significant increase in fasting C-peptide concentration from mean baseline of 2.00 ng/mL to 2.38 ng/mL *1490*

Erythrocytes *Blood Decrease Physiological* Leukopenia, agranulocytosis, thrombocytopenia, hemolytic and aplastic anemias and pancytopenia have been reported to occur with sulfonylureas *2639*

Glucose *Serum Decrease Physiological* Therapeutic intent of drug is to reduce blood glucose concentration but it may cause hypoglycemia (glucose below 60 mg/dL). An incidence of 0.9 - 1.7% was observed in two large well controlled 1-year studies *2639*

Serum Increase Physiological In 465 type 2 diabetics treatment with glimepiride over 12 months caused nonsignificant increase in fasting glucose concentration from mean baseline of 8.8 mmol/L to 9.7 mmol/L *1490*

Granulocytes *Blood Decrease Physiological* Leukopenia, agranulocytosis, thrombocytopenia, hemolytic and aplastic anemias and pancytopenia have been reported to occur with sulfonylureas *2639*

HDL-Cholesterol *Serum No Effect Physiological* In 455 type 2 diabetics treatment for 12 months caused no significant change in concentration *1490*

Hematocrit *Blood Decrease Physiological* Leukopenia, agranulocytosis, thrombocytopenia, hemolytic and aplastic anemias and pancytopenia have been reported to occur with sulfonylureas *2639*

Hemoglobin A_{1c} *Blood Increase Physiological* In 455 type 2 diabetics treatment with glimepiride over 12 months caused increase from mean baseline of 8.03% to 8.39% *1490*

Insulin *Plasma Increase Physiological* In 429 type 2 diabetics treatment with glimepiride over 12 months caused significant increase in fasting insulin concentration from mean baseline of 15.29 µU/mL to 17.47 µU/mL *1490*

LDL-Cholesterol *Serum No Effect Physiological* In 455 type 2 diabetics treatment for 12 months caused no significant change in concentration *1490*

Leukocytes *Blood Decrease Physiological* Leukopenia, agranulocytosis, thrombocytopenia, hemolytic and aplastic anemias and pancytopenia have been reported to occur with sulfonylureas *2639*

Platelets *Blood Decrease Physiological* Leukopenia, agranulocytosis, thrombocytopenia, hemolytic and aplastic anemias and pancytopenia have been reported to occur with sulfonylureas *2639*

Prothrombin Time *Plasma Decrease Physiological* Concomitant administration of glimepiride (4 mg once daily) with warfarin caused a reduction in the mean AUC of the prothrombin time and maximum prothrombin time of 3.3% and 9.9% respectively *2639*

Sodium *Serum Decrease Physiological* Hyponatremia reported to occur with sulfonylureas most often in patients receiving other drugs reported to cause hyponatremia or with medical conditions known to cause hyponatremia or cause release of antidiuretic hormone *2639*

Triglycerides *Serum No Effect Physiological* In 455 type 2 diabetics treatment for 12 months caused no significant change in concentration *1490*

Warfarin *Plasma No Effect Physiological* Concomitant administration of glimepiride (4 mg once daily) had no effect on the pharmacokinetic parameters of R- or S-warfarin *2639*

Glipizide

Albumin *Urine No Effect Analytical* Using a fluorimetric assay with Albumin Blue 580 on a Cobas Fara centrifugal analyzer for the detection of microalbuminuria no significant interference was detected at a concentration of 2 mg/L *3117*

Cyclosporine *Blood Increase Physiological* Coadministration of glipizide with cyclosporine caused 150% increase in cyclosporine concentration despite a 10% reduction in its dose possibly due to inhibition of the microsomal drug hydroxylating enzymes in the liver *859*

Serum Increase Physiological Coadministration of glipizide with cyclosporine caused 150% increase in cyclosporine concentration despite a 10% reduction in its dose possibly due to inhibition of the microsomal drug hydroxylating enzymes in the liver *859*

Glucose *Serum Decrease Physiological* Fasting concentrations gradually decreased in 5 patients with noninsulin dependent diabetes mellitus following ingestion of glipizide but concentration increased in 3 patients *1776* At dose of 2.5-5.0 mg produces rapid decrease *4539* In 15 patients with NIDDM treatment caused decrease from mean baseline of 10.1 ± 2.7 mmol/L to 9.1 ± 2.1 mmol/L after 3 months and 9.3 ± 2.4 mmol/L after 15 months *579* Incidence of 11.3% observed in French Pharmacovigilance database *4106*

Glycated Hemoglobin *Blood No Effect Analytical* At a concentration of 500 mg/L had an insignificant 0.4% interference with method on Abbott Vision *1885*

Hemoglobin A_{1c} *Blood Decrease Physiological* Glipizide improves glucose homeostasis in both young and old diabetics *4648*

Histamine *Plasma No Effect Analytical* Improbable inhibition of radio-enzyme assay at therapeutic concentrations *2492*

Insulin *Plasma Increase Physiological* In 15 patients with NIDDM treatment caused increase from mean baseline of 124 ± 55 pmol/L to 139 ± 74 pmol/L after 3 months and 173 ± 70 pmol/L after 15 months *579* Stimulated beta cells in pancreas *4539*

Lovastatin *Serum No Effect Physiological* In patients with hypercholesterolemia and noninsulin-dependent diabetes mellitus coadministration of lovastatin and oral hypoglycemics had no interactions *3982*

Water Clearance, Free *Urine Increase Physiological* Glipizide caused slight increase in free water clearance in one placebo-controlled cross-over study *4648*

Glisoxepide

Fatty Acids (FFA), Free *Serum Decrease Physiological* Small immediate rise then fall to 25% at 90 minutes *2511*

Glycerol *Serum Decrease Physiological* Response similar to that of free fatty acids *2511*

Insulin *Plasma Increase Physiological* Immediate sharp increase lasting for 20 minutes *2511*

γ-Globulin

Alanine Aminotransferase *Serum Increase Physiological* In 18 patients with primary immunodeficiency treated with intravenous γ-globulin for 6 to 15 months serial measurements showed transient minor increases in 5 patients on 8 occasions *5121*

Albumin *Serum Increase Physiological* Significant increase from existing low concentration observed in 8 patients with systemic juvenile rheumatoid arthritis following intravenous γ-globulin *5558*

Urine No Effect Analytical Using a fluorimetric assay with Albumin Blue 580 on a Cobas Fara centrifugal analyzer for the detection of microalbuminuria no significant interference was detected at a concentration of 1000 mg/L *3117*

Anti-Cytomegalovirus Antibodies
Serum Positive Analytical In 165 lots of intravenous immune γ globulin 96% tested positive for anti-CMV antibodies *3562* In 165 lots of intravenous immune γ-globulin 96% tested positive for anti-CMV antibodies *3562*

Anti-Hepatitis A Antibodies *Serum Positive Analytical* In all of 165 lots of intravenous immune γ globulin test for anti-HAV was positive *3562*

Anti-Hepatitis B Core Antibodies
Serum Positive Analytical In 97% of 165 lots of intravenous immune γ globulin test for antibodies was positive *3562*

Anti-Hepatitis B Surface Antigen
Serum Positive Analytical In all of 165 lots of intravenous immune γ globulin test for anti-HBs Ag was positive *3562*

Anti-HIV-1 Antibodies *Serum Positive Analytical* In 39% of 165 lots of intravenous immune γ globulin positive reaction observed *3562*

C-Reactive Protein *Serum No Effect Analytical* No significant effect observed at concentrations up to 100 g/L with liposome turbidimetric assay of Nissui Pharmaceutical Co *6126*

Creatinine *Serum Increase Physiological* Transient increase observed in 6 nephrotic patients with glomerular nephritis treated with high dose intravenous IgG not associated with symptoms or change in urinary deposit *5340*

Erythrocyte Sedimentation Rate
Blood Decrease Physiological Following intravenous γ-globulin reduction observed from high pretreatment concentration in 8 patients with systemic juvenile rheumatoid arthritis *5558*

Ethanol *Serum No Effect Analytical* No significant interference observed at a concentration of 3 g/L with method developed for use with Roche Cobas Bio, Fara or Mira *5098*

Ferritin *Serum No Effect Analytical* At abnormal concentrations no significant interference observed with Microgenics method using recombinant enzyme fragments *5520*

Hemoglobin *Blood Increase Physiological* Significant increase from low existing concentration observed with intravenous γ-globulin in 8 patients with systemic juvenile rheumatoid arthritis *5558*

Immunoglobulin G *Serum Decrease Physiological* Significant decrease observed from high pretreatment concentration following intravenous γ-globulin treatment in 8 patients with systemic juvenile rheumatoid arthritis *5558*

Lactate Dehydrogenase *Serum Decrease Physiological* With successful response to treatment in patients with AIDS activity declined, decreasing to normal in 9 of 12 patients given drug intravenously *5557*

Platelets *Blood Decrease Physiological* Significant reduction from high pretreatment concentration observed in 7 of 8 patients with systemic juvenile rheumatoid arthritis following intravenous γ-globulin *5558*

Potassium *Serum Increase Analytical* Concentration as much as 10% higher on Kodak Ektachem® 400 when measured with one generation of reference fluid but not observed with another generation *1646*

Protein *Urine Increase Analytical* 77% recovery observed when analyzed by method on Du Pont aca *1553*

Rapid Plasma Reagin Test *Serum Positive Analytical* In 165 lots of intravenous immune γ globulin 29% tested positive *3562*

γ-Globulin *(continued)*

Sodium *Serum Increase Analytical* Falsely high concentration observed (by about 10%) in specimens from patients with above normal serum γ-globulin concentrations when measured on Kodak Ektachem® 400 although discrepancy when a new generation of reference fluid used *1646* Concentration as much as 10% higher in specimens measured on Kodak Ektachem® 400 analyzer when one generation of reference fluid used, but not observed with another generation *1646*
Serum No Effect Analytical No significant difference observed in specimens containing above-normal γ-globulin concentrations when measured on Beckman Astra® when compared against flame photometry *1646*

Glucocorticoids

Aldosterone *Urine Decrease Physiological* May inhibit aldosterone production *5085*

Amino Acids *Plasma Increase Physiological* Due to breakdown of tissue proteins *128*

Amylase *Serum Increase Physiological* Well documented early and late pancreatitis *4014*

Angiotensinogen *Plasma Increase Physiological* May increase concentration but effect is much less than that of estrogen, rarely causing more than a twofold increase *5422*

Basal Metabolic Rate *Patient Decrease Physiological* Metabolic action of hormones *3669*

Calcium *Serum Decrease Physiological* Glucocorticoids cause hypocalcemia through impairment of intestinal cell calcium transport processes, including decreased synthesis of calcium-binding proteins *6526* Effective if hypercalcemia due to sarcoid, vitamin D *128*
Urine Increase Physiological Promote renal excretion *128* Glucocorticoids cause increased excretion of calcium initially because of rapid decrease in bone formation: in patients undergoing long term treatment increased excretion is due to increased skeletal mobilization of calcium and decreased renal tubular reabsorption *6526*

1,25-Dihydroxy Vitamin D *Serum Increase Physiological* Glucocorticoids cause a transient increase in the serum concentration of 1,25-$(OH)_2D$ after the initiation of therapy *6526*

Eosinophils *Blood Decrease Physiological* Characteristic finding as a result of redistribution of cells rather than cell lysis. Effect usually transient lasting less than 24 h *648* Reduced inflammatory response *128*

Erythrocytes *Blood Increase Physiological* Stimulate erythropoiesis *128*

Glucagon *Plasma Increase Physiological* Increase basal and stimulated concentrations and promote gluconeogenesis *648* After 4 d fasting level increased 24 pg/mL *3787*
Plasma No Effect Physiological Intravenous injection failed to modify concentration *3787*

Glucose *Serum Increase Physiological* Diabetogenic action (increased gluconeogenesis) *3810* After i.v. 6 mg/dL at 150 minutes to 15 at 4 h *3787*
Urine Increase Physiological Due to hyperglycemia *3810*

Glucose Tolerance *Serum Decrease Physiological* In majority of nondiabetic patients although adaptive response usually occurs with time and glucose concentrations revert to pretreatment values *648*

25-Hydroxy Vitamin D *Serum Decrease Physiological* Glucocorticoids do not alter the conversion of vitamin D to active metabolites and do not alter serum concentrations of 25-OHD or the clearance of vitamin D metabolites *6526*

3-Hydroxyanthranilic Acid *Urine Increase Physiological* Induce tryptophan pyrrolase *5085*

3-Hydroxykynurenine *Urine Increase Physiological* Induce tryptophan pyrrolase *5085*

Hydroxyproline *Urine Decrease Physiological* In rheumatoids under treatment *4865*

^{131}I Uptake *Serum Decrease Physiological* Associated with reduced BMR *3669*

Immunoglobulin A *Serum Decrease Physiological* Less marked effect than with IgG *648*

Immunoglobulin G *Serum Decrease Physiological* May be reduced by 50% for up to 3 mo after 1 week treatment *648*

Immunoglobulin M *Serum No Effect Physiological* No effect seen, although other immunoglobulins affected *648*

Insulin *Plasma No Effect Physiological* Intravenous injection failed to modify concentration *3787*

Insulin-like Growth Factor-I *Serum No Effect Physiological* Glucocorticoids have no effect on plasma concentration of IGF-I although local tissue production may be reduced by glucocorticoids *6526*

Kynurenine *Urine Increase Physiological* Induce tryptophan pyrrolase *5085*

Lymphocytes *Blood Decrease Physiological* Characteristic finding as a result of redistribution of cells rather than cell lysis. Effect usually transient lasting less than 24 h *648* Also decrease in lymphoid tissue *128*

Monocytes *Blood Decrease Physiological* Characteristic finding as a result of redistribution of cells rather than cell lysis. Effect usually transient lasting less than 24 h *648*

Neutrophils *Blood Increase Physiological* Characteristic finding as a result of redistribution of cells rather than cell lysis. Effect usually transient lasting less than 24 h *648*

Occult Blood *Feces Increase Physiological* May cause lower intestinal ulceration, perforation and hemorrhage *648*

Osteocalcin *Serum Decrease Physiological* In individuals treated with glucocorticoids significant decrease of about 50% observed due to reduction in rate of bone formation *5948* In 9 patients receiving glucocorticoid therapy mean concentration of 17 ± 5 μg/L (2.9 nmol/L) significantly different from that in healthy adults (men 25 ± 5 μg/L, women 20 ± 6 μg/L) *668*

Parathyroid Hormone, Intact
Plasma Increase Physiological Glucocorticoids cause increased excretion of calcium initially because of rapid decrease in bone formation: in patients undergoing long term treatment increased excretion is due to increased skeletal mobilization of calcium and decreased renal tubular reabsorption. The resulting negative calcium balance leads to secondary hyperthyroidism and increased plasma PTH *6526*

Phosphate *Urine Increase Physiological* Glucocorticoids cause secondary hyperthyroidism and increased urinary phosphate *6526*

Platelets *Blood Increase Physiological* Stimulate production of platelets *128*

Potassium *Serum Decrease Physiological* May cause potassium loss *128*

Sodium *Serum Increase Physiological* May cause sodium retention *128*

Thyroid Stimulating Hormone
Serum Decrease Physiological In euthyroidism and hypothyroidism with diminished response to TRH due to hypophyseal inhibition *6412* Potent inhibitors of pituitary TSH secretion: concentrations often reduced to below reference range *1269*

Thyroxine (T4) *Serum Decrease Physiological* Concentration reduced due to reduction of TBG *2412* Or no change typically with inhibition of conversion *6412*
Serum Increase Physiological In Hashimoto's disease typically with inhibition of conversion *6412*
Serum No Effect Physiological Commonly observed typically with inhibition of conversion *6412*

Tri-iodothyronine (T3) *Serum Decrease Physiological* Concentration reduced due to decreased TBG *2412* Typically with inhibition of conversion *6412*

Triglycerides *Serum Increase Physiological* Mean 16% increase observed with low dose *1448* Concentration increased in patients receiving glucocorticoids *4989*

TSH response to TRH *Serum Decrease Physiological* Potent inhibitors of TSH response to TRH especially with high doses *1269*

Xanthurenic Acid *Urine Increase Physiological* Induce tryptophan pyrrolase *5085*

Glucosulfone

Erythrocytes *Blood Decrease Physiological* Hemolytic anemia *4017*

Hematocrit *Blood Decrease Physiological* Hemolytic anemia *1212*

Hemoglobin *Blood Decrease Physiological* Hemolytic anemia *1212*

Leukocytes *Blood Decrease Physiological* Leukopenia *3810*

Methemoglobin *Blood Increase Physiological* Hemolytic anemia *1212*

Sulfhemoglobin *Blood Increase Physiological* Hemolytic anemia *4017*

Gludopa

Aldosterone *Urine Decrease Physiological* Reduction observed in comparison with placebo in 12 healthy salt replete men at 7 hours when drug or placebo infused i.v. for 10 hours *3712*

Amphetamine *Serum Decrease Physiological* Gastrointestinal acidifying agents, such as glutamic acid hydrochloride, lower absorption of amphetamines including dextroamphetamine *5641*

Atrial Natriuretic Peptide *Plasma No Effect Physiological* No significant difference in 12 healthy salt replete men given i.v. infusion for 12 hours of either gludopa or placebo *3712*

Kallikrein *Urine No Effect Physiological* No significant difference between excretion following gludopa and with placebo infusion in 12 healthy men *3712*

Potassium *Urine No Effect Physiological* No significant alteration in excretion in 12 healthy salt replete men given i.v. infusion for 10 hours *3712*

Renin Activity *Plasma No Effect Physiological* No significant difference over 12 hours in 12 men infused i.v. either gludopa or placebo for 10 hours *3712*

Sodium *Urine Increase Physiological* Cumulative natriuresis of 46.5 mmol over 12 hours compared with placebo in 12 healthy salt replete men given i.v. infusion for 10 hours *3712*

Glutethimide

Alanine Aminotransferase *Serum No Effect Analytical* At acute overdose concentration (5 mg/dL) on Technicon SMAC® method *6266*

Albumin *Serum No Effect Analytical* At concentration of 50 mg/L had no effect on BCG method *5704* At acute overdose concentration (5 mg/dL) on Technicon SMAC® method *6266*

Alkaline Phosphatase *Serum No Effect Analytical* At acute overdose concentration (5 mg/dL) on Technicon SMAC® method *6266*

δ-Aminolevulinic Acid *Urine Increase Physiological* May induce acute intermittent porphyria *1384* May precipitate acute porphyria *2210*

Aspartate Aminotransferase *Serum No Effect Analytical* At acute overdose concentration (5 mg/dL) on Technicon SMAC® method *6266*

Barbiturate *Serum No Effect Analytical* No significant interference observed at a concentration of 100 µg/mL (0.46 mmol/L) with method on Du Pont aca *1511*
Urine No Effect Analytical Negative result obtained at a concentration of 25 µg/mL (0.12 mmol/L) with method on Du Pont aca *1555*

Benzodiazepine Screen *Serum No Effect Analytical* No significant interference observed at a concentration of 200 µg/mL (0.92 mmol/L) with method on Du Pont aca *1512*

Bilirubin *Serum No Effect Analytical* At concentration of 50 mg/L had no effect on Jendrassik and Grof method *5704* At acute overdose concentration (5 mg/dL) on Technicon SMAC® method *6266*
Serum No Effect Physiological Insignificant protein-displacement effect in neonates *6314*

Calcium *Serum No Effect Analytical* At acute overdose concentration (5 mg/dL) on Technicon SMAC® method *6266* At concentration of 50 mg/L had no effect on cresolphthalein method *5704*

Cannabinoids *Urine No Effect Analytical* No effect on Roche Abuscreen method *5006*

Carbamazepine *Serum No Effect Analytical* No cross-reactivity observed with method on Du Pont aca *1513*

Cholesterol *Serum Increase Physiological* Significant effect from about 15 d of treatment with 500 mg drµg/d in 6 volunteers *642*
Serum No Effect Analytical At concentration of 50 mg/L had no effect on Liebermann-Burchard method *5704* At acute overdose concentration (5 mg/dL) on Technicon SMAC® method *6266*

Color *Urine Increase Physiological* May impart red color in association with induced acute intermittent porphyria *1384*

Coproporphyrin *Feces Increase Physiological* May cause modest increase in association with induced acute intermittent porphyria *1384* May precipitate acute porphyria *2210*
Urine Increase Physiological May induce acute intermittent porphyria *1384* May precipitate acute porphyria *2210*

Creatine Kinase *Serum No Effect Analytical* At acute overdose concentration (5 mg/dL) on Technicon SMAC® method *6266*

Creatinine *Serum No Effect Analytical* At concentration of 50 mg/L had no effect on Technicon AutoAnalyzer® Jaffe method *5704* At acute overdose concentration (5 mg/dL) on Technicon SMAC® method *6266*

Drugs of Abuse Screen *Urine No Effect Analytical* No effect at concentration of 100 µg/mL on EZ-SCREEN procedure for cannabinoids and cocaine *1739*

Erythrocytes *Blood Decrease Physiological* May cause aplastic/megaloblastic anemia *128* May occasionally cause aplastic anemia *1384*

Ethanol *Serum Increase Physiological* Coadministration observed to increase ethanol concentration probably due to effect on hepatic metabolism *4143* Concomitant ingestion of both compounds may cause ethanol concentration by approximately 10% probably due to an effect on hepatic enzymes *1384*

Ethosuximide *Serum Increase Analytical* At concentrations above 100 µg/mL (460 µmol/L) cross-reacts with method used on Du Pont aca but at clinically relevant concentrations probably no significant interference occurs *1523*

Folate *Red Blood Cells Decrease Physiological* Characteristic with anticonvulsant intake, possibly due to enhanced catabolism *5055*
Serum Decrease Physiological Characteristic with anticonvulsant intake, possibly due to enhanced catabolism *5055*

Glucaric Acid *Urine Increase Physiological* Manifestation of hepatic enzyme induction when 500 mg daily ingested for 21 d by 6 volunteers *642*

Glucose *Serum No Effect Analytical* No effect on method on Kodak Ektachem® at concentrations up to 17.5 mg/L *5706* At acute overdose concentration (5 mg/dL) on Technicon SMAC® method *6266*

Glutethimide *Blood Increase Physiological* 1 g orally may produce concentration of 7 mg/L *3868*

HDL-Cholesterol *Serum Increase Physiological* Significant effect from about 15 d of treatment with 500 mg drµg/d in 6 volunteers *642*

HDL-Triglycerides *Serum No Effect Physiological* No significant effect with 21 d of 500 mg daily in 6 volunteers *642*

Hematocrit *Blood Decrease Physiological* May occasionally cause aplastic anemia *1384*

Hemoglobin *Blood Decrease Physiological* May occasionally cause aplastic anemia *1384*

Iron *Serum No Effect Analytical* At acute overdose concentration (5 mg/dL) on Technicon SMAC® method *6266* At concentration of 50 mg/L had no effect on Ferrozine method *5704*

17-Ketogenic Steroids *Urine No Effect Analytical* Probably minimum interference with Zimmermann reaction *5869*

Lactate Dehydrogenase *Serum No Effect Analytical* At acute overdose concentration (5 mg/dL) on Technicon SMAC® method *6266*

LDL-Cholesterol *Serum Increase Physiological* Significant effect from about 15 d of treatment with 500 mg drµg/d in 6 volunteers *642*

LDL-Triglycerides *Serum No Effect Physiological* No significant effect with 21 d of 500 mg daily in 6 volunteers *642*

Leukocytes *Blood Decrease Physiological* May cause aplastic anemia *128* May occasionally cause leukopenia or aplastic anemia *1384*

Glutethimide *(continued)*

MCV *Blood Increase Physiological* May cause megaloblastic anemia *2242*

Methemoglobin *Blood Increase Physiological* Bleeding associated with overdosage *4014*

p-Aminophenol *Urine No Effect Analytical* With addition of drugs at a concentration of 100 mg/L and of related compounds at 50 mg/L no significant effect observed on colorimetric method of van Bocxlaer on Cobas Mira analyzer which involves reacting free p-aminophenol with resorcinol in the presence of magnesium ions to form an indophenol dye measured at 550 nm *6163*

Phosphate *Serum No Effect Analytical* At acute overdose concentration (5 mg/dL) on Technicon SMAC® method *6266* At concentration of 50 mg/L had no effect on phosphomolybdate method *5704*

Platelets *Blood Decrease Physiological* May cause aplastic anemia or thrombocytopenic purpura occasionally *1384* Thrombocytopenia or aplastic anemia *128*

Porphobilinogen *Urine Increase Physiological* May precipitate acute porphyria *2210* May cause acute intermittent porphyria *1384*

Porphyrin, Total *Urine Increase Physiological* May precipitate attack of acute porphyria *3669*

Potassium *Serum No Effect Analytical* At concentration of 10 mg/L had no effect on measurement by ISE with predilution *5704*

Primidone *Serum No Effect Analytical* No significant cross-reactivity with method on Du Pont aca *1541*

Protein *Serum No Effect Analytical* At acute overdose concentration (5 mg/dL) on Technicon SMAC® method *6266* At concentration of 50 mg/L had no effect on biuret method with blank correction *5704*

Prothrombin Time *Plasma Decrease Physiological* In 10 patients receiving 0.5 g/d when on warfarin due to hepatic microsomal enzyme Induction *6118* Increases rate of degradation of administered coumarins *4998*
Plasma Increase Physiological Effect observed with overdosage *4014*

Protoporphyrin *Feces Increase Physiological* May precipitate acute porphyria *2210* May cause increase in association with induced acute intermittent porphyria *1384*

Sodium *Serum No Effect Analytical* At concentration of 10 mg/L had no effect on measurement by ISE with predilution *5704*

Triglycerides *Serum No Effect Analytical* At acute overdose concentration (5 mg/dL) on Technicon SMAC® method *6266* At concentration of 50 mg/L had no effect on lipase/esterase method *5704*
Serum No Effect Physiological No significant effect with 21 d of 500 mg daily in 6 volunteers *642*

Urea Nitrogen *Serum No Effect Analytical* At acute overdose concentration (5 mg/dL) on Technicon SMAC® method *6266* At concentration of 50 mg/L had no effect on diacetylmonoxime method *5704* At concentrations up to 17.5 mg/L had no effect on method on Kodak Ektachem® *5706*

Uric Acid *Serum No Effect Analytical* At concentration of 17.5 mg/L had no effect on Kageyama-Hantzsch method *5704* At concentration of 50 mg/L had no effect on phosphotungstate reduction method *5704* At acute overdose concentration (5 mg/dL) on Technicon SMAC® method *6266*

Uroporphyrin *Urine Increase Physiological* May cause acute intermittent porphyria *1384*

VLDL-Cholesterol *Serum Increase Physiological* Significant effect from about 15 d of treatment with 500 mg drµg/d in 6 volunteers *642*

VLDL-Triglycerides *Serum No Effect Physiological* No significant effect with 21 d of 500 mg daily in 6 volunteers *642*

Warfarin *Plasma Decrease Physiological* In a study of normal individuals significant reduction in concentration probably due to induction of hepatic metabolizing microsomal enzymes: hypoprothrombinemic response to warfarin greatly reduced as a consequence *3711*

Glyburide

Alanine Aminotransferase *Serum Increase Physiological* Rare and reverts to normal if therapy continued *197* Intrahepatic cholestasis described in 61 y old diabetic *6536* Cholestatic jaundice and abnormalities of liver function tests rarely observed with glyburide administration *4676* Cholestatic jaundice and hepatitis may occur rarely with treatment *2646*
Serum No Effect Analytical No effect at therapeutic concentration on Boehringer Mannheim Reflotron method *3231* No effect at 1 mg/L on Boehringer Mannheim Reflotron method *5706*

Alkaline Phosphatase *Serum Increase Physiological* Intrahepatic cholestasis described in 61 y old diabetic *6536* Cholestatic jaundice and hepatitis may occur rarely with treatment *2646* Cholestatic jaundice and abnormalities of liver function tests rarely observed with glyburide administration *4676* Rare and reverts to normal if therapy continued *197*

Amylase *Serum No Effect Analytical* At a concentration of 1 mg/L had no effect on method on Boehringer Mannheim Reflotron system *5706*

Amylase, Pancreatic Isoenzyme
Serum No Effect Analytical No significant effect observed at toxic concentration of 1 mg/L on method on Boehringer Mannheim Reflotron *3647*

Antidiuretic Hormone *Urine Increase Physiological* Slight (not significant) effect *4136*

Aspartate Aminotransferase *Serum Increase Physiological* Intrahepatic cholestasis described in 61 y old diabetic *6536* Rare and reverts to normal if therapy continued *197* Cholestatic jaundice and abnormalities of liver function tests rarely observed with glyburide administration *4676* Cholestatic jaundice and hepatitis may occur rarely with treatment *2646*
Serum No Effect Analytical No effect at therapeutic concentration on Boehringer Mannheim Reflotron method *3231* No effect at 1 mg/L on Boehringer Mannheim Reflotron method *5706*

Bilirubin *Serum Increase Physiological* Cholestatic jaundice and hepatitis may occur rarely with treatment *2646* Intrahepatic cholestasis described in 61 y old diabetic *6536*
Serum No Effect Analytical No effect at 0.4 mg/L on Ames Seralyzer method *5706* At concentration of 1 mg/L had no effect on method on Boehringer Mannheim Reflotron system *5706*

Carvedilol *Serum No Effect Physiological* In 12 healthy individuals coadministration of drugs had no clinically relevant effect on pharmacokinetics of either compound *5639*

Cholesterol *Serum Decrease Physiological* Average reduction of 0.21 mmol/L in 16 diabetic patients treated for 9 months *4229* Similar effect to that of insulin in study of group of 31 noninsulin-dependent diabetics *4229* Fall by over 50 mg/dL in treated diabetics *197*
Serum Increase Physiological In 28 noninsulin-dependent diabetics treatment with 14 mg/d caused mean increase of 0.10 mmol/L after 4 months and 0.16 mmol/L after 6 months *2570*
Serum No Effect Analytical At concentration of 32 mg/L had no effect on method using catalase-Hantzsch reaction *5704* At concentration of 32 mg/L had no effect on catalase-AIDH method *5704* At concentration of 32 mg/L had no effect on Liebermann-Burchard method *5704* At concentration of 32 mg/L had no effect on CHOD-PAP method *5704* At concentration of 32 mg/L had no effect on CHOD-Iodide method *5704* No effect at 0.4 mg/L on Ames Seralyzer method *5706* No effect at therapeutic concentration on Boehringer Mannheim Reflotron method *3231* At concentration of 1 mg/L no effect on method on Boehringer Mannheim Reflotron system *5706*
Serum No Effect Physiological In 12 normotensive patients with NIDDM treatment for one month caused nonsignificant mean decrease of 0.2 mmol/L from baseline of 5.4 ± 0.2 mmol/L *959*

Cortisol *Plasma Increase Physiological* Occasional slightly higher, no significant change after glucose *197*
Plasma No Effect Analytical At a concentration of 1 mg/L no significant effect observed on CEDIA or Enzymun methods *1097*

C-Peptide *Plasma Increase Physiological* In one patient who had taken an overdose of glibenclamide concentration on admission was 839 pmol/L *3355*

Plasma No Effect Physiological Response to standardized meal unaffected by prior administration of 10 mg glyburide. Fasting concentration unchanged in 10 patients with noninsulin dependent diabetes mellitus following ingestion of 10 mg glyburide *1776* No significant effect in 11 noninsulin dependent diabetics treated for 6-10 weeks although blood glucose concentration reduced *5472*

Creatine Kinase *Serum No Effect Analytical* No effect at 0.4 mg/L on method on Ames Seralyzer *5706*

Creatinine *Serum No Effect Analytical* At 10 mg/L on reversed phase liquid chromatographic procedure of Zhiri et al *6656* At concentration of 3 mg/L had no effect on kinetic Jaffe method on BKA-2 *5704* Apparently no significant effect on Jaffe methods performed manually or on Technicon SMAC® , Beckman Astra® , Du Pont aca, or Roche Cobas-Bio at 5 times therapeutic concentration *4976* No effect at 0.4 mg/L on Ames Seralyzer method *5706* At concentration of 3 mg/L had no effect on Jaffe-Fading-Fraction method *5704* At concentration of 3 mg/L had no effect on Jaffe-Fuller's earth method *5704*

Serum No Effect Physiological No significant effect observed *197*

Fatty Acids (FFA), Free *Serum Decrease Physiological* Protracted fall maximal at 4.5 h *2511*

Fluvastatin *Serum No Effect Physiological* In 16 healthy individuals coadministration of glyburide with fluvastatin had no significant effect on the latter's concentration *227*

Fructosamine *Serum No Effect Physiological* In 12 normotensive patients with NIDDM treatment for one month caused nonsignificant mean decrease of 3.2 mmol/L from mean baseline of 329 ± 11 mmol/L *959*

Glucose *Serum Decrease Physiological* Fasting concentration reduced in 10 patients with noninsulin dependent diabetes mellitus *1776* Long acting sulfonylurea has effect comparable to that of insulin secretion *3659* Significant reduction in 16 diabetics treated for 9 months but not quite to extent in those treated with insulin *4229* Study involving comparison of insulin and glyburide showed glyburide effective in obtaining normoglycemia in group of noninsulin-dependent diabetics, with improvement similar to that obtained with insulin *4229* In 15 patients with NIDDM treatment caused reduction from mean baseline of 9.5 ± 2.4 mmol/L to 7.7 ± 1.7 mmol/L after 3 months and 8.4 ± 3.1 mmol/L after 15 months *579* After 6-10 weeks treatment in 11 patients with noninsulin-dependent diabetes mellitus fasting concentration decreased from mean of 12.3 mmol/L to 6.8 mmol/L *5472* In 12 normotensive patients with NIDDM treatment for one month caused mean decrease of 2.4 mmol/L from baseline of 10.5 ± 0.7 mmol/L *959* Therapeutic intent is to reduce blood glucose concentration but has the potential to cause hypoglycemia *2646*

Serum No Effect Analytical No effect at 0.4 mg/L on glucose oxidase method on Ames Seralyzer *5706* At concentration of 0.3 mg/L had no effect on Kodak Ektachem® method *5704* At concentration of 1 mg/L no effect on method on Boehringer Mannheim Reflotron system *5706* No effect on glucose oxidase method of Boehringer Mannheim *5480* No effect at therapeutic concentration on Boehringer Mannheim Reflotron method *3231*

Serum No Effect Physiological Response to a standardized meal during first hours following ingestion of 10 mg glyburide unaffected *1776*

Glucose Tolerance *Serum Increase Physiological* Marked improvement noted *3659*

γ-Glutamyltransferase *Serum No Effect Analytical* At concentration of 1 mg/L no effect on method on Boehringer Mannheim Reflotron system *5706* No effect at therapeutic concentration on Boehringer Mannheim Reflotron method *3231*

Glycated Hemoglobin *Blood No Effect Analytical* At a concentration of 500 mg/L had an insignificant - 0.7% interference with method on Abbott Vision *1885*

Glycerol *Serum Decrease Physiological* Response similar to that of free fatty acids *2511*

Granulocytes *Blood Decrease Physiological* Agranulocytosis rarely observed with sulfonylurea administration *4676* Agranulocytosis may occur rarely with treatment *2646*

Growth Hormone *Plasma No Effect Physiological* No effect observed *197*

HDL-Cholesterol *Serum Increase Physiological* Lesser effect than that of insulin in study of 31 noninsulin-dependent diabetics, but still marked effect. Ratio of HDL-cholesterol to total cholesterol increased *4229* Average increase of 0.21 mmol/L in 16 diabetic patients treated for 9 months *4229*

Serum No Effect Analytical At a concentration up to 1 mg/L had no significant effect on Reflotron method for whole blood cholesterol *6352*

Serum No Effect Physiological In 12 normotensive patients with NIDDM treatment for 4 weeks caused nonsignificant mean decrease of 0.05 mmol/L from mean baseline of 1.3 ± 0.1 mmol/L *959*

Hematocrit *Blood Decrease Physiological* Hemolytic or aplastic anemia rarely observed with sulfonylurea administration *4676* Hemolytic or aplastic anemia may occur rarely with treatment *2646*

Hemoglobin *Blood Decrease Physiological* Hemolytic or aplastic anemia rarely observed with sulfonylurea administration *4676* Hemolytic or aplastic anemia may occur rarely with treatment *2646*

Hemoglobin A_{1c} *Blood Decrease Physiological* Similar to insulin in extent of effect in 31 noninsulin-dependent diabetics *4229* In 12 normotensive patients with NIDDM treatment for 4 weeks caused mean decrease of 0.3% from mean baseline of 7.5 ± 0.2% *959* Marked effect in diabetic patients comparable to that in patients treated with insulin after 9 months treatment *4229*

Histamine *Plasma No Effect Analytical* Improbable inhibition of radio-enzyme assay at therapeutic concentrations *2492*

β-Hydroxybutyrate *Serum Decrease Physiological* In one patient who had taken an overdose of glibenclamide concentration on admission was 300 μmol/L in the presence of glucose concentration of 0.7 mmol/L *3355*

Indomethacin *Serum No Effect Analytical* No effect on HPLC method of Roberts and Smith *4978*

Insulin *Plasma Increase Physiological* Concentration remains increased longer (although of the same magnitude) in patients with NIDDM after test meal when glibenclamide coadministered probably by inhibiting the degradation of insulin in the vascular endothelial cells of the liver *4159* In 15 patients with NIDDM treatment caused increase from baseline of 103 ± 53 pmol/L to 114 ± 72 pmol/L after 3 months and 127 ± 60 pmol/L after 15 months *579* Significant increase reported *3659* Mean fasting concentration increased relative to nondiabetic control subjects during chronic treatment with glyburide *1776* In one patient with an overdose of glibenclamide concentration on admission 27 pmol/L inappropriately hogh for glucose concentration of 0.7 mmol/L *3355*

Plasma No Effect Physiological Response to standardized meal unaffected by ingestion of 10 mg glyburide. Fasting concentration unchanged by ingestion of 10 mg glyburide *1776* No significant effect observed with treatment for 6-10 weeks in 11 noninsulin dependent diabetics although blood glucose concentration reduced *5472*

Lactate Dehydrogenase *Serum No Effect Analytical* No effect at 0.4 mg/L on method on Ames Seralyzer *5706*

LDL-Cholesterol *Serum Decrease Physiological* In 28 noninsulin-dependent diabetics treatment with 14 mg/d for 4 months caused a mean decrease of 0.03 mmol/L *2570*

Serum Increase Physiological In 28 noninsulin-dependent diabetics treatment with 14 mg/d caused mean increase of 0.13 mmol/L after 6 months *2570*

Serum No Effect Physiological In 12 normotensive patients with NIDDM treatment for 4 weeks caused nonsignificant mean decrease of 0.2 mmol/L from mean baseline of 3.4 ± 0.2 mmol/L *959*

Leukocytes *Blood Decrease Physiological* Leukopenia rarely observed with sulfonylurea administration *4676* Leukopenia may occur rarely with treatment *2646*

Metformin *Serum No Effect Physiological* In a single dose study during which glyburide and metformin were coadministered no effect observed on pharmacokinetics or pharmacodynamics of metformin *726*

Osmolality *Urine Decrease Physiological* Normal diuretic response *4136*

Phenprocoumon *Plasma No Effect Physiological* No effect noted on plasma concentration nor drug half-life with coadministration *2538*

Glyburide *(continued)*

Platelets *Blood Decrease Physiological* Rare thrombocytopenia reported *197* Thrombocytopenia, which may occasionally present as purpura, may occur rarely with treatment *2646* Thrombocytopenia rarely observed with sulfonylurea administration *4676*

Potassium *Serum No Effect Analytical* At concentration of 3 mg/L had no effect on measurement by ISE with predilution *5704*

Proinsulin *Plasma No Effect Physiological* No significant effect after 6 mo *1612*

Protein *Urine Increase Analytical* Significant effect with Ponceau S dye method in comparison with sulfosalicylic method in 12 patients receiving up to 15 mg daily *6611*
Urine No Effect Analytical No significant difference in 12 patients receiving up to 15 mg daily with sulfosalicylic acid and trichloracetic acid methods *6611*

Protein Electrophoresis *Serum No Effect Analytical* At concentration of 3 mg/L had no effect on automated Olympus-Hite method *5704*

Prothrombin Time *Plasma Decrease Physiological* Possible interactions reported between glyburide and coumarin derivatives either potentiating or weakening the effects of the coumarin derivatives but the mechanism of these interactions not known *2646*
Plasma Increase Physiological Possible interactions reported between glyburide and coumarin derivatives either potentiating or weakening the effects of the coumarin derivatives but the mechanism of these interactions not known *2646*

Simvastatin *Serum No Effect Physiological* In 16 healthy individuals coadministration of glyburide with simvastatin had no significant effect on the latter's concentration *227*

Sodium *Serum Decrease Physiological* Hyponatremia rarely observed with glyburide administration *4676* Hyponatremia may occur rarely with treatment with glyburide or other sulfonylureas *2646*
Serum No Effect Analytical At concentration of 3 mg/L had no effect on measurement by ISE with predilution *5704*

Tirofiban *Serum No Effect Physiological* Coadministration had no significant effect on plasma clearance of tirofiban *3957*

Triglycerides *Serum Decrease Physiological* Fall by 50% in treated diabetics *197* Average reduction of 0.36 mmol/L in 16 diabetic patients treated for 9 months *4229* Similar effect to that of insulin in group of 31 noninsulin-dependent diabetics *4229*
Serum No Effect Analytical No effect at therapeutic concentration on Boehringer Mannheim Reflotron method *3231* No effect at 1 mg/L on Boehringer Mannheim Reflotron method *5706*
Serum No Effect Physiological In 12 normotensive patients with NIDDM treatment for 4 weeks caused nonsignificant mean decrease of 0.14 mmol/L from mean baseline of 1.5 ± 0.3 mmol/L *959*

Troglitazone *Serum No Effect Physiological* Coadministration of glyburide with troglitazone had no significant effect on the pharmacokinetics of either drug but may further decrease plasma glucose concentration *4532*

Urea Nitrogen *Serum No Effect Analytical* At concentration of 0.3 mg/L had no effect on Kodak Ektachem® method *5704* No effect at 1 mg/L on Boehringer Mannheim Reflotron method *5706* No effect at therapeutic concentration on Boehringer Mannheim Reflotron method *3231* No effect at 0.4 mg/L on method on Ames Seralyzer *5706*
Serum No Effect Physiological No significant effect observed *197*

Uric Acid *Serum No Effect Analytical* At concentration of 3 mg/L had no effect on Kageyama-Hantzsch method *5704* No effect at 1 mg/L on method on Boehringer Mannheim Reflotron *5706* At concentration of 3 mg/L had no effect on catalase-AIDH method *5704* No effect at therapeutic concentration on Boehringer Mannheim Reflotron method *3231* At 10 mg/L on reversed phase liquid chromatographic procedure of Zhiri et al *6656*

Volume *Urine Increase Physiological* Normal diuretic response *4136*

Water Clearance, Free *Urine Increase Physiological* Normal diuretic response *4136*

Glyceraldehyde

Lactate *Plasma No Effect Analytical* No significant effect observed at a concentration of 300 mg/dL with method on Kodak Ektachem® systems *2519*

Triglycerides *Serum Increase Analytical* Measured as glycerol with enzymatic procedures *4953*

Glyceric Acid

Lactate *Plasma Decrease Analytical* High concentrations interfere with enzymatic method *1887*

Glycerin

Acid Phosphatase *Serum No Effect Analytical* No interference observed at a concentration of 1 mmol/L with method on Kodak Ektachem® *2519*

1,2-Butanediol *Serum Increase Analytical* At an ethylene glycol concentration of 20 mmol/L 1,2-BD reacts on an equimolar basis with enzymatic method using glycerol dehydrogenase *3747*

2,3-Butanediol *Serum Increase Analytical* At an ethylene glycol concentration of 20 mmol/L 2,3-BD reacts slowly at a rate comparable to that of ethylene glycol with enzymatic method using glycerol dehydrogenase *3747*

Creatinine *Serum Increase Analytical* 100 mg/L of glycerin is equivalent to 0.03 mg/dL creatinine with method of Heinegard *2539*
Serum No Effect Analytical No interference observed at a concentration of 25 mg/L with HPLC method of Rosano et al *5083*

Ethanol *Serum No Effect Analytical* At a concentration of 1 mmol/L had no significant effect on method on Kodak Ektachem® *2519*

Ethylene Glycol *Serum Decrease Analytical* At an ethylene glycol concentration of 20 mmol/L reduction of 19% observed in the presence of 5 mmol/L glycerol with enzymatic method using glycerol dehydrogenase due to rapid NADH formation *3747*
Serum No Effect Analytical No significant effect observed at a concentration of 100 mmol/L with method of Standefer and Blackwell *5770* No significant interference observed with enzymatic method of Hansson and Masson since complete oxidation of the compound occurs in less than 1 minute *4299*

Glucose *Serum No Effect Physiological* No effect of ingestion of glycerol *6063*

Glycerol *Serum Increase Physiological* Rose from normal 0.51 mmol/L to 20 mmol/L *6063*

Hematocrit *Blood Decrease Physiological* Hemolysis may occur after i.v. administration *2400* Maximum decrease about 80 minutes after ingestion *6063*

Hemoglobin *Blood Decrease Physiological* Hemolysis may occur after i.v. administration *2400*
Plasma Increase Physiological Hemolysis may occur after i.v. administration *2400*
Urine Increase Physiological Rare transient effect after i.v. infusion *6063* Isolated cases after 20% solution i.v *2474*

ionized Calcium *Serum Decrease Analytical* At 0.1-1.0 mol/L with calcium specific electrode *820*

Lactate *Plasma No Effect Analytical* No significant effect observed at a concentration of 0.75 mmol/L with method on Kodak Ektachem® systems *2519*

Lipase *Serum No Effect Analytical* No effect of concentrations up to 2.85 mmol/L on method on Kodak Ektachem® *5706* No significant effect observed at concentrations of 0.85 and 2.85 mmol/L with method on Kodak Ektachem® systems *2519*

Lithium *Serum No Effect Analytical* No significant effect observed at a concentration of 1 mmol/L with method on Kodak Ektachem® systems *2519*

Osmolality *Serum Increase Physiological* Rose an average of 19 mosm/kg *6063*

Phosphatidylglycerol *Amniotic Fluid Increase Analytical* Since glycerol content 20 times that of analyte results inaccurate by enzymatic method unless glycerol removed *2573*

Amniotic Fluid *No Effect* *Analytical* At a concentration of 1000 µmol/L had no significant effect on enzymatic method of Jones and Ashwood *2969*

Protein *Test Conditions* *Increase* *Analytical* Interferes with Lowry and biuret methods *6674*
Urine *Increase* *Physiological* Hemolysis may occur after i.v. administration *2400*

Sodium *Serum* *Decrease* *Physiological* Maximum effect of less than 5% *6063*

Triglycerides *Serum* *Increase* *Analytical* When enzymatic procedure used is end product of reaction *6028* At a concentration of 0.75 mmol/L caused positive bias of 33 mg/dL at triglyceride concentration of 80 mg/dL with method on Kodak Ektachem® systems *2519* Reacts in method on Du Pont Dimension *1592* Will react in method on Du Pont aca and cause positive interference *1551*

Volume *Urine* *Increase* *Physiological* Weak osmotic diuretic action *4311*

Glycerophosphate

Phosphate *Serum* *No Effect* *Analytical* No interference observed from α- and β-glycerophosphates at concentration of 55 mg/dL (3.0 mmol/L) with method on Du Pont aca *1539*

Triglycerides *Serum* *No Effect* *Analytical* No significant effect observed with α-glycerophosphate at a concentration of 2 mg/dL (59 µmol/L) on method on Du Pont aca *1551*

Glycine Xylidide

Lidocaine *Serum* *No Effect* *Analytical* At a concentration of 1250 mg/L had less than 10% effect on method on Baxter Stratus *5705* No significant interference observed at a concentration of 100 µg/mL (561 µmol/L) with method on Du Pont aca *1534*

N-Acetylprocainamide *Serum* *No Effect* *Analytical* No significant interference observed at a concentration of 100 µg/mL (561 µmol/L) with method on Du Pont aca *1536*

Procainamide *Serum* *No Effect* *Analytical* No significant interference observed at a concentration of 100 µg/mL (561 µmol/L) with method on Du Pont aca *1542*

Glycine Xylidine

Lidocaine *Serum* *No Effect* *Analytical* No significant interference observed at a concentration of 100 µg/mL (561 µmol/L) with method on Du Pont aca *1534*

N-Acetylprocainamide *Serum* *No Effect* *Analytical* No significant interference observed at a concentration of 100 µg/mL (561 µmol/L) with method on Du Pont aca *1536*

Procainamide *Serum* *No Effect* *Analytical* No significant interference observed at a concentration of 100 µg/mL (561 µmol/L) with method on Du Pont aca *1542*

Glycocholate

Lipase *Serum* *Increase* *Analytical* Sodium salts prevent inactivation of enzyme *6027*

Glycocyamidine

Creatinine *Serum* *Increase* *Analytical* Reacts to give false increase with Jaffe reagent *5869*
Urine *Increase* *Analytical* 1 mg equivalent to 0.30 mg with automated Jaffe procedure *4222*

Glycolic Acid

Ethanol *Serum* *No Effect* *Analytical* At a concentration of 700 mg/dL had no significant effect on method on Kodak Ektachem® *2519*

β-Hydroxybutyrate *Urine* *No Effect* *Analytical* At concentration of 100-200 mmol/L did not affect enzymatic procedure of GDS Diagnostics *1824*

Glycopyrrolate

Alanine Aminotransferase *Serum* *Increase* *Physiological* Hepatotoxicity *3810*

Alkaline Phosphatase *Serum* *Increase* *Physiological* Hepatotoxicity *3810*

Aspartate Aminotransferase *Serum* *Increase* *Physiological* Hepatotoxicity *3810*

Bile *Urine* *Increase* *Physiological* Hepatotoxicity *3810*

Bilirubin *Serum* *Increase* *Physiological* Hepatotoxicity *3810*

BSP Retention *Serum* *Increase* *Physiological* Hepatotoxicity *3810*

Histamine *Plasma* *No Effect* *Analytical* No effect at physiological concentrations on radio-enzyme assay *2492*

Glycylglycine

Protein *Test Conditions* *Decrease* *Analytical* Lowry procedure due to chelation of chemicals *2936*

Glymidine

Erythrocyte Sedimentation Rate
Blood *Increase* *Physiological* Slight rise in mean rate reported *4014*

Glucose *Serum* *Decrease* *Physiological* Plasma half-life approximately 4 h *4227*

Gold

Alanine Aminopeptidase *Urine* *Increase* *Physiological* In 13% (not significant) increase of microsomal enzyme in 31 patients treated with parenteral gold *4889*

Alanine Aminotransferase *Serum* *Increase* *Physiological* Due to toxic effect on drug on liver *2741* Hepatotoxicity with centrolobular necrosis *3810*

Alkaline Phosphatase *Serum* *Increase* *Physiological* Rare side effect with liver damage (reversible) *139* Cholestatic jaundice in 3 patients with rheumatoid arthritis given gold sodium thiomalate: all patients recovered spontaneously *1814* In 3 patients with rheumatoid arthritis during chrysotherapy *1656* In 17 women with rheumatoid arthritis treatment for 24 months caused a significant increase in activity *6011*

Alkaline Phosphatase, Bone Isoenzyme
Serum *Increase* *Physiological* In 17 women with rheumatoid arthritis treatment for 24 months caused a significant increase in activity *6011*

δ-Aminolevulinic Acid *Urine* *Increase* *Physiological* Occurs with panmyelopathy *2242*

Aspartate Aminotransferase *Serum* *Increase* *Physiological* Due to toxic effect of drug on liver *2741* Cholestatic jaundice in 3 patients with rheumatoid arthritis given gold sodium thiomalate: all patients recovered spontaneously *1814* Hepatotoxicity with centrolobular necrosis *3810* In 3 patients with rheumatoid arthritis during chrysotherapy *1656*

Bile *Urine* *Increase* *Physiological* Hepatotoxicity with centrolobular necrosis *3810*

Bilirubin *Serum* *Increase* *Physiological* Cholestatic jaundice in 3 patients with rheumatoid arthritis given gold sodium thiomalate: all patients recovered spontaneously *1814* Due to toxic effect of drug on liver *2741* In 3 patients with rheumatoid arthritis during chrysotherapy *1656* Rare side effect with liver damage *4014*

Bilirubin, Direct *Serum* *Increase* *Physiological* Cholestatic jaundice in 3 patients with rheumatoid arthritis given gold sodium thiomalate; all patients recovered spontaneously *1814* In 3 patients with rheumatoid arthritis during chrysotherapy *1656*

BSP Retention *Serum* *Increase* *Physiological* Hepatotoxicity with centrolobular necrosis *3810*

Cholesterol *Serum* *Increase* *Physiological* May cause hypersensitive cholestasis *2377*

Coproporphyrin *Urine* *Increase* *Physiological* Occurs with panmyelopathy *2242*

Gold (continued)

Creatinine Clearance *Urine Decrease Physiological* In 11 patients who showed glomerular injury, including minimal change nephrotic syndrome with a membranous pattern of immune complex deposition as well as other patterns of deposition *1934*

Diclofenac *Serum No Effect Physiological* Coadministration of gold with diclofenac did not significantly affect the peak concentration or AUC of diclofenac *1025*

Eosinophils *Blood Increase Physiological* Occurred in 21% patients taking gold sodium thiomalate and in 13% taking auranofin. Occurred in 24% and 30% respectively with toxicity *1655* Transient allergic response *209* Observed in 11% of 64 treated patients *5617*

Erythrocyte Sedimentation Rate
Blood Decrease Physiological With 200 mg aurothioglucose at 4 weeks intervals mean ESR fell from 46 to 26 mm/h in 30 patients *4330*

Erythrocytes *Blood Decrease Physiological* Blood dyscrasias major side effect as reported to UK Committee on safety of Medicines *1204* 7 cases out of 246 treated cases *1278* Occasional case of aplastic anemia reported *6264* Aplastic anemia *209*
Urine Increase Physiological Produces actual bleeding *1714*

γ-Globulin *Serum Decrease Physiological* Single case reported *4014*

γ-Glutamyltransferase *Serum No Effect Physiological* No significant changes of microsomal enzyme in patients treated with parenteral drug *4889*
Urine Increase Physiological In 6.5% (not significant) in 31 patients treated with parenteral gold *4889*

Gold *Red Blood Cells Increase Physiological* Up to 45% of blood concentration in RBC *5626*

Hematocrit *Blood Decrease Physiological* Aplastic anemia *209*

Hemoglobin *Blood Decrease Physiological* Aplastic anemia *209*
Urine Increase Physiological Produces actual bleeding *1714*

^{131}I Uptake *Serum No Effect Physiological* No effect observed *3107*

immunoglobulin A *Serum Decrease Physiological* Substantial lowering at 3 mo in 25 patients with rheumatoid arthritis treated with gold *6193*

Immunoglobulin G *Serum Decrease Physiological* Substantial lowering at 3 mo in 25 patients with rheumatoid arthritis treated with gold *6193*

Immunoglobulin M *Serum Decrease Physiological* Substantial lowering at 12 mo in 25 patients with rheumatoid arthritis treated with gold *6193*

Lactate Dehydrogenase *Serum Increase Physiological* Cholestatic jaundice in 3 patients with rheumatoid arthritis given gold sodium thiomalate: all patients recovered spontaneously *1814*

LE Cells *Blood Positive Physiological* SLE may occur, usually normalizes when stopped *5102*

Leukocytes *Blood Decrease Physiological* Significant reduction observed in 10 cases through action on bone marrow *6588* Occasional case of aplastic anemia reported *6264* Aplastic anemia/Leukopenia/agranulocytosis *209* Reported in 6 patients: brief self-limiting process *2266* 7 cases out of 246 treated cases *1278* Blood dyscrasias major side effect as reported to UK Committee on Safety of Medicines *1204* In 3% of 90 patients with rheumatoid arthritis *2413*
Blood Increase Physiological Due to eosinophilia of hypersensitivity *3810*

Lymphocytes *Blood No Effect Physiological* No effect observed with megadose supplementation *2245*

N-Acetyl-Glucosaminidase *Serum No Effect Physiological* No significant changes of microsomal enzyme in patients treated with parenteral drug *4889*
Urine Increase Physiological In 77% in 31 patients treated with parenteral gold *4889*

Neutrophils *Blood Decrease Physiological* Occasional case of sodium aurothiomalate induced neutropenia *241* Reported in 6 patients: brief self-limiting process *2266*
Blood No Effect Physiological No effect observed with megadose supplementation *2245*

Occult Blood *Feces Increase Physiological* Associated with thrombocytopenia *4014* Rare side effect as reported to UK Committee on Safety of Medicines *1204*

Partial Thromboplastin Time
Plasma Increase Physiological In one 3 y old with rheumatoid arthritis *2741*

Platelets *Blood Decrease Physiological* 7 cases out of 246 treated cases *1278* Occasional case of aplastic anemia reported *6264* Severe thrombocytopenia observed 18 mo after end of gold therapy for rheumatoid arthritis *5766* Significant reduction observed with treatment observed in 10 cases *6588* In 23 patients treated for 25 y: apparently associated with HLA-DR3 alloantigen *1066* Several cases of platelet-associated IgG and thrombocytopenia *3102* In 3% of 90 patients with rheumatoid arthritis *2413* Aplastic anemia (thrombocytopenia) *209* Blood dyscrasias major side effect as reported to UK Committee on Safety of Medicines *1204*

Protein *Urine Increase Physiological* Observed in 16% of 90 patients with rheumatoid arthritis in one study *1204* HLA DR3 positive patients had 3 times risk of this side effect than those without antigen *2289* Observed in 3% of 1283 patients ranging from mild to heavy: did not persist beyond 12 mo. Some patients showed membranous glomerulonephritis *3066* May cause nephrotoxicity *4014* In 11 patients who showed glomerular injury, including minimal change nephrotic syndrome with a membranous pattern of immune complex deposition as well as other patterns of deposition *1934* Nephrotoxic effect (at least in 50% cases) *1714* Good correlation between amount of protein and duration of proteinuria. Moderate proteinuria does not preclude reinstitution of therapy once protein has cleared *4270* Prevalence of gold nephropathy about 1 in 500. Nephropathy not necessarily related to other side effects *1278* In 16% of 90 patients with rheumatoid arthritis *2413*

Prothrombin Time *Plasma Increase Physiological* In one 3 year old with rheumatoid arthritis *2741*

Soluble Interleukin-2 Receptor
Serum Decrease Physiological In37 patients with rheumatoid arthritis treatment with parenteral gold for 37 weeks caused mean concentration to decrease from 928 ± 372 U/mL to 854 ± 370 U/mL *3999*

T3-Uptake *Serum No Effect Physiological* No effect observed with resin *3107*

Urea Nitrogen *Serum Increase Physiological* May cause nephrotoxicity *5377*

Xylose *Urine Decrease Physiological* May produce gastrointestinal irritation, impaired absorption and subsequent reduced excretion *929*

Gold Sodium Thiomalate

Alanine Aminotransferase *Serum Increase Physiological* Hepatitis, jaundice (with/without cholestasis) may occur as a consequence of gold toxicity *3986*

Alkaline Phosphatase *Serum Increase Physiological* Hepatitis, jaundice (with/without cholestasis) may occur as a consequence of gold toxicity *3986*

Aspartate Aminotransferase *Serum Increase Physiological* Hepatitis, jaundice (with/without cholestasis) may occur as a consequence of gold toxicity *3986*

Bilirubin *Serum Increase Physiological* Hepatitis, jaundice (with/without cholestasis) may occur as a consequence of gold toxicity *3986*

Blood *Urine Increase Physiological* Hematuria or proteinuria may occur with a glomerulitis or nephrotic type syndrome, although the complications are usually relatively mild *3986*

Eosinophils *Blood Increase Physiological* Blood dyscrasias, including eosinophilia are rare but may have serious consequences *3986*

γ-Glutamyltransferase *Serum Increase Physiological* Hepatitis, jaundice (with/without cholestasis) may occur as a consequence of gold toxicity *3986*

Granulocytes *Blood Decrease Physiological* Blood dyscrasias, including hypoplastic and aplastic anemia, are rare but may have serious consequences *3986*

Hematocrit *Blood Decrease Physiological* Blood dyscrasias, including hypoplastic and aplastic anemia, are rare but may have serious consequences *3986*

Hemoglobin *Blood Decrease Physiological* Blood dyscrasias, including hypoplastic and aplastic anemia, are rare but may have serious consequences *3986*

Phenylalanine *Plasma No Effect Analytical* No inteference observed with rapid quantitative whole blood method of Campbell et al using phenylalanine dehydrogenase *867*

Platelets *Blood Decrease Physiological* Blood dyscrasias are rare but may have serious consequences. Thrombocytopenia may occur with or without purpura *3986*

Protein *Urine Increase Physiological* Hematuria or proteinuria may occur with a glomerulitis or nephrotic type syndrome, although the complications are usually relatively mild *3986*

Testosterone *Serum No Effect Physiological* In a group of male patients with rheumatoid arthritis taking gold sodium thiomalate mean concentration not significantly different from concentration in untreated male patients *3808*

Gold Thioglucose

Chondrex *Serum No Effect Analytical* Concentrations up to 10 g/L had no significant effect on sandwich-type ELISA procedure of Harvey et al *2491*

Gonadotropin-Releasing Hormone

Follicle Stimulating Hormone
Plasma Increase Physiological 100 µg i.v. bolus injection caused significant increase in both normal cycling women and perimenopausal women with dysfunctional uterine bleeding but increase greater in control group *872*

Luteinizing Hormone *Plasma Increase Physiological* Significant increase in both normal cycling women and perimenopausal women with dysfunctional uterine bleeding following i.v. bolus injection of 100 µg, but effect greater in control women *872* After bolus of 100 µg i.v. concentration rose from about 5 mIU/mL to 25 mIU/mL at 45 minutes after injection in 3 lean children but peak much lower in obese children *517*

Polyamines *Serum Increase Physiological* After i.v. bolus of 100 µg in 6 normal children rose from mean of 12.6 to 19.3 nmol/mL at 60 minutes but no significant change observed in obese children *517*

Prolactin *Plasma Increase Physiological* Effect observed in both normal cycling women and perimenopausal women with dysfunctional uterine bleeding following 100 µg i.v. bolus injection *872*

Spermidine *Serum Increase Physiological* Increases in parallel to total polyamine concentration in normal children following i.v. injection of bolus of 100 µg with peak at 60 minutes *517*

Spermine *Serum Increase Physiological* Increases in parallel with total polyamine concentration in normal children following i.v. bolus of 100 µg with peak concentration at 60 minutes *517*

Goserelin

Alanine Aminotransferase *Serum Increase Physiological* Reported to cause increased activity in fewer than 1% treated women *6652*

Androsterone *Plasma No Effect Physiological* Nonsignificant reduction from mean of 7.4 nmol/L to 6.4 nmol/L in 6 nonobese women with minimal endometriosis treated with 3.6 mg subcutaneously every 28 days *2233*

Antithrombin III *Plasma Decrease Physiological* Decrease observed in 22 patients with metastatic prostatic cancer but not as marked as when DES used *1731*

Aspartate Aminotransferase *Serum Increase Physiological* Reported to cause increased activity in fewer than 1% treated women *6652*

Blood *Urine Increase Physiological* Reported to cause hematuria in 1 to 5% treated patients *6652*

Cholesterol *Serum No Effect Physiological* No effect observed in patients with pelvic endometriosis *1173*

C-Peptide *Plasma No Effect Physiological* Nonsignificant increase from mean of 330 pmol/L to 350 pmol/L in fasting concentration in 6 nonobese women with minimal endometriosis treated with 3.6 mg subcutaneously every 28 days: also no change in summed concentration with OGTT *2233*

Dehydroepiandrosterone Sulfate
Plasma No Effect Physiological No significant change observed in 6 nonobese women with minimal endometriosis treated with 3.6 mg subcutaneously every 28 days *2233*

Estradiol *Plasma Decrease Physiological* Castrate levels produced in majority of patients with premenopausal advanced breast cancer. When combined with tamoxifen effect even more marked *4992* Sharp suppression of estradiol-17β concentration observed in 32 women with laparoscopic diagnosis of endometriosis when treated with drug for 6 months *6226*

17β-Estradiol *Plasma Decrease Physiological* Sharp suppression observed in 32 women with laparoscopic diagnosis of endometriosis when treated with drug for 6 months *6226*

Follicle Stimulating Hormone
Plasma Decrease Physiological Significant reduction from mean of 6.3 IU/L to 3.4 IU/L in 6 nonobese women with minimal endometriosis treated with 3.6 mg subcutaneously every 28 days *2233*
Plasma No Effect Physiological After initial decrease reverted to pretreatment concentration in 32 women with laparoscopic diagnosis of endometriosis when treated for 6 months *6226*

Glucagon *Plasma No Effect Physiological* Nonsignificant increase in fasting concentration from mean of 16 pmol/L to 22 pmol/L in 6 nonobese women with minimal endometriosis treated with 3.6 mg subcutaneously every 28 days with increase in summed concentration from 62 to 81 pmol/L with OGTT *2233*

Glucose *Serum Increase Physiological* Reported to cause diabetes mellitus in 1 to 5% treated patients *6652*
Serum No Effect Physiological No significant change in fasting concentration or in summed concentration in 6 nonobese women with minimal endometriosis following treatment with 3.6 mg subcutaneously every 28 days *2233*

HDL_3-Cholesterol *Serum Increase Physiological* Subfraction increased in response to treatment in patients with pelvic endometriosis *1173*

HDL-Cholesterol *Serum Increase Physiological* Reported to cause mean increase of 2.7 mg/dL in treated women *6652*

Hematocrit *Blood Decrease Physiological* Reported to cause anemia in 1 to 5% treated patients *6652*

Hemoglobin *Blood Decrease Physiological* Reported to cause anemia in 1 to 5% treated patients *6652*

Insulin *Plasma No Effect Physiological* Nonsignificant increase from 40 pmol/L to 49 pmol/L in fasting concentration in 6 nonobese women with minimal endometriosis treated with 3.6 mg subcutaneously every 28 days: Likewise no significant change observed in summed concentration following OGTT *2233*

Insulin-like Growth Factor-I *Serum Increase Physiological* In 8 out of 12 premenopausal women mean concentration decreased from 23.3 nmol/L to 19.4 nmol/L during treatment *3566*

LDL-Cholesterol *Serum Increase Physiological* Reported to cause mean increase of 21.3 mg/dL in treated women *6652*

Luteinizing Hormone *Plasma Decrease Physiological* Depressed concentrations observed in 32 women with laparoscopic diagnosis of endometriosis treated for 6 months *6226* Significant decrease from mean baseline concentration of 8.0 IU/L to 3.8 IU/L in 6 nonobese women with minimal endometriosis treated with 3.6 mg subcutaneously every 28 days *2233*
Plasma Increase Physiological Observed during first month of treatment *1384*

Progesterone *Plasma Decrease Physiological* Castrate levels produced in majority of premenopausal women with advanced breast cancer *4992*

Prostate-specific Antigen, Free *Serum No Effect Analytical* Goserelin acetate at a concentration of 2.5 mg/L had no significant effect on the Hybritech Tandem® -R free PSA immunoassay *4286*

Goserelin *(continued)*

Sex-Hormone Binding Globulin
Serum No Effect Physiological Nonsignificant reduction from mean of 62 nmol/L to 51 nmol/L in 6 nonobese women with minimal endometriosis treated with 3.6 mg subcutaneously every 28 days *2233*

Testosterone *Serum Decrease Physiological* Median concentration reduced to below 50 ng/dL in 81 men with stage D_2 prostate cancer with 4 weeks treatment with 3.6 mg goserelin acetate (zoladex) and remained suppressed for up to 60 weeks *5681* Only androgenic hormone observed to be decreased in 32 women with laparoscopic diagnosis of endometriosis when treated for 6 months *6226*
Serum Increase Physiological Transient increases in concentration with initiation of treatment *6652* Observed during first month of treatment *1384*
Serum No Effect Physiological Insignificant reduction from mean of 2.2 nmol/L to 1.8 nmol/L in 6 nonobese women with minimal endometriosis treated with 3.6 mg subcutaneously every 28 days *2233*

Testosterone Index, Free *Serum No Effect Physiological* No significant change observed in 6 nonobese women with minimal endometriosis treated with 3.6 mg subcutaneously every 28 days *2233*

Triglycerides *Serum Increase Physiological* Reported to cause mean increase of 8.0 mg/dL in treated women *6652*
Serum No Effect Physiological No effect observed in patients with pelvic endometriosis *1173*

Uric Acid *Serum Increase Physiological* Reported to cause gout rarely *6652*

Gossypol

Cortisol *Plasma No Effect Physiological* No significant effect observed when 10 mg/day given for 3 months *1961*

Estradiol *Plasma No Effect Physiological* No significant effect observed when 10 mg/day given for 3 months *1961*

Follicle Stimulating Hormone
Plasma No Effect Physiological No significant effect observed when 10 mg/day given for 3 months *1961*

Luteinizing Hormone *Plasma No Effect Physiological* No significant effect observed when 10 mg/day given for 3 months *1961*

β_2-Microglobulin *Serum No Effect Physiological* No significant effect observed when 10 mg/day given for 3 months *1961*

Potassium *Serum No Effect Physiological* No significant effect observed when 10 mg/day given for 3 months *1961*

Prolactin *Plasma No Effect Physiological* No significant effect observed when 10 mg/day given for 3 months *1961*

Protein *Urine No Effect Physiological* No significant effect observed when 10 mg/day given for 3 months. No effect observed on other urinalyses *1961*

Sperm Count *Semen Decrease Physiological* After 2 months of treatment with 10 mg/day significant effect noted although increase actually observed during first month in this study *1961*

Sperm Motility *Semen Decrease Physiological* Significant reduction observed after incubation with gossypol although no effect observed immediately after incubation *2696* Significant reduction observed within first month of treatment with 10 mg/day *1961*

Testosterone *Serum No Effect Physiological* No significant effect observed when 10 mg daily given for 3 months *1961*

Urea Nitrogen *Serum No Effect Physiological* No significant effect observed when 10 mg/day given for 3 months *1961*

GPA-1714

Alanine Aminotransferase *Serum Increase Physiological* In 4 of 11 patients increased when dose of approximately 3 g given *5566*

Granisetron

Alanine Aminotransferase *Serum Increase Physiological* Increases of more than two times the upper limit of normal observed in 6% of treated patients *5649*

Aspartate Aminotransferase *Serum Increase Physiological* Increases of more than two times the upper limit of normal observed in 5% of treated patients *5649*

Hematocrit *Blood Decrease Physiological* Anemia observed in 4% of treated patients *5649*

Hemoglobin *Blood Decrease Physiological* Anemia observed in 4% of treated patients *5649*

Leukocytes *Blood Decrease Physiological* Leukopenia observed in 11% of treated patients *5649*

Platelets *Blood Decrease Physiological* Thrombocytopenia observed in 3% of treated patients *5649*

Granulocyte Colony Stimulating Factor

Alkaline Phosphatase *Serum Increase Physiological* Reversible spontaneous increases observed in 27 to 58% of 98 patients receiving drug in a blinded manner following cytotoxic chemotherapy. Increases were mild to moderate *147* Increase observed following administration *3567*
White Blood Cells Increase Physiological Consistent increase in score to above 200 (normal 60 to 140) observed in 6 patients with cyclic neutropenia treated for 3 to 15 months *2430*

Basophils *Blood No Effect Physiological* No significant change observed in patients receiving drug with counts remaining within normal range *147*

Cholesterol *Serum Decrease Physiological* Decrease observed after initiation of treatment *3567*

Eosinophil Cationic Protein *Serum Increase Physiological* In 14 healthy volunteers administration of G-CSF for 6 days at a dose of 7.5 or 10 µg/kg body weight caused four-fold increase of mean concentration on day 2 and reached a maximum concentration of 61.82 ± 7.38 µg/L on day 4 from basal concentration of 12.39 ± 2.45 µg/L *3040*

Eosinophil Peroxidase *Serum Increase Physiological* In 14 healthy volunteers administration of G-CSF for 6 days at a dose of 7.5 or 10 µg/kg body weight caused a significant increase of mean concentration on day 3 and reached a maximum concentration of 19.98 ± 5.1 µg/L on day 5 from basal concentration of 8.89 ± 2.2 µg/L *3040*

Eosinophil Protein X *Serum Increase Physiological* In 14 healthy volunteers administration of G-CSF for 6 days at a dose of 7.5 or 10 µg/kg body weight caused a significant increase of mean concentration on day 2 and reached a maximum concentration of 87.86 ± 9.8 µg/L on day 5 from basal concentration of 28.05 ± 4.54 µg/L *3040*

Eosinophils *Blood Increase Physiological* In 14 healthy volunteers administration of G-CSF for 6 days at a dose of 7.5 or 10 µg/kg body weight caused increase of mean concentration to $0.37 \pm 0.19 \times 10^9$/L on day 2 and $0.61 \pm 0.10 \times 10^9$/L from basal concentration of $0.22 \pm 0.04 \times 10^9$/L *3040*
Blood No Effect Physiological No significant effect observed in patients receiving drug with count remaining within the normal range *147*

Glucose *Serum Decrease Physiological* Rate of decrease of blood glucose concentration increased in patients receiving granulocyte-colony stimulating factor (0.29 mmol/L/h) compared with 0.17 mmol/L/h in 10 controls probably due to increased glucose uptake by WBC and through induction of energy processes *265*

Lactate Dehydrogenase *Serum Increase Physiological* Increased lactate dehydrogenase observed after administration *3567* Spontaneous reversible increases observed in 27 to 58% of 98 patients receiving filgrastim in a blinded manner following cytotoxic chemotherapy. Increases were mild to moderate *147*

Leukocytes *Blood Decrease Physiological* Administration results in immediate transient leukopenia with nadir occurring 5-15 min after intravenous administration and 30-60 min after subcutaneous administration *3567*
Blood Increase Physiological Leukocytosis of 100,000 /µL or more observed in approximately 2% patients receiving doses above 5 µg/kg/d *147*

Lymphocytes *Blood Increase Physiological* With doses of about 10 μg/kg body weight/d concentration increases slightly *3567*

Lysozyme *Serum Increase Physiological* After initiation of treatment significant increase in activity observed *3567*

Magnesium *Granulocyte No Effect Physiological* Mean concentration in patients receiving granulocyte-colony stimulating factor 4.45 ± 0.55 fmol/cell not significantly different from 4.35 ± 0.62 fmol/cell in healthy controls *3660*
Monocytes No Effect Physiological Mean concentration in patients receiving granulocyte-colony stimulating factor 3.82 ± 0.39 fmol/cell not significantly different from 3.74 ± 0.66 fmol/cell in healthy controls *3660*

Monocytes *Blood Decrease Physiological* Transient reduction observed 5-15 min after intravenous administration and 30-60 min after subcutaneous administration *3567*
Blood Increase Physiological Dose-dependent increase observed in most patients receiving drug although percentage of monocytes in the differential count remained within the normal range *147* With doses of about 10 μg/kg body weight /d monocyte concentration increased slightly *3567*

Myeloblasts *Blood Increase Physiological* Observed usually during neutrophil recovery from chemotherapy-induced nadir *147*

Neutrophils *Blood Decrease Physiological* After administration transient reduction observed occurring 5-15 min after intravenous administration and 30-60 min after subcutaneous administration *3567*
Blood Increase Physiological Significant in vivo effect observed in one patient with idiopathic neutropenia treated with 3 μg/kg per day for about 5 months with count increasing from less than 500 /μL to over 10000 /μL *2892* In 6 individuals with cyclic neutropenia i.v. or s.c. for 3 to 15 months increased mean count from 717 /μL to 9814 /μL with reduced cycling period in 5 of the 6 patients *2430* In 8 patients with chronic neutropenia mean concentration increased from baseline of 400 to 1600 cells /μL to 1800 to 11000 cells /μL after several weeks treatment with doses from 10 to 30 μg/sq m/d *3000* In 14 healthy volunteers administration of G-CSF for 6 days at a dose of 7.5 or 10 μg/kg body weight caused six-fold increase of mean concentration after 2 days with decrease occurring after day 7 *3040* Caused dose-dependent increase in absolute neutrophil count when given to patients prior to chemotherapy. If given to patients after chemotherapy reduced the number of days during which the absolute neutrophil count was less than 1000 /μL *6034* Administration for 2 weeks showed sustained dose-dependent increase with stabilization or slight decrease during second week (generally about 8-fold increase. Neutrophilia is characterized by 'left shift' to more immature forms. After cessation of treatment concentration reverts to baseline in 4-7 days *3567* In a phase I study involving 96 patients with various non-myeloid malignancies administration of drug resulted in a dose-dependent increase in circulating neutrophils over dose range of 1-70 μg/kg/d regardless of route of administration *147*

Promyelocytes *Blood Increase Physiological* Observed with treatment with shift towards granulocyte progenitor cells (left shift) usually during neutrophil recovery following the chemotherapy induced nadir *147*

Soluble E-selectin *Serum Increase Physiological* In 12 neutropenic patients with hematological malignancies administration of G-CSF given 50 μg/m²/d subcutaneously for 4 days caused significant increase from mean baseline of 51 ± 20 ng/mL to 78 ± 20 ng/mL *4385*

Soluble L-selectin *Serum Increase Physiological* In 12 neutropenic patients with hematological malignancies administration of G-CSF given 50 μg/m²/d subcutaneously for 4 days caused significant increase from mean baseline of 514 ± 56 ng/mL to 746 ± 64 ng/mL *4385*

Soluble P-selectin *Serum Increase Physiological* In 12 neutropenic patients with hematological malignancies administration of G-CSF given 50 μg/m²/d subcutaneously for 4 days caused significant increase from mean baseline of 638 ± 115 ng/mL to 921 ± 107 ng/mL *4385*

Uric Acid *Serum Increase Physiological* After initiation of treatment increased concentration observed *3567* Spontaneously reversible increases in concentration observed in from 27% of 98 patients receiving filgrastim in a blinded manner following cytotoxic chemotherapy. Increases were mild to moderate *147*

Griseofulvin

Alanine Aminotransferase *Serum Increase Physiological* Hepatoxicity occurred rarely in treated patients *5330* May be hepatotoxic *3669*

Alkaline Phosphatase *Serum Increase Physiological* Hepatoxicity occurred rarely in treated patients *5330* May be hepatotoxic *3669*

δ-Aminolevulinic Acid *Urine Increase Physiological* May precipitate acute porphyria attack *2210*

Aspartate Aminotransferase *Serum Increase Physiological* Hepatoxicity occurred rarely in treated patients *5330* May be hepatotoxic *3669*

Bilirubin *Serum Increase Physiological* Hepatoxicity occurred rarely in treated patients *5330*

Casts *Urine Increase Physiological* Cylindruria may occur without renal insufficiency *2242*

Coproporphyrin *Feces Increase Physiological* May precipitate acute porphyria attack *2210*
Urine Increase Physiological May precipitate acute porphyria attack *2210*

Creatinine *Serum Increase Physiological* Rare renal damage reported *198*

Creatinine Clearance *Urine Decrease Physiological* Rare renal damage reported *198*

γ-Glutamyltransferase *Serum Increase Physiological* Hepatoxicity occurred rarely in treated patients *5330*

Granulocytes *Blood Decrease Physiological* Administration associated with rare granulocytopenia *111*

LE Cells *Blood Positive Physiological* May produce LE-like syndrome *5870*

Leukocytes *Blood Decrease Physiological* May cause leukopenia/neutropenia *4014* Administration associated with rare leukopenia *111* Leukopenia may occur rarely with treatment *4447* Leukopenia occurred rarely in treated patients *5330*

Lymphocytes *Blood Increase Physiological* (relative lymphocytosis) *4014*

Monocytes *Blood Increase Physiological* Causes relative monocytosis *4014*

Neutrophils *Blood Decrease Physiological* Occasional case of agranulocytosis reported *6264* May cause decrease by up to 20% with fall in total count *3883*

Porphobilinogen *Urine Increase Physiological* May precipitate acute porphyria attack *2210*

Porphyrin, Total *Blood Increase Physiological* May precipitate acute porphyria attack *4691*
Urine Increase Physiological Stimulates formation of ALA-synthetase *2242*

Protein *Urine Increase Physiological* ?nephrotoxic effect (transient and reversible) *1714* Proteinuria may occur rarely with treatment *4447* May cause nephrotoxicity *965* Administration associated with rare proteinuria *111* Proteinuria occurred rarely in treated patients *5330*

Prothrombin Time *Plasma Decrease Physiological* When coadministered with warfarin increases its metabolic clearance *2625* Reduces prothrombin time when coadministered with warfarin probably through increased metabolic clearance *2625* Induces hepatic metabolism of anticoagulants *1191*

Protoporphyrin *Feces Increase Physiological* May precipitate acute porphyria attack *2210*

Urea Nitrogen *Serum Increase Physiological* Rare renal damage reported *198*

Uric Acid *Serum Decrease Physiological* Effective in treatment of gout ?mechanism *6326*

Growth Hormone Releasing Hormone

Fatty Acids (FFA), Free *Serum Increase Physiological* Administration of 1 μg/kg GHRH [GRF-(1-29)NH_2] caused increase to peak concentration of about 470 μEq/L from baseline of about 450 μEq/L in 7 healthy controls and to about 1100 μEq/L from about 1000 μEq/L in 6 hyperthyroid individuals 30 min after infusion, with increases to about 800 μEq/L and 1300 μEq/L respectively after 120 min *3475*

Growth Hormone Releasing Hormone *(continued)*

Follicle Stimulating Hormone
Plasma Increase Physiological Following intravenous injection of 1 µg/kg into 20 short prepubertal children short-term small increase noted *2075*

Growth Hormone *Plasma Increase Physiological* Effect observed with both GHRH 1-29 and GHRH 1-40 in 20 short prepubertal children. Mean maximal peak concentration similar (of the order of 90 mU/L) after each hormone given as 1 µg/kg body weight intravenously *2075* Administration of 1 µg/kg GHRH [GRF-(1-29)NH_2] caused increase to peak concentration of 25 µg/L in 7 healthy controls and 8 µg/L in 6 hyperthyroid individuals 30 min after infusion *3475*

Luteinizing Hormone *Plasma Increase Physiological* Following intravenous injection of 1 µg/kg into 20 short prepubertal children short-term small increase noted *2075*

Prolactin *Plasma Increase Physiological* Following intravenous injection of 1 µg/kg of GHRH 1-29 into 20 short prepubertal children short-term small increase noted *2075* In patients with pituitary dwarfism administration of 1 µg/kg of synthetic human pancreatic GH-releasing hormone (hpGRF-44) caused increase of 120% at 15 minutes *2495*

Thyroid Stimulating Hormone
Serum Decrease Physiological 1 µg/kg body weight intravenously of synthetic human pancreatic GH-RH caused decrease from mean basal concentration of 1.22 /µU/mL to 1.00 /µU/mL at 30 minutes to 1.07 /µU/mL at 60 min and 0.95 /µU/mL at 90 min in patients with pituitary dwarfism *2495*
Serum No Effect Physiological No effect observed in healthy individuals when 1 µg/kg injected intravenously *2495*

Guaiacol

Color *Urine Increase Analytical* May produce green color *1957*

5-Hydroxyindoleacetic Acid *Urine No Effect Analytical* No effect of guaiacol glyceryl ether on FPIA method on Abbott TDx *695*

Guaifenesin

Cannabinoids *Urine No Effect Analytical* No effect on Roche Abuscreen method *5006*

Guaiacols Spot Test *Urine Positive Analytical* False reaction with screening test of Rogers *5061*

5-Hydroxyindoleacetic Acid *Urine Increase Analytical* Interferes with nitrosonaphthol method *2024* Affects quantitative method of Udenfriend *882* Reported interference with some analytical procedures *939*
Urine No Effect Analytical No effect on TLC method of McGregor *3899* No effect *in vivo* dose on method of Goldenberg *2220*

2-Methoxyphenoxy-Lactic Acid
Urine Increase Physiological Major metabolite (44% of 1 g in 3 h) *6206*

p-Aminophenol *Urine No Effect Analytical* With addition of drugs at a concentration of 100 mg/L and of related compounds at 50 mg/L no significant effect observed on colorimetric method of van Bocxlaer on Cobas Mira analyzer which involves reacting free p-aminophenol with resorcinol in the presence of magnesium ions to form an indophenol dye measured at 550 nm *6163*

Platelet Aggregation *Blood Decrease Physiological* Reported effect *5560*

Theophylline *Serum No Effect Analytical* At concentration of 200 mg/L produced no interference with methods on Kodak DT60, Abbott TDx, Abbott Vision with either whole blood or serum, 3M Diagnostics TheoFAST, Syntex AccµLevel or Ames Seralyzer *1122*

Uric Acid *Serum Decrease Physiological* Modest hypouricemic effect, with fall of up to 3 mg/dL over 3 d in some patients *4847*

Vanillylmandelic Acid *Urine Increase Analytical* Reported interference with some analytical procedures *939* Affects p-nitraniline in initial part of reaction *1174*

Guanabenz

Apolipoprotein A-I *Serum No Effect Physiological* Increase by 5 mg/dL in patients given 4 to 8 mg daily for 12 to 16 weeks *4213*

Apolipoprotein B *Serum No Effect Physiological* Increase by 2 mg/dL in patients given 4 to 8 mg daily for 12 to 16 weeks *4213*

Apolipoprotein C-II *Serum No Effect Physiological* No change in patients given 4 to 8 mg daily for 12 to 16 weeks *4213*

Apolipoprotein C-III *Serum No Effect Physiological* No change in patients given 4 to 8 mg daily for 12 to 16 weeks *4213*

Apolipoprotein E *Serum Decrease Physiological* No change in patients given 4 to 8 mg daily for 12 to 16 weeks *4213*

Cholesterol *Serum Decrease Physiological* Decrease by -10 mg/dL in patients given 4 to 8 mg daily for 12 to 16 weeks *4213* Mean concentration in 480 patients treated for up to 2 y decreased by 10 mg/dL. Decrease maintained throughout subsequent therapy *3036*

Glucagon *Plasma Increase Physiological* In 30 hypertensives: effect most marked in individuals with higher doses. No change observed on withdrawal of drug *1689*

Growth Hormone *Plasma No Effect Physiological* In 30 patients treated with twice daily doses of from 4 to 32 mg *1689*

HDL-Cholesterol *Serum No Effect Physiological* Increase by 1 mg/dL in patients given 4 to 8 mg daily for 12 to 16 weeks *4213* No effect in 39 hypertensives treated for 2 y *3036*

Insulin *Plasma No Effect Physiological* In 30 patients treated with twice daily doses of from 4 to 32 mg *1689*

LDL-Cholesterol *Serum Decrease Physiological* In 39 patients treated for 2 y: approximately 23 mg/dL decrease *3036*

Prolactin *Plasma No Effect Physiological* In 30 patients treated with twice daily doses of from 4 to 32 mg *1689*

Triglycerides *Serum No Effect Physiological* Decrease by -13 mg/dL in patients given 4 to 8 mg daily for 12 to 16 weeks *4213* No effect in 39 hypertensives treated for 2 y *3036*

Guanazole

Leukocytes *Blood Decrease Physiological* Observed in approximately 80% patients *2584*

Platelets *Blood Decrease Physiological* Observed in almost all patients *2584*

Guancydine

Aspartate Aminotransferase *Serum Increase Physiological* Transient increases observed in some cases *1049*

Chloride *Urine Decrease Physiological* Reduced renal blood flow causes retention *3516*

Creatinine Clearance *Urine Decrease Physiological* Due to decreased renal blood flow *3516*

Effective Renal Plasma Flow
Patient Decrease Physiological Due to hypotensive action of drug *3516*

Sodium *Urine Decrease Physiological* Probable action on renal tubules *6261*

Volume *Urine Decrease Physiological* Probable action on renal tubules *6261*

Guanethidine

Alanine Aminotransferase *Serum Increase Physiological* Possible myopathic complication *3669*

Amphetamine *Serum Decrease Physiological* Gastrointestinal acidifying agents lower absorption of amphetamines including dextroamphetamine *5641*

Aspartate Aminotransferase *Serum Increase Physiological* Possible myopathic complication *3669*

Catecholamines *Urine Decrease Physiological* Inhibits release of norepinephrine *6277*

Chloride *Serum Increase Physiological* Salt retention ?due to tubular effect *2242*

Epinephrine *Urine Increase Physiological* Slight increased output reported *5147*

Glucose *Serum Decrease Physiological* Antidiabetic activity (rise once stop therapy) *2370*

Glucose Tolerance *Serum Increase Physiological* Antidiabetic activity (change at end of treatment) *2370*

Norepinephrine *Urine Decrease Physiological* Nonsignificant decrease reported *5147*

Prothrombin Time *Plasma Increase Physiological* Enhances anticoagulant activity *2242*

Quinidine *Serum No Effect Analytical* No significant interference observed at a concentration of 100 µg/mL (504 µmol/L) with method on Du Pont aca *1543*

Sodium *Serum Increase Physiological* Salt retention ?due to tubular effect *2242*

Tyramine Test *Patient Increase Physiological* Increased response to tyramine due to MAO inhibition *2213*

Urea Nitrogen *Serum Increase Analytical* Due to chemical similarity to urea *139*
Serum Increase Physiological Rare increase in urea nitrogen concentration observed *1029* Associated with blood pressure reduction, decreased blood flow *2754*

Vanillylmandelic Acid *Urine Decrease Physiological* 30% reduction seen if given therapeutically *6540*
Urine Increase Physiological Initial pharmacological response (changes later) *1444*

Guanfacine

Aldosterone *Plasma Decrease Physiological* Nonsignificant reduction from mean baseline with placebo of 6.32 ng/dL to 5.73 ng/dL in 11 patients with untreated and uncomplicated essential hypertension when treated with 1 g daily for 4 weeks *510*

Antidiuretic Hormone *Plasma Decrease Physiological* In 11 patients with untreated and uncomplicated essential hypertension administration of 1 mg daily for 4 weeks reduced mean vasopressin concentration with placebo from 8.21 ng/L to 2.81 ng/L with drug *510*

Catecholamines *Urine Decrease Physiological* Reduction from mean of 209 µg/24 h to 140 µg/24 h in 20 patients with hypertension following single oral dose of 3 mg *3840*

Cholesterol *Serum Decrease Physiological* Increase by 14% in 30 patients treated for 2 y *142*

Dopamine *Plasma Decrease Physiological* Significant reduction in 20 patients with hypertension from baseline of 188 pg/mL to 150 pg/mL at 60 minutes and 143 pg/mL at 120 minutes following single oral dose of 3 mg *3840*

Epinephrine *Plasma Decrease Physiological* Significant reduction in 20 hypertensive patients given single oral dose of 3 mg from mean of 395 pg/mL at baseline to 311 pg/mL at 60 minutes and 299 pg/mL at 120 minutes *3840*

5-Hydroxyindoleacetic Acid *Urine Decrease Physiological* Reduction from mean baseline concentration of 4.7 mg/24 h to 3.3 mg/24 h in 20 hypertensive patients following single oral dose of 3 mg *3840*

5-Hydroxytryptamine *Urine Decrease Physiological* Reduction from mean baseline excretion of 5.0 mg/24 h to 4.0 mg/24 h in 20 patients with hypertension following single oral dose of 3 mg *3840*

Metanephrine *Urine No Effect Analytical* No effect at 2 mg/L on HPLC method *557*

Norepinephrine *Plasma Decrease Physiological* Significant reduction from mean of 693 pg/mL to 526 pg/mL at 60 minutes and 474 pg/mL at 120 minutes in 20 patients with hypertension given single oral dose of 3 mg *3840*

Normetanephrine *Urine No Effect Analytical* No effect at 2 mg/L on HPLC method *557*

Osmolality *Serum No Effect Physiological* No significant change from mean baseline with placebo of 289 mOsm/kg to 290 mOsm/kg with 1 g drug daily for 4 weeks in 11 patients with untreated and uncomplicated essential hypertension *510*

Renin Activity *Plasma Decrease Physiological* Nonsignificant reduction from mean activity of 0.75 ng/mL/h to 0.68 ng/mL/h in 11 patients with untreated and uncomplicated essential hypertension treated with 1 mg daily for 4 weeks *510*

Triglycerides *Serum Decrease Physiological* Increase by 15% in 30 patients treated for 2 y *142*

Vanillylmandelic Acid *Urine Decrease Physiological* Reduction from mean baseline excretion of 3.5 µg/24 h to 2.1 µg/24 h in 20 hypertensive patients following single oral dose of 3 mg *3840*

Guanoclor

Alanine Aminotransferase *Serum Increase Physiological* Possible effect on liver *3669*

Aspartate Aminotransferase *Serum Increase Physiological* Possible effect on liver *3669*

Glucose *Serum Decrease Analytical* Affects glucose oxidase method of Boehringer *5480*

Urea Nitrogen *Serum Increase Physiological* May decrease renal blood flow *1714*

Guanoxan

Alanine Aminotransferase *Serum Increase Physiological* May cause hepatic toxicity *3810*

Alkaline Phosphatase *Serum Increase Physiological* May cause hepatic toxicity *3810*

Aspartate Aminotransferase *Serum Increase Physiological* May cause hepatic toxicity *3810*

Bile *Urine Increase Physiological* May cause hepatic toxicity *3810*

Bilirubin *Serum Increase Physiological* May cause hepatic toxicity *3810*

BSP Retention *Serum Increase Physiological* May cause hepatic toxicity *1975*

LE Cells *Blood Positive Physiological* SLE may occur, usually normalizes when stopped *5102*

Norepinephrine *Urine Decrease Physiological* Decreased output reported *5147*

Urea Nitrogen *Serum Increase Physiological* Due to decreased blood flow *3669*

Gum Tragacanth

Cholesterol *Serum No Effect Physiological* In 5 male volunteers consuming 9.9 g daily for 21 d *1650*

Fat *Feces Increase Physiological* In 5 male volunteers consuming 9.9 g daily for 21 d *1650*

Glucose Tolerance *Serum No Effect Physiological* In 5 male volunteers consuming 9.9 g daily for 21 d *1650*

Hydrogen *Breath No Effect Physiological* In 5 male volunteers consuming 9.9 g daily for 21 d *1650*

Methane *Breath No Effect Physiological* In 5 male volunteers consuming 9.9 g daily for 21 d *1650*

Phospholipids *Serum No Effect Physiological* In 5 male volunteers consuming 9.9 g daily for 21 d *1650*

Triglycerides *Serum No Effect Physiological* In 5 male volunteers consuming 9.9 g daily for 21 d *1650*

Haemaccel

Amylase *Serum No Effect Analytical* At a concentration of 7,000 mg/L had no effect on p-nitrophenylmaltoheptoside/hexoside method *5704* At a concentration of 7,000 mg/L had no effect on p-nitrophenylmaltoheptoside method *5704* At a concentration of 7,000 mg/L had no effect on maltotetrose method *5704*

Halazepam

Benzodiazepine *Urine Positive Analytical* At concentrations of 0.3 μg/mL or greater produces positive result with Syva EMIT II assay *1785*

Halofenate

Alanine Aminotransferase *Serum Increase Physiological* Mild transient effect observed. ?origin *250*

Aspartate Aminotransferase *Serum Increase Physiological* Mild transient effect observed. ?origin *250*

Bilirubin *Serum Decrease Physiological* No reversal of early effect with long treatment *2798*

Cholesterol *Serum Decrease Physiological* Irregular effect, mean decrease up to 9% *511*
Serum No Effect Physiological No significant effect observed in hyperlipemics *250*

Creatine Kinase *Serum Increase Physiological* Mild transient effect observed. ?origin *250*

Prealbumin *Serum No Effect Physiological* No effect observed after 3 weeks *4114*

Propranolol *Serum Decrease Physiological* Concomitant administration of both drugs although mechanism not established *2755*

T3-Uptake *Serum Increase Physiological* Resin uptake increased by 20% after 3 weeks *4114*

Thyroxine Binding Globulin *Serum No Effect Physiological* No effect observed after 3 weeks *4114*

Thyroxine (T4) *Serum Decrease Physiological* Interferes with binding of T4 to thyroxine binding globulin *4114*
Serum Increase Physiological Associated with competition for transport proteins *6412*

Thyroxine (T4), Free *Serum Increase Physiological* Associated with competition for transport proteins *6412* Interferes with binding of T4 to thyroxine binding globulin *4114*

Thyroxine (T4), Free Dialyzable
Serum Increase Physiological Lowers binding to thyroxine binding globulin and albumin *1280*

Thyroxine (T4) Index, Free *Serum Increase Physiological* Associated with competition for transport proteins *6412*

Thyroxine (T4) (Murphy-Pattee)
Serum Increase Physiological Significant increase observed *4114*

Tolbutamide *Serum Increase Physiological* Effect observed in 6 of 9 diabetics receiving halofenate with reduction in glucose concentration: mechanism not yet understood *2889*

Tri-iodothyronine (T3) *Serum Increase Physiological* Associated with competition for transport proteins *6412*

Triglycerides *Serum Decrease Physiological* Reduced by up to 50% *4114*

Uric Acid *Serum Decrease Physiological* Uricosuric action *4114* 500 mg/d/48 weeks causes reduction of 35% *250*
Urine Increase Physiological Effect independent of GFR *4114*

Haloperidol

Alanine Aminotransferase *Serum Increase Physiological* In 71 patients treated with haloperidol 45.8% had activity greater than the upper limit of normal *2773* Reports of impaired liver function and/or jaundice *3915* In isolated case producing cholestatic liver disease: typical frequency of liver disease is 0.2% *1433* May cause hepatocellular changes *3810*

Alkaline Phosphatase *Serum Increase Physiological* May cause hepatocellular changes *3810* In isolated case producing cholestatic liver disease: typical frequency of liver disease is 0.2% *1433* Reports of impaired liver function and/or jaundice *3915* In 71 patients treated with haloperidol 13.6% had activity greater than the upper limit of normal *2773*

Antidiuretic Hormone *Plasma No Effect Physiological* No effect of intravenous injection *4866*

Aspartate Aminotransferase *Serum Increase Physiological* In 71 patients treated with haloperidol 37.1% had activity greater than the upper limit of normal *2773* Reports of impaired liver function and/or jaundice *3915* In isolated case producing cholestatic liver disease: typical frequency of liver disease is 0.2% *1433* May cause hepatocellular changes *3810*

Bile *Urine Increase Physiological* May cause hepatocellular changes *3810*

Bilirubin *Serum Increase Physiological* Reports of impaired liver function and/or jaundice *3915* In 71 patients treated with haloperidol 16.2% had a concentration greater than the upper limit of normal *2773* In isolated case producing cholestatic liver disease: typical frequency of liver disease is 0.2% In isolated case producing cholestatic liver disease: typical frequently of liver disease is 0.2% *1433* May cause hepatocellular changes *3810*

Bilirubin, Direct *Serum Increase Physiological* In isolated case producing cholestatic liver disease; typical frequency of liver disease is 0.2% *1433*

BSP Retention *Serum Increase Physiological* May cause hepatocellular changes *3810*

Calcium *Serum No Effect Physiological* In 10 patients treatment with 30 to 45 mg/d for 2 weeks caused nonsignificant change from mean baseline of 4.71 ± 0.41 mEq/L to 4.68 ± 0.48 mEq/L *2366*

Carbamazepine *Serum Decrease Physiological* In 14 patients treated with haloperidol and carbamazepine mean concentration of carbamazepine 6.4 ± 1.8 μg/mL significantly higher than 4.5 ± 1.5 μg/mL in 8 patients treated with carbamazepine alone *2852*

Catecholamines *Plasma No Effect Analytical* No effect on HPLC method of Koller for dopamine, epinephrine, and norepinephrine *3230*

Cholesterol *Serum Decrease Physiological* Inhibits cholesterol biosynthesis *3810*
Serum No Effect Physiological No detectable effect observed in man *5565*

Clomipramine *Serum Increase Physiological* Coadministration with clomipramine has been reported to increase the plasma concentration of clomipramine *1021*

Corticotropin-releasing Hormone
Cerebrospinal Fluid Increase Physiological Concentration in 18 of 21 male chronic schizophrenics rose significantly on withdrawal of haloperidol *1915*

Creatine Kinase *Serum Increase Physiological* In 35 acutely psychotic patients treatment with olanzapine and haloperidol (2 - 33 determinations per patient) was associated with 4 marked elevations (in 11.4% of the patients) *3947*
Serum No Effect Physiological In 3 of 4 individuals injected with 2 mL fluid intramuscularly CK activity not increased *309*

Desmosterol *Serum Increase Physiological* Further metabolism inhibited so accumulates *2242*

Eosinophils *Blood Increase Physiological* In isolated case producing cholestatic liver disease: typical frequency of liver disease is 0.2% *1433*

Erythrocytes *Blood Decrease Physiological* Reports of minimal decreases in erythrocyte count and anemia *3915* May cause anemia *3810*

Glucose *Serum Decrease Physiological* Insulin like action of drug reported in one case *2451* Reports of both hypoglycemia and hyperglycemia *3915*
Serum Increase Physiological Observed endocrinological disorder *2754* Reports of both hypoglycemia and hyperglycemia *3915*

γ-Glutamyltransferase *Serum Increase Physiological* In 71 patients treated with haloperidol 17.5% had activity greater than the upper limit of normal *2773* In isolated case producing cholestatic liver disease: typical frequency of liver disease is 0.2% *1433*

Granulocytes *Blood Decrease Physiological* In 218 patients with refractory schizophrenia treated for one year neutropenia of less than 1500 granulocytes/μL observed in 9 patients *5100*

Hematocrit *Blood Decrease Physiological* Reports of minimal decreases in erythrocyte count and anemia *3915*

Hemoglobin *Blood Decrease Physiological* Reports of minimal decreases in erythrocyte count and anemia *3915*

Histamine *Plasma No Effect Analytical* Improbable inhibition of radio-enzyme assay at physiological concentrations *2492*

Homovanillic Acid *Plasma Decrease Physiological* Study of 14 schizophrenic subjects showed good correlation between reduction from day 4 to day 28 and degree of improvement after 4 weeks of treatment *1272*

Immunoglobulin M *Serum No Effect Physiological* In 14 patients with schizophrenia treatment for 5 years did not increase IgM concentrations *0*

Indocyanine Green *Serum Decrease Physiological* Mechanism not yet established *3942*

Leukocytes *Blood Decrease Physiological* Several cases reported but none of agranulocytosis *407* In 218 patients with refractory schizophrenia treated for one year leukopenia of less than 3000 leukocytes/μL observed in 2 patients *5100* Reports of both transient leukopenia or leukocytosis *3915* May cause anemia *3810*

Blood Increase Physiological Reports of both transient leukopenia or leukocytosis *3915* Rarely reported leukocytosis *128*

Lymphocytes *Blood Increase Physiological* Slight effect may occur *2754*

Lysergic Acid Diethylamide *Urine Increase Analytical* Minimum concentration that caused a positive result with EMIT method to measure LSD 0.07 mg/L *4968*

Magnesium *Serum Decrease Physiological* In 4 patients treatment with 30 to 45 mg/d for 2 days caused reduction from mean baseline of 2.10 ± 0.40 mEq/L to 1.80 ± 0.25 mEq/L after 2 weeks of treatment *2856*

Monoamine Oxidase *Platelets Decrease Physiological* Significant reduction in both acute and chronic schizophrenics. Effect seen after 14 d and results did not correlate with response to treatment *3742*

Monocytes *Blood Increase Physiological* Slight effect may be observed *2754*

Nefazodone *Serum No Effect Physiological* Administration of 5 mg haloperidol to individuals dosed with nefazodone to steady state led to no significant pharmacokinetic interaction of haloperidol on the pharmacokinetics of nefazodone and its metabolites *365*

Peptides, Low-molecular Weight

Urine Decrease Physiological In one schizophrenic patient treatment with 8 mg/d for 5 weeks caused significant reduction from 47 μmol/d to 13 μmol/d *4901*

Phosphate *Serum No Effect Physiological* In 10 patients treatment with 30 to 45 mg/d for 2 weeks caused nonsignificant change from mean baseline of 1.10 ± 0.25 mEq/L to 1.17 ± 0.20 mEq/L *2856*

Platelets *Blood No Effect Physiological* No significant reduction, in contrast to phenothiazines, in psychiatric patients treated for more than 1 y *2684*

Prolactin *Plasma Increase Physiological* Repeated administration of 1 mg i.m. to 19 normal men produced reproducible dose-response curve *3402* Without prior treatment prolactin concentration increased in response to oral or intramuscular haloperidol in schizophrenics. After treatment for 1 month with haloperidol effect no longer seen *3797* In schizophrenic population treated with fluphenazine by injection half of the patients exhibited increased concentration *6454*

Prothrombin Time *Plasma Decrease Physiological* May shorten action of anticoagulants *2753*

Sodium *Serum Decrease Physiological* Reports of hyponatremia in association with other medications *3915*

Testosterone *Serum No Effect Physiological* Has no effect, unlike some other neuroleptics *2836*

Tricyclic Antidepressants *Serum Increase Physiological* Interacts pharmacokinetically to inhibit metabolism of tricyclic antidepressants *3590*

Valproic Acid *Serum No Effect Physiological* In a study involving the coadministration of a 6 to 10 mg/d doses of haloperidol to schizophrenics with 400 mg/d dose of valproate resulted in no significant effect on the trough plasma concentrations of valproate *15* Administration of 6 - 10 mg/d of haloperidol to schizophrenic patients already receiving 200 mg b.i.d. revealed no significant change in trough valproic acid concentration *17*

Zolpidem *Serum No Effect Physiological* Coadministration of haloperidol had no effect on the pharmacokinetics or pharmacodynamics of zolpidem *2062*

Halothane

Alanine Aminotransferase *Serum Increase Physiological* Mild, moderate and severe hepatic dysfunction, including hepatic necrosis, have observed as adverse effects *6556*

Alkaline Phosphatase *Serum Increase Physiological* Mild, moderate and severe hepatic dysfunction, including hepatic necrosis, have observed as adverse effects *6556*

Aspartate Aminotransferase *Serum Increase Physiological* Mild, moderate and severe hepatic dysfunction, including hepatic necrosis, have observed as adverse effects *6556*

Bilirubin *Serum Increase Physiological* Mild, moderate and severe hepatic dysfunction, including hepatic necrosis, have observed as adverse effects *6556*

Bromide *Serum Increase Physiological* Theoretical possibility if halothane hydrobromide is administered since it contains 81% bromide *5116*

γ-Glutamyltransferase *Serum Increase Physiological* Mild, moderate and severe hepatic dysfunction, including hepatic necrosis, have observed as adverse effects *6556*

Glutathione S-Transferase *Serum Increase Physiological* In 16 of 20 patients who received halothane as anesthetic for mild urological procedures small transient rise observed 1-3 hours after anesthesia *2796* Halothane anesthesia caused a significant increase in GST concentration with peak concentrations occurring 3 h after anesthesia (by 20 - 50%) *4880*

Phenytoin *Serum Increase Physiological* When halothane ingested with fosphenytoin concentration of phenytoin may be increased *4519* Coadministration with phenytoin may increase plasma phenytoin concentration *4522*

Hemoglobin Substitute

Alanine Aminotransferase *Serum Decrease Analytical* At any concentration tested caused unacceptable results with Ektachem® and Hitachi procedures *1007*

Albumin *Serum No Effect Analytical* At concentrations less than 2 g/dL had no effect on Beckman method *1007*

Alkaline Phosphatase *Serum Decrease Analytical* At any concentration studied caused unacceptable results with Kodak Ektachem® and Hitachi procedures *1007*

Aspartate Aminotransferase *Serum Decrease Analytical* At any concentration tested caused unacceptable results with Kodak Ektachem® and Hitachi procedures *1007*

Bicarbonate *Serum No Effect Analytical* No effect observed on Beckman method at any concentrations tested *1007*

Bilirubin *Serum Increase Analytical* At any concentration tested caused unacceptable results with Kodak Ektachem® and Hitachi procedures *1007*

Calcium *Serum No Effect Analytical* At concentrations less than 0.44 g/dL had no significant effect on Kodak Ektachem® and Hitachi methods *1007*

Creatine Kinase *Serum No Effect Analytical* With dilution had no effect at any concentration tested with Kodak Ektachem® method *1007*

Creatine Kinase Isoenzymes *Serum No Effect Analytical* At any concentration tested after dilution had no significant effect on Baxter Stratus CK-MB method *1007*

Creatinine *Serum No Effect Analytical* At any concentration tested no significant effect observed on Beckman method *1007*

Glucose *Serum No Effect Analytical* No effect observed at any concentration tested with Beckman procedure *1007*

Phosphate *Serum No Effect Analytical* At concentrations tested had no significant effect on Kodak Ektachem® and Hitachi procedures *1007*

Potassium *Serum No Effect Analytical* At any concentration tested had no effect on Beckman method *1007*

Protein *Serum No Effect Analytical* At any concentration tested had no effect on Kodak Ektachem® procedure *1007*

Hemoglobin Substitute *(continued)*

Sodium *Serum* *No Effect* *Analytical* At any concentration tested had no effect on Beckman method *1007*

Urea Nitrogen *Serum* *No Effect* *Analytical* No effect observed at any concentration tested on Beckman method *1007*

Hepatitis A Vaccine, Inactivated

Alanine Aminotransferase *Serum* *Increase* *Physiological* In post-marketing reports jaundice and hepatitis observed *5647* Isolated reports of abnormal liver function tests following treatment *3996*

Alkaline Phosphatase *Serum* *Increase* *Physiological* Isolated reports of abnormal liver function tests following treatment *3996* In post-marketing reports jaundice and hepatitis observed *5647*

Aspartate Aminotransferase *Serum* *Increase* *Physiological* Isolated reports of abnormal liver function tests following treatment *3996* In post-marketing reports jaundice and hepatitis observed *5647*

Bilirubin *Serum* *Increase* *Physiological* Isolated reports of abnormal liver function tests following treatment *3996* In post-marketing reports jaundice and hepatitis observed *5647*

Eosinophils *Blood* *Increase* *Physiological* Isolated reports of eosinophilia following treatment *3996*

γ-Glutamyltransferase *Serum* *Increase* *Physiological* In post-marketing reports jaundice and hepatitis observed *5647*

Protein *Urine* *Increase* *Physiological* Isolated reports of increased excretion of protein following treatment *3996*

Hepatitis B Vaccine

Alanine Aminotransferase *Serum* *Increase* *Physiological* In clinical practice some cases of abnormal liver function reported *5644*

Alkaline Phosphatase *Serum* *Increase* *Physiological* In clinical practice some cases of abnormal liver function reported *5644*

Aspartate Aminotransferase *Serum* *Increase* *Physiological* In clinical practice some cases of abnormal liver function reported *5644*

Bilirubin *Serum* *Increase* *Physiological* In clinical practice some cases of abnormal liver function reported *5644*

Platelets *Blood* *Decrease* *Physiological* In clinical practice some cases of thrombocytopenia reported *5644*

HEPES

Protein *Test Conditions* *Increase* *Analytical* Interferes with Folin-Ciocalteu of Lowry *6104*

Heptabarbital

Prothrombin Time *Plasma* *Decrease* *Physiological* Induces hepatic metabolism of anticoagulants *3669*

Heptachlor

Alanine Aminotransferase *Serum* *Increase* *Physiological* Liver damage occurs as late effect of poisoning *2183*

Aspartate Aminotransferase *Serum* *Increase* *Physiological* Liver damage occurs as late effect of poisoning *2183*

Hetacillin

Aspartate Aminotransferase *Serum* *Increase* *Physiological* Observed with other penicillins (cause?) *2754*

Eosinophils *Blood* *Increase* *Physiological* Probably allergic response *2754*

Erythrocytes *Blood* *Decrease* *Physiological* Occasional anemia reported with penicillins *2754*

Leukocytes *Blood* *Decrease* *Physiological* Probably allergic response (rare) *2754*

Occult Blood *Feces* *Increase* *Physiological* Caused bleeding with dose of 4 g *1342*

Platelets *Blood* *Decrease* *Physiological* Thrombocytopenia may occur occasionally *2754*

Hetastarch

Amylase *Serum* *Increase* *Physiological* Administration of multiple doses has been associated with temporary increases in activity although no association with pancreatitis has been reported. The increased activity persists longer in patients with renal impairment *1597*

Bilirubin *Serum* *No Effect* *Physiological* Administration of multiple doses had no effect on total bilirubin concentration although indirect bilirubin transiently increased *1597*

Bilirubin, Indirect *Serum* *Increase* *Physiological* Administration of multiple doses caused increases to 8.3 mg/L in 2 of 20 normal individuals (normal 0,0 to 7.0 mg/L) but returned to normal within 96 hours after cessation of treatment *1597*

Bleeding Time *Patient* *Increase* *Physiological* Administration causes hemodilution and may result in transient prolongation of time *1597*

Factor VIII *Plasma* *Decrease* *Physiological* Administration causes hemodilution and a mild inhibitory action on factor VIII *1597*

Hematocrit *Blood* *Decrease* *Physiological* Anemia may occur in conjunction with hemodilution *1597* Large doses decrease hematocrit *1384* Administration causes hemodilution and may result in reduced hematocrit *1597*

Hemoglobin *Blood* *Decrease* *Physiological* Anemia may occur in conjunction with hemodilution *1597*

Lipase *Serum* *No Effect* *Physiological* Administration of multiple doses has been associated with temporary increases in amylase activity although no effect on lipase activity has been reported *1597*

Partial Thromboplastin Time *Plasma* *Increase* *Physiological* Administration causes hemodilution and may result in transient prolongation of time *1597*

pH *Blood* *Decrease* *Physiological* Metabolic acidosis may occur with administration *1597*

Protein *Serum* *Decrease* *Physiological* Large doses decrease concentration through dilution *1384* Administration causes hemodilution and may result in reduced hematocrit *1597*

Prothrombin Time *Plasma* *Increase* *Physiological* Administration causes hemodilution and may result in transient prolongation of time *1597*

Specific Gravity *Urine* *Increase* *Physiological* One report described an increase in urinary specific gravity in patients with renal glomerular damage due to leakage of large molecules into the urine *1597*

Volume *Plasma* *Increase* *Physiological* Administration causes hemodilution *1597*

Hexachlorobenzene

Erythrocytes *Blood* *Decrease* *Physiological* Pancytopenia (AMA Blood dyscrasias) *4017*

Leukocytes *Blood* *Decrease* *Physiological* Pancytopenia (AMA Blood dyscrasias) *4017*

Platelets *Blood* *Decrease* *Physiological* Pancytopenia (AMA Blood dyscrasias) *4017*

Porphyrin, Total *Urine* *Increase* *Physiological* Stimulates formation of ALA-synthetase *2242*

Hexamethylenetetramine

Histamine *Plasma* *No Effect* *Analytical* Improbable inhibition of radio-enzyme assay at therapeutic concentrations *2492*

Potassium *Urine* *Increase* *Analytical* At a concentration of 1 tablet per 30 mL urine causes 34% increase with method on Kodak Ektachem® systems *2519*

Sodium *Urine No Effect Analytical* At a concentration of 1 tablet/30 mL urine causes 6% increase with method on Kodak Ektachem® systems *2519*

Hexaprazol

Gastric Inhibitory Polypeptide
Plasma No Effect Physiological No significant effect in 13 healthy volunteers over 2 hours following intravenous injection of 300 mg *6252*

Gastrin *Serum No Effect Physiological* No significant change observed in 13 healthy volunteers over 2 hours following intravenous injection of 300 mg *6252*

Pancreatic Polypeptide *Plasma Increase Physiological* Increase from mean of 170 μg/L to peak of 187 μg/L at 20 minutes in 13 healthy volunteers given 300 mg injection intravenously *6252*

Pepsinogen I *Serum No Effect Physiological* No effect observed in 13 healthy volunteers over 2 hours following intravenous injection of 300 mg *6252*

Secretin *Plasma No Effect Physiological* No effect observed in 13 healthy volunteers over 2 hours following intravenous injection of 300 mg *6252*

Somatostatin *Plasma No Effect Physiological* No significant effect observed in 13 healthy volunteers over 2 hours following intravenous injection of 300 mg *6252*

Vasoactive Intestinal Polypeptide
Plasma No Effect Physiological No significant change observed in 13 healthy volunteers for 2 hours following intravenous injection of 300 mg *6252*

Hexarelin

C-terminal Propeptide of Type I Collagen
Serum Increase Physiological In healthy individuals 16 weeks of twice-daily subcutaneous hexarelin (1.5 μg/kg body weight) had a significant effect on the plasma concentration of 75.1 ± 6.1 ng/mL at baseline changing to 93 ± 9.2 ng/mL at 16 weeks *4834*

Deoxypyridinoline *Urine No Effect Physiological* In healthy individuals 16 weeks of twice-daily subcutaneous hexarelin (1.5 μg/kg body weight) had no significant effect on the plasma concentration of 81.9 ± 8.6 nmol/L at baseline changing to 89.6 ± 9.5 nmol/L at 16 weeks *4834*

Growth Hormone *Plasma Decrease Physiological* In healthy individuals 16 weeks of twice-daily subcutaneous hexarelin (1.5 μg/kg body weight) caused a reduction in the plasma growth hormone area under the curve from 19.1 ± 2.4 μg/L/h at baseline to 13.1 ± 2.3 μg/L/h at 1 week and 12.3 ± 2.4 μg/L/h at 4 weeks, 10.5 ± 1.8 μg/L/h at 16 weeks and 19.4 ± 3.7 μg/L/h at 20 weeks *4834*

Insulin-like Growth Factor-I *Serum No Effect Physiological* In healthy individuals 16 weeks of twice-daily subcutaneous hexarelin (1.5 μg/kg body weight) had no significant effect on the plasma concentration of 115 ± 12 μg/L at baseline changing to 121 ± 10 μg/L at 1 week and 113 ± 12 μg/L at 4 weeks, 130 ± 10 μg/L at 16 weeks and 124 ± 12 μg/L at 20 weeks *4834*

Insulin-like Growth Factor Binding Protein-3
Serum No Effect Physiological In healthy individuals 16 weeks of twice-daily subcutaneous hexarelin (1.5 μg/kg body weight) had no significant effect on the plasma concentration of 3.7 ± 0.2 μg/L at baseline changing to 3.7 ± 0.3 μg/L at 1 week and 3.9 ± 0.3 μg/L at 4 weeks, 3.7 ± 0.2 μg/L at 16 weeks and 3.5 ± 12 μg/L at 0.2 weeks *4834*

Osteocalcin *Serum No Effect Physiological* In healthy individuals 16 weeks of twice-daily subcutaneous hexarelin (1.5 μg/kg body weight) had no significant effect on the plasma concentration of 15.6 ± 2.2 ng/mL at baseline changing to 16.5 ± 3.1 ng/mL at 16 weeks *4834*

Procollagen III Peptide *Serum No Effect Physiological* In healthy individuals 16 weeks of twice-daily subcutaneous hexarelin (1.5 μg/kg body weight) had no significant effect on the plasma concentration of 3.4 ± 0.26 μg/L at baseline changing to 3.5 ± 0.37 μg/L at 16 weeks *4834*

Prolactin *Plasma Increase Physiological* Hexarelin 2 μg/kg intravenously caused significant increase from mean baseline of 10 mU/L to 150 mU/L after 2 hours in 14 healthy individuals and from 6 μg/kg to 190 μg/kg in 8 patients with active acromegaly *1043*

Pyridinoline *Urine No Effect Physiological* In healthy individuals 16 weeks of twice-daily subcutaneous hexarelin (1.5 μg/kg body weight) had no significant effect on the plasma concentration of 334 ± 30 nmol/L at baseline changing to 360 ± 35 nmol/L at 16 weeks *4834*

Hexobarbital

Erythromycin *Serum Increase Physiological* Concomitant administration of hexobarbital with erythromycin may increase its plasma concentration through its effect on cytochrome P450 *20*

p-Aminophenol *Urine No Effect Analytical* With addition of drugs at a concentration of 100 mg/L and of related compounds at 50 mg/L no significant effect observed on colorimetric method of van Bocxlaer on Cobas Mira analyzer which involves reacting free p-aminophenol with resorcinol in the presence of magnesium ions to form an indophenol dye measured at 550 nm *6163*

Phenobarbital *Serum No Effect Analytical* Cross-reactivity of 2.4% only observed with method on Baxter Stratus *5705*

Phenylalanine *Plasma No Effect Analytical* No interference observed with rapid quantitative whole blood method of Campbell et al using phenylalanine dehydrogenase *867*

Primidone *Serum No Effect Analytical* At a concentration of 680 mg/L causes 25% increase with method on Baxter Stratus but physiological concentration only up to 5 mg/L *5705*

Hexocyclium

Hydrochloric Acid *Gastric Fluid Decrease Physiological* Effective anticholinergic action *2753*

Volume *Gastric Fluid Decrease Physiological* Effective anticholinergic action *2753*

Hexoprenaline

Estriol *Plasma Decrease Physiological* Significant effect when given to women in premature labor *2510*

Hirudin

Hemoglobin *Blood Decrease Physiological* Incidence of serious bleeding in 1028 patients not different from that in 1023 patients treated with an LMW heparin (enoxaprin) *1747*

Histrelin

Blood *Urine Increase Physiological* Hematuria observed as a complication in 1% of 183 treated children *4983*

Glucose *Urine Increase Physiological* Glycosuria observed as a complication in 1% of 183 treated children *4983*

Lipids *Serum Increase Physiological* Hyperlipidemia observed as a complication in 1% of 183 treated children *4983*

HMG CoA Reductase Inhibitors

Cholesterol *Serum Decrease Physiological* In 35 patients with primary hypercholesterolemia treatment with diet and HMG CoA reductase inhibitors caused significant reduction from mean baseline of 8.9 ± 0.27 mmol/L to 6.9 ± 0.24 mmol/L after 6 months, 7.0 ± 0.22 mmol/L after 12 months and 6.4 ± 0.24 mmol/L after 24 months *4153*

HDL-Cholesterol *Serum No Effect Physiological* In 37 patients with primary hypercholesterolemia treatment with diet and HMG CoA reductase inhibitors caused nonsignificant change from mean baseline of 1.34 ± 0.07 mmol/L to 1.34 ± 0.06 mmol/L after 6 months, 1.37 ± 0.07 mmol/L after 12 months and 1.29 ± 0.05 mmol/L after 24 months *4153*

HMG CoA Reductase Inhibitors *(continued)*

LDL-Cholesterol *Serum Decrease Physiological* In 37 patients with primary hypercholesterolemia treatment with diet and HMG CoA reductase inhibitors caused significant change from mean baseline of 6.7 ± 0.24 mmol/L to 5.0 ± 0.23 mmol/L after 6 months, 5.1 ± 0.24 mmol/L after 12 months and 4.4 ± 0.21 mmol/L after 24 months *4153* In 105 patients without history of coronary artery disease treated with HMG-CoA reductase inhibitors for 1 year mean concentration decreased to 114 ± 23 mg/dL compared with 147 ± 22 mg/dL in untreated controls *849*

Retinol *Serum Increase Physiological* In 35 patients with primary hypercholesterolemia treatment with diet and HMG CoA reductase inhibitors caused significant increase from mean baseline of 3.29 ± 0.11 mmol/L to 3.71 ± 0.13 mmol/L after 24 months *4153*

Triglycerides *Serum Decrease Physiological* In 37 patients with primary hypercholesterolemia treatment with diet and HMG CoA reductase inhibitors caused significant change from mean baseline of 1.71 ± 0.17 mmol/L to 1.37 ± 0.11 mmol/L after 6 months, 1.30 ± 0.08 mmol/L after 12 months and 1.61 ± 0.16 mmol/L after 24 months *4153*

HMW Heparin

α_2-Antiplasmin *Plasma No Effect Physiological* In 12 healthy male volunteers administration of a single intravenous bolus dose of 7500 IU had no significant effect on α_2-antiplasmin concentration over 120 minutes *1337*

Antithrombin III *Plasma No Effect Physiological* In 12 healthy male volunteers administration of a single intravenous bolus of 7500 IU had no significant effect on AT-III concentration over 120 minutes *1337*

Factor XII *Plasma No Effect Physiological* In 12 healthy male volunteers administration of 7500 IU had no significant effect on heparin-cofactor II concentration over 120 minutes *1337*

Heparin-Cofactor II *Plasma No Effect Physiological* In 12 healthy male volunteers administration of a single intravenous bolus of 7500 IU had no significant effect on heparin-cofactor II concentration over 120 minutes *1337*

Plasminogen *Plasma No Effect Physiological* In 12 healthy male volunteers administration of a single intravenous bolus dose of 7500 IU had no significant effect on plasminogen concentration over 120 minutes *1337*

Prekallikrein *Plasma No Effect Physiological* In 12 healthy male volunteers administration of 7500 IU had no significant effect on heparin-cofactor II concentration over 120 minutes *1337*

Protein C Activity *Plasma No Effect Physiological* In 12 healthy male volunteers administration of 7500 IU had no significant effect on heparin-cofactor II concentration over 120 minutes *1337*

Protein S Antigen *Plasma No Effect Physiological* In 12 healthy male volunteers administration of 7500 IU had no significant effect on heparin-cofactor II concentration over 120 minutes *1337*

Tissue Plasminogen Activator-1
Plasma No Effect Physiological In 12 healthy male volunteers administration of 7500 IU had no significant effect on heparin-cofactor II concentration over 120 minutes *1337*

Homatropine

Bromide *Serum Increase Physiological* Theoretical possibility if methylbromide compound is administered since it contains 29% bromide *5116*

Homoharringtonine

Erythrocytes *Blood Decrease Physiological* Myelosuppression has been reported as a side effect *1384*

Glucose *Serum Increase Physiological* Hyperglycemia has been reported as a significant side effect *1384*

Leukocytes *Blood Decrease Physiological* Myelosuppression has been reported as a significant side effect *1384*

Platelets *Blood Decrease Physiological* Myelosuppression has been reported as a significant side effect *1384*

Hormone Replacement Therapy

Acid Phosphatase, Tartrate Resistant
Serum Decrease Physiological In 11 recently postmenopausal women treatment with HRT for 24 weeks, 6 cycles, caused 15.1% reduction in activity *2436*

Alkaline Phosphatase, Bone Isoenzyme
Serum Decrease Physiological In 236 healthy women 1 to 3 years postmenopause treatment with estrogen plus progesterone with calcium correlation coefficient of -0.22 with serum activity after 3 months and -0.32 after 6 months *986* In 11 recently postmenopausal women treatment with HRT for 24 weeks, 6 cycles, caused 22.0% reduction in activity *2436*

Amino-terminal Propeptide of Type I Procollagen
Serum Decrease Physiological In 11 recently postmenopausal women treatment with HRT for 24 weeks, 6 cycles, caused 40.3% reduction in concentration *2436*

Calcium *Urine Decrease Physiological* In 11 recently postmenopausal women treatment with HRT for 24 weeks, 6 cycles, caused 22.8% reduction in calcium excretion per unit of creatinine *2436*

Cholesterol *Serum Decrease Physiological* In 109 postmenopausal women treatment with 0.625 mg conjugated equine estrogens daily for 25 days and with 10 mg medroxyprogesterone acetate from 16th to 25th day of the month caused a significant change from mean baseline of 5.36 ± 0.87 mmol/L to 5.13 ± 0.87 mmol/L after 12 months and treatment with estradiol valerate and norgestrel cyclically in 71 women caused a significant decrease from 5.28 ± 0.81 mmol/L to 4.61 ± 0.78 mmol/L *3138*

C-terminal Propeptide of Type I Collagen
Serum Decrease Physiological In 11 recently postmenopausal women treatment with HRT for 24 weeks, 6 cycles, caused 19.5% reduction in concentration *2436*

C-terminal Telopeptide of Type I Collagen
Urine Decrease Physiological In 11 recently postmenopausal women treatment with HRT for 24 weeks, 6 cycles, caused 66.9% reduction in C-terminal telopeptides of type I collagen excretion per unit of creatinine *2436*

Deoxypyridinoline *Urine Decrease Physiological* In 11 recently postmenopausal women treatment with HRT for 24 weeks, 6 cycles, caused 48.3% reduction in total deoxypyridinoline excretion per unit of creatinine *2436*

Deoxypyridinoline, Free *Urine Decrease Physiological* In 11 recently postmenopausal women treatment with HRT for 24 weeks, 6 cycles, caused 26.7% reduction in free deoxypyridinoline excretion per unit of creatinine *2436*

Estrone Sulfate *Plasma Increase Physiological* In 22 postmenopausal women receiving hormone replacement therapy mean concentration of 2.56 ± 0.47 pmol/L significantly higherer than mean of 0.96 ± 0.17 pmol/L in 20 women in follicular phase and mean of 1.74 ± 0.32 µg/L in 20 women during luteal phase, and 0.13 ± 0.03 pmol/L in 21 untreated postmenopausal women *4849*

Glutathione S-Transferase *Serum Decrease Physiological* Treatment of 64 postmenopausal women with 17β-estradiol and norethisterone acetate for 78 dayscaused significant decrease to 1.81 µg/L from mean baseline of 1.94 µg/L *4162*

HDL-Cholesterol *Serum Increase Physiological* In 109 postmenopausal women treatment with 0.625 mg conjugated equine estrogens daily for 25 days and with 10 mg medroxyprogesterone acetate from 16th to 25th day of the month caused a significant change from mean baseline of 1.69 ± 0.41 mmol/L to 1.92 ± 0.43 mmol/L after 12 months and treatment with estradiol valerate and norgestrel cyclically in 71 women caused a nonsignificant change from 1.62 ± 0.38 mmol/L to 1.65 ± 0.43 mmol/L *3138*

Hydroxyproline *Urine Decrease Physiological* In 236 healthy women 1 to 3 years postmenopause treatment with estrogen plus progesterone with calcium correlation coefficient of -0.14 with urine excretion after 3 months and -0.20 after 6 months *986*

Urine Increase Physiological In 11 recently postmenopausal women treatment with HRT for 24 weeks, 6 cycles, caused 16.3% increase in hydroxyproline excretion per unit of creatinine *2436*

LDL-Cholesterol *Serum Decrease Physiological* In 109 postmenopausal women treatment with 0.625 mg conjugated equine estrogens daily for 25 days and with 10 mg medroxyprogesterone acetate from 16th to 25th day of the month caused a significant change from mean baseline of 3.28 ± 0.63 mmol/L to 2.91 ± 0.62 mmol/L after 12 months and treatment with estradiol valerate and norgestrel cyclically in 71 women caused a significant decrease from 3.24 ± 0.68 mmol/L to 2.67 ± 0.57 mmol/L *3138*

Lipoprotein Lp(a) *Serum Decrease Physiological* In 109 postmenopausal women treatment with 0.625 mg conjugated equine estrogens daily for 25 days and with 10 mg medroxyprogesterone acetate from 16th to 25th day of the month caused a significant change from mean baseline of 25.1 ± 20.7 mg/dL to 17.6 ± 17.3 mg/dL after 12 months and treatment with estradiol valerate and norgestrel cyclically in 71 women caused a significant decrease from 25.2 ± 21.1 mg/dL to 17.6 ± 17.3 mg/dL *3138*

Osteocalcin *Serum Decrease Physiological* In 11 recently postmenopausal women treatment with HRT for 24 weeks, 6 cycles, caused 25.9% reduction in concentration *2436* In 236 healthy women 1 to 3 years postmenopause treatment with estrogen plus progesterone with calcium correlation coefficient of -0.23 with serum concentration after 3 months and -0.11 after 6 months *986*

Pyridinoline, Free *Urine Decrease Physiological* In 11 recently postmenopausal women treatment with HRT for 24 weeks, 6 cycles, caused 20.5% reduction in free pyridinoline excretion per unit of creatinine *2436*

Triglycerides *Serum Decrease Physiological* In 109 postmenopausal women treatment with 0.625 mg conjugated equine estrogens daily for 25 days and with 10 mg medroxyprogesterone acetate from 16th to 25th day of the month caused a nonsignificant change from mean baseline of 1.49 ± 0.85 mmol/L to 1.33 ± 0.67 mmol/L after 12 months and treatment with estradiol valerate and norgestrel cyclically in 71 women caused a significant decrease from 1.51 ± 1.00 mmol/L to 1.02 ± 0.55 mmol/L *3138*

Type I Collagen Cross-linked N-telopeptide
Urine Decrease Physiological In 236 healthy women 1 to 3 years postmenopause treatment with estrogen plus progesterone with calcium correlation coefficient of -0.30 with urine excretion after 3 months and -0.39 after 6 months *986* In 11 recently postmenopausal women treatment with HRT for 24 weeks, 6 cycles, caused 38.5% reduction in cross-linked N-telopeptides of type I collagen excretion per unit of creatinine *2436*

Type I Collagen Teleopeptide
Serum Decrease Physiological In 11 recently postmenopausal women treatment with HRT for 24 weeks, 6 cycles, caused 9.9% reduction in concentration *2436*

VLDL-Cholesterol *Serum Decrease Physiological* In 109 postmenopausal women treatment with 0.625 mg conjugated equine estrogens daily for 25 days and with 10 mg medroxyprogesterone acetate from 16th to 25th day of the month caused a significant change from mean baseline of 0.39 ± 0.31 mmol/L to 0.30 ± 0.21 mmol/L after 12 months and treatment with estradiol valerate and norgestrel cyclically in 71 women caused a significant decrease from 0.42 ± 0.38 mmol/L to 0.29 ± 0.22 mmol/L *3138*

Hycanthone

Alanine Aminotransferase *Serum Increase Physiological* Transient change in liver function *128*

Aspartate Aminotransferase *Serum Increase Physiological* Transient change in liver function *128*

Bilirubin *Serum Increase Physiological* Induces form of acute toxic hepatitis *1799*

BSP Retention *Serum Increase Physiological* Induces form of acute toxic hepatitis *1799*

Hydantoin Derivatives

Alanine Aminotransferase *Serum Increase Physiological* Severe delayed hypersensitivity reported *4014*

Alkaline Phosphatase *Serum Increase Physiological* Severe delayed hypersensitivity reported *4014*

δ-Aminolevulinic Acid *Urine Increase Physiological* May precipitate attack of acute porphyria *1687*

Amylase *Serum Increase Physiological* Pancreatitis may occur as an adverse reaction *3978*

Bilirubin *Serum Increase Physiological* Severe delayed hypersensitivity reported *4014*

γ-Globulin *Serum Increase Physiological* Observed in cases of hypersensitivity *4014*

LE Cells *Blood Positive Physiological* May cause appearance of LE cells *3669*

Methemoglobin *Blood Increase Physiological* Reported effect *3669*

Platelets *Blood Decrease Physiological* Thrombocytopenia (immunologically induced) *3810*

Porphyrin, Total *Urine Increase Physiological* May precipitate attack of acute porphyria *1687*

Urea Nitrogen *Serum Increase Analytical* Absorbance relative to urea = 0.3 in diacetyl procedure *882*

Hydralazine

Alanine Aminotransferase *Serum Increase Physiological* Isolated case with moderate hepatomegaly, abnormal findings resolved when drug discontinued *1921* Centrilobular necrosis observed in 3 patients 2 to 4 months after drug therapy for hypertension *2847*

Albumin *Serum Decrease Physiological* Centrilobular necrosis observed in 3 patients 2 to 4 months after drug therapy for hypertension *2847*

Aldosterone *Plasma Increase Physiological* Significant effect following 20 mg i.v. in 30 to 60 minutes *2619*
Plasma No Effect Physiological In 18 patients with NIDDM and proteinuria greater than 500 mg/d treatment with hydralazine (40 - 200 mg/d) for 18 months caused a nonsignificant change from mean baseline of 13.59 ± 0.89 ng/mL to 14.26 ± 1.23 ng/mL *3601*

Alkaline Phosphatase *Serum Increase Physiological* Cholestatic jaundice observed in one patient *5823* Isolated case with moderate hepatomegaly, abnormal findings resolved when drug discontinued *1921* Asymptomatic or symptomatic reversible hepatitis-like reaction or granulomatous hepatitis *3904* Centrilobular necrosis observed in 3 patients 2 to 4 months after drug therapy for hypertension *2847*

Anti-ds DNA Antibodies *Serum No Effect Physiological* Observed in one patient with induced systemic lupus erythematosus *6389*

Anti-Histone Antibodies *Serum Positive Physiological* Observed in 9 patients developing rapidly progressive glomerulonephritis during treatment *590*

Antinuclear Antibodies *Serum Increase Physiological* More common in slow acetylators *4614* Raised in patients who developed symptoms of lupus, unrelated to dose of drug *569*

Aspartate Aminotransferase *Serum Increase Analytical* At 1 mmol/L affects Technicon SMA 12/60 method *5576*
Serum Increase Physiological Centrilobular necrosis observed in 3 patients 2 to 4 months after drug therapy for hypertension *2847* Asymptomatic or symptomatic reversible hepatitis-like reaction or granulomatous hepatitis *3904* Isolated case with moderate hepatomegaly, abnormal findings resolved when drug discontinued *1921* Cholestatic jaundice observed in one patient *5823*

Bicarbonate *Serum No Effect Analytical* At concentration of 6 mg/L had no effect on method using phenolphthalein *5704*

Bilirubin *Serum Increase Physiological* Centrilobular necrosis observed in 3 patients 2 to 4 months after drug therapy for hypertension *2847* Observed in a case of obstructive jaundice with pancytopenia *5823* Asymptomatic or symptomatic reversible hepatitis-like reaction or granulomatous hepatitis *3904*

Hydralazine *(continued)*

Bilirubin *(continued)*

Serum No Effect Analytical At concentration of 160 mg/L had no effect on Jendrassik and Grof method *5704*

Serum No Effect Physiological Isolated case with moderate hepatomegaly, abnormal findings resolved when drug discontinued *1921*

Bilirubin, Direct *Serum Increase Physiological* Centrilobular necrosis observed in 3 patients 2 to 4 months after drug therapy for hypertension *2847*

Calcium *Serum Increase Analytical* At 1 mmol/L has slight effect on Technicon SMA 12/60 method *5576* At concentrations above 150 mg/L (normal therapeutic concentration 2.3 mg/L) raised concentration as measured by cresolphthalein method *5704*

Urine No Effect Physiological No change in 15 normo- or hypertensive individuals given 75 mg daily for 3 days *5429*

Catecholamines *Urine No Effect Physiological* No effect observed *1444*

Chloride *Serum No Effect Analytical* At concentration of 6 mg/L had no effect on mercurimetric method *5704*

Cholesterol *Serum Decrease Physiological* 12% reduction in 7 patients treated for 4 mo *141* When given to patients with essential hypertension as monotherapy caused significant reduction *6470* Increase by 12% in 7 individuals treated for 4 mo *142*

Serum No Effect Analytical At concentration of 160 mg/L had no effect on Liebermann-Burchard method *5704* At concentration of 0.5 mg/L had no effect on CHOD-PAP method *5704*

Color *Feces Increase Analytical* Black color reported with hydralazine ingestion *3388*

Complement C_1q *Serum Decrease Physiological* Observed in one patient with induced systemic lupus erythematosus *6389*

Complement C_3 *Serum Decrease Physiological* Observed in one patient with induced systemic lupus erythematosus *6389*

Complement C_4 *Serum No Effect Physiological* Observed in one patient with induced systemic lupus erythematosus *6389*

Complement CH50 *Serum Decrease Physiological* Observed in one patient with induced systemic lupus erythematosus *6389*

Complement Factor B *Serum Decrease Physiological* Observed in one patient with induced systemic lupus erythematosus *6389*

Coombs' Test *Blood Positive Physiological* Mechanism obscure *2453*

Coombs' Test, Direct *Blood Positive Physiological* Observed in one patient receiving low dose of drug for hypertension. Mechanism involved in producing erythrocyte-reacting antibody not known *4432* May occur if SLE induced *2452*

Creatine Kinase *Serum No Effect Physiological* In one individual injection of 2 mL fluid intramuscularly had no effect on plasma CK activity *3377*

Creatinine *Serum Increase Physiological* In 18 patients with NIDDM and proteinuria greater than 500 mg/d treatment with hydralazine (40 - 200 mg/d) for 18 months caused a significant increase from mean baseline of 2.2 ± 0.3 mg/dL to 2.9 ± 0.4 mg/dL *3601* Insignificant increase from mean of 71 µmol/L to 80 µmol/L in 15 normo- or hypertensive individuals given 75 mg daily for 3 days *5429*

Serum No Effect Analytical At concentration of 6 mg/L had no effect on Technicon AutoAnalyzer® Jaffe method *5704*

Cyclosporine *Blood No Effect Analytical* At a concentration of 32 mg/L had no effect on Syva EMIT method *495*

Digoxin *Serum Decrease Physiological* Reduces plasma concentration by increasing renal clearance of glycoside *1384*

Drugs of Abuse Screen *Urine No Effect Analytical* No effect at concentration of 100 µg/mL on EZ-SCREEN procedure for cannabinoids and cocaine *1739*

Effective Renal Plasma Flow

Patient Decrease Physiological In 18 patients with NIDDM and proteinuria greater than 500 mg/d treatment with hydralazine (40 - 200 mg/d) for 18 months caused a nonsignificant change from mean baseline of 228 ± 23 mL/min to 231 ± 23 mL/min after 6 months, 226 ± 24 mL/min after 12 months and 203 ± 18 mL/min after 18 months *3601*

Eosinophils *Blood Increase Physiological* Blood eosinophilia reported with a hypersensitivity reaction *1023*

Erythrocyte Sedimentation Rate

Blood Increase Physiological Observed in 9 patients developing rapidly progressive glomerulonephritis during treatment *590*

Erythrocytes *Blood Decrease Physiological* Pancytopenia may occur *84* Blood dyscrasias have been reported with administration *1023* Observed in 9 patients developing rapidly progressive glomerulonephritis during treatment *590* Blood dyscrasias may occur with treatment *5680*

Urine Increase Physiological Reported finding *4014*

Filtration Fraction *Urine Decrease Physiological* In 18 patients with NIDDM and proteinuria greater than 500 mg/d treatment with hydralazine (40 - 200 mg/d) for 18 months caused a nonsignificant change from mean baseline of 32 ± 4% to 29 ± 3% after 6 months, 29 ± 3% after 12 months and 28 ± 3% after 18 months *3601*

γ-Globulin *Serum Increase Physiological* Reported finding *4014*

Glomerular Filtration Rate *Urine Decrease Physiological* In 18 patients with NIDDM and proteinuria greater than 500 mg/d treatment with hydralazine (40 - 200 mg/d) for 18 months caused a significant change from mean baseline of 66 ± 5 mL/min to 62 ± 5 mL/min after 6 months, 60 ± 5 mL/min after 12 months and 54 ± 5 mL/min after 18 months *3601*

Urine No Effect Physiological In 8 hypertensive patients treated with up to 200 mg daily for up to 6 months when also treated with a diuretic *889*

Glucose *Serum Decrease Analytical* At concentrations above 115 mg/L (normal therapeutic concentration 2.3mg/L) lowered concentration as measured by GOD-PERID method *5704* Affects glucose oxidase method of Boehringer *5480*

Serum Increase Analytical At 1 mmol/L affects Technicon SMA 12/60 method *5576* 150.4% increase in absorbance with 10 mmol/L and 14.3% increase with 1 mmol/L on glucokinase based assay of Scott *5414*

Serum No Effect Analytical At concentration of 0.5 mg/L had no effect on GOD/POD-PAP method *5704* Affects Boehringer GOD-PERID method *5480*

Granulocytes *Blood Decrease Physiological* Blood dyscrasias have been reported with administration *1023* Blood dyscrasias, including agranulocytosis, may occur with treatment *5680*

HDL-Cholesterol *Serum No Effect Physiological* No effect observed in patients with essential hypertension when given as monotherapy *6470*

Hematocrit *Blood Decrease Physiological* May cause hemolytic anemia *84*

Hemoglobin *Blood Decrease Physiological* Blood dyscrasias have been reported with administration *1023* Observed in a case of obstructive jaundice with pancytopenia *5823* Observed in 9 patients developing rapidly progressive glomerulonephritis during treatment *590* Observed in one patient receiving low dose of drug for hypertension. Mechanism involved in producing erythrocyte-reacting antibody not known *4432* May cause hemolytic anemia *84*

Urine Increase Physiological Microscopic hematuria observed in 9 patients developing rapidly progressive glomerulonephritis during treatment *590* Reported finding *4014*

Hemoglobin A_{1c} *Blood No Effect Physiological* In 18 patients with NIDDM and proteinuria greater than 500 mg/d treatment with hydralazine (40 - 200 mg/d) for 18 months caused a nonsignificant change from mean baseline of 8.4 ± 0.4% to 8.8 ± 0.5% *3601*

Histamine *Plasma No Effect Analytical* No inhibition of radio-enzyme assay at therapeutic concentrations *2492*

Homocysteine *Plasma Increase Physiological* As a vitamin B_6 antagonist causes increased concentration *6123*

Inulin Clearance *Urine No Effect Physiological* No change in 15 normo- or hypertensive individuals given 75 mg daily for 3 days *5429*

Ionized Calcium *Serum No Effect Physiological* No change in 15 normo- or hypertensive individuals given 75 mg daily for 3 days *5429*

17-Ketogenic Steroids *Urine Increase Analytical* Glucuronide interferes with Zimmermann reaction *5869*

Lactate Dehydrogenase *Serum Increase Physiological* Isolated case with moderate hepatomegaly, abnormal findings resolved when drug discontinued *1921* Asymptomatic or symptomatic reversible hepatitis-like reaction or granulomatous hepatitis *3904*

LDL-Cholesterol *Serum Decrease Physiological* Reduction observed in patients with essential hypertension when given as monotherapy *6470*

LE Cells *Blood Positive Physiological* More common in slow acetylators *4614* Observed in one patient with induced systemic lupus erythematosus *6389* 3% patients developed lupus-like syndrome all of whom were slow acetylators and receiving less than 200 mg drμg/d *569*

Leukocytes *Blood Decrease Physiological* Blood dyscrasias have been reported with administration *1023* Agranulocytosis/pancytopenia/Leukopenia *84* Blood dyscrasias may occur with treatment *5680* Observed in a case of obstructive jaundice with pancytopenia *5823*

Magnesium *Serum No Effect Physiological* No change in 15 normo- or hypertensive individuals given 75 mg daily for 3 days *5429*

Urine No Effect Physiological No change in 15 normo- or hypertensive individuals given 75 mg daily for 3 days *5429*

Metoprolol *Serum Increase Physiological* In 10 pregnant hypertensive women addition of 25 mg hydralazine twice daily increased area under curve and maximum concentration by average of 38% and 88% respectively, but had no effect on circulating concentration of α-hydroxy-metoprolol *3587*

Midazolam *Serum No Effect Analytical* On GC-ECD method of Ha et al *2387*

Neutrophils *Blood Decrease Physiological* Occasional case of agranulocytosis reported *6264*

Occult Blood *Feces Increase Physiological* Rare gastrointestinal hemorrhage *2242*

PAH Clearance *Urine No Effect Physiological* Insignificant increase from mean of 553 mL/min/1.73 sq m to 599 mL/min/1.73 sq m in 15 normo- or hypertensive individuals given 75 mg daily for 3 days *5429*

Parathyroid Hormone *Plasma No Effect Physiological* In 15 normo- or hypertensive individuals given 75 mg drug daily for 3 days insignificant reduction of midmolecule PTH from mean of 1.09 pg/L to 1.06 pg/mL *5429*

Phenylalanine *Plasma No Effect Analytical* No interference observed with rapid quantitative whole blood method of Campbell et al using phenylalanine dehydrogenase *867*

Phosphate *Serum No Effect Analytical* At concentration of 6 mg/L had no effect on phosphomolybdate method *5704*

Serum No Effect Physiological No significant change in 15 normo- or hypertensive individuals given 75 mg daily for 3 days *5429*

Urine No Effect Physiological Insignificant reduction from mean of 32 mmol/24 h to 26 mmol/24 h in 15 normo- or hypertensive individuals given 75 mg daily for 3 days *5429*

Platelets *Blood Decrease Physiological* Rare finding in patients treated for hypertension: also observed in neonates *6437* Blood dyscrasias including purpura have been reported with administration *1023* Blood dyscrasias including purpura may occur with treatment *5680* Pancytopenia may occur with purpura *84*

Potassium *Serum No Effect Analytical* At concentration of 0.5 mg/L had no effect on flame-photometric method *5704* At concentration of 6 mg/L had no effect on measurement by ISE with predilution *5704*

Serum No Effect Physiological In 18 patients with NIDDM and proteinuria greater than 500 mg/d treatment with hydralazine (40 - 200 mg/d) for 18 months caused a nonsignificant change from mean baseline of 4.12 ± 0.11 mmol/L to 4.19 ± 0.10 mmol/L *3601*

Protein *Serum No Effect Analytical* At concentration of 6 mg/L had no effect on biuret method with blank correction *5704*

Urine Increase Physiological May cause nephrotoxicity *5377*

Urine No Effect Physiological In 18 patients with NIDDM and proteinuria greater than 500 mg/d treatment with hydralazine (40 - 200 mg/d) for 18 months caused a nonsignificant change from mean baseline of 2.89 ± 0.57 g/d to 2.69 ± 0.45 g/d after 6 months, 2.62 ± 0.52 g/d after 12 months and 2.62 ± 0.59 g/d after 18 months *3601*

Quinidine *Serum No Effect Analytical* No significant interference observed at a concentration of 100 μg/mL (624 μmol/L) with method on Du Pont aca *1543*

Renin Activity *Plasma Decrease Physiological* May be suppressed activity *3940*

Plasma Increase Physiological Significant effect following 20 mg i.v. in 30 to 120 minutes *2619* Drug administration usually increases plasma renin activity, presumably through increased secretion by the renal juxtaglomerular cells in response to reflex sympathetic discharge *1023*

Plasma No Effect Physiological In 18 patients with NIDDM and proteinuria greater than 500 mg/d treatment with hydralazine (40 - 200 mg/d) for 18 months caused a nonsignificant change from mean baseline of 1.11 ± 0.11 ng/mL/h to 1.31 ± 0.16 ng/mL/h *3601*

Reticulocytes *Blood Increase Physiological* Observed in one patient receiving low dose of drug for hypertension. Mechanism involved in producing erythrocyte-reacting antibody not known *4432*

Sodium *Serum No Effect Analytical* At concentration of 6 mg/L had no effect on measurement by ISE with predilution *5704* At concentration of 0.5 mg/L had no effect on flame-photometric method *5704*

Urine No Effect Physiological In 18 patients with NIDDM and proteinuria greater than 500 mg/d treatment with hydralazine (40 - 200 mg/d) for 18 months caused a nonsignificant change from mean baseline of 130 ± 2 mmol/L to 128 ± 3 mmol/L *3601* No change in 15 normo- or hypertensive individuals given 75 mg daily for 3 days *5429*

Triglycerides *Serum No Effect Analytical* At concentration of 6 mg/L had no effect on lipase/esterase method *5704*

Serum No Effect Physiological No effect observed in patients with essential hypertension when given as monotherapy *6470*

Tyramine Test *Patient Increase Physiological* Increased responsiveness *2451*

Urea Nitrogen *Serum Increase Physiological* In 18 patients with NIDDM and proteinuria greater than 500 mg/d treatment with hydralazine (40 - 200 mg/d) for 18 months caused a significant increase from mean baseline of 33 ± 5 mg/dL to 38 ± 5 mg/dL *3601* May cause nephrotoxicity *5377*

Serum No Effect Analytical At concentration of 160 mg/L had no effect on diacetylmonoxime method *5704*

Uric Acid *Serum Increase Analytical* At concentrations above 6 mg/L (normal therapeutic concentration 2.3mg/L) raised concentration as measured by phosphotungstate reduction method *5704* At 1 mmol/L affects Technicon SMA 12/60 and Henry methods *5576*

Vanillylmandelic Acid *Urine No Effect Physiological* No effect observed *1444*

Wassermann Reaction *Serum Positive Physiological* False positive reaction reported *4014*

Hydrazine Derivatives

Alanine Aminotransferase *Serum Increase Physiological* May cause hepatotoxicity *3810*

Alkaline Phosphatase *Serum Increase Physiological* May cause hepatotoxicity *3810*

Aspartate Aminotransferase *Serum Increase Physiological* May cause hepatotoxicity *3810*

Bile *Urine Increase Physiological* May cause hepatotoxicity *3810*

Bilirubin *Serum Increase Physiological* May cause hepatotoxicity *3810*

BSP Retention *Serum Increase Physiological* May cause hepatotoxicity *3810*

Erythrocyte Sedimentation Rate

Blood Increase Physiological Augmentation with SLE-like syndrome *1475*

Hydrazine Derivatives *(continued)*

Glucose *Serum* *Decrease* *Physiological* May potentiate action of insulin in diabetics *3669*

5-Hydroxyindoleacetic Acid *Urine* *Decrease* *Physiological* May potentiate action of drugs on CNS *3669*

LE Cells *Blood* *Positive* *Physiological* May activate lupus erythematosus *944*

Lymphocytes *Blood* *Decrease* *Physiological* Significant effect observed with megadose supplementation *2245*

Metanephrines, Total *Urine* *Increase* *Physiological* May potentiate action of drugs on CNS *3669*

Neutrophils *Blood* *No Effect* *Physiological* No effect observed with megadose supplementation *2245*

Normetanephrine *Urine* *Increase* *Physiological* May potentiate action of drugs on CNS *3669*

Vanillylmandelic Acid *Urine* *Decrease* *Physiological* May potentiate action of drugs on CNS *3669*

Hydrochlorothiazide

Adenosine Monophosphate *Urine* *No Effect* *Physiological* No effect observed in patients with previous thiazide-induced hyponatremia, elderly hypertensives and healthy young controls following single dose of combination of hydrochlorothiazide and amiloride *1964*

Alanine Aminotransferase *Serum* *Increase* *Physiological* May cause cholestasis or cholangiolitic hepatitis *2754*

Aldosterone *Plasma* *Increase* *Physiological* In 28 mild to moderate hypertensives treatment with 25 mg/d for 2 weeks caused significant increase *3213* In 2 children with nephrogenic diabetes insipidus baseline concentration of about 370 pmol/L significantly increased to about 900 pmol/L after treatment with 2 mg/kg/d for 2 weeks *2891* In 9 patients with mild to moderate hypertension treatment with up to 50 mg/d for 8 weeks caused significant increase from mean baseline of 285 ± 185 pmol/L to 442 ± 229 pmol/L *1919*
Plasma *No Effect* *Physiological* No significant change observed in 10 patients with essential hypertension treated with 25 mg hydrochlorothiazide only for 4 weeks but significant increase (46%) when 4 mg perindopril daily combined with hydrochlorothiazide *757* In 2 children with partial nephrogenic diabetes insipidus baseline concentration of about 370 pmol/L not significantly increased to about 400 pmol/L after treatment with 2 mg/kg/d for 2 weeks *2891*
Urine *Increase* *Physiological* Significant increase observed in 6 volunteers given 100 mg/day for 3 days *1813*

Amantadine *Serum* *Decrease* *Physiological* In one patient dyazide (triamterene/hydrochlorothiazide) reported to cause increased amantadine concentration but not known which component of drug was responsible *1600*

Amylase *Serum* *Increase* *Physiological* Acute pancreatitis may occur *6001*

Angiotensin-converting Enzyme
Serum *No Effect* *Physiological* No significant change observed in 10 patients with essential hypertension treated with 25 mg daily for 4 weeks but when perindopril 4 mg daily also given reduction of 49.4% observed 24 hours after last dose *757*

Antidiuretic Hormone *Plasma* *Increase* *Physiological* Secreted in response to hyponatremia *1856*
Plasma *No Effect* *Physiological* No effect observed on already low concentration following single dose of combination of hydrochlorothiazide and amiloride in patients with previous thiazide-induced hyponatremia, elderly hypertensives and young healthy controls *1964*
Urine *No Effect* *Physiological* No significant effect in 6 volunteers given 100 mg/day for 3 days *1813*

Apolipoprotein A *Serum* *No Effect* *Physiological* In 9 hypertensive patients treated with 25 mg/d (as Moduretic) no significant change from mean baseline of 2.1 ± 0.7 g/dL observed after 3 months and 12 months *4460*

Apolipoprotein A-I *Serum* *No Effect* *Physiological* Usual observation when thiazides given to patients *6384*

Apolipoprotein A-II *Serum* *No Effect* *Physiological* Usual observation when thiazides given to patients *6384*

Apolipoprotein B *Serum* *No Effect* *Physiological* In 9 hypertensive patients treated with 25 mg/d (as Moduretic) no significant change from mean baseline of 2.1 ± 0.7 g/dL observed at 3 months and 12 months *4460*

Aspartate Aminotransferase *Serum* *Increase* *Physiological* May cause cholestasis or cholangiolitic hepatitis *2754*

Atrial Natriuretic Peptide *Plasma* *No Effect* *Physiological* In 9 patients with mild to moderate hypertension treatment with up to 50 mg/d for 8 weeks caused nonsignificant decrease from mean baseline of 15 ± 19 pg/mL to 13 ± 12 pg/mL *1919*

Benazepril *Serum* *No Effect* *Physiological* No clinically important pharmacokinetic interactions observed when drugs coadministered *1033*

Betaxolol *Serum* *No Effect* *Physiological* Coadministration had no effect on pharmacokinetics of betaxolol *2067*

Bicarbonate *Serum* *Increase* *Physiological* May cause metabolic alkalosis *1856* Significant increase observed in 33 mild-to-moderate essential hypertensives treated with 25 mg/d for 4 weeks *4131*

Bilirubin *Serum* *Increase* *Physiological* Cholestatic jaundice reported effect of thiazides *4555*

Calcium *Feces* *Decrease* *Physiological* Accentuates positive calcium balance *4014*
Serum *Decrease* *Physiological* Increase by 0.13 mg/dL in approximately 175 patients with essential hypertension treated for 1 y *6248*
Serum *Increase* *Physiological* Impaired excretion (probably also released from bone) *5869* Increase by 0.3 mg/dL in 343 patients with hypertension given drug for 10 weeks *6247* Increased renal tubular reabsorption, usually associated with mild primary hyperparathyroidism *1769* In 9 patients treated with mean dose of 72 mg/d concentration increased from mean baseline of 2.30 mmol/L to 2.42 mmol/L at 12 weeks although it subsequently declined to an overall nonsignificant increase over 1 year *4809* With hydrochlorothiazide use hypercalcemia may occur rarely with concentration returning to normal when drug withdrawn *24*
Urine *Decrease* *Physiological* Observed effect *697* In 9 patients treated with mean dose of 72 mg/d for 1 year excretion reduced when expressed as calcium to creatinine ratio and as the fractional excretion of calcium *4809*

Cannabinoids *Urine* *No Effect* *Analytical* No effect on Roche Abuscreen method *5006*

Carvedilol *Serum* *No Effect* *Physiological* In 12 patients with hypertension coadministration of 25 mg carvedilol and 25 mg hydrochlorothiazide had no clinically relevant effect on pharmacokinetics of either compound *5639*

Casts *Urine* *No Effect* *Physiological* Normally but augments effects of acidifying agents *2814*

Chloride *Serum* *Decrease* *Physiological* May cause marked reduction *1856*
Serum *Increase* *Physiological* Hyperchloremic alkalosis with prolonged therapy *3669*
Urine *Increase* *Physiological* Significant effect in 5 h after 150 mg orally *1959*

Cholesterol *Serum* *Decrease* *Physiological* In MRFIT study when given with chlorthalidone involving many patients *141* In 436 patients with serum cholesterol concentration greater than 200 mg/dL treatment with hydrochlorothiazide for 24 months caused significant decrease from mean baseline of 180 mg/dL to 146 mg/dL (34 mg/dL, 8%) *2968*
Serum *Increase* *Physiological* 4-7% in short term study *141* In 16 patients with normolipidemia but with essential hypertension treatment with 25 mg/d hydrochlorothiazide for 5 months caused a significant 15.8 ± 33.1 mg/dL increase in concentration *321* In short term studies administration of hydrochlorothiazide increased concentration of cholesterol by 10 to 20% within a year *3730* Increase by 7 mg/dL in 343 patients with hypertension given drug for 10 weeks *6247* In 188 hypertensive patients treated with up to 50 mg/d for 8 weeks mean concentration increased by 3.3 mg/dL (0.086 mmol/L) *3841* In 9 patients treated with mean dose of 72 mg/d for 1 year mean concentration increased significantly from baseline of 5.14 mmol/L to 5.84 mmol/L *4809* In 10 patients with mild hypertension treatment with 12.5 mg/d for 6 months caused significant increase from mean baseline of 185 ± 7 mg/dL to 198 ± 9 mg/dL *1306* 7% change in individuals given drug alone for less than 1 y *2337* Observed with 100 mg/d *6156*

Serum No Effect Physiological In 9 patients with mild to moderate hypertension treatment with up to 50 mg/d for 8 weeks caused nonsignificant increase from mean baseline of 5.76 ± 1.3 mmol/L to 5.93 ± 1.2 mmol/L *1919* No significant change observed in 37 hypertensives treated with up to 100 mg/d for 1 year *4098* No effect with 25 or 50 mg/d in hypertensive patients *3225* Nonsignificant increase in 85 patients with hypertension treated with 25 or 50 mg daily for 8 weeks *4115* In 10 hypertensive men administration of 25 mg hydrochlorothiazide (in Moduretic) caused insignificant increase from mean baseline of 7.3 ± 2.1 mmol/L decreased nonsignificantly to 7.2 ± 1.4 mmol/L at 3 months and nonsignificant increase to 7.5 ± 2.2 mmol/L after 12 months *4460* In long term involving many patients *141* In approximately 175 patients with essential hypertension treated for 1 y *6248*

Cholesterol Esters *Serum Increase Physiological* In 16 patients with normolipidemia but with essential hypertension treatment with 25 mg/d hydrochlorothiazide for 5 months caused a significant 12.2 ± 22.6 mg/dL increase in concentration *321*

Cholesterol, Free *Serum No Effect Physiological* In 16 patients with normolipidemia but with essential hypertension treatment with 25 mg/d hydrochlorothiazide for 5 months caused a nonsignificant 3.6 ± 18.6 mg/dL increase in concentration *321*

Cholinesterase *Serum No Effect Analytical* No effect observed at concentration of 2 µg/mL with butyrylthiocholine methoa on Kodak Ektachem® *2504*

Citrate *Urine Decrease Physiological* By up to 30% reported *5436*

Cortisol *Urine Decrease Physiological* Possibly altered cortisol secretion *2452*

C-Peptide *Urine No Effect Physiological* In 14 hypertensives men with type 2 diabetes treated for 2 weeks with or without propranolol *1476*

Creatinine *Serum Increase Physiological* But by less than 0.1 mg/dL in 33 patients with hypertension given drug for 10 weeks to reduce diastolic blood pressure to less than 90 mm Hg *6247*

Serum No Effect Analytical At concentration of 1.4 mg/L had no effect on creatinine iminohydrolase method *5704*

Serum No Effect Physiological No effect observed in patients with previous thiazide-induced hyponatremia, elderly hypertensives or healthy young controls following single dose of combination of hydrochlorothiazide and amiloride *1964* In approximately 175 patients with essential hypertension treated for 1 y *6248* In 9 patients with mild to moderate hypertension treatment with up to 50 mg/d caused nonsignificant change from mean baseline of 90.1 ± 17.6 µmol/L to 94.1 ± 14.4 µmol/L *1919*

Creatinine Clearance *Urine Decrease Physiological* Reported effect *3669*

Urine No Effect Physiological No significant effect observed in 6 volunteers given 100 mg/day for 3 days *1813*

Cyclosporine *Blood No Effect Analytical* At a concentration of 40 mg/L had no effect on Syva EMIT method *495*

Doxazosin *Serum No Effect Physiological* Coadministration with doxazosin had no effect on its pharmacokinetics *4642*

Drugs of Abuse Screen *Urine No Effect Analytical* No effect at concentration of 100 µg/mL on EZ-SCREEN procedure for cannabinoids and cocaine *1739*

Effective Renal Plasma Flow

Patient No Effect Physiological In 4 patients with nephrogenic diabetes insipidus treatment with 2 mg/kg/d for 2 weeks had no significant effect *2891*

Enalapril *Serum Increase Physiological* In 6 hypertensive patients coadministration of 12.5 mg hydrochlorothiazide with 20 mg enalapril daily for 7 days had no significant effect on pharmacokinetics of enalapril regardless of degree of renal function impairment *2577*

Epinephrine *Plasma No Effect Physiological* In 28 mild to moderate hypertensives treatment with 25 mg/d for 2 weeks had no significant effect *3213*

Erythrocyte Aggregation *Blood Decrease Physiological* In 39 patients with mild to moderate hypertension treatment with 25 mg/d for 4 weeks caused reduction from mean baseline of 2.00 ± 0.47 s to 1.92 ± 0.39 s *6630*

Blood No Effect Physiological In 28 mild to moderate hypertensives treatment with 25 mg/d for 2 weeks caused nonsignificant change from baseline of 10.5 ± 0.1 units to 11.3 ± 0.47 units *3215*

Erythrocyte Disaggregation Shear Rate

Blood Increase Physiological In 39 patients with mild to moderate hypertension treatment with 25 mg/d for 4 weeks caused increase from mean baseline of 181 ± 54 s to 196 ± 82 s *6630*

Erythrocyte Disaggregation Shear Stress

Blood Increase Physiological In 39 patients with mild to moderate hypertension treatment with 25 mg/d for 4 weeks caused increase from mean baseline of 813 ± 268 mPa to 868 ± 392 mPa *6630*

Erythrocytes *Blood Decrease Physiological* Aplastic anemia may occur *2754* Occasional case of aplastic anemia reported *6264*

Blood Increase Physiological Average increase of 0.1 million /µL in 85 patients with hypertension treated with 25 or 50 mg daily for 8 weeks *4115*

Estriol *Urine Decrease Analytical* Interferes in hydrolysis of conjugates stage *5105* Destroys estriol during acid hydrolysis *882*

Urine No Effect Analytical At 4 times normal concentration with enzyme hydrolysis and Kober procedure *1177*

Estrogens *Urine Increase Physiological* In pregnant but mechanism unknown *54*

Filterability Index *Blood Increase Physiological* In 39 patients with mild to moderate hypertension treatment with 25 mg/d for 4 weeks caused nonsignificant increase from 19.13 ± 3.34 to 19.97 ± 3.83 *6630*

Fluconazole *Serum No Effect Physiological* Concomitant administration of hydrochlorothiazide 50 mg with fluconazole 100 mg for 10 days to 10 healthy men resulted in a significant increase in the plasma fluconazole AUC (45 ± 31%) and maximum concentration of 43 ± 31% due to reduced renal clearance *4645*

Glomerular Filtration Rate *Urine No Effect Physiological* In 4 patients with nephrogenic diabetes insipidus treatment with 2 mg/kg/d for 2 weeks had no significant effect *2891*

Glucagon *Plasma Increase Physiological* Higher in 15 hypertensives during treatment with 50 mg twice daily than before treatment and after withdrawal *1689*

Glucose *Serum Increase Physiological* Increase from mean baseline of 5.3 mmol/L to 5.9 mmol/L in 50 patients with hypertension treated with mean dose of 40 mg/day for 18 weeks *4735* Significant increase from mean baseline of 5.1 mmol/L to 5.3 mmol/L after 3 months treatment with up to 100 mg daily in 37 hypertensives, and from 5.2 to 5.5 mmol/L at 6 months and at 12 months *4098* Diabetogenic-like action of drug *5869* To extent of coma in 2 diabetics given hydrochlorothiazide with propranolol: exact mechanism not known *4223* In 186 patients with essential hypertension treated with up to 50 mg/d for 8 weeks mean concentration increased by 6.7 mg/dL (0.37 mmol/L) and persisted for 2 years *3841* Increase by 6 mg/dL in 343 patients with hypertension given drug for 10 weeks *6247* Increase by 4.7 mg/dL in approximately 175 patients with essential hypertension treated for 1 y *6248* In 16 patients with normolipidemia but with essential hypertension treatment with 25 mg/d hydrochlorothiazide for 5 months caused a significant 0.9 ± 2.2 mmol/L increase in concentration *321* Average increase of 7 mg/dL in 85 patients with hypertension treated with 25 or 50 mg daily for 8 weeks *4115* In 14 hypertensive men with type 2 diabetes by 31% over 3 weeks: effect augmented by coadministered propranolol *1476*

Serum No Effect Analytical At concentration of 7 mg/L had no effect on GOD/POD-PAP method *5704*

Serum No Effect Physiological In 147 hypertensive men treatment with 50 mg/d for 2 months caused nonsignificant change in fasting concentration from mean baseline of 5.1 mmol/L to 5.2 mmol/L *5544* No effect in hypertensives given potassium supplement if demonstrated no effect in response to hydrochlorothiazide alone *3893* In 9 patients with mild to moderate hypertension treatment with up to 50 mg/d for 8 weeks caused insignificant change from mean baseline of 5.3 ± 0.38 mmol/L to 5.4 ± 0.60 mmol/L *1919*

Urine Increase Physiological Diabetogenic-like action of drug due to hyperglycemia if produced *5869*

Hydrochlorothiazide *(continued)*

Glucose Tolerance *Serum Decrease Physiological* Diabetogenic-like action of drug *4555*

γ-Glutamyltransferase *Serum Increase Physiological* Average increase of 8 U/L in 85 patients with hypertension treated with 25 or 50 mg daily for 8 weeks *4115*

Glycated Hemoglobin *Blood No Effect Analytical* At a concentration of 50 mg/L had an insignificant 1.9% interference with method on Abbott Vision *1885*

Granulocytes *Blood Decrease Physiological* Apparent association between use and agranulocytosis in Israel but effect not observed in other countries and importance of observation uncertain *3098*

Growth Hormone *Plasma No Effect Physiological* In 15 hypertensives treated with 50 mg twice daily *1689*

HDL_2-Cholesterol *Serum No Effect Physiological* In 16 patients with normolipidemia but with essential hypertension treatment with 25 mg/d hydrochlorothiazide for 5 months caused a nonsignificant 0.2 ± 3.0 mg/dL decrease in concentration *321*

HDL_2-Cholesterol, Esterified
Serum No Effect Physiological In 16 patients with normolipidemia but with essential hypertension treatment with 25 mg/d hydrochlorothiazide for 5 months caused a nonsignificant 0.01 ± 1.7 mg/dL decrease in concentration *321*

HDL_2-Cholesterol, Free *Serum No Effect Physiological* In 16 patients with normolipidemia but with essential hypertension treatment with 25 mg/d hydrochlorothiazide for 5 months caused a nonsignificant 0.2 ± 1.4 mg/dL decrease in concentration *321*

HDL_2-Lecithin *Serum No Effect Physiological* In 16 patients with normolipidemia but with essential hypertension treatment with 25 mg/d hydrochlorothiazide for 5 months caused a nonsignificant 0.1 ± 1.04 U/mL increase in concentration *321*

HDL_2-Lysolecithin *Serum No Effect Physiological* In 16 patients with normolipidemia but with essential hypertension treatment with 25 mg/d hydrochlorothiazide for 5 months caused a nonsignificant 0.0 ± 0.01 U/mL change in concentration *321*

HDL_2-Phosphatidylethanolamine
Serum No Effect Physiological In 16 patients with normolipidemia but with essential hypertension treatment with 25 mg/d hydrochlorothiazide for 5 months caused a nonsignificant 0.0 ± 0.01 U/mL change in concentration *321*

HDL_2-Phosphatidylinositol *Serum No Effect Physiological* In 16 patients with normolipidemia but with essential hypertension treatment with 25 mg/d hydrochlorothiazide for 5 months caused a nonsignificant 0.0 ± 0.01 U/mL change in concentration *321*

HDL_2-Sphingomyelin *Serum No Effect Physiological* In 16 patients with normolipidemia but with essential hypertension treatment with 25 mg/d hydrochlorothiazide for 5 months caused a nonsignificant 0.0 ± 0.01 U/mL change in concentration *321*

HDL_2-Triglycerides *Serum Increase Physiological* In 16 patients with normolipidemia but with essential hypertension treatment with 25 mg/d hydrochlorothiazide for 5 months caused a nonsignificant 1.0 ± 4.2 mg/dL increase in concentration *321*

HDL_3-Cholesterol *Serum No Effect Physiological* In 16 patients with normolipidemia but with essential hypertension treatment with 25 mg/d hydrochlorothiazide for 5 months caused a nonsignificant 0.32 ± 6.8 mg/dL decrease in concentration *321*

HDL_3-Cholesterol, Esterified
Serum No Effect Physiological In 16 patients with normolipidemia but with essential hypertension treatment with 25 mg/d hydrochlorothiazide for 5 months caused a nonsignificant 0.19 ± 4.7 mg/dL decrease in concentration *321*

HDL_3-Cholesterol, Free *Serum No Effect Physiological* In 16 patients with normolipidemia but with essential hypertension treatment with 25 mg/d hydrochlorothiazide for 5 months caused a nonsignificant 0.13 ± 3.2 mg/dL decrease in concentration *321*

HDL_3-Lecithin *Serum No Effect Physiological* In 16 patients with normolipidemia but with essential hypertension treatment with 25 mg/d hydrochlorothiazide for 5 months caused a nonsignificant 0.01 ± 0.11 U/mL increase in concentration *321*

HDL_3-Lysolecithin *Serum No Effect Physiological* In 16 patients with normolipidemia but with essential hypertension treatment with 25 mg/d hydrochlorothiazide for 5 months caused a nonsignificant 0.01 ± 0.03 U/mL increase in concentration *321*

HDL_3-Phosphatidylethanolamine
Serum No Effect Physiological In 16 patients with normolipidemia but with essential hypertension treatment with 25 mg/d hydrochlorothiazide for 5 months caused a nonsignificant 0.0 ± 0.01 U/mL change in concentration *321*

HDL_3-Phosphatidylinositol *Serum No Effect Physiological* In 16 patients with normolipidemia but with essential hypertension treatment with 25 mg/d hydrochlorothiazide for 5 months caused a nonsignificant 0.0 ± 0.01 U/mL change in concentration *321*

HDL_3-Sphingomyelin *Serum No Effect Physiological* In 16 patients with normolipidemia but with essential hypertension treatment with 25 mg/d hydrochlorothiazide for 5 months caused a nonsignificant 0.0 ± 0.02 U/mL change in concentration *321*

HDL_3-Triglycerides *Serum Increase Physiological* In 16 patients with normolipidemia but with essential hypertension treatment with 25 mg/d hydrochlorothiazide for 5 months caused a nonsignificant 2.0 ± 5.3 mg/dL decrease in concentration *321*

HDL-Cholesterol *Serum Decrease Physiological* In 10 patients with mild hypertension treatment with 12.5 mg/d for 6 months caused significant reduction from mean baseline of 47 ± 4 mg/dL to 42 ± 3 mg/dL *1306*
Serum Increase Physiological Insignificant increase from mean baseline of 1.27 mmol/L to 1.49 mmol/L in 9 patients treated with mean dose of 72 mg/d for 1 year *4809*
Serum No Effect Physiological No significant change in 39 individuals given drug alone for less than 1 y *2337* No effect with 25 or 50 mg/d in hypertensive patients *3225* In long term over 1 y in many patients *141* In 9 hypertensive men treatment with 25 mg/d (in Moduretic) caused insignificant decrease from mean baseline of 1.02 ± 0.24 mmol/L to 0.95 ± 0.24 mmol/L after 3 months and increase to 1.16 ± 0.18 mmol/L after 12 months *4460*

HDL-Cholesterol:Cholesterol Ratio
Serum No Effect Physiological In 9 hypertensive men administration of 25 mg/d (in Moduretic) caused insignificant decrease to 0.14 ± 0.05 from mean 0.16 ± 0.05 after 3 months and insignificant increase to 0.18 ± 0.07 after 12 months *4460*

Hematocrit *Blood Increase Physiological* Average increase of 0.8% in 85 patients with hypertension treated with 25 or 50 mg daily for 8 weeks *4115*
Blood No Effect Physiological In 39 patients with mild to moderate hypertension treatment with 25 mg/d for 4 weeks caused no change from mean baseline of 43.7 ± 2.5% *6630* In 28 mild to moderate hypertensives treatment with 25 mg/d for 2 weeks caused nonsignificant reduction from mean baseline of 45.2 ± 0.91% to 45.5 ± 0.34% observed *3215*

Hemoglobin *Blood No Effect Physiological* In 9 patients with mild to moderate hypertension treatment with up to 50 mg/d for 8 weeks caused nonsignificant change from mean baseline of 143 ± 13.9 g/L to 144 ± 18.4 g/L *1919*

Hemoglobin A_{1c} *Blood Increase Physiological* Increase by 6% in 14 hypertensive type 2 diabetic men over 3 weeks: effect augmented by coadministered propranolol *1476* Mean increase from 4.6% to 5.3% in 50 hypertensive patients treated with mean dose of 40 mg/day for 18 weeks *4735*

Histamine *Plasma No Effect Analytical* Improbable inhibition of radio-enzyme assay at therapeutic concentrations *2492*

^{131}I Uptake *Serum No Effect Physiological* No change observed *882*

Initial Blood Filterability *Blood Decrease Physiological* In 39 patients with mild to moderate hypertension treatment with 25 mg/d for 4 weeks caused nonsignificant reduction from 29.6 ± 8.9 to 24.4 ± 8.6 *6630*

Insulin *Plasma Decrease Physiological* Intravenous injection has effect with little effect on blood sugar concentration *4014*

Plasma Increase Physiological In 16 patients with normolipidemia but with essential hypertension treatment with 25 mg/d hydrochlorothiazide for 5 months caused a significant 3.4 ± 5.0 pmol/L increase in concentration *321* In 147 hypertensive men treatment with 50 mg/d for 2 months caused non-significant increase of fasting concentration from mean baseline of 141.3 pmol/L to 150.7 pmol/L *5544* Increase from mean fasting concentration of 54 pmol/L to 71 pmol/L in 50 hypertensive patients treated with mean dose of 40 mg/day for 18 weeks. Steady state insulin concentration unchanged *4735*
Plasma No Effect Physiological In 15 hypertensives treated with 50 mg twice daily *1689*

Iodide *Urine Increase Physiological* Significant effect in 5 h after 150 mg orally *1959*

Ionized Calcium *Serum Increase Physiological* Observed effect *697* Increased for up to 2 weeks after drug withdrawal *5840*

Irbesartan *Serum No Effect Physiological* Coadministration of hydrochlorothiazide with irbesartan had no effect on the pharmacokinetics of irbesartan *725*

Isradipine *Serum No Effect Physiological* Concomitant administration of both drugs in healthy individuals had no effect on the pharmacokinetics of either drug *5230*

LDL-Cholesterol *Serum Increase Physiological* Transient but significant increase in LDL-cholesterol after 3 months treatment with up to 100 mg daily in 37 hypertensive patients (4.45 mmol/L versus 4.05 mmol/L at baseline) *4098* Observed with 100 mg/d *6156* In short term studies administration of hydrochlorothiazide increased concentration of LDL-cholesterol by 10 to 20% within a year *3730* Significant increase from mean baseline concentration of 142 to 153 mg/dL in 87 hypertensive patients treated with up to 50 mg daily for 8 weeks *1441*
Serum No Effect Physiological In 10 patients with mild hypertension treatment with 12.5 mg/d for 6 months caused nonsignificant change from mean baseline of 115 ± 6 mg/dL to 117 ± 6 mg/dL *1306* In short term study involving many patients *141* No significant change in 39 individuals given drug alone for less than 1 y *2337* In 9 hypertensive men administration of 25 mg/d (in Moduretic) caused insignificant change from mean baseline of 5.5 ± 1.8 mmol/L to 5.4 ± 1.5 mmol/L after 3 months and 5.6 ± 1.8 mmol/L after 2 months *4460*

Lecithin *Serum No Effect Physiological* In 16 patients with normolipidemia but with essential hypertension treatment with 25 mg/d hydrochlorothiazide for 5 months caused a nonsignificant 0.12 ± 0.22 U/mL increase in concentration *321*

Leukocytes *Blood Decrease Physiological* Occasional case of aplastic anemia reported *6264* May cause leukopenia/agranulocytosis *1322*
Blood Increase Physiological In 9 patients with mild to moderate hypertension treatment with up to 50 mg/d for 8 weeks caused significant increase from mean baseline of 5500 ± 1400 /µL to 6700 ±1400 /µL *1919*

Lidocaine *Serum No Effect Analytical* No significant interference observed at a concentration of 100 µg/mL (336 µmol/L) with method on Du Pont aca *1534* At a concentration of 1250 mg/L (normal therapeutic concentration up to 0.45 mg/L) had effect of less than 10% on method on Baxter Stratus *5705*

Lisinopril *Serum No Effect Physiological* Coadministration of lisinopril with hyrochlorothiazide appears to have no effect on the pharmacokinetics of either drug *3990*

Lithium *Serum Increase Physiological* Significant increase with 50 mg/d over 2 weeks possible effect on reabsorption in loop of Henle *2916* Reported in 2 cases taking lithium: drug also given with triamterene: due to reduced clearance of lithium *3934*

Losartan *Serum No Effect Physiological* Coadministration had no effect on the pharmacokinetics of losartan and that of its active metabolite *3979* Coadministration of losartan with hydrochlorothiazide had no effect on the pharmacokinetics of either drug *3965* Coadministration of losartan with hydrochlorothiazide had no significant effect on the concentration of either drug *1596* No significant interaction when hydrochlorothiazide coadministered with losartan *3881*

Lysolecithin *Serum No Effect Physiological* In 16 patients with normolipidemia but with essential hypertension treatment with 25 mg/d hydrochlorothiazide for 5 months caused a nonsignificant 0.01 ± 0.03 U/mL increase in concentration *321*

Magnesium *Red Blood Cells No Effect Physiological* No significant change observed in 9 patients treated with mean dose of 72 mg/d for 1 year: baseline 0.04 pmol/100 cells, post-treatment 0.03 pmol/100 cells *4809*
Serum Decrease Physiological In 10% patients receiving diuretics, but majority had diseases likely also to hypomagnesemia *3350*
Serum No Effect Physiological No significant change from mean baseline of 0.86 mmol/L to 0.79 mmol/L in 9 patients treated with mean dose of 72 mg/d for 1 year *4809* No significant difference in hypertensive patients with 50 mg/d *3225* No effect observed in patients with previous thiazide-induced hyponatremia, elderly hypertensive patients and young healthy controls following single dose of combination of hydrochlorothiazide and amiloride *1964*
Urine Increase Physiological 60% increase after 200 mg in 1 dose orally *2452*
Urine No Effect Physiological No significant change observed in 9 patients treated with mean dose of 72 mg/d for 1 year: baseline 137 mmol/d, post-treatment 129 mmol/d *4809* No effect observed in patients with previous thiazide-induced hyponatremia, elderly hypertensives or healthy young controls following single dose of combination of hydrochlorothiazide and amiloride *1964* No significant effect on clearance noted with i.v. infusion of 50 mg, although long-term oral studies suggest some increased loss and reduction of plasma concentration *5169*

Malondialdehyde *Blood Increase Physiological* In 38 patients with mild to moderate hypertension treatment with 25 mg/d for 4 weeks caused increase from mean baseline of 5.73 ± 2.74 nmol/L per 10^9 platelets to 6.57 ± 2.48 nmol/L per 10^9 platelets *6630*

N-Acetylprocainamide *Serum No Effect Analytical* No significant interference observed at a concentration of 100 µg/mL (336 µmol/L) with method on Du Pont aca *1536*

Neutrophils *Blood Decrease Physiological* Occasional case of agranulocytosis reported *6264* Occasionally observed *4014*

Norepinephrine *Plasma No Effect Physiological* In 28 mild to moderate hypertensives treatment with 25 mg/d for 2 weeks had no significant effect on concentration *3213*

Osmolality *Serum Decrease Physiological* In 4 patients with nephrogenic diabetes insipidus treatment with 2 mg/kg/d for 2 weeks caused significant reduction of concentration *2891* Decreased by as much as 14 mmol/kg within 6 to 8 hours in patients with previous thiazide-induced hyponatremia following single dose of combination of hydrochlorothiazide and amiloride *1964* Due to hyponatremia of diuretic action *1856*
Urine Increase Physiological In 4 patients with nephrogenic diabetes insipidus treatment with 2 mg/kg/d for 2 weeks caused significant increase from about 65 mosmol/kg to 85 mosmol/kg *2891*

Parathyroid Hormone *Plasma No Effect Physiological* No effect (?mechanism of effect on calcium) *5840*

Phosphate *Serum Decrease Physiological* Observed in some cases with prolonged treatment *2754*
Serum Increase Physiological Altered parathyroid metabolism *718*
Urine Increase Physiological Altered parathyroid metabolism *718*

Phosphatidylinositol *Serum No Effect Physiological* In 16 patients with normolipidemia but with essential hypertension treatment with 25 mg/d hydrochlorothiazide for 5 months caused a nonsignificant 0.0 ± 0.01 U/mL change in concentration *321*

Platelet Aggregation *Blood No Effect Physiological* In 34 patients with mild to moderate hypertension treatment with 25 mg/d for 4 weeks had no significant effect on arachidonic acid-induced aggregation *6630* In 35 patients with mild to moderate hypertension treatment with 25 mg/d for 4 weeks had no significant effect on ADP-induced aggregation *6630*

Platelets *Blood Decrease Physiological* Occasional case of aplastic anemia reported *6264* Several cases of immune mediated thrombocytopenia reported *4139* Thrombocytopenia reported *4555*
Blood No Effect Physiological In 39 patients with mild to moderate hypertension treatment with 25 mg/d for 4 weeks caused nonsignificant decrease from baseline of 225025 ± 92170 /µL to 216769 ± 79026 /µL *6630*

Hydrochlorothiazide *(continued)*

Potassium *Red Blood Cells No Effect Physiological* No significant change from mean baseline of 0.78 pmol/100 cells to 0.74 pmol/100 cells in 9 patients treated with mean dose of 72 mg/d for 1 year *4809*
Serum Decrease Physiological Increase by 0.6 mmol/L in approximately 175 patients with essential hypertension treated for 1 y *6248* Increase by 0.6 mmol/L in 343 patients with hypertension given drug for 10 weeks *6247* Diuretic action *5869* During 3 mo treatment in hypertensive patients with either 25 or 50 mg/d, but only significant statistically with 50 mg *3225* Slight decrease in 6 volunteers given 100 mg/day for 3 days *1813* Significant reduction observed from 4.4 mmol/L to 4.0 mmol/L in 87 hypertensive patients treated with up to 50 mg daily for 8 weeks *1441* Significant decrease from mean baseline of 4.2 mmol/L to 3.8 mmol/L in 9 patients treated with mean dose of 72 mg/d for 1 year *4809* With hydrochlorothiazide use hypokalemia may occur, especially if brisk diuresis takes place *24* Average reduction of 0.6 mmol/L in 85 patients with hypertension treated with 25 or 50 mg daily for 8 weeks *4115* Significant reduction observed in 33 patients with mild-to-moderate essential hypertension treated with 25 mg/d for 4 weeks *4131* 28% patients with hypokalemia given long term 25-100 mg/d *506*
Serum Increase Physiological Marked effect when given with amiloride to 3 patients with renal failure (creatinine 0.2 - 0.7 mmol/L) *6430*
Serum No Effect Analytical At concentration of 50 mg/L caused nonsignificant 1.1% interference with method on Abbott Vision *681*
Serum No Effect Physiological If potassium supplement coadministered with hydrochlorothiazide in hypertensive women *3893* In 9 patients with mild to moderate hypertension treatment with up to 50 mg/d for 8 weeks caused nonsignificant decrease to 3.7 ± 0.4 mmol/L from mean baseline of 3.9 ± 0.4 mmol/L *1919* No effect observed following single dose of combination of hydrochlorothiazide and amiloride in patients with previous thiazide-induced hyponatremia, elderly hypertensive patients and young healthy controls *1964*
Urine Increase Physiological Significant effect in 5 h after 150 mg orally *1959* In hypokalemic patients receiving drug over initial period of therapy: Increase of up to 41 mmol/d *4502* Peak excretion in patients with previous thiazide-induced hyponatremia as well as in young and elderly controls 6 to 8 hours after single dose of combination of hydrochlorothiazide and amiloride *1964* Significant increase from mean baseline of 69 mmol/d to 98 mmol/d in 9 patients treated with mean dose of 72 mg/d for 1 year *4809*
Urine No Effect Physiological In patients who were normokalemic after receiving drug for treatment for uncomplicated systemic hypertension *4502*

Pramipexole *Serum No Effect Physiological* Coadministration of hydrochlorothiazide with pramipexole presumed to have no effect on the oral clearance of pramipexole *4680*

Procainamide *Serum No Effect Analytical* No significant interference observed at a concentration of 100 µg/mL (336 µmol/L) with method on Du Pont aca *1542*

Prolactin *Plasma No Effect Physiological* In 15 hypertensives treated with 50 mg twice daily *1689*

Prostaglandin $F_{2\alpha}$ *Urine No Effect Physiological* No effect observed in 6 volunteers given 100 mg daily for 3 days *1813*

Prostaglandins *Urine No Effect Physiological* No effect observed in 6 volunteers given 100 mg daily for 3 days *1813*

Pyrophosphate *Urine Increase Physiological* Associated with increased orthophosphate also *4481*

Quinidine *Serum Increase Physiological* Drugs that alkalinize the urine reduce the renal elimination of quinidine *5996* Alkalinizes urine, increases reabsorption *2452*
Serum No Effect Analytical Hydrochlorothiazide at a concentration of 100 µg/mL had no significant cross-reactivity with quinidine at a concentration of 2.0 µg/mL in method on Bayer Technicon Immuno 1® *431* No significant interference observed at a concentration of 100 µg/mL (336 µmol/L) with method on Du Pont aca *1543*

Red Cell Transit Time *Blood No Effect Physiological* In 28 mild to moderate hypertensives treatment with 25 mg/d for 2 weeks caused nonsignificant increase from mean baseline of 14.5 ± 0.58 units to 16.1 ± 0.73 units *3215*

Relative Filtration Rate *Blood Decrease Physiological* In 28 mild to moderate hypertensives treatment for 2 weeks with 25 mg/d caused significant reduction from mean baseline of 0.25 ± 0.009 units to 0.23 ± 0.008 units *3215*

Renin Activity *Plasma Increase Physiological* In 33 mild-to-moderate essential hypertensives treatment with 25 mg/d for 4 weeks caused increase from mean baseline of 2.8 ng/mL/h to 4.5 ng/mL/h *4131* In 2 children with nephrogenic diabetes insipidus baseline renin activity of 2 and 5 µg/L/h significantly increased to 22 and 50 µg/L/h after treatment with 2 mg/kg/d for 2 weeks *2891* Significant increase in 6 volunteers given 100 mg daily for 3 days *1813*
Plasma No Effect Physiological No significant change observed in 10 patients with essential hypertension treated with 25 mg hydrochlorothiazide alone daily for 4 weeks but when combined with perindopril increase of mean concentration from 2.31 to 7.33 ng AI/mL/h *757* In 9 patients with mild to moderate hypertension treatment with up to 50 mg/d for 8 weeks caused nonsignificant increase from mean baseline of 2.27 ± 0.90 ng/mL to 2.73 ± 0.98 ng/mL *1919* In 28 mild to moderate hypertensives treatment with 25 mg/d for 2 weeks caused significant increase *3213*

Sodium *Serum Decrease Physiological* In 4 patients with nephrogenic diabetes insipidus treatment with 2 mg/kg/d for 2 weeks caused significant reduction of serum concentration *2891* May cause hyponatremia *1856* Reduction of up to 5.5 mmol/L in patients with previous thiazide-induced hyponatremia within 6 hours of administration of single dose of combination of hydrochlorothiazide and amiloride *1964* Severe hyponatremia observed in several cases *260* With hydrochlorothiazide use dilutional hyponatremia may occur in edematous patients in hot weather *24*
Serum No Effect Physiological No effect of 100 mg/day for 3 days in 6 volunteers *1813*
Urine Increase Physiological Diuretic action of drug *3669* Peak excretion in patients with previous thiazide-induced hyponatremia as well as in young and elderly controls 6 to 8 hours after administration of a single dose of combination of hydrochlorothiazide and amiloride *1964*

Sphingomyelin *Serum No Effect Physiological* In 16 patients with normolipidemia but with essential hypertension treatment with 25 mg/d hydrochlorothiazide for 5 months caused a nonsignificant 0.02 ± 0.04 U/mL increase in concentration *321*

Theophylline *Serum No Effect Analytical* At concentration of 1.0 mg/L produced no interference with methods used on Kodak DT-60, Abbott TDx, Abbott Vision with either whole blood or serum, 3M Diagnostics TheoFAST, Syntex AccµLevel or Ames Seralyzer *1122*

Triglycerides *Serum Increase Physiological* 17% in short term, and increase in MRFIT study when given with chlorthalidone *141* In short term studies administration of hydrochlorothiazide increased concentration of triglycerides by as much as 50% within a year *3730* Nonsignificant increase from mean baseline of 1.32 mmol/L to 1.54 mmol/L in 9 patients treated with mean dose of 72 mg/d for 1 year *4809* In 16 patients with normolipidemia but with essential hypertension treatment with 25 mg/d hydrochlorothiazide for 5 months caused a nonsignificant 37.8 ± 83.2 mg/dL increase in concentration *321* Observed with 100 mg/d *6156* In 9 patients with mild to moderate hypertension treatment with up to 50 mg/d for 8 weeks caused significant increase from mean baseline of 1.28 ± 0.59 mmol/L to 1.59 ± 0.61 mmol/L *1919* 17% change in 39 individuals given drug alone for less than 1 y *2337*
Serum No Effect Analytical At concentration of 7 mg/L had no effect on GPO-PAP method *5704*
Serum No Effect Physiological Nonsignificant change by 7 mg/dL in 33 patients with hypertension given drug for 10 weeks to reduce diastolic blood pressure to less than 90 mm Hg *6247* In approximately 175 patients with essential hypertension treated for 1 y *6248* In 9 hypertensive men administration of 25 mg/d (in Moduretic) caused insignificant decrease from mean baseline of 2.3 ± 1.0 mmol/L to 2.2 ± 1.1 mmol/L after 3 months and 2.1 ± 1.3 mmol/L after 12 months *4460* Nonsignificant increase in 85 patients with hypertension treated with 25 or 50 mg daily for 8 weeks *4115* No effect with 25 or 50 mg/d in hypertensive patients *3225* No significant change observed in 37 hypertensives treated with up to 100 mg daily for 1 year *4098* In short term, and long term involving many patients *141*

Urea Nitrogen *Serum Increase Physiological* May occur with prolonged therapy *3669* Average increase of 2.3 mg/dL in 85 patients with hypertension treated with 25 or 50 mg daily for 8 weeks *4115* Increase by 2.7 mg/dL in 343 patients with hypertension given drug for 10 weeks to reduce diastolic blood pressure to less than 90 mm Hg *6247* Increase by 2.5 mg/dL in approximately 175 patients with essential hypertension treated for 1 y *6248*
Serum No Effect Physiological No effect observed in patients with previous thiazide-induced hyponatremia or in elderly hypertensive patients or healthy young controls following single dose of combination of hydrochlorothiazide and amiloride *1964*

Uric Acid *Serum Increase Physiological* Slight effect in hypertensive patients given either 25 or 50 mg/d *3225* Significant increase observed in 33 patients with mild-to-moderate hypertension treated with 25 mg/d for 4 weeks *4131* Significant increase from mean baseline concentration of 4.8 mg/dL to 5.7 mg/dL in 87 hypertensive patients treated with up to 50 mg/d for 8 weeks *1441* In 2 patients with hypertension diuretic induced gout observed *5416* Average increase of 0.8 mg/dL in 85 patients with hypertension treated with 25 or 50 mg daily for 8 weeks *4115* In 37 hypertensives treatment with up to 100 mg daily caused change from mean baseline concentration of 325 µmol/L to 380 µmol/L at 3 months, from 315 to 376 µmol/L at 6 months and 314 µmol/L to 367 µmol/L at 1 year *4098* Decreased urate clearance *5869* Increase by 2.0 mg/dL in 343 patients with hypertension given drug for 10 weeks *6247* Increase by 1.37 mg/dL in approximately 175 patients with essential hypertension treated for 1 y *6248* In 9 patients with mild to moderate hypertension treatment with up to 50 mg/d for 8 weeks caused significant increase from mean baseline of 272 ± 116 µmol/L to 309 ± 109 µmol/L *1919* With hydrochlorothiazide use hyperuricemia or even frank gout may occur in certain patients *24*
Serum No Effect Analytical At concentration of 7 mg/L had no effect on uricase-PAP method *5704*
Urine Decrease Physiological Decreased urate clearance *3669*

Viscosity *Blood No Effect Physiological* In 39 patients with mild to moderate hypertension treatment with 25 mg/d for 4 weeks caused no significant effect at shear rates from 0.2 s^{-1} to 128 s^{-1}*6630*
Plasma No Effect Physiological In 39 patients with mild to moderate hypertension treatment with 25 mg/d for 4 weeks caused no change from mean baseline of 1.29 ± 0.06 $m^2/s \times 10^{-2}$*6630* In 28 mild to moderate hypertensives treatment with 25 mg/d for 2 weeks caused significant increase from mean baseline of 1.28 ± 0.02 mPa/s to 1.31 ± 0.01 mPa/s *3215*

VLDL + LDL-Cholesterol *Serum Increase Physiological* In 16 patients with normolipidemia but with essential hypertension treatment with 25 mg/d hydrochlorothiazide for 5 months caused a significant 10.7 ± 29.3 mg/dL increase in concentration *321*

VLDL + LDL-Cholesterol Ester
Serum Increase Physiological In 16 patients with normolipidemia but with essential hypertension treatment with 25 mg/d hydrochlorothiazide for 5 months caused a significant 7.4 ± 19.4 mg/dL increase in concentration *321*

VLDL + LDL-Cholesterol, Free
Serum Increase Physiological In 16 patients with normolipidemia but with essential hypertension treatment with 25 mg/d hydrochlorothiazide for 5 months caused a nonsignificant 3.4 ± 19.6 mg/dL increase in concentration *321*

VLDL + LDL-Lecithin *Serum Increase Physiological* In 16 patients with normolipidemia but with essential hypertension treatment with 25 mg/d hydrochlorothiazide for 5 months caused a significant 0.1 ± 0.14 U/mL increase in concentration *321*

VLDL + LDL-Lysolecithin *Serum No Effect Physiological* In 16 patients with normolipidemia but with essential hypertension treatment with 25 mg/d hydrochlorothiazide for 5 months caused a nonsignificant 0.0 ± 0.03 U/mL change in concentration *321*

VLDL + LDL-Phosphatidylinositol
Serum No Effect Physiological In 16 patients with normolipidemia but with essential hypertension treatment with 25 mg/d hydrochlorothiazide for 5 months caused a nonsignificant 0.0 ± 0.01 U/mL change in concentration *321*

VLDL + LDL-Sphingomyelin *Serum No Effect Physiological* In 16 patients with normolipidemia but with essential hypertension treatment with 25 mg/d hydrochlorothiazide for 5 months caused a nonsignificant 0.01 ± 0.07 U/mL increase in concentration *321*

VLDL + LDL-Triglycerides *Serum Increase Physiological* In 16 patients with normolipidemia but with essential hypertension treatment with 25 mg/d hydrochlorothiazide for 5 months caused a significant 22.9 ± 40.6 mg/dL increase in concentration *321*

VLDL-Cholesterol *Serum Increase Physiological* In short term studies administration of hydrochlorothiazide increased concentration of VLDL-cholesterol by as much as 50% within a year *3730* 13% in a short term involving many patients *141* 13% change in individuals given drug alone for less than 1 y *2337*
Serum No Effect Physiological No significant change observed in 37 hypertensives treated with up to 100 mg daily for 1 year *4098* In 10 patients with mild hypertension treatment with 12.5 mg/d for 6 months caused nonsignificant decrease from mean baseline of 22 ± 6 mg/dL to 19 ± 5 mg/dL *1306*

VLDL-Triglycerides *Serum Increase Physiological* Observed with 100 mg/d *6156*

Volume *Urine Decrease Physiological* In 4 patients with nephrogenic diabetes insipidus treatment with 2 mg/kg/d for 2 weeks caused reduction of urinary volume by 25% *2891*
Urine Increase Physiological Significant effect in 5 h after 150 mg orally *1959*

Zinc *Serum Increase Physiological* Slight effect observed or no effect *4484*
Urine Increase Physiological Twice normal reached on fifth day *4484* Increase by 60% in 9 patients with hypertension over 2 weeks *6418*

Hydrocodone

Cannabinoids *Urine No Effect Analytical* No effect on Roche Abuscreen method *5006*

Opiates *Urine Positive Analytical* At concentration of 1.0 µg/mL (3.34 µmol/L) on method on Du Pont aca *1559* Cross-reactivity of over 50% observed with Roche Abuscreen Online procedure when adapted for use with Roche Cobas Fara II analyzers *5547* Significant cross-reactivity observed with Roche Abuscreen method adapted for use with Olympus AU 5121 and 5131 analyzers *214*

p-Aminophenol *Urine No Effect Analytical* With addition of drugs at a concentration of 100 mg/L and of related compounds at 50 mg/L no significant effect observed on colorimetric method of van Bocxlaer on Cobas Mira analyzer which involves reacting free p-aminophenol with resorcinol in the presence of magnesium ions to form an indophenol dye measured at 550 nm *6163*

Hydrocortisone

Amino Acids *Urine Increase Physiological* Glucocorticoid hormonal action *2999*

Bicarbonate *Serum Increase Physiological* May cause hypochloremic hypokalemic alkalosis *2242*

Chloride *Serum Decrease Physiological* May cause hypochloremic hypokalemic alkalosis *2242*
Serum Increase Physiological May cause retention and edema *128*

Color *Feces Increase Analytical* Black color reported with hydrocortisone ingestion *3388*

Cortisol *Plasma Increase Physiological* In 8 healthy male volunteers intravenous administration of 20 mg produced peak of about 520 µg/L, after oral administration of 20 mg 300 µg/L and after rectal administration of 100 mg 30 µg/L *6095* In 5 adult patients with active acromegaly bolus injection followed by infusion caused concentration to increase above 2000 nmol/L at all time points studied in all individuals *2142* Effect lasts for at least 24 h *2895* In 10 healthy young individuals infusion of 100 or 300 mg over 24 hours caused increase comparable to that seen in moderate to severe stress with increase from 298 ± 50 nmol/L to 704 ± 116 nmol/L with low dose and from 364 ± 52 nmol/L to 1082 ± 77 nmol/L with high dose *5216*

Hydrocortisone *(continued)*

Cortisol *(continued)*

Saliva Increase Physiological In 8 healthy men after intravenous administration of 20 mg mean peak of about 100 µg/L observed, after 20 mg orally peak of about 75 µg/L and after 100 mg rectally less than 10 µg/L *6095*

Dexamethasone *Serum Increase Analytical* Very slight cross reactivity in procedure of Hichens *2588*

Eosinophils *Blood Decrease Physiological* Due to hormonal action on adrenals *393*

Estradiol *Plasma No Effect Physiological* In 4 female volunteers infusion of 100 mg/24 h caused nonsignificant change from 173 ± 70nmol/L to 176 ± 44 nmol/L and of 300 mg/24 h from 228 ± 103 nmol/L to 165 ± 66 nmol/L *5216*

Follicle Stimulating Hormone

Plasma Increase Physiological In 9 girls with 21-hydroxylase deficiency aged 61.7 ± 28.1 days mean concentration of about 2.0 IU/L significantly increased to about 3.6 IU/L when treated with 20 mg/sq m/d for a mean duration of 45.7 ± 20.8 days *459*

Plasma No Effect Physiological In 10 healthy individuals infusion of 100 mg or 300 mg had no effect on mean or pulsatile secretion of FSH *5216*

Glucose *Serum No Effect Physiological* In 5 adults with active acromegaly bolus injection followed by steady infusion had no significant effect on concentration *2142*

Glucose Tolerance *Serum Decrease Physiological* Decreased carbohydrate tolerance may occur as an adverse reaction *3978*

Growth Hormone *Plasma Decrease Physiological* In 5 adults with active acromegaly infusion of hydrocortisone caused decrease of 18.4- 50.5% compared with saline with mean decrease to 9.0 ± 3.9 µg/L compared with baseline of 21 ± 7.9 µg/L *2142* Marked effect of 100 mg i.v. by 4 h *4893*

Histamine *Plasma No Effect Analytical* Insignificant inhibition of radio-enzyme assay even at concentrations much greater than physiological *2492*

3-Hydroxyanthranilic Acid *Urine Increase Physiological* Causes induction of tryptophan pyrrolase *5086*

3-Hydroxykynurenine *Urine Increase Physiological* Causes induction of tryptophan pyrrolase *5086*

Kynurenine *Urine Increase Physiological* Causes induction of tryptophan pyrrolase *5086*

Leukotriene C_4 *Plasma Decrease Physiological* In 6 asthmatic patients treatment with 100 mg hydrocortisone succinate reduced mean baseline concentration from 284 pg/mL to 249 pg/mL *5529* Treatment of 4 asthmatics with only 100 mg hydrocortisone intravenously caused decrease of mean concentration from 284 ng/L to 249 ng/L *5529*

Plasma Increase Physiological 100 mg hydrocortisone given with 250 mg aminophylline intravenously to 6 asthmatics caused decrease of mean concentration from 181 ng/L to 132 ng/L *5529*

Lipase *Serum Increase Physiological* Pancreatitis may occur as an adverse reaction *3978*

Luteinizing Hormone *Plasma Increase Physiological* In 9 girls with 21-hydroxylase deficiency aged 61.7 ± 28.1 days mean concentration of about 1.4 IU/L significantly increased to 3.4 ± 4.82 IU/L when treated with 20 mg/sq m/d for a mean duration of 45.7 ± 20.8 days *459*

Plasma No Effect Physiological Infusion of 100 mg or 300 mg to 10 healthy volunteers had no effect on mean or pulsatile luteinizing concentration *5216*

Lymphocytes *Blood Decrease Physiological* Due to hormonal action on adrenals *393*

Neutrophils *Blood Increase Physiological* Due to hormonal action on adrenals *393*

Nitrogen Balance *Patient Negative Physiological* Negative nitrogen balance due to protein catabolism may occur as an adverse reaction *3978*

Occult Blood *Feces Increase Physiological* May cause hemorrhage or ulceration of gastrointestinal tract *929* Peptic ulcer with possible subsequent perforation and hemorrhage may occur as an adverse reaction *3978*

PAH Clearance *Urine Increase Physiological* Increases GFR *2242*

Parathyroid Hormone *Plasma Increase Physiological* If given i.v. stimulates secretion *6467*

pH *Blood Increase Physiological* Hypokalemic alkalosis may occur as an adverse reaction *3978*

Platelet Aggregation *Blood Decrease Physiological* Inhibits streptokinase induced aggregation *5173*

Potassium *Serum Decrease Physiological* Potassium loss may occur as an adverse reaction *3978* Promotes urinary elimination *128*

Urine Increase Physiological Increases elimination in urine *128*

Progesterone *Plasma No Effect Analytical* 1% or less cross reactivity with RIA *858*

Protein *Cerebrospinal Fluid No Effect Analytical* No significant effect when added in vitro to concentration of 10.0 mg/dL on Kodak Ektachem® slide method *3654*

Sodium *Serum Increase Physiological* May cause retention and edema *128*

Urine Increase Physiological Enhances excretion especially if prior loading *2242*

α-Subunit of Glycoprotein Hormones

Plasma No Effect Physiological In 10 healthy volunteers neither the infusion of 100 mg or 300 mg hydrocortisone had any effect on mean or pulsatile secretion *5216*

T3-Uptake *Serum No Effect Physiological* In 10 healthy volunteers infusion of 100 mg/24 h caused nonsignificant change from 0.30 ± 0.01 to 0.30 ± 0.02 and after 300 mg/24 h from 0.30 ± 0.01 to 0.32 ± 0.02 *5216*

Testosterone *Serum No Effect Physiological* In 6 male volunteers infusion of 100 mg/24 h caused nonsignificant change from 17.0 ± 2.7 nmol/L to 19.8 ± 1.0 nmol/L and of 300 mg/24 h from 18.9 ± 1.9 nmol/L to 17.9 ± 2.5 nmol/L *5216*

Theophylline *Serum No Effect Analytical* At concentration of 15 mg/L produced no interference with methods on Kodak DT-60, Abbott TDx, Abbott Vision with either whole blood or serum, 3M Diagnostics TheoFAST, Syntex AccµLevel, and Ames Seralyzer *1122*

Serum No Effect Physiological No documented significant interaction with theophylline reported *6117* No clinically significant effect on theophylline concentration observed when drugs coadministered *5999*

Thromboxane *Plasma No Effect Physiological* No effect of up to 100 µmol/L on formation during clotting *4817*

Thyroid Stimulating Hormone

Serum Decrease Physiological Infusion of 100 mg over 24 hours in 10 healthy individuals caused decrease in TSH pulse amplitude by 60% and reduced mean concentration from 2.58 ± 0.42 mU/L to 1.04 ± 0.76 mU/L and abolished nocturnal TSH surge although TSH pulse frequency not affected. 300 mg/24 h caused decrease to 0.88 mU/L *5216*

Thyroxine (T4) *Serum No Effect Physiological* In 10 healthy volunteers infusion of 100 mg/24 h caused nonsignificant change from mean baseline of 82.4 ± 6.4 nmol/L to 70.8 ± 9.0 nmol/L and with 300 mg/24 h from 75.9 ± 7.7 nmol/L to 68.2 ± 6.4 nmol/L *5216*

Tri-iodothyronine (T3) *Serum Decrease Physiological* In 10 healthy volunteers infusion of 100 mg/24 h caused nonsignificant reduction from mean baseline of 1.50 ± 0.16 nmol/L to 1.29 ± 0.14 nmol/L and significant decrease from mean of 1.72 ± 0.10 nmol/L to 1.10 ± 0.06 nmol/L *5216*

Tyrosine *Plasma Decrease Physiological* Hormonal effect observed in 2 weeks *1313*

Xanthurenic Acid *Urine Increase Physiological* Causes induction of tryptophan pyrrolase *5086*

Hydroflumethiazide

Alanine Aminotransferase *Serum Increase Physiological* May cause intrahepatic cholestasis *2754*

Alkaline Phosphatase *Serum Increase Physiological* May cause intrahepatic cholestasis *2754*

Ammonia *Plasma Increase Physiological* May occur especially if pre-existing hepatic impairment *2754*

Amylase *Serum Increase Physiological* Acute pancreatitis may occur with thiazides *2754*

Aspartate Aminotransferase *Serum Increase Physiological* May cause intrahepatic cholestasis *2754*

Bicarbonate *Serum Increase Physiological* May cause hypochloremic alkalosis *2754*

Bilirubin *Serum Increase Physiological* May cause intrahepatic cholestatic jaundice *2754* Concentration may be increased by displacement of bilirubin from albumin binding sites *6553*

BSP Retention *Serum Increase Physiological* May cause intrahepatic cholestasis *2754*

Chloride *Serum Decrease Physiological* Diuretic action *2754*

Urine Increase Physiological Diuretic action *2754*

Erythrocytes *Blood Decrease Physiological* Pancytopenia, aplastic anemia *6474*

Glucose *Serum Increase Physiological* Thiazide diuretics may increase plasma concentration *6553* May occur (similar action to other thiazides) *2754*

Urine Increase Physiological Excretion may be increased in patients with a predisposition to glucose intolerance *6553* May occur as consequence of hyperglycemia *2754*

Glucose Tolerance *Serum Decrease Physiological* Diabetogenic like action of drug *2754*

Hematocrit *Blood Decrease Physiological* Pancytopenia *6474*

Hemoglobin *Blood Decrease Physiological* Pancytopenia *6474*

Leukocytes *Blood Decrease Physiological* Pancytopenia, agranulocytosis or aplastic anemia *6474*

Lithium *Serum Increase Physiological* Lithium plasma concentration may be increased because of reduced renal clearance *6553*

Lithium Clearance *Urine Decrease Physiological* Lithium plasma concentration may be increased because of reduced renal clearance *6553*

Magnesium *Serum Decrease Physiological* Concentration may be decreased by administration of hydroflumethiazide *6553*

Serum Increase Physiological Concentration may be decreased by administration of hydroflumethiazide, except in uremic patients in whom concentration may be increased *6553*

Mezlocillin *Serum Increase Analytical* Cannot be assayed by HPLC method used at Mayo Clinic in presence of hydroflumethiazide *3858*

Platelets *Blood Decrease Physiological* Pancytopenia or thrombocytopenia with purpura *6474*

Potassium *Serum Decrease Physiological* Diuretic action *2754* Concentration may be decreased by administration of hydroflumethiazide *6553*

Prothrombin Time *Plasma Decrease Physiological* Anticoagulant effect may be decreased when anticoagulants used with thiazide diuretics *6553*

Sodium *Serum Decrease Physiological* Diuretic action *2754* Concentration may be decreased by administration of hydroflumethiazide *6553*

Urine Increase Physiological Diuretic action *2754*

Urea Nitrogen *Serum Increase Physiological* May occur especially if pre-existing renal disease *2754*

Uric Acid *Serum Increase Physiological* Probably due to impaired clearance *2754* Thiazide diuretics may increase plasma concentration *6553*

Hydromorphone

Cannabinoids *Urine No Effect Analytical* No effect on Roche Abuscreen method *5006*

Carbon Dioxide Partial Pressure

Blood Increase Physiological 10 times as potent as morphine *758*

Morphine *Urine Increase Analytical* Cross reactivity equal (or more) with RIA procedures. Substantial cross reactivity with hemagglutination inhibition *4163*

Opiates *Urine Positive Analytical* Significant cross-reactivity observed with Roche Abuscreen method adapted for use with Olympus AU 5121 and 5131 analyzers *214* Significant cross-reactivity observed with Roche Abuscreen method adapted for use with Olympus AU 1521 and 5131 analyzers *214* At concentration of 3.0 μg/mL (10.5 μmol/L) on method on Du Pont aca *1559*

Hydroquinone

Glucose *Urine Decrease Analytical* Reported to inhibit glucose oxidase Stix reactions *134* May inhibit peroxidase reaction on Clinistix® *4206*

1α-Hydroxy Vitamin D_3

Calcium *Serum No Effect Physiological* Mean concentration in 14 patients with chronic renal failure undergoing regular hemodialysis increased nonsignificantly from 8.8 ± 0.2 mg/dL to 8.9 ± 0.2 mg/dL after 8 weeks of treatment with 0.5 μg/d *2457*

1,25-Dihydroxy Vitamin D_3 *Serum Increase Physiological* In 14 patients with chronic renal failure undergoing regular hemodialysis treatment with 0.5 μg/d for 8 weeks caused significant increase from mean baseline of 7.2 ± 1.2 pg/mL to 25 ± 3.5 pg/mL *2457*

Parathyroid Hormone *Plasma Decrease Physiological* Mean concentration in 14 patients with chronic renal failure undergoing regular hemodialysis decreased significantly from mean baseline of 325 ± 44 pg/mL to 271 ± 44 pg/mL after treatment with 0.5 μg/d for 8 weeks *2457*

Phosphate *Serum Decrease Physiological* In 14 patients with chronic renal failure undergoing regular hemodialysis mean concentration decreased significantly from 6.0 ± 0.3 mg/dL to 5.8 ± 0.3 mg/dL after 8 weeks treatment with 0.5 μg/d *2457*

Soluble Tumor Necrosis Factor Receptor-A

Serum Decrease Physiological In 14 patients with chronic renal failure undergoing regular hemodialysis treatment with 0.5 μg/d for 8 weeks caused a significant reduction in concentration from mean baseline of 25 ± 2 ng/mL to 20 ± 2 ng/mL *2457*

Soluble Tumor Necrosis Factor Receptor-B

Serum No Effect Physiological In 14 patients with chronic renal failure undergoing regular hemodialysis treatment with 0.5 μg/d for 8 weeks caused nonsignificant change from mean baseline of 22 ± 1 ng/mL to 24 ± 1 ng/mL *2457*

Tumor Necrosis Factor-α *Serum No Effect Physiological* Mean concentration of 0.5 ± 0.2 ng/mL in 14 patients with chronic renal failure undergoing regular hemodialysis treatment with 0.5 μg/d for 8 weeks caused nonsignificant decrease from mean baseline of 0.9 ± 0.2 ng/mL *2457*

25-Hydroxy-Vitamin D_3

Vitamin D Binding Globulin *Serum No Effect Analytical* No significant effect observed when added in 1000-fold excess with method on Behring nephelometer *2509*

25-Hydroxy-Vitamin D

1,25-Dihydroxy Vitamin D_3 *Serum Increase Physiological* In 5 patients with hypomagnesemic hypocalcemia circulating concentration rose within 48 hours to normal when patients treated orally *1995*

25-Hydroxy Vitamin D_3 *Serum Increase Physiological* Expected increase observed in 5 patients with hypomagnesemic hypocalcemia when treated with oral replacement compound *1995*

Magnesium *Serum Increase Physiological* In patients with hypomagnesemic hypocalcemia oral administration caused reversion towards normal concentration *1995*

Parathyroid Hormone *Plasma Increase Physiological* Oral administration to 5 patients with hypomagnesemic hypocalcemia caused increase *1995*

Hydroxyacetamide

Alanine Aminotransferase *Serum Increase Physiological* Toxicity effect *3810*

Alkaline Phosphatase *Serum Increase Physiological* Hepatotoxicity *1714*

Aspartate Aminotransferase *Serum Increase Physiological* Toxicity effect *3810*

Bile *Urine Increase Physiological* Hepatotoxicity *3810*

Bilirubin *Serum Increase Physiological* Hepatotoxicity *3810*

BSP Retention *Serum Increase Physiological* Hepatotoxicity *3810*

4-Hydroxyacetanilide

5-Hydroxyindoleacetic Acid *Urine No Effect Analytical* No effect with 10 mg/dL on method of Goldenberg *2220*

4-Hydroxyandrostenedione

Estrogens *Plasma Decrease Physiological* In postmenopausal women with breast cancer treatment with doses from 250 mg per 2 weeks to 500 mg/wk caused significant reduction *736*

Insulin-like Growth Factor-I *Serum Increase Physiological* In 17 women with breast cancer treatment with 500 mg intramuscularly every two weeks caused a significant change from median baseline concentration of 176.0 ng/mL to 182.9 ng/mL after 1 month and 194.9 ng/mL after 3 months *1846*

Serum No Effect Physiological In 16 women with breast cancer treatment with 250 mg intramuscularly every two weeks caused no significant change from median baseline concentration of 170.2 ng/mL to 157.7 ng/mL after 1 month and 155.5 ng/mL after 3 months *1846*

2-Hydroxybutyrate

β-Hydroxybutyrate *Urine No Effect Analytical* At concentrations of 100-200 mmol/L did not affect enzymatic procedure of GDS Diagnostics *1824*

Hydroxychloroquine

Cholesterol *Serum Decrease Physiological* Significant reduction in mean concentration to 181 mg/dL in 58 women with SLE or rheumatoid arthritis treated with mean dose of 386 mg/d for at least 3 months compared with 205 mg/dL in 44 untreated control women *6318*

Chondrex *Serum No Effect Analytical* Concentrations up to 5 g/L had no significant effect on sandwich-type ELISA procedure of Harvey et al *2491*

Digoxin *Serum Decrease Physiological* Observed effect *1384*

Serum Increase Physiological Significant increase observed in two patients when drugs coadministered, possibly due to effect on absorption or renal and nonrenal clearance *3460*

Erythrocyte Sedimentation Rate
Blood Decrease Physiological In 35 patients with rheumatoid arthritis treatment with 1000 mg/d sulfasalazine and 400 mg/d hydroxychloroquine caused significant reduction from mean baseline of 45 ± 27 mm/h to 36 ± 29 mm/h after 9 mo and 16 ± 12 mm/h after 24 h *4361*

Erythrocytes *Blood Decrease Physiological* Anemia *3810*

HDL-Cholesterol *Serum Increase Physiological* Mean concentration of 59 mg/dL in 58 women patients with SLE or rheumatoid arthritis treated with mean dose of 386 mg/d for 3 months compared with 54 mg/dL in 44 controls *6318*

Hemoglobin *Blood Decrease Physiological* Hemolytic anemia may develop in patients with glucose-6-phosphate deficiency *1384*

LDL-Cholesterol *Serum Decrease Physiological* Mean concentration of 101 mg/dL in 58 women with SLE or rheumatoid arthritis when treated with mean dose of 386 mg/d for 3 months compared with mean concentration of 128 mg/dL in 44 controls *6318*

Leukocytes *Blood Decrease Physiological* Leukopenia *3810*

Neutrophils *Blood Decrease Physiological* Occasional case of agranulocytosis reported *6264*

Platelet Aggregation *Blood Increase Physiological* Significant interference with platelet aggregation reported *6557*

Platelets *Blood Decrease Physiological* Thrombocytopenia *4803*

Porphyrin, Total *Urine Increase Physiological* Acute intermittent porphyria may rarely occur *1384*

Testosterone *Serum No Effect Physiological* In a group of male patients with rheumatoid arthritis taking hydroxychloroquine mean concentration not significantly different from concentration in untreated male patients *3808*

Triglycerides *Serum Decrease Physiological* Mean concentration of 106 mg/dL in 58 women with SLE or rheumatoid arthritis treated with mean dose of 386 mg/d for 3 months compared with 129 mg/dL in 44 untreated control patients *6318*

Hydroxydione

Glucose *Serum Increase Physiological* Significant increase 1 h after anesthesia *483*

Hydroxyethyltheophylline

Theophylline *Serum No Effect Analytical* No effect at 20 mg/L of β-hydroxyethyltheophylline on method on Ames Seralyzer *5706*

Hydroxyhexamide

Glucose *Serum Decrease Physiological* Mild effect (stimulates release of insulin) *6622*

Uric Acid *Serum Decrease Physiological* Mild uricosuric action *6622*

Urine Increase Physiological Mild uricosuric action *6622*

2-Hydroxyisobutyric Acid

β-Hydroxybutyrate *Urine No Effect Analytical* At concentration of 100-200 mmol/L did not affect enzymatic procedure of GDS Diagnostics *1824*

Hydroxymethadone

Methadone *Urine No Effect Analytical* Significant cross-reactivity of 60% observed with Roche Abuscreen ONTRAK method *3279*

Hydroxymethotrexate

Methotrexate *Serum No Effect Analytical* No significant interference from 7-hydroxymethotrexate at a concentration of 3 µmol/L with method on Du Pont aca *1535*

Hydroxyphenobarbital

Cannabinoids *Urine No Effect Analytical* No effect on Roche Abuscreen method *5006*

Phenobarbital *Serum No Effect Analytical* At maximum physiological or pharmacological concentrations no cross-reactivity observed with phenobarbital method on Bayer Technicon Immuno 1® *427* Cross-reactivity of p-hydroxyphenobarbital less than 0.5% observed with CEDIA phenobarbital assay adapted for use with Hitachi 704 *2924*

4-Hydroxyphenylacetic Acid

5-Hydroxyindoleacetic Acid *Urine No Effect Analytical* No effect with 10 mg/dL on method of Goldenberg *2220*

17-Hydroxyprogesterone

Progesterone *Plasma No Effect Analytical* 17-hydroxyprogesterone at a concentration of up to 1000 ng/mL had a cross-reactivity of only 1.3% in progesterone method on Bayer Technicon Immuno 1® *429* Cross-reactivity of 0.9% observed with method on Ciba Corning ACS:180 *1113* No significant cross-reactivity observed with method on Organon Teknika AuraFlex random access immunoassay analyzer *3520*

Hydroxypropylmethylcellulose

Glucose *Serum Decrease Physiological* Administration of 10 g high viscosity hydroxypropylmethylcellulose to patients with NIDDM caused maximum reduction of 24% over 150 minutes following its administration *4918*

Insulin *Plasma Decrease Physiological* Following administration of 10 g to patients with NIDDM significant reduction observed at 120 minutes compared with controls *4918*

3-Hydroxyquinidine

Quinidine *Serum No Effect Analytical* No significant interference observed at a concentration of 5 µg/mL (14.6 µmol/L) with method on Du Pont aca *1543*

Hydroxyquinoline

Angiotensin-converting Enzyme
Serum Decrease Analytical 100% inhibition with method using benzyloxycarbonyl-phenylalanyl-histidyl-leucine as substrate with 8 hydroxyquinolone *5409*

5-Hydroxytryptophan

Protein *Cerebrospinal Fluid Increase Analytical* 1.0 mg = 3.9 mg in Folin-Ciocalteu procedure *882*

Hydroxyurea

Bilirubin *Serum Decrease Physiological* Reduction in 3 patients with sickle cell anemia from 27 to 17 µmol/L, 60 to 36 µmol/L and 43 to 23 µmol/L respectively when treated with hydroxyurea for 3-5 months *2214*

BSP Retention *Serum Increase Physiological* Abnormal retention reported *2754*

Cholinesterase *Serum No Effect Analytical* No effect observed at concentration of 1 µg/mL with butyrylthiocholine method on Kodak Ektachem® *2504*

Creatinine *Serum Increase Physiological* ?related to impaired tubular function *2754*

Erythrocyte Survival *Blood Increase Physiological* Half-life of cells labeled with radioactive chromium increased in 3 patients with sickle cell anemia from 9 to 17 days, 6 to 12 days, and 10 to 14 days respectively following treatment for 3-5 months with hydroxyurea *2214*
Blood No Effect Physiological Although reduces rate of iron utilization *2754*

Erythrocytes *Blood Decrease Physiological* Anemia (may be transient megaloblastic) *128*

Erythropoietin *Serum Increase Physiological* Nonsignificant increase in 3 patients with sickle cell anemia when treated with hydroxyurea for 3-5 months *2214*

F Reticulocytes *Blood Increase Physiological* Significant increase in 3 patients with sickle cell anemia when treated with hydroxyurea for 3-5 months (from 13.0 to 39.4%, 10.9 to 32.1%, and 1.3 to 32.1%) *2214*

Hemoglobin *Blood Decrease Physiological* Decreases of from 0.5 to 6.0 g/dL common *4264*
Blood Increase Physiological In 14 thalassemic patients treatment for 20 - 35 weeks caused significant increase from mean baseline of 9.0 ± 1.2 g/dL to 9.0 ± 1.1 g/dL *6279* Significant increase observed in 3 patients with sickle cell anemia following treatment with hydroxyurea for 3 to 5 months *2214*

Hemoglobin F *Blood Increase Physiological* In 10 hospitalized patients with sickle cell disease treatment for 3 months caused 2- to 10-fold increase in fetal hemoglobin from mean of 1.6 ± 1.6% of total hemoglobin to 6.8 ± 4.7%, with 3 patients having concentrations of 10 to 15% of toal hemoglobin although 3 patients did not respond to hydroxyurea *5044* Significant increases in 3 patients with sickle cell anemia when treated with hydroxyurea for 3-5 months (from 8.5 to 19.5%, 6.7 to 17.0%, and 0.7 to 11.0%) *2214* In 14 thalassemic patients treatment for 20 - 35 weeks caused significant increase from mean baseline of 3.6 ± 2.1% (3.0 ± 2.0 g/dL) to 22.9 ± 7.7% (21.1 ± 7.4 g/dL) *6279*

Irreversibly Sickled Erythrocytes
Blood Decrease Physiological In 3 patients with sickle cell anemia reduction from 8.1 to 4.3%, 4.4 to 1.6%, and 15.0 to 3.6% respectively following treatment with hydroxyurea for 3-5 months *2214*

Lactate Dehydrogenase *Serum Decrease Physiological* Significant reductions observed in 3 patients with sickle cell anemia from 490 to 313 U/L, 673 to 456 U/L, and 707 to 490 U/L respectively following 3-5 months treatment with hydroxyurea *2214*

Leukocytes *Blood Decrease Physiological* Leukopenia may occur *4014*

Lipase *Serum Decrease Analytical* At concentrations above 300 mg/L causes decreased result as determined by method on Kodak Ektachem® *5706*

MCHC *Blood Increase Physiological* In 14 thalassemic patients treatment for 20 - 35 weeks caused nonsignificant increase from mean baseline of 30.8 ± 0.9% to 31.8 ± 1.0% *6279*

MCV *Blood Increase Physiological* In 14 thalassemic patients treatment for 20 - 35 weeks caused significant increase from mean baseline of 71.9 ± 5.7 fL to 95.0 ± 14.1 fL *6279* Significant increase in 3 patients with sickle cell anemia treated with hydroxyurea for 3-5 months *2214*

Neutrophils *Blood Decrease Physiological* May cause agranulocytosis *4265* Significant reduction in 2 of 3 patients with sickle cell anemia, and nonsignificant reduction in the third, when examined 3-5 months following treatment with hydroxyurea *2214*

Platelets *Blood Decrease Physiological* Significant reduction in one and nonsignificant reduction in two patients with sickle cell anemia when treated with hydroxyurea for 3-5 months *2214* In 56 patients treated with hydroxyurea for 6 months mean count decreased from 870000 /µL to 500000 µL compared with continued increase in untreated patients *1141* Thrombocytopenia *128*

Reticulocytes *Blood Decrease Physiological* Significant reduction observed in 3 patients with sickle cell anemia treated with hydroxyurea for 3-5 months *2214*

Triglycerides *Serum Decrease Analytical* Inhibits action of glycerol oxidase included as part of Technicon RA-1000 method but no effect on procedure used on Beckman Astra® 8 *3922*

Urea Nitrogen *Serum Increase Physiological* ?related to impaired tubular function *2754* Probably associated with tissue destruction *4264*

Uric Acid *Serum Increase Physiological* Probable effect of cell catabolism *2451*

3-Hydroxyvalproic Acid

Valproic Acid *Serum Increase Analytical* Cross-reactivity of 3.8% observed with competitive immunoassay used with PB Diagnostics OPUS analyzer *41*
Serum No Effect Analytical No significant interference observed at a concentration of 100 µg/mL (620 µmol/L) with method on Du Pont aca *1560* No significant interference observed at a concentration of 100 µ.g/mL (620 µmol/L) with method on Du Pont aca *1560*

4-Hydroxyvalproic Acid

Valproic Acid *Serum Increase Analytical* Cross-reactivity of 8% observed with competitive immunoassay used with PB Diagnostics OPUS analyzer *41*
Serum No Effect Analytical No significant interference observed at a concentration of 100 µg/mL (620 µmol/L) with method on Du Pont aca *1560*

5-Hydroxyvalproic Acid

Valproic Acid *Serum Increase Analytical* Cross-reactivity of 50% observed with competitive immunoassay used with PB Diagnostics OPUS analyzer *41*
Serum No Effect Analytical No significant interference observed at a concentration of 100 µg/mL (620 µmol/L) with method on Du Pont aca *1560*

Hydroxyzine

Albumin *Urine No Effect Analytical* Using a fluorimetric assay with Albumin Blue 580 on a Cobas Fara centrifugal analyzer for the detection of microalbuminuria no significant interference was detected at a concentration of 20 mg/L *3117*

Carbon Dioxide Partial Pressure
Blood No Effect Physiological In 13 patient volunteers with COPD (mean age 63.4 years) infusion of 1.5 mg/kg intravenously caused no increase for up to 60 minutes post-infusion *6683*

Cholinesterase *Serum No Effect Analytical* No effect observed at concentration of 500 mg/dL with butyrylthiocholine method on Kodak Ektachem® *2504*

17-Hydroxycorticosteroids *Urine Increase Analytical* Interferes with Porter-Silber reaction *4012*

17-Ketogenic Steroids *Urine Increase Analytical* Interferes with Zimmermann reaction *4245*

Oxygen Partial Pressure *Blood No Effect Physiological* In 13 patient volunteers with COPD at concentration of 1.5 mg/kg intravenously no significant decrease observed for up to 60 minutes post-infusion *6683*

pH *Blood No Effect Physiological* After infusion of 1.5 mg/kg intravenously in 13 patient volunteers with COPD (mean age 63.4 years) no significant decrease observed over 60 minutes after infusion *6683*

Prothrombin Time *Plasma Increase Physiological* Prolongs action of anticoagulants *6515*
Plasma No Effect Physiological Reported to have no effect *2452*

Hyoscine-N-Butylbromide

Cholesterol *Serum No Effect Analytical* At concentration of 300 mg/L had no effect on CHOD-PAP method *5704* At concentration of 300 mg/L had no effect on Liebermann-Burchard method *5704* At concentration of 300 mg/L had no effect on catalase-AIDH method *5704* At concentration of 300 mg/L had no effect on method using catalase-Hantzsch reaction method *5704* At concentration of 300 mg/L had no effect on CHOD-Iodide method *5704*

Creatinine *Serum No Effect Analytical* At concentration of 12 mg/L had no effect on Jaffe-Fuller's earth method *5704* At concentration of 12 mg/L had no effect on Jaffe-Fading-Fraction method *5704*

Glucose *Serum No Effect Analytical* At concentration of 2 mg/L had no effect on Kodak Ektachem® method *5704*

Potassium *Serum No Effect Analytical* At concentration of 20 mg/L had no effect on measurement by ISE without predilution *5704*

Protein Electrophoresis *Serum No Effect Analytical* At concentration of 20 mg/L had no effect on automated Olympus-Hite method *5704*

Sodium *Serum Decrease Analytical* At concentrations above 20 mg/L lowered concentration as measured by ISE without predilution *5704*

Urea Nitrogen *Serum No Effect Analytical* At concentration of 2 mg/L had no effect on Kodak Ektachem® method *5704*

Uric Acid *Serum No Effect Analytical* At concentration of 60 mg/L had no effect on Kageyama-Hantzsch method *5704* At concentration of 12 mg/L had no effect on catalase-AIDH method *5704*

Ibandronate

Albumin *Serum No Effect Physiological* In 6 patients with various malignant diseases treatment with ibandronate 0.5 to 2 mg intravenously for 2 h caused nonsignificant change from mean baseline of 40.0 ± 2.8 g/L to 42.2 ± 2.2 g/L when measured after 24 h and 41.6 ± 2.5 g/L at 48 h *5294*

Calcium, Albumin-corrected *Serum No Effect Physiological* In 6 patients with various malignant diseases treatment with ibandronate 0.5 to 2 mg intravenously for 2 h caused nonsignificant change from mean baseline of 2.33 ± 0.10 mmol/L to 2.32 ± 0.07 mmol/L when measured after 48 h *5294*

C-terminal Telopeptides of Type I Collagen Degradation Products *Serum Decrease Physiological* In 180 healthy postmenopausal women at least 10 years postmenopause those receiving either 0.25 mg/d to 5 mg/d showed decreases in concentration of 60 - 80% after 3 months treatment which was sustained with continuing treatment *1008*
Urine Decrease Physiological In 180 healthy postmenopausal women at least 10 years postmenopause those receiving either 0.25 mg/d to 5 mg/d showed decreases in concentration of 40 - 80% after 3 months treatment which was sustained with continuing treatment *1008*

Interleukin-6 *Serum No Effect Physiological* In 6 patients with various malignant diseases treatment with ibandronate 60 mg intravenously for 4 h caused nonsignificant change from mean baseline in 5 of 6 patients *5294*

Leukocytes *Blood No Effect Physiological* In 6 patients with various malignant diseases treatment with ibandronate 0.5 to 2 mg intravenously for 2 h caused nonsignificant change from mean baseline of 6,003 ± 910 /µL to 6,260 ± 739 /µL when measured after 24 h and 6,272 ± 1035 /µL at 48 h *5294*

Lymphocytes *Blood No Effect Physiological* In 6 patients with various malignant diseases treatment with ibandronate 0.5 to 2 mg intravenously for 2 h caused nonsignificant change from mean baseline of 1016 ± 161 /µL to 1203 ± 135 /µL when measured after 24 h and 982 ± 195 /µL at 48 h *5294*

Monocytes *Blood No Effect Physiological* In 6 patients with various malignant diseases treatment with ibandronate 0.5 to 2 mg intravenously for 2 h caused nonsignificant change from mean baseline of 259 ± 48 /µL to 265 ± 104 /µL when measured after 24 h and 250 ± 66 /µL at 48 h *5294*

Platelets *Blood No Effect Physiological* In 6 patients with various malignant diseases treatment with ibandronate 0.5 to 2 mg intravenously for 2 h caused nonsignificant change from mean baseline of 223,000 ± 37,000 /µL to 226,000 ± 40,000 /µL when measured after 24 h and 219,000 ± 35,000 /µL at 48 h *5294*

Ibopamine

Aldosterone *Plasma Decrease Physiological* Oral administration of 100 mg significantly inhibited aldosterone secretion in 8 of 13 men with chronic heart failure 30 minutes after administration *4069*
Plasma No Effect Physiological In 10 healthy volunteers administration of 100 mg had no significant effect on concentration *2132* No significant effect observed in 10 patients with severe congestive heart failure following a single oral dose of 100 mg *2133*

Creatinine Clearance *Urine Increase Physiological* Reported to increase clearance in normal man without effect on heart rate and blood pressure *2133*
Urine No Effect Physiological Reportedly no effect observed in normal man *2133*

Dopamine *Plasma No Effect Physiological* In 10 healthy volunteers administration of 100 mg had no significant effect on concentration *2132*
Urine No Effect Physiological Administration of 100 mg to 10 healthy volunteers had no significant effect on excretion *2132*

Effective Renal Plasma Flow
Patient Increase Physiological In 10 patients with severe congestive heart failure administration of 100 mg ibopamine caused mean increase of 11% after 2 hours *2133*
Patient No Effect Physiological In 10 healthy volunteers administration of 100 mg had no significant effect on ERPF *2132*

Epinephrine *Plasma Decrease Physiological* Effect observed with long-term treatment due to presynaptic DA_2 effect *2846*
Plasma No Effect Physiological Administration of 100 mg had no significant effect in 10 healthy volunteers *2132*
Urine No Effect Physiological Administration of 100 mg to 10 healthy volunteers had no significant effect on excretion *2132*

Glomerular Filtration Rate *Urine Increase Physiological* In 10 patients with severe congestive heart failure after administration of 100 mg ibopamine increase of 15% observed after 3 hours *2133* In 10 healthy volunteers administration of 100 mg caused significant increase to 109 - 134 mL/min/1.73 sq m one hour later compared with mean baseline of 99 - 124 mL/min/sq m *2132*

Glucagon *Plasma No Effect Physiological* 300 mg drug had no effect over period of 90 minutes *5712*

Glucose *Serum Increase Physiological* Peaked after 45 minutes in all subjects: normalized in 90 minutes *5712*

Insulin *Plasma Increase Physiological* Peaked after 45 minutes in all subjects: normalized in 90 minutes *5712*

Norepinephrine *Plasma Decrease Physiological* Single oral dose decreases concentration due to presynaptic DA_2 effect *2846* Single oral dose decreases concentration due to presynaptic DA2 effect *2846* Increased concentration observed in patients with congestive heart failure reduced by administration of drug possibly due to stimulation of DA2-receptor and α_2-receptor or improved hemodynamics *2133*
Plasma No Effect Physiological No significant change observed in 6 patients with severe congestive heart failure following a single oral dose of 100 mg *2133* In 10 healthy volunteers administration of 100 mg had no significant effect on concentration *2132*
Urine No Effect Physiological Administration of 100 mg to 10 healthy volunteers had no effect on excretion *2132*

Potassium *Urine No Effect Physiological* No significant change observed in 10 patients with severe congestive heart failure treated with 100 mg ibopamine *2133* In 10 healthy volunteers administration of 100 mg caused no significant change in excretion *2132*

Prolactin *Plasma No Effect Physiological* 300 mg drug had no effect over period of 90 minutes *5712*

Renin Activity *Plasma Decrease Physiological* Nonsignificant reduction at 60 minutes from mean baseline of 3.08 ng/mL/h to 2.46 ng/mL/h in 13 men with chronic cardiac failure following oral dose of 100 mg *4069* Observed after a single oral dose due to presynaptic DA_2 effect *2846* Single oral dose of drug can decrease activity *2846*
Plasma No Effect Physiological In 10 healthy volunteers administration of 100 mg had no significant effect on activity *2132* No significant effect observed after 100 mg ibopamine in 10 patients with severe congestive heart failure *2133*

Sodium *Urine Increase Physiological* In 10 healthy volunteers administration of 100 mg caused significant increase over next 4 hours *2132* Reported to increase urinary excretion in normal man without changes in heart rate and blood pressure *2133*
Urine No Effect Physiological Reportedly no effect observed in normal man *2133* No significant change observed in 10 patients with severe congestive heart failure following administration of 100 mg ibopamine except after 4 hours *2133*

Ibufenac

Alanine Aminotransferase *Serum Increase Physiological* Hepatotoxic effect *3810*

Alkaline Phosphatase *Serum Increase Physiological* Hepatotoxic effect *3810*

Aspartate Aminotransferase *Serum Increase Physiological* Hepatotoxic effect *3810*

Bile *Urine Increase Physiological* Hepatotoxic effect *3810*

Bilirubin *Serum Increase Physiological* Probable effect as bilirubin clearance reduced *2466*

BSP Retention *Serum Increase Physiological* Hepatotoxic effect *3810*

Glucose *Urine Increase Physiological* Augmentation of diabetic glycosuria seen *4014*

Occult Blood *Feces Increase Physiological* May cause gastrointestinal tract bleeding *3810*

Platelet Aggregation *Blood Decrease Physiological* Observed *in vitro*, may cause gastrointestinal bleeding etc *915*

Uric Acid *Serum Increase Physiological* Side effect similar to that of aspirin *3810*

Ibuprofen

Alanine Aminotransferase *Serum Decrease Analytical* On colorimetric method at 10 times maximal therapeutic concentration *2919*
Serum Increase Physiological Incidence of acute liver injury of 1.6 per 100,000 treated patients with reported in United Kingdom. Liver damage among all cases primarily hepatocellular in some and primarily cholestatic in others *5049* Rare hepatotoxicity reported: associated in one case with Stevens-Johnson syndrome *5814* Borderline increased activity of one or more liver enzymes increased in 15% of treated patients. Increases of more than 3 times the upper limit of normal occurred in less than 1% patients *3913* Hepatorenal syndrome, liver necrosis, liver failure, hepatitis, jaundice or abnormal liver function observed in less than 1% patients *3913* As with NSAIDs borderline increases of liver enzymes occur in up to 15% patients. Increases above 3 times the upper limit of normal occurred in less than 1% of patients *3200* Occasional hypersensitivity reaction observed, especially in women *1384*
Serum No Effect Analytical On continuous method at 10 times maximal therapeutic concentration *2919* At 5 times upper limit of therapeutic range on methods on Technicon SMAC® , Abbott-VP, Du Pont aca, Roche Cobas-Bio and KDA *3525*

Albumin *Serum Decrease Physiological* Significantly lower in patients receiving drug than in controls (4.0 g/dL vs 4.2 g/dL); same effect noted before and after treatment started *2922*
Serum No Effect Analytical At concentration of 200 mg/L had no effect on Kodak Ektachem® method *5706* At 5 times upper limit of therapeutic range on methods on Technicon SMAC® , Kodak Ektachem® , Hitachi® 705 and KDA *3525* At concentration of 200 mg/L had no effect on BCG method *5704* On bromocresol green method on Technicon SMA II at physiological concentrations *2922*
Urine Decrease Physiological 400 mg t.i.d. administered to 20 volunteers caused decrease from mean baseline excretion of 10.35 µg/min to 5.43 µg/min after 3 days treatment and a further reduction when sulfasalazine coadministered *2259*

Alkaline Phosphatase *Serum Increase Analytical* At 5 times upper limit of therapeutic range on method on Technicon SMAC® *3525*
Serum Increase Physiological Rare case of hepatotoxicity: in one case associated with Stevens-Johnson syndrome *5814* Hepatorenal syndrome, liver necrosis, liver failure, hepatitis, jaundice or abnormal liver function observed in less than 1% patients *3913* Minimal increase observed occasionally, most often in women, as part of a hypersensitivity reaction *1384* Borderline increased activity of one or more liver enzymes increased in 15% of treated patients *3913*
Serum No Effect Analytical On continuous method at 10 times maximal therapeutic concentrations *2919* At 5 times upper limit of therapeutic range on methods on Abbott-VP, Du Pont aca, Roche Cobas-Bio, Hitachi® 705 and KDA *3525*

Alkaline Phosphatase, Bone Isoenzyme
Serum No Effect Analytical At a concentration of 400 mg/L had no effect on Tandem-MP Ostase method *777* At a concentration of 150 mg/L had no effect on EIA method of Gomez et al *2234*

Amphetamine *Urine No Effect Analytical* Improbable interference reported with Syva EMIT procedure *6469*

Amylase *Serum Increase Physiological* Pancreatitis observed in less than 1% patients *3913*

Ibuprofen *(continued)*

Amylase *(continued)*
Serum No Effect Analytical At 5 times upper limit of therapeutic range on methods on Du Pont aca, Kodak Ektachem® and Hitachi® 705 *3525*

Aspartate Aminotransferase *Serum Decrease Analytical* On continuous method at 10 times maximal therapeutic concentrations *2919*
Serum Increase Physiological Borderline increased activity of one or more liver enzymes increased in 15% of treated patients. Increases of more than 3 times the upper limit of normal occurred in less than 1% patients *3913* Incidence of acute liver injury of 1.6 per 100,000 treated patients with reported in United Kingdom. Liver damage among all cases primarily hepatocellular in some and primarily cholestatic in others *5049* As with NSAIDs borderline increases of liver enzymes occur in up to 15% patients. Increases above the upper limit of normal occurred in less than 1% patients *3200* Rare hepatotoxicity reported: associated in one case with Stevens-Johnson syndrome *5814* Occasional hypersnsitivity reaction observed, especially in women *1384*
Serum No Effect Analytical At 5 times upper limit of therapeutic range on methods on Technicon SMAC®, Abbott-VP, Du Pont aca, Roche Cobas-Bio, Hitachi® 705 and KDA *3525* On colorimetric method at 10 times maximal therapeutic concentrations *2919*

Barbiturate *Urine Increase Analytical* Probable false positive result obtained in one urine from a patient who had ingested chronic doses of ibuprofen when measured by Abbott TDx. Positive result not confirmed by GC/MS *5070*
Urine No Effect Analytical Improbable interference with Syva EMIT assay reported *6469*

Benzodiazepine *Urine No Effect Analytical* No false positive observed in 2 patients ingesting ibuprofen chronically as measured by Syva EMIT and Abbott TDx methods *5070* No significant interference observed in urines of people taking ibuprofen with new Syva EMIT assay *3370* Improbable interference reported with Syva EMIT procedure *6469*
Urine Positive Analytical . At concentration occurring in urine following ingestion positive result obtained with Abbott TDx procedure *3420*

Bilirubin *Serum Increase Physiological* Rare hepatotoxicity reported: associated in one case with Stevens-Johnson syndrome *5814* As with NSAIDs borderline increases of liver enzymes occur in up to 15% patients. Increases above the upper limit of normal occurred in less than 1% patients. Severe hepatic reactions, including jaundice and cases of fatal hepatitis, have been reported *3200* Hepatorenal syndrome, liver necrosis, liver failure, hepatitis, jaundice or abnormal liver function observed in less than 1% patients *3913* Minimal increase observed as part of a hypersensitivity reaction, most often in women *1384*
Serum No Effect Analytical On diazo method on Technicon SMA II at physiological concentration *2922* At concentration of 200 mg/L had no effect on Jendrassik and Grof method *5704* At 5 times upper limit of therapeutic range on methods on Technicon SMAC®, Du Pont aca, Roche Cobas-Bio, Kodak Ektachem®, Hitachi® 705 and KDA *3525* No effect at therapeutic concentrations on Jendrassik-Grof,dimethylsulfoxide and spectrophotometric methods *2920*
Serum No Effect Physiological No effect seen in patients undergoing treatment *2922* At pharmacological concentrations has little or no protein displacement effect *6314*

Bilirubin, Conjugated *Serum No Effect Analytical* At concentration of 200 mg/L had no effect on method on Kodak Ektachem® *5706*

Bilirubin, Direct *Serum Increase Physiological* Rare hepatotoxicity reported; associated in one case with Stevens-Johnson syndrome *5814*

Bilirubin, Unconjugated *Serum No Effect Analytical* At concentration of 200 mg/L had no effect on method on Kodak Ektachem® *5706*

Blood *Urine Increase Physiological* Occasional reports in humans of interstitial nephritis with hematuria, proteinuria and even nephrotic syndrome *3200*

Calcium *Serum No Effect Analytical* At concentration of 200 mg/L had no effect on cresolphthalein method *5704* On cresolphthalein complexone method on Technicon SMA II at physiological concentration *2922* At 5 times upper limit of therapeutic range on methods on Technicon SMAC®, Abbott-VP, Du Pont aca, Kodak Ektachem®, Hitachi® 705 and KDA *3525*
Serum No Effect Physiological No effect seen in patients undergoing treatment *2922*

Cannabinoids *Urine No Effect Analytical* Improbable interference with Syva EMIT procedure reported *6469*
Urine Positive Analytical Probable false positive screen obtained with Roche Abuscreen and Abbott TDx assay in patients taking ibuprofen chronically. Positives not confirmed by GC/MS *5070*

Catecholamines *Plasma No Effect Analytical* No effect on HPLC method of Koller for dopamine, epinephrine, and norepinephrine *3230*

Cholesterol *Serum Increase Physiological* Significantly higher in patients receiving drug than in controls (5.26 mmol/L vs 4.60 mmol/L) *2922*
Serum No Effect Analytical No effect at therapeutic concentrations on Liebermann-Burchard and enzymatic methods *2920* At concentration of 200 mg/L had no effect on CHOD-PAP method *5704* At 5 times upper limit of therapeutic range on methods on Technicon SMAC®, Abbott-VP, Roche Cobas-Bio, Kodak Ektachem®, Hitachi® 705 and KDA *3525* On enzymatic method on Technicon SMA II at physiological concentration *2922*

Cholinesterase *Serum No Effect Analytical* No effect observed at concentration of 20 mg/dL with butyrylthiocholine method on Kodak Ektachem® *2504*

Chondrex *Serum No Effect Analytical* Concentrations up to 10 g/L had no significant effect on sandwich-type ELISA procedure of Harvey et al *2491*

Color *Urine Increase Analytical* Pink, red, purple and rust color *2024*

Coombs' Test *Blood Positive Physiological* Hemolytic anemia, sometimes Coombs' positive, observed in less than 1% patients *3913* Coombs' positive hemolytic anemia observed as a complication of treatment is less than 1% treated cases *3200*

Creatine Kinase *Serum No Effect Analytical* On continuous method at 10 times maximal therapeutic concentrations *2919* At 5 times upper limit of therapeutic range on methods on Technicon SMAC®, Abbott-VP, Roche Cobas-Bio, Du Pont aca, and Hitachi® 705 *3525*

Creatinine *Serum Decrease Physiological* Significant reduction in patients receiving medication *2922*
Serum Increase Physiological Acute renal failure may occur in patients with pre-existing impaired renal function may result in decreased creatinine clearance, polyuria, azotemia, cystitis and hematuria *3200* In 2 patients with systemic lupus erythematosus *1904* Increase by 40% in patients with chronic glomerular disease *1018* In one study a decrease of hemoglobin concentration was observed with positive occult blood tests and increased serum creatinine concentration *3913*
Serum No Effect Analytical On alkaline picrate method on Technicon SMA II at physiological concentrations *2922* No effect at therapeutic concentrations on alkaline picrate and Slot methods *2920* At concentration of 200 mg/L had no effect on Technicon AutoAnalyzer® method *5704* No effect of concentrations up to 200 mg/L on 2-slide method on Kodak Ektachem® *5706* At 5 times upper limit of therapeutic range on methods on Technicon SMAC®, Abbott-VP, Du Pont aca, Roche Cobas-Bio, Kodak Ektachem®, Hitachi® 705 and KDA *3525*
Serum No Effect Physiological No effect during coadministration with digoxin *4825*

Creatinine Clearance *Urine Decrease Physiological* Acute renal failure may occur in patients with pre-existing impaired renal function may result in decreased creatinine clearance, polyuria, azotemia, cystitis and hematuria *3200* Increase by 28% in patients with chronic glomerular disease but no effect in healthy people *1018*
Urine No Effect Physiological No effect observed in 8 healthy volunteers given 800 mg three times daily for 3 days *4549*

Digoxin *Serum Increase Physiological* In one study of 12 patients mean serum concentration increased by 60% after one week's treatment *4822* Significant increase after 7 d treatment with average effect of 59% *4825*

2,3-Dinor-6-Keto-Prostaglandin $F_{1\alpha}$
Urine Decrease Physiological Reduction observed in mildly hypertensive patients when treated for 1 week following two weeks without antihypertensive medications *4065*

2,3-Dinor-Thromboxane B_2 *Urine Decrease Physiological* Reduction observed in mildly hypertensive patients after 7 days therapy following two weeks without antihypertensive medications *4065*

Doxazosin *Serum No Effect Physiological* Coadministration with doxazosin had no effect on its pharmacokinetics *4642*

Drugs of Abuse Screen *Urine Increase Analytical* Following acute dose of ibuprofen probable false positive obtained in one patient with Syva EMIT d.a.u. screen. Positvity not confirmed by GC/MS *5070*
Urine No Effect Analytical No effect at concentration of 100 µg/mL on EZ-SCREEN procedure for cannabinoids and cocaine *1739*

β-Endorphin *Plasma Increase Physiological* In 15 patients undergoing approximately 30 min surgery mean concentration increased from baseline of 4.3 fmol/mL by 2.6 fold 5 minutes after start significantly greater than with placebo *6075*

Eosinophils *Blood Increase Physiological* Eosinophilia observed in less than 1% patients *3913* Eosinophilia observed as a complication of treatment is less than 1% treated cases *3200*

Erythrocytes *Blood Decrease Physiological* In 3% of patients with juvenile rheumatoid arthritis *386*
Urine Increase Physiological In 2 patients with systemic lupus erythematosus *1904*

Felbamate *Serum No Effect Analytical* No significant interference observed with GLC method of Rifai et al *4958*

Fractional Excretion of Potassium
Urine Decrease Physiological In individuals treated with 800 mg three times daily caused 8.5% reduction, 11.5% in elderly and 12.5% in elderly with renal insufficiency *4189*

Fractional Excretion of Sodium
Urine Decrease Physiological In individuals treated with 800 mg three times daily caused 0.5% reduction, 0.7% in elderly and 1.5% in elderly with renal insufficiency *4189*

Glomerular Filtration Rate *Urine No Effect Physiological* At doses up to 800 mg three times daily for 3 days had no effect in 8 healthy volunteers as measured by inulin clearance *4549*

Glucose *Serum No Effect Analytical* On hexokinase method on Technicon SMA II at physiological concentration *2922* No effect at therapeutic concentrations on hexokinase, glucose dehydrogenase ABTS, 2,4-dichlorophenol or o-toluidine methods *2920* At 5 times upper limit of therapeutic range on methods on Technicon SMAC® , Abbott-VP, Du Pont aca, Roche Cobas-Bio, Kodak Ektachem® , Hitachi® 705 and KDA *3525* At concentration of 200 mg/L had no effect on hexokinase/G-6-PDH method *5704*
Serum No Effect Physiological No effect seen in patients undergoing treatment *2922*

γ-Glutamyltransferase *Serum Increase Physiological* Hepatorenal syndrome, liver necrosis, liver failure, hepatitis, jaundice or abnormal liver function observed in less than 1% patients *3913* Rare case of hepatotoxicity: in one case associated with Stevens-Johnson syndrome *5814*
Serum No Effect Analytical At 5 times upper limit of therapeutic range on methods on Technicon SMAC® , Abbott-VP, and Hitachi® 705 *3525*

Granular Casts *Urine Increase Physiological* In 2 patients with systemic lupus erythematosus *1904*

Granulocytes *Blood Decrease Physiological* Agranulocytosis been reported very rarely *1384* Agranulocytosis observed as a complication of treatment is less than 1% treated cases *3200* Agranulocytosis observed in less than 1% patients *3913*

Hematocrit *Blood Decrease Physiological* Slight but probably clinically insignificant decrease reported, sometimes as a result of hemolytic anemia *1384* Aplastic or hemolytic anemia observed in less than 1% patients *3913* In studies with doses of 1200 to 3200 mg/d for several weeks a slight dose-related decrease was observed *3200* Aplastic or hemolytic anemia observed as a complication of treatment is less than 1% treated cases *3200*

Hemoglobin *Blood Decrease Physiological* Slight and probably clinically insignificant decrease observed, sometimes as a result of hemolytic anemia *1384* Slight dose response decrease in hemoglobin/hematocrit observed but even with daily doses of 3200 mg total decrease in hemoglobin is less than 1 g/dL. However, in one study a decrease of 1 g/dL was observed in 17.1% of 193 arthritis patients receiving 1600 mg/d and in 22.8% of 189 patients receiving 2400 mg/d *3913* In studies with doses of 1200 to 3200 mg/d for several weeks a slight dose-related decrease was observed *3200* Aplastic or hemolytic anemia observed as a complication of treatment is less than 1% treated cases *3200*
Urine Increase Physiological In 3% of patients with juvenile rheumatoid arthritis *386*

Histamine *Plasma No Effect Analytical* Improbable inhibition of radio-enzyme assay at physiological concentrations *2492*

Hydroxybutyrate Dehydrogenase
Serum No Effect Analytical On continuous method at 10 times maximal therapeutic concentration *2919*

Iron *Serum No Effect Analytical* On Ferrozine method on Technicon SMA II at physiological concentrations *2922* No effect at therapeutic concentrations on Ramsay and bathophenanthroline methods *2920* At 5 times upper limit of therapeutic range on Ferrozine method on Technicon SMAC® *3525* At concentration of 200 mg/L had no effect on Ferrozine method *5704*
Serum No Effect Physiological No effect seen in patients undergoing treatment *2922*

6-Keto-Prostaglandin $F_{1\alpha}$ *Urine Decrease Physiological* Observed in mildly hypertensive patients after one week treatment following two weeks without antihypertensive medication *4065* Reduced by 80% in patients with chronic glomerular disease and in healthy people *1018*

Ketorolac *Serum No Effect Physiological* At therapeutic concentrations had no effect on ketorolac-protein binding *5035*

Lactate *Blood Increase Physiological* In 224 patients with sepsis and acute failure of at least one organ system treatment with 10 mg/kg given intravenously every 6 hours for 8 doses caused mean decrease of 22% from mean baseline concentration of 3.0 ± 3.0 mmol/L *516*

Lactate Dehydrogenase *Serum Increase Physiological* Rare case of hepatotoxicity: in one case associated with Stevens-Johnson syndrome *5814*
Serum No Effect Analytical On continuous method with lactate or pyruvate as substrate at 10 times maximal therapeutic concentration. On colorimetric method at 10 times maximal therapeutic concentration *2919* At 5 times upper limit of therapeutic range on methods on Technicon SMAC® , Abbott-VP, Roche Cobas-Bio, Hitachi® 705 and KDA *3525*

Leukocytes *Blood Decrease Physiological* In one elderly man associated with a complement-dependent IgG antibody: reversible with cessation of treatment *1769* Rare adverse reactions reported by physicians to UK Committee on Safety of Medicines *1204*
Cerebrospinal Fluid Increase Physiological Few cases of aseptic meningitis described *2102*

Lipase *Serum Increase Physiological* Pancreatitis observed in less than 1% patients *3913*

Lithium *Serum Increase Physiological* Coadministration of ibuprofen with lithium increases its plasma concentration (by 15%) and decreases its renal clearance (by 19%) *3913* In 11 normal volunteers ibuprofen has been shown to reduce the renal clearance of lithium (by 19%) and an increase in its plasma concentration (15%) *3200* Mean concentration increased by 15% when ibuprofen co-administered with increased RBC to plasma ratio *3295* 1800 mg/day increased serum lithium concentration within 6 days of ibuprofen administration in 9 patients by an average of 34% but with marked individual variation ranging from 12-67% *4831*
Serum No Effect Physiological No observed effect on lithium concentration, unlike effects reported after indomethacin and phenylbutazone *1384* Inconsistent change when drug added to therapeutic regime in 3 patients *4832*
Urine Decrease Physiological Total body and renal clearance significantly reduced during co-administration *3295*

Lithium Clearance *Urine Decrease Physiological* Reduction in clearance observed in association with increased serum concentration in 9 patients in whom ibuprofen was administered concomitantly with lithium. Normalized with withdrawal of

Ibuprofen *(continued)*

Lithium Clearance *(continued)*
ibuprofen *4831* Coadministration of ibuprofen with lithium increases its plasma concentration (by 15%) and decreases its renal clearance (by 19%) *3913* In 11 normal volunteers ibuprofen has been shown to reduce the renal clearance of lithium (by 19%) and an increase in its plasma concentration (15%) *3200*

Lymphocytes *Blood Decrease Physiological* Observed in one child with juvenile rheumatoid arthritis when dose of drug increased. At same time altered liver function occurred. Resolved with cessation of treatment *5809* Rare lymphopenia reported *1384*

Metformin *Serum No Effect Physiological* In a single dose study during which ibuprofen and metformin were coadministered ibuprofen appeared to have no effect on the pharmacokinetics of metformin *726*

Neutrophils *Blood Decrease Physiological* Neutropenia observed in less than 1% patients *3913* Neutropenia observed as a complication of treatment is less than 1% treated cases *3200* In one elderly man associated with a complement-dependent IgG antibody: reversible with cessation of treatment *1769* Occasional case of agranulocytosis reported *6264*

Occult Blood *Feces Increase Physiological* May produce gastric irritation and activate ulcer *2671* Occasional case of gastrointestinal bleeding reported but much less frequent than with aspirin *1384* Serious gastrointestinal ulceration and bleeding may occur without warning symptoms *3200* In one study a decrease of hemoglobin concentration was observed with positive occult blood tests. Gastric or duodenal ulcer bleeding with/without gastrointestinal hemorrhage or hematemesis observed in less than 1% patients *3913* Rare adverse reactions reported by physicians to UK Committee on Safety of Medicines *1204*
Feces No Effect Physiological In 6 healthy volunteers treatment with 1200 mg/d for 5 days caused nonsignificant increase from mean baseline of 0.376 ± 0.097 mL/d to 0.894 ± 0.342 mL/d *548*

p-Aminophenol *Urine No Effect Analytical* With addition of drugs at a concentration of 100 mg/L and of related compounds at 50 mg/L no significant effect observed on colorimetric method of van Bocxlaer on Cobas Mira analyzer which involves reacting free p-aminophenol with resorcinol in the presence of magnesium ions to form an indophenol dye measured at 550 nm *6163*

PAH Clearance *Urine Decrease Physiological* Increase by 35% in patients with chronic glomerular disease *1018*

Phosphate *Serum No Effect Analytical* At 5 times upper limit of therapeutic range on methods on Technicon SMAC® , Du Pont aca, Hitachi® 705 and KDA *3525* At concentration of 200 mg/L had no effect on phosphomolybdate method *5704*
Serum No Effect Physiological No effect seen in patients undergoing treatment *2922*

Platelet Aggregation *Blood Decrease Physiological* Administration to healthy women of 3 x 200 mg/d or 3 x 400 mg/d caused 3% and 22% reduction respectively in arachidonic acid induced platelet aggregation compared with controls *5826* Effect less marked that observed with treatment with aspirin *3694* Reported to reversibly inhibit platelet aggregation *3913* Effect is considerably less than aspirin or indomethacin *1384*
Blood Increase Physiological Significant interference with platelet aggregation reported *6557*

Platelets *Blood Decrease Physiological* Thrombocytopenia, with/without purpura, observed in less than 1% patients *3913* Rare adverse reactions reported by physicians to UK Committee on Safety of Medicines *1204* Thrombocytopenia with or without purpura observed as a complication of treatment is less than 1% treated cases *3200*

Potassium *Urine No Effect Physiological* Insignificant increase in 8 healthy volunteers given 800 mg three times daily for 3 days *4549*

Prostaglandin E-M *Urine Decrease Physiological* Administration to healthy women of 3 x 400 mg/d caused a 53% reduction in 24-hour excretion *5826*

Prostaglandins *Urine Decrease Physiological* Reduced by 80% in patients with chronic glomerular disease and in healthy people *1018*

Protein *Cerebrospinal Fluid Increase Physiological* Few cases of aseptic meningitis described *2102*
Serum No Effect Analytical At 5 times upper limit of therapeutic range on methods on Technicon SMAC® , Abbott-VP, Kodak Ektachem® , Hitachi® 705 and KDA *3525* On biuret method on Technicon SMA II at physiological concentrations *2922* No effect at therapeutic concentrations on biuret and spectrophotometric methods *2920* At concentration of 200 mg/L had no effect on biuret method with blank correction *5704*
Serum No Effect Physiological No effect seen in patients undergoing treatment *2922*
Urine Increase Physiological In 2 patients with systemic lupus erythematosus *1904* Occasional reports in humans of interstitial nephritis with hematuria, proteinuria and even nephrotic syndrome *3200*

Prothrombin Time *Plasma No Effect Physiological* Ibuprofen not observed to affect prothrombin time in patients receiving coumarin anticoagulants *3200* Several short term studies failed to show an effect of ibuprofen on prothrombin times *3913*

Renal Blood Flow *Patient No Effect Physiological* At doses of up to 800 mg three times daily for 3 days had no effect in 8 healthy volunteers as measured by PAH clearance *4549*

Renin Activity *Plasma Decrease Physiological* 59% reduction in patients being treated *1018*
Plasma No Effect Physiological Insignificant reduction in 8 healthy volunteers given 800 mg daily for 3 days (mean control 1.7 ng/mL/h, post-ibuprofen mean 1.2 ng/mL/h) *4549*

Sodium *Serum No Effect Analytical* No interference observed at concentration of 500 mg/L with Technicon Chromolyte method *969*
Urine Decrease Physiological Ibuprofen has been shown to reduce the natriuretic effect of furosemide and thiazides *3200*
Urine No Effect Physiological Insignificant reduction in 8 healthy volunteers given 800 mg three times daily for 3 days *4549*

Sucrose *Serum No Effect Analytical* Using automated procedure involving sucrose phosphorylase, phosphoglutamase and glucose-6-phosphatase of Vinet et al no significant interference observed at a concentration of 1 mmol/L *6267*
Urine No Effect Analytical Using automated procedure involving sucrose phosphorylase, phosphoglutamase and glucose-6-phosphatase of Vinet et al no significant interference observed at a concentration of 1 mmol/L *6267*

Thromboxane B_2 *Plasma Decrease Physiological* Significant reduction in patients during treatment *1018*
Urine Decrease Physiological In 11 healthy volunteers in randomized trial *698* Reduction observed in mildly hypertensive patients with 7 days treatment following two weeks without antihypertensive medication *4065*

Thromboxane B_2 Production
Plasma Decrease Physiological Administration to healthy women of 3 x 200 mg/d caused 23% a nonsignificant reduction in thromboxane B_2 synthesis *5826*

Thyroid Stimulating Hormone
Serum No Effect Physiological In 11 patients treated with a mean dose of 1473 mg/d for at least 3 weeks mean concentration of 1.6 ± 0.2 mU/L not significantly different from 1.5 ± 0.2 mU/L in 22 controls *585*

Thyroxine (T4) *Serum No Effect Physiological* In 11 individuals treated with a mean dose of 1473 mg/d for at least 3 weeks mean concentration of 95 ± 4 nmol/L not significantly different from 94 ± 4 nmol/L in 22 controls *585*

Thyroxine (T4) Index, Free *Serum No Effect Physiological* In 11 individuals treated with a mean dose of 1473 mg/d for at least 3 weeks mean FTI of 91 ± 4 not significantly different from 93 ± 4 in 22 controls *585*

Tri-iodothyronine, Free (fT3) *Serum No Effect Analytical* At a concentration of 0.4 g/L cross-reactivity of 0.0% with free triiodothyronine method on Bayer Technicon Immuno 1® system *425*

Tri-iodothyronine (T3) *Serum No Effect Physiological* In 11 individuals treated with a mean dose of 1473 mg/d for at least 3 weeks mean concentration of 2.0 ± 0.1 nmol/L not different from 2.0 ± 0.1 nmol/L in 22 controls *585*

Triglycerides *Serum No Effect Analytical* No effect at therapeutic concentrations on enzymatic methods *2920* On enzymatic method on Technicon SMA II at physiological concentra-

tions *2922* At 5 times upper limit of therapeutic range on methods on Technicon SMAC® , Abbott-VP, Kodak Ektachem® , Hitachi® 705 and KDA *3525*
Serum *No Effect* *Physiological* No effect seen in patients undergoing treatment *2922*

Urea Nitrogen *Serum* *Increase* *Physiological* Significant effect in group of patients with rheumatoid arthritis, although most values remained within normal range *1388* In 2 patients with systemic lupus erythematosus *1904* Acute renal failure may occur in patients with pre-existing impaired renal function may result in decreased creatinine clearance, polyuria, azotemia, cystitis and hematuria *3200*
Serum *No Effect* *Analytical* No effect at therapeutic concentrations on glutamate, dehydrogenase, phenol- hypochlorite, and diacetyl monoxime methods *2920* No effect at therapeutic concentrations on glutamate dehydrogenase-based method *2920* At concentrations up to 200 mg/L had no effect on method on Kodak Ektachem® *5706* At concentration of 200 mg/L had no effect on diacetylmonoxime method *5704* On diacetyl monoxime method on Technicon SMA II at physiological concentrations *2922* On diacetylmonoxime method on Technicon SMA II at physiological concentrations *2922*

Uric Acid *Serum* *Decrease* *Physiological* Significantly less in drug treated group than in controls. Same effect noted with initiation of therapy *2922*
Serum *Increase* *Physiological* Significant effect in group of patients with rheumatoid arthritis, although most values remained within normal range *1388*
Serum *No Effect* *Analytical* At concentration of 200 mg/L had no effect on phosphotungstate reduction method *5704* At 5 times upper limit of therapeutic range on methods on Technicon SMAC® , Abbott-VP, Du Pont aca, Roche Cobas-Bio, Kodak Ektachem® , Hitachi® 705 and KDA *3525* On phosphotungstate method on Technicon SMA II at physiological concentrations *2922* No effect at therapeutic concentrations on uricase-catalase, aldehyde dehydrogenase direct UV-test and phosphotungstate methods *2920*

Vitamin B_{12} *Serum* *No Effect* *Analytical* At concentrations up to 40 mg/dL had no clinically significant cross-reactivity in vitamin B_{12} method on Bayer Technicon Immuno 1® *439*

Volume *Urine* *No Effect* *Physiological* No significant effect observed in 8 healthy volunteers given 800 mg three times daily for 3 days *4549*

Icterogenin

Alanine Aminotransferase *Serum* *Increase* *Physiological* Causes intrahepatic cholestasis *239*

Alkaline Phosphatase *Serum* *Increase* *Physiological* Causes intrahepatic cholestasis *239*

Aspartate Aminotransferase *Serum* *Increase* *Physiological* Causes intrahepatic cholestasis *239*

Bile *Urine* *Increase* *Physiological* Causes intrahepatic cholestasis *239*

Bilirubin *Serum* *Increase* *Physiological* Causes intrahepatic cholestasis *239*

BSP Retention *Serum* *Increase* *Physiological* Causes intrahepatic cholestasis *239*

Idarubicin

Alanine Aminotransferase *Serum* *Increase* *Physiological* Transient increases may occur with idarubicin, often when potentially hepatotoxic drugs were coadministered *4679*

Alkaline Phosphatase *Serum* *Increase* *Physiological* Transient increases may occur with idarubicin, often when potentially hepatotoxic drugs were coadministered *4679*

Aspartate Aminotransferase *Serum* *Increase* *Physiological* Transient increases may occur with idarubicin, often when potentially hepatotoxic drugs were coadministered *4679*

Bilirubin *Serum* *Increase* *Physiological* Transient increases may occur with idarubicin, often when potentially hepatotoxic drugs were coadministered *4679*

Creatinine *Serum* *Increase* *Physiological* Transient increases may occur with idarubicin, often when potentially nephrotoxic antibiotics were coadministered *4679*

Erythrocytes *Blood* *Decrease* *Physiological* Severe bone marrow suppression may occur with idarubicin *4679*

Hematocrit *Blood* *Decrease* *Physiological* Severe bone marrow suppression may occur with idarubicin *4679*

Hemoglobin *Blood* *Decrease* *Physiological* Severe bone marrow suppression may occur with idarubicin *4679*

Leukocytes *Blood* *Decrease* *Physiological* Severe bone marrow suppression may occur with idarubicin *4679*

Platelets *Blood* *Decrease* *Physiological* Severe bone marrow suppression and bleeding may occur with idarubicin *4679*

Urea Nitrogen *Serum* *Increase* *Physiological* Transient increases may occur with idarubicin, often when potentially nephrotoxic antibiotics were coadministered *4679*

Vanillylmandelic Acid *Serum* *Increase* *Physiological* Transient increases may occur with idarubicin, often when potentially hepatotoxic drugs were coadministered *4679*

Idoxuridine

Alkaline Phosphatase *Serum* *Increase* *Physiological* Cholestatic jaundice reported in one case *1297*

Aspartate Aminotransferase *Serum* *Increase* *Physiological* Cholestatic jaundice reported in one case *1297*

Bilirubin *Serum* *Increase* *Physiological* Cholestatic jaundice reported in one case *1297*

Leukocytes *Blood* *Decrease* *Physiological* Effect of high concentration only *3810*

Ifosfamide

Adenosine Deaminase Binding Protein
Urine *Increase* *Physiological* Manifestation of nephrotoxicity in 12 children given drug 1.6 g/m^2 for 5 d *2255*

Alanine Aminopeptidase *Urine* *Increase* *Physiological* Manifestation of nephrotoxicity in 12 children given drug 1.6 g/m^2 for 5 d *2255*

Alanine Aminotransferase *Serum* *Increase* *Physiological* Manifestation of hepatotoxicity *6182*

Alkaline Phosphatase *Serum* *Increase* *Physiological* Manifestation of hepatotoxicity *6182*

Amino Acids *Urine* *Increase* *Physiological* Increased excretion of selected free amino acids in comparison with controls in 2 of 4 patients with malignant lymphoma treated only with ifosfamide, suggesting the presence of a proximal tubular defect *4562*

Aspartate Aminotransferase *Serum* *Increase* *Physiological* Manifestation of hepatotoxicity *6182*

Bicarbonate *Serum* *Decrease* *Physiological* Decreased serum bicarbonate observed in two patients with malignant lymphoma treated only with ifosfamide with increased urinary pH suggesting inappropriate urinary loss of alkali *4562*

Casts *Urine* *Increase* *Physiological* Large number of granular casts in all patients *6182*

Erythrocytes *Urine* *Increase* *Physiological* Urotoxicity may occur manifested as hemorrhagic cystitis or with other symptoms of bladder irritation *1384* Occurs in one third patients within 2 d *6182*

Glucose *Urine* *Increase* *Physiological* Two of 4 patients with malignant lymphoma treated only with ifosfamide had increased urinary excretion without concomitant hyperglycemia or history of diabetes - suggestive of proximal tubular defect *4562*

Hemoglobin *Blood* *Decrease* *Physiological* Occurs in 32% patients after 150 mg/kg *6182*
Urine *Increase* *Physiological* Microscopic hematuria observed in all four patients with malignant lymphoma treated only with ifosfamide *4562* Occurs in one third patients within 2 d *6182*

Ketones *Urine* *Increase* *Analytical* Four patients with malignant lymphoma treated solely with ifosfamide had false positive results *4562*

Leukocytes *Blood* *Decrease* *Physiological* Dose limiting toxicity is marrow suppression *1384* Occurs in 80% patients after 150 mg/kg *6182*

Ifosfamide *(continued)*

N-Acetyl-Glucosaminidase *Urine Increase Physiological* Commonly observed: seen in all patients in one study in spite of concomitant therapy *2254* Manifestation of nephrotoxicity in 12 children given drug 1.6 g/m² for 5 d *2255*
Urine No Effect Analytical At 1 g/L had no effect on 2 colorimetric analytical methods *2254*

pH *Urine Increase Physiological* Urinary pH increased in general in all four patients with malignant lymphoma treated only with ifosfamide, usually to pH 7 but pH of 8 or 9 observed without concomitant alkali administration *4562*

Phosphate *Urine Increase Physiological* Increased excretion observed in one of 4 patients with malignant lymphoma which decreased after cessation of therapy, possibly as result of proximal tubular damage *4562*

Platelets *Blood Decrease Physiological* Occurs in 13% patients after 150 mg/kg *6182* Dose limiting toxicity is bone marrow suppression *1384*

Protein *Urine Increase Physiological* 3 of 4 patients with malignant lymphoma had excretions ranging from trace to 100 mg/dL when treated solely with ifosfamide but not observed in fourth individual who had fewer courses *4562*

Retinol-binding Protein *Urine Increase Physiological* In 10 patients aged 15 - 59 years with soft tissue sarcoma or Ewing's sarcoma excretion increased from mean baseline of 30 µg/mmol creatinine or less to 58 to 8400 µg/mmol creatinine after 72 hours *3411*

Sodium *Urine Increase Physiological* Increased excretion observed in one of 4 patients with malignant lymphoma treated solely with ifosfamide which subsided with cessation of treatment *4562*

Urea Nitrogen *Serum Increase Physiological* Common toxic manifestation *6182*

Uric Acid *Urine Increase Physiological* Increased excretion observed in one of 4 patients with malignant lymphoma treated only with ifosfamide which lessened with cessation of treatment *4562*

Imidapril

Angiotensin-converting Enzyme
Serum Decrease Physiological In 40 patients with acute myocardial infarction treatment with imidapril caused a significant reduction of activity after 24 h to 3.6 ± 0.6 U/L compared with placebo treated group, in whom activity was 7.4 ± 0.8 U/L *4453*

Plasminogen Activator Inhibitor
Serum Decrease Physiological In 40 patients with acute myocardial infarction treatment with imidapril caused a significant reduction of activity after 48 h to 7.9 ± 1.9 U/mL compared with placebo treated group, in whom activity was 18.4 ± 3.5 U/mL *4453*

Imipenem/Cilastatin

Alanine Aminotransferase *Serum Increase Physiological* Mild and reversible increase observed in 1.2% patients treated with imipenem/cilastatin *1384*

Alkaline Phosphatase *Serum Increase Physiological* Mild and reversible increase observed in 0.8% patients treated with imipenem/cilastatin *1384*

δ-Aminolevulinic Acid *Urine Increase Analytical* In one child administration of Tienam caused a significant increase to 556 µmol/L with colorimetric procedure of Mauzerall and Granick which declined to 39 µmol/L 3 days after withdrawal of treatment *6240*

Aspartate Aminotransferase *Serum Increase Physiological* Mild and reversible increase observed in 1.1% patients treated with imipenem and cilastatin *1384*

Bilirubin *Serum No Effect Analytical* No effect of mixture of imipenem and cilastatin at concentration up to 1000 mg/L on DPD method on Hitachi 717 or Kodak Ektachem® analyzers *4695*
Serum No Effect Physiological Probably clinically insignificant displacement from protein in neonates *6314*

Clindamycin *Serum Positive Analytical* Interferes with bioassays *3858*

Colistin *Serum Positive Analytical* Interferes with bioassays *3858*

Coombs' Test *Blood Positive Physiological* Observed in some patients treated with imipenem/cilastatin *1384*

Cyclosporine *Blood Increase Physiological* 150% increase in concentration in one renal transplant patient after only two doses of imipenem/cilastatin (but note same combination of drugs reduced concentration in rats) *6637* Coadministration with cyclosporine appeared to cause a significant increase in cyclosporine concentration *859*
Serum Increase Physiological Coadministration with cyclosporine appeared to cause a significant increase in cyclosporine concentration *859* When given in conjunction with cilastatin reported to inhibit hepatic metabolism of cyclosporine although this combination of drugs is also suspected of being nephrotoxic *1069* In a 62-year old renal transplant patient 130% increase in blood cyclosporine concentration with neurotoxicity observed after 2 doses of imipenem/cilastatin *6596*

Eosinophils *Blood Increase Physiological* Observed in some patients treated with imipenem/cilastatin *1384*

Erythromycin *Serum Increase Analytical* Interferes with bioassays *3858*

Ketone Body Ratio *Serum No Effect Analytical* When added at a concentration of 0.75 g/L imipenem cilastatin sodium had no significant effect on AKBR method of Uno et al *6131*

Metronidazole *Serum Increase Analytical* Interferes with bioassays *3858*

Neutrophils *Blood Decrease Physiological* Reversible neutropenia observed in some patients treated with imipenem/cilastatin *1384*

Platelets *Blood Decrease Physiological* Reversible thrombocytopenia observed in some patients treated with imipenem/cilastatin *1384*
Blood Increase Physiological Rare reports of thrombocytosis (0.6% patients) when treated with imipenem/cilastatin *1384*

Polymyxin *Serum Increase Analytical* Interferes with bioassays *3858*

Porphobilinogen *Urine Increase Analytical* In one child administration of Tienam caused a significant increase to 66 µmol/L with Mauzerall and Granick colorimetric procedure which declined to 1.3 µmol/L 3 days after withdrawal of treatment *6240*

Prothrombin Time *Plasma Increase Physiological* Rare reports of hypoprothrombinemia following treatment with imipenem/cilastatin *1384*

Tacrolimus *Serum No Effect Analytical* In HPLC/MS method of Christians et al no significant interference observed with measurement of FK 506 *1010*

Tetracycline *Serum Increase Analytical* Interferes with bioassays *3858*

Trimethoprim *Serum Increase Analytical* Interferes with bioassays *3858*

Imipramine

Acetaminophen *Serum No Effect Analytical* No interference observed at a concentration of 2000 µg/mL (713 µmol/L) with method on Du Pont aca *1506*

Alanine Aminotransferase *Serum Increase Physiological* May cause cholestatic jaundice *3045* Jaundice, simulating obstructive, and altered liver function may occur as side effects of treatment *1040* Either due to hepatotoxicity or hypersensitivity in 33 year old woman *4138*

Alkaline Phosphatase *Serum Increase Physiological* Either due to hepatotoxicity or hypersensitivity in 33 year old woman *4138* Jaundice, simulating obstructive, and altered liver function may occur as side effects of treatment *1040* May cause cholestatic jaundice *3045*

Amitriptyline *Serum Increase Analytical* May cause false positive reaction in EMIT immunoassay for amitriptyline *3590*

Antidiuretic Hormone *Urine Increase Physiological* Mean excretion of 10.6 mU/h in 7 normal and 10 depressive patients when given 75 mg/d compared to control of 2.6 mU/h *4816*

Aspartate Aminotransferase *Serum Increase Physiological* Either due to hepatotoxicity or hypersensitivity in 33 year old woman *4138* Jaundice, simulating obstructive, and altered liver function may occur as side effects of treatment *1040* May cause cholestatic jaundice *3045*

Benzodiazepine Screen *Serum No Effect Analytical* No significant interference observed at a concentration of 100 µg/mL (0.36 mmol/L) with method on Du Pont aca *1512*

Bile *Urine Increase Physiological* May cause cholestatic jaundice *3810*

Bilirubin *Serum Increase Physiological* Jaundice, simulating obstructive, and altered liver function may occur as side effects of treatment *1040* May cause cholestatic jaundice *3045*
Serum No Effect Physiological Insignificant protein displacement effect in neonates *6314*
Urine Increase Physiological May cause cholestatic jaundice *3045*

BSP Retention *Serum Increase Physiological* May cause cholestatic jaundice *4048*

Cannabinoids *Urine No Effect Analytical* No effect on Roche Abuscreen method *5006*

Carbamazepine *Serum Increase Analytical* Cross-reactivity of 8.3% observed with competitive fluorescence immunoassay used with PB Diagnostics OPUS analyzer *1153*

Catecholamines *Plasma No Effect Analytical* No effect on HPLC method of Koller for dopamine, epinephrine, and norepinephrine *3230*

Cholesterol *Serum Increase Physiological* Possible cholestatic effect *4909*

Citalopram *Serum No Effect Physiological* Coadministration to healthy volunteers had no significant effect on concentration of citalopram or its major metabolites *2288*

Cocaethylene *Urine Increase Analytical* Possible interference observed with TLC method of Bailey *328*

Creatinine *Serum Increase Physiological* Observed in one psychiatric case *5287*

Digoxin *Serum No Effect Physiological* No effect on serum concentration reported *558*

Drugs of Abuse Screen *Urine No Effect Analytical* No effect at concentration of 100 µg/mL on EZ-SCREEN procedure for cannabinoids and cocaine *1739*

Eosinophils *Blood Increase Physiological* Bone marrow depression may occur as a side effect of treatment *1040* Allergic response (may produce Loffler's syndrome) *5483*

Ethosuximide *Serum No Effect Analytical* Insignificant cross-reactivity with method on Du Pont aca *1523*

Glucose *Serum Decrease Physiological* Reported effect *51* Hypoglycemia or hyperglycemia may occur as a side effect of treatment *1040*
Serum Increase Physiological Hypoglycemia or hyperglycemia may occur as a side effect of treatment *1040* Reported effect *51*

Glucose Tolerance *Serum Decrease Physiological* Preliminary observations only reported *243*

Granulocytes *Blood Decrease Physiological* Bone marrow depression may occur as a side effect of treatment *1040*

Hemoglobin *Blood Decrease Physiological* Bone marrow depression may occur as a side effect of treatment *1040*

Histamine *Plasma No Effect Analytical* Although 50% inhibition of radio-enzyme assay occurs at 29 µg/mL clinical effects unlikely since physiological concentration 0.1-0.5 µg/mL *2492*

Homovanillic Acid *Urine No Effect Physiological* In 9 depressed outpatients treatment with up to 196 ± 63 mg/d for 6 weeks mean excretion increased from baseline of 25.3 ± 5.8 µmol/d to 25.8 ± 7.3 µmol/d *2958*

4-Hydroxy-3-Methoxy-Phenylglycol
Urine Decrease Physiological In 9 depressed outpatients treated with up to 196 ± mg/d for 6 weeks significant reduction from mean baseline of 10.5 ± 2.9 µmol/d to 8.1 ± 3.1 µmol/d *2958*
Urine No Effect Physiological In 20 patients with depression treatment with up to 300 mg/d for 12 weeks caused nonsignificant change from mean baseline of 1747 ± 698 µg/d to 1878 ± 754 µg/d *2039*

5-Hydroxyindoleacetic Acid *Urine Decrease Analytical* May inhibit color development in reaction *1444*
Urine Decrease Physiological May decrease up to 50%: decrease cell permeability to 5-HT *2498*

^{131}I Uptake *Serum Decrease Physiological* Tofranil® contains tetraiodofluorescein *4360*

Imipramine *Serum Increase Physiological* After 150-300 mg/d blood concentration ranged from 0.1 to 0.6 mg/L *3868*

Lactate Dehydrogenase *Serum Increase Physiological* May cause cholestatic jaundice *3045*

Leukocytes *Blood Decrease Physiological* May cause leukopenia/agranulocytosis *5483*
Blood Increase Physiological (transient 1-6 h) (possibly Loffler's syndrome) *5483*

Lysergic Acid Diethylamide *Urine Increase Analytical* Minimum concentration that caused a positive result with EMIT method to measure LSD 50 mg/L *4968*

Metanephrine *Urine No Effect Physiological* In 9 depressed outpatients treatment with up to 196 ± 63 mg/d for 6 weeks nonsignificant reduction from mean baseline of 0.69 ± 0.22 µmol/d to 0.65 ± 0.29 µmol/d *2958*

Metanephrines, Total *Urine No Effect Analytical* At 15 mg/L on modified Pisano procedure *2372*

Mycophenolic Acid *Serum No Effect Analytical* No significant interference observed with HPLC method of Shipkova et al *5526*

Mycophenolic Acid Glucuronide
Serum No Effect Analytical No significant interference observed with HPLC method of Shipkova et al *5526*

Neutrophils *Blood Decrease Physiological* Occasional case of agranulocytosis reported *6264*

Norepinephrine *Plasma Increase Physiological* In 9 depressed outpatients treatment with up to 194 ± 21 mg/d for 6 weeks caused increase from mean baseline of 2.01 ± 0.71 pmol/L to 2.52 ± 0.57 pmol/L *2958*

Normetanephrine *Urine Increase Physiological* In 9 depressed outpatients treatment with up to 196 ± 63 mg/d for 6 weeks caused nonsignificant increase from mean baseline of 1.41 ± 0.36 µmol/d to 1.62 ± 0.64 µmol/d *2958*

5'-Nucleotidase *Serum Increase Physiological* Due to cholestasis *2911*

p-Aminophenol *Urine No Effect Analytical* With addition of drugs at a concentration of 100 mg/L and of related compounds at 50 mg/L no significant effect observed on colorimetric method of van Bocxlaer on Cobas Mira analyzer which involves reacting free p-aminophenol with resorcinol in the presence of magnesium ions to form an indophenol dye measured at 550 nm *6163*

Phenylalanine *Plasma No Effect Analytical* No interference observed with rapid quantitative whole blood method of Campbell et al using phenylalanine dehydrogenase *867*

Platelets *Blood Decrease Physiological* Bone marrow depression and purpura may occur as a side effect of treatment *1040* May be marrow depression and purpura *2754*

Potassium *Serum No Effect Analytical* At concentration of 30 mg/L had no effect on measurement by ISE with predilution *5704*

Prolactin *Plasma Increase Physiological* Marked increase in male and female psychiatric patients treated for up to 4 weeks *6098*
Plasma No Effect Physiological Like other tricyclic antidepressants no effect *1126*

Protein *Cerebrospinal Fluid Increase Analytical* 1.0 mg = 3.5 mg in Folin-Ciocalteu procedure *882*

Riluzole *Serum No Effect Physiological* No effect on riluzole binding observed *4941*

Sodium *Serum No Effect Analytical* At concentration of 30 mg/L had no effect on measurement by ISE with predilution *5704*

Urea Nitrogen *Serum Increase Physiological* Observed in one psychiatric case *5287*
Test Conditions Increase Analytical Produces turbidity with Berthelot's reagent *3144*

Urobilinogen *Urine Increase Physiological* May cause cholestatic jaundice *3045*

Vanillylmandelic Acid *Urine Decrease Physiological* In 9 depressed outpatients treatment with up to 196 ± 63 mg/d for 6 weeks caused nonsignificant reduction from mean baseline of

Imipramine *(continued)*

Vanillylmandelic Acid *(continued)*
18.1 ± 4.3 μmol/d to15.6 ± 5.0 μmol/d *2958* Approximately 30% decrease, block of uptake into cells *2498*

Immune Globulin

Creatinine *Serum Increase Physiological* Administration may potentially cause acute renal failure which, if it occurs, usually begins within one hour of administration *936*

Cyclosporine *Blood No Effect Analytical* At a concentration of 5000 mg/L had no effect on Syva EMIT method *495*

Immunoglobulin G *Serum Increase Physiological* Intravenous globulin produced concentrations well above normally accepted level considered to be therapeutic in immunodeficient patients *212*

Interleukin-10 *Serum Decrease Physiological* Mean concentration in 23 patients with Kawasaki disease of 125.037 ± 111.161 pg/mL significantly reduced with IVIG treatment to 32.437 ± 54.716 pg/mL *4313*

Platelets *Blood Decrease Physiological* Fall observed several days after injection *4014*
Blood Increase Physiological In 19 children with idiopathic thrombocytopenic purpura treatment with 0.5 g/kg for 5 days caused increase from mean baseline of about 10 x10^9 /L to peak of 210 x10^9 /L at 8 days *89*

Urea Nitrogen *Serum Increase Physiological* Administration may potentially cause acute renal failure which, if it occurs, usually begins within one hour of administration *936* Nephritis may occur with serum sickness *4014*

Immunotherapy

D. farinae-specific IgE Antibodies
Serum Decrease Physiological In 39 patients with perennial allergic rhinitis treatment with up to 3000 AU with weekly injections for up to 8 weeks caused a significant reduction from mean baseline of 90.8 ± 136.2 ARU/mL to 22.3 ± 38.3 ARU/mL (31.0 ± 130.7%) *4381*
Serum No Effect Physiological In 25 patients with perennial allergic rhinitis treatment with weekly specific injections caused a nonsignificant change from mean baseline of 31.3 ± 24.1 ARU/mL at baseline to 30.4 ± 20.6 ARU/mL after 1 y, 31.2 ± 20.9 ARU/mL after 3 y, 29.4 ± 19.1 ARU/mL after 5 y and 31.3 ± 21.3 ARU/mL after 8 y *4380*

D. farinae-specific IgG_4 Antibodies
Serum No Effect Physiological In 25 patients with perennial allergic rhinitis treatment with weekly specific injections caused a nonsignificant change from mean baseline of 0.52 ± 0.28 U/mL at baseline to 0.54 ± 0.28 U/mL after 1 y, 0.49 ± 0.29 U/mL after 3 y, 0.57 ± 0.33 U/mL after 5 y and 0.58 ± 0.33 U/mL after 8 y *4380*

Interleukin-4 *Serum Decrease Physiological* In 39 patients with perennial allergic rhinitis treatment with corticosteroids for up to 8 weeks caused a significant change from mean baseline of 13.3 ± 10.7 pg/mL by 58.8 ± 40.6% *4381*

Soluble Interleukin-2 Receptor
Serum Decrease Physiological In 48 patients with perennial allergic rhinitis mean concentration of 490 ± 189 U/mL before specific immunotherapy with D farinae extracts decreased by 30.5 ± 65.0% to 351 ± 97 U/mL after treatment by 20.8 ± 30.3% *4382*

Indandione Derivatives

Alanine Aminotransferase *Serum Increase Physiological* Hepatocellular damage with cholestasis *3810*

Aspartate Aminotransferase *Serum Increase Physiological* Hepatocellular damage with cholestasis *3810*

Bile *Urine Increase Physiological* May cause hepatotoxicity *3810*

Bilirubin *Serum Increase Physiological* As result of hypersensitivity *4014*

BSP Retention *Serum Increase Physiological* May cause hepatotoxicity *3810*

Color *Urine Increase Analytical* May be orange to red in color *4012*

Eosinophils *Blood Increase Physiological* With other signs of hypersensitivity *4014*

Erythrocytes *Urine Increase Physiological* May cause hematuria: manifestation of overdose *2024*

Hemoglobin *Urine Increase Physiological* May cause hematuria: manifestation of overdose *2024*

Leukocytes *Blood Decrease Physiological* With other evidence of hypersensitivity *3810*

Indapamide

Albumin *Urine Decrease Physiological* Regression of microalbuminuria observed after long-term treatment *2017*

Apolipoprotein A-I *Serum No Effect Physiological* In 13 hypertensive patients with diabetes treated for 24 weeks *4452*

Apolipoprotein B *Serum No Effect Physiological* In 18 patients treated for 6 weeks *141*

Apolipoprotein B-100 *Serum Decrease Physiological* In 13 hypertensives patients with diabetes treated for 24 weeks *4452*

Calcium *Serum No Effect Physiological* Insignificant mean increase of 0.1 mmol/L in 18 black women with essential hypertension treated 2.5 mg daily for 12 weeks *4788*

Cholesterol *Serum Increase Physiological* Increase by 17 mg/dL in 17 patients with essential hypertension treated with 2.5 mg daily for 3 mo *3280* Slight and insignificant in 13 hypertensive diabetics treated for 24 weeks *4452* Significant mean increase of 0.98 mmol/L in 18 black women with essential hypertension treated with 2.5 mg daily for 12 weeks *4788*
Serum No Effect Physiological In 27 subjects treated for less than 1 y with this drug only *1085* No significant change in 24 hypertensive patients treated for 60 days with 2.5 mg daily *5682* In various studies involving more than 30 patients when used as sole drug for less than 1 y *141*

C-Peptide *Plasma Increase Physiological* Both mean fasting and stimulated in 13 hypertensive diabetics *4452*

Creatinine *Serum No Effect Analytical* At 10 mg/L on reversed phase liquid chromatographic procedure of Zhiri et al *6656*

Glucose *Serum Increase Physiological* And after 75 g load in 13 hypertensive diabetics *4452* Insignificant mean increase of 0.4 mmol/L in 16 black women with essential hypertension treated with 2.5 mg daily for 12 weeks *4788* Increase by 7 mg/dL in 17 patients with essential hypertension treated with 2.5 mg daily for 3 mo *3280*

HDL-Cholesterol *Serum Decrease Physiological* Slight effect in 13 hypertensive diabetics treated for 24 weeks *4452*
Serum Increase Physiological Significant mean increase of 0.23 mmol/L in 18 black women with essential hypertension treated with 2.5 mg daily for 12 weeks *4788*
Serum No Effect Physiological In various studies involving more than 30 patients when used as sole drug for less than 1 y *141* Slight but not significant increase in 24 hypertensive patients treated with 2.5 mg daily for 60 days *5682* In 43 subjects treated with this drug for less than 1 y *6384*

Hemoglobin A_{1c} *Blood Increase Physiological* After 24 weeks in 13 hypertensive diabetics *4452* Insignificant mean increase of 0.4% in 16 nondiabetic black women with essential hypertension treated with 2.5 mg daily for 12 weeks *4788*

ionized Calcium *Serum No Effect Physiological* Insignificant mean increase of 0.02 mmol/L in 15 black women with essential hypertension treated for 12 weeks with 2.5 mg daily *4788*

LDL-Cholesterol *Serum Increase Physiological* Slight and insignificant in 13 hypertensive diabetics treated for 24 weeks *4452* Significant mean increase of 0.70 mmol/L in 18 black women with essential hypertension treated with 2.5 mg daily for 12 weeks *4788*
Serum No Effect Physiological In 27 subjects treated for less than 1 y with this drug only *1085* In various studies involving more than 30 patients when used as sole drug for less than 1 y *141* No significant change in 24 hypertensive patients treated with 2.5 mg daily for 60 days *5682*

Magnesium *Red Blood Cells No Effect Physiological* No effect observed in group of elderly mildly hypertensive patients following 2.5 mg *5963*
Serum Increase Physiological Insignificant mean increase of 0.04 mmol/L in 18 black women with essential hypertension treated with 2.5 mg daily for 12 weeks *4788*
Serum No Effect Physiological No effect observed with 2.5 mg in a group of elderly patients with mild hypertension *5963*

Norepinephrine *Plasma Increase Physiological* Insignificant mean increase of 0.59 nmol/L in 17 black women with essential hypertension treated with 2.5 mg daily for 12 weeks *4788*

Potassium *Serum Decrease Physiological* In 3 of 13 hypertensive patients with diabetes treated for 24 weeks *4452* Mean fall from 4.2 to 3.4 mmol/L in 8 hypertensives treated for 16 weeks *568* Increase by 0.4 mmol/L in 17 patients with essential hypertension treated with 2.5 mg daily for 3 mo *3280* Effect observed in group of elderly hypertensive patients following 2.5 mg, associated with loss of sodium into red cells *5963*
Serum No Effect Physiological Insignificant mean increase of 0.1 mmol/L in 16 black women with essential hypertension treated with 2.5 mg daily for 12 weeks *4788* No significant change in 24 hypertensive patients treated with 2.5 mg daily for 60 days *5682*

Renin Activity *Plasma Increase Physiological* But not significant in 8 hypertensives treated for 16 weeks *568* Significant increase to mean of 0.87 ng/L/s from mean baseline of 0.20 ng/L/s 17 black women with essential hypertension treated with 2.5 mg daily for 12 weeks *4788*

Selenium *Serum Increase Physiological* Insignificant mean increase of 0.08 µmol/L in 19 black women with essential hypertension treated with 2.5 mg daily for 12 weeks *4788*

Sodium *Serum No Effect Physiological* No significant change in 24 hypertensive patients treated with 2.5 mg daily for 60 days *5682* In 8 hypertensives treated for 16 weeks *568*

Triglycerides *Serum Increase Physiological* Slight and insignificant in 13 hypertensive diabetics treated for 24 weeks *4452*
Serum No Effect Physiological In 27 subjects treated for less than 1 y with this drug only *1085* In various studies involving more than 30 patients when used as sole drug for less than 1 y *141* Insignificant mean increase of 0.12 mmol/L in 18 black women with essential hypertension treated with 2.5 mg daily for 12 weeks *4788* No significant change in 24 hypertensive patients treated with 2.5 mg daily for 60 days *5682*

Urea Nitrogen *Serum No Effect Physiological* In 8 hypertensives treated for 16 weeks *568*

Uric Acid *Serum Increase Physiological* Observed in normal men and those with mild essential hypertension *6384* Increase by 1.4 mg/dL in 17 patients with essential hypertension treated with 2.5 mg daily for 3 mo *3280* Insignificant mean increase of 48 µmol/L in 18 black women with essential hypertension treated with 2.5 mg daily for 12 weeks *4788*
Serum No Effect Analytical At 10 mg/L on reversed phase liquid chromatographic procedure of Zhiri et al *6656*
Serum No Effect Physiological No significant change in 24 hypertensive patients treated with 2.5 mg daily for 60 days *5682*

VLDL-Cholesterol *Serum No Effect Physiological* In various studies involving more than 30 patients when used as sole drug for less than 1 y *141* In 27 subjects treated for less than 1 y with this drug only *1085*

Indenolol

Albumin *Urine No Effect Physiological* No significant change observed in 133 hypertensive diabetics when treated with up to 120 mg/d for 6 months *3746*

Cholesterol *Serum No Effect Physiological* No significant change observed in 133 hypertensive diabetics treated with up to 120 mg/d for 6 months *3746*

C-Peptide *Urine No Effect Physiological* No significant change observed in 133 diabetic hypertensives when tretaed with up to 120 mg/d for 6 months *3746*

Glucose *Serum No Effect Physiological* No significant change observed in mean fasting concentration and concentrations at 11:30 a.m. and 3:00 p.m. in 133 hypertensive diabetics treated with up to 120 mg/d for 6 months *3746*

Hemoglobin A_{1c} *Blood No Effect Physiological* No significant change observed in 133 hypertensive diabetics tretaed with up to 120 mg/d for 6 months *3746*

Triglycerides *Serum No Effect Physiological* No significant effect observed in 133 hypertensive diabetics treated with up to 120 mg/d for 6 months *3746*

Indigo Blue

Color *Urine Increase Analytical* May produce blue color *1957*

Indigotin

Crystals *Urine Increase Physiological* Amorphous blue or small crystals (all pH) *684*

Indigotindisulfonate

Color *Urine Increase Analytical* Blue-green, decolorized with alkali *684* Color used to measure kidney function *128*

Indinavir

Alanine Aminotransferase *Serum Increase Physiological* In 31 HIV-infected patients previously treated with zidovudine for at least 6 months treatment with 800 mg indinavir every 8 h for 24 weeks caused aminotransferase activity to increase above 5 times the upper limit of normal in one patient *2364* Administration of indinavir may cause asymptomatic bilirubinemia (concentration greater than 2.5 mg/dL), predominantly indirect bilirubin, in approximately 10% patients. In less than 1% of patients this was associated with increased hepatic enzyme activity. In two studies of 196 patients activity was increased above 5 times the upper limit of normal in 3.1% *3966* Increased activity observed in in fewer than 10% treated patients, but occurring at least twice as often as in control individuals *1891*

Amylase *Serum Increase Physiological* Administration of indinavir may cause hyperamylasemia with an activity of greater than twice the upper limit of normal in 1.0% patients *3966*

Aspartate Aminotransferase *Serum Increase Physiological* In 31 HIV-infected patients previously treated with zidovudine for at least 6 months treatment with 800 mg indinavir every 8 h for 24 weeks caused aminotransferase activity to increase above 5 times the upper limit of normal in one patient *2364* Administration of indinavir may cause asymptomatic bilirubinemia (concentration greater than 2.5 mg/dL), predominantly indirect bilirubin, in approximately 10% patients. In less than 1% of patients this was associated with increased hepatic enzyme activity. In two studies of 196 patients activity was increased above 5 times the upper limit of normal in 2.1% *3966* Increased activity observed in in fewer than 10% treated patients, but occurring at least twice as often as in control individuals *1891*

Astemizole *Serum Increase Physiological* Decreased metabolism with increased risk of cardiac toxicity or arrhythmia *886*

Bilirubin *Serum Increase Physiological* Increased concentration observed in in fewer than 10% treated patients, but occurring at least twice as often as in control individuals *1891* In 31 HIV-infected patients previously treated with zidovudine for at least 6 months treatment with 800 mg indinavir every 8 h for 24 weeks caused serum bilirubin concentration to increase above 2.5 mg/dL in 8 patients, but in none of them did the bilirubin concentration increase above 5.0 mg/dL *2364* Administration of indinavir may cause asymptomatic bilirubinemia (concentration greater than 2.5 mg/dL), predominantly indirect bilirubin, in approximately 10% treated patients. In two studies of 196 patients concentration increased above 2.5 mg/dL in 7.5% patients treated with indinavir *3966*

Indinavir *(continued)*

Bilirubin, Indirect *Serum Increase Physiological* Administration of indinavir may cause asymptomatic bilirubinemia (concentration greater than 2.5 mg/dL), predominantly indirect bilirubin, in approximately 10% patients *3966*

Blood *Urine Increase Physiological* Administration of indinavir may precipitate nephrolithiasis with or without hematuria. This has been observed in approximately 4% of all treated patients *3966*

CD3⁺ Lymphocytes *Blood No Effect Physiological* In 20 HIV-infected patients treatment with indinavir caused a nonsignificant change from mean baseline of 62.7 ± 3.8% (363 ± 51 cells/µL) to 64.2 ± 3.8% after 2 weeks, 66.2 ± 3.6% after 6 weeks and 69.9 ± 3.1% (764 ± 58 cells/µL) after 12 weeks *587*

CD4⁺ Lymphocytes *Blood Increase Physiological* In 31 HIV-infected patients previously treated with zidovudine for at least 6 months treatment with 800 mg indinavir every 8 h for 24 weeks caused CD4⁺ cell count to increase by 100.6 ± 12.5 cells/µL *2364* In 20 HIV-infected patients treatment with indinavir caused a significant change from mean baseline of 2.7 ± 0.6% (14 ± 3 cells/µL) to 6.4 ± 1.5% after 2 weeks, 7.1 ± 1.1% after 6 weeks and 8.9 ± 1.6% (97 ± 16 cells/µL) after 12 weeks *587*

CD8⁺/CD38⁺ Lymphocytes *Blood Decrease Physiological* In 20 HIV-infected patients treatment with indinavir caused a nonsignificant change from mean baseline of 41.2 ± 3.4% to 35.7 ± 3.5% after 2 weeks, but a significant change to 34.9 ± 3.1% after 6 weeks and 30.7 ± 3.3% after 12 weeks *587*
Blood No Effect Physiological In 20 HIV-infected patients treatment with indinavir caused a nonsignificant change from mean baseline of 41.2 ± 3.4% to 35.7 ± 3.5% after 2 weeks *587*

CD8⁺/CD45RO⁺ Lymphocytes *Blood Increase Physiological* In 20 HIV-infected patients treatment with indinavir caused a nonsignificant change from mean baseline of 26.9 ± 2.5% to 28.3 ± 2.9% after 2 weeks, but a significant change to 32.1 ± 2.5% after 6 weeks and a nonsignificant change to 29.9 ± 1.9% after 12 weeks *587*
Blood No Effect Physiological In 20 HIV-infected patients treatment with indinavir caused a nonsignificant change from mean baseline of 26.9 ± 2.5% (152 ± 3 cells/µL) to 28.3 ± 2.9% after 2 weeks, but a significant change to 32.1 ± 2.5% after 6 weeks and a nonsignificant change to 29.9 ± 1.9% (346 ± 34 cells/µL) after 12 weeks *587*

CD8⁺/HLA-DR⁺ Lymphocytes *Blood Increase Physiological* In 20 HIV-infected patients treatment with indinavir caused a nonsignificant change from mean baseline of 15.9 ± 1.9% to 16.2 ± 2.0% after 2 weeks, but a significant change to 19.7 ± 2.5% after 6 weeks and a nonsignificant change to 17.7 ± 1.8% after 12 weeks *587*
Blood No Effect Physiological In 20 HIV-infected patients treatment with indinavir caused a nonsignificant change from mean baseline of 15.9 ± 1.9% (94 ± 15 cells/µL) to 16.2 ± 2.0% after 2 weeks, but a significant change to 19.7 ± 2.5% (221 ± 41 cells/µL) after 6 weeks and a nonsignificant change to 17.7 ± 1.8% after 12 weeks *587*

CD8⁺ Lymphocytes *Blood No Effect Physiological* In 20 HIV-infected patients treatment with indinavir caused a nonsignificant change from mean baseline of 55.3 ± 3.8% (323 ± 47 cells/µL) to 53.6 ± 3.4% after 2 weeks, 54.3 ± 3.2% after 6 weeks and 56.7 ± 2.8% (616 ± 49 cells/µL) after 12 weeks *587*

Cisapride *Serum Increase Physiological* Decreased metabolism with increased risk of cardiac toxicity or arrhythmia *886*

Clarithromycin *Serum Increase Physiological* Causes a 53% increase in area under the concentration curve when indinavir coadministered *1891* Administration of indinavir 800 mg every 8 hours with clarithromycin 500 mg every 12 hours for 1 week resulted in a 29 ± 42% increase in indinavir AUC and a 53 ± 36% increase in clarithromycin AUC *3966*

Ethinyl Estradiol *Serum Increase Physiological* Administration of indinavir 800 mg every 8 hours with Ortho-Novum 1/35 for 1 week resulted in a 24 ± 17% increase in ethinyl estradiol AUC and a 26 ± 14% increase in norethindrone AUC *3966* Causes a 24% increase in area under the concentration curve when indinavir coadministered *1891*

Fluconazole *Serum No Effect Physiological* Administration of indinavir 1000 mg every 6 hours with fluconazole 400 mg/d for 1 week resulted in a 19 ± 33% decrease in indinavir AUC but had no effect on fluconazole AUC *3966*

Glucose *Serum Increase Physiological* Increased concentration observed in in fewer than 10% treated patients, but occurring at least twice as often as in control individuals *1891*

Hematocrit *Blood Decrease Physiological* Administration of indinavir may cause anemia *3966*

Hemoglobin *Blood Decrease Physiological* Administration of indinavir may cause anemia with a hemoglobin concentration of less than 80 g/L in 0.6% patients *3966*
Blood No Effect Physiological In 31 HIV-infected patients previously treated with zidovudine for at least 6 months treatment with 800 mg indinavir every 8 h for 24 weeks caused hemoglobin concentration to decrease below 8.5 g/dL in no patients *2364*

HIV-1 RNA *Serum Decrease Physiological* In 20 HIV-infected patients treatment with indinavir caused a significant reduction from mean baseline of 4.45 ± 0.27 $\log_{10}$ copies/mL to 3.23 ± 0.29 $\log_{10}$ copies/mL after 2 weeks, 2.57 ± 0.43 $\log_{10}$ copies/mL after 6 weeks and 2.45 ± 0.48 $\log_{10}$ copies/mL after 12 weeks *587*
Serum Increase Physiological In 31 HIV-infected patients previously treated with zidovudine for at least 6 months treatment with 800 mg indinavir every 8 h for 24 weeks caused HIV-RNA to decrease by 1.24 ± 0.11 $\log_{10}$*2364*

Indinavir *Urine Increase Physiological* Since indinavir introduced as a treatment for HIV-1-positive patients more than 100 patients developed renal colic or passed radiolucent stones containing indinavir 1 to 20 weeks after start of treatment *1248*

Interleukin-16 *Serum Increase Physiological* In 20 HIV-infected patients treatment with indinavir caused a significant change from mean baseline of 114.7 ± 22.3 pg/mL to 402.9 ± 154.0 pg/mL after 2 weeks, 600.9 ± 202.5 pg/mL after 6 weeks and 1506.2 ± 461.7 pg/mL after 12 weeks *587*

Isoniazid *Serum Increase Physiological* Causes a 13% increase in area under the concentration curve when indinavir coadministered *1891* Administration of indinavir 800 mg every 8 hours with isoniazid 300 mg/d for 1 week resulted in a 13 ± 15% increase in isoniazid AUC but had no effect on indinavir AUC *3966*

Ketoconazole *Serum Increase Physiological* Causes a 68% increase in area under the concentration curve when indinavir coadministered *1891*

Lamivudine *Serum Decrease Physiological* Administration of indinavir 800 mg every 8 hours with zidovudine 200 mg every 8 hours in combination with lamivudine 150 mg twice daily for 1 week resulted in no change in indinavir AUC a 36% increase in zidovudine AUC and a 6% decrease in lamivudine AUC *3966* Causes a 6% decrease in area under the concentration curve when indinavir coadministered *1891*

Macrophage Inflammatory Protein-1α
Serum Increase Physiological In 20 HIV-infected patients treatment with indinavir caused a nonsignificant change from mean baseline of 24.7 ± 1.1 pg/mL to 25.6 ± 1.6 pg/mL after 2 weeks, but a significant increase to 28.7 ± 1.5 pg/mL after 6 weeks and 29.3 ± 2.1 pg/mL after 12 weeks *587*
Serum No Effect Physiological In 20 HIV-infected patients treatment with indinavir caused a nonsignificant change from mean baseline of 24.7 ± 1.1 pg/mL to 25.6 ± 1.6 pg/mL after 2 weeks *587*

Macrophage Inflammatory Protein-1β
Serum Increase Physiological In 20 HIV-infected patients treatment with indinavir caused a significant change from mean baseline of 77.0 ± 6.3 pg/mL to 88.1 ± 5.1 pg/mL after 2 weeks *587*
Serum No Effect Physiological In 20 HIV-infected patients treatment with indinavir caused a significant change from mean baseline of 77.0 ± 6.3 pg/mL to 88.1 ± 5.1 pg/mL after 2 weeks, but a nonsignificant change to 81.1 ± 4.6 pg/mL after 6 weeks and 78.5 ± 7.2 pg/mL after 12 weeks *587*

Monocyte Chemotactic Protein-1
Serum Decrease Physiological In 20 HIV-infected patients treatment with indinavir caused a significant reduction from mean baseline of 701 ± 61 pg/mL to 578 ± 45 pg/mL after 2 weeks, 528 ± 47 pg/mL after 6 weeks and 478 ± 38 pg/mL after 12 weeks *587*

Nelfinavir *Serum Increase Physiological* Coadministration of Indinavir with nelfinavir caused a 83% increase in AUC of nelfinavir *66* Causes a 83% increase in area under the concentration curve when indinavir coadministered *1891*

Neutrophils *Blood Decrease Physiological* Administration of indinavir may cause neutropenia with a count of less than 750 /µL in 1.1% patients *3966* In 31 HIV-infected patients previously treated with zidovudine for at least 6 months treatment with 800 mg indinavir every 8 h for 24 weeks caused a decrease in absolute neutrophil count to below 500 cells/µL in one patient *2364*

Norethindrone *Serum Increase Physiological* Causes a 26% increase in area under the concentration curve when indinavir coadministered *1891* Administration of indinavir 800 mg every 8 hours with Ortho-Novum 1/35 for 1 week resulted in a 24 ± 17% increase in ethinyl estradiol AUC and a 26 ± 14% increase in norethindrone AUC *3966*

Platelets *Blood Decrease Physiological* Administration of indinavir may cause thrombocytopenia with a platelet count of less than 50,000 /µL in 0.5% patients *3966*

Blood Increase Physiological In 18 thrombocytopenic patients treatment with indinavir caused an increase from mean baseline of 117,000 /µL to 173,000 /µL: in 44 nonthrombocytopenic patients mean concentration increased from baseline of 240,000 /µL to 252,000 /µL with indinavir treatment *3764*

Blood No Effect Physiological In 31 HIV-infected patients previously treated with zidovudine for at least 6 months treatment with 800 mg indinavir every 8 h for 24 weeks caused platelet numbers to decrease below 50,000 cells/µL in no patients *2364*

Protein *Urine Increase Physiological* Administration of indinavir may cause proteinuria with various forms of renal disease *3966*

RANTES *Serum Increase Physiological* In 20 HIV-infected patients treatment with indinavir caused a nonsignificant change from mean baseline of 15.6 ± 0.5 ng/mL to 17.3 ± 0.8 ng/mL after 2 weeks, but a significant increase to 18.0 ± 0.7 ng/mL after 6 weeks and 17.6 ± 0.6 pg/mL after 12 weeks *587*

Serum No Effect Physiological In 20 HIV-infected patients treatment with indinavir caused a nonsignificant change from mean baseline of 15.6 ± 0.5 ng/mL to 17.3 ± 0.8 ng/mL after 2 weeks *587*

Rifabutin *Serum Increase Physiological* Increased serum concentration *886* Causes a 204% increase in area under the concentration curve when indinavir coadministered *1891* Administration of indinavir 800 mg every 8 hours with rifabutin 300 mg/d for 10 days resulted in a 32 ± 19% decrease in indinavir AUC and a 204 ± 142% increase in rifabutin AUC *3966*

Saquinavir *Serum Increase Physiological* Increases the area under the concentration curve by 500% when indinavir coadministered *1891*

Stavudine *Serum Increase Physiological* Causes a 25% increase in area under the concentration curve when indinavir coadministered *1891* Administration of indinavir 800 mg every 8 hours with stavudine 40 mg every 12 hours for 1 week resulted in no change in indinavir AUC and a 25 ± 26% increase in stavudine AUC *3966*

Sulfamethoxazole *Serum No Effect Physiological* Administration of indinavir 400 mg every 6 hours with trimethoprim/sulfamethoxazole (one double strength tablet every 12 hours) for 1 week resulted in no change in indinavir AUC, a 19 ± 31% increase in trimethoprim AUC and no change in sulfamethoxazole AUC *3966* Has no effect on area under the concentration curve when indinavir coadministered *1891*

Terfenadine *Serum Increase Physiological* Decreased metabolism with increased risk of cardiac toxicity or arrhythmia *886*

Trimethoprim *Serum Increase Physiological* Causes a 19% increase in area under the concentration curve when indinavir coadministered *1891* Administration of indinavir 400 mg every 6 hours with trimethoprim/sulfamethoxazole (one double strength tablet every 12 hours) for 1 week resulted in no change in indinavir AUC, a 19 ± 31% increase in trimethoprim AUC and no change in sulfamethoxazole AUC *3966*

Zidovudine *Serum Increase Physiological* Administration of indinavir 1000 mg every 8 hours with zidovudine 200 mg every 8 hours for 1 week resulted in a 13 ± 48% increase in indinavir AUC and a 17 ± 23% increase in zidovudine AUC *3966* Causes a 17 to 36% increase in area under the concentration curve when indinavir coadministered *1891*

Indocyanine Green

Bilirubin *Serum Increase Analytical* At concentration of dye of 100 mg/L interference with Kodak Ektachem® 700 method calculated to be 56 mmol/L *1468*

Bilirubin, Unconjugated *Serum No Effect Analytical* At concentration of 100 mg/L added in vitro had no effect on Kodak Ektachem® 700 method *1468*

γ-Glutamyltransferase *Serum No Effect Analytical* No effect of concentrations up to 100 mg/L on method on Kodak Ektachem® *5706* No significant effect observed at a concentration of 10 mg/dL with method on Kodak Ektachem® systems *2519*

^{131}I Uptake *Serum Decrease Physiological* Contains iodine, inhibits further uptake *3669*

Indomethacin

Alanine Aminotransferase *Serum Increase Physiological* Cytotoxic and cholestatic liver damage *3100* Toxic hepatitis and jaundice may occur in less than 1% treated patients *3980*

Serum No Effect Analytical No effect at therapeutic concentration on Boehringer Mannheim Reflotron method *3231* On continuous method at 10 times maximal therapeutic concentration. On colorimetric method at 10 times maximal therapeutic concentration *2919* No effect at 100 mg/L on Boehringer Mannheim Reflotron method *5706*

Albumin *Serum No Effect Analytical* At concentration of 13 mg/L had no effect on BCG method *5704* On bromocresol green method on Technicon SMA II at physiological concentration *2922* No interference observed at a concentration of 3 mg/L (8.4 µmol/L) with method on Du Pont aca *1507*

Serum No Effect Physiological No effect seen in patients undergoing treatment *2922*

Urine No Effect Analytical Using a fluorimetric assay with Albumin Blue 580 on a Cobas Fara centrifugal analyzer for the detection of microalbuminuria no significant interference was detected at a concentration of 10 mg/L *3117*

Aldosterone *Plasma Decrease Physiological* Significant reduction from mean baseline concentration of 177 pmol/L to 100 pmol/L at 30 min, 89 pmol/L at 60 min, 104 pmol/L at 90 min and 94 pmol/L at 120 minutes in 7 healthy male volunteers following 50 mg orally *4303* Marked reversal on withdrawal of drug in one young woman *5939*

Plasma Increase Physiological Administration of 50 mg t.i.d. for one day was associated with a significant increase in concentration from 383 ± 41 pmol/L to 692 ± 75 pmol/L, not significantly different from controls *6167*

Plasma No Effect Physiological Insignificant change with 1 week treatment *4076*

Urine Decrease Physiological With 1 week treatment fell from 43 to 18 µg/24 h *4076* Marked reversal on withdrawal of drug in one young woman *5939*

Alkaline Phosphatase *Serum Increase Physiological* Toxic hepatitis and jaundice may occur in less than 1% treated patients *3980* Cytotoxic and cholestatic liver damage *3100*

Serum No Effect Analytical On continuous method *2919*

Aminoglycosides *Serum Increase Physiological* Concurrent administration may cause increased concentrations because of reduced clearance *1384*

Amylase *Serum Increase Physiological* Single case reported (?correct implication) *2358*

Serum No Effect Analytical At a concentration of 100 mg/L had no effect on method on Boehringer Mannheim Reflotron system *5706*

Amylase, Pancreatic Isoenzyme

Serum No Effect Analytical No significant effect observed at toxic concentration of 10 mg/L on method on Boehringer Mannheim Reflotron *3647*

Angiotensin-II *Plasma No Effect Physiological* In 12 patients with coronary artery disease, although systolic blood pressure increased and coronary blood flow decreased *1914*

Angiotensin-converting Enzyme

Serum No Effect Physiological No change observed over 120 minutes in 7 healthy volunteers given either 25 or 50 mg

Indomethacin *(continued)*

Angiotensin-converting Enzyme *(continued)* orally *4303* In 9 uncomplicated essential hypertensives receiving chronic enalapril treatment *5208*

Apolipoprotein A-I *Serum Decrease Physiological* In proteinuric patients treatment with indomethacin augmented the effect of lisinopril alone in reducing both protein excretion and plasma concentration of apolipoprotein A-I: subsequent treatment with indomethacin alone had a comparable effect to that of lisinopril alone *4235*

Apolipoprotein B *Serum Decrease Physiological* In proteinuric patients treatment with indomethacin augmented the effect of lisinopril alone in reducing both protein excretion and plasma concentration of apolipoprotein B: subsequent treatment with indomethacin alone had a comparable effect to that of lisinopril alone *4235*

Apolipoprotein Lp(a) *Serum Decrease Physiological* In proteinuric patients treatment with indomethacin augmented the effect of lisinopril alone in reducing both protein excretion and plasma concentration of apolipoprotein Lp(a): subsequent treatment with indomethacin alone had a comparable effect to that of lisinopril alone *4235*

Aspartate Aminotransferase *Serum Increase Physiological* Cytotoxic and cholestatic liver damage *3100* Toxic hepatitis and jaundice may occur in less than 1% treated patients *3980*
Serum No Effect Analytical On continuous method at 10 times maximal therapeutic concentration. On colorimetric method at 10 times maximal therapeutic concentration *2919* No effect at therapeutic concentration on Boehringer Mannheim Reflotron method *3231* No effect at 100 mg/L on Boehringer Mannheim Reflotron method *5706*

Bicarbonate *Serum No Effect Analytical* At concentration of 13 mg/L had no effect on method using phenolphthalein *5704*

Bile *Urine Increase Physiological* Cytotoxic and cholestatic liver damage *139*

Bilirubin *Serum Increase Physiological* Cytotoxic and cholestatic types of liver damage *3100* Toxic hepatitis and jaundice may occur in less than 1% treated patients *3980*
Serum No Effect Analytical No effect at therapeutic concentrations on Jendrassik-Grof, dimethylsulfoxide and spectrophotometric methods *2920* On diazo method on Technicon SMA II at physiological concentration *2922* At concentration of 100 mg/L no effect on method on Boehringer Mannheim Reflotron system *5706* No effect at 10 mg/L on Ames Seralyzer method *5706* At concentration of 13 mg/L had no effect on Jendrassik and Grof method *5704*
Serum No Effect Physiological Although tightly bound to protein at pharmacological concentrations has little or no displacement effect *6314* No effect seen in patients undergoing treatment *2922*

Bilirubin, Direct *Serum Increase Physiological* Cytotoxic and cholestatic liver damage *3100*

Bilirubin, Unconjugated *Serum Increase Physiological* Displaces bilirubin from albumin *1384*

Blood *Urine Increase Physiological* Hematuria may occur in less than 1% treated patients *3980*

BSP Retention *Serum Increase Physiological* Cytotoxic and cholestatic liver damage *3100*

Calcium *Serum No Effect Analytical* On cresolphthalein complexone method on Technicon SMA II at physiological concentrations *2922* At concentration of 13 mg/L had no effect on cresolphthalein method *5704*
Serum No Effect Physiological No effect seen in patients undergoing treatment *2922*

Casts *Urine Increase Physiological* Granular casts in one patient *779*

Catecholamines *Plasma No Effect Physiological* In 12 patients with coronary artery disease, although systolic blood pressure increased and coronary blood flow decreased *1914*

Chloride *Serum No Effect Analytical* At concentration of 13 mg/L had no effect on mercurimetric method *5704*
Urine Increase Physiological Administration of 50 mg t.i.d. for one day was associated with a significant increase in urinary chloride excretion from 7.9 ± 2.7 μmol/min to 157.6 ± 16.6 μmol/min, but significantly less than in controls *6167*

Cholesterol *Serum Decrease Physiological* In proteinuric patients treatment with indomethacin augmented the effect of lisinopril alone in reducing both protein excretion and plasma concentration of cholesterol: subsequent treatment with indomethacin alone had a comparable effect to that of lisinopril alone *4235*
Serum No Effect Analytical At concentration of 30 mg/L had no effect on CHOD-PAP method *5704* At concentration of 30 mg/L had no effect on catalase-AIDH method *5704* At concentration of 30 mg/L had no effect on CHOD-Iodide method *5704* At concentration of 30 mg/L had no effect on Liebermann-Burchard method *5704* No effect at 10 mg/L on Ames Seralyzer method *5706* No effect at therapeutic concentrations on enzymatic and Liebermann-Burchard methods *2920* On enzymatic method on Technicon SMA II at physiological concentration *2922* At concentration of 30 mg/L had no effect on method using catalase-Hantzsch reaction *5704* No effect at therapeutic concentration on Boehringer Mannheim Reflotron method *3231* At concentration of 100 mg/L no effect on method on Boehringer Mannheim Reflotron system *5706*
Serum No Effect Physiological No effect seen in patients undergoing treatment *2922*

Cholinesterase *Serum No Effect Analytical* No effect observed at concentration of 1 mg/dL with butyrylthiocholine method on Kodak Ektachem® *2504*

Chondrex *Serum No Effect Analytical* Concentrations up to 10 g/L had no significant effect on sandwich-type ELISA procedure of Harvey et al *2491*

Color *Feces Increase Analytical* Green color reported with ingestion of indomethacin *3388*
Urine Increase Analytical Indirect result of hepatic toxicity, green urine *1832*

Cortisol *Plasma Decrease Physiological* Nonsignificant reduction from mean baseline concentration of 264 nmol/L to 217 nmol/L at 30 min, 215 nmol/L at 60 min, 240 nmol/L at 90 min and 234 nmol/L at 120 minutes in 7 healthy male volunteers following 50 mg orally *4303*
Plasma No Effect Analytical At concentration of 10 mg/L no significant effect observed on CEDIA method (worst case recovey 95.2%) *1097*

Creatine Kinase *Serum No Effect Analytical* On continuous method *2919* No effect at 10 mg/L on method on Ames Seralyzer *5706*

Creatinine *Serum Increase Physiological* Oliguric renal failure developed in one man during treatment: reversible *2041* Associated with increasing risk of renal insufficiency in cirrhosis, nephrotic syndrome, decompensated congestive heart failure and chronic renal disease *595* Associated with decreased secretion of renin and aldosterone, decreased sodium delivery to distal tubule and reduction of urinary flow rate *2013*
Serum No Effect Analytical At concentration of 40 mg/L had no effect on kinetic Jaffe method on BKA-2 *5704* No effect at therapeutic concentrations on alkaline picrate and Slot methods *2920* At concentration of 6 mg/L had no effect on creatinine iminohydrolase method *5704* At concentration of 30 mg/L had no effect on Jaffe-Fading-Fraction method *5704* On alkaline picrate method on Technicon SMA II at physiological concentration *2922* At concentration of 13 mg/L had no effect on Technicon AutoAnalyzer® Jaffe method *5704* No effect up to 1.5 mg/L on Ames Seralyzer method but at higher concentrations apparently clinically significant reduction in creatinine concentration *5706* At concentration of 30 mg/L had no effect on Jaffe-Fuller's earth method *5704*
Serum No Effect Physiological No effect seen in patients undergoing treatment *2922*

Creatinine Clearance *Urine Decrease Physiological* Reduced by about 50% in states of diminished circulatory blood volume *5457*
Urine No Effect Physiological No significant change observed in 8 healthy volunteers given 50 mg three times daily for 3 days *4549*

Dexamethasone Suppression
Patient Abnormal Physiological False negative results have been reported when indomethacin administered *3969*

Digoxin *Serum Increase Physiological* Coadministration with digoxin may increase the digoxin concentration *2161* Coadministration of indomethacin with digoxin reported to increase the serum concentration and prolong the half life of digoxin *3980* Intravenous administration decreases renal excretion in premature infants *1384*

Doxazosin *Serum No Effect Physiological* Coadministration with doxazosin had no effect on its pharmacokinetics *4642*

Eosinophils *Blood Decrease Physiological* Occasional effect *617*
Blood Increase Physiological Oliguric renal failure developed in one man during treatment: reversible *2041*

Erythrocyte Sedimentation Rate
Blood Increase Physiological Oliguric renal failure developed in one man during treatment: reversible *2041*

Erythrocytes *Blood Decrease Physiological* Secondary to gastrointestinal bleed/agranulocytosis/pancytopenia *605* Occasional case of aplastic anemia reported *6264*
Urine Increase Physiological Oliguric renal failure developed in one man during treatment: reversible *2041* May cause actual bleeding *1714*

Felodipine *Serum No Effect Physiological* No significant effect observed on either felodipine or indomethacin concentrations when drugs coadministered *266*

Fibrin Degradation Products *Urine Decrease Physiological* In 2/3 patients with proliferative glomerulonephritis *1053*

Glomerular Filtration Rate *Urine Decrease Physiological* Transient reduction in individuals during sustained diuresis (fell from 114 mL/minute to 100 mL/min) *4076*
Urine No Effect Physiological In 23 hypertensive patients treated with 75 mg/d for 3 weeks mean flow 81.76 ± 7.41 mL/min not significantly different from 73.79 ± 6.11 mL/min in placebo-treated patients *4790*

Glucagon *Plasma No Effect Physiological* Ingestion of 100 mg daily by 7 healthy volunteers had no effect on plasma glucagon concentration *5354*

Glucose *Serum Increase Physiological* Rare side effect *2451* Hyperglycemia and glycosuria may occur in less than 1% treated patients *3980* In one patient with psoriatic arthritis, reverted to normal with drug withdrawal *6042*
Serum No Effect Analytical At concentration of 100 mg/L no effect on method on Boehringer Mannheim Reflotron system *5706* At concentration of 40 mg/L had no effect on hexokinase/G-6-PDH method *5704* At concentration of 25 mg/L had no effect on GOD/POD-PAP method *5704* At concentration of 4 mg/L had no effect on Kodak Ektachem® method *5704* No effect at therapeutic concentration on Boehringer Mannheim Reflotron method *3231* On hexokinase method on Technicon SMA II at physiological concentrations *2922* No effect at therapeutic concentrations on hexokinase, glucose dehydrogenase 2,4-dichlorophenol, ABTS and o-toluidine methods *2920* No effect up to 10 mg/L on glucose oxidase method on Ames Seralyzer but above this concentration apparent reduction in glucose concentration although not of clinical significance *5706*
Serum No Effect Physiological No effect seen in patients undergoing treatment *2922*
Urine Increase Physiological Rare side effect. As result of rare hyperglycemia *2451* Hyperglycemia and glycosuria may occur in less than 1% treated patients *3980*

γ-Glutamyltransferase *Serum No Effect Analytical* No effect at therapeutic concentration on Boehringer Mannheim Reflotron method *3231* At concentration of 100 mg/L no effect on method on Boehringer Mannheim Reflotron system *5706*
Urine No Effect Physiological No significant effect on excretion in 18 patients with degenerative arthritis and normal renal function when treated with 150 mg/24 hours for 7 days *5284*

Granulocytes *Blood Decrease Physiological* Agranulocytosis may occur in less than 1% treated patients *3980*

Growth Hormone *Plasma Increase Physiological* In 7 healthy volunteers 100 mg indomethacin daily caused increase from mean baseline concentration of 1.7 ng/mL to 5.4 ng/mL *5354*

Haptoglobin *Serum Decrease Physiological* May cause hemolytic anemia *128*

HDL-Cholesterol *Serum Decrease Physiological* In proteinuric patients treatment with indomethacin augmented the effect of lisinopril alone in reducing both protein excretion and plasma concentration of HDL-cholesterol: subsequent treatment with indomethacin alone had a comparable effect to that of lisinopril alone *4235*
Serum No Effect Analytical At a concentration up to 100 mg/L had no significant effect on Reflotron method for whole blood cholesterol *6352*

Hematocrit *Blood Decrease Physiological* Aplastic or hemolytic anemia may occur in less than 1% treated patients *3980* Secondary to gastrointestinal bleeding: agranulocytosis/pancytopenia *605*

Hemoglobin *Blood Decrease Physiological* Aplastic or hemolytic anemia may occur in less than 1% treated patients *3980* Secondary to gastrointestinal bleeding: agranulocytosis/pancytopenia *605*
Urine Increase Physiological Produces actual bleeding *1714*

Histamine *Plasma No Effect Analytical* Improbable inhibition of radio-enzyme assay at physiological concentrations *2492*

Hydroxybutyrate Dehydrogenase
Serum No Effect Analytical On continuous method at 10 times maximal therapeutic concentrations *2919*

Iron *Serum No Effect Analytical* No effect at therapeutic concentrations on bathophenanthroline and Ramsay methods *2920* On Ferrozine method on Technicon SMA II at physiological concentrations *2922*
Serum No Effect Physiological No effect seen in patients undergoing treatment *2922*

6-Keto-Prostaglandin $F_{1\alpha}$ *Urine Decrease Physiological* Reduction by about 40% in 18 patients with degenerative arthritis and normal renal function treated with 150 mg/24 hours for 7 days *5284* In 9 uncomplicated essential hypertensives receiving chronic enalapril treatment *5208*

Lactate *Plasma No Effect Analytical* At concentration of 40 mg/L had no effect on enzymatic method *5704*

Lactate Dehydrogenase *Serum No Effect Analytical* On colorimetric method at 10 times maximal therapeutic concentrations *2919* With lactate or pyruvate as substrate on continuous method *2919* No effect at 10 mg/L on method on Ames Seralyzer *5706*

Lecithin:Cholesterol Acyltransferase
Serum Decrease Physiological In proteinuric patients treatment with indomethacin augmented the effect of lisinopril alone in reducing both protein excretion and the increased plasma activity of LCAT: subsequent treatment with indomethacin alone had a comparable effect to that of lisinopril alone *4235*

Leukocytes *Blood Decrease Physiological* Leukopenia may occur in less than 1% treated patients *3980* Agranulocytosis/pancytopenia *5001* Occasional case of aplastic anemia reported *6264* Rare side effect reported to UK Committee on Safety of Medicines *1204*
Urine Increase Physiological Oliguric renal failure developed in one man during treatment: reversible *2041*

Lipase *Serum Increase Physiological* Associated with cholestatic liver damage *2024*

Lithium *Serum Increase Physiological* Lithium toxicity reported with the concomitant administration of indomethacin *4399* 7 days treatment with 150 mg/day in three manic patients caused increase of plasma lithium by 59% at steady state. In four other volunteers average increase of 30% observed with reduction of lithium clearance *4831* Concomitant administration caused clinically relevant increase and delirium in one patient *1384* Concentration increased due to reduction of lithium clearance *1384* Coadministration of indomethacin with lithium reported to cause a clinically relevant increase of plasma lithium concentration and reduction of its renal clearance in normal and psychiatric patients *3980* Concentration increased from 0.9 to 1.4 mEq/L within 6 d of indomethacin administration in 3 patients due to reduced lithium excretion possibly by inhibition of prostaglandin action *4832*

Lithium Clearance *Urine Decrease Physiological* Lithium toxicity reported with the concomitant administration of indomethacin *4399* Average reduction of 31% observed in healthy volunteers in whom plasma concentration increased by 30% *4831* Coadministration of indomethacin with lithium reported to cause a clinically relevant increase of plasma lithium concentration and reduction of its renal clearance in normal and psychiatric patients *3980*

Methotrexate *Serum Increase Physiological* Coadministration of indomethacin with methotrexate reported to increase methotrexate concentration by decreasing its tubular secretion *3980*

Indomethacin *(continued)*

N-Acetyl-Glucosaminidase *Urine No Effect Physiological* No significant effect in 18 patients with degenerative arthritis and normal renal function when treated with 150 mg/24 hours for 7 days *5284*

Neutrophils *Blood Decrease Physiological* Occasional case of agranulocytosis reported *6264* Rare neutropenia/may also cause aplastic anemia *2242* Occasional case of drug-induced neutropenia *241*

Nitroblue Tetrazolium Test *Blood Increase Physiological* Mechanism not discussed *1483*

5'-Nucleotidase *Serum Increase Physiological* Due to cholestasis *2911*

Occult Blood *Feces Increase Physiological* May cause ulceration of stomach, duodenum, gut with rectal bleeding in less than 1% treated patients *3980* Rare side effect reported to UK Committee on Safety of Medicines *1204*

2',5'-Oligoadenylate Synthetase
Serum Increase Physiological 2.8-fold increase to 115.5 ± 21 pg/dL from mean baseline of 40.2 ± 7.9 pg/dL observed 8 hours after administration in 21 patients with chronic active hepatitis B or C *177*

p-Aminophenol *Urine No Effect Analytical* With addition of drugs at a concentration of 100 mg/L and of related compounds at 50 mg/L no significant effect observed on colorimetric method of van Bocxlaer on Cobas Mira analyzer which involves reacting free p-aminophenol with resorcinol in the presence of magnesium ions to form an indophenol dye measured at 550 nm *6163*

Phenylalanine *Plasma No Effect Analytical* No interference observed with rapid quantitative whole blood method of Campbell et al using phenylalanine dehydrogenase *867*

Phosphate *Serum No Effect Analytical* At concentration of 13 mg/L had no effect on phosphomolybdate method *5704*

Platelet Aggregation *Blood Decrease Physiological* Effect less marked that observed with treatment with aspirin *3694* Observed *in vitro*, might cause gastrointestinal bleeding etc *915* Aggregation reduced: dose and plasma concentration related. Effect is shorter than with aspirin *1384*
Blood Increase Physiological Significant interference with platelet aggregation reported *6557*

Platelets *Blood Decrease Physiological* Thrombocytopenic purpura may occur in less than 1% treated patients *3980* Rare agranulocytosis/pancytopenia/aplastic anemia *5001* Occasional case of aplastic anemia reported *6264* Rare side effect reported to UK Committee on Safety of Medicines *1204*

Potassium *Serum Increase Physiological* Associated with increasing risk of renal insufficiency in cirrhosis, nephrotic syndrome, decompensated congestive heart failure and chronic renal disease *595* Significant increase from mean baseline concentration of 3.9 mmol/L to 4.1 mmol/L at 30 minutes and subsequently in 7 healthy male volunteers given 50 mg orally but, in effect, no change when given only 25 mg orally *4303* Observed in 3 patients with gouty arthritis who developed renal insufficiency *1863* Associated with decreased secretion of renin and aldosterone, decreased sodium delivery to distal tubule and reduction of urinary flow rate *2013* Rise from 4.3 to 4.6 mmol/L with treatment for 1 week *4076* Marked reversal on withdrawal of drug in one young woman *5939* Hyperkalemia may occur in less than 1% treated patients *3980* Administration of 50 mg t.i.d. for one day was associated with a significant increase in plasma potassium concentration from 3.93 ± 0.08 mmol/L to 5.05 ± 0.06 mmol/L, not significantly different from controls *6167*
Serum No Effect Analytical At concentration of 40 mg/L had no effect on measurement by ISE without predilution *5704* At concentration of 13 mg/L had no effect on measurement by ISE with predilution *5704*
Urine Increase Physiological Administration of 50 mg t.i.d. for one day was associated with a significant increase in urinary potassium excretion from 75.8 ± 9.6 µmol/min to 301.7 ± 20.5 µmol/min, not significantly different from controls *6167*
Urine No Effect Physiological No significant change observed in 8 healthy volunteers given 50 mg three times daily for 3 days *4549*

Pramipexole *Serum No Effect Physiological* Coadministration of indomethacin with pramipexole presumed to have no effect on the oral clearance of pramipexole *4680*

Prazosin *Serum No Effect Physiological* Coadministration of prazosin with indomethacin had no apparent adverse drug interaction in limited clinical experience *4649*

Prolactin *Plasma No Effect Physiological* In up to 35 healthy men given 100 mg/d for 1 week in response to TRH stimulation *4841*

Prostaglandin E *Plasma Decrease Physiological* Decrease by 67% in rats at least *2880* In up to 35 healthy men given 100 mg/d for 1 week *4841*

Prostaglandin E_2 *Plasma Decrease Physiological* Significant reduction from mean baseline concentration of 5.3 pg/mL to 4.1 pg/mL at 45 min, 3.8 pg/mL at 60 and 90 min, and 4.4 pg/mL at 120 min in 7 healthy male volunteers following 50 mg orally but no significant change observed after 25 mg orally *4303*
Urine No Effect Physiological Administration of 50 mg t.i.d. for one day was associated with no significant change in excretion from 0.17 ± 0.08 pmol/min to 0.18 ± 0.07 pmol/min, not significantly different from controls *6167*

Prostaglandin F *Plasma Decrease Physiological* In up to 35 healthy men given 100 mg/d for 1 week *4841*

Prostaglandins *Urine Decrease Physiological* Marked reversal on withdrawal of drug in one young woman *5939* Reduction by about 70% in 18 patients with degenerative arthritis and normal renal function treated with 150 mg/24 hours for 7 days *5284*

Protein *Serum Decrease Physiological* Nephrotic syndrome or interstitial nephritis may occur in less than 1% treated patients *3980*
Serum No Effect Analytical At concentration of 13 mg/L had no effect on biuret method with blank correction *5704* No effect at therapeutic concentrations on biuret and spectrophotometric methods *2920* On biuret method on Technicon SMA II at physiological concentrations *2922*
Serum No Effect Physiological No effect seen in patients undergoing treatment *2922*
Urine Increase Physiological Reported in one patient *779* Oliguric renal failure developed in one man during treatment: reversible *2041* Proteinuria may occur in less than 1% treated patients *3980*

Protein Electrophoresis *Serum No Effect Analytical* At concentration of 40 mg/L had no effect on automated Olympus-Hite method except for slight displacement of fractions *5704*

Prothrombin Time *Plasma Increase Physiological* Displaces anticoagulants from binding protein *4144*
Plasma No Effect Physiological Coadministration of indomethacin with oral anticoagulants had no effect on prothrombin time *3980*

Renal Blood Flow *Patient Decrease Physiological* Associated with decreased secretion of renin and aldosterone, decreased sodium delivery to distal tubule and reduction of urinary flow rate *2013*
Patient No Effect Physiological No significant effect observed in 8 healthy volunteers given 50 mg three times daily for 3 days *4549*

Renal Plasma Flow *Patient No Effect Physiological* In 23 hypertensive patients treated with 75 mg/d for 3 weeks mean flow 335.38 ± 31.81 mL/min not significantly different from 309.16 ± 29.41 mL/min in placebo-treated patients *4790*

Renin Activity *Plasma Decrease Physiological* In 9 uncomplicated essential hypertensives receiving chronic enalapril treatment *5208* Significant reduction from mean of 1.7 ng/mL/h to mean of 0.7 ng/mL/h in 8 healthy volunteers given 50 mg three times daily for 3 days *4549* Marked reversal on withdrawal of drug in one young woman *5939* In 7 healthy male volunteers 25 mg orally caused reduction from mean baseline of 0.28 ng/L/s to 0.21 ng/L/s at 30 min, 0.19 ng/L/s at 60 min and 0.14 ng/L/s at 120 min. With 50 mg reduction of similar magnitude *4303* Administration of indomethacin reduces basal PRA as well as increases induced by furosemide or salt or volume depletion *3980*
Plasma No Effect Physiological In 12 patients with coronary artery disease, although systolic blood pressure increased and coronary blood flow decreased *1914* Administration of 50 mg t.i.d. for one day was associated with no significant change in concentration from 493 ± 124 fmol/L/s to 459 ± 127 fmol/L/s, not significantly different from controls *6167* Insignificant change with 1 week treatment *4076*

Sodium *Serum Decrease Physiological* Marked reduction in some neonates (to below 130 mmol/L) within 48 h of administration to close patent ductus arteriosus *2427*
Serum No Effect Analytical At concentration of 13 mg/L had no effect on measurement by ISE with predilution *5704* At concentration of 40 mg/L had no effect on measurement by ISE without predilution *5704*
Serum No Effect Physiological No significant change observed over next 120 minutes in 7 healthy male volunteers given either 25 mg or 50 mg orally *4303*
Urine Decrease Physiological Caused by increased tubular absorption with marked oliguria as a result *5457*
Urine Increase Physiological Administration of 50 mg t.i.d. for one day was associated with a significant increase in urinary sodium excretion from 19.9 ± 6.1 µmol/min to 123.7 ± 25.1 µmol/min, but significantly less than in controls *6167*
Urine No Effect Physiological Insignificant reduction in 8 healthy volunteers given 50 mg three times daily for 3 days *4549*

Sucrose *Serum No Effect Analytical* Using automated procedure involving sucrose phosphorylase, phosphoglutamase and glucose-6-phosphatase of Vinet et al no significant interference observed at a concentration of 0.1 mmol/L *6267*
Urine No Effect Analytical Using automated procedure involving sucrose phosphorylase, phosphoglutamase and glucose-6-phosphatase of Vinet et al no significant interference observed at a concentration of 0.1 mmol/L *6267*

Thromboxane B_2 *Plasma Decrease Physiological* In 9 uncomplicated essential hypertensives receiving chronic enalapril treatment *5208* Marked fall from 191 ng/mL to 1.4 ng/mL in 12 patients with coronary artery disease, although systolic blood pressure increased and coronary blood flow decreased *1914*
Urine Decrease Physiological Reduction by about 40% in 18 patients with degenerative arthritis and normal renal function treated with 150 mg/24 hours for 7 days *5284*

Thyroid Stimulating Hormone
Serum No Effect Physiological No effect on TSH secretion *6412* In 10 individuals treated with a mean dose of 108 mg/d for at least 3 weeks mean concentration of 1.9 ± 0.2 mU/L not significantly different from 1.5 ± 0.2 mU/L in 22 controls *585*

Thyroxine (T4) *Serum Increase Analytical* Using the Ciba-Corning ACS:180 analyzer mean concentration not significantly changed in 1 specimen whose concentration differed by +10% compared with the concentration measured by the Amerlex-M method *5621*
Serum No Effect Physiological In 10 individuals treated with a mean dose of 108 mg/d for at least 3 weeks mean concentration of 93 ± 6 nmol/L not significantly different from 94 ± 4 nmol/L in 22 controls *585* In up to 35 healthy men given 100 mg/d for 1 week *4841*

Thyroxine (T4) Index, Free *Serum No Effect Physiological* In 10 individuals treated with a mean dose of 108 mg/d for at least 3 weeks mean FTI of 88 ± 6 not significantly from 93 ± 4 in 22 controls *585*

Tiludronate *Serum Increase Physiological* Bioavailabilty of tiludronate is increased 2 - 4-fold by indomethacin *5258*

Tri-iodothyronine (T3) *Serum No Effect Physiological* In up to 35 healthy men given 100 mg/d for 1 week *4841*

Triglycerides *Serum Decrease Physiological* In proteinuric patients treatment with indomethacin augmented the effect of lisinopril alone in reducing both protein excretion and plasma concentration of triglycerides: subsequent treatment with indomethacin alone had a comparable effect to that of lisinopril alone *4235*
Serum No Effect Analytical No effect at therapeutic concentration on Boehringer Mannheim Reflotron method *3231* No effect at 100 mg/L on Boehringer Mannheim Reflotron method *5706* On enzymatic method on Technicon SMA II at physiological concentrations *2922* No effect on enzymatic methods at therapeutic concentrations *2920* At concentration of 13 mg/L had no effect on lipase/esterase method *5704*
Serum No Effect Physiological No effect seen in patients undergoing treatment *2922*

Tryptophan *Plasma Decrease Physiological* (total measured) in rheumatoids on therapy *303*

Tryptophan, Free *Plasma Increase Physiological* In rheumatoids on therapy *303*

TSH response to TRH *Serum Increase Physiological* In up to 35 healthy men given 100 mg/d for 1 week *4841*
Serum No Effect Physiological In up to 35 healthy men given 100 mg/d for 1 week *4841*

Urea Nitrogen *Serum Increase Physiological* Occasional increase usually to upper normal limit *4023* Associated with increasing risk of renal insufficiency in cirrhosis, nephrotic syndrome, decompensated congestive heart failure and chronic renal disease *595* Associated with decreased secretion of renin and aldosterone, decreased sodium delivery to distal tubule and reduction of urinary flow rate *2013* Oliguric renal failure developed in one man during treatment: reversible *2041* Increased plasma urea nitrogen, renal insufficiency (including renal failure) may occur in less than 1% treated patients *3980*
Serum No Effect Analytical On diacetyl monoxime method on Technicon SMA II at physiological concentration *2922* No effect at therapeutic concentrations on glutamate dehydrogenase, phenol- hypochlorite and diacetyl monoxime methods *2920* No effect at 10 mg/L on method on Ames Seralyzer *5706* At concentration of 4 mg/L had no effect on Kodak Ektachem® method *5704* No effect at therapeutic concentration on Boehringer Mannheim Reflotron method *3231* At concentration of 13 mg/L had no effect on diacetylmonoxime method *5704* No effect of concentrations up to 4 mg/L on method on Kodak Ektachem® *5706* No effect at 100 mg/L on Boehringer Mannheim Reflotron method *5706*
Serum No Effect Physiological No effect seen in patients undergoing treatment *2922*

Uric Acid *Serum Decrease Physiological* Of some value in treatment of gouty arthritis *2222*
Serum Increase Physiological Oliguric renal failure developed in one man during treatment: reversible *2041*
Serum No Effect Analytical No effect at 100 mg/L on method on Boehringer Mannheim Reflotron *5706* At concentration of 13 mg/L had no effect on phosphotungstate reduction method *5704* At concentration of 25 mg/L had no effect on uricase-PAP method *5704* At concentration of 30 mg/L had no effect on Kageyama-Hantzsch method *5704* At concentration of 30 mg/L had no effect on catalase-AIDH method *5704* On phosphotungstate method on Technicon SMA II at physiological concentration *2922* No effect at therapeutic concentration on Boehringer Mannheim Reflotron method *3231* No effect at therapeutic concentrations on uricase-catalase, aldehyde dehydrogenase, direct UV-test, phosphotungstate methods *2920*
Serum No Effect Physiological No effect seen in patients undergoing treatment *2922*

VLDL + LDL-Cholesterol *Serum Decrease Physiological* In proteinuric patients treatment with indomethacin augmented the effect of lisinopril alone in reducing both protein excretion and plasma concentration of VLDL and LDL-cholesterol: subsequent treatment with indomethacin alone had a comparable effect to that of lisinopril alone *4235*

Volume *Urine Decrease Physiological* Caused by increased tubular absorption with marked oliguria as a result *5457*
Urine No Effect Physiological Insignificant reduction in 8 healthy volunteers given 50 mg three times daily for 3 days *4549*

Xylose *Urine Decrease Physiological* ?due to increased motility of gut *3105*

Influenza Virus Vaccine

Theophylline *Serum Increase Physiological* May prolong half-life of theophylline *1384*
Serum No Effect Physiological No documented significant interaction with theophylline reported *6117* No clinically significant effect on theophylline concentration observed when drugs coadministered *5999*

Inositol

Ketones *Urine Increase Analytical* Possible reported effect *2999*

Phosphate *Urine No Effect Analytical* No effect at a concentration of 20 mg/dL in method of Jung/Parekh *2992*

Insulin

Albumin *Serum No Effect Analytical* At concentration of 3 mg/L had no effect on BCG method *5704*

Amino Acids *Plasma Decrease Physiological* Metabolic effects *570*
Urine Decrease Physiological Metabolic effects *2024*
Urine Increase Physiological Metabolic effects *1714*

α-Amino-Nitrogen *Plasma Decrease Physiological* Increased uptake by tissues *2024*

Bicarbonate *Serum No Effect Analytical* At concentration of 3 mg/L had no effect on method using phenolphthalein *5704*

Bilirubin *Serum No Effect Analytical* At concentration of 3 mg/L had no effect on Jendrassik and Grof method *5704*

Calcium *Serum Decrease Physiological* Reported effect *570*
Serum No Effect Analytical At concentration of 3 mg/L had no effect on cresolphthalein method *5704*

Chloride *Serum No Effect Analytical* At concentration of 3 mg/L had no effect on mercurimetric method *5704*

Cholesterol *Serum Decrease Physiological* Average reduction of 0.36 mmol/L in 15 diabetic patients treated for 9 months *4229* Therapeutic goal *5869* In 14 patients with NIDDM treatment with insulin caused significant reduction from mean baseline of 6.29 ± 0.42 mmol/L to 4.98 ± 0.24 mmol/L after 3 months and 4.76 ± 0.26 mmol/L after 6 months *2561*
Serum No Effect Analytical At concentration of 3 mg/L had no effect on Liebermann-Burchard method *5704*

Corticosteroids *Plasma Increase Physiological* Large effect at 60 minutes after i.v. injection *5778*

Corticotropin *Plasma Increase Physiological* Significant effect after i.v. in normals 45-90 minutes *5778* Response to stress *4039* Mean concentration rose from baseline of 7.1 ng/L to 263 ng/L in 6 healthy volunteers following 0.2 mg intravenously with peak concentration occurring about 1 hour after administration *3612*

Cortisol *Plasma Increase Physiological* Marked effect in insulin induced hypoglycemia *5991* Increase from mean of 280 nmol/L to 602 nmol/L in 6 volunteers following 0.2 U/kg intravenously with peak occurring about 1 hour after administration *3612*

Creatine Kinase *Serum Increase Physiological* Is an activator of enzyme *1079*

Creatinine *Serum No Effect Analytical* At concentration of 3 mg/L had no effect on Technicon AutoAnalyzer® Jaffe method *5704*
Serum No Effect Physiological In 72 insulin treated patients with NIDDM mean concentration of 88 ± 31 μmol/L not significantly different from 92 ± 25 μmol/L in 20 diet treated patients *2532*

Dihydroxyphenylalanine *Plasma Decrease Physiological* Infusion at rate of 200 mU/m²/mL caused reduction of 233 pg/mL in obese and 376 pg/mL in lean individuals (difference between groups not significant) *4378*

Epinephrine *Plasma Increase Physiological* Stimulation of adrenal medulla, ?by hypoglycemia *4039* Marked effect in insulin induced hypoglycemia *5991* Markedly increased in 10 volunteers following insulin-induced hypoglycemia in 10 volunteers *1189*
Urine Increase Physiological Hypoglycemia produces up to tenfold increase *467*

Fatty Acids (FFA), Free *Serum Decrease Physiological* Effect similar in normals and diabetics *4742*

Gastrin *Serum Increase Physiological* Similar response (fairly marked) *6572*

Glucagon *Plasma Decrease Physiological* In 14 patients with NIDDM treatment with insulin caused significant reductions from mean baseline of 250 ± 20 ng/L to 190 ± 20 ng/L after 1 month, 200 ± 20 ng/L after 3 months and 200 ± 20 ng/L after 6 months *2561*
Plasma Increase Physiological Marked increase at 45 minutes after injection *4419*

Glucose *Serum Decrease Physiological* Natural action of hormone *3810* Anticipated reduction in 15 diabetics treated with drug for 9 months *4229* In 14 patients with NIDDM treatment with insulin caused significant reduction of fasting glucose from mean baseline of 15.7 ± 0.7 mmol/L to 6.4 ± 0.5 mmol/L after 1 month, 6.6 ± 0.4 mmol/L after 3 months and 6.3 ± 0.2 mmol/L after 6 months *2561* Incidence of 8.1% observed in French Pharmacovigilance database *4106*
Serum Increase Physiological In 72 insulin patients with NIDDM mean concentration of 8.9 ± 3.6 mmol/L significantly higher than 6.5 ± 1.9 mmol/L in 20 diet treated patients *2532*
Serum No Effect Analytical No effect of 1 U/L on hexokinase method on Ames Seralyzer *5706*
Urine Decrease Physiological In 14 patients with NIDDM treatment with insulin caused significant reduction from mean baseline of 600 ± 125 mmol/d to 33 ± 28 mmol/d after 1 month, 12 ± 8 mmol/d after 3 months and 5 ± 2 mmol/d after 6 months *2561*

Glycated Hemoglobin *Blood Increase Physiological* in 72 insulin treated patients with NIDDM mean concentration 8.4 ± 1.5% significantly higher than 6.6 ± 1.2% in 20 diet treated patients *2532*

Growth Hormone *Plasma Increase Physiological* In 12 healthy short stature children administration of 0.1 unit/kg intravenously caused mean increase of 0.8 nmol/L presumably by some mechanism other than GHRH release *2111* Occurs only when glucose down to 10 mg/dL *6492* Marked effect in insulin induced hypoglycemia *5991* In 12 healthy male volunteers significant increase at 30 to 60 minutes following injection *3825* Increase of 22 ng/mL after 0.1 U/kg *3584*

Growth Hormone Releasing Hormone
Plasma No Effect Physiological Insignificant mean increase of 0.5 pmol/L observed in 12 healthy short stature children given 0.1 U/kg intravenously *2111*

HDL-Cholesterol *Serum Increase Physiological* Average increase of 0.22 mmol/L in 15 diabetic patients treated for 15 months *4229*
Serum No Effect Physiological In 14 patients with NIDDM treatment with insulin caused nonsignificant from mean baseline of 0.97 ± 0.08 mmol/L to 1.05 ± 0.07 mmol/L after 3 months and 1.02 ± 0.07 mmol/L after 6 months *2561* In 72 patients with NIDDM mean concentration with insulin treatment 1.24 ± 0.42 mmol/L compared with 1.14 ± 0.48 mmol/L in 20 diet treated patients *2532*

Hemoglobin A_{1c} *Blood Decrease Physiological* In 14 patients with NIDDM mean concentration at baseline of 7.7 ± 0.3% significantly reduced to 6.1 ± 0.2% after 1 month, 5.3 ± 0.2% after 3 months and 5.1 ± 0.2% after 6 months *2561* Marked reduction in 15 diabetic patients treated for 9 months with drug *4229*

Histamine *Plasma No Effect Analytical* No inhibition of radio-enzyme assay at therapeutic concentrations *2492*

Hydrochloric Acid *Gastric Fluid Decrease Physiological* Absolute amount decreased by injection or infusion *902*
Gastric Fluid Increase Physiological Hypoglycemia is powerful stimulant *1252*

IgG Insulin Antibodies *Serum Positive Physiological* Observed in 47% of 45 children at mean level of 0.96 mU/mL treated long-term with porcine insulin but significant decrease of both number of patients and amount of antibodies when switched to semisynthetic human insulin (11% patients, mean 0.53 mU/mL) *1472*

Insulin *Plasma Increase Physiological* In 14 patients with NIDDM mean baseline of 308 ± 80 pmol/L increased to 392 ± 57 pmol/L after 1 month of insulin therapy, 513 ± 102 pmol/L after 3 months and 510 ± 102 pmol/L after 6 months *2561* In 12 healthy male volunteers significant increase at 30 to 60 minutes following injection *3825*

Ketones *Urine Increase Physiological* Occurs especially if low liver glycogen stores *2240*

LDL-Cholesterol *Serum No Effect Physiological* In 14 patients with NIDDM treatment with insulin caused no significant change from mean baseline of 2.98 ± 0.31 mmol/L to 3.01 ± 0.23 mmol/L after 3 months and 2.95 ± 0.21 mmol/L after 6 months *2561*

LDL-Receptor Activity *Tissue Increase Physiological* Increased activity observed with insulin administration *3730*

Lipoprotein Lp(a) *Serum No Effect Physiological* In 72 insulin treated patients with NIDDM mean concentration of 251 U/L not significantly higher than 190 U/L in 20 diet treated patients *2532*

Magnesium *Red Blood Cells Increase Physiological* Significant effect observed at 180 and 210 minutes of glucose tolerance test and when incubated with insulin *in vitro* due to shift of magnesium from plasma to erythrocytes *4501*

Serum Decrease Physiological Effect seen in treatment of diabetic coma *6285* Significant effect observed at 180 and 210 minutes of glucose tolerance test and when incubated with insulin *in vitro* due to shift of magnesium from plasma to erythrocytes *4501*

Norepinephrine *Plasma Increase Physiological* Infusion at rate of 200 mU/m²/min caused increase of 85 pg/mL in obese and 109 pg/mL in lean individuals *4378* Marked effect in insulin induced hypoglycemia *5991* Markedly increased in 10 volunteers following insulin-induced hypoglycemia *1189*
Urine No Effect Physiological Not appreciably affected by hypoglycemia *467*

Pepsin *Gastric Material Increase Physiological* Hypoglycemia is powerful stimulant *1252*

Phenprocoumon *Plasma No Effect Physiological* No effect noted with coadministration on half-life or plasma concentration *2538*

Phosphate *Serum Decrease Physiological* Increased phosphorylation of glucose *6515*
Serum No Effect Analytical At concentration of 3 mg/L had no effect on phosphomolybdate method *5704*

Potassium *Serum Decrease Physiological* Therapeutic effect, causes intracellular shift *2240*
Serum No Effect Analytical At concentration of 3 mg/L had no effect on measurement by ISE with predilution *5704*

Prazosin *Serum No Effect Physiological* Coadministration of prazosin with insulin had no apparent adverse drug interaction in limited clinical experience *4649*

Prolactin *Plasma Increase Physiological* In post vagotomy patients marked if i.v. or single injection *6492* Marked effect in insulin induced hypoglycemia *5991*
Plasma No Effect Physiological No significant effect with hypoglycemia *2382*

Protein *Serum Increase Physiological* Associated with increased protein synthesis *1095*
Serum No Effect Analytical At concentration of 3 mg/L had no effect on biuret method with blank correction *5704*

Sodium *Serum No Effect Analytical* At concentration of 3 mg/L had no effect on measurement by ISE with predilution *5704*
Urine Decrease Physiological Antinatriuresis with/without acidosis may be marked *5220* Infusion at rate of 200 mU/m²/mL caused reduction of excretion by 2.2 mmol/h in lean subjects *4378*
Urine Increase Physiological Infusion at rate of 200 mU/m²/mL caused increased excretion at rate of 5.3 mmol/L in obese individuals *4378*

Thyroid Stimulating Hormone
Serum No Effect Physiological No effect observed *4468*

Thyroxine (T4) *Serum Increase Physiological* Probable enhanced release from liver *6412*
Serum No Effect Physiological No change during insulin induced hypoglycemia *5991*

Tirofiban *Serum No Effect Physiological* Coadministration had no significant effect on plasma clearance of tirofiban *3957*

Tri-iodothyronine, Reverse (rT3)
Serum Decrease Physiological Fell from mean of 0.184 to 0.171 µg/L but not significant after i.v. injection *5991*

Tri-iodothyronine (T3) *Serum Increase Physiological* Mean increase from 1.86 to 2.51 µg/L at 45 minutes after injection *5991*

Triglycerides *Serum Decrease Physiological* In 14 patients with NIDDM treatment with insulin caused significant reduction from mean baseline of 5.02 ± 1.22 mmol/L to 2.16 ± 0.46 mmol/L after 3 months and 2.00 ± 0.30 mmol/L after 6 months *2561* Average reduction of 0.34 mmol/L in 15 diabetics treated for 9 months *4229*
Serum No Effect Analytical At concentration of 3 mg/L had no effect on lipase/esterase method *5704*
Serum No Effect Physiological In 72 insulin treated patients with NIDDM mean concentration of 1.86 mmol/L not significantly different from 1.93 mmol/L in 20 diet treated patients *2532*

TSH response to TRH *Serum No Effect Physiological* Hypoglycemia had no effect on TRH-stimulated TSH release *6412*

Urea Nitrogen *Serum No Effect Analytical* At concentration of 3 mg/L had no effect on diacetylmonoxime method *5704*

Uric Acid *Serum No Effect Analytical* At concentration of 3 mg/L had no effect on phosphotungstate reduction method *5704*

Vanillylmandelic Acid *Urine Increase Physiological* Increase after insulin shock, none with normal dose *5871*

Volume *Gastric Fluid Decrease Physiological* In response to injection or infusion *902*

Interferon

Alanine Aminotransferase *Serum Decrease Physiological* In patients with hepatitis C successful treatment was associated with a reduction in ALT activity *6593* Significant reduction observed in 15 of 23 patients with chronic non-A, non-B hepatitis treated for 4 to 6 weeks with interferon-α or β *4398*

Anti-Hepatitis C Antibodies *Serum Decrease Physiological* In patients with hepatitis C successful treatment was associated with a decrease in the concentration of anti-c100-3 antibody *6593*

Hepatitis C Virus RNA *Serum Decrease Physiological* In patients with hepatitis C treated with interferon RNA concentration disappeared from serum for at least 24 months in those who responded. In partial responders RNA disappeared transiently and in transient or nonresponders RNA remained persistently positive *6593*

Interleukin-1α-Autoantibody *Serum Increase Physiological* In 3 patients with chronic active hepatitis with IL-1α autoantibody concentration greater than 2000 ng/mL during treatment concentration increased significantly although returning to lower levels on completion of treatment *2849*

2',5'-Oligoadenylate Synthetase
Neutrophils Increase Physiological Activity increased 2 - 41 times in 23 patients with chronic non-A, non-B hepatitis treated with either interferon-α or beta for 4 to 6 weeks *4398*

Theophylline *Serum Increase Physiological* Recombinant human α-A decreases theophylline clearance, increasing theophylline concentration by about 100% *5999*

Interferon-Alfa

Alanine Aminotransferase *Serum Decrease Physiological* In 20 patients with chronic hepatitis who had a sustained response over 12 months mean activity decreased to 85 ± 15 U/L compared with 112 ± 18 U/L in 20 nonresponders *6577*

Albumin *Serum Increase Physiological* In 20 patients with chronic hepatitis who had a sustained response over 12 months mean concentration increased to 4.11 ± 0.10 g/dL compared with 3.93 ± 0.10 g/dL in 20 nonresponders *6577*

Aspartate Aminotransferase
Serum Decrease Physiological In 20 patients with chronic hepatitis who had a sustained responseover 12 months mean activity decreased to 54 ± 8 U/L compared with 78 ± 15 U/L in 20 nonresponders *6577*

5-Fluorouracil *Serum Increase Physiological* Administration of interferon-α with 5-fluorouracil causes inhibition of dihydropyridimine dehydrogenase which is responsible for more than 80% of the metabolism of 5-FU leading to a significant increase in its plasma AUC *3909*

Procollagen III Peptide *Serum Decrease Physiological* In 20 patients with chronic hepatitis who had a sustained response over 12 months mean concentration decreased to 0.94 ± 0.05 U/mL compared with 1.07 ± 0.06 U/mL in 20 nonresponders *6577*

7S Collagen *Serum Decrease Physiological* In 20 patients with chronic hepatitis who had a sustained response over 12 months mean concentration decreased to 6.09 ± 0.40 ng/mL compared with 6.51 ± 0.67 ng/mL in 20 nonresponders *6577*

Vitronectin *Serum Increase Physiological* In 20 patients with chronic hepatitis who had a sustained response over 12 months mean concentration increased to 215 ± 16 µg/mL compared with 145 ± 10 µg/mL in 20 nonresponders *6577*

Interferon Alfa-2

Aspartate Aminotransferase *Serum Increase Physiological* Hepatotoxicity occurred at median of 6 to 9 days in patients with cancer treated with 10 MU/day intramuscularly *3157*

Cortisol *Plasma Increase Physiological* At dose level of 5 x 10^6 units significant increase observed in 5 healthy controls and 5 patients with hepatitis C *6441*

Immunoglobulin A *Serum Increase Physiological* In 15 patients with hepatitis C with cryoglobulinemia treatment for 24 weeks caused mean to increase from 191 mg/dL to 200 mg/dL (+6 ± 3%) *4068*

Leukocytes *Blood Decrease Physiological* At doses above 10 MU/day intramuscularly in patients with cancer, toxicity occurred at a median of 6 to 9 days *3157*

Thyroid Stimulating Hormone
Serum Decrease Physiological At dose of 5 x 10^6 units significant reduction observed in 5 healthy controls and 5 patients with hepatitis C. Effect occurred 12 h after injection with maximum suppression observed 24 h after injection *6441*

Thyroxine (T4) *Serum Decrease Physiological* Concentration maximally decreased 24 h after subcutaneous injection of 5 x 10^6 units in 5 healthy controls and 5 patients with hepatitis C *6441*

Tri-iodothyronine (T3) *Serum Decrease Physiological* Maximal suppression observed 24 hours after subcutaneous injection of 5 x 10^6 units in 5 healthy controls and 5 patients with hepatitis C *6441*

Interferon Alfa-2a

α_1-Acid Glycoprotein *Serum No Effect Physiological* In 7 cancer patients treatment with 3 x 10^6 units 3 times weekly for 2 weeks caused nonsignificant change from mean baseline of 125 ± 31 mg/dL to 140 ± 43 mg/dL *2843*

Alanine Aminotransferase *Serum Decrease Physiological* Significant reduction observed in patients with hepatitis C when treated with 3 MU three times per week with recombinant human α-interferon for 24 weeks although activity increased in many patients once treatment was stopped *3785* In 15 patients with hepatitis C with cryoglobulinemia who responded to 24 weeks treatment mean activity decreased from 62 U/L to 45 U/L (-2 ± 18%) *4068* In 30 patients with chronic non-A, non-B hepatitis treatment for 12 months caused reduction to normal in 70% with reduction to less than 50% baseline in another 10% *4882* May normalize serum ALT acyivity in patients with chronic hepatitis C *5032* Probability of normalization in patients with chronic hepatitis C treated with interferon-alfa three times weekly for 24 weeks 46% when dose of 3 million units used and 28% when dose of 1 million units used although relapse occurred in many later *1274* Rapid decrease observed in most patients with chronic hepatitis C frequently falling to within normal range and in other patients falling by as much as 50%. Average decrease with 6 months treatment was 62% *1410* In 10 of 14 patients (71%) with chronic hepatitis D treated with 9 million units intramuscularly 3 times weekly for 48 weeks activity became normal compared with 1 of 13 untreated controls and in 4 of 14 treated with 3 million units *1797* In 36% of 64 patients with chronic hepatitis B infection reduction in activity observed in response to treatment although some relapses observed when treatment withdrawn *3249* Reduction observed in 15 patients with chronic non-A, non-B hepatitis with normal activities observed in 40% after 1 month and after 18 months *2236*
Serum Increase Physiological Hepatotoxicity occurred in patients with cancer with 10 MU/day intramuscularly at median of 6 to 9 days *3157* Dose dependent effect in 3 of 81 patients with malignant disease *5508* In 147 patients with metastatic renal cell carcinoma treatment with recombinant human interferon alfa-2a caused increased activity in 4 *4242*
Serum No Effect Physiological In 7 patients with cancer treatment with 3 x 10^6 units on each of two days caused nonsignificant increase from mean baseline of 18 ± 10 U/L to 26 ± 16 U/L and when the same dose was given 3 times weekly for 2 weeks mean activity increased nonsignificantly to 27 ± 12 U/L *2843* In 11 patients with active cirrhosis treatment for one month caused nonsignificant change from mean baseline of 58 U/L to 56 U/L *6679*

Albumin *Serum No Effect Physiological* Concentration usually normal in patients with chronic hepatitis C and unchanged with therapy *1410* In 7 patients with cancer treatment with 3 x 10^6 units on each of two consecutive days mean concentration was unchanged at 34 ± 6 g/L as it was after the same dose was given 3 times weekly for 2 weeks *2843*

Alkaline Phosphatase *Serum Increase Physiological* In 203 patients with chronic hepatitis C treatment with 3 MIU t.i.w. caused increased activity in 0%. In 218 patients with hairy cell leukemia treatment caused increased activity in 3%. In 241 patients with Kaposi's sarcoma treatment caused increased activity in 11%. In a US study of 91 patients and a non-US study of 219 patients treatment caused increased activity in 3% and 1% cases respectively *5032*
Serum No Effect Physiological In 7 cancer patients treatment with 3 x 10^6 units for 2 consecutive days caused nonsignificant increase from mean baseline of 138 ± 79 U/L to 149 ± 87 U/L and when the same dose was given 3 times weekly for 2 weeks mean activity increased nonsignificantly to 164 ± 129 U/L *2843* In 203 patients with chronic hepatitis C treatment with 3 MIU t.i.w. caused increased activity in 0% *5032*

Amino-terminal Propeptide of Type III Procollagen
Serum Decrease Physiological In patients with active cirrhosis who responded to treatment for serum concentration decreased significantly after 6 and 12 months although no significant difference from nonresponders to that time with decrease paralleling that of AST activity *6679*
Serum Increase Physiological In 11 patients with active cirrhosis treatment for one month caused serum concentration to increase from median of 25 to 40 μg/L while AST and ALT activities remained the same *6679*
Serum No Effect Physiological In 4 healthy volunteers treatment with a single dose of 3 MU IFN-α_{-2a} caused no significant change from mean baseline of 4.7 μg/L over next 3 days *6679* In 46 patients treatment for one month had no effect on serum concentration in those with either chronic persistent hepatitis or chronic active hepatitis *6679*

Antinuclear Antibodies *Serum Increase Physiological* Although 5 of 32 patients with chronic hepatitis B had antinuclear antibodies before treatment with α-interferon ANA appeared in another 5 (18%) of 28 previously negative patients following treatment with titer becoming negative after end of therapy *1810*

Antipyrine *Serum No Effect Physiological* In 7 cancer patients treatment with 3 x 10^6 units 3 times weekly for 2 weeks caused nonsignificant change in oral clearance from mean baseline of 2.94 ± 1.3 L/h to 2.35 ± 1.1 L/h *2843*

Apolipoprotein A-I *Serum Decrease Physiological* In 9 patients with chronic myeloid leukemia and hypertriglyceridemia treatment with IFN-α caused a decrease from median in 53% patients *4593*
Serum No Effect Physiological In 16 patients with chronic active hepatitis C treatment with 3 megaU t.i.w. SQ for 3 months had no significant effect on concentration *2238*

Apolipoprotein B *Serum Decrease Physiological* In 9 patients with chronic myeloid leukemia and hypertriglyceridemia treatment with IFN-α caused a decrease from median in 13% patients *4593*
Serum No Effect Physiological In 16 patients with chronic active hepatitis C treatment with 3 megaU t.i.w. SQ for 3 months had no significant effect on concentration *2238*

Aspartate Aminotransferase
Serum Decrease Physiological Marked decrease observed in patients with chronic hepatitis C (43% reduction in treated group versus 11% in placebo group) over 6 months *1410* In 36% of 64 patients who were HBeAg positive negative reaction obtained together with reduction in aminotransferase activity in response to treatment although some relapses observed when treatment stopped *3249*
Serum Increase Physiological In 147 patients with metastatic renal cell carcinoma treatment with recombinant human interferon alfa-2a caused increased activity in 4 *4242* In 218 patients with hairy cell leukemia treatment caused increased activity in 9%. In 241 patients with Kaposi's sarcoma treatment caused increased activity in 46%. In a US study of 91 patients and a non-US study of 219 patients treatment caused increased activity in 5% and 1% cases respectively *5032* Dose dependent effect in 3 of 81 patients with malignant disease *5508*

Serum *No Effect* *Physiological* In 11 patients with active cirrhosis treatment for one month caused nonsignificant change from mean baseline activity *6679* In 7 cancer patients treatment with 3 x 10^6 units on two consecutive days caused nonsgnificant change from mean baseline of 32 ± 21 U/L to 38 ± 25 U/L and when the same dose was given 3 times weekly for 2 weeks activity to increase to 42 ± 34 U/L *2843*

Bilirubin *Serum* *No Effect* *Physiological* In 147 patients with metastatic renal cell carcinoma treatment with recombinant human interferon alfa-2a had no effect on bilirubin concentrations *4242* In 7 cancer patients treatment with 3 x 10^6 units on each of two days caused no change from 6.8 ± 3.4 μmol/L and administration of the same dose 3 times weekly for 2 weeks caused nonsignificant reduction to 5.1 ± 3.4 μmol/L *2843* Concentration usually normal in patients with chronic hepatitis C and unchanged with therapy *1410*

Calcium *Serum* *Decrease* *Physiological* In 10 patients with amyotrophic lateral sclerosis intravenous infusion of high dose human leukocyte IFN-α caused significant reduction from mean of 2.28 ± 0.03 mmol/L to 2.01 ± 0.06 mmol/L *1802*

Complement C_3 *Serum* *No Effect* *Physiological* In 15 patients with hepatitis C and cryoglobulinemia who responded to treatment for 24 weeks nonsignificant change from mean baseline of 95 mg/dL to 96 mg/dL (+1 ± 2 mg/dL) occurred *4068*

Complement C_4 *Serum* *No Effect* *Physiological* In 15 patients with hepatitis C and cryoglobulinemia who responded to treatment for 24 weeks nonsignificant increase from mean baseline of 9.1 mg/dL to 9.2 mg/dL (+1 ± 1%) observed *4068*

Cortisol *Plasma* *Increase* *Physiological* 3 million IU injected twice intramuscularly in 8 healthy volunteers caused increased concentration *3226*

C-Reactive Protein *Serum* *No Effect* *Physiological* In 7 cancer patients treatment with 3 x 10^6 units 3 times weekly for 2 weeks caused nonsignificant decrease from mean baseline of 25 ± 28 μg/mL to 16 ± 15 μg/mL *2843*

Creatinine *Serum* *Decrease* *Physiological* In patients with hepatitis C who responded to treatment for 24 weeks mean concentration decreased from 1.3 mg/dL to 1.15 mg/dL (-13 ± 5%) *4068*

Serum *No Effect* *Physiological*, In 147 patients with metastatic renal cell carcinoma treatment with recombinant human interferon alfa-2a had no effect on concentration *4242*

Cryoprecipitate *Serum* *Decrease* *Physiological* In 15 patients with hepatitis C related cryoglobulinemia mean concentration decreased from 4.6 mg/mL to 1.7 mg/mL with 24 weeks treatment *4068*

Eosinophils *Blood* *Decrease* *Physiological* Marked reduction produced in one patient with hypereosinophilic syndrome after therapy with hydroxyurea, aspirin, prednisone and dipyridamole had failed. Dose of 8 million U/d required to achieve effect *6661*

Glucagon *Plasma* *Increase* *Physiological* 3 million IU injected intramuscularly caused increased concentration in 8 healthy volunteers *3226*

Glucose *Serum* *Increase* *Physiological* 3 million IU injected intramuscularly twice overnight in 8 healthy volunteers caused increased concentration *3226*

Glucose Tolerance *Serum* *Decrease* *Physiological* Area under curve 2.6 fold greater in 8 healthy volunteers following 3 million IU injected intramuscularly. With intravenous glucose tolerance test rate of glucose disappearance reduced by 28% *3226*

Growth Hormone *Plasma* *Increase* *Physiological* 3 million IU injected twice intramuscularly in 8 healthy volunteers caused increased concentration *3226*

HDL_3-Cholesterol *Serum* *Decrease* *Physiological* In 16 patients with chronic active hepatitis C treatment with 3 megaU t.i.w. SQ which decreased from mean baseline of 29.3 ± 10.8 mg/dL to 26.0 ± 10.6 mg/dL after 30 days and to 25.2 ± 11.9 mg/dL after 90 days *2238*

HDL-Cholesterol *Serum* *Decrease* *Physiological* In 9 patients with chronic myeloid leukemia and hypertriglyceridemia treatment with IFN-α caused a decrease from median in 81% patients *4593*

Hematocrit *Blood* *Decrease* *Physiological* In 147 patients with metastatic renal cell carcinoma treatment with recombinant human interferon alfa-2a caused anemia in 9 *4242*

Blood *No Effect* *Physiological* In 7 cancer patients acute administration of 3 x 10^6 units on two days caused nonsignificant change from mean baseline of 38 ± 6.3% to 37 ± 5.6% and to 37 ± 5.5% when given the same dose 3 times weekly for 2 weeks *2843* In 3 patients with hepatitis C receiving hemodialysis and recombinant erythropoietin mean concentration changed insignificantly from baseline of 29% to 28.7% with α-interferon treatment for 8 months *5872*

Hemoglobin *Blood* *Decrease* *Physiological* In 147 patients with metastatic renal cell carcinoma treatment with recombinant human interferon alfa-2a caused anemia in 9 *4242* In 203 patients with chronic hepatitis C treatment with 3 MIU t.i.w. caused anemia in 0%. In 218 patients with hairy cell leukemia treatment caused anemia in 31%. In 241 patients with Kaposi's sarcoma treatment caused anemia in 27%. In a US study of 91 patients and a non-US study of 219 patients treatment caused anemia in 15% and 4% cases respectively *5032*

Blood *No Effect* *Physiological* In 3 patients with hepatitis C receiving hemodialysis and recombinant erythropoietin mean concentration changed insignificantly from baseline of 9.5 g/dL to 9.4 g/dL with α-interferon treatment for 8 months *5872* In 203 patients with chronic hepatitis C treatment with 3 MIU t.i.w. caused anemia in 0% *5032*

Hepatitis B Virus DNA *Serum* *Decrease* *Physiological* Significantly greater disappearance in patients with hepatitis B when treated with prednisone and interferon alfa-2b or 5 million units interferon alfa-2b alone daily for 16 weeks than in patients given 1 million units only daily or in controls *4613*

Hepatitis Be Antigen *Serum* *Decrease* *Physiological* Disappearance from serum significantly greater in patients with hepatitis B given interferon alfa-2b with prednisone or 5 million units daily of interferon alfa-2b alone than in controls or those given only 1 million units daily for 16 weeks *4613* In 64 patients with chronic hepatitis B infection 36% responded to treatment with loss of HBeAg *3249*

Hepatitis D Virus RNA *Serum* *Decrease* *Physiological* In 10 of 14 patients with chronic hepatitis D treatment with 9 million units 3 times weekly intramuscularly for 48 weeks HDV RNA became undetectable as compared with 0 of 13 controls and 5 of 14 patients treated with 3 million units *1797*

Hexobarbital *Serum* *No Effect* *Physiological* In 7 cancer patients treatment with 3 x 10^6 units 3 times weekly for 2 weeks caused nonsignificant decrease in oral clearance from mean baseline of 15.0 ± 4.7 L/h to 14.0 ± 6.0 L/h *2843*

High Density Lipoproteins *Serum* *Decrease* *Physiological* In 16 patients with chronic viral hepatitis C treatment with 3 megaU t.i.w. SQ caused decrease from mean baseline of 42.9 ± 16.2 mg/dL to 39.6 ± 14.4 mg/dL after 3 days and 37.7 ± 13.4 mg/dL after 1 month but returned to 40.7 ± 14.7 mg/dL after 3 months but in responders (10 out of 16 in whom transaminases normalized) concentration decreased by 6.1 ± 7.4 mg/dL compared with baseline, whereas in nonresponders concentration increased by 4.2 ± 4.3 mg/dL *2238*

Hyaluronic Acid *Serum* *Decrease* *Physiological* In 42 patients with hepatitis C in the 8 who responded completely to treatment the mean concentration decreased to 36.8 ± 8.6 μg/L, compared with 74.1 ± 16.7 μg/L in 13 who partially responded and 134.6 ± 37.4 μg/L in 21 who failed to respond *3845*

Serum *Increase* *Physiological* In 46 patients with chronic hepatitis B virus infection treatment for one month increased the serum hyaluronic acid concentration by up to 150 μg/L in 44, but with cessation of treatment concentration reverted to the pre-therapy level. Concentration, both pretreatment and during treatment, higher in patients with active cirrhosis (+ 220 μg/L during treatment) than in those with chronic persistent hepatitis (+52 μg/L). Mean increase of 120 g/L in patients with chronic active hepatitis *6679*

Serum *No Effect* *Physiological* In 4 healthy volunteers treatment with a single dose of 3 MU IFN-α_{2a} caused no significant change from mean baseline of 18 μg/L over next 3 days *6679*

Immunoglobulin E *Serum* *No Effect* *Physiological* In 4 children with asthma receiving 2 million U/m^2 recombinant IFN-α2athree times a week for 4 weeks no significant difference from baseline value observed *395*

Immunoglobulin G *Serum* *Increase* *Physiological* In 15 patients with hepatitis C with cryoglobulinemia who responded to treatment for 24 weeks mean activity increased from 1437 mg/dL to 1506 mg/dL (+8 ± 6%) *4068*

Interferon Alfa-2a *(continued)*

Immunoglobulin M *Serum Decrease Physiological* In 15 patients with hepatitis C with cryoglobulinemia who responded to treatment for 24 weeks mean concentration decreased from 630 mg/dL to 379 mg/dL (-26 ± 5%) *4068*

Insulin *Plasma Increase Physiological* 3 million IU injected twice intramuscularly caused increased concentration in 8 healthy volunteers *3226*

Interleukin-4 *Serum No Effect Physiological* In 4 children with asthma receiving 2 million U/m^2 recombinant IFN-α2athree times a week for 4 weeks no significant difference from baseline value observed *395*

Interleukin-6 *Serum No Effect Physiological* In 7 cancer patients treatment with 3 x 10^6 units 3 times weekly for 2 weeks caused nonsignificant change from mean baseline of 3.8 ± 2.5% of maximal count to 4.1 ± 2.9% of maximal count *2843* In 14 HIV-1 infected patients with Kaposi's sarcoma treatment with high-dose human recombinant interferon-α had no consistent effect on serum IL-6 concentrations *1328* In 16 patients with chronic active hepatitis C treatment with 3 megaU t.i.w. sq for 3 months had no effect on IL-6 concentration (which was initially normal) *2238*

Lactate Dehydrogenase *Serum Increase Physiological* In 218 patients with hairy cell leukemia treatment caused increased activity in less than 1%. In 241 patients with Kaposi's sarcoma treatment caused increased activity in 10% *5032*

Leukocytes *Blood Decrease Physiological* In 147 patients with metastatic renal cell carcinoma treatment with recombinant human interferon alfa-2a caused leukopenia in one *4242* In 203 patients with chronic hepatitis C treatment with 3 MIU t.i.w. caused leukopenia in 1.5%. In 218 patients with hairy cell leukemia treatment caused leukopenia in 45%. In 241 patients with Kaposi's sarcoma treatment caused leukopenia in 49%. In a US study of 91 patients and a non-US study of 219 patients treatment caused leukopenia in 20% and 3% cases respectively *5032* In 7 cancer patients administration of 3 x 10^6 units 3 times weekly for 2 weeks caused significant reduction from mean baseline of 7500 ± 1800 /μL to 5300 ± 1000 /μL *2843* Dose dependent leukopenia in 3 of 81 patients with malignant disease *5508*

Blood Increase Physiological In 3 patients with hepatitis C receiving hemodialysis and recombinant erythropoietin mean concentration changed insignificantly from baseline of 4400 /μL to 5600 /μL with α-interferon treatment for 8 months *5872*

Blood No Effect Physiological In 7 cancer patients administration of 3 x 10^6 units on each of two days caused nonsignificant change from 7500 ± 1800 /μL to 7100 ± 1300 /μL *2843*

Lipoprotein Lp(a) *Serum No Effect Physiological* In 16 patients with chronic active hepatitis C treatment with 3 megaU t.i.w. SQ for 3 months had no significant effect on concentration *2238*

Magnesium *Urine Decrease Physiological* In 10 patients with amyotrophic lateral sclerosis treatment with intravenous infusion of high-dose human leukocyte IFN-α caused significant reduction from mean baseline of 5.32 ± 2.04 mmol/L to 2.65 ± 1.68 mmol/L *1802*

β_2-Microglobulin *Serum Increase Physiological* In 24 patients with AIDS-associated Kaposi's sarcoma concentration increased regardless of response to treatment but most increased in responders. Increase only found during initial 8 weeks of treatment but thereafter concentrations declined with continuing treatment but change may have been due to dose modification at this time *1327* In 4 healthy volunteers treatment with a single dose of 3 MU IFN-α_{2a} caused significant change from mean baseline of 1.05 mg/L to 1.7 and 1.9 mg/L on second and third day but with decrease to 1.7 mg/L on fourth day *6679* Mean increase of 109% (range 29 to 185%) observed in 8 patients with multiple myeloma treated with 6 million IU daily for 1-2 weeks before chemotherapy. Effect most marked when both serum β_2-microglobulin and creatinine concentrations high initially *6025*

Neutrophils *Blood Decrease Physiological* May be dose limiting adverse event *1384* In 203 patients with chronic hepatitis C treatment with 3 MIU t.i.w. caused neutropenia in 10%. In 218 patients with hairy cell leukemia treatment caused neutropenia in 68%. In 241 patients with Kaposi's sarcoma treatment caused neutropenia in 52%. In a US study of 91 patients and a non-US study of 219 patients treatment caused neutropenia in 22% and 0% cases respectively *5032* Dose dependent leukopenia in 3 of 81 patients with malignant disease *5508*

2',5'-Oligoadenylate Synthetase *Serum Increase Physiological* 1.5-fold increase to 63.4 ± 11 pg/dL from mean baseline of 40.2 ± 7.9 pg/dL observed 8 hours after administration of the drug in 21 patients with chronic active hepatitis B or C *177*

Osmolality *Serum Decrease Physiological* In 10 patients with amyotrophic lateral aclerosis intravenous infusion of high dose human leukocyte IFN-α for 4 days caused significant reduction from mean of 296 ± 9.9 mosmol/kg to 281 ± 2.5 mosmol/kg *1802*

Platelets *Blood Decrease Physiological* In 203 patients with chronic hepatitis C treatment with 3 MIU t.i.w. caused thrombocytopenia in 4.5%. In 218 patients with hairy cell leukemia treatment caused thrombocytopenia in 62%. In 241 patients with Kaposi's sarcoma treatment caused thrombocytopenia in 35%. In a US study of 91 patients and a non-US study of 219 patients treatment caused thrombocytopenia in 27% and 5% cases respectively *5032* Low value occurred in one patient heavily pretreated with nitrosoureas *5508*

Blood Increase Physiological In 11 of 13 patients with steroid-unresponsive idiopathic immune thrombocytopenic purpura 3 MU of recombinant-α IIb interferon for 12 doses caused significant increase *4802* In 3 patients with hepatitis C receiving hemodialysis and recombinant erythropoietin mean concentration changed insignificantly from baseline of 122000 /μL to 158000 /μL with α-interferon treatment for 8 months *5872*

Blood No Effect Physiological In 147 patients with metastatic renal cell carcinoma treatment with recombinant human interferon alfa-2a had no effect on concentration *4242*

Protein *Serum No Effect Physiological* Concentration usually normal in patients with chronic hepatitis and unchanged with therapy *1410*

Urine Decrease Physiological In 15 patients with hepatitis C and cryoglobulinemia and who responded to treatment for 24 weeks mean protein-creatinine index decreased from 0.81 to 0.55 (-9 ± 13) *4068*

Urine Increase Physiological 1 to 2 g/24 h in 2 patients receiving relatively large amount of drug: normalized 1 to 2 weeks after treatment stopped *5508* In 218 patients with hairy cell leukemia treatment caused increased excretion in 10%. In 241 patients with Kaposi's sarcoma treatment caused increased excretio in less than 1% *5032*

Urine No Effect Physiological In 203 patients with chronic hepatitis C treatment with 3 MIU t.i.w. caused increased increased excretion in 0% *5032*

Prothrombin Time *Plasma No Effect Physiological* Usually normal in patients with chronic hepatitis C and unchanged by therapy *1410*

Rheumatoid Factor *Serum Decrease Physiological* In 15 patients with hepatitis C and cryoglobulinemia who responded to treatment for 24 weeks reduction from mean baseline of 1148 IU/mL to 543 IU/mL occurred (-31 ± 6%) *4068*

Soluble CD23$^+$ *Serum No Effect Physiological* In 4 children with asthma receiving 2 million U/m^2 recombinant IFN-α_{2a} three times a week for 4 weeks no significant difference from baseline value observed *395*

Soluble Interleukin-2 Receptor *Serum No Effect Analytical* T Cell Diagnostics assay not affected by therapeutic concentrations of α-interferon *5908* No significant effect at therapeutic concentrations *5909*

Theophylline *Serum Increase Physiological* In 11 adults significant increase of approximately 15% in mean values of the terminal elimination half-life, area under the curve and mean residence time in association with similar decrease in plasma clearance when given i.m. before i.v. aminophylline *2978* 1 d after i.m. injection in 5 patients with hepatitis and 4 healthy volunteers significantly reduced clearance and significant increase of elimination half- life *6472* Decreases theophylline clearance and increases serum theophylline concentration by 100% *3125* Reported to reduce clearance of theophylline *5032* In 7 cancer patients treatment with 3 x 10^6 units 3 times weekly for 2 weeks caused significant reduction in clearance from mean baseline of 3.31 ± 1.3 L/h to 2.23 ± 0.7 L/h *2843*

Triglycerides *Serum Increase Physiological* In 22 patients with chronic myeloid leukemia treatment with IFN-α caused increase from median baseline of 150 mg/dL observed in 73% patients with increase maximal in first months of treatment *4593*

Serum No Effect Physiological In 16 patients with chronic active hepatitis C treatment with 3 megaU t.i.w. SQ had no significant effect over 3 months *2238*

Tumor Necrosis Factor *Serum Decrease Physiological* In 7 cancer patients treatment with 3 x 10^6 units 3 times weekly for 2 weeks caused significant reduction from mean baseline of 4.4 ± 3.2 U/L to 2.6 ± 2.9 U/L *2843*

Tumor Necrosis Factor-α *Serum No Effect Analytical* At a concentration of up to 1000 pg/mL had no significant effect on third generation T Cell Diagnostics procedure *4054*

Serum No Effect Physiological In 16 patients with chronic active hepatitis C although tendency for serum TNF to be higher at baseline in nonresponding patients treatment with 3 megaU t.i.w. SQ for 3 months had no significant effect on concentration in either nonresponders or responders *2238*

Interferon Alfa-2b

Alanine Aminotransferase *Serum Decrease Physiological* In patients with chronic active hepatitis C treatment with inteferon-alfa2b caused a complete response with marked reduction of ALT in 70% patients and partial response with 25% reduction of AST in remainder *1806* In 98 of 172 patients with chronic hepatitis B treated with interferon alfa-2b alone serum alanine aminotransferase decreased to within the normal range after treatment for 24 weeks. In 154 of 173 patients treated with interferon alfa-2b and ribovirin activity decreased to normal *1275* Serum ALT normalized in 77% of patients with chronic non-A, non-B hepatitis treated with interferon-alfa2b whereas no effect observed in control group *2028* Serum ALT normalized in 77% of patients with chronic non-A, non-B hepatitis treated with interferon-$alfa_{2b}$ whereas no effect observed in control group *2028* In patients with chronic active hepatitis C treatment with inteferon-$alfa_{2b}$ caused a complete response with marked reduction of ALT in 70% patients and partial response with 25% reduction of AST in remainder *1806* Significant reduction (from mean baseline of 187 U/L to 113 U/L at 12 months and 98 U/L at 24 months) in 8 patients with chronic active HBsAg-positive hepatitis treated for 12 months *5989*

Alkaline RNase *Serum Increase Physiological* Significant increase in mean concentration in 9 patients with chronic hepatitis B from 66 U/L to 84 U/L following one week of therapy. Increase persisted until two weeks after end of therapy *6084*

Aspartate Aminotransferase

Serum Decrease Physiological Significant reduction (from mean baseline of 95 U/L to 72 U/L at 12 months and 65 U/L at 24 months) in 8 patients with chronic active HBsAg-positive hepatitis treated for 12 months *5989*

Serum Increase Physiological Increased activity occurred in 63% treated patients with malignant melanoma, with life-threatening associated increases observed in 14% treated patients *5333*

5-Fluorouracil *Serum Increase Physiological* In 12 patients with gastric carcinoma coadministration of 9 MU IFN after intravenous administration of 5-FU caused doubling of its concentration from 27 µg/mL to 49 µg/mL *1206*

γ-Globulin *Serum No Effect Physiological* No change observed over 24 months in 8 patients with chronic active HBsAg-positive hepatitis treated with interferon for 12 months *5989*

Hematocrit *Blood Decrease Physiological* Anemia occurred in 22% treated patients with malignant melanoma *5333*

Hemoglobin *Blood Decrease Physiological* Anemia occurred in 22% treated patients with malignant melanoma *5333*

Hepatitis C Virus RNA *Serum Decrease Physiological* In only 18 of 164 patients with chronic hepatitis B treated with interferon alfa-2b alone was HCV RNA detectable after treatment for 24 weeks. In 10 of 89 treated with interferon alfa-2b HCV RNA detectable after 24 weeks *1275*

Histamine *Plasma No Effect Analytical* Minimal inhibition of radio-enzyme assay at concentration half to one third therapeutic concentration *2492*

5-Hydroxyindoleacetic Acid *Urine Decrease Physiological* 24% patients with midgut carcinoid after removal of primary tumor responded with more than a 50% reduction in excretion *2449*

Leukocytes *Blood Decrease Physiological* Leukopenia occurred in 26% treated patients with malignant melanoma *5333*

Neutrophils *Blood Decrease Physiological* Neutropenia developed in more than 20% treated patients with malignant melanoma *5333*

2',5'-Oligoadenylate Synthetase

Serum Decrease Physiological In patients with chronic hepatitis C treatment with 3 MU three times weekly for 6 months caused reduction in activity with mean values fluctuating between 145 and 50 fmol/50 µL *5671*

Serum Increase Physiological In patients with chronic hepatitis C who failed to respond to up to 6 MU three times weekly mean concentration increased with peak of about 440 fmol/50 µL after 3 months *5671* Mean concentration in 9 patients with chronic hepatitis B 6.3 pmol/min/L before treatment but increased to 52 pmol/min/L with first week of therapy to 85 pmol/min/L at second week but declined thereafter to just above initial concentration at sixth week *6084*

Proline Hydroxylase *Serum Decrease Physiological* No significant change observed during treatment for 12 months of 8 patients with chronic active HBsAg-positive hepatitis, but significant reduction 3 months later which was maintained *5989*

Thyroglobulin Autoantibodies

Serum No Effect Physiological In 5 patients with hepatitis C infection treatment for 6 months caused nonsignificant change from mean baseline of 11.8 ± 1.4 mIU/L to 11.8 ± 2.2 mIU/L after 6 months and 12.0 ± 2.9 mIU/L after 12 months *384*

Thyroid Microsomal Autoantibodies

Serum No Effect Physiological In 5 patients with hepatitis C infection treatment for 6 months caused nonsignificant change from mean baseline of 11.7 ± 1.5 mIU/L to 10.0 ± 1.1 mIU/L after 6 months and 12.4 ± 1.9 mIU/L after 12 months *384*

Thyroid Stimulating Hormone

Serum No Effect Physiological In 5 patients with hepatitis C infection treatment for 6 months caused nonsignificant change from mean baseline of 2.4 ± 1.2 mIU/L to 1.7 ± 0.7 mIU/L after 6 months and 1.8 ± 1.2 mIU/L after 12 months *384*

Thyroxine Binding Globulin *Serum No Effect Physiological* In 5 patients with hepatitis C infection treatment for 6 months caused nonsignificant change from mean baseline of 28.2 ± 9.3 mg/L to 27.4 ± 8.4 mg/L after 6 months and 26.0 ± 7.8 mg/L after 12 months *384*

Thyroxine (T4) *Serum Decrease Physiological* Both hyper- and hypothyroidism observed in fewer than 1% patients treated with interferon alfa-2b for chronic hepatitis NANB/C *5333*

Serum Increase Physiological Both hyper- and hypothyroidism observed in fewer than 1% patients treated with interferon alfa-2b for chronic hepatitis NANB/C *5333*

Serum No Effect Physiological In 5 patients with hepatitis C infection treatment for 6 months caused nonsignificant change from mean baseline of 156 ± 38 nmol/L to 138 ± 41 nmol/L after 6 months and 160 ± 46 nmol/L after 12 months *384*

Thyroxine (T4), Free *Serum No Effect Physiological* In 5 patients with hepatitis C infection treatment for 6 months caused nonsignificant change from mean baseline of 10.8 ± 2.4 pmol/L to 11.7 ± 1.3 pmol/L after 6 months and 13.0 ± 1.5 pmol/L after 12 months *384*

Tri-iodothyronine (T3) *Serum No Effect Physiological* In 5 patients with hepatitis C infection treatment for 6 months caused nonsignificant change from mean baseline of 2.4 ± 0.7 nmol/L to 2.1 ± 0.5 nmol/L after 6 months and 2.6 ± 0.8 nmol/L after 12 months *384*

Interferon Alfa-A

Theophylline *Serum Increase Physiological* Up to 100% increase in serum theophylline concentration due to decreased theophylline clearance *6117*

Interferon Alfa-n3

Alkaline Phosphatase *Serum Increase Physiological* Increased activity observed in 8% of 31 patients with cancer *5995*

Aspartate Aminotransferase *Serum Increase Physiological* Increased activity observed in 3% of 31 patients with cancer *5995*

Bilirubin *Serum Increase Physiological* Increased concentration observed in 4% of 31 patients with cancer *5995*

γ-Glutamyltransferase *Serum Increase Physiological* Increased activity observed in 6% of 31 patients with cancer *5995*

Hemoglobin *Blood Decrease Physiological* Decreased concentration observed in 7% of 31 patients with cancer *5995*

Leukocytes *Blood Decrease Physiological* Decreased leukocyte count observed in 11% of treated patients compared with 4% of placebo-treated controls *5995*

Platelets *Blood Decrease Physiological* Decreased concentration observed in 3% of 31 patients with cancer *5995*

Interferon β-1b

Alanine Aminotransferase *Serum Decrease Physiological* At up to 3 MIU/day in patients with chronic non-A non-B hepatitis effective response observed in 9 of 12 patients. Activity increased in 6 of the 9 patients once treatment stopped *3168*

Apolipoprotein B *Serum Decrease Physiological* In 4 normal individuals intravenous administration of 4.5 x 10^6 units daily for at least 3 weeks caused mean reduction of 27% but in 6 with mild hypercholesterolemia no significant decrease observed *5317*

Corticotropin *Plasma Increase Physiological* In 18 patients with inoperable cancer intravenous administration of 90 x 10^6 IU 3 times/week for 15 days caused significant increase from mean baseline of 6.9 pmol/L to peak of 14.8 pmol/L: administration of 450 x 10^6 IU with same schedule to 10 of these patients caused increase from 8.8 pmol/L to peak of 24.6 pmol/L *4317*

Cortisol *Plasma Increase Physiological* In 18 patients with inoperable cancer treatment with 90 x 10^6 IU intravenously caused significant increase from mean baseline of 367 nmol/L to peak of 731 nmol/L and after 450 x 10^6 IU in 10 of these patients from 356 nmol/L to 935 nmol/L *4317*

Urine Increase Physiological In 10 patients with inoperable cancer intravenous administration of 450 x 10^6 IU caused significant increase from mean baseline of 115 nmol/d to 171 nmol/d on the following day *4317*

DR+ Cells *Cerebrospinal Fluid Increase Physiological* In 16 patients with multiple sclerosis treatment with intrathecal natural β-interferon for 6 months caused increase suggesting activation of the intrathecal immune response *4032*

Growth Hormone *Plasma Increase Physiological* In 18 patients with inoperable cancer intravenous administration of 90 x 10^6 IU caused significant increase from mean baseline of 2.2 µg/L to peak of 4.3 µg/L and after 450 x 10^6 IU in 10 of these from 2.5 µg/L to a peak of 4.6 µg/L *4317*

IgG Index *Cerebrospinal Fluid Increase Physiological* Increase observed in 16 patients with multiple sclerosis treated with intrathecal natural β-interferon for 6 months *4032*

LDL-Cholesterol *Serum Decrease Physiological* In 4 healthy individuals intravenous administration of 4.5 x 10^6 units daily for at least 3 weeks caused a mean reduction of 25% but in 6 individuals with hypercholesterolemia concentration reduced by 38% *5317*

Myelin Basic Protein
Cerebrospinal Fluid Increase Physiological Increase observed in 16 patients with multiple sclerosis treated with intrathecal natural interferon-β for 6 months *4032*

Prolactin *Plasma Increase Physiological* In 18 patients with inoperable cancer treatment with 90 x 10^6 IU intravenously caused significant increase from mean baseline of 5.2 µg/L to peak of 11.0 µg/L and in 10 of these given 450 x 10^6 IU increase from 6.8 µg/L to peak of 10.2 µg/L observed *4317*

Soluble Interleukin-2 Receptor
Serum Increase Physiological In 26 patients with chronic hepatitis B infection following 4 weeks treatment with prednisone which caused concentration to decrease to 384.8 ± 39.4 U/mL which then increased to 733.4 ± 45.7 U/mL with 4 weeks treatment with interferon but returned to pretreatment concentration on completion of the interferon course *3528*

Interferon γ

Anti-Smooth Muscle Antibodies
Serum Increase Physiological In 4 of 11 patients with chronic active hepatitis B treated with recombinant γ-interferon antibodies for 16 weeks antibodies developed during or after treatment *3321*

Antinuclear Antibodies *Serum Increase Physiological* In 4 of 11 patients with chronic active hepatitis B treated with recombinant γ-interferon for 16 weeks with follow-up for 1 year antibodies developed during or after treatment *3321*

C_1-Inhibitor Antigen *Serum No Effect Physiological* In 6 normal volunteers treated with 25 µg/sq m daily for 4 days no significant change in concentration observed *2195*

Complement C_1 Inhibitor *Serum Increase Physiological* Increased concentration reported in patients with colon cancer when treated with γ-interferon *2195*

Serum No Effect Physiological Increased concentrations observed in patients with colon cancer when treated with γ-interferon but when recombinant human γ-interferon administered at a dose of 25 µg/sq m subcutaneously for 4 days no significant effect observed *2195*

Cortisol *Plasma Increase Physiological* In a small number of patients with inoperable cancer intravenous administration of 30 x 10^6 IU caused increase from mean baseline of 419 nmol/L to 855 nmol/L and after 100 x 10^6 IU from 163 nmol/L to 759 nmol/L 60 to 120 minutes later *4317*

Factor XII *Plasma No Effect Physiological* In 6 healthy volunteers administration of 25 µg/sq m rHuIFN-γ for 4 consecutive days had no significant effect on plasma concentration *2195*

Fibrinogen Degradation Products
Plasma No Effect Physiological In 37 patients following traumatic injuries treatment with interferon-γ caused mean concentration to change insignificantly from 4600 ng/mL at baseline to 5000, 7400 and 5100 ng/mL respectively after 3, 8 and 22 days treatment with 100 µg for 21 days *1498*

HMW-Kininogen *Plasma No Effect Physiological* Administration of 25 µg/sq m rHuIFN-γ subcutaneously for 4 days to 6 healthy volunteers had no significant effect on concentration *2195*

Immunoglobulin E *Serum No Effect Physiological* In 22 patients with chronic severe atopic dermatitis treatment with up to 0.05 mg/sq m for up to 14 nonths had no effect on concentration *638*

Kallikrein *Plasma No Effect Physiological* In 6 volunteers treatment with 25 µg/sq m rHuIFN-γ subcutaneously for 4 days had no significant effect on concentration *2195*

Lymphocyte T-Cells *Blood Increase Physiological* Significant increase observed in 11 patients with chronic active hepatitis B treated for 16 weeks with follow-up for one year *3321*

Plasminogen Activator Inhibitor
Plasma Increase Physiological In 6 healthy volunteers administration of 25 µg/sq m rHuIFN-γ subcutaneously for 4 days caused significant increase in concentration *2195*

Plasma No Effect Physiological In 10 volunteers treated with 25 µg/sq m/d subcutaneously for 4 days no significant variation in concentration observed *2195*

Plasminogen Activator Inhibitor-1
Plasma Increase Physiological In 37 patients following traumatic injuries treatment with interferon-γ caused mean concentration to decrease significantly from 84 ng/mL at baseline to 44, 68 and 53 ng/mL respectively after 3, 8 and 22 days treatment with 100 µg for 21 days *1498*

Plasminogen Activator Inhibitor-1 Antigen
Plasma Decrease Physiological In 6 healthy volunteers administration of 25 µg/sq m rHuIFN-γ subcutaneously for 4 days caused significant decrease *2195*

Prekallikrein *Plasma No Effect Physiological* In 6 healthy volunteers treated with 25 µg/d/sq m subcutaneously for 4 days no significant effect observed on concentration *2195*

Thrombin/Antithrombin III Complex
Plasma Increase Physiological In 37 patients following traumatic injuries treatment with interferon-γ caused mean concentration to be significantly greater than in control trauma patients after 3, 8 and 22 days treatment with 100 µg for 21 days *1498*

Thyroid Stimulating Hormone
Serum No Effect Physiological No significant effect observed in 11 patients with chronic active hepatitis B treated for 16 weeks with recombinant γ-interferon with follow-up for one year *3321*

Thyroxine (T4) *Serum No Effect Physiological* No significant effect observed in 11 patients with chronic active hepatitis B treated with 1 million U/sq m/d i.m. 3 times/week for 16 weeks with follow-up for 1 year *3321*

Thyroxine (T4) Index, Free *Serum No Effect Physiological* No significant effect observed in 11 patients with chronic active hepatitis B treated for 16 weeks with recombinant γ-interferon with follow-up for 1 year *3321*

Tissue Factor Pathway Inhibitor
Plasma No Effect Physiological In 37 patients following traumatic injuries treatment with interferon-γ caused mean concentration to change insignificantly from 115 ng/mL at baseline to 135, 175 and 170 ng/mL respectively after 3, 8 and 22 days treatment with 100 µg for 21 days *1498*

Tissue Plasminogen Activator
Plasma Decrease Physiological In 5 healthy volunteers treated with 25 µg/sq m/d for 4 days nonsignificant change from mean baseline of 5.34 ± 3.2 U/mL to 2.06 ± 0.6 U/mL observed with Kabi assay but significant decrease observed in another 5 individuals from 1.23 ± 0.56 U/mL to < 0.5 U/mL with the Biopool assay *2195*
Plasma Increase Physiological In 37 patients following traumatic injuries treatment with interferon-γ caused mean concentration to decrease significantly from 22 ng/mL at baseline to 12, 16 and 14 ng/mL respectively after 3, 8 and 22 days treatment with 100 µg for 21 days *1498*

Tissue Plasminogen Activator Antigen
Plasma No Effect Physiological In 6 healthy volunteers administration of 25 µg/sq m rHuIFN-γ subcutaneously for 4 days had no significant effect on concentration *2195*

Tri-iodothyronine (T3) *Serum No Effect Physiological* No significant change observed in 11 patients with chronic active hepatitis B treated for 16 weeks with recombinant γ-inteferon with follow-up for 1 year *3321*

Tumor Necrosis Factor-α *Serum No Effect Physiological* In 73 patients following traumatic injuries treated with 100 µg for 21 days concentration higher but not significantly greater than in control trauma patients *1498*

Interferon γ-1b

Alanine Aminotransferase *Serum Increase Physiological* Rare side effect of hepatic insufficiency observed *2080*

Alkaline Phosphatase *Serum Increase Physiological* Rare side effect of hepatic insufficiency observed *2080*
Serum No Effect Physiological In 14 patients with osteopetrosis with mean baseline of 366 ± 501 U/L activity changed nonsignificantly to 282 ± 339 U/L after 6 months and 431 ± 719 U/L after 18 months *3123*

Amylase *Serum Increase Physiological* Rare side effect of pancreatitis observed *2080*

Aspartate Aminotransferase *Serum Increase Physiological* Rare side effect of hepatic insufficiency observed *2080*

Bilirubin *Serum Increase Physiological* Rare side effect of hepatic insufficiency observed *2080*

Calcium *Serum Increase Physiological* In 14 patients with osteopetrosis with mean baseline of 9.0 ± 0.8 mg/dL concentration increased nonsignificantly to 9.4 ± 0.7 mg/dL after 6 months and 9.1 ± 0.3 mg/dL after 18 months *3123*
Urine Increase Physiological In 14 patients with osteopetrosis with mean baseline of 0.19 ± 0.26 g/g creatinine increased excretion significantly to 0.71 ± 0.79 g/g creatinine after 6 months and 0.50 ± 0.60 g/g creatinine after 18 months *3123*

Glucose *Serum Increase Physiological* Rare side effect of treatment observed *2080*

Hemoglobin *Blood Increase Physiological* In 14 patients with osteopetrosis with mean baseline of 7.5 ± 2.9 g/dL concentration increased significantly to 9.4 ± 0.4 g/dL after 6 months and 10.5 ± 0.3 g/dL after 18 months *3123*

Hydroxyproline *Urine Increase Physiological* In 14 patients with osteopetrosis with mean baseline of 0.18 ± 0.15 mg/g creatinine excretion increased significantly to 0.51 ± 0.33 mg/g creatinine after 6 months and 0.31 ± 0.16 mg/g creatinine after 18 months *3123*

Leukocytes *Blood Increase Physiological* In 14 patients with osteopetrosis with mean baseline of 7800 ± 4900 /µL concentration increased significantly to 11700 ± 10900 /µL after 6 months and 13500 ± 13900 /µL after 18 months *3123*

Lipase *Serum Increase Physiological* Rare side effect of pancreatitis observed *2080*

Occult Blood *Feces Increase Physiological* Rare gastrointestinal bleeding observed *2080*

Platelets *Blood Increase Physiological* In 14 patients with osteopetrosis with mean baseline of 63000 ± 54000 /µL concentration increased significantly to 135000 ± 97000 /µL after 6 months and 187000 ± 127000 /µL after 18 months *3123*

Sodium *Serum Decrease Physiological* Rare side effect of treatment observed *2080*

Type I Collagen Cross-linked N-telopeptide
Urine Increase Physiological In 14 patients with osteopetrosis with mean baseline of 305 ± 486 µmol/mol creatinine excretion increased significantly to 1209 ± 914 µmol/mol creatinine after 6 months and 773 ± 571 µmol/mol creatinine after 18 months *3123*

Interleukin-2

Alanine Aminotransferase *Serum Increase Physiological* Median increase to 91 U/L in over 200 patients with cancer treated with mean of 11.7 doses. Effect due to reversible cholestasis *1877* Liver function abnormalities reported as a side effect *1384* Liver function abnormalities reported *1384* Mean 6.2 fold increase in 21 patients with cancer treated with IL-2 for 5 days *2746* In 138 patients with metastatic renal cell carcinoma treatment with recombinant human IL-2 caused increased ALT or AST activity in 15 *4242*

Albumin *Serum Decrease Physiological* Median decrease to 3.0 g/dL in over 200 patients with cancer treated with mean of 11.7 doses. Effect due to reversible cholestasis *1877*

Alkaline Phosphatase *Serum Increase Physiological* Median increase to 256 U/L in over 200 patients with cancer treated with mean of 11.7 doses. Effect due to reversible cholestasis *1877* Mean 4.8 fold increase in 21 patients with cancer treated with IL-2 for 5 days *2746*

Aspartate Aminotransferase *Serum Increase Physiological* In 138 patients with metastatic renal cell carcinoma treatment with recombinant human IL-2 caused increased ALT or AST activity in 15 *4242* Median increase to 80 U/L in over 200 patients with cancer treated with mean of 11.7 doses. Effect due to reversible cholestasis *1877* Mean 6.1 fold increase in 21 patients with cancer treated for 5 days with IL-2 *2746*

Bilirubin *Serum Increase Physiological* In 138 patients with metastatic renal cell carcinoma treatment with recombinant human IL-2 caused increased creatinine concentration in one *4242* Mean 15.4 fold increase in 21 patients with cancer treated with IL-2 for 5 days *2746* Median increase to 4.5 mg/dL in over 200 cancer patients treated with mean of 11.7 doses: reversible cholestatsis *1877*

Bilirubin, Direct *Serum Increase Physiological* Mean 52.1 fold increase in 14 patients with cancer treated with IL-2 for 5 days *2746*

CD4+ Lymphocytes *Blood Decrease Physiological* Marked reduction observed in 6 patients with severe atopic dermatitis refractory to conventional therapy when given up to 60000 U/kg/d for 9-12 days *2743*

Cholylglycine *Serum Increase Physiological* Increase from mean of 32.3 mg/mL to 1556.0 mg/mL in prospectively evaluated group of 10 cancer patients. Effect due to reversible cholestasis *1877*

Interleukin-2 *(continued)*

Cortisol *Plasma Increase Physiological* Mean concentrations significantly increased in patients with metastatic renal cancer during 24-hour infusion of IL-2. Circadian rhythm completely abolished *3606*
Plasma No Effect Physiological Nonsignificant transient increase observed in 6 men with renal cancer or melanoma treated with large dose intravenous boluses for 5 days *3937*

C-Reactive Protein *Serum Increase Physiological* Mean 7.7 fold increase in 15 patients with cancer treated with IL-2 for 5 days *2746*

Creatine Kinase *Serum Increase Physiological* Mean 2.4 fold increase in 21 patients with cancer treated with IL-2 for 21 days *2746*

Creatinine *Serum Increase Physiological* Mean 2.0 fold increase in 21 patients with cancer treated for 5 days with IL-2 *2746* Nephrotoxicity occurs as rare side effect *1384* In 138 patients with metastatic renal cell carcinoma treatment with recombinant human IL-2 caused increased creatinine concentration in five *4242*

Dehydroepiandrosterone *Plasma Decrease Physiological* Significant decrease observed in 6 men with renal cancer or melanoma treated with large dose intravenous boluses intravenously for 5 days. Mean baseline about 7.5 nmol/L reduced to 1.5 nmol/L at day 6 but then returned to baseline after day 10 *3937*

Dehydroepiandrosterone Sulfate
Plasma No Effect Physiological No significant effect observed in 6 men with renal cancer or melanoma treated with large dose intravenous boluses for 5 days *3937*

β-Endorphin *Plasma Increase Physiological* Significant increase observed during 24-hour intravenous infusion in patients with metastatic renal cancer. Circadian rhythm completely abolished *3606*

Eosinophils *Blood Increase Physiological* Reported as a side effect *1384* Invariably observed in patients treated with IL-2: in 5 patients with cancer without initial eosinophilia concentration rose to 2328 to 15958 /μL *6183*

Estradiol *Plasma Increase Physiological* In 6 men with renal cancer or melanoma treatment with large doses boluses intravenously for 5 days caused decrease from mean baseline of about 50 pmol/L to mean of about 430 pmol/L on day 4 after treatment started but then declined to baseline at day 8 *3937*

Follicle Stimulating Hormone
Plasma No Effect Physiological No significant effect observed in 6 men with renal cancer or melanoma given high dose intravenous bolus drug for 5 days *3937*

γ-Glutamyltransferase *Serum Increase Physiological* Mean 11.5 fold increase in 17 patients with cancer treated for 5 days with IL-2 *2746*

Growth Hormone *Plasma Increase Physiological* Nonsignificant increase observed during 24-hour intravenous infusion in patients with metastatic renal cancer *3606*

Hematocrit *Blood Decrease Physiological* In 138 patients with metastatic renal cell carcinoma treatment with recombinant human IL-2 caused anemia in 24 *4242*

Hemoglobin *Blood Decrease Physiological* Anemia reported as a side effect *1384* In 138 patients with metastatic renal cell carcinoma treatment with recombinant human IL-2 caused anemia in 24 *4242*

Immunoglobulin E *Serum No Effect Physiological* No significant effect observed in 6 patients with severe atopic dermatitis refractory to conventional therapy when treated with up to 60000 U/kg/d for 9-12 days *2743*

Interleukin-2 *Serum No Effect Physiological* No significant change observed in 6 patients with severe atopic dermatitis treated with up to 60000 U/kg/d for 9 - 12 days *2743*

Interleukin-2 Receptor (CD25+) Lymphocytes
Blood Increase Physiological Marked increase observed in 6 patients with severe atopic dermatitis refractory to conventional therapy given up to 60000 U/kg/d for 9-12 days *2743*

Interleukin-5 *Serum Increase Physiological* Temporal relationship observed between infusion of interleukin-2 and increase in concentration of IL-5 in 5 patients with advanced malignancy *6183*

Lactate Dehydrogenase *Serum Increase Physiological* Mean 1.8 fold increase in 21 patients with cancer treated with IL-2 for 5 days *2746*

Leukocytes *Blood Decrease Physiological* In 138 patients with metastatic renal cell carcinoma treatment with recombinant human IL-2 caused decreased leukocyte count in one *4242*

Luteinizing Hormone *Plasma No Effect Physiological* No significant change observed in 6 men with renal cancer or melanoma treated with intravenous bolus dose of interleukin-2 for 5 days although mean concentrations increased on days 2 and 4 after beginning treatment *3937*

Major Basic Protein *Serum Increase Physiological* In 5 patients with advanced malignancy by time of third infusion of IL-2 high concentrations, up to 5600 ng/mL, observed in all patients before eosinophilia became apparent *6183*

Melatonin *Plasma Decrease Physiological* Significant decrease observed during 24-hour infusion in patients with metastatic renal cancer *3606*

Platelets *Blood Decrease Physiological* In 138 patients with metastatic renal cell carcinoma treatment with recombinant human IL-2 caused decreased platelet concentration in five *4242*

Prolactin *Plasma Increase Physiological* Nonsignificant increase observed in patients with metastatic renal cancer during 24-hour intravenous infusion of IL-2 *3606*

Prothrombin Time *Plasma Increase Physiological* Median increase to 13.4 s in over 200 patients with cancer given mean of 11.7 doses. Effect due to reversible cholestasis *1877*

Testosterone *Serum Decrease Physiological* In 6 men with renal cancer or melanoma high dose bolus injection for 5 days caused significant decrease from mean baseline of about 21 nmol/L to about 2 nmol/L at 6 days after treatment begun *3937*

Tumor Necrosis Factor-α *Serum No Effect Analytical* T Cell Diagnostics assay unaffected by presence of interleukin 2 *5908*

Urea Nitrogen *Serum Increase Physiological* Mean 2.4 fold increase in 16 patients with cancer treated with IL-2 for 5 days *2746* Nephrotoxicity occurs as rare side effect *1384*

Intra-Amniotic Saline

Chloride *Serum Increase Physiological* Increased by approximately 3 mEq/L after 1 h *6534*
Urine Increase Physiological Significant effect for 24 h *6534*

Potassium *Serum Increase Physiological* No change until 8 h after then by 0.6 mEq/L *6534*
Urine Increase Physiological Significant effect for 24 h *6534*

Sodium *Serum Increase Physiological* Increased by approximately 4 mEq/L after 1 h *6534*
Urine Increase Physiological Significant effect for 24 h *6534*

Volume *Urine Increase Physiological* Significant increase over next 24 h *6534*

Inulin

Cholesterol *Serum No Effect Physiological* In 64 healthy young women consuming 40 g low fat spread containing 14 g inulin mean concentration of 4.24 ± 0.75 mmol/L not significantly different from 4.28 ± 0.76 mmol/L when they were consuming their habitual diet *4579*

Estrogens *Urine Decrease Analytical* Affects hydrolysis of estrogen conjugates *55*

HDL-Cholesterol *Serum Increase Physiological* In 64 healthy young women consuming 40 g low fat spread containing 14 g inulin mean concentration of 1.38 ± 0.30 mmol/L significantly different from 1.32 ± 0.28 mmol/L when they were consuming their habitual diet *4579*

LDL-Cholesterol *Serum No Effect Physiological* In 64 healthy young women consuming 40 g low fat spread containing 14 g inulin mean concentration of 2.38 ± 0.67 mmol/L not significantly different from 2.48 ± 0.72 mmol/L when they were consuming their habitual diet *4579*

LDL-Cholesterol:HDL-Cholesterol Ratio
Serum Decrease Physiological In 64 healthy young women consuming 40 g low fat spread containing 14 g inulin mean concentration of 1.82 ± 0.69 significantly different from 1.97 ± 0.73 when they were consuming their habitual diet *4579*

Osmolality *Serum Increase Physiological* Massive doses have marked effect *128*

p-Aminohippurate *Serum No Effect Analytical* No significant interference observed at concentration of 25 mg/dL with method of Ramey et al using Roche Cobas Mira *4842*
Urine No Effect Analytical No significant interference observed at concentrations up to 300 mg/dL with method of Ramey et al using Roche Cobas Mira *4842*

Triglycerides *Serum No Effect Physiological* In 64 healthy young women consuming 40 g low fat spread containing 14 g inulin mean concentration of 0.97 ± 0.39 mmol/L not significantly different from 0.95 ± 0.31 mmol/L when they were consuming their habitual diet *4579*

Volume *Urine Increase Physiological* Massive doses produce marked diuresis *128*

Invermectin

Alanine Aminotransferase *Serum Increase Physiological* In controlled clinical trials involving 109 patients given either one or two doses of 170 - 200 µg/kg increased activity observed in 2% patients *3993*

Aspartate Aminotransferase *Serum Increase Physiological* In controlled clinical trials involving 109 patients givem either one or two doses of 170 - 200 µg/kg increased activity observed in 2% patients *3993*

Eosinophils *Blood Increase Physiological* In controlled clinical trials increased concentration observed in 3% patients *3993*

Hemoglobin *Blood Decrease Physiological* In one patient leukopenia and anemia observed *3993*
Blood Increase Physiological In controlled clinical trials increased concentration observed in 1% patients *3993*

Leukocytes *Blood Decrease Physiological* In controlled clinical trials involving 109 patients given either one or two doses of 170 - 200 µg/kg decreased concentration observed in 3% patients *3993*

Iobenzamic Acid

Thyroid Stimulating Hormone
Serum Increase Physiological Blocks intrahypophyseal conversion of T4 to T3 *6412*

Thyroxine (T4) *Serum Increase Physiological* Impaired conversion of T4 to T3 *6412*

Tri-iodothyronine (T3) *Serum Decrease Physiological* Impaired conversion of T4 to T3 *6412*

Iodates

Cholesterol *Serum Increase Analytical* Interference with Zlatkis-Zak reaction *5869*

Iodide

Bicarbonate *Serum Increase Analytical* Increases result with method on Kodak Ektachem® systems *2519*

Bilirubin, Conjugated *Serum No Effect Analytical* At concentration of 500 mg/L had no effect on method on Kodak Ektachem® *5706*

Bilirubin, Unconjugated *Serum No Effect Analytical* At concentration of 500 mg/L had no effect on method on Kodak Ektachem® *5706*

Chloride *Serum Increase Analytical* Increases serum chloride concentration by 0.51 mEq/L at an iodide concentration of 20 mEq/L in the method of Fingerhut *1865* At concentrations greater than 1 mmol/L causes increased measurement as determined by Kodak Ektachem® : of probable clinical significance *5706*

Cholesterol *Serum Increase Analytical* Interference with Zlatkis-Zak reaction *5869*
Serum No Effect Analytical No effect at concentrations up to 254 mg/L on method on Kodak Ektachem® *5706*

Color *Feces Increase Analytical* Black color reported with ingestion of iodide containing drugs *3388*

Creatinine *Serum No Effect Analytical* No effect of concentrations up to 5000 mg/L on single slide method on Kodak Ektachem® *5706*
Urine No Effect Analytical Causes less than 2% effect on single-slide method on Kodak Ektachem® systems *2519*

Eosinophils *Blood Increase Physiological* Allergic response *3810*

Glucose *Serum No Effect Analytical* No effect of concentrations up to 254 mg/L on method on Kodak Ektachem® *5706* At a concentration of 2 mEq/L had no significant effect on method on Kodak Ektachem® systems *2519*

Hemoglobin *Urine Increase Analytical* Interferes with guaiac and benzidine tests *2024*

17-Hydroxycorticosteroids *Urine Increase Analytical* Interferes with Porter-Silber reaction *5869*

^{131}I Uptake *Serum Decrease Physiological* Massive doses increase pool *882*

Iodide *Serum Increase Physiological* With supplements of 1500 µg or more per day caused significant increase of total iodide within 15 days *2030*
Urine Increase Physiological Significant increase noted within 15 days in volunteers given 500 µg or more per day *2030*

Iodide, Inorganic *Serum Increase Physiological* Significant increase in volunteers given as little as 500 µg per day for 15 days *2030*

ionized Calcium *Serum Increase Analytical* Observed interference with ion specific electrode *820*

Lactate *Plasma No Effect Analytical* No significant effect observed at a concentration of 2 mEq/L with method on Kodak Ektachem® systems *2519*

Leukocytes *Blood Increase Physiological* Due to eosinophilia *3810*

Occult Blood *Feces Increase Analytical* Interferes with benzidine test *879* *In vitro* reaction, ?high enough concentration *in vivo882*
Feces Increase Physiological Chronic poisoning may cause bloody diarrhea *2242*

Potassium *Serum Increase Analytical* Of clinical significance since presence of iodide at any concentration increases result as determined by method on Kodak Ektachem® *5706*

Salicylate *Serum No Effect Analytical* No significant effect observed at a concentration of 2 mEq/L with method on Kodak Ektachem® systems *2519*

T3-Uptake *Serum No Effect Physiological* No significant change in volunteers over 15 days even when given as much as 4500 µg daily *2030*

Thyroid Stimulating Hormone
Serum Increase Physiological Also increased response to TRH related to decreased T4 and T3 concentrations *6412* No effect at 500 µg per day in volunteers when given for 15 days, but significant increase with 1500 µg or more per day for same time period *2030*

Thyroxine (T4) *Serum Decrease Physiological* Associated with inhibition of conversion *6412* Decrease synthesis if diagnostic or therapeutic ^{131}I *5869* No significant effect of 500 µg per day for 15 days in volunteers, but significant reduction when 1500 µg give daily over same time period *2030*

Thyroxine (T4) Index, Free *Serum Decrease Physiological* No significant change at dose of 500 µg per day in volunteers but significant reduction when 1500 µg given daily for 15 days *2030*

Tri-iodothyronine (T3) *Serum Decrease Physiological* Associated with inhibition of conversion *6412*
Serum No Effect Physiological No significant effect in volunteers even when given as much as 4500 µg daily for 15 days *2030*

Triglycerides *Serum No Effect Analytical* No significant effect observed at a concentration of 2 mEq/L with method on Kodak Ektachem® systems *2519*

Iodide *(continued)*

TSH response to TRH *Serum Increase Physiological* Significant increase in volunteers given 500 µg or more per day for 15 days *2030*

Urea Nitrogen *Serum No Effect Analytical* No effect of concentrations up to 500 mg/dL on method on Kodak Ektachem® *5706*

Uric Acid *Serum No Effect Analytical* No significant effect observed at a concentration of 2 mEq/L with method on Kodak Ektachem® systems *2519*

Iodinated Glycerol

Thyroid Stimulating Hormone
Serum Increase Physiological In 8 elderly nursing home residents taking iodinated glycerol as an expectorant concentration significantly increased in five *1500*

Thyroxine (T4) *Serum Decrease Physiological* In one of 8 elderly nursing home residents taking iodinated glycerol as an expectorant concentration significantly decreased *1500*

Thyroxine (T4) Index, Free *Serum Decrease Physiological* In one of eight elderly nursing home residents taking iodinated glycerol as an expectorant index significantly decreased *1500*

Iodine

Amylase *Serum No Effect Analytical* No effect at concentration of 500 mg/L on method on Kodak Ektachem® *5706*

Cholinesterase *Serum No Effect Analytical* No effect observed at concentration of 2 mEq/L with butyrylthiocholine method on Kodak Ektachem® *2504*

Creatinine *Serum No Effect Analytical* No effect of concentrations up to 5000 mg/L on 2-slide method on Kodak Ektachem® *5706*

Thyroxine (T4) *Serum Increase Analytical* Some organic iodine may elute (odd pattern) *882*

Triglycerides *Serum No Effect Analytical* No effect of concentrations up to 5000 mg/L on method on Kodak Ektachem® *5706*

Uric Acid *Serum No Effect Analytical* At concentrations up to 500 mg/L had no effect on method on Kodak Ektachem® *5706*

Zinc *Serum No Effect Analytical* At 50 to 1 with flameless atomic absorption *3333*
Urine No Effect Analytical At 50 to 1 with flameless atomic absorption *3333*

^{131}Iodine

Glutathione S-Transferase *Serum Decrease Physiological* Treatment of hyperthyroid patients caused initially high activity to be reduced *448*

Iodine Containing Drugs

Casts *Urine Increase Physiological* Hemorrhagic nephritis with toxic doses *2183*

Erythrocytes *Urine Increase Physiological* Hemorrhagic nephritis with toxic doses *2183*

^{131}I Uptake *Serum Decrease Physiological* Small doses may affect but not PBI *882*

Iodine *Serum Increase Physiological* Iodine contamination increases total iodine concentration *2024*

Occult Blood *Feces Negative Physiological* May occur with toxicological doses *2183*

Protein *Urine Increase Physiological* Result of hemorrhagic nephritis at toxic doses *2183*

T3-Uptake *Serum No Effect Physiological* No effect on resin test observed *3107*

Iodipamide

Bilirubin *Serum Increase Physiological* Clinically significant displacement from protein potentially in neonates *6314*

BSP Retention *Serum Increase Physiological* Reported without evidence of liver damage *3669*

Cholinesterase *Serum Decrease Physiological* Fairly powerful inhibitor *3428*

^{131}I Uptake *Serum Decrease Physiological* Due to iodine component of material *3669*

17-Ketogenic Steroids *Urine Decrease Analytical* Interferes with reaction *4245*

Uric Acid *Serum Decrease Physiological* Uricosuric effect *4151*
Urine Increase Physiological Uricosuric effect *4151*

Iodixanol

Albumin *Urine No Effect Physiological* In 10 healthy men injection had no significant effect on excretion *2890*

Alkaline Phosphatase *Urine Increase Physiological* In 10 healthy men injection was followed 375% increase after 4 hours and increase at lower level persisted over next 48 hours *2890*

Glomerular Filtration Rate *Urine No Effect Physiological* In 10 healthy men injection of contrast medium had no significant effect on GFR *2890*

β_2-Microglobulin *Urine Increase Physiological* In 10 healthy men injection was followed by increase of 150% from 0 - 4 hours after injection *2890*

N-Acetyl-Glucosaminidase *Urine No Effect Physiological* In 10 healthy men no significant change observed after injection *2890*

Iodized Oil

^{131}I Uptake *Serum Decrease Physiological* Interferes with uptake *128*

Iodoalphionic Acid

BSP Retention *Serum Increase Physiological* Effect reported without abnormal liver function *3669*

Creatinine Clearance *Urine Decrease Physiological* Reported to cause renal failure *116*

^{131}I Uptake *Serum Decrease Physiological* Organic iodine contamination *2024*

Protein *Urine Increase Analytical* Affects acid precipitation methods *116*

Thyroxine (T4) *Serum Increase Analytical* Interferes with direct bromination *882*

Urea Nitrogen *Serum Increase Physiological* Reported to cause renal failure *116*

Iodoamide

Thyroid Stimulating Hormone
Serum Decrease Physiological In 17 euthyroid men following arteriography: maximum effect of more than 50% and at 10-12 weeks *1729*

Thyroxine (T4) *Serum No Effect Physiological* In 17 euthyroid men following arteriography for up to 14 weeks *1729*

Tri-iodothyronine, Reverse (rT3)
Serum No Effect Physiological In 17 euthyroid men following arteriography for up to 14 weeks *1729*

Tri-iodothyronine (T3) *Serum No Effect Physiological* In 17 euthyroid men following arteriography for up to 14 weeks, although initial slight reduction *1729*

Iodochlorhydroxyquin

Ferric Chloride Test *Urine Positive Analytical* If on diaper may give false positive *2754*

^{131}I Uptake *Serum Decrease Physiological* Contains organically bound iodine *3537*

Neutrophils *Blood Increase Physiological* Toxic effect reported *5987*

Phenylketones *Urine Positive Analytical* Green with $FeCl_3$ *1195*

Iodoform

^{131}I Uptake *Serum Decrease Physiological* Organically bound iodine, inhibits further uptake *3669*

Iodopyracet

^{131}I Uptake *Serum Decrease Physiological* Due to iodine component of material *3669*

Protein *Urine Increase Analytical* If acid precipitation methods used *4917* Gives false positive with turbidity tests *1174*

PSP Excretion *Urine Decrease Physiological* May compete for excretion through renal tubules *1622*

Uric Acid *Serum Decrease Physiological* Uricosuric action *2378*
Urine Increase Physiological Uricosuric action *2378*

Iodoquinol

Erythrocytes *Blood Decrease Physiological* May cause anemia *3810*

^{131}I Uptake *Serum Decrease Physiological* Effect lasts for several weeks *2451*

Leukocytes *Blood Decrease Physiological* May cause leukopenia *3810*

Iohexol

Alanine Aminopeptidase *Urine Increase Physiological* Observed in 20 patients with normal renal function following intravenous urography with 0.6-3.3 g/kg body weight with maximum effect observed after one day: typically reverted to normal by 3 days *1463*

Alkaline Phosphatase *Urine Increase Physiological* In 20 patients with normal renal function intravenous pyelography with 0.6-3.3 g/kg body weight: maximal effect at one day with reversion to normal by 3 days *1463*

Clotting Time *Blood Increase Physiological* Normal clotting time of venous blood prolonged from 15 minutes to 160 minutes *4870*

γ-Glutamyltransferase *Urine Increase Physiological* Observed in 20 patients with normal renal function following intravenous pyelography with 0.6-3.3 g/kg body weight with maximal effect observed after one day, but typical reversion to normal by 3 days *1463*

Lactate Dehydrogenase *Urine Increase Physiological* Observed in 20 patients with normal renal function following intravenous pyelography with 0.6-3.3 g/kg body weight. Maximal effect observed at one day with reversion to normal by 3 days *1463*

N-Acetyl-Glucosaminidase *Urine Increase Physiological* Observed in 20 patients with normal renal function following intravenous pyelography with 0.6-3.3 g/kg body weight with maximal effect at 1 day and reversion to normal by 3 days *1463*

Partial Thromboplastin Time
Plasma Increase Physiological Insignificant prolongation of normal 36 second partial thromboplastin time of platelet-poor plasma to 40 seconds *4870*

Ion Exchange Resins

Ammonia *Plasma Increase Physiological* Mechanism not reported: ?depends on resin *2451*

Chloride *Serum Increase Physiological* Mechanism not cited: ?depends on resin *1009*

Iopamidol

Bilirubin *Serum No Effect Analytical* No effect at 100 mg/L on Ames Seralyzer method *5706*

Cholesterol *Serum No Effect Analytical* No effect at 100 mg/L on Ames Seralyzer method *5706*

Creatine Kinase *Serum No Effect Analytical* No effect at 100 mg/L on method on Ames Seralyzer *5706*

Creatinine *Serum Increase Physiological* Transient increase at 3rd day after i.v. administration for angiography *1768* Significant effect (0.5 mg/dL) in 8.2% of 208 patients receiving compound for cardiac catheterization, but in 15% patients with diabetes mellitus, heart failure or pre-existing renal insufficiency *5389*
Serum No Effect Analytical No effect at 100 mg/L on Ames Seralyzer method *5706*

Glucose *Serum No Effect Analytical* No effect at 100 mg/L on glucose oxidase method on Ames Seralyzer *5706*

Lactate Dehydrogenase *Serum No Effect Analytical* No effect at 100 mg/L on method on Ames Seralyzer *5706*

Urea Nitrogen *Serum No Effect Analytical* No effect at 100 mg/L on method on Ames Seralyzer *5706*

Iopanoic Acid

Alanine Aminotransferase *Serum Increase Physiological* May cause hepatotoxicity *3810*

Aspartate Aminotransferase *Serum Increase Physiological* May cause hepatotoxicity *3810*

Bilirubin *Serum Increase Physiological* May cause hepatotoxicity *3810* Clinically significant displacement from protein observable in neonates *6314*

BSP Retention *Serum Increase Physiological* Competes for hepatocellular protein binding sites *5370*

Cholinesterase *Serum Decrease Physiological* Potent inhibitor at 0.06 mmol/L *3428*

Creatinine Clearance *Urine Decrease Physiological* Reported cause of acute renal failure *116*

^{131}I Uptake *Serum Decrease Physiological* Due to iodine component of material *3669*

Platelets *Blood Decrease Physiological* 3 episodes in one patient occurring from 8 to 40 d after drug ingestion, resolution occurred after drug withdrawn *2802* Few cases transient thrombocytopenia noted *6513*

Protein *Urine Increase Analytical* Causes false positive with turbidity tests *116* Gives turbidity if acid precipitation tests used *4917*
Urine No Effect Analytical No effect on heat and acetic acid test. No effect on Albustix, Labstix® *2452*

Thyroid Stimulating Hormone
Serum Increase Physiological Still increased 1 week after course of agent *5883* Blocks intrahypophyseal conversion of T4 to T3 *6412* Two-fold increase observed in 8 morbidly obese men given 600 kcal/d diet for 6 weeks after iopanoic acid added for 2 weeks *3067*

Thyroxine (T4) *Serum Increase Analytical* Contaminating iodine affects test *5401*
Serum Increase Physiological Inhibition of conversion of thyroxine to tri-iodothyronine *6412*

Thyroxine (T4), Free *Serum Increase Physiological* Inhibition of conversion of thyroxine to tri-iodothyronine *6412*

Tri-iodothyronine, Reverse (rT3)
Serum Increase Physiological When combined for 2 weeks with 600 kcal/d diet for 6 weeks mean increase of 289% observed in 8 morbidly obese men compared with situation when only low calorie diet given *3067*

Tri-iodothyronine (T3) *Serum Decrease Physiological* When combined with low calorie diet in 8 morbidly obese men mean reduction from baseline of 49.5% observed *3067* Inhibition of conversion of thyroxine to tri-iodothyronine *6412*

Uric Acid *Serum Decrease Physiological* Uricosuric effect *4151*
Urine Increase Physiological Uricosuric effect *4151*

Urobilinogen *Urine Increase Analytical* Produce white cloudy precipitate with Ehrlich's reagent *882*

Iopentol

Albumin *Urine No Effect Physiological* Injection had no significant effect on excretion *2890*

Alkaline Phosphatase *Urine Increase Physiological* Following injection ncrease in excretion greater than after mannitol (500% versus 175%) and persisted longer *2890*

Glomerular Filtration Rate *Urine No Effect Physiological* In 10 healthy volunteer men no significant effect observed after injection of contrast medium *2890*

β_2-Microglobulin *Urine Increase Physiological* In 10 healthy men injection caused 300% increase from 0 - 4 h with lower increasing persisting over next 24 hours *2890*

N-Acetyl-Glucosaminidase *Urine Increase Physiological* In 10 healthy men injection of contrast medium caused increase of 121% from 4 to 24 hours after injection, with increase persisting for 24-48 hours *2890*

Iophenoxic Acid

^{131}I Uptake *Serum Decrease Physiological* Due to iodine component of material *3669*

Protein *Urine Increase Analytical* Affects turbidity tests for up to 3 d *116*

Iopydone

^{131}I Uptake *Serum Decrease Physiological* Due to iodine component of material *3669*

Iothalamate

Alanine Aminopeptidase *Urine Increase Physiological* After appropriate clinical indication in children 19-fold increase in excretion observed *3187*

Protein *Urine Increase Analytical* Precipitated as if protein in turbidimetric method on Du Pont aca *4274*
Urine No Effect Analytical No interference observed with Ames N-Multistix *4274*

Iothiouracil

^{131}I Uptake *Serum Decrease Physiological* Drug consists of organically bound iodine *1279*

Leukocytes *Blood Decrease Physiological* Agranulocytosis *3810*

T3-Uptake *Serum Decrease Physiological* Depresses thyroid function *882*

Thyroxine (T4) *Serum Decrease Physiological* Depresses thyroid function *882*
Serum Increase Analytical Organic iodine compound (no effect with Murphy-Pattee procedure) *572*

Thyroxine (T4) (Murphy-Pattee)
Serum Decrease Physiological Depresses thyroid function *882*
Serum No Effect Analytical No effect on method *3669*

Ioxaglate

Alanine Aminopeptidase *Urine Increase Physiological* After appropriate diagnostic indication 10-fold increase in excretion of enzyme observed *3187*

Clotting Time *Blood Increase Physiological* Normal clotting time of venous blood prolonged from 15 minutes to 330 minutes *4870*

Partial Thromboplastin Time
Plasma Increase Physiological Normal partial thromboplastin time of 36 seconds in venous platelet-poor plasma prolonged to 54 seconds *4870*

Protein *Urine Increase Analytical* Contrast medium precipitated as if protein in turbidimetric method on Du Pont aca *4274*
Urine No Effect Analytical No interference observed with Ames N-Multistix *4274*

Ioxitalamic Acid

Histamine *Plasma Increase Physiological* Major increase in arterial and mixed venous blood in 30 s following injection for translumbar arterial aortography in 16 patients *2269*

Osmolality *Serum Increase Physiological* Major increase in arterial osmolality within 30 s following injection of 77 ± 16 mL Telebrix 38 for translumbar arterial aortography in 16 patients *2269*

Thyroxine (T4) *Serum No Effect Analytical* No effect observed after i.v. injection *230*

Ipecac

Lysergic Acid Diethylamide
Gastric Material Increase Analytical Fluorescent spectrum may interfere *4152*

Ipodate

Bilirubin *Serum Increase Physiological* Probably due to competition for excretion *1009*

Creatinine *Serum Increase Physiological* Nephrotoxic effect *1298*

Erythrocytes *Urine Increase Physiological* Nephrotoxic effect *1298*

Hemoglobin *Urine Increase Physiological* Nephrotoxic effect *1298*

^{131}I Uptake *Serum Decrease Physiological* Interferes with uptake *128*

Protein *Urine Increase Physiological* Nephrotoxic effect *1298*

T3-Uptake *Serum No Effect Physiological* Significant increase unrelated to I_2 content *882*

Thyroid Stimulating Hormone
Serum Increase Physiological Affects intrahypophyseal conversion of T4 to T3 *6412*

Thyroxine (T4) *Serum Increase Physiological* Inhibition of T4 to T3 conversion *6412*

Tri-iodothyronine (T3) *Serum Decrease Physiological* Inhibition of T4 to T3 conversion *6412*

Urea Nitrogen *Serum Increase Physiological* Nephrotoxic effect *1298*

Uric Acid *Serum Decrease Physiological* Uricosuric effect *4151*
Urine Increase Physiological Uricosuric effect *4151*

Urobilin *Urine Increase Physiological* Nephrotoxic effect *1298*

Ipriflavone

Alkaline Phosphatase *Serum Decrease Physiological* In patients with Paget's disease of the bone administration of two 30-day courses (600 and 1200 mg/d) resulted in significant 35% decrease in activity *4897*

Hydroxyproline *Urine Decrease Physiological* In patients with Paget's disease of the bone treatment with two courses of 600 mg/d and 1200 mg/d for 30 days caused significant 25% reduction in mean excretion *4897*

Iprindole

Alanine Aminotransferase *Serum Increase Physiological* Hepatic cholestasis without inflammation *78*

Alkaline Phosphatase *Serum Increase Physiological* Mild elevation with cholestasis *78*

Aspartate Aminotransferase *Serum Increase Physiological* Hepatic toxicity *5869*

Bile *Urine Increase Physiological* Due to hepatic toxicity *78*

Bilirubin *Serum Increase Physiological* Associated with low serum phosphate *78*

Bilirubin, Direct *Serum Increase Physiological* Associated with low serum phosphate *78*

Eosinophils *Blood Increase Physiological* Allergic response reported *78*

Iproniazid

Alanine Aminotransferase *Serum Increase Physiological* Prolonged use may cause hepatotoxicity *6461*

Albumin *Serum No Effect Analytical* At concentration of 40 mg/L had no effect on BCG method *5704*

Alkaline Phosphatase *Serum Increase Physiological* May cause cholestatic jaundice *3810*

Aspartate Aminotransferase *Serum Increase Physiological* Prolonged use may cause hepatotoxicity *6461*

Bicarbonate *Serum No Effect Analytical* At concentration of 40 mg/L had no effect on method using phenolphthalein *5704*

Bile *Urine Increase Physiological* Prolonged use may cause hepatotoxicity *3810*

Bilirubin *Serum Increase Physiological* May cause cholestatic and cytotoxic jaundice *402*
Serum No Effect Analytical At concentration of 40 mg/L had no effect on Jendrassik and Grof method *5704*

BSP Retention *Serum Increase Physiological* May cause cholestatic jaundice *3810*.

Calcium *Serum No Effect Analytical* At concentration of 40 mg/L had no effect on cresolphthalein method *5704*

Chloride *Serum No Effect Analytical* At concentration of 40 mg/L had no effect on mercurimetric method *5704*

Cholesterol *Serum No Effect Analytical* At concentration of 40 mg/L had no effect on Liebermann-Burchard method *5704*

Creatinine *Serum No Effect Analytical* At concentration of 40 mg/L had no effect on Technicon AutoAnalyzer® Jaffe method *5704*

Erythrocytes *Blood Decrease Physiological* Pancytopenia (AMA Blood dyscrasias) *4017*

Glucose *Serum Decrease Analytical* At concentrations above 110 mg/L lowered concentration as measured by GOD-PERID method *5704* Depresses glucose oxidase method of Boehringer *5480*
Serum No Effect Analytical No effect at 100 mg/L on hexokinase method on Ames Seralyzer *5706* Affects Boehringer GOD-PERID method *5480*

β-Glucuronidase *Serum Increase Physiological* Effect of toxic hepatitis *6461*

Guanase *Serum Increase Physiological* May cause cholestatic and cytotoxic jaundice *402*

Isocitrate Dehydrogenase *Serum Increase Physiological* May cause cholestatic and cytotoxic jaundice *402*

Leukocytes *Blood Decrease Physiological* Pancytopenia (AMA Blood dyscrasias) *4017*

Ornithine Carbamoyltransferase
Serum Increase Physiological May cause cholestatic and cytotoxic jaundice *402*

Phosphate *Serum No Effect Analytical* At concentration of 40 mg/L had no effect on phosphomolybdate method *5704*

Platelets *Blood Decrease Physiological* Pancytopenia (AMA Blood dyscrasias) *4017*

Potassium *Serum No Effect Analytical* At concentration of 40 mg/L had no effect on measurement by ISE with predilution *5704*

Protein *Serum No Effect Analytical* At concentration of 40 mg/L had no effect on biuret method with blank correction *5704*

Pyridoxal *Serum Decrease Physiological* Observed in patient with toxicity *1148*

Pyridoxine *Serum Decrease Physiological* Observed in patient with toxicity *1148*

Sodium *Serum No Effect Analytical* At concentration of 40 mg/L had no effect on measurement by ISE with predilution *5704*

Triglycerides *Serum No Effect Analytical* At concentration of 40 mg/L had no effect on lipase/esterase method *5704*

Urea Nitrogen *Serum No Effect Analytical* At concentration of 40 mg/L had no effect on diacetylmonoxime method *5704*

Uric Acid *Serum No Effect Analytical* At concentration of 40 mg/L had no effect on phosphotungstate reduction method *5704*

Iproplatin

Alkaline Phosphatase *Urine No Effect Physiological* Overall no significant increase in patients with solid tumors given several courses of treatment *5594*

Creatinine Clearance *Urine No Effect Physiological* No overall effect in patients with solid tumors given several course of treatment *5594*

Lactate Dehydrogenase *Urine No Effect Physiological* Overall no significant increase in patients with solid tumors given several courses of treatment *5594*

β_2-Microglobulin *Urine No Effect Physiological* No effect observed overall in patients with solid tumors given several courses of treatment *5594*

N-Acetyl-Glucosaminidase *Urine No Effect Physiological* Overall no significant increase in patients with solid tumors given several courses of treatment *5594*

Platelets *Blood Decrease Physiological* Thrombocytopenia is often dose limiting *1384*

Protein *Urine No Effect Physiological* Transient increases observed in patients with solid tumors given several courses of treatment but overall no change *5594*

Ipsapirone

Corticotropin *Plasma No Effect Physiological* In 6 healthy volunteers treatment with up to 30 mg/d had no significant effect *477*

Corticotropin-releasing Hormone
Plasma No Effect Physiological In 6 healthy volunteers treatment with up to 30 mg/d had no significant effect *477*

Cortisol *Plasma No Effect Physiological* In 6 healthy volunteers treatment with up to 30 mg/d had no significant effect on concentration *477*

Melatonin *Plasma No Effect Physiological* In 8 healthy volunteers administration of 20 mg ipsapirone at 20:00 h caused no significant effect on nocturnal plasma melatonin concentration *4230*

Irbesartan

Creatinine *Serum Increase Physiological* Minor increases in patients with essential hypertension observed in less than 0.7% patients compared with 0.9% of placebo-treated controls *725*

Digoxin *Serum No Effect Physiological* Administration of irbesartan for 7 days had no effect on the pharmacokinetics of digoxin *725*

Hemoglobin *Blood No Effect Physiological* Mean decreases of 0.2 g/dL in patients with essential hypertension observed in 0.2% patients compared with 0.3% of placebo-treated controls *725*

Hydrochlorothiazide *Serum No Effect Physiological* Administration of irbesartan for 7 days had no effect on the pharmacodynamics of hydrochlorothiazide *725*

Neutrophils *Blood No Effect Physiological* Mean decreases below 1000 cells/μL in patients with essential hypertension observed in 0.3% patients compared with 0.5% of placebo-treated controls *725*

Prothrombin Time *Plasma No Effect Physiological* Administration of irbesartan for 7 days had no effect on the pharmacodynamics of warfarin *725*

Urea Nitrogen *Serum Increase Physiological* Minor increases in patients with essential hypertension observed in less than 0.7% patients compared with 0.9% of placebo-treated controls *725*

Uric Acid *Serum Increase Physiological* Gout reported as rare complication of treatment *725*

Warfarin *Plasma No Effect Physiological* Administration of irbesartan for 7 days had no effect on the pharmacodynamics of warfarin *725*

Irinotecan

Alkaline Phosphatase *Serum Increase Physiological* Reported to occur as a side effect within 24 hours of administration in 3.9% of patients with NCI grades 3 and 4 disease and in 13.2% of patients with grades 1 to 4 disease *4666*

Aspartate Aminotransferase *Serum Increase Physiological* Reported to occur as a side effect within 24 hours of administration in 1.3% of patients with NCI grades 3 and 4 disease and in 10.5% of patients with grades 1 to 4 disease *4666*

Glucose *Serum Increase Physiological* Hyperglycemia has been reported to occur as a side effect but usually only in patients with a prior history of diabetes mellitus or evidence of glucose intolerance *4666*

Hematocrit *Blood Decrease Physiological* Severe myelosuppression may occur as a side effect. Anemia occurred in 6.9% of patients with NCI grades 3 and 4 disease and in 60.5% of patients with grades 1 to 4 disease *4666*

Hemoglobin *Blood Decrease Physiological* Severe myelosuppression may occur as a side effect. Anemia occurred in 6.9% of patients with NCI grades 3 and 4 disease and in 60.5% of patients with grades 1 to 4 disease *4666*

Leukocytes *Blood Decrease Physiological* Severe myelosuppression may occur as a side effect. Leukopenia occurred in 28.0% of NCI grades 3 and 4 disease and 63.2% of patients with grades 1 to 4 disease *4666*

Lymphocytes *Blood Decrease Physiological* Lymphocytopenia has been reported to occur as a side effect *4666*

Neutrophils *Blood Decrease Physiological* Severe myelosuppression may occur as a side effect. Neutropenia occurred in 26.3% of patients with NCI grades 3 and 4 disease and in 53.9% patients with grades 1 to 4 disease *4666*

Platelets *Blood Decrease Physiological* Severe myelosuppression may occur as a side effect *4666*

Iron

Acetaminophen *Serum Decrease Physiological* Has functional chemical group in a configuration which will result in stable iron-drug complex possibly resulting in reduced serum drug concentration due to impaired gastrointestinal absorption *863*

Alanine Aminotransferase *Serum Increase Physiological* May cause severe liver damage with poisoning *467*

Ampicillin *Serum Decrease Physiological* Drug has functional chemical group in a configuration that results in stable iron-drug complex that might reduce gastrointestinal absorption and result in reduced serum concentration *863*

Antazoline *Serum Decrease Physiological* Potential problem with oral administration because of possible strong binding to iron because of known ability to bind copper or because of functional groups present *863*

Aspartate Aminotransferase *Serum Increase Physiological* May cause severe liver damage with poisoning *467*

Bephenium *Serum Decrease Physiological* Potential problem with oral administration because of known strong binding to copper or because of functional groups present *863*

Bilirubin *Serum Increase Physiological* With poisoning 3-4 d after ingestion *6432*

Bilirubin, Conjugated *Serum No Effect Analytical* Over the concentration range of 98 - 500 µg/dL had no significant effect on method on Kodak Ektachem® systems *2519*

Bilirubin, Direct *Serum Increase Physiological* With poisoning 3-4 d after ingestion *6432*

Bilirubin, Unconjugated *Serum No Effect Analytical* Over the concentration range of 98 - 500 µg/dL had no significant effect on method on Kodak Ektachem® systems *2519*

Calcium *Serum Increase Analytical* Interfere with direct EDTA titration *2559*

Captopril *Serum Decrease Physiological* Drug has functional chemical configuration that results in stable iron-drug complex that impairs gastrointestinal absorption and might ultimately result in reduced serum concentration *863*

Carbidopa *Serum Decrease Physiological* Drug has functional chemical group in a configuration that results in stable iron-drug complex that results in impaired gastrointetinal absorption with 75% reduction in bioavailability. Iron catalyzed oxidation of carbidopa occurs in vitro *863*

Cefdinir *Serum Decrease Physiological* Concomitant administration of 60 mg elemental iron as ferrous sulfate or vitamins supplemented with 10 mg of elemental iron with cefdinir reduced its absorption by 80% and 31% respectively *4528*

Chlorpheniramine *Serum Decrease Physiological* Potential problem with oral administration because of known strong binding to copper or because of functional groups present *863*

Ciprofloxacin *Serum Decrease Physiological* Decreased oral bioavailability *886* Drug has functional chemical group in a configuration that causes stable iron-drug complex that impairs gastrointestinal absorption and might ultimately result in reduced serum concentration *863*

Color *Feces Increase Analytical* Black (gray-black) darkens in air with about 70 mg *3810*

Urine Increase Analytical Iron Sorbitex can cause brown urine (Fe sulfide) *2024*

Cyclosporine *Serum Decrease Physiological* Potential problem with oral administration because of known strong binding with copper or because of functional groups present *863*

Diagnex Blue Excretion *Urine Increase Physiological* Heavy metal displacement of diagnex blue *6515*

Dicumarol *Plasma Decrease Physiological* Potential problem with oral administration because of known strong binding to copper or because of functional groups present *863*

Diethylstilbestrol *Serum Decrease Physiological* Potential problem with oral administration because of known binding of drug with copper or because of functional groups present *863*

Digoxin *Serum Decrease Physiological* Potential problem with oral administration because of known strong binding with copper or because of functional groups present *863*

Diphenhydramine *Serum Decrease Physiological* Potential problem because of known strong binding of drug with copper or because of functional groups present *863*

Doxycycline *Serum Decrease Physiological* Stable iron-drug complex formed in gastrointestinal tract reducing absorption of drug *863*

Erythrocytes *Urine Increase Physiological* Hematuria reported after chronic administration Fe sorbitol *2754*

Ethambutol *Serum Decrease Physiological* Drug has functional chemical group in a configuration that results in stable iron-drug complex that impairs gastrointestinal absorption and might ultimately result in reduced serum concentration *863*

17-Ethinylestradiol *Serum Decrease Physiological* Potential problem because of known strong binding of drug with copper or because of functional groups present *863*

Ferritin *Serum Increase Physiological* With 200 mg iron daily, most patients serum ferritin increased as well as bone marrow stainable iron *2469*

Fibrinogen *Plasma Decrease Physiological* One case reported with poisoning *6432*

Folate *Serum Decrease Physiological* Drug has functional chemical group in a configuration that results in stable iron-drug complex that might impair gastrointestinal absorption and ultimately reduce serum concentration *863*

Furosemide *Serum Decrease Physiological* Potential problem with oral administration because of known strong binding of drug with copper or because of functional groups present *863*

Glucose Tolerance *Serum Decrease Physiological* As Fe ascorbate before glucose tolerance test *2452*

Hemoglobin *Urine Increase Physiological* Hematuria reported after iron Sorbitex *4014*

Hexylresorcinol *Serum Decrease Physiological* Potential problem with oral administration because of known strong binding with copper or because of functional groups present *863*

Indomethacin *Serum Decrease Physiological* Drug has a functional chemical group in a configuration that results in a stable iron-drug complex that might impair gastrointestinal absorption and ultimately cause reduced serum concentration *863*

Iron *Serum Increase Physiological* Effect of i.m. iron *2024*

Iron-Binding Capacity, Total *Serum Increase Physiological* Effect of intramuscular iron *2024*

Iron-Binding Capacity, Unsaturated *Serum Decrease Physiological* Effect of i.m. iron *2024*

Isoprenaline *Serum Decrease Physiological* Drug has functional chemical group in a configuration that forms a stable iron-drug complex that might impair gastrointestinal absorption and ultimately result in a reduced serum concentration *863*

Levodopa *Serum Decrease Physiological* Drug has a functional chemical group in a configuration that forms a stable 3:1 levodopa:iron complex that impairs gastrointestinal absorption and reduces bioavailability by 51% and 55% reduction in peak serum concentration *2601*

Lithium *Serum No Effect Analytical* No significant effect observed at a concentration of 124 μmol/L with method on Kodak Ektachem® systems *2519*

Magnesium *Serum No Effect Analytical* No interference observed with calmagite method with EDTA blank adapted for use with Technicon SMAC® *771* No significant effect at concentration of 280 μg/dL on calmagite method on Beckman Synchron CX 4/5 *4701* No effect of concentrations up to 5 mg/L on method on Kodak Ektachem® *5706* At a concentration of 500 μg/dL had no significant effect on method on Kodak Ektachem® systems *2519*

Methacycline *Serum Decrease Physiological* Stable iron-drug complex formed in gastrointestinal tract thereby reducing absorption of drug *863*

Methotrexate *Serum Decrease Physiological* Potential problem with oral administration because of known strong binding with copper or because of functional groups present *863*

Methyldopa *Serum Decrease Physiological* Stable iron-drug complex formed in g.i. tract reducing absorption (73% with $FeSO_4$ and 61% with Fe gluconate). Metabolism of drug altered in vivo so that 88% reduction in renal excretion of unmetabolized drug with $FeSO_4$ and 79% with Fe gluconate *863*

Minoxidil *Serum Decrease Physiological* Stable iron-drug complex formed in gastrointestinal tract thereby limiting availability for absorption *863*

Nalidixic Acid *Serum Decrease Physiological* Stable iron-drug complex formed in gastrointestinal tract thereby limiting availability of drug for absorption *863*
Urine Decrease Physiological Divalent or trivalent cations such as iron may interfere with the absorption of nalidixic acid resulting in lower urine concentrations than desired *5255*

Nickel *Test Conditions Increase Analytical* If ferrous and atomic absorption used *5866*

Norfloxacin *Serum Decrease Physiological* Stable iron-drug complex formed in gastrointestinal tract thereby limiting availability for absorption *863* Multivitamins, or other products containing iron or zinc, may interfere with the absorption of norfloxacin resulting in lower plasma and urine concentrations *4981* Decreased oral bioavailability *886*
Urine Decrease Physiological Multivitamins, or other products containing iron or zinc, may interfere with the absorption of norfloxacin resulting in lower plasma and urine concentrations *4981*

Occult Blood *Feces Increase Analytical* Interferes with guaiac test (?benzidine) *6021*
Feces Increase Physiological With poisoning may cause gastrointestinal hemorrhage *6432*
Feces No Effect Analytical If 3,3-dimethylnaphthidine used as chromogen *1331* No effect on Hemoquant procedure *6172*

Ofloxacin *Serum Decrease Physiological* Quinolines form chelates with alkaline earth and transition metal cations resulting in reduced absorption *3914*

Oxazepam *Serum Decrease Physiological* Potential problem with oral administration because of known strong binding to copper or because of functional groups present *863*

Oxytetracycline *Serum Decrease Physiological* Stable iron-drug complex formed in gastrointestinal tract thereby reducing absorption of drug *863*

Penicillamine *Serum Decrease Physiological* Forms stable iron-drug complex (2 drug molecules with 1 of iron) in gastrointestinal tract thereby limiting availability for absorption. Bioavailability of penicillamine reduced by 80% with 300 mg ferrous sulfate and peak serum concentration by 67% *863*

Pheniramine *Serum Decrease Physiological* Potential problem with oral administration because of known strong binding to copper or because of functional groups present *863*

Phosphate *Serum No Effect Analytical* At concentration of 100 mg/dL (17.9 mmol/L) no interference observed with method on Du Pont aca *1539*

Protein *Cerebrospinal Fluid No Effect Analytical* No effect of concentrations up to 8 mg/L on method on Kodak Ektachem® *5706* No significant effect observed at a concentration of 27 μg/dL with method on Kodak Ektachem® systems *2519*
Urine Increase Physiological May cause nephrotoxicity *2451*
Urine No Effect Analytical No effect of concentrations up to 8 mg/L on method on Kodak Ektachem® *5706*

Rifampin *Serum Decrease Physiological* Forms stable drug-iron complex in gastrointestinal tract thereby limiting availability for absorption *863*

Salicylate *Serum Decrease Physiological* Forms stable iron-drug complex in gastrointestinal tract thereby limiting availability for absorption *863*

Sedoheptulose *Urine Decrease Analytical* Ferric iron inhibits cysteine-H_2SO_4 reaction *3865*

Sparfloxacin *Serum Decrease Physiological* Iron and zinc salts significantly reduce the absorption of sparfloxacin and must be taken 4 hours after the ingestion of sparfloxacin to avoid reducing its bioavailability *4943*

Tetracycline *Serum Decrease Physiological* Decreased oral bioavailability *886* Marked reduction in gastrointestinal absorption occurs due to stable iron-drug complex formation. Two molecules of tetracycline combine with one of iron. Tetracycline plasma levels may be reduced by as much as 50%. Problem avoided if Fe given 3 h before *863*

Thonzylamine *Serum Decrease Physiological* Potential problem with oral administration because of known strong binding with copper or because of functional groups present *863*

Thyroxine (T4) *Serum Decrease Physiological* Forms stable iron-drug complex in gastrointestinal tract thereby limiting availability for absorption *863*

Trovafloxacin *Serum Decrease Physiological* Coadministration of iron as ferrous salts significantly reduces the absorption of trovafloxacin *4663*

Urea Nitrogen *Serum Increase Physiological* May cause nephrotoxicity *5377*

Urobilin *Urine Increase Physiological* May exacerbate urinary tract infections *4014*

Vitamin B_{12} *Red Blood Cells Increase Physiological* During treatment of iron-deficient anemia *2482*

Zinc *Serum No Effect Analytical* At 50 to 1 with flameless atomic absorption *3333*
Urine No Effect Analytical At 50 to 1 with flameless atomic absorption *3333*

Iron Dextran

Bilirubin *Serum Increase Analytical* May cause falsely increased values with certain methods *5320*

Calcium *Serum Decrease Analytical* May cause falsely decreased values with certain methods *5320*

Color *Serum Increase Physiological* Large doses of iron dextran (5 mL or more) reported to give a brown color to serum from a blood specimen drawn 4 hours after administration *5320*
Urine Increase Analytical Black urine on standing reported *2753*

Creatinine Clearance *Urine No Effect Physiological* No effect if prior normal renal function *2753*

Erythrocytes *Urine Increase Physiological* Reversible after chronic administration in one patient *2753*

Ferritin *Serum Increase Physiological* Concentration peaks approximately 7 to 9 days after an intravenous dose of INFeD and slowly returns to baseline after 3 weeks following administration *5320* Concentration of 2840 ng/mL observed in one woman who had received 100 mg elemental iron intramuscularly every 2 weeks for 20 years *5297* In two individuals 40 and 20 mL of intravenously infused iron dextran caused peak concentrations of about 230 μg/L at 7 and 9 days respectively *614*

Iron Dextran *(continued)*

Glucose *Serum Increase Analytical* At 5 g Fe/dL on glucose oxidase procedure (slight). 5 g Fe/dL equivalent to 15.5 mmol/L with o-toluidine procedure. 5 g Fe/dL equivalent to 3.5 mmol/L with p-HBAH procedure. Slight effect at 5 g Fe/dL on alkaline ferricyanide procedure *3531*

Hematocrit *Blood Increase Physiological* Effect observed in 7 individuals with chronic disease given total dose intravenous infusion *290*

Hemoglobin *Blood Increase Physiological* In two individuals 40 and 20 mL of intravenously infused iron dextran caused peak concentrations of about 3.6 g/dL over 25 days in one and somewhat slower response in the other *614* Effect observed in 7 individuals with chronic disease following total dose intravenous infusion *290*

Urine Increase Physiological Reversible after chronic administration in one patient *2753*

Iron *Serum Increase Analytical* 20-30% of iron added (10-225 µmol/L) recovered when colorimetric procedure on Roche Cobas-Bio used with commercial reagents from Baker. At 1 hour after iron dextran administration to 4 patients significant increase in iron but only 26% of that with AAS *6228* 89-120% of added iron (10-225 µmol/L) recovered when measured by atomic absorption spectrometry and significant increase observed at 1 hour after administration to 4 patients *6228* Less than 6% added iron (10-225 µmol/L) recovered when iron dextran added in vitro but significant effect at 1 hour after in vivo administration to 4 patients but only 5% of that when iron measured by AAS *6228* Minimal effect of iron in iron-dextran as only 3% not tightly bound to dextran when method on Kodak Ektachem® 700 used *2865*

Serum Increase Physiological Concentration of 227 µg/dL observed in one woman who had received 100 mg elemental iron intramuscularly every 2 weeks for 20 years *5297* Increased iron stores *3810* May cause increased values for 3 weeks following administration *5320* In two individuals 40 and 20 mL of intravenously infused iron dextran caused peak concentrations of about 8000 and 4750 µmol/L immediately after infusion *614*

Urine Increase Physiological Approximately 30% Fe Sorbitex in urine in 24 h *2753*

Iron-Binding Capacity, Total *Serum Increase Analytical* Addition of iron dextran both in vivo or in vitro caused increase when measured by AAS, Ferrozine method on Roche Cobas-Bio and by method on Kodak Ektachem® but changes appear to be completely related to effect of added iron and not effect on UIBC *6228*

Iron-Binding Capacity, Unsaturated

Serum Decrease Physiological Due to increased availability of iron *3810*

Serum No Effect Analytical Neither in vivo or in vitro did the addition of iron dextran affect the unsaturated binding capacity as measured by atomic absorption spectrometry, colorimetrically using Ferrozine on Roche Cobas-Bio or on method on Kodak Ektachem® 700 *6228*

Leukocytes *Blood Increase Physiological* Leukemoid reaction reported *4014* May cause leukocytosis *5320*

Protein *Urine Increase Physiological* Reversible after chronic administration in one patient *2753*

Iron-Protein-Succinylate

Iron *Serum Increase Physiological* Increased concentration noted after oral administration of compound *1462*

Iron Sorbitex

Color *Urine Increase Analytical* Complex with citrate produce black urine *1957*

Glucose *Serum Increase Analytical* 5 g Fe/dL equivalent to 7.1 mmol/L o-toluidine. 5 g Fe/dL equivalent to 1.9 mmol/L p-HBAH procedure. 5 g Fe/dL equivalent to 1.0 mmol/L alkaline ferricyanide. 5 g Fe/dL equivalent to 1/6 mmol/L glucose oxidase *3531*

Irtemazole

Uric Acid *Serum Decrease Physiological* Increasing doses up to 37.5 mg caused proprtional decrease in plasma concentration with decrease of about 40% observed with 37.5 mg. With 25 mg in 6 healthy individuals decrease from about 4.9 mg/dL at baseline to about 3.7 mg/dL after 8 hours *2326*

Urine Increase Physiological In 6 healthy volunteers excretion increased with maximum reached 30 to 120 min after administration. After single oral dose of 12.5 maximal excretion was 41.9 to 145.0 mg/h (average 86.0 mg/h), after 25 mg 82.1 to 140.5 mg/h (average 105.9 mg/h) and after 37.5 mg 102.3 to 155.0 mg/h (average 134.2 mg/h). After 50 mg an increase of 150.8 mg/h observed *2326*

Isocarbazide

Glucose *Serum No Effect Analytical* At concentration of 55 mg/L had no effect on GOD-PERID method *5704*

Isocarboxazid

Alanine Aminotransferase *Serum Increase Physiological* Cholestatic effect *3810*

Alkaline Phosphatase *Serum Increase Physiological* Cholestatic effect *3810*

Ammonia *Plasma Decrease Physiological* Reportedly effective in reducing NH_3 intoxication *2451*

Aspartate Aminotransferase *Serum Increase Physiological* Cholestatic effect *3810*

Bile *Urine Increase Physiological* Cholestatic effect *3810*

Bilirubin *Serum Increase Physiological* Cholestatic effect *3810*

BSP Retention *Serum Increase Physiological* Intrahepatic cholestasis reported *834*

Erythrocytes *Blood Decrease Physiological* Rare agranulocytosis with anemia *3810*

Glucose *Serum Decrease Analytical* Affects glucose oxidase method of Boehringer Mannheim *5480*

Serum Decrease Physiological MAO inhibitors have slight effect *2451*

Serum No Effect Analytical Affects Boehringer GOD-PERID method *5480*

Hematocrit *Blood Decrease Physiological* May occasionally produce anemia *4014*

Hemoglobin *Blood Decrease Physiological* May occasionally produce anemia *4014*

5-Hydroxyindoleacetic Acid *Urine Decrease Physiological* Due to inhibition of conversion of 5-HT to 5-HIAA *2451*

Leukocytes *Blood Decrease Physiological* Rare agranulocytosis with leukopenia *2629*

Vanillylmandelic Acid *Urine Decrease Physiological* Inhibition of formation *2451*

Xylose *Urine Decrease Physiological* Decreased gastrointestinal tract absorption with consequent reduced excretion *6192*

Isoflurane

Aldosterone *Plasma Increase Physiological* In 8 patients administered isoflurane plasma aldosterone changed significantly with 60 minutes middle ear surgery, although increased during recovery phase, as did controls *3844*

Arginine Vasopressin *Plasma No Effect Physiological* In 8 patients administered isoflurane plasma AVP changed insignificantly with 60 minutes middle ear surgery, although increased during recovery phase, as did controls *3844*

Corticotropin *Plasma No Effect Physiological* In 8 patients administered lisoflurane plasma cortiicotropin changed insignificantly with 60 minutes middle ear surgery, although increased during recovery phase, as did controls *3844*

Cortisol *Plasma Decrease Physiological* In 8 patients administered lisoflurane plasma cortisol changed significantly with 60 minutes middle ear surgery *3844*

Fluoride *Serum Increase Physiological* In 4 patients given isoflurane as sedative highest concentration observed 24.9 µmol/L in patients not undergoing dialysis and 13.7 ± 3.6 µmol/L in those undergoing peritoneal or hemodialysis *1984* In 11 patients given isoflurane anesthesia mean concentration changed to a peak of 4.8 ± 0.5 µmol/L 16 hours after anesthesia *2599*

F Protein *Serum Increase Physiological* In 13 patients following surgery with isoflurane mean concentration increased 6 days later, but changes unrelated to duration of anesthesia, quantity of delivered volatile agent or mode of ventilation *1124*

Hematocrit *Blood No Effect Physiological* In 8 patients administered isoflurane hematocrit changed insignificantly from 41% at induction to 37% at end of 60 minutes middle ear surgery, not significantly different from controls *3844*

Histamine *Plasma No Effect Analytical* No inhibition of radio-enzyme assay of clinical significance likely to occur at physiological concentrations *2492*

Leukocytes *Blood Increase Physiological* Normal response to anesthesia *5818*

Osmolality *Serum No Effect Physiological* In 8 patients administered isoflurane serum osmolality changed insignificantly from 282 mosmol/kg at induction to 293 mosmol/kg at end of 60 minutes middle ear surgery, not significantly different from controls *3844*

pH *Blood No Effect Physiological* In 8 patients administered isoflurane arterial pH changed insignificantly from 7.39 at induction to 7.42 at end of 60 minutes middle ear surgery not significantly different from controls *3844*

Remifentanil *Serum No Effect Physiological* Remifentanil clearance is not altered when isoflurane coadministered *2165*

Theophylline *Serum No Effect Physiological* No clinically significant effect on theophylline concentration observed when drugs coadministered *5999* No documented significant interaction with theophylline reported *6117*

Isoflurophate

Cholinesterase *Serum Decrease Physiological* Therapeutic action of drug *128*

Isometheptene

Amphetamine *Urine Positive Analytical* Reacts as if amphetamine in EMIT screening and confirmatory assays (Note compound is a component of Midrin® used to treat migraine) *3539*

Drugs of Abuse Screen *Urine Increase Analytical* False positive produced with Abbott ADx method for amphetamine/methamphetamine *4279*

Isomil®

Amino Acids *Urine Increase Analytical* Reddish-pink spot with DL-methionine with ninhydrin on thin-layer chromatography *2109*

Isoniazid

Acetaminophen *Serum Increase Physiological* Severe hepatic and renal toxicity in one woman who had ingested no more than 11.5 g acetaminophen. Concentration of 150 µmol/L observed. Toxicity suggested to be due to induction of P-450IIEI in liver and conversion of drug to toxic metabolites *4186*

Alanine Aminotransferase *Serum Increase Physiological* In 72 patients with tuberculosis all receiving isoniazid and rifampin and, in addition, pyrazinamide in 72.2%, ethambutol in 80% and streptomycin in 16.7% drug-induced hepatitis observed with AST activity reaching mean of 330.2 ± 425.5 U/L *5577* Risk of hepatitis caused by or exacerbated by drug over 12 mo 5.2 per 1,000 patients; clinically picture resembles viral hepatitis *2135* Liver toxicity occurred in 18% patients receiving combined isoniazid and rifampin: effect slight in 14% and severe in 4% *2345* Probable intrahepatic cholestatic jaundice *3669* In 3.3% children also treated with rifampin: all reactions occurring in first 10 weeks *4350* Observed in up to 0.5% patients slightly greater than in placebo treated group *2824* Most common adverse reactions of ioniazid involve the nervous system and liver *223* 15 of 89 patients developed significant liver disease, typically hepatitis, although one developed cholestasis, in patients taking drug for at least 2 mo *1422* Mild liver injury occurs in approximately 10% patients taking drug, possibly due to conversion of drug to acetylhydrazine or related hepatotoxic derivatives *3725*

Albumin *Serum No Effect Analytical* At concentration of 100 mg/L had no effect on BCG method *5704*
Urine No Effect Analytical At concentration of 500 mg/dL had no significant effect on Boehringer Mannheim Tina-quant method *2799*

Alkaline Phosphatase *Serum Increase Physiological* Probable cholestatic effect *3669* 15 of 89 patients developed significant liver disease, typically hepatitis, although one developed cholestasis, in patients taking drug for at least 2 mo *1422*

Amino-4-Imidazole-5-Carboxamide Ribotide
Urine Increase Physiological Occurs if megaloblastic anemia *6370*

Ammonia *Plasma Increase Physiological* Due to metabolism of isonicotinic acid *6670*
Plasma No Effect Physiological No effect observed in most studies *2452*

Amylase *Serum Increase Physiological* Reported cause of acute pancreatitis, much doubt *2451*

Antinuclear Antibodies *Serum Increase Physiological* Up to 78% tuberculous patients develop antibodies *83*

Aspartate Aminotransferase *Serum Increase Analytical* At therapeutic concentration may affect Technicon SMA 12/60 method *5576*
Serum Increase Physiological Mild liver injury occurs in approximately 10% patients taking drug, possibly due to conversion of drug to acetylhydrazine or related hepatotoxic derivatives *3725* In 3.3% children also treated with rifampin: all reactions occurring in first 10 weeks *4350* In 18.3% versus 6.7% of controls in adult patients receiving drug for prophylaxis *836* Risk of hepatitis caused by or exacerbated by drug over 12 mo 5.2 per 1,000 patients; clinically picture resembles viral hepatitis *2135* Probable intrahepatic cholestatic jaundice *3669* Observed in up to 0.5% patients slightly greater than in placebo treated group *2824* Liver toxicity occurred in 18% patients receiving combined isoniazid and rifampin: effect slight in 14% and severe in 4% *2345* 15 of 89 patients developed significant liver disease, typically hepatitis, although one developed cholestasis, in patients taking drug for at least 2 mo *1422* In 72 patients with tuberculosis all receiving isoniazid and rifampin and, in addition, pyrazinamide in 72.2%, ethambutol in 80% and streptomycin in 16.7% drug-induced hepatitis observed with AST activity reaching mean of 428.4 ± 666.0 U/L *5577* Most common adverse reactions of ioniazid involve the nervous system and liver *223* Occurs in about 20% of treated patients due to acetylhydrazine metabolite: higher incidence in older and in consumers of excess alcohol *98*

Bicarbonate *Serum No Effect Analytical* At concentration of 100 mg/L had no effect on method using phenolphthalein *5704*

Bile *Urine Increase Physiological* Intrahepatic cholestatic jaundice *139*

Bile Acids *Serum Increase Physiological* In 72% of 61 patients studied for 80 d when treatment combined with rifampin but most other liver function tests including bilirubin could be normal *498* 15 of 89 patients developed significant liver disease, typically hepatitis, although one developed cholestasis, in patients taking drug for at least 2 mo *1422*

Bilirubin *Serum Increase Physiological* In 72 patients with tuberculosis all receiving isoniazid and rifampin and, in addition, pyrazinamide in 72.2%, ethambutol in 80% and streptomycin in 16.7% drug-induced hepatitis observed with bilirubin concentration reaching mean of 5.34 ± 4.68 mg/dL *5577* Intrahepatic cholestasis *1714* Most common adverse reactions of ioniazid involve the nervous system and liver *223* 15 of 89 patients developed significant liver disease, typically hepatitis, although one developed cholestasis, in patients taking drug for at least 2 mo *1422*
Serum No Effect Analytical At concentration of 100 mg/L had no effect on Jendrassik and Grof method *5704*

Isoniazid *(continued)*

Bilirubin *(continued)*
Urine Increase Physiological Most common adverse reactions of ioniazid involve the nervous system and liver *223*

BSP Retention *Serum Increase Physiological* Intrahepatic cholestatic jaundice *139*

Calcium *Serum Decrease Physiological* Reduction from mean of 2.35 mmol/L to 2.22 mmol/L in 8 healthy volunteers given 300 mg/d for 14 days *737*
Serum No Effect Analytical At concentration of 100 mg/L had no effect on cresolphthalein method *5704*

Carbamazepine *Serum Increase Physiological* Due to inhibition of liver enzymes by drug: caused intoxication in 10 of 13 epileptic patients *6159* Increased plasma concentration *886* Drugs that inhibit CYP 3A4 inhibit metabolism of carbamazepine producing clinically meaningful effect *1039* Concomitant administration with carbamazepine causes marked increase of plasma carbamazepine concentration resulting in toxicity in some cases *282* Due to effect on hepatic metabolism *1384* Inhibits carbamazepine metabolism and increases plasma concentration *3119* Metabolism inhibitsd and may produce neurotoxicity and synergistic hepatotoxicity *3118* Metabolism inhibited and may produce neurotoxicity and synergistic hepatotoxicity *3118*

Casts *Urine Increase Physiological* Nephrotoxic effect *3810*

Chloride *Serum No Effect Analytical* At concentration of 100 mg/L had no effect on mercurimetric method *5704* No effect of concentrations up to 4 mg/L with method on Kodak Ektachem® *5706*

Cholesterol *Serum Decrease Physiological* Probable hepatotoxic effect *3669*
Serum No Effect Analytical At concentration of 100 mg/L had no effect on Liebermann-Burchard method *5704* No effect at concentrations up to 4 mg/L on method on Kodak Ektachem® *5706*

Coombs' Test *Blood Positive Physiological* Immunological response to drug *2453*

Coombs' Test, Direct *Blood Positive Physiological* Complement type of positive response *2452*

Corticosteroids *Plasma Increase Physiological* Decreased metabolism *886*

Creatine Kinase *Serum No Effect Analytical* No effect of concentrations up to 5 mg/L on method on Kodak Ektachem® systems *5706*

Creatinine *Serum No Effect Analytical* At 20 mg/L on reversed phase liquid chromatographic procedure of Zhiri et al *6656* Although elutes at the same time as creatinine with HPLC method of Rosano et al concentration is sufficiently low clinically that it would cause no interference in practice *5083* No effect of concentrations up to 15 mg/L on single slide method on Kodak Ektachem® *5706* At concentration of 100 mg/L had no effect on Technicon AutoAnalyzer® method *5704*

Cyclosporine *Blood No Effect Analytical* At a concentration of 70 mg/L had no effect on Syva EMIT method *495*
Serum Decrease Physiological Enhances metabolism by hepatic enzyme induction *6288*

Diazepam *Serum Increase Physiological* Inhibition of hepatic metabolism observed in 9 healthy volunteers. Total clearance reduced from 0.54 to 0.40 mL/min/kg *4354* Probably through inhibition of hepatic microsomal enzymes prolongs elimination half-life of diazepam by 30% *1384*

1,25-Dihydroxy Vitamin D_3 *Serum Decrease Physiological* Mean fall of 47% observed in 8 healthy volunteers treated with 300 mg/d for 14 days *737*

Eosinophils *Blood Increase Physiological* Eosinophilia may occur as an adverse reaction *223* Allergic phenomenon *2484*

Erythrocytes *Blood Decrease Physiological* Hemolytic anemia (rare complication) *3810*

Ethosuximide *Serum Increase Physiological* Inhibits metabolism and increases plasma concentration *1384*

Folate *Serum Decrease Physiological* Low incidence of impaired absorption *6370*

Glucose *Serum Decrease Analytical* At concentrations above 55 mg/L (normal therapeutic concentration 10 mg/L) lowered concentration as measured by GOD-PERID method *5704* At concentrations above 500 mg/L (normal therapeutic concentration 10 mg/L) lowered concentration as measured by Ames Seralyzer method *5704* Affects glucose oxidase method of Boehringer Mannheim *5480*
Serum Increase Physiological Large doses cause hyperglycemia by glycogenolysis *2451* Hyperglycemia may occur as an adverse reaction *223*
Serum No Effect Analytical No effect of concentrations up to 4 mg/L on method on Kodak Ektachem® *5706* No effect at 5000 mg/L on hexokinase method on Ames Seralyzer *5706* Affects Boehringer GOD-PERID method *5480*
Urine Increase Physiological Due to hyperglycemia *3669* Glycosuria may follow induced hyperglycemia *2451*
Urine No Effect Analytical Has no effect on Ames Keto-Diastix, Diastix, Multistix, Clinistix and Clinitest procedures *4034*

γ-Glutamyltransferase *Serum Increase Physiological* Increase in activity from mean of 12.6 U/L to 14.5 U/L in 8 healthy volunteers treated with 300 mg/d for 14 days *737*

Glycated Hemoglobin *Blood No Effect Analytical* At a concentration of 25 mg/L had an insignificant 2.0% interference with method on Abbott Vision *1885*

Granulocytes *Blood Decrease Physiological* Agranulocytosis may occur as an adverse reaction *223*

Guanase *Serum Increase Physiological* Cytotoxic hepatocellular damage *402*

Haptoglobin *Serum Decrease Physiological* Hemolytic anemia *3810*

HDL-Cholesterol *Serum No Effect Analytical* No effect of concentrations up to 4 mg/L on method on Kodak Ektachem® *5706*

Hematocrit *Blood Decrease Physiological* Hemolytic anemia/rare megaloblastic anemia *3810*

Hemoglobin *Blood Decrease Physiological* Very rare cases of pure red cell aplasia, other cases of hemolytic anemia pyridoxine-responsive sideroblastic anemia also reported *1048* Rare hemolytic anemia in patients with glucose-6-phosphate deficiency *2135* Hemolytic anemia/rare megaloblastic anemia *3810* Hemolytic, sideroblastic or aplastic anemia may occur as an adverse reaction *223*
Blood No Effect Analytical No effect of concentrations up to 4 mg/L on method on Kodak Ektachem® *5706*

Histamine *Plasma No Effect Analytical* No inhibition of radio-enzyme assay at concentration 10 times therapeutic *5706*

Homocysteine *Plasma Increase Physiological* As a vitamin B_6 antagonist causes increased concentration *6123*

25-Hydroxy Vitamin D_3 *Serum Decrease Physiological* Concentration declined, and to below normal range in 6 of 8 healthy volunteers treated with 300 mg/d for 14 days *737*

5-Hydroxyindoleacetic Acid *Urine Decrease Physiological* Causes decarboxylase inhibition with reduced 5-HT *1281*

3-Hydroxykynurenine *Urine Increase Physiological* Induces pyridoxal PO_4 deficiency *5085*

^{131}I Uptake *Serum Decrease Physiological* Reduces uptake *3669*

Indinavir *Serum No Effect Physiological* Administration of indinavir 800 mg every 8 hours with isoniazid 300 mg/d for 1 week resulted in a 13 ± 15% increase in isoniazid AUC but had no effect on indinavir AUC *3966*

INH-Ketoglutarate *Urine Increase Physiological* Major metabolite in urine *5160*

INH-Pyruvate *Urine Increase Physiological* Major metabolite in urine *5160*

Iron *Serum No Effect Analytical* At a concentration of 50 μg/mL had no significant effect on mean concentration (10.00 μmol/L) compared with control (9.91 μmol/L) as measured by Ferrochem II analyzer and 11.20 μmol/L versus 11.40 μmol/L as measured by atomic absorption *5217* Insignificant reduction of iron concentration at therapeutic concentration on method on Ferrochem II instrument *4489*

Isocitrate Dehydrogenase *Serum Increase Physiological* Cytotoxic hepatocellular jaundice *402*

itraconazole *Serum Decrease Physiological* Itraconazole and its major metabolite hydroxyitraconazole inhibit the cytochrome P450 3A enzyme system thereby affecting the metabolism of drugs by this system: isoniazid reduces the concentration of itraconazole *2905*

Ketones *Urine Increase Physiological* Mechanism not listed *2451*

Kynurenine *Urine Increase Physiological* Induces pyridoxal PO_4 deficiency *5085*

Lactate *Plasma Increase Physiological* If overdose with inhibition of NAD activity *2452*
Plasma No Effect Physiological Probable effect of normal dose and renal function *2452*

Lactate Dehydrogenase *Serum No Effect Analytical* No effect of concentrations up to 4 mg/L on method on Kodak Ektachem® systems *5706*

LE Cells *Blood Positive Physiological* More common in slow acetylators *3827*

Leukocytes *Blood Decrease Physiological* Rare agranulocytosis observed *359* Occasional case of agranulocytosis reported *6197*
Blood Increase Physiological Due to eosinophilia *3810*

MCV *Blood Increase Physiological* If megaloblastic anemia occurs *3810*

Methemoglobin *Blood Increase Physiological* Reported effect *2242*

Mexiletine *Serum Increase Physiological* Decreases clearance and prolongs half-life *3281*

N-Acetyl-Glucosaminidase *Urine No Effect Analytical* At concentration of 500 mg/dL no significant effect observed on Boehringer Mannheim CPR method *3174*

Neutrophils *Blood Decrease Physiological* May cause neutropenia *4265* Occasional case of agranulocytosis reported *6264*

N-Formiminoglutamic Acid *Urine Increase Physiological* Occurs if megaloblastic anemia *6370*

Ornithine Carbamoyltransferase
Serum Increase Physiological Cytotoxic hepatocellular damage *402*

Parathyroid Hormone *Plasma Increase Physiological* Mean increase of 36% in 8 healthy volunteers treated with 300 mg/d for 14 days *737*

pH *Blood Decrease Physiological* Large doses may produce severe acidosis *2242*

Phenytoin *Serum Increase Physiological* Isoniazid may decrease the excretion of phenytoin or enhance its effects *223* Significant increase in concentration when drugs coadministered *1384* Causes increase in concentration when drugs coadministered through enzyme inhibition *6350* Coadministration with phenytoin may increase plasma phenytoin concentration *4522* Increased serum concentration *886* Increases blood concentration and toxicity *6197* Drug shown to inhibit metabolism of phenytoin in many studies. Effect seems to be more important in individuals who are slow metabolizers of isoniazid and in those taking isoniazid with para-aminosalicylic acid *4188* From 12 to 42 µg/mL (with dose of 300 mg) *3339* When isoniazid ingested with fosphenytoin concentration of phenytoin may be increased *4519* Impairs metabolism in approximately 10% *3340*

Phosphate *Serum Decrease Physiological* Reduction from mean of 1.26 mmol/L to mean of 1.05 mmol/L in 8 healthy volunteers given 300 mg/d for 14 days *737*
Serum No Effect Analytical At concentration of 100 mg/L had no effect on phosphomolybdate method *5704*

Platelets *Blood Decrease Physiological* May rarely cause bone marrow aplasia *359* Thrombocytopenia may occur as an adverse reaction *223*

Potassium *Serum Increase Physiological* Reported effect of overdose *2451*
Serum No Effect Analytical At concentration of 25 mg/L non-significant interference of 1.1% observed with method on Abbott Vision *681*

Protein *Serum No Effect Analytical* At concentration of 100 mg/L had no effect on biuret method with blank correction *5704*
Urine Increase Physiological Nephrotoxic effect *1714* May have nephrotoxic effect *2451*

Prothrombin Time *Plasma Increase Physiological* Probable interaction with warfarin when drugs coadministered *2625*

Pyridoxine *Serum Decrease Physiological* Observed in 13% of 38 children when measured with protozoan procedure: also reported in 2% of adults after 6 mo *4592*
Urine Increase Physiological Particularly prevalent with use of large doses of drug or in nutritionally deficient persons such as alcoholics *6197* Dose related effect *5054*

Quinine *Serum No Effect Physiological* In 9 healthy individuals mean maximum concentration of 4.6 ± 1.0 mg/L following a single oral dose of 600 mg quinine sulfate reduced insignificantly to 4.4 ± 1.6 mg/L when volunteers pretreated with isoniazid *6346*

Sodium *Serum No Effect Analytical* No effect of concentrations up to 4 mg/L on method on Kodak Ektachem® systems *5706*

Spermidine Oxidase *Serum No Effect Analytical* At concentration of 0.2 mmol/L had no effect on method of Tabor and Kellogg *1884*

Sugar *Urine Increase Analytical* False positive with Benedict's and Clinitest® *1825*

Theophylline *Serum Increase Physiological* Reduces clearance so plasma concentration increases with 400 mg/d for 2 weeks *5212*
Serum No Effect Physiological No documented significant interaction with theophylline reported *6117* No clinically significant effect on theophylline concentration observed when drugs coadministered *5999*

Triazolam *Serum Increase Physiological* Concentration increased due to inhibition of hepatic metabolism *4353*

Triglycerides *Serum No Effect Analytical* No effect of concentrations up to 4 mg/L on method on Kodak Ektachem® systems *5706* At concentration of 100 mg/L had no effect on lipase/esterase method *5704*

Urea Nitrogen *Serum No Effect Analytical* At concentration of 100 mg/L had no effect on diacetylmonoxime method *5704*

Uric Acid *Serum Increase Analytical* At concentrations above 14 mg/L (normal therapeutic concentration 10 mg/L) raised concentration as measured by phosphotungstate reduction method *5704*
Serum No Effect Analytical At 20 mg/L on reversed phase liquid chromatographic procedure of Zhiri et al *6656*

Xanthurenic Acid *Urine No Effect Physiological* Initial response may be decreased later *5085*

Zidovudine *Serum No Effect Analytical* No effect on liquid chromatographic method of Hedaya and Sawchuk *2525*

Isonicotinic Acid

Glucose *Serum No Effect Analytical* At concentration of 5 mg/L had no effect on Ektachem® method *5704*

Isopropamide

^{131}I Uptake *Serum Decrease Physiological* Contains iodine: reduces further uptake *2451*

Isopropyl Dipyrone

δ-Aminolevulinic Acid *Urine Increase Physiological* May precipitate attack of acute porphyria *1687*

Porphyrin, Total *Urine Increase Physiological* May precipitate attack of acute porphyria *1687*

Isoproterenol

Adenosine Monophosphate *Plasma Increase Physiological* No effect unless β-blocking agent also given. Response to i.v. infusion in normals *350*
Urine Decrease Physiological In normals but increased in hypertensives *2422*
Urine Increase Physiological Effect less marked than in blood *350*

Aspartate Aminotransferase *Serum Increase Analytical* At 1 mmol/L affects Technicon SMA 12/60 method *5576*

Isoproterenol *(continued)*

Bilirubin *Serum Increase Analytical* At 1 mmol/L affects Technicon SMA 12/60 method *5576*

Calcium *Serum No Effect Analytical* At concentration of 211 mg/L had no effect on cresolphthalein method *5704*

Catecholamines *Plasma Increase Physiological* Due to inhalation: effect slight *1175*

Plasma No Effect Analytical No effect on HPLC method of Koller for measurement of dopamine, epinephrine, or norepinephrine *3230*

Urine Increase Physiological Observed for up to 4 d after drug stopped *1444*

C-Peptide *Plasma Increase Physiological* Intravenous infusion in 8 healthy female volunteers caused increase but with reduction of plasma C-peptide/insulin molar ratio *2258*

Cyclosporine *Blood No Effect Analytical* At a concentration of 0.06 mg/L had no effect on Syva EMIT method *495*

Epinephrine *Plasma Increase Analytical* Interference observed because of co-elution when HPLC with electrochemical detection method of Meineke et al used. Interference can be avoided by use of buffer with acetonitrile (95:5, v/v) as mobile phase *3938*

Urine Increase Physiological Probably small effect with usual doses *1175*

Fatty Acids (FFA), Free *Serum Decrease Analytical* At a concentration of 62.5 µmol/L caused reduction to 46.4% of control, at 125 µmol/L 21.1%, at 250 µmol/L 2.9% and at 500 µmol/L caused reduction to 0% of control when measured by Wako NEFA C test kit *898*

Serum Increase Physiological As effective as epinephrine *2242*

Glomerular Filtration Rate *Urine Decrease Physiological* Frequently observed to be diminished *5379*

Glucose *Serum Increase Analytical* At 1 mmol/L affects Technicon SMA 12/60 method *5576* 7.1% increase in absorbance with 10 mmol/L on glucokinase based assay of Scott *5414*

Serum Increase Physiological Not as marked as with epinephrine *2242*

Serum No Effect Physiological Infusion intravenously had no effect on concentration in 8 healthy volunteers *2258*

Insulin *Plasma Increase Physiological* Intravenous infusion had similar effect to that of glucose in raising concentration in 8 healthy female volunteers *2258*

Lidocaine *Serum No Effect Analytical* At a concentration of 1250 mg/L had effect of less than 10% on method on Baxter Stratus *5705* No significant interference observed at a concentration of 100 µg/mL (473 µmol/L) with method on Du Pont aca *1534*

Myosin *Serum Increase Physiological* All patients receiving intravenous infusion had increases of cardiac-specific myosin light-chains up to 42 ng/mL during administration *981*

N-Acetylprocainamide *Serum No Effect Analytical* No significant interference observed at a concentration of 100 µg/mL (473 µmol/L) with method on Du Pont aca *1536*

Oxygen Partial Pressure *Blood Decrease Physiological* By approximately 10 mm Hg in chronic lung disease *4014*

Phenylalanine *Plasma No Effect Analytical* No interference observed with rapid quantitative whole blood method of Campbell et al using phenylalanine dehydrogenase *867*

Phosphate *Serum No Effect Analytical* At concentration of 211 mg/L had no effect on phosphomolybdate method *5704*

Procainamide *Serum No Effect Analytical* No significant interference observed with method on Du Pont aca at a concentration of 100 µg/mL (473 µmol/L) with method on Du Pont aca *1542*

Protein *Serum No Effect Analytical* At concentration of 211 mg/L had no effect on biuret method with blank correction *5704*

Quinidine *Serum No Effect Analytical* No significant interference observed at a concentration of 100 µg/mL (473 µmol/L) with method on Du Pont aca *1543*

Theophylline *Serum Decrease Physiological* Coadministration of theophylline with isoproterenol increases theophylline clearance and decreases theophylline concentration by about 20% *5999* Up to 20% decrease in serum theophylline concentration due to increased theophylline clearance with intravenous isoproterenol *6117*

Serum Increase Physiological Decreases theophylline clearance and increases serum theophylline concentration by 20% *3125*

Serum No Effect Analytical No effect on Kodak Ektachem® 700 method *1716*

Urea Nitrogen *Serum No Effect Analytical* At concentration of 211 mg/L had no effect on diacetylmonoxime method *5704*

Uric Acid *Serum No Effect Analytical* At concentration of 211 mg/L had no effect on phosphotungstate reduction method *5704*

Vanillylmandelic Acid *Urine Increase Physiological* Pharmacological effect (still seen 4 d after stopping) *1444*

Urine No Effect Analytical No apparent methodological effect *2452*

Urine No Effect Physiological No apparent physiological effect *2452*

Volume *Urine Decrease Physiological* Antidiuretic effect mediated through ADH release *5379*

Isosorbide

Chloride *Urine Increase Physiological* Similar to natriuretic effect *4311*

Cortisol *Plasma No Effect Analytical* At a concentration of 5 mg/L had no significant effect on Enzymun method *1097*

Creatinine Clearance *Urine Increase Physiological* ?due to decreased tubular reabsorption *4311*

Epinephrine *Plasma Decrease Physiological* In 12 healthy volunteers ingestion of 20 mg caused insignificant reduction from mean baseline of 0.30 ± 0.09 nmol/L to 0.22 ± 0.02 nmol/L *6330*

Granulocytes *Blood Decrease Physiological* Agranulocytosis observed in 4.8% of patients versus 1.8% of controls but not of significance (multivariate risk estimate of 1.5) *3098*

Guanosine Monophosphate

Plasma Decrease Physiological Administration of a single oral dose of 40 mg caused transient reduction of cGMP from 16.7 ± 9.7 pmol/mL to 13.0 ± 6.6 pmol/mL at 1 hour *5538*

Hematocrit *Blood No Effect Physiological* In 10 healthy volunteers oral ingestion of 20 mg caused nonsignificant reduction from mean baseline of 42.7 ± 0.5% to 42.0 ± 0.5% *6330*

Histamine *Plasma No Effect Analytical* Improbable inhibition of radio-enzyme assay at therapeutic concentrations *2492*

Indomethacin *Serum No Effect Physiological* No effect on HPLC method of Roberts and Smith *4978*

Leukocytes *Blood No Effect Physiological* In 10 healthy volunteers oral ingestion of 20 mg caused nonsignificant change from mean baseline of 5300 ± 300 /µL to 5400 ± 300 /µL *6330*

Mean Platelet Volume *Blood No Effect Physiological* In 8 healthy volunteers ingestion of 20 mg caused nonsignificant increase from mean baseline of 9.3 fL to 9.6 fL *6330*

Methemoglobin *Blood Increase Physiological* Significant increase in angina patients but probably not of routine significance, but may be important in anemics or in patients with coronary insufficiency (difference = 1.13 vs 0.99 in controls) *3442* Commonly used nitrates at regular doses capable of causing usually clinically insignificant increases *253*

Norepinephrine *Plasma Decrease Physiological* In 12 healthy individuals ingestion of 20 mg caused significant increase from mean baseline of 1.31 ± 0.11 nmol/L to 1.72 ± 0.08 nmol/L *6330*

Osmolar Clearance *Urine Increase Physiological* Diuretic action alone, potentiates others *4311*

Plasminogen Activator Inhibitor-1 Activity

Plasma No Effect Physiological In 12 healthy volunteers oral ingestion of 20 mg caused nonsignificant reduction from mean baseline of 2.43 ± 0.77 arb U/mL to 1.36 ± 0.47 arb U/mL compared with placebo *6330*

Plasminogen Activator Inhibitor-1 Antigen

Plasma No Effect Physiological In 12 healthy volunteers oral ingestion of 20 mg caused nonsignificant reduction from mean baseline of 7.04 ± 0.98 ng/mL to 4.75 ± 0.65 ng/mL when compared with placebo *6330*

Platelets *Blood No Effect Physiological* In 12 healthy volunteers oral ingestion of 20 mg caused nonsignificant increase from mean baseline of 217,000 /µL to 222,000 /µL *6330*

Potassium *Urine Increase Physiological* Slight effect only if given alone *4311*

Renal Blood Flow *Patient No Effect Physiological* In 8 cirrhotic patients 20 mg isosorbide nitrate caused an insignificant reduction from 302.5 ± 49.4 mL/min to 301.7 ± 58.8 mL/min *5772*

Sodium *Serum Increase Physiological* Dehydration with overdosage *5539*
Urine Increase Physiological Diuretic action alone, potentiates others *4311*

β-Thromboglobulin *Plasma No Effect Physiological* In 12 healthy volunteers oral ingestion of 20 mg caused nonsignificant change from mean baseline of 1.27 ± 0.03 ng/mL to 1.29 ± 0.06 ng/mL *6330*
Urine Increase Physiological In 12 healthy volunteers oral ingestion of 20 mg caused significant increase from mean baseline of 0.30 ± 0.04 ng/mmol creatinine to 0.43 ± 0.07 ng/mmol creatinine *6330*

Tirofiban *Serum No Effect Physiological* Coadministration had no significant effect on plasma clearance of tirofiban *3957*

Tissue Plasminogen Activator
Plasma No Effect Physiological In 11 healthy volunteers oral ingestion of 20 mg caused nonsignificant increase from 0.36 ± 0.04 arb U/mL to 0.47 ± 0.05 arb U/mL when compared with effect of placebo *6330*

Tissue Plasminogen Activator Antigen
Plasma No Effect Physiological In 12 healthy volunteers oral ingestion of 20 mg caused nonsignificant decrease from 2.05 ± 0.44 ng/mL to 1.98 ± 0.46 ng/mL compared with placebo ingesting controls *6330*

Urea Nitrogen *Serum Increase Physiological* Dehydration with overdosage *5539*

Volume *Urine Increase Physiological* Diuretic action alone, potentiates others *4311*

von Willebrand Factor *Plasma No Effect Physiological* In 12 healthy volunteers ingestion of 20 mg caused nonsignificant reduction from basal concentration of 0.84 ± 0.10 IU/mL to 0.77 ± 0.10 IU/mL *6330*

Isosorbide Dinitrate

Alanine Aminotransferase *Serum Increase Physiological* Increased enzyme activity observed in less than 5% of all patients to whom drug was administered *3124*

Aspartate Aminotransferase *Serum Increase Physiological* Increased enzyme activity observed in less than 5% of all patients to whom drug was administered *3124*

Cholesterol *Serum Decrease Analytical* Nitrates and nitrites may interfere with Zlatkis-Zak color reaction causing falsely low results *3124*

Granulocytes *Blood Decrease Physiological* Agranulocytosis observed in 4.8% of patients versus 1.8% of controls but not of significance (multivariate risk estimate of 1.5) *3098*

Hematocrit *Blood Decrease Physiological* Hypochromic anemia observed in less than 5% of all patients to whom drug was administered *3124*

Hemoglobin *Blood Decrease Physiological* Hypochromic anemia observed in less than 5% of all patients to whom drug was administered *3124*

Methemoglobin *Blood Increase Physiological* Very rarely may cause methemoglobinemia *6649*

Occult Blood *Feces Increase Physiological* Melena and gastrointestinal bleeding observed in less than 5% of all patients to whom drug was administered *3124*

Platelets *Blood Decrease Physiological* Thrombocytopenia and purpura observed in less than 5% of all patients to whom drug was administered *3124*

Sodium *Serum Decrease Physiological* Hyponatremia observed in less than 5% of all patients to whom drug was administered *3124*

Uric Acid *Serum Increase Physiological* Hyperuricemia observed in less than 5% of all patients to whom drug was administered *3124*

Isotretinoin

Alanine *Plasma No Effect Physiological* In 13 patients with severe acne treatment with 1.0 mg/kg/d for 16 weeks had no significant effect on concentration *3368*

Alanine Aminotransferase *Serum Increase Physiological* In 10 - 20% patients increased activity observed *5014* In 10 of 523 patients with mean daily dose of 109 mg for 150 d *6500* In 1 of 11 patients given drug orally *6500*
Serum No Effect Physiological Significant effect at 6 weeks in 7 patients with severe rosacea treated with 1 mg/kg/d *3804* In 18 patients with severe acne given 0.8 mg/kg daily for 3 mo: changes reverted to normal after treatment stopped *3699*

Albumin *Serum No Effect Physiological* In 18 patients with severe acne given 0.8 mg/kg daily for 3 mo: changes reverted to normal after treatment stopped *3699*

Alkaline Phosphatase *Serum Increase Physiological* In 1 of 11 patients given drug orally *6500* In 7 patients with severe rosacea treated with 1 mg/kg/d for 12 weeks. Effects possibly due to induction of hepatic microsomal enzymes *3804* In 10 - 20% patients increased activity observed *5014* In 10 of 523 patients with mean daily dose of 109 mg for 150 d *6500*
Serum No Effect Physiological In 11 children with cystic acne no significant effect observed with 2 months treatment *5047*

Apolipoprotein A-I *Serum No Effect Physiological* In 12 patients with hyperkeratotic disorders given 40 mg daily for 2 mo *6150* In 13 patients with severe acne mean concentration unchnaged with treatment with 1.0 mg/kg/d for 16 weeks *3368*

Apolipoprotein A-II *Serum No Effect Physiological* In 12 patients with hyperkeratotic disorders given 40 mg daily for 2 mo *6150*

Apolipoprotein B *Serum Increase Physiological* In 13 patients with severe acne mean concentration increased significantly when treated with 1.0 mg/kg/d for 16 weeks *3368* From 132 to 157% in 12 patients with hyperkeratotic disorders given 40 mg daily for 2 mo *6150*

Aspartate Aminotransferase *Serum Increase Physiological* In 10 - 20% patients increased activity observed *5014* Reversible dose-related effect noted in patients with myelodysplastic syndrome and leukemia at high doses *2208* In 1 of 11 patients given drug orally *6500* In 7 patients with severe rosacea treated with 1 mg/kg/d for 12 weeks. Effects possibly due to induction of hepatic microsomal enzymes *3804* Mean increase of 17.8% at 20 weeks in 150 patients with acne given 0.1 mg/kg/d, with 15.2% after 0.5 mg/kg/d and 18.4% after 1.0 mg/kg/d *5760*
Serum No Effect Physiological In 18 patients with severe acne given 0.8 mg/kg daily for 3 mo: changes reverted to normal after treatment stopped *3699*

Bilirubin *Serum Decrease Physiological* Significant at 12 weeks in 7 patients with severe rosacea treated with 1 mg/kg/d *3804* In 7 patients with severe rosacea treated with 1 mg/kg/d for 12 weeks effect possibly due to induction of hepatic microsomal enzymes *3804*
Serum Increase Physiological Reversible dose-related effect noted in patients with myelodysplastic syndrome and leukemia at high doses *2208*
Serum No Effect Physiological In 18 patients with severe acne given 0.8 mg/kg daily for 3 mo: changes reverted to normal after treatment stopped *3699*

Blasts *Bone Marrow Decrease Physiological* Therapeutic response is normalization but effect not usually observed until after 2 weeks *2208*

Blood *Urine Increase Physiological* In fewer than 10% treated patients microscopic or gross hematuria observed *5014*

Calcium *Serum No Effect Physiological* In 11 patients with cystic acne treated for 2 weeks no significant change in concentration observed *5047*

Carbamazepine *Serum Decrease Physiological* Concentration of both carbamazepine and carbamazepine epoxide reduced in a patient in whom drugs were coadministered *3119*

Carnitine *Serum No Effect Physiological* In 13 patients with severe acne treatment with 1.0 mg/kg/d for 16 weeks had no significant effect on concentration *3368*

Cholesterol *Serum Decrease Physiological* Significant effect observed in patients with acne during first 6 weeks of treatment *6310*

Isotretinoin *(continued)*

Cholesterol *(continued)*
Serum Increase Physiological Increase in both men and women with 1 mg/kg/d for 20 weeks when given for nodulocystic acne *524* In 7 patients with severe rosacea treated with 1 mg/kg/d for 12 weeks. Effects possibly due to induction of hepatic microsomal enzymes *3804* In 150 patients with acne significant increase at 20 weeks in patients given 0.1 and 1.0 mg/kg/d but not when 0.5 mg/kg/d given *5760* During treatment but not to abnormal levels *2967* From 0.8 to 1.6 mmol/L at 6 weeks in 7 patients with severe rosacea treated with mg/kg/d *3804* In 116 patients with acne treatment with 1 mg/kg day caused cholesterol concentrations to increase during first 6 weeks of treatment at which point they stabilized *6310* From 5.75 to 6.49 mmol/L in 12 patients with hyperkeratotic disorders given 40 mg daily for 2 mo *6150* From 0.9 to 2.2 mmol/L in 18 patients with severe acne given 0.8 mg/kg daily for 3 mo: changes reverted to normal after treatment stopped *3699* Significant increase observed in 13 patients with severe acne when treated for 16 weeks with 1.0 mg/kg/d *3368* Approximately 7% of treated patients develop mild increases in concentration, reversible with cessation of treatment *5014*

Creatine Kinase *Serum Increase Physiological* Increase observed in less than 1% of all patients receiving drug *1384* Increase observed in 10 of 63 patients *535* In fewer than 10% treated patients increased activity observed *5014*

Creatinine *Serum Increase Physiological* Observed in one man treated with topical drug over two months, associated with decreased creatinine clearance *4569*

1,25-Dihydroxy Vitamin D *Serum Decrease Physiological* In 11 patients with cystic acne treated for 2 months significant decrease observed *5047*

24,25-Dihydroxy Vitamin D *Serum No Effect Physiological* In 11 patients with cystic acne treatment for 2 months had no significant effect observed on concentration *5047*

Erythrocyte Sedimentation Rate
Blood Increase Physiological Approximately 40% of treated patients develop increased ESR, often from increased baseline rate *5014* In 50 of 523 patients with mean daily dose of 109 mg for 150 d *6500*

Erythrocytes *Blood Decrease Physiological* In 10 of 523 patients with mean daily dose of 109 mg for 150 d *6500* In 10 - 20% patients reduction in red cell parameters observed *5014*

Euglobulin Fibrinolytic Activity
Plasma No Effect Physiological In 12 patients with skin disorders administration of 20 - 60 mg/d for 1 month caused non-significant change from mean baseline of 2.9 ± 4.8 U/mL to 3.0 ± 5.7 U/mL *1339*

Fatty Acids (FFA), Free *Serum No Effect Physiological* In 13 patients with severe acne treatment with 1.0 mg/kg/d for 16 weeks had no significant effect *3368*

Follicle Stimulating Hormone
Plasma No Effect Physiological In 7 patients with severe rosacea treated with 1 mg/kg/d for 12 weeks. Effects possibly due to induction of hepatic microsomal enzymes *3804* With 12 weeks treatment with 1 mg/kg/d *3804*

FSH response to LHRH *Plasma No Effect Physiological* In 7 patients with severe rosacea treated with 1 mg/kg/d for 12 weeks. Effects possibly due to induction of hepatic microsomal enzymes *3804*

Glucose *Serum Increase Physiological* Increase observed in less than 1% of all patients receiving drug *1384* In fewer than 10% treated patients increased fasting blood glucose concentration observed *5014*
Serum No Effect Physiological In 13 patients with severe acne no significant effect observed on concentration when patients treated with 1.0 mg/kg/d for 16 weeks *3368*

γ-Glutamyltransferase *Serum Increase Physiological* Slight increase with high dose treatment *2967* In 10 - 20% patients increased activity observed *5014* From 13.0 to 21.1 U/L in 18 patients with severe acne given 0.8 mg/kg daily for 3 mo: changes reverted to normal after treatment stopped *3699* In 7 patients with severe rosacea treated with 1 mg/kg/d for 12 weeks. Effects possibly due to induction of hepatic microsomal enzymes *3804*

Glycerol *Serum No Effect Physiological* In 13 patients with severe acne treatment with 1.0 mg/kg/d for 16 weeks had no significant effect on concentration *3368*

HDL-Cholesterol *Serum Decrease Physiological* From 1.30 to 1.04 mmol/L at 6 weeks in 7 patients with severe rosacea treated with 1 mg/kg/d *3804* From 1.1 to 0.9 mmol/L in 18 patients with severe acne given 0.8 mg/kg daily for 3 mo: changes reverted to normal after treatment stopped *3699* Approximately 16% of treated patients develop mild to moderate decreases in concentration, reversible with cessation of treatment *5014* Mean decrease of 13.6% in 150 patients with acne treated with 0.1 mg/kg/d for 20 weeks, 20.5% when treated with 0.5 mg/kg/d and 16.7% when treated with 1.0 mg/kg/d *5760* From 1.28 to 1.14 mmol/L in 12 patients with hyperkeratotic disorders given 40 mg daily for 2 mo *6150* Increase in both men and women with 1 mg/kg/d for 20 weeks when given for nodulocystic acne *524* In both men and women with 1 mg/kg/d for 20 weeks when given for nodulocystic acne *524* In 7 patients with severe rosacea treated with 1 mg/kg/d for 12 weeks. Effects possibly due to induction of hepatic microsomal enzymes *3804*

HDL-Triglycerides *Serum Increase Physiological* Effects possibly due to induction of hepatic microsomal enzymes *3804* From 0.14 to 0.31 mmol/L at 6 weeks in 7 patients with severe rosacea treated with 1 mg/kg/d for 12 weeks *3804*
Serum No Effect Physiological From 0.28 to 0.26 mmol/L in 12 patients with hyperkeratotic disorders given 40 mg daily for 2 mo *6150*

Hematocrit *Blood Decrease Physiological* Anemia has been reported to occur in fewer than 1% of treated patients *5014*

Hemoglobin *Blood Decrease Physiological* Anemia has been reported to occur in fewer than 1% of treated patients *5014*
Blood Increase Physiological Therapeutic response is normalization but effect not usually observed until after 3 weeks *2208*
Urine Increase Physiological Microscopic or macroscopic increase observed in less than 1% of all patients receiving drug *1384*

Hepatic Triglyceride Lipase *Serum No Effect Physiological* Increase in both men and women with 1 mg/kg/d for 20 weeks when given for nodulocystic acne *524*

25-Hydroxy Vitamin D *Serum No Effect Physiological* No significant effect observed in 11 patients with cystic acne after treatment for 2 months *5047*

β-Hydroxybutyrate *Serum No Effect Physiological* In 13 patients with severe acne treatment with 1.0 mg/kg/d for 16 weeks had no significant effect on concentration *3368*

Insulin *Plasma No Effect Physiological* In 13 patients with severe acne treatment with 1.0 mg/kg/d for 16 weeks had no significant effect on plasma concentration *3368*

Lactate *Plasma No Effect Physiological* In 13 patients with severe acne treatment with 1.0 mg/kg/d for 16 weeks had no significant effect on concentration *3368*

Lactate Dehydrogenase *Serum Increase Physiological* Mean increase of 25.0% in 150 patients with acne when treated with 0.1 mg/kg/d for 20 weeks, 23.9% when treated with 0.5 mg/kg/d and 20.4% when treated with 1.0 mg/kg/d *5760* In 10 - 20% patients increased activity observed *5014*

LDL-Cholesterol *Serum Increase Physiological* Increase in both men and women with 1 mg/kg/d for 20 weeks when given for nodulocystic acne *524* From 3.92 to 5.33 mmol/L at 6 weeks in 7 patients with severe rosacea treated with 1 mg/kg/d *3804*

LDL-Triglycerides *Serum Increase Physiological* From 0.45 to 0.61 mmol/L in 12 patients with hyperkeratotic disorders given 40 mg daily for 2 mo *6150* From 0.26 to 0.56 mmol/L at 6 weeks in 7 patients with severe rosacea treated with 1 mg/kg/d for 12 weeks. Effects possibly due to induction of hepatic microsomal enzymes *3804*

Leukocytes *Blood Decrease Physiological* In 10 - 20% patients reduction in cell count observed *5014* In 10 of 523 patients with mean daily dose of 109 mg for 150 d *6500*
Blood Increase Physiological Therapeutic response is normalization but effect not usually observed until after 3 weeks *2208*
Urine Increase Physiological In 10 - 20% patients increased urinary excretion of leukocytes observed *5014* In 10 of 523 patients with mean daily dose of 109 mg for 150 d *6500*

Mean increase of 4.4% in 150 patients with acne treated with 0.1 mg/kg/d for 20 weeks, 4.4% when treated with 0.5 mg/kg/d and 15.2% when treated with 1.0 mg/kg/d *5760*

LH response to LHRH *Plasma No Effect Physiological* In 7 patients with severe rosacea treated with 1 mg/kg/d for 12 weeks. Effects possibly due to induction of hepatic microsomal enzymes *3804*

Lipoprotein Lipase *Serum No Effect Physiological* Increase in both men and women with 1 mg/kg/d for 20 weeks when given for nodulocystic acne *524*

Luteinizing Hormone *Plasma No Effect Physiological* In 7 patients with severe rosacea treated with 1 mg/kg/d for 12 weeks. Effects possibly due to induction of hepatic microsomal enzymes *3804*

Parathyroid Hormone *Plasma No Effect Physiological* In 11 patients with cystic acne no significant effect observed on concentration *5047*

Phosphate *Serum No Effect Physiological* In 11 patients with cystic acne treated for 2 months no significant effect observed on concentration *5047*

Plasminogen Activator Inhibitor-1
Plasma Increase Physiological In 12 patients with skin disorders administration of 20 - 60 mg/d for 1 month caused non-significant increase from mean baseline of 4.4 ± 4.0 ng/mL to 6.1 ± 6.4 ng/mL *1339*

Platelets *Blood Decrease Physiological* One case of thrombocytopenia verified by rechallenge reported *1384* In fewer than 10% treated patients decreased concentration observed *5014*
Blood Increase Physiological In 10 - 20% patients increase in cell count observed *5014* In 10 of 523 patients with mean daily dose of 109 mg for 150 d *6500* Therapeutic response is normalization but effect not usually observed until after 3 weeks *2208* Mean 4.4% increase after 20 weeks in 150 acne patients treated with 0.1 mg/kg/d but 11.4% increase with 0.5 mg/kg/d and 8.3% increase with 1.0 mg/kg/d also at 20 weeks *5760*

Protein *Serum Increase Physiological* Mean increase of 17.8% in 150 patients with acne when treated with 0.1 mg/kg/d for 20 weeks, 4.3% with 0.5 mg/kg/d and 10.2 mg/kg/d when treated with 1.0 mg/kg/d *5760*
Serum No Effect Physiological In 18 patients with severe acne given 0.8 mg/kg daily for 3 mo: changes reverted to normal after treatment stopped *3699*
Urine Increase Physiological In fewer than 10% treated patients proteinuria observed *5014* Increase observed in less than 1% of all patients receiving drug *1384*

Pyruvate *Plasma No Effect Physiological* In 13 patients with severe acne treatment with 1.0 mg/kg/d for 16 weeks had no significant effect on concentration *3368*

Specific Gravity *Urine Increase Physiological* Significant mean increase of 6.7% in 150 patients with acne treated with 0.1 mg/kg/d for 20 weeks, 11.8% when given 0.5 mg/kg/d and 15.6% when given 1.0 mg/kg/d *5760*

Thyroid Stimulating Hormone
Serum No Effect Physiological Or no significant change in 24 healthy men given 1 mg/kg/d for 16 weeks *4403* In 7 patients with severe rosacea treated with 1 mg/kg/d for 12 weeks. Effects possibly due to induction of hepatic microsomal enzymes *3804* In 7 patients given 1 mg/kg/d for 12 weeks *3804* In 18 patients with severe acne given 0.8 mg/kg daily for 3 mo: changes reverted to normal after treatment stopped *3699*

Thyroxine (T4) *Serum Decrease Physiological* In 7 patients with severe rosacea treated with 1 mg/kg/d for 12 weeks. Effects possibly due to induction of hepatic microsomal enzymes *3804* From 98 to 85 nmol/L in 18 patients with severe acne given 0.8 mg/kg daily for 3 mo: changes reverted to normal after treatment stopped *3699* Significant at 12 weeks in 7 patients with severe rosacea treated with 1 mg/kg/d *3804*

Thyroxine (T4), Free *Serum Decrease Physiological* In 7 patients given 1 mg/kg/d for 12 weeks *3804*
Serum No Effect Physiological No significant change in 24 healthy men given 1 mg/kg/d for 16 weeks *4403*

Thyroxine (T4) Index, Free *Serum Decrease Physiological* Significant at 12 weeks in 7 patients with severe rosacea treated with 1 mg/kg/d *3804* From 91 to 78 in 18 patients with severe acne given 0.8 mg/kg daily for 3 mo: changes reverted to normal after treatment stopped *3699*

Tissue Plasminogen Activator
Plasma Increase Physiological In 12 patients with skin disorders administration of 20 - 60 mg/d for 1 month caused significant increase from mean baseline of 2.6 ± 1.3 ng/mL to 3.3 ± 1.6 ng/mL *1339*

Tri-iodothyronine (T3) *Serum Decrease Physiological* In 7 patients with severe rosacea treated with 1 mg/kg/d for 12 weeks. Effects possibly due to induction of hepatic microsomal enzymes *3804*
Serum No Effect Physiological No significant change in 24 healthy men given 1 mg/kg/d for 16 weeks *4403*

Triglycerides *Serum Increase Physiological* From 5.4 to 6.8 mmol/L at 6 weeks in 7 patients with severe rosacea treated with 1 mg/kg/d for 12 weeks *3804* Approximately 25% of treated patients develop hypertriglyceridemia with triglyceride concentration above 500 mg/dL, reversible with cessation of treatment. Magnitude of effect usually dose related *5014* During treatment but not to abnormal levels *2967* In 13 patients with severe acne mean concentration increased significantly when treated with 1.0 mg/kg/d for 16 weeks *3368* In 25 of 523 patients with mean daily dose of 109 mg for 150 d *6500* Treatment with 1 mg/kg/day of 116 patients with acne caused concentration to increase at 6 weeks but it continued to increase thereafter while therapy was continued *6310* Reversible dose-related effect noted in patients with myelodysplastic syndrome and leukemia at high doses *2208* Increase in both men and women with 1 mg/kg/d for 20 weeks when given for nodulocystic acne *524* From 5.1 to 6.1 mmol/L in 18 patients with severe acne given 0.8 mg/kg daily for 3 mo: changes reverted to normal after treatment stopped *3699* Mean increase of 4.4% in 150 patients with acne when treated with 0.1 mg/kg/d for 20 weeks, 10.9% when treated with 0.5 mg/kg/d and 24.5% with 1.0 mg/kg/d *5760*
Serum No Effect Physiological From 2.12 to 2.72 mmol/L in 12 patients with hyperkeratotic disorders given 40 mg *6150*

TSH response to TRH *Serum No Effect Physiological* In 7 patients with severe rosacea treated with 1 mg/kg/d for 12 weeks. Effects possibly due to induction of hepatic microsomal enzymes *3804*

Uric Acid *Serum Increase Physiological* In fewer than 10% treated patients increased concentration observed *5014* Increased concentration observed in less than 1% of all patients receiving drug *1384*

VLDL-Cholesterol *Serum Increase Physiological* From 0.17 to 0.39 mmol/L at 6 weeks in 7 patients with severe rosacea treated with 1 mg/kg/d *3804* In 7 patients with severe rosacea treated with 1 mg/kg/d for 12 weeks. Effects possibly due to induction of hepatic microsomal enzymes *3804* From 0.69 to 0.93 mmol/L in 12 patients with hyperkeratotic disorders given 40 mg daily for 2 mo *6150*

VLDL-Triglycerides *Serum Increase Physiological* From 0.43 to 0.77 mmol/L at 6 weeks in 7 patients with severe rosacea treated with 1 mg/kg/d for 12 weeks. Effects possibly due to induction of hepatic microsomal enzymes *3804* From 1.34 to 1.81 mmol/L in 12 patients with hyperkeratotic disorders given 40 mg daily for 2 mo *6150*

Isoxicam

γ-Glutamyltransferase *Urine No Effect Physiological* No effect observed on excretion in 18 patients with degenerative arthritis and normal renal function when treated with 200 mg/24 hours for 7 days *5284*

6-Keto-Prostaglandin $F_{1\alpha}$ *Urine Decrease Physiological* Reduction by about 40% in 18 patients with degenerative arthritis and normal renal function when treated with 200 mg/24 hours for 7 days *5284*

N-Acetyl-Glucosaminidase *Urine No Effect Physiological* No effect in 18 patients with degenerative arthritis and normal renal function when treated with 200 mg/24 hours for 7 days *5284*

Prostaglandins *Urine Decrease Physiological* Reduction by about 70% in 18 patients with degenerative arthritis and normal renal function when treated with 200 mg/24 hours for 7 days *5284*

Isoxicam *(continued)*

Thromboxane B_2 *Urine Decrease Physiological* Reduction by about 40% in 18 patients with degenerative arthritis and normal renal function treated with 200 mg/24 hours for 7 days *5284*

Isoxsuprine

Amphetamine *Urine Positive Analytical* At concentrations above 6.0 µg/mL (19.90 µmol/L) with method on Du Pont aca *1554*

Drugs of Abuse Screen *Urine Increase Analytical* False positive produced with Abbott ADx method for amphetamine/methamphetamine *4279*

Histamine *Plasma No Effect Analytical* 50% inhibition of radio-enzyme assay observed at 28 µg/mL but not necessarily of clinical significance since physiological concentration less than 10 µg/mL *2492*

Isradipine

Alanine Aminotransferase *Serum Increase Physiological* Administration has been reported to cause abnormal function tests *5230*

Albumin *Urine No Effect Physiological* No significant change observed in 10 healthy men following 5 mg orally *3269*

Alkaline Phosphatase *Serum Increase Physiological* Administration has been reported to cause abnormal function tests *5230*

Aspartate Aminotransferase *Serum Increase Physiological* Administration has been reported to cause abnormal function tests *5230*

Bilirubin *Serum Increase Physiological* Administration has been reported to cause abnormal function tests *5230*

Cholesterol *Serum Decrease Physiological* Mean reduction of 9 mg/dL observed in 13 hypertensive patients treated with up to 20 mg daily for 6 weeks compared with increase of 9 mg/dL in placebo treated controls *6503* Mean reduction of 3.6 mg/dL at 6 months and 7.5 mg/dL at 12 months in 56 elderly patients with benign essential hypertension treated with a mean dose of 11 mg/day *5797*

Creatinine Clearance *Urine No Effect Physiological* No significant effect observed in 10 healthy men given single oral dose of 5 mg *3269*

Digoxin *Serum Increase Physiological* In single dose study in healthy volunteers caused 9% decrease in volume of distribution, which is unlikely to be of clinical significance *2956* Concomitant administration of single doses of both drugs in healthy individuals did not affect renal, non-renal and total body clearance of digoxin *5230* In healthy volunteers coadministration was associated with a 25% increase in the maximum concentration of digoxin *5345*

Effective Renal Plasma Flow *Patient No Effect Physiological* No significant effect observed in 10 healthy men following single oral dose of 5 mg *3269*

Erythrocytes *Blood No Effect Physiological* No significant effect observed in 78 mild to moderately severe hypertensives treated with up to 20 mg daily for 6 weeks *6503*

Glomerular Filtration Rate *Urine No Effect Physiological* Apart from transient decrease one hour after oral administration of 5 mg in 10 healthy men no effect observed *3269*

γ-Glutamyltransferase *Serum Increase Physiological* Administration has been reported to cause abnormal function tests *5230*

HDL-Cholesterol *Serum Increase Physiological* Mean increase of 1.3 mg/dL in 56 elderly patients with benign essential hypertension after 6 months treatment with mean dose of 11 mg/day and mean increase in concentration of 3.9 mg/dL after 12 months *5797*

Hydrochlorothiazide *Serum No Effect Physiological* Concomitant administration of both drugs in healthy individuals had no effect on the pharmacokinetics of either drug *5230*

Indocyanine Green Clearance *Serum Increase Physiological* In 18 patients administration of 5 mg b.i.d. for 4 days caused modest increase from 0.484 ± 0.087 L/h/kg to 0.574 ± 0.109 L/h/kg (19% increase) *5345*

LDL-Cholesterol *Serum Increase Physiological* Mean increase of 4.3 mg/dL at 6 months but mean decrease of 6.2 mg/dL in 56 elderly patients with benign essential hypertension when treated with mean dose of 11 mg/day *5797*

Leukocytes *Blood Decrease Physiological* Administration has been reported to cause leukopenia *5230*

β_2-Microglobulin *Urine No Effect Physiological* No significant effect observed in 10 healthy men following a single oral dose of 5 mg *3269*

Occult Blood *Feces No Effect Physiological* Administration has not been reported to cause gastrointestinal bleeding *5230*

Platelet Aggregation *Blood No Effect Physiological* No change in response to adenosine diphosphate, collagen or epinephrine in healthy male individuals compared with control state *5692*

Propranolol *Serum Increase Physiological* Concomitant administration of single doses of both drugs in healthy individuals increased the area under the concentration curve by 27% and the maximum plasma concentration of propranolol by 58% *5230*

Protein *Urine No Effect Physiological* No significant change observed in 78 mild to moderately hypertensive patients treated with up to 20 mg daily for 6 weeks *6503*

Sodium Clearance *Urine Increase Physiological* Significant increase observed from 1-2 h after 5 mg orally in 10 healthy men (3.3 mL/min versus 2.2 mL/min after placebo) and from 2-3 hours (2.8 mL/min versus 2.2 mL/min after placebo) *3269*

Theophylline *Serum No Effect Physiological* No clinically significant effect on theophylline concentration observed when drugs coadministered *5999* No documented significant interaction with theophylline reported *6117*

Volume *Urine Increase Physiological* Significant increase 1-2 hours after 5 mg orally in 10 healthy men *3269*

Itraconazole

Alanine Aminotransferase *Serum Increase Physiological* Mild reversible increases without serious hepatotoxicity *5985* Itraconazole caused increased activity (more than twice ULN) in 4% of 112 treated patients *2905* Observed in 10 of 189 patients treated for mean of 5 months *6086* In 36 patients with HIV infection and superimposed P. marneffei infection treated with 200 mg/d itraconazole in a maintenance study 17 of 33 developed increased activity compared with 12 of 29 treated with placebo *5875* In one patient with fungal toenails being treated with simvastatin 40 mg/d for type IIa hyperlipidemia addition of 200 mg/d itraconazole caused rhabdomyolysis with enzyme activity increased to 446,000 U/L *2718*

Aldolase *Serum Increase Physiological* In one patient with fungal toenails being treated with simvastatin 40 mg/d for type IIa hyperlipidemia addition of 200 mg/d itraconazole caused rhabdomyolysis with enzyme activity increased to 423,600 U/L *2718*

Alkaline Phosphatase *Serum Increase Physiological* In 36 patients with HIV infection and superimposed P. marneffei infection treated with 200 mg/d itraconazole in a maintenance study 15 of 30 developed increased activity compared with 13 of 31 treated with placebo *5875* Observed in 3 of 189 patients treated for mean of 5 months *6086*

Alprazolam *Serum Increase Physiological* By inhibiting CYP 3A itraconazole may cause a two-fold increase in alprazolam concentration *4685*

Aspartate Aminotransferase *Serum Increase Physiological* Mild reversible increases without serious hepatotoxicity *5985* In 36 patients with HIV infection and superimposed P. marneffei infection treated with 200 mg/d itraconazole in a maintenance study 12 of 26 developed increased activity compared with 19 of 28 treated with placebo *5875* In one patient with fungal toenails being treated with simvastatin 40 mg/d for type IIa hyperlipidemia addition of 200 mg/d itraconazole caused rhabdomyolysis with enzyme activity increased to 990,000 U/L *2718* Itraconazole caused increased activity (more than twice

ULN) in 4% of 112 treated patients *2905* Observed in 10 of 189 patients treated for mean of 5 months *6086*

Astemizole *Serum Increase Physiological* Decreased metabolism with increased risk of cardiac toxicity or arrhythmia *886* Itraconazole and its major metabolite hydroxyitraconazole inhibit the cytochrome P450 3A enzyme system thereby affecting the metabolism of drugs by this system and increasing the plasma concentrations of both astemizole and desmethylastemizole *2905* Concomitant administration of ketoconazole with astemizole causes increased astemizole concentration because ketoconazole inhibits the metabolism of astemizole and itraconazole has a similar chemical structure *2901*

Bilirubin *Serum Increase Physiological* Observed in 2 of 189 patients treated for mean of 5 months *6086*

Blood *Urine Increase Physiological* In one patient with fungal toenails being treated with simvastatin 40 mg/d for type IIa hyperlipidemia addition of 200 mg/d itraconazole caused rhabdomyolysis with positive occult blood *2718*

Carbamazepine *Serum Increase Physiological* Drugs that inhibit CYP 3A4 inhibit metabolism of carbamazepine producing clinically meaningful effect *1039*

Cisapride *Serum Increase Physiological* By inhibiting cytochrome P450 3A4 inhibits metabolism of cisapride and increases its plasma concentration *2903* Ketoaconazole potently inhibits the cytochrome P450 3A enzyme system thereby affecting the metabolism of drugs by this system, raising their concentration: itraconazole probably has a similar effect *2905* Decreased metabolism with increased risk of cardiac toxicity or arrhythmia *886*

Clozapine *Serum No Effect Physiological* In 7 schizophrenic volunteers coadministration of 200 mg itraconazole with clozapine caused no significant effect on the concentration of clozapine changing it only from 913 nmol/L to 887 nmol/L *4827*

Creatine Kinase *Serum Increase Physiological* In one patient with fungal toenails being treated with simvastatin 40 mg/d for type IIa hyperlipidemia addition of 200 mg/d itraconazole caused rhabdomyolysis with enzyme activity increased to 22,800,000 U/L *2718*

Cyclosporine *Blood Increase Physiological* Coadministration may cause greater than two-fold increase in cyclosporine trough concentration but severe nephrotoxicity is rare *859*

Blood No Effect Physiological No significant change observed in mean weekly concentration in 14 bone marrow transplant patients compared with controls in whom only cyclosporine given *4338*

Serum Increase Physiological Two studies, each involving one patient, showed substantial increase when 200 mg/d itraconazole coadministered. Effect possibly associated with deterioration of renal function *6595* Increased concentrations reported when drugs coadministered *1384* Coadministration may cause greater than two-fold increase in cyclosporine trough concentration but severe nephrotoxicity is rare *859* May increase cyclosporine concentration by inhibiting hepatic cytochrome P-450 III A which metabolizes cyclosporine *5236* In one patient considerable increase in concentration observed (more than double) when drugs coadministered: probably related to effect on hepatic metabolism *3346*

Serum No Effect Physiological No effect reported on metabolism *5985* In one study involving 20 patients who had received bone marrow transplants no difference observed in mean whole blood weekly measurements *6595*

Cyclosporine A *Blood Increase Physiological* Itraconazole potently inhibits the cytochrome P450 3A enzyme system thereby affecting the metabolism of drugs by this system, raising their concentration *2905* Coadministration with cyclosporine A increases its concentration *5240*

Digoxin *Serum Increase Physiological* Itraconazole inhibits the metabolism of digoxin increasing its plasma concentration *2905* Coadministration with digoxin may increase the digoxin concentration *2161* Itraconazole and its major metabolite hydroxyitraconazole inhibit the cytochrome P450 3A enzyme system thereby affecting the metabolism of drugs by this system, raising their concentration *2905*

Granular Casts *Urine Increase Physiological* In one patient with fungal toenails being treated with simvastatin 40 mg/d for type IIa hyperlipidemia addition of 200 mg/d itraconazole caused rhabdomyolysis with 1 to 4 granular casts/hpf *2718*

Hematocrit *Blood Decrease Physiological* In 36 patients with HIV infection and superimposed P. marneffei infection treated with 200 mg/d itraconazole in a maintenance study 17 of 30 developed anemia compared with 10 of 28 treated with placebo *5875*

Hemoglobin *Blood Decrease Physiological* In 36 patients with HIV infection and superimposed P. marneffei infection treated with 200 mg/d itraconazole in a maintenance study 17 of 30 developed anemia compared with 10 of 28 treated with placebo *5875*

Hyaline Casts *Urine Increase Physiological* In one patient with fungal toenails being treated with simvastatin 40 mg/d for type IIa hyperlipidemia addition of 200 mg/d itraconazole caused rhabdomyolysis with 1 to 4 hyaline casts/hpf *2718*

Indinavir *Serum Increase Physiological* Itraconazole and its major metabolite hydroxyitraconazole inhibit the cytochrome P450 3A enzyme system thereby affecting the metabolism of drugs by this system and increasing their plasma concentrations *2905*

Lactate Dehydrogenase *Serum Increase Physiological* Observed in 3 of 189 patients treated for mean of 5 months *6086* In one patient with fungal toenails being treated with simvastatin 40 mg/d for type IIa hyperlipidemia addition of 200 mg/d itraconazole caused rhabdomyolysis with enzyme activity increased to 927,000 U/L *2718*

Leukocytes *Blood Decrease Physiological* In 36 patients with HIV infection and superimposed P. marneffei infection treated with 200 mg/d itraconazole in a maintenance study 16 of 28 developed leukopenia compared with 10 of 28 treated with placebo *5875*

Lovastatin *Serum Increase Physiological* Itraconazole and its major metabolite hydroxyitraconazole inhibit the cytochrome P450 3A enzyme system thereby affecting the metabolism of drugs by this system, raising their concentration *2905* In a study of normal volunteers plasma concentrations of lovastatin were increased about 20-fold when administered concomitantly with itraconazole, probably related to the metabolism of both drugs by the same P450 isoform *3982*

Methylprednisolone *Serum Increase Physiological* Itraconazole potently inhibits the cytochrome P450 3A enzyme system thereby affecting the metabolism of drugs by this syste *2905*

Midazolam *Serum Increase Physiological* Administration of itraconazole caused the AUC of midazolam to increase 8- or 2.6-fold *317* Itraconazole and its major metabolite hydroxyitraconazole inhibit the cytochrome P450 3A enzyme system thereby affecting the metabolism of drugs by this system, raising their concentration *2905* By inhibiting cytochrome P450 3A4 may reduce plasma clearance of midazolam when drugs coadministered *5037*

Myoglobin *Urine Increase Physiological* In one patient with fungal toenails being treated with simvastatin 40 mg/d for type IIa hyperlipidemia addition of 200 mg/d itraconazole caused rhabdomyolysis with 222 ng/mL myoglobin *2718*

N-Desethyloxybutynin *Serum No Effect Physiological* Administration of 5 mg oxybutynin to 10 patients who had consumed 200 mg itraconazole daily for 4 days caused a significant in AUC of itraconazole and a two-fold increase in the peak concentration of oxybutenin but had no effect on the AUC or peak concentration of its major active metabolite *3678*

N-Desmethylclozapine *Serum No Effect Physiological* In 7 schizophrenic volunteers coadministration of 200 mg itraconazole with clozapine caused no significant effect on the concentration of clozapine changing it only from 543 nmol/L to 582 nmol/L *4827*

Oral Hypoglycemic Agents *Serum Increase Physiological* Itraconazole potently inhibits the cytochrome P450 3A enzyme system thereby affecting the metabolism of drugs by this system, raising their concentration and causing severe hypoglycemia *2905*

Oxybutynin *Serum Increase Physiological* Administration of 5 mg oxybutynin to 10 patients who had consumed 200 mg itraconazole daily for 4 days caused a significant in AUC of itraconazole and a two-fold increase in the peak concentration of oxybutenin *3678*

Itraconazole *(continued)*

Phenytoin *Serum No Effect Physiological* In healthy males coadministration of phenytoin with itraconazole caused an insignificant change in the diphenylhydantoin concentration from 4.6 ± 0.6 µg/mL to 4.6 ± 0.5 µg/mL but a significant reduction in area under the curve from 144 ± 39 µg.h/mL to 159 ± 50 µg.h/mL *1610*

Platelets *Blood Decrease Physiological* Observed in 1 of 189 patients treated for mean of 5 months *6086*

Potassium *Serum Decrease Physiological* Observed in 6% of 189 patients treated for mean of 5 months *6086*

Prothrombin Time *Plasma Increase Physiological* Coadministration of Itraconazole with coumarin anticoagulants enhances the anticoagulant action of these drugs by inhibiting their metabolism *2905* Increased INR observed in patients receiving warfarin *886*

Quinidine *Serum Increase Physiological* Administration of 200 mg/d itraconazole by 9 healthy individuals with 100 mg quinidine sulfate caused an increase of 1.6-fold in quinidine concentration and a 2.4 in its AUC *3071* Itraconazole potently inhibits the cytochrome P450 3A enzyme system thereby affecting the metabolism of drugs by this system *2905*

Ritonavir *Serum Increase Physiological* Itraconazole and its major metabolite hydroxyitraconazole inhibit the cytochrome P450 3A enzyme system thereby affecting the metabolism of drugs by this system and increasing their plasma concentrations *2905*

Sildenafil *Serum Increase Physiological* Theoretical effect: drug likely to increase area under concentration curve of sildenafil due to CYP3A4 inhibition *4657*

Simvastatin *Serum Increase Physiological* Itraconazole and its major metabolite hydroxyitraconazole inhibit the cytochrome P450 3A enzyme system thereby affecting the metabolism of drugs by this system, raising their concentration *2905*

Sodium *Serum Decrease Physiological* Observed in 1 of 189 patients treated for mean of 5 months *6086*

Tacrolimus *Serum Increase Physiological* Itraconazole potently inhibits the cytochrome P450 3A enzyme system thereby affecting the metabolism of drugs by this system, raising their concentration *2905* By inhibiting cytochrome P-450 IIIA enzyme systems may inhibit the metabolism of tacrolimus *1987*

Terfenadine *Serum Increase Physiological* Decreased metabolism with increased risk of cardiac toxicity or arrhythmia *886* Itraconazole and its major metabolite hydroxyitraconazole inhibit the cytochrome P450 3A enzyme system thereby affecting the metabolism of drugs by this system and increasing their plasma concentrations *2905* In 6 healthy volunteers 200 mg itraconazole for 7 days coadministered with 120 mg terfenadine area under curve for acid metabolite increased from mean of 2732 ± 603 ng/h/mL to 3549 ± 622 ng/h/mL *2699* Itraconazole markedly inhibits the metabolism of terfenadine *2653*

Thyroxine (T4) *Serum Decrease Physiological* Observed in 1 of 189 patients treated for mean of 5 months *157*

Triazolam *Serum Increase Physiological* Itraconazole and its major metabolite hydroxyitraconazole inhibit the cytochrome P450 3A enzyme system thereby affecting the metabolism of drugs by this system, raising their concentration *2905*

Triglycerides *Serum Increase Physiological* Hypertriglyceridemia observed in 9% of 189 patients treated for a mean of 5 months *6086*

Vinca Alkaloids *Serum Increase Physiological* Itraconazole and its major metabolite hydroxyitraconazole inhibit the cytochrome P450 3A enzyme system thereby affecting the metabolism of drugs by this system, raising the concentration of vinca alkaloids *2905*

Warfarin *Plasma Increase Physiological* Itraconazole and its major metabolite hydroxyitraconazole inhibit the cytochrome P450 3A enzyme system thereby affecting the metabolism of drugs by this system: prothrombin time would also be affected *2905*

Zidovudine *Serum No Effect Physiological* Itraconazole and its major metabolite hydroxyitraconazole inhibit the cytochrome P450 3A enzyme system thereby affecting the metabolism of drugs by this system but coadministration of 100 mg b.i.d. of itraconazole with 8 ± 0.4 mg/kg/d to 8 HIV-infected patients had no effect on its pharmacokinetics *2905* Coadministration of Itraconazole with zidovudine has no effect on the pharmacokineitics of zidovudine *2905*

Zolpidem *Serum Increase Physiological* In 10 healthy volunteers coadministration of 200 mg itraconazole with 10 mg zolpidem caused a 34% increase in the zolpidem AUC from 567 ng/h/mL to 759 ng/h/mL and increase in its mean serum concentration from 163 ng/mL to 180 ng/mL *3695*

Josamycin

Alanine Aminotransferase *Serum No Effect Physiological* Mean activity 27 U/L after 10 days of 2 g/d in 6 healthy male volunteers compared with activity of 30 U/L after placebo *6146*

Alkaline Phosphatase *Serum Increase Physiological* Mean activity 184 U/L after 2 g/d for 10 days in 6 healthy male volunteers compared with 170 U/L after placebo *6146*

Aspartate Aminotransferase *Serum No Effect Physiological* Mean activity 24 U/L after 2 g/d for 10 days in 6 healthy male volunteers compared with 26 U/L after placebo *6146*

Bilirubin *Serum No Effect Physiological* Nonsignificant increase to mean concentration of 14.8 µmol/L in 6 healthy male volunteers given 2 g/d compared with 13.2 µmol/L after placebo *6146*

Carbamazepine *Serum Increase Physiological* Inhibits metabolism and increases plasma concentration *3118*

Cortisol *Plasma No Effect Physiological* No significant change observed in 6 healthy male volunteers given 2 g/d for 10 days *6146*

Cortisol, Free *Urine Decrease Physiological* Nonsignificant reduction from mean baseline of 121 nmol/d to 92 nmol/d in 6 healthy male volunteers given 2 g/d for 10 days *6146*

Cyclosporine *Blood Increase Physiological* Coadministration of josamycin with cyclosporine caused a ≤400% increase in cyclosporine concentration probably due to competitive inhibition of cyclosporine metabolism *859*
Serum Increase Physiological Increased concentrations reported in two renal transplant patients after both oral and intravenous administration at a dose of 1 or 2 g/day *3284* In 2 renal transplant patients after both intravenous and oral josamycin at a dose of 2 g/d increased concentration of cyclosporine observed but mechanism not discussed *6595* Probably related to inhibition of hepatic degradation but may also be alteration in absorption or distribution *1069* Coadministration of josamycin with cyclosporine caused a ≤400% increase in cyclosporine concentration probably due to competitive inhibition of cyclosporine metabolism *859*

Dehydroepiandrosterone Sulfate *Plasma No Effect Physiological* Nonsignificant increase from mean baseline of 9.4 µmol/L to 10.8 µmol/L in 6 healthy male volunteers given 2 g/d for 10 days *6146*

Estradiol *Plasma No Effect Physiological* Nonsignificant reduction from mean baseline of 83 pmol/L to 90 pmol/L in 6 healthy male volunteers given 2 g/d for 10 days *6146*

Follicle Stimulating Hormone *Plasma No Effect Physiological* Nonsignificant increase from mean baseline of 1.50 IU/L to 1.63 IU/L in 10 healthy male volunteers given 2 g/d for 10 days *6146*

γ-Glutamyltransferase *Serum Increase Physiological* Nonsignificant increase to 20 U/L in 6 healthy male volunteers given 2 g/d for 10 days compared with 15 U/L after placebo *6146*

6-β-Hydroxycortisol *Urine Decrease Physiological* Significant reduction from mean baseline of 500 nmol/d to 384 nmol/d in 6 healthy male volunteers given 2 g/d for 10 days *6146*

Luteinizing Hormone *Plasma No Effect Physiological* Nonsignificant increase from mean baseline of 1.45 IU/L to 1.93 IU/L in 6 healthy male volunteers given 2 g/d for 10 days *6146*

Testosterone, Free *Serum No Effect Physiological* Nonsignificant reduction from mean baseline of 96 pmol/L to 92 pmol/L in 6 healthy male volunteers given 2 g/d for 10 days *6146*

Thyroid Stimulating Hormone *Serum Decrease Physiological* Nonsignificant reduction in 6 healthy men from mean of 1.72 mU/L to 1.64 mU/L following 2 g/d for 10 days *6146*

Thyroxine (T4) *Serum No Effect Physiological* In 6 healthy male volunteers 2 g/d for 10 days caused nonsignificant increase from mean 99 nmol/L to 104 nmol/L *6146*

Thyroxine (T4), Free *Serum No Effect Physiological* Nonsignificant increase observed in 6 healthy male volunteers given 2 g/d for 10 days *6146*

Tri-iodothyronine, Free (fT3)
Serum No Effect Physiological Nonsignificant increase from mean baseline of 6.76 pmol/L to 7.00 pmol/L in 6 healthy male volunteers following 2 g/d for 10 days *6146*

Tri-iodothyronine, Reverse (rT3)
Serum No Effect Physiological Nonsignificant increase from baseline of 0.42 nmol/L to 0.45 nmol/L in 6 healthy male volunteers given 2 g/d for 10 days *6146*

K 12.148

Apolipoprotein A-I *Serum No Effect Physiological* No significant change observed in healthy male volunteers treated with up to 900 mg daily for 12 weeks *2496*

Apolipoprotein A-I:Apolipoprotein B Ratio
Serum Increase Physiological Significant increase observed in dose-dependent manner when healthy male volunteers treated with between 300 mg and 900 mg daily for 12 weeks *2496*

Apolipoprotein B *Serum Decrease Physiological* At doses of 300 mg, 600 mg and 900 mg daily for 12 weeks significant reduction in concentration observed in healthy male volunteers *2496*

Cholesterol *Serum Decrease Physiological* In 40 healthy young males divided into groups of 8 treatment for 14 days caused mean reduction of 13.4% with 300 mg daily, 23.8% with 600 mg daily and 25.6% with 900 mg daily *2496*

Cortisol *Plasma No Effect Physiological* No significant change observed in healthy male volunteers treated with up to 900 mg daily for 12 weeks *2496*

HDL-Cholesterol *Serum Decrease Physiological* Nonsignificant reduction of 13.4% observed in 8 healthy male volunteers given 900 mg daily for 12 weeks but almost no change observed at lower doses *2496*

17-Hydroxyprogesterone *Plasma No Effect Physiological* No significant change in 17α-hydroxyprogesterone concentration observed in healthy male volunteers treated with up to 900 mg daily for 12 weeks *2496*

17α-Hydroxyprogesterone *Plasma No Effect Physiological* No significant change observed in healthy male volunteers treated with up to 900 mg daily for 12 weeks *2496*

LDL-Cholesterol *Serum Decrease Physiological* In 40 healthy young male volunteers divided into groups of 8 treatment for 14 days with 300 mg daily caused mean reduction of 14.7%, with 600 mg daily a reduction of 33.3% and with 900 mg daily a reduction of 34.8% *2496*

Testosterone *Serum No Effect Physiological* No significant change observed in healthy male volunteers treated with doses up to 900 mg daily for 12 weeks *2496*

Triglycerides *Serum Decrease Physiological* Although nonsignificant increase observed at a dose level of 150 mg daily for 12 weeks nonsignificant decrease observed with increasing doses up to 900 mg daily in healthy male volunteers *2496*

Kanamycin

Alanine Aminotransferase *Serum Increase Physiological* May cause hepatotoxicity *3810*

Alkaline Phosphatase *Serum Increase Physiological* May cause hepatotoxicity *3810*
Urine Increase Physiological Due to nephrotoxic effect of drug *4826*

Amikacin *Serum Increase Analytical* Interferes with method on Abbott TDx *3858* At a concentration of 4 mg/L causes 25% error when added to a specimen containing 15 mg/L and measured on a Baxter Stratus analyzer *5705*

Amino Acids *Urine Increase Analytical* Unusual ninhydrin positive spot observed with TLC *2605* Reacts with ninhydrin; extra spot TLC, high voltage electrophoresis *4760*

Ammonia *Plasma Decrease Physiological* Impairs NH_3 production by gut bacteria *2452*

Aspartate Aminotransferase *Serum Increase Physiological* May cause hepatotoxicity *3810*

Bilirubin *Serum Increase Physiological* May cause hepatotoxicity *3810*
Serum No Effect Physiological Clinically insignificant displacement from protein in neonates *6314*

BSP Retention *Serum Increase Physiological* May cause hepatotoxicity *1714*

Carotene *Serum Decrease Physiological* May induce malabsorption with diarrhea *2754*

Casts *Urine Increase Physiological* Nephrotoxic effect (cylindruria and granular casts) *128*

Cholesterol *Serum Decrease Physiological* Forms salts with bile acids in gut *1773*

Creatinine *Serum Increase Physiological* Nephrotoxic effect (common but slight) *3669*
Serum No Effect Analytical No effect of concentrations up to 15 mg/L on single slide method on Kodak Ektachem® *5706*

Eosinophils *Blood Increase Physiological* Allergic reaction *2484*

Erythrocytes *Urine Increase Physiological* Actual bleeding may occur *1714*

Fat *Feces Increase Physiological* Steatorrhea produced probably by causing mucosal damage *5055* May induce malabsorption with diarrhea *2754*

Fibrinogen *Plasma Decrease Physiological* May occur at beginning of therapy *2242*

Gentamicin *Serum No Effect Analytical* No interference observed at concentrations up to 500 µg/mL (1035 µmol/L) with method on Du Pont aca *1526* Has cross-reactivity of less than 0.1% with method on Baxter Stratus *5705* Specimens containing kanamycin showed no cross-reactivity when gentamicin measured by method on Bayer Technicon Immuno 1® system *426* No interference observed with method on Abbott TDx *3858*

Hemoglobin *Urine Increase Physiological* Actual bleeding occurs *1714*

Ketone Body Ratio *Serum No Effect Analytical* When added at a concentration of 5 g/L had no significant effect on AKBR method of Uno et al *6131*

Leucine Aminopeptidase *Urine Increase Physiological* Associated with proximal renal tubular injury *135*

Leukocytes *Blood Increase Physiological* Due to eosinophilia *3810*

Neomycin *Serum No Effect Analytical* No interference observed with method on Abbott TDx *3858*

Netilmicin *Serum No Effect Analytical* No interference observed with method on Abbott TDx *3858*

Nonprotein Nitrogen *Serum Increase Physiological* Nephrotoxic effect *3810*

Phenylalanine *Plasma No Effect Analytical* No interference observed with rapid quantitative whole blood method of Campbell et al using phenylalanine dehydrogenase *867*

Potassium *Serum No Effect Analytical* At concentration of 10 mg/L had no effect on measurement by ISE with predilution *5704*

Protein *Urine Increase Physiological* Nephrotoxic effect *1714*

Prothrombin Time *Plasma Decrease Physiological* Effect noted at beginning of therapy *4014*
Plasma Increase Physiological May decrease vitamin K synthesis by gut bacteria *2452*

Sodium *Serum No Effect Analytical* At concentration of 10 mg/L had no effect on measurement by ISE with predilution *5704*

Streptomycin *Serum No Effect Analytical* No interference observed with method on Abbott TDx *3858*

Tobramycin *Serum Increase Analytical* At a concentration of 5 mg/L causes 25% increase of tobramycin concentration as measured by method on Baxter Stratus with therapeutic concentration up to 25 mg/L *5705* Cross-reacts with reagents in method on Du Pont aca *1547* Interferes with method on Abbott TDx *3858*

Kanamycin *(continued)*

Tobramycin *(continued)*
Serum No Effect Analytical Cross-reactivity of 1.3% observed with tobramycin method on Bayer Technicon Immuno 1® *435*

Urea Nitrogen *Serum Increase Physiological* Nephrotoxic effect (common slight elevation) *129*

Urobilin *Urine Increase Physiological* Nephrotoxic effect *2754*

Vancomycin *Serum No Effect Analytical* No interference observed with method on Abbott TDx *3858*

Volume *Urine Decrease Physiological* Nephrotoxicity may occur with oliguria, azotemia *2754*

Xylose *Urine Decrease Physiological* Due to impaired gastrointestinal absorption *2754*

Kaolin-Pectin

Chloroquine *Serum Decrease Physiological* Gastrointestinal absorption reduced *3891*

Clindamycin *Serum Decrease Physiological* With pectin causes delayed absorption *6403*

Diagnex Blue Excretion *Urine Increase Physiological* Kaolin causes displacement of diagnex blue from resin *6515*

Digoxin *Serum Decrease Physiological* Gastrointestinal absorption inhibited by binding in gastrointestinal tract *760* Bioavailability reduced with concomitant administration *1384* By decreasing intestinal digoxin absorption may decrease the digoxin concentration *2161*

Lincomycin *Serum Decrease Physiological* Kaolin inhibits gastrointestinal absorption *2452* Plasma concentration markedly reduced when drugs coadministered due to inhibition of gastrointestinal absorption *3870*

Pseudoephedrine *Serum Decrease Physiological* Delayed absorption due to adsorption onto kaolin *6403*

Quinidine *Serum Decrease Physiological* Coadministration causes reduction of plasma concentration of quinidine due to reduced gastrointestinal absorption because of adsorption of quinidine onto kaolin-pectin. Maximum concentration of quinidine reduced by 53% and area under curve by 5% *4147*

Ketamine

Alanine Aminotransferase *Serum Increase Physiological* In 14 of 34 individuals who had drug as anesthetic for intermediate operations *1621*

Alkaline Phosphatase *Serum Increase Physiological* In 14 of 34 individuals who had drug as anesthetic for intermediate operations *1621*

Aspartate Aminotransferase *Serum Increase Physiological* In 14 of 34 individuals who had drug as anesthetic for intermediate operations *1621*

γ-Glutamyltransferase *Serum Increase Physiological* In 14 of 34 individuals who had drug as anesthetic for intermediate operations *1621*

Histamine *Plasma No Effect Analytical* Although 50% inhibition of radio-assay at 38 µg/mL no clinical effects likely since physiological concentration less than 2.2 µg/mL *2492*

Ketanserin

Albumin *Urine No Effect Physiological* Nonsignificant reduction from mean of 257 mg/d to 230 mg/d in 10 hypertensive patients treated with up to 80 mg daily for 8 weeks *906*

Aldosterone *Plasma No Effect Physiological* No significant effect of treatment with 40 mg/d for 4 weeks observed in 10 patients with uncomplicated mild essential hypertension *2018*

Apolipoprotein A-I *Serum Increase Physiological* Significant increase from mean concentration of 1.54 g/L to 1.67 g/L in 10 patients with mild to moderate essential hypertension treated with up to 80 mg daily for 8 weeks *3650*
Serum No Effect Physiological Insignificant change observed in 34 patients with mild to moderate hypertension treated with up to 60 mg daily for 12 weeks *4214* No significant change from mean baseline of 145.8 mg/dL in 13 patients with essential hypertension when treated with 80 mg daily for 12 weeks *3778*

Apolipoprotein A-II *Serum No Effect Physiological* Insignificant change observed in 34 patients treated for 12 weeks with up to 60 mg daily *4214*

Apolipoprotein B *Serum Decrease Physiological* Significant decrease observed in 34 patients with mild to moderate hypertension treated with up to 60 mg daily for 12 weeks *4214* Significant decrease from mean of 1.33 g/L to 1.16 g/L in 10 patients with mild to moderate essential hypertension treated with up to 80 mg daily for 8 weeks *3650*
Serum Increase Physiological Significant increase after 12 weeks treatment of 15 mild to moderate hypertensives treated with 40 mg daily (baseline 149 mg/dL, 6 weeks 150 mg/dL, 12 weeks 161 mg/dL) but increase not significant in 14 hypertensives given 80 mg daily *551*
Serum No Effect Physiological No significant change from mean baseline of 136.4 mg/dL in 13 patients with essential hypertension when treated with 80 mg daily for 12 weeks *3778*

Apolipoprotein C-II *Serum No Effect Physiological* Insignificant change observed in 34 patients with mild to moderate hypertension treated for 12 weeks with up to 60 mg daily *4214*

Apolipoprotein C-III *Serum No Effect Physiological* Insignificant change observed in 34 patients with mild to moderate hypertension treated with up to 60 mg daily for 12 weeks *4214*

Apolipoprotein E *Serum Decrease Physiological* Significant reduction observed in 34 patients with mild to moderate hypertension treated for 12 weeks with up to 60 mg daily *4214*

Atrial Natriuretic Peptide *Plasma Increase Physiological* In 15 mild to moderate hypertensives treatment with 40 mg daily caused increase from mean concentration of 19 ng/L to 32 ng/L after 24 weeks and from 22 ng/L to 41 ng/L in 14 hypertensives treated with 80 mg daily for 24 weeks *551*

Cholesterol *Serum Decrease Physiological* Significant decrease in 10 patients with mild to moderate essential hypertension treated with up to 80 mg daily for 8 weeks from mean of 6.22 mmol/L to 5.74 mmol/L *3650* With up to 60 mg daily for 12 weeks in 34 patients with mild or moderate hypertension average reduction of 6.3% observed *4214*
Serum No Effect Physiological No significant change from mean baseline of 219 mg/dL in 13 patients with essential hypertension treated with 80 mg daily for 12 weeks *3778* No significant effect of treatment with either 40 mg/d or 80 mg/d for 12 weeks in 15 and 14 mild to moderate hypertensives respectively *551* In 50 hypertensive patients given 80 mg/daily for 3 mo *3574*

Filtration Fraction *Urine No Effect Physiological* Nonsignificant increase from 21% to 22% in 10 hypertensive patients treated with up to 80 mg daily for 8 weeks *906*

Glomerular Filtration Rate *Urine No Effect Physiological* Insignificant increase from 96 to 101 mL/min/1.73 sq m in 10 hypertensive patients treated with up to 80 mg daily for 8 weeks *906*

Glucose *Serum No Effect Physiological* No significant change from mean baseline of 94.6 mg/dL in 13 patients with essential hypertension when treated with 80 mg daily for 12 weeks *3778*

HDL-Cholesterol *Serum Decrease Physiological* Insignificant change observed in 34 patients with mild to moderate hypertension treated for 12 weeks with up to 60 mg daily *4214*
Serum Increase Physiological Increase from mean concentration of 1.44 mmol/L to 1.65 mmol/L in 10 patients with mild to moderate essential hypertension treated with up to 80 mg daily for 8 weeks *3650* In 50 hypertensive patients given 80 mg/daily for 3 mo *3574*
Serum No Effect Physiological No significant effect observed in 15 mild to moderate hypertensives treated with 40 mg/d for 12 weeks or in 14 patients treated with 80 mg daily for 12 weeks *551* No significant change from mean baseline of 47.6 mg/dL in 13 patients with essential hypertension when treated with 80 mg daily for 12 weeks *3778*

6-Keto-Prostaglandin $F_{1\alpha}$ *Urine No Effect Physiological* No significant effect observed on nocturnal excretion in 10 patients with mild essential hypertension when treated with 40 mg/d for 4 weeks *2018*

LDL-Cholesterol *Serum Decrease Physiological* Average reduction of 8.8% observed in 34 patients with mild to moderate hypertension treated with up to 60 mg daily for 12 weeks *4214* Insignificant reduction observed in 15 patients with mild to moderate hypertension treated with 40 mg/d for 12 weeks or in 14 patients treated with 80 mg/d for 12 weeks *551* Significant decrease from mean concentration of 4.15 mmol/L to 3.76 mmol/L in 10 patients with mild to moderate essential hypertension treated with up to 80 mg daily for 8 weeks *3650* In 50 hypertensive patients given 80 mg/daily for 3 mo *3574*
Serum No Effect Physiological No significant change from mean baseline of 155.5 mg/dL in 13 patients with essential hypertension when treated with 80 mg daily for 12 weeks *3778*

Phospholipids *Serum No Effect Physiological* Insignificant change observed in 34 patients with mild to moderate hypertension treated for 12 weeks with up to 60 mg daily *4214*

Platelet Aggregation *Blood Decrease Physiological* Significant reduction in aggregation induced by arachidonic acid and collagen in 10 patients with mild to moderate essential hypertension treated with up to 80 mg daily for 8 weeks *3650*
Blood No Effect Physiological No significant effect observed in response to ADP in 10 patients with mild to moderate essential hypertension treated with up to 80 mg daily for 8 weeks *3650*

Potassium *Serum No Effect Physiological* No significant change observed in 10 hypertensive patients treated with up to 80 mg daily for 8 weeks *906*

Renal Plasma Flow *Patient No Effect Physiological* Nonsignificant reduction from mean 456 mL/min/sq m to 445 mL/min/1.73 sq m in 10 hypertensive patients treated with up to 80 mg daily for 8 weeks *906*

Renin Activity *Plasma No Effect Physiological* Small but insignificant decrease observed over 24 weeks in 15 mild to moderate hypertensives treated with 40 mg daily or 14 treated with 80 mg daily *551* No significant effect of 4 weeks treatment with 40 mg/d observed in 10 patients with uncomplicated essential hypertension *2018*

Sodium *Serum No Effect Physiological* No significant change in 10 hypertensive patients treated with up to 80 mg daily for 8 weeks *906*

Thromboxane B_2 *Urine No Effect Physiological* No significant effect observed on nocturnal excretion in 10 patients with mild essential hypertension when treated with 40 mg/d for 4 weeks *2018*

Triglycerides *Serum Decrease Physiological* Significant decrease from mean 1.83 mmol/L to 1.30 mmol/L observed in 10 patients with mild to moderate essential hypertension treated with up to 80 mg daily for 8 weeks *3650*
Serum No Effect Physiological No significant change from mean baseline of 108.6 mg/dL in 13 patients with essential hypertension when treated with 80 mg daily for 12 weeks *3778* No significant effect of treatment of 15 mild to moderate hypertensives for 12 weeks with 40 mg/d or in 14 with 80 mg/d *551* Insignificant change observed in 34 patients with mild to moderate hypertension treated for 12 weeks with up to 60 mg daily *4214*

Uric Acid *Serum No Effect Physiological* No significant change from mean baseline of 5.3 mg/dL in 13 patients with essential hypertension when treated with 80 mg daily for 12 weeks *3778*

VLDL-Cholesterol *Serum Decrease Physiological* Significant reduction from baseline of 33 mg/dL to 26 mg/dL after 6 weeks treatment with 40 mg/d in 15 mild to moderate hypertensives but no longer significant after 12 weeks: no significant change observed in 14 patients who received 80 mg/d for 12 wk *551*
Serum No Effect Physiological No significant change from mean baseline of 13.3 mg/dL in 13 patients with essential hypertension treated with 80 mg daily for 12 weeks *3778*

Volume *Plasma No Effect Physiological* In 10 patients with hypertension and normal renal function treatment with up to 80 mg daily for 8 weeks had no effect *906*

Ketazolam

Benzodiazepine *Urine Positive Analytical* At concentrations of 3.0 µg/mL or greater produces positive result with Syva EMIT II assay *1785*

α-Ketobutyric Acid

Ferric Chloride Test *Urine Positive Analytical* Purple: fades to red brown *684*

Ketoconazole

Acid Phosphatase, Prostatic
Serum Decrease Physiological In men with prostatic cancer with 400 mg every 8 h and prolonged treatment *5701*

Adenosine Monophosphate *Urine Increase Physiological* In one patient with sarcoidosis treatment with 800 mg/d for 6 days caused nonsignificant increase from 1.96 nmol/dL GFR to 2.18 nmol/dL GFR *2147*
Urine No Effect Physiological No effect on excretion in patients with primary hyperparathyroidism and hypercalcemia *2149*

Alanine Aminotransferase *Serum Increase Physiological* Rapidly developing liver failure in 67 year old woman taking 200 mg drug daily for 2 mo *1604* Reported incidence of hepatotoxicity in 1:10000 exposed patients *2902* Delayed reaction to drug after withdrawal in single case of chronic candidiasis in 61 y old woman *5886* Transient abnormalities of liver function observed in 10% patients but true hepatic injury in only 0.1 to 1%. Probably idiosyncrasy involved but may be immune hypersensitivity in some cases *5701* In 4 of 36 patients treated with 200 mg daily over 8 mo *5071*

Aldosterone *Plasma Decrease Physiological* In 3 patients with primary hyperaldosteronism reduced concentration to near normal values. Effect apparent within one week *3451*

Alkaline Phosphatase *Serum Increase Physiological* Reported incidence of hepatotoxicity in 1:10000 exposed patients *2902* Rapidly developing liver failure in 67 year old woman taking 200 mg drug daily for 2 mo *1604* Delayed reaction to drug after withdrawal in single case of chronic candidiasis in 61 y old woman *5886*
Serum No Effect Physiological No effect in patients with primary hyperparathyroidism and hypercalcemia *2149* In 9 healthy men given up to 1200 mg/d for 1 week *2148*

Alprazolam *Serum Increase Physiological* By inhibiting CYP 3A ketoconazole may cause a significant increase in alprazolam concentration *4685*

Androstenedione *Plasma Decrease Physiological* Significant reduction from mean baseline of 4.05 nmol/L to 2.70 nmol/L in 12 normotensive men given 6 doses of 300 mg over 48 hours but insignificant increase observed in 12 hypertensive men with same protocol *2758* Nonsignificant reduction from mean baseline of 258.7 ng/dL observed at 2 months but significant reduction to 191.0 ng/dL observed at 6 months in 7 hirsute women treated with 200 mg/12 h p.o *1107* Observed in 2 h after single 200 mg dose in normal men *5701* In 37 women with polycystic ovary disease treatment with 200 mg/12 h for 9 months caused significant decrease from mean baseline of 4.3 ± 0.3 nmol/L to 3.3 ± 0.3 nmol/L after 3 months and 2.5 ± 0.2 nmol/L after 9 months *6255*

δ_4-Androstenedione *Plasma Decrease Physiological* Reduction of plasma concentration of δ-4-androstenedione from mean baseline of 2.17 µg/L to 2.06 µg/L in 9 hyperandrogenic women treated with 400 mg/d for 10 days and from 2.98 µg/L to 1.94 µg/L in another 9 treated with 800 mg/d for 10 days *933* Reduction from mean baseline of 2.17 µg/L to 2.06 µg/L in 9 hyperandrogenic women treated with 400 mg/d for 10 days and from 2.98 µg/L to 1.94 µg/L in another 9 treated with 800 mg/d for 10 days *933*

Androstenedione, Free *Plasma Decrease Physiological* Observed in 2 h after single 200 mg dose in normal men *5701*

Apolipoprotein A-I *Serum Increase Physiological* Increase from mean baseline of 131 mg/dL to 140 mg/dL in 9 hyperandrogenic women treated with 400 mg/d for 10 days and from 137 mg/dL to 154 mg/dL in another 9 treated with 800 mg/d for 10 days *933*

Apolipoprotein B *Serum Decrease Physiological* Reduction from mean baseline of 98 mg/dL to 93 mg/dL in 9 hyperandrogenic women treated with 400 mg/d for 10 days and from 120 mg/dL to 94 mg/dL in another 9 treated with 800 mg/d for 10 days *933* Observed in hyperandrogenic women *933*

Aspartate Aminotransferase *Serum Increase Physiological* Delayed reaction to drug after withdrawal in single case of

Ketoconazole *(continued)*

Aspartate Aminotransferase *(continued)* chronic candidiasis in 61 y old woman *5886* Reported incidence of hepatotoxicity in 1:10000 exposed patients *2902* Rapidly developing liver failure in 67 year old woman taking 200 mg drug daily for 2 mo *1604* Transient abnormalities of liver function observed in 10% patients but true hepatic injury in only 0.1 to 1%. Probably idiosyncrasy involved but may be immune hypersensitivity in some cases *5701* In 4 of 36 patients treated with 200 mg daily over 8 mo *5071*

Astemizole *Serum Increase Physiological* Concomitant administration of ketoconazole with astemizole causes increased astemizole concentration because ketoconazole inhibits the metabolism of astemizole *2901* Ketoconazole inhibits the metabolism of astemizaloe increasing its plasma concentration and that of its metabolite desmethylastemizole *2905* Through inhibition of cytochrome P450IIIA4, ketoconazole blocks the metabolism of astemizole leading to a higher plasma concentration *5684* Coadministration of ketoconazole with astemizole caused increases in the concentration of astemizole *2902* Coadministration of ketoconazole with astemizole caused significant increase in terfenadine concentration due to inhibition of cytochrome P450IIIA4 in the liver *729*

Azelastine *Serum Increase Analytical* Coadministration of ketoconazole (200 mg b.i.d. for 7 days) interfered with the measurement of azelastine *6320*

Bilirubin *Serum Increase Physiological* Delayed reaction to drug after withdrawal in single case of chronic candidiasis in 61 y old woman *5886* Reported incidence of hepatotoxicity in 1:10000 exposed patients *2902* Rapidly developing liver failure in 67 year old woman taking 200 mg drug daily for 2 mo *1604*

Bilirubin, Direct *Serum Increase Physiological* Rapidly developing liver failure in 67 year old woman taking 200 mg drug daily for 2 mo *1604*

Calcium *Serum Decrease Physiological* In one patient with sarcoidosis and hypercalcemia oral treatment with 800 mg/day caused reduction of 15% in serum concentration within 4 days *48* In a patient with hypercalcemia and sarcoidosis treatment with oral ketoconazole 800 mg/d caused plasma concentration to decrease by 15% within 4 days *48* Slight but significant reduction in patients with primary hyperparathyroidism and hypercalcemia not correlated with change in 1,25-dihydroxyvitamin D *2149*

Serum No Effect Physiological In one patient with sarcoidosis treatment with 800 mg/d for 6 days changed baseline concentration insignificantly from 3.80 mmol/L to 3.73 mmol/L. In a second patient treatment with 800 mg/d for 4 days caused nonsignificant change from 2.86 mmol/L to 2.71 mmol/L *2147* In 9 healthy men given up to 1200 mg/d for 1 week *2148*

Urine Decrease Physiological In one patient with sarcoidosis treatment with 800 mg/d for 6 days caused reduction from 21.3 mmol/d to 17.5 mmol/d. In a second patient excretion decreased from 16.3 mmol/d to 9.3 mmol/d after 4 days of 800 mg/d *2147* Reduction of fractional urinary excretion rate by 57% in a patient with sarcoidosis and hypercalcemia when treated with 800 mg/day for 4 days *48*

Carbamazepine *Serum Increase Physiological* Drugs that inhibit CYP 3A4 inhibit metabolism of carbamazepine producing clinically meaningful effect *1039*

Cetirizine *Serum No Effect Physiological* No clinically significant effect observed *4661*

Chlordiazepoxide *Serum Increase Physiological* Clearance reduced when drugs coadministered *1384*

Cholesterol *Serum Decrease Physiological* Reduces serum cholesterol concentration by about 20% by inhibiting 14α-demethylation of lanosterol to reduce synthesis and also inhibits gastrointestinal absorption *3114* In 7 patients with heterozygous familial hypercholesterolemiz and 3 patients with primary hypercholesterolemia treatment with 400 mg/d for 3 weeks caused significant reduction from mean of 9.26 ± 0.63 mmol/ L to 7.03 ± 0.66 mmol/L *2383* Mean reduction of 19% observed in 9 women with xanthomatous familial hypercholesterolemia treated with 400 mg/d *2384* In patients with prostatic cancer high doses cholesterol synthesis from lanosterol (reduction typically of the order of 20-30%) *1384* After high dose treatment in patients with advanced prostatic cancer; appears to be dose related *5701* Effect observed in hyperandrogenic women *933* Reduction from mean of 164 mg/dL to 147 mg/dL in 9 hyperandrogengic women treated with 400 mg/d for 10 days and from 182 mg/dL to 143 mg/dL in another 9 treated with 800 mg/d for 10 days *933*

Cisapride *Serum Increase Physiological* Through inhibition of cytochrome P450IIIA4, ketoconazole blocks the metabolism of cisapride leading to a higher plasma concentration *5684* Coadministration of ketoconazole with cisapride caused significant increase in terfenadine concentration due to inhibition of cytochrome P450IIIA4 in the liver *729* Ketoconazole inhibits the metabolism of cisapride increasing its plasma concentration *2905* By inhibiting cytochrome P450 3A4 inhibits metabolism of cisapride and increases its plasma concentration *2903* Coadministration of ketoconazole with cisapride caused increases in the concentration of cisapride *2902*

Corticotropin *Plasma Increase Physiological* In 37 women with polycystic ovary disease treatment with 200 mg/12 h for 9 months caused increase from mean baseline of 16.3 ± 1.9 ng/L to 41.7 ± 8.1 ng/L after 3 months (significant) and 32.8 ± 6.8 ng/L after 9 months (nonsignificant) *6255*

Cortisol *Plasma Decrease Physiological* Marked reduction of mean 24-hour concentration observed in 3 patients with Cushing's disease without expected rise of ACTH *5988* Significant reduction in patients receiving 800 mg or more daily *4744* In critically ill patients relative hypoadrenalism observed with ketoconazole therapy because of its effect on cortisol synthesis *3381*

Plasma No Effect Physiological No blunting of basal or GnRH-stimulated concentration observed in 9 hirsute women treated with 600 mg/d for 6 months *80* No significant change observed in 7 hirsute women treated with 200 mg/12 h p.o. for 6 months. No change observed in cortisol increment after ACTH *1107* Observed in 2 h after single 200 mg dose in normal men *5701* No significant effect observed of 6 oral doses of 300 mg in either 12 normotensive or 12 hypertensive men *2758*

Urine Decrease Physiological In 5 of 6 patients with Cushing's Disease treatment with 800 mg daily caused excretion to fall to within normal range but evidence of drug toxicity developed in 4 of them as demonstrated by reversible hepatotoxicity *3871* Blocks adrenal response to corticotropin and related to serum concentration of drug *4744* Significant reduction in 6 patients receiving 1.2 g daily for prostatic cancer, also blunted plasma cortisol response to Synacthen *6424*

Cortisol, Free *Plasma No Effect Physiological* In 37 women with polycystic ovary disease treatment with 200 mg/12 h for 9 months caused no significant change from mean baseline of 0.52 ± 0.03 μmol/L to 0.54 ± 0.0 μmol/L after 3 months and 0.53 ± 0.05 μmol/L after 9 months *6255*

Urine Decrease Physiological Approximate 50% reduction in patients receiving 800 mg daily *4744*

Creatinine Clearance *Urine Decrease Physiological* In one patient with sarcoidosis treatment with 800 mg/d for 6 days caused decrease from 79 mL/min to 42 mL/min. In a second patient decrease was from 59 mL/min to 27 mL/min with 800 mg/d for 4 days *2147*

Cyclosporine *Blood Increase Physiological* Inhibits function of cytochrome P-450 hepatic enzymes inhibiting clearance of cyclosporine *1835* Coadministration may cause dramatic increase in cyclosporine concentration allowing potential dose reduction of nearly 80%. Ketoconazole acts by inhibiting CYP or other hepatic enzymes *859*

Blood No Effect Analytical At a concentration of 70 mg/L had no effect on Syva EMIT method *495*

Serum Increase Physiological In 3 renal transplant patients and 6 marrow transplant recipients as well as 3 cardiac transplant recipients cyclosporine concentration increased probably due to inhibitory effect on microsomal enzyme activity *6595* Effect observed in one patient possibly related to decreased hepatic metabolism but mechanism not yet fully established *1835* Coadministration may cause dramatic increase in cyclosporine concentration allowing potential dose reduction of nearly 80%. Ketoconazole acts by inhibiting CYP or other hepatic enzymes *859* Prolongs half-life, probably by competing for metabolizing enzymes *6422* May increase cyclosporine concentration by inhibiting hepatic cytochrome P-450 III A which metabolizes cyclosporine *5236*

Cyclosporine A *Blood Increase Physiological* Coadministration with cyclosporine A increases its concentration *5240*

Coadministration of ketoconazole with cyclosporine caused increases in the concentration of cyclosporine *2902*
Serum Increase Physiological Coadministration of ketoconazole or other CYP3A4 inhibitors with cyclosporine to transplant recipients been demonstrated to increase the plasma concentration of cyclosporine so that its dosage may be reduced *3909*

Dehydroepiandrosterone Sulfate
Plasma Decrease Physiological Significant reduction from mean baseline concentration of 2.82 µg/mL to 2.05 µg/mL at 2 months in 7 hirsute women treated with 200 mg/12 h p.o. but reduction at 6 months not significant *1107* In 37 women with polycystic ovary disease treatment with 200 mg/12 h for 9 months caused decrease from mean baseline of 8.3 ± 0.8 µmol/L to 6.4 ± 0.8 µmol/L after 3 months (nonsignificant) and 5.1 ± 0.6 µmol/L after 9 months (significant) *6255* Reduction from mean baseline of 11.2 nmol/L to 7.1 nmol/L in 12 male normotensives after 6 doses of 300 mg orally but only from 3.08 nmol/L to 2.31 nmol/L in 12 hypertensives *2758* Decrease from mean baseline of 444.95 mg/L to 365.18 mg/L in 9 hyperandrogenic women treated with 400 mg/d for 10 days and from 443.00 mg/L to 280.82 mg/L in another 9 treated with 800 mg/d for 10 days *933* Significant reduction observed in 9 hirsute women treated 600 mg/d for 6 months *80*

11-Deoxycortisol *Plasma Increase Physiological* Significant increase observed following 6 oral doses of 300 mg in 12 normotensive men (from mean baseline of 8.42 nmol/L to 34.4 nmol/L) and in 12 hypertensive men (from mean baseline of 30.8 nmol/L to 149.1 nmol/L) *2758*

Didanosine *Serum No Effect Physiological* No significant effect observed on the concentration of either drug when two drugs coadministered *730*

Digoxin *Serum Increase Physiological* Coadministration of ketoconazole with digoxin caused rare increases in the concentration of digoxin *2902*

1,25-Dihydroxy Vitamin D *Serum Decrease Physiological* In one patient with sarcoidosis and hypercalcemia 800 mg/day orally decreased serum concentration of 1,25-dihydroxyvitamin D by 73% within 4 days. Effect probably due to direct action on enzymatic synthesis of 1,25-dihydroxyvitamin D *48* In one patient with sarcoidosis treatment with 600 mg/d for 6 days caused significant decrease from 336 pmol/L to 129 pmol/L. In a second patient 800 mg/d for 4 days caused reduction from 154 pmol/L to 102 pmol/L *2147*

1,25-Dihydroxy Vitamin D_3 *Serum Decrease Physiological* Effect observed with treatment in two patients with sarcoidosis-associated hypercalcemia *48* Dose dependent effect after administration to normal volunteers *5701* Observed in normal subjects, also observed in patients with primary hyperparathyroidism *2149* In 9 healthy men given up to 1200 mg/d for 1 week *2148*

Donepezil *Serum Increase Physiological* Ketoconazole inhibits CYP450 3A4 inhibiting donepezil metabolism in vitro although in vivo inhibition has not yet been demostrated *0*

Estradiol *Plasma Decrease Physiological* In 12 hypertensive men 300 mg orally for 6 doses caused reduction from mean baseline concentration of 104 pmol/L to 57 pmol/L *2758* Mild effect in 4 volunteer males with 600 mg doses. Bound and free ratio unchanged in 5 males receiving high doses for long time effect variable but estradiol testosterone ratio persistently increased *4743*
Plasma Increase Physiological Increase from mean baseline of 44.93 ng/L to 99.80 ng/L in 9 hyperandrogenic women treated with 400 mg/d for 10 days and from 42.46 ng/L to 94.05 ng/L in another 9 treated with 800 mg/d for 10 days *933* In 12 normotensive men 300 mg orally for 6 doses caused increase from mean baseline concentration of 79 pmol/L to 160 pmol/L *2758* In 37 women with polycystic ovary disease treatment with 200 mg/12 h for 9 months caused significant increase from mean baseline of 139 ± 10.6 pmol/L to 244 ± 34 pmol/L after 3 months and 277 ± 23 pmol/L after 9 months *6255* Effect observed in hyperandrogenic women with treatment *933*
Plasma No Effect Physiological No significant change observed in 7 hirsute women treated with 200 mg/12 h p.o. for 6 months *1107* In men with prostatic cancer with 400 mg every 8 h and prolonged treatment *5701* No significant effect observed in 9 hirsute women treated with 600 mg/d for 6 months although estradiol:testosterone ratio significantly higher because of reduction in testosterone concentration *80*

Estrone *Plasma Decrease Physiological* 6 doses of 300 mg caused reduction from mean baseline concentration of 283 pmol/L to 162 pmol/L in 12 hypertensive men *2758*
Plasma Increase Physiological 6 doses of 300 mg caused increase from mean baseline concentration of 87 pmol/L to 105 pmol/L in 12 normotensive men *2758*

Fexofenadine *Serum Increase Physiological* Coadministration of ketoconazole 400 mg once daily with 7 days of fexofenadine 120 mg every 12 hours (twice recommended dose) caused an 135% increase in concentration and 164% increase in area under time-concentration curve *2637*

Follicle Stimulating Hormone
Plasma Increase Physiological Increase by 63% approximately in normal men with dose effect maximal at 900 mg/d. Due to stimulatory effect of dose dependent fall of testosterone *2146*
Plasma No Effect Physiological No significant change observed in 7 hirsute women treated with 200 mg/12 h p.o. for 6 months *1107*

HDL-Cholesterol *Serum Decrease Physiological* In 7 patients with heterozygous familial hypercholesterolemia and 3 with primary hypercholesterolemia treatment with 400 mg/d for 3 weeks caused nonsignificant reduction from 1.25 ± 0.07 mmol/L to 1.16 ± 0.04 mmol/L *2383*
Serum Increase Physiological Increase from mean of 42 mg/dL to 48 mg/dL in 9 hyperandrogenic women treated with 800 mg/d for 10 days but insignificant reduction from mean of 50 mg/dL to 49 mg/dL in another 9 treated with 400 mg/d for 10 days *933*
Serum No Effect Physiological No significant change observed in 9 women with xanthomatous familial hypercholesterolemia treated with 400 mg/d nor when combined with 12 g/d cholestyramine *2384* No effect of treatment in hyperandrogenic women *933*

HDL-Triglycerides *Serum No Effect Physiological* In 7 patients with heterozygous familial hypercholesterolemia and 3 with primary hypercholesterolemia treatment with 400 mg/d for 3 weeks caused insignificant reduction from mean 0.17 ± 0.03 mmol/L to 0.14 ± 0.01 mmol/L *2383*

Histamine *Plasma No Effect Analytical* Moderate inhibition of radio-enzyme assay at 20 times therapeutic concentration *2492*

25-Hydroxy Vitamin D_3 *Serum No Effect Physiological* No effect in patients with primary hyperparathyroidism and hypercalcemia *2149* After administration to normal volunteers *5701* In 9 healthy men given up to 1200 mg/d for 1 week *2148*

25-Hydroxy Vitamin D *Serum Decrease Physiological* In one patient with sarcoidosis treatment with 800 mg/d for 6 days caused nonsignificant reduction from 50 mmol/L to 43 mmol/L. In a second patient treatment with 800 mg/d for 4 days caused decrease from 55 mmol/L to 41 mmol/L *2147*

17-Hydroxyprogesterone *Plasma Increase Physiological* Significant increase from mean baseline concentration of 17α-hydroxyprogesterone of 0.60 ng/mL to 1.85 ng/mL after 2 months and 1.39 ng/mL after 6 months in 7 hirsute women when treated with 200 mg/12 h p.o *1107* Observed in normal men due to blockade of 17,20-desmolase by drug, with inconsistent effect on serum estradiol *2146* Both basal and GnRH-stimulated concentration significantly increased in 9 hirsute women treated with 600 mg/d for 6 months *80* 6 oral doses of 300 mg were followed by an increase in mean concentration of 17α-hydroxyprogesterone concentration from baseline of 3.15 nmol/L to 8.80 nmol/L in 12 normotensive men and from 2.14 nmol/L to 4.70 nmol/L in 12 hypertensive men *2758* In 37 women with polycystic ovary disease treatment with 200 mg/12 h for 9 months caused significant increase from mean baseline of 4.2 ± 0.3 nmol/L to 8.4 ± 0.9 nmol/L after 3 months and 8.1 ± 0.9 nmol/L after 9 months *6255*

17α-Hydroxyprogesterone *Plasma Increase Physiological* Significant increase from mean baseline of 0.60 ng/mL to 1.85 ng/mL after 2 months and 1.39 ng/mL after 6 months in 7 hirsute women when treated with 200 mg/12 h p.o *1107* 6 oral doses of 300 mg were followed by an increase in mean concentration from baseline of 3.15 nmol/L to 8.80 nmol/L in 12 normotensive men and from 2.14 nmol/L to 4.70 nmol/L in 12 hypertensive men *2758*

Ketoconazole *(continued)*

IDL-Cholesterol *Serum Decrease Physiological* In 7 patients with heterozygous familial hypercholesterolemia and 3 patients with primary hypercholesterolemia treatment with 400 mg/d for 3 weeks caused significant decrease from 0.41 ± 0.08 mmol/L to 0.30 ± 0.04 mmol/L *2383*

IDL-Triglycerides *Serum No Effect Physiological* In 7 patients with heterozygous familial hypercholesterolemia and 3 with primary hypercholesterolemia treatment with 400 mg/d for 3 weeks caused nonsignificant reduction from 0.10 ± 0.01 mmol/L to 0.09 ± 0.01 mmol/L *2383*

Indinavir *Serum Increase Physiological* Causes a 62% increase in area under the concentration curve when ketoconazole coadministered *1891* Administration of indinavir 400 mg with ketoconazole 400 mg resulted in a 68 ± 48% increase in indinavir AUC *3966*

ionized Calcium *Serum No Effect Physiological* In one patient with sarcoidosis treatment with 800 mg/d for 6 days caused insigniicant change from 1.91 mmol/L to 1.97 mmol/L. In a second after 800 mg/d for 4 days insignificant change from 1.56 mmol/L to 1.49 mmol/L *2147* No effect observed in patients with primary hyperparathyroidism although total calcium reduced *2149*

Lanosterol *Serum Increase Physiological* Increase occurs because of inhibition of conversion of lanosterol to cholesterol *1384*

LDL-Apolipoprotein B *Serum Decrease Physiological* Treatment with 400 mg/d for 3 weeks caused reduction of 21% in 7 patients with heterozygous familial hypercholesterolemia and by 28% in 3 patients with primary hypercholesterolemia *2383*

LDL-Cholesterol *Serum Decrease Physiological* In 7 patients with heterozygous familial hypercholesterolemia and 3 with primary hypercholesterolemia treatment with 400 mg/d for 3 weeks caused significant decrease from mean 7.10 ± 0.81 mmol/L to 5.05 ± 0.51 mmol/L *2383* Reduction of plasma cholesterol in patients treated with ketoconazole almost entirely due to reduction of LDL-cholesterol *1384* Reduction from mean baseline of 96 mg/dL to 57 mg/dL in 9 hyperandrogenic women treated with 400 mg/d for 10 days and from 114 mg/dL to 72 mg/dL in another 9 treated with 800 mg/d for 10 days *933* Effect observed with treatment in hyperandrogenic women *933* Mean reduction of 22% observed in 9 women with xanthomatous familial hypercholesterolemia treated with 400 mg/d *2384*

LDL-Triglycerides *Serum No Effect Physiological* In 7 patients with heterozygous familial hypercholesterolemia and 3 with primary hypercholesterolemia treatment with 400 mg/d for 3 weeks caused insignificant reduction from 0.36 ± 0.04 mmol/L to 0.33 ± 0.03 mmol/L *2383*

Loratadine *Serum Increase Physiological* With coadministration increased plasma concentrations (24 hour AUC) of loratidine (307%) and descarboethoxyloratidine (73%) observed in normal volunteers but without clinical effects *5327* Coadministration of oral ketoconazole 200 mg b.i.d. with one 20 mg dose of loratadine in 11 individuals the AUC and maximum concentration of loratadine averaged 302 ± 142% and 251 ± 68% of those obtained after placebo. The concentration of its main metabolite was also substantially increased *2902*

Luteinizing Hormone *Plasma Decrease Physiological* In 37 women with polycystic ovary disease treatment with 200 mg/12 h for 9 months caused significant decrease from mean baseline of 12.4 ± 0.6 IU/L to 9.6 ± 1.9 IU/L after 9 months *6255*

Plasma Increase Physiological Increase by 127% approximately in normal men with dose effect maximal at 900 mg/d. Due to stimulatory effect of dose dependent fall of testosterone *2146*

Plasma No Effect Physiological No significant change observed in 7 hirsute women treated with 200 mg/12 h p.o. for 6 months *1107* In 37 women with polycystic ovary disease treatment with 200 mg/12 h for 9 months caused nonsignificant increase from mean baseline of 12.4 ± 0.6 IU/L to 13.5 ± 1.5 IU/L after 3 months *6255*

Methylprednisolone *Serum Increase Physiological* Coadministration of ketoconazole with methylprednisolone caused increases in the concentration of methylprednisolone *2902*

Midazolam *Serum Increase Physiological* By inhibiting cytochrome P450 3A4 may reduce plasma clearance of midazolam when drugs coadministered *5037* Coadministration of ketoconazole with midazolam caused increases in the concentration of midazolam *2902*

Nelfinavir *Serum Increase Physiological* Causes a 35% increase in area under the concentration curve when ketoconazole coadministered *1891* Coadministration of ketoconazole with nelfinavir caused a 35% increase in AUC of nelfinavir, but not considered significantly large to warrant changing dose of nelfinavir *66*

Osmolality *Serum Decrease Physiological* To 248 mosmol/kg in 73 year old man with prostatic cancer treated with 600 mg daily for 2.5 mo *4706*

Parathyroid Hormone *Plasma Increase Physiological* In one patient with sarcoidosis treatment with 800 mg/d for 6 days caused increase from 0.42 pmol/L to 0.53 pmol/L. In a second patient concentration increased from 4.7 pmol/L to 6.1 pmol/L after 800 mg/d for 4 days *2147*

Plasma No Effect Physiological No effect in patients with primary hyperparathyroidism with hypercalcemia *2149* After administration to normal volunteers *5701* In 9 healthy men given up to 1200 mg/d for 1 week *2148*

Phenytoin *Serum Decrease Physiological* Due to stimulated drug metabolism *1384*

Phosphate *Serum No Effect Physiological* No effect in patients with primary hyperparathyroidism and hypercalcemia *2149* In 9 healthy men given up to 1200 mg/d for 1 week *2148*

Potassium *Serum Increase Physiological* In 3 patients with primary hyperaldosteronism treatment caused considerable change starting within one week *3451*

Urine Decrease Physiological In 3 patients with primary hyperaldosteronism reduction began within one week of beginning treatment *3451*

Prednisolone *Serum No Effect Physiological* No significant effect observed with coadministration on prednisolone clearance, mean residence time, volume of distribution or plasma protein binding *6586*

Progesterone *Plasma Increase Physiological* In men with prostatic cancer with 400 mg every 8 h and prolonged treatment *5701*

Prolactin *Plasma No Effect Physiological* In men with prostatic cancer with 400 mg every 8 h and prolonged treatment *5701*

Prothrombin Time *Plasma Increase Physiological* Coadministration of ketoconazole with coumarin-type anticoagulants caused increases in the prothrombin time *2902* Effect observed in some patients receiving coumarin derivatives *1384* Rapidly developing liver failure in 67 year old woman taking 200 mg drug daily for 2 mo *1604* Probable interaction with warfarin when drugs coadministered *2625*

Quinidine *Serum Decrease Physiological* Hepatic elimination of quinidine accelerated when ketoconazole coadministered probably because of competition for cytochrome P450IIIA4 metabolic pathway *5996*

Rifampin *Serum Decrease Physiological* When rifampin is taken with ketoconazole both the rifampin and ketoconazole concentrations may decrease due to augmented hepatic metabolism *2652* Increased metabolism of ketoconazole and decreased serum concentration of rifampin *886* Due to stimulated hepatic metabolism *1384*

Saquinavir *Serum Increase Physiological* Coadministration of saquinavir 600 mg t.i.d. with ketoconazole 200 mg q.d. to 12 healthy volunteers produced 3-fold increase of AUC and maximum concentration compared when saquinavir was given alone *5024* Increases the area under the concentration curve by 300% when ketoconazole coadministered *1891*

Sex-Hormone Binding Globulin

Serum Increase Physiological In 37 women with polycystic ovary disease treatment with 200 mg/12 h for 9 months caused nonsignificant increase from mean baseline of 26.6 ± 3.5 nmol/L to 32.3 ± 3.4 μmol/L after 3 months and 41.4 ± 2.9 nmol/L after 9 months *6255*

Serum No Effect Physiological No significant change observed in 7 hirsute women treated with 200 mg/12 h p.o. for 6 months *1107*

Sibutramine *Serum Increase Physiological* Concomitant administration of 200 mg ketoconazole b.i.d. with 20 mg sibutramine per day for 7 days to 12 obese but otherwise healthy individuals caused increases of AUC and concentration of metabolite M_1 of 58% and 36% respectively and of concentration of M_2 of 20% and 19% respectively *3203*

Sildenafil *Serum Increase Physiological* Theoretical effect: drug likely to increase area under concentration curve of sildenafil due to CYP3A4 inhibition *4657*

Sodium *Serum Decrease Physiological* To 121 mmol/L in 73 year old man with prostatic cancer treated with 600 mg daily for 2.5 mo *4706*

Sperm Count *Semen Decrease Physiological* With prolonged treatment with 800-1200 mg/d *5701* Azospermia common in patients receiving drug *4744*

Tacrolimus *Serum Increase Analytical* In HPLC/MS method of Christians et al interference observed with measurement of FK 506 because of similar retention time *1010*
Serum Increase Physiological By inhibiting cytochrome P-450 IIIA enzyme systems may inhibit the metabolism of tacrolimus *1987* Coadministration of ketoconazole with tacrolimus caused increases in the concentration of tacrolimus *2902*

Terfenadine *Serum Increase Physiological* Coadministration of ketoconazole with terfenadine caused significant increase in terfenadine concentration due to inhibition of cytochrome P450IIIA4 in the liver *729* In 6 healthy volunteers taking terfenadine 60 mg/12 h for 7 days, daily concomitant administration of oral ketoconazole, 200 mg/12 h, caused significant increase in area under the the curve of the acid metabolite of tefenadine *2700* Through inhibition of cytochrome P450IIIA4, ketoconazole blocks the metabolism of terfenadine leading to a higher plasma concentration *5684* Coadministration of ketoconazole with terfenadine caused increases in the concentration of terfenadine *2902* Ketoconazole markedly inhibits the metabolism of terfenadine *2653*

Testosterone *Serum Decrease Physiological* Significant reduction observed in 9 hirsute women treated with 600 mg/d for 6 months *80* Transiently blocks testosterone synthesis. Doses above 800 mg/d may cause more prolonged blockade *4744* In 37 women with polycystic ovary disease treatment with 200 mg/12 h for 9 months caused decrease from mean baseline of 2.7 ± 0.2 nmol/L to 2.0 ± 0.1 nmol/L after 3 months (nonsignificant) and 1.7 ± 0.2 nmol/L after 9 months (significant) *6255* When 300 mg administered for six doses to 12 normal men mean reduction from baseline of 19.6 nmol/L to 4.7 nmol/L and in 12 hypertensives from 11.8 nmol/L to 2.1 nmol/L. Similar change observed when transdermal patch with estradiol used at same time *2758* Significant reduction from mean baseline of 56.42 ng/dL to 33.57 ng/dL at 2 months and 32 ng/dL at 6 months in 7 hirsute women treated with 200 mg/12 h p.o *1107* Marked effect in 4 volunteer males with 600 mg doses. With long term high dose treatment same effect observed *4743*

Testosterone, Free *Serum Decrease Physiological* Observed in 2 h after single 200 mg dose in normal men *5701* Equally reduced with bound testosterone *4744* Significant reduction from mean baseline concentration of 0.67 nmol/L to 0.14 nmol/L in 12 normotensive men given 300 mg orally for 6 doses and from 0.31 nmol/L to 0.06 nmol/L in 12 hypertensive men *2758* Reduction from mean baseline of 12.15 ng/L to 6.38 ng/L in 9 hyperandrogenic women treated with 400 mg/d for 10 days and from 14.91 ng/L to 4.33 ng/L in another 9 treated with 800 mg/d for 10 days *933*

Testosterone Index, Free *Serum Decrease Physiological* In 37 women with polycystic ovary disease treatment with 200 mg/12 h for 9 months caused decrease from mean baseline of 4.4 ± 0.6 to 2.8 ± 0.1 after 3 months (nonsignificant) and 1.5 ± 0.4 after 9 months (significant) *6255*

Theophylline *Serum Increase Physiological* Reduced clearance reported when drugs coadministered *1384*
Serum No Effect Physiological No documented significant interaction with theophylline reported *6117* No clinically significant effect on theophylline concentration observed when drugs coadministered *5999*

Thyroxine (T4) *Serum Decrease Physiological* Hypothyroidism may occur as a result of a genetic determined influence *1384*

Tolbutamide *Serum Increase Physiological* In 7 healthy volunteers treatment with for 1 week with 200 mg oral ketoconazole caused elimination half-life from mean of 3.7 ± 0.4 h to 12.3 ± 1.9 h and area under the curve (0.12 h) of tolbutamide from 309 ± 27 μg/mL/h to 546 ± 20 μ.g/mL/h *3289*

Triazolam *Serum Increase Physiological* Coadministration of ketoconazole with triazolam caused increases in the concentration of trirazolam *2902*

Triglycerides *Serum Decrease Physiological* Reduction from mean of 92 mg/dL to 84 mg/dL in 9 hyperandrogenic women treated with 400 mg/d for 10 days and from 133 mg/dL to 112 mg/dL in another 9 treated with 800 mg/d for 10 days *933*
Serum No Effect Physiological No significant change observed in 9 women with xanthomatous familial hypercholesterolemia treated with 400 mg/d or when combined with 12 g/d cholestyramine *2384* In 7 patients with heterozygous familial hypercholesterolemia and 3 with primary hypercholesterolemia treatment with 400 mg/d for 3 weeks caused nonsignificant reduction from 1.63 ± 0.22 mmol/L to 1.55 ± 0.19 mmol/L *2383*

VLDL-Cholesterol *Serum No Effect Physiological* In 7 patients with heterozygous familial hypercholesterolemia and 3 patients with primary hypercholesterolemia treatment with 400 mg/d for 3 weeks caused nonsignificant increase from 0.50 ± 0.08 mmol/L to 0.52 ± 0.09 mmol/L *2383* No significant effect observed in 9 women with xanthomatous familial hypercholesterolemia treated with 400 mg/d or when combined with 12 g/d cholestyramine *2384*

VLDL-Triglycerides *Serum No Effect Physiological* In 7 patients with heterozygous familial hypercholesterolemia and 3 with primary hypercholesterolemia treatment with 400 mg/d for 3 weeks had no effect on basal concentration of 0.92 ± 0.18 mmol/L *2383*

Zidovudine *Serum No Effect Analytical* No effect on liquid chromatographic method of Hedaya and Sawchuk *2525*

Ketoprofen

Acetylsalicylic Acid *Serum No Effect Physiological* Ketoprofen has no effect on aspirin absorption *6564*

Alanine Aminotransferase *Serum Decrease Analytical* On continuous method *2919*
Serum Increase Physiological Incidence of acute liver injury of 8.8 per 100,000 treated patients with reported in United Kingdom. Liver damage among all cases primarily hepatocellular in some and primarily cholestatic in others *5049* Ketoprofen may cause hepatic dysfunction in fewer than 1% treated patients *6564*
Serum No Effect Analytical On colorimetric method at 10 times maximal therapeutic concentration *2919*

Albumin *Serum No Effect Analytical* At concentration of 60 mg/L had no effect on BCG method *5704* On bromocresol green method on Technicon SMA II at physiological concentration *2922*
Serum No Effect Physiological No effect seen in patients undergoing treatment *2922*
Urine No Effect Analytical Using a fluorimetric assay with Albumin Blue 580 on a Cobas Fara centrifugal analyzer for the detection of microalbuminuria no significant interference was detected at a concentration of 40 mg/L *3117*

Alkaline Phosphatase *Serum Increase Physiological* Ketoprofen may cause hepatic dysfunction in fewer than 1% treated patients *6564*
Serum No Effect Analytical On continuous method at 10 times maximal therapeutic concentration *2919*

Aspartate Aminotransferase *Serum Decrease Analytical* On continuous method *2919*
Serum Increase Physiological Ketoprofen may cause hepatic dysfunction in fewer than 1% treated patients *6564* Incidence of acute liver injury of 8.8 per 100,000 treated patients with reported in United Kingdom. Liver damage among all cases primarily hepatocellular in some and primarily cholestatic in others *5049*
Serum No Effect Analytical On colorimetric method at 10 times maximal therapeutic concentration *2919*

Bilirubin *Serum Increase Physiological* Ketoprofen may cause hepatic dysfunction in fewer than 1% treated patients *6564*

Ketoprofen *(continued)*

Bilirubin *(continued)*
Serum No Effect Analytical At concentration of 60 mg/L had no effect on Jendrassik and Grof method *5704* On diazo method on Technicon SMA II at physiological concentration *2922* No effect at therapeutic concentrations on Jendrassik-Grof, dimethylsulfoxide and spectrophotometric methods *2920*
Serum No Effect Physiological No effect seen in patients undergoing treatment *2922*

Bleeding Time *Patient No Effect Physiological* In acute studies but prolonged in subacute in 11 patients given drug intravenously *2019*

Blood *Urine Increase Physiological* Ketoprofen may cause hematuria and renal failure, interstitial nephritis or nephrotic syndrome in fewer than 1% treated patients *6564*

Calcium *Serum No Effect Analytical* At concentration of 60 mg/L had no effect on cresolphthalein method *5704* On cresolphthalein complexone method on Technicon SMA II at physiological concentration *2922*
Serum No Effect Physiological No effect seen in patients undergoing treatment *2922*

Chloride *Serum Decrease Physiological* When coadministered with hydrochlorothiazide, ketoprofen produces a reduction in excretion compared with hydrochlorothiazide alone *6564*

Cholesterol *Serum No Effect Analytical* At concentration of 60 mg/L had no effect on Liebermann-Burchard method *5704* No effect on Liebermann-Burchard and enzymatic methods at therapeutic concentrations *2920* On enzymatic method on Technicon SMA II at physiological concentration *2922*
Serum No Effect Physiological No effect seen in patients undergoing treatment *2922*

Chondrex *Serum No Effect Analytical* Concentrations up to 1 g/L had no significant effect on sandwich-type ELISA procedure of Harvey et al *2491*

Creatine Kinase *Serum No Effect Analytical* On continuous method at 10 times maximal therapeutic concentration *2919*

Creatinine *Serum Increase Physiological* Case reported of irreversible renal failure following 10 days treatment with drug *4571* Ketoprofen may cause renal failure, interstitial nephritis or nephrotic syndrome in fewer than 1% treated patients *6564*
Serum No Effect Analytical On alkaline picrate method on Technicon SMA II at physiological concentration *2922* No effect at therapeutic concentrations on alkaline picrate and Slot methods *2920* At concentration of 60 mg/L had no effect on Technicon AutoAnalyzer® Jaffe method *5704*
Serum No Effect Physiological No effect seen in patients undergoing treatment *2922*
Urine Decrease Physiological Excretion reduced without concomitant increase in serum concentration in 6 healthy men given 200 mg daily for 3 days suggesting diminished tubular secretion *6190*

Digoxin *Serum No Effect Physiological* When coadministered with digoxin, ketoprofen produces no effect on the digoxin concentration *6564*

Effective Renal Plasma Flow
Patient No Effect Physiological No significant effect observed in 6 healthy male volunteers given 200 mg daily for 3 days *6190*

Glomerular Filtration Rate *Urine No Effect Physiological* No significant effect observed in 6 healthy male volunteers given 200 mg daily for 3 days with and without a low sodium diet *6190*

Glucose *Serum Increase Physiological* Ketoprofen may aggravate diabetes mellitus in fewer than 1% treated patients *6564*
Serum No Effect Analytical On hexokinase method on Technicon SMA II at physiological concentration *2922* No effect at therapeutic concentrations on hexokinase, glucose dehydrogenase 2,4-dichlorophenol, ABTS and o-toluidine methods *2920*
Serum No Effect Physiological No effect seen in patients undergoing treatment *2922*

γ-Glutamyltransferase *Serum Increase Physiological* Ketoprofen may cause hepatic dysfunction in fewer than 1% treated patients *6564*

Granulocytes *Blood Decrease Physiological* Ketoprofen may cause agranulocytosis in fewer than 1% treated patients *6564*

Hematocrit *Blood Decrease Physiological* Ketoprofen may cause anemia in fewer than 1% treated patients *6564*

Hemoglobin *Blood Decrease Physiological* Ketoprofen may cause anemia in fewer than 1% treated patients *6564*

Hydroxybutyrate Dehydrogenase
Serum No Effect Analytical On continuous method at 10 times maximal therapeutic concentration *2919*

Iron *Serum No Effect Analytical* No effect at therapeutic concentrations on Ramsay and bathophenanthroline methods *2920* At concentration of 60 mg/L had no effect on Ferrozine method *5704* On Ferrozine method on Technicon SMA II at physiological concentration *2922*
Serum No Effect Physiological No effect seen in patients undergoing treatment *2922*

Lactate Dehydrogenase *Serum Decrease Analytical* With lactate as substrate on continuous method. Marked effect on colorimetric method at 10 times maximal therapeutic concentration *2919*
Serum No Effect Analytical With pyruvate as substrate on continuous method *2919*

Lithium *Serum Increase Physiological* Single case report of lithium toxicity in one patient who had ingested 400 mg/d of ketoprofen *4831* When coadministered with lithium, ketoprofen may increase the steady-state concentration of lithium *6564*

Methotrexate *Serum Increase Physiological* When coadministered with methotrexate, ketoprofen may increase the plasma concentration of methotrexate and induce toxicity *6564* Concomitant administration caused severe methotrexate toxicity when high dose of methotrexate given *1384*

Occult Blood *Feces Increase Physiological* Gastrointestinal irritation is probably major side effect as reported to UK Committee on Safety of Medicines *1204* Ketoprofen may cause melena or rectal hemorrhage in fewer than 1% treated patients *6564*

Partial Thromboplastin Time
Plasma No Effect Physiological In 11 patients given drug intravenously *2019*

Phosphate *Serum No Effect Analytical* At concentration of 60 mg/L had no effect on phosphomolybdate method *5704*

Platelet Aggregation *Blood Decrease Physiological* In 11 patients given drug intravenously *2019* Administration to healthy women of 3 x 25 mg/d or 3 x 50 mg/d caused 57% and 85% reduction respectively in arachidonic acid induced platelet aggregation compared with controls *5826*

Platelets *Blood Decrease Physiological* Ketoprofen may cause purpura or thrombocytopenia in fewer than 1% treated patients *6564*

Potassium *Serum Decrease Physiological* When coadministered with hydrochlorothiazide, ketoprofen produces a reduction in excretion compared with hydrochlorothiazide alone *6564*

Prostaglandin E-M *Urine Decrease Physiological* Administration to healthy women of 3 x 25 mg/d caused a 39% reduction in 24-hour excretion *5826*

Protein *Serum No Effect Analytical* No effect at therapeutic concentrations on biuret and spectrophotometric methods *2920* On biuret method on Technicon SMA II at physiological concentration *2922* At concentration of 60 mg/L had no effect on biuret method with blank correction *5704*
Serum No Effect Physiological No effect seen in patients undergoing treatment *2922*

Prothrombin Time *Plasma No Effect Physiological* In 11 patients given drug intravenously *2019* When coadministered with warfarin, ketoprofen produces no effect on the prothrombin time *6564*

Sodium *Serum Decrease Physiological* Ketoprofen may cause hyponatremia in fewer than 1% treated patients *6564*

Thromboxane B_2 Production
Plasma Decrease Physiological Administration to healthy women of 3 x 25 mg/d or 3 x 50 mg/d caused 72% and 97% reduction respectively in thromboxane B_2 synthesis *5826*

Thyroxine (T4) *Serum No Effect Analytical* Using the Ciba-Corning ACS:180 analyzer mean concentration not significantly changed in 1 specimen whose concentration differed by -1% compared with the concentration measured by the Amerlex-M method *5621*

Triglycerides *Serum No Effect Analytical* On enzymatic method on Technicon SMA II at physiological concentration *2922* No effect at therapeutic concentrations on enzymatic methods *2920*

Serum No Effect Physiological No effect seen in patients undergoing treatment *2922*

Urea Nitrogen *Serum Increase Physiological* Ketoprofen may impair renal function in 3 to 9% treated patients *6564* Case report of irreversible renal failure in a man given drug for 10 days *4571* Ketoprofen may cause renal failure, interstitial nephritis or nephrotic syndrome in fewer than 1% treated patients *6564*

Serum No Effect Analytical No effect at therapeutic concentrations on glutamate dehydrogenase, phenol- hypochlorite and diacetyl monoxime methods *2920* On diacetyl monoxime method on Technicon SMA II at physiological concentration *2922* At concentration of 60 mg/L had no effect on diacetylmonoxime method *5704*

Serum No Effect Physiological No effect seen in patients undergoing treatment *2922*

Uric Acid *Serum No Effect Analytical* On phosphotungstate method on Technicon SMA II at physiological concentration *2922* No effect at therapeutic concentrations on uricase-catalase, aldehyde dehydrogenase, direct UV-test and phosphotungstate methods *2920* At concentration of 60 mg/L had no effect on phosphotungstate reduction method *5704*

Serum No Effect Physiological No effect seen in patients undergoing treatment *2922*

Ketorolac

Alanine Aminotransferase *Serum Increase Physiological* In post-marketing studies ketorolac reported to cause hepatitis, liver failure or cholestatic jaundice *5035*

Alkaline Phosphatase *Serum Increase Physiological* In post-marketing studies ketorolac reported to cause hepatitis, liver failure or cholestatic jaundice *5035*

Aspartate Aminotransferase *Serum Increase Physiological* In post-marketing studies ketorolac reported to cause hepatitis, liver failure or cholestatic jaundice *5035*

Bilirubin *Serum Increase Physiological* In post-marketing studies ketorolac reported to cause hepatitis, liver failure or cholestatic jaundice *5035*

Bleeding Time *Patient Increase Physiological* Inhibits platelet aggregation and thromboxane production *1384*

Patient No Effect Physiological Ketorolac, when coadministered with heparin, had no effect on bleeding time *5035*

Blood *Urine Increase Physiological* Ketorolac reported to cause hematuria in fewer than 1% of all patients *5035*

Creatinine *Serum Increase Physiological* In 3 patients treated with ketorolac acute renal failure developed with hyperkalemia *2456* In post-marketing studies ketorolac reported to cause acute renal failure with/wiyhout hematuria and/or nephritis, hyponatremia, hyperkalemia or hemolytic uremia syndrome *5035*

Digoxin *Serum No Effect Physiological* Ketorolac has no significant effect on digoxin binding to plasma plasma proteins *5035*

Eosinophils *Blood Increase Physiological* Ketorolac reported to cause eosinophilia in fewer than 1% of all patients *5035*

Hematocrit *Blood Decrease Physiological* Ketorolac reported to cause anemia in fewer than 1% of all patients *5035*

Hemoglobin *Blood Decrease Physiological* Ketorolac reported to cause anemia in fewer than 1% of all patients *5035*

Lithium *Red Blood Cells Increase Physiological* Administration of 40 mg/d ketorolac to healthy volunteers receiving 900 mg/d lithium caused significant increase in serum lithium AUC (24%) and erythrocyte lithium AUC (27%) *1087*

Serum Increase Physiological In a few cases reports that when ketorolac is coadministered with lithium the clearance of lithium was reduced resulting in an increase in its plasma concentration *5035* Reported to increase concentration *3590* Administration of 40 mg/d ketorolac to healthy volunteers receiving 900 mg/d lithium caused significant increase in serum lithium AUC (24%) and erythrocyte lithium AUC (27%) *1087*

Lithium Clearance *Urine Decrease Physiological* In a few case reports, ketorolac, when coadministered with lithium, reduced the clearance of lithium resulting in an increase in its plasma concentration *5035*

Occult Blood *Feces Increase Physiological* Ketorolac reported to cause rectal bleeding in fewer than 1% of all patients *5035*

Partial Thromboplastin Time

Plasma No Effect Physiological Has no significant effect on partial thromboplastin time *1384*

Potassium *Serum Increase Physiological* In post-marketing studies ketorolac reported to cause acute renal failure with/without hematuria and/or nephritis, hyponatremia, hyperkalemia or hemolytic uremia syndrome *5035* In 3 patients treated with ketorolac acute renal failure developed with hyperkalemia *2456*

Protein *Urine Increase Physiological* Ketorolac reported to cause proteinuria in fewer than 1% of all patients *5035*

Prothrombin Time *Plasma No Effect Physiological* Has no significant effect on prothrombin time *1384*

Sodium *Serum Decrease Physiological* In post-marketing studies ketorolac reported to cause acute renal failure with/wiyhout hematuria and/or nephritis, hyponatremia, hyperkalemia or hemolytic uremia syndrome *5035*

Urine Decrease Physiological Ketorolac, when coadministered with furosemide, reduced the excretion of sodium and water induced by furosemide, by approximately 17% *5035*

Urea Nitrogen *Serum Increase Physiological* In 3 patients treated with ketorolac acute renal failure developed with hyperkalemia *2456* In post-marketing studies ketorolac reported to cause acute renal failure with/wiyhout hematuria and/or nephritis, hyponatremia, hyperkalemia or hemolytic uremia syndrome *5035*

Volume *Urine Decrease Physiological* Ketorolac, when coadministered with furosemide, reduced the excretion of sodium and water induced by furosemide, by approximately 17% *5035*

Warfarin *Plasma No Effect Physiological* Ketorolac has no significant effect on warfarin binding to plasma plasma proteins *5035*

3-Ketovalproic Acid

Valproic Acid *Serum No Effect Analytical* No significant interference observed at a concentration of 100 µg/mL (620 µmol/L) with method on Du Pont aca *1560*

L-α-Acetylmethadol

Luteinizing Hormone *Plasma No Effect Physiological* In 9 male heroin addicts maintained on drug and in 2 weeks following abrupt withdrawal *3952*

Methadone *Urine No Effect Analytical* Significant cross-reactivity of 50% observed with Roche Abuscreen ONTRAK method *3279*

Testosterone *Serum No Effect Physiological* In 9 male heroin addicts maintained on drug and in 2 weeks following abrupt withdrawal *3952*

Labetalol

Alanine Aminotransferase *Serum Increase Physiological* Hepatic necrosis, hepatitis, cholestatic jaundice and abnormal liver function tests have been reported as complications of treatment *5335* Hepatic necrosis, hepatitis or cholestatic jaundice may occur as a complication of treatment *2164* Rare cases of increased activity reported probably in association with cholestatsis *1384*

Aldosterone *Plasma Increase Physiological* In 8 patients administered labetolol plasma aldosterone changed significantly with 60 minutes middle ear surgery, although increased during recovery phase, as did controls *3844*

Labetalol *(continued)*

Aldosterone *(continued)*
Urine Decrease Physiological With treatment for 4 mo in 15 patients with essential hypertension variable effect observed *6376*
Urine Increase Physiological With treatment for 4 mo in 15 patients with essential hypertension variable effect observed *6376*
Urine No Effect Physiological With treatment for 4 mo in 15 patients with essential hypertension variable effect observed *6376*

Alkaline Phosphatase *Serum Increase Physiological* Hepatic necrosis, hepatitis or cholestatic jaundice may occur as a complication of treatment *2164* Hepatic necrosis, hepatitis, cholestatic jaundice and abnormal liver function tests have been reported as complications of treatment *5335*

Amphetamine *Urine Increase Analytical* May give false positive reaction with Toxi-Lab A® and EMIT-d.a.u.® method *5335*
Urine Positive Analytical At concentrations above 39 µmol/L (119 µmol/L) with method on Du Pont aca *1554*

Antimitochondrial Antibodies
Serum Increase Physiological Hepatic necrosis, hepatitis or cholestatic jaundice may occur as a complication of treatment *2164* Some patients have developed antimitochondrial antibodies in response to treatment *1384*

Antinuclear Antibodies *Serum Increase Physiological* In one patient previously treated with methyldopa and atenolol *2329*

Arginine Vasopressin *Plasma No Effect Physiological* In 8 patients administered labetolol plasma AVP changed insignificantly with 60 minutes middle ear surgery, although increased during recovery phase, as did controls *3844*

Aspartate Aminotransferase *Serum Increase Physiological* Hepatic necrosis, hepatitis or cholestatic jaundice may occur as a complication of treatment *2164* Hepatic necrosis, hepatitis, cholestatic jaundice and abnormal liver function tests have been reported as complications of treatment *5335* Rare increase of activity reported, possibly in association with cholestasis *1384*

Bilirubin *Serum Increase Physiological* Hepatic necrosis, hepatitis, cholestatic jaundice and abnormal liver function tests have been reported as complications of treatment *5335* Rare cholestasis reported *1384*

Catecholamines *Plasma No Effect Analytical* No effect on HPLC method of Koller for dopamine, epinephrine, and norepinephrine *3230*
Urine Decrease Analytical Using reversed-phase HPLC-ECD large peak occurs at about twice the retention time of internal standard dihydroxybenzylamine although problem can be avoided by use of a different internal standard *1257*
Urine Increase Analytical With fluorometric method of Crout et al *4018* Metabolites may give false positive reaction with some fluorometric or photometric methods leading to apparently increased excretion *5335*

Cholesterol *Serum No Effect Physiological* No significant effect in 20 hypertensive patients treated with up to 800 mg daily for 4 weeks *1808* In several studies from 1 to 12 mo *141* In 8 patients given 600-1200 mg daily for 4 mo *2953* No significant change in several studies with patients treated for 1-12 mo *142*

Corticotropin *Plasma No Effect Physiological* In 8 patients administered labetolol plasma cortiicotropin changed insignificantly with 60 minutes middle ear surgery, although increased during recovery phase, as did controls *3844*

Cortisol *Plasma Decrease Physiological* In 8 patients administered labetolol plasma cortisol changed significantly with 60 minutes middle ear surgery *3844*

C-Peptide *Plasma No Effect Physiological* In response to i.v. infusion of 100 mg over 10 minutes *367*

Creatine Kinase *Serum Increase Physiological* In 3 of 9 patients with essential hypertension. Note MM isoenzyme most affected *5275*

Creatinine *Serum Increase Physiological* Transient increases observed in 8 of 100 patients, associated with decreases in blood pressure *5335*
Serum No Effect Physiological No significant effect in 15 patients with essential hypertension treated for 1 mo *6376*

Dopamine *Urine No Effect Analytical* On HPLC method with electrochemical detection *669*

Drugs of Abuse Screen *Urine Increase Analytical* False positive result produced with Abbott ADx method for amphetamine/methamphetamine *4279*

Epinephrine *Plasma Increase Analytical* Elutes simultaneously with epinephrine with HPLC and electrochemical detection detection using method of Krstulovic et al *670*
Plasma No Effect Physiological No significant effect of acute i.v. administration (as measured by HPLC) *4949*
Urine Increase Analytical On HPLC method with electrochemical detection *669* Metabolites may give false positive reaction with some photometric or fluorometric methods leading to apparently increased excretion *5335*

Fatty Acids (FFA), Free *Serum No Effect Physiological* In response to i.v. infusion of 100 mg over 10 minutes *367*

Glucose *Serum Increase Physiological* Probably in response to norepinephrine release in response to i.v. infusion of 100 mg over 10 minutes *367*

γ-Glutamyltransferase *Serum Increase Physiological* Hepatic necrosis, hepatitis, cholestatic jaundice and abnormal liver function tests have been reported as complications of treatmen *5335*

Growth Hormone *Plasma No Effect Physiological* In response to i.v. infusion of 100 mg over 10 minutes *367*

HDL-Cholesterol *Serum No Effect Physiological* No significant change in 20 hypertensive patients treated with up to 800 mg daily for 4 weeks *1808* No significant change in several studies with patients treated for 1-12 mo *142* Although values reported from -12 to +23% in several studies from 1 to 12 mo *141*

Hematocrit *Blood No Effect Physiological* In 8 patients administered labetalol hematocrit changed insignificantly from 39% at induction to 35% at end of 60 minutes middle ear surgery, not significantly different from controls *3844*

High Density Lipoproteins *Serum Increase Physiological* In 15 patients with essential hypertension, also decreased total cholesterol: HDL ratio *6376*

LDL-Cholesterol *Serum No Effect Physiological* No significant change in several studies with patients treated for 1-12 mo *142* No significant effect in 20 hypertensive patients treated with up to 800 mg daily for 4 weeks *1808*

Leukocytes *Blood Decrease Physiological* In one patient previously treated with methyldopa and atenolol *2329*

Metanephrine *Urine Increase Analytical* Metabolites may give false positive reaction with some fluorometric or photometric methods leading to apparently increased excretion *5335*

Metanephrines, Total *Urine Increase Analytical* With photometric method of Pisano et al and method of Crout et al *4018* Especially when combined with other antihypertensive drugs and HPLC method unless toluene extraction used *1162*
Urine No Effect Analytical On method of Bigelow and Weil-Malherbe *4018*

Norepinephrine *Plasma Increase Physiological* In response to i.v. infusion of 100 mg over 10 minutes *367*
Plasma No Effect Physiological No significant effect of acute i.v. administration (as measured by HPLC) *4949*
Urine Increase Analytical Metabolites may give false positive reaction with some fluorometric or photometric methods leading to apparently increased excretion *5335*
Urine No Effect Analytical On HPLC method with electrochemical detection *669*

Normetanephrine *Urine Increase Analytical* Metabolites may give false positive reaction with some fluorometric or photometric methods leading to apparently increased excretion *5335*

Osmolality *Serum No Effect Physiological* In 8 patients administered labetolol serum osmolality changed insignificantly from 290 mosmol/kg at induction to 290 mosmol/kg at end of 60 minutes middle ear surgery, not significantly different from controls *3844*

pH *Blood No Effect Physiological* In 8 patients administered labetalol arterial pH changed insignificantly from 7.40 at induction to 7.43 at end of 60 minutes middle ear surgery not significantly different from controls *3844*

Platelet Aggregation *Blood No Effect Physiological* In 15 hypertensives treated with up to 600 mg/d for up to 8 weeks had no significant effect on collagen-induced platelet aggregation *3583* In 15 hypertensives treatment with up to 600 mg/d for up to 8 weeks had no significant effect on ADP-induced aggregation *3583* In 15 hypertensives treatment with up to 600 mg/d for up to 8 weeks had no significant effect on epinephrine-induced aggregation *3583*

Potassium *Serum Increase Physiological* Intravenous administration caused significant increase in three renal transplant recipients *255*

Prolactin *Plasma Increase Physiological* Marked in women,less so in men: possibly due to antidopaminergic effect of drug in response to i.v. infusion of 100 mg over 10 minutes *367*

Renin Activity *Plasma Decrease Physiological* With treatment for 4 mo in 15 patients with essential hypertension variable effect observed *6376*

Plasma Increase Physiological With treatment for 4 mo in 15 patients with essential hypertension variable effect observed *6376*

Plasma No Effect Physiological With treatment for 4 mo in 15 patients with essential hypertension variable effect observed *6376*

Triglycerides *Serum Increase Physiological* Increase by 27% in 8 patients given 600-1200 mg daily for 4 mo *2953*

Serum No Effect Physiological No significant change in several studies with patients treated for 1-12 mo *142* In several studies from 1 to 12 mo *141*

Urea Nitrogen *Serum Increase Physiological* Transient increases observed in 8 of 100 patients, associated with decreases in blood pressure *5335*

Serum No Effect Physiological No significant effect in 15 patients with essential hypertension treated for 1 mo *6376*

Vanillylmandelic Acid *Urine Increase Analytical* Metabolites may give false positive reaction with some fluorometric or photometric methods leading to apparently increased excretion *5335*

Urine No Effect Analytical On method of Pisano et al *4018*

VLDL-Cholesterol *Serum No Effect Physiological* No significant change in several studies with patients treated for 1-12 mo *142* No significant effect in 20 hypertensive patients treated with up to 800 mg daily for 4 weeks *1808*

Labetolol

Lysergic Acid Diethylamide *Urine Increase Analytical* Minimum concentration that caused a positive result with EMIT method to measure LSD 60 mg/L *4968*

Lacidipine

Aldosterone *Plasma Increase Physiological* In 11 patients with essential hypertension treatment with 4 mg/d caused increase from mean baseline of 218 ± 15 pg/mL to 227 ± 34 pg/mL after 1 day and 262 ± 28 pg/mL after 30 days *4861*

Plasma No Effect Physiological In 25 outpatients with symptoms of mild to moderate heart failure treatment with 4 mg/d for 8 weeks had no significant effect on concentration *1325*

Cholesterol *Serum No Effect Physiological* No significant change observed in 6 patients with uncomplicated mild to moderate essential hypertension treated with up to 6 mg/d for 14 months (mean baseline concentration 5.1 mmol/L: concentration at 14 months 5.3 mmol/L) *5715*

Glomerular Filtration Rate *Urine Increase Physiological* In 11 patients with essential hypertension treatment with 4 mg/d caused increase from mean baseline of 110.3 ± 6.9 mL/min/1.73 sq m to 101.6 ± 6.9 mL/min/1.73 sq m after one day and 142.6 ± 30 mL/min/1.73 sq m *4861*

HDL-Cholesterol *Serum No Effect Physiological* Mean baseline concentration 1.1 mmol/L in 6 mild to moderate essential hypertensives treated with up to 6 mg/d for 14 months (mean baseline concentration 1.1 mmol/L, final concentration 1.2 mmol/L) *5715*

LDL-Cholesterol *Serum Increase Physiological* Mean baseline concentration 3.5 mmol/L in 6 patients with mild to moderate essential hypertension which increased to 3.7 mmol/L after treatment with up to 6 mg/d for 14 months *5715*

Norepinephrine *Plasma No Effect Physiological* In 25 outpatients with symptoms of mild to moderate heart failure treatment with 4 mg/d for 8 weeks had no significant effect on concentration *1325*

Renal Plasma Flow *Patient Increase Physiological* In 11 patients with essential hypertension treatment with 4 mg/d caused significant increase from mean baseline of 375.3 ± 32 mL/min/1.73 sq m to 458.0 ± 47 mL/min/1.73 sq m after one day but nonsignificant decrease to 334.7 ± 51 mL/min/1.73 sq m *4861*

Renin Activity *Plasma Increase Physiological* In 11 patients with essential hypertension treatment with 4 mg/d caused increase from mean baseline of 1.6 ± 0.4 ng/mL/h to 2.4 ± 0.5 ng/mL/h after 1 day and 2.1 ± 0.4 ng/mL/h after 30 days *4861*

Plasma No Effect Physiological In 25 outpatients with symptoms of mild to moderate heart failure treatment with 4 mg/d for 8 weeks had no significant effect on concentration *1325*

Sodium *Urine Increase Physiological* In 11 patients with essential hypertension treatment with 4 mg/d caused increase from mean baseline of 153 ± 23 mmol/d to 203 ± 48 mmol/d but decreased to 128 ± 13 mmol/d on day 30 *4861*

Triglycerides *Serum No Effect Physiological* Mean baseline concentration in 6 mild to moderate essential hypertensives 1.1 mmol/L reduced to 1.0 mmol/L after treatment with up to 6 mg/d for 14 months *5715* No significant change observed in 8 patients with mild to moderate hypertension treated with drug for up to 14 months *5715*

Volume *Urine Increase Physiological* In 11 patients with essential hypertension treated with 4 mg/d after one day increase from mean baseline of 1552 ± 239 mL to 1741 ± 282 mL observed but decreased to 1508 ± 277 mL after 30 days *4861*

Lactobacillus Acidophilus

Ammonia *Plasma Decrease Physiological* Causes reduction in hepatic encephalopathy *3709*

Lamivudine

Alanine Aminotransferase *Serum Increase Physiological* In studies of several thousand patients with HIV infection treated with 150 mg lamivudine b.i.d with zidovudine for 24 weeks ALT activity greater than 5.0 ULN observed in 3.7%. In 97 pediatric patients in those with normal baseline increased activity observed in 4% and in 29% of those with abnormal baseline *2174* In 2 of 143 patients treated with 100 mg/d for one year AST or ALT activity increased, although incidence less than in placebo-treated controls *3365*

Amylase *Serum Decrease Physiological* In studies of 656 patients with HIV infection treated with 300 mg lamivudine b.i.d alone or with zidovudine for 24 weeks pancreatitis observed in 3 (< 0.5%). In a larger study of several thousand patients treated with lamivudine and zidovudine 4.2% patients had amylase concentrations above 2.0 ULN *2174*

Serum Increase Physiological In 97 children with HIV infection treated with lamivudine abnormal activity (increased above 2 times ULN) observed in 3% of those with normal baseline and in 23% of those with abnormal baseline *2174*

Aspartate Aminotransferase *Serum Increase Physiological* In 2 of 143 patients treated with 100 mg/d for one year AST or ALT activity increased, although incidence less than in placebo-treated controls *3365* In studies of several thousand patients with HIV infection treated with 150 mg lamivudine b.i.d with zidovudine for 24 weeks AST activity greater than 5.0 ULN observed in 1.7%. In 97 children abnormal activity observed in 0% of those with normal baseline and in 19% of those with abnormal baseline *2174*

Serum No Effect Physiological In 97 children with HIV infection treated with lamivudine abnormal activity observed in 0% of those with normal baseline and in 19% of those with abnormal baseline *2174*

Bilirubin *Serum Increase Physiological* In studies of several thousand patients with HIV infection treated with 150 mg lamivudine b.i.d with zidovudine for 24 weeks bilirubin concentration greater than 2.5 ULN observed in 0.8% *2174*

Lamivudine *(continued)*

CD4+ Lymphocytes *Blood Increase Physiological* In a study of 366 previously untreated patients with HIV infection treated with 300 mg lamivudine b.i.d alone for 24 weeks mean concentration increased by about 30 cells/μL *2174*

Creatine Kinase *Serum Increase Physiological* In 3 of 143 patients treated with 100 mg/d for one year activity increased, compared with one in placebo-treated controls *3365*

Hemoglobin *Blood Decrease Physiological* In studies of several thousand patients with HIV infection treated with 150 mg lamivudine b.i.d with zidovudine for 24 weeks anemia with hemoglobin concentration of less than 8.0 g/dL observed in 2.9%. In 97 pediatric patients anemia observed in 2% of those with normal baseline and 24% of those with abnormal baseline *2174*

HIV-1 RNA *Serum Decrease Physiological* In a study of 366 previously untreated patients with HIV infection treated with 300 mg lamivudine b.i.d alone for 24 weeks mean HIV RNA decreased by about 0.5 copies/mL with a greater response when coadministered with zidovudine *2174*

Indinavir *Serum No Effect Physiological* Causes no significant effect on area under the concentration curve when lamivudine coadministered *1891*

Nelfinavir *Serum No Effect Physiological* Coadministration of lamivudine with nelfinavir had no effect on the pharmacokinetics of either drug *66*

Neutrophils *Blood Decrease Physiological* In studies of several thousand patients with HIV infection treated with 150 mg lamivudine b.i.d with zidovudine for 24 weeks neutrophil counts of less than 750 /μL observed in 7.2%. In 97 pediatric patients neutropenia observed in 22% of those with normal baseline and 45% of those with abnormal baseline *2174*

Platelets *Blood Decrease Physiological* In studies of several thousand patients with HIV infection treated with 150 mg lamivudine b.i.d with zidovudine for 24 weeks platelet counts of less than 50,000 /μL observed in 0.4%. In 97 pediatric patients thrombocytopenia observed in 0% of those with normal baseline and 25% of those with abnormal baseline *2174*

Blood No Effect Physiological In 97 pediatric patients with HIV infection thrombocytopenia (platelet count of less than 40,000 /μL) observed in 0% of those with normal baseline and 25% of those with abnormal baseline *2174*

Sulfamethoxazole *Serum No Effect Physiological* Coadministration of trimethoprim/sulfamethoxazole (TMP 160 mg/SMX 800 mg) once daily for 5 days with 300 mg lamivudine had no effect on the pharmacokinetic properties of trimethoprim and sulfamethoxazole *2174*

Trimethoprim *Serum No Effect Physiological* Coadministration of trimethoprim/sulfamethoxazole (TMP 160 mg/SMX 800 mg) once daily for 5 days with 300 mg lamivudine had no effect on the pharmacokinetic properties of trimethoprim and sulfamethoxazole *2174*

Zidovudine *Serum Increase Physiological* Coadministration of lamovudine with zidovudine increased the plasma maximum concentration of zidovudine by 39 ± 62% *2163* Coadministration of lamivudine with zidovudine caused a significant 39 ± 62% increase in the maximum plasma concentration of zidovudine *2174*

Lamotrigine

Alanine Aminotransferase *Serum Increase Physiological* Rare hepatitis reported as a complication of treatment *2160*

Alkaline Phosphatase *Serum Increase Physiological* Rare hepatitis reported as a complication of treatment *2160*

Aspartate Aminotransferase *Serum Increase Physiological* Rare hepatitis reported as a complication of treatment *2160*

Bilirubin *Serum Increase Physiological* Rare hepatitis reported as a complication of treatment *2160*

Blood *Urine Decrease Physiological* Infrequently hematuria occurs as a complication of treatment *2160*

Carbamazepine *Serum No Effect Physiological* Coadministration of lamotrigine with carbamazepine has no effect on the latter's concentration *2160*

Cortisol, Free *Urine No Effect Analytical* No significant interference observed with HPLC method of Turpeinen et al *6105*

Creatinine *Serum Increase Physiological* Rarely concentration increases as a complication of treatment *2160*

Eosinophils *Blood Increase Physiological* Infrequently eosinophilia reported as a complication of treatment *2160*

Fibrinogen *Plasma Decrease Physiological* Infrequently hypofibrinogenemia reported as a complication of treatment *2160*

Hematocrit *Blood Decrease Physiological* Infrequently anemia reported as a complication of treatment. Rarely iron deficiency anemia or macrocytic anemia occurs *2160*

Hemoglobin *Blood Decrease Physiological* Infrequently anemia reported as a complication of treatment Rarely iron deficiency or macrocytic anemia occurs *2160* A single case of pure red cell aplasia observed in a 32-year old man with a history of β-thalassemia. The patient had a microcytic anemia (hemoglobin 11 g/dL) which was stable while receiving carbamazepine but became more severe after receiving lamotrigine *2160*

Leukocytes *Blood Decrease Physiological* Infrequently leukocytosis or leukopenia reported as a complication of treatment *2160*

Blood Increase Physiological Infrequently leukocytosis or leukopenia reported as a complication of treatment *2160*

MCV *Blood Increase Physiological* Rarely macrocytic anemia occurs as a complication of treatment *2160*

Mycophenolic Acid *Serum No Effect Analytical* No significant interference observed with HPLC method of Shipkova et al *5526*

Mycophenolic Acid Glucuronide
Serum No Effect Analytical No significant interference observed with HPLC method of Shipkova et al *5526*

Occult Blood *Feces Increase Physiological* Rare gastrointestinal hemorrhage and melena reported as a complication of treatment *2160*

Phenytoin *Serum No Effect Physiological* Coadministration of lamotrigine with phenytoin has no effect on the latter's concentration *2160*

Platelets *Blood Decrease Physiological* Rarely thrombocytopenia occurs as a complication of treatment *2160*

Thyroxine (T4) *Serum Decrease Physiological* Rare goiter and hypothyroidism reported as a complication of treatment *2160*

Valproic Acid *Serum Decrease Physiological* Coadministration of lamotrigine with valproic acid caused a significant reduction in the plasma concentration of valproic acid *2160*

Lanatoside

Digoxin *Serum Increase Analytical* Lanatoside had a significant cross-reactivity of 60% with method on Bayer Technicon Immuno 1® *421*

Lanreotide

Bile Salts *Gastric Fluid Decrease Physiological* In 8 healthy male volunteers infusion of lanreotide (100 μg/h after a bolus of 100 μg 15 min before the beginning of the study) caused a significant decrease in output from 3.9 ± 0.5 mmol/3 h with placebo to 0.26 ± 0.03 mmol/3 h *3387*

Follicle Stimulating Hormone
Plasma No Effect Physiological In 13 patients with acromegaly treatment with 30 mg intramuscularly twice monthly for 9 months caused no significant change in concentration from median baseline *3793*

Fructosamine *Serum Increase Physiological* In 10 patients with acromegaly treatment with 30 mg intramuscularly twice monthly caused significant decrease from median baseline of 0.80 ± 0.12 mmol/L to 1.02 ± 0.16 mmol/L after 3 months and to 1.14 ± 0.22 mmol/L after 9 months *3793*

Glucose *Serum Decrease Physiological* In 10 patients with acromegaly treatment with 30 mg intramuscularly twice monthly caused nonsignificant decrease from median baseline of 4.1 ± 0.2 mmol/L to 4.5 ± 0.1 mmol/L after 3 months and to 3.8 ± 0.2 mmol/L after 9 months *3793*

Growth Hormone *Plasma Decrease Physiological* In 13 patients with acromegaly treatment with 30 mg intramuscularly twice monthly caused significant decrease from median baseline of 32.0 ± 29.4 μg/L to 10.0 ± 3.6 μg/L after 3 months and to 19.1 ± 5.7 μg/L after 9 months *3793*

Plasma Increase Physiological In 10 patients with advanced breast cancer treatment with 30 mg i.m. fortnightly caused mean concentration to increase from baseline of 0.51 ± 0.78 ng/mL to 0.85 ± 1.18 ng/mL after 14 days, 1.06 ± 2.32 ng/mL after 1 month and 2.13 ± 3.35 ng/mL after 3 months *1411*

Hydrochloric Acid *Gastric Fluid Decrease Physiological* In 8 healthy male volunteers infusion of lanreotide (100 μg/h after a bolus of 100 μg 15 min before the beginning of the study) caused a significant decrease in acid secretion from 39.7 ± 7 mmol/3 h with placebo to 4.2 ± 0.6 mmol/3 h *3387*

Insulin *Plasma Decrease Physiological* In 10 patients with acromegaly treatment with 30 mg intramuscularly twice monthly caused significant decrease from median baseline of 25.5 ± 4.0 μU/mL to 5.0 ± 4.0 μU/mL after 3 months and to 9.6 ± 2.5 μU/mL after 9 months *3793*

Plasma Increase Physiological In 20 patients who had received PTCA and subcutaneous continuous infusion of lanreotide concentration of insulin changed insignificantly from baseline one day after PTCA from 29 ± 4 mU/L to 40 ± 6 mU/L *1980* In a population of 38 patients who received a continuous subcutaneous infusion of lanreotide for 4 days following PTCA caused insignificant change from mean baseline of 29 ± 4 mU/L to 40 ± 6 mU/L on day 1, and 51 ± 8 mU/L on day 2 *1980*

Insulin-like Growth Factor-I *Serum Decrease Physiological* In a population of 38 patients who received a continuous subcutaneous infusion of lanreotide for 4 days following PTCA caused a significant reduction from mean baseline of 112 ± 37 μg/L to 104 ± 37 μg/L after 1 day, 104 ± 32 μg/L after 2 days and 98 ± 24 μg/L on follow-up days 6 to 11 *1980* In 13 patients with acromegaly treatment with 30 mg intramuscularly twice monthly caused significant decrease from median baseline of 1193 ± 73 μg/L to 782 ± 99 μg/L after 3 months and to 621 ± 103 μg/L after 9 months *3793*

Serum No Effect Physiological In 10 patients with advanced breast cancer treatment with 30 mg i.m. fortnightly caused mean concentration to change nonsignificantly from baseline of 183.1 ± 69.7 ng/mL to 147.2 ± 52.5 ng/mL after 14 days, 162.1 ± 72.2 ng/mL after 1 month and 172.9 ± 64.8 ng/mL after 3 months *1411*

Insulin-like Growth Factor-I, Free

Serum Decrease Physiological In 20 patients who had received PTCA concentration of free IGF-I decreased significantly by 22 - 27% one day after initiation of continuous subcutaneous infusion of lanreotide from 680 ± 400 ng/L to 530 ± 380 ng/L *1980*

Serum No Effect Physiological In a population of 38 patients who received a continuous subcutaneous infusion of lanreotide for 4 days following PTCA caused no significant change from mean baseline of 730 ± 240 ng/L to 530 ± 380 ng/L on day 1, and 500 ± 370 ng/L on day 2 *1980*

Insulin-like Growth Factor-II

Serum Decrease Physiological In 20 patients who had received PTCA concentration of total IGF-II decreased significantly at days 6 through 11 after initiation of continuous subcutaneous infusion of lanreotide for 4 days from 784 ± 176 μg/L to 728 ± 117 μg/L *1980* In a population of 38 patients who received a continuous subcutaneous infusion of lanreotide for 4 days following PTCA caused a significant reduction from mean baseline of 784 ± 176 μg/L to 750 ± 173 μg/L on day 6, 766 ± 228 μg/L on day 8 and 728 ± 117 μg/L on day 11 *1980*

Insulin-like Growth Factor-II, Free

Serum No Effect Physiological In a population of 38 patients who received a continuous subcutaneous infusion of lanreotide for 4 days following PTCA caused no significant change from mean baseline of 1300 ± 670 ng/L to 1060 ± 800 ng/L on day 1, and 1100 ± 700 ng/L on day 2 *1980* In 20 patients who had received PTCA concentration of free IGF-II changed insignificantly at day 1 after initiation of continuous subcutaneous infusion of lanreotide for 4 days from 1300 ± 670 ng/L to 1060 ± 800 ng/L *1980*

Insulin-like Growth Factor Binding Protein-1

Serum Increase Physiological In a population of 38 patients who received a continuous subcutaneous infusion of lanreotide for 4 days following PTCA caused significant change from mean baseline of 2.5 ± 2.7 μg/L to 6.7 ± 4.2 μg/L on day 1, and 6.3 ± 3.6 μg/L on day 2 *1980* In 20 patients who had received PTCA concentration of IGFBP-1 increased significantly by 168% at day 1 after initiation of continuous subcutaneous infusion of lanreotide for 4 days from 2.5 ± 2.7 μg/L to 6.7 ± 4.2 μg/L *1980* Subcutaneous administration of up to 80 μg/kg caused dose-dependent increase starting 1 - 2 hours after administration and remaining increased for 5 hours *6530* Admnistration causes increased concentration *4439*

Insulin-like Growth Factor Binding Protein-3

Serum Decrease Physiological In 12 patients with acromegaly treatment with 30 mg intramuscularly twice monthly caused significant decrease from median baseline of 8.7 ± 1.5 mg/L to 6.4 ± 0.8 mg/L after 3 months and to 5.4 ± 1.0 mg/L after 9 months *3793*

Serum No Effect Physiological In 20 patients who had received PTCA concentration of IGFBP-3 changed insignificantly at day 1 after initiation of continuous subcutaneous infusion of lanreotide for 4 days from 3.14 ± 0.93 mg/L to 3.87 ± 0.93 mg/L *1980* In a population of 38 patients who received a continuous subcutaneous infusion of lanreotide for 4 days following PTCA caused no significant change from mean baseline of 4.22 ± 1.08 mg/L to 3.90 ± 1.05 mg/L on day 0, 4.01 ± 1.07 mg/L on day 1, 4.33 ± 1.06 mg/L on day 2 and 4.21 ± 1,24 mg/L on days 6 through 11 *1980*

Lipase *Gastric Fluid Decrease Physiological* In 8 healthy male volunteers infusion of lanreotide (100 μg/h after a bolus of 100 μg 15 min before the beginning of the study) caused a significant decrease in output from 173 ± 20 kIU/3 h with placebo to 33 ± 10 kIU/3 h *3387*

Luteinizing Hormone *Plasma No Effect Physiological* In 13 patients with acromegaly treatment with 30 mg intramuscularly twice monthly for 9 months caused no significant change in concentration from median baseline *3793*

Somatomedin *Plasma Decrease Physiological* In 9 patients with acromegaly treatment with 30 mg intramuscularly twice monthly caused significant decrease from median baseline of 1.56 ± 0.06 kIU/L to 1.16 ± 0.13 kIU/L after 3 months and to 1.08 ± 0.16 kIU/L after 9 months *3793*

Thyroid Stimulating Hormone

Serum No Effect Physiological In 13 patients with acromegaly treatment with 30 mg intramuscularly twice monthly for 9 months caused no significant change in concentration from median baseline *3793*

Thyroxine (T4) *Serum No Effect Physiological* In 13 patients with acromegaly treatment with 30 mg intramuscularly twice monthly for 9 months caused no significant change in concentration from median baseline *3793*

Volume *Gastric Fluid Decrease Physiological* In 8 healthy male volunteers infusion of lanreotide (100 μg/h after a bolus of 100 μg 15 min before the beginning of the study) caused a nonsignificant decrease in fluid volume from 3722 ± 301 mL/15 min with placebo to 2933 ± 275 mL/15 min *3387*

Lansoprazole

Abnormal Leukocytes *Blood Increase Physiological* Abnormal cells reported as an adverse event *5946*

Alanine Aminotransferase *Serum Increase Physiological* Isolated cases of increased activity reported but no greater than in patients treated with placebo *5946*

Albumin *Urine Increase Physiological* Albuminuria reported in both short term and long term studies in fewer than 1% patients *5946*

Albumin:Globulin Ratio *Serum Decrease Physiological* Isolated cases of increased concentration of globulins reported leading to abnormal A/G ratio *5946* Decreased ratio reported as an adverse event *5946*

Lansoprazole *(continued)*

Aldosterone *Plasma No Effect Physiological* Treatment for up to 8 weeks had no significant effect on concentration *5946*

Alkaline Phosphatase *Serum Increase Physiological* Isolated cases of increased activity reported *5946* Increased activity reported as an adverse event *5946*

Amoxicillin *Serum No Effect Physiological* No clinically significant interaction with amoxicillin observed *5946*

Antipyrine *Serum No Effect Physiological* Although lansoprazole is metabolized by the cytochrome P450 system, it does not clinically significantly affect the metabolism of other drugs metabolized by the same system *5946*

Aspartate Aminotransferase *Serum Increase Physiological* Increased activity reported as an adverse event *5946* Isolated cases of increased activity reported but no greater than in patients treated with placebo *5946*

Bilirubin *Serum Increase Physiological* Isolated cases of increased concentration reported *5946* Increased concentration reported as an adverse event *5946*

Blood *Urine Increase Physiological* Hematuria reported in both short term and long term studies in fewer than 1% patients *5946*

Cholesterol *Serum Decrease Physiological* Isolated cases of decreased concentration reported *5946* Hypocholesterolemia reported as an adverse event *5946*

Serum Increase Physiological Isolated cases of increased concentration reported *5946* Hypercholesterolemia reported as an adverse event *5946*

Clarithromycin *Serum No Effect Physiological* Although lansoprazole is metabolized by the cytochrome P450 system, it does not clinically significantly affect the metabolism of other drugs metabolized by the same system *5946*

Cortisol *Plasma No Effect Physiological* Treatment for up to 8 weeks had no significant effect on concentration *5946*

Creatinine *Serum Increase Physiological* Isolated cases of increased concentration reported *5946*

Dehydroepiandrosterone Sulfate

Plasma No Effect Physiological Treatment for up to 8 weeks had no significant effect on concentration *5946*

Diazepam *Serum No Effect Physiological* Although lansoprazole is metabolized by the cytochrome P450 system, it does not clinically significantly affect the metabolism of other drugs metabolized by the same system *5946* Coadministration of lansoprazole with diazepam plasma elimination half-life, clearance and volume of distribution not significantly different from control values of 26.0 ± 1.6 h, 22.5 ± 1.1 mL/h/kg and 0.82 ± 0.04 L/kg respectively *3490*

Eosinophils *Blood Increase Physiological* Isolated cases of increased concentration reported *5946*

Erythrocytes *Blood Abnormal Physiological* Abnormal cells reported as an adverse event *5946*

Estradiol *Plasma No Effect Physiological* Treatment for up to 8 weeks had no significant effect on concentration *5946*

Follicle Stimulating Hormone

Plasma No Effect Physiological Treatment for up to 8 weeks had no significant effect on concentration *5946*

Gastrin *Serum Increase Physiological* In one study of 2100 patients treatment with 15 - 60 mg/d caused increase from mean baseline of 50 - 100% but remained within normal range, reching a plateau within two months of therapy and returning to baseline within 4 weeks after discontinuation of therapy *5946*

Globulin *Serum Increase Physiological* Isolated cases of increased concentration reported *5946* Increased concentration reported as an adverse event *5946*

Glucagon *Plasma No Effect Physiological* Treatment for up to 8 weeks had no significant effect on concentration *5946*

Glucose *Serum Decrease Physiological* Hypoglycemia reported in both short term and long term studies in fewer than 1% patients *5946* Both hyperglycemia and hypoglycemia observed in fewer than 1% of treated patients *5946*

Serum Increase Physiological Both hyperglycemia and hypoglycemia observed in fewer than 1% of treated patients *5946*

Urine Increase Physiological Glycosuria reported in both short term and long term studies in fewer than 1% patients *5946*

γ-Glutamyltransferase *Serum Increase Physiological* Isolated cases of increased activity reported *5946* Increased activity reported as an adverse event *5946*

Granulocytes *Blood Decrease Physiological* Agranulocytosis observed in fewer than 1% of treated patients *5946*

Hematocrit *Blood Decrease Physiological* Anemia and hemolysis reported in both short term and long term studies in fewer than 1% patients *5946*

Hemoglobin *Blood Decrease Physiological* Anemia, including aplastic or hemolytic anemia, observed in fewer than 1% of treated patients *5946* Anemia and hemolysis reported in both short term and long term studies in fewer than 1% patients *5946*

Ibuprofen *Serum No Effect Physiological* Although lansoprazole is metabolized by the cytochrome P450 system, it does not clinically significantly affect the metabolism of other drugs metabolized by the same system *5946*

Indomethacin *Serum No Effect Physiological* Although lansoprazole is metabolized by the cytochrome P450 system, it does not clinically significantly affect the metabolism of other drugs metabolized by the same system *5946*

Insulin *Plasma No Effect Physiological* Treatment for up to 8 weeks had no significant effect on concentration *5946*

Lactate Dehydrogenase *Serum Increase Physiological* Isolated cases of increased activity reported *5946* Increased activity reported as an adverse event *5946*

Leukocytes *Blood Decrease Physiological* Leukopenia or pancytopenia observed in fewer than 1% of treated patients *5946*

Blood Increase Physiological Increased concentration reported as an adverse event *5946*

Lipids *Serum Increase Physiological* Hyperlipidemia reported as an adverse event *5946*

Luteinizing Hormone *Plasma No Effect Physiological* Treatment for up to 8 weeks had no significant effect on concentration *5946*

Neutrophils *Blood Decrease Physiological* Neutropenia or pancytopenia observed in fewer than 1% of treated patients *5946*

Occult Blood *Feces Increase Physiological* Melena reported in both short term and long term studies in fewer than 1% patients *5946*

Parathyroid Hormone *Plasma No Effect Physiological* Treatment for up to 8 weeks had no significant effect on concentration *5946*

pH *Gastric Fluid Increase Physiological* In one extensive study treatment with 15 mg/d cause increase of mean 24-hour pH from 2.1 to 2.7 on day 1 to 4.0 on day 5 and with 30 mg/d to 3.6 on day 1 and 4.9 on day 5 *5946*

Phenytoin *Serum No Effect Physiological* Although lansoprazole is metabolized by the cytochrome P450 system, it does not clinically significantly affect the metabolism of other drugs metabolized by the same system *5946*

Platelets *Blood Abnormal Physiological* Reported as an adverse event *5946*

Blood Decrease Physiological Thrombocytopenia, thrombotic thrombocytopenic purpura or pancytopenia observed in fewer than 1% of treated patients *5946*

Blood Increase Physiological Reported as an adverse event *5946* Isolated cases of increased concentration reported *5946*

Prednisone *Serum No Effect Physiological* Although lansoprazole is metabolized by the cytochrome P450 system, it does not clinically significantly affect the metabolism of other drugs metabolized by the same system *5946*

Prolactin *Plasma No Effect Physiological* Treatment for up to 8 weeks had no significant effect on concentration *5946*

Propranolol *Serum No Effect Physiological* Although lansoprazole is metabolized by the cytochrome P450 system, it does not clinically significantly affect the metabolism of other drugs metabolized by the same system *5946*

Sex-Hormone Binding Globulin

Serum No Effect Physiological Treatment for up to 8 weeks had no significant effect on concentration *5946*

Somatotropin *Serum No Effect Physiological* Treatment for up to 8 weeks had no significant effect on concentration *5946*

Terfenadine *Serum No Effect Physiological* Although lansoprazole is metabolized by the cytochrome P450 system, it does not clinically significantly affect the metabolism of other drugs metabolized by the same system *5946*

Testosterone *Serum No Effect Physiological* Treatment for up to 8 weeks had no significant effect on concentration *5946*

Theophylline *Serum Decrease Physiological* Although lansoprazole is metabolized by the cytochrome P450 system, it generally does not clinically significantly affect the metabolism of other drugs metabolized by the same system, although the clearance of theophylline is increased by about 10% *5946*

Thyroid Stimulating Hormone
Serum No Effect Physiological Treatment for up to 8 weeks had no significant effect on concentration *5946*

Thyroxine (T4) *Serum No Effect Physiological* Treatment for up to 8 weeks had no significant effect on concentration *5946*

Tri-iodothyronine (T3) *Serum No Effect Physiological* Treatment for up to 8 weeks had no significant effect on concentration *5946*

Uric Acid *Serum Increase Physiological* Gout reported in both short term and long term studies in fewer than 1% patients *5946*

Warfarin *Plasma No Effect Physiological* Although lansoprazole is metabolized by the cytochrome P450 system, it does not clinically significantly affect the metabolism of other drugs metabolized by the same system *5946*

Laxatives

Aldosterone *Plasma Increase Physiological* Marked increase in chronic abuser with dehydration *6195*

Bicarbonate *Serum Increase Physiological* If chronic abuse occurs *6195*

Calcium *Serum Decrease Physiological* Excessive use may have effect *3810*

Chloride *Serum Decrease Physiological* If chronic abuse occurs *6195*

Cyclosporine *Blood Decrease Physiological* With coadministration of GoLytely Lavage Solution whole blood concentration was observed to be reduced by 80% in one patient *859*
Serum Decrease Physiological With coadministration of GoLytely Lavage Solution whole blood concentration was observed to be reduced by 80% in one patient *859*

Estriol *Urine Decrease Analytical* If contain phenolphthalein reduce hydrolysis *641*

pH *Blood Increase Physiological* If chronic abuse may cause metabolic alkalosis *6195*

Potassium *Serum Decrease Physiological* Excessive use may have effect *3810*

Protein *Serum Decrease Physiological* May occur with continued use *3669*

Prothrombin Time *Plasma Increase Physiological* Accelerated gastrointestinal passage and decrease absorption of vitamin K *2452*

Renin Activity *Plasma Increase Physiological* Marked increase in chronic abuser with dehydration *6195*

Sodium *Serum Decrease Physiological* Excessive use may have effect *3810*

Lebenin®

Indican *Serum Decrease Physiological* In 10 uremic patients undergoing regular hemodialysis 4 weeks administration of Lebenin® caused mean concentration of phenol to change significantly from 215 ± 30 nmol/mL to 140 ± 25 nmol/mL *2592*

Indole *Feces Decrease Physiological* In 10 uremic patients undergoing regular hemodialysis 2 weeks administration of Lebenin® caused mean concentration of p-cresol to decrease significantly from 220 ± 40 nmol/mg feces to 95 ± 40 nmol/mg feces *2592*

p-Cresol *Feces Decrease Physiological* In 10 uremic patients undergoing regular hemodialysis 2 weeks administration of Lebenin® caused mean concentration of p-cresol to decrease significantly from 860 ± 160 nmol/mg feces to 550 ± 110 nmol/mg feces *2592*
Serum No Effect Physiological In 10 uremic patients undergoing regular hemodialysis 4 weeks administration of Lebenin® caused mean concentration of phenol to change insignificantly from 165 ± 30 nmol/mL to 160 ± 40 nmol/mL *2592*

Phenol *Feces Decrease Physiological* In 10 uremic patients undergoing regular hemodialysis 2 weeks administration of Lebenin® caused mean concentration of phenol to decrease nonsignificantly from 67 ± 23 nmol/mg feces to 62 ± 32 nmol/mg feces *2592*
Serum No Effect Physiological In 10 uremic patients undergoing regular hemodialysis 4 weeks administration of Lebenin® caused mean concentration of phenol to change insignificantly from 19 ± 9 nmol/mL to 22 ± 7 nmol/mL *2592*

Leflunomide

Alanine Aminotransferase *Serum Increase Physiological* In 100 patients with rheumatoid arthritis treatment with 10 mg/d for 24 weeks and of 101 patients with 25 mg/d caused significant effects on activity although activities remained within normal range *5139*

Alkaline Phosphatase *Serum Increase Physiological* In 100 patients with rheumatoid arthritis treatment with 10 mg/d for 24 weeks and of 101 patients with 25 mg/d caused significant effects on activity although activities remained within normal range *5139*

Aspartate Aminotransferase *Serum Increase Physiological* In 100 patients with rheumatoid arthritis treatment with 10 mg/d for 24 weeks and of 101 patients with 25 mg/d caused significant effects on activity although activities remained within normal range *5139*

C-Reactive Protein *Serum Decrease Physiological* In 100 patients with rheumatoid arthritis treatment with 10 mg/d for 24 weeks and of 101 patients with 25 mg/d caused significant effects on concentration with significant decreases of 14.9 and 9.5 mg/dL respectively compared with 3.1 mm/h in 102 placebo-treated controls *5139*
Serum No Effect Physiological In 95 patients with rheumatoid arthritis treatment with 5 mg/d for 24 weeks had no significant effect on concentration with insignificant increase of 2.4 mg/dL compared with 5.3 mg/dL in 102 placebo-treated controls *5139*

Erythrocyte Sedimentation Rate
Blood Decrease Physiological In 100 patients with rheumatoid arthritis treatment with 10 mg/d for 24 weeks and of 101 patients with 25 mg/d caused significant effects on rate with significant decreases of 5.2 and 5.4 mm/h respectively compared with 3.1 mm/h in 102 placebo-treated controls *5139*
Blood No Effect Physiological In 95 patients with rheumatoid arthritis treatment with 5 mg/d for 24 weeks had no significant effect on rate with insignificant increase of 4.2 mm/h compared with 3.1 mm/h in 102 placebo-treated controls *5139*

Letrozole

Aldosterone *Plasma No Effect Physiological* In two studies of women with breast cancer doses from 0.1 to 2.5 mg had no significant effect on concentration *6076*

Androstenedione *Plasma No Effect Physiological* In two studies of women with breast cancer doses from 0.1 to 2.5 mg had no significant effect on concentration *6076*

Corticotropin *Plasma Decrease Physiological* In one study of women with breast cancer doses of 5 mg had no significant effect on concentration *6076*

Cortisol *Plasma No Effect Physiological* In two studies of women with breast cancer doses from 0.1 to 2.5 mg had no significant effect on concentration *6076*

Letrozole *(continued)*

Dehydroepiandrosterone Sulfate
Plasma Decrease Physiological In one study of women with breast cancer doses of 5 mg had no significant effect on concentration *6076*

Estradiol *Plasma Decrease Physiological* In two studies of women with breast cancer doses from 0.1 to 2.5 mg caused decrease in concentration by 74-90% to below 3 pmol/L in some patients *6076*
Urine Decrease Physiological In one study of women with breast cancer doses of 5 mg caused a significant decrease in concentration *6076*

Estrone *Plasma Decrease Physiological* In two studies of women with breast cancer doses from 0.1 to 2.5 mg caused decrease in concentration by 79-90% to below 10 pmol/L in some patients *6076*
Urine Decrease Physiological In one study of women with breast cancer doses of 5 mg caused a significant decrease in concentration *6076*

Estrone Sulfate *Plasma Decrease Physiological* In one study of women with breast cancer doses of 5 mg caused a significant decrease in concentration *6076*

Follicle Stimulating Hormone
Plasma No Effect Physiological In two studies of women with breast cancer doses from 0.1 to 2.5 mg had no significant effect on concentration *6076*

17α-Hydroxyprogesterone *Plasma No Effect Physiological* In two studies of women with breast cancer doses from 0.1 to 2.5 mg had no significant effect on concentration *6076*

Luteinizing Hormone *Plasma No Effect Physiological* In two studies of women with breast cancer doses from 0.1 to 2.5 mg had no significant effect on concentration *6076*

Testosterone *Serum Decrease Physiological* In one study of women with breast cancer doses of 5 mg had no significant effect on concentration *6076*

Thyroid Stimulating Hormone
Serum No Effect Physiological In two studies of women with breast cancer doses from 0.1 to 2.5 mg had no significant effect on concentration *6076*

Thyroxine (T4) *Serum Decrease Physiological* In one study of women with breast cancer doses of 5 mg had no significant effect on concentration *6076*

Leucovorin

Folate *Serum No Effect Analytical* At concentration of 500 ng/mL cross-reactivity of less than 1.6% on method on Stratus family of analyzers *4141*

Methotrexate *Serum No Effect Analytical* No significant interference observed at a concentration of 100 μmol/L with method on Du Pont aca *1535*

Leukotriene B_4

Eosinophils *Blood Decrease Physiological* In 6 asthmatic individuals given a mean inhaled dose of LTB_4 of 17.6 μg significant reduction of eosinophil count to 81.2 ± 31.5% of baseline at 6 h and 74.3 ± 36.5% of baseline at 24 h *5213*

Leukocytes *Blood Increase Physiological* In 6 healthy individuals and 6 patients with mild asthma given a mean inhaled dose of LTB_4 of 17.6 μg significant increase in leukocyte count observed in both healthy individuals and asthmatics *5213*

Monocytes *Blood Decrease Physiological* In 6 healthy individuals given a mean inhaled dose of LTB_4 of 17.6 μg significant reduction of monocyte count to 58% of baseline at 5 minutes *5213*
Blood Increase Physiological In 6 healthy individuals given a mean inhaled dose of LTB_4 of 17.6 μg significant reduction of monocyte count to 58% of baseline at 5 minutes rising to 553% of baseline at 30 min *5213*

Neutrophils *Blood Decrease Physiological* In 6 healthy individuals given a mean inhaled dose of LTB_4 of 17.6 μg significant reduction of neutrophil count to 19.8 ± 6.3% of baseline at 5 minutes *5213*
Blood Increase Physiological In 6 healthy individuals given a mean inhaled dose of LTB_4 of 17.6 μg significant reduction of neutrophil count to 19.8 ± 6.3% of baseline at 5 minutes followed by a neutrophilia of 183 ± 17.2% of baseline at 30 min, with return to baseline after 6 h. Response less in asthmatics *5213*

Leuprolide

Acid Phosphatase, Prostatic
Serum Decrease Physiological Administration of 30 mg intramuscularly every 16 weeks to 49 men with stage D2 prostate cancer caused reduction from mean baseline concentration of 161.5 ng/mL to 27.5 ng/mL at 16 weeks and 21.9 ng/mL after 32 weeks *5474*

Androstanediol Glucuronide
Plasma Decrease Physiological Mean reduction of 14% in 10 hirsute women with polycystic ovarian syndrome and of 7% in 8 women with idiopathic hirsutism treated with up to 20 μg/kg/d for 5-6 months *4972*

Androstenedione *Plasma Decrease Physiological* Mean reduction of 53% in 10 hirsute women with polycystic ovarian syndrome and of 31% in 9 women with idiopathic hirsutism when treated with up to 20 μg/kg/d for 5-6 months *4972* In 26 men with benign prostatic cancer treatment with 3.75 mg leuprolide depot intramuscularly every 28 days for 24 weeks caused a 48% reduction in plasma concentration during treatment *1744*

Androstenedione Sulfate *Plasma No Effect Physiological* In 10 women with hirsutism due to polycystic ovarian syndrome and in 9 with idiopathic hirsutism treatment with leuprolide for 5-6 months had no significant effect *4972*

Blood *Urine Increase Physiological* Hematuria observed in 6 of 98 treated patients *5945*

Calcitonin *Plasma No Effect Physiological* In 6 women with endometriosis treatment with 3.75 mg depot leuprolide acetate monthly over 24 weeks had no effect on the plasma calcitonin concentration *1286*

Calcium *Serum Increase Physiological* Increased concentration observed in fewer than 5% of treated patients *5945*

Creatinine *Serum Increase Physiological* Increased concentration observed in fewer than 5% of treated patients *5945*

Dehydroepiandrosterone Sulfate
Plasma Decrease Physiological In 26 men with benign prostatic cancer treatment with 3.75 mg leuprolide depot intramuscularly every 28 days for 24 weeks caused a 24% reduction in plasma concentration during treatment *1744*
Plasma No Effect Physiological No change observed in either 10 hirsute women with polycystic ovarian syndrome or 9 women with idiopathic hirsutism when treated with up to 20 μg/kg/d for 5 - 6 months *4972*

Dihydrotestosterone *Serum Decrease Physiological* In 26 men with benign prostatic cancer treatment with 3.75 mg leuprolide depot intramuscularly every 28 days for 24 weeks caused a 90% reduction in plasma concentration during treatment *1744*

Estradiol *Plasma Decrease Physiological* In 26 men with benign prostatic cancer treatment with 3.75 mg leuprolide depot intramuscularly every 28 days for 24 weeks caused a reduction in plasma concentration during treatment, typically to a nondetectable level *1744* In 6 women with endometriosis treatment with 3.75 mg depot leuprolide acetate monthly concentration decreased from mean baseline of about 60 pg/mL to < 25 pg/mL after about 8 weeks *1286* Mean concentration reduced in women with endometriosis following intranasal administration of 1.6 mg/day. Effect greater than with danazol *6093*
Plasma Increase Physiological In 5 healthy men administration of 10 μg/kg subcutaneously caused a significant change from mean baseline of 166 ± 21 pmol/L to 405 ± 44 pmol/L after 16 - 24 h, and from baseline of 312 ± 56 pmol/L to 1200 ± 165 pmol/L after 16 - 24 h *5099*

Estrone *Plasma Decrease Physiological* In 26 men with benign prostatic cancer treatment with 3.75 mg leuprolide depot intramuscularly every 28 days for 24 weeks caused a 35% reduction in plasma concentration during treatment *1744*

Follicle Stimulating Hormone
Plasma Decrease Physiological In 26 men with benign prostatic cancer treatment with 3.75 mg leuprolide depot intramuscularly every 28 days for 24 weeks caused a 55% reduction in plasma concentration during treatment *1744*
Plasma Increase Physiological In 5 healthy men administration of 10 µg/kg subcutaneously caused a significant increase from mean baseline of 2.6 ± 0.5 IU/L to 6.1 ± 1.2 IU/L at peak and 5.2 ± 0.8 IU/L after 24 h, and from baseline of 6.2 ± 0.5 IU/L to 22 ± 1.3 IU/L at peak and 16 ± 2.0 IU/L after 24 h in 5 normal women *5099*
Plasma No Effect Physiological No effect on cumulative concentration although at times concentration lower in women with endometriosis receiving 1.6 mg/day intranasal drug *6093*

Glucose *Serum Decrease Physiological* Diabetes or hypoglycemia observed in fewer than 5% of treated patients *5945*
Serum Increase Physiological Diabetes or hypoglycemia observed in fewer than 5% of treated patients *5945*

Hematocrit *Blood Decrease Physiological* Anemia observed in 5 of 98 treated patients *5945*

Hemoglobin *Blood Decrease Physiological* Anemia observed in 5 of 98 treated patients *5945*

Leukocytes *Blood Decrease Physiological* Decreased concentration observed as an adverse event *5945*

Luteinizing Hormone *Plasma Decrease Physiological* In 26 men with benign prostatic cancer treatment with 3.75 mg leuprolide depot intramuscularly every 28 days for 24 weeks caused a 90% reduction in plasma concentration during treatment *1744* Administration of 30 mg intramuscularly every 16 weeks to 49 men with stage D2 prostate cancer caused reduction from mean baseline concentration of 19.5 mIU/mL to a higher value at 4 days then fell to 13.4 mIU/mL by 1 week and then declined further to the lower end of normal range (3 to 10 mIU/mL) after 3 weeks *5474*
Plasma Increase Physiological In 5 healthy men administration of 10 µg/kg subcutaneously caused a significant increase from mean baseline of 6.4 ± 0.2 IU/L to 42 ± 2.2 IU/L at peak and 31 ± 1.0 IU/L after 24 h, and from baseline of 8.6 ± 0.9 IU/L to 60 ± 9.2 IU/L at peak and 45 ± 8.2 IU/L after 24 h in 5 normal women *5099* Administration of 30 mg intramuscularly every 16 weeks to 49 men with stage D2 prostate cancer caused reduction from mean baseline concentration of 19.5 mIU/mL to a higher value at 4 days then fell to 13.4 mIU/mL by 1 week and then declined further to the lower end of normal range (3 to 10 mIU/mL) after 3 weeks *5474*
Plasma No Effect Physiological No cumulative effect in women with endometriosis receiving 1.6 mg/day intranasally although at times concentration lower *6093*

Occult Blood *Feces Increase Physiological* Gastrointestinal bleeding observed in fewer than 5% of treated patients *5945*

Progesterone *Plasma Decrease Physiological* Mean concentration in women with endometriosis reduced following intranasal administration of 1.6 mg/day. Effect greater than with danazol *6093*

Prolactin *Plasma No Effect Physiological* In 26 men with benign prostatic cancer treatment with 3.75 mg leuprolide depot intramuscularly every 28 days for 24 weeks had no significant effect on plasma concentration during treatment *1744*

Prostate-specific Antigen *Serum Decrease Physiological* Administration of 30 mg intramuscularly every 16 weeks to 49 men with stage D2 prostate cancer caused reduction from mean baseline concentration of 1096 ng/dL to 93 ng/dL at 16 weeks and 104 ng/dL after 32 weeks *5474*
Serum No Effect Analytical Leuprolide at a concentration of up to 1 µg/mL caused less than 0.1% cross-reactivity with method on PSA method on Bayer Technicon Immuno 1® *430*

Prostate-specific Antigen, Free *Serum No Effect Analytical* Leuprolide acetate at a concentration of 8.0 µg/L had no significant effect on the Hybritech Tandem® -R free PSA immunoassay *4286*

Protein *Serum Decrease Physiological* Decreased concentration observed as an adverse event *5945*

Sex-Hormone Binding Globulin
Serum No Effect Physiological In 26 men with benign prostatic cancer treatment with 3.75 mg leuprolide depot intramuscularly every 28 days for 24 weeks had no significant effect on plasma concentration during treatment *1744*

Testosterone *Serum Decrease Physiological* In 10 hirsute women with polycystic ovarian syndrome and 9 with idiopathic hirsutism treatment with leuprolide for 5-6 months testosterone concentration decreased by 54 ± 6% and 36 ± 3% respectively *4972* Administration of 30 mg intramuscularly every 16 weeks to 49 men with stage D2 prostate cancer caused reduction from mean baseline concentration of 423.7 ng/dL to 659.6 ng/dL at 4 days then fell to below 50 ng/mL by 3 weeks *5474* In 26 men with benign prostatic cancer treatment with 3.75 mg leuprolide depot intramuscularly every 28 days for 24 weeks caused a 96% reduction in plasma concentration during treatment to 0.7 nmol/L *1744*
Serum Increase Physiological In the majority of treated patients concentration increased above baseline during first week of treatment, declining to baseline concentrations by the end of the second week *5945* Administration of 30 mg intramuscularly every 16 weeks to 49 men with stage D2 prostate cancer caused reduction from mean baseline concentration of 423.7 ng/dL to 659.6 ng/dL at 4 days then fell to below 50 ng/mL by 3 weeks *5474*
Serum No Effect Physiological In 10 healthy men administration of 100 µg caused an insignificant change from mean baseline of 20 ± 2.0 nmol/L to 28 ± 2.9 nmol/L after 16 - 24 h, and from baseline of 1.2 ± 0.1 nmol/L to 1.25 ± 0.1 nmol/L after 16 - 24 h *5099*

Urea Nitrogen *Serum Increase Physiological* Transient increases observed in a few patients *1384* Increased concentration observed in fewer than 5% of treated patients *5945*

Uric Acid *Serum Increase Physiological* Increased concentration observed as an adverse event *5945*

Levamisole

Acetylsalicylic Acid *Serum No Effect Physiological* Coadministration had no effect on salicylate pharmacokinetics *4062*

Alanine Aminotransferase *Serum Increase Physiological* In 1 of 11 patients receiving postoperative radiation treatment following breast cancer *4921*

Aspartate Aminotransferase *Serum Increase Physiological* Mild increase in 2 of 11 patients at 2 and 6 mo respectively after start of treatment. Normalized with withdrawal of treatment *4503* In 1 of 11 patients receiving postoperative radiation treatment following breast cancer *4921*

Bilirubin *Serum Increase Physiological* Administration of levamisole alone to 440 patients caused hyperbilirubinemia in < 1% patients and when also given with fluorouracil to 599 patients the incidence was 1% *2900*

Creatine Kinase *Serum Increase Physiological* In one man with stage B2 colon cancer activity began to increase dramatically 4 weeks after initiation of combined therapy with levamisole and 5-fluorouracil: increased activity due to CK-MM *942*

Creatine Kinase MM-Isoenzyme
Serum Increase Physiological In one man with stage B2 colon cancer activity began to increase dramatically 4 weeks after initiation of combined therapy with levamisole and 5-fluorouracil: increased activity due to CK-MM *942*

Granulocytes *Blood Decrease Physiological* Administration of levamisole alone to 440 patients caused granulocytopenia in < 1% patients and when also given with fluorouracil to 599 patients the incidence was 2% *2900* Most severe adverse reaction involves agranulocytosis especially in individuals with HLA B_{27} *1384*

Hematocrit *Blood Decrease Physiological* Administration of levamisole alone to 440 patients caused anemia in 0% patients and when also given with fluorouracil to 599 patients the incidence was 6% *2900*
Blood No Effect Physiological Administration of levamisole alone to 440 patients caused anemia in 0% patients and when also given with fluorouracil to 599 patients the incidence was 6% *2900*

Hemoglobin *Blood Decrease Physiological* Administration of levamisole alone to 440 patients caused anemia in 0% patients and when also given with fluorouracil to 599 patients the incidence was 6% *2900*

Levamisole *(continued)*

Hemoglobin *(continued)*
Blood No Effect Physiological Administration of levamisole alone to 440 patients caused anemia in 0% patients and when also given with fluorouracil to 599 patients the incidence was 6% *2900*

Leukocytes *Blood Decrease Physiological* In 4 of 11 patients with breast cancer and radiation treatment *4921* In 16% of 201 patients treated for rheumatoid arthritis had to be withdrawn from study. Occurred after mean treatment time of 7.4 mo *6251* Administration of levamisole alone to 440 patients caused the leukocyte count to fall below 2000 cells/µL in < 1% patients, between 2000 and 4000 cells/µL in 4% and above 4000 cells/µL in 2%. When also given with fluorouracil to 599 patients the incidence was 1, 19 and 33% respectively *2900* In 2 of 60 patients: sufficiently severe to warrant withdrawal from treatment *4401*

Neutrophils *Blood Decrease Physiological* Observed in 17 of 174 patients with breast cancer *5976* 16% of 201 patients treated for rheumatoid arthritis had to be withdrawn from study. Occurred after mean treatment time of 7.4 mo *6251* Occasional case of agranulocytosis reported *6264* In 35% of 60 patients treated for rheumatoid arthritis, reversed with withdrawal of drug *6468* In one patient with acute lymphoblastic leukemia receiving drug with methotrexate *6478* Causally related to presence of autoantibodies in serum. Granulocytoxins found in 6 of 20 patients *1495* In one patient with herpes simplex but also receiving other drugs *3034* In 4 of 11 patients with breast cancer and radiation treatment *4921*

Phenytoin *Serum Increase Physiological* Concomitant administration of levamisole with phenytoin and fluorouracil significantly increased the plasma concentration of phenytoin *2900*

Platelets *Blood Decrease Physiological* Administration of levamisole alone to 440 patients caused the platelet count to fall below 50,000 cells/µL in 0% patients, between 50,000 and 130,000 cells/µL in 1% and above 130,000 cells/µL in 1%. When also given with fluorouracil to 599 patients the incidence was 0, 8 and 10% respectively *2900* Marked reduction in one patient, recovered on withdrawal of drug, but fell with rechallange *1690*
Blood No Effect Physiological Administration of levamisole alone to 440 patients caused the platelet count to fall below 50,000 cells/µL in 0% patients, between 50,000 and 130,000 cells/µL in 1% and above 130,000 cells/µL in 1%. When also given with fluorouracil to 599 patients the incidence was 0, 8 and 10% respectively *2900*

Prothrombin Time *Plasma Increase Physiological* Concomitant administration of levamisole with warfarin was associated with a prolongation of prothrombin time *2900*

Levarterenol

Adenosine Monophosphate *Plasma Increase Physiological* Response to i.v. infusion in normals. No effect unless β-blocking agent also given *350*
Urine Increase Physiological Effect less marked than in blood *350*

Amino Acids *Plasma Increase Physiological* Catabolic effect *1714*
Urine Increase Analytical Reacts with ninhydrin; extra spot TLC, high voltage electrophoresis *4760*

Basal Metabolic Rate *Patient Increase Physiological* Normal metabolic response *1944*

Chloride *Urine Decrease Physiological* Increased tubular resistance and reabsorption *1944*

Cholesterol *Serum Increase Physiological* Reported effect ?mechanism *2452*

Effective Renal Plasma Flow
Patient Decrease Physiological Slight fall after i.v. infusion *4014* Blood flow reduced, filtration rate unchanged *2242*

Fatty Acids (FFA), Free *Serum Increase Physiological* Metabolic response *1944* Marked increase observed after i.v. infusion *5186*

Glomerular Filtration Rate *Urine Decrease Physiological* Slight fall after i.v. infusion *4014*
Urine No Effect Physiological After i.v. but increased filtration fraction *1944*

Glucose *Serum Increase Analytical* At 10 mg/dL affects alkaline ferricyanide procedure *2197*
Serum Increase Physiological Slight increase observed after i.v. infusion *5186*
Serum No Effect Analytical At 10 mg/dL no effect on glucose oxidase procedure of Gochman *2197*

Guaiacols Spot Test *Urine Negative Analytical* Action on procedure of Rogers *5061*

Metanephrines, Total *Urine No Effect Analytical* At 50 mg/L on modified Pisano procedure *2372*

Norepinephrine *Plasma Increase Physiological* After i.v. infusion *6691*

Occult Blood *Feces Increase Physiological* Diffuse hemorrhagic enteritis with vasoconstriction *5864*

Potassium *Urine Decrease Physiological* Increased tubular resistance and reabsorption *1944*

Renal Blood Flow *Patient Increase Physiological* After i.v. but increased filtration fraction *1944*

Sodium *Urine Decrease Physiological* Increased tubular resistance and reabsorption *1944*

Thyroxine (T4) *Serum Increase Physiological* Metabolic response *1944*

Urea Nitrogen *Test Conditions Increase Analytical* Brown with Berthelot's reagent *3144*

Uric Acid *Serum Increase Physiological* Result of decreased urate clearance *1851*
Urine Decrease Physiological Decreases urate excretion and renal plasma flow *1851*

Uric Acid Clearance *Urine Decrease Physiological* 20% reduction with infusion *1852*

Vanillylmandelic Acid *Urine Increase Physiological* Normal metabolite, effect slight usually *5871*

Volume *Plasma Decrease Physiological* Due to loss of protein-free fluid to tissues *2242*
Urine Decrease Physiological Slight fall after i.v. infusion *4014*
Urine No Effect Physiological Observed after i.v. 0.2-44.0 µg/min *1944*

Levocarnitine

Acylcarnitine, Long Chain *Serum Increase Physiological* Significant increase in 18 patients with hyperlipidemia being treated by hemodialysis when given 1 mg L-carnitine/kg body weight after dialysis for 3 months *6345*

Acylcarnitine, Short Chain *Serum Increase Physiological* Treatment with 1 mg L-carnitine/kg body weight after dialysis for 3 months of 18 patients with hyperlipidemia being treated with hemodialysis caused significant increase *6345*

Carnitine *Serum Increase Physiological* Low dose treatment with 1 mg L-carnitine/kg body weight after dialysis for 3 months of 18 patients with hyperlipidemia being treated by hemodialysis caused increase in plasma total carnitine *6345*

Carnitine, Free *Serum Increase Physiological* Observed in responders (significant reduction in serum triglyceride concentration) among 18 patients with hyperlipidemia being treated with hemodialysis when given 1 mg L-carnitine/kg body weight after dialysis for 3 months *6345*

HDL-Triglycerides *Serum Increase Physiological* Increase observed in 13 of 15 patients with hyperlipidemia being treated with hemodialysis and 1 mg L-carnitine/kg body weight following dialysis for 3 months *6345*

Triglycerides *Serum Decrease Physiological* Observed in responders among patients with hyperlipidemia being treated by hemodialysis and receiving 1 mg L-carnitine/kg body weight after dialysis for 3 months *6345*

VLDL-Cholesterol *Serum Decrease Physiological* Observed among responders with hyperlipidemia who were being treated with hemodialysis and 1 mg L-carnitine/kg body weight after dialysis for 3 months *6345*

VLDL-Phospholipids *Serum Decrease Physiological* Observed among responding patients with hyperlipidemia being treated with hemodialysis and 1 mg L-carnitine/kg body weight given after dialysis for 3 months *6345*

VLDL-Triglycerides *Serum Decrease Physiological* Observed among responders among patients with hyperlipidemia being treated with hemodialysis and 1 mg L-carnitine/kg body weight after dialysis for 3 months *6345*
Serum Increase Physiological Observed in 5 of 15 patients with hyperlipidemia being treated with hemodialysis and 1 mg L-carnitine/kg body weight after dialysis for 3 months *6345*

Levodopa

Alanine Aminotransferase *Serum Increase Physiological* Transient effect returns to normal *2754* Increase by 17% for 2 mo although later normalized, in patients with Parkinson's disease *2353* Administration of levodopa has been associated with increased activity, but significance unknown *5027*
Serum No Effect Analytical No effect at 0.3 mg/L on method on Ames Seralyzer *5706*

Alkaline Phosphatase *Serum Increase Physiological* Rare elevation reported *128* Administration of levodopa has been associated with increased activity, but significance unknown *5027*

Amino Acids *Urine Increase Analytical* Reacts with ninhydrin; extra spot TLC, high voltage electrophoresis *4760*

Ammonia *Plasma Decrease Physiological* Observed in one case: ?unrelated *2452*

Amylase *Serum No Effect Analytical* At a concentration of 1,000 mg/L had no effect on maltotetrose method *5704*

Aspartate Aminotransferase *Serum Increase Analytical* At 1 mmol/L affects Technicon SMA 12/60 method *5576*
Serum Increase Physiological Administration of levodopa has been associated with increased activity, but significance unknown *5027* Transient effect, normalizes despite continuation *128* Increase by 30% for 2 mo although later normalized, in patients with Parkinson's disease *2353*

Bilirubin *Serum Increase Analytical* Increase at concentration of 100 mg/L with method on Kodak Ektachem® but effect of no clinical significance since normal therapeutic range 0.5-1.5 mg/L *5706* Theoretically reacts with diazo reagent *5407* At concentrations above 80 mg/L raised concentration as measured by Jendrassik and Grof method *5704* At 1 mmol/L affects Technicon SMA 12/60 method *5576*
Serum Increase Physiological Administration of levodopa has been associated with increased concentration, but significance unknown *5027* Rare elevation reported *128*
Serum No Effect Analytical At concentration of 6 mg/L had no effect on Kodak Ektachem® method *5704*

Bilirubin, Conjugated *Serum Increase Analytical* At concentrations above 60 mg/L significant effect on method on Kodak Ektachem® but not of clinical significance since therapeutic concentration of drug 0.5-1.5 mg/L *5706*

Bilirubin, Unconjugated *Serum Decrease Analytical* Effect observed at concentrations above 60 mg/L with method on Kodak Ektachem® but not of clinical significance since therapeutic concentration 0.5-1.5 mg/L *5706*

Biotin *Serum Decrease Physiological* Associated with burning feet syndrome *1276*

BSP Retention *Serum Increase Physiological* Mild and transient effect *1276*

Calcium *Serum No Effect Analytical* At concentration of 197 mg/L had no effect on cresolphthalein method *5704*

Catecholamines *Plasma Increase Analytical* Measured as epinephrine/norepinephrine by ethylenediamine *3766*

Chloride *Serum No Effect Analytical* No effect of concentrations up to 80 mg/L with method on Kodak Ektachem® *5706*

Cholesterol *Serum No Effect Analytical* No effect at concentrations up to 6 mg/L on method on Kodak Ektachem® *5706*

Cholinesterase *Serum Increase Analytical* At activity of 4.5 kU/L activity increased by 1.13 kU/L at concentration of levodopa of 300 µg/mL with butyrylthiocholine method on Kodak Ektachem® *2504*

Color *Saliva Increase Analytical* Brown color reported with treatment *1226*
Sweat Increase Physiological Dark-colored sweat observed *1384*
Urine Increase Analytical Red-tinged on voiding, blackens on standing *5227*

Coombs' Test *Blood Positive Physiological* Administration of levodopa has been occasionally associated with positive reaction during extended therapy *5027* Autoimmune phenomenon (occurs after several months) *2453*

Coombs' Test, Direct *Blood Positive Physiological* Possible dose related without hemolysis *2452*

Coombs' Test, Indirect *Blood Positive Physiological* Observed in fewer than 1% of patients *1276*

Corticotropin *Plasma Increase Physiological* Magnitude variable, stress effect *5563*

Cortisol *Plasma Decrease Physiological* Probably diminished ACTH secretion *2310*

Creatine Kinase *Serum No Effect Analytical* No effect of concentrations up to 6 mg/L on method on Kodak Ektachem® *5706*

Creatinine *Serum Increase Analytical* Acts as reducing agent (probable effect) *189*
Serum No Effect Analytical No interference observed at a concentration of 0.1 mg/L with HPLC method of Rosano et al *5083* At concentration of 6 mg/L had no effect on creatinine iminohydrolase method *5704*
Urine Increase Analytical Probable action as reducing agent *189*
Urine No Effect Physiological In 5 healthy volunteers given 300 mg nonsignificant increase to 16 ± 1 mmol/d from 15 ± 1 mmol/d at baseline *2890*

Creatinine Clearance *Urine Increase Analytical* Reducing properties affect Jaffe method *1867*

Dihydroxyphenylalanine
Cerebrospinal Fluid Increase Physiological Concentrations in 4 patients with tyrosine hydroxylase deficiency increased to higher limit of reference interval (10 nmol/L) or above with treatment with 2.9 - 4.4 mg/kg/d over one year but remained below the reference interval *788*
Plasma Increase Physiological In 12 drug-treated patients with Parkinson's disease mean concentration 280 ± 230 µg/L compared with 1.5 ± 0.7 µg/L in 10 geriatric controls *1637*
Urine Increase Physiological In 8 levodopa treated patients with Parkinson's disease mean excretion 1900 ± 1600 mg/mol creatinine compared with 7 ± 6 mg/mol creatinine in 12 geriatric controls *1637*

Dopamine *Plasma Increase Physiological* In 12 drug-treated patients with Parkinson's disease mean concentration 1± 0.5 µg/L compared with < 0.1 µ.g/L in 10 healthy geriatric controls *1637*
Urine Increase Physiological In 8 drug-treated patients with Parkinson's disease mean excretion 3000 ± 2000 mg/mol creatinine compared with 30 ± 20 mg/mol creatinine in 12 healthy geriatric controls *1637* Response to therapy in Parkinsonism *4504* In 5 healthy volunteers given 300 mg significant increase 18,533 ± 3,425 µg/d from 1,209 ± 375 µg/d *389*

Dopamine, Conjugated *Urine Increase Physiological* In 5 healthy volunteers ingestion of 300 mg caused significant increase from mean baseline of 16630 ± 3428 µg/d from mean baseline of 959 ± 346 µg/d and proportion of total dopamine excreted increased from 76 ± 5 % to 88 ± 4 % *389*

Dopamine, Free *Urine Increase Physiological* In 5 healthy volunteers ingestion of 300 mg was followed by significant increase to 1903 ± 464 µg/d from mean baseline of 249 ± 53 µg/d *389*

Eosinophils *Blood Increase Physiological* Occasionally observed without symptoms *1276*

Epinephrine *Plasma No Effect Physiological* In 36 patients with essential hypertension treatment with 250 mg/d had no significant effect on concentration *5188* In 12 levodopa-treated patients with Parkinson's disease no significant effect observed *1637*

Erythrocytes *Blood Decrease Physiological* One case of hemolytic anemia reported *2754*
Urine Increase Physiological Occasional report of hematuria *128*

Fatty Acids (FFA), Free *Serum Increase Physiological* Significant increase if levodopa high in serum (i.v. greater effect) *4975*

Ferric Chloride Test *Urine Positive Analytical* When 1-5 g/d ingested black/brown color observed *882*

Folate *Serum Decrease Physiological* Associated with burning feet syndrome *1276*

Levodopa *(continued)*

Follicle Stimulating Hormone
Plasma Increase Physiological Possible increase over fluctuations in controls *4607*

Glucose *Serum Decrease Analytical* At concentrations above 3 mg/L lowered concentration as measured by GOD-PERID method *5704* May cause marked decrease with glucose oxidase method *4240* At concentrations above 100 mg/L lowered concentration as measured by Ektachem® method *5704* At concentrations above 300 mg/L lowered concentration as measured by Ames Seralyzer method *5704*
Serum Increase Analytical 29.4% increase with 10 mmol/L and 6.2% increase with 1 mmol/L and glucokinase based assay of Scott *5414* At 1 mmol/L affects Technicon SMA 12/60 method *5576* At 10 mg/dL affects alkaline ferricyanide procedure *2197*
Serum Increase Physiological Probably converted to dopamine which acts *741*
Serum No Effect Analytical No effect on hexokinase method *4240* No effect at 500 mg/L on hexokinase method on Ames Seralyzer *5706* At concentrations up to 500 mg/L no effect on method on Fuji Drichem 1000 *5706* At 10 mg/dL on MBTH procedure of Neeley *4241* At 10 mg/dL no effect on glucose oxidase procedure of Gochman *2197*
Serum No Effect Physiological No effect observed although increased plasma insulin *3031*
Urine Decrease Analytical False negative, inhibition of glucose oxidase method. False negative if Clinistix® used (no effect on TesTape®) *1825*
Urine No Effect Analytical No effect on TesTape® *1825*

Glycated Hemoglobin *Blood No Effect Analytical* At a concentration of 100 mg/L had an insignificant - 3.9% interference with method on Abbott Vision *1885*

Gonadotropins *Plasma Increase Physiological* Reported metabolic effect *2310*

Growth Hormone *Plasma Increase Physiological* In normals single dose cause increase in 1-2 h *3031* After i.v. infusion mean rose to 15.5 ng/mL *2821*

Guaiacols Spot Test *Urine Negative Analytical* Action on procedure of Rogers *5061*

HDL-Cholesterol *Serum No Effect Analytical* No effect of concentrations up to 6 mg/L on method on Kodak Ektachem® *5706*

Hematocrit *Blood Decrease Physiological* Administration of levodopa has been occasionally associated with decreased value *5027* Mild not related to hemolysis *128*

Hemoglobin *Blood Decrease Physiological* Administration of levodopa has been occasionally associated with decreased concentration *5027* Mild not related to hemolysis *128*
Urine Increase Physiological Occasional report of hematuria *128*

Histamine *Plasma No Effect Analytical* Concentrations at which inhibition of radio-enzyme assay occurs greatly exceed physiological concentrations *693*

Homovanillic Acid
Cerebrospinal Fluid Increase Physiological Concentrations in 4 patients with tyrosine hydroxylase deficiency increased 35 - 51% with treatment with 2.9 - 4.4 mg/kg/d over one year but remained below the reference interval *788* ?metabolic response (variable between individuals) *4505*
Urine Increase Physiological In Parkinsonian patients is response to therapy *850*

4-Hydroxy-3-Methoxy-Phenylglycol
Cerebrospinal Fluid Increase Physiological Concentrations in 4 patients with tyrosine hydroxylase deficiency increased 28 - 61% with treatment with 2.9 - 4.4 mg/kg/d over one year but remained below the reference interval *788*

Hydroxy-Methoxymandelic Acid *Urine Increase Analytical* In a patient given Sinemet® (levodopa/carbidopa) using Pisano method. Note high blank *1096*

17-Hydroxycorticosteroids *Urine Decrease Physiological* Possible inhibition of ACTH secretion *55*

5-Hydroxyindoleacetic Acid
Cerebrospinal Fluid Decrease Physiological Inhibition of 5-hydroxytryptophan hydroxylase *4505*
Urine Decrease Physiological In Parkinson's disease. ?increased tryptophan pyrrolase activity *782*

^{131}I Uptake *Serum Decrease Physiological* Larodopa® contains tetraiodofluorescein *4360*

Insulin *Plasma Increase Physiological* During therapy of Parkinsonism *3031*

Inulin Clearance *Urine Increase Physiological* ?secondary to renal vasodilatation or direct action on tubules *1867*

Isohomovanillic Acid *Urine Increase Physiological* Response to therapy in Parkinson patients *1105*

Ketones *Urine Increase Analytical* May produce false positive (trace or less) result with Ames Multistix and other reagent strip tests. Similar false positive result may occur with Ames Acetest reagent tablets *4034* Affects alkaline nitroprusside procedure *882* Intermittent false positive if Ketostix® or Phenistix® used *6523*

Lactate Dehydrogenase *Serum Increase Physiological* Rare instance of elevation, ?origin *128* Administration of levodopa has been associated with increased activity, but significance unknown *5027*
Serum No Effect Analytical No effect of concentrations up to 6 mg/L on method on Kodak Ektachem® systems *5706*

Leukocytes *Blood Decrease Physiological* Transitory depression in a few patients *128* Administration of levodopa has been occasionally associated with decreased concentration *5027*
Blood Increase Physiological Unassociated with fever or infection reported *1276*

Luteinizing Hormone *Plasma No Effect Physiological* No effect after 2 weeks in males *5580*

Lymphocytes *Blood Increase Physiological* Observed with hemolytic anemia *1276*

Metanephrines, Total *Urine Decrease Physiological* ?dopamine as neurotransmitter suppresses normetanephrine *2787*

Methionine *Cerebrospinal Fluid Decrease Physiological* In Parkinson patients significant effect after 2 weeks *2462*
Cerebrospinal Fluid No Effect Physiological No significant change observed in 6 dopamine-deficient children treated with levodopa *5877*

3-Methoxytyrosine
Cerebrospinal Fluid Increase Physiological Treatment with levodopa of 6 children with dopamine deficiency caused significant increase in CSF 3-methoxytyrosine concentration *5877*
Serum Increase Physiological Observed after 1 week when given levodopa *1831*

5-Methyltetrahydrofolate
Cerebrospinal Fluid No Effect Physiological No significant effect observed in 6 dopamine-deficient children treated with levodopa *5877*

Midazolam *Serum No Effect Analytical* On GC-ECD method of Ha et al *2387*

Monoamine Oxidase *Serum Increase Physiological* Increased activity after 2-3 mo therapy *6079*

Neutrophils *Blood Decrease Physiological* Occasional case of agranulocytosis reported *6264*

Norepinephrine *Plasma No Effect Physiological* In 36 patients with essential hypertension treatment with 250 mg orally had no significant effect on concentration *5188* In 12 levodopa-treated patients with Parkinson's disease no significant efect observed on plasma concentration *1637*
Urine Increase Physiological No effect on epinephrine excretion *5269*

Normetanephrine *Urine Decrease Physiological* Sharp decrease in normal after 3 g dose *4375*

3-o-Methyldihydrophenylalanine
Cerebrospinal Fluid Increase Physiological Concentrations in 4 patients with tyrosine hydroxylase deficiency increased to above reference interval (0 - 50 nmol/L) with treatment with 2.9 - 4.4 mg/kg/d over one year but remained below the reference interval *788*

Occult Blood *Feces Increase Physiological* Single case of gastritis with melena *4954*

PAH Clearance *Urine Increase Physiological* ?secondary to renal vasodilatation or direct action on tubules *1867*

Phenylalanine *Plasma No Effect Analytical* No interference observed with rapid quantitative whole blood method of Campbell et al using phenylalanine dehydrogenase *867*

Plasma No Effect Physiological In patients after 1 week given levodopa *1831*

Phosphate *Serum No Effect Analytical* At concentration of 197 mg/L had no effect on phosphomolybdate method *5704* No effect of concentrations up to 520 mg/L on method on Kodak Ektachem® *5706*

Platelets *Blood Decrease Physiological* Slight effect observed with hemolytic anemia *1276*

Potassium *Serum Decrease Physiological* Large doses may cause hypokalemia in association with increased plasma aldosterone concentrations *1384* Reduction of up to 0.9 mmol/L in normal subjects with inhalation of drug *2389*
Serum No Effect Analytical No effect at 20 mg/L on method on Ames Seralyzer but at higher concentrations potassium concentration appears to be increased although of no clinical significance *5706* No effect of concentrations up to 6 mg/L on method on Kodak Ektachem® *5706* At concentration of 200 mg/L had no effect on measurement by ISE with predilution *5704* At concentration of 100 mg/L caused nonsignificant 1.1% interference with method on Abbott Vision *681*
Urine Increase Physiological ?secondary to renal vasodilatation or direct action on tubules *1867*

Pramipexole *Serum No Effect Physiological* Coadministration of pramipexole with levodopa/carbidopa did not affect the pharmacokinetics of pramipexole *4680*

Prolactin *Plasma Decrease Physiological* Completely suppressed for 1-4 h after 250 mg orally *2382* In 36 patients with essential hypertension treatment with 250 mg/d caused significant reduction *5188* Transient effect in nonpuerperal galactorrhea *3748* Fall to 8.7% of baseline after 2 h in normals *796*

Proline *Plasma Increase Physiological* In Parkinson patients significant effect after 2 weeks *2462*

Protein *Serum No Effect Analytical* At concentration of 197 mg/L had no effect on biuret method with blank correction *5704*

PSP Excretion *Urine Increase Physiological* Increased plasma flow *1867*

Pyridoxine *Serum Decrease Physiological* Associated with burning feet syndrome *1276*

Renin Activity *Plasma Decrease Physiological* Mean concentration fell by 50% in 6 subjects given 7 µg/kg/min intravenously in contrast to slight rise following saline infusion *6542* In 36 patients with essential hypertension treatment with 250 mg/d caused significant reduction *5188*

Reticulocytes *Blood Increase Physiological* Hemolytic anemia when decarboxylase inhibitor also *741*

S-Adenosylmethionine *Blood Decrease Physiological* O-methylation of catecholamines slowed *3849*
Cerebrospinal Fluid Decrease Physiological Administration of levodopa to 6 children with dopamine deficiency caused significant decrease in CSF S-adenosylmethionine *5877*

Sodium *Serum No Effect Analytical* At concentration of 200 mg/L had no effect on measurement by ISE with predilution *5704*
Urine Increase Physiological Significant increase in excretion following intravenous infusion of 7 µg/kg/min in 6 subjects *6542* ?secondary to renal vasodilatation or direct action on tubules *1867*
Urine No Effect Physiological In 8 levodopa-treated patients with Parkinson's disease excretion of sodium not affected significantly *1637* In 5 volunteers after ingestion of 300 mg nonsignificant increase to 196 ± 18 mmol/d from baseline of 187 ± 14 mmol/d *389*

Sugar *Urine Increase Analytical* False positive with Clinitest® . Produces trace positive if Clinitest® used *1825*

T3-Uptake *Serum No Effect Physiological* No effect observed in chronic treatment *3031*

Testosterone *Serum No Effect Physiological* No significant effect observed after 2 weeks in males *5580*

Thyroid Stimulating Hormone
Serum Decrease Physiological In hypothyroidism but no change in euthyroid: is dopamine precursor. Diminishes response to TRH in hypothyroidism *6412*
Serum No Effect Physiological No effect observed *5563*

Thyroxine (T4) *Serum Increase Physiological* During therapy of Parkinsonism *3031*
Serum No Effect Physiological No effect observed *1276*

Triglycerides *Serum Decrease Analytical* At concentrations above 6 mg/L lowered concentration as measured by GPO-PAP method *5704*
Serum No Effect Analytical No effect of concentrations up to 6 mg/L on method on Kodak Ektachem® *5706*

Trihydroxyphenylacetate *Urine Increase Physiological* Observed in treatment of Parkinsonian patients *5226*

Tyrosine *Plasma No Effect Physiological* In patients after 1 week given levodopa *1831*

Urea Nitrogen *Serum Decrease Analytical* At concentrations above 100 mg/L lowered concentration as measured by Ames Seralyzer method *5704*
Serum Increase Physiological Affects hepatic enzymes, probably not dehydration *3815* Administration of levodopa has been associated with increased concentration, but significance unknown *5027*
Serum No Effect Analytical At concentration of 197 mg/L had no effect on diacetylmonoxime method *5704*

Uric Acid *Serum Decrease Analytical* At concentrations above 3 mg/L lowered concentration as measured by uricase-PAP method *5704*
Serum Increase Analytical Administration of levodopa has been associated with increased concentrations when some colorimetric procedures have been used *5027* Falsely high values with phosphotungstate methods *2197* At concentrations above 20 mg/L raised concentration as measured by phosphotungstate reduction method *5704*
Serum Increase Physiological Two cases reported, exaggerated by fructose *102*
Serum No Effect Analytical Administration of levodopa has been associated with increased concentrations when some colorimetric procedures have been used but not when uricase methods have been used *5027* No effect observed at a concentration of 10 mg/dL (0.5 mmol/L) on method on Du Pont aca *1552* At concentration of 3 mg/L had no effect on uricase method on Du Pont aca *5704* No increase reported when uricase used *128* No effect up to 100 mg/L on uricase method on Ames Seralyzer but at higher concentrations apparently reduced concentration of uric acid observed although not of clinical significance *5706* At concentrations up to 6 mg/L had no effect on method on Kodak Ektachem® *5706*
Urine Increase Analytical Falsely high values with phosphotungstate methods *2197*

Urobilin *Urine Increase Physiological* Usually minor and unimportant *1276*

Vanillylmandelic Acid *Urine Decrease Physiological* ?dopamine as neurotransmitter suppresses normetanephrine *2787*
Urine Increase Physiological Small increase, larger increase HVA *850*

Volume *Urine No Effect Physiological* In 5 volunteers following ingestion of 300 mg nonsignificant increase in excretion from mean 2200 ± 189 mL/d to 2550 ± 140 mL/d *389*

Levofloxacin

Cyclosporine *Serum No Effect Physiological* Concurrent administration of levofloxacin with cyclosporine A had no significant effect on the peak plasma concentration, or AUC of cyclosporine in healthy volunteers *3916* No significant effect observed on plasma concentration or AUC of cyclosporine in healthy volunteers *4448*

Cyclosporine A *Blood No Effect Physiological* No significant effect observed of levofloxacin on plasma concentration, AUC, and other disposition parameters of cyclosporine observed in healthy volunteers *3916*

Digoxin *Serum No Effect Physiological* No significant effect observed on plasma concentration or AUC of digoxin in healthy volunteers *4448* Concurrent administration of levofloxacin with digoxin had no significant effect on the peak plasma concentration, or AUC of digoxin in healthy volunteers *3916* No significant effect observed of levofloxacin on plasma concentration, AUC, and other disposition parameters of digoxin observed in healthy volunteers *3916*

Glucose *Serum Decrease Physiological* Both hyperglycemia and hypoglycemia observed in individuals receiving antidiabetic agents including insulin when levofloxacin *4448* Administration of levofloxacin in multiple doses was associated with a reduced glucose concentration in 1.9% patients *3916*

Levofloxacin *(continued)*

Glucose *(continued)*
Reduction in concentration observed in 1.9% when multiple doses of levofloxacin administered *3916*
Serum Increase Physiological Both hyperglycemia and hypoglycemia observed in individuals receiving antidiabetic agents including insulin when levofloxacin *4448*

Lymphocytes *Blood Decrease Physiological* Reduction in concentration observed in 1.9% patients when multiple doses of levofloxacin administered *3916* Administration of levofloxacin in multiple doses was associated with a reduced lymphocyte count in 1.9% patients *3916*

Prothrombin Time *Plasma No Effect Physiological* No significant effect observed when levofloxacin coadministered with warfarin *4448* No significant effect observed of levofloxacin on prothrombin time in patients receiving heparin concomitantly with levofloxacin *3916*

Theophylline *Serum No Effect Physiological* Concurrent administration of levofloxacin with theophylline had no significant effect on the plasma concentration and AUC of theophylline *3916* No significant effect observed of levofloxacin on plasma concentration, AUC, and other disposition parameters of theophylline observed in 14 healthy volunteers *3916* In 14 healthy volunteers no effect on plasma concentration or AUC of theophylline observed *4448*

Warfarin *Plasma No Effect Physiological* No significant effect observed on plasma concentration or AUC of R- or S-warfarin observed *4448* No significant effect observed of levofloxacin on plasma concentration, AUC, and other disposition parameters of R- and S-warfarin observed in healthy volunteers *3916* Concurrent administration of levofloxacin with warfarin had no significant effect on the plasma concentrations of either R- or S-warfarin *3916*

Levoglutamide

Ammonia *Plasma Decrease Analytical* Inhibits indophenol color in Berthelot reaction *4368*
Plasma Increase Physiological Potential source of additional ammonia *3161*
Plasma No Effect Analytical On indophenol reaction with 5,000 nmoles *2131*

Urea Nitrogen *Test Conditions Increase Analytical* Blue color with Berthelot's reagent *3144*

Levomepromazine

Amphetamine/Methamphetamine
Urine No Effect Analytical No false positive results observed in 15 urines from 14 patients taking drug when measured by Syva EMIT II procedure *5634*

Citalopram *Serum No Effect Physiological* Coadministration had no significant effect on citalopram kinetics although 10-20% increase in concentration of desmethylcitalopram from initial steady-state concentration *2288*

Levomethadyl Acetate

Alanine Aminotransferase *Serum Increase Physiological* Hepatitis and abnormal liver function observed in less than 1% of treated patients but causal relationship not established *5132*

Aspartate Aminotransferase *Serum Increase Physiological* Hepatitis and abnormal liver function observed in less than 1% of treated patients but causal relationship not established *5132*

Bilirubin *Serum Increase Physiological* Hepatitis and abnormal liver function observed in less than 1% of treated patients but causal relationship not established *5132*

γ-Glutamyltransferase *Serum Increase Physiological* Hepatitis and abnormal liver function observed in less than 1% of treated patients but causal relationship not established *5132*

Levonorgestrel

Albumin *Serum Increase Physiological* In a group of women using levonorgestrel covered rods versus controls using copper IUD *1419*
Serum No Effect Physiological No significant difference over 3 y between implant recipients and IUD users *1179*

Alkaline Phosphatase *Serum No Effect Physiological* In a group of women using levonorgestrel covered rods versus controls using copper IUD *1419* No significant difference over 3 y between implant recipients and IUD users *1179*

Androstenedione *Plasma Decrease Physiological* In 17 women using Norplant implants *2943*
Plasma Increase Physiological After 1 mo in 25 female volunteers when given as subdermal implant *4456*

Apolipoprotein A-I *Serum No Effect Physiological* No significant effect observed with levonorgestrel-only formulations. Mean concentration 1230 mg/L versus 1266 mg/L in nonuser controls *2201* When 150 µg levonorgestrel given with 30 µg ethinyl estradiol for 3 mo. Results normal within 2 mo after treatment stopped *504*

Apolipoprotein A-II *Serum No Effect Physiological* No significant effect with levonorgestrel-only formulations: mean concentration 338 mg/L versus 336 mg/L in nonuser controls *2201*

Apolipoprotein B *Serum Increase Physiological* Increase by 19% (apo B: apo A-I increased by 18%) when 150 µg levonorgestrel given with 30 µg ethinyl estradiol for 3 mo. Results normal within 2 mo after treatment stopped *504*
Serum No Effect Physiological No effect observed with either 30 or 37.5 mg regime. Mean concentration 598 mg/L versus 572 mg/L in nonuser controls *2201*

Aspartate Aminotransferase
Serum No Effect Physiological In a group of women using levonorgestrel covered rods versus controls using copper IUD *1419* No significant difference over 3 y between implant recipients and IUD users *1179*

Bilirubin *Serum No Effect Physiological* In a group of women using levonorgestrel covered rods versus controls using copper IUD *1419* No significant difference over 3 y between implant recipients and IUD users *1179*

Calcium *Serum No Effect Physiological* In a group of women using levonorgestrel covered rods versus controls using copper IUD *1419* No significant difference over 3 y between implant recipients and IUD users *1179*

Ceruloplasmin *Serum Decrease Physiological* Significant decrease throughout cycle in women ingesting 150 µg daily *5700* Slight effect with daily dose of 0.125 mg in 30 healthy female volunteers when given alone. Values normal within 30 d of end of treatment *5157*

Cholesterol *Serum Decrease Physiological* In 20 women receiving 250 µg/d on days 15 to 28 of cycle *6032* Significant reduction in patients over 3 y compared with patients with IUDs for 2 1/2 y *1179*
Serum No Effect Physiological Insignificant decrease in 11 normolipoproteinemic women given 250 µg/d for 2 weeks *6032* In a group of women using levonorgestrel covered rods versus controls using copper IUD *1419* When 150 µg levonorgestrel given with 30 µg ethinyl estradiol for 3 mo. Results normal within 2 mo after treatment stopped *504*

Corticosteroid-Binding Globulin
Serum No Effect Physiological With daily dose of 0.125 mg in 30 healthy female volunteers when given alone. Values normal within 30 d of end of treatment *5157*

Cortisol *Plasma No Effect Physiological* In a group of women using levonorgestrel versus control group with copper IUD *5304* No effect observed in group of women 20 and 65 mo after levonorgestrel treated rods inserted in uterus *1419*

Cyclosporine *Serum Increase Physiological* Observed effect presumed to be due to inhibition of hepatic microsomal enzymes although levonorgestrel known to stimulate some hepatic enzymes *1069*

Estradiol *Plasma Decrease Physiological* In a group of women using levonorgestrel versus control group with copper IUD *1419*
Plasma No Effect Physiological No effect observed in group of women 20 and 65 mo after levonorgestrel treated rods inserted in uterus *1419*

Glucose *Serum Increase Physiological* In implant users in comparison with IUD users (average difference of 5 mg/dL) *1179*
Serum No Effect Physiological In a group of women using levonorgestrel covered rods versus controls using copper IUD *1419*

Glucose Tolerance *Serum Decrease Physiological* Levonorgestrel-only preparations increased incremental area to 9.3 mmol/L/min compared with 7.3 mmol/L/min in non-oral contraceptive user controls *2201*

Glycated Protein *Serum No Effect Physiological* When 150 µg levonorgestrel given with 30 µg ethinyl estradiol for 3 mo. Results normal within 2 mo after treatment stopped *504*

HDL_2-Cholesterol *Serum Decrease Physiological* Oral contraceptive combinations containing levonorgestrel reduced concentration by 15 to 43% with the highest dose causing the greatest effect *2201* Decrease of 50% observed in women when estradiol added to regime with levonorgestrel *6032*

HDL_3-Cholesterol *Serum No Effect Physiological* No effect observed when estradiol added to regime involving levonorgestrel *6032*

HDL-Cholesterol *Serum Decrease Physiological* Significant reduction in 20 women receiving 250 µg/d on days 15 to 18 of cycle *6032* With daily dose of 0.125 mg in 30 healthy female volunteers when given alone. Values normal within 30 d of end of treatment *5157* Decrease of 27% observed in women when estradiol added to regime with levonorgestrel *6032*
Serum No Effect Physiological When 150 µg levonorgestrel given with 30 µg ethinyl estradiol for 3 mo. Results normal within 2 mo after treatment stopped *504* No difference between implant recipients and IUD users *1179*

HDL-Triglycerides *Serum Decrease Physiological* Significant effect in 20 women receiving 250 µg/d on days 15 to 28 of cycle *6032*
Serum No Effect Physiological Insignificant increase in 11 normolipoproteinemic women given 250 µg/d for 2 weeks *6032*

Lactate Dehydrogenase *Serum No Effect Physiological* No significant difference over 3 y between implant recipients and IUD users *1179* In a group of women using levonorgestrel covered rods versus controls using copper IUD *1419*

LDL-Cholesterol *Serum Decrease Physiological* Significant reduction in patients over 3 y compared with patients with IUDs for 2 1/2 y *1179*
Serum No Effect Physiological Insignificant increase in 11 normolipoproteinemic women given 250 µg/d for 2 weeks *6032*

LDL-Triglycerides *Serum Decrease Physiological* By about 14 % in 11 normolipoproteinemic women given 250 µg/d for 2 weeks *6032*

Phosphate *Serum Decrease Physiological* Significant slight reduction in implant recipients compared with IUD users over 3 y *1179*
Serum No Effect Physiological In a group of women using levonorgestrel covered rods versus controls using copper IUD *1419*

Postheparin Hepatic Lipase *Plasma Increase Physiological* Increase by 64% in 11 normolipoproteinemic women given 250 µg/d for 2 weeks *6032* Increase by 64% in 20 women receiving 250 µg/d on days 15 to 28 of cycle. Increase of 97% observed when estradiol added to levonorgestrel regime *6032*

Postheparin Lipoprotein Lipase
Plasma No Effect Physiological No effect observed in 20 women receiving 250 µg/d during days 15 to 28 of cycle *6032* Insignificant increase in 11 normolipoproteinemic women given 250 µg/d for 2 weeks *6032*

Protein *Serum Increase Physiological* In a group of women using levonorgestrel covered rods versus controls using copper IUD *1419*
Serum No Effect Physiological No significant difference over 3 y between implant recipients and IUD users *1179*

Sex-Hormone Binding Globulin
Serum Decrease Physiological With daily dose of 0.125 mg in 30 healthy female volunteers when given alone. Values normal within 30 d of end of treatment *5157* In 17 women using Norplant implants *2943* In women receiving 150 µg daily concentration decreased throughout a cycle of treatment *5700*

Sperm Count *Semen Decrease Physiological* When combined with testosterone enanthate may cause oligospermia *1499*

Testosterone *Serum Decrease Physiological* In 17 women using Norplant implants *2943* In a group of women using levonorgestrel versus control group with copper IUD *1419*
Serum Increase Physiological Approximately 24% increase after 6 mo use of subdermal implant *4456*
Serum No Effect Physiological No effect observed in group of women 20 and 65 mo after levonorgestrel treated rods inserted in uterus *1419*

Testosterone, Free *Serum No Effect Physiological* In 17 women using Norplant implants *2943*

Thyroid Stimulating Hormone
Serum No Effect Physiological No effect observed in group of women 20 and 65 mo after levonorgestrel treated rods inserted in uterus *1419*

Thyroxine (T4) *Serum No Effect Physiological* In a group of women using levonorgestrel versus control group with copper IUD *1419* No effect observed in group of women 20 and 65 mo after levonorgestrel treated rods inserted in uterus *1419*

Tri-iodothyronine (T3) *Serum No Effect Physiological* No effect observed in group of women 20 and 65 mo after levonorgestrel treated rods inserted in uterus versus control group with copper IUD *1419*

Triglycerides *Serum Decrease Physiological* Significant reduction in patients over 3 y compared with patients with IUDs for 2 1/2 y *1179* Increase by 32 % in 11 normolipoproteinemic women given 250 µg/d for 2 weeks *6032*
Serum Increase Physiological Increase by 48% when 150 µg levonorgestrel given with 30 µg ethinyl estradiol for 3 mo. Results normal within 2 mo after treatment stopped *504*

Urea Nitrogen *Serum No Effect Physiological* In a group of women using levonorgestrel covered rods versus controls using copper IUD *1419* No significant difference over 3 y between implant recipients and IUD users *1179*

Uric Acid *Serum No Effect Physiological* In a group of women using levonorgestrel covered rods versus controls using copper IUD *1419* No significant difference over 3 y between implant recipients and IUD users *1179*

VLDL-Cholesterol *Serum Decrease Physiological* By more than 50% in 11 normolipoproteinemic women given 250 µg/d for 2 weeks *6032*

VLDL-Triglycerides *Serum Decrease Physiological* Increase by 45% in 11 normolipoproteinemic women given 250 µg/d for 2 weeks *6032*

Levorphanol

Creatinine *Serum Increase Physiological* Administration of levodopa has been associated with kidney failure *5028*

Morphine *Urine Increase Analytical* Cross reacts equally (or more) with RIA procedures *4163*
Urine No Effect Analytical Insignificant cross react with hemagglutination inhibition *4163*

Opiates *Urine Positive Analytical* At concentration of 3.0 µg/mL (11.65 µmol/L) on method on Du Pont aca *1559*

Urea Nitrogen *Serum Increase Physiological* Administration of levodopa has been associated with kidney failure *5028*

Levothyroxine

Alanine Aminotransferase *Serum Increase Physiological* Increase observed with therapy in individuals whose hypothyroidism occurred spontaneously but no change observed in those whose hypothyroidism was due to prior radioiodine *2273*

Alkaline Phosphatase *Serum Increase Physiological* Administration of levothyroxine may increase activity as a result of enhanced bone turnover *6526*

Apolipoprotein A *Serum No Effect Physiological* Insignificant change from 2.7 to 2.8 g/L in 11 hypothyroid women treated with 0.1 to 0.2 mg daily *1969*

Apolipoprotein A-I *Serum Decrease Physiological* In 12 patients with hypothyroidism mean concentration decreased significantly from 1.38 ± 0.09 g/L to 1.25 ± 0.08 g/L after one month's treatment with up to 150 µg/d levothyroxine *4572*

Levothyroxine *(continued)*

Apolipoprotein A-I *(continued)*
Serum No Effect Physiological No significant effect observed over 4 months in 13 stable subclinical hypothyroid patients given thyroxine to restore euthyroid state *238* In 19 hypothyroid patients in whom initial FTI was 0 - 15 treatment to change FTI to 55 - 65 caused nonsignificant change in apolipoprotein A-I concentration from 1.72 ± 0.37 g/L to 1.79 ± 0.46 g/L *1303*

Apolipoprotein B *Serum Decrease Physiological* In 12 patients with hypothyroidism mean concentration decreased significantly from 1.89 ± 0.02 g/L to 1.52 ± 0.17 g/L after one month's treatment with up to 150 µg/d levothyroxine *4572* In 19 overtly hypothyroid individuals treatment starting with 25 µg/d and causing change of FTI from 0 - 15 to 45 - 55 caused significant change from 1174 ± 268 mg/L to 701 ± 207 mg/L *1303* In 13 stable subclinical hypothyroid patients treatment to restore euthyroid state caused decrease from mean baseline concentration of 91 mg/dL to 74 mg/dL and 75 mg/dL at 4 months *238*

Basal Metabolic Rate *Patient Increase Physiological* Metabolic effect of hormone (maximum at 1 week) *3669*

Carbonic Anhydrase I
Red Blood Cells Decrease Physiological In patients with thyroid nodules receiving suppresive doses of thyroxine mean concentration 300 ± 53 nmol/g hemoglobin significantly reduced compared with those with primary hypothyroidism receiving replacement doses of thyroxine (340 ± 57 nmol/g hemoglobin) *6604*

Catechol-O-Methyltransferase
Test Conditions Decrease Physiological Heavy doses inhibit *in vivo1944*

Cholesterol *Serum Decrease Physiological* In 70 patients with primary hypothyroidism treatment caused median concentration to decrease significantly from 272 mg/dL to 225 mg/dL *4351* In 29 thyroidectomized patients treatment with thyroxine caused significant reduction from mean baseline of 342 ± 78 mg/dL to 193 ± 46 mg/dL *5735* In 13 patients with stable subclinical hypothyroidism treatment to restore euthyroid state caused decrease from mean baseline concentration of 5.5 mmol/L to 4.8 mmol/L at 2 months *238* Often therapeutic intent *5869* In 12 patients with hypothyroidism mean concentration decreased significantly from 8.04 ± 0.57 mmol/L to 6.43 ± 0.41 mmol/L after one month's treatment with up to 150 µg/d levothyroxine *4572* From 7.8 to 6.1 mmol/L in 11 hypothyroid women treated with 0.1 to 0.2 mg daily *1969* In 26 patients with hypothyroidism treatment caused concentration to decrease significantly from mean pretreatment concentration of 6.29 mmol/L to 5.40 mmol/L *2963*

2,3-Diphosphoglycerate Mutase
Blood No Effect Physiological No effect on amount of 2,3-DPG produced *6057*

Epidermal Growth Factor *Urine Decrease Physiological* In 23 patients following total thyroidectomy for papillary carcinoma of the thyroid treated with thyroxine mean concentration of EGF decreased substantially and was inversely correlated with TSH concentrations and positively associated with serum thyroxine concentrations *2748*

Estriol *Urine Decrease Physiological* Decreased formation due to metabolic action *54*

Fatty Acids (FFA), Free *Serum Decrease Physiological* Correction of hypothyroid state *5869*

γ-Glutamyltransferase *Serum Increase Physiological* Increased activity observed in individuals whose hypothyroidism had occurred spontaneously although not in those in whom it followed radioiodine treatment *2273*

Glutathione S-Transferase *Serum Increase Physiological* Dose-dependent increase observed in individuals being treated for hypothyroidism due to either radioiodine therapy or when it had occurred spontaneously *2273* In hypothyroid patients treated with thyroxine significant increase in activity observed *448*

HDL_2-Cholesterol *Serum Decrease Physiological* In 12 patients with hypothyroidism mean concentration decreased significantly from 0.65 ± 0.09 mmol/L to 0.52 ± 0.07 mmol/L after one month's treatment with up to 150 µg/d levothyroxine *4572*
Serum Increase Physiological Slight tendency to increase in 13 stable subclinical hypothyroid patients treated with thyroxine over 4 months *238*

HDL_2-Phospholipids *Serum Decrease Physiological* In 12 patients with hypothyroidism mean concentration changed significantly from 0.67 ± 0.08 mmol/L to 0.59 ± 0.08 mmol/L after one month's treatment with up to 150 µg/d levothyroxine *4572*

HDL_2-Triglycerides *Serum Decrease Physiological* In 12 patients with hypothyroidism mean concentration decreased nonsignificantly from 0.07 ± 0.01 mmol/L to 0.05 ± 0.01 mmol/L after one month's treatment with up to 150 µg/d levothyroxine *4572*

HDL_3-Cholesterol *Serum Decrease Physiological* In 12 patients with hypothyroidism mean concentration decreased nonsignificantly from 0.81 ± 0.04 mmol/L to 0.80 ± 0.06 mmol/L after one month's treatment with up to 150 µg/d levothyroxine *4572*
Serum No Effect Physiological No significant change observed in 13 stable subclinical hypothyroid patients given thyroxine to restore euthyroid state over 4 months *238*

HDL_3-Phospholipids *Serum No Effect Physiological* In 12 patients with hypothyroidism mean concentration changed nonsignificantly from 0.90 ± 0.07 mmol/L to 0.91 ± 0.07 mmol/L after one month's treatment with up to 150 µg/d levothyroxine *4572*

HDL_3-Triglycerides *Serum No Effect Physiological* In 12 patients with hypothyroidism mean concentration changed nonsignificantly from 0.26 ± 0.03 mmol/L to 0.26 ± 0.03 mmol/L after one month's treatment with up to 150 µg/d levothyroxine *4572*

HDL-Cholesterol *Serum Decrease Physiological* In 44 patients with primary hypothyroidism treatment caused median concentration to decrease from 58 mg/dL to 51 mg/dL *4351* In 12 patients with hypothyroidism mean concentration decreased nonsignificantly from 1.46 ± 0.13 mmol/L to 1.32 ± 0.10 mmol/L after one month's treatment with up to 150 µg/d levothyroxine *4572* In 29 hypothyroid patients treatment with levothyroxine caused significant reduction from mean baseline of 75 ± 22 mg/dL to 56 ± 18 mg/dL *5735* In 13 stable subclinical hypothyroid patients given thyroxine to restore euthyroid state increase from mean baseline concentration of 4.8 mmol/L to 4.5 mmol/L at 2 months and 3.9 mmol/L at 4 months *238* From 1.6 to 1.4 mmol/L in 11 hypothyroid women treated with 0.1 to 0.2 mg daily *1969*
Serum No Effect Physiological In 19 hypothyroid individuals with FTI 0 - 15 treatment to bring FTI to 55 - 65 caused nonsignificant change from mean baseline of 1.12 ± 0.28 mmol/L to 1.14 ± 0.23 mmol/L *1303*

HDL-Phospholipids *Serum Decrease Physiological* In 12 patients with hypothyroidism mean concentration changed nonsignificantly from 1.57 ± 0.14 mmol/L to 1.50 ± 0.13 mmol/L after one month's treatment with up to 150 µg/d levothyroxine *4572*

HDL-Triglycerides *Serum Decrease Physiological* In 12 patients with hypothyroidism mean concentration decreased nonsignificantly from 0.33 ± 0.03 mmol/L to 0.30 ± 0.03 mmol/L after one month's treatment with up to 150 µg/d levothyroxine *4572*

2-Hydroxyestrone *Urine Increase Physiological* Metabolic effect of hormone administration *54*

Hydroxyproline *Urine Increase Physiological* Administration of levothyroxine may increase concentration as a result of enhanced bone turnover *6526*

^{131}I Uptake *Serum Decrease Physiological* Due to metabolic effect of drug *3669*

immunoglobulin A *Serum Decrease Physiological* In all 5 children with infantile hypothyroidism soon after start of treatment in 4 concentration returned to normal *5421*

Immunoglobulin G *Serum No Effect Physiological* No significant effect in children with infantile hypothyroidism *5421*

Immunoglobulin M *Serum No Effect Physiological* No significant effect in children with infantile hypothyroidism *5421*

LDL-Cholesterol *Serum Decrease Physiological* In 42 patients with primary hypothyroidism treatment caused median concentration to decrease significantly from 195 mg/dL to 160 mg/dL *4351* From 5.5 to 4.1 mmol/L in 11 hypothyroid women treated with 0.1 to 0.2 mg daily *1969* In 13 patients with stable subclinical hypothyroidism treatment to restore euthyroidism caused decrease from mean baseline concentration of 3.7 mmol/L to 2.9 mmol/L at 2 months and 4 months *238* In 12 patients with hypothyroidism mean concentration decreased significantly from 5.71 ± 0.62 mmol/L to 4.37 ± 0.44 mmol/L after one month's treatment with up to 150 µg/d levothyroxine *4572* In 19 hypothyroid individuals treatment to bring FTI from 0 - 15 to 55 - 65 caused change in LDL-cholesterol concentration from 6.45 ± 1.13 mmol/L to 4.28 ± 1.11 mmol/L *1303* In 29 thyroidectomized patients treatment with thyroxine caused significant reduction from mean baseline of 225 ± 72 mg/dL to 111 ± 43 mg/dL *5735*

LDL-Cholesterol:HDL-Cholesterol Ratio
Serum Decrease Physiological In 13 stable subclinical hypothyroid patients treatment with thyroxine to restore euthyroid state caused decrease from mean baseline ratio of 3.3 to 2.9 at 2 months and 2.5 at 4 months *238*

Lipoprotein Lp(a) *Serum Decrease Physiological* In 29 thyroidectomized patients treatment with levothyroxine caused nonsignificant reduction from mean baseline of 80 mg/L to 55 mg/L *5735* In 19 hypothyroid individuals treatment with 25 µg/d caused a 55% decrease from 255 to 116 mg/L after 4 weeks *1303* In 12 patients with hypothyroidism mean concentration decreased nonsignificantly from 496 ± 123 mg/L to 464 ± 128 mg/L after one month's treatment with up to 150 µg/d levothyroxine *4572*
Serum Increase Physiological In 8 of 19 hypothyroid patients after initial treatment with 25 µg/d for 4 weeks which reduced concentration to 116 mg/L with increased doses concentration increased to 196 mg/L (69%) associated with increase of FTI from 15 - 25 to 25 - 35 *1303*

2-Methoxyestrone *Urine Increase Physiological* Metabolic effect on hormone administration *54*

Monoamine Oxidase *Serum Decrease Physiological* Observed *in vitro* and *in vivo1944*

Neutrophils *Blood Decrease Physiological* May cause neutropenia *4265*

Norepinephrine *Plasma Decrease Physiological* From high pretreatment values to normal range with 30-60 d treatment of 7 hypothyroid women with dry thyroid extract *3770*

Osteocalcin *Serum Increase Physiological* Administration of levothyroxine may increase concentration as a result of enhanced bone turnover *6526*

Phospholipids *Serum Decrease Physiological* Correction of hypothyroid state *5869*

Prothrombin Time *Plasma Increase Physiological* May potentiate action of anticoagulants *2754*

Pyridinium Crosslinks *Urine Increase Physiological* Administration of levothyroxine may increase concentration as a result of enhanced bone turnover *6526*

Sex-Hormone Binding Globulin
Serum Increase Physiological In 19 hypothyroid individuals with initial FTI 0 - 15 and SHBG concentration of 15.4 ± 12.6 nmol/L treatment to change FTI to 55 - 65 caused SHBG to increase to 46.8 ± 29.2 nmol/L *1303* Concentration significantly increased in patients treated with thyroid hormone *1804*

Soluble Interleukin-2 Receptor
Serum Increase Physiological In 22 patients with hypothyroid autoimmune thyroiditis in whom mean concentration was 48.6 pmol/L treatment with L-thyroxine caused significant increase to 85.1 pmol/L similar to 86.4 pmol/L in 21 age and sex-matched healthy controls *3665*

T3-Uptake *Serum Increase Physiological* From 0.59 to 0.98 arbitrary units in 11 hypothyroid women treated with 0.1 to 0.2 mg daily *1969*

Thyroid Stimulating Hormone
Serum Decrease Physiological In 13 patients with stable subclinical hypothyroidism treatment to restore euthyroid state caused decrease from mean baseline concentration of 16.6 mU/L to 3.1 mU/L at 2 months and 3.2 mU/L at 4 months *238* In 62 patients with primary hypothyroidism treatment caused median concentration to decrease significantly from 43 mIU/L to 1.2 mIU/L *4351* In 27 euthyroid individuals significant reduction compared with controls *2761* In 26 hypothyroid patients treatment caused decrease of mean concentration from 39.0 mU/L to 2.01 mU/L *2963* Suppressed concentration in many patients taking drug *5109* In hypothyroidism in response to T4 analog *6412*
Serum Increase Physiological 50% premenopausal clinically euthyroid women taking replacement or suppressive doses of L-thyroxine had increased indices *6526*
Serum No Effect Physiological In euthyroid patients treatment with T4 therapy caused concentration to decrease to low or low-normal level *2412*

Thyroxine Binding Globulin *Serum No Effect Analytical* On radioimmunoassay procedure of Van Herle *6188*

Thyroxine (T4) *Serum Increase Physiological* From 24 to 124 nmol/L 11 hypothyroid women treated with 0.1 to 0.2 mg daily *1969* 62% of 27 euthyroid individuals receiving L-thyroxine had concentrations in hyperthyroid range *2761* Patients taking replacement or suppressive doses of L-thyroxine may increase concentration *6526* In euthyroid patients treatment with T4 therapy caused slight increase in concentration or no change *2412* Endogenous hormone suppressed, exogenous measured *572* Slight effect observed in many patients taking customary doses of drug without clinical symptoms of hyperthyroidism *5109* Raised but still less than controls with 30-60 d treatment of 7 hypothyroid women with dry thyroid extract *3770* In 26 hypothyroid patients treatment caused significant increase of mean concentration from 61.5 nmol/L to 129.9 nmol/L *2963* In 65 patients with primary hypothyroidism treatment caused median concentration to increase significantly from 4.1 µg/dL to 8.5 µg/dL *4351*

Thyroxine (T4), Free *Serum Decrease Physiological* Falls with therapy of hypothyroid state *2754*
Serum Increase Physiological In 27 clinically euthyroid individuals concentration increased as measured by 3 different analog assays with percentage of individuals in hyperthyroid range varying from 41-63% *2761* Raised but still less than controls with 30-60 d treatment of 7 hypothyroid women with dry thyroid extract *3770* In 29 hypothyroid patients treatment caused significant increase to 20 ± 3 pg/mL from mean baseline of 2.4 ± 0.4 pg/mL *5735* In euthyroid patients treatment with T4 therapy caused slight increase in concentration or no change *2412* Patients taking replacement or suppressive doses of L-thyroxine may increase concentration *6526*

Thyroxine (T4) Index, Free *Serum Increase Physiological* in premenopausal clinically euthyroid women taking replacement or suppressive doses of L-thyroxine had increased indices *6526*

Tirofiban *Serum Decrease Physiological* Coadministration with tirofiban increased the rate of plasma clearance of tirofiban *3957*

Tri-iodothyronine, Free (fT3) *Serum Increase Physiological* In 29 treated hypothyroid patients mean concentration increased significantly from 1.2 ± 3.0 pg/mL to 5.2 ± 1 pg/mL *5735*
Serum No Effect Physiological In euthyroid patients treatment with T4 therapy had no effect on plasma concentration *2412*

Tri-iodothyronine, Reverse (rT3)
Serum No Effect Physiological In euthyroid patients treatment with T4 therapy had no effect on plasma concentration *2412*

Tri-iodothyronine (T3) *Serum Increase Analytical* 33% cross reactivity if product from Cyclo *5438*
Serum Increase Physiological In 26 patients with hypothyroidism treatment caused increase from mean pretreatment concentration of 1.37 nmol/L to 1.78 nmol/L *2963* From 0.7 to 17 nmol/L in 11 hypothyroid women treated with 0.1 to 0.2 mg daily *1969*
Serum No Effect Analytical Cross-reactivity of 0.4% observed with method on Baxter Stratus *5705*
Serum No Effect Physiological In euthyroid patients treatment with T4 therapy had no effect on plasma concentration *2412* In 27 euthyroid individuals receiving L-thyroxine no significant difference from controls *2761* Apparently normal concentration in many patients although T4 may be slightly increased *5109* Patients taking replacement or suppressive doses of L-thyroxine have on effect on concentration *6526*

Triglycerides *Serum Decrease Physiological* In 12 patients with hypothyroidism mean concentration decreased from 1.91 ± 0.38 mmol/L to 1.60 ± 0.21 mmol/L after one month's treatment with up to 150 µg/d levothyroxine *4572* In 29 thyroidectomized patients mean concentration decreased

Levothyroxine *(continued)*

Triglycerides *(continued)*
from baseline of 182 ± 87 mg/dL to 112 ± 42 mg/dL *5735* In 19 hypothyroid individuals with FTI 0 - 15 treatment to bring FTI 55 - 65 caused significant reduction of triglyceride concentration from 3.03 ± 1.61 mmol/L to 1.30 ± 0.75 mmol/L *1303* In 13 stable subclinical hypothyroid patients treatment with levothyroxine caused decrease from mean baseline concentration of 1.3 mmol/L to 0.9 mmol/L at 4 months *238* In 69 patients with primary hypothyroidism treatment caused median concentration to decrease from 108 mg/dL to 101 mg/dL *4351*
Serum Increase Physiological Effect observed in hypothyroid patients *4074*
Serum No Effect Physiological Insignificant effect in 11 hypothyroid women treated with 0.1 to 0.2 mg daily *1969*

Lidocaine

Acetaminophen *Serum No Effect Analytical* No interference observed at a concentration of 2000 µg/mL (853 µmol/L) with method on Du Pont aca *1506*

Alanine Aminotransferase *Serum No Effect Analytical* No effect Technicon SMA 12/60 method with 3.5 mg/dL *4390*

Albumin *Serum No Effect Analytical* No effect on Technicon SMA 12/60 method with 3.5 mg/dL *4390*

Alkaline Phosphatase *Serum No Effect Analytical* No effect Technicon SMA 12/60 method with 3.5 mg/dL *4390*

Bilirubin *Serum No Effect Analytical* No effect Technicon SMA 12/60 method with 3.5 mg/dL *4390*

Calcium *Serum No Effect Analytical* No effect Technicon SMA 12/60 method with 3.5 mg/dL *4390*

Cholesterol *Serum No Effect Analytical* No effect Technicon SMA 12/60 method with 3.5 mg/dL *4390*

Cholinesterase *Serum No Effect Analytical* No effect observed at concentration of 4 mg/dL with butyrylthiocholine method on Kodak Ektachem® *2504*

Cocaethylene *Urine No Effect Analytical* No interference observed with TLC method of Bailey *328*

Creatine Kinase *Serum Increase Physiological* Intramuscular injection may increase plasma activity of creatine kinase *280*

Creatine Kinase Isoenzymes *Serum No Effect Analytical* No interference observed at a concentration of 40 mg/L (170.7 µmol/L) with CK-MB method on Du Pont aca *1519*

Creatinine *Serum Increase Analytical* Some interference in some specimens with Gen02 slides for Kodak Ektachem® system, but rarely more than 3 mg/L *2261* Lidocaine per se does not interfere but positive bias due to metabolite N-ethylglycine. Effect less marked with generations 2 onwards than with first generation. In this study less than 2% creatinine results had a clinically significant bias *5444*
Serum No Effect Analytical No effect on Technicon SMA 12/60 method with 3.5 mg/dL *4390*

Cyclosporine *Blood No Effect Analytical* At a concentration of 60 mg/L had no effect on Syva EMIT method *495*

D-Dimer *Plasma Increase Physiological* In 10 apparently healthy men administration of lidocaine 3 mg/kg into a vein in the hand at a rate of 20 mL/min caused a significant change in concentration from the ipsolateral arm (80 ng/mL at baseline, 193 ng/mL after 20 min, 111 ng/mL after 50 min) *4292*

Drugs of Abuse Screen *Urine No Effect Analytical* No effect at concentration of 100 µg/mL on EZ-SCREEN procedure for cannabinoids and cocaine *1739*

Glucose *Serum No Effect Analytical* No effect Technicon SMA 12/60 method with 3.5 mg/dL *4390* At concentration of 3.2 mg/L had no effect on Kodak Ektachem® method *5704*

Hematocrit *Blood No Effect Physiological* In 10 apparently healthy men administration of lidocaine 3 mg/kg into a vein in the hand at a rate of 20 mL/min caused no significant change in blood from the contralateral arm *4292*

Histamine *Plasma No Effect Analytical* Improbable inhibition of radio-enzyme assay at physiological concentrations *2492*

Lactate Dehydrogenase *Serum No Effect Analytical* No effect Technicon SMA 12/60 method with 3.5 mg/dL *4390*

Midazolam *Serum No Effect Analytical* On GC-ECD method of Ha et al *2387*

Mycophenolic Acid *Serum No Effect Analytical* No significant interference observed with HPLC method of Shipkova et al *5526*

Mycophenolic Acid Glucuronide
Serum No Effect Analytical No significant interference observed with HPLC method of Shipkova et al *5526*

N-Acetylprocainamide *Serum No Effect Analytical* No significant interference observed at a concentration of 100 µg/mL (427 µmol/L) with method on Du Pont aca *1536*

p-Aminophenol *Urine No Effect Analytical* With addition of drugs at a concentration of 100 mg/L and of related compounds at 50 mg/L no significant effect observed on colorimetric method of van Bocxlaer on Cobas Mira analyzer which involves reacting free p-aminophenol with resorcinol in the presence of magnesium ions to form an indophenol dye measured at 550 nm *6163*

Phenylalanine *Plasma No Effect Analytical* No interference observed with rapid quantitative whole blood method of Campbell et al using phenylalanine dehydrogenase *867*

Phosphate *Serum No Effect Analytical* No effect Technicon SMA 12/60 method with 3.5 mg/dL *4390*

Plasminogen Activator Inhibitor
Plasma No Effect Physiological In 10 apparently healthy men administration of lidocaine 3 mg/kg into a vein in the hand at a rate of 20 mL/min caused an insignificant change in concentration from the ipsolateral arm (6.4 AU/mL at baseline, 5.0 AU/mL after 20 min, 5.0 AU/mL after 50 min) *4292*

Platelet Aggregation response to ADP
Blood No Effect Physiological In 10 apparently healthy men administration of lidocaine 3 mg/kg into a vein in the hand at a rate of 20 mL/min caused an insignificant change in concentration from the ipsolateral arm (0.6 µmol/L at baseline, 0.7 µmol/L after 20 min, 0.7 µmol/L after 50 min) *4292*

Platelets *Blood No Effect Physiological* In 10 apparently healthy men administration of lidocaine 3 mg/kg into a vein in the hand at a rate of 20 mL/min caused no significant change in blood platelets from the contralateral arm (baseline 253,000 /µL, 248,000 /µL after 20 min, and 256,000 /µL after 50 min) *4292*

Potassium *Serum No Effect Analytical* At concentration of 0.5 mg/L had no effect on measurement by ISE with predilution *5704*

Procainamide *Serum Decrease Analytical* Superpharmacologic doses of lidocaine may inhibit the fluorescence of procainamide and NAPA *4530*
Serum No Effect Analytical No significant interference observed at a concentration of 100 µg/mL (427 µmol/L) with method on Du Pont aca *1542*

Protein *Cerebrospinal Fluid Increase Analytical* Reacts with Folin-Ciocalteu reagent *2024*
Serum No Effect Analytical No effect Technicon SMA 12/60 method with 3.5 mg/dL *4390*

Protein C Activity *Plasma Decrease Physiological* In 10 apparently healthy men administration of lidocaine 3 mg/kg into a vein in the hand at a rate of 20 mL/min caused a significant change in concentration from the ipsolateral arm (96% at baseline, 83% after 20 min, 94% after 50 min) *4292*

Quinidine *Serum No Effect Analytical* Lidocaine at a concentration of 100 µg/mL had no significant cross-reactivity with quinidine at a concentration of 2.0 µg/mL in method on Bayer Technicon Immuno 1® *431* At concentrations of greater than 5000 mg/L causes 30% increase in concentration as measured by method on Baxter Stratus but physiological concentrations are up to 6 mg/L only *5705* No significant interference observed at a concentration of 100 µg/mL (427 µmol/L) with method on Du Pont aca *1543*

SDZ PSC 833 *Blood No Effect Analytical* At a concentration of 6.5 mg/L had no effect on HPLC method of Scott et al when used to measure PSC (with CsD as internal standard) at a concentration of 5 mg/L *5418*

Sodium *Serum No Effect Analytical* At concentration of 0.5 mg/L had no effect on measurement by ISE with predilution *5704*

Tacrolimus *Blood No Effect Analytical* No significant effect observed at a concentration of 5 mg/L with MEIA method on Abbott IMx analyzer *1871*

Serum *Increase* *Analytical* In HPLC/MS method of Christians et al interference observed with measurement of metabolites of FK 506 because of similar retention time *1010*
Serum *No Effect* *Analytical* At a concentration of 5 mg/L had no significant effect on ELISA method *6329*

β-Thrombomodulin *Plasma* *No Effect* *Physiological* In 10 apparently healthy men administration of lidocaine 3 mg/kg into a vein in the hand at a rate of 20 mL/min caused a significant change in concentration from the ipsolateral arm (19.7 IU/mL at baseline, 25.6 IU/mL after 20 min, 19.1 IU/mL after 50 min) *4292*

Tissue Plasminogen Activator
Plasma *Increase* *Physiological* In 10 apparently healthy men administration of lidocaine 3 mg/kg into a vein in the hand at a rate of 20 mL/min caused a significant change in concentration from the ipsolateral arm (0.5 IU/mL at baseline, 2.1 IU/mL after 20 min, 0.6 IU/mL after 50 min) *4292*

Tissue Plasminogen Activator Antigen
Plasma *Increase* *Physiological* In 10 apparently healthy men administration of lidocaine 3 mg/kg into a vein in the hand at a rate of 20 mL/min caused a significant change in concentration from the ipsolateral arm (3.8 ng/mL at baseline, 7.1 ng/mL after 20 min, 3.4 ng/mL after 50 min) *4292*

Urea Nitrogen *Serum* *No Effect* *Analytical* At concentration of 3.2 mg/L had no effect on Kodak Ektachem® method *5704*

Uric Acid *Serum* *No Effect* *Analytical* No effect Technicon SMA 12/60 method with 3.5 mg/dL *4390*

Lidoflazine

Digoxin *Serum* *No Effect* *Physiological* Reportedly no effect on serum concentration *558*

γ-Glutamyltransferase *Serum* *Increase* *Physiological* ?due to changes in vasculature *1771* Positive correlation with clinical state (normal liver function tests) *520*

Lifibrol

Apolipoprotein A-I *Serum* *No Effect* *Physiological* In 168 patients with primary hypercholesterolemia treatment for one month with 150, 300, 450 or 600 mg/d caused mean changes of +6.9%, -2.8%, -6.6% and -3.2% respectively *5390*

Apolipoprotein B *Serum* *Decrease* *Physiological* In 168 patients with primary hypercholesterolemia treatment for one month with 150, 300, 450 or 600 mg/d caused mean reductions of 9.2%, 24.3%, 28.2% and 34.3% respectively *5390* In about 90 patients with primary hypercholesterolemia treatment with 150 mg/d and 300 mg/d for 4 weeks caused mean reductions of 15 ± 2% and 25 ± 2% respectively *3630*

Campesterol *Serum* *Decrease* *Physiological* In about 90 patients with primary hypercholesterolemia treatment with 150 mg/d and 300 mg/d for 4 weeks caused mean reductions of 10 ± 5% and 16 ± 4% respectively from mean baseline of about 3.7 mg/mL with greater effects at higher concentrations *3630*

Cholesterol *Serum* *Decrease* *Physiological* In 168 patients with primary hypercholesterolemia treatment for one month with 150, 300, 450 or 600 mg/d caused mean reductions of 9.4%, 21.8%, 26.4% and 28.4% respectively *5390* In about 90 patients with primary hypercholesterolemia treatment with 150 mg/d and 300 mg/d for 4 weeks caused mean reductions of 10 ± 2% and 22 ± 3% respectively *3630*

Creatinine Clearance *Urine* *No Effect* *Physiological* In about 90 patients with primary hypercholesterolemia treatment with 150 to 900 mg/d for 4 weeks caused nonconsistent nonsignificant reduction from mean baseline *3630*

Desmosterol *Serum* *Decrease* *Physiological* In about 90 patients with primary hypercholesterolemia treatment with 150 mg/d and 300 mg/d for 4 weeks caused mean reductions of 8 ± 4% and 13 ± 4% respectively from mean baseline of about 1.60 mg/mL with greater effects at higher concentrations *3630*

Fibrinogen *Plasma* *Decrease* *Physiological* In 168 patients with primary hypercholesterolemia treatment for one month with 150, 300, 450 or 600 mg/d caused mean reductions of 7.0%, 6.1%, 17.8% and 13.5% respectively *5390*

Glycochenodeoxycholic Acid
Serum *Increase* *Physiological* In about 90 patients with primary hypercholesterolemia treatment with 300 mg/d for 4 weeks caused significant mean change of 144 ± 56% from mean baseline of 1121 ± 299 mg/mL with greater effects at higher concentrations, but change with 150 mg/d not significant *3630*

Glycocholic Acid *Serum* *Increase* *Physiological* In about 90 patients with primary hypercholesterolemia treatment with 300 mg/d for 4 weeks caused significant mean change of 263 ± 107% from mean baseline of 420 ± 133 mg/mL with greater effects at higher concentrations, but change with 150 mg/d not significant *3630*

Glycodeoxycholic Acid *Serum* *Increase* *Physiological* In about 90 patients with primary hypercholesterolemia treatment with 300 mg/d for 4 weeks caused significant mean change of 79 ± 36% from mean baseline of 520 ± 141 mg/mL with greater effects at higher concentrations, but change with 150 mg/d not significant *3630*

HDL-Cholesterol *Serum* *No Effect* *Physiological* In 168 patients with primary hypercholesterolemia treatment for one month with 150, 300, 450 or 600 mg/d caused mean changes of +8.1%, -4.5%, -5.3% and -1.5% respectively *5390*

Hypoxanthine *Urine* *No Effect* *Physiological* In about 90 patients with primary hypercholesterolemia treatment with 150 to 900 mg/d for 4 weeks caused nonconsistent nonsignificant change from mean baseline *3630*

Lanosterol *Serum* *Decrease* *Physiological* In about 90 patients with primary hypercholesterolemia treatment with 150 mg/d and 300 mg/d for 4 weeks caused mean reductions of 24 ± 6% and 27 ± 7% respectively from mean baseline of about 0.30 mg/mL *3630*

Lathosterol *Serum* *Decrease* *Physiological* In about 90 patients with primary hypercholesterolemia treatment with 150 mg/d and 300 mg/d for 4 weeks caused mean reductions of 16 ± 4% and 28 ± 5% respectively from mean baseline of about 2.45 mg/mL with greater effects at higher concentrations *3630*

LDL-Cholesterol *Serum* *Decrease* *Physiological* In 168 patients with primary hypercholesterolemia treatment for one month with 150, 300, 450 or 600 mg/d caused mean reductions of 11.1%, 27.7%, 34.5% and 35.0% respectively *5390* In about 90 patients with primary hypercholesterolemia treatment with 150 mg/d and 300 mg/d for 4 weeks caused mean reductions of 14 ± 3% and 27 ± 4% respectively *3630*

LDL-Cholesterol:HDL-Cholesterol Ratio
Serum *Decrease* *Physiological* In about 90 patients with primary hypercholesterolemia treatment with 150 mg/d and 300 mg/d for 4 weeks caused mean reductions of 11 ± 6% and 28 ± 3% respectively *3630*

Lipoprotein Lp(a) *Serum* *Decrease* *Physiological* In 168 patients with primary hypercholesterolemia treatment for one month with 150, 300, 450 or 600 mg/d caused mean reductions of 8.1%, 9.7%, 16.6% and 13.4% respectively *5390*

Mevalonate *Urine* *No Effect* *Physiological* In about 90 patients with primary hypercholesterolemia treatment with 150 to 900 mg/d for 4 weeks caused nonconsistent nonsignificant change from mean baseline *3630*

β-Sitosterol *Serum* *Decrease* *Physiological* In about 90 patients with primary hypercholesterolemia treatment with 150 mg/d and 300 mg/d for 4 weeks caused mean reductions of 13 ± 4% and 16 ± 4% respectively from mean baseline of about 2.7 mg/mL with similar effects at higher concentrations *3630*

Squalene *Serum* *No Effect* *Physiological* In about 90 patients with primary hypercholesterolemia treatment with doses from 150 mg/d to 900 mg/d for 4 weeks caused variable responses from a reduction of 23% to an increase of 48% *3630*

Triglycerides *Serum* *Decrease* *Physiological* In 168 patients with primary hypercholesterolemia treatment for one month with 150, 300, 450 or 600 mg/d caused mean changes of -9.5%, -10.3%, +0.8% and -27.9% respectively *5390* In about 80 patients with primary hypercholesterolemia treatment with 300 mg/d and 900 mg/d for 4 weeks caused mean reductions of 15 to 23% *3630*

Uric Acid *Urine* *No Effect* *Physiological* In about 90 patients with primary hypercholesterolemia treatment with 150 to 900 mg/d for 4 weeks caused nonconsistent nonsignificant change from mean baseline *3630*

Lifibrol *(continued)*

Xanthine *Urine No Effect Physiological* In about 90 patients with primary hypercholesterolemia treatment with 150 to 900 mg/d for 4 weeks caused nonconsistent nonsignificant change from mean baseline *3630*

Lincomycin

Alanine Aminotransferase *Serum Increase Physiological* Hepatotoxic-cholestatic effect *3669*

Alkaline Phosphatase *Serum Increase Physiological* Hepatotoxic-cholestatic effect *1714*

Aspartate Aminotransferase *Serum Increase Physiological* Hepatotoxic-cholestatic effect *3669*

Bile *Urine Increase Physiological* Occurs with hepatotoxicity *3810*

Bilirubin *Serum Increase Physiological* Hepatotoxic-cholestatic effect *3669*

Serum No Effect Physiological Clinically insignificant displacement from protein in neonates *6314*

Chloramphenicol *Serum No Effect Analytical* No effect at 100 mg/L on coupled enzymatic method *4122*

Cholesterol *Serum Decrease Physiological* Hepatotoxic effect *3669*

Creatinine *Serum No Effect Analytical* No effect of concentrations up to 15 mg/L on single slide method on Kodak Ektachem® systems *5706*

Fat *Feces Increase Physiological* Steatorrhea may result from mucosal damage *5055*

Folate *Serum Decrease Analytical* Inhibits growth of *L. Casei5870*

Glucose *Serum Decrease Physiological* May occur with hepatotoxicity *3669*

^{131}I Uptake *Serum Decrease Physiological* Lincocin® contains tetraiodofluorescein *4360*

Leukocytes *Blood Decrease Physiological* Agranulocytosis/Leukopenia/neutropenia *131*

Neutrophils *Blood Decrease Physiological* Occasional case of agranulocytosis reported *6264*

5'-Nucleotidase *Serum Increase Physiological* Due to cholestasis *2911*

Occult Blood *Feces Increase Physiological* Occasional case of pseudomembranous colitis reported with bloody or mucus diarrhea *689* May cause severe enterocolitis *5540*

Phenylalanine *Plasma No Effect Analytical* No interference observed with rapid quantitative whole blood method of Campbell et al using phenylalanine dehydrogenase *867*

Platelets *Blood Decrease Physiological* Rare reversible thrombocytopenia *2242*

Linoleamide

Cholesterol *Serum Decrease Physiological* Inhibits sterol absorption *1480*

Linseed Oil

HDL-Cholesterol *Serum Decrease Physiological* Significant decrease observed in 11 mildly hypercholesterolemic men fed 9 g/d for 6 weeks *7*

LDL-Cholesterol *Serum Decrease Physiological* Mean decrease of 0.10 mmol/L in 11 mildly hypercholesterolemic men fed 9 g/d for 6 weeks *7*

Triglycerides *Serum No Effect Physiological* In 11 mildly hypercholesterolemic men supplement of 9 g/d for 6 weeks *7*

Liothyronine

Basal Metabolic Rate *Patient Increase Physiological* Metabolic effect of hormone *3669*

Digitalis-like Immunoreactivity

Serum Decrease Physiological Thyroid hormone replacement increases the metabolic rate of digitalis requiring an increase in digitalis dosage *5640*

Glucose *Serum Increase Physiological* Initially treatment may cause an increase in insulin or oral hypoglycemic agent requirement *5640*

^{131}I Uptake *Serum Decrease Physiological* Except in hyperthyroidism *3669*

Thyroxine (T4) *Serum Decrease Physiological* Depression of endogenous hormone *3669*

Liotrix

Cholesterol *Serum Decrease Physiological* In hypothyroids falls to within normal range *2754*

Prothrombin Time *Plasma Increase Physiological* May potentiate action of oral anticoagulants *2754*

T3-Uptake *Serum Increase Physiological* Increases but remains within normal range *2754*

Lipid Emulsion

Fibronectin *Plasma No Effect Physiological* No effect of 10 hour infusion observed over 24 hours in 10 patients *674*

Lipomul®

Bicarbonate *Serum Decrease Physiological* Nephrotoxic effect with azotemia *1714*

BSP Retention *Serum Increase Physiological* Part of fat-overloading syndrome *4014*

Creatinine *Serum Increase Physiological* Nephrotoxic effect *3810*

Erythrocytes *Blood Decrease Physiological* May be progressive anemia with excess *4014*

Urine Increase Physiological May cause actual bleeding *1714*

Hemoglobin *Blood Decrease Physiological* May be severe hemolytic anemia *4014*

Urine Increase Physiological Produces actual bleeding *1714*

Nonprotein Nitrogen *Serum Increase Physiological* Nephrotoxic effect *3810*

Occult Blood *Feces Increase Physiological* May be severe gastrointestinal tract bleeding *4014*

Phosphate *Serum Increase Physiological* May occur with azotemia *3810*

Platelets *Blood Decrease Physiological* Thrombocytopenia with fat-overloading *3810*

Potassium *Serum Increase Physiological* Nephrotoxic effect *3810*

Protein *Urine Increase Physiological* Nephrotoxic effect *1714*

Urea Nitrogen *Serum Increase Physiological* Possible nephrotoxic effect *1009*

Uric Acid *Serum Increase Physiological* Decreased clearance *3810*

Liposyn

Alanine Aminotransferase *Serum No Effect Analytical* No effect of concentrations up to 30,000 mg/L on method on Kodak Ektachem® *5706*

Aspartate Aminotransferase *Serum No Effect Analytical* No effect of concentrations up to 30,000 mg/L on method on Kodak Ektachem® *5706*

Bicarbonate *Serum No Effect Analytical* With 2% Liposyn® given as total parenteral nutrition no effect on nonenzymatic method on Kodak Ektachem® *2519*

Bilirubin *Serum No Effect Analytical* At a concentration of 10% causes no significant effect on method on Kodak Ektachem® systems *2519*

Cholesterol *Serum No Effect Analytical* At a concentration of 10% causes no significant effect on method on Kodak Ektachem® systems *2519*

Creatinine *Serum No Effect Analytical* At a concentration of 10% causes no significant effect on method on Kodak Ektachem® systems *2519*

Lactate Dehydrogenase *Serum No Effect Analytical* No effect of concentrations up to 30,000 mg/L on method on Kodak Ektachem® *5706*

Lipase *Serum Increase Analytical* 3.3% Liposyn® will give a DP error at a concentration of 7.9 mmol/L, as does 6.6% Liposyn® at 15.8 mmol/L and 10% Liposyn® at 23.1 mmol/L with method on Kodak Ektachem® systems *2519*

Phosphate *Serum No Effect Analytical* At a concentration of 10% causes no significant effect on method on Kodak Ektachem® systems *2519*

Triglycerides *Serum Increase Physiological* Infusion will cause increase which typically will revert to normal within 18 - 24 hours *2519*

Lisinopril

Alanine Aminotransferase *Serum Increase Physiological* Hepatitis (hepatocellular or cholestatic jaundice) reported as infrequent complication of treatment *3990* May cause hepatocellular hepatitis or cholestatic jaundice in 0.3 to 1.0% treated patients *6651*

Aldosterone *Plasma Decrease Physiological* In 15 hypertensives treatment with lisinopril for 6 months caused significant decrease of plasma aldosterone concentration *3436*

Alkaline Phosphatase *Serum Increase Physiological* Hepatitis (hepatocellular or cholestatic jaundice) reported as infrequent complication of treatment *3990*

Amino-terminal Propeptide of Type III Procollagen
Serum Decrease Physiological In 15 hypertensives treatment with lisinopril for 6 months caused significant decrease from mean baseline of 11.76 ng/mL to 8.47 ± 0.66 ng/mL *3436*

Amylase *Serum Increase Physiological* Pancreatitis reported as infrequent complication of treatment *3990* May cause pancreatitis in 0.3 to 1.0% treated patients *6651*

Angiotensin-I *Plasma Increase Physiological* Significant increase from mean baseline concentration of 30.2 pg/mL to 161 pg/mL at 6 hours with concentration remaining high up to 24 hours in 8 healthy volunteers following a single oral dose of 20 mg *3075*

Angiotensin-II *Plasma Decrease Physiological* Significant decrease from mean baseline concentration of 6.76 pg/mL to 1.84 pg/mL at 4 hours, 2.10 pg/mL at 8 hours but returned to 5.84 pg/mL at 24 hours following a single oral dose of 20 mg in 8 healthy volunteers *3075*

Angiotensin-converting Enzyme
Serum Decrease Physiological Decrease from mean baseline activity of 13.2 mU/mL to 5.69 mU/mL at 2 hours, 0.99 mU/mL at 6 hours and 3.58 mU/mL at 24 hours in 8 healthy volunteers following a single oral dose of 20 mg *3075*

Angiotensinogen *Plasma No Effect Physiological* No significant change from mean baseline concentration of 1.22 µg/mL over subsequent 24 hours in 8 healthy volunteers given a single oral dose of 20 mg *3075*

Apolipoprotein A-I *Serum Decrease Physiological* In proteinuric patients treatment with lisinopril reduced both protein excretion and plasma concentration of apolipoprotein A-I *4235*

Apolipoprotein B *Serum Decrease Physiological* In proteinuric patients treatment with lisinopril reduced both protein excretion and plasma concentration of apolipoprotein B *4235*

Apolipoprotein Lp(a) *Serum Decrease Physiological* In proteinuric patients treatment with lisinopril reduced both protein excretion and plasma concentration of apolipoprotein Lp(a) *4235*

Aspartate Aminotransferase *Serum Increase Physiological* May cause hepatocellular hepatitis or cholestatic jaundice in 0.3 to 1.0% treated patients *6651* Hepatitis (hepatocellular or cholestatic jaundice) reported as infrequent complication of treatment *3990*

Bilirubin *Serum Increase Physiological* Rare increases of serum bilirubin concentration observed *6651* Hepatitis (hepatocellular or cholestatic jaundice) reported as infrequent complication of treatment *3990*

Cholesterol *Serum Decrease Physiological* Significant change observed from mean baseline of 177 ± 8 mg/dL to 161 ± 8 mg/dL in 16 young adults with mild hypertension treated with lisinopril for 12 weeks *1791* In proteinuric patients treatment with lisinopril reduced both protein excretion and plasma concentration of total cholesterol *4235* In 19 middle-aged patients with essential hypertension treatment with up to 40 mg/d for up to 12 weeks caused decrease of 0.26 ± 0.24 mmol/L from mean baseline of 5.03 ± 0.17 mmol/L *4397* In 19 patients with essential hypertension treatment with up to 8 mg/d for 8 - 12 weeks caused reduction of 0.26 ± 0.24 mmol/L from mean baseline of 5.03 ± 0.17 mmol/L *4397*
Serum Increase Physiological Nonsignificant increase from mean baseline concentration of 208 mg/dL to 213 mg/dL in 13 nondiabetic hypertensives treated for mean of 9.0 months and from 214 mg/dL to 219 mg/dL in 15 diabetic hypertensives treated for a mean of 8.3 months *5525*
Serum No Effect Physiological No effect observed when given as monotherapy to patients with essential hypertension *6470* In 10 patients with mild hypertension treatment with 10 mg/d for 6 months caused nonsignificant change from mean baseline of 190 ± 8 mg/dL to 193 ± 7 mg/dL *1306*

Creatinine *Serum Decrease Physiological* Significant reduction from mean baseline concentration of 1.0 mg/dL to 0.8 mg/dL in 13 nondiabetic hypertensives treated for mean of 9.0 months and from 1.1 mg/dL to 0.9 mg/dL in 15 diabetic hypertensives treated for a mean of 8.3 months *5525*
Serum Increase Physiological In one of 66 patients treated with up to 40 mg/d serum creatinine concentration increased to 156 µmol/L from 93 µmol/L *454* May cause uremia, progressive azotemia or renal dysfunction *6651* Minor increase observed, reversible on discontinuation of lisinopril, observed in about 2.0% of hypertensive patients and in 11.6% patients with heart failure also receiving diuretics *3990* Administration of lisinopril was asssociated with an increased concentration in about 2.0% patients with essential hypertension *3990*
Serum No Effect Physiological No significant effect of treatment of 8 non-insulin dependent hypertensive diabetics treated with mean dose of 32 mg daily for 6 weeks *339* Nonsignificant increase from mean baseline concentration of 93.7 µmol/L to 95.4 µmol/L in 66 patients with essential hypertension treated with up to 40 mg/d for 8 weeks *454*

Creatinine Clearance *Urine No Effect Physiological* No significant effect of treatment with mean dose of 32 mg daily for 6 weeks in 8 non-insulin dependent hypertensive diabetics *339*

Digoxin *Serum No Effect Physiological* No clinically significant interaction observed when drugs coadministered *6651* Coadministration of lisinopril with digoxin appears to have no effect on plasma digoxin concentration *3990*

Erythrocyte Aggregation Time
Blood Increase Physiological In 41 patients with mild to moderate hypertension treated with 20 mg/d for 4 weeks caused significant increase from mean baseline of 1.98 ± 0.50 s to 2.08 ± 0.52 s *6630*

Erythrocyte Disaggregation Shear Rate
Blood Decrease Physiological In 41 mild to moderate hypertensives treatment with 20 mg/d for 4 weeks caused significant decrease from mean baseline of 159 ± 46 s to 153 ± 40 s *6630*

Erythrocyte Disaggregation Shear Stress
Blood Decrease Physiological In 41 patients with mild to moderate hypertension treatment with 20 mg/d for 4 weeks caused reduction from 705 ± 257 mPa to 659 ± 204 mPa *6630*

Filterability Index *Blood No Effect Physiological* In 41 patients with mild to moderate hypertension treatment with 20 mg/d for 4 weeks caused nonsignificant increase from 16.99 ± 4.11 to 17.31 ± 3.22 *6630*

Filtration Fraction *Urine Decrease Physiological* In 12 patients with mild to moderate essential hypertension administration of 20 mg caused significant reduction from mean baseline of 27 ± 1% to 23 ± 1% after 4 h and 24 ± 1% after 6 h *1347*
Urine No Effect Physiological In 12 patients with mild to moderate essential hypertension treatment with 20 mg/d for 3 months caused nonsignificant reduction from 27 ± 1% to 25 ± 1% *1347*

Lisinopril *(continued)*

Glomerular Filtration Rate *Urine No Effect Physiological* In 12 patients with mild to moderate essential hypertension administration of 20 mg caused no significant change from baseline of 57 mL/min/sq m. When given the same dose daily for 3 months mean rate changed nonsignificantly from 57 ± 2 mL/min/sq m to 58 mL/min/sq m *1347*

Glucose *Serum Decrease Physiological* Incidence of 0.6% observed in French Pharmacovigilance database *4106* Reduction from mean baseline concentration of 137 mg/dL to 121 mg/dL in 15 diabetic hypertensives treated with lisinopril for a mean of 8.3 months *5525*

Serum Increase Physiological Diabetes mellitus reported as rare complication of treatment *3990* May cause diabetes mellitus *6651* In 19 middle-aged patients with essential hypertension treatment with up to 40 mg/d for up to 12 weeks caused increase of 0.3 ± 0.2 mmol/L from mean baseline of 6.2 ± 0.2 mmol/L *4397*

Serum No Effect Physiological No significant change observed from mean baseline of 98 ± 3 mg/dL to 98 ± 3 mg/dL in 16 young adults with mild hypertension treated with lisinopril for 12 weeks *1791* Insignificant reduction from 98 mg/dL to 95 mg/dL in 13 nondiabetic hypertensives treated with lisinopril for mean of 9.0 months *5525*

Urine Increase Physiological Diabetes mellitus reported as rare complication of treatment *3990*

Glucose Tolerance *Serum Increase Physiological* Significant improvement in tolerance in response to 75 g oral glucose *4397*

γ-Glutamyltransferase *Serum Increase Physiological* Hepatitis (hepatocellular or cholestatic jaundice) reported as infrequent complication of treatment *3990*

HDL-Cholesterol *Serum Decrease Physiological* In 19 middle-aged patients with essential hypertension treatment with up to 40 mg/d for up to 12 weeks caused decrease of 0.10 ± 0.07 mmol/L from mean baseline of 0.96 ± 0.07 mmol/L *4397* In proteinuric patients treatment with lisinopril reduced both protein excretion and plasma concentration of HDL-cholesterol *4235*

Serum No Effect Physiological Nonsignificant increase from mean of 48.8 mg/dL to 51.0 mg/dL in 13 nondiabetic hypertensives treated for a mean of 9.0 months and from 43.6 mg/dL to 47.6 mg/dL in 15 diabetic hypertensives treated for a mean of 8.3 months *5525* No effect observed when given as monotherapy to patients with essential hypertension *6470* In 10 patients with mild hypertension treatment with 10 mg/d for 6 months caused nonsignificant change from mean baseline of 41 ± 3 mg/dL to 42 ± 5 mg/dL *1306* Nonsignificant change observed from mean baseline of 47 ± 4 mg/dL to 46 ± 3 mg/dL in 16 young adults with mild hypertension treated with lisinopril for 12 weeks *1791*

Hematocrit *Blood Decrease Physiological* May cause rare cases of bone marrow depression or hemolytic anemia: mean decrease of approximately 1.3% observed frequently *6651* Administration of lisinopril was asssociated with a mean decrease of 1.3% *3990* Bone marrow depression, neutropenia and thrombocytopenia reported as rare complications of treatment. Hematocrit may decrease by as much as 1.3% commonly without clinical impact *3990*

Blood No Effect Physiological In 41 patients with mild to moderate hypertension treatment with 20 mg/d for 4 weeks nonsignificant reduction from 43.0 ± 3.7% to 42.6 ± 3.8% observed *6630*

Hemoglobin *Blood Decrease Physiological* Mean decrease of about 0.4 g/dL observed frequently in treated patients *3990* May cause rare cases of bone marrow depression or hemolytic anemia: mean decrease of 0.4 g/dL observed frequently *6651* Bone marrow depression, neutropenia and thrombocytopenia reported as rare complications of treatment. Concentration may decrease commonly by as much as 0.4 g/dL without clinical impact *3990* Administration of lisinopril was asssociated with a mean decrease of 0.4 g/dL *3990*

Hemoglobin A_{1c} *Blood Decrease Physiological* Significant reduction from mean baseline concentration of 7.9% to 7.2% in 15 diabetic hypertensives treated for a mean of 8.3 months *5525*

Blood No Effect Physiological No significant change observed in 13 nondiabetic hypertensives treated for a mean of 9.0 months *5525*

Hydrochlorothiazide *Serum No Effect Physiological* No clinically significant interaction observed when drugs coadministered *6651* Coadministration of lisinopril with hydrochlorothiazide appears to have no effect on the pharmacokinetics of either drug *3990*

Initial Blood Filterability *Blood No Effect Physiological* In 41 patients with mild to moderate hypertension treatment with 20 mg/d for 4 weeks caused nonsignificant change from 29.2 ± 8.0 to 29.3 ± 9.3 *6630*

Insulin *Plasma Increase Physiological* In 19 patients with essential hypertension treatment with up to 8 mg/d caused significant increase of 0.0 ± 1.5 μU/mL in fasting insulin concentration from mean baseline of 11.9 ± 0.9 μU/mL *4397*

Plasma No Effect Physiological No significant change observed from mean baseline of 14.3 ± 1.7 μU/mL to 19.3 ± 4.1 μU/mL in 16 young adults with mild hypertension treated with lisinopril for 12 weeks *1791* In 19 middle-aged patients with essential hypertension treatment with up to 40 mg/d for up to 12 weeks caused no change in fasting basal concentration from mean baseline of 11.9 ± 0.9 μU/mL *4397*

LDL-Cholesterol *Serum Decrease Physiological* Significant change observed from mean baseline of 107 ± 7 mg/dL to 91 ± 7 mg/dL in 16 young adults with mild hypertension treated with lisinopril for 12 weeks *1791*

Serum No Effect Physiological In 10 patients with mild hypertension treatment with 10 mg/d for 6 months caused nonsignificant change from mean baseline of 119 ± 5 mg/dL to 118 ± 6 mg/dL *1306* No effect observed in patients with essential hypertension when given as monotherapy *6470*

Lecithin:Cholesterol Acyltransferase
Serum Decrease Physiological In proteinuric patients treatment with lisinopril reduced both protein excretion and the increased plasma activity of LCAT *4235*

Leukocytes *Blood Decrease Physiological* May cause rare cases of bone marrow depression with leukopenia *6651*

Lipase *Serum Increase Physiological* May cause pancreatitis in 0.3 to 1.0% treated patients *6651* Pancreatitis reported as infrequent complication of treatment *3990*

Lithium *Serum Increase Physiological* Coadministration of lisinopril with lithium probably increases its plasma concentration as been reported for other ACE inhibitors which cause elimination of sodium *3990*

Lithium Clearance *Urine Decrease Physiological* Coadministration of lisinopril with lithium probably increases its plasma concentration as been reported for other ACE inhibitors which cause elimination of sodium *3990*

Malondialdehyde *Blood Increase Physiological* In 41 patients with mild to moderate hypertension treatment with 20 mg/d for 4 weeks caused increase from mean baseline of 5.52 ± 2.25 nmol/L per 10^9 platelets to 6.98 ± 2.45 nmol/L per 10^9 platelets *6630*

Neutrophils *Blood Decrease Physiological* Post-marketing experience suggests that there may be occasional neutropenia and bone marrow depression as with captopril *3990* May cause rare cases of bone marrow depression with neutropenia *6651*

Nifedipine *Serum No Effect Physiological* Coadministration produced no effect on kinetics of nifedipine *3485*

Nitrate *Serum No Effect Physiological* No clinically significant interaction observed when drugs coadministered *6651*

Platelet Aggregation *Blood No Effect Physiological* In 41 patients with mild to moderate hypertension treatment with 20 mg/d for 4 weeks had no significant effect on arachidonic acid-induced aggregation *6630* No sgnificant change in ADP-induced aggregation observed in 39 patients with mild to moderate hypertension after treatment for 4 weeks with 20 mg *6630*

Platelets *Blood Decrease Physiological* Bone marrow depression, neutropenia and thrombocytopenia reported as rare complications of treatment *3990* May cause rare cases of bone marrow depression with thrombocytopenia *6651*

Blood No Effect Physiological In 41 patients with mild to moderate hypertension treatment with 20 mg/d for 4 weeks caused nonsignificant change from mean baseline of 232,048 ± 8,956 /μL to 255,804 ± 85,085 /μL *6630*

Potassium *Red Blood Cells No Effect Physiological* Nonsignificant change observed from mean baseline of 100 ± 3.0 mmol/L cells to 98 ± 3.5 mmol/L cells in 16 young adults with mild hypertension treated with lisinopril for 12 weeks *1791*

Serum Increase Physiological May cause hyperkalemia *6651* Administration of lisinopril was asssociated with increase of serum potassium to greater than 5.7 mmol/L observed in approximately 4.8% patients with heart failure and in 2.2% patients with hypertension *3990* In clinical trials hyperkalemia (concentration greater than 5.7 mmol/L) observed in approximately 2.2% hypertensive patients and 4.8% patients with heart failure *3990* In two of 66 patients receiving up to 40 mg/d for 8 weeks serum potassium concentrations increased to 5.1 and 5.3 mmol/L *454*

Serum No Effect Physiological No significant change observed in 66 patients with essential hypertension treated with up to 40 mg/d for 8 weeks *454*

Propranolol *Serum No Effect Physiological* Coadministration of lisinopril with propranolol appears to have no effect on the pharmacokinetics of either drug *3990* No clinically significant interaction observed when drugs coadministered *6651*

Protein *Urine Decrease Physiological* In proteinuric patients treatment with lisinopril reduced excretion from mean baseline of 8.1 ± 1.5 g/d to 3.7 ± 1.3 g/d *4235* Reduction from mean of 3.8 g/d to 2.6 g/d in 8 non-insulin dependent hypertensive diabetics treated with mean dose of 32 mg daily for 6 weeks *339*

Renal Plasma Flow *Patient Increase Physiological* In 12 patients with mild to moderate essential hypertension adminiistration of 20 mg caused significant increase from baseline of 216 ± 11 mL/min/sq m to 227 mL/min/sq m at 2 h, 245 mL/min/sq m at 4 h and 236 mL/min/sq m at 6 h *1347*

Patient No Effect Physiological In 12 patients with mild to moderate essential hypertension treatment with 20 mg/d for 3 months caused nonsignificant mean change from 216 ± 11 mL/min/sq m to 231 mL/min/sq m *1347*

Renin Activity *Plasma Increase Physiological* In 15 hypertensives treatment with lisinopril for 6 months caused significant increase in renin activity concomitant with decrease in PIIIP *3436* Significant reduction from mean baseline of 1.97 ng/mL/h to 10.8 ng/mL/h at 6 hours which remained increased to 10.3 ng/mL/h in 8 healthy volunteers given single oral dose of 20 mg *3075*

Sodium *Red Blood Cells No Effect Physiological* Nonsignificant change observed from mean baseline of 8.3 ± 0.44 mmol/L cells to 8.9 ± 0.49 mmol/L cells in 16 young adults with mild hypertension treated with lisinopril for 12 weeks *1791*

Serum Decrease Physiological Administration of lisinopril was asssociated with hyponatremia in a small proportion of patients *3990* Hyponatremia reported as rare complication of treatment *3990* May cause hyponatremia *6651*

Urine No Effect Physiological No significant effect in 8 non-insulin dependent hypertensive diabetics treated with mean dose of 32 mg daily for 6 weeks *339*

Triglycerides *Serum Decrease Physiological* In 19 middle-aged patients with essential hypertension treatment with up to 40 mg/d for up to 12 weeks caused decrease of 0.05 ± 0.18 mmol/L from mean baseline of 1.56 ± 0.17 mmol/L *4397* In proteinuric patients treatment with lisinopril reduced both protein excretion and plasma concentration of triglycerides *4235*

Serum No Effect Physiological Nonsignificant increase from mean baseline concentration of 152 mg/dL to 162 mg/dL in 13 nondiabetic hypertensives treated for a mean of 9.0 months and decrease from 222 mg/dL to 192 mg/dL in 15 diabetic hypertensives treated for a mean of 8.3 months *5525* No effect noted when given as monotherapy in patients with essential hypertension *6470* In 19 patients with essential hypertension treatment with up to 8 mg/d for 8 - 12 weeks caused nonsignificant decrease of 0.05 ± 0.18 mmol/L from mean baseline of 1.56 ± 0.17 mmol/L *4397* Nonsignificant change observed from mean baseline of 132 ± 27 mg/dL to 134 ± 27 mg/dL in 16 young adults with mild hypertension treated with lisinopril for 12 weeks *1791*

Urea Nitrogen *Serum Increase Physiological* Administration of lisinopril was asssociated with an increased concentration in about 2.0% patients with essential hypertension *3990* Minor increase observed, reversible on discontinuation of lisinopril, observed in about 2.0% of hypertensive patients and in 11.6% patients with heart failure also receiving diuretics *3990* May cause uremia, progressive azotemia or renal dysfunction *6651* In one of 66 patients with essential hypertension serum concentration increased from baseline of 9.6 mmol/L to 14.6 mmol/L following treatment with up to 40 mg/d for 8 weeks *454*

Serum No Effect Physiological Nonsignificant increase from mean baseline concentration of 5.5 mmol/L to 5.8 mmol/L in 66 patients with essential hypertension treated with up to 40 mg/d for 8 weeks *454*

Uric Acid *Serum Decrease Physiological* Significant reduction from mean baseline concentration of 5.5 mg/dL to 5.1 mg/dL in 13 nondiabetic hypertensives treated for a mean of 9.0 months and from 6.2 mg/dL to 5.5 mg/dL in 15 diabetic hypertensives treated for a mean of 8.3 months *5525*

Serum Increase Physiological May cause gout *6651*

Viscosity *Blood No Effect Physiological* No significant difference from baseline at shear rates from 0.2 s^{-1} to 128 s^{-1} in 41 patients with mild to moderate hypertension treated with 20 mg/d for 4 weeks *6630*

Plasma No Effect Physiological In 41 patients with mild to moderate hypertension treatment with 20 mg/d for 4 weeks caused no significant change from mean baseline of 1.29 ± 0.07 $m^2/s \times 10^{-2}$*6630*

VLDL + LDL-Cholesterol *Serum Decrease Physiological* In proteinuric patients treatment with lisinopril reduced both protein excretion and plasma concentration of VLDL and LDL-cholesterol *4235*

VLDL-Cholesterol *Serum No Effect Physiological* Nonsignificant change observed from mean baseline of 22 ± 3 mg/dL to 23 ± 4 mg/dL in 16 young adults with mild hypertension treated with lisinopril for 12 weeks *1791* In 10 patients with mild essential hypertension treatment with 10 mg/d for 6 months caused nonsignificant change from mean baseline of 20 ± 5 mg/dL to 21 ± 4 mg/dL *1306*

Lisuride

Thyroid Stimulating Hormone

Serum Decrease Physiological Can lower basal and TRH-stimulated values *6412*

Lithium

Adipate *Urine Increase Physiological* May be considerable effect *3473*

Albumin *Serum No Effect Physiological* No difference between treated manic depressives and controls *3356*

Aldosterone *Plasma No Effect Physiological* No significant effect observed in 15 healthy volunteers following ingestion of either 300 or 600 mg lithium carbonate *5530*

Urine Increase Physiological Occurs after initial fall *4181*

Alkaline Phosphatase *Serum Increase Physiological* Effect in 20% manic depressives treated for minimum of 20 mo. Markedly increased effect on bone isoenzyme observed in 66% manic depressives treated for minimum of 20 mo *751* Significant increase noted in drug treated population and bone isoenzyme increased in 27 of 41 such patients. In 19 patients bone isoenzyme increased although total normal *751*

Alprazolam *Serum No Effect Physiological* No significant difference observed in 10 normal subjects. Steady state alprazolam clearance unaffected by multiple lithium dosing *1770*

Aluminum *Serum Increase Physiological* Concentration higher in 32 patients on long-term treatment compared with 32 age- and sex- matched controls *860*

Antidiuretic Hormone *Plasma Increase Physiological* Concentration doubled during treatment *4595* Occurs in majority of patients with polyuria consistent with defect in water balance at level of kidney (lithium administration now most common cause of nephrogenic diabetes insipidus) *5198* Also acts like vasopressin *2927*

Atrial Natriuretic Peptide *Plasma No Effect Physiological* No significant effect observed in 7 healthy volunteers following ingestion of either 300 or 600 mg lithium carbonate *5530*

Bicarbonate *Urine Increase Physiological* Occurs on first day of treatment only *2927*

Calcium *Serum Increase Physiological* Increased above normal in about 13% patients, reversible *5198* 8% higher than in controls in 12 patients taking drug for 2 to 13 y *1940* Probably due to unmasking of primary hyperparathyroidism *1769* Increase observed for next few hours when drug given at 10 p.m *3944* In 7 of 97 patients not necessarily attributable to

Lithium *(continued)*

Calcium *(continued)*
drug *1099* Mean effect in 130 manic depressives versus controls (about 2% increase) *3356*
Serum No Effect Physiological Mean concentration (2.39 ± 0.09 mmol/L) within normal range in all of 26 patients with bipolar or unipolar affective disorders treated with lithium for 10 years or longer *4322* No significant effect observed with chronic treatment *751*
Urine Decrease Physiological Picture of primary hyperparathyroidism observed in patients given treatment for long time, but mechanism not fully understood *5198* Reduced at night in lithium treated patients versus other psychiatric patients and healthy controls *3944* ?Affects calcium dependent catecholamine system *3750*

Carbamazepine *Serum No Effect Physiological* No apparent pharmacodynamic interactions when drugs coadministered *3119*

Chloride *Serum Increase Physiological* Significant increase in men who had received lithium for mean of 103 months compared with controls probably due to effect of increased PTH *3756*

Cholesterol *Serum Increase Physiological* Reported to induce myxedema *3670*

Choline *Red Blood Cells Increase Physiological* In 16 patients receiving oral lithium concentration significantly increased compared with 9 age-matched control *4042*

Cholinesterase *Serum No Effect Analytical* No effect observed at concentration of 3.5 mEq/L with butyrylthiocholine method on Kodak Ektachem® *2504*

Citalopram *Serum No Effect Physiological* Coadministration had no significant effect on kinetics of citalopram or of its major metabolites *2288*

Citrate *Urine No Effect Physiological* No effect observed after administration *647* No consistent effect observed *3473*

Cobalt *Serum Decrease Physiological* Concentration lower in 32 patients on long-term treatment than in 32 age- and sex-matched controls *860*

Cortisol *Plasma Decrease Physiological* Lower in morning and less diurnal variation *2417* Significant decrease in a.m. cortisol after 1 y in 48 depressed patients; p.m. values also affected in individuals with greatest change in response to treatment *5611*
Plasma Increase Physiological In 29 patients with bipolar affective disorder mean concentration increased from baseline of 11.7 ± 1.0 µg/dL to 13.7 ± 1.1 µg/dL after 3 days, 15.8 ± 0.6 µg/dL and 10 days but decrease to 10.9 ± 0.8 µg/dL after 6 months *4473* Observed in some patients *4721*

Creatine Kinase *Serum Increase Physiological* May be high sustained increase although disease controlled *2260*

Creatinine *Serum Increase Analytical* 5 mmol/L of lithium lactate reacts as if it were 0.01 mg/dL creatinine with method of Heinegard *2539*
Serum Increase Physiological Observed in a few patients but risk of renal insufficiency is remote even in patients given drug for many years *5375* Mean increase from 92 µmol/L to 102 µmol/L in 37 psychiatric outpatients treated with lithium with or without other drugs for 7 years. Increase greater in women who are treated with thyroxine *4296* Average increase from 0.94 to 1.08 mg/dL in 237 patients on long term treatment *6246* In lithium treated patients than healthy subjects *794* In 3 of 97 patients not necessarily attributable to drug *1099*
Serum No Effect Analytical No interference observed with lithium acetate at a concentration of 13 mg/L with HPLC method of Rosano et al *5083*

Creatinine Clearance *Urine Decrease Physiological* Slight decrease: significant negative regression on serum lithium concentration with long-term treatment *6246*

1,25-Dihydroxy Vitamin D_3 *Serum Increase Physiological* Observed in male patients who had received lithium for mean of 103 months compared with controls. Effect probably due to increased concentration of PTH *3756*

Fumarate *Urine Increase Physiological* May be considerable effect *3473*

Glucose *Serum Increase Physiological* Hyperglycemia been reported after use (transient) *6180* In two patients glycosuria and hyperglycemia occurred when lithium started: tests previously normal *2961*
Serum No Effect Analytical No effect of concentrations up to 9.7 mg/L on method on Kodak Ektachem® *5706*
Urine Increase Physiological Reported effect of lithium therapy in some cases consequence of hyperglycemia *2451* In two patients glycosuria and hyperglycemia occurred when lithium started: tests previously normal *2961*

Glucose Tolerance *Serum Decrease Physiological* Associated with hyperglycemia (?mechanism) *2754*

Glutarate *Urine Increase Physiological* Reversible inhibition of renal transport *647*

Glycerophosphorylcholine
Red Blood Cells Decrease Physiological In 16 patients receiving oral lithium mean concentration significantly reduced compared with that in 9 age-matched controls *4042*

4-Hydroxy-3-Methoxy-Phenylglycol
Cerebrospinal Fluid Decrease Physiological Significant reduction with treatment of manic patients. Initial high values correlates with severity of disease *5894*

2-Hydroxy-4-Ketoglutarate *Urine Increase Physiological* May be considerable effect *3473*

α-Hydroxyglutarate *Urine Increase Physiological* May be considerable effect *3473*

^{131}I Uptake *Serum Decrease Physiological* Lithionate contains tetraiodofluorescein *4360*
Serum Increase Physiological Mechanism unclear *823*

ionized Calcium *Serum Increase Physiological* 9% higher than in controls in 12 patients taking drug for 2 to 13 y *1940* Higher by 0.03-0.04 mmol/L in men who had received lithium for mean of 1.7 months than in normal subjects *3756* Mean concentration of 1.29 ± 0.03 mmol/L increased above upper limit of normal (range 1.24 ± 0.03 mmol/L) in 11 of 26 patients with bipolar or unipolar affective disorders treated with lithium for 10 years or longer *4322*

α-Ketoglutarate *Urine Increase Physiological* Reversible inhibition of renal transport *647*

Lactate *Plasma No Effect Analytical* No significant effect observed at a concentration of 1 mEq/L with method on Kodak Ektachem® systems *2519*
Urine No Effect Physiological No effect observed after administration *647*

Lecithin *Red Blood Cells Decrease Physiological* In 16 patients treated with oral lithium concentration significantly decreased in comparison with 9 age-matched controls *4042*

Leukocytes *Blood Decrease Physiological* Severe leukopenia may occur as a result of lithium toxicity *4399*
Blood Increase Physiological Mean increase of 2.2 thousand /µL with treatment *3409* ?Drug associated endocrine effect (may double) *3857* After 4 weeks treatment increase in 21 patients on average from 6.3 to 8.6 thousand /µL *2941* In 29 patients with bipolar affective disorder mean concentration increased from baseline of 7221 ± 250 /µL to 9548 ± 291 /µL after 3 days, 8934 ± 359 /µL after 10 days, and 7128 ± 238 /µL after 6 months *4473*

Lithium *Cerebrospinal Fluid Increase Physiological* Concentration about half in serum *2242*
Red Blood Cells Increase Physiological But only to maximum of 50% in plasma *2392* In 29 patients with bipolar affective disorder treatment caused increase from mean baseline of 0.0 mEq/L to 1.45 ± 0.06 mEq/L after 3 days, 1.73 ± 0.04 mEq/L after 10 days, and 1,75 ± 0.05 mEq/L after 6 months *4473*
Serum Increase Physiological In 29 patients with bipolar affective disorder mean concentration increased from baseline of 0.0 mEq/L to 0.52 ± 0.03 mEq/L after 3 days, 0.67 ± 0.02 mEq/L after 10 days and 0.62 ± 0.23 mEq/L after treatment for 6 months *4473* In 15 healthy volunteers ingestion of 300 mg lithium carbonate produced mean concentration of 120 µmol/L and of 600 mg produced concentration of 241 µmol/L *5530* Therapeutic level between 0.5 and 1.0 mEq/L *2242*
Urine Increase Physiological Excretion proportional to plasma concentration *2754*

Lymphocytes *Blood Decrease Physiological* ?Drug associated endocrine effect *5537*
Blood No Effect Physiological No change observed although WBC count changed *3409*

Magnesium *Cerebrospinal Fluid Decrease Physiological* Significant effect (reverse of serum) *2392*
Cerebrospinal Fluid No Effect Physiological In 13 patients treated until steady-state concentration achieved nonsignificant change in concentration from mean baseline of 1.15 ± 0.09 mmol/L to 1.11 ± 0.05 mmol/L observed *2091*
Serum Increase Physiological Picture of primary hyperparathyroidism observed in patients given treatment for long term, but mechanism not fully understood *5198* Increased for 24 h after drug administered *3944* ?Affects membrane transport systems *5869*
Serum No Effect Analytical No effect of concentrations up to 1 mmol/L on method on Kodak Ektachem® *5706*
Urine Increase Physiological Following administration of therapy *3750* Increased during day in lithium treated patients versus other psychiatric patients and healthy controls *3944*

Malate *Urine Increase Physiological* May be considerable effect *3473*

Methylmalonate *Urine No Effect Physiological* No consistent effect observed *3473*

β2-Microglobulin *Serum Increase Physiological* In 10 of 53 patients treated with lithium up to 32 mEq/d mean concentration increased above upper limit of normal of 2.5 µg/mL without signs of pathologyprobably reflecting early impairment of glomerular tubular function *2376*

Neutrophils *Blood Decrease Physiological* Treatment of 6 healthy adults with 2400 mg/d for 5 days caused nonsignificant increase from mean of 3675 /µL to 4945 /µL *531*
Blood Increase Physiological Increase largely responsible for increase in WBC count *3409* ?drug associated endocrine effect *5537*

Norepinephrine *Urine Decrease Physiological* Significant reduction with treatment of manic patients. Initial high values correlated with severity of disease *5894*

o-Desmethylvenlafaxine *Serum No Effect Physiological* When 600 mg lithium administered to 12 healthy men no effect observed on steady state pharmacokinetics of venlafaxine or o-desmethylvenlafaxine when venlafaxine administered 50 mg every 8 hours *6555*

Osmolality *Urine Decrease Physiological* Reduced concentrating ability in lithium treated patients than in healthy subjects *794*

Parathyroid Hormone *Plasma Increase Physiological* Concentration of both intact and midregion iPTH increased compared with normal controls in individuals who had received lithium for mean of 103 months *3756* Mean concentration of 37 ± 16 ng/L increased above upper limit of normal (30 ± 11 ng/L) in 5 of 26 patients with bipolar or unipolar affective disorders treated with lithium for 10 years or longer *4322* Observed in 21% psychiatric patients given compound, positively correlated with serum lithium concentration *5198* 38% higher than in controls in 12 patients taking drug for 2 to 13 y *1940*
Plasma No Effect Physiological Neither intact PTH nor midregion iPTH increased in men who had received lithium for mean of 1.7 months compared with normal subjects *3756*

Phenylalanine *Plasma No Effect Analytical* No interference observed from lithium carbonate with rapid quantitative whole blood method of Campbell et al using phenylalanine dehydrogenase *867*

Phosphate *Serum Decrease Physiological* Significant reduction in patients who had received lithium for mean of 103 months probably from biological action of increased PTH *3756* Picture of primary hyperparathyroidism observed in patients given treatment for long time, but mechanism not fully understood *5198* When given at 10 p.m. drug caused decrease for next few hours *3944*
Serum No Effect Physiological Mean concentration (1.0 ± 0.1 mmol/L) within normal range of 0.8 - 1.2 mmol/L in all of 26 patients with bipolar or unipolar affective disorders treated with lithium for 10 years or longer *4322* No significant effect observed with chronic treatment *751*
Urine No Effect Physiological No effect observed in lithium treated patients versus other psychiatric patients and healthy controls *3944*

Phosphorylcholine *Red Blood Cells Decrease Physiological* In 16 patients treated with oral lithium mean concentration significantly reduced compared with that in 9 age-matched controls *4042*

Pimelate *Urine No Effect Physiological* No consistent effect observed *3473*

Platelets *Blood Increase Physiological* After 4 weeks treatment increase in 21 patients on average from 302 to 342 thousand /µL *2941*

Potassium *Serum Decrease Physiological* Slight decreases observed only *804*
Serum Increase Physiological ?By displacing from cells *3750*
Serum No Effect Analytical No significant effect observed on colorimetric enzymatic method of Kimura et al using urea amidohydrolase at a concentraton of 3.0 mmol/L *3139* No effect up to 100 mmol/L on method on Ames Seralyzer although at higher concentrations apparently increased potassium concentration *5706* Negligible effect of lithium chloride at a concentration of 5 mmol/L on spectrophotometric enzymatic method of Berry et al *523* No effect of lithium chloride at concentrations up to 1 mmol/L on method on Kodak Ektachem® *5706*
Serum No Effect Physiological No significant effect observed with chronic treatment *751* Isolated case of hyperkalemia reported but usually no effect reported *4739*
Urine Increase Physiological 600 mg lithium carbonate administered to 15 healthy volunteers caused increase of 19 mmol in first 16 hours after ingestion *5530*
Urine No Effect Physiological No significant effect of 300 mg lithium carbonate observed in 15 healthy volunteers *5530*

Prolactin *Plasma No Effect Physiological* No significant effect with up to 8 g daily orally *2352*

Protein *Urine Increase Physiological* May have slight nephrotoxic effect *2451*

Pyruvate *Urine No Effect Physiological* No effect observed after administration *647*

Renin Activity *Plasma Increase Physiological* Concentration increased in 15 healthy volunteers after ingestion of 600 mg lithium carbonate from control of 2.02 pmol Ang-I/h/mL to 3.40 pmol Ang-I/h/mL *5530*
Plasma No Effect Physiological No significant effect observed in 15 healthy volunteers following ingestion of 300 mg lithium carbonate *5530*

Sodium *Serum Decrease Physiological* Due to initial natriuresis and diuresis *3750*
Serum No Effect Analytical No interference observed at concentration of 5 mol/L with Technicon Chromolyte method *969* No practical interference observed with kinetic enzymatic procedure on Roche Cobas Fara analyzer *2853*
Urine Decrease Physiological Due to action of aldosterone (initial increase) *4181*
Urine Increase Physiological Impairs reabsorption by tubules *2754* In 15 healthy individuals 300 mg lithium carbonate increased sodium excretion by 17 mmol in 24 hours with almost all effect occuring in first 16 hours. 600 mg caused increase of 48 mmol/d again occuring in first 16 hours *5530*

Specific Gravity *Urine Decrease Physiological* Large proportion of patients with polyuria with long term treatment *6246*

Suberate *Urine No Effect Physiological* No consistent effect observed *3473*

Succinate *Urine Increase Physiological* May be considerable effect *3473*

T3-Uptake *Serum Decrease Physiological* Reported to induce myxedema *3670* Irreversible myxedema observed in 2 patients treated for 1 y *4597*
Serum No Effect Physiological Observed in one patient who developed thyrotoxicosis without pre-existing goiter *4003*

Thyroid Antibodies *Serum Positive Physiological* In two thirds women with hypothyroidism treated for 2 y *3596* Observed in 19% of patients in association with subclinical hypothyroidism *618*

Thyroid Stimulating Hormone
Serum Increase Physiological Hypophyseal influence responsible for augmented TRH-induced values *6412* Increase observed in 19% of patients in one study *618* Approximately 10% of 219 patients treated with drug had some evidence of hypothyroidism with 5% sufficiently severe to require treatment, apparently unrelated to serum concentration of drug *76* Compensatory response to reduced peripheral hormone concentrations. Observed in about 15% patients given long-term treatment. TSH response to TRH is increased *5198* Irreversible myxedema observed in 2 patients treated for 1 y

Lithium *(continued)*

Thyroid Stimulating Hormone *(continued)*
4612 In 20% of women, but no men among 53 psychiatric patients treated for 2 y *3596* Mechanism unclear *823* Observed in long-term therapy in manic depressives *3595* In 10 of 237 patients with smaller increases in others treated for more than 6 mo: normalized in most cases on withdrawal *138* In 50 Chinese psychiatric patients 50% had goiters and mean concentration in population as a whole 1.95 ± 1.05 mIU/L compared with 1.24 ± 0.72 mIU/L in healthy controls *1001*

Thyroxine (T4) *Serum Decrease Physiological* Hypothyroidism observed in 1-2% of 2590 psychiatric patients treated with lithium *4718* In 20% of women, but no men among 53 psychiatric patients treated for 2 y *3596* In 10 of 237 patients with smaller increases in others treated for more than 6 mo: normalized in most cases on withdrawal *138* Reduces thyroidal iodine uptake, iodination of tyrosine, release of T4, to T3 and hepatic metabolism of T4 to T3 *5198* Reported to induce myxedema *3670* Irreversible myxedema observed in 2 patients treated for 1 y *4612*
Serum Increase Physiological Observed in one patient who developed thyrotoxicosis without pre-existing goiter *4003*

Thyroxine (T4), Free *Serum Decrease Physiological* Mechanism unclear, non toxic goiter may occur *5536*

Titratable Acidity *Urine Decrease Physiological* Falls on first day of treatment *2927*

Tri-iodothyronine (T3) *Serum Decrease Physiological* In 10 of 237 patients with smaller increases in others treated for more than 6 mo: normalized in most cases on withdrawal *138* Reduces thyroidal iodine uptake, iodination of tyrosine, release of T4, to T3 and hepatic metabolism of T4 to T3 *5198*

Triglycerides *Serum No Effect Analytical* No significant effect observed at concentration of 12.5 mg/dL (12.5 mmol/L) on method on Du Pont aca *1551*

Urea Nitrogen *Serum No Effect Analytical* No effect of concentrations up to 9.7 mg/L on method on Kodak Ektachem® *5706*

Uric Acid *Serum Decrease Physiological* Reported to have uricosuric effect *218*
Urine Increase Physiological Reported effect of $LiCO_3$ in manic-depressives *2452*

Vanadium *Serum Decrease Physiological* Concentration lower in 32 patients on long-term treatment compared with 32 age- and sex- matched controls *860*

Vanillylmandelic Acid *Urine Increase Physiological* Slight increase only, mechanism not clear *2451*

Venlafaxine *Serum No Effect Physiological* When 600 mg lithium administered to 12 healthy men no effect observed on steady state pharmacokinetics of venlafaxine or o-desmethylvenlafaxine when venlafaxine administered 50 mg every 8 hours *6555*

Volume *Urine Increase Physiological* Occurs in about 60% patients with start of treatment and persists in about 20- -25% *5198* Significant increase observed over 24 hours following ingestion of 600 mg lithium carbonate by 15 healthy volunteers *5530* Rare inhibition of vasopressin action on tubules *4848* Large proportion of patients with polyuria with long term treatment *6246* Polyuria identified as side effect of lithium toxicity *4399*
Urine No Effect Physiological Nonsignificant increase observed over 24 hours in 15 healthy volunteers following ingestion of 300 mg *5530*

Zinc *Serum No Effect Analytical* At 50 to 1 with flameless atomic absorption *3333*
Urine No Effect Analytical At 50 to 1 with flameless atomic absorption *3333*

Lithium Carbonate

Albumin *Urine Increase Physiological* Reported as a non-dose related side effect in some patients *5130* Increased excretion observed in some treated patients *5645*

Aldosterone *Plasma No Effect Physiological* No significant effect observed in 15 healthy volunteers following ingestion of either 300 or 600 mg *5530*

Antimicrosomal Antibodies *Serum No Effect Physiological* In 27 normal individuals treatment with lithium carbonate 1200 - 1500 mg/d for 4 weeks caused no significant change in concentration *4858*

Antithyroglobulin Antibodies
Serum No Effect Physiological In 27 normal individuals treatment with lithium carbonate 1200 - 1500 mg/d for 4 weeks caused no significant change in concentration *4858*

Atrial Natriuretic Peptide *Plasma No Effect Physiological* No significant effect observed in 7 healthy volunteers following ingestion of either 300 or 600 mg *5530*

Calcium *Serum Increase Physiological* Hypercalcemia observed in some treated patients *5645*

Creatinine Clearance *Urine Decrease Physiological* Decreased clearance observed in some treated patients *5645*

Glucose *Serum Increase Physiological* Transient hyperglycemia may be observed in some treated patients *5130* Transient hyperglycemia observed in some treated patients *5645*
Urine Increase Physiological Glycosuria observed in some treated patients *5645* Reported as a non-dose related side effect in some patients *5130*

^{131}I Uptake *Serum Increase Physiological* Euthyroid goiter or hypothyroidism (even myxedema) observed in some treated patients. ^{131}I uptake may be increased *5645* Euthyroid goiter and'or hypothyroidism reported as a side effect with reduced plasma T3 and T4 concentrations in some patients. ^{131}iodine uptake may be increased *5130*

Leukocytes *Blood Increase Physiological* Leukocytosis observed in some treated patients *5645*

Lithium *Serum Increase Physiological* In 15 healthy volunteers ingestion of 300 mg produced mean concentration of 120 µmol/L and of 600 mg produced concentration of 241 µmol/L *5530*

Parathyroid Hormone *Plasma Increase Physiological* Hyperparathyroidism observed in some treated patients *5645*

Paroxetine *Serum No Effect Physiological* No significant effect on the pharmacokinetics of either lithium carbonate or paroxetine observed when the drugs coadministered *5654*

Potassium *Urine Increase Physiological* 600 mg administered to 15 healthy volunteers caused increase of 19 mmol in first 16 hours after ingestion *5530*
Urine No Effect Physiological No significant effect of 300 mg observed in 15 healthy volunteers *5530*

Renin Activity *Plasma Increase Physiological* Concentration increased in 15 healthy volunteers after ingestion of 600 mg from control of 2.02 pmol Ang I/h/mL to 3.40 pmol Ang I/h/mL *5530*
Plasma No Effect Physiological No significant effect observed in 15 healthy volunteers following ingestion of 300 mg *5530*

Sodium *Urine Increase Physiological* In 15 healthy individuals 300 mg increased sodium excretion by 17 mmol in 24 hours with almost all effect occuring in first 16 hours. 600 mg caused increase of 48 mmol/d again occuring in first 16 hours *5530*

Soluble Interleukin-2 Receptor
Serum Increase Physiological In 27 normal individuals treatment with lithium carbonate 1200 - 1500 mg/d caused a significant increase from mean baseline of 446 ± 177 U/mL to 498 ± 232 U/mL after 4 weeks *4858*

Thyroxine (T4) *Serum Decrease Physiological* Euthyroid goiter or hypothyroidism (even myxedema) observed in some treated patients *5645* Euthyroid goiter and'or hypothyroidism reported as a side effect with reduced plasma T3 and T4 concentrations in some patients *5130*

Tri-iodothyronine (T3) *Serum Decrease Physiological* Euthyroid goiter or hypothyroidism (even myxedema) observed in some treated patients *5645* Euthyroid goiter and'or hypothyroidism reported as a side effect with reduced plasma T3 and T4 concentrations in some patients *5130*

Volume *Urine Increase Physiological* Significant increase observed over 24 hours following ingestion of 600 mg by 15 healthy volunteers *5530* Polyuria observed in some treated patients with symptoms of nephrogenic diabetes insipidus *5645*
Urine No Effect Physiological Nonsignificant increase observed over 24 hours in 15 healthy volunteers following ingestion of 300 mg *5530*

LMW Heparin

Activated Factor X inhibition
Plasma Increase Physiological Effect of both 7500 AXaU and 15000 AXaU subcutaneously in 30 healthy volunteers substantially higher and longer lasting than with 5000 IU calcium heparin *5074*

Alanine Aminotransferase *Serum Increase Physiological* Observed in 17% of 43 patients after 8 days of prophylactic treatment *4099* Observed in one of 49 patients after 8 days prophylactic treatment *4099*
Serum No Effect Physiological In 24 patients with chronic renal failure undergoing hemodialysis mean activity changed nonsignificantly from baseline of 7.11 ± 5.08 U/L to 7.98 ± 4.42 U/L after 6 months *3302*

Albumin *Urine No Effect Physiological* In 11 IDDM patients treatment with low molecular weight heparin for 3 months caused nonsignificant change from mean baseline of 54 ng/min to 54 ng/min *4201*

Aldosterone *Plasma Decrease Physiological* Mean reduction to 182 pmol/L during and 267 pmol/L from baseline of 333 pmol/L in 12 patients receiving enoxaparin and to 174 pmol/L during and 230 pmol/L after from baseline of 285 pmol/L in 15 patients receiving fraxiparine *3532*

α_2-Antiplasmin *Plasma No Effect Physiological* In 12 healthy male volunteers administration of a single intravenous bolus dose of 2500 IU had no significant effect on α_2-antiplasmin concentration over 120 minutes *1337*

Antithrombin III *Plasma No Effect Physiological* In 12 healthy male volunteers administration of a single intravenous bolus of 2500 IU had no significant effect on AT-III concentration over 120 minutes *1337*

Apolipoprotein A-I *Serum Decrease Physiological* In 22 patients on chronic hemodialysis switching to LMW heparin from conventional heparin for 6 months caused significant reduction *5361*
Serum No Effect Physiological In 24 patients with chronic renal failure undergoing hemodialysis mean concentration changed nonsignificantly from baseline of 115.7 ± 33.4 mg/dL to 117.5 ± 24.9 mg/dL after 6 months *3302*

Apolipoprotein A-IV *Serum No Effect Physiological* In 24 patients with chronic renal failure undergoing hemodialysis mean concentration changed nonsignificantly from baseline of 27.0 ± 11.9 mg/dL to 30.8 ± 7.0 mg/dL after 6 months *3302*

Apolipoprotein B *Serum Decrease Physiological* In 22 patients on chronic hemodialysis switching to LMW heparin from conventional heparin for 6 months caused significant reduction *5361*
Serum No Effect Physiological In 24 patients with chronic renal failure undergoing hemodialysis mean concentration changed nonsignificantly from baseline of 99.6 ± 40.2 mg/dL to 100.0 ± 35.3 mg/dL after 6 months *3302*

Aspartate Aminotransferase *Serum Increase Physiological* Observed in 14% of 43 patients after 8 days of prophylactic treatment *4099*
Serum No Effect Physiological In 24 patients with chronic renal failure undergoing hemodialysis mean activity changed nonsignificantly from baseline of 6.81 ± 3.52 U/L to 6.97 ± 3.09 U/L after 6 months *3302*

Cholesterol *Serum Decrease Physiological* In 22 patients on chronic hemodialysis switch to LMW heparin for 6 months from conventional heparin caused significant decrease *5361* In patients on chronic hemodialysis significant reduction observed compared with time when standard heparin used *1399*
Serum No Effect Physiological In 24 patients with chronic renal failure undergoing hemodialysis mean concentration changed nonsignificantly from baseline of 159.1 ± 44.0 mg/dL to 168.6 ± 42.2 mg/dL after 6 months *3302*

Cortisol *Plasma No Effect Physiological* No significant effect observed in 27 patients with potential for thromboembolic complications when treated with either enoxaparin or fraxiparine *3532*

Creatinine *Serum No Effect Physiological* In 24 patients with chronic renal failure undergoing hemodialysis mean concentration changed nonsignificantly from baseline of 10.49 ± 2.10 mg/dL to 10.76 ± 2.37 mg/dL after 6 months *3302*

D-Dimer *Plasma No Effect Physiological* In 5 patients with chronic renal failure undergoing hemodialysis using 3000 - 7250 IU bolus of low molecular weight heparin mean arterial concentration of 690 ± 199 ng/mL at baseline changed insignificantly overall to 719 ± 231 ng/mL after 10 min, 885 ± 312 ng/mL after 60 min, 730 ± 196 ng/mL after 120 min and 712 ± 186 ng/mL after 180 min *4337*

2,3-Dinor-6-Keto-Prostaglandin $F_{1\alpha}$
Urine No Effect Physiological No effect on excretion observed in 6 volunteers following intravenous injection of LMW heparin suggesting no effect on endothelial release of prostacyclin *3619*

2,3-Dinor-Thromboxane B_2 *Urine No Effect Physiological* No effect of intravenous injection on excretion suggesting no effect on platelet activation *3619*

Factor XII *Plasma No Effect Physiological* In 12 healthy male volunteers administration of 2500 IU had no significant effect on heparin-cofactor II concentration over 120 minutes *1337*

Fibrinogen *Plasma No Effect Physiological* In 5 patients with chronic renal failure undergoing hemodialysis using 3000 - 7250 IU bolus of low molecular weight heparin mean arterial concentration of 411 ± 60 mg/dL at baseline changed insignificantly to 415 ± 55 mg/dL after 120 min and 5.6 ± 2.7 ng/mL after 180 min *4337*

Fibrinopeptide *Plasma Decrease Physiological* Significant reduction of fibrinopeptide concentration with infusion in patients on maintenance hemodialysis with no significant difference when patients were receiving commercial unfractionated heparin *153*

γ-Glutamyltransferase *Serum No Effect Physiological* In 24 patients with chronic renal failure undergoing hemodialysis mean activity changed nonsignificantly from baseline of 11.79 ± 5.55 U/L to 13.52 ± 7.12 U/L after 6 months *3302*

HDL-Cholesterol *Serum No Effect Physiological* In 22 patients on chronic hemodialysis a switch to LMW heparin for 6 months from conventional heparin had no significant effect on concentration *5361* In 24 patients with chronic renal failure undergoing hemodialysis mean concentration changed nonsignificantly from baseline of 31.0 ± 13.0 mg/dL to 32.8 ± 12.5 mg/dL after 6 months *3302*

Hemoglobin A_{1c} *Blood No Effect Physiological* In 11 IDDM patients treatment with low molecular weight heparin for 3 months caused nonsignificant change from mean baseline of 10.0% to 10.2% *4201*

Heparin-Cofactor II *Plasma No Effect Physiological* In 12 healthy male volunteers administration of a single intravenous bolus of 2500 IU had no significant effect on heparin-cofactor II concentration over 120 minutes *1337*

Heptest *Plasma Increase Physiological* Dose dependent increase in clotting time observed with peak of 85 s after 60 mg subcutaneously after 3 hours *2709*

LDL-Cholesterol *Serum Decrease Physiological* In 22 patients on chronic hemodialysis switch to LMW heparin for 6 months after conventional heparin caused significant reduction in concentration *5361*
Serum No Effect Physiological In 24 patients with chronic renal failure undergoing hemodialysis mean concentration changed nonsignificantly from baseline of 94.1 ± 38.0 mg/dL to 106.4 ± 35.2 mg/dL after 6 months *3302*

Leukocytes *Blood No Effect Physiological* In 24 patients with chronic renal failure undergoing hemodialysis mean concentration changed nonsignificantly from baseline of 7880 ± 2320 /µL to 7490 ± 2170 /µL after 6 months *3302*

Lipoprotein Lp(a) *Serum No Effect Physiological* In 24 patients with chronic renal failure undergoing hemodialysis mean concentration changed nonsignificantly from baseline of 23.2 ± 33.2 mg/dL to 19.2 ± 24.4 mg/dL after 6 months *3302*

Partial Thromboplastin Time
Plasma Decrease Physiological Less inhibited with low molecular heparin than with unfractionated heparin *2463*
Plasma Increase Physiological Significant increase in 30 healthy volunteers following single subcutaneous injection of 1500 AXaU. No effect observed after injection of 7500 AXaU *5074*

LMW Heparin *(continued)*

Plasmin-Plasmin Inhibitor Complex
Plasma Increase Physiological In 5 patients with chronic renal failure undergoing hemodialysis using 3000 - 7250 IU bolus of low molecular weight heparin mean arterial concentration of 424 ± 112 ng/mL at baseline changed significantly overall to 376 ± 100 ng/mL after 10 min, 485 ± 157 ng/mL after 60 min, 493 ± 154 ng/mL after 120 min and 560 ± 163 ng/mL after 180 min *4337*

Plasminogen *Plasma No Effect Physiological* In 12 healthy male volunteers administration of a single intravenous bolus dose of 2500 IU had no significant effect on plasminogen concentration over 120 minutes *1337*

Platelet Aggregation *Blood Decrease Physiological* In 22 patients on chronic hemodialysis switching to LMW heparin from conventional heparin for 6 months caused significant improvement in aggregation induced by collagen *5361*
Blood Increase Physiological Aggregation potentiated in platelet rich plasma from 6 volunteers given intravenous injection of LMW heparin *3619*

Platelet Distribution Width *Blood No Effect Physiological* No effect observed in 6 volunteers following intravenous injection of LMW heparin *3619*

Platelet Factor 4 *Plasma Increase Physiological* Intravenous injection increased concentration in volunteers but did not induce platelet activation *3619*

Platelet Volume *Blood No Effect Physiological* No effect observed in 6 volunteers given intravenous injection of LMW heparin *3619*

Platelets *Blood No Effect Physiological* In none of 333 patients receiving low molecular weight heparin for up to 14 days was thrombocytopenia observed *970* No effect observed in 6 volunteers following intravenous injection of LMW heparin *3619*

Potassium *Serum Increase Physiological* In 12 patients with potential for thromboembolic complications during treatment with enoxaparin mean potassium concentration increased from baseline of 4.0 mmol/L to 4.4 mmol/L and in patients treated with fraxiparine increased from 4.1 to 4.5 mmol/L *3532*

Prekallikrein *Plasma No Effect Physiological* In 12 healthy male volunteers administration of 2500 IU had no significant effect on heparin-cofactor II concentration over 120 minutes *1337*

Protein *Serum No Effect Physiological* In 24 patients with chronic renal failure undergoing hemodialysis mean concentration changed nonsignificantly from baseline of 63.9 ± 7.7 g/L to 65.6 ± 6.2 g/L after 6 months *3302*

Protein C Activity *Plasma No Effect Physiological* In 12 healthy male volunteers administration of 2500 IU had no significant effect on heparin-cofactor II concentration over 120 minutes *1337*

Protein S Antigen *Plasma No Effect Physiological* In 12 healthy male volunteers administration of 2500 IU had no significant effect on heparin-cofactor II concentration over 120 minutes *1337*

Renin Activity *Plasma No Effect Physiological* No significant effect observed during or following treatment with enoxaparin or fraxiparine in 27 patients with potential for thromboembolic complications *3532*

Sodium *Serum No Effect Physiological* No significant effect observed during or after treatment of 27 patients with potential for thromboembolic complications when treated with either enoxaparin of fraxiparine *3532*

Thrombin Time *Blood Decrease Physiological* Less inhibited with low molecular weight heparin than with unfractionated heparin *2463*
Blood No Effect Physiological No significant effect of either 7500 AXaU or 15000 AXaU subcutaneously in 30 healthy volunteers *5074*

Thrombin/Antithrombin III Complex
Plasma Increase Physiological In 5 patients with chronic renal failure undergoing hemodialysis using 3000 - 7250 IU bolus of low molecular weight heparin mean arterial concentration of 2.3 ± 0.4 ng/mL at baseline changed significantly overall to 2.3 ± 0.3 ng/mL after 10 min, 2.4 ± 0.4 ng/mL after 60 min, 3.1 ± 0.9 ng/mL after 120 min and 5.6 ± 2.7 ng/mL after 180 min *4337*

β-Thromboglobulin *Plasma No Effect Physiological* No effect on concentration following intravenous injection suggesting no effect on platelet activation *3619*
Urine No Effect Physiological No effect following intravenous injection suggesting no effect on platelet activation *3619*

Tissue Factor Pathway Inhibitor
Plasma Increase Physiological Dose dependent increase in concentration observed with peak of 220 ng/mL after 60 mg subcutaneously after 1 hour *2709*

Tissue Plasminogen Activator
Plasma No Effect Physiological No effect observed in 6 volunteers following intravenous injection of LMW heparin *3619*

Tissue Plasminogen Activator-1
Plasma No Effect Physiological In 12 healthy male volunteers administration of 2500 IU had no significant effect on heparin-cofactor II concentration over 120 minutes *1337*

Tissue Plasminogen Inhibitor
Plasma No Effect Physiological No effect observed in 6 volunteers following intravenous injection of LMW heparin *3619*

Triglycerides *Serum Decrease Physiological* In patients on chronic hemodialysis receiving LMW heparin significant reduction observed compared with standard heparin *1399*
Serum Increase Physiological In 22 patients on chronic hemodialysis switching to LMW heparin from conventional heparin caused significant increase after 2 months but then decreased to baseline concentration within another 4 months *5361*
Serum No Effect Physiological In 24 patients with chronic renal failure undergoing hemodialysis mean concentration changed nonsignificantly from baseline of 148.9 ± 94.3 mg/dL to 148.7 ± 85.0 mg/dL after 6 months *3302*

Urea *Serum No Effect Physiological* In 24 patients with chronic renal failure undergoing hemodialysis mean concentration changed nonsignificantly from baseline of 149.2 ± 38.7 mg/dL to 138.2 ± 39.4 mg/dL after 6 months *3302*

von Willebrand Factor *Plasma No Effect Physiological* No effect observed in 6 volunteers following intravenous injection of LMW heparin *3619*

Local Anesthetics

Erythrocytes *Blood Decrease Physiological* Bone marrow depression reported *4014*

Leukocytes *Blood Decrease Physiological* Bone marrow depression and agranulocytosis reported *4014*

Methemoglobin *Blood Increase Physiological* Reported effect *4014*

Lofepramine

Alkaline Phosphatase *Serum Increase Physiological* Slight increase observed in one patient treated with up to 210 mg daily for 12 weeks *3358*

Aspartate Aminotransferase *Serum Increase Physiological* Significant increase observed in one patient treated with up to 210 mg daily for up to 12 weeks *3358*

Bilirubin *Serum Increase Physiological* Slight increase observed in one patient treated with up to 210 mg daily for 12 weeks *3358*

γ-Glutamyltransferase *Serum Increase Physiological* Significant increase observed in one patient treated with up to 210 mg daily after 12 weeks *3358*

Tricyclic Antidepressants Screen
Serum No Effect Analytical No significant effect observed at a concentration of 1000 μg/mL (2.4 mmol/L) with method on Du Pont aca *1550*

Lomefloxacin

Caffeine *Serum No Effect Physiological* Minimal effect observed on clearance *2704*

Theophylline *Serum No Effect Physiological* No significant effect observed on clearance in 9 male volunteers when 400 mg lomefloxacin (400 mg 12 hourly) administered while volunteers also receiving theophylline 125 mg 8 hourly *5003* No significant effect on elimination half-life in 12 healthy male volunteers when drugs coadministered *5767* No clinically significant effect on theophylline concentration observed when drugs coadministered *5999* Coadministration of lomefloxacin with theophylline in 15 volunteers did not affect theophylline clearance after either single or multiple doses of lomefloxacin. Urinary excretion of theophylline and major metabolites remained stable during study *3455* No documented significant interaction with theophylline reported *6117*

Lomerfloxacin

Alanine Aminotransferase *Serum Increase Physiological* Increased activity reported as side effect in 0.4% treated patients *2068*

Albumin *Serum Decrease Physiological* Decreased concentration reported as side effect in ≤0.1% treated patients *2068*

Alkaline Phosphatase *Serum Increase Physiological* Increased activity reported as side effect in 0.1% treated patients *2068*

Aspartate Aminotransferase *Serum Increase Physiological* Increased activity reported as side effect in 0.3% treated patients *2068*

Bilirubin *Serum Increase Physiological* Increased concentration reported as side effect in 0.1% treated patients *2068*

Blood *Urine Increase Physiological* Hematuria reported as occasional side effect *2068*

Caffeine *Serum No Effect Physiological* Concomitant administration of caffeine with lomerfloxacin had no effect on the pharmacokinetics of either compound *2068*

Eosinophils *Blood Increase Physiological* Eosinophilia reported as side effect in ≤0.1% treated patients *2068*

Erythrocyte Sedimentation Rate
Blood Increase Physiological Increased rate reported as side effect in 0.1% treated patients *2068*

Glucose *Serum Decrease Physiological* Hypoglycemia reported as side effect in ≤0.1% treated patients *2068* Hypoglycemia reported as occasional side effect *2068*

γ-Glutamyltransferase *Serum Increase Physiological* Increased activity reported as side effect in ≤0.1% treated patients *2068*

Hematocrit *Blood Decrease Physiological* Anemia reported as side effect in ≤0.1% treated patients *2068*

Hemoglobin *Blood Decrease Physiological* Anemia reported as side effect in ≤0.1% treated patients *2068*

Leukocytes *Blood Decrease Physiological* Leukopenia reported as side effect in ≤0.1% treated patients *2068*

Monocytes *Blood Increase Physiological* Increased concentration reported as side effect in 0.3% treated patients *2068*

Occult Blood *Feces Increase Physiological* Gastrointestinal bleeding reported as occasional side effect *2068*

Platelets *Blood Decrease Physiological* Thrombocytopenia reported as side effect in ≤0.1% treated patients *2068*
Blood Increase Physiological Thrombocythemia reported as occasional side effect *2068*

Potassium *Serum Decrease Physiological* Decreased concentration reported as side effect in 0.1% treated patients *2068*

Protein *Serum Decrease Physiological* Decreased concentration reported as side effect in ≤0.1% treated patients *2068*

Prothrombin Time *Plasma Increase Physiological* Prolonged prothrombin time reported as side effect in ≤0.1% treated patients *2068*
Plasma No Effect Physiological Concomitant administration of lomerfloxacin with warfarin may enhance its effects and prolong the prothrombin time *2068*

Specific Gravity *Urine Increase Physiological* Abnormalities of specific gravity reported as side effect in ≤0.1% treated patients *2068*

Theophylline *Serum No Effect Physiological* In three studies theophylline clearance and concentration not affected by administration of lomerfloxacin *2068*

Urea Nitrogen *Serum Increase Physiological* Increased concentration reported as side effect in 0.1% treated patients *2068*

Uric Acid *Serum Increase Physiological* Gout reported as occasional side effect *2068*

Lomustine

Leukocytes *Blood Decrease Physiological* Most severe adverse reaction is bone marrow suppression: leukopenia may develop about 6 weeks after a dose of lomustine. Bone marrow suppression is dose related and dose limiting *1384*

Platelets *Blood Decrease Physiological* Most severe adverse reaction is bone marrow suppression with thrombocytopenia developing about 4 weeks after a dose of lomustine: bone marrow suppression is delayed, dose related, dose limiting and cumulative *1384*

Loperamide

Didanosine *Serum No Effect Physiological* No significant effect observed on the concentration of either drug when two drugs coadministered *730*

Hydrochloric Acid *Gastric Fluid Decrease Physiological* Effect on both basal and submaximal pentagastrin-stimulated gastric acid secretion. Effect dose related *844*

Volume *Gastric Fluid Decrease Physiological* Effect on both basal and submaximal pentagastrin-stimulated gastric acid secretion. Effect dose related *844*

Zalcitabine *Serum No Effect Physiological* Coadministration of loperamide and single doses of zalcitabine 1.5 mg to 12 HIV-positive patients had no significant effect on pharmacokinetics of either drug *5023*

Loprazolam

Cortisol *Urine Decrease Physiological* Observed in 9 poor sleepers given up to 1 mg/d for 3 weeks: overnight urinary cortisol measured. Rebound increase on withdrawal *45*

Loracarbef

Alanine Aminotransferase *Serum Increase Physiological* Transient increases in enzyme activity have been observed with administration of loracarbef *1701*

Alkaline Phosphatase *Serum Increase Physiological* Transient increases in enzyme activity have been observed with administration of loracarbef *1701*

Aspartate Aminotransferase *Serum Increase Physiological* Transient increases in enzyme activity have been observed with administration of loracarbef *1701*

Creatinine *Serum Increase Physiological* Transient increases in concentration have been observed with administration of loracarbef *1701*

Eosinophils *Blood Increase Physiological* Transient eosinophilia has been observed with administration of loracarbef *1701*

Leukocytes *Blood Decrease Physiological* Transient leukopenia has been observed with administration of loracarbef *1701*

Platelets *Blood Decrease Physiological* Transient thrombocytopenia has been observed with administration of loracarbef *1701*

Urea Nitrogen *Serum Increase Physiological* Transient increases in concentration have been observed with administration of loracarbef *1701*

Loratadine

Alanine Aminotransferase *Serum Increase Physiological* Hepatic function abnormalities reported as a side effect *5327*

Alkaline Phosphatase *Serum Increase Physiological* Hepatic function abnormalities reported as a side effect *5327*

Aspartate Aminotransferase *Serum Increase Physiological* Hepatic function abnormalities reported as a side effect *5327*

Carbamazepine *Serum Increase Physiological* Drugs that inhibit CYP 3A4 inhibit metabolism of carbamazepine producing clinically meaningful effect *1039*

Cimetidine *Serum No Effect Physiological* Coadministration of loratidine with cimetidine had no effect on cimetidine concentration *5327*

Loratadine *(continued)*

Erythromycin *Serum Decrease Physiological* Coadministration of loratidine with erythromycin caused a 15% reduction of 0 - 24 h AUC of erythromycin *5327*

γ-Glutamyltransferase *Serum Increase Physiological* Hepatic function abnormalities reported as a side effect *5327*

Ketoconazole *Serum No Effect Physiological* Coadministration of loratidine with ketoconazole had no effect on ketoconazole concentration *5327*

Lorazepam

Albumin *Serum No Effect Analytical* At concentration of 0.05 mg/L had no effect on BCG method *5704*
Urine No Effect Analytical Using a fluorimetric assay with Albumin Blue 580 on a Cobas Fara centrifugal analyzer for the detection of microalbuminuria no significant interference was detected at a concentration of 0.8 mg/L *3117*

Benzodiazepine *Urine Positive Analytical* Detectable limit 0.7 µg/mL with improved EMIT assay and Syva ETS system compared with 2.0 µg/mL of former d.a.u. assay *3370* Positive result observed at a concentration of 3.0 µg/mL (9.34 µmol/L) with method on Du Pont aca *1556* At concentrations of 1.0 µg/mL or greater produces positive result with Syva EMIT II assay *1785*

Bicarbonate *Serum No Effect Analytical* At concentration of 0.05 mg/L had no effect on method using phenolphthalein *5704*

Bilirubin *Serum No Effect Analytical* At concentration of 0.05 mg/L had no effect on Jendrassik and Grof method *5704*

Calcium *Serum No Effect Analytical* At concentration of 0.05 mg/L had no effect on cresolphthalein method *5704*

Catecholamines *Plasma No Effect Analytical* No effect on HPLC method of Koller for dopamine, epinephrine, and norepinephrine *3230*

Chloride *Serum No Effect Analytical* At concentration of 0.05 mg/L had no effect on mercurimetric method *5704*

Cholesterol *Serum No Effect Analytical* At concentration of 0.05 mg/L had no effect on Liebermann-Burchard method *5704*

Creatinine *Serum No Effect Analytical* At 10 mg/L on reversed phase liquid chromatographic procedure of Zhiri et al *6656* At concentration of 0.05 mg/L had no effect on Technicon AutoAnalyzer® Jaffe method *5704*

Glucose *Serum No Effect Analytical* At concentration of 0.05 mg/L had no effect on GOD/POD-PAP method *5704*

Indomethacin *Serum No Effect Analytical* No effect on HPLC method of Roberts and Smith *4978*

Nefazodone *Serum No Effect Physiological* Administration of 200 mg nefazodone twice daily to individuals dosed with 2 mg lorazepam had no effect on the steady state pharmacokinetics of nefazodone or its metabolites *2317*

Phosphate *Serum No Effect Analytical* At concentration of 0.05 mg/L had no effect on phosphomolybdate method *5704*

Potassium *Serum No Effect Analytical* At concentration of 0.05 mg/L had no effect on flame-photometric method *5704*

Protein *Serum No Effect Analytical* At concentration of 0.05 mg/L had no effect on biuret method with blank correction *5704*

Sodium *Serum No Effect Analytical* At concentration of 0.05 mg/L had no effect on flame-photometric method *5704*

Tirofiban *Serum No Effect Physiological* Coadministration had no significant effect on plasma clearance of tirofiban *3957*

Triglycerides *Serum No Effect Analytical* At concentration of 0.05 mg/L had no effect on lipase/esterase method *5704*

Urea Nitrogen *Serum No Effect Analytical* At concentration of 0.05 mg/L had no effect on diacetylmonoxime method *5704*

Uric Acid *Serum No Effect Analytical* At concentration of 0.05 mg/L had no effect on phosphotungstate reduction method *5704* At 10 mg/L on reversed phase liquid chromatographic procedure of Zhiri et al *6656*

Lorcainide

Osmolality *Serum Decrease Physiological* Significant effect in 16 of 33 patients with organic heart disease and ventricular arrhythmias. Effect observed after single i.v. dose *5687*

Sodium *Serum Decrease Physiological* Increase by 8 mEq/L significant effect in 16 of 33 patients with organic heart disease and ventricular arrhythmias. Effect observed after single i.v. dose *5687*

Lormetazepam

Benzodiazepine *Urine Positive Analytical* Produces positive result at concentrations of 1.0 µg/mL or greater with Syva EMIT II assay *1785*

Lornoxicam

Prothrombin Time *Plasma Increase Physiological* Significant increase in prothrombin time in 12 healthy nonsmoking male volunteers when drug coadministered with warfarin (23.6 s) than when warfarin only administered (19.5 s) *4878*

Warfarin *Plasma Increase Physiological* When coadministered with warfarin mean concentration 0.25 µg/mL higher than when only warfarin administered in 12 nonsmoking male volunteers *4878*

Losartan

Alanine Aminotransferase *Serum Increase Physiological* Administration of losartan has been reported to cause minor increases in activity in fewer than 0.1% of treated patients with essential hypertension when treated with losartan alone *3965*
Serum No Effect Physiological Administration of losartan to patients with essential hypertension was rarely associated with an increase in activity *1596*

Albumin *Serum No Effect Physiological* In 11 patients with nephrotic syndrome treatment with 100 mg/d for 1 month caused nonsignificant change from baseline of 35.8 ± 1.9 g/L to 36.1 ± 1.5 g/L *1330*

Aldosterone *Plasma Decrease Physiological* In 20 normotensive and 7 hypertensive individuals treatment with 25 mg significantly decreased plasma renin activity from a mean of 17.7 ± 1.6 ng/dL to 6.4 ± 0.7 ng/dL in controls *2004*

Apolipoprotein A-I *Serum Decrease Physiological* In 11 patients with nephrotic syndrome treatment with 100 mg/d for 1 month caused nonsignificant change from baseline of 1.71 ± 0.12 g/L to 1.64 ± 0.10 g/L *1330*

Apolipoprotein A-I:Apolipoprotein B Ratio
Serum Increase Physiological In 13 nondiabetic patients with proteinuria treatment with losartan reduced the plasma apolipoprotein B concentration, and protein excretion from mean baseline of 6.2 ± 1.3 g/d to 4.2 ± 1.3 g/d, resulting in an increase in the apolipoprotein A-I:apolipoprotein B ratio *4235* In 11 patients with nephrotic syndrome treatment with 100 mg/d for 1 month caused significant change from baseline of 1.77 ± 0.15 to 2.00 ± 0.20 *1330*

Apolipoprotein B *Serum Decrease Physiological* In 13 nondiabetic patients with proteinuria treatment with losartan reduced the plasma apolipoprotein B concentration and protein excretion from mean baseline of 6.2 ± 1.3 g/d to 4.2 ± 1.3 g/d *4235* In 11 patients with nephrotic syndrome treatment with 100 mg/d for 1 month caused significant change from baseline of 1.02 ± 0.09 g/L to 0.86 ± 0.05 g/L *1330*

Apolipoprotein Lp(a) *Serum Decrease Physiological* In 11 patients with nephrotic syndrome treatment with 100 mg/d for 1 month caused nonsignificant change from baseline of 287 ± 57 mg/L to 218 ± 35 mg/L *1330*

Aspartate Aminotransferase *Serum Increase Physiological* Administration of losartan has been reported to cause minor increases in activity in fewer than 0.1% of treated patients with essential hypertension when treated with losartan alone *3965*
Serum No Effect Physiological Administration of losartan to patients with essential hypertension was rarely associated with an increase in activity *1596*

Bilirubin *Serum Increase Physiological* Administration of losartan has been reported to cause minor increases in concentration in fewer than 0.1% of treated patients with essential hypertension when treated with losartan alone *3965*
Serum No Effect Physiological Administration of losartan to patients with essential hypertension was rarely associated with an increase in concentration *1596*

Cholesterol *Serum Decrease Physiological* In 11 patients with nephrotic syndrome treatment with 100 mg/d for 1 month caused significant change from baseline of 6.67 ± 0.46 mmol/L to 6.08 ± 0.42 mmol/L *1330* In 13 nondiabetic patients with proteinuria treatment with losartan reduced the plasma cholesterol concentration mainly due to a reduction of VLDL and LDL-cholesterol and protein excretion from mean baseline of 6.2 ± 1.3 g/d to 4.2 ± 1.3 g/d *4235*

Cimetidine *Serum No Effect Physiological* Coadministration of losartan with cimetidine had no significant effect on the concentration of either drug *1596*

Creatinine *Serum Increase Physiological* Administration of losartan has been reported to cause minor increases in concentration in fewer than 0.1% of treated patients with hypertension when treated with losartan alone *3965*
Serum No Effect Physiological Administration of losartan to patients with essential hypertension was associated with an increase in serum concentration in less than 0.1% patients *1596*

Digoxin *Serum No Effect Physiological* Losartan coadministered with digoxin had no effect on its pharmacokinetics *3965* Coadministration had no effect on on the pharmacokinetics of oral or intravenous digoxin *3979* Coadministration of losartan with digoxin had no significant effect on the concentration of either drug *1596*

2,3-Dinor-6-Keto-Prostaglandin $F_{1\alpha}$
Urine Increase Physiological In 20 normotensive and 7 hypertensive individuals treatment with 75 mg had no significant effect on excretion *2004*

HDL-Cholesterol *Serum No Effect Physiological* In 11 patients with nephrotic syndrome treatment with 100 mg/d for 1 month caused nonsignificant change from baseline of 1.06 ± 0.09 mmol/L to 1.00 ± 0.09 mmol/L *1330*

Hematocrit *Blood Decrease Physiological* Administration of losartan has been reported to cause anemia in fewer than 1% of treated patients (mean decrease of approximately 0.11 g/dL) *3965*
Blood No Effect Physiological Administration of losartan to patients with essential hypertension was frequently associated with an insignificant decrease in concentration of 0.09% *1596*

Hemoglobin *Blood Decrease Physiological* Administration of losartan to patients was frequently associated with a decrease in concentration of 0.11 g/dL *1596* Administration of losartan has been reported to cause anemia in fewer than 1% of treated patients (mean decrease of approximately 0.09%) *3965*

Hydrochlorothiazide *Serum No Effect Physiological* Coadministration of losartan with hydrochlorothiazide had no effect on the pharmacokinetics of either drug *3965* Coadministration of losartan with hydrochlorothiazide had no significant effect on the concentration of either drug *1596* Coadministration had no effect on the pharmacokinetics of hydrochlorothiazide *3979* No significant interaction when hydrochlorothiazide coadministered with losartan *3881*

Phenobarbital *Serum No Effect Physiological* Coadministration of losartan with phenobarbital had no significant effect on the concentration of either drug *1596*

Protein *Serum Decrease Physiological* In 13 nondiabetic patients with proteinuria treatment with losartan reduced protein excretion from mean baseline of 6.2 ± 1.3 g/d to 4.2 ± 1.3 g/d *4235*
Serum No Effect Physiological In 11 patients with nephrotic syndrome treatment with 100 mg/d for 1 month caused nonsignificant change from baseline of 57.4 ± 2.2 g/L to 58.2 ± 1.9 g/L *1330*
Urine Decrease Physiological In 11 patients with nephrotic syndrome treatment with 100 mg/d for 1 month caused significant change from baseline of 6.2 ± 1.3 g/d to 4.1 ± 1.3 g/d *1330*

Prothrombin Time *Plasma No Effect Physiological* Losartan administered for 12 days had no effect on the pharmacodynamics/pharmacokinetics of a single dose of warfarin *3965* Coadministration of losartan with warfarin had no significant effect on the prothrombin time *1596*

Renal Plasma Flow *Patient Increase Physiological* In 20 normotensive and 7 hypertensive individuals treatment with 75 mg significantly increased renal plasma flow *2004*

Renin Activity *Plasma Increase Physiological* In 20 normotensive and 7 hypertensive individuals treatment with 75 mg significantly increased plasma renin activity by a mean of 2.0 ± 0.7 ng angiotensin I/mL/h compared with -0.2 ± 0.2 ng angiotensin I/mL/h in controls *2004*

Sodium *Urine Increase Physiological* In 20 normotensive and 7 hypertensive individuals treatment with 75 mg caused a significant increase in urinary excretion to 19.3 ± 2.0 mmol compared with 11.9 ± 1.7 mmol in controls *2004*

Triglycerides *Serum No Effect Physiological* In 11 patients with nephrotic syndrome treatment with 100 mg/d for 1 month caused nonsignificant change from baseline of 2.25 ± 0.60 mmol/L to 2.36 ± 0.73 mmol/L *1330*

Urea Nitrogen *Serum Increase Physiological* Administration of losartan has been reported to cause minor increases in concentration in fewer than 0.1% of treated patients with hypertension when treated with losartan alone *3965*
Serum No Effect Physiological Administration of losartan to patients with essential hypertension was associated with an increase in serum concentration in less than 0.1% patients *1596*

Uric Acid *Serum Increase Physiological* Gout has been reported as a side effect of administration *3979* Administration of losartan has been reported to cause gout in fewer than 1% of treated patients *3965*

VLDL + LDL-Cholesterol *Serum Decrease Physiological* In 13 nondiabetic patients with proteinuria treatment with losartan reduced the plasma cholesterol concentration mainly due to a reduction of VLDL and LDL-cholesterol and protein excretion from mean baseline of 6.2 ± 1.3 g/d to 4.2 ± 1.3 g/d *4235* In 11 patients with nephrotic syndrome treatment with 100 mg/d for 1 month caused significant change from baseline of 5.61 ± 0.51 mmol/L to 5.08 ± 0.46 mmol/L *1330*

Warfarin *Plasma No Effect Physiological* Losartan administered for 12 days had no effect on the pharmacodynamics/pharmacokinetics of a single dose of warfarin *3965* Coadministration had no effect on on the pharmacokinetics or pharmacodynamics of warfarin *3979*

Lovastatin

Alanine Aminotransferase *Serum Increase Physiological* Tendency to rise especially with higher doses but not increased above 3 times upper limit of normal *2514* In 2 patients treated with lovastatin activity increased to 8 times the upper limit of normal after 6 weeks in one and increased with the addition of lovastatin to the therapeutic regime and decreased with its withdrawal *2333* In one woman with hypercholesterolemia treatment with 80 mg/d caused significant increase from mean baseline of 44 U/L to 296 U/L *4877* In 8245 hypercholesterolemic patients increase observed in 0.1% (same as in placebo group) when given 20 mg/d for 48 weeks and 1.5% in patients receiving 80 mg daily for duration of study *682* Observed increase above three times upper limit of normal in 1.9% of patients treated for at least one year: slowly reverted to normal when drug discontinued. Increase usually observed 3-12 months following start of treatment *3982* Marked persistent increases to more than 3 times the upper limit of normal observed in 1.9% of adult patients treated for at least one year. Increase usually occurred 3 to 12 months after the start of treatment. Activity slowly returned to normal when treatment stopped *3982*
Serum No Effect Physiological No significant effect in 11 patients with renal transplants treated with 20 mg daily for 6 weeks *3055*

Albumin *Serum Increase Physiological* In 7 patients with nephrotic syndrome treatment with up to 40 mg/d for two years caused significant change from mean baseline of 25 ± 7 g/L to 39 ± 7 g/L *4771* In 20 nondiabetic nephrotic patients treatment with diet and up to 0.06 g/d for up to 30 months caused a significant increase from mean baseline of 25.9 ± 1.5 g/L to 35.5 ± 1.9 g/L *4263*

Lovastatin *(continued)*

Albumin *(continued)*

Serum No Effect Physiological In 12 patients with nephrotic syndrome and initially increased serum Lp(a) concentration treatment with lovastatin (40 mg/d) for 8 weeks caused a non-significant change from mean baseline of 25 ± 6 g/L to 28 ± 5 g/L. In 8 patients with initially normal Lp(a) concentration mean concentration changed non significantly from 28 ± 6 g/L to 27 ± 6 g/L *755* No significant effect in 11 patients with renal transplants treated with 20 mg daily for 6 weeks *3055*

Aldolase *Serum Increase Physiological* Rhabdomyolysis may occur in patients treated with lovastatin alone or when combined with immunosuppressive therapy including cyclosporine or lipid-lowering doses of nicotinic acid. May occur with or without renal impairment *3982*

Alkaline Phosphatase *Serum Increase Physiological* In one female patient with hypercholesterolemia administration of lovastatin (80 mg/d) was associated with marked increase from mean baseline of 66 U/L to 626 U/L *4877* In 2 patients treated with lovastatin activity increased to 1.5 times the upper limit of normal after 6 weeks in one and increased with the addition of lovastatin to the therapeutic regime and decreased with its withdrawal *2333*

α_2-Antiplasmin *Plasma No Effect Physiological* In 20 patients with type IIa hypercholesterolemia treatment for 12 months had no significant effect on concentration *3856*

Antipyrine *Serum No Effect Physiological* Lovastatin had no effect on the pharmacokinetics or metabolism of antipyrine *3982* Coadministration of lovastatin with antipyrine had no effect on its pharmacokinetics *3982*

Antithrombin III *Plasma No Effect Physiological* In 20 patients with type IIa hypercholesterolemia treatment for 12 months had no signiicant effect on concentration *3856*

Apolipoprotein A *Serum Decrease Physiological* In 7 patients with nephrotic syndrome treatment with up to 40 mg/d for two years caused nonsignificant change from mean baseline of 171 ± 65 mg/dL to 156 ± 30 mg/dL *4771*

Apolipoprotein A-I *Serum Decrease Physiological* In 32 patients in the Monitored Atherosclerosis Regression Study treatment with 80 mg/d for 2 years caused significant change of -8.5 ± 5.5 mg/dL from mean baseline of 135.6 ± 6.2 mg/dL (6%) *85*

Serum Increase Physiological Slight effect in clinical trial of 101 patients with heterozygous familial hypercholesterolemia *2514* In 59 patients with hypercholesterolemia treatment with up to 80 mg/d for 24 weeks caused significant increase of 9 ± 17% from mean baseline of 131 ± 23 mg/dL *2833* In 17 patients with hypercholesterolemia treated with 20 mg/d for 4 weeks caused increase from mean baseline of 148 ± 6 mg/dL to 154 ± 7 mg/dL (nonsignificant) and with treatment with 40 mg/d for another 4 weeks significant increase to 161 ± 8 mg/dL (9%), and with 80 mg/d for 8 weeks concentration increased to 160 ± 7 mg/dL (8%) *2862* In 35 patients with primary hyperlipoproteinemia administration of up to 80 mg/d for 3 months caused change from mean of 170 ± 8 mg/dL to 176 ± 11 mg/dL (4%) *3214*

Serum No Effect Physiological In 80 patients with primary hypercholesterolemia treated with up to 80 mg/d for 12 weeks no change from initial concentration of 1.4 ± 0.2 g/L *1651* No significant change in 11 patients with renal transplants following treatment with 20 mg daily for 6 weeks *3055* Nonsignificant increase in 30 patients with nonfamilial primary hypercholesterolemia treated with up to 80 mg/day with appropriate diet for 6 months *1572* Nonsignificant increase from mean baseline concentration of 165 mg/dL to 175 mg/dL in 19 patients with primary hypercholesterolemia treated with up to 80 mg/d for 12 weeks *3848*

Apolipoprotein A-II *Serum Decrease Physiological* In 17 patients with primary hypercholesterolemia treatment with 20 mg/d for 4 weeks caused significant decrease from mean baseline of 96 ± 6 mg/dL to 82 ± 3 mg/dL (15%), after another 4 weeks with 40 mg/d mean concentration decreased to 80 ± 4 mg/dL (17%) and after 8 weeks with 80 mg/d mean concentration reduced to 79 ± 3 mg/dL (18%) *2862* in 35 patients with primary hyperlipoproteinemia treatment with up to 80 mg/d for 3 months caused change from mean of 65 ± 4 mg/dL to 59 ± 3 mg/dL (9%) *3214*

Serum Increase Physiological Slight effect in clinical trial of 101 patients with heterozygous familial hypercholesterolemia *2514*

Serum No Effect Physiological Nonsignificant increase in 30 patients with primary nonfamilial hypercholesterolemia treated with up to 80 mg/day with appropriate diet for 6 months *2850* No change from mean baseline concentration of 54 mg/dL observed in 19 patients with primary hypercholesterolemia treated with up to 80 mg/d for 12 weeks *3848*

Apolipoprotein B *Serum Decrease Physiological* In 35 patients with primary hyperlipoproteinemia treatment with up to 80 mg/d for 3 months caused decrease of mean from 122 ± 6 mg/dL to 96 ± 4 mg/dL (21%) *3214* Significant reduction from mean baseline concentration of 273 mg/dL to 190 mg/dL observed in 19 patients with primary hypercholesterolemia treated with up to 80 mg/d for 12 weeks *3848* In 80 patients with primary hypercholesterolemia treated with up to 80 mg/d for 12 weeks significant reduction of 33.3% from mean baseline of 1.8 ± 0.3 g/L to 1.2 ± 0.2 g/L *1651* Significant reduction of 11.8% in 17 hypercholesterolemic patients treated with 20 mg/day for 6 weeks and of 28.5% in 23 patients with serum cholesterols above 7.8 mmol/L treated with 40 mg/day for 6 weeks *4387* In 7 patients with nephrotic syndrome treatment with up to 40 mg/d for two years caused significant change from mean baseline of 162 ± 60 mg/dL to 108 ± 42 mg/dL *4771* In one study of 191 hypercholesterolemic patients treatment with 20 mg/d for 16 weeks caused a 20% reduction in concentration *4534* In 32 patients in the Monitored Atherosclerosis Regression Study treatment with 80 mg/d for 2 years caused significant change of -16.5 ± 4.5 mg/dL from mean baseline of 96.2 ± 4.4 mg/dL (17%) *85* In 14 patients with nephrotic syndrome treatment with up to 80 mg/d for 6 months caused normalization to 1.11 ± 0.09 g/L from mean baseline of 1.51 ± 0.0 g/L (mean 26% reduction) *961* In 17 patients with hypercholesterolemia treatment with 20 mg/d for 4 weeks caused 21% reduction from mean baseline of 244 ± 12 mg/dL to 194 ± 11 mg/dL, to 178 ± 10 mg/dL after another 4 weeks with 40 mg/d (27% reduction) and to 178 ± 10 mg/dL after another 8 weeks with 80 mg/d (27% reduction) *2862* In 59 patients with hypercholesterolemia treatment with up to 80 mg/d for 24 weeks caused significant decrease of 29 ± 12% from mean baseline of 200 ± 27 mg/dL *2833* In 19 hypercholesterolemic patients on 43% high fat diet for 3 weeks lovastatin 40 mg/day caused mean reduction of 30% versus placebo. In 16 patients on 25% low fat diet the same dose of lovastatin caused a mean reduction of 26% *1064* Increase by 23% at 40 mg b.i.d. in clinical trial of 101 patients with heterozygous familial hypercholesterolemia *2514*

Serum No Effect Physiological Insignificant reduction by 9% in 11 patients with renal transplants when treated with 20 mg daily for 6 weeks *3055*

Apolipoprotein B-I *Serum Decrease Physiological* Significant reduction in 29 of 30 patients with primary nonfamilial hypercholesterolemia after 1 month treatment with 20 mg/day or more *2850*

Apolipoprotein C-III *Serum Decrease Physiological* In 32 patients in the Monitored Atherosclerosis Regression Study treatment with 80 mg/d for 2 years caused significant change of -1.3 ± 0.5 mg/dL from mean baseline of 12.3 ± 0.7 mg/dL (11%) *85*

Apolipoprotein E *Serum Decrease Physiological* In 17 patients with primary hypercholesterolemia treatment with 20 mg/d for 4 weeks significant 28% reduction from mean baseline of 33 ± 3 mg/dL to 24 ± 3 mg/dL with reduction to 23 ± 4 mg/dL (30%) after another 4 weeks with 40 mg/d and further reduction to 22 ± 4 mg/dL (33%) after another 8 weeks with 80 mg/d *2862* In 32 patients in the Monitored Atherosclerosis Regression Study treatment with 80 mg/d for 2 years caused significant change of -1.8 ± 0.8 mg/dL from mean baseline of 13.5 ± 0.7 mg/dL (13%) *85* Significant reduction from mean baseline concentration of 5.1 mg/dL to 3.8 mg/dL in 19 patients with primary hypercholesteroiemia treated with up to 80 mg/d for 12 weeks *3848*

Aspartate Aminotransferase *Serum Increase Physiological* In one patient with hypercholesterolemia treatment with 80 mg/d caused significant increase from mean baseline of 15 U/L to 256 U/L *4877* Incidence of increased activity 0.1% in hypercholesterolemic patients receiving 20 mg/d for 48 weeks and 1.5% in patients receiving 80 mg/d for duration of study (incidence of increased activity in placebo-treated patients 0.1%) *682* Lovastatin administration has been associated with marked persistent increases in activity *3982* Marked persistent increases to more than 3 times the upper limit of normal observed in 1.9% of adult patients treated for at least one year. Increase usually occurred 3 to 12 months after start of treatment. Activity slowly returned to normal when treatment stopped *3982* In 2 patients treated with lovastatin activity increased to 6 times the upper limit of normal after 6 weeks in one and increased with the addition of lovastatin to the therapeutic regime and decreased with its withdrawal *2333*

Serum No Effect Physiological No significant effect in 11 patients with renal transplants treated with 20 mg daily for 6 weeks *3055*

Bilirubin *Serum Increase Physiological* In one patient with hypercholesterolemia treatment with 80 mg/d caused significant increase from mean baseline of 6 µmol/L to 12 µmol/L *4877* In 2 patients treated with lovastatin bilirubin increased to 200 µmol/L after 6 weeks in one and increased with the addition of lovastatin to the therapeutic regime and decreased with its withdrawal *2333*

Serum No Effect Physiological No significant effect in 11 renal transplant patients treated with 20 mg/day for 6 weeks *3055*

C_1-Esterase Inhibitor *Serum No Effect Physiological* In 20 patients with type IIa hypercholesterolemia treatment for 12 months had no significant on concentration *3856*

Campesterol *Serum Increase Physiological* In 7 patients with familial hypercholesterolemia treatment with 40 mg/d caused increase from mean baseline of 214 ± 26 100 x mmol/mol cholesterol by 21 ± 8, 23 ± 12 and 38 ± 22 100 x mmol/mol cholesterol after 1, 2 and 4 weeks respectively *6209*

$CD57^+$ Lymphocytes *Blood No Effect Physiological* in 25 patients with primary hypercholesterolemia treatment with 40 mg/d for 8 weeks caused nonsignificant change from mean baseline of 10.7% to 11.8% of total lymphocytes *3921*

Chlorpropamide *Serum No Effect Physiological* In patients with hypercholesterolemia and noninsulin-dependent diabetes mellitus coadministration of lovastatin and oral hypoglycemics had no interactions *3982*

Cholestanol *Serum Decrease Physiological* In 7 patients with familial hypercholesterolemia treatment with 40 mg/d caused significant reduction of δ8-cholestenol concentration from mean baseline of 207± 78 100 x mmol/mol cholesterol by 101 ± 23, 101 ± 20 and 98 ± 26 100 x mmol/mol cholesterol after 1, 2 and 4 weeks respectively *6209*

Serum No Effect Physiological In 7 patients with familial hypercholesterolemia insignificant change from mean baseline of 107 ± 14 100 x mmol/mol cholesterol after treatment with 40 mg/d of - 19 ± 16, - 1 +/ 22 and + 11 ± 30 100 x mmol/mol cholesterol after treatment for 1, 2 and 4 weeks respectively *6209*

Cholesterol *Serum Decrease Physiological* In 30 hypercholesterolemic patients treated for 5 years mean reduction of 25-31% attained and sustained with reversible myopathy as only significant side effect *3739* In 35 patients with primary hyperlipoproteinemia administration of up to 80 mg/d for 3 months caused significant decrease from mean of 326 ± 12 mg/dL to 244 ± 8 mg/dL (25%) *3214* In 12 individuals with hypertriglyceridemia treatment with lovastatin for 6 weeks caused reduction to 193 ± 26 mg/dL compared with 271 ± 43 mg/dL after placebo *2103* In 20 patients with primary hypercholesterolemia treatment with mean dose of 70.5 mg/d caused reduction of 21% at 4 weeks, 23% at 6 weeks, 28% at 10 weeks and 27% at 12 weeks *458* 21% reduction in 11 postrenal transplant patients with hypercholesterolemia when treated with 20 mg/day for 6 weeks *3055* In 17 patients with primary hypercholesterolemia treatment with 20 mg/d for 4 weeks caused significant (18%) decrease from 9.66 ± 0.37 mmol/L to 7.89 ± 0.44 mmol/L: after 40 mg/d for 4 weeks mean concentration decreased to 7.42 ± 0.40 mmol/L (23% from baseline) and to 6.86 ± 0.41 mmol/L (29%) after another 8 weeks *2862* In 56 patients with type IIa and IIb hyperlipoproteinemia treated with 20 mg daily for 6 weeks mean concentration fell by an average of 26% from 8.12 mmol/L to 6.03 mmol/L *401* Significant decrease from mean baseline of 365 mg/dL to 256 mg/dL in 19 patients with primary hypercholesterolemia treated with up to 80 mg/d for 12 weeks *3848* Reduction from mean baseline concentration of 310 mg/dL to 217 mg/dL in 15 patients with type II hyperlipoproteinemia treated with lovastatin for 3 months *3245* Significant reduction from mean of 284 mg/dL to 210 mg/dL in 7 patients with combined hyperlipidemia treated with 40 mg daily for 6 weeks to 3 months and from 401 mg/dL to 293 mg/dL in 3 patients with familial hypercholesterolemia *232* In 80 patients with primary hypercholesterolemia treatment with up to 80 mg/d for 12 weeks caused significant reduction (33.4%) from mean of 10.1 ± 2.0 mmol/L to 6.7 ± 1.4 mmol/L *1651* In 29 of 30 patients with nonfamilial primary hypercholesterolemia treatment with 20 mg/day for 1 month caused significant reduction *2850* Transient decrease in one patient with diabetes mellitus, goitrous hypothyroidism due to Hashimoto's thyroiditis and Type IIa hyperlipoproteinemia when lovastatin added to thyroxine regime on which she had been stabilized *1379* In 9 hyperlipidemic men treatment with 40 mg/d for 48 weeks caused a 20.8% decrease from mean baseline of 273 mg/dL to 216 mg/dL *1450* In 59 patients with hypercholesterolemia treatment with up to 80 mg/d for 24 weeks caused significant decrease of 27 ± 11% from mean baseline of 299 ± 49 mg/dL *2833* In 19 hypercholesterolemic patients receiving 43% high fat diet lovastatin 40 mg/day for 3 weeks caused mean reduction of 23%. In 16 patients receiving 25% low fat diet for 3 weeks the same dose of lovastatin also caused a mean reduction of 23% *1064* Increase by 14 to 34% in clinical trial of 101 patients with heterozygous familial hypercholesterolemia *2514* In 919 asymptomatic men and women treatment with up to 40 mg/d for 3 years caused a change from mean baseline of 235 ± 22 mg/dL to 193 ± 27 mg/dL after 1 year and 195 ± 29 mg/dL after 3 years *4795* Reduction by 27% after 3 months at which level it remained stable in 11 cardiac transplant patients with hypercholesterolemia treated with up to 60 mg/day for 1 year *3329* In 14 patients with nephrotic syndrome treatment with up to 80 mg/d for 6 months caused significant reduction of 31% from mean baseline of 8.24 ± 0.49 mmol/L to 5.7 ± 0.18 mmol/L *961* Mean decrease of 17% in 8 hypercholesterolemic patients treated with 20 mg in evening for 48 weeks and decrease of 29% when 20 mg given with breakfast and dinner to 9 patients for same time *682* In 12 patients with nephrotic syndrome and initially increased serum Lp(a) concentration treatment with lovastatin (40 mg/d) for 8 weeks caused a significant change from mean baseline of 380.0 ± 90.0 mg/dL to 243.3 ± 39.6 mg/dL. In 8 patients with initially normal Lp(a) concentration mean change from 323.0 ± 90.0 mg/dL to 223.4 ± 28.3 mg/dL *755* In 20 patients with type IIa hypercholesterolemia treated with up to 80 mg/d for 12 months mean reduction of 66 mg/dL (from 320 ± 12.6 to 254 ± 12.0 mg/dL) observed *3856* In 32 patients in the Monitored Atherosclerosis Regression Study treatment with 80 mg/d for 2 years caused significant reduction of 73.1 ± 3.5 mg/dL from mean baseline of 226.3 ± 4.3 mg/dL (32%) *85* In 17 hypercholesterolemic patients significant reduction at 6 weeks of 16.4% with 20 mg/day and 27.2% reduction with 40 mg/day in 23 hypercholesterolemic patients *4387* In 85 patients with hypercholesterolemia treatment with 40 mg/d for 12 weeks caused a mean decrease of 27%, and in 88 treated with 80 mg/d for 12 weeks caused a mean 34% decrease *3982* In 17 patients treatment with 40 mg/d for 6 weeks caused decrease from mean of 6.53 ± 0.44 mmol/L at baseline to 4.78 ± 0.55 mmol/L *3905* In 25 patients with primary hypercholesterolemia treatment with 40 mg/d caused significant decrease of 30 ± 2% after 4 weeks and 29 ± 2% after 8 weeks from mean baseline of 7.7 ± 0.3 mmol/L *3921* In one study of 191 hypercholesterolemic patients treatment with 20 mg/d for 16 weeks caused a 19% reduction in concentration *4534* In 7 patients with familial hypercholesterolemia treatment with 40 mg/d caused significant decrease from mean baseline of 11.0 ± 0.67 mmol/L by 2.5 ± 0.47 mmol/L after 1 week, 3.3 ± 0.47 mmol/L after 2 weeks and 3.4 ± 0.59 mmol/L after 4 weeks *6209* Mean reduction of 20.0% in 50 noninsulin dependent diabetics with primary hypercholesterolemia treated for 24 weeks with 20 mg daily *2215* In 7 patients with nephrotic syndrome treatment with up to 40 mg/d for two years caused significant change from mean baseline of 446 ± 165 mg/dL to 250 ± 57 mg/dL *4771* In 27 patients with hypercholesterolemia 3 months of treatment with 20 mg daily concentration 28% less than in controls (208 mg/dL versus 289 mg/dL) *2354* In 15 non-diabetic type II hypercholesterolemic patients 80 mg/d for 6 weeks caused mean 30% reduction *3880* In 20 nondiabetic nephrotic patients treatment with diet and up to 0.06 g/d for up to 30 months caused a significant decrease from mean baseline of

Lovastatin *(continued)*

Cholesterol *(continued)*
350.1 ± 17.5 mg/dL to 229.3 ± 16.65 mg/dL *4263* In 28 individuals with plasma cholesterol concentrations between 200 and 240 mg/dL treatment with 10 mg/d for 20 weeks caused a 24% decrease from baseline *5144*

Cholesterol:HDL-Cholesterol Ratio
Serum Decrease Physiological In 17 patients treated with 40 mg/d for 6 weeks caused significant reduction from mean baseline of 7.50 ± 0.76 to 4.88 ± 0.94 *3905* In 85 patients with hypercholesterolemia treatment with 40 mg/d for 12 weeks caused a mean decrease of 31%, and in 88 treated with 80 mg/d for 12 weeks caused a mean 37% decrease *3982* Reduction of 21% when 12 hypercholesterolemic patients treated with 20 mg daily for 48 weeks and reduction of 34% when treated with 40 mg at breakfast and 40 mg at dinner for 48 weeks *682*

Cortisol *Plasma No Effect Physiological* Lovastatin administration has no effect on basal concentration of cortisol or effect on adrenal reserve *3982* No significant change even in patients with familial hypercholesterolemia receiving 40 mg b.i.d *2514*

C-Reactive Protein *Serum No Effect Physiological* In 20 patients with type IIa hypercholesterolemia treatment with drug for 12 months did not cause concentration to exceed normal range *3856*

Creatine Kinase *Serum Increase Physiological* Marked increase to 1500 to 2000 U/L in one man with familial hypercholesterolemia receiving 40 mg daily but also receiving an angiotensin-converting enzyme inhibitor. Myositis and creatine kinase increases due to lovastatin previously reported *1657* Severe cases of rhabdomyolysis observed when lovastatin given alone or more often when combined with cyclosporine, gemfibrozil or large doses of nicotinic acid: also observed in patients taking erythromycin. Increased CK seen in about 11% patients *3982* Rhabdomyolysis may occur in patients treated with lovastatin alone or when combined with immunosuppressive therapy including cyclosporine or lipid-lowering doses of nicotinic acid. May occur with or without renal impairment. About 11% patients have demonstrated increased activity on one or more occasions *3982* Increase of more than 10 times the upper limit of normal observed in 5 of 8245 hypercholesterolemic patients treated with doses of from 20 mg/d to 80 mg/d for 48 weeks. One of the 5 received 40 mg/d, the other 4 received 80 mg/d *682* Increase of more than 10 times the upper limit of normal observed in 5 of 8245 hypercholesterolemic patients treated with doses of from 20 mg/d to 80 mg/d for 48 weeks. One of the 5 received 40 mg/d, the other 4 received 80 mg/d *682* In 2 men total creatine kinase activity increased by 183% and 242% respectively 24 hours after exercise whereas average response of creatine kinase to exercise in 18 other individuals did not differ before and after lovastatin treatment *6013* Significant increase to above 1000 U/L observed in one of 50 noninsulin dependent diabetics with primary hypercholesterolemia treated with 20 mg daily for 24 weeks but no sign of myopathy and value returned to baseline in spite of continued therapy *2215*
Serum No Effect Physiological No significant effect in 11 patients with renal transplants treated with 20 mg daily for 6 weeks *3055*

Creatine Kinase MM-Isoenzyme
Serum Increase Physiological About 11% patients have demonstrated increased activity on one or more occasions attributable to the CK-MM fraction *3982*

Creatinine *Serum Increase Physiological* In 7 patients with nephrotic syndrome treatment with up to 40 mg/d for two years caused nonsignificant change from mean baseline of 1.03 ± 0.4 mg/dL to 1.90 ± 2.9 mg/dL *4771* In 20 nondiabetic nephrotic patients treatment with diet and up to 0.06 g/d for up to 30 months caused a significant increase from mean baseline of 1.67 ± 0.22 mg/dL to 1.93 ± 0.44 mg/dL *4263*
Serum No Effect Physiological No effect observed in 8245 hypercholesterolemic patients receiving 20-80 mg/d for 48 weeks *682* No significant effect in 11 patients with renal transplants treated with 20 mg daily for 6 weeks *3055*

Creatinine Clearance *Urine Decrease Physiological* In 12 patients with nephrotic syndrome and initially increased serum Lp(a) concentration treatment with lovastatin (40 mg/d) for 8 weeks caused a significant change from mean baseline of 70.0 ± 41.9 mL/min to 60.4 ± 39.8 mL/min *755*
Urine No Effect Physiological In 8 patients with nephrotic syndrome and initially normal serum Lp(a) concentration treatment with lovastatin (40 mg/d) for 8 weeks caused a nonsignificant change from mean baseline of 77.4 ± 20.8 mL/min to 75.3 ± 22.7 mL/min *755*

Cyclosporine *Blood No Effect Analytical* At a concentration of 4 mg/L had no effect on Syva EMIT method *495*

Desmosterol *Serum No Effect Physiological* In 7 patients with familial hypercholesterolemia treatment with 40 mg/d caused reduction (but not significant) from mean baseline of 48 ± 13 100 x mmol/mol cholesterol after 4 weeks *6209*

Digoxin *Serum No Effect Physiological* In patients with hypercholesterolemia coadministration of lovastatin and digoxin had no effect on the plasma concentration of digoxin *3982* No effect observed on digoxin concentration of concomitant administration of lovastatin *3982*

Erythrocyte Aggregation *Blood No Effect Physiological* In 35 patients with primary hyperlipoproteinemia treatment with up to 80 mg/d for 3 months caused nonsignificant decrease fro 3.3 ± 0.2 units to 3.2 ± 0.2 units (3%) *3214*

Erythrocyte Transit Time *Blood No Effect Physiological* In 35 patients with primary hyperlipoproteinemia treatment with up to 80 mg/d for 3 months caused nonsignificant reduction from 14.4 ± 0.7 units to 13.7 ± 0.4 units *3214*

Fibrinogen *Plasma Decrease Physiological* Insignificant reduction from mean baseline concentration of 346 mg/dL to 331 mg/dL in 15 patients with type II hyperlipoproteinemia treated for 3 months with lovastatin *3245* In 20 patients with type IIa hypercholesterolemia treated for 12 months significant decrease observed. Long term treatment was associated with reduction of concentration *3856*
Plasma Increase Physiological In 59 patients with hypercholesterolemia treatment with up to 80 mg/d for 24 weeks caused significant increase of 19 ± 52% from mean baseline of 337 ± 98 mg/dL *2833*
Plasma No Effect Physiological In 35 patients with primary hyperlipoproteinemia treated with up to 80 mg/d for 3 months caused no change from baseline concentration of 2.5 g/L *3214*

Glipizide *Serum No Effect Physiological* In patients with hypercholesterolemia and noninsulin-dependent diabetes mellitus coadministration of lovastatin and oral hypoglycemics had no interactions *3982*

Glucose *Serum No Effect Physiological* No significant difference observed after 6 weeks treatment with 80 mg/d for 6 weeks in 15 type II hypercholesterolemic patients *3880* Insignificant increase of 4.9% in 50 noninsulin dependent diabetics with primary hypercholesterolemia treated with 20 mg daily for 24 weeks *2215* No effect observed in 8245 hypercholesterolemic patients receiving doses of from 20 mg/d to 80 mg/d for 48 weeks *682*

Glucose Tolerance *Serum No Effect Physiological* In 15 nondiabetic patients with type II hypercholesterolemia treatment with 80 mg/d for weeks had no significant effect on glucose tolerance *3880*

γ-Glutamyltransferase *Serum Increase Physiological* In one woman with hypercholesterolemia treatment with 80 mg/d caused significant increase from mean baseline of 25 U/L to 612 U/L *4877*

HDL_2-Cholesterol *Serum No Effect Physiological* In 7 patients with nephrotic syndrome treatment with up to 40 mg/d for two years caused nonsignificant change from mean baseline of 8.3 ± 5.1 mg/dL to 9.3 ± 2.9 mg/dL *4771*

HDL_3-Cholesterol *Serum Increase Physiological* In 7 patients with nephrotic syndrome treatment with up to 40 mg/d for two years caused significant change from mean baseline of 23 ± 15 mg/dL to 30 ± 12 mg/dL *4771*

HDL-Apolipoprotein A-I *Serum Increase Physiological* Nonsignificant increase from mean baseline concentration of 114 mg/dL to 121 mg/dL in 19 patients with primary hypercholesterolemia treated with up to 80 mg/d for 12 weeks *3848*

HDL-Apolipoprotein E *Serum Decrease Physiological* Nonsignificant decrease from mean baseline concentration of 3.27 mg/dL to 2.75 mg/dL in 19 patients with primary hypercholesterolemia treated with up to 80 mg/d for 12 weeks *3848*

HDL-Cholesterol *Serum Increase Physiological* Nonsignificant increase from mean baseline concentration of 48 mg/dL to 56 mg/dL in 19 patients with primary hypercholesterolemia treated with up to 80 mg/d for 12 weeks *3848* In 17 patients treatment with 40 mg/d for 6 weeks caused increase from mean baseline of 0.88 ± 0.09 mmol/L to 1.01 ± 0.13 mmol/L *3905* Nonsignificant increase from mean of 29 mg/dL to 35 mg/dL in 7 patients with combined hyperlipidemia and from 30 mg/dL to 33 mg/dL in 3 patients with familial hypercholesterolemia when treated with 40 mg daily for 6 weeks to 3 months *232* Mean increase of 13.6% in 50 noninsulin dependent diabetics with primary hypercholesterolemia treated with 20 mg daily for 24 weeks *2215* In 17 type IIb hyperlipoproteinemic patients with moderately increased cholesterol treatment with 20 mg/d for 6 weeks caused mean increase of 5% and in 23 with high cholesterol treatment caused increase of 10% *6033* In 27 hypercholesterolemics treatment with 20 mg daily for 3 months caused increase of 12% (change from 43 mg/dL to 48 mg/dL) *2354* Slight effect in clinical trial of 101 patients with heterozygous familial hypercholesterolemia *2514* In 25 patients with hypercholesterolemia treatment with 40 mg/d caused nonsignificant increase of 7 ± 5% after 4 weeks and 4 ± 5% after 8 weeks from mean baseline of 1.3 ± 0.1 mmol/L *3921* In 20 patients with primary hypercholesterolemia treatment with mean dose of 70.5 mg/d for 4 weeks caused mean increase of 7% with an increase of 15% at 6 weeks, 17% at 10 weeks and 21% at 12 weeks *458* In 80 patients with primary hypercholesterolemia treated with up to 80 mg/d for 12 weeks significant 13.5% increase from mean of 1.16 ± 0.33 mmol/L to 1.29 ± 0.7 mmol/L *1651* In 12 individuals with hypertriglyceridemia treatment with lovastatin for 6 weeks caused nonsignificant increase to 33.3 ± 9.5 mg/dL compared with 29.4 ± 6.2 mg/dL after placebo *2103* In 12 patients with nephrotic syndrome and initially increased serum Lp(a) concentration treatment with lovastatin (40 mg/d) for 8 weeks caused a significant change from mean baseline of 40.8 ± 9.6 mg/dL to 48.8 ± 12.9 mg/dL *755* In 59 patients with hypercholesterolemia treatment with up to 80 mg/d for 24 weeks caused significant increase of 13 ± 17% from mean baseline of 46 ± 9 mg/dL *2833* In 19 patients receiving 43% high fat diet for 3 weeks with 40 mg lovastatin daily concentration increased concentration by 8%: in 16 patients receiving 25% low fat diet the same dose of lovastatin caused increase of 7% *1064* Insignificant increase of 7.6% in 56 patients with type IIa and type IIb hyperlipoproteinemia treated with 20 mg daily for 6 weeks. Concentration increased in 89% patients with a mild decrease noted in 11% *401* Treatment of 73 type IIa hyperlipoproteinemic patients with average of 71 mg/d for 12 weeks caused mean increase of about 5% *6033* In 9 hyperlipidemic men treatment with 40 mg/d for 48 weeks caused a 10.9% increase from mean baseline of 33.9 mg/dL to 37.5 mg/dL *1450* In one study of 191 hypercholesterolemic patients treatment with 20 mg/d for 16 weeks caused a 7% increase in concentration *4534* In 17 patients with primary hypercholesterolemia treatment with 20 mg/d for 4 weeks caused significant increase (11%) to 1.28 ± 0.10 mmol/L from baseline of 1.15 ± 0.07 mmol/L and to 1.37 ± 0.12 mmol/L (19%) after another 4 weeks with 40 mg/d with no further increase in spite of increase of dose to 80 mg/d for 8 weeks *2862* In over 8000 patients with moderately severe hypercholesterolemia treated for 2 years mean concentration increased by 12% with 20 mg/d, 14% with 40 mg/d and 17% with 80 mg/d *683* Increase of 6.6% when 20 mg given with evening meal and increase of 9.5% when 40 mg given at breakfast and 40 mg given at dinner in 13 hypercholesterolemic patients treated for 48 weeks *682* In 7 patients with nephrotic syndrome treatment with up to 40 mg/d for two years caused nonsignificant change from mean baseline of 34 ± 17 mg/dL to 41 ± 12 mg/dL *4771* In 61 middle-aged men with low HDL concentration treatment increased mean concentration by 6% *6219* In 446 asymptomatic women treatment with up to 40 mg/d for 3 years caused an insignificant change from mean baseline of 58 ± 14 mg/dL to 61 ± 15 mg/dL after 1 year and 58 ± 15 mg/dL after 3 years *4795* In 85 patients with hypercholesterolemia treatment with 40 mg/d for 12 weeks caused a mean increase of 9%, and in 88 treated with 80 mg/d for 12 weeks caused a mean 8% increase *3982* Insignificant increase of 4.7% in 17 patients with hypercholesterolemia treated with 20 mg/day for 6 weeks but significant increase in 23 patients with serum cholesterols above 7.8 mmol/L treated with 40 mg/day for 6 weeks *4387* In 35 patients with primary hyperlipoproteinemia treatment with up to 80 mg/d for 3 months caused nonsignificant increase from mean of 50 ± 4 mg/dL to 54 mg/dL (7%) *3214*

Serum No Effect Physiological No significant effect in 11 postcardiac transplant patients with hypercholesterolemia treated with up to 60 mg/day for 1 year *3329* Insignificant increase in 11 patients with postrenal transplant hypercholesterolemia when treated with 20 mg/day for 6 weeks *3055* In 7 patients with familial hypercholesterolemia treatment with 40 mg/d for up to 4 weeks caused insignificant change from mean baseline of 1.27 ± 0.13 mmol/L *6209* In 32 patients in the Monitored Atherosclerosis Regression Study treatment with 80 mg/d for 2 years caused nonsignificant change of +2.3 ± 0.6 mg/dL from mean baseline of 42.0 ± 1.3 mg/dL (5%) *85* Nonsignificant increase from mean baseline of 48 mg/dL to 52 mg/dL in 19 patients with primary hypercholesterolemia treated with up to 80 mg/d for 12 weeks *3848* In 8 patients with nephrotic syndrome and initially normal serum Lp(a) concentration treatment with lovastatin (40 mg/d) for 8 weeks caused a nonsignificant change from mean baseline of 56.8 ± 18.6 mg/dL to 56.4 ± 17.4 mg/dL *755* Nonsignificant increase in 20 patients with nonfamilial primary hypercholesterolemia treated with up to 80 mg/day and appropriate diet for 6 months *2850* No effect of up to 80 mg daily for 3 months in 5 patients with hypertriglyceridemia and in 5 with normal concentrations of triglycerides *6391* In 473 asymptomatic men treatment with up to 40 mg/d for 3 years caused an insignificant change from mean baseline of 46 ± 10 mg/dL to 48 ± 15 mg/dL after 1 year and 47 ± 12 mg/dL after 3 years *4795*

HDL-Cholesterol:LDL-Cholesterol Ratio
Serum Increase Physiological Significant increase of 38.6% in 17 hypercholesterolemic patients treated with 20 mg/day for 6 weeks and of 71.0% in 23 patients with serum cholesterols initially above 7.8 mmol/L treated with 40 mg/day for 6 weeks *4387*

Hematocrit *Blood No Effect Physiological* No significant change observed in 15 patients with type II hyperlipoproteinemia treated with lovastatin for 3 months *3245* In 35 patients with primary hyperlipoproteinemia treatment with up to 80 mg/d for 3 months caused insignificant change from 0.466 ± 0.011 to 0.476 ± 0.012 (2%) *3214*

Hemoglobin *Blood No Effect Physiological* No effect observed in 8245 hypercholesterolemic patients receiving doses of 20-80 mg/d for 48 weeks *682* No effect observed in 11 patients with renal transplants treated with 20 mg daily for 6 weeks *3055*

Hemoglobin A_{1c} *Blood Increase Physiological* Mean increase of 7.2% in 49 noninsulin dependent diabetics with primary hypercholesterolemia treated with 20 mg daily for 24 weeks *2215*

IDL-Apolipoprotein B *Serum Decrease Physiological* Nonsignificant reduction from mean of 104 mg/dL to 55 mg/dL in 7 patients with combined hyperlipidemia and from 61 mg/dL to 36 mg/dL in 3 patients with familial hypercholesterolemia when treated with 40 mg daily for 6 weeks to 3 months *232*

IDL-Cholesterol *Serum Decrease Physiological* Nonsignificant reduction from mean of 22 mg/dL to 14 mg/dL in 7 patients with combined hyperlipidemia and from 18 mg/dL to 7 mg/dL in 3 patients with familial hypercholesterolemia when treated with 40 mg daily for 6 weeks to 3 months *232* In 12 individuals treated with lovastatin for 6 weeks mean concentration decreased to 12.3 mg/dL compared with 20.8 ± 5.9 mg/dL after placebo *2103*

Immunoglobulin A *Serum Decrease Physiological* In 25 patients with hypercholesterolemia treatment with 40 mg/d for 8 weeks caused marginally significant decrease from mean baseline of 4% from mean baseline of 2.3 g/L *3921*

Immunoglobulin G *Serum Decrease Physiological* In 25 patients with primary hypercholesterolemia treatment with 40 mg/d for 8 weeks caused marginally significant decrease of 2% from mean baseline of 11.6 g/L *3921*

Immunoglobulin M *Serum Decrease Physiological* In 25 patients with primary hypercholesterolemia treatment with 40 mg/d for 8 weeks caused nonsignificant decrease of 8% from mean baseline of 1.3 g/L *3921*

Lovastatin *(continued)*

Insulin *Plasma No Effect Physiological* In 15 nondiabetic patients with type II hypercholesterolemia mean concentration of 15 mIU/L after treatment with 80 mg/d for 6 weeks not significantly different from 14 mIU/L pretreatment *3880*

Lactate Dehydrogenase *Serum No Effect Physiological* No significant effect in 11 patients with renal transplants treated with 20 mg daily for 6 weeks *3055*

Lathosterol *Serum Decrease Physiological* In 7 patients with familial hypercholesterolemia significant reduction from mean baseline of 207 ± 78 100 x mmol/mol cholesterol of 101 ± 23, 101 ± 20 and 98 ± 26 100 x mmol/mol cholesterol observed after treatment with 40 mg/d for 1, 2 and 4 weeks respectively *3235*

LDL-Apolipoprotein B *Serum Decrease Physiological* Nonsignificant reduction from mean baseline concentration of 167 mg/dL to 120 mg/dL in 19 patients with primary hypercholesterolemia treated with up to 80 mg/d for 12 weeks *3848* Reduction from mean of 1328 mg/L to 797 mg/L in 7 patients with combined hyperlipidemia when treated with 40 mg daily for 6 weeks to 3 months and from 1916 mg/dL to 1391 mg/dL in 3 patients with familial hypercholesterolemia *232*

LDL-Apolipoprotein E *Serum Decrease Physiological* Nonsignificant reduction from mean baseline concentration of 0.91 mg/dL to 0.51 mg/dL in 19 patients with primary hypercholesterolemia treated with up to 80 mg/d for 12 weeks *3848*

LDL-Cholesterol *Bile Decrease Physiological* In 9 normolipidemic volunteers treatment with 20 mg/d caused mean 30% reduction *1603*

Serum Decrease Physiological In 12 adults with well-characterized heterozygous familial hypercholesterolemia decrease from mean of 321 mg/dL when diet only treatment to 207 mg/dL when 80 mg drug given daily (reduction of 35.5%) *2812* In 59 patients with hypercholesterolemia treatment with up to 80 mg/d for 24 weeks caused significant decrease of 34 ± 13% from mean baseline of 213 ± 32 mg/dL *2833* Reduction in 5 patients with normal triglyceride concentration from mean of 8.9 mmol/L to 4.5 mmol/L with up to 80 mg/day for 3 months and from 7.1 mmol/L to 4.5 mmol/L in 5 patients with hypertriglyceridemia *6391* Reduction from 189 mg/dL to 135 mg/dL in single case with long-standing Type I diabetes and mild renal insufficiency and familial hypercholesterolemia *1657* In 27 hypercholesterolemic patients treatment with 20 mg daily for 3 months caused reduction by 40% (from 215 mg/dL to 130 mg/dL) *2354* In 61 middle-aged men with low HDL treatment effectively reduced LDL-cholesterol concentration *6219* In 80 patients with primary hypercholesterolemia treatment with up to 80 mg/d for 12 weeks caused significant reduction (40.7%) from mean of 8.0 ± 2.2 mmol/L to 4.7 mmol/L *1651* In 73 type IIa hyperlipoproteinemic patients with serum cholesterol greater than 7.8 mmol/L lovastatin reduced LDL-cholesterol by more than 40% with 12 weeks treatment with average of 71 mg/d *6033* Significant reduction observed in 29 of 30 patients with nonfamilial hypercholesterolemia after 1 month treatment with 20 mg/day or more *2850* In 9 normolipidemic volunteers treatment with 80 mg/d caused mean approximate 50% reduction *1603* In 17 patients with type IIb hyperlipoproteinemia and moderate hypercholesterolemia treatment with 20 mg/d for 6 weeks caused mean reduction of 23% and in 23 patients with very high cholesterol reduction of 34% observed *6033* In 28 men with plasma concentrations between 200 and 240 mg/dL treatment with 10 mg/d for 20 weeks caused 24% decrease from baseline after 20 weeks *5144* Increase by 17 to 39% in clinical trial of 101 patients with heterozygous familial hypercholesterolemia *2514* In 17 patients with primary hypercholesterolemia treatment with 20 mg/d for 4 weeks caused significant decrease (21%) from mean baseline of 7.76 ± 0.33 mmol/L to 6.10 ± 0.38 mmol/L and to 5.47 ± 0.35 mmol/L (30%) after another 4 weeks when treated with 40 mg/d and to 4.96 ± 0.36 mmol/L (36%) after 80 mg/d for another 8 weeks *2862* In one study of 191 hypercholesterolemic patients treatment with 20 mg/d for 16 weeks caused a 27% reduction in concentration *4534* In 7 patients with nephrotic syndrome treatment with up to 40 mg/d for two years caused significant change from mean baseline of 343 ± 121 mg/dL to 174 ± 49 mg/dL *4771* In 85 patients with hypercholesterolemia treatment with 40 mg/d for 12 weeks caused a mean decrease of 32%, and in 88 treated with 80 mg/d for 12 weeks caused a mean 42% decrease *3982* 28% reduction in 11 patients with postrenal transplant hypercholesterolemia when treated with 20 mg/day for 6 weeks *3055* In 12 patients with nephrotic syndrome and initially increased serum Lp(a) concentration treatment with lovastatin (40 mg/d) for 8 weeks caused a significant change from mean baseline of 242.0 ± 66.0 mg/dL to 138.7 ± 36.5 mg/dL. In 8 patients in whom Lp(a) concentration was initially normal mean concentration decreased from 225.0 ± 84.0 mg/dL to 132.0 ± 29.3 mg/dL *755* In 11 hypercholesterolemic patients treated with up to 80 mg daily reduction of 40% observed versus reduction of 24% when 20 mg given with evening meal only. Study continued for 48 weeks *682* In 32 patients in the Monitored Atherosclerosis Regression Study treatment with 80 mg/d for 2 years caused significant reduction of 68.0 ± 3.5 mg/dL from mean baseline of 151.6 ± 4.3 mg/dL (45%) *85* In 35 patients with primary hyperlipoproteinemia treatment with up to 80 mg/d for 3 months caused significant decrease from mean of 248 ± 15 mg/dL to 159 ± 8 mg/dL (36%) *3214* In 7 patients with familial hypercholesterolemia treatment with 40 mg/d for 1 week caused significant decrease of 2.3 ± 0.31 mmol/L from mean baseline of 8.7 ± 0.65 mmol/L, and by 2.7 ± 0.52 mmol/L after 2 weeks, 3.5 ± 0.44 mmol/L after 4 weeks *3235* In 9 hyperlipidemic men treatment with 40 mg/d for 48 weeks caused a 29.0% decrease from mean baseline of 198 mg/dL to 141 mg/dL *1450* In 14 patients with nephrotic syndrome treatment with up to 80 mg/d for 6 months caused normalization to 3.26 ± 0.21 mmol/L from pretreatment concentration of 5.76 ± 0.48 mmol/L (43% reduction) *961* In 42 patients with noninsulin dependent diabetes and primary hypercholesterolemia mean reduction of 26.2% after treatment for 24 weeks with 20 mg daily *2215* In 12 individuals with hypertriglyceridemia treatment with lovastatin for 6 weeks caused significant reduction to 99.4 ± 26.1 mg/dL compared with 149.4 ± 42.3 mg/dL after placebo *2103* Significant reduction from mean of 142 mg/dL to 93 mg/dL observed in 7 patients with combined hyperlipidemia when treated with 40 mg daily for 6 weeks to 3 months and from 304 mg/dL to 218 mg/dL in 3 patients with familial hypercholesterolemia *232* In over 8000 patients with moderately severe hypercholesterolemia treated for 2 years mean concentration decreased by 27% with 20 mg/d, 31% with 40 mg/d and 40% with 80 mg/d *683* In 919 asymptomatic men and women treatment with up to 40 mg/d for 3 years caused a change from mean baseline of 157 ± 17 mg/dL to 119 ± 22 mg/dL after 1 year and 117 ± 25 mg/dL after 3 years *4795* Compared with placebo in 19 hypercholesterolemic patients receiving 43% high fat diet 40 mg lovastatin daily caused mean reduction of 30% over 3 weeks. In 16 patients on 25% low fat diet the same regime of lovastatin also caused mean reduction of 30% *1064* In 28 patients with heterozygous familial hypercholesterolemia mean decrease from baseline of 22%, 26%, 30%, and 35% respectively after treatment for 6 weeks with each of 10, 20, 40, and 80 mg daily *4507* In 25 patients with primary hypercholesterolemia treatment with 40 mg/d caused significant 38 ± 3% after 4 weeks and 36 ± 4% after 8 weeks from mean baseline of 5.6 ± 0.2 mmol/L *3921* In 17 patients treatment with 40 mg/d for 6 weeks caused significant reduction from mean baseline of 4.67 ± 0.36 mmol/L to 3.08 ± 0.46 mmol/L *3905* Treatment of patients with familial hypercholesterolemia with 80 mg/day caused mean reduction of 40% *4506* In 15 nondiabetic type II hypercholesterolemic patients treated with 80 mg/d for 6 weeks caused mean 36% reduction *3880* In 20 patients with type IIa hypercholesterolemia treated with lovastatin for 12 months mean concentration decreased by 56 mg/dL (from 244 ± 11.4 to 188 ± 12.1 mg/dL) *3856* Significant reduction from mean baseline of 287 mg/dL to 178 mg/dL in 19 patients with primary hypercholesterolemia treated with up to 80 mg/d for 12 weeks *3848* Nonsignificant reduction from mean baseline concentration of 327 mg/dL to 214 mg/dL in 19 patients with primary hypercholesterolemia treated with up to 80 mg/d for 12 weeks *3848* In 17 patients with hyperlipidemia type IIb and serum cholesterol between 6.2 and 7.8 mmol/L treatment with 20 mg/d for 6 weeks caused mean reduction of 23%: in 23 patients with cholesterol above 7.9 mmol/L treatment with 40 mg/d caused decrease of 34% *4387* In 56 patients with either type IIa or type IIb hyperlipoproteinemia mean concentration fell from 5.48 mmol/L to 3.72 mmol/L (32%) following treatment with 20 mg daily for 6 weeks *401* Significant reduction of 22.8% in 17 patients with hypercholesterolemia treated with 20 mg/day for 6 weeks and of 33.7% in 23 hypercholesterolemic patients treated with 40 mg/day for 6 weeks *4387* Reduction by 34% after 3 months at which concentration it remained stable in 11 postcardiac transplant patients with hypercholesterolemia when treated with up to 60 mg/day for 1 year *3329* In 20 patients with primary hypercholesterolemia treatment with average dose of 70.5 mg/d caused mean reduction of 28% at 4 weeks, 30% at 6 weeks, 36% at 10 weeks and 35% at 12 weeks *458*

LDL-Cholesterol:HDL-Cholesterol Ratio

Serum Decrease Physiological In 85 patients with hypercholesterolemia treatment with 40 mg/d for 12 weeks caused a mean decrease of 36%, and in 88 treated with 80 mg/d for 12 weeks caused a mean 44% decrease *3982* In 14 hypercholesterolemic patients treatment with 20 mg daily with evening meal caused decrease of 27% and when 40 mg given twice daily caused reduction of 44% when treatment continued for 48 weeks *682* In 80 patients treated with up to 80 mg/d for 12 weeks significant reduction of 46.6% from mean of 7.5 ± 3.3 to 3.9 ± 1.8 *1651* In 17 patients treatment with 40 mg/d for 6 weeks caused significant reduction from 5.36 ± 0.58 to 3.18 ± 0.81 *3905*

Leukocytes *Blood Increase Physiological* Significant increase (27%) observed in 11 patients with renal transplants receiving azothioprine when treated with 20 mg daily of lovastatin for 6 weeks. Effect possibly due to reduced azathioprine bone marrow suppression *3055*

Blood No Effect Physiological No significant effect observed in 8245 hypercholesterolemic patients receiving 20-80 mg/d for 48 weeks *682*

Lipoprotein Lp(a) *Serum Decrease Physiological* In 24 patients with primary hyperlipoproteinemia treatment with up to 80 mg/d for 3 months caused decrease of median from 9.5 mg/dL to 6 mg/dL *3214*

Serum Increase Physiological In 7 hyperlipidemic men treatment with 40 mg/d for 48 weeks caused a 3% increase from mean baseline of 13.6 mg/dL *1450* In 12 patients with nephrotic syndrome and initially increased serum Lp(a) concentration treatment with lovastatin (40 mg/d) for 8 weeks caused a significant change from mean baseline of 101.5 mg/dL to 74.0 mg/dL *755*

Serum No Effect Physiological In 59 patients with hypercholesterolemia treatment with up to 80 mg/d for 24 weeks caused nonsignificant increase of 7 ± 36% from mean baseline of 32 ± 32 mg/dL *2833* In 8 patients with nephrotic syndrome and initially normal serum Lp(a) concentration treatment with lovastatin (40 mg/d) for 8 weeks caused a nonsignificant change from mean baseline of 22.5 mg/dL to 21.0 mg/dL *755* Nonsignificant increase from mean baseline on 41 mg/dL to 43 mg/dL in 19 patients with primary hypercholesterolemia treated with up to 80 mg/d for 12 weeks *3848*

Luteinizing Hormone *Plasma No Effect Physiological* No significant change even in patients with familial hypercholesterolemia receiving 40 mg b.i.d *2514*

Lymphocyte B-Cells *Blood No Effect Physiological* In 25 patients with primary hypercholesterolemia treatment with 40 mg/d for 8 weeks caused nonsignificant change from mean baseline of 8.7% to 9.6% of total lymphocytes *3921*

Lymphocyte T-Cells *Blood No Effect Physiological* In 25 patients with primary hypercholesterolemia treatment with 40 mg/d for 8 weeks caused nonsignificant change to 69.5% of total lymphocytes from mean baseline of 69.7% *3921*

Lymphocytes *Blood No Effect Physiological* No significant effect in 11 patients with renal transplants also receiving azathioprine treated with 20 mg daily for 6 weeks *3055* No significant effect observed in white cell differential count in 8245 hypercholesterolemic patients treated with 20-80 mg/d for 48 weeks *682*

Methylmalonate *Urine Decrease Physiological* In patients with familial hypercholesterolemia treatment with 80 mg/day caused reduction by 34% *4506*

Mevalonate *Urine Decrease Physiological* In 20 patients with primary hypercholesterolemia treatment with an average dose of 70.5 mg/d caused mean reduction of 31% at 4 weeks, 39% reduction at 10 weeks and 38% at 12 weeks *458* In 28 patients with heterozygous familial hypercholesterolemia mean decrease of 19% from baseline after 4 weeks on 10 mg daily, 35% on 20 mg daily, 31% on 40 mg daily and 31% also on 80 mg daily after successive 6 week periods of treatment *4507*

Natural Killer Cells *Blood No Effect Physiological* In 25 patients with primary hypercholesterolemia treatment with 40 mg/d for 8 weeks caused nonsignificant change from mean baseline of 15.8% of total to 15.7% of lymphocytes *3921*

Neutrophils *Blood Increase Physiological* 45% increase observed in 11 patients with renal transplants receiving azathioprine with added treatment of 20 mg daily for 6 weeks of lovastatin *3055*

Blood No Effect Physiological No significant change observed in white cell differential count observed in 8245 hypercholesterolemic patients treated with 20-80 mg/d for 48 weeks *682*

Partial Thromboplastin Time

Plasma No Effect Physiological In 20 patients with type IIa hypercholesterolemia treatment for 12 months had no significant effect *3856*

Plasminogen *Plasma No Effect Physiological* In 20 patients with type IIa hypercholesterolemia treatment for 12 months had no significant effect on concentration *1737*

Plasminogen Activator Inhibitor-1

Plasma Decrease Physiological In 59 patients with hypercholesterolemia treatment with up to 80 mg/d for 24 weeks caused significant decrease of 22 ± 39% from mean baseline of 53 ± 30 ng/mL *2833*

Platelet Aggregation *Blood Decrease Physiological* In 20 patients with type IIa hypercholesterolemia treatment for 12 months was associated with a significant decrease in the initial slope of ADP-induced platelet aggregation. Long term treatment was associated with significant reduction of ADP-induced aggregation *3856*

Blood No Effect Physiological No significant change observed in 15 patients with type II hyperlipoproteinemia treated with lovastatin for 3 months *3245*

Platelets *Blood Decrease Physiological* Slight decrease observed in comparison with placebo-treated group among 8245 patients treated with doses from 20-80 mg/d for 48 weeks *682*

Blood No Effect Physiological In 20 patients with type IIa hypercholesterolemia treatment for 12 months had no effect on concentration which remained within normal range *3856*

Potassium *Serum Increase Physiological* Increase to above 8.0 mmol/L in one patient with familial hypercholesterolemia also receiving angiotensin-converting enzyme inhibitor. Effect probably due to muscle cell breakdown with release of intracellular potassium *1657*

Propranolol *Serum No Effect Physiological* Coadministration of single doses of lovastatin and propranolol had no effect on the pharmacokinetics of either drug *3982* No effect observed in normal volunteers with concomitant administration of single doses of lovastatin and propranolol *3982*

Protein *Serum No Effect Physiological* No significant effect in 11 patients with renal transplants treated with 20 mg daily for 6 weeks *3055*

Urine Decrease Physiological In 7 patients with nephrotic syndrome treatment with up to 40 mg/d for two years caused significant change from mean baseline of 8.6 ± 4.6 g/d to 5.0 ± 3.7 g/d *4771* In 20 nondiabetic nephrotic patients treatment with diet and up to 0.06 g/d for up to 30 months caused a significant decrease from mean baseline of 11.85 ± 1.43 g/d to 4.38 ± 0.78 g/d *4263* In 12 patients with nephrotic syndrome and initially increased serum Lp(a) concentration treatment with lovastatin (40 mg/d) for 8 weeks caused a nonsignificant change from mean baseline of 8.5 ± 4.8 g/d to 6.9 ± 4.2 g/d *755*

Urine No Effect Physiological In 8 patients with nephrotic syndrome and initially normal serum Lp(a) concentration treatment with lovastatin (40 mg/d) for 8 weeks caused a nonsignificant change from mean baseline of 7.3 ± 3.6 g/d to 7.1 ± 5.4 g/d *755*

Protein C *Plasma No Effect Physiological* Concentration in 20 type IIa hypercholesterolemic patients treated for 12 months remained within normal range *3856*

Protein S *Plasma No Effect Physiological* In 20 patients with type IIa hypercholesterolemia treatment for 12 months did not cause concentration to exceed normal limits *3856*

Prothrombin Time *Plasma Increase Physiological* Coadministration of lovastatin with warfarin reported to cause bleeding and/or increased prothrombin time in a few patients *3982*

Lovastatin *(continued)*

Prothrombin Time *(continued)*
Plasma No Effect Physiological In 20 patients with type IIa hypercholesterolemia treatment for 12 months had no significant effect on time *3856* Coadministration of lovastatin with warfarin had no effect on prothrombin time *3982*

Sitosterol *Serum Increase Physiological* In 7 patients with familial hypercholesterolemia treatment with 40 mg/d caused increase from mean baseline of 151 ± 17 100 x mmol/mol cholesterol by 12 ± 7, 33 ± 10 and 23 ± 13 100 x mmol/mol cholesterol after 1, 2 and 4 weeks respectively *6209*

Squalene *Serum No Effect Physiological* In 7 patients with familial hypercholesterolemia treatment with 40 mg/d for 4 weeks caused insignificant change from mean baseline of 15 ± 2 100 x mmol/mol cholesterol *6209*

Testosterone *Serum No Effect Physiological* Lovastatin administration has no effect on basal concentration of testosterone *3982* No significant change even in patients with familial hypercholesterolemia receiving 40 mg b.i.d *2514*

Testosterone response to hCG
Serum No Effect Physiological Lovastatin administration 40 mg/d for 16 weeks to 21 men caused a slight but not significant reduction *3982*

Thrombin Time *Blood No Effect Physiological* In 20 patients with type IIa hypercholesterolemia treatment for 12 months had no effect on thrombin clotting time *3856*

Thyroid Stimulating Hormone
Serum Increase Physiological Marked increase when lovastatin added to thyroxine regime on which a woman with diabetes mellitus, hypothyroidism and Type IIa hyperlipoproteinemia had been stabilized *1379*

Thyroxine (T4) *Serum Decrease Physiological* Marked reduction in thyroxine concentration observed in one patient with diabetes mellitus, goitrous hypothyroidism due to Hashimoto's thyroiditis and type IIa hyperlipoproteinemia receiving oral thyroxine *1379*
Serum Increase Physiological One case with insulin-dependent diabetes and Hashimoto's thyroiditis became hyperthyroxinemic and possibly thyrotoxic when lovastatin added to thyroxine regime she was receiving. In most cases added lovastatin had no effect on thyroxine concentration *3690*

Thyroxine (T4) Index, Free *Serum Decrease Physiological* Simultaneous reduction when thyroxine decreased in one patient with diabetes mellitus, hypothyroidism and type IIa hyperlipoproteinemia when lovastatin added to thyroxine regime on which she had been stabilized *1379*

Tirofiban *Serum No Effect Physiological* Coadministration had no significant effect on plasma clearance of tirofiban *3957*

Tissue Plasminogen Activator
Plasma No Effect Physiological In 59 patients with hypercholesterolemia treatment with up to 80 mg/d for 24 weeks caused nonsignificant change of 1 ± 44% from mean baseline of 20 ± 8 IU/mL *2833*

Triglyceride:LDL-Cholesterol Ratio
Serum Increase Physiological In a group of hypertriglyceridemic patients treatment with 20 mg/d for 4 weeks caused significant increase in ratio to 1.08, with 40 mg/d causing an increase to 1.12 and 80 mg/d an increase to 1.31 *5796*

Triglycerides *Serum Decrease Physiological* Mean decrease of 12% in 56 patients with type IIa and type IIb hyperlipoproteinemia treated with 20 mg daily for 6 weeks *401* In 12 patients with nephrotic syndrome and initially increased serum Lp(a) concentration treatment with lovastatin (40 mg/d) for 8 weeks caused a significant change from mean baseline of 342.0 ± 273.0 mg/dL to 166.1 ± 72.5 mg/dL *755* In 15 nondiabetic type II hypercholesterolemic patients treatment with 80 mg/d for 6 weeks caused mean 26% reduction *3880* In 25 patients with primary hypercholesterolemia treatment with 40 mg/d caused significant decrease of 23 ± 6% after 4 weeks and 13 ± 8% after 8 weeks from mean baseline of 1.9 ± 0.2 mmol/L *3921* In 20 patients with primary hypercholesterolemia treatment with average dose of 70.5 mg/d for 6 weeks caused mean decrease of 2%, with a decrease of 6% at 10 weeks and 16% at 12 weeks *458* In 27 hypercholesterolemics treatment with 20 mg daily for 3 months caused reduction by 15% (decrease from 166 mg/dL to 142 mg/dL) *2354* In a group of hypertriglyceridemic patients treatment with 20 mg/d for 4 weeks caused significant 32% decrease, with 40 mg/d causing 36% decrease and 80 mg/d a 44% decrease *5796* Increase by 14% at 40 mg b.i.d. in clinical trial of 101 patients with heterozygous familial hypercholesterolemia *2514* Insignificant reduction of 6.7% in 17 hypercholesterolemic patients treated with 20 mg/day for 6 weeks but significant reduction of 26.1% in 23 patients treated with 40 mg daily for 6 weeks *4387* Fell from mean of 145 mg/dL to 105 mg/dL in 12 adults with well-characterized heterozygous familial hypercholesterolemia (decrease of 27.6%) with 80 mg daily *2812* In 7 patients with nephrotic syndrome treatment with up to 40 mg/d for two years caused significant change from mean baseline of 336 ± 273 mg/dL to 182 ± 71 mg/dL *4771* About 4% reduction observed in 73 type IIa hyperlipoproteinemic patients treated with average of 71 mg/d for 12 weeks *6033* In 17 type IIb hyperlipoproteinemic patients with moderately high serum cholesterol treatment with 20 mg/d for 6 weeks caused mean decrease of 7%: treatment of 23 patients with high serum cholesterol caused mean decrease of 26% *6033* In 59 patients with hypercholesterolemia treatment with up to 80 mg/d for 24 weeks caused significant decrease of 23 ± 29% from mean baseline of 214 ± 105 mg/dL *2833* Nonsignificant reduction from mean baseline of 143 mg/dL to 129 mg/dL in 19 patients with primary hypercholesterolemia treated with up to 80 mg/d for 12 weeks *3848* In 32 patients in the Monitored Atherosclerosis Regression Study treatment with 80 mg/d for 2 years caused significant reduction of 37.0 ± 8.4 mg/dL from mean baseline of 163.9 ± 14.4 mg/dL (23%) *85* In 17 patients with primary hypercholesterolemia treatment with 20 mg/d for 4 weeks caused significant decrease (17%) from mean baseline of 1.74 ± 0.22 mmol/L to 1.44 ± 0.21 mmol/L and treatment for another 4 weeks caused further decrease to 1.36 ± 0.14 mmol/L (21%): treatment with 80 mg/d for another 8 weeks caused reduction to 1.40 ± 0.15 mmol/L (20%) *2862* In 19 hypercholesterolemic patients receiving 43% high fat diet for 3 weeks lovastatin 40 mg/day reduced triglyceride concentration by mean of 11%: in 16 patients receiving 25% low fat diet with same dose of lovastatin concentration reduced by 7% *1064* In 61 middle-aged men with low HDL concentrations treatment effectively lowered plasma triglyceride concentration *6219* Reduction from mean of 11.1 mmol/L to 6.6 mmol/L in 5 patients with increased LDL-cholesterol and normal triglyceride concentration and from 9.7 to 6.4 mmol/L in 5 patients with triglyceride concentration above 1.8 mmol/L with up to 80 mg/d for 3 months *6391* In over 8000 patients with moderately severe hypercholesterolemia treated for 2 years mean concentration decreased by 3% with 20 mg/d, 9% with 40 mg/d and 18% with 80 mg/d *683* Mean reduction of 10% observed in hypercholesterolemic patients given 20 mg daily for 48 weeks and reduction of 19% observed in those receiving 80 mg daily for 48 weeks *682* In 919 asymptomatic men and women treatment with up to 40 mg/d for 3 years caused a change from mean baseline of 136 ± 60 mg/dL to 127 ± 64 mg/dL after 1 year and 129 ± 66 mg/dL after 3 years *4795* In 17 patients treatment with 40 mg/d for 6 weeks caused significant reduction from mean baseline of 2.02 ± 0.77 mmol/L to 1.52 ± 0.81 mmol/L *3905* In 12 individuals with hypertriglyceridemia treated with lovastatin for 6 weeks mean concentration reduced to 309 ± 99 mg/dL compared with 431 ± 130 mg/dL with placebo *2103* In 80 patients with primary hypercholesterolemia treatment with up to 80 mg/d mean concentration decreased significantly by 26.0% from 2.2 ± 0.9 mmol/L to 1.6 ± 0.7 mmol/L *1651* In 9 hyperlipidemic men treatment with 40 mg/d for 48 weeks caused a 28.0% decrease from mean baseline of 188 mg/dL to 136 mg/dL *1450* In one study of 191 hypercholesterolemic patients treatment with 20 mg/d for 16 weeks caused a 6% reduction in concentration *4534* In 20 nondiabetic nephrotic patients treatment with diet and up to 0.06 g/d for up to 30 months caused a significant decrease from mean baseline of 403.3 ± 53.2 mg/dL to 258 ± 60.6 mg/dL *4263* In 85 patients with hypercholesterolemia treatment with 40 mg/d for 12 weeks caused a mean decrease of 21%, and in 88 treated with 80 mg/d for 12 weeks caused a mean 27% decrease *3982* Nonsignificant reduction from mean of 316 mg/dL to 248 mg/dL in 7 patients with combined hyperlipidemia treated with 40 mg daily for 6 weeks to 3 months and from 123 mg/dL to 97 mg/dL in 3 patients with familial hypercholesterolemia *232* In 35 patients with primary hyperlipoproteinemia treatment with up to 80 mg/d for 3 months caused reduction from mean of 155 ± 9 mg/dL to 136 ± 9 mg/dL (12%) *3214*

Serum Increase Physiological Treatment of 20 patients with primary hypercholesterolemia with average dose of 70.5 mg/d for 4 weeks caused mean increase of 4.1% although further treatment produced a significant reduction *458*
Serum No Effect Physiological No significant effect in 11 postcardiac transplant patients with hypercholesterolemia treated with up to 60 mg/day for 1 year *3329* Nonsignificant reduction in 30 patients with primary nonfamilial hypercholesterolemia treated with up to 80 mg/day and appropriate diet for 6 months *2850* Nonsignificant reduction in 11 patients with renal transplants from mean baseline of 203 mg/dL to 169 mg/dL after 6 weeks treatment with 20 mg/day *3055* In 12 patients with nephrotic syndrome and initially increased serum Lp(a) concentration treatment with lovastatin (40 mg/d) for 8 weeks caused a nonsignificant change from mean baseline of 173.0 ± 86.0 mg/dL to 161.8 ± 96.4 mg/dL *755* In 7 patients with familial hypercholesterolemia treatment with 40 mg/d caused insignificant reduction of 0.03 ± 0.19 mmol/L from mean baseline of 1.34 ± 0.19 mmol/L after 1 week, of 0.26 ± 0.20 mmol/L after 2 weeks and of 0.37 ± 0.20 mmol/L after 4 weeks *6209* Insignificant increase (1.8%) in 50 noninsulin dependent diabetics with primary hypercholesterolemia treated with 20 mg daily for 24 weeks *2215*

Viscosity *Plasma Decrease Physiological* 3 months treatment of 15 patients with type II hyperlipoproteinemia caused significant reduction from mean baseline concentration of 1.74 mPa/s to 1.65 mPa/s *3245*
Plasma No Effect Physiological In 35 patients with primary hyperlipoproteinemia treatment with up to 80 mg/d for 3 months caused nonsignificant reduction from 1.34 ± 0.01 mPa/s to 1.29 ± 0.01 mPa/s (4%) *3214*

VLDL-Apolipoprotein B *Serum Decrease Physiological* Nonsignificant reduction from mean of 194 mg/dL to 134 mg/dL in 7 patients with combined hyperlipidemia and from 50 mg/dL to 37 mg/dL in 3 patients with familial hypercholesterolemia when treated with 40 mg daily for 6 weeks to 3 months *232* Nonsignificant reduction from mean baseline concentration of 8.0 mg/dL to 6.5 mg/dL in 19 patients with primary hypercholesterolemia treated with up to 80 mg/d for 12 weeks *3848*

VLDL-Apolipoprotein E *Serum No Effect Physiological* No significant effect observed in 19 patients with primary hypercholesterolemia treated with up to 80 mg/d for 12 weeks *3848*

VLDL-Cholesterol *Serum Decrease Physiological* Nonsignificant reduction from mean of 66 mg/dL to 52 mg/dL in 7 patients with combined hyperlipidemia and from 20 mg/dL to 16 mg/dL in 3 patients with familial hypercholesterolemia when treated with 40 mg daily for 6 weeks to 3 months *232* In 12 individuals with hypertriglyceridemia treatment with lovastatin for 6 weeks caused a significant reduction to 48.7 ± 29.5 mg/dL compared with 72.3 ± 27.2 mg/dL with placebo *2103* Mean reduction of 27.9% in 42 noninsulin dependent diabetics with primary hypercholesterolemia treated with 20 mg daily for 24 weeks *2215* Nonsignificant reduction observed in 19 patients with primary hypercholesterolemia from mean baseline concentration of 18.4 mg/dL to 6.5 mg/dL after treatment with up to 80 mg/d for 12 weeks *3848* In 19 hypercholesterolemic patients 43% high fat diet with 40 mg lovastatin daily for 3 weeks reduced concentration by 13%: in 16 patients receiving 25% low fat diet lovastatin caused 21% reduction *1064* In 85 patients with hypercholesterolemia treatment with 40 mg/d for 12 weeks caused a mean decrease of 34%, and in 88 treated with 80 mg/d for 12 weeks caused a mean 31% decrease *3982* Reduction from mean of 1.7 mmol/L to 0.8 mmol/L in 5 patients with hypertriglyceridemia treated with up to 80 mg daily for 3 months but no effect observed in 5 patients with normal triglyceride concentration *6391* In 17 patients with primary hypercholesterolemia treatment with up to 40 mg/d for 8 weeks mean concentration decreased from 0.68 ± 0.11 mmol/L to 0.49 ± 0.09 mmol/L (28%) and to 0.44 ± 0.05 mmol/L (36%) after another 8 weeks of treatment with 80 mg/d *2862* In 17 patients treated with 40 mg/d for 6 weeks mean concentration decreased from mean baseline of 0.93 ± 0.35 mmol/L to 0.69 ± 0.37 mmol/L *3905*
Serum No Effect Physiological Nonsignificant reduction in 30 patients with primary nonfamilial hypercholesterolemia treated with up to 80 mg/day and appropriate diet for 6 months *2850*

VLDL-Triglycerides *Serum Decrease Physiological* In 17 patients with primary hypercholesterolemia treatment with 20 mg/d for 4 weeks caused significant decrease from mean baseline of 1.33 ± 0.19 mmol/L to 1.04 ± 0.18 mmol/L (22%) and to 0.94 ± 0.12 mmol/L (29%) after another 4 weeks treatment with 40 mg/d: after another 8 weeks with 80 mg/d concentration reduced to 1.04 ± 0.14 mmol/L (reduced by 21% from baseline) *2862* Nonsignificant reduction from mean of 212 mg/dL to 166 mg/dL in 7 patients with combined hyperlipidemia treated with 40 mg daily for 6 weeks to 3 months and from 51 mg/dL to 42 mg/dL in 3 patients with hypercholesterolemia *232*

Loxapine

Alanine Aminotransferase *Serum Increase Physiological* Hepatocellular injury has been reported as a rare side effect with jaundice or hepatitis rarely questionably associated with loxapine administration *3464*

Aspartate Aminotransferase *Serum Increase Physiological* Hepatocellular injury has been reported as a rare side effect with jaundice or hepatitis rarely questionably associated with loxapine administration *3464*

Bilirubin *Serum Increase Physiological* Hepatocellular injury has been reported as a rare side effect with jaundice or hepatitis rarely questionably associated with loxapine administration *3464*

Clara Cell Protein *Serum No Effect Physiological* In 24 schizophrenics treated with loxapine mean concentration of 18.5 ± 6.0 ng/mL not significantly different from that in 14 untreated schizophrenics in whom the mean concentration was 19.3 ± 5.2 ng/mL *3732*

Creatine Kinase *Serum Increase Physiological* In 11 acutely psychotic patients treatment with loxapine (1 - 11 determinations per patient) was associated with 3 marked elevations (in 27.3% of the patients) *3947*

Granulocytes *Blood Decrease Physiological* Thrombocytopenia has been reported as a rare side effect *3464*

Interleukin-1 Receptor Antagonist
Serum No Effect Physiological In 24 schizophrenics treated with loxapine mean concentration of 0.27 ± 0.18 U/mL not significantly different from that in 14 untreated schizophrenics in whom the mean concentration was 0.29 ± 0.18 U/mL *3732*

Leukocytes *Blood Decrease Physiological* Leukopenia has been reported as a rare side effect *3464*

p-Aminophenol *Urine No Effect Analytical* With addition of drugs at a concentration of 100 mg/L and of related compounds at 50 mg/L no significant effect observed on colorimetric method of van Bocxlaer on Cobas Mira analyzer which involves reacting free p-aminophenol with resorcinol in the presence of magnesium ions to form an indophenol dye measured at 550 nm *6163*

Platelets *Blood Decrease Physiological* Thrombocytopenia has been reported as a rare side effect *3464*

Prolactin *Plasma Increase Physiological* Significant change in response to 10 mg orally *2352*

Soluble CD8$^+$ *Serum No Effect Physiological* In 24 schizophrenics treated with loxapine mean concentration of 490 ± 196 U/mL not significantly different from that in 14 untreated schizophrenics in whom the mean concentration was 82 ± 82 U/mL *3732*

Soluble Interleukin-2 Receptor
Serum No Effect Physiological In 24 schizophrenics treated with loxapine mean concentration of 94 ± 103 U/mL not significantly higher than that in 14 untreated schizophrenics in whom the mean concentration was 82 ± 82 U/mL *3732*

Lucanthone

Alanine Aminotransferase *Serum Increase Physiological* Chronic toxicity may cause liver damage *2242*

Protein *Urine Increase Physiological* Chronic toxicity may cause renal damage *2242*

Lugol's Iodine

Bilirubin *Serum Increase Physiological* Occasional hypersensitive response to iodines *128*

Eosinophils *Blood Increase Physiological* Rare allergic response to iodines *128*

Platelets *Blood Decrease Physiological* Rare possible response with purpura *128*

Thyroxine (T4) *Serum No Effect Analytical* No effect on methods *5401*

Lynestrenol

Ceruloplasmin *Serum Increase Physiological* When 5 mg daily given alone to 30 healthy female volunteers. Normal values observed 30 d after treatment stopped *5157*

Corticosteroid-Binding Globulin
Serum Increase Physiological When 5 mg daily given alone to 30 healthy female volunteers. Normal values observed 30 d after treatment stopped *5157*

HDL-Cholesterol *Serum Decrease Physiological* Icrease by 32% due to progestational activity in 6 women with endometriosis given 5 to 10 mg daily for 6 mo *3754* When 5 mg daily given alone to 30 healthy female volunteers. Normal values observed 30 d after treatment stopped *5157*

LDL-Cholesterol *Serum Increase Physiological* Increase by 19% due to progestational activity in 6 women with endometriosis given 5 to 10 mg daily for 6 mo *3754*

Sex-Hormone Binding Globulin
Serum Decrease Physiological When 5 mg daily given alone to 30 healthy female volunteers. Normal values observed 30 d after treatment stopped *5157*

Lysergide

Chromosomes *Test Conditions Abnormal Physiological* Clastogenic in human cells *in vitro* (?*in vitro*) *5484*

Creatinine Clearance *Urine Decrease Physiological* Temporary effect observed *2677*

Fatty Acids (FFA), Free *Serum Increase Physiological* 73% after 1.5 µg/kg orally *2675*

Glucose *Serum Increase Physiological* Reported effect *192*

Phosphate Clearance *Urine Decrease Physiological* Temporary effect observed *2677*

Lysine Clonixinate

Occult Blood *Feces No Effect Physiological* In 6 healthy volunteers treatment with 375 mg/d for 5 days caused non-significant increase from mean baseline of 0.627 ± 0.245 mL/d to 0.947 ± 0.429 mL/d *548*

Macrolides

Astemizole *Serum Increase Physiological* Significantly decreased metabolism resulting in cardiac toxicity or arrhythmias, especially torsade des pointes *886*

Carbamazepine *Serum Increase Physiological* Significantly decreased metabolism and increased plasma concentration *886* Drugs that inhibit CYP 3A4 inhibit metabolism of carbamazepine producing clinically meaningful effect *1039*

Prothrombin Time *Plasma Increase Physiological* Increased INR observed in patients receiving warfarin *886*

Rifabutin *Serum Increase Physiological* Decreased metabolism and increased risk of uveitis *886*

Terfenadine *Serum Increase Physiological* Significantly decreased metabolism resulting in cardiac toxicity or arrhythmias, especially torsade des pointes *886*

Theophylline *Serum Increase Physiological* Decreased metabolism *886*

Mafenide

Amino Acids *Urine Increase Analytical* Reacts with ninhydrin; extra spot TLC, high voltage electrophoresis *4760*

Ammonia *Urine Decrease Physiological* Inhibits carbonic anhydrase if applied topically *6425*

Bicarbonate *Urine Increase Physiological* Inhibits carbonic anhydrase if applied topically *6425*

Carbon Dioxide Partial Pressure
Blood Decrease Physiological Inhibits carbonic anhydrase if applied topically *6425*

Chloride *Urine Decrease Physiological* Selective retention *201*

Leukocytes *Blood Decrease Physiological* Probable effect observed in one child *201*

pH *Blood Decrease Physiological* If respiratory impairment as reduced renal buffering *201*
Blood Increase Physiological Usual finding with respiratory alkalosis *201*
Urine Increase Physiological Inhibits carbonic anhydrase if applied topically *6425*

Potassium *Urine Increase Physiological* Inhibits carbonic anhydrase if applied topically *6425*

Magaldrate

Isoniazid *Serum Decrease Physiological* Inhibits gastrointestinal absorption to some extent *2789*

Magnesium Antacids

Cefdinir *Serum Decrease Physiological* Concomitant administration of aluminum or magnesium-containing antacids with 300 mg cefdinir reduce absorption of cefdinir. Problem can be avoided by giving cefdinir two hours before or after antacid administration *4528*

Magnesium Carbonate

Salicylate *Serum No Effect Analytical* At a concentration of 14.6 mg/dL has no significant effect on method on Kodak Ektachem® systems *2519*

Magnesium Hydroxide

Cefaclor *Serum Decrease Physiological* Absorption reduced if taken within one hour of ingestion of magesium or aluminum hydroxide containing antacids *1627*

Ciprofloxacin *Serum Decrease Physiological* Concurrent administration of ciprofloxacin with antacids containing magnesium, aluminum, or calcium may substantially interfere with the absorption of ciprofloxacin and plasma and urine concentrations less than desired *416* Magnesium containing antacids bind ciprofloxacin in gastrointestinal tract thereby reducing its bioavailability and reducing serum concentration by 50-65% *4774*
Urine Decrease Physiological Concurrent administration of ciprofloxacin with antacids containing magnesium, aluminum, or calcium may substantially interfere with the absorption of ciprofloxacin and plasma and urine concentrations less than desired *416*

Diclofenac *Serum No Effect Physiological* Neither rate of absorption affected in 6 healthy volunteers with coadministration of magnesium hydroxide and diclofenac *4256*

Dicumarol *Plasma Increase Physiological* Peak concentration higher and reached earlier when drug given with antacids due to readily absorbed magnesium chelate of dicumarol *136* 75% increase in peak concentration if coadministered *136* Increased absorption due to chelation *6403*

Digoxin *Serum Decrease Physiological* Gastrointestinal absorption reduced by about 30% *760*

Enoxacin *Serum Decrease Physiological* Antacids containing aluminum hydroxide and magnesium hydroxide reduce the oral absorption of enoxacin by 75% *4940*

Glipizide *Serum No Effect Physiological* Area under concentration-time curve from 0 to 0.5 h and from 0 to 1 h increased by 180% but peak plasma concentration, total area under curve, elimination half-life and mean residence time remained unchanged *3166*

Glucose *Serum No Effect Physiological* Over 21 weeks treatment with 500 mg/d in 16 insulin dependent diabetics no change in fasting glucose concentration observed although insulin requirement significantly reduced *5590*

Hemoglobin A_{1c} *Blood No Effect Physiological* In 16 insulin-dependent diabetics treatment with 500 mg/d had no effect on blood concentration but caused significantly reduced insulin requirement over 21 week study period *5590*

Ibuprofen *Serum Increase Physiological* Area under curve between 0 and 1 h by 65% and peak concentration in plasma by 31% in 6 healthy volunteers after 400 mg ibuprofen and 850 mg magnesium hydroxide *4256*

Ketoprofen *Serum No Effect Physiological* Neither rate nor extent of absorption affected by coadministration of magnesium hydroxide in 6 healthy volunteers *4256*

Magnesium *Muscle Increase Physiological* Administration of 500 mg/d increased previously low concentration in muscle biopsies in insulin-dependent diabetics to normal concentration *5590*

Serum Increase Physiological Administration of 500 mg daily increased previously low concentration in insulin-dependent diabetics to normal concentration after 7 and 14 weeks but not after 21 weeks *5590*

Urine Increase Physiological Transient increase observed in 16 patients with insulin dependent diabetes mellitus when fed 500 mg/d significant at 7 weeks but not thereafter *5590*

Mefenamic Acid *Serum Increase Physiological* Dose-dependent increased absorption from gastrointestinal tract with reduced time to peak concentration *4259*

Norfloxacin *Urine Decrease Physiological* When magnesium hydroxide coingested with 400 mg norfloxacin excretion of norfloxacin over next 24 hours reduced by 90% due to interference with absorption *865*

Potassium *Muscle Increase Physiological* Significant increase observed in 16 insulin-dependent diabetics treated with 500 mg daily for 21 weeks *5590*

Prothrombin Time *Plasma Increase Physiological* Theoretically if bishydroxycoumarin co-administered *136*

Salicylate *Serum No Effect Analytical* At a concentration of 215 mg/dL has no significant effect on method on Kodak Ektachem® systems *2519*

Sparfloxacin *Serum Decrease Physiological* Magnesium and aluminum containing antacids form chelation complexes with sparfloxacin and must be given either 2 hours before or after sparfloxacin to avoid reducing its bioavailability *4943*

Tiludronate *Serum Decrease Physiological* Bioavailabilty of tiludronate reduced by 60% when some aluminum or calcium containing antacids are administered one hour before tiludronate *5258*

Tolfenamic Acid *Serum Increase Physiological* Dose-dependent increased absorption from gastrointestinal tract with reduced time to peak concentration *4259*

Valproic Acid *Serum No Effect Physiological* Coadministration of valproate 500 mg with commonly administered antacids (Maalox, Trisogel, Titralac - 160 mEq doses) had no effect on the absorption of valproic acid *17*

Warfarin *Plasma No Effect Physiological* No effect observed *6403* Coadministration had no effect on plasma concentration *136*

Magnesium Nitrate

Bilirubin *Serum No Effect Analytical* No effect at concentration of 100 mmol/L on method on Kodak Ektachem® *5706*

Bilirubin, Conjugated *Serum No Effect Analytical* No effect at concentration of 100 mmol/L on method on Kodak Ektachem® *5706*

Bilirubin, Unconjugated *Serum No Effect Analytical* No effect at concentration of 100 mmol/L on method on Kodak Ektachem® *5706*

Potassium *Serum No Effect Analytical* No effect of concentrations up to 2.0 mmol/L on method on Kodak Ektachem® *5706*

Magnesium Salts

Alkaline Phosphatase *Serum Increase Analytical* Activators of enzyme in laboratory procedures *6026*

Calcium *Serum Decrease Physiological* Competes with calcium for gastrointestinal tract absorption *3272*

Serum Increase Analytical Measured as calcium in some EDTA procedures *2559*

Diagnex Blue Excretion *Urine Increase Physiological* Heavy metal displacement of diagnex blue *6515*

Magnesium *Serum Increase Physiological* Absorbed from gastrointestinal tract from antacids etc *2451*

Magnesium Sulfate

Angiotensin-converting Enzyme

Serum Decrease Physiological Decreased in 16 women with pregnancy induced hypertension 1-8 h after treatment then plateaued *1981*

Calcium *Serum Increase Physiological* In one woman given i.v. drug because of Crohn's disease for which she was receiving calcium supplements *4217*

Serum No Effect Physiological In 10 healthy men infusion of 3 g over one hour caused insignificant change from mean baseline of 2.34 ± 0.04 mmol/L to 2.32 ± 0.04 mmol/L *6677*

Cortisol *Plasma Decrease Physiological* In 10 healthy men infusion of 3 g over 60 minutes caused significantly reduction from mean baseline of 444 ± 36 nmol/L to 306 ± 41 nmol/L *6677*

Dopamine *Plasma No Effect Physiological* In 10 healthy men infusion of 3 g over 60 minutes caused nonsignificant reduction from mean baseline of 0.26 ± 0.04 nmol/L to 0.19 ± 0.02 nmol/L *6677*

Urine No Effect Physiological In 10 healthy men infusion of 6 g caused excretion of 1.62 ± 0.36 μmol/min not significantly different from 1.12 ± 0.21 μmol/min following infusion of saline *6677*

Epinephrine *Plasma No Effect Physiological* In 10 healthy men infusion of 3 g over 60 minutes caused nonsignificant reduction from mean baseline of 0.36 ± 0.05 nmol/L to 0.31 ± 0.06 nmol/L *6677*

Urine No Effect Physiological In 10 healthy men infusion of 6 g over 160 minutes caused excretion of 0.04 ± 0.005 μmol/min not significantly different from 0.03 ± 0.01 μmol/min following saline infusion *6677*

Follicle Stimulating Hormone

Plasma No Effect Physiological In 10 healthy men infusion of 3 g over one hour had no significant effect on concentration *6677*

Luteinizing Hormone *Plasma No Effect Physiological* In 10 healthy men intravenous infusion of 3 g over one hour had no significant effect on concentration *6677*

Magnesium *Serum Increase Physiological* No effect of a single oral dose of 30 g, but 9 of 14 subjects had significantly higher concentration following multiple doses at 4 hour intervals (2.61 mEq/L versus 1.80 mEq/L) *5613*

Norepinephrine *Plasma No Effect Physiological* In 10 healthy men infusion of 3 g over 60 minutes caused nonsignificant reduction from mean baseline of 1.65 ± 0.21 nmol/L to 1.59 ± 0.27 nmol/L *6677*

Urine No Effect Physiological In 10 healthy men nonsignificant difference observed over 160 minutes of 6 g infusion compared with saline infusion over same timeframe (0.18 ± 0.03 μmol/min compared with 0.13 ± 0.02 μmol/min) *6677*

Orthophosphate *Test Conditions No Effect Analytical* No effect up to 1 mol/L *2713*

Parathyroid Hormone *Plasma Decrease Physiological* In 10 healthy men infusion of 3 g caused significant decrease from mean baseline of 34.2 ± 3.5 ng/L to 20.5 ± 1.4 ng/L *6677*

Phosphate *Serum No Effect Physiological* In 10 healthy men infusion of 3 g over one hour caused insignificant change from mean baseline of 0.82 ± 0.04 mmol/L to 0.83 ± 0.03 mmol/L *6677*

Magnesium Sulfate *(continued)*

Potassium *Serum No Effect Analytical* Negligible effect at a concentration of 2 mmol/L on enzymatic spectrophotometric method of Berry et al *523*

Salicylate *Serum No Effect Analytical* At a concentration of 4.5 mg/dL (0.37 mmol/L) has no significant effect on method on Kodak Ektachem® systems *2519*

Sodium *Serum No Effect Analytical* Negligible effect at a concentration of 2 mmol/L on spectrophotometric enzymatic method of Berry et al *523*

Testosterone *Serum Decrease Physiological* In 10 healthy men infusion of 3 g over one hour caused significant reduction from mean baseline of about 2.0 nmol/L to 1.7 nmol/L *6677*

Tetracycline *Serum Decrease Physiological* Reduced absorption noted *6403*

Magnesium Trisilicate

Digoxin *Serum Decrease Physiological* Gastrointestinal absorption reduced by about 30% *760*

Nitrofurantoin *Serum Decrease Physiological* Absorbs nitrofurantoin and may decrease its gastrointestinal absorption *1384* Absorption reduced due to adsorption *6403* Antacids containing magnesium trisilicate when administered concomitantly with with nitrofurantoin reduce both the rate and extent of absorption of nitrofurantoin, probably due to adsorption of nitrofurantoin onto the surface of magnesium trisilicate *4800*

Osmolality *Serum Increase Physiological* In a single case large doses over a long period of time caused hyperosmolality and cerebral dehydration with coma *1796*

Maleinimide

Glucose *Serum No Effect Analytical* At concentration of 2000 mg/L no effect on method on Boehringer Mannheim Reflotron system *5706*

Mannitol

Albumin *Serum No Effect Analytical* No effect on Technicon SMA 12/60 method at 445 mg/dL *4390*
Urine No Effect Physiological No significant increase observed after injection of 5.2% or 11.1% solution in 10 healthy men *2890*

Alkaline Phosphatase *Serum No Effect Analytical* No effect on Technicon SMA 12/60 method at 445 mg/dL *4390*
Urine Increase Physiological In 10 healthy men after injection of 5.2% mean excretion increased significantly from 0.21 ± 0.04 U/mmol creatinine to 0.37 ± 0.06 U/mmol creatinine over next 4 hours and after 11.1% mannitol increased from 0.20 ± 0.03 U/mmol creatinine to 0.63 ± 0.21 U/mmol creatinine *2890*

Ammonia *Feces Increase Physiological* Modest rise observed *65*

Amylase *Serum No Effect Analytical* At a concentration of 40,000 mg/L had no effect on maltotetrose method *5704* At concentration of 40,000 mg/L had no effect on p-nitrophenylmaltoheptoside method *5704* At a concentration of 40,000 mg/L had no effect on p-nitrophenylmaltopentoside/hexoside method *5704*

Aspartate Aminotransferase *Serum No Effect Analytical* No effect on Technicon SMA 12/60 method at 445 mg/dL *4390*

Bilirubin *Serum No Effect Analytical* No effect on Technicon SMA 12/60 method at 445 mg/dL *4390*

Calcium *Serum No Effect Analytical* No effect on Technicon SMA 12/60 method at 445 mg/dL *4390*
Urine Increase Physiological Initial diuretic response *174*

Chloride *Serum Decrease Physiological* Effect if marked diuresis *128*

Cholesterol *Serum No Effect Analytical* No effect on Technicon SMA 12/60 method at 445 mg/dL *4390*

Cholinesterase *Serum No Effect Analytical* No effect observed at concentration of 35 mg/dL with butyrylthiocholine method on Kodak Ektachem® *2504*

Creatinine *Serum Increase Physiological* Due to dehydration *3810*
Serum No Effect Analytical No effect on Technicon SMA 12/60 method at 445 mg/dL *4390*
Serum No Effect Physiological Injection of either 5.2% or 11.1% mannitol had no significant effect on concentration *2890*

Creatinine Clearance *Urine Increase Physiological* In 10 healthy men after injection of 5.2% mannitol clearance increased from mean baseline of 142 ± 34 mL/min to 148 ± 19 mL/min over next 4 hours and after 11.1% mannitol increased from 130 ± 22 mL/min to 145 ± 20 mL/min *2890*

Glucose *Serum No Effect Analytical* No effect on Technicon SMA 12/60 method at 445 mg/dL *4390*

5-Hydroxyindoleacetic Acid *Urine No Effect Physiological* No significant effect observed in healthy volunteers following intravenous infusion *1187*

Lactate Dehydrogenase *Serum No Effect Analytical* No effect on Technicon SMA 12/60 method at 445 mg/dL *4390*

Lipase *Serum No Effect Analytical* No effect of concentrations up to 4555 mg/L on method on Kodak Ektachem® *5706*

β_2-Microglobulin *Serum No Effect Physiological* Injection of 5.2% or 11.1% mannitol had no effect in 10 healthy men *2890*
Urine Increase Physiological In 10 healthy men injection of 5.2% mannitol caused increase from mean baseline of 142 ± 45 µg/d to 177 ± 61 µg/d over next 4 hours and no change from 173 ± 72 µg/d to 172 ± 49 µg/d after 11.1% mannitol over next 4 hours *2890*

Midazolam *Serum No Effect Analytical* On GC-ECD method of Ha et al *2387*

N-Acetyl-Glucosaminidase *Urine Increase Physiological* In 10 healthy men after injection of 5.2% mannitol mean excretion increased from baseline of 2.4 ± 0.8 nmol/h/µmol creatinine to 3.2 ± 1.1 nmol/h/µmol creatinine over next 4 hours and from 2.8 ± 1.0 nmol/h/µmol creatinine to 3.7 ± 0.9 nmol/h/µmol creatinine after 11.1% mannitol *2890*

Osmolality *Serum Increase Analytical* Concentration related increase: 6% at 3.1 g/L and 12.3% at 6.2 g/L *3391*
Serum Increase Physiological May cause marked dehydration *3669*
Urine Increase Physiological In 10 healthy male volunteers mean excretion increased from 2.5 ± 0.6 mL/min to 4.8 ± 0.8 mL/min during first 4 hours with 5.2% mannitol and from 2.6 ± 0.4 mL/min to 6.4 ± 1.1 mL/min with 11.1% mannitol *2890*

pH *Feces No Effect Physiological* No effect observed *65*

Phosphate *Serum Decrease Analytical* 19% reduction at 6.2 g/L on normal phosphate concentration: 23% reduction at 3.1 g/L on increased phosphate specimen on Du Pont aca method affecting also other methods in which Elon used as reducing agent *3391* At concentrations above 3100 mg/L lowered concentration as measured by Du Pont aca method *5704* Inhibition of color development *881* Concentration related reduction, possibly related to nature of reducing agent, on Dade® Paramax and Du Pont aca *1679*
Serum Increase Analytical Concentrations above 6400 mg/L increase results as determined by method on Kodak Ektachem® : of probable clinical importance since concentrations may exceed 7300 mg/L in actual practice *5706*
Serum No Effect Analytical No effect on Technicon SMA 12/60 method at 445 mg/dL *4390* No effect on method on Technicon AutoAnalyzer® even at 15.5 g/L *3391* Usually not high enough concentration to interfere *882*
Urine Decrease Analytical Complexes molybdate, decreases color develop *882*

Potassium *Serum Increase Physiological* Mechanism not discussed *4112*

Protein *Cerebrospinal Fluid No Effect Analytical* No significant effect when added in vitro to concentration of 200 mg/dL when measured by Kodak Ektachem® slide method *3654*
Serum No Effect Analytical No effect on Technicon SMA 12/60 method at 445 mg/dL *4390*

Sodium *Serum Decrease Physiological* Effect if marked diuresis *128*
Serum Increase Physiological May cause marked dehydration *3669*
Urine Increase Physiological In 10 healthy men injection of 5.2% mannitol caused significant increase from mean baseline of 146 ± 84 mmol/d to 207 ± 97 mmol/d over next 4 hours and from 174 ± 65 mmol/d to 319 ± 123 mmol/d after injection of 11.1% mannitol *2890* Slight increase occurs only *3669*

Uric Acid *Serum Decrease Physiological* Reported to have uricosuric action *1967*
Serum No Effect Analytical No effect on Technicon SMA 12/60 method at 445 mg/dL *4390*
Urine Increase Physiological Intravenously produces uricosuria *2452*

Volume *Urine Increase Physiological* In 20 healthy male volunteers injection of mannitol caused increased excretion by 327% to 373% in following 4 hours, but returned to normal within 24 hours *2890*

MAO Inhibitors

Alanine Aminotransferase *Serum Increase Physiological* Intrahepatic cholestasis *3669*

Alkaline Phosphatase *Serum Increase Physiological* Cholestatic effect *3669*

Ammonia *Plasma Decrease Physiological* Reported effect in exogenous NH_3 toxicity *3160*

Amphetamine *Serum Increase Physiological* MAO antidepressants slow metabolism of amphetamines increasing their effect on the release of norepinehrine and other monoamines from adrenergic nerve endings *5641*

Aspartate Aminotransferase *Serum Increase Physiological* Intrahepatic cholestasis *3669*

Bile *Urine Increase Physiological* Hepatotoxic effect *3810*

Bilirubin *Serum Increase Physiological* Viral hepatitis-like jaundice in some patients *5464*

BSP Retention *Serum Increase Physiological* Intrahepatic cholestasis with possible cell damage *2024*

Catecholamines *Plasma Increase Physiological* Prevent deamination but not degradation by catechol-o-methyl transferase *189*

Cholesterol *Serum Decrease Physiological* Hepatotoxic effect *3669*

Dopamine *Plasma Increase Physiological* Effect observed after single large dose *2242*

Epinephrine *Plasma Increase Physiological* Effect observed after single large dose *2242*

Erythrocytes *Blood Decrease Physiological* Anemia may occasionally occur *3810*

Glucose *Serum Decrease Physiological* Mechanism not clear (possible hepatotoxicity) *57*

Glucose Tolerance *Serum Increase Physiological* Seen in diabetics treated with insulin *3669*

Guaiacols Spot Test *Urine Positive Analytical* False reaction with screening test of Rogers *5061*

Hematocrit *Blood Decrease Physiological* Occasional anemia may occur *4014*

Hemoglobin *Blood Decrease Physiological* Occasional anemia may develop *4014*

Histamine Test *Patient Increase Physiological* Enhanced responsiveness *2213*

4-Hydroxy-3-Methoxy-Phenylglycol
Urine Decrease Physiological Inhibition of amine oxidase *660*

17-Hydroxycorticosteroids *Urine Decrease Physiological* Probably due to depressed central synthesis *55*

5-Hydroxyindoleacetic Acid *Urine Decrease Physiological* Inhibition of conversion of 5-HT to 5-HIAA *3145*

5-Hydroxytryptamine *Plasma Increase Physiological* Effect observed after single large dose *2242*

5-Hydroxytryptamine Glucuronide
Urine Increase Physiological Due to inhibition of conversion of 5-HT to 5-HIAA *2242*

Leukocytes *Blood Decrease Physiological* Occasional leukopenia/agranulocytosis *3810*

Metanephrines, Total *Urine Increase Physiological* Prevent deamination *2242*

N-Acetylmetanephrine *Urine Increase Physiological* Due to inhibition of amine oxidase *660*

N-Acetylnormetanephrine *Urine Increase Physiological* Due to inhibition of amine oxidase *660*

Norepinephrine *Plasma Increase Physiological* Effect observed after single large dose *2242*

Normetanephrine *Urine Increase Physiological* Prevent deamination *2242*

Phentolamine Test *Patient Increase Physiological* Enhanced responsiveness *2213*

Phenylethylamine *Urine Increase Physiological* Prevent deamination *2242*

Prothrombin Time *Plasma Increase Physiological* May prolong action of anticoagulants *2753*

Tryptamine *Urine Increase Physiological* Due to utilization of alternative pathways *2242*

Tyramine *Urine Increase Physiological* Prevent deamination *2242*

Tyramine Test *Patient Increase Physiological* Enhanced responsiveness *2213*

Vanillylmandelic Acid *Urine Decrease Physiological* Inhibition of normetanephrine conversion to VMA *2451*

Xylose *Urine Decrease Physiological* Decreased gastrointestinal tract absorption with subsequent reduced excretion *2024*

Maprotiline

Alanine Aminotransferase *Serum Increase Physiological* Slight reversible rise in approximately 1% patients *348*

Albumin *Urine No Effect Analytical* Using a fluorimetric assay with Albumin Blue 580 on a Cobas Fara centrifugal analyzer for the detection of microalbuminuria no significant interference was detected at a concentration of 10 mg/L *3117*

Aspartate Aminotransferase *Serum Increase Physiological* Slight reversible rise in approximately 1% patients *348*

Bilirubin *Serum No Effect Physiological* Insignificant displacement from protein in neonates *6314*

Catecholamines *Plasma No Effect Analytical* No effect on HPLC method of Koller for dopamine, epinephrine, and norepinephrine *3230*

Creatinine *Serum No Effect Analytical* No interference observed with liquid chromatographic method of Paroni *4540*

Eosinophils *Blood Increase Physiological* Bone marrow depression including agranulocytosis and thrombocytopenia or eosinophilia observed as isolated event *1034*

Glucose *Serum Decrease Physiological* Rare instances of increased or decreased glucose concentration *1034*
Serum Increase Physiological Rare instances of increased or decreased glucose concentration *1034*

Granulocytes *Blood Decrease Physiological* Bone marrow depression including agranulocytosis and thrombocytopenia observed as isolated event *1034*

Midazolam *Serum No Effect Analytical* On GC-ECD method of Ha et al *2387*

Platelets *Blood Decrease Physiological* Bone marrow depression including agranulocytosis and thrombocytopenia with purpura observed as isolated event *1034*

Tricyclic Antidepressants Screen
Serum Negative Analytical Not detected at concentrations up to 1000 µg/mL (3.67 mmol/L) by method on Du Pont aca *1550*

Marimastat

Alanine Aminotransferase *Serum Increase Physiological* At an oral dose of 50 mg caused increased activity to just above upper limit of normal in 1 of 12 treated volunteers *4036*

Albumin *Urine Increase Physiological* At an oral dose of 25 mg caused albuminuria in 1 of 12 treated volunteers *4036*

Bilirubin *Serum Increase Physiological* At an oral dose of 25 mg caused hyperbilirubinemia in 1 of 12 treated volunteers *4036*

Glucose *Serum Increase Physiological* Repeat oral doses caused hyperglycemia and/or glycosuria in 4 of 12 treated volunteers *4036*
Urine Increase Physiological Repeat oral doses caused hyperglycemia and/or glycosuria in 4 of 12 treated volunteers *4036*

Marimastat *(continued)*

Lymphocytes *Blood Increase Physiological* At an oral dose of 100 mg caused lymphocytosis in 1 of 12 treated volunteers 24 h after dosing *4036*

Platelets *Blood Decrease Physiological* At oral doses of 50 mg caused small decreases in platelet count in 12 treated volunteers *4036*

Marophen

Eosinophils *Blood Increase Physiological* Low incidence reported *4014*

Marvelon

Follicle Stimulating Hormone *Plasma Decrease Physiological* In 20 patients with idiopathic hirsutism treatment for at least 1 year caused a significant decrease in plasma FSH concentration *1443*

Luteinizing Hormone *Plasma Decrease Physiological* In 20 patients with idiopathic hirsutism treatment for at least 1 year caused a significant decrease in plasma LH concentration *1443*

Sex-Hormone Binding Globulin *Serum Increase Physiological* In 20 patients with idiopathic hirsutism treatment for at least 1 year caused a significant increase in SHBG concentration *1443*

Testosterone *Serum No Effect Physiological* In 20 patients with idiopathic hirsutism treatment for at least 1 year caused no significant change in total testosterone concentration *1443*

Testosterone, Free *Serum Decrease Physiological* In 20 patients with idiopathic hirsutism treatment for at least 1 year caused a significant decrease in % free testosterone concentration *1443*

Mayo Enema

Bicarbonate *Serum Increase Physiological* May cause retention from bicarbonate in enema *1129*

pH *Blood Increase Physiological* Due to bicarbonate in enema *1129*

Sodium *Serum Increase Physiological* High sodium content; sodium may be retained *1129*

Mazindol

Amobarbital *Urine No Effect Analytical* No interference on TLC using ethyl acetate: methanol: water: ammonium hydroxide and modified Dragendorff's reagent for detection *6502*

Amphetamine *Urine No Effect Analytical* No interference on TLC using ethyl acetate: methanol: water: ammonium hydroxide and modified Dragendorff's reagent for detection *6502*

Chlordiazepoxide *Urine Positive Analytical* Same R_f and color reaction on TLC using ethyl acetate: methanol: water: ammonium hydroxide and modified Dragendorff's reagent *6502*

Flurazepam *Urine Positive Analytical* Same R_f and color reaction on TLC using ethyl acetate: methanol: water: ammonium hydroxide and modified Dragendorff's reagent *6502*

Growth Hormone *Plasma Decrease Physiological* Apparent diminution in mean concentration after 3 and 6 months in 40 patients with Duchenne muscular dystrophy but effect not significant after 9 and 12 months treatment *6634*

Hydromorphone *Urine No Effect Analytical* No interference on TLC using ethyl acetate: methanol: water: ammonium hydroxide and modified Dragendorff's reagent for detection *6502*

Mescaline *Urine No Effect Analytical* No interference on TLC using ethyl acetate: methanol: water: ammonium hydroxide and modified Dragendorff's reagent for detection *6502*

Methadone *Urine Increase Analytical* Same R_f and color reaction on TLC using ethyl acetate: methanol: water: ammonium hydroxide and modified Dragendorff's reagent *6502*

Methamphetamine *Urine No Effect Analytical* No interference on TLC using ethyl acetate: methanol: water: ammonium hydroxide and modified Dragendorff's reagent for detection *6502*

Methapyrilene *Urine Positive Analytical* Same R_f and color reaction on TLC using ethyl acetate: methanol: water: ammonium hydroxide and modified Dragendorff's reagent *6502*

Methylphenidate *Urine Positive Analytical* Same R_f and color reaction on TLC using ethyl acetate: methanol: water: ammonium hydroxide and modified Dragendorff's reagent *6502*

Morphine *Urine No Effect Analytical* No interference on TLC using ethyl acetate: methanol: water: ammonium hydroxide and modified Dragendorff's reagent for detection *6502*

Pentobarbital *Urine No Effect Analytical* No interference on TLC using ethyl acetate: methanol: water: ammonium hydroxide and modified Dragendorff's reagent for detection *6502*

Phendimetrazine *Urine Positive Analytical* Same R_f and color reaction on TLC using ethyl acetate: methanol: water: ammonium hydroxide and modified Dragendorff's reagent *6502*

Phenobarbital *Urine No Effect Analytical* No interference on TLC using ethyl acetate: methanol: water: ammonium hydroxide and modified Dragendorff's reagent for detection *6502*

Phenylpropanolamine *Urine No Effect Analytical* No interference on TLC using ethyl acetate: methanol: water: ammonium hydroxide and modified Dragendorff's reagent for detection *6502*

Secobarbital *Urine No Effect Analytical* No interference on TLC using ethyl acetate: methanol: water: ammonium hydroxide and modified Dragendorff's reagent for detection *6502*

MDEA

p-Aminophenol *Urine No Effect Analytical* With addition of drugs at a concentration of 100 mg/L and of related compounds at 50 mg/L no significant effect observed on colorimetric method of van Bocxlaer on Cobas Mira analyzer which involves reacting free p-aminophenol with resorcinol in the presence of magnesium ions to form an indophenol dye measured at 550 nm *6163*

Measles Virus Vaccine

Platelets *Blood Decrease Physiological* May cause thrombocytopenic purpura *4014*

Mebanazine

Glucose *Serum Decrease Physiological* Appears to potentiate insulin in diabetics *4014*

Mebendazole

Histamine *Plasma No Effect Analytical* Improbable inhibition of radio-enzyme assay at therapeutic concentrations *2492*

Theophylline *Serum No Effect Physiological* No clinically significant effect on theophylline concentration observed when drugs coadministered *5999* No documented significant interaction with theophylline reported *6117*

Mebhydrolin

Neutrophils *Blood Decrease Physiological* Occasional case of agranulocytoisis reported *6264*

Mebutamate

Platelets *Blood Decrease Physiological* Rare thrombocytopenic purpura *2754*

Mecamylamine

Catecholamines *Urine No Effect Physiological* No effect observed *1444*

Uric Acid *Serum Increase Physiological* ?Due to reduced renal blood flow *1461*

Vanillylmandelic Acid *Urine No Effect Physiological* No effect observed *1444*

Mechlorethamine

Alanine Aminotransferase *Serum Increase Physiological* May cause cytotoxic (hepatocellular) damage *402*

Alkaline Phosphatase *Serum Increase Physiological* Hepatotoxic effect *402*

Aspartate Aminotransferase *Serum Increase Physiological* May cause cytotoxic (hepatocellular) damage *402*

Bile *Urine Increase Physiological* Hepatotoxic effect *402*

BSP Retention *Serum Increase Physiological* Hepatotoxic effect *402*

Cholinesterase *Serum Decrease Physiological* Observed activity *in vitro*, probable *in vivo6684*

Erythrocytes *Blood Decrease Physiological* Mild effect *128*

Granulocytes *Blood Decrease Physiological* Significant granulocytopenia may occur within 6 to 8 days and last for 10 days to 3 weeks. Leukopenia may resolve within two weeks of the maximum reduction *3985*

Guanase *Serum Increase Physiological* May cause cytotoxic (hepatocellular) damage *402*

Hematocrit *Blood Decrease Physiological* Hemolytic anemia may occur occasionally in patients with lymphoma or chronic lymphocytic leukemia *3985*

Hemoglobin *Blood Decrease Physiological* Hemolytic anemia may occur occasionally in patients with lymphoma or chronic lymphocytic leukemia *3985*

Isocitrate Dehydrogenase *Serum Increase Physiological* May cause cytotoxic (hepatocellular) damage *402*

Leukocytes *Blood Decrease Physiological* Leukopenia may resolve within two weeks of the maximum reduction *3985*

Lymphocytes *Blood Decrease Physiological* Occurs within 24 h *2242* Significant lymphocytopenia may occur within 24 hours of the first injection *3985*

Occult Blood *Feces Increase Physiological* Thrombcytopenia is variable but may lead to bleeding from the gums and gastrointestinal tract *3985*

Ornithine Carbamoyltransferase *Serum Increase Physiological* May cause cytotoxic (hepatocellular) damage *402*

Platelet Aggregation *Blood Decrease Physiological* Observed *in vitro*, might cause gastrointestinal bleeding etc *915*

Platelets *Blood Decrease Physiological* Bone marrow depression *128* Thrombcytopenia is variable but may lead to bleeding from the gums and gastrointestinal tract *3985*

Sperm Count *Semen Decrease Physiological* Impaired spermatogenesis, azospermia and total germinal aplasia have been reported, with spermatogenesis ultimately returning in some patients in remission *3985*

Uric Acid *Serum Decrease Physiological* More effective than several uricosuric agents *5002*
Serum Increase Physiological Leucocyte destruction, catabolism of nucleic acids *5869* Hyperuricemia may occur as a result of cellular destruction *3985*

Meclofenamate

Alanine Aminotransferase *Serum Increase Physiological* Rare increase in activity reported *1384*

Alkaline Phosphatase *Serum Increase Physiological* Rare increase in activity observed *1384*

Aspartate Aminotransferase *Serum Increase Physiological* Rare increase in activity reported *1384*

Bleeding Time *Patient No Effect Physiological* In contrast to aspirin had no effect on bleeding time *1384*

Chondrex *Serum No Effect Analytical* Concentrations up to 1 g/L had no significant effect on sandwich-type ELISA procedure of Harvey et al *2491*

Creatinine *Serum Increase Physiological* Rare increase in concentration observed *1384*

Erythrocytes *Blood Decrease Physiological* Reduced in about 10% treated patients but not necessary to discontinue treatment *1384*

Hematocrit *Blood Decrease Physiological* Reduced in about 10% treated patients but not necessary to discontinue treatment *1384*

Hemoglobin *Blood Decrease Physiological* Reduced in about 10% treated patients but not necessary to discontinue treatment *1384*

Leukocytes *Blood Decrease Physiological* Rare reduction observed *1384*

Platelet Aggregation *Blood No Effect Physiological* Repeated administration had no effect on collagen induced aggregation *1384*

Prothrombin Time *Plasma Increase Physiological* Observed in patients already receiving warfarin *1384*

Salicylate *Serum No Effect Physiological* When aspirin and meclofenamate given together no effect on salicylate concentration observed *1384*

Urea Nitrogen *Serum Increase Physiological* Rare increase in concentration observed *1384*

Medazepam

Benzodiazepine *Urine Positive Analytical* At concentrations of 0.3 µg/mL or greater produces positive result with Syva EMIT II assay *1785*

Catecholamines *Plasma No Effect Analytical* No effect on HPLC method of Koller for dopamine, epinephrine, and norepinephrine after extraction with alumina *3230*

5-Hydroxyindoleacetic Acid *Urine Increase Analytical* Slight effect when added *in vitro* in method of Udenfriend *1051*

Medrogesterone

Apolipoprotein A-I *Serum No Effect Physiological* In 59 postmenopausal women receiving conjugated estrogens with medrogesterone mean concentration of 1.51 ± 0.19 mg/dL not significantly different from 1.51 ± 0.24 mg/dL in 55 postmenopausal women receiving conjugated estrogens alone *3529*

Apolipoprotein B *Serum No Effect Physiological* In 59 postmenopausal women receiving conjugated estrogens with medrogesterone mean concentration of 1.31 ± 0.27 mg/dL not significantly different from 1.26 ± 0.23 mg/dL in 55 postmenopausal women receiving conjugated estrogens alone *3529*

Cholesterol *Serum No Effect Physiological* In 59 postmenopausal women receiving conjugated estrogens with medrogesterone mean concentration of 5.94 ± 0.73 mmol/L not significantly different from 5.78 ± 0.70 mmol/L in 55 postmenopausal women receiving conjugated estrogens alone *3529*

HDL_2-Cholesterol *Serum No Effect Physiological* In 59 postmenopausal women receiving conjugated estrogens with medrogesterone mean concentration of 0.40 ± 0.19 mmol/L not significantly different from 0.41 ± 0.17 mmol/L in 55 postmenopausal women receiving conjugated estrogens alone *3529*

HDL_3-Cholesterol *Serum No Effect Physiological* In 59 postmenopausal women receiving conjugated estrogens with medrogesterone mean concentration of 0.99 ± 0.16 mmol/L not significantly different from 0.99 ± 0.20 mmol/L in 55 postmenopausal women receiving conjugated estrogens alone *3529*

HDL-Cholesterol *Serum No Effect Physiological* In 59 postmenopausal women receiving conjugated estrogens with medrogesterone mean concentration of 1.47 ± 0.28 mmol/L not significantly different from 1.47 ± 0.32 mmol/L in 55 postmenopausal women receiving conjugated estrogens alone *3529*

LDL-Cholesterol *Serum No Effect Physiological* In 59 postmenopausal women receiving conjugated estrogens with medrogesterone mean concentration of 3.80 ± 0.69 mmol/L not significantly different from 3.77 ± 0.61 mmol/L in 55 postmenopausal women receiving conjugated estrogens alone *3529*

Medrogesterone *(continued)*

Lipoprotein Lp(a) *Serum* *No Effect* *Physiological* In 59 postmenopausal women receiving conjugated estrogens with medrogesterone mean concentration of 10 mg/dL (range 3.7 - 25) not significantly different from 15 mg/dL (range 4.4 - 38) in 55 postmenopausal women receiving conjugated estrogens alone *3529*

Triglycerides *Serum* *Increase* *Physiological* In 59 postmenopausal women receiving conjugated estrogens with medrogesterone mean concentration of 1.35 ± 0.58 mmol/L significantly different from 1.17 ± 0.51 mmol/L in 55 postmenopausal women receiving conjugated estrogens alone *3529*

VLDL-Cholesterol *Serum* *Increase* *Physiological* In 59 postmenopausal women receiving conjugated estrogens with medrogesterone mean concentration of 0.67 ± 0.28 mmol/L significantly different from 0.53 ± 0.49 mmol/L in 55 postmenopausal women receiving conjugated estrogens alone *3529*

Medroxyprogesterone

Alanine Aminotransferase *Serum* *Increase* *Physiological* Administration may cause abnormal liver function tests *4683* Liver function tests may become abnormal during treatment *4671*

Alkaline Phosphatase *Serum* *Increase* *Physiological* Administration may cause abnormal liver function tests *4683* Liver function tests may become abnormal during treatment *4671*

Androgens *Urine* *Decrease* *Physiological* Inhibition of steroid biosynthesis in adrenals *6099*

Angiotensinogen *Plasma* *Increase* *Physiological* In 23 healthy postmenopausal women treatment with conjugated estrogens 0.625 mg and 5 mg medroxyprogesterone acetate in 21-day sequences over 12 cycles caused significant change in concentration from 1889 ± 80 ng/mL to 4341 ± 271 ng/mL *588*

Antithrombin III *Plasma* *Decrease* *Physiological* In 21 healthy postmenopausal women treatment with conjugated estrogens 0.625 mg and 5 mg medroxyprogesterone acetate in 21-day sequences over 12 cycles caused significant change in concentration from 1.11 ± 0.024 mg/L to 1.05 ± 0.024 mg/L *588*

Apolipoprotein A-I *Serum* *Decrease* *Physiological* Increase by 7% in 11 men with sexual deviation syndrome given approximately 1273 mg over a total of approximately 17 d *978*

Apolipoprotein B *Serum* *Decrease* *Physiological* Increase by 15% in 11 men with sexual deviation syndrome given approximately 1273 mg over a total of approximately 17 d *978*

Aspartate Aminotransferase *Serum* *Increase* *Physiological* Liver function tests may become abnormal during treatment *4671* Administration may cause abnormal liver function tests *4683*

Bilirubin *Serum* *Increase* *Physiological* Liver function tests may become abnormal during treatment *4671*

BR-MA *Serum* *Decrease* *Physiological* In 14 patients with advanced breast cancer treated with 1000 mg/d medroxyprogesterone acetate significant change observed at 12 weeks *4187*
Serum *No Effect* *Physiological* In 11 patients with advanced breast cancer treated with 500 mg/d medroxyprogesterone acetate no significant change in concentration observed at 2, 6 and 12 weeks, and in 14 treated with 1000 mg/d no significant change observed at 2 and 6 weeks *4187*

Calcium *Serum* *No Effect* *Physiological* No difference observed compared with controls *5567*

Carcinoembryonic Antigen *Serum* *Increase* *Physiological* In 11 patients with advanced breast cancer treated with 500 mg/d medroxyprogesterone acetate no significant change in concentration observed at 12 weeks, and in 14 receiving 1000 mg/d no significant change observed after 2, 6 and 12 weeks *4187*

Cholesterol *Serum* *Decrease* *Physiological* Both transient increases and decreases have been reported during treatment *4671* Increase by 14% effects observed in 15 postmenopausal women with endometrial cancer after 2 weeks treatment *3503* Increase by 12% in 11 men with sexual deviation syndrome given approximately 1273 mg over a total of approximately 17 d *978* In 30 healthy postmenopausal women aged 56 ± 5 years treatment with oral 2.5 medroxyprogesterone acetate with 0.625 mg conjugated estrogen daily for one month caused significant change from mean baseline of 238 ± 39 mg/dL to 221 ± 35 mg/dL *3219* In both short and long-term users of depot medroxyprogesterone moderate but not significant decrease observed *2042*
Serum *Increase* *Physiological* Both transient increases and decreases have been reported during treatment *4671*
Serum *No Effect* *Physiological* Concentration unchanged by i.m. administration of 150 mg depot preparation to either chronic or first time recipients *2042* In 20 healthy postmenopausal women treatment with conjugated estrogens 0.625 mg and 5 mg medroxyprogesterone acetate in 21-day sequences over 12 cycles caused nonsignificant change in concentration from 5.00 ± 0.17 mmol/L to 5.07 ± 0.16 mmol/L in estrogenic phase and 4.90 ± 0.13 mmol/L in progestogenic phase *588* Concentration unchanged by I.M. administration of 150 mg depot preparation to either chronic or first time recipients *2042*

Color *Feces* *Increase* *Analytical* Green color reported with ingestion of medroxyprogesterone *3388*

Cortisol *Plasma* *Decrease* *Physiological* Significant reduction of previously increased concentration observed in patients with carcinoma of the bronchus and cachexia with gain of 3 kg body weight with 4 weeks treatment with medroxyprogesterone *1684* In critically ill patients relative hypoadrenalism observed with medroxyprogesterone therapy *3381* Plasma concentration and urinary excretion reduced during treatment *4671*
Urine *Decrease* *Physiological* Plasma concentration and urinary excretion reduced during treatment *4671*

C-terminal Telopeptide of Type I Collagen
Urine *Decrease* *Physiological* In 33 postmenopausal women treated with 0.625 mg/d conjugated equine estrogens and 2.5 mg/d medroxyprogesterone acetate for 12 months caused significant change from mean baseline of 280 µg/mmol creatinine to 120 µg/mmol creatinine after 6 momths and 70 µg/mmol creatinine after one year *5912*

Cytokeratin 8/18 *Serum* *Decrease* *Physiological* In 11 patients with advanced breast cancer treated with 1000 mg/d medroxyprogesterone acetate significant change in concentration observed at 2, 6 and 12 weeks *4187*
Serum *No Effect* *Physiological* In 11 patients with advanced breast cancer treated with 500 mg/d medroxyprogesterone acetate no significant change in concentration observed at 2, 6 and 12 weeks *4187*

Dehydroepiandrosterone Sulfate
Plasma *Decrease* *Physiological* In 23 healthy postmenopausal women treatment with conjugated estrogens 0.625 mg and 5 mg medroxyprogesterone acetate in 21-day sequences over 12 cycles caused nonsignificant decrease in concentration from 3.17 ± 0.43 µmol/L to 2.82 ± 0.75 µmol/L *588*

Deoxypyridinoline *Urine* *Decrease* *Physiological* In 33 postmenopausal women treated with 0.625 mg/d conjugated equine estrogens and 2.5 mg/d medroxyprogesterone acetate for 12 months caused significant change from mean baseline of 6.7 pmol/µmol creatinine to 4.2 pmol/µmol creatinine after 6 momths and 3.6 pmol/µmol creatinine after one year *5912*

Epithelial Mucin Core Antigen
Serum *Decrease* *Physiological* In 14 patients with advanced breast cancer treated with 1000 mg/d medroxyprogesterone acetate significant change observed at 12 weeks *4187*
Serum *Increase* *Physiological* In 11 patients with advanced breast cancer treated with 500 mg/d medroxyprogesterone acetate significant increase in concentration observed after two weeks *4187*
Serum *No Effect* *Physiological* In 11 patients with advanced breast cancer treated with 500 mg/d medroxyprogesterone acetate no significant change in concentration observed at 6 and 12 weeks, and in 14 treated with 1000 mg/d no significant change observed at 2 and 6 weeks *4187*

Epithelial Mucin Core Antigen-2
Serum *Decrease* *Physiological* In 14 patients with advanced breast cancer treated with 1000 mg/d medroxyprogesterone acetate significant change observed at 12 weeks *4187*
Serum *Increase* *Physiological* In 11 patients with advanced breast cancer treated with 500 mg/d medroxyprogesterone acetate significant increase in concentration observed after two weeks *4187*

Serum No Effect Physiological In 11 patients with advanced breast cancer treated with 500 mg/d medroxyprogesterone acetate no significant change in concentration observed at 6 and 12 weeks, and in 14 treated with 1000 mg/d no significant change observed at 2 and 6 weeks *4187*

Estradiol *Plasma Decrease Physiological* Plasma concentration and urinary excretion reduced during treatment *4671*
Plasma Increase Physiological In 28 healthy postmenopausal women treatment with conjugated estrogens 0.625 mg and 5 mg medroxyprogesterone acetate in 21-day sequences over 12 cycles caused significant increase in concentration from 62 ± 17 pmol/L to 313 ± 40 pmol/L *588*
Urine Decrease Physiological Plasma concentration and urinary excretion reduced during treatment *4671*

17β-Estradiol *Plasma Increase Physiological* In 30 healthy postmenopausal women aged 56 ± 5 years treatment with oral 2.5 medroxyprogesterone acetate with 0.625 mg conjugated estrogen daily for one month caused significant increase from mean baseline of 16 ± 7 pg/mL to 68 ± 32 pg/mL *3219*

Estrone *Plasma Decrease Physiological* In 20 healthy postmenopausal women treatment with conjugated estrogens 0.625 mg and 5 mg medroxyprogesterone acetate in 21-day sequences over 12 cycles caused significant decrease in concentration from 2361 ± 17 pmol/L to 729 ± 64 pmol/L *588*
Plasma Increase Physiological In 30 healthy postmenopausal women aged 56 ± 5 years treatment with oral 2.5 medroxyprogesterone acetate with 0.625 mg conjugated estrogen daily for one month caused significant increase from mean baseline of 22 ± 12 pg/mL to 113 ± 60 pg/mL *3219*

Factor VII *Plasma Increase Physiological* Plasma concentration may increase during treatment *4671* Administration may cause increase in concentration *4683*

Factor VIII *Plasma Increase Physiological* Administration may cause increase in concentration *4683* Plasma concentration may increase during treatment *4671*

Factor IX *Plasma Increase Physiological* Plasma concentration may increase during treatment *4671* Administration may cause increase in concentration *4683*

Factor X *Plasma Increase Physiological* Plasma concentration may increase during treatment *4671*

Fibrinogen *Plasma Decrease Physiological* In 23 healthy postmenopausal women treatment with conjugated estrogens 0.625 mg and 5 mg medroxyprogesterone acetate in 21-day sequences over 12 cycles caused significant change in concentration from 3.01 ± 0.11 g/L to 2.82 ± 0.08 g/L *588*

Follicle Stimulating Hormone
Plasma Decrease Physiological In 29 healthy postmenopausal women treatment with conjugated estrogens 0.625 mg and 5 mg medroxyprogesterone acetate in 21-day sequences over 12 cycles caused significant decrease in concentration from 70.3 ± 6.8 IU/L to 22.8 ± 2.2 IU/L *588* Plasma concentration and urinary excretion reduced during treatment *4671*

Glucose *Serum Increase Physiological* Metabolic effect observed after 1 y *5742*

Glucose Tolerance *Serum Decrease Physiological* Abnormal in 15% may not return to normal in 1 y *5742*

γ-Glutamyltransferase *Serum Increase Physiological* Administration may cause abnormal liver function tests *4683* Liver function tests may become abnormal during treatment *4671*

Growth Hormone *Plasma Decrease Physiological* In patients with carcinoma of the bronchus and cachexia with regain of 3 kg body weight with 4 weeks treatment with medroxyprogesterone 60% decrease in plasma concentration observed *1684*
Plasma No Effect Physiological No effect observed after 1 y *5742*

HDL_2-Cholesterol *Serum Decrease Physiological* Increase by 15% at 2 weeks and more after longer treatment: dose-dependent correlation with results *1784* Increase by 35% effects observed in 15 postmenopausal women with endometrial cancer after 2 weeks treatment *3503*

HDL_3-Cholesterol *Serum Decrease Physiological* Increase by 15% effects observed in 15 postmenopausal women with endometrial cancer after 2 weeks treatment *3503*
Serum No Effect Physiological No effect although changes in other fractions *1784*

HDL-Cholesterol *Serum Decrease Physiological* Significant decrease observed after 3 and 15 months treatment *1781* Increase by 8% at 2 weeks and more after longer treatment: dose-dependent correlation with results *1784* In both short and long-term users after depot insertion moderate but not significant decrease observed *2042* Nonsignificant progessive decline observed in both chronic and first time recipients following i.m. injection of 150 mg depot preparation *2042* Increase by 33% effects observed in 15 postmenopausal women with endomentrial cancer after 2 weeks treatment *3503* Both transient increases and decreases have been reported during treatment *4671* Effect observed when combined with testosterone enanthate *6319*
Serum Increase Physiological Both transient increases and decreases have been reported during treatment *4671* In 30 healthy postmenopausal women aged 56 ± 5 years treatment with oral 2.5 medroxyprogesterone acetate with 0.625 mg conjugated estrogen daily for one month caused significant change from mean baseline of 60 ± 16 mg/dL to 65 ± 18 mg/dL *3219*
Serum No Effect Physiological No significant effect in 11 men with sexual deviation syndrome given approximately 1273 mg over a total of approximately 17 d *978* In 20 healthy postmenopausal women treatment with conjugated estrogens 0.625 mg and 5 mg medroxyprogesterone acetate in 21-day sequences over 12 cycles caused nonsignificant change in concentration from 1.60 ± 0.08 mmol/L to 1.62 ± 0.07 mmol/L in estrogenic phase and 1.57 ± 0.07 mmol/L in progestogenic phase *588*

17-Hydroxycorticosteroids *Urine Decrease Physiological* Inhibition of steroid biosynthesis in adrenals *6099*

Hydroxyproline *Urine Decrease Physiological* In 33 postmenopausal women treated with 0.625 mg/d conjugated equine estrogens and 2.5 mg/d medroxyprogesterone acetate for 12 months caused significant change from mean baseline of 20 mg/g creatinine to 13 mg/g creatinine after 6 momths and 12 mg/g creatinine after one year *5912*

Insulin *Plasma Increase Physiological* Metabolic effect (?glucocorticoid) *5742* In patients with carcinoma of bronchus and cachexia treatment with medroxyprogesterone acetate for 4 weeks caused 50% increase in fasting immunoreactive insulin concentration *1684*
Plasma No Effect Physiological In 30 healthy postmenopausal women aged 56 ± 5 years treatment with oral 2.5 medroxyprogesterone acetate with 0.625 mg conjugated estrogen daily for one month caused nonsignificant change from mean baseline of 8.3 ± 6.2 μU/mL to 8.7 ± 6.2 μU/mL *3219*

Insulin-like Growth Factor-I *Serum Increase Physiological* In patients previously with cachexia and with carcinoma of the bronchus and who put on more than 3 kg in weight with treatment 4 weeks of treatment with medroxyprogesterone mean concentration significantly increased *1684*

Interleukin-6 *Serum Decrease Physiological* In 21 women with metastatic breast cancer treatment with 600 - 1200 mg/d medroxyprogesterone acetate for 4 weeks caused a significant reduction from mean baseline of 9.83 ± 2.10 pg/mL to 4.66 ± 1.33 pg/mL *6585*

LDL-Cholesterol *Serum Decrease Physiological* Both transient increases and decreases have been reported during treatment *4671* In 30 healthy postmenopausal women aged 56 ± 5 years treatment with oral 2.5 medroxyprogesterone acetate with 0.625 mg conjugated estrogen daily for one month caused significant change from mean baseline of 155 ± 33 mg/dL to 134 ± 29 mg/dL *3219* Increase by 13% in 11 men with sexual deviation syndrome given approximately 1273 mg over a total of approximately 17 d *978*
Serum Increase Physiological Significant increase observed after 3 and 15 months use of depot medroxyprogesterone *1781* Both transient increases and decreases have been reported during treatment *4671*
Serum No Effect Physiological No significant effect observed in either short or long term depot users 92 days after intramuscular injection of 150 mg *2042* In 20 healthy postmenopausal women treatment with conjugated estrogens 0.625 mg and 5 mg medroxyprogesterone acetate in 21-day sequences over 12 cycles caused nonsignificant change in concentration from 2.84 ± 0.17 mmol/L to 2.87 ± 0.15 mmol/L in estrogenic phase and 2.88 ± 0.15 mmol/L in progestogenic phase *588* Concentration unchanged in both chronic and first time recipients following i.m. injection of 150 mg depot preparation *2042*

Medroxyprogesterone *(continued)*

Lecithin:Cholesterol Acyltransferase
Serum Decrease Physiological Significant reduction after treatment. Effects observed in 15 postmenopausal women with endometrial cancer after 2 weeks treatment *3503*

Lipoprotein Lp(a) *Serum Decrease Physiological* Significant reduction observed with administration to postmenopausal women *5699* In 30 healthy postmenopausal women aged 56 ± 5 years treatment with oral 2.5 medroxyprogesterone acetate with 0.625 mg conjugated estrogen daily for one month caused significant change from mean baseline of 32.2 ± 22.8 mg/dL to 25.6 ± 16.1 mg/dL *3219*

Luteinizing Hormone *Plasma Decrease Physiological* In 29 healthy postmenopausal women treatment with conjugated estrogens 0.625 mg and 5 mg medroxyprogesterone acetate in 21-day sequences over 12 cycles caused significant decrease in concentration from 58.6 ± 8.0 IU/L to 34.0 ± 3.1 IU/L *588* Plasma concentration and urinary excretion reduced during treatment *4671*

Magnesium *Serum Increase Physiological* Estrogen type of response *5567*

Occult Blood *Feces Increase Physiological* Ischemic colitis reported in one case *2076*

Partial Thromboplastin Time
Plasma No Effect Physiological In 21 healthy postmenopausal women treatment with conjugated estrogens 0.625 mg and 5 mg medroxyprogesterone acetate in 21-day sequences over 12 cycles caused nonsignificant change in concentration from 90.7 ± 2.4% to 89.4 ± 2.5% *588*

Phosphate *Serum Increase Physiological* Observed effect (unlike oral contraceptives) *5567*

Phospholipids *Serum Decrease Physiological* Concentration reduced in first time and chronic recipients following I.M. injection of 150 mg. Initial concentration in chronic users 2.80 mmol/L decreased to 2.56 mmol/L at 29 days: in first time users declined from 2.91 mmol/L to 2.51 mmol/L at 92 days *2042* In both short term and long term users of depot medroxyprogesterone significant reduction observed 92 days after intramuscular injection of 150 mg *2042*

Plasminogen Activator Inhibitor-1
Plasma Decrease Physiological In 30 healthy postmenopausal women aged 56 ± 5 years treatment with oral 2.5 medroxyprogesterone acetate with 0.625 mg conjugated estrogen daily for one month caused significant change from mean baseline of 31 ± 29 ng/mL to 15 ± 11 ng/mL *3219*
Plasma No Effect Physiological In 30 healthy postmenopausal women aged 56 ± 5 years treatment with oral 2.5 medroxyprogesterone acetate with 0.625 mg conjugated estrogen daily for one month caused nonsignificant change from mean baseline of 530 ± 654 ng/mL to 503 ± 460 ng/mL *3219*

Pregnanediol *Plasma Decrease Physiological* Plasma concentration and urinary excretion reduced during treatment *4671*
Urine Decrease Physiological Induces anovulatory state *6099* Plasma concentration and urinary excretion reduced during treatment *4671*

Progesterone *Plasma Decrease Physiological* Plasma concentration and urinary excretion reduced during treatment *4671*
Plasma No Effect Analytical Medroxyprogesterone at a concentration of up to 1000 ng/mL had a cross-reactivity of only 0.9% in progesterone method on Bayer Technicon Immuno 1® *429*
Urine Decrease Physiological Plasma concentration and urinary excretion reduced during treatment *4671*

Prothrombin *Plasma Increase Physiological* Plasma concentration may increase during treatment *4671*

Prothrombin Time *Plasma No Effect Physiological* In 22 healthy postmenopausal women treatment with conjugated estrogens 0.625 mg and 5 mg medroxyprogesterone acetate in 21-day sequences over 12 cycles caused nonsignificant change in concentration from 96.8 ± 0.7% to 96.9 ± 0.9% *588*

Pyridinoline *Urine Decrease Physiological* In 33 postmenopausal women treated with 0.625 mg/d conjugated equine estrogens and 2.5 mg/d medroxyprogesterone acetate for 12 months caused significant change from mean baseline of 30 pmol/μmol creatinine to 22 pmol/μmol creatinine after 6 momths and 20 pmol/μmol creatinine after one year *5912*

Renin Activity *Plasma No Effect Physiological* In 23 healthy postmenopausal women treatment with conjugated estrogens 0.625 mg and 5 mg medroxyprogesterone acetate in 21-day sequences over 12 cycles caused nonsignificant change in concentration from 4.1 ± 0.53 ng/mL/h to 3.9 ± 0.66 ng/mL/h *588*

Sex-Hormone Binding Globulin
Serum Decrease Physiological Concentration reduced in patients receiving combined treatment with testosterone enanthate *6319* Plasma concentration and urinary excretion reduced during treatment *4671*
Serum Increase Physiological In 21 healthy postmenopausal women treatment with conjugated estrogens 0.625 mg and 5 mg medroxyprogesterone acetate in 21-day sequences over 12 cycles caused significant increase in concentration from 50.6 ± 4.2 nmol/L to 117.2 ± 9.9 nmol/L *588*

Sulfobromophthalein *Serum Increase Physiological* Administration may cause BSP retention *4683* Retention may become abnormal during treatment *4671*

T3-Uptake *Serum Decrease Physiological* Administration may cause decreased uptake *4683* Decreased uptake has been reported during treatment *4671*
Serum No Effect Physiological In 25 healthy postmenopausal women treatment with conjugated estrogens 0.625 mg and 5 mg medroxyprogesterone acetate in 21-day sequences over 12 cycles caused nonsignificant change in concentration from 0.53 ± 0.10 to 0.48 ± 0.09 *588*

Testosterone *Serum Decrease Physiological* In 17 healthy postmenopausal women treatment with conjugated estrogens 0.625 mg and 5 mg medroxyprogesterone acetate in 21-day sequences over 12 cycles caused nonsignificant decrease in concentration from 1.39 ± 0.15 nmol/L to 1.27 ± 0.13 nmol/L *588* Plasma concentration and urinary excretion reduced during treatment *4671* Significant reduction after treatment. Effects observed in 15 postmenopausal women with endometrial cancer after 2 weeks treatment *3503*
Urine Decrease Physiological Plasma concentration and urinary excretion reduced during treatment *4671*

Theophylline *Serum No Effect Physiological* No documented significant interaction with theophylline reported *6117* No clinically significant effect on theophylline concentration observed when drugs coadministered *5999*

Thyroid Stimulating Hormone
Serum Increase Physiological In 28 healthy postmenopausal women treatment with conjugated estrogens 0.625 mg and 5 mg medroxyprogesterone acetate in 21-day sequences over 12 cycles caused nonsignificant increase in concentration from 2.11 ± 0.52 mIU/L to 2.82 ± 0.75 mIU/L *588*

Thyroxine (T4) *Serum Increase Physiological* In 29 healthy postmenopausal women treatment with conjugated estrogens 0.625 mg and 5 mg medroxyprogesterone acetate in 21-day sequences over 12 cycles caused significant increase in concentration from 101.5 ± 5.6 mmol/L to 132.8 ± 3.7 mmol/L *588*

Triglycerides *Serum Decrease Physiological* Both transient increases and decreases have been reported during treatment *4671* Increase by 24% in 11 men with sexual deviation syndrome given approximately 1273 mg over a total of approximately 17 d *978* Slight and transient decrease observed at 29 days after 150 mg given i.m. as depot to 14 chronic recipients and at 15 days in first time recipients *2042* Significant reduction. Effects observed in 15 postmenopausal women with endometrial cancer after 2 weeks treatment *3503*
Serum Increase Physiological Moderate increase observed in chronic depot medroxyprogesterone users *2042* Both transient increases and decreases have been reported during treatment *4671* In 20 healthy postmenopausal women treatment with conjugated estrogens 0.625 mg and 5 mg medroxyprogesterone acetate in 21-day sequences over 12 cycles caused significant change in concentration from 0.98 ± 0.09 mmol/L to 1.45 ± 0.17 mmol/L in estrogenic phase and 1.18 ± 0.11 mmol/L in progestogenic phase *588*

Serum *No Effect* *Physiological* In 30 healthy postmenopausal women aged 56 ± 5 years treatment with oral 2.5 medroxyprogesterone acetate with 0.625 mg conjugated estrogen daily for one month caused nonsignificant change from mean baseline of 110 ± 69 mg/dL to 108 ± 54 mg/dL *3219*

Tumor Necrosis Factor *Serum* *Decrease* *Physiological* In patients with carcinoma of the bronchus and cachexia weight gain associated with treatment with medroxyprogesterone for 4 weeks caused significant decrease of previously increased concentration *1684*

Type I Collagen Cross-linked N-telopeptide
Urine *Decrease* *Physiological* In 33 postmenopausal women treated with 0.625 mg/d conjugated equine estrogens and 2.5 mg/d medroxyprogesterone acetate for 12 months caused significant change from mean baseline of 54 nMBCE/mmol creatinine to 33 nMBCE/mmol creatinine after 6 momths and 24 nMBCE/mmol creatinine after one year *5912*

Vitamin B_{12} *Serum* *No Effect* *Physiological* No effect seen in Africans at least *722*

VLDL-Cholesterol *Serum* *No Effect* *Physiological* In 20 healthy postmenopausal women treatment with conjugated estrogens 0.625 mg and 5 mg medroxyprogesterone acetate in 21-day sequences over 12 cycles caused nonsignificant change in concentration from 0.56 ± 0.06 mmol/L to 0.58 ± 0.07 mmol/L in estrogenic phase and 0.46 ± 0.05 mmol/L in progestogenic phase *588* Concentration unchanged in both first time and chronic recipients after administration of 150 mg I.M. depot preparation *2042*

Mefenamic Acid

Alanine Aminotransferase *Serum* *Increase* *Physiological* Incidence of acute liver injury of 2.5 per 100,000 treated patients with reported in United Kingdom. Liver damage among all cases primarily hepatocellular in some and primarily cholestatic in others *5049*

Aspartate Aminotransferase *Serum* *Increase* *Physiological* Incidence of acute liver injury of 2.5 per 100,000 treated patients with reported in United Kingdom. Liver damage among all cases primarily hepatocellular in some and primarily cholestatic in others *5049*

Bile *Urine* *Increase* *Analytical* Reported interference with testing procedure *3061*

Bilirubin *Serum* *Increase* *Physiological* May cause autoimmune hemolytic anemia *1798*

Blood *Urine* *Increase* *Physiological* Renal failure, including papillary necrosis, has been reported to occur in elderly individuals after treatment for as short as 2 to 6 weeks. Hematuria also reported as a side effect *4529*

Chondrex *Serum* *No Effect* *Analytical* Concentrations up to 0.1 g/L had no significant effect on sandwich-type ELISA procedure of Harvey et al *2491*

Coombs' Test *Blood* *Positive* *Physiological* Autoimmune phenomenon (occurs after several months) *2453* Continuous administration for more than 12 months has been reported to cause autoimmune hemolytic anemia with positive Coombs' test *4529*

Coombs' Test, Direct *Blood* *Positive* *Physiological* Drug induces autoimmune phenomenon *2452*

Creatinine *Serum* *Increase* *Physiological* Renal failure, including papillary necrosis, has been reported to occur in elderly individuals after treatment for as short as 2 to 6 weeks *4529*

Drugs of Abuse Screen *Urine* *Decrease* *Analytical* False negative results observed in 2 specimens using Syva EMIT drug of abuse screening method due to high background absorbance *2437*

Eosinophils *Blood* *Increase* *Physiological* Eosinophilia has been reported as side effect *4529* Allergic reactions noted *2754*

Erythrocytes *Blood* *Decrease* *Physiological* Pancytopenia *3810*
Urine *Increase* *Physiological* Actual bleeding caused by drug *3810*

Glucose Tolerance *Serum* *Decrease* *Physiological* Effect noted in a diabetic *2754*

Granulocytes *Blood* *Decrease* *Physiological* Agranulocytosis, pancytopenia and bone marrow hypoplasia have been reported as side effects *4529*

Hematocrit *Blood* *Decrease* *Physiological* Continuous administration for more than 12 months has been reported to cause autoimmune hemolytic anemia. Noted in 2 - 5% patients on long term treatment *4529* May cause autoimmune hemolytic anemia *1798*

Hemoglobin *Blood* *Decrease* *Physiological* Continuous administration for more than 12 months has been reported to cause autoimmune hemolytic anemia *4529* May cause autoimmune hemolytic anemia *1798*
Urine *Increase* *Physiological* Actual bleeding caused by the drug *1714*

Leukocytes *Blood* *Decrease* *Physiological* Pancytopenia (temporary depression may occur often) *3810* Leukopenia has been reported as side effect *4529*

Lithium *Serum* *Increase* *Physiological* In 3 patients administration of 1-2 g/d reprted to produce signs of lithium toxicity with, in one, lithium concentration increasing from 0.5 mEq/L to 2.0 mEq/L within 6 days of starting treatment with 1.5 g/d *4831*

MCV *Blood* *Increase* *Physiological* Megaloblastic anemia reported *128*

Midazolam *Serum* *No Effect* *Analytical* On GC-ECD method of Ha et al *2387*

Occult Blood *Feces* *Increase* *Physiological* Occurs less frequently than with aspirin *128* Mefenamic acid administration may cause severe gastrointestinal ulceration *4529*

Platelet Aggregation *Blood* *Decrease* *Physiological* Observed *in vitro*, might cause gastrointestinal bleeding etc *915*

Platelets *Blood* *Decrease* *Physiological* Pancytopenia *1212* Thrombocytopenic purpura has been reported as side effect *4529*

Protein *Urine* *Increase* *Physiological* Nephrotoxic effect *2024* *1714*

Prothrombin Time *Plasma* *Increase* *Physiological* Mefenamic acid administration may prolong prothrombin time *4529* Displaces coumarins from albumin *5440*

Urea Nitrogen *Serum* *Increase* *Physiological* Reported in one study with normal volunteers *128* Renal failure, including papillary necrosis, has been reported to occur in elderly individuals after treatment for as short as 2 to 6 weeks *4529*

Uric Acid *Serum* *Decrease* *Physiological* Uricosuric action of drug *5002*

Mefloquine

Alanine Aminotransferase *Serum* *Increase* *Physiological* Occasional transient increases reported *1384* Administration of mefloquine has been associated with transient increases of aminotransferase activity *5026*

Aspartate Aminotransferase *Serum* *Increase* *Physiological* Occasional transient increases reported *1384* Administration of mefloquine has been associated with transient increases of aminotransferase activity *5026*

Hematocrit *Blood* *Decrease* *Physiological* Occasionally observed *1384* Administration of mefloquine has been associated with decreased hematocrit *5026*

Leukocytes *Blood* *Decrease* *Physiological* Occasional leukopenia reported *1384* Administration of mefloquine has been associated with leukopenia *5026*

Platelets *Blood* *Decrease* *Physiological* Occasional thrombocytopenia reported *1384* Administration of mefloquine has been associated with thrombocytopenia *5026*

Valproic Acid *Serum* *Decrease* *Physiological* Administration of mefloquine with valproic acid was associated with loss of seizure control and lower than expected plasma valproate concentrations *5026*

Mefruside

Chloride *Urine* *Increase* *Physiological* Diuretic action *291*

Potassium *Serum* *Decrease* *Physiological* Diuretic action less effective than thiazides *6484*
Urine *Increase* *Physiological* Diuretic action, acts up to 20 h *6484*

Mefruside *(continued)*

Sodium *Urine Increase Physiological* Diuretic action, less effective than thiazides *6484*

Uric Acid *Serum Increase Physiological* Inhibits excretion of urate *6484*

Volume *Urine Increase Physiological* Diuretic action, less effective than thiazides *291*

Megestrol

Albumin *Serum Decrease Physiological* In 11 patients with gastrointestinal cancer with weight loss treatment with 480 mg/d megestrol acetate for 12 weeks caused decrease from mean baseline of 40 g/L (35 - 43 g/L) to 37 g/L (32 - 42 g/L) *3912*

CA549 *Serum No Effect Analytical* No interference observed at concentrations from 2.6 - 39.6 mg/L with immunoradiometric BRESMARQ procedure *958* No statistically significant effect observed over a concentration range of 2.6 to 39.6 mg/L with BRESMARQ assay *958*

Cortisol *Plasma Decrease Physiological* In critically ill patients relative hypoadrenalism observed with megestrol acetate therapy *3381*

C-Reactive Protein *Serum No Effect Physiological* In 11 patients with gastrointestinal cancer with weight loss treatment with 480 mg/d megestrol acetate for 12 weeks caused nonsignificant change from mean baseline of 15 mg/L (range < 10 - 170 mg/L) to mean of 16 mg/L (< 10 - 94 mg/L) *3912*

11-Deoxycortisol *Plasma Decrease Physiological* In 18 postmenopausal women with breast cancer *99*

Estradiol *Plasma Decrease Physiological* In 18 postmenopausal women with breast cancer *99*

Follicle Stimulating Hormone
Plasma Decrease Physiological In 18 postmenopausal women with breast cancer *99*

Glucose *Serum Decrease Physiological* In 18 postmenopausal women with breast cancer *99*

Growth Hormone *Plasma No Effect Physiological* In 18 postmenopausal women with breast cancer *99*

Hemoglobin *Blood Decrease Physiological* In 11 patients with gastrointestinal cancer with weight loss treatment with 480 mg/d megestrol acetate for 12 weeks caused decrease from mean baseline of 134 g/L (range 91 - 154 g/L) to mean of 120 g/L (range 94 - 140 g/L) *3912*

Insulin *Plasma Increase Physiological* In 18 postmenopausal women with breast cancer *99*

Leukocytes *Blood Increase Physiological* In 11 patients with gastrointestinal cancer with weight loss treatment with 480 mg/d megestrol acetate for 12 weeks caused increase from mean baseline of 7800 /µL (range 4400 - 18700 /µL) to 9400 /µL (5300 - 24000 /µL) *3912*

Luteinizing Hormone *Plasma Decrease Physiological* Suppresses LH peak *5424* In 18 postmenopausal women with breast cancer *99*

Megestrol *Serum Increase Physiological* Progressive increase in concentration with time, regardless of dose given *99*

Nitroblue Tetrazolium Test *Blood Increase Physiological* With 0.5 mg/d 6-9% with positive levels *252*

Platelets *Blood Increase Physiological* In 11 patients with gastrointestinal cancer with weight loss treatment with 480 mg/d megestrol acetate for 12 weeks caused increase from mean baseline of 352000 /µL (156000 - 663000 /µL) to 390000 /µL (range 213000 - 562000 /µL) *3912*

Prolactin *Plasma Increase Physiological* Affects both basal and TRH-stimulated concentration in 18 postmenopausal women with breast cancer *99*

Prostate-specific Antigen, Free *Serum No Effect Analytical* Megestrol acetate at a concentration of 39.6 mg/L had no significant effect on the Hybritech Tandem® -R free PSA immunoassay *4286*

Sex-Hormone Binding Globulin
Serum Decrease Physiological In 18 postmenopausal women with breast cancer *99*

Thyroid Stimulating Hormone
Serum No Effect Physiological In 18 postmenopausal women with breast cancer *99*

Transferrin *Serum Decrease Physiological* In 11 patients with gastrointestinal cancer with weight loss treatment with 480 mg/d megestrol acetate for 12 weeks caused decrease from mean baseline of 2.8 g/L (range 2.3 - 3.4 g/L) to mean 2.5 g/L (1.6 - 3.2 g/L) *3912*

Meglumine

Cholesterol *Serum No Effect Analytical* At concentration of 1200 mg/L had no effect on method using catalase-Hantzsch reaction *5704* At concentration of 1200 mg/L had no effect on catalase-AIDH method *5704* At concentration of 1200 mg/L had no effect on CHOD-PAP method *5704* At concentration of 1200 mg/L had no effect on Liebermann-Burchard method *5704* At concentration of 1200 mg/L had no effect on CHOD-Iodide method *5704*

Cortisol *Plasma No Effect Analytical* No effect on concentration either physiologically or on RIA procedure *3073*
Plasma No Effect Physiological No effect on concentration either physiologically or on RIA procedure *3073*
Urine No Effect Analytical No effect either physiologically or on RIA analytical method *3073*
Urine No Effect Physiological No effect either physiologically or on RIA analytical method *3073*

Creatinine *Serum No Effect Analytical* At concentration of 1200 mg/L had no effect on Jaffe-Fuller's earth method *5704* At concentration of 6,000 mg/L had no effect on kinetic Jaffe method on BKA-2 *5704* At concentration of 1200 mg/L had no effect on Jaffe-Fading-Fraction method *5704*

Glucose *Serum No Effect Analytical* At concentration of 2,000 mg/L had no effect on hexokinase/G-6-PDH method *5704* At concentration of 200 mg/L had no effect on Kodak Ektachem® method *5704*

17-Ketogenic Steroids *Urine Decrease Analytical* Marked decrease observed probably because drug interferes in the periodate oxidation step of the measurement *3073*

17-Ketosteroids *Urine No Effect Analytical* No effect following intravenous injection in contrast to effect on 17-KGS *3073*

Lactate *Plasma No Effect Analytical* At concentration of 1200 mg/L had no effect on enzyme method *5704*

Potassium *Serum No Effect Analytical* At concentration of 2,000 mg/L had no effect on ISE measurement without predilution *5704*

Protein Electrophoresis *Serum No Effect Analytical* At concentration of 2,000 mg/L had no effect on automated Olympus-Hite method *5704*

Sodium *Serum No Effect Analytical* At concentration of 1200 mg/L had no effect on ISE measurement without predilution *5704*

Urea Nitrogen *Serum No Effect Analytical* At concentration of 200 mg/L had no effect on Kodak Ektachem® method *5704*

Uric Acid *Serum No Effect Analytical* At concentration of 2,000 mg/L had no effect on Kageyama-Hantzsch method *5704* At concentration of 1200 mg/L had no effect on catalase-AIDH method *5704*

Meglumine Adipionate

Bilirubin *Serum No Effect Analytical* No effect at 350 mg/L on Ames Seralyzer method *5706*

Cholesterol *Serum No Effect Analytical* No effect at 350 mg/L on Ames Seralyzer method *5706*

Creatine Kinase *Serum No Effect Analytical* No effect at 350 mg/L on method on Ames Seralyzer *5706*

Creatinine *Serum No Effect Analytical* No effect at 350 mg/L on Ames Seralyzer method *5706*

Glucose *Serum No Effect Analytical* No effect at 350 mg/L on glucose oxidase method on Ames Seralyzer *5706* No effect at concentrations up to 200 mg/L on method on Kodak Ektachem® *5706*

Lactate Dehydrogenase *Serum No Effect Analytical* No effect at 350 mg/L on method on Ames Seralyzer *5706*

Urea Nitrogen *Serum* *No Effect* *Analytical* No effect at 350 mg/L on method on Ames Seralyzer *5706*

Meglumine Amidotrizoate

Bilirubin *Serum* *No Effect* *Analytical* No effect at 1500 mg/L on Ames Seralyzer method *5706*

Cholesterol *Serum* *No Effect* *Analytical* No effect at 1500 mg/L on Ames Seralyzer method *5706*

Creatine Kinase *Serum* *No Effect* *Analytical* No effect at 1500 mg/L on method on Ames Seralyzer *5706*

Creatinine *Serum* *No Effect* *Analytical* No effect at 1500 mg/L on Ames Seralyzer method *5706*

Glucose *Serum* *No Effect* *Analytical* No effect at 1500 mg/L on glucose oxidase method on Ames Seralyzer *5706*

Lactate Dehydrogenase *Serum* *No Effect* *Analytical* No effect at 1500 mg/L on method on Ames Seralyzer *5706*

Urea Nitrogen *Serum* *No Effect* *Analytical* No effect at 1500 mg/L on method on Ames Seralyzer *5706*

Meglumine Diatrizoate

Cholesterol *Serum* *No Effect* *Analytical* No effect at concentrations up to 5000 mg/L on method on Kodak Ektachem® *5706*

Meglumine Ioglycamate

Bilirubin *Serum* *Increase* *Physiological* Possible clinically significant displacement from protein in neonates *6314*

Meglumine Iothalomate

Bilirubin *Serum* *No Effect* *Analytical* No effect at 300 mg/L on Ames Seralyzer method *5706*

Cholesterol *Serum* *No Effect* *Analytical* No effect at 300 mg/L on Ames Seralyzer method *5706*

Creatine Kinase *Serum* *No Effect* *Analytical* No effect at 300 mg/L on method on Ames Seralyzer *5706*

Creatinine *Serum* *No Effect* *Analytical* No effect at 300 mg/L on Ames Seralyzer method *5706*

Glucose *Serum* *No Effect* *Analytical* No effect at 300 mg/L on glucose oxidase method on Ames Seralyzer *5706*

Lactate Dehydrogenase *Serum* *No Effect* *Analytical* No effect at 300 mg/L on method on Ames Seralyzer *5706*

Urea Nitrogen *Serum* *No Effect* *Analytical* No effect at 300 mg/L on method on Ames Seralyzer *5706*

Meglumine Iotroxinate

Bilirubin *Serum* *No Effect* *Analytical* No effect at 190 mg/L on Ames Seralyzer method *5706*

Cholesterol *Serum* *No Effect* *Analytical* No effect at 190 mg/L on Ames Seralyzer method *5706*

Creatine Kinase *Serum* *No Effect* *Analytical* No effect at 190 mg/L on method on Ames Seralyzer *5706*

Creatinine *Serum* *No Effect* *Analytical* No effect at 190 mg/L on Ames Seralyzer method *5706*

Glucose *Serum* *No Effect* *Analytical* No effect at 190 mg/L on glucose oxidase method on Ames Seralyzer *5706*

Lactate Dehydrogenase *Serum* *No Effect* *Analytical* No effect at 190 mg/L on method on Ames Seralyzer *5706*

Urea Nitrogen *Serum* *No Effect* *Analytical* No effect at 190 mg/L on method on Ames Seralyzer *5706*

Melarsonyl

Alanine Aminotransferase *Serum* *Increase* *Physiological* May produce hepatotoxicity *128*

Aspartate Aminotransferase *Serum* *Increase* *Physiological* May produce hepatotoxicity *128*

Casts *Urine* *Increase* *Physiological* Nephrotoxic effect *128*

Erythrocytes *Blood* *Decrease* *Physiological* May cause hemolytic anemia in G-6-PD deficiency *128*

Hematocrit *Blood* *Decrease* *Physiological* May cause hemolytic anemia in G-6-PD deficiency *128*

Hemoglobin *Blood* *Decrease* *Physiological* May cause hemolytic anemia in G-6-PD deficiency *128*

Protein *Urine* *Increase* *Physiological* Nephrotoxic effect *128*

Melarsoprol

Alanine Aminotransferase *Serum* *Increase* *Physiological* May produce hepatotoxicity *128*

Aspartate Aminotransferase *Serum* *Increase* *Physiological* May produce hepatotoxicity *128*

Casts *Urine* *Increase* *Physiological* Nephrotoxic effect *3810*

Protein *Urine* *Increase* *Physiological* Nephrotoxic effect *3810*

Melitracen

Albumin *Urine* *No Effect* *Analytical* Using a fluorimetric assay with Albumin Blue 580 on a Cobas Fara centrifugal analyzer for the detection of microalbuminuria no significant interference was detected at a concentration of 8 mg/L *3117*

Melperone

Creatine Kinase *Serum* *Increase* *Physiological* In 47 acutely psychotic patients treatment with loxapine (1 - 51 determinations per patient) was associated with 12 marked elevations (in 2.1% of the patients) *3947*

Melphalan

Alanine Aminotransferase *Serum* *Increase* *Physiological* Hepatic toxicity, including veno-occlusive disease has been reported *2172*

Alkaline Phosphatase *Serum* *Increase* *Physiological* Hepatic toxicity, including veno-occlusive disease has been reported *2172*

Aspartate Aminotransferase *Serum* *Increase* *Physiological* Hepatic toxicity, including veno-occlusive disease has been reported *2172*

Bilirubin *Serum* *Increase* *Physiological* May cause hemolytic anemia *3895* Hepatic toxicity, including veno-occlusive disease has been reported *2172*

Bilirubin, Direct *Serum* *Increase* *Physiological* May cause hemolytic anemia *3895*

Color *Feces* *Increase* *Analytical* Black color reported with ingestion of melphalan *3388*

Coombs' Test *Blood* *Positive* *Physiological* Immunological response to drug (γ antibody) *2453*

Cyclosporine *Blood* *No Effect* *Physiological* Coadministration of melphalan with cyclosporine had no significant effect on the cyclosporine concentration but was associated with a high incidence of renal impairment *859*
Serum *No Effect* *Physiological* Coadministration of melphalan with cyclosporine had no significant effect on the cyclosporine concentration but was associated with a high incidence of renal impairment *859*

Erythrocytes *Blood* *Decrease* *Physiological* May cause bone marrow depression (dose related) *822*

Hematocrit *Blood* *Decrease* *Physiological* Anemia may occur rarely *4014*

Hemoglobin *Blood* *Decrease* *Physiological* Anemia may occur rarely *4014*

5-Hydroxyindoleacetic Acid *Urine* *Increase* *Physiological* Probably due to tissue destruction if carcinoid *3652*

Melphalan *(continued)*

Leukocytes *Blood Decrease Physiological* May cause bone marrow depression (dose related) *822* Most common side effect is bone marrow suppression with nadir occurring about 2 to 3 weeks after treatment with recovery in 4 to 5 weeks after treatment *2172*
Blood Increase Physiological 4 cases of acute leukemia in 474 patients with ovarian carcinoma: all cases in patients who had received at least 300 mg for 3 y *1678*

Occult Blood *Feces Increase Physiological* May cause gastrointestinal hemorrhage *128*

Platelets *Blood Decrease Physiological* May cause bone marrow depression (dose related) *822* Most common side effect is bone marrow suppression with nadir occurring about 2 to 3 weeks after treatment with recovery in 4 to 5 weeks after treatment *2172*

Protein Electrophoresis *Serum No Effect Analytical* At concentration of 1.5 mg/L had no effect on automated Olympus-Hite method but with slight displacement of fractions *5704*

Urea Nitrogen *Serum Increase Physiological* Azotemia may occur *128*

Menadione Sodium Bisulfite

Cholinesterase *Serum No Effect Analytical* No effect observed at concentration of 2 μg/mL with butyrylthiocholine method on Kodak Ektachem® *2504*

Mepartricin

Estradiol *Plasma Decrease Physiological* Significant effect on estradiol-17β concentration in men with benign prostatic hypertrophy treated for 30 days *3655*

Estriol *Plasma Decrease Physiological* Significant reduction in men with benign prostatic hypertrophy treated for 30 days *3655*

Estrone *Plasma Decrease Physiological* Significant reduction over 30 days in patients with benign prostatic hypertrophy *3655*

Mepazine

Alanine Aminotransferase *Serum Increase Physiological* Cholestatic effect (up to 6 times normal) *2803*

Alkaline Phosphatase *Serum Increase Physiological* May alter liver function (cholestasis) *3810*

Aspartate Aminotransferase *Serum Increase Physiological* Cholestatic effect (up to 6 times normal) *2803*

Bile *Urine Increase Physiological* May alter liver function (cholestasis) *3810*

Bilirubin *Serum Increase Physiological* Cholestatic effect *2803*

BSP Retention *Serum Increase Physiological* Cholestatic effect *2803*

Cholesterol *Serum Increase Physiological* Cholestatic effect *2803*

Erythrocytes *Blood Decrease Physiological* Pancytopenia/aplastic anemia *3810*

Leukocytes *Blood Decrease Physiological* Agranulocytosis *1869*

Neutrophils *Blood Decrease Physiological* Occasional case of agranulocytosis reported *6264*

Platelets *Blood Decrease Physiological* Pancytopenia *3810*

Prothrombin Time *Plasma Increase Physiological* Associated with failure of excretion of bile salts *2803*

Urobilinogen *Feces Decrease Physiological* Due to cholestasis (pale stools result) *2803*
Urine Decrease Physiological Cholestatic effect *2803*

Mepenzolate

Volume *Urine Decrease Physiological* Rare urinary retention may occur *2754*

Meperidine

Alanine Aminotransferase *Serum Increase Physiological* May cause rise in intrabiliary pressure *5869*
Serum No Effect Analytical At acute overdose concentration (5 mg/dL) on Technicon SMAC® method *6266*

Albumin *Serum No Effect Analytical* At acute overdose concentration (5 mg/dL) on Technicon SMAC® method *6266* At concentration of 50 mg/L had no effect on BCG method *5704*

Alkaline Phosphatase *Serum No Effect Analytical* At acute overdose concentration (5 mg/dL) on Technicon SMAC® method *6266*

Amylase *Serum Increase Physiological* May cause spasm of sphincter of Oddi *5540*

Aspartate Aminotransferase *Serum Increase Physiological* May cause rise in intrabiliary pressure *402*
Serum No Effect Analytical At acute overdose concentration (5 mg/dL) on Technicon SMAC® method *6266*

Bicarbonate *Serum No Effect Analytical* At concentration of 60 mg/L had no effect on method using phenolphthalein *5704*

Bilirubin *Serum No Effect Analytical* At acute overdose concentration (5 mg/dL) on Technicon SMAC® method *6266* At concentration of 60 mg/L had no effect on Jendrassik and Grof method *5704*

BSP Retention *Serum Increase Physiological* Due to spasm of sphincter of Oddi *834*

Calcium *Serum No Effect Analytical* At acute overdose concentration (5 mg/dL) on Technicon SMAC® method *6266* At concentration of 60 mg/L had no effect on cresolphthalein method *5704*

Cannabinoids *Urine No Effect Analytical* No effect on Roche Abuscreen method *5006* No effect observed at a concentration of 500 μg/mL (2.02 mmol/L) on method on Du Pont aca *1557*

Carbon Dioxide Partial Pressure
Blood Increase Physiological Depresses responsiveness of respiratory center to CO_2*2242* In 14 volunteer patients with COPD (mean age 49.4 years) infusion of 1.5 mg/kg intravenously caused significant increase from mean baseline of 36.4 ± 3.6 mm Hg to 44.0 ± 3.9 mm Hg after 5 minutes with gradual decline towards baseline thereafter *6683* Significant increase in concentration 5 minutes after intravenous administration of 1.5 mg/kg in 19 volunteers *6682*

Chloride *Serum No Effect Analytical* At concentration of 60 mg/L had no effect on mercurimetric method *5704*

Cholesterol *Serum No Effect Analytical* At concentration of 60 mg/L had no effect on Liebermann-Burchard method *5704* At acute overdose concentration (5 mg/dL) on Technicon SMAC® method *6266*

Cocaethylene *Urine No Effect Analytical* No interference observed with TLC method of Bailey *328*

Creatine Kinase *Serum Increase Physiological* Increase of 2-fold after single i.m. injection of 50 mg *5092*
Serum No Effect Analytical At acute overdose concentration (5 mg/dL) on Technicon SMAC® method *6266*
Serum No Effect Physiological No reported effect *4014*

Creatinine *Serum No Effect Analytical* At concentration of 60 mg/L had no effect on Technicon AutoAnalyzer® method *5704* At acute overdose concentration (5 mg/dL) on Technicon SMAC® method *6266*

Glucose *Serum Increase Physiological* Central effect also involves epinephrine release *2242*
Serum No Effect Analytical At acute overdose concentration (5 mg/dL) on Technicon SMAC® method *6266*

Histamine *Plasma Increase Physiological* Associated with dose associated with anesthesia *3648*
Plasma No Effect Analytical Although 50% inhibition of radio-enzyme assay at 42 μg/mL no clinical effect likely to occur since physiological concentration 0.2-0.8 μg/mL *2492*

Hydroxybutyrate Dehydrogenase
Serum Increase Physiological May cause spasm of sphincter of Oddi *4014*

17-Hydroxycorticosteroids *Urine Decrease Physiological* Probable effect (inhibits ACTH and PGH release) *2242*

Indocyanine Green *Serum Decrease Physiological* Observed in small series, normal liver function tests *3942*

Iron *Serum No Effect Analytical* At acute overdose concentration (5 mg/dL) on Technicon SMAC® method *6266*

17-Ketosteroids *Urine Decrease Physiological* Probable effect (inhibits ACTH and PGH release) *2242*

Lactate Dehydrogenase *Serum Increase Physiological* May cause rise in intrabiliary pressure *402*
Serum No Effect Analytical At acute overdose concentration (5 mg/dL) on Technicon SMAC® method *6266*

Lipase *Serum Increase Physiological* May cause spasm of sphincter of Oddi *5540*

Meperidine *Serum Increase Physiological* 100 mg i.m. produces 1 mg/L *3868*
Urine Increase Physiological Main excretion product in neonates and pregnant *4014*

Normeperidine *Urine Positive Physiological* Main metabolite in normals *4014*

Opiates *Urine No Effect Analytical* No effect observed at a concentration of 20 µg/mL (81 µmol/L) on method on Du Pont aca *1559*

Oxygen Partial Pressure *Blood Decrease Physiological* Intravenous infusion of 1.5 mg/kg in 19 volunteers caused significant decrease within 5 minutes *6682* In 14 patient volunteers with COPD (mean age 49.4 years) infusion of 1.5 mg/kg intravenously caused significant decrease from mean baseline of 69.2 ± 6.7 mm Hg to 62.0 ± 4.7 mm Hg after 20 minutes with return to baseline by 60 minutes *6683* Significant reduction in arterial oxygen pressure *4014*

p-Aminophenol *Urine No Effect Analytical* With addition of drugs at a concentration of 100 mg/L and of related compounds at 50 mg/L no significant effect observed on colorimetric method of van Bocxlaer on Cobas Mira analyzer which involves reacting free p-aminophenol with resorcinol in the presence of magnesium ions to form an indophenol dye measured at 550 nm *6163*

pH *Blood Decrease Physiological* Significant reduction in 19 volunteers 5 minutes after intravenous infusion of 1.5 mg/kg *6682*
Blood No Effect Physiological Insignificant effect observed *4014* In 14 volunteer patients with COPD (mean age 49.4 years) infusion of 1.5 mg/kg intravenously was not associated with significant changes over the following hour *6683*

Phosphate *Serum No Effect Analytical* At concentration of 60 mg/L had no effect on phosphomolybdate method *5704* At acute overdose concentration (5 mg/dL) on Technicon SMAC® method *6266*

Protein *Cerebrospinal Fluid No Effect Analytical* No significant effect when added in vitro to concentration of 10.0 mg/dL when measured by Kodak Ektachem® slide method *3654*
Serum No Effect Analytical At acute overdose concentration (5 mg/dL) on Technicon SMAC® method *6266* At concentration of 60 mg/L had no effect on biuret method with blank correction *5704*

Triglycerides *Serum No Effect Analytical* At concentration of 60 mg/L had no effect on lipase/esterase method *5704* At acute overdose concentration (5 mg/dL) on Technicon SMAC® method *6266*

Urea Nitrogen *Serum No Effect Analytical* At concentration of 60 mg/L had no effect on diacetylmonoxime method *5704* At acute overdose concentration (5 mg/dL) on Technicon SMAC® method *6266*

Uric Acid *Serum No Effect Analytical* At concentration of 60 mg/L had no effect on phosphotungstate reduction method *5704* At acute overdose concentration (5 mg/dL) on Technicon SMAC® method *6266*

Volume *Urine Decrease Physiological* Causes release of ADH *2242*

Mephenesin

Albumin *Serum No Effect Analytical* At concentration of 100 mg/L had no effect on BCG method *5704*

Bicarbonate *Serum No Effect Analytical* At concentration of 100 mg/L had no effect on method using phenolphthalein *5704*

Bilirubin *Serum No Effect Analytical* At concentration of 100 mg/L had no effect on Jendrassik and Grof method *5704*

Calcium *Serum No Effect Analytical* At concentration of 100 mg/L had no effect on cresolphthalein method *5704*

Chloride *Serum No Effect Analytical* At concentration of 100 mg/L had no effect on mercurimetric method *5704*

Cholesterol *Serum No Effect Analytical* At concentration of 100 mg/L had no effect on Liebermann-Burchard method *5704*

Creatinine *Serum No Effect Analytical* At concentration of 100 mg/L had no effect on Technicon AutoAnalyzer® Jaffe method *5704*

Erythrocytes *Urine Increase Physiological* Actual bleeding may be caused by drug *1714*

Hemoglobin *Urine Increase Physiological* Actual bleeding caused by drug *1714*

5-Hydroxyindoleacetic Acid *Urine Increase Analytical* Interferes with nitrosonaphthol reaction *6515* Metabolite reacts in quantitative Udenfriend procedure *882*
Urine No Effect Analytical No effect of *in vivo* dose on method of Goldenberg *2220* No effect observed with FPIA method on Abbott TDx *695*

Leukocytes *Blood Decrease Physiological* May cause leukopenia *3810*

Phosphate *Serum No Effect Analytical* At concentration of 100 mg/L had no effect on phosphomolybdate method *5704*

Potassium *Serum No Effect Analytical* At concentration of 100 mg/L had no effect on measurement by ISE with predilution *5704*

Protein *Serum No Effect Analytical* At concentration of 100 mg/L had no effect on biuret method with blank correction *5704*

Sodium *Serum No Effect Analytical* At concentration of 100 mg/L had no effect on measurement by ISE with predilution *5704*

Triglycerides *Serum No Effect Analytical* At concentration of 100 mg/L had no effect on lipase/esterase method *5704*

Urea Nitrogen *Serum Increase Physiological* Fatal anuria with intravascular hemolysis *2242*
Serum No Effect Analytical At concentration of 100 mg/L had no effect on diacetylmonoxime method *5704*

Uric Acid *Serum No Effect Analytical* At concentration of 100 mg/L had no effect on phosphotungstate reduction method *5704*

Mephenoxalone

Eosinophils *Blood Increase Physiological* Rare side effect *128*

Erythrocytes *Blood Decrease Physiological* May cause anemia *3810*

Leukocytes *Blood Decrease Physiological* Mild and transitory *128*

Mephentermine

Amphetamine *Urine Positive Analytical* At concentrations above 0.5 µg/mL (3.07 µmol/L) with method on Du Pont aca *1554*

Drugs of Abuse Screen *Urine Increase Analytical* False positive with Abbott ADx method for amphetamine/methamphetamine *4279*

Mephenytoin

Alanine Aminotransferase *Serum Increase Physiological* Hepatotoxicity *3810*

Alkaline Phosphatase *Serum Increase Physiological* Hepatotoxicity *3810*

Mephenytoin *(continued)*

Aspartate Aminotransferase *Serum Increase Physiological* Hepatotoxicity *3810*

Bile *Urine Increase Physiological* Hepatotoxicity *3810*

Bilirubin *Serum Increase Physiological* May cause hemolytic anemia *3895*

Bilirubin, Direct *Serum Increase Physiological* May cause hemolytic anemia *3895*

BSP Retention *Serum Increase Physiological* Hepatotoxicity *3810*

Carbamazepine *Serum No Effect Analytical* No cross-reactivity observed with method on Du Pont aca *1513*

Coombs' Test, Direct *Blood Positive Physiological* Mechanism obscure *2453*

Coombs' Test, Indirect *Blood Positive Physiological* Mechanism obscure *2453*

Eosinophils *Blood Increase Physiological* Rare cases described *2754* Administration of mephenytoin reported to cause eosinophilia *5234*

Erythrocytes *Blood Decrease Physiological* Occasional case of aplastic anemia reported *6264* Hemolytic anemia *4995*

Ethosuximide *Serum No Effect Analytical* Insignificant cross-reactivity in method used on Du Pont aca *1523*

Felbamate *Serum No Effect Analytical* No significant interference observed with GLC method of Rifai et al *4958*

Granulocytes *Blood Decrease Physiological* Administration of mephenytoin reported to cause agranulocytosis *5234*

Haptoglobin *Serum Decrease Physiological* May cause hemolytic anemia *3895*

Hematocrit *Blood Decrease Physiological* Hemolytic/aplastic/megaloblastic anemia *4995* Administration of mephenytoin reported to cause simple anemia, aplastic anemia, megaloblastic anemia or hemolytic anemia *5234*

Hemoglobin *Blood Decrease Physiological* Hemolytic/aplastic/megaloblastic anemia *4995* Administration of mephenytoin reported to cause simple anemia, aplastic anemia, megaloblastic anemia or hemolytic anemia *5234*

^{131}I Uptake *Serum Decrease Physiological* Mesantoin® contains tetraiodofluorescein *4360*
Serum No Effect Physiological No effect reported *3669*

LE Cells *Blood Positive Physiological* SLE may occur, usually normalized when stopped *5102*

Leukocytes *Blood Decrease Physiological* Administration of mephenytoin reported to cause leukopenia *5234* Occasional case of aplastic anemia reported *6264* Agranulocytosis/aplastic anemia *4995*
Blood Increase Physiological Rare cases described *2754* Administration of mephenytoin reported to cause monocytosis *5234*

MCV *Blood Increase Physiological* May cause megaloblastic anemia *128*

Monocytes *Blood Increase Physiological* Administration of mephenytoin reported to cause monocytosis *5234* Rare cases described *2754*

Neutrophils *Blood Decrease Physiological* Administration of mephenytoin reported to cause neutropenia *5234* May occur with/without pancytopenia *2754* Occasional case of agranulocytosis reported *6264*

Phenobarbital *Serum No Effect Analytical* At concentration of 100 μg/mL (458 μmol/L) has no effect on method on Du Pont Dimension *1582*

Phenytoin *Serum Decrease Analytical* Slight effect only at 4 μg/mL *6029*
Serum No Effect Analytical At a concentration of 35 μg/mL no cross-reactivity observed with phenytoin at a concentration of 10 μg/mL when measured by the method on Bayer Technicon Immuno 1® *428* No significant interference observed at a concentration of 250 μg/mL (1.15 mmol/L) with method on Du Pont aca *1538* No effect at concentration of 250 μg/mL (1145 μmol/L) on method on Du Pont Dimension *1583* Cross-reactivity of less than 1% at a concentration of 100 μg/mL observed with phenytoin II procedure run on Abbott AxSYM analyzer *356*

Platelets *Blood Decrease Physiological* Secondary to aplastic anemia/pancytopenia *4995* Occasional case of aplastic anemia reported *6264* Administration of mephenytoin reported to cause thrombocytopenia *5234*

Potassium *Serum No Effect Analytical* At concentration of 20 mg/L had no effect on measurement by ISE with predilution *5704*

Primidone *Serum No Effect Analytical* No significant cross-reactivity with method on Du Pont aca *1541*

Sodium *Serum No Effect Analytical* At concentration of 20 mg/L had no effect on measurement by ISE with predilution *5704*

Mephobarbital

Acenocoumarol *Plasma Decrease Physiological* May reduce plasma concentration of acenocoumarol and causes a decrease in anticoagulant activity as measured by reduced prothrombin time *5254*

Albumin *Serum No Effect Analytical* At concentration of 150 mg/L had no effect on BCG method *5704*

Bilirubin *Serum No Effect Analytical* At concentration of 150 mg/L had no effect on Jendrassik and Grof method *5704*

Calcium *Serum No Effect Analytical* At concentration of 150 mg/L had no effect on cresolphthalein method *5704*

Carbamazepine *Serum No Effect Analytical* No cross-reactivity observed with method on Du Pont aca *1513*

Chloride *Serum No Effect Analytical* At concentration of 150 mg/L had no effect on mercurimetric method *5704*

Cholesterol *Serum No Effect Analytical* At concentration of 150 mg/L had no effect on Liebermann-Burchard method *5704*

Creatinine *Serum No Effect Analytical* At concentration of 150 mg/L had no effect on Technicon AutoAnalyzer® Jaffe method *5704*

Dicumarol *Plasma Decrease Physiological* May reduce plasma concentration of dicumarol and causes a decrease in anticoagulant activity as measured by reduced prothrombin time *5254*

Doxycycline *Serum Decrease Physiological* May reduce plasma concentration of doxycycline by shortening its half-life, even for as long as 3 weeks after mephobarbital withdrawn, probably through induction of hepatic microsomal enzymes *5254*

Erythrocytes *Blood Decrease Physiological* Megaloblastic anemia *3810*

Estradiol *Plasma Decrease Physiological* May decrease the effect of estradiol by increasing its metabolism *5254*

Felbamate *Serum No Effect Analytical* No significant interference observed with GLC method of Rifai et al even though co-extracted *4958*

Glucose *Serum No Effect Analytical* At concentration of 41 mg/L had no effect on Kodak Ektachem® method *5704*

Griseofulvin *Serum Decrease Physiological* May reduce plasma concentration of griseofulvin by interfering with its gastrointestinal absorption *5254*

Hematocrit *Blood Decrease Physiological* May cause megaloblastic anemia *3810*

Hemoglobin *Blood Decrease Physiological* May cause megaloblastic anemia *3810*

MCV *Blood Increase Physiological* May cause megaloblastic anemia *3810*

Phenobarbital *Serum Increase Analytical* At concentration of 5 μg/mL (22 μmol/L) falsely increases result by more than 4 μg/mL (17 μmol/L) with method on Du Pont Dimension *1582* 73% cross-reactivity observed with Kodak thin-film assay *2601* At concentration of 5 μg/mL (22 μmol/L) increases concentration as measured on Du Pont aca by 4 μg/mL (17 μmol/L) *1537* Cross-reactivity of 412% observed with method on Baxter Stratus *5705*
Serum Increase Physiological Metabolic conversion *in vivo5093*

Phenprocoumon *Plasma Decrease Physiological* May reduce plasma concentration of phenprocoumon and causes a decrease in anticoagulant activity as measured by reduced prothrombin time *5254*

Phenytoin *Serum No Effect Analytical* No significant interference observed at a concentration of 1000 μg/mL (4.06

mmol/L) with method on Du Pont aca *1538* No effect at concentration of 1000 µg/mL (4060 µmol/L) on method on Du Pont Dimension *1583*

Phosphate *Serum No Effect Analytical* At concentration of 150 mg/L had no effect on phosphomolybdate method *5704*

Primidone *Serum Increase Analytical* At a concentration of 63 mg/L causes 25% increase with method on Baxter Stratus but unlikely to be significant since physiological concentration up to 40 mg/L *5705*
Serum No Effect Analytical No significant cross-reactivity with method on Du Pont aca *1541*

Protein *Serum No Effect Analytical* At concentration of 150 mg/L had no effect on biuret method with blank correction *5704*

Prothrombin Time *Plasma Decrease Physiological* May reduce plasma concentration of dicumarol and causes a decrease in anticoagulant activity as measured by reduced prothrombin time *5254*

Urea Nitrogen *Serum No Effect Analytical* At concentration of 41 mg/L had no effect on Kodak Ektachem® method *5704*

Uric Acid *Serum No Effect Analytical* At concentration of 150 mg/L had no effect on phosphotungstate reduction method *5704*

Warfarin *Plasma Decrease Physiological* May reduce plasma concentration of warfarin and causes a decrease in anticoagulant activity as measured by reduced prothrombin time *5254*

Mepindolol

Cholesterol *Serum No Effect Physiological* No significant effect in about 20 mild to moderate hypertensive men treated with 10 mg/day for 2 years *1899*

HDL-Cholesterol *Serum No Effect Physiological* Insignificant effect in about 20 mild to moderate hypertensive men treated with 10 mg/day for 2 years *1899*

LDL-Cholesterol *Serum No Effect Physiological* No significant effect in about 20 mild to moderate hypertensive men treated with 10 mg/day for 2 years *1899*

Triglycerides *Serum Increase Physiological* Increase of 14-25% in about 20 mild to moderate hypertensive men treated with 10 mg/day for 2 years *1899*

Meprednisone

Glucose *Serum Increase Physiological* Alteration of carbohydrate metabolism *2754*
Urine Increase Physiological Alteration of carbohydrate metabolism *2754*

Hydrochloric Acid *Gastric Fluid Increase Physiological* Steroid effect *2754*

Nitrogen Balance *Patient Negative Physiological* Due to protein catabolism *2754*

Occult Blood *Feces Increase Physiological* Activation or complication of ulcer *2754*

Meprobamate

Alanine Aminotransferase *Serum Increase Physiological* May cause cholestatic (hepatocanalicular) jaundice *402*
Serum No Effect Analytical At acute overdose concentration (20 mg/dL) on Technicon SMAC® method *6266*

Albumin *Serum No Effect Analytical* At concentration of 200 mg/L had no effect on BCG method *5704* At acute overdose concentration (20 mg/dL) on Technicon SMAC® method *6266*
Urine No Effect Analytical Using a fluorimetric assay with Albumin Blue 580 on a Cobas Fara centrifugal analyzer for the detection of microalbuminuria no significant interference was detected at a concentration of 80 mg/L *3117*

Alkaline Phosphatase *Serum Increase Physiological* May cause cholestatic (hepatocanalicular) jaundice *402*
Serum No Effect Analytical At acute overdose concentration (20 mg/dL) on Technicon SMAC® method *6266*

δ-Aminolevulinic Acid *Urine Increase Physiological* May precipitate acute porphyria *2210*

Ammonia *Plasma No Effect Analytical* At concentration of 20 mg/L had no effect on Kodak Ektachem® method *5704*

Aspartate Aminotransferase *Serum Increase Physiological* May cause cholestatic (hepatocanalicular) jaundice *402*
Serum No Effect Analytical At acute overdose concentration (20 mg/dL) on Technicon SMAC® method *6266*

Bicarbonate *Serum No Effect Analytical* At concentration of 25 mg/L had no effect on method using phenolphthalein *5704*

Bilirubin *Serum Increase Physiological* May cause cholestatic (hepatocanalicular) jaundice *402*
Serum No Effect Analytical At acute overdose concentration (20 mg/dL) on Technicon SMAC® method *6266* At concentration of 200 mg/L had no effect on Jendrassik and Grof method *5704*
Serum No Effect Physiological Insignificant displacement from protein in neonates *6314*

Calcium *Serum No Effect Analytical* At concentration of 200 mg/L had no effect on cresolphthalein method *5704* At acute overdose concentration (20 mg/dL) on Technicon SMAC® method *6266*

Catecholamines *Urine No Effect Analytical* No effect observed *1444*
Urine No Effect Physiological No effect observed *1444*

Chloride *Serum No Effect Analytical* At concentration of 25 mg/L had no effect on mercurimetric method *5704* No effect of concentrations up to 20 mg/L with method on Kodak Ektachem® *5706*

Cholesterol *Serum Increase Physiological* May cause cholestatic (hepatocanalicular) jaundice *402*
Serum No Effect Analytical At acute overdose concentration (20 mg/dL) on Technicon SMAC® method *6266* At concentration of 25 mg/L had no effect on CHOD-PAP method *5704* At concentration of 200 mg/L had no effect on Liebermann-Burchard method *5704*

Chromosomes *Test Conditions Abnormal Physiological* Clastogenic in human lymphocytes *in vitro5484*

Coproporphyrin *Feces Increase Physiological* May precipitate acute porphyria *2210*
Urine Increase Physiological May precipitate acute porphyria *2210*

Creatine Kinase *Serum No Effect Analytical* At acute overdose concentration (20 mg/dL) on Technicon SMAC® method *6266*

Creatinine *Serum No Effect Analytical* At 200 mg/L on reversed phase liquid chromatographic procedure of Zhiri et al *6656* At acute overdose concentration (20 mg/dL) on Technicon SMAC® method *6266* No interference observed at a concentration of 2 mg/L with HPLC method of Rosano et al *5083* At concentration of 200 mg/L had no effect on Technicon AutoAnalyzer® method *5704* No effect of concentrations up to 20 mg/L on 2-slide method on Kodak Ektachem® *5706* No effect of concentrations up to 20 mg/L on single slide method on Kodak Ektachem® *5706* At concentration of 20 mg/L had no effect on Kodak Ektachem® method *5704*

Eosinophils *Blood Increase Physiological* Rare allergic manifestation *2754*

Erythrocytes *Blood Decrease Physiological* Aplastic anemia/erythroid hypoplasia *4017*

Glucose *Serum No Effect Analytical* At acute overdose concentration (20 mg/dL) on Technicon SMAC® method *6266* At concentration of 484 mg/L had no effect on Kodak Ektachem® method *5704* At concentration of 25 mg/L had no effect on GOD/POD-PAP method *5704*

Hematocrit *Blood Decrease Physiological* May cause aplastic anemia *536*

Hemoglobin *Blood Increase Physiological* May cause aplastic anemia *536*

Histamine *Plasma No Effect Analytical* Improbable inhibition of radio-enzyme assay likely at physiological concentrations *2492*

17-Hydroxycorticosteroids *Urine Increase Analytical* Glucuronide interferes with Porter-Silber reaction *3669* Small effect on modified Glenn-Nelson method *6515*

Iron *Serum No Effect Analytical* At acute overdose concentration (20 mg/dL) on Technicon SMAC® method *6266* At concentration of 200 mg/L had no effect on Ferrozine method *5704*

Meprobamate *(continued)*

17-Ketogenic Steroids *Urine Increase Analytical* Glucuronide interferes with Zimmermann reaction *5869*

Lactate Dehydrogenase *Serum No Effect Analytical* At acute overdose concentration (20 mg/dL) on Technicon SMAC® method *6266*

Leukocytes *Blood Decrease Physiological* Pancytopenia (may be agranulocytosis) *133*

Meprobamate *Serum Increase Physiological* 0.4 to 1.2 g orally produces blood concentrations of 5-15 mg/L *3868*

Neutrophils *Blood Decrease Physiological* occasional case of agranulocytosis reported *6264*

p-Aminophenol *Urine No Effect Analytical* With addition of drugs at a concentration of 100 mg/L and of related compounds at 50 mg/L no significant effect observed on colorimetric method of van Bocxlaer on Cobas Mira analyzer which involves reacting free p-aminophenol with resorcinol in the presence of magnesium ions to form an indophenol dye measured at 550 nm *6163*

Phenylalanine *Plasma No Effect Analytical* No interference observed with rapid quantitative whole blood method of Campbell et al using phenylalanine dehydrogenase *867*

Phosphate *Serum No Effect Analytical* At acute overdose concentration (20 mg/dL) on Technicon SMAC® method *6266* At concentration of 200 mg/L had no effect on phosphomolybdate method *5704*

Platelets *Blood Decrease Physiological* Rare bone marrow aplasia, thrombocytopenia *133*

Porphobilinogen *Urine Increase Physiological* May precipitate acute porphyria *2210*

Porphyrin, Total *Urine Increase Physiological* May precipitate attack of acute porphyria *3669*

Potassium *Serum No Effect Analytical* At concentration of 25 mg/L had no effect on flame-photometric method *5704* At concentration of 160 mg/L had no effect on measurement by ISE with predilution *5704*

Procainamide *Serum Decrease Analytical* Superpharmacologic doses of meprobamate may inhibit the fluorescence of procainamide and NAPA *4530*

Protein *Serum No Effect Analytical* At concentration of 200 mg/L had no effect on biuret method with blank correction *5704* At acute overdose concentration (20 mg/dL) on Technicon SMAC® method *6266*

Prothrombin Time *Plasma Decrease Physiological* Induces hepatic metabolism of anticoagulants *2242*
Plasma No Effect Physiological Probably no significant effect clinically *2452*

Protoporphyrin *Feces Increase Physiological* May precipitate acute porphyria *2210*

Sodium *Serum No Effect Analytical* At concentration of 160 mg/L had no effect on measurement by ISE with predilution *5704* At concentration of 25 mg/L had no effect on flame-photometric method *5704*

Triglycerides *Serum No Effect Analytical* At concentration of 200 mg/L had no effect on lipase/esterase method *5704* At acute overdose concentration (20 mg/dL) on Technicon SMAC® method *6266*

Urea Nitrogen *Serum No Effect Analytical* At concentration of 484 mg/L had no effect on Kodak Ektachem® method *5704* At acute overdose concentration (20 mg/dL) on Technicon SMAC® method *6266* At concentration of 200 mg/L had no effect on diacetylmonoxime method *5704*

Uric Acid *Serum No Effect Analytical* At concentration of 200 mg/L had no effect on phosphotungstate reduction method *5704* At acute overdose concentration (20 mg/dL) on Technicon SMAC® method *6266* At 200 mg/L on reversed phase liquid chromatographic procedure of Zhiri et al *6656*

Vanillylmandelic Acid *Urine No Effect Analytical* No effect observed *1444*
Urine No Effect Physiological No effect observed *1444*

Meptazinol

Epinephrine *Plasma Increase Physiological* Almost 2 fold increase in 20 minutes with up to 1.4 mg/kg i.v *3771*

Norepinephrine *Plasma Increase Physiological* Almost 2 fold increase in 20 minutes with up to 1.4 mg/kg i.v *3771*

Meralluride

Albumin *Serum No Effect Analytical* No effect at 0.07 mL/dL on Technicon SMA 12/60 method *4390*

Alkaline Phosphatase *Serum No Effect Analytical* No effect at 0.07 mL/dL on Technicon SMA 12/60 method *4390*

Aspartate Aminotransferase *Serum No Effect Analytical* No effect at 0.07 mL/dL on Technicon SMA 12/60 method *4390*

Bicarbonate *Serum Increase Physiological* Alkalosis may occur with loss of chloride *2754*

Bilirubin *Serum No Effect Analytical* No effect at 0.07 mg/dL on Technicon SMA 12/60 method *4390*

Calcium *Serum No Effect Analytical* No effect at 0.07 mL/dL on Technicon SMA 12/60 method *4390*
Urine Increase Physiological Reabsorption impaired *4555*

Chloride *Serum Decrease Physiological* Diuretic action *6515*

Cholesterol *Serum No Effect Analytical* No effect at 0.07 mL/dL on Technicon SMA 12/60 method *4390*

Creatinine *Serum No Effect Analytical* No effect at 0.07 mL/dL on Technicon SMA 12/60 method *4390*

Glucose *Serum No Effect Analytical* No effect at 0.07 mL/dL on Technicon SMA 12/60 method *4390*
Urine Decrease Analytical Interferes with glucose oxidase method *4012*

^{131}I Uptake *Serum No Effect Physiological* No effect on thyroid function *3669*

Lactate Dehydrogenase *Serum No Effect Analytical* No effect at 0.07 mL/dL on Technicon SMA 12/60 method *4390*

Leukocytes *Blood Decrease Physiological* May cause bone marrow depression *2754*

Magnesium *Serum Decrease Physiological* Hypomagnesemia especially if NH_4Cl also given *3811*

Neutrophils *Blood Decrease Physiological* May cause bone marrow depression *2754*

pH *Blood Increase Physiological* Alkalosis may occur with massive diuresis *2754*

Phosphate *Serum No Effect Analytical* No effect at 0.07 mL/dL on Technicon SMA 12/60 method *4390*

Potassium *Serum Decrease Physiological* Diuretic action *5869*

Protein *Serum No Effect Analytical* No effect at 0.07 mL/dL on Technicon SMA 12/60 method *4390*

Sodium *Serum Decrease Physiological* Diuretic action *6515*

Urea Nitrogen *Serum Increase Physiological* May cause transient neutropenia *2754*

Uric Acid *Serum Increase Physiological* May cause occasional hyperuricemia *2754*
Serum No Effect Analytical No effect at 0.07 mL/dL on Technicon SMA 12/60 method *4390*

Merbarone

Uric Acid *Serum Decrease Physiological* Reduced from mean of 5.7 mg/dL to 1.3 mg/dL in 20 patients given up to 750 mg/sq meter for 5 days by increasing urinary excretion *6355*
Urine Increase Physiological Substantial increase observed to start within 24 hours of treatment being initiated and maximal by 48 to 72 hours probably due to direct effect on renal tubules *6355*

Merbromin

Color *Urine Increase Analytical* Fluorescent pink staining of cells *703*

Gentamicin *Serum Decrease Analytical* Significant reduction with Abbott TDx method due to background fluorescence from dye that is structurally similar to the TDx tracer dye *916*

Urobilin *Urine Increase Analytical* Yields pink color and mauve fluorescence *2559*

Mercaptoethane

N-Acetyl-Glucosaminidase *Urine* *No Effect* *Analytical* At 60 mmol/L on 2 colorimetric analytical methods *2254*

Mercaptoethanol

Chromosomes *Test Conditions* *Abnormal* *Physiological* Clastogenic in human cells *5484*

Mercaptomerin

Bilirubin *Serum* *No Effect* *Analytical* At concentration of 58 mg/L had no effect on Jendrassik and Grof method *5704*

Calcium *Serum* *No Effect* *Analytical* At concentration of 58 mg/L had no effect on cresolphthalein method *5704*
Urine *Increase* *Physiological* Reabsorption impaired *4555*

Magnesium *Urine* *Increase* *Physiological* Excretion increased by up to 30% *5633*

Phosphate *Serum* *No Effect* *Analytical* At concentration of 58 mg/L had no effect on phosphomolybdate method *5704*

Protein *Serum* *No Effect* *Analytical* At concentration of 58 mg/L had no effect on biuret method with blank correction *5704*

Urea Nitrogen *Serum* *No Effect* *Analytical* At concentration of 58 mg/L had no effect on diacetylmonoxime method *5704*

Uric Acid *Serum* *No Effect* *Analytical* At concentration of 58 mg/L had no effect on phosphotungstate reduction method *5704*

Zinc *Urine* *No Effect* *Physiological* No effect observed on excretion *4484*

Mercaptopurine

Alanine Aminotransferase *Serum* *Increase* *Physiological* Intrahepatic cholestasis observed in several patients *3949* May cause hepatotoxicity (centrolobular necrosis) *326*

Alkaline Phosphatase *Serum* *Increase* *Physiological* Hepatotoxicity (centrolobular necrosis) *3810* Intrahepatic cholestasis observed in several patients *3949*

Ammonia *Plasma* *No Effect* *Analytical* At concentration of 150 mg/L had no effect on Kodak Ektachem® method *5704*

Amylase *Serum* *Increase* *Physiological* An increased risk of pancreatitis may be associated with the investigational use of mercaptopurine in inflammatory bowel disease *2179* One case of hemorrhagic pancreatitis *4014*

Aspartate Aminotransferase *Serum* *Increase* *Physiological* May cause hepatotoxicity (centrolobular necrosis) *326* Intrahepatic cholestasis observed in several patients *3949* Picture of cholestasis in 10 of 19 leukemic patients, but drug co-administered with Adriamycin® in all and additional drugs in others *5051*

Bile *Urine* *Increase* *Physiological* Hepatotoxic effect *3810*

Bilirubin *Serum* *Increase* *Physiological* Reported in up to 53% leukemic patients treated with drug *3949* Picture of cholestasis in 10 of 19 leukemic patients, but drug co-administered with Adriamycin® in all and additional drugs in others *5051* May cause increase, especially if prior damage *5502*
Serum *No Effect* *Analytical* At concentration of 152 mg/L had no effect on Jendrassik and Grof method *5704*

BSP Retention *Serum* *Increase* *Physiological* Hepatotoxicity (centrolobular necrosis) *3810*

Calcium *Serum* *No Effect* *Analytical* At concentration of 152 mg/L had no effect on cresolphthalein method *5704*

Chloride *Serum* *No Effect* *Analytical* At concentration of 15 mg/L had no effect on Kodak Ektachem® method *5704*

Cholesterol *Serum* *No Effect* *Analytical* No effect at concentrations up to 15 mg/L on method on Kodak Ektachem® *5706*

Chromosomes *Test Conditions* *Abnormal* *Physiological* Clastogenic in human cells *5484*

Creatine Kinase *Serum* *No Effect* *Analytical* No effect of concentrations up to 15 mg/L on method on Kodak Ektachem® *5706*

Creatinine *Serum* *No Effect* *Analytical* No effect of concentrations up to 150 mg/L on 2-slide method on Kodak Ektachem® *5706* At concentration of 150 mg/L had no effect on Kodak Ektachem® method *5704* No effect of concentrations up to 15 mg/L on single slide method on Kodak Ektachem® *5706* No interference observed at a concentration of 1 mg/L with HPLC method of Rosano et al *5083*

Crystals *Urine* *Increase* *Physiological* Direct renal damage with doses over 750 mg/sq m *1636*

Erythrocytes *Blood* *Decrease* *Physiological* May occur with bone marrow depression *4014* The most frequent adverse reactions to mercaptopurine is marrow suppression *2179*
Urine *Increase* *Physiological* Direct renal damage with doses over 750 mg/sq m *1636*

Glucose *Serum* *Increase* *Analytical* 8.8% increase in absorbance with 10 mmol/L and glucokinase based assay of Scott *5414* At 1 mmol/L affects Technicon SMA 12/60 method *5576*
Serum *No Effect* *Analytical* At concentrations up to 100 mg/L no effect on method on Fuji Drichem 1000 *5706* At concentration of 20 mg/L had no effect on Kodak Ektachem® method *5704*

HDL-Cholesterol *Serum* *No Effect* *Analytical* No effect of concentrations up to 15 mg/L on method on Kodak Ektachem® *5706*

Hematocrit *Blood* *Decrease* *Physiological* The most frequent adverse reactions to mercaptopurine is marrow suppression *2179* May occur with bone marrow depression *4014*

Hemoglobin *Blood* *Decrease* *Physiological* The most frequent adverse reactions to mercaptopurine is marrow suppression *2179* May occur with bone marrow depression *4014*
Blood *No Effect* *Analytical* No effect of concentrations up to 15 mmol/L on method on Kodak Ektachem® *5706*
Urine *Increase* *Physiological* Direct renal damage with doses over 750 mg/sq m *1636*

Histamine *Plasma* *No Effect* *Analytical* No inhibition of radio-enzyme assay at much higher than therapeutic concentrations *2492*

Lactate Dehydrogenase *Serum* *No Effect* *Analytical* No effect of concentrations up to 15 mg/L on method on Kodak Ektachem® *5706*

Leukocytes *Blood* *Decrease* *Physiological* Agranulocytosis *4013* The most frequent adverse reactions to mercaptopurine is marrow suppression *2179*

Lipase *Serum* *Increase* *Physiological* An increased risk of pancreatitis may be associated with the investigational use of mercaptopurine in inflammatory bowel disease *2179*

Phosphate *Serum* *No Effect* *Analytical* At concentration of 152 mg/L had no effect on phosphomolybdate method *5704*

Platelets *Blood* *Decrease* *Physiological* The most frequent adverse reactions to mercaptopurine is marrow suppression *2179* May cause bone marrow depression *4013*

Potassium *Serum* *No Effect* *Analytical* No effect of concentrations up to 15 mg/L on method on Kodak Ektachem® *5706*

Protein *Cerebrospinal Fluid* *No Effect* *Analytical* No significant effect when added in vitro to concentration of 10.0 mg/dL on Kodak Ektachem® slide method *3654*
Serum *No Effect* *Analytical* At concentration of 152 mg/L had no effect on biuret method with blank correction *5704*

Prothrombin Time *Plasma* *Increase* *Physiological* Depresses clotting factor synthesis *5674*

Sodium *Serum* *No Effect* *Analytical* No effect of concentrations up to 15 mg/L on method on Kodak Ektachem® *5706*

Triglycerides *Serum* *No Effect* *Analytical* No effect of concentrations up to 15 mg/L on method on Kodak Ektachem® *5706*

Urea Nitrogen *Serum* *No Effect* *Analytical* At concentration of 152 mg/L had no effect on diacetylmonoxime method *5704* At concentration of 15 mg/L had no effect on Kodak Ektachem® method *5704*

Uric Acid *Serum* *Increase* *Analytical* At concentrations above 14 mg/L raised concentration as measured by phosphotungstate reduction method *5704* At 1 mmol/L affects Technicon SMA 12/60 method *5576*
Serum *Increase* *Physiological* May occur as a result of rapid cell lysis accompanying the antineoplastic effect *2179* Leucocyte destruction, catabolism of nucleic acids *5869*

Mercaptopurine *(continued)*

Uric Acid *(continued)*
Serum *No Effect* *Analytical* No effect of concentrations up to 15 mg/L on method on Kodak Ektachem® *5706*
Urine *Increase* *Physiological* May occur as a result of rapid cell lysis accompanying the antineoplastic effect *2179* Increased nuclear protein breakdown *2024*

Mercurial Diuretics

Ammonia *Plasma* *Increase* *Physiological* Presumed effect as may precipitate hepatic coma *2452*

Calcium *Serum* *Decrease* *Physiological* Enhances excretion reducing serum concentration *174*
Urine *Increase* *Physiological* Reabsorption impaired *4555*

Chloride *Serum* *Decrease* *Physiological* May cause hypochloremic alkalosis and diuresis *4555*
Urine *Increase* *Physiological* Therapeutic intent (dominant urinary anion) *4555*

Erythrocytes *Blood* *Decrease* *Physiological* Anemia may occur *3810*

Glucose *Urine* *Decrease* *Analytical* May cause false negative results with glucose oxidase methods *2451* May produce false negative with glucose oxidase based Stix *3805*

^{131}I Uptake *Serum* *No Effect* *Physiological* No effect in euthyroid subjects *882*

Leukocytes *Blood* *Decrease* *Physiological* Neutropenia/agranulocytosis reported *3260*

Magnesium *Serum* *Decrease* *Physiological* Effect most marked if NH_4Cl also given *3811*
Urine *Increase* *Physiological* Excretion increased by up to 30% *5633*

pH *Blood* *Increase* *Physiological* May cause systemic alkalosis especially if hypochloremia *2242*

Phosphate *Urine* *Increase* *Physiological* Reported effect *5377*

Platelets *Blood* *Decrease* *Physiological* Thrombocytopenia reported (sensitization) *2242*

Potassium *Serum* *Decrease* *Physiological* May induce hypokalemia in some cases *1958*

Protein *Urine* *Increase* *Physiological* May produce nephrotic syndrome *1958*

Sodium *Serum* *Decrease* *Physiological* Diuretic action with sodium depletion *3810*
Urine *Increase* *Physiological* Therapeutic intent *2242*

Urea Nitrogen *Serum* *Increase* *Physiological* May produce renal failure or nephrotic syndrome *1958*

Uric Acid *Serum* *Increase* *Physiological* May precipitate attacks of gout *711*

Volume *Urine* *Decrease* *Physiological* May produce oliguria and tubular necrosis *1958*
Urine *Increase* *Physiological* Therapeutic intent *2242*

Mercury Compounds

Acetoacetate Decarboxylase *Serum* *Decrease* *Analytical* $HgCl_2$ causes denaturation *6198*

α-Amino-Nitrogen *Urine* *Increase* *Physiological* Fanconi syndrome with laxative overuse *3474*

Bicarbonate *Serum* *Decrease* *Physiological* May be depressed in established poisoning *1647*

Calcium *Serum* *Decrease* *Physiological* Induced with chronic laxative ingestion *3474*

Casts *Urine* *Increase* *Physiological* May cause severe nephritis if absorbed *128*

Color *Feces* *Increase* *Analytical* Green with about 130 mg of calomel *3810*
Urine *Increase* *Analytical* Red brown due to hematuria *3810*

Erythrocytes *Urine* *Increase* *Physiological* May cause severe nephritis if absorbed *128*

Glucose *Urine* *Increase* *Physiological* May cause Fanconi syndrome *3474*

Hemoglobin *Urine* *Increase* *Physiological* May cause severe nephritis if absorbed *128*

^{131}I Uptake *Serum* *No Effect* *Physiological* No effect observed *3107*

Leukocytes *Blood* *Increase* *Physiological* May induce leukocytosis *409*

Magnesium *Serum* *Decrease* *Physiological* Induced with chronic laxative ingestion *3474*

Mercury *Urine* *Increase* *Physiological* Due to ingestion of compound and if poisoning *5892*

Occult Blood *Feces* *Increase* *Physiological* Bloody diarrhea occurs with poisoning *2242*

pH *Blood* *Decrease* *Physiological* Induced with chronic laxative ingestion *3474*

Phosphate *Urine* *Increase* *Physiological* Occurs with Fanconi syndrome *3474*

Potassium *Serum* *Decrease* *Physiological* Induced with chronic laxative ingestion *3474*

Protein *Cerebrospinal Fluid* *Increase* *Physiological* May produce Guaillain-Barre like syndrome *5892*
Serum *Decrease* *Physiological* Due to albuminuria and starvation *3810*
Urine *Increase* *Physiological* Nephrotoxic effect *2024*

Sodium *Serum* *Decrease* *Physiological* May occur with established mercury poisoning *1647*

T3-Uptake *Serum* *No Effect* *Physiological* No effect on resin uptake *3107*

Uric Acid *Serum* *Decrease* *Physiological* Occurs with Fanconi syndrome *3474*
Urine *Increase* *Physiological* Occurs with Fanconi syndrome *3474*

Meropenem

Alanine Aminotransferase *Serum* *Increase* *Physiological* May cause hepatotoxic jaundice or cholestatic jaundice *6647*

Alkaline Phosphatase *Serum* *Increase* *Physiological* May cause hepatotoxic jaundice or cholestatic jaundice *6647*

Aspartate Aminotransferase *Serum* *Increase* *Physiological* May cause hepatotoxic jaundice or cholestatic jaundice *6647*

Bilirubin *Serum* *Increase* *Physiological* May cause hepatotoxic jaundice or cholestatic jaundice *6647*

Coombs' Test, Direct *Blood* *Positive* *Physiological* May cause positive direct or indirect Coomb's test *6647*

Coombs' Test, Indirect *Blood* *Positive* *Physiological* May cause positive direct or indirect Coomb's test *6647*

Creatinine *Serum* *Increase* *Physiological* May cause kidney failure *6647*

Eosinophils *Blood* *Increase* *Physiological* May cause eosinophilia *6647*

Erythrocytes *Urine* *Increase* *Physiological* May cause increased number of red blood cells in urine *6647*

γ-Glutamyltransferase *Serum* *Increase* *Physiological* May cause hepatotoxic jaundice or cholestatic jaundice *6647*

Hematocrit *Blood* *Decrease* *Physiological* May cause anemia *6647*

Hemoglobin *Blood* *Decrease* *Physiological* May cause anemia *6647*

Leukocytes *Blood* *Decrease* *Physiological* May cause leukopenia *6647*

Occult Blood *Feces* *Increase* *Physiological* Reported to cause gastrointestinal hemorrhage, melena and other bleeding in 0.7% of treated patients *6647*

Partial Thromboplastin Time
Plasma *Decrease* *Physiological* May cause shortened partial thromboplastin time *6647*
Plasma *Increase* *Physiological* May cause prolonged partial thromboplastin time *6647*

Platelets *Blood* *Decrease* *Physiological* May cause thrombocytopenia *6647*
Blood *Increase* *Physiological* May cause thrombocythemia *6647*

Prothrombin Time *Plasma* *Decrease* *Physiological* May cause shortened prothrombin time *6647*

Plasma *Increase* *Physiological* May cause prolonged prothrombin time *6647*

Urea Nitrogen *Serum* *Increase* *Physiological* May cause increased concentration *6647* May cause kidney failure *6647*

Mersalyl

Calcium *Urine* *Increase* *Physiological* Reabsorption impaired *4555*

Chloride *Serum* *Decrease* *Physiological* Consequence of diuretic action *4555*

Erythrocytes *Urine* *Increase* *Physiological* Actual bleeding may be caused by drug *1714*

Hemoglobin *Urine* *Increase* *Physiological* Actual bleeding caused by drug *1714*

Uric Acid *Serum* *Decrease* *Physiological* Uricosuric action *2378*

Urine *Increase* *Physiological* Uricosuric action *2378*

Mesalamine

Alanine Aminotransferase *Serum* *Increase* *Physiological* Administration of mesalamine has been reportedly rarely to be associated with hepatitis *4796* Adverse effect observed in less than 1% of treated patients *2651*

Albumin *Urine* *Increase* *Physiological* Adverse effect observed in less than 1% of treated patients *2651*

Alkaline Phosphatase *Serum* *Increase* *Physiological* Administration of mesalamine has been reportedly rarely to be associated with hepatitis *4796* Adverse effect observed in less than 1% of treated patients *2651*

Amylase *Serum* *Increase* *Physiological* Administration of mesalamine has been reportedly rarely to be associated with pancreatitis *4796* Pancreatitis observed in less than 1% of treated patients *2651*

Aspartate Aminotransferase *Serum* *Increase* *Physiological* Adverse effect observed in less than 1% of treated patients *2651* Administration of mesalamine has been reportedly rarely to be associated with hepatitis *4796*

Bilirubin *Serum* *Increase* *Physiological* Administration of mesalamine has been reportedly rarely to be associated with hepatitis *4796*

Serum *No Effect* *Analytical* No effect at concentration of 40 mg/L on method on Kodak Ektachem® *5706*

Bilirubin, Conjugated *Serum* *No Effect* *Analytical* No effect at concentration of 40 mg/L on method on Kodak Ektachem® *5706*

Bilirubin, Unconjugated *Serum* *No Effect* *Analytical* No effect at concentration of 40 mg/L on method on Kodak Ektachem® *5706*

Blood *Urine* *Increase* *Physiological* Adverse effect observed in less than 1% of treated patients *2651*

Cortisol *Plasma* *Decrease* *Physiological* Morning concentration in 46 patients with Crohn's disease who completed 16 weeks of treatment 15.3 ± 7.9 µg/dL with 83% of patients having normal values *6018*

Creatinine *Serum* *Increase* *Physiological* Administration of mesalamine has been reportedly associated with minimal change nephropathy, and acute and chronic interstitial nephritis *4796*

Eosinophils *Blood* *Increase* *Physiological* Administration of mesalamine has been reportedly rarely to be associated with eosinophilia *4796*

γ-Glutamyltransferase *Serum* *Increase* *Physiological* Adverse effect observed in less than 1% of treated patients *2651*

Granulocytes *Blood* *Decrease* *Physiological* Administration of mesalamine has been reportedly rarely to be associated with agranulocytosis *4796*

Hematocrit *Blood* *Decrease* *Physiological* Aplastic anemia, anemia, leukopenia and pancytopenia observed as adverse effects in post-marketing reports *2651* Administration of mesalamine has been reportedly rarely to be associated with aplastic anemia or anemia *4796*

Hemoglobin *Blood* *Decrease* *Physiological* Administration of mesalamine has been reportedly rarely to be associated with aplastic anemia or anemia *4796* Aplastic anemia, anemia, leukopenia and pancytopenia observed as adverse effects in post-marketing reports *2651*

Lactate Dehydrogenase *Serum* *Increase* *Physiological* Adverse effect observed in less than 1% of treated patients *2651*

Leukocytes *Blood* *Decrease* *Physiological* Administration of mesalamine has been reported to be associated with leukopenia *4796* Aplastic anemia, anemia, leukopenia and pancytopenia observed as adverse effects in post-marketing reports *2651*

Lipase *Serum* *Decrease* *Analytical* At concentrations above 150 mg/L causes decreased activity with method on Kodak Ektachem® *5706*

Serum *Increase* *Physiological* Pancreatitis observed in less than 1% of treated patients *2651* Administration of mesalamine has been reportedly rarely to be associated with pancreatitis *4796*

Neutrophils *Blood* *Decrease* *Physiological* Aplastic anemia, anemia, leukopenia and pancytopenia observed as adverse effects in post-marketing reports *2651*

Occult Blood *Feces* *Increase* *Physiological* Gastrointestinal bleeding observed in less than 1% of treated patients *2651*

Platelets *Blood* *Decrease* *Physiological* Administration of mesalamine has been reportedly rarely to be associated with thrombocytopenia *4796* Thrombocythemia and thrombocytopenia observed as adverse effects in less than 1% of treated patients *2651*

Blood *Increase* *Physiological* Thrombocythemia and thrombocytopenia observed as adverse effects in less than 1% of treated patients *2651*

Protein *Urine* *Increase* *Physiological* Administration of mesalamine has been reportedly associated with minimal change nephropathy, and acute and chronic interstitial nephritis *4796*

Sperm Count *Semen* *No Effect* *Physiological* No effect observed and indeed has reversed hypospermia and disturbances of motility caused by sulfasalazine *1384*

Urea Nitrogen *Serum* *Increase* *Physiological* Administration of mesalamine has been reportedly associated with minimal change nephropathy, and acute and chronic interstitial nephritis *4796*

Uric Acid *Serum* *Increase* *Physiological* Administration of mesalamine has been reportedly to cause gout *4796*

Mescaline

Chromosomes *Test Conditions* *Abnormal* *Physiological* Teratogenic in experimental animals *5484*

Fatty Acids (FFA), Free *Serum* *Increase* *Physiological* 115% increase after 5 mg/kg body weight orally *2675*

Mesna

β-Hydroxybutyrate *Urine* *Increase* *Analytical* False positive result observed with enzymatic procedure of GDS Diagnostics but to a lesser extent than with nitroprusside dipstick ketone test *1824*

Ketones *Urine* *Increase* *Analytical* False positive result obtained with this and other compounds containing free sulfhydryl groups with Legal method *1185* Common if not invariable in patients given i.v. mesna *875* Concentration of 10 mmol/L causes +++/++ reaction with Boehringer Mannheim Chemstrip but addition of 9 volumes of 500 g/L iodoacetate to 1 volume of urine eliminates effect within 2 minutes *4749* False-positive with Multistix® and Chemstrip® but red color can be discharged with glacial acetic acid *1185* False positive or atypical reaction may be observed with Ames Multistix and other reagent strip tests *4034* Positive correlation with sulfhydryl concentrations in 931 urine specimens following infusion of mesna with Boehringer Mannheim Chemstrip. Color can be removed from test strip by a drop of glacial acetic acid *2253*

Platelet Aggregation *Blood* *No Effect* *Physiological* Not impaired after stimulation with epinephrine, ADP or arachidonic acid *2560*

Mesoglycan

Alanine Aminotransferase *Serum No Effect Physiological* In 30 patients who previously had had a stroke treatment with 100 mg/d for 90 days caused nonsignificant increase from mean baseline of 16.9 ± 5.7 U/L to 17.5 ± 5.3 U/L *4424*

Alkaline Phosphatase *Serum No Effect Physiological* In 30 patients who previously had had a stroke treatment with 100 mg/d for 90 days caused insignificant reduction from mean baseline of 70.3 ± 10.3 U/L to 68.5 ± 10.9 U/L *4424*

Antithrombin III *Plasma No Effect Physiological* In 30 patients with previous strokes treatment with 100 mg/d caused nonsignificant increase from mean baseline of 10.9 ± 1.2 IU/mL to 11.2 ± 1.0 IU/mL after 30 days and 11.1 ± 1.2 IU/mL after 90 days *4424*

Aspartate Aminotransferase
Serum No Effect Physiological In 30 patients who previously had had a stroke treatment with 100 mg/d for 90 days caused nonsignificant increase from mean baseline of 15.4 ± 10.6 U/L to 16.3 ± 8.1 U/L *4424*

Creatinine *Serum No Effect Physiological* In 30 patients who previously had had a stroke treatment with 100 mg/d for 90 days had no effect on basal concentration of 0.9 ± 0.04 mg/dL *4424*

Erythrocytes *Blood No Effect Physiological* In 30 patients with previous strokes treatment with 100 mg/d for 90 days caused insignificant reduction from mean baseline of 5.0 ± 0.7 million/ μL to 4.8 ± 0.5 million/ μL *4424*

Fibrinogen *Plasma Decrease Physiological* In 30 patients who previously had an atherothrombotic stroke receiving 100 mg/d for 3 months significant reduction from baseline of 361 ± 77 mg/dL to 280 ± 53 mg/dL at 30 days and 257 ± 63 mg/dL at 90 days *4424*

Glucose *Serum No Effect Physiological* In 30 patients who previously had had a stroke treatment with 100 mg/d for 90 days caused nonsignificant reduction from mean baseline of 105 ± 26 mg/dL to 101 ± 24 mg/dL *4424*

γ-Glutamyltransferase *Serum No Effect Physiological* In 30 patients who previously had had a stroke treatment with 100 mg/d for 90 days caused nonsignificant increase from mean baseline of 19.4 ± 9.2 U/L to 21.0 ± 11.9 U/L *4424*

Leukocytes *Blood No Effect Physiological* In 30 patients with previous strokes treatment with 100 mg/d for 90 days caused nonsignificant reduction from mean baseline of 7700 ± 1600 /μL to 6800 +/ 1400 /μL *4424*

Partial Thromboplastin Time
Plasma No Effect Physiological In 30 patients with previous strokes treatment with 100 mg/d caused nonsignificant reduction from mean baseline of 25.2 ± 9.1 seconds to 25.0 ± 6.8 seconds after 30 days and increase to 25.5 ± 10.2 seconds after 90 days *4424*

Platelets *Blood No Effect Physiological* In 30 patients with previous strokes treated with 100 mg/d caused nonsignificant reduction from mean baseline of 278,000 /μL to 259,000 /μL after 30 days and 253,000 /μL after 90 days *4424*

Prothrombin Time *Plasma No Effect Physiological* In 30 patients with previous strokes treatment with 100 mg/d caused insignificant reduction from mean baseline of 94.0 ± 6.7% to 90.8 ± 6.5% after 30 days and 91.2 ± 7.6% after 90 days *4424*

Urea Nitrogen *Serum No Effect Physiological* In 30 patients who previously had had a stroke treatment with 100 g/d caused nonsignificant reduction from mean baseline of 21 ± 5 mg/dL to 20 ± 4 mg/dL after 90 days *4424*

Mesoridazine

Alanine Aminotransferase *Serum No Effect Analytical* At acute overdose concentration (20 mg/dL) on Technicon SMAC® method *6266*

Albumin *Serum No Effect Analytical* At acute overdose concentration (20 mg/dL) on Technicon SMAC® method *6266*

Alkaline Phosphatase *Serum No Effect Analytical* At acute overdose concentration (20 mg/dL) on Technicon SMAC® method *6266*

Aspartate Aminotransferase *Serum Increase Physiological* Transient effect noted *128*
Serum No Effect Analytical At acute overdose concentration (20 mg/dL) on Technicon SMAC® method *6266*

Bilirubin *Serum Increase Physiological* Jaundice as manifestation of hepatotoxicity *2754*
Serum No Effect Analytical At acute overdose concentration (20 mg/dL) on Technicon SMAC® method *6266*

Calcium *Serum No Effect Analytical* At acute overdose concentration (20 mg/dL) on Technicon SMAC® method *6266*

Cholesterol *Serum No Effect Analytical* At acute overdose concentration (20 mg/dL) on Technicon SMAC® method *6266*

Creatine Kinase *Serum No Effect Analytical* At acute overdose concentration (20 mg/dL) on Technicon SMAC® method *6266*

Creatinine *Serum No Effect Analytical* At acute overdose concentration (20 mg/dL) on Technicon SMAC® method *6266*

Eosinophils *Blood Increase Physiological* Manifestation of allergic reaction *2754*

Erythrocytes *Blood Decrease Physiological* Anemia/aplastic anemia/pancytopenia *2754*

Glucose *Serum No Effect Analytical* At acute overdose concentration (20 mg/dL) on Technicon SMAC® method *6266*

^{131}I Uptake *Serum Decrease Physiological* Serentil® contains tetraiodofluorescein *4360*

Iron *Serum No Effect Analytical* At acute overdose concentration (20 mg/dL) on Technicon SMAC® method *6266*

Lactate Dehydrogenase *Serum No Effect Analytical* At acute overdose concentration (20 mg/dL) on Technicon SMAC® method *6266*

Leukocytes *Blood Decrease Physiological* Transient agranulocytosis reported *128*

Phosphate *Serum No Effect Analytical* At acute overdose concentration (20 mg/dL) on Technicon SMAC® method *6266*

Platelets *Blood Decrease Physiological* Thrombocytopenia may occur *2754*

Protein *Serum No Effect Analytical* At acute overdose concentration (20 mg/dL) on Technicon SMAC® method *6266*

Triglycerides *Serum No Effect Analytical* At acute overdose concentration (20 mg/dL) on Technicon SMAC® method *6266*

Urea Nitrogen *Serum No Effect Analytical* At acute overdose concentration (20 mg/dL) on Technicon SMAC® method *6266*

Uric Acid *Serum No Effect Analytical* At acute overdose concentration (20 mg/dL) on Technicon SMAC® method *6266*

Mesterolone

Tyrosine *Plasma Decrease Physiological* Hormonal effect (?exact mechanism) *1313*

Mestranol

Albumin *Serum Decrease Physiological* Metabolic effect *5454*

Antithrombin III *Plasma Decrease Physiological* In over 20%: not dose related *6685*

BSP Retention *Serum Increase Physiological* Depresses hepatic secretory transport maximum *2452*

Calcium *Serum Decrease Physiological* Increased sensitivity to calcitonin in postmenopausal women *74*
Urine Decrease Physiological Increased sensitivity to calcitonin in postmenopausal women *74*

Cortisol, Free *Plasma Increase Physiological* Slight effect if over 0.1 mg *815*

Follicle Stimulating Hormone
Plasma Decrease Physiological Hormonal effect (inhibitory action of estrogen) *5424*

α_2-Globulin *Serum Increase Physiological* Metabolic effect *5454*

β-Globulin *Serum Increase Physiological* Metabolic effect *5454*

Glucose Tolerance *Serum Decrease Physiological* May provoke mild to moderate deterioration *3012*

Iron-Binding Capacity, Total *Serum Increase Physiological* 20% rise on average *2719*

Luteinizing Hormone *Plasma Increase Physiological* Estrogen exerts stimulatory action *6598*

α_2-Macroglobulin *Serum Increase Physiological* Maximum effect 1 week after treatment *2719*

Phosphate *Serum Decrease Physiological* Increased sensitivity to calcitonin in postmenopausal women *74*
Urine Increase Physiological Increased response to calcitonin *74*

Prolactin *Plasma Increase Physiological* In 31 of 88 oophorectomized women treated for 3 to 11 y *377*

Thyroid Stimulating Hormone
Serum No Effect Physiological Insignificant difference in 19 post-menopausal women receiving mean of 24 µg/d versus controls *31*

Thyroxine Binding Globulin *Serum Increase Physiological* From 24 to 47 mg/L in 19 post-menopausal women receiving mean of 24 µg/d versus controls *31*

Thyroxine (T4) *Serum Increase Physiological* From 100 to 133 nmol/L in 19 post-menopausal women receiving mean of 24 µg/d versus controls *31*

Thyroxine (T4), Free *Serum Decrease Physiological* From 19.2 to 15.7 pmol/L in 19 post-menopausal women receiving mean of 24 µg/d versus controls *31*

Transferrin *Serum Increase Physiological* Maximum effect 1 week after treatment *2719*

Tri-iodothyronine (T3) *Serum Increase Physiological* From 2.22 to 2.72 nmol/L in 19 post-menopausal women receiving mean of 24 µg/d versus controls *31*

Triglycerides *Serum Increase Physiological* ?Impaired triglyceride removal from circulation *5869*

Tyrosine *Plasma Decrease Physiological* Effect of both estrogen and progestogen *1313*

Metahexamide

Alanine Aminotransferase *Serum Increase Physiological* Hepatotoxicity (viral hepatitis type) *3810*

Alkaline Phosphatase *Serum Increase Physiological* Hepatotoxicity (viral hepatitis type) *3810*

Aspartate Aminotransferase *Serum Increase Physiological* Hepatotoxicity (viral hepatitis type) *3810*

Bile *Urine Increase Physiological* Hepatotoxicity (viral hepatitis type) *3810*

Bilirubin *Serum Increase Physiological* Hepatotoxicity (viral hepatitis type) *3810*

BSP Retention *Serum Increase Physiological* Hepatotoxicity (viral hepatitis type) *3810*

Protein *Urine Increase Analytical* Interference by drug metabolite *1714 6284*

Metamizole

Albumin *Urine No Effect Analytical* Using a fluorimetric assay with Albumin Blue 580 on a Cobas Fara centrifugal analyzer for the detection of microalbuminuria no significant interference was detected at a concentration of 100 mg/L *3117*

Metaoxedrine

Histamine *Plasma No Effect Analytical* 50% inhibition of radio-enzyme assay observed at 27 µg/mL but unlikely to be of clinical significance *2492*

Metaproterenol

Sugar *Urine Increase Analytical* Interferes with Benedict's reagent *1714*

Theophylline *Serum No Effect Analytical* At concentration of 15 mg/L produced no interference with methods used on Kodak DT60, Abbott TDx, Abbott Vision with either whole blood or serum, 3M Diagnostics TheoFAST, Syntex AccµLevl or Ames Seralyzer *1122*

Metaraminol

Histamine *Plasma No Effect Analytical* No evidence of clinically significant inhibition of radio-enzyme assay *2492*

Metaxalone

Alanine Aminotransferase *Serum Increase Physiological* Hepatotoxic effect *3810*

Alkaline Phosphatase *Serum Increase Physiological* Hepatotoxic effect *3810*

Aspartate Aminotransferase *Serum Increase Physiological* Hepatotoxic effect *3810*

Bile *Urine Increase Physiological* Hepatotoxic effect *3810*

Bilirubin *Serum Increase Physiological* Hepatotoxic effect *3810*

BSP Retention *Serum Increase Physiological* Hepatotoxic effect *1714*

Glucose *Urine No Effect Analytical* No effect on glucose oxidase methods *2452*

Protein *Urine Increase Physiological* May have nephrotoxic effect *1714*

Sugar *Urine Increase Analytical* False positive with copper reduction procedures. False positive with Benedict's, Fehling's reactions *5869*

Metformin

Albumin *Urine No Effect Analytical* Using a fluorimetric assay with Albumin Blue 580 on a Cobas Fara centrifugal analyzer for the detection of microalbuminuria no significant interference was detected at a concentration of 340 mg/L *3117*

Amino-4-Imidazole-5-Carboxamide Ribotide
Urine Increase Physiological May cause megaloblastic anemia *6050*

Androgen Index, Free (FAI)
Plasma Decrease Physiological In 26 women with polycystic ovary syndrome treatment with 1.5 g/d for 8 weeks caused significant decrease from mean baseline of 6.02 ± 4.1 to 2.09 ± 1.8 *6221*

Androstanediol Glucuronide
Plasma No Effect Physiological In 12 hirsute, obese women treatment with up to 1700 mg/d caused a nonsignificant change from mean baseline of 8.26 ± 2.15 nmol/L to 7.54 ± 1.60 nmol/L after 4 months *1161*

Androstenedione *Plasma Decrease Physiological* In 26 women with polycystic ovary syndrome treatment with 1.5 g/d for 8 weeks caused significant decrease from mean baseline of 1.76 ± 0.6 ng/mL to 1.15 ± 0.4 ng/mL *6221*

δ_4-Androstenedione *Plasma Decrease Physiological* In 12 hirsute, obese women treatment with up to 1700 mg/d caused a significant change from mean baseline of 6.21 ± 0.76 nmol/L to 4.08 ± 0.38 nmol/L after 4 months *1161*

Apolipoprotein A-I *Serum Decrease Physiological* Non-significant reduction from mean baseline placebo concentration of 1.45 mg/dL to 1.39 mg/dL in 24 nondiabetic patients with type IIb hyperlipidemia treated with 2.0 g/d for 9 weeks *4598*
Serum Increase Physiological In 26 women with polycystic ovary syndrome treatment with 1.5 g/d for 8 weeks caused significant increase from mean baseline of 120 ± 14 mg/dL to 126 ± 12 mg/dL *6221*
Serum No Effect Physiological Nonsignificant increase from mean baseline of 140 mg/dL to 142 mg/dL at 4 weeks, 151 mg/dL at 8 and 12 weeks in 40 patients with NIDDM and hyperlipoproteinemia when treated with metformin *5362* In 12 hirsute, obese women treatment with up to 1700 mg/d caused a nonsignificant change from mean baseline of 1.23 ± 0.06 g/L to 1.30 ± 0.09 g/L after 2 months and 1.29 ± 0.08 g/L after 4 months *1161*

Apolipoprotein A-II *Serum No Effect Physiological* No significant change from mean baseline of 55 mg/dL observed in 40 patients with NIDDM and hyperlipoproteinemia when treated with metformin for 12 weeks *5362*

Apolipoprotein B *Serum No Effect Physiological* In 12 hirsute, obese women treatment with up to 1700 mg/d caused a nonsignificant change from mean baseline of 1.06 ± 0.06 g/L to 1.02 ± 0.04 g/L after 2 months and 1.13 ± 0.08 g/L after 4

Metformin *(continued)*

Apolipoprotein B *(continued)*
months *1161* In 26 women with polycystic ovary syndrome treatment with 1.5 g/d for 8 weeks caused nonsignificant reduction from mean baseline of 79 ± 13 mg/dL to 73 ± 11 mg/dL *6221* No significant change observed from mean baseline of 104 mg/dL in 40 patients with NIDDM and hyperlipoproteinemia when treated with metformin for 12 weeks *5362* Nonsignificant increase from mean placebo concentration of 1.28 mg/dL to 1.32 mg/dL in 24 nondiabetic type IIb hyperlipidemic patients treated with 2.0 g/d for 9 weeks *4598*

Bicarbonate *Serum Decrease Physiological* May cause marked acidosis (lactic acidosis) *1714*

Carotene *Serum Decrease Physiological* Probably associated with malabsorption *6050*

Cholesterol *Serum Decrease Physiological* In 143 obese patients with NIDDM treatment with 2550 mg/d for 29 weeks caused significant reduction from 211 ± 3 mg/dL to 201 ± 4 mg/dL *1345* Significant reduction from mean baseline of 242 mg/dL to 232 mg/dL at 4 weeks and 8 weeks, and 233 mg/dL at 12 weeks in 40 patients with NIDDM and hyperlipoproteinemia treated for 12 weeks *5362* In 12 normotensive patients with NIDDM treatment for 4 weeks caused significant mean decrease of 0.7 mmol/L from mean baseline of 5.4 ± 0.2 mmol/L *959* Significant reduction observed in the absence of change in plasma insulin concentration in 6 noninsulin-dependent diabetics treated with 1700 mg/d for 4 weeks *4948* Significant reduction observed in 24 nondiabetics with type iib hyperlipidemia treated with 2.0 g/d for 9 weeks with reduction from mean of 8.54 mmol/L to 7.79 mmol/L but reduction not significant when 1 g/d given instead *4598* Significant reduction observed in 24 nondiabetics with type IIB hyperlipidemia treated with 2.0 g/d for 9 weeks with reduction from mean of 8.54 mmol/L to 7.79 mmol/L but reduction not significant when 1 g/d given instead *4598* Treatment with 3 g/d in 28 noninsulin-dependent diabetics caused mean decrease of 0.24 mmol/L at 4 months and 0.07 mmol/L at 6 months *2570*
Serum No Effect Physiological No correlation between serum concentration of drug and concentration of analyte in 20 type II diabetics *3786* In 26 women with polycystic ovary syndrome treatment with 1.5 g/d for 8 weeks caused nonsignificant reduction from mean baseline of 207 ± 56 mg/dL to 204 ± 40 mg/dL *6221* In 12 hirsute, obese women treatment with up to 1700 mg/d caused a nonsignificant change from mean baseline of 4.8 ± 0.2 mmol/L to 4.5 ± 0.2 mmol/L after 2 months and 4.9 ± 0.2 mmol/L after 4 months *1161* In 68 type II diabetic patients treated with sulfonylureas addition of metformin to regime for 6 months caused a nonsignificant change in concentration from mean baseline of 218.07 ± 9.32 mg/dL to 206.63 ± 8.73 mg/dL *2323* No effect although phenformin causes decrease *2452*

Cimetidine *Serum No Effect Physiological* In both single and multiple dose studies during which cimetidine and metformin were coadministered metformin appeared to have no effect on the pharmacokinetics of cimetidine *726*

Clot Retraction *Blood No Effect Physiological* No change observed in 24 nondiabetic patients with type IIb hyperlipidemia treated with 2.0 g/d for 9 weeks when compared with values with placebo *4598*

C-Peptide *Plasma No Effect Physiological* In 68 type II diabetic patients treated with sulfonylureas addition of metformin to regime for 6 months caused a nonsignificant reduction in concentration from mean baseline of 1.05 ± 0.23 ng/mL to 0.97 ± 0.18 ng/mL *2323*

Creatinine *Serum No Effect Analytical* At 2 g/L on reversed phase liquid chromatographic procedure of Zhiri et al *6656*
Serum No Effect Physiological Nonsignificant change from mean placebo baseline concentration of 79.6 μmol/L to 78.6 μmol/L in 24 nondiabetic patients with type IIb hyperlipidemia treated with 2.0 g/d for 9 weeks *4598*

Dehydroepiandrosterone Sulfate
Plasma Decrease Physiological In 26 women with polycystic ovary syndrome treatment with 1.5 g/d for 8 weeks caused significant decrease from mean baseline of 250 ± 112 μg/mL to 189 ± 89 μg/mL *6221*
Plasma Increase Physiological In 12 hirsute, obese women treatment with up to 1700 mg/d caused a significant change from mean baseline of 6.35 ± 0.44 μmol/L to 7.25 ± 0.47 μmol/L after 4 months *1161*

Estradiol *Plasma No Effect Physiological* In 26 women with polycystic ovary syndrome treatment with 1.5 g/d for 8 weeks caused nonsignificant change from mean baseline of 45.3 ± 18 pg/mL to 45.2 ± 27 pg/mL *6221*

Euglobulin Fibrinolytic Activity
Plasma Increase Physiological Activity lower in obese women than in control women (4.95 mm versus 9.0 mm) but after 15 days with 1.7 g/day increased to 6.5 mm *6149*

Fatty Acids (FFA), Free *Serum Decrease Physiological* In 68 type II diabetic patients treated with sulfonylureas addition of metformin to regime for 6 months caused a nonsignificant change in concentration from mean baseline of 682.2 ± 22.06 μmol/L to 607.2 ± 19.4 μmol/L after 3 months and 622.6 ± 18.3 μmol/L after 6 months *2323* In 9 patients with NIDDM treatment with 2.5 g/d for 3 months caused significant reduction in mean hourly concentration from 502 ± 45 μmol/L to 460 ± 35 μmol/L *2673* Significant reduction observed in 6 noninsulin-dependent diabetics treated with 1700 mg/d for 4 weeks. Plasma turnover rate and oxidation also lower after metformin *4948*
Serum No Effect Physiological No change observed in 24 nondiabetic patients with type IIb hyperlipidemia treated with 2.0 g/d for 9 weeks *4598*

Fibrinogen *Plasma No Effect Physiological* Nonsignificant increase from mean placebo concentration of 26.8 g/L to 27.3 g/L in 24 nondiabetic patients with type IIb hyperlipidemia treated with 2.0 g/d for 9 weeks *4598*

Folate *Serum Decrease Physiological* Due to decreased absorption of dietary folate *493*
Serum Increase Physiological High in patients if B_{12} malabsorption *6050*
Serum No Effect Physiological In 143 obese patients with NIDDM treatment with 2550 mg/d for 29 weeks caused nonsignificant change from mean baseline *1345* In controlled clinical trials of 29 weeks duration no significant effect on serum folic acid concentration observed although serum vitamin B_{12} concentration reduced in 9% patients *726*

Follicle Stimulating Hormone
Plasma Increase Physiological In 26 women with polycystic ovary syndrome treatment with 1.5 g/d for 8 weeks caused significant increase from mean baseline of 7.9 ± 4.4 mIU/mL to 10.3 ± 4.0 mIU/mL *6221*
Plasma No Effect Physiological In 20 obese women with polycystic ovary syndrome and hyperandrogenemia treatment with up to 2550 mg/d for 12 weeks caused nonsignificant change from mean baseline of 9.2 ± 1.8 IU/L to 9.3 ± 2.9 IU/L *1673*

Fructosamine *Serum No Effect Physiological* In 12 normotensive patients with NIDDM treatment for 4 weeks caused nonsignificant mean decrease of 0.6 mmol/L from mean baseline of 329 ± 11 mmol/L *959*

Furosemide *Serum Decrease Physiological* In a single dose study during which furosemde and metformin were coadministered the maximun concentration and AUC of furosemide were decreased by 31% and 12% respectively *726*

Glucagon *Plasma No Effect Physiological* In 10 healthy obese patients with NIDDM treatment with 2550 mg/d for 12 weeks caused no significant change from mean baseline of 108 ± 21 pg/mL to 112 ± 13 pg/mL *5854*

Glucose *Serum Decrease Physiological* During metformin treatment of 15 type II diabetics for 3 months blood glucose concentration decreased by 3.2 mmol/L (20%) *2827* In 6 noninsulin-dependent diabetics 4 weeks treatment with 1700 mg/d caused significant reduction in the absence of a change in plasma insulin concentration. Glucose oxidation increased *4948* In 10 healthy obese patients with NIDDM treatment with 2550 mg/d for 12 weeks caused significant reduction from mean baseline of 220 ± 41 mg/dL to 155 ± 28 mg/dL *5854* Nonsignificant reduction from mean baseline placebo concentration of 4.99 mmol/L to 4.74 mmol/L in 24 nondiabetic patients with type IIb hyperlipidemia treated with 2.0 g/d for 9 weeks *4598* In 12 normotensive patients with NIDDM treatment for 4 weeks caused decrease from mean baseline of 10.5 ± 0.7 mmol/L by average of 2.2 mmol/L *959* In 9 patients with NIDDM treatment with 2.5 g/d for 3 months caused significant reduction of mean hourly blood glucose concentration from 7.5

± 0.5 mmol/L to 6.5 ± 0.4 mmol/L *2673* In 68 type II diabetic patients treated with sulfonylureas addition of metformin to regime for 6 months caused a significant reduction in plasma glucose concentration from mean baseline of 219.13 ± 6.78 mg/dL to 155.64 ± 4.15 mg/dL *2323* Mode of action uncertain (occurs with overdose) *1952* In 143 obese patients with NIDDM treatment with 2550 mg/d for 29 weeks caused significant reduction to below 140 mg/dL in 22% of the patients *1345* Incidence of 5.2% observed in French Pharmacovigilance database *4106* In 143 obese patients with NIDDM treatment with 2550 mg/d for 29 weeks caused significant reduction of 52 ± 5 mg/dL from mean baseline of 241 ± 5 mg/dL *1345* Hypoglycemia does not usually occur when metformin administered alone, but could occur when caloric intake is insufficient, or when strenuous exercise is not compensated for by increased caloric intake *726*

Serum No Effect Analytical No effect at 10 mmol/L on glucokinase based assay of Scott *5414*

Serum No Effect Physiological Hypoglycemia does not usually occur when metformin administered alone, but could occur when caloric intake is insufficient, or when strenuous exercise is not compensated for by increased caloric intake *726* In 12 hirsute, obese women treatment with up to 1700 mg/d caused a nonsignificant change from mean baseline of 4.94 ± 0.15 mmol/L to 5.1 ± 0.1 mmol/L after 2 months and 4.9 ± 0.1 mmol/L after 4 months *1161*

Glucose Tolerance *Serum Increase Physiological* Mode of action uncertain *1952* In 143 obese patients with NIDDM treatment with 2550 mg/d for 29 weeks caused significant reduction of mean glucose after glucose ingestion from 347 ± 7 mg/dL to 275 ± 7 mg/dL *1345*

Glyburide *Serum Decrease Physiological* When metformin coadministered with glyburide its AUC and plasma concentration reduced but to a variable extent *4676* In a single dose study during which glyburide and metformin were coadministered highly variable decrease of AUC and maximum concentration of glyburide observed *726*

Glycated Hemoglobin *Blood Decrease Physiological* In 9 patients with NIDDM treatment with 2.5 g/d for 3 months caused significant reduction from mean baseline of 7.0 ± 0.5% to 6.2 ± 0.2% *2673* In 143 obese patients with NIDDM treatment with 2550 mg/d for 29 weeks caused significant reduction of 1.4 ± 0.1% from mean baseline of 8.4 ± 0.1% *1345* In 10 healthy obese patients with NIDDM treatment with 2550 mg/d for 12 weeks caused significant reduction from mean baseline of 13.2 ± 2.2% to 10.5 ± 1.6% *5854*

Blood No Effect Physiological During metformin treatment of 15 type II diabetics for 3 months no significant effect observed on glycated hemoglobin concentration *2827*

HDL_2-Apolipoprotein A-I *Serum No Effect Physiological* Nonsignificant increase from mean baseline of 30 mg/dL to 37 mg/dL after 12 weeks treatment with metformin in 40 patients with NIDDM and hyperlipoproteinemia *5362*

HDL_2-Apolipoprotein A-II *Serum No Effect Physiological* No significant change from mean baseline concentration of 14 mg/dL observed in 40 patients with NIDDM and hyperlipoproteinemia when treated with metformin for 12 weeks *5362*

HDL_2-Cholesterol *Serum Increase Physiological* Nonsignificant increase from placebo baseline concentration of 0.64 mmol/L to 0.72 mmol/L after 9 weeks treatment with 2.0 g/d in 24 nondibetics with type IIb hyperlipidemia *4598* Significant correlation between serum concentration of drug and concentration of analyte in 20 type II diabetics *3786*

Serum No Effect Physiological No significant change from mean baseline of 24 mg/dL observed in 40 patients with NIDDM and hyperlipoproteinemia when treated with metformin for 12 weeks *5362*

HDL_2-Phospholipids *Serum No Effect Physiological* Nonsignificant reduction from mean baseline of 41 mg/dL to 37 mg/dL after 12 weeks treatment with metformin in 40 patients with NIDDM and hyperlipoproteinemia *5362*

HDL_2-Triglycerides *Serum No Effect Physiological* No significant change from mean baseline of 11 mg/dL observed in 40 patients with NIDDM and hyperlipoproteinemia when treated with metformin for 12 weeks *5362*

HDL_3-Cholesterol *Serum Decrease Physiological* Nonsignificant reduction from mean baseline of 0.49 mmol/L to 0.46 mmol/L in 24 nondiabetic patients with type IIb hyperlipidemia treated with 2.0 g/d for 9 weeks *4598*

Serum No Effect Physiological No correlation between serum concentration of drug in 20 type II diabetics and concentration of analyte *3786*

HDL-Apolipoprotein A-I *Serum Increase Physiological* Significant increase from mean baseline of 98 mg/dL to 110 mg/dL in 40 patients with NIDDM and hyperlipoproteinemia when treated with metformin for 12 weeks *5362*

HDL-Apolipoprotein A-II *Serum Increase Physiological* Significant increase from mean baseline of 39 mg/dL to 44 mg/dL in 40 patients with NIDDM and hyperlipoproteinemia when treated with metformin for 12 weeks *5362*

HDL-Cholesterol *Serum Increase Physiological* Slight increase observed *2569* In 68 type II diabetic patients treated with sulfonylureas addition of metformin to regime for 6 months caused a significant change in concentration from mean baseline of 47.16 ± 2.28 mg/dL to 49.32 ± 1.90 mg/dL *2323* In 9 patients with NIDDM treatment with 2.5 g/d for 3 months caused significant increase in concentration *2673* Significant increase observed in 12 patients with noninsulin dependent diabetes treated for 4 months *6548* Significant positive correlation between serum concentration of drug and analyte concentration in 20 type II diabetics *3786* Nonsignificant increase from 1.13 mmol/L to 1.18 mmol/L in 24 nondiabetics with type IIb hyperlipidemia treated with 2.0 g/d for 9 weeks with no change at all observed when 1.0 g/d administered *4598*

Serum No Effect Physiological In 26 women with polycystic ovary syndrome treatment with 1.5 g/d for 8 weeks caused nonsignificant increase from mean baseline of 44 ± 11 mg/dL to 50 ± 11 mg/dL *6221* In 12 normotensive patients with NIDDM treatment for 4 weeks caused nonsignificant mean decrease of 0.02 mmol/L from mean baseline of 1.3 ± 0.1 mmol/L *959* No significant change observed from mean baseline of 47 mg/dL observed in 40 patients with NIDDM and hyperlipoproteinemia when treated with metformin for 12 weeks *5362* In 12 hirsute, obese women treatment with up to 1700 mg/d caused a nonsignificant change from mean baseline of 0.92 ± 0.05 mmol/L to 0.99 ± 0.07 mmol/L after 2 months and 0.98 ± 0.05 mmol/L after 4 months *1161* In 143 obese patients with NIDDM treatment with 2550 mg/d for 29 weeks caused nonsignificant change from 39 ± 1 mg/dL to 40 ± 1 mg/dL *1345*

HDL-Phospholipids *Serum No Effect Physiological* Nonsignificant reduction from mean baseline of 89 mg/dL to 84 mg/dL after 12 weeks treatment with metformin in 40 patients with NIDDM and hyperlipoproteinemia *5362*

HDL-Triglycerides *Serum No Effect Physiological* Nonsignificant reduction from mean baseline of 24 mg/dL to 19 mg/dL in 40 patients with NIDDM and hyperlipoproteinemia when treated with metformin for 12 weeks *5362* In 68 type II diabetic patients treated with sulfonylureas addition of metformin to regime for 6 months caused a nonsignificant change in concentration from mean baseline of 18.96 ± 1.63 mg/dL to 18.87 ± 1.76 mg/dL *2323* Nonsignificant reduction from mean placebo concentration of 0.15 mmol/L to 0.14 mmol/L in 24 nondiabetic patients with type IIb hyperlipidemia treated with 2.0 g/d for 9 weeks *4598*

Hematocrit *Blood Decrease Physiological* May be associated with megaloblastic anemia *6050*

Hemoglobin *Blood Decrease Physiological* Associated with impaired B_{12} absorption *6050*

Hemoglobin A_{1c} *Blood Decrease Physiological* In 68 type II diabetic patients treated with sulfonylureas addition of metformin to regime for 6 months caused a significant reduction in concentration from mean baseline of 9.98 ± 0.19% to 8.02 ± 0.18% *2323* Significant reduction observed in 6 noninsulin-dependent diabetics treated with 1700 mg/d for 4 weeks without change in insulin concentration *4948*

Blood No Effect Physiological In 12 normotensive patients with NIDDM treatment for 4 weeks caused nonsignificant mean decrease of 0.2% from mean baseline of 7.5 ± 0.2% *959*

Histamine *Plasma No Effect Analytical* Improbable inhibition of radio-enzyme assay at therapeutic concentrations *2492*

Ibuprofen *Serum No Effect Physiological* In single dose studies during which ibuprofen and metformin were coadministered metformin appeared to have no effect on the pharmacokinetics of ibuprofen *726*

Insulin *Plasma Decrease Physiological* Nonsignificant reduction from mean baseline placebo concentration of 15.8 mU/L to 14.1 mU/L after 9 weeks treatment with 2.0 g/d in 24

Metformin *(continued)*

Insulin *(continued)*
nondiabetic patients with type IIb hyperlipidemia *4598* Significant decrease from 24.5 to 18.5 µU/mL in obese women following treatment with 1.7 g/day for 15 days *6149* Slight efect with all hyperlipoproteinemias but marked with type IV hyperlipoproteinemia *2374* In 9 patients with NIDDM treatment with 2.5 g/d caused significant reduction in mean hourly concentration from 519 ± 81 pmol/L to 364 ± 64 pmol/L *2673* In 12 hirsute, obese women treatment with up to 1700 mg/d caused a significant change from mean baseline of 166 ± 21 pmol/L to 146 ± 18 pmol/L after 2 months and 124 ± 16 pmol/L after 4 months *1161* In 10 healthy obese patients with NIDDM treatment with 2550 mg/d for 12 weeks caused no significant change from mean baseline of 12 ± 5 µU/mL to 10 ± 3 µU/mL *5854*
Plasma *No Effect* *Physiological* In 68 type II diabetic patients treated with sulfonylureas addition of metformin to regime for 6 months caused a nonsignificant reduction in concentration from mean baseline of 31.68 ± 3.48 µU/mL to 29.27 ± 3.11 µU/mL *2323*

Iron *Serum* *Decrease* *Physiological* Associated with impaired B_{12} absorption *6050*

6-Keto-Prostaglandin $F_{1\alpha}$ *Urine* *No Effect* *Physiological* Nonsignificant reduction from mean placebo concentration of 0.20 µg/L to 0.19 µg/L in 24 nondiabetic patients with type IIb hyperlipidemia treated with 2.0 g/d for 9 weeks *4598*

Ketones *Urine* *Increase* *Physiological* Associated with lactic acidosis *1714*

Lactate *Plasma* *Increase* *Physiological* Lactic acidosis observed is a rare but serious metabolic complication of metformin treatment, generally with metformin concentrations greater than 5 mmol/L *726* Possibly always with predisposing condition *3454*
Plasma *No Effect* *Physiological* In 143 obese patients with NIDDM treatment with 2550 mg/d for 29 weeks caused nonsignificant change from 1.41 ± 0.04 mmol/L to 1.46 ± 0.05 mmol/L *1345* Nonsignificant increase in blood lactate concentration from mean baseline concentration of 1.16 mmol/L to 1.24 mmol/L in 24 nondiabetic patients with type IIb hyperlipidemia treated with 2.0 g/d for 9 weeks *4598* In 10 healthy obese patients with NIDDM treatment with 2550 mg/d for 12 weeks caused nonsignificant change from mean baseline of 1.06 ± 0.32 mmol/L to 0.99 ± 0.28 mmol/L *5854* In 68 type II diabetic patients treated with sulfonylureas addition of metformin to regime for 6 months caused a nonsignificant change in concentration from mean baseline of 1.39 ± 0.18 mmol/L to 1.40 ± 0.21 mmol/L *2323*

LDL-Apolipoprotein B *Serum* *No Effect* *Physiological* No significant change from mean baseline of 72 mg/dL in 40 patients with NIDDM and hyperlipoproteinemia when treated with metformin for 12 weeks *5362*

LDL-Cholesterol *Serum* *Decrease* *Physiological* Mean decrease of 0.13 mmol/L after 4 months and 0.02 mmol/L after 6 months in 28 patients with noninsulin-dependent diabetes treated with 3 g daily *2570* Significant reduction from mean of 5.52 mmol/L to 4.88 mmol/L observed in 24 nondiabetics with type IIb hyperlipidemia treated with 2.0 g/d for 9 weeks but reduction not significant after 1.0 g/d for same time *4598* In 143 obese patients with NIDDM treatment with 2550 mg/d for 29 weeks caused significant reduction from 136 ± 3 mg/dL to 123 ± 3 mg/dL *1345* In 12 normotensive patients with NIDDM treatment for 4 weeks caused mean decrease of 0.5 mmol/L from mean baseline of 3.4 ± 0.2 mmol/L *959* In 68 type II diabetic patients treated with sulfonylureas addition of metformin to regime for 6 months caused a significant change in concentration from mean baseline of 184.63 ± 5.97 mg/dL to 172.46 ± 5.59 mg/dL *2323*
Serum *No Effect* *Physiological* In 26 women with polycystic ovary syndrome treatment with 1.5 g/d for 8 weeks caused nonsignificant change from mean baseline of 127 ± 44 mg/dL to 128 ± 35 mg/dL *6221* Nonsignificant increase from mean baseline of 133 mg/dL to 147 mg/dL in 40 patients with NIDDM and hyperlipoproteinemia when treated with metformin for 12 weeks *5362*

LDL-Phospholipids *Serum* *Increase* *Physiological* Significant increase from mean baseline of 96 mg/dL in 40 patients with NIDDM and hyperlipoproteinemia to 106 mg/dL at 8 weeks and 107 mg/dL at 12 weeks when treated with metformin *5362*

LDL-Triglycerides *Serum* *Decrease* *Physiological* Significant reduction from mean placebo concentration of 0.55 mmol/L to 0.41 mmol/L following treatment for 9 weeks with 2.0 g/d in 24 nondiabetic patients with type IIb hyperlipidemia *4598*
Serum *No Effect* *Physiological* In 68 type II diabetic patients treated with sulfonylureas addition of metformin to regime for 6 months caused a nonsignificant change in concentration from mean baseline of 39.83 ± 2.13 mg/dL to 39.45 ± 1.95 mg/dL *2323* Nonsignificant reduction from mean baseline of 56 mg/dL to 45 mg/dL after 12 weeks treatment with metformin in 40 patients with NIDDM and hyperlipoproteinemia *5362*

Lipoprotein Lp(a) *Serum* *No Effect* *Physiological* In 68 type II diabetic patients treated with sulfonylureas addition of metformin to regime for 6 months caused a nonsignificant change in concentration from mean baseline of 18.42 mg/dL to 18.83 mg/dL *2323*

Luteinizing Hormone *Plasma* *Decrease* *Physiological* In 26 women with polycystic ovary syndrome treatment with 1.5 g/d for 8 weeks caused significant reduction from mean baseline of 17.3 ± 8.3 mIU/mL to 9.7 ± 5.6 mIU/mL *6221*
Plasma *No Effect* *Physiological* In 20 obese women with polycystic ovary syndrome and hyperandrogenemia treatment with up to 2550 mg/d for 12 weeks caused nonsignificant change from mean baseline of 11.1 ± 9.7 IU/L to 10.3 ± 9.5 IU/L *1673*

Luteinizing Hormone:Follicle Stimulating Hormone Ratio
Plasma *No Effect* *Physiological* In 20 obese women with polycystic ovary syndrome and hyperandrogenemia treatment with up to 2550 mg/d for 12 weeks caused nonsignificant change from mean baseline of 1.2 ± 0.9 to 1.2 ± 1.0 *1673*

MCV *Blood* *Increase* *Physiological* Occurs if megaloblastic anemia *6050*

N-Formiminoglutamic Acid *Urine* *Increase* *Physiological* May cause megaloblastic anemia *6050*

Nifedipine *Serum* *Decrease* *Physiological* In a single dose study during which nifedipine and metformin were coadministered metformin appeared to have minimal effect on the metabolism of nifedipine *726*

Non-Sex Hormone Binding Globulin-bound Testosterone
Serum *No Effect* *Physiological* In 12 hirsute, obese women treatment with up to 1700 mg/d caused a nonsignificant change from mean baseline of 0.22 ± 0.03 nmol/L to 0.19 ± 0.02 nmol/L after 4 months *1161*

Partial Thromboplastin Time
Plasma *No Effect* *Physiological* No change compared with placebo when given 2.0 g/d for 9 weeks in 24 nondiabetic patients with type IIb hyperlipidemia *4598*

Phenylalanine *Plasma* *No Effect* *Analytical* No interference observed with rapid quantitative whole blood method of Campbell et al using phenylalanine dehydrogenase *867*

Phospholipids *Serum* *No Effect* *Physiological* Nonsignificant reduction from mean baseline of 305 mg/dL to 284 mg/dL at 4 and 8 weeks, and 290 mg/dL at 12 weeks observed in 40 patients with NIDDM and hyperlipoproteinemia when treated with metformin *5362*

Plasminogen Activator Inhibitor Activity
Plasma *Decrease* *Physiological* Significant effect on plasminogen activator inhibitor capacity in obese women following 15 days treatment with 1.7 g/day for 15 days (decrease from 9.48 to 5.51) *6149*

Platelet Aggregation *Blood* *No Effect* *Physiological* No significant change compared with placebo in response to ADP, epinephrine and collagen in 24 nondiabetic patients with type IIb hyperlipidemia treated with 2.0 g/d for 9 weeks *4598*

Platelets *Blood* *Decrease* *Physiological* Nonsignificant reduction from placebo concentration of 205000 /µL to 190000 /µL in 24 nondiabetic patients with type IIb hyperlipidemia treated with 2.0 g/d for 9 weeks *4598*

Propranolol *Serum* *No Effect* *Physiological* In single dose studies during which propranolol and metformin were coadministered metformin appeared to have no effect on the pharmacokinetics of propranolol *726*

Prostaglandin E_2 *Urine* *Decrease* *Physiological* Nonsignificant reduction from mean placebo concentration of 1.55 µg/L to 1.31 µg/L in 24 nondiabetic patients with type IIb hyperlipidemia treated with 2.0 g/d for 9 weeks *4598*

Prostaglandin $F_{2\alpha}$ *Urine Decrease Physiological* Nonsignificant reduction from mean baseline placebo concentration of 0.18 µg/L to 0.16 µg/L in 24 nondiabetic patients with type IIb hyperlipidemia treated with 2.0 g/d for 9 weeks *4598*

Sex-Hormone Binding Globulin
Serum Decrease Physiological In 20 obese women with polycystic ovary syndrome and hyperandrogenemia treatment with up to 2550 mg/d for 12 weeks caused significant reduction from mean baseline of 13.8 ± 13.1 nmol/L to 8.7 ± 7.0 nmol/L *1673*
Serum Increase Physiological In 26 women with Polycystic Ovary Syndrome treatment with 1.5 g/d for 8 weeks caused significant increase from mean baseline of 40 ± 14 nmol/L to 52 ± 22 nmol/L *6221* In 12 hirsute, obese women treatment with up to 1700 mg/d caused a significant change from mean baseline of 17.6 ± 1.6 nmol/L to 21.6 ± 2.1 nmol/L after 4 months *1161*

Testosterone *Serum Decrease Physiological* In 26 women with polycystic ovary syndrome treatment with 1.5 g/d for 8 weeks caused significant decrease from mean baseline of 0.6 ± 0.3 ng/mL to 0.26 ± 0.16 ng/mL *6221* In 20 obese women with polycystic ovary syndrome and hyperandrogenemia treatment with up to 2550 mg/d for 12 weeks caused reduction from mean baseline of 83.3 ± 29.0 ng/dL to 68.4 ± 28.7 ng/dL *1673*
Serum No Effect Physiological In 12 hirsute, obese women treatment with up to 1700 mg/d caused a nonsignificant change from mean baseline of 1.18 ± 0.18 nmol/L to 1.2 ± 0.12 nmol/L after 4 months *1161*

Testosterone, Free *Serum Decrease Physiological* In 26 women with polycystic ovary syndrome treatment with 1.5 g/d for 8 weeks caused significant decrease from mean baseline of 11.3 ± 6.97 pg/mL to 4.24 ± 3.19 pg/mL *6221* In 20 obese women with polycystic ovary syndrome and hyperandrogenemia treatment with up to 2550 mg/d for 12 weeks caused reduction from mean baseline of 26.6 ± 12.7 pg/mL to 22.4 ± 9.8 pg/mL *1673*

Thromboxane B_2 *Urine No Effect Physiological* Nonsignificant decrease from mean placebo concentration of 0.26 µg/mL to 0.23 µg/mL in 24 nondiabetic patients with type IIb hyperlipidemia treated with 2.0 g/d for 9 weeks *4598*

Triglycerides *Serum Decrease Physiological* Significant negative correlation between serum concentration of drug and triglycerides concentration in 20 type II diabetics *3786* Significant effect observed in 12 patients with noninsulin-dependent diabetes mellitus treated for 4 months *6548* Significant reduction observed in 6 noninsulin-dependent diabetics treated with 1700 mg/d for 4 weeks *4948* Significant reduction from mean baseline of 340 mg/dL to 250 mg/dL at 4 weeks, 259 mg/dL at 8 weeks and 242 mg/dL at 12 weeks in 40 patients with NIDDM and hyperlipoproteinemia treated with metformin *5362* Average of 26% in type IV hyperlipoproteinemia *2374* In 9 patients with NIDDM treatment with 2.5 g/d for 3 months caused significant reduction in mean hourly concentration from 3.60 ± 0.33 mmol/L to 3.02 ± 0.31 mmol/L. Fasting concentration also significantly reduced *2673* Significant reduction in obese women from 1.47 mmol/L to 1.08 mmol/L following treatment with 1.7 g/day for 15 days *6149* Significant hypotriglyceridemic effect exerted in nondiabetic patients possibly related to reduced liver/intestinal biosynthesis of VLDL *5586*
Serum No Effect Physiological Nonsignificant reduction from 3.22 mmol/L to 2.76 mmol/L observed in 24 nondiabetic patients with type IIb hyperlipidemia treated with 2.0 g/d for 9 weeks *4598* In 26 women with polycystic ovary syndrome treatment with 1.5 g/d for 8 weeks caused nonsignificant reduction from mean of 176 ± 104 mg/dL to 134 ± 64 mg/dL *6221* In 143 obese patients with NIDDM treatment with 2550 mg/d for 29 weeks caused nonsignificant change from 209 ± 15 mg/dL to 193 ± 10 mg/dL *1345* In 12 normotensive patients with NIDDM treatment for one month caused nonsignificant decrease of 0.32 mmol/L from mean baseline of 1.5 ± 0.3 mmol/L *959* In 12 hirsute, obese women treatment with up to 1700 mg/d caused a nonsignificant change from mean baseline of 1.18 ± 0.20 mmol/L to 0.94 ± 0.11 mmol/L after 2 months and 1.04 ± 0.18 mmol/L after 4 months *1161* In 68 type II diabetic patients treated with sulfonylureas addition of metformin to regime for 6 months caused a nonsignificant change in concentration from mean baseline of 160.32 ± 13.27 mg/dL to 149.83 ± 12.84 mg/dL *2323*

Uric Acid *Serum No Effect Analytical* At 2 g/L on reversed phase liquid chromatographic procedure of Zhiri et al *6656*
Serum No Effect Physiological Insignificant increase from mean baseline placebo concentration of 3.26 µmol/L to 3.37 µmol/L in 24 nondiabetic patients with type IIb hyperlipidemia treated with 2.0 g/d for 9 weeks *4598*

Vitamin B_{12} *Serum Decrease Physiological* Due to impaired B_{12} absorption *6050* Reported to cause ileal malabsorption *5055* A decrease to subnormal concentrations without clinical manifestations may occur in approximately of 7% of patients treated with metformin as occurred in controlled clinical trials of 29 weeks duration, possibly due to interference with B_{12} absorption *726*
Serum No Effect Physiological In 143 obese patients with NIDDM treatment with 2550 mg/d for 29 weeks caused significant change of 22% from mean baseline *1345*
Urine Decrease Physiological May cause megaloblastic anemia *6050*

VLDL-Apolipoprotein B *Serum Decrease Physiological* Significant reduction from mean baseline of 15 mg/dL to 9 mg/dL at 4 weeks, 13 mg/dL at 8 weeks and 10 mg/dL at 12 weeks in 40 patients with NIDDM and hyperlipoproteinemia when treated with metformin *5362*

VLDL-Cholesterol *Serum Decrease Physiological* In 9 patients with NIDDM treatment with 2.5 g/d for 3 months caused significant reduction in concentration *2673* Nonsignificant decrease from mean placebo baseline of 1.83 mmol/L to 1.56 mmol/L in 24 nondiabetic patients with type IIb hyperlipidemia treated with 2.0 g/d for 9 weeks *4598* Significant reduction from mean baseline of 56 mg/dL to 38 mg/dL at 4 weeks, 35 mg/dL at 8 weeks and 34 mg/dL at 12 weeks in 40 patients with NIDDM and hyperlipoproteinemia when treated with metformin *5362*
Serum No Effect Physiological In 68 type II diabetic patients treated with sulfonylureas addition of metformin to regime for 6 months caused a nonsignificant change in concentration from mean baseline of 35.84 ± 2.83 mg/dL to 35.16 ± 2.46 mg/dL *2323*

VLDL-Phospholipids *Serum Decrease Physiological* Significant reduction from mean baseline of 68 mg/dL to 40 mg/dL at 4 and 8 weeks and 38 mg/dL at 12 weeks in 40 patients with NIDDM and hyperlipoproteinemia when treated with metformin *5362*

VLDL-Triglycerides *Serum Decrease Physiological* Significant reduction from mean baseline of 243 mg/dL to 173 mg/dL at 4 weeks, 186 mg/dL at 8 weeks and 170 mg/dL at 12 weeks in 40 patients with NIDDM and hyperlipoproteinemia when treated with metformin *5362* In 9 patients with NIDDM treatment for 3 months with 2.5 g/d caused significant reduction in concentration *2673* Nonsignificant reduction from mean placebo concentration of 2.54 mmol/L to 2.22 mmol/L in 24 nondiabetic patients with type iib hyperlipidemia treated with 2.0 g/d for 9 weeks *4598* Nonsignificant reduction from mean placebo concentration of 2.54 mmol/L to 2.22 mmol/L in 24 nondiabetic patients with type IIb hyperlipidemia treated with 2.0 g/d for 9 weeks *4598*
Serum No Effect Physiological In 68 type II diabetic patients treated with sulfonylureas addition of metformin to regime for 6 months caused a nonsignificant change in concentration from mean baseline of 152.61 ± 6.66 mg/dL to 148.31 ± 7.39 mg/dL *2323*

Xylose *Urine Decrease Physiological* Probably dose related malabsorption *6050*

Methacholine

Amylase *Serum Increase Physiological* Stimulates pancreatic secretion, constricts ampulla *2242* Pancreatic stimulation, constriction of ampulla *2024*

Aspartate Aminotransferase *Serum Increase Physiological* Impairs excretion by spasm of sphincter of Oddi *1009*

Bilirubin *Serum Increase Physiological* Impairs excretion through biliary tract *1009*

BSP Retention *Serum Increase Physiological* Impairs excretion by spasm of sphincter of Oddi *1009*

Epinephrine *Urine No Effect Physiological* No effect observed *467*

Lipase *Serum Increase Physiological* Constricts sphincter of Oddi *1009*

Methacholine *(continued)*

Norepinephrine *Urine Increase Physiological* Slight increase observed *467*

Methacycline

Alanine Aminotransferase *Serum Increase Physiological* Possible hepatotoxicity *128*

Aspartate Aminotransferase *Serum Increase Physiological* Possible hepatotoxicity *128*

Eosinophils *Blood Increase Physiological* May cause allergic response *2754*

Erythrocytes *Blood Decrease Physiological* May cause hemolytic anemia *2754*

Neutrophils *Blood Decrease Physiological* Neutropenia reported *2754*

Platelets *Blood Decrease Physiological* Thrombocytopenia may occur *2754*

Urea Nitrogen *Serum Increase Physiological* Possible nephrotoxicity *128*

Methadol

Methadone *Urine No Effect Analytical* Significant cross-reactivity of 120% observed with Roche Abuscreen ONTRAK method *3279*

Methadone

Acetaminophen *Serum No Effect Analytical* No interference observed with methadone hydrochloride at a concentration of 2000 µg/mL (572 µmol/L) with method on Du Pont aca *1506*

Activated T Lymphocytes *Blood Increase Physiological* Mean proportion in 54 methadone treated HIV positive drug users 11.9 ± 7.2% and 4.5 ± 5.4% in 52 HIV negative drug users significantly higher than 9.9 ± 6.5% and 3.6 ± 2.3% in 67 untreated HIV positive and 47 HIV negative drug users respectively *883*

Blood No Effect Physiological Mean concentration in 54 methadone treated HIV positive drug users 217.8 ± 176.8 /µL and 104.2 ± 292.5 /µL in 52 HIV negative drug users not significantly different from 184.0 ± 156.4 /µL and 90.3 ± 61.2 /µL in 67 untreated HIV positive and 47 HIV negative drug users respectively *883*

Alanine Aminotransferase *Serum No Effect Analytical* At acute overdose concentration (2.5 mg/dL) on Technicon SMAC® method *6266*

Serum No Effect Physiological No toxicity if liver function tests normal initially *3282*

Albumin *Serum No Effect Analytical* At concentration of 25 mg/L had no effect on BCG method *5704* At acute overdose concentration (2.5 mg/dL) on Technicon SMAC® method *6266*

Alkaline Phosphatase *Serum No Effect Analytical* At acute overdose concentration (2.5 mg/dL) on Technicon SMAC® method *6266*

Serum No Effect Physiological No toxicity if liver function tests normal initially *3282*

Amphetamine *Urine No Effect Analytical* Negative result observed with Du Pont aca at a concentration of 1000 µg/L (3.23 mmol/L) *1554*

Aspartate Aminotransferase *Serum No Effect Analytical* At acute overdose concentration (2.5 mg/dL) on Technicon SMAC® method *6266*

Serum No Effect Physiological No evidence of toxicity if initially normal liver function test *3282*

Barbiturate *Urine No Effect Analytical* Negative result obtained at a concentration of 1000 µg/mL (3.23 mmol/L) with method on Du Pont aca *1555*

Benzodiazepine *Urine No Effect Analytical* Negative result observed at a concentration of 1000 µg/mL (3.23 mmol/L) with method on Du Pont aca *1556*

Benzoylecgonine *Urine No Effect Analytical* Negative result obtained at a concentration of 500 µg/mL (1.61 mmol/L) with method on Du Pont aca *1558* No significant interference observed at a concentration of 1615 µmol/L with Sung and Neely modification of Syva EMIT procedure *148*

Bilirubin *Serum No Effect Analytical* At acute overdose concentration (2.5 mg/dL) on Technicon SMAC® method *6266* At concentration of 25 mg/L had no effect on Jendrassik and Grof method *5704*

Serum No Effect Physiological No toxicity if liver function tests normal initially *3282*

BSP Retention *Serum Increase Physiological* Hepatotoxic effect or spasm of sphincter of Oddi *6515*

Calcium *Serum No Effect Analytical* At concentration of 25 mg/L had no effect on cresolphthalein method *5704* At acute overdose concentration (2.5 mg/dL) on Technicon SMAC® method *6266*

Cannabinoids *Urine No Effect Analytical* No effect on Roche Abuscreen method *5006*

Carbon Dioxide Partial Pressure
Blood Increase Physiological May cause diminished pulmonary ventilation *2242*

CD4⁺:CD8⁺ Lymphocyte Ratio
Blood Decrease Physiological Mean ratio in 54 methadone treated HIV positive drug users 0.42 ± 0.34 and 1.38 ± 0.57 in 52 HIV negative drug users significantly lower than 0.55 ± 0.39 and 1.82 ± 0.72 in 67 untreated HIV positive and 47 HIV negative drug users respectively *883*

CD4⁺ Lymphocytes *Blood Decrease Physiological* In 52 HIV negative drug users treated with methadone mean proportion of lymphocytes 40.0 ± 7.9% and in 54 HIV positive drug users mean proportion 19.7 ± 11.1% significantly different from 45.5 ± 7.2% in 47 untreated HIV negative drug users and 24.1 ± 10.6% in 67 HIV positive drug users *883*

Blood No Effect Physiological In 52 HIV negative drug users treated with methadone mean concentration 1040 ± 342 /µL and in 54 HIV positive drug users mean concentration 377 ± 311/µL not significantly different from 1110 ± 345 /µL in 47 untreated HIV negative drug users and 440 ± 267 /µL in 67 HIV positive drug users *883*

CD8⁺ Lymphocytes *Blood Increase Physiological* Mean concentration in 54 methadone treated HIV positive drug users 1017 ± 546 /µL (55.2 ± 13.8%) and 920 ± 577 /µL (32.5 ± 9.8%) in 52 HIV negative drug users significantly higher than 930 ± 578 /µL (49.5 ± 12.0%) and 693 ± 336 /µL (27.6 ± 7.7%) in 67 untreated HIV positive and 47 HIV negative drug users respectively *883*

Chloride *Serum No Effect Analytical* At concentration of 7 mg/L had no effect on mercurimetric method *5704*

Cholesterol *Serum No Effect Analytical* At acute overdose concentration (2.5 mg/dL) on Technicon SMAC® method *6266* At concentration of 25 mg/L had no effect on Liebermann-Burchard method *5704*

Chromosomes *Test Conditions No Effect Physiological* No effect on human leucocytes at concentrations 1/6-3 times normal *1790*

Cocaethylene *Urine No Effect Analytical* No interference observed with TLC method of Bailey *328*

Cortisol *Plasma Increase Physiological* Significant response to cold not seen in controls *4915*

Creatine Kinase *Serum No Effect Analytical* At acute overdose concentration (2.5 mg/dL) on Technicon SMAC® method *6266*

Creatinine *Serum No Effect Analytical* At acute overdose concentration (2.5 mg/dL) on Technicon SMAC® method *6266* At concentration of 25 mg/L had no effect on Technicon AutoAnalyzer® Jaffe method *5704*

Doxepin *Serum Increase Analytical* Methadone metabolite may cause false positive reaction for doxepin when measured by HPLC *3590*

Drugs of Abuse Screen *Urine No Effect Analytical* No effect at concentration of 100 µg/mL on EZ-SCREEN procedure for cannabinoids and cocaine *1739*

Follicle Stimulating Hormone
Plasma No Effect Physiological Normal concentration in male heroin addicts receiving methadone *4833*

Glucose *Serum No Effect Analytical* At acute overdose concentration (2.5 mg/dL) on Technicon SMAC® method *6266*

Immunoglobulin G *Serum Increase Physiological* Commonly seen in response to treatment *1202*

Indocyanine Green *Serum Decrease Physiological* Observed in small series, normal liver function tests *3942*

Iron *Serum No Effect Analytical* At concentration of 25 mg/L had no effect on Ferrozine method *5704* At acute overdose concentration (2.5 mg/dL) on Technicon SMAC® method *6266*

Lactate Dehydrogenase *Serum No Effect Analytical* At acute overdose concentration (2.5 mg/dL) on Technicon SMAC® method *6266*

Luteinizing Hormone *Plasma No Effect Physiological* Normal concentration in male heroin addicts receiving methadone *4833*

Methadone *Urine No Effect Analytical* Significant cross-reactivity of 100% observed with dl-methadone with Roche Abuscreen ONTRAK method *3279*

Morphine *Urine Increase Analytical* Significant positive result observed at a concentration of 646 µmol/L with Sung and Neely modification of Syva EMIT method *148*
Urine No Effect Analytical Insignificant cross reactivity with RIA procedures Insignificant cross reactivity with EMIT procedure for opiates *4163*

Nortriptyline *Serum Increase Analytical* May cause false positive reaction for nortriptyline when measured by HPLC *3590*

Opiates *Urine No Effect Analytical* No effect observed at a concentration of 500 µg/mL (1.61 mmol/L) on method on Du Pont aca *1559*

p-Aminophenol *Urine No Effect Analytical* With addition of drugs at a concentration of 100 mg/L and of related compounds at 50 mg/L no significant effect observed on colorimetric method of van Bocxlaer on Cobas Mira analyzer which involves reacting free p-aminophenol with resorcinol in the presence of magnesium ions to form an indophenol dye measured at 550 nm *6163*

Phenylalanine *Plasma No Effect Analytical* No interference observed with rapid quantitative whole blood method of Campbell et al using phenylalanine dehydrogenase *867*

Phosphate *Serum No Effect Analytical* At concentration of 25 mg/L had no effect on phosphomolybdate method *5704* At acute overdose concentration (2.5 mg/dL) on Technicon SMAC® method *6266*

Pregnancy Tests *Urine Positive Analytical* Highest incidence with Gravindex™ *2727*

Prolactin *Plasma No Effect Physiological* Normal concentration observed in male addicts receiving methadone *4833*

Protein *Serum No Effect Analytical* At concentration of 25 mg/L had no effect on biuret method with blank correction *5704* At acute overdose concentration (2.5 mg/dL) on Technicon SMAC® method *6266*

Testosterone *Serum No Effect Physiological* In treated/untreated male addicts *1201* Normal concentration in male heroin addicts receiving methadone *4833*

Thyroid Stimulating Hormone
Serum No Effect Physiological No significant effect observed *307*

Thyroxine (T4) *Serum Increase Physiological* Slight but not significant increase *307* Increased binding capacity (augmentation of transport proteins) *6412*

Thyroxine (T4), Free *Serum Decrease Physiological* Significantly lower percentage *307*

Tri-iodothyronine (T3) *Serum Increase Physiological* Increased binding capacity (augmentation of transport proteins) *6412* Significant increase observed compared with normals *307*

Triglycerides *Serum No Effect Analytical* At acute overdose concentration (2.5 mg/dL) on Technicon SMAC® method *6266* At concentration of 25 mg/L had no effect on lipase/esterase method *5704*

Urea Nitrogen *Serum No Effect Analytical* At concentration of 25 mg/L had no effect on diacetylmonoxime method *5704* At acute overdose concentration (2.5 mg/dL) on Technicon SMAC® method *6266*

Uric Acid *Serum No Effect Analytical* At concentration of 25 mg/L had no effect on phosphotungstate reduction method *5704* At acute overdose concentration (2.5 mg/dL) on Technicon SMAC® method *6266*

Zidovudine *Serum Increase Physiological* Methadone appears to increase concentration when drugs coadministered in drug-using patients with HIV infection *5393* Decreased metabolism and increased serum concentration *886*

Methamphetamine

Albumin *Serum No Effect Analytical* At concentration of 2 mg/L had no effect on BCG method *5704*

Amino Acids *Urine Increase Analytical* Reacts with ninhydrin; extra spot TLC, high voltage electrophoresis *4760*

Amphetamine *Urine Positive Analytical* At concentration of 1.0 µg/mL (6.71 µmol/L) with method on Du Pont aca *1554*

Amphetamine/Methamphetamine
Serum Increase Analytical d-amphetamine at a concentration of 1000 ng/mL caused 107.6% cross-reactivity with method on Abbott AxSYM and 105.6% with method on TDx: dl-methamphetamine at a concentration of 8000 ng/mL caused cross-reactivities of 21.2% and 20.2% respectively *6404*

Bicarbonate *Serum No Effect Analytical* At concentration of 2 mg/L had no effect on method using phenolphthalein *5704*

Bilirubin *Serum No Effect Analytical* At concentration of 2 mg/L had no effect on Jendrassik and Grof method *5704*

Calcium *Serum No Effect Analytical* At concentration of 2 mg/L had no effect on cresolphthalein method *5704*

Cannabinoids *Urine No Effect Analytical* No effect on Roche Abuscreen method *5006*

Chloride *Serum No Effect Analytical* At concentration of 2 mg/L had no effect on mercurimetric method *5704*

Cholesterol *Serum No Effect Analytical* At concentration of 2 mg/L had no effect on Liebermann-Burchard method *5704* At concentration of 2 mg/L had no effect on CHOD-PAP method *5704*

Cocaethylene *Urine No Effect Analytical* No interference observed with TLC method of Bailey *328*

Corticosteroids *Plasma Increase Physiological* Effect most marked in am when given i.v *2451* Amphetamine administration associated with significant increases of plasma corticosteroids *18*

Creatinine *Serum No Effect Analytical* At concentration of 2 mg/L had no effect on Technicon AutoAnalyzer® Jaffe method *5704*

Drugs of Abuse Screen *Urine No Effect Analytical* No effect at concentration of 100 µg/mL on EZ-SCREEN procedure for cannabinoids and cocaine *1739*

Epinephrine *Urine Increase Physiological* For 3 h after administration (slight) *2452*

Growth Hormone *Plasma Increase Physiological* Significant rise *532*

5-Hydroxyindoleacetic Acid *Urine Increase Physiological* Single instance reported *3534*

Lidocaine *Serum No Effect Analytical* No significant interference observed at a concentration of 100 µg/mL (670 µmol/L) with method on Du Pont aca *1534* At a concentration of 1250 mg/L (normal therapeutic concentration up to 0.05 mg/L) had effect of less than 10% on method on Baxter Stratus *5705*

Methamphetamine *Urine Decrease Analytical* Cross-reactivity of -10% observed with L-methamphetamine in D-methamphetamine assay of Roche Abuscreen Online as performed on Roche Cobas Mira *6347*

Norepinephrine *Urine No Effect Physiological* No effect observed *2452*

Phosphate *Serum No Effect Analytical* At concentration of 2 mg/L had no effect on phosphomolybdate method *5704*

Protein *Serum No Effect Analytical* At concentration of 2 mg/L had no effect on biuret method with blank correction *5704*

Quinidine *Serum No Effect Analytical* No significant interference observed at a concentration of 100 µg/mL (670 µmol/L) with method on Du Pont aca *1543*

Triglycerides *Serum No Effect Analytical* At concentration of 2 mg/L had no effect on lipase/esterase method *5704*

Urea Nitrogen *Serum No Effect Analytical* At concentration of 2 mg/L had no effect on diacetylmonoxime method *5704*

Methamphetamine *(continued)*

Uric Acid *Serum No Effect Analytical* At concentration of 2 mg/L had no effect on phosphotungstate reduction method *5704*

Methandriol

Alanine Aminotransferase *Serum Increase Physiological* Intrahepatic cholestatic jaundice *2242*

Alkaline Phosphatase *Serum Increase Physiological* Intrahepatic cholestatic jaundice *2242*

Aspartate Aminotransferase *Serum Increase Physiological* Intrahepatic cholestatic jaundice *2242*

Bile *Urine Increase Physiological* Intrahepatic cholestatic jaundice *2242*

Bilirubin *Serum Increase Physiological* Intrahepatic cholestatic jaundice *2242*

BSP Retention *Serum Increase Physiological* Intrahepatic cholestatic jaundice *2242*

Methandrostenolone

Alanine Aminotransferase *Serum Increase Physiological* Up to 3-6 times normal due to cholestasis *2803*

Alkaline Phosphatase *Serum Increase Physiological* Intrahepatic cholestatic jaundice *2242*

Aspartate Aminotransferase *Serum Increase Physiological* Up to 3-6 times normal due to cholestasis *2803* In 2 of 6 body-builders taking up to 20 mg/d intermittently for a year or more *5498*

Bile *Urine Increase Physiological* Intrahepatic cholestatic jaundice *2242*

Bilirubin *Serum Increase Physiological* Due to cholestasis *2803*

BSP Retention *Serum Increase Physiological* Cholestatic phenomenon *1174* Hepatotoxic effect (common) *3810*

Calcium *Serum Increase Physiological* May occur spontaneously, but especially if breast cancer *2754*

Cholesterol *Serum Decrease Physiological* Reported effect (may increase as alternative) *2754*
Serum Increase Physiological Due to cholestasis *2803*

Creatine *Urine Increase Physiological* May persist up to 2 weeks after treatment *51*

Creatinine *Urine Increase Physiological* May persist up to 2 weeks after treatment *51*

Factor II *Plasma Increase Physiological* Metabolic effect *51*

Factor V *Plasma Increase Physiological* Metabolic effect *51*

Factor VII *Plasma Increase Physiological* Metabolic effect *51*

Factor X *Plasma Increase Physiological* Metabolic effect *51*

Glucose *Serum Decrease Physiological* Anabolic effect *51*

Glucose Tolerance *Serum Decrease Physiological* Alters curve in diabetic direction *4014*
Serum Increase Physiological Anabolic effect *51*

β-Glucuronidase *Serum Increase Physiological* Metabolic effect *368*

Haptoglobin *Serum Increase Physiological* Metabolic effect *368*

17-Hydroxycorticosteroids *Urine Decrease Physiological* Inhibits response to metyrapone *55*

^{131}I Uptake *Serum Decrease Physiological* Also modifies binding of thyroid hormones *4014*

17-Ketosteroids *Urine Decrease Physiological* Metabolic action of drug *51*

Luteinizing Hormone *Plasma Decrease Physiological* In 4 of 6 body-builders taking up to 20 mg/d intermittently for a year or more *5498*

Metyrapone Test *Patient Positive Physiological* Anabolic effect *4433*

Oxyphenbutazone *Serum Increase Physiological* Possibly due to inhibition of metabolism *2452*

Phenylbutazone *Serum No Effect Physiological* Unaffected by concomitant administration *2452*

Plasminogen *Plasma Increase Physiological* Metabolic effect *368*

Prothrombin Time *Plasma Increase Physiological* Also seen with other 17-alkyl substituted steroids *1667* Prolongs action of anticoagulants *3810*

Sialic Acid *Serum Increase Physiological* Metabolic effect *368*

Sodium *Serum Increase Physiological* May be affected but water also retained *51*

T3-Uptake *Serum Increase Physiological* Affects RBC and resin uptakes *51* In 6 body-builders taking up to 20 mg/d intermittently for a year or more *5498*

Testosterone *Serum Decrease Physiological* In 4 of 6 body-builders taking up to 20 mg/d intermittently for a year or more *5498*

Thyroxine Binding Globulin
Serum Decrease Physiological Metabolic effect *51*

Thyroxine (T4) *Serum No Effect Physiological* In 6 body-builders taking up to 20 mg/d intermittently for a year or more *5498*

Thyroxine (T4), Free *Serum No Effect Physiological* No change observed *51*

Triglycerides *Serum Decrease Physiological* Metabolic (anabolic) effect *5833*

Urobilinogen *Feces Decrease Physiological* Light stools, due to cholestasis *2803*
Urine Decrease Physiological Due to cholestasis *2803*

Methantheline

^{131}I Uptake *Serum Decrease Physiological* Reported to decrease results *882*

Methapyrilene

Albumin *Serum No Effect Analytical* At concentration of 13 mg/L had no effect on BCG method *5704*

Bicarbonate *Serum No Effect Analytical* At concentration of 13 mg/L had no effect on method using phenolphthalein *5704*

Bilirubin *Serum No Effect Analytical* At concentration of 13 mg/L had no effect on Jendrassik and Grof method *5704*

Calcium *Serum No Effect Analytical* At concentration of 13 mg/L had no effect on cresolphthalein method *5704*

Chloride *Serum No Effect Analytical* At concentration of 13 mg/L had no effect on mercurimetric method *5704*

Cholesterol *Serum No Effect Analytical* At concentration of 13 mg/L had no effect on Liebermann-Burchard method *5704*

Creatinine *Serum No Effect Analytical* At concentration of 13 mg/L had no effect on Technicon AutoAnalyzer® Jaffe method *5704*

Erythrocytes *Blood Decrease Physiological* Anemia (AMA Blood dyscrasias) *4017*

Glucose *Urine Increase Analytical* Methapyrilene compounds may may give positive result with Ames 2-drop Clinitest method at concentrations less than 0.5 g/dL *4034*
Urine No Effect Analytical Methapyrilene compounds have no effect on Ames Keto-Diastix, Diastix, Multistix and Clinistix methods *4034*

Phosphate *Serum No Effect Analytical* At concentration of 13 mg/L had no effect on phosphomolybdate method *5704*

Potassium *Serum No Effect Analytical* At concentration of 13 mg/L had no effect on measurement by ISE with predilution *5704*

Protein *Serum No Effect Analytical* At concentration of 13 mg/L had no effect on biuret method with blank correction *5704*

Sodium *Serum No Effect Analytical* At concentration of 13 mg/L had no effect on measurement by ISE with predilution *5704*

Triglycerides *Serum* *No Effect* *Analytical* At concentration of 13 mg/L had no effect on lipase/esterase method *5704*

Urea Nitrogen *Serum* *No Effect* *Analytical* At concentration of 13 mg/L had no effect on diacetylmonoxime method *5704*

Uric Acid *Serum* *No Effect* *Analytical* At concentration of 13 mg/L had no effect on phosphotungstate reduction method *5704*

Methaqualone

Alanine Aminotransferase *Serum* *No Effect* *Analytical* No effect at therapeutic concentration on Boehringer Mannheim Reflotron method *3231* At acute overdose concentration (2.5 mg/dL) on Technicon SMAC® method *6266* No effect at 50 mg/L on Boehringer Mannheim Reflotron method *5706*

Albumin *Serum* *No Effect* *Analytical* At concentration of 25 mg/L had no effect on BCG method *5704* At acute overdose concentration (2.5 mg/dL) on Technicon SMAC® method *6266*

Alkaline Phosphatase *Serum* *No Effect* *Analytical* At acute overdose concentration (2.5 mg/dL) on Technicon SMAC® method *6266*

Amylase *Serum* *No Effect* *Analytical* At a concentration of 50 mg/L had no effect on method on Boehringer Mannheim Reflotron system *5706*

Antipyrine *Serum* *No Effect* *Physiological* No significant effect on half-life *5820*

Aspartate Aminotransferase *Serum* *No Effect* *Analytical* No effect at 50 mg/L on Boehringer Mannheim Reflotron method *5706* No effect at therapeutic concentration on Boehringer Mannheim Reflotron method *3231* At acute overdose concentration (2.5 mg/dL) on Technicon SMAC® method *6266*

Barbiturate *Serum* *No Effect* *Analytical* No significant interference observed at a concentration of 100 µg/mL (0.40 mmol/L) with method on Du Pont aca *1511*

Benzodiazepine *Urine* *No Effect* *Analytical* Negative result obtained at a concentration of 1000 µg/mL (4.00 mmol/L) with method on Du Pont aca *1556*

Benzodiazepine Screen *Serum* *No Effect* *Analytical* No significant interference observed at a concentration of 100 µg/mL (0.40 mmol/L) with method on Du Pont aca *1512*

Benzoylecgonine *Urine* *No Effect* *Analytical* No significant interference observed at a concentration of 400 µmol/L with Sung and Neely modification of Syva EMIT procedure *148* Negative result obtained at a concentration of 100 µg/mL (0.40 mmol/L) with method on Du Pont aca *1558*

Bilirubin *Serum* *No Effect* *Analytical* At concentration of 50 mg/L no effect on method on Boehringer Mannheim Reflotron system *5706* At concentration of 25 mg/L had no effect on Jendrassik and Grof method *5704* At acute overdose concentration (2.5 mg/dL) on Technicon SMAC® method *6266*

Calcium *Serum* *No Effect* *Analytical* At acute overdose concentration (2.5 mg/dL) on Technicon SMAC® method *6266* At concentration of 25 mg/L had no effect on cresolphthalein method *5704*

Cannabinoids *Urine* *No Effect* *Analytical* No effect on Roche Abuscreen method *5006* No effect observed at a concentration of 100 µg/mL (0.40 mmol/L) on method on Du Pont aca *1557*

Cholesterol *Serum* *No Effect* *Analytical* At acute overdose concentration (2.5 mg/dL) on Technicon SMAC® method *6266* At concentration of 25 mg/L had no effect on Liebermann-Burchard method *5704* No effect at therapeutic concentration on Boehringer Mannheim Reflotron method *3231* At concentration of 50 mg/L no effect on method on Boehringer Mannheim Reflotron system *5706*

Cocaethylene *Urine* *No Effect* *Analytical* No interference observed with TLC method of Bailey *328*

Cortisol *Plasma* *No Effect* *Analytical* At concentration of 20 mg/L no significant effect on CEDIA method (worst case recovery 89.9% with one specimen and 104.8% with a second) *1097*

Creatine Kinase *Serum* *No Effect* *Analytical* At acute overdose concentration (2.5 mg/dL) on Technicon SMAC® method *6266*

Creatinine *Serum* *No Effect* *Analytical* At concentration of 25 mg/L had no effect on Technicon AutoAnalyzer® Jaffe method *5704* At acute overdose concentration (2.5 mg/dL) on Technicon SMAC® method *6266*

Drugs of Abuse Screen *Urine* *No Effect* *Analytical* No effect at concentration of 100 µg/mL on EZ-SCREEN procedure for cannabinoids and cocaine *1739*

Erythrocytes *Blood* *Decrease* *Physiological* One possible case of aplastic anemia reported *3810*

Glucose *Serum* *No Effect* *Analytical* At concentration of 50 mg/L no effect on method on Boehringer Mannheim Reflotron system *5706* At acute overdose concentration (2.5 mg/dL) on Technicon SMAC® method *6266* No effect at therapeutic concentration on Boehringer Mannheim Reflotron method *3231* At concentration of 80 mg/L had no effect on hexokinase/G-6-PDH method *5704*

γ-Glutamyltransferase *Serum* *No Effect* *Analytical* At concentration of 50 mg/L no effect on method on Boehringer Mannheim Reflotron system *5706* No effect at therapeutic concentration on Boehringer Mannheim Reflotron method *3231*

^{131}I Uptake *Serum* *Decrease* *Physiological* Parest® contains tetraiodofluorescein *4360*

Iron *Serum* *No Effect* *Analytical* At acute overdose concentration (2.5 mg/dL) on Technicon SMAC® method *6266* At concentration of 25 mg/L had no effect on Ferrozine method *5704*

Lactate *Plasma* *No Effect* *Analytical* At concentration of 25 mg/L had no effect on enzymatic method *5704*

Lactate Dehydrogenase *Serum* *No Effect* *Analytical* At acute overdose concentration (2.5 mg/dL) on Technicon SMAC® method *6266*

Leukocytes *Blood* *Decrease* *Physiological* 1 case of pancytopenia reported *2754*

Methaqualone *Serum* *Increase* *Physiological* 250 mg orally produced plasma concentration of 2 mg/L in 30 minutes *3868*

Morphine *Urine* *No Effect* *Analytical* No significant interference observed at a concentration of 400 µmol/L with Sung and Neely modification of Syva EMIT method *148*

p-Aminophenol *Urine* *No Effect* *Analytical* With addition of drugs at a concentration of 100 mg/L and of related compounds at 50 mg/L no significant effect observed on colorimetric method of van Bocxlaer on Cobas Mira analyzer which involves reacting free p-aminophenol with resorcinol in the presence of magnesium ions to form an indophenol dye measured at 550 nm *6163*

Phenylbutazone *Serum* *No Effect* *Physiological* No significant effect on half-life *5820*

Phosphate *Serum* *No Effect* *Analytical* At acute overdose concentration (2.5 mg/dL) on Technicon SMAC® method *6266* At concentration of 25 mg/L had no effect on phosphomolybdate method *5704*

Platelets *Blood* *Decrease* *Physiological* 1 case of pancytopenia reported *2754*

Potassium *Serum* *No Effect* *Analytical* At concentration of 6,000 mg/L had no effect on measurement by ISE with predilution *5704*

Protein *Serum* *No Effect* *Analytical* At acute overdose concentration (2.5 mg/dL) on Technicon SMAC® method *6266*

Prothrombin Time *Plasma* *Decrease* *Physiological* In 10 patients receiving 0.3 g/d also on warfarin: effect mild and not significant. Weak inducer of hepatic microsomal enzymes *6118*

Sodium *Serum* *No Effect* *Analytical* At concentration of 6,000 mg/L had no effect on measurement by ISE with predilution *5704*

Tricyclic Antidepressants Screen *Serum* *No Effect* *Analytical* No significant effect observed at a concentration of 100 µg/mL (0.40 mmol/L) with method on Du Pont aca *1550*

Triglycerides *Serum* *No Effect* *Analytical* No effect at therapeutic concentration on Boehringer Mannheim Reflotron method *3231* At concentration of 25 mg/L had no effect on lipase/esterase method *5704* No effect at 50 mg/L on Boehringer Mannheim Reflotron method *5706* At acute overdose concentration (2.5 mg/dL) on Technicon SMAC® method *6266*

Urea Nitrogen *Serum* *No Effect* *Analytical* At concentration of 25 mg/L had no effect on diacetylmonoxime method *5704* No effect at therapeutic concentration on Boehringer Mannheim Reflotron method *3231* At acute overdose concentration (2.5

Methaqualone *(continued)*

Urea Nitrogen *(continued)*
mg/dL) on Technicon SMAC® method *6266* No effect at 50 mg/L on Boehringer Mannheim Reflotron method *5706*

Uric Acid *Serum No Effect Analytical* At acute overdose concentration (2.5 mg/dL) on Technicon SMAC® method *6266* No effect at 50 mg/L on method on Boehringer Mannheim Reflotron *5706* At concentration of 25 mg/L had no effect on phosphotungstate reduction method *5704* No effect at therapeutic concentration on Boehringer Mannheim Reflotron method *3231*

Metharbital

Barbital *Serum Increase Physiological* Metabolic conversion *in vivo5093*

Felbamate *Serum No Effect Analytical* No significant interference observed with GLC method of Rifai et al *4958*

Prothrombin Time *Plasma Decrease Physiological* Theoretical possibility due to enzyme induction *2754*

Methazolamide

Erythrocytes *Blood Decrease Physiological* Two cases of possible drug-associated aplastic anemia reported *4088*

Hematocrit *Blood Decrease Physiological* Two cases of possible drug-associated aplastic anemia reported *4088*

Hemoglobin *Blood Decrease Physiological* Some cases of aplastic anemia, and leukopenia reported when used in treatment for glaucoma *6413* Two cases of possible drug-associated aplastic anemia reported *4088*

Leukocytes *Blood Decrease Physiological* Two cases of possible drug-associated aplastic anemia reported *4088* Some cases of aplastic anemia, and leukopenia reported when used in treatment for glaucoma *6413* Probable effect as like acetazolamide *3810*

Neutrophils *Blood Decrease Physiological* Occasional case of agranulocytosis reported *6264*

Platelets *Blood Decrease Physiological* Some cases of aplastic anemia, and leukopenia reported when used in treatment for glaucoma *6413* Two cases of possible drug-associated aplastic anemia reported *4088* Probable effect as like acetazolamide *3810*

Potassium *Serum Decrease Physiological* With prolonged use (carbonic anhydrase inhibition) *3810*

Methchlorethamine

Uric Acid *Serum Increase Physiological* Hyperuricemia may occur particularly in lymphoma patients *1384*

Methdilazine

Alanine Aminotransferase *Serum Increase Physiological* Rare case of cholestasis *2754*

Aspartate Aminotransferase *Serum Increase Physiological* Rare case of cholestasis *2754*

Bilirubin *Serum Increase Physiological* Rare case of cholestasis *2754*

Methenamine

Alanine Aminotransferase *Serum Increase Physiological* Mild transient effect in some cases *2754*

Ammonia *Urine Increase Physiological* Hydrolyzed in acid urine (to formaldehyde also) *2753*

Amphetamine *Urine Increase Physiological* Urinary excretion of amphetamine is increased and efficacy is reduced by acidifying agents used in methenamine therapy *5641*

Aspartate Aminotransferase *Serum Increase Physiological* Mild transient effect in some cases *2754*

Catecholamines *Plasma Increase Analytical* Interference with fluorescence *189*

Crystals *Urine Increase Physiological* Mandelate may occasionally cause crystalluria *2242*

Erythrocytes *Urine Increase Physiological* May cause actual bleeding *1714*

Estriol *Urine Decrease Analytical* Interferes with hydrolysis stage of methods *1740*
Urine No Effect Analytical At 1 g/dL with enzyme hydrolysis and Oakey procedure *1177*

Estrogens *Urine Decrease Analytical* Affects hydrolysis of estrogen conjugates *55*

Hemoglobin *Urine Increase Physiological* Actual bleeding produced by drug *1714*

Hippuric Acid *Urine Increase Physiological* If given as hippurate salt *2753*

^{131}I Uptake *Serum Decrease Physiological* Mandelamine® contains tetraiodofluorescein *4360*

pH *Urine Decrease Physiological* Mandelate is an acidifying agent *2242*

Protein *Urine Increase Physiological* Nephrotoxic in large doses *2242 1714*

PSP Excretion *Urine Increase Analytical* Produces interfering color in urine *1174*

Sugar *Urine Increase Analytical* False positive with Benedict's reagent *3530*

Urobilinogen *Urine Increase Analytical* Produces formaldehyde which interferes *408*

Methergoline

Thyroid Stimulating Hormone
Serum Decrease Physiological In hypothyroidism: is a serotonin antagonist *6412*

Methicillin

Alanine Aminotransferase *Serum No Effect Analytical* At 5 times upper limit of therapeutic range on methods on Technicon SMAC® , Abbott-VP, Roche Cobas-Bio, Du Pont aca, and KDA *3525*

Albumin *Serum No Effect Analytical* At 5 times upper limit of therapeutic range on Technicon SMAC® , Abbott-VP, Kodak Ektachem® , Hitachi® 705 and KDA *3525* At concentration of 900 mg/L had no effect on BCG method *5704*

Alkaline Phosphatase *Serum No Effect Analytical* At 5 times upper limit of therapeutic range on methods on Technicon SMAC® , Abbott-VP, Du Pont aca, Roche Cobas-Bio, Hitachi® 705 and KDA *3525*

Amylase *Serum No Effect Analytical* At 5 times upper limit of therapeutic range on methods on Du Pont aca, Cobas-Bio and Kodak Ektachem® *3525*

Aspartate Aminotransferase *Serum No Effect Analytical* At 5 times upper limit of therapeutic range on methods on Technicon SMAC® , Abbott-VP, Du Pont aca, Roche Cobas-Bio, Hitachi® 705 and KDA *3525*

Bicarbonate *Serum Decrease Physiological* Nephrotoxicity may cause azotemia *3810*
Serum No Effect Analytical At concentration of 900 mg/L had no effect on method using phenolphthalein *5704*

Bilirubin *Serum No Effect Analytical* At concentration of 900 mg/L had no effect on Jendrassik and Grof method *5704* At 5 times upper limit of therapeutic range on Technicon SMAC® , Du Pont aca, Roche Cobas-Bio, Kodak Ektachem® , Hitachi® 705 and KDA *3525*
Serum No Effect Physiological Clinically insignificant displacement from protein in neonates *6314*

Bilirubin, Conjugated *Serum No Effect Analytical* No effect at concentration of 1100 mg/L on method on Kodak Ektachem® *5706*

Bilirubin, Unconjugated *Serum No Effect Analytical* No effect at concentration of 1100 mg/L on method on Kodak Ektachem® *5706*

Bleeding Time *Patient No Effect Physiological* Even at 300 mg/kg/d had no effect in volunteers *756*

Calcium *Serum Decrease Physiological* Reported effect (?mechanism) *3810*

Serum *No Effect* *Analytical* No effect of concentrations up to 1100 mg/L with method on Kodak Ektachem® *5706* At concentration of 900 mg/L had no effect on cresolphthalein method *5704* At 5 times upper limit of therapeutic range on methods on Technicon SMAC®, Abbott-VP, Du Pont aca *3525*

Casts *Urine* *Increase* *Physiological* Nephrotoxic effect (cylindruria observed) *3810*

Chloride *Serum* *No Effect* *Analytical* At concentration of 900 mg/L had no effect on mercurimetric method *5704*

Cholesterol *Serum* *No Effect* *Analytical* At concentration of 20 mg/L had no effect on CHOD-PAP method *5704* At 5 times upper limit of therapeutic range on methods on Technicon SMAC®, Abbott-VP, Roche Cobas-Bio, Kodak Ektachem®, Hitachi® 705 and KDA *3525* At concentration of 900 mg/L had no effect on Liebermann-Burchard method *5704*

Clot Retraction *Blood* *No Effect* *Physiological* No effect with doses as high as 300 mg/kg/d in volunteers *756*

Coombs' Test, Direct *Blood* *Positive* *Physiological* In 31% of 45 patients receiving drug (hypersensitivity reaction) *3195*

Creatine Kinase *Serum* *No Effect* *Analytical* At 5 times upper limit of therapeutic range on methods on Technicon SMAC®, Abbott-VP, Roche Cobas-Bio, Du Pont aca and Hitachi® 705 *3525*

Creatinine *Serum* *Increase* *Physiological* Nephrotoxic effect *3810*

Serum *No Effect* *Analytical* At concentration of 900 mg/L had no effect on Technicon AutoAnalyzer® Jaffe method *5704* No effect of concentrations up to 1100 mg/L on 2-slide method on Kodak Ektachem® *5706* No effect of concentrations up to 15 mg/L on single slide method on Kodak Ektachem® *5706* At 5 times upper limit of therapeutic range on Technicon SMAC®, Abbott-VP, Roche Cobas-Bio, Du Pont aca, Kodak Ektachem®, Hitachi® 705 and KDA *3525*

Eosinophils *Blood* *Increase* *Physiological* In 31% of 45 patients receiving drug (hypersensitivity reaction) *3195* In 3 of 28 children within 5 to 8 d *4212* Hypersensitivity reaction *345*

Urine *Increase* *Physiological* Observed with methicillin-induced nephrotoxicity (interstitial nephritis) observed 2-37 days after initiation of therapy *1384*

Erythrocytes *Blood* *Decrease* *Physiological* May rarely cause bone marrow depression *4691*

Urine *Increase* *Physiological* Observed with methicillin-induced nephrotoxicity (interstitial nephritis) *1384* Hypersensitivity reaction, nephrotoxicity *345* Associated with allergic response and interstitial nephritis *1384*

Fibrinogen *Plasma* *No Effect* *Physiological* No effect with doses as high as 300 mg/kg/d in volunteers *756*

Glucose *Serum* *No Effect* *Analytical* At 5 times upper limit of therapeutic range on Technicon SMAC®, Abbott-VP, Roche Cobas-Bio, Du Pont aca, Kodak Ektachem®, Hitachi® 705 and KDA *3525* At concentration of 20 mg/L had no effect on GOD/POD-PAP method *5704*

γ-Glutamyltransferase *Serum* *No Effect* *Analytical* At 5 times upper limit of therapeutic range on methods on Technicon SMAC®, Abbott-VP and Hitachi® 705 *3525*

Haptoglobin *Serum* *Decrease* *Physiological* One doubtful case of hemolytic anemia *128*

Hemoglobin *Urine* *Increase* *Physiological* Hypersensitivity reaction, nephrotoxicity *345* Associated with interstitial nephritis and allergic reaction *1384*

Iron *Serum* *Increase* *Physiological* If erythrocyte maturation depressed *4928*

Serum *No Effect* *Analytical* At 5 times upper limit of therapeutic range on Ferrozine method on Technicon SMAC® *3525*

Iron-Binding Capacity, Unsaturated

Serum *Decrease* *Physiological* If erythrocyte maturation depressed *4928*

Lactate Dehydrogenase *Serum* *No Effect* *Analytical* At 5 times upper therapeutic range on methods on Technicon SMAC®, Abbott-VP, Roche Cobas-Bio, Hitachi® 705 and KDA *3525*

Leukocytes *Blood* *Decrease* *Physiological* May cause bone marrow depression *3810*

Blood *Increase* *Physiological* Due to eosinophilia/Leukocytosis *3810*

Urine *Increase* *Physiological* Associated with interstitial nephritis following allergic reaction *1384*

Methemoglobin *Blood* *Increase* *Physiological* One doubtful case of hemolytic anemia *128*

Neutrophils *Blood* *Decrease* *Physiological* Neutropenia with granulocytopenia may occur *2754*

Nonprotein Nitrogen *Serum* *Increase* *Physiological* Nephrotoxic effect *3810*

Partial Thromboplastin Time

Plasma *No Effect* *Physiological* No effect with doses as high as 300 mg/kg/d in volunteers *756*

Phosphate *Serum* *Increase* *Analytical* At concentrations above 500 mg/L (normal therapeutic concentration 21 mg/L) raised concentration as measured by phosphomolybdate method *5704* At 5 times upper limit of therapeutic range on methods on Technicon SMAC®, Du Pont aca, and Hitachi® 705 *3525*

Serum *Increase* *Physiological* Occurs with nephrotoxicity *3810*

Serum *No Effect* *Analytical* At 5 times upper limit of therapeutic range on method on KDA *3525*

Platelet Aggregation *Blood* *Decrease* *Physiological* In response to ADP in 1 of 5 volunteers receiving up to 300 mg/kg/d *756*

Platelets *Blood* *Decrease* *Physiological* May rarely cause bone marrow depression *4691*

Blood *No Effect* *Physiological* No effect with doses as high as 300 mg/kg/d in volunteers *756*

Potassium *Serum* *Increase* *Physiological* Possible result of nephrotoxicity *3810*

Serum *No Effect* *Analytical* At concentration of 20 mg/L had no effect on flame-photometric method *5704*

Protein *Cerebrospinal Fluid* *Increase* *Analytical* At concentration of 16 mg/L on SDS/Coomassie Blue method of Huang caused positive interference of 11% when compared against method on Du Pont aca *2745* At concentrations greater than 10 μg/dL (248 mmol/L) increases result as determined by method on Du Pont aca *1515*

Cerebrospinal Fluid *No Effect* *Analytical* No significant effect when added in vitro to concentration of 100 mg/dL on Kodak Ektachem® slide method *3654*

Serum *Increase* *Analytical* At concentrations above 500 mg/L (normal therapeutic concentration 21 mg/L) raised concentration as measured by biuret method with blank correction *5704*

Serum *No Effect* *Analytical* At 5 times upper limit of therapeutic range on methods on Technicon SMAC®, Abbott-VP, Kodak Ektachem®, Hitachi® 705 and KDA *3525*

Urine *Increase* *Physiological* Nephrotoxicity may occur *128* Nephrotoxic effect *4134* Associated with interstitial nephritis following allergic reaction *1384*

Prothrombin Time *Plasma* *No Effect* *Physiological* No effect with doses as high as 300 mg/kg/d in volunteers *756*

Sodium *Serum* *No Effect* *Analytical* At concentration of 20 mg/L had no effect on flame-photometric method *5704*

Thrombin Time *Blood* *No Effect* *Physiological* No effect with doses as high as 300 mg/kg/d in volunteers *756*

Triglycerides *Serum* *Increase* *Analytical* At 5 times upper limit of therapeutic range on enzymatic method on Abbott-VP *3525*

Serum *No Effect* *Analytical* At 5 times upper limit of therapeutic range on Technicon SMAC®, Kodak Ektachem®, Hitachi® 705 and KDA *3525* At concentration of 900 mg/L had no effect on lipase/esterase method *5704*

Urea Nitrogen *Serum* *Increase* *Physiological* May cause azotemia with nephrotoxicity *128*

Serum *No Effect* *Analytical* At concentration of 900 mg/L had no effect on diacetylmonoxime method *5704* At 5 times upper limit of therapeutic range on methods on echnicon SMAC®, Abbott-VP, Roche Cobas-Bio, Kodak Ektachem®, Hitachi® 705 and KDA *3525*

Uric Acid *Serum* *Increase* *Physiological* Nephrotoxic effect *3810*

Serum *No Effect* *Analytical* At concentration of 900 mg/L had no effect on phosphotungstate reduction method *5704* At 5 times upper limit of therapeutic range on Technicon SMAC®, Abbott-VP, Roche Cobas-Bio, Du Pont aca, Kodak Ektachem®, Hitachi® 705 and KDA *3525*

Urobilin *Urine* *Increase* *Physiological* Pyuria reported as complication *2754*

Methicillin *(continued)*

Vancomycin *Serum* *No Effect* *Analytical* No significant interference observed at a concentration of 500 µg/mL (1318 µmol/L) with method on Du Pont aca *1561*

Methimazole

Alanine Aminotransferase *Serum* *Increase* *Physiological* Rare reports of fulminant hepatitis, hepatic necrosis indicate serious side effects of treatment *2971* Rare case of cholestatic jaundice reported *2898* May affect liver function (cholestasis) *3810*

Albumin *Serum* *No Effect* *Analytical* At concentration of 114 mg/L had no effect on BCG method *5704*

Alkaline Phosphatase *Serum* *Increase* *Physiological* Rare case of cholestatic jaundice reported *2898* Rare reports of fulminant hepatitis, hepatic necrosis indicate serious side effects of treatment *2971* May affect liver function (cholestasis) *3810*

Antithyroglobulin Antibodies
Serum *Decrease* *Physiological* In 23 patients with Graves' disease mean concentration decreased to 83.0 U/mL (range 5.1 - 417.1) from 191.5 U/mL (range 22.0 - 1196.0) after treatment with 40 mg/d for 8 weeks *6406*

Antithyroid Peroxidase Antibodies
Serum *Decrease* *Physiological* In 23 patients with Graves' disease mean concentration decreased to 1064 U/mL (range 25 - 2056) from 2348 U/mL (range 230 - 9996) after treatment with 40 mg/d for 8 weeks *6406*

Antithyroid Receptor Antibodies
Serum *Decrease* *Physiological* In 23 patients with Graves' disease mean concentration decreased to 11 U/mL (range 0.9 - 66.9) from 45.1 U/mL (range 14.4 - 173.1) after treatment with 40 mg/d for 8 weeks *6406*

Aspartate Aminotransferase *Serum* *Increase* *Physiological* Rare reports of fulminant hepatitis, hepatic necrosis indicate serious side effects of treatment *2971* May affect liver function (cholestasis) *3810* Rare case of cholestatic jaundice reported *2898*

Atrial Natriuretic Peptide *Plasma* *Decrease* *Physiological* In 5 patients with thyrotoxicosis caused by toxic nodular goitre with sinus cardiac rhythm treatment with methimazole 60 mg/d for 10 days caused a significant reduction of median from 20.0 pmol/L to 9.2 pmol/L *1207*

B-Cell Differentiation Factor
Monocytes *No Effect* *Physiological* No effect on production when cells from normal individuals stimulated with mitogens *6379*

Bile *Urine* *Increase* *Physiological* May affect liver function *3810*

Bilirubin *Serum* *Increase* *Physiological* Toxic effect associated with bone marrow depression *445* Rare case of cholestatic jaundice reported *2898* May affect liver function (cholestasis) *3810* Rare reports of fulminant hepatitis, hepatic necrosis indicate serious side effects of treatment *2971*
Serum *No Effect* *Analytical* No effect at 20 mg/L on Ames Seralyzer method *5706* At concentration of 114 mg/L had no effect on Jendrassik and Grof method *5704*

BSP Retention *Serum* *Increase* *Physiological* May affect liver function (cholestasis) *3810*

Calcium *Serum* *No Effect* *Analytical* At concentration of 114 mg/L had no effect on cresolphthalein method *5704*

Cholesterol *Serum* *Decrease* *Physiological* In 25 patients with hyperthyroidism mean concentration of 194.8 ± 54.2 mg/dL was significantly different from 226.9 ± 68.0 mg/dL during treatment with 60 mg/d methimazole and 60 mg/d propranolol *2710*
Serum *Increase* *Physiological* In 14 hyperthyroid patients treatment caused significant increase of concentration from mean baseline of 148 ± 49 mg/dL to 254 ± 67 mg/dL *5735* Cholestatic effect *2803*
Serum *No Effect* *Analytical* No effect at 20 mg/L on Ames Seralyzer method *5706*

Cortisol *Plasma* *No Effect* *Analytical* At a concentration of 40 mg/L had no significant effect on Enzymun method *1097*

Creatine Kinase *Serum* *No Effect* *Analytical* No effect at 20 mg/L on method on Ames Seralyzer *5706*

Creatinine *Serum* *No Effect* *Analytical* No effect at 20 mg/L on Ames Seralyzer method *5706*

Erythrocytes *Blood* *Decrease* *Physiological* Occasional case of aplastic anemia reported *6504* Aplastic anemia *3810* Leukopenia, thrombocytopenia and aplastic anemia (pancytopenia) are potentially serious side effects of treatment *2971*

Ferritin *Serum* *Decrease* *Physiological* Values significantly lower in patients with Graves disease following treatment with drug *6694*

Fibronectin *Plasma* *Increase* *Physiological* Mean fasting concentration in 10 hyperthyroid patients of 68.9 ± 14.8 mg/dL significantly decreased to 32.2 ± 7.2 mg/dL after normalization of thyroid function after treatment with methimazole *5527*

γ-Globulin *Serum* *Increase* *Physiological* Polyclonal hypergammagloblulinemia reported possibly as result of production of nonspecific drug-stimulated polyclonal antibodies *6504*

Glucose *Serum* *Increase* *Analytical* At 1 mmol/L affects Technicon SMA 12/60 method *5576*
Serum *No Effect* *Analytical* No effect at 20 mg/L on glucose oxidase method on Ames Seralyzer *5706* No effect at 10 mmol/L on glucokinase based assay of Scott *5414* No effect at 400 mg/L on hexokinase method on Ames Seralyzer *5706*

Granulocytes *Blood* *Decrease* *Physiological* Agranulocytosis is a potentially serious side effect of treatment *2971*

Guanosine Monophosphate
Plasma *Decrease* *Physiological* In 5 patients with thyrotoxicosis caused by toxic nodular goitre with sinus cardiac rhythm treatment with methimazole 60 mg/d for 10 days caused a significant reduction of median from 6.5 nmol/L to 4.2 nmol/L *1207*

HDL-Cholesterol *Serum* *Decrease* *Physiological* In 25 patients with hyperthyroidism mean concentration of 42.7 ± 9.04 mg/dL was significantly different from 51.6 ± 21.2 mg/dL during treatment with 60 mg/d methimazole and 60 mg/d propranolol *2710*
Serum *Increase* *Physiological* In 14 hyperthyroid patients mean concentration increased from baseline of 39 ± 9 mg/dL to 50 ± 15 mg/dL *5735*

Hematocrit *Blood* *Decrease* *Physiological* Leukopenia, thrombocytopenia and aplastic anemia (pancytopenia) are potentially serious side effects of treatment *2971* Occasional case of aplastic anemia reported *6504*

Hemoglobin *Blood* *Decrease* *Physiological* Leukopenia, thrombocytopenia and aplastic anemia (pancytopenia) are potentially serious side effects of treatment *2971* Occasional case of aplastic anemia reported *6504*

^{131}I Uptake *Serum* *Decrease* *Physiological* Effect may last from 2 to 8 d *2396*
Serum *No Effect* *Physiological* No effect on uptake by thyroid *3669*

Insulin-like Growth Factor-I *Serum* *Decrease* *Physiological* Administration of 10 - 15 mg/d for 11 - 21 weeks to a group of patients with hyperthyroidism caused significant reduction from mean baseline of 1410 ± 200 U/L to 990 ± 90 U/L *6151*

Interferon-γ *Monocytes* *No Effect* *Physiological* No effect on production when cells from normal individuals stimulated with mitogens *6379*

Interleukin-1 *Monocytes* *No Effect* *Physiological* No effect on production when cells from normal individuals stimulated with mitogens *6379*

Interleukin-2 *Monocytes* *Increase* *Physiological* Increased activity in culture supernatants when mononuclear cells from normals stimulated with mitogens. Effect apparent between 24 h and 60 h *6379*

Interleukin-2 Receptor Expression
Monocytes *No Effect* *Physiological* No effect of the drug on mitogen stimulated mononuclear cells from normal individuals *6379*

Iron *Serum* *Increase* *Physiological* Significant increase in 60 women with Graves disease following treatment with drug *6694*

Lactate Dehydrogenase *Serum* *No Effect* *Analytical* No effect at 20 mg/L on method on Ames Seralyzer *5706*

Laminin *Plasma* *Decrease* *Physiological* In 23 patients with Graves' disease mean concentration decreased to 742 ng/mL (range 282 - 1180) from 1376 ng/mL (range 712 - 2042) after treatment with 40 mg/d for 8 weeks *6406*

LDL-Cholesterol *Serum Decrease Physiological* In 25 patients with hyperthyroidism mean concentration of 122.1 ± 48.6 mg/dL was significantly different from 146.8 ± 56.0 mg/dL during treatment with 60 mg/d methimazole and 60 mg/d propranolol *2710*
Serum Increase Physiological In 14 hyperthyroid patients treatment with metimazole caused significant increase from mean baseline of 87 ± 38 mg/dL to 178 ± 51 mg/dL *5735*

LE Cells *Blood Positive Physiological* Lupus-like syndrome reported *2754*

Leukocytes *Blood Decrease Physiological* Rare agranulocytosis or pancytopenia *4014* Twelve of 7000 patients receiving treatment for hyperthyroidism developed agranulocytosis. Effect is unrelated to dose, patient age, duration of treatment and second exposure *5936* Occasional case of aplastic anemia reported *6504* Agranulocytosis *133* Leukopenia, thrombocytopenia and aplastic anemia (pancytopenia) are potentially serious side effects of treatment *2971*

Lipoprotein Lp(a) *Serum Increase Physiological* In 14 hyperthyroid patients treatment with metimazole caused significant increase from median baseline of 57 mg/L to 84 mg/L *5735*
Serum No Effect Physiological In 25 patients with hyperthyroidism mean concentration of 7.60 ± 7.66 mg/dL was not significantly different from 7.73 ± 7.13 mg/dL during treatment with 60 mg/d methimazole and 60 mg/d propranolol *2710*

Neutrophils *Blood Decrease Physiological* Agranulocytosis observed in 12 of 7000 patients treated with methimazole for hyperthyroidism. Effect unrelated to dose, duration of treatment, patient's age and second course of treatment *5936* Occasional case of drug-induced neutropenia *241*

Osteocalcin *Serum No Effect Physiological* In 8 postmenopausal women with endogenous subclinical hyperthyroidism treatment with at least 30 mg/d to produce TSH concentration of 1 - 3.5 mU/L caused nonsignificant change of osteocalcin to 13.2 ± 1.1 µg/L compared with 13.6 ± 0.7 µg/L in 8 controls *4150*
Urine No Effect Physiological In 8 postmenopausal women with endogenous subclinical hyperthyroidism treatment with at least 30 mg/d to produce TSH concentration of 1 - 3.5 mU/L caused nonsignificant change of hydroxyproline excretion to 22.8 ± 2.4 mmol/mol creatinine compared with 20.4 ± 2.4 mmol/mol creatinine in 8 controls *4150*

Phosphate *Serum No Effect Analytical* At concentration of 114 mg/L had no effect on phosphomolybdate method *5704*

Platelets *Blood Decrease Physiological* Leukopenia, thrombocytopenia and aplastic anemia (pancytopenia) are potentially serious side effects of treatment *2971* Thrombocytopenia *4013* Occasional case of aplastic anemia reported *6504*

Protein *Serum No Effect Analytical* At concentration of 114 mg/L had no effect on biuret method with blank correction *5704*

Prothrombin Time *Plasma Increase Physiological* Anti-vitamin K activity of tapazole may potentiate the activity of anticoagulants *2971*

T3-Uptake *Serum Decrease Physiological* Therapeutic result *2396*
Serum No Effect Analytical At concentration of 10 µg/dL (876 nmol/L) has no effect on method on Du Pont Dimension *1586*

Thyroid Stimulating Hormone
Serum Increase Physiological In 23 patients with Graves' disease mean concentration increased to 0.1 µU/mL (range < 0.01 - 3.5) from < 0.01 µU/mL after treatment with 40 mg/d for 8 weeks *6406* In 14 hyperthyroid patients treatment with metimazole caused significant increase in concentration from mean baseline of < 0.1 µU/mL to 4 ± 3 µU/mL *5735* In 5 patients with thyrotoxicosis caused by toxic nodular goitre with sinus cardiac rhythm treatment with methimazole 60 mg/d for 10 days caused a significant increase of median from 0.15 mU/L to 1.2 mU/L *1207*

Thyroxine (T4) *Serum Decrease Physiological* Therapeutic intent (stops iodination of tyrosine) *2396* In 5 patients with thyrotoxicosis caused by toxic nodular goitre with sinus cardiac rhythm treatment with methimazole 60 mg/d for 10 days caused a significant reduction of median from 232.8 ng/mL to 166.6 ng/mL *1207* Reduction from mean of 274 nmol/L to 54 nmol/L with 40 days treatment with 40 mg drug daily in 9 patients with hyperthyroidism. Effect marginally greater when given in divided doses rather than in single dose *5118*
Serum Increase Analytical Slightly increased concentration observed when added in vitro with CEDIA method *2717*
Serum No Effect Analytical At concentration of 10 µg/dL (876 nmol/L) has no effect on method on Du Pont Dimension *1587*

Thyroxine (T4), Free *Serum Decrease Physiological* In 23 patients with Graves' disease mean concentration decreased to 12.2 pg/mL (range 8.3 - 21.2) from 58.2 pg/mL (range 24.3 - 92.2) after treatment with 40 mg/d for 8 weeks *6406* In 11 patients with hyperthyroidism treatment with 10 - 15 mg/d for 11 - 21 weeks caused significant decrease from mean baseline of 52.9 ± 7.6 pmol/L to 11.8 ± 1.5 pmol/L *6151*
Serum Increase Physiological In 14 hyperthyroid patients treatment with metimazole caused significant reduction from mean baseline of 35 ± 15 pg/mL to 14 ± 6 pg/mL *5735* In 25 patients with hyperthyroidism mean concentration of 60.10 ± 30.19 U/L was significantly higher than 18.37 ± 10.39 U/L during treatment with 60 mg/d methimazole and 60 mg/d propranolol *2710*
Serum No Effect Analytical Toxic concentration caused change of less than 0.01 ng/dL with method on Technicon Immuno-1 *1296* Methimazole at a concentration of 100 µg/dL had no cross-reactivity FT4 in method on Bayer Technicon Immuno 1® *424*
Serum No Effect Physiological In 8 postmenopausal women with endogenous subclinical hyperthyroidism treatment with at least 30 mg/d to produce TSH concentration of 1 - 3.5 mU/L caused nonsignificant increase of FT4 to 16.7 ± 0.4 pmol/L compared with 14.8 ± 1.2 pmol/L in 8 controls *4150*

Thyroxine (T4) Index, Free *Serum Decrease Physiological* From 23.8 to 17.0 after 4 weeks treatment with 30 mg daily *306*

Tri-iodothyronine, Free (fT3)
Serum Decrease Physiological In 23 patients with Graves' disease mean concentration decreased to 2.6 pg/mL (range 1.3 - 5.6) from 16.1 pg/mL (range 5.4 - 32.6) after treatment with 40 mg/d for 8 weeks *6406* In 14 hyperthyroid patients treatment with metimazole caused significant reduction from mean baseline of 15 ± 9 pg/mL to 5 ± 2 pg/mL *5735* In 11 hyperthyroid patients treatment with 10 - 15 mg/d for 11 - 21 weeks caused significant decrease from mean baseline of 13.1 ± 2.2 pmol/L to 3.1 ± 0.3 pmol/L *6151*
Serum No Effect Analytical At a concentration of 1.0 x 10^{-3} g/L cross-reactivity of 0.0% with free triiodothyronine method on Bayer Technicon Immuno 1® system *425*

Tri-iodothyronine (T3) *Serum Decrease Physiological* In 5 patients with thyrotoxicosis caused by toxic nodular goitre with sinus cardiac rhythm treatment with methimazole 60 mg/d for 10 days caused a significant reduction of median from 4.0 ng/mL to 1.8 ng/mL *1207* Reduction from mean of 5.8 nmol/L to 1.9 nmol/L in 9 patients with hyperthyroidism given 40 mg/day for 40 days. Effect slightly greater with divided doses than with single dose *5118*
Serum No Effect Physiological In 8 postmenopausal women with endogenous subclinical hyperthyroidism treatment with at least 30 mg/d to produce TSH concentration of 1 - 3.5 mU/L caused nonsignificant change of T3 to 2.6 ± 0.2 nmol/L compared with 2.7 ± 0.1 nmol/L in 8 controls *4150*

Tri-iodothyronine (T3) Index, Free
Serum Decrease Physiological From 512 to 368 after 4 weeks treatment with 30 mg daily *306*

Triglycerides *Serum Decrease Analytical* At concentrations above 100 mg/L lowered concentration as measured by GPO-PAP method *5704*
Serum Decrease Physiological In 25 patients with hyperthyroidism mean concentration of 118.0 ± 62.4 mg/dL was significantly different from 144.6 ± 83.6 mg/dL during treatment with 60 mg/d methimazole and 60 mg/d propranolol *2710*
Serum No Effect Physiological In 14 hyperthyroid patients treatment with metimazole caused nonsignificant change from mean baseline of 124 ± 40 mg/dL to 138 ± 43 mg/dL *5735*

Urea Nitrogen *Serum No Effect Analytical* At concentration of 114 mg/L had no effect on diacetylmonoxime method *5704* No effect at 20 mg/L on method on Ames Seralyzer *5706*

Methimazole *(continued)*

Uric Acid *Serum No Effect Analytical* At concentration of 114 mg/L had no effect on phosphotungstate reduction method *5704*

Urobilinogen *Feces Decrease Physiological* Cholestatic effect *2803*
Urine Decrease Physiological Cholestatic effect *2803*

Methocarbamol

Color *Urine Increase Analytical* Brown, green, blue or black on standing *606* Green color observed *4325*

Erythrocytes *Urine Increase Physiological* May cause intravascular hemolysis *2242*

Hemoglobin *Urine Increase Physiological* May cause intravascular hemolysis *2242*

5-Hydroxyindoleacetic Acid *Urine Increase Analytical* Affects quantitative method of Udenfriend *882* Metabolite allegedly reacts with nitrosonaphthol *2695*
Urine No Effect Analytical No effect observed on FPIA method on Abbott TDx *695*

Leukocytes *Blood Decrease Physiological* May cause leukopenia *3810*

Phenylalanine *Plasma No Effect Analytical* No interference observed with rapid quantitative whole blood method of Campbell et al using phenylalanine dehvdrogenase *867*

Vanillylmandelic Acid *Urine Increase Analytical* False positive with screening, no effect quantitative method *1714*

Methohexital

Albumin *Serum No Effect Analytical* At concentration of 50 mg/L had no effect on BCG method *5704*

Bicarbonate *Serum No Effect Analytical* At concentration of 50 mg/L had no effect on method using phenolphthalein *5704*

Bilirubin *Serum No Effect Analytical* At concentration of 50 mg/L had no effect on Jendrassik and Grof method *5704*
Serum No Effect Physiological Insignificant protein-displacing effect in neonates *6314*

Calcium *Serum No Effect Analytical* At concentration of 50 mg/L had no effect on cresolphthalein method *5704*

Chloride *Serum No Effect Analytical* At concentration of 50 mg/L had no effect on mercurimetric method *5704*

Cholesterol *Serum No Effect Analytical* At concentration of 50 mg/L had no effect on Liebermann-Burchard method *5704*

Creatinine *Serum No Effect Analytical* At concentration of 50 mg/L had no effect on Technicon AutoAnalyzer® Jaffe method *5704*

Phosphate *Serum No Effect Analytical* At concentration of 50 mg/L had no effect on phosphomolybdate method *5704*

Protein *Serum No Effect Analytical* At concentration of 50 mg/L had no effect on biuret method with blank correction *5704*

Triglycerides *Serum No Effect Analytical* At concentration of 50 mg/L had no effect on lipase/esterase method *5704*

Urea Nitrogen *Serum No Effect Analytical* At concentration of 50 mg/L had no effect on diacetylmonoxime method *5704*

Uric Acid *Serum No Effect Analytical* At concentration of 50 mg/L had no effect on phosphotungstate reduction method *5704*

Methopterin

Methotrexate *Serum No Effect Analytical* No significant interference observed at a concentration of 1 µmol/L with method on Du Pont aca *1535*

Methotrexate

α_1-Acid Glycoprotein *Serum Increase Physiological* In 94 patients with Crohn's disease treatment with methotrexate for 4 weeks caused reduction to 82 ± 3 mg/dL compared with 97 ± 6 mg/dL in 47 placebo treated patients *1817*

Adenosine Deaminase Binding Protein *Urine Increase Physiological* Manifestation of nephrotoxicity in 12 children receiving chemotherapy; up to 5-fold increase in excretion *2255*

Alanine Aminopeptidase *Urine Increase Physiological* Manifestation of nephrotoxicity in 12 children receiving chemotherapy: up to 5 fold increase in excretion *2255*

Alanine Aminotransferase *Serum Decrease Analytical* At 5 times upper limit of therapeutic range on method on Technicon SMAC® *3525*
Serum Increase Physiological Methotrexate has the potential to cause acute (increased aminotransferase activity) and chronic (fibrosis and cirrhosis) hepatic toxicity *2818* In 152 of 250 courses of treatment but most regressed *3949* May cause cytotoxic hepatocellular damage *402* In 117 patients with rheumatoid arthritis mean value 18.0 U/L compared with reference range of 10 - 41 U/L with 5.1% outside reference range, increasing to 10.8% outside reference range when treated with methotrexate for several years *538*
Serum No Effect Analytical At 5 times upper limit of therapeutic range on method on Abbott-VP, Du Pont aca, Roche Cobas-Bio, Hitachi® 705 and KDA *3525*
Serum No Effect Physiological In 20 patients with psoriasis on long-term therapy *2551*

Albumin *Serum Decrease Physiological* In 117 patients with rheumatoid arthritis mean value 31.6 g/L compared with reference range of 32 - 52 g/L with 41.6% outside reference range, decreasing to 18.2% with treatment with methotrexate for several years *538*
Serum No Effect Analytical At 5 times upper limit of therapeutic range on method on Technicon SMAC® , Kodak Ektachem® , Hitachi® 705, and KDA *3525*

Alkaline Phosphatase *Serum Increase Analytical* At 5 times upper limit of therapeutic range on method on Technicon SMAC® *3525*
Serum Increase Physiological Strong correlation between abnormal activity and abnormal liver biopsy in patients with psoriasis *4359* Hepatotoxic effect (seen in 5% cases psoriasis) *4318* In psoriatic patients receiving drug in comparison with topically treated and controls *582* Methotrexate has the potential to cause acute (increased aminotransferase activity) and chronic (fibrosis and cirrhosis) hepatic toxicity *2818* In 117 patients with rheumatoid arthritis mean value 98.3 U/L compared with reference range of 36 - 120 U/L with 17.9% outside reference range, increasing to 18.3% when treated with methotrexate for several years *538*
Serum No Effect Analytical At 5 times upper limit of therapeutic range on method on Abbott-VP, Du Pont aca, Roche Cobas-Bio, Hitachi® 705 and KDA *3525*
Serum No Effect Physiological No effect in long-term treatment of 20 patients with psoriasis noted *2551* In 20 patients with psoriasis on long-term therapy *2551*

Amino-4-Imidazole-5-Carboxamide Ribotide *Urine Increase Physiological* Occurs with induced folic acid deficiency *6370*

Amylase *Serum No Effect Analytical* At 5 times upper limit of therapeutic range on methods on Du Pont aca, Roche Cobas-Bio and Kodak Ektachem® *3525*

Aspartate Aminotransferase *Serum Increase Physiological* In 152 of 250 courses of treatment but most regressed *3949* Hepatotoxicity (drug induced cirrhosis) *3810* Strong correlation between abnormal activity and abnormal liver biopsy observed in patients with psoriasis *4359* Methotrexate has the potential to cause acute (increased aminotransferase activity) and chronic (fibrosis and cirrhosis) hepatic toxicity *2818* In 117 patients with rheumatoid arthritis mean value 15.5 U/L compared with reference range of 11 - 36 U/L with 0.8% outside reference range, but increased to 7.6% outside reference range when treated with methotrexate for several years *538*
Serum No Effect Analytical At 5 times upper limit of therapeutic range on methods on Technicon SMAC® , Abbott-VP, Du Pont aca, Roche Cobas-Bio, Hitachi® 705 and KDA *3525*
Serum No Effect Physiological No effect in long-term treatment of 20 patients with psoriasis noted *2551*

Bile *Urine Increase Physiological* Hepatotoxicity *3810*

Bile Acids *Serum Decrease Physiological* In 117 patients with rheumatoid arthritis mean value 2.3 µmol/L compared with reference range of 0 - 6 µmol/L with 3.4% outside reference range, decreasing to 2.4% when treated with methotrexate for several months *538*

Bilirubin *Serum Increase Analytical* Clinically significant effect at upper limit of therapeutic range on method on Ektachem® *3525*
Serum Increase Physiological In 117 patients with rheumatoid arthritis mean value 7.6 µmol/L compared with reference range of 3 - 26 µmol/L with 0.0% outside reference range, increasing to 0.8% with treatment with methotrexate for several years *538* Strong correlation between increased concentration and abnormal liver biopsy in patients with psoriasis *4359* In 10 of 250 courses of treatment but most regressed *3949* Methotrexate has the potential to cause acute (increased aminotransferase activity) and chronic (fibrosis and cirrhosis) hepatic toxicity *2818* May cause cytotoxic hepatocellular damage *402*
Serum No Effect Analytical No significant effect at 5 times upper limit of therapeutic range on Technicon SMAC® , Du Pont aca, Roche Cobas-Bio, Hitachi® 705 and KDA *3525* No effect at 0.13 mg/L on Ames Seralyzer method *5706*

Bilirubin, Conjugated *Serum Increase Analytical* At concentration of 1,000 µmol/L as much as 38 mg/L increase in concentration on Kodak Ektachem® 400 *5895*

Bilirubin, Unconjugated *Serum Decrease Analytical* Falsely low values in serum of patients containing large amount of drug following i.v. infusion *5895*

BSP Retention *Serum Increase Physiological* Hepatotoxicity, may be post-necrotic cirrhosis *2578*

CA549 *Serum No Effect Analytical* No statistically significant effect observed over a concentration range of 0.9 to 13.2 mg/L with BRESMARQ assay *958* No interference observed over concentration range of 0.9 - 13.2 mg/L with immunoradiometric BRESMARQ method *958*

Calcium *Serum No Effect Analytical* At 5 times upper limit of therapeutic range on method on Technicon SMAC® , Abbott-VP, Du Pont aca, Kodak Ektachem® , Hitachi® 705 and KDA *3525*

Carcinoembryonic Antigen *Serum No Effect Analytical* At a concentration of up to 16.0 µg/mL caused less than 10% error in the concentration of CEA as measured by the method on Bayer Technicon Immuno 1® *418*

Cholesterol *Serum Increase Analytical* At 5 times upper limit of therapeutic range on enzymatic method on KDA At 5 times upper limit of therapeutic range on enzymatic method on KDA *3525*
Serum No Effect Analytical At concentration of 500 mg/L had no effect on catalase-AIDH method *5704* At concentration of 500 mg/L had no effect on method using catalase-Hantzsch reaction *5704* No effect at 0.13 mg/L on Ames Seralyzer method *5706* At 5 times upper limit of therapeutic range on methods on Technicon SMAC® , Abbott-VP, Roche Cobas-Bio, Kodak Ektachem® and Hitachi® 705 *3525* At concentration of 500 mg/L had no effect on CHOD-Iodide method *5704* No effect at concentrations up to 500 mg/L on method on Kodak Ektachem® *5706* At concentration of 500 mg/L had no effect on Liebermann-Burchard method *5704* At concentration of 500 mg/L had no effect on CHOD-PAP method *5704*

Cholinesterase *Serum No Effect Analytical* No effect observed at concentrations of 5 and 50 µg/mL with butyrylthiocholine method on Kodak Ektachem® *2504*

Chondrex *Serum No Effect Analytical* Concentrations up to 10 g/L had no significant effect on sandwich-type ELISA procedure of Harvey et al *2491*

Chromosomes *Test Conditions Abnormal Physiological* Clastogenic in human lymphocytes in culture *5484*

Cisplatin *Serum Increase Physiological* Increased area under the curve in 5 patients when methotrexate coadministered with cisplatin over 8 hours after injection. Associated with reduced renal excretion (by as much as 50%) in the first 3 hours *4775*

Cobalamin *Serum No Effect Physiological* In 6 patients with cancer but with plasma homocysteine concentration within reference interval each given six courses of high dose methotrexate caused nonsignificant change from mean baseline of 475 ± 255 pmol/L to 476 ± 123 pmol/L *2380*

Color *Feces Increase Analytical* Black color reported with ingestion of methotrexate *3388*

C-Reactive Protein *Serum Decrease Physiological* In 8 patients with rheumatoid arthritis treatment with 15 mg intravenously weekly for 4 months caused significant reduction from mean baseline of 46.01 mg/L to 22.88 mg/L *6359*

Creatine Kinase *Serum No Effect Analytical* At 5 times upper limit of therapeutic range on methods on Technicon SMAC® , Abbott-VP, Du Pont aca, Roche Cobas-Bio, and Hitachi® 705 *3525* No effect at 0.13 mg/L on method on Ames Seralyzer *5706*
Serum No Effect Physiological In one patient injection of 0.3 mL fluid caused no significant change from mean baseline of 104 U/L to 107 U/L after 12 h, 58 U/L after 24 h and 43 U/L after 36 h *309*

Creatinine *Serum Increase Physiological* Methotrexate in high doses may cause renal damage leading to acute renal failure *2818*
Serum No Effect Analytical No effect of concentrations up to 500 mg/L on 2-slide method on Kodak Ektachem® *5706* At concentration of 1 mg/L had no effect on Jaffe-Fuller's earth method *5704* No effect at 0.13 mg/L on Ames Seralyzer method *5706* At concentration of 55 mg/L had no effect on kinetic Jaffe method on BKA-2 *5704* At 5 times upper limit of therapeutic range on method on Technicon SMAC® , Abbott-VP, Roche Cobas-Bio, Kodak Ektachem® , Hitachi® 705 and KDA *3525* At concentration of 1 mg/L had no effect on Jaffe-Fading-Fraction method *5704*
Serum No Effect Physiological In 6 patients with cancer but with plasma homocysteine concentration within reference interval each given six courses of high dose methotrexate caused nonsignificant change from mean baseline of 98 ± 13 µmol/L to 93 ± 7 µmol/L *2380*
Urine Increase Physiological Manifestation of nephrotoxicity *2255*

Crystals *Urine Increase Physiological* Crystals of unknown identity (probably drug) *1635*

Erythrocyte Sedimentation Rate
Blood Decrease Physiological In 8 patients with rheumatoid arthritis treatment with 15 mg intravenously weekly for 4 months caused significant decrease from mean baseline of 53.25 mm/h to 25.13 mm/h *6359* In 36 patients with rheumatoid arthritis treatment with 7.5 to 17.5 mg/wk caused significant reduction from mean baseline of 39 ± 29 mm/h to 19 ± 16 mm/h after 9 mo and 16 ± 13 mm/h after 24 h *4361*

Erythrocytes *Blood Decrease Physiological* May cause megaloblastic anemia (folic acid antagonist) *6370*

Fat *Feces Increase Physiological* Probably due to mucosal damage with impaired regeneration of epithelial cells of small intestine *5055*

Folate *Red Blood Cells Decrease Physiological* Significantly lower in patients with psoriasis with long term treatment reflecting low polyglutamate storage *2551*
Red Blood Cells Increase Analytical At therapeutic concentrations may have a significant effect on method on Bayer Technicon Immuno 1® because of inherent cross-reactivity of folate binding proteins for folate analogs *432*
Red Blood Cells No Effect Analytical Cross-reactivity of less than 2% observed at a concentration of 1 µg/mL with method on Bio-Rad Radias *3557*
Serum Decrease Physiological Inhibits folate reductase *5054* Significantly higher in patients with psoriasis reflecting decreased dihydrofolate reductase activity. Both oxidized forms pteroylglutamate and dihydrofolate affected *2551*
Serum Increase Analytical At therapeutic concentrations may have a significant effect on method on Bayer Technicon Immuno 1® because of inherent cross-reactivity of folate binding proteins for folate analogs *423*
Serum No Effect Analytical At concentration of 500 ng/mL no clinically significant effect observed on method on Stratus family of analyzers *4141*
Serum No Effect Physiological In 6 patients with cancer but with plasma homocysteine concentration within reference interval each given six courses of high dose methotrexate caused change from below 45.3 nmol/L to above 45.3 nmol/L *2380*

γ-Globulin *Serum Decrease Physiological* Possible immunosuppressive response *2754*

Glucose *Serum No Effect Analytical* At concentration of 25 mg/L had no effect on GOD/POD-PAP method *5704* At concentration of 1200 mg/L had no effect on Kodak Ektachem®

Methotrexate *(continued)*

Glucose *(continued)*
method *5704* No effect at 0.13 mg/L on glucose oxidase method on Ames Seralyzer *5706* At 5 times upper limit of therapeutic range on method on Technicon SMAC®, Abbott-VP, Roche Cobas-Bio, Kodak Ektachem®, Hitachi® 705 and KDA *3525*

γ-Glutamyltransferase *Serum Decrease Physiological* In 117 patients with rheumatoid arthritis mean value 50.8 U/L compared with reference range of 8 - 45 U/L with 33.0% outside reference range, decreasing to 23.1% outside normal range when treated with methotrexate for several months *538*
Serum Increase Physiological In psoriatic patients receiving drug in comparison with topically treated and controls *582*
Serum No Effect Analytical At 5 times upper limit of therapeutic range on methods on Technicon SMAC®, Abbott-VP, and Hitachi® 705 *3525*

Guanase *Serum Increase Physiological* May cause cytotoxic hepatocellular damage *402*

Hematocrit *Blood Decrease Physiological* Methotrexate may suppress hematopoiesis and cause anemia, leukopenia and/or thrombocytopenia *2818* May cause megaloblastic anemia (folic acid antagonist) *6370*

Hemoglobin *Blood Decrease Physiological* May cause megaloblastic anemia (folic acid antagonist) *6370* Methotrexate may suppress hematopoiesis and cause anemia, leukopenia and/or thrombocytopenia *2818*
Blood No Effect Physiological No effect in long-term treatment of 20 patients with psoriasis noted *2551* In 20 patients with psoriasis on long-term therapy *2551*
Urine Increase Physiological May cause hematuria *6612*

Histamine *Plasma No Effect Analytical* No inhibition of radio-enzyme assay at much higher than therapeutic concentrations *2492*

Homocysteine *Plasma Increase Physiological* Mean increase of 62% with very high dose methotrexate at 36 hours and of 56% at 24 hours with high dose methotrexate after infusion begun *776* In 6 patients with cancer but with plasma homocysteine concentration within reference interval each given six courses of high dose methotrexate caused change from mean baseline of 8.6 ± 2.7 μmol/L to 9.7 ± 6.2 μmol/L *2380*

Homocystine *Plasma Increase Physiological* At doses of 25 mg to 8 g/m^2 rapid and transient increase in concentration observed *6123*

Hydantoin-5-Propionic Acid *Urine Increase Physiological* Major effect of treatment observed *6194*

Indocyanine Green Clearance
Serum Decrease Physiological In psoriatic patients receiving drug in comparison with topically treated and controls *582*

Iron *Serum Increase Physiological* Sharp increase 8-12 h after end of cycle. Maximum value of 295% at 48-60 h; after 108 h had returned to normal in only 50% *5312*
Serum No Effect Analytical At 5 times upper limit of therapeutic range on Ferrozine method on Technicon SMAC® *3525*

Isocitrate Dehydrogenase *Serum Increase Physiological* May cause cytotoxic hepatocellular damage *402*

Lactate Dehydrogenase *Serum Decrease Analytical* At 5 times upper limit of therapeutic range on method on Technicon SMAC® *3525*
Serum Increase Physiological Effect in 40% cases of psoriasis (reversible) *4318*
Serum No Effect Analytical At 5 times upper limit of therapeutic range on method on Abbott-VP, Roche Cobas-Bio, Hitachi® 705 and KDA *3525* No effect at 0.13 mg/L on method on Ames Seralyzer *5706*

Leukocytes *Blood Decrease Physiological* Agranulocytosis/Lymphocytopenia *4013* Methotrexate may suppress hematopoiesis and cause anemia, leukopenia and/or thrombocytopenia *2818*

Lipase *Serum No Effect Analytical* No effect of concentrations up to 500 mg/L on method on Kodak Ektachem® *5706*

MCV *Blood Increase Physiological* Occurs with megaloblastic anemia *6370*
Blood No Effect Physiological No effect in long-term treatment of 20 patients with psoriasis noted *2551*

Methionine *Plasma Decrease Physiological* Mean reduction of 73% with high dose treatment at 4.5 hours and 70% at 24 hours after start of infusion *776*

N-Acetyl-Glucosaminidase *Urine Increase Physiological* Manifestation of nephrotoxicity in 12 children receiving chemotherapy: up to 5 fold increase in excretion *2255*
Urine No Effect Analytical At 1 mmol/L on 2 colorimetric analytical methods *2254*

N-Formiminoglutamic Acid *Urine Increase Physiological* Large effect of treatment observed *6194*

Occult Blood *Feces Increase Physiological* May cause hemorrhagic enteritis *202*

Ornithine Carbamoyltransferase
Serum Increase Physiological May cause cytotoxic hepatocellular damage *402*

Phenylalanine *Plasma Increase Physiological* Infusion of 5-8 g/sq meter to 46 patients caused significant increase in 95% methotrexate cycles probably due to inhibition of dihydropteridine reductase *1409*
Plasma No Effect Analytical No interference observed with rapid quantitative whole blood method of Campbell et al using phenylalanine dehydrogenase *867*

Phosphate *Serum Increase Analytical* At upper limit of therapeutic range on methods on Du Pont aca and Hitachi® 705 and at 5 times this on method on Technicon SMAC® *3525*
Serum No Effect Analytical At 5 times upper limit of therapeutic range on KDA method *3525*

Platelets *Blood Decrease Physiological* Methotrexate may suppress hematopoiesis and cause anemia, leukopenia and/or thrombocytopenia *2818* May occur with megaloblastic anemia *6370*

Potassium *Serum No Effect Analytical* At concentration of 80 mg/L had no effect on measurement by ISE without predilution *5704*

Prostate-specific Antigen *Serum No Effect Analytical* Methotrxate at a concentration of up to 30 μg/mL caused less than 0.1% cross-reactivity with method on PSA method on Bayer Technicon Immuno 1® *430*

Prostate-specific Antigen, Free *Serum No Effect Analytical* Methotrexate at a concentration of 13.2 mg/L had no significant effect on the Hybritech Tandem® -R free PSA immunoassay *4286*

Protein *Cerebrospinal Fluid Increase Analytical* High absorbance with turbidimetric methods. Reacts as if phenol with Folin-Ciocalteu *6693* Marked effect on Du Pont aca method (up to 40 times actual concentration) even at therapeutic concentration; if concentration low enough not to produce yellow color protein concentration not significantly affected *6241*
Cerebrospinal Fluid No Effect Analytical No significant effect when added in vitro to concentration of 0.3 mg/dL when measured by Kodak Ektachem® slide method *3654*
Serum No Effect Analytical At 5 times upper limit of therapeutic range on methods on Technicon SMAC®, Abbott-VP, Hitachi® 705 and KDA *3525* No effect of concentrations up to 500 mg/L on method on Kodak Ektachem® *5706*

Protein Electrophoresis *Serum No Effect Analytical* At concentration of 80 mg/L had no effect on automated Olympus-Hite method *5704*

Prothrombin Time *Plasma Increase Physiological* May occur with hepatic malfunction *2452*

Reticulocytes *Blood Decrease Physiological* Affects hematopoiesis *2242*

Rheumatoid Factor *Serum Decrease Physiological* In 8 patients with rheumatoid arthritis treatment with 15 mg intravenously weekly for 4 months caused significant reduction from mean baseline of 576.98 IU/mL to 115.63 IU/mL *6359*

SDZ PSC 833 *Blood No Effect Analytical* At a concentration of 8 μmol/L had no effect on HPLC method of Scott et al when used to measure PSC (with CsD as internal standard) at a concentration of 5 mg/L *5418*

Sodium *Serum No Effect Analytical* At concentration of 80 mg/L had no effect on measurement by ISE without predilution *5704*

Soluble Interleukin-2 Receptor
Serum Decrease Physiological In 41 patients with rheumatoid arthritis treatment with methotrexate caused significant reduction of mean concentration from mean baseline of 910 ± 422 units to 681 ± 335 units *4729*

Sperm Count *Semen Decrease Physiological* Oligospermia occurs without altering plasma hormone concentrations *1499*

Testosterone *Serum No Effect Physiological* In a group of male patients with rheumatoid arthritis taking methotrexate mean concentration not significantly different from concentration in untreated male patients *3808*

Theophylline *Serum Increase Physiological* Decreases theophylline clearance, increasing theophylline concentration by about 20% after low dose treatment with a greater effect with higher doses *5999* Methotrexate may decrease the clearance of theophylline thereby increasing its serum concentration *2818* Up to 20% increase in serum theophylline concentration due to decreased theophylline clearance with low dose methotrexate, possibly greater effect at higher concentrations *6117* Decreases theophylline clearance and increases serum theophylline concentration by 20% agter low dose methotrexate so higher doses are likely to have a greater effect *3125*

Triglycerides *Serum Decrease Analytical* At 5 times upper limit of therapeutic range on Technicon SMAC® method *3525*
Serum No Effect Analytical At concentration of 25 mg/L had no effect on GPO-PAP method *5704* At 5 times upper limit of therapeutic range on methods on Abbott-VP, Kodak Ektachem®, Hitachi® 705 and KDA *3525*

Urea Nitrogen *Serum Increase Physiological* May cause severe nephropathy, azotemia *2754* Methotrexate in high doses may cause renal damage leading to acute renal failure *2818*
Serum No Effect Analytical At concentration of 1100 mg/L had no effect on Kodak Ektachem® method *5704* At 5 times upper limit of therapeutic range on method on Technicon SMAC®, Abbott-VP, Roche Cobas-Bio, Kodak Ektachem®, Hitachi® 705 and KDA *3525* No effect at 0.13 mg/L on method on Ames Seralyzer *5706*

Uric Acid *Serum Decrease Analytical* At 5 times upper limit of therapeutic range on enzymatic method on Hitachi® 705 *3525*
Serum Decrease Physiological Inhibits synthesis *5402*
Serum Increase Physiological Seen in gouty patients and also some decrease in leukemics *3812*
Serum No Effect Analytical At concentration of 25 mg/L had no effect on uricase-PAP method *5704* At 5 times upper limit of therapeutic range on methods on Technicon SMAC®, Abbott-VP, Du Pont aca, Roche Cobas-Bio, Kodak Ektachem® and KDA *3525* At concentration of 1 mg/L had no effect on Kageyama-Hantzsch method *5704* At concentration of 1 mg/L had no effect on catalase-AIDH method *5704*
Urine Increase Physiological Increased excretion associated with cell destruction *2209*

Urocanic Acid *Urine Increase Physiological* With treatment of folic acid/B_{12} deficiency *6194*

Urocanylglycine *Urine Increase Physiological* Large effect of treatment observed *6194*

Methotrimeprazine

Alanine Aminotransferase *Serum Increase Physiological* Jaundice and hepatotoxicity have been reported as complications of long-term high-dose drug administration *2817*

Alkaline Phosphatase *Serum Increase Physiological* Jaundice and hepatotoxicity have been reported as complications of long-term high-dose drug administration *2817*

Aspartate Aminotransferase *Serum Increase Physiological* Jaundice and hepatotoxicity have been reported as complications of long-term high-dose drug administration *2817*

Bicarbonate *Serum No Effect Analytical* At concentration of 1 mg/L had no effect on method using phenolphthalein *5704*

Bilirubin *Serum Increase Physiological* Jaundice and hepatotoxicity have been reported as complications of long-term high-dose drug administration *2817* Three cases reported *2451*
Serum No Effect Analytical At concentration of 1 mg/L had no effect on Jendrassik and Grof method *5704*

Calcium *Serum No Effect Analytical* At concentration of 1 mg/L had no effect on cresolphthalein method *5704*

Carbon Dioxide Partial Pressure
Blood No Effect Physiological In dose of 0.15 mg/kg intravenously had no significant increase in concentration *6682*

Chloride *Serum No Effect Analytical* At concentration of 1 mg/L had no effect on mercurimetric method *5704*

Cholesterol *Serum No Effect Analytical* At concentration of 1 mg/L had no effect on CHOD-PAP method *5704*

Creatinine *Serum No Effect Analytical* At concentration of 1 mg/L had no effect on Technicon AutoAnalyzer® Jaffe method *5704*

Eosinophils *Blood Increase Physiological* Noted with other phenothiazines *2754* Leukopenia, pancytopenia, eosinophilia and thrombocytopenia have been reported as complications of long-term high-dose drug administration *2817*

Ferric Chloride Test *Urine Positive Analytical* Positive if more than 100 mg/d for 6 d *4014*

Glucose *Serum No Effect Analytical* At concentration of 1 mg/L had no effect on GOD/POD-PAP method *5704*

γ-Glutamyltransferase *Serum Increase Physiological* Jaundice and hepatotoxicity have been reported as complications of long-term high-dose drug administration *2817*

Granulocytes *Blood Decrease Physiological* Agranulocytosis has been reported as complication of long-term high-dose drug administration *2817*

Hematocrit *Blood Decrease Physiological* Leukopenia, pancytopenia, eosinophilia and thrombocytopenia have been reported as complications of long-term high-dose drug administration *2817*

Hemoglobin *Blood Decrease Physiological* Leukopenia, pancytopenia, eosinophilia and thrombocytopenia have been reported as complications of long-term high-dose drug administration *2817*

Leukocytes *Blood Decrease Physiological* Leukopenia, pancytopenia, eosinophilia and thrombocytopenia have been reported as complications of long-term high-dose drug administration *2817* Agranulocytosis with long-term high-dose use *2754*

Neutrophils *Blood Decrease Physiological* Occasional case of drug-induced neutropenia *241*

Oxygen Partial Pressure *Blood No Effect Physiological* In dose of 0.15 mg/kg intravenously had no significant effect in 6 healthy volunteers *6682*

Phenylketones *Urine Positive Analytical* Phenistix® positive if more than 100 mg/d for 6 d *4014*

Pheochromocytoma Test *Patient Positive Physiological* May cause false test as produces hypotension *2451*

Platelets *Blood Decrease Physiological* Noted with other phenothiazines *2754* Leukopenia, pancytopenia, eosinophilia and thrombocytopenia have been reported as complications of long-term high-dose drug administration *2817*

Potassium *Serum No Effect Analytical* At concentration of 1 mg/L had no effect on flame-photometric method *5704*

Protein *Cerebrospinal Fluid Increase Physiological* May occur if cerebral edema etc *2754*
Serum No Effect Analytical At concentration of 1 mg/L had no effect on biuret method with blank correction *5704*

Sodium *Serum No Effect Analytical* At concentration of 1 mg/L had no effect on flame-photometric method *5704*

Triglycerides *Serum No Effect Analytical* At concentration of 1 mg/L had no effect on lipase/esterase method *5704*

Urea Nitrogen *Serum No Effect Analytical* At concentration of 1 mg/L had no effect on diacetylmonoxime method *5704*

Uric Acid *Serum No Effect Analytical* At concentration of 1 mg/L had no effect on phosphotungstate reduction method *5704*

Methoxamine

Corticotropin *Plasma Increase Physiological* Drug may increase the concentration of corticotropin *2166*

Cortisol *Plasma Increase Physiological* Drug may increase the concentration of cortisol *2166*

Methoxsalen

Alanine Aminotransferase *Serum Increase Physiological* Hepatotoxic effect *3810*

Alkaline Phosphatase *Serum Increase Physiological* Hepatotoxic effect *3810*

Aspartate Aminotransferase *Serum Increase Physiological* Hepatotoxic effect *3810*

Bile *Urine Increase Physiological* Hepatotoxic effect *3810*

Bilirubin *Serum Increase Physiological* Hepatotoxic effect *3810*

BSP Retention *Serum Increase Physiological* Hepatotoxic effect *3810*

Caffeine *Serum No Effect Physiological* Peak concentration and time to reach this not affected although mean elimination greatly increased *3859*

Methoxyflurane

Alanine Aminotransferase *Serum Increase Physiological* Hepatic toxicity *5503* In 2 pregnant women when used as analgesia for labor: hepatitis observed *1369*

Alkaline Phosphatase *Serum Increase Physiological* In 2 pregnant women when used as analgesia for labor: hepatitis observed *1369* Hepatic toxicity *5503*

Aspartate Aminotransferase *Serum Increase Physiological* Hepatic toxicity *5503* In 2 pregnant women when used as analgesia for labor: hepatitis observed *1369*

Bile *Urine Increase Physiological* Hepatotoxic effect *3810*

Bilirubin *Serum Increase Physiological* Hepatic toxicity *5503* In 2 pregnant women when used as analgesia for labor: hepatitis observed *1369*

BSP Retention *Serum Increase Physiological* Hepatotoxicity *3810*

Calcium *Serum Decrease Physiological* Slight lowering reported in one case *4801*

Chloride *Serum Increase Physiological* Toxic nephropathy reported *4952*

Creatinine *Serum Increase Physiological* Impaired renal tubular function *3887*

Creatinine Clearance *Urine No Effect Physiological* No effect observed with high or low concentrations *2290*

Effective Renal Plasma Flow
Patient Decrease Physiological Decrease noted during normal anesthesia *4014*

Fluoride *Serum Increase Physiological* Metabolic degradation product of anesthetic *1946*
Urine Increase Physiological Persisting high concentration many days with renal impairment *5960*

Glomerular Filtration Rate *Urine Decrease Physiological* Decrease noted during normal anesthesia *4014*
Urine No Effect Physiological No effect observed with high or low concentrations *2290*

Osmolality *Serum Increase Physiological* Associated with high-output renal failure after administration for long time without dose reduction and dehydration *1384* Impaired renal tubular function *1159*
Urine Decrease Physiological Nephrotoxic effect of drug (dose dependent) *4029*

Oxalate *Serum Increase Physiological* Metabolic degradation product of drug *4801*
Urine Increase Physiological Metabolic degradation product of drug *4801*

Proline Hydroxylase *Serum Increase Physiological* Marked elevation observed due to liver cell injury *5799*

Prothrombin Time *Plasma Increase Physiological* In 2 pregnant women when used as analgesia for labor: hepatitis observed *1369*

Sodium *Serum Increase Physiological* Impaired renal tubular function *1159*

Specific Gravity *Urine Decrease Physiological* Impaired renal tubular function (dose dependent) Impaired renal tubular function *1159*

Thyroid Stimulating Hormone
Serum No Effect Physiological No effect observed with anesthesia *4469*

Thyroxine (T4) *Serum No Effect Physiological* No effect observed with anesthesia *4469*

Urea Nitrogen *Serum Increase Physiological* Impaired renal tubular function *1159*

Uric Acid *Serum Increase Physiological* Decreased urate clearance: contraction of extracellular fluid volume *3887*

Volume *Urine Increase Physiological* After administration for long periods without time-dependent dose reductions may be vasopressin-resistant high-output renal failure *1384* Impaired distal renal tubular function *1159*

Water Clearance, Free *Urine No Effect Physiological* No effect observed with high or low concentrations *2290*

4-Methoxyphenol

5-Hydroxyindoleacetic Acid *Urine No Effect Analytical* No effect with 5 mg/dL on method of Goldenberg *2220*

Methsuximide

Albumin *Serum No Effect Analytical* At concentration of 40 mg/L had no effect on BCG method *5704*

Bicarbonate *Serum No Effect Analytical* At concentration of 40 mg/L had no effect on method using phenolphthalein *5704*

Bilirubin *Serum Increase Physiological* Hepatic damage reported *128*
Serum No Effect Analytical At concentration of 40 mg/L had no effect on Jendrassik and Grof method *5704*

Calcium *Serum No Effect Analytical* At concentration of 40 mg/L had no effect on cresolphthalein method *5704*

Chloride *Serum No Effect Analytical* At concentration of 40 mg/L had no effect on Kodak Ektachem® method *5704*

Creatinine *Serum No Effect Analytical* At concentration of 40 mg/L had no effect on Kodak Ektachem® method *5704*

Cyclosporine *Serum Decrease Physiological* Reported effect presumably as result of induction of hepatic microsomal enzymes *1069*

Eosinophils *Blood Increase Physiological* Methsuximide may cause eosinophilia as an adverse reaction *4518* Reported effect *2754*

Erythrocytes *Blood Decrease Physiological* Rare aplastic anemia reported *3810*

Ethosuximide *Serum Increase Analytical* Compound metabolized to N-desmethylmethsuximide which cross-reacts with method used on Du Pont aca *1523*

Felbamate *Serum No Effect Analytical* No significant interference observed with GLC method of Rifai et al *4958*

Glucose *Serum No Effect Analytical* At concentration of 40 mg/L had no effect on Kodak Ektachem® method *5704*

LE Cells *Blood Positive Physiological* Cause of SLE reported *2754*

Leukocytes *Blood Decrease Physiological* Methsuximide may cause leukopenia and pnacytopenia with or without bone marrow suppression as an adverse reaction *4518* Rare aplastic anemia or reversible leukopenia *3810*

Monocytes *Blood Increase Physiological* Reported observation *2754* Methsuximide may cause monocytosis as an adverse reaction *4518*

Phenobarbital *Serum Increase Physiological* Coadministration of methsuximide with phenobarbital may increase the latter's concentration *4518*
Serum No Effect Analytical At concentration of 1.00 mg/mL (4.92 mmol/L) has no effect on method on Du Pont Dimension *1582* No significant cross-reactivity observed with method on Du Pont aca *1537*

Phenytoin *Serum Increase Physiological* Coadministration of methsuximide with phenytoin may increase the latter's concentration *4518*
Serum No Effect Analytical No effect at concentration of 1000 μg/mL (4920 μmol/L) on method on Du Pont Dimension

1583 No significant interference observed at a concentration of 1000 µg/mL (4.92 mmol/L) with method on Du Pont aca *1538*

Phosphate *Serum No Effect Analytical* At concentration of 40 mg/L had no effect on phosphomolybdate method *5704*

Platelets *Blood Decrease Physiological* May rarely cause bone marrow aplasia *2385*

Protein *Serum No Effect Analytical* At concentration of 40 mg/L had no effect on biuret method with blank correction *5704*
Urine Increase Physiological Renal damage reported *2024*

Triglycerides *Serum No Effect Analytical* At concentration of 40 mg/L had no effect on lipase/esterase method *5704*

Urea Nitrogen *Serum Increase Physiological* Renal damage reported *128*
Serum No Effect Analytical At concentration of 40 mg/L had no effect on diacetylmonoxime method *5704*

Uric Acid *Serum No Effect Analytical* At concentration of 40 mg/L had no effect on phosphotungstate reduction method *5704*

Methyclothiazide

Amylase *Serum Increase Physiological* Pancreatitis may occur with thiazide therapy *2754*

Antidiuretic Hormone *Plasma Increase Physiological* Secreted in response to hyponatremia *1856*

Apolipoprotein A-I *Serum Increase Physiological* Statistically significant increase in 65 mildly hypertensive patients treated with 5 mg daily for 10 weeks *3691*

Apolipoprotein B *Serum Increase Physiological* Statistically significant increase in 65 mildly hypertensive patients treated with 5 mg daily for 10 weeks *3691*

Bicarbonate *Serum Increase Physiological* Diuretic action (hypochloremic alkalosis) *2251*
Urine Increase Physiological Slight effect only *2754*

Bilirubin *Serum Increase Physiological* Jaundice may occur with thiazide therapy *2754*

Calcium *Serum Increase Physiological* Thiazides may cause intermittent and slight increase of plasma calcium in the absence of known calcium disorders *19* ?related to decreased excretion *2754*
Urine Decrease Physiological Impairs excretion *2754* Significant reduction compared with placebo in normal volunteers *3354*
Urine Increase Physiological Thiazides may decrease urinary calcium excretion *19*

Chloride *Serum Decrease Physiological* Diuretic action (hypochloremic alkalosis) *2251*
Serum Increase Physiological Chloride deficit, if it occurs in response to methyclothiazide, is generally mild and usually does not require treatment *19*
Urine Increase Physiological Intended diuretic action (maximum in 6 h) *2754*

Cholesterol *Serum Increase Physiological* Statistically significant increase in 67 mildly hypertensive patients treated with 5 mg daily for 10 weeks *3691* Thiazides may cause increased concentration of plasma cholesterol *19*

Creatinine *Serum No Effect Analytical* No interference observed with liquid chromatographic method of Paroni *4540*

Erythrocytes *Blood Decrease Physiological* Aplastic anemia may occur with thiazides *2754*

Glucose *Serum Increase Physiological* Diabetogenic action of thiazides *2754* Latent diabetes mellitus may become apparent during thiazide administration *19*
Urine Increase Physiological May occur as result of hyperglycemia *2754*

HDL-Cholesterol *Serum No Effect Physiological* No significant change in 66 mildly hypertensive patients treated with 5 mg daily for 10 weeks *3691*

Leukocytes *Blood Decrease Physiological* Agranulocytosis or aplastic anemia may occur *2754*

Lithium Clearance *Urine Decrease Physiological* Thiazides may reduce renal clearance of lithium *19*

Low Density Lipoprotein *Serum Increase Physiological* Thiazides may cause increased concentration of plasma low density lipoproteins *19*

Magnesium *Urine Increase Physiological* Small but significant increase in excretion in 8 normal volunteers when given alone (2 mg) or with triamterene. Effect prevented by only smallest dose (25 mg) of triamterene *3354*

Osmolality *Serum Decrease Physiological* With ADH secretion due to hyponatremia *1856*

pH *Urine No Effect Physiological* No significant effect usually observed *2754*

Platelets *Blood Decrease Physiological* Thrombocytopenia with purpura may occur *2754*

Potassium *Serum Decrease Physiological* Diuretic action *2251*
Serum Increase Physiological Hypokalemia may develop with treatment, especially with brisk diuresis, when severe cirrhosis is present, during concomitant use of corticosteroids or ACTH, or after prolonged therapy *19*
Urine Increase Physiological Small but significant effect in normal volunteers *3354*

Renin Activity *Plasma Increase Physiological* Stimulates plasma renin activity *2251*

Sodium *Serum Decrease Physiological* Diuretic action *2251*
Serum Increase Physiological Dilutional hyponatremia may occur in edematous patients in cold weather *19*
Urine Increase Physiological Intended diuretic action (maximum in 6 h) *2754*

Triglycerides *Serum Increase Physiological* Thiazides may cause increased concentration of plasma triglycerides *19* Statistically significant increase in 67 mildly hypertensive patients treated with 5 mg daily for 10 weeks *3691*

Urea Nitrogen *Serum Increase Physiological* Slight change only *2251*

Uric Acid *Serum Increase Physiological* Reduces clearance *2251*

VLDL + LDL-Cholesterol *Serum Increase Physiological* Significant increase observed in 66 mildly hypertensive patients treated with 5 mg daily for 10 weeks *3691*

Volume *Urine Increase Physiological* Intended diuretic action (maximum in 6 h) *2754*

Methylaminoantipyrine

Cholesterol *Serum Decrease Analytical* At concentrations above 120 mg/L lowered concentration as measured by CHOD-PAP method *5704*

Methylbromide

Casts *Urine Increase Physiological* Due to tubular necrosis *2183*

Erythrocytes *Urine Increase Physiological* Due to tubular necrosis *2183*

Protein *Urine Increase Physiological* Due to tubular necrosis *2183*

Urea Nitrogen *Serum Increase Physiological* Late effect with tubular necrosis of poisoning *2183*

Methyldopa

Alanine Aminotransferase *Serum Increase Physiological* Chronic active hepatitis associated with immune hemolytic anemia in one case *5468* Drug induced hepatitis with severe, chronic, aggressive inflammation *343* Disturbances in liver function in 5 to 35% of patients treated for hypertension. Hepatocellular injury may occur after short or long-term exposure *251* Methyldopa administration may cause hepatitis *3958* Result of hepatocellular damage or cholestasis *6515*
Serum No Effect Analytical No effect up to 2 mg/L on Boehringer Mannheim Reflotron method but above this inhibition of enzyme activity but not of clinical significance *5706* No effect at therapeutic concentration on Boehringer Mannheim Reflotron method *3231*

Albumin *Serum Decrease Physiological* Disturbances in liver function in 5 to 35% of patients treated for hypertension. Hepatocellular injury may occur after short- or long-term exposure *251*

Methyldopa *(continued)*

Albumin *(continued)*
Serum No Effect Analytical At concentration of 80 mg/L had no effect on BCG method *5704*
Urine No Effect Analytical At concentration of 150 mg/dL had no significant effect on Boehringer Mannheim Tina-quant method *2799*

Alkaline Phosphatase *Serum Increase Physiological* Drug induced hepatitis with severe, chronic, aggressive inflammation *343* Intrahepatic cholestatic jaundice *1715* Disturbances in liver function in 5 to 35% of patients treated for hypertension. Hepatocellular injury may occur after short or long-term exposure *251* Methyldopa administration may cause hepatitis *3958*

Amino Acids *Urine Increase Analytical* Reacts with ninhydrin; extra spot TLC, high voltage electrophoresis *4760*

δ-Aminolevulinic Acid *Urine Increase Physiological* May precipitate acute porphyria attack *2210*

Amylase *Serum No Effect Analytical* At a concentration of 1 mg/L had no effect on method on Boehringer Mannheim Reflotron system *5706*

Amylase, Pancreatic Isoenzyme
Serum No Effect Analytical No significant effect observed at toxic concentration of 20 mg/L on method on Boehringer Mannheim Reflotron *3647*

Anti-Smooth Muscle Antibodies
Serum Increase Physiological Disturbances in liver function in 5 to 35% of patients treated for hypertension. Hepatocellular injury may occur after short- or long-term exposure *251* Chronic active hepatitis associated with immune hemolytic anemia in one case *5468*

Antinuclear Antibodies *Serum Increase Physiological* Observed in one patient with hepatocellular damage of moderate severity due to sensitization by drug *1373* More common in females than males *2780* Methyldopa administration may cause positive test for antinuclear antibody *3958*
Serum No Effect Physiological In a study of 9 hypertensives *3101*

Apolipoprotein A-I *Serum No Effect Physiological* In several patients treated for 2-4 mo *142* Decrease by -2 mg/dL in 11 patients given 750 mg daily for 8 weeks *4213*

Apolipoprotein A-II *Serum No Effect Physiological* In several patients treated for 2-4 mo *142*

Apolipoprotein B *Serum No Effect Physiological* Increase by 1 mg/dL in 11 patients given 750 mg daily for 8 weeks *4213* In several patients treated for 2-4 mo *142*

Apolipoprotein C-II *Serum No Effect Physiological* Increase by 2 mg/dL in 11 patients given 750 mg daily for 8 weeks *4213*

Apolipoprotein C-III *Serum Increase Physiological* Increase by 3 mg/dL in 11 patients given 750 mg daily for 8 weeks *4213*

Apolipoprotein E *Serum No Effect Physiological* Increase by 1 mg/dL in 11 patients given 750 mg daily for 8 weeks *4213*

Aspartate Aminotransferase *Serum Increase Analytical* Methyldopa may interfere with colorimetric methods *3958* At 1 mmol/L affects Technicon SMA 12/60 method *5576*
Serum Increase Physiological Chronic active hepatitis associated with immune hemolytic anemia in one case *5468* Drug induced hepatitis with severe, chronic, aggressive inflammation *343* Result of hepatocellular damage or cholestasis *6515* Methyldopa administration may cause hepatitis *3958* Disturbances in liver function in 5 to 35% of patients treated for hypertension. Hepatocellular injury may occur after short or long-term exposure *251*
Serum No Effect Analytical No effect at therapeutic concentration on Boehringer Mannheim Reflotron method *3231* Methyldopa has no effect on spectrophotometric methods *3958* At up to 2 mg/L no effect on Boehringer Mannheim Reflotron method but above this decreased enzyme activity although of no clinical significance since normal concentration less than 2 mg/L *5706*

Bicarbonate *Serum No Effect Analytical* At concentration of 80 mg/L had no effect on method using phenolphthalein *5704*

Bile *Urine Increase Physiological* Occurs as result of hepatocellular damage *6114*

Bilirubin *Serum Increase Analytical* At 1 mmol/L affects Technicon SMA 12/60 method *5576* At concentrations above 65 mg/L (normal therapeutic concentration 2 mg/L) raised concentration as measured by Jendrassik and Grof method *5704* Theoretically reacts with diazo reagent *5407*
Serum Increase Physiological Chronic active hepatitis associated with immune hemolytic anemia in one case *5468* Methyldopa administration may cause hepatitis *3958* Mild hepatocellular jaundice in about 1% cases *1715* Disturbances in liver function in 5 to 35% of patients treated for hypertension. Hepatocellular injury may occur after short or long-term exposure *251*
Serum No Effect Analytical No effect of α-methyldopa at concentration of 3 mg/L on Ames Seralyzer method *5706* At concentration of 1 mg/L no effect on method on Boehringer Mannheim Reflotron system *5706*
Urine Increase Physiological Occurs as result of hepatocellular damage *6114*

Bilirubin, Direct *Serum Increase Physiological* Mild hepatocellular jaundice may occur *2024*

BSP Retention *Serum Increase Physiological* Result of hepatocellular damage (cholestasis also) *6515*

Calcium *Serum No Effect Analytical* At concentration of 80 mg/L had no effect on cresolphthalein method *5704*

Catecholamines *Plasma Increase Analytical* Interference with fluorometric methods *5269* Reacts like catecholamines, may persist for days *2242*
Plasma Increase Physiological Pronounced increase observed, reduced by barbiturates *3009*
Plasma No Effect Analytical No effect on HPLC method of Koller to measure dopamine, epinephrine, and norepinephrine *3230*
Urine Decrease Physiological Depletion of tissue stores *3669*
Urine Increase Analytical Using reversed-phase HPLC-ECD large peak with retention time of epinephrine and even larger peak with retention time of about twice that of dopamine *1257* Methyldopa may interfere with analytical methods because of its fluorescence *3958* Has similar fluorescence *2999* With trihydroxyindole fluorometric procedures *4172*
Urine No Effect Analytical In volunteers with HPLC methods using electrochemical detection *4172*

Chloride *Serum Increase Physiological* May cause salt retention and edema *2242*
Serum No Effect Analytical At concentration of 80 mg/L had no effect on mercurimetric method *5704*

Cholesterol *Serum Decrease Analytical* At concentrations above 50 mg/L (normal therapeutic concentration 2 mg/L) lowered concentration as measured by CHOD-PAP method *5704* At high concentrations of methyldopa cholesterol concentration reduced when measured by method on Roche Cobas Ready *5705* At concentrations above 200 mg/L (normal therapeutic concentration 2 mg/L) lowered concentration as measured by CHOD-Iodide method *5704*
Serum Decrease Physiological In 17 hypertensive patients given drug for 3 mo *1614*
Serum No Effect Analytical At concentration of 400 mg/L had no effect on method using catalase-Hantzsch reaction *5704* No effect up to 1 mg/L on Ames Seralyzer method although above this concentration apparently clinically significant increase *5706* At concentration of 400 mg/L had no effect on Liebermann-Burchard method *5704* At concentrations up to 2 mg/L no effect on method on Boehringer Mannheim Reflotron system but at concentrations above this cholesterol concentration decreased *5706* At concentration of 400 mg/L had no effect on catalase-AIDH method *5704* No effect at therapeutic concentration on Boehringer Mannheim Reflotron method *3231*
Serum No Effect Physiological In 3 studies of 7 to 17 patients for up to 3 mo *141* In several patients treated for 2-4 mo *142* Increase by 2 mg/dL in 11 patients given 750 mg daily for 8 weeks *4213*

Color *Urine Increase Analytical* May produce brown-black on standing *684*

Complement C_3 *Serum Decrease Physiological* Observed in one patient with hepatocellular damage of moderate severity due to sensitization by drug *1373*

Complement C_4 *Serum Decrease Physiological* Observed in one patient with hepatocellular damage of moderate severity due to sensitization by drug *1373*

Coombs' Test *Blood Positive Physiological* Methyldopa administration may cause positive Coombs' tests *3958*

Coombs' Test, Direct *Blood Positive Physiological* Observed in 5 of 9 patients typically seen in 20% of treated patients. Probably due to impaired F_c-dependent reticuloendothelial function *3101* Autoimmune phenomenon (occurs with weeks of treatment) *2453*

Coombs' Test, Indirect *Blood Positive Physiological* Autoimmune phenomenon (occurs with weeks of treatment) *2453*

Coproporphyrin *Feces Increase Physiological* May precipitate acute porphyria attack *2210*

Urine Increase Physiological May precipitate acute porphyria attack *2210*

Cortisol *Plasma No Effect Analytical* No significant effect at a concentration of 20 mg/L on CEDIA or Enzymun methods (worst case 94.8% recovery) *1097*

Creatine Kinase *Serum No Effect Analytical* No effect at 3 mg/L on method on Ames Seralyzer *5706*

Creatine Kinase Isoenzymes *Serum No Effect Analytical* No interference observed at a concentration of 15 mg/L (71 µmol/L) with CK-MB method on Du Pont aca *1519*

Creatinine *Serum Decrease Analytical* At high concentrations may cause falsely lowered result as measured by method on Roche Cobas Ready *5705*

Serum Increase Analytical Methyldopa may interfere with methods using alkaline picrate *3958* At concentrations above 200 mg/L (normal therapeutic concentration 2 mg/L) raised concentration as measured by Technicon AutoAnalyzer® Jaffe method *5704* At concentrations above 2,000 mg/L (normal therapeutic concentration 2 mg/L) raised concentration as measured by Jaffe-Fuller's earth method *5704* Readily oxidized and affects alkaline picrate method *3810* Above 2 mg/mL even affects Fuller's earth procedures *3724*

Serum No Effect Analytical At concentration of 320 mg/L had no effect on Jaffe-Fading-Fraction method *5704* At 30 mg/L on reversed phase liquid chromatographic procedure of Zhiri et al *6656* At concentration of 20 mg/L had no effect on creatinine iminohydrolase method *5704* At concentrations above 50 mg/L (normal therapeutic concentration 2 mg/L) raised concentration as measured by kinetic Jaffe method on BKA-2 *5704* No effect up to 1.5 mg/L on Ames Seralyzer method but at higher concentrations apparently clinically significant increase in creatinine concentration *5706* No interference observed at a concentration of 10 mg/L with HPLC method of Rosano et al *5083*

Urine Increase Analytical Acts as reducing agent with alkaline picrate *1174*

Dopamine *Urine No Effect Physiological* No effect when methyldopa administered and HPLC used to measure catecholamines *4172*

Effective Renal Plasma Flow

Patient Increase Physiological Slight increase or normal in normo- or hypertensives *2242*

Endoplasmic Reticulum Antibody

Serum Increase Physiological Observed in one patient with chronic active hepatitis and cirrhosis *442*

Eosinophils *Blood Increase Physiological* Allergic response *3810*

Epinephrine *Urine No Effect Physiological* No effect when methyldopa administered and HPLC used to measure catecholamines *4172*

Erythrocytes *Blood Decrease Physiological* On rare occasion may produce hemolysis. Great majority of patients do not show this *3101* Autoimmune hemolytic anemia/aplastic anemia *900*

Ferric Chloride Test *Urine Positive Analytical* At 0.2 mg/mL in alkaline urine *3401*

Follicle Stimulating Hormone

Plasma No Effect Physiological No effect in patient on long term treatment who had drug-induced hyperprolactinemia *256*

Glomerular Filtration Rate *Urine Increase Physiological* Slight increase or normal in normo- and hyper-tensives *2242*

Glucose *Serum Decrease Analytical* At concentrations above 200 mg/L (normal therapeutic concentration 2 mg/L) lowered concentration as measured by GOD-PERID method *5704* At concentrations above 100 mg/L (normal therapeutic concentration 2 mg/L) lowered concentration as measured by Kodak Ektachem® method *5704* At concentrations above 7 mg/L (normal therapeutic concentration 2 mg/L) lowered concentration as measured by GOD/POD-PAP method *5704*

Serum Increase Analytical 14.6% increase in absorbance in glucokinase based assay of Scott *5414* At 1 mmol/L affects Technicon SMA 12/60 method *5576*

Serum No Effect Analytical At concentrations up to 2 mg/L no effect on method on Boehringer Mannheim Reflotron system but above this glucose concentration reduced *5706* No effect up to 0.6 mg/L on glucose oxidase method on Ames Seralyzer but above this concentration apparent reduction of glucose concentration of sufficient magnitude to be of clinical significance *5706* At concentration of 400 mg/L had no effect on hexokinase/G-6-PDH method *5704* No effect at therapeutic concentration on Boehringer Mannheim Reflotron method *3231*

Urine No Effect Analytical No effect on glucose oxidase methods *1825*

γ-Glutamyltransferase *Serum Increase Physiological* Drug induced hepatitis with severe, chronic, aggressive inflammation *343*

Serum No Effect Analytical At concentration of 100 mg/L no effect on method on Boehringer Mannheim Reflotron system *5706* No effect at therapeutic concentration on Boehringer Reflotron method *3231*

Granulocytes *Blood Decrease Physiological* Methyldopa administration may cause bone marrow depression and granulocytopenia *3958*

Blood No Effect Physiological No significant association between ingestion and agranulocytosis *3098*

Growth Hormone *Plasma Decrease Physiological* Slight effect on basal concentration after many mo of treatment for hypertension. Concentration increased to greater extent in response to insulin in short-term treated individuals than in controls or long-term treated *5805*

Guaiacols Spot Test *Urine Positive Analytical* False reaction with screening test of Rogers *5061*

Haptoglobin *Serum Decrease Physiological* May cause hemolytic anemia *3810*

HDL-Cholesterol *Serum Decrease Physiological* By up to 15% in 3 studies of 7 to 17 patients for up to 3 mo *141* Increase by 10% in 32 middle-aged hypertensive males treated for 6 weeks *3515* Decrease by -4 mg/dL in 11 patients given 750 mg daily for 8 weeks *4213*

Serum No Effect Analytical At a concentration up to 100 mg/L had no significant effect on Reflotron method for whole blood cholesterol *6352*

Serum No Effect Physiological In 17 hypertensive patients given drug for 3 mo *1614* In several patients treated for 2-4 mo *142*

Hematocrit *Blood Decrease Physiological* Autoimmune hemolytic anemia *900* Methyldopa administration may cause hemolytic anemia *3958*

Hemoglobin *Blood Decrease Physiological* Autoimmune hemolytic anemia *900* Methyldopa administration may cause hemolytic anemia *3958* On rare occasion may produce hemolysis. Great majority of patients do not show this *3101*

Blood No Effect Analytical No effect on method on Boehringer Mannheim Reflotron *5706*

4-Hydroxy-3-Methoxy-Phenylglycol

Urine Decrease Physiological By more than VMA, ?affects aldehyde reductase. Inhibition of dopa decarboxylase, ?also aldehyde reductase *660*

5-Hydroxyindoleacetic Acid *Urine Decrease Physiological* Inhibition of aromatic amino acid decarboxylation *1281*

Immune Complexes *Serum No Effect Physiological* In a study of 9 hypertensives *3101*

immunoglobulin A *Serum Increase Physiological* Observed in one patient with hepatocellular damage of moderate severity due to sensitization by drug *1373*

Immunoglobulin G *Serum Increase Physiological* Observed in one patient with hepatocellular damage of moderate severity due to sensitization by drug *1373*

Immunoglobulin M *Serum Increase Physiological* Observed in one patient with hepatocellular damage of moderate severity due to sensitization by drug *1373*

Indomethacin *Serum No Effect Analytical* No effect on HPLC method of Roberts and Smith *4978*

Methyldopa *(continued)*

Ketones *Urine Increase Analytical* Affects alkaline nitroprusside procedure *882*

Lactate *Plasma No Effect Analytical* At concentration of 400 mg/L had no effect on enzymatic method *5704*

Lactate Dehydrogenase *Serum Increase Physiological* Chronic active hepatitis associated with immune hemolytic anemia in one case *5468*
Serum No Effect Analytical No effect at 15 mg/L on method on Ames Seralyzer *5706*

LDL-Cholesterol *Serum Decrease Physiological* In 17 hypertensive patients given drug for 3 mo *1614*
Serum No Effect Physiological In several patients treated for 2-4 mo *142*

LE Cells *Blood Positive Physiological* Autoimmune phenomenon *5505* Methyldopa administration may cause positive test for LE cells *3958*

Leukoagglutinins *Serum Positive Physiological* Observed in one patient with hepatocellular damage of moderate severity due to sensitization by drug *1373*

Leukocytes *Blood Decrease Physiological* Very rare, may cause granulocytopenia *3155* Methyldopa administration may cause bone marrow depression and leukopenia *3958*
Blood Increase Physiological Due to eosinophilia *3810*
Urine No Effect Analytical At concentration of 1,000 mg/L had no effect on Cytur-Test *5704*

Luteinizing Hormone *Plasma No Effect Physiological* No effect in patient on long term treatment who had drug-induced hyperprolactinemia *256*

Magnesium *Serum No Effect Analytical* No significant effect at concentration of 0.3 mg/mL on calmagite method on Beckman Synchron CX 4/5 *4701*

Melanogen *Urine Positive Analytical* At 0.2 mg/mL in alkaline urine *3401*

Metanephrines, Total *Urine Increase Analytical* Questionable interference with fluorometric methods *6515*

N-Acetyl-Glucosaminidase *Urine No Effect Analytical* At concentration of 150 mg/dL no significant effect observed on Boehringer Mannheim CPR method *3174*

Neutrophils *Blood Decrease Physiological* Occasional case of agranulocytosis reported *6264*

Norepinephrine *Urine No Effect Physiological* No effect when methyldopa administered and HPLC used to measure catecholamines *4172*

p-Aminophenol *Urine Increase Analytical* With addition of drug at a concentration of 100 mg/L significant increase of 5.0% observed on colorimetric method of van Bocxlaer on Cobas Mira analyzer which involves reacting free p-aminophenol with resorcinol in the presence of magnesium ions to form an indophenol dye measured at 550 nm *6163*

Phenylalanine *Plasma No Effect Analytical* No interference observed with rapid quantitative whole blood method of Campbell et al using phenylalanine dehydrogenase *867*

Phosphate *Serum No Effect Analytical* At concentration of 211 mg/L had no effect on phosphomolybdate method *5704*

Platelet-associated IgG *Serum No Effect Physiological* In a study of 9 hypertensives *3101*

Platelets *Blood Decrease Physiological* Very rare occurs within days or months *3155* Methyldopa administration may cause bone marrow depression and granulocytopenia *3958*

Porphobilinogen *Urine Increase Physiological* May precipitate acute porphyria attack *2210*

Porphyrin, Total *Urine Increase Physiological* May precipitate attack of acute porphyria *1687*

Potassium *Serum No Effect Analytical* At concentration of 7 mg/L had no effect on flame-photometric method *5704* At concentration of 100 mg/L had no effect on measurement by ISE with predilution *5704* At concentration of 800 mg/L had no effect on measurement by ISE without predilution *5704*

Prolactin *Plasma Increase Physiological* Methyldopa administration may cause hyperprolactinemia *3958* Marked effect in male and female hypertensives treated for up to 6 weeks *6098* Increased concentration after single doses of drug during long-term treatment *256* After single doses of 750 or 1,000 mg peak reached 4 to 6 h after administration. With long term administration 3 to 4 fold increase over normal noted *5805*

Protein *Serum No Effect Analytical* At concentration of 211 mg/L had no effect on biuret method with blank correction *5704*

Protein Electrophoresis *Serum No Effect Analytical* At concentration of 800 mg/L had no effect on automated Olympus-Hite method *5704*

Prothrombin Time *Plasma Increase Physiological* Decreased synthesis of prothrombin associated with hepatitis in some cases *3726* Enhances anticoagulant activity *6515*

Quinidine *Serum No Effect Analytical* No significant interference observed at a concentration of 100 µg/mL (473 µmol/L) with method on Du Pont aca *1543*

Red Cell-associated IgG *Blood Positive Physiological* Observed in 5 of 9 patients typically seen in 20% of treated patients. Probably due to impaired F_c-dependent reticuloendothelial function *3101*

Reticulocytes *Blood Increase Physiological* Hemolytic anemia of autoimmune type occurring in fewer than 1% of treated patients *707*

Rheumatoid Factor *Serum Increase Physiological* Methyldopa administration may cause positive test for rheumatoid factor *3958* Reported effect *2242*

Sodium *Serum Increase Physiological* May cause salt retention and edema *3810*
Serum No Effect Analytical At concentration of 100 mg/L had no effect on measurement by ISE with predilution *5704* At concentration of 800 mg/L had no effect on measurement by ISE without predilution *5704* At concentration of 7 mg/L had no effect on flame-photometric method *5704*

Sugar *Urine Increase Analytical* False positive with Clinitest® , no effect glucose oxidase method *1825*
Urine No Effect Analytical No effect reported at 0.2 mg/mL *3401*

Thormahlen Test *Urine Positive Analytical* At 0.2 mg/mL in alkaline urine *3401*

Triglycerides *Serum Decrease Analytical* At concentrations above 8 mg/L (normal therapeutic concentration 2 mg/L) lowered concentration as measured by GPO-PAP method *5704*
Serum Increase Physiological Increase by 20 mg/dL in 11 patients given 750 mg daily for 8 weeks *4213* Increase by 28% in 32 middle-aged hypertensive males treated for 6 weeks *3515*
Serum No Effect Analytical No effect at 5 mg/L on Boehringer Mannheim Reflotron method *5706* At concentration of 80 mg/L had no effect on lipase/esterase method *5704* No effect at therapeutic concentration on Boehringer Mannheim Reflotron method *3231*
Serum No Effect Physiological In several patients treated for 2-4 mo *142* In 3 studies of 7 to 17 patients for up to 3 mo *141*

Tyramine Test *Patient Increase Physiological* Enhanced responsiveness reported *2451*

Urea Nitrogen *Serum Increase Physiological* Methyldopa administration may cause increased concentration *3958* ?due to decreased renal blood flow *6515*
Serum No Effect Analytical At concentration of 80 mg/L had no effect on Kodak Ektachem® method *5704* No effect at 2 mg/L on Boehringer Mannheim Reflotron method *5706* At concentration of 211 mg/L had no effect on diacetylmonoxime method *5704* No effect at therapeutic concentration on Boehringer Mannheim Reflotron method *3231* No effect at 3 mg/L on method on Ames Seralyzer *5706*

Uric Acid *Serum Decrease Analytical* At concentrations above 3mg/L (normal therapeutic concentration 2 mg/L) lowered concentration as measured by uricase-PAP method *5704* At concentrations above 300 mg/L (normal therapeutic concentration 2 mg/L) lowered concentration as measured by Kageyama-Hantzsch method *5704*
Serum Increase Analytical Interferes with phosphotungstate procedure *2451* Methyldopa may interfere with methods using phosphotungstate reduction *3958* At concentrations above 20 mg/L (normal therapeutic concentration 2 mg/L) raised concentration as measured by phosphotungstate reduction method *5704*
Serum No Effect Analytical No effect up to 2 mg/L on method on Boehringer Mannheim Reflotron but above this concentration reduced uric acid concentration although unlikely to

be of clinical significance *5706* No effect at therapeutic concentration on Boehringer Mannheim Reflotron method *3231* At 30 mg/L on reversed phase liquid chromatographic procedure of Zhiri et al *6656* At concentration of 320 mg/L had no effect on catalase-AIDH method *5704*
Urine Increase Analytical Interferes with phosphotungstate procedure *2024*

Urobilinogen *Urine Increase Physiological* Autoimmune hemolytic anemia *900*

Vanillylmandelic Acid *Urine Decrease Physiological* Depletion of tissue stores *1460*
Urine Increase Analytical Interference by 5-HIAA with nonspecific diazo reaction *5401*
Urine Increase Physiological Initial physiological response, changes later *1444*
Urine No Effect Analytical Methyldopa does not interfere with analytical methods that convert VMA to vanillin *3958*

VLDL-Cholesterol *Serum Decrease Physiological* In 17 hypertensive patients given drug for 3 mo *1614*

Volume *Plasma Increase Physiological* Occurs with sodium retention if sole agent *4479*

Methyldopa Hydrazine

Dihydroxyphenylalanine *Plasma Increase Physiological* 5 fold potentiation with pretreatment *3803*

Growth Hormone *Plasma Increase Physiological* 2 fold increase when given with Dopa *3803*

Homovanillic Acid *Plasma Decrease Physiological* 65% reduction when given with Dopa *3803*

Methylene Blue

Bacteria *Urine Negative Analytical* May interfere with color on Microstix *203*

Bilirubin *Serum Increase Physiological* May cause hemolysis with G-6-PD deficiency *402*

Color *Feces Increase Analytical* Blue especially on exposure to air with 130-140 mg *1424*
Urine Increase Analytical Blue color *2240*

Diagnex Blue Excretion *Urine Increase Analytical* Detection of methylene blue *6515*

Erythrocytes *Blood Decrease Physiological* May cause hemolysis with G-6-PD deficiency *402*

Haptoglobin *Serum Decrease Physiological* May cause hemolysis *3810*

Heinz Body Formation *Blood Positive Physiological* Early stage of hemolytic anemia *536*

Hematocrit *Blood Decrease Physiological* May cause hemolysis with G-6-PD deficiency *402*

Hemoglobin *Blood Decrease Physiological* May cause hemolysis with G-6-PD deficiency *402*

Lactate *Plasma Decrease Physiological* Variable response when lactic acidosis *2452*

Methemoglobin *Blood Increase Physiological* May cause hemolysis (also used as treatment) *623*

Methylenedioxyamphetamine

Aspartate Aminotransferase *Serum Increase Physiological* Reported effect ,?of muscle origin *4950*

Bicarbonate *Serum Decrease Physiological* Respiratory acidosis *4950*

Carbon Dioxide Partial Pressure
Blood Increase Physiological Respiratory acidosis *4950*

pH *Blood Decrease Physiological* Respiratory acidosis *4950*

Methylethinylestradiol

17-Hydroxycorticosteroids *Urine Decrease Physiological* Decreased excretion of cortisol metabolites *55*

Methylparaben

Bicarbonate *Serum No Effect Analytical* No interference observed from methylparaben in bacteriostatic saline flush used with Kodak Ektachem® 700 *5941*

Chloride *Serum No Effect Analytical* No interference observed with chloride measurements on Kodak Ektachem® 700 from methylparaben in bacteriostatic saline flush *5941*

Lithium *Serum Decrease Analytical* Negative bias of 0.17 mmol/L at a concentration of 150 mg/dL at a lithium concentration of 1.0 mmol/L with method on Kodak Ektachem® systems *2519*

Potassium *Serum No Effect Analytical* No interference observed from methylparaben in bacteriostatic saline flush with potassium measurement in Ektachem,rg] 700 *5941*

Sodium *Serum Increase Analytical* Bacteriostatic saline flush containing methylparaben and propylparaben used with Kodak Ektachem® 700 caused 7-15 mmol/L increase in sodium concentration with specimens from patients with indwelling catheters. Benzalkonium chloride used as coating in central lines has been shown to increase sodium concentrations as measured by Kodak Ektachems® *5941*

Volume *Urine Increase Physiological* Hypercalcemia of malignancy common with this type of cancer which leads to diminished capacity of renal tubules to concentrate urine which, in turn, decreases the ECF and the kidney's ability to eliminate excess calcium. Renal impairment eventually causes nitrogen retention, acidosis and renal failure and a further decrease in calcium excretion *4015*

Methylphenidate

Alanine Aminotransferase *Serum Increase Physiological* Abnormal liver function or even hepatic coma has been probably associated with methylphenidate administration *1038*
Serum No Effect Analytical At acute overdose concentration (20 mg/dL) on Technicon SMAC® method *6266*

Albumin *Serum No Effect Analytical* At concentration of 200 mg/L had no effect on BCG method *5704* At acute overdose concentration (20 mg/dL) on Technicon SMAC® method *6266*

Alkaline Phosphatase *Serum No Effect Analytical* At acute overdose concentration (20 mg/dL) on Technicon SMAC® method *6266*

Amitriptyline *Serum Increase Physiological* Inhibits metabolism of tricyclic antidepressants *2452*

Amphetamine *Urine Positive Analytical* At concentrations above 120 µg/mL (514 µmol/L) with method on Du Pont aca *1554*

Aspartate Aminotransferase *Serum Increase Physiological* Abnormal liver function or even hepatic coma has been probably associated with methylphenidate administration *1038*
Serum No Effect Analytical At acute overdose concentration (20 mg/dL) on Technicon SMAC® method *6266*

Bilirubin *Serum No Effect Analytical* At concentration of 200 mg/L had no effect on Jendrassik and Grof method *5704* At acute overdose concentration (20 mg/dL) on Technicon SMAC® method *6266*

Calcium *Serum No Effect Analytical* At concentration of 200 mg/L had no effect on cresolphthalein method *5704* At acute overdose concentration (20 mg/dL) on Technicon SMAC® method *6266*

Cholesterol *Serum No Effect Analytical* At concentration of 200 mg/L had no effect on Liebermann-Burchard method *5704* At acute overdose concentration (20 mg/dL) on Technicon SMAC® method *6266*

Clomipramine *Serum Increase Physiological* Methylphenidate may inhibit metabolism of tricyclic antidepressants *1038*

Coumarin *Plasma Increase Physiological* Methylphenidate may inhibit metabolism of coumarin anticoagulants *1038*

Creatine Kinase *Serum No Effect Analytical* At acute overdose concentration (20 mg/dL) on Technicon SMAC® method *6266*

Creatinine *Serum No Effect Analytical* At concentration of 200 mg/L had no effect on Technicon AutoAnalyzer® Jaffe method *5704* At acute overdose concentration (20 mg/dL) on Technicon SMAC® method *6266*

Methylphenidate *(continued)*

Desipramine *Serum Increase Physiological* Methylphenidate may inhibit metabolism of tricyclic antidepressants *1038*

Dopamine *Urine No Effect Physiological* In children with attention deficit disorder and hyperactivity treatment with methylphenidate had no effect on excretion *6628*

Epinephrine *Urine Increase Physiological* For 3 h after administration (slight) *2452*

Glucose *Serum No Effect Analytical* At acute overdose concentration (20 mg/dL) on Technicon SMAC® method *6266*

Hemoglobin *Blood Decrease Physiological* Isolated cases of anemia reported with methylphenidate administration *1038*

4-Hydroxy-3-Methoxy-Phenylglycol
Urine Increase Physiological In children with attention deficit disorder and hyperactivity 22% excretion observed with treatment with methylphenidate *6628*
Urine No Effect Physiological No significant effect on urinary excretion in children with attention deficit disorder with hyperactivity when treated with 0.74 mg/kg/day for 2 weeks *6627*

5-Hydroxyindoleacetic Acid *Urine No Effect Physiological* Administration to children with attention deficit disorder and hyperactivity had no effect on excretion of 5-HIAA *6628*

5-Hydroxytryptamine *Urine No Effect Physiological* In children with attention deficit disorder and hyperactivity treatment with methylphenidate had no effect observed on excretion *6628*

Imipramine *Serum Increase Physiological* Methylphenidate may inhibit metabolism of tricyclic antidepressants *1038*

Iron *Serum No Effect Analytical* At acute overdose concentration (20 mg/dL) on Technicon SMAC® method *6266* At concentration of 200 mg/L had no effect on Ferrozine method *5704*

Lactate Dehydrogenase *Serum No Effect Analytical* At acute overdose concentration (20 mg/dL) on Technicon SMAC® method *6266*

Leukocytes *Blood Decrease Physiological* Isolated cases of leukopenia reported with methylphenidate administration *1038*

Mexiletine *Serum Increase Physiological* Decreases clearance and prolongs half-life *3281*

Norepinephrine *Urine Increase Physiological* In children with attention deficit disorder and hyperactivity administration of methylphenidate increased urinary excretion of norepinephrine *6628*
Urine No Effect Physiological No effect observed *2452*

Normetanephrine *Urine Increase Physiological* In children with attention deficit disorder and hyperactivity administration of methylphenidate caused significantly greater excretion of normetanephrine *6628*

Phenobarbital *Serum Increase Physiological* Methylphenidate may inhibit metabolism of anticonvulsants *1038* May increase serum concentration *1384*

Phenylbutazone *Serum Increase Physiological* Methylphenidate may inhibit metabolism of anticonvulsants *1038* May increase plasma concentration *1384*

Phenylethylamine *Urine No Effect Physiological* In children with attention deficit disorder and hyperactivity administration of methylphenidate had no effect on excretion *6628*

Phenytoin *Serum Increase Physiological* When methylphenidate ingested with fosphenytoin concentration of phenytoin may be increased *4519* Coadministration with phenytoin may increase plasma phenytoin concentration *4522* May increase serum concentration *1384* May increase from 9 to 28 µg/mL (at 20-40 mg/d) *3339* Methylphenidate may inhibit metabolism of anticonvulsants *1038*
Serum No Effect Physiological No effect observed in 11 patients in one study *2452*

Phosphate *Serum No Effect Analytical* At acute overdose concentration (20 mg/dL) on Technicon SMAC® method *6266* At concentration of 200 mg/L had no effect on phosphomolybdate method *5704*

Platelets *Blood Decrease Physiological* Occasional thrombocytopenic purpura reported *2753*

Primidone *Serum Increase Physiological* Methylphenidate may inhibit metabolism of anticonvulsants *1038* May increase serum concentration *1384*

Protein *Serum No Effect Analytical* At concentration of 200 mg/L had no effect on biuret method with blank correction *5704* At acute overdose concentration (20 mg/dL) on Technicon SMAC® method *6266*

Prothrombin Time *Plasma Increase Physiological* Inhibits metabolism of coumarins and phytonadione *2037*

Tricyclic Antidepressants *Serum Increase Physiological* Interacts pharmacokinetically to inhibit metabolism of tricyclic antidepressants *3590* May increase plasma concentrations *1384*

Triglycerides *Serum No Effect Analytical* At acute overdose concentration (20 mg/dL) on Technicon SMAC® method *6266* At concentration of 200 mg/L had no effect on lipase/esterase method *5704*

Urea Nitrogen *Serum No Effect Analytical* At acute overdose concentration (20 mg/dL) on Technicon SMAC® method *6266* At concentration of 200 mg/L had no effect on diacetylmonoxime method *5704*

Uric Acid *Serum No Effect Analytical* At concentration of 200 mg/L had no effect on phosphotungstate reduction method *5704* At acute overdose concentration (20 mg/dL) on Technicon SMAC® method *6266*

Warfarin *Plasma Increase Physiological* May increase the concentration of coumarin anticoagulants *1384*

Methylprednisolone

Alkaline Phosphatase, Bone Isoenzyme
Serum No Effect Physiological In 7 patients with severe rheumatic disease in whom concentrations were within reference range of 3.6 - 21.2 µg/L a single pulse injection of methylprednisolone caused no significant change from mean baseline of 9.7 ± 1.6 µg/L *4604*

Aluminum *Urine No Effect Physiological* Although excretion increased in renal transplant patients to about 5 times basal state no further increase observed with pulsed methylprednisolone treatment *1251*

Amylase *Serum Increase Physiological* To well above normal in 10 patients given 1 g/d i.v. for 3 d. Maximum effect on days 5 to 8 *1231*

Amylase, Pancreatic Isoenzyme
Serum Increase Physiological To well above normal in 10 patients given 1 g/d i.v. for 3 d. Maximum effect days 5 to 8. Possible subclinical damage of pancreatic acinar cells *1231*

Amylase, Salivary Isoenzyme
Serum No Effect Physiological No effect in patients given drug i.v. although pancreatic component significantly affected *1231*

Angiotensin-converting Enzyme
Serum Decrease Analytical Moderate inhibition by doses generally greater than used clinically *5077* After 96 h incubation *in vitro* at high concentrations but no effect under normal measurement conditions *5119*

Bicarbonate *Serum Increase Physiological* May cause hypokalemic alkalosis *2754*

Color *Feces Increase Analytical* Black color reported with ingestion of methylprednisolone *3388*

Corticotropin *Plasma Decrease Physiological* Suppression for 3 weeks following single injection in 12 patients *2867*

Cortisol *Plasma Decrease Physiological* Suppression for 2 weeks following single lumbar extradural injection in 12 patients *2867*

Creatinine *Serum Increase Physiological* In 52 patients with renal or collagen disease administration of bolus doses of 1 g on each of 3 days increase from mean baseline of 1.25 ± 0.92 mg/dL to 1.42 ± 1.31 mg/dL observed *5192*

Creatinine Clearance *Urine Increase Physiological* Varies with inulin clearance *6373*
Urine No Effect Physiological In 15 patients with renal or collagen disease pulse intravenous administration of 1 g on each of 3 days causes insignificant reduction to 73.1 ± 34.1 mL/min from 79.1 ± 36.0 mL/min *5192*

C-terminal Propeptide of Type I Procollagen
Serum Decrease Physiological In 7 patients with severe rheumatic disease in whom concentrations were within reference range of 55 - 165 μg/L a single pulse injection of methylprednisolone caused significant decrease from mean baseline of 93 ± 8 μg/L to nadir to 55 ± 5 μg/L. Concentration began to decrease later than Gla protein but nadir still reached at 24 h *4604*

Cyclosporine *Serum Decrease Physiological* In one study of post-transplant patients significant increase of cyclosporine clearance observed with reduction of plasma concentration. Cytochrome P-450 enzyme that metabolizes cyclosporine is glucocorticoid-inducible *6596*
Serum Increase Physiological High dose therapy reduces clearance of cyclosporine *1069* High doses produce effect probably due to effect on hepatic enzymes *1075* May increase cyclosporine concentration by inhibiting hepatic cytochrome P-450 III A which metabolizes cyclosporine *5236* Large doses given intravenously increase cyclosporine concentrations in renal transplant patients *1384*
Serum No Effect Physiological In one study doses above 250 mg/d intravenously caused no change in blood trough concentrations *6596*

Cyclosporine A *Blood Increase Physiological* Coadministration with cyclosporine A increases its concentration *5240*

Digoxin *Serum Increase Analytical* At 50 ng/mL equals 0.2 ng/mL by RIA *6638*

2,3-Diphosphoglycerate
Red Blood Cells No Effect Physiological No significant effect following i.v. infusion of drug in patients with myocardial infarction compared with controls *2555*

β-Endorphin *Plasma Decrease Physiological* In 15 patients undergoing approximately 30 min surgery mean concentration increased from baseline of 3.2 fmol/mL significantly less (to about 3.5 fmol/mL) than with placebo when concentration rose to about 5.8 fmol/mL *6075*

Follicle Stimulating Hormone
Plasma No Effect Physiological No apparent effect, unlike that on testosterone, in 67 y old males with chronic pulmonary disease taking drug for more than 1 mo *3707*

Glucose Tolerance *Serum Decrease Physiological* Decreased carbohydrate tolerance *2754*

Granulocyte Colony Stimulating Factor
Serum Increase Physiological In children with ALL and 9 episodes of neutropenia with mean concentration of 13.3 ± 11.7 pg/mL when treated with 30 mg/kg/d for 3 - 5 days rose to 83.3 ± 86.8 pg/mL and in children with AML with 6 episodes of neutropenia in whom mean concentration was 6.6 ± 12.1 pg/mL before therapy rose to 28.3 ± 11.3 pg/mL with same therapy *6094*

Granulocyte-Macrophage Colony Stimulating Factor
Serum Increase Physiological In children with ALL and 9 episodes of neutropenia with mean concentration of 12.2 ± 10.9 pg/mL when treated with 30 mg/kg/d for 3 - 5 days rose to 36 ± 24.7 pg/mL and in children with AML with 6 episodes of neutropenia in whom mean concentration was 13.3 ± 4 pg/mL before therapy rose to 45 ± 48.1 pg/mL with same therapy *6094*

immunoglobulin A *Serum Decrease Physiological* Significant effect in 43% of individuals *832*

Immunoglobulin G *Serum Decrease Physiological* After 96 mg/d for 5 d *832*

Immunoglobulin M *Serum Decrease Physiological* Noted in 14% of individuals *832*

Intercellular Adhesion Molecule-1
Serum No Effect Physiological In 13 patients (7 with bullous pemphigoid and 6 with pemphigus vulgaris) variable response observed after 4 - 6 weeks treatment with methylprednisolone *1250*

Interferon-γ *Serum Decrease Physiological* In children with ALL and 9 episodes of neutropenia with mean concentration of 204.1 ± 210.3 pg/mL when treated with 30 mg/kg/d for 3 - 5 days decreased to 28.6 ± 50.5 pg/mL and in children with AML with 6 episodes of neutropenia in whom mean concentration was 130.8 ± 138.3 pg/mL before therapy decreased to 23.3 ± 20.4 pg/mL with same therapy *6094*

Inulin Clearance *Urine Increase Physiological* At 24 h after 1 g i.v. in normals *6373*

Lactate *Plasma Increase Physiological* Significant effect in 10 of 13 patients with myocardial infarction. Effect observed in 1 h, maximum at 3 h, persisted for 24 h *2555*

Lipase *Serum Increase Physiological* To well above normal in 10 patients given 1 g/d i.v. for 3 d. Maximum effect days 5 to 8, possible subclinical damage of pancreatic acinar cell *1231*

Luteinizing Hormone *Plasma No Effect Physiological* No apparent effect, unlike that on testosterone, in 67 y old males with chronic pulmonary disease taking drug for more than 1 mo *3707*

Neutrophils *Blood Increase Physiological* In children with ALL and 9 episodes of neutropenia with mean absolute neutrophil count 611 ± 335.6 /μL when treated with 30 mg/kg/d for 3 - 5 days mean count rose to 1282.9 ± 2082 /μL and in children with AML with 6 episodes of neutropenia in whom mean absolute neutrophil count was 611 ± 335.6 /μL before therapy mean count rose to 1217 ± 520.7 /μL with same therapy *6094*

Nitroblue Tetrazolium Test *Blood Decrease Physiological* False negative in one patient on 1 g/d *4276*

Nitrogen Balance *Patient Negative Physiological* Due to protein catabolism *2754*

Osmolality *Serum No Effect Physiological* No significant effect following i.v. infusion of drug in patients with myocardial infarction compared with controls *2555*

Osteocalcin *Serum Decrease Physiological* In 7 patients with severe rheumatic disease in whom concentrations were within reference range of 1.6 - 4.8 μg/L a single pulse injection of methylprednisolone caused significant decrease from mean baseline of 1.7 ± 0.5 μg/L to nadir to 0.7 ± 0.1 μg/L. Concentration began to decrease within 6 h of pulse and nadir reached at 24 h *4604*

Oxygen Partial Pressure *Blood Decrease Physiological* Initial reduction in myocardial infarction patients compared with placebo treated controls (112 mm Hg to 88 mm Hg on average) *2555*

PAH Clearance *Urine Increase Physiological* At 24 h after 1 g i.v. in normals *6373*

pH *Blood No Effect Physiological* No significant effect following i.v. infusion of drug in patients with myocardial infarction compared with controls *2555*

Platelets *Blood Increase Physiological* In 19 children with idiopathic thrombocytopenic purpura treatment with 50 mg/kg for 7 days caused increase from mean baseline of about 10 $x10^9$ /L to peak of 350 $x10^9$ /L at 8 days *89* In 8 patients with autoimmune thrombocytopenic purpura treatment with 15 mg/kg/d caused mean count to increase from 12 ± 10 x 10^9/L to > 50 x 10^9/L in 7 and to 34 x 10^9/L in the eighth *2198*

Potassium *Serum Decrease Physiological* May cause potassium loss *2754*
Serum No Effect Analytical At concentration of 100 mg/L had no effect on measurement by ISE with predilution *5704*

Protein *Cerebrospinal Fluid No Effect Analytical* No significant effect when added in vitro to concentration of 10.0 mg/dL when measured by Kodak Ektachem® slide method *3654*
Urine Decrease Physiological In 28 children with severe Schönlein-Henoch purpura treated with intravenous pulses of methylprednisolone and subsequently oral prednisone decreasing to 15 mg/m^2 for 5 months caused mean baseline excretion of 162 ± 68 mg/kg/d to decrease to 38 ± 15 mg/kg/d and 17 ± 6 mg/kg/d after one year *4278*

Sodium *Serum Decrease Physiological* In 48 patients with renal or collagen disease intravenous administration of bolus doses of 1 g on each of 3 days caused significant decrease from mean baseline of 140.4 ± 2.8 mmol/L to 138.7 ± 3.6 mmol/L *5192*
Serum No Effect Analytical At concentration of 100 mg/L had no effect on measurement by ISE with predilution *5704*
Urine Decrease Physiological In 15 patients with renal or collagen disease intravenous administration of pulses of 1 g on each of 3 days caused significant reduction from mean baseline of 103.5 ± 51.8 mmol/d to 86.4 ± 51.5 mmol/d on first day, 42.3 ± 23.4 mmol/d on second day and 57.1 ± 36.6 mmol/d on third day *5192*

Methylprednisolone *(continued)*

Sodium Excretion, Free *Urine Decrease Physiological* In 15 patients with renal or collagen disease intravenous administration of 1 g boluses on 3 days caused significant reduction from mean baseline of 0.59 ± 0.31% to 0.50 ± 0.31% after 1 day, 0.27 ± 0.14% after 2 days and 0.38 ± 0.19% after 3 days *5192*

Soluble E-selectin *Serum Decrease Physiological* In 13 patients (7 with bullous pemphigoid and 6 with pemphigus vulgaris) median concentration 55.8 ng/mL (range 34.5 - 109.6) decreased to 24 ng/mL (range 11 - 68.9) after 4 - 6 weeks treatment with methylprednisolone paralleling the reduction in the number of lesions *1250*

Soluble Interleukin-2 Receptor
Serum Decrease Physiological In 2 patients with active rheumatoid arthritis intravenous pulses of 1 g methylprednisolone caused marked reduction in IL-2R concentration *1142*

Tacrolimus *Blood No Effect Analytical* No significant effect observed at a concentration of 5 mg/L with MEIA method on Abbott IMx analyzer *1871*
Serum Increase Physiological By inhibiting cytochrome P-450 IIIA enzyme systems may inhibit the metabolism of tacrolimus *1987*
Serum No Effect Analytical At a concentration of 5 mg/L had no significant effect on ELISA method *6329*

Testosterone *Serum Decrease Physiological* Reduced by more than 50% in 14 of 16 67 y old men with chronic pulmonary disease receiving drug for more than 1 mo. Testosterone concentration inversely correlated with dose of drug. Serum protein-binding unaffected. Effect probably due to suppression of secretion of gonadotropin releasing hormone by hypothalamus *3707*

Trypsin *Serum Increase Physiological* Increase by 35-109% in 10 patients given 1 g/d i.v. for 3 d. Maximum effect days 5 to 8 possible subclinical damage of pancreatic acinar cells *1231*

Tumor Necrosis Factor-α *Serum Decrease Physiological* In children with ALL and 9 episodes of neutropenia with mean concentration of 93.5 ± 161 pg/mL when treated with 30 mg/kg/d for 3 - 5 days decreased to 76.1 ± 160 pg/mL and in children with AML with 6 episodes of neutropenia in whom mean concentration was 78.3 ± 61.4 pg/mL before therapy decreased to 19.1 ± 39.8 pg/mL with same therapy *6094*

Volume *Blood Decrease Physiological* Transient but significant effect observed in patients given i.v. infusion after myocardial infarction in comparison with placebo treated control population *2555*
Plasma Increase Physiological May cause fluid retention *2754*
Urine Increase Physiological In 52 patients with renal or collagen disease administration of boluses of 1 g intravenously on each of 3 days caused significant increase from mean baseline of 4026 ± 1523 mL to 4456 ± 1641 mL *5192*

6α-Methylprednisolone

Cortisol *Plasma Increase Analytical* At concentration of 4.0 mg/L caused 24.4% cross reactivity with method on Baxter Stratus *5705*

Cortisol, Free *Urine No Effect Analytical* No significant interference observed with HPLC method of Turpeinen et al *6105*

Methylprednisone

Cyclosporine *Blood No Effect Analytical* At a concentration of 12 mg/L had no effect on Syva EMIT method *495*
Blood No Effect Physiological Coadministration of methylprednisolone (intravenously) with cyclosporine had no effect on whole blood cyclosporine concentration or volume of distribution, but increase in blood cyclosporine clearance from 5.5 to 6.6 mL/min/kg *859*
Serum No Effect Physiological Coadministration of methylprednisolone (intravenously) with cyclosporine had no effect on whole blood cyclosporine concentration or volume of distribution, but increase in blood cyclosporine clearance from 5.5 to 6.6 mL/min/kg *859*

Insulin *Plasma Increase Physiological* In 30 healthy young men with a body mass index of 22.7 ± 0.4 kg/m^2 mean fasting concentration increased significantly from 46 ± 6 pmol/L to 91 ± 13 pmol/L after 7 days treatment with 0.5 mg/kg/d methylprednisolone orally *518*

Leptin *Serum Increase Physiological* In 30 healthy young men with a body mass index of 22.7 ± 0.4 kg/m^2 mean fasting concentration increased significantly from 2.3 ng/mL to 2.9 ng/mL after 7 days treatment with 0.5 mg/kg/d methylprednisolone orally *518*

Theophylline *Serum No Effect Physiological* No documented significant interaction with theophylline reported *6117* No clinically significant effect on theophylline concentration observed when drugs coadministered *5999*

Methylpromazine

Leukocytes *Blood Decrease Physiological* Leukopenia (AMA Blood dyscrasias) *4017*

Neutrophils *Blood Decrease Physiological* Occasional case of agranulocytosis reported *6264*

Methylsuccimide

Felbamate *Serum No Effect Analytical* No significant interference observed with GLC method of Rifai et al *4958*

Methylsulfonal

δ-Aminolevulinic Acid *Urine Increase Physiological* May precipitate acute porphyria *2210*

Color *Urine Increase Analytical* Red (may provoke porphyria) *3810*

Coproporphyrin *Feces Increase Physiological* May precipitate acute porphyria *2210*
Urine Increase Physiological May precipitate acute porphyria *2210*

Methemoglobin *Blood Increase Physiological* May cause hemolytic anemia *4017*

Porphobilinogen *Urine Increase Physiological* May precipitate acute porphyria *2210*

Protoporphyrin *Feces Increase Physiological* May precipitate acute porphyria *2210*

Methyltestosterone

Alanine Aminotransferase *Serum Increase Physiological* May cause cholestatic jaundice, alterations in liver function tests, rarely hepatic neoplasms and peliosis hepatitis *2805*

Alkaline Phosphatase *Serum Increase Physiological* May cause cholestatic jaundice, alterations in liver function tests, rarely hepatic neoplasms and peliosis hepatitis *2805*

Aspartate Aminotransferase *Serum Increase Physiological* May cause cholestatic jaundice, alterations in liver function tests, rarely hepatic neoplasms and peliosis hepatitis *2805*

Bilirubin *Serum Increase Physiological* May cause cholestatic jaundice, alterations in liver function tests, rarely hepatic neoplasms and peliosis hepatitis *2805*

Calcium *Serum Increase Physiological* May cause retention of chloride, potassium, sodium, calcium, inorganic phosphate and water *2805*

Chloride *Serum Increase Physiological* May cause retention of chloride, potassium, sodium, calcium, inorganic phosphate and water *2805*

Cholesterol *Serum Increase Physiological* May cause increased serum cholesterol as a complication of treatment *2805*

Cyclosporine *Blood Increase Physiological* Coadministration of methyltestosterone with cyclosporine caused increase in cyclosporine concentration possibly due to inhibition of the microsomal drug hydroxylating enzymes in the liver *859*
Serum Increase Physiological Coadministration of methyltestosterone with cyclosporine caused increase in cyclosporine concentration possibly due to inhibition of the microsomal drug hydroxylating enzymes in the liver *859*

Glucose *Serum Decrease Physiological* In diabetic patients the metabolic effect of methyltestosterone may reduce insulin requirements *2806*

Hematocrit *Blood Increase Physiological* May cause polycythemia as a complication of treatment *2805*

Hemoglobin *Blood Increase Physiological* May cause polycythemia as a complication of treatment *2805*

Oxyphenbutazone *Serum Increase Physiological* Coadministration of methyltestosterone with oxyphenbutazone may cause increased plasma concentration of oxyphenbutazone *2806*

Phosphate *Serum Increase Physiological* May cause retention of chloride, potassium, sodium, calcium, inorganic phosphate and water *2805*

Potassium *Serum Increase Physiological* May cause retention of chloride, potassium, sodium, calcium, inorganic phosphate and water *2805*

Prothrombin Time *Plasma Increase Physiological* In patients receiving anticoagulants C-17 substituted derivatives of testosterone have been reported to decrease anticoagulant requirements *2806*

Sodium *Serum Increase Physiological* May cause retention of chloride, potassium, sodium, calcium, inorganic phosphate and water *2805*

T3-Uptake *Serum Increase Physiological* Androgens like methyltestosterone may reduce concentration of thyroxine binding globulin and thus total thyroxine concentration but increase T3-uptake *2806*

Testosterone *Serum Increase Analytical* With INCSTAR solid phase radioimmunoassay 3.7% cross-reactivity observed *3020*
Serum No Effect Analytical Cross-reactivity of 1.0% observed with methyltestosterone in testosterone method on Bayer Technicon Immuno 1® *433*

Thyroxine Binding Globulin
Serum Decrease Physiological Androgens like methyltestosterone may reduce concentration of thyroxine binding globulin *2806*

Thyroxine (T4) *Serum Decrease Physiological* Androgens like methyltestosterone may reduce concentration of thyroxine binding globulin and thus total thyroxine concentration *2806*

Thyroxine (T4), Free *Serum No Effect Physiological* Androgens like methyltestosterone may reduce concentration of thyroxine binding globulin and thus total thyroxine concentration but have no effect on free hormone concentration *2806*

Volume *Plasma Increase Physiological* May cause retention of chloride, potassium, sodium, calcium, inorganic phosphate and water *2805*

Methyltetrahydrofolic Acid

Methotrexate *Serum No Effect Analytical* No significant interference observed from 5-methyltetrahydrofolic acid at a concentration of 100 μmol/L with method on Du Pont aca *1535*

Methylthiouracil

Alanine Aminotransferase *Serum Increase Physiological* Hepatotoxic effect *3810*

Alkaline Phosphatase *Serum Increase Physiological* Hepatotoxic effect *3810*

Aspartate Aminotransferase *Serum Increase Physiological* Hepatotoxic effect *3810*

Bile *Urine Increase Physiological* Hepatotoxic effect *3810*

Bilirubin *Serum Increase Physiological* Hepatotoxic effect *3810*

BSP Retention *Serum Increase Physiological* Hepatotoxic effect *3810*

Cortisol *Plasma No Effect Analytical* At a concentration of 600 mg/L had no significant effect on Enzymun method *1097*

Erythrocytes *Blood Decrease Physiological* Occasional case of aplastic anemia reported *6264*

^{131}I Uptake *Serum No Effect Physiological* No effect on uptake by thyroid *3669*

LE Cells *Blood Positive Physiological* May produce LE-like syndrome *5869*

Leukocytes *Blood Decrease Physiological* Occasional case of aplastic anemia reported *6264* Occasional leukopenia or agranulocytosis *3810*

Neutrophils *Blood Decrease Physiological* Occasional case of agranulocytosis reported *6264*

Platelets *Blood Decrease Physiological* Occasional case of aplastic anemia reported *6264*

Prothrombin Time *Plasma Increase Physiological* Also exaggerated response to anticoagulants *3210*

Thyroxine (T4) *Serum Decrease Physiological* Inhibits synthesis, stops iodination of tyrosine *128*

Methyprylon

Alanine Aminotransferase *Serum No Effect Analytical* At acute overdose concentration (10 mg/dL) on Technicon SMAC® method *6266*

Albumin *Serum No Effect Analytical* At acute overdose concentration (10 mg/dL) on Technicon SMAC® method *6266* At concentration of 100 mg/L had no effect on BCG method *5704*

Alkaline Phosphatase *Serum No Effect Analytical* At acute overdose concentration (10 mg/dL) on Technicon SMAC® method *6266*

δ-Aminolevulinic Acid *Urine Increase Physiological* Ala-synthetase stimulated in animals *2242*

Aspartate Aminotransferase *Serum No Effect Analytical* At acute overdose concentration (10 mg/dL) on Technicon SMAC® method *6266*

Bilirubin *Serum No Effect Analytical* At concentration of 100 mg/L had no effect on Jendrassik and Grof method *5704* At acute overdose concentration (10 mg/dL) on Technicon SMAC® method *6266*

Calcium *Serum No Effect Analytical* At acute overdose concentration (10 mg/dL) on Technicon SMAC® method *6266* At concentration of 100 mg/L had no effect on cresolphthalein method *5704*

Cannabinoids *Urine No Effect Analytical* No effect on Roche Abuscreen method *5006*

Cholesterol *Serum No Effect Analytical* At concentration of 100 mg/L had no effect on Liebermann-Burchard method *5704* At acute overdose concentration (10 mg/dL) on Technicon SMAC® method *6266*

Creatine Kinase *Serum No Effect Analytical* At acute overdose concentration (10 mg/dL) on Technicon SMAC® method *6266*

Creatinine *Serum No Effect Analytical* At concentration of 100 mg/L had no effect on Technicon AutoAnalyzer® Jaffe method *5704* At acute overdose concentration (10 mg/dL) on Technicon SMAC® method *6266*

Glucose *Serum No Effect Analytical* At acute overdose concentration (10 mg/dL) on Technicon SMAC® method *6266*

Iron *Serum No Effect Analytical* At concentration of 100 mg/L had no effect on Ferrozine method *5704* At acute overdose concentration (10 mg/dL) on Technicon SMAC® method *6266*

17-Ketogenic Steroids *Urine Increase Analytical* Interferes with Zimmermann reaction *5869*

Lactate Dehydrogenase *Serum No Effect Analytical* At acute overdose concentration (10 mg/dL) on Technicon SMAC® method *6266*

Leukocytes *Blood Decrease Physiological* Due to toxic action of metabolite *3810*

Phosphate *Serum No Effect Analytical* At acute overdose concentration (10 mg/dL) on Technicon SMAC® method *6266* At concentration of 100 mg/L had no effect on phosphomolybdate method *5704*

Methyprylon *(continued)*

Platelets *Blood Decrease Physiological* Isolated reports (?actually responsible) *2754*

Protein *Serum No Effect Analytical* At concentration of 100 mg/L had no effect on biuret method with blank correction *5704* At acute overdose concentration (10 mg/dL) on Technicon SMAC® method *6266*

Sugar *Urine Increase Analytical* Excreted as glucuronide, acts as reducing substance *2242*

Triglycerides *Serum No Effect Analytical* At concentration of 100 mg/L had no effect on lipase/esterase method *5704* At acute overdose concentration (10 mg/dL) on Technicon SMAC® method *6266*

Urea Nitrogen *Serum No Effect Analytical* At acute overdose concentration (10 mg/dL) on Technicon SMAC® method *6266* At concentration of 100 mg/L had no effect on diacetylmonoxime method *5704*

Uric Acid *Serum No Effect Analytical* At concentration of 100 mg/L had no effect on phosphotungstate reduction method *5704* At acute overdose concentration (10 mg/dL) on Technicon SMAC® method *6266*

Methysergide

Coombs' Test, Direct *Blood Positive Physiological* Single case with retroperitoneal fibrosis *2452*

Eosinophils *Blood Decrease Physiological* Starts to occur within 1 h (up to 100% decrease) *4014*

Blood Increase Physiological Eosinophilia may occur as a complication *5242* Transient effect up to 36 h after i.m. injection *2100*

Erythrocyte Sedimentation Rate

Blood Increase Physiological Retroperitoneal fibrosis may occur with increased ESR and low grade fever *5242*

Hydrochloric Acid *Gastric Fluid Increase Physiological* Affects basal juice and after histamine *3669*

5-Hydroxytryptamine *Plasma Decrease Physiological* Noted in migraine subjects *1194*

LE Cells *Blood Positive Physiological* Observed effect in some cases *1475*

Leukocytes *Blood Decrease Physiological* Neutropenia reported *3810*

Blood Increase Physiological Due to neutrophilia *3810*

Lymphocytes *Blood Decrease Physiological* Average decrease of 29% noted *4014*

Neutrophils *Blood Decrease Physiological* Neutropenia may occur as a complication *5242* Reported side effect *2754*

Blood Increase Physiological Average increase of 23% noted *4014*

Platelets *Blood Decrease Physiological* Thrombocytopenia may occur as a complication *5242*

Urea Nitrogen *Serum Increase Physiological* Retroperitoneal fibrosis may occur with increased plasma urea concentration *5242* Possible decrease in already impaired renal function *139*

Metiamide

Neutrophils *Blood Decrease Physiological* Occasional case of agranulocytosis reported *6264*

Metiazinic Acid

Uric Acid *Serum Decrease Physiological* Possible interference with tubular reabsorption *3716*

Metoclopramide

Acetaminophen *Serum Increase Physiological* Absorption from the small bowel may be increased *4982* Increased rate of absorption with faster gastric emptying *6403*

Acetylsalicylic Acid *Serum Increase Physiological* Pretreatment with metoclopramide either orally or intramuscularly prompted earlier absorption and a higher serum concentration although rates of absorption and elimination were not affected *4062*

Alanine Aminotransferase *Serum Increase Physiological* Rarely hepatotoxicity may occur with jaundice and altered liver function tests, when metoclopramide administered with other drugs with known hepatotoxic potential *4982*

Aldosterone *Plasma Increase Physiological* Fluid retention secondary to transient increase in aldosterone concentration may occur *4982* Administration to both normal individuals and acromegalics caused increased concentration *6625* Secretion increased but mechanism mediating effect not elucidated but probably through a factor whose concentration is increased in serum *861* Increase by 99% 15 minutes after 1 mg/kg intravenously in healthy volunteers *5765* Peak 15 minutes after injection: 3 fold higher than control at peak *769* Increased by single i.v. bolus of 10 mg: probably related to basal activity of renin angiotensin aldosterone system *4204* Observed in normal subjects after 10 mg drug over 2 h; higher response in patients with primary aldosteronism *6520*

Alkaline Phosphatase *Serum Increase Physiological* Rarely hepatotoxicity may occur with jaundice and altered liver function tests, when metoclopramide administered with other drugs with known hepatotoxic potential *4982*

Androsterone *Urine No Effect Physiological* No significant influence of drug on excretion in menstruating women *156*

Aspartate Aminotransferase *Serum Increase Physiological* Rarely hepatotoxicity may occur with jaundice and altered liver function tests, when metoclopramide administered with other drugs with known hepatotoxic potential *4982*

Bilirubin *Serum Increase Physiological* Rarely hepatotoxicity may occur with jaundice and altered liver function tests, when metoclopramide administered with other drugs with known hepatotoxic potential *4982*

Serum No Effect Physiological No significant displacement from protein observed in neonates *6314*

Chlorothiazide *Serum Decrease Physiological* Decreased absorption due to absorption window or dissolution *6403*

Cimetidine *Serum Decrease Physiological* Oral availability reduced by 25-30% if given together *1384*

Corticosterone *Plasma No Effect Physiological* No effect even though other constituents affected by i.v. bolus of 10 mg *4204* No change observed in normal individuals or in patients with primary aldosteronism after 10 mg drug *6520*

Corticotropin *Plasma Increase Physiological* Increase by 55% 15 minutes after 1 mg/kg intravenously in healthy volunteers *5765*

Cortisol *Plasma Increase Physiological* Increase by 75% 15 minutes after 1 mg/kg intravenously in healthy volunteers *5765*

Plasma No Effect Physiological No effect even though other constituents affected by i.v. bolus of 10 mg *4204* No change observed in normal individuals or in patients with primary aldosteronism after 10 mg drug *6520* No significant change following i.v. injection *769*

Cyclosporine *Blood Increase Physiological* Coadministered drug causes increased absorption, area under curve and blood concentration *6288* With coadministration of drugs modest increase in area under concentration-time curve and maximum concentration suggesting an increase in rate and extent of absorption of about 30% *859*

Blood No Effect Analytical At a concentration of 4 mg/L had no effect on Syva EMIT method *495*

Serum Increase Physiological In 14 renal transplant patients addition of metoclopramide to therapeutic regime caused increase in area under the concentration curve with other evidence to suggest that oral absorption of cyclosporine increased *6596* With coadministration of drugs modest increase in area under concentration-time curve and maximum concentration suggesting an increase in rate and extent of absorption of about 30% *859* May increase cyclosporine concentration by inhibiting hepatic cytochrome P-450 III A which metabolizes cyclosporine *5236* Reported effect since bioavailability increased through alteration of gastric transit time *1069*

Cyclosporine A *Blood Increase Physiological* Absorption from the small bowel may be increased *4982* Coadministration with cyclosporine A increases its concentration *5240*

Dehydroepiandrosterone Sulfate
Plasma No Effect Physiological No significant differences in either cycling or post-menopausal woman receiving drug *156*
Urine No Effect Physiological No significant influence of drug on excretion in menstruating women *156*

Deoxycorticosterone *Plasma No Effect Physiological* No effect even though other constituents affected by i.v. bolus of 10 mg *4204*

Didanosine *Serum No Effect Physiological* No significant effect observed on the concentration of either drug when two drugs coadministered *730*

Digoxin *Serum Decrease Physiological* Gastrointestinal absorption of slowly dissolving brands reduced due to reduced gastrointestinal motility *3772* Absorption from the stomach may be impaired *4982* With tablets of low bioavailability due to stimulation of bowel motility *4631* Reduced absorption with limited dissolution *6403*

Estradiol *Plasma No Effect Physiological* No significant baseline differences in cycling women before and after drug *156*

Ethanol *Serum Increase Physiological* Increased rate of absorption with faster gastric emptying *6403* Absorption from the small bowel may be increased *4982*

Etiocholanolone *Urine No Effect Physiological* No significant influence of drug on excretion in menstruating women *156*

Follicle Stimulating Hormone
Plasma No Effect Physiological No significant baseline differences in cycling women before and after drug *156*

Fosfomycin *Serum Decrease Physiological* When coadministered with fosfomycin reported to lower the serum concentration and urinary excretion of fosfomycin through its action of increasing gastrointestinal motility *1912*
Urine Decrease Physiological When coadministered with fosfomycin reported to lower the serum concentration and urinary excretion of fosfomycin through its action of increasing gastrointestinal motility *1912*

Granulocytes *Blood Decrease Physiological* A few cases of agranulocytosis reported with administration of metoclopramide *4982*

Growth Hormone *Plasma Increase Physiological* In 5 of 9 cirrhotic male patients after single injection of 10 mg *6276* 5 fold increase at 30-45 minutes after 0.17 mg/kg bolus i.v. in 10 children *3834* Increased from 30 to 60 minutes after single i.v. injection in 6 normal women *996*
Plasma No Effect Physiological In normal subjects after single i.v. injection of 10 mg *6276* With pharmacological doses in normal men, but increased in hypogonadal men *996*

18-Hydroxycorticosterone *Plasma Increase Physiological* Increased by single i.v. bolus of 10 mg: probably related to basal activity of renin angiotensin aldosterone system *4204* Observed in normal subjects after 10 mg drug over 2 h; higher response in patients with primary aldosteronism *6520*
Plasma No Effect Physiological No change observed in normal individuals or in patients with primary aldosteronism after 10 mg drug *6520*

Leukocytes *Blood Decrease Physiological* A few cases of leukopenia reported with administration of metoclopramide, although without clear relationship to metoclopramide *4982*

Levodopa *Serum Increase Physiological* Increased rate of absorption with faster gastric emptying *6403* Absorption from the small bowel may be increased *4982*

Lithium *Serum Increase Physiological* Increased rate of absorption with faster gastric emptying *6403*

Luteinizing Hormone *Plasma No Effect Physiological* After administration of 10 mg orally no significant effect observed on concentration in either patients with anorexia nervosa or control individuals *2217* No significant baseline differences in cycling women before and after drug *156*

Lysergic Acid Diethylamide *Urine Increase Analytical* Minimum concentration that caused a positive result with EMIT method to measure LSD < 0.8 mg/L *4968*

Methemoglobin *Blood Increase Physiological* Methemoglobinemia has been reported with administration of metoclopramide, especially with overdose in neonates *4982* Observed in neonates who received excessive doses *1384*

Neutrophils *Blood Decrease Physiological* A few cases of neutropenia reported with administration of metoclopramide, although without clear relationship to metoclopramide *4982*

Occult Blood *Feces Increase Analytical* No effect on Hemoquant method *6172*

p-Aminophenol *Urine No Effect Analytical* With addition of drugs at a concentration of 100 mg/L and of related compounds at 50 mg/L no significant effect observed on colorimetric method of van Bocxlaer on Cobas Mira analyzer which involves reacting free p-aminophenol with resorcinol in the presence of magnesium ions to form an indophenol dye measured at 550 nm *6163*

Phenylalanine *Plasma No Effect Analytical* No interference observed with rapid quantitative whole blood method of Campbell et al using phenylalanine dehydrogenase *867*

Potassium *Serum Decrease Physiological* At dose of 10 mg causes decrease of about 0.3 mmol/L *4739*
Serum No Effect Physiological No significant change following i.v. injection *769*

Progesterone *Plasma No Effect Physiological* No significant baseline differences in cycling women before and after drug *156*

Prolactin *Plasma Decrease Physiological* In patients with anorexia nervosa response to 10 mg orally metoclopramide significantly reduced concentration compared with normal individuals *2217*
Plasma Increase Physiological Administration to either normal or acromegalics caused significant increase in concentration *6625* Significant increase in some menstruating women compared with control cycle *156* 11 fold increase after i.v. injection (0.04 mg/kg) *769* Increased by single i.v. bolus of 10 mg: probably related to basal activity of renin angiotensin aldosterone system *4204* Observed in normal subjects after 10 mg drug over 2 h; higher response in patients with primary aldosteronism *6520* In both hyperthyroid and euthyroid subjects in response to oral drug *5300* Response smaller in thyrotoxic than euthyroid patients with long term treatment *5897*

Propranolol *Serum No Effect Physiological* Coadministration of metoclopramide with propranolol had no effect on circulating propranolol concentration *972*

Renal Blood Flow *Patient Decrease Physiological* In 20 patients given 1 to 2.5 mg/kg (from mean 443 mL/min to 387 mL/min) *2844*

Renin Activity *Plasma No Effect Physiological* No significant change following i.v. injection *769* No effect even though other constituents affected by i.v. bolus of 10 mg *4204* No change observed in normal individuals or in patients with primary aldosteronism after 10 mg drug *6520*

Tacrolimus *Serum Increase Physiological* By inhibiting cytochrome P-450 IIIA enzyme systems may inhibit the metabolism of tacrolimus *1987*

Tetracycline *Serum Increase Physiological* Absorption from the small bowel may be increased *4982*

Thyroid Stimulating Hormone
Serum Increase Physiological Following 10 mg orally marked increase within 1 h in euthyroid subjects: effect most marked in patients with primary hypothyroidism *5305* Increased in euthyroidism and hyperthyroidism; maximum effect 3 to 6 h after administration *6412*
Serum No Effect Physiological Basal values did not change as result of long-term treatment *5897* In either hyperthyroid or euthyroid subjects in response to oral drug *5300*

Tirofiban *Serum No Effect Physiological* Coadministration had no significant effect on plasma clearance of tirofiban *3957*

Zalcitabine *Serum Decrease Physiological* Coadministration of 20 mg metoclopramide and single doses of zalcitabine 1.5 mg to 12 HIV-positive patients decreased AUC from 69 ng.h/mL to 62 ng.h/mL, resulting in a 10% decrease in bioavailability *5023*

Metolazone

Alanine Aminotransferase *Serum Increase Physiological* Metolazone may cause hepatitis or intrahepatic cholestasis *3928*

Alkaline Phosphatase *Serum Increase Physiological* Metolazone may cause hepatitis or intrahepatic cholestasis *3928*

Ammonia *Urine No Effect Physiological* No effect on carbonic anhydrase *5611*

Metolazone *(continued)*

Amylase *Serum Increase Physiological* Metolazone may cause pancreatitis *3928*

Angiotensin-II *Plasma Increase Physiological* 2 to 3 fold increase after 6 weeks treatment with 5 mg daily in 5 or 6 hypertensives *6499*

Aspartate Aminotransferase *Serum Increase Physiological* Metolazone may cause hepatitis or intrahepatic cholestasis *3928*

Bicarbonate *Serum Increase Physiological* Diuretic action of drug acting on distal tubules *4705* Increase by about 3-5 mmol/L after 6 weeks treatment with 5 mg daily in 5 or 6 hypertensives *6499*

Urine No Effect Physiological No effect on carbonic anhydrase *5611*

Bilirubin *Serum Increase Physiological* Metolazone may cause hepatitis or intrahepatic cholestasis *3928*

Calcium *Serum Increase Physiological* Metolazone may occasionally cause hypercalcemia, especially in patients taking high doses of vitamin D or with high bone turnover states *3928*

Urine Increase Physiological Maximum diuretic response of 0.4 µEq/min *5611*

Chloride *Serum Decrease Physiological* Diuretic action of drug acting on distal tubules *4705*

Urine Increase Physiological Diuretic action of drug *2369*

Effective Renal Plasma Flow

Patient No Effect Physiological No effect observed *5611*

Glomerular Filtration Rate *Urine Decrease Physiological* Diuretic action *5859*

Urine No Effect Physiological No effect observed *5611*

Glucose *Serum Increase Physiological* Metolazone may increase both blood and urinary concentrations in patients with overt or latent diabetes *3928* Diabetic-like action of diuretics *4705*

Urine Increase Physiological Metolazone may increase both blood and urinary concentrations in patients with overt or latent diabetes *3928*

Lipase *Serum Increase Physiological* Metolazone may cause pancreatitis *3928*

Lithium *Serum Increase Physiological* Metolazone may increase the serum lithium concentration *3928*

Magnesium *Serum Decrease Physiological* In isolated case as result of marked diuresis *5490*

Urine Increase Physiological Maximum diuretic response of 0.4 µEq/min *5611*

Osmolality *Urine Increase Physiological* Diuretic action *5859*

Osmolar Clearance *Urine Increase Physiological* Diuretic action of drug *5859*

pH *Urine Decrease Physiological* Associated with diuretic response *5611*

Phosphate *Urine Increase Physiological* Maximum diuretic response up to 8 µEq/min *5611*

Potassium *Serum Decrease Physiological* Mean decrease of 0.5-0.6 mmol/L in group of patients as hypertension controlled *4130* Metolazone may cause hypokalemia with consequent weakness. It is a particular hazard in patients who are digitalized. Hypokalemia is dose related *3929* Significant reduction after 6 weeks treatment of 5 hypertensives given 5 mg daily *6499* Hypokalemia may occur with large doses of the drug, when diuresis is rapid, when severe liver disease is present, when corticosteroids are administered, when oral intake is inadequate, or when excessive loss of potassium occurs as with vomiting or diarrhea *3928* Potassium loss in urine *2369*

Urine Increase Physiological Slight diuretic response *5611*

Renin Activity *Plasma Increase Physiological* Approximately doubled after 6 weeks treatment with 5 mg daily in 5 or 6 hypertensives *6499*

Sodium *Serum Decrease Physiological* Metolazone may cause hyponatremia rapidly as with other diuretics *3929* Diuretic action of drug acting on distal tubules *4705* Hyponatremia may occur at any time during long term treatment *3928*

Urine Increase Physiological Diuretic action of drug *2369*

Titratable Acidity *Urine Increase Physiological* Associated with diuretic response *5611*

Urea Nitrogen *Serum Increase Physiological* Diuretic action of drug acting on distal tubules *4705* Metolazone may precipitate prerenal azotemia. Renal impairment may occur *3928*

Uric Acid *Serum Increase Physiological* Metolazone may increase the plasma uric acid concentration and may occasionally induce gout attacks, even in patients without a history of them *3928* Increase by 3-5 mmol/L after 6 weeks treatment with 5 mg daily in 5 or 6 hypertensives *6499* Diuretic action of drug acting on distal tubules *4705*

Volume *Urine Increase Physiological* Diuretic action *2369*

Water Clearance, Free *Urine Decrease Physiological* Diuretic action of drug *5859*

Metoprolol

Acetylsalicylic Acid *Serum Increase Physiological* In one study coadministration of metoprolol and aspirin increased total serum concentration of acetylsalicylic acid by 30% but mechanism not clear *4062*

Adenosine Monophosphate

Plasma No Effect Physiological Significantly less than in patients receiving pindolol but significantly greater than in patients receiving propranolol *6511*

Platelets Increase Physiological Significantly higher in patients receiving this drug than in those receiving propranolol *6511*

β-Adrenergic Receptors

Lymphocytes No Effect Physiological No change in number observed in 8 patients with chronic congestive cardiac failure treated with 75-100 mg daily for 8 weeks *4247*

Alanine Aminotransferase *Serum Increase Physiological* Acute drug-induced hepatitis observed in one patient treated with drug for 17 days, reversible on withdrawal *3417* Increases may occur as a result of treatment *279* Occasional increased enzyme activity may be observed *1032*

Albumin *Serum No Effect Analytical* At concentration of 0.34 mg/L had no effect on BCG method *5704*

Aldosterone *Urine Decrease Physiological* In 15 patients with essential hypertension treated for 4 weeks, associated with reduction in sympathetic tone and reduced activity of renin-aldosterone system *1974*

Alkaline Phosphatase *Serum Increase Physiological* Increases may occur as a result of treatment *279* Occasional increased enzyme activity may be observed *1032*

Apolipoprotein A-I *Serum Decrease Physiological* In 39 hypertensives treatment with 200 mg/d for 9 months caused 7% reduction from mean baseline of 1.53 ± 0.08 g/L to 1.43 ± 0.07 g/L *1423*

Serum No Effect Physiological No significant change from mean baseline of 134.1 mg/dL observed in 13 patients with essential hypertension treated with 200 mg daily for 12 weeks *3778*

Apolipoprotein A-I:Apolipoprotein B Ratio

Serum Decrease Physiological In 39 hypertensive patients treatment with 200 mg/d for 9 months caused significant 25% reduction from mean baseline of 1.49 ± 0.09 to 1.15 ± 0.08 *1423*

Apolipoprotein A-II *Serum No Effect Physiological* In 39 patients with hypertension treatment with 200 mg/d for 9 months caused 3% increase from mean baseline of 0.38 ± 0.03 g/L to 0.39 ± 0.03 g/L *1423*

Apolipoprotein B *Serum Increase Physiological* In 39 hypertensives treatment with 200 mg/d for 9 months caused significant increase from mean baseline of 1.14 ± 0.09 g/L to 1.32 ± 0.09 g/L *1423*

Serum No Effect Physiological No significant change from mean baseline of 141.9 mg/dL in 13 patients with essential hypertension treated with 200 mg daily for 12 weeks *3778* No significant effect in 15 hypertensive patients given 200 mg/d for 10 weeks *1840*

Aspartate Aminotransferase *Serum Increase Physiological* Occasional increased enzyme activity may be observed *1032* Increases may occur as a result of treatment *279*

Atrial Natriuretic Peptide *Plasma No Effect Physiological* In 14 hypertensive patients treatment with an average of 200 mg/d caused nonsignificant increase to 26.2 ± 3.7 pg/mL after 6 weeks from mean baseline of 21.5 ± 2.7 pg/mL and decrease to 20.8 ± 3.5 pg/mL after 12 weeks *553*

Bicarbonate *Serum No Effect Analytical* At concentration of 0.34 mg/L had no effect on method using phenolphthalein *5704*

Bilirubin *Serum No Effect Analytical* At concentration of 0.34 mg/L had no effect on Jendrassik and Grof method *5704*

Calcium *Serum No Effect Analytical* At concentration of 0.34 mg/L had no effect on cresolphthalein method *5704*

Chloride *Serum No Effect Analytical* At concentration of 0.34 mg/L had no effect on mercurimetric method *5704*

Cholesterol *Serum Decrease Physiological* Treatment for 6 months caused mean reduction in 37 hypertensive patients of 0.3 mmol/L (5%) from pretreatment value *3609*
Serum No Effect Analytical At concentration of 0.34 mg/L had no effect on CHOD-PAP method *5704*
Serum No Effect Physiological No significant effect observed with treatment with up to 300 mg daily for 1 year *4098* In 20 hypertensives given 200 mg/d for 3 mo *5115* No significant change from mean baseline of 223.0 mg/dL in 13 patients with essential hypertension treated with 200 mg daily for 12 weeks *3778* No effect in 1 or 3 mo study *3499* In 42 mild to moderate hypertensives treatment with up to 200 mg/d for 24 weeks had no significant effect *1923* Insignificant reduction in men (baseline 6.11 mmol/L, after treatment 6.01 mmol/L) and in women (baseline 5.78 mmol/L, after treatment 5.53 mmol/L) with up to 300 mg daily for 2 months *5907* In 20 hypertensive diabetic patients *6544* In 10 patients with chronic stable angina mean concentration changed nonsignificantly with 6 months treatment from mean baseline of 7.1 ± 1.2 mmol/L to 7.1 ± 0.7 mmol/L *6547* In several studies for up to 3 mo *142* In 39 patients with mild to moderate hypertension treatment with 200 mg/d for 9 months caused nonsignificant change from mean baseline of 6.24 ± 0.25 mmol/L to 6.45 ± 0.35 mmol/L *1423* No significant effect in 24 noninsulin dependent diabetic hypertensives treated with 100 mg daily for 8 weeks *1671*

Corticosterone *Urine No Effect Physiological* In 15 patients with essential hypertension treated for 4 weeks, associated with reduction in sympathetic tone and reduced activity of renin-aldosterone system *1974*

Cortisol *Urine No Effect Physiological* In 15 patients with essential hypertension treated for 4 weeks, associated with reduction in sympathetic tone and reduced activity of renin-aldosterone system *1974*

Creatinine *Serum Increase Physiological* Treatment of 42 mild to moderate hypertensives with up to 200 mg/d for 24 weeks caused slight mean increase of 3.9% *1923*
Serum No Effect Analytical At concentration of 0.34 mg/L had no effect on Technicon AutoAnalyzer® Jaffe method *5704*
Serum No Effect Physiological In 12 hypertensive post-renal transplant patients treatment with up to 200 mg/d for 12 weeks caused no change from mean baseline of 1.5 ± 0.1 mg/dL *3482*

Cyclosporine *Serum Decrease Physiological* Reported effect in end stage renal failure but mechanism not discussed. Note overall profile of plasma curve not affected *1069*

Deoxycorticosterone *Urine No Effect Physiological* In 15 patients with essential hypertension treated for 4 weeks, associated with reduction in sympathetic tone and reduced activity of renin-aldosterone system *1974*

Diazepam *Serum Increase Physiological* 200 mg daily increased area under diazepam concentration curve by about 25% *2517*

Effective Renal Plasma Flow
Patient Increase Physiological In 13 healthy male volunteers administration of a single oral dose of 100 mg caused a mean increase of 10.4 ± 5.2% in the fasting state *639*

Epinephrine *Plasma Decrease Physiological* In 8 patients with chronic congestive cardiac failure treated with 75-100 mg/day for 8 weeks caused reduction from mean concentration of 613 to 303 pg/mL *4247*
Plasma No Effect Physiological No consistent effect but effect generally high when drug concentration high in 11 healthy young men studied under variety of conditions *1432*

Fatty Acids (FFA), Free *Serum Decrease Physiological* Significant effect over 3 mo in 53 patients given 100 mg twice daily *1292* Observed with pharmacological doses in nondiabetic hypertensives *2346*

Felodipine *Serum No Effect Physiological* Coadministration of metoprolol with felodipine had no significant on the area under the curve or its maximum plasma concentration *266*

Glomerular Filtration Rate *Urine Increase Physiological* In 12 hypertensive post-renal transplant patients treatment with up to 200 mg/d caused significant increase from mean baseline of 39 ± 3 mL/min to 42 ± 2 mL/min *3482* Administration of a single oral dose of 100 mg caused a mean increase of 9.0 ± 2.7% in 13 healthy male volunteers *639*

Glucagon *Plasma Decrease Physiological* Lower in nondiabetic hypertensives when receiving drug compared with placebo *2346*

Glucose *Serum Increase Physiological* Small but significant increase in nondiabetic hypertensives *2346* Increase by 1.0 to 1.5 mmol/L in 20 hypertensive diabetic patients *6544*
Serum No Effect Analytical At concentration of 3 mg/L had no effect on GOD/POD-PAP method *5704*
Serum No Effect Physiological No significant change from mean baseline of 97.6 mg/dL in 13 patients with essential hypertension treated with 200 mg daily for 12 weeks *3778* No significant effect observed in 37 hypertensive patients treated with up to 300 mg daily for 1 year *4098* In 10 patients with chronic stable angina mean fasting concentration changed nonsignificantly with 6 months treatment from mean baseline of 5.0 ± 0.4 mmol/L to 5.5 ± 0.8 mmol/L *6547* No significant effect on either fasting or postprandial glucose in 24 noninsulin dependent hypertensive patients treated with 100 mg daily for 8 weeks *1671*

Glucose Tolerance *Serum Decrease Physiological* During early part of i.v. glucose tolerance test *2346*
Serum Increase Physiological Compared with placebo caused improvement with 200 mg/day for 3 weeks in 22 patients with primary hypertension and impaired or diabetic glucose tolerance when controlled-release preparation used *1778*

γ-Glutamyltransferase *Serum Increase Physiological* Acute drug-induced hepatitis observed in one patient treated for 17 days, reversible on withdrawal *3417*

Granulocytes *Blood Decrease Physiological* Occasional reversible agranulocytosis may be observed *1032* Rare reversible agranulocytosis may occur as a result of treatment *279*

HDL_2-Cholesterol *Serum Decrease Physiological* Significant reduction in men (baseline 0.75 mmol/L, after treatment 0.53 mmol/L) and in women (baseline 0.69 mmol/L, after treatment 0.49 mmol/L) with up to 300 mg daily for 2 months *5907*

HDL_3-Cholesterol *Serum Increase Physiological* Significant increase in men (baseline 0.73 mmol/L, after treatment 0.94 mmol/L) and in women (baseline 0.76 mmol/L, after treatment 0.88 mmol/L) with up to 300 mg daily for 2 months *5907*

HDL-Cholesterol *Serum Decrease Physiological* Increase by 13% after 1 mo in one study and 8% (nonsignificant) in another *3499* From 43 to 35 mg/dL in 18 hypertriglyceridemic hypertensives after 12 weeks *552* Mean decrease from 37 to 31 mg/dL in 15 hypertensives patients given 200 mg/d for 10 weeks *1840* Treatment of 42 mild to moderate hypertensives for 24 weeks with up to 200 mg/d caused mean reduction of 5.6% (change from 1.34 mmol/L to 1.26 mmol/L) *1923* Increase by 6 to 13% in several studies of 2 to 4 mo with up to 400 mg drμg/d *2953* Significant reduction in 22 patients with primary hypertension and impaired or diabetic glucose tolerance when controlled-release preparation administered 200 mg/day for 3 weeks *1778* No effect observed in 37 hypertensives treated with up to 300 mg daily at 3 or 6 months but at one year reduction from mean baseline concentration of 1.27 mmol/L to 1.17 mmol/L *4098* Insignificant reduction in men (baseline 1.48 mmol/L, after treatment 1.41 mmol/L) and in women (baseline 1.45 mmol/L, after treatment 1.35 mmol/L) with up to 300 mg daily for 2 months *5907* In 14 hypertensive patients treatment with an average of 200 mg/d for 3 months caused significant decrease from mean baseline of 45 ± 2 mg/dL to 38 ± 2 mg/dL *553* Fell from 1.42 to 1.31 mmol/L in 20 hypertensives given 200 mg/d for 3 mo *5115*
Serum No Effect Physiological No significant effect in 24 noninsulin dependent hypertensive diabetics treated with 100 mg daily for 8 weeks *1671* No significant change from mean baseline of 37.1 mg/dL observed in 13 patients with essential

Metoprolol *(continued)*

HDL-Cholesterol *(continued)*
hypertension treated with 200 mg daily for 12 weeks *3778* In 10 patients with chronic stable angina mean concentration changed nonsignificantly with 6 months treatment from mean baseline of 1.2 ± 0.3 mmol/L to 1.1 ± 0.2 mmol/L *6547* In 39 hypertensive patients treatment with 5 mg/d for 9 months caused nonsignificant reduction from mean baseline of 1.13 ± 0.10 mmol/L to 1.00 ± 0.07 mmol/L *1423* Typically although slight reduction in 1 study *142*

HDL-Cholesterol: VLDL + LDL-Cholesterol Ratio
Serum No Effect Physiological Treatment of 42 mild to moderate hypertensives for 24 weeks with up to 200 mg/d caused no significant change *1923*

HDL-Triglycerides *Serum No Effect Physiological* In 20 hypertensives given 200 mg/d for 3 mo *5115* In 18 hypertriglyceridemic-hypertensives after 12 weeks *552*

Hemoglobin A_{1c} *Blood No Effect Physiological* No significant effect in 24 noninsulin dependent hypertensive diabetics treated with 100 mg daily for 8 weeks *1671*

18-Hydroxycorticosterone *Urine No Effect Physiological* In 15 patients with essential hypertension treated for 4 weeks, associated with reduction in sympathetic tone and reduced activity of renin-aldosterone system *1974*

18-Hydroxydeoxycorticosterone
Urine No Effect Physiological In 15 patients with essential hypertension treated for 4 weeks, associated with reduction in sympathetic tone and reduced activity of renin-aldosterone system *1974*

Insulin *Plasma Increase Physiological* In 10 patients with chronic stable angina mean fasting concentration changed significantly with 6 months treatment from mean baseline of 7.2 ± 3.6 mmol/L to 15.0 ± 0.8 mU/L *6547*
Plasma No Effect Physiological In 20 hypertensive diabetic patients *6544* Insignificant change although plasma concentration of glucose changed *2346*

Kallikrein *Urine Decrease Physiological* In 15 patients with essential hypertension treated for 4 weeks, associated with reduction in sympathetic tone and reduced activity of renin-aldosterone system *1974*

Lactate Dehydrogenase *Serum Increase Physiological* Increases may occur as a result of treatment *279* Occasional increased enzyme activity may be observed *1032*

LDL-Apolipoprotein B *Serum No Effect Physiological* In 14 patients with hypertension treatment with an average of 200 mg/d for 3 months nonsignificant decrease from mean baseline of 134 ± 8 mg/dL to 127 ± 9 mg/dL observed *553*

LDL-Cholesterol *Serum Decrease Physiological* Increase by 7 to 8.5% in several studies of 2 to 4 mo with up to 400 mg drµg/d *2953* Small but significant decrease observed in 22 patients with primary hypertension and impaired or diabetic glucose tolerance given 200 mg of controlled-release preparation daily for 3 weeks *1778*
Serum No Effect Physiological In 39 hypertensive patients treatment with 200 mg/d for 9 months caused nonsignificant increase from mean baseline of 4.29 ± 0.27 mmol/L to 4.40 ± 0.33 mmol/L *1423* In 14 hypertensives treatment with average dose of 200 mg/d for 3 months caused nonsignificant decrease from mean baseline of 160 mg/dL to 151 ± 12 mg/dL *553* In 20 hypertensives given 200 mg/d for 3 mo *5115* No significant change observed in 37 hypertensive patients treated with up to 300 mg daily for 1 year *4098* No significant change after 12 weeks in 18 hypertriglyceridemic hypertensives *552* Insignificant change after 1 or 3 mo studies *3499* No significant change from mean baseline of 163.3 mg/dL observed in 13 patients with essential hypertension treated with 200 mg daily for 12 weeks *3778* Although slight reduction in one study *142* No significant effect in 24 noninsulin dependent diabetic hypertensives treated with 100 mg daily for 8 weeks *1671*

LDL-Triglycerides *Serum Increase Physiological* From 24 to 32 mg/dL after 12 weeks in 18 hypertriglyceridemic hypertensives *552*
Serum No Effect Physiological Rose from 1 to 1.29 mmol/L in 20 hypertensives given 200 mg/d for 3 mo *5115*

Lecithin:Cholesterol Acyltransferase
Serum Decrease Physiological At concentration of 0.5 µmol/L in vitro reduction of activity to 66.5 ± 19.6% observed *5316*

Lidocaine *Serum Increase Physiological* Clearance reduced by more than 20% with coadministration of metoprolol due to inhibition of hepatic metabolizing enzymes *1114*

Lipoprotein Lipase *Serum No Effect Physiological* No significant effect in 15 hypertensive patients given 200 mg/d for 10 weeks *1840*

Melatonin *Urine Decrease Physiological* After 4 weeks of treatment with up to 400 mg daily of 13 hypertensive patients significant reduction observed *724*

Mibefradil *Serum No Effect Physiological* Metoprolol coadministration had no significant effect on pharmacokinetics of mibefradil *5009*

Norepinephrine *Plasma Decrease Physiological* In 8 patients with chronic congestive cardiac failure mean resting concentration reduced from 71 to 40 pg/mL when patients treated with 75-100 mg daily for 8 weeks *4247*
Plasma Increase Physiological Significant effect in 11 healthy young men studied under variety of conditions *1432*

Phosphate *Serum No Effect Analytical* At concentration of 0.34 mg/L had no effect on phosphomolybdate method *5704*

Plasminogen Activator Inhibitor-1
Plasma No Effect Physiological In 10 patients with chronic stable angina mean concentration did not change significantly with 6 months treatment from mean baseline of 65 ng/mL *6547*

Platelet Aggregation *Blood Increase Physiological* Higher in patients receiving 100 mg b.i.d. than in those receiving either pindolol or propranolol *6511*
Blood No Effect Physiological No effect observed on basal level nor on morning increase in 10 patients with coronary artery disease *6475* No effect observed in response ADP compared with placebo in healthy volunteers *6260*

Platelets *Blood Decrease Physiological* Both thrombocytopenic and nonthrombocytopenic purpura may occur as a result of treatment *279*
Blood Increase Physiological When given twice per day for 1 week in healthy volunteers, also after single dose *6260*

Potassium *Serum Increase Physiological* Significant increase in patients with suspected myocardial infarction compared with placebo on first day after admission (4.27 mmol/L vs 4.14 mmol/L) *2567*
Serum No Effect Analytical At concentration of 0.34 mg/L had no effect on flame-photometric method *5704*
Serum No Effect Physiological Treatment of 42 mild to moderate hypertensives with up to 200 mg/d for 24 weeks caused no significant effect *1923*

Protein *Serum No Effect Analytical* At concentration of 0.34 mg/L had no effect on biuret method with blank correction *5704*

Renal Blood Flow *Patient No Effect Physiological* In 12 hypertensive post-renal transplant patients treatment with up to 200 mg/d for 8 weeks caused nonsignificant change from mean baseline of 311 ± 27 mL/min to 316 ± 14 ml/min *3482*

Renin Activity *Plasma Decrease Physiological* In 15 patients with essential hypertension treated for 4 weeks, associated with reduction in sympathetic tone and reduced activity of renin-aldosterone system *1974* In 14 hypertensive patients treatment with an average of 200 mg/d caused significant decrease from mean baseline of 1.02 ± 0.30 ng/mL/h to 0.38 ± 0.14 ng/mL/h after 6 weeks and 0.28 ± 0.11 bg/mL/h after 12 weeks *553*

Sodium *Serum No Effect Analytical* At concentration of 0.34 mg/L had no effect on flame-photometric method *5704*
Serum No Effect Physiological Treatment of 42 mild to moderate hypertensives for 24 weeks with up to 200 mg/d caused no significant effect *1923*
Urine Increase Physiological In 12 hypertensive post-renal transplant patients treatment with up to 200 mg/d caused nonsignificant increase from mean baseline of 80 ± 11 mmol/d to 87 ± 14 mmol/d *3482*

T3-Uptake *Serum Increase Physiological* Significant increase from mean baseline of 1.15 arbitrary units to 1.21 arbitrary units after 1 week and 1.22 arbitrary units after 3 weeks treatment with 200 mg/d in 8 healthy young normotensive men *3076*
Serum No Effect Physiological No significant effect in 16 hyperthyroid patients treated with 100 mg daily for 7 days *4610*

Theophylline *Serum Increase Physiological* Clearance reduced by 30-50% in healthy individuals given 200 mg or more per day: possibly due to a metabolite binding to cytochrome P-450 *1116*
Serum No Effect Physiological No clinically significant effect on theophylline concentration observed when drugs coadministered *5999* No documented significant interaction with theophylline reported *6117*

Thyroid Stimulating Hormone
Serum Increase Physiological Nonsignificant increase observed from mean baseline concentration of 1.67 mU/L to 1.81 mU/L after 1 week and 1.83 mU/L after 3 weeks treatment with 200 mg/d in 8 healthy normotensive men *3076*

Thyroxine (T4) *Serum Decrease Physiological* Nonsignificant decrease with treatment with 200 mg/d from mean baseline concentration of 93 nmol/L to 82 nmol/L after 1 week and 84 nmol/L after 3 weeks in 8 healthy normotensive young men *3076*
Serum No Effect Physiological No effect observed in 16 patients with hyperthyroidism treated with 100 mg daily for 7 days *4610*

Thyroxine (T4), Free *Serum No Effect Physiological* Nonsignificant increase from mean baseline concentration of 16.5 pmol/L to 17.1 pmol/L after 1 week with reversion to baseline after 3 weeks in 8 healthy young normotensive men treated with 200 mg/d *3076*

Thyroxine (T4) Index, Free *Serum No Effect Physiological* Nonsignificant increase from mean baseline of 99 arbitrary units to 100 arbitrary units after 1 week and 103 arbitrary units after 3 weeks in 8 healthy young normotensive men treated with 200 mg/d *3076*

Tirofiban *Serum No Effect Physiological* Coadministration had no significant effect on plasma clearance of tirofiban *3957*

Tissue Plasminogen Activator Antigen
Plasma No Effect Physiological In 10 patients with chronic stable angina mean concentration did not change significantly with 6 months treatment from mean baseline of 8.3 ng/mL *6547*

Tri-iodothyronine, Reverse (rT3)
Serum Decrease Physiological Decrease from mean of 1.20 nmol/L to 1.10 nmol/L in 16 hyperthyroid patients treated with 100 mg daily for 7 days: effect probably due to inhibition of 5-deiodinase enzyme *4610* Nonsignificant decrease from mean baseline concentration of 0.46 nmol/L to 0.44 nmol/L at 1 week and 0.43 nmol/L at 3 weeks in 8 healthy young normotensive men treated with 200 mg/d *3076*

Tri-iodothyronine (T3) *Serum Decrease Physiological* Reduction from mean of 7.8 nmol/L to 7.2 nmol/L in 16 hyperthyroid patients treated with 100 mg daily for 7 days *4610*
Serum No Effect Physiological No significant change from mean baseline concentration of 2.1 nmol/L after treatment for 1 week and for 3 weeks with 200 mg/d in 8 healthy young normotensive men *3076*

Triglycerides *Serum Increase Physiological* Treatment of 42 mild to moderate hypertensives with up to 200 mg/d for 24 weeks caused mean increase of 10.3% (change from 1.65 mmol/L to 1.82 mmol/L) *1923* Significant effect in men (baseline 2.08 mmol/L, after treatment 2.51 mmol/L) but not in women (baseline 2.08 mmol/L, after treatment 2.14 mmol/L) with up to 300 mg daily for 2 months *5907* In 15 hypertensive patients given 200 mg/d for 10 weeks caused mean increase from 122 to 142 mg/dL *1840* Significant increase from mean of 168 mg/dL to 227 mg/dL in 24 noninsulin dependent diabetic hypertensives treated with 100 mg daily for 8 weeks *1671* Insignificant in 20 hypertensive diabetic patients *6544* Up to 34% in some studies but no effect in almost as many *142* Significant effect of 33% and 14% for 1 mo and 3 mo studies respectively *3499* No effect observed in 37 hypertensives with up to 300 mg daily for 3 months but increase from mean baseline of 1.10 mmol/L to 1.40 mmol/L at 6 months and from 1.14 mmol/L to 1.38 mmol/L at 12 months *4098* Rose from 2.51 to 3.41 mmol/L in 20 hypertensives given 200 mg/d for 3 mo *5115*
Serum No Effect Analytical At concentration of 0.34 mg/L had no effect on lipase/esterase method *5704* At concentration of 3 mg/L had no effect on GPO-PAP method *5704*
Serum No Effect Physiological No significant change from mean baseline of 130.3 mg/dL observed in 13 patients with essential hypertension treated for 12 weeks with 200 mg daily *3778* In 10 patients with chronic stable angina mean concentration changed nonsignificantly with 6 months treatment from mean baseline of 2.2 ± 0.9 mmol/L to 2.1 ± 1.0 mmol/L *6547* Mean concentration of 2.01 ± 0.27 mmol/L in 39 hypertensive patients increased 13% to 2.27 ± 0.16 mmol/L after treatment with 200 mg/d for 9 months *1423* Insignificant increase after 12 weeks treatment in hypertriglyceridemic hypertensives *552*

Urea Nitrogen *Serum Increase Physiological* Insignificant in 20 hypertensive diabetic patients *6544*
Serum No Effect Analytical At concentration of 0.34 mg/L had no effect on diacetylmonoxime method *5704*

Uric Acid *Serum No Effect Analytical* At concentration of 3 mg/L had no effect on uricase-PAP method *5704* At concentration of 0.34 mg/L had no effect on phosphotungstate reduction method *5704*
Serum No Effect Physiological No significant effect observed in 37 hypertensive patients treated with up to 300 mg daily for 1 year *4098* No significant change from mean baseline of 5.0 mg/dL in 13 patients with essential hypertension treated with 200 mg daily for 12 weeks *3778*

Verapamil *Serum No Effect Physiological* No effect observed on plasma concentration when drugs coadministered *6358*

VLDL + LDL-Cholesterol *Serum No Effect Physiological* Treatment of 42 mild to moderate hypertensives for 24 weeks with up to 200 mg/d caused no significant change *1923*

VLDL-Apolipoprotein B *Serum Increase Physiological* In 14 hypertensive patients treated with an average dose of 200 mg/d for 3 months nonsignificant increase from mean baseline of 20 ± 5 mg/dL to 32 ± 10 mg/dL *553*

VLDL-Cholesterol *Serum Decrease Physiological* Increase by 6 to 7% in several studies of 2 to 4 mo with up to 400 mg drµg/d *2953*
Serum Increase Physiological In 14 hypertensive patients treated with an average of 200 mg/d for 3 months caused significant increase from mean baseline of 33 ± 4 mg/dL to 40 ± 6 mg/dL *553* Increase by 30% in one study *142* Rose from 1.00 to 1.29 mmol/L in 20 hypertensives given 200 mg/d for 3 mo *5115*
Serum No Effect Physiological Nonstatistically significant increase from 61 to 67 mg/dL after 12 weeks in 18 hypertriglyceridemic hypertensives *552* In 39 hypertensive patients treatment with 200 mg/d for 9 months caused nonsignificant increase from mean baseline of 0.85 ± 0.13 mmol/L to 0.88 ± 0.09 mmol/L *1423* No significant effect observed in 37 hypertensive patients treated with up to 300 mg daily for 1 year *4098* No significant change from mean baseline of 15.9 mg/dL observed in 13 patients with essential hypertension treated with 200 mg daily for 12 weeks *3778*

VLDL-Triglycerides *Serum Increase Physiological* 36% in one study *142*
Serum No Effect Physiological Non-statistically significant increase from 203 to 232 mg/dL after 12 weeks in 18 hypertriglyceridemic hypertensives *552* In 20 hypertensives given 200 mg/d for 3 mo *5115*

Metrifonate

Alanine Aminotransferase *Serum No Effect Physiological* No effect reported on hepatic function *4014*

Cholinesterase *Serum Decrease Physiological* Decreased to 5% of pretreatment value within 6 hours of drug administration but returns to normal within 4-6 weeks *1384* A single oral dose of 10 mg/kg body weight administered to primary school children caused activity to be reduced to less than 70% of normal for a period of at least 5 days in 43% of individuals *4277* Powerful inhibitor of enzyme *4014*

Urea Clearance *Urine No Effect Physiological* No effect reported on renal function *4014*

Metrizamide

Bilirubin *Serum No Effect Physiological* Probably nonclinically significant protein displacement effect in neonates *6314*

Protein *Cerebrospinal Fluid Increase Analytical* At concentrations greater than 10 mmol/L significantly increased result obtained with method on Du Pont aca *1515*

Metrizoate

Bilirubin *Serum Increase Physiological* Theoretically possible effect in neonates because of high circulating concentration *6314*

γ-Glutamyltransferase *Serum Increase Physiological* Effect observed in subjects with liver tumors *115*

Metronidazole

Alanine Aminotransferase *Serum Decrease Analytical* With certain reactions involving enzymatic coupling with oxidation-reduction of NAD. Interference may occur due to the similarity of absorbance peaks of NADH (340 nm) and metronidazole (322 nm) at pH 7. Values of zero may be observed *4446* Metronidazole reported to interfere with certain enzymatic assays with values of zero being observed sometimes. Affected methods involving the coupling of the assay to oxidation reduction of NAD. Interference is due to the similarity in absorbance peaks of NADH (300 nm) and metronidazole (322 nm) at pH 7 *2066* Reported to reduce activity, even to zero, with certain methods that involve enzymatic coupling to NAD or NADH, due to similarity of absorbance peaks of NADH (340 nm) and metronidazole (322 nm) at pH 7 *5420*

Alprazolam *Serum No Effect Physiological* No effect on clearance observed when metronidazole coadministered *616*

Amylase *Serum Increase Physiological* Isolated cases of metronidazole-induced pancreatitis reported *1384*

Aspartate Aminotransferase *Serum Decrease Analytical* With continuous flow endpoint reaction method because of drug's high absorbance at 340 nm, although no effect on kinetic methods *1382* Metronidazole reported to interfere with certain enzymatic assays with values of zero being observed sometimes. Affected methods involve the coupling of the assay to oxidation reduction of NAD. Interference is due to the similarity in absorbance peaks of NADH (300 nm) and metronidazole (322 nm) at pH 7 *2066* Reported to reduce activity, even to zero, with certain methods that involve enzymatic coupling to NAD or NADH, due to similarity of absorbance peaks of NADH (340 nm) and metronidazole (322 nm) at pH 7 *5420* With certain reactions involving enzymatic coupling with oxidation-reduction of NAD. Interference may occur due to the similarity of absorbance peaks of NADH (340 nm) and metronidazole (322 nm) at pH 7. Values of zero may be observed *4446* Artifactual depression of activity in almost all patients with NADH-coupled analytical methods *5097*
Serum No Effect Analytical On continuous flow procedure if blank correction incorporated *2667* No effect noted on coupled NADH procedure on Technicon SMA II if appropriate blanking used *2667*

Bilirubin *Serum No Effect Analytical* No effect at 250 mg/L on Ames Seralyzer method *5706*

Chloramphenicol *Serum No Effect Analytical* No effect at 100 mg/L on coupled enzymatic method *4122*

Cholesterol *Serum Decrease Physiological* Reported effect but mechanism and clinical significance unknown *1384*
Serum No Effect Analytical No effect at 250 mg/L on Ames Seralyzer method *5706*

Clindamycin *Serum Positive Analytical* Interferes with bioassays *3858*

Colistin *Serum Positive Analytical* Interferes with bioassays *3858*

Color *Urine Increase Analytical* Brown color probably due to metabolite *2024* Darkened urine reported, probably due to a metabolite of metronidazole, but of no clinical significance *5420*

Creatine Kinase *Serum No Effect Analytical* No effect at 250 mg/L on method on Ames Seralyzer *5706*

Creatinine *Serum No Effect Analytical* No effect at 250 mg/L on method on Ames Seralyzer *5706*

Erythromycin *Serum Increase Analytical* Interferes with bioassays *3858*

Glucose *Serum Decrease Analytical* At concentrations above 100 mg/L (normal therapeutic concentration 47.5 mg/L) lowered concentration as measured by hexokinase/G-6-PDH method *5704* At concentrations above 200 mg/L (normal therapeutic concentration 47.5 mg/L) lowered concentration as measured by Du Pont aca method *5704* With hexokinase reaction involving enzymatic coupling with oxidation-reduction of NAD. Interference may occur due to the similarity of absorbance peaks of NADH (340 nm) and metronidazole (322 nm) at pH 7. Values of zero may be observed *4446* Reported to reduce activity, even to zero, with certain hexokinase methods that involve enzymatic coupling to NAD or NADH, due to similarity of absorbance peaks of NADH (340 nm) and metronidazole (322 nm) at pH 7 *5420* Metronidazole reported to interfere with certain enzymatic assays with values of zero being observed sometimes. Affected methods involve the coupling of the assay to oxidation reduction of NAD. Interference is due to the similarity in absorbance peaks of NADH (300 nm) and metronidazole (322 nm) at pH 7. Hexokinase glucose methods reported to be affected *2066*
Serum Increase Analytical Increased values observed with Technicon SMAC® and Du Pont aca hexokinase methods. Normal drug concentration increased glucose by about 60 mg/L *1477* On hexokinase method on Technicon SMAC® at therapeutic concentration *1478*
Serum No Effect Analytical No effect at 10 mmol/L on glucokinase based assay of Scott *5414* No effect up to 15 mg/L on glucose oxidase method on Ames Seralyzer apparent reduction of glucose concentration but since this concentration is within the therapeutic range is of probable clinical significance *5706* On glucose oxidase method on Beckman Astra® at therapeutic concentration *1478*

Glyoxal *Urine Increase Analytical* Derived from 2-hydroxyethyl side-chain after cleavage from imidazole ring during analysis. Probably some also derived from endogenous glyoxylic acid *4057*

Histamine *Plasma No Effect Analytical* No inhibition of radio-enzyme assay at 10 times therapeutic concentration *2492*

^{131}I Uptake *Serum No Effect Physiological* 1200 mg/d for 1 week no effect *882*

Indomethacin *Serum No Effect Analytical* No effect on HPLC method of Roberts and Smith *4978*

17-Ketosteroids *Urine Decrease Physiological* If previously elevated, ?depresses adrenal cortex *2242*

Lactate Dehydrogenase *Serum Decrease Analytical* Reported to reduce activity, even to zero, with certain methods that involve enzymatic coupling to NAD or NADH, due to similarity of absorbance peaks of NADH (340 nm) and metronidazole (322 nm) at pH 7 *5420* Metronidazole reported to interfere with certain enzymatic assays with values of zero being observed sometimes. Affected methods involve the coupling of the assay to oxidation reduction of NAD. Interference is due to the similarity in absorbance peaks of NADH (300 nm) and metronidazole (322 nm) at pH 7 *2066* With certain reactions involving enzymatic coupling with oxidation-reduction of NAD. Interference may occur due to the similarity of absorbance peaks of NADH (340 nm) and metronidazole (322 nm) at pH 7. Values of zero may be observed *4446*
Serum No Effect Analytical No effect at 3 mg/L but reduced activity at 15 mg/L on method on Ames Seralyzer. Effect of possible clinical significance since therapeutic range from 6.8-47.5 mg/L *5706*

Leukocytes *Blood Decrease Physiological* Leukopenia and reduction of polymorphs *3810* Reversible leukopenia may occur with treatment *4446* Reversible neutropenia (leukopenia) reported with metronidazole treatment *5420* A mild leukopenia has been observed during administration *2066* Administration of metronidazole may cause a mild leukopenia *4446* Occasional leukopenia reported with neutrophils most affected *1384*

Lipase *Serum Increase Physiological* Isolated cases of metronidazole-induced pancreatitis reported *1384*
Serum No Effect Analytical No effect of concentrations up to 40 mg/L on method on Kodak Ektachem® *5706*

Lithium *Serum Increase Physiological* In patients stabilized on relatively high doses pf lithium administration of metronidazole has been reported to increase plasma lthium concentration *4446* When patients stabilized on relatively high doses of lithium short term metronidazole administration may increase lithium concentration *2066*

Lorazepam *Serum No Effect Physiological* No effect observed on plasma clearance when drugs coadministered *616*

Neutrophils *Blood Decrease Physiological* Occasional case of agranulocytosis reported *6264* Reversible neutropenia (leukopenia) reported with metronidazole treatment *5420* Reversible neutropenia may occur with treatment *4446* Transient neutropenia may occur *4014*

Partial Thromboplastin Time
Plasma Increase Physiological In one patient stabilized on warfarin to whose therapeutic regime metronidazole was added *1332*

Phenylalanine *Plasma No Effect Analytical* No interference observed with rapid quantitative whole blood method of Campbell et al using phenylalanine dehydrogenase *867*

Phenytoin *Serum Increase Physiological* Moderate increase in plasma concentration observed due to inhibition of phenytoin metabolism: clearance reduced by 15% *616* Administration of metronidazole with phenytoin may impair clearance of phenytoin *4446* When drugs that induce hepatic microsomal enzymes coadministered elimination of metronidazole may be accelerated, but metronidazole may impair the clearance of phenytoin *2066* Increased concentration reported in several patients *4693* Reported to impair clearance of phenytoin, increasing its blood concentration *5420*

Platelets *Blood Decrease Physiological* Rarely reversible thrombocytopenia reported with metronidazole treatment *5420* Reversible rare thrombocytopenia may occur with treatment *4446*

Polymyxin *Serum Increase Analytical* Interferes with bioassays *3858*

Prothrombin Time *Plasma Increase Physiological* In one patient stabilized on warfarin to whose therapeutic regime metronidazole was added *1332* When warfarin coadministered prolongs prothrombin time through stereoselective inhibition of clearance of S isomer *2625* Marked effect reported in a single patient previously stabilized on warfarin but to whose regime metronidazole was added *3079* Potentiates effect on warfarin *3079* Reported to prolong anticoagulant effect of warfarin when drugs coadministered *2066* Reported to potentiate the anticoagulant effect of warfarin and other oral coumarin anticoagulants *5420* Significant increase in concentration of warfarin and prolongation of prothrombin time. Effect noted with S (-) warfarin but not R (+) warfarin *4429* Administration of metronidazole may potentiate anticoagulant effect of coumarin and warfarin *4446*

Short-Chain Fatty Acids *Feces No Effect Physiological* No significant effect when given orally for 6 d *2734*

T3-Uptake *Serum No Effect Physiological* 1200 mg/d for 1 week producing no effect *882*

Terfenadine *Serum Increase Physiological* Because of similar chemical structure to ketoconazole and itraconazole which markedly inhibit the metabolism of terfenadine, probably has similar effect *2653*

Tetracycline *Serum Increase Analytical* Interferes with bioassays *3858*

Theophylline *Serum No Effect Physiological* No clinically significant effect on theophylline concentration observed when drugs coadministered *5999* No documented significant interaction with theophylline reported *6117*

Triglycerides *Serum Decrease Analytical* Metronidazole reported to interfere with certain enzymatic assays with values of zero being observed sometimes. Affected methods involve the coupling of the assay to oxidation reduction of NAD. Interference is due to the similarity in absorbance peaks of NADH (300 nm) and metronidazole (322 nm) at pH 7 *2066* Reported to reduce activity, even to zero, with certain methods that involve enzymatic coupling to NAD or NADH, due to similarity of absorbance peaks of NADH (340 nm) and metronidazole (322 nm) at pH 7 *5420* With certain reactions involving enzymatic coupling with oxidation-reduction of NAD. Interference may occur due to the similarity of absorbance peaks of NADH (340 nm) and metronidazole (322 nm) at pH 7. Values of zero may be observed *4446*
Serum Decrease Physiological Reported effect but mechanism and clinical significance unknown *1384*

Trimethoprim *Serum Increase Analytical* Interferes with bioassays *3858*

Urea Nitrogen *Serum No Effect Analytical* No effect at 250 mg/L on method on Ames Seralyzer *5706*

Warfarin *Plasma Increase Physiological* May potentiate effects by effect on metabolism *5096*

Zidovudine *Serum Decrease Analytical* Eluted at same retention time as one of the internal standards in liquid chromatographic method of Hedaya and Sawchuk, but effect can be avoided by use of other internal standard only *2525*

Metyrapone

Acetaminophen *Serum Increase Physiological* Metyrapone may inhibit glucuronidation of acetaminophen enhancing its toxicity *1035*

Aldosterone *Urine Decrease Physiological* May inhibit aldosterone production *4605*

Androstenedione *Plasma Increase Physiological* Increase in 3-8 h in men, marked increase in women *4298*

Corticotropin *Plasma Increase Physiological* Response to stress *3395* Significant increase observed in 9 normal individuals and 12 patients with Cushing's disease following 6 doses of 750 mg orally every 4 hours *6059*

Cortisol *Plasma Decrease Physiological* In critically ill patients relative hypoadrenalism observed with metyrapone therapy because of its effect on cortisol synthesis *3381* Normal response to test *3939* Administration of 750 mg orally every 4 hours for 1 day caused decrease in concentration in 9 normal individuals and 12 patients with Cushing's disease *6059*

Cortisol, Free *Urine No Effect Analytical* No significant interference observed with HPLC method of Turpeinen et al *6105*

11-Deoxycortisol *Plasma Increase Physiological* Normal response to test *789*

Growth Hormone *Plasma No Effect Physiological* No significant effect with 750 mg orally *3584*

17-Hydroxycorticosteroids *Plasma Increase Physiological* Indirectly stimulates ACTH production *3646*
Urine Decrease Physiological Direct effect on adrenal steroidogenesis *55*
Urine Increase Physiological Normal response to injection is 2-4 times increase *3646* In normal individuals metyrapone administration causes a 2 - 4-fold increase in excretion *1035*

17-Ketogenic Steroids *Urine Decrease Analytical* Interferes with Zimmermann reaction *5869*
Urine Increase Physiological Normal response to injection is doubling of output *2754* In normal individuals metyrapone administration causes a doubling of excretion *1035*

17-Ketosteroids *Urine Decrease Analytical* Interferes with Zimmermann reaction *5869*

Porphyrin, Total *Urine Increase Physiological* Reported to precipitate attack of acute porphyria *3669*

Testosterone *Serum Decrease Physiological* Fall in 2 h in men, minor increase in women *4298*

Metyrosine

Aspartate Aminotransferase *Serum Increase Physiological* Increased activity has been reported in a few patients *3970* Increased activity observed in some patients *1384*

Blood *Urine Increase Physiological* Transient increases have been observed in a few patients *3970*

Catecholamines *Urine Increase Analytical* Spurious increases may occur due to the presence of the drug *3970*

Crystals *Urine Increase Physiological* Crystalluria observed in some patients *1384* Administration has been reported to cause crystalluria in a few patients *3970*

Dihydroxyphenylalanine *Plasma Increase Physiological* In patients with malignant pheochromocytoma treatment caused increase in concentration *3313*

Dihydroxyphenylalanine Sulfate Esters
Plasma Increase Physiological Treatment of patients with malignant pheochromocytoma with metyrosine caused significant increase in concentration *3313*

Dihydroxyphenylethanol *Urine Increase Physiological* In patients with malignant pheochromocytoma treatment with metyrosine caused significant increase even in the absence of a change in plasma dopamine concentration *3313*

Metyrosine *(continued)*

Dopamine *Plasma Increase Physiological* In patients with malignant pheochromocytoma with metyrosine caused significant increase in concentration *3313*
Urine Increase Physiological In patients with malignant pheochromocytoma treatment with metyrosine caused progressive increase even in the absence of an increase in plasma dopamine concentration *3313*

Eosinophils *Blood Increase Physiological* Eosinophilia observed in some patients *1384* Eosinophilia has been reported in a few patients *3970*

Epinephrine *Plasma Decrease Physiological* In patients with malignant pheochromocytoma treatment with metyrosine caused marked suppression *3313*

Hematocrit *Blood Decrease Physiological* Anemia has been reported in a few patients *3970*

Hemoglobin *Blood Decrease Physiological* Anemia has been reported in a few patients *3970*
Urine Increase Physiological Hemoglobinuria observed in some patients *1384*

Platelets *Blood Decrease Physiological* Both thrombocytopenia and thrombocytosis have been reported in a few patients *3970*
Blood Increase Physiological Both thrombocytopenia and thrombocytosis have been reported in a few patients *3970*

Tyrosine *Plasma Increase Physiological* In patients with malignant pheochromocytoma treatment with metyrosine caused increase in concentration *3313*

Mexiletine

Alanine Aminotransferase *Serum Increase Physiological* Hepatitis occurs as rare reaction *1384* Occurs in fewer than 1% treated patients *3281*

Antinuclear Antibodies *Serum Increase Physiological* Occurs as rare reaction *1384* Occurs in fewer than 1% treated patients *3281*

Aspartate Aminotransferase *Serum Increase Physiological* Hepatitis occurs as rare reaction *1384* Occurs in fewer than 1% treated patients *3281*

Digoxin *Serum No Effect Physiological* No significant effect when drug coadministered *3449*

Histamine *Plasma No Effect Analytical* Improbable inhibition of radio-enzyme assay at therapeutic concentrations *2492*

Leukocytes *Blood Decrease Physiological* Occurs in fewer than 1% treated patients *3281*

Neutrophils *Blood Decrease Physiological* Occurs in fewer than 1% treated patients *3281*

p-Aminophenol *Urine No Effect Analytical* With addition of drugs at a concentration of 100 mg/L and of related compounds at 50 mg/L no significant effect observed on colorimetric method of van Bocxlaer on Cobas Mira analyzer which involves reacting free p-aminophenol with resorcinol in the presence of magnesium ions to form an indophenol dye measured at 550 nm *6163*

Platelets *Blood Decrease Physiological* Occurs in fewer than 1% treated patients *3281* Thrombocytopenia occurs as rare reaction *1384*

Theophylline *Serum Increase Physiological* Up to 80% increase in serum theophylline concentration due to decreased theophylline clearance caused by inhibition of hydroxylation and demethylation *6117* Decreases theophylline clearance by inhibiting hydroxylation and demethylation, increasing theophylline concentration by about 80% *5999* Decreases theophylline clearance by inhibiting hydroxylation and demethylation and increases serum theophylline concentration by 80% *3125* In 3 patients when mexiletine added to therapeutic regime with theophylline alone theophylline concentration increased about 2-fold *6125* Reported to increase plasma concentration and combined therapy may cause adverse effects on cardiac rhythm *1384* In 8 healthy men pretreated with mexilitine trough increased from 8.1 ± 0.1 µg/mL to 13.4 ± 0.6 µg/mL and reduced plasma clearance from 44.7 ± 5.1 to 25.4 +/ 1.2 mL/h. Both N-demethylated metabolites of theophylline decreased by 60% with mexiletine. Theophylline concentrations returned to pre-mexiletine values when mexiletine discontinued *2790*

Mezlocillin

Creatinine *Serum No Effect Analytical* No effect at therapeutic concentrations on Beckman Astra® and Technicon SMAC® *1181*

Glucose *Urine Increase Analytical* Falsely elevated values with Clinitest® *3446*
Urine No Effect Analytical Concentrations measured accurately by Diastix® . Concentration measured accurately by TesTape® *3446*

Penicillin V *Serum Positive Analytical* Cannot be assayed by HPLC method used at Mayo Clinic in presence of mezlocillin *3858*

Protein *Urine Increase Analytical* False positive reaction with biuret following precipitation with trichloracetic acid and resuspension *4422*

Tacrolimus *Serum No Effect Analytical* In HPLC/MS method of Christians et al no significant interference observed with measurement of FK 506 *1010*

Vancomycin *Serum No Effect Analytical* Negligible interference at up to 500 mg/L on Abbott TD_x*4002*

Mianserin

Albumin *Urine No Effect Analytical* Using a fluorimetric assay with Albumin Blue 580 on a Cobas Fara centrifugal analyzer for the detection of microalbuminuria no significant interference was detected at a concentration of 12 mg/L *3117*

Catecholamines *Plasma No Effect Analytical* No effect on HPLC method of Koller for dopamine, epinephrine, and norepinephrine *3230*

Leukocytes *Blood Decrease Physiological* Decreased concentration reported in 4 individuals who were also receiving other drugs *60*

Neutrophils *Blood Decrease Physiological* Decreased concentration reported in 4 individuals who were also receiving other drugs *60*

Mibefradil

Alanine Aminotransferase *Serum No Effect Physiological* During administration of mibefradil no significant change observed *5009*

Aspartate Aminotransferase
Serum No Effect Physiological During administration of mibefradil no significant change observed *5009*

Astemizole *Serum Increase Physiological* Mibefradil inhibits its metabolism of drugs metabolized by cytochrome P450 3A4. Although no studies of the effect of mibefradil on astemizole have been conducted an increase of astemizole concentration could be predicted *5009*

Atenolol *Serum No Effect Physiological* No significant interaction observed between mibefradil and atenolol at recommended doses *5009*

Bilirubin *Serum No Effect Physiological* During administration of mibefradil no significant change observed *5009*

Calcium *Serum No Effect Physiological* During administration of mibefradil no significant change observed *5009*

Cholesterol *Serum No Effect Physiological* During administration of mibefradil no significant change observed *5009*

Cimetidine *Serum No Effect Physiological* No significant interaction observed between mibefradil and cimetidine at recommended doses *5009*

Cisapride *Serum Increase Physiological* Mibefradil inhibits metabolism of drugs metabolized by cytochrome P450 3A4. Although no studies of the effect of mibefradil on cisapride have been conducted an increase of cisapride concentration could be predicted *5009*

Creatinine *Serum No Effect Physiological* During administration of mibefradil no significant change observed *5009*

Cyclosporine A *Blood Increase Physiological* Mibefradil inhibits metabolism of drugs metabolized by cytochrome P450 3A4. Cyclosporine A concentration increased twofold when cyclosporine A coadministered with mibefranil 50 mg/d for 8 days *5009*

Desipramine *Serum Increase Physiological* Mibefradil inhibits metabolism of drugs metabolized by cytochrome P450 2D6 in the liver such as desipramine *5009*

Dextromethorphan *Serum Increase Physiological* Mibefradil inhibits metabolism of drugs metabolized by cytochrome P450 2D6 in the liver such as dextromethorphan *5009*

Digoxin *Serum No Effect Physiological* Insignificant clinical interaction observed between mibefradil at doses of 50 or 100 mg/d and digoxin but with the concentration of digoxin increasing 20 to 30%. Trough concentrations and concentrations in patients with congestive cardiac failure *5009*

Enalapril *Serum No Effect Physiological* No significant interaction observed between mibefradil and enalapril at recommended doses *5009*

Erythrocytes *Blood No Effect Physiological* During administration of mibefradil no significant change observed *5009*

Flecainamide *Serum Increase Physiological* Mibefradil inhibits metabolism of drugs metabolized by cytochrome P450 2D6 in the liver such as flecainamide *5009*

Glucose *Serum No Effect Physiological* During administration of mibefradil no significant change observed *5009*

Hematocrit *Blood No Effect Physiological* During administration of mibefradil no significant change observed *5009*

Hemoglobin *Blood No Effect Physiological* During administration of mibefradil no significant change observed *5009*

Imipramine *Serum Increase Physiological* Mibefradil inhibits its metabolism of drugs metabolized by cytochrome P450 2D6 in the liver such as imipramine *5009*

Metoprolol *Serum Increase Physiological* Mibefradil inhibits its metabolism of drugs metabolized by cytochrome P450 2D6. Peak plasma concentration of R- and S-enantiomers of metoprolol in healthy individuals increased twofold and about a four- to fivefold increase of AUC. Elimination half-life increased from 3 hours to 7 to 8 hours. The increase in the pharmacologically active S-entantiomer was only 30% so that the pharmacological effect was little changed *5009*

Mexiletine *Serum Increase Physiological* Mibefradil inhibits metabolism of drugs metabolized by cytochrome P450 2D6 in the liver such as mexiletine *5009*

Phenytoin *Serum No Effect Physiological* Insignificant clinical interaction observed with mibefradil which is 99.5% protein bound, mainly to α_1-acid glycoprotein (95%) *5009*

Potassium *Serum No Effect Physiological* During administration of mibefradil no significant change observed *5009*

Propafenone *Serum Increase Physiological* Mibefradil inhibits metabolism of drugs metabolized by cytochrome P450 2D6 in the liver such as propafenone *5009*

Quinidine *Serum Increase Physiological* Mibefradil inhibits metabolism of drugs metabolized by cytochrome P450 3A4. Peak quinidine concentration increased by 15 to 19% and AUC increased by 50% when single doses of quinidine coadministered with either 50 mg or 100 mg of mibefranil but the concentration of the active metabolite of quinidine markedly reduced *5009*

Sildenafil *Serum Increase Physiological* Theoretical effect: drug likely to increase area under concentration curve of sildenafil due to CYP3A4 inhibition *4657*

Sodium *Serum No Effect Physiological* During administration of mibefradil no significant change observed *5009*

Terfenadine *Serum Increase Physiological* Mibefradil inhibits metabolism of drugs metabolized by cytochrome P450 3A4. Coadministration of terfenadine to healthy individuals resulted in an increase in plasma concentration of terfenadine to 40 µg/L with twice daily dosing of terfenadine of 60 mg *5009*

Theophylline *Serum No Effect Physiological* No significant clinical interaction observed between mibefradil and theophylline, a CYP 450 1A2 substrate, although inhibition observed in vitro *5009*

Triglycerides *Serum No Effect Physiological* During administration of mibefradil no significant change observed *5009*

Urea Nitrogen *Serum No Effect Physiological* During administration of mibefradil no significant change observed *5009*

Uric Acid *Serum No Effect Physiological* During administration of mibefradil no significant change observed *5009*

Warfarin *Plasma No Effect Physiological* Insignificant clinical interaction observed with mibefradil which is 99.5% protein bound, mainly to α_1-acid glycoprotein (95%) *5009*

Miconazole

Chlorpropamide *Serum Increase Physiological* Possible interaction of miconazole with chlorpropamide reported leading to severe hypoglycemia *4644*

Cholesterol *Serum Increase Physiological* Commonly observed but due to vehicle (polyethoxylated castor oil) rather than to drug itself *1384*

Cisapride *Serum Increase Physiological* By inhibiting cytochrome P450 3A4 inhibits metabolism of cisapride and increases its plasma concentration *2903*

Creatine Kinase *Serum Increase Physiological* Observed as isolated finding in patients given drug i.v *5815*

Cyclosporine *Blood Increase Physiological* Coadministration caused a 40% increase in cyclosporine trough concentration in one case report *859*

Serum Increase Physiological Coadministration caused a 40% increase in cyclosporine trough concentration in one case report *859* Increased concentrations reported when drugs coadministered *1384*

Hematocrit *Blood Decrease Physiological* By more than 4% in 44% treated patients *5815*

Hemoglobin *Blood Decrease Physiological* Anemia occurs quite frequently as a side effect *1384*

Leukocytes *Blood Decrease Physiological* Observed as isolated finding in patients given drug i.v *5815*

Phenytoin *Serum Increase Physiological* Isolated case reported with phenytoin concentration markedly increased after miconazole given i.v., probably due to inhibition of hepatic cytochrome P-450 *5066*

Platelets *Blood Decrease Physiological* Thrombocytopenia occurs quite often as a side effect *1384*

Blood Increase Physiological Occurred in 31% of courses followed *5815*

Protein *Cerebrospinal Fluid No Effect Analytical* No significant effect when added in vitro to concentration of 10.0 mg/dL when measured by Kodak Ektachem® slide method *3654*

Prothrombin Time *Plasma Increase Physiological* In patients receiving warfarin, probably due to displacement from plasma protein *6365* In patients receiving warfarin whose hepatic metabolism is inhibited *5816*

Sodium *Serum Decrease Physiological* Hyponatremia due to inappropriate secretion of antidiuretic hormone occurs quite frequently *1384* Occurred in 46% of courses followed, with average decrease of 10 mmol/L *5815*

Terfenadine *Serum Increase Physiological* Because of similar chemical structure to ketoconazole and itraconazole which markedly inhibit the metabolism of terfenadine, probably has similar effect *2653*

Triglycerides *Serum Increase Physiological* Commonly observed but due to vehicle (polyethoxylated castor oil) rather than to the drug itself *1384*

Midazolam

Albumin *Urine No Effect Analytical* Using a fluorimetric assay with Albumin Blue 580 on a Cobas Fara centrifugal analyzer for the detection of microalbuminuria no significant interference was detected at a concentration of 20 mg/L *3117*

Carbon Dioxide Partial Pressure
Blood Increase Physiological In healthy volunteers but of short duration *1748*

Cortisol *Plasma Decrease Physiological* In 8 healthy individuals undergoing cholecystectomy mean concentration significantly less during surgery to 830 nmol/L after 30 minutes compared with 1155 nmol/L when no midazolam given and increase to 1034 nmol/L after 90 minutes compared to 1465 nmol/L when no drug given *1397*

Midazolam *(continued)*

Glucose *Serum Decrease Physiological* In patients undergoing cholecystectomy mean concentration rose more slowly from mean baseline of 4.90 mmol/L in patients receiving midazolam to 6.64 mmol/L at 90 minutes than in those not so doing (increase from 4.79 mmol/L at baseline to 7.30 mmol/L after 60 minutes) *1397*

Growth Hormone *Plasma Increase Physiological* In patients undergoing cholecystectomy with administration of midazolam as well as anesthesia mean concentration increased to 23.2 mU/L after 30 minutes compared with 16.4 mU/L when no midazolam given with increase being maintained until 90 minutes *1397*

Histamine *Cerebrospinal Fluid Increase Physiological* Mean concentration increased to about 0.8 pmol/L from baseline of about 0.6 pmol/L in 10 patients about one hour after they were given 0.015 mg/kg orally *5724*
Plasma No Effect Analytical Improbable inhibition of radioenzyme assay at physiological concentrations *2492*

Insulin *Plasma Decrease Physiological* In patients undergoing cholecystectomy induction of anesthesia when midazolam also given caused decrease from mean of 14.1 mU/L to 7.1 mU/L *1397*

Mepivacaine *Serum No Effect Physiological* No significant effect observed in 10 children who had received 0.4 mg/kg midazolam rectally as premedication following a lumbar block with 0.4 mL/kg mepivacaine 2.0% *2104*

Oxygen Partial Pressure *Blood Decrease Physiological* In healthy volunteers but of short duration *1748*

Tacrolimus *Serum Increase Analytical* In HPLC/MS method of Christians et al interference observed with measurement of FK 506 because of similar retention time *1010*

Mifepristone

Aldosterone *Plasma Decrease Physiological* Nonsignificant reduction from mean of about 250 pmol/L to about 190 pmol/L in 11 healthy men given 10 mg/kg/d for 7-14 days *3431*
Urine Decrease Physiological Significant reduction observed in 11 healthy male volunteers from mean baseline of about 16.6 nmol/L to about 2.0 nmol/L when given 10 mg/kg/d for 7-14 days *3431*

Androstenedione *Plasma Increase Physiological* Following long term administration of 200 - 400 mg/d to patients with breast cancer or inoperable mengioma significant increases in concentration observed *5754* Significant increase observed in 4 patients not receiving other treatment when receiving 200 mg/d for 12 months *3380*

Bicarbonate *Serum No Effect Physiological* No significant change observed in 11 healthy male volunteers given 10 mg/kg/d for 7-14 days *3431*

Chloride *Serum No Effect Physiological* No significant change observed in 11 healthy male volunteers given 10 mg/kg/d for 7-14 days *3431* No significant change observed in 10 patients with meningiomas treated with 200 mg/d for 12 months *3380*

β-Chorionic Gonadotropin *Plasma Decrease Physiological* Concentration of β-hCG decreases in pregnant woman with expulsion of fetus *412*

Corticosteroid-Binding Globulin
Serum No Effect Physiological No significant change observed in 11 healthy male volunteers given 10 mg/kg/d for 7-14 days *3431*

Corticotropin *Plasma Increase Physiological* Administration to healthy individuals of 6 mg/kg at midnight augmented increase in serum corticotropin during subsequent morning but not when the same dose was given at 10:00 h. Long-term administration causes persistent increase. Diurnal variation unaffected *5755* Following long term administration of 200 - 400 mg/d to patient with breast cancer or inoperable meningioma significant increases in concentration observed. Administration of single doses of 4.5 mg/kg in women and 6 mg/kg in men caused significant increases in concentration although smaller doses did not *5754* Significant increase from mean baseline of about 3.2 pmol/L to about 9.0 pmol/L in 11 healthy men given 10 mg/kg/d for 7-14 days *3431*

Corticotropin response to CRH
Plasma No Effect Physiological Even with long-term administration to healthy individuals which causes increased corticotropin concentration response to CRH is unchanged *5755*

Cortisol *Plasma Decrease Physiological* In critically ill patients relative hypoadrenalism observed with mifepristone therapy because of its blockade of peripheral glucocorticoid receptors *3381*
Plasma Increase Physiological Increase at time of expulsion of fetus in pregnant woman but soon reverts to normal *412* Significant increase from mean baseline of about 300 nmol/L to about 850 nmol/L in 11 healthy men given 10 mg/kg/d for 7-14 days *3431* Following long term administration of 200 - 400 mg/d to patients with breast cancer or inoperable meningioma significant increases in concentration observed. Single doses of 4.5 mg/kg in wmen and 6 mg/kg in men caused significant increase although smaller doses did not *5754* In healthy individuals administration of 6 mg/kg at midnight augments the increase in serum concentration during the subsequent morning but not observed when the same dose is given at 10:00 h. Long-term administration causes persistent increase. Diurnal variation unaffected *5755*
Urine Increase Physiological Significant increase observed from mean baseline of about 15 nmol/mmol creatinine to about 100 nmol/mmol creatinine in 11 healthy male volunteers given 10 mg/kg/d for 7-14 days *3431* Excretion doubled after 2 days in 10 patients with meningiomas treated with 200 mg/d for 12 months: increased further to maximum after 3 weeks and remained at same high level for duration of treatment *3380*

Dehydroepiandrosterone *Plasma Increase Physiological* Significant increase observed in 4 patients with meningiomas not treated with other drugs when receiving 200 mg/d for 12 months *3380*

Dehydroepiandrosterone Sulfate
Plasma Increase Physiological Following long term administration of 200 - 400 mg/d in patients with breast cancer or inoperable meningioma significant increases in concentration observed *5754* Significant increase in 4 patients with meningiomas not treated with other drugs when receiving 200 mg/d for 12 months *3380*

Deoxycortisol *Plasma Increase Physiological* Significant increase observed in 4 patients with meningiomas treated with 200 mg/d for 12 months *3380*

11-Deoxycortisol *Plasma Increase Physiological* Significant increase observed in 4 patients with meningiomas treated with 200 mg/d for 12 months *3380*

Eosinophils *Blood No Effect Physiological* No significant change observed in 11 healthy men given 10 mg/kg/d for 7-14 days *3431* Although transient increase in first three days of treatment reverted to pretreatment concentration after 3 weeks of treatment in 10 patients with meningiomas treated with 200 mg/d for 12 months *3380*

Erythrocyte Sedimentation Rate
Blood No Effect Physiological No significant effect observed in 11 healthy men given 10 mg/kg/d for 7-14 days *3431*

Estradiol *Plasma Decrease Physiological* Concentration rapidly decreases in pregnant woman with expulsion of fetus *412*
Plasma Increase Physiological Significant increase observed in 4 patients with meningiomas and not receiving any other drug when receiving 200 mg/d for 12 months *3380* Following long term administration of 200 - 400 mg/d to patients with breast cancer significant increases in concentration observed probably due to aromatization of adrenal androgens in nonendocrine tissues *5754*
Plasma No Effect Physiological Following administration of 200 mg/d to patients with inoperable meningioma no significant change in concentration observed as with 100 mg/d for 3 months in patients with endometriosis *5754*

Glucose *Serum No Effect Physiological* No significant change observed in 10 patients with meningiomas treated with 200 mg/d for 12 months *3380*

Gravidin *Plasma Decrease Physiological* In 28 women in first trimester administration of RU-486 with successful abortion caused mean decrease from 100% to 94% after 2 days *6494*

Growth Hormone *Plasma Increase Physiological* In 10 patients with meningiomas increase from mean baseline concentration of 32 ng/L to 59 ng/L after 3 days and 89 ng/L after 3 weeks of treatment with 200 mg/d of mifepristone *3380*

17-Hydroxycorticosteroids *Urine Increase Physiological* Significant increase from mean baseline of about 18 µmol/d to about 70 µmol/d in 11 healthy men given 10 mg/kg/d for 7-14 days *3431*

immunoglobulin A *Serum No Effect Physiological* No significant effect observed in 11 healthy male volunteers given 10 mg/kg/d for 7-14 days *3431*

Immunoglobulin G *Serum No Effect Physiological* No significant effect observed in 11 healthy male volunteers given 10 mg/kg/d for 7-14 days *3431*

Immunoglobulin M *Serum No Effect Physiological* No significant effect observed in 11 healthy male volunteers given 10 mg/kg/d for 7-14 days *3431*

Leukocytes *Blood No Effect Physiological* No significant effect observed in 11 healthy male volunteers given 10 mg/kg/d for 7-14 days *3431*

Lymphocytes *Blood No Effect Physiological* No significant change observed in 11 healthy male volunteers given 10 mg/kg/d for 7-14 days *3431*

Neutrophils *Blood No Effect Physiological* No significant effect observed in 11 healthy male volunteers given 10 mg/kg/d for 7-14 days *3431*

Potassium *Serum Decrease Physiological* In individuals receiving 100 to 200 mg daily for a long time slight decrease in concentration observed *5755*
Serum No Effect Physiological No significant change observed in 10 patients with meningiomas treated with 200 mg/d for 12 months *3380* No significant change observed in 11 healthy men given 10 mg/kg/d for 7-14 days *3431*

Progesterone *Plasma Increase Physiological* Concentration begins to increase within 1 day of treatment of pregnant woman rapidly decreasing with expulsion of fetus *412* Significant increase observed in 4 patients with meningiomas treated with 200 mg/d for 12 months and no other drugs: Effect less marked than with most other hormones *3380*

Prostaglandin $F_{2\alpha}$ *Plasma Increase Physiological* Concentration begins to increase in pregnant women within 12 to 24 hours of administration *412*

Sodium *Serum No Effect Physiological* No significant change observed in 10 patients with meningiomas treated with 200 mg/d for 12 months *3380* No significant change observed in 11 healthy men given 10 mg/kg/d for 7-14 days *3431*

Testosterone *Serum Increase Physiological* Significant increase observed in 4 patients with meningiomas when treated with 200 mg/d for 12 months and no other drugs but effect less marked than with most other hormones *3380*

Miglitol

C-Peptide *Plasma Decrease Physiological* 300 mg/day for 8 weeks caused reduction in postprandial increase in noninsulin-dependent diabetics *5355*

Glucose *Serum Decrease Physiological* Drug (300 mg/day for 8 weeks) caused reduction in postprandial glucose concentration in noninsulin-dependent diabetics although had no effect on basal glucose concentration *5355*

Glycated Hemoglobin *Blood Decrease Physiological* Slight effect noted in 15 noninsulin-dependent diabetics given 300 mg/day for 8 weeks (from mean of 10.0% to 9.50%) with effect more marked in insulin-treated patients than in those treated with oral hypoglycemic agents *5355*

Milrinone

Captopril *Serum No Effect Physiological* No untoward clinical effects observed when drugs are taken concurrently *5257*

Chlorthalidone *Serum No Effect Physiological* No untoward clinical effects observed when drugs are taken concurrently *5257*

Diazepam *Serum No Effect Physiological* No untoward clinical effects observed when drugs are taken concurrently *5257*

Digoxin *Serum No Effect Physiological* No effect on serum concentration when milrinone coadministered *1420* No untoward clinical effects observed when drugs are taken concurrently *5257*

Furosemide *Serum No Effect Physiological* No untoward clinical effects observed when drugs are taken concurrently *5257*

Heparin *Plasma No Effect Physiological* No untoward clinical effects observed when drugs are taken concurrently *5257*

Hydralazine *Serum No Effect Physiological* No untoward clinical effects observed when drugs are taken concurrently *5257*

Hydrochlorothiazide *Serum No Effect Physiological* No untoward clinical effects observed when drugs are taken concurrently *5257*

Insulin *Plasma No Effect Physiological* No untoward clinical effects observed when drugs are taken concurrently *5257*

Isosorbide *Serum No Effect Physiological* No untoward clinical effects observed when drugs are taken concurrently *5257*

Lidocaine *Serum No Effect Physiological* No untoward clinical effects observed when drugs are taken concurrently *5257*

Nitroglycerin *Serum No Effect Physiological* No untoward clinical effects observed when drugs are taken concurrently *5257*

Platelets *Blood Decrease Physiological* Decreased concentration reported in 0.4% treated patients *5257*

Potassium *Serum Decrease Physiological* Low potassium observed in one of 60 patients receiving combination of milrinone and digoxin, but no similar case in 59 patients receiving milrinone alone *1420* Decreased concentration reported in 0.6% treated patients *5257*

Prazosin *Serum No Effect Physiological* No untoward clinical effects observed when drugs are taken concurrently *5257*

Quinidine *Serum No Effect Physiological* No untoward clinical effects observed when drugs are taken concurrently *5257*

Spironolactone *Serum No Effect Physiological* No untoward clinical effects observed when drugs are taken concurrently *5257*

Warfarin *Plasma No Effect Physiological* No untoward clinical effects observed when drugs are taken concurrently *5257*

Minocycline

Alanine Aminotransferase *Serum Increase Physiological* Rarely hepatitis and liver failure have been reported as side effects *3465*

Alkaline Phosphatase *Serum Increase Physiological* Conceivable complication of therapy *204* Rarely hepatitis and liver failure have been reported as side effects *3465*

Amylase *Serum Increase Physiological* Pancreatitis has been reported as a side effect *3465*

Aspartate Aminotransferase *Serum Increase Physiological* Conceivable complication of therapy *204* Rarely hepatitis and liver failure have been reported as side effects *3465*

Bilirubin *Serum Increase Physiological* Rarely hepatitis and liver failure have been reported as side effects *3465*

Chloramphenicol *Serum No Effect Analytical* No effect at 100 mg/L on coupled enzymatic method *4122*

Creatinine *Serum No Effect Analytical* No effect of concentrations up to 15 mg/L on single slide method on Kodak Ektachem® systems *5706*

Eosinophils *Blood Increase Physiological* Eosinophilia has been reported as a side effect *3465* Allergic response *2794*

Erythrocyte Sedimentation Rate
Blood Decrease Physiological In 23 patients with rheumatoid arthritis ESR decreased from mean baseline of 26 ± 18 mm/h decreased to 15 ± 17 mm/h following treatment with 200 mg/d for 6 months *4362*

Minocycline *(continued)*

Hematocrit *Blood Decrease Physiological* Hemolytic anemia has been reported as a side effect *3465* May cause hemolytic anemia (rare) *2754*

Hemoglobin *Blood Decrease Physiological* Hemolytic anemia has been reported as a side effect *3465* Reported cases of hemolytic anemia *2754*

LE Cells *Blood Positive Physiological* May cause exacerbation of SLE *2754*

Leukocytes *Blood Decrease Physiological* Reported as side effects *2754*

Lipase *Serum Increase Physiological* Pancreatitis has been reported as a side effect *3465*

Neutrophils *Blood Decrease Physiological* Neutropenia has been reported as a side effect *3465* May cause hypersensitivity reaction *2794*

pH *Blood Decrease Physiological* May occur if impaired renal function *2754*

Phosphate *Serum Increase Physiological* If impaired renal function *2754*

Platelets *Blood Decrease Physiological* Reported as side effects *2754* Thrombocytopenia has been reported as a side effect *3465*

Potassium *Serum No Effect Analytical* At concentration of 6 mg/L had no effect on measurement by ISE with predilution *5704*

Prothrombin Time *Plasma Increase Physiological* May prolong action of anticoagulants *2794*

Sodium *Serum No Effect Analytical* At concentration of 6 mg/L had no effect on measurement by ISE with predilution *5704*

Urea Nitrogen *Serum Increase Physiological* Antianabolic action of class of drugs *2754*

Minoxidil

Bilirubin *Serum No Effect Analytical* No effect at concentration of 2 mg/L on method on Kodak Ektachem® *5706*

Bilirubin, Conjugated *Serum No Effect Analytical* No effect at concentration of 2 mg/L on method on Kodak Ektachem® *5706*

Bilirubin, Unconjugated *Serum No Effect Analytical* No effect at concentration of 2 mg/L on method on Kodak Ektachem® *5706*

Coombs' Test, Direct *Blood Positive Physiological* Occurred without hemolysis in one patient *3579*

HDL-Cholesterol *Serum Increase Physiological* Slight effect (order of 10%) after 3 or 6 mo treatment *2954*

Histamine *Plasma No Effect Analytical* Although 50% inhibition of radio-enzyme assay at 30 µg/mL unlikely to be of clinical significance since therapeutic concentration 0.04 - 0.25 µg/mL *2492*

LDL-Cholesterol *Serum Decrease Physiological* Approximately 10% reduction after 3 mo and 20% after 6 mo *2954*

Renin Activity *Plasma No Effect Physiological* No significant effect when given alone or with added diuretics at 3 or 6 mo *2954*

Mirtazepine

Acid Phosphatase *Serum Increase Physiological* Infrequently increased activity may occur with continuing treatment *4434*

Alanine Aminotransferase *Serum Increase Physiological* Increases of greater than 3 times the upper limit of normal were observed in 2.0% of patients (8 of 42) treated with mirtazepine in short-term clinical trials compared with 0.3% for placebo-treated patients (1 of 328) *4434*

Alkaline Phosphatase *Serum Increase Physiological* Infrequently cholecystitis or cirrhosis of the liver may occur with continuing treatment *4434*

Amylase *Serum Increase Physiological* Infrequently pancreatitis may occur with continuing treatment *4434*

Aspartate Aminotransferase *Serum Increase Physiological* Infrequently cholecystitis or cirrhosis of the liver may occur with continuing treatment *4434*

Bilirubin *Serum Increase Physiological* Infrequently cholecystitis or cirrhosis of the liver may occur with continuing treatment *4434*

Blood *Urine Increase Physiological* Rarely hematuria may occur with continuing treatment *4434*

Cholesterol *Serum Increase Physiological* Nonfasting increases of up to 20% above normal were observed in 15% of patients treated with mirtazepine compared with 7% for placebo-treated patients *4434*

Glucose *Serum Increase Physiological* Infrequently diabetes mellitus may occur with continuing treatment *4434*
Urine Increase Physiological Infrequently diabetes mellitus may occur with continuing treatment *4434*

Granulocytes *Blood Decrease Physiological* Agranulocytosis has been reported as a side effect *4434*

Hematocrit *Blood Decrease Physiological* Infrequently anemia or pancytopenia may occur with continuing treatment *4434*

Hemoglobin *Blood Decrease Physiological* Infrequently anemia or pancytopenia may occur with continuing treatment *4434*

Leukocytes *Blood Decrease Physiological* Infrequently leukopenia or pancytopenia may occur with continuing treatment *4434*

Lipase *Serum Increase Physiological* Infrequently pancreatitis may occur with continuing treatment *4434*

Lymphocytes *Blood Decrease Physiological* Infrequently lymphocytopenia or pancytopenia may occur with continuing treatment *4434*

Platelets *Blood Decrease Physiological* Infrequently thrombocytopenia or pancytopenia may occur with continuing treatment *4434*

Thyroxine (T4) *Serum Increase Physiological* Rarely goiter or hypothyroidism may occur with continuing treatment *4434*

Triglycerides *Serum Increase Physiological* Nonfasting increases of up to 500 mg/dL were observed in 6% of patients treated with mirtazepine compared with 3% for placebo-treated patients *4434*

Misoprostol

Alkaline Phosphatase *Serum Increase Physiological* Possible causal relationship to increased activity *2064*

Blood *Urine Increase Physiological* Possible causal relationship to hematuria *2064*

Cortisol *Plasma No Effect Physiological* Has no significant effect on concentration *2064*

Creatinine *Serum No Effect Physiological* Has no significant effect on concentration *2064*

Cyclosporine *Blood Increase Physiological* Coadministration of misoprostol with cyclosporine caused an increase of the cyclosporine concentration *859*
Blood No Effect Analytical At a concentration of 0.015 mg/L had no effect on Syva EMIT method *495*
Serum Increase Physiological Coadministration of misoprostol with cyclosporine caused an increase of the cyclosporine concentration *859*

Erythrocyte Sedimentation Rate
Blood Increase Physiological Possible causal relationship with increased erythrocyte sedimentation rate *2064*

Follicle Stimulating Hormone
Plasma No Effect Physiological Has no significant effect on concentration *2064*

Gastrin *Serum No Effect Physiological* Produces no significant effect on fasting or postprandial gastrin concentration *2064*

Glomerular Filtration Rate *Urine No Effect Physiological* When admistered with diclofenac no significant effect observed on renal function in 24 patients with rheumatoid arthritis *634*

Glucose *Urine Increase Physiological* Possible causal relationship to glycosuria *2064*

Growth Hormone *Plasma No Effect Physiological* Has no significant effect on concentration *2064*

Hematocrit *Blood Decrease Physiological* Possible causal relationship to anemia *2064*

Hemoglobin *Blood Decrease Physiological* Possible causal relationship to anemia *2064*

Hydrochloric Acid *Gastric Fluid Decrease Physiological* Over the range of 50 to 200 µg produces a reduction of basal and nocturnal gastric acid secretion, and acid secretion in response to a variety of stimuli, including meals, histamine, pentagastrin and coffee *2064*

Indomethacin *Serum Increase Physiological* In 16 healthy volunteers 200 µg misoprostol as a single dose or q.i.d. as a multiple dose had no effect on absorption of indomethacin but caused 32% increase in its steady state maximum concentration *4837*

Leukocyte Differential *Blood Abnormal Physiological* Possible causal relationship with abnormal leukocyte differential *2064*

Luteinizing Hormone *Plasma No Effect Physiological* Has no significant effect on concentration *2064*

Motilin *Plasma No Effect Physiological* Has no significant effect on concentration *2064*

Occult Blood *Feces Increase Physiological* Possible causal relationship to gastrointestinal bleeding *2064*

Pepsin *Gastric Material Decrease Physiological* Produces a moderate decrease in concentration during basal conditions, but not during histamine stimulation *2064*

Pepsin response to Histamine *Gastric Material No Effect Physiological* Produces a moderate decrease in concentration during basal conditions, but not during histamine stimulation *2064*

Platelet Aggregation *Blood No Effect Physiological* Has no significant effect on aggregation *2064*

Platelets *Blood Decrease Physiological* Possible causal relationship with thrombocytopenia and purpura *2064*

Prolactin *Plasma No Effect Physiological* Has no significant effect on concentration *2064*

Salicylate *Serum No Effect Physiological* Has no significant effect on the absorption, blood concentration and antiplatelet effects of aspirin *2064*

Somatostatin *Plasma No Effect Physiological* Has no significant effect on concentration *2064*

Thyroid Stimulating Hormone *Serum No Effect Physiological* Has no significant effect on concentration *2064*

Thyroxine (T4) *Serum No Effect Physiological* Has no significant effect on concentration *2064*

Urea Nitrogen *Serum Increase Physiological* Possible causal relationship to increased concentration *2064*

Uric Acid *Serum Increase Physiological* Possible causal relationship to gout *2064*

Vasoactive Intestinal Polypeptide *Plasma No Effect Physiological* Has no significant effect on concentration *2064*

Mitoguazone

Glucose *Serum Decrease Physiological* Delayed hypoglycemia observed as adverse side effect *1384*

Mitolactol

Alanine Aminotransferase *Serum Increase Physiological* Hepatic complications rarely noted *1384*

Aspartate Aminotransferase *Serum Increase Physiological* Hepatic complications rarely observed *1384*

Leukocytes *Blood Decrease Physiological* Leukopenia may be observed as a result of myelosuppression *1384*

Platelets *Blood Decrease Physiological* Thrombocytopenia may be observed as a result of myelosuppression *1384*

Mitomycin

Alanine Aminotransferase *Serum Increase Physiological* Centrilobular stasis in 5 of 6 patients and toxic hepatitis in the other *3949*

Aspartate Aminotransferase *Serum Increase Physiological* Centrilobular stasis in 5 of 6 patients and toxic hepatitis in the other *3949*

CA549 *Serum No Effect Analytical* No interference observed at concentrations ranging from 1.0 - 12.7 mg/L with immunoradiometric BRESMARQ procedure *958* No statistically significant effect observed over a concentration range of 1 to 12.7 mg/L with BRESMARQ assay *958*

Carcinoembryonic Antigen *Serum No Effect Analytical* At a concentration of up to 13.84 µg/mL caused less than 10% error in the concentration of CEA as measured by the method on Bayer Technicon Immuno 1® *418*

Chromosomes *Test Conditions Abnormal Physiological* Clastogenic in human cells *5484*

Creatinine *Serum Increase Physiological* Nephrotoxic effect *3615*

Creatinine Clearance *Urine Decrease Physiological* Due to nephrotoxicity *3615*

Erythrocytes *Blood Decrease Physiological* Pancytopenia *3615*

Leukocytes *Blood Decrease Physiological* Pancytopenia *3615* Bone marrow suppression as major dose limiting toxicity: nadir of thrombocytopenia observed in about 3.5 weeks after a single dose of 20 mg per square meter persisting at a low level for 1-2 weeks but then typically recovering *1384*

Lipase *Serum No Effect Analytical* No effect of concentrations up to 2.4 mg/L on method on Kodak Ektachem® *5706*

Platelets *Blood Decrease Physiological* Pancytopenia *3615* Delayed and unpredictable bone marrow suppression with effect on platelets observed about 4 weeks after a single dose of 20 mg per sq m: persists for 2-3 weeks then typically recovers *1384*

Protein *Urine Increase Physiological* Nephrotoxic effect *3615*

Urea Nitrogen *Serum Increase Physiological* Nephrotoxic effect *3615*

Uric Acid *Serum Increase Physiological* Due to nephrotoxicity *3615*

Mitotane

Cortisol *Plasma Decrease Physiological* In critically ill patients relative hypoadrenalism observed with mitotane therapy because of its effect on cortisol synthesis *3381*

Erythrocytes *Urine Increase Physiological* May occasionally produce hematuria *2754*

Hemoglobin *Urine Increase Physiological* May occasionally produce hematuria *2754*

17-Hydroxycorticosteroids *Urine Decrease Physiological* Stimulates extra-adrenal hydroxylation of cortisol *1112*

6-β-Hydroxycortisol *Urine Increase Physiological* Altered cortisol metabolism induced by drug *4126*

Protein *Urine Increase Physiological* May rarely produce hematuria, renal damage *2754*

T3-Uptake *Serum Increase Physiological* Competes for sites on thyroxine binding globulin *882*

Thyroxine (T4) *Serum Decrease Physiological* Competes with T4 for thyroxine binding globulin *882* Inhibits binding of T4 to TBG *2412*

Thyroxine (T4) (Murphy-Pattee) *Serum Decrease Physiological* Competes with T4 for thyroxine binding globulin *882*

Tri-iodothyronine (T3) *Serum Decrease Physiological* Inhibits binding of T3 to TBG *2412*

Mitoxantrone

Alanine Aminotransferase *Serum Increase Physiological* When used in the induction of treatment for patients with ALL abnormal liver function tests occurred in 16% and jaundice in 3% *2819* Mild transient effects in 11 of 26 patients *4476*

Alkaline Phosphatase *Serum Increase Physiological* When used in the induction of treatment for patients with ALL abnormal liver function tests occurred in 16% and jaundice in 3% *2819*

Aspartate Aminotransferase *Serum Increase Physiological* Mild transient effects in 11 of 26 patients *4476* When used in the induction of treatment for patients with ALL abnormal liver function tests occurred in 16% and jaundice in 3% *2819*

Bilirubin *Serum Increase Physiological* When used in the induction of treatment for patients with ALL abnormal liver function tests occurred in 16% and jaundice in 3% *2819* Mild transient effects in 11 of 26 patients *4476*

Color *Urine Increase Analytical* Transient blue-green color may occur during first 24 hours after administration *1384*

Creatinine *Serum Increase Physiological* Infrequent renal toxicity observed *1384* When used in the induction of treatment for patients with ALL renal failure occurred in 8% *2819*

Erythrocytes *Blood Decrease Physiological* Erythrocytes not acutely affected but mild anemia in most patients with successive courses *5497*

Leukocytes *Blood Decrease Physiological* Granulocytopenia is dose-limiting toxicity. In phase II studies nadir between 8 and 15 d. Less than 5% patients had nadir below 1,000 /µL. Granulocyte concentration falls with each treatment until 5th or 6th course *5497*

Occult Blood *Feces Increase Physiological* When used in the induction of treatment for patients with ALL gastrointestinal bleeding occurred in 16% *2819*

Platelets *Blood Decrease Physiological* Less than 10% patients develop count of less than 100,000 /µL. Count usually falls to 5th to 6th course *5497*

Urea Nitrogen *Serum Increase Physiological* When used in the induction of treatment for patients with ALL renal failure occurred in 8% *2819*

MK-270

Glucose *Serum Decrease Physiological* Slight nonsignificant decrease in fasting value *5165*

Glucose Tolerance *Serum Increase Physiological* Produces flattening of curve *5165*

MK-0434

Dihydrotestosterone *Serum Decrease Physiological* In 16 healthy men administration of single doses of more than 5 mg caused significant 50% reduction in concentration maximal at 24 h and maintained through 48 h post-treatment *6186*

MK-677

Amino-terminal Propeptide of Type III Procollagen
Serum Increase Physiological In 24 healthy obese men aged 19 - 49 years treatment with 25 mg/d caused significant increase from mean baseline of 0.46 ± 0.04 kU/L to 0.59 ± 0.05 kU/L after 2 weeks and 0.63 ± 0.04 kU/L after 8 weeks *5890*

Calcium *Serum Increase Physiological* In 24 healthy obese men aged 19 - 49 years treatment with 25 mg/d caused increase from mean baseline of 2.31 ± 0.03 mmol/L to 2.34 ± 0.03 mmol/L (significant) after 2 weeks and 2.39 ± 0.02 mmol/L after 8 weeks (insignificant) *5890*
Urine Increase Physiological In 24 healthy obese men aged 19 - 49 years treatment with 25 mg/d caused significant increase from mean baseline of 0.26 ± 0.02 mmol/mmol creatinine to 0.43 ± 0.04 mmol/mmol creatinine after 2 weeks and 0.35 ± 0.03 mmol/mmol creatinine after 8 weeks *5890*

C-terminal Propeptide of Type I Procollagen
Serum Increase Physiological In 24 healthy obese men aged 19 - 49 years treatment with 25 mg/d caused significant increase from mean baseline of 108.5 ± 27.1 µg/L to 132.2 ± 23.4 µg/L after 2 weeks and 147.8 ± 39.8 µg/L after 8 weeks *5890*

C-terminal Telopeptide of Type I Collagen
Serum Increase Physiological In 24 healthy obese men aged 19 - 49 years treatment with 25 mg/d caused significant increase from mean baseline of 3.97 ± 0.54 µg/L to 4.69 ± 0.62 µg/L after 2 weeks and 4.84 ± 0.57 µg/L after 8 weeks *5890*

Hydroxyproline *Urine Increase Physiological* In 24 healthy obese men aged 19 - 49 years treatment with 25 mg/d caused significant increase from mean baseline of 12.00 ± 0.71 mmol/mmol creatinine to 15.83 ± 1.50 mmol/mmol creatinine after 2 weeks and 14.42 ± 0.71 mmol/mmol creatinine after 8 weeks *5890*

Insulin-like Growth Factor-I *Serum Increase Physiological* In 24 healthy obese men aged 19 - 49 years treatment with 25 mg/d caused significant change from mean baseline of 150.3 ± 12.1 ng/mL to 208.5 ± 12.2 ng/mL after 2 weeks and 212.8 ± 13.6 ng/mL after 8 weeks *5890*

Insulin-like Growth Factor Binding Protein-3
Serum Increase Physiological In 24 healthy obese men aged 19 - 49 years treatment with 25 mg/d caused significant change from mean baseline of 2.8 ± 0.1 mg/L to 3.5 ± 0.1 mg/L after 2 weeks and 3.2 ± 0.2 mg/L after 8 weeks *5890*

Insulin-like Growth Factor Binding Protein-4
Serum Increase Physiological In 24 healthy obese men aged 19 - 49 years treatment with 25 mg/d caused change from mean baseline of 358.5 ± 21.6 ng/mL to 443.1 ± 25.7 ng/mL (significant) after 2 weeks and 406.3 ± 18.1 ng/mL after 8 weeks (insignificant) *5890*

Insulin-like Growth Factor Binding Protein-5
Serum Increase Physiological In 24 healthy obese men aged 19 - 49 years treatment with 25 mg/d caused significant change from mean baseline of 390.2 ± 24.5 ng/mL to 549.0 ± 18.6 ng/mL after 2 weeks and 545.7 ± 17.8 ng/mL after 8 weeks *5890*

Interleukin-1β *Serum No Effect Physiological* In 24 healthy obese men aged 19 - 49 years treatment with 25 mg/d caused change from mean baseline of 0.82 ± 0.20 pg/mL to 0.86 ± 0.23 pg/mL after 2 weeks and 0.79 ± 0.20 pg/mL after 8 weeks *5890*

Interleukin-6 *Serum No Effect Physiological* In 24 healthy obese men aged 19 - 49 years treatment with 25 mg/d caused change from mean baseline of 1.61 ± 0.29 pg/mL to 1.64 ± 0.23 pg/mL after 2 weeks and 1.47 ± 0.18 pg/mL after 8 weeks *5890*

Osteocalcin *Serum Increase Physiological* In 24 healthy obese men aged 19 - 49 years treatment with 25 mg/d caused increase from mean baseline of 9.09 ± 0.66 µg/L to 9.12 ± 0.65 µg/L after 2 weeks (insignificant) and 10.38 ± 0.73 µg/L after 8 weeks (significant) *5890*

Parathyroid Hormone, Intact
Plasma No Effect Physiological In 24 healthy obese men aged 19 - 49 years treatment with 25 mg/d caused nonsignificant change from mean baseline of 40.6 ± 4.7 ng/L to 38.2 ± 3.2 ng/L after 2 weeks and 44.1 ± 4.9 ng/L after 8 weeks *5890*

Soluble Interleukin-6 Receptor
Serum No Effect Physiological In 24 healthy obese men aged 19 - 49 years treatment with 25 mg/d caused change from mean baseline of 35.0 ± 2.3 pg/µL to 35.2 ± 2.0 pg/µL after 2 weeks and 35.6 ± 2.3 pg/µL after 8 weeks *5890*

MK-886

Leukotriene B_4 *Plasma Decrease Physiological* Following dose of 300 mg/d mean concentration decreased to 98% on day 1, 62% on day 4 and 61% on day 11 2 h after morning dose in 12 healthy men. With 750 mg/d concentrations decreased to 73%, 46% and 38% respectively 2 h after morning dose in 24 healthy men *1387*

MK-906

Alanine Aminotransferase *Serum No Effect Physiological* No significant effect observed in 10 healthy men given doses of up to 25 mg/d *1323*

Androstanediol Glucuronide *Plasma Decrease Physiological* Near maximal suppression in 12 healthy volunteers with dose of 10 mg with significant dose response correlation *4971*

Androsterone Glucuronide *Plasma Decrease Physiological* Near maximal suppression with single dose of 10 mg but significant dose response correlation *4971*

Aspartate Aminotransferase *Serum No Effect Physiological* No significant effect observed in 10 healthy men given doses of up to 25 mg/d *1323*

Creatine Kinase *Serum No Effect Physiological* No significant effect observed in 10 healthy men given doses up to 25 mg/d *1323*

Dihydrotestosterone *Serum Decrease Physiological* Single dose of 10 mg in 12 healthy men caused near maximal suppression with significant dose response relationship *4971* In 10 healthy men mean concentration decreased by 56% 24 hours after treatment with a single dose of 25 mg. Effect continued for 72 hours with a decrease in conversion of testosterone to dihydrotestosterone *1323*

Erythrocytes *Blood No Effect Physiological* No significant effect observed in 10 healthy men given doses of up to 25 mg/d *1323*

Hematocrit *Blood No Effect Physiological* No significant effect observed in 10 healthy men given up to 25 mg/d *1323*

Hemoglobin *Blood No Effect Physiological* No significant effect observed in 10 healthy men given doses up to 25 mg/d *1323*

Lactate Dehydrogenase *Serum No Effect Physiological* No significant effect observed in 10 healthy men given doses of up to 25 mg/d *1323*

Leukocyte Differential *Blood No Effect Physiological* No significant effect observed in 10 healthy men given doses up to 25 mg/d *1323*

Leukocytes *Blood No Effect Physiological* No significant effect observed in 10 healthy men given doses of up to 25 mg/d *1323*

Peripheral Smear *Blood No Effect Physiological* No significant effect observed on white blood cell differential count in 10 healthy men given doses up to 25 mg/d *1323*

Testosterone *Serum No Effect Physiological* Possible slight increase although considerable variability observed following doses of 25 mg in 10 healthy men *1323* In 12 healthy men a single dose of up to 100 mg had no effect on concentration *4971*

Moclobemide

Albumin *Urine No Effect Analytical* Using a fluorimetric assay with Albumin Blue 580 on a Cobas Fara centrifugal analyzer for the detection of microalbuminuria no significant interference was detected at a concentration of 4 mg/L *3117*

Cortisol *Plasma Increase Physiological* Administration of 300 mg to healthy individuals had a significant effect on nocturnal secretion with an increase from mean baseline of 65 ng/mL from 23:00 h to 07:00 h to 88 ng/mL from 23:00 h to 07:00 h *5791*

Estradiol *Plasma Decrease Physiological* After 28 days treatment in 12 depressed men decrease from mean baseline concentration of 109 pmol/L to 91 pmol/L *3796*

Follicle Stimulating Hormone *Plasma No Effect Physiological* No significant change from mean baseline of 4.7 mIU/mL at either 14 or 28 days in 12 depressed men with treatment with moclobemide *3796* Administration of 300 mg to healthy individuals had no significant effect on nocturnal secretion *5791*

Growth Hormone *Plasma No Effect Physiological* Administration of 300 mg to healthy individuals had no significant effect on nocturnal secretion *5791*

Homovanillic Acid *Urine Decrease Physiological* Reduction observed in 12 depressed male patients after 14 and 28 days treatment *3796* Significant reduction from mean baseline concentration of 17.0 nmol/mg creatinine to 12.2 nmol/mg at 14 days and 12.5 nmol/mg at 28 days in 12 depressed men with treatment. Absolute excretion also decreased *3796*

4-Hydroxy-3-Methoxy-Phenylglycol *Urine Decrease Physiological* Significant change observed after both 14 and 28 days in 12 depressed men when treated with moclobemide and concentration expressed in terms of nmol/mg creatinine and absolute amount in μmol/24 h *3796* Significant reduction in excretion observed in 12 male depressed patients after 14 and 28 days treatment *3796*

5-Hydroxyindoleacetic Acid *Urine Decrease Physiological* Reduction observed in 12 depressed male patients after 14 and 28 days treatment *3796* Significant decrease from mean baseline concentration of 13.7 nmol/mg to 10.8 nmol/mg at 14 days and 10.2 nmol/mg creatinine at 28 days in 12 depressed men when treated with moclobemide. Absolute excretion also reduced *3796*

Luteinizing Hormone *Plasma No Effect Physiological* Administration of 300 mg to healthy individuals had no significant effect on nocturnal secretion *5791* No significant change from mean baseline concentration of 6.5 mIU/mL in 12 depressed men treated for 14 and 28 days *3796*

Prolactin *Plasma No Effect Physiological* No significant change observed from mean baseline of 6.0 ng/mL in 12 depressed men following treatment for 14 or 28 days *3796* Administration of 300 mg to healthy individuals had no significant effect on nocturnal secretion *5791*

Sex-Hormone Binding Globulin *Serum Decrease Physiological* Significant reduction observed in 12 depressed male patients treated for 14 and 28 days *3796* Decrease from mean baseline concentration of 51.1 nmol/L to 43.6 nmol/L at both 14 and 28 days in 12 depressed men when treated with moclobemide *3796*

Testosterone *Serum Increase Physiological* Significant increase in 12 depressed men from mean baseline concentration of 14.3 nmol/L to 19.4 nmol/L at 14 days and 21.9 nmol/L at 28 days with treatment with moclobemide *3796* Significant increase observed in 12 depressed male patients treated for 14 and 28 days *3796*
Serum No Effect Physiological Administration of 300 mg to healthy individuals had no significant effect on nocturnal secretion *5791*

Moexipiril

Alanine Aminotransferase *Serum Increase Physiological* Administration may cause increased liver enzyme activity in some patients *5405*

Alkaline Phosphatase *Serum Increase Physiological* Administration may cause increased liver enzyme activity in some patients *5405*

Aspartate Aminotransferase *Serum Increase Physiological* Administration may cause increased liver enzyme activity in some patients *5405*

Creatinine *Serum Increase Physiological* Administration may cause increased concentration in about 1% patients, as with other ACE inhibitors, reversible with discontinuation of treatment *5405*

γ-Glutamyltransferase *Serum Increase Physiological* Administration may cause increased liver enzyme activity in some patients *5405*

Urea Nitrogen *Serum Increase Physiological* Administration may cause increased concentration in about 1% patients, as with other ACE inhibitors, reversible with discontinuation of treatment *5405*

Molindone

Alanine Aminotransferase *Serum Increase Physiological* Alterations of enzyme activity observed rarely in patients receiving molindone *2048* Single case report (?cause) *3097*

Alkaline Phosphatase *Serum Increase Physiological* Alterations of enzyme activity observed rarely in patients receiving molindone *2048*

Molindone *(continued)*

Aspartate Aminotransferase *Serum Increase Physiological* Alterations of enzyme activity observed rarely in patients receiving molindone *2048*

Bilirubin *Serum Increase Physiological* Alterations of bilirubin concentration observed rarely in patients receiving molindone *2048*

Fatty Acids (FFA), Free *Serum Increase Physiological* Sustained and significant rise *2676*

Glucose *Serum Increase Physiological* Nonsignificant alterations of glucose concentration observed rarely in patients receiving molindone *2048*
Serum No Effect Physiological Relatively unaffected over short term *2676*

Leukocytes *Blood Decrease Physiological* Leukopenia observed rarely in patients receiving molindone *2048*
Blood Increase Physiological Leukocytosis observed rarely in patients receiving molindone *2048*

Phenytoin *Serum Decrease Physiological* Coadministration of Moban® brand of molindone with phenytoin may decrease plasma phenytoin concentration because it contains calcium ions which interfere with the absorption of phenytoin *4522*

Prolactin *Plasma Increase Physiological* Significant response to 5 mg given orally *2352*

Urea Nitrogen *Red Blood Cells No Effect Physiological* Nonsignificant alterations of erythrocyte concentration observed rarely in patients receiving molindone *2048*
Serum Increase Physiological Nonsignificant alterations of urea nitrogen concentration observed rarely in patients receiving molindone *2048*

Vanillylmandelic Acid *Urine No Effect Physiological* Relatively unaffected over short term *2676*

Molsidomine

Guanosine Monophosphate
Plasma No Effect Physiological No significant change from baseline observed in 10 volunteers following single intravenous injection of 60 µg/kg body weight *3052*

Platelet Aggregation *Blood Decrease Physiological* Addition of platelet-activating factor at higher concentration was necessary to cause aggregation. Extent of aggregation significantly reduced *3052*

Monatepil

Apolipoprotein A-I *Serum No Effect Physiological* In 39 patients with mild to moderate hypertension treatment with mean dose of 38.5 mg/d for 12 weeks caused no significant decrease from mean baseline *5279*

Apolipoprotein B *Serum Decrease Physiological* In 39 patients with mild to moderate hypertension treatment with mean dose of 38.5 mg/d for 12 weeks caused significant decrease from mean baseline of 127 ± 18 mg/dL to 121 ± 19 mg/dL *5279*

Apolipoprotein E *Serum No Effect Physiological* In 39 patients with mild to moderate hypertension treatment with mean dose of 38.5 mg/d for 12 weeks caused no significant decrease from mean baseline *5279*

Cholesterol *Serum Decrease Physiological* In 39 patients with mild to moderate hypertension treatment with mean dose of 38.5 mg/d for 12 weeks caused significant decrease from mean baseline of 253 ± 23 mg/dL to 240 ± 26 mg/dL *5279*

C-Peptide *Plasma No Effect Physiological* In 39 patients with mild to moderate hypertension treatment with mean dose of 38.5 mg/d for 12 weeks caused nonsignificant decrease from mean baseline of 2.82 ± 1.23 ng/mL to 2.50 ± 1.10 ng/mL *5279*

Glucose *Serum No Effect Physiological* In 39 patients with mild to moderate hypertension treatment with mean dose of 38.5 mg/d for 12 weeks caused nonsignificant decrease from mean baseline of 104.6 ± 12.3 mg/dL to 102.1 ± 9.8 mg/dL *5279*

HDL-Cholesterol *Serum No Effect Physiological* In 39 patients with mild to moderate hypertension treatment with mean dose of 38.5 mg/d for 12 weeks caused no significant decrease from mean baseline *5279*

Hemoglobin A_{1c} *Blood Decrease Physiological* In 39 patients with mild to moderate hypertension treatment with mean dose of 38.5 mg/d for 12 weeks caused significant decrease from mean baseline of 5.46 ± 0.42% to 5.32 ± 0.45% *5279*

Insulin *Plasma No Effect Physiological* In 39 patients with mild to moderate hypertension treatment with mean dose of 38.5 mg/d for 12 weeks caused nonsignificant decrease from mean baseline of 7.20 ± 4.60 µU/mL to 7.08 ± 4.25 µU/mL *5279*

LDL-Cholesterol *Serum Decrease Physiological* In 39 patients with mild to moderate hypertension treatment with mean dose of 38.5 mg/d for 12 weeks caused significant decrease from mean baseline of 169 ± 25 mg/dL to 158 ± 25 mg/dL *5279*

LDL-Cholesterol:HDL-Cholesterol Ratio
Serum Decrease Physiological In 39 patients with mild to moderate hypertension treatment with mean dose of 38.5 mg/d for 12 weeks caused significant decrease from mean baseline of 3.27 ± 0.93 to 3.02 ± 0.83 *5279*

Lipoprotein Lp(a) *Serum Decrease Physiological* In 39 patients with mild to moderate hypertension treatment with mean dose of 38.5 mg/d for 12 weeks caused significant decrease from mean baseline of 34 mg/dL to 31 mg/dL *5279*

Triglycerides *Serum Decrease Physiological* In 39 patients with mild to moderate hypertension treatment with mean dose of 38.5 mg/d for 12 weeks caused significant decrease from mean baseline of 143 ± 66 mg/dL to 137 ± 65 mg/dL *5279*

Monoamine Oxidase Inhibitors

Chlorpropamide *Serum Increase Physiological* Drugs that are highly protein-bound compete with chlorpropamide for binding sites and may potentiate hypoglycemic action of sulfonylurea *4644*

Phenobarbital *Serum Increase Physiological* Coadministration of monoamine oxidase inhibitors with phenobarbital causes an increase in plasma phenobarbital concentration because monoamine oxidase inhibitors inhibit its metabolism *1706*

Secobarbital *Serum Increase Physiological* Coadministration of monoamine oxidase inhibitors with secobarbital probably causes an increase in plasma secobarbital concentration because monoamine oxidase inhibitors inhibit its metabolism as has been reported for phenobarbital *1708*

Sumatriptan *Serum No Effect Physiological* Concomitant administration of MAO-A inhibitors with sumatriptan caused a 2-fold increase of sumatriptan concentration if the MAO-A inhibitor was given subcutaneously and 7-fold if given orally *2158*

Monoethylglycine Xylidine

Benzoylecgonine *Urine No Effect Analytical* Negative result obtained at a concentration of 1000 µg/mL (4.87 mmol/L) with method on Du Pont aca *1558*

Lidocaine *Serum No Effect Analytical* At a concentration of 1250 mg/L (normal serum concentration up to 0.2 mg/L) had less than 10% effect on method on Baxter Stratus *5705* No significant interference observed at a concentration of 30 µg/mL (146 µmol/L) with method on Du Pont aca *1534*

N-Acetylprocainamide *Serum No Effect Analytical* No significant interference observed at a concentration of 100 µg/mL (485 µmol/L) with method on Du Pont aca *1536*

Procainamide *Serum No Effect Analytical* No significant interference observed at a concentration of 100 µg/mL (485 µmol/L) with method on Du Pont aca *1542*

Quinidine *Serum No Effect Analytical* No significant interference observed at a concentration of 100 µg/mL (485 µmol/L) with method on Du Pont aca *1543*

Montelukast

Alanine Aminotransferase *Serum Increase Physiological* In 1995 treated patients increased activity observed in 2.1% compared with 2.0% in placebo-treated controls *3992* One of 54 treated asthmatics and one of placebo-treated patients demonstrated increased activity to above three times upper limit of normal. Effect transient and self-limiting *3492*

Aspartate Aminotransferase *Serum Increase Physiological* One of 54 treated asthmatics and one of placebo-treated patients demonstrated increased activity to above three times upper limit of normal. Effect transient and self-limiting *3492* In 1995 treated patients increased activity observed in 1.6% compared with 1.2% in 1180 placebo-treated controls *3992*

Digoxin *Serum No Effect Physiological* Has no clinically important effect on the pharmacokinetics of digoxin *3992*

Ethinyl Estradiol *Serum No Effect Physiological* Has no clinically important effect on the pharmacokinetics of northindrone and ethinyl estradiol when administered as components of oral contraceptives *3992*

Leukocytes *Urine Increase Physiological* In 1924 treated patients pyuria observed in 1.0% compared with 0.9% in 1159 placebo-treated controls *3992*

Norethindrone *Serum No Effect Physiological* Has no clinically important effect on the pharmacokinetics of northindrone and ethinyl estradiol when administered as components of oral contraceptives *3992*

Prednisolone *Serum No Effect Physiological* Has no clinically important effect on the pharmacokinetics of prednisolone *3992*

Prednisone *Serum No Effect Physiological* Has no clinically important effect on the pharmacokinetics of prednisone *3992*

Terfenadine *Serum No Effect Physiological* Has no clinically important effect on the pharmacokinetics of terfenadine *3992*

Theophylline *Serum No Effect Physiological* Has no clinically important effect on the pharmacokinetics of theophylline *3992*

Warfarin *Plasma No Effect Physiological* Has no clinically important effect on the pharmacokinetics of warfarin *3992*

MOPP

MCV *Blood Increase Physiological* Reflection of bone marrow reaction to cytotoxic therapy in people with malignant disease *1310*

Moricizine

Alanine Aminotransferase *Serum Increase Physiological* Hepatitis reported to occur rarely *1384* Clinically significant alteration of liver function tests reported rarely, but consistent with hepatitis *4980*

Aspartate Aminotransferase *Serum Increase Physiological* Clinically significant alteration of liver function tests reported rarely, but consistent with hepatitis *4980* Hepatitis reported to occur rarely *1384*

Bilirubin *Serum Increase Physiological* Clinically significant alteration of liver function tests reported rarely, but consistent with hepatitis *4980*

Digoxin *Serum No Effect Physiological* Concomitant administration of moricizine with digoxin had no effect on its plasma concentration *1062*

Platelets *Blood Decrease Physiological* Thrombocytopenia reported occasionally *1384* Administration reported to cause thrombocytopenia in two patients *4980*

Prothrombin Time *Plasma No Effect Physiological* Although moricizine may slightly shorten the elimination half-life of warfarin, neither the prothrombin time nor the warfarin osage requirement changes significantly sfter moricizine therapy is begun *1062*

Theophylline *Serum Decrease Physiological* In 12 healthy volunteers coadministration of moricizine with theophylline caused area under the theophylline concentration curve by 36% after theophylline and by 32% after aminophylline probably due to enzyme induction by moricizine *4696* Concomitant administration increased clearance of theophylline by 44-66% and plasma half-life decreased by 19-33% *1384* Increases theophylline clearance and decreases serum theophylline concentration by 25% *3125* Coadministration of theophylline with moricizine increases theophylline clearance and substantially decreases theophylline concentration by about 25% *5999* Up to 25% decrease in serum theophylline concentration due to increased theophylline clearance *6117*
Serum Increase Physiological Concomitant administration of moricizine with theophylline increased its plasma concentration by 46 to 68% and decreases its elimination half-life by 20 to 34% *1062*

Morinamide

Bilirubin *Serum Increase Physiological* Jaundice reported as side effect *4014*

Hydrochloric Acid *Gastric Fluid Increase Physiological* Hyperacidity reported *4014*

Uric Acid *Serum Increase Physiological* Decreased renal clearance *4014*

Morphine

Alanine Aminotransferase *Serum Increase Physiological* May cause rise in intrabiliary pressure *5869*
Serum No Effect Analytical At acute overdose concentration (20 mg/dL) on Technicon SMAC® method *6266*

Albumin *Serum No Effect Analytical* At concentration of 200 mg/L had no effect on BCG method *5704* At acute overdose concentration (20 mg/dL) on Technicon SMAC® method *6266*

Alkaline Phosphatase *Serum Increase Physiological* Associated with abnormal liver function *3810*
Serum No Effect Analytical At acute overdose concentration (20 mg/dL) on Technicon SMAC® method *6266*

Amphetamine *Urine No Effect Analytical* Negative result with method on Du Pont aca at a concentration of 1000 μg/L (3.50 mmol/L) *1554*

Amylase *Serum Increase Physiological* Causes spasm of sphincter of Oddi for 48 h *5869*
Urine Increase Physiological Observed in some patients after administration *2321*

Aspartate Aminotransferase *Serum Increase Physiological* May cause rise in intrabiliary pressure *5869*
Serum No Effect Analytical At acute overdose concentration (20 mg/dL) on Technicon SMAC® method *6266*

Atrial Natriuretic Peptide *Plasma Increase Physiological* Near doubling of immunoreactive peptide observed in 21 individuals for elective surgery 5 minutes after intravenous injection of either 0.15 or 0.30 mg/kg but concentration already had begun to fall after 10 min when 0.15 mg dose *4376*

Barbiturate *Serum No Effect Analytical* No significant interference observed at a concentration of 100 μg/mL (0.35 mmol/L) with method on Du Pont aca *1511* No interference with UV absorption methods *4953*
Urine No Effect Analytical Negative result obtained at a concentration of 1000 μg/mL (3.50 mmol/L) with method on Du Pont aca *1555*

Basal Metabolic Rate *Patient Decrease Physiological* Metabolic effect of drug *3669*

Benzodiazepine *Urine No Effect Analytical* Negative result observed at a concentration of 1000 μg/mL (3.50 mmol/L) with method on Du Pont aca *1556*

Benzodiazepine Screen *Serum No Effect Analytical* No significant effect observed at a concentration of 25 μg/mL (88 μmol/L) with method on Du Pont aca *1512*

Benzoylecgonine *Urine No Effect Analytical* No significant interference observed at a concentration of 700 μmol/L with Sung and Neely modification of Syva EMIT procedure *148* Negative result obtained at a concentration of 200 μg/mL (0.70 mmol/L) with method on Du Pont aca *1558*

Bicarbonate *Serum No Effect Analytical* At concentration of 1 mg/L had no effect on method using phenolphthalein *5704*

Bilirubin *Serum Increase Physiological* Associated with abnormal liver function *3810*

Morphine *(continued)*

Bilirubin *(continued)*
Serum No Effect Analytical At acute overdose concentration (20 mg/dL) on Technicon SMAC® method *6266* At concentration of 200 mg/L had no effect on Jendrassik and Grof method *5704*

BSP Retention *Serum Increase Physiological* Abnormal liver function tests reported *6515*

Calcium *Serum No Effect Analytical* At concentration of 200 mg/L had no effect on cresolphthalein method *5704* At acute overdose concentration (20 mg/dL) on Technicon SMAC® method *6266*

Cannabinoids *Urine No Effect Analytical* No effect on Roche Abuscreen method *5006* No effect observed at a concentration of 200 μg/mL (0.70 mmol/L) on method on Du Pont aca *1557*

Carbon Dioxide Partial Pressure
Blood Increase Physiological Diminishes ventilation, causes hypercapnia *128*

Chloride *Serum No Effect Analytical* At concentration of 1 mg/L had no effect on mercurimetric method *5704*

Cholesterol *Serum No Effect Analytical* At concentration of 200 mg/L had no effect on Liebermann-Burchard method *5704* At acute overdose concentration (20 mg/dL) on Technicon SMAC® method *6266*

Chromosomes *Test Conditions No Effect Physiological* No effect on human leucocytes at concentrations 1/6-3 times normal *1790*

Cocaethylene *Urine No Effect Analytical* No interference observed with TLC method of Bailey *328*

Cortisol *Plasma Decrease Physiological* In 14 volunteer subjects given 5 mg intravenously *6672* Administration to patients with anorexia nervosa caused progressive decrease of raised basal concentration. Similar reduction observed in normal individuals and in depressed patients *6673* With 4 mg extradurally administered in 10 postoperative patients significant reduction observed and to a greater extent than with 150 μg clonidine *3682*

Creatine Kinase *Serum Increase Physiological* Response to frequent i.m. injections *403*
Serum No Effect Analytical At acute overdose concentration (20 mg/dL) on Technicon SMAC® method *6266*
Serum No Effect Physiological No change, although other enzymes increased *4014*

Creatinine *Serum No Effect Analytical* At acute overdose concentration (20 mg/dL) on Technicon SMAC® method *6266* At concentration of 200 mg/L had no effect on Technicon AutoAnalyzer® Jaffe method *5704*

Cyclosporine *Blood No Effect Analytical* at a concentration of 6 mg/L had no effect on Syva EMIT method *495*

Drugs of Abuse Screen *Urine No Effect Analytical* No effect at concentration of 100 μg/mL on EZ-SCREEN procedure for cannabinoids and cocaine *1739*

Enteroglucagon *Plasma Decrease Physiological* Postprandial secretion abolished in 6 volunteers after drug given i.v *956*

Epinephrine *Plasma Increase Physiological* Mechanism obscure also involved in glucose release *2854*

Gastric Inhibitory Polypeptide
Plasma Decrease Physiological Reduction in secretion following test meal and drug in 6 healthy volunteers *956*

Gastrin *Serum Increase Physiological* Secretion prolonged following test meal and drug i.v. in 6 healthy volunteers *956*

Glucagon, Pancreatic *Plasma No Effect Physiological* No effect observed in 6 healthy volunteers after test meal and drug i.v *956*

Glucose *Serum Increase Physiological* Significant increase following 4 mg extradurally in 10 postoperative patients *3682* Minor, clinically insignificant increase *2242*
Serum No Effect Analytical At acute overdose concentration (20 mg/dL) on Technicon SMAC® method *6266*

Guaiacols Spot Test *Urine Positive Analytical* False reaction with screening test of Rogers *5061*

Hematocrit *Blood Decrease Physiological* May cause anemia as an adverse event *6646*

Hemoglobin *Blood Decrease Physiological* May cause anemia as an adverse event *6646*

Histamine *Cerebrospinal Fluid Increase Physiological* Mean concentration increased to about 1.2 pmol/L from baseline of about 0.6 pmol/L in 11 patients about one hour following 0.14 mg/kg intramuscularly *5724*
Plasma Increase Physiological Observed with injection associated with anesthesia *3648*

Hydrochloric Acid *Gastric Fluid Decrease Physiological* Slight decrease in secretion of acid *2242*

Hydroxybutyrate Dehydrogenase
Serum Increase Physiological Probably due to spasm of sphincter of Oddi *4014*

17-Hydroxycorticosteroids *Plasma Decrease Physiological* Inhibits ACTH and pituitary gonadotropin release *2242*
Urine Decrease Physiological Inhibits ACTH and pituitary gonadotropin release *2242*

Indocyanine Green *Serum Decrease Physiological* Observed in small series, normal liver function tests *3942*

Insulin *Plasma Decrease Physiological* Reduction in secretion following test meal and drug in 6 healthy volunteers *956*

Iron *Serum No Effect Analytical* At acute overdose concentration (20 mg/dL) on Technicon SMAC® method *6266* At concentration of 200 mg/L had no effect on Ferrozine method *5704*

17-Ketosteroids *Plasma Decrease Physiological* Inhibits ACTH and pituitary gonadotropin release *2242*
Urine Decrease Physiological Inhibits ACTH and pituitary gonadotropin release *2242*
Urine Increase Analytical Due to chemical structure affects Zimmermann procedure *5402*

Lactate *Plasma Decrease Physiological* Intravenous administration of 0.33 mg/kg caused 50% decrease *2452*

Lactate Dehydrogenase *Serum Increase Physiological* May cause rise in intrabiliary pressure *5869*
Serum No Effect Analytical At acute overdose concentration (20 mg/dL) on Technicon SMAC® method *6266*

Lactate Dehydrogenase Isoenzymes
Serum Increase Physiological Hepatic fraction increased. ?due to spasm of sphincter *4014*

Leucine Aminopeptidase *Serum Increase Physiological* Possibly due to spasm of sphincter of Oddi *4014*

Leukocytes *Blood Decrease Physiological* May cause leukopenia as an adverse event *6646*

Lipase *Serum Increase Physiological* Causes spasm of sphincter of Oddi *5869*

Methylhistamine *Cerebrospinal Fluid Increase Physiological* Detectable in CSF of 5 of 11 patients after they were given 0.14 mg/kg intramuscularly (mean concentration 1.92 pmol/L) *5724*

Midazolam *Serum No Effect Analytical* On GC-ECD method of Ha et al *2387*

Morphine *Serum Increase Physiological* After 10 mg i.v. concentration is 0.1 mg/L in 1 h *3868*
Urine Increase Analytical Significant interference observed at a concentration of 0.07 μmol/L with Sung and Neely modification of Syva EMIT procedure *148*

Motilin *Plasma Decrease Physiological* Postprandial secretion abolished in 6 volunteers after drug given i.v *956*

Neurotensin *Plasma Decrease Physiological* Reduction in secretion following test meal and drug in 6 healthy volunteers *956*

Norepinephrine *Plasma Decrease Physiological* Mechanism obscure *2854*

p-Aminophenol *Urine No Effect Analytical* With addition of drugs at a concentration of 100 mg/L and of related compounds at 50 mg/L no significant effect observed on colorimetric method of van Bocxlaer on Cobas Mira analyzer which involves reacting free p-aminophenol with resorcinol in the presence of magnesium ions to form an indophenol dye measured at 550 nm *6163*

Pancreatic Polypeptide *Plasma Decrease Physiological* Postprandial secretion abolished in 6 volunteers after drug given i.v *956*

Phosphate *Serum No Effect Analytical* At concentration of 200 mg/L had no effect on phosphomolybdate method *5704*

At acute overdose concentration (20 mg/dL) on Technicon SMAC® method *6266*

Platelets *Blood Decrease Physiological* May cause thrombocytopenia as an adverse event *6646*

Prolactin *Plasma Decrease Physiological* Normal response to administration is reduction in concentration. This effect was also observed in patients with anorexia nervosa but response significantly attenuated in patients with depression *6673*

Plasma Increase Physiological 10 mg i.v. produced prompt and significant increase in 7 hypothyroid and 5 healthy individuals *1400* In 14 volunteer subjects given 5 mg intravenously *6672*

Protein *Serum No Effect Analytical* At acute overdose concentration (20 mg/dL) on Technicon SMAC® method *6266* At concentration of 200 mg/L had no effect on biuret method with blank correction *5704*

Test Conditions Increase Analytical Reacts with Folin-Ciocalteu method of Lowry *1102*

Sodium *Serum Decrease Physiological* May cause hyponatremia due to inappropriate secretion of antidiuretic hormone *6646*

Somatostatin *Plasma No Effect Physiological* No effect observed in 6 healthy volunteers after test meal and drug i.v *956*

Sugar *Urine Increase Analytical* Interferes with copper reduction method *4012*

Thyroid Stimulating Hormone

Serum Increase Physiological 10 mg i.v. produced prompt and significant increase in 7 hypothyroid and 5 healthy individuals *1400*

Tirofiban *Serum No Effect Physiological* Coadministration had no significant effect on plasma clearance of tirofiban *3957*

Tricyclic Antidepressants Screen

Serum No Effect Analytical No significant effect observed at a concentration of 100 µg/mL (0.35 mmol/L) with method on Du Pont aca *1550*

Triglycerides *Serum No Effect Analytical* At acute overdose concentration (20 mg/dL) on Technicon SMAC® method *6266* At concentration of 200 mg/L had no effect on lipase/esterase method *5704*

Trovafloxacin *Serum Decrease Physiological* Coadministration of intravenous morphine significantly reduces the absorption of oral trovafloxacin *4663*

Urea Nitrogen *Serum No Effect Analytical* At acute overdose concentration (20 mg/dL) on Technicon SMAC® method *6266* At concentration of 200 mg/L had no effect on diacetylmonoxime method *5704*

Uric Acid *Serum No Effect Analytical* At concentration of 200 mg/L had no effect on phosphotungstate reduction method *5704* At acute overdose concentration (20 mg/dL) on Technicon SMAC® method *6266*

Vanillylmandelic Acid *Urine Decrease Physiological* Clinically significant but small effect *3888*

Vasoactive Intestinal Polypeptide

Plasma No Effect Physiological No effect observed in 6 healthy volunteers after test meal and drug i.v *956*

Volume *Urine Decrease Physiological* May stimulate release of ADH *128*

Morphine Glucuronide

Cannabinoids *Urine No Effect Analytical* No effect on Roche Abuscreen method *5006*

Morphine *Urine Increase Analytical* Significant interference observed at a concentration of 6.5 µmol/L with Sung and Neely modification of Syva EMIT procedure *148*

Opiates *Urine Positive Analytical* At concentration of 3.0 µg/mL (6.51 µmol/L) on method on Du Pont aca *1559* Significant cross-reactivity observed with Roche Abuscreen method adapted for use with Olympus AU 5121 and 5131 analyzers *214* Cross-reactivity of over 50% observed with Roche Abuscreen Online procedure when adapted for use with Roche Cobas Fara II analyzer *5547*

Morpholine

ionized Calcium *Serum Decrease Analytical* At concentrations > 0.1 mmol/L on calcium specific electrode *820*

Moxalactam

Alanine Aminotransferase *Serum Increase Physiological* In about 3% patients as reported from several studies *893*

Albumin *Serum No Effect Analytical* At concentration of 96 mg/L had no effect on BCG method *5704*

Alkaline Phosphatase *Serum Increase Physiological* In about 3% patients as reported from several studies *893*

Aspartate Aminotransferase *Serum Increase Physiological* In about 3% patients as reported from several studies *893*

Bilirubin *Serum Increase Physiological* Clinically significant displacement from protein in neonates *6314*

Serum No Effect Analytical No effect at 10,000 mg/L on Ames Seralyzer method *5706* At concentration of 96 mg/L had no effect on Jendrassik and Grof method *5704* At 2.50 mmol/L on method on Eppendorf Epos *2351*

Bleeding Time *Patient Increase Physiological* Reversible bleeding diathesis observed in 5 patients *6401* Occurs due to dose-dependent inhibition of platelet function *1384* Because it affects bleeding time in its own right has potential to increase risk of warfarin-associated bleeding *2625* In 10 healthy volunteers 8 g intravenously daily for 6 days caused increase from mean of 4.2 minutes to 7.4 minutes *4629*

Cholesterol *Serum No Effect Analytical* At 2.50 mmol/L on method on Eppendorf Epos *2351* No effect at 10,000 mg/L on Ames Seralyzer method *5706*

Clindamycin *Serum Positive Analytical* Interferes with bioassays because cannot be inactivated *3858*

Colistin *Serum Positive Analytical* Interferes with bioassays because cannot be inactivated *3858*

Coombs' Test *Blood Positive Physiological* Observed in some cases with all cephalosporins *4327*

Coombs' Test, Indirect *Blood Positive Physiological* In up to 0.5% patients as reported from several studies *893*

Creatine Kinase *Serum No Effect Analytical* No effect at 10,000 mg/L on method on Ames Seralyzer *5706*

Creatinine *Serum Increase Analytical* Slow and slight reaction in Jaffe methods *2351*

Serum Increase Physiological In about 2% patients as reported from several studies *893*

Serum No Effect Analytical No effect of concentrations up to 500 mg/L on 2-slide method on Kodak Ektachem® *5706* No effect at concentrations of 1000 mg/L on Jaffe methods on IL Monarch, Technicon SMAC® , or Serono Centrifichem, or on enzymatic Boehringer Mannheim Creatinine PAP, Wako Creatinine B and Kodak Ektachem® methods *2302* No effect at 1000 mg/L on Ames Seralyzer method *5706* No effect on Jaffe methods *3299* At concentration of 400 mg/L had no effect on Technicon AutoAnalyzer® Jaffe method *5704* At concentration of 400 mg/L had no effect on kinetic Jaffe method on Du Pont aca *5704* At up to 1,000 µg/mL on Technicon SMAC® Jaffe procedure *5729*

Eosinophils *Blood Increase Physiological* In about 2.5% patients as reported from several studies *893*

Erythrocytes *Urine Increase Physiological* In about 2% patients as reported from several studies *893*

Erythromycin *Serum Increase Analytical* Interferes with bioassays because cannot be inactivated *3858*

Factor II *Plasma Decrease Physiological* Depression in 40 preoperative surgical patients: effects mild *5202*

Factor VII *Plasma Decrease Physiological* Depression in 40 preoperative surgical patients: effects mild *5202*

Glucose *Serum No Effect Analytical* No effect up to 830 mg/L on glucose oxidase method on Ames Seralyzer but above this concentration apparent reduction of glucose concentration although probably not of clinical significance *5706*

Urine No Effect Analytical No effect on copper reduction procedures such as Clinitest® *4327*

Ketone Body Ratio *Serum No Effect Analytical* When added at a concentration of 0.7 g/L had no significant effect on AKBR method of Uno et al *6131*

Moxalactam *(continued)*

Lactate Dehydrogenase *Serum No Effect Analytical* No effect at 10,000 mg/L on method on Ames Seralyzer *5706*

Leukocytes *Blood Decrease Physiological* Reported in fewer than 0.5% treated patients *4327* In up to 0.5% patients as reported from several studies *893*
Blood Increase Physiological In up to 0.5% patients as reported from several studies *893*
Urine Increase Physiological In about 2% patients as reported from several studies *893*

Metronidazole *Serum Increase Analytical* Interferes with bioassays because cannot be inactivated *3858*

Neutrophils *Blood Decrease Physiological* Counts below 500 /μL reported in some cases *4327*

Partial Thromboplastin Time
Plasma No Effect Physiological Insignificant change noted in preoperative patients *5202*

Platelet Aggregation *Blood Decrease Physiological* Reduced response to ADP demonstrated *in vitro6401* Amount of ADP required to induce platelet aggregation substantially increased when 10 healthy volunteers given 8 g intravenously daily for 6 days *4629* Reduced in response to ADP in some patients *4327*

Platelets *Blood Decrease Physiological* In up to 0.5% patients as reported from several studies *893*
Blood Increase Physiological In up to 0.5% patients as reported from several studies *893*
Blood No Effect Physiological Insignificant changes in preoperative surgical patients *5202*

Polymyxin *Serum Increase Analytical* Interferes with bioassays because cannot be inactivated *3858*

Potassium *Serum Decrease Physiological* Common when coadministered with amikacin *893*

Protein *Serum No Effect Analytical* At 2.50 mmol/L on method on Eppendorf Epos *2351* At concentration of 96 mg/L had no effect on biuret method with blank correction *5704*
Urine Increase Physiological In about 2% patients as reported from several studies *893*
Urine No Effect Analytical No effect of 1 g/L on sulfosalicylic acid and Albustix methods *3927*

Prothrombin Time *Plasma Increase Physiological* May interfere with hepatic vitamin K metabolism. A bleeding event occurred in 2.5% of clinical trial patients treated for 4 or more days *1384* In up to 0.5% patients as reported from several studies *893* Caused transient plasma appearance of Vitamin K_1 2,3-epoxide in response to intravenous dose of Vitamin K_1*5488* Bleeding tendency may occur especially in debilitated patients, also impaired platelet function may occur *5291* Persistent mild increase of 0.7s in 40 preoperative patients *5202* Observed in some patients especially malnourished *4327*
Plasma No Effect Physiological 4 g intravenously 12 hourly had no effect in 6 subjects *4341*

Tetracycline *Serum Increase Analytical* Interferes with moxalactam because cannot be inactivated *3858*

Trimethoprim *Serum Increase Analytical* Interferes with bioassays because cannot be inactivated *3858*

Urea Nitrogen *Serum Increase Physiological* In about 2% patients as reported from several studies *893*
Serum No Effect Analytical At concentration of 96 mg/L had no effect on diacetylmonoxime method *5704* At 2.50 mmol/L on method on Eppendorf Epos *2351* No effect at 10000 mg/L on method on Ames Seralyzer *5706*

Uric Acid *Serum No Effect Analytical* At concentration of 96 mg/L had no effect on phosphotungstate reduction method *5704* At 2.50 mmol/L on method on Eppendorf Epos *2351*

Moxonidine

Calcium *Urine Decrease Physiological* In a group of individuals given 0.2 mg moxonidine intravenously calcium excretion changed nonsignificantly from 0.4 ± 0.1 mmol/2 h to 0.5 ± 0.2 mmol/2 h 2 hours later, 0.5 ± 0.3 mmol/2 h after 4 h and 0.5 ± 0.3 mmol/2 h after 6 h. Results were similar in placebo treated patients *6439*

Fractional Distal Reabsorption of Sodium
Urine No Effect Physiological In a group of individuals given 0.2 mg moxonidine intravenously fractional distal reabsorption of sodium changed nonsignificantly from 96 ± 2% to 95 ± 3% 2 hours later and 95 ± 4% after 4 h *6439*

Fractional Excretion of Sodium
Urine No Effect Physiological In a group of individuals given 0.2 mg moxonidine intravenously sodium excretion increased nonsignificantly from 0.5 ± 0.3% to 0.6 ± 0.4% 2 hours later, 0.6 ± 0.4% after 4 h and 0.6 ± 0.4% *6439*

Fractional Proximal Reabsorption of Sodium
Urine No Effect Physiological In a group of individuals given 0.2 mg moxonidine intravenously fractional proximal reabsorption of sodium changed nonsignificantly from 87 ± 5% to 88 ± 3% 2 hours later and 88 ± 3% after 4 h *6439*

Lithium Clearance *Urine No Effect Physiological* In a group of individuals given 0.2 mg moxonidine intravenously lithium clearance changed nonsignificantly from 15 ± 7% to 14 ± 5% 2 hours later, 13 ± 3% after 4 h and 16 ± 8% *6439*

Norepinephrine *Plasma Decrease Physiological* In a group of individuals given 0.2 mg moxonidine intravenously plasma norepinephrine concentration decreased significantly from mean baseline of 1.03 ± 0.44 nmol/L to 0.86 ± 0.25 nmol/L after 2 hours whereas no significant change was observed in patients given placebo *6439*

Phosphate *Urine Decrease Physiological* In a group of individuals given 0.2 mg moxonidine intravenously phosphate excretion changed nonsignificantly from 1.3 ± 0.5 mmol/2 h to 1.3 ± 0.7 mmol/2 h 2 hours later, 1.2 ± 0.6 mmol/2 h after 4 h and 1.3 ± 0.7 mmol/2 h after 6 h. Results were similar in placebo treated patients *6439*

Potassium *Urine Decrease Physiological* In a group of individuals given 0.2 mg moxonidine intravenously potassium excretion changed nonsignificantly from 13.4 ± 6.6 mmol/2 h to 11.0 ± 3.1 mmol/2 h 2 hours later, 11.2 ± 3.5 mmol/2 h after 4 h and 8.6 ± 3.1 mmol/2 h after 6 h. Results were similar in placebo treated patients *6439*

Renin Activity *Plasma Increase Physiological* In a group of individuals given 0.2 mg moxonidine intravenously plasma norepinephrine concentration increased significantly from mean baseline of 1.17 ± 0.56 ng angiotensin I/mL/h to 1.50 ± 0.76 ng angiotensin I/mL/h after 2 hours whereas no significant change was observed in patients given placebo *6439*

Sodium *Urine No Effect Physiological* In a group of individuals given 0.2 mg moxonidine intravenously sodium excretion increased nonsignificantly from 0.07 ± 0.05 mmol/min to 0.09 ± 0.07 mmol/min 2 hours later, 0.09 ± 1.6 mmol/min after 4 h and 0.10 ± 0.07 mmol/min *6439*

Volume *Urine No Effect Physiological* In a group of individuals given 0.2 mg moxonidine intravenously urine flow increased nonsignificantly from 3.4 ± 1.4 mL/min to 3.7 ± 1.3 mL/min 2 hours later, 3.3 ± 1.6 mL/min after 4 h and 3.6 ± 1.9 mL/min *6439*

MPCA

Acetoacetate *Serum Decrease Physiological* Anti-lipolytic effect of drug *2515*

Cholesterol *Serum No Effect Physiological* No significant change after 1 mo treatment (270 mg t.i.d.) *2367*

Fatty Acids (FFA), Free *Serum Decrease Physiological* Anti-lipolytic effect of drug (acts for 4 h) *2515*

β-Hydroxybutyrate *Serum Decrease Physiological* Anti-lipolytic effect of drug *2515*

Triglycerides *Serum No Effect Physiological* No significant change when given in fed state *2367*

Multivitamins

Dehydroepiandrosterone Sulfate
Plasma Decrease Physiological Significant negative correlation of r = -0.16 in healthy men with multivitamin use *5209*

Ferritin *Serum No Effect Physiological* In 31 women not taking oral contraceptives administration of multivitamins with folic acid for at least 28 days caused nonsignificant change of -0.51 ± 2.16 μg/L *4103*

Hematocrit *Blood Decrease Physiological* In 31 women not taking oral contraceptives administration of multivitamins with folic acid for at least 28 days caused nonsignificant reduction of 0.004 ± 0.004 *4103*

Hemoglobin *Blood Decrease Physiological* In 31 women not taking oral contraceptives administration of multivitamins with folic acid for at least 28 days caused significant reduction of 0.25 ± 0.07 mmol/L *4103*

Iron *Serum Increase Physiological* In 31 women not taking oral contraceptives administration of multivitamins with folic acid for at least 28 days caused significant change of 2.33 ± 0.95 µmol/L *4103*

Iron-Binding Capacity, Total
Serum No Effect Physiological In 31 women not taking oral contraceptives administration of multivitamins with folic acid for at least 28 days caused nonsignificant change of 1.07 ± 0.98 µmol/L *4103*

MCH *Blood No Effect Physiological* In 31 women not taking oral contraceptives administration of multivitamins with folic acid for at least 28 days caused nonsignificant change of -0.002 ± 0.019 fmol *4103*

MCHC *Blood Decrease Physiological* In 31 women not taking oral contraceptives administration of multivitamins with folic acid for at least 28 days caused significant change of -0.40 ± 0.14 mmol/L *4103*

MCV *Blood Increase Physiological* In 31 women not taking oral contraceptives administration of multivitamins with folic acid for at least 28 days caused nonsignificant increase of 1.79 ± 0.80 fL *4103*

Nalidixic Acid *Urine Decrease Physiological* Multivitamins containing zinc may interfere with the absorption of nalidixic acid resulting in lower urine concentrations than desired *5255*

Norfloxacin *Serum Decrease Physiological* Coadministration of multiviamins containing iron or zinc within two hours of norfloxacin reported to reduce gastrointestinal absorption of norfloxacin with reduction of plasma and urinary concentrations *3987*
Urine Decrease Physiological Coadministration of multiviamins containing iron or zinc within two hours of norfloxacin reported to reduce gastrointestinal absorption of norfloxacin with reduction of plasma and urinary concentrations *3987*

Ofloxacin *Serum Decrease Physiological* Quinolines form chelates with multivitamins containing zinc resulting in reduced absorption *3914*

Mumps Virus Vaccine

Platelets *Blood Decrease Physiological* May cause thrombocytopenic purpura *2754*

Muromonab-CD3

Alanine Aminotransferase *Serum Increase Physiological* Increased activity with hepato/splenomegaly or hepatitis, usually secondary to viral infection or lymphoma reported as an adverse event in clinical trials *4444*

Aspartate Aminotransferase *Serum Increase Physiological* Increased activity with hepato/splenomegaly or hepatitis, usually secondary to viral infection or lymphoma reported as an adverse event in clinical trials *4444*

Cyclosporine *Serum No Effect Analytical* No interference observed from variations with Incstar RIA procedure *2930*

Hematocrit *Blood Decrease Physiological* Aplastic anemia and pancytopenia reported as adverse events in clinical trials *4444*

Hemoglobin *Blood Decrease Physiological* Aplastic anemia and pancytopenia reported as adverse events in clinical trials *4444*

Leukocytes *Blood Decrease Physiological* Leukopenia and pancytopenia reported as adverse events in clinical trials *4444*
Blood Increase Physiological Leukocytosis and pancytopenia reported as adverse events in clinical trials *4444*

Lymphocytes *Blood Decrease Physiological* Lymphocytopenia and pancytopenia reported as adverse events in clinical trials *4444*

Neutrophils *Blood Decrease Physiological* Neutropenia and pancytopenia reported as adverse events in clinical trials *4444*

Occult Blood *Feces Increase Physiological* Gastrointestinal hemorrhage reported as an adverse event in clinical trials *4444*

Platelets *Blood Decrease Physiological* Thrombocytopenia and pancytopenia reported as adverse events in clinical trials *4444*

Muscarine

Histamine *Plasma No Effect Analytical* Probably clinically insignificant inhibition of radio-enzyme assay at physiological concentrations *2492*

Mustard

4-Hydroxybenzylamine *Urine Increase Physiological* Excreted after mustard eaten *4616*

Mustard Gas

Erythrocytes *Blood Decrease Physiological* May cause aplastic anemia *4017*

Muzolimine

Creatinine Clearance *Urine No Effect Physiological* Not changed in 10 hypertensive patients given 30 mg daily for 16 weeks *2015*

Glucose Tolerance *Serum Decrease Physiological* Significant reduction in 10 hypertensive patients given 30 mg daily for 16 weeks *2015*

Potassium *Red Blood Cells No Effect Physiological* Not appreciably affected in 10 hypertensive patients given 30 mg daily for 16 weeks *2015*
Serum No Effect Physiological No significant change in 10 hypertensive patients given 30 mg daily for 16 weeks *2015*

Renin Activity *Plasma Increase Physiological* Statistically significant increase in 10 hypertensive patients given 30 mg daily *2015*

Sodium *Serum No Effect Physiological* No significant change in 10 hypertensive patients given 30 mg daily for 16 weeks *2015*

Triglycerides *Serum No Effect Physiological* Insignificant change in 10 hypertensive patients given 30 mg daily for 16 weeks *2015*

Uric Acid *Serum Increase Physiological* Average 26 µmol/L in 10 hypertensive patients given 30 mg daily for 16 weeks *2015*

Mycophenolate

Acyclovir *Serum Increase Physiological* Coadministration of mycophenolate mofentil (1 g) with acyclovir (800 mg) in 12 healthy volunteers caused a 21.9% increase in acyclovir AUC *5017*

Alanine Aminotransferase *Serum Increase Physiological* Administration of 2 g/d or 3 g/d mycophenolate to over 660 renal transplant patients caused increased activity in ≥3% patients *5017*

Albumin *Urine Increase Physiological* Administration of 2 g/d or 3 g/d mycophenolate to over 660 renal transplant patients caused albuminuria in ≥3% patients *5017*

Alkaline Phosphatase *Serum Increase Physiological* Administration of 2 g/d or 3 g/d mycophenolate to over 660 renal transplant patients caused increased activity in ≥3% patients *5017*

Aspartate Aminotransferase *Serum Increase Physiological* Administration of 2 g/d or 3 g/d mycophenolate to over 660 renal transplant patients caused increased activity in ≥3% patients *5017*

Mycophenolate *(continued)*

Blood *Urine Increase Physiological* Administration of 2 g/d mycophenolate mofentil to 336 renal transplant patients and 3 g/d to 330 renal transplant patients caused hematuria in 14.0% and 12.1% patients respectively *5017*

Calcium *Serum Decrease Physiological* Administration of 2 g/d or 3 g/d mycophenolate to over 660 renal transplant patients caused decreased concentration in ≥3% patients *5017*
Serum Increase Physiological Administration of 2 g/d or 3 g/d mycophenolate to over 660 renal transplant patients caused increased concentration in > 3% patients *5017*

Cholesterol *Serum Increase Physiological* Administration of 2 g/d mycophenolate mofentil to 336 renal transplant patients and 3 g/d to 330 renal transplant patients caused hypercholesterolemia in 12.8% and 8.5% patients respectively *5017*

Creatinine *Serum Increase Physiological* Administration of 2 g/d or 3 g/d mycophenolate to over 660 renal transplant patients caused increased concentration in ≥3% patients *5017*

Cyclosporine A *Blood Increase Physiological* Coadministration of mycophenolate mofentil (1.5 g b.i.d.) in single or multiple doses with acyclovir (275 - 415 mg/d) in 10 stable renal transplant patients had no effect on AUC *5017*

Erythrocytes *Blood Increase Physiological* Administration of 2 g/d or 3 g/d mycophenolate to over 660 renal transplant patients caused polycythemia in ≥3% patients *5017*

Ganciclovir *Serum No Effect Physiological* Coadministration of single doses of mycophenolate mofentil with ganciclovir (1.5 mg/d) in 12 stable renal transplant patients had no significant effect on AUC and concentration of ganciclovir *5017*

Glucose *Serum Decrease Physiological* Administration of 2 g/d or 3 g/d mycophenolate to over 660 renal transplant patients caused decreased concentration in ≥3% patients *5017*
Serum Increase Physiological Administration of 2 g/d mycophenolate mofentil to 336 renal transplant patients and 3 g/d to 330 renal transplant patients caused hyperglycemia in 8.6% and 12.4% patients respectively *5017*

γ-Glutamyltransferase *Serum Increase Physiological* Administration of 2 g/d or 3 g/d mycophenolate to over 660 renal transplant patients caused increased activity in ≥3% patients *5017*

Hematocrit *Blood Decrease Physiological* Administration of 2 g/d mycophenolate mofentil to 336 renal transplant patients and 3 g/d to 330 renal transplant patients caused anemia in 25.6% and 25.8% patients respectively, with hypochromic anemia observed in 7.4% and 11.5% respectively *5017*

Hemoglobin *Blood Decrease Physiological* Administration of 2 g/d mycophenolate mofentil to 336 renal transplant patients and 3 g/d to 330 renal transplant patients caused anemia in 25.6% and 25.8% patients respectively, with hypochromic anemia in 7.4% and 11.5% respectively *5017*

Lactate Dehydrogenase *Serum Increase Physiological* Administration of 2 g/d or 3 g/d mycophenolate to over 660 renal transplant patients caused increased activity in ≥3% patients *5017*

Leukocytes *Blood Decrease Physiological* Administration of 2 g/d mycophenolate mofentil to 336 renal transplant patients and 3 g/d to 330 renal transplant patients caused leukopenia in 23.2% and 34.5% patients respectively *5017*
Blood Increase Physiological Administration of 2 g/d mycophenolate mofentil to 336 renal transplant patients and 3 g/d to 330 renal transplant patients caused leukocytosis in 7.1% and 10.9% patients respectively *5017*

Lipids *Serum Increase Physiological* Administration of 2 g/d or 3 g/d mycophenolate to over 660 renal transplant patients caused hyperlipemia in ≥3% patients *5017*

Occult Blood *Feces Increase Physiological* Administration of 2 g/d or 3 g/d mycophenolate to over 660 renal transplant patients caused gastrointestinal hemorrhage in ≥3% patients *5017*

pH *Blood Decrease Physiological* Administration of 2 g/d or 3 g/d mycophenolate to over 660 renal transplant patients caused acidosis in ≥3% patients *5017*

Phosphate *Serum Decrease Physiological* Administration of 2 g/d mycophenolate mofentil to 336 renal transplant patients and 3 g/d to 330 renal transplant patients caused hypophosphatemia in 12.5% and 15.8% patients respectively *5017*

Platelets *Blood Decrease Physiological* Administration of 2 g/d mycophenolate mofentil to 336 renal transplant patients and 3 g/d to 330 renal transplant patients caused leukopenia in 10.1% and 8.2% patients respectively *5017*

Potassium *Serum Decrease Physiological* Administration of 2 g/d mycophenolate mofentil to 336 renal transplant patients and 3 g/d to 330 renal transplant patients caused hypokalemia in 10.1% and 10.0% patients respectively *5017*
Serum Increase Physiological Administration of 2 g/d mycophenolate mofentil to 336 renal transplant patients and 3 g/d to 330 renal transplant patients caused hyperkalemia in 8.9% and 10.3% patients respectively *5017*

Protein *Serum Decrease Physiological* Administration of 2 g/d or 3 g/d mycophenolate to over 660 renal transplant patients caused decreased concentration in ≥3% patients *5017*

Uric Acid *Serum Increase Physiological* Administration of 2 g/d or 3 g/d mycophenolate to over 660 renal transplant patients caused increased concentration in ≥3% patients *5017*

Nabumetone

Alanine Aminotransferase *Serum Increase Physiological* Meaningful increases of more than 3 times the upper limit of normal have occurred with treatment in fewer than 1% patients. Cholestatic jaundice observed in fewer than 1% treated patients *5652*

Albumin *Urine Increase Physiological* Azotemia, nephrotic syndrome, or interstitial nephritis observed in fewer than 1% treated patients *5652*

Alkaline Phosphatase *Serum Increase Physiological* Cholestatic jaundice observed in fewer than 1% treated patients *5652*

Amylase *Serum Increase Physiological* Pancreatitis possibly related to drug use observed in fewer than 1% treated patients *5652*

Aspartate Aminotransferase *Serum Increase Physiological* Meaningful increases of more than 3 times the upper limit of normal have occurred with treatment in fewer than 1% patients. Cholestatic jaundice observed in fewer than 1% treated patients *5652*

Bilirubin *Serum Increase Physiological* Cholestatic jaundice observed in fewer than 1% treated patients *5652*
Urine Increase Physiological Bilirubinuria possibly related to drug use observed in fewer than 1% treated patients *5652*

Chondrex *Serum No Effect Analytical* Concentrations up to 0.1 g/L had no significant effect on sandwich-type ELISA procedure of Harvey et al *2491*

Glucose *Serum Increase Physiological* Hyperglycemia possibly related to drug use observed in fewer than 1% treated patients *5652*

γ-Glutamyltransferase *Serum Increase Physiological* Cholestatic jaundice observed in fewer than 1% treated patients *5652*

Granulocytes *Blood Decrease Physiological* Granulocytopenia possibly related to drug use observed in fewer than 1% treated patients *5652*

Hematocrit *Blood Decrease Physiological* Anemia possibly related to drug use observed in fewer than 1% treated patients *5652*

Hemoglobin *Blood Decrease Physiological* Anemia possibly related to drug use observed in fewer than 1% treated patients *5652*

Leukocytes *Blood Decrease Physiological* Leukopenia possibly related to drug use observed in fewer than 1% treated patients *5652*

Lipase *Serum Increase Physiological* Pancreatitis possibly related to drug use observed in fewer than 1% treated patients *5652*

Occult Blood *Feces Increase Physiological* Positive guaiac test, probably causally related, observed in more than 1% patients *5652*

Platelets *Blood Decrease Physiological* Thrombocytopenia possibly related to drug use observed in fewer than 1% treated patients *5652*

Potassium *Serum Decrease Physiological* Hypokalemia possibly related to drug use observed in fewer than 1% treated patients *5652*

Urea Nitrogen *Serum Increase Physiological* Azotemia, nephrotic syndrome, or interstitial nephritis observed in fewer than 1% treated patients *5652*
Urine Increase Physiological Hematuria possibly related to drug use observed in fewer than 1% treated patients *5652*

Uric Acid *Serum Increase Physiological* Hyperuricemia observed in fewer than 1% treated patients *5652*

N-Acetylprocainamide

Acetaminophen *Serum No Effect Analytical* No interference observed at a concentration of 2000 µg/mL (7220 µmol/L) with method on Du Pont aca *1506*

Creatine Kinase MB-Isoenzyme *Serum No Effect Analytical* At a concentration of 7.5 mg/dL has no significant effect on method on Kodak Ektachem® systems *2519*

Lidocaine *Serum No Effect Analytical* No significant interference observed at a concentration of 100 µg/mL (342 µmol/L) with method on Du Pont aca *1534* At a concentration of 1250 mg/L (normal serum concentration with therapy up to 12 mg/L) caused less than 10% effect on method on Baxter Stratus *5705*

Lithium *Serum Increase Analytical* May cause positive bias at high concentrations when lithium measured by an ion-specific electrode *3590*

Procainamide *Serum No Effect Analytical* No significant interference observed at a concentration of 40 µg/mL (144 µmol/L) with method on Du Pont aca *1542*

Quinidine *Serum No Effect Analytical* No significant interference observed at a concentration of 100 µg/mL (342 µmol/L) with method on Du Pont aca *1543* N-acetylprocainamide at a concentration of 100 µg/mL had no significant cross-reactivity with quinidine at a concentration of 2.0 µg/mL in method on Bayer Technicon Immuno 1® *431* Although concentrations of more than 10000 mg/L produce 30% increas in concentration as measured by method on Baxter Stratus clinical concentrations are up to 12 mg/L only *5705*

SDZ PSC 833 *Blood No Effect Analytical* At a concentration of 10.5 mg/L had no effect on HPLC method of Scott et al when used to measure PSC (with CsD as internal standard) at a concentration of 5 mg/L *5418*

Theophylline *Serum No Effect Analytical* No significant effect observed at a concentration of 15 µg/mL with method on Kodak Ektachem® systems *2519*

Nadolol

Cholesterol *Serum No Effect Physiological* In 94 patients treated for 3 mo *6249* In 13 patients given 50-200 mg daily for 10 weeks *2953*

HDL-Cholesterol *Serum Decrease Physiological* Increase by 3% in 13 patients given 50-200 mg daily for 10 weeks *2953* In hypertensive patients while fasting and during and after a meal and an exercise test. ?secondary to reduction of lipoprotein lipase *4578* Primarily observed effect with nonselective β-blockers is decrease of HDL-cholesterol concentration *3730*

LDL-Cholesterol *Serum No Effect Physiological* In 13 patients given 50-200 mg daily for 10 weeks *2953* No difference between treatment with drug and placebo *4578*

Lidocaine *Serum Increase Physiological* Clearance reduced by more than 20% due to inhibition of hepatic drug metabolizing enzymes when two drugs coadministered *5359*

Theophylline *Serum No Effect Physiological* No documented significant interaction with theophylline reported *6117* No clinically significant effect on theophylline concentration observed when drugs coadministered *5999* No significant effect of pretreatment with 80 mg/day for 7 days in 6 healthy male smokers *1139*

Thyroid Stimulating Hormone
Serum No Effect Physiological No effect over 2 weeks in 10 healthy volunteers *4895*

Thyroxine (T4) *Serum No Effect Physiological* No effect over 2 weeks in 10 healthy volunteers *4895*

Tri-iodothyronine, Reverse (rT3)
Serum No Effect Physiological No effect over 2 weeks in 10 healthy volunteers *4895*

Tri-iodothyronine (T3) *Serum No Effect Physiological* No effect over 2 weeks in 10 healthy volunteers *4895*

Triglycerides *Serum Increase Physiological* Increase by 15% in 13 patients given 50-200 mg daily for 10 weeks *2953* Primarily observed effect with nonselective β-blockers is increase of triglyceride concentration *3730* Higher in fasting state in patients on treatment, but not significantly higher, maybe secondary to reduction in lipoprotein lipase activity *4578* In hypertensive patients though not significantly, further increased post- prandially and after exercise *4578* In 94 patients treated for 3 mo *6249*

VLDL-Cholesterol *Serum Increase Physiological* Increase by 29% in 13 patients given 50-200 mg daily for 10 weeks *2953*

Nadrolone

Cholesterol *Serum No Effect Physiological* No significant effect of treatment with 50 mg intramuscularly every 3 weeks for one year in 39 healthy osteoporotic women *2501*

Creatinine *Urine Increase Physiological* 20% increase due to increase in muscle mass observed in 39 healthy osteoporotic women receiving 50 mg drug intramuscularly every 3 weeks for one year *2501*

HDL-Cholesterol *Serum Decrease Physiological* Slight decrease observed in 39 healthy osteoporotic women receiving 50 mg intramuscularly every 3 weeks for one year *2501*

LDL-Cholesterol *Serum No Effect Physiological* No significant effect of treatment with 50 mg intramuscularly every 3 weeks for one year in 39 healthy osteoporotic women *2501*

Triglycerides *Serum No Effect Physiological* No significant effect of treatment with 50 mg intramuscularly for one year in 39 healthy osteoporotic women *2501*

Nafamostat

Ketone Body Ratio *Serum No Effect Analytical* When added at a concentration of 30 mg/L had no significant effect on AKBR method of Uno et al *6131*

Potassium *Serum Increase Physiological* In one patient treated with 150 mg/d nafamostat mesylate (containing 30 - 50 mmol/d potassium) for 9 days mean concentration increased from 4.2 mmol/L to 6.3 mmol/L probably due to blockage of sodium conductance in the cortical collecting ducts leading to reversible hyperkalemia *3164*

Nafarelin

Alanine Aminotransferase *Serum Increase Physiological* During clinical trials activity increased above twice upper limit of normal in only one patient, and activity returned to normal when treatment stopped *2070*

Alkaline Phosphatase *Serum Increase Physiological* Mean increase of 20.5% in almost 100 women with endometriosis treated with 400 µg daily for 6 months due to increase in bone metabolism as typically observed in women receiving gonadotropin-releasing hormone agonist therapy *5069* Significant effect observed in patients with endometriosis treated with 400 or 800 µg by nasal spray for 6 months *2562* In 20 women with endometriosis treatment with 200 µg intranasally twice daily caused significant change from mean baseline of 100% to 165% after 3 months and 190% after 6 months *1866*

Alkaline Phosphatase, Bone Isoenzyme
Serum Increase Physiological Increase of 30-40% observed in 12 women with confirmed endometriosis treated with 400 µg/day intranasally for 6 months: still increased 3 months after end of treatment *6600*

Aminoterminal Propeptide of Type III Collagen
Serum No Effect Physiological No significant effect of treatment with 400 µg/day intranasally for 6 months in 12 women with confirmed endometriosis *6600*

Nafarelin *(continued)*

Androstenedione *Plasma Decrease Physiological* Reduction from mean of 8.3 nmol/L at baseline to 6.3 nmol/L at 3 months and 6.3 nmol/L at 6 months also in 12 women with endometriosis treated with 400 μg daily *6157*
Plasma Increase Physiological After 100 μg subcutaneously, rose between 16 and 24 hours in normal women and women with polycystic ovary syndrome and at 24 hours in men *381*

Apolipoprotein A-I *Serum No Effect Physiological* No change observed in 12 women with endometriosis when treated with 400 μg daily for 6 months *6157*

Apolipoprotein A-II *Serum No Effect Physiological* No change observed in 12 women with endometriosis treated with 400 μg daily for 6 months *6157*

Aspartate Aminotransferase *Serum Increase Physiological* Increase commonly observed in almost 100 patients with endometriosis treated with 400 μg daily for 6 months *5069* During clinical trials activity increased above twice upper limit of normal in only one patient and activity returned to normal once treatment stopped *2070*

Calcidiol *Serum No Effect Physiological* In 20 women with endometriosis treatment with 200 μg intranasally twice daily caused nonsignificant change from mean baseline of 30 ± 20 ng/mL to 35 ± 31 ng/mL after 3 months and 37 ± 34 ng/mL after 6 months *1866*

Calcitonin *Plasma No Effect Physiological* No significant change observed in 12 women with confirmed endometriosis treated with 400 μg/day intranasally for 6 months *6600*

Calcium *Serum Increase Physiological* In 20 women with endometriosis treatment with 200 μg intranasally twice daily caused significant change from mean baseline of 9.0 ± 0.4 mg/dL to 9.2 ± 0.4 mg/dL after 3 months and 9.4 ± 0.4 mg/dL after 6 months *1866* During clinical trials of patients 10 - 15% had decreases in concentration *2070*
Serum No Effect Physiological No significant change observed in 12 women with confirmed endometriosis treated with 400 μg/day intranasally for 6 months *6600*
Urine No Effect Physiological Insignificant change in excretion observed in 12 women with confirmed endometriosis treated with 400 μg/day intranasally for 6 months *6600*

Cholesterol *Serum Increase Physiological* During clinical trials of patients who had cholesterol concentrations initially below 250 mg/dL 6% demonstrated increased cholesterol concentration after treatment *2070* Increase in almost 100 patients with endometriosis treated with 400 μg daily for 6 months *5069* In 20 women with endometriosis treatment with 200 μg intranasally twice daily caused nonsignificant change from mean baseline of 174 ± 27 mg/dL to 182 ± 28 mg/dL after 3 months and 179 ± 30 mg/dL after 6 months *1866*
Serum No Effect Physiological No significant effect in 12 women with endometriosis treated with 400 μg daily for 6 months *6157* During clinical trials 9% of patients had initially increased cholesterol concentration which was unaffected by treatment *2070*

Corticotropin *Plasma No Effect Physiological* In 11 women intranasal administration of 200 μg twice daily for 3 months caused no significant change from mean baseline (all values remaining within the normal range) *4463*

Cortisol *Plasma No Effect Physiological* In 11 women given 200 μg twice daily for 3 months no significant effect observed on plasma concentration *4463*

Dehydroepiandrosterone *Plasma Increase Physiological* Effect observed in women with polycystic ovary syndrome after 100 μg subcutaneously but not in normal men and women *381*

1,25-Dihydroxy Vitamin D *Serum No Effect Physiological* In 20 women with endometriosis treatment with 200 μg intranasally twice daily caused nonsignificant change from mean baseline of 35 ± 10 pg/mL to 36 ± 11 pg/mL after 3 months and 36 ± 12 pg/mL after 6 months *1866*

Eosinophils *Blood Increase Physiological* During clinical trials of patients 10 - 15% had increases in concentration *2070*

Estradiol *Plasma Decrease Physiological* In 20 women with endometriosis treatment with 200 μg intranasally twice daily caused significant decrease from mean baseline of 84 ± 53 pg/mL to 31 ± 16 pg/mL after 3 months and 33 ± 14 pg/mL after 6 months *1866* In 12 patients with confirmed endometriosis 400 μg/day intranasally caused reduction of concentration below 21.6 pg/mL after 3 months *6600* Mean decrease of about 55% in mean early follicular concentration in almost 100 women with endometriosis treated with 400 μg/day for 6 months *5069* Reduction from mean baseline concentration of 0.50 nmol/L in 12 women with endometriosis treated with 400 μg daily to 0.11 nmol/L at 3 months and 0.08 nmol/L at 6 months *6157*
Plasma Increase Physiological In 10 healthy men administration of 100 μg caused a significant change from mean baseline of 113 ± 13 pmol/L to 284 ± 20 pmol/L after 16 - 24 h, and from baseline of 195 ± 26 pmol/L to 822 ± 87 pmol/L after 16 - 24 h *5099* After 100 μg subcutaneously, normal women, women with polycystic ovary syndrome and men all had significant increases *381*

Estrone *Plasma Increase Physiological* Significant increase observed in normal women and men following 100 μg subcutaneously, but no significant change observed in women with polycystic ovary syndrome *381*

Follicle Stimulating Hormone
Plasma Increase Physiological Rapid increase observed in 16 normal women following 100 μg subcutaneously. Lower peak response observed in men and women with polycystic ovary syndrome *381* In 10 healthy men administration of 100 μg caused a significant increase from mean baseline of 5.0 ± 0.6 IU/L to 20 ± 3.5 IU/L at peak and 18 ± 3.0 IU/L after 24 h, and from baseline of 9.7 ± 0.9 IU/L to 39 ± 3.8 IU/L at peak and 20 ± 1.6 IU/L after 24 h in 20 normal women *5099*

HDL_3-Cholesterol *Serum No Effect Physiological* Insignificant change in 12 women with endometriosis treated with 400 μg daily for 6 months *6157*

HDL_3-Phospholipids *Serum No Effect Physiological* Insignificant change in 12 women with endometriosis treated with 400 μg daily for 6 months *6157*

HDL_3-Triglycerides *Serum Decrease Physiological* Very slight fall in concentration at 6 months in 12 women with endometriosis treated with 400 μg daily *6157*

HDL-Cholesterol *Serum Increase Physiological* In 20 women with endometriosis treatment with 200 μg intranasally twice daily caused nonsignificant change from mean baseline of 55 ± 17 mg/dL to 59 ± 17 mg/dL after 3 months and 58 ± 14 mg/dL after 6 months *1866* Increase by 15% at 3 months in 12 women with endometriosis treated with 400 μg daily. 3 months after treatment stopped concentration had reverted to baseline *6157* Increase observed in almost 100 women with endometriosis treated with 400 μg daily for 6 months *5069*
Serum No Effect Physiological During clinical trials of patients none had abnormal concentrations below 30 mg/dL at the end of treatment *2070*

17-Hydroxypregnenolone *Plasma Increase Physiological* Significant rise observed in women with polycystic ovary syndrome after 100 μg subcutaneously, but not observed in normal women and men *381*

17-Hydroxyprogesterone *Plasma Increase Physiological* Significant increase of 17αhydroxyprogesterone concentration in normal men and women and in women with polycystic ovary syndrome, but greater in men and in women with polycystic ovary syndrome *381*

Hydroxyproline *Urine Increase Physiological* In 20 women with endometriosis treatment with 200 μg intranasally twice daily caused significant change from mean baseline of 100% to 180% after 3 months and 230% after 6 months *1866* In 12 patients with confirmed endometriosis intranasal administration of 400 μg/day for 6 months caused approximate 50% increase in excretion: still increased 3 months after end of treatment *6600*

LDL-Cholesterol *Serum Increase Physiological* In 20 women with endometriosis treatment with 200 μg intranasally twice daily caused nonsignificant change from mean baseline of 105 ± 20 mg/dL to 108 ± 23 mg/dL after 3 months and 108 ± 20 mg/dL after 6 months *1866* Mean 6% increase (not significant) in 12 women with endometriosis treated with 400 μg daily for 6 months *6157*
Serum No Effect Physiological Little or no effect observed in almost 100 women with endometriosis treated with 400 μg daily for 6 months *5069* During clinical trials of patients none had abnormal concentrations above 190 mg/dL at the end of treatment *2070*

LDL-Cholesterol:HDL-Cholesterol Ratio
Serum *No Effect* *Physiological* During clinical trials of patients none had increases in the ratio at the end of treatment *2070*

Leukocytes *Blood* *Increase* *Physiological* During clinical trials of patients 10 - 15% had decreases in concentration *2070*

Luteinizing Hormone *Plasma* *Increase* *Physiological* Rapid increase in 16 normal women following 100 µg subcutaneously (within 4 hours). Women with polycystic ovary disease and men had greater earlier response (30 min to 1 hour) *381* In 10 healthy men administration of 100 µg caused a significant increase from mean baseline of 7.4 ± 0.5 IU/L to 51 ± 3.8 IU/L at peak and 42 ± 3.9 IU/L after 24 h, and from baseline of 7.7 ± 0.5 IU/L to 88 ± 9.3 IU/L at peak and 52 ± 3.4 IU/L after 24 h in 20 normal women *5099*

Osteocalcin *Serum* *Increase* *Physiological* In 20 women with endometriosis treatment with 200 µg intranasally twice daily caused significant change from mean baseline of 100% to 290% after 3 months and 330% after 6 months *1866* Mean increase of 80-120% observed in 12 women with confirmed endometriosis treated with 400 µg/day intranasally for 6 months: still increased 3 months after end of treatment *6600*

Parathyroid Hormone *Plasma* *No Effect* *Physiological* In 20 women with endometriosis treatment with 200 µg intranasally twice daily caused nonsignificant change from mean baseline of 25 ± 10 pg/mL to 26 ± 13 pg/mL after 3 months and 27 ± 11 pg/mL after 6 months *1866* No significant change observed in 12 women with confirmed endometriosis treated with 400 µg/day intranasally for 6 months *6600*

Phosphate *Serum* *Increase* *Physiological* In 20 women with endometriosis treatment with 200 µg intranasally twice daily caused significant change from mean baseline of 3.4 ± 0.5 mg/dL to 3.8 ± 0.5 mg/dL after 3 months and 3.9 ± 0.8 mg/dL after 6 months *1866* During clinical trials of patients 10 - 15% had increases in plasma phosphate concentration *2070*

Progesterone *Plasma* *No Effect* *Physiological* No significant effect observed in normal women, normal men and women with polycystic ovary syndrome *381*

Pyridinoline *Urine* *Increase* *Physiological* In 20 women with endometriosis treatment with 200 µg intranasally twice daily caused significant change from mean baseline of 100% to 200% after 3 months and 230% after 6 months *1866*

Sex-Hormone Binding Globulin
Serum *Decrease* *Physiological* Reduction from mean baseline concentration of 68.5 nmol/L in 12 women with endometriosis receiving 400 µg daily to mean of 53.8 nmol/L at 3 months and 52.6 nmol/L at 6 months *6157*

Testosterone *Serum* *Decrease* *Physiological* In 12 women with endometriosis receiving 400 µg daily reduction from mean of 3.1 nmol/L at baseline to 2.3 nmol/L at 3 months and 1.8 nmol/L at 6 months *6157* In all 9 patients with benign prostatic hypertrophy treated with nafarelin acetate: due to reduced production in testes by inhibition of pituitary release of gonadotropins. Concentration reversibly reduced from normal to castration level *4628*
Serum *Increase* *Physiological* Significant increase observed in men, but not in women, following 100 µg subcutaneously *381*
Serum *No Effect* *Physiological* In 10 healthy men administration of 100 µg caused an insignificant change from mean baseline of 21 ± 1.6 nmol/L to 25 ± 1.6 nmol/L after 16 - 24 h, and from baseline of 1.1 ± 0.1 nmol/L to 0.9 ± 0.2 nmol/L after 16 - 24 h *5099*

Testosterone, Free *Serum* *Decrease* *Physiological* Insignificant reduction from mean baseline of 35.7 pmol/L to 30.2 pmol/L at 3 months and 24.8 pmol/L at 6 months in 12 women with endometriosis receiving 400 µg daily *6157*

Triglycerides *Serum* *Increase* *Physiological* During clinical trials of patients who had triglycerides concentrations measured 12% demonstrated increased concentration after treatment *2070*

VLDL-Cholesterol *Serum* *No Effect* *Physiological* No change observed in 12 women with endometriosis treated with 400 µg daily for 6 months *6157*

VLDL-Phospholipids *Serum* *No Effect* *Physiological* No change observed in 12 women with endometriosis treated with 400 µg daily for 6 months *6157*

VLDL-Triglycerides *Serum* *No Effect* *Physiological* No change observed in 12 women with endometriosis treated for 6 months with 400 µg daily *6157*

Nafcillin

Alanine Aminotransferase *Serum* *Increase* *Physiological* 1 of 32 patients developed abnormal liver function on 3rd day of treatment *4212*

Albumin *Serum* *No Effect* *Analytical* At concentration of 50 mg/L had no effect on BCG method *5704*

Aspartate Aminotransferase *Serum* *Increase* *Physiological* 1 of 32 patients developed abnormal liver function on 3rd day of treatment *97* Possibly due to trauma of injection *3810*

Bicarbonate *Serum* *No Effect* *Analytical* At concentration of 50 mg/L had no effect on method using phenolphthalein *5704*

Bilirubin *Serum* *No Effect* *Analytical* No effect at concentration of 30 mg/L on method on Kodak Ektachem® systems *5706* At concentration of 50 mg/L had no effect on Jendrassik and Grof method *5704*

Bilirubin, Conjugated *Serum* *No Effect* *Analytical* No effect at concentration of 30 mg/L on method on Kodak Ektachem® *5706*

Bilirubin, Unconjugated *Serum* *No Effect* *Analytical* No effect at concentration of 30 mg/L on method on Kodak Ektachem® *5706*

Bleeding Time *Patient* *Increase* *Physiological* Reportedly 4 times normal in two patients, reverted to normal on withdrawal *97*

BSP Retention *Serum* *Increase* *Physiological* Reported effect (?hepatotoxicity) *128*

Calcium *Serum* *No Effect* *Analytical* At concentration of 50 mg/L had no effect on cresolphthalein method *5704*

Chloride *Serum* *No Effect* *Analytical* At concentration of 50 mg/L had no effect on mercurimetric method *5704*

Cholesterol *Serum* *No Effect* *Analytical* At concentration of 50 mg/L had no effect on Liebermann-Burchard method *5704*

Cloxacillin *Serum* *Increase* *Analytical* Cannot be assayed by HPLC method used at Mayo Clinic in presence of nafcillin *3858*

Creatinine *Serum* *No Effect* *Analytical* At concentration of 50 mg/L had no effect on Technicon AutoAnalyzer® Jaffe method *5704* No effect of concentrations up to 15 mg/L on single slide method on Kodak Ektachem® *5706*

Cyclosporine *Blood* *Decrease* *Physiological* When given intravenously to one renal transplant patient reduction noted by third day but concentration returned to baseline after treatment discontinued *6230* Coadministration of nafcillin with cyclosporine caused a gradual reduction of cyclosporine concentration to about 50% of its baseline concentration *859*
Serum *Decrease* *Physiological* Coadministration of nafcillin with cyclosporine caused a gradual reduction of cyclosporine concentration to about 50% of its baseline concentration *859* May decrease cyclosporine concentration by inducing hepatic cytochrome P-450 III A which metabolizes cyclosporine *5236* Intravenous nafcillin reported to reduce plasma concentration of cyclosporine, probably by induction of hepatic enzymes *6595* Observed effect probably due to induction of hepatic microsomal enzymes *1069*

Dicloxacillin *Serum* *Positive* *Analytical* Cannot be assayed by HPLC method used at Mayo Clinic in presence of nafcillin *3858*

Eosinophils *Blood* *Increase* *Physiological* 3 of 32 children developed eosinophilia within 1-4 d *4212*

Neutrophils *Blood* *Decrease* *Physiological* Reported in 10-20% patients receiving 150 to 200 mg/kg per day for 10 to 14 days or longer (reversible on discontinuation of drug) *1384* 2 of 32 children developed neutropenia within 4 to 13 d *4212*

Phenytoin, Free *Serum* *Increase* *Physiological* In vivo, in presence of nafcillin, concentration of free phenytoin increased from calculated concentrations of 3.4-7.7 µmol/L to 3.9-9.3 µmol/L in four patients treated with phenytoin *1242*

Phosphate *Serum* *No Effect* *Analytical* At concentration of 50 mg/L had no effect on phosphomolybdate method *5704*

Nafcillin *(continued)*

Platelet Aggregation *Blood Decrease Physiological* Reduced response to ADP collagen and epinephrine *97*

Platelets *Blood No Effect Physiological* Unchanged in spite of abnormal bleeding time and aggregation *97*

Protein *Cerebrospinal Fluid No Effect Analytical* At concentration of 10 mg/L on SDS/Coomassie Blue method of Huang *2745*
Serum Increase Analytical At concentrations above 500 mg/L raised concentration as measured by biuret method with blank correction *5704*

Triglycerides *Serum No Effect Analytical* At concentration of 50 mg/L had no effect on lipase/esterase method *5704*

Urea Nitrogen *Serum No Effect Analytical* At concentration of 50 mg/L had no effect on diacetylmonoxime method *5704*

Uric Acid *Serum No Effect Analytical* At concentration of 50 mg/L had no effect on phosphotungstate reduction method *5704*

Valproic Acid, Free *Serum No Effect Physiological* No statistically significant increase in concentration of free drug in the presence of low albumin concentrations even at toxic concentrations of nafcillin *1241*

Warfarin *Plasma Decrease Physiological* Warfarin elimination halflife increased from 5.3 hours during nafcillin coadministration to 14.5 hours when nafcillin was discontinued in one patient *1282* In one patient concomitant administration of drugs caused decrease in warfarin half-life but it returned to normal after discontinuation of nafcillin *1384*

Nafenopin

Cholesterol *Serum Decrease Physiological* More effective than clofibrate *1480*

Triglycerides *Serum Decrease Physiological* More effective than clofibrate *1480*

Nalidixic Acid

Alanine Aminotransferase *Serum Increase Physiological* Rarely cholestasis may occur with treatment *5255* May cause cholestatic jaundice *4691*

Alkaline Phosphatase *Serum Increase Physiological* May cause cholestatic jaundice *4691* Rarely cholestasis may occur with treatment *5255*

Aspartate Aminotransferase *Serum Increase Physiological* Rarely cholestasis may occur with treatment *5255* May cause cholestatic jaundice *4691*

Bilirubin *Serum Increase Physiological* Rarely cholestasis may occur with treatment *5255* May cause cholestatic jaundice *4691*
Serum No Effect Physiological No clinically significant displacement from protein likely in neonates *6314*

Bilirubin, Direct *Serum Increase Physiological* Hemolytic anemia especially if G-6-PD deficiency *6512*

Chromosomes *Test Conditions Abnormal Physiological* Clastogenic in human cells *5484*

Coombs' Test, Direct *Blood Positive Physiological* May cause hemolytic anemia with normal G-6-PD *2113*

Coproporphyrin I *Urine No Effect Analytical* At a concentration of 0.35 mmol/L no effect observed on HPLC method with fluorescence detection *5366*

Coproporphyrin III *Urine No Effect Analytical* At a concentration of 0.35 mmol/L had no effect on HPLC method with fluorescence detection *5366*

Creatinine *Serum Increase Physiological* May cause nitrogen retention *4691*
Serum No Effect Analytical At concentration of 60 mg/L had no effect on creatinine iminohydrolase method *5704* No effect of concentrations up to 15 mg/L on single slide method on Kodak Ektachem® *5706*

Eosinophils *Blood Increase Physiological* Allergic response *2484*

Erythrocytes *Blood Decrease Physiological* Hemolytic anemia with G-6-PD deficiency *467*

Glucose *Serum Increase Analytical* Copper reduction methods affected *5869*
Serum No Effect Analytical No effect at 1 g/L on glucokinase based assay of Scott *5414* At concentration of 50 mg/L had no effect on GOD/POD-PAP method *5704*
Urine Increase Analytical May cause false positive with Ames Clinitest tablet procedure *4034* May cause false positive reaction with Benedict's or Fehling's test or with Clinitest® reagent strip *5255*
Urine No Effect Analytical No effect with Clinistix® , Tes-Tape® *6512* Has no effect on Ames Keto-Diastix, Diastix, Multistix and Clinistix methods *4034* Has no effect on Clinistix® or TesTape® reagent strips *5255*

Haptoglobin *Serum Decrease Physiological* May cause hemolytic anemia especially if G-6-PD deficiency *6512*

Hematocrit *Blood Decrease Physiological* Rarely hemolytic anemia may occur with treatment *5255* Hemolytic anemia with G-6-PD deficiency *467*

Hemoglobin *Blood Decrease Physiological* Rarely hemolytic anemia may occur with treatment *5255* Hemolytic anemia with G-6-PD deficiency *467*

Histamine *Plasma No Effect Analytical* No inhibition of radio-enzyme assay at concentration 3 times therapeutic *2492*

17-Hydroxycorticosteroids *Urine No Effect Analytical* No effect with Porter-Silber reaction *6512*

Hydroxynalidixic Acid *Urine Increase Physiological* Major metabolites with glucuronide conjugates *2753*

17-Ketogenic Steroids *Urine Increase Analytical* May cause falsely increased concentration because of an interaction between the drug and m-nitrobenzene used in most reactions *5255* Interferes with Zimmermann reaction *3623*
Urine No Effect Analytical Drug has no effect on apparent concentration when Porter-Silber reaction used to measure the steroids *5255*

17-Ketosteroids *Urine Increase Analytical* May cause falsely increased concentration because of an interaction between the drug and m-nitrobenzene used in most reactions *5255* Interferes with Zimmermann reaction *3623*
Urine No Effect Analytical Drug has no effect on apparent concentration when Porter-Silber reaction used to measure the steroids *5255*

Leukocytes *Blood Decrease Physiological* Rarely leukopenia may occur with treatment *5255*
Blood Increase Physiological Due to eosinophilia *3810*

Nalidixic Acid *Serum Increase Physiological* After 1 g orally 25-35 µg/mL in 2 h *2753*
Urine Increase Physiological Major metabolites with glucuronide conjugates *2753*

Nonprotein Nitrogen *Serum Increase Physiological* May cause nitrogen retention *4691*

5'-Nucleotidase *Serum Increase Physiological* Due to cholestasis *2911*

Occult Blood *Feces Increase Physiological* May cause bleeding from gastrointestinal tract *128*

pH *Blood Decrease Physiological* Rarely metabolic acidosis may occur with treatment *5255*

Phenylalanine *Plasma No Effect Analytical* No interference observed with rapid quantitative whole blood method of Campbell et al using phenylalanine dehydrogenase *867*

Platelets *Blood Decrease Physiological* Rarely thrombocytopenia may occur with treatment *5255* Thrombocytopenia *6512* Thrombocytopenia occurred in 6 cases in Netherlands characteristically within 10-15 d after 4 g daily. Recovered rapidly once drug stopped but reaction could be severe *4010*

Porphyrin, Total *Urine Increase Analytical* At a concentration of 0.35 mmol/L 2-fold increase observed with screening method of Porphyrin Products *5366*
Urine No Effect Analytical At a concentration of 0.35 mmol/L had no effect on HPLC method with fluorescence detection *5366*

Potassium *Serum No Effect Analytical* At concentration of 10 mg/L had no effect on measurement by ISE with predilution *5704*

Prothrombin Time *Plasma Increase Physiological* May increase plasma concentration of warfarin and prolong prothrombin time *5255* Displaces coumarins from albumin *5440*

Sodium *Serum No Effect Analytical* At concentration of 10 mg/L had no effect on measurement by ISE with predilution *5704*

Sugar *Urine Increase Analytical* False positive with Fehlings, Benedict's, Clinitest® *6512*

Theophylline *Serum Increase Physiological* May increase plasma concentration of theophylline *5255*

Triglycerides *Serum No Effect Analytical* At concentration of 50 mg/L had no effect on GPO-PAP method *5704*

Urea Nitrogen *Serum Increase Physiological* May cause nitrogen retention *4691*

Uric Acid *Serum No Effect Analytical* At concentration of 50 mg/L had no effect on uricase-PAP method *5704*

Urobilinogen *Feces Decrease Physiological* May occur with cholestasis *4691*
Urine Increase Physiological May occur if cholestasis *4691*

Uroporphyrin *Urine No Effect Analytical* At a concentration of 0.35 mmol/L had no effect on HPLC method with fluorescence detection *5366*

Vanillylmandelic Acid *Urine Increase Analytical* Apparent 4 fold increase with normal regime *882* Affects Pisano procedure *199*

Xylose *Urine Decrease Physiological* May cause gastrointestinal irritation, impaired absorption *929*

Nalmefene

Luteinizing Hormone *Plasma Increase Physiological* In 5 of 9 oligo-amenorrheic women and in one of 5 controls a significant response to nalmefene occurred *3867* In 6 normal men ingestion of 10 mg over 6 hours caused significant increase from mean baseline of 3.9 ± 0.3 mIU/mL to 8.4 ± 0.5 mIU/mL *2297*

Testosterone *Serum Increase Physiological* In 6 normal men ingestion of 10 mg over 6 hours caused significant increase from mean baseline of 4.9 ± 0.4 ng/mL to 7.5 ± 0.7 ng/mL *2297*

Nalmfene

Opiates *Urine No Effect Analytical* In spite of structural similarity to morphine has no effect on EMIT II assay on Syva ETS® for 24 h after 2 mg intravenous dose *5839*

Nalorphine

Morphine *Urine No Effect Analytical* Insignificant cross reactivity with EMIT procedure for opiates. Insignificant cross reactivity with hemagglutination inhibition *4163*

Opiates *Urine No Effect Analytical* No effect observed at a concentration of 20 µg/mL (64 µmol/L) on method on Du Pont aca *1559*

Protein *Test Conditions Increase Analytical* Reacts with Folin-Ciocalteu method of Lowry *1102*

Naloxone

Antidiuretic Hormone *Plasma No Effect Physiological* No effect of 10 mg on basal values *286*

Corticotropin *Plasma No Effect Physiological* In patients with normal ACTH concentration or high concentration of untreated Cushing's disease with infusion for 90 min of 0.8 mg/h *4110*

Cortisol *Plasma Increase Physiological* Concentration increased by 50% in men of all ages following 4 mg given in an intravenous bolus with 10 mg subsequently infused over 2 hours *1084* Peak at 60 minutes after start of infusion remained high for duration *1365* Administration intravenously of a single dose of 20 mg naloxone caused increase of same magnitude in healthy controls at 30 to 60 minutes and in short term abstinent alcoholics and alcoholics at 3 days and 1 month after last alcohol *3104*
Plasma No Effect Physiological In patients with Cushing's or Addison's diseases or in controls given low dose infusion *4110*

β-Endorphin *Plasma Increase Physiological* Similar increase in about 30 to 60 minutes after intravenous administration of 20 mg in healthy controls, in short term abstinent alcohol abusers and in alcoholics after 3 days and 4 weeks *3104*

Follicle Stimulating Hormone
Plasma Increase Physiological Significant effect within 60 minutes of start of i.v. infusion *1365* Slight but significant increase in men aged 22-59 years but not in those over age 62 years following intravenous bolus of 4 mg and subsequent infusion of 10 mg over 2 hours *1084*
Plasma No Effect Physiological Infusion did not affect concentration of hormone at concentrations varying from 0.02 to 0.5 mg/kg *3207*

Gastric Inhibitory Polypeptide
Plasma No Effect Physiological In 6 healthy volunteers after ingestion of test meal and intravenous administration of drug *956*

Gastrin *Serum No Effect Physiological* In 6 healthy volunteers after ingestion of test meal and intravenous administration of drug *956*

Glucagon *Plasma No Effect Physiological* In 6 healthy volunteers after ingestion of test meal and intravenous administration of drug *956* With infusion in normal and obese subjects *286*

Glucagon, Pancreatic *Plasma No Effect Physiological* In 6 healthy volunteers after ingestion of test meal and intravenous administration of drug *956*

Glucose *Serum No Effect Physiological* In 6 healthy volunteers after ingestion of test meal and intravenous administration of drug *956*

Growth Hormone *Plasma No Effect Physiological* No significant effect with i.v. infusion *1365*

Hydrochloric Acid *Gastric Fluid Decrease Physiological* Reduces basal and meal stimulated concentration *286*

Insulin *Plasma No Effect Physiological* No significant change observed on increased concentration in obese and low concentration in nonobese patients with polycystic ovary disease following intravenous bolus of 10 mg *3353* With infusion in normal and obese subjects *286* In 6 healthy volunteers after ingestion of test meal and intravenous administration of drug *956*

Insulin-like Growth Factor-I *Serum No Effect Physiological* No significant effect observed in either obese or lean individuals with polycystic ovary disease following single intravenous bolus of 10 mg *3353*

Insulin-like Growth Factor Binding Protein-1
Serum Decrease Physiological After intravenous bolus of 10 mg decrease observed in nonobese patients with polycystic ovarian disease and concentration remained low in obese patients with polycystic disease although no effect observed in healthy individuals *3353*

Luteinizing Hormone *Plasma Increase Physiological* Striking increase observed in men aged 22 - 59 years but not in those aged over 62 years following single bolus intravenously of 4 mg with infusion of 10 mg over 2 hours *1084* In 5 normal men infusion of 2 mg/h over 6 hours caused significant increase from mean baseline of 3.9 ± 0.3 mIU/mL to 6.0 ± 1.1 mIU/mL *2297* Significant increase observed in 7 obese women with polycystic ovarian disease varying from 8% to 60% of starting value at 30 to 40 minutes after 10 mg intravenous bolus but no change observed in nonobese women. Slight increase in healthy individuals *3353* In 8 healthy men boluses of naloxone caused significant increase from mean baseline of 7.6 ± 0.4 IUL to 10.0 ± 0.9 IUL during saline infusion *3185* Significant effect within 30 minutes of start of i.v. infusion *1365* After 0.08 mg/kg body weight i.v. in girls and boys at most advanced stage of gonadal maturation: ineffective in prepubertal and early pubertal children *4638* Effect observed regardless of amount infused *3207*
Plasma No Effect Physiological No effect of low dose infusion in patients with Cushing's or Addison's disease or in controls *4110*

Morphine *Urine No Effect Analytical* Insignificant cross reactivity with RIA procedures. Insignificant cross reactivity with EMIT procedure for opiates *4163*

Motilin *Plasma No Effect Physiological* In 6 healthy volunteers after ingestion of test meal and intravenous administration of drug *956*

Naloxone *(continued)*

Neurotensin *Plasma No Effect Physiological* In 6 healthy volunteers after ingestion of test meal and intravenous administration of drug *956*

Opiates *Urine No Effect Analytical* No effect observed at a concentration of 150 µg/mL (0.46 mmol/L) on method on Du Pont aca *1559*

Oxytocin *Plasma No Effect Physiological* No effect observed for 120 minutes in healthy male volunteers after intravenous injection of 10 mg *2694*

Pancreatic Polypeptide *Plasma No Effect Physiological* In 6 healthy volunteers after ingestion of test meal and intravenous administration of drug *956*

Partial Thromboplastin Time
Plasma Increase Physiological With multiple doses effect observed (no bleeding) *51*

Prolactin *Plasma No Effect Physiological* No significant effect with i.v. infusion *1365* Basal and stimulated levels not affected *286* Infusion did not affect concentration of hormone at concentrations varying from 0.02 to 0.5 mg/kg *3207* In 5 normal men infusion of 2 mg/h over 6 hours caused nonsignificant decrease from mean baseline of 6.9 ± 1.2 ng/mL to 5.3 ± 0.8 ng/mL *2297* In 6 normal men ingestion of 10 mg over 6 hours caused nonsignificant decrease from mean baseline of 6.9 ± 1.2 ng/mL to 5.9 ± 0.4 ng/mL *2297*

Somatostatin *Plasma No Effect Physiological* In 6 healthy volunteers after ingestion of test meal and intravenous administration of drug *956*

Testosterone *Serum Increase Physiological* In 5 normal men infusion of 2 mg/h over 6 hours caused significant increase from mean baseline of 4.9 ± 0.4 ng/mL to 6.8 ± 0.5 ng/mL *2297*

Thyroid Stimulating Hormone
Serum No Effect Physiological No significant effect with i.v. infusion *1365*

Vasoactive Intestinal Polypeptide
Plasma No Effect Physiological In 6 healthy volunteers after ingestion of test meal and intravenous administration of drug *956*

Naltrexone

Alanine Aminotransferase *Serum Increase Physiological* Dose related hepatotoxicity is most severe adverse reaction usually reversible. Most severe hepatotoxicity usually observed in obese individuals in whom peak enzyme activity observed to be 3-19 times upper limit of normal after 3-8 weeks treatment *1384* Administration was associated with increased activity of aminotransferase activity although activities eventually reverted to normal after several weeks *1599*

Aspartate Aminotransferase
Serum Decrease Physiological Significant fall over 3 months in 53 patients, especially in those in whom initial values were above normal range. This finding is different from previous perceptions of potential hepatotoxicity *686*
Serum Increase Physiological Most severe adverse reaction is dose-related hepatotoxicity but usually reversible *1384* Administration was associated with increased activity in 5 of 26 patients in a placebo controlled study with values increasing 3 to 19 times the baseline activity after 3 to 8 weeks of treatment *1599*

Cortisol *Plasma No Effect Physiological* No change in unstimulated values observed *286*

C-Peptide *Plasma No Effect Physiological* In 9 obese individuals treated with 50 mg/d for 6 days mean fasting concentration of 860.6 ± 198.6 pmol/L changed nonsignificantly to 865.2 ± 200.9 pmol/L *6250*

Drugs of Abuse Screen *Urine No Effect Analytical* No effect at concentration of 100 µg/mL on EZ-SCREEN procedure for cannabinoids and cocaine *1739*

Estradiol *Plasma No Effect Physiological* With 50 to 100 mg administered daily to obese subjects over 8 weeks *286*

Follicle Stimulating Hormone
Plasma No Effect Physiological With 50 to 100 mg administered daily to obese subjects over 8 weeks *286*

Glucose *Serum No Effect Physiological* In 9 obese individuals treated with 50 mg/d for 6 days mean fasting concentration of 3.8 ± 0.1 mmol/L changed nonsignificantly to 4.1 ± 0.1 mmol/L *6250* No effect of long-term administration to obese individuals *286*

Insulin *Plasma No Effect Physiological* In 9 obese individuals treated with 50 mg/d for 6 days mean fasting concentration of 138.4 ± 26.0 pmol/L changed nonsignificantly to 118.3 ± 3.5 pmol/L *6250* No effect of long-term administration to obese individuals *286*

Lactate Dehydrogenase *Serum Decrease Physiological* Significant decrease observed in 53 patients over 3 months, most marked in individuals whose initial values were above normal range. This effect does not support previous reports of hepatic toxicity *686*

Luteinizing Hormone *Plasma No Effect Physiological* With 50 to 100 mg administered daily to obese subjects over 8 weeks *286*

Methadone *Urine No Effect Analytical* Administration has no effect on thin-layer, gas-liquid or high pressure liquid chromatographic methods to measure methadone *1599*

Morphine *Urine No Effect Analytical* Administration has no effect on thin-layer, gas-liquid or high pressure liquid chromatographic methods to measure morphine *1599*

Quinine *Urine No Effect Analytical* Administration has no effect on thin-layer, gas-liquid or high pressure liquid chromatographic methods to measure quinine *1599*

Testosterone *Serum No Effect Physiological* With 50 to 100 mg administered daily to obese subjects over 8 weeks *286*

Nandrolone

Alanine Aminotransferase *Serum Increase Physiological* Reported to affect liver function *3669*

Alkaline Phosphatase *Serum Increase Physiological* Reported to affect liver function *3669*

Aspartate Aminotransferase *Serum Increase Physiological* Reported to affect liver function *3669*

Calcium *Serum Increase Physiological* May occur in women with neoplasm of breast *4433*
Urine Increase Physiological Due to hypercalcemia *4433*

Cholesterol *Serum Decrease Physiological* Due to action on liver *4433*
Serum Increase Physiological Due to action on liver *4433*

Creatine *Urine Decrease Physiological* Anabolic effect *4433*

Creatinine *Urine Decrease Physiological* Anabolic effect *4433*

Estradiol *Plasma Decrease Physiological* In 11 healthy men treatment with 300 mg intramuscularly weekly for 6 weeks caused nonsignificant decrease from mean baseline of 143.1 ± 27.5 pmol/L to 92.5 ± 20.2 pmol/L *2634*

Estrogens *Urine Increase Physiological* Normal route of metabolism *55*

Factor II *Plasma Increase Physiological* Metabolic effect *4433*

Factor V *Plasma Increase Physiological* Metabolic effect *4433*

Factor VII *Plasma Increase Physiological* Metabolic effect *4433*

Factor X *Plasma Increase Physiological* Metabolic effect *4433*

Glucose *Serum Decrease Physiological* Anabolic effect *4433*

Glucose Tolerance *Serum Increase Physiological* Anabolic effect *4433*

Growth Hormone *Plasma No Effect Physiological* In 11 healthy men treatment with 300 mg intramuscularly weekly for 6 weeks caused nonsignificant change from mean baseline of 1.7 ± 0.7 µg/L to 1.9 ± 0.6 µg/L *2634*

Hematocrit *Blood Increase Physiological* Due to decreased plasma volume *530*

^{131}I Uptake *Serum Decrease Physiological* Anabolic effect *4433*

Insulin-like Growth Factor Binding Protein-3
Serum Decrease Physiological In 11 healthy men treatment with 300 mg intramuscularly weekly for 6 weeks caused significant decrease from mean baseline of 3.89 ± 0.16 mg/L to 3.33 ± 0.16 mg/L *2634*
17-Ketosteroids *Urine Increase Physiological* Anabolic effect *4433*
Metyrapone Test *Patient Positive Physiological* Anabolic effect *4433*
Prothrombin Time *Plasma Increase Physiological* May increase sensitivity to anticoagulants *4433*
Sex-Hormone Binding Globulin
Serum Decrease Physiological In 11 healthy men treatment with 300 mg intramuscularly weekly for 6 weeks caused significant reduction from mean baseline of 25.6 ± 2.2 nmol/L to 20.2 nmol/L *2634*
T3-Uptake *Serum Increase Physiological* Anabolic effect *4433*
Testosterone *Serum Decrease Physiological* In 11 healthy men treated with 300 mg intramuscularly weekly for 6 weeks caused significant decrease from mean baseline of 16.5 ± 2.4 nmol/L to 10.0 ± 1.3 nmol/L *2634*
Testosterone, Free *Serum Decrease Physiological* In 11 healthy men treatment with 300 mg intramuscularly weekly for 6 weeks caused significant decrease of calculated free testosterone from mean baseline of 352.4 ± 60.4 pmol/L to 233.0 ± 31.6 pmol/L *2634*
Thyroxine Binding Globulin
Serum Decrease Physiological Anabolic effect *4433*
Volume *Plasma Decrease Physiological* May occur from 10 weeks onwards (anabolic effect) *530*

Naphazoline

Histamine *Plasma No Effect Analytical* 50% inhibition of radio-enzyme assay at 13 µg/mL but clinical significance of this unknown *2492*

Naphthalene

Bilirubin *Serum Increase Physiological* May cause hemolysis with G-6-PD deficiency *402*
Casts *Urine Increase Physiological* Nephrotoxic effect *2183*
Color *Urine Increase Analytical* Brown or black due to blood and hemoglobin *2183*
Erythrocytes *Blood Decrease Physiological* May cause hemolysis with G-6-PD deficiency *402*
Urine Increase Physiological Occurs occasionally following inhalation of vapor *2183*
Haptoglobin *Serum Decrease Physiological* May cause hemolysis *402*
Heinz Body Formation *Blood Positive Physiological* Early stage of hemolytic anemia *536*
Hematocrit *Blood Decrease Physiological* May cause hemolysis with G-6-PD deficiency *402*
Hemoglobin *Blood Decrease Physiological* Hemolysis in glucose-6-phosphate dehydrogenase deficiency or methemoglobin reductase deficiency may be caused by drug *2873* May cause hemolysis with G-6-PD deficiency *402*
Urine Increase Physiological Due to G-6-PD related hemolysis or poisoning *2183*
Leukocytes *Blood Increase Physiological* Leukocytosis may occur following ingestion *2183*
Methemoglobin *Blood Increase Physiological* May cause hemolysis with G-6-PD deficiency *6015*
α-Naphthol *Urine Positive Physiological* Present as metabolite *2183*
Protein *Urine Increase Physiological* Nephrotoxic effect *2183*

Naphthol

Color *Urine Increase Analytical* Dark color on standing *3810*

Naphthoxyacetic Acid

Platelets *Blood Decrease Physiological* Reported effect (AMA Blood dyscrasias committee) *4017*

Naproxen

Abnormal Erythrocytes *Blood Increase Physiological* Administration of naproxen has been reported to cause abnormal erythrocytes in fewer than 1% patients *6560*
Abnormal Leukocytes *Blood Increase Physiological* Administration of naproxen has been reported to cause abnormal leukocytes in fewer than 1% patients *6560*
Alanine Aminotransferase *Serum Increase Physiological* Incidence of acute liver injury of 3.8 per 100,000 treated patients with reported in United Kingdom. Liver damage among all cases primarily hepatocellular in some and primarily cholestatic in others *5049* In 6% of patients receiving drug for juvenile rheumatoid arthritis *386* Administration of naproxen has been reported to cause borderline increases in activity in up to 15% patients. Increases above three times the upper limit of normal occur in only about 1% of all patients, but severe hepatic reactions have also been reported including jaundice and fatal hepatitis *6560* Occasional cholestatic jaundice observed, most often in women, usually after several months of treatment *1384*
Serum No Effect Analytical At 5 times upper limit of therapeutic range on methods on Technicon SMAC® , Abbott-VP, Du pont aca, Roche Cobas-Bio, and KDA *3525*
Albumin *Serum No Effect Analytical* At 5 times upper limit of therapeutic range on methods on Technicon SMAC® , Kodak Ektachem® , Hitachi® 705 and KDA *3525*
Urine Increase Physiological Administration of naproxen has been associated with albuminuria in fewer than 1% patients *6560*
Aldosterone *Plasma No Effect Physiological* In 10 furosemide treated patients with well controlled congestive heart failure *1749*
Alkaline Phosphatase *Serum Increase Analytical* At 5 times upper limit of therapeutic range on methods on Technicon SMAC® *3525*
Serum Increase Physiological Administration of naproxen has been reported to cause severe hepatic reactions occasionally including jaundice and fatal hepatitis *6560*
Serum No Effect Analytical At 5 times upper limit of therapeutic range on methods on Abbott-VP, Du Pont aca, Roche Cobas-Bio, Hitachi® 705 and KDA *3525*
Amphetamine *Urine No Effect Analytical* Improbable interference reported with Syva EMIT procedure *6469*
Amylase *Serum Increase Physiological* Pancreatitis observed in less than 1% treated patients *5030*
Serum No Effect Analytical At 5 times upper limit of therapeutic range on methods on Du Pont aca, Roche Cobas-Bio and Kodak Ektachem® *3525*
Aspartate Aminotransferase *Serum Increase Physiological* Incidence of acute liver injury of 3.8 per 100,000 treated patients with reported in United Kingdom. Liver damage among all cases primarily hepatocellular in some and primarily cholestatic in others *5049* In 6% of patients receiving drug for juvenile rheumatoid arthritis *386* Administration of naproxen has been reported to cause borderline increases in activity in up to 15% patients. Increases above three times the upper limit of normal occur in only about 1% of all patients, but severe hepatic reactions have also been reported including jaundice and fatal hepatitis *6560* Occasional cholestatic jaundice observed, most often in women and after several months of treatment *1384*
Serum No Effect Analytical At 5 times upper limit of therapeutic range on methods on Technicon SMAC® , Abbott-VP, Du pont aca, Roche Cobas-Bio, Hitachi® 705 and KDA *3525*

Naproxen *(continued)*

Barbiturate *Urine Increase Analytical* Probable false positive result in urine of one patient who had ingested chronic doses of naproxen. Positive result not confirmed by GC/MS *5070*
Urine No Effect Analytical Improbable interference reported with Syva EMIT procedure *6469*

Benazepril *Serum No Effect Physiological* No clinically important pharmacokinetic interactions observed when drugs coadministered *1033*

Benzodiazepine *Urine No Effect Analytical* Improbable interference reported with Syva EMIT procedure *6469* No significant interference observed in urine of patients taking naproxen with new Syva EMIT assay *3370* No false positives in urines identified as being negative by Syva EMIT assay and Abbott TDx procedure as confirmed by GC/MS *5070*

Bicarbonate *Serum Increase Analytical* Falsely high value, linearly correlated with serum drug concentration with Technicon® RA-1000 ion-specific electrode *2483*

Bilirubin *Serum Increase Physiological* Isolated case of hemolytic anemia: one other case reported previously *2760* Occasional cholestatic jaundice observed, most often in women, after several months treatment *1384* Jaundice observed in less than 1% treated patients *5030*
Serum No Effect Analytical At 5 times upper limit of therapeutic range on methods on Technicon SMAC® , Du Pont aca, Roche Cobas-Bio, Kodak Ektachem® , Hitachi® 705 and KDA *3525*
Serum No Effect Physiological At pharmacological concentration has little or no protein displacement effect *6314*

Bilirubin, Conjugated *Serum No Effect Analytical* No effect at concentration of 600 mg/L on method on Kodak Ektachem® *5706*

Bilirubin, Unconjugated *Serum No Effect Analytical* No effect at concentration of 600 mg/L on method on Kodak Ektachem® *5706*

Bleeding Time *Patient Increase Physiological* Bleeding time may be increased in some treated patients *5030* Administration of naproxen has been reported to prolong bleeding time *6560* Like aspirin prolongs bleeding time *1384*

Blood *Urine Increase Physiological* Hematuria observed in less than 1% treated patients *5030* Administration of naproxen has been reported to cause acute interstitial nephritis with hematuria and proteinuria, but with occasionally nephrotic syndrome occurring *6560*

Calcium *Serum No Effect Analytical* At 5 times upper limit of therapeutic range on methods on Technicon SMAC® , Abbott-VP, Du Pont aca, Kodak Ektachem® , Hitachi® 705 and KDA *3525*

Cannabinoids *Urine No Effect Analytical* No effect on Roche Abuscreen method *5006* Improbable interference reported with Syva EMIT procedure *6469*

Chloride *Urine Decrease Physiological* Increase by 26% in 10 furosemide treated patients with well controlled congestive heart failure *1749*

Cholesterol *Serum Increase Physiological* Administration of naproxen has been associated with hypercholesterolemia in fewer than 1% patients *6560*
Serum No Effect Analytical At 5 times upper limit of therapeutic range on methods on Technicon SMAC® , Abbott-VP, Roche Cobas-Bio, Kodak Ektachem® , Hitachi® 705 and KDA *3525*

Chondrex *Serum No Effect Analytical* Concentrations up to 5 g/L had no significant effect on sandwich-type ELISA procedure of Harvey et al *2491*

Cortisol, Free *Urine No Effect Analytical* No significant interference observed with HPLC method of Turpeinen et al *6105*

C-Reactive Protein *Serum No Effect Physiological* In 93 patients with rheumatoid arthritis treatment for up to 20 weeks had no significant effect on concentration *1083*

Creatine Kinase *Serum No Effect Analytical* At 5 times upper limit of therapeutic range on methods on Technicon SMAC® , Abbott-VP, Du Pont aca, Roche Cobas-Bio and Hitachi® 705 *3525*

Creatinine *Serum Increase Physiological* Several cases reported in whom protracted use of naproxen was associated with renal failure *3597* Administration of naproxen has been reported to cause interstitial nephritis, nephrotic syndrome, renal disease, renal failure or renal papillary necrosis in fewer than 1% patients *6560* In isolated case of patient with arthritis in the absence of hypertension *715*
Serum No Effect Analytical No effect of concentrations up to 600 mg/L on 2-slide method on Kodak Ektachem® *5706* At 5 times upper limit of therapeutic range on methods on Technicon SMAC® , Abbott-VP, Du Pont aca, Roche Cobas-Bio, Kodak Ektachem® , Hitachi® 705 and KDA *3525*

Creatinine Clearance *Urine No Effect Physiological* When given for 14 d to patients with rheumatoid arthritis and heart failure *5889*

Cyclosporine *Blood No Effect Analytical* At a concentration of 1000 mg/L had no effect on Syva EMIT method *495*

Diflunisal *Serum No Effect Physiological* No significant effect observed on plasma concentration with coadministration *1384* Concomitant administration of diflunisal with naproxen had no effect on the plasma concentration of diflunisal *3972*

Drugs of Abuse Screen *Urine Increase Analytical* Probable false positive in one patient when measured by Syva EMIT d.a.u. screen, Roche Abuscreen and Abbott TDx but positivity not confirmed by GC/MS *5070*
Urine No Effect Analytical No effect at concentration of 100 µg/mL on EZ-SCREEN procedure for cannabinoids and cocaine *1739*

Eosinophils *Blood Increase Physiological* Administration of naproxen has been reported to cause eosinophilia in fewer than 1% patients *6560* Eosinophilia observed in less than 1% treated patients *5030* Hypersensitivity reaction in 3 women with pulmonary infiltrates: resolved when drug discontinued *826*

Erythrocyte Sedimentation Rate
Blood No Effect Physiological In 93 patients with rheumatoid arthritis treatment with naproxen for up to 20 weeks had no significant effect *1083*

Erythrocytes *Blood Decrease Physiological* In 4% of patients receiving drug for juvenile rheumatoid arthritis *386*

Glucose *Serum Increase Physiological* Administration of naproxen has been reported to cause hyperglycemia in more than 1% patients *6560*
Serum No Effect Analytical At 5 times upper limit of therapeutic range on methods on Technicon SMAC® , Abbott-VP, Du Pont aca, Roche Cobas-Bio, Kodak Ektachem® , Hitachi® 705 and KDA *3525*
Urine Increase Physiological Administration of naproxen has been associated with glycosuria in fewer than 1% patients *6560*

Glucose Tolerance *Serum Decrease Physiological* Administration of naproxen has been associated with decreased glucose tolerance in fewer than 1% patients *6560*

γ-Glutamyltransferase *Serum Increase Physiological* Administration of naproxen has been reported to cause severe hepatic reactions occasionally including jaundice and fatal hepatitis *6560*
Serum No Effect Analytical At 5 times upper limit of therapeutic range on methods on Technicon SMAC® , Abbott-VP, and Hitachi® 705 *3525*

Granulocytes *Blood Decrease Physiological* Agranulocytosis or granulocytopenia observed in less than 1% treated patients *5030* Administration of naproxen has been reported to cause agranulocytosis or granulocytopenia in fewer than 1% patients *6560*

Hematocrit *Blood Decrease Physiological* Aplastic or hemolytic anemia probably associated with drug administration observed in less than 1% treated patients *5030* Administration of naproxen has been reported to cause anemia in more than 1% patients *6560*

Hemoglobin *Blood Decrease Physiological* Isolated case of hemolytic anemia: one other case reported previously *2760* Aplastic or hemolytic anemia probably associated with drug administration observed in less than 1% treated patients *5030* Administration of naproxen has been reported to cause anemia in more than 1% patients *6560*
Urine Increase Physiological In 2% of patients receiving drug for juvenile rheumatoid arthritis *386*

Histamine *Plasma No Effect Analytical* No inhibition of radio-enzyme assay at concentrations twice physiological *2492*

19-Hydroxy-Prostaglandin E
Semen Decrease Physiological Significant effect but returned to prior level 1 week after treatment stopped *476*

19-Hydroxy-Prostaglandin F
Semen Decrease Physiological Significant effect but returned to prior level 1 week after treatment stopped *476*

17-Hydroxycorticosteroids *Urine No Effect Analytical* Administration of naproxen has been reported to have no effect on the apparent excretion of 17-OHCS *6560* No significant effect observed in analytical methods using Porter-Silber reaction *5030*

5-Hydroxyindoleacetic Acid *Urine Increase Analytical* Due to metabolite desmethylnaproxen on spectrophotometric assays but compound is thermolabile and can be destroyed by heat *6315* Apparently increased concentration observed in some methods *5030* Administration of naproxen has been reported to increase apparent excretion because of interference with some methods *6560*
Urine No Effect Analytical No effect observed with FPIA method on Abbott TDx *695*

Interleukin-6 *Serum No Effect Physiological* In 93 patients treated for up to 20 weeks with naproxen no significant effect observed on mean serum concentration *1083*

Iron *Serum No Effect Analytical* At 5 times upper limit of therapeutic range on Ferrozine method of Technicon SMAC® *3525*

6-Keto-Prostaglandin $F_{1\alpha}$ *Urine Decrease Physiological* Increase by 76% in 10 furosemide treated patients with well controlled congestive heart heart failure *1749*

17-Ketogenic Steroids *Urine Increase Analytical* Administration of naproxen has been reported to increase apparent excretion because of interaction between the drug and/or its metabolites with m-dinitrobenzene *6560* Apparently increased concentration observed in some methods because of interaction of naproxen with m-dinitrobenzene *5030*

Ketorolac *Serum No Effect Physiological* At therapeutic concentrations had no effect on ketorolac-protein binding *5035*

Lactate Dehydrogenase *Serum No Effect Analytical* At 5 times upper limit of therapeutic range on methods on Technicon SMAC® , Abbott-VP, Roche Cobas-Bio, Hitachi® 705 and KDA *3525*

Leukocytes *Blood Decrease Physiological* Administration of naproxen has been reported to cause leukopenia in fewer than 1% patients *6560* Leukopenia observed in less than 1% treated patients *5030*

Lipase *Serum Increase Physiological* Pancreatitis observed in less than 1% treated patients *5030*

Lithium *Serum Increase Physiological* Administration of 750 mg/d to 7 patients with median age of 60 years caused increase of serum lithium concentration by average of 16% but with marked individual variation from no increase to 42% increase *4831*

Nicardipine *Serum No Effect Physiological* Had no effect on plasma protein binding in vitro and presumed to have no effect on nicardipine concentration in vivo *5016*

Occult Blood *Feces Increase Physiological* Gastrointestinal hemorrhage or melena observed in less than 1% treated patients *5030* Administration of naproxen has been reported to cause gastric ulceration and bleeding occasionally *6560* Several cases of gastrointestinal bleeding reported to UK Committee on Safety of Medicines *1204*

pH *Blood Increase Physiological* Administration of naproxen has been associated with alkalosis in fewer than 1% patients *6560*

Phosphate *Serum Increase Analytical* At 5 times upper limit of therapeutic range on methods on Du Pont aca and Hitachi® 705 *3525*
Serum No Effect Analytical At 5 times upper limit of therapeutic range on methods on Technicon SMAC® and KDA *3525*

Platelet Aggregation *Blood Decrease Physiological* Like aspirin inhibits aggregation *1384* Effect less marked that observed with treatment with aspirin *3694* Administration of naproxen has been reported to decrease platelet aggregation *6560*

Platelets *Blood Decrease Physiological* Administration of naproxen has been reported to cause thrombocytopenia in fewer than 1% patients *6560* Thrombocytopenia observed in less than 1% treated patients *5030*

Potassium *Serum Decrease Physiological* Administration of naproxen has been associated with hypokalemia in fewer than 1% patients *6560*
Serum Increase Physiological Hyperkalemia observed in less than 1% treated patients *5030* Administration of naproxen has been reported to cause hyperkalemia in fewer than 1% patients *6560*

Prostaglandin E *Semen Decrease Physiological* Significant effect but returned to prior level 1 week after treatment stopped *476*

Prostaglandin F *Semen Decrease Physiological* Significant effect but returned to prior level 1 week after treatment stopped *476*

Prostaglandin $F_{2\alpha}$ *Urine Decrease Physiological* When given for 14 d to patients with rheumatoid arthritis and heart failure. Marked effect *5889*

Prostaglandins *Urine Decrease Physiological* When given for 14 d days to patients with rheumatoid arthritis and heart failure. Marked effect *5889*
Urine No Effect Physiological In 11 volunteers in randomized trial *698*

Protein *Serum No Effect Analytical* At 5 times upper limit of therapeutic range on methods on Technicon SMAC® , Abbott-VP, Kodak Ektachem® , Hitachi® 705 and KDA *3525*
Urine Increase Physiological In isolated case of patient with arthritis in the absence of hypertension *715* Administration of naproxen has been reported to cause acute interstitial nephritis with hematuria and proteinuria, but with occasionally nephrotic syndrome occurring *6560* Several cases reported in whom several months treatment caused renal failure *3597*

Renin Activity *Plasma Decrease Physiological* When given for 14 d to patients with rheumatoid arthritis and heart failure. Marked effect *5889*
Plasma No Effect Physiological In 10 furosemide treated patients with well controlled congestive heart failure *1749*

Reticulocytes *Blood Increase Physiological* Isolated case of hemolytic anemia: one other case reported previously *2760*

Sodium *Urine Decrease Physiological* Increase by 26% in 10 furosemide treated patients with well controlled congestive heart failure *1749*

Sperm Count *Semen No Effect Physiological* No change with treatment although prostaglandin concentration reduced *476*

Sperm Motility *Semen No Effect Physiological* No change with treatment although prostaglandin concentration reduced *476*

Thromboxane B_2 *Urine Decrease Physiological* In 11 volunteers in randomized trial *698*

Thyroid Stimulating Hormone
Serum No Effect Physiological In 12 individuals treated with a mean dose of 927 mg/d for at least 3 weeks mean concentration of 2.0 ± 0.3 mU/L not significantly different from 1.5 ± 0.2 mU/L in 22 controls *585*

Thyroxine (T4) *Serum No Effect Analytical* Using the Ciba-Corning ACS:180 analyzer mean concentration not significantly changed in 1 specimen whose concentration differed by +8% compared with the concentration measured by the Amerlex-M method *5621*
Serum No Effect Physiological In 12 individuals treated with a mean dose of 927 mg/d for at least 3 weeks mean concentration of 93 ± 3 nmol/L not significantly different from 94 ± 4 nmol/L in 22 controls *585*

Thyroxine (T4) Index, Free *Serum No Effect Physiological* In 12 individuals treated with a mean dose of 927 mg/d for at least 3 weeks mean FTI of 96 ± 5 not significantly different from 93 ± 4 in 22 controls *585*

Tri-iodothyronine (T3) *Serum Decrease Physiological* In 12 individuals treated with a mean dose of 927 mg/d for at least 3 weeks mean concentration of 1.7 ± 0.1 nmol/L significantly less than 2.0 ± 0.1 nmol/L in 22 controls *585*

Triglycerides *Serum Decrease Analytical* At 5 times upper limit of therapeutic range on enzymatic method on Technicon SMAC® *3525*
Serum No Effect Analytical At 5 times upper limit of therapeutic range on methods on Abbott-VP, Kodak Ektachem® , Hitachi® 705 and KDA *3525*

Naproxen *(continued)*

Urea Nitrogen *Serum Increase Physiological* Administration of naproxen has been reported to cause interstitial nephritis, nephrotic syndrome, renal disease, renal failure or renal papillary necrosis in fewer than 1% patients *6560*
Serum No Effect Analytical At 5 times upper limit of therapeutic range on methods on Technicon SMAC®, Abbott-VP, Roche Cobas-Bio, Kodak Ektachem®, Hitachi® 705 and KDA *3525*

Uric Acid *Serum Increase Analytical* At 5 times upper limit of therapeutic range on method on Hitachi® 705 *3525*
Serum Increase Physiological Administration of naproxen has been associated with hyperuricemia in fewer than 1% patients *6560*
Serum No Effect Analytical At 5 times upper limit of therapeutic range on methods on Technicon SMAC®, Abbott-VP, Du Pont aca, Kodak Ektachem® and KDA *3525*

Volume *Urine Decrease Physiological* Increase by 19% in 10 furosemide treated patients with well controlled congestive heart failure *1749*

Zidovudine *Serum No Effect Physiological* In 12 HIV-positive men coadministration of naproxen with zidovudine had no significant effect on zidovudine pharmacokinetics *5185*

Zinc *Serum No Effect Physiological* Mean increase of 35% in 10 healthy volunteers receiving 250 mg 3 times per day for 1 week, but mechanism not known *1719*
Urine Increase Physiological Mean increase of 35% in 10 healthy volunteers receiving 250 mg 3 times per day for 1 week, but mechanism not known *1719*

Narcotic Antagonists

Prothrombin Time *Plasma Increase Physiological* Reported enhancement of anticoagulant activity *2452*

Narcotics

Amylase *Serum Increase Physiological* Cause spasm of sphincter of Oddi *189*

Aspartate Aminotransferase *Serum Increase Physiological* Impaired excretion due to spasm of sphincter of Oddi *1009*

Basal Metabolic Rate *Patient Decrease Physiological* Metabolic effect of drugs *3669*

BSP Retention *Serum Increase Physiological* Impaired excretion because of spasm of sphincter of Oddi *1009*

Creatine Kinase *Serum Increase Physiological* Response to i.m. injections *403*

Glucose *Serum Increase Physiological* May be rare insignificant increases *2452*

Immunoglobulin G *Serum Increase Physiological* Often elevated in addicts (?liver problem) *3282*

Immunoglobulin M *Serum Increase Physiological* Frequently elevated in addicts (?liver problem) *3282*

Lipase *Serum Increase Physiological* Impaired excretion because of spasm of sphincter of Oddi *1009*

Lymphocytes *Blood Increase Physiological* Frequent absolute and relative increase in addicts *3282*

Prothrombin Time *Plasma Increase Physiological* Prolonged use may have effect *2753*

N-Desmethyldiazepam

Benzodiazepine *Urine Positive Analytical* Positive result observed at a concentration of 2.0 µg/mL (7.41 µmol/L) with method on Du Pont aca *1556*

N-Dimethyldiazepam

Albumin *Serum No Effect Analytical* At concentration of 6 mg/L had no effect on BCG method *5704*

Bicarbonate *Serum No Effect Analytical* At concentration of 6 mg/L had no effect on method using phenolphthalein *5704*

Bilirubin *Serum No Effect Analytical* At concentration of 6 mg/L had no effect on Jendrassik and Grof method *5704*

Calcium *Serum No Effect Analytical* At concentration of 6 mg/L had no effect on cresolphthalein method *5704*

Chloride *Serum No Effect Analytical* At concentration of 6 mg/L had no effect on mercurimetric method *5704*

Cholesterol *Serum No Effect Analytical* At concentration of 6 mg/L had no effect on Liebermann-Burchard method *5704*

Creatinine *Serum No Effect Analytical* At concentration of 6 mg/L had no effect on Technicon AutoAnalyzer® Jaffe method *5704*

Phosphate *Serum No Effect Analytical* At concentration of 6 mg/L had no effect on phosphomolybdate method *5704*

Protein *Serum No Effect Analytical* At concentration of 6 mg/L had no effect on biuret method with blank correction *5704*

Triglycerides *Serum No Effect Analytical* At concentration of 6 mg/L had no effect on lipase/esterase method *5704*

Urea Nitrogen *Serum No Effect Analytical* At concentration of 6 mg/L had no effect on diacetylmonoxime method *5704*

Uric Acid *Serum No Effect Analytical* At concentration of 6 mg/L had no effect on phosphotungstate reduction method *5704*

Nedocromil

Amino-terminal Propeptide of Type I Procollagen
Serum No Effect Physiological In 14 prepubertal children with newly detected perennial asthma mean baseline concentration of 13.8 nmol/L when first treated with budesonide for 6 months with significant reduction in concentration, rose to 13.2 nmol/L after 6 months treatment with 4 mg t.i.d. inhaled nedocromil *5719*

Amino-terminal Propeptide of Type III Procollagen
Serum No Effect Physiological In 14 prepubertal children with newly detected perennial asthma mean baseline concentration of 1.22 nmol/L when first treated with budesonide for 6 months with significant reduction in concentration, rose to 1.26 nmol/L after 6 months treatment with 4 mg t.i.d. inhaled nedocromil *5719*

C-terminal Propeptide of Type I Collagen
Serum No Effect Physiological In 14 prepubertal children with newly detected perennial asthma mean baseline concentration of 3.2 nmol/L first treated with budesonide for 6 months with significant reduction in concentration rose to 2.9 nmol/L after 6 months treatment with 4 mg t.i.d. inhaled nedocromil *5719*

Dipyridinoline *Urine No Effect Physiological* In 14 prepubertal children with newly detected perennial asthma mean baseline concentration of 18.4 nmol/mmol creatinine when first treated with budesonide for 6 months with significant reduction in excretion, rose to 19.3 nmol/mmol creatinine after 6 months treatment with 4 mg t.i.d. inhaled nedocromil *5719*

Osteocalcin *Serum Increase Physiological* In 14 prepubertal children with newly detected perennial asthma mean baseline concentration of 11.5 µg/L when first treated with budesonide for 6 months with significant reduction in concentration, rose to 21 µg/L after 6 months treatment with 4 mg t.i.d. inhaled nedocromil *5719*

Pyridinoline *Urine No Effect Physiological* In 14 prepubertal children with newly detected perennial asthma mean baseline concentration of 150 nmol/mmol creatinine when first treated with budesonide for 6 months with significant reduction in concentration, rose to 132 nmol/mmol creatinine after 6 months treatment with 4 mg t.i.d. inhaled nedocromil *5719*

Type I Collagen Cross-linked N-telopeptide
Urine No Effect Physiological In 14 prepubertal children with newly detected perennial asthma mean baseline concentration of 532 nmol/mmol creatinine when first treated with budesonide for 6 months with significant reduction in concentration rose to 578 nmol/mmol creatinine after 6 months treatment with 4 mg t.i.d. inhaled nedocromil *5719*

Nefazodone

Alanine Aminotransferase *Serum Increase Physiological* Administration of nefazodone was associated with infrequent increases of ALT activity *729*

Alprazolam *Serum Increase Physiological* By inhibiting CYP 3A inefazodone may cause a significant increase in alprazolam concentration *4685* Administration of 200 mg nefazodone twice daily to individuals dosed with 1 mg alprazolam caused mean concentration of alprazolam to increase approximately twofold *2316*

Aspartate Aminotransferase *Serum Increase Physiological* Administration of nefazodone was associated with infrequent increases of AST activity *729*

Cholesterol *Serum Increase Physiological* Administration of nefazodone was associated with rare increases of cholesterol concentration *729*

Cimetidine *Serum No Effect Physiological* When nefazodone coadministered with cimetidine no significant effect observed on the concentrations of nefazodone or its principal metabolite hydroxynefazodone *363* Coadministration of nefazodone 200 mg b.i.d. with 300 mg q.i.d. cimetadine for 1 week had no effect on the concentration of either drug *729*

Digoxin *Serum Increase Physiological* In 18 healthy male volunteers phenotyped as P450IID6 extensive metabolizers coadministration of nefazodone 200 mg b.i.d. with 0.2 mg q.i.d. digoxin for 9 days caused a 29% increase in the maximum concentration of digoxin *729*
Serum No Effect Physiological In 18 healthy male volunteers treatment with 400 mg/d nefazodone together with 0.2 mg/d digoxin for 8 days caused increases of digoxin concentration of from 15% to 29% *1454*

Glucose *Serum Decrease Physiological* Administration of nefazodone was associated with rare decreases of plasma glucose concentration *729*

Haloperidol *Serum Increase Physiological* Administration of 5 mg haloperidol to individuals dosed with nefazodone to steady state led to a moderate pharmacokinetic interaction with increases of 36%, 13% and 37% respectively in mean AUC, highest concentration and 12 h concentration of haloperidol *365*

Lactate Dehydrogenase *Serum Increase Physiological* Administration of nefazodone was associated with infrequent increases of lactate dehydrogenase activity *729*

Lorazepam *Serum No Effect Physiological* Administration of 200 mg nefazodone twice daily to individuals dosed with 2 mg lorazepam had no effect on the steady state pharmacokinetics of lorazepam *2317*

Propranolol *Serum Increase Physiological* In 18 healthy male volunteers phenotyped as P450IID6 extensive metabolizers coadministration of nefazodone 200 mg b.i.d. with 40 mg b.i.d. propranolol for 5.5 days caused a 30% decrease in the maximum concentration of propranolol and a 14% reduction in the concentration of 4-hydroxypropranolol *729*

Triazolam *Serum Increase Physiological* Administration of 200 mg nefazodone twice daily to individuals dosed with triazolam caused mean concentration of triazolam to increase from 2.33 ng/mL to 3.88 ng/mL primarily to the inhibition of cytochrome P450 3A4 metabolism by nefazodone *364*

Nelfinavir

Alanine Aminotransferase *Serum Increase Physiological* Increased activity observed in in fewer than 10% treated patients, but occurring at least twice as often as in control individuals *1891* Administration of nelfinavir caused an increase in the plasma activity of alanine aminotransferase in less than 2% of all patients receiving the drug *66*

Alkaline Phosphatase *Serum Increase Physiological* Administration of nelfinavir caused an increase in the plasma activity of alkaline phosphatase in less than 2% of all patients receiving the drug *66*

Amylase *Serum Increase Physiological* Administration of nelfinavir caused an increase in the plasma activity of amylase in less than 2% of all patients receiving the drug *66*

Aspartate Aminotransferase *Serum Increase Physiological* Increased activity observed in in fewer than 10% treated patients, but occurring at least twice as often as in control individuals *1891* Administration of nelfinavir caused an increase in the plasma activity of aspartate aminotransferase in less than 2% of all patients receiving the drug *66*

Creatine Kinase *Serum Increase Physiological* Administration of nelfinavir caused an increase in the plasma activity of creatine kinase in less than 2% of all patients receiving the drug *66*

Ethinyl Estradiol *Serum Decrease Physiological* Coadministration of OVOCON-35 (oral contraceptive) with nelfinavir caused a 47% decrease in the plasma concentration of ethinyl estradiol *66* Decreases area under the concentration curve by 47% when nelfinavir coadministered *1891*

Glucose *Serum Decrease Physiological* Administration of nelfinavir caused an decrease in the plasma concentration of glucose in less than 2% of all patients receiving the drug *66*
Serum Increase Physiological Increased concentration observed in in fewer than 10% treated patients, but occurring at least twice as often as in control individuals *1891*

γ-Glutamyltransferase *Serum Increase Physiological* Administration of nelfinavir caused an increase in the plasma activity of γ-glutamyltransferase in less than 2% of all patients receiving the drug *66*

Hemoglobin *Blood Decrease Physiological* Administration of nelfinavir caused an decrease in the blood hemoglobin concentration in less than 2% of all patients receiving the drug *66*

Indinavir *Serum Increase Physiological* Causes a 51% increase in area under the concentration curve when nelfinavir coadministered *1891* Coadministration of indinavir with nelfinavir caused a 51% increase in AUC of indinavir *66*

Lactate Dehydrogenase *Serum Increase Physiological* Administration of nelfinavir caused an increase in the plasma activity of lactate dehydrogenase in less than 2% of all patients receiving the drug *66*

Lamivudine *Serum Increase Physiological* Increases area under the concentration curve by 10% when nelfinavir coadministered *1891*
Serum No Effect Physiological Coadministration of lamivudine with nelfinavir had no effect on the pharmacokinetics of either drug *66*

Lymphocytes *Blood Decrease Physiological* Administration of nelfinavir caused an decrease in the blood lymphocyte concentration in less than 2% of all patients receiving the drug *66*

Neutrophils *Blood Decrease Physiological* Administration of nelfinavir caused an decrease in the blood neutrophil concentration in less than 2% of all patients receiving the drug *66*

Norethindrone *Serum Decrease Physiological* Decreases area under the concentration curve by 18% when nelfinavir coadministered *1891* Coadministration of OVOCON-35 (oral contraceptive) with nelfinavir caused a 18% decrease in the plasma concentration of norethindrone *66*

Rifabutin *Serum Increase Physiological* Increases area under the concentration curve by 207% when nelfinavir coadministered *1891* Coadministration of rifabutin with nelfinavir caused a 207% increase in the plasma AUC of rifabutin *66*

Ritonavir *Serum Increase Physiological* Increases area under the concentration curve by 9% when nelfinavir coadministered *1891*
Serum No Effect Physiological Coadministration of ritonavir with nelfinavir caused an insignificant increase in AUC of ritonavir *66*

Saquinavir *Serum Increase Physiological* Increases the area under the concentration curve by 392% when nelfinavir coadministered *1891* Coadministration of saquinavir with nelfinavir caused a 392% increase in AUC of saquinavir *66*

Stavudine *Serum No Effect Physiological* Coadministration of stavudine with nelfinavir had no effect on the pharmacokinetics of either drug *66* Has no effect on the concentration curve when nelfinavir coadministered *1891*

Terfenadine *Serum Increase Physiological* Coadministration of Nelfinavir with terfenadine caused unchanged terfenadine to appear in plasma *66*

Uric Acid *Serum Increase Physiological* Administration of nelfinavir caused an increase in the plasma concentration of uric acid in less than 2% of all patients receiving the drug *66*

Zidovudine *Serum Decrease Physiological* Decreases area under the concentration curve by 35% when nelfinavir coadministered *1891* Coadministration of zidovudine with nelfinavir caused a 35% decrease in plasma AUC of zidovudine, not necessitating an alteration in dosage *66*

Neo-Mull-Soy®

Amino Acids *Urine Increase Analytical* Reddish-pink spot with DL-methionine with ninhydrin on thin-layer chromatography *2109*

Methionine *Urine Increase Physiological* Contained in large amount in infant formula *2859*

Neoarsphenamine

Hemoglobin *Blood Decrease Physiological* May cause hemolysis *3094*

Neocinchophen

Sugar *Urine Increase Analytical* Affects Benedict's, Clinitest® tests *882*

Neomycin

Amikacin *Serum No Effect Analytical* Error of less than 5% observed when added at a concentration of 100 mg/L to a specimen containing 15 mg/L amikacin and measured on Baxter Stratus *5705* No interference observed at a concentration of 500 µg/mL (1032 µmol/L) with method on Du Pont aca *1508* No interference observed with method on Abbott TDx *3858*

Amino-4-Imidazole-5-Carboxamide Ribotide
Urine Increase Physiological If megaloblastic anemia develops *6370*

Amino Acids *Urine Increase Analytical* Reacts with ninhydrin; extra spot TLC, high voltage electrophoresis *4760* Purple spot with ninhydrin on thin-layer chromatography when combined with triamcinolone and nystatin in Kenacomb *2109*

Ammonia *Plasma Decrease Physiological* Reduces NH_3 producing bacteria in gastrointestinal tract *6529*
Urine Increase Physiological May occur if hypokalemia induced *1793*

Apolipoprotein A-I *Serum Decrease Physiological* In 9 healthy individuals treated with neomycin mean concentration decreased from 147 ± 14 mg/dL to 118 ± 9.8 mg/dL after 13 days and 120 ± 13 mg/dL after 42 days *2409*

Apolipoprotein B *Serum Decrease Physiological* In 9 healthy individuals treated with neomycin mean concentration decreased from 127 ± 23 mg/dL to 107 ± 16 mg/dL after 13 days and 99 ± 16 mg/dL after 42 days *2409*

Bile Acids *Feces Increase Physiological* Precipitates bile salts in gastrointestinal tract *1793*

Calcium *Feces Increase Physiological* Occurs independent of steatorrhea *1793*
Urine Decrease Physiological Occurs when fecal calcium increased *1793*

Carotene *Serum Decrease Physiological* Striking effect even if oral supplements *1793*

Casts *Urine Increase Physiological* Nephrotoxic effect *3810*

Chenodeoxycholic Acid *Feces Increase Physiological* Due to altered intestinal flora *1793*

Chloramphenicol *Serum No Effect Analytical* No effect at 100 mg/L on coupled enzymatic method *4122*

Cholesterol *Serum Decrease Physiological* Neomycin appears to perturb the formation of micelles of bile acids and neutral sterols leading to a significant loss of neutral sterols in the feces *5586* Forms salts with bile acids in gut *5869* Neomycin inhibits cholesterol absorption in man and also reduces serum concentration *3114* In 20 subjects with type II hyperlipoproteinemia given 2 g/d for 9 mo caused 15% decline in cholesterol *2656* In 9 healthy individuals treated with neomycin mean concentration decreased from 222 ± 34 mg/dL to 175 ± 24 mg/dL after 13 days and 168 ± 18 mg/dL after 42 days *2409* Marked effect over diet in 20 patients with type II hyperlipoproteinemia treated over several months *2656*

Cholic Acid *Feces Increase Physiological* Due to altered intestinal flora *1793*

Cholinesterase *Serum No Effect Analytical* No effect observed at concentration of 12 µg/mL with butyrylthiocholine method on Kodak Ektachem® *2504*

Creatinine *Serum Increase Physiological* Nephrotoxic effect *4691*
Serum No Effect Analytical No effect of concentrations up to 15 mg/L on single slide method on Kodak Ektachem® *5706*

Deoxycholic Acid *Feces Decrease Physiological* Due to alteration of intestinal flora *1793*

Digoxin *Serum Decrease Physiological* Oral neomycin appears to inhibit gastrointestinal absorption of digoxin *1384* Reduced absorption due to sprue-like syndrome *6403* At doses of 1-3 g decreased serum concentration and urinary excretion, also prolonged time to peak concentration. Gastrointestinal absorption decreased *3588* By decreasing intestinal digoxin absorption may decrease the digoxin concentration *2161* At doses of 3 g/d reduces bioavailability *4631*

Erythrocytes *Blood Decrease Physiological* Megaloblastic anemia (impaired vitamin B_{12} absorption) *6370*

Estriol *Urine Decrease Physiological* Possibly affects integrity of intestinal microflora *54*

Estriol-3-Glucuronide *Urine Decrease Physiological* Possibly affects integrity of intestinal microflora *54*

Estrogens *Urine Decrease Physiological* In pregnant women due to alteration of gut flora *4812*

Fat *Feces Increase Physiological* Alters intestinal villi, inhibits triglyceride hydrolysis *6486* Steatorrhea produced because of mucosal damage and rendering bile salts less available for fat absorption *5055*

Fatty Acids (FFA), Free *Serum Decrease Physiological* Probably related to altered fat absorption *1793*

5-Fluorouracil *Serum Decrease Physiological* Slight reduction observed when drugs coadministered due to reduction of absorption *780*

Gentamicin *Serum No Effect Analytical* No interference observed at concentrations up to 500 µg/mL (815 µmol/L) with method on Du Pont aca *1526* No interference observed with method on Abbott TDx *3858* Has cross-reactivity of less than 0.1% with method on Baxter Stratus *5705*

HDL-Cholesterol *Serum Decrease Physiological* In 9 healthy individuals treated with neomycin mean concentration decreased from 43 ± 5 mg/dL to 32 ± 4 mg/dL after 13 days and 33 ± 5 mg/dL after 42 days *2409*
Serum No Effect Physiological No significant effect in 20 patients with type II hyperlipoproteinemia treated over several months *2656* No significant effect in 20 type II hyperlipoproteinemic subjects given 2 g/d for 9 mo *2656* No significant effect usually observed *264*

Hematocrit *Blood Decrease Physiological* Megaloblastic anemia (impaired vitamin B_{12} absorption) *6370*

Hemoglobin *Blood Decrease Physiological* Megaloblastic anemia (impaired vitamin B_{12} absorption) *6370*

Kanamycin *Serum No Effect Analytical* No interference observed with method on Abbott TDx *3858*

Lactose Tolerance *Serum Decrease Physiological* Significantly lowered glucose response noted *1793*

LDL-Cholesterol *Serum Decrease Physiological* In 20 subjects with type II hyperlipoproteinemia given 2 g/d for 9 mo caused 16% decrease *2656* In 9 healthy individuals treated with neomycin mean concentration decreased from 162 ± 32 mg/dL to 128 ± 23 mg/dL after 13 days and 121 ± 23 mg/dL after 42 days *2409*

Leukocytes *Blood Decrease Physiological* If severe megaloblastic anemia *6370*

Lithocholic Acid *Feces Decrease Physiological* Due to alteration of intestinal flora *1793*

Magnesium *Serum Decrease Physiological* May be loss in stools due to steatorrhea *2242*

MCV *Blood Increase Physiological* If megaloblastic anemia develops *6370*

Nadolol *Serum Increase Physiological* Coadministration of neomycin with erythromycin orally together with oral nadolol caused approximate doubling of nadolol concentration with single dose: effect probably related to augmented bioavailability *1601*

Netilmicin *Serum No Effect Analytical* No interference observed with method on Abbott TDx *3858*

N-Formiminoglutamic Acid *Urine Increase Physiological* If megaloblastic anemia develops *6370*

Nitrogen *Feces Increase Physiological* Alters intestinal villi, inhibits triglyceride hydrolysis *6486*
Urine Decrease Physiological Due to reduced absorption of amino acids etc *1793*

Nonprotein Nitrogen *Serum Increase Physiological* Nephrotoxic effect *3810*

Penicillin *Serum Decrease Physiological* Decrease by 50% when given orally *2452* Serum concentration of penicillin V reduced due to inhibition of absorption *983* Oral neomycin observed to decrease gastrointestinal absorption of penicillin V *1384* Reduced absorption due to sprue-like syndrome *6403*

Phenylalanine *Plasma No Effect Analytical* No interference observed with rapid quantitative whole blood method of Campbell et al using phenylalanine dehydrogenase *867*

Platelets *Blood Decrease Physiological* If severe megaloblastic anemia *6370*

Potassium *Feces Increase Physiological* Induced by steatorrhea *1793*
Serum Decrease Physiological May occur with neomycin induced malabsorption *1793*

Protein *Urine Increase Physiological* Nephrotoxic effect *1714*

Prothrombin Time *Plasma Increase Physiological* Reduces availability of vitamin K *6119*

Sodium *Feces Increase Physiological* Induced by steatorrhea *1793*

Sterols *Feces Increase Physiological* Precipitates bile salts in gastrointestinal tract *1793*

Streptomycin *Serum No Effect Analytical* No interference observed with method on Abbott TDx *3858*

Thyroglobulin *Serum Decrease Physiological* Mean decrease from 17.3 to 11.7 ng/mL when given 2.0 g/d orally for 7 d *1602*

Thyroxine (T4) *Serum No Effect Physiological* When given 2.0 g/d orally for 7 d *1602*

Tobramycin *Serum No Effect Analytical* At concentrations less than 1000 µg/mL (1.63 mmol/L) no significant effect observed on method on Du Pont aca *1547* At a concentration of 1250 mg/L increased concentration by 15% when measured by method on Baxter Stratus but therapeutic concentration only up to 20 mg/L *5705* No interference observed with method on Abbott TDx *3858*

Tri-iodothyronine, Reverse (rT3)
Serum No Effect Physiological When given 2.0 g/d orally for 7 d *1602*

Tri-iodothyronine (T3) *Serum Decrease Physiological* Mean decrease from 104 to 92 ng/dL when given 2.0 g/d for 7 d orally *1602*

Triglycerides *Serum Decrease Physiological* In 9 healthy individuals treated with neomycin mean concentration decreased from 137 ± 49 mg/dL to 118 ± 38 mg/dL after 13 days and 94 ± 33 mg/dL after 42 days *2409* Consistent but insignificant decrease in concentration in 20 subjects with type II hyperlipoproteinemia given 2 g/d for 9 mo *2656*
Serum No Effect Physiological No effect in 20 patients with type II hyperlipoproteinemia treated over several months *2656*

Urea Nitrogen *Serum Increase Physiological* Nephrotoxic effect *1714*

Urobilinogen *Feces Decrease Physiological* Reduces flora in gastrointestinal tract *2451*
Urine Decrease Physiological Reduces flora in gastrointestinal tract *2451*

Vancomycin *Serum No Effect Analytical* No interference observed with method on Abbott TDx *3858*

Vanillylmandelic Acid *Urine No Effect Physiological* No effect on excretion observed *660*

Vitamin A *Serum Decrease Physiological* Probably related to reduced absorption bile salts *1793* Value lowered with bile acid sequestration but probably remains within normal range *5055* Reduced absorption due to sprue-like syndrome *6403*

Vitamin B_{12} *Serum Decrease Physiological* Reduced absorption due to sprue-like syndrome *6403* Impairs absorption *6370*
Urine Decrease Physiological With impaired absorption *6370*

VLDL-Cholesterol *Serum No Effect Physiological* No significant effect in 20 patients with type II hyperlipoproteinemia treated over several months *2656*

Xylose *Urine Decrease Physiological* Affects intestinal absorption with mucosal damage *2869*
Urine No Effect Physiological Single doses did not affect absorption of D-xylose *3588*

Neostigmine

Bicarbonate *Serum No Effect Analytical* Insignificant increase on method on Kodak Ektachem® but no effect on method on Beckman Astra® 8 *3233*

Bromide *Serum Increase Physiological* Theoretical possibility if bromide salt is administered since it contains 38% bromide *5116*

Chloride *Serum Increase Analytical* Significant effect on method on Kodak Ektachem® but without significant effect on method on Beckman Astra® 8 *3233*

Cholinesterase *Serum Decrease Physiological* Direct effect of drug *5900*
Test Conditions Decrease Analytical Inhibitory effect observed *4821*

Cholinesterase (True)
Red Blood Cells Decrease Physiological In healthy individuals administration of 0.036 mg/kg and 0.071 mg/kg caused significant decrease to 11.3 ± 1.2% and 11.4 ± 0.8% of baseline after 2 minutes but recovery to 43.2 ± 6.2% and 27.9 ± 2.9% respectively after 60 minutes *5197*

Histamine *Plasma No Effect Analytical* Probably no inhibition of radio-enzyme assay at physiological concentrations *2492*

Midazolam *Serum No Effect Analytical* On GC-ECD method of Ha et al *2387*

Neridronate

Deoxypyridinoline *Urine Decrease Physiological* In 6 postmenopausal women treated with 400 mg/d neridronate for 4 weeks caused significant reduction from mean baseline of 17.7 ± 4.7 nmol/mmol creatinine to 14.9 ± 6.9 nmol/mmol creatinine after 1 week, 10.5 ± 5.5 nmol/mmol creatinine after 2 weeks and 8.6 ± 4.2 nmol/mmol creatinine after 4 weeks *6043*

Deoxypyridinoline, Free *Urine Decrease Physiological* In 6 postmenopausal women treated with 400 mg/d neridronate for 4 weeks caused a nonsignificant reduction from mean baseline of 5.7 ± 1.5 nmol/mmol creatinine to 5.4 ± 1.7 nmol/mmol creatinine after 1 week, 4.4 ± 1.7 nmol/mmol creatinine after 2 weeks and 4.2 ± 1.7 nmol/mmol creatinine after 4 weeks *6043*

Deoxypyridinoline, Peptide-bound
Urine Decrease Physiological In 6 postmenopausal women treated with 400 mg/d neridronate for 4 weeks caused significant reduction from mean baseline of 12.1 ± 3.4 nmol/mmol creatinine to 9.6 ± 5.5 nmol/mmol creatinine after 1 week, 6.2 ± 4.0 nmol/mmol creatinine after 2 weeks and 4.4 ± 2.6 nmol/mmol creatinine after 4 weeks *6043*

Pyridinoline *Urine Decrease Physiological* In 6 postmenopausal women treated with 400 mg/d neridronate for 4 weeks caused nonsignificant reduction from mean baseline of 59.1 ± 13.3 nmol/mmol creatinine to 57.5 ± 22.3 nmol/mmol creatinine after 1 week, 50.4 ± 22.2 nmol/mmol creatinine after 2 weeks and 43.3 ± 14.2 nmol/mmol creatinine after 4 weeks *6043*

Pyridinoline, Free *Urine Decrease Physiological* In 6 postmenopausal women treated with 400 mg/d neridronate for 4 weeks caused nonsignificant reduction from mean baseline of 19.2 ± 4.1 nmol/mmol creatinine to 18.7 ± 5.5 nmol/mmol creatinine after 1 week, 16.9 ± 5.5 nmol/mmol creatinine after 2 weeks and 14.7 ± 5.4 nmol/mmol creatinine after 4 weeks *6043*

Pyridinoline, Peptide-bound *Urine Decrease Physiological* In 6 postmenopausal women treated with 400 mg/d neridronate for 4 weeks caused nonsignificant reduction from mean baseline of 39.9 ± 9.9 nmol/mmol creatinine to 38.8 ± 18.3 nmol/mmol creatinine after 1 week, 33.5 ± 17.1 nmol/mmol creatinine after 2 weeks and 28.5 ± 9.7 nmol/mmol creatinine after 4 weeks *6043*

Netilmicin

Alanine Aminotransferase *Serum Increase Physiological* Adverse hepatic effects observed in 15 of 100 treated patients *5334*

Alkaline Phosphatase *Serum Increase Physiological* Adverse hepatic effects observed in 15 of 100 treated patients *5334*

Amikacin *Serum No Effect Analytical* No interference observed with method on Abbott TDx *3858* No interference observed at a concentration of 100 µg/mL (210 µmol/L) with method on Du Pont aca *1508*

Aspartate Aminotransferase *Serum Increase Physiological* Adverse hepatic effects observed in 15 of 100 treated patients *5334*

Bilirubin *Serum Increase Physiological* Adverse hepatic effects observed in 15 of 100 treated patients *5334*
Serum No Effect Analytical No effect at 1000 mg/L on Ames Seralyzer method *5706*

Casts *Urine Increase Physiological* Adverse renal effects observed in 7 of 100 treated patients *5334*

Cells *Urine Increase Physiological* Adverse renal effects observed in 7 of 100 treated patients *5334*

Cholesterol *Serum No Effect Analytical* No effect at 1000 mg/L on Ames Seralyzer method *5706*

Creatine Kinase *Serum No Effect Analytical* No effect at 1000 mg/L on method on Ames Seralyzer *5706*

Creatinine *Serum Increase Physiological* Observed in one of 60 cancer patients receiving drug q.d. and in 3 receiving drug t.i.d *6175 6176* Adverse renal effects observed in 7 of 100 treated patients *5334* 44% increase on average in elderly population with initial clearance of 81 mL/min (increase significant) *1971*
Serum No Effect Analytical No effect at therapeutic concentration on Jaffe procedure on Beckman Astra® and Technicon SMAC® *1181* No effect at 1000 mg/L on method on Ames Seralyzer *5706*

Creatinine Clearance *Urine Decrease Physiological* Adverse renal effects observed in 7 of 100 treated patients *5334*

Eosinophils *Blood Increase Physiological* Eosinophilia observed in 4 of 100 treated patients *5334*

Gentamicin *Serum Increase Analytical* Specimens containing netilmicin showed 45.2% cross-reactivity when gentamicin measured by method on Bayer Technicon Immuno 1® system, invalidating the use of the method for such specimens *426* Significant cross-reactivity observed with method on Du Pont aca *1526* Interferes with method on Abbott TDx *3858*

Glucose *Serum No Effect Analytical* No effect at 1000 mg/L on glucose oxidase method on Ames Seralyzer *5706*
Urine No Effect Analytical On Clinitest®, Diastix® and TesTape® at physiological concentrations *4538*

Hematocrit *Blood Decrease Physiological* Side effect observed in fewer than 1 per 1000 treated patients *5334*

Hemoglobin *Blood Decrease Physiological* Side effect observed in fewer than 1 per 1000 treated patients *5334*

Immature Leukocytes *Blood Decrease Physiological* Side effect observed in fewer than 1 per 1000 treated patients *5334*

Kanamycin *Serum No Effect Analytical* No interference observed with method on Abbott TDx *3858*

Lactate Dehydrogenase *Serum No Effect Analytical* No effect at 1000 mg/L on method on Ames Seralyzer *5706*

Leukocytes *Blood Decrease Physiological* Side effect observed in fewer than 1 per 1000 treated patients *5334*

Mycophenolic Acid *Serum No Effect Analytical* No significant interference observed with HPLC method of Shipkova et al *5526*

Mycophenolic Acid Glucuronide
Serum No Effect Analytical No significant interference observed with HPLC method of Shipkova et al *5526*

Neomycin *Serum No Effect Analytical* No interference observed with method on Abbott TDx *3858*

Platelets *Blood Decrease Physiological* Side effect observed in fewer than 1 per 1000 treated patients *5334*
Blood Increase Physiological Thrombocytosis observed in 2 of 100 treated patients *5334*

Potassium *Serum Increase Physiological* Side effect observed in fewer than 1 per 1000 treated patients *5334*

Protein *Urine Increase Physiological* Adverse renal effects observed in 7 of 100 treated patients *5334*

Prothrombin Time *Plasma Increase Physiological* Prolonged prothrombin time observed in 1 of 1000 treated patients *5334*

Streptomycin *Serum No Effect Analytical* No interference observed with method on Abbott TDx *3858*

Tacrolimus *Blood No Effect Analytical* No significant effect observed at a concentration of 10 mg/L with MEIA method on Abbott IMx analyzer *1871*
Serum No Effect Analytical No significant effect of netilmicin at a concentration of 10 mg/L on ELISA method *6329*

Theophylline *Serum No Effect Analytical* No effect at 11 mg/L on method on Ames Seralyzer *5706*

Thyroxine (T4) *Serum No Effect Physiological* No effect when given i.v. with cloxacillin *1602*

Tobramycin *Serum No Effect Analytical* No significant effect observed with method on Du Pont aca at concentrations less than 100 µg/mL (210 µmol/L) *1547* No detectable cross-reactivity of observed with tobramycin method on Bayer Technicon Immuno 1® *435* No interference observed with method on Abbott TDx *3858*

Tri-iodothyronine, Reverse (rT3)
Serum No Effect Physiological No effect when given i.v. with cloxacillin *1602*

Tri-iodothyronine (T3) *Serum Decrease Physiological* Mean decrease from 114 ng/dL to 75 ng/dL when combined with cloxacillin given i.v., probably because of increased clearance. Free T3 proportion increased *1602*

Urea Nitrogen *Serum Increase Physiological* About 2 mg/dL increase in elderly patients with initial poor renal function *1971* Adverse renal effects observed in 7 of 100 treated patients *5334*
Serum No Effect Analytical No effect at 1000 mg/L on method on Ames Seralyzer *5706*

Vancomycin *Serum No Effect Analytical* No significant interference observed at a concentration of 100 µg/mL (210 µmol/L) with method on Du Pont aca *1561* No interference observed with method on Abbott TDx *3858*

Neuroleptics

Interleukin-1β *Serum Decrease Physiological* In 20 schizophrenics treated for 5 - 6 weeks with neuroleptics IL-1β concentration decreased nonsignificantly from mean concentration of 100.6 ± 45.7 pg/mL to 80.3 ± 32.6 pg/mL *3063*

Interleukin-6 *Serum Decrease Physiological* In 104 previously medicated schizophrenics mean concentration of 0.60 ± 1.02 pg/mL not significantly less than 1.04 ± 1.07 pg/mL in 24 neuroleptic naive schizophrenics *2022*

Oxytocin *Cerebrospinal Fluid No Effect Physiological* In 20 schizophrenics treated with neuroleptics mean concentration 10.58 ± 4.23 pg/mL not significantly different from 8.05 ± 4.46 pg/mL in 31 neuroleptic free schizophrenics *2189*

Neuromuscular Relaxants

Carbon Dioxide Partial Pressure
Blood Decrease Physiological Secondary to hyperventilation postoperatively *2242*

Cholinesterase *Serum Decrease Physiological* If enzyme deficiency may cause toxicity *2242*

Potassium *Serum Decrease Physiological* If potassium deficiency potentiates effect *2242*

Neutral Red

Chromosomes *Test Conditions Abnormal Physiological* Clastogenic in human cells *5484*

Nevirapine

Alanine Aminotransferase *Serum Increase Physiological* Increase of activity to above 250 U/L described in 3.4% treated patients, similar to 3.5% in control population *5134*

Aspartate Aminotransferase *Serum Increase Physiological* Increase of activity to above 250 U/L described in 2.0% treated patients, similar to 2.4% in control population *5134*

Bilirubin *Serum Increase Physiological* Increase of activity to above 2.5 mg/dL described in 0.4% treated patients, similar to 1.2% in control population *5134*

γ-Glutamyltransferase *Serum Increase Physiological* Increase of activity to above 450 U/L described in 2.4% treated patients, similar to 1.2% in control population *5134*

Hemoglobin *Blood Decrease Physiological* Decrease of blood hemoglobin to below 8.0 g/dL described in 1.2% treated patients, compared with incidence of 2.0% in control population *5134*

Indinavir *Serum Decrease Physiological* Causes a 28% decrease in area under the concentration curve when nevirapine coadministered *1891*

Neutrophils *Blood Decrease Physiological* Decrease of neutrophil count to below 750 /μL described in 11.1% treated patients, similar to 10.2% in control population *5134*

Platelets *Blood Decrease Physiological* Decrease of platelet count to below 50,000 /μL described in 0.8% treated patients, no different from control population *5134*

Ritonavir *Serum No Effect Physiological* Has no effect on the area under the concentration curve when nevirapine coadministered *1891*

Saquinavir *Serum Decrease Physiological* The area under the concentration curve decreased by 27% when nevirapine coadministered *1891*

Niacin

Alanine Aminotransferase *Serum Increase Physiological* In 7 of 14 patients receiving sustained release niacin reversible hepatitis developed although no cases of hepatitis observed in those taking R-niacin *2554* Cases of severe hepatic toxicity, including fulminant hepatic necrosis, have occurred in patients who have substituted sustained-release niacin products for immediate-release (crystalline) niacin at equivalent doses *3253* In 39 patients with hypercholesterolemia treatment with 1 g/d caused increase of 104.1% after 4 weeks and 45.2% after 8 weeks following 3.5% reduction after 2 weeks *1271* Large doses may produce liver damage *1384* Intrahepatic cholestasis observed rarely *2056* Occasionally abnormal liver function reported following treatment and on rare occasions toxic hepatitis may occur *5586* 5 cases of reversible hepatitis reported following low dose (e.g. 2 g daily for several weeks) sustained-release niacin *1764*

Serum No Effect Analytical No effect at therapeutic concentration on Boehringer Mannheim Reflotron method *3231* No effect up to 400 mg/L on Boehringer Mannheim Reflotron method but above this concentration inhibition of enzyme activity although not of clinical significance since normal concentration 4-10 mg/L *5706*

Albumin *Serum Decrease Physiological* Decreased synthesis due to liver damage *5365*

Aldolase *Serum Increase Physiological* Rare cases of rhabdomyolysis reported in patients receiving more than 1 g/d of niacin with HMG-CoA inductase inhibitors *3253*

Alkaline Phosphatase *Serum Increase Physiological* May cause impairment of hepatic function *4508* Cases of severe hepatic toxicity, including fulminant hepatic necrosis, have occurred in patients who have substituted sustained-release niacin products for immediate-release (crystalline) niacin at equivalent doses *3253* 5 cases of low-dose (about 2 g/d for several weeks) sustained-release niacin-induced hepatitis reported which resolved on withdrawal of therapy *1764*

Amylase *Serum Increase Physiological* Increased activity observed in some patients *3253*

Serum No Effect Analytical At a concentration of 400 mg/L had no effect on method on Boehringer Mannheim Reflotron system *5706*

Amylase, Pancreatic Isoenzyme

Serum No Effect Analytical No significant effect observed at toxic concentration of 100 mg/L on method on Boehringer Mannheim Reflotron *3647*

Apolipoprotein A-I *Serum Increase Physiological* Increase by 12% in 34 hypercholesterolemic individuals with 1.5 g/d for 1 mo then 3.0 g/d up to 6 mo *3205* Decreased catabolism *264*

Serum No Effect Analytical At a concentration of 20 mmol/L no significant effect observed on automated immunoturbidimetric method on Baxter Paramax analyzer *3005*

Apolipoprotein A-II *Serum Decrease Physiological* Decreased synthesis *264*

Serum No Effect Physiological In 34 hypercholesterolemic individuals with 1.5 g/d for 1 mo, then 3.0 g/d up to 6 mo *3205*

Apolipoprotein B *Serum Decrease Physiological* Highly significant reduction of concentration in 24 hyperlipoproteinemic patients treated with 4 g daily for 6 weeks *6297*

Serum No Effect Analytical At a concentration of 20 mmol/L no significant effect observed on automated immunoturbidimetric method on Baxter Paramax analyzer *3005*

Apolipoprotein C-I *Serum Decrease Physiological* Highly significant reduction observed in 24 patients with hyperlipoproteinemia treated with 4 g daily for 6 weeks *6297*

Apolipoprotein C-II *Serum Decrease Physiological* Highly significant reduction observed in 24 patients with hyperlipoproteinemia treated with 4 g daily for 6 weeks *6297*

Apolipoprotein C-III *Serum Decrease Physiological* Highly significant reduction in 24 patients with hyperlipoproteinemia treated with 4 g daily for 6 weeks *6297*

Apolipoprotein E *Serum Decrease Physiological* Highly significant reduction observed in 24 patients with hyperlipoproteinemia treated with 4 g daily for 6 weeks *6297*

Aspartate Aminotransferase *Serum Increase Physiological* In 39 patients with hypercholesterolemia treatment with 1 g/d caused increase of 3.3% after 2 weeks and significant increases of 63.8% after 4 weeks and 30.8% after 8 weeks *1271* Cases of severe hepatic toxicity, including fulminant hepatic necrosis, have occurred in patients who have substituted sustained-release niacin products for immediate-release (crystalline) niacin at equivalent doses *3253* Intrahepatic cholestasis observed rarely *2056* Reversible hepatitis developed in 7 of 14 patients receiving sustained release niacin compared with none in patients taking R-niacin *2554* 5 cases reversible hepatitis reported following treatment for hypercholesterolemia with low dose (about 2 g/d for several weeks) sustained-release niacin *1764* Abnormal liver function may occur in response to treatment and even toxic hepatitis may occur *5586* Large doses may produce liver damage *1384*

Serum No Effect Analytical No effect at therapeutic concentration on Boehringer Mannheim Reflotron method *3231* At up to 400 mg/L no effect on Boehringer Mannheim Reflotron method but above this concentration decreased enzyme activity. However, this is of no clinical significance since normal concentration is 4-10 mg/L *5706*

Bile *Urine Increase Physiological* May be impaired hepatic function *3810*

Bilirubin *Serum Increase Physiological* May cause impairment of hepatic function *4508* 7 of 14 patients receiving sustained release niacin developed reversible hepatitis although no cases observed in patients taking R-niacin *2554* Cases of severe hepatic toxicity, including fulminant hepatic necrosis, have occurred in patients who have substituted sustained-release niacin products for immediate-release (crystalline) niacin at equivalent doses *3253* 5 cases reported of reversible hepatitis reported following low-dose (about 2 g/d) sustained-release niacin for several weeks *1764*

Serum No Effect Analytical At concentration of 400 mg/L no effect on method on Boehringer Mannheim Reflotron system *5706*

BSP Retention *Serum Increase Physiological* Liver function impairment, ?competition for conjugated *4508*

Serum No Effect Physiological Usual unless liver previously damaged *2658*

Catecholamines *Plasma Increase Analytical* Occurs with large doses, interfering fluorescence *2451* Niacin administration may produce falsely increased test results with some fluorometric methods *3253*

Niacin *(continued)*

Catecholamines *(continued)*

Urine Increase Analytical Niacin administration may produce falsely increased test results with some fluorometric methods *3253* May produce interfering fluorescence *2452*

Cholesterol *Serum Decrease Physiological* In 13 dyslipidemic noninsulin dependent diabetics treated with 4.5 g daily for 8 weeks mean concentration decreased by 24% *2033* In 47 nontransplant dyslipidemic patients and in 17 heart transplant dyslipidemic patients treatment with an average dose of 2.5 g/d caused mean decrease of 17% per gram of niacin in nontransplant patients and 32% in heart transplant recipients *2554* In 39 patients with hypercholesterolemia treatment with nicotinic acid 1 g/d caused 4.8% decrease after 2 weeks, 15.8% decrease after 4 weeks and 11.3% decrease after 8 weeks *1271* When 4 g given daily for 6 weeks to 41 weight-stable patients with type IIa, type IIb or type IV hyperlipoproteinemia reduction from mean concentration of 8.37 mmol/L to 6.58 mmol/L *6298* Therapeutic goal (rebound increase when discontinued) *5869* Concentration typically reduced by 15-20% in patients with combined hyperlipidemias when treated with 2-8 g/d *5586* In 14 patients with type II hyperlipidemia treatment with 3 g/d for 2 months caused reduction from mean of 7.30 ± 0.56 mmol/L to 6.00 ± 0.24 mmol/L (16.3%) *5427*

Serum No Effect Analytical No effect at therapeutic concentration on Boehringer Mannheim Reflotron method *3231* No effect at concentrations up to 1000 mg/L on method on Kodak Ektachem® *5706* No effect at concentration of 400 mg/L on method on Boehringer Mannheim Reflotron system *5706*

Cortisol *Plasma No Effect Analytical* At concentration of 100 mg/L no significant effect observed on CEDIA method (worst case 92.7% recovery). At a concentration of 400 mg/L had no significant effect on Enzymun method (recoveries 95.4% and 95.7% on female and male sera respectively) *1097*

Plasma No Effect Physiological No effect either if patient is fed or starved *1019*

Creatine Kinase *Serum Increase Physiological* In 39 patients with hypercholesterolemia treatment with 1 g/d caused increase of 0.7% after 2 weeks and significant increases of 25.8% after 4 weeks and 19.8% after 8 weeks *1271* Rare cases of rhabdomyolysis reported in patients receiving more than 1 g/d of niacin with HMG-CoA inductase inhibitors *3253*

Diagnex Blue Excretion *Urine Increase Physiological* Displaces diagnex blue from resin *6515*

Eosinophils *Blood Decrease Physiological* By up to 60% in 2 h, increased after 24 h *2658*

Fatty Acids (FFA), Free *Serum Decrease Physiological* In 6 healthy individuals infusion of nicotinic acid at a rate of 2.8 mg/min for 4 hours caused a decrease from a mean of about 550 μmol/L to 250 μmol/L after 60 minutes with a continuing decrease to 150 μmol/L at 4 hours *3389* Marked reduction observed due to suppression of lipolysis in adipose tissue *878* Marked fall then progressive secondary rise *2831*

Fibrinolytic Time *Plasma Increase Physiological* Significant effect if given parenterally *658*

Fluvastatin *Serum No Effect Physiological* Administration of niacin with fluvastatin to patients with hypercholesterolemia had no effect on the metabolism and excretion of fluvastatin *5232*

Glucagon *Plasma No Effect Physiological* No significant change observed in 5 healthy individuals after infusion of 2.8 mg/min for 4 hours *3389*

Glucose *Serum Decrease Physiological* In 6 healthy individuals infusion of 2.8 mg/min for 4 hours had no effect at 60 minutes but a mean decrease of 6% after 120 minutes and 12% after 4 hours *3389*

Serum Increase Physiological Mean increase of 16% observed in 13 dyslipidemic noninsulin dependent diabetics treated with 4.5 g/d for 8 weeks *2033* Diabetic patients may experience a dose related increase in glucose intolerance *3253* Mechanism not discussed *2242*

Serum No Effect Analytical At concentration of 400 mg/L no effect on method on Boehringer Mannheim Reflotron system *5706* No effect at therapeutic concentration on Boehringer Mannheim Reflotron method *3231*

Urine Increase Analytical Niacin administration may produce falsely increased test results with methods using Benedicts' reagent *3253*

Urine Increase Physiological Due to hyperglycemia *2056* As result of hyperglycemia *2242* Diabetic patients may experience a dose related increase in glucose intolerance *3253*

Glucose Tolerance *Serum Decrease Physiological* Reduced tolerance observed in diabetics *3669* Major drawback of treatment with niacin in patients with hyperlipidemias *5586* Glucose intolerance may be aggravated as important side-effect *878* Large doses may impair glucose tolerance *1384*

Serum Increase Physiological Increases glucose disappearance after i.v. glucose tolerance test *1260*

γ-Glutamyltransferase *Serum Increase Physiological* Cases of severe hepatic toxicity, including fulminant hepatic necrosis, have occurred in patients who have substituted sustained-release niacin products for immediate-release (crystalline) niacin at equivalent doses *3253*

Serum No Effect Analytical At concentration of 400 mg/L no effect on method on Boehringer Mannheim Reflotron system *5706* No effect at therapeutic concentration on Boehringer Mannheim Reflotron method *3231*

Glycine *Urine Decrease Physiological* 2 g causes 30% decrease at 2 h *2658*

Growth Hormone *Plasma Increase Physiological* Produced by fall in free fatty acids *2831*

HDL_2-Cholesterol *Serum Increase Physiological* Mean increase of 135% in 41 weight-stable patients with type IIa, type IIb or type IV hyperlipoproteinemia when treated with 4 g daily for 6 weeks *6298* Increase by 36% in 34 hypercholesterolemic individuals with 1.5 g/d for 1 mo then 3.0 g/d up to 6 mo *3205*

HDL_{2b}-Cholesterol *Serum Increase Physiological* Increase observed in 23 hyperlipidemic patients given 4 g/d for 6 weeks almost entirely due to increase in the HDL_{2b} fraction: significant inverse correlation with VLDL-triglyceride concentration observed both before and after treatment *2947*

HDL_3-Cholesterol *Serum Increase Physiological* Increase by 35% in 34 hypercholesterolemic individuals with 1.5 g/d for 1 mo then 3.0 g/d up to 6 mo *3205*

Serum No Effect Physiological No significant effect in 41 weight-stable patients with type IIa, type IIb or type IV hyperlipoproteinemia when treated with 4 g daily for 6 weeks *6298*

HDL_{3b}-Cholesterol *Serum Decrease Physiological* 25% reduction observed in 23 hyperlipidemic patients given 4 g/d for 6 weeks *2947*

HDL_{3c}-Cholesterol *Serum Decrease Physiological* 25% reduction observed in concentration in 23 hyperlipidemic patients given 4 g/d for 6 weeks *2947*

HDL-Cholesterol *Serum Increase Physiological* In 14 patients with type II hyperlipidemia treatment with 3 g/d for 2 months caused significant increase from mean baseline of 1.15 ± 0.10 mmol/L to 1.55 ± 0.11 mmol/L (37.3%) *5427* Slight effect observed in 31 patients with hypertriglyceridemia *6053* In 37 middle-aged men with low HDL concentration treatment with 4.5 g/d caused significant 30% increase *6219* Mean increase of 37% in 41 weight-stable patients with type IIa, type IIb or type IV hyperlipoproteinemia when treated with 4 g daily for 6 weeks *6298* Significant increase observed as result of therapy *878* Increase by 26% in 34 hypercholesterolemic individuals with 1.5 g/d for 1 mo then 3.0 g/d up to 6 mo *3205* Expected increase observed in 23 hyperlipidemic patients given 4 g/d for 6 weeks: actual increase of 45% *2947* In 83% of 65 dyslipidemic patients an average dose of 2.5 g/d caused mean 12% increase per gram of niacin *2554* Decreased apo A-I catabolism and decreased apo A-II synthesis. Increased activity of lipoprotein lipase *264* Mean increase of 34% observed in 13 dyslipidemic noninsulin dependent diabetics treated with 4.5 g/d for 8 weeks *2033* In 39 patients with hypercholesterolemia treatment with nicotinic acid 1 g/d caused increase of 4.9% after 2 weeks, 2.5% after 4 weeks and 12.2% after 8 weeks *1271*

Hemoglobin *Plasma No Effect Physiological* No effect observed with increased blood flow *2868*

Hemoglobin A_{1c} *Blood Increase Physiological* Mean increase of 21% observed in 13 dyslipidemic noninsulin dependent diabetics treated for 8 weeks with 4.5 g/d *2033*

Hydrochloric Acid *Gastric Fluid Increase Physiological* Increase up to 230% in patients after 0.5 g orally *168*

Insulin *Plasma Decrease Physiological* In 5 healthy individuals after infusion of 2.8 mg/min for 4 hours mean significant decrease of 40% observed *3389*
Plasma Increase Physiological ?response to increased glucose output *2056*

Ketones *Urine Increase Physiological* ?due to hepatic mobilization of ketogenic amino acids *2056*

LDL-Cholesterol *Serum Decrease Physiological* In 14 patients with type II hyperlipidemia treatment with 3 g/d for 2 months caused mean concentration of 5.45 ± 0.63 mmol/L to decrease to 4.16 ± 0.28 mmol/L (23.7% reduction) *5427* Concentration typically reduced by 20% or more in patients with combined hyperlipidemias when treated with 2-8 g/d *5586* Increase by 21% in 34 hypercholesterolemic individuals with 1.5 g/d for 1 mo then 3.0 g/d up to 6 mo *3205* Reduction from mean concentration of 5.92 mmol/L to 3.94 mmol/L in 41 weight-stable patients with type IIa, type IIb or type IV hyperlipoproteinemia when treated with 4 g daily for 6 weeks *6298* Highly significant reduction in concentration in 24 hyperlipoproteinemic patients treated with 4 g daily for 6 weeks *6297* Expected reduction observed in 23 hyperlipidemic patients given 4 g/d for 6 weeks *2947* With 3-5 weeks treatment reduction observed. Reduction of the order of 10-15% is the consequence of the decrease of VLDL *878* In 39 patients with hypercholesterolemia treatment with nicotinic acid 1 g/d caused reduction of 7.5% after 2 weeks, 21.1% after 4 weeks and 16.1% after 8 weeks *1271* Mean reduction of 15% observed in 13 dyslipidemic noninsulin dependent diabetics treated with 4.5 g/d for 8 weeks *2033* In 17 dyslipidemic heart transplant recipients avreage dose of 2.5 g/d caused mean decrease of 19% and in 47 non transplant dyslipidemic patients the same dose caused mean decrease of 14% per gram niacin *2554*
Serum No Effect Physiological In 37 middle-aged men with low HDL treated with 4.5 g/d no significant effect observed *6219*

LDL-Triglycerides *Serum Decrease Physiological* Reduction from mean concentration of 0.56 mmol/L to 0.36 mmol/L in 41 weight-stable patients with type IIa, type IIb or type IV hyperlipoproteinemia treated with 4 g daily for 6 weeks *6298* Marked reduction observed in 24 patients with hyperlipoproteinemia treated with 4 g daily for 6 weeks: positive correlation with reduction of serum apolipoprotein concentrations *6297*

Lipids *Serum Decrease Physiological* Prompt and sustained hypolipemic action *2754*

β-Lipoprotein *Serum Decrease Physiological* Chronic administration has slight effect *2242*

Lipoprotein Lp(a) *Serum Decrease Physiological* Unlike most lipid lowering agents high dose niacin may have marked effect on plasma concentration *5586* In 14 patients with type II hyperlipidemia treatment with 3 g/d for 2 months caused significant reduction of antilog of mean log values of 63.2 mg/dL to 38.3 mg/dL (36.4% reduction) *5427*

Lipoproteins, Pre-β *Serum Decrease Physiological* Therapeutic effect *2242*

Lymphocytes *Blood Decrease Physiological* By up to 20% in 2 h, ?normal at 24 h *2658* Significant effect with megadose supplementation *2245*

Neutrophils *Blood Increase Physiological* By up to 100% in 2 h, high at 24 h *2658*
Blood No Effect Physiological No effect with megadose supplementation *2245*

pH *Urine Decrease Physiological* Increases acidity at 4 h *2658*

Phosphate *Serum Decrease Physiological* Niacin administration has been associated with small but statistically significant transient reduction in phosphate concentration (mean 13% reduction with 2000 mg) *3253*

Phospholipids *Serum Decrease Physiological* Prompt and sustained hypolipemic action *2754*

Platelets *Blood Decrease Physiological* Niacin administration has been associated with small but statistically significant reduction in platelet counts (mean 11% reduction with 2000 mg) *3253*

Potassium *Urine Decrease Physiological* With 1 g, no change with 2 g *2658*

Pravastatin *Serum No Effect Physiological* Coadministration with pravastatin caused no significant effect on bioavailability of pravastatin *728*

Prothrombin Time *Plasma Increase Physiological* Niacin administration has been associated with small but statistically significant increase in prothrombin time (mean 4% increase with 2000 mg) *3253* Due to hepatocellular and obstructive liver damage *5365*

Sodium *Urine Increase Physiological* 20% increase at 4 h after 2 g *2658*

Sugar *Urine Increase Analytical* Interferes with Benedict's reagent *1714*

Triglycerides *Serum Decrease Physiological* In 39 patients with hypercholesterolemia treatment with nicotinic acid 1 g/d caused decrease of 3.6% after 2 weeks, 13.3% after 4 weeks and 11.4% after 8 weeks *1271* Concentration typically reduced by 30-40% in patients with combined hyperlipidemias when treated with 2-8 g/d *5586* In 14 patients with type II hyperlipidemia treatment with 3 g/d for 2 months caused significant reduction of mean from 1.51 ± 0.25 mmol/L to 0.87 ± 0.38 mmol/L (25.5%) *5427* Therapeutic intent *4543* Effect due to increased catabolism caused by increase in triglyceride fractional removal rate. Decreased hepatic synthesis also observed. Triglyceride concentration typically reduced 20-80% *878* Increase by 27% in 34 hypercholesterolemic individuals with 1.5 g/d for 1 mo then 3.0 g/d up to 6 mo *3205* Mean reduction of 45% observed in 13 dyslipidemic noninsulin dependent diabetics treated with 4.5 g/d for 8 weeks *2033* When 4 g given daily for 6 weeks to 41 weight-stable patients with type IIa, type IIb or type IV hyperlipoproteinemia reduction of mean concentration from 2.64 mmol/L to 1.48 mmol/L *6298*
Serum No Effect Analytical No effect at 400 mg/L on Boehringer Mannheim Reflotron method *5706* No effect at therapeutic concentration on Boehringer Mannheim Reflotron method *3231*

Urea Nitrogen *Serum No Effect Analytical* No effect at therapeutic concentration on Boehringer Mannheim Reflotron method *3231* No effect at 400 mg/L on Boehringer Mannheim Reflotron method *5706*

Uric Acid *Serum Increase Physiological* May rise by up to 1.5 mg/dL if large doses *4543* Observed as important side-effect of treatment *878* Large doses reported to increase serum concentration *1384* Serious side effect of treatment with niacin in patients with combined hyperlipidemias *5586* Hyperuricemia may occur with niacin therapy *3253*
Serum No Effect Analytical No effect at 400 mg/L on Boehringer Mannheim Reflotron method *5706* No effect at therapeutic concentration on Boehringer Reflotron method *3231*
Urine Decrease Physiological Decreases by approximately 50% *2056*

Uric Acid Clearance *Urine Decrease Physiological* Decreases by 75%, ?due to altered tubular handling *2056*

VLDL-Cholesterol *Serum Decrease Physiological* In 47 non transplant dyslipidemic patients administration of an average of 2.5 g/d caused mean decrease of 15% per gram of niacin and in 17 heart transplant dyslipidemic recipients the same dose caused mean decrease of 18% per gram niacin *2554* Expected reduction observed in 23 hyperlipidemic patients given 4 g daily for 6 weeks *2947* Reduction from mean concentration of 1.29 mmol/L to 0.48 mmol/L in 41 weight-stable patients with type IIa, type IIb or type IV hyperlipoproteinemia when treated with 4 g daily for 6 weeks *6298* In 47 non transplant dyslipidemic patients administration of an acerage of 2.5 g/d caused mean decrease of 15% per gram of niacin and in 17 heart transplant dyslipidemic recipients the same dose caused mean decrease of 18% per gram niacin *2554* Mean 58% reduction observed in 13 noninsulin dependent dyslipidemic diabetics treated with 4.5 g/d for 8 weeks *2033*

VLDL-Triglycerides *Serum Decrease Physiological* Concentration reduced with treatment. Triglyceride concentration reduced in proportion to the initial plasma concentration of VLDL *878* When 4 g given daily for 6 weeks to 41 weight-stable patients with type IIa, type IIb or type IV hyperlipoproteinemia reduction from mean basal concentration of 1.90 mmol/L to 0.77 mmol/L *6298*

Niacinamide

Alanine Aminotransferase *Serum Increase Physiological* Rare probable reversible toxic effect *6508* Large doses may produce liver damage *1384*

Alkaline Phosphatase *Serum Increase Physiological* Rare probable reversible toxic effect *6508*

Aspartate Aminotransferase *Serum Increase Physiological* Rare probable reversible toxic effect *6508* Large doses may produce liver damage *1384*

Bilirubin *Serum Increase Physiological* Rare probable reversible toxic effect *6508*

Bilirubin, Direct *Serum Increase Physiological* Rare probable reversible toxic effect *6508*

Cannabinoids *Urine No Effect Analytical* No effect on Roche Abuscreen method *5006*

Carbamazepine *Serum Increase Physiological* Drugs that inhibit CYP 3A4 inhibit metabolism of carbamazepine producing clinically meaningful effect *1039* Plasma concentration of carbamazepine may be increased with coadministration of drugs *3119* Large doses increase plasma concentrations in children *1384*

Cholesterol *Serum No Effect Analytical* At concentration of 40 mg/L had no effect on CHOD-Iodide method *5704* At concentration of 40 mg/L had no effect on CHOD-PAP method *5704* At concentration of 40 mg/L had no effect on Liebermann-Burchard method *5704* At concentration of 40 mg/L had no effect on catalase-AIDH method *5704* At concentration of 400 mg/L had no effect on catalase-Hantzsch reaction *5704*
Serum No Effect Physiological No effect observed in normals *2658*

Creatinine *Serum No Effect Analytical* At concentration of 120 mg/L had no effect on kinetic Jaffe method on BKA-2 *5704* At concentration of 40 mg/L had no effect on Jaffe-Fuller's earth method *5704* At concentration of 40 mg/L had no effect on Jaffe-Fading-Fraction method *5704*

Drugs of Abuse Screen *Urine No Effect Analytical* No effect at concentration of 100 µg/mL on EZ-SCREEN procedure for cannabinoids and cocaine *1739*

Eosinophils *Blood Decrease Physiological* No change after 2 h, marked at 4 h *2658*

Glucose *Serum No Effect Analytical* At concentration of 12 mg/L had no effect on Kodak Ektachem® method *5704*

Glucose Tolerance *Serum Decrease Physiological* Large doses may impair glucose tolerance *1384*

Glycine *Urine Increase Physiological* Increased up to 80% with 1 g at 4 h *2658*

Histamine *Plasma No Effect Analytical* Improbable inhibition of radio-enzyme assay at therapeutic concentrations *2492*

Leukocytes *Blood Increase Physiological* Marked elevation noted at 24 h *2658*

Lipids *Serum No Effect Physiological* No lowering effect observed *2242*

Lymphocytes *Blood Increase Physiological* Up by 25% at 4 h, 40% at 24 h *2658*

Neutrophils *Blood Increase Physiological* Up by 40% after 2 g at 4 h *2658*

pH *Urine Increase Physiological* Reduces acidity at 2-4 h *2658*

Potassium *Serum No Effect Analytical* At concentration of 120 mg/L had no effect on measurement by ISE without predilution *5704*
Urine Increase Physiological 1 g causes marked excretion *2658*

Protein Electrophoresis *Serum No Effect Analytical* At concentration of 120 mg/L had no effect on automated Olympus-Hite method *5704*

Prothrombin Time *Plasma Increase Physiological* Rare probable reversible toxic effect *6508*

Sodium *Serum No Effect Analytical* At concentration of 120 mg/L had no effect on measurement by ISE without predilution *5704*
Urine Increase Physiological 1 g causes up to 40% increase at 4 h *2658*

Urea Nitrogen *Serum No Effect Analytical* At concentration of 12 mg/L had no effect on Kodak Ektachem® method *5704*

Uric Acid *Serum Increase Physiological* Large doses reported to increase serum concentration *1384*
Serum No Effect Analytical At concentration of 40 mg/L had no effect on catalase-AIDH method *5704* At concentration of 40 mg/L had no effect on Kageyama-Hantzsch method *5704*
Urine Increase Physiological By up to 40% at 2 h maximum at 4 h *2658*

Nialamide

Alkaline Phosphatase *Serum Increase Physiological* Probable hypersensitive hepatitis *128*

Aspartate Aminotransferase *Serum Increase Physiological* Probable hypersensitive hepatitis *128*

Bile *Urine Increase Physiological* Probable hypersensitive hepatitis *128*

Bilirubin *Serum Increase Physiological* Probable hypersensitive hepatitis *128*

BSP Retention *Serum Increase Physiological* Hepatotoxic/cholestatic syndromes *2242*

Bufotenin *Urine Increase Physiological* In one man oral administration 300 mg or 1000 mg caused significant increase above mean baseline of 0.089 nmol/mmol creatinine, range 0.002-1.78 nmol/mmol creatinine. Maximum excretion 16.5 nmol/mmol creatinine and maximum urinary output 495 nmol/d *3046*

Glucose *Serum Decrease Physiological* May prolong action of insulin in diabetics *4014*

Leukocytes *Blood Decrease Physiological* Leukopenia reported *128*

Phenylketones *Urine Positive Analytical* Fading green with $FeCl_3$, green with Phenistix® *1195*

Urea Nitrogen *Test Conditions Increase Analytical* Bilious yellow-green with Berthelot's reagent *3144*

Vanillylmandelic Acid *Urine Decrease Physiological* Effect observed in schizophrenics *4014*

Nicardipine

Alanine Aminotransferase *Serum Increase Physiological* Rare abnormalities of liver function tests observed *5016*

Albumin *Serum No Effect Physiological* In 9 patients with essential hypertension treated with nicardipine for 6 months baseline value of 41 ± 4 g/L not significantly changed to 42 ± 3 g/L *2237*

Aldosterone *Plasma Decrease Physiological* Significant reduction in hypertensive patients with initially high plasma renin activity within one month of starting treatment with 60 mg/day *5458*
Plasma No Effect Physiological No significant effect observed in 18 mild to moderate hypertensives treated with drug for 2 months *5714* Nonsignificant increase in hypertensive patients with initially low/normal plasma renin activity with treatment with 60 mg/day for 3 months *5458*

Alkaline Phosphatase *Serum Increase Physiological* Rare abnormalities of liver function tests observed *5016*

Angiotensin-converting Enzyme
Serum Decrease Physiological Significant reduction in hypertensive patients with initially high plasma renin activity within one month of starting treatment with 60 mg/day *5458*
Serum Increase Physiological Significant effect observed in hypertensive patients with initially low/normal plasma renin activity within one month of starting treatment with 60 mg/day *5458*

Apolipoprotein A-I *Serum No Effect Physiological* No significant change observed in 9 type II diabetics with slight hypertension treated with nicardipine for 120 days *1780*

Apolipoprotein A-II *Serum No Effect Physiological* No significant effect observed in 9 type II diabetics with mild hypertension treated with nicardipine for 120 days *1780*

Apolipoprotein B *Serum No Effect Physiological* No significant change observed in 9 type II diabetics with slight hypertension treated with nicardipine for 120 days *1780*

Aspartate Aminotransferase *Serum Increase Physiological* Rare abnormalities of liver function tests observed *5016*

Bilirubin *Serum Increase Physiological* Rare abnormalities of liver function tests observed *5016*

Calcium *Serum No Effect Physiological* No significant change observed in 18 mild to moderate hypertensives treated with 60 mg/d drug for 2 months *5714*

Urine No Effect Physiological No significant effect observed with 60 mg/d for 2 months observed in 18 mild to moderate hypertensives *5714*

Carbamazepine *Serum Increase Physiological* Concomitant administration of calcium channel blockers with carbamazepine causes marked increase of plasma carbamazepine concentration resulting in toxicity in some cases *282*

Cholesterol *Serum No Effect Physiological* In 9 patients with essential hypertension treated with nicardipine for 6 months baseline value of 5.7 ± 0.8 mmol/L not significantly changed to 5.8 ± 1.3 mmol/L *2237* In 23 patients with mild to moderate hypertension treatment with up to 120 mg/d caused nonsignificant change from 5.10 ± 0.16 mmol/L to 5.29 ± 0.13 mmol/L after 12 weeks *6340* No significant change observed in 9 type II diabetics with mild hypertension treated with nicardipine for 120 days *1780* No significant effect observed in 18 mild to moderate hypertensives when treated with 60 mg/d for 2 months *5714*

C-Peptide *Plasma No Effect Physiological* No significant change observed in 23 patients with mild to moderate hypertension treated with up to 120 mg/d for 12 weeks from mean baseline of 761 ± 66 pmol/L to 695 ± 36 pmol/L after treatment *6340*

Creatinine *Serum Decrease Physiological* In 9 patients with essential hypertension treated with nicardipine for 6 months baseline value of 78 ± 18 µmol/L significantly changed to 69 ± 22 µmol/L *2237*

Serum No Effect Physiological No significant effect observed in 18 mild to moderate hypertensives when treated with 60 mg/d for 2 months *5714*

Urine No Effect Physiological No significant effect observed in 18 mild to moderate hypertensives when treated with 60 mg/d for 2 months *5714*

Creatinine Clearance *Urine No Effect Physiological* In 22 hypertensive patients given 60 mg daily for 3 months *5458*

Cyclosporine *Serum Increase Physiological* Doubling in concentration observed when two drugs coadministered due to inhibition of metabolism *672* Concentration reported to increase in 38 renal transplant patients. Concentration started to increase from 1 day to 1 month after treatment started, not always associated with changes in renal function *6596* May increase cyclosporine concentration by inhibiting hepatic cytochrome P-450 III A which metabolizes cyclosporine *5236* Increased concentration reported when drugs coadministered *1384* After introduction of nicardipine 20 mg three times daily blood cyclosporine concentration increased an average of 110% (range 24 to 341%) *5411* Doubling of concentration (trough levels) when added to therapeutic regime *6288*

Cyclosporine A *Blood Increase Physiological* Coadministration with cyclosporine A increases its concentration *5240* When administered concomitantly increases cyclosporine concentration *5016*

Blood No Effect Physiological Nicardipine administration has been shown not to increase cyclosporine concentration *6551*

Digoxin *Serum No Effect Physiological* When administered concomitantly does not usually affect digoxin concentration *5016* Addition of nicardipine for 5 days in 20 patients who had received digoxin for at least 3 weeks caused no significant change in concentration at 7 control times during 24-hour period *1335* Nicardipine administration has been shown not to affect digoxin concentration *6551* When two drugs coadministerd in two trials of patients with atrial fibrillation or congestive heart failure no significant effect on pharmacokinetics observed, except in one patient in whom the steady state concentration increased by 77%. Average increase in plasma steady state concentration 23% *5345*

Fibrinogen *Plasma No Effect Physiological* In 9 patients with essential hypertension treated with nicardipine for 6 months baseline value of 2.71 ± 1.05 g/L not significantly changed to 2.86 ± 1.03 g/L *2237*

Filtration Rate *Red Blood Cells No Effect Physiological* In 9 patients with essential hypertension treated with nicardipine for 6 months baseline value of 65 ± 9 µL/s not significantly changed to 57 ± 13 µL/s *2237*

Glomerular Filtration Rate *Urine Increase Physiological* Increase by 35% after 0.5 mg i.v. in 7 patients with mild to moderate hypertension *310*

Glucagon *Plasma No Effect Physiological* No significant effect in 10 healthy volunteers on basal concentration following 20 mg drug *5916*

Glucose *Serum Decrease Physiological* Incidence of 0.7% observed in French Pharmacovigilance database *4106*

Serum No Effect Physiological In 9 patients with essential hypertension treated with nicardipine for 6 months baseline value of 5.6 ± 0.7 mmol/L not significantly changed to 5.5 ± 0.8 mmol/L *2237* No significant effect observed in 18 mild to moderate hypertensives treated for 2 months with 60 mg/d *5714* No effect of 20 mg drug on basal concentration or on glucose tolerance following 75 g oral glucose in 10 healthy volunteers *5916* In 23 patients with mild to moderate hypertension treatment with up to 120 mg/d caused for 12 weks had no significant effect on conentration which was 5.9 ± 0.2 mmol/L before treatment and 5.9 ± 0.1 mmol/L after *6340* No significant change observed in fasting or postprandial glucose in 9 patients with type II diabetes and slight hypertension treated for 120 days with nicardipine *1780*

Glucose Tolerance *Serum No Effect Physiological* Tolerance largely unchanged in 42 patients at a dose of 60 or 120 mg/d for an average of 7.8 weeks *3135* In 23 patients with mild to moderate hypertension treatment with up to 120 mg/d for 12 weeks caused nonsignificant change in total area under the curve from 18.4 ± 1.0 mmol/L/h to 18.6 ± 0.9 mmol/L/h after an oral dose of 75 g. Change in insulin concentration equally small *6340*

γ-Glutamyltransferase *Serum Increase Physiological* Rare abnormalities of liver function tests observed *5016*

HDL-Cholesterol *Serum Increase Physiological* Significant increase observed in 42 patients when given 60 or 120 mg/d for an average of 7.8 weeks *3135* Significant increase in mild to moderate hypertensive patients given 30 mg t.i.d. for 2 years *4232*

Serum No Effect Physiological No significant change observed in 9 type II diabetics with mild hypertension treated with nicardipine for 120 days *1780* In 9 patients with essential hypertension treated with nicardipine for 6 months baseline value of 1.3 ± 0.1 mmol/L not significantly changed to 1.6 ± 0.5 mmol/L *2237* No significant effect observed in 18 mild to moderate hypertensives treated with 60 mg/d for 2 months *5714* In 23 patients with mild to moderate hypertension treatment with up to 120 mg/d for 12 weeks caused nonsignificant change from mean baseline of 1.21 ± 0.06 mmol/L to 1.25 ± 0.06 mmol/L *6340*

HDL-Triglycerides *Serum No Effect Physiological* In 23 patients with mild to moderate hypertension treatment with up to 120 mg/d caused no change from mean baseline of 0.18 ± 0.01 mmol/L *6340*

Hematocrit *Blood No Effect Physiological* In 9 patients with essential hypertension treated with nicardipine for 6 months baseline value of 0.42 ± 0.04 not significantly changed to 0.42 ± 0.03 *2237*

Hemoglobin A_{1c} *Blood Increase Physiological* In 9 patients with NIDDM and hypertension treatment with β-blockers caused mean concentration to increase by 0.29 ± 0.15% (nonsignificant) after 1 month, 0.56 ± 0.19% after 3 months and 0.80 ± 0.28% after 6 months *5276*

Blood No Effect Physiological No significant change observed in 9 patients with type II diabetes and mild hypertension treated with nicardipine for 120 days *1780* In 23 patients with mild to moderate hypertension treatment with up to 120 mg/d for 12 weeks caused nonsignificant change from 5.5 ± 0.2% to 5.7 ± 0.1% *6340*

Insulin *Plasma No Effect Physiological* Concentration largely unchanged in 42 patients treated with 60 or 120 mg/d for an average of 7.8 weeks *3135* No significant change observed in 9 patients with type II diabetes and mild hypertension treated with nicardipine for 120 days *1780* In 23 patients with mild to moderate hypertension treatment with up to 120 mg/d for 12 weeks caused nonsignificant reduction from baseline of 106 ± 1.9 pmol/L to 100 ± 9 pmol/L *6340* No significant effect on basal concentration following 20 mg drug in 10 healthy volunteers *5916*

Ketone Body Ratio *Serum No Effect Analytical* When added at a concentration of 20 mg/L had no significant effect on AKBR method of Uno et al *6131*

Nicardipine *(continued)*

LDL-Cholesterol *Serum No Effect Physiological* In 23 patients with mild to moderate hypertension treatment with up to 120 mg/d for 12 weeks caused nonsignificant change from mean baseline of 2.93 ± 0.16 mmol/L to 3.13 ± 0.13 mmol/L *6340*

LDL-Triglycerides *Serum No Effect Physiological* In 23 patients with mild to moderate hypertension treatment with up to 120 mg/d for 12 weeks caused nonsignificant increase from mean baseline of 0.36 ± 0.02 mmol/L to 0.37 ± 0.02 mmol/L *6340*

Magnesium *Serum No Effect Physiological* No significant effect observed in 18 mild to moderate hypertensives treated with 60 mg/d drug for 2 months *5714*
Urine No Effect Physiological No significant effect observed in 18 mild to moderate hypertensives when treated with 60 mg/d for 2 months *5714*

Norepinephrine *Plasma Increase Physiological* Increase in sympathetic tone soon after administration causes increase in concentration *2528*

PAH Clearance *Urine Increase Physiological* After 0.5 mg i.v. increased renal blood flow in 7 patients with mild to moderate hypertension by average of 27% *310*

Parathyroid Hormone *Plasma No Effect Physiological* No significant change observed in 18 mild to moderate hypertensives treated with drug for 2 months *5714*

Phosphate *Serum Decrease Physiological* Nicardipine administration has been shown to cause hypophosphatemia *6551*
Serum No Effect Physiological No significant change observed in 18 mild to moderate hypertensives when treated with 60 mg/d drug for 2 months *5714*
Urine No Effect Physiological No significant effect observed with 60 mg/d for 2 months in 18 mild to moderate hypertensives *5714*

Platelets *Blood Decrease Physiological* Nicardipine administration has been shown to cause thrombocytopenia *6551*

Potassium *Serum No Effect Physiological* In hypertensive patients with either high or low/normal plasma renin activity given 60 mg/day for 3 months *5458* No significant effect observed in 18 patients with mild to moderate hypertensives treated with 60 mg/d drug for 2 months *5714*
Urine No Effect Physiological In 22 hypertensive patients given 60 mg/day for 3 months *5458* No significant effect observed in 18 mild to moderate hypertensives when treated with 60 mg/d for 2 months *5714*

Propranolol *Serum Increase Physiological* Administration of a single dose of 30 mg nicardipine to 12 healthy volunteers after prior administration of 80 mg propranolol caused doubling of the area under the curve and the maximum concentration of propranolol *6229* Single oral dose of 30 mg in 12 healthy volunteers caused increase in area under curve and mean maximal concentration (from 73 to 131 µg/L) by impairing hepatic first-pass clearance *5374*

Renin Activity *Plasma Decrease Physiological* In hypertensive patients with initially high plasma renin activity. Significant change observed within one month of start of treatment with 60 mg/day *5458*
Plasma Increase Physiological In hypertensive patients with initially low/normal PRA. Significant change observed within one month of start of treatment with 60 mg/day *5458*
Plasma No Effect Physiological No significant effect observed in 18 mild to moderate hypertensives treated with drug for 2 months *5714*

Sodium *Serum Decrease Physiological* Significant reduction in hypertensive patients with high plasma renin activity, but not in those with low/normal plasma renin activity, given 60 mg/day. Effect noticeable within one month *5458*
Serum No Effect Physiological No significant effect observed in 18 mild to moderate hypertensives treated with 60 mg/d drug for 2 months *5714*
Urine Increase Physiological Increase by 56% after 0.5 mg i.v. in 7 patients with mild to moderate hypertension *310* In hypertensive patients with increased plasma renin activity within first month of treatment with 60 mg/day of drug *5458*
Urine No Effect Physiological No significant effect observed in 18 mild to moderate hypertensives when treated with 60 mg/d for 2 months *5714*

Tacrolimus *Serum Increase Analytical* In HPLC/MS method of Christians et al interference observed with measurement of FK 506 because of similar retention time *1010*
Serum Increase Physiological By inhibiting cytochrome P-450 IIIA enzyme systems may inhibit the metabolism of tacrolimus *1987*

Triglycerides *Serum Decrease Physiological* In association with nicardipine administration at a dose of 60 or 120 mg/d for average of 7.8 weeks significant decrease observed *3135*
Serum No Effect Physiological No significant change observed in 9 type II diabetics with slight hypertension treated with nicardipine for 120 days *1780* No significant effect observed in 18 mild to moderate hypertensives when treated with 60 mg/d for 2 months *5714* In 9 patients with essential hypertension treated with nicardipine for 6 months baseline value of 1.6 ± 0.6 mmol/L not significantly changed to 1.7 ± 0.7 mmol/L *2237* In 23 patients with mild to moderate hypertension treatment with up to 120 mg/d for 12 weeks caused nonsignificant increase from mean baseline of 1.42 ± 0.10 mmol/L to 1.55 ± 0.17 mmol/L *6340*

Viscosity *Blood Decrease Physiological* In 9 patients with essential hypertension treated with nicardipine for 6 months significant reduction observed over shear rate from 2.25 to 22.5 /s *2237*
Plasma No Effect Physiological In 9 patients with essential hypertension treated with nicardipine for 6 months no significant change over shear rate from 2.25 to 450 /s *2237*

VLDL-Cholesterol *Serum No Effect Physiological* In 23 patients with mild to moderate hypertension treatment with up to 120 mg/d for 12 weeks caused nonsignificant change from mean baseline of 1.01 ± 0.14 mmol/L to 0.90 ± 0.14 mmol/L *6340*

VLDL-Triglycerides *Serum No Effect Physiological* In 23 patients with mild to moderate hypertension treatment with up to 120 mg/d for 12 weeks caused nonsigignificant increase from mean baseline of 0.91 ± 0.09 mmol/L to 0.99 ± 0.15 mmol/L *6340*

Volume *Urine Increase Physiological* Significant increase in glomerular filtration rate in 22 hypertensives given 60 mg daily for 3 months associated with natriuresis *5458*
Urine No Effect Physiological No significant effect observed in 18 mild to moderate hypertensives when treated with 60 mg/d for 2 months *5714*

Nicergoline

Creatinine *Serum No Effect Analytical* At 10 mg/L on reversed phase liquid chromatographic procedure of Zhiri et al *6656*

Erythrocyte Deformability *Blood Decrease Physiological* Passing time of 1 mL and 2 mL significantly reduced at 8 weeks and passing volume in 10 and 20 seconds significantly reduced at 8 weeks also when 11 geriatric patients with cerebral infarction treated with 15 mg daily *4205*

Platelet Aggregation *Blood Decrease Physiological* Collagen, arichidonic acid and PAF-induced platelet aggregation significantly reduced in 11 geriatric patients with cerebral infarction when 15 mg nicergoline given daily for 8 weeks *4205*
Blood No Effect Physiological No significant effect observed on ADP-induced platelet aggregation in 11 patients with cerebral infarction treated with 15 mg daily for 8 weeks *4205*

Platelets *Blood No Effect Physiological* No significant effect observed in 11 geriatric patients with cerebral infarction treated with 15 mg daily for 8 weeks *4205*

Uric Acid *Serum No Effect Analytical* At 10 mg/L on reversed phase liquid chromatographic procedure of Zhiri et al *6656*

Viscosity *Plasma Decrease Physiological* Significant reduction of viscosity of EDTA plasma and citrated plasma after both 4 and 8 weeks treatment of 11 geriatric patients with cerebral infarction with 15 mg nicergoline daily *4205*

Niceritrol

Cholesterol *Serum Decrease Physiological* Significant reduction from 239 mg/dL to 213 mg/dL in group of type II diabetics treated with 750 mg daily for 4 weeks *5447*

Glucose *Serum Decrease Physiological* Significant reduction in type II diabetics when treated with 750 mg daily for 4 weeks (mean value of 154 mg/dL declined to 140 mg/dL) *5447*

Glucose Tolerance *Serum Increase Physiological* Significant improvement in type II diabetics treated with 750 mg daily for 4 weeks. Overall reduction of blood glucose associated with no significant change in total immunoreactive insulin *5447*

HDL-Cholesterol *Serum No Effect Physiological* No significant change in type II diabetics when treated with 750 mg daily for 4 weeks *5447*

Hemoglobin A_1 *Blood Decrease Physiological* Reduction of mean proportion from 9.2% to 8.1% in group of type II diabetics treated with 750 mg daily for 4 weeks *5447*

Lipoprotein Lp(a) *Serum Decrease Physiological* In 15 male patients with gout and Lp(a) concentration greater than 20 mg/dL treatment with 750 mg/d caused significant reduction from mean baseline of 42.5 ± 5.5 mg/dL to 35.8 ± 6.7 mg/dL after 1 month, 36.7 ± 6.8 mg/dL after 3 months and 33.3 ± 4.6 mg/dL after 5 months *5923*

Triglycerides *Serum Decrease Physiological* Significant reduction from mean of 217 mg/dL to 186 mg/dL in group of type II diabetics treated with 750 mg daily for 4 weeks *5447*

Nicotine Patch

Cotinine *Serum Decrease Physiological* In 24 smokers mean concentration while smoking and wearing 22 mg nicotine patch about 130 ng/mL, reached after 4 days, compared with 260 ng/mL while smoking and not wearing patch *2788*

Nicotine *Serum Decrease Physiological* In 24 smokers mean concentration while smoking and wearing 22 mg nicotine patch approximately 12 ng/mL compared with 25 ng/mL while smoking but without patch *2788*

Nicotinic Acid

Alkaline Phosphatase *Serum No Effect Physiological* In 15 normolipidemic men (cholesterol less than 6 mmol/L, triglycerides less than 2.75 mmol/L) treated with up to 3 g/d for 12 weeks mean activity changed nonsignificantly from baseline of 106.3 ± 48.8 U/L to 113.4 ± 70.6 U/L *3142*

Amylase, Pancreatic Isoenzyme
Serum No Effect Analytical No significant effect observed at toxic concentration of 100 mg/L on method on Boehringer Mannheim Reflotron *3647*

Apolipoprotein A-I *Serum Increase Physiological* Decreased catabolism *264* In 15 normolipidemic men (cholesterol less than 6 mmol/L, triglycerides less than 2.75 mmol/L) treated with up to 3 g/d for 12 weeks mean concentration increased significantly from baseline of 108.4 ± 22.9 mg/dL to 119.1 ± 27.2 mg/dL *3142*

Apolipoprotein A-II *Serum Decrease Physiological* Decreased synthesis *264*

Apolipoprotein B *Serum Decrease Physiological* In 15 normolipidemic men (cholesterol less than 6 mmol/L, triglycerides less than 2.75 mmol/L) treated with up to 3 g/d for 12 weeks mean concentration decreased significantly from baseline of 84.8 ± 23.1 mg/dL to 57.8 ± 14.1 mg/dL *3142*

Aspartate Aminotransferase *Serum Increase Physiological* In 15 normolipidemic men (cholesterol less than 6 mmol/L, triglycerides less than 2.75 mmol/L) treated with up to 3 g/d for 12 weeks mean activity changed significantly from baseline of 26.7 ± 9.5 U/L to 33.2 ± 11.7 U/L *3142*

Cholesterol *Serum Decrease Physiological* In 15 normolipidemic men (cholesterol less than 6 mmol/L, triglycerides less than 2.75 mmol/L) treated with up to 3 g/d for 12 weeks mean concentration decreased significantly from baseline of 4.97 ± 0.76 mmol/L to 4.26 ± 0.77 mmol/L *3142* In 13 dyslipidemic noninsulin dependent diabetics treated with 4.5 g daily for 8 weeks mean concentration decreased by 24% *2033* In the Stockholm Ischemic Heart Study of 555 myocardial infarction patients treatment with clofibrate and nicotinic acid caused mean decrease of 13% *3115* When 4 g given daily for 6 weeks to 41 weight-stable patients with type IIa, type IIb or type IV hyperlipoproteinemia reduction from mean concentration of 8.37 mmol/L to 6.58 mmol/L *6298*

C-Peptide *Plasma No Effect Physiological* In 12 healthy individuals treatment with up to 2 g/d caused a nonsignificant change from mean baseline of 0.57 ± 0.04 nmol/L to 0.59 ± 0.06 nmol/L on day 3, 0.61 ± 0.05 nmol/L on day 7 and 0.59 ± 0.05 nmol/L on day 14 *125*

Fatty Acids (FFA), Free *Serum Decrease Physiological* Marked reduction observed due to suppression of lipolysis in adipose tissue *878* In 12 healthy individuals treatment with up to 2 g/d caused a significant change from mean baseline of 0.66 ± 0.07 mmol/L to 0.41 ± 0.05 mmol/L on day 3, 0.44 ± 0.06 mmol/L on day 7 but an insignificant change to 0.61 ± 0.09 mmol/L on day 14 *125*

Glucagon *Plasma No Effect Physiological* In 12 healthy individuals treatment with up to 2 g/d caused a nonsignificant change from mean baseline of 187 ± 44 ng/L to 180 ± 48 ng/L on day 3, 192 ± 59 ng/L on day 7 and 181 ± 32 ng/L on day 14 *125*

Glucose *Serum Increase Physiological* Mean increase of 16% observed in 13 dyslipidemic noninsulin dependent diabetics treated with 4.5 g/d for 8 weeks *2033*
Serum No Effect Physiological In 15 normolipidemic men (cholesterol less than 6 mmol/L, triglycerides less than 2.75 mmol/L) treated with up to 3 g/d for 12 weeks mean concentration changed nonsignificantly from baseline of 5.23 ± 0.48 mmol/L to 5.44 ± 0.54 mmol/L *3142* In 12 healthy individuals treatment with up to 2 g/d caused a nonsignificant change from mean baseline of 4.57 ± 0.15 mmol/L to 4.77 ± 0.16 mmol/L on day 3, 4.60 ± 0.12 mmol/L on day 7 and 4.69 ± 0.15 mmol/L on day 14 *125*

Glucose Tolerance *Serum Decrease Physiological* Glucose intolerance may be aggravated as important side-effect *878*

HDL_2-Cholesterol *Serum Increase Physiological* Mean increase of 135% in 41 weight-stable patients with type IIa, type IIb or type IV hyperlipoproteinemia when treated with 4 g daily for 6 weeks *6298* Increase observed in 23 hyperlipidemic patients given 4 g/d for 6 weeks almost entirely due to increase in the HDL_2b fraction: significant inverse correlation with VLDL-triglyceride concentration observed both before and after treatment *2947* In 15 normolipidemic men (cholesterol less than 6 mmol/L, triglycerides less than 2.75 mmol/L) treated with up to 3 g/d for 12 weeks mean concentration increased significantly from baseline of 0.12 ± 0.006 mmol/L to 0.24 ± 0.14 mmol/L *3142*

HDL_3-Cholesterol *Serum Increase Physiological* In 15 normolipidemic men (cholesterol less than 6 mmol/L, triglycerides less than 2.75 mmol/L) treated with up to 3 g/d for 12 weeks mean concentration increased significantly from baseline of 0.70 ± 0.10 mmol/L to 0.85 ± 0.16 mmol/L *3142*
Serum No Effect Physiological No significant effect in 41 weight-stable patients with type IIa, type IIb or type IV hyperlipoproteinemia when treated with 4 g daily for 6 weeks *6298*

HDL_{3b}-Cholesterol *Serum Decrease Physiological* 25% reduction observed in 23 hyperlipidemic patients given 4 g/d for 6 weeks *2947*

HDL_{3c}-Cholesterol *Serum Decrease Physiological* 25% reduction observed in concentration in 23 hyperlipidemic patients given 4 g/d for 6 weeks *2947*

HDL-Cholesterol *Serum Increase Physiological* Mean increase of 37% in 41 weight-stable patients with type IIa, type IIb or type IV hyperlipoproteinemia when treated with 4 g daily for 6 weeks *6298* Significant increase observed as result of therapy *878* In 15 normolipidemic men (cholesterol less than 6 mmol/L, triglycerides less than 2.75 mmol/L) treated with up to 3 g/d for 12 weeks mean concentration increased significantly from baseline of 0.82 ± 0.16 mmol/L to 1.07 ± 0.26 mmol/L *3142* Expected increase observed in 23 hyperlipidemic patients given 4 g/d for 6 weeks: actual increase of 45% *2947* Mean increase of 34% observed in 13 dyslipidemic noninsulin dependent diabetics treated with 4.5 g/d for 8 weeks *2033* Decreased apo A-I catabolism and decreased apo A-II synthesis. Increased activity of lipoprotein lipase *264*
Serum No Effect Analytical At a concentration up to 400 mg/L had no significant effect on Reflotron method for whole blood cholesterol *6352*

Hemoglobin A_{1c} *Blood Increase Physiological* Mean increase of 21% observed in 13 dyslipidemic noninsulin dependent diabetics treated for 8 weeks with 4.5 g/d *2033*

Nicotinic Acid *(continued)*

Insulin *Plasma Increase Physiological* In 12 healthy individuals treatment with up to 2 g/d caused a nonsignificant change from mean baseline of 79 ± 7 pmol/L to 83 ± 9 pmol/L on day 3, 86 ± 9 pmol/L on day 7 and 93 ± 12 pmol/L on day 14 *125*

LDL-Cholesterol *Serum Decrease Physiological* Reduction from mean concentration of 5.92 mmol/L to 3.94 mmol/L in 41 weight-stable patients with type IIa, type IIb or type IV hyperlipoproteinemia when treated with 4 g daily for 6 weeks *6298* Mean reduction of 15% observed in 13 dyslipidemic noninsulin dependent diabetics treated with 4.5 g/d for 8 weeks *2033* With 3-5 weeks treatment reduction observed. Reduction of the order of 10-15% is the consequence of the decrease of VLDL *878* Expected reduction observed in 23 hyperlipidemic patients given 4 g/d for 6 weeks *2947* In 15 normolipidemic men (cholesterol less than 6 mmol/L, triglycerides less than 2.75 mmol/L) treated with up to 3 g/d for 12 weeks mean concentration decreased significantly from baseline of 3.17 ± 0.69 mmol/L to 2.60 ± 0.68 mmol/L *3142*

LDL-Triglycerides *Serum Decrease Physiological* Reduction from mean concentration of 0.56 mmol/L to 0.36 mmol/L in 41 weight-stable patients with type IIa, type IIb or type IV hyperlipoproteinemia treated with 4 g daily for 6 weeks *6298*

Proinsulin *Plasma Increase Physiological* In 12 healthy individuals treatment with up to 2 g/d caused a nonsignificant change from mean baseline of 2.7 ± 0.6 pmol/L to 2.7 ± 0.5 pmol/L on day 3, 2.8 ± 0.7 pmol/L on day 7 and 3.1 ± 0.7 pmol/L on day 14 *125*

Triglycerides *Serum Decrease Physiological* When 4 g given daily for 6 weeks to 41 weight-stable patients with type IIa, type IIb or type IV hyperlipoproteinemia reduction of mean concentration from 2.64 mmol/L to 1.48 mmol/L *6298* In 15 normolipidemic men (cholesterol less than 6 mmol/L, triglycerides less than 2.75 mmol/L) treated with up to 3 g/d for 12 weeks mean concentration decreased significantly from baseline of 2.17 ± 0.83 mmol/L to 1.31 ± 0.51 mmol/L *3142* In the Stockholm Ischemic Heart Study of 555 myocardial infarction patients treatment with clofibrate and nicotinic acid caused mean decrease of 19% *3115* Mean reduction of 45% observed in 13 dyslipidemic noninsulin dependent diabetics treated with 4.5 g/d for 8 weeks *2033* Effect due to increased catabolism caused by increase in triglyceride fractional removal rate. Decreased hepatic synthesis also observed. Triglyceride concentration typically reduced 20-80% *878*

Uric Acid *Serum Increase Physiological* Observed as important side-effect of treatment *878* In 15 normolipidemic men (cholesterol less than 6 mmol/L, triglycerides less than 2.75 mmol/L) treated with up to 3 g/d for 12 weeks mean concentration changed significantly from baseline of 391.8 ± 73.4 µmol/L to 488.3 ± 114.9 µmol/L *3142*

VLDL-Cholesterol *Serum Decrease Physiological* Reduction from mean concentration of 1.29 mmol/L to 0.48 mmol/L in 41 weight-stable patients with type IIa, type IIb or type IV hyperlipoproteinemia when treated with 4 g daily for 6 weeks *6298* Expected reduction observed in 23 hyperlipidemic patients given 4 g daily for 6 weeks *2947* Mean 58% reduction observed in 13 noninsulin dependent dyslipidemic diabetics treated with 4.5 g/d for 8 weeks *2033*

VLDL-Triglycerides *Serum Decrease Physiological* Concentration reduced with treatment. Triglyceride concentration reduced in proportion to the initial plasma concentration of VLDL *878* When 4 g given daily for 6 weeks to 41 weight-stable patients with type IIa, type IIb or type IV hyperlipoproteinemia reduction from mean basal concentration of 1.90 mmol/L to 0.77 mmol/L *6298*

Nifedipine

Alanine Aminotransferase *Serum Increase Physiological* Rare, usually transient, but occasionally significant increase in enzyme activity observed following drug administration *415* Rare, usually transient but occasionally significantly increased activity observed *4652*
Serum No Effect Physiological Nonsignificant increase from mean baseline activity of 19.6 U/L to 20.3 U/L following 16 weeks treatment with long-acting nifedipine in 76 mild to moderate hypertensives *2263*

Albumin *Urine Increase Physiological* Increase from 14 to 28 µg/min 40 to 60 minutes after single oral dose of 20 mg sublingually *1003*

Aldosterone *Plasma Decrease Physiological* General tendency to decrease observed in 11 hypertensive patients given 40 mg/d for 4 days but effect not significant *4079*
Plasma Increase Physiological Significant increase from mean baseline of 58.3 pg/mL to 72.6 pg/mL at 7 days in 10 patients with uncomplicated essential hypertension treated with 30 mg/d (no significant change observed at day 3) *1086*
Plasma No Effect Physiological Possibly due to drug's calcium antagonizing action since calcium is required to secrete aldosterone *2619* Insignificant change from 108 to 121 pg/mL in young hypertensives after 3 h *2619*
Urine Increase Physiological In 25 patients with mild to moderate primary hypertension given up to 80 mg daily *4383*

Alkaline Phosphatase *Serum Increase Physiological* Rare, usually transient but occasionally significantly increased activity observed. A small (5.4%) increase observed in patients treated with nifedipine *4652* Rare, usually transient, but occasionally significant increase in enzyme activity observed following drug administration. An increase of less than 5% observed in mean activity *415*
Serum No Effect Physiological Nonsignificant increase from mean baseline activity of 150.3 U/L to 153.5 U/L in 71 patients with mild to moderate hypertension treated with long-acting nifedipine for 16 weeks *2263*

Angiotensin-I *Plasma Increase Physiological* In young but not old people within 3 h of 10 mg orally *2619* From 1923 to 2669 pg/mL in young hypertensives after 3 h *2619*

Angiotensin-II *Plasma Increase Physiological* From 167 to 215 pg/mL in young hypertensives after 3 h *2619* General tendency to increase observed in 11 hypertensive patients given 40 mg/d for 4 days but effect not significant *4079* In young but not old people within 3 h of 10 mg orally *2619*

Angiotensin-converting Enzyme
Serum No Effect Physiological No significant effect within 3 h after 10 mg orally *2619*

Antidiuretic Hormone *Plasma No Effect Physiological* No significant effect observed in 11 hypertensive patients given 40 mg/d for 4 days *4079*

Antipyrine *Serum No Effect Physiological* In contrast to effects of diltiazem and verapamil had no effect on antipyrine kinetics *411*

Apolipoprotein A-I *Serum Increase Physiological* In 49 individuals with mild to moderate hypertension treatment for 21 weeks caused significant increase *2733* In 11 patients with 80 mg daily for 6 weeks *6242* Increase by 5 % in 11 individuals treated for 1.5 mo *142*
Serum No Effect Analytical At a concentration of 17 µmol/L no significant effect observed on automated immunoturbidimetric method on Baxter Paramax analyzer *3005*
Serum No Effect Physiological In 52 patients with NIDDM and hypertension treatment with up to 80 mg/d for 12 weeks caused nonsignificant increase of 5.3 mg/dL *960* Insignificant reduction observed with treatment with 40 mg long-acting drug daily for 16 weeks in over 30 patients with mild to moderate hypertension *2263* No significant effect in either diabetic or nondiabetic hypertensives treated with 40 mg daily for 16 weeks *3083* Increase by 3 mg/dL in patients given 30 to 60 mg daily for 8 weeks *4213*

Apolipoprotein A-II *Serum Increase Physiological* In 49 individuals with mild to moderate hypertension treatment for 21 weeks caused significant increase in concentration *2733* Increase by 7 % in 11 individuals treated for 1.5 mo *142* In 11 patients with 80 mg daily for 6 weeks *6242*
Serum No Effect Physiological Insignificant reduction observed after treatment for 4 to 12 weeks with 40 mg long-acting drug daily in over 30 patients with mild to moderate hypertension *2263*

Apolipoprotein B *Serum Decrease Physiological* Significant reduction in both diabetic and nondiabetic hypertensives when given 40 mg daily for 16 weeks *3083* Significant reduction of 2.6 mg/dL after 4 weeks treatment with 40 mg long-acting drug daily in over 30 patients with mild to moderate hypertension: significant reduction of 4.7 mg/dL also observed after 8 weeks but reduction thereafter nonsignificant *2263*
Serum No Effect Analytical At a concentration of 17 µmol/L no significant effect observed on automated immunoturbidimetric method on Baxter Paramax analyzer *3005*

Serum No Effect Physiological In 11 patients with 80 mg daily for 6 weeks *6242* In 52 patients with NIDDM and hypertension treatment with up to 80 mg/d for 12 weeks caused nonsignificant decrease of 2.3 mg/dL *960* Decrease by -6 mg/dL in patients given 30 to 60 mg daily for 8 weeks *4213* In 49 patients with mild to moderate hypertension treatment for 21 weeks had no significant effect on concentration *2733*

Apolipoprotein C-II *Serum No Effect Physiological* No significant change observed in over 30 patients with mild to moderate hypertension treated with 40 mg long-acting drug daily for 16 weeks *2263* No change in patients given 30 to 60 mg daily for 8 weeks *4213*

Apolipoprotein C-III *Serum No Effect Physiological* No change in patients given 30 to 60 mg daily for 8 weeks *4213* No significant effect observed in over 30 patients with mild to moderate hypertension treated with 40 mg long-acting drug daily for 16 weeks *2263*

Apolipoprotein E *Serum No Effect Physiological* No change in patients given 30 to 60 mg daily for 8 weeks *4213* Insignificant reduction observed in over 30 patients treated with 40 mg long-acting drug daily for 16 weeks *2263*

Aspartate Aminotransferase *Serum Increase Physiological* Rare, usually transient but occasionally significantly increased activity observed *4652* Rare, usually transient, but occasionally significant increase in enzyme activity observed following drug administration *415*

Serum No Effect Physiological No significant change from mean baseline activity of 20.2 U/L to 20.7 U/L after 16 weeks treatment of 76 mild to moderate hypertensives with long-acting nifedipine *2263*

Atenolol *Serum No Effect Physiological* Coadministration had no effect on kinetics of atenolol in 8 healthy individuals *2020* In healthy volunteers coadministration of nifedipine (10 mg every 8 h) with atenolol (100 mg/d for 3 days) had no effect on maximum atenolol concentration, half-life, and area under the concentration curve *5411*

Atrial Natriuretic Peptide *Plasma Increase Physiological* After 10 mg sublingually increased from mean 19.4 pg/mL to 24.1 pg/mL at 90 minutes *4862* 10 mg sublingually caused increase from mean of 19.4 pg/mL at baseline to 23.9 pg/mL at 60 minutes and 24.1 pg/mL at 90 minutes *4863*

Plasma No Effect Physiological Insignificant reduction observed after 7 days treatment in 10 patients with uncomplicated essential hypertension treated with 30 mg/d (no change observed after 3 days) *1086* No effect of 200 mg in 6 normal men when effect compared against that of placebo *6433* No significant change observed in 11 hypertensive patients given 40 mg/d for 4 days *4079*

Betaxolol *Serum No Effect Physiological* Coadministration had no effect on pharmacokinetics of betaxolol *2067* In study of 6 healthy volunteers coadministration of drugs did not affect betaxolol kinetics *6262* Coadministration of nifedipine with betaxolol had no effect on its pharmacokinetics *5411*

Bleeding Time *Patient Increase Physiological* Observed 1 h after ingestion of 20 mg in 20 people *1224* Increase in bleeding time observed in some patients possibly due to inhibition of calcium transport across the platelet membrane *4652* Increase in bleeding time observed in some patients with administration of nifedipine *415*

Calcium *Serum No Effect Physiological* No effect of 80 mg/d for 2 d *6227* In both normals and hypertensives following 10 mg orally *2298*

Carbamazepine *Serum Increase Physiological* Concomitant administration of calcium channel blockers with carbamazepine causes marked increase of plasma carbamazepine concentration resulting in toxicity in some cases *282*

Serum No Effect Physiological No significant effect observed on plasma concentration during coadministration of drugs *3119*

Catecholamines *Urine Increase Physiological* Significant increase from mean baseline excretion of 39.7 µg/d to 45.2 µg/d in 10 patients with uncomplicated essential hypertension treated with 30 mg/d although increase at day 3 considerably less *1086*

Chloride *Serum Increase Physiological* Nonsignificant increase from mean baseline concentration of 99.5 mmol/L to 101.5 mmol/L in 73 patients with mild to moderate hypertension treated with long-acting nifedipine for 16 weeks *2263*

Cholesterol *Serum Decrease Physiological* Significant decrease in 11 hypertensive diabetics with mild to moderate hypertension treated with 40 mg daily for 16 weeks. Significant effect also observed in 8 nondiabetic hypertensive controls *3083* In over 30 patients with mild to moderate hypertension treatment with 40 mg long-acting drug daily 7 mg/dL reduction after 4 and 8 weeks treatment but reverted no normal by 16 weeks *2263* In 23 patients over 60 y old with essential mild to moderate hypertension *5356* Transient decrease observed in patients with essential hypertension *2265* Significant reduction 8 weeks after about 30 mg/day in group of individuals with hyperlipoproteinemia but then reverted to normal *5282*

Serum No Effect Physiological In 49 patients with mild to moderate hypertension treatment for 21 weeks had no significant effect on concentration *2733* In 52 patients with NIDDM and hypertension treatment with up to 80 mg/d for 12 weeks caused nonsignificant decrease of 0.16 mmol/L *960* No effect observed in 14 patients with essential hypertension treated over 2 mo with 20 mg twice daily *3505* No significant effect in 101 hypertensive patients treated with up to 80 mg daily for 12 weeks *2996* Insignificant change in 15 male patients with mild to moderate hypertension from mean concentration of 6.28 mmol/L before nifedipine 30-60 mg/d for 6 weeks to 6.35 mmol/L after treatment *4458* No effect on concentration observed with administration of nifedipine *415* Decrease by -5 mg/dL in patients given 30 to 60 mg daily for 8 weeks *4213*

Cholesterol:HDL-Cholesterol Ratio

Serum Decrease Physiological Significant reduction observed in diabetic hypertensives although not in nondiabetic hypertensives when given 40 mg daily for 16 weeks *3083*

Clopidogrel *Serum No Effect Physiological* Nifedipine administration does not appear to affect the pharmacodynamics of clopidogrel *5256*

Coombs' Test, Direct *Blood Positive Physiological* Positive reaction, with or without hemolytic anemia, observed in some patients with administration of nifedipine but relationship not conclusively established *415*

Cortisol *Plasma Decrease Physiological* Slight but progressive decrease over 3 h after oral administration of 10 mg in young people but not in old *2619*

Plasma No Effect Physiological No effect of 200 mg in 6 normal men when compared against effect of placebo *6433*

Creatine Kinase *Serum Increase Physiological* Rare, usually transient, but occasionally significant increase in enzyme activity observed following drug administration *415* Rare, usually transient but occasionally significantly increased activity observed *4652*

Creatinine *Serum Increase Physiological* At end of 6 weeks treatment with mean 45 mg/d long-acting nifedipine concentration increased and persisted over 14 weeks, increasing from baseline of 159 µmol/L to 212 µmol/L *1376* Acute reversible deterioration of renal function in 4 patients with chronic renal failure *1417*

Serum No Effect Physiological In 12 hypertensive patients treatment with nifedipine GTIS for 5 weeks caused insignificant change to 2.8 ± 1.3 mg/dL from 2.7 ± 1.4 mg/dL during placebo period *4883* No significant change observed in 80 patients with mild to moderate hypertension treated with long-acting nifedipine for 16 weeks *2263*

Creatinine Clearance *Urine Increase Physiological* After 10 mg sublingually in next 2 h *4862* In 12 hypertensive patients treatment with nifedipine GTIS for 5 weeks caused significant increase to 45 ± 19 mL/min/1.73 sq m compared with 41 ± 18 mL/min/1.73 sq m during placebo period *4883* Effect observed over the next 2 hours in 8 hypertensive patients following administration of 10 mg sublingually *4863*

Urine No Effect Physiological Neither single doses of 20 mg of slow-release formulation or 10 mg of conventional formulation nor 2 weeks treatment with either had any effect in healthy volunteers *53*

Cyclosporine *Blood No Effect Physiological* Appears to have little effect, if any, on blood concentration as observed from several studies *6596*

Serum No Effect Physiological No significant change observed in cyclosporine concentration when cyclosporine and nifedipine coadministered *6596* Coadministration of nifedipine with cyclosporine had minimal effect on cyclosporine concentration *5411* No significant effect observed on area under curve, maximum and steady-state concentration and trough concentration in 7 patients following renal transplant. No significant

Nifedipine *(continued)*

Cyclosporine *(continued)*
effect observed on major metabolites either *6058* No effect on concentration when drug added (20-30 mg/d) to therapeutic regime *6288*

Digitoxin *Serum No Effect Physiological* No significant effect observed on serum concentration when two drugs coadministered *3318* No evidence for interactions occurring when the two drugs coadministered *5345* Coadministration of nifedipine with digitoxin had no effect on digitoxin steady state concentration or clearances *5345*

Digoxin *Serum Increase Physiological* Increased concentration observed in some patients with administration of nifedipine but relationship not conclusively established *415* In patients receiving doses of nifedipine from 15 to 90 mg/d area under curve, renal clearance and minimal and steady state concentrations either increased or remained unchanged: total digoxin clearance either decreased or remained unchanged. Minimum concentrations in two different studies increased by 18% and 33% respectively *5345* In 12 healthy volunteers increase of 45% observed when 0.125 mg t.i.d. digoxin given with 10 mg t.i.d. nifedipine for 14 days. Renal clearance reduced by 30% *472* Increase by 15% in patients to whom 20 mg b.i.d. were added to a stable digoxin regime *3180* 45% increase in volunteers given both drugs compared with digoxin alone, but mechanism uncertain *470* Coadministration of nifedipine with digoxin caused an average 45% increase in 9 of 12 normal volunteers *4652*
Serum No Effect Physiological Coadministration of nifedipine with digoxin caused no significant effect in 13 patients with coronary artery disease *4652* Probably does not cause a clinically important increase *1384* Insignificant effect on serum concentration when two drugs coadministered *5396*

1,25-Dihydroxy Vitamin D_3 *Serum No Effect Physiological* No effect of 80 mg/d for 2 d *6227*

Effective Renal Plasma Flow
Patient Increase Physiological In 13 healthy men a single oral dose of 10 mg caused a mean increase of 6.8 ± 8.2% in ERPF in the fasting state *639* In 11 patients with well compensated alcoholic cirrhosis administration of 10 mg nifedipine caused significant increase from mean baseline of 450 ± 32 mL/min to 545 ± 39 mL/min over one hour due to a substantial decrease in renal vascular resistance *6531* In 12 hypertensives treatment with nifedipine GTIS for 5 weeks caused significant 40% increase compared with placebo period (PAH clearance increased from 106 ± 56 mL/min/1.73 sq m to 127 ± 66 mL/min/1.73 sq m) *4883*

Epinephrine *Plasma No Effect Physiological* No significant change observed in 11 hypertensive patients given 40 mg/d for 4 days *4079*

Fatty Acids (FFA), Free *Serum Decrease Physiological* Nonsignificant reduction from mean of 0.73 mEq/L to 0.63 mEq/L in 20 mild to moderate hypertensives treated with long-acting nifedipine for 16 weeks *2263*

Filtration Fraction *Urine Decrease Physiological* In 11 patients with well compensated alcoholic cirrhosis administration of 10 mg nifedipine caused nonsignificant change from mean baseline of 26 ± 3% to 22 ± 3% over one hour *6531*

Fructosamine *Serum No Effect Physiological* In 52 patients with NIDDM and hypertension treatment with up to 80 mg/d for 12 weeks caused nonsignificant decrease of 0.03 mmol/L *960*

Glomerular Filtration Rate *Urine Increase Physiological* In 13 healthy individuals administration of a single dose of 10 mg caused a mean increase of 12.8 ± 3.5% in the fasting state *639*
Urine No Effect Physiological Insignificant difference in 12 hours following a single oral dose of 20 mg in 10 elderly hypertensives *5412* In 11 patients with well compensated alcoholic cirrhosis administration of 10 mg nifedipine caused nonsignificant change from mean baseline of 120 ± 20 mL/min to 119 ± 17 mL/min over one hour *6531*

Glucagon *Plasma Increase Physiological* Significant effect in normal subjects (0.045 vs 0.034 nmol/L) *974*

Glucose *Serum Decrease Physiological* Incidence of 1.0% observed in French Pharmacovigilance database *4106* From 102 to 95 mg/dL in 15 hypertensive patients undergoing hemodialysis after 3 weeks treatment *4956*
Serum Increase Physiological Fasting concentration increased by 10% in normal subjects *974*
Serum No Effect Physiological No effect on concentration observed with administration of nifedipine *415* In 11 patients with 80 mg daily for 6 weeks *6242* In 52 patients with NIDDM and hypertension treatment with up to 80 mg/d for 12 weeks caused nonsignificant increase of 0.01 mmol/L *960* No significant effect in 11 diabetic outpatients with mild to moderate hypertension and 8 nondiabetic hypertensives treated with 40 mg daily for 16 weeks *3083* Insignificant reduction from 103 mg/dL to 102 mg/dL in 60 mild to moderate hypertensives treated with long-acting nifedipine for 16 weeks *2263*

Glucose Tolerance *Serum Decrease Physiological* Both in normal subjects and those with already impaired glucose tolerance but in normals improved tolerance after 60 minutes *2140* Significantly higher concentrations of glucose at 60 and 90 minutes and area under curve greater at the 5% level in 8 males with mild hypertension studied before and after 12 weeks of therapy *4490*
Serum No Effect Physiological In 11 patients with 80 mg daily for 6 weeks *6242* In 15 hypertensive patients undergoing hemodialysis after 3 weeks treatment *4956*

Granulocytes *Blood Decrease Physiological* Agranulocytosis observed in 4.4% of patients taking nifedipine compared with 1.9% in controls (relative risk estimate 2.8 - of borderline significance) *3098*

HDL_2-Cholesterol *Serum Increase Physiological* In 49 patients with mild to moderate hypertension treatment for 21 weeks caused significant increase in concentration *2733*
Serum No Effect Physiological Overall no significant change observed in about 30 patients with mild to moderate hypertension treated with 40 mg daily for 16 weeks *2263*

HDL_2-Phospholipids *Serum No Effect Physiological* No significant effect observed in 11 diabetics with mild to moderate hypertension treated with 40 mg daily for 16 weeks, but significant reduction in 8 nondiabetic hypertensive with same therapeutic regime at 16 weeks *3083*

HDL_3-Cholesterol *Serum Increase Physiological* Nonsignificant increase observed after 21 weeks treatment in 49 patients with mild to moderate hypertension *2733*
Serum No Effect Physiological No significant change observed in about 30 patients with mild to moderate hypertension treated with long-acting drug daily for 16 weeks *2263*

HDL_3-Triglycerides *Serum No Effect Physiological* No significant effect in 11 diabetics with mild to moderate hypertension treated with 40 mg daily for 16 weeks. Also no effect observed in 8 nondiabetic hypertensive controls *3083*

HDL-Cholesterol *Serum Increase Physiological* Increase of 7-8% in 101 hypertensive patients treated with up to 80 mg daily for 12 weeks *2996* In 49 patients with mild to moderate hypertension treated for 21 weeks significant increase in HDL-cholesterol observed *2733* In 100 patients in a double-blind randomized trial *6690* Treatment of 40 patients over 8 weeks caused a statistically significant increase in concentration probably due to stimulation of lysosomal and cytoplasmic cholesterase *3730*
Serum No Effect Physiological No effect observed in 14 patients with essential hypertension treated over 2 mo with 20 mg twice daily *3505* Insignificant change from mean baseline concentration of 1.18 mmol/L to 1.21 mmol/L in 15 male patients with mild to moderate hypertension treated with 30-60 mg/d for 6 weeks *4458* In 52 patients with NIDDM and hypertension treatment with up to 80 mg/d for 12 weeks caused nonsignificant increase of 0.07 mmol/L *960* No significant change observed in over 30 patients with mild to moderate hypertension treated with 40 mg long-acting drug daily for 16 weeks *2263* Increase by 1 mg/dL in patients given 30 to 60 mg daily for 8 weeks *4213* In 11 patients with 80 mg daily for 6 weeks *6242* Nonsignificant reduction in 11 diabetics with mild to moderate hypertension treated with 40 mg daily for 16 weeks. Similar findings in 8 nondiabetic hypertensive controls *3083* No significant effect in patients with hyperlipoproteinemia treated with about 30 mg/day for 20 weeks *5282*

HDL-Phospholipids *Serum No Effect Physiological* Nonsignificant increase in 11 diabetics with mild to moderate hypertension treated with 40 mg daily for 16 weeks. Similar findings in 8 nondiabetic hypertensive controls *3083*

HDL-Triglycerides *Serum Decrease Physiological* In 11 patients with 80 mg daily for 6 weeks *6242*

Serum No Effect Physiological No significant effect in 11 diabetics with mild to moderate hypertension treated with 40 mg daily for 16 weeks. Also no effect in 8 nondiabetic hypertensive controls with same therapeutic regime *3083*

Hemoglobin A_{1c} *Blood No Effect Physiological* In 52 patients with NIDDM and hypertension treatment with up to 80 mg/d for 12 weeks caused nonsignificant decrease of 0.20% *960* No significant effect in 11 diabetics with mild to moderate hypertension and 8 nondiabetics with hypertension treated with 40 mg daily for 16 weeks *3083*

High Density Lipoproteins *Serum No Effect Physiological* No significant change in either diabetic or nondiabetic hypertensive patients treated with 40 mg daily for 16 weeks *3083*

Histamine *Plasma No Effect Analytical* Improbable inhibition of radio-enzyme assay at therapeutic concentrations *2492*

Indocyanine Green Clearance
Serum Increase Physiological In 9 healthy male volunteers administration of 20 mg nifedipine orally followed by 0.5 mg/kg indocyanine green by intravenous bolus injection caused increase by 104% (mean 95% confidence interval 60 - 162%) *1302*

Indomethacin *Serum No Effect Analytical* No effect on HPLC method of Roberts and Smith *4978*

Insulin *Plasma Decrease Physiological* Response to glucose challenge significantly reduced in subjects taking drug *2140* Basal insulin concentration reduced by 26% in normals *974* From 20 to 14 µU/mL in 15 hypertensive patients undergoing hemodialysis after 3 weeks treatment *4956*
Plasma No Effect Physiological In 11 patients with 80 mg daily for 6 weeks *6242*

Inulin Clearance *Urine No Effect Physiological* Nonsignificant increase observed in normal subjects but not in hypertensives following 10 mg orally *2298*

Irbesartan *Serum No Effect Physiological* Coadministration of nifedipine with irbesartan had no effect on the pharmacokinetics of irbesartan *725*

Ketone Body Ratio *Serum No Effect Analytical* When added at a concentration of 10 mg/L had no significant effect on AKBR method of Uno et al *6131*

Ketones *Serum Increase Physiological* In 15 hypertensive patients undergoing hemodialysis after 3 weeks treatment *4956*

Lactate *Plasma No Effect Physiological* In 15 hypertensive patients undergoing hemodialysis after 3 weeks treatment *4956*

Lactate Dehydrogenase *Serum Increase Physiological* Rare, usually transient, but occasionally significant increase in enzyme activity observed following drug administration *415* Rare, usually transient but occasionally significantly increased activity observed *4652*
Serum No Effect Physiological Nonsignificant change from mean baseline activity of 297.9 U/L to 296.1 U/L in 76 patients with mild to moderate hypertension treated with long-acting nifedipine for 16 weeks *2263*

LDL-Cholesterol *Serum Decrease Physiological* In over 30 patients with mild to moderate hypertension treatment with 40 mg long-acting drug daily for 16 weeks caused significant reduction of 8 mg/dL at 8 weeks but not at other times *2263*
Serum No Effect Physiological Nonsignificant reduction in 11 diabetics with mild to moderate hypertension treated with 40 mg daily for 16 weeks. With same therapeutic regime significant reduction observed in 8 nondiabetic hypertensive controls at 4 and 16 weeks *3083* In 49 patients with mild to moderate hypertension treatment for 21 weeks had no significant effect on concentration *2733* In 52 patients with NIDDM and hypertension treatment with up to 80 mg/d for 12 weeks caused nonsignificant decrease of 0.07 mmol/L *960* No significant effect in patients with hyperlipoproteinemia given about 30 mg/day for 20 weeks *5282* No effect observed in 14 patients with essential hypertension treated over 2 mo with 20 mg twice daily *3505* Insignificant change in 15 male patients with mild to moderate hypertension from mean baseline of 4.21 mmol/L to 4.38 mmol/L after 6 weeks treatment with 30-60 mg/d *4458*

LDL-Phospholipids *Serum No Effect Physiological* Nonsignificant reduction in 11 diabetics with mild to moderate hypertension treated with 40 mg daily for 16 weeks. With same therapeutic regime significant reduction observed at 4 and 16 weeks in 8 nondiabetic hypertensive controls *3083*

LDL-Triglycerides *Serum No Effect Physiological* Nonsignificant reduction in 11 diabetics with mild to moderate hypertension treated with 40 mg daily for 16 weeks and in 8 nondiabetic hypertensive controls *3083*

Lisinopril *Serum No Effect Physiological* Coadministration produced no effect on kinetics of lisinopril *3485*

Magnesium *Serum Increase Physiological* Treatment of 54 patients with essential hypertension caused correction to within normal range after 7-10 days in patients in whom concentration was low although treatment had no effect when concentration initially within normal range *6144*
Serum No Effect Physiological In both normals and hypertensives given 10 mg orally *2298*

Metformin *Serum Increase Physiological* In a single dose study during which nifedipine and metformin were coadministered nifedipine increased the maximum concentration and AUC of metformin by 20% and 9% respectively *726*
Urine Increase Physiological In a single dose study during which nifedipine and metformin were coadministered nifedipine increased the maximum concentration and AUC of metformin by 20% and 9% respectively and also increased its urinary excretion. probably as a result of enhanced gastrointestinal absorption *726*

Metoprolol *Serum No Effect Physiological* In healthy volunteers coadministration of nifedipine with 200 mg/day metoprolol for 3 days had no effect on metoprolol maximum concentration, half-life, and area under the curve although plasma concentrations were not at steady state when blood specimens were drawn *5411* Coadministration had no effect on kinetics of metoprolol in 8 healthy volunteers *2020*

β_2-Microglobulin *Urine Increase Physiological* Increase from 0.12 to 0.74 µg/min 40 to 60 minutes after single oral dose of 20 mg sublingually *1003*

Midazolam *Serum No Effect Analytical* On GC-ECD method of Ha et al *2387*

Norepinephrine *Plasma Increase Physiological* Increase observed soon after administration due to increase in sympathetic tone *2528* In 11 hypertensive patients 40 mg/d for 4 days caused significant increase *4079*
Plasma No Effect Physiological No significant effect observed in hypertensive patients with chronic administration *2528*

Occult Blood *Feces Increase Physiological* In fewer than 1% of all treated patients melena reported as a complication *4652*

PAH Clearance *Urine Increase Physiological* Significant effect observed in normal subjects but not in hypertensives following 10 mg orally *2298*

Parathyroid Hormone *Plasma Increase Physiological* In 15 premenopausal women given 30 mg sustained release nifedipine parathyroid concentration increased significantly from mean baseline of about 16.5 ng/L to 18.5 ng/L although no significant change observed after 28 days treatment *6372*

Phenytoin *Serum Increase Physiological* Increase in plasma concentration and signs of phenytoin toxicity observed when drugs coadministered *1384* Observation reported in one epileptic patient previously stabilized on a constant dose of phenytoin but whose serum concentration was markedly increased four weeks after nifedipine was coadministered: effect probably due to impairment of metabolism *71*

Phosphate *Serum Increase Physiological* Treatment for 7-10 days of 54 patients with essential hypertension caused increase into normal range in those patients in whom concentration was initially low although no effect was observed when concentration was initially within normal range *6144*
Serum No Effect Physiological No effect of 80 mg/d for 2 d *6227*

Phospholipids *Serum No Effect Physiological* Nonsignificant decrease over 16 weeks in 11 diabetics with mild to moderate hypertension treated with 40 mg daily but significant reduction observed in 8 nondiabetic hypertensive controls *3083*

Platelet Aggregation *Blood Decrease Physiological* Significant reduction observed in epinephrine and collagen induced aggregation in 15 male patients with mild to moderate hypertension given 30-60 mg/d for 6 weeks. Reduction in ADP-stimulated aggregation also occurred but not statistically significant *4458* Maximal rate in response to ADP reduced by 20-26% and by 23% in response to collagen *1224* In a limited number of clinical trials a moderate but statistically significant

Nifedipine *(continued)*

Platelet Aggregation *(continued)*
decrease in platelet aggregation observed *4652* Significant reduction of collagen-induced and ADP-induced aggregation probably by inhibiting increase of intracytoplasmic calcium by blocking calcium channel through platelet membrane: also inhibits platelet aggregability induced by exercise *5920* Oral nifedipine, 20 mg sustained release, reduced aggregation by collagen by 15%. No effect observed with intravenous nifedipine *6331*
Blood Increase Physiological Moderate but statistically significant decrease in platelet aggregation observed with administration of nifedipine *415*
Blood No Effect Physiological No significant change in threshold for ADP-induced aggregation in 12 healthy volunteers given 10 or 20 mg t.i.d *1668* No significant change in threshold for epinephrine-induced aggregation in 12 healthy volunteers given either 10 mg t.i.d. or 20 mg t.i.d *6510*

Platelet Factor 4 *Plasma Decrease Physiological* Reduction of about 3 ng/mL in 12 healthy volunteers given 10 mg t.i.d. but nonsignificant increase observed when given 20 mg t.i.d *6510*

Platelets *Blood No Effect Physiological* No effect in 20 people following ingestion of 20 mg *1224*

Potassium *Serum Decrease Physiological* Single case of drug induced hypokalemia reported *6039*
Serum Increase Physiological In 23 patients over 60 y old with essential mild to moderate hypertension *5356* At dose of 40 mg/d caused increase of 0.3 mmol/L when also treated with propranolol *4739*
Serum No Effect Physiological in both normals and hypertensives following 10 mg orally *2298* In 12 hypertensives treatment with nifedipine GITS for 5 weeks caused nonsignificant reduction to 4.2 ± 0.6 mmol/L from 4.4 ± 0.6 mmol/L during placebo period *4883* No significant change from baseline concentration of 4.13 mmol/L to 4.10 mmol/L after 16 weeks treatment with long-acting nifedipine in 72 mild to moderate hypertensives *2263* No effect on concentration observed with administration of nifedipine *415*
Urine Increase Physiological Nonsignificant increase at 3 and 7 days observed in 10 patients with uncomplicated essential hypertension treated with 30 mg/d *1086*
Urine No Effect Physiological No effect following single 20 mg sublingual dose *1003* In 12 hypertensives treatment with nifedipine GITS for 5 weeks caused nonsignificant change from 38 ± 19 mmol/g creatinine in placebo period to 40 ± 25 mmol/g creatinine *4883* Neither single doses of 20 mg of slow-release formulation nor 10 mg of conventional formulation nor 2 weeks treatment with either had any effect in healthy individuals *53* No significant change over 12 hours in 10 elderly hypertensives given a single oral dose of 20 mg *5412*

Prolactin *Plasma Decrease Physiological* Peak value and area under the curve in response to TRH significantly reduced in 10 mildly hypertensive patients treated with 30 mg daily for 1 week *6153*
Plasma No Effect Physiological No effect of 80 mg/d for 2 d *6227*

Propranolol *Serum Decrease Physiological* Single oral dose of 20 mg reduced steady-state plasma concentration by about 40% but did not alter unbound fraction *3181*
Serum Increase Physiological In study of 6 healthy volunteers coadministration of drugs increased propranolol bioavailability and plasma concentration probably because of increased gastrointestinal absorption *6262* In a study using healthy volunteers receiving propranolol 80 mg every 12 hours the addition of nifedipine 10 mg three times daily increased mean total maximum plasma propranolol concentration by 56% compared with propranolol alone. In addition there was a 23% increase in propranolol area under the curve and a 15% reduction of the propranolol half-life *5411*
Serum No Effect Physiological In controlled studies in healthy volunteers nifedipine had no effect on pharmacokinetics or pharmacodynamics of propranolol *5411*

Protein *Serum No Effect Physiological* Insignificant reduction from mean baseline of 74.2 g/L to 73.8 g/L in 74 patients with mild to moderate hypertension treated with 20-40 mg long-acting drug daily for 16 weeks *2263*
Urine Increase Physiological Acute reversible deterioration of renal function in 4 patients with chronic renal failure *1417* Increase from mean of 2.8 g/d at baseline to 5.3 g/d after 6 weeks treatment with mean 45 mg/d long-acting nifedipine in 14 noninsulin-dependent diabetics *1376*
Urine No Effect Physiological In 12 hypertensives treatment with nifedipine GTIS for 5 weeks caused nonsignificant decrease to 1.60 ± 1.43 g/g creatinine from baseline of 1.63 ± 1.28 g/g creatinine *4883*

Prothrombin Time *Plasma Increase Physiological* Increased prothrombin time observed in some patients taking warfarin with administration of nifedipine but relationship not conclusively established *415* Rare reports of increased prothrombin times in patients taking coumarins and nifedipine *4652*

Pyruvate *Plasma Increase Physiological* In 15 hypertensive patients undergoing hemodialysis after 3 weeks treatment *4956*

Quinidine *Serum Decrease Physiological* Rare reports of decreased concentration observed in some patients with administration of nifedipine but relationship not conclusively established *415* Increased concentrations of quinidine observed when drugs coadministered and then nifedipine withdrawn *1384* Unusually low concentrations of quinidine noted when nifedipine coadministered with rebound increase of quinidine concentration (up to 112%) on withdrawal of nifedipine *5345* By mechanisms not understood concentration of quinidine decreased when nifedipine coadministered *5996* Reduction of concentration by 20-40% in several patients when quinidine coadministered but mechanism not yet established *1807* One case reported in whom coadministration of drugs caused reduced quinidine concentration which increased when nifedipine withdrawn but mechanism not yet determined *2305*
Serum Increase Physiological Marked effect observed once drug discontinued, probably hemodynamically induced interaction *1384*
Serum No Effect Physiological In one study of 12 patients no interaction between nifedipine and quinidine observed and change in clearance observed in only one patient *5345* Insignificant increase of maximum plasma concentration from mean baseline of 747 ± 52 ng/mL to 859 ± 77 ng/mL when nifedipine coadministered with quinidine *327*

Renin Activity *Plasma Increase Physiological* Slight increase of 0.3 ng/mL/h in 11 hypertensive patients given 40 mg/d for 4 days *4079* Significant increase from mean baseline of 1.77 ng/mL/h to 2.44 ng/mL/h at 7 days in 10 patients with uncomplicated essential hypertension treated with 30 mg/d (no significant change observed at 3 days) *1086* From 2.26 to 3.72 ng/mL/h in young hypertensives after 3 h *2619* In 25 patients with mild to moderate primary hypertension given up to 80 mg daily *4383*

Renin Substrate *Plasma No Effect Physiological* No effect of 200 mg when compared against effect of placebo *6433*

Sodium *Serum Decrease Physiological* In 23 patients over 60 y old with essential mild to moderate hypertension *5356* Significant reduction from mean concentration of 142.4 mmol/L to 141.5 mmol/L with 16 weeks treatment with long-acting nifedipine in 72 mild to moderate hypertensives *2263*
Serum No Effect Physiological In 7 normal and 7 hypertensives given 10 mg drug orally with specimens collected over the following hour *2298* In 12 hypertensive patients with renal insufficiency treatment with nifedipine GITS for 5 weeks had no significant effect (mean concentration 135 ± 5 mmol/L) *4883*
Urine Decrease Physiological In 11 patients with well compensated alcoholic cirrhosis administration of 10 mg nifedipine caused nonsignificant change from mean baseline of 137 ± 19 µmol/min to 122 ± 30 µmol/min over one hour *6531*
Urine Increase Physiological After 10 mg sublingually in next 2 h *4862* Increase observed in excretion over subsequent two hours in 8 hypertensive men treated with 10 mg sublingually *4863* Single dose of 20 mg of slow release formulation caused an increase in 8-hour excretion. Effect similar with 10 mg of normal formulation. Natriuresis similar in individuals treated with 20 mg slow-release formulation for 2 weeks and controls *53* Mean excretion of 163 µmol/min in 10 elderly hypertensives versus 89 µmol/min in controls during 12 hours following administration of a single dose of 20 mg *5412* Significant effect following 20 mg sublingually *1003* Nonsignificant increase observed in 10 patients with uncomplicated essential hypertension treated with 30 mg/d *1086*

Urine *No Effect* *Physiological* In 12 hypertensive patients treatment with nifedipine GITS for 5 weeks had no significant effect on urinary excretion (decrease to 103 ± 26 mmol/g creatinine versus 117 ± 41 mmol/g creatinine in controls) *4883*

Tacrolimus *Serum* *No Effect* *Analytical* In HPLC/MS method of Christians et al no significant interference observed with measurement of FK 506 *1010*

Theophylline *Serum* *Decrease* *Physiological* Although no effect observed at 15 days when 13 hypertensive women took 20 mg/d nifedipine on top of their prior regime of 400 mg/d theophylline (trough theophylline concentration 11.2 µg/mL) but after 45 days concentration reduced to 7.3 µg/mL *6601*

Serum *No Effect* *Physiological* No documented significant interaction with theophylline reported *6117* In 8 healthy volunteers administration of 20 mg nifedipine orally twice daily and theophylline intravenously had no effect on theophylline clearance, area under the curve and elimination half-life *2860* No clinically significant effect on theophylline concentration observed when drugs coadministered *5999* Concomitant administration of nifedipine with theophylline had no effect on area under theophylline concentration curve, theophylline clearance or half-life *5345*

β-Thromboglobulin *Plasma* *Decrease* *Physiological* Significant reduction by about 20 ng/mL in 12 healthy volunteers given 10 mg t.i.d. but nonsignificant increase observed in volunteers when given 80 mg t.i.d *6510*

Thyroid Stimulating Hormone

Serum *Decrease* *Physiological* Peak value and release in response to TRH significantly reduced in 10 mildly hypertensive patients treated with 30 mg daily for 1 week *6153*

Serum *No Effect* *Physiological* No effect on either basal or TRH-stimulated concentration in 10 mildly hypertensive patients treated with 30 mg daily for 1 week *6153*

Thyroxine (T4) *Serum* *No Effect* *Physiological* Neither basal nor TRH-stimulated concentrations modified in 10 hypertensive patients given 30 mg daily for 1 week *6153*

Tirofiban *Serum* *No Effect* *Physiological* Coadministration had no significant effect on plasma clearance of tirofiban *3957*

Tissue Plasminogen Activator Antigen

Plasma *No Effect* *Physiological* Administration of 20 mg nifedipine orally to 9 healthy men did not affect the concentration of t-PA antigen administered as 35 mg of rt-PA or activity of rt-PA *1302*

Tri-iodothyronine, Reverse (rT3)

Serum *No Effect* *Physiological* No effect on either basal or TRH-stimulated concentration in 10 mildly hypertensive patients treated with 30 mg daily for 1 week *6153*

Tri-iodothyronine (T3) *Serum* *No Effect* *Physiological* No effect on either basal or TRH-stimulated concentration in 10 mildly hypertensive individuals treated with 30 mg daily for 1 week *6153*

Triglycerides *Serum* *Decrease* *Physiological* In 49 patients with mild to moderate hypertension treatment for 21 weeks caused nonsignificant decrease *2733* Nonsignificant decrease in mean concentration from baseline of 1.98 mmol/L to 1.71 mmol/L in 15 male patients with mild to moderate hypertension treated with 30-60 mg/d for 6 weeks *4458* In 100 patients in a double-blind randomized trial *6690* In 23 patients over 60 y old with essential mild to moderate hypertension *5356*

Serum *No Effect* *Physiological* No significant effect in patients with hyperlipoproteinemia treated with about 30 mg/day for 20 weeks *5282* In 52 patients with NIDDM and hypertension treatment with up to 80 mg/d for 12 weeks caused significant decrease of 0.27 mmol/L *960* No significant effect in 101 hypertensive patients treated with up to 80 mg daily for 12 weeks *2996* Nonsignificant decrease in 11 diabetics with mild to moderate hypertension treated with 40 mg daily for 16 weeks. After reduction at 4 weeks in 8 nondiabetic hypertensive controls return to starting concentration at 16 weeks *3083* Increase by 4 mg/dL in patients given 30 to 60 mg daily for 8 weeks *4213* No effect observed in 14 patients with essential hypertension treated over 2 mo with 20 mg twice daily *3505* No significant change observed in over 30 patients with mild to moderate hypertension treated with 40 mg long-acting drug daily although mean concentration fell by 6 mg/dL after 4 weeks and increased by 11 mg/dL at 8 weeks and 8 mg/dL at 8 weeks *2263*

Urea Nitrogen *Serum* *Increase* *Physiological* Acute reversible deterioration of renal function in 4 patients with chronic renal failure *1417*

Serum *No Effect* *Physiological* Nonsignificant change from mean baseline concentration of 15.3 mg/dL to 15.1 mg/dL in 80 patients with mild to moderate hypertension treated with long-acting nifedipine for 16 weeks *2263*

Uric Acid *Serum* *Decrease* *Physiological* Nonsignificant reduction from mean concentration of 5.61 mg/dL to 5.44 mg/dL in 72 mild to moderate hypertensives treated with long-acting nifedipine for 16 weeks *2263*

Serum *No Effect* *Physiological* No effect on concentration observed with administration of nifedipine *415*

Urine *Increase* *Physiological* Significant effect following 20 mg sublingual dose *1003*

Vanillylmandelic Acid *Urine* *Increase* *Analytical* Interference observed with spectrophotometric Pisano procedure *602*

VLDL-Cholesterol *Serum* *Decrease* *Physiological* Significant and progressive fall in patients with hyperlipoproteinemia treated with about 30 mg/day for 20 weeks *5282*

Serum *No Effect* *Physiological* No effect observed in 14 patients with essential hypertension treated over 2 mo with 20 mg twice daily *3505* Nonsignificant decrease in 11 diabetics with mild to moderate hypertension treated with 40 mg daily for 16 weeks. No effect observed in 8 nondiabetic hypertensive controls *3083*

VLDL-Phospholipids *Serum* *No Effect* *Physiological* Nonsignificant decrease in diabetics with mild to moderate hypertension treated with 40 mg daily for 16 weeks. No effect observed in 8 nondiabetic hypertensive controls *3083*

VLDL-Triglycerides *Serum* *Decrease* *Physiological* Significant reduction in 11 diabetics with mild to moderate hypertension treated with 40 mg daily for 16 weeks. Nonsignificant reduction observed in 8 nondiabetic hypertensive controls *3083*

Serum *No Effect* *Physiological* No consistent effect in patients with hyperlipoproteinemia treated with about 30 mg/day over 20 weeks *5282*

Volume *Urine* *Decrease* *Physiological* In 11 patients with well compensated alcoholic cirrhosis administration of 10 mg nifedipine caused nonsignificant change from mean baseline of 127 ± 19 mL/h to 124 ± 24 mL/h over one hour *6531*

Urine *Increase* *Physiological* In 10 volunteers 20 mg of slow-release formulation caused increased excretion over 8 hours. Effect similar with 10 mg of normal formulation. Diuresis similar to that in controls when slow-release formulation taken for 2 weeks *53* Increase from mean of 0.84 mL/min to 1.14 mL/min in 10 elderly hypertensives over 12 hours following a single oral dose of 20 mg *5412* After 10 mg sublingually in next 2 h *4862* Nonsignificant increase observed at 3 and 7 days in 10 patients with uncomplicated essential hypertension treated with 30 mg/d *1086* Increase observed in 8 hypertensive patients in the 2 hours following administration of 10 mg sublingually *4863*

Niflumic Acid

Cholesterol *Serum* *No Effect* *Analytical* At concentration of 200 mg/L had no effect on CHOD-PAP method *5704*

Creatinine *Serum* *No Effect* *Analytical* At 200 mg/L on reversed phase liquid chromatograhic procedure of Zhiri et al *6656* At concentration of 150 mg/L had no effect on Jaffe-Fading-Fraction method *5704* At concentration of 150 mg/L had no effect on Jaffe-Fuller's earth method *5704*

Uric Acid *Serum* *No Effect* *Analytical* At concentration of 150 mg/L had no effect on catalase-AIDH method *5704* At concentration of 200 mg/L had no effect on Kageyama-Hantzsch method *5704* At 200 mg/L on reversed phase liquid chromatographic procedure of Zhiri et al *6656*

Nifurtimox

Glucose *Serum* *Decrease* *Physiological* May cause decline *128*

Nilutamide

Alanine Aminotransferase *Serum Increase Physiological* Administration has been reported to cause marked increase in enzyme activity in 1% of patients in controlled clinical trials *2648*

Alkaline Phosphatase *Serum Increase Physiological* Administration has been reported to cause increase in activity in 3% of patients in controlled clinical trials *2648*

Androstenedione *Plasma No Effect Physiological* In 12 men with prostatic cancer treatment with 300 mg/d had no significant effect over 6 months *1336*

Aspartate Aminotransferase *Serum Increase Physiological* Administration has been reported to cause marked increase in enzyme activity in 1% of patients in controlled clinical trials *2648*

Creatinine *Serum Increase Physiological* Administration has been reported to cause increase in concentration in 2% of patients in controlled clinical trials *2648*

Dehydroepiandrosterone *Plasma No Effect Physiological* Treatment of 12 men with prostatic cancer had no significant effect over 6 months *1336*

Dehydroepiandrosterone Sulfate
Plasma No Effect Physiological In 12 men with prostatic cancer treatment for 6 months had no significant effect on concentration *1336*

Estradiol *Plasma Increase Physiological* In 12 men with prostatic cancer treatment with 300 mg/d for 6 months caused significant increase from mean baseline of 29.5 ± 4.1 pg/mL to 51.1 ± 6.5 pg/mL *1336*

Follicle Stimulating Hormone
Plasma Increase Physiological In 12 men with prostatic cancer treatment with 300 mg/d for 6 months caused significant increase from mean baseline of 13.8 ± 1.9 mIU/mL to 31.5 ± 6.2 mIU/mL *1336*

Glucose *Serum Increase Physiological* Administration has been reported to cause increase in concentration in 4% of patients in controlled clinical trials *2648*

Haptoglobin *Serum Increase Physiological* Administration has been reported to cause increase in concentration in 2% of patients in controlled clinical trials *2648*

Leukocytes *Blood Decrease Physiological* Administration has been reported to cause decrease in concentration in 3% of patients in controlled clinical trials *2648*

Luteinizing Hormone *Plasma Increase Physiological* Mean concentration in 12 men with prostatic cancer treated with 300 mg/d for 6 months caused significant increase from mean baseline of 17.5 ± 1.6 mIU/mL to 55.4 ± 6.2 mIU/mL *1336*

Prolactin *Plasma No Effect Physiological* In 12 men with prostatic cancer treatment with 300 mg/d for 6 months caused nonsignificant change from mean baseline of 9.9 ± 1.3 ng/mL to 10.9 ± 1.4 ng/mL *1336*

Testosterone *Serum Increase Physiological* In 12 men with prostatic cancer treatment with 300 mg/d for 6 months caused significant increase from mean baseline of 3.7 ± 0.5 ng/mL to 5.2 ± 0.6 ng/mL *1336*

Urea Nitrogen *Serum Increase Physiological* Administration has been reported to cause increase in concentration in 2% of patients in controlled clinical trials *2648*

Nilvadipine

Aldosterone *Plasma No Effect Physiological* Administration of a single oral dose of 2 mg to 9 patients with mild to moderate hypertension had no effect on plasma concentration. Treatment for one week also had no effect *5929*

Norepinephrine *Plasma Increase Physiological* Slight effect only in 10 individuals with mild hypertension *5918*

Renin Activity *Plasma Increase Physiological* A single oral dose of 2 mg in 9 patients with mild to moderate essential hypertension increased mean renin activity from 1.5 ng/mL/h to 2.5 ng/mL/h at one hour and activity remained increased for 4 hours. No effect with one week's treatment *5929*
Plasma No Effect Physiological In 10 patients with mild essential hypertension *5918*

Nimodipine

Carbamazepine *Serum Increase Physiological* Concomitant administration of calcium channel blockers with carbamazepine causes marked increase of plasma carbamazepine concentration resulting in toxicity in some cases *282*
Serum No Effect Physiological No significant effect observed on concentration with coadministration *3119*

Growth Hormone *Plasma No Effect Physiological* No significant effect observed in 8 patients with migraine when treated for 4 months *1916*

Luteinizing Hormone *Plasma No Effect Physiological* No significant effect observed in 8 patients with migraine when treated with nimodipine for 4 months *1916*

Nifedipine *Serum Increase Analytical* 96.5% cross-reactivity observed with STC microplate assay *6275*

Prolactin *Plasma No Effect Physiological* No significant effect observed in 8 patients with migraine when treated for 4 months *1916*

Nipagin

Glucose *Serum No Effect Analytical* At 2 g/dL on glucose oxidase procedure. At 2 g/dL on p-HBAH procedure of Lever. At 2 g/dL on alkaline ferricyanide procedure. At 2 g/dL on o-toluidine procedure *3531*

Niridazole

Color *Urine Increase Analytical* Urine becomes dark *2242*

Eosinophils *Blood Increase Physiological* Quite common allergic response *4014*

Erythrocytes *Blood Decrease Physiological* May cause hemolysis if G-6-PD deficiency *2242*

Hematocrit *Blood Decrease Physiological* Occurs with marked hemolysis *2242*

Hemoglobin *Blood Decrease Physiological* Occurs with marked hemolysis *2242* Hemolysis in glucose-6-phosphate dehydrogenase deficiency or methemoglobin reductase deficiency may be caused by drug *2873* Hemolytic anemia may occur in patients with glucose-6-phosphate dehydrogenase deficiency *1384*

Methemoglobin *Blood Increase Physiological* May cause hemolysis if G-6-PD deficiency *2242*

Nirvanol

Ethosuximide *Serum No Effect Analytical* Insignificant cross-reactivity observed with method on Du Pont aca *1523*

Nisoldipine

Alanine Aminotransferase *Serum Increase Physiological* May cause abnormal liver function tests in fewer than 1% treated patients *6650*

Aldosterone *Plasma Decrease Physiological* Decrease observed in both normo- and hypertensives despite increase in renin activity and angiotensin II concentrations without change in urinary excretion *4461*
Urine No Effect Physiological No reduction observed in 29 hypertensives although plasma concentration decreased when treatment continued for up to 6 months with 10-40 mg daily *4461*

Angiotensin-II *Plasma Increase Physiological* Considerable variation observed in both normo- and hypertensives after administration of nisoldipine *4461*

Apolipoprotein A *Serum Increase Physiological* Treatment of a small number of patients over 4 weeks caused a statistically significant 12% increase in concentration *3730*

Apolipoprotein B *Serum No Effect Physiological* Treatment of a small number of patients over 4 weeks had no statistically significant effect on concentration *3730*

Aspartate Aminotransferase *Serum Increase Physiological* May cause abnormal liver function tests in fewer than 1% treated patients *6650*

Bilirubin *Serum No Effect Physiological* In 14 mild to moderately hypertensive noninsulin dependent diabetic patients *4363*

Blood *Urine Increase Physiological* May cause hematuria concentration in fewer than 1% treated patients *6650*

Calcium *Serum Increase Physiological* Change from average of 2.4 to 2.5 mmol/L in 14 mild to moderately hypertensive noninsulin dependent diabetic patients *4363*

Carbamazepine *Serum Increase Physiological* Concomitant administration of calcium channel blockers with carbamazepine causes marked increase of plasma carbamazepine concentration resulting in toxicity in some cases *282*

Cholesterol *Serum No Effect Physiological* In 14 mild to moderately hypertensive noninsulin dependent diabetic patients *4363* Treatment of a small number of patients over 4 weeks had no statistically significant effect on concentration *3730*

Creatine Kinase *Serum Increase Physiological* May cause increased activity in fewer than 1% treated patients *6650*

Creatinine *Serum Increase Physiological* May cause increased creatinine concentration in fewer than 1% treated patients *6650*

Serum No Effect Physiological In 14 mild to moderately hypertensive noninsulin dependent diabetic patients *4363*

Digoxin *Serum Increase Physiological* Increase of serum concentration of up to 20% observed when two drugs coadministered. Hemodynamic effects altered in patients with congestive heart failure *3154* In patients with cardiac insufficiency coadministration of nisoldipine with digoxin caused increases of both maximal (26%) and minimal (36%) concentrations of digoxin *5345*

Serum No Effect Physiological No significant interaction observed between nisoldipine and digoxin *6650*

Effective Renal Plasma Flow

Patient No Effect Physiological No significant effect in patients with hypertension with normal renal function but 12% reduction in patients with renal insufficiency *6489*

Epinephrine *Plasma No Effect Physiological* No effect observed following administration of a dose in either normo- or hypertensives *4461*

Glomerular Filtration Rate *Urine No Effect Physiological* No significant effect in hypertensive patients with or without renal impairment with 6 weeks treatment *6489*

Glucose *Serum Increase Physiological* May cause diabetes mellitus in fewer than 1% treated patients *6650*

Serum No Effect Physiological In 14 mild to moderately hypertensive noninsulin dependent diabetic patients *4363*

γ-Glutamyltransferase *Serum Increase Physiological* May cause abnormal liver function tests in fewer than 1% treated patients *6650*

HDL_3-Cholesterol *Serum Increase Physiological* Treatment of a small number of patients over 4 weeks caused a statistically significant 13% increase in concentration *3730*

HDL-Cholesterol *Serum Increase Physiological* Treatment of a small number of patients over 4 weeks caused a statistically significant 14% increase in concentration probably due to stimulation of lysosomal and cytoplasmic cholesterase *3730*

Hematocrit *Blood Decrease Physiological* May cause anemia in fewer than 1% treated patients *6650*

Hemoglobin *Blood Decrease Physiological* May cause anemia in fewer than 1% treated patients *6650* From 14.7 to 14.0 g/dL in 14 mild to moderately hypertensive noninsulin dependent diabetic patients *4363*

Hemoglobin A_{1c} *Blood Decrease Physiological* From 14.7 to 14.0 g/dL in 14 mild to moderately hypertensive noninsulin dependent diabetic patients *4363*

LDL-Cholesterol *Serum No Effect Physiological* Treatment of a small number of patients over 4 weeks had no statistically significant effect on concentration *3730*

Leukocytes *Blood Decrease Physiological* May cause leukopenia in fewer than 1% treated patients *6650*

Nifedipine *Serum Increase Analytical* 100% cross-reactivity observed with STC microplate assay *6275*

Nonprotein Nitrogen *Serum Increase Physiological* May cause increased NPN in fewer than 1% treated patients *6650*

Norepinephrine *Plasma Increase Physiological* Slight increase observed for 2-4 hours after administration in both normo- and hypertensives but then decrease *4461*

Plasma No Effect Physiological No significant change observed in 20 patients with severe heart failure 30 min following intravenous bolus of 0.2 mg then continuous infusion of 0.2 µg/kg/min *1752*

Occult Blood *Feces Increase Physiological* May cause gastrointestinal hemorrhage and melena in fewer than 1% treated patients *6650*

Potassium *Serum Decrease Physiological* May cause hypokalemia in fewer than 1% treated patients *6650*

Propranolol *Serum Increase Physiological* Area under curve increased by mean of 43% and peak plasma concentration increased by 68% when drugs coadministered *3542* Following a single oral dose of nisoldipine (20 mg) a single dose of propranolol (40 mg) was given one hour later: area under the concentration curve of propranolol was increased by 43% and its maximum concentration was increased by 68%. Effect due to increased absorption of propranolol thereby increasing its bioavailability *5411*

Quinidine *Serum Increase Physiological* Administration of quinidine 648 mg twice daily with immediate release, but not coat-core formulated nisoldipine caused a 20% increase in the plasma concentration of quinidine *6650*

Renin Activity *Plasma Increase Physiological* Nonsignificant increase observed in both normal individuals and hypertensives 1 hour after first dose but effect not significant: return to normal observed after 2 hours *4461*

Plasma No Effect Physiological No significant effect in hypertensive patients with or without renal impairment with 6 weeks treatment *6489* No significant change observed in 20 patients with severe heart failure after 30 min following infusion of nisoldipine after initial intravenous bolus *1752*

Sodium *Serum Decrease Physiological* Fell by average of 3 mmol/L in 14 mild to moderately hypertensive noninsulin dependent diabetic patients *4363*

Triglycerides *Serum Decrease Physiological* From 1.9 to 1.6 mmol/L in 14 mild to moderately hypertensive noninsulin dependent diabetic patients *4363*

Serum No Effect Physiological Treatment of a small number of patients over 4 weeks had no statistically significant effect on concentration *3730*

Urea Nitrogen *Serum Increase Physiological* May cause increased urea nitrogen concentration in fewer than 1% treated patients *6650*

Serum No Effect Physiological In 14 mild to moderately hypertensive noninsulin dependent diabetic patients *4363*

Uric Acid *Serum Increase Physiological* May cause gout in fewer than 1% treated patients *6650*

Serum No Effect Physiological In 14 mild to moderately hypertensive noninsulin dependent diabetic patients *4363*

Warfarin *Plasma No Effect Physiological* No significant interaction observed between nisoldipine and warfarin *6650*

Nitrazepam

Acetaminophen *Serum No Effect Analytical* At 2 mg/L no effect on HPLC method *5775*

Albumin *Urine No Effect Analytical* Using a fluorimetric assay with Albumin Blue 580 on a Cobas Fara centrifugal analyzer for the detection of microalbuminuria no significant interference was detected at a concentration of 4 mg/L *3117*

Amitriptyline *Serum No Effect Physiological* No effect on serum concentration if given together *5559*

Antipyrine *Serum No Effect Physiological* No significant effect on half-life *5820*

Benzodiazepine *Urine Positive Analytical* Positive result observed at a concentration of 2.0 µg/mL (7.10 µmol/L) with method on Du Pont aca *1556* At concentrations of 0.5 µg/mL or greater produces positive result with Syva EMIT II assay *1785*

Bilirubin *Serum No Effect Physiological* Insignificant displacement from protein in neonates *6314*

Calcium *Serum No Effect Physiological* No effect when given in normal therapeutic amounts to elderly *6618*

Catecholamines *Plasma No Effect Analytical* No effect on HPLC method of Koller for dopamine, epinephrine, and norepinephrine *3230*

Nitrazepam *(continued)*

Glucose *Serum Decrease Analytical* Slight effect glucose oxidase method of Boehringer *5480*

Histamine *Plasma No Effect Analytical* Improbable inhibition of radio-enzyme assay at physiological concentrations *2492*

17-Hydroxycorticosteroids *Urine No Effect Physiological* No effect although 6-hydroxycortisol increased *5820*

6-β-Hydroxycortisol *Urine No Effect Physiological* No significant effect *5820*

5-Hydroxyindoleacetic Acid *Urine Increase Analytical* Slight effect when added *in vitro* in method of Udenfriend *1051*

Nortriptyline *Serum No Effect Physiological* No effect on serum concentration if given together *5559*

Phenylbutazone *Serum No Effect Physiological* No significant effect on half-life *5820*

Phenytoin *Serum Increase Physiological* Probably inhibits metabolism in liver *2452*

Platelets *Blood Decrease Physiological* May cause thrombocytopenia *4265*

Prothrombin Time *Plasma No Effect Physiological* No effect observed with phenprocoumon *550*

Warfarin *Plasma No Effect Physiological* No effect observed on plasma concentration in one individual when drugs coadministered also no effect seen on prothrombin time *6428*

Nitrendipine

Acebutolol *Serum No Effect Physiological* Coadministration had no significant effect on drug kinetics *3147*

Albumin *Urine Decrease Physiological* In 12 patients with essential hypertension and albuminuria treatment for 8 weeks caused nonsignificant reduction *545*

Aldosterone *Plasma No Effect Physiological* In 20 hypertensive type I diabetic patients treatment with 20 mg/d for 6 weeks caused insignificant change fro 77.1 ± 44.4 pg/mL to 79.0 ± 56.4 pg/mL *3496*

Apolipoprotein A-I *Serum No Effect Physiological* In 33 patients with mild to moderate hypertension treatment with mean dose of 6.8 mg/d for 12 weeks caused no significant change from mean baseline *5279* No significant change observed in 15 noninsulin-dependent diabetic hypertensives and 15 nondiabetic hypertensives treated with 20-40 mg/d for 24 weeks *2141*

Apolipoprotein B *Serum No Effect Physiological* In 33 patients with mild to moderate hypertension treatment with mean dose of 6.8 mg/d for 12 weeks caused no significant change from mean baseline *5279* No significant change observed in 15 noninsulin-dependent diabetic hypertensives and 15 nondiabetic hypertensives treated with 20-40 mg/d for 24 weeks *2141*

Apolipoprotein E *Serum No Effect Physiological* In 33 patients with mild to moderate hypertension treatment with mean dose of 6.8 mg/d for 12 weeks caused no significant change from mean baseline *5279*

Atenolol *Serum No Effect Physiological* Coadministration had no significant effect on drug pharmacokinetics *3147*

Atrial Natriuretic Peptide *Plasma Decrease Physiological* In 20 hypertensive type I diabetics treatment with 20 mg/d for 6 weeks caused reduction of mean from 106.7 ± 112.8 pg/mL to 89.7 ± 107.4 pg/mL but change not statistically significant due to influence of grossly abnormal results in 2 patients *3496*

Cholesterol *Serum No Effect Physiological* In 38 mild to moderate hypertensives treatment for 12 months caused nonsignificant decrease from 220 ± 35.8 mg/dL to 196 ± 31.3 mg/dL *1415* No effect observed in patients with essential hypertension when given as monotherapy *6470* In hypertensives treated with 20 mg/d mean concentration changed insignificantly from 182 ± 36 mg/dL to 173 ± 28 mg/dL *1841* In 33 patients with mild to moderate hypertension treatment with mean dose of 6.8 mg/d for 12 weeks caused no significant change from mean baseline *5279* In hypertensives treated with 20 mg/d mean concentration increased insignificantly from 192 ± 33 mg/dL to 200 ± 43 mg/dL *3800* No significant change observed in 15 noninsulin diabetic hypertensives and 15 nondiabetic hypertensives treated with 20-40 mg/d for 24 weeks *2141*

Cholesterol:HDL-Cholesterol Ratio *Serum No Effect Physiological* In 38 mild to moderate hypertensives treatment for 12 months caused nonsignificant increase from 23 ± 9.7 mg/dL to 29 ± 12.7 mg/dL *1415*

C-Peptide *Plasma Decrease Physiological* In 33 patients with mild to moderate hypertension treatment with mean dose of 6.8 mg/d for 12 weeks caused nonsignificant change from mean baseline of 3.25 ± 1.73 ng/mL to 2.57 ± 1.13 ng/mL *5279*
Plasma No Effect Physiological No significant change observed in 15 noninsulin-dependent diabetic hypertensives and 15 nondiabetic hypertensives treated with 20-40 mg/d for 24 weeks *2141*

Creatinine Clearance *Urine No Effect Physiological* In 12 patients with essential hypertension treatment for 8 weeks caused nonsignificant increase from mean baseline of 99.1 ± 2.3 mL/min to 102 ± 3.0 mL/min *545*

Cyclosporine *Blood No Effect Physiological* No significant change observed during treatment with 20 mg/d in 16 hypertensive renal transplant patients over 3 weeks *1130*
Serum No Effect Physiological Coadministration of nitrendipine 20 to 30 mg daily with cyclosporine (8 mg/kg) had no effect on cyclosporine concentration *5411* In 16 hypertensive renal transplant patients treatment with 20 mg/d for 3 weeks had no significant effect on plasma cyclosporine concentration *6596*

Dehydroepiandrosterone Sulfate *Plasma Increase Physiological* In 8 insulin-resistant obese and hypertensive men treatment with 20 mg/d for 7 days caused significant increase of 63% from mean baseline of 4.21 ± 0.17 µmol/L to 6.84 ± 0.21 µmol/L *452*

Digoxin *Serum Increase Physiological* At a daily dose of 20 mg/d caused area under curve to increase by 16% and reduced clearance by 13% although pharmacokinetics were not altered with a 10 mg/d dose *5345* Dose-dependent increase in serum concentration in patients in whom drugs coadministered *3150*

Fructosamine *Serum No Effect Physiological* In 20 hypertensive type I diabetics treatment with 20 mg/d for 6 weeks caused insignificant change from 3.21 ± 0.56 mg/dL to 3.25 ± 0.59 mg/dL *3496* No significant effect observed in 15 noninsulin-dependent diabetic hypertensives and 15 nondiabetic hypertensives treated with 20-40 mg/d for 24 weeks *2141*

Glipizide *Serum No Effect Physiological* A single dose of nitrendipine had no effect on disposition of glipizide in 6 NIDD patients treated for at least 2 months, although mean postprandial insulin decreased by 18.5% *5345*

Glucose *Serum Decrease Physiological* Incidence of 0.3% observed in French Pharmacovigilance database *4106*
Serum No Effect Physiological In hypertensives treated with 20 mg/d mean concentration changed insignificantly from 70 ± 11 mg/dL to 73 ± 14 mg/dL *1841* In 38 mild to moderate hypertensives treatment for 12 months caused nonsignificant decrease from mean baseline of 94 +/ 8.7 mg/dL to 92 ± 5.4 mg/dL *1415* In hypertensive patients treatment with 20 mg/d caused no change from mean baseline of 75 ± 12 mg/dL *3800* No significant change observed in 15 noninsulin-dependent diabetic hypertensive diabetics and 15 nondiabetic hypertensives treated with 20-40 mg/d for 24 weeks *2141* In 33 patients with mild to moderate hypertension treatment with mean dose of 6.8 mg/d for 12 weeks caused nonsignificant change from mean baseline of 107.4 ± 13.4 mg/dL to 104.6 ± 12.5 mg/dL *5279*

Glucose Tolerance *Serum Increase Physiological* In 8 insulin-resistant obese and hypertensive men treatment with 20 mg/d for 7 days caused a reduction in the area under the curve from 1246 ± 31 mmol/L.min to 1091 ± 26 mmol/L.min. Area under insulin curve also reduced *452*

Glycated Hemoglobin *Blood No Effect Physiological* In 20 hypertensive type I diabetic patients treatment with 20 mg/d for 6 weeks caused insignificant change from 9.48 ± 1.73% to 9.17 ± 1.66% *3496*

HDL-Cholesterol *Serum No Effect Physiological* No effect observed in patients with essential hypertension when given as monotherapy *6470* In hypertensive patients treated with 20 mg/d insignificant decrease from 44 ± 13 mg/dL to 40 ± 8 mg/dL *1841* In 38 mild to moderate hypertensives treatment for 12 months caused nonsignificant increase from mean baseline of 52 ± 15.2 mg/dL to 54 ± 15.0 mg/dL *1415* In 33 patients with mild to moderate hypertension treatment with mean dose of 6.8 mg/d for 12 weeks caused no significant change from mean baseline *5279* No significant change observed in 15 noninsulin-dependent diabetic hypertensives and 15 nondiabetic hypertensives treated with 20-40 mg/d for 24 weeks *2141* In hypertensives treated with 20 mg/d mean concentration changed insignificantly from 46 ± 9 mg/dL to 50 ± 14 mg/dL *3800*

Hemoglobin A_{1c} *Blood No Effect Physiological* In 33 patients with mild to moderate hypertension treatment with mean dose of 6.8 mg/d for 12 weeks caused nonsignificant change from mean baseline of 5.55 ± 0.55% to 5.52 ± 0.55% *5279* In 38 mild to moderate hypertensives treatment for 12 months caused nonsignificant increase from mean baseline of 5.2 ± 1.0% to 5.5 +/ 1.2% *1415* No significant change observed in 15 noninsulin-dependent diabetic hypertensives and 15 nondiabetic hypertensives treated with 20-40 mg/d for 24 weeks *2141*

Insulin *Plasma Decrease Physiological* In 8 insulin-resistant obese and hypertensive men treatment with 20 mg/d for 7 days caused reduction of mean concentration from 265 ± 24 pmol/L to 194 ± 22 pmol/L without changing the plasma glucose concentration *452*
Plasma Increase Physiological In hypertensives treatment with 20 mg/d caused change from mean baseline of 8.5 ± 2.7 µU/mL to 10.9 ± 4.7 µU/mL *3800*
Plasma No Effect Physiological In 33 patients with mild to moderate hypertension treatment with mean dose of 6.8 mg/d for 12 weeks caused nonsignificant change from mean baseline of 8.87 ± 6.64 µU/mL to 7.47 ± 4.26 µU/mL *5279*

LDL-Cholesterol *Serum Decrease Physiological* In 38 mild to moderate hypertensives treatment for one month caused significant decrease from mean baseline of 141 ± 33.5 mg/dL to 113 ± 33.2 mg/dL *1415*
Serum No Effect Physiological In 33 patients with mild to moderate hypertension treatment with mean dose of 6.8 mg/d for 12 weeks caused no significant change from mean baseline *5279* No effect observed in patients with essential hypertension when given as monotherapy *6470*

LDL-Cholesterol:HDL-Cholesterol Ratio
Serum No Effect Physiological In 33 patients with mild to moderate hypertension treatment with mean dose of 6.8 mg/d for 12 weeks caused no significant change from mean baseline *5279*

Lipoprotein Lp(a) *Serum No Effect Physiological* In 33 patients with mild to moderate hypertension treatment with mean dose of 6.8 mg/d for 12 weeks caused no significant change from mean baseline *5279*

Metoprolol *Serum No Effect Physiological* Coadministration had no significant effect on kinetics of drug *3147*

Midazolam *Serum No Effect Physiological* Coadministration had no effect on pharmacokinetics and pharmacodynamics of midazolam *5345*

Na/K-ATPase *Red Blood Cells Increase Physiological* In 15 middle-aged hypertensives treatment with 20 mg/d for 4 weeks caused significant increase in 15 middle-aged hypertensives from mean baseline of 104.60 ± 29.37 nmol P/mg protein/h to 158.13 ± 26.80 nmol P/g protein/h *6130*

Nifedipine *Serum Increase Analytical* 99.7% cross-reactivity observed with STC microplate assay *6275*

Norepinephrine *Plasma Increase Physiological* Increase observed shortly after administration in hypertensives during chronic therapy due to increase in sympathetic tone *2528*

Renin Activity *Plasma Increase Physiological* In 20 hypertensive diabetic patients treatment with 20 mg/d for 6 weeks caused significant increase from mean of 1.28 ± 0.98 ng angiotensin-I/mL/h to 1.91 ± 0.88 ng angiotensin-I/mL/h *3496*

Sodium *Urine No Effect Physiological* In 12 patients with essential hypertension treatment for 8 weeks caused nonsignificant change from mean baseline of 138 ± 2.9 mL/min to 135 ± 3.4 mmol/d *545*

Triglycerides *Serum Decrease Physiological* In 33 patients with mild to moderate hypertension treatment with mean dose of 6.8 mg/d for 12 weeks caused significant change from mean baseline of 150 ± 84 mg/dL to 130 ± 45 mg/dL *5279*
Serum Increase Physiological In hypertensives treated with 20 mg/d insignificant increase from 111 ± 40 mg/dL to 130 ± 50 mg/dL observed *1841*
Serum No Effect Physiological In hypertensives treatment with 20 mg/d caused insignificant change from 83 ± 57 mg/dL to 84 ± 37 mg/dL *3800* No significant change observed in 15 noninsulin-dependent hypertensives and 15 nondiabetic hypertensives treated with 20-40 mg/d for 24 weeks *2141* No effect observed in patients with essential hypertension when given as monotherapy *6470* In 38 mild to moderate hypertensives treatment for 12 months caused nonsignificant increase from mean baseline of 113 ± 49.4 mg/dL to 128 ± 53.3 mg/dL *1415*

Uric Acid *Serum No Effect Physiological* In 38 mild to moderate hypertensives treatment for 12 months caused no change from mean baseline of 5.2 ± 1.1 mg/dL *1415*

Nitrofurans

Alanine Aminotransferase *Serum Increase Physiological* Hepatotoxicity *3810*

Alkaline Phosphatase *Serum Increase Physiological* Hepatotoxicity *3810*

Aspartate Aminotransferase *Serum Increase Physiological* Hepatotoxicity *3810*

Bile *Urine Increase Physiological* Hepatotoxicity *3810*

Bilirubin *Serum Increase Physiological* Hepatotoxicity or due to hemolytic anemia *3810*

BSP Retention *Serum Increase Physiological* Hepatotoxicity *3810*

Color *Urine Increase Analytical* Brown, green, blue color *2024*

Creatinine *Urine Increase Analytical* Reacts with color reagent in Jaffe procedures *3669*

Eosinophils *Blood Increase Physiological* May be serious anaphylactoid reaction *128*

Folate *Serum Decrease Physiological* May induce folate deficiency- megaloblastic anemia *4014*

Glutathione, Reduced
Red Blood Cells Decrease Physiological Occurs with hemolysis *3094*

Heinz Body Formation *Blood Positive Physiological* Occurs initially with hemolysis *3094*

Hematocrit *Blood Decrease Physiological* May cause hemolytic anemia if G-6-PD deficiency *128*

Hemoglobin *Blood Decrease Physiological* May cause hemolytic anemia if G-6-PD deficiency *128*
Plasma Increase Physiological Occurs with intravascular hemolysis *4013*
Urine Increase Physiological May occur with severe hemolytic anemia *3094*

Leukocytes *Blood Decrease Physiological* May occasionally cause agranulocytosis *4014*

MCV *Blood Increase Physiological* May cause megaloblastic anemia *4014*

Methemoglobin *Blood Increase Physiological* May cause hemolytic anemia if G-6-PD deficiency *128*

Reticulocytes *Blood Increase Physiological* Occurs during recovery after hemolysis *3094*

Sugar *Urine Increase Analytical* Metabolites reduce Benedict's reagent *3669*

Nitrofurantoin

Alanine Aminotransferase *Serum Increase Physiological* May cause cholestatic jaundice *4691* Moderate increase chronic active hepatitis, much more common in women than men, but still rare *4041* Hepatic reactions, including hepatitis, cholestatic jaundice, chronic active hepatitis and hepatic necrosis occur rarely *4800* Hepatic reactions, including hepatitis, cholestatic jaundice, chronic active hepatitis and hepatic necrosis reported as adverse reactions (in about 1 - 5% treated patients) *4799*
Serum No Effect Analytical No effect at 16 mg/L on Boehringer Mannheim Reflotron method *5706* No effect at therapeutic concentration on Boehringer Mannheim Reflotron

Nitrofurantoin *(continued)*

Alanine Aminotransferase *(continued)*
method *3231* On routine methods in use on Technicon SMAC® , Kodak Ektachem® , Abbott-VP, Roche Cobas-Bio, Du Pont aca, Hitachi® 705, KDA at 5 times normal upper therapeutic concentration *3525*

Albumin *Serum Decrease Physiological* In association with chronic active hepatitis *5851*
Serum No Effect Analytical At concentration of 4 mg/L had no effect on BCG method *5704* On routine methods in use on Technicon SMAC® , Kodak Ektachem® , Abbott-VP, Roche Cobas-Bio, Du Pont aca, Hitachi® 705, KDA at 5 times normal upper therapeutic concentration *3525*
Urine No Effect Analytical At concentration of 18 mg/dL had no significant effect on Boehringer Mannheim Tina-quant method *2799*

Alkaline Phosphatase *Serum Increase Analytical* 19% increase on p-nitrophenyl phosphate method on Technicon SMAC® at 5 times normal therapeutic concentration *3525*
Serum Increase Physiological May follow acute hepatitis with or without cholestasis or as chronic active hepatitis or chronic granulomatous reaction *3904* Moderate increase chronic active hepatitis, much more common in women than men, but still rare *4041* Hepatic reactions, including hepatitis, cholestatic jaundice, chronic active hepatitis and hepatic necrosis reported as adverse reactions *4799* Hepatic reactions, including hepatitis, cholestatic jaundice, chronic active hepatitis and hepatic necrosis occur rarely *4800* May cause cholestatic jaundice *4691*
Serum No Effect Analytical On routine methods in use on Abbott-VP, Roche Cobas-Bio, Du Pont aca, Hitachi® 705, KDA at 5 times normal therapeutic concentration *3525*
Urine Decrease Analytical Interference with determination method *4331*

Amylase *Serum Increase Physiological* Isolated case confirmed by rechallenge, rapidly resolved on withdrawal of drug. Edema of pancreatic head also caused jaundice *4244* Pancreatitis reported as an adverse reaction *4799* Sialadenitis and pancreatitis have been reported as complications of treatment *4800*
Serum No Effect Analytical On routine methods in use on Technicon SMAC® , Kodak Ektachem® , Abbott-VP, Roche Cobas-Bio, Du Pont aca, Hitachi® 705, KDA at 5 times normal upper therapeutic concentration *3525* At a concentration of 16 mg/L had no effect on method on Boehringer Mannheim Reflotron system *5706*
Urine Increase Physiological Isolated case confirmed by rechallenge, rapidly resolved on withdrawal of drug. Edema of pancreatic head also caused jaundice *4244*

Amylase, Pancreatic Isoenzyme
Serum No Effect Analytical No effect observed at toxic concentration of 18 mg/L on method on Boehringer Mannheim Reflotron *3647*

Anti-Smooth Muscle Antibodies
Serum Increase Physiological Increased to 1:640 chronic active hepatitis, much more common in women than men, but still rare *4041*

Antinuclear Antibodies *Serum Increase Physiological* Increased to 1:640 chronic active hepatitis, much more common in women than men, but still rare *4041*

Antithyroglobulin Antibodies
Serum Increase Physiological Mild increase developed lupus-like syndrome associated with pulmonary reaction *5442*

Aspartate Aminotransferase *Serum Increase Analytical* 36% increase on kinetic MDH procedure on KDA at 5 times normal therapeutic concentration *3525*
Serum Increase Physiological Hepatic reactions, including hepatitis, cholestatic jaundice, chronic active hepatitis and hepatic necrosis reported as adverse reactions (in about 1 - 5% treated patients) *4799* Hepatic reactions, including hepatitis, cholestatic jaundice, chronic active hepatitis and hepatic necrosis occur rarely *4800* May follow acute hepatitis with or without cholestasis or as chronic active hepatitis or chronic granulomatous reaction *3904* Moderate increase with chronic active hepatitis, much more common in women than men, but still rare *4041* May cause cholestatic jaundice *4691*
Serum No Effect Analytical On routine methods in use on Technicon SMAC® , Abbott-VP, Du Pont aca, Roche Cobas-Bio, Hitachi® 705 at 5 times normal therapeutic concentration *3525* No effect at therapeutic concentration on Boehringer Mannheim Reflotron method *3231* No effect at 16 mg/L on Boehringer Mannheim Reflotron method *5706*

Bicarbonate *Serum Decrease Physiological* Nephrotoxicity may cause azotemia *1714*
Serum No Effect Analytical At concentration of 4 mg/L had no effect on method using phenolphthalein *5704*

Bile *Urine Increase Physiological* May cause cholestatic jaundice *3810*

Bilirubin *Serum Increase Analytical* Clinically significant effect at upper limit of normal therapeutic range on Ektachem® 400/700 method *3525*
Serum Increase Physiological Hepatic reactions, including hepatitis, cholestatic jaundice, chronic active hepatitis and hepatic necrosis reported as adverse reactions *4799* May follow acute hepatitis with or without cholestasis or as chronic active hepatitis or chronic granulomatous reaction *3904* Chronic active hepatitis much more common in women than men, but still rare *4041* May cause hemolytic anemia or cholestasis *3211* Hepatic reactions, including hepatitis, cholestatic jaundice, chronic active hepatitis and hepatic necrosis occur rarely *4800*
Serum No Effect Analytical No effect at 5 mg/L on Ames Seralyzer method *5706* On routine methods in use on Technicon SMAC® , Abbott-VP, Roche Cobas-Bio, Du Pont aca, Hitachi® 705, KDA at 5 times normal upper therapeutic concentration *3525* At concentration of 16 mg/L no effect on method on Boehringer Mannheim Reflotron system *5706* At concentration of 4 mg/L had no effect on Jendrassik and Grof method *5704*

Bilirubin, Conjugated *Serum Increase Analytical* At concentrations above 1 mg/L increases result as measured by method on Kodak Ektachem® . Effect of clinical significance since therapeutic range 1.8-5.5 mg/L *5706*

Bilirubin, Unconjugated *Serum Decrease Analytical* Result lower at concentrations above 1 mg/L when measured on Kodak Ektachem® . Effect of clinical significance since therapeutic range 1.8-5.5 mg/L *5706*

BSP Retention *Serum Increase Physiological* Intrahepatic cholestatic jaundice *1753*

Calcium *Serum No Effect Analytical* On routine methods in use on Technicon SMAC® , Kodak Ektachem® , Abbott-VP, Roche Cobas-Bio, Du Pont aca, Hitachi® 705, KDA at 5 times normal upper therapeutic concentration *3525* At concentration of 4 mg/L had no effect on cresolphthalein method *5704*

Chloride *Serum No Effect Analytical* At concentration of 4 mg/L had no effect on mercurimetric method *5704*

Cholesterol *Serum No Effect Analytical* At concentration of 98 mg/L had no effect on catalase-AIDH method *5704* At concentration of 98 mg/L had no effect on Liebermann-Burchard method *5704* At concentration of 98 mg/L had no effect on CHOD-PAP method *5704* At concentration of 98 mg/L had no effect on CHOD-Iodide method *5704* No effect at 5 mg/L on Ames Seralyzer method *5706* At concentration of 16 mg/L no effect on method on Boehringer Mannheim Reflotron system *5706* At concentration of 98 mg/L had no effect on method using catalase-Hantzsch reaction *5704* No effect at therapeutic concentration on Boehringer Mannheim Reflotron method *3231* On routine methods in use on Technicon SMAC® , Kodak Ektachem® , Abbott-VP, Roche Cobas-Bio, Du Pont aca, Hitachi® 705, KDA at 5 times normal upper therapeutic concentration *3525*

Cholinesterase *Serum No Effect Analytical* No effect observed at concentration of 20 µg/mL with butyrylthiocholine method on Kodak Ektachem® *2504*

Color *Urine Increase Analytical* Brown, yellow color *1714*

Coombs' Test, Direct *Blood Positive Physiological* Developed lupus-like syndrome. Syndrome associated with pulmonary reaction *5442*

Cortisol *Plasma No Effect Analytical* At a concentration of 18 mg/L no significant effect observed on CEDIA or Enzymun methods *1097*

Creatine Kinase *Serum No Effect Analytical* On routine methods in use on Technicon SMAC® , Kodak Ektachem® , Abbott-VP, Roche Cobas-Bio, Du Pont aca, Hitachi® 705, KDA at 5 times normal upper therapeutic concentration *3525* No effect at 5 mg/L on method on Ames Seralyzer *5706*

Creatinine *Serum Increase Analytical* At concentrations above 5 mg/L (normal therapeutic concentration 5.5 mg/L) raised concentration as measured by Jaffe-Fuller's earth method *5704* At concentrations above 5 mg/L (normal therapeutic concentration 5.5 mg/L) raised concentration as measured by Jaffe-Fading-Fraction method *5704* At concentrations above 18 mg/L (normal therapeutic concentration 5.5 mg/L) raised concentration as measured by kinetic Jaffe method on BKA-2 *5704*
Serum Increase Physiological Nephrotoxic effect *3669* In 8 of 56 acute and 3 of 22 chronic drug induced pulmonary reactions *2679*
Serum No Effect Analytical At concentration of 4 mg/L had no effect on Technicon AutoAnalyzer® Jaffe method *5704* No effect of concentrations up to 15 mg/L on single slide method on Kodak Ektachem® *5706* No effect at 5 mg/L on method on Ames Seralyzer *5706* No effect of concentrations up to 20 mg/L on 2-slide method on Kodak Ektachem® *5706* On routine methods in use on Technicon SMAC® , Kodak Ektachem® , Abbott-VP, Roche Cobas-Bio, Du Pont aca, Hitachi® 705, KDA at 5 times normal upper therapeutic concentration *3525*

Eosinophils *Blood Increase Physiological* In 158 of 191 acute and 14 of 32 chronic drug induced pulmonary reactions *2679* Allergic response (greater than 1%) *3211* Mild increase developed lupus-like syndrome associated with pulmonary reaction *5442* Eosinophilia has been reported rarely as the most common adverse reaction, in 1 - 5% treated patients *4799* Eosinophilia may occur, but more frequently in acute form than in subacute form: usually occurs in first week of treatment and reversible with cessation of therapy *4800*

Erythrocyte Sedimentation Rate
Blood Increase Physiological Developed lupus-like syndrome associated with pulmonary reaction *5442*

Erythrocytes *Blood Decrease Physiological* Hypersensitivity (G-6-PD)/megaloblastic anemia *3890*

Folate *Serum Decrease Physiological* Inhibits intestinal conjugase *5101*

γ-Globulin *Serum Increase Physiological* In 3 of 9 acute and 16 of 20 chronic pulmonary reactions *2680*

Glucose *Serum No Effect Analytical* At concentration of 60 mg/L had no effect on hexokinase/G-6-PDH method *5704* At concentration of 5 mg/L had no effect on Kodak Ektachem® method *5704* At concentration of 2.5 mg/L had no effect on GOD/POD-PAP method *5704* No effect at therapeutic concentration on Boehringer Mannheim Reflotron method *3231* At concentration of 16 mg/L no effect on method on Boehringer Mannheim Reflotron system *5706* On routine methods in use on Technicon SMAC® , Kodak Ektachem® , Abbott-VP, Roche Cobas-Bio, Du Pont aca, Hitachi® 705, KDA at 5 times normal upper therapeutic concentration *3525* No effect at 5 mg/L on glucose oxidase method on Ames Seralyzer *5706*
Urine Increase Analytical False positive reactions observed with Benedict's and Fehling's reagents *4799* False positive reaction may occur with Benedict's and Fehling's reagents *4800*
Urine No Effect Analytical No effect observed with glucose enzymatic methods but false positive reaction may occur with Benedict's and Fehling's reagents *4800* At concentration of 500 mg/L had no effect on Diabur-test *5704* No effect observed on glucose oxidase reagent strips *4799*

Glucose Tolerance *Serum Decrease Physiological* Single case reported *2415*

γ-Glutamyltransferase *Serum Increase Physiological* Hepatic reactions, including hepatitis, cholestatic jaundice, chronic active hepatitis and hepatic necrosis occur rarely *4800* Hepatic reactions, including hepatitis, cholestatic jaundice, chronic active hepatitis and hepatic necrosis reported as adverse reactions *4799*
Serum No Effect Analytical On routine methods in use on Technicon SMAC® , Kodak Ektachem® , Abbott-VP, Roche Cobas-Bio, Du Pont aca, Hitachi® 705, KDA at 5 times normal upper therapeutic concentration *3525* No effect at therapeutic concentration on Boehringer Mannheim Reflotron method *3231* At concentration of 16 mg/L no effect on method on Boehringer Mannheim Reflotron system *5706*

Granulocytes *Blood Decrease Physiological* Agranulocytosis has been reported as complication of treatment *4800* Agranulocytosis and granulocytopenia have been reported rarely as adverse reactions *4799*

Haptoglobin *Serum Decrease Physiological* Hemolytic anemia *3810*

HDL-Cholesterol *Serum No Effect Analytical* At a concentration up to 16 mg/L had no significant effect on Reflotron method for whole blood cholesterol *6352*

Heinz Body Formation *Blood Positive Physiological* May cause hemolytic anemia *536*

Hematocrit *Blood Decrease Physiological* Hemolytic anemia of the primaquine-sensitivity type may be induced by nitrofurantoin: hemolysis may be linked to glucose-6-dehydrogenase deficiency *4800* Hemolytic or megaloblastic anemia have been reported rarely as adverse reactions *4799* Megaloblastic anemia/hypersensitivity (G-6-PD) *3890*

Hemoglobin *Blood Decrease Physiological* Hemolytic or megaloblastic anemia have been reported rarely as adverse reactions *4799* Hemolysis in glucose-6-phosphate dehydrogenase deficiency or methemoglobin reductase deficiency may be caused by drug *2873* Megaloblastic anemia/hypersensitivity (G-6-PD) *3890* Hemolytic anemia of the primaquine-sensitivity type may be induced by nitrofurantoin: hemolysis may be linked to glucose-6-dehydrogenase deficiency *4800*

Histamine *Plasma No Effect Analytical* No inhibition of radio-enzyme assay at concentration 200 times therapeutic *2492*

Immunoglobulin G *Serum Increase Physiological* Chronic active hepatitis, much more common in women than men, but still rare *4041*

Indocyanine Green *Serum Decrease Physiological* Mechanism not yet established *3942*

Iron *Serum No Effect Analytical* On routine methods in use on Technicon SMAC® , Kodak Ektachem® , Abbott-VP, Roche Cobas-Bio, Du Pont aca, Hitachi® 705, KDA at 5 times normal upper therapeutic concentration *3525*

Lactate *Plasma No Effect Analytical* At concentration of 60 mg/L had no effect on enzymatic method *5704*

Lactate Dehydrogenase *Serum Increase Physiological* May cause hemolytic anemia *3211* In 16 of 1756 acute and 12 of 19 chronic drug induced pulmonary reactions *2679* In 6 of 17 acute and 12 of 19 chronic drug induced pulmonary reactions *2679* May follow acute hepatitis with or without cholestasis or as chronic active hepatitis or chronic granulomatous reaction *3904*
Serum No Effect Analytical No effect at 5 mg/L on method on Ames Seralyzer *5706* On routine methods in use on Technicon SMAC® , Kodak Ektachem® , Abbott-VP, Roche Cobas-Bio, Du Pont aca, Hitachi® 705, KDA at 5 times normal upper therapeutic concentration *3525*
Urine Decrease Analytical Interference with determination method *4331*

Leukocytes *Blood Decrease Physiological* Leukopenia has been reported as complication of treatment *4800* Leukopenia/agranulocytosis may occur *1658* Leukopenia has been reported rarely as an adverse reaction *4799*
Blood Increase Physiological In 80 of 153 acute and 5 of 33 chronic drug induced pulmonary reactions *2679*

Lipase *Serum Increase Physiological* Sialadenitis and pancreatitis have been reported as complications of treatment *4800* Pancreatitis reported as an adverse reaction *4799*

MCV *Blood Decrease Physiological* Megaloblastic anemia/hypersensitivity (G-6-PD) *3890*
Blood Increase Physiological Megaloblastic anemia has been reported as complication of treatment *4800*

Methemoglobin *Blood Increase Physiological* Cyanosis secondary to methemoglobinemia has been reported rarely as an adverse reaction *4799* May cause hemolysis with G-6-PD deficiency *6015* Cyanosis secondary to methemoglobinemia has been reported rarely *4800*

N-Acetyl-Glucosaminidase *Urine No Effect Analytical* At concentration of 18 mg/dL had no significant effect on Boehringer Mannheim CPR method *3174*

Neutrophils *Blood Decrease Physiological* Occasional case of agranulocytosis reported *6264*

Nonprotein Nitrogen *Serum Increase Physiological* Nephrotoxic effect *3810*

5'-Nucleotidase *Serum Increase Physiological* Due to cholestasis *2911*

Nitrofurantoin *(continued)*

Phenylalanine *Plasma No Effect Analytical* No interference observed with rapid quantitative whole blood method of Campbell et al using phenylalanine dehydrogenase *867*

Phenytoin *Serum Decrease Physiological* Reported occurrence in one patient but not confirmed *1384*

Phosphate *Serum Increase Physiological* Reported as an adverse reaction (in about 1 - 5% treated patients) *4799* Increased concentration has been reported as complication of treatment *4800*

Serum No Effect Analytical On routine methods in use on Technicon SMAC® , Kodak Ektachem® , Abbott-VP, Roche Cobas-Bio, Du Pont aca, Hitachi® 705, KDA at 5 times normal upper therapeutic concentration *3525* At concentration of 4 mg/L had no effect on phosphomolybdate method *5704*

Platelet Aggregation *Blood Decrease Physiological* Significant effect on ADP induced aggregation *5112*

Platelets *Blood Decrease Physiological* Thrombocytopenia *1658* Thrombocytopenia has been reported rarely as an adverse reaction *4799* Thrombocytopenia has been reported as complication of treatment *4800*

Potassium *Serum No Effect Analytical* At concentration of 14 mg/L had no effect on measurement by ISE with predilution *5704* At concentration of 50 mg/L had no effect on measurement by ISE without predilution *5704* At concentration of 2.5 mg/L had no effect on flame-photometric method *5704*

Protein *Serum No Effect Analytical* On routine methods in use on Technicon SMAC® , Kodak Ektachem® , Abbott-VP, Roche Cobas-Bio, Du Pont aca, Hitachi® 705, KDA at 5 times normal upper therapeutic concentration *3525* At concentration of 4 mg/L had no effect on biuret method with blank correction *5704*

Protein Electrophoresis *Serum No Effect Analytical* At concentration of 50 mg/L had no effect on automated Olympus-Hite method *5704*

Sodium *Serum Increase Analytical* At concentrations above 40 mg/L (normal therapeutic concentration 5.5 mg/L) raised concentration as measured by ISE without predilution *5704*

Serum No Effect Analytical At concentration of 14 mg/L had no effect on method using ISE with predilution *5704* At concentration of 2.5 mg/L had no effect on flame-photometric method *5704*

Sugar *Urine Increase Analytical* Metabolites may reduce Benedict's, yield false positive *3669*

Triglycerides *Serum No Effect Analytical* On routine methods in use on Technicon SMAC® , Kodak Ektachem® , Abbott-VP, Roche Cobas-Bio, Du Pont aca, Hitachi® 705, KDA at 5 times normal upper therapeutic concentration *3525* No effect at 16 mg/L on Boehringer Mannheim Reflotron method *5706* At concentration of 4 mg/L had no effect on lipase/esterase method *5704* At concentration of 0.5 mg/L had no effect on GPO-PAP method *5704* No effect at therapeutic concentration on Boehringer Mannheim Reflotron method *3231*

Urea Nitrogen *Serum Increase Physiological* Possible decrease in already impaired renal function *139*

Serum No Effect Analytical At concentration of 4 mg/L had no effect on diacetylmonoxime method *5704* At concentration of 5 mg/L had no effect on Kodak Ektachem® method *5704* No effect at therapeutic concentration on Boehringer Mannheim Reflotron method *3231* No effect at 5 mg/L on method on Ames Seralyzer *5706* No effect at 16 mg/L on Boehringer Mannheim Reflotron method *5706* On routine methods in use on Technicon SMAC® , Kodak Ektachem® , Abbott-VP, Roche Cobas-Bio, Du Pont aca, Hitachi® 705, KDA at 5 times normal upper therapeutic concentration *3525*

Uric Acid *Serum No Effect Analytical* At concentration of 4 mg/L had no effect on phosphotungstate reduction method *5704* At concentration of 0.5 mg/L had no effect on uricase-PAP method *5704* No effect at therapeutic concentration on Boehringer Mannheim Reflotron method *3231* At concentration of 30 mg/L had no effect on catalase-AIDH method *5704* On routine methods in use on Technicon SMAC® , Kodak Ektachem® , Abbott-VP, Roche Cobas-Bio, Du Pont aca, Hitachi® 705, KDA at 5 times normal upper therapeutic concentration *3525* No effect at 16 mg/L on Boehringer Mannheim Reflotron method *5706* At concentration of 30 mg/L had no effect on Kageyama-Hantzsch method *5704*

Urobilinogen *Urine Decrease Physiological* Intrahepatic cholestatic jaundice *1753*

Nitrofurazone

Bilirubin *Serum Increase Physiological* May cause hemolysis with G-6-PD deficiency *402*

Creatinine *Urine Increase Analytical* React with color reagent *2024*

Erythrocytes *Blood Decrease Physiological* May cause hemolysis with G-6-PD deficiency *402*

Haptoglobin *Serum Decrease Physiological* May cause hemolysis *402*

Heinz Body Formation *Blood Positive Physiological* May occur in early stages of hemolytic anemia *536*

Hematocrit *Blood Decrease Physiological* May cause hemolysis with G-6-PD deficiency *402*

Hemoglobin *Blood Decrease Physiological* May cause hemolysis with G-6-PD deficiency *402*

Methemoglobin *Blood Increase Physiological* May cause hemolytic anemia *536*

Sugar *Urine Increase Analytical* Metabolites may reduce Benedict's reagent due to reducing action of metabolites *2024*

Nitroglycerin

Catecholamines *Plasma Increase Physiological* Effect dosage dependent *189*

Urine Increase Physiological 2 fold increase of catecholamines *2452*

Cholesterol *Serum Decrease Analytical* Nitroglycerin may cause a false negative measurement with Zlatkis-Zak method for measuring cholesterol *4527*

Cyclosporine *Blood No Effect Analytical* At a concentration of 5 mg/L had no effect on Syva EMIT method *495*

Epinephrine *Urine Increase Physiological* ?Due to adrenergic stimulation of hypotension *6258*

Granulocytes *Blood No Effect Physiological* Agranulocytosis observed in 1.5% patients versus 1.3% controls *3098*

Ketone Body Ratio *Serum No Effect Analytical* When added at a concentration of 50 mg/L had no significant effect on AKBR method of Uno et al *6131*

Methemoglobin *Blood Increase Physiological* Case reports of significant methemoglobinemia in association with moderate overdoses of organic nitrates *2649* May cause hemolysis *4013* Reports of some cases in whom concentration increased with moderate doses of organic nitrates but incidence comparable to that in individuals receiving placebo when normal doses administered *3703* Reported occasional complication of i.v. drug *2607*

Midazolam *Serum No Effect Analytical* On GC-ECD method of Ha et al *2387*

Nitroglycerin *Serum Decrease Physiological* Enhanced metabolism when phenobarbital coadministered *2607*

Norepinephrine *Urine Increase Physiological* ?Due to adrenergic stimulation of hypotension *6258*

Platelets *Blood Decrease Physiological* Immunologic response occurs after 5 mo *2385*

Triglycerides *Serum Increase Analytical* Because of propylene glycol content of intravenous nitroglycerin serum triglyceride measurements using glycerol oxidase may give falsely high results *2649* In method on Technicon RA-1000 using glycerol oxidase *4273*

Serum No Effect Analytical No effect on method using glycerol kinase and glycerol-3-phosphate on RA-1000 and Kodak DT-60 *4273*

Vanillylmandelic Acid *Urine Increase Physiological* Effect greater than that on catecholamines *6258*

Nitromethane

Creatinine *Serum Increase Analytical* Linear correlation between concentration and increased creatinine concentration when measured by Jaffe procedure but no effect on enzymatic methods *1314*

Nitroprusside

Creatinine Clearance *Urine No Effect Physiological* No significant effect observed in 5-6 patients with severe hypertension in whom a men of 0.93 µg/kg/min was infused for 2 hours *2133* In 10 hypertensive patients with impaired renal function given intravenous infusion until blood pressure fell to 100 to 110 mm Hg caused nonsignificant change from mean baseline of 38 ± 7 mL/min to 44 ± 9 mL/min *5542*

Digoxin *Serum Decrease Physiological* Acute administration reduces serum concentration by increasing renal clearance of glycoside *1384*

^{131}I Uptake *Serum Decrease Physiological* Single case reported (?due to thiocyanate) *4336*

Potassium *Urine No Effect Physiological* In 10 hypertensive patients with impaired renal function intravenous infusion of drug until diastolic blood pressure fell to 100 to 110 mm Hg caused nonsignificant increase from mean baseline of 24.4 ± 4.4 µEq/min to 27.2 µEq/min *5542*

Sodium *Urine No Effect Physiological* Infusion of a mean of 0.93 µg/kg/min for 2 hours in 5-6 patients with severe hypertension had no effect on urine excretion rate *2133* In 10 hypertensive patients with impaired renal function intravenous infusion of drug until diastolic blood pressure fell to 100 to 110 mm Hg caused nonsignificant reduction from 86 ± 28 µEq/min to 83 ± 47 µEq/min *5542*

Thyroxine (T4) *Serum Decrease Physiological* Due to thyroidal inhibition especially in patients with some renal impairment *6412*

Volume *Urine No Effect Physiological* Infusion of a mean of 0.93 µg/kg/min for 2 hours in 5-6 patients with severe hypertension had no effect on urinary flow rate *2133* In 10 hypertensive patients with impaired renal function intravenous infusion until diastolic blood pressure decreased to 100 to 110 mm Hg caused nonsignificant reduction from mean baseline of 110 ± 37 mL/h to 99 ± 36 mL/h *5542*

Nitrous Oxide

Alanine Aminotransferase *Serum No Effect Physiological* No evidence of liver damage observed in 100 having total hip replacement 1-3 days after surgery *3386*

Alkaline Phosphatase *Serum No Effect Physiological* No evidence of liver damage observed in 100 patients 1-3 days following hip surgery when nitrous oxide used as one of the anesthetic agents *3386*

Bilirubin *Serum No Effect Physiological* No evidence of liver damage in 100 patients 1-3 days after hip surgery when nitrous oxide used as one of anesthetic agents *3386*

Corticotropin *Plasma No Effect Physiological* No significant effect observed in 6 healthy male volunteers at concentration of 48.8% *2121*

Cortisol *Plasma Decrease Physiological* Statistically significant decrease produced in 6 healthy male volunteers at concentration of 48.8% *2121*

Erythrocytes *Blood Decrease Physiological* Bone marrow depress (of no significance normally) *2242*
Blood No Effect Physiological No discernible effect of nitrous oxide anesthesia observed *6302*

Folate *Serum Increase Physiological* If intraoperative exposure of patient is greater than 6 h, but unchanged if exposure for less than 1 h *3236*

Follicle Stimulating Hormone
Plasma No Effect Physiological No significant effect observed in 6 healthy male volunteers at concentration of 48.8% *2121*

Growth Hormone *Plasma No Effect Physiological* No significant effect in 6 healthy male volunteers at concentration of 48.8% *2121*

Hemoglobin *Blood No Effect Physiological* No discernible effect of nitrous oxide anesthesia noted *6302*

Homocystine *Plasma Increase Physiological* Nitrous oxide anesthesia causes rapid but transient increase *6123*

Luteinizing Hormone *Plasma No Effect Physiological* No significant effect in 6 healthy male volunteers at concentration of 48.8% *2121*

MCV *Blood No Effect Physiological* No discernible effect of nitrous oxide anesthesia noted *6302*

N-Formiminoglutamic Acid *Urine Increase Physiological* In 50 surgical patients receiving nitrous oxide anesthesia for limb surgery 22 had a dose-dependent increase in excretion for 2 days after the operation. Exposure to 70% nitrous oxide for more than 90 min appeared to cause abnormal metabolism of folate *240*

Platelets *Blood No Effect Physiological* No difference between effects of nitrous oxide and other anesthetics on platelet count *6302*

Prolactin *Plasma Increase Physiological* Statistically significant increase produced in 6 healthy male individuals at concentration of 48.8% *2121*

Red Cell Distribution Width *Blood No Effect Physiological* No discernible effect of nitrous oxide anesthesia noted *6302*

Reticulocytes *Blood No Effect Physiological* No effect of nitrous oxide anesthesia noted *6302*

Thyroid Stimulating Hormone
Serum No Effect Physiological No significant effect in 6 healthy male volunteers at concentration of 48.8% *2121*

Thyroxine (T4) *Serum No Effect Physiological* No significant effect in 6 healthy male volunteers at concentration of 48.8% *2121*

Vitamin B_{12} *Serum No Effect Physiological* With intraoperative exposure for as long as 6 h *3236*

Nizatidine

Alanine Aminotransferase *Serum Increase Physiological* Hepatocellular injury occurre in some patients and was possibly or probably related to nizatadine. In some cases the enzyme increase was substantial, although overall incidence of increased enzyme activity not significantly different between drug and placebo treated groups *1691* In one man treated with nizatidine for 28 days on admission to hospital ALT activity observed to be 229 U/L: subsequently patient developed subfulminant hepatic failure and even later cirrhosis *990*

Alkaline Phosphatase *Serum Increase Physiological* In one man treated with nizatidine for 28 days on admission to hospital alkaline phosphatase activity observed to be 188 U/L: subsequently patient developed subfulminant hepatic failure and even later cirrhosis *990* Hepatocellular injury occurre in some patients and was possibly or probably related to nizatadine. In some cases the enzyme increase was substantial, although overall incidence of increased enzyme activity not significantly different between drug and placebo treated groups *1691*

Aspartate Aminotransferase *Serum Increase Physiological* In one man treated with nizatidine for 28 days on admission to hospital AST activity observed to be 255 U/L: subsequently patient developed subfulminant hepatic failure and even later cirrhosis *990* Hepatocellular injury occurre in some patients and was possibly or probably related to nizatadine. In some cases the enzyme increase was substantial, although overall incidence of increased enzyme activity not significantly different between drug and placebo treated groups *1691*

Bicarbonate *Gastric Material No Effect Physiological* In 18 men with duodenal ulcer after pentagastrin stimulation intravenous administration of 300 mg nizatidine had no effect on bicarbonate concentration although it reduced the volume of bicarbonate secretion *6253*

Bilirubin *Serum Increase Physiological* In one man treated with nizatidine for 28 days on admission to hospital bilirubin concentration observed to be 16.8 mg/dL: subsequently patient developed subfulminant hepatic failure and even later cirrhosis *990*

Chlordiazepoxide *Serum No Effect Physiological* No interaction observed when drugs coadministered *1384* Administration had no effect on steady-state plasma concentration *316*

Nizatidine *(continued)*

Diazepam *Serum No Effect Physiological* No interaction observed when drugs coadministered *1384* Administration had no effect on steady-state plasma concentration *316*

Eosinophils *Blood Increase Physiological* Eosinophilia has been reported with drug administration *1691*

Gonadotropin, Pituitary *Plasma No Effect Physiological* Administration had no effect on steady-state plasma concentration *316*

Hematocrit *Blood Decrease Physiological* Anemia was significantly more common in drug treated group than in placebo treated individuals *1691*

Hemoglobin *Blood Decrease Physiological* Anemia was significantly more common in drug treated group than in placebo treated individuals *1691*

Hydrochloric Acid *Gastric Fluid Decrease Physiological* In 18 men with duodenal ulcer administration of 300 mg intravenously caused significant reduction from maximum pentagastrin stimulated excretion of 34.6 ± 19.0 mmol/h to minimum of 1.2 ± 1.2 mmol/h 60 min after nizatidine *6253* Progressive reduction in acid secretion with increasing concentration of nizatidine in 5 healthy male volunteers. Mean inhibition of acid secretion 54% at niztaidine concentration of 69 µg/L, 84% at 247 µg/L, and 94% at 575 µg/L *5358*

Lidocaine *Serum No Effect Physiological* No interaction observed when drugs coadministered *1384*

Lorazepam *Serum No Effect Physiological* Administration had no effect on steady-state plasma concentration *316* No interaction observed when drugs coadministered *1384*

pH *Gastric Fluid Increase Physiological* Mean pH of basal gastric secretion was 1.6 during placebo infusion and 4.6 when mean plasma nizatadine concentration was 575 µg/L in 5 healthy male volunteers *5358*

Gastric Material Increase Physiological Mean pH of basal gastric secretion was 1.6 during placebo infusion and 4.6 when mean plasma nizatadine concentration was 575 µg/L in 5 healthy male volunteers *5358*

Platelets *Blood Decrease Physiological* Rare cases of thrombocytopenic purpura reported *1691*

Prothrombin Time *Plasma Increase Physiological* In one man treated with nizatidine for 28 days on admission to hospital prothrombin time observed to be 20 s: subsequently patient developed subfulminant hepatic failure and even later cirrhosis *990*

Plasma No Effect Physiological Administration had no effect on time in patients with steady-state plasma concentration of warfarin *316*

Theophylline *Serum No Effect Physiological* No clinically significant effect on theophylline concentration observed when drugs coadministered *5999* No documented significant interaction with theophylline reported *6117* No interaction observed when drugs coadministered *1384* In 17 patients with COPD given theophylline for 42 days coadministration of cimetidine caused nonsignificant change in mean AUC_{0-12} from 113.95 mg/h/L to 113.41 mg/h/L and mean maximum concentration from 9.5 mg/L to 9.5 mg/L *316*

Uric Acid *Serum Increase Physiological* Hyperuricemia not associated with gout or nephrolithiasis has been reported with administration of drug *1691*

Volume *Gastric Fluid Decrease Physiological* In 18 men with duodenal ulcer 300 mg nizatidine intravenously caused decrease from maximum stimulated volume of 75.8 ± 39.6 mL/15 min to minimum of 17.0 ± 14.3 mL/min 45 min after nizatidine administration *6253*

Warfarin *Plasma No Effect Physiological* Administration had no effect on steady-state plasma concentration *316* No interaction observed when drugs coadministered *1384*

N-Methylephedrine

Methamphetamine *Urine No Effect Analytical* Less than 0.05% cross-reactivity with Hycor accuPINCH method *162*

N-Methylformamide

Alanine Aminotransferase *Serum Increase Physiological* Reversible hepatotoxicity has been observed *1384*

Aspartate Aminotransferase *Serum Increase Physiological* Reversible hepatotoxicity has been observed *1384*

Nocloprost

pH *Gastric Material No Effect Physiological* Nocloprost given 100 µg three times daily 30 min before meals did not affect gastric pH significantly *3241*

Nonaluminum-containing Antacids

Alkaline Phosphatase *Serum No Effect Physiological* In 10 men aged from 60 - 80 y taking nonaluminum containing antacids mean activity of 88.2 ± 29.6 U/L not significantly different from 87 ± 22.7 U/L in healthy age-matched controls. In 5 women older than 50 y taking nonaluminum antacids mean activity of 100 ± 37 U/L not significantly different from 88.1 ± 22.3 U/L in age-matched controls *5479*

Aluminum *Serum Increase Physiological* In women younger than 50 y taking nonaluminum antacids mean concentration of 7.3 ± 4 µg/L not significantly higher but in those aged over 50 y significantly higher than 4.0 ± 2.8 µg/L in 128 women not taking antacids *5479*

Dicyclomine *Serum Decrease Physiological* May interfere with the absorption of anticholinergic agents *2640*

Digoxin *Serum Decrease Physiological* By decreasing intestinal digoxin absorption may decrease the digoxin concentration *2161*

Felbamate *Serum No Effect Physiological* The rate and extent of absorption of felbamate not affected by coadministration of antacids *6324*

Osteocalcin *Serum Decrease Physiological* In 10 men aged from 60 - 80 y taking nonaluminum containing antacids mean concentration of 11.9 ± 5.4 ng/mL not significantly less than 15.7 ± 7 ng/mL in healthy age-matched controls. In 7 women older than 50 y taking nonaluminum antacids mean concentration of 11.5 ± 4.2 µg/mL not significantly less than 14.9 ± 4.7 ng/mL in age-matched controls *5479*

Procollagen I Peptide *Serum Decrease Physiological* In 10 men aged from 60 - 80 y taking nonaluminum containing antacids mean concentration of 162 ± 65.5 (?units) significantly less than 219 ± 84 (?units) in healthy age-matched controls. In 7 women older than 50 y taking nonaluminum antacids mean concentration of 153 ± 40 (?units) not significantly less than 177 ± 75 (?units) in age-matched controls *5479*

Nonsteroidal Antiinflammatory Drugs

Aldosterone *Plasma Decrease Physiological* Associated with inhibition of prostaglandin synthesis *2556*

Bleeding Time *Patient Increase Physiological* Prolong bleeding time in their own right but increase potential risk warfarin-associated bleeding *2625*

Chlorpropamide *Serum Increase Physiological* Drugs that are highly protein-bound compete with chlorpropamide for binding sites and may potentiate hypoglycemic action of sulfonylurea *4644*

C-Reactive Protein *Serum Decrease Physiological* In 9 patients with rheumatoid arthritis who responded to NSAID treatment for 8 weeks mean concentration decreased from 4.4 ± 3.3 mg/dL *1469*

Serum No Effect Physiological In 17 patients with rheumatoid arthritis who failed to respond to NSAID treatment for 8 weeks meam concentration changed nonsignificantly from 2.9 ± 2.4 mg/dL to 3.4 ± 2.9 mg/dL *1469*

Creatinine *Serum Increase Physiological* Reversible acute renal failure associated with many drugs *2556*

Eosinophils *Blood Increase Physiological* Observed in 9% of 56 patients treated with these drugs alone for rheumatoid arthritis *1834*

Erythrocyte Sedimentation Rate
Blood Decrease Physiological In 9 patients with rheumatoid arthritis who responded to 8 weeks treatment mean concentration decreased from 72 ± 47 mm/h to 52 ± 32 mm/h *1469*
Blood No Effect Physiological In 17 patients with rheumatoid arthritis who failed to respond to 8 weeks treatment mean concentration changed nonsignificantly from 71 ± 35 mm/h to 76 ± 32 mm/h *1469*

Hemoglobin *Urine No Effect Physiological* No association observed between ingestion of nonsteroidal anti-inflammatory drugs and presence of dipstick hematuria in over 1000 men aged 60 years and older *732*

Lipoprotein Lp(a) *Serum No Effect Physiological* In 116 individuals ingesting NSAIDs mean and median concentrations of 170 and 96 mg/L not significantly different from 181 and 106 mg/L in 1411 controls *5604*

Lithium *Serum Increase Physiological* Lithium toxicity reported with the concomitant administration of NSAIDs *4399* Increase concentration by reducing renal elimination *3590*

Methotrexate *Serum Increase Physiological* Concomitant administration of NSAIDs with high dose methotrexate reportedly increases and prolongs concentration of methotrexate *2818*

Osteocalcin *Serum No Effect Physiological* No significant effect of nonsteroidal anti-inflammatory drugs observed on plasma concentration *5948*

Potassium *Serum Increase Physiological* Associated with inhibition of prostaglandin synthesis *2556*

Protein *Urine Increase Physiological* Most of drugs have been associated with reversible clinical syndrome of heavy proteinuria and renal insufficiency *2556*

Renin Activity *Plasma Decrease Physiological* Associated with inhibition of prostaglandin synthesis *2556*

Rheumatoid Factor *Serum Decrease Physiological* In 9 patients with rheumatoid arthritis who responded to NSAID treatment for 8 weeks mean concentration decreased from 1342 ± 1117 IU/mL to 1074 ± 821 IU/mL *1469*
Serum No Effect Physiological In 17 patients with rheumatoid arthritis who failed to respond to treatment for 8 weeks with NSAID mean concentration changed nonsignificantly from 1289 ± 1570 IU/mL to 1180 ± 1255 IU/mL *1469*

Sodium *Serum Decrease Physiological* May be associated with water retention *2556*

Soluble Interleukin-2 Receptor
Serum Decrease Physiological In 9 patients with rheumatoid arthritis who responded to NSAID treatment over 8 weeks mean concentration decreased from mean baseline of 1000 U/mL to 850 U/mL *1469*
Serum Increase Physiological In 17 patients with rheumatoid arthritis who failed to respond to treatment with NSAIDs for 8 weeks mean concentration increased from 750 U/mL to 900 U/mL *1469*

Noramidopyrine

Alanine Aminotransferase *Serum No Effect Analytical* No effect at 200 mg/L on Boehringer Mannheim Reflotron method *5706*

Cholesterol *Serum No Effect Analytical* At concentration of 20 mg/L no effect on method on Boehringer Mannheim Reflotron system *5706*

HDL-Cholesterol *Serum No Effect Analytical* At a concentration up to 200 mg/L had no significant effect on Reflotron method for whole blood cholesterol *6352*

Uric Acid *Serum No Effect Analytical* No effect at 200 mg/L on Boehringer Mannheim Reflotron method *5706*

Norcocaine

Benzoylecgonine *Urine No Effect Analytical* No significant interference observed with 5000 ng/mL l-norcocaine with Roche Abuscreen ONTRAK assay *1106*

Nordiazepam

Benzodiazepine *Urine Increase Analytical* Cross-reactivity of 30-100% observed with Roche Abuscreen method adapted for use with Roche Cobas Mira analyzer *231*
Urine Positive Analytical Cross-reactivity of 30-100% observed with Roche Abuscreen method adapted for use with Roche Cobas Mira analyzer *231*

Norethandrolone

Alanine Aminotransferase *Serum Increase Physiological* Usually reversible cholestasis *2112*

Alkaline Phosphatase *Serum Increase Physiological* Cholestasis produced without cholangiolitis *2522*

Aspartate Aminotransferase *Serum Increase Physiological* Cholestasis produced without cholangiolitis *5311*

Bile *Urine Increase Physiological* Cholestatic effect *5311*

Bilirubin *Serum Increase Physiological* Intrahepatic cholestasis produced (up to 20%) *2112*
Urine Increase Physiological Cholestasis produced without cholangiolitis *5311*

Bilirubin, Direct *Serum Increase Physiological* Reversible cholestasis produced *2112*

BSP Retention *Serum Increase Physiological* Transport and conjugation of BSP impaired *239*

Cholesterol *Serum Increase Physiological* Due to cholestasis *2803*

Fibrinogen *Plasma Increase Physiological* Metabolic effect *368*

β-Glucuronidase *Serum Increase Physiological* Metabolic effect *368*

Haptoglobin *Serum Increase Physiological* Metabolic effect *368*

Lactate Dehydrogenase *Serum Increase Physiological* ?Part of cholestatic syndrome *882*

5'-Nucleotidase *Serum Increase Physiological* Due to cholestasis *2911*

Plasminogen *Plasma Increase Physiological* Metabolic effect *368*

Prealbumin *Serum Increase Physiological* Decreases thyroxine binding globulin however *102*

Prothrombin Time *Plasma Increase Physiological* Also seen with other 17-alkyl substituted steroids *1667*

Thyroxine Binding Globulin
Serum Decrease Physiological Decreases concentration of thyroxine binding globulin, increases thyroxine binding prealbumin *5869*

Urobilinogen *Feces Decrease Physiological* Light stools due to cholestasis *2803*
Urine Decrease Physiological Manifestation of cholestasis *2112*

Norethandrostenolone

Alkaline Phosphatase *Serum Increase Physiological* Intrahepatic cholestatic jaundice *5367*

Bile *Urine Increase Physiological* Intrahepatic cholestatic jaundice *5367*

Bilirubin *Serum Increase Physiological* Intrahepatic cholestatic jaundice *5367*

BSP Retention *Serum Increase Physiological* Impaired hepatic uptake and excretion *1009*

Norethindrone

α_1-Acid Glycoprotein *Serum Decrease Physiological* Metabolic estrogen effect *723*

Alanine Aminotransferase *Serum Increase Physiological* Intrahepatic cholestatic jaundice *3810* In 5.6% patients being treated for advanced or recurrent breast cancer *3404*

Albumin *Serum No Effect Physiological* No effect observed *723*

Norethindrone *(continued)*

Alkaline Phosphatase *Serum Decrease Physiological* Significant fall in postmenopausal women. At 16 weeks both liver and bone isoenzymes affected, but after 24 weeks only bone component below pretreatment value *1341*
Serum Increase Physiological In 5.6% patients being treated for advanced or recurrent breast cancer *3404* Intrahepatic cholestatic jaundice *2242*

Antithrombin III *Plasma No Effect Physiological* In 75 women who had received up to 24 intragluteal injections of 200 mg every 56 d *2735*

Apolipoprotein A-I *Serum Decrease Physiological* Significant reduction to 1167 mg/L in norethindrone-only users compared with 1266 mg/L in nonuser controls *2201* Some patients may experience slight reduction in concentration *4442*
Serum No Effect Physiological Usually no effect observed in patients receiving 0.35 mg daily *4442*

Apolipoprotein A-II *Serum Decrease Physiological* Some patients may experience slight reduction in concentration *4442* Significant reduction to 313 mg/L in norethindrone-only users compared with 336 mg/L in nonuser controls *2201*
Serum No Effect Physiological Usually no effect observed in patients receiving 0.35 mg daily *4442*

Apolipoprotein B *Serum No Effect Physiological* Nonsignificant reduction to 533 mg/L in norethindrone-only users compared with 572 mg/L in nonuser controls *2201*

Aspartate Aminotransferase *Serum Increase Physiological* Intrahepatic cholestatic jaundice *3810*

Bile *Urine Increase Physiological* Intrahepatic cholestatic jaundice *2242*

Bilirubin *Serum Increase Physiological* Intrahepatic cholestatic jaundice *2242* In 5.6% patients being treated for advanced or recurrent breast cancer *3404*

BSP Retention *Serum Increase Physiological* Cholestatic phenomenon (occurs in 20%) *5570*

Cannabinoids *Urine No Effect Analytical* No effect on Roche Abuscreen method *5006*

Carotene *Serum Decrease Physiological* Hormonal influence *2005*

Ceruloplasmin *Serum Increase Physiological* Metabolic estrogen effect *723*

Cholesterol *Serum No Effect Physiological* In 75 women who had received up to 24 intragluteal injections of 200 mg every 56 d *2735* Insignificant reduction to 4.34 mmol/L in norethindrone only users from 4.50 mmol/L in nonuser controls *2201* Usually no effect observed in patients receiving 0.35 mg daily *4442* No significant effect with 0.4 mg/d *2193*

Cortisol *Plasma Decrease Physiological* Slight effect compared with controls *444*
Urine Decrease Physiological When results compared with normal menstrual cycle *444*

C-Peptide *Plasma No Effect Physiological* Norethindrone-only formulations had no effect on carbohydrate metabolism *2201*

Cyclosporine *Serum Increase Physiological* Observed effect presumed to be due to inhibition of hepatic microsomal enzymes *1069*

Factor X *Plasma No Effect Physiological* In 75 women who had received up to 24 intragluteal injections of 200 mg every 56 d *2735*

Glucose *Serum Increase Physiological* Some patients may experience slight deterioration in glucose tolerance *4442*
Serum No Effect Physiological Norethindrone-only formulations had no effect on carbohydrate metabolism *2201*

Glucose Tolerance *Serum Decrease Physiological* Some patients may experience slight deterioration in glucose tolerance *4442* After 6 mo treatment compared with control *5739*
Serum Increase Physiological In 75 women who had received up to 24 intragluteal injections of 200 mg every 56 d *2735*

Haptoglobin *Serum Decrease Physiological* Metabolic estrogen effect *723*
Serum Increase Physiological With high dose, prolonged treatment *723*

HDL_2-Cholesterol *Serum Decrease Physiological* Some patients may experience slight reduction in concentration *4442* High dose (1000 µg) with 35 µg estrogen combination caused reduction of HDL_2-cholesterol by 27% *2201* Nonsignificant reduction to 0.68 mmol/L in norethindrone-only users compared with 0.72 mmol/L in nonuser controls *2201* High dose (1000 ug) with 35 µg estrogen combination caused reduction of HDL_2-cholesterol by 27% *2201*

HDL_3-Cholesterol *Serum No Effect Physiological* Usually no effect observed in patients receiving 0.35 mg daily *4442* Nonsignificant reduction to 0.98 mmol/L in norethindrone-only users compared with 1.01 mmol/L in nonuser controls *2201*

HDL-Cholesterol *Serum Decrease Physiological* In 75 women who had received up to 24 intragluteal injections of 200 mg every 56 d *2735* Norethindrone-only users had mean concentration of 1.65 mmol/L significantly less than 1.73 mmol/L in nonuser controls *2201* Some patients may experience slight reduction in concentration *4442*

Insulin *Plasma Increase Physiological* During glucose tolerance test after 6 mo treatment compared with controls *5739* Some patients may experience slight deterioration in glucose tolerance with increase in plasma insulin concentration *4442*
Plasma No Effect Physiological Norethindrone-only formulations had no effect on carbohydrate metabolism *2201*

LDL-Cholesterol *Serum Decrease Physiological* Nonsignificant reduction to 2.35 mmol/L in norethindrone-only users versus 2.40 mmol/L in nonuser controls *2201*
Serum No Effect Physiological Usually no effect observed in patients receiving 0.35 mg daily *4442* In 75 women who had received up to 24 intragluteal injections of 200 mg every 56 d *2735*

Lipase, Hepatic *Serum Increase Physiological* Increase may be observed in patients receiving 0.35 mg daily *4442*

Luteinizing Hormone *Plasma Decrease Physiological* Apparent suppression of production or release *4109*

Sex-Hormone Binding Globulin *Serum Decrease Physiological* Concentration may be decreased in patients receiving 0.35 mg daily *4442*

T3-Uptake *Serum No Effect Physiological* When treatment results compared with controls *443*

Thyroxine Binding Globulin *Serum Decrease Physiological* Concentration may be decreased in patients receiving 0.35 mg daily *4442*

Thyroxine (T4) *Serum Decrease Physiological* Concentration may be decreased in patients receiving 0.35 mg daily due to decrease in TBG concentration *4442* When treatment results compared with controls *443*

Thyroxine (T4), Free *Serum Decrease Physiological* Slight effect when compared with controls *443*

Triglyceride Lipase *Serum Increase Physiological* In normal and hyperlipemic women *2193*

Triglycerides *Serum Decrease Physiological* In normal and hyperlipemic women *2193*
Serum No Effect Physiological No change observed in norethindrone-only users versus nonuser controls *2201* In 75 women who had received up to 24 intragluteal injections of 200 mg every 56 d *2735*

Vitamin A *Serum Increase Physiological* Due to alteration in concentration of binding globulin *2005*

VLDL-Cholesterol *Serum No Effect Physiological* In 75 women who had received up to 24 intragluteal injections of 200 mg every 56 d *2735* Usually no effect observed in patients receiving 0.35 mg daily *4442*

Norethynodrel

Alanine Aminotransferase *Serum Increase Physiological* Cholestatic effect *3810*

Alkaline Phosphatase *Serum Increase Physiological* Due to cholestasis *2911*

Aspartate Aminotransferase *Serum Increase Physiological* Cholestatic effect *3810*

Bile *Urine Increase Physiological* Intrahepatic cholestatic jaundice *2242*

Bilirubin *Serum Increase Physiological* Intrahepatic cholestatic jaundice *2242*

BSP Retention *Serum Increase Physiological* Cholestatic phenomenon *1174*

Glucose Tolerance *Serum Decrease Physiological* Gluconeogenetic effect of steroids *2024*

17-Hydroxycorticosteroids *Urine Decrease Physiological* Decreased excretion of cortisol metabolites *55*

5'-Nucleotidase *Serum Increase Physiological* Due to cholestasis *2911*

Thyroxine Binding Globulin *Serum Increase Physiological* Direct effect of drug *42*

Norfenefrin

Cholesterol *Serum No Effect Analytical* At concentration of 2.4 mg/L had no effect on CHOD-PAP method *5704* At concentration of 2.4 mg/L had no effect on method using catalase-Hantzsch reaction *5704* At concentration of 2.4 mg/L had no effect on Liebermann-Burchard method *5704* At concentration of 2.4 mg/L had no effect on catalase-AIDH method *5704* At concentration of 2.4 mg/L had no effect on CHOD-Iodide method *5704*

Creatinine *Serum Decrease Analytical* At concentrations above 4 mg/L (normal therapeutic concentration 0.4 mg/L) lowered concentration as measured by kinetic Jaffe method on BKA-2 *5704*

Serum No Effect Analytical At concentration of 6 mg/L had no effect on Jaffe-Fading-Fraction method *5704* At concentration of 6 mg/L had no effect on Jaffe-Fuller's earth method *5704*

Glucose *Serum No Effect Analytical* At concentration of 0.48 mg/L had no effect on Kodak Ektachem® method *5704*

Potassium *Serum No Effect Analytical* At concentration of 3 mg/L had no effect on measurement by ISE without predilution *5704*

Protein Electrophoresis *Serum No Effect Analytical* At concentration of 4.8 mg/L had no effect on automated Olympus-Hite method *5704*

Sodium *Serum Increase Analytical* At concentrations above 4.8 mg/L (normal therapeutic concentration 0.4 mg/L) raised concentration as measured by ISE without predilution *5704*

Urea Nitrogen *Serum No Effect Analytical* At concentration of 0.48 mg/L had no effect on Kodak Ektachem® method *5704*

Uric Acid *Serum No Effect Analytical* At concentration of 6 mg/L had no effect on Kageyama-Hantzsch method *5704* At concentration of 6 mg/L had no effect on catalase-AIDH method *5704*

Norfloxacin

Alanine Aminotransferase *Serum Increase Physiological* In 2 of 1540 patients in clinical trials *1138* Increased activity reported in 1.6% treated patients in single dose studies and in 1.4% patients in multiple dose studies *4981* In chronic studies of more than 2000 individuals with urinary tract infections or prostatitis significant increases in activity observed in 1.4% *3987*

Albumin *Urine Increase Physiological* Reported as an adverse event with quinolone treatment *3987*

Alkaline Phosphatase *Serum Increase Physiological* In chronic studies of more than 2000 individuals with urinary tract infections or prostatitis significant increases in activity observed in 1.1% *3987* Increased activity reported in 1.1% patients in multiple dose studies *4981*

Amylase *Serum Increase Physiological* In postmarketing reports rare cases of pancreatitis reported *3987* Rare pancreatitis reported in patients in multiple dose studies *4981*

Aspartate Aminotransferase *Serum Increase Physiological* In single dose studies in 220 healthy individuals or in patients with gonorrhea 1.6% had significant increases in activity. In chronic studies of 2000 individuals with urinary tract infections or prostatitis significant increases in activity observed in 1.4% *3987* In 2 of 1540 patients in clinical trials *1138* Increased activity reported in 1.4% patients in multiple dose studies *4981*

Blood *Urine Increase Physiological* Reported as an adverse event with quinolone treatment *3987*

Caffeine *Serum Increase Physiological* Administration of systemic norfloxacin has been associated with interference with the metabolism of caffeine *3962* Significant increase of area under curve and decreased plasma clearance following ingestion of single dose of caffeine after pretreatment with norfloxacin *884*

Serum No Effect Physiological Minimal effect on clearance *2704*

Cholesterol *Serum Increase Physiological* Reported as an adverse event with quinolone treatment *3987*

Ciprofloxacin *Serum Increase Analytical* Cannot be assayed by HPLC method used at Mayo Clinic in presence of norfloxacin *3858*

Coproporphyrin I *Urine Increase Analytical* In urine to which norfloxacin added to a concentration of 0.25 mmol/L peak area increased by 2% measured by HPLC method with fluorescence detection *5366*

Coproporphyrin III *Urine Increase Analytical* In urine to which norfloxacin added to a concentration of 0.25 mmol/L peak area increased by 2% as measured by HPLC method with fluorescence detection *5366*

Creatinine *Serum Increase Physiological* Rare complication of treatment *6316* Increased concentration reported infrequently in patients in multiple dose studies *4981* In chronic studies of more than 2000 individuals with urinary tract infections or prostatitis significant increases in concentration observed in fewer than 0.6% *3987*

Crystals *Urine Increase Physiological* Reported as an adverse event with quinolone treatment *3987* May occur with high doses of drug *6316*

Cyclosporine *Blood Increase Physiological* Coadministration of norfoxacin with cyclosporine to one heart transplant patient caused the cyclosporine concentration to double two days after the start of the treatment *859*

Serum Increase Physiological Well documented case reported: Cytochrome P-450 inhibition caused by this drug *1069* Coadministration of norfoxacin with cyclosporine to one heart transplant patient caused the cyclosporine concentration to double two days after the start of the treatment *859* Administration of systemic norfloxacin has been associated with increased plasma concentration of cyclosporine *3962* Concentration rapidly doubled in one cardiac transplant patient after receiving norfloxacin 800 mg/d for 5 days *6596* Rapid doubling of concentration observed in one cardiac transplant patient after receiving 800 mg norfloxacin daily for 5 days *6020*

Serum No Effect Physiological In one study of 6 renal transplant patients and one of 4 cardiac transplants no significant change in trough concentrations observed *6596* No significant change observed in trough concentrations in 6 renal transplant patients and 4 cardiac transplant patients when norfloxacin coadministered *5000*

Cyclosporine A *Blood Increase Physiological* Clinically significant increases in concentration have been reported when cyclosporine has been administered with norfloxacin *4981* Norfloxacin reported to increase concentration of cyclosporine *3987*

Cylinders *Urine Increase Physiological* Reported as an adverse event with quinolone treatment *3987*

Eosinophils *Blood Decrease Physiological* Increased concentration reported in 0.6% treated patients in single dose studies and in 1.5% of patients in multiple dose studies *4981*

Blood Increase Physiological In 2 of 1540 patients in clinical trials *1138* In single dose studies in 220 healthy individuals or in patients with gonorrhea 0.6% had significantly increased concentration. In chronic studies of more than 2000 individuals eosinophilia observed in 1.5% *3987*

Erythrocytes *Blood Decrease Physiological* Rare complication of treatment *6316*

Glucose *Serum Decrease Physiological* Symptomatic hypoglycemia reported as an adverse event with quinolone treatment *3987*

Serum Increase Physiological Reported as an adverse event with quinolone treatment *3987*

Urine Increase Physiological In chronic studies of more than 2000 individuals with urinary tract infections or prostatitis significant increases in concentration observed in fewer than 0.6% *3987* Increased excretion reported infrequently in patients in multiple dose studies *4981*

Granulocytes *Blood Decrease Physiological* Reported as an adverse event with quinolone treatment *3987*

Norfloxacin (continued)

Hematocrit *Blood Decrease Physiological* Decreased value reported in 0.6% treated patients *4981* In single dose studies in 220 healthy individuals or in patients with gonorrhea 0.6% had significantly decreased value *3987*

Hemoglobin *Blood Decrease Physiological* Decreased concentration reported in 0.6% treated patients *4981* In single dose studies in 220 healthy individuals or in patients with gonorrhea 0.6% had significantly decreased concentration. In chronic studies of more than 2000 individuals with urinary tract infections or prostatitis decreased concentration observed in fewer than 0.6% *3987*

Lactate Dehydrogenase *Serum Increase Physiological* In chronic studies of more than 2000 individuals with urinary tract infections or prostatitis significant increases in activity observed in fewer than 0.6% *3987* In 2 of 1540 patients in clinical trials *1138* Increased activity reported infrequently in patients in multiple dose studies *4981*

Leukocytes *Blood Decrease Physiological* In single dose studies in 220 healthy individuals or in patients with gonorrhea 1.3% had significantly decreased concentrations. In 2000 individuals in chronic studies significant increases in concentration observed in 1.4% *3987* Occurs in about 1% treated cases probably via an immunologic mechanism *4557* Leukopenia reported in 1.3% treated patients in single dose studies and in 1.4% patients in multiple dose studies *4981* Reduction but not to below 1,000 /μL in 6 of 1540 patients, usually plateaued between 3,000-4,000 /μL *1138*

Lipase *Serum Increase Physiological* In postmarketing reports rare cases of pancreatitis reported *3987* Rare pancreatitis reported in patients in multiple dose studies *4981*

Neutrophils *Blood Decrease Physiological* Occurs in about 1% treated cases probably via an immunologic mechanism *4557* Decreased concentration reported in 1.4% of patients in multiple dose studies *4981* In 2000 individuals in chronic studies significant decreases in concentration of leukocytes and/or neutrophils observed in 1.4% *3987*

Platelets *Blood Decrease Physiological* Throbocytopenia reported in 1.0% treated patients in single dose studies *4981* In single dose studies in 220 healthy individuals or in patients with gonorrhea 1.0% had significantly decreased concentrations *3987*

Porphyrin, Total *Urine Increase Analytical* In urine to which norfloxacin added to a concentration of 0.25 mmol/L peak area increased by 2% with HPLC method with fluorescence detection *5366* At a concentration of 0.25 mmol/L 2-fold increase observed with screening method of Porphyrin Products *5366*

Potassium *Serum Increase Physiological* Reported as an adverse event with quinolone treatment *3987*

Protein *Urine Increase Physiological* Increased urinary protein excretion reported in 1.0% treated patients *4981* In single dose studies in 220 healthy individuals or in patients with gonorrhea 1.0% had significantly increased excretion *3987*

Prothrombin Time *Plasma Increase Physiological* Norfloxacin reported to enhance the effect of oral anticoagulants *3987* Administration of systemic norfloxacin has been associated with enhancing the effects of warfarin and its derivatives *3962* Clinically significant increases in prothrombin time have been observed when warfarin has been administered with norfloxacin *4981*

Theophylline *Serum Increase Physiological* Administration of systemic norfloxacin has been associated with increases in the plasma concentration of theophylline *3962* Increases plasma theophylline concentration *3125* Quinolones reported to increase concentration of theophylline *3987* Mean clearance decreased when drugs coadministered for 3 days although not enough to cause clinically important effects *1283* Clinically significant increases in concentration have been reported when theophylline has been administered with quinolones *4981*

Serum No Effect Physiological Minimal effect observed on clearance *2704* No clinically significant effect on theophylline concentration observed when drugs coadministered *5999* No documented significant interaction with theophylline reported *6117*

Triglycerides *Serum Increase Physiological* Reported as an adverse event with quinolone treatment *3987*

Urea Nitrogen *Serum Increase Physiological* Increased concentration reported infrequently in patients in multiple dose studies *4981* In chronic studies of more than 2000 individuals with urinary tract infections or prostatitis significant increases in concentration observed in fewer than 0.6% *3987* Rare complication of treatment *6316*

Uroporphyrin *Urine Increase Analytical* In urine to which norfloxacin added to a concentration of 0.25 mmol/L peak area increased by 2% as measured by HPLC method with fluorescence detection *5366*

Norgestrel

Creatinine *Serum No Effect Analytical* At 10 mg/L on reversed phase liquid chromatographic procedure of Zhiri et al *6656*

Uric Acid *Serum No Effect Analytical* At 10 mg/L on reversed phase liquid chromatographic procedure of Zhiri et al *6656*

Normorphine

Morphine *Urine No Effect Analytical* Insignificant cross react with hemagglutination inhibition Insignificant cross react with EMIT procedure for opiates *4163*

Norplant

Alanine Aminotransferase *Serum No Effect Physiological* No significant change observed in 47 normal healthy women after 6 months use *5462*

Albumin *Serum Increase Physiological* Transient increases observed in first and third month of use in 47 healthy normal women studied over 6 months *5462*

Alkaline Phosphatase *Serum No Effect Physiological* No significant effect observed in 47 healthy normal women after 6 months use *5462*

Antithrombin III *Plasma Decrease Physiological* In 47 normal healthy women mean concentration decreased after 6 months of use *5461*

α_1-Antitrypsin *Serum No Effect Physiological* No significant effect observed in 47 normal healthy women after 6 months use *5461*

Aspartate Aminotransferase

Serum No Effect Physiological In 47 normal healthy women no effect observed after 6 months use *5462*

Bile Acids *Serum Increase Physiological* Significant increase observed in first month of use but thereafter decline to normal range for remaining 5 months of study in 47 normal healthy women *5462*

Bilirubin *Serum Increase Physiological* Significant increase observed in first month of use but thereafter reversion to normal concentration in 47 healthy normal women *5462*

Ceruloplasmin *Serum Decrease Physiological* In 47 normal healthy women studied for 6 months serum ceruloplasmin concentration decreased significantly during the sixth month *5462*

Cholesterol *Serum Decrease Physiological* Significant reduction observed in 47 normal healthy women during 12 months of use *5460* In 180 norplant users mean concentration rose from baseline of 165 .1 ± 27.7 mg/dL to 178.3 ± 65.1 mg/dL after 6 months use but decreased progressively to 132.8 ± 21.8 mg/dL after 24 months *4312*

Serum Increase Physiological In 180 norplant users mean concentration rose from baseline of 165 .1 ± 27.7 mg/dL to 178.3 ± 65.1 mg/dL after 6 months use *4312*

Cholesterol:HDL-Cholesterol Ratio

Serum Decrease Physiological In 180 norplant users mean ratio rose from baseline of 3.75 ± 0.71 to 4.20 ± 1.14 after 6 months, before decreasing to 3.51 ± 0.58 after 24 months *4312*

Serum Increase Physiological In 180 norplant users mean ratio rose from baseline of 3.75 ± 0.71 to 4.20 ± 1.14 after 6 months *4312*

Closure Time by Thrombostat
Plasma *No Effect* *Physiological* In 19 women using Norplant contraceptive mean closure of 82 ± 10 s not significantly different from 90 ± 14 s in 29 healthy controls *5199*

Factor I *Plasma* *No Effect* *Physiological* No significant effect observed in 47 normal healthy women after 6 months use *5461*

Factor II *Plasma* *No Effect* *Physiological* No significant effect observed in 47 normal healthy women after 6 months use *5461*

Factor V *Plasma* *No Effect* *Physiological* No significant effect observed in 47 normal healthy women after 6 months use *5461*

Factor VI *Plasma* *No Effect* *Physiological* No significant effect observed in 47 normal healthy women after 6 months use *5461*

Factor VII *Plasma* *Increase* *Physiological* Significant increase observed in 47 normal healthy women during 6 months use *5461*

Factor VIII *Plasma* *No Effect* *Physiological* No significant effect observed in 47 healthy normal women after 6 months use *5461*

Factor IX *Plasma* *No Effect* *Physiological* No significant effect observed in 47 normal healthy women after 6 months use *5461*

Factor X *Plasma* *No Effect* *Physiological* No significant effect observed in 47 normal healthy women after 6 months use *5461*

Factor XI *Plasma* *No Effect* *Physiological* No significant effect observed in 47 normal healthy women after 6 months use *5461*

Factor XII *Plasma* *No Effect* *Physiological* No significant effect observed in 47 normal healthy women after 6 months use *5461*

Factor XIII *Plasma* *No Effect* *Physiological* No significant effect observed in 47 normal healthy women after 6 months use *5461*

Fibrin Degradation Products
Plasma *No Effect* *Physiological* No significant effect observed in 47 normal healthy women after 6 months use *5461*

γ-Glutamyltransferase *Serum* *No Effect* *Physiological* No significant effect observed in 47 healthy normal women after 6 months use *5462*

Haptoglobin *Serum* *No Effect* *Physiological* No significant effect observed in 47 normal healthy women studied over 6 months *5462*

HDL-Cholesterol *Serum* *Decrease* *Physiological* In 180 norplant users mean concentration rose from baseline of 45.6 ± 14.4 mg/dL to 51.6 ± 27.5 mg/dL after 6 months use then decreasing to 38.9 ± 5.8 mg/dL for 24 months *4312*
Serum *Increase* *Physiological* In 180 norplant users mean concentration rose from baseline of 45.6 ± 14.4 mg/dL to 51.6 ± 27.5 mg/dL after 6 months use *4312*
Serum *No Effect* *Physiological* No significant change observed in 47 normal healthy women studied over 12 months until 12th month when a significant increase observed *5460*

Hematocrit *Blood* *No Effect* *Physiological* After 12 months use hematocrit remained relatively unchanged *1787*

Hemoglobin *Blood* *No Effect* *Physiological* After 12 months use concentration of hemoglobin remained relatively unchanged *1787*

Hemopexin *Serum* *No Effect* *Physiological* No significant effect observed in 47 normal healthy women studied over 6 months *5462*

immunoglobulin A *Serum* *No Effect* *Physiological* No significant effect observed in 47 normal healthy women studied over 6 months *5462*

Immunoglobulin G *Serum* *No Effect* *Physiological* No significant effect observed in 47 normal healthy women studied over 6 months *5462*

Immunoglobulin M *Serum* *No Effect* *Physiological* No significant effect observed in 47 normal healthy women studied over 6 months *5462*

LDL-Cholesterol *Serum* *Decrease* *Physiological* Significant reduction observed in 47 normal healthy women during 12 months use *5460* In 180 norplant users mean concentration rose from baseline of 105.8 ± 27.6 mg/dL to 78.6 ± 19.9 mg/dL after 24 months *4312*

α_2-Macroglobulin *Serum* *No Effect* *Physiological* No significant effect observed in 47 normal healthy women after 6 months use *5461*

Mean Platelet Volume *Blood* *No Effect* *Physiological* In 19 women using Norplant contraceptive mean concentration of 7.43 ± 0.6 /µL not significantly different from 7.68 ± 0.9 /µL in 29 healthy controls *5199*

Partial Thromboplastin Time
Plasma *No Effect* *Physiological* No significant effect observed in 47 normal healthy women after 6 months use *5461*

Plasminogen *Plasma* *No Effect* *Physiological* No significant effect observed in 47 normal healthy women after 6 months use *5461*

Platelet Aggregation response to ADP
Blood *No Effect* *Physiological* In 19 women using Norplant contraceptive mean release of 0.44 ± 0.24 nmol/L not significantly different from 0.47 ± 0.34 nmol/L in 29 healthy controls *5199* In 19 women using Norplant contraceptive mean aggregation of 18 ± 12 ohms not significantly different from 19.2 ± 12 ohms in 29 healthy controls *5199*

Platelet Aggregation response to Collagen
Blood *No Effect* *Physiological* In 19 women Norplant contraceptive mean release of 1.01 ± 0.35 nmol/L not significantly different from 0.95 ± 0.29 nmol/L in 29 healthy controls *5199* In 19 women using Norplant contraceptive mean aggregation of 40.7 ± 7.8 ohms not significantly different from 39 ± 8.5 ohms in 29 healthy controls *5199*

Platelets *Blood* *Decrease* *Physiological* Administration has been associated with thrombotic thrombocytopenic purpura in fewer that 1% of treated patients *6562*
Blood *No Effect* *Physiological* In 19 women taking using Norplant contraceptive mean concentration of 231 ± 53 x 10^9/L not significantly different from 232 ± 55 x 10^9/L in 29 healthy controls *5199* No significant effect observed in 47 normal healthy women after 6 months use *5461*

Protein *Serum* *No Effect* *Physiological* No significant effect observed in 47 normal healthy women studied over 6 months *5462*

Prothrombin Time *Plasma* *No Effect* *Physiological* No significant effect observed in 47 normal healthy women after 6 months use *5461*

Sex-Hormone Binding Globulin
Serum *Decrease* *Physiological* Administration has been associated with reduced concentration *6562*

T3-Uptake *Serum* *Increase* *Physiological* Administration has been associated with increased uptake *6562*

Thrombin Time *Blood* *No Effect* *Physiological* In 47 normal healthy women no significant effect observed after 6 months use *5461*

Thyroxine (T4) *Serum* *Decrease* *Physiological* Administration has been associated with reduced concentration *6562*

Transferrin *Serum* *No Effect* *Physiological* No significant effect observed in 47 normal healthy women studied over 6 months *5462*

Triglycerides *Serum* *Decrease* *Physiological* In 180 norplant users mean concentration rose from baseline of 76.2 ± 29.8 mg/dL to 92.3 ± 57.0 mg/dL after 6 months use then fluctuating around baseline for 24 months *4312* Significant decrease observed in 47 normal healthy women when studied over 12 months *5460*

Nortriptyline

Acid Phosphatase *Serum* *No Effect* *Analytical* At concentration of 1000 ng/mL (3.8 µmol/L) had no effect on method on Du Pont Dimension *1562*

Alanine Aminotransferase *Serum* *Increase* *Physiological* May cause cholestasis *128* Reported to cause jaundice, including obstructive, and altered liver function *5237*
Serum *No Effect* *Analytical* At acute overdose concentration (20 mg/dL) on Technicon SMAC® method *6266* No effect at concentration of 1.00 µg/mL (3.8 µmol/L) on method on Du Pont Dimension *1563*

Nortriptyline *(continued)*

Albumin *Serum No Effect Analytical* At concentration of 200 mg/L had no effect on BCG method *5704* At concentration of 1.00 µg/mL (3.8 µmol/L) had no effect on method on Du Pont Dimension *1564* At acute overdose concentration (20 mg/dL) on Technicon SMAC® method *6266*

Alkaline Phosphatase *Serum Increase Physiological* May cause cholestatic jaundice *128* Reported to cause jaundice, including obstructive, and altered liver function *5237*
Serum No Effect Analytical At acute overdose concentration (20 mg/dL) on Technicon SMAC® method *6266* At concentration of 1.00 µg/mL (3.8 µmol/L) no effect on method on Du Pont Dimension *1565*

Ammonia *Plasma No Effect Analytical* No effect at concentration of 1.0 µg/mL (3.8 µmol/L) on method on Du Pont Dimension *1566*

Amylase *Serum No Effect Analytical* At concentration of 1.00 µg/mL (3.8 µmol/L) had no effect on method on Du Pont Dimension *1567*

Antipyrine *Serum Increase Physiological* Impairs metabolism *4426*

Aspartate Aminotransferase *Serum Increase Physiological* Reported to cause jaundice, including obstructive, and altered liver function *5237* May cause cholestasis *128*
Serum No Effect Analytical At acute overdose concentration (20 mg/dL) on Technicon SMAC® method *6266* No effect at concentration of 1.00 µg/mL (3.8 µmol/L) on method on Du Pont Dimension *1568*

Bicarbonate *Serum No Effect Analytical* At concentration of 2 mg/L had no effect on method using phenolphthalein *5704*

Bile *Urine Increase Physiological* May cause cholestatic jaundice *128*

Bilirubin *Serum Increase Physiological* Reported to cause jaundice, including obstructive, and altered liver function *5237* May cause cholestatic jaundice *128*
Serum No Effect Analytical At concentration of 200 mg/L had no effect on Jendrassik and Grof method *5704* No effect at concentration of 1000 ng/mL (3.8 µmol/L) on method on Du Pont Dimension *1589* At acute overdose concentration (20 mg/dL) on Technicon SMAC® method *6266*
Serum No Effect Physiological Insignificant protein-displacement effect in neonates *6314*

Bilirubin, Direct *Serum No Effect Analytical* At concentration of 1.00 µg/mL (3.8 µmol/L) had no effect on method on Du Pont Dimension *1574*

Calcium *Serum No Effect Analytical* No effect at concentration of 1.00 µg/mL (3.8 µmol/L) on method on Du Pont Dimension *1569* At concentration of 200 mg/L had no effect on cresolphthalein method *5704* At acute overdose concentration (20 mg/dL) on Technicon SMAC® method *6266*

Carbamazepine *Serum Increase Analytical* 9.1% cross-reactivity observed with competitve fluorescence immunoassay used with PB Diagnostics OPUS analyzer *1153*
Serum No Effect Analytical No cross-reactivity observed with method on Du Pont aca *1513*

Chloride *Serum No Effect Analytical* At concentration of 2 mg/L had no effect on mercurimetric method *5704*

Chlorpromazine *Serum Increase Physiological* When nortriptyline coadministered concentration of chlorpromazine increased probably as a result of inhibition of metabolism *3634*

Cholesterol *Serum No Effect Analytical* At acute overdose concentration (20 mg/dL) on Technicon SMAC® method *6266* At concentration of 1.00 µg/mL (3.8 µmol/L) had no effect on method on Du Pont Dimension *1570* At concentration of 200 mg/L had no effect on Liebermann-Burchard method *5704*

Cholinesterase *Serum No Effect Analytical* Minimal interference observed with method on Du Pont Dimension *3271*

Cocaethylene *Urine No Effect Analytical* No interference observed with TLC method of Bailey *328*

Creatine Kinase *Serum No Effect Analytical* At acute overdose concentration (20 mg/dL) on Technicon SMAC® method *6266*

Creatine Kinase Isoenzymes *Serum No Effect Analytical* At concentration of 1.00 µg/mL (3.8 µmol/L) had no effect on method to measure CK-MB on Du Pont Dimension *1571*

Creatinine *Serum No Effect Analytical* No effect at concentration of 1.00 µg/mL (3.8 µmol/L) on method on Du Pont Dimension *1572* At concentration of 200 mg/L had no effect on Technicon AutoAnalyzer® Jaffe method *5704* At acute overdose concentration (20 mg/dL) on Technicon SMAC® method *6266*

Desipramine *Serum Increase Analytical* May cause false positive reaction in EMIT immunoassay for desipramine *3590*

Dicumarol *Plasma Increase Physiological* Impairs metabolism *4426*

Eosinophils *Blood Decrease Physiological* May cause bone marrow depression, including agranulocytosis, eosinophilia, purpura or thrombocytopenia *5237*
Blood Increase Physiological Presumed allergic response *2754*

Ethosuximide *Serum No Effect Analytical* Insignificant cross-reactivity observed with method on Du Pont aca *1523*

Glucose *Serum Decrease Physiological* Endocrine response *2754* Reported to cause hypoglycemia or hyperglycemia *5237*
Serum Increase Physiological Endocrine response *2754* Reported to cause hypoglycemia or hyperglycemia *5237*
Serum No Effect Analytical At concentration of 1.00 µg/mL (3.8 µmol/L) has no effect on method on Du Pont Dimension *1575* At acute overdose concentration (20 mg/dL) on Technicon SMAC® method *6266*

γ-Glutamyltransferase *Serum Increase Physiological* Reported to cause jaundice, including obstructive, and altered liver function *5237*
Serum No Effect Analytical At concentration of 1.00 µg/mL (3.8 µmol/L) has no effect on method on Du Pont Dimension *1579*

Granulocytes *Blood Decrease Physiological* May cause bone marrow depression, including agranulocytosis, eosinophilia, purpura or thrombocytopenia *5237*

HDL-Cholesterol *Serum No Effect Analytical* No effect at concentration of 1.00 µg/mL (3.8 µmol/L) on method on Du Pont Dimension *1576*

Hematocrit *Blood Decrease Physiological* May cause bone marrow depression, including agranulocytosis, eosinophilia, purpura or thrombocytopenia *5237*

Hemoglobin *Blood Decrease Physiological* May cause bone marrow depression, including agranulocytosis, eosinophilia, purpura or thrombocytopenia *5237*

5-Hydroxyindoleacetic Acid
Cerebrospinal Fluid Decrease Physiological Increase by 4.8 ng/mL in depressed patients *257*

Indoleacetic Acid
Cerebrospinal Fluid Decrease Physiological Increase by 2 ng/mL in depressed patients *257*

Iron *Serum No Effect Analytical* At acute overdose concentration (20 mg/dL) on Technicon SMAC® method *6266* No effect at concentration of 1.00 µg/mL (3.8 µmol/L) on method on Du Pont Dimension *1577* At concentration of 200 mg/L had no effect on Ferrozine method *5704*

Iron-Binding Capacity, Total *Serum No Effect Analytical* No effect at concentration of 1.00 µg/mL (3.80 µmol/L) on method on Du Pont Dimension *1590*

Lactate Dehydrogenase *Serum No Effect Analytical* At acute overdose concentration (20 mg/dL) on Technicon SMAC® method *6266* At concentration of 1.00 µg/mL (3.8 µmol/L) has no effect on method on Du Pont Dimension *1578*

Leukocytes *Blood Decrease Physiological* May cause agranulocytosis *128*

Lipase *Serum No Effect Analytical* At concentration of 1.00 µg/mL (3.8 µmol/L) has no effect on method on Du Pont Dimension *1580*

Magnesium *Serum No Effect Analytical* No effect at concentration of 1.00 µg/mL (3.8 µmol/L) on method on Du Pont Dimension *1581*

Nortriptyline *Serum Increase Physiological* 30-160 µg/L after 75-225 mg for 4 d *3868*

Phenytoin *Serum No Effect Analytical* No significant interference observed at a concentration of 100 µg/mL (380 µmol/L) with method on Du Pont aca *1538* No effect at concentration of 1.00 µg/mL (3.8 µmol/L) on method on Du Pont Dimension *1583*

Phosphate *Serum No Effect Analytical* At acute overdose concentration (20 mg/dL) on Technicon SMAC® method *6266*

At concentration of 200 mg/L had no effect on phosphomolybdate method *5704* At concentration of 1.00 μg/mL (3.8 μmol/L) has no effect on method on Du Pont Dimension *1584*

Platelets *Blood Decrease Physiological* May cause bone marrow depression, including agranulocytosis, eosinophilia, purpura or thrombocytopenia *5237* Purpura and thrombocytopenia observed *2754*

Primidone *Serum No Effect Analytical* No significant cross-reactivity with method on Du Pont aca *1541*

Prolactin *Plasma No Effect Physiological* In 10 patients with depression treatment with nortriptyline (up to 125 mg/d) for 2 weeks had no significant effect on prolactin concentration (12.1 ± 3.7 ng/mL pretreatment and 13.8 ± 5.9 ng/mL posttreatment) with no change in ratio of concentration by RIA to that by bioassay *6351*

Protein *Serum No Effect Analytical* At concentration of 200 mg/L had no effect on biuret method with blank correction *5704* At concentration of 1.00 μg/mL (3.8 μmol/L) had negligible effect on method on Du Pont Dimension *1591* At acute overdose concentration (20 mg/dL) on Technicon SMAC® method *6266*

Prothrombin Time *Plasma Increase Physiological* Patients on coumarins (unconfirmed clinically) *6244*

T3-Uptake *Serum No Effect Analytical* No significant effect observed at a concentration of 1.0 μg/mL (3.80 μmol/L) with method on Du Pont aca *1545*

Theophylline *Serum No Effect Analytical* At concentration of 1.00 μg/mL (3.8 μmol/L) had no effect on method on Du Pont Dimension *1585*

Thyroxine (T4) *Serum No Effect Analytical* No significant effect observed at a concentration of 1000 ng/mL (3.80 μmol/L) with method on Du Pont aca *1546 1588*

Triglycerides *Serum No Effect Analytical* At concentration of 1.00 μg/mL (3.8 μmol/L) has no effect on method on Du Pont Dimension *1592* At concentration of 200 mg/L had no effect on lipase/esterase method *5704* At acute overdose concentration (20 mg/dL) on Technicon SMAC® method *6266*

Urea Nitrogen *Serum No Effect Analytical* At concentration of 200 mg/L had no effect on diacetylmonoxime method *5704* At acute overdose concentration (20 mg/dL) on Technicon SMAC® method *6266* No effect at concentration of 1.0 μg/mL (3.8 μmol/L) on method on Du Pont Dimension *1593*

Uric Acid *Serum No Effect Analytical* At concentration of 200 mg/L had no effect on phosphotungstate reduction method *5704* At acute overdose concentration (20 mg/dL) on Technicon SMAC® method *6266* No effect at concentration of 1.00 μg/mL (3.80 μmol/L) on method on Du Pont Dimension *1594*

Noscapine

Histamine *Plasma No Effect Analytical* Improbable inhibition of radio-enzyme assay since therapeutic concentration 0.2 - 0.35 μg/mL and minimal effect observed at 100 μg/mL *2492*

Novaminsulfon

Cholesterol *Serum Decrease Analytical* At concentrations above 150 mg/L (normal therapeutic concentration 15 mg/L) lowered concentration as measured by CHOD-PAP method *5704*

Serum No Effect Analytical At concentration of 900 mg/L had no effect on Liebermann-Burchard method *5704* At concentration of 900 mg/L had no effect on CHOD-lodide method *5704* At concentration of 900 mg/L had no effect on catalase-AIDH method *5704* At concentration of 1160 mg/L had no effect on catalase-Hantzsch method *5704*

Creatinine *Serum Increase Analytical* At concentrations above 8,000 mg/L (normal therapeutic concentration 15 mg/L) raised concentration as measured by Jaffe-Fuller's earth method *5704*

Serum No Effect Analytical At concentration of 8,000 mg/L had no effect on Jaffe-Fading-Fraction method *5704* At concentration of 100 mg/L had no effect on creatinine iminohydrolase method *5704*

Glucose *Serum Decrease Analytical* At concentrations above 200 mg/L (normal therapeutic concentration 15 mg/L) lowered concentration as measured by GOD-PAP method *5704* At concentrations above 400 mg/L (normal therapeutic concentration 15 mg/L) lowered concentration as measured by GOD-PERID method *5704*

Serum No Effect Analytical At concentration of 80 mg/L had no effect on Kodak Ektachem® method *5704* At concentration of 800 mg/L had no effect on hexokinase/G-6-PDH method *5704*

Lactate *Plasma No Effect Analytical* At concentration of 800 mg/L had no effect on enzymatic method *5704*

Potassium *Serum No Effect Analytical* At concentration of 800 mg/L had no effect on measurement by ISE without predilution *5704*

Protein Electrophoresis *Serum No Effect Analytical* At concentration of 800 mg/L had no effect on automated Olympus-Hite method *5704*

Sodium *Serum No Effect Analytical* At concentration of 800 mg/L had no effect on measurement by ISE without predilution *5704*

Triglycerides *Serum Decrease Analytical* At concentrations above 100 mg/L (normal therapeutic concentration 15 mg/L) lowered concentration as measured by GPO-PAP method *5704*

Urea Nitrogen *Serum No Effect Analytical* At concentration of 80 mg/L had no effect on Kodak Ektachem® method *5704*

Uric Acid *Serum Decrease Analytical* At concentrations above 100 mg/L (normal therapeutic concentration 15 mg/L) lowered concentration as measured by Kageyama-Hantzsch method *5704*

Serum No Effect Analytical At concentration of 800 mg/L had no effect on catalase-AIDH method *5704*

Novobiocin

Alanine Aminotransferase *Serum Increase Physiological* Intrahepatic cholestasis may occur *3810*

Alkaline Phosphatase *Serum Increase Physiological* Intrahepatic cholestatic jaundice can occur *2242*

Aspartate Aminotransferase *Serum Increase Physiological* Intrahepatic cholestasis may occur *3810*

Bile *Urine Increase Physiological* Intrahepatic cholestatic jaundice can occur *2242*

Bilirubin *Serum Increase Analytical* Yellow metabolite affects direct methods *882* Interference by metabolite (Evelyn-Malloy) *3810*

Serum Increase Physiological Especially in newborn: inhibits its conjugating mechanism *565*

Bilirubin, Direct *Serum Increase Physiological* Competes for conjugation in liver *563*

BSP Retention *Serum Increase Physiological* Competition for excretion, may be actual damage *565*

Eosinophils *Blood Increase Physiological* Allergic reaction *2484*

Erythrocytes *Blood Decrease Physiological* Hemolytic anemia, usually mild *1117*

Hematocrit *Blood Decrease Physiological* Hemolytic anemia, usually mild *1117*

Hemoglobin *Blood Decrease Physiological* Hemolytic anemia, usually mild *1117*

^{131}I Uptake *Serum Decrease Physiological* Albamycin contains tetraiodofluorescein *4360*

Icteric Index *Serum Increase Physiological* Competition for conjugation mechanism *4012*

Leukocytes *Blood Decrease Physiological* May induce blood dyscrasias *3810*

Blood Increase Physiological Due to eosinophilia *3810*

Occult Blood *Feces Increase Physiological* Intestinal hemorrhage may occur *2242*

Platelets *Blood Decrease Physiological* Thrombocytopenia (immunologically induced) *2242*

PSP Excretion *Urine Decrease Physiological* ?Nephrotoxic effect *1714*

Novobiocin *(continued)*

Urobilinogen *Urine Increase Physiological* Hemolytic anemia in G-6-PD deficiency *2242*

NSD 3004

Bicarbonate *Serum Decrease Physiological* Long acting carbonic anhydrase inhibitor *3683*

Carbon Dioxide Partial Pressure
Blood Decrease Physiological Arterial blood long acting carbonic anhydrase inhibition *3683*

Standard Bicarbonate *Blood Decrease Physiological* Arterial blood long acting carbonic anhydrase inhibition *3683*

Nylidrin

Amphetamine *Urine Positive Analytical* At concentrations above 2.0 µg/mL (6.68 µmol/L) with method on Du Pont aca *1554*

Drugs of Abuse Screen *Urine Increase Analytical* False positive result with Abbott ADx method for amphetamine/methamphetamine *4279*

Hydrochloric Acid *Gastric Fluid Increase Physiological* 10 mg caused significant increase in 20 healthy volunteers *2357*

Volume *Gastric Fluid Increase Physiological* In 20 healthy volunteers 10 mg produced significant increase *2357*

Nystatin

Amino Acids *Urine Increase Analytical* Purple spot on thin-layer chromatography with ninhydrin when combined with neomycin and triamcinolone in Kenacomb *2109*

Eosinophils *Blood Increase Physiological* May cause allergic reaction *4691*

Platelets *Blood Decrease Physiological* Thrombocytopenia (AMA Blood dyscrasias) *4017*

Protein *Urine No Effect Analytical* At concentration of 1200 kU/L had no effect as measured by benzethonium chloride method *1171*

Zidovudine *Serum No Effect Analytical* No effect on liquid chromatographic method of Hedaya and Sawchuk *2525*

OAP

Amino Acids *Urine No Effect Physiological* Mean excretion of 28.0 mmol/d in 16 patients with leukemia undergoing chemotherapy not different from 29.1 ± 23.4 mmol/d in 52 patients with acute leukemia and 19.8 ± 10.4 mmol/d in 29 healthy controls of both sexes *6517*

Octreotide

Alanine Aminotransferase *Serum Increase Physiological* Hepatitis, jaundice, and increased liver enzymes have been observed as side effects in fewer than 1% treated patients *5241*
Serum No Effect Physiological No significant effect observed in 10 patients with acromegaly treated with up to 1500 µg/d for up to 2 years *5513*

Albumin *Urine No Effect Physiological* In 15 IDDM patients infusion of a 20 µg bolus followed by 10 µg/h for 2 hours caused nonsignificant increase to 38 µg/dL GFR during first hour from baseline of 32 µg/dL GFR *5785* In 13 normoalbuminuric, normotensive diabetics intravenous infusion of 8 µg/h had no significant effect on excretion *4585*

Aldosterone *Plasma Decrease Physiological* In 13 normoalbuminuric, normotensive dabetics intravenous infusion of 8 µg/h had no effect on plasma concentration *4585*
Plasma No Effect Physiological In 15 patients with IDDM infusion of bolus of 20 µg followed by 10 µg/h for 2 hours caused no significant effect on plasma concentration *5785*

Alkaline Phosphatase *Serum Increase Physiological* Hepatitis, jaundice, and increased liver enzymes have been observed as side effects in fewer than 1% treated patients *5241*
Serum No Effect Physiological No significant effect observed in 10 patients with acromegaly treated with up to 1500 µg/d for up to 2 years *5513*

Amino-terminal Propeptide of Type III Procollagen
Serum Decrease Physiological Mean reduction of 40% in 10 patients with active acromegaly when treated with up to 1500 µg daily subcutaneously for up to 15 months. In all patients with initially increased concentration normalized *5205*

Amylase *Duodenal Fluid Decrease Physiological* In 18 volunteers during secretin stimulation amylase inhibited between 41 and 59% with up to 80 µg/h octreotide: during secretin and ceruletide stimulation amylase inhibited by 84%, 78% and 81% respectively with 5, 20 and 80 µg/h octreotide *3103*
Serum Increase Physiological Several cases of pancreatitis reported in patients receiving octreotide *5241*

Androstenedione *Plasma Decrease Physiological* Decrease from mean concentration over 4 hours in 10 amenorrheic women with polycystic ovary syndrome from 7.39 nmol/L to 5.95 nmol/L following treatment with 200 µg subcutaneously daily for 7 days *4776*

Angiotensin-II *Plasma No Effect Physiological* In 13 normalbuminuric, normotensive diabetics intravenous infusion of 8 µg/h had no significant effect on concentration *4585*

Antidiuretic Hormone *Plasma No Effect Physiological* In 13 normoalbuminuric, normotensive diabetics intravenous infusion of 8 µg/h had no significant effect on arginine vasopressin concentration *4585*

Aspartate Aminotransferase *Serum Increase Physiological* Hepatitis, jaundice, and increased liver enzymes have been observed as side effects in fewer than 1% treated patients *5241*
Serum No Effect Physiological No significant effect observed in 10 patients with acromegaly treated with up to 1500 µg/d for up to 2 years *5513*

Atrial Natriuretic Peptide *Plasma No Effect Physiological* In 13 normoalbuminuric, normotensive diabetics intravenous infusion of 8 µg/h had no significant effect on concentration *4585*

Bicarbonate *Duodenal Fluid Decrease Physiological* In 18 volunteers secretin stimulated secretion reduced by up to 31% with up to 80 µg/h octreotide: with secretin and ceruletide secretion reduced by 25%, 11% and 19% respectively with 5, 20 and 80 µg/h octreotide *3103*

Bilirubin *Serum Increase Physiological* Hepatitis, jaundice, and increased liver enzymes have been observed as side effects in fewer than 1% treated patients *5241*

Bleeding Time *Patient No Effect Physiological* No significant effect observed in 15 patients with metastatic carcinoid or islet cell tumor following 1500 µg subcutaneously daily for 14 days *6521*

Blood *Urine Increase Physiological* Hematuria may be observed in fewer than 1% of treated patients *5241*

Calcitonin *Plasma Decrease Physiological* In group of patients with medullary carcinoma of thyroid generally higher concentrations both before treatment and after it was stopped although considerable variations of concentration measured throughout study *2363*

Calcium *Serum No Effect Physiological* In 10 patients with active acromegaly treatment with up to 300 µg/d subcutaneously caused insignificant change from mean baseline of 9.48 ± 0.12 mg/dL to 9.24 ± 0.22 mg/dL (significant) after 1 month, 9.32 ± 0.27 mg/dL after 6 months and 9.39 ± 0.31 mg/dL after 12 months *3494* In 10 volunteers given 100 µg subcutaneously concentration did not change significantly from mean baseline of 2.32 mmol/L over next 3 hours *664* No significant effect observed in 10 patients with acute acromegaly when treated with up to 1500 µg subcutaneously for up to 15 months *5205* No significant effect observed in 10 patients with acromegaly treated with up to 1500 µg/d for up to 2 years *5513*
Urine Decrease Physiological Reduction by 66% in healthy volunteers under conditions of mild diuresis 2 hours following subcutaneous injection of 100 µg *526*

Carcinoembryonic Antigen *Serum No Effect Physiological* No significant change observed with 60 days treatment in 18 patients with medullary carcinoma of thyroid *2363*

Carotene *Serum Decrease Physiological* In 98 patients with acromegaly treatment with 100 μg every 8 h increasing to 1,500 μg/d octreotide subcutaneously for an average of 24 months caused a change in mean concentration from 2.9 ± 0.1 μmol/L at baseline to 2.3 ± 0.1 μmol/L (significant) after 6 months, 2.3 ± 0.1 μmol/L (significant) at 12 months, 2.3 ± 0.1 μmol/L (significant) at 18 months and 2.4 ± 0.1 μmol/L (significant) at 24 months *4267*

Chloride *Serum No Effect Physiological* No significant effect observed in 10 patients with acromegaly treated with up to 1500 μg/d for up to 2 years *5513*

Urine Decrease Physiological Reduction by 28% in healthy volunteers under conditions of mild diuresis 2 hours following single subcutaneous injection of 100 μg *526*

Cholesterol *Serum No Effect Physiological* No significant change observed in 10 patients with acromegaly treated with up to 1500 μg/d for up to 2 years *5513*

β-Chorionic Gonadotropin *Plasma Decrease Physiological* Treatment in one woman with an α-subunit increase due to a pituitary adenoma caused fall in concentration but only partial reduction in 3 acromegalics *5286*

Chymotrypsin *Duodenal Fluid Decrease Physiological* In 18 volunteers inhibition of secretin stimulated secretion between 55 and 70% with up to 80 μg/h octreotide: with octreotide and ceruletide inhibition of 77%, 55%, and 60% observed with 5, 20, and 80 μg/h octreotide respectively *3103*

Corticotropin *Plasma Decrease Physiological* Treatment of one patient with Nelson's syndrome with 300 μg daily for 2 years caused significant decrease also observed in two other patients with Nelson's syndrome but no effect observed in patients with untreated Cushing's disease *3382*

Plasma Increase Physiological In one patient with Nelson's syndrome treatment with 100 μg t.i.d. for 7 days caused the plasma ACTH concentration to decrease by approximately 54% from 67 pmol/L to 36 pmol/L *3093*

Plasma No Effect Physiological In 5 patients with Cushing's disease administration of 100 μg octreotide subcutaneously had no effect on basal ACTH concentration *5769*

Cortisol *Plasma Increase Physiological* In 8 patients undergoing abdominal hysterectomy pretreatment with 100 μg subcutaneously had no effect on normal response from mean baseline of 330 ± 55 nmol/L to 787 ± 32 nmol/L *1396*

Plasma No Effect Physiological In 5 patients with Cushing's disease administration of 100 μg subcutaneously had no significant effect on basal plasma cortisol concentration *5769* No significant effect observed in 10 patients with acromegaly treated with up to 1500 μg/d for up to 2 years *5513* No effect observed in three patients with untreated Cushing's disease *3382*

Cortisol, Free *Urine No Effect Analytical* No significant interference observed with HPLC method of Turpeinen et al *6105*

C-Peptide *Plasma No Effect Physiological* No significant change observed in 4 patients with insulinomas when treated with octreotide for 3 weeks *6038* No significant change observed in 10 amenorrheic women with polycystic ovary syndrome treated with 200 μg subcutaneously daily for 7 days but response during glucose tolerance test significantly less *4776*

Creatinine *Serum No Effect Physiological* No significant effect observed in 10 patients with acromegaly treated with up to 1500 μg/d for up to 2 years *5513*

Creatinine Clearance *Urine Decrease Physiological* In 8 volunteers given 100 μg subcutaneously clearance fell significantly from mean baseline of 124 ± 10 mL/min to 66 ± 6 mL/min 2 to 4 hours later with gradual return to baseline after 10 to 12 hours *6090*

Urine Increase Physiological Significant effect in 9 cirrhotic patients with ascites and low urine output with infusion of 40 μg/h for 2 hours. Effect persisted for 24 hours *4145*

Urine No Effect Physiological Single subcutaneous injection of 100 μg had no effect at 2 hours in healthy volunteers *526*

Cyclosporine *Blood Decrease Physiological* With coadministration of drugs absorption of oral cyclosporine decreased with decease in maximal concentration but mechanism unclear *859* Rapid decrease reported within 24 to 48 hours in 9 pancreatic transplant patients probably due to reduced of absorption of cyclosporine by inhibition of pancreatic lipase or bile acids *3392*

Serum Decrease Physiological In patients after pancreatic transplant cyclosporine concentration rapidly reduced possibly by decreasing cyclosporine absorption through inhibition of the secretion of pancreatic lipase or bile acids *6595* With coadministration of drugs absorption of oral cyclosporine decreased with decease in maximal concentration but mechanism unclear *859* May decrease cyclosporine concentration by inducing hepatic cytochrome P-450 III A which metabolizes cyclosporine *5236* Effect probably occurs as result of inhibition of pancreatic exocrine function which inhibits fat absorption which also reduces cyclosporine absorption *1069*

Cyclosporine A *Blood Decrease Physiological* Depressed concentrations have been reported in patients receiving octreotide *5241*

1,25-Dihydroxy Vitamin D_3 *Serum No Effect Physiological* No significant effect observed in 10 patients with active acromegaly following treatment with up to 1500 μg daily subcutaneously for up to 15 months *5205*

Dopamine *Urine Decrease Physiological* In 8 healthy volunteers administration of 100 μg subcutaneously caused significant reduction from mean baseline of 5692 ± 850 pmol/min to 1096 ± 221 pmol/min after 2 to 4 hours, and 1023 ± 206 pmol/min after 8 to 10 hours with return to 4260 ± 708 pmol/min after 10 to 12 hours *6090*

Effective Renal Plasma Flow

Patient Decrease Physiological In 15 patients with IDDM infusion of a bolus of 20 μg followed by 10 μg/h for 2 hours mean flow rate decreased by 43.9 mL/min/1.73 sq m from baseline *5785* In 13 normoalbuminuric, normotensive diabetic patients intravenous infusion of 8 μg/h caused significant reduction from mean baseline of 550 ± 69 mL/min/1.73 sq m to 492 ± 73 mL/min/1.73 sq m *4585*

Epidermal Growth Factor *Urine No Effect Physiological* In 9 male volunteers administration of 100 μg subcutaneously caused no significant change from baseline excretion of 20.41 ± 8.2 ng/mg creatinine but with excretion decreasing to 14.27 ± 8.38 ng/mg creatinine during hours 2 to 3 after drug administration *664*

Epinephrine *Plasma Decrease Physiological* Infusion of 50 μg over 120 min in 6 patients with chromaffin cell tumors caused nonsignificant reduction at 120 min but decrease to 76.1 ± 13.8% of baseline at 240 min *2825*

Plasma No Effect Physiological In 15 patients with IDDM infusion of 20 μg bolus followed by 10 μg/h for 2 hours had no significant effect on concentration *5785*

Urine Decrease Physiological In 8 healthy volunteers administration of 100 μg subcutaneously caused significant reduction from mean baseline of 65 ± 12 pmol/min to 31 ± 4 pmol/min after 2 to 4 hours, 23 ± 4 pmol/min after 8 to 10 hours with return to 50 ± 11 pmol/min after 10 to 12 hours *6090*

Erythrocytes *Blood No Effect Physiological* No significant effect observed in 10 patients with acromegaly treated with up to 1500 μg/d for up to 2 years *5513*

Estradiol *Plasma Decrease Physiological* Decrease from mean baseline concentration of 0.165 nmol/L to 0.116 nmol/L in 10 amenorrheic women with polycystic ovary syndrome treated with 200 μg subcutaneously daily for 7 days *4776*

Factor VIII Coagulant *Plasma No Effect Physiological* No significant effect observed in 15 patients with metastatic carcinoid or islet cell tumor treated with 1500 μg subcutaneously daily for 14 days *6521*

Fat *Feces No Effect Physiological* No significant effect observed in 10 patients with active acromegaly treated with up to 1500 μg subcutaneously daily for up to 15 months *5205*

Follicle Stimulating Hormone

Plasma Decrease Physiological Partial reduction in response to treatment by one woman with menopausal concentration *5286*

Plasma No Effect Physiological No significant change in integrated concentration, number of peaks, peak amplitude or average nadir observed in 10 amenorrheic women with polycystic ovary syndrome treated with 200 μg subcutaneously daily for 7 days *4776*

Octreotide *(continued)*

Gastric Inhibitory Polypeptide
Plasma No Effect Physiological Increase from 100 to 220 ng/L observed in 7 patients with dumping syndrome in response to glucose tolerance test not seen when 50 µg octreotide administered subcutaneously 15 minutes before glucose ingested *6091*

Glomerular Filtration Rate *Urine Decrease Physiological* In 13 normoalbuminuric, normotensive diabetics intravenous infusion of octreotide (8 µg/h) caused reduction from 140 ± 15 mL/min/1.73 sq m to 131 ± 14 mL/min/1.73 sq m *4585* In 15 patients with IDDM infusion of 20 µg bolus followed by 10 µg/h for 2 hours caused mean decrease of GFR by 6.3 mL/min/1.73 sq m from baseline *5785* Significant reduction observed in 5 patients with insulin-dependent diabetes mellitus treated with 300 µg subcutaneously per day for 12 weeks from mean baseline 136 mL/min compared with control of 157 mL/min *5452*

Glucagon *Plasma Decrease Physiological* In 15 patients with IDDM infusion of bolus of 20 µg followed by 10 µg/h for 2 hours significant reduction observed during first and second hour *5785* In 13 normoalbuminuric, normotensive diabetics intravenous infusion of 8 µg/h caused significant suppression of plasma glucagon concentration *4585*
Plasma No Effect Physiological No significant change observed in 5 insulin-dependent diabetics treated with 300 µg subcutaneously per day for 12 weeks *5452* No significant effect observed in 4 patients with insulinomas treated with octreotide when treated for 3 weeks *6038*

Glucose *Serum Decrease Physiological* May cause hypo- or hyperglycemia which occurred in 3% or 16% acromegalic patients *5241* Transient decrease in glucose concentration and symptomatic hypoglycemia in two patients with insulinomas *5788* Single subcutaneous injection appears to reduce postprandial and nocturnal hyperglycemia *4234* In 15 patients with IDDM infusion of 20 µg bolus followed by 10 µg/h caused significant reduction beginning during first hour *5785*
Serum Increase Physiological Suppresses hormone secretion in many tissues and can alter the homeostatic balance in hormone secretion affecting insulin, growth hormone and glucagon resulting in either hyperglycemia or hypoglycemia *1384* In 8 patients undergoing abdominal hysterectomy pretreatment with 100 µg subcutaneously caused slowing and reduction of normal response from mean baseline of 4.1 ± 0.4 mmol/L to 5.5 ± 0.6 mmol/L *1396* May cause hypo- or hyperglycemia which occurred in 3% or 16% acromegalic patients *5241*
Serum No Effect Physiological In 13 normoalbuminuric, normotensive diabetics intravenous infusion of 8 µg/h had no significant effect on plasma glucose concentration *4585* No significant change observed in 5 insulin-dependent diabetics treated with 300 µg subcutaneously per day for 12 weeks *5452* In 10 patients with pheochromocytoma treatment with 3 100 µg subcutaneous doses of octreotide caused no significant change from mean baseline of 5.9 ± 0.41 nmol/L to 5.9 ± 0.31 nmol/L *4723* Insignificant reduction from mean of 5.9 mmol/L to 5.6 mmol/L in 10 patients with active acromegaly when treated with up to 1500 µg/day subcutaneously for up to 15 months *5205* Insignificant increase of fasting concentration but significant increase of mean concentration in 8 patients with active acromegaly when treated with 100 µg twice daily for 6 weeks with no effect observed with higher doses *2633* No effect observed with 3 weeks treatment in 4 patients with insulinoma *6038*
Urine No Effect Physiological No significant effect observed in 10 patients with acromegaly treated with up to 1500 µg/d for up to 2 years *5513*

Glucose Tolerance *Serum Decrease Physiological* Glucose intolerance may develop as a result of suppression of secretion of many hormones *1384* After 7 days of 200 µg subcutaneously daily for 7 days 6 of 10 amenorrheic women with polycystic ovary syndrome, all with initially normal glucose tolerance, showed intolerance with peak glucose concentrations above 10.0 mmol/L *4776*
Serum Increase Physiological In patients with acromegaly treatment with octreotide for several weeks caused decreases of 40-50% in nadir with oral glucose tolerance test *5513*

γ-Glutamyltransferase *Serum Increase Physiological* Hepatitis, jaundice, and increased liver enzymes have been observed as side effects in fewer than 1% treated patients *5241*

Glycated Hemoglobin *Blood No Effect Physiological* In 94 patients with acromegaly treatment with 100 µg every 8 h increasing to 1,500 µg/d octreotide subcutaneously for an average of 24 months caused a nonsignificant change in mean concentration from 6.8 ± 0.1% at baseline to 6.8 ± 0.1% after 6 months, 6.9 ± 0.2% at 12 months, 6.7 ± 0.2% at 18 months and 6.7 ± 0.3% at 24 months *4267* Treatment of 9 tall children aged 7 - 14 years with a nocturnal infusion of 1 - 1.5 µg/kg body weight caused no significant change from mean baseline concentration during course of treatment *2611*

Growth Hormone *Plasma Decrease Physiological* Basal mean concentration in 10 acromegalics of 44 ng/mL fell to within normal range after daily treatment with 200 to 300 µg for average of 64 weeks *3379* Significant reduction in 2 men with acromegaly secondary to ectopic GHRH secretion by metastatic carcinoid tumors with either s.c. or i.v. treatment *4093* In 13 normoalbuminuric, normotensive diabetics intravenous infusion of 8 µg/h caused marked suppression of GH concentration *4585* Reduces plasma concentrations of growth hormone and IGF-I in acromegalics who have not responded to other forms of therapy *5241* Treatment of 9 tall children aged 7 - 14 years with a nocturnal infusion of 1 - 1.5 µg/kg body weight caused a decrease in the 24-hour serum GH concentration by 50% *2611* Subcutaneous injection of 50 µg caused significant reduction in concentration for up to 4 hours in 20 patients with midgut carcinoid tumors and liver metastases *4344* In 17 acromegalic patients following one month treatment with 100 µg subcutaneously mean concentration decreased from 19 ± 5 µg/L to 3 ± 0.6 µg/L *1774* In 103 patients with acromegaly treatment with 100 µg every 8 h increasing to 1,500 µg/d octreotide subcutaneously for an average of 24 months caused a decrease in mean concentration from 30.9 µg/L to 5.7 µg/L after 3 months *4267* In 15 patients with IDDM infusion of bolus of 20 µg followed by 10 µg/h for 2 hours caused significant reduction beginning during first hour *5785* In 8 acromegalics in whom mean daytime serum growth hormone concentration was increased and ranged from 16.2 ± 4.8 µg/L pretreatment, treatment with nasal octreotide powder caused a decrease to 8.3 ± 2.3 µg/L on day 2 *2826* In one woman who had acromegaly mean concentration decreased with treatment from 9.1 µg/L to 6.6 µg/L but one month after treatment stopped concentration increased to 24.4 µg/L although it subsequently declined after 8 months to intratreatment level *971* Following single injection of 100 µg caused significant decrease in most patients with acromegaly treated with drug. Continuing treatment caused further decrease with most patients showing a greater than 50% reduction after 6-12 months *5513* 100 µg twice daily for 6 to 12 weeks significantly reduced mean or nadir concentration in 8 patients with active acromegaly (mean baseline 23.3 mIU/mL to 14.9 mIU/mL and nadir from 13.7 mIU/mL to 3.8 mIU/mL) *2633* In 10 patients with active acromegaly treatment with up to 300 µg/d caused reduction from mean baseline of 33.90 ± 36.00 ng/mL to 4.64 ± 3.11 ng/mL after 1 month, 3.08 ± 1.38 ng/mL after 6 months and significantly to 2.54 ± 1.58 ng/mL after 12 months *3494* Daily injections of 50 to 300 µg subcutaneously in 37 acromegalics produced progressive decrease *6046* In acromegalic patients 15 had 75% of their values below 2 µg/L although in some patients no reduction below 10 µg/L occurred *5052* In 10 patients with active acromegaly treatment with up to 1500 µg/day for up to 15 months caused mean reduction of 64% with normalization in 3 patients *5205*
Plasma No Effect Physiological No significant effect observed in 5 insulin-dependent diabetics treated with 300 µg subcutaneously per day for 12 weeks *5452* In 8 patients who received abdominal hysterectomy 100 µg subcutaneously prevented normal increase in concentration from baseline seen 60 minutes after start of surgery *1396*

Growth Hormone Releasing Hormone
Plasma Decrease Physiological Significant reduction observed in 2 men with acromegaly secondary to ectopic GHRH secretion by metastatic carcinoid tumors following either s.c. or i.v. treatment *4093*

Hematocrit *Blood Decrease Physiological* Iron-deficiency anemia may be observed in fewer than 1% of treated patients *5241*
Blood No Effect Physiological In patients with dumping syndrome increase observed in response to glucose tolerance test from 0.36 to 0.43 not seen when 50 µg was injected subcutaneously 15 minutes before glucose ingested *6091*

Hemoglobin *Blood* *Decrease* *Physiological* Iron-deficiency anemia may be observed in fewer than 1% of treated patients *5241*

Hemoglobin A_{1c} *Blood* *No Effect* *Physiological* No significant effect observed in 5 insulin-dependent diabetics treated with 300 µg subcutaneously daily for 12 weeks *5452*

5-Hydroxyindoleacetic Acid *Urine* *Decrease* *Physiological* Twice daily subcutaneous injection of 50 µg caused mean reduction of excretion by 26% in 20 patients with midgut carcinoid tumors and liver metastases *4344*

Insulin *Plasma* *Decrease* *Physiological* Significant reduction from mean of 254 pmol/L to 134 pmol/L in 10 patients with active acromegaly when treated with up to 1500 µg daily subcutaneously for up to 15 months *5205* In 8 acromegalics in whom mean insulin concentration was increased and ranged from 22.3 ± 6.3 mU/L pretreatment, treatment with nasal octreotide powder caused a decrease to 10.5 ± 2.2 mU/L on day 2 *2826* Subcutaneous injection of 50 µg caused significant reduction for up to 4 hours in 20 patients with midgut carcinoid tumors and liver metastases *4344* In 6 patients with chromaffin cell tumors infusion of 50 µg over 120 minutes caused decrease of insulin concentration to 49.7 +- 4.6% of baseline after 60 min and to 68.7 ± 7.2% of baseline after 120 min *2825* Insignificant reduction in 8 patients with active acromegaly treated with 100 µg twice daily for 6-12 weeks from mean of 38.4 mU/L to 30.9 mU/L with no effect observed with higher doses *2633* In 10 volunteers given 100 µg octreotide subcutaneously mean concentration decreased significantly from baseline of 9.15 µU/mL to 2.02 µU/mL at 1 hour, 2.6 µU/mL at 2 hours and 3.34 µU/mL at 3 hours *664*

Plasma *No Effect* *Physiological* Increase from 10 µU/mL to 40 µU/mL observed in 7 patients with dumping syndrome in response to glucose tolerance test not seen when 50 µg octreotide injected subcutaneously 15 minutes before glucose ingested *6091* No significant effect observed in 4 patients with insulinomas when treated with octreotide for 3 weeks *6038* No significant change observed in fasting concentration in 10 amenorrheic women with polycystic ovary syndrome treated with 200 µg subcutaneously daily for 7 days but responses during glucose tolerance test significantly lower *4776* In 8 patients undergoing abdominal hysterectomy pretreatment with 100 µg octreotide subcutaneously prevented normal increase observed 60 minutes after start of surgery *1396*

Insulin-like Growth Factor-I *Serum* *Decrease* *Physiological* Treatment of 17 acromegalics with 100 µg for one month caused decrease from mean baseline of 1021 ± 168 µg/L to 467 ± 75 µg/L *1774* In 10 adolescent children with constitutionally tall stature treatment for 12 months caused decrease of plasma concentration of somatomedin C (IGF-I) as well as reduction of 24-hour growth hormone pulsatility *5956* In 103 patients with acromegaly treatment with 100 µg every 8 h increasing to 1,500 µg/d octreotide subcutaneously for an average of 24 months caused a decrease in mean concentration from 5,200 ± 300 U/L to 2,300 ± 200 U/L after 6 months *4267* Substantial reduction in 10 acromegalics treated with 200 to 300 µg daily for average of 64 weeks *3379* Daily administration of 50 to 300 µg subcutaneously to 37 acromegalics produced reduction in parallel with reduction of growth hormone concentration *6046* In 10 individuals with active acromegaly treatment with up to 300 µg subcutaneously daily caused reduction from mean baseline of 7,857 ± 6,541 U/L to 2,541 ± 1,787 U/L after 1 month, 2,548 ± 1,583 U/L after 6 months and significantly to 2,479 ± 1,065 U/L after 12 months *3494* Decrease from 5,900 to 2,500 U/L in 1 of 2 men with acromegaly secondary to ectopic GHRH secretion by metastatic carcinoid tumors following chronic continuous s.c. therapy *4093* In 8 acromegalics in whom mean daytime serum IGF-I concentration was increased and ranged from 737 ± 50 µg/L pretreatment, treatment with nasal octreotide powder caused a decrease to 560 ± 69 µg/L on day 2 *2826* Concentration normalized in 17 of 31 patients with acromegaly with treatment *5052* Reduces plasma concentrations of growth hormone and IGF-I in acromegalics who have not responded to other forms of therapy *5241* Concentration reduced by average of 40% in 10 patients with active acromegaly when treated with up to 1500 µg daily subcutaneously for up to 15 months. Concentration normalized in 8 patients *5205* Significant reduction with 100 µg twice daily for 6 to 12 weeks in 8 patients with active acromegaly from mean of 122 U/mL to 83 U/mL *2633* Significant reduction observed at 3 weeks (concentration 0.50 U/mL) from baseline (0.96 U/mL) in 5 insulin-dependent diabetics and at 12 weeks (0.57 U/mL) after 300 µg subcutaneously per day *5452* In patients with acromegaly concentration returned to normal in 8 patients and was decreased by more than 50% in another patient while having no effect in another when treated for up to 1 year *5513*

Serum *No Effect* *Physiological* Treatment of 9 tall children aged 7 - 14 years with a nocturnal infusion of 1 - 1.5 µg/kg body weight caused an insignificant change from 1.05 ± 0.06 U/mL prior to treatment to 1.15 ±0.7 U/mL on therapy *2611*

Insulin-like Growth Factor Binding Protein-1

Serum *Increase* *Physiological* In 17 acromegalic patients treatment with 100 µg for one month caused increase from mean baseline of 36 ± 8 µg/L to 95 ± 16 µg/L *1774* Administration causes increased concentration *4439*

Serum *No Effect* *Physiological* In 8 acromegalics in whom mean daytime serum IGFBP-1 concentration was measured no consistent change observed with octreotide treatment *2826*

Insulin-like Growth Factor Binding Protein-3

Serum *Decrease* *Physiological* In 8 acromegalics in whom mean daytime serum IGFBP-3 concentration was increased and ranged from 5.7 ± 0.5 mg/L pretreatment, treatment with nasal octreotide powder caused a decrease to 4.4 ± 0.4 mg/L on day 29 *2826*

ionized Calcium *Serum* *No Effect* *Physiological* In 10 volunteers given 100 µg subcutaneously mean concentration did not change significantly from baseline of 1.26 mmol/L *664*

Leukocytes *Blood* *No Effect* *Physiological* No significant effect observed in 10 patients with acromegaly treated with up to 1500 µg/d for up to 2 years *5513*

Lipase *Serum* *Increase* *Physiological* Several cases of pancreatitis reported in patients receiving octreotide *5241*

Luteinizing Hormone *Plasma* *Decrease* *Physiological* In 10 amenorrheic women with polycystic ovary syndrome treated with 200 µg subcutaneously daily for 7 days significant decreases observed in mean pulse amplitude, average nadir concentration, and integrated concentration over 4 hours *4776* Partial reduction in woman with menopausal concentration in response to treatment *5286*

Neuropeptide Y *Plasma* *No Effect* *Physiological* In 10 patients with pheochromocytoma treatment with 3 100 µg subcutaneous doses of octreotide caused no significant change in area under the concentration curve from mean baseline of 29.6 ± 9.54 pmol/1 h to 32.0 ± 10.2 pmol/1 h *4723*

Norepinephrine *Plasma* *Decrease* *Physiological* In 15 patients with IDDM infusion of a bolus of 20 µg followed by 10 µg/h for 2 hours caused slight but significant decrease at end of first hour *5785* Infusion over 120 min of 50 µg octreotide in 6 patients with chromaffin cell tumors caused significant decrease to 51.3 ± 11.5% after 120 min and 72.4 ± 11.5% of baseline after 240 min *2825*

Plasma *No Effect* *Physiological* In 10 patients with pheochromocytoma treatment with 3 100 µg subcutaneous doses of octreotide caused no significant change in area under the concentration curve from mean baseline of 10.8 ± 3.85 nmol/1 h to 10.8 ± 3.09 nmol/1 h *4723*

Urine *Decrease* *Physiological* In 8 healthy volunteers significant reduction observed from mean baseline of 374 ± 50 pmol/min to 74 ± 11 pmol/min after 2 to 4 hours, 112 pmol/min after 8 to 10 hours and restoration to 234 ± 46 pmol/min after 10 to 12 hours *6090*

Urine *No Effect* *Physiological* In 10 patients with pheochromocytoma treatment with 3 100 µg subcutaneous doses of octreotide caused no significant change from mean baseline of 1.66 ± 0.52 µmol/d to 1.63 ± 0.49 µmol/d *4723*

N-terminal Propiomelanocortin

Serum *No Effect* *Physiological* No significant effect observed in 10 patients with acromegaly treated with up to 1500 µg/d for up to 2 years *5513*

Occult Blood *Feces* *Increase* *Physiological* Gastrointestinal bleeding may be observed in fewer than 1% of treated patients *5241*

Feces *No Effect* *Physiological* No significant effect observed in 10 patients with acromegaly treated with up to 1500 µg/d for up to 2 years *5513*

Octreotide *(continued)*

Osmolality *Serum No Effect Physiological* No difference compared with placebo-treated controls in healthy volunteers 2 hours after single subcutaneous injection of 100 μg *526*
Urine Decrease Physiological Significant reduction in 9 cirrhotic patients with ascites and low urine output with infusion of 40 μg/h for 2 hours. Effect persisted for 24 hours *4145*
Urine Increase Physiological In 13 normoalbuminuric, normotensive diabetics intravenous infusion of 8 μg/h caused significant increase in osmolality *4585* In 8 healthy volunteers administration of 100 μg subcutaneously caused significant increase from mean baseline of 312 ± 11 mosmol/L to 528 ± 46 mosmol/L after 2 to 4 hours, 556 mosmol/L after 4 to 6 hours, 449 mosmol/L after 6 to 8 hours, 424 mosmol/L after 8 to 10 hours with return to 331 mosmol/L after 10 to 12 hours *6090*
Urine No Effect Physiological No difference compared with placebo 2 hours following single subcutaneous injection of 100 μg in healthy volunteers *526*

Osmolar Clearance *Urine Decrease Physiological* Significant reduction in normal volunteers under conditions of mild diuresis 2 hours following single subcutaneous injection of 100 μg *526*

Osteocalcin *Serum Decrease Physiological* In 10 patients with active acromegaly treatment with octreotide up to 300 μg subcutaneously each day caused change from mean baseline of 11.78 ± 2.84 mgL to 9.72 ± 3.47 mg/L (significant) after 1 month, to 10.38 ± 4.46 mg/L (nonsignificant) after 6 months and 9.22 ± 4.92 mg/L (significant) after 12 months *3494*
Serum No Effect Physiological In 10 volunteers given 100 μg subcutaneously concentration did not change significantly from mean baseline of 3.81 ± 1.23 ng/mL over the next 3 hours *664*

Pancreatic Polypeptide *Plasma Decrease Physiological* Subcutaneous injection of 50 μg caused significant reduction for up to 4 hours in 20 patients with midgut carcinoid tumors and liver metastases *4344*

Parathyroid Hormone *Plasma Increase Physiological* In 10 patients with active acromegaly treatment with up to 300 μg/d administered subcutaneously caused significant increase from mean baseline of 30.50 ± 11.02 mg/L to 43.00 ± 14.11 mg/L after 1 month, 51.60 ± 17.28 mg/L after 6 months and 61.80 ± 22.86 mg/L after 12 months *3494*
Plasma No Effect Physiological In 10 healthy volunteers subcutaneous injection of 100 μg octreotide caused insignificant change from baseline of 31.11 ± 13.7 pg/mL to 41.77 ± 17.48 pg/mL 3 hours later *664*

Partial Thromboplastin Time
Plasma No Effect Physiological No significant effect observed in 15 patients with metastatic carcinoid or islet cell tumor treated with 1500 μg subcutaneously daily for 14 days *6521*

Phosphate *Serum No Effect Physiological* No significant effect observed in 10 patients with acromegaly treated with up to 1500 μg/d for up to 2 years *5513* In 10 patients with active acromegaly treatment with up to 300 μg/d subcutaneously caused nonsignificant change from mean baseline of 3.90 ± 0.41 mg/dL to 3.93 ± 0.33 mg/dL after 1 month, 3.72 ± 0.42 mg/dL after 6 months and 3.94 ± 0.44 mg/dL after 12 months *3494* No significant effect observed in 10 patients with active acromegaly when treated with up to 1500 μg daily subcutaneously for up to 15 months *5205*
Urine No Effect Physiological Single subcutaneous injection of 100 μg had no effect at 2 hours in healthy volunteers *526*

Platelets *Blood No Effect Physiological* No significant effect observed in 10 patients with acromegaly treated with up to 1500 μg/d for up to 2 years *5513* No significant effect observed in 15 patients with metastatic carcinoid or islet cell tumor following treatment with 1500 μg subcutaneously daily for 14 days *6521*

Potassium *Serum No Effect Physiological* No significant effect observed in 10 patients with acromegaly treated with up to 1500 μg/d for up to 2 years *5513*
Urine No Effect Physiological In healthy volunteers single subcutaneous injection of 100 μg had no effect after 2 hours *526*

Prolactin *Plasma Decrease Physiological* High plasma concentration not affected in 4 microprolactinoma patients but reduced in patients with mixed GH/PRL tumors *3379*
Plasma No Effect Physiological Basal concentration unchanged by treatment for up to 15 months with up to 1500 μg daily subcutaneously in 10 patients with active acromegaly but peak response to TRH stimulation significantly reduced during therapy *5205*

Protein *Urine No Effect Physiological* no significant effect observed in 10 patients with acromegaly treated with up to 1500 μg/d for up to 2 years *5513*

Prothrombin Time *Plasma No Effect Physiological* No significant change observed in majority of 15 patients with metastatic carcinoid or islet cell tumor treated with 1500 μg subcutaneously daily for 14 days *6521*

Renin Activity *Plasma Decrease Physiological* In 15 patients with IDDM infusion of bolus of 20 μg followed by 10 μg/h over next 2 hours caused slight but significant reduction at end of first hour *5785*

Sodium *Serum No Effect Physiological* No significant effect in 9 cirrhotic patients with ascites with infusion of 40 μg/h for 2 hours *4145* No significant effect observed in 10 patients with acromegaly treated with up to 1500 μg/d for up to 2 years *5513*
Urine Decrease Physiological In 8 healthy volunteers administration of 100 μg subcutaneously caused significant decrease from mean baseline of 320 ± 26 μmol/min to 155 ± 17 μmol/min from 2 to 4 hours later, 156 μmol/min from 4 to 6 hours later, 189 μmol/min from 6 to 8 hours later and 223 μmol/min 8 to 10 hours later with restoration to 339 ± 21 μmol/min from 10 to 12 hours after administration *6090* Reduction by 49% 2 hours following single subcutaneous injection of 100 μg in healthy volunteers under conditions of mild diuresis *526*
Urine No Effect Physiological No significant effect in 9 cirrhotic patients with ascites with infusion of 40 μg/h for 2 hours *4145*

Tachykinins *Plasma Decrease Physiological* Subcutaneous injection of 50 μg caused significant reduction for up to 4 hours in 20 patients with midgut carcinoid tumors and liver metastases *4344*

Testosterone *Serum Decrease Physiological* Decrease from 4 hour mean of 4.27 nmol/L to 3.13 nmol/L in 10 amenorrheic women with polycystic ovary disease following treatment with 200 μg subcutaneously daily for 7 days *4776*

Thrombin Time *Blood No Effect Physiological* No significant change observed in 15 patients with metastatic carcinoid or islet cell tumor treated with 1500 μg subcutaneously daily for 14 days *6521*

Thyroid Stimulating Hormone
Serum Decrease Physiological Dose-dependent suppression lasting for 8 hours observed in 4 normal male subjects *2848* In 97 patients with acromegaly treatment with 100 μg every 8 h increasing to 1,500 μg/d octreotide subcutaneously for an average of 24 months caused a change in mean concentration from 1.4 ± 0.1 mIU/L at baseline to 1.0 ± 0.09 mIU/L (significant) after 6 months, 1.1 ± 0.1 mIU/L (significant) at 12 months, 1.2 ± 0.1 mIU/L (nonsignificant) at 18 months and 1.1 ± 0.1 mIU/L (nonsignificant) at 24 months *4267* Inhibitory effect on thyrotropin secretion reported, observed both in people whose initially high concentration was due to neoplasia and to a lesser extent in patients whose high concentration was due to non-neoplastic resistance to thyroid hormone *449* Reduction observed in one woman with thyrotropic adenoma *5286* Treatment of 9 tall children aged 7 - 14 years with a nocturnal infusion of 1 - 1.5 μg/kg body weight caused the nocturnal TSH concentration to decrease to that observed during the day *2611*
Serum No Effect Physiological No significant change observed in patients with active acromegaly with a variety of treatment doses ranging up to 333 μg three times daily regardless of whether patients were receiving thyroid replacement therapy or not *2633* No effect observed on basal concentration in 10 patients with active acromegaly when treated with up to 1500 μg subcutaneously for up to 15 months although peak response to TRH stimulation significantly reduced during therapy *5205* No significant effect observed in 10 patients with acromegaly treated with up to 1500 μg/d for up to 2 years *5513*

Thyroxine (T4) *Serum Decrease Physiological* In treated acromegalic patients 12% developed biochemical hypothyroidism and 8% developed goiter *5241*

Serum *No Effect* *Physiological* Treatment of 9 tall children aged 7 - 14 years with a nocturnal infusion of 1 - 1.5 μg/kg body weight caused no significant change from mean baseline of 104 ± 5.6 nmol/L to 104 ± 5.8 nmol/L *2611* No significant change in patients with active acromegaly when treated with doses up to 333 μg three times daily for up to 12 weeks *2633* No significant change observed in 10 patients with acromegaly treated with up to 1500 μg/d for up to 2 years *5513*

Thyroxine (T4), Free *Serum* *Decrease* *Physiological* In 93 patients with acromegaly treatment with 100 μg every 8 h increasing to 1,500 μg/d octreotide subcutaneously for an average of 24 months caused a change in mean concentration from 27 ± 1.3 pmol/L at baseline to 24 ± 0.8 pmol/L (nonsignificant) after 6 months, 24 ± 0.9 pmol/L (significant) at 12 months, 24 ± 0.8 pmol/L (significant) at 18 months and 30 ± 1.0 pmol/L (significant) at 24 months *4267* Normalization observed in 4 patients with neoplastic disease treated with 100 μg daily for up to 1 month. Parallel decrease in serum TSH observed *449*

Serum *No Effect* *Physiological* No significant effect observed in 10 patients with active acromegaly when treated with up to 1500 μg subcutaneously daily for up to 15 months *5205*

Tri-iodothyronine (T3) *Serum* *No Effect* *Physiological* No significant effect observed in 10 patients with acromegaly treated with up to 1500 μg/d for up to 2 years *5513* No significant change in patients with active acromegaly when treated with doses up to 333 μg three times daily for up to 12 weeks regardless of whether they were receiving thyroid replacement therapy or not *2633*

Triglycerides *Serum* *No Effect* *Physiological* No significant change observed in 10 patients with acromegaly treated with up to 1500 μg/d for up to 2 years *5513*

Trypsin *Duodenal Fluid* *Decrease* *Physiological* In 18 healthy volunteers during secretin stimulation trypsin inhibited between 28 and 72% with up to 80 μg/h octreotide: during secretin and ceruletide stimulation inhibition of 76%, 55%, and 52% observed with 5, 20 and 80 μg/h octreotide *3103*

Urea Nitrogen *Serum* *No Effect* *Physiological* No significant effect observed in 10 patients with acromegaly treated with up to 1500 μg/d for up to 2 years *5513*

Uric Acid *Serum* *No Effect* *Physiological* No significant change observed in 10 patients with acromegaly treated with up to 1500 μg/d for up to 2 years *5513*

Vasoactive Intestinal Polypeptide
Plasma *No Effect* *Physiological* Increase from 3.0 to 10.2 pmol/L observed in patients with dumping syndrome in response to glucose tolerance test not observed when 50 μg octreotide injected subcutaneously 15 minutes before glucose ingested *6091*

Vitamin A *Serum* *No Effect* *Physiological* No significant effect observed in 10 patients with active acromegaly when treated with up to 1500 μg subcutaneously daily for up to 15 months *5205*

Vitamin B_{12} *Serum* *Decrease* *Physiological* Depressed concentrations have been reported in patients receiving octreotide *5241*

Volume *Urine* *Decrease* *Physiological* In 15 patients with IDDM bolus infusion of 20 μg followed by 10 μg/h for 2 hours caused significant reduction from mean baseline of 7.8 mL/min to 3.7 mL/min during first hour and 4.5 mL/min in second hour *5785* In 13 normoalbuminuric, normotensive diabetics intravenous infusion of 8 μg/h caused marked reduction of urinary flow rate *4585* Marked reduction (45%) in healthy volunteers within 2 hours of single subcutaneous injection of 100 μg *526* In 8 healthy volunteers 100 μg octreotide administered subcutaneously caused a significant reduction from mean baseline of 3.5 ± 0.3 mL/min to 1.7 ± 0.1 mL/min from hours 2 to 4, 1.8 mL/min from hours 4 to 6, 2.0 mL/min from hours 6 to 8 and 2.4 mL/min from hours 8 to 10 with return to 3.4 mL/min from hours 10 to 12 *6090*

Urine *Increase* *Physiological* Significant increase with infusion of 40 μg/h for 2 hours in 9 cirrhotic patients with ascites and low urine output. Effect persisted for 24 hours *4145*

von Willebrand Factor Antigen
Plasma *No Effect* *Physiological* No significant effect observed in 15 patients with metastatic carcinoid or islet cell tumor treated with 1500 μg subcutaneously daily for 14 days *6521*

von Willebrand Ristocetin Cofactor
Plasma *No Effect* *Physiological* No significant effect observed in 15 patients with metastatic carcinoid or islet cell tumor treated with 1500 μg subcutaneously daily for 14 days *6521*

Water Clearance, Free *Urine* *Decrease* *Physiological* In 15 patients with IDDM infusion of 20 μg bolus followed by 10 μg/h for 2 hours mean clearance decreased to 1.4 mL/min during first hour and to 1.6 mL/min during second hour from mean baseline of 4.6 mL/min *5785* In 8 volunteers administration of 100 μg subcutaneously caused significant decrease from mean baseline of -0.16 ± 0.12 mol/min to -1.26 ± 0.20 2 to 4 hours later, -1.54 ± 0.18 mol/min 4 to 6 hours later with return to -0.29 ± 0.14 mol/min 10 to 12 hours later *6090*

Urine *No Effect* *Physiological* No effect observed in 9 cirrhotic patients with ascites with infusion of 40 μg/h for 2 hours *4145*

Ofloxacin

Alanine Aminotransferase *Serum* *Increase* *Physiological* Occasional associations with hepatitis, jaundice or acute hepatic necrosis/failure reported *3914* Very infrequent side effect observed during many courses of treatment *2995*

Albumin *Urine* *Increase* *Physiological* Increased excretion reported in some patients in post-marketing studies *3914*

Urine *No Effect* *Analytical* At concentration of 40 mg/dL had no significant effect on Boehringer Mannheim Tina-quant method *2799*

Alkaline Phosphatase *Serum* *Increase* *Physiological* Occasional associations with hepatitis, jaundice or acute hepatic necrosis/failure reported *3914*

Aspartate Aminotransferase *Serum* *Increase* *Physiological* Occasional associations with hepatitis, jaundice or acute hepatic necrosis/failure reported *3914* Very infrequent side effect observed during many courses of treatment *2995*

Bands *Blood* *Increase* *Physiological* Occasional associations with increased band forms reported *3914*

Bilirubin *Serum* *Increase* *Physiological* Occasional associations with hepatitis, jaundice or acute hepatic necrosis/failure reported *3914*

Blood *Urine* *Increase* *Physiological* Hematuria reported in more than 1% of treated patients *3914*

Caffeine *Serum* *No Effect* *Physiological* Minimal effect observed on clearance *2704* No interaction between caffeine and ofloxacin reported *3914*

Cholesterol *Serum* *Increase* *Physiological* Hypercholesterolemia reported in some patients in post-marketing studies *3914*

Coproporphyrin I *Urine* *Increase* *Analytical* In urine collected 3 days after start of 400 mg/d ofloxacin mean apparent excretion 550 nmol/d as measured by HPLC method with fluorescence detection significantly increased compared with 154 nmol/d 1 week after end of treatment *5366*

Coproporphyrin III *Urine* *Increase* *Analytical* In urine collected 3 days after start of treatment with 400 mg/d ofloxacin apparent excretion of 841 nmol/d as measured by HPLC method with fluorecence detection as compared with 280 nmol/d 1 week after end of treatment *5366*

Creatinine *Serum* *Increase* *Physiological* Very infrequent side effect observed during many courses of treatment *2995* Occasional associations with interstitial nephritis or acute renal failure/insufficiency reported *3914*

Creatinine Clearance *Urine* *Decrease* *Physiological* Very infrequent side effect observed during many courses of treatment *2995*

Cyclosporine *Blood* *No Effect* *Physiological* Coadministration of ofloxacin with cyclosporine to 39 renal transplant patients had no effect on cyclosporine concentration or renal function *859* In one study of 39 renal transplant patients, no significant change in trough blood cyclosporine concentrations or serum creatinine concentrations *6274*

Serum *No Effect* *Physiological* In one study of 39 renal transplant patients no change in either plasma cyclosporine or creatinine concentrations observed *6596* Coadministration of ofloxacin with cyclosporine to 39 renal transplant patients had no effect on cyclosporine concentration or renal function *859*

Ofloxacin *(continued)*

Eosinophils *Blood Increase Physiological* Eosinophilia reported in more than 1% of treated patients *3914*

Erythrocyte Sedimentation Rate
Blood Increase Physiological Increased ESR reported in more than 1% of treated patients *3914*

Glucose *Serum Decrease Physiological* Both hyperglycemia and hypoglycemia reported in more than 1% of treated patients *3914*
Serum Increase Physiological Both hyperglycemia and hypoglycemia reported in more than 1% of treated patients *3914*
Urine Increase Physiological Glycosuria reported in more than 1% of treated patients *3914*

γ-Glutamyltransferase *Serum Increase Physiological* Very infrequent side effect observed during many courses of treatment *2995* Occasional associations with hepatitis, jaundice or acute hepatic necrosis/failure reported *3914*

Granulocytes *Blood Decrease Physiological* Occasional associations with agranulocytosis reported *3914*

Hematocrit *Blood Decrease Physiological* Occasional associations with anemia, including hemolytic and aplastic, reported *3914*

Hemoglobin *Blood Decrease Physiological* Occasional associations with anemia, including hemolytic and aplastic, reported *3914*

Lactate Dehydrogenase *Serum Increase Physiological* Increased activity reported in some patients in post-marketing studies *3914*

Leukocytes *Blood Decrease Physiological* Occasional associations with leukopenia reported *3914*
Blood Increase Physiological Occasional leukocytosis reported (in more than 1.0% patients) *3914*
Urine Increase Physiological Pyuria reported in more than 1% of treated patients *3914*

Lymphocytes *Blood Decrease Physiological* Both lymphocytopenia and lymphocytosis reported in more than 1% of treated patients *3914*
Blood Increase Physiological Both lymphocytopenia and lymphocytosis reported in more than 1% of treated patients *3914*

N-Acetyl-Glucosaminidase *Urine No Effect Analytical* At concentration of 500 mg/dL no significant effect observed on Boehringer Mannheim CPR method *3174*

Neutrophils *Blood Decrease Physiological* Occasional associations with neutropenia reported *3914*
Blood Increase Physiological Occasional neutrophilia reported (in more than 1% treated patients) *3914*

pH *Blood Decrease Physiological* Acidosis reported in some patients in post-marketing studies *3914*
Urine Increase Physiological Alkalinuria reported in more than 1% of treated patients *3914*

Platelets *Blood Decrease Physiological* Occasional associations with thrombocytopenia, including thrombotic thrombocytopenic purpura, reported *3914*
Blood Increase Physiological Thrombocytosis reported in more than 1% of treated patients *3914*

Porphyrin, Total *Urine Increase Analytical* In urine collected 3 days after the start of treatment with 400 mg/d mean concentration as measured by HPLC method with fluorescence detection apparently increased to 1533 nmol/d compared with 564 nmol/d 1 week after the end of treatment *5366*

Potassium *Serum Increase Physiological* Hyperkalemia reported in some patients in post-marketing studies *3914*

Theophylline *Serum Increase Physiological* Steady state concentration of theophylline may be increased (9%) and AUC increased by approximately 15% when ofloxacin coadministered due to inhibition of P450 cytochrome *3914* Effect appears to be minimal and of no clinical significance *1384* Increases plasma theophylline concentration *3125*
Serum No Effect Physiological No clinically significant effect on theophylline concentration observed when drugs coadministered *5999* Minimal effect observed on clearance *2704* No documented significant interaction with theophylline reported *6117*

Triglycerides *Serum Increase Physiological* Hypertriglyceridemia reported in some patients in post-marketing studies *3914*

Urea Nitrogen *Serum Increase Physiological* Occasional associations with interstitial nephritis or acute renal failure/insufficiency reported *3914* Increased serum urea nitrogen concentration reported in more than 1% of treated patients *3914*

Uroporphyrin *Urine Increase Analytical* In urine collected 3 days after start of 400 mg/d ofloxacin mean apparent excretion of 142 nmol/d as measured by HPLC method with fluorescence detection significantly increased as compared with 130 nmol/d 1 week after therapy *5366*

Ohio 469

Bilirubin *Serum Increase Physiological* Preliminary finding of significant increase post operatively *2687*

Glucose *Serum Increase Physiological* 10-30% higher in postoperative period *2687*

Lactate Dehydrogenase *Serum Increase Physiological* Preliminary finding of significant increase postoperatively *2687*

Leukocytes *Blood Increase Physiological* Significant rise postoperatively especially of segmented neutrophils *2687*

OKY-246

Theophylline *Serum No Effect Physiological* No significant effect observed on elimination half-life, total body clearance or volume of distribution observed in 8 hospitalized patients following either single intravenous dose or oral administration of 200 mg twice daily for 7 days *3074*

Olanzapine

Creatine Kinase *Serum Increase Physiological* In 35 acutely psychotic patients treatment with olanzapine and haloperidol (2 - 33 determinations per patient) was associated with 4 marked elevations (in 11.4% of the patients) *3947*

Oleandomycin

Alanine Aminotransferase *Serum Increase Physiological* May cause hepatotoxicity (cholestatic syndrome) *3810*

Alkaline Phosphatase *Serum Increase Physiological* Cholestatic jaundice reported *129*

Aspartate Aminotransferase *Serum Increase Physiological* May cause hepatotoxicity (cholestatic syndrome) *3810*

Bile *Urine Increase Physiological* Hepatotoxic effect *3810*

Bilirubin *Serum Increase Physiological* May cause intrahepatic cholestatic jaundice *2024*

BSP Retention *Serum Increase Physiological* May cause intrahepatic cholestasis *2024*

Eosinophils *Blood Increase Physiological* Associated with allergic cholestasis *2753*

Erythrocytes *Blood Decrease Physiological* Probably due to hemolytic anemia *3810*

17-Hydroxycorticosteroids *Urine Increase Analytical* Interferes with Porter-Silber reaction *4340*

^{131}I Uptake *Serum Decrease Physiological* Cyclamycin contains tetraiodofluorescein *4360*

17-Ketogenic Steroids *Urine Increase Analytical* Interferes with Zimmermann reaction *5869*

17-Ketosteroids *Urine Increase Analytical* Interferes with Zimmermann reaction *4340*

Leukocytes *Blood Increase Physiological* Occasional leukocytosis after 2 weeks *2753*

Olestra

Ethinyl Estradiol *Serum No Effect Physiological* No significant effect noted on days 12 to 14 of treatment cycle in 28 women taking 18 g/day for 28 days when taking oral contraceptive containing 300 µg norgestrel and 30 µg ethinyl estradiol *4046*

Norgestrel *Serum No Effect Physiological* No significant effect observed in 28 women taking 18 g/day for 28 days when concentration measured during days 12 to 14 of treatment cycle when also taking oral contraceptive containing 300 µg norgestrel and 30 µg ethinyl estradiol *4046*

Olsalazine

Alanine Aminotransferase *Serum Increase Physiological* Rare cases of granulomatous hepatitis and nonspecific reactive hepatitis observed in patients taking olsalazine. A single case of mild cholestatic hepatitis reported *4672*

Alkaline Phosphatase *Serum Increase Physiological* Rare cases of granulomatous hepatitis and nonspecific reactive hepatitis observed in patients taking olsalazine. A single case of mild cholestatic hepatitis reported *4672*

Aspartate Aminotransferase *Serum Increase Physiological* Rare cases of granulomatous hepatitis and nonspecific reactive hepatitis observed in patients taking olsalazine. A single case of mild cholestatic hepatitis reported *4672*

Blood *Urine Increase Physiological* Rare cases of hematuria, proteinuria, nephrotic syndrome or interstitial nephritis observed in patients taking olsalazine *4672*

Creatinine *Serum Increase Physiological* Rare cases of hematuria, proteinuria, nephrotic syndrome or interstitial nephritis observed in patients taking olsalazine *4672*

Eosinophils *Blood Decrease Physiological* Rare cases of leukopenia, neutropenia, lymphopenia, thrombocytopenia, anemia or hemolytic anemia, eosinophilia and reticulocytosis observed in patients taking olsalazine *4672*

γ-Glutamyltransferase *Serum Increase Physiological* Rare cases of granulomatous hepatitis and nonspecific reactive hepatitis observed in patients taking olsalazine. A single case of mild cholestatic hepatitis reported *4672*

Hematocrit *Blood Decrease Physiological* Rare cases of leukopenia, neutropenia, lymphopenia, thrombocytopenia, anemia or hemolytic anemia, eosinophilia and reticulocytosis observed in patients taking olsalazine *4672*

Hemoglobin *Blood Decrease Physiological* Rare cases of leukopenia, neutropenia, lymphopenia, thrombocytopenia, anemia or hemolytic anemia, eosinophilia and reticulocytosis observed in patients taking olsalazine *4672*

Leukocytes *Blood Decrease Physiological* Rare cases of leukopenia, neutropenia, lymphopenia, thrombocytopenia, anemia or hemolytic anemia, eosinophilia and reticulocytosis observed in patients taking olsalazine *4672*

Lymphocytes *Blood Decrease Physiological* Rare cases of leukopenia, neutropenia, lymphopenia, thrombocytopenia, anemia or hemolytic anemia, eosinophilia and reticulocytosis observed in patients taking olsalazine *4672*

Neutrophils *Blood Decrease Physiological* Rare cases of leukopenia, neutropenia, lymphopenia, thrombocytopenia, anemia or hemolytic anemia, eosinophilia and reticulocytosis observed in patients taking olsalazine *4672*

Occult Blood *Feces Increase Physiological* Rectal bleeding observed in 1 of 441 patients taking olsalazine *4672*

Platelets *Blood Decrease Physiological* Rare cases of leukopenia, neutropenia, lymphopenia, thrombocytopenia, anemia or hemolytic anemia, eosinophilia and reticulocytosis observed in patients taking olsalazine *4672*

Protein *Serum Decrease Physiological* Rare cases of hematuria, proteinuria, nephrotic syndrome or interstitial nephritis observed in patients taking olsalazine *4672*

Urine Increase Physiological Rare cases of hematuria, proteinuria, nephrotic syndrome or interstitial nephritis observed in patients taking olsalazine *4672*

Prothrombin Time *Plasma Increase Physiological* Increased time observed in patients taking warfarin *4672*

Reticulocytes *Blood Decrease Physiological* Rare cases of leukopenia, neutropenia, lymphopenia, thrombocytopenia, anemia or hemolytic anemia, eosinophilia and reticulocytosis observed in patients taking olsalazine *4672*

Urea Nitrogen *Serum Increase Physiological* Rare cases of hematuria, proteinuria, nephrotic syndrome or interstitial nephritis observed in patients taking olsalazine *4672*

Omeprazole

Acid *Gastric Fluid Decrease Physiological* After multiple daily dosing with 20 mg/d minimum decrease of 80 - 97% in intragastric acidity. With 40 mg doses decrease was 92 - 94% *267*

Alanine Aminotransferase *Serum Increase Physiological* Pronounced rise in activity in one patient on eighth day of treatment *2375* Mild and rarely marked increased activity observed. In rare cases overt liver disease has occurred, including hepatocellular, cholestatic or mixed hepatitis, liver necrosis, hepatic failure and hepatic encephalopathy *267*

Alkaline Phosphatase *Serum Increase Physiological* Mild and rarely marked increased activity observed. In rare cases overt liver disease has occurred, including hepatocellular, cholestatic or mixed hepatitis, liver necrosis, hepatic failure and hepatic encephalopathy *267*

Aminophenazone *Serum No Effect Physiological* No significant effect of coadministration observed on concentration *169*

Aspartate Aminotransferase *Serum Increase Physiological* Mild and rarely marked increased activity observed. In rare cases overt liver disease has occurred, including hepatocellular, cholestatic or mixed hepatitis, liver necrosis, hepatic failure and hepatic encephalopathy *267*

Basal Acid Output *Gastric Fluid Decrease Physiological* After multiple daily dosing with 20 mg/d maximum decrease of 78% in BAO and 58 - 80% decrease in minimum BAO. With 40 mg doses decreases were 94% and 80 - 93% respectively *267* In 10 healthy male volunteers administration of 20 mg/d for 2 weeks caused decrease from mean baseline of 2.6 mEq/h to 0.7 mEq/h and 40 mg/d caused decrease from 2.6 mEq/h to 0.2 mEq/h *3790*

Gastric Fluid Increase Physiological After multiple daily dosing with 20 mg/d maximum decrease of 78% in BAO and 58 - 80% decrease in minimum BAO. With 40 mg doses decreases were 94% and 80-93% respectively *267*

Bilirubin *Serum Increase Physiological* Mild and rarely marked increased concentration observed. In rare cases overt liver disease has occurred, including hepatocellular, cholestatic or mixed hepatitis, liver necrosis, hepatic failure and hepatic encephalopathy *267*

Blood *Urine Increase Physiological* Most commonly reported side effect is bleeding, usually mild. Incidence of 10.7% reported *3957*

Caffeine *Serum No Effect Physiological* Metabolism of caffeine unaltered by coadministration *169*

Clotting Time *Blood No Effect Physiological* In 28 patients coadministration of omeprazole with warfarin caused no significant effect. Thrombotest time 106 s with omeprazole and 98 s with placebo *6128*

Cortisol *Plasma No Effect Physiological* No effect observed in 8 volunteers given 30 mg/d for 28 d *4165*

C-Peptide *Plasma No Effect Physiological* No effect observed in 8 volunteers given 30 mg/d for 28 d *4165*

Creatinine Clearance *Urine No Effect Physiological* No effect observed in 8 healthy men given 60 mg/day for 9 days *5981*

Cyclosporine *Blood Increase Physiological* With coadministration of omeprazole absorption of cyclosporine is delayed and dosage:concentration ratio decreased leading to increased cyclosporine concentration *859*

Blood No Effect Analytical At a concentration of 14 mg/L had no effect on Syva EMIT method *495*

Blood No Effect Physiological No significant effect observed with coadministration in patients with renal grafts *169* In 10 men 1 to 7 years after renal transplantation mean concentration with omeprazole treatment 102 µg/L when measured by HPLC and 81 µg/L when measured by RIA compared with 100 µg/L and 95 µg/L respectively during placebo treatment *607*

Omeprazole *(continued)*

Cyclosporine *(continued)*
Serum Decrease Physiological One case reported but details not discussed *1069*
Serum Increase Physiological With coadministration of omeprazole absorption of cyclosporine is delayed and dosage:concentration ratio decreased leading to increased cyclosporine concentration *859*

Dehydroepiandrosterone *Plasma No Effect Physiological* No effect observed in 8 volunteers given 30 mg/d for 28 d *4165*

Diazepam *Serum Increase Physiological* Mean clearance of diazepam reduced by 27% and half-life increased by 36% in 8 healthy males when a single dose of diazepam (0.1 mg/kg intravenously) was given after one week of omeprazole (20 mg once daily) *170* Mean clearance of omeprazole decreased by 26% in rapid metabolizers of omeprazole after 1 week of oral treatment with 20 mg daily and single dose of 0.1 mg/kg diazepam intravenously. No apparent interaction observed in slow metabolizers of omeprazole *171* 40 mg omeprazole in the morning for one week in 8 healthy volunteers caused mean decrease of 54% in plasma clearance of intravenously administered diazepam. At lower doses of omeprazole clearance still decreased but not to same extent *169*

Digoxin *Serum Increase Physiological* Area under concentration curve increased by 10% when drugs coadministered but probably of no clinical significance. Effect due to increased absorption resulting from decreased hydrolysis of digoxin within the stomach because of higher pH *169*

Erythrocytes *Blood Decrease Physiological* Rare pancytopenia or anemia observed with treatment *267*

Estradiol *Plasma No Effect Physiological* No effect observed in 8 volunteers given 30 mg/d for 28 d *4165*

Ethanol *Serum No Effect Physiological* No significant effect observed on area under curve with coadministration of omeprazole and alcohol *169* Administration of omeprazole with alcohol has no influence on ethanol concentration *5064*

Fluvastatin *Serum Increase Physiological* Administration of omeprazole with fluvastatin to patients with hypercholesterolemia caused a significant increase of 50% in the AUC of fluvastatin and 24 - 33% in its maximum concentration and 18 - 23% decrease in its plasma clearance *5232*

Folate *Serum No Effect Physiological* In 5 patients receiving 20 mg/d for 2 weeks mean concentration changed non-significantly from 52 ± 14 ng/mL to 50 ± 12 ng/mL and in those receiving 40 mg/d from 43 ± 13 ng/mL to 45 ± 14 ng/mL *3790*

Gastrin *Serum Increase Physiological* In 10 healthy male volunteers administration of 20 mg/d for 2 weeks caused significant increase from 48 mg/L to 94 mg/L and after 40 mg/d increased from 42 mg/L to 105 mg/L *3790* In 10 healthy men after ingestion of 40 mg/d for 10 days mean concentrations in phases I, II, and III of the migrating motor complex were 18.8, 23.3 and 19.9 pmol/L respectively compared with 9.3, 9.6 and 9.5 pmol/L in placebo group respectively *4868* In 19 healthy male volunteers receiving omeprazole 40 mg q a.m. mean gastrin concentration 108 ± 16 pg/mL, on 40 mg q p.m. 132 ± 23 pg/mL and on 20 mg b.i.d. 113 ± 15 pg/mL, compared with 41 ± 4 pg/mL prior to treatment *3328* After 1 to 2 weeks of therapeutic doses of omeprazole in more than 200 individuals serum gastrin concentration increased. Median increase with 20 mg doses of omeprazole were 1.3 to 3.6-fold *267* Moderate increase in concentration observed in 10 elderly patients with duodenal ulcer when peak acid output was suppressed by more than 80%. Moderate increase observed with dose of 20-40 mg *3585* In 5 patients receiving 40 mg omeprazole daily for 2 weeks caused significant increase from mean baseline of 42 ± 4 ng/L to 105 ± 15 ng/L. In those receiving 20 mg/d concentration increased from 49 ± 8 ng/L to 96 ± 30 ng/L *3790* Raised to 80.9 pg/mL from 55.5 pg/mL in 8 volunteers after 29 d but reversible *4165* Significantly increased after 7 and 14 d treatment but not after a single dose *1853*
Serum No Effect Physiological Basal and integrated bombesin-stimulated values not significantly affected but bombesin-stimulated peak secretion significantly increased with intermittent treatment schedule *1169*

Glucagon *Plasma No Effect Physiological* No effect observed in 8 volunteers given 30 mg/d for 28 d *4165*

Glucose *Serum Decrease Physiological* Rare hypoglycemia observed with treatment *267*

γ-Glutamyltransferase *Serum Increase Physiological* Mild and rarely marked increased activity observed. In rare cases overt liver disease has occurred, including hepatocellular, cholestatic or mixed hepatitis, liver necrosis, hepatic failure and hepatic encephalopathy *267*

Granulocytes *Blood Decrease Physiological* Rare pancytopenia or agranulocytosis observed with treatment *267*

Hematocrit *Blood Decrease Physiological* Most commonly reported side effect is bleeding, usually mild. Frequency of reduced hematocrit about 2.2% *3957*

Hemoglobin *Blood Decrease Physiological* Most commonly reported side effect is bleeding, usually mild. Frequency of reduced hemoglobin about 2.1% *3957* Rare pancytopenia, hemolytic anemia or anemia observed with treatment *267*

Hydrochloric Acid *Gastric Fluid Decrease Physiological* When stimulated acid output reduced from 27.4 mmol H^+/h to 7.8 mmol H^+/h after 29 d in 8 volunteers but reversible *4165* Marked reduction of both basal and either bombesin or pentagastrin stimulated secretion *1169* In 10 elderly patients with duodenal ulcers doses up to 40 mg/d for 7 days caused suppression of peak output of up to 85%. A minimum dose of 20 mg was required to obtain a marked inhibitary effect in all patients *3585*

Hydroxy-Diphenylhydantoin *Urine No Effect Physiological* No significant effect observed in 8 epileptic patients when omeprazole 20 mg/day coadministered with phenytoin for 3 weeks *172*

Indocyanine Green Clearance
Serum No Effect Physiological No significant difference from normal observed in individuals receiving omeprazole *169*

Insulin *Plasma No Effect Physiological* No effect observed in 8 volunteers given 30 mg/d for 28 d *4165*

Itraconazole *Serum Decrease Physiological* Decreased oral bioavailability *886*

Ketoconazole *Serum Decrease Physiological* Decreased oral bioavailability *886*

Leukocytes *Blood Increase Physiological* Rare leukocytosis observed with treatment *267*

Lidocaine *Serum No Effect Physiological* Metabolism unaffected by treatment with 40 mg once daily in the morning *169*

Maximal Acid Output *Gastric Fluid Decrease Physiological* After multiple daily dosing with 20 mg/d maximum decrease of 79% in MAO and 50 - 59% decrease in minimum MAO. With 40 mg doses decreases were 88% and 62 - 68% respectively *267*
Gastric Fluid No Effect Physiological In 10 healthy adult males administration of 20 mg/d for 2 weeks caused significant reduction from mean baseline of 24 mEq/h to 5 mEq/h and after 40 mg/d from 18 mEq/h to 0 mEq/h *3790*

Metoprolol *Serum No Effect Physiological* When given 40 mg/d for 8 days had no significant effect on serum concentration of metoprolol given 100 mg daily *173* Concomitant administration of omeprazole and metoprolol had no significant influence on the steady-state plasma concentrations of either the R or S-enantiomers of metoprolol *169*

Neutrophils *Blood Decrease Physiological* Rare pancytopenia or neutropenia observed with treatment *267*

Nifedipine *Serum Increase Physiological* Although area under concentration curve unaffected by single administration, it was increased 21% after one week pretreatment with omeprazole *169*

Occult Blood *Feces Increase Physiological* Most commonly reported side effect is bleeding, usually mild. Incidence of 18.3% *3957*

Osmolality *Serum Decrease Physiological* In one patient inappropriate secretion of antidiuretiic hormone followed administration of omeprazole so serum osmolality decreased to 249 and 232 mOsm/kg which corrected with withdrawal of omeprazole *1631*
Urine Decrease Physiological In one patient inappropriate secretion of antidiuretiic hormone followed administration of omeprazole so urine osmolality decreased to 278 and 287 mOsm/kg which corrected with withdrawal of omeprazole *1631*

Parathyroid Hormone *Plasma No Effect Physiological* No effect observed in 8 volunteers given 30 mg/d for 28 d *4165*

Pepsin *Gastric Material Increase Physiological* Pepsin concentration in gastric secretion increased although basal and pentagastrin-stimulated pepsin output unchanged in 8 healthy male volunteers given 60 mg/day orally for 9 days. Concentration increased because of reduced volume *5981*

Pepsinogen *Serum Increase Physiological* Significant increase in pepsinogens A and C observed in 8 healthy volunteers given 60 mg daily for 9 days due to release of more pepsinogen into circulation, possibly due to back diffusion from gastric mucosa *5981*

Urine Increase Physiological Increased excretion of pepsinogen A but that of pepsinogen C unchanged in response to ingestion of 60 mg daily by 8 healthy volunteers. Renal clearance of pepsinogen C decreased *5981*

Pepsinogen A *Serum Increase Physiological* Administration of 20 mg/d for 3 days induces significant increase in concentration which rapidly declined on cessation of therapy *554*

Pepsinogen C *Serum Increase Physiological* Significant increase observed in both normal individuals and in patients with duodenal ulcer following 3 days treatment with 20 mg/d with rapid reversion to baseline with cessation of treatment *554*

pH *Gastric Fluid Increase Physiological* In one extensive study treatment with 15 mg/d cause increase of mean 24-hour pH from 2.1 to 2.5 on day 1 to 4.2 on day 5 *5946*

Gastric Material Decrease Physiological In 19 healthy male volunteers receiving omeprazole 40 mg q a.m. mean total time pH was greater than 4 was 68%, on 40 mg q p.m. 67% and on 20 mg b.i.d. 76%, compared with 15% prior to treatment *3328*

Gastric Material Increase Physiological Basal and pentagastrin-stimulated acid secretion reduced in 8 healthy men given 60 mg/day for 9 days *5981*

Phenazone *Serum No Effect Physiological* No significant effect observed on concentration when drugs coadministered *169*

Phenytoin *Serum Increase Physiological* 40 mg daily in the morning for one week caused 15% decrease in plasma clearance of intravenously administered phenytoin. After a single oral dose of 300 mg phenytoin area under concentration curve increased by 19% *169* Half-life prolonged in patients treated with omeprazole because it inhibits the drug metabolizing hepatic microsomal P-450 monooxygenase system *1384*

Serum No Effect Physiological No significant change observed in 8 epileptic patients with unchanged dose of phenytoin when treated for 3 weeks with 20 mg omeprazole daily *172*

Urine No Effect Physiological No significant change observed in 8 epileptic patients when 20 mg/day omeprazole coadministered with phenytoin for 3 weeks *172*

Platelets *Blood Decrease Physiological* When combined with heparin incidence of platelet counts below 90,000 /µL 1.5%, and to below 50,000 /µL 0.3% *3957* Rare pancytopenia or thrombocytopenia observed with treatment *267*

Prolactin *Plasma No Effect Physiological* No effect observed in 8 volunteers given 30 mg/d for 28 d *4165* In cases of gynecomastia and impotence associated with omeprazole no effect observed on plasma prolactin concentration *3594*

Propranolol *Serum No Effect Physiological* Area under concentration curve and peak and trough steady-state plasma concentrations unaffected by coadministration *169*

Prothrombin Time *Plasma Increase Physiological* Causes minimal prolongation of prothrombin time through stereoselective inhibition of clearance of R isomer of warfarin when it is coadministered *2625*

Quinidine *Serum No Effect Physiological* Omeprazole has no effect on the pharmacokinetics of quinidine *5996* Concentration unaffected by coadministration of omeprazole *169*

Secretin *Plasma Decrease Physiological* In 10 healthy men after ingestion of 40 mg/d omeprazole mean concentrations in phases I, II and III of migrating motor complex were 1.6, 1.4 and 1.1 pmol/L compared with 2.0, 1.7 and 2.2 pmol/L respectively in placebo ingesting controls *4868*

Sodium *Serum Decrease Physiological* In one patient inappropriate secretion of antidiuretiic hormone followed administration of omeprazole so sodium concentration decreased to 126 and 124 mmol/L which corrected with withdrawal of omeprazole *1631* Rare hyponatremia observed with treatment *267*

Urine Decrease Physiological In one patient inappropriate secretion of antidiuretiic hormone followed administration of omeprazole so urine sodium concentration decreased to 42 mmol/L which corrected with withdrawal of omeprazole *1631*

Tacrolimus *Serum Increase Analytical* In HPLC/MS method of Christians et al interference observed with measurement of metabolites of FK 506 because of similar retention time *1010*

Testosterone *Serum No Effect Physiological* No effect observed in 8 volunteers given 30 mg/d for 28 d *4165*

Theophylline *Serum No Effect Physiological* No clinically significant effect on theophylline concentration observed when drugs coadministered *5999* No effect observed on clearance or metabolism of coadministered omeprazole *169* No documented significant interaction with theophylline reported *6117*

Thrombotest *Plasma Decrease Physiological* Reduction from mean of 21.1% to 18.7% when omeprazole administered concomitantly with warfarin in 21 healthy young men *5879*

Thyroid Stimulating Hormone
Serum No Effect Physiological No effect observed in 8 volunteers given 30 mg/d for 28 d *4165*

Thyroxine Binding Globulin *Serum No Effect Physiological* No effect observed in 8 volunteers given 30 mg/d for 28 d *4165*

Thyroxine (T4) *Serum No Effect Physiological* No effect observed in 8 volunteers given 30 mg/d for 28 d *4165*

Tirofiban *Serum Decrease Physiological* Coadministration with tirofiban increased the rate of plasma clearance of tirofiban *3957*

Tri-iodothyronine (T3) *Serum No Effect Physiological* No effect observed in 8 volunteers given 30 mg/d for 28 d *4165*

Vitamin B_{12} *Serum Increase Physiological* In 10 healthy young male volunteers administration of 20 mg/d for 2 weeks caused increase from mean baseline of 300 pmol/L to 340 pmol/L and after 40 mg/d from 270 pmol/L to 290 pmol/L *3790*

Serum No Effect Physiological In 5 patients given 20 mg/d for 2 weeks mean concentration changed nonsignificantly from 300 ± 40 pmol/L to 340 ± 50 pmol/L and with 40 mg/d from 270 ± 40 pmol/L to 400 ± 20 pmol/L. Note, however, that these changes may solely be due to administration of intramuscular vitamin B_{12} for Schilling test *3790*

Volume *Gastric Fluid Decrease Physiological* Basal and pentagastrin-stimulated volume decreased in 8 healthy male volunteers given 60 mg/day orally for 9 days *5981*

Warfarin *Plasma Increase Physiological* In 28 patients coadministration of omeprazole with warfarn caused the mean plasma concentration of R-warfarin to increase by 9.5% although the concentration of S-warfarin unaffected *6128*

Plasma No Effect Physiological No effect observed on concentration of S-isomer but increased concentration of R-isomer by 12%. Metabolism of warfarin minimally affected by coadministered omeprazole and effects not of clinical significance *169* No effect of concomitant administration on mean plasma concentration of (S)-warfarin (379 ng/mL with and 387 ng/mL without) but caused slight significant increase of (R)-warfarin concentration (490 ng/mL to 548 ng/mL) *5879*

Ondansetron

Alanine Aminotransferase *Serum Increase Physiological* In 723 patients receiving cyclophosphamide-based chemotherapy and also receiving ondansetron ALT activity increased to above twice ULN in 1 to 2% patients. On repeat exposure a similar transient increase occurred but symptomatic liver disease did not occur *2181* Small number of probable drug related increases in patients taking drug but increases declined with withdrawal of drug *596*

Aspartate Aminotransferase *Serum Increase Physiological* Small number of mild increases in patients receiving drug: increases declined with withdrawal of drug *596* In 723 patients receiving cyclophosphamide-based chemotherapy and also receiving ondansetron AST activity increased to above twice ULN in 1 to 2% patients. On repeat administration a similar transient increase was observed but no symptomatic hepatic disease occurred *2181*

Potassium *Serum Decrease Physiological* Rare cases of hypokalemia observed following administration of ondansetron *2181*

Opiates

Aldosterone *Plasma Increase Physiological* Significant increase within 1 h of i.m. injection of hyoscine, meperidine or omnopon *3133*

Atrial Natriuretic Peptide *Plasma No Effect Physiological* No effect either with or without anesthesia or surgery *3133*

Carbohydrate-deficient Transferrin
Serum Decrease Physiological Opiate therapy or abuse has no effect on concentration *1906*

Cortisol *Plasma Increase Physiological* Significant increase within 1 h of i.m. injection of hyoscine, meperidine or omnopon *3133*

Epinephrine *Plasma Increase Physiological* Significant increase within 1 h of i.m. injection of hyoscine, meperidine or omnopon *3133*

Norepinephrine *Plasma Increase Physiological* Significant increase within 1 h of i.m. injection of hyoscine, meperidine or omnopon *3133*

Renin Activity *Plasma Increase Physiological* Significant increase within 1 h of i.m. injection of hyoscine, meperidine or omnopon *3133*

Thyroxine (T4) *Serum Increase Physiological* Increase observed due to increased thyroxine-binding globulin *2412*

Tri-iodothyronine (T3) *Serum Increase Physiological* Increase observed due to increased thyroxine-binding globulin *2412*

Opipramol

Glucose *Serum No Effect Analytical* No effect on glucose oxidase method of Boehringer *5480*

Opium Alkaloids

Amylase *Serum Increase Physiological* Impaired excretion spasm of sphincter of Oddi *1009*

Aspartate Aminotransferase *Serum Increase Physiological* Possibly due to spasm of sphincter of Oddi *1009*

BSP Retention *Serum Increase Physiological* Impaired excretion spasm of sphincter of Oddi *1009*

Cholinesterase *Serum Decrease Physiological* May cause inhibition of activity *2754*

Indocyanine Green *Serum Decrease Physiological* Mechanism not yet established *3942*

Xylose *Urine Decrease Physiological* Some may produce gastrointestinal irritation with impaired absorption and excretion *929*

Optimax

Creatinine *Serum No Effect Analytical* No effect at therapeutic concentrations on Beckman Astra® and Technicon SMAC® methods *1181*

Oral Contraceptives

Acetaminophen *Serum Decrease Physiological* Coadministration of acetaminophen with oral contraceptives causes reduction of acetaminophen concentration due to enhanced glucuronidation *34* Metabolic clearance may be increased requiring increased dose of acetaminophen to acheive the same effect *1384*

Acetylsalicylic Acid *Serum Decrease Physiological* Coadministration reduces concentration in women due to probable enhanced glucuronidation and activation of CoA-synthetases *4062*

α_1-Acid Glycoprotein *Serum Decrease Physiological* Metabolic changes in liver synthesis (estrogen) *3604*

Activated Factor VII *Plasma Increase Physiological* In 20 healthy women administration of Cileste (35 μg ethinyl estradiol and 250 μg norgestimate) for 3 cycles caused significant change of concentration from mean baseline of 35.1 ± 15.7 mU/mL to 99.7 ± 111 mU/mL *4823* In 20 healthy women administration of Tri-Cileste (35 μg ethinyl estradiol and 180 or 250 μg norgestimate) for 3 cycles caused significant change of concentration from mean baseline of 50.6 ± 46.1 mU/mL to 71.2 ± 47.8 mU/mL *4823* In 20 healthy women administration of Triodena (30 or 40 μg ethinyl estradiol, 50, 70 or 100 μg gestodene) for 3 cycles caused significant change of concentration from mean baseline of 70.8 ± 90 mU/mL to 99.4 ± 78.3 mU/mL *4823*

Adenosine Monophosphate *Urine No Effect Physiological* No significant effect of oral contraceptives on excretion *6103*

Alanine *Plasma Decrease Physiological* Hormonal effect (second part of cycle) *1154*

Alanine Aminopeptidase *Serum Increase Physiological* The use of oral contraceptives increased activity by 12% *5223*

Alanine Aminotransferase
Red Blood Cells Decrease Physiological Possibly associated with vitamin B_6 deficiency *852*
Red Blood Cells Increase Physiological Significantly higher than in women not using oral contraceptives *1501*
Red Blood Cells No Effect Physiological No effect even if treated for 3 y *5087* No effect, but stimulated *in vivo* by vitamin B_6*5088*
Serum Increase Physiological Significant increase observed within 3 mo usually continuing for several y *5308* Cholestatic-hepatotoxic effect *3810*

Albumin *Serum Decrease Physiological* Mean concentration in 52 pill-users 44 ± 3.3 g/L significantly different from 46 ± 2.9 g/L in 156 healthy controls *2035* 10% fall if used for several months *2698* Not significant after 3 mo cessation, significant after 3 y *5249*
Urine Increase Physiological Mean excretion in 15 healthy women taking Minulet/Femovan 9.76 μg/min, in 16 taking Marvelon 9.34 μg/min and in 15 taking Diane 12.0 μg/min not significantly different from 4.51 μg/min in 28 healthy controls *691*

Aldosterone *Plasma No Effect Physiological* No effect observed in women on low dose oral contraceptives *1256* Normal activity in users in spite of changes in renin substrate concentration *2223* Inconsistent response after 4 weeks *6393*
Urine Increase Physiological Estrogen effect (in small number of people) *887*

Alkaline DNase *Serum No Effect Physiological* No influence of oral contraceptives observed *294*

Alkaline Phosphatase *Serum Decrease Physiological* Significant effect observed within 3 mo usually continuing for several y *5308* But effects less marked with low estrogen preparations *2564* Slight decrease reported in one study *4014*
Serum Increase Physiological May cause cholestasis, rare hepatocellular degeneration *2803*
White Blood Cells Increase Physiological Observed effect *2452*

Alkaline Phosphatase, Bone Isoenzyme
Serum Decrease Physiological In 52 oral contraceptive pill users mean activity of 7.5 ± 2.3 ng/mL significantly different from 8.8 ± 2.7 ng/mL in 156 age matched controls *2035*

Alprazolam *Serum Increase Physiological* Oxidative metabolism inhibited by coadministration of oral contraceptives *5831* Concomitant administration of propoxyphene with alprazolam caused a increase in the maximum concentration of alprazolam of 18%, decreased its plasma clearance by 2% and increased its half-life by 29% *4685*

Amino-4-Imidazole-5-Carboxamide Ribotide
Urine Increase Physiological Occurs if megaloblastic anemia develops *6370*

α-Amino-Nitrogen *Plasma Decrease Physiological* Anabolic effect of synthetic steroids (progestogen) *1155*

δ-Aminolevulinic Acid *Urine Decrease Physiological* In one patient with acute intermittent porphyria mean excretion of 402 μmol/d significantly different from reference range of 2 - 49 μmol/d but reduced to 56 μmol/d after 3 months treatment with oral contraceptives *2341* In one patient with hereditary coproporphyria mean excretion of 727 μmol/d significantly different from reference range of 2 - 49 μmol/d but reduced to 87 μmol/d after 4 months treatment with oral contraceptives *2341*
Urine Increase Physiological May precipitate porphyria attack *2210*

Amylase *Serum Increase Physiological* Isolated case of acute pancreatitis reported *4170* In approximately 23%: probably of liver origin *56*
Urine No Effect Physiological Although high in serum, suggestive of hepatic origin *56*

Androgen Index, Free (FAI)
Plasma Decrease Physiological Significant reduction observed in 34 women with micropolycystic ovary syndrome treated with ethinyl estradiol and desogestrel or gestodene for 6 cycles *5666* In 22 patients with polycystic ovary syndrome treatment for 6 weeks caused significant reduction from mean baseline of 11.7 ± 0.86 to 1.75 ± 0.13 *3367*

Androstanediol Glucuronide
Plasma Decrease Physiological Concentration significantly reduced in 28 women receiving oral contraceptives (0.6 ± 0.4 nmol/L) compared with mean of 2.2 ± 0.8 nmol/L in 20 healthy young women *5306*

Androstenedione *Plasma Decrease Physiological* Treatment of 7 women with polycystic disease of the ovaries and 5 healthy women with oral contraceptives for 3 months caused significant decrease in concentration *5858* Significant reduction observed in 34 women with micropolycystic ovary syndrome treated with ethinyl estradiol and desogestrel or gestodene for 6 cycles *5666* In 22 patients with polycystic ovary syndrome treatment for 6 weeks caused significant reduction from mean 14.1 ± 0.95 nmol/L to 7.7 ± 0.52 nmol/L *3367*
Plasma No Effect Physiological Insignificant reduction over 9 months in 33 women receiving cycles of 35 μg ethinyl estradiol and 1 mg norethindrone when measured at 3, 6, and 9 months *4180*

Androstenedione, Free *Plasma Decrease Physiological* Equally reduced in women taking ethinyl estradiol with either levonorgestrel or desogestrel *5901*
Saliva No Effect Physiological No difference in concentrations in women taking ethinyl estradiol with either levonorgestrel or desogestrel in comparison with controls *5901*

Androsterone *Urine Decrease Physiological* Compared with controls, but details not discussed *802*

Angiotensin *Plasma Increase Physiological* Twofold increase *887*

Angiotensin-II *Plasma Increase Physiological* Elevated to 3 times normal during administration *840*

Angiotensinogen *Plasma Increase Physiological* Threefold increase with 0.5 mg mestranol *887* Increases in plasma estrogen concentrations associated with increased plasma angiotensinogen concentration *5422*

Antinuclear Antibodies *Serum Increase Analytical* False positive test for antinuclear antibodies observed *1384*
Serum Increase Physiological Slight effect in users *3843*

α_2-Antiplasmin/Plasmin Complex
Plasma Increase Physiological In 25 healthy women using oral contraceptives mean concentration 412 ± 132 μg/L not significantly higher than 312 ± 140 μg/L in 31 healthy women not using oral contraceptives *3936*

Antipyrine *Serum Increase Physiological* Coadministration impairs antipyrine metabolism *4417*

Antithrombin III *Plasma Decrease Physiological* Insignificant decrease from mean of 107 to 97% in 14 healthy premenopausal women given low-dose oral contraceptives for either one or two cycles *3327* In 20 healthy women administration of Tri-Cileste (35 μg ethinyl estradiol and 180 or 250 μg norgestimate) for 3 cycles caused significant change of concentration from mean baseline of 99 ± 10% to 92 ± 10% *4823* ?Predisposing cause of thrombosis *6686* Slight reduction during treatment with drug low in estrogen content: note effect not as marked as reported when high estrogens content preparations used *2934* In 20 healthy women administration of Triodena (30 or 40 μg ethinyl estradiol, 50, 70 or 100 μg gestodene) for 3 cycles caused significant change of concentration from mean baseline of 108 ± 9% to 101 ± 9% *4823* Reduced concentration observed with use *3694* In 20 healthy women administration of Cileste (35 μg ethinyl estradiol and 250 μg norgestimate) for 3 cycles caused significant change from mean baseline of 99 ± 12% to 93 ± 7% *4823*
Plasma No Effect Physiological In patients receiving 20 μg ethinyl estradiol and 150 μg desogestrel mean concentration changed over 12 months from 96% to 99% and in those receiving 30 μg ethinyl estradiol and 75 μg gestodene mean concentration changed from 101% to 100% over 12 months *5214* No effect observed in women taking either desogestrel/ethinyl estradiol or levonorgestrel/ethinyl estradiol *3191* No effect observed in 25 fertile women even after 15 treatment cycles with desogestrel/ethinyl estradiol preparation *6089* No significant changes at various intervals during treatment compared with controls *2355*

Antithrombin III Antigen *Plasma Decrease Physiological* By activity unchanged in women given low dose ethinyl estradiol and norethindrone *4334*

α_1-Antitrypsin *Serum Increase Physiological* Metabolic changes in liver synthesis (estrogen) *3604* In women given low dose ethinyl estradiol and norethindrone *4334* But effects less marked with low estrogen preparations *2564*
Serum No Effect Physiological No significant changes at various intervals during treatment compared with controls *2355*

Apolipoprotein A *Serum Increase Physiological* Mean concentration of 1.24 g/L at baseline in 22 women with IDDM changed significantly to 1.38 g/L after 1 month, 1.38 g/L after 3 months, 1.39 g/L after 6 months and 1.40 g/L after 12 months during treatment with 30 μg ethinyl estradiol and 75 μg gestodene *4633*

Apolipoprotein A-I *Serum Decrease Physiological* Concentration decreased by high dose monophasic levonorgestrel combination (250 μg progestin with 30 μg estrogen) to 1169 mg/L compared with 1266 mg/L in controls *2201* Between ages 18 and 35 years concentrations decreased by 7% (non-significant) but after age 35 years no variation was observed *5807*
Serum Increase Physiological Increase of from 5-12% after 6 months treatment with three different triphasic contraceptive regimes in 150 women *4560* Increased by all combination preparations except high dose monophasic levonorgestrel combination. Typical concentration observed 1350 to 1560 mg/L compared with 1266 mg/L in nonuser controls *2201* In 58 healthy women receiving for 3 months ethinyl estradiol with either desogestrel, gestodene or levonorgestrel actual increase or tendency to increase observed *5794* Significant increase observed in women taking either ethinyl estradiol/norgestrel or ethinyl estradiol/norethindrone over 12 months although concentration did not exceed clinically acceptable limits *4333* Increased by all combination preparations except high dose monophasic levonorgestrel combination. Typical concentration observed 1350 to 1560 mg/L compared with 1266 mg/L in nonuser controls *2201* Significant increase over 6 months in women taking 35 μg ethinyl estradiol (EE) + 1 mg ethynodiol, 30 μg EE + 0.15 mg levonorgestrel, 35 μg EE + 1 mg norethindrone, and 35 μg EE + 0.5 and 1 mg norethindrone. Average increase 20 mg/dL *816* With low-dose ethinyl estradiol and desogestrel 35.5% increase after 3 months use and 23.3% increase after 6 months in 18 healthy young women *2489* Insignificant increase from mean baseline concentration of 146 mg/dL to 149 mg/dL after 1 treatment cycle but marked increase after 10 cycles to 170 mg/dL in 20 women *3689* Significant increase observed over 3 cycles in 60 nonpregnant women taking either of 2 low-dose regimes *3504* Small but significant increase in concentration in 25 fertile women treated with desogestrel/ethinyl estradiol preparation for up to 15 cycles *6089* Significant increase from mean baseline value of 170 mg/dL to 185 mg/dL at 3 months, 178 mg/dL at 6 months and 171 mg/dL at 9 months in women taking 50 μg ethinyl estradiol and 1.0 mg norethindrone and similar changes with other combinations of same drugs *817* In 19 healthy women treated for 6 cycles with biphasic oral contraceptive containing ethinylestradiol and desogestrel mean concentration increased significantly from baseline of 141.7 ± 19.2 mg/dL to 174.2 ± 22.2 mg/dL *3316* In 16 healthy young women with normal menstrual cycles treatment with a combination of 30 μg ethinyl estradiol and 150 μg 3-keto-desogestrel caused a significant change from mean baseline of 146 ± 25 mg/dL to 171± 25 mg/dL on day 21 of the third cycle *3315* In 16 healthy young women with normal menstrual cycles treatment with a combination of 30 μg ethinyl estradiol and 150 μg desogestrel caused a nonsignificant change from mean baseline of 146 ± 25 mg/dL to 168 ± 35 mg/dL on day 21 of the third cycle *3315*
Serum No Effect Physiological No significant effect observed in 22 women taking 30 μg ethinyl estradiol with either

Oral Contraceptives *(continued)*

Apolipoprotein A-I *(continued)*
75 µg gestodene or 150 µg desogestrel for 12 cycles *3317* In 16 healthy young women with normal menstrual cycles treatment with a combination of 30 µg ethinyl estradiol and 150 µg desogestrel caused a nonsignificant change from mean baseline of 146 ± 25 mg/dL to 138 ± 20 mg/dL on day 3 of the first cycle *3315* Typically insignificant change over 6 cycles in women with low dose ethinyl estradiol with low dose levonorgestrel or desogestrel *2047* Insignificant increase from mean baseline of 1.63 g/L to 1.86 g/L in 28 women treated for 12 cycles with ethinyl estradiol/gestodene and from 1.63 g/L to 1.92 g/L in 25 women treated with ethinyl estradiol/desogestrel for 12 cycles *2099* In 16 healthy young women with normal menstrual cycles treatment with a combination of 30 µg ethinyl estradiol and 150 µg 3-keto-desogestrel caused a nonsignificant change from mean baseline of 146 ± 25 mg/dL to 143 ± 18 mg/dL on day 3 of the first cycle *3315*

Apolipoprotein A-II *Serum Decrease Physiological* In 16 healthy young women with normal menstrual cycles treatment with a combination of 30 µg ethinyl estradiol and 150 µg desogestrel caused a slight but significant decrease from mean baseline on day 3 of the first cycle *3315*
Serum Increase Physiological Significant increase observed in 60 nonpregnant women over 3 cycles taking either of 2 low-dose regimes *3797* Concentration increased by all combination drugs, typically in the range of 379 mg/L to 409 mg/L, compared with 336 mg/L in nonuser controls *2201* Significant increase from mean baseline concentration of 42 mg/dL to 47 mg/dL after 1 treatment cycle and 55 mg/dL after 10 cycles in 20 women receiving triphasic preparation *3689* In 58 healthy women treated for 3 months with ethinyl estradiol with either desogestrel, gestodene or levonorgestrel actual increase or tendency to increase observed *5794* Significant increase from mean baseline of 0.63 g/L to 0.74 g/L in 28 women treated with ethinyl estradiol/gestodene for 12 cycles and insignificant increase from 0.67 g/L to 0.81 g/L in 25 women treated with ethinyl estradiol/desogestrel for 12 cycles *2099* In 11 women taking 30 µg ethinyl estradiol with 150 µg desogestrel for 12 cycles significant increase of about 15% after 3 cycles, 18% after 6 cycles and 20% after 12 cycles *3317* Significant increase of 20% after 3 cycles, 25% after 6 cycles and 22% after 12 cycles in 11 women taking 30 µg ethinyl estradiol with 75 µg gestodene for 12 cycles *3317* With low-dose ethinyl estradiol preparation transient increase of 21.4 % at 3 months but reverted to normal by 6 months in 18 healthy young women *2489* In 19 healthy women treated for 6 cycles with biphasic oral contraceptive containing ethinyl estradiol and desogestrel mean concentration increased significantly from mean baseline of 33.2 ± 6.9 mg/dL to 45.6 ± 7.1 mg/dL *3316*

Apolipoprotein A-IV *Serum No Effect Physiological* In 58 healthy women receiving for 3 months either ethinyl estradiol/desogestrel, ethinyl estradiol/gestodene or ethinyl estradiol/Levonorgestrel no significant change observed *5794*

Apolipoprotein B *Serum Increase Physiological* Concentration increased by levonorgestrel combinations and by high dose and triphasic norethindrone combinations typically to above 620 mg/L versus 572 mg/L in controls *2201* Significant increase observed (15% at third cycle, 20% at sixth and 22% at twelfth) in 11 women taking 30 µg ethinyl estradiol with 75 µg gestodene *3317* Significant increase from mean baseline 0.89 g/L to 1.13 g/L in 28 women treated with ethinyl estradiol/gestodene for 12 cycles and from 0.92 g/L to 1.14 g/L in 25 women treated with ethinyl estradiol/desogestrel for 12 cycles *2099* In 19 healthy women treated with biphasic oral contraceptive containing ethinylestradiol and desogestrel for 6 cycles mean concentration increased significantly from baseline of about 58 mg/dL to about 68 mg/dL *3316* Increase from mean baseline concentration of 89 mg/dL to 98 mg/dL after 1 month and 108 mg/dL after 10 months in 20 women taking triphasic preparation *3689* Significant effect in 10 women after 3 treatment cycles with desogestrel/ethinyl estradiol preparation *3190* Mean concentration of 0.86 g/L at baseline in 22 women with IDDM changed nonsignificantly to 0.87 g/L after 1 month, 0.92 g/L after 3 months, 0.86 g/L after 6 months and 0.91 g/L after 12 months during treatment with 30 µg ethinyl estradiol and 75 µg gestodene *4633* Significant increase observed (23% at sixth cycle and 25% at twelfth) in 11 women taking 30 µg ethinyl estradiol and 150 µg desogestrel *3317* Significant increase after 6 months of from 20-23% in 150 nonsmoking normolipidemic women receiving three different triphasic regimes *4560* Significant increase over 12 months observed in women taking either ethinyl estradiol/norgestrel or ethinyl estradiol/norethindrone although concentration did not exceed clinically acceptable limits *4333*
Serum No Effect Physiological No significant effect observed in 58 women randomized into 3 groups of monophasic ethinyl estradiol with desogestrel, ethinyl estradiol and gestodene or triphasic ethinyl estradiol with levonorgestrel *376* No significant change observed in 58 healthy women receiving for 3 months either ethinyl estradiol/desogestrel, ethinyl estradiol/gestodene or ethinyl estradiol/Levonorgestrel *5794* Typically insignificant change over 6 cycles in women with low dose ethinyl estradiol with low dose levonorgestrel or desogestrel *2047*

Apolipoprotein C-III *Serum No Effect Physiological* No significant effect observed in 58 women randomized into three groups of monophasic ethinyl estradiol with desogestrel, ethinyl estradiol with gestodene and triphasic ethinyl estradiol with levonorgestrel *376*

Apolipoprotein E *Serum Decrease Physiological* In 19 healthy women treated for 6 cycles with biphasic oral contraceptive containing ethinyl estradiol and desogestrel mean concentration decreased significantly from baseline of about 6.7 mg/dL to about 4.9 mg/dL *3316* Highly significant decrease observed in 58 healthy women treated for 3 months with ethinyl estradiol with either desogestrel, gestodene or levonorgestrel *5794* Significant reduction observed in all 3 groups into which 58 women were randomized. Groups were monophasic ethinyl estradiol with desogestrel, monophasic ethinyl estradiol with gestodene and triphasic ethinyl estradiol with levonorgestrel *376*
Serum No Effect Physiological Although significant reduction after 1 cycle in 20 women receiving triphasic preparation no significant change after 10 cycles *3689*

Ascorbic Acid *Serum Decrease Physiological* Maximum effect at 2 weeks, greater effect in platelets *3010*
Urine Decrease Physiological Significant effect 50% decrease on comparable diets *2477*
White Blood Cells Decrease Physiological Mean 19 mg/100 g (control 25.7 mg/100 g) *3910*

Aspartate Aminotransferase
Red Blood Cells Increase Physiological Increased when women treated for 6 mo or longer *5087* Compared with normal, vitamin B_6 stimulation had no effect *5088*
Serum Increase Physiological Significant increase observed within 3 mo usually continuing for several y *5308* Hepatotoxic effect (cholestasis induced) *3425*

Atrial Natriuretic Peptide *Plasma Increase Physiological* Enhanced concentration observed in women on low dose oral contraceptives *1256*

Basal Metabolic Rate *Patient No Effect Physiological* In 24 young women receiving oral contraceptives mean rate 5841 ± 471 kJ/d not significantly different from that in 22 healthy young women not receiving drugs in whom mean BMR was 5601 ± 614 kJ/d *1426*

Bilirubin *Serum Increase Physiological* Interferes with canalicular excretion *563*

Bilirubin, Direct *Serum Increase Physiological* Hypersensitivity to estrogen component *2451*

BSP Retention *Serum Increase Physiological* Occurs in 40%, estrogen depresses secretory mechanism *3425*

Caffeine *Serum Increase Physiological* Half-life increased and total plasma clearance reduced when oral contraceptives taken but exact mechanism not established *4563*

Calcium *Serum Decrease Physiological* Seen in osteoporosis, ?due to fall in albumin *6616* Isolated case of acute pancreatitis reported *4170*
Serum Increase Physiological Increased ingestion would increase concentration *1009*
Serum No Effect Physiological In 52 oral contraceptive pill users mean concentration of 2.32 ± 0.09 mmol/L not significantly different from 2.32 ± 0.10 mmol/L in 156 age matched controls *2035* No effect observed over 24 months in 17 women given low-dose estrogen preparation *3618*
Urine Decrease Physiological Occurs with fall in serum concentration *6616*

Carbonic Anhydrase
Red Blood Cells Increase Physiological Measured as B isoenzyme (hormonal effect) *5324*

β-Carotene *Serum Decrease Physiological* Significant reduction to 9.4 ± 7.1 μg/dL in 88 oral contraceptive users compared with 14.9 ± 10.0 μg/dL in 58 nonusers *4485*

Catechol-O-Methyltransferase
Red Blood Cells Increase Physiological When high in estrogen content *2330*

Catecholamines *Urine No Effect Physiological* No effect observed with ingestion *5402*

Cephalin Time *Blood Decrease Physiological* Metabolic effect *4737*

Ceruloplasmin *Serum Increase Physiological* In 10 healthy women aged 20 - 29 years taking oral contraceptives mean concentration of 612 ± 140 mg/L (enzymatically) and 372 ± 70 mg/L (by RID) not significantly increased compared with 502 ± 128 mg/L (enzymatically) and 330 ± 61 mg/L (by RID) in 10 healthy women aged 20 - 29 years not taking oral contraceptives *2959* Significant increase observed in 34 women with micropolycystic ovary disease treated with ethinyl estradiol and desogestrel or gestodene for 6 cycles *5666* Increase by 115 to 123% after 3 mo with different preparations *503* Significant increase in 17 healthy women given low-dose estrogen preparation over 17 months *3617* Estrogen effect on liver, no change in activity *3604* At age 20-29 years mean concentration in 4 women receiving oral contraceptives 371 (270-460) mg/L compared with 330 (260-440) mg/L in 10 healthy controls when measured by RID and 503 (330-690) mg/L and 612 (342-790) mg/L when measured enzymatically. In women aged 30-39 years concentration measured enzymatically 744 (480-1030) mg/L in oral contraceptive users and 516 (380-930) mg/L in control women *3519* In 7 women receiving oral contraceptives mean "concentration" of 92 ± 7.1 sq mm significantly higher than 52 ± 7.3 sq mm in 22 healthy controls *5517*

Cervical Secretion *Patient Increase Physiological* Leukorrhea due to estrogen in 20% women *3869*
Patient No Effect Physiological Leucorrhea due to estrogen in 20% women *3869*

Chenodeoxycholic Acid *Serum No Effect Physiological* No effect observed over 12 mo in 29 women given combination of ethinyl estradiol and norgestrel *2537*

Chlordiazepoxide *Serum Increase Physiological* In women receiving oral contraceptives half-life prolonged as result of inhibition of oxidative metabolism *4987*

Chlordiazepoxide, Free *Serum Increase Physiological* Concentration may be increased in oral contraceptive users although no difference in clinical effect have been demonstrated *1384*

Cholesterol *Serum Decrease Physiological* Mean concentration of 4.93 mmol/L at baseline in 22 women with IDDM changed nonsignificantly to 4.64 mmol/L after 1 month, 4.64 mmol/L after 3 months, 4.74 mmol/L after 6 months and 4.53 mmol/L after 12 months during treatment with 30 μg ethinyl estradiol and 75 μg gestodene *4633* In 16 healthy young women with normal menstrual cycles treatment with a combination of 30 μg ethinyl estradiol and 150 μg desogestrel caused a significant decrease from mean baseline of 15% on day 3 of the first cycle *3315*
Serum Increase Physiological Significant increase at 3, 6, and 9 months in women taking either 50 μg ethinyl estradiol and 1.0 mg norethindrone, 35 μg ethinyl estradiol and 1.0 mg norethindrone or 35 μg ethinyl estradiol and 0.5 mg norethindrone *817* Increase of from 3-10% after 6 months in 150 women receiving three different triphasic regimes *4560* Extent of effect varies with exact composition of oral contraceptive *2410* Significant increase at 6 months in users but no significant difference between those taking 35 μg ethinyl estradiol (EE) + 1 mg ethynodiol, 30 μg EE + 0.15 mg levonorgestrel, 35 μg EE + 1 mg norethindrone, and 35 μg EE + 0.5 and 1 mg norethindrone *816* Increase observed in women taking either ethinyl estradiol/Levonorgestrel or ethinyl estradiol/norethindrone over 12 months but concentration did not exceed clinically acceptable limits *4333* May result with oral contraceptive containing more than 75 μg estrogen *50* In 19 healthy women treated for 6 cycles with biphasic oral contraceptive containing ethinyl estradiol and desogestrel mean concentration increased significantly from mean baseline of 189.6 ± 29.6 mg/dL to 209.4 +/ 33.4 mg/dL *3316* In 10 women receiving ethinyl estradiol with norethindrone *3278* If initially low (no effect if about 200 mg/dL) *887* Increase by 4 to 15% depending on preparation used *4768* Slight effect with high-dose combination drugs *2046* In women users significant correlation observed (r = 0.104) *2399*
Serum No Effect Physiological In 16 healthy young women with normal menstrual cycles treatment with a combination of 30 μg ethinyl estradiol and 150 μg 3-keto-desogestrel caused a significant reduction from mean baseline of 9% on day 3 of the first cycle *3315* In 16 healthy young women with normal menstrual cycles treatment with a combination of 30 μg ethinyl estradiol and 150 μg desogestrel caused a nonsignificant change from mean baseline of 180 mg/dL *3315* In 16 healthy young women with normal menstrual cycles treatment with a combination of 30 μg ethinyl estradiol and 150 μg 3-keto-desogestrel caused a significant increase from mean baseline by day 21 of the third cycle *3315* Mean concentration of 4.98 ± 0.88 mmol/L in 9 desogestrel users and 4.61 ± 0.45 mmol/L in 9 levonorgestrel users not significantly different from 4.49 ± 0.61 mmol/L in 41 controls *1309* No effect even after 15 treatment cycles with desogestrel/ethinyl estradiol preparation in 25 fertile women *6089* Typically insignificant change over 6 cycles in women with low dose ethinyl estradiol with low dose levonorgestrel or desogestrel *2047* Observed in 60 nonpregnant women for 3 cycles with either of 2 low-dose regimes *2098* In 58 healthy women receiving either ethinyl estradiol/desogestrel, ethinyl estradiol/gestodene or ethinyl estradiol/Levonorgestrel for 3 months no significant change observed *5794* No difference between treated women and others *2184* Combination oral contraceptives had no effect on concentration *2201* No significant effect observed in 925 women using 150 or 250 μg of levonorgestrel, 500 or 1000 μg of norethindrone, or 150 μg desogestrel as progestin *2202* No significant change observed over 6 months in 18 healthy young women receiving low-dose ethinyl estradiol with levonorgestrel *2489* No effect observed usually *4014* Insignificant increase in 20 women after 10 cycles of treatment with triphasic preparation, but with no effect after first cycle *3689* May occur due to opposing effects of estrogen and progestogen components *50* No significant change observed in 58 healthy women randomized into groups taking either monophasic ethinyl estradiol with desogestrel, ethinyl estradiol and gestodene or triphasic ethinyl estradiol with levonorgestrel *376* In 10 women receiving ethinyl estradiol with norgestrel *3278* No significant effect observed in 11 women followed for 12 cycles while receiving 30 μg ethinyl estradiol and 150 μg desogestrel *3317* No significant effect observed in 11 women followed for 12 cycles while receiving 30 μg ethinyl estradiol with 75 μg gestodene *3317*

Cholesterol, α-Lipoprotein *Serum Decrease Physiological* Increase by 19 mg/dL in white girl drug users vs controls *6278*

Cholesterol:HDL-Cholesterol Ratio
Serum Increase Physiological In 10 women receiving ethinyl estradiol with norgestrel *3278*
Serum No Effect Physiological In 10 women receiving ethinyl estradiol with norethindrone *3278*

Cholic Acid *Serum No Effect Physiological* No effect observed over 12 mo in 29 women given combination of ethinyl estradiol and norgestrel *2537*

Cholinesterase *Serum Decrease Physiological* Significant reduction by about 12% in drug users versus controls *3518* Significant effect observed within 3 mo usually continuing for several years *5308* Estrogen effect *5869*

Clofibrate *Serum Decrease Physiological* Oral contraceptives may increase clofibrate clearance when taken together *3668*

Clonazepam *Serum Increase Physiological* Reported to increase plasma concentration *1384*

Closure Time by Thrombostat
Plasma No Effect Physiological In 25 women taking low dose oral contraceptives mean closure of 88 ± 12 s not significantly different from 90 ± 14 s in 29 healthy controls *5199*

Clotting Time *Blood Decrease Physiological* (Silicone clotting time) associated with clot problems *1176* Nonsignificant reduction from mean of 409 to 365 seconds in whole blood clotting time, from 522 to 378 seconds (significant) in platelet-rich plasma in 14 healthy premenopausal women treated with low-dose oral contraceptives for one or two cycles *3327*

Color *Serum Increase Analytical* Concentration of ceruloplasmin may be so high blue-green color observed *5869*

Oral Contraceptives *(continued)*

Complement APH$_{50}$ *Serum No Effect Physiological* Compared with nonusers in first year of use; largely influence of progestogen *1358*

Complement C$_3$ *Serum Increase Physiological* Compared with nonusers in first year of use: largely influence of progestogen *1358*

Complement C$_4$ *Serum Increase Physiological* Compared with nonusers in first year of use: largely influence of progestogen *1358*

Complement CH50 *Serum Increase Physiological* Compared with nonusers in first year of use: largely influence of progestogen *1358*

Complement Factor B *Serum Increase Physiological* Compared with nonusers in first year of use: largely influence of progestogen *1358*

Copper *Hair No Effect Physiological* No significant effect in young women studied for at least 3 mo *6270*
Red Blood Cells No Effect Physiological In 22 women ingesting combination type contraceptives *2613*
Serum Increase Physiological In women receiving oral contraceptives concentration versus control women: at age 20 to 29 years 21.2 µmol/L versus 15.9 µmol/L, at age 30 to 39 years 25.3 µmol/L versus 15.5 µmol/L *3519* In 7 women receiving oral contraceptives mean concentration of 194 ± 22.9 µg/dL significantly higher than 105 ± 12.6 µg/dL in 22 healthy controls *5517* Significant increase observed in 17 healthy women given low-dose estrogen preparation over 24 months, but returned to initial value after discontinuation of contraception *3618* In 22 women ingesting combination type contraceptives *2613* Estrogens increase concentration of binding protein (maybe x 2) *5954* In 10 healthy women aged 20 - 29 years taking oral contraceptives mean concentration of 21.2 ± 2.8 µmol/L significantly increased compared with 15.9 ± 4.2 µmol/L in 10 healthy women aged 20 - 29 years not taking oral contraceptives *2959*
White Blood Cells No Effect Physiological In 22 women ingesting combination type contraceptives *2613*

Coproporphyrin *Blood Increase Physiological* May precipitate porphyria attack *2210*
Feces Decrease Physiological In one patient with hereditary coproporphyria mean excretion of 15450 nmol/g dry weight significantly different from reference range of 5 - 37 nmol/g dry weight but reduced to 525 nmol/g dry weight after 4 months treatment with oral contraceptives *2341*
Feces Increase Physiological May precipitate porphyria attack *2210*
Urine Decrease Physiological In one patient with hereditary coproporphyria mean excretion of 29715 nmol/d significantly different from reference range of 37 - 159 nmol/d but reduced to 204 nmol/d after 4 months treatment with oral contraceptives *2341* In one patient with acute intermittent porphyria mean excretion of 1166 nmol/d significantly different from reference range of 37 - 159 nmol/d but reduced to 362 nmol/d after 3 months treatment with oral contraceptives *2341* In 40 healthy female volunteers treatment with either 75 µg gestoden and 30 µg ethinylestradiol or 150 µg desogestrel and 30 µg ethinylestradiol caused nonsignificant decrease from 107 ± 38 nmol/d to 98 ± 39 nmol/d and from 99 ± 40 nmol/d to 86 ± 24 nmol/d respectively over 6 cycles *2341*
Urine Increase Physiological May induce porphyria cutanea tarda *5059*

Corticosteroid-Binding Globulin
Serum Increase Physiological Significant increase to mean of 89 µg/mL in 38 women given 75 µg gestodene/d and 30 µg ethinyl estradiol/d for mean of 11 months and to 93 µg/mL in 28 women given 30 µg ethinyl estradiol/d and 150 µg desogestrel/d for mean of 38 months *2774* Due to estrogenic component *128* All of seven oral contraceptive preparations caused a significant increase over 6 months with monophasic cyproterone acetate inducing a higher concentration than any other preparation *6179* Increase by 115 to 140% after 3 mo with different preparations *503* 2-fold increase observed in women taking either desogestrel/ethinyl estradiol and in those taking levonorgestrel/ethinyl estradiol *3191* Significant effect in 17 healthy women given low-dose estrogen preparation over 24 months, but effect more marked with ethinyl estradiol-desogestrel than with ethinyl estradiol-levonorgestrel *3617* Metabolic changes in liver synthesis *3604*

Corticosteroids *Plasma Increase Physiological* With increased total plasma cortisol *5913*

Corticosterone *Plasma No Effect Physiological* Inconsistent response after 4 weeks *6393*

Cortisol *Plasma Increase Analytical* Estrogens, as in oral contraceptives, may cause a clinically significant effect with method on Bayer Technicon Immuno 1® *419*
Plasma Increase Physiological Decreases cortisol clearance (estrogen effect) *5570* Early morning concentration higher than in controls and pregnant women although evening concentration similar to that observed in pregnant women *4009* On combined therapy at 9 a.m. compared with female controls and men *2737* Significant increase to mean of 281 ng/mL in 37 women treated with 75 µg/d gestodene and 30 µg/d ethinyl estradiol for mean of 11 months and to 280 ng/mL in 27 women treated with 30 µg/d ethinyl estradiol and 150 µg/d desogestrel for a mean of 38 months *2774*
Saliva Increase Physiological Significantly higher on combined therapy versus control women and men *2737* Concentration increased and peak shifted to later in the morning in oral contraceptive users *4009*
Urine Decrease Physiological When results during therapy compared with normal *444*
Urine Increase Physiological Significant hormonal effect *3591*
Urine No Effect Physiological No significant difference when referenced to creatinine in women on combined therapy versus controls *2737*

Cortisol, Free *Plasma Increase Physiological* Significant hormonal effect *3591* In 27 women using an estrogen oral contraceptive measured at 37 °C using Abbott TDx median concentration 31.6 nmol/L (range 11 to 53) and percentage of free cortisol 1.5 to 4.5% compared with 21.7 nmol/L (range 12 to 39) and percentage of free cortisol 3.7 to 9.0% in 57 healthy women aged 18 to 60 year old women *3514* Estrogen effect *887*
Urine Increase Physiological 50% increase with oral contraceptives *5402*

Cortisol, Protein Bound *Plasma Increase Physiological* When results on therapy compared with normal *444*

Cortisone *Plasma Increase Physiological* Concentration higher than in control women although less than in pregnant women. Little cyclical change observed from morning to evening *4009*
Saliva Increase Physiological Concentration higher and peak shifted until later in morning in oral contraceptive users compared with controls *4009*

C-Peptide *Plasma Increase Physiological* Generally increased by combination oral contraceptives. Typically levonorgestrel combinations had greater effect than those containing norethindrone or desogestrel *2201* Slight but statistically significant increase in healthy women volunteers over 3 treatment cycles with low-dose ethinyl estradiol-desogestrel preparation *6174*

C-Reactive Protein *Serum Decrease Physiological* Progestogen effect *5869*
Serum Increase Physiological Estrogen effect *5570*

Creatine Kinase *Serum Increase Physiological* Slight effect only (2 U/L) *4554*

Creatinine *Serum No Effect Physiological* Mean concentration in 52 pill-users 84 ± 11 µmol/L not significantly different from 83 ± 10 µmol/L in 156 healthy controls *2035* In 52 oral contraceptive pill users mean concentration of 84 ± 11 µmol/L not significantly different from 83 ± 10 µmol/L in 156 age matched controls *2035*

Creatinine Clearance *Urine Increase Physiological* In control women mean clearance 81 mL/min increased significantly to 96 mL/min in 6 women taking Minulet/Femovan, 95 mL/min in 6 taking Marvelon and 110 mL/min in 6 taking Diane *691*

Crosslaps *Urine Decrease Physiological* Mean excretion in 52 pill-users of 175 ± 91 µg/mmol creatinine significantly less than 211 ± 105 µg/mmol creatinine in 156 healthy controls *2035*

Cryofibrinogen *Plasma Increase Physiological* Incidence much higher than in controls *3923*

C-terminal Propeptide of Type I Collagen
Serum Decrease Physiological In 52 oral contraceptive pill users mean activity of 77.2 ± 23.7 ng/mL significantly different from 93.1 ± 31.9 ng/mL in 156 age matched controls *2035*

C-terminal Propeptide of Type I Procollagen
Serum Decrease Physiological Mean concentration in 52 pill-users 77.2 ± 23.7 ng/mL not significantly less than 93.1 ± 31.9 ng/mL in 156 healthy controls *2035*

Cyclosporine *Blood Increase Physiological* Coadministration of desogestrel 150 µg with ethinyl estradiol 0.03 µg with cyclosporine caused 3-fold increase in cyclosporine concentration possibly due to inhibition of the microsomal drug hydroxylating enzymes in the liver *859*
Serum Increase Physiological Two-fold increase reported in one patient with uveitis with abnormal liver and renal function tests. Also observed in other patients with a variety of oral contraceptive preparations *6596* Coadministration of desogestrel 150 µg with ethinyl estradiol 0.03 µg with cyclosporine caused 3-fold increase in cyclosporine concentration possibly due to inhibition of the microsomal drug hydroxylating enzymes in the liver *859* Possible increase to toxic concentrations in patients when oral contraceptives added to treatment regime, possibly due to inhibition of cyclosporine metabolism in the liver *1384*

Cytochrome c Oxidase *Monocytes Decrease Physiological* In 5 healthy women aged 20 - 29 years taking oral contraceptives mean concentration of 0.266 ± 0.065 U/mg protein not significantly decreased compared with 0.294 ± 0.136 U/mg protein in 6 healthy women aged 20 - 29 years not taking oral contraceptives *2959*
Platelets Increase Physiological In 9 healthy women aged 20 - 29 years taking oral contraceptives mean concentration of 2.87 ± 1.16 U/10^6 platelets not significantly increased compared with 2.36 ± 1.40 U/10^6 platelets in 9 healthy women aged 20 - 29 years not taking oral contraceptives *2959*

D-Dimer *Plasma Increase Physiological* In 20 healthy women administration of Cileste (35 µg ethinyl estradiol and 250 µg norgestimate) for 3 cycles caused significant change of concentration from mean baseline of 213 ± 88 ng/mL to 393 ± 288 ng/mL *4823* In 20 healthy women administration of Tri-Cileste (35 µg ethinyl estradiol and 180 or 250 µg norgestimate) for 3 cycles caused significant change of concentration from mean baseline of 328 ± 133 ng/mL to 584 ± 744 ng/mL *4823* In 20 healthy women administration of Triodena (30 or 40 µg ethinyl estradiol, 50, 70 or 100 µg gestodene) for 3 cycles caused significant change of concentration from mean baseline of 276 ± 130 ng/mL to 548 ± 471 ng/mL *4823*

Dehydroepiandrosterone *Plasma Decrease Physiological* Significant reduction observed in 34 women with micropolycystic ovary syndrome treated with ethinyl estradiol and desogestrel or gestodene for 6 cycles *5666*
Urine Decrease Physiological Compared with controls, but details not discussed *802*

Dehydroepiandrosterone Sulfate
Plasma Decrease Physiological In 22 patients with polycystic ovary syndrome mean concentration decreased from 8.3 ± 0.40 µmol/L to 5.9 ± 0.37 µmol/L after 6 weeks treatment *3367* Usually reduced in response to most regimes *3757* Significant reduction in 33 women receiving cycle of 35 µg ethinyl estradiol and 1 mg norethindrone for 9 cycles with reduction from about 280 µg/dL to 200 µg/dL at 3 months which remained suppressed *4180* Significant reduction observed in 34 women with micropolycystic ovary syndrome treated with ethinyl estradiol and desogestrel or gestodene for 6 cycles *5666* Time dependent reduction in women taking ethinyl estradiol with either gestodene or desogestrel with reduction from mean of about 2400 ng/mL at all stages of control cycle to 1650 ng/mL after 6 cycles with EE/G and from 2000 ng/mL to 1300 ng/mL with EE/D *2994*

Deoxycholic Acid *Serum No Effect Physiological* No effect observed over 12 mo in 29 women given combination of ethinyl estradiol and norgestrel *5789*

Dexamethasone Suppression
Patient Abnormal Physiological False positive results for dexamethasone suppression test may be observed due to increased corticosteroid binding globulin concentration in the circulation. Lack of suppression of cortisol noted in 50% of normal individuals *6538*

Diazepam *Serum Increase Physiological* Low-dose estrogen-containing prolong elimination half-life probably by inhibiting hepatic microsomal enzymes *1384* Half-life prolonged and reduced metabolic clearance associated with reduced oxidative metabolism *35*

1,25-Dihydroxy Vitamin D, Free
Serum Increase Physiological Mean concentration of 235 ± 47 fg/mL observed in 3 women taking oral contraceptives compared with 174 ± 46 fg/mL in normal women *561*

Epidermal Growth Factor *Urine Decrease Physiological* Mean concentration decreased in 5 women on low dose oral contraceptives (19.5 ± 6.0 µg/g creatinine) compared with 37.2 ± 6.0 µg/g creatinine in 8 normal menstruating women although difference not significant *2661*

Erythrocyte Sedimentation Rate
Blood Increase Physiological Associated with increased fibrinogen *5913*

Erythrocytes *Blood Decrease Physiological* In 46 oral contraceptive users compared with controls studied over at least 2 y *1951* May cause megaloblastic anemia *6370*

Estradiol *Plasma Decrease Physiological* Inhibits physiological rise *3163*
Urine Decrease Physiological Hormonal effect *3646*

Estradiol Binding Globulin *Serum Increase Physiological* Metabolic changes in liver synthesis *3604*

Estriol *Urine Decrease Physiological* Hormonal effect *3646*

Estrogen Binding Globulin *Serum Increase Physiological* Metabolic effect *3923*

Estrogens *Plasma Increase Physiological* Often related to nausea *887*
Urine Decrease Physiological Hormonal effect (decreased by 40%) *5402*

Estrone Sulfate *Plasma Decrease Physiological* In 20 women receiving oral contraceptives mean concentration of 0.74 ± 0.11 pmol/L significantly lower than 0.96 ± 0.17 pmol/L in 20 women in follicular phase and mean concentration of 1.74 ± 0.32 µg/L in 20 women during luteal phase *4849*

Ethinyl Estradiol *Serum Increase Physiological* Mean increase to 106-129 pg/mL in 37 women taking 30 µg/d ethinyl estradiol with 75 µg/d gestodene for mean of 11 mo and in 27 women taking 30 µg/d ethinyl estradiol with 150 µg/d desogestrel for mean of 38 mo. Peak at 1.6-1.8 h after pill ingestion *2774*

Etiocholanolone *Urine Decrease Physiological* Compared with controls, but details not discussed *802*

Expiratory Volume *Patient No Effect Physiological* No significant effect observed *1955*

Factor I *Plasma No Effect Physiological* Usually no effect observed *547*

Factor II *Plasma Increase Physiological* Reported effect of estrogens *666*

Factor V *Plasma Increase Physiological* Significant effect of combined oral contraceptives *4063*
Plasma No Effect Physiological Usually no effect observed *547*

Factor VII *Plasma Decrease Physiological* Metabolic effect *4737*
Plasma Increase Physiological In patients receiving 20 µg ethinyl estradiol and 150 µg desogestrel mean concentration changed over 12 months from 80% to 126% and in those receiving 30 µg ethinyl estradiol and 75 µg gestodene mean concentration changed from 87% to 137% over 12 months *5214* Estrogen effect (higher than in pregnancy) *5570*

Factor VII Antigen *Plasma Increase Physiological* In 20 healthy women administration of Triodena (30 or 40 µg ethinyl estradiol, 50, 70 or 100 µg gestodene) for 3 cycles caused significant change of concentration from mean baseline of 112 ± 25% to 156 ± 16% *4823* In 20 healthy women administration of Tri-Cileste (35 µg ethinyl estradiol and 180 or 250 µg norgestimate) for 3 cycles caused significant change of concentration from mean baseline of 95 ± 27% to 123 ± 44% *4823* In 20 healthy women administration of Cileste (35 µg ethinyl estradiol and 250 µg norgestimate) for 3 cycles caused significant change of activity from mean baseline of 92 ± 12% to 138 ± 29% *4823*

Factor VII Clotting Assay *Plasma Increase Physiological* In 20 healthy women administration of Tri-Cileste (35 µg ethinyl estradiol and 180 or 250 µg norgestimate) for 3 cycles caused significant change of concentration from mean baseline of 101 ± 34% to 117 ± 32% *4823* In 20 healthy women administration of Cileste (35 µg ethinyl estradiol and 250 µg norgestimate) for 3 cycles caused significant change of activity from

Oral Contraceptives *(continued)*

Factor VII Clotting Assay *(continued)*
mean baseline of 96 ± 20% to 137 ± 31% *4823* In 20 healthy women administration of Triodena (30 or 40 µg ethinyl estradiol, 50, 70 or 100 µg gestodene) for 3 cycles caused significant change of concentration from mean baseline of 114 ± 42% to 201 ± 192% *4823*

Factor VIII *Plasma Increase Physiological* Slight effect observed *2414*

Factor IX *Plasma Increase Physiological* Estrogen effect *5570*

Factor X *Plasma Decrease Physiological* Metabolic effect *4737*
Plasma Increase Physiological Slight effect observed *2414*

Factor XII *Plasma Increase Physiological* Reported effect *3923*

Fatty Acids (FFA), Free *Serum Increase Physiological* If given for 3 mo *5869*
Serum No Effect Physiological Mean concentration of 0.86 mmol/L in 22 women with IDDM during treatment with 30 µg ethinyl estradiol and 75 µg gestodene not significantly different from 0.88 mmol/L before treatment started *4633*

Ferritin *Serum Increase Physiological* Mean of 40 ng/mL vs 25 ng/mL in control population followed for at least 2 y *1951*
Serum No Effect Physiological Smaller proportion of contraceptive users had low values than controls *2275*

Fibrinogen *Plasma Decrease Physiological* When combined estrogen and progestogen *4014*
Plasma Increase Physiological In 20 healthy women administration of Tri-Cileste (35 µg ethinyl estradiol and 180 or 250 µg norgestimate) for 3 cycles caused significant change of concentration from mean baseline of 278 ± 58 ng/mL to 296 ± 55 mg/dL *4823* In 20 healthy women administration of Triodena (30 or 40 µg ethinyl estradiol, 50, 70 or 100 µg gestodene) for 3 cycles caused significant change of concentration from mean baseline of 256 ± 48 mg/dL to 300 ± 60 mg/dL *4823* Increase observed in young women *5546* In 20 healthy women administration of Cileste (35 µg ethinyl estradiol and 250 µg norgestimate) for 3 cycles caused significant change from mean baseline of 260 ± 26 mg/dL to 283 ± 36 mg/dL *4823* Insignificant increase in 14 premenopausal women from mean of 249 to 279 mg/dL when low-dose oral contraceptives given for one or two cycles *3327* Mean concentration in women younger than 30 years taking oral contraceptives 17 mg/dL higher than in those not taking oral contraceptives *1903* In patients receiving 20 µg ethinyl estradiol and 150 µg desogestrel mean concentration changed over 12 months from 7.2 µmol/L to 8.7 µmol/L and in those receiving 30 µg ethinyl estradiol and 75 µg gestodene mean concentration changed from 7.7 µmol/L to 8.4 µmol/L over 12 months *5214* Metabolic changes in liver synthesis (estrogen) *3604*

Fibrinogen Degradation Products
Plasma No Effect Physiological In patients receiving 20 µg ethinyl estradiol and 150 µg desogestrel mean concentration changed over 12 months from 0.18 µg/mL to 0.15 µg/mL and in those receiving 30 µg ethinyl estradiol and 75 µg gestodene mean concentration changed from 0.16 µg/mL to 0.15 µg/mL over 12 months *5214*

Folate *Red Blood Cells Decrease Physiological* Mild effect in oral contraceptive users *5534* Impaired metabolism due to hormonal factors *5535*
Red Blood Cells No Effect Physiological A monophasic sub-50 oral contraceptive (Marvelon) administered to 26 healthy women during both the high and low-hormonal phase of their cycle had no significant effect on concentration compared with 15 control women *5780*
Serum Decrease Physiological Interferes with gastrointestinal absorption *6416* Mild effect in oral contraceptive users *5534* Greater proportion of contraceptive users had low values than controls *2275*
Serum No Effect Physiological A monophasic sub-50 oral contraceptive (Marvelon) administered to 26 healthy women during both the high and low-hormonal phase of their cycle had no significant effect on concentration compared with 15 control women *5780*

Follicle Stimulating Hormone
Plasma Decrease Physiological Over years depressed to 70% of control values *2231* Significant reduction in 33 women receiving 35 µg ethinyl estradiol and 1 mg norethindrone starting within days 1-5 of each cycle for 9 cycles with maximum decrease of 61% at 3 months *4180*
Urine Decrease Physiological Marked depression in normal subjects *5817*

Gastrin *Serum No Effect Physiological* No significant effect observed with treatment with low-dose oral contraceptives *5554*

α_1-Globulin *Serum Increase Physiological* Metabolic change with combined contraceptive *3809*
Serum No Effect Physiological No significant effect at 3 mo cessation or 3 y *5249*

α_2-Globulin *Serum Increase Physiological* After 3 y, not after 3 mo cessation *5249* May be increased by as much as 8 times *887*

β-Globulin *Serum Increase Physiological* After 3 y but not after 3 mo cessation *5249* Metabolic changes in liver synthesis *5454*

γ-Globulin *Serum Increase Physiological* After 3 y, not after 3 mo cessation *5249*

Glucaric Acid *Urine Increase Physiological* Reported induction of hepatic enzymes *2782*

Glucocorticoids *Plasma Increase Physiological* Expected effect observed *1261*

Glucose *Serum Decrease Physiological* Concentration generally lower in low-dose monophasic levonorgestrel and triphasic norethindrone combinations (about 4.7 mmol/L) versus about 4.8 mmol/L in nonuser controls *2201* Estrogen effect of combined oral contraceptive *50* Significantly lower in drug users *2046*
Serum Increase Physiological Three different types of triphasic oral contraceptives produced statistically but not clinically significant increases in a population of 130 women *675* Mean concentration of 11.6 mmol/L in 22 women with IDDM during treatment with 30 µg ethinyl estradiol and 75 µg gestodene higher than 9.9 mmol/L before treatment started *4633* Does not affect fasting glucose but alters glucose tolerance test *5869*
Serum No Effect Physiological No significant effect in healthy women volunteers over 3 treatment cycles with low-dose ethinyl estradiol-desogestrel *6174*

Glucose Tolerance *Serum Decrease Physiological* Glucose higher by 11 mg/dL at 1 h in drug users *2046* Slight but significant effect observed over 3 treatment cycles in women volunteers with low-dose ethinyl estradiol-desogestrel *6174* Mainly estrogen effect (reversible in 3 out 4) *2414* Observed in 925 women receiving a variety of different monophasic and triphasic preparations but greatest effect observed with formulations containing levonorgestrel *2202* Significant increase observed in 29 women given ethinyl estradiol and levonorgestrel over 3 month study period *5741*
Serum No Effect Physiological Estrogen effect of combined oral contraceptive *50* No significant effect in 130 women receiving 3 different types of triphasic preparations *675*

Glucuronic Acid *Urine Increase Physiological* Extent of effect varies with exact composition of oral contraceptive *2410*

β-Glucuronidase *Serum Increase Physiological* Altered metabolism (estrogen effect) *368* Significant effect observed within 3 mo usually continuing for several years *5308*

Glutamate Dehydrogenase *Serum Increase Physiological* Significant effect observed within 3 mo usually continuing for several years *5308*

Glutamic Acid *Plasma Decrease Physiological* Hormonal effect (second part of cycle) *1154*

γ-Glutamyltransferase *Serum Increase Physiological* Extent of effect varies with exact composition of oral contraceptive *2410* Positive association between activity and oral contraceptive use (average 28% Increase) *242* But effects less marked with low estrogen preparations *2564* Significant effect observed within 3 mo usually continuing for several years *5308*

Glutathione *Blood Decrease Physiological* Nonsignificant difference observed between mean concentrations in 27 individuals who ingested oral contraceptives (871 ± 152 µmol/L) and 51 nonusers (935 ± 150 µmol/L) *4020*

Glutathione, Reduced *Blood Decrease Physiological* Nonsignificant difference observed between mean concentrations in 27 individuals who ingested oral contraceptives (794 ± 125 µmol/L) and 51 nonusers (843 ± 167 µmol/L) *4020*

Glutathione Reductase
Red Blood Cells Decrease Physiological Manifestation of poor riboflavin status in women of low socioeconomic status *5056*

Glycated Protein *Serum No Effect Physiological* No effect even after 15 treatment cycles with desogestrel/ethinyl estradiol preparation in 25 fertile women *6089* No significant effect over 3 treatment cycles in healthy women volunteers with low-dose ethinyl estradiol-desogestrel *6174*

Glycine *Plasma Decrease Physiological* Hormonal effect (second part of cycle) *1154*

Gonadotropins *Urine Decrease Physiological* Hormonal effect *3646*

Growth Hormone *Plasma Increase Physiological* During first year of use (may be increased 3 fold) *128*
Plasma No Effect Physiological No overall effect observed on concentration in 9 healthy young women receiving a combination of 30 µg ethinyl estradiol and 150 µg levonorgestrel for 3 months although mean peak amplitude, mean peak areaand mean interpeak interval decreased *3049*

Guanosine Monophosphate *Urine No Effect Physiological* No significant effect of oral contraceptives observed on mean excretion *6103*

Haptoglobin *Serum Decrease Physiological* Metabolic changes in liver synthesis (estrogen) *3604*

HDL$_2$-Cholesterol *Serum Decrease Physiological* High dose monophasic norethindrone (1000 µg) with 35 µg estrogen combination lowered HDL$_2$-cholesterol concentration by 27% *2201* High dose monophasic norethindrone (1000 ug) with 35 µg estrogen combination lowered HDL$_2$-cholesterol concentration by 27% *2201* Decrease by 29-33% after 6 months in 150 women receiving three different triphasic contraceptive regimes *4560* Reduction from mean of 25 mg/dL to 18 mg/dL with 10 cyles of triphasic preparation in 20 women *3689* Triphasic levonorgestrel combination (50-125 µg progestin with 30-40 µg estrogen) reduced concentration by 15% and triphasic norethindrone combination (500-1000 µg progestin with 35 µg estrogen) reduced concentration by 8% *2201* Decrease greater than that of HDL-cholesterol in women taking either ethinyl estradiol/norgestrel or ethinyl estradiol/norethindrone over 12 months *4333*
Serum Increase Physiological 15% increase after one cycle then subsequent decline by third cycle and no change from baseline after 6 and 12 cycles in 11 women taking 30 µg ethinyl estradiol with 75 µg gestodene for 12 cycles *3317*
Serum No Effect Physiological Monophasic desogestrel combination (150 µg progestin with 30 µg estrogen) had no effect on concentrations *2201* Low dose monophasic combination (500 µg norethindrone plus 35 µg estrogen) had no effect *2201* No significant change observed in 11 women taking 30 µg ethinyl estradiol with 150 µg desogestrel for 12 cycles *3317* In 19 healthy women treated for 6 cycles with biphasic oral contraceptive containing ethinyl estradiol and desogestrel mean concentration increased nonsignificantly from mean baseline of 22.0 ± 8.1 mg/dL to 25.1 ± 7.3 mg/dL *3316* Mean concentration of 0.64 mmol/L at baseline in 22 women with IDDM changed nonsignificantly to 0.67 mmol/L after 1 month, 0.59 mmol/L after 3 months, 0.67 mmol/L after 6 months and 0.50 mmol/L after 12 months during treatment with 30 µg ethinyl estradiol and 75 µg gestodene *4633* No significant change observed in 58 women randomized into 3 groups of either monophasic ethinyl estradiol with desogestrel, ethinyl estradiol with gestodene, or triphasic ethinyl estradiol with levonorgestrel *376*

HDL$_2$-Phospholipids *Serum Increase Physiological* Significant increase of 20% observed after one cycle but thereafter increase, if any, not significant in 11 women taking 30 µg ethinyl estradiol with 75 µg gestodene for 12 cycles *3317* Slight significant increase of about 10% after 6 cycles but not before or after in 11 women taking 30 µg ethinyl estradiol with 150 µg desogestrel for 12 cycles *3317*

HDL$_{2a}$-Cholesterol *Serum No Effect Physiological* In 10 women receiving ethinyl estradiol with norethindrone. In 10 women receiving ethinyl estradiol with norgestrel *3278*

HDL$_{2b}$-Cholesterol *Serum Decrease Physiological* In 10 women receiving ethinyl estradiol with norethindrone *3278*
Serum Increase Physiological In 10 women receiving ethinyl estradiol with norethindrone *3278*

HDL$_3$-Cholesterol *Serum Increase Physiological* Concentrations increased by all combination oral contraceptives except high dose monophasic levonorgestrel combination (250 µg progestin with 30 µg estrogen) *2201* Significant increase of 15% after 3 cycles, 12% after 6 cycles, and 12% after 12 cycles in 11 women taking 30 µg ethinyl estradiol with 150 µg desogestrel *3317* In 10 women receiving ethinyl estradiol with norethindrone *3278* Significant increase over 12 months in women taking either ethinyl estradiol/norgestrel or ethinyl estradiol/norethindrone but did not exceed clinically acceptable limits *4333* In 11 women taking 30 µg ethinyl estradiol with 75 µg gestodene significant increase (about 12%) after 3 cycles, 15% after 6 cycles and 5% after 12 cycles *3317* Increase by 20-23% in 150 women after 6 months on 3 different triphasic contraceptive regimes *4560* Increase from mean of 28 mg/dL to 35 mg/dL in 20 women after 10 cycles when receiving triphasic preparation *3689* Mean concentration of 0.75 mmol/L at baseline in 22 women with IDDM changed significantly to 0.80 mmol/L after 1 month, 0.86 mmol/L after 3 months, 0.88 mmol/L after 6 months and 1.00 mmol/L after 12 months during treatment with 30 µg ethinyl estradiol and 75 µg gestodene *4633*
Serum No Effect Physiological In 19 healthy women treated for 6 cycles with a biphasic contraceptive containing ethinyl estradiol and desogestrel mean concentration increased nonsignificantly from mean baseline of 37.2 ± 4.5 mg/dL to 40.3 ± 9.3 mg/dL *3316* In 10 women receiving ethinyl estradiol with norgestrel *3278*

HDL$_3$-Phospholipids *Serum Increase Physiological* In 11 women taking 30 µg ethinyl estradiol with 75 µg gestodene significant increase of 10% observed after 3 cycles, and 15% after 6 cycles when followed for 12 cycles *3317* In 11 women taking 30 µg ethinyl estradiol with 150 µg desogestrel significant increase of 15% after 3 cycles, 12% after 6 cycles and 8% after 12 cycles *3317*

HDL-Cholesterol *Serum Decrease Physiological* Slight but not significant decrease observed over 6 months in 18 healthy young women receiving low-dose ethinyl estradiol with levonorgestrel *2489* If oral contraceptive contains more than 50 µg estrogen *50* Significant decrease observed in women taking either ethinyl estradiol/norgestrel or ethinyl estradiol/norethindrone over 12 months *4333* Observed with monophasic preparations containing levonorgestrel *2202* Depending on preparation used *4768* In women taking estrogen/high or low progestin combination *6295* Slight reduction after 6 months in patients taking 30 µg ethinyl estradiol (EE) + 0.15 mg levonorgestrel, 35 µg EE + 1 mg norethindrone and 35 µg EE + 0.5 and 1 mg norethindrone but slight increase with 35 µg EE + 1 mg ethynodiol *816* Monophasic, but not triphasic, levonorgestrel combinations reduced concentrations (1.73 mmol/L in controls, 1.46 mmol/L in women taking 250 µg levonorgestrel and 30 µg estrogen) *2201* Levonorgestrel combinations lowered concentration by 15 to 43% with the highest dose inducing the greatest decrease *2201* Increase by 20% with high dose compound containing 500 µg norgestrel *2046*
Serum Increase Physiological Increased concentration observed in patients taking gestodene with ethinyl estradiol *2143* Increase by 35% with high-dose oral contraceptives that are overly estrogenic *2046* If oral contraceptive contains more than 80 µg estrogen *50* Significant increase from baseline of 67 mg/dL to 73 mg/dL at 3 months, 70 mg/dL at 6 months and 71 mg/dL at 9 months with 35 µg ethinyl estradiol and 0.5 mg norethindrone whereas no significant change with other combinations of same drugs *817* Observed with monophasic preparations containing 500 µg norethindrone or 150 µg desogestrel but not affected by other progestins *2202* With low-dose ethinyl estradiol transient increase of 24% after 3 months use but normal concentration after 6 months in 18 healthy young women *2489* In women taking high estrogen/Low progestin combination *6295* Low dose monophasic norethindrone (500 µg) with 35 µg estrogen as well as desogestrel (150 µg) with 30 µg estrogen increased concentration to means of 1.90 mmol/L and 1.94 mmol/L respectively compared with 1.73 mmol/L in controls *2201* In 10 women receiving ethinyl estradiol with norethindrone *3278* Small but significant increase in 25 women treated with up to 15 cycles of desogestrel/ethinyl estradiol preparation *6089* In 58 healthy women receiving for 3 months ethinyl estradiol with either desogestrel. gestodene or levonorgestrel actual increase or tendency to increase observed *5794* Depending on preparation used. Increase by 17 to 81% depending on preparation used *4768*

Oral Contraceptives *(continued)*

HDL-Cholesterol *(continued)*
In 19 healthy women treated for 6 cycles with biphasic oral contraceptive containing ethinyl estradiol and desogestrel mean concentration increased significantly from mean baseline of 59.2 ± 10.9 mg/dL to 65.4 ± 7.5 mg/dL *3316* Mean concentration of 1.36 mmol/L at baseline in 22 women with IDDM changed nonsignificantly to 1.43 mmol/L after 1 month, 1.47 mmol/L after 3 months, 1.47 mmol/L after 6 months and 1.52 mmol/L after 12 months during treatment with 30 µg ethinyl estradiol and 75 µg gestodene *4633* In 11 women taking 30 µg ethinyl estradiol with 75 µg gestodene significant increase of about 10% observes after 6 cycles and 5% after 12 cycles *3317* In 11 women taking 30 µg ethinyl estradiol with 150 µg desogestrel significant increase observed of about 5% after 3 cycles, 10% after 6 cycles and 15% after 12 cycles *3317* Significant increase of about 20% observed in 60 nonpregnant women taking either of 2 low-dose regimes *3797*
Serum No Effect Physiological Insignificant reduction of from 2 to 4% after 6 months in 150 women receiving three different triphasic regimes *4560* In 16 healthy young women with normal menstrual cycles treatment with a combination of 30 µg ethinyl estradiol and 150 µg 3-keto-desogestrel caused a nonsignificant change from mean baseline of 60.3 ± 11.0 mg/dL to 57.5 ± 12.1 mg/dL on day 3 of the first cycle *3315* In 16 healthy young women with normal menstrual cycles treatment with a combination of 30 µg ethinyl estradiol and 150 µg desogestrel caused a nonsignificant change from mean baseline of 60.3 ± 11.0 mg/dL to 66.7 ± 14.6 mg/dL on day 21 of the third cycle *3315* In 16 healthy young women with normal menstrual cycles treatment with a combination of 30 µg ethinyl estradiol and 150 µg 3-keto-desogestrel caused a nonsignificant change from mean baseline of 60.3 ± 11.0 mg/dL to 61.4± 7.4 mg/dL on day 21 of the third cycle *3315* No change with 10 treatment cycles in 20 women *3689* In 16 healthy young women with normal menstrual cycles treatment with a combination of 30 µg ethinyl estradiol and 150 µg desogestrel caused a nonsignificant change from mean baseline of 60.3 ± 11.0 mg/dL to 54.7 ± 9.1 mg/dL on day 3 of the first cycle *3315* In 9 desogestrel users mean concentration of 1.66 ± 0.34 mmol/L and 1.66 ± 0.39 mmol/L in 9 levonorgestrel users not significantly different from 1.57 ± 0.38 mmol/L in 41 healthy controls *1309* No significant effect in 10 women after 3 treatment cycles with desogestrel/ethinyl estradiol preparation *3190* No significant correlation observed between oral contraceptive use and HDL-cholesterol concentration *2399* Triphasic preparations containing 50-125 µg levonorgestrel or 500-1000 µg norethindrone had no effect on HDL-cholesterol concentration *2202* Triphasic norethindrone (500-1000 ug) with 35 µg estrogen had no effect on concentration *2201* Triphasic norethindrone (500-1000 µg) with 35 µg estrogen had no effect on concentration *2201* No effect of monophasic high dose (1000 ug) norethindrone plus 35 µg estrogen *2201* No effect of monophasic high dose (1000 µg) norethindrone plus 35 µg estrogen *2201* No difference between treated women and others *2184* Insignificant increase from mean baseline of 1.32 mmol/L to 1.49 mmol/L in 29 women after treatment for 12 cycles with ethinyl estradiol/gestodene and from 1.38 mmol/L to 1.48 mmol/L in 26 women treated with ethinyl estradiol/desogestrel for 12 cycles *2099* In 10 women receiving ethinyl estradiol with norgestrel *3278* With high dose drugs containing norethisterone or ethynodiol *2046* Typically insignificant change over 6 cycles in women with low dose ethinyl estradiol with low dose levonorgestrel or desogestrel *2047*

HDL-Cholesterol:Cholesterol Ratio
Serum No Effect Physiological Mean ratio of 0.31 at baseline in 22 women with IDDM changed nonsignificantly to 0.33 after 1 month, 0.33 after 3 months, 0.33 after 6 months and 0.34 after 12 months during treatment with 30 µg ethinyl estradiol and 75 µg gestodene *4633*

HDL-Phospholipids *Serum Increase Physiological* In 11 women taking 30 µg ethinyl estradiol with 150 µg desogestrel significant increase of about 15% observed after 3, 6 and 12 cycles *3317* Significant increase of 5% after 3 cycles and 12% after 6 cycles in 11 women taking 30 µg ethinyl estradiol with 75 µg gestodene for 12 cycles *3317*

HDL-Triglycerides *Serum Increase Physiological* In 11 women taking 30 µg ethinyl estradiol with 150 µg desogestrel significant increase observed (75% after one cycle, 55% after 3 cycles, 65% after 6 cycles, and 85% after 12 cycles) *3317* In 11 women taking 30 µg ethinyl estradiol with 75 µg gestodene significant increase observed (65% after one cycle, 85% after 3 cycles, 75% after 6 cycles and 115% after 12 cycles) *3317* In 16 healthy young women with normal menstrual cycles treatment with a combination of 30 µg ethinyl estradiol and 150 µg desogestrel caused a significant change from mean baseline of 12.4 ± 3.6 mg/dL to 19.9 ± 6.0 mg/dL on day 21 of the third cycle *3315* In 16 healthy young women with normal menstrual cycles treatment with a combination of 30 µg ethinyl estradiol and 150 µg 3-keto-desogestrel caused a significant change from mean baseline of 12.4 ± 3.6 mg/dL to 22.7± 5.8 mg/dL on day 21 of the third cycle *3315* Increase by 17 to 81% depending on preparation used *4768* In 19 healthy women treated for 6 cycles with biphasic oral contraceptive containing ethinyl estradiol and desogestrel concentration increased significantly from mean baseline of 11.6 ± 2.5 mg/dL to 20.7 ± 6.4 mg/dL *3316*
Serum No Effect Physiological In 16 healthy young women with normal menstrual cycles treatment with a combination of 30 µg ethinyl estradiol and 150 µg desogestrel caused a nonsignificant change from mean baseline of 12.4 ± 3.6 mg/dL to 14.5 ± 5.4 mg/dL on day 3 of the first cycle *3315* In 16 healthy young women with normal menstrual cycles treatment with a combination of 30 µg ethinyl estradiol and 150 µg 3-keto-desogestrel caused a nonsignificant change from mean baseline of 12.4 ± 3.6 mg/dL to 13.4 ± 4.5 mg/dL on day 3 of the first cycle *3315*

Hematocrit *Blood Decrease Physiological* May cause megaloblastic anemia *5054* In 46 oral contraceptive users compared with controls studied over at least 2 y *1951*
Blood Increase Physiological Probably progestogen effect *5954*
Blood No Effect Physiological No significant difference between oral contraceptive users and control adolescents *2275* No significant effect in oral contraceptive users *5534*

Hemoglobin *Blood Decrease Physiological* May cause megaloblastic anemia *5054*
Blood Increase Physiological Increase after 12 mo with low base combined pill regime *4974*
Blood No Effect Physiological In 46 oral contraceptive users compared with controls studied over at least 2 y *1951* No significant difference between oral contraceptive users and control adolescents *2275* No significant effect in oral contraceptive users *5534*

Hemoglobin A_{1c} *Blood No Effect Physiological* Mean concentration of 8.4% in 22 women with IDDM during treatment with 30 µg ethinyl estradiol and 75 µg gestodene not significantly different from 8.2% before treatment started *4633*

High Density Lipoproteins *Serum Increase Physiological* In 10 women receiving ethinyl estradiol with norethindrone *3278*
Serum No Effect Physiological In 10 women receiving ethinyl estradiol with norgestrel *3278*

Histidine-rich Glycoprotein *Serum Decrease Physiological* In patients receiving 20 µg ethinyl estradiol and 150 µg desogestrel mean concentration changed over 12 months from 98% to 82% and in those receiving 30 µg ethinyl estradiol and 75 µg gestodene mean concentration changed from 112% to 74% over 12 months *5214*

Homocysteine *Plasma Increase Physiological* A monophasic sub-50 oral contraceptive (Marvelon) administered to 26 healthy women during the low-hormonal phase of their cycle caused median concentration to increase to 11.0 µmol/L significantly higher than 6.6 µmol/L in 15 control women *5780*
Plasma No Effect Physiological A monophasic sub-50 oral contraceptive (Marvelon) administered to 26 healthy women during the high-hormonal phase of their cycle had no effect on median concentration of 7.8 µmol/L compared with 6.4 µmol/L in 15 control women *5780*

25-Hydroxy Vitamin D *Serum Increase Physiological* In 52 oral contraceptive pill users mean concentration of 101 ± 36 nmol/L significantly different from 91 ± 40 nmol/L in 156 age matched controls *2035*

3-Hydroxyanthranilic Acid *Urine Increase Physiological* After 2 g tryptophan load *5089* Estrogen component induces tryptophan pyrrolase *5085*

17-Hydroxycorticosteroids *Urine Decrease Physiological* Probably due to estrogen decreasing cortisol secretion *4288*

6-β-Hydroxycortisol *Urine* *Increase* *Physiological* Mean excretion in women receiving oral contraceptives 34.1 ± 27.7 μg/h compared with 24.8 ± 19.7 μg/h in control women *2016*

3-Hydroxykynurenine *Urine* *Increase* *Physiological* After 2 g tryptophan load *5089* Estrogen component induces tryptophan pyrrolase *5085*

17-Hydroxyprogesterone *Plasma* *Decrease* *Physiological* Significant reduction observed in 34 women with micropolycystic ovary syndrome treated with ethinyl estradiol and desogestrel or gestodene for 6 cycles *5666*

3-Hydroxyxanthurenic Acid *Urine* *Increase* *Physiological* After 2 g tryptophan load *5089*

^{131}I Uptake *Serum* *No Effect* *Physiological* Thyroid function unaffected *128*

IDL-Cholesterol *Serum* *No Effect* *Physiological* In 10 women receiving ethinyl estradiol with norethindrone. In 10 women receiving ethinyl estradiol with norgestrel *3278* In 19 healthy women treated for 6 cycles with biphasic contraceptive containing ethinylestradiol and desogestrel mean concentration increased nonsignificantly from baseline of about 4.6 mg/dL to about 6.2 mg/dL *3316*

IDL-Triglycerides *Serum* *Increase* *Physiological* In 19 healthy women treated for 6 cycles with biphasic oral contraceptive containing ethinyl estradiol and desogestrel mean concentration increased significantly from baseline of 4.9 ± 3.7 mg/dL to 10.5 ± 5.2 mg/dL *3316*

Imidazolepyruvic Acid *Urine* *Increase* *Physiological* Mechanism not yet established *6194*

Imipramine *Serum* *Increase* *Physiological* Increased bioavailability probably due to inhibition of oxidation in the liver *1384*

immunoglobulin A *Serum* *Decrease* *Physiological* Estrogen effect *5869*

Immunoglobulins *Serum* *Decrease* *Physiological* Estrogen effect *5570*
Serum *Increase* *Physiological* Metabolic changes in liver synthesis *3604*

Insulin *Plasma* *Increase* *Physiological* Fasting concentration generally higher in users of combination oral contraceptive users compared with nonuser controls. Levonorgestrel combinations had greater effect than those containing norethindrone or desogestrel *2201* Significant increase in mean concentration in 130 women at 3 months, but not at 6 months, in 130 women receiving 3 different types of triphasic preparations *675* In women in whom insulin was initially normal *5740* Concentration increased with low-dose oral contraceptives *5554*
Plasma *No Effect* *Physiological* No significant effect in healthy women volunteers over 3 treatment cycles with low-dose ethinyl estradiol-desogestrel combination *6174* No significant effect in response to glucose challenge in 29 women given ethinyl estradiol and levonorgestrel combination for 3 months *5741*

Insulin-like Growth Factor-I *Serum* *Decrease* *Physiological* In 7 women with polycystic disease of the ovaries treated with oral contraceptives mean concentration decreased from baseline of 326 μg/L to 199 μg/L *5858*
Serum *No Effect* *Physiological* No change observed in 5 healthy women treated with oral contraceptives for 3 months (baseline mean concentration 235 μg/L, after oral contraceptives 226 μg/L) *5858*

Insulin-like Growth Factor Binding Protein-1
Serum *Increase* *Physiological* In 7 women with polycystic ovaries disease treatment with oral contraceptives for 3 months caused increase from mean baseline of 24 μg/L to 73 μg/L *5858*
Serum *No Effect* *Physiological* Insignificant increase from mean baseline of 44 μg/L to 61 μg/L observed in 5 healthy women treated with oral contraceptives for 3 months *5858*

Iodine *Serum* *Increase* *Physiological* Altered metabolism increases plasma total iodine concentration *2414*

Iron *Serum* *Increase* *Physiological* Increase after 12 mo with low base combined pill regime *4974* Increase in available binding protein (plus 20% increase) *5954* In 46 oral contraceptive users compared with controls studied over at least 2 y *1951*
Serum *No Effect* *Physiological* No significant change observed in 17 healthy women given low-dose estrogen preparations over 24 months *3618*

Iron-Binding Capacity, Total *Serum* *Increase* *Physiological* In 46 oral contraceptive users compared with controls studied over at least 2 y *1951* May increase TIBC to 90 μmol/L from typical reference range of 50 - 70 μmol/L *5510* Estrogen or progestogen effect (usually plus 20%) *5954*

Isoleucine *Plasma* *Decrease* *Physiological* Hormonal effect (second part of cycle) *1154*

Kaolin-Cephalin Time *Blood* *Decrease* *Physiological* Metabolic effect *4737*

17-Ketogenic Steroids *Urine* *Decrease* *Physiological* Probably due to estrogen decreasing cortisol secretion *4288*

17-Ketosteroids *Urine* *Decrease* *Physiological* Probable decrease in cortisol secretion *4288*

Kynurenine *Urine* *Increase* *Physiological* Estrogen component induces tryptophan pyrrolase *5085*

Lactate *Plasma* *Increase* *Physiological* Alteration in carbohydrate metabolism *3923*

Lactate Dehydrogenase *Serum* *No Effect* *Physiological* No significant effect observed *5548*

LDL+HDL-Triglycerides *Serum* *Increase* *Physiological* Increase from mean of 20 mg/dL at baseline to 35 mg/dL after 1 cycle and 37 mg/dL after 10 cycles in 20 women taking triphasic preparation *3689*

LDL_1-Cholesterol *Serum* *Decrease* *Physiological* In 20 desogestrel or levonorgestrel users mean proportion of 27 ± 8% significantly less than 34 ± 10% in 41 healthy controls *1309*

LDL_2-Cholesterol *Serum* *No Effect* *Physiological* Mean proportion of 41 ± 5% in 20 oral contraceptive users not significantly different from 40 ± 9% in 41 healthy controls *1309*

LDL_3-Lipoprotein *Serum* *Increase* *Physiological* In 20 desogestrel and levonorgestrel users mean proportion of 32 ± 8% significantly higher than 26 ± 13% in 41 healthy controls *1309*

LDL-Apolipoprotein B *Serum* *Increase* *Physiological* Substantial increase in women taking for 6 months either 35 μg ethinyl estradiol (EE) + 1 mg ethynodiol, 30 μg EE + 0.15 levonorgestrel, and 35 μg EE + 0.5 and 1 mg norethindrone, but no change in those taking 30 μg EE + 1 mg norethindrone *816* Marked increase (typically by 20 mg/dL) after 6 months in women taking 30 μg ethinyl estradiol (EE) + 1 mg ethynodiol, 30 μg EE + 0.15 mg levonorgestrel, 35 mg EE + 1 mg norethindrone, and 35 μg EE + 0.5 and 1 mg norethindrone *816* Increase from mean baseline of 86 mg/dL to 110 mg/dL at 3 and 6 months and 107 mg/dL at 9 months in women taking 50 μg ethinyl estradiol and 1.0 mg norethindrone and similar changes on other combinations of same drugs *817* Increase from mean baseline of 79 mg/dL to 92 mg/dL after 1 month and 100 mg/dL after 10 cycles in 20 women taking triphasic preparation *3689*
Serum *No Effect* *Physiological* In 9 desogestrel users mean concentration of 1.28 ± 0.27 mmol/L and 1.16 ± 0.21 mmol/L not significantly different from 1.10 ± 0.24 mmol/L in 41 healthy controls *1309*

LDL-Cholesterol *Serum* *Decrease* *Physiological* In 11 women taking 30 μg ethinyl estradiol and 75 μg gestodene significant reduction (8%) and in 11 taking 30 μg ethinyl estradiol with 150 μg desogestrel 15% reduction after one cycle: thereafter concentrations reverted to normal *3317* Slight reduction observed in 60 nonpregnant women over 3 cycles taking either of 2 low-dose regimes *3797* Monophasic contraceptives containing 500 μg norethindrone or 150 μg desogestrel decreased LDL-cholesterol which was not affected by other progestins *2202* Reduced by 14% in users of monophasic desogestrel combination (150 μg progestin and 30 μg estrogen) and by 12% in low-dose norethindrone (500 ug) plus 35 μg estrogen users *2201* Mean concentration of 3.16 mmol/L at baseline in 22 women with IDDM changed significantly to 2.56 mmol/L after 1 month, 2.55 mmol/L after 3 months, 2.55 mmol/L after 6 months and 2.46 mmol/L after 12 months during treatment with 30 μg ethinyl estradiol and 75 μg gestodene *4633* Reduced by 14% in users of monophasic desogestrel combination (150 μg progestin and 30 μg estrogen) and by 12% in low-dose norethindrone (500 μg) plus 35 μg estrogen users *2201*
Serum *Increase* *Physiological* Mainly estrogen response *5913* 24% higher median concentration using combination with relatively low estrogen and medium or high progestin *6295*

Oral Contraceptives *(continued)*

LDL-Cholesterol *(continued)*
Significant increase observed at 6 months observed in women taking 35 μg ethinyl estradiol (EE) + 1 mg ethynodiol, 30 μg EE + 0.15 mg levonorgestrel, 35 μg EE + 1 mg norethindrone, and 35 μg EE + 0.5 and 1 mg norethindrone *816* Increase of 24% when high progestogen compounds ingested *2046* Increase by 8 to 15% depending on preparation used *4768* Increase of up to 11% after 6 months in 150 women receiving three different triphasic oral contraceptive regimes *4560* Significant increase over 12 months in women taking either ethinyl estradiol/norgestrel or ethinyl estradiol/norethindrone but increase did not exceed clinically acceptable limits *4333* In 10 women receiving ethinyl estradiol with norethindrone *3278* Significant positive correlation between oral contraceptive use and LDL-cholesterol concentration *2399*
Serum No Effect Physiological In 10 women receiving ethinyl estradiol with norethindrone. In 10 women receiving ethinyl estradiol with norgestrel *3278* Triphasic preparations containing 50-125 μg levonorgestrel or 500-1000 μg norethindrone had no effect on LDL-cholesterol concentration *2202* No change with 10 cycles of treatment with triphasic preparation in 20 women *3689* No significant change over 9 months in women taking various combinations of ethinyl estradiol and norethindrone *817* No change with high-dose oral contraceptives that are overly estrogenic *2046* No difference between treated women and others *2184* No significant effect in 18 healthy young women receiving low-dose ethinyl estradiol with levonorgestrel for 6 months *2489* No significant effect observed in women taking gestodene with ethinyl estradiol *2143* In 9 desogestrel users mean concentration of 2.79 ± 0.71 mmol/L and 2.50 ± 0.35 mmol/L in 9 levonorgestrel users not significantly different from 2.53 ± 0.57 mmol/L in 41 healthy controls *1309* Typically insignificant change over 6 cycles in women with low dose ethinyl estradiol with low dose levonorgestrel or desogestrel *2047* In 19 healthy women treated for 6 cycles with biphasic oral contraceptive containing ethinylestradiol and desogestrel nonsignificant change observed from mean baseline of about 115 mg/dL to about 120 mg/dL *3316* Insignificant change from mean of 2.92 mmol/L to 2.79 mmol/L after 12 cycles treatment with ethinyl estradiol/gestodene in 29 women and from mean baseline of 3.01 mmol/L to 2.74 mmol/L in 26 women treated with ethinyl estradiol/desogestrel for 12 cycles *2099*

LDL-Phospholipids *Serum Decrease Physiological* Significant reduction of 20% at first cycle and 15% reduction at third cycle observed in 11 women taking 30 μg ethinyl estradiol with 75 μg gestodene with progressive lessening of reduction thereafter *3317* Significant reduction observed in 11 women treated with 30 μg ethinyl estradiol and 150 μg desogestrel for 12 cycles. Reduction of 30% in first cycle, 25% in third and sixth but reduction not significant by twelfth cycle *3317*

LDL-Triglycerides *Serum Increase Physiological* Increase by 42 to 60% depending on preparation used *4768* In 16 healthy young women with normal menstrual cycles treatment with a combination of 30 μg ethinyl estradiol and 150 μg 3-keto-desogestrel caused a significant change from mean baseline of 22.6 ± 7.5 mg/dL to 28.3± 9.7 mg/dL on day 21 of the third cycle *3315* In 19 healthy women treated with biphasic oral contraceptive containing ethinyl estradiol and desogestrel for 6 cycles mean concentration increased significantly from mean baseline of about 16 mg/dL to about 36 mg/dL *3316* Significant increase observed (26% at third cycle and 22% at sixth cycle) in 11 women taking 30 μg ethinyl estradiol with 75 μg gestodene for 12 cycles *3317*
Serum No Effect Physiological In 16 healthy young women with normal menstrual cycles treatment with a combination of 30 μg ethinyl estradiol and 150 μg 3-keto-desogestrel caused a nonsignificant change from mean baseline of 22.6 ± 7.5 mg/dL to 19.0 ± 6.0 mg/dL on day 3 of the first cycle *3315* Nonsignificant increase observed in 11 women taking 30 μg ethinyl estradiol with 150 μg desogestrel for 12 cycles *3317* In 16 healthy young women with normal menstrual cycles treatment with a combination of 30 μg ethinyl estradiol and 150 μg desogestrel caused a nonsignificant change from mean baseline of 22.6 ± 7.5 mg/dL to 26.6 ± 11.9 mg/dL on day 21 of the third cycle *3315*

LDL-Triglycerides:HDL-Triglycerides Ratio
Serum Increase Physiological Increase from mean of 20 mg/dL at baseline to 35 mg/dL after 1 cycle and 37 mg/dL after 10 cycles in 20 women taking triphasic preparation *3689*

LE Cells *Blood Positive Analytical* False positive test for LE cells been reported *1384*
Blood Positive Physiological May precipitate or exaggerate LE-like syndrome *5869*

Leucine *Plasma Decrease Physiological* Hormonal effect (second part of cycle) *1154*

Leucine Aminopeptidase *Serum Increase Physiological* Possible liver damage *2414*

Leucine Aminopeptidase Isoenzymes
Serum Increase Physiological Increased slow component. ?liver involvement *5155*

Leukocytes *Blood Increase Physiological* ?Stimulating effect of steroids on bone marrow *1873*

Lipase *Serum Increase Physiological* Isolated case of acute pancreatitis reported *4170*

Lipids *Cerebrospinal Fluid Increase Physiological* Altered metabolism *2609*
Serum Increase Physiological 155% higher in pill-users than controls *4457*

Lipoprotein A-I *Serum Decrease Physiological* Nonsignificant decrease of 7% observed in women under age 35 years taking oral contraceptives but no difference observed in those after age 35 years *5795*
Serum Increase Physiological Effect observed in group of healthy young women receiving triphasic ethinyl estradiol with levonorgestrel but not in women receiving monophasic ethinyl estradiol with either gestodene or desogestrel *376*
Serum No Effect Physiological No significant effect observed in 58 women randomized to receive either monophasic ethinyl estradiol with desogestrel, ethinyl estradiol with gestodene or triphasic ethinyl estradiol with levonorgestrel *376*

β-Lipoprotein *Serum Increase Physiological* Extent of effect varies with exact composition of oral contraceptive *2410* Affects cholesterol (approximately 20% increase after 6 mo) *887*

Lipoprotein Cholesterol *Serum No Effect Physiological* No difference between treated women and others *1965*

β-Lipoprotein Cholesterol *Serum Increase Physiological* Icrease by 34 mg/dL in white girl drug users vs controls *6278*

Lipoprotein Lipase *Serum Decrease Physiological* Reduced response to heparin injection *887*

Lipoprotein Lp(a) *Serum No Effect Physiological* Median concentration in women on oral contraceptives the same as in those not receiving oral contraceptives (92 mg/L) *5604* No significant association observed in children between oral contraceptive use and serum Lp(a) concentration *5762*

Lipoproteins *Serum Increase Physiological* 50% increase after 6 mo use *5869*

α-Lipoproteins *Serum Increase Physiological* Responsible for increased phospholipids *887*

Lipoproteins, Pre-β *Serum Increase Physiological* Probably due to increased apoprotein synthesis *3923*

Lorazepam *Serum Decrease Physiological* Half-life reduced and metabolic clearance increased due to enhanced glucuronidation *5831*

Low Density Lipoprotein B *Serum Increase Physiological* Significant increase observed in 60 nonpregnant women over 3 cycles treated with either of 2 low-dose regimes: increase continued over additional treated cycles *3797*

Luteinizing Hormone *Plasma Decrease Physiological* Combination type pill lowered value to 20% control *2231* In 7 women with polycystic disease of the ovaries and 5 healthy women treatment with oral contraceptives for 3 months caused significant decrease in concentration *5858* Reduction to about 15 pg/mL at day 10 versus 73 pg/mL in control and to 12 pg/mL at day 21 versus 158 pg/mL in control in women taking 30 μg ethinyl estradiol with either 75 μg gestodene or 150 μg desogestrel reproducible over several cycles *2994* In 33 women receiving cycle of 35 μg ethinyl estradiol and 1 mg norethindrone for 9 cycles maximum suppression of 30% at 3 months with continued suppression at 6 and 9 months *4180*
Urine Decrease Physiological Marked depression in normal subjects *5817*

Lymphocyte Mitotic Index
Test Conditions Decrease Physiological Hormonal action *1881*

Lymphocyte response to Phytohemagglutinin
Blood Decrease Physiological Hormonal action *1881*

Lysolecithin *Serum Decrease Physiological* If administered for long period *4281*

α_2-Macroglobulin *Serum Increase Physiological* Metabolic changes in liver synthesis *3604*
Serum No Effect Physiological No significant changes at various intervals during treatment compared with controls *2355*

Magnesium *Serum Decrease Physiological* Generally significant reduction in all women taking oral contraceptives versus age-matched controls *5773* 0.15 mEq/L decrease reported (estrogen effect) *2227* In black women mean concentration 1.59 mEq/L compared with 1.62 mEq/L in same age controls and 1.65 mEq/L in white oral contraceptive users compared with 1.67 mEq/L in same age controls *3667*
Serum No Effect Physiological No difference from normal observed *807*
Urine Decrease Physiological Associated with fall in serum concentration *2227*

MCH *Blood Increase Physiological* In 46 oral contraceptive users compared with controls studied over at least 2 y *1951* Slight increase with continuing use *1873*

MCHC *Blood Increase Physiological* In 46 oral contraceptive users compared with controls studied over at least 2 y *1951* Significant effect in users for less than 5 y *1873*
Blood No Effect Physiological No significant difference between oral contraceptive users and control adolescents *2275*

MCV *Blood Increase Physiological* Occurs if megaloblastic anemia develops *5054*
Blood No Effect Physiological No significant difference between oral contraceptive users and control adolescents *2275* In 46 oral contraceptive users compared with controls studied over at least 2 y *1951*

Mean Platelet Volume *Blood No Effect Physiological* In 25 women taking low dose oral contraceptives mean concentration of 7.52 ± 0.8 /µL not significantly different from 7.68 ± 0.9 /µL in 29 healthy controls *5199*

Melatonin *Plasma Increase Physiological* In 36 women aged 19 to 40 years no significant change induced with treatment with either monophasic or triphasic oral contraceptives *1363*

Metoprolol *Serum Increase Physiological* In 12 women taking oral contraceptives area under metoprolol concentration curve was 70% higher than in control women probably due to inhibition of metabolism of metoprolol *3106*

Mycophenolate *Serum No Effect Physiological* Coadministration of single doses of mycophenolate mofentil with oral contraceptives in 15 healthy women had no significant effect on the pharmacokinetics of mycophenolate *5017*

Natural Killer Cells *Blood Decrease Physiological* Statistically significant decrease in activity after 3 months which disappeared by 6 months due to greater variability *333*

N-Formiminoglutamic Acid *Urine Increase Physiological* Response to histidine tolerance test *5535* Mild effect in oral contraceptive users *5534*

Nitroblue Tetrazolium Test *Blood Increase Physiological* Observed in 4 out of 6 subjects (?mechanism) *4321*

Nitrogen *Urine No Effect Physiological* In 15 healthy women taking Minulet/Femovan mean excretion 8.66 g/d, in 16 taking Marvelon 8.96 g/d and in 15 taking Diane 9.41 g/d not significantly differ from 8.04 g/d in 28 healthy controls *691*

Ornithine Carbamoyltransferase
Serum Increase Physiological Often raised during first month of treatment *2465*

Osteocalcin *Serum Decrease Physiological* In 52 oral contraceptive pill users mean concentration of 7.7 ± 2.7 ng/mL significantly different from 10.1 ± 3.1 ng/mL in 156 age matched controls *2035*
Serum No Effect Physiological No significant difference observed between age and weight matched women taking oral contraceptives (4.3 ± 3.3 µg/L) and those not (5.0 ± 2.4 µg/L) *5948*

Oxazepam *Serum Decrease Physiological* Half-life reduced and metabolic clearance increased as result of stimulated glucuronidation *5831*

Oxytocin *Plasma Increase Physiological* Significant increase observed with low-dose oral contraceptive medication *5554* Significant effect in women taking oral contraceptives *5553*

Parathyroid Hormone *Plasma Decrease Physiological* Mean concentration in 52 pill-users 29 ± 10 ng/L not significantly different from 32 ± 10 ng/L in 156 healthy controls *2035*
Plasma No Effect Physiological In 52 oral contraceptive pill users mean concentration of intact parathyroid hormone of 29 ± 10 ng/L not significantly different from 32 ± 10 ng/L in 156 age matched controls *2035*

Partial Thromboplastin Time
Plasma Decrease Physiological Associated with disordered clotting *1176* In women given low dose ethinyl estradiol and norethindrone *4334* Slight but significant reduction (from mean of 30.2 seconds to 28,0 seconds) in 14 healthy premenopausal women given low-dose oral contraceptives for one or two cycles *3327*

Phenprocoumon *Plasma Decrease Physiological* Clearance increased in 7 healthy women from mean of 1.6 mL/min/kg to 2.0 mL/min/kg and urinary recovery of phenprocoumon glucuronide significantly increased. Plasma protein binding of phenprocoumon unchanged *4094*

Phenytoin *Serum Increase Physiological* Higher concentrations observed in plasma in relation to dose in oral contraceptive users but not quite statistically significant *1315*

Phosphate *Serum Decrease Physiological* Reduction of approximately 2 mg/dL *4813*
Serum Increase Physiological 18% increase reported in some patients *4014*
Serum No Effect Physiological In 52 oral contraceptive pill users mean concentration of 1.07 ± 0.12 mmol/L not significantly different from 1.10 ± 0.12 mmol/L in 156 age matched controls *2035*

Phosphatides, Total *Serum Increase Physiological* Altered metabolism *2609*

Phospholipids *Serum Increase Physiological* About 20% higher in pill-users after 6 mo *887* Significant effect in 10 women after 3 treatment cycles with desogestrel/ethinyl estradiol preparations *3190* With low-dose ethinyl estradiol and desogestrel 21.9% increase after 3 months use and 16.8% increase after 6 months use in 18 healthy young women *2489* In 19 healthy women treated for 6 cycles with biphasic oral contraceptive containing ethinyl estradiol and desogestrel concentration increased significantly from mean baseline of 201.3 ± 33.3 mg/dL to 246.8 ± 33.9 mg/dL *3316*
Serum No Effect Physiological No significant change observed in 18 healthy young women over 6 months who had received low-dose ethinyl estradiol with levonorgestrel *2489* Typically insignificant change over 6 cycles in women with low dose ethinyl estradiol with low dose levonorgestrel or desogestrel *3659* No significant change observed in 22 women taking either 30 µg ethinyl estradiol and 75 µg gestodene or 30 µg ethinyl estradiol and 150 µg desogestrel for 12 cycles *3317*

Plasmin *Plasma Increase Physiological* Associated also with increased plasminogen (common effect) *547*

Plasminogen *Plasma Increase Physiological* Metabolic changes in liver synthesis (estrogen) *3604* Mean concentration in 694 women taking oral contraceptives 122.5 % (mean ± 2 SD 68-126%) significantly greater than 97.2 % (mean ± 2 SD 81-163%) in 1724 no pill taking control women *5917*

Plasminogen Activator Inhibitor-1
Plasma Decrease Physiological In women who took oral contraceptives PAI activity significantly less than in women who did not *5546*

Plasminogen Activator Inhibitor Activity
Plasma Decrease Physiological In patients receiving 20 µg ethinyl estradiol and 150 µg desogestrel mean activity changed over 12 months from 4.7 U/mL to 4.1 U/mL and in those receiving 30 µg ethinyl estradiol and 75 µg gestodene mean activity changed from 8.1 U/mL to 4.6 U/mL over 12 months *5214*

Plasminogen Activator Inhibitor Antigen
Plasma Decrease Physiological In patients receiving 20 µg ethinyl estradiol and 150 µg desogestrel mean concentration changed over 12 months from 7.6 ng/mL to 5.2 ng/mL and in those receiving 30 µg ethinyl estradiol and 75 µg gestodene mean concentration changed from 7.9 ng/mL to 3.8 ng/mL over 12 months *5214*

Oral Contraceptives *(continued)*

Plasminogen Antigen *Plasma Increase Physiological* In patients receiving 20 µg ethinyl estradiol and 150 µg desogestrel mean concentration changed over 12 months from 94% to 136% and in those receiving 30 µg ethinyl estradiol and 75 µg gestodene mean concentration changed from 106% to 139% over 12 months *5214* In women given low dose ethinyl estradiol and norethindrone *4334*

Platelet Aggregation *Blood Increase Physiological* In response to ADP *887* Increased aggregation observed with use *3694*

Platelet Aggregation response to ADP
Blood No Effect Physiological In 25 women taking low dose oral contraceptives mean release of 0.33 ± 0.22 nmol/L not significantly different from 0.47 ± 0.34 nmol/L in 29 healthy controls *5199* In 25 women taking low dose oral contraceptives mean aggregation of 12.5 ± 10 ohms not significantly different from 19.2 ± 12 ohms in 29 healthy controls *5199*

Platelet Aggregation response to Collagen
Blood No Effect Physiological In 25 women taking low dose oral contraceptives mean aggregation of 35.6 ± 9.9 ohms not significantly different from 39 ± 8.5 ohms in 29 healthy controls *5199* In 25 women taking low dose oral contraceptives mean release of 0.95 ± 0.44 nmol/L not significantly different from 0.95 ± 0.29 nmol/L in 29 healthy controls *5199*

Platelets *Blood Increase Physiological* Slight effect during treatment period *2934* Reported effect *128*
Blood No Effect Physiological In 25 women taking low dose oral contraceptives mean concentration of 223 ± 56 x 10^9/L not significantly different from 232 ± 55 x 10^9/L in 29 healthy controls *5199* Insignificant reduction from mean of 234 G/L to 224 G/L in 14 healthy premenopausal women given low-dose oral contraceptives for either one or two cycles *3327*

Porphobilinogen *Urine Decrease Physiological* In one patient with acute intermittent porphyria mean excretion of 409 µmol/d significantly different from reference range of 1 - 8 µmol/d but reduced to 16 µmol/d after 3 months treatment with oral contraceptives *2341* In one patient with hereditary coproporphyria mean excretion of 409 µmol/d significantly different from reference range of 1 - 8 µmol/d but reduced to 2 µmol/d after 4 months treatment with oral contraceptives *2341*
Urine Increase Physiological May precipitate porphyria attack *2210*

Porphyrin, Total *Feces Decrease Physiological* In one patient with hereditary coproporphyria mean excretion of 17186 nmol/g dry weight significantly different from reference range of 27 - 224 nmol/g dry weight but reduced to 653 nmol/g dry weight after 4 months treatment with oral contraceptives *2341*
Urine Decrease Physiological In one patient with hereditary coproporphyria mean excretion of 35598 nmol/d significantly different from reference range of 63 - 205 nmol/d but reduced to 226 nmol/d after 4 months treatment with oral contraceptives *2341* In one patient with acute intermittent porphyria mean excretion of 9581 nmol/d significantly different from reference range of 63 - 205 nmol/d but reduced to 1233 nmol/d after 3 months treatment with oral contraceptives *2341* May occur in patients with established disease *4014*

Postheparin Hepatic Triglyceride Lipase
Plasma Decrease Physiological Reduced by 46% in oral contraceptive treated women *2184*

Potassium *Serum No Effect Physiological* In 28 healthy controls mean concentration 4.31 mmol/L not significantly different from 4.38 mmol/L in 15 women taking Minulet/Femovan, 4.32 mmol/L in 16 taking Marvelon and 4.42 mmol/L in 15 taking Diane *691*
Urine Increase Physiological In 16 healthy women taking Marvelon mean excretion of 70.2 mmol/d significantly increased as in 15 women taking Diane in whom excretion was 85.6 mmol/d compared with 54.3 mmol/d in 28 healthy controls *691*
Urine No Effect Physiological In 15 women taking Minulet/Femovan mean excretion 60.3 mmol/d not significantly different from 54.3 mmol/d in 28 healthy controls *691*

Prealbumin *Serum Increase Physiological* Metabolic changes in liver synthesis *3604*

Prednisolone *Serum Increase Physiological* Plasma clearance of total prednisolone about 50% less than in men and in women not receiving oral contraceptives. Area under curve for unbound prednisolone about double that in men and in women not receiving oral contraceptives *631*

Pregnancy-associated Protein
Serum Increase Physiological Significant effect observed in 17 women given low-dose estrogen preparation over 24 months *3617*

Pregnanediol *Urine Decrease Physiological* Hormonal effect (may be absent excretion) *3646*

Progesterone *Plasma Decrease Physiological* Slight reduction during early part of cycle but reduced from mean of 13.2 ng/mL during control cycle at day 21 to 1.3 pg/mL with ethinyl estradiol/gestodene and from 4.8 ng/mL to 0.8 ng/mL in women taking ethinyl estradiol/desogestrel *2994* Less than 100 ng/dL throughout cycle *1378*

Prolactin *Plasma Increase Physiological* Mean concentration in 54 oral contraceptive users 356 mU/L compared with 168 mU/L in healthy hospital personnel *1151* In 30% women to varying extent, not correlated with dose of estrogen or duration of treatment *4929* Mean change from 8.9 ng/mL to 10.2 ng/mL at 3 mo in 120 women with low estrogen pills *2800*
Plasma No Effect Physiological No significant effect of meals or oral contraceptives *5553*

Proline *Plasma Decrease Physiological* Hormonal effect (second part of cycle) *1154*

Prorenin *Plasma Decrease Physiological* Concentration decreased in women taking oral contraceptives compared with healthy normal controls *1391*

Protein *Serum Decrease Physiological* Estrogen effect *5570*
Serum Increase Physiological Significant increase 3 y after administration, after 3 mo cessation *5249*
Serum No Effect Physiological In 15 healthy women taking Minulet/Femovan mean concentration 67.3 g/L, in 16 taking Marvelon 70.2 g/L and in 15 taking Diane 73.5 g/L compared with 71.5 g/L in 28 healthy controls *691*

Protein C *Plasma Increase Physiological* Significantly higher concentration in women using oral contraceptives and during pregnancy than in control women *3759* In patients receiving 20 µg ethinyl estradiol and 150 µg desogestrel mean concentration changed over 12 months from 86% to 103% and in those receiving 30 µg ethinyl estradiol and 75 µg gestodene mean concentration changed from 88% to 93% over 12 months *5214*

Protein C Activity *Plasma Increase Physiological* In 20 healthy women administration of Triodena (30 or 40 µg ethinyl estradiol, 50, 70 or 100 µg gestodene) for 3 cycles caused significant change of concentration from mean baseline of 113 ± 22% to 131 ± 24% *4823* In 20 healthy women administration of Cileste (35 µg ethinyl estradiol and 250 µg norgestimate) for 3 cycles caused significant change from mean baseline of 102 ± 17% to 117 ± 18% *4823* In 20 healthy women administration of Tri-Cileste (35 µg ethinyl estradiol and 180 or 250 µg norgestimate) for 3 cycles caused significant change of concentration from mean baseline of 100 ± 17% to 111 ± 20% *4823*

Protein S *Plasma Decrease Physiological* In 20 healthy women administration of Triodena (30 or 40 µg ethinyl estradiol, 50, 70 or 100 µg gestodene) for 3 cycles caused significant change of concentration from mean baseline of 94 ± 23% to 76 ± 18% *4823* In patients receiving 20 µg ethinyl estradiol and 150 µg desogestrel mean concentration changed over 12 months from 94% to 84% and in those receiving 30 µg ethinyl estradiol and 75 µg gestodene mean concentration changed from 101% to 84% over 12 months *5214* In 20 healthy women administration of Cileste (35 µg ethinyl estradiol and 250 µg norgestimate) for 3 cycles caused significant change of protein S activity from mean baseline of 96 ± 26% to 71 ± 23% *4823* Mean concentration in women receiving oral contraceptives 17.7 mg/L compared with 23.5 mg/L in control population of women *3759* In 20 healthy women administration of Tri-Cileste (35 µg ethinyl estradiol and 180 or 250 µg norgestimate) for 3 cycles caused significant change of concentration from mean baseline of 104 ± 24% to 79 ± 19% *4823*

Protein S Antigen *Plasma Decrease Physiological* In 20 healthy women administration of Triodena (30 or 40 µg ethinyl estradiol, 50, 70 or 100 µg gestodene) for 3 cycles caused significant change of concentration from mean baseline of 98 ± 24% to 82 ± 24% *4823* In 20 healthy women administration of Cileste (35 µg ethinyl estradiol and 250 µg norgestimate) for 3 cycles caused significant change of total protein S antigen from mean baseline of 109 ± 38% to 92 ± 30% *4823* In 20 healthy women administration of Tri-Cileste (35 μg ethinyl estradiol and 180 or 250 μg norgestimate) for 3 cycles caused significant change of concentration from mean baseline of 99 ± 26% to 80 ± 18% *4823*

Protein S Antigen, Free *Plasma Decrease Physiological* In 20 healthy women administration of Cileste (35 μg ethinyl estradiol and 250 μg norgestimate) for 3 cycles caused significant change of free protein S antigen from mean baseline of 95 ± 25% to 75 ± 15% *4823* In 20 healthy women administration of Tri-Cileste (35 μg ethinyl estradiol and 180 or 250 μg norgestimate) for 3 cycles caused significant change of concentration from mean baseline of 85 ± 17% to 71 ± 16% *4823* In 20 healthy women administration of Triodena (30 or 40 μg ethinyl estradiol, 50, 70 or 100 μg gestodene) for 3 cycles caused significant change of concentration from mean baseline of 83 ± 17% to 77 ± 15% *4823*

Protein S, Free *Plasma Decrease Physiological* Mean concentration reduced to 6.6 mg/L compared with mean concentration of 8.3 mg/L in control population of women *3759*

Prothrombin Fragment 1.2 *Plasma Increase Physiological* In 20 healthy women administration of Triodena (30 or 40 μg ethinyl estradiol, 50, 70 or 100 μg gestodene) for 3 cycles caused significant change of concentration from mean baseline of 1.1 ± 0.5 nmol/L to 1.4 ± 0.6 nmol/L *4823* In 20 healthy women administration of Tri-Cileste (35 μg ethinyl estradiol and 180 or 250 μg norgestimate) for 3 cycles caused significant change of concentration from mean baseline of 1.2 ± 0.8 nmol/L to 1.5 ± 0.4 nmol/L *4823* In 20 healthy women administration of Cileste (35 μg ethinyl estradiol and 250 μg norgestimate) for 3 cycles caused significant change of concentration from mean baseline of 0.8 ± 0.2 nmol/L to 1.3 ± 0.2 nmol/L *4823*

Prothrombin Time *Plasma Decrease Physiological* Decreases response to oral anticoagulants *1405*
Plasma Increase Physiological Associated with failure of excretion of bile salts *2803*
Plasma No Effect Physiological Insignificant increase from mean of 91.6 to 92.9% in 14 healthy premenopausal women given low-dose oral contraceptives for one or two cycles *3327*

Protoporphyrin *Blood Increase Physiological* May precipitate porphyria attack *2210*
Feces Decrease Physiological In one patient with hereditary coproporphyria mean excretion of 742 nmol/g dry weight significantly different from reference range of 21 - 151 nmol/g dry weight but reduced to 111 nmol/g dry weight after 4 months treatment with oral contraceptives *2341*
Feces Increase Physiological May precipitate porphyria attack *2210*

Pyridinoline *Urine Decrease Physiological* In 52 oral contraceptive pill users mean excretion of 175 ± 91 μg/mmoL creatinine significantly different from 211 ± 105 μg/mmoL creatinine in 156 age matched controls as measured by Crosslaps procedure *2035*

Pyridoxal Phosphate *Blood Decrease Physiological* A monophasic sub-50 oral contraceptive (Marvelon) administered to 26 healthy women during the low-hormonal phase of their cycle caused median concentration to decrease to 43 pmol/L significantly lower than 47 pmol/L in 15 control women. During high-hormonal phase median concentration of 43 pmol/L also significantly lower than 47 pmol/L in controls *5780*

Pyruvate *Plasma Increase Physiological* Estrogen effect of combined oral contraceptive *50* Greater increase than normal during glucose tolerance test *887*

Renin *Plasma Decrease Physiological* Mean concentration 131, range 41-415 pg/mL in women receiving oral contraceptives compared with 248, 101-562 pg/mL in normal women *1391*

Renin Activity *Plasma Decrease Physiological* Significantly reduced in women taking oral contraceptives compared with healthy controls *1391* Metabolic changes in liver synthesis *3604* From 30 ng/mL/h to 13 ng/mL/h at 1 week onwards *446*
Plasma Increase Physiological Activity increased although concentration lowered *840* Enhanced concentration observed in women on low dose oral contraceptives *1256* Estrogen effect *5570* Significant increase in women in 3 month study taking low dose estrogen-progestogen (30-35 μg estrogen) oral contraceptives *3749*
Plasma No Effect Physiological Normal activity in users in spite of changes in renin substrate concentration *2223*

Renin Concentration *Plasma Decrease Physiological* Mean concentration 131 pg/mL, range 41-415 pg/mL in women receiving oral contraceptives compared with 248 pg/mL, range 101-562 pg/mL in normal women *1391*

Renin Substrate *Plasma Decrease Physiological* Almost 4 fold increase in oral contraceptive users compared with nonusers probably due to stimulated hepatic synthesis *2223*
Plasma Increase Physiological Hormonal effect *128* From 1.3 μg/mL to 4 μg/mL at 1 week, 6 μg/mL at 3 mo *446* Metabolic changes in liver synthesis *3604* Significant effect in women in 3 month trial of low dose estrogen-progestogen (30-35 μg estrogen) oral contraceptives *3749*

Respiratory Peak Flow *Patient No Effect Physiological* No significant effect observed *1955*

Retinol *Serum Increase Physiological* Significant increase to 84.9 ± 20.5 μg/dL in 88 oral contraceptive users compared with 70.6 ± 16.1 μg/dL in 58 nonusers *4485*

Retinol-binding Protein *Serum Increase Physiological* Values doubled in 6 mo in 8 women taking estrogenic combination but diminished to some extent after 4 y *1192* Increased to about 150% of controls in women on a variety of oral contraceptives *2184* Due to direct effect on synthesis of protein *5055*

Retinol Esters *Serum Increase Physiological* Minimally increased fasting concentration in treated women *2184*

Rheumatoid Factor *Serum Increase Physiological* Slight effect in users *3843*

Sex-Hormone Binding Globulin
Serum Increase Physiological Marked increase in concentration in 25 fertile women treated with desogestrel/ethinyl estradiol preparation for up to 15 cycles *6089* All of 7 oral contraceptive preparations caused a significant increase over 6 mo with monophasic cyproterone acetate producing a greater effect than any other. Monophasic norethisterone had least effect with monophasic levonorgestrel next lowest *6179* Significant effect in 8 healthy women given low-estrogen preparation (ethinyl estradiol-desogestrel) over 24 months, but no effect with ethinyl estradiol-levonorgestrel in another 9 women *3617* Highly significant increase induced by ethinyl estradiol *3757* Increase by 80 to 213% after 3 mo with different preparations *503* Significantly higher concentration observed in women taking desogestrel/ethinyl estradiol than when taking levonorgestrel/ethinyl estradiol due to lower intrinsic androgenicity of 3-keto desogestrel (biologically active metabolite of desogestrel) *3191* Concentration increased and higher in women taking ethinyl estradiol with desogestrel than with levonorgestrel *5901* Increase by 250 to 300% in women taking 30 μg ethinyl estradiol with either 30 μg gestodene or 150 μg desogestrel with initial marked increase in first cycle but thereafter slight progressive increase for 12 cycles of study *2994* Increase from mean baseline of 65.1 nmol/L in 33 women receiving cycle of 35 μg ethinyl estradiol and 1 mg norethindrone for 9 cycles to about 120 nmol/L at 3 months and subsequently *4180* Significant increase observed in 34 women with micropolycystic ovary syndrome treated with ethinyl estradiol and desogestrel or gestodene for 6 cycles *5666* Treament of 7 women with polycystic disease of the ovaries and 5 healthy women caused substantial increase in concentration in both groups *5858* Significant increase observed from baseline to mean concentrations of 186 to 226 nmol/L in 65 women treated with 30 μg ethinyl estradiol and either 75 μg gestodene or 150 μg desogestrel daily for mean of 11 to 38 months *2774* In 22 patients with polycystic ovary syndrome 6 weeks treatment caused significant increase from mean baseline of 34.9 ± 3 nmol/L to 160 ± 21 nmol/L *3367*

Sialic Acid *Serum Decrease Physiological* Metabolic alteration (estrogen effect) *368*

Sodium *Serum Increase Physiological* May cause sodium retention *3810*
Serum No Effect Physiological In 28 healthy control women mean concentration 149 mmol/L not significantly different from 147 mmol/L in 15 taking Minulet/Femovan, 146 mmol/L in 16 taking Marvelon and in 15 taking Diane *691*
Urine Increase Physiological In 15 healthy women taking Minulet/Femovan mean excretion 136 mmol/d, in 16 taking Marvelon 121 mmol/d (not significantly increased) and 145 mmol/d in 15 taking Diane compared with 107 mol/d in 28 healthy controls *691*

Oral Contraceptives *(continued)*

Somatostatin *Plasma Decrease Physiological* Postprandial concentrations reduced in patients receiving low-dose oral contraceptives *5554*

Superoxide Dismutase
Red Blood Cells Increase Physiological In 8 healthy women aged 20 - 29 years taking oral contraceptives mean concentration of 3381 ± 674 U/g hemoglobin not significantly increased compared with 2839 ± 464 U/g hemoglobin in 10 healthy women aged 20 - 29 years not taking oral contraceptives *2959*
Red Blood Cells No Effect Physiological In women users aged 30-39 years no significant difference between activity of 2890 U/g hemoglobin compared with 3170 U/g hemoglobin in non-user controls *3519*

T3-Uptake *Serum Decrease Physiological* Falls from 80-100% to 55-90% (resin test) *887* Similar values to those of first trimester of pregnancy *5726*

Temazepam *Serum Decrease Physiological* Stimulated glucuronidation reduces half-life and increases metabolic clearance *5831*

Testosterone *Serum Decrease Physiological* Significant decrease observed in 34 women with micropolycystic ovary syndrome treated with ethinyl estradiol and desogestrel or gestodene for 6 cycles *5666* Marked and significant reduction in 33 women receiving cycles of 35 µg ethinyl estradiol and 1 mg norethindrone for 9 months with reduction from baseline of about 27 pg/dL to 16 pg/dL at 3 months, 14 pg/dL and 17 pg/dL at 9 months *4180* Reduction by about 20 to 30% in women receiving 30 µg ethinyl estradiol with either 75 µg gestodene or 150 µg desogestrel without further reduction after first cycle *2994* In 22 patients with polycystic ovary syndrome mean concentration reduced from 3.7 ± 0.25 nmol/L to 2.7 ± 0.56 nmol/L after 6 weeks treatment *3367* All of 7 oral contraceptive preparations studied produced a reduction in concentration over 6 months with the exception of monophasic cyproterone acetate *6179*
Serum Increase Physiological Metabolic changes in liver synthesis *3604* Higher in women taking ethinyl estradiol with desogestrel than in those taking ethinyl estradiol with levonorgestrel *5901*

Testosterone Binding Globulin
Serum Increase Physiological Metabolic effect *3923*

Testosterone, Free *Saliva No Effect Physiological* No difference in concentrations in women taking ethinyl estradiol with either levonorgestrel or desogestrel in comparison with controls *5901*
Serum Decrease Physiological Significant reduction observed with all of 7 oral contraceptives studied over 6 months *6179* Equally reduced in women taking ethinyl estradiol and either levonorgestrel or desogestrel *5901* Treatment of 7 women with polycystic disease of the ovaries and 5 healthy women with oral contraceptives for 3 months caused significant decrease in concentration *5858* As a result of markedly increased sex hormone binding globulin *3757* Significant reduction observed in 34 women with micropolycystic ovary syndrome treated with ethinyl estradiol and desogestrel or gestodene for 6 cycles *5666* Reduction of 50 to 70% observed in women taking 30 µg ethinyl estradiol with either 30 µg gestodene or 150 µg desogestrel. Reduction occurred with first cycle of treatment and concentration remained lowered during other cycles with further treatment *2994*

Theophylline *Serum Increase Physiological* Metabolism may be reduced *1384* Up to 30% increase in serum theophylline concentration with oral contraceptives containing estrogens in a dose-related manner *6117* Estrogen-containing oral contraceptives decrease theophylline clearance in a dose-dependent manner, increasing theophylline concentration by about 30% *5999* Estrogens decrease theophylline clearance in a dose-dependent manner and increases serum theophylline concentration by 30% *3125*

Thrombin/Antithrombin III Complex
Plasma No Effect Physiological In patients receiving 20 µg ethinyl estradiol and 150 µg desogestrel mean concentration changed over 12 months from 2.7 µg/L to 3.1 µg/L and in those receiving 30 µg ethinyl estradiol and 75 µg gestodene mean concentration changed from 2.9 µg/L to 3.0 µg/L over 12 months *5214*

Thrombomodulin *Plasma Decrease Physiological* In 20 healthy women administration of Cileste (35 µg ethinyl estradiol and 250 µg norgestimate) for 3 cycles caused significant change of concentration from mean baseline of 41.7 ± 17.0 ng/mL to 34.4 ± 12.0 ng/mL *4823* In 20 healthy women administration of Triodena (30 or 40 µg ethinyl estradiol, 50, 70 or 100 µg gestodene) for 3 cycles caused significant change of concentration from mean baseline of 46.2 ± 33.9 ng/mL to 37.3 ± 22.8 ng/mL *4823*
Plasma Increase Physiological In 20 healthy women administration of Tri-Cileste (35 µg ethinyl estradiol and 180 or 250 µg norgestimate) for 3 cycles caused significant change of concentration from mean baseline of 42.1 ± 9.6 ng/mL to 34.4 ± 6.5 ng/mL *4823*

Thromboplastin Generation *Blood Increase Physiological* Significant effect observed *4063*

Thyro-Binding Index *Serum Increase Physiological* For up to 1 mo after stopping treatment *1444*

Thyroid Stimulating Hormone
Serum No Effect Physiological No significant difference from nonpregnant values *5726* Hypophyseal mediated effect; results generally contradictory *6412*

Thyroxine Binding Globulin *Serum Increase Physiological* Increased concentration observed as a physiological response to estrogen-containing oral contraceptives *277* Estrogen activation of carrier protein *622* In response to amount of circulating estrogen *887*

Thyroxine (T4) *Serum Increase Physiological* Similar values to those in late first trimester *5726* Increased concentration observed as a physiological response to estrogen-containing oral contraceptives *277* Increased binding protein available *5869* Increased binding capacity (augmentation of transport proteins) *6412*

Thyroxine (T4), Free *Serum Decrease Physiological* When treatment results compared with controls *443*
Serum No Effect Physiological No effect observed although PBI may be increased *4014* No significant difference from nonpregnant values *5726*

Thyroxine (T4) Index, Free *Serum Increase Physiological* May be slightly increased even 1 mo after treatment *1444*
Serum No Effect Physiological Thyroid function unaffected *128*

Thyroxine (T4) (Murphy-Pattee)
Serum Increase Physiological Increased binding protein available (effect 2-4 weeks) *5315*

Tissue Plasminogen Activator
Plasma Increase Physiological In patients receiving 20 µg ethinyl estradiol and 150 µg desogestrel mean activity changed over 12 months from 0.10 U/mL to 0.15 U/mL and in those receiving 30 µg ethinyl estradiol and 75 µg gestodene mean activity changed from 0.09 U/mL to 0.13 U/mL over 12 months *5214*

Tissue Plasminogen Activator Antigen
Plasma Decrease Physiological In patients receiving 20 µg ethinyl estradiol and 150 µg desogestrel mean concentration changed over 12 months from 2.9 ng/mL to 2.4 ng/mL and in those receiving 30 µg ethinyl estradiol and 75 µg gestodene mean concentration changed from 4.0 ng/mL to 2.0 ng/mL over 12 months *5214*

Transferrin *Serum Increase Physiological* Metabolic changes in liver synthesis (estrogen) *3604* Refence interval for women using estrogens 2.25 - 3.85 g/L compared with upper limit of normal in noncontraceptive-taking women of 3.26 g/L *2545* In 46 oral contraceptive users compared with controls studied over at least 2 y *1951*

Tri-iodothyronine (T3) *Serum Decrease Physiological* Due to increase in thyroxine binding globulin *5315*
Serum Increase Physiological Similar values to those in late first trimester *5726* Increased binding capacity (augmentation of transport proteins) *6412*

Triazolam *Serum Increase Physiological* Oxidative metabolism inhibited by coadministration of oral contraceptives *5831*

Triglycerides *Serum Increase Physiological* In 10 women receiving ethinyl estradiol with norgestrel *3278* Significant increase (about 40%) observed by third cycle in 11 women taking 30 µg ethinyl estradiol with 75 µg gestodene but slight decline from peak observed during ninth and twelfth cycle *3317* Increase by 40 mg/dL in white girl drug users vs controls *6278*

In 16 healthy young women with normal menstrual cycles treatment with a combination of 30 µg ethinyl estradiol and 150 µg desogestrel caused a significant change from mean baseline of 66.6 ± 22.7 mg/dL to 91.2 ± 39.9 mg/dL on day 21 of the third cycle *3315* In 19 healthy women treated for 6 cycles with biphasic oral contraceptive containing ethinyl estradiol and desogestrel caused significant increase from mean baseline of about 60 mg/dL to about 125 mg/dL *3316* Significant increase from baseline of 66 mg/dL to 100 mg/dL after 1 cycle and 106 mg/dL after 10 cyles of a triphasic preparation in 20 women *3689* Significant increase of about 20% observed in 60 non-pregnant women over three cycles when taking either of 2 low-dose regimes *3797* Positive correlation with serum γ-glutamyltransferase activity suggesting involvement of hepatic enzyme induction *3813* Significant increase in women taking either ethinyl estradiol/norgestrel or ethinyl estradiol/norethindrone over 12 months although did not exceed clinically acceptable limits *4333* Significant increase of from 28-52% in 150 non-smoking normolipidemic women on three different triphasic contraceptive regimes *4560* Mean concentration of 0.88 mmol/L at baseline in 22 women with IDDM changed significantly to 1.03 mmol/L after 1 month, 1.23 mmol/L after 3 months, 1.14 mmol/L after 6 months and 1.10 mmol/L after 12 months during treatment with 30 µg ethinyl estradiol and 75 µg gestodene *4633* Increase by 25 to 62% depending on preparation used *4768* In 16 healthy young women with normal menstrual cycles treatment with a combination of 30 µg ethinyl estradiol and 150 µg 3-keto-desogestrel caused a significant change from mean baseline of 66.6 ± 22.7 mg/dL to 98.7 ± 33.5 mg/dL on day 21 of the third cycle *3315* Concentration increased in patients taking oral contraceptives *4989* Estrogen effect of combined oral contraceptive *50* In 58 healthy women receiving for 3 months ethinyl estradiol with either desogestrel, gestodene or levonorgestrel actual increase or tendency to increase observed *5794* With low-dose ethinyl estradiol and desogestrel 39.3% increase after 3 months and 45.6% increase after 6 months use of preparation in 18 healthy young women *2489* Significant effect after 3 treatment cycles with desogestrel/ethinyl estradiol preparation in 10 women *3190* If given for 3 mo impaired removal (estrogen) *5869* After 12 cycles in 29 women taking ethinyl estradiol/gestodene increase from median concentration of 0.73 mmol/L to 1.24 mmol/L and in 26 women taking ethinyl estradiol/desogestrel increase of median from 0.73 mmol/L to 1.28 mmol/L after 12 cycles *2099* With high-dose combination drugs. With drug with high progestogen component induce greater than 50% increase on average *2046* Significant increase from baseline of about 55 mg/dL to 84 mg/dL at 3 months, 90 mg/dL at 6 months and 91 mg/dL in women taking 50 µg ethinyl estradiol and 1.0 mg norethindrone and with other combinations of same drugs *817* Mean concentration of 1.08 ± 0.45 mmol/L in 9 desogestrel users and 1.04 ± 0.28 mmol/L in 9 levonorgestrel users significantly different from 0.83 mmol/L in 41 healthy controls *1309* Significant increase observed in women taking gestodene with ethinyl estradiol *2143* Increased in response to a variety of different preparations *2184* Significant increase at 6 mo in all users but effect greater in those taking 35 µg ethinyl estradiol (EE) + 1 mg ethynodiol, 35 µg EE + 1 mg norethindrone, and 35 µg EE + 05 and 1 mg norethindrone than in those receiving 30 µg EE + 0.15 mg levonorgestrel *816* Effect observed with all oral contraceptives studied in this study - including those with 150 or 250 µg levonorgestrel, 500 or 1000 µg of norethindrone or 150 µg desogestrel as the progestin *2202* Increase of 13 to 75% observed in combination oral contraceptive users *2201* Increase by 80% with high dose oral contraceptives that are overly estrogenic *2046*

Serum No Effect Physiological No significant correlation observed between oral contraceptive use and plasma triglyceride concentration *2399* Extent of effect varies with exact composition of oral contraceptive *2410* In 16 healthy young women with normal menstrual cycles treatment with a combination of 30 µg ethinyl estradiol and 150 µg desogestrel caused a nonsignificant change from mean baseline of 66.6 ± 22.7 mg/dL to 64.5 ± 19.1 mg/dL on day 3 of the first cycle *3315* No significant change observed over 6 months in 18 healthy young women receiving low-dose ethinyl estradiol with levonorgestrel *2489* Nonsignificant increase observed in 11 women taking 30 µg ethinyl estradiol with 75 µg gestodene over 12 cycles *3317* In 10 women receiving ethinyl estradiol with norethindrone *3278* Typically insignificant change over 6 cycles in women with low dose ethinyl estradiol with low dose levonorgestrel or desogestrel *2047* In 16 healthy young women with normal menstrual cycles treatment with a combination of 30 µg ethinyl estradiol and 150 µg 3-keto-desogestrel caused a nonsignificant change from mean baseline of 66.6 ± 22.7 mg/dL to 60.5 ± 20.2 mg/dL on day 3 of the first cycle *3315*

Type I Collagen Cross-linked N-telopeptide
Urine Decrease Physiological Mean excretion in 52 pill-users of 16.2 ± 5.9 nmol bone collagen equivalent/mmol creatinine significantly less than 22.5 ± 9.4 nmol bone collagen equivalent/mmol creatinine in 156 healthy controls *2035* In 52 oral contraceptive pill users mean excretion of 16.2 ± 5.9 µg/mmoL creatinine significantly different from 22.5 ± 9.4 µg/mmoL creatinine in 156 age matched controls *2035*

Tyrosine *Plasma Decrease Physiological* Hormonal effect (second part of cycle) *1154*

Urobilinogen *Feces Decrease Physiological* Pale stools, due to cholestasis *2803*
Urine Decrease Physiological May induce cholestasis *2803*

Uroporphyrin *Urine Decrease Physiological* In one patient with hereditary coproporphyria mean excretion of 822 nmol/d significantly different from reference range of 4 - 29 nmol/d but reduced to 10 nmol/d after 4 months treatment with oral contraceptives *2341* In one patient with acute intermittent porphyria mean excretion of 7605 nmol/d significantly different from reference range of 4 - 29 nmol/d but reduced to 761 nmol/d after 3 months treatment with oral contraceptives *2341*
Urine Increase Physiological May induce porphyria cutanea tarda *5059*
Urine No Effect Physiological In 40 healthy female volunteers treatment with either 75 µg gestoden and 30 µg ethinylestradiol or 150 µg desogestrel and 30 µg ethinylestradiol caused nonsignificant decrease from 9.7 ± 4.9 nmol/d to 9.5 ± 5.8 nmol/d and from 10.2 ± 4.1 nmol/d to 8.4 ± 3.7 nmol/d respectively over 6 cycles *2341*

Valine *Plasma Decrease Physiological* Hormonal effect (second part of cycle) *1154*

Valproic Acid *Serum No Effect Physiological* Administration of a single dose of ethinyl estradiol (50µg) with levonorgestrel (250 µg) to 6 women receiving valproic acid (250 µg b.i.d.) for 2 months had no effect on the pharmacokinetics of valproic acid *17*

Vanillylmandelic Acid *Urine No Effect Physiological* No effect observed with ingestion *5402*

Vital Capacity *Patient No Effect Physiological* No significant effect observed *1955*

Vitamin A *Serum Increase Physiological* Increased to about 150% of controls in women on a variety of oral contraceptives *2184* Values doubled in 6 mo in 8 women taking estrogenic combination but diminished to some extent after 4 y *1192* Due to influence on binding protein *5055*

Vitamin B_{12} *Serum Decrease Physiological* Probable interference with gastrointestinal absorption *6416* Mild effect in oral contraceptive users *5534*
Serum No Effect Physiological A monophasic sub-50 oral contraceptive (Marvelon) administered to 26 healthy women during both the high and low-hormonal phase of their cycle had no significant effect on concentration compared with 15 control women *5780* No significant difference between oral contraceptive users and control adolescents *2275*

Vitamin B Binding Protein *Serum Increase Physiological* Mean concentration of 603 ± 228 µg/dL observed in 3 women taking oral contraceptives compared with 404 ± 124 µg/dL in 24 normal individuals *561*

VLDL-Apolipoprotein B *Serum No Effect Physiological* No significant change over 10 cycles in 20 women taking triphasic preparation *3689*

VLDL-Cholesterol *Serum Increase Physiological* In 16 healthy young women with normal menstrual cycles treatment with a combination of 30 µg ethinyl estradiol and 150 µg 3-keto-desogestrel caused a significant change from mean baseline of 9.6 ± 4.4 mg/dL to 15.4 ± 7.0 mg/dL on day 21 of the third cycle *3315* Increase by 16 to 40% depending on preparation used *4768* Mean concentration of 0.53 ± 0.32 mmol/L in 9 desogestrel users and 0.45 ± 0.16 mmol/L in 9 levonorgestrel users not significantly different from 0.40 ± 0.21 mmol/L in 41 healthy controls *1309* Slightly increased (from mean of 16 mg/dL to 20 mg/dL) after 10 cycles of treatment with triphasic

Oral Contraceptives *(continued)*

VLDL-Cholesterol *(continued)*
preparation in 20 women *3689* In 16 healthy young women with normal menstrual cycles treatment with a combination of 30 µg ethinyl estradiol and 150 µg desogestrel caused a significant change from mean baseline of 9.6 ± 4.4 mg/dL to 14.2 ± 8.0 mg/dL on day 21 of the third cycle *3315* Mean concentration of 0.41 mmol/L at baseline in 22 women with IDDM changed significantly to 0.47 mmol/L after 1 month, 0.56 mmol/L after 3 months, 0.53 mmol/L after 6 months and 0.51 mmol/L after 12 months during treatment with 30 µg ethinyl estradiol and 75 µg gestodene *4633* Slow increase with time so that by twelfth cycle significant increase of about 18% observed in 11 women taking 30 µg ethinyl estradiol with 150 µg desogestrel *3317* In 19 healthy women treated for 6 cycles with biphasic contraceptive containing ethinyl estradiol and desogestrel mean concentration increased significantly from baseline of about 10 mg/dL to about 15 mg/dL *3316* Steady increase over time so that at twelfth cycle increase of 50% observed in 11 women taking 30 µg ethinyl estradiol with 75 µg gestodene *3317*
Serum No Effect Physiological No difference between treated women and others *2184* In 16 healthy young women with normal menstrual cycles treatment with a combination of 30 µg ethinyl estradiol and 150 µg desogestrel caused a nonsignificant change from mean baseline of 9.6 ± 4.4 mg/dL to 8.9 ± 4.2 mg/dL on day 3 of the first cycle *3315* In 16 healthy young women with normal menstrual cycles treatment with a combination of 30 µg ethinyl estradiol and 150 µg 3-keto-desogestrel caused a nonsignificant change from mean baseline of 9.6 ± 4.4 mg/dL to 9.6 ± 5.6 mg/dL on day 3 of the first cycle *3315*

VLDL-Phospholipids *Serum Increase Physiological* Significant increase (30% at third cycle, 35% at sixth and 25% at twelfth) in 11 women taking 30 µg ethinyl estradiol with 75 µg gestodene *3317* Significant increase of almost 40% at sixth cycle and 20% at twelfth cycle in 11 women taking 30 µg ethinyl estradiol with 150 µg desogestrel *3317*

VLDL-Triglycerides *Serum Increase Physiological* Increase from mean of 45 mg/dL at baseline to 65 mg/dL after 1 cycle and 68 mg/dL after 10 cycles in 20 women receiving triphasic preparation *3689* Increase by 16 to 52% depending on preparation used *4768* In 16 healthy young women with normal menstrual cycles treatment with a combination of 30 µg ethinyl estradiol and 150 µg 3-keto-desogestrel caused a significant change from mean baseline of 31.6 ± 15.1 mg/dL to 52.0± 23.6 mg/dL on day 21 of the third cycle *3315* In 19 healthy women treated for 6 cycles with biphasic oral contraceptive containing ethinyl estradiol and desogestrel mean concentration increased significantly from baseline of about 28 mg/dL to about 60 mg/dL *3316* Significant increase (about 35%) observed at the first cycle but steady decline thereafter in 11 women taking 30 µg ethinyl estradiol with 75 µg gestodene when followed for 12 cycles *3317* In 16 healthy young women with normal menstrual cycles treatment with a combination of 30 µg ethinyl estradiol and 150 µg desogestrel caused a significant change from mean baseline of 31.6 ± 15.1 mg/dL to 44.6 ± 34.2 mg/dL on day 21 of the third cycle *3315*
Serum No Effect Physiological In 16 healthy young women with normal menstrual cycles treatment with a combination of 30 µg ethinyl estradiol and 150 µg 3-keto-desogestrel caused a nonsignificant change from mean baseline of 31.6 ± 15.1 mg/dL to 27.9 ± 13.9 mg/dL on day 3 of the first cycle *3315* Mean concentrations of 0.59 ± 0.34 mmol/L in 9 desogestrel users and 0.53 ± 0.23 mmol/L in 9 levonorgestrel users not significantly different from 0.45 ± 0.24 mmol/L in 41 healthy controls *1309* No significant change observed over 12 cycles in 11 women taking 30 µg ethinyl estradiol with 150 µg desogestrel *3317* In 16 healthy young women with normal menstrual cycles treatment with a combination of 30 µg ethinyl estradiol and 150 µg desogestrel caused a nonsignificant change from mean baseline of 31.6 ± 15.1 mg/dL to 27.9 ± 13.9 mg/dL on day 3 of the first cycle *3315*

Xanthurenic Acid *Urine Increase Physiological* Estrogen component induces tryptophan pyrrolase *5085*

Zinc *Hair No Effect Physiological* No significant effect in young women studied for at least 3 mo *6270*
Red Blood Cells No Effect Physiological In 22 women ingesting combination type contraceptives *2613*
Serum Decrease Physiological Duration of use unrelated to zinc concentration *2418*
Serum Increase Physiological In 18 pregnant or pill users median concentration 28.2 µmol/L significantly higher than 18.6 µmol/L in 82 other women *2291*
Serum No Effect Physiological No significant difference observed in nursing mothers following ingestion of a variety of different oral contraceptives *1474* No difference from normal observed *807* In 22 women ingesting combination type contraceptives *2613* No effect observed in 17 healthy women given low-dose estrogen preparation over 24 months *3618*
White Blood Cells No Effect Physiological In 22 women ingesting combination type contraceptives *2613*

Oral Hypoglycemics

Alkaline Phosphatase *Serum Increase Physiological* Mean activity as observed in 28 individuals in a population of 6000 adults taking oral hypoglycemic agents of 78.3 U/L significantly higher than 62.7 U/L in those not taking such drugs when corrected for the influence of age, sex, relative weight and glucose concentration *2252*

Oral Resins

Ammonia *Plasma Increase Physiological* Exchanged for other ions in gastrointestinal tract *1714*

Ornidazole

Midazolam *Serum No Effect Analytical* On GC-ECD method of Ha et al *2387*

Orphenadrine

Albumin *Serum No Effect Analytical* At concentration of 9 mg/L had no effect on BCG method *5704*

Bicarbonate *Serum No Effect Analytical* At concentration of 9 mg/L had no effect on method using phenolphthalein *5704*

Bilirubin *Serum No Effect Analytical* At concentration of 9 mg/L had no effect on Jendrassik and Grof method *5704*

Calcium *Serum No Effect Analytical* At concentration of 9 mg/L had no effect on cresolphthalein method *5704*

Chloride *Serum No Effect Analytical* At concentration of 9 mg/L had no effect on mercurimetric method *5704*

Chlorpromazine *Serum Decrease Physiological* Gastrointestinal absorption of chlorpromazine is presumed to be reduced when two drugs given concomitantly *3633*

Cholesterol *Serum No Effect Analytical* At concentration of 9 mg/L had no effect on Liebermann-Burchard method *5704*

Creatinine *Serum No Effect Analytical* At concentration of 9 mg/L had no effect on Technicon AutoAnalyzer® Jaffe method *5704*

Erythrocytes *Blood Decrease Physiological* Very rare cases of aplastic anemia have been reported in association with the use of orphenadrine *3701* 2 cases of aplastic anemia reported *2754*

Hematocrit *Blood Decrease Physiological* Very rare cases of aplastic anemia have been reported in association with the use of orphenadrine *3701*

Hemoglobin *Blood Decrease Physiological* Very rare cases of aplastic anemia have been reported in association with the use of orphenadrine *3701*

Histamine *Plasma No Effect Analytical* Although 50% inhibition of radio-enzyme assay occurs at 26 µg/mL unlikely to be relevant clinically since physiological concentration 0.1 - 0.2 µg/mL *2492*

Leukocytes *Blood Decrease Physiological* Very rare cases of aplastic anemia have been reported in association with the use of orphenadrine *3701* 2 cases of aplastic anemia reported *2754*

p-Aminophenol *Urine No Effect Analytical* With addition of drugs at a concentration of 100 mg/L and of related compounds at 50 mg/L no significant effect observed on colorimetric method of van Bocxlaer on Cobas Mira analyzer which involves reacting free p-aminophenol with resorcinol in the presence of magnesium ions to form an indophenol dye measured at 550 nm *6163*

Phosphate *Serum No Effect Analytical* At concentration of 9 mg/L had no effect on phosphomolybdate method *5704*

Platelets *Blood Decrease Physiological* Very rare cases of aplastic anemia have been reported in association with the use of orphenadrine *3701* 2 cases of aplastic anemia reported *2754*

Potassium *Serum No Effect Analytical* At concentration of 9 mg/L had no effect on measurement by ISE with predilution *5704*

Protein *Serum No Effect Analytical* At concentration of 9 mg/L had no effect on biuret method with blank correction *5704*

Prothrombin Time *Plasma Decrease Physiological* May enhance metabolism of anticoagulants *2753*

T3-Uptake *Serum Increase Physiological* Observed in 10 of 13 psychiatric patients treated with drug without evidence of thyroid disorders also observed in 15 psychiatric patients in matched control study *4083*

Thyroxine (T4) *Serum Increase Physiological* Reported in two studies *6412*

Thyroxine (T4) Index, Free *Serum Increase Physiological* Observed in 10 of 13 psychiatric patients receiving drug. Value gradually increased with start of therapy and fell on withdrawal *4083* Reported in two studies *6412*

Tri-iodothyronine (T3) *Serum No Effect Physiological* Reported in two studies *6412*

Triglycerides *Serum No Effect Analytical* At concentration of 9 mg/L had no effect on lipase/esterase method *5704*

Urea Nitrogen *Serum No Effect Analytical* At concentration of 9 mg/L had no effect on diacetylmonoxime method *5704*

Uric Acid *Serum No Effect Analytical* At concentration of 9 mg/L had no effect on phosphotungstate reduction method *5704*

Orthophosphate

Ammonium *Urine Decrease Physiological* In 12 patients with primary hyperoxaluria treatment with orthophosphate and pyridoxine for 2 days caused significant reduction from mean baseline of 0.64 ± 0.39 mg/mg creatinine to 0.31 ± 0.11 mg/mg creatinine *4056*

Bicarbonate *Urine Increase Physiological* In 12 patients with primary hyperoxaluria treatment with orthophosphate and pyridoxine for 2 days caused significant increase from mean baseline of 0.26 ± 0.14 mg/mg creatinine to 0.83 ± 0.40 mg/mg creatinine *4056*

Calcium *Urine Decrease Physiological* In 12 patients with primary hyperoxaluria treatment with orthophosphate and pyridoxine for 2 days caused significant reduction from mean baseline of 0.11 ± 0.07 mg/mg creatinine to 0.04 ± 0.02 mg/mg creatinine *4056*

Citrate *Urine No Effect Physiological* In 12 patients with primary hyperoxaluria treatment with orthophosphate and pyridoxine for 2 days caused nonsignificant increase from mean baseline of 0.47 ± 0.41 mg/mg creatinine to 0.56 ± 0.29 mg/mg creatinine *4056*

Magnesium *Urine Decrease Physiological* In 12 patients with primary hyperoxaluria treatment with orthophosphate and pyridoxine for 2 days caused significant reduction from mean baseline of 0.12 ± 0.04 mg/mg creatinine to 0.08 ± 0.03 mg/mg creatinine *4056*

Oxalate *Urine Decrease Physiological* In 12 patients with primary hyperoxaluria treatment with orthophosphate and pyridoxine for 2 days caused significant reduction from mean baseline of 0.18 ± 0.13 mg/mg creatinine to 0.13 ± 0.08 mg/mg creatinine *4056*

pH *Urine Increase Physiological* In 12 patients with primary hyperoxaluria treatment with orthophosphate and pyridoxine for 2 days caused significant increase from mean baseline of 5.71 ± 0.28 to 6.34 ± 0.28 *4056*

Phosphate *Urine Increase Physiological* In 12 patients with primary hyperoxaluria treatment with orthophosphate and pyridoxine for 2 days caused significant increase from mean baseline of 0.82 ± 0.28 mg/mg creatinine to 1.73 ± 0.56 mg/mg creatinine *4056*

Pyrophosphate *Urine Increase Physiological* In 12 patients with primary hyperoxaluria treatment with orthophosphate and pyridoxine for 2 days caused significant increase from mean baseline of 0.0058 ± 0.0053 mg/mg creatinine to 0.0124 ± 0.0079 mg/mg creatinine *4056*

Ouabain

Albumin *Serum No Effect Analytical* At 0.02 mg/dL had no effect on Technicon SMA 12/60 method *4390*

Alkaline Phosphatase *Serum No Effect Analytical* At 0.02 mg/dL had no effect on Technicon SMA 12/60 method *4390*

Aspartate Aminotransferase *Serum No Effect Analytical* At 0.02 mg/dL had no effect on Technicon SMA 12/60 method *4390*

Bilirubin *Serum No Effect Analytical* At 0.02 mg/dL had no effect on Technicon SMA 12/60 method *4390*

Calcium *Serum No Effect Analytical* At 0.02 mg/dL had no effect on Technicon SMA 12/60 method *4390*

Catecholamines *Urine Decrease Physiological* Marked effect but mechanism unexplained *5303*

Cholesterol *Serum No Effect Analytical* At 0.02 mg/dL had no effect on Technicon SMA 12/60 method *4390*

Creatinine *Serum No Effect Analytical* At 0.02 mg/dL hsd no effect on Technicon SMA 12/60 method *4390*

Digitoxin *Serum Increase Analytical* Cross-reactivity of 3% observed with method on Du Pont aca *1521*
Serum No Effect Analytical At concentrations of 0.01 mg/L has no cross reactivity with method on Baxter Stratus *5705*

Digoxin *Serum Increase Analytical* Reported to affect RIA methods *6638*
Serum No Effect Analytical Ouabain had no detectable cross-reactivity with method on Bayer Technicon Immuno 1® *421* At concentrations up to 50 µg/mL no significant effect observed with method on Ciba Corning ACS:180 *1412* Cross reactivity of less than 10% observed with method on Baxter Stratus *5705*

Glucose *Serum No Effect Analytical* At 0.02 mg/dL had no effect on Technicon SMA 12/60 method *4390*
Serum No Effect Physiological No effect with i.v. infusion for 1 h *5303*

Insulin *Plasma No Effect Physiological* No effect with i.v. infusion for 1 h *5303*

Lactate Dehydrogenase *Serum No Effect Analytical* At 0.02 mg/dL had no effect on Technicon SMA 12/60 method *4390*

Phosphate *Serum No Effect Analytical* At 0.02 mg/dL had no effect on Technicon SMA 12/60 method *4390*

Protein *Serum No Effect Analytical* At 0.02 mg/dL had no effect on Technicon SMA 12/60 method *4390*

Quinidine *Serum No Effect Analytical* No significant interference observed at a concentration of 1 µg/mL (1.71 µmol/L) with method on Du Pont aca *1543*

Uric Acid *Serum No Effect Analytical* At 0.02 mg/dL had no effect on Technicon SMA 12/60 method *4390*

Oxacillin

Alanine Aminotransferase *Serum Increase Physiological* Abnormal liver function in 1 of 8 treated patients on day 15 *4212* Typically occurring 3 to 14 d after treatment started, may occur without eosinophilia *3904* Drug associated hepatitis in patients given high dose drug i.v *4418* Asymptomatic hepatic dysfunction in 5 cases following high dose treatment: reversible *4738* Possible hepatotoxic effect *3669* Reversible high-dose associated liver injury *4021* Reversible phenomenon observed in 8 patients given drug i.v *4400*

Alkaline Phosphatase *Serum Increase Physiological* Asymptomatic hepatic dysfunction in 5 cases following high dose treatment: reversible *4738* Cholestatic jaundice reported

Oxacillin *(continued)*

Alkaline Phosphatase *(continued)*
in one case *1714* Reversible high-dose associated liver injury *4021*

Aspartate Aminotransferase *Serum Increase Physiological* Typically occurring 3 to 14 d after treatment started, may occur without eosinophilia *3904* Possible hepatotoxic effect *3669* Asymptomatic hepatic dysfunction in 5 cases following high dose treatment: reversible *4738* Hypersensitivity reaction observed in one patient with Staphylococcus Aureus endocarditis *1383* Drug associated hepatitis in patients given high dose drug i.v *4418* Abnormal liver function in 1 of 8 treated patients on day 15 *4212* Reversible high-dose associated liver injury *4021* Reversible phenomenon observed in 8 patients given drug i.v *4400*

Bile *Urine Increase Physiological* Reversible hepatocellular dysfunction *3810*

Bilirubin *Serum Increase Physiological* Cholestatic jaundice reported in one case *4544* Reversible high-dose associated liver injury *4021*
Serum No Effect Analytical At concentration of 40 mg/L had no effect on Jendrassik and Grof method *5704*
Serum No Effect Physiological Asymptomatic hepatic dysfunction in 5 cases following high dose treatment: reversible *4738*

BSP Retention *Serum Increase Physiological* Cholestatic jaundice reported in one case *1714*

Calcium *Serum No Effect Analytical* At concentration of 40 mg/L had no effect on cresolphthalein method *5704*

Coombs' Test, Direct *Blood No Effect Physiological* 0 of 10 patients demonstrated hypersensitivity reaction *3195*

Creatinine *Serum Increase Physiological* Transient azotemia with large doses *128*
Serum No Effect Analytical No effect of concentrations up to 15 mg/L on single slide method on Kodak Ektachem® *5706*

Cyclosporine *Blood No Effect Physiological* Coadministration with cyclosporine appeared to have no significant effect on its concentration *859*
Serum No Effect Physiological Coadministration with cyclosporine appeared to have no significant effect on its concentration *859*

Eosinophils *Blood Increase Physiological* Reversible phenomenon observed in 8 patients given drug i.v *4400* Reported effect (?allergic) *128* Suggestive of hypersensitivity reaction *3904*
Blood No Effect Physiological 0 of 10 patients demonstrated hypersensitivity reaction *3195*

Erythrocytes *Blood Decrease Physiological* Large doses parenteral penicillin may have effect *2754*
Urine Increase Physiological Nephrotoxicity with hematuria *128*

Hemoglobin *Urine Increase Physiological* Nephrotoxicity with hematuria *128*

Iron *Serum No Effect Analytical* No interference observed with method on Kodak Ektachem® *2792*

Lactate *Plasma No Effect Analytical* No effect at final concentration of 100 µg/mL on method on Kodak Ektachem® *2793*

Lactate Dehydrogenase *Serum Increase Physiological* Reversible high-dose associated liver injury *4021*

Leukocytes *Blood Decrease Physiological* In 2 patients receiving 12-15 g/d intravenously *2686* Observed in one man, recovery began within 2 d of withdrawal *3003* May cause bone marrow depression *3810* In two cases in one of which abnormalities developed within 48 h and in other in 17 d *745* Single case of drug-related agranulocytosis in patient with prior history of penicillin sensitivity *5304*

Lymphocytes *Blood No Effect Physiological* In 2 patients receiving 12-15 g/d intravenously *2686*

Mezlocillin *Serum Increase Analytical* Cannot be assayed by HPLC method used at Mayo Clinic in presence of oxacillin *3858*

Neutrophils *Blood Decrease Physiological* Granulocytopenia in 2 cases within 2 d of treatment being started *1792* In two cases in one of which abnormalities developed within 48 h and in other in 17 d *745* Case observed after i.v. drug in 1 y old child: postulated that mechanism due to toxic effect on maturation of cells *1015* Observed in one man, recovery began within 2 d of withdrawal *3003* Abnormal liver function in 1 of 8 treated patients on day 15 *4212* Single case of drug-related agranulocytosis in patient with prior history of penicillin sensitivity *5304* Observed in 5 patients given high doses intravenously: reversible with cessation of therapy *69*

5'-Nucleotidase *Serum Increase Physiological* Due to cholestasis *2911*

Phosphate *Serum No Effect Analytical* At concentration of 40 mg/L had no effect on phosphomolybdate method *5704*

Platelets *Blood Decrease Physiological* Usually only associated with large parenteral doses *2754*

Protein *Cerebrospinal Fluid No Effect Analytical* No effect observed at concentration of 100 µg/mL with method on Kodak Ektachem® *2791*
Serum Increase Analytical At concentrations above 500 mg/L (normal therapeutic concentration 6 mg/L) raised concentration as measured by biuret method with blank correction *5704*
Urine Increase Physiological Nephrotoxic effect *128*

Urea Nitrogen *Serum Increase Physiological* Transient azotemia with large doses *128*
Serum No Effect Analytical At concentration of 40 mg/L had no effect on diacetylmonoxime method *5704*

Uric Acid *Serum No Effect Analytical* At concentration of 40 mg/L had no effect on phosphotungstate reduction method *5704*

Oxametacin

Uric Acid Clearance *Urine No Effect Physiological* Treatment of 8 healthy volunteers with 200 mg had no effect on clearance over 24 hours *740*

Oxamniquine

Alanine Aminotransferase *Serum Increase Physiological* Liver function abnormalities reported as a side effect *1384*

Aspartate Aminotransferase *Serum Increase Physiological* Liver function abnormalities reported as side effect *1384*

Bilirubin *Serum Increase Physiological* Liver function abnormalities reported as a side effect *1384*

Eosinophils *Blood Increase Physiological* Eosinophilia reported as one of the most common side-effects *1384*

Oxandrolone

BSP Retention *Serum Increase Physiological* Slight increase in one child (other liver function tests normal) *2861*

Cholesterol *Serum Decrease Physiological* Anabolic effect *2192*

Fibrinogen *Plasma Increase Physiological* Metabolic effect *368*

Glucose *Serum Decrease Physiological* Anabolic effect *2192*

Growth Hormone *Plasma No Effect Physiological* Administration to 15 patients with prepubertal Turner's syndrome had no effect on secretion *3835*

Haptoglobin *Serum Increase Physiological* Metabolic effect *368*

Plasminogen *Plasma Increase Physiological* Metabolic effect *368*

Sialic Acid *Serum Increase Physiological* Metabolic effect *368*

Triglycerides *Serum Decrease Physiological* Increases triglyceride hydrolysis peripherally *2192*

Oxaprotiline

Melatonin *Plasma Increase Physiological* In 10 healthy men treatment with (+)oxaprotiline caused increased concentrations at night on days 1, 7, and 21 compared with concentrations when (-)oxaprotiline administered due to sustained increase in noradrenergic activity within the pineal gland *4486*

Oxaprozin

Alanine Aminotransferase *Serum Increase Physiological* As with other NSAIDs borderline increases in activity may occur in 15% of recipients. Increases above 3 times the upper limit of normal occurred in 1% of patients *2065*

Aldosterone *Plasma No Effect Physiological* No significant change observed in 7 volunteers treated for up to 1 week *4076*
Urine No Effect Physiological No significant change observed in 7 volunteers treated for up to 1 week *4076*

Alkaline Phosphatase *Serum Increase Physiological* As with other NSAIDs borderline increases in activity may occur in 15% of recipients *2065*

Amylase *Serum Increase Physiological* Pssible causal association of oxaprozin with pancreatitis has been reported as side effect *2065*

Aspartate Aminotransferase *Serum Increase Physiological* As with other NSAIDs borderline increases in activity may occur in 15% of recipients *2065*

Benzodiazepine *Urine Increase Physiological* In 10 specimens negative by GC/MS concentrations ranged from 460 - < 1000 µg/L by Du Pont EMIT, 232 - 728 µg/L by Abbott TDx FPIA with several positive results with Biosite Triage and Cedia procedure on Hitachi 717 *855*

Bleeding Time *Patient Increase Physiological* Decreased platelet aggregation with increased bleeding time has been reported as side effect, as with other NSAIDs *2065*

Blood *Urine Increase Physiological* Acute interstitial nephritis, hematuria, and proteinuria have been reported as side effects as with other NSAIDs *2065*

Creatinine *Serum Increase Physiological* Acute interstitial nephritis, hematuria, and proteinuria have been reported as side effects as with other NSAIDs *2065*

Glomerular Filtration Rate *Urine No Effect Physiological* No significant change observed in 7 volunteers treated for up to 1 week *4076*

Hematocrit *Blood Decrease Physiological* Anemia has been reported as side effect as with other NSAIDs, due to gastrointestinal bleeding or an incompletely described effect upon erythrogenesis *2065*

Hemoglobin *Blood Decrease Physiological* Anemia has been reported as side effect as with other NSAIDs, due to gastrointestinal bleeding or an incompletely described effect upon erythrogenesis *2065*

Lactate Dehydrogenase *Serum Increase Physiological* As with other NSAIDs borderline increases in activity may occur in 15% of recipients *2065*

Leukocytes *Blood Decrease Physiological* Pssible causal association of oxaprozin with leukopenia has been reported as side effect *2065*

Lipase *Serum Increase Physiological* Pssible causal association of oxaprozin with pancreatitis has been reported as side effect *2065*

Occult Blood *Feces Increase Physiological* Gastrointestinal bleeding has been reported as side effect, as with other NSAIDs *2065*

Phenytoin *Serum Increase Analytical* At a concentrations of 200 mg/L and higher caused a slight cross-reactivity with Abbott TDX method *1247* At a concentration of 200 mg/L caused a 50% cross-reactivity with Abbott TDXII method but at higher concentrations concentrations, 300 and 400 mg/L, cross-reactivities were 99% and 131% respectively *1247*
Serum No Effect Analytical At a concentration of 200 mg/L and higher had no significant cross-reactivity with Chiron ACS:180 method *1247*

Platelet Aggregation *Blood Decrease Physiological* Decreased platelet aggregation has been reported as side effect as with other NSAIDs *2065*

Potassium *Serum No Effect Physiological* No significant change observed in 7 volunteers treated for up to 1 week *4076*

Protein *Urine Increase Physiological* Acute interstitial nephritis, hematuria, and proteinuria have been reported as side effects as with other NSAIDs *2065*

Prothrombin Time *Plasma No Effect Physiological* Coadministration with warfarin had no effect on its anticoagulation effects *2065*

Renin Activity *Plasma No Effect Physiological* No significant change observed in 7 volunteers treated for up to 1 week *4076*

Urea Nitrogen *Serum Increase Physiological* Acute interstitial nephritis, hematuria, and proteinuria have been reported as side effects as with other NSAIDs *2065*

Oxazepam

Acetaminophen *Serum No Effect Analytical* At 2 mg/L had no effect on HPLC method *5775*

Alanine Aminotransferase *Serum Increase Physiological* Possible hepatotoxicity *3810* A small number of cases develop hepatic dysfunction with treatment *6570*
Serum No Effect Analytical No effect at 10 mg/L on Boehringer Mannheim Reflotron method *5706* No effect at therapeutic concentration on Boehringer Mannheim Reflotron method *3231*

Albumin *Serum No Effect Analytical* At concentration of 1 mg/L had no effect on BCG method *5704*
Urine No Effect Analytical Using a fluorimetric assay with Albumin Blue 580 on a Cobas Fara centrifugal analyzer for the detection of microalbuminuria no significant interference was detected at a concentration of 4 mg/L *3117*

Alkaline Phosphatase *Serum Increase Physiological* Possible hepatotoxicity *3810* A small number of cases develop hepatic dysfunction with treatment *6570*

Amitriptyline *Serum No Effect Physiological* No effect on serum concentration if given together *5559*

Amphetamine *Urine No Effect Analytical* Negative result with method on Du Pont aca at a concentration of 300 µg/L (1.05 mmol/L) *1554*

Amylase *Serum No Effect Analytical* No effect of concentrations up to 10 mg/L on method on Boehringer Mannheim Reflotron *5706*

Aspartate Aminotransferase *Serum Increase Physiological* Possible hepatotoxicity *3810* A small number of cases develop hepatic dysfunction with treatment *6570*
Serum No Effect Analytical No effect at 10 mg/L on Boehringer Mannheim Reflotron method *5706* No effect at therapeutic concentration on Boehringer Mannheim Reflotron method *3231*

Barbiturate *Urine No Effect Analytical* Negative result obtained at a concentration of 250 µg/mL (0.87 mmol/L) with method on Du Pont aca *1555*

Benzoylecgonine *Urine No Effect Analytical* Negative result obtained at a concentration of 250 µg/mL (0.87 mmol/L) with method on Du Pont aca *1558* No interference observed at a concentration of 872 µmol/L with Sung and Neely modification of Syva EMIT procedure *148*

Bicarbonate *Serum No Effect Analytical* At concentration of 1 mg/L had no effect on method using phenolphthalein *5704*

Bile *Urine Increase Physiological* Possible hepatotoxicity *3810*

Bilirubin *Serum Increase Physiological* Possible hepatotoxicity *3810* A small number of cases develop hepatic dysfunction with treatment *6570*
Serum No Effect Analytical At concentration of 10 mg/L no effect on method on Boehringer Mannheim Reflotron system *5706* At concentration of 1 mg/L had no effect on Jendrassik and Grof method *5704* No effect at 5 mg/L on Ames Seralyzer method *5706*
Serum No Effect Physiological Insignificant displacement from protein in neonates *6314*

BSP Retention *Serum Increase Physiological* Possible hepatotoxicity *3810*

Calcium *Serum No Effect Analytical* At concentration of 1 mg/L had no effect on cresolphthalein method *5704*

Cannabinoids *Urine No Effect Analytical* No effect observed at a concentration of 100 µg/mL (0.35 mmol/L) on method on Du Pont aca *1557* No effect on Roche Abuscreen method *5006*

Catecholamines *Plasma No Effect Analytical* No effect on HPLC method of Koller for dopamine, epinephrine, and norepinephrine *3230*

Chloride *Serum No Effect Analytical* At concentration of 1 mg/L had no effect on mercurimetric method *5704*

Oxazepam *(continued)*

Cholesterol *Serum No Effect Analytical* At concentration of 1 mg/L had no effect on Liebermann-Burchard method *5704* No effect at therapeutic concentration on Boehringer Mannheim Reflotron method *3231* No effect at 5 mg/L on Ames Seralyzer method *5706* At concentration of 10 mg/L no effect on method on Boehringer Mannheim Reflotron system *5706*

Cortisol *Plasma Decrease Physiological* Effect of either 45 or 60 mg less than that of dexamethasone on spontaneous afternoon cortisol in group of hospitalized depressed patients *1006*

Plasma No Effect Analytical At a concentration of 10 mg/L no significant effect observed on CEDIA or Enzymun methods *1097*

Cortisol, Free *Urine No Effect Analytical* No significant interference observed with HPLC method of Turpeinen et al *6105*

Creatine Kinase *Serum No Effect Analytical* No effect at 5 mg/L on method on Ames Seralyzer *5706*

Creatinine *Serum No Effect Analytical* At concentration of 1 mg/L had no effect on Technicon AutoAnalyzer® method *5704* At 10 mg/L on reversed phase liquid chromatographic procedure of Zhiri et al *6656* No effect at 5 mg/L on method on Ames Seralyzer *5706*

Drugs of Abuse Screen *Urine No Effect Analytical* No effect at concentration of 100 µg/mL on EZ-SCREEN procedure for cannabinoids and cocaine *1739*

Eosinophils *Blood Increase Physiological* Rare allergic response *128*

Glucose *Serum Increase Analytical* Filler affects o-toluidine, Neocuproin methods *4005*

Serum No Effect Analytical At concentration of 30 mg/L had no effect on hexokinase/G-6-PDH method *5704* No effect at therapeutic concentration on Boehringer Mannheim Reflotron method *3231* No effect at 5 mg/L on glucose oxidase method on Ames Seralyzer *5706* No effect on glucose oxidase method of Boehringer *5480* At concentration of 10 mg/L no effect on method on Boehringer Mannheim Reflotron system *5706*

γ-Glutamyltransferase *Serum No Effect Analytical* At concentration of 10 mg/L no effect on method on Boehringer Mannheim Reflotron system *5706* No effect at therapeutic concentration on Boehringer Mannheim Reflotron method *3231*

5-Hydroxyindoleacetic Acid *Urine No Effect Analytical* Slight effect when added *in vitro* in method of Udenfriend *1051*

^{131}I Uptake *Serum Decrease Physiological* Serax® contains tetraiodofluorescein *4360*

Lactate *Plasma No Effect Analytical* At concentration of 30 mg/L had no effect on enzymatic method *5704*

Lactate Dehydrogenase *Serum No Effect Analytical* No effect at 5 mg/L on method on Ames Seralyzer *5706*

Leukocytes *Blood Decrease Physiological* Leukopenia occurs rarely *3810* A small number of cases develop leukopenia with treatment *6570*

Midazolam *Serum No Effect Analytical* On GC-ECD method of Ha et al *2387*

Morphine *Urine No Effect Analytical* Significant interference observed at a concentration of 872 µmol/L with Sung and Neely modification of Syva EMIT procedure *148*

Nortriptyline *Serum No Effect Physiological* No effect on serum concentration if given together *5559*

Opiates *Urine No Effect Analytical* No effect observed at a concentration of 250 µg/mL (0.87 mmol/L) on method on Du Pont aca *1559*

Phosphate *Serum No Effect Analytical* At concentration of 1 mg/L had no effect on phosphomolybdate method *5704*

Protein *Serum No Effect Analytical* At concentration of 1 mg/L had no effect on biuret method with blank correction *5704*

Tirofiban *Serum No Effect Physiological* Coadministration had no significant effect on plasma clearance of tirofiban *3957*

Triglycerides *Serum No Effect Analytical* At concentration of 1 mg/L had no effect on lipase/esterase method *5704* No effect at therapeutic concentration on Boehringer Mannheim Reflotron method *3231* No effect at 10 mg/L on Boehringer Mannheim Reflotron method *5706*

Urea Nitrogen *Serum No Effect Analytical* No effect at 10 mg/L on Boehringer Mannheim Reflotron method *5706* At concentration of 1 mg/L had no effect on diacetylmonoxime method *5704* No effect at 5 mg/L on method on Ames Seralyzer *5706* No effect at therapeutic concentration on Boehringer Mannheim Reflotron method *3231*

Uric Acid *Serum No Effect Analytical* No effect at 10 mg/L on Boehringer Mannheim Reflotron method *5706* At concentration of 1 mg/L had no effect on phosphotungstate reduction method *5704* No effect at therapeutic concentration on Boehringer Mannheim Reflotron method *3231* At 10 mg/L on reversed phased liquid chromatographic procedure of Zhiri et al *6656*

Oxcarbazepine

Albumin *Urine No Effect Analytical* Using a fluorimetric assay with Albumin Blue 580 on a Cobas Fara centrifugal analyzer for the detection of microalbuminuria no significant interference was detected at a concentration of 8 mg/L *3117*

Androgen Index, Free (FAI) *Plasma No Effect Physiological* Insignificant change from mean baseline concentration of 58.8% to 56.1% after 8 days treatment and 56.6% after 15 days but significant increase to 65.4% post-study *3413* In 12 epileptic men aged 21 to 40 years treated with oxcarbazepine for 6 months mean concentration of 65.8 ± 25.9 not significantly different from concentration when treated with carbamazepine (mean concentration of 61.5 ± 34.0 not significantly different from normal) *2841*

Androstenedione *Plasma Decrease Physiological* Significant reduction from mean baseline of 7.3 nmol/L to 5.3 nmol/L after 8 days chronic treatment in 8 healthy volunteers but reversion to 7.5 nmol/L after 15 days and 6.7 nmol/L post-study *3413*

Antipyrine *Saliva No Effect Physiological* Half-life and clearance not affected by chronic dosing in 8 healthy men *3413*

Antipyrine Clearance *Patient Increase Physiological* In 12 epileptic men aged 21 to 40 years treated with oxcarbazepine for 2 months mean clearance of 71.4 ± 20.8 mL/min significantly different from normal of 23.8 - 51.2 mL/min *2841*

Chloride *Serum Decrease Physiological* Review of 48 patients who had received oxcarbazepine showed that 4 had developed hypochloremia *662*

Cortisol, Free *Urine No Effect Analytical* No significant interference observed with HPLC method of Turpeinen et al *6105*

Dehydroepiandrosterone Sulfate

Plasma Decrease Physiological Insignificant decrease from mean baseline concentration of 8.3 µmol/L to 8.1 µmol/L after 8 days chronic treatment and 7.7 µmol/L after 15 days but with increase to 9.9 µmol/L after study *3413*

Plasma No Effect Physiological In 12 epileptic men aged 21 to 40 years treated with oxcarbazepine for 6 months mean concentration of 8.6 ± 3.0 µmol/L significantly different from concentration when treated with carbamazepine (mean concentration of 5.4 ± 1.7 µmol/L) but not different from normal of 0.8 - 16.0 µmol/L *2841*

Felodipine *Serum Decrease Physiological* Repeated doses of oxcarbazepine caused significant reduction of area under the curve by 28% and maximum plasma concentration from mean baseline of 16.0 ± 4.4 nmol/L to 10.4 ± 4.1 nmol/L (34%) with 900 mg/d *6623*

Follicle Stimulating Hormone

Plasma Increase Physiological Significant increase from mean baseline concentration of 3.2 U/L to 4.2 U/L after 8 days and 4.6 U/L after 15 days chronic treatment in 8 healthy men with continuing increase post-study *3413*

Plasma No Effect Physiological In 12 epileptic men aged 21 to 40 years treated with oxcarbazepine for 6 months mean concentration of 5.3 ± 4.0 IU/L significantly different from concentration when treated with carbamazepine (mean concentration of 5.4 ± 4.0 IU/L and not different from normal) *2841*

6-β-Hydroxycortisol *Urine No Effect Physiological* Excretion unaltered by chronic dosing in 8 healthy male volunteers *3413*

Luteinizing Hormone *Plasma Increase Physiological* Insignificant increase from mean baseline of 6.3 IU/L to 7.2 IU/L after 8 and 15 days chronic treatment but significant increase to 8.1 IU/L post-study in 8 healthy men *3413*
Plasma No Effect Physiological In 12 epileptic men aged 21 to 40 years treated with oxcarbazepine for 6 months mean concentration of 4.9 ± 1.9 IU/L significantly different from concentration when treated with carbamazepine (mean concentration of 5.0 ± 2.3 IU/L and not different from normal) *2841*

Prolactin *Plasma Increase Physiological* Significant increase from mean baseline concentration of 118 mU/L to 170 mU/L after 8 days chronic treatment and 131 mU/L (insignificant) after 15 days with further rise to 186 mU/L post-study in 8 healthy men *3413*
Plasma No Effect Physiological In 12 epileptic men aged 21 to 40 years treated with oxcarbazepine for 6 months mean concentration of 9.9 ± 3.6 µg/L significantly different from concentration when treated with carbamazepine (mean concentration of 11.9 ± 4.5 µg/L and not different from normal) *2841*

Sex-Hormone Binding Globulin
Serum No Effect Physiological In 12 epileptic men aged 21 to 40 years treated with oxcarbazepine for 6 months mean concentration of 39.3 ± 15.6 nmol/L not significantly different from normal concentration of 11.2 - 42.0 nmol/L but significantly less than when the patients were treated with carbamazepine (mean concentration of 50.5 ± 20.6 nmol/L) *2841* Insignificant change from baseline concentration of 24.9 nmol/L to 25.4 nmol/L after 8 days, 22.9 nmol/L after 15 days chronic treatment and 22.4 nmol/L post-treatment in 8 healthy men *3413*

Sodium *Serum Decrease Physiological* Review of 48 patients who had received oxcarbazepine showed that 9 had developed hyponatremia *662*

Testosterone *Serum No Effect Physiological* Insignificant reduction from mean baseline concentration of 14.3 nmol/L to 13.3 nmol/L after 8 days and 12.6 nmol/L after 15 days chronic treatment in 8 healthy men but with slight rise to 13.9 nmol/L following the study *3413* In 12 epileptic men aged 21 to 40 years treated with oxcarbazepine for 6 months mean concentration of 23.4 ± 8.9 nmol/L not significantly different from concentration when treated with carbamazepine (mean concentration of 25.8 ± 4.6 nmol/L not significantly different from normal) *2841*

Testosterone, Free *Serum No Effect Physiological* In 12 epileptic men aged 21 to 40 years treated with oxcarbazepine for 6 months mean concentration of 70.8 ± 16.5 pmol/L not significantly different from concentration when treated with carbamazepine (mean concentration of 76.4 ± 20.8 pmol/L not significantly different from normal) *2841*

Oxedrine

Glucose *Serum No Effect Analytical* At concentration of 60 mg/L had no effect on GOD/POD-PAP method *5704*

Triglycerides *Serum No Effect Analytical* At concentration of 60 mg/L had no effect on GPO-PAP method *5704*

Uric Acid *Serum No Effect Analytical* At concentration of 60 mg/L had no effect on uricase-PAP method *5704*

Oxmetidine

pH *Gastric Material Increase Physiological* pH 5 reached 80 minutes after 200 mg drug *4253*

Prolactin *Plasma No Effect Physiological* No significant effect during treatment *4253*

Volume *Gastric Fluid Decrease Physiological* Significant inhibition following treatment *4253*

Oxolinic Acid

Ciprofloxacin *Serum Increase Analytical* Cannot be assayed by HPLC method used at Mayo Clinic in presence of oxolinic acid *3858*

Norfloxacin *Serum Increase Analytical* Cannot be assayed by HPLC method used at Mayo Clinic in presence of oxolinic acid *3858*

Oxoprogesterone

Progesterone *Plasma Increase Analytical* 22% cross reactivity with RIA method of Cameron *858*

2-Oxoquinidinone

Quinidine *Serum No Effect Analytical* No significant interference observed from 2'-oxoquinidinone at a concentration of 20 µg/mL (58.8 µmol/L) with method on Du Pont aca *1543*

Oxprenolol

Albumin *Serum Decrease Physiological* Significant decrease from mean baseline concentration of 655 µmol/L to 617 µmol/L at four hours and insignificant decrease to 625 µmol/L in 6 patients with hyperthyroidism treated with 160 mg daily for one week *3077*

Cholesterol *Serum Increase Physiological* Mild effect as possessed relatively weak intrinsic sympathomimetic activity *3499*
Serum No Effect Physiological In several studies treated for more than 1 mo *142* In 20 hypertensive men given 160 mg/d for 5 weeks *3521* Insignificant effect in 12 patients receiving 160 mg/d for 2 weeks *2953*

Fatty Acids (FFA), Free *Serum Decrease Physiological* Marked effect in 53 patients given 80 mg twice daily for 3 mo *1292*

Glomerular Filtration Rate *Urine Decrease Physiological* Observed with acute experiments *2804*

Growth Hormone *Plasma Increase Physiological* Observed with chronic treatment of 5 active hypertensive patients *1819*

HDL-Cholesterol *Serum Decrease Physiological* Significant effect in 53 patients given 80 mg/twice daily for 3 mo *1292* Mild effect as possessed relatively weak intrinsic sympathomimetic activity *3499*
Serum No Effect Physiological In 20 hypertensive men given 160 mg/d for 5 weeks *3521* In several studies of 1-4 mo *142*

5-Hydroxyindoleacetic Acid *Urine Increase Analytical* Interferes with screening tests with nitrosonaphthol *2950*

17-Ketosteroids *Urine No Effect Analytical* No effect of treatment on concentration as measured by Zimmermann method *4421*

LDL-Cholesterol *Serum Increase Physiological* Mild effect as possessed relatively weak intrinsic sympathomimetic activity *3499*
Serum No Effect Physiological In several studies of 1-4 mo *142*

Metanephrines, Total *Urine Increase Analytical* Especially when combined with other antihypertensive drugs and HPLC method used unless toluene extraction used *1162*

Phosphate *Serum Increase Physiological* In 6 patients with hyperthyroidism given 160 mg daily for 1 week: Baseline concentration was 0.98 mmol/L, with concentration of 1.36 mmol/L 4 hours after start of treatment and 1.36 mmol/L after one week *3077*

Platelets *Blood Decrease Physiological* Observed in one patient after slow release drug normalized within 7 d of withdrawal of drug *1455* Observed with regular preparation in one individual *2461*

Potassium *Serum Increase Physiological* Slight rise observed in patients treated with moderate doses *4739*

Renin Activity *Plasma Decrease Physiological* In 10 patients with essential hypertension treated over 5 weeks: significant effect with plasma concentration of about 1,000 ng/mL *1836*

Terbutaline *Serum Increase Physiological* Decreased clearance and increased area under curve when co-administered *2977*

Triglycerides *Serum Increase Physiological* Increase by 22-27% in several studies treated for more than 1 mo *142* Marked effect in 53 patients given 80 mg twice daily for 3 mo *1292* Increase by 22% in 20 hypertensive men given 160 mg/d for 5 weeks *3521* Mild effect as possessed relatively weak intrinsic sympathomimetic activity *3499*

Oxprenolol *(continued)*

Triglycerides *(continued)*
Serum No Effect Physiological Insignificant effect in 12 patients receiving 160 mg/d for 2 weeks *2953* In several studies treated for more than 1 mo *142*

Uric Acid *Serum No Effect Physiological* In 20 hypertensive men given 160 mg/d for 5 weeks *3521*

VLDL-Cholesterol *Serum No Effect Physiological* In several studies of 1-4 mo *142* In 20 hypertensive men given 160 mg/d for 5 weeks *3521*

VLDL-Triglycerides *Serum Increase Physiological* In several studies of 1-4 mo *142* Significant effect in 53 patients given 80 mg twice daily for 3 mo *1292*

Oxybutyrin

Cortisol, Free *Urine No Effect Analytical* No significant interference observed with HPLC method of Turpeinen et al *6105*

Oxycodone

Blood *Urine Increase Physiological* May occur as a side effect in less than 1% of patients treated in clinical trials *5997*

Cannabinoids *Urine No Effect Analytical* No effect on Roche Abuscreen method *5006*

Histamine *Plasma No Effect Analytical* No inhibition of radio-enzyme assay likely at physiological concentrations *2492*

Opiates *Urine Positive Analytical* At concentration of 50 µg/mL (159 µmol/L) on method Du Pont aca *1559*

Sodium *Serum Decrease Physiological* May occur as a side effect in less than 1% of patients treated in clinical trials *5997*

Oxycycline

Prostate-specific Antigen, Free *Serum No Effect Analytical* Goserelin acetate at a concentration of 2.6 µg/mL had no significant effect on the Hybritech Tandem® -R free PSA immunoassay *4286*

Oxymetazoline

Corticosteroids *Plasma Decrease Physiological* Clear suppression when induction compared with induction by thiopentone *113*

Oxymetholone

α_1-Acid Glycoprotein *Serum Increase Physiological* Anabolic metabolic effect *368*

Alanine Aminotransferase *Serum Increase Physiological* Cholestatic effect (increased up to 6 times normal) *2803*

Alkaline Phosphatase *Serum Increase Physiological* Cholestatic effect *2803* One case of peliosis hepatitis reported *3886* Cholestatic hepatitis developed in two patients *6613*

α_1-Antitrypsin *Serum Increase Physiological* Metabolic effect *368*

Aspartate Aminotransferase *Serum Increase Physiological* One case of peliosis hepatitis reported *3886* Cholestatic hepatitis developed in two patients *6613* Cholestatic effect (increased up to 6 times normal) *2803*

Bilirubin *Serum Increase Physiological* Cholestatic hepatitis developed in two patients *6613* One case of peliosis hepatitis reported *3886* Cholestatic effect *2803*

BSP Retention *Serum Increase Physiological* Cholestatic hepatitis developed in two patients *6613* Cholestatic effect *2803*

Calcium *Serum Increase Physiological* May occur spontaneously or if carcinoma of breast *2753*

Ceruloplasmin *Serum No Effect Physiological* No metabolic effect *368*

Cholesterol *Serum Decrease Physiological* May cause decrease with therapy *2753*
Serum Increase Physiological Cholestatic effect *2803*

Creatine *Urine Increase Physiological* Anabolic effect (possible for 2 weeks after stopping drug) *2753*

Creatinine *Urine Increase Physiological* Anabolic effect (possible for 2 weeks after stopping drug) *2753*

Erythropoietin *Urine Increase Physiological* Enhances production and excretion if anemia *2753*

Factor II *Plasma Increase Physiological* Anabolic effect increasing factors *2753*

Factor V *Plasma Increase Physiological* Anabolic effect increasing factors *2753*

Factor VII *Plasma Increase Physiological* Anabolic effect increasing factors *2753*

Factor X *Plasma Increase Physiological* Anabolic effect increasing factors *2753*

Fibrinogen *Plasma Increase Physiological* Metabolic effect *368*

Glucose *Serum Decrease Physiological* Anabolic effect (possible for 2 weeks after stopping drug) *2753*

β-Glucuronidase *Serum Increase Physiological* Metabolic effect *368*

Haptoglobin *Serum Increase Physiological* Metabolic effect *368*

^{131}I Uptake *Serum Increase Physiological* Anabolic effect (possible for 2 weeks after stopping drug) *2753*

Iron *Serum Decrease Physiological* Iron deficiency anemia may occur *2753*

Iron-Binding Capacity, Unsaturated
Serum Increase Physiological Decreases percentage saturation of transferrin *2753*

17-Ketosteroids *Urine Decrease Physiological* Anabolic effect (possible for 2 weeks after stopping drug) *2753*

Metyrapone Test *Patient Positive Physiological* Anabolic effect (possible for 2 weeks after stopping drug) *2753*

Plasminogen *Plasma Increase Physiological* Metabolic effect *368*

Prothrombin Time *Plasma Increase Physiological* May increase sensitivity to anticoagulants *2753* Also seen with other 17-alkyl substituted steroids *1667*

Sialic Acid *Serum Increase Physiological* Metabolic effect *368*

T3-Uptake *Serum Increase Physiological* Anabolic effect (possible for 2 weeks after stop) *2753*

Thyroxine Binding Globulin
Serum Decrease Physiological Direct effect of drug *42*

Thyroxine (T4), Free *Serum No Effect Physiological* Anabolic effect (possible for 2 weeks after stop) *2753*

Triglycerides *Serum Decrease Physiological* Anabolic effect *513*

Urobilinogen *Feces Decrease Physiological* Cholestatic effect *2803*
Urine Decrease Physiological Cholestatic effect *2803*

Oxyphenbutazone

Alanine Aminotransferase *Serum Increase Physiological* Possible hepatotoxicity *3810*

Alkaline Phosphatase *Serum Increase Physiological* Possible hepatotoxicity *3810*

Amylase *Serum Increase Physiological* Parotitis is rare complication of therapy *2348* Occasional case of acute swelling of salivary glands *977*

Aspartate Aminotransferase *Serum Increase Physiological* Possible hepatotoxicity *3810*

Bile *Urine Increase Physiological* Possible hepatotoxicity *3810*

Bilirubin *Serum Increase Physiological* Possible hepatotoxicity *3810*
Serum No Effect Analytical No effect at 24 mg/L on Ames Seralyzer method *5706*
Serum No Effect Physiological Probably little or no effect on displacement from protein *6314*

BSP Retention *Serum Increase Physiological* Possible hepatotoxicity *3810*

Chloride *Serum Increase Physiological* May cause marked salt retention *3810*

Cholesterol *Serum No Effect Analytical* At concentration of 600 mg/L had no effect on catalase-AIDH method *5704* At concentration of 600 mg/L had no effect on Liebermann-Burchard method *5704* At concentration of 600 mg/L had no effect on method using catalase-Hantzsch reaction *5704* No effect at 24 mg/L on Ames Seralyzer method *5706* At concentration of 600 mg/L had no effect on CHOD-PAP method *5704* At concentration of 600 mg/L had no effect on CHOD-Iodide method *5704*

Color *Feces Increase Analytical* Pink/red color reported with oxyphenbutazone administration *3388*
Urine Increase Analytical Red color observed following ingestion of oxyphenbutazone *3388*

Creatine Kinase *Serum No Effect Analytical* No effect at 24 mg/L on method on Ames Seralyzer *5706*

Creatinine *Serum Increase Physiological* Numerous reports of kidney damage up to acute renal failure following therapeutic use of drug *4777*
Serum No Effect Analytical At concentration of 600 mg/L had no effect on kinetic Jaffe method on BKA-2 *5704* No effect at 24 mg/L on method on Ames Seralyzer *5706* At concentration of 120 mg/L had no effect on Jaffe-Fading-Fraction method *5704* At concentration of 120 mg/L had no effect on Jaffe-Fuller's earth method *5704* At concentration of 220 mg/L had no effect on creatinine iminohydrolase method *5704*

Creatinine Clearance *Urine Decrease Physiological* Numerous reports of kidney damage up to acute renal failure following therapeutic use of drug *4777*

Crystals *Urine Increase Physiological* May cause crystallization of uric acid *51*

Erythrocytes *Blood Decrease Physiological* Aplastic anemia with death in 38 per 100,000 users *2822* Occasional case of aplastic anemia reported *6264* May cause blood dyscrasias *3810*
Urine Increase Physiological May cause actual bleeding *1714* Numerous reports of kidney damage up to acute renal failure following therapeutic use of drug *4777*

Glucose *Serum Decrease Analytical* At concentrations above 25 mg/L (normal therapeutic concentration 20 mg/L) lowered concentration as measured by GOD-PERID method *5704*
Serum Increase Physiological Metabolic/endocrine response *2754*
Serum No Effect Analytical At concentration of 12 mg/L had no effect on Kodak Ektachem® method *5704* At concentration of 200 mg/L had no effect on hexokinase/G-6-PDH method *5704* No effect of concentrations up to 12 mg/L on method on Kodak Ektachem® *5706* No effect at 24 mg/L on glucose oxidase method on Ames Seralyzer *5706*

Hematocrit *Blood Decrease Physiological* Dilutional effect of water retention *2242*

Hemoglobin *Blood Decrease Physiological* Dilutional effect of water retention *2242*
Urine Increase Physiological Actual bleeding caused by drug *1714*

^{131}I Uptake *Serum Decrease Physiological* Impaired synthesis of thyroxine *3107*

Lactate *Plasma No Effect Analytical* At concentration of 120 mg/L had no effect on enzymatic method *5704*

Lactate Dehydrogenase *Serum No Effect Analytical* No effect at 24 mg/L on method on Ames Seralyzer *5706*

Leukocytes *Blood Decrease Physiological* Rare side effect reported to UK Committee on Safety of Medicines *1204* Occasional case of aplastic anemia reported *6264* Agranulocytosis/Leukopenia *3810*
Blood Increase Physiological May cause leukemia type of reaction *51*

Lithium *Serum Increase Physiological* Single case report of lithium toxicity in one patient following the administration of 500 mg/day of oxyphenbutazone *4831*

Neutrophils *Blood Decrease Physiological* May cause neutropenia *4265* Occasional case of drug-induced neutropenia *241* Occasional case of agranulocytosis reported *6264*

Occult Blood *Feces Increase Physiological* May cause gastrointestinal bleeding *128* Rare side effect reported to UK Committee on Safety of medicines *1204*

Platelets *Blood Decrease Physiological* Thrombocytopenia may occur after 1 week therapy *3810* Rare side effect reported to UK Committee on Safety of Medicines *1204* Occasional case of aplastic anemia reported *6264*

Potassium *Serum No Effect Analytical* At concentration of 120 mg/L had no effect on measurement by ISE without predilution *5704*

Protein *Urine Increase Physiological* May be nephrotoxicity *2754* May cause renal damage *51*

Protein Electrophoresis *Serum No Effect Analytical* At concentration of 120 mg/L had no effect on automated Olympus-Hite method *5704*

Prothrombin Time *Plasma Increase Physiological* Displaces anticoagulants from albumin *3810*

Sodium *Serum Increase Physiological* May cause marked salt retention *3810*
Serum No Effect Analytical At concentration of 120 mg/L had no effect on measurement by ISE without predilution *5704*

T3-Uptake *Serum Increase Physiological* Impaired synthesis of thyroxine *3107*

Thyroxine (T4) *Serum Decrease Analytical* Yellow eluate persists in reaction mixture *882*
Serum Decrease Physiological Impaired synthesis may occur *3107*

Tolbutamide *Serum Increase Physiological* Half-life increased from 8.1 to 30.2 hours in 2 volunteers with coadministration of drugs, probably due to induction of a form of cytochrome P-450 *4740*

Triglycerides *Serum No Effect Analytical* At concentration of 120 mg/L had no effect on GPO-PAP method *5704*

Urea Nitrogen *Serum Increase Physiological* Numerous reports of kidney damage up to acute renal failure following therapeutic use of drug *4777* May occur with renal damage *3669*
Serum No Effect Analytical At concentration of 12 mg/L had no effect on Kodak Ektachem® method *5704* No effect at 24 mg/L on method on Ames Seralyzer *5706*

Uric Acid *Serum Decrease Physiological* Uricosuric effect *1112*
Serum Increase Analytical At concentrations above 200 mg/L (normal therapeutic concentration 20 mg/L) raised concentration as measured by Kageyama-Hantzsch method *5704*
Serum No Effect Analytical At concentration of 120 mg/L had no effect on catalase-AIDH method *5704*

Volume *Plasma Increase Physiological* May cause marked salt and water retention *2242*
Urine Decrease Physiological May cause marked water retention *2242*

Oxyphencyclimine

Hydrochloric Acid *Gastric Fluid Decrease Physiological* Absolute decrease by 60%, but not concentration *4200*

Pepsin *Gastric Material Decrease Physiological* Absolute decrease by 60%, but not concentration *4200*

Volume *Gastric Fluid Decrease Physiological* Basal output decreased by 60% *4200*

Oxyphenisatin

Alanine Aminotransferase *Serum Increase Physiological* May cause hypersensitivity reaction *4934* Liver damage may present as acute hepatitis or as more advanced chronic disease: usual liver disease is chronic active hepatitis *3725*

Albumin *Serum Decrease Physiological* May cause hypersensitivity reaction *4934* Observed with chronic active hepatitis induced by drug *1425*

Alkaline Phosphatase *Serum Increase Physiological* Observed with chronic active hepatitis induced by drug *1425* Hepatic toxicity if over prolonged period *4574*

Anti-Smooth Muscle Antibodies
Serum Increase Physiological As component of hypersensi-

Oxyphenisatin *(continued)*

Anti-Smooth Muscle Antibodies *(continued)*
tivity response *2144* Liver damage may present as acute hepatitis or as more advanced chronic disease: usual liver disease is chronic active hepatitis *3725*

Antimitochondrial Antibodies
Serum Increase Physiological Very rare observation with chronic hepatitis *2144*

Antinuclear Antibodies *Serum Increase Physiological* Liver damage may present as acute hepatitis or as more advanced chronic disease: usual liver disease is chronic active hepatitis *3725* May cause hypersensitivity reaction *4934*

Aspartate Aminotransferase *Serum Increase Physiological* Observed with chronic active hepatitis induced by drug *1425* Liver damage may present as acute hepatitis or as more advanced chronic disease: usual liver disease is chronic active hepatitis *3725* Hepatic toxicity if over prolonged period *4574*

Bile *Urine Increase Physiological* May cause hypersensitivity reaction *4934*

Bilirubin *Serum Increase Physiological* Observed with chronic active hepatitis induced by drug *1425* Liver damage may present as acute hepatitis or as more advanced chronic disease: usual liver disease is chronic active hepatitis *3725* Hepatic toxicity if over prolonged period *4574*

BSP Retention *Serum Increase Physiological* May cause hypersensitivity reaction *4934*

Coombs' Test *Blood Positive Physiological* May cause hypersensitivity reaction *4934*

Coombs' Test, Direct *Blood Positive Physiological* Single case with positive LE cell test *2452*

γ-Globulin *Serum Increase Physiological* May cause hypersensitivity reaction *4934*

^{131}I Uptake *Serum Decrease Physiological* Dialose contains tetraiodofluorescein *4360*

immunoglobulin A *Serum Increase Physiological* As component of hypersensitivity response *2144*

Immunoglobulin G *Serum Increase Physiological* Observed with chronic active hepatitis induced by drug *1425*

Lactate Dehydrogenase *Serum Increase Physiological* Increase observed with active hepatitis *120*

LE Cells *Blood Positive Physiological* Liver damage may present as acute hepatitis or as more advanced chronic disease: usual liver disease is chronic active hepatitis *3725* May cause lupoid hepatitis *4934*

Ornithine Carbamoyltransferase
Serum Increase Physiological Rare increase with chronic active hepatitis *2144* Observed when combined with iron preparation *2145*

Prothrombin Time *Plasma Increase Physiological* May cause hypersensitivity reaction *4934*

Rheumatoid Factor *Serum Increase Physiological* Liver damage may present as acute hepatitis or as more advanced chronic disease: usual liver disease is chronic active hepatitis *3725*

Oxypurinol

Chloride *Serum Decrease Analytical* At concentrations above 200 mg/L apparently reduces concentration of chloride as measured by Kodak Ektachem® *5706*

Lipase *Serum No Effect Analytical* No significant effect observed at a concentration of 9 μg/mL with method on Kodak Ektachem® systems *2519*

11-Oxysteroids

Amino Acids *Plasma Increase Physiological* Promote tissue catabolism *570*

α-Amino-Nitrogen *Plasma Increase Physiological* Promote tissue catabolism *1714*
Urine Increase Physiological Promote tissue catabolism *3810*

Oxytetracycline

Alanine Aminotransferase *Serum No Effect Analytical* No effect at therapeutic concentration on Boehringer Mannheim Reflotron method *3231* No effect at 160 mg/L on Boehringer Mannheim Reflotron method *5706*

Albumin *Urine No Effect Analytical* At concentration of 32 mg/dL had no significant effect on Boehringer Mannheim Tinaquant method *2799*

Amylase *Serum No Effect Analytical* No effect of concentrations up to 160 mg/L on method on Boehringer Mannheim Reflotron *5706*

Amylase, Pancreatic Isoenzyme
Serum No Effect Analytical No significant effect observed at toxic concentration of 100 mg/L on method on Boehringer Mannheim Reflotron *3647*

Aspartate Aminotransferase *Serum No Effect Analytical* No effect at therapeutic concentration on Boehringer Mannheim Reflotron method *3231* No effect at 160 mg/L on Boehringer Mannheim Reflotron method *5706*

Bilirubin *Serum Increase Analytical* At concentrations above 50 mg/L raised concentration as measured by Jendrassik and Grof method *5704*
Serum No Effect Analytical At concentration of 160 mg/L no effect on method on Boehringer Mannheim Reflotron system *5706*
Serum No Effect Physiological Clinically insignificant displacement from protein in neonates *6314*

Calcium *Serum No Effect Analytical* At concentration of 50 mg/L had no effect on cresolphthalein method *5704*

Catecholamines *Plasma Increase Analytical* Interferes with fluorometric methods *6515*

Chloramphenicol *Serum No Effect Analytical* No effect at 100 mg/L on coupled enzymatic method *4122*

Cholesterol *Serum No Effect Analytical* No effect at therapeutic concentration on Boehringer Mannheim Reflotron method *3231* At concentration of 160 mg/L no effect on method on Boehringer Mannheim Reflotron system *5706*
Serum No Effect Physiological No effect seen even when administered orally *2452*

Cortisol *Plasma No Effect Analytical* At concentration of 100 mg/L no significant effect observed on CEDIA or Enzymun methods (worst case 95.0% recovery) *1097*

Creatinine *Serum No Effect Analytical* No effect of concentrations up to 15 mg/L on single slide method on Kodak Ektachem® *5706*

Dehydroepiandrosterone Sulfate
Plasma No Effect Physiological Despite decreased urine excretion and increased fecal excretion of estrogens due to decreased hydrolysis by β-glucuronidase in gastrointestinal tract *2420*

Eosinophils *Blood Increase Physiological* Hemolytic anemia, thrombocytopenia, neutropenia and eosinophilia have been reported as adverse reactions *4656*

Estradiol *Plasma No Effect Physiological* Despite decreased urine excretion and increased fecal excretion of estrogens due to decreased hydrolysis by β-glucuronidase in gastrointestinal tract *2420*

Estriol *Urine Decrease Physiological* Probably due to decreased hydrolysis by β-glucuronidase of estrogen conjugates in intestinal tract, with increased fecal loss *2420*

Estriol-3-Glucuronide *Urine Decrease Physiological* Probably due to decreased hydrolysis by β-glucuronidase of estrogen conjugates in intestinal tract with increased fecal loss *2420*

Estrone *Plasma No Effect Physiological* Despite decreased urine excretion and increased fecal excretion of estrogens due to decreased hydrolysis by β-glucuronidase in gastrointestinal tract *2420*

Folate *Urine Increase Physiological* With dose of 2.5 g/d *2242*

Glucose *Serum Decrease Physiological* Mild hypoglycemic effect observed in diabetics *5443*
Serum No Effect Analytical At concentration of 160 mg/L no effect on method on Boehringer Mannheim Reflotron system *5706* At concentration of 600 mg/L had no effect on hexokinase/G-6-PDH method *5704* No effect at therapeutic concentration on Boehringer Mannheim Reflotron method *3231*

Urine Decrease Analytical Affects dipsticks if buffered with ascorbic acid *2559*

γ-Glutamyltransferase *Serum No Effect Analytical* No effect at therapeutic concentration on Boehringer Mannheim Reflotron method *3231* At concentration of 160 mg/L no effect on method on Boehringer Mannheim Reflotron system *5706*

HDL-Cholesterol *Serum No Effect Analytical* At a concentration up to 160 mg/L had no significant effect on Reflotron method for whole blood cholesterol *6352*

Hematocrit *Blood Decrease Physiological* Hemolytic anemia, thrombocytopenia and eosinophilia have been reported as adverse reactions *4656*

Hemoglobin *Blood Decrease Physiological* Hemolytic anemia, thrombocytopenia and eosinophilia have been reported as adverse reactions *4656*

^{131}I Uptake *Serum Decrease Physiological* Terramycin® contains tetraiodofluorescein *4360*

Lactate *Plasma No Effect Analytical* At concentration of 600 mg/L had no effect on enzymatic method *5704*

Luteinizing Hormone *Plasma No Effect Physiological* Despite decreased urine excretion and increased fecal excretion of estrogens due decreased hydrolysis by β-glucuronidase in gastrointestinal tract *2420*

Metanephrines, Total *Urine Increase Analytical* Interferes with fluorometric methods *6515*

N-Acetyl-Glucosaminidase *Urine No Effect Analytical* At concentration of 32 mg/dL no significant effect observed on Boehringer Mannheim CPR method *3174*

Neutrophils *Blood Decrease Physiological* Hemolytic anemia, thrombocytopenia, neutropenia and eosinophilia have been reported as adverse reactions *4656*

Nitrogen *Urine Increase Physiological* Observed in malnourished *2242*

N-Methylnicotinamide *Urine Increase Physiological* With dose of 2.5 g/d *2242*

Phenylalanine *Plasma No Effect Analytical* No interference observed with rapid quantitative whole blood method of Campbell et al using phenylalanine dehydrogenase *867*

Phosphate *Serum No Effect Analytical* At concentration of 50 mg/L had no effect on phosphomolybdate method *5704*

Platelets *Blood Decrease Physiological* Thrombocytopenia reported to occur *2385* Hemolytic anemia, thrombocytopenia, neutropenia and eosinophilia have been reported as adverse reactions *4656*

Porphyrin, Total *Urine Increase Analytical* Produces interfering fluorescence *2025*

Protein *Cerebrospinal Fluid Increase Analytical* Reacts as if phenol with Folin-Ciocalteu procedure *6681*
Serum No Effect Analytical At concentration of 50 mg/L had no effect on biuret method with blank correction *5704*

Prothrombin Time *Plasma Decrease Physiological* May depress prothrombin activity *4656*

Riboflavin *Urine Increase Physiological* With dose of 2.5 g/d *2242*

Sugar *Urine Increase Analytical* Acts as reducing agent *6515*

Testosterone *Serum No Effect Physiological* Despite decreased urine excretion and increased fecal excretion of estrogens due to decreased hydrolysis by β-glucuronidase in gastrointestinal tract *2420*

Testosterone, Free *Serum No Effect Physiological* Despite decreased urine excretion and increased fecal excretion of estrogens due to decreased hydrolysis by β-glucuronidase in gastrointestinal tract *2769*

Triglycerides *Serum No Effect Analytical* No effect at therapeutic concentration on Boehringer Mannheim Reflotron method *3231* No effect at 160 mg/L on Boehringer Mannheim Reflotron method *5706*

Urea Nitrogen *Serum Increase Physiological* Dose related nephrotoxicity occurs rarely *4656*
Serum No Effect Analytical No effect at therapeutic concentration on Boehringer Mannheim Reflotron method *3231* No effect at 160 mg/L on Boehringer Mannheim Reflotron method *5706* At concentration of 50 mg/L had no effect on diacetylmonoxime method *5704*

Uric Acid *Serum Increase Analytical* At concentrations above 50 mg/L raised concentration as measured by phosphotungstate reduction method *5704*
Serum No Effect Analytical No effect at therapeutic concentration on Boehringer Mannheim Reflotron method *3231* No effect at 160 mg/L on Boehringer Mannheim Reflotron method *5706*

Vanillylmandelic Acid *Urine Increase Analytical* Produces interfering color in reaction *6515*

p-Aminophenol

Aspartate Aminotransferase *Serum Increase Analytical* At 1 mmol/L affects Technicon SMA 12/60 method *5576*

Bilirubin *Serum Increase Analytical* At 1 mmol/L affects Technicon SMA 12/60 method *5576*
Serum No Effect Analytical At concentration of 109 mg/L had no effect on Jendrassik and Grof method *5704*

Calcium *Serum Increase Analytical* At concentrations above 10 mg/L raised concentration as measured by cresolphthalein method *5704* At 0.1 mmol/L affects Technicon SMA 12/60 method *5576*

Chloride *Serum No Effect Analytical* At concentration of 5 mg/L had no effect on mercurimetric method *5704*

Glucose *Serum Decrease Analytical* At concentrations above 25 mg/L lowered concentration as measured by GOD-PERID method *5704*
Serum Increase Analytical At 1 mmol/L affects Technicon SMA 12/60 method *5576*
Serum No Effect Analytical At concentration of 200 mg/L had no effect on hexokinase/G-6-PDH method *5704* No effect on method on Fuji Drichem 1000 at concentration up to 200 mg/L *5706* At concentration of 50 mg/L had no effect on Kodak Ektachem® method *5704*

Phosphate *Serum No Effect Analytical* At concentration of 109 mg/L had no effect on phosphomolybdate method *5704*

Protein *Serum No Effect Analytical* At concentration of 109 mg/L had no effect on biuret method with blank correction *5704*

Urea Nitrogen *Serum Increase Analytical* May react in Berthelot procedure *3033*
Serum No Effect Analytical At concentration of 109 mg/L had no effect on diacetylmonoxime method *5704*

Uric Acid *Serum Increase Analytical* At 1 mmol/L affects Technicon SMA 12/60 and Henry methods *5576* At concentrations above 5 mg/L raised concentration as measured by phosphotungstate reduction method *5704*

p-Aminosalicylic Acid

Acid Phosphatase *Serum Increase Analytical* Positive bias of 1.8 U/L observed at a concentration of 40 mg/dL with method on Kodak Ektachem® *2519*

Calcium *Serum No Effect Analytical* At a concentration of 23 mg/dL caused no significant effect on method on Kodak Ektachem® systems *2519*

Glucose *Urine No Effect Analytical* Has no effect on Ames Keto-Diastix, Diastix, Multistix, Clinistix and Clinitest methods *4034*

Protein *Urine Increase Analytical* PAS in urines containing certain preservatives may cause false positive with Sulfosalicylic Acid and Exton's reagent tests *4034*
Urine No Effect Analytical PAS in urine containing certain preservatives has no effect on protein test areas of Ames Multistix and other reagent strip tests *4034*

Rifampin *Serum Decrease Physiological* When drugs coadministered rifampin concentration may be decreased so drugs should be administered 4 hours apart *1037*

Urobilinogen *Urine Increase Analytical* May react with urobilinogen test area on Ames Multistix and other reagent test strips *4034*
Urine No Effect Analytical Has no effect on Watson semi-quantitative test if blank is used *4034*

p-Hydroxy-phenylhydantoin

Carbamazepine *Serum No Effect Analytical* No cross-reactivity observed with method on Du Pont aca *1513*

Ethosuximide *Serum No Effect Analytical* Insugnificant cross-reactivity observed with method on Du Pont aca *1523*

Phenytoin *Serum Increase Analytical* Less than 10% cross-reactivity observed with whole blood enzyme inhibition immunoassay used with Abbott Vision analyzer *5348*

Primidone *Serum No Effect Analytical* No significant cross-reactivity with method on Du Pont aca *1541*

p-Hydroxyamphetamine

Amphetamine/Methamphetamine
Serum Increase Analytical At a concentration of 10000 ng/mL caused 25.9% cross-reactivity with method on Abbott AxSYM and 38.5% with method on TDx *6404*

p-Hydroxyphenobarbital

Phenobarbital *Serum No Effect Analytical* Cross-reactivity of less than 1.3% observed with method on Baxter Stratus *5705*

Primidone *Serum No Effect Analytical* At a concentration of 940 mg/L causes 25% increase with method on Baxter Stratus but this probably exceeds physiological concentration *5705*

p-Hydroxyphenyl-phenylhydantoin

Phenytoin *Serum Decrease Analytical* Reacts quantitatively in radioimmunoassay *6029*
Serum Increase Analytical 2.2% cross-reactivity observed with Kodak thin-film method *347*

Paclitaxel

Granulocytes *Blood Decrease Physiological* In 15 patients with advanced gastric cancer treatment with paclitaxel up to 225 mg/m^2 caused grade 1-2 leukopenia in 5 patients, 1 at 175 mg/m^2, 2 at 200 mg/m^2 and 2 at 225 mg/m^2*910*

Hematocrit *Blood Decrease Physiological* In 15 patients with advanced gastric cancer treatment with paclitaxel 225 mg/m^2 caused grade 1-2 anemia in 1 patient *910* Anemia reported in 9 of 95 patients when pacitaxel only administered *2079*

Hemoglobin *Blood Decrease Physiological* In 15 patients with advanced gastric cancer treatment with paclitaxel 225 mg/m^2 caused grade 1-2 anemia in 1 patient *4528* Anemia reported in 9 of 95 patients when pacitaxel only administered *2079*

Leukocytes *Blood Decrease Physiological* Leukopenia reported in 17 of 95 patients when pacitaxel only administered *2079*

Neutrophils *Blood Decrease Physiological* Principal toxic effect noted, particularly when combined with cisplatin administered before paclitaxel due to decreased plasma clearance of paclitaxel possibly caused by the modulating effects of cisplatin on cytochrome P-450 enzymes *5125* Neutropenia is common although of brief duration *1384*

Platelets *Blood Decrease Physiological* In 15 patients with advanced gastric cancer treatment with paclitaxel 225 mg/m^2 caused grade 1-2 thrombocytopenia in 1 patient *910*

Pamabrom

Bromide *Serum Increase Physiological* Theoretical possibility since compound contains 23% bromide *5116*

Pamaquine

Bilirubin *Serum Increase Physiological* May cause hemolysis in G-6-PD deficiency *402*

Color *Urine Increase Analytical* Brown color *1714*

Erythrocytes *Blood Decrease Physiological* Hemolytic anemia in G-6-PD deficient persons *1212* May cause hemolytic anemia *3810*

Haptoglobin *Serum Decrease Physiological* May cause hemolytic anemia *1212*

Heinz Body Formation *Blood Positive Physiological* May occur in early stages of hemolysis *536*

Hematocrit *Blood Decrease Physiological* Hemolytic anemia in G-6-PD deficient persons *1212* May cause hemolytic anemia *3810*

Hemoglobin *Blood Decrease Physiological* Hemolytic anemia in G-6-PD deficient persons *1212* May cause hemolytic anemia *3810*

Methemoglobin *Blood Increase Physiological* May cause hemolysis in G-6-PD deficiency *6015* May cause hemolytic anemia *3810*

Pamidronate

Acid Phosphatase, Tartrate Resistant
Serum Decrease Physiological In 14 patients with Paget's disease treatment with 15 mg pamidronate for 5 days caused significant change from mean baseline of 6.1 ± 0.9 U/L to 5.1 ± 0.7 U/L on day 8, 4.5 ± 0.5 U/L on day 15 and 4.2 ± 0.7 U/L on day 30 *3819*

Albumin *Serum Decrease Physiological* In 29 patients with various malignant diseases treatment with pamidronate 60 mg intravenously for 4 h caused decrease from mean baseline of 40.6 ± 1.1 g/L to 40.7 ± 1.2 g/L when measured after 24 h and significant change to 39.2 ± 1.1 g/L at 48 h *5294*

Alkaline Phosphatase *Serum Decrease Physiological* In 13 patients with Paget's disease of the bone treatment with up to 6 weekly infusions of 60 mg caused reduction from mean baseline of 436 U/L to 353 U/L after 2 weeks and 189 U/L after 6 weeks *4850* In 71 patients with Paget's disease treatment with either mild, moderate or severe disease were treated with a total of 120, 180 or 240 mg causing a significant decrease in activity, with return to reference range by 6 months in 43 of 49 patients with mildest disease and in 3 of 13 in those with severest disease *2379* In patients with Paget's disease and alkaline phosphatase 3 times the upper limit of normal administration of pamidronate caused reduction of activity by 50% in 50% of patients and by 30% in 80% patients *271* In 30 children with osteogenesis imperfecta treatment with a mean of 6.8 ± 1.1 mg/kg/y over 4 to 12 cycles of treatment sustained decrease in activity of 14 ± 18% observed over a 3 to 4 month period, with steady decrease of 13 ± 8% per year *2188* In 24 patients with Paget's disease significant decrease observed with treatment from log 2.9 to log 2.6 with daily infusions for 10 days and to log 2.0 after 6 months *1403* Marked reduction observed in two cases of Paget's disease with fall from about 30 times the upper limit of the normal range to within the normal range *3755* Fall from 900 U/L to 250 U/L following 30 mg/d intravenously in one patient with calcitonin-resistant Paget's disease *1491* In 14 patients with Paget's disease treatment with 15 mg pamidronate for 5 days caused significant change from mean baseline of 2967 ± 737 U/L to 2716 ± 754 U/L on day 8, 1977 ± 513 U/L on day 15 and 1514 ± 421 U/L on day 30 *3819*

Alkaline Phosphatase, Bone Isoenzyme
Serum No Effect Analytical At a concentration of 180 mg/L had no effect on Tandem-MP Ostase method *777*

Calcium *Serum Decrease Physiological* In patients with hypercalcemia of malignancy treatment with a single intravenous infusion of 90 mg caused normalization in 70-10% patients *562* In 30 children with osteogenesis imperfecta treatment with a mean of 6.8 ± 1.1 mg/kg/y over 4 to 12 cycles of treatment transient decrease in serum calcium of 12 ± 7% observed following each infusion cycle *2188* In 3 clinical trials doses of 60 mg/4 h, 60 mg/24 h and 90 mg/24 h caused hypocalcemia in 0%, 1% and 12% respectively *271* Transient fall in one patient with calcitonin-resistant Paget's disease following intravenous infusion of 30 mg/d for 3 days *1491*
Urine Decrease Physiological Effect noted after 3 days of 30 mg/d intravenously in one patient with calcitonin-resistant Paget's disease *1491* In 30 children with osteogenesis imperfecta treatment with a mean of 6.8 ± 1.1 mg/kg/y over 4 to 12 cycles of treatment sustained decrease in activity of 66 ± 49% observed over a 3 to 4 month period *2188*

Calcium, Albumin-corrected
Serum Decrease Physiological In 29 patients with various malignant diseases treatment with pamidronate 60 mg intravenously for 4 h caused significant decrease from mean baseline of 2.43 ± 0.03 mmol/L to 2.19 ± 0.03 mmol/L when measured after 48 h *5294*

C-Reactive Protein *Serum Increase Physiological* In 29 patients with various malignant diseases treatment with pamidronate 60 mg intravenously for 4 h caused significant change from mean baseline of 24 mg/L to 25 pg/mL when measured after 24 h and 30 pg/mL at 48 h in those with normal body temperature and increase from 27 pg/mL to 41 mg/L after 24 h and 58 mg/L after 48 h in those with fever *5294*

Creatinine *Serum Increase Physiological* In 3 clinical trials involving 113 patients a dose of 60 mg/4 h in 23 patients was associated with uremia in 4 patients *271*

Deoxypyridinoline *Urine Decrease Physiological* In 13 patients with Paget's disease of the bone treatment with up to 6 weekly infusions of 60 mg caused reduction from mean baseline of 96 μmol/mol creatinine to 29 μmol/mol creatinine after 2 weeks and 19 μmol/mol creatinine after 6 weeks *4850*

Deoxypyridinoline, Free *Urine Decrease Physiological* In 23 patients with untreated Paget's disease of the bone treatment with pamidronate caused mean excretion of 13.6 ± 10.1 μmol/mol creatinine to decrease to 7.6 ± 3.8 μmol/mol creatinine *5084*

1,25-Dihydroxy Vitamin D *Serum Increase Physiological* In 24 patients with Paget's disease treatment for 2-10 days caused 3-fold increase from about 100 pmol/L to 300 ± 20 pmol/L remaining above the reference limits for 4 - 8 weeks after therapy (188 ± 15 pmol/L) and returning to normal of 134 ± 11 pmol/L only after 12 weeks *1403*

1,25-Dihydroxy Vitamin D_3 *Serum Increase Physiological* In 14 patients with Paget's disease treatment with 15 mg pamidronate for 5 days caused significant change from mean baseline of 85 pmol/L to 108 pmol/L on day 8, 150 pmol/L on day 15 and 90 pmol/L on day 30 *3819*

24,25-Dihydroxy Vitamin D *Serum Decrease Physiological* In 24 patients with Paget's disease treatment for 2 - 10 days caused significant reduction to 2.44 ± 0.25 nmol/L from already low pretreatment concentration of 3.93 ± 0.5 nmol/L, returning to pretreatment concentrations after 12 weeks (4.14 ± 0.35 nmol/L) *1403*

Hemoglobin *Blood Decrease Physiological* In 3 clinical trials doses of 60 mg/4 h, 60 mg/24 h and 90 mg/24 h caused anemia in 0%, 0% and 6% respectively *271*

25-Hydroxy Vitamin D *Serum No Effect Physiological* No significant effect observed with daily intravenous infusions for 2 - 10 days in 24 patients with Paget's disease *1403*

Hydroxyproline *Urine Decrease Physiological* In patients with Paget's disease and alkaline phosphatase 3 times the upper limit of normal administration of pamidronate caused reduction of concentration by 50% in 50% of patients and by 30% in 80% patients *271* In 71 patients with Paget's disease treatment with either mild, moderate or severe disease were treated with a total of 120, 180 or 240 mg causing a significant decrease in excretion, with return to reference range in all patients with mildest disease and in many of those with severe disease *2379* In 24 patients with Paget's disease treatment for 2 - 10 days caused significant decrease in urinary hydroxyproline:creatinine ratio from 0.12 ± 0.02 above reference limits to 0.04 ± 0.008 (reference range in women 0.006 - 0.027 and 0.005 - 0.020 in men) remaining at this level for 6 months after therapy *1403* 30 mg/d intravenously for 3 days caused normalization of urinary excretion in one patient with calcitonin-resistant Paget's disease *1491* In 13 patients with Paget's disease treatment with up to 6 weekly infusions of 60 mg caused reduction from mean baseline of 55 mmol/mol creatinine to 16 mmol/mol creatinine after 2 weeks and 20 mmol/mol creatinine after 6 weeks *4850*

Hydroxypyridinoline, Free *Urine Decrease Physiological* In 14 patients with Paget's disease treatment with 15 mg pamidronate for 5 days caused nonsignificant change from mean baseline of 123 ± 54.3 nmol/mmol creatinine to 101 ± 29.4 nmol/mmol creatinine on day 8, 64.3 ± 32.3 nmol/mmol creatinine on day 15 and 66 ± 17.6 nmol/mmol creatinine on day 30 *3819*

Interleukin-6 *Serum Increase Physiological* In 29 patients with various malignant diseases treatment with pamidronate 60 mg intravenously for 4 h caused significant change from mean baseline of 24 pg/mL to 33 pg/mL when measured after 24 h and 20 pg/mL at 48 h in those with normal body temperature and increase from 35 pg/mL to 100 pg/mL after 24 h and 40 pg/mL after 48 h in those with fever *5294*

ionized Calcium *Serum Decrease Physiological* In 24 patients with Paget's disease treatment with daily infusons for 2 to 10 days caused significant decrease from mean baseline of 1.26 mmol/L to 1.14 mmol/L but with rapid rebound to initial concentration thereafter *1403* In 14 patients with Paget's disease treatment with 15 mg pamidronate for 5 days caused significant change from mean baseline of 1.31 mmol/L to 1.23 mmol/L on day 8, 1.24 mmol/L on day 15 and 1.27 mmol/L on day 30 *3819*

Leukocytes *Blood Decrease Physiological* In 3 clinical trials doses of 60 mg/4 h, 60 mg/24 h and 90 mg/24 h caused leukopenia in 4%, 0% and 0% respectively *271* In 29 patients with various malignant diseases treatment with pamidronate 60 mg intravenously for 4 h caused change from mean baseline of 5,940 ± 397 /μL to 6,033 ± 429 /μL when measured after 24 h and significant change to 4,823 ± 417 /μL at 48 h *5294*
Blood No Effect Physiological In 29 patients with various malignant diseases treatment with pamidronate 60 mg intravenously for 4 h caused change from mean baseline of 5,940 ± 397 /μL to 6,033 ± 429 /μL when measured after 24 h and significant change to 4,823 ± 417 /μL at 48 h *5294*

Lymphocytes *Blood Decrease Physiological* In 29 patients with various malignant diseases treatment with pamidronate 60 mg intravenously for 4 h caused significant change from mean baseline of 1078 ± 130 /μL to 693 ± 94 /μL when measured after 24 h and 706 ± 83 /μL at 48 h *5294*

Magnesium *Serum Decrease Physiological* In 3 clinical trials doses of 60 mg/4 h, 60 mg/24 h and 90 mg/24 h caused hypomagnesemia in 4%, 10% and 12% respectively *271*

Monocytes *Blood No Effect Physiological* In 29 patients with various malignant diseases treatment with pamidronate 60 mg intravenously for 4 h caused change from mean baseline of 198 ± 20 /μL to 179 ± 18 /μL when measured after 24 h and 206 ± 24 /μL at 48 h *5294*

Neutrophils *Blood Decrease Physiological* In 3 clinical trials doses of 60 mg/4 h, 60 mg/24 h and 90 mg/24 h caused neutropenia in 0%, 1% and 0% respectively *271*

Osteocalcin *Serum Decrease Physiological* In 71 patients with Paget's disease treatment with either mild, moderate or severe disease were treated with a total of 120, 180 or 240 mg causing a significant decrease in concentration with a nadir reached between days 4 and 10 *2379* In 71 patients with Paget's disease treatment with either mild, moderate or severe disease were treated with a total of 120, 180 or 240 mg causing a significant decrease in concentration with a nadir reached between 12 and 24 months *2379*
Serum Increase Physiological Rise by 10th week in one patient with calcitonin-resistant Paget's disease following intravenous infusion of 30 mg/d for 3 days. return to pretreatment value by 16th week *1491* In 29 patients with Paget's disease treatment for 2 to 10 days caused significant increase from mean baseline of 22.3 ± 2.98 μg/L to 40.5 ± 5.6 μg/L *1403* In 14 patients with Paget's disease treatment with 15 mg pamidronate for 5 days caused significant change from mean baseline of 9.2 ± 1.1 ng/mL to 11.0 ± 1.2 ng/mL on day 8, 10.8 ± 1.3 ng/mL on day 15 and 10.1 ± 1.2 ng/mL on day 30 *3819*
Serum No Effect Physiological In 24 patients with Paget's disease treatment caused initial significant increase to mean 40.5 ± 5.6 μg/L from baseline of 22.3 ± 2.98 μg/L but decreased to 18.7 ± 5.4 μg/L, not significantly different from baseline when treatment discontinued for 6 months *1403*

Parathyroid Hormone *Plasma Increase Physiological* In 14 patients with Paget's disease treatment with 15 mg pamidronate for 5 days caused significant change from mean baseline of 4.0 pmol/L to 8.6 pmol/L on day 8, 8.0 pmol/L on day 15 and 5.6 pmol/L on day 30 *3819* Transient increase in one patient with calcitonin-resistant Paget's disease following treatment with 30 mg/d intravenously for 3 days *1491* In 24 patients with Paget's disease treatment with daily infusions for 2 to 10 days caused significant increase to 86 ± 11 pmol/L twice the mean baseline concentration falling to the reference range (46 ± 4 pmol/L) 4 - 8 weeks after treatment *1403*

Pamidronate *(continued)*

Parathyroid Hormone, Intact
Plasma Increase Physiological In 71 patients with Paget's disease treatment with either mild, moderate or severe disease were treated with a total of 120, 180 or 240 mg causing a significant increase in concentration from 2.3 ± 0.3 pmol/L to 3.3 ± 0.3 pmol/L in the mild group, from 3.2 ± 0.3 pmol/L to 3.8 ± 0.3 pmol/L in the moderate group and from 2.6 ± 0.4 pmol/L to 3.5 ± 0.5 pmol/L in the severe group after one year *2379*

Phosphate *Serum Decrease Physiological* In 3 clinical trials doses of 60 mg/4 h, 60 mg/24 h and 90 mg/24 h caused hypophosphatemia in 0%, 9% and 18% respectively *271* In 24 patients with Paget's disease treatment with daily intravenous infusions for 2 to 10 days caused sigificant decrease from mean baseline of 1.11 ± 0.12 mmol/L to 0.81 ± 0.14 mmol/L (even though concentration remained within normal range of 0.80 - 1.40 mmol/L) *1403* In 30 children with osteogenesis imperfecta treatment with a mean of 6.8 ± 1.1 mg/kg/y over 4 to 12 cycles of treatment transient decrease in serum calcium of 23 ± 18% observed following each infusion cycle *2188*

Platelets *Blood Decrease Physiological* In 3 clinical trials doses of 60 mg/4 h, 60 mg/24 h and 90 mg/24 h caused thrombocytopenia in 0%, 1% and 0% respectively *271* In 29 patients with various malignant diseases treatment with pamidronate 60 mg intravenously for 4 h caused significant change from mean baseline of 254,000 ± 16,000 /µL to 234,000 ± 14,000 /µL when measured after 24 h and 230,000 ± 14,000 /µL at 48 h *5294*

Potassium *Serum Decrease Physiological* In 3 clinical trials doses of 60 mg/4 h, 60 mg/24 h and 90 mg/24 h caused hypokalemia in 4%, 4% and 18% respectively *271*

Pyridinoline *Urine Decrease Physiological* In 13 patient's with Paget's disease of the bone treatment with up to 6 weekly infusions of 60 mg caused reduction from mean baseline of 249 µmol/mol creatinine to 75 µmol/mol creatinine after 2 weeks and 74 µmol/mol creatinine after 6 weeks *4850*

Pyridinoline Crosslinked Telopeptide of Type I Collagen
Serum No Effect Physiological In 13 patients with Paget's disease of the bone treatment with up to 6 weekly infusions of 60 mg caused nonsignificant change from mean baseline of 6.7 µg/L to 7.0 µg/L after 2 weeks and 5.7 µg/L after 6 weeks *4850*

Pyridinoline, Free *Urine Decrease Physiological* In 14 patients with Paget's disease treatment with 15 mg pamidronate for 5 days caused significant change from mean baseline of 142 ± 41.3 nmol/mmol creatinine to 86 ± 17.1 nmol/mmol creatinine on day 8, 106 ± 16.1 nmol/mmol creatinine on day 15 and 98 ± 6.0 nmol/mmol creatinine on day 30 *3819*

Thyroxine (T4) *Serum Decrease Physiological* In 3 clinical trials involving 113 patients doses of 60 mg/4 h, 60 mg/24 h and 90 mg/24 h was associated with hypothyroidism in 3 patients at the highest dose level *271*

Tumor Necrosis Factor-α *Serum Increase Physiological* In 29 patients with various malignant diseases treatment with pamidronate 60 mg intravenously for 4 h caused significant change from mean baseline of 13 pg/mL to 22 pg/mL when measured after 24 h and 22 pg/mL at 48 h in those with normal body temperature and increase from 15 pg/mL to 32 pg/mL after 24 h and 36 pg/mL after 48 h in those with fever *5294*

Type I Collagen Cross-linked N-telopeptide
Urine Decrease Physiological In 28 patients with thyroid cancer treatment with thyroxine and pamidronate 30 mg intravenously every 3 months for 2 years caused significant decrease in excretion of N-telopeptide cross-links of type I collagen after one month by 58% and by 32% after 12 months *5094* In 30 children with osteogenesis imperfecta treatment with a mean of 6.8 ± 1.1 mg/kg/y over 4 to 12 cycles of treatment sustained decrease in activity of 43 ± 31% observed over a 3 to 4 month period, with steady decrease in excretion of 26 ± 17% per year *2188*

Urea Nitrogen *Serum Increase Physiological* In 3 clinical trials involving 113 patients a dose of 60 mg/4 h in 23 patients was associated with uremia in 4 patients *271*

Pancrelipase

Uric Acid *Serum Increase Physiological* Very high doses reported to cause hyperuricemia *5683* High doses have been associated with hyperuricemia and hyperuricosuria *4985*
Urine Increase Physiological High doses have been associated with hyperuricemia and hyperuricosuria *4985* Very high doses reported to cause uricosuria *5683*

Pancreozymin

Amylase *Serum Increase Analytical* Preparation contains amylase *2024*
Serum Increase Physiological Effect seen when pancreatic disorders,?in normals *5575*

Glucagon *Plasma No Effect Physiological* No effect of 1 unit/kg body weight *4419*

Glucose *Serum Increase Physiological* Intravenous infusion causes increase *2909*
Serum No Effect Physiological No change after 1 unit/kg i.v *4419*

Insulin *Plasma Increase Physiological* Intravenous infusion causes increase *2909*
Plasma No Effect Physiological No effect of 1 unit/kg body weight *4419*

Lipase *Serum Increase Analytical* Preparation contains lipase *2024*

Protein *Pancreatic Fluid Increase Physiological* Increase in response to challenge *746*

Pancuronium

Bromide *Serum Increase Physiological* Theoretical possibility if bromide salt is administered since it contains 37% bromide *5116*

Cholinesterase *Serum Decrease Physiological* ?*in vivo*, but *in vitro* 25 µmol causes 80% inhibition *5737*

Epinephrine *Plasma Increase Physiological* During halothane anesthesia if also given *5737*

Histamine *Plasma No Effect Analytical* Probably insignificant effect on radio-enzyme assay since 50% inhibition at 3.8 µg/mL whereas physiological concentration is less than 0.6 µg/mL *2492*

Midazolam *Serum No Effect Analytical* On GC-ECD method of Ha et al *2387*

Norepinephrine *Plasma Increase Physiological* During halothane anesthesia if also given *5737*

Panthetine

Cholesterol *Serum Decrease Physiological* In many clinical trials been shown to reduce plasma concentration by about 10-12% *5586*

LDL-Cholesterol *Serum Decrease Physiological* In many clinical trials been shown to reduce concentration by about 12-15% due to reduced activation of HMG-CoA reductase in the presence of high concentrations of cholesterol precursors *5586*

Triglycerides *Serum Decrease Physiological* Some effect observed in hypertriglyceridemias *5586*

Pantoprazole

Gastrin *Serum Increase Physiological* After 5 days treatment with 40 mg/d mean preprandial increase of 41% in H. pylori positive duodenal ulcer patients and 45% in H. pylori-eradicated patients. Rise in postprandial rise 81% in H. pylori-positive and 69% in H. pylori-eradicated patients *3877*

Pepsinogen I *Serum Increase Physiological* In duodenal ulcer patients treated with pantoprazole 40 mg/d for 5 days caused 114% increase in H.pylori-postive patients and 8% in H. pylori-eradicated patients *3877*

Theophylline *Serum No Effect Physiological* In 8 healthy male volunteers administration of pantoprazole with theophylline had no significant effect on the area under the concentration/time curve *5384*

Papaverine

Alanine Aminotransferase *Serum Increase Physiological* Probable hypersensitivity reaction *5080* Hepatitis, probably related to an immune mechanism, has been reported infrequently with rare progression to cirrhosis *1705*

Albumin *Serum No Effect Analytical* At concentration of 10 mg/L had no effect on BCG method *5704*

Alkaline Phosphatase *Serum Increase Physiological* In 2 patients: fever anorexia and jaundice 4 to 5 weeks after start of treatment due to pericholangitis: reversible *5663* In 6 of 14 patients abnormal liver function, possibly due to allergic response and to metabolic aberration in host *4556* Hepatitis, probably related to an immune mechanism, has been reported infrequently with rare progression to cirrhosis *1705* Reversible hepatotoxic effect *5080*

Aspartate Aminotransferase *Serum Increase Physiological* Probable hypersensitivity reaction *5080* In 6 of 14 patients abnormal liver function, possibly due to allergic response and to metabolic aberration in host *4556* Hepatitis, probably related to an immune mechanism, has been reported infrequently with rare progression to cirrhosis *1705* In 2 patients: fever anorexia and jaundice 4 to 5 weeks after start of treatment due to pericholangitis: reversible *5663*

Bicarbonate *Serum No Effect Analytical* At concentration of 10 mg/L had no effect on method using phenolphthalein *5704*

Bilirubin *Serum Increase Physiological* Small effect, reversible hypersensitivity reaction *5465* In 2 patients: fever anorexia and jaundice 4 to 5 weeks after start of treatment due to pericholangitis reversible *5663* Hepatitis, probably related to an immune mechanism, has been reported infrequently with rare progression to cirrhosis *1705* In 6 of 14 patients abnormal liver function, possibly due to allergic response and to metabolic aberration in host *4556*
Serum No Effect Analytical At concentration of 10 mg/L had no effect on Jendrassik and Grof method *5704*

Calcium *Serum No Effect Analytical* At concentration of 10 mg/L had no effect on cresolphthalein method *5704*

Chloride *Serum No Effect Analytical* At concentration of 10 mg/L had no effect on mercurimetric method *5704*

Cholesterol *Serum No Effect Analytical* At concentration of 10 mg/L had no effect on Liebermann-Burchard method *5704*

Creatinine *Serum No Effect Analytical* At concentration of 10 mg/L had no effect on Technicon AutoAnalyzer® Jaffe method *5704*

Eosinophils *Blood Increase Physiological* Allergic response reported to occur *2754*

γ-Glutamyltransferase *Serum Increase Physiological* In 6 of 14 patients abnormal liver function, possibly due to allergic response and to metabolic aberration in host *4556*

Histamine *Plasma No Effect Analytical* Improbable inhibition of radio-enzyme assay at therapeutic concentrations *2492*

Phosphate *Serum No Effect Analytical* At concentration of 10 mg/L had no effect on phosphomolybdate method *5704*

Potassium *Serum No Effect Analytical* At concentration of 10 mg/L had no effect on measurement by ISE with predilution *5704*

Protein *Serum No Effect Analytical* At concentration of 10 mg/L had no effect on biuret method with blank correction *5704*

Sodium *Serum No Effect Analytical* At concentration of 10 mg/L had no effect on measurement by ISE with predilution *5704*

Triglycerides *Serum No Effect Analytical* At concentration of 10 mg/L had no effect on lipase/esterase method *5704*

Urea Nitrogen *Serum No Effect Analytical* At concentration of 10 mg/L had no effect on diacetylmonoxime method *5704*

Uric Acid *Serum No Effect Analytical* At concentration of 10 mg/L had no effect on phosphotungstate reduction method *5704*

Paraldehyde

Alanine Aminotransferase *Serum Increase Physiological* Possible hepatotoxicity *3810*

Albumin *Serum No Effect Analytical* At concentration of 2,000 mg/L had no effect on BCG method *5704*

Alkaline Phosphatase *Serum Increase Physiological* Possible hepatotoxicity *3810*

Aspartate Aminotransferase *Serum Increase Physiological* Possible hepatotoxicity *3810*

Bicarbonate *Serum Decrease Physiological* Metabolic acidosis in paraldehyde habitues *2242*
Serum No Effect Analytical At concentration of 2,000 mg/L had no effect on method using phenolphthalein *5704*

Bile *Urine Increase Physiological* Possible hepatotoxicity *3810*

Bilirubin *Serum Increase Physiological* Possible hepatotoxicity *3810*
Serum No Effect Analytical At concentration of 2,000 mg/L had no effect on Jendrassik and Grof method *5704*

BSP Retention *Serum Increase Physiological* Possible hepatotoxicity *3810*

Calcium *Serum No Effect Analytical* At concentration of 2,000 mg/L had no effect on cresolphthalein method *5704*

Chloride *Serum No Effect Analytical* At concentration of 2,000 mg/L had no effect on mercurimetric method *5704*

Cholesterol *Serum No Effect Analytical* At concentration of 2,000 mg/L had no effect on Liebermann-Burchard method *5704*

Creatine Kinase *Serum Increase Physiological* In individulas receiving a single intramuscular injection significant increase in activity observed with maximum observed at about 24 h with magnitude of increase loosely linked to the volume of fluid injected *3377*

Creatinine *Serum Increase Physiological* Possible nephrotoxicity *2395*
Serum No Effect Analytical At concentration of 2,000 mg/L had no effect on Technicon AutoAnalyzer® Jaffe method *5704*

Glucose *Serum Increase Physiological* Has caused transient hyperglycemia *3669*

17-Hydroxycorticosteroids *Urine Increase Analytical* Interferes with Porter-Silber reaction *5869*

Ketones *Serum Increase Physiological* Transient hyperglycemia and ketosis *3669*
Urine Increase Analytical False positive when drug combined with ethanol *2395* Affects alkaline nitroprusside procedure *882*

Leukocytes *Blood Increase Physiological* Leukocytosis in severe acute or chronic poisoning *2242*

Occult Blood *Feces Increase Physiological* Bleeding gastritis in acute or chronic poisoning *2242*

Paraldehyde *Blood Increase Physiological* Usually fatal at 500 mg/L *3868*

pH *Blood Decrease Physiological* Acidotic action (decomposes to acetic acid) *3810*

Phosphate *Serum No Effect Analytical* At concentration of 2,000 mg/L had no effect on phosphomolybdate method *5704*

Protein *Serum No Effect Analytical* At concentration of 2,000 mg/L had no effect on biuret method with blank correction *5704*
Urine Increase Physiological Nephrotoxic effect (nephrosis with poisoning) *2395*

Prothrombin Time *Plasma Decrease Physiological* May shorten action of anticoagulants *2753*

Triglycerides *Serum No Effect Analytical* At concentration of 2,000 mg/L had no effect on lipase/esterase method *5704*

Urea Nitrogen *Serum Increase Physiological* Possible nephrotoxicity in poisoning *2395*
Serum No Effect Analytical At concentration of 2,000 mg/L had no effect on diacetylmonoxime method *5704*

Uric Acid *Serum No Effect Analytical* At concentration of 2,000 mg/L had no effect on phosphotungstate reduction method *5704*

Paramethadione

Alanine Aminotransferase *Serum Increase Physiological* Possible hepatotoxicity *3810*

Alkaline Phosphatase *Serum Increase Physiological* Possible hepatotoxicity *3810*

Paramethadione *(continued)*

Aspartate Aminotransferase *Serum Increase Physiological* Possible hepatotoxicity *3810*

Bile *Urine Increase Physiological* Possible hepatotoxicity *3810*

Bilirubin *Serum Increase Physiological* Possible hepatotoxicity *3810*

BSP Retention *Serum Increase Physiological* Possible hepatotoxicity *3810*

Calcium *Serum Decrease Physiological* Theoretical effect of type of drug *2403*

Casts *Urine Increase Physiological* May have nephrotoxic effect *3810*

Cholesterol *Serum Increase Physiological* Possible liver damage *3810*

Creatinine *Serum Increase Physiological* Possible nephrotoxicity *3810*

Erythrocytes *Blood Decrease Physiological* Aplastic anemia may occur rarely *3810*

Felbamate *Serum No Effect Analytical* No significant interference observed with GLC method of Rifai et al *4958*

Glucaric Acid *Urine Increase Physiological* Probable effect as reported to induce hepatic enzymes *6518*

25-Hydroxy Vitamin D_3 *Serum Decrease Physiological* Theoretical effect of type of drug *2403*

LE Cells *Blood Positive Physiological* Rare idiosyncratic response *3340*

Leukocytes *Blood Decrease Physiological* Aplastic anemia/neutropenia *128*

Neutrophils *Blood Decrease Physiological* May occur without overall effect on WBC *2754*

Occult Blood *Feces Increase Physiological* Gastrointestinal bleeding may occur (can affect many organs) *2754*

Platelets *Blood Decrease Physiological* Aplastic anemia may occur rarely *128*

Protein *Urine Increase Physiological* May have nephrotoxic effect *4134*

Urea Nitrogen *Serum Increase Physiological* Possible nephrotoxicity *3810*

Paramethasone

Amylase *Serum Increase Physiological* May cause pancreatitis occasionally *2754*

Bicarbonate *Serum Increase Physiological* May cause hypokalemic alkalosis *2754*

Glucose Tolerance *Serum Decrease Physiological* Decreased carbohydrate tolerance *2754*

Occult Blood *Feces Increase Physiological* May cause peptic ulcer with hemorrhage *2754*

Potassium *Serum Decrease Physiological* May cause potassium loss *2754*

Sodium *Urine Increase Physiological* May be excreted although edema may occur *128*

Urea Nitrogen *Serum Decrease Physiological* Negative nitrogen balance, protein catabolism *2754*

Paraquat

Creatinine *Serum Increase Analytical* In one patient who had ingested paraquat significant increase observed with modified Jaffe rate reaction on Hitachi 911 analyzer. 1000 mg/L paraquat appeared to increase plasma creatinine concentration by 1000 µmol/L *75*

Parathiazine

Leukocytes *Blood Decrease Physiological* May occur with prolonged use *3810*

Parathion

Cholinesterase *Red Blood Cells Decrease Physiological* Specific inhibitor of enzyme *6479*

Serum Decrease Physiological Inhibitory action of drug with poisoning *2183*

Leukocytes *Blood Decrease Physiological* Leukopenia (AMA Blood dyscrasias) *4017*

p-Nitrophenol *Urine Increase Physiological* Roughly increased in proportion to inhibitor of cholinesterase *6479*

Parathyroid Extract

Amino Acids *Urine Increase Physiological* Hormonal action *2242*

Bicarbonate *Urine Increase Physiological* Inhibits tubular exchange of Na^+ for H^+ *4323*

Calcium *Serum Increase Physiological* Increased calcium mobilization from bone *1009*

Urine Decrease Physiological Increases tubular reabsorption *128*

Urine Increase Physiological Due to mobilization from bone *2999*

Chloride *Urine Increase Physiological* Hormonal action *2242*

Citrate *Urine Increase Physiological* Hormonal action *2242*

Magnesium *Serum Increase Physiological* Due to decreased renal excretion *2242*

Urine Decrease Physiological Decreased clearance *2391*

pH *Urine Increase Physiological* Inhibits tubular exchange of Na^+ for H^+ *4323*

Phosphate *Serum Increase Physiological* Due to increased excretion in urine *3810*

Urine Increase Physiological Increased clearance *2391*

Potassium *Urine Increase Physiological* Increased clearance *2391*

Sodium *Urine Increase Physiological* Increased clearance *2391*

Sulfate *Urine Increase Physiological* Hormonal action *2242*

Volume *Urine Increase Physiological* Hormonal action *2242*

Parathyroid Hormone

Adenosine Monophosphate *Plasma Increase Physiological* Causes immediate increase in concentration following i.v. injection with maximum reached in 5 to 10 minutes *1950*

Alkaline Phosphatase *Serum Increase Physiological* In 20 patients with osteoporosis aged 50 to 78 years treatment for 14 days with hPTH 1-38 caused increase still detectable for 90 days afterwards *2635*

Calcitonin *Plasma No Effect Physiological* In response to infusion of 150 units in 10 normal subjects *717*

Calcium *Serum Increase Physiological* Infusion of 1.76 µg PTH(1-38)/kg body weight/24 h caused nonsignificant increases from mean baselines of 2.34 ± 0.07 mmol/L to 2.63 ± 0.13 mmol/L in 15 healthy controls and from 2.42 ± 0.09 mmol/L to 2.87 ± 0.15 mmol/L in 13 patients with rheumatoid arthritis and high ESR *2944* 15% increase observed in 15 healthy women with infusion of synthetic 1-38 human PTH subcutaneously over 24 hours. Increase greater in postmenopausal women *2939* In 20 patients with osteoporosis aged 50 to 78 years given synthetic hPTH 1-38 for 2 weeks mean concentration increased from 2.20 ± 0.07 mmol/L to 2.56 ± 0.16 mmol/L during PTH infusion but not significantly increased during intermittent treatment *2635*

Urine Increase Physiological In 20 patients aged 50-78 years with osteoporosis treatment with hPTH 1-38 for 14 days significant increase in excretion observed *2635* Mean 55% increase observed in 15 women with infusion subcutaneously over 24 hours of 1-38 synthetic human PTH *2939*

1,25-Dihydroxy Vitamin D *Serum Increase Physiological* In 20 patients aged 50 to 78 years with osteoporosis treatment for 14 days with hPTH 1-38 caused significant increase from mean baseline of 22.8 ± 8.2 pg/mL to 52.2 ± 25.1 pg/mL during infusion and remained significantly higher than baseline after 14 days intermittent treatment (33.1 ± 19.4 pg/mL) *2635*

Hydroxyproline *Urine Increase Physiological* Mean 80% increase observed in 15 healthy women in whom synthetic 1-38 human parathyroid hormone infused subcutaneously over 24 hours. Increase greater in postmenopausal women *2939* Due to catabolic action *6111* In 20 patients with osteoporosis aged 50 to 78 years treatment with hPTH 1-38 years caused significant increase in excretion from 30.5 ± 13.9 μmol/mmol creatinine to 43.4 ± 17.5 μmol/mmol creatinine immediately after infusion and mean excretion persistently higher than baseline during intermittent treatment *2635*

Insulin-like Growth Factor-I *Serum No Effect Physiological* In 15 healthy controls and 13 patients with active rheumatoid arthritis infusion of 1.76 μg PTH(1-38)/kg body weight/24 h had no significant effect on concentration *2944*

Insulin-like Growth Factor-II *Serum No Effect Physiological* In 13 patients with active rheumatoid arthritis and 15 healthy controls infusion of 1.76 μg PTH(1-38)/kg body weight/24 h had no significant effect on plasma concentration *2944*

Insulin-like Growth Factor Binding Protein-3
Serum Increase Physiological Infusion of 1.76 μg PTH(1-38)/kg body weight/24 h in 15 healthy individuals caused significant increase from mean baseline of about 4500 μg/L to about 6000 μg/L *2944*
Serum No Effect Physiological In 13 patients with actve rheumatoid arthritis infusion of 1.76 μg PTH(1-38)/kg body weight/24 h had no significant effect on concentration but as inflammation subsided infusion tended to cause an increase in concentration *2944*

ionized Calcium *Serum Increase Physiological* Infusion of 1.76 μg PTH(1-38)/kg body weight/24 h caused nonsignificant increase from mean baseline of 1.18 ± 0.02 mmol/L to 1.36 ± 0.06 mmol/L in 15 healthy controls and from 1.20 ± 0.04 mmol/L to 1.49 ± 0.11 mmol/L in 13 patients with rheumatoid arthritis and high ESR *2944*

Osteocalcin *Serum Decrease Physiological* Mean 15% decrease observed in 15 healthy women in whom synthetic 1-38 human parathyroid hormone infused subcutaneously over 24 hours *2939*
Serum Increase Physiological In 20 patients with osteoporosis aged 50-78 years treatment for 2 weeks with hPTH 1-38 caused significant increase still detectable 90 days later *2635*

Parathyroid Hormone *Plasma Decrease Physiological* Infusion of 1.76 μg PTH(1-38)/kg body weight/24 h caused decrease from mean baseline of 29.6 ± 6.3 ng/L to 11.8 ± 2.3 ng/L in 15 healthy controls and from 22.2 ± 5.0 ng/L to 9.4 ± 1.2 ng/L in 13 patients with rheumatoid arthritis and high ESR *2944*

Prolactin *Plasma Increase Physiological* From 5.1 ng/mL to 14.9 ng/mL on average in 10 normal subjects after infusion of 150 units *717*

Thyroid Stimulating Hormone
Serum No Effect Physiological In response to infusion of 150 units in 10 normal subjects *717*

Paraxanthine

Theophylline *Serum No Effect Analytical* No significant interference observed with Syva EMIT 2000 assay *413*

Pargyline

Alanine Aminotransferase *Serum Increase Physiological* Possible hepatotoxicity (reversible) *3810*

Alkaline Phosphatase *Serum Increase Physiological* Possible hepatotoxicity (reversible) *3810*

Aspartate Aminotransferase *Serum Increase Physiological* Possible hepatotoxicity (reversible) *3810*

Bile *Urine Increase Physiological* Possible hepatotoxicity (reversible) *3810*

Bilirubin *Serum Increase Physiological* Possible hepatotoxicity (reversible) *3810*

BSP Retention *Serum Increase Physiological* Possible hepatotoxicity (reversible) *3810*

Glucose *Serum Decrease Physiological* Possible hepatotoxic effect *3810*

Glucose Tolerance *Serum Increase Physiological* Flat curve may be produced *3669*

Peripheral Smear *Blood Abnormal Physiological* Poikilocytosis and inisocytosis common *4014*

Urea Nitrogen *Serum Increase Physiological* Possible decrease in already impaired renal function *139*

Paromomycin

Cholesterol *Serum Decrease Physiological* Reduction up to 18%. ?mechanism *5215*

Creatinine *Serum Increase Physiological* Frequently observed renal damage *198*

Creatinine Clearance *Urine Decrease Physiological* Frequently observed renal damage *198*

Protein *Urine Increase Physiological* Potentially nephrotoxic if given parenterally *128*

Urea Nitrogen *Serum Increase Physiological* Potentially nephrotoxic if given parenterally *128*

Paroxetine

Abnormal Erythrocytes *Blood Increase Physiological* Rarely abnormal erythrocytes observed with treatment *5654*

Alanine Aminotransferase *Serum Increase Physiological* Infrequent increased activity observed with treatment *5654*

Albumin *Urine No Effect Analytical* Using a fluorimetric assay with Albumin Blue 580 on a Cobas Fara centrifugal analyzer for the detection of microalbuminuria no significant interference was detected at a concentration of 4 mg/L *3117*

Alkaline Phosphatase *Serum Increase Physiological* Rare increased activity observed with treatment *5654*

Amitriptyline *Serum Increase Physiological* When coadministered, by inhibiting cytochrome P450 2D6, may increase the concentration of amitriptyline *6645*

Aspartate Aminotransferase *Serum Increase Physiological* Infrequent increased activity observed with treatment *5654*

Atypical Lymphocytes *Blood Increase Physiological* Rarely abnormal lymphocytes observed with treatment *5654*

Basophils *Blood Increase Physiological* Rarely basophilia observed with treatment *5654*

Bilirubin *Serum Increase Physiological* Rare increased concentration observed with treatment *5654*

Blood *Urine Increase Physiological* Rarely observed with treatment *5654*

Calcium *Serum Decrease Physiological* Rare hypocalcemia observed with treatment *5654*
Serum Increase Physiological Rare hypercalcemia observed with treatment *5654*

Cholesterol *Serum Increase Physiological* Rare increased concentration observed with treatment *5654*

Creatine Kinase *Serum Increase Physiological* Rarely increased activity observed with treatment *5654*

Desipramine *Serum Increase Physiological* In 9 extensive metabolizers of sparteine 20 mg/d paroxetine concomitantly with 100 mg/d desipramine caused significant increase in the plasma concentrations in both fast and slow metabolizers but with no significant change in poor metabolizers *750*

Digoxin *Serum Decrease Physiological* When the drugs coadministered mean digoxin AUC at steady state decreased by 15% *5654*

Eosinophils *Blood Increase Physiological* Rarely eosinophilia observed with treatment *5654*

γ-Globulin *Serum Increase Physiological* Rare increased concentration observed with treatment *5654*

Glucose *Serum Decrease Physiological* Infrequent hypoglycemia observed with treatment *5654*

Paroxetine *(continued)*

Glucose *(continued)*
Serum Increase Physiological Infrequent hyperglycemia observed with treatment *5654*

Hemoglobin *Blood Decrease Physiological* Infrequent hypochromic, iron-deficiency; or microcytic anemia observed with treatment *5654*

Ketones *Serum Increase Physiological* Rare increased concentration observed with treatment *5654*

Lactate Dehydrogenase *Serum Increase Physiological* Rare increased activity observed with treatment *5654*

Leukocytes *Blood Decrease Physiological* Infrequent leukopenia observed with treatment *5654*
Blood Increase Physiological Rare leukocytosis observed with treatment *5654*

Lymphocytes *Blood Increase Physiological* Rare lymphocytosis observed with treatment *5654*

Melatonin *Plasma No Effect Physiological* In 8 healthy volunteers administration of 20 mg paroxetine at 20:00 h caused no significant effect on nocturnal plasma melatonin concentration *4230*

Monocytes *Blood Increase Physiological* Rarely monocytosis observed with treatment *5654*

Phenytoin *Serum Decrease Physiological* When a single oral dose of paroxetine was given orally with phenytoin a decrease of 12% in the AUC of phenytoin occurred *5654*

Phosphate *Serum Increase Physiological* Rare increased concentration observed with treatment *5654*

Platelets *Blood Increase Physiological* Rarely thrombocythemia observed with treatment *5654*

Potassium *Serum Decrease Physiological* Rare decreased concentration observed with treatment *5654*
Serum Increase Physiological Rare increased concentration observed with treatment *5654*

Procyclidine *Serum Increase Physiological* When daily doses of paroxetine were given orally with procyclidine steady state increases of 35%, 37% and 67% occurred in the AUC, maximum and minimum concentrations of procyclidine respectively *5654*

Propranolol *Serum No Effect Physiological* When daily doses of paroxetine (30 mg q.i.d.) were given orally with propranolol (80 mg b.i.d.) no change was observed in the steady state concentration of propranolol *5654*

Sodium *Serum Decrease Physiological* Rare decreased concentration observed with treatment *5654*

Terfenadine *Serum No Effect Physiological* Coadministration of paroxetine with terfenadine had no effect on the pharmacokinetics of terfenadine *5654*

Theophylline *Serum No Effect Physiological* Paroxetine reportedly increases the concentration of theophyliine *5654*

Thyroxine (T4) *Serum Decrease Physiological* Rarely hyperthyroidism, hypothyroidism or thyroiditis observed with treatment *5654*
Serum Increase Physiological Rarely hyperthyroidism, hypothyroidism or thyroiditis observed with treatment *5654*

Tricyclic Antidepressants *Serum Increase Physiological* Interacts pharmacokinetically to inhibit metabolism of tricyclic antidepressants *3590*

Urea Nitrogen *Serum Increase Physiological* Rare increased concentration observed with treatment *5654*

Uric Acid *Serum Increase Physiological* Rarely increased concentration observed with treatment *5654*

PCMPS

Cholesterol *Serum No Effect Analytical* Insignificant increase observed on enzymatic method of Allain et al when 2 mmol/L added in vitro *2481*

Triglycerides *Serum Decrease Analytical* Marked reduction observed, e.g. from 88 mg/dL to 20 mg/dL, 180 mg/dL to 38 mg/dL and 269 mg/dL to 64 mg/dL when added at concentration of 2 mmol/L on method of Bucolo and David with glycerol blanking *2481*

PCNU

Alanine Aminotransferase *Serum Increase Physiological* Hepatic toxicity is rare *1384*

Aspartate Aminotransferase *Serum Increase Physiological* Hepatic toxicity is rare *1384*

Erythrocytes *Blood Decrease Physiological* Myelosuppression is dose limiting *1384*

Leukocytes *Blood Decrease Physiological* Myelosuppression is dose-limiting *1384*

Platelets *Blood Decrease Physiological* Myelosuppression is dose-limiting *1384*

Urea Nitrogen *Serum Increase Physiological* Renal toxicity is rare *1384*

Pefloxacin

Caffeine *Serum Increase Physiological* Clearance inhibited to some extent *2704*

Cyclosporine *Serum No Effect Physiological* In one study of renal transplant patients coadministration of pefloxacin had no effect on concentration *6596* No significant interaction observed in renal transplant recipients *3400*

Theophylline *Serum Increase Physiological* Clearance inhibited to some extent *2704*

Pegaspargase

Alanine Aminotransferase *Serum Increase Physiological* Increased activity has been reported as complication of treatment in more than 5% of treated patients *4939*

Albumin *Serum Decrease Physiological* Hypoproteinemia with hypoalbuminemia has been reported as complication of treatment in more than 1% of treated patients *4939*

Alkaline Phosphatase *Serum Increase Physiological* Jaundice and abnormal liver function tests have been reported as complication of treatment in more than 1% of treated patients *4939*

Ammonia *Plasma Increase Physiological* Increased concentration has occurred with the conversion of L-asparagine to aspartic acid by pegaspargase *4939*

Amylase *Serum Increase Physiological* Pancreatitis is major complication of treatment *4939*

Antithrombin III *Plasma Decrease Physiological* Decreased concentration has been reported as complication of treatment in more than 1% of treated patients *4939*

Aspartate Aminotransferase *Serum Increase Physiological* Jaundice and abnormal liver function tests have been reported as complication of treatment in more than 1% of treated patients *4939*

Bilirubin *Serum Increase Physiological* Jaundice and abnormal liver function tests have been reported as complication of treatment in more than 1% of treated patients *4939*

Blood *Urine Increase Physiological* Hematuria has been reported as complication of treatment in less than 1% of treated patients, probably due to thrombocytopenia *4939*

Clotting Time *Blood Increase Physiological* Increased coagulation time has been reported as complication of treatment in more than 1% of treated patients *4939*

Creatinine *Serum Increase Physiological* Abnormal renal function has been reported as complication of treatment in less than 1% of treated patients *4939*

Fibrinogen *Plasma Decrease Physiological* Decreased anticoagulant effect has been reported as complication of treatment in more than 1% of treated patients *4939*

Glucose *Serum Decrease Physiological* Hypoglycemia has been reported as complication of treatment in more than 1% of treated patients *4939*
Serum Increase Physiological Hyperglycemia may occur as complication of treatment *4939*

γ-Glutamyltransferase *Serum Increase Physiological* Increased activity has been reported as complication of treatment *4939*

Granulocytes *Blood Decrease Physiological* Agranulocytosis has been reported as complication of treatment *4939*

Hematocrit *Blood Decrease Physiological* Hemolytic anemia has been reported as complication of treatment in more than 1% of treated patients *4939*

Hemoglobin *Blood Decrease Physiological* Hemolytic anemia has been reported as complication of treatment in more than 1% of treated patients *4939*

Leukocytes *Blood Decrease Physiological* Leukopenia or pancytopenia have been reported as complications of treatment in more than 1% of treated patients *4939*

Lipase *Serum Increase Physiological* Pancreatitis is major complication of treatment *4939*

Lymphoblasts *Blood Decrease Physiological* A fall in concentration may occur after treatment is initiated *4939*

Partial Thromboplastin Time
Plasma Decrease Physiological Decreased anticoagulant effect has been reported as complication of treatment in more than 1% of treated patients *4939*

pH *Blood Decrease Physiological* Metabolic acidosis has been reported as complication of treatment *4939*

Platelets *Blood Decrease Physiological* Thrombocytopenia or pancytopenia have been reported as complication of treatment in more than 1% of treated patients *4939*

Protein *Serum Decrease Physiological* Hypoproteinemia has been reported as complication of treatment in more than 1% of treated patients *4939*
Urine Increase Physiological Proteinuria has been reported as complication of treatment *4939*

Prothrombin Time *Plasma Decrease Physiological* Decreased anticoagulant effect has been reported as complication of treatment in more than 1% of treated patients *4939*

Thromboplastin Generation *Blood Increase Physiological* Increased thromboplastin has been reported as complication of treatment in more than 1% of treated patients *4939*

Urea Nitrogen *Serum Increase Physiological* Abnormal renal function has been reported as complication of treatment in less than 1% of treated patients *4939*

Uric Acid *Serum Increase Physiological* An increase may occur in association with a fall in lymphoblast concentration may occur after treatment is initiated *4939*

Pemoline

Acid Phosphatase *Serum Increase Physiological* In one 63-year old man with prostatic enlargement treatment with pemoline caused an increase in activity which declined with withdrawal of the drug and recurred when the drug was readministered *14*

Alanine Aminotransferase *Serum Increase Physiological* Delayed hypersensitivity reaction observed in a small number of patients after several months treatment, usually reversible *1384* Use has been associated with hepatic dysfunction, including increased enzyme activity, hepatitis and jaundice *14*

Aspartate Aminotransferase *Serum Increase Physiological* Occasional hypersensitivity reaction observed after several weeks of treatment but usually reversible *1384* Use has been associated with hepatic dysfunction, including increased enzyme activity, hepatitis and jaundice *14*

Bilirubin *Serum Increase Physiological* Use has been associated with hepatic dysfunction, including increased enzyme activity, hepatitis and jaundice *14* Occasional jaundice observed as result of delayed hypersensitivity reaction which is usually reversible *1384*
Serum No Effect Analytical No significant effect observed in long-term studies *1384*

Erythrocytes *Blood Decrease Physiological* Use has been associated with aplastic anemia *14*
Blood No Effect Physiological No significant effect observed in long-term studies *1384*

Hemoglobin *Blood Decrease Physiological* Use has been associated with aplastic anemia *14*
Blood No Effect Physiological No significant effect observed in long-term studies *1384*

Lactate Dehydrogenase *Serum Increase Physiological* Occasional delayed hypersensitivity reaction observed but usually reversible *1384*

Leukocytes *Blood Decrease Physiological* Use has been associated with aplastic anemia *14*
Blood No Effect Physiological No significant effect observed in long-term studies *1384*

Platelets *Blood Decrease Physiological* Use has been associated with aplastic anemia *14*
Blood No Effect Physiological No significant effect observed in long-term studies *1384*

Urea Nitrogen *Serum No Effect Physiological* No significant effect observed in long-term studies *1384*

Uric Acid *Serum No Effect Physiological* No significant effect observed in long-term studies *1384*

Pempidine

Uric Acid *Serum Increase Physiological* ?Due to reduced renal blood flow *1461*

Penicillamine

Acetylcholine Receptor Antibodies
Serum Increase Physiological Myasthenia gravis may occur as autoimmune syndrome, possibly as result of direct binding of drug to receptor *2881*

α_1-Acid Glycoprotein *Serum Decrease Physiological* In 21 patients with rheumatoid arthritis treated for 48 weeks given 250 to 750 mg daily *3864*

Alanine Aminotransferase *Serum Increase Physiological* Administration of penicillamine has been associated with intrahepatic cholestasis or toxic hepatitis *3967* Case of acute cholestatic jaundice in patient with systemic lupus erythematosus *5433* Increase by 45% in 3 patients with Wilson's disease although effect disappeared after 12 mo *2353* In 6 of 99 patients treated for rheumatoid arthritis: evidence of toxic liver necrosis observed in two cases *6527* Isolated cases of hepatic dysfunction or intrahepatic cholestasis and toxic hepatitis may occur with treatment *6321* Possible hepatotoxicity *3810*

Albumin *Serum No Effect Physiological* In 21 patients with rheumatoid arthritis treated for 48 weeks given 250 to 750 mg daily *3864*

Alkaline Phosphatase *Serum Decrease Physiological* In rheumatoid arthritis patients when treated for 6 mo. Changes not related to activity of disease *2932*
Serum Increase Physiological Case of acute cholestatic jaundice in patient with systemic lupus erythematosus *5433* Isolated cases of hepatic dysfunction or intrahepatic cholestasis and toxic hepatitis may occur with treatment *6321* Administration of penicillamine has been associated with intrahepatic cholestasis or toxic hepatitis *3967* In 6 of 99 patients treated for rheumatoid arthritis: evidence of toxic liver necrosis observed in two cases *6527* Possible hepatotoxicity *1714* In 15 women with rheumatoid arthritis treatment for 24 months caused a significant increase in activity *6011*
Serum No Effect Physiological In rheumatoid arthritis patients when treated for 6 mo. Changes not related to activity of disease *2932* But decreased in granulocytes related to transient changes in zinc metabolism *2932*

Alkaline Phosphatase, Bone Isoenzyme
Serum Increase Physiological In 15 women with rheumatoid arthritis treatment for 24 weeks caused a significant increase in activity *6011*

Amino Acids *Urine Increase Analytical* Reacts with ninhydrin; extra spot TLC, high voltage electrophoresis *4760* 2 unusual purple spots with ninhydrin on thin-layer chromatography of urine from patients with Wilson's disease. Spots stain gray with isatin *2605*

Amylase *Serum Increase Physiological* Isolated cases of pancreatitis may occur with treatment *6321*

Anti-DNA Antibodies *Serum Increase Physiological* In 6 patients with rheumatoid arthritis developed systemic lupus erythematosus-like syndrome *951*

Antinuclear Antibodies *Serum Increase Physiological* In 6 patients with rheumatoid arthritis developed systemic lupus erythematosus-like syndrome *951*

Aspartate Aminotransferase
Serum Decrease Physiological Increase by 47% in 3 patients with Wilson's disease although effect disappeared after 12 mo *2353*

Penicillamine *(continued)*

Aspartate Aminotransferase *(continued)*
Serum Increase Physiological Possible hepatotoxicity *3810* Isolated cases of hepatic dysfunction or intrahepatic cholestasis and toxic hepatitis may occur with treatment *6321* Administration of penicillamine has been associated with intrahepatic cholestasis or toxic hepatitis *3967* In 6 of 99 patients treated for rheumatoid arthritis: evidence of toxic liver necrosis observed in two cases *6527* Case of acute cholestatic jaundice in patient with systemic lupus erythematosus *5433*

Bilirubin *Serum Increase Physiological* Administration of penicillamine has been associated with intrahepatic cholestasis or toxic hepatitis *3967* Case of acute cholestatic jaundice in patient with systemic lupus erythematosus *5433* Isolated cases of hepatic dysfunction or intrahepatic cholestasis and toxic hepatitis may occur with treatment *6321*

Blood *Urine Increase Physiological* Administration of penicillamine has been associated with proteinuria which may herald membranous glomerulopathy *3967* Hematuria may occur with treatment and may be a warning sign of membranous glomerulonephropathy *6321*

Carbonic Anhydrase
Red Blood Cells Decrease Physiological In rheumatoid arthritis patients when treated for 6 mo. Changes not related to activity of disease *2932*

Cholesterol *Serum Decrease Analytical* At concentrations above 10 mg/L (normal therapeutic concentration 11 mg/L) lowered concentration as measured by CHOD-Iodide method *5704*
Serum Increase Physiological Single case reported *2451*
Serum No Effect Analytical At concentration of 960 mg/L had no effect on Liebermann-Burchard method *5704* At concentration of 960 mg/L had no effect on catalase-AIDH method *5704* At concentration of 960 mg/L had no effect on CHOD-PAP method *5704* At concentration of 960 mg/L had no effect on method using catalase-Hantzsch reaction *5704*

Chondrex *Serum No Effect Analytical* Concentrations of D-penicillamine up to 1 g/L had no significant effect on sandwich-type ELISA procedure of Harvey et al *2491*

Complement C_4 *Serum Decrease Physiological* In 6 patients with rheumatoid arthritis developed systemic lupus erythematosus-like syndrome *951*

Coombs' Test *Blood Positive Physiological* In 6 patients with rheumatoid arthritis developed systemic lupus erythematosus-like syndrome *951*

Copper *Serum No Effect Analytical* No effect at concentration of 250 mg/L on colorimetric DiBr-PAESA method of Abe et al *32*
Urine Increase Physiological Administration of penicillamine is intended to remove excess copper in Wilson's disease *3967* In selected patients with Wilson's disease previously treated with penicillamine for one year after a single dose of 500 mg excretion increased from baseline of 17 µg/6 h to 320 µg/6 h. In 7 patients not previously treated a single dose of 500 mg caused a significant increase from mean baseline of 68 µg/6 h to 1074 µg/6 h *3994* If poisoning due to copper (also in normals) *128*

C-Reactive Protein *Serum Decrease Physiological* Significant reduction observed in 163 patients with active rheumatoid arthritis treated for 3-6 months but with continued reduction observed for up to 60 months *5587*

Creatine Kinase *Serum Increase Physiological* Marked increase observed in one patient with rheumatoid arthritis after 1 mo treatment *1489*

Creatinine *Serum Increase Physiological* Possible nephrotoxicity *2024*
Serum No Effect Analytical At concentration of 55 mg/L had no effect on kinetic Jaffe method on BKA-2 *5704* At concentration of 480 mg/L had no effect on Jaffe-Fuller's earth method *5704* At concentration of 480 mg/L had no effect on Jaffe-Fading-Fraction method *5704*

Crystals *Urine Decrease Physiological* Administration of penicillamine decreases cystine excretion in cystinosis and reduces crystalluria *3967*

Cystine *Urine Decrease Physiological* Administration of penicillamine decreases cystine excretion in cystinosis *3967*
Urine Increase Physiological If a patient has cystinuria *128*

Diclofenac *Serum No Effect Physiological* Coadministration of D-penicillamine with diclofenac did not significantly affect the peak concentration or AUC of diclofenac *1025*

Digoxin *Serum Decrease Physiological* Reduced concentrations observed in one study when penicillamine coadministered *4086*

Eosinophils *Blood Increase Physiological* May occur with rash *128* In 14% patients treated with up to 750 mg daily (63 patients studied who had taken penicillamine) *5617* Administration of penicillamine has been associated with eosinophilia in a very small number of cases *3967* Eosinophilia may or may not occur with treatment *6321*

Erythrocyte Sedimentation Rate
Blood Decrease Physiological In 21 patients with rheumatoid arthritis treated for 48 weeks given 250 to 750 mg daily *3864*

Erythrocytes *Blood Decrease Physiological* Rare blood dyscrasias as reported to UK Committee on Safety of Medicines *1204* Hypochromic anemia in child, menstruating woman *130*
Blood No Effect Physiological In 21 patients with rheumatoid arthritis treated for 48 weeks given 250 to 750 mg daily *3864*
Urine Increase Physiological In 1 of 21 patients with rheumatoid arthritis treated for 48 weeks given 250 to 750 mg daily *3864*

Fructosamine *Serum Decrease Analytical* Negative interference at concentration of 0.5 mmol/L with Roche reagents on Cobas-Bio but effect highly albumin dependent with positive interference at low concentrations. However concentration of drug at which interference occurs above therapeutic range *5153* When D-penicillamine added at a concentration of 0.5 mmol/L 10% reduction observed and at 1.0 mmol/L 13% reduction observed in concentration as measured by Roche method on Cobas Fara although these concentrations are much higher than therapeutic of about 70 µmol/L *5152*

Glucose *Serum Decrease Physiological* Administration of penicillamine has been associated with rare hypoglycemia and anti-insulin antibodies *3967*
Serum No Effect Analytical At concentration of 36 mg/L had no effect on Kodak Ektachem® method *5704*
Serum No Effect Physiological In 21 patients with rheumatoid arthritis treated for 48 weeks given 250 to 750 mg daily *3864*
Urine No Effect Physiological In 21 patients with rheumatoid arthritis treated for 48 weeks given 250 to 750 mg daily *3864*

Gold *Blood No Effect Physiological* No effect in patients with rheumatoid arthritis previously treated with gold *2212*
Urine Increase Physiological Slight effect when given to patients with rheumatoid arthritis previously treated with gold *2212*

Hematocrit *Blood Decrease Physiological* Hypochromic anemia in child, menstruating woman *130*

Hemoglobin *Blood Decrease Physiological* Hypochromic anemia in child, menstruating woman *130*
Blood No Effect Physiological In 21 patients with rheumatoid arthritis treated for 48 weeks given 250 to 750 mg daily *3864*

Histamine *Plasma No Effect Analytical* Improbable inhibition of radio-enzyme assay at therapeutic concentrations *2492*

Homocysteine *Plasma Increase Physiological* As a vitamin B_6 antagonist causes increased concentration *6123*

immunoglobulin A *Serum Decrease Physiological* But not significantly in 21 patients with rheumatoid arthritis treated for 48 weeks given 250 to 750 mg daily *3864* Reported reversible or permanent deficiency induced by penicillamine *2426*

Immunoglobulin G *Serum Decrease Physiological* But not significantly in 21 patients with rheumatoid arthritis treated for 48 weeks given 250 to 750 mg daily *3864*

Immunoglobulin M *Serum Decrease Physiological* But not significantly in 21 patients with rheumatoid arthritis treated for 48 weeks given 250 to 750 mg daily *3864*

Insulin Antibodies *Serum Increase Physiological* Administration of penicillamine has been associated with rare hypoglycemia and anti-insulin antibodies *3967*

Iron *Urine Increase Physiological* If poisoning due to iron *128*

Ketones *Urine Increase Analytical* Like other compounds with free sulfhydryl groups can give false positive reaction with Legal reaction *1185*

Kynurenine *Urine Increase Physiological* Induces pyridoxine antagonism *2242*

Lactate Dehydrogenase *Serum Increase Physiological* In 6 of 99 patients treated for rheumatoid arthritis: evidence of toxic liver necrosis observed in two cases *6527* Administration of penicillamine has been associated rarely with increased activity *3967*

LE Cells *Blood Positive Physiological* Observed effect in some cases *1475* In 6 patients with rheumatoid arthritis developed systemic lupus erythematosus-like syndrome *951*

Lead *Urine Increase Physiological* Administration of penicillamine is intended to remove excess copper in Wilson's disease but will also remove excess zinc *3967* If poisoning due to lead *128*

Leukocytes *Blood Decrease Physiological* Leukopenia may occur with rash *130* Leukopenia observed in up to 5% treated patients *6321* Toxicity observed in some patients with rheumatoid disease *3084* Rare blood dyscrasias as reported to UK Committee on Safety of Medicines *1204* In 3% of 90 patients with rheumatoid arthritis previously treated with gold *2413* Administration of penicillamine has been associated with reduced count in up to 5% of patients. Penicillamine can cause bone marrow depression with leukopenia in 2% patients *3967* Most serious and potentially life-threatening effect of drug. Either idiosyncratic response seen in first year of treatment. Independent of dosage or more commonly dose related with gradual onset *2881*

Blood Increase Physiological Administration of penicillamine has been associated with leukocytosis in a very small number of cases *3967*

Blood No Effect Physiological In 21 patients with rheumatoid arthritis treated for 48 weeks given 250 to 750 mg daily *3864*

Levodopa *Serum Increase Physiological* In one man with Parkinson's disease who had low concentrations of copper and ceruloplasmin coadministration of penicillamine increased the plasma concentration of levodopa from 3015 ng/mL/h to 4760 ng/mL/h probably by facilitating its gastrointestinal absorption *4082*

Lipase *Serum Increase Physiological* Isolated cases of pancreatitis may occur with treatment *6321*

MCHC *Blood Decrease Physiological* Hypochromic anemia in child, menstruating woman *130*

Mercury *Urine Increase Physiological* Related to drug dosage in toxicity cases *5892* Administration of penicillamine is intended to remove excess copper in Wilson's disease but will also remove excess zinc *3967*

Monocytes *Blood Increase Physiological* Administration of penicillamine has been associated with monocytosis in a very small number of cases *3967*

N-Acetyl-Glucosaminidase *Urine No Effect Analytical* At 20 mmol/L on 2 colorimetric analytical methods *2254*

Neutrophils *Blood Decrease Physiological* Occasional case of drug-induced neutropenia *241* In 14 of 84 patients occurring typically in first 6 mo of treatment *3085*

Occult Blood *Feces Increase Physiological* Occasional side effect as reported to UK Committee on Safety of Medicines *1204*

Platelets *Blood Decrease Physiological* In 3% of 90 patients with rheumatoid arthritis previously treated with gold *2413* Administration of penicillamine has been associated with reduced count in up to 5% of patients. In other reports thrombocytopenia has occurred in 4% patients *3967* Rare blood dyscrasias as reported to UK Committee on Safety of Medicines *1204* Significant effect from 36th week in 21 patients with rheumatoid arthritis treated for 48 weeks given 250 to 750 mg daily *3864* Toxicity observed in some patients with rheumatoid disease *3084* Thrombocytopenia observed in up to 5% treated patients *6321* Most serious and potentially life-threatening effect of drug. Either idiosyncratic response seen in first year of treatment. Independent of dosage or more commonly dose related with gradual onset *2881* Thrombocytopenia may occur with rash *130* Apparently some bone marrow depression in some patients but normal lifespan of cells *6006* In 14 of 84 patients occurring typically in first 6 mo of treatment *3085*

Blood Increase Physiological Administration of penicillamine has been associated with thrombocytosis in a very small number of cases *3967*

Potassium *Serum No Effect Analytical* At concentration of 360 mg/L had no effect on measurement by ISE without predilution *5704*

Protein *Urine Increase Physiological* In 16% of 90 patients with rheumatoid arthritis previously treated with gold *2413* Administration of penicillamine has been associated with proteinuria which may herald membranous glomerulopathy (occurs in about 6% patients) *3967* May be minimal and asymptomatic or lead to nephrotic syndrome due to immune complex glomerulitis *2881* In 30% patients with rheumatoid arthritis or cystinuria and 4% in patients with Wilson's disease *205* In 3 of 21 patients with rheumatoid arthritis treated for 48 weeks given 250 to 750 mg daily *3864* In 15 of 84 patients occurring most often in 6 to 12 mo after treatment started *3085* Nephrotoxic effect *2024* Toxicity observed in some patients with rheumatoid disease *3084* Proteinuria may occur with treatment and may be a warning sign of membranous glomerulonephropathy *6321* In 10 to 20% of patients with rheumatoid arthritis in first year, of which one third may proceed to nephrotic syndrome *1166*

Protein Electrophoresis *Serum No Effect Analytical* At concentration of 360 mg/L had no effect on automated Olympus-Hite method *5704*

Rheumatoid Factor *Serum No Effect Physiological* In 21 patients with rheumatoid arthritis treated for 48 weeks given 250 to 750 mg daily *3864*

Sodium *Serum No Effect Analytical* At concentration of 360 mg/L had no effect on measurement by ISE without predilution *5704*

Thyroxine (T4) *Serum Decrease Physiological* Inhibits binding of T4 to TBG *2412*

Serum No Effect Physiological In 21 patients with rheumatoid arthritis treated for 48 weeks given 250 to 750 mg daily *3864*

Tri-iodothyronine (T3) *Serum Decrease Physiological* Inhibits binding of T3 to TBG *2412*

Urea Nitrogen *Serum Increase Physiological* Possible nephrotoxicity *2024*

Serum No Effect Analytical At concentration of 36 mg/L had no effect on Kodak Ektachem® method *5704*

Uric Acid *Serum No Effect Analytical* At concentration of 480 mg/L had no effect on catalase-AIDH method *5704*

Xanthurenic Acid *Urine Increase Physiological* Induces pyridoxine antagonism *2242*

Zinc *Red Blood Cells Increase Physiological* But granulocyte concentration decreased related to transient changes in zinc metabolism *2932* In rheumatoid arthritis patients when treated for 6 mo. Changes not related to activity of disease *2932*

Serum Increase Physiological Related to transient changes in zinc metabolism *2932* In rheumatoid arthritis patients when treated for 6 mo. Changes not related to activity of disease *2932*

Urine Increase Physiological If poisoning due to zinc *2242* Administration of penicillamine is intended to remove excess copper in Wilson's disease but will also remove excess zinc *3967* Related to transient changes in zinc metabolism *2932* In rheumatoid arthritis patients when treated for 6 mo. Changes not related to activity of disease *2932*

White Blood Cells Decrease Physiological In rheumatoid arthritis patients when treated for 6 mo. Changes not related to activity of disease *2932*

Penicillin

Albumin *Serum Decrease Analytical* At concentrations above 18,000 mg/L (normal therapeutic concentration about 12 mg/L) lowered concentration as measured by BCG method *5704*

Amikacin *Serum Decrease Analytical* Concentration as measured on Baxter Stratus reduced if specimen stored for a prolonged period *5705*

Serum No Effect Analytical No imterference observed at a concentration of 1000 µg/mL (2917 µmol/L) with method on Du Pont aca *1508*

δ-Aminolevulinic Acid *Urine Increase Analytical* Derivative reacts with Ehrlich's reagent *3252*

Penicillin *(continued)*

Antithrombin III *Plasma No Effect Analytical* At concentration of 100 mg/L had no effect on Du Pont aca method *5704*

Aspartate Aminotransferase *Serum Increase Physiological* Nonspecific hepatitis without cholestasis *6515*

Bilirubin *Serum Decrease Physiological* In newborn combined with sulfisoxazole has effect *5869*
Serum Increase Physiological Nonspecific hepatitis without cholestasis *6515*

Bilirubin, Conjugated *Serum No Effect Analytical* At concentration of 34.8 U/mL (62 µmol/L) had no effect on method on Du Pont aca *1517*

Bleeding Time *Patient Increase Physiological* Because of binding to adenosine diphosphate receptors may inhibit platelet aggregation and cause increased bleeding time, most marked with carbenicillin and ticarcillin *1384*

Casts *Urine Increase Physiological* Renal cell and other types *2242*

Cholesterol *Serum No Effect Analytical* No effect at concentrations up to 1070 mg/L on method on Kodak Ektachem® *5706*

Chromosomes *Test Conditions No Effect Physiological* Not clastogenic in human cells *5484*

Clindamycin *Serum No Effect Analytical* If inactivated do not interfere with bioassays *3858*

Colistin *Serum No Effect Analytical* If inactivated do not interfere with bioassays *3858*

Coombs' Test, Direct *Blood Positive Physiological* Combines to RBC, immunoglobulins develop to drug *2453*

Coombs' Test, Indirect *Blood Positive Physiological* Combines to RBC, immunoglobulins develop to drug *2453*

Creatine Kinase *Serum Increase Physiological* Frequent injections may cause increase up to 5 times *2583*

Creatine Kinase Isoenzymes *Serum No Effect Analytical* No interference observed at a concentration of 5 MU/L with CK-MB method on Du Pont aca *1519*

Creatinine *Serum Increase Physiological* Hypersensitivity reaction or nephropathy *2242*

Eosinophils *Blood Increase Physiological* Associated with allergic reaction *1384* Allergic reaction (may be up to 20% of all WBC) *1659*
Urine Increase Physiological Associated with interstitial nephritis arising from allergic response *1384*

Erythrocytes *Blood Decrease Physiological* Hemolytic anemia due to binding to erythrocytes *1659* Coombs' positive hemolytic anemia is rare adverse reaction with all penicillins *1384*
Urine Increase Physiological Hypersensitivity reaction, nephrotoxicity *345* Associated with interstitial nephritis and allergic reaction *1384*

Erythromycin *Serum No Effect Analytical* If inactivated do not interfere with bioassays *3858*

Estriol *Plasma Decrease Physiological* In pregnant women due to alteration of gut flora *4812*

Estrogens *Urine Decrease Physiological* In pregnant women due to alteration of gut flora *4812*
Urine Increase Analytical Activates enzyme used for hydrolysis *55*

Factor VIII Antibodies *Serum Decrease Physiological* Induction of factor VIII antibodies observed after high-dose penicillin therapy *3694*

Fibrinogen *Plasma No Effect Analytical* At concentration of 100 mg/L had no effect on Du Pont aca method *5704*

Folate *Serum Decrease Analytical* Inhibits growth of *L. casei5869*
Serum No Effect Analytical Allegedly no effect on autoclave method *2965*

Gentamicin *Serum Decrease Analytical* Penicillin and its analogs reduce stability of gentamicin so concentration reduced when penicillin added for long time and measured by Baxter Stratus and other analyzers *5705*
Serum Increase Analytical At concentrations up to 750 mg/L (normal clinical concentration up to 24 mg/L) caused 25% increase in concentration with method on Baxter Stratus but not clinically significant because concentration not clinically relevant *5705*
Serum No Effect Analytical No interference observed at concentrations up to 500 µg/mL (1459 µmol/L) with method on Du Pont aca *1526*

Glucose *Urine Increase Analytical* In massive doses may react positively with Ames Clinitest tablets *4034*
Urine No Effect Analytical No effect observed with Tes-Tape® . No effect on Clinistix® or TesTape® *4174* Even massive doses have no effect on Ames Keto-Diastix, Diastix, Multistix and Clinistix procedures *4034*

Haptoglobin *Serum Decrease Physiological* May cause hemolytic anemia *3810*

Hematocrit *Blood Decrease Physiological* Hemolytic anemia due to binding to erythrocytes *1659*

Hemoglobin *Blood Decrease Physiological* Hemolytic anemia due to binding to erythrocytes *1659*
Urine Increase Physiological Hypersensitivity reaction, nephrotoxicity *345* Associated with interstitial nephritis associated with allergic reaction *1384*

Histamine *Plasma No Effect Analytical* No effect observed at concentration 20 times higher than therapeutic with radioenzyme assay *2492*

17-Hydroxycorticosteroids *Urine No Effect Analytical* No effect on modified Glenn-Nelson procedure *2452*

^{131}I Uptake *Serum Decrease Physiological* V-cillin contains tetraiodofluorescein *4360* If hydriodide salt given decreases further uptake *3669*

17-Ketogenic Steroids *Urine Increase Analytical* Interferes with Zimmermann (Norymberski) reaction *5869*

17-Ketosteroids *Urine Increase Analytical* Interferes with Zimmermann reaction *5869*

LE Cells *Blood Positive Physiological* Allergic response with urticaria in one case *2242*

Leukocytes *Blood Decrease Physiological* Agranulocytosis/Leukopenia *4467*
Urine Increase Physiological Associated with interstitial nephritis arising from allergic reaction *1384*

Mercury *Urine Increase Physiological* Acts as chelating agent in acrodynia at least *3432*

Methotrexate *Serum Increase Physiological* Observed in one patient probably as result of interference with renal secretion *601* Penicillins may reduce the renal clearance of methotrexate thereby increasing its serum concentration *2818*

Metronidazole *Serum No Effect Analytical* If inactivated do not interfere with bioassays *3858*

Neutrophils *Blood Decrease Physiological* Agranulocytosis/Leukopenia *4467* Neutropenia observed occasionally after administration of all penicillins, particularly with large doses: reversible with discontinuation of therapy (immune mediated or direct toxic effect on proliferation of myeloid precursor cells) *1384*

Phosphate *Serum No Effect Analytical* No effect of concentrations up to 4000 U/L on method on Kodak Ektachem® *5706*

Plasminogen *Plasma No Effect Analytical* At concentration of 100 mg/L had no effect on Du Pont aca method *5704*

Platelet Aggregation *Blood Decrease Physiological* High concentrations of all penicillins bind adenosine diphosphate receptors in platelets and prevent normal platelet aggregation *1384*

Platelets *Blood Decrease Physiological* Effect observed after high-dose penicillin therapy *3694* Agranulocytosis/thrombocytopenia *1659* Rarely reported side effect (probably immune mediated) *1384*

Polymyxin *Serum No Effect Analytical* If inactivated do not interfere with bioassays *3858*

Potassium *Serum Decrease Physiological* If i.v. sodium penicillin infused *5869* Large doses of any penicillin given intravenously, but especially carbenicillin and ticarcillin, may cause hypokalemia due to the large amount of nonreabsorbable anion in the distal renal tubules *1384*
Serum Increase Physiological May occur if K salt given i.v. also alkalosis *5869*
Serum No Effect Analytical At concentration of 15,000 mg/L had no effect on measurement by ISE with predilution *5704*
Urine Increase Physiological If i.v. sodium penicillin infused *5869*

Pramipexole *Serum No Effect Physiological* Coadministration of penicillins with pramipexole presumed to have no effect on the oral clearance of pramipexole *4680*

Protein *Cerebrospinal Fluid Increase Analytical* Causes turbidity if sulfosalicylic acid used *5869* Reacts as if phenol with Folin-Ciocalteu procedure *6681*
Cerebrospinal Fluid No Effect Analytical At concentration of 0.7 mg/L on SDS/Coomassie Blue method of Huang *2745*
Test Conditions Increase Analytical Massive doses may cause turbidity with acid tests *3810*
Urine Increase Analytical Massive doses may cause false positive with Sulfosalicylic Acid and Exton's reagent tests *4034* Massive doses may produce turbidity with acid *703* Causes turbidity if sulfosalicylic acid used *5869* With sulfosalicylic acid and acetic acid tests *684*
Urine Increase Physiological Associated with allergic reaction associated with interstitial nephropathy *1384* Nephrotoxicity may occur with large doses *2242*
Urine No Effect Analytical No effect on Albustix even with massive doses *703* Even massive doses have no effect on protein test areas of Ames Multistix and other reagent strip tests *4034*

Protein Electrophoresis *Serum Positive Analytical* Causes bisalbuminemia *5869*

Prothrombin Time *Plasma Decrease Physiological* Penicillins reduce prothrombin time when coadministered with warfarin *2625*
Plasma Increase Physiological Occasional effect *51*

PSP Excretion *Urine Decrease Physiological* Interference with PSP excretion *6515*

Reticulocytes *Blood Decrease Physiological* Rarely reported side effect (probably immune mediated) *1384*
Blood Increase Physiological Consequence of hemolytic anemia *1659*

Sodium *Serum No Effect Analytical* At concentration of 15,000 mg/L had no effect on measurement by ISE with predilution *5704*

Sugar *Urine Increase Analytical* False positive with copper reduction procedures *5869* Drug and metabolites act as red substances in high concentrations *882*

T3-Uptake *Serum Increase Physiological* Competes for thyroxine binding prealbumin sites *882*

Tetracycline *Serum No Effect Analytical* If inactivated do not interfere with bioassays *3858*

Theophylline *Serum No Effect Physiological* No effect observed on half-life *1384*

Thyroxine (T4) *Serum Decrease Physiological* Competes for thyroxine binding prealbumin binding sites *882*

Thyroxine (T4) (Murphy-Pattee)
Serum Decrease Physiological Binds with thyroxine binding prealbumin but not thyroxine binding globulin *882*

Tobramycin *Serum Decrease Analytical* When specimens containing penicillin or its analogs are stored for a long period tobramycin concentration decreases *5705*
Serum No Effect Analytical No significant effect observed at concentrations less than 1000 µg/mL (2.92 mmol/L) with method on Du Pont aca *1547* No detectable cross-reactivity observed with tobramycin method on Bayer Technicon Immuno 1® *435*

Trimethoprim *Serum No Effect Analytical* If inactivated do not interfere with bioassays *3858*

Urea Nitrogen *Serum Increase Physiological* Rare reaction to large doses given parenterally *2754*

Penicillin G

Alanine Aminotransferase *Serum No Effect Analytical* At 5 times upper limit of therapeutic range on methods on Technicon SMAC® , Abbott-VP, Roche Cobas-Bio, Du Pont aca, and KDA *3525*

Albumin *Serum No Effect Analytical* At concentration of 2,000 mg/L had no effect as measured by BCG method *5704* No effect at concentration of 1070 mg/L on Kodak Ektachem® method *5706* At 5 times upper limit of therapeutic range on methods on Technicon SMAC® , Kodak Ektachem® , Hitachi® 705 and KDA *3525*

Alkaline Phosphatase *Serum No Effect Analytical* At 5 times upper limit of therapeutic range on methods on Technicon SMAC® , Abbott-VP, Roche Cobas-Bio, Du Pont aca, Hitachi® 705 and KDA *3525*

Amdinocillin *Serum Increase Analytical* Cannot be assayed by HPLC method used at Mayo Clinic in presence of penicillin G *3858*

Amino Acids *Urine No Effect Analytical* No reaction observed with ninhydrin in paper chromatography, paper electrophoresis and ion-exchange chromatography *4761*

δ-Aminolevulinic Acid *Urine Increase Analytical* In method of Mauzerall and Granick interacts with acetylacetone which reacts with p-dimethylmenine benzaldehyde *6107*

Amylase *Serum No Effect Analytical* At 5 times upper limit of therapeutic range on methods on Du Pont aca, Roche Cobas-Bio and Kodak Ektachem® *3525* No effect at concentration of 1070 mg/L on method on Kodak Ektachem® *5706*

Aspartate Aminotransferase *Serum No Effect Analytical* At 5 times upper limit of therapeutic range on methods on Technicon SMAC® , Abbott-VP, Roche Cobas-Bio, Du Pont aca, Hitachi® 705 and KDA *3525*

Bicarbonate *Serum No Effect Analytical* At concentration of 2,000 mg/L had no effect as measured by method using phenolphthalein *5704*

Bilirubin *Serum No Effect Analytical* At 5 times upper limit of therapeutic range on methods on Technicon SMAC® , Du Pont aca, Abbott-VP, Kodak Ektachem® , Hitachi® 705 and KDA *3525* At concentration of 2,000 mg/L had no effect as measured by Jendrassik and Grof method *5704*
Serum No Effect Physiological Insignificant displacement from protein in neonates *6314*

Bilirubin, Conjugated *Serum No Effect Analytical* No effect at concentration of 1070 mg/L on method on Kodak Ektachem® *5706*

Bilirubin, Unconjugated *Serum No Effect Analytical* No effect at concentration of 1070 mg/L on method on Kodak Ektachem® *5706*

Bleeding Time *Patient Increase Physiological* Progressive lengthening with dose of 24 million U/d from 3.2 to 6.1 minutes on average, longer with higher dose *756*

Calcium *Serum No Effect Analytical* No effect at concentrations up to 1070 mg/L with method on Kodak Ektachem® *5706* At concentration of 2,000 mg/L had no effect as measured by cresolphthalein method *5704* At 5 times upper limit of therapeutic range on methods on Technicon SMAC® , Abbott-VP, Du Pont aca, Kodak Ektachem® , Hitachi® 705 and KDA *3525*

Cannabinoids *Urine No Effect Analytical* No effect on Roche Abuscreen method *5006*

Chloride *Serum No Effect Analytical* At concentration of 2,000 mg/L had no effect as measured by mercurimetric method *5704*

Cholesterol *Serum No Effect Analytical* At 5 times upper limit of therapeutic range on methods on Technicon SMAC® , Abbott-VP, Roche Cobas-Bio, Kodak Ektachem® , Hitachi® 705 and KDA *3525* At concentration of 2,000 mg/L had no effect as measured by Liebermann-Burchard method *5704*

Clot Retraction *Blood No Effect Physiological* No effect with doses as high as 48 million U/d *756*

Coombs' Test, Direct *Blood Positive Physiological* 44% of 39 patients demonstrated hypersensitivity reaction *3195*

Creatine Kinase *Serum No Effect Analytical* At 5 times upper limit of therapeutic range on methods on Technicon SMAC® , Abbott-VP, Du Pont aca, Roche Cobas-Bio and Hitachi® 705 *3525*

Creatinine *Serum No Effect Analytical* At concentration of 2,000 mg/L had no effect as measured by Technicon AutoAnalyzer® Jaffe method *5704* No effect of concentrations up to 15 mg/L on single slide method on Kodak Ektachem® *5706* No effect of concentrations up to 1070 mg/L on 2-slide method on Kodak Ektachem® *5706* At 5 times upper limit of therapeutic range on methods on Technicon SMAC® , Abbott-VP, Roche Cobas-Bio, Du Pont aca, Kodak Ektachem® , Hitachi® 705 and KDA *3525*

Drugs of Abuse Screen *Urine No Effect Analytical* No effect at concentration of 100 µg/mL on EZ-SCREEN procedure for cannabinoids and cocaine *1739*

Penicillin G *(continued)*

Eosinophils *Blood Increase Physiological* 44% of 39 patients demonstrated hypersensitivity reaction *3195*

Fibrinogen *Plasma No Effect Physiological* No effect with doses as high as 48 million U/d *756*

Glucose *Serum No Effect Analytical* At 5 times upper limit of therapeutic range on methods on Technicon SMAC® , Abbott-VP, Roche Cobas-Bio, Du Pont aca, Kodak Ektachem® , Hitachi® 705 and KDA *3525* At concentration of 90 mg/L had no effect as measured by GOD/POD-PAP method *5704* No effect of concentrations up to 1070 mg/L on method on Kodak Ektachem® *5706*
Urine Increase Analytical At 16.2 mg/mL gave false positive with negative urine but at higher concentrations gave occasional falsely low value *3710*
Urine No Effect Analytical At concentration of 3.6 mg/L had no effect as measured by Diabur-test *5704* No effect at up to 16.2 mg/mL on any glucose concentration as measured by Diastix® or TesTape® *3710*

γ-Glutamyltransferase *Serum No Effect Analytical* At 5 times upper limit of therapeutic range on methods on Technicon SMAC® , Abbott-VP and Hitachi® 705 *3525*

Glycated Hemoglobin *Blood No Effect Analytical* At a concentration of 10000 U/L had an insignificant 0.0% interference with method on Abbott Vision *1885*

Histamine *Plasma No Effect Analytical* No inhibition of radio-enzyme assay at concentration 50 times therapeutic *2492*

Immunoglobulin E *Serum Increase Physiological* Present in some patients with drug-induced acute interstitial nephritis *225*

Iron *Serum No Effect Analytical* At 5 times upper limit of therapeutic range on methods on Technicon SMAC® *3525*

Lactate Dehydrogenase *Serum No Effect Analytical* At 5 times upper limit of therapeutic range on methods on Technicon SMAC® , Abbott-VP, Roche Cobas-Bio, Hitachi® 705 and KDA *3525*

Leukocytes *Blood Decrease Physiological* In 2 patients receiving 140-150 mg/kg/d intravenously *2686* Occasional case of drug associated leukopenia *2997*

Lymphocytes *Blood No Effect Physiological* In 2 patients receiving 140-150 mg/kg/d intravenously *2686*

Methicillin *Serum Increase Analytical* Cannot be assayed by HPLC method used at Mayo Clinic in presence of penicillin G *3858*

Neutrophils *Blood Decrease Physiological* Occasional case of drug associated leukopenia *2997*

Partial Thromboplastin Time
Plasma No Effect Physiological No effect with doses as high as 48 million U/d *756*

Phenylalanine *Plasma No Effect Analytical* No interference observed with quantiative rapid whole blood method of Campbell et al using phenylalanine dehydrogenase *867*

Phosphate *Serum No Effect Analytical* At 5 times upper limit of therapeutic range on methods on Technicon SMAC® , Du Pont aca, Hitachi® 705, and KDA *3525* At concentration of 2,000 mg/L had no effect as measured by phosphomolybdate method *5704*

Platelet Aggregation *Blood Decrease Physiological* Defective aggregation in response to ADP at 24 million U/d *756*

Platelets *Blood Decrease Physiological* Isolated case of platelet-associated IgG and thrombocytopenia *3102*
Blood No Effect Physiological No effect with doses as high as 48 million U/d *756*

Potassium *Serum Decrease Physiological* Nonreabsorbable anion in distal nephron promoting potassium loss especially with high doses. Effect quite marked in leukemia *984*
Serum Increase Physiological If massive doses of penicillin G potassium salt (containing 1.7 mmol potassium per 1 million units) are infused hyperkalemia may occur *1384*
Serum No Effect Analytical At concentration of 18 mg/L had no effect as measured by flame-photometric method *5704* At concentration of 10000 U/L nonsignificant interference of -0.7% observed with method on Abbott Vision *681*

Protein *Serum Increase Analytical* At concentrations above 500 mg/L (normal therapeutic concentration 12 mg/L) raised concentration as measured by biuret method with blank correction *5704*
Serum No Effect Analytical No effect of concentrations up to 1070 mg/L on method on Kodak Ektachem® *5706* At 5 times upper limit of therapeutic range on methods on Technicon SMAC® , Abbott-VP, Kodak Ektachem® , Hitachi® 705 and KDA *3525*
Urine Increase Analytical When measured by Ponceau S dye method in comparison with sulfosalicylic acid or trichloracetic acid methods in 5 patients receiving therapeutic doses *6611*

Prothrombin Time *Plasma No Effect Physiological* No effect with doses as high as 48 million U/d *756*

Sodium *Serum No Effect Analytical* At concentration of 18 mg/L had no effect as measured by flame-photometric method *5704*

Sugar *Urine Increase Analytical* Reacts positively with Clinitest *4761*

Thrombin Time *Blood No Effect Physiological* No effect with doses as high as 48 million U/d *756*

Triglycerides *Serum No Effect Analytical* At 5 times upper limit of therapeutic range on methods on Technicon SMAC® , Abbott-VP, Kodak Ektachem® , Hitachi® 705 and KDA *3525* At concentration of 90 mg/L had no effect as measured by GPO-PAP method *5704* No effect of concentrations up to 1070 mg/L on method on Kodak Ektachem® *5706* At concentration of 2,000 mg/L had no effect as measured by lipase/esterase method *5704*

Urea Nitrogen *Serum No Effect Analytical* At 5 times upper limit of therapeutic range on methods on Technicon SMAC® , Abbott-VP, Roche Cobas-Bio, Kodak Ektachem® , Hitachi® 705 and KDA *3525* No effect of concentrations up to 1070 mg/L on method on Kodak Ektachem® *5706* At concentration of 2,000 mg/L had no effect as measured by diacetylmonoxime method *5704*

Uric Acid *Serum No Effect Analytical* At concentration of 2,000 mg/L had no effect as measured by phosphotungstate reduction method *5704* At concentration of 90 mg/L had no effect as measured by uricase-PAP method *5704* No effect of concentrations up to 1070 mg/L on method on Kodak Ektachem® *5706* At 5 times upper limit of therapeutic range on methods on Technicon SMAC® , Abbott-VP, Roche Cobas-Bio, Du Pont aca, Kodak Ektachem® , Hitachi® 705 and KDA *3525*

Penicillin V

Bilirubin *Serum Increase Physiological* Possible clinically significant displacement from protein especially in especially in critically ill neonates *6314* Possible clinically significant displacement from protein especially in critically ill neonates *6314* Isolated case of hemolytic anemia with IgM antibody *576*

Chloramphenicol *Serum No Effect Analytical* No effect at 100 mg/L on coupled enzymatic method *4122*

Coombs' Test, Direct *Blood Positive Physiological* Isolated case of hemolytic anemia with IgM antibody *576*

Hemoglobin *Blood Decrease Physiological* Isolated case of hemolytic anemia with IgM antibody *576*

Histamine *Plasma No Effect Analytical* No inhibition of radio-enzyme assay at 20 times therapeutic concentration *2492*

Methemalbumin *Serum Increase Physiological* Isolated case of hemolytic anemia with IgM antibody *576*

Phenylalanine *Plasma No Effect Analytical* No interference observed with rapid quantitative whole blood method of Campbell et al using phenylalanine dehydrogenase *867*

Piperacillin *Serum Increase Analytical* Cannot be assayed by HPLC method used at Mayo Clinic in presence of penicillin V *3858*

Pentaerythritol

Granulocytes *Blood No Effect Physiological* Agranulocytosis observed in 1.9% of patients versus 2.9% controls *3098*

Pentagastrin

Calcitonin *Plasma Increase Physiological* Slight effect seen in hypocalcemics if given i.v *1346*

Plasma *No Effect* *Physiological* Intravenous infusion had no effect in normals *1346*

Calcium *Serum* *No Effect* *Physiological* Intravenous infusion had no effect in normals *1346*

Growth Hormone *Plasma* *Increase* *Physiological* In 3 of 9 women to 4.87 ng/mL from 1.96 ng/mL, but increase not significant *6116*

Histamine *Urine* *Increase* *Physiological* All gastric stimulants produce effect *1252*

Hydrochloric Acid *Gastric Fluid* *Increase* *Physiological* If infused i.v *1081*

Pepsin *Gastric Material* *Increase* *Physiological* If infused i.v *1081*

Prolactin *Plasma* *Increase* *Physiological* Increased in 63% of 9 women: mean concentration increased from 9.67 ng/mL to 16.08 ng/mL in 5 to 10 minutes *6116*

Pentamidine

Amino-4-Imidazole-5-Carboxamide Ribotide
Urine *Increase* *Physiological* If megaloblastic anemia develops *6370*

Bicarbonate *Serum* *Decrease* *Physiological* Observed in 19 of 20 admissions of patients with AIDS when treated with drug. Concentrations observed varied from 14 to 21 mmol/L *3357*

Calcium *Serum* *Decrease* *Physiological* Reported side effect on occasion *1384*

Creatinine *Serum* *Increase* *Physiological* Increased concentrations observed (from 1.5 to 11.8 mg/dL) in 19 of 20 admissions of patients with AIDS when receiving drug *3690* Renal toxicity observed in about 25% patients *5541* Renal toxicity possibly due to formation of insoluble precipitates of pentamidine with nucleic acids, also associated with hypovolemia *5789*

Erythrocytes *Blood* *Decrease* *Physiological* Megaloblastic anemia: inhibits dihydrofolate reductase *6370*
Urine *Increase* *Physiological* Gross hematuria observed in a single patient *5541*

Folate *Serum* *Decrease* *Physiological* Inhibits dihydrofolate reductase *6370*

Glucose *Serum* *Decrease* *Physiological* Four patients with pneumocystis carinii developed severe fasting hypoglycemia *667* Hypoglycemia occurred in 10 to 30% patients with pneumocystis carinii pneumonia, usually 5 to 13 d after treatment, but fatal case described after 2 weeks *5290* Hypoglycemia is a possible effect *2242*
Serum *Increase* *Physiological* Paradoxical effect observed *2242*

Hematocrit *Blood* *Decrease* *Physiological* Megaloblastic anemia may occur: inhibits dihydrofolate reductase *6370*

Hemoglobin *Blood* *Decrease* *Physiological* Megaloblastic anemia may occur: inhibits dihydrofolate reductase *6370*
Urine *Increase* *Physiological* Gross hematuria observed in a single patient *5541*

Leukocytes *Blood* *Decrease* *Physiological* Occasional leukopenia reported *1384*

Magnesium *Serum* *Decrease* *Physiological* Marked reduction observed in one patient with AIDS *2276*

MCV *Blood* *Increase* *Physiological* Megaloblastic anemia *6370*

N-Formiminoglutamic Acid *Urine* *Increase* *Physiological* If megaloblastic anemia develops *6370*

Platelets *Blood* *Decrease* *Physiological* Occasional thrombocytopenia reported *1384*

Potassium *Serum* *Increase* *Physiological* In 19 of 20 patients with AIDS potassium concentration increased (5.1 to 8.7 mmol/L) which was not observed in same patients when admitted but when not receiving pentamidine due to nephrotoxicity of drug *3357*

Urea Nitrogen *Serum* *Increase* *Physiological* Renal toxicity possibly due to formation of insoluble precipitates of pentamidine with nucleic acids, also associated with hypovolemia *5789* Reversible renal dysfunction reported *2242* Increase observed in 19 of 20 admissions of patients with AIDS when they were treated with drug *3357* Renal toxicity observed in about 25% patients *5541*

Pentaquine

Bilirubin *Serum* *Increase* *Physiological* May cause hemolysis with G-6-PD deficiency *402*

Erythrocytes *Blood* *Decrease* *Physiological* May cause hemolysis with G-6-PD deficiency *402*

Haptoglobin *Serum* *Decrease* *Physiological* May cause hemolysis *402*

Heinz Body Formation *Blood* *Positive* *Physiological* May cause hemolysis with G-6-PD deficiency *536*

Hematocrit *Blood* *Decrease* *Physiological* May cause hemolysis with G-6-PD deficiency *402*

Hemoglobin *Blood* *Decrease* *Physiological* May cause hemolysis with G-6-PD deficiency *402*

Methemoglobin *Blood* *Increase* *Physiological* May cause hemolysis in G-6-PD deficiency *6015*

Pentastarch

Albumin *Serum* *Decrease* *Physiological* Hemodilution observed in patients undergoing repeated leukapheresis using pentastarch *1598*

Amylase *Serum* *Increase* *Physiological* Large amounts of pentastarch may cause transient increases of serum amylase activity without there being any obvious pancreatitis *1598*

Calcium *Serum* *Decrease* *Physiological* Hemodilution with reduction of protein concentration observed in patients undergoing repeated leukapheresis using pentastarch *1598*

Clotting Time *Blood* *Increase* *Physiological* Large amounts of pentastarch may cause transient slight prolongation of time due to hemodilution *1598*

Fibrinogen *Plasma* *Decrease* *Physiological* Hemodilution with reduction of protein concentration observed in patients undergoing repeated leukapheresis using pentastarch *1598*

Hematocrit *Blood* *Decrease* *Physiological* Effect observed with large doses *1384*

Hemoglobin *Blood* *Decrease* *Physiological* Slight decrease in hemoglobin concentration observed in patients undergoing repeated leukapheresis using pentastarch. Usually returns to normal within 24 hours *1598*

Partial Thromboplastin Time
Plasma *Increase* *Physiological* Large amounts of pentastarch may cause transient slight prolongation of time due to hemodilution *1598*

Platelets *Blood* *Decrease* *Physiological* Slight decrease in platelet concentration observed in patients undergoing repeated leukapheresis using pentastarch *1598*

Protein *Serum* *Decrease* *Physiological* Hemodilution observed in patients undergoing repeated leukapheresis using pentastarch *1598* Dilutes plasma and reduces concentration *1384*

Prothrombin Time *Plasma* *Increase* *Physiological* Large amounts of pentastarch may cause transient slight prolongation of time due to hemodilution *1598*

Volume *Plasma* *Decrease* *Physiological* Hemodilution observed in patients undergoing repeated leukapheresis using pentastarch *1598*

Pentazocine

δ-Aminolevulinic Acid *Urine* *Increase* *Physiological* May precipitate acute porphyria attack *2210*

Amphetamine *Urine* *Increase* *Physiological* Interferes with colorimetric methyl orange method *1972*

Amylase *Serum* *Increase* *Physiological* Causes spasm of sphincter of Oddi *2615*

Carbon Dioxide Partial Pressure
Blood *Increase* *Physiological* High doses produce marked respiratory depression *2242*

Coproporphyrin *Feces* *Increase* *Physiological* May precipitate acute porphyria attack *2210*

Pentazocine *(continued)*

Coproporphyrin *(continued)*
Urine Increase Physiological May precipitate acute porphyria attack *2210*

Cyclosporine *Serum Increase Physiological* Reported effect although no details discussed *1069*

Effective Renal Plasma Flow
Patient Decrease Physiological Observed in normal individuals *2242*

Eosinophils *Blood Increase Physiological* Eosinophilia reported as a complication *5259*

Epinephrine *Plasma Increase Physiological* Significant effect after 0.6 mg/kg i.v. in 20 minutes *3771*

Granulocytes *Blood Decrease Physiological* Decreased concentration of granulocytes reported, which is usually reversible *5259*

11-Hydroxycorticosteroids *Urine Decrease Physiological* ?Due to depression of adrenocortical secretion *1184*

17-Hydroxycorticosteroids *Urine Decrease Physiological* ?Due to depression of adrenocortical secretion *1184*

Leukocytes *Blood Decrease Physiological* Effect observed in 3 patients although taking other drugs, but effect recurred with reinstitution of treatment *2711* Decreased concentration reported, especially of granulocytes, which is usually reversible *5259*

Lipase *Serum Increase Physiological* Causes spasm of sphincter of Oddi *4012*

Neutrophils *Blood Decrease Physiological* Occasional case of agranulocytosis reported *6264*

Norepinephrine *Plasma Increase Physiological* After up to 0.6 mg/kg i.v. almost 2-fold increase in 10-20 minutes *3771*

Pentazocine *Blood Increase Physiological* Concentration of 150 µg/L achieved *3868*

pH *Blood Decrease Physiological* Slight fall (average 0.05) 15 minutes after i.v *4045*

Porphobilinogen *Urine Increase Physiological* May precipitate acute porphyria attack *2210*

Porphyrin, Total *Urine Increase Physiological* May precipitate attack of acute porphyria *1687*

Protoporphyrin *Feces Increase Physiological* May precipitate acute porphyria attack *2210*

Pentobarbital

Alanine Aminotransferase *Serum No Effect Analytical* At acute overdose concentration (20 mg/dL) on Technicon SMAC® method *6266*

Albumin *Serum No Effect Analytical* At concentration of 340 mg/L had no effect on BCG method *5704* At acute overdose concentration (20 mg/dL) on Technicon SMAC® method *6266*

Alkaline Phosphatase *Serum No Effect Analytical* At acute overdose concentration (20 mg/dL) on Technicon SMAC® method *6266*

Alprenolol *Serum Decrease Physiological* In 6 healthy volunteers pretreatment with pentobarbital for 10 days caused reduction of concentrations of both alprenolol and its major metabolite, 4-hydroxyalprenolol by about 40% over 7 hours *1098*

Aspartate Aminotransferase *Serum No Effect Analytical* At acute overdose concentration (20 mg/dL) on Technicon SMAC® method *6266*

Barbiturate *Urine Increase Analytical* Positive result obtained at a concentration of 1.0 µg/mL (4.4 µmol/L) with method on Du Pont aca *1555*

Bicarbonate *Serum No Effect Analytical* At concentration of 340 mg/L had no effect on method using phenolphthalein method *5704*

Bilirubin *Serum No Effect Analytical* At acute overdose concentration (20 mg/dL) on Technicon SMAC® method *6266* At concentration of 340 mg/L had no effect on Jendrassik and Grof method *5704*

Calcium *Serum No Effect Analytical* At acute overdose concentration (20 mg/dL) on Technicon SMAC® method *6266* At concentration of 340 mg/L had no effect on cresolphthalein method *5704*

Cannabinoids *Urine No Effect Analytical* No effect on Roche Abuscreen method *5006*

Carbamazepine *Serum No Effect Analytical* No cross-reactivity observed with method used with Du Pont aca *1513*

Chloride *Serum No Effect Analytical* At concentration of 340 mg/L had no effect on mercurimetric method *5704*

Cholesterol *Serum No Effect Analytical* At acute overdose concentration (20 mg/dL) on Technicon SMAC® method *6266* At concentration of 340 mg/L had no effect on Liebermann-Burchard method *5704*

Corticosteroids *Plasma Decrease Physiological* Barbiturates enhance the metabolism of exogenous corticosteroids *22*

Creatine Kinase *Serum No Effect Analytical* At acute overdose concentration (20 mg/dL) on Technicon SMAC® method *6266*

Creatinine *Serum No Effect Analytical* At acute overdose concentration (20 mg/dL) on Technicon SMAC® method *6266* At concentration of 340 mg/L had no effect on Technicon AutoAnalyzer® method *5704*

Dicumarol *Plasma Decrease Physiological* Phenobarbital, and presumably pentobarbital, lowers the plasma concentration of dicumarol, reducing its anticoagulant activity *22*

Doxycycline *Serum Decrease Physiological* Phenobarbital shortens the half-life of doxycycline for as long as 2 weeks after barbiturate therapy is discontinued, probably through induction of hepatic microsomal enzymes *22*

Drugs of Abuse Screen *Urine No Effect Analytical* No effect at concentration of 100 µg/mL on EZ-SCREEN procedure for cannabinoids and cocaine *1739*

Estradiol *Plasma Decrease Physiological* Pretreatment or concurrent administration of pentobarbital with estradiol may reduce its effects by increasing its metabolism *22*

Estrone *Plasma Decrease Physiological* Pretreatment or concurrent administration of pentobarbital with estrone may reduce its effects by increasing its metabolism *22*

Glucose *Serum No Effect Analytical* At acute overdose concentration (20 mg/dL) on Technicon SMAC® method *6266*

Griseofulvin *Serum Decrease Physiological* Phenobarbital interferes with the absorption of orally administered griseofulvin thus decreasing its blood concentration *22*

^{131}I Uptake *Serum Decrease Physiological* Lilly product contains tetraiodofluorescein *4360*

Iron *Serum No Effect Analytical* At concentration of 340 mg/L had no effect on Ferrozine method *5704* At acute overdose concentration (20 mg/dL) on Technicon SMAC® method *6266*

Lactate Dehydrogenase *Serum No Effect Analytical* At acute overdose concentration (20 mg/dL) on Technicon SMAC® method *6266*

Pentobarbital *Serum Increase Physiological* 600 mg orally produces concentration of 3.3 mg/L *3868*

Phenobarbital *Serum No Effect Analytical* No significant cross-reactivity observed with method on Du Pont aca *1537* At concentration of 1.00 mg/mL (4.028 mmol/L) has no effect on method on Du Pont Dimension *1582* No interference observed at a concentration of 200 µmol/L with Sung and Neely modification of Syva EMIT procedure *148* Cross-reactivity of less than 1.3% observed with method on Baxter Stratus *5705* At maximum physiological or pharmacological concentrations no cross-reactivity observed with phenobarbital method on Bayer Technicon Immuno 1® *427*

Phenytoin *Serum Decrease Physiological* Phenobarbital administration with phenytoin reported to accelerate its metabolism or to have no effect *22*
Serum No Effect Analytical No effect at concentration of 1000 µg/mL (4420 µmol/L) on method on Du Pont Dimension *1583* No significant interference observed at a concentration of 1000 µg/mL (4.03 mmol/L) with method on Du Pont aca *1538*
Serum No Effect Physiological Phenobarbital administration with phenytoin reported to accelerate its metabolism or to have no effect *22*

Phosphate *Serum No Effect Analytical* At acute overdose concentration (20 mg/dL) on Technicon SMAC® method *6266*

At concentration of 340 mg/L had no effect on phosphomolybdate method *5704*

Primidone *Serum No Effect Analytical* At concentrations above 1250 mg/L causes 25% increase as measured by method on Baxter Stratus but physiological concentrations up to 15 mg/L only *5705* No significant cross-reactivity with method on Du Pont aca *1541*

Progesterone *Plasma Decrease Physiological* Pretreatment or concurrent administration of pentobarbital with progesterone may reduce its effects by increasing its metabolism *22*

Protein *Serum No Effect Analytical* At concentration of 340 mg/L had no effect on biuret method with blank correction *5704* At acute overdose concentration (20 mg/dL) on Technicon SMAC® method *6266*

Theophylline *Serum Decrease Physiological* Total plasma clearance increased by mean of 40% in 9 healthy volunteers after 10 days of treatment with 100 mg pentobarbital each night. Renal clearance remained unchanged *1215*

Serum No Effect Analytical No effect of concentrations up to 20 mg/L on method on Kodak Ektachem® *5706*

Urine Decrease Physiological Fraction of theophylline excreted unchanged in urine reduced during simultaneous administration of theophylline and pentobarbital *1215*

Triglycerides *Serum No Effect Analytical* At concentration of 340 mg/L had no effect on lipase/esterase method *5704* At acute overdose concentration (20 mg/dL) on Technicon SMAC® method *6266*

Urea Nitrogen *Serum No Effect Analytical* At concentration of 340 mg/L had no effect on diacetylmonoxime method *5704* At acute overdose concentration (20 mg/dL) on Technicon SMAC® method *6266*

Uric Acid *Serum No Effect Analytical* At concentration of 340 mg/L had no effect on phosphotungstate reduction method *5704* At acute overdose concentration (20 mg/dL) on Technicon SMAC® method *6266*

Valproic Acid *Serum Decrease Physiological* Phenobarbital administration with valproic acid reported to accelerate its metabolism or to have no effect *22*

Serum No Effect Physiological Phenobarbital administration with valproic acid reported to accelerate its metabolism or to have no effect *22*

Pentopril

Alkaline Phosphatase *Serum No Effect Physiological* No effect attributable to drug observed in 15 patients with rheumatoid arthritis treated with up to 150 mg daily for up to 24 weeks *577*

Angiotensin-converting Enzyme
Serum Decrease Physiological Consistent reduction in relation to dosing observed in 15 patients with active rheumatoid arthritis treated with up to 150 mg daily for up to 24 weeks *577*

Aspartate Aminotransferase
Serum No Effect Physiological No effect attributable to drug observed in 15 patients with rheumatoid arthritis treated with up to 150 mg daily for up to 24 weeks *577*

Bilirubin *Serum No Effect Physiological* No effect attributable to drug observed in 15 patients with rheumatoid arthritis treated with up to 150 mg daily for up to 24 weeks *577*

C-Reactive Protein *Serum Decrease Physiological* Significant, but unexplained, reduction of concentration at week 16 in 15 patients with rheumatoid arthritis treated with up to 150 mg daily for up to 24 weeks *577*

Creatinine *Serum No Effect Physiological* No effect attributable to drug observed in 15 patients with rheumatoid arthritis treated with up to 150 mg daily for up to 24 weeks *577*

Erythrocyte Sedimentation Rate
Blood No Effect Physiological No significant change observed in 15 patients with rheumatoid arthritis treated with up to 150 mg daily for up to 24 weeks *577*

Erythrocytes *Blood No Effect Physiological* No effect attributable to drug observed in 15 patients with rheumatoid arthritis treated with up to 150 mg daily for up to 24 weeks *577*

Hemoglobin *Blood Decrease Physiological* Reduction noted, although it remained within the normal range, observed in 15 patients with rheumatoid arthritis treated with up to 150 mg daily for up to 24 weeks *577*

Histidine *Plasma No Effect Physiological* No significant change observed in 15 patients with rheumatoid arthritis treated with up to 150 mg daily for up to 24 weeks *577*

Leukocytes *Blood No Effect Physiological* No effect attributable to drug observed in 15 patients with rheumatoid arthritis treated with up to 150 mg daily for up to 24 weeks *577*

Platelets *Blood No Effect Physiological* No effect attributable to drug observed in 15 patients with rheumatoid arthritis treated with up to 150 mg daily for up to 24 weeks *577*

Potassium *Serum No Effect Physiological* No effect attributable to drug observed in 15 patients with rheumatoid arthritis treated with up to 150 mg daily for up to 24 weeks *577*

Rheumatoid Factor *Serum No Effect Physiological* No significant effect observed in 15 patients with rheumatoid arthritis treated with up to 150 mg/d for up to 24 weeks *577*

Sodium *Serum No Effect Physiological* No effect attributable to drug observed in 15 patients with rheumatoid arthritis treated with up to 150 mg daily for up to 24 weeks *577*

Sulfhydryl *Serum No Effect Physiological* No significant change observed in 15 patients with rheumatoid arthritis treated with up to 150 mg daily for up to 24 weeks *577*

Urea Nitrogen *Serum No Effect Physiological* No effect attributable to drug observed in 15 patients treated with up to 150 mg daily for up to 24 weeks *577*

Viscosity *Plasma No Effect Physiological* No significant change observed in 15 patients with rheumatoid arthritis treated with up to 150 mg daily for up to 24 weeks. Actual deterioration observed at week 4 *577*

Pentosan Polysulfate

Partial Thromboplastin Time
Plasma No Effect Physiological In 24 healthy male volunteers doses up to 1200 mg/d for 8 days had no effect *336*

Prothrombin Time *Plasma No Effect Physiological* In 24 healthy male volunteers doses up to 1200 mg/d for 8 days had no effect *336*

Pentostatin

Calcium *Serum Increase Physiological* Hypercalcemia occurred in less than 3% of pentostatin-treated hairy cell leukemia patients *5873*

Creatinine *Serum Increase Physiological* Increased concentration occurred in 3 to 10% of pentostatin-treated hairy cell leukemia patients *5873*

Erythrocytes *Blood Decrease Physiological* Toxicity has included myelosuppression *1384*

Granulocytes *Blood Decrease Physiological* Agranulocytosis occurred in 3 to 10% of pentostatin-treated hairy cell leukemia patients *5873*

Hematocrit *Blood Decrease Physiological* Aplastic or hemolytic anemia occurred in less than 3% of pentostatin-treated hairy cell leukemia patients *5873*

Hemoglobin *Blood Decrease Physiological* Aplastic or hemolytic anemia occurred in less than 3% of pentostatin-treated hairy cell leukemia patients *5873*

Leukocytes *Blood Decrease Physiological* Myelosuppression observed as manifestation of toxicity *1384*

Lymphocytes *Blood Decrease Physiological* Myelosuppression observed as sign of toxicity with lymphopenia being pronounced *1384*

2',5'-Oligoadenylate Synthetase
Monocytes Increase Physiological In 10 patients with hairy cell leukemia and seven patients with other B-cell chronic leukemias, in those with hairy cell leukemia increased 4.6 fold at 4 h and 11.5 fold at 24 h compared to the pretreatment value but in some patients with B-cell chronic leukemia activity remained unchanged *2630*

Serum Increase Physiological In patients with hairy cell leukemia activity in plasma followed same respose as observed in monocytes *2630*

Platelets *Blood Decrease Physiological* Toxicity includes myelosuppression *1384*

Pentostatin *(continued)*

Sodium *Serum Decrease Physiological* Hyponatremia occurred in less than 3% of pentostatin-treated hairy cell leukemia patients *5873*

Urea Nitrogen *Serum Increase Physiological* Renal toxicity observed as an adverse effect *1384* Renal failure or renal insufficiency occurred in less than 3% of pentostatin-treated hairy cell leukemia patients *5873*

Uric Acid *Serum Increase Physiological* Hypercalcemia occurred in less than 3% of pentostatin-treated hairy cell leukemia patients *5873* Renal toxicity includes hyperuricemia *1384*

Pentoxifylline

Alanine Aminotransferase *Serum Increase Physiological* Occasional case of hepatitis reported *1384* Cholecystitis has been reported as a complication with a frequency of less than 1% *2654*

Aspartate Aminotransferase *Serum Increase Physiological* Occasional case of hepatitis reported *1384* Cholecystitis has been reported as a complication with a frequency of less than 1% *2654*

Bilirubin *Serum Increase Physiological* Occasional case of hepatitis and jaundice reported *1384*

CD4+ Lymphocytes *Blood No Effect Physiological* In 17 patients with AIDS treatment with 1200 mg/d for 8 weeks caused nonsignificant reduction from mean baseline of 69 (median 32) cells /µL to 57 (median 34) cells /µL *1407*

Erythrocytes *Blood Decrease Physiological* Occasional pancytopenia reported and even more rarely aplastic anemia *1384*

Fibrinogen *Plasma Decrease Physiological* Reduction of concentration observed *1384* Inhibitory effect observed *3186*

Hematocrit *Blood Decrease Physiological* In 2 patients receiving other drugs concomitantly but for considerable time previously without ill effects *3705*

Leukocytes *Blood Decrease Physiological* In 2 patients receiving other drugs concomitantly but for considerable time previously without ill effects *3705* Leukopenia has been reported as a complication with a frequency of less than 1% *2654*

β_2-Microglobulin *Serum Increase Physiological* In 17 patients with AIDS treatment with 1200 mg/d for 8 weeks caused increase from mean baseline of 2.71 µg/L to 2.88 µg/L *1407*

Neopterin *Serum Increase Physiological* In 17 patients with AIDS treatment with 1200 mg/d for 8 weeks caused significant increase from mean baseline of 16.8 nmol/L to 18.6 nmol/L *1407*

Platelets *Blood Decrease Physiological* In 2 patients receiving other drugs concomitantly but for considerable time previously without ill effects *3705*

Sperm Count *Semen No Effect Physiological* No effect observed when pentoxifylline administered to patients who had had asthenozoospermia for 3 months *5495*

Sperm Motility *Semen Increase Physiological* Sperm motility significantly increased in patients with asthenozoospermia for 3 months when pentoxifylline administered *5495* Motility increased by 1.5-fold compared with controls at 120, 180 and 240 minutes after pentoxifylline treatment *1993*

Theophylline *Serum Increase Physiological* Decreases theophylline clearance increases plasma theophylline concentration by 30% *3125* Decreases theophylline clearance increasing theophylline concentration by about 30% *5999* Up to 30% increase in serum theophylline concentration due to decreased theophylline clearance *6117*
Serum No Effect Analytical Although structurally similar, pentoxifylline and its metabolites appear to have no effect at normal doses on theophylline measurement by the Abbott TDx *4128* No effect observed on immunoassay measurement systems *5999*

Triglycerides *Serum Decrease Physiological* In 17 patients with AIDS treatment with 1200 mg/d for 8 weeks caused significant decrease from mean baseline of 254 mg/dL to 188 mg/dL *1407*

Tumor Necrosis Factor-α *Serum Decrease Physiological* In 14 patients with advanced cancer with abnormally high concentrations of TNF-α treatment for 7 days (300 mg/d intravenously) caused significant decrease from mean baseline of 44 ± 7 mg/mL to 21 ± 4 mg/mL *3605* In 3 of 5 patients with AIDS related wasting in whom TNF-α concentration was increased treatment for 4 - 8 weeks caused reductions of from 113 to 10 pg/mL, 35 to 6 pg/mL and 21 to 15 pg/mL respectively *3394*

Tumor Necrosis Factor-α mRNA *Lymphocytes Decrease Physiological* In 16 patients with AIDS treatment with 1200 mg/d pentoxifyline for 8 weeks caused decrease in concentration in lymphocytes and monocytes in 10 of the patients. No change was observed in 4 patients and the concentration increased in 2. Median change in all 16 patients 29% decrease *1407*

Pentylenetetrazole

Cholesterol *Serum Decrease Physiological* Maximal effect seen after 2 weeks *533*

Histamine *Plasma No Effect Analytical* Improbable inhibition of radio-enzyme assay at therapeutic concentrations *2492*

Pregnancy Tests *Urine Positive Analytical* In one patient affected hCG and Pregslide tests *2452*

Perfenazine

Tricyclic Antidepressants *Serum Increase Analytical* May cause false positive reaction in immunoassays for tricyclic antidepressants *3590*

Pergolide

Cholesterol *Serum Increase Physiological* Hypercholesterolemia has been reported to occur as an infrequent side effect *283*

Eosinophils *Blood Increase Physiological* Eosinophilia has been reported to occur as a rare side effect *283*

Erythrocytes *Urine Increase Physiological* Hematuria has been reported to occur as a frequent side effect *283*

Glucose *Serum Decrease Physiological* Hypoglycemia has been reported to occur as an infrequent side effect *283*
Serum Increase Physiological Hyperglycemia has been reported to occur as an infrequent side effect *283*

Hemoglobin *Blood Decrease Physiological* Anemia has been reported to occur frequently as a side effect *283*
Urine Increase Physiological Hematuria has been reported to occur as a frequent side effect *283*

Iron *Serum Decrease Physiological* Iron deficiency anemia has been reported to occur as an infrequent side effect *283*

Leukocytes *Blood Decrease Physiological* Leukopenia has been reported to occur infrequently as a side effect *283*
Blood Increase Physiological Leukocytosis has been reported to occur infrequently as a side effect *283*

Lymphocytes *Blood Increase Physiological* Lymphocytosis has been reported to occur as a rare side effect *283*

MCH *Blood Increase Physiological* Megaloblastic anemia has been reported to occur as an infrequent side effect *283*

MCV *Blood Increase Physiological* Megaloblastic anemia has been reported to occur as an infrequent side effect *283*

pH *Blood Decrease Physiological* Acidosis has been reported to occur as a rare side effect *283*

Platelets *Blood Decrease Physiological* Thrombocytopenia has been reported to occur infrequently as a side effect *283*
Blood Increase Physiological Thrombocythemia has been reported to occur as a rare side effect *283*

Potassium *Serum Decrease Physiological* Hypokalemia has been reported to occur as an infrequent side effect *283*

Prolactin *Plasma Decrease Physiological* Marked reduction in patients with Parkinson's disease to low or undetectable levels *3178* Single dose reduced concentration for 24 h in normal subjects, multiple doses reduced concentration by 80% *3513*

Thyroxine (T4) *Serum Decrease Physiological* Hypothyroidism has been reported to occur infrequently as a side effect *283*

Uric Acid *Serum Increase Physiological* Gout has been reported to occur as an infrequent side effect *283*

Urine Increase Physiological Increased excretion has been reported to occur as a rare side effect *283*

Perhexilene

Alkaline Phosphatase *Serum Increase Physiological* Transient elevation observed *2657*

Aspartate Aminotransferase *Serum Increase Physiological* Transient elevation observed *2657*

Peribedil

Thyroid Stimulating Hormone

Serum Decrease Physiological Effect noted in hypothyroid subjects *6412*

Perindopril

Albumin *Urine Decrease Physiological* In mild hypertensive diabetics controlled with insulin, perindopril reduced albumin excretion. In those with albuminuria of 15-150 mg/day mean excretion reduced from 59 mg/24 h to 32 mg/24 h after 1 month; effect sustained for 9 months of study *716* In mild hypertensive diabetics controlled with insulin, perindopril reduced albumin excretion. In those with albuminuria of 15-150 mg/day mean excretion reduced from 59 mg/24 h to 32 mg/24 h after 1 month; effect sustained for 9 months of study *716*

Urine No Effect Physiological In mild to moderate hypertensive diabetics no change observed over 9 months in those patients excreting less than 15 mg/24 h or more than 150 mg/24 h at start of study *716*

Aldosterone *Plasma Decrease Physiological* Maximal effect observed 4-6 hours after single oral dose of 4-8 mg but substantial effect still observed after 24 hours *3714* 51% reduction (from mean concentration of 145.4 pg/mL to 70.6 pg/mL) in 10 patients with essential hypertension treated with 4 mg daily for 4 weeks *757* Significant reduction observed 4 hours after single dose of 4 mg in 6 volunteers but effect more marked after 8 days treatment *6289* After doses of 4 mg twice daily within 4 h of administration *829*

Angiotensin-I *Plasma Increase Physiological* Maximal effect observed 4-6 hours after single oral dose of 4-8 mg with substantial effect still observed after 24 hours *3714* After doses of 4 mg twice daily within 4 h of administration *829* Concentration increased at same time as decrease in angiotensin II concentration in 6 healthy volunteers following single dose of 4 mg with increase being more marked after last dose of 8 days treatment *6289*

Angiotensin-II *Plasma Decrease Physiological* Maximal effect observed 4-6 hours after a single oral dose of 4-8 mg but with substantial effect still seen at 24 hours *3714* After doses of 4 mg twice daily within 4 h of administration *829* Significant reduction 4 hours after single dose of 4 mg. Concentration remained reduced for 24 hours after first dose but not after dose at end of 8 days treatment *6289*

Angiotensin-converting Enzyme

Serum Decrease Physiological At doses of 4 to 8 mg maximal effect observed 4-6 hours after administration with substantial effect still apparent at 24 hours *3714* Sustained inhibition following intravenous administration *3484* With doses of up to 16 mg daily for 1 week reduction observed maximal 4 to 8 hours after drug intake but still markedly reduced after 24 hours. Reduction of up to 95% with single dose of 16 mg *6289* After 3 months treatment of 40 mild to moderate hypertensive insulin-treated diabetic patients marked inhibition of enzyme observed (decrease from mean of 9.82 U/L to 2.35 U/L) *716* With single doses of 8 to 16 mg produced reduction to less than 10% of control in 4 h with lasting effect for 72 h *829* After 3 months treatment with up to 8 mg/d of 40 mild to moderate hypertensive insulin-treated diabetic patients marked inhibition of enzyme observed (decrease from mean of 9.82 U/L to 2.35 U/L) *716* In 10 patients with essential hypertension treatment with 4 mg daily for 4 weeks caused 59.4% reduction in activity 24 hours after last dose administered *757*

Calcium *Serum No Effect Physiological* No effect in 11 healthy volunteers over 24 h when given 16 mg *4926*

Urine No Effect Physiological No effect in 11 healthy volunteers for 24 h when given up to 16 mg *4926*

Chloride *Serum No Effect Physiological* No effect in 11 healthy volunteers over 24 h when given 16 mg *4926*

Urine No Effect Physiological No effect for up to 24 h in 11 healthy volunteers given up to 16 mg *4926*

Cholesterol *Serum Decrease Physiological* In 10 patients with essential hypertension treatment with up to 8 mg/d for 8 - 12 weeks caused decrease of 0.26 ± 0.24 mmol/L from mean baseline of 4.71 ± 0.21 mmol/L *4397* In 10 middle-aged patients with essential hypertension treatment with up to 8 mg/d for up to 12 weeks caused decrease of 0.26 ± 0.24 mmol/L from mean baseline of 4.71 ± 0.21 mmol/L *4397*

Creatinine *Serum No Effect Physiological* No significant change observed over 18 months treatment in hypertensive patients *5267* No clinically significant effect in 11 healthy volunteers over 24 h when given 16 mg *4926*

Urine No Effect Physiological No effect in 11 healthy volunteers for 24 h when given up to 16 mg *4926*

Creatinine Clearance *Urine No Effect Physiological* No significant change observed in 40 insulin controlled diabetics with mild to moderate hypertension when treated with up to 8 mg/d over 9 months *716* No significant change observed in 40 insulin controlled diabetics with mild to moderate hypertension when treated over 9 months *716*

Fructosamine *Serum No Effect Physiological* No significant effect (concentration remained within range of 3.6-3.7 mmol/L) observed when perindopril given for 9 months to 40 insulin controlled diabetics with mild to moderate hypertension *716*

Glucose *Serum Decrease Physiological* Incidence of 0.6% observed in French Pharmacovigilance database *4106*

Serum Increase Physiological In 10 middle-aged patients with essential hypertension treatment with up to 8 mg/d for up to 12 weeks caused increase of 0.4 ± 1.2 mmol/L from mean baseline of 6.2 ± 0.4 mmol/L *4397*

Serum No Effect Physiological No significant alteration of insulin requirements in 40 insulin controlled diabetics when their mild to moderate hypertension treated with perindopril over 9 months *716*

Glucose Tolerance *Serum No Effect Physiological* In patients with essential hypertension treatment for 8 - 12 weeks had no significant effect on tolerance to 75 g glucose *4397*

HDL-Cholesterol *Serum Increase Physiological* In 10 middle-aged patients with essential hypertension treatment with up to 8 mg/d for up to 12 weeks caused increase of 0.08 ± 0.07 mmol/L from mean baseline of 1.16 ± 0.10 mmol/L *4397*

Serum No Effect Physiological In 10 patients with essential hypertension treatment with up to 8 mg/d for 8 - 12 weeks caused nonsignificant increase of 0.08 ± 0.07 mmol/L from mean baseline of 1.16 ± 0.10 mmol/L *4397*

Hemoglobin A_{1c} *Blood No Effect Physiological* No effect observed on concentration (about 7%) when 40 mild to moderate hypertensive insulin controlled diabetics were treated with perindopril over 9 months *716*

Insulin *Plasma Increase Physiological* In 10 middle-aged patients with essential hypertension treatment with up to 8 mg/d for up to 12 weeks caused increase of 0.6 ± 3.0 µU/mL from mean baseline of 14.4 ± 2.6 µU/mL *4397*

Magnesium *Serum No Effect Physiological* No clinically significant effect in 11 healthy volunteers over 24 h when given 16 mg *4926*

Urine No Effect Physiological No effect in 11 healthy volunteers for 24 h when given up to 16 mg *4926*

Phosphate *Serum No Effect Physiological* No effect in 11 healthy volunteers over 24 h after 16 mg *4926*

Urine No Effect Physiological No effect in 11 healthy volunteers for 24 h when given up to 16 mg *4926*

Potassium *Serum Increase Physiological* Nonclinically significant increase in hypertensive patients treated for 18 months with drug as sole therapeutic agent *5267*

Serum No Effect Physiological No effect in 11 healthy volunteers over 24 h when given 16 mg *4926*

Perindopril *(continued)*

Potassium *(continued)*
Urine *No Effect* *Physiological* No effect in 11 healthy volunteers for 24 h when given up to 16 mg *4926*

Prolidase *Serum* *No Effect* *Analytical* Slight inhibitory effect observed in vitro but at much higher concentration than therapeutic *4197*

Renin Activity *Plasma* *Increase* *Physiological* Significant increase from mean concentration of 2.15 to 3.26 ng AI/mL/h in 10 patients with essential hypertension treated with 4 mg daily for 4 weeks *757* After doses of 4 mg twice daily within 4 h of administration *829* After 3 months treatment with up to 8 mg/d of 40 mild to moderate hypertensive insulin-controlled diabetic patients with perindopril activity increased from mean of 2.33 ng/mL/h to 7.49 ng/mL/h *716* Significant increase in 6 normal volunteers following single dose of 4 mg but even more marked increase after 8 days treatment with 4 mg daily *6289* Maximal effect after dose of 4-8 mg seen 4-6 hours later with substantial effect still apparent after 24 hours *3714* After 3 months treatment of 40 mild to moderate hypertensive insulin-controlled diabetic patients with perindopril activity increased from mean of 2.33 ng/mL/h to 7.49 ng/mL/h *716*

Sodium *Serum* *No Effect* *Physiological* No effect in 11 healthy volunteers for 24 h after 16 mg *4926*
Urine *No Effect* *Physiological* No effect in 11 healthy volunteers for 24 h when given up to 16 mg *4926*

Triglycerides *Serum* *Increase* *Physiological* In 10 middle-aged patients with essential hypertension treatment with up to 8 mg/d for up to 12 weeks caused increase of 0.16 ± 0.16 mmol/L from mean baseline of 1.48 ± 0.12 mmol/L *4397*
Serum *No Effect* *Physiological* In 10 patients with essential hypertension treatment with up to 8 mg/d for 8 - 12 weeks caused nonsignificant increase of 0.16 ± 0.16 mmol/L from mean baseline of 1.48 ± 0.12 mmol/L *4397*

Urea Nitrogen *Serum* *No Effect* *Physiological* No effect in 11 healthy volunteers over 24 h when given 16 mg *4926*
Urine *No Effect* *Physiological* No effect in 11 healthy volunteers for 24 h when given up to 16 mg *4926*

Uric Acid *Serum* *No Effect* *Physiological* No effect in 11 healthy volunteers over 24 h when given 16 mg *4926*
Urine *No Effect* *Physiological* No effect in 11 healthy volunteers for 24 h when given up to 16 mg *4926*

Volume *Urine* *No Effect* *Physiological* No effect for up to 24 h in healthy volunteers given up to 16 mg *4926*

Zinc *Serum* *No Effect* *Physiological* No effect in 11 healthy volunteers over 24 h when given 16 mg *4926*
Urine *No Effect* *Physiological* No effect in 11 healthy volunteers for 24 h when given up to 16 mg *4926*

Perphenazine

Alanine Aminotransferase *Serum* *Increase* *Physiological* Administration may cause biliary stasis or jaundice *5338*
Serum *No Effect* *Analytical* At acute overdose concentration (20 mg/dL) on Technicon SMAC® method *6266*

Albumin *Serum* *No Effect* *Analytical* At concentration of 200 mg/L had no effect on BCG method *5704* At acute overdose concentration (20 mg/dL) on Technicon SMAC® method *6266*

Alkaline Phosphatase *Serum* *Increase* *Physiological* Administration may cause biliary stasis or jaundice *5338*
Serum *No Effect* *Analytical* At acute overdose concentration (20 mg/dL) on Technicon SMAC® method *6266*

Aspartate Aminotransferase *Serum* *Increase* *Physiological* Administration may cause biliary stasis or jaundice *5338*
Serum *No Effect* *Analytical* At acute overdose concentration (20 mg/dL) on Technicon SMAC® method *6266*

Bicarbonate *Serum* *No Effect* *Analytical* At concentration of 1 mg/L had no effect on measurement by phenolphthalein method *5704*

Bile *Urine* *Increase* *Physiological* Low incidence of jaundice reported *3810*

Bilirubin *Serum* *Increase* *Physiological* Administration may cause biliary stasis or jaundice *5338* Low incidence of jaundice reported *128*
Serum *No Effect* *Analytical* At acute overdose concentration (20 mg/dL) on Technicon SMAC® method *6266* At concentration of 200 mg/L had no effect on Jendrassik and Grof method *5704*
Urine *Increase* *Physiological* Low incidence of jaundice reported *3810*

Calcium *Serum* *No Effect* *Analytical* At concentration of 200 mg/L had no effect on cresolphthalein method *5704* At acute overdose concentration (20 mg/dL) on Technicon SMAC® method *6266*

Catecholamines *Plasma* *Increase* *Physiological* Increased metabolism, decreased organ uptake of norepinephrine *2024*

Chloride *Serum* *No Effect* *Analytical* At concentration of 1 mg/L had no effect on mercurimetric method *5704*

Cholesterol *Serum* *No Effect* *Analytical* At concentration of 200 mg/L had no effect on Liebermann-Burchard method *5704* At concentration of 1 mg/L had no effect on CHOD-PAP method *5704* At acute overdose concentration (20 mg/dL) on Technicon SMAC® method *6266*

Creatine Kinase *Serum* *No Effect* *Analytical* At acute overdose concentration (20 mg/dL) on Technicon SMAC® method *6266*

Creatinine *Serum* *No Effect* *Analytical* At concentration of 200 mg/L had no effect on Technicon AutoAnalyzer® method *5704* At acute overdose concentration (20 mg/dL) on Technicon SMAC® method *6266*

Eosinophils *Blood* *Increase* *Physiological* Administration may cause agranulocytosis, eosinophilia, leukopenia, hemolytic anemia, thrombocytopenic purpura and pancytopenia *5338*

Glucose *Serum* *Decrease* *Physiological* Administration may cause hyperglycemia or hypoglycemia *5338*
Serum *Increase* *Physiological* May cause hyperglycemia *2754* Administration may cause hyperglycemia or hypoglycemia *5338*
Serum *No Effect* *Analytical* At acute overdose concentration (20 mg/dL) on Technicon SMAC® method *6266* At concentration of 1 mg/L had no effect on GOD/POD-PAP method *5704*
Urine *Increase* *Physiological* Administration may cause hyperglycemia or hypoglycemia *5338*

Glucose Tolerance *Serum* *Decrease* *Physiological* Abnormal curves in 35% subjects *4014*

Granulocytes *Blood* *Decrease* *Physiological* Administration may cause agranulocytosis, eosinophilia, leukopenia, hemolytic anemia, thrombocytopenic purpura and pancytopenia *5338*

Hematocrit *Blood* *Decrease* *Physiological* Administration may cause agranulocytosis, eosinophilia, leukopenia, hemolytic anemia, thrombocytopenic purpura and pancytopenia *5338*

Hemoglobin *Blood* *Decrease* *Physiological* Administration may cause agranulocytosis, eosinophilia, leukopenia, hemolytic anemia, thrombocytopenic purpura and pancytopenia *5338*

Histamine *Plasma* *No Effect* *Analytical* Improbable inhibition of radio-enzyme assay at physiological concentrations *2492*

17-Hydroxycorticosteroids *Urine* *Decrease* *Physiological* Acts on hypothalamus to depress ACTH secretion *661*

^{131}I Uptake *Serum* *Decrease* *Physiological* Depresses uptake *882*
Serum *No Effect* *Physiological* No effect observed in euthyroid subjects *3669*

Iron *Serum* *No Effect* *Analytical* At acute overdose concentration (20 mg/dL) on Technicon SMAC® method *6266* At concentration of 200 mg/L had no effect on Ferrozine method *5704*

Lactate Dehydrogenase *Serum* *No Effect* *Analytical* At acute overdose concentration (20 mg/dL) on Technicon SMAC® method *6266*

Leukocytes *Blood* *Decrease* *Physiological* Administration may cause agranulocytosis, eosinophilia, leukopenia, hemolytic anemia, thrombocytopenic purpura and pancytopenia *5338* Suspected of causing agranulocytosis *4714*

Neutrophils *Blood* *Decrease* *Physiological* May cause neutropenia/agranulocytosis *4265*

Nortriptyline *Serum Increase Physiological* In 25 elderly patients addition of perphenazine to a treatment regime involving nortriptyline caused median quotient of nortriptyline plasma level to dose to increase from 6.1 to 8.6 due to inhibition of cytochrome P450 2D6 *4168*

Peptides, Low-molecular Weight
Urine Decrease Physiological In one schizophrenic patient treatment with 12 mg/d for 5 weeks caused significant reduction from 34.3 μmol/d to 9.4 μmol/d *4901*

Phosphate *Serum No Effect Analytical* At concentration of 200 mg/L had no effect on phosphomolybdate method *5704* At acute overdose concentration (20 mg/dL) on Technicon SMAC® method *6266*

Platelets *Blood Decrease Physiological* Administration may cause agranulocytosis, eosinophilia, leukopenia, hemolytic anemia, thrombocytopenic purpura and pancytopenia *5338*

Potassium *Serum No Effect Analytical* At concentration of 1 mg/L had no effect on flame-photometric method *5704*

Pregnancy Tests *Urine Positive Analytical* Administration may cause false positive pregnancy tests *5338*

Prolactin *Plasma Increase Physiological* Marked effect in male and female psychiatric patients treated for up to 4 weeks *6098* By approximately 800% in women after 8 mg *797* Typical dose-related response to i.m. administered drug due to antidopaminergic action *3402*

Protein *Cerebrospinal Fluid Increase Physiological* Altered proteins reported *2754*
Serum No Effect Analytical At acute overdose concentration (20 mg/dL) on Technicon SMAC® method *6266* At concentration of 200 mg/L had no effect on biuret method with blank correction *5704*

Sodium *Serum No Effect Analytical* At concentration of 1 mg/L had no effect on flame-photometric method *5704*

T3-Uptake *Serum Decrease Physiological* Occurs with prolonged use *3810*

Thyroxine Binding Globulin *Serum Increase Physiological* Direct effect of drug *42*

Tricyclic Antidepressants Screen
Serum No Effect Analytical No significant effect observed at a concentration of 350 ng/mL (0.87 μmol/L) with method on Du Pont aca *1550*

Triglycerides *Serum No Effect Analytical* At concentration of 200 mg/L had no effect on lipase/esterase method *5704* At acute overdose concentration (20 mg/dL) on Technicon SMAC® method *6266*

Urea Nitrogen *Serum No Effect Analytical* At acute overdose concentration (20 mg/dL) on Technicon SMAC® method *6266* At concentration of 200 mg/L had no effect on diacetylmonoxime method *5704*

Uric Acid *Serum No Effect Analytical* At acute overdose concentration (20 mg/dL) on Technicon SMAC® method *6266* At concentration of 200 mg/L had no effect on phosphotungstate reduction method *5704*

Phenacemide

Alanine Aminotransferase *Serum Increase Physiological* Hepatitis has been observed with fatalities in 2 of 100 patients *25* May affect liver function in about 2% cases *3810*

Alkaline Phosphatase *Serum Increase Physiological* May affect liver function in about 2% cases *3810* Hepatitis has been observed with fatalities in 2 of 100 patients *25*

Aspartate Aminotransferase *Serum Increase Physiological* May affect liver function in about 2% cases *3810* Hepatitis has been observed with fatalities in 2 of 100 patients *25*

Bile *Urine Increase Physiological* May affect liver function in about 2% cases *3810*

Bilirubin *Serum Increase Physiological* Hepatitis has been observed with fatalities in 2 of 100 patients *25* May affect liver function in about 2% cases *3810*

BSP Retention *Serum Increase Physiological* May alter liver function in about 2% cases *3810*

Creatinine *Serum Decrease Analytical* Positive interference with kinetic Jaffe reaction within 21 s but negative result thereafter *3300* As measured by Du Pont aca due to decrease of absorbance of product with picrate with time *3300*
Serum Increase Physiological Rise in serum creatinine or nephritis observed in fewer than 1 in 100 patients *25*

Erythrocytes *Blood Decrease Physiological* Leukopenia is main blood dyscrasia but fatal aplastic anemia occurred in two of 100 patients *25* Aplastic anemia/agranulocytosis *3810*

Felbamate *Serum No Effect Analytical* No significant interference observed with GLC method of Rifai et al *4958*

Hematocrit *Blood Decrease Physiological* Aplastic anemia *128*

Hemoglobin *Blood Decrease Physiological* Aplastic anemia *128*

Leukocytes *Blood Decrease Physiological* Leukopenia is main blood dyscrasia but fatal aplastic anemia occurred in two of 100 patients *25* Aplastic anemia (leukopenia reported most often) *128*

Platelets *Blood Decrease Physiological* Aplastic anemia may occur rarely *128* Leukopenia is main blood dyscrasia but fatal aplastic anemia occurred in two of 100 patients *25*

Protein *Urine Increase Physiological* Occasional nephropathy *1714* *128*

Urea Nitrogen *Serum Increase Physiological* Occasional nephropathy *128*

Phenacetin

Alanine Aminotransferase *Serum No Effect Analytical* No effect at 200 mg/L on method on Ames Seralyzer *5706*

α-Fetoprotein *Serum Decrease Physiological* Administration of drug to pregnant women is associated with reduction in concentration *2229*

5-Hydroxyindoleacetic Acid *Urine No Effect Analytical* No effect observed with FPIA method on Abbott TDx *695*

p-Aminophenol *Urine No Effect Analytical* With addition of drugs at a concentration of 100 mg/L and of related compounds at 50 mg/L no significant effect observed on colorimetric method of van Bocxlaer on Cobas Mira analyzer which involves reacting free p-aminophenol with resorcinol in the presence of magnesium ions to form an indophenol dye measured at 550 nm *6163*

Phenylalanine *Plasma No Effect Analytical* No interference observed with rapid quantitative whole blood method of Campbell et al using phenylalanine dehydrogenase *867*

Phenaglycodol

Cortisol *Plasma No Effect Analytical* No physiological effect observed *2452*

17-Ketogenic Steroids *Urine Increase Analytical* Interferes with Zimmermann reaction *5869*

17-Ketosteroids *Urine Increase Analytical* Interferes with Zimmermann reaction *5869*

Phenanthroline

Angiotensin-converting Enzyme
Serum Decrease Analytical 80% inhibition of method using benzyloxycarbonyl-phenylalanyl-histidyl-leucine as substrate *5409*

Phenazocine

Carbon Dioxide Partial Pressure
Blood Increase Physiological May produce respiratory depression *2242*

Phenazone

Glucose *Serum No Effect Analytical* No effect of concentrations up to 1000 mg/L on method on Kodak Ektachem® *5706*

Histamine *Plasma No Effect Analytical* Insignificant inhibition of radio-enzyme assay at concentrations five times physiological *2492*

Phenazone *(continued)*

Salicylate *Serum Increase Analytical* At 100 mg/L has slight effect (8%) on method of Keller but 22% on that of Trinder, also observed in one patient who had taken overdose of drug *2910*

Urea Nitrogen *Serum No Effect Analytical* No effect of concentrations up to 1000 mg/L on method on Kodak Ektachem® *5706*

Phenazopyridine

Alanine Aminotransferase *Serum Increase Physiological* May cause hepatic toxicity as a side effect *4531* Hepatotoxic effect *3810*
Serum No Effect Analytical No effect at 25 mg/L on Boehringer Mannheim Reflotron method *5706* No effect at therapeutic concentration on Boehringer Mannheim Reflotron method *3231*

Albumin *Serum Increase Analytical* Contributes to absorption binding procedure *882*

Alkaline Phosphatase *Serum Increase Physiological* Hepatotoxic effect *3810* May cause hepatic toxicity as a side effect *4531*

Amylase *Serum No Effect Analytical* No effect of concentrations up to 25 mg/L on method on Boehringer Mannheim Reflotron *5706*

Amylase, Pancreatic Isoenzyme
Serum No Effect Physiological No significant effect observed at a toxic concentration of 25 mg/L with method on Boehringer Mannheim Reflotron *3647*

Aspartate Aminotransferase *Serum Increase Physiological* Hepatotoxic effect *3810* May cause hepatic toxicity as a side effect *4531*
Serum No Effect Analytical No effect at 25 mg/L on Boehringer Mannheim Reflotron method *5706* No effect at therapeutic concentration on Boehringer Mannheim Reflotron method *3231*

Bacteria *Urine Negative Analytical* May interfere with color on Microstix *203*

Bile *Urine Increase Analytical* False positive with Ictotest®, BiliLabstix® *4233*
Urine Increase Physiological Hepatotoxic effect *3810*

Bilirubin *Serum Decrease Physiological* Atypical color causes interference with some assays *3810*
Serum Increase Analytical Postulated increased color with diazotization *1009*
Serum Increase Physiological Single report of jaundice (?due to hemolysis) *2701* May cause hepatic toxicity as a side effect *4531*
Serum No Effect Analytical No effect at concentration of 80 mg/L on method on Kodak Ektachem® *5706* No effect at 20 mg/L on Ames Seralyzer method *5706*

Bilirubin, Conjugated *Serum No Effect Analytical* No effect at concentration of 80 mg/L on method on Kodak Ektachem® *5706*

Bilirubin, Unconjugated *Serum No Effect Analytical* No effect at concentration of 80 mg/L on method on Kodak Ektachem® *5706*

BSP Retention *Serum Decrease Analytical* High absorbancy in blank if acidified *882*
Serum Increase Analytical Increased spectral absorbancy in colorimetric reading *6515*
Serum Increase Physiological Hepatic damage reported in one case *2701*

Cholesterol *Serum No Effect Analytical* At concentration of 25 mg/L no effect on method on Boehringer Mannheim Reflotron system *5706* No effect at 20 mg/L on Ames Seralyzer method *5706* No effect at therapeutic concentration on Boehringer Mannheim Reflotron method *3231*

Color *Feces Increase Analytical* Orange red *3810*
Urine Increase Analytical Yellow orange increases with HCl *684*
Urine Increase Physiological May cause an orange to red color which may interfere with photometric measurements *4531*

Creatinine *Serum Increase Physiological* May cause renal toxicity as a side effect *4531*
Serum No Effect Analytical No effect at 20 mg/L on method on Ames Seralyzer *5706*

Diagnex Blue Excretion *Urine Increase Analytical* Orange color produces interference *6515*

Erythrocytes *Blood Decrease Physiological* Hemolytic anemia (sensitivity dependent) *4013*

Glucose *Serum Decrease Analytical* Delays coupled glucose oxidase reaction *882*
Serum No Effect Analytical No effect at therapeutic concentration on Boehringer Mannheim Reflotron method *3231* At concentration of 20 mg/dL (800 µmol/L) has no effect on method on Du Pont Dimension *1575* At concentration of 25 mg/L no effect on method on Boehringer Mannheim Reflotron system *5706* At concentration of 120 mg/L had no effect on hexokinase/G-6-PDH method *5704*
Urine Decrease Analytical False negative with glucose oxidase methods *4233*
Urine Increase Analytical False positive reported with Tes-Tape® *4233*

γ-Glutamyltransferase *Serum Increase Physiological* May cause hepatic toxicity as a side effect *4531*
Serum No Effect Analytical No effect at therapeutic concentration on Boehringer Mannheim Reflotron method *3231* At concentration of 25 mg/L no effect on method on Boehringer Mannheim Reflotron system *5706*

HDL-Cholesterol *Serum No Effect Analytical* At a concentration up to 25 mg/L had no significant effect on Reflotron method for whole blood cholesterol *6352*

Heinz Body Formation *Blood Positive Physiological* Associated with hemolytic anemia, methemoglobinemia *4014*

Hematocrit *Blood Decrease Physiological* Hemolytic anemia (sensitivity dependent) *1212* May cause hemolytic anemia as a side effect *4531*

Hemoglobin *Blood Decrease Physiological* Hemolytic anemia (sensitivity dependent) *1212* May cause hemolytic anemia as a side effect *4531*

^{131}I Uptake *Serum Decrease Physiological* Donnasep contains tetraiodofluorescein *4360*

17-Ketogenic Steroids *Urine Increase Analytical* Interferes with Zimmermann reaction *5869*

Ketones *Urine Decrease Analytical* Nitroprusside reaction masked by color *882*
Urine Increase Analytical False positive with Ketostix® or $FeCl_3$*4233*

17-Ketosteroids *Urine Increase Analytical* Interferes with Zimmermann reaction *5869*

Lactate *Plasma No Effect Analytical* At concentration of 120 mg/L had no effect on enzymatic method *5704*

Methemoglobin *Blood Increase Physiological* May cause hemolysis *4013* May cause methemoglobinemia *4531*

N-Acetyl-Glucosaminidase *Urine No Effect Analytical* At 40 µmol/L on 2 colorimetric analytical methods *2254*

Porphyrin, Total *Urine Increase Analytical* Interference with fluorescence (in screening test) *6515*

Potassium *Serum No Effect Analytical* At concentration of 20 mg/L had no effect on measurement by ISE with predilution *5704*

Pregnanediol *Urine Increase Analytical* Mechanism unknown *3669*

Protein *Serum Increase Analytical* Orange-brown color affects absorbance *882*
Urine Increase Analytical False positive with Labstix® etc *4233*
Urine No Effect Analytical No effect on sulfosalicylic acid, heat tests *2452*

PSP Excretion *Urine Increase Analytical* False color reaction at alkaline pH *6515*

Sodium *Serum No Effect Analytical* At concentration of 20 mg/L had no effect on measurement by ISE with predilution *5704*

Sulfhemoglobin *Blood Increase Physiological* Positive with severe oxidative hemolysis *1998*

Triglycerides *Serum No Effect Analytical* No effect at therapeutic concentration on Boehringer Mannheim Reflotron method *3231* No effect at 25 mg/L on Boehringer Mannheim Reflotron method *5706*

Urea Nitrogen *Serum Increase Physiological* Transient acute renal failure reported *128* May cause renal toxicity as a side effect *4531*
Serum No Effect Analytical No effect at 25 mg/L on Boehringer Mannheim Reflotron method *5706* No effect at therapeutic concentration on Boehringer Mannheim Reflotron method *3231*

Uric Acid *Serum No Effect Analytical* No effect at therapeutic concentration on Boehringer Mannheim Reflotron method *3231* No effect at 25 mg/L on Boehringer Mannheim Reflotron method *5706*

Urobilinogen *Urine Increase Analytical* Gives false positive reaction with Ehrlich's reagent *409* Orange-red with Ehrlich's aldehyde reaction *6515*

Vanillylmandelic Acid *Urine Increase Analytical* Yields similar color in reaction *3669*

Xylose *Urine Increase Analytical* Due to interfering background color *4908*

Phencyclidine

Albumin *Serum No Effect Analytical* At concentration of 6 mg/L had no effect on BCG method *5704*

Amphetamine *Urine No Effect Analytical* Negative result with method on Du Pont aca at a concentration of 1000 µg/L (4.10 mmol/L) *1554*

Barbiturate *Urine No Effect Analytical* Negative result obtained at a concentration of 1000 µg/mL (4.10 mmol/L) with method on Du Pont aca *1555*

Benzodiazepine *Urine No Effect Analytical* Negative result observed at a concentration of 1000 µg/mL (4.10 mmol/L) with method on Du Pont aca *1556*

Benzodiazepine Screen *Serum No Effect Analytical* No significant effect observed at a concentration of 1.0 mg/mL (4.11 mmol/L) with method on Du Pont aca *1512*

Benzoylecgonine *Urine No Effect Analytical* Negative result obtained at a concentration of 750 µg/mL (3.08 mmol/L) with method on Du Pont aca *1558* No significant interference observed at a concentration of 3080 µmol/L with Sung and Neely modification of Syva EMIT procedure *148*

Bilirubin *Serum No Effect Analytical* At concentration of 6 mg/L had no effect on Jendrassik and Grof method *5704*

Calcium *Serum No Effect Analytical* At concentration of 6 mg/L had no effect on cresolphthalein method *5704*

Cannabinoids *Urine No Effect Analytical* No effect observed at a concentration of 750 µg/mL (3.08 mmol/L) on method on Du Pont aca *1557* No effect on Roche Abuscreen method *5006*

Chloride *Serum No Effect Analytical* At concentration of 6 mg/L had no effect on mercurimetric method *5704*

Cholesterol *Serum No Effect Analytical* At concentration of 6 mg/L had no effect on Liebermann-Burchard method *5704*

Cocaethylene *Urine No Effect Analytical* No interference observed with TLC method of Bailey *328*

Creatinine *Serum No Effect Analytical* At concentration of 6 mg/L had no effect on Technicon AutoAnalyzer® Jaffe method *5704*

Drugs of Abuse Screen *Urine No Effect Analytical* No effect at concentration of 100 µg/mL on EZ-SCREEN procedure for cannabinoids and cocaine *1739*

Morphine *Urine No Effect Analytical* No interference observed at a concentration of 3080 µmol/L with Sung and Neely modification of Syva EMIT procedure *148*

Opiates *Urine No Effect Analytical* No effect observed at a concentration of 1000 µg/mL (4.10 mmol/L) on method on Du Pont aca *1559*

Phosphate *Serum No Effect Analytical* At concentration of 6 mg/L had no effect on phosphomolybdate method *5704*

Protein *Serum No Effect Analytical* At concentration of 6 mg/L had no effect on biuret method with blank correction *5704*

Tricyclic Antidepressants Screen
Serum No Effect Analytical No significant effect observed at a concentration of 1000 µg/mL (4.11 mmol/L) with method on Du Pont aca *1550*

Urea Nitrogen *Serum No Effect Analytical* At concentration of 6 mg/L had no effect on diacetylmonoxime method *5704*

Uric Acid *Serum No Effect Analytical* At concentration of 6 mg/L had no effect on phosphotungstate reduction method *5704*

Phendimetrazine

Amobarbital *Urine No Effect Analytical* No interference with TLC using ethyl acetate: methanol: water: ammonium hydroxide and modified Dragendorff's reagent for detection *6502*

Amphetamine *Urine No Effect Analytical* No interference with TLC using ethyl acetate: methanol: water: ammonium hydroxide and modified Dragendorff's reagent for detection *6502*

Chlordiazepoxide *Urine Positive Analytical* Same R_f and color reaction on TLC using ethyl acetate: methanol: water: ammonium hydroxide and modified Dragendorff's reagent *6502*

Hydromorphone *Urine No Effect Analytical* No interference with TLC using ethyl acetate: methanol: water: ammonium hydroxide and modified Dragendorff's reagent for detection *6502*

Mazindol *Urine Positive Analytical* Same R_f and color reaction on TLC using ethyl acetate: methanol: water: ammonium hydroxide and modified Dragendorff's reagent *6502*

Mescaline *Urine No Effect Analytical* No interference with TLC using ethyl acetate: methanol: water: ammonium hydroxide and modified Dragendorff's reagent for detection *6502*

Methadone *Urine Increase Analytical* Same R_f and color reaction on TLC using ethyl acetate: methanol: water: ammonium hydroxide and modified Dragendorff's reagent *6502*

Methamphetamine *Urine No Effect Analytical* No interference with TLC using ethyl acetate: methanol: water: ammonium hydroxide and modified Dragendorff's reagent for detection *6502*

Methapyrilene *Urine Positive Analytical* Same R_f and color reaction on TLC using ethyl acetate: methanol: water: ammonium hydroxide and modified Dragendorff's reagent *6502*

Morphine *Urine No Effect Analytical* No interference with TLC using ethyl acetate: methanol: water: ammonium hydroxide and modified Dragendorff's reagent for detection *6502*

Nicotine *Urine Positive Analytical* Same R_f and color reaction on TLC using ethyl acetate: methanol: water: ammonium hydroxide and modified Dragendorff's reagent *6502*

Pentobarbital *Urine No Effect Analytical* No interference with TLC using ethyl acetate: methanol: water: ammonium hydroxide and modified Dragendorff's reagent for detection *6502*

Phenobarbital *Urine No Effect Analytical* No interference with TLC using ethyl acetate: methanol: water: ammonium hydroxide and modified Dragendorff's reagent for detection *6502*

Phenylpropanolamine *Urine No Effect Analytical* No interference with TLC using ethyl acetate: methanol: water: ammonium hydroxide and modified Dragendorff's reagent for detection *6502*

Secobarbital *Urine No Effect Analytical* No interference with TLC using ethyl acetate: methanol: water: ammonium hydroxide and modified Dragendorff's reagent for detection *6502*

Phenelzine

Alanine Aminotransferase *Serum Increase Physiological* Increased activity may be observed without signs and symptoms *4525* May cause hypersensitive hepatitis *128*

Aspartate Aminotransferase *Serum Increase Analytical* At 1 mmol/L affects Technicon SMA 12/60 method *5576*
Serum Increase Physiological Increased activity may be observed as a common side effect without signs and symptoms *4525* May cause hypersensitive hepatitis *128*

Bile *Urine Increase Physiological* May cause hypersensitive hepatitis *128*

Bilirubin *Serum Increase Analytical* At 1 mmol/L affects Technicon SMA 12/60 method slightly *5576*

Phenelzine *(continued)*

Bilirubin *(continued)*
Serum Increase Physiological May cause hypersensitive hepatitis *128* Fatal necrotizing hepatocellular damage has been reported but more commonly reversible jaundice may occur *4525*
Serum No Effect Analytical At concentration of 136 mg/L had no effect on Jendrassik and Grof method *5704*

BSP Retention *Serum Increase Physiological* Hepatotoxic/cholestatic syndromes *2242*

Calcium *Serum No Effect Analytical* At concentration of 136 mg/L had no effect on cresolphthalein method *5704*

Carbamazepine *Serum No Effect Physiological* No apparent effect observed on the plasma concentration of either drug *3118*

Cholinesterase *Serum Decrease Physiological* May cause hypersensitive hepatitis *5869*

Creatine Kinase *Serum Increase Physiological* Increased activity has been reported as a rare side effect *4525*

Glucose *Serum Increase Physiological* Decreases glucose tolerance *6192*

Homocysteine *Plasma Increase Physiological* As a vitamin B_6 antagonist causes increased concentration *6123*

4-Hydroxy-3-Methoxy-Phenylglycol
Urine Decrease Physiological Nonsignificant reduction of 28% observed in 6 healthy men during third week of treatment with 60 mg/day. Reduction of 39% during week after treatment stopped *549*

Leukocytes *Blood Decrease Physiological* May cause leukopenia *128* Leukopenia has been reported as a rare side effect *4525*

pH *Blood Increase Physiological* Metabolic acidosis has been reported as a rare side effect *4525*

Phosphate *Serum No Effect Analytical* At concentration of 136 mg/L had no effect on phosphomolybdate method *5704*

Protein *Serum No Effect Analytical* At concentration of 136 mg/L had no effect on biuret method with blank correction *5704*

Sodium *Serum Increase Physiological* Rare hypernatremia reported *2754* Hypernatremia has been reported as a common side effect *4525*

Tryptamine *Urine Increase Physiological* In 6 healthy men 45 mg daily caused 3.1 fold increase and 60 mg/day caused 12.7 fold increase (from 0.047 to 0.597 mg/g creatinine) during 2 week's administration. Concentration still about twice normal 2 weeks after treatment stopped *549*

Urea Nitrogen *Serum No Effect Analytical* At concentration of 136 mg/L had no effect on diacetylmonoxime method *5704*

Uric Acid *Serum Increase Analytical* At 1 mmol/L slightly affects Technicon SMA 12/60, Henry methods *5576*
Serum No Effect Analytical At concentration of 136 mg/L had no effect on phosphotungstate reduction method *5704*

Vanillylmandelic Acid *Urine Decrease Physiological* Nonsignificant reduction of about 28% in 6 healthy men given 60 mg/day during third week of treatment, but with further reduction to 39% in week after treatment stopped *549*

Xylose *Urine Decrease Physiological* Decreased absorption of xylose from gastrointestinal tract *6192*

Phenethicillin

Eosinophils *Blood Increase Physiological* Few cases reported only (minor effect) *2754*

Erythrocytes *Blood Decrease Physiological* Theoretically may cause hemolytic anemia *2754*

Hemoglobin *Blood Decrease Physiological* Theoretical effect of penicillins *2754*

Leukocytes *Blood Decrease Physiological* Theoretically leukopenia may occur *2754*

Phenethylamine

Amphetamine *Urine No Effect Analytical* Less than 1% cross-reactivity observed with Roche Abuscreen method when adapted for use with Roche Cobas Mira analyzer *5120*

Methamphetamine *Urine No Effect Analytical* Less than 1% cross-reactivity with Roche Abuscreen Online assay as performed on Roche Cobas Mira *6347*

Phenformin

Glucose *Serum No Effect Analytical* No effect at 4,000 mg/L on hexokinase method on Ames Seralyzer *5706*

Prazosin *Serum No Effect Physiological* Coadministration of prazosin with phenformin had no apparent adverse drug interaction in limited clinical experience *4649*

Phenindione

Alanine Aminotransferase *Serum Increase Physiological* May modify liver function (cholestasis) *3810*

Alkaline Phosphatase *Serum Increase Physiological* May modify liver function (cholestasis) *3810*

Aspartate Aminotransferase *Serum Increase Physiological* May modify liver function (cholestasis) *3810*

Bile *Urine Increase Physiological* May modify liver function (cholestasis) *3810*

Bilirubin *Serum Increase Physiological* Probable effect as bilirubin clearance reduced *2466*

Bilirubin, Direct *Serum Increase Physiological* Probable effect as bilirubin conjugation affected *2466*

BSP Retention *Serum Increase Physiological* May modify liver function (cholestasis) *3810*

Color *Urine Increase Analytical* Red-orange color produced in alkaline urine *1123*

Eosinophils *Blood Increase Physiological* Allergic response after treatment for 15 d in one patient *2575*

Erythrocytes *Urine Increase Physiological* May cause actual bleeding *1714*

Hemoglobin *Urine Increase Physiological* Actual bleeding caused by drug *1714*

^{131}I Uptake *Serum Decrease Physiological* Uncommon reported effect *3669*

Leukocytes *Blood Decrease Physiological* Agranulocytosis/Leukopenia *3810*
Blood Increase Physiological Occasional leukocytosis may occur *2242*

Phenytoin *Serum No Effect Physiological* No effect on metabolism due to different chemical configuration from other coumarins *5966*

Protein *Urine Increase Physiological* Nephrotoxicity may occur *4134*

Tolbutamide *Serum No Effect Physiological* No effect apparent on plasma concentration or metabolism *5595*

Urea Nitrogen *Serum Increase Physiological* Nephrotoxicity may occur with tubular necrosis *2242*

Uric Acid *Serum Decrease Physiological* Uricosuric action *2378*
Urine Increase Physiological Uricosuric action *2378*

Pheniprazine

Alanine Aminotransferase *Serum Increase Physiological* May cause hepatocellular jaundice *3810*

Alkaline Phosphatase *Serum Increase Physiological* May cause hepatocellular jaundice *3810*

Aspartate Aminotransferase *Serum Increase Physiological* May cause hepatocellular jaundice *3810*

Bile *Urine Increase Physiological* May affect liver function *3810*

Bilirubin *Serum Increase Physiological* Hypersensitive hepatitis *3810*

BSP Retention *Serum Increase Physiological* May affect liver function *3810*

Phenmetrazine

Amobarbital *Urine No Effect Analytical* No interference on TLC using ethyl acetate: methanol: water: ammonium hydroxide and modified Dragendorff's reagent for detection *6502*

Amphetamine *Urine No Effect Analytical* No interference on TLC using ethyl acetate: methanol: water: ammonium hydroxide and modified Dragendorff's reagent for detection *6502*

Urine Positive Analytical At concentrations above 1.0 μg/mL (5.65 μmol/L) with method on Du Pont aca *1554*

Chlorphentermine *Urine Positive Analytical* Similar R_f and color reaction on TLC using ethyl acetate: methanol: water: ammonium hydroxide and modified Dragendorff's reagent *6502*

Drugs of Abuse Screen *Urine Increase Analytical* False positive result with Abbott ADx method for amphetamine/methylamphetamine *4279*

Epinephrine *Urine Increase Physiological* For 3 h after administration (slight) *2452*

Hydromorphone *Urine No Effect Analytical* No interference with TLC using ethyl acetate: methanol: water: ammonium and modified Dragendorff's reagent for detection *6502*

5-Hydroxyindoleacetic Acid *Urine Increase Physiological* Reported effect *3534*

^{131}I Uptake *Serum Decrease Physiological* Preludin® contains tetraiodofluorescein *4360*

Mescaline *Urine No Effect Analytical* No interference with TLC using ethyl acetate: methanol: water: ammonium and modified Dragendorff's reagent for detection *6502*

Methamphetamine *Urine No Effect Analytical* No interference on TLC using ethyl acetate: methanol: water: ammonium hydroxide and modified Dragendorff's reagent for detection *6502*

Morphine *Urine No Effect Analytical* No interference on TLC using ethyl acetate: methanol: water: ammonium hydroxide and modified Dragendorff's reagent for detection *6502*

Norepinephrine *Urine No Effect Physiological* No effect observed *2452*

Pentobarbital *Urine No Effect Analytical* No interference on TLC using ethyl acetate: methanol: water: ammonium hydroxide and modified Dragendorff's reagent for detection *6502*

Phenobarbital *Urine No Effect Analytical* No interference on TLC using ethyl acetate: methanol: water: ammonium hydroxide and modified Dragendorff's reagent for detection *6502*

Phentermine *Urine Positive Analytical* Similar R_f and color reaction on TLC using ethyl acetate: methanol: water: ammonium hydroxide and modified Dragendorff's reagent *6502*

Phenylpropanolamine *Urine No Effect Analytical* No interference on TLC using ethyl acetate: methanol: water: ammonium hydroxide and modified Dragendorff's reagent for detection *6502*

Quinine *Urine Increase Analytical* Similar R_f and color reaction on TLC using ethyl acetate: methanol: water: ammonium hydroxide and modified Dragendorff's reagent *6502*

Secobarbital *Urine No Effect Analytical* No interference on TLC using ethyl acetate: methanol: water: ammonium hydroxide and modified Dragendorff's reagent for detection *6502*

Phenobarbital

Acenocoumarol *Plasma Decrease Physiological* In 9 healthy volunteers when 10 mg acenocoumarol given after one week pretreatment with phenobarbital *3305* Coadministration of phenobarbital with acenocoumarol reduces its plasma concentration and decreases its anticoagulant effect *1706*

Acetaminophen *Serum No Effect Analytical* No interference observed at a concentration of 2000 μg/mL (861 μmol/L) with method on Du Pont aca *1506* At 10 mg/L had no effect on HPLC method *5775*

Acid Phosphatase *Serum No Effect Analytical* At concentration of 80 μg/mL (340 μmol/L) had no effect on method on Du Pont Dimension *1562*

Alanine Aminotransferase *Serum Increase Physiological* Hepatotoxicity with centrolobular necrosis *3171*

Serum No Effect Analytical No effect at 250 mg/L on Boehringer Mannheim Reflotron method *5706* On continuous method at 10 times maximal therapeutic concentration. On colorimetric method at 10 times maximal therapeutic concentration *2919* At acute overdose concentration (20 mg/dL) on Technicon SMAC® method *6266* No effect at therapeutic concentration on Boehringer Mannheim Reflotron method *3231* No effect at concentration of 80 μg/mL (344 μmol/L) on method on Du Pont Dimension *1563*

Serum No Effect Physiological In 75 epileptic patients of mean age of 17.1 ± 13.4 y mean activity of 14.9 ± 5.8 U/L not significantly different from 13.5 ± 5.5 U/L in 42 healthy controls *6234*

Albumin *Serum Increase Physiological* Concentration increased in epileptic patients but less than when patients treated with carbamazepine *4347*

Serum No Effect Analytical At acute overdose concentration (20 mg/dL) on Technicon SMAC® method *6266* At concentration of 250 mg/L had no effect on BCG method *5704* At concentration of 80 μg/mL (340 μmol/L) had no effect on method on Du Pont Dimension *1564* No significant effect on BCG method at 25 mg/L *4335*

Alkaline Phosphatase *Serum Increase Physiological* Increased activity occurs early in epileptic children *3555* May cause osteomalacia (?also liver effect) *2320*

Serum No Effect Analytical At concentration of 80 μg/mL (345 μmol/L) had no effect on method on Du Pont Dimension *1565* At acute overdose concentration (20 mg/dL) on Technicon SMAC® method *6266* On continuous method *2919*

Serum No Effect Physiological No effect observed in 14 adult epileptic inpatients given drug alone (dose and duration of treatment alone) *1922*

Amino-4-Imidazole-5-Carboxamide Ribotide
Urine Increase Physiological If megaloblastic anemia develops *5054*

Amino Acids *Urine Increase Analytical* Unusual ninhydrin positive spot in all systems adjacent to threonine and orange in color *2605*

δ-Aminolevulinic Acid *Serum Increase Physiological* Slight but not significant increase (112 nmol/L versus 99 nmol/L in controls) *2246*

Aminopyrine *Serum Decrease Physiological* Reported interaction due to alteration of metabolism *3340*

Ammonia *Plasma No Effect Analytical* No effect at concentration of 30 mg/L on method on Kodak Ektachem® *5706* At concentration of 30 mg/L had no effect on Kodak Ektachem® method *5704* No effect at concentration of 80 μg/mL (340 μmol/L) on method on Du Pont Dimension *1566*

Plasma No Effect Physiological No striking abnormality when given to epileptics *6233*

Amylase *Serum No Effect Analytical* No effect of concentrations up to 250 mg/L on method on Boehringer Mannheim Reflotron *5706* At concentration of 80 μg/mL (340 μmol/L) had no effect on method on Du Pont Dimension *1567*

δ_4-Androstenedione *Plasma Increase Physiological* In 21 epileptic patients treated with phenobarbital for a median of 14.0 years median concentration higher than in controls *4178*

Apolipoprotein A *Serum Increase Physiological* Significantly higher concentration observed in chronically treated epileptics compared with age and sex matched controls *843*

Apolipoprotein A-I *Serum Increase Physiological* Mean concentration of 140 mg/dL in 21 female epileptic patients treated with up to 300 mg/day for at least 5 years versus 129 mg/dL in appropriate controls *6583*

Apolipoprotein A-II *Serum No Effect Physiological* No significant difference between 21 female epileptic patients treated with up to 300 mg/day for at least 5 years compared with appropriate controls *6583*

Apolipoprotein B *Serum Decrease Physiological* Mean concentration of 92 mg/dL in 21 female epileptic patients treated with up to 300 mg/day for at least 5 years compared with 92 mg/dL in appropriate controls *6583*

Serum Increase Physiological Significantly increased concentration observed in chronically treated epileptics compared with age and sex matched controls *843*

Phenobarbital *(continued)*

Aspartate Aminotransferase *Serum Increase Physiological* Hepatotoxicity with centrolobular necrosis *3171* In 75 epileptic patients of mean age of 17.1 ± 13.4 y mean activity of 22.4 ± 8.6 U/L significantly different from 15.1 ± 5.6 U/L in 42 healthy controls *6234*
Serum No Effect Analytical At acute overdose concentration (20 mg/dL) on Technicon SMAC® method *6266* No effect at therapeutic concentration on Boehringer Mannheim Reflotron method *3231* On continuous method at 10 times maximal therapeutic concentration. On colorimetric method at 10 times maximal therapeutic concentration *2919* No effect at concentration of 80 µg/mL (344 µmol/L) on method on Du Pont Dimension *1568* No effect at 250 mg/L on Boehringer Mannheim Reflotron method *5706*

Aspirin Esterase *Serum Increase Physiological* Significantly higher activity in treated epileptics than in controls *4806*

Barbiturate *Urine Increase Analytical* Positive result obtained at a concentration of 3.0 µg/mL (12.9 µmol/L) with method on Du Pont aca *1555*

Bicarbonate *Serum No Effect Analytical* At concentration of 250 mg/L had no effect on method using phenolphthalein *5704*

Bilirubin *Serum Decrease Physiological* Induces hepatic microsomal enzymes especially in pregnant women *5869* Mean reduction of 3.5 µmol/L in 18 epileptic patients treated for several years compared with control population *2267*
Serum Increase Physiological Hepatotoxicity with centrolobular necrosis *3171*
Serum No Effect Analytical At concentration of 250 mg/L had no effect on Jendrassik and Grof method *5704* No effect at 20 mg/L on Ames Seralyzer method *5706* At concentration of 250 mg/L no effect on method on Boehringer Mannheim Reflotron system *5706* No effect at therapeutic concentrations on Jendrassik-Grof, dimethylsulfoxide and spectrophotometric methods *2920* At acute overdose concentration (20 mg/dL) on Technicon SMAC® method *6266* No effect at concentration of 80 µg/mL (344 µmol/L) on method on Du Pont Dimension *1589*
Serum No Effect Physiological Insignificant protein-displacement effect in neonates *6314*

Bilirubin, Direct *Serum No Effect Analytical* At concentration of 80 µg/mL (344 µmol/L) had no effect on method on Du Pont Dimension *1574*

Biotin *Serum Decrease Physiological* Dose related in long-term treated epileptics compared with controls *3275*

BSP Retention *Serum Decrease Physiological* Increased clearance by liver in newborns *6599*

Bupropion *Serum Decrease Physiological* May induce the metabolism of bupropion due to effect on CYP2B6 isoenzyme *2171*

Calcium *Serum Decrease Physiological* Slight but significant reduction compared with untreated elderly at doses other than for treatment of epilepsy *6618* Metabolic effect with chronic therapy (osteomalacia) *2403*
Serum Increase Analytical Value more than 3% high when test performed on Technicon SRA-2000 with concentration 10 times therapeutic *4348*
Serum No Effect Analytical At acute overdose concentration (20 mg/dL) on Technicon SMAC® method *6266* No effect at concentration of 80 µg/mL (340 µmol/L) on method on Du Pont Dimension *1569* At concentration of 250 mg/L had no effect on cresolphthalein method *5704*

Cannabinoids *Urine No Effect Analytical* No effect on Roche Abuscreen method *5006*

Carbamazepine *Serum Decrease Physiological* Induces hepatic metabolism thereby reducing plasma concentration *3118* Simultaneous administration causes marked reduction of plasma carbamazepine concentration *282* Slight reduction of total concentration from mean of 7.6 µg/mL to 6.5 µg/mL in 14 epileptics when phenobarbital coadministered *4846* Drugs that induce CYP 3A4 enhance metabolism of carbamazepine producing clinically meaningful effect *1039* Usually slight decrease when drugs coadministered due to hepatic enzyme induction but may be slight increase *1384* Causes decreased concentration by stimulating P450 enzymes which enhance metabolism *6350*
Serum Increase Physiological In 123 patients receiving carbamazepine mean concentration in those receiving phenobarbital 5.5 mg/L compared with 6.7 mg/L in those not receiving phenobarbital *1012*
Serum No Effect Analytical No cross-reactivity observed with method on Du Pont aca *1513* At a concentration of 500 µg/mL had no significant cross-reactivity with carbamazepine at a concentration of 4.0 µg/mL when measured by method on Bayer Technicon Immuno 1® system *417* Cross reactivity of about 0.05% observed with method on Baxter Stratus *5705*

Carbamazepine-10,11-Epoxide
Serum Decrease Physiological Significant reduction in half life observed and increased plasma clearance observed in 6 epileptic patients stabilized on phenobarbital monotherapy. Effect probably due to phenobarbital-induced hepatic metabolism of carbamazepine epoxide *5750*
Serum Increase Physiological Slight increase from mean of 1.2 µg/mL to 2.3 µg/mL in 14 patients with epilepsy when phenobarbital coadministered *4846*

Carbamazepine-10,11-Epoxide, Free
Serum Increase Physiological Slight increase from mean of 0.5 µg/mL in controls treated only with carbamazepine to 0.9 µg/mL when phenobarbital coadministered *4846*

Carbamazepine, Free *Serum Decrease Physiological* Slight reduction from mean of 1.7 µg/mL to 1.5 µg/mL in 14 epileptic patients when phenobarbital coadministered *4846*

Carnitine *Serum Decrease Physiological* In 119 young epileptics receiving phenobarbital mean concentration 32.7 ± 15.3 nmol/L significantly less than 57.8 ± 15.4 nmol/mL in 32 healthy control children *2757*

Carnitine, Free *Serum No Effect Physiological* In 119 epileptic children mean concentration 24.6 ± 12.3 nmol/mL not significantly less than 42.5 ± 14.1 nmol/mL in 32 healthy control children *2757*

Catecholamines *Plasma No Effect Analytical* No effect on HPLC method of Koller for dopamine, epinephrine, and norepinephrine *3230*
Urine No Effect Physiological No effect short term ingestion of 120 mg/d *1184*

Ceruloplasmin *Serum Increase Physiological* Observed in both hospitalized and home-living patients with long-term administration *6417*
Serum No Effect Physiological No significant effect observed in 28 epileptic patients receiving phenobarbital as sole therapy *4346*

Chenodeoxycholic Acid *Serum No Effect Physiological* No effect on increased concentration in patients with intrahepatic cholestasis of pregnancy *2536*

Chloramphenicol *Serum Decrease Physiological* Due to hepatic enzyme induction *1384* Enhances hepatic clearance and reduces clinical effectiveness *1384*

Chloride *Serum No Effect Analytical* No effect of concentrations up to 30 mg/L with method on Kodak Ektachem® *5706* At concentration of 250 mg/L had no effect on mercurimetric method *5704*

Chlorpromazine *Serum Decrease Physiological* Concomitant administration of barbiturate with chlorpromazine caused reduction in chlorpromazine concentration due to induction of hepatic microsomal enzymes *3633* Induces hepatic microsomal enzymes *2452*
Urine Increase Physiological Induces hepatic microsomal enzymes *2452*

Cholesterol *Serum Increase Physiological* Significantly increased concentration observed in chronically treated epileptics compared with age and sex matched controls *843*
Serum No Effect Analytical At concentration of 250 mg/L on method on Boehringer Mannheim Reflotron system *5706* No effect on enzymatic and Liebermann-Burchard methods at therapeutic concentrations *2920* No effect at 20 mg/L on Ames Seralyzer method *5706* No effect at therapeutic concentration on Boehringer Mannheim Reflotron method *3231* At concentration of 80 µg/mL (340 µmol/L) had no effect on method on Du Pont Dimension *1570* At concentration of 520 mg/L had no effect on method using catalase-Hantzsch reaction *5704* At concentration of 352 mg/L had no effect on CHOD-Iodide method *5704* At concentration of 650 mg/L had no effect on CHOD-PAP method *5704* At concentration of 352 mg/L had no effect on catalase-AIDH method *5704* At concentration of 352 mg/L had no effect on Liebermann-Burchard method *5704*

At acute overdose concentration (20 mg/dL) on Technicon SMAC® method *6266*
Serum No Effect Physiological No significant difference between 21 phenobarbital treated epileptics receiving up to 300 mg/day for at least 5 years and appropriate controls *6583*

Cholic Acid *Serum No Effect Physiological* No effect on increased concentration in patients with intrahepatic cholestasis increased of pregnancy *2536*

Cholinesterase *Serum No Effect Analytical* Insignificant decrease of 0.43 U/mL at a concentration of 80 µg/mL with method on Du Pont Dimension *3271* No effect observed at concentration of 15 mg/dL with butyrylthiocholine method on Kodak Ektachem® *2504* Insignificant decrease of 0.04 U/mL at a concentration of 80 µg/mL with method on Du Pont aca *3271*

Cholinesterase (True) *Serum Increase Physiological* Substantially higher activity in treated epileptics than in controls *4806*

Cimetidine *Serum Decrease Physiological* Slight reduction in concentration observed in healthy individuals when drugs coadministered due to enhanced hepatic metabolism *5698*

Clonazepam *Serum Decrease Physiological* May decrease plasma concentration through effect on hepatic metabolism *1384* One study showed slight increase in clonazepam clearance when phenobarbital coadministered due to increased hepatic metabolism *3130*

Clopidogrel *Serum No Effect Physiological* Phenobarbital administration does not appear to affect the pharmacodynamics of clopidogrel *5256*

Copper *Serum Increase Physiological* In 28 epileptics treated for 1 month mean concentration of 101.9 ± 36.4 µg/dL significantly increased to 101.9 ± 36.4 µg/dL compared with 74.7 ± 9.4 µg/dL In 30 healthy controls *3344* Observed in both hospitalized and home-living patients with long-term administration *6417*

Cortisol *Plasma Decrease Physiological* In critically ill patients relative hypoadrenalism observed with phenobarbital therapy because of its effect of increasing the metabolism of cortisol *3381*
Plasma No Effect Analytical At concentration of 250 mg/L no significant effect on CEDIA method (worst case recovery 95.0%) recovery *1097*

Cortisol, Free *Urine No Effect Analytical* No significant interference observed with HPLC method of Turpeinen et al *6105*

C-Reactive Protein *Serum No Effect Analytical* No interference observed at concentrations up to 100 µg/mL (431 µmol/L) with method on Du Pont aca *1518* At concentration of 100 mg/L (431 µmol/L) had no effect on method on Du Pont aca *5403*

Creatine Kinase *Serum No Effect Analytical* No effect at 20 mg/L on method on Ames Seralyzer *5706* On continuous method at 10 times maximal therapeutic concentration *2919* At acute overdose concentration (20 mg/dL) on Technicon SMAC® method *6266*

Creatine Kinase Isoenzymes *Serum No Effect Analytical* At concentration of 80 µg/mL (340 µmol/L) had no effect on method to measure CK-MB isoenzyme on Du Pont Dimension *1571*

Creatinine *Serum No Effect Analytical* No effect at 20 mg/L on Ames Seralyzer method *5706* At concentration of 60 mg/L had no effect on kinetic Jaffe method on BKA-2 *5704* No effect of concentrations up to 30 mg/L on 2-slide method on Kodak Ektachem® *5706* At 50 mg/L on reversed phase liquid chromatographic procedure of Zhiri et al *6656* At concentration of 80 mg/L had no effect on Jaffe-Fuller's earth method *5704* At concentration of 30 mg/L had no effect on Kodak Ektachem® method *5704* No effect at concentration of 80 µg/mL (344 µmol/L) on method on Du Pont Dimension *1572* At acute overdose concentration (20 mg/dL) on Technicon SMAC® method *6266* At concentration of 250 mg/L had no effect on Technicon AutoAnalyzer® Jaffe method *5704* No effect of concentrations up to 30 mg/L on single slide method on Kodak Ektachem® *5706* At concentration of 80 mg/L had no effect on Jaffe-Fading-Fraction method *5704* Although elutes at 6.2 min compared with 8.9 min for creatinine with HPLC method of Rosano et al difference is sufficiently great so as not to cause interference *5083* No effect on alkaline picrate and Slot methods at therapeutic concentrations *2920* At concentration of 80 mg/L had no effect on creatinine iminohydrolase method *5704*

Cyclosporine *Blood Decrease Physiological* Induces cytochrome P-450 hepatic enzymes thereby increasing clearance of cyclosporine *808* Coadministration with cyclosporine caused a significant decrease in cyclosporine concentrations *859*
Blood Increase Physiological Impaired metabolism observed in neonates following cardiac transplantation when phenobarbital coadministered with cyclosporine. Effect possibly due to metabolism by same P-450 system *457*
Blood No Effect Analytical At a concentration of 150 mg/L had no effect on Syva EMIT method *495*
Serum Decrease Physiological Dose related reduction observed when phenobarbital coadministered with cyclosporine: associated with increased plasma clearance but main effect probably due to hepatic enzyme induction *6595* May decrease cyclosporine concentration by inducing hepatic cytochrome P-450 III A which metabolizes cyclosporine *5236* Enhances hepatic clearance and reduces clinical effectiveness *1384* Coadministration with cyclosporine caused a significant decrease in cyclosporine concentrations *859* Effect occurs as result of induction of hepatic cytochrome P-450 *1069*
Serum Increase Physiological Clearance enhanced when drugs coadministered *1384*

Cyclosporine A *Blood Decrease Physiological* Coadministration with cyclosporine A decreases its concentration *5240*

Dehydroepiandrosterone Sulfate
Plasma Decrease Physiological In 21 epileptic patients treated with phenobarbital for a median of 14.0 years median concentration in both follicular and luteal phases significantly lower than that in controls *4178*

Deoxycholic Acid *Serum No Effect Physiological* No effect on increased concentration in patients with intrahepatic cholestasis increased of pregnancy *2536*

Desipramine *Serum Decrease Physiological* Enhances hepatic clearance and decreases clinical effectiveness *1384*

Dexamethasone *Serum Decrease Physiological* 88% increase in metabolic clearance rate with substantial reduction in half-life *2985* May enhance metabolic clearance resulting in decreased plasma concentrations and lessened physiologic effects *3969*
Serum Increase Physiological Coadministration with dexamethasone led to more rapid clearance of dexamethasone due to enhanced hepatic enzyne activity possibly leading to an increase in the false positive rate with the dexamethasone suppression test for the diagnosis of Cushing's syndrome *6538*

Dicumarol *Plasma Decrease Physiological* Coadministration of phenobarbital with dicumarol reduces its plasma concentration and decreases its anticoagulant effect *1706*

Digitoxin *Serum Decrease Physiological* May depress to subtherapeutic value due to induction of mixed function oxidases *4631* Enhances hepatic clearance and reduces clinical effectiveness *1384* Stimulates metabolism, induces hepatic microsomal enzymes *2452* Metabolism of digitoxin increased by induction of hepatic microsomal enzymes *5673*

Disopyramide *Serum Decrease Physiological* When drugs that induce hepatic microsomal enzymes are coadministered with disopyramide concentration of disopyramide significantly reduced *2069*
Serum No Effect Physiological Concentration unaffected at level used to induce hepatic enzymes *3032*

Doxorubicin *Serum Decrease Physiological* Enhances hepatic metabolism and reduces clinical effectiveness *1384* Coadministration may cause increased elimination of doxorubicin *273*

Doxycycline *Serum Decrease Physiological* Enhances hepatic clearance and reduces plasma concentration *1384* Hepatic metabolism stimulated by barbiturates *4261* Coadministration of phenobarbital with doxycycline shortens its half-life for as long as 2 weeks after barbiturate therapy is discontinued *1706*

Drugs of Abuse Screen *Urine No Effect Analytical* No effect at concentration of 100 µg/mL on EZ-SCREEN procedure for cannabinoids and cocaine *1739*

Epinephrine *Urine No Effect Physiological* No effect short term ingestion of 120 mg/d *1184*

Erythrocytes *Blood Decrease Physiological* Megaloblastic anemia secondary to disturbance in folic acid metabolism *3122*

Phenobarbital *(continued)*

Estradiol *Plasma Decrease Physiological* Coadministration of phenobarbital with estradiol reduces its concentration by increasing its metabolism *1706* In 21 epileptic patients treated with phenobarbital for a median of 14.0 years median concentration in follicular phase significantly lower than median in 20 age-matched controls *4178*
Plasma Increase Physiological In 21 epileptic patients treated with phenobarbital for a median of 14.0 years median concentration in luteal phase significantly higher than median in 20 age-matched controls *4178*

Ethanol *Serum Decrease Physiological* Hepatic enzyme induction probably responsible for slight reduction in blood concentration *4143*

Ethosuximide *Serum Decrease Physiological* Reported to decrease plasma concentrations *1384*
Serum No Effect Analytical Insignificant cross-reactivity observed with method on Du Pont aca *1523*

Etoposide *Serum Decrease Physiological* Administration of anticonvulsants with etoposide causes significant reduction in etoposide AUC due to increased clearance caused by induction of hepatic enzymes *3909*

Felbamate *Serum Decrease Physiological* With coadministration of phenobarbital concentration of felbamate at steady-state decreased by 29% in patients receiving 2400 mg/d felbamate *6324*
Serum No Effect Analytical No significant interference observed with GLC method of Rifai et al *4958*

Felodipine *Serum Decrease Physiological* Marked reduction of area under under curve when phenobarbital coadministered due to hepatic enzyme induction *876* Coadministration of phenobarbital with felodipine caused a reduction in the maximal plasma concentration of felodipine and a significant reduction to 6% of the area under the time-concentration curve in healthy individuals *266*

Fenoprofen *Serum Decrease Physiological* Chronic administration of phenobarbital decreases biological half-life of fenoprofen probably because of its hepatic enzyme induction action *1439*

Ferroxidase *Serum Increase Physiological* Significant effect in 40 adult epileptics receiving long term treatment *6108*

Fibrin Degradation Products *Plasma No Effect Analytical* No interference observed with concentrations up to 100 mg/dL (431 µmol/L) with method on Du Pont aca *1525*

Flecainide *Serum Decrease Physiological* 30% increase in the rate of plasma elimination when drug coadministered with flecainide *3702*

Folate *Cerebrospinal Fluid Decrease Physiological* Low serum folate in from 27 to 91% of treated epileptics in different studies *3383* Occurs in many long-treated epileptics *4931*
Red Blood Cells Decrease Physiological Low serum folate in from 27 to 91% of treated epileptics in different studies *3383* Inverse correlation with drug concentration *4930*
Serum Decrease Physiological May cause megaloblastic anemia *5054* Low serum folate in from 27 to 91% of treated epileptics in different studies *3383*
Test Conditions No Effect Analytical No effect on *L. casei* or *S. fecalis4014*

Follicle Stimulating Hormone
Plasma No Effect Physiological In 21 epileptic patients treated with phenobarbital for a median of 10.0 years median concentration of 14.0 mIU/mL in follicular phase and 7.1 mIU/mL in luteal phase not markedly different from medians of 8.1 and 9.4 mIU/mL in 20 age-matched controls *4178*

Gabapentin *Serum No Effect Physiological* Coadministration of phenobarbital with gabapentin to 12 patients had no effect on the pharmacokinetics of gabapentin *4526*

Glucaric Acid *Urine Increase Physiological* Due to induction of hepatic enzymes *3669* In 98% of patients with epilepsy receiving long term treatment *6108* Dose dependent effect, greater than other anticonvulsants *4623*

Glucose *Serum No Effect Analytical* No effect at therapeutic concentrations on hexokinase, glucose dehydrogenase 2,4-dichlorophenol, ABTS and o-toluidine methods *2920* At concentration of 80 µg/mL (344 µmol/L) has no effect on method on Du Pont Dimension *1575* At concentration of 250 mg/L no effect on method on Boehringer Mannheim Reflotron system *5706* At concentration of 100 mg/L had no effect on GOD/POD-PAP method *5704* No effect at 20 mg/L on glucose oxidase method on Ames Seralyzer *5706* At concentration of 30 mg/L had no effect on Kodak Ektachem® method *5704* At acute overdose concentration (20 mg/dL) on Technicon SMAC® method *6266* At concentration of 60 mg/L had no effect on hexokinase/G-6-PDH method *5704* No effect at therapeutic concentration on Boehringer Mannheim Reflotron method *3231*
Serum No Effect Physiological No significant effect observed in epileptic patients receiving phenobarbital *4077*
Urine Decrease Analytical Low with Clinistix®, Diastix® *1826*
Urine No Effect Analytical No effect observed on TesTape® *1826*

Glutamine *Plasma Increase Physiological* Significant effect noted in children, possibly due to inhibition of carbamoylphosphate synthase *6109*
Plasma No Effect Physiological No striking abnormality when given to epileptics *6233*

γ-Glutamyltransferase *Serum Increase Physiological* Observed 2 times upper limit of normal in 2 of 15 adult epileptic inpatients (dose and duration of treatment unknown) *1922* ?Induction or damage of hepatic microsomes *5082* In epileptic patients increase in proportion to amount of administered drug *4078*
Serum No Effect Analytical No effect at therapeutic concentration on Boehringer Mannheim Reflotron method *3231* At concentration of 80 µg/mL (344 µmol/L) has no effect on method on Du Pont Dimension *1579* At concentration of 250 mg/L no effect on method on Boehringer Mannheim Reflotron system *5706*

Glycine *Plasma No Effect Physiological* No striking abnormality when given to epileptics *6233*

Griseofulvin *Serum Decrease Physiological* Absorption from gastrointestinal tract reduced *4957* Enhances hepatic clearance and reduces plasma concentration *1384* Impairs gastrointestinal absorption *2452* Coadministration of phenobarbital with griseofulvin reduces its absorption and decreases its plasma concentration *1706*

Guanfacine *Serum Decrease Physiological* Enhances hepatic clearance and reduces clinical effectiveness. Decreases half-life of drug *1384*

Haloperidol *Serum Decrease Physiological* Enhances hepatic clearance and decreases clinical effectiveness *1384*

HDL_2-Cholesterol *Serum Increase Physiological* Mean of 20.9 mg/dL in 21 female epileptics treated with up to 300 mg/day for at least 5 years compared with 12.4 mg/dL in appropriate controls *6583*

HDL_3-Phospholipids *Serum Increase Physiological* Mean concentration of 77.7 mg/dL in 21 female epileptics treated with up to 300 mg/day for at least 5 years versus 67.7 mg/dL in appropriate controls *6583*
Serum No Effect Physiological Insignificant increase in 21 female epileptics treated with up to 300 mg/day for at least 5 years compared with appropriate controls *6583*

HDL-Cholesterol *Serum Increase Physiological* Significantly increased concentration observed in chronically treated epileptics compared with age and sex matched controls *843* Mean concentration of 39.0 mg/dL in 21 female epileptics treated with up to 300 mg/day for up to 5 years compared with 34.0 mg/dL in appropriate controls *6583*
Serum No Effect Analytical No effect at concentration of 80 µg/mL (344 µmol/L) on method on Du Pont Dimension *1576*

Hematocrit *Blood Decrease Physiological* Megaloblastic anemia secondary to disturbance in folic acid metabolism *4932*

Hemoglobin *Blood Decrease Physiological* Megaloblastic anemia secondary to disturbance in folic acid metabolism *3122*

Hemopexin *Serum Increase Physiological* Significant effect in 40 adult epileptics receiving long term treatment *6108*

25-Hydroxy Vitamin D_3 *Serum Decrease Physiological* Positive correlation with calcium level *2403* Observed effect in some children *5055*

Hydroxybutyrate Dehydrogenase
Serum Decrease Analytical On continuous method at 10 times maximal therapeutic concentration *2919*

11-Hydroxycorticosteroids *Urine No Effect Physiological* No effect short term ingestion of 120 mg/d *1184*

17-Hydroxycorticosteroids *Urine Decrease Physiological* With chronic ingestion cortisol is metabolized to 6-β-hydroxycortisol *825*
Urine No Effect Physiological No significant change in response to chronic treatment *6657* No effect short term ingestion of 120 mg/d *1184*

6-β-Hydroxycortisol *Urine Increase Physiological* Chronic treatment leads to substantially increased excretion compared with controls (approximately 9 fold increase) *6657* Alteration of steroid excretory pattern (long term) *1184* Increased conversion of cortisol produced *55*

5-Hydroxyindoleacetic Acid *Urine Increase Analytical* May cause false high colorimetric values *1444*
Urine No Effect Analytical No effect observed with FPIA method on Abbott TDx *695*

Hydroxyproline *Urine Increase Physiological* Increased excretion occurred early in epileptic children without obvious bone changes suggestive of rickets *3555*

Imipramine *Serum Decrease Physiological* Plasma concentration of drug may be decreased when hepatic enzyme inducers given concomitantly *1040*

Indocyanine Green *Serum Decrease Physiological* Mechanism not yet established *3942*

Indomethacin *Serum No Effect Analytical* No effect on HPLC method of Roberts and Smith *4978*

Iron *Serum No Effect Analytical* At concentration of 200 mg/L had no effect on Ferrozine method *5704* No effect at concentration of 80 µg/mL (344 µmol/L) on method on Du Pont Dimension *1577* No effect at therapeutic concentrations on bathophenanthroline and Ramsay methods *2920*

Iron-Binding Capacity, Total *Serum No Effect Analytical* No effect at concentration of 80 µg/mL (344 µmol/L) on method on Du Pont Dimension *1590*

itraconazole *Serum Decrease Physiological* Itraconazole potently inhibits the cytochrome P450 3A enzyme system thereby affecting the metabolism of drugs by this system: the concentration of itraconazole is substantially reduced with coadministration of phenobarbital *2905*

17-Ketosteroids *Urine No Effect Physiological* No effect short term ingestion of 120 mg/d *1184*

Lactate *Plasma Increase Physiological* Dose related in long-term treated epileptics compared with controls *3275*
Plasma No Effect Analytical At concentration of 60 mg/L had no effect on enzymatic method *5704*
Plasma No Effect Physiological No significant effect observed in epileptic patients receiving phenobarbital *4077*

Lactate Dehydrogenase *Serum Increase Analytical* With lactate as substrate on continuous method *2919*
Serum No Effect Analytical With pyruvate as substrate on continuous method. On colorimetric method at 10 times maximal therapeutic concentration *2919* At concentration of 80 µg/mL (344 µmol/L) has no effect on method on Du Pont Dimension *1578* No effect at 20 mg/L on method on Ames Seralyzer *5706* At acute overdose concentration (20 mg/dL) on Technicon SMAC® method *6266*

Lamotrigine *Serum Decrease Physiological* Coadministration of phenobarbital with lamotrigine caused a significant approximately 40% reduction in the plasma concentration of lamotrigine *2160*

LE Cells *Blood Positive Physiological* Rare idiosyncratic response *3340*

Lecithin:Cholesterol Acyltransferase
Serum No Effect Physiological Insignificant difference between 21 female epileptic patients treated with up to 300 mg/day for at least 5 years compared with appropriate controls *6583*

Leucine Aminopeptidase Isoenzymes
Serum No Effect Physiological No effect observed *5155*

Leukocytes *Blood Decrease Physiological* Pancytopenia (AMA Blood dyscrasias) *4017*

Lipase *Serum No Effect Analytical* At concentration of 80 µg/mL (344 µmol/L) has no effect on method on Du Pont Dimension *1580*

Long-chain Fatty Acid Carnitine Esters
Serum No Effect Physiological In 119 epileptic children treated with phenobarbital mean concentration of 2.2 ± 1.3 nmol/mL not significantly less than 3.1 ± 2.5 nmol/mL in 32 healthy control children *2757*

Losartan *Serum Decrease Physiological* Coadministration of phenobarbital with losartan caused an decrease of about 20% in the AUC of losartan and that of its active metabolite *3965* Coadministration caused a 20% decrease in the AUC of losartan and that of its active metabolite *3979*
Serum No Effect Physiological Coadministration of losartan with phenobarbital had no significant effect on the concentration of either drug *1596*

Luteinizing Hormone *Plasma Increase Physiological* In 21 epileptic patients treated with phenobarbital for a median of 14.0 years median concentration of 10.7 mIU/mL in follicular phase and 9.0 mIU/mL in luteal phase not markedly higher than medians of 7.4 and 9.4 mIU/mL in 20 age-matched controls *4178*

Luteinizing Hormone:Follicle Stimulating Hormone Ratio
Plasma No Effect Physiological In 21 epileptic patients treated with sodium valproate for a median of 14.0 years median 1.0 in follicular phase and 1.4 in luteal phase not markedly different from medians of 0.9 and 1.0 in 20 age-matched controls *4178*

Magnesium *Serum No Effect Analytical* No effect at concentration of 80 µg/mL (344 µmol/L) on method on Du Pont Dimension *1581*

Maprotiline *Serum Decrease Physiological* Concentration may be decreased when hepatic enzyme inducers are coadministered *1034*

MCV *Blood Increase Physiological* Megaloblastic anemia secondary to disturbance in folic acid metabolism *3122*

Methylprednisolone *Serum Decrease Physiological* 90% increase in metabolic clearance rate with substantial reduction in half-life *2985* Half-life reduced as result of hepatic enzyme induction *5828*

Metoprolol *Serum Decrease Physiological* Increases hepatic clearance and decreases plasma concentration *1384*

Metronidazole *Serum Decrease Physiological* Administration of drugs that induce microsomal liver enzymes may accelerate the elimination of metronidazole *4446* By inducing microsomal hepatic enzymes may accelerate the elimination of metronidazole with reduction of its plasma concentration *5420* In one case presumed reduction of serum concentration due to enhanced hepatic metabolism of metronidazole *3926* Due to induction of hepatic metabolizing enzymes *1384*
Serum Increase Physiological When drugs that induce hepatic microsomal enzymes coadministered elimination of metronidazole may be accelerated *2066*

Mexiletine *Serum Decrease Physiological* Induces hepatic enzymes: may reduce elimination half-life by 50% *3281*

Montelukast *Serum Decrease Physiological* Phenobarbital induces hepatic metabolism and the area under the curve after a single dose of 10 mg of montelukast was reduced 40% by phenobarbital *3992*

Mycophenolic Acid *Serum No Effect Analytical* No significant interference observed with HPLC method of Shipkova et al *5526*

Mycophenolic Acid Glucuronide
Serum No Effect Analytical No significant interference observed with HPLC method of Shipkova et al *5526*

N-Formiminoglutamic Acid *Urine Increase Physiological* If megaloblastic anemia develops *5054*

Nitroglycerin *Serum Decrease Physiological* When coadministered with nitroglycerin because of enhanced metabolism *2607*

Norepinephrine *Urine No Effect Physiological* No effect short term ingestion of 120 mg/d *1184*

Nortriptyline *Serum Decrease Physiological* Enhances hepatic clearance and reduces clinical effectiveness *1384*

5'-Nucleotidase *Serum No Effect Physiological* No effect observed in 12 adult epileptic in patients given drug alone (dose and duration of treatment unknown) *1922*

Organic Acids *Urine Increase Physiological* Dose related in long-term treated epileptics compared with controls *3275*

Ornithine *Plasma No Effect Physiological* No striking abnormality when given to epileptics *6233*

Phenobarbital *(continued)*

p-Aminophenol *Urine No Effect Analytical* With addition of drugs at a concentration of 100 mg/L and of related compounds at 50 mg/L no significant effect observed on colorimetric method of van Bocxlaer on Cobas Mira analyzer which involves reacting free p-aminophenol with resorcinol in the presence of magnesium ions to form an indophenol dye measured at 550 nm *6163*

Paroxetine *Serum Decrease Physiological* When a single oral dose of paroxetine was given orally with phenobarbital a decrease of 25% in the AUC of paroxetine occurred *5654*

Phenobarbital *Cerebrospinal Fluid Increase Physiological* Concentration about half serum level *5093*
Serum Increase Physiological 600 mg orally produces concentration of 23 mg/L in blood *3868*

Phenprocoumon *Plasma Decrease Physiological* Coadministration of phenobarbital with phenprocoumon reduces its plasma concentration and decreases its anticoagulant effect *1706*

Phenylalanine *Plasma No Effect Analytical* No interference observed with rapid quantitative whole blood method of Campbell et al using phenylalanine dehydrogenase *867*

Phenylbutazone *Serum Decrease Physiological* Reported interaction due to alteration of metabolism *3340* Concentration reduced in healthy individuals when drugs coadministered probably due to stimulation of hepatic microsomal enzymes *6431*

Phenytoin *Serum Decrease Physiological* Coadministration of phenobarbital with phenytoin has been reported to decrease its concentration or have no effect on it *1706* Causes decreased concentration by stimulating P450 enzymes which enhance metabolism *6350*
Serum Increase Physiological Competitive inhibition of metabolism *2452*
Serum No Effect Analytical No detectable inhibition at 125 µg/mL *6029* No significant interference observed at a concentration of 80 µg/mL (345 µmol/L) with method on Du Pont aca *1538* No effect at concentration of 80 µg/mL (344 µmol/L) on method on Du Pont Dimension *1583* At a concentration of 120 µg/mL no cross-reactivity observed with phenytoin at a concentration of 10 µg/mL when measured by the method on Bayer Technicon Immuno 1® *428* Cross-reactivity of less than 1.0% observed with method on Baxter Stratus *5705*
Serum No Effect Physiological Coadministration of phenobarbital with phenytoin has been reported to decrease its concentration or have no effect on it *1706*

Phosphate *Serum Decrease Physiological* Increases clearance (secondary hyperparathyroidism) *2320*
Serum No Effect Analytical At concentration of 80 µg/mL (344 µmol/L) has no effect on method on Du Pont Dimension *1584* At acute overdose concentration (20 mg/dL) on Technicon SMAC® method *6266* At concentration of 250 mg/L had no effect on phosphomolybdate method *5704*

Phospholipids *Serum No Effect Physiological* No significant difference between 21 female epileptics treated with up to 300 mg/day for at least 5 years and appropriate controls *6583*

Platelets *Blood Decrease Physiological* Thrombocytopenia may occur after some time *4017*

Potassium *Serum No Effect Analytical* At concentration of 10 mg/L had no effect on flame-photometric method *5704* At concentration of 250 mg/L had no effect on measurement by ISE with predilution *5704* At concentration of 60 mg/L had no effect on measurement by ISE without predilution *5704* No effect of concentrations up to 30 mg/L on method on Kodak Ektachem® *5706*

Prazosin *Serum No Effect Physiological* Coadministration of prazosin with phenobarbital had no apparent adverse drug interaction in limited clinical experience *4649*

Prealbumin *Serum Increase Physiological* Mean concentration increased above upper reference limit in epileptic patients treated with phenobarbital alone *4347*

Prednisone *Serum Decrease Physiological* Concentration reduced in asthmatics when phenobarbital coadministered due to hepatic enzyme induction: with withdrawal of phenobarbital effect reversed *749*

Primidone *Serum Decrease Physiological* Causes decreased concentration by stimulating P450 enzymes which enhance metabolism *6350*
Serum No Effect Analytical No significant cross-reactivity with method on Du Pont aca *1541* At concentrations up to 185 mg/L causes 25% increase with method on Baxter Stratus but physiological concentrations up to 40 mg/L so effect likely to be insignificant *5705*

Progesterone *Plasma Decrease Physiological* In 21 epileptic patients treated with phenobarbital for a median of 14.0 years median concentration in luteal phase lower than 12.7 nmol/L in 23.8% *4178*
Plasma No Effect Physiological In 21 epileptic patients treated with phenobarbital for a median of 14.0 years median concentration in follicular phase not significantly different from that in controls *4178*

Prolactin *Plasma No Effect Physiological* In 21 epileptic patients treated with sodium valproate for a median of 14.0 years median concentration of 11.9 ng/mL in follicular phase and 15.4 ng/mL in luteal phase not markedly different from medians of 15.1 and 14.2 ng/mL in 20 age-matched controls *4178*

Propranolol *Serum Decrease Physiological* Enhances hepatic clearance and decreases plasma concentration *1384* Clearance greatly increased when drugs coadministered *6558*

Protein *Serum Increase Analytical* Value more than 3% high when added at 10 times therapeutic concentration and test performed on Technicon SRA-2000 *4348*
Serum No Effect Analytical At concentration of 250 mg/L had no effect on biuret method with blank correction *5704* No effect at therapeutic concentrations on biuret and spectrophotometric method *2920* At acute overdose concentration (20 mg/dL) on Technicon SMAC® method *6266* At concentration of 80 µg/mL (344 µmol/L) had negligible effect on method on Du Pont Dimension *1591*

Protein Electrophoresis *Serum No Effect Analytical* At concentration of 60 mg/L had no effect on automated Olympus-Hite method *5704*

Prothrombin Time *Plasma Decrease Physiological* Coadministration of phenobarbital with dicumarol reduces its plasma concentration and decreases its anticoagulant effect *1706* Metabolism enhanced by barbiturates *128* With 0.1 g/d in 10 patients receiving warfarin due to induction of hepatic microsomal enzymes *6118*

Pyruvate *Plasma No Effect Physiological* No significant effect observed in epileptic patients receiving phenobarbital *4077*

Quinidine *Serum Decrease Physiological* Enhances hepatic clearance and reduces clinical effectiveness *1384* Phenobarbital appears to be capable of enhancing metabolism of quinidine in liver *1245* Hepatic elimination of quinidine accelerated when phenobarbital coadministered because of increased production of cytochrome P450IIIA4 *5996*

Retinol-binding Protein *Serum Increase Physiological* In comparison with untreated cognitively delayed children 4.0 mg/dL on average versus 3.3 mg/dL *3266*

Saquinavir *Serum Decrease Physiological* Coadministration of phenobarbital with saquinavir reduced the latter's concentration by inducing CYP3A4 in the liver *5024*

SDZ PSC 833 *Blood No Effect Analytical* At a concentration of 35 mg/L had no effect on HPLC method of Scott et al when used to measure PSC (with CsD as internal standard) at a concentration of 5 mg/L *5418*

Sex-Hormone Binding Globulin
Serum No Effect Physiological In 21 epileptic patients treated with phenobarbital for a median of 14.0 years median concentration in both follicular and luteal phases not significantly different from that in controls because of wide dispersion of results *4178*

Short-chain Fatty Acid Carnitine Esters
Serum No Effect Physiological In 119 epileptic children treated with phenobarbital mean concentration of 8.6 ± 6.8 nmol/mL not significantly less than 15.4 ± 9.1 nmol/mL in 32 healthy control children *2757*

Sodium *Serum No Effect Analytical* At concentration of 250 mg/L had no effect on measurement by ISE with predilution *5704* At concentration of 10 mg/L had no effect on flame-photometric method *5704* At concentration of 60 mg/L had no effect on measurement by ISE without predilution *5704*

Sucrose *Serum No Effect Analytical* Using automated procedure involving sucrose phosphorylase, phosphoglutamase and glucose-6-phosphatase of Vinet et al no significant interference observed at a concentration of 1 mmol/L *6267*
Urine No Effect Analytical Using automated procedure involving sucrose phosphorylase, phosphoglutamase and glucose-6-phosphatase of Vinet et al no significant interference observed at a concentration of 1 mmol/L *6267*

Sulfa as Sulfanilamide *Urine Increase Analytical* Positive reaction but delayed with usual amount present *409*

T3-Uptake *Serum No Effect Analytical* At concentration of 80 µg/mL (344 µmol/L) has no effect on method on Du Pont Dimension *1586* No significant effect observed at a concentration of 80 µg/mL (344 µmol/L) with method on Du Pont aca *1545*
Serum No Effect Physiological In 18 epileptic patients of mean age of 17.1 ± 13.4 y mean ratio of 0.89 ± 0.1 not significantly different from 0.91 ± 0.1 in 32 healthy controls *6234*

Tacrolimus *Blood No Effect Analytical* No significant effect observed at a concentration of 40 mg/L with MEIA method on Abbott IMx analyzer *1871* No interference observed with radioreceptor assay of Murthy et al *4191*
Serum Decrease Physiological By inducing cytochrome P-450 IIIA enzyme systems may stimulate the metabolism of tacrolimus *1987*
Serum No Effect Analytical At concentration of 40 mg/L had no significant effect on ELISA method *6329*

Tamoxifen *Serum Decrease Physiological* When coadministered with tamoxifen may cause decreased steady-state concentration, 26 ng/mL versus 122 ng/mL in patients receiving tamoxifen only *6648*

Teniposide *Serum Decrease Physiological* Administration of anticonvulsants with teniposide causes significant reduction in teniposide AUC due to increased clearance caused by induction of hepatic enzymes *3909*

Theophylline *Serum Decrease Physiological* Enhances hepatic clearance and decreases clinical effectiveness *1384* Significant reduction observed in some patients probably due to enhanced metabolism caused by hepatic enzyme induction *3390* Increases theophylline clearance by induction of microsomal enzyme activity and decreases serum theophylline concentration by 25% after two weeks of treatment *3125* Increases theophylline clearance by induction of microsomal enzyme activity, decreasing theophylline concentration by about 25% after two weeks of phenobarbital treatment *5999* Up to 25% decrease in serum theophylline concentration after 2 weeks of treatment due to increased theophylline clearance caused by induction of microsomal enzyme activity *6117*
Serum Increase Analytical At concentration of 80 mg/L produced positive bias of 5.20 mg/L at a concentration of 20 mg/L when measured by method on 3M Diagnostics TheoFAST *1122*
Serum No Effect Analytical At concentration of 80 µg/mL (344 µmol/L) had no effect on method on Du Pont Dimension *1585* No effect at 26 mg/L on method on Ames Seralyzer *5706* No effect of concentrations up to 20 mg/L on method on Kodak Ektachem® *5706* At concentration of 80 mg/L produced no interference with methods used with Kodak DT-60, Abbott TDx, Abbott Vision with both whole blood and serum, Syntex AccµLevel and Ames Seralyzer *1122* No effect on Kodak Ektachem® 700 method *1716*

Thyroxine (T4) *Serum Decrease Physiological* In comparison with untreated cognitively delayed children 7.2 µg/dL on average versus 8.4 µg/dL *3266* Reduction observed in the absence of an increase in TSH or clinical features of hypothyroidism. Effect also observed in hyperthyroid patients *1269* Concentration reduced due to hepatic enzyme induction *2412* Both significant and nonsignificant changes noted, associated with enzyme induction *6412* In 18 epileptic patients of mean age of 17.1 ± 13.4 y mean concentration of 91 ± 18 nmol/L not significantly different from 99 ± 19 nmol/L in 32 healthy controls *6234*
Serum No Effect Analytical No significant effect observed at a concentration of 80 µg/mL (344 µmol/L) with method on Du Pont aca *1546* At concentration of 80 µg/mL (344 µmol/L) has no effect on method on Du Pont Dimension *1587* No significant effect observed at a concentration of 80 µg/mL (344 µmol/L) with method on Du Pont aca *1588*

Thyroxine (T4), Free *Serum Decrease Physiological* Reduction observed in the absence of an increase in TSH or clinical features of hypothyroidism. Effect also observed in hyperthyroid patients *1269*
Serum No Effect Analytical Phenobarbital at a concentration of 3000 µg/dL had no cross-reactivity FT4 in method on Bayer Technicon Immuno 1® *424*

Thyroxine (T4) Index, Free *Serum Decrease Physiological* Both significant and nonsignificant changes noted, associated with enzyme induction *6412*
Serum Increase Physiological In 75 epileptic patients of mean age of 17.1 ± 13.4 y mean index of 101.7 ± 14.2 nmol/L not significantly different from 106.8 ± 15.4 nmol/L in 32 healthy controls *6234*

Toremifene *Serum Decrease Physiological* Cytochrome P450 3A4 inducers increase the rate of toremifene metabolism thereby reducing its serum concentration *5329*

Transferrin *Serum No Effect Physiological* No significant effect observed in epileptic patients receiving phenobarbital as sole therapy *4346*

Tri-iodothyronine, Free (fT3) *Serum No Effect Analytical* At a concentration of 0.2 g/L cross-reactivity of 0.0% with free triiodothyronine method on Bayer Technicon Immuno 1® system *425*

Tri-iodothyronine (T3) *Serum Decrease Physiological* Concentration reduced due to hepatic enzyme induction *2412* Changes less marked than with thyroxine in treated patients *1269*

Tricyclic Antidepressants *Serum Decrease Physiological* Interacts pharmacokinetically to induce metabolism of tricyclic antidepressants *3590*

Triglycerides *Serum No Effect Analytical* No effect at 250 mg/L on Boehringer Mannheim Reflotron method *5706* No effect at therapeutic concentrations on enzymatic methods *2920* No effect at therapeutic concentration on Boehringer Mannheim Reflotron method *3231* At concentration of 100 mg/L had no effect on GPO-PAP method *5704* At concentration of 80 µg/mL (344 µmol/L) has no effect on method on Du Pont Dimension *1592* At acute overdose concentration (20 mg/dL) on Technicon SMAC® method *6266* At concentration of 250 mg/L had no effect on lipase/esterase method *5704*
Serum No Effect Physiological No significant difference between 21 female epileptics treated with up to 300 mg/day for at least 5 years and appropriate controls *6583*

Urea Nitrogen *Serum No Effect Analytical* No effect at 20 mg/L on method on Ames Seralyzer *5706* No effect at therapeutic concentration on Boehringer Mannheim Reflotron method *3231* At concentration of 30 mg/L had no effect on Kodak Ektachem® method *5704* At concentration of 250 mg/L had no effect on diacetylmonoxime method *5704* No effect at 250 mg/L on Boehringer Mannheim Reflotron method *5706* No effect at therapeutic concentrations on glutamate dehydrogenase, phenol- hypochlorite and diacetyl monoxime methods *2920* At acute overdose concentration (20 mg/dL) on Technicon SMAC® method *6266* No effect at concentration of 80 µg/mL (340 µmol/L) on method on Du Pont Dimension *1593*

Uric Acid *Serum No Effect Analytical* No effect at 250 mg/L on Boehringer Mannheim Reflotron method *5706* At 50 mg/L on reversed phase liquid chromatographic procedure of Zhiri et al *6656* At concentration of 100 mg/L had no effect on uricase-PAP method *5704* At concentration of 250 mg/L had no effect on phosphotungstate reduction method *5704* At concentration of 80 mg/L had no effect on Kageyama-Hantzsch method *5704* No effect at concentration of 80 µg/mL (344 µmol/L) on method on Du Pont Dimension *1594* No effect at therapeutic concentration on Boehringer Mannheim Reflotron method *3231* At acute overdose concentration (20 mg/dL) on Technicon SMAC® method *6266* No effect at therapeutic concentrations on uricase-catalase, aldehyde dehydrogenase, direct UV-test and phosphotungstate methods *2920*

Valproic Acid *Serum Decrease Physiological* Significant reduction in half-life from 10.9 h to 8.2 h due to enzyme induction *3684* Concentration reduced to about 75% when phenobarbital coadministered *3855* Causes decreased concentration by stimulating P450 enzymes which enhance metabolism *6350* Through induction of hepatic enzymes may increase the

Phenobarbital *(continued)*

Valproic Acid *(continued)*
plasma clearance of valproate *15* By increasing the expression of hepatic enzymes, especially those that increase the amount of glucuronosyl transferases, may increase the clearance of valproate twofold *17:*
Serum No Effect Analytical At concentrations up to 750 µg/mL had no significant cross-reactivity in valproic acid method on Bayer Technicon Immuno 1® *437* No significant interference observed at a concentration of 750 µg/mL (3229 µmol/L) with method on Du Pont aca *1560*

Verapamil *Serum Decrease Physiological* Enhances hepatic clearance and reduces clinical effectiveness *1384* Coadministration may increase verapamil clearance *3201* Coadministration of phenobarbital with verapamil may markedly increase verapamil clearance *3470* When drugs coadministered phenobarbital may increase clearance of verapamil *2063*

Vitamin A *Serum No Effect Physiological* No difference between treated and untreated cognitively delayed children *3266*

Vitamin B_{12} *Cerebrospinal Fluid Decrease Physiological* Significantly lower with long term therapy *1960*
Serum No Effect Analytical At concentrations up to 20 mg/dL had no clinically significant cross-reactivity in vitamin B_{12} method on Bayer Technicon Immuno 1® *439*

Vitamin E *Serum Decrease Physiological* Mean of 0.58 mg/dL versus 0.67 mg/dL in untreated control of handicapped children *2596*

Warfarin *Plasma Decrease Physiological* Coadministration of phenobarbital with warfarin reduces its plasma concentration and decreases its anticoagulant effect *1706*

Zinc *Serum No Effect Physiological* No significant difference on average between treated and untreated handicapped children, although hypozincemia in 7 of 32 treated children and 0 of 13 controls *2596* In 28 epileptic patients treated for 1 month insignificant reduction to 73.6 ± 9.4 µg/dL compared with 78.4 ± 12.8 µg/dL in 30 healthy controls *3344* Observed in both hospitalized and home-living patients with long-term administration *6417*

Phenolphthalein

BSP Retention *Serum Increase Analytical* Color development on alkalinization of sample *6515*

Color *Feces Increase Analytical* Imparts red color *128*
Urine Increase Analytical Pink, red, purple (alkaline), orange, rust (acid) *606*

Erythrocytes *Urine Increase Physiological* May cause acute nephrosis (K deficiency) *4014*

Estriol *Urine Decrease Analytical* Interferes with acidic and enzyme hydrolysis *641*

Estrogens *Urine Decrease Analytical* Competes for enzyme used for hydrolysis *55*

Fat *Feces Increase Physiological* Steatorrhea observed in some laxative abusers *5055*

Glucose *Serum Increase Physiological* Impaired glucose tolerance may occur due to potassium loss *1108*

Glucose Tolerance *Serum Decrease Physiological* Result of hypokalemia *1108*

Hemoglobin *Urine Increase Physiological* May cause acute nephrosis (K deficiency) *4014*

^{131}I Uptake *Serum Decrease Physiological* Phenolax contains tetraiodofluorescein *4360*

Ketones *Urine Increase Analytical* Pink with Rothera, Ketostix® and Acetest® tests *199* Presumed false positive from color *2452*

LE Cells *Blood Positive Physiological* Associated with hypersensitivity *4014*

Occult Blood *Feces Increase Physiological* Protracted treatment may cause ulceration *929*

Platelets *Blood Decrease Physiological* Immunologically induced thrombocytopenia *3051*

Potassium *Serum Decrease Physiological* If chronic laxative abuse and aldosteronism *1886*

Protein *Urine Increase Analytical* Similar interference to that of phenolphthalein with Du Pont aca benzethonium chloride method *3261*
Urine Increase Physiological May cause acute nephrosis (K deficiency) *4014*

Prothrombin Time *Plasma Increase Physiological* Patients on coumarins *4014*

PSP Excretion *Urine Increase Analytical* Color development on alkalinization of urine *6515*

Phenolsulfonphthalein

Acetone *Urine Increase Analytical* Chromogenicity in color reaction (Rothera test) *6515*

BSP Retention *Serum Increase Analytical* May increase colorimetric reading *2451*

Color *Urine Increase Analytical* Purple red or pink in alkaline urine *1957*

Creatine *Urine Increase Analytical* Chromogenicity in color reaction *3810*

Creatinine *Serum Increase Analytical* Chromogenicity in color reaction *5869*
Serum No Effect Analytical No interference observed at a concentration of 10 mg/L with HPLC method of Rosano et al *5083*
Urine Increase Analytical Interference with Jaffe procedure *1009*

Ketones *Urine Increase Analytical* Presumed false positive from color *2452* Red-purple color with alkaline nitroprusside *882*

Leucine Aminopeptidase *Urine Increase Physiological* Facilitates permeation of enzyme into tubules *4826*

Protein *Urine Increase Analytical* Marked increase in absorption, linearly related to dye concentration, with benzethonium chloride method on Du Pont aca *3261*

Uric Acid *Serum Decrease Physiological* Uricosuric action *2378*
Urine Increase Physiological Uricosuric action *2378*

Vanillylmandelic Acid *Urine Increase Analytical* May interfere with colorimetric method *140*

Phenothiazine

Acetoacetate *Urine Increase Analytical* Metabolites react with $FeCl_3$*6515*

Alanine Aminotransferase *Serum Decrease Physiological* Observed in treatment of female schizophrenics *480*
Serum Increase Physiological May cause cholestatic hepatitis (in up to 4% patients) *3810* Liver damage observed after different phenothiazines administered in succession *3108*

Aldolase *Serum Decrease Physiological* In schizophrenics with high initial values *4014*

Alkaline Phosphatase *Serum Increase Physiological* Liver damage observed after different phenothiazines administered in succession *3108* Intrahepatic cholestatic syndrome *2559*

Amitriptyline *Serum Increase Physiological* When coadministered, by inhibiting cytochrome P450 2D6, may increase the concentration of amitriptyline *6645*

Aspartate Aminotransferase *Serum Increase Physiological* May cause cholestatic hepatitis (in up to 4% patients) *3810*

Bile *Urine Increase Analytical* Alleged interference with BiliLabstix® *2451*
Urine Increase Physiological May cause cholestatic hepatitis *3810*
Urine No Effect Analytical Ictotest® unaffected *2452*

Bilirubin *Serum Increase Physiological* Liver damage observed after different phenothiazines administered in succession *3108* Hypersensitivity cholestatic reaction may occur *2242*
Urine Increase Physiological May cause cholestatic hepatitis *3810*

Bilirubin, Direct *Serum Increase Physiological* Relatively large increase compared with total *2242*

BSP Retention *Serum Increase Physiological* May cause cholestatic hepatitis (in up to 4% patients) *3810*

Cannabinoids *Urine No Effect Analytical* No effect on Roche Abuscreen method *5006*

Catecholamines *Plasma Increase Physiological* Increased metabolism, decreased organ uptake of norepinephrine *189*

Cholesterol *Serum Increase Physiological* Frequently reported effect, ?mechanism *4909*
Serum No Effect Analytical At concentration of 150 mg/L had no effect on Liebermann-Burchard method *5704* At concentration of 150 mg/L had no effect on CHOD-Iodide method *5704* At concentration of 150 mg/L had no effect on CHOD-PAP method *5704* At concentration of 150 mg/L had no effect on method using catalase-Hantzsch reaction *5704* At concentration of 150 mg/L had no effect on catalase-AIDH method *5704*

Cholinesterase *Serum Decrease Physiological* Also affects erythrocyte enzyme *2452*

Color *Urine Increase Analytical* Pink, red, purple, orange, rust color *4012*

Creatine Kinase *Serum Decrease Physiological* In schizophrenics with high initial values *4014*
Serum Increase Physiological Probable effect of i.m. injection *2451*

Creatinine *Serum No Effect Analytical* At concentration of 200 mg/L had no effect on kinetic Jaffe method on BKA-2 *5704* At concentration of 30 mg/L had no effect on Jaffe-Fuller's earth method *5704* At concentration of 30 mg/L had no effect on Jaffe-Fading-Fraction method *5704*

Eosinophils *Blood Increase Physiological* Allergic response *3810*

Erythrocytes *Blood Decrease Physiological* Hemolytic anemia (sensitivity dependent) *1212*

Estrogens *Urine Decrease Physiological* Blocks ovulation, inhibits decidual reaction *1714*

Ferric Chloride Test *Urine Positive Analytical* Pink/purple color from metabolites *882*

Follicle Stimulating Hormone
Plasma Decrease Physiological Stimulation effect of gonadotropins inhibited *3669*

Glucose *Serum Increase Physiological* Probable effect, adrenergic response *2452*
Serum No Effect Analytical At concentration of 20 mg/L had no effect on Kodak Ektachem® method *5704*
Urine Increase Physiological Long term effect in some patients *2452* Effect seen especially in long term therapy of diabetics *4132*

Glucose Tolerance *Serum Decrease Physiological* May produce diabetic type of curve in normals *3669*

γ-Glutamyltransferase *Serum Increase Physiological* Liver damage observed after different phenothiazines administered in succession *3108*

Gonadotropins *Urine Decrease Physiological* Associated with other endocrinological changes *4014*

Hematocrit *Blood Decrease Physiological* Hemolytic anemia (sensitivity dependent) *1212*

Hemoglobin *Blood Decrease Physiological* Hemolytic anemia (sensitivity dependent) *1212*

17-Hydroxycorticosteroids *Urine Decrease Physiological* Inhibit release of steroid hormones *3669*

5-Hydroxyindoleacetic Acid *Urine Decrease Analytical* False decrease if nitrosonaphthol used *6515*
Urine No Effect Analytical No effect observed with FPIA method on Abbott TDx *695*

^{131}I Uptake *Serum Increase Physiological* Reported effect in hyperthyroidism *2451*
Serum No Effect Physiological No effect observed even with prolonged use *3107*

17-Ketogenic Steroids *Urine Increase Analytical* Yield similar color with Zimmermann reaction *3669*

Ketones *Urine Increase Analytical* Pink or purple with Gerhardt's test *882*

17-Ketosteroids *Urine Decrease Physiological* Inhibit release of steroid hormones *3669*

Leukocytes *Blood Decrease Physiological* Agranulocytosis/Leukopenia especially if low initially *3491*
Blood Increase Physiological Due to eosinophilia or generalized leukocytosis *3810*

Luteinizing Hormone *Plasma Decrease Physiological* Stimulation effect of gonadotropins inhibited *3669*

5'-Nucleotidase *Serum Increase Physiological* Due to cholestasis *2911*

Phenobarbital *Serum Decrease Physiological* But not to quite same extent as for phenytoin *2407*

Phenothiazines *Urine Positive Physiological* Some detectable up to 18 mo after therapy *2242*

Phenylketones *Urine Positive Analytical* Pink/red-purple with $FeCl_3$, same with Phenistix® *1195*

Phenytoin *Serum Decrease Physiological* Decreased by more than 40% with start of drug or increased dose *2407*
Serum Increase Physiological Coadministration of phenothiazines with phenytoin may increase plasma phenytoin concentration *4522* When phenothiazines ingested with fosphenytoin concentration of phenytoin may be increased *4519*

Phosphate *Serum Decrease Analytical* Affect methods using phosphomolybdate *1688*

Platelets *Blood Decrease Physiological* Hemolytic anemia (sensitivity dependent) *1212*

Porphobilinogen *Urine Increase Analytical* May react with Ehrlich's aldehyde reagent *4912*

Potassium *Serum No Effect Analytical* At concentration of 200 mg/L had no effect on measurement by ISE without predilution *5704*

Pregnanediol *Urine Decrease Physiological* Reported effect *3669*

Primidone *Serum No Effect Physiological* No significant effect on serum concentration *2407*

Progesterone *Urine Decrease Physiological* Associated with other endocrinological changes *4014*

Protein *Cerebrospinal Fluid Increase Analytical* False positive with Folin-Ciocalteu reagent *2024*

Protein Electrophoresis *Serum No Effect Analytical* At concentration of 200 mg/L had no effect on automated Olympus-Hite method *5704*

Sodium *Serum No Effect Analytical* At concentration of 200 mg/L had no effect on measurement by ISE without predilution *5704*

Sorbitol Dehydrogenase *Serum Decrease Physiological* Observed with therapy of female schizophrenics *480*

T3-Uptake *Serum Decrease Physiological* Due to increased thyroxine binding globulin with prolonged use *3107*

Thyroxine Binding Globulin *Serum Increase Physiological* Occurs with prolonged use *3107*

Thyroxine (T4) *Serum Decrease Physiological* Observed with long-term treatment but cause not clear *6412*
Serum Increase Physiological Increase observed due to increased thyroxine-binding globulin *2412*

Tri-iodothyronine (T3) *Serum Increase Physiological* Increase observed due to increased thyroxine-binding globulin *2412*

Urea Nitrogen *Serum Decrease Physiological* Decreased urea production if hepatic cirrhosis occurs *1009*
Serum No Effect Analytical At concentration of 20 mg/L had no effect on Kodak Ektachem® method *5704*

Uric Acid *Serum Decrease Physiological* Reported uricosuric action *3669*
Serum Increase Physiological Reported effect *4567*
Serum No Effect Analytical At concentration of 30 mg/L had no effect on catalase-AIDH method *5704* At concentration of 30 mg/L had no effect on Kageyama-Hantzsch method *5704*
Urine Increase Physiological Reported uricosuric action *3669*

Urobilinogen *Urine Increase Analytical* May react with Ehrlich's aldehyde reagent *4912*

Vanillylmandelic Acid *Urine Decrease Physiological* Alters blood concentration *189*

Phenoxybenzamine

Catecholamines *Urine No Effect Physiological* No effect observed *1444*

Phenoxybenzamine *(continued)*

Sodium *Serum Decrease Physiological* Isolated case. Presumed to be due to drug-induced inappropriate release of vasopressin *248*

Vanillylmandelic Acid *Urine No Effect Physiological* No effect observed *1444*

Phenoxypropazine

Alanine Aminotransferase *Serum Increase Physiological* Produced fatal hepatotoxicity *4014*

Alkaline Phosphatase *Serum Increase Physiological* Produced fatal hepatotoxicity *4014*

Aspartate Aminotransferase *Serum Increase Physiological* Produced fatal hepatotoxicity *4014*

Bilirubin *Serum Increase Physiological* Produced fatal hepatotoxicity *4014*

Phenprocoumon

Alanine Aminotransferase *Serum Increase Physiological* Mild effect but recurrently in 2 patients having repeated exposure to drug *5597*
Serum No Effect Analytical No effect at 20 mg/L on Boehringer Mannheim Reflotron method *5706* No effect at therapeutic concentration on Boehringer Mannheim Reflotron method *3231*

Alkaline Phosphatase *Serum Increase Physiological* Mild effect but recurrently in 2 patients having repeated exposure to drug *5597*

Amylase *Serum No Effect Analytical* No effect of concentrations up to 20 mg/L on method on Boehringer Mannheim Reflotron *5706*

Amylase, Pancreatic Isoenzyme
Serum No Effect Analytical No significant effect observed at a toxic concentration of 40 mg/L with method on Boehringer Mannheim Reflotron *3647*

Aspartate Aminotransferase *Serum Increase Physiological* Mild effect but recurrently in 2 patients having repeated exposure to drug *5597*
Serum No Effect Analytical No effect at 20 mg/L on Boehringer Mannheim Reflotron method *5706* No effect at therapeutic concentration on Boehringer Mannheim Reflotron method *3231*

Bilirubin *Serum Increase Physiological* Mild effect but recurrently in 2 patients having repeated exposure to drug *5597*
Serum No Effect Analytical At concentration of 20 mg/L no effect on method on Boehringer Mannheim Reflotron system *5706* No effect at 5 mg/L on Ames Seralyzer method *5706*

Bilirubin, Direct *Serum Increase Physiological* Mild effect but recurrently in 2 patients having repeated exposure to drug *5597*

BSP Retention *Serum Increase Physiological* Mild effect but recurrently in 2 patients having repeated exposure to drug *5597*

Cholesterol *Serum No Effect Analytical* No effect at therapeutic concentration on Boehringer Mannheim Reflotron method *3231* At concentration of 20 mg/L no effect on method on Boehringer Mannheim Reflotron system *5706* At concentration of 80 mg/L had no effect on method using catalase-Hantzsch reaction *5704* No effect at 5 mg/L on Ames Seralyzer method *5706* At concentration of 80 mg/L had no effect on catalase-AIDH method *5704* At concentration of 80 mg/L had no effect on Liebermann-Burchard method *5704* At concentration of 80 mg/L had no effect on CHOD-Iodide method *5704* At concentration of 80 mg/L had no effect on CHOD-PAP method *5704*

Cortisol *Plasma No Effect Analytical* At a concentration of 40 mg/L no significant effect observed on CEDIA method *1097*

Creatine Kinase *Serum No Effect Analytical* No effect at 5 mg/L on method on Ames Seralyzer *5706*

Creatinine *Serum No Effect Analytical* At concentration of 6 mg/L had no effect on Jaffe-Fuller's earth method *5704* No effect at 5 mg/L on Ames Seralyzer method *5706* At concentration of 6 mg/L had no effect on Jaffe-Fading-Fraction method *5704* At concentration of 26 mg/L had no effect on kinetic Jaffe method on BKA-2 *5704*

Glucose *Serum No Effect Analytical* At concentration of 20 mg/L no effect on method on Boehringer Mannheim Reflotron system *5706* No effect at 5 mg/L on glucose oxidase method on Ames Seralyzer *5706* At concentration of 2 mg/L had no effect on hexokinase/G-6-PDH method *5704* At concentration of 0.36 mg/L had no effect on Kodak Ektachem® method *5704* No effect at therapeutic concentration on Boehringer Mannheim Reflotron method *3231*

γ-Glutamyltransferase *Serum Increase Physiological* Mild effect but recurrently in 2 patients having repeated exposure to drug *5597*
Serum No Effect Analytical At concentration of 20 mg/L no effect on method on Boehringer Mannheim Reflotron system *5706* No effect at therapeutic concentration on Boehringer Mannheim Reflotron method *3231*

HDL-Cholesterol *Serum No Effect Analytical* At a concentration up to 20 mg/L had no significant effect on Reflotron method for whole blood cholesterol *6352*

Lactate *Plasma No Effect Analytical* At concentration of 2 mg/L had no effect on enzymatic method *5704*

Lactate Dehydrogenase *Serum Increase Physiological* Mild effect but recurrently in 2 patients having repeated exposure to drug *5597*
Serum No Effect Analytical No effect at 5 mg/L on method on Ames Seralyzer *5706*

Phenytoin *Serum Increase Physiological* Half-life increased by 40% in three patients *5966*

Potassium *Serum No Effect Analytical* At concentration of 3.6 mg/L had no effect on measurement by ISE without predilution *5704*

Protein Electrophoresis *Serum No Effect Analytical* At concentration of 3.6 mg/L had no effect on automated Olympus-Hite method *5704*

Sodium *Serum No Effect Analytical* At concentration of 3.6 mg/L had no effect on measurement by ISE without predilution *5704*

Tolbutamide *Serum No Effect Physiological* No effect apparent on plasma concentration or metabolism of drug *5595*

Triglycerides *Serum No Effect Analytical* No effect at therapeutic concentration on Boehringer Mannheim Reflotron method *3231* No effect at 20 mg/L on Boehringer Mannheim Reflotron method *5706*

Urea Nitrogen *Serum No Effect Analytical* At concentration of 0.36 mg/L had no effect on Kodak Ektachem® method *5704* No effect at 20 mg/L on Boehringer Mannheim Reflotron method *5706* No effect at therapeutic concentration on Boehringer Mannheim Reflotron method *3231* No effect at 5 mg/L on method on Ames Seralyzer *5706*

Uric Acid *Serum No Effect Analytical* No effect at therapeutic concentration on Boehringer Mannheim Reflotron method *3231* At concentration of 6 mg/L had no effect on Kageyama-Hantzsch method *5704* No effect at 20 mg/L on Boehringer Mannheim Reflotron method *5706* At concentration of 6 mg/L had no effect on catalase-AIDH method *5704*

Phensuximide

Albumin *Serum No Effect Analytical* At concentration of 120 mg/L had no effect on BCG method *5704*

Bicarbonate *Serum No Effect Analytical* At concentration of 120 mg/L had no effect on method using phenolphthalein *5704*

Bilirubin *Serum No Effect Analytical* At concentration of 120 mg/L had no effect on Jendrassik and Grof method *5704*

Calcium *Serum No Effect Analytical* At concentration of 120 mg/L had no effect on cresolphthalein method *5704*

Chloride *Serum No Effect Analytical* At concentration of 120 mg/L had no effect on mercurimetric method *5704*

Cholesterol *Serum No Effect Analytical* At concentration of 120 mg/L had no effect on Liebermann-Burchard method *5704*

Color *Urine Increase Analytical* Pink, red, purple, orange and rust color *4012*

Creatinine *Serum No Effect Analytical* At concentration of 120 mg/L had no effect on Technicon AutoAnalyzer® Jaffe method *5704*

Erythrocytes *Urine Increase Physiological* Hematuria and renal damage reported *2754*

Ethosuximide *Serum No Effect Analytical* Insignificant cross-reactivity observed with method on Du Pont aca *1523*

Felbamate *Serum No Effect Analytical* No significant interference observed with GLC method of Rifai et al *4958*

^{131}I Uptake *Serum Decrease Physiological* Milontin® contains tetraiodofluorescein *4360*

Leukocytes *Blood Decrease Physiological* Possible agranulocytosis (very rare) *128*

Phosphate *Serum No Effect Analytical* At concentration of 120 mg/L had no effect on phosphomolybdate method *5704*

Potassium *Serum No Effect Analytical* At concentration of 120 mg/L had no effect on measurement by ISE with predilution *5704*

Protein *Serum No Effect Analytical* At concentration of 120 mg/L had no effect on biuret method with blank correction *5704*
Urine Increase Physiological Reversible nephropathy (especially in children) *128*

Sodium *Serum No Effect Analytical* At concentration of 120 mg/L had no effect on measurement by ISE with predilution *5704*

Triglycerides *Serum No Effect Analytical* At concentration of 120 mg/L had no effect on lipase/esterase method *5704*

Urea Nitrogen *Serum Increase Physiological* Reversible nephropathy (especially in children) *128*
Serum No Effect Analytical At concentration of 120 mg/L had no effect on diacetylmonoxime method *5704*

Uric Acid *Serum No Effect Analytical* At concentration of 120 mg/L had no effect on phosphotungstate reduction method *5704*

Phentermine

Amobarbital *Urine No Effect Analytical* No interference on TLC using ethyl acetate: methanol: water: ammonium hydroxide and modified Dragendorff's reagent for detection *6502*

Amphetamine *Urine No Effect Analytical* No interference on TLC using ethylacetate: methanol: water: ammonium hydroxide and modified Dragendorff's reagent for detection *6502*
Urine Positive Analytical At concentrations above 0.5 µg/mL (3.35 µmol/L) with method on Du Pont aca *1554*

Chlorphenmetrazine *Urine Positive Analytical* Similar R_f and color reaction on TLC using ethyl acetate: methanol: water: ammonium hydroxide and modified Dragendorff's reagent *6502*

Drugs of Abuse Screen *Urine Increase Analytical* False positive result with Abbott ADx method for amphetamine/methamphetamine *4279*

Hydromorphone *Urine No Effect Analytical* No interference on TLC using ethylacetate: methanol: water: ammonium hydroxide and modified Dragendorff's reagent for detection *6502*

Mescaline *Urine No Effect Analytical* No interference on TLC using ethylacetate: methanol: water: ammonium hydroxide and modified Dragendorff's reagent for detection *6502*

Methamphetamine *Urine No Effect Analytical* No interference on TLC using ethylacetate: methanol: water: ammonium hydroxide and modified Dragendorff's reagent for detection *6502*

Morphine *Urine No Effect Analytical* No interference on TLC using ethylacetate: methanol: water: ammonium hydroxide and modified Dragendorff's reagent for detection *6502*

p-Aminophenol *Urine No Effect Analytical* With addition of drugs at a concentration of 100 mg/L and of related compounds at 50 mg/L no significant effect observed on colorimetric method of van Bocxlaer on Cobas Mira analyzer which involves reacting free p-aminophenol with resorcinol in the presence of magnesium ions to form an indophenol dye measured at 550 nm *6163*

Pentobarbital *Urine No Effect Analytical* No interference on TLC using ethylacetate: methanol: water: ammonium hydroxide and modified Dragendorff's reagent for detection *6502*

Phenmetrazine *Urine Positive Analytical* Similar R_f and color reaction on TLC using ethyl acetate: methanol: water: ammonium hydroxide and modified Dragendorff's reagent *6502*

Phenobarbital *Urine No Effect Analytical* No interference on TLC using ethylacetate: methanol: water: ammonium hydroxide and modified Dragendorff's reagent for detection *6502*

Phenylpropanolamine *Urine No Effect Analytical* No interference on TLC using ethylacetate: methanol: water: ammonium hydroxide and modified Dragendorff's reagent for detection *6502*

Quinine *Urine Increase Analytical* Similar R_f and color reaction on TLC using ethyl acetate: methanol: water: ammonium hydroxide and modified Dragendorff's reagent *6502*

Secobarbital *Urine No Effect Analytical* No interference on TLC using ethylacetate: methanol: water: ammonium hydroxide and modified Dragendorff's reagent for detection *6502*

Phentolamine

Catecholamines *Plasma Increase Physiological* ?Due to releasing action or to altered metabolism *2242*
Urine No Effect Physiological No effect observed *1444*

Glucose *Serum Decrease Physiological* Toxic doses over long period of time *2242*

5-Hydroxyindoleacetic Acid *Urine Increase Analytical* May cause falsely high colorimetric values *1444*

Midazolam *Serum No Effect Analytical* On GC-ECD method of Ha et al *2387*

Vanillylmandelic Acid *Urine No Effect Physiological* No effect observed *1444*

Phenyl Salicylate

Color *Urine Increase Analytical* Dark green *3810*

Phenylbutazone

Alanine Aminotransferase *Serum Increase Physiological* May cause cholestatic and cytotoxic jaundice *402* Frequent hypersensitivity reaction but also with hepatotoxic potential: may be hepatocellular injury or systemic vasculitis *482*

Albumin *Serum No Effect Analytical* At concentration of 750 mg/L had no effect on BCG method *5704* No interference observed at a concentration of 100 mg/L (324 µmol/L) with method on Du Pont aca *1507*

Alkaline Phosphatase *Serum Increase Physiological* Observed in one patient: clear evidence of intrahepatic cholestasis *6169* In 2 patients subsided after drug withdrawn associated with granulomas and cholestatic-hepatocellular injury *2834* Frequent hypersensitivity reaction but also with hepatotoxic potential: may be hepatocellular injury or systemic vasculitis *482* Observed in 7 patients with side effects due to drug *5736* Hepatitis may occur as complication of therapy *4192*

Amylase *Serum Increase Physiological* Parotitis may occur as rare complication *2348* Sialadenitis reported to occur occasionally, but in 5 of 7 patients in this study *5736*

Aspartate Aminotransferase *Serum Increase Physiological* Frequent hypersensitivity reaction but also with hepatotoxic potential: may be hepatocellular injury or systemic vasculitis *482* In 2 patients subsided after drug withdrawn associated with granulomas and cholestatic-hepatocellular injury *2834* Observed in 7 patients with side effects due to drug *5736* May cause cholestatic and cytotoxic jaundice *402*

Bicarbonate *Serum No Effect Analytical* At concentration of 750 mg/L had no effect on method using phenolphthalein *5704*

Bilirubin *Serum Increase Physiological* Observed in one patient: clear evidence of intrahepatic cholestasis *6169* In 2 patients subsided after drug withdrawn associated with granulomas and cholestatic-hepatocellular injury *2834* Granulomatous reaction in liver *2228* Observed in 7 patients with side

Phenylbutazone *(continued)*

Bilirubin *(continued)*
effects due to drug *5736* Clinically significant displacement from protein in neonates *6314* Frequent hypersensitivity reaction but also with hepatotoxic potential: may be hepatocellular injury or systemic vasculitis *482*
Serum No Effect Analytical At concentration of 750 mg/L had no effect on Jendrassik and Grof method *5704*

Bilirubin, Direct *Serum Increase Physiological* In 2 patients subsided after drug withdrawn, associated with granulomas and cholestatic-hepatocellular injury *2834* Observed in one patient; clear evidence of intrahepatic cholestasis *6169*

BSP Retention *Serum Increase Physiological* May cause cholestasis *3810*

Calcium *Serum No Effect Analytical* At concentration of 750 mg/L had no effect on cresolphthalein method *5704*

Cannabinoids *Urine No Effect Analytical* No effect on Roche Abuscreen method *5006*

Chloride *Serum Increase Physiological* May cause salt retention (?tubular dysfunction) *6201*
Serum No Effect Analytical At concentration of 750 mg/L had no effect on mercurimetric method *5704*

Cholesterol *Serum Increase Physiological* Observed in one patient: clear evidence of intrahepatic cholestasis *6169*
Serum No Effect Analytical At concentration of 280 mg/L had no effect on method using catalase-Hantzsch reaction *5704* At concentration of 280 mg/L had no effect on catalase-AlDH method *5704* At concentration of 750 mg/L had no effect on Liebermann-Burchard method *5704* At concentration of 280 mg/L had no effect on CHOD-Iodide method *5704* At concentration of 280 mg/L had no effect on CHOD-PAP method *5704*

Color *Feces Increase Analytical* Pink/red color reported with phenylbutazone ingestion *3388*
Urine Increase Analytical Red color observed following ingestion of phenylbutazone *3388*

Coombs' Test *Blood Positive Physiological* Immunological response to drug *2453*

Coombs' Test, Direct *Blood Positive Physiological* Single case after 2 weeks therapy *2452*

Creatinine *Serum Increase Physiological* May increase especially if coexisting renal damage *4014*
Serum No Effect Analytical At concentration of 120 mg/L had no effect on Jaffe-Fading-Fraction method *5704* At concentration of 750 mg/L had no effect on Technicon AutoAnalyzer® Jaffe method *5704* At concentration of 400 mg/L had no effect on kinetic Jaffe method on BKA-2 *5704* At concentration of 120 mg/L had no effect on Jaffe-Fuller's earth method *5704*

Digitoxin *Serum Decrease Physiological* Due to induction of mixed function oxidases which may reduce to subtherapeutic level *4631*

Eosinophils *Blood Increase Physiological* In 2 patients subsided after drug withdrawn associated with granulomas and cholestatic-hepatocellular injury *2834*

Erythrocyte Sedimentation Rate
Blood Increase Physiological Observed in 7 patients with side effects due to drug *5736*

Erythrocytes *Blood Decrease Physiological* Bone marrow depression/secondary to Na and H_2O retention *857* Fatal aplastic anemia in 2.2 per 100,000 *2822* Occasional case of aplastic anemia reported *6264*
Urine Increase Physiological Observed effect, may occasionally be marked with oliguria or renal failure *4777* Actual bleeding caused by drug *1714*

Etodolac, Free *Serum Increase Physiological* Administration of phenylbutazone with etodolac causes an increase in the free fraction of etodolac (about 80%) *6559*

γ-Globulin *Serum Increase Physiological* Observed in 2 cases (?due to antibodies) *3554*

Glucaric Acid *Urine Increase Physiological* May induce hepatic enzymes *4*

Glucose *Serum Increase Physiological* Metabolic/endocrine response *2754*
Serum No Effect Analytical At concentration of 200 mg/L had no effect on GOD/POD-PAP method *5704* At concentration of 12 mg/L had no effect on Kodak Ektachem® method *5704* At concentration of 200 mg/L had no effect on GOD-PERID method *5704* At concentration of 200 mg/L had no effect on hexokinase/G-6-PDH method *5704*
Urine Increase Physiological Observed effect, may occasionally be marked with oliguria or renal failure *4777*

Granulocytes *Blood Decrease Physiological* Indicative of toxicity developing *2754*

Guanase *Serum Increase Physiological* May cause cholestatic and cytotoxic jaundice *402*

Hematocrit *Blood Decrease Physiological* Bone marrow depression/secondary to Na and H_2O retention *857*

Hemoglobin *Blood Decrease Physiological* Bone marrow depression/secondary to Na and H_2O retention *857*
Urine Increase Physiological Actual bleeding caused by drug *1714*

Histamine *Plasma No Effect Analytical* Insignificant inhibition of radio-enzyme assay at physiological concentrations *2492*

17-Hydroxycorticosteroids *Urine Decrease Physiological* Cortisol metabolism diverted to 6-β-hydroxycortisol *3325*

6-β-Hydroxycortisol *Urine Increase Physiological* Long term change in steroid excretory pattern *3325*

^{131}I Uptake *Serum Decrease Physiological* May last up to 2 weeks *5382*

Indocyanine Green *Serum Decrease Physiological* Mechanism not yet established *3942*

Isocitrate Dehydrogenase *Serum Increase Physiological* May cause cholestatic and cytotoxic jaundice *402*

Lactate Dehydrogenase *Serum Increase Physiological* In 2 patients subsided after drug withdrawn associated with granulomas and cholestatic-hepatocellular injury *2834*

LE Cells *Blood Positive Physiological* May precipitate or exaggerate LE-like syndrome *5869*

Leukocytes *Blood Decrease Physiological* Occasional case of aplastic anemia reported *6264* Rare side effects reported to UK Committee on Safety of Medicines *1204* Agranulocytosis/aplastic anemia/Leukopenia *4885*
Blood Increase Physiological Leukemia drug induced *4014*

Lithium *Serum Increase Physiological* Concentration increased due to reduction of lithium clearance *1384*
Serum No Effect Physiological Nonsignificant increase reported when 500 mg/d administered to 5 patients (11.1% increase after 6 days) *4831*

Neutrophils *Blood Decrease Physiological* Occasional case of aplastic anemia reported *6264*

Nitroblue Tetrazolium Test *Blood Decrease Physiological* Mechanism not discussed *1483*

Occult Blood *Feces Increase Physiological* Rare side effects reported to UK Committee on Safety of Medicines *1204* May cause gastrointestinal tract bleeding *3810*

Ornithine Carbamoyltransferase
Serum Increase Physiological May cause cholestatic and cytotoxic jaundice *402*

p-Aminophenol *Urine No Effect Analytical* With addition of drugs at a concentration of 100 mg/L and of related compounds at 50 mg/L no significant effect observed on colorimetric method of van Bocxlaer on Cobas Mira analyzer which involves reacting free p-aminophenol with resorcinol in the presence of magnesium ions to form an indophenol dye measured at 550 nm *6163*

pH *Blood Increase Physiological* May cause respiratory or metabolic alkalosis *2754*

Phenprocoumon *Plasma Increase Physiological* Increased concentration of anticoagulant displaced from protein with increase of free component *4427*

Phenylalanine *Plasma No Effect Analytical* No interference observed with rapid quantitative whole blood method of Campbell et al using phenylalanine dehydrogenase *867*

Phenytoin *Serum Increase Physiological* Reported impairment of metabolism *3340* Coadministration with phenytoin may increase plasma phenytoin concentration *4522* When phenylbutazone ingested with fosphenytoin concentration of phenytoin may be increased *4519*

Phenytoin, Free *Serum Increase Physiological* Causes increase in free fraction when drugs coadministered *6350*

Phosphate *Serum No Effect Analytical* At concentration of 750 mg/L had no effect on phosphomolybdate method *5704*

Platelet Aggregation *Blood Decrease Physiological* Lack second phase ADP agglutination *1291* Effect less marked that observed with treatment with aspirin *3694*
Blood Increase Physiological Significant interference with platelet aggregation reported *6557*

Platelets *Blood Decrease Physiological* Rare side effects reported to UK Committee on Safety of Medicines *1204* May cause aplastic anemia or thrombocytopenia *1639* Several cases of immune-mediated thrombocytopenia reported *4139* Occasional case of aplastic anemia reported *6264*

Potassium *Serum No Effect Analytical* At concentration of 120 mg/L had no effect on measurement by ISE without predilution *5704* At concentration of 750 mg/L had no effect on measurement by ISE with predilution *5704*

Prazosin *Serum No Effect Physiological* Coadministration of prazosin with phenylbutazone had no apparent adverse drug interaction in limited clinical experience *4649*

Protein *Serum No Effect Analytical* At concentration of 750 mg/L had no effect on biuret method with blank correction *5704*
Urine Increase Physiological Observed effect, may occasionally be marked with oliguria or renal failure *4777* Reported nephrotoxic effect *2451*

Protein Electrophoresis *Serum No Effect Analytical* At concentration of 120 mg/L had no effect on automated Olympus-Hite method *5704*

Prothrombin Time *Plasma Increase Physiological* Potentiates action of anticoagulants *62* Displaces warfarin from protein binding sites *4881* When warafrin administered prolongs prothrombin time through stereoselective inhibition of clearance of S isomer *2625* Increased concentration of anticoagulant displaced from protein with increase of free component *4427*

Sodium *Serum Increase Physiological* May cause salt retention *6201*
Serum No Effect Analytical At concentration of 750 mg/L had no effect on measurement by ISE with predilution *5704* At concentration of 120 mg/L had no effect on measurement by ISE without predilution *5704*

Sucrose *Serum No Effect Analytical* Using automated procedure involving sucrose phosphorylase, phosphoglutamase and glucose-6-phosphatase of Vinet et al no significant interference observed at a concentration of 0.1 mmol/L *6267*
Urine No Effect Analytical Using automated procedure involving sucrose phosphorylase, phosphoglutamase and glucose-6-phosphatase of Vinet et al no significant interference observed at a concentration of 0.1 mmol/L *6267*

T3-Uptake *Serum Increase Physiological* Resin and red cell uptake affected *5382*

Taurine *Urine Decrease Physiological* Reduces increased output in rheumatoids *5171*

Thyro-Binding Index *Serum Decrease Physiological* For up to 3 weeks after therapy *1444*

Thyroxine (T4) *Serum Decrease Physiological* Drug inhibits binding of T4 to TBG *2412* Due to impaired synthesis, competes for thyroxine binding albumin *3107* Reported in two studies due to competition for transport proteins *6412*
Serum No Effect Analytical Cross-reactivity of less than 0.1% observed with method on Baxter Stratus *5705*

Thyroxine (T4), Free *Serum Decrease Physiological* Long-term effect due to thyroidal inhibition *6412*
Serum Increase Physiological Initial increase after start of treatment but after a few days reverts to normal *1269* Insignificant short-term increase associated with competition for transport proteins *6412*
Serum No Effect Analytical At concentrations up to 0.3 mg/L had no effect on method on Baxter Stratus *5705* Phenylbutazone at a concentration of 1000 µg/dL had no cross-reactivity FT4 in method on Bayer Technicon Immuno 1® *424* Toxic concentration caused change of less than 0.01 ng/dL with method on Technicon Immuno-1 *1296*

Thyroxine (T4) Index, Free *Serum Decrease Physiological* Low normal or slight decrease for 3 weeks after therapy *1444*

Thyroxine (T4) (Murphy-Pattee)
Serum Decrease Physiological Binds to thyroxine binding albumin, has antithyroid activity *882*

Tolbutamide *Serum Increase Physiological* Increased half-life (from 7.9 to 23.1 hours) observed in 8 healthy volunteers *4740* Displaces from protein inhibits carboxylation *2452*

Tri-iodothyronine, Free (fT3) *Serum Increase Physiological* Initial increase observed at start of treatment but reverts to normal after a few days of treatment *1269*
Serum No Effect Analytical At a concentration of 0.01 g/L cross-reactivity of 0.0% with free triiodothyronine method on Bayer Technicon Immuno 1® system *425*

Tri-iodothyronine (T3) *Serum Decrease Physiological* Inhibits binding of T3 to TBG *2412*
Serum No Effect Analytical No cross-reactivity observed with method on Baxter Stratus *5705*

Triglycerides *Serum No Effect Analytical* At concentration of 200 mg/L had no effect on GPO-PAP method *5704* At concentration of 750 mg/L had no effect on lipase/esterase method *5704*

Urea Nitrogen *Serum Increase Physiological* Reported nephrotoxic effect *3810*
Serum No Effect Analytical At concentration of 750 mg/L had no effect on diacetylmonoxime method *5704* At concentration of 12 mg/L had no effect on Kodak Ektachem® method *5704*

Uric Acid *Serum Decrease Physiological* Uricosuric action at high doses *2378*
Serum Increase Physiological Antiuricosuric action at low doses *2378*
Serum No Effect Analytical At concentration of 120 mg/L had no effect on catalase-AIDH method *5704* At concentration of 200 mg/L had no effect on Kageyama-Hantzsch method *5704* At concentration of 750 mg/L had no effect on phosphotungstate reduction method *5704* At concentration of 200 mg/L had no effect on uricase-PAP method *5704*
Urine Increase Physiological Uricosuric action *2378*

Volume *Plasma Increase Physiological* May increase by 50% due to salt and water retention *2242*
Urine Decrease Physiological Causes significant water retention *2242*

Warfarin *Plasma Increase Physiological* Displaces warfarin from protein binding sites *803*

Phenylephrine

Acetaminophen *Serum No Effect Analytical* No interference observed at a concentration of 1000 µg/mL (960 µmol/L) with method on Du Pont aca *1506*

Albumin *Serum No Effect Analytical* At concentration of 4 mg/L had no effect on BCG method *5704*

Amino Acids *Urine Increase Analytical* Reacts with ninhydrin; extra spot TLC, high voltage electrophoresis *4760* Orange-brown spot with ninhydrin on thin-layer chromatography *2109*

Bilirubin *Serum No Effect Analytical* At concentration of 4 mg/L had no effect on Jendrassik and Grof method *5704*

Calcium *Serum No Effect Analytical* At concentration of 4 mg/L had no effect on cresolphthalein method *5704*

Chloride *Serum No Effect Analytical* At concentration of 4 mg/L had no effect on mercurimetric method *5704*

Cholesterol *Serum No Effect Analytical* At concentration of 4 mg/L had no effect on Liebermann-Burchard method *5704*

Color *Feces Increase Analytical* Black color reported with ingestion of phenylephrine *3388*

Creatinine *Serum No Effect Analytical* At concentration of 4 mg/L had no effect on Technicon AutoAnalyzer® Jaffe method *5704*

Glucose *Serum Increase Physiological* Reported to increase sugar *4508*

Growth Hormone *Plasma No Effect Physiological* No effect with/without propranolol *3833*

Metanephrines, Total *Urine Increase Analytical* At concentration possibly 10 times higher than would be encountered when measured by Pisano method *5747*
Urine No Effect Analytical At 5 mg/L on modified Pisano procedure *2372*

Midazolam *Serum No Effect Analytical* On GC-ECD method of Ha et al *2387*

Phenylephrine *(continued)*

Occult Blood *Feces Increase Physiological* May cause hemorrhagic enteritis with vasoconstriction *5864*

Phenylalanine *Plasma No Effect Analytical* No interference observed with rapid quantitative whole blood method of Campbell et al using phenylalanine dehydrogenase *867*

Phosphate *Serum No Effect Analytical* At concentration of 4 mg/L had no effect on phosphomolybdate method *5704*

Protein *Serum No Effect Analytical* At concentration of 4 mg/L had no effect on biuret method with blank correction *5704*

Urea Nitrogen *Serum No Effect Analytical* At concentration of 4 mg/L had no effect on diacetylmonoxime method *5704*

Uric Acid *Serum No Effect Analytical* At concentration of 4 mg/L had no effect on phosphotungstate reduction method *5704*

Phenylhydrazine

Bilirubin *Serum Increase Physiological* Causes hemolysis *563*

Bilirubin, Direct *Serum Increase Physiological* Causes hemolysis *563*

Color *Urine Increase Analytical* May produce dark brown urine *1957*

Erythrocytes *Blood Decrease Physiological* Hemolytic anemia *4014*

Haptoglobin *Serum Decrease Physiological* May cause hemolysis (hemolytic anemia) *4014*

Heinz Body Formation *Blood Positive Physiological* May occur in early stages of hemolysis *536*

Hematocrit *Blood Decrease Physiological* Hemolytic anemia *1212*

Hemoglobin *Blood Decrease Physiological* Hemolysis in glucose-6-phosphate dehydrogenase deficiency or methemoglobin reductase deficiency may be caused by drug *2873* Hemolytic anemia *1212*

Methemoglobin *Blood Increase Physiological* May cause hemolysis *4014*

Porphyrin, Total *Urine Increase Physiological* May occasionally precipitate attack of porphyria *6515*

Phenylpropanolamine

Amino Acids *Urine Increase Analytical* Reacts with ninhydrin; extra spot TLC, high voltage electrophoresis *4760* Unusual ninhydrin reacting spot observed on TLC *2605* False positive because of peak appearing after arginine in next chromatogram when short-column postcolumn derivitization used with HPLC. Results likely to be similar regardless of whether o-phthaldehyde or ninhydrin used as detection system *714*

Amphetamine *Urine No Effect Analytical* Less than 1% cross-reactivity observed with Roche Abuscreen method when adapted for use with Roche Cobas Mira analyzer *5120*
Urine Positive Analytical At concentrations above 1.0 µg/mL (5.33 µmol/L) with method on Du Pont aca *1554* False positive observed in patients with large amounts of phenylpropanolamine in their urine with Syva® EMIT monoclonal assay although not with polyclonal assay *2339*

Amphetamine/Methamphetamine
Serum No Effect Analytical At a concentration of 1000 mg/mL caused no detectable cross-reactivity with methods on Abbott AxSYM and TDx *6404*

Cannabinoids *Urine No Effect Analytical* No effect on Roche Abuscreen method *5006*

Cholinesterase *Serum No Effect Analytical* No effect observed at concentration of 1.25 mg/dL with butyrylthiocholine method on Kodak Ektachem® *2504*

Drugs of Abuse Screen *Urine No Effect Analytical* No effect at concentration of 100 µg/mL on EZ-SCREEN procedure for cannabinoids and cocaine *1739*

Felbamate *Serum No Effect Analytical* No significant interference observed with GLC method of Rifai et al *4958*

Histamine *Plasma No Effect Analytical* No effect on radioenzyme assay likely at physiological concentrations *2492*

Methamphetamine *Urine No Effect Analytical* Less than 0.5% cross-reactivity with Hycor accuPINCH method *162* Less than 1% cross-reactivity observed with Roche Abuscreen Online assay as performed on Roche Cobas Mira analyzer *6347*

Phentolamine Test *Patient Increase Physiological* Single case reported *1638*

Theophylline *Serum No Effect Analytical* No effect on method on Kodak Ektachem® 700 *1716*

Phenylthiourea

Protein *Test Conditions Increase Analytical* Reacts with Folin-Ciocalteu method of Lowry *1102*

Phenyramidol

Cholesterol *Serum Decrease Physiological* Probable inhibition of hepatic microsomal enzymes *5380*

Glucose *Serum Decrease Physiological* Reported effect *192*

Phenytoin *Serum Increase Physiological* May increase concentration from 7 to 12 µg/mL (dose of 1.2 g/d) *3339*

Prothrombin Time *Plasma Increase Physiological* Inhibits metabolism of bishydroxycoumarin *903*

Tolbutamide *Serum Increase Physiological* Probably impairs metabolism of drug *2452*

Phenytoin

Acetaminophen *Serum No Effect Analytical* No interference observed at a concentration of 2000 µg/mL (793 µmol/L) with method on Du Pont aca *1506*
Urine Increase Physiological Significantly greater proportion excreted as glucuronide in response to coadministration of drug *621*

α_1-Acid Glycoprotein *Serum No Effect Physiological* In 10 epileptic patients mean concentration increased to 0.61 g/L from baseline of 0.59 g/L *5944*

Acid Phosphatase *Serum No Effect Analytical* At concentration of 30 µg/mL (120 µmol/L) had no effect on method on Du Pont Dimension *1562*

Adenosine Monophosphate *Urine Increase Physiological* In epileptic children in comparison with controls *3309*

Alanine Aminotransferase *Serum Increase Physiological* Intrahepatic cholestatic jaundice *3810* In 56 epileptics with mean age of 37.6 treatment with phenytoin caused mean activity of 21.1 ± 9.2 U/L significantly increased compared with 13.5 ± 5.5 U/L in 42 healthy controls *6234*
Serum No Effect Analytical No effect at therapeutic concentration on Boehringer Mannheim Reflotron method *3231* No effect at concentration of 30 µg/mL (119 µmol/L) on method on Du Pont Dimension *1563* No effect at 200 mg/L on Boehringer Mannheim Reflotron method *5706* At acute overdose concentration (20 mg/dL) on Technicon SMAC® method *6266*

Albumin *Serum Decrease Physiological* Significant reduction observed in epileptic patients with a negative correlation between the phenytoin and albumin concentrations *4347*
Serum No Effect Analytical No interference observed at a concentration of 21 mg/L (83 µmol/L) with method on Du Pont aca *1507* No effect at 1.8 mg/dL on Technicon SMA 12/60 method *4390* At concentration of 30 µg/mL (120 µmol/L) had no effect on method on Du Pont Dimension *1564* At acute overdose concentration (20 mg/dL) on Technicon SMAC® method *6266* At concentration of 240 mg/L had no effect on BCG method *5704*
Serum No Effect Physiological In about 20 patients treated for 2 y *1370*

Alkaline Phosphatase *Serum Increase Physiological* Observed 2 times upper limit of normal in 6 of 112 adult epileptic in patients *1922* In 42% of 60 epileptics treated for 10 y or more *4129* Hepatotoxicity with centrolobular necrosis *3810*
Serum No Effect Analytical At acute overdose concentration (20 mg/dL) on Technicon SMAC® method *6266* At concentration of 30 µg/mL (120 µmol/L) had no effect on method on

Du Pont Dimension *1565* No effect at 1.8 mg/dL on Technicon SMA 12/60 method *4390*

Alkaline Phosphatase Isoenzymes
Serum Increase Physiological Hepatic isoenzyme relatively greater increase than bone fraction in association with increased total enzyme activity (bone still largest single component) *2404*

Amino-4-Imidazole-5-Carboxamide Ribotide
Urine Increase Physiological Occurs with impaired absorption of folic acid *6370*

δ-Aminolevulinic Acid *Serum Increase Physiological* Significant increase to 124 nmol/L from 99 nmol/L in controls *2246*
Urine Increase Physiological May precipitate acute porphyria *2210*

Amiodarone *Serum Decrease Physiological* Concurrent administration with amiodarone has been reported to decrease concentration of amiodarone *6552* Sharp decrease in concentration observed in 5 healthy volunteers when 2-4 mg/kg/d phenytoin administered during administration of 200 mg/d amiodarone for 6.5 weeks *4315*

Ammonia *Plasma No Effect Analytical* No effect at concentration of 30 µg/mL (120 µmol/L) on method on Du Pont Dimension *1566* At concentration of 20 mg/L had no effect on Kodak Ektachem® method *5704* No effect at concentration of 20 mg/L on method on Kodak Ektachem® *5706*

Amylase *Serum No Effect Analytical* At concentration of 30 µg/mL (120 µmol/L) had no effect on method on Du Pont Dimension *1567* No effect of concentrations up to 20 mg/L on method on Boehringer Mannheim Reflotron *5706*

Amylase, Pancreatic Isoenzyme
Serum No Effect Analytical No significant effect observed at a toxic concentration of 100 mg/L with method on Boehringer Mannheim Reflotron *3647*

Androgen Index, Free (FAI)
Plasma Decrease Physiological Significant reduction to mean of 61 in 17 male epileptic patients treated for mean of 10.4 years compared with 87 in healthy control subjects *2840* In 11 epileptic patients treatment with phenytoin caused a significant change in concentration to 60.6 ± 9.2 after 5 years compared with 86.5 ± 21.8 in 18 control subjects *2842*

Antinuclear Antibodies *Serum Increase Physiological* Related to number of drugs, higher in women *6411* Occasional increase; possible subclinical collagen-vascular disorder *2471* Elicited in 25% subjects treated *944*
Serum No Effect Physiological Same frequency before and after drug therapy *373*

Apolipoprotein A *Serum Increase Physiological* In 100 chronic epileptics treated with phenytoin mean concentration increased to 234 ± 49 mg/dL compared with 222 ± 31 mg/dL in 100 controls. Effect more marked in women than men *842*

Apolipoprotein A-I *Serum Increase Physiological* Mean of 2.1 g/L versus 1.8 g/L in controls in 28 patients treated with 200-300 mg/d for 1 to 35 y *4294* In 100 chronic epileptics treated with phenytoin mean concentration increased to 186 ± 39 mg/dL compared with 165 ± 17 mg/dL in 100 controls. Effect more marked in women than men *842* In 5 healthy individuals ingestion of 100 mg/d for 2 weeks caused nonsignificant change to 168.9 ± 8.2 mg/dL and of 300 mg/d for 2 weeks to 172.5 ± 8.8 mg/dL (significant) from mean baseline of 156.6 ± 8.7 mg/dL *1931*
Serum No Effect Physiological In 5 patients with hypoalphalipoproteinemia ingestion of 100 mg/d for 2 weeks caused nonsignificant change to 117.1 ± 4.2 mg/dL and of 300 mg/d for 2 weeks to 113.7 ± 3.8 mg/dL (nonsignificant) from mean baseline of 112.2 ± 4.9 mg/dL *1931*

Apolipoprotein A-II *Serum Increase Physiological* In 5 healthy individuals ingestion of 100 mg/d for 2 weeks caused nonsignificant change to 43.7 ± 1.3 mg/dL and of 300 mg/d for 2 weeks to 46.3 ± 2.1 mg/dL (significant) from mean baseline of 40.8 ± 2.5 mg/dL *1931*
Serum No Effect Physiological In 5 patients with hypoalphalipoproteinemia ingestion of 100 mg/d for 2 weeks caused nonsignificant change to 31.4 ± 1.2 mg/dL and of 300 mg/d for 2 weeks to 30.0 ± 1.0 mg/dL (nonsignificant) from mean baseline of 29.8 ± 1.9 mg/dL *1931* No significant difference between treated epileptics and controls *4294*

Apolipoprotein B *Serum Decrease Physiological* In 100 chronic epileptics treated with phenytoin mean concentration significantly reduced to 67 ± 18 mg/dL compared with 81 ± 18 mg/dL in 100 controls. Effect more marked in women than men *842*

Aspartate Aminotransferase *Serum Increase Physiological* Intrahepatic cholestatic jaundice *3810*
Serum No Effect Analytical No effect at concentration of 30 µg/mL (119 µmol/L) on method on Du Pont Dimension *1568* No effect at 200 mg/L on Boehringer Mannheim Reflotron method *5706* No effect at 1.8 mg/dL on Technicon SMA 12/60 method *4390* No effect at therapeutic concentration on Boehringer Mannheim Reflotron method *3231* At acute overdose concentration (20 mg/dL) on Technicon SMAC® method *6266*
Serum No Effect Physiological In 56 epileptics with mean age of 37.6 treatment with phenytoin caused activity of 18.5 ± 5.7 U/L compared with 15.1 ± 5.6 U/L in 42 healthy controls *6234*

Aspirin Esterase *Serum Increase Physiological* Significant increase from mean of 186 µg/mL/h in controls to 317 µg/mL/h in epileptics receiving phenytoin only *4807* Substantially higher activity in treated epileptics than in controls *4806*

Barbiturate *Serum No Effect Analytical* No significant interference observed at a concentration of 100 µg/mL (0.40 mmol/L) with method on Du Pont aca *1511*
Urine Increase Analytical False positive reaction with Abbott fluorescence polarization immunoassay used in TDx due to drug and its major metabolite *5549* With Abbott ADx 50% of false positive barbiturates due to cross-reactivity from phenytoin *4535*

Benzodiazepine Screen *Serum No Effect Analytical* No significant effect observed on method on Du Pont aca at a concentration of 100 µg/mL (0.40 mmol/L) *1512*

Bicarbonate *Serum No Effect Analytical* At concentration of 240 mg/L had no effect on method using phenolphthalein *5704*

Bile *Urine Increase Physiological* Hepatotoxicity *3810*

Bilirubin *Serum Decrease Physiological* Mean reduction of 3.4 µmol/L in 41 epileptic patients treated for several years versus control population *2267*
Serum Increase Physiological Rare hypersensitivity reaction *2451*
Serum No Effect Analytical No effect at 12 mg/L on Ames Seralyzer method *5706* At concentration of 20 mg/L no effect on method on Boehringer Mannheim Reflotron system *5706* No effect at concentration of 30 µg/mL (119 µmol/L) on method on Du Pont Dimension *1589* No effect at 1.8 mg/dL on Technicon SMA 12/60 method *4390* At concentration of 240 mg/L had no effect on Jendrassik and Grof method *5704* At acute overdose concentration (20 mg/dL) on Technicon SMAC® method *6266*
Serum No Effect Physiological Insignificant protein displacement effect in neonates *6314* In about 20 patients treated for 2 y *1370*

Bilirubin, Direct *Serum No Effect Analytical* At concentration of 30 µg/mL (119 µmol/L) had no effect on method on Du Pont Dimension *1574*

Biotin *Serum Decrease Physiological* Dose related in long-term treated epileptics compared with controls *3275*

BSP Retention *Serum Increase Physiological* Due to hypersensitivity or intrahepatic cholestasis *2451*

Bupropion *Serum Decrease Physiological* May induce the metabolism of bupropion due to effect on CYP2B6 isoenzyme *2171*

Busulphan *Serum Decrease Physiological* In 17 patients coadministration of phenytoin with busulphan caused increased mean clearance, 3.32 mL/min/kg versus 3.03 mL/min/kg in controls, lower mean area under the concentration-time curve, 5412 ng/h/mL versus 6475 ng/h/mL in controls and reduced mean elimination half-life, 3.03 h compared with 3.94 h in controls *2503*

Calcitonin *Plasma Decrease Physiological* In epileptic children in comparison with controls *3309*

Calcium *Serum Decrease Physiological* With or without osteoporosis in chronic users *3340* Metabolic effect with chronic therapy *2403* In about 20 patients treated for 2 y *1370* In 7% of 60 epileptics treated for 10 y or more *4129* May produce osteomalacia with protracted treatment *199*

Phenytoin (continued)

Calcium *(continued)*
Serum No Effect Analytical At acute overdose concentration (20 mg/dL) on Technicon SMAC® method *6266* No effect at 1.8 mg/dL on Technicon SMA 12/60 method *4390* At concentration of 240 mg/L had no effect on cresolphthalein method *5704* No effect at concentration of 30 µg/mL (120 µmol/L) on method on Du Pont Dimension *1569*
Urine Decrease Physiological In 60 epileptic patients treated for 10 y or more *4129*

Cannabinoids *Urine No Effect Analytical* No effect on Roche Abuscreen method *5006*

Carbamazepine *Serum Decrease Physiological* Concentration in plasma reduced probably due to hepatic enzyme induction as carbamazepine binding is unchanged *3118* Total serum concentration increased by a mean of 48% four weeks after discontinuation in 22 epileptic patients *1619* Drugs that induce CYP 3A4 enhance metabolism of carbamazepine producing clinically meaningful effect *1039* Due to hepatic enzyme induction when drugs coadministered typically reduction of concentration of both drugs but may be slight increase *1384* Significant reduction observed in total concentration from 7.6 µg/mL when carbamazepine only given to 4.4 µg/mL when phenytoin coadministered in 49 epileptics *4846* Simultaneous administration causes marked reduction of plasma carbamazepine concentration *282*
Serum No Effect Analytical No cross-reactivity observed with method on Du Pont aca *1513* At a concentration of 500 µg/mL had no significant cross-reactivity with carbamazepine at a concentration of 4.0 µg/mL when measured by method on Bayer Technicon Immuno 1® system *417*

Carbamazepine-10,11-Epoxide
Serum No Effect Physiological No significant effect observed in 22 epileptic patients with discontinuation of phenytoin treatment for 3 weeks *1619* No significant change noted in 49 epileptics when phenytoin coadministered *4846*

Carbamazepine-10,11-Epoxide, Free
Serum No Effect Physiological No significant change in 49 epileptics when phenytoin coadministered *4846* No significant effect observed in 22 epileptic patients with discontinuation of phenytoin for 3 weeks *1619*

Carbamazepine, Free *Serum Decrease Physiological* Significant reduction (from mean of 1.7 µg/mL to 1.1 µg/mL) observed in 49 epileptic patients when phenytoin coadministered *4846* Mean increase of 30% observed in 22 epileptic patients within 4 weeks of discontinuation of phenytoin *1619*

Carnitine *Serum No Effect Physiological* In 92 epileptic children treated with valproic acid mean concentration of 39.7 ± 12.2 nmol/mL not significantly less than 57.8 ± 15.4 nmol/mL in 32 healthy control children *2757*

Carnitine, Free *Serum Decrease Physiological* In 92 epileptic children treated with phenytoin mean concentration of 31.4 ± 10.4 nmol/mL significantly less than 42.5 ± 14.1 nmol/mL in 32 healthy control children *2757*

Ceruloplasmin *Serum Increase Physiological* Observed in both hospitalized and home-living individuals with long-term administration *6417* Effect on synthesis of protein in liver *5869*
Serum No Effect Physiological In 15 epileptic patients receiving only phenytoin as therapy no significant difference from controls observed *4346*

Chloramphenicol *Serum Decrease Physiological* Due to hepatic enzyme induction *1384*

Chloride *Serum No Effect Analytical* No effect with concentrations up to 20 mg/L on method on Kodak Ektachem® *5706* At concentration of 240 mg/L had no effect on mercurimetric method *5704*

Cholesterol *Serum Decrease Physiological* In 100 chronic epileptics treated with phenytoin mean concentration reduced to 200 ± 46 mg/dL compared with 213 ± 33 mg/dL in controls *842*
Serum Increase Analytical At 10 times therapeutic concentration caused statistically significant increase with method used on Technicon SRA-2000 *4348*
Serum Increase Physiological Hepatotoxicity with centrolobular necrosis *6191* Possibly due to subclinical hypothyroidism caused by drug or due to hepatic synthesis stimulation with increase of pool size of bile acids (increase of 6 to 48% in 11 patients) *4591* In 5 healthy individuals ingestion of 100 mg/d for 2 weeks caused nonsignificant increase to 212.3 ± 42.4 mg/dL and of 300 mg/d for 2 weeks to 233.0 ± 47.8 mg/dL (nonsignificant) from mean baseline of 209.7 ± 52.4 mg/dL *1931* In men in 27 patients with transient brain ischemia *3058*
Serum No Effect Analytical At concentration of 200 mg/L no effect on method on Boehringer Mannheim Reflotron system *5706* No effect at therapeutic concentration on Boehringer Mannheim Reflotron method *3231* At concentration of 30 µg/mL (120 µmol/L) had no effect on concentration on Du Pont Dimension *1570* At concentration of 20 mg/L had no effect on CHOD-PAP method *5704* No effect at 1.8 mg/dL on Technicon SMA 12/60 method *4390* At concentration of 240 mg/L had no effect on Liebermann-Burchard method *5704* At acute overdose concentration (20 mg/dL) on Technicon SMAC® method *6266* No effect at 12 mg/L on Ames Seralyzer method *5706*
Serum No Effect Physiological In women in 27 patients with transient brain ischemia *3058* In 5 patients with hypoalphalipoproteinemia ingestion of 100 mg/d for 2 weeks caused nonsignificant increase to 223.6 ± 9.7 mg/dL and of 300 mg/d for 2 weeks to 237.5 ± 11.1 mg/dL (nonsignificant) from mean baseline of 232.0 ± 15.7 mg/dL *1931* No significant difference between epileptics given 200-300 mg/d for 1 to 35 y and controls *4294*

Cholesterol Ester Transfer Protein
Serum Decrease Physiological In 5 healthy individuals treatment with phenytoin caused mean concentration of 1.18 ± 0.12 µg/mL to change significantly to 0.68 ± 0.10 µg/mL *1931*
Serum No Effect Physiological In 5 patients with primary hypoalphalipoproteinemia treatment with phenytoin caused mean concentration of 0.97 ± 0.27 µg/mL to change nonsignificantly to 1.18 ± 0.33 µg/mL *1931*

Cholinesterase *Serum Increase Physiological* Significant increase from mean of 4.77 U/L in controls to 6.27 U/L in epileptics receiving phenytoin only *4807*
Serum No Effect Analytical No change observed at a concentration of 30 µg/mL with method on Du Pont Dimension *3271* Insignificant decrease of 0.06 U/mL at a concentration of 30 µg/mL with method on Du Pont aca *3271*

Cholinesterase (True) *Serum Increase Physiological* Substantially higher activity in treated epileptics than in controls *4806*

Chromosomes *Test Conditions Abnormal Physiological* One case reported with an abnormal Y chromosome *3549*

Clonazepam *Serum Decrease Physiological* Slight but probably not clinically significant reduction in clonazepam when drugs coadministered probably due to enhanced hepatic metabolism *3130* May decrease plasma concentration through stmulation of hepatic metabolism *1384*

Clozapine *Serum Decrease Physiological* Phenytoin administration with clozapine may decrease the plasma concentration of clozapine resulting in a decrease in the effectiveness of the drug *5229*

Color *Urine Increase Analytical* Pink, red or red-brown color may occur *2451*

Complement C_3 *Serum Decrease Physiological* Observed in 50% patients *1649*
Serum No Effect Physiological In about 118 treated epileptics *373*

Complement C_3c *Serum Decrease Physiological* Observed in 50% patients *1649*

Complement C_4 *Serum No Effect Physiological* In about 118 treated epileptics *373*

Complement CH50 *Serum No Effect Physiological* No effect of treatment of epileptics *373*

Coombs' Test *Blood Positive Physiological* Immunological response to drug *2453*

Coombs' Test, Direct *Blood Positive Physiological* Few cases with hemolytic anemia *2452*

Copper *Serum Increase Physiological* In 27 epileptics treated for 1 month mean concentration significantly increased to 103.8 ± 39.0 µg/dL compared with 74.7 ± 9.4 µg/dL in 30 healthy controls *3344* In 20 female epileptics treated with a mean of 220 mg/d of phenytoin mean concentration of 126 ± 36 µg/dL significantly different from 98 ± 17 µg/dL in 20 healthy controls *3613* Observed in both hospitalized and home-living individuals with long-term administration *6417*

Serum No Effect Physiological No significant effect in 22 patients being treated for epilepsy *4710*

Copper Zinc Superoxide Dismutase
Serum Increase Physiological In 20 female epileptics treated with a mean of 220 mg/d of phenytoin mean activity of 178 ± 64 U/dL significantly different from 97 ± 36 U/dL in 20 healthy controls *3613*

Coproporphyrin *Feces Increase Physiological* May precipitate acute porphyria *2210*
Urine Increase Physiological May precipitate acute porphyria *2210*

Corticosteroid-Binding Globulin
Serum Increase Physiological In 10 women receiving anticonvulsants, mainly phenytoin versus 10 controls, drug taken on average for 15 y *441*

Corticosteroids *Plasma Decrease Physiological* Increased metabolism and loss of efficacy *886*
Plasma Increase Physiological Alters steroid metabolism *6239*

Cortisol *Plasma Decrease Physiological* In 10 women receiving anticonvulsants, mainly phenytoin versus 10 controls, drug taken on average for 15 y *441* In critically ill patients relative hypoadrenalism observed with phenytoin therapy because of its effect of increasing the metabolism of cortisol *3381* Chronic administration effect in Cushing's syndrome *3669*
Plasma No Effect Analytical At a concentration of 100 mg/L no significant effect on CEDIA or Enzymun methods (worst case 103.6% recovery) *1097*
Plasma No Effect Physiological Although increases hepatic turnover but serum concentration remains in normal range due to increased secretion *1712*

Cortisol, Free *Urine No Effect Analytical* No significant interference observed with HPLC method of Turpeinen et al *6105*

C-Reactive Protein *Serum No Effect Analytical* No interference observed at concentrations up to 50 µg/dL (198 µmol/L) with method on Du Pont aca *1518* At concentration of 50 mg/L (198 µmol/L) had no effect on method on Du Pont aca *5403*

Creatine Kinase *Serum Increase Physiological* Myopathy observed in one case as part of hypersensitivity reaction *2471*
Serum No Effect Analytical No effect at 12 mg/L on method on Ames Seralyzer *5706* At acute overdose concentration (20 mg/dL) on Technicon SMAC® method *6266*

Creatine Kinase Isoenzymes *Serum Increase Physiological* Myopathy observed in one case as part of hypersensitivity reaction. Increase of M33 isoenzyme *2471*
Serum No Effect Analytical At concentration of 30 µg/mL (120 µmol/L) had no effect on method for measuring CK-MB on Du Pont Dimension *1571* No interference observed at a concentration of 15 mg/L (59.5 µmol/L) with CK-MB method on Du Pont aca *1519*

Creatinine *Serum No Effect Analytical* No effect at 1.8 mg/dL on Technicon SMA 12/60 method *4390* No interference observed at a concentration of 1 mg/L with HPLC method of Rosano et al *5083* No effect at concentration of 30 µg/mL (119 µmol/L) on method on Du Pont Dimension *1572* At acute overdose concentration (20 mg/dL) on Technicon SMAC® method *6266* No effect at 12 mg/L on Ames Seralyzer method *5706* No effect of concentrations up to 20 mg/L on single slide method on Kodak Ektachem® *5706* At concentration of 240 mg/L had no effect on Technicon AutoAnalyzer® method *5704* At concentration of 20 mg/L had no effect on Kodak Ektachem® method *5704* no effect of concentrations up to 20 mg/L on 2-slide method on Kodak Ektachem® *5706*

Cyclosporine *Blood Decrease Physiological* Coadministration with cyclosporine caused a significant decrease in whole blood and serum cyclosporine concentrations, 37% and 64% respectively, probably due to induction of hepatic CYP enzymes by phenytoin. Concentrations of metabolites also reduced. Interaction resolved about 1 week after withdrawal of phenytoin *859* With coadministration of drugs absorption of oral cyclosporine decreased with decease in area under concentration-time curve of 50%, possibly related to reduction in bile salt concentration *859* Induces cytochrome P-450 hepatic enzymes thereby increasing clearance of cyclosporine *1956*
Blood No Effect Analytical At a concentration of 100 mg/L had no effect on Syva EMIT method *495*
Serum Decrease Physiological Marked lowering of serum or blood concentration, presumably due to hepatic enzyme induction *1075* With coadministration of drugs absorption of oral cyclosporine decreased with decease in area under concentration-time curve of 50%, possibly related to reduction in bile salt concentration *859* Clearance enhanced when drugs coadministered *1384* Coadministration with cyclosporine caused a significant decrease in whole blood and serum cyclosporine concentrations, 37% and 64% respectively, probably due to induction of hepatic CYP enzymes by phenytoin. Concentrations of metabolites also reduced. Interaction resolved about 1 week after withdrawal of phenytoin *859* Effect occurs as result of hepatic cytochrome P-450 induction. Note also that phenytoin has been reported to decrease absorption of cyclosporine *1069* May decrease cyclosporine concentration by inducing hepatic cytochrome P-450 III A which metabolizes cyclosporine *5236* Significant reduction usually observed when phenytoin coadministered with cyclosporine probably due to increased metabolism of cyclosporine through induction of P-450 enzymes *6595*

Cyclosporine A *Blood Decrease Physiological* Coadministration with cyclosporine A decreases its concentration *5240*

DDT (Chlorophenothane) *Serum Decrease Physiological* Reported interaction due to alteration of metabolism *3340*

Dehydroepiandrosterone Sulfate
Plasma Decrease Physiological Mean reduced to 3.4 µmol/L in 17 male epileptic patients treated for mean of 10.4 years compared with 8.0 µmol/L in healthy control subjects *2840* Significant reduction in both men and women compared with untreated epileptics. Same effect observed when combined with carbamazepine *3533*

Dexamethasone *Serum Decrease Physiological* Due to accelerated hepatic clearance of steroid: may given false impression of Cushing's syndrome *2985* May enhance metabolic clearance resulting in decreased plasma concentrations and lessened physiologic effects *3969*
Serum Increase Physiological Coadministration with dexamethasone led to more rapid clearance of dexamethasone due to enhanced hepatic enzyme activity possibly leading to an increase in the false positive rate with the dexamethasone suppression test for the diagnosis of Cushing's syndrome *6538*

Dexamethasone Suppression
Patient Abnormal Physiological Alters steroid metabolism *2451*

Dicumarol *Plasma Decrease Physiological* Average decrease from 29-21 µg/mL (DPH dose approximately 1 g/d) *3339* With long-term therapy: in one study decreased from 20 to 5 µg/mL *5966*

Digitoxin *Serum Decrease Physiological* May be reduced to subtherapeutic concentration due to induction of mixed function oxidases *4631* In one case reduced concentration of digitoxin observed when phenytoin coadministered: occurs as a result of enhanced hepatic metabolism *5675* Average decrease from 25 to 10 µg/mL (DPH dose 900 mg/d) *3339*

Digoxin *Serum Decrease Physiological* In 6 healthy volunteers administration of 400 mg phenytoin following intravenous digoxin caused 22% reduction in mean serum digoxin concentration and 27% increase in digoxin clearance *4839*
Serum Increase Analytical At 10 mg/mL equals 0.2 ng/mL by RIA *6638*

Disopyramide *Serum Decrease Physiological* When drugs that induce hepatic microsomal enzymes are coadministered with disopyramide concentration of disopyramide significantly reduced *2069* In 10 volunteers mean decrease of 52% in area under curve and 51% reduction in half-life when administration of disopyramide preceded by 14 days therapy with phenytoin. Effect due to stimulated hepatic metabolism and associated with increased metabolism *4293*

Doxycycline *Serum Decrease Physiological* Decreased plasma concentration *886* Observed to decrease half-life of doxycycline *4357* Decreased half-life observed because of increased hepatic metabolism *1384* Observed in one study. Half-life increased probably due to increased hepatic metabolism *4262*

Drugs of Abuse Screen *Urine No Effect Analytical* No effect at concentration of 100 µg/mL on EZ-SCREEN procedure for cannabinoids and cocaine *1739*

Eosinophils *Blood Increase Physiological* General feature of hepatotoxicity (although this occurs rarely), hypersensitivity

Phenytoin *(continued)*

Eosinophils *(continued)*
usually responsible *1494* Rare hypersensitivity reaction *2451* Associated with several cases of hepatotoxicity due to hypersensitivity reaction *3248* In 89% patients who developed hepatotoxicity *4166*

Erythrocytes *Blood Decrease Physiological* Occasional case of aplastic anemia reported *6264* Single case of marked aplasia, apparently mediated through an IgG inhibitor requiring the presence of drug to suppress erythroid colony formation *in vitro* inhibitor appears to exert effect on erythroid progenitors at or beyond stage of differentiation of CFU-E. But not on erythroblasts *1398* Megaloblastic/hemolytic/aplastic anemia/pancytopenia *5569*

Erythromycin *Serum Increase Physiological* Concomitant administration of phenytoin with erythromycin may increase its plasma concentration through its effect on cytochrome P450 *20*

Estradiol *Plasma Increase Physiological* In 20 men receiving phenytoin monotherapy mean concentration 56.3 pg/mL compared with 32.4 pg/mL in 21 untreated epileptic men and 34.3 pg/mL in 20 age-matched controls *2574* Mean increased to 0.22 nmol/L in 17 male epileptic patients treated for mean of 10.4 years compared with 0.15 nmol/L in healthy control subjects *2840* In 20 epileptic men receiving phenytoin mean concentration of 56.3 ± 29.4 pg/mL significantly higher than 32.4 ± 27.4 pg/mL in 21 untreated men with complex epilepsy and 34.3 ± 12.7 pg/mL in 20 age matched controls *2581*
Plasma No Effect Physiological In 10 women receiving anticonvulsants, mainly phenytoin versus 10 controls, drug taken on average for 15 y *441*

Estradiol, Free *Plasma Increase Physiological* In 20 epileptic men treatment with phenytoin caused increase of physiologically active non-SHBG bound estradiol to 45.1 ± 21.7 pg/mL compared with 29.9 ± 17.2 pg/mL in 20 untreated men and 31.1 ± 11.4 pg/mL in controls *2581*

Ethosuximide *Serum Decrease Physiological* Reported to decrease plasma concentration *1384*
Serum No Effect Analytical No significant cross-reactivity with method on Du Pont aca *1523*

Etoposide *Serum Decrease Physiological* Administration of anticonvulsants with etoposide causes significant reduction in etoposide AUC due to increased clearance caused by induction of hepatic enzymes *3909*

Factor VII *Plasma Decrease Physiological* May cross placenta (vitamin K dependent) *5672*

Felbamate *Serum Decrease Physiological* Addition of phenytoin to felbamate regime caused an approximate 45% decrease in steady state felbamate concentration *6323*
Serum No Effect Analytical No significant interference observed with GLC method of Rifai et al even though it is co-extracted *4958*

Felodipine *Serum Decrease Physiological* Coadministration of phenytoin with felodipine caused a reduction in the maximal plasma concentration of felodipine and a significant reduction to 6% of the area under the time-concentration curve in healthy individuals *266* Area under curve in several epileptics markedly reduced when phenytoin coadministered due to hepatic enzyme induction *876*

Fibrin Degradation Products *Plasma No Effect Analytical* No interference observed at concentrations up to 5 µg/dL (19.8 µmol/L) with method on Du Pont aca *1525*

Flecainide *Serum Decrease Physiological* 30% increase in the rate of plasma elimination when drug coadministered with flecainide *3702*

Fludrocortisone *Serum Decrease Physiological* Decreased concentration observed when drugs coadministered due increased metabolic clearance of fludrocortisone because of induction of hepatic enzymes *221*

Folate *Cerebrospinal Fluid Decrease Physiological* Occurs in many long-treated epileptics *4931* Low folate in from 27 to 91% of treated epileptics in different studies *3383*
Red Blood Cells Decrease Physiological Low folate in from 27 to 91% of treated epileptics in different studies *3383* Impaired deconjugation of polyglutamates in gut *5870*
Serum Decrease Physiological Low folate in from 27 to 91% of treated epileptics in different studies *3383* May cause megaloblastic anemia (impairs absorption) *6370*
Test Conditions Decrease Analytical Mild depressant effect on *L. casei4014*

Follicle Stimulating Hormone
Plasma Decrease Physiological Insignificant reduction of mean to 4.8 U/L in 17 male epileptic patients treated for mean of 10.4 years compared with mean of 6.2 U/L in healthy control subjects *2840*
Plasma Increase Physiological Mean 3.7 U/L versus 1.9 in controls in approximately 24 male patients given phenytoin alone or with primidone or phenobarbital *6055*

Gabapentin *Serum No Effect Physiological* Coadministration of phenytoin with gabapentin had no effect on pharmacokinetics of gabapentin *4526*

α_2-Globulin *Serum Increase Physiological* Related to duration of therapy *4014*

β_1-α-Globulin *Serum Decrease Physiological* Observed in 50% patients *1649*

β_1-Globulin C/A *Serum Decrease Physiological* Probable drug induced immunological effect *2340*

Glucaric Acid *Urine Increase Physiological* Equipotent with phenobarbital *3430* Dose dependent effect next to phenobarbital in potency *4623* Induces hepatic enzymes *2782*

Glucose *Serum Increase Physiological* Metabolic effect of drug *199* Small number of cases with hyperglycemia; occasional convulsions and coma reported. Probably due to decreased insulin secretion *901* Administration of phenytoin may increase plasma glucose concentration *4522* Inhibitory effect on insulin secretion *1213*
Serum No Effect Analytical At concentration of 200 mg/L no effect on method on Boehringer Mannheim Reflotron system *5706* At concentration of 36 mg/L had no effect on Kodak Ektachem® method *5704* No effect at therapeutic concentration on Boehringer Mannheim Reflotron method *3231* At acute overdose concentration (20 mg/dL) on Technicon SMAC® method *6266* No effect at 1.8 mg/dL on Technicon SMA 12/60 method *4390* At concentration of 20 mg/L had no effect on GOD/POD-PAP method *5704* At concentration of 30 µg/mL (119 µmol/L) has no effect on method on Du Pont Dimension *1575* At concentration of 160 mg/L had no effect on hexokinase/G-6-PDH method *5704* No effect at 12 mg/L on glucose oxidase method on Ames Seralyzer *5706*
Serum No Effect Physiological No significant effect observed in epileptic patients receiving phenytoin *4077* No significant difference between drug treated epileptics and controls *4617*
Urine Increase Physiological Occurs with inhibition of insulin secretion. Occurs with hyperglycemia *1213*

Glucose Tolerance *Serum Decrease Physiological* Decreases insulin excretion *3669*
Serum Increase Physiological Lower in chronic patients than in controls *919*
Serum No Effect Physiological No significant difference between drug treated epileptics and controls *4617* No consistent change seen in patients on long-term treatment *4591*

Glucuronic Acid *Urine Increase Physiological* Due to hepatic enzyme induction in liver *1329*

Glutamine *Plasma Increase Physiological* Significant increase in children possibly due to inhibition of carbamoylphosphate synthase *6109*

γ-Glutamyltransferase *Serum Increase Physiological* Administration of phenytoin may increase plasma activity *4522* Possibly due to enzyme induction *6429* Mean 3 fold increase in 90% patients after 6 mo treatment: not influenced by age or sex or additional anticonvulsant therapy, accentuated by regular consumption of alcohol *3089* In 100 chronic epileptics treated with phenytoin mean activity significantly increased to 51 ± 21 U/L compared with 31 ± 10 U/L in 100 healthy controls. Effect more marked in women than men *842* Observed 2 times upper limit of normal in 58 of 125 adult epileptic inpatients and 5 times upper limit in 9 of 125 (dose and duration of therapy not known) *1922*
Serum No Effect Analytical No effect at therapeutic concentration on Boehringer Mannheim Reflotron method *3231* At concentration of 30 µg/mL (119 µmol/L) has no effect on method on Du Pont Dimension *1579* At concentration of 200 mg/L no effect on method on Boehringer Mannheim Reflotron system *5706*

Glutathione Peroxidase
Red Blood Cells No Effect Physiological No significant effect in 22 patients being treated for epilepsy *4710*

Glutathione, Reduced *Plasma Decrease Physiological* In 20 female epileptics treated with a mean of 220 mg/d of phenytoin mean concentration of 28 ± 7 μmol/L significantly different from 32 ± 6 μmol/L in 20 healthy controls *3613*

Glycated Hemoglobin *Blood No Effect Analytical* At a concentration of 80 mg/L had an insignificant 0.0% interference with method on Abbott Vision *1885*

Growth Hormone *Plasma Increase Physiological* Release of hormone in response to diazepam and glucagon much greater in epileptics treated with phenytoin than when other antiepileptics used *1164*

HDL_2-Cholesterol *Serum Increase Physiological* In 5 healthy individuals ingestion of 100 mg/d for 2 weeks caused nonsignificant change to 18.6 ± 4.1 mg/dL and of 300 mg/d for 2 weeks to 25.0 ± 3.6 mg/dL (significant) from mean baseline of 16.7 ± 3.9 mg/dL *1931*
Serum No Effect Physiological In 5 patients with hypoalphalipoproteinemia ingestion of 100 mg/d for 2 weeks caused nonsignificant change to 6.1 ± 0.6 mg/dL and of 300 mg/d for 2 weeks to 6.1 ± 2.1 mg/dL (nonsignificant) from mean baseline of 6.7 ± 1.3 mg/dL *1931*

HDL_3-Cholesterol *Serum Increase Physiological* In 5 healthy individuals ingestion of 100 mg/d for 2 weeks caused significant change to 44.0 ± 6.4 mg/dL and of 300 mg/d for 2 weeks to 50.0 ± 5.2 mg/dL (significant) from mean baseline of 36.3 ± 6.3 mg/dL *1931*
Serum No Effect Physiological In 5 patients with hypoalphalipoproteinemia ingestion of 100 mg/d for 2 weeks caused nonsignificant change to 27.3 ± 2.1 mg/dL and of 300 mg/d for 2 weeks to 27.4 ± 1.7 mg/dL (nonsignificant) from mean baseline of 26.5 ± 2.2 mg/dL *1931*

HDL-Cholesterol *Serum Increase Physiological* In both men and women in 27 patients with transient brain ischemia *3058* In 100 chronic epileptics treated with phenytoin concentration significantly increased to 72 ± 27 mg/dL compared with 59 ± 12 mg/dL in controls. Effect more marked in women than men *842* In 5 healthy individuals ingestion of 100 mg/d for 2 weeks caused significant change to 62.6 ± 5.8 mg/dL and of 300 mg/d for 2 weeks to 75.0 ± 6.7 mg/dL (significant) from mean baseline of 53.0 ± 5.2 mg/dL *1931* In 92 men with low HDL-cholesterol concentration treatment with 100 mg/d for 14 weeks raised concentration by 2% , with 200 mg/d by 12% and with 300 mg/d 9% *2204* In 43% of 28 patients treated with 200-300 mg/d for 1 to 35 y (1.87 mmol/L vs 1.51 mmol/L in controls) *4294*
Serum No Effect Analytical At a concentration up to 200 mg/L had no significant effect on Reflotron method for whole blood cholesterol *6352* No effect at concentration of 30 μg/mL (119 μmol/L) on method on Du Pont Dimension *1576*
Serum No Effect Physiological In 5 patients with hypoalphalipoproteinemia ingestion of 100 mg/d for 2 weeks caused nonsignificant change to 33.4 ± 1.3 mg/dL and of 300 mg/d for 2 weeks to 33.5 ± 1.2 mg/dL (nonsignificant) from mean baseline of 33.2 ± 2.1 mg/dL *1931*

HDL-Triglycerides *Serum Increase Physiological* In both men and women in 27 patients with transient brain ischemia *3058*

Hematocrit *Blood Decrease Physiological* Megaloblastic/hemolytic/aplastic anemia, pancytopenia *5569*

Hemoglobin *Blood Decrease Physiological* Megaloblastic/hemolytic/aplastic anemia,pancytopenia *5569*
Blood No Effect Analytical No effect of concentrations up to 20 mg/L on method on Kodak Ektachem® *5706*

Histamine *Plasma No Effect Analytical* Improbable inhibition of radio-enzyme assay at physiological concentrations *2492*

Homocysteine *Plasma Increase Physiological* Treatment causes increased concentration probably by interfering with folate functions *6123*

Hydrocortisone *Serum Decrease Physiological* 25% increase in metabolic clearance rate with much reduced half-life *2985*

Hydroxy-Diphenylhydantoin *Urine Increase Physiological* Normal metabolite (absolute amount variable in individuals) *2094*

25-Hydroxy Vitamin D_3 *Serum Decrease Physiological* Positive correlation with calcium level *2403* Reduced by approximately 50% in long term treatment in children: most marked with combination therapy *2404* Observed effect in some children *5055*
Serum No Effect Physiological In 10 women receiving anticonvulsants, mainly phenytoin, versus 10 controls, drug taken on average for 15 y *441*

17-Hydroxycorticosteroids *Urine Decrease Analytical* Inhibit β-glucuronidase during hydrolysis *55*
Urine Decrease Physiological With chronic ingestion cortisol is metabolized to 6-β-hydroxycortisol *6414*

6-β-Hydroxycortisol *Urine Increase Physiological* Manifestation of drug induced 6-β-hydroxylase activity *1712* Alters steroid metabolism *6414* Marked increase reflecting hepatic enzyme induction *621*

Hydroxyitraconazole *Serum Decrease Physiological* In healthy males coadministration of phenytoin with itraconazole caused a decrease of its area under the concentration-time curve from 6224 to 315 ng.h/mL and a decrease in its half-life from 11.3 to 2.9 h due to induction of itraconazole metabolism *1610*

Hydroxyproline *Urine Increase Physiological* In epileptic children in comparison with controls *3309*

^{131}I Uptake *Serum No Effect Physiological* No effect observed *3107*

Imipramine *Serum Decrease Physiological* Plasma concentration of drug may be decreased when hepatic enzyme inducers given concomitantly *1040*

immunoglobulin A *Serum Decrease Physiological* Observed in 21% (mechanism not elucidated) *5716* Reported permanent or reversible deficiency induced by phenytoin *2426* Further decrease from typical low values of epilepsy with drug treatment *373*

Immunoglobulin D *Serum No Effect Physiological* No effect of treatment of epileptics *373* In about 118 treated epileptics *373*

Immunoglobulin E *Serum Decrease Physiological* Significant decreases in patients with different types of epilepsy *373* In about 118 treated epileptics *373*

Immunoglobulin G *Serum Decrease Physiological* Significant effect due to immunosuppressive action *3718* Minor effect in about 118 treated epileptics *373*

Immunoglobulin M *Serum Decrease Physiological* Minor effect in about 118 treated epileptics *373*

Indomethacin *Serum No Effect Analytical* No effect on HPLC method of Roberts and Smith *4978*

Insulin *Plasma Decrease Physiological* Lower values in drug treated group than in controls reached significant level at 90 minutes after glucose *4617* Reduces insulin response to glucose challenge *3751*
Plasma No Effect Physiological No significant difference from controls during glucose tolerance test *919*

Iron *Serum No Effect Analytical* No effect at concentration of 30 μg/mL (119 μmol/L) on method on Du Pont Dimension *1577* No interference observed with method on Kodak Ektachem® *2792* At acute overdose concentration (20 mg/dL) on Technicon SMAC® method *6266* At concentration of 200 mg/L had no effect on Ferrozine method *5704*

Iron-Binding Capacity, Total *Serum No Effect Analytical* No effect at concentration of 30 μg/mL (119 μmol/L) on method on Du Pont Dimension *1590*

itraconazole *Serum Decrease Physiological* Itraconazole potently inhibits the cytochrome P450 3A enzyme system thereby affecting the metabolism of drugs by this system: the concentration of itraconazole is substantially reduced with coadministration of phenytoin *2905* In healthy males coadministration of phenytoin with itraconazole caused a decrease of its area under the concentration-time curve by more than 90%, from 3203 to 224 ng.h/mL and a decrease in its half-life from 22.3 to 3.8 h due to induction of itraconazole metabolism *1610*
Serum Increase Physiological Coadministration of phenytoin with Itraconazole inhibits its metabolism thereby increasing the plasma concentration of itraconazole *2905*

Ketoconazole *Serum Decrease Physiological* Due to reciprocal stimulated hepatic metabolism *1384*

Phenytoin *(continued)*

Ketorolac *Serum No Effect Physiological* At therapeutic concentrations had no effect on ketorolac-protein binding *5035*

17-Ketosteroids *Urine Decrease Physiological* Alters steroid metabolism *2451*

Lactate *Plasma Increase Physiological* Dose related in long-term treated epileptics compared with controls *3275*
Plasma No Effect Analytical No effect at final concentration of 17 µg/mL with method on Kodak Ektachem® *2793* At concentration of 160 mg/L had no effect on enzymatic method *5704*
Plasma No Effect Physiological No significant effect observed in epileptic patients receiving phenytoin *4077*

Lactate Dehydrogenase *Serum No Effect Analytical* No effect at 12 mg/L on method on Ames Seralyzer *5706* No effect at 1.8 mg/dL on Technicon SMA 12/60 method *4390* At concentration of 30 µg/mL (119 µmol/L) has no effect on method on Du Pont Dimension *1578* At acute overdose concentration (20 mg/dL) on Technicon SMAC® method *6266*

Lamotrigine *Serum Decrease Physiological* Coadministration of phenytoin with lamotrigine caused a significant reduction in the steady state plasma concentration of lamotrigine by approximately 45 to 54% depending on the total daily dose of phenytoin (100 to 400 mg) *2160*

LDL-Cholesterol *Serum Decrease Physiological* In 100 chronic epileptics treated with phenytoin mean concentration 108 ± 58 mg/dL compared with 135 ± 29 mg/dL in 100 controls. Effect more marked in women than men *842*
Serum No Effect Physiological In 5 healthy individuals ingestion of 100 mg/d for 2 weeks caused nonsignificant change to 124.8 ± 34.9 mg/dL and of 300 mg/d for 2 weeks to 134.4 ± 34.8 mg/dL (nonsignificant) from mean baseline of 136.7 ± 40.5 mg/dL. In 5 patients with hypoalphalipoproteinemia changes to 154.5 ± 8.7 mg/dL and 166.0 ± 12.0 mg/dL from 170.4 ± 14.6 mg/dL also not significant *1931* In both men and women in 27 patients with transient brain ischemia In 27 patients with transient brain ischemia *3058*

LDL-Triglycerides *Serum No Effect Physiological* In both men and women in 27 patients with transient brain ischemia *3058*

LE Cells *Blood Positive Physiological* May activate lupus erythematosus *944*

Lecithin:Cholesterol Acyltransferase
Serum No Effect Physiological In 5 patients with primary hypoalphalipoproteinemia treatment with phenytoin caused mean concentration of 4.65 ± 1.45 µg/mL to change nonsignificantly to 4.05 ± 1.46 µg/mL and in 5 healthy individuals from 4.93 ± 1.03 µg/mL to 4.32 ± 1.42 µg/mL *1931*

Leucine Aminopeptidase Isoenzymes
Serum Increase Physiological Increased slower running components *5155*

Leukocytes *Blood Decrease Physiological* Megaloblastic/hemolytic/aplastic anemia/pancytopenia *133* Occasional case of aplastic anemia reported *6264*
Blood Increase Physiological General feature of hepatotoxicity (although this occurs rarely), hypersensitivity usually responsible *1494* Due to eosinophilia *3810*

Levonorgestrel *Serum Decrease Physiological* Markedly lessened concentrations when drug co-administered due to enhanced metabolism *4366*

Lidocaine *Serum Decrease Physiological* Bioavailability of orally administered lidocaine reduced by phenytoin and rate of elimination increased in patients in whom lidocaine given intravenously *4620*
Serum No Effect Analytical No significant interference observed at a concentration of 100 µg/mL (396 µmol/L) with method on Du Pont aca *1534* At a concentration of 1250 mg/L (normal therapeutic concentration up to 20 mg/L) had less than 10% effect on method on Baxter Stratus *5705*

Lipase *Serum No Effect Analytical* At concentration of 30 µg/mL (119 µmol/L) has no effect on method on Du Pont Dimension *1580*

Long-chain Fatty Acid Carnitine Esters
Serum No Effect Physiological In 92 epileptic children treated with phenytoin mean concentration of 2.4 ± 1.1 nmol/mL not significantly different from 3.1 ± 1.1 nmol/mL in 32 healthy control children *2757*

Luteinizing Hormone *Plasma Decrease Physiological* Mean decreased to 6.6 IU/L in 17 male epileptic patients treated for mean of 10.4 years compared with mean of 8.0 IU/L in healthy control subjects *2840*
Plasma Increase Physiological Mean 10.0 IU/L versus 4.6 in controls in approximately 24 male patients given phenytoin alone or with primidone or phenobarbital *6055*

Lymphocytes *Blood Decrease Physiological* Dose related associated with decreased DNA synthesis *3718*

Magnesium *Serum No Effect Analytical* No effect at concentration of 30 µg/mL (119 µmol/L) on method on Du Pont Dimension *1581*

Malondialdehyde *Serum Increase Physiological* In 20 female epileptics treated with a mean of 220 mg/d of phenytoin mean concentration of 2.6 ± 0.7 µmol/L significantly different from 1.8 ± 0.7 µmol/L in 20 healthy controls *3613*

Maprotiline *Serum Decrease Physiological* Concentration may be decreased when hepatic enzyme inducers are coadministered *1034*

MCV *Blood Increase Physiological* In 100 patients with macrocytosis (MCV greater than 110 fL) one had been treated with phenytoin *5664* In about 20 patients treated for 2 y *1370* May occur with megaloblastic anemia *5569*

Mebendazole *Serum Decrease Physiological* Plasma concentration reduced when phenytoin coadministered probably as result of stimulated hepatic metabolism *3675*

Meperidine *Serum Decrease Physiological* Hepatic metabolism appears to be increased as evidenced by one study of 4 healthy individuals *4741*

Methadone *Serum Decrease Physiological* Decreased plasma concentration, loss of pain control, risk of withdrawal *886*

Methemoglobin *Blood Increase Physiological* Occurs with hemolytic anemia *3669*

Methotrexate *Serum Increase Physiological* Displaces from plasma protein binding *2452*

Methylprednisolone *Serum Decrease Physiological* 130% increase in metabolic clearance rate with much reduced half-life *2985*

Metronidazole *Serum Decrease Physiological* By inducing microsomal hepatic enzymes may accelerate the elimination of metronidazole with reduction of its plasma concentration *5420* Administration of drugs that induce microsomal liver enzymes may accelerate the elimination of metronidazole *4446*
Serum Increase Physiological When drugs that induce hepatic microsomal enzymes coadministered elimination of metronidazole may be accelerated *2066*

Metyrapone *Serum Decrease Physiological* Metabolism of metapyrone accelerated by phenytoin so phenytoin should be withdrawn for 2 weeks before metyrapone test is performed *1035* Reduced concentrations invalidating metyrapone test as result of increased hepatic metabolism *4052* Average decrease from 48 to 7 µg/dL (with 3.5 g DPH) *3339*

Mexiletine *Serum Decrease Physiological* In 6 healthy volunteers administration of 300 mg phenytoin daily caused reduction of area under curve by 54% and half-life reduced from 17.2 to 8.4 hours. Effect due to stimulation of hepatic metabolism *456* Hepatic enzyme induction may reduce elimination half-life by 50% *3281*

Mycophenolic Acid *Serum No Effect Analytical* No significant interference observed with HPLC method of Shipkova et al *5526*

Mycophenolic Acid Glucuronide
Serum No Effect Analytical No significant interference observed with HPLC method of Shipkova et al *5526*

N-Acetylprocainamide *Serum No Effect Analytical* No significant interference observed at a concentration of 100 µg/mL (396 µmol/L) with method on Du Pont aca *1536*

N-Desethylamiodarone *Serum Increase Physiological* Significant increase observed when phenytoin coadministered to 5 healthy volunteers receiving amiodarone: probably due to induction of amiodarone metabolism *4315*

Neutrophils *Blood Decrease Physiological* Megaloblastic/hemolytic/aplastic anemia,pancytopenia *133* Rare cases of neutropenia reported *241* Occasional case of aplastic anemia reported *6264*

N-Formiminoglutamic Acid *Urine Increase Physiological* Occurs with impaired absorption of folic acid *6370*

Non-Sex Hormone Binding Globulin-bound Estradiol *Serum Increase Physiological* In 20 epileptic men treated with phenytoin monotherapy mean concentration 45.1 pg/mL compared with 31.1 pg/mL in 20 normal controls and 29.9 pg/mL in 21 untreated male epileptics *2574*

5'-Nucleotidase *Serum Increase Physiological* Observed 2 times upper limit of normal in 10 of 127 adult epileptic inpatients *1922*

Organic Acids *Urine Increase Physiological* Dose related in long-term treated epileptics compared with controls *3275*

p-Aminophenol *Urine No Effect Analytical* With addition of drugs at a concentration of 100 mg/L and of related compounds at 50 mg/L no significant effect observed on colorimetric method of van Bocxlaer on Cobas Mira analyzer which involves reacting free p-aminophenol with resorcinol in the presence of magnesium ions to form an indophenol dye measured at 550 nm *6163*

Parathyroid Hormone *Plasma Increase Physiological* In epileptic children in comparison with controls *3309*

Paroxetine *Serum Decrease Physiological* When a single oral dose of paroxetine was given orally with phenytoin a decrease of 50% in the AUC of paroxetine occurred *5654*

Partial Thromboplastin Time *Plasma Increase Physiological* May cross placenta (vitamin K dependent) *5672*

Phenobarbital *Serum Increase Analytical* Significant interference observed at a concentration of 250 µmol/L with Sung and Neely modification of Syva EMIT procedure *148*
Serum Increase Physiological Concentration decreased by mean of 30% after 4 weeks discontinuation of treatment in 22 epileptic patients *1619* Average increase from 22 to 48 µg/mL (DPH dose 900 mg/d) *3339* Concentration decreased by mean of 30% after 4 weeks discontinuation of treatment in 22 epileptic patient *1619* Enhances the conversion of primidone to phenobarbital when primidone coadministered with phenytoin *6350*
Serum No Effect Analytical At concentration of 500 µg/mL (1980 µmol/L) has no effect on method on Du Pont Dimension *1582* At maximum physiological or pharmacological concentrations no cross-reactivity observed with phenobarbital method on Bayer Technicon Immuno 1® *427* No significant cross-reactivity observed with method on Du Pont aca *1537*

Phenylalanine *Plasma No Effect Analytical* No interference observed with rapid quantitative whole blood method of Campbell et al using phenylalanine dehydrogenase *867*

Phenytoin *Cerebrospinal Fluid Increase Physiological* Concentration same as unbound concentration in plasma *5093*
Serum Increase Physiological Therapeutic plasma concentrations obtained within 24 h in most patients: peaking of concentration occurred between 48 and 96 h after loading *6451* 600 mg orally produces concentration of 10 mg/L *3868*

Phosphate *Serum Decrease Physiological* In about 20 patients treated for 2 y *1370*
Serum No Effect Analytical At concentration of 30 µg/mL (119 µmol/L) has no effect on method on Du Pont Dimension *1584* No effect of concentrations up to 20 mg/L on method on Kodak Ektachem® *5706* At concentration of 240 mg/L had no effect on phosphomolybdate method *5704* No effect at 1.8 mg/dL on Technicon SMA 12/60 method *4390* At acute overdose concentration (20 mg/dL) on Technicon SMAC® method *6266*
Serum No Effect Physiological In 60 epileptic patients treated for 10 y or more *4129*

Platelets *Blood Decrease Physiological* Megaloblastic/hemolytic/aplastic anemia/pancytopenia *133* Several cases of immune-mediated thrombocytopenia reported *4139* Occasional case of aplastic anemia reported *6264*

Porphobilinogen *Urine Increase Physiological* May precipitate acute porphyria *2210*

Potassium *Serum No Effect Analytical* At concentration of 240 mg/L had no effect on measurement by ISE with predilution *5704* At concentration of 80 mg/L nonsignificant interference of -0.2% observed with method on Abbott Vision *681* At concentration of 20 mg/L had no effect on flame-photometric method *5704*

Prednisolone *Serum Decrease Physiological* 77% increase in metabolic clearance rate with much reduced half-life *2985*

Primidone *Serum No Effect Analytical* At concentrations above 1250 mg/L causes 25% increase as measured by the method on Baxter Stratus but physiological concentration only up to 20 mg/L *5705* No significant cross-reactivity with method on Du Pont aca *1541*

Procainamide *Serum No Effect Analytical* No significant interference observed at a concentration of 100 µg/mL (396 µmol/L) with method on Du Pont aca *1542*

Progesterone *Plasma Decrease Physiological* Insignificant reduction to mean of 0.81 nmol/L in 17 male epileptic patients treated for mean of 10.4 years compared with 1.01 nmol/L in healthy control subjects *2840*

Prolactin *Plasma Decrease Physiological* Mean decreased to 5.1 µg/L in 17 male epileptic patients treated for mean of 10.4 years compared with mean of 9.5 µg/L in healthy control subjects *2840*
Plasma Increase Physiological Mean 312 mU/L versus 207 in controls in approximately 24 male patients given phenytoin alone or with primidone or phenobarbital *6055*

Propranolol *Serum Decrease Physiological* Clearance greatly increased when drugs coadministered *6558*

Protein *Cerebrospinal Fluid No Effect Analytical* No effect observed at final concentration of 8 µg/mL with method on Kodak Ektachem® *2791*
Serum No Effect Analytical At acute overdose concentration (20 mg/dL) on Technicon SMAC® method *6266* At concentration of 240 mg/L had no effect on biuret method with blank correction *5704* At concentration of 30 µg/mL (119 µmol/L) had negligible effect on method on Du Pont Dimension *1591* No effect at 1.8 mg/dL on Technicon SMA 12/60 method *4390*
Serum No Effect Physiological In about 20 patients treated for 2 y *1370*

Prothrombin Time *Plasma Increase Physiological* Probable interaction with warfarin when drugs coadministered *2625* Significant increase when drug added to regime of warfarin on which previously stabilized *4220* Patients on coumarins which inhibit its metabolism *3669*

Protoporphyrin *Feces Increase Physiological* May precipitate acute porphyria *2210*

Pyridoxal Phosphate *Serum Decrease Physiological* Increase by 20% at 4 weeks, 60% at 12 weeks *4910*

Pyruvate *Plasma No Effect Physiological* No significant effect observed in epileptic patients receiving phenytoin *4077*

Quinidine *Serum Decrease Physiological* Reduces half-life by more than 50% due to induction of hepatic cytochrome P-450 activity *3296* Hepatic elimination of quinidine accelerated when phenytoin coadministered because of increased production of cytochrome P450IIIA4 *5996*
Serum No Effect Analytical No significant interference observed at a concentration of 100 µg/mL (396 µmol/L) with method on Du Pont aca *1543*

Retinol-binding Protein *Serum Increase Physiological* In comparison with untreated cognitively delayed children 4.0 mg/dL versus 3.3 mg/dL *3266*

Ritonavir *Serum Decrease Physiological* Increased metabolism *886*

Saquinavir *Serum Decrease Physiological* Coadministration of phenytoin with saquinavir reduced the latter's concentration by inducing CYP3A4 in the liver *5024*

SDZ PSC 833 *Blood No Effect Analytical* At a concentration of 22 mg/L had no effect on HPLC method of Scott et al when used to measure PSC (with CsD as internal standard) at a concentration of 5 mg/L *5418*

Selenium *Serum Decrease Physiological* Reduction from mean of 15.9 µg/dL to 13.1 µg/dL in 22 patients being treated for epilepsy *4710*

Sex-Hormone Binding Globulin *Serum Increase Physiological* In 10 women receiving anticonvulsants, mainly phenytoin versus 10 controls, drug taken on average for 15 y *441* Significant increase of mean to 57.4 nmol/L in 17 male epileptic patients treated for mean of 10.4 years compared with healthy control subjects (27.2 nmol/L) *2840* Mean 8.3 mol/L versus 5.0 mol/L in controls in approximately 24 male patients given phenytoin alone or with

Phenytoin *(continued)*

Sex-Hormone Binding Globulin *(continued)*
primidone or phenobarbital *6055* In 11 epileptic patients treatment with phenytoin caused a significant change in concentration to 57.3 ± 23.4 nmol/L after 5 years compared with 26.9 ± 8.2 nmol/L in 18 control subjects *2842*

Short-chain Fatty Acid Carnitine Esters
Serum No Effect Physiological In 92 epileptic children treated with phenytoin mean concentration of 8.3 ± 4.2 nmol/mL not significantly less than 15.4 ± 4.2 nmol/mL in 32 healthy control children *2757*

Sodium *Serum No Effect Analytical* At concentration of 240 mg/L had no effect on measurement by ISE with predilution *5704* At concentration of 20 mg/L had no effect on flame-photometric method *5704*

Sperm Motility *Semen Decrease Physiological* In 10 epileptic patients on long term therapy mean transmembrane ratio at 0 time 19.1 ± 10.5 and at 2 h 11.6 ± 7.3 significantly less than 42.6 ± 12.5 and 35.2 ± 7.0 respectively in 45 healthy donors *980*

Superoxide Dismutase
Red Blood Cells No Effect Physiological No significant effect in 22 patients being treated for epilepsy *4710*

T3-Uptake *Serum Increase Physiological* Affects both resin and red cell uptake *2451*
Serum No Effect Analytical At concentration of 30 µg/mL (119 µmol/L) has no effect on method on Du Pont Dimension *1586* No significant effect observed at a concentration of 30 µg/mL (119 µmol/L) with method on Du Pont aca *1545*
Serum No Effect Physiological No effect of 300 mg/d for 1 week *882* With long-term treatment due to accelerated thyroxine clearance via stimulation of hepatic microsomal enzymes *3568* In 83 epileptics with mean age of 37.6 treatment with phenytoin caused mean ratio of 0.87 ± 0.1 not significantly different from 0.91 ± 0.1 in 32 healthy controls *6234*

Tacrolimus *Blood No Effect Analytical* No interference observed with radioreceptor assay of Murthy et al *4191* No significant effect observed at a concentration of 25 mg/L with MEIA method on Abbott IMx analyzer *1871*
Serum Decrease Physiological By inducing cytochrome P-450 IIIA enzyme systems may stimulate the metabolism of tacrolimus *1987*
Serum No Effect Analytical At concentration of 25 mg/L had no significant effect on ELISA method *6329*

Teniposide *Serum Decrease Physiological* Administration of anticonvulsants with teniposide causes significant reduction in teniposide AUC due to increased clearance caused by induction of hepatic enzymes *3909*

Testosterone *Serum Increase Physiological* Mean increase to 32.4 nmol/L in 17 male epileptic patients treated for mean of 10.4 years compared with mean of 23.3 nmol/L in healthy control subjects *2840* In 11 epileptic patients treatment with phenytoin caused a significant change in concentration to 33.3 ± 12.1 nmol/L after 5 years compared with 23.2 ± 8.3 nmol/L in 18 control subjects *2842* Mean 30.7 nmol/L versus 17.8 in controls in approximately 24 male patients given phenytoin alone or with primidone or phenobarbital *6055*
Serum No Effect Physiological Usual effect *2836*

Testosterone, Free *Serum Decrease Physiological* In 20 men with epilepsy mean concentration decreased due to induction of aromatase enhancing conversion of free testosterone to estradiol, as well as SHBG synthetase *2581* Observed effect *2836*
Serum No Effect Physiological No difference in concentrations (mean 91 pmol/L) between 17 male epileptic patients treated for mean of 10.4 years and healthy control subjects *2840*

Theophylline *Serum Decrease Physiological* Decreases serum theophylline concentration by about 40% due to increased theophylline clearance caused by induction of microsomal enzyme activity *6117* Concomitant administration may reduce half-life of theophylline through induction of hepatic drug metabolizing enzymes *1384* Increases theophylline clearance by induction of microsomal enzyme activity and decreases serum theophylline concentration by about 40% *3125* In one study of 10 normal individuals half-life of theophylline reduced by about 50% when both drugs coadministered. Effect probably due to enhanced hepatic metabolism. Total body clearance almost doubled *3802* Increases theophylline clearance by induction of microsomal enzyme activity, decreasing theophylline absorption and its concentration by about 40% *5999*
Serum Increase Analytical At concentration of 40 mg/L caused display of "interfering substance" message *1122*
Serum No Effect Analytical At concentration of 30 µg/mL (119 µmol/L) had no effect on method on Du Pont Dimension *1585* No effect observed at concentration of 40 mg/L with methods used with Kodak DT-60, Abbott TDx, Abbott Vision when serum used, 3M Diagnostics TheoFAST, Syntex Accµ Level or Ames Seralyzer *1122* No effect at 24 mg/L on method on Ames Seralyzer *5706* At concentration of 169 µg/mL had no effect on method on Kodak Ektachem® *6100*

Thyro-Binding Index *Serum Decrease Physiological* For up to 3 weeks after therapy *1444*

Thyroid Stimulating Hormone
Serum Increase Physiological Slight effect observed in 50% patients at dose of 3 mg/kg/d with normal serum concentration *2136*
Serum No Effect Physiological Therapeutic concentrations of phenytoin have no effect on plasma TSH concentration *5876* No increase observed in treated individuals *1269* Basal concentration usually unaffected in spite of decreased T4 and T3, suggesting that phenytoin may function as a thyroid hormone agonist *2412* No change or in response to TRH: probably central regulation involved *6412* Mean concentration of 1.4 mU/L in 17 male epileptic patients treated for mean of 10.4 years, same as in healthy control subjects *2840* In 26 chronic epileptic patients treatment with phenytoin caused mean concentration of 1.7 ± 1.3 mU/L not significantly different from 1.7 ± 0.8 mU/L in 28 healthy controls *2839* In euthyroid patients treatment with phenytoin had no effect on concentration *2412* With long-term treatment due to accelerated thyroxine clearance via stimulation of hepatic microsomal enzymes *3568*

Thyroxine Binding Globulin
Serum Decrease Physiological 19.6 µg/mL in treated epileptics vs 23.4 µg/mL in controls *5884*
Serum No Effect Physiological In 10 women receiving anticonvulsants, mainly phenytoin versus 10 controls, drug taken on average for 15 y *441*

Thyroxine (T4) *Serum Decrease Physiological* In 83 epileptics with mean age of 37.6 treatment with phenytoin caused mean concentration of 75 ± 11 nmol/L significantly reduced compared with 99 ± 19 nmol/L in 32 healthy controls *6234* Slight effect observed in 50% patients at dose of 3 mg/kg/d with normal serum concentration *2136* 5.5 µg/dL in treated epileptics vs 8.1 µg/dL in controls *5884* Displaces thyroxine from binding sites *5869* Therapeutic concentrations of phenytoin displace thyroxine from its binding proteins with increased free T4 but decreased total thyroxine to 60% of untreated values *5876* With long-term treatment due to accelerated thyroxine clearance via stimulation of hepatic microsomal enzymes *3568* Inhibits binding to TBG. Phenytoin induces hepatic enzymes thereby affecting metabolism. Phenytoin probably acts as a thyroid hormone agonist *2412* In comparison with untreated cognitively delayed children 7.1 µg/dL versus 8.4 µg/dL *3266* Mean reduction to 73 nmol/L in 17 male epileptic patients treated for mean of 10.4 years compared with 93 nmol/L in healthy control subjects *2840* In 26 chronic epileptics treated with long term phenytoin mean concentration reduced to 71.0 ± 12.9 nmol/L compared with 91.6 ± 12.9 nmol/L in 28 controls *2839* 15-30% reduction observed in individuals receiving therapeutic doses of drug *1269*
Serum Increase Physiological In 10 women receiving anticonvulsants, mainly phenytoin versus 10 controls, drug taken on average for 15 y *441*
Serum No Effect Analytical No significant effect observed at a concentration of 30 µg/mL (119 µmol/L) with method on Du Pont aca *1588* Cross-reactivity of less than 0.05% observed with EIA method on Bio-Rad RADIAS analyzer *4819* No significant effect observed at a concentration of 30 µg/mL (119 µmol/L) with method on Du Pont aca *1546* Cross-reactivity of less than 0.1% observed with method on Baxter Stratus *5705*
Urine Increase Physiological Increases during therapy (as binds to thyroxine binding globulin) *963*

Thyroxine (T4), Free *Serum Decrease Physiological* Competes with T4 for thyroxine binding globulin, increased liver degradation *42* 1.2 ng/dL in treated epileptics vs 1.5 ng/dL in controls *5884* As measured by equilibrium dialysis and analog-type radioimmunoassays: not due to displacement from binding proteins *3569* Concentraton possibly affected by hepatic enzyme induction. Phenytoin probably acts as a thyroid hormone agonist *2412* In 28 chronic epileptics treated with long term phenytoin mean concentration significantly reduced to 13.4 ± 2.3 pmol/L compared with 16.3 ± 2.4 pmol/L in 28 healthy controls *2839* 15-30% reduction observed in individuals receiving therapeutic doses of drug *1269* In euthyroid patients treatment with phenytoin causes low or low-normal concentration *2412* Mean decrease to 13.8 pmol/L in 17 male epileptic patients treated for mean of 10.4 years compared with 16.5 pmol/L in healthy control subjects *2840*

Serum Increase Analytical As measured by addition of drug to control sera and measured by analog radioimmunoassay *3569*

Serum Increase Physiological In 10 women receiving anticonvulsants, mainly phenytoin versus 10 controls, drug taken on average for 15 y *441*

Serum No Effect Analytical Phenytoin at a concentration of 3000 µg/dL had no cross-reactivity FT4 in method on Bayer Technicon Immuno 1® *424* Toxic concentration caused change of less than 0.01 ng/dL with method on Technicon Immuno-1 *1296* At concentrations up to 30 mg/L had no effect on method on Baxter Stratus *5705*

Thyroxine (T4), Free Dialyzable

Serum No Effect Physiological Therapeutic concentrations of phenytoin displace thyroxine from its binding proteins with increased proportion of free T4 but absolute amount of free thyroxine normal *5876*

Thyroxine (T4) Index, Free *Serum Decrease Physiological* Low normal or decrease for up to 3 weeks after therapy *1444* With long-term treatment due to accelerated thyroxine clearance via stimulation of hepatic microsomal enzymes *3568*

Serum No Effect Physiological In 83 epileptics with mean age of 37.6 treatment with phenytoin caused mean decrease of 86.2 ± 11.6 nmol/L significantly reduced compared with 106.8 ± 15.4 nmol/L in 32 healthy controls *6234*

Thyroxine (T4) (Murphy-Pattee) *Serum Increase Analytical* Extractable with ethanol, false increase *882*

Toremifene *Serum Decrease Physiological* Cytochrome P450 3A4 inducers increase the rate of toremifene metabolism thereby reducing its serum concentration *5329*

Tri-iodothyronine, Free (fT3)

Serum Decrease Physiological Concentration reduced due to hepatic enzyme induction. Phenytoin probably also acts as a thyroid hormone agonist *2412* Observed in treated individuals, often to below reference range *1269* In euthyroid patients treatment with phenytoin caused concentration to fall to low or low-normal level *2412* As measured by equilibrium dialysis and analog-type radioimmunoassays: not due to displacement from binding proteins *3569*

Serum Increase Analytical As measured by addition of drug to control sera and measured by analog radioimmunoassay *3569*

Serum No Effect Analytical At a concentration of 0.7 g/L cross-reactivity of less than 0.1% with free triiodothyronine method on Bayer Technicon Immuno 1® system *425*

Serum No Effect Physiological Therapeutic concentrations of phenytoin displace tri-iodothyronine from its binding proteins with increased proportion of free T3 but amount of free tri-iodothyronine unchanged *5876*

Tri-iodothyronine, Reverse (rT3)

Serum Decrease Physiological Observed in treated individuals but effect less marked than on thyroxine *1269*

Serum No Effect Physiological With long-term treatment due to accelerated thyroxine clearance via stimulation of hepatic microsomal enzymes *3568*

Tri-iodothyronine (T3) *Serum Decrease Physiological* Drug inhibits binding of tri-iodothyronine to TBG. Phenytoin inhibits nuclear binding of T3 in a dose dependent manner. Concentration probably also affected by stimulation of hepatic enzymes *2412* With long-term treatment due to accelerated thyroxine clearance via stimulation of hepatic microsomal enzymes *3568* In euthyroid patients treatment with phenytoin caused concentration to decrease to low or low-normal level *2412* Slight effect observed in 50% patients at dose of 3 mg/kg/d with normal serum concentration *2136* Therapeutic concentrations of phenytoin displace tri-iodothyronine from its binding proteins with increased free T3 but total tri-iodothyronine concentration reduced *5876* Reduction observed in treated individuals compared with controls but effect less marked than on thyroxine *1269*

Serum Increase Physiological In 10 women receiving anticonvulsants, mainly phenytoin versus 10 controls, drug taken on average for 15 y *441*

Serum No Effect Physiological Mean concentration of 1.8 nmol/L in 17 male epileptic patients treated for mean of 10.4 years compared with mean of 1.7 nmol/L in healthy control subjects *2840* In 26 chronic epileptic patients treatment with long term phenytoin mean concentration 1.7 ± 0.3 nmol/L not significantly different from concentration in controls *2839*

Tricyclic Antidepressants *Serum Decrease Physiological* Interacts pharmacokinetically to induce metabolism of tricyclic antidepressants *3590*

Tricyclic Antidepressants Screen

Serum No Effect Analytical No significant effect observed at a concentration of 100 µg/mL (0.40 mmol/L) with method on Du Pont aca *1550*

Triglycerides *Serum Increase Physiological* In 5 healthy individuals ingestion of 100 mg/d for 2 weeks caused non-significant increase to 124.3 ± 30.8 mg/dL and of 300 mg/d for 2 weeks to 117.7 ± 48.2 mg/dL (nonsignificant) from mean baseline of 100.0 ± 28.5 mg/dL In 5 patients with hypoalphalipoproteinemia concentrations increased nonsignificantly to 178.5 ± 14.3 mg/dL and 189.9 ± 20.1 mg/dL from baseline of 142.0 ± 17.0 mg/dL *1931*

Serum No Effect Analytical At concentration of 30 µg/mL (119 µmol/L) has no effect on method on Du Pont Dimension *1592* No effect at 200 mg/L on Boehringer Mannheim Reflotron method *5706* At acute overdose concentration (20 mg/dL) on Technicon SMAC® method *6266* No effect at therapeutic concentration on Boehringer Mannheim Reflotron method *3231* At concentration of 240 mg/L had no effect on lipase/esterase method *5704*

Serum No Effect Physiological No overall significant difference between treated epileptics and controls but higher proportion of males had high concentrations than controls *4294* No consistent change seen in patients on long-term treatment *4591* In both men and women in 27 patients with transient brain ischemia *3058* In 100 chronic epileptics treated with phenytoin mean concentration nonsignificantly increased to 97 ± 38 mg/dL compared with 93 ± 47 mg/dL in 100 healthy controls *842*

TSH response to TRH *Serum Increase Physiological* Major stimulation when patients given 3 mg/kg/d with normal serum concentration *2136*

Serum No Effect Physiological No augmented response observed in treated individuals *1269* Response usually normal or reduced *2412*

Urea Nitrogen *Serum No Effect Analytical* No effect at 12 mg/L on method on Ames Seralyzer *5706* No effect at 200 mg/L on Boehringer Mannheim Reflotron method *5706* At acute overdose concentration (20 mg/dL) on Technicon SMAC® method *6266* No effect at concentration of 30 µg/mL (120 µmol/L) on method on Du Pont Dimension *1593* No effect at therapeutic concentration on Boehringer Mannheim Reflotron method *3231* At concentration of 240 mg/L had no effect on diacetylmonoxime method *5704* At concentration of 36 mg/L had no effect on Kodak Ektachem® method *5704*

Uric Acid *Serum No Effect Analytical* No effect at 200 mg/L on Boehringer Mannheim Reflotron method *5706* At concentration of 240 mg/L had no effect on phosphotungstate reduction method *5704* At acute overdose concentration (20 mg/dL) on Technicon SMAC® method *6266* No effect at concentration of 30 µg/mL (119 µmol/L) on method on Du Pont Dimension *1594* No effect at 1.8 mg/dL on Technicon SMA 12/60 method *4390* No effect at therapeutic concentration on Boehringer Mannheim Reflotron method *3231*

Valproic Acid *Serum Decrease Physiological* Concentration approximately 50% less when phenytoin co-administered *3855* Four weeks after discontinuation of phenytoin treatment in 22 epileptic patients mean increase of 19% observed *1619* Significant reduction of half-life from 10.9 h to 6.9 h when drugs coadministered *3684* By increasing the expression of hepatic enzymes, especially those that increase the amount of glucuronosyl transferases, may increase the clearance of valproate twofold *17* Through induction of hepatic enzymes may increase the plasma clearance of valproate *15*

Phenytoin *(continued)*

Valproic Acid *(continued)*
Serum No Effect Analytical No significant interference observed at a concentration of 1000 µg/mL (3964 µmol/L) with method on Du Pont aca *1560* At concentrations up to 1000 µg/mL had no significant cross-reactivity in valproic acid method on Bayer Technicon Immuno 1® *437*

Verapamil *Serum Decrease Physiological* Marked reduction to below therapeutic concentration observed when drugs coadministered: probably due to induction of hepatic metabolizing enzymes *6539*

Vitamin A *Serum Increase Physiological* In comparison with untreated cognitively delayed children 28.8 µg/dL versus 19.4 µg/dL *3266*

Vitamin B_{12} *Cerebrospinal Fluid Decrease Physiological* Significantly lower with long term therapy *1960*
Serum No Effect Analytical At concentrations up to 70 mg/dL had no clinically significant cross-reactivity in vitamin B_{12} method on Bayer Technicon Immuno 1® *439*

Vitamin D Binding Globulin *Serum No Effect Physiological* In 10 women receiving anticonvulsants mainly phenytoin versus 10 controls, drug taken on average for 15 y *441*

Vitamin E *Serum Decrease Physiological* Significantly reduced values in treated handicapped children *2596* Mean of 0.58 mg/dL versus 0.67 mg/dL in untreated control of handicapped children *2596*

VLDL-Cholesterol *Serum No Effect Physiological* In both men and women in 27 patients with transient brain ischemia *3058* In 100 chronic epileptics treated with phenytoin mean concentration 19.5 ± 7.5 mg/dL compared with 18.7 ± 9.4 mg/dL in 100 controls *842*

VLDL-Triglycerides *Serum No Effect Physiological* In both men and women in 27 patients with transient brain ischemia *3058*

Zidovudine *Serum Increase Physiological* Coadministration of phenytoin with zidovudine may increase the concentration of zidovudine by causing a 30% decrease in its oral clearance *2163*

Zinc *Serum Decrease Physiological* Reduction from mean of 670.0 µg/dL to 592.5 µg/dL in 22 patients being treated with drug for epilepsy *4710*
Serum Increase Physiological In 20 female epileptics treated with a mean of 220 mg/d of phenytoin mean concentration of 92 ± 14 µg/dL not significantly different from 87 ± 12 µg/dL in 20 healthy controls *3613*
Serum No Effect Physiological Observed in both hospitalized and home-living individuals with long-term administration *6417* No significant difference in average values between treated and untreated handicapped children although hypozincemia in 7 of 32 treated children and 0 of 13 controls *2596* In 27 epileptic patients treated with phenytoin for 1 month mean concentration of 73.9 ± 13.0 µg/dL not significantly less than 78.4 ± 12.8 µg/dL in 30 healthy controls *3344*

Phetharbital

Glucaric Acid *Urine Increase Physiological* Potent enzyme-inducing agent *2782*

6-β-Hydroxycortisol *Urine Increase Physiological* Increased to over 400 µg/d *5501*

Phleomycin

Chromosomes *Test Conditions Abnormal Physiological* Clastogenic in human cells *5484*

Phloridzin

Glucose *Urine Increase Physiological* Decreases glucose reabsorption *5592* Increases clearance *3810*

Glucose Clearance *Urine Increase Physiological* Due to decreased reabsorption *5592*

Inulin Clearance *Urine Decrease Physiological* Decrease of up to 30% *5592*

Osmolality *Urine Increase Physiological* Due to increased excretion of glucose etc *5592*

Phosphate *Urine Decrease Physiological* Probably due to increased reabsorption *5592*

Phosphate Clearance *Urine Decrease Physiological* Due to reduced excretion *5592*

Uric Acid *Urine Increase Physiological* Uricosuric action in man *5592*

Uric Acid Clearance *Urine Increase Physiological* Probably inhibits tubular reabsorption *5592*

Pholcodine

p-Aminophenol *Urine No Effect Analytical* With addition of drugs at a concentration of 100 mg/L and of related compounds at 50 mg/L no significant effect observed on colorimetric method of van Bocxlaer on Cobas Mira analyzer which involves reacting free p-aminophenol with resorcinol in the presence of magnesium ions to form an indophenol dye measured at 550 nm *6163*

Phospho-Soda®

Phosphate *Serum Increase Physiological* High concentration of phosphate absorbed from gut *5869*

Phosphorus

Alanine Aminotransferase *Serum Increase Physiological* Hepatotoxic effect with necrosis *3810*

Alkaline Phosphatase *Serum Increase Physiological* Hepatotoxic effect with necrosis *3810*

α-Amino-Nitrogen *Urine Increase Physiological* Due to nephrotoxicity *2183*

Aspartate Aminotransferase *Serum Increase Physiological* Hepatotoxic effect with necrosis *3810*

Bile *Urine Increase Physiological* Hepatotoxic effect with necrosis *3810*

Bilirubin *Serum Increase Physiological* Hepatotoxic effect with necrosis *3810*

BSP Retention *Serum Increase Physiological* Hepatotoxic effect with necrosis *3810*

Casts *Urine Increase Physiological* Nephrotoxic effect *2183*

Clotting Time *Blood Increase Physiological* Due to toxicity *2242*

Creatinine *Serum Increase Physiological* Nephrotoxic effect with necrosis *2024*

Erythrocytes *Blood Decrease Physiological* Occurs with chronic poisoning *2183*
Urine Increase Physiological Nephrotoxic effect *1714*

Fibrinogen *Plasma Decrease Physiological* Probable hepatotoxic effect *2183*

Glucose *Serum Decrease Physiological* Toxic effect *3810*

Hemoglobin *Urine Increase Physiological* Actual bleeding caused by drug *1714*

Icteric Index *Serum Increase Physiological* Due to nephrotoxicity *2183*

Leukocytes *Blood Decrease Physiological* Reported effect with poisoning *2183*
Blood Increase Physiological Reported leukocytosis with poisoning *2183*

Monocytes *Blood Increase Physiological* Reported effect of poisoning *2183*

Nonprotein Nitrogen *Serum Increase Physiological* Due to nephrotoxicity *2183*

Occult Blood *Feces Increase Physiological* Bloody diarrhea may occur with poisoning *2242*

Platelets *Blood Increase Physiological* Reported effect with poisoning *2183*

Protein *Serum No Effect Physiological* Decreased synthesis due to liver damage *467*
Urine Increase Physiological Renal toxic effect *2024*

Prothrombin Time *Plasma Increase Physiological* Toxicity effect (hypoprothrombinemia) *3810*

Silicon *Test Conditions Increase Analytical* Above 60 mg/L affects Jolles/Neurath method *2897*

Urea Nitrogen *Serum Increase Physiological* Nephrotoxic effect *3810*

Volume *Urine Decrease Physiological* Toxicity effect *2242*

Phthalylsulfathiazole

Estriol *Urine Decrease Physiological* Possibly affects integrity of intestinal microflora *54*

Estriol-3-Glucuronide *Urine Decrease Physiological* Possibly affects integrity of intestinal microflora *54*

Phylloerythrinogen

Urobilin *Urine Increase Analytical* Produces red fluorescence *2559*

Urobilinogen *Urine Increase Analytical* Produces red color with Ehrlich's reagent *2559*

Physostigmine

Antidiuretic Hormone
Cerebrospinal Fluid No Effect Physiological No effect observed in 11 normal volunteers following acute intravenous injection of up to 15 µg/kg *521*

Cholinesterase *Serum Decrease Physiological* Direct effect of drug *5900*

Corticotropin-releasing Hormone
Cerebrospinal Fluid No Effect Physiological No effect observed in 11 normal volunteers following acute intravenous injection of up to 15 µg/kg *521*

Galanin *Cerebrospinal Fluid No Effect Physiological* No significant effect observed in 11 normal volunteers following acute intravenous administration of up to 15 µg/kg *521*

Growth Hormone Releasing Hormone
Cerebrospinal Fluid No Effect Physiological No significant effect observed in 11 normal volunteers following acute intravenous injection of up to 15 µg/kg *521*

Histamine *Plasma No Effect Analytical* 50% inhibition of radio-enzyme assay at 10 µg/mL but improbable at physiological concentration of 4 - 9 pg/mL *2492*

β-Lipoprotein *Cerebrospinal Fluid No Effect Physiological* No effect observed in 11 normal volunteers following acute intravenous injection of up to 15 µg/kg *521*

Neuropeptide Y *Cerebrospinal Fluid Increase Physiological* Significant increase (10%) in 11 normal volunteers following acute intravenous injection of 15 µg/kg dose with increase occurring within 60 minutes of administration *521*

Somatostatin *Cerebrospinal Fluid No Effect Physiological* No significant effect observed in 11 normal volunteers following acute intravenous injection of up to 15 µg/kg *521*

Vasoactive Intestinal Polypeptide
Cerebrospinal Fluid No Effect Physiological No effect observed in 11 normal volunteers following acute intravenous injection of up to 15 µg/kg *521*

Phytonadione

Bilirubin *Serum Increase Physiological* Large dose effect, or with G-6-PD deficiency *1714*
Serum No Effect Analytical No effect at concentration of 8.3 mg/L on method on Kodak Ektachem® *5706*

Bilirubin, Conjugated *Serum No Effect Analytical* No effect at concentration of 8.3 mg/L on method on Kodak Ektachem® *5706*

Bilirubin, Unbound *Serum Increase Physiological* Parenteral administration in neonates can cause significant increase in plasma unbound bilirubin *1384*

Bilirubin, Unconjugated *Serum No Effect Analytical* No effect at concentration of 8.3 mg/L on method on Kodak Ektachem® *5706*

Erythrocytes *Blood Decrease Physiological* Hemolysis may occur with G-6-PD deficiency *3810*
Urine Increase Physiological Actual bleeding caused by drug *3810*

Hematocrit *Blood Decrease Physiological* Hemolysis may occur with G-6-PD deficiency *3810*

Hemoglobin *Blood Decrease Physiological* Hemolysis may occur with G-6-PD deficiency *3810* Parenteral administration in neonates can cause hemolytic anemia *1384*
Urine Increase Physiological Hemoglobinuria may occur in neonates given phytonadione parenterally *1384* Actual bleeding caused by drug *1714*

Prothrombin Time *Plasma Decrease Physiological* Stimulates synthesis of clotting factors *5674*

Picoline

ionized Calcium *Serum Increase Analytical* At concentrations > 0.1 mmol/L on calcium specific electrode *820*

Picotamide

Cyclosporine *Blood No Effect Physiological* Coadministration of picotamide with cyclosporine caused no effect on cyclosporine concentration having no effect on its pharmacokinetics or bioavailability *859*
Serum No Effect Physiological Coadministration of picotamide with cyclosporine caused no effect on cyclosporine concentration having no effect on its pharmacokinetics or bioavailability *859*

2,3-Dinor-6-Keto-Prostaglandin $F_{1\alpha}$
Urine No Effect Physiological No significant effect observed in 8 healthy controls and 8 patients with peripheral arteriopathy treated with 900 mg/d for 7 days *4066*

2,3-Dinor-Thromboxane B_2 *Urine No Effect Physiological* No effect observed in 8 patients with peripheral arteriopathy and healthy controls given 900 mg/d for 7 days *4066*

6-Keto-Prostaglandin $F_{1\alpha}$ *Urine No Effect Physiological* No effect of treatment with 900 mg/d for 7 days observed in 8 healthy controls and 8 patients with peripheral arteriopathy treated with 900 mg/d for 7 days *4066*

Platelet Aggregation *Blood Decrease Physiological* Significant reduction observed in ADP-induced platelet aggregation in 8 patients with peripheral arteriopathy and 8 healthy controls given 900 mg/d for 7 days but no effect observed on arachidonic acid or U46619-induced aggregation *4066*

PIDH

Glucose *Serum Decrease Physiological* Significant reduction after glucose load *5167*

Insulin *Plasma Decrease Physiological* Reduces insulin response to glucose load *5167*

Pilocarpine

Erythrocytes *Blood Increase Physiological* Probably due to contraction of spleen *2242*

Histamine *Plasma No Effect Analytical* 50% inhibition in radio-enzyme assay at concentration of 52 µg/mL but improbable at clinical concentrations *2492*

Hydrochloric Acid *Gastric Fluid Increase Physiological* Produces secretion like that of vagal stimulation *2242*

Leukocytes *Blood Decrease Physiological* Leukopenia observed in a small number of treated patients *4016*
Blood Increase Physiological Probably due to contraction of spleen *2242*

Pepsin *Gastric Material Increase Physiological* Produces secretion like that of vagal stimulation *2242*

Potassium *Saliva Decrease Physiological* Produces secretion like plasma ultrafiltrate *2242*

Pimobendan

Glomerular Filtration Rate *Urine No Effect Physiological* In 8 healthy men given 5 mg orally no significant change from mean baseline of 101.2 mL/min/1.73 sq m observed *3814*

Renal Plasma Flow *Patient No Effect Physiological* In 8 healthy men given 5 mg orally no significant change from mean baseline of 311.6 mL/min/1.73 sq m *3814*

Pimozide

Catecholamines *Plasma No Effect Analytical* No effect on HPLC method of Koller for dopamine, epinephrine, and norepinephrine *3230*

Follicle Stimulating Hormone
Plasma Decrease Physiological Statistically significant decline when given to acutely psychotic males although still within normal range *5584*

Hematocrit *Blood Decrease Physiological* Hemolytic anemia observed occasionally in postmarketing reports *2049*

Hemoglobin *Blood Decrease Physiological* Hemolytic anemia observed occasionally in postmarketing reports *2049*

Histamine *Plasma No Effect Analytical* Improbable inhibition of radio-enzyme assay at physiological concentrations *2492*

Luteinizing Hormone *Plasma Decrease Physiological* Statistically significant decline when given to acutely psychotic males although *5584*

Prolactin *Plasma Increase Physiological* General effect observed *2836* In acutely psychotic males *5584*

Sodium *Serum Decrease Physiological* Hyponatremia observed occasionally in postmarketing reports *2049*

Testosterone *Serum No Effect Physiological* In acutely psychotic males *5584* General effect observed *2836*

Thyroid Stimulating Hormone
Serum Decrease Physiological But effect contrary to assumed mechanism of a dopamine blocker *6412*

Pinacidil

Alkaline Phosphatase *Serum No Effect Physiological* No significant effect in 71 hypertensive patients treated with up to 100 mg daily for 20 weeks *5813*

Apolipoprotein A-I *Serum Increase Physiological* In 52 pinacidil treated hypertensives previously stabilized on hydrochlorothiazide mean concentration increased significantly by 9.0 ± 25.6 mg/dL after 8 weeks *1132*

Apolipoprotein B *Serum Decrease Physiological* In 52 hypertensives previously stabilized on hydrochlorothiazide treatment with pinacidil caused significant decrease of 6.3 ± 22.5 mg/dL from baseline *1132*

Apolipoprotein C-III *Serum Decrease Physiological* In 52 hypertensives previously stabilized on hydrochlorothiazide addition of pinacidil for 8 weeks caused significant decrease of 2.3 ± 5.5 mg/dL *1132*

Apolipoprotein E *Serum Decrease Physiological* In 52 hypertensives previously stabilized on hydrochlorothiazide addition of pinacidil caused significant decrease of 2.0 ± 4.9 mg/dL from mean baseline after 8 weeks *1132*

Aspartate Aminotransferase
Serum No Effect Physiological No significant effect in 71 patients with hypertension treated with up to 100 mg daily for 20 weeks *5813*

Cholesterol *Serum Decrease Physiological* Significant reduction by mean of 8 mg/dL in 199 patients treated with up to 150 mg/day for up to 5 months *5041* In 52 placidil treated hypertensives previously stabilized on hydrochlorothiazide mean concentration decreased significantly by 11.8 ± 34.8 mg/dL after 8 weeks *1132*
Serum No Effect Physiological No significant change in 96 hypertensive patients treated with up to 100 mg daily for 12 weeks *2996*

Creatinine *Serum No Effect Physiological* No difference in 8 hypertensive patients treated with up to 50 mg daily for up to 6 months together with a diuretic *889* No significant effect in 71 hypertensive patients treated with up to 100 mg daily for 20 weeks *5813*

Glomerular Filtration Rate *Urine No Effect Physiological* No difference in 8 hypertensive patients treated for up to 6 months with up to 50 mg daily together with a diuretic *889*

Glucose *Serum No Effect Physiological* No significant change observed in 6 healthy volunteers following two weeks treatment with up to 50 mg daily on either basal concentration or in comparison with controls during oral glucose tolerance test *4291*

Glucose Tolerance *Serum No Effect Physiological* No significant difference in comparison with controls in 6 healthy volunteers given up to 50 mg pinacidil daily for 2 weeks *4291*

HDL_2-Cholesterol *Serum Increase Physiological* Concentration increased in patients undergoing treatment for mild to moderate hypertension *5195*

HDL-Cholesterol *Serum Increase Physiological* Increased by 7-8% in 96 hypertensive patients treated with up to 100 mg daily for 12 weeks *2996* Significant increase by mean of 4 mg/dL in 199 patients treated for up 5 months with up to 150 mg daily *5041*
Serum No Effect Physiological In 52 pinacidil treated hypertensives previously stabilized on hydrochlorothiazide mean concentration decreased nonsignificantly by 5.9 ± 22.7 mg/dL after 8 weeks *1132*

Hemoglobin *Blood Decrease Physiological* Mean reduction of 0.2 mmol/L in 71 hypertensive patients treated with up to 100 mg daily for 20 weeks possibly related to fluid retention *5813*

Insulin *Plasma No Effect Physiological* After two weeks treatment with up to 50 mg daily in 6 healthy volunteers no effect observed on basal insulin concentration or difference from control during oral glucose tolerance test *4291*

LDL-Cholesterol *Serum Decrease Physiological* Significant reduction by mean of 8 mg/dL in 194 patients treated with up to 150 mg/day for up to 5 months *5041*
Serum No Effect Physiological In 52 pinacidil treated hypertensives previously stabilized on hydrochlorothiazide treatment for 8 weeks caused nonsignificant decrease of 5.9 ± 22.7 mg/dL *1132*

Leukocytes *Blood No Effect Physiological* No significant effect in 71 hypertensive patients treated with up to 100 mg daily for 20 weeks *5813*

Potassium *Serum No Effect Physiological* No significant effect in 71 hypertensive patients treated with up to 100 mg daily for 20 weeks *5813*

Triglycerides *Serum Decrease Physiological* Significant reduction by mean of 15 mg/dL in 199 patients treated with up to 150 mg/day for up to 5 months *5041* Concentration reduced in mild to moderate hypertensives with treatment *5195* In 52 placidil treated hypertensives previously stabilized on hydrochlorothiazide mean concentration decreased by 54.1 ± 157.9 mg/dL after 8 weeks *1132*
Serum No Effect Physiological No significant change in 96 hypertensive patients treated with up to 100 mg daily for 12 weeks *2996*

Pindolol

Adenosine Monophosphate *Plasma Increase Physiological* Substantially higher in patients receiving drug 5 mg b.i.d. than in those receiving either propranolol or metoprolol *6511*
Platelets Increase Physiological Significantly higher in patients receiving this drug than in those receiving propranolol *6511*

Alanine Aminotransferase *Serum Increase Physiological* Minor persistent increases reported in about 7% patients but not progressive *1880*

Albumin *Serum No Effect Physiological* No significant change either at 4 hours or after one week's treatment with 160 mg daily in in 9 patients with hyperthyroidism *3077*

Alkaline Phosphatase *Serum Increase Analytical* At 5 mg/L conventional methods when added to serum *2877*
Serum Increase Physiological Increased alkaline phosphatase activity during pindolol administration may be observed on rare occasions *5244*

Apolipoprotein A-I *Serum No Effect Physiological* No significant changes found during 12 mo treatment *3500* No significant change in 20 normolipidemic patients with mild to moderate hypertension treated with 10 mg daily for 12 weeks *5280* Nonsignificant increase from mean baseline concentration of 115 mg/dL to 121 mg/dL in 21 patients with mild to moderate hypertension treated with up to 15 mg/d for 6 months *966* No significant changes after 12 mo treatment *3499*

Apolipoprotein A-II *Serum Increase Physiological* Significant increase in 20 normolipidemic patients with mild to moderate hypertension given 10 mg daily for 12 weeks *5280*
Serum No Effect Physiological Nonsignificant increase from mean baseline concentration of 34 mg/dL to 35 mg/dL in 21 patients with mild to moderate hypertension treated with up to 15 mg/d for 6 months *966* No significant effect observed in normolipemic or moderately hyperlipemic patients with moderate hypertension when treated for 6 months *966* No significant changes after 12 mo treatment *3499* No significant changes found during 12 mo treatment *3500*

Apolipoprotein B *Serum No Effect Physiological* Nonsignificant increase from mean baseline concentration of 123 mg/dL to 127 mg/dL in 21 normolipemic or hyperlipidemic patients with mild to moderate hypertension treated with up to 15 mg/d for 6 months *966* No significant change in 20 normolipidemic patients with mild to moderate hypertension treated with 10 mg daily for 12 weeks *5280*

Apolipoprotein B:Apolipoprotein A-I Ratio
Serum Decrease Physiological Significant reduction observed in 20 normolipidemic patients with mild to moderate hypertension treated with 10 mg daily for 12 weeks *5280*

Apolipoprotein C-II *Serum No Effect Physiological* No significant effect in 20 normolipidemic patients with mild to moderate hypertension treated with 10 mg daily for 12 weeks *5280*

Apolipoprotein C-III *Serum No Effect Physiological* No significant effect in 20 normolipidemic patients with mild to moderate hypertension treated with 10 mg daily for 12 weeks *5280*

Apolipoprotein E *Serum No Effect Physiological* No significant effect in 20 patients with mild to moderate hypertension treated with 10 mg daily for 12 weeks *5280*

Aspartate Aminotransferase *Serum Decrease Analytical* At 5 mg/L with conventional methods when pindolol added to serum *2877*
Serum Increase Physiological Minor persistent increases in enzyme activity observed in 7% treated patients during pindolol administration *5244* Minor persistent increases reported in about 7% patients but not progressive *1880*

Bicarbonate *Serum No Effect Physiological* No significant change observed in 21 patients with mild to moderate hypertension treated with up to 15 mg/d for 6 months *966*

Bilirubin *Serum Decrease Analytical* At 5 mg/L conventional methods when added to serum *2877*

Calcium *Serum No Effect Physiological* No significant effect even with 6 weeks treatment *5482*

Catecholamines *Plasma No Effect Analytical* No effect on HPLC method of Koller for dopamine, epinephrine, and norepinephrine *3230*

Chloride *Serum No Effect Physiological* No significant change observed in 21 patients with mild to moderate hypertension treated with up to 15 mg/d for 6 months *966*

Cholesterol *Serum Decrease Physiological* Significant reduction in men (baseline 6.11 mmol/L, after treatment 5.81 mmol/L) but reduction in women (baseline 5.78 mmol/L, after treatment 5.56 mmol/L) not significant with up to 15 mg daily for 2 months *5907* Lower after 6 mo of therapy than after one *3500*
Serum Increase Physiological Increase by 5.5% in one study of 4 weeks with 15-30 mg/d *2953*
Serum No Effect Physiological Nonsignificant increase from mean baseline concentration of 5.8 mmol/L to 6.0 mmol/L in 21 normolipemic or moderately hyperlipemic patients with mild to moderate hypertension treated with up to 15 mg/d for 6 months *966* No significant effect in 34 elderly hypertensive patients treated with up to 15 mg daily for 12 weeks *5768* No significant change typically seen with treatment for 1 mo or more *142* No significant change observed in 22 patients with mild previously untreated hypertension treated with average of 11.7 mg/day for 50 weeks *894* No effect in short-term study of 10 hypertensive men with 15 mg/d *3521* No significant change in four studies of 1 to 12 mo *3499* Nonsignificant reduction in 82 hypertensive men at 6 and 12 months following average dose of 7.7 mg daily *5983* No significant change in total cholesterol in 20 normolipidemic patients with mild to moderate hypertension treated with 10 mg daily for 12 weeks *5280* No significant change observed in either normolipemic or hyperlipemic moderately hypertensive patients after 6 months treatment *966*

Creatine Kinase *Serum Decrease Analytical* At 5 mg/L conventional methods when added to serum *2877*
Serum Increase Physiological In 20 of 25 patients with essential hypertension with increase of 20 to 760% compared with pretreatment values. MM isoenzyme most affected, but 8 of 25 showed slight increase of MB *5275*

Creatinine *Serum No Effect Physiological* No significant change observed in 21 patients with mild to moderate hypertension treated with up to 15 mg/d for 6 months *966*

Erythrocytes *Blood No Effect Physiological* No significant effect observed in 21 patients with mild to moderate hypertension treated with up to 15 mg/d for 6 months *966*

Fatty Acids (FFA), Free *Serum No Effect Physiological* No significant changes after 12 mo treatment *3499* Remained constant during 12 mo therapy *3500*

Glucagon *Plasma Decrease Physiological* In 18 patients with mild essential hypertension treated with chlorothiazide concomitantly over 4 weeks *1734*

Glucose *Serum No Effect Physiological* In 18 patients with mild essential hypertension treated with chlorothiazide concomitantly over 4 weeks *1734* No significant change observed in 21 patients with mild to moderate hypertension treated with up to 15 mg/d for 6 months *966* No significant changes found during 12 mo treatment *3500*

Glucose Tolerance *Serum Decrease Physiological* Slight effect after 60 minutes, significant effect at 120 minutes during oral glucose tolerance test *3500*

γ-Glutamyltransferase *Serum No Effect Physiological* No significant change observed in 21 patients with mild to moderate hypertension treated with up to 15 mg/d for 6 months *966*

Granulocytes *Blood Decrease Physiological* Agranulocytosis may occur as a complication during pindolol administration *5244*

HDL_2-Apolipoprotein A-II *Serum Decrease Physiological* Insignificant reduction in men (baseline 0.75 mmol/L, after treatment 0.58 mmol/L) and in women (baseline 0.69 mmol/L, after treatment 0.63 mmol/L) with up to 15 mg daily for 2 months *5907*

HDL_2-Cholesterol *Serum Decrease Physiological* Insignificant reduction in men (baseline 0.75 mmol/L, after treatment 0.58 mmol/L) and in women (baseline 0.69 mmol/L, after treatment 0.63 mmol/L) with up to 15 mg daily for 2 months *5907*
Serum No Effect Physiological Nonsignificant increase from mean baseline of 0.49 mmol/L to 0.52 mmol/L in 21 patients with mild to moderate hypertension treated with up to 15 mg/d for 6 months *966* No significant change in 20 patients with mild to moderate hypertension treated with 10 mg daily for 12 weeks *5280*

HDL_3-Cholesterol *Serum Increase Physiological* Insignificant increase in men (baseline 0.73 mmol/L, after treatment 0.78 mmol/L) but significant increase in women (baseline 0.76 mmol/L, after treatment 0.91 mmol/L) with up to 15 mg daily for 2 months *5907*
Serum No Effect Physiological No significant change in 20 normolipidemic patients treated with 10 mg daily for 12 weeks *5280* No change from mean baseline concentration of 0.79 mmol/L in 21 patients with mild to moderate hypertension treated with up to 15 mg/d for 6 months *966*

HDL-Cholesterol *Serum Decrease Physiological* Insignificant reduction in men (baseline 1.48 mmol/L, after treatment 1.36 mmol/L) and no change in women (baseline 1.45 mmol/L, after treatment 1.50 mmol/L) with up to 15 mg daily for 2 months *5907*
Serum Increase Physiological Significant increase in 20 normolipidemic patients with mild to moderate hypertension given 10 mg daily for 12 weeks *5280* 20% increase in one 3 mo study *3499* Concentration increased after 5 mg twice daily for 12 weeks *5283* Significant increase during first month of therapy *3500*
Serum No Effect Physiological No effect observed in 22 patients with previously untreated mild hypertension treated with average of 11.7 mg/day for 50 weeks *894* No significant

Pindolol *(continued)*

HDL-Cholesterol *(continued)*
change in 2 studies of 2 to 12 mo *3499* No significant effect in 34 elderly hypertensive patients treated with up to 15 mg daily for 12 weeks *5768* No significant change from mean baseline concentration of 1.22 mmol/L in 21 patients with mild to moderate hypertension treated with up to 15 mg/d for 6 months *966* No significant change from baseline concentration of 1.31 mmol/L 6 and 12 months after receiving mean daily dose of 7.7 mg daily in 82 hypertensive men *5983* No effect in short-term study of 10 hypertensive men with 15 mg/d *3521* No significant change typically seen with treatment for 1 mo or more *142*

HDL-Triglycerides *Serum Decrease Physiological* Nonsignificant decrease from mean baseline concentration of 0.21 mmol/L to 0.19 mmol/L in 21 patients with mild to moderate hypertension treated with up to 15 mg/d for 6 months *966*
Serum Increase Physiological Increase from mean baseline value of 0.16 mmol/L to 0.18 mmol/L at 6 months and 0.17 mmol/L in 82 hypertensive men receiving mean daily dose of 7.7 mg daily *5983*

Histamine *Plasma No Effect Analytical* Improbable inhibition of radio-enzyme assay at therapeutic concentrations *2492*

Insulin *Plasma No Effect Physiological* In 18 patients with mild essential hypertension treated with chlorothiazide *1734* No significant change in concentration during glucose tolerance test after drug *3500*

Lactate Dehydrogenase *Serum Increase Physiological* Increased lactate dehydrogenase activity during pindolol administration may be observed on rare occasions *5244*

LDL-Cholesterol *Serum Decrease Physiological* Decrease from mean baseline of 4.36 mmol/L to 4.16 mmol/L at 6 months and 4.21 mmol/L in 82 hypertensive men receiving mean daily dose of 7.7 mg *5983*
Serum Increase Physiological Slight tendency to rise during treatment *3500* Significant increase in 20 normolipidemic mild to moderate hypertensive patients given 10 mg daily for 12 weeks *5280*
Serum No Effect Physiological No significant change typically seen with treatment for 1 mo or more *142* No significant effect in 34 elderly hypertensive patients treated with up to 15 mg daily for 12 weeks *5768* No significant change in 3 studies of 2 to 12 mo *3499* Nonsignificant increase from mean baseline of 4.01 mmol/L to 4.16 mmol/L in 21 patients with mild to moderate hypertension treated with up to 15 mg/d for 6 months *966*

LDL-Triglycerides *Serum Decrease Physiological* Nonsignificant decrease from mean baseline of 0.68 mmol/L to 0.59 mmol/L in 21 patients with mild to moderate hypertension treated with up to 15 mg/d for 6 months *966*
Serum Increase Physiological Slight increase from baseline of 0.38 mmol/L to 0.39 mmol/L after 12 months treatment with mean daily dose of 7.7 mg daily in 82 hypertensive men *5983*

LE Cells *Blood Positive Physiological* Drug induced systemic lupus erythematosus reported in one case *488*

Lecithin:Cholesterol Acyltransferase
Serum No Effect Physiological At in vitro concentration of 0.5 µmol/L nonsignificant reduction of activity to 97.8 ± 3.9% observed *5316*

Leukocytes *Blood No Effect Physiological* No significant change observed in 21 patients with mild to moderate hypertension treated with up to 15 mg/d for 6 months *966*

Lidocaine *Serum No Effect Physiological* No apparent effect on clearance of lidocaine when both drugs coadministered *5888*

Magnesium *Serum No Effect Physiological* No significant effect even with 6 weeks treatment *5482*

Neutrophils *Blood Decrease Physiological* Occasional case of agranulocytosis reported *6264*

Parathyroid Hormone *Plasma Decrease Physiological* Observed within 3 h of treatment: significant effect over 6 weeks *5482*

Phosphate *Serum Increase Physiological* Significant increase in 9 patients with hyperthyroidism treated with 10 mg daily for one week. Baseline concentration 1.01 mmol/L, with concentration of 1.36 mmol/L after 4 hours and 1.21 mmol/L after one week *3077*
Serum No Effect Physiological No significant effect even with 6 weeks treatment *5482*

Platelet Aggregation *Blood Increase Physiological* Significantly higher threshold in patients receiving 5 mg drug b.i.d. than in those receiving propranolol 80 mg b.i.d *6511*

Platelets *Blood Decrease Physiological* Thrombocytopenic or nonthrombocytopenic purpura may occur as a complication during pindolol administration *5244*

Potassium *Serum Increase Physiological* Slight rise in patients treated with moderate doses of drug *4739*
Serum No Effect Physiological No significant change observed in 21 patients with mild to moderate hypertension treated with up to 15 mg/d for 6 months *966* No significant effect even with 6 weeks treatment *5482*

Sodium *Serum No Effect Physiological* No significant effect even with 6 weeks treatment *5482* No significant change observed in 21 patients with mild to moderate hypertension treated with up to 15 mg/d for 6 months *966*

Thioridazine *Serum Increase Physiological* When drugs coadministered plasma thioridazine concentration may be increased *5244*

Triglycerides *Serum Decrease Physiological* Concentration reduced in individuals when treated with 5 mg twice daily for 12 weeks *5283*
Serum Increase Physiological In 18 patients with mild essential hypertension treated with chlorothiazide concomitantly over 4 weeks *1734* Significant increase in 82 hypertensive men at 6 months after treatment with mean dose of 7.7 mg daily (change from 1.83 mmol/L to 2.10 mmol/L) although fall to a nonsignificant increase at 1 year *5983* 28% increase in one 1 mo study *3499* Increase by 28 % in one study of 4 weeks with 15-30 mg/d *2953* Slight increase in men (rose from 2.08 mmol/L to 2.25 mmol/L) and in women (baseline 2.08 mmol/L, with treatment 2.39 mmol/L) with 2 months of treatment with up to 15 mg/day *5907*
Serum No Effect Physiological No effect observed in 22 patients with previously untreated mild hypertension treated with average of 11.7 mg/day for 50 weeks *894* No significant change typically seen with treatment for 1 mo or more *142* No significant effect in 34 elderly hypertensive patients treated with up to 15 mg daily for 12 weeks *5768* Remained constant during 12 mo therapy *3500* No effect in short-term study of 10 hypertensive men with 15 mg/d *3521* No significant change in 20 patients with mild to moderate hypertension treated with 10 mg daily for 12 weeks *5280* Insignificant change in 3 studies of 2 to 12 mo *3499* Nonsignificant increase from mean baseline of 1.6 mmol/L to 1.7 mmol/L in 21 normolipemic or moderately hyperlipemic patients with mild to moderate hypertension treated with up to 15 mg/d for 6 months *966*

Uric Acid *Serum Increase Physiological* Concentration may be increased during pindolol administration on rare occasions *5244*
Serum No Effect Physiological No effect in short-term study of 10 hypertensive men with 15 mg/d *3521* No significant effect observed in 21 patients with mild to moderate hypertension treated with up to 15 mg/d for 6 months *966*

VLDL-Cholesterol *Serum Decrease Physiological* 35% reduction in concentration after 2 mo in 11 hypertensive patients but after 16 mo treatment had reverted to normal *2327* Significant decrease in 20 normolipidemic patients with mild to moderate hypertension given 10 mg daily for 12 weeks *5280*
Serum Increase Physiological Insignificant increase from baseline of 0.81 mmol/L to 0.90 mmol/L at 6 months and 0.85 mmol/L at 12 months in 82 hypertensive men receiving mean daily dose of 7.7 mg *5983*
Serum No Effect Physiological No effect in short-term study of 10 hypertensive men with 15 mg/d *3521* Nonsignificant increase from mean baseline of 0.48 mmol/L to 0.57 mmol/L in 21 patients with mild to moderate hypertension treated with up to 15 mg/d for 6 months *966*

VLDL-Triglycerides *Serum Decrease Physiological* 35% reduction in concentration after 2 mo in 11 hypertensive patients but after 16 mo treatment had reverted to normal *2327*
Serum Increase Physiological Nonsignificant increase from mean baseline of 0.73 mmol/L to 0.93 mmol/L in 21 patients with mild to moderate hypertension when treated with up to 15 mg/d for 6 months *966* Nonsignificant increase from baseline of 1.27 mmol/L in 82 hypertensive men at 6 months (1.47 mmol/L) and 12 months (1.41 mmol/L) given mean daily dose of 7.7 mg *5983*

Pipamazine

Erythrocytes *Blood Decrease Physiological* Pancytopenia (AMA Blood dyscrasias) *4017*

Leukocytes *Blood Decrease Physiological* Pancytopenia (AMA Blood dyscrasias) *4017*

Platelets *Blood Decrease Physiological* Pancytopenia (AMA Blood dyscrasias) *4017*

Pipamperone

p-Aminophenol *Urine No Effect Analytical* With addition of drugs at a concentration of 100 mg/L and of related compounds at 50 mg/L no significant effect observed on colorimetric method of van Bocxlaer on Cobas Mira analyzer which involves reacting free p-aminophenol with resorcinol in the presence of magnesium ions to form an indophenol dye measured at 550 nm *6163*

Pipemidic Acid

Alanine Aminopeptidase *Urine No Effect Physiological* No significant effect in healthy individuals and those with infections of lower urinary tract but reduction in patients with pyelonephritis when given for 10 d *1057*

Caffeine *Serum Increase Physiological* After single dose of caffeine following pretreatment with pipemidic acid significant increase of area under curve and decreased plasma clearance *884*

N-Acetyl-Glucosaminidase *Urine No Effect Physiological* No significant effect in healthy individuals and those with infections of lower urinary tract but reduction in patients with pyelonephritis when given for 10 d *1057*

Theophylline *Serum No Effect Physiological* Insignificant increase in concentration of parent drug although significant increase of elimination half-life from mean of 5.7 h to 10.8 h in 12 healthy male volunteers when two drugs coadministered with increased conversion to 1-methylxanthine *5767*

Piperacetazine

Alanine Aminotransferase *Serum Increase Physiological* Transient reversible effect *2012*

Aspartate Aminotransferase *Serum Increase Physiological* Transient reversible increase *2012*

Bilirubin *Serum Increase Physiological* Rare reversible jaundice (like infectious hepatitis) *128*

Eosinophils *Blood Increase Physiological* Occasional allergic response *2754*

Erythrocytes *Blood Decrease Physiological* Rare hemolytic anemia/pancytopenia *51*

Glucose *Serum Decrease Physiological* Disordered endocrine response *51*

Serum Increase Physiological Disordered endocrine response *51*

Urine Increase Physiological Due to induced hyperglycemia *51*

Hematocrit *Blood Decrease Physiological* Mild transient decrease with hypotension *2012*

Hemoglobin *Blood Decrease Physiological* Mild transient decrease with hypotension *2012*

Leukocytes *Blood Decrease Physiological* Rare leukopenia/agranulocytosis (reversible) *128*

Platelets *Blood Decrease Physiological* Rare thrombocytopenia (reversible) *128*

Pregnancy Tests *Urine Positive Analytical* Associated with endocrine disorders *51*

Protein *Cerebrospinal Fluid Increase Physiological* Abnormality produced *51*

Piperacillin

Alanine Aminotransferase *Serum Increase Physiological* In 1 of 29 patients given 181 mg/kg i.v. for 6 d *5475* Occasional increases in liver enzyme activity observed with less frequent hyperbilirubinemia or cholestatic hepatitis *3467*

Alkaline Phosphatase *Serum Increase Physiological* In 1 of 29 patients given 181 mg/kg i.v. for 6 d *5475*

Aspartate Aminotransferase *Serum Increase Physiological* Occasional increases in liver enzyme activity observed with less frequent hyperbilirubinemia or cholestatic hepatitis *3467* Transient increase in 1 of 20 treated patients *5221* In 1 of 59 patients given drug as sole agent with many patients with severe illness *6507* In 1 of 29 patients given 181 mg/kg i.v. for 6 d *5475*

Bilirubin *Serum Increase Physiological* Occasional increases in liver enzyme activity observed with less frequent hyperbilirubinemia or cholestatic hepatitis *3467*

Serum No Effect Analytical No effect at 2000 mg/L on Ames Seralyzer method *5706*

Cephalothin *Serum Increase Analytical* Cannot be assayed by HPLC method used at Mayo Clinic in presence of piperacillin *3858*

Cholesterol *Serum No Effect Analytical* No effect up to 200 mg/L on Ames Seralyzer method but at higher concentrations disproportionately increased cholesterol concentration of possible clinical significance since therapeutic concentration of drug is 200-500 mg/L *5706*

Coombs' Test, Direct *Blood Positive Physiological* In 1 of 59 patients given drug as sole agent with many patients with severe illness *6507*

Creatine Kinase *Serum No Effect Analytical* No effect at 2000 mg/L on method on Ames Seralyzer *5706*

Creatinine *Serum Increase Physiological* In 1 of 59 patients given drug as sole agent with many patients with severe illness *6507* Infrequent increased concentration of creatinine with rarely interstitial nephritis *3467*

Serum No Effect Analytical No effect up to 200 mg/L on method on Ames Seralyzer but at higher concentrations apparently clinically significant increase in creatinine concentration *5706*

Cyclosporine *Blood No Effect Analytical* At a concentration of 8 mg/L had no effect on Syva EMIT method *495*

Eosinophils *Blood Increase Physiological* In 1 of 29 patients given 181 mg/kg i.v. for 6 d *5475* Reversible leukopenia, neutropenia, thrombocytopenia and/or eosinophilia have been reported *3467* In 5 of 59 patients given drug as sole agent with many patients with severe illness *6507*

Glucose *Serum No Effect Analytical* No effect at 2000 mg/L on glucose oxidase method on Ames Seralyzer *5706*

Urine Increase Analytical Falsely elevated values with Clinitest® *3446*

Urine No Effect Analytical Concentrations accurately measured by Diastix® . Concentrations accurately measured by TesTape® *3446*

Ketone Body Ratio *Serum No Effect Analytical* When added at a concentration of 5 g/L had no significant effect on AKBR method of Uno et al *6131*

Lactate Dehydrogenase *Serum Increase Physiological* Occasional increases in liver enzyme activity observed with less frequent hyperbilirubinemia or cholestatic hepatitis *3467* In 1 of 59 patients given drug as sole agent with many patients with severe illness *6507*

Serum No Effect Analytical No effect up to 200 mg/L on method on Ames Seralyzer but at higher concentrations clinically significant inhibition of enzyme activity *5706*

Leukocytes *Blood Decrease Physiological* Reversible leukopenia, neutropenia, thrombocytopenia and/or eosinophilia have been reported *3467* 6 of 20 patients had small drop in leukocyte count *5221*

Monocytes *Blood Increase Physiological* In 1 of 29 patients given 181 mg/kg i.v. for 6 d *5475*

Neutrophils *Blood Decrease Physiological* In 1 of 59 patients given drug as sole agent with many patients with severe illness *6507* Reversible leukopenia, neutropenia, thrombocytopenia and/or eosinophilia have been reported *3467*

Occult Blood *Feces Increase Physiological* Bloody diarrhea observed as an infrequent side effect *3467*

Piperacillin *(continued)*

OVX1 *Blood Decrease Physiological* Reversible leukopenia, neutropenia, thrombocytopenia and/or eosinophilia have been reported *3467*

Penicillin G *Serum Positive Analytical* Cannot be assayed by HPLC method used at Mayo Clinic in presence of piperacillin *3858*

Potassium *Serum Decrease Physiological* Individuals with liver disease or receiving cytotoxic therapy or diuretics may rarely demonstrate decreases in potassium concentration when given high doses of piperacillin *3467*

Protein *Urine Increase Analytical* False positive reaction with biuret following precipitation with trichloracetic acid and resuspension *4422*

Tacrolimus *Serum No Effect Analytical* In HPLC/MS method of Christians et al no significant interference observed with measurement of FK 506 *1010*

Urea Nitrogen *Serum Increase Physiological* Infrequent increased concentration of urea nitrogen with rarely interstitial nephritis *3467*

Serum No Effect Analytical No effect at 2000 mg/L on method on Ames Seralyzer *5706*

Vancomycin *Serum No Effect Analytical* Negligible interference at up to 500 mg/L on Abbott TD_x *4002*

Piperazine

Bilirubin *Serum Increase Physiological* May cause hemolytic anemia *3895*

Chromosomes *Test Conditions Abnormal Physiological* Clastogenic to bone marrow and leukocytes *5484*

Erythrocytes *Blood Decrease Physiological* May cause hemolytic anemia *3895*

Hematocrit *Blood Decrease Physiological* May cause hemolytic anemia *3895*

Hemoglobin *Blood Decrease Physiological* May cause hemolytic anemia *3895*

Histamine *Plasma No Effect Analytical* No inhibition of radio-enzyme assay at twice therapeutic concentrations *2492*

Uric Acid *Serum Decrease Analytical* Reported observation *570*

Piperidine

ionized Calcium *Serum Decrease Analytical* At concentrations greater than 0.1 mmol/L on calcium specific electrode *820*

Pipobroman

Bilirubin *Serum Increase Physiological* May cause hemolytic anemia *1714*

Erythrocytes *Blood Decrease Physiological* May cause anemia (bone marrow depression) *128*

Hematocrit *Blood Decrease Physiological* Intended effect when polycythemia present *2754*

Hemoglobin *Blood Decrease Physiological* Hemolytic anemia has been described *129*

Leukocytes *Blood Decrease Physiological* Bone marrow depression may occur after 4 weeks *2754*

Platelets *Blood Decrease Physiological* May cause bone marrow depression *2754*

Reticulocytes *Blood Increase Physiological* Hemolytic anemia has been described *129*

Urobilinogen *Urine Increase Physiological* Hemolytic anemia has been described *129*

Pipothiazine

Amphetamine *Urine Increase Analytical* 2 false positive results observed in 4 assays using Syva EMIT amphatamine method using a monoclonal antibody *1160*

Urine No Effect Analytical No false positive results observed in 4 assays using Syva EMIT amphatamine method using a polyclonal antibody *1160*

Piracetam

p-Aminophenol *Urine No Effect Analytical* With addition of drugs at a concentration of 100 mg/L and of related compounds at 50 mg/L no significant effect observed on colorimetric method of van Bocxlaer on Cobas Mira analyzer which involves reacting free p-aminophenol with resorcinol in the presence of magnesium ions to form an indophenol dye measured at 550 nm *6163*

Pirenzepine

Amoxicillin *Serum No Effect Physiological* No significant effect observed in 10 volunteers when 4 doses of 50 mg given together with 1000 mg amoxicillin *1386*

Cephalexin *Serum No Effect Physiological* No significant change in 10 healthy volunteers given 4 doses of 50 mg concomitantly with 1000 mg of cephalexin *1386*

Doxycycline *Serum No Effect Physiological* No significant effect in 10 healthy volunteers given 4 doses each of 50 mg concomitantly with 200 mg doxycycline *1386*

Glucagon *Plasma No Effect Physiological* Treatment for 1 week had no effect on basal concentrations *6624*

Growth Hormone *Plasma Decrease Physiological* Nocturnal secretion (area under curve from 23:00 to 08:00) significantly decreased in 13 diabetic patients following treatment with 100 mg/day orally for 1 month *3816*

Hemoglobin A_{1c} *Blood Decrease Physiological* Significant reduction in 13 diabetic patients treated with 100 mg/day orally for 1 month *3816*

Insulin *Plasma No Effect Physiological* Treatment for 1 week had no effect on basal concentrations *6624*

Leukocytes *Blood Decrease Physiological* In isolated cases even though other drugs also being ingested *5845*

Lysergic Acid Diethylamide *Urine Increase Analytical* Mucolytics such as ambroxol or pirenzepin cause false positive reaction with Boehringer-Mannheim CEDIA® DAU LSD procedure, not confirmed by HPLC *3658*

Neutrophils *Blood Decrease Physiological* In isolated cases even though other drugs also being ingested *5845*

Pancreatic Polypeptide *Plasma Decrease Physiological* Borderline significant reduction from basal mean value of 37 ng/L to 26.2 ng/L after treatment with 100 mg/d for 7 d *6624*

Platelets *Blood Decrease Physiological* In isolated cases even though other drugs also being ingested *5845*

Piretanide

Cholesterol *Serum Increase Physiological* Effect observed with 12 mg/d *6156*

Cobalt *Serum No Effect Physiological* No significant effect with up to 12 mg/d for 3 mo *6232*

Copper *Serum No Effect Physiological* No significant effect with up to 12 mg/d for 3 mo *6232*

C-Peptide *Plasma Increase Physiological* 61% higher than pretreatment level after 8 weeks in 12 male patients with mild hypertension (6 mg b.i.d.) *2472*

Glucose Tolerance *Serum No Effect Physiological* In 12 male patients with mild hypertension (6 mg b.i.d.) *2472*

Hemoglobin A_{1c} *Blood No Effect Physiological* In 12 male patients with mild hypertension (6 mg b.i.d.) *2472*

Insulin *Plasma No Effect Physiological* In 12 male patients with mild hypertension (6 mg b.i.d.) *2472*

Iron *Serum Decrease Physiological* Slight drop with 12 mg/d for 3 mo *6232*

LDL-Cholesterol *Serum Increase Physiological* Effect observed with 12 mg/d *6156*

Manganese *Serum No Effect Physiological* No significant effect with up to 12 mg/d for 3 mo *6232*

Triglycerides *Serum Increase Physiological* Effect observed with 12 mg/d *6156*

VLDL-Triglycerides *Serum Increase Physiological* Effect observed with 12 mg/d *6156*

Zinc *Serum No Effect Physiological* No significant effect with up to 12 mg/d for 3 mo *6232*

Piribedil

Corticotropin *Plasma No Effect Physiological* No consistent effect observed in 12 healthy women at least 5 years post menopause treated with daily oral doses of 40-100 mg *1318*

Follicle Stimulating Hormone
Plasma No Effect Physiological No consistent change observed in 12 healthy women at least 5 years postmenopause treated with 40-100 mg orally daily *1318*

Growth Hormone *Plasma Increase Physiological* Effect observed in 12 healthy women at least 5 years postmenopause treated with daily oral doses from 40-100 mg *1318*

Luteinizing Hormone *Plasma No Effect Physiological* No consistent change observed in 12 healthy women at least 5 years postmenopause treated with 40-100 mg orally daily *1318*

Prolactin *Plasma Decrease Physiological* Decrease observed in 12 healthy women at least 5 years after menopause with daily doses from 40-100 mg orally *1318*

Thyroid Stimulating Hormone
Serum No Effect Physiological No consistent change observed in 12 healthy women postmenopausal for at least 5 years treated with 40-100 mg orally daily *1318*

Pirmenol

Prothrombin Time *Plasma No Effect Physiological* Coadministration with warfarin had no effect on prothrombin time during administration or following it *5848*

Warfarin *Plasma No Effect Physiological* Coadministration appears to have no effect on concentration or metabolism of warfarin *5848*

Piroxicam

Alanine Aminotransferase *Serum Increase Physiological* Incidence of acute liver injury of 6.0 per 100,000 treated patients with reported in United Kingdom. Liver damage among all cases primarily hepatocellular in some and primarily cholestatic in others *5049* Severe hepatic reactions including jaundice and cases of fatal hepatitis have been reported with piroxicam *4646* Some transient increases reported *4465* Occasional case of liver damage reported *4716*

Alkaline Phosphatase *Serum Increase Physiological* Severe hepatic reactions including jaundice and cases of fatal hepatitis have been reported with piroxicam *4646* Occasional case of liver damage reported *4716*

Amylase *Serum Increase Physiological* Possible pancreatitis reported as complication in less than 1% treated patients *4646*

Antinuclear Antibodies *Serum Increase Physiological* Possible positive ANA test reported as complication in less than 1% treated patients *4646*

Aspartate Aminotransferase *Serum Increase Physiological* Severe hepatic reactions including jaundice and cases of fatal hepatitis have been reported with piroxicam *4646* Incidence of acute liver injury of 6.0 per 100,000 treated patients with reported in United Kingdom. Liver damage among all cases primarily hepatocellular in some and primarily cholestatic in others *5049* Some transient increases reported *4465* Occasional case of liver damage reported *4716*

Bilirubin *Serum Increase Physiological* Occasional case of liver damage reported *4716* Severe hepatic reactions including jaundice and cases of fatal hepatitis have been reported with piroxicam *4646*
Serum No Effect Analytical No effect at concentration of 10 mg/L on method on Kodak Ektachem® *5706*

Bilirubin, Conjugated *Serum Increase Analytical* Increased value observed with concentrations above 5 mg/L with method on Kodak Ektachem® . Effect unlikely to be of clinical significance since therapeutic concentration is 3-5 mg/L *5706*

Bilirubin, Unconjugated *Serum Decrease Analytical* Decreased value observed at concentrations above 5 mg/L with method on Kodak Ektachem® . Effect unlikely to be of clinical significance since therapeutic concentration 3-5 mg/L *5706*

Bleeding Time *Patient Increase Physiological* Prolongs bleeding time and decreases platelet aggregation *4465* Like aspirin prolongs bleeding time *1384*

Blood *Urine Increase Physiological* Occasional reports of acute interstitial nephritis with hematuria, proteinuria and occasionally nephrotic syndrome *4646*

Cholinesterase *Serum No Effect Analytical* No effect observed at concentration of 10 µg/mL with butyrylthiocholine method on Kodak Ektachem® *2504*

Chondrex *Serum No Effect Analytical* Concentrations up to 5 g/L had no significant effect on sandwich-type ELISA procedure of Harvey et al *2491*

Creatinine *Serum Increase Physiological* Increased concentration related to interstitial nephritis or nephrotic syndrome reported as complication in more than 1% treated patients *4646* Occasional drug induced nephrotoxicity, with isolated azotemia, acute interstitial nephritis or nephrotic syndrome *4716* Possible increase due to drug in some patients *6438*
Serum No Effect Physiological No effect in spite of effect on urea nitrogen *4465*

Drugs of Abuse Screen *Urine No Effect Analytical* No effect at concentration of 100 µg/mL on EZ-SCREEN procedure for cannabinoids and cocaine *1739*

Eosinophils *Blood Increase Physiological* Eosinophilia reported as complication in more than 1% treated patients *4646*

Erythrocytes *Blood Decrease Physiological* Has been reported to cause aplastic anemia *1384*
Urine Increase Physiological Occasional drug induced nephrotoxicity, with isolated azotemia, acute interstitial nephritis or nephrotic syndrome *4716*

Fractional Excretion of Potassium
Urine Decrease Physiological In individuals treated with 20 mg daily caused 10% reduction, 9% in elderly and 13% in elderly with renal insufficiency *4189*

Fractional Excretion of Sodium
Urine Decrease Physiological In individuals treated with 20 mg daily caused 0.3% reduction, 0.8% in elderly and 1.3% in elderly with renal insufficiency *4189*

Glucose *Serum Decrease Physiological* Both hyperglycemia and hypoglycemia reported as complications in less than 1% treated patients *4646*
Serum Increase Physiological Both hyperglycemia and hypoglycemia reported as complications in less than 1% treated patients *4646*

γ-Glutamyltransferase *Serum Increase Physiological* Severe hepatic reactions including jaundice and cases of fatal hepatitis have been reported with piroxicam *4646*

Granular Casts *Urine Increase Physiological* Few: occasional drug induced nephrotoxicity, with isolated azotemia, acute interstitial nephritis or nephrotic syndrome *4716*

Granulocytes *Blood Decrease Physiological* Has been reported to cause aplastic anemia *1384*

Hematocrit *Blood Decrease Physiological* Reported, unassociated with obvious gastrointestinal bleeding *4465* Possibly related to drug administration or concomitant therapy in patients with osteoarthrosis *5978* Although at the recommended dose of 30 mg/d increased fecal blood loss did not occur reductions occurred in about 4% treated patients *4646*

Hemoglobin *Blood Decrease Physiological* Reported, unassociated with obvious gastrointestinal bleeding *4465* Possibly related to drug administration or concomitant therapy in patients with osteoarthrosis *5978* Although at the recommended dose of 30 mg/d increased fecal blood loss did not occur reductions occurred in about 4% treated patients *4646*
Urine Increase Physiological Occasional drug induced nephrotoxicity, with isolated azotemia, acute interstitial nephritis or nephrotic syndrome *4716*

Piroxicam *(continued)*

Histamine *Plasma No Effect Analytical* No inhibition of radio-enzyme assay at concentration 6 times physiological *2492*

Hyaline Casts *Urine Increase Physiological* Many: occasional drug induced nephrotoxicity, with isolated azotemia, acute interstitial nephritis or nephrotic syndrome *4716*

Ketorolac *Serum No Effect Physiological* At therapeutic concentrations had no effect on ketorolac-protein binding *5035*

Leukocytes *Blood Decrease Physiological* Has been reported to cause aplastic anemia *1384* Leukopenia reported as complication in more than 1% treated patients *4646*

Lipase *Serum Increase Physiological* Possible pancreatitis reported as complication in less than 1% treated patients *4646*

Lithium *Serum Increase Physiological* Lithium toxicity reported with the concomitant administration of piroxicam *4399* Concomitant administration increases lithium concentration because its elimination is reduced *1384* Toxicity reported with 20-40 mg/d in four cases: piroxicam noted to delay elimination of lithium following discontinuation of lithium therapy *4831*

Occult Blood *Feces Increase Physiological* Gastrointestinal bleeding most common severe problem *3351*
Feces No Effect Physiological At the recommended dose of 30 mg/d increased fecal blood loss did not occur *4646*

p-Aminophenol *Urine No Effect Analytical* With addition of drugs at a concentration of 100 mg/L and of related compounds at 50 mg/L no significant effect observed on colorimetric method of van Bocxlaer on Cobas Mira analyzer which involves reacting free p-aminophenol with resorcinol in the presence of magnesium ions to form an indophenol dye measured at 550 nm *6163*

Platelet Aggregation *Blood Decrease Physiological* Like aspirin inhibits platelet aggregation *1384*

Platelets *Blood Decrease Physiological* Has been reported to cause aplastic anemia *1384* Throbocytopenia reported as complication in less than 1% treated patients *4646*

Potassium *Serum Increase Physiological* Hyperkalemia reported as complication in less than 1% treated patients *4646*

Protein *Serum Decrease Physiological* Occasional reports of acute interstitial nephritis with hematuria, proteinuria and occasionally nephrotic syndrome *4646*
Urine Increase Physiological Occasional drug induced nephrotoxicity, with isolated azotemia, acute acute interstitial nephritis or nephrotic syndrome *4716* Occasional reports of acute interstitial nephritis with hematuria, proteinuria and occasionally nephrotic syndrome *4646*

Prothrombin Time *Plasma Increase Physiological* Probable interaction with warfarin when drugs coadministered *2625*

Thyroid Stimulating Hormone
Serum No Effect Physiological In 11 individuals treated with a mean dose of 20 mg/d for at least 3 weeks mean concentration of 1.4 ± 0.2 mU/L not significantly different from 1.5 ± 0.2 mU/L in 22 controls *585*

Thyroxine (T4) *Serum No Effect Analytical* Using the Ciba-Corning ACS:180 analyzer mean concentration not significantly changed in 1 specimen whose concentration differed by -1% compared with the concentration measured by the Amerlex-M method *5621*
Serum No Effect Physiological In 11 individuals treated with a mean dose of 20 mg/d mean concentration of 91 ± 5 nmol/L not significantly different from 94 ± 4 nmol/L in 22 controls *585*

Thyroxine (T4) Index, Free *Serum No Effect Physiological* In 11 individuals treated with a mean dose of 20 mg/d for at least 3 weeks mean of FTI 90 ± 5 not significantly different from 93 ± 4 in 22 controls *585*

Tri-iodothyronine (T3) *Serum No Effect Physiological* In 11 patients treated with 20 mg/d for at least 3 weeks mean concentration of 2.0 ± 0.2 nmol/L not different from 2.0 ± 0.1 nmol/L in 22 controls *585*

Urea Nitrogen *Serum Increase Physiological* Possible increase due to drug in some patients *6438* Increased concentration related to interstitial nephritis or nephrotic syndrome reported as complication in more than 1% treated patients *4646* Occasional increase noted not progressive *4465*

Uric Acid *Serum Increase Physiological* In patients with normal concentrations pretreatment. Variable effect in people with initial high concentrations *6438*

Pizotyline

Fatty Acids (FFA), Free *Serum No Effect Physiological* No effect after 2 mg i.v *5738*

Glucose *Serum Decrease Physiological* 10% reduction after 3-5 h with 2 mg i.v *5738*

Insulin *Plasma No Effect Physiological* No effect after 2 mg i.v *5738*

PK-11195

Glucaric Acid *Urine Increase Physiological* Twofold increase observed in excretion of D-glucaric acid in 16 healthy men and women volunteers when treated with 400 mg/day for 5 days with increase continuing as long as drug treatment continued *1954*

γ-Glutamyltransferase *Serum Increase Physiological* Twofold increase in 16 healthy men and women volunteers given 400 mg/day for 5 days with elevation persisting as long as drug continued *1954*

6-β-Hydroxycortisol *Urine Increase Physiological* 3.5 fold increase observed in 16 healthy men and women on 5th day of treatment with 400 mg/day orally remaining increased as long as treatment continued but reverting to normal with withdrawal of drug *1954*

Plantago Ovata

Cholesterol *Serum No Effect Physiological* Insignificant reduction observed in 9 hyperlipoproteinemic individuals treated with 30 g/day for 11 days compared with low fiber diet *4027*

Cholesterol, Free *Serum Decrease Physiological* Reduction from mean of 2.1 mmol/L to 1.9 mmol/L in 9 hyperlipoproteinemic individuals treated with 30 g/day for 11 days compared with low fiber diet *4027*

HDL-Cholesterol *Serum Increase Physiological* Significant increase from mean of 1.0 mmol/L to 1.2 mmol/L in 9 patients with hyperlipoproteinemia when treated with 30 g/day for 11 days when compared against low fiber treatment *4027*

LDL-Cholesterol *Serum Decrease Physiological* Significant reduction from mean of 6.6 mmol/L to 6.0 mmol/L in 9 patients with hyperlipoproteinemia treated with 30 g/day for 11 days compared with low fiber treatment *4027*

Triglycerides *Serum No Effect Physiological* Insignificant reduction in 9 hyperlipoproteinemic individuals treated with 30 g/day for 11 days compared with low fiber diet *4027*

Plaunotol

Amylase *Pancreatic Fluid Increase Physiological* In 8 healthy volunteers intrajejunal injection of doses from 80 to 320 mg/30 min caused nondose related but significant increase *5528*

Bicarbonate *Pancreatic Fluid Increase Physiological* In 8 healthy volunteers intrajejunal injection of doses from 80 to 320 mg/30 min caused significant increase and correlated well with plasma secretin concentration *5528*

Secretin *Plasma Increase Physiological* Intrajejunal injection of doses from 80 to 320 mg/30 min in 8 healthy volunteers caused significant increase in dose related manner *5528*

Plicamycin

Alanine Aminotransferase *Serum Increase Physiological* Abnormal results have been associated with treatment *1384* Hepatocellular damage observed *128* Consistent moderate increase in most cases *3949*

Alkaline Phosphatase *Serum Increase Physiological* Noted in approximately 50% of treated patients *3949*

Aspartate Aminotransferase *Serum Increase Physiological* Consistent moderate increase in most cases *3949* Hepatocellular damage observed *128* Abnormal results have been associated with treatment *1384*

Bleeding Time *Patient Increase Physiological* Observed in association with hemorrhagic diathesis *1384* Reversible effect *128*

Calcium *Serum Decrease Physiological* Reported to often be decreased *1384* Inhibition of bone resorption of calcium *5600*

Urine Increase Physiological Inhibition of bone resorption of calcium *5600*

Clot Retraction *Blood Decrease Physiological* Reversible poor retraction *128*

Clotting Time *Blood Increase Physiological* Reversible effect *128*

Creatinine *Serum Increase Physiological* Nephrotoxic effect *128* Abnormal results have been associated with treatment *1384*

Factor II *Plasma Decrease Physiological* Observed in association with bleeding diathesis *1384*

Factor V *Plasma Decrease Physiological* Observed in association with hemorrhagic diathesis *1384*

Factor VII *Plasma Decrease Physiological* Observed in association with hemorrhagic diathesis *1384*

Factor X *Plasma Decrease Physiological* Observed in association with hemorrhagic diathesis *1384*

Hemoglobin *Blood Decrease Physiological* Reversible effect *128*

Hydroxyproline *Urine Decrease Physiological* Inhibition of bone resorption of calcium *5600*

Lactate Dehydrogenase *Serum Increase Physiological* Hepatocellular damage observed *128*

Leukocytes *Blood Decrease Physiological* Observed less frequently than thrombocytopenia *1384* Reversible effect *128*

Phosphate *Serum Decrease Physiological* Inhibition of bone resorption of calcium *5600*

Platelets *Blood Decrease Physiological* Dose related bleeding syndrome with hemorrhagic diathesis observed: first manifestation often epistaxis *1384* Thrombocytopenia *128*

Potassium *Serum Decrease Physiological* Depression of level reported *128*

Protein *Urine Increase Physiological* Nephrotoxic effect *128*

Prothrombin Time *Plasma Increase Physiological* Reversible decreased prothrombin level *128*

Urea Nitrogen *Serum Increase Physiological* Nephrotoxic effect *128* Abnormal results have been associated with treatment *1384*

Poliovirus Vaccine

Platelets *Blood Decrease Physiological* May rarely cause thrombocytopenia *4014*

Protein *Cerebrospinal Fluid Increase Physiological* May rarely cause Guaillain-Barre syndrome *4014*

Polyestradiol Phosphate

Cholesterol *Serum No Effect Physiological* In 17 prostatic cancer patients treatment with up to 160 mg/month for 6 months had no effect on concentration *247*

HDL_2-Cholesterol *Serum Increase Physiological* In 17 men with prostatic cancer treatment with up to 160 mg/month for 6 months caused an average 26% increase *247*

HDL-Cholesterol *Serum Increase Physiological* In 17 men with prostatic cancer treatment with up to 160 mg/month for 6 months caused an average 11% increase *247*

LDL-Triglycerides *Serum Decrease Physiological* In 17 men with prostatic cancer treatment with up to 160 mg/month for 6 months caused an average 27% decrease *247*

Triglycerides *Serum Decrease Physiological* In 17 men with prostatic cancer treatment with up to 160 mg/month for 6 months caused an average 24% decrease *247*

Polymethylmethacrylate

γ-Glutamyltransferase *Serum Increase Physiological* 11 of 90 total hip arthroplasty and 7 of 23 knee arthroplasty patients had abnormal GGT increases 5-10 d post-surgery: not observed in controls *4969*

Polymyxin B

Creatinine *Serum No Effect Analytical* No effect of concentrations up to 15 mg/L on single slide method on Kodak Ektachem® *5706*

Polystyrene Sulfonate

Calcium *Feces Increase Physiological* Causes impaired absorption *1714*

Serum Decrease Physiological Exchanged for potassium, increased fecal loss *3810* May also cause hypocalcemia as it reduces plasma potassium concentration in patients with hyperkalemia *5253*

Serum Increase Physiological Increased administered calcium (if in calcium form) *5869*

Potassium *Serum Decrease Physiological* Exchanges for sodium (if sodium form used) *3810* Therapeutic intent in patients with hyperkalemia *5253*

Sodium *Serum Increase Physiological* May cause sodium retention as it reduces plasma potassium concentration in patients with hyperkalemia *5253*

Polysucrose

Protein *Test Conditions Increase Analytical* Affects Lowry, Folin-Ciocalteu procedures *3626*

Polythiazide

Alanine Aminotransferase *Serum Increase Physiological* May affect liver function *3810*

Alkaline Phosphatase *Serum Increase Physiological* May affect liver function *3810*

Amylase *Serum Increase Physiological* Rare pancreatitis reported with other thiazides *2754*

Antidiuretic Hormone *Plasma Increase Physiological* Secreted in response to hyponatremia *1856*

Aspartate Aminotransferase *Serum Increase Physiological* May affect liver function *3810*

Bicarbonate *Serum Increase Physiological* Metabolic alkalosis with marked diuresis *1856*

Urine Increase Physiological But effect minimal *2754*

Bile *Urine Increase Physiological* May affect liver function *3810*

Bilirubin *Serum Increase Physiological* May affect liver function *3810*

BSP Retention *Serum Increase Physiological* May affect liver function *3810*

Calcium *Feces Decrease Physiological* Accentuates positive calcium balance *4014*

Serum Increase Physiological May be increased by up to 0.35 mEq/L *4014*

Urine Decrease Physiological Excretion decreased by up to 50% *4014*

Chloride *Serum Decrease Physiological* Diuretic effect *1856*

Cholesterol *Serum Increase Physiological* 4% change in 20 people when treated only with drug for less tan 1 y *2957*

Citrate *Urine Decrease Physiological* Excretion decreased by up to 30% *4014*

Creatinine *Serum No Effect Analytical* No interference observed with liquid chromatographic method of Paroni *4540*

Glucose *Serum Increase Physiological* Diabetogenic action *3810*

Urine Increase Physiological Consequence of hyperglycemia *3810*

Polythiazide *(continued)*

Glucose Tolerance *Serum Decrease Physiological* Impaired tolerance may occur *2754*

HDL-Cholesterol *Serum No Effect Physiological* Not significant change in 20 people when treated only with drug for less than 1 year *2957*

LDL-Cholesterol *Serum No Effect Physiological* Not significant change in 20 people when treated only with drug for less than 1 year *2957*

Leukocytes *Blood Decrease Physiological* Rare reported side effect *2754*

Neutrophils *Blood Decrease Physiological* Rare reported side effect *2754*

Osmolality *Serum Decrease Physiological* ADH secretion with hyponatremia *1856*

Platelets *Blood Decrease Physiological* With/without purpura may occur *2754*

Potassium *Serum Decrease Physiological* Diuretic action *1856*

Sodium *Serum Decrease Physiological* Diuretic action, with potassium deficiency *1856* Severe hyponatremia noted in one patient with mild hypertension *260*
Urine Increase Physiological Therapeutic intent (peak effect at 6 h) *2754*

Triglycerides *Serum Increase Physiological* 14% change in 20 people when treated only with drug for less than 1 y *2957*

Uric Acid *Serum Increase Physiological* Due to impaired renal clearance *2754*

VLDL-Cholesterol *Serum No Effect Physiological* Not significant change in 20 people when treated only with drug for less than 1 year *2957*

POMP

Amino Acids *Urine No Effect Physiological* Mean excretion of 21.2 mmol/d in 10 patients with leukemia undergoing chemotherapy not different from 29.1 ± 23.4 mmol/d in 52 patients with acute leukemia and 19.8 ± 10.4 mmol/d in 29 healthy controls of both sexes *6517*

Ponsinomycin

Carbamazepine *Serum Increase Physiological* Inhibits metabolism and increases plasma concentration *3118* In healthy volunteers 13% increase (statistically significant) in area under curve observed but 26% decrease in active 10,11-epoxycarbamazepine metabolite. Tendency to increase in area under curve of unbound carbamazepine, although not significant *1145*

Cyclosporine *Blood Increase Physiological* Coadministration of ponsinomycin with cyclosporine caused a 2-fold increase in the area under the concentration-time curve and in nadir blood concentration *859*
Serum Increase Physiological Coadministration of ponsinomycin with cyclosporine caused a 2-fold increase in the area under the concentration-time curve and in nadir blood concentration *859*

Posterior Pituitary

Basal Metabolic Rate *Patient Increase Physiological* Temporary effect after injection *409*

Potassium Aminobenzoate

Glucose *Serum Decrease Physiological* Reported effect *3810*

Potassium Bromide

Bromide *Serum Increase Physiological* Theoretical possibility since compound contains 67% bromide *5116*

Potassium Chlorate

Methemoglobin *Blood Increase Physiological* May cause hemolytic anemia *4017*

Potassium Iodide

Amylase *Serum Increase Physiological* Parotitis reported as result of treatment *2754*

Eosinophils *Blood Increase Physiological* Allergic response *2549*

Leukocytes *Blood Increase Physiological* Due to eosinophilia *3810*

Orthophosphate *Test Conditions Decrease Analytical* Total inhibition at 0.1 mol/L on method of Horder *2713*

Platelets *Blood Decrease Physiological* Thrombocytopenia reported to occur *2385*

Thyroid Stimulating Hormone
Serum Increase Physiological Increase by 2.3 µU/mL over 11 d in normals *6148*

Thyroxine (T4) *Serum Decrease Physiological* In normals by 1 µg/dL over 11 d *6148*

Tri-iodothyronine (T3) *Serum Decrease Physiological* In normals by 15 ng/dL over 11 d *6148*

Potassium Perchlorate

Cortisol *Plasma No Effect Analytical* At a concentration of 300 mg/L had no significant effect on Enzymun method *1097*

Practolol

Alkaline Phosphatase *Serum Increase Physiological* After 4 y treatment 2 cases of primary biliary cirrhosis *768*

Bilirubin *Serum Increase Physiological* After 4 y treatment 2 cases of primary biliary cirrhosis *768*

Cholesterol *Serum No Effect Physiological* Insignificant changes in 2 studies of 2 weeks and 6 mo *2953*

Triglycerides *Serum Increase Physiological* Increase by 8 to 16% in 2 studies of 2 weeks to 6 mo respectively *2953*

Pralidoxime

Alanine Aminotransferase *Serum Increase Physiological* Increased activity observed in one of six normal volunteers given 1200 mg pralidoxime intramuscularly and in 4 of 6 given 1800 mg intramuscularly. Activity returned to normal after 2 weeks *6567*

Aspartate Aminotransferase *Serum Increase Physiological* Increased activity observed in one of six normal volunteers given 1200 mg pralidoxime intramuscularly and in 4 of 6 given 1800 mg intramuscularly. Activity returned to normal after 2 weeks *6567*

Pramipexole

Carbidopa *Serum No Effect Physiological* Coadministration of pramipexole with carbidopa did affect its AUC or its elimination *4680*

Creatine Kinase *Serum Increase Physiological* Increased activity (10,631 U/L) observed in a single patient with Parkinson's disease aged 49 years *4680*

Levodopa *Serum Increase Physiological* Coadministration of pramipexole with levodopa/carbidopa caused an increase in the maximal concentration of levodopa of 40% and a decrease in its T_{max} 2.5 to 0.5 h *4680*

Prasterone

Alanine Aminotransferase
Red Blood Cells Decrease Physiological Effect observed when given orally *3645*

Estriol *Urine Increase Physiological* SO_4 compound also affects if i.v. or oral in pregnant women *54*

Pravastatin

Alanine Aminotransferase *Serum Increase Physiological* In 82 patients with primary hypercholesterolemia treatment with 40 mg/d for 16 weeks caused increased enzyme activity in 2 (3.5%) *5140* In 359 hypercholesterolemic patients under age 65 years treatment for 48 weeks caused 14% increase, whereas in 44 individuals older than 65 years activity increased by only 6% *3945* Occasional toxicity observed *3924* In 39 patients with hypercholesterolemia treatment with 40 mg/d caused significant increases of 11.9% and 22.0% after 2 and 8 weeks respectively and nonsignificant increase of 5.6% after 4 weeks *1271*
Serum No Effect Physiological In 91 patients with type 2 diabetes mellitus treatment pravastatin caused nonsignificant change from mean baseline of 20.2 ± 1.4 U/L to 21.6 ± 2.5 U/L after 4 weeks and 19.9 ± 1.7 U/L after 12 weeks *5961*

Albumin *Serum No Effect Physiological* In 16 patients with type II hyperproteinemia mean value of 41 ± 3 g/L not significantly changed to 40 ± 2 g/L following treatment with 10-15 mg/d for an average of 10.2 weeks *6083*

Aldosterone *Plasma Increase Physiological* In 35 hypercholesterolemic patients treated with up to 80 mg/d caused increase from mean baseline of 8.7 ± 0.8 ng/dL to 9.9 ± 1.1 ng/dL *1451*

Alkaline Phosphatase *Serum No Effect Physiological* In 91 patients with type 2 diabetes mellitus treatment pravastatin caused nonsignificant change from mean baseline of 161.9 ± 7.2 U/L to 162.8 ± 11.5 U/L after 4 weeks and 162.3 ± 8.8 U/L after 12 weeks *5961*

γ-Aminotransferase *Serum No Effect Physiological* In 91 patients with type 2 diabetes mellitus treatment pravastatin caused nonsignificant change from mean baseline of 29.9 ± 4.0 U/L to 33.4 ± 6.5 U/L after 4 weeks and 25.7 ± 4.3 U/L after 12 weeks *5961*

Androstenedione *Plasma No Effect Physiological* In a group of patients with heterozygous familial hypercholesterolemia treatment for 12 weeks had no significant effect on concentration *2912*

Apolipoprotein A-I *Serum Decrease Physiological* In 24 hypercholesterolemic patients treatment with up to 40 mg/d for 18 weeks caused significant decrease from mean baseline of 140.5 ± 4.7 mg/dL to 131.7 ± 5.1 mg/dL *3599* Treatment of 7 patients with familial hypercholesterolemia with 40 mg/d for 4 weeks was associated with nonsignificant reduction from mean of 166 ± 13 mg/dL to 146 ± 11 mg/dL *6208* In 75 patients with coronary artery disease treatment with up to 40 mg/d for 3 years caused an insignificant change from mean baseline of 162.2 ± 4.29 mg/dL to 151.5 ± 2.86 mg/dL after 3 years *835*
Serum Increase Physiological In 16 patients with primary hypercholesterolemia treatment with 10 mg/d for 8 weeks caused significant increase from mean baseline of 133.3 ± 19.1 mg/dL to 140.5 ± 16.8 mg/dL *988* Slight increase observed with treatment with 40 mg/d for 12 weeks *372* In 79 patients treatment for 12 weeks caused significant reduction from mean baseline of 137 mg/dL to 155 mg/dL and to 156 mg/dL after 48 weeks *2779* In 18 patients with primary hypercholesterolemia mean concentration increased from mean baseline of 142 ± 6 mg/dL to 152 ± 7 mg/dL (7%) after treatment with 20 mg/d for 4 weeks and to 150 ± 6 mg/dL (6%) after a further 4 weeks treatment with 40 mg/d *2862* Mean increase of 7% in 10 patients with gallstone disease treated with 40 mg daily for 3 weeks *4904* In 82 patients with primary hypercholesterolemia treatment with 40 mg/d for 16 weeks caused 10% increase from mean baseline of 118 mg/dL to 130 mg/dL *5140* In 137 diabetic patients with hypercholesterolemia treatment for 12 weeks caused 4 mg/dL increase from mean baseline of 133 mg/dL and in 51 nondiabetic patients caused increase of 10 mg/dL from baseline of 136 mg/dL *3080* In 63-69 patients with hypercholesterolemia treatment for 12 weeks caused increase from mean baseline of 1.45 ± 0.04 g/L to 1.50 ± 0.04 g/L (3.3%) *6463*
Serum No Effect Physiological No significant effect of treatment with 40 mg daily for 16 weeks in 9 patients with familial hypercholesterolemia *1930* No significant effect observed in 30 patients with type IIa or IIb hyperlipoproteinemia treated with up to 40 mg daily for 24 weeks *5302* In 30 patients with familial defective apolipoprotein B-100 treatment with 40 mg/d for 8 weeks caused an insignificant change from mean baseline of 1.09 ± 0.03 g/L to 1.08 ± 0.02 g/L *2445*

Apolipoprotein A-II *Serum Decrease Physiological* Slight effect observed with treatment with 40 mg/d for 12 weeks *372*
Serum Increase Physiological In 16 patients with primary hypercholesterolemia treatment with 10 mg/d for 8 weeks caused significant increase from mean baseline of 34.0 ± 4.2 mg/dL to 36.1 ± 5.1 mg/dL *988* In 24 hypercholesterolemic patients treatment with up to 40 mg/d caused significant increase from mean baseline of 39.6 ± 2.2 mg/dL to 44.0 ± 2.1 mg/dL *3599*
Serum No Effect Physiological In 79 patients treated for 12 weeks significant increase to 43 mg/dL from mean baseline of 38 mg/dL and nonsignificant reduction to 37 mg/dL after 48 weeks *2779* No significant change observed in 30 patients with type IIa or IIb hyperlipoproteinemia treated with up to 40 mg daily for 24 weeks *5302* In 18 patients with primary hypercholesterolemia treatment with 20 mg/d for 4 weeks caused insignificant change from mean baseline of 70 ± 3 mg/dL to 70 ± 4 mg/dL and to 66 ± 2 mg/dL after 40 mg/d for another 4 weeks *2862* No significant effect of treatment with 40 mg daily for 16 weeks in 9 patients with familial hypercholesterolemia *1930*

Apolipoprotein B *Serum Decrease Physiological* In 16 patients with primary hypercholesterolemia treatment with 10 mg/d for 8 weeks caused significant reduction from mean baseline of 168.6 ± 22.2 mg/dL to 141.3 ± 19.8 mg/dL *988* Significant reduction from mean of 283 mg/dL to 211 mg/dL in 9 patients with familial hypercholesterolemia after treatment with 40 mg daily for 16 weeks *1930* In 137 diabetic patients with hypercholesterolemia treatment for 12 weeks caused 21 mg/dL decrease from mean baseline of 126 mg/dL and in 51 nondiabetic patients caused reduction of 23 mg/dL from baseline of 127 mg/dL *3080* In 18 patients with primary hypercholesterolemia treatment with 20 mg/d for 4 weeks caused significant reduction from 235 ± 12 mg/dL to 192 ± 9 mg/dL (18%), and with 40 mg/d for another 4 weeks concentration decreased to 174 ± 7 mg/dL (26% reduction) *2862* In 79 patients treatment for 12 weeks caused significant reduction from mean baseline of 148 mg/dL to 119 mg/dL which decreased further to 99 mg/dL after 48 weeks *2779* In 10 patients with heterozygous familial hypercholesterolemia treatment with 40 mg/d for 6 months caused mean decrease of 29.1% *2002* In one study of 77 hypercholesterolemic patients treatment with 20 mg/d for 16 weeks caused a 17% reduction in concentration *4534* In 75 patients with coronary artery disease treatment with up to 40 mg/d for 3 years caused a significant change from mean baseline of 122.9 ± 4.08 mg/dL to 92.4 ± 2.70 mg/dL after 3 years *835* Reduction of 27.7 - 37.4% observed with 4-12 weeks treatment with 40 mg/d *372* Reduction of 27.7-37.4% observed with 4-12 weeks treatment with 40 mg/d *372* In 24 hypercholesterolemic patients treatment with up to 40 mg/dL for 18 weeks caused significant decrease from mean baseline of 150.8 ± 5.4 mg/dL to 116.7 ± 4.7 mg/dL *3599* In normocholesterolemic individuals treatment for 10 days with 20 mg/day caused reduction of 18%, with 40 mg/day 24% and with 80 mg/day 37% reduction *4493* In 13 patients with heterozygous familial hypercholesterolemiawith and without ileal bypass surgery treatment with 40 mg daily for 4 weeks caused mean decrease of 34% in those without and 31% in those with bypass surgery *4491* Mean reduction of 29% in 10 pateints with gallstone disease treated with 40 mg daily for 3 weeks *4904* Reduction of 23% in 30 patients with type IIa or IIb hyperlipoproteinemia treated with up to 40 mg daily for 24 weeks *5302* Treatment of 7 patients with familial hypercholesterolemia without ileal bypass with 40 mg/d for 4 weeks was associated with significant reduction from mean baseline of 201 ± 12 mg/dL to 132 ± 8 mg/dL *6208* In 63-69 patients with hypercholesterolemia treatment for 12 weeks caused significant decrease from mean baseline of 1.56 ± 0.06 g/L to 1.13 ± 0.04 g/L (28.8%) *6463* In 30 patients with familial defective apolipoprotein B-100 treatment with 40 mg/d for 8 weeks caused a significant change from mean baseline of 1.55 ± 0.06 g/L to 1.22 ± 0.05 g/L *2445*

Apolipoprotein B-100 *Serum Decrease Physiological* In 82 patients with primary hypercholesterolemia given first 20 mg/d for 8 weeks then 40 mg/d for 8 weeks mean concentration by 23% (from 118 mg/dL to 91 mg/dL) *5140*

Pravastatin *(continued)*

Apolipoprotein B:Apolipoprotein A-I Ratio
Serum Decrease Physiological In 137 diabetic patients with hypercholesterolemia treatment for 12 weeks caused 0.20 decrease from mean baseline of 1.00 and in 51 nondiabetic patients caused reduction of 0.24 from baseline of 0.98 *3080*

Apolipoprotein C-III *Serum Decrease Physiological* Slight effect observed with treatment with 40 mg/d for 12 weeks *372*

Apolipoprotein E *Serum Decrease Physiological* In 18 patients with primary hypercholesterolemia treatment with 20 mg/d for 4 weeks caused reduction from mean baseline of 26 ± 2 mg/dL to 23 ± 12 mg/dL (12%, nonsignificant) and significantly to 20 ± 1 mg/dL (23%) after a further 4 weeks treatment with 40 mg/d *2862* Mean reduction of 16% observed in 30 patients with type IIa or IIb hyperlipoproteinemia treated with up to 40 mg daily for 24 weeks *5302* Slight effect observed with treatment with 40 mg/d for 12 weeks *372*
Serum No Effect Physiological In 16 patients with primary hypercholesterolemia treatment with 10 mg/d for 8 weeks caused nonsignificant change from mean baseline of 4.5 ± 2.0 mg/dL to 4.7 ± 1.3 mg/dL *988*

Apolipoprotein Lp(a) *Serum Increase Physiological* In 30 patients with familial defective apolipoprotein B-100 treatment with 40 mg/d for 8 weeks caused an insignificant change from mean baseline of 9.22 mg/dL to 10.13 mg/dL *2445*

Aspartate Aminotransferase *Serum Increase Physiological* In 359 hypercholesterolemic patients under age 65 years treatment for 48 weeks caused mean 20% increase in activity and in 53 aged over 65 years mean increase of 17% observed *3945* In 39 patients with hypercholesterolemia treatment with 40 mg/d caused nonsignificant increases of 7.1%, 5.6% and 9.6% after 2, 4 and 8 weeks respectively *1271*
Serum No Effect Physiological In 91 patients with type 2 diabetes mellitus treatment pravastatin caused nonsignificant change from mean baseline of 19.6 ± 0.9 U/L to 23.8 ± 2.4 U/L after 4 weeks and 21.1 ± 2.0 U/L after 12 weeks *5961*

Bile Acids *Bile Decrease Physiological* Concentration reduced to about 60% of basal values after a single oral dose of 80 mg *4175*
Feces Decrease Physiological In 7 patients with familial hypercholesterolemia treatment with 40 mg/d for 4 weeks caused significant decrease from mean 7.2 ± 1.8 mg/kg/d to 4.8 ± 0.6 mg/d/kg *6208*

Bilirubin *Serum No Effect Physiological* In 91 patients with type 2 diabetes mellitus treatment pravastatin caused nonsignificant change from mean baseline of 0.6 ± 0.03 mg/dL to 1.0 ± 0.26 mg/dL after 4 weeks and 0.7 ± 0.06 mg/dL after 12 weeks *5961*

Campesterol *Serum Increase Physiological* In 7 patients with familial hypercholesterolemia treatment with 40 mg/d caused significant increase from mean baseline of 201 ± 18 100 x mmol/mol cholesterol of 39 ± 15, 21 ± 9 and 43 ± 16 100 x mmol/mol cholesterol after 1, 2 and 4 weeks respectively *6209*

Cholestanol *Feces No Effect Physiological* In 7 patients with familial hypercholesterolemia treatment with 40 mg/d for 4 weeks caused nonsignificant reduction from mean 0.18 ± 0.02 mg/d/kg to 0.16 ± 0.02 mg/d/kg *6208*
Serum No Effect Physiological In 7 patients with familial hypercholesterolemia treatment with 40 mg/d caused insignificant increase from mean baseline of 99 ± 10 100 x mmol/mol cholesterol by 8 ± 7, 7 ± 9 and 15 ± 7 100 x mmol/mol cholesterol after 1, 2 and 4 weeks respectively *6209* In 7 patients with familial hypercholesterolemia treatment with 40 mg/d 4 weeks caused insignificant reduction from mean baseline concentration of δ8-cholestenol of 42 ± 21 100 x mmol/mol cholesterol *6209*

Cholesterol *Bile Decrease Physiological* In patients with biliary fistula significant reduction to about 70% of basal concentration observed between 5 and 7 hours after a single oral dose of 80 mg *4175*
Serum Decrease Physiological Mean reduction of 26% in 10 patients with gallstone disease treated with 40 mg daily for 3 weeks *4904* In 13 patients with heterozygous familial hypercholesterolemia with and without ileal bypass surgery treatment with 40 mg daily for 4 weeks caused mean decrease of 25% in those without bypass surgery and 35% in those without *4491* In 58 patients with types IIa and IIb primary hypercholesterolemia treated with up to 40 mg/d pravastatin for 12 weeks mean concentration fell from 364 mg/dL to 281 mg/dL *245* Concentration reduced by mean of 22% in 30 patients with type IIa or IIb hyperlipoproteinemia treated with up to 40 mg daily for 24 weeks *5302* Treatment of 31 hypercholesterolemic patients for 4 weeks with 24 mg cholestyramine daily and 10-40 mg/d pravastatin caused decrease of about 50% *4491* In 90 individuals aged 64 - 90 y with primary (type II) hypercholesterolemia treatment with up to 40 mg/d caused significant change (-21.9%) from mean baseline of 271.6 ± 28.2 mg/dL to 213.6 ± 31.1 mg/dL after 16 weeks *5266* In 33 hypercholesterolemic patients treatment for 4 weeks with 10, 20 and 40 mg daily caused mean decreases of 17%, 20% and 24% respectively *4491* In 450 patients with coronary atherosclerosis treatment with pravastatin caused significant change from baseline of 6.02 mmol/L to 4.72 mmol/L after 2 months, 4.82 mmol/L after 12 months and 4.90 mmol/L after 24 months *2987* In 24 hypercholesterolemic patients treatment with up to 40 mg/d for 18 weeks caused significant reduction from mean baseline of 8.4 ± 0.3 mmol/L to 6.7 ± 0.2 mmol/L *3599* Concentration reduced by mean of 22% in 30 patients with type IIa or IIb hyperlipoprtoeinemia treated with up to 40 mg daily for 24 weeks *5302* In 10 normocholesterolemic patients with gallstone disease treatment with 40 mg daily for 3 weeks caused 26% reduction *4491* In 67 previously untreated type II hyperlipidemic patients treatment with 10 mg/d for 6 weeks caused significant reduction from mean baseline of 7.98 ± 1.25 mmol/L to 6.14 ± 1.05 mmol/L. In 32 treated with 20 mg/d mean concentration decreased from 9.50 ± 1.34 mmol/L to 6.83 ± 1.48 mmol/L *5806* In 39 patients with hypercholesterolemia treatment with 40 mg/d caused 19.6% decrease after 2 weeks, 23.2% decrease after 4 weeks and 23.1% after 8 weeks *1271* Treatment of 7 people with familial hypercholesterolemia without ileal bypass for 4 weeks with 40 mg/d caused significant decrease of 29% from mean baseline of 12.8 ± 0.7 mmol/L with return to baseline 4 weeks after treatment stopped *6208* In 9014 patients with a history of myocardial infarction or hospitalization for unstable angina treated with 40 mg/d 12% with cholesterol concentrations < 213 mg/dL, 13% with cholesterols between 213 and 250 mg/dL, and 12% with concentrations ≥251 mg/dL died compared with 14%, 17% and 16% with same concentrations in control group *5994* In 7 patients with familial hypercholesterolemia treatment with 40 mg/d caused significant decrease from mean baseline of 10.8 ± 0.75 mmol/L by 2.5 ± 0.34 mmol/L after 1 week, 3.5 ± 0.57 mmol/L after 2 weeks and 3.4 ± 0.54 mmol/L after 4 weeks *6209* In 51 patients with hypercholesterolemia treatment with 10 mg/d for more than 3 months caused reduction from mean baseline of 336 ± 58 mg/dL to 231 ± 37 mg/dL *6286* In 16 patients with type II hyperproteinemia mean concentration of 270 mg/dL pretreatment significantly reduced to 225 mg/dL following treatment with 10 - 15 mg/d for an average of 10.2 weeks *6083* In 16 patients with primary hypercholesterolemia treatment with 10 mg/d for 8 weeks caused significant reduction from mean baseline of 264.9 ± 22.4 mg/dL to 225.3 ± 21.2 mg/dL *988* In the Cholesterol and Recurrent Events Trial of 4,159 patients treatment with 40 mg/d for 5.0 years caused mean decrease of 20% and the West of Scotland Trial of 6,595 patients treatment with 40 mg/d for 4.9 years caused mean decrease of 20% *3115* In 23 patients with hypercholesterolemia resistant to dietary modification treatment for one year caused 22% reduction in concentration *1452* In 10 patients with heterozygous familial hypercholesterolemia treatment with 40 mg/d for 6 months caused mean decrease of 19.7% *2002* In patients with nephrotic syndrome treatment with 20 mg pravastatin caused a 22% decrease in concentration *4440* In 82 patients with primary hypercholesterolemia 20 mg/d pravastatin for 8 weeks caused mean reduction of 20% (from 6.85 mmol/L to 5.48 mmol/L). When given 40 mg/d for another 8 weeks concentration reduced to 5.30 mmol/L *5140* In healthy normocholesterolemic individuals treatment for 10 days with 20 mg/day caused reduction of 18%, with 40 mg/day caused 23% reduction and with 80 mg/day 30% reduction *4493* In 75 patients with coronary artery disease treatment with up to 40 mg/d for 3 years caused a change from mean baseline of 236 mg/dL to 186 mg/dL after 3 years *835* In 63-69 patients with hypercholesterolemia treatment for 12 weeks caused significant reduction from mean baseline of 7.41 ± 0.13 mmol/L to 5.44 ± 0.11 mmol/L (26.25%) *6463* 20% reduction observed in in 20 patients with types IIa and IIb hyperlipidemias treated with 10-

20 mg/d for 8 to 16 weeks *2716* After 4 weeks of treatment with doses of from 5 mg to 40 mg daily total cholesterol decreased significantly by mean of 17 to 24% in 33 patients with primary hypercholesterolemia. Effect enhanced when cholestyramine also administered *4492* In one study of 77 hypercholesterolemic patients treatment with 20 mg/d for 16 weeks caused a 17% reduction in concentration *4534* Dose-dependent reductions of 14.3-25.1% in 150 patients with primary hypercholesterolemia treated with doses from 5-40 mg/d for 8 weeks *2974* In 79 patients treated for 12 weeks mean concentration decreased significantly from mean baseline of 302 mg/L to 249 mg/dL after 12 weeks treatment and 225 mg/dL after 48 weeks *2779* Significant reduction from mean of 425 mg/dL to 325 mg/dL in 9 patients with familial hypercholesterolemia treated with 40 mg daily for 16 weeks *1930* In 6 patients with IDDM treatment for 1 year caused significant decrease from mean baseline of 231 mg/dL to 165 mg/dL *4104* In 18 patients with primary hypercholesterolemia treatment with 20 mg/d for 4 weeks caused significant decrease from mean baseline of 9.66 ± 0.43 mmol/L to 7.76 ± 0.38 mmol/L (20%) and to 7.36 ± 0.26 mmol/L (24%) after another 4 weeks of treatment with 40 mg/d *2862* In 7 hyperlipidemic men treatment with 40 mg/d for 48 weeks caused a 22.6% decrease from mean baseline of 260 mg/dL to 201 mg/dL *1450* In 20 patients with type IIa hypercholesterolemia treatment with 40 mg/d for 4 weeks caused mean 23% decrease from mean baseline of 301 ± 40 mg/dL *4033* In 30 patients with familial defective apolipoprotein B-100 treatment with 40 mg/d for 8 weeks caused a significant change from mean baseline of 8.30 ± 0.27 mmol/L to 6.62 ± 0.20 mmol/L *2445* In 10 patients with primary moderate hypercholesterolemia reduced concentration by 25% compared with placebo *6220* 20 mg/d for 8-16 weeks reduced serum cholesterol in hypercholesterolemic patients caused reduction from mean baseline of 286.2 ± 2.6 mg/dL to 230.7 ± 2.3 mg/dL (19%) in nonelderly patients and from 288.5 ± 8.7 mg/dL to 234.5 ± 7.8 mg/dL (19%) in elderly. 40 mg/d reduced serum cholesterol from 309.0 ± 3.6 mg/dL to 238.2 ± 3.3 mg/dL (23%) in the nonelderly and from 298.4 ± 6.5 mg/dL to 223.6 ± 6.3 mg/dL (23%) in the elderly. With 48 weeks treatment 25% reduction observed in both elderly and nonelderly *3945* In 137 diabetic patients with hypercholesterolemia treatment for 12 weeks caused 50 mg/dL decrease from mean baseline of 261 mg/dL and in 51 nondiabetic patients caused reduction of 55 mg/dL from baseline of 269 mg/dL *3080*

Serum Increase Physiological In 10 patients with recent pancreatic transplants (6 with kidney transplants also) treatment with pravastatin (mean 11.7 ± 0.8 mg/d) initiated 250 ± 53 days after the transplant and continued for an average of 143 ± 18 days caused a significant decrease from 278 ± 10 mg/dL to 231 ± 10 mg/dL comparable to the preoperative concentration *100*

Cholesterol Ester Transfer Protein
Serum No Effect Physiological In 16 patients with primary hypercholesterolemia treatment with 10 mg/d for 8 weeks caused nonsignificant increase from mean baseline of 2.42 ± 0.70 µg/mL to 2.54 ± 1.07 µg/mL *988*

Cholesterol:HDL-Cholesterol Ratio
Serum Decrease Physiological In 20 patients with type IIa hypercholesterolemia treatment with 40 mg/d for 4 weeks caused mean decrease of 28% *4033* In 137 diabetic patients with hypercholesterolemia treatment for 12 weeks caused 1.4 decrease from mean baseline of 5.7 and in 51 nondiabetic patients caused reduction of 1.4 from baseline of 5.5 *3080*

Corticotropin *Plasma Decrease Physiological* Significant decrease from mean baseline concentration of 42.4 ng/L to 30.8 ng/L in 12 hypercholesterolemic men treated with 40 mg/d for 24 years *1859* In 35 hypercholesterolemic patients treated with up to 80 mg/d for 12 months caused reduction from 69.0 ± 7.6 pg/mL to 48.2 ± 4.8 pg/mL *1451*

Cortisol *Plasma Decrease Physiological* In 35 hypercholesterolemic patients treatment with up to 80 mg/d caused nonsignificant reduction from mean baseline of 14.3 ± 0.9 µg/dL to 12.3 ± 0.7 µg/dL *1451*
Plasma No Effect Physiological Nonsignificant reduction from mean baseline of 15.5 µg/dL to 14.4 µg/dL in 12 male hypercholesterolemic patients after treatment with 40 mg/d for 24 months *1859*

Cortisol response to Tetracosactrin
Plasma No Effect Physiological In 12 patients with heterozygous familial hypercholesterolemia receiving pravastatin for 12 weeks no change observed in response compared with controls *2912*

C-Reactive Protein *Serum No Effect Physiological* No consistent change observed in 14 hypercholesterolemic patients treated over 2 years *1858*

Creatine Kinase *Serum Increase Physiological* In 39 patients with hypercholesterolemia treatment with 40 mg/d caused nonsignificant increases of 6.0% and 4.2% after 2 and 4 weeks respectively but nonsignificant 2.0% decrease after 8 weeks *1271* Minor transient increase observed in some patients *3924* In 359 hypercholesterolemic patients aged less than 65 years treatment for 48 weeks caused significant 4% *3945*
Serum No Effect Physiological In 53 hypercholesterolemic patients aged 65 years or more treatment for 48 weeks caused nonsignificant 2% increase *3945* In 91 patients with type 2 diabetes mellitus treatment pravastatin caused nonsignificant change from mean baseline of 61.3 ± 4.4 U/L to 52.6 ± 5.3 U/L after 4 weeks and 73.4 ± 6.3 U/L after 12 weeks *5961*

Creatine Kinase Isoenzymes *Serum Increase Physiological* In 82 patients with primary hypercholesterolemia treatment with 40 mg/d for 16 weeks was associated with increased CK-MM in 3 (5.3%) *5140*

Creatinine *Serum No Effect Physiological* In 412 hypercholesterolemic patients treatment for 48 weeks caused no significant change *3945* In 91 patients with type 2 diabetes mellitus treatment pravastatin caused nonsignificant change from mean baseline of 0.9 ± 0.03 mg/dL to 0.8 ± 0.07 mg/dL after 4 weeks and 0.8 ± 0.06 mg/dL after 12 weeks *5961*

Creatinine Clearance *Urine No Effect Physiological* In 14 normolipidemic patients treated with 20 mg/d for 17 days nonsignificant change from mean baseline of 117.95 ± 27.09 mL/min to 122.83 ± 43.99 mL/min observed *2725*

Cyclosporine *Serum No Effect Physiological* Concurrent administration of cyclosporine with pravastatin caused no meaningful increase in the plasma cyclosporine concentration *728*

D-Dimer *Plasma Decrease Physiological* In 51 patients with hypercholesterolemia treatment with 10 mg/d for at least 3 months caused significant reduction from mean baseline of 114 ± 60 ng/mL to 57 ± 38 ng/mL *6286*

Dehydroepiandrosterone Sulfate
Plasma No Effect Physiological In a group of patients with heterozygous familial hypercholesterolemia treatment for 12 weeks had no significant effect on concentration *2912* In 35 hypercholesterolemic patients treatment for 12 months with up to 80 mg/d caused nonsignificant change from mean baseline of 101.6 ± 12.6 µg/dL to 101.1 ± 13.2 µg/dL *1451*

Desmosterol *Serum Decrease Physiological* In 7 patients with familial hypercholesterolemia significant reductions from mean baseline of 62 ± 24 100 x mmol/mol cholesterol observed of 15 ± 6, 21 ± 6 and 16 ± 6 100 x mmol/mol cholesterol after 1, 2 and 4 weeks respectively with treatment with 40 mg/d *6209*

Dolichol *Serum Decrease Physiological* Small but significant decrease of 16% observed after 12 weeks of treatment in 6 patients with heterozygous familial hypercholesterolemia *1725*

Erythrocytes *Blood No Effect Physiological* In 91 patients with type 2 diabetes mellitus treatment pravastatin caused nonsignificant change from mean baseline of 4.52 ± 0.05 million/µL to 4.45 ± 0.10 million/µL after 4 weeks and 4.48 ± 0.09 million/µL after 12 weeks *5961*

Estradiol *Plasma Decrease Physiological* In 12 hypercholesterolemic women treatment with 40 mg/d for 6 months caused reduction from mean baseline of 24.6 ± 10.3 pg/mL to 17.1 ± 6.0 pg/mL *1451*
Plasma No Effect Physiological In a group of patients with heterozygous familial hypercholesterolemia treatment for 12 weeks had no significant effect on concentration *2912* In 22 hypercholesterolemic men treatment with 40 mg/d for 6 months caused nonsignificant change from mean baseline of 28.8 ± 3.3 pg/mL to 27.2 ± 2.7 pg/mL *1451*

Pravastatin *(continued)*

Fibrin Degradation Products
Plasma No Effect Physiological In 51 patients with hypercholesterolemia treatment with 10 mg/d for at least 3 months caused nonsignificant change in fibrin degradation products concentration from mean baseline of 3.7 ± 1.4 µg/dL to 3.4 ± 0.9 µg/dL *6286*

Fibrinogen *Plasma Decrease Physiological* In 16 patients with type II hyperproteinemia mean concentration of 270 mg/dL significantly reduced to 309 mg/dL following treatment with 10 - 15 mg/d for an average of 10.2 weeks *6083*
Plasma No Effect Physiological In 51 patients with hypercholesterolemia treatment with 10 mg/d for at least 3 months caused nonsignificant reduction from 349 ± 101 mg/dL to 328 ± 112 mg/dL *6286*

Fibrinopeptide A *Plasma Decrease Physiological* In 51 patients with hypercholesterolemia treatment with 10 mg/d for at least 3 months caused significant reduction from mean baseline of 5.06 ± 6.42 ng/mL to 2.27 ± 2.11 ng/mL *6286*

Follicle Stimulating Hormone
Plasma Decrease Physiological Significant reduction from mean baseline concentration of 6.7 U/L to 5.9 U/L in 12 hypercholesterolemic men treated with 40 mg/d for 24 months *1859* Significant reduction from mean baseline concentration of 6.7 IU/L to 5.9 IU/L in 12 hypercholesterolemic men treated with 40 mg/d for 24 months *1859*
Plasma Increase Physiological In 22 hypercholesterolemic men treatment with 40 mg/d for 6 months caused increase from mean baseline of 4.8 ± 0.7 mIU/mL to 11.2 ± 6.8 mIU/mL *1451*
Plasma No Effect Physiological In 12 hypercholesterolemic women treatment with 40 mg/d for 6 months caused nonsignificant change from mean baseline of 37.3 ± 4.1 IU/mL to 37.7 ± 4.9 mIU/mL *1451*

Glucose *Serum Increase Physiological* In 412 hypercholesterolemic patients treatment for 48 weeks caused significant 2% mean increase in those under age 65 years and nonsignificant increase of 3% in those over age 65 years *3945*
Serum No Effect Physiological In 137 diabetic patients with hypercholesterolemia treatment for 12 weeks caused no significant change from mean baseline of 150 ± 4 mg/dL to 153 ± 5 mg/dL and in 51 nondiabetic patients caused no significant change from baseline of 99 ± 2 mg/dL to 103 ± 2 mg/dL *3080* In 91 patients with type 2 diabetes mellitus treatment pravastatin caused nonsignificant change from mean baseline of 147 ± 7.4 mg/dL to 149 ± 8.5 mg/dL after 4 weeks and 135 ± 7.2 mg/dL after 12 weeks *5961*

HDL_2-Cholesterol *Serum Decrease Physiological* In 75 patients with coronary artery disease treatment with up to 40 mg/d for 3 years caused a significant change from mean baseline of 7.29 ± 0.51 mg/dL to 6.14 ± 0.24 mg/dL after 3 years *835*
Serum Increase Physiological In 82 patients with primary hypercholesterolemia treatment with 40 mg/d for 16 weeks caused 60% increase from mean baseline of 0.13 mmol/L to 0.21 mmol/L *5140* In 16 patients with primary hypercholesterolemia treatment with 10 mg/d for 8 weeks caused nonsignificant decrease from mean baseline of 10.2 ± 4.7 mg/dL to 9.2 ± 4.4 mg/dL *988*
Serum No Effect Physiological No significant change in 9 patients with familial hypercholesterolemia following 16 weeks treatment with 40 mg daily *1930*

HDL_3-Cholesterol *Serum Increase Physiological* In 82 patients with primary hypercholesterolemia treatment with 40 mg/d for 16 weeks caused 7% increase from mean baseline of 0.98 mg/dL to 1.06 mg/dL *5140* In 16 patients with primary hypercholesterolemia treatment with 10 mg/d for 8 weeks caused significant increase from mean baseline of 39.1 ± 8.2 mg/dL to 41.4 ± 6.0 mg/dL *988*
Serum No Effect Physiological No significant change in 9 patients with familial hypercholesterolemia following treatment with 40 mg daily for 16 weeks *1930* In 75 patients with coronary artery disease treatment with up to 40 mg/d for 3 years caused an insignificant change from mean baseline of 35.4 ± 0.79 mg/dL to 34.8 ± 0.47 mg/dL after 3 years *835*

HDL-Cholesterol *Serum Increase Physiological* Treatment of 33 hypercholesterolemic patients for 4 weeks with 10, 20 and 40 mg daily caused mean increases of 8-9% *4491* In 31 hypercholesterolemic patients treatment for 4 weeks with 24 mg cholestyramine and 10-40 mg pravastatin daily caused mean increase of 11-18% *4491* Increase by mean of 8 to 9% in 33 patients with primary hypercholesterolemia treated with doses from 5 mg to 40 mg daily for 4 weeks. Effect enhanced when cholestyramine coadministered *4492* In 450 patients with coronary atherosclerosis treatment with pravastatin caused significant change from baseline of 0.93 mmol/L to 1.03 mmol/L after 2 months, 1.05 mmol/L after 12 months and 1.01 mmol/L after 24 months *2987* In hypercholesterolemic patients 20 mg/d for 8-16 weeks caused 5% increase in nonelderly and 6% increase in elderly: with 40 mg/d 7% increase observed in nonelderly and 10% increase in elderly. Treatment for 48 weeks caused 7% increase in nonelderly and 8% increase in elderly *3945* Consistent non-dose-dependent increase observed with treatment of both familial and nonfamilial hypercholesterolemia *3924* Treatment of 10 normocholesterolemic patients with gallstone disease with 40 mg daily for 3 weeks caused mean increase of 27% *4491* Slight increase observed with treatment with 40 mg/d for 12 weeks *372* Mean increase of 24% in 10 patients with gallstone disease treated with 40 mg daily for 3 weeks *4904* In 82 patients with primary hypercholesterolemia treatment with 40 mg/d for 16 weeks caused 11% increase from mean baseline of 1.22 mmol/L to 1.24 mmol/L *5140* In one study of 77 hypercholesteroleic patients treatment with 20 mg/d for 16 weeks caused a 8% increase in concentration *4534* Mean increases of up to 11.7% observed in 150 patients with primary hypercholesterolemia treated with doses of from 5 mg/d to 40 mg/d for 8 weeks *2974* In 90 individuals aged 64 - 90 y with primary (type II) hypercholesterolemia treatment with up to 40 mg/d caused significant increase (11.3%) from mean baseline of 50.2 ± 12.6 mg/dL to 55.4 ± 14.2 mg/dL after 16 weeks *5266* In 79 patients treatment caused significant increase from mean baseline of 46 mg/dL to 49 mg/dL after 12 weeks and 49 mg/dL after 48 weeks *2779* In 7 hyperlipidemic men treatment with 40 mg/d for 48 weeks caused a 4.0% increase from mean baseline of 43.6 mg/dL to 45.4 mg/dL *1450* Treatment of 13 patients with primary hypercholesterolemia for 6 weeks with 40 mg daily caused mean increase of 2% *4491* In 137 diabetic patients with hypercholesterolemia treatment for 12 weeks caused 2.8 mg/dL increase from mean baseline of 51.0 mg/dL and in 51 nondiabetic patients caused increase of 3.8 mg/dL from baseline of 53.0 mg/dL *3080* In 58 patients with primary hypercholesterolemia types IIa or IIb treatment with up to 40 mg/d for 12 weeks caused mean increase of 8.4% *245* In 9014 patients with a history of myocardial infarction or hospitalization for unstable angina treated with 40 mg/d 13% with HDL-cholesterol concentrations < 39 mg/dL and 10% with concentrations ≥39 mg/dL died compared with 17% and 14% with same concentrations in control group *5994* In the Cholesterol and Recurrent Events Trial of 4,159 patients treatment with 40 mg/d for 5.0 years caused mean increase of 5% and the West of Scotland Trial of 6,595 patients treatment with 40 mg/d for 4.9 years caused mean increase of 5% *3115* Mean increase of 11% in 30 patients with type IIa or IIb hyperlipoproteinemia treated with up to 40 mg daily for 24 weeks *5302* In 63-69 patients with hypercholesterolemia treatment for 12 weeks caused significant increase from mean baseline of 1.25 ± 0.05 mmol/L to 1.32 ± 0.04 mmol/L (5.9%) *6463* In patients with nephrotic syndrome treatment with 20 mg pravastatin caused a increasing trend in concentration *4440* In 39 patients with hypercholesterolemia treatment with 40 mg/d caused increase of 3.4% after 2 weeks, 8.3% after 4 weeks and 13.5% after 8 weeks *1271* In 7 patients with familial hypercholesterolemia treatment with 40 mg/d for 4 weeks caused nonsignificant increase from mean of 1.23 ± 0.16 mmol/L to 1.34 ± 0.16 mmol/L *6208* In 67 patients with type II hyperlipidemia treatment with 10 mg/d for 6 weeks caused nonsignificant increase from 1.13 ± 0.39 mmol/L to 1.14 ± 0.32 mmol/L but significant increase from 1.09 ± 0.36 mmol/L to 1.18 ± 0.35 mmol/L observed when 32 patients treated with 20 mg/d for 6 weeks *5806* Mean concentration of 52.7 ± 14.4 mg/dL in 51 patients with hypercholesterolemia increased to 57.5 ± 14.1 mg/dL after treatment with 10 mg/d for more than 3 months *6286*
Serum No Effect Physiological In 18 patients with primary hypercholesterolemia treatment with either 20 or 40 mg/d for 4 weeks caused no significant change from mean baseline of 1.16 ± 0.09 mmol/L *2862* No significant change observed in 9 patients with familial hypercholesterolemia treated with 40 mg daily for 16 weeks *1930* In 7 patients with familial hypercholesterolemia treatment with 40 mg/d for 4 weeks caused insignificant change from mean baseline of 0.14 ± 0.02

mmol/L to 0.12 ± 0.01 mmol/L *6208* In 10 patients with recent pancreatic transplants (6 with kidney transplants also) treatment with pravastatin (mean 11.7 ± 0.8 mg/d) initiated 250 ± 53 days after the transplant and continued for an average of 143 ± 18 days caused a nonsignificant decrease from 63 ± 6 mg/dL to 61 ± 5 mg/dL *100* No significant effect observed in 20 patients with types IIa and IIb hyperlipidemias treated with 10-20 mg/d for 8-16 weeks *2716* In 24 hypercholesterolemic patients treatment with up to 40 mg/d for 18 weeks caused nonsignificant increase from mean baseline of 1.1 ± 0.1 mmol/L to 1.2 ± 0.1 mmol/L *3599* In 16 patients with type II hyperproteinemia mean concentration of 44 mg/dL following treatment with 10 - 15 mg/d for an average of 10.2 weeks *6083* In 30 patients with familial defective apolipoprotein B-100 treatment with 40 mg/d for 8 weeks caused no significant change from mean baseline of 1.33 ± 0.07 mmol/L to 1.38 ± 0.07 mmol/L *2445* In 16 patients with primary hypercholesterolemia treatment with 10 mg/d for 8 weeks caused nonsignificant change from mean baseline of 49.5 ± 12.1 mg/dL to 50.8 ± 10.2 mg/dL *988* In 75 patients with coronary artery disease treatment with up to 40 mg/d for 3 years caused an insignificant change from mean baseline of 42.3 ± 1.11 mg/dL to 40.7 ± 0.42 mg/dL after 3 years *835* In 23 patients with dietary-resistant hypercholesterolemia treatment for one year had no significant effect *1452* In 10 patients with heterozygous familial hypercholesterolemia treatment with 40 mg/d for 6 months had no significant effect on concentration *2002* In 7 patients with familial hypercholesterolemia treatment with 40 mg/ for 1 week caused insignificant reduction of 0.08 ± 0.08 mmol/L from mean baseline of 1.29 ± 0.18 mmol/L, and by 0.05 ± 0.05 mmol/L after 2 weeks and increase of 0.05 ± 0.10 mmol/L after 4 weeks *3235*

HDL-Triglycerides *Serum Increase Physiological* In 16 patients with primary hypercholesterolemia treatment with 10 mg/d for 8 weeks caused significant increase from mean baseline of 9.6 ± 3.2 mg/dL to 11.2 ± 3.0 mg/dL *988*

Hematocrit *Blood No Effect Physiological* In 12 patients with type II hyperproteinemia mean value of 41.9 ± 2.9% not significantly changed to 40.9 ± 3.3% following treatment with 5-19 mg/d for an average of 13.9 weeks *6083* In 16 patients with type II hyperproteinemia mean value of 42.6 ± 3.3% not significantly changed to 41.9 ± 4.0% following treatment with 10-15 mg/d for an average of 10.2 weeks *6083* In 91 patients with type 2 diabetes mellitus treatment pravastatin caused nonsignificant change from mean baseline of 41.1 ± 0.6% to 41.0 ± 0.9% after 4 weeks and 41.6 ± 0.7% after 12 weeks *5961*

Hemoglobin *Blood No Effect Physiological* In 91 patients with type 2 diabetes mellitus treatment pravastatin caused nonsignificant change from mean baseline of 138 ± 2 g/L to 133 ± 3 g/L after 4 weeks and 138 ± 2 g/L after 12 weeks *5961*

Hemoglobin A_{1c} *Blood Decrease Physiological* In 91 patients with type 2 diabetes mellitus treatment pravastatin caused nonsignificant change from mean baseline of 8.5 ± 1.4% to 8.2 ± 1.2% after 4 weeks and 8.1 ± 1.2% (significant) after 12 weeks *5961*

Blood No Effect Physiological In 137 diabetic patients with hypercholesterolemia treatment for 12 weeks caused no significant change from mean baseline of 7.8 ± 0.1% to 7.6± 0.1% and in 51 nondiabetic patients caused no significant change from baseline of 6.3 ± 0.1% to 6.4 ± 0.1% *3080*

17-Hydroxycorticosteroids *Urine No Effect Physiological* In 14 normolipidemic patients treatment with 20 mg/d for 17 days caused nonsignificant increase from mean baseline of 5.92 ± 2.12 mg/d to 6.95 ± 3.11 mg/d *2725*

6-β-Hydroxycortisol *Urine Increase Physiological* In 14 normolipidemic patients treated with 20 mg/d for 17 days caused nonsignificant increase from mean baseline of 281.6 ± 142.6 μg/d to 318.6 ± 179.4 μg/d *2725*

17-Hydroxyprogesterone *Plasma No Effect Physiological* In a group of patients with heterozygous familial hypercholesterolemia treatment for 12 weeks had no significant effect on concentration of 17α-hydroxyprogesterone *2912*

IDL-Cholesterol *Serum Decrease Physiological* In 7 patients with familial hypercholesterolemia treatment with 40 mg/d for 4 weeks caused reduction from mean of 0.50 ± 0.10 mmol/L to 0.34 ± 0.05 mmol/L *6208* Reduced concentration by 47% in 10 patients with primary moderate hypercholesterolemia compared with placebo-treated controls *6220*

IDL-Triglycerides *Serum Decrease Physiological* In 7 patients with familail hypercholesterolemia treatment with 40 mg/d for 4 weeks was associated with nonsignificant reduction from mean 0.13 ± 0.03 mmol/L to 0.08 ± 0.01 mmol/L *6208*

Lactate Dehydrogenase *Serum No Effect Physiological* In 91 patients with type 2 diabetes mellitus treatment pravastatin caused nonsignificant change from mean baseline of 345.4 ± 7.8 U/L to 372.7 ± 15.4 U/L after 4 weeks and 354.9 ± 8.8 U/L after 12 weeks *5961*

Lanostanol *Feces Decrease Physiological* In 7 patients with familial hypercholesterolemia treatment with 40 mg/d for 4 weeks caused significant reduction from mean 0.12 ± 0.02 mg/d/kg to 0.08 ± 0.01 mg/d/kg *6208*

Lathosterol *Feces Decrease Physiological* In 7 patients with familial hypercholesterolemia treatment with 40 mg/d for 4 weeks caused significant decrease from mean of 0.16 ± 0.04 mg/d/kg to 0.10 ± 0.02 mg/d/kg *6208*

Serum Decrease Physiological Treatment of 6 patients with heterozygous familial hypercholesterolemia for 12 weeks with pravastatin caused mean decrease of 46% *1725* Decrease of free latherosterol from mean of 2.4 mg/L to 0.9 mg/L in 9 patients with gallstone disease treated with 40 mg daily for 3 weeks. Ratio of free latherosterol to free cholesterol reduced by 47% *4904* In 7 patients with familial hypercholesterolemia treated with 40 mg/d significant reduction from mean baseline of 248 ± 102 100 x mmol/mol cholesterol of 101 ±33, 96 ± 41, and 73 ± 31 100 x mmol/mol cholesterol observed after 1,2 and 4 weeks respectively *6209*

LDL-Cholesterol *Serum Decrease Physiological* In 63-69 patients with hypercholesterolemia treatment for 12 weeks caused significant reduction from mean baseline of 5.19 ± 0.14 mmol/L to 3.44 ± 0.11 mmol/L (33.54%) *6463* Compared with placebo reduced concentration in 10 patients with primary moderate hypercholesterolemia by 29% *6220* Reduction from baseline by 27% in 30 patients with type IIa or IIb hyperlipoproteinemia treated with up to 40 mg daily for 24 weeks *5302* In 7 patients with familial hypercholesterolemia treatment with 40 mg/d for 4 weeks caused significant reduction of 34% from mean baseline of 7.47 ± 0.71 mmol/L to 4.90 ± 0.34 mmol/L *6208* In 67 patients with type II hyperlipidemia treatment with 10 mg/d for 6 weeks caused significant decrease from mean baseline of 5.91 ± 0.95 mmol/L to 4.30 ± 0.96 mmol/L. In 32 treated with 20 mg/d mean concentration decreased from 7.65 ± 1.33 mmol/L to 4.98 ± 1.53 mmol/L *5806* In 90 individuals aged 64 - 90 y with primary (type II) hypercholesterolemia treatment with up to 40 mg/d caused significant change (-30.9%) from mean baseline of 198.4 ± 23.6 mg/dL to 138.7 ± 24.4 mg/dL after 16 weeks *5266* In 30 patients with familial defective apolipoprotein B-100 treatment with 40 mg/d for 8 weeks caused a significant change from mean baseline of 6.25 ± 0.25 mmol/L to 4.64 ± 0.18 mmol/L *2445* In 51 patients with hypercholesterolemia treatment with 10 mg/d for at least 3 months was associated with decrease from mean baseline of 231 ± 51 mg/dL to 131 ± 45 mg/dL *6286* In 137 diabetic patients with hypercholesterolemia treatment for 12 weeks caused 46 mg/dL decrease from mean baseline of 175 mg/dL and in 51 nondiabetic patients caused reduction of 56 mg/dL from baseline of 189 mg/dL *3080* In 7 patients with familial hypercholesterolemia treatment with 40 mg/d caused significant reduction from mean baseline of 8.3 ± 0.70 mmol/L by 1.7 ± 0.44 mmol/L after 1 week, 2.6 ± 0.52 mmol/L after 2 weeks, and 3.0 ± 0.44 mmol/L after 4 weeks *3235* In 82 patients with primary hypercholesterolemia treatment with 20 mg/d for 8 weeks caused mean 28% reduction from 5.17 mmol/L to 3.75 mmol/L. When given 40 mg/d for another 8 weeks mean concentration reduced by 31% to 3.59 mmol/L *5140* Mean reduction of 39% in 10 patients with gallstone disease treated with 40 mg daily for 3 weeks *4904* When combined with 24 mg cholestyramine daily treatment of 31 hypercholesterolemic patients with 10-40 mg daily for 4 weeks caused mean decrease of 47-56% *4491* In 450 patients with coronary atherosclerosis treatment with pravastatin caused significant change from baseline of 4.30 mmol/L to 2.95 mmol/L after 2 months, 3.04 mmol/L after 12 months and 3.24 mmol/L after 24 months *2987* In 75 patients with coronary artery disease treatment with up to 40 mg/d for 3 years caused a change from mean baseline of 168 mg/dL to 120 mg/dL after 3 years *835* Treatment with 40 mg daily for 3 weeks in 10 normocholesterolemic patients with gallstone dis-

Pravastatin *(continued)*

LDL-Cholesterol *(continued)*
ease caused mean reduction of 38% *4491* Dose-dependent reductions of 19.2-34.1% with doses from 5-40 mg/d for 8 weeks in 150 patients with primary hypercholesterolemia *2974* In 7 hyperlipidemic men treatment with 40 mg/d for 48 weeks caused a 30.6% decrease from mean baseline of 186 mg/dL to 129 mg/dL *1450* Treatment for 6 weeks with 40 mg daily caused mean reduction of 36% in 13 patients with primary moderate hypercholesterolemia *4491* In 196 patients 8 weeks treatment with 40 mg once daily in the morning caused mean reduction of 30%, 40 mg once daily in the evening caused mean reduction of 33% and 20 mg b.i.d. once in the morning and once in the evening caused mean decrease of 34% *2777* In 10 patients with recent pancreatic transplants (6 with kidney transplants also) treatment with pravastatin (mean 11.7 ± 0.8 mg/d) initiated 250 ± 53 days after the transplant and continued for an average of 143 ± 18 days caused a significant decrease from 178 ± 7 mg/dL to 134 ± 8 mg/dL comparable to the pre-operative concentration *100* In 33 hypercholesterolemic patients with mean baseline concentration of 222 mg/dL treatment for 4 weeks with 10, 20 and 40 mg daily caused mean decreases of 23%, 28% and 35% respectively *4491* In one study of 77 hypercholesterolemic patients treatment with 20 mg/d for 16 weeks caused a 23% reduction in concentration *4534* In 18 hypercholesterolemic patients treatment for 4 weeks with 10 mg b.i.d. caused mean reduction of 28% and with 20 mg b.i.d. mean reduction of 35% *4491* In 10 patients with heterozygous familial hypercholesterolemia treatment with 40 mg/d for 6 months caused mean reduction of 25.4% *2002* In 18 hypercholesterolemic patients for 8 weeks treatment with either 20 or 40 mg in one dose each day caused decrease of 27% and 32% respectively *4491* In the Cholesterol and Recurrent Events Trial of 4,159 patients treatment with 40 mg/d for 5.0 years caused mean decrease of 28% and the West of Scotland Trial of 6,595 patients treatment with 40 mg/d for 4.9 years caused mean decrease of 26% *3115* In 58 patients with types IIa and IIb primary hypercholesterolemia 4 wk treatment with 20 mg/d decreased LDL-cholesterol to 190 mg/dL or less in 27 patients. With treatment up to 40 mg/d for 12 wk mean fell from 288 mg/dL to 206 mg/dL in all patients *245* In 9014 patients with a history of myocardial infarction or hospitalization for unstable angina treated with 40 mg/d 12% with LDL-cholesterol concentrations < 135 mg/dL, 12% with triglycerides between 135 and 173 mg/dL, and 13% with concentrations ≥174 mg/dL died compared with 14%, 16% and 18% with same concentrations in control group *5994* In 13 patients with heterozygous familial hypercholesterolemia with and without ileal bypass surgery 4 weeks treatment with 40 mg daily caused mean decrease of 29% in those without surgery and 47% in those with bypass surgery *4491* Treatment for 10 days in normocholesterolemic individuals caused 13% reduction with 20 mg/day, with 40 mg/day 28% and with 80 mg/day 40% reduction *4493* In 16 patients with primary hypercholesterolemia treatment with 10 mg/d for 8 weeks caused significant reduction from mean baseline of 184.9 ± 16.0 mg/dL to 151.5 ± 22.0 mg/dL *988* In 39 patients with hypercholesterolemia treatment with pravastatin 40 mg/d caused 25.3% decrease after 2 weeks, 30.7% after 4 weeks and 32.7% after 8 weeks *1271* Significant decrease by mean of 25 to 35% in 33 patients with primary hypercholesterolemia when treated with doses from 5 to 40 mg daily for 4 weeks. Effect increased 1.5 to 2.0 fold when cholestyramine coadministered *4492* In 20 patients with type IIa hypercholesterolemia treatment with 40 mg/d for 4 weeks caused mean 31% decrease from mean baseline of 212 ± 40 mg/dL *4033* In hypercholesterolemic patients treated with 20 mg/d for 8-16 weeks in nonelderly 27% reduction observed and in elderly 26%: with 40 mg/d reductions of 32% and 34% respectively observed. With treatment for 48 weeks reductions of 35% observed in both elderly and nonelderly *3945* In 35 hypercholesterolemic patients treatment with up to 80 mg/d for 12 months caused reduction from mean baseline of 42 ± 3% *1451* In patients with either familial or nonfamilial hypercholesterolemia reductions were on average 18% with 10 mg/d, 23% with 20 mg/d and 31% with 30 mg/d after 12 weeks *3924* In 23 patients with dietary-resistant hypercholesterolemia treatment for one year caused 30% reduction *1452* In 24 patients with hypercholesterolemia treated with up to 40 mg/d for 18 weeks significant decrease from mean baseline of 6.3 ± 0.3 mmol/L to 4.6 ± 0.2 mmol/L observed *3599* In 79 patients treatment for 12 weeks caused significant reduction to 173 mg/dL from mean baseline of 227 mg/dL and further reduction to 151 mg/dL after 48 weeks treatment *2779* Decrease of 26.2-30.7% observed with 4-12 weeks treatment with 40 mg/d *372* In 18 patients with primary hypercholesterolemia treatment with 20 mg/d for 4 weeks caused significant decrease from mean baseline of 7.95 ± 0.43 mmol/L to 6.00 ± 0.34 mmol/L (24%) and to 5.54 ± 0.26 mmol/L (30%) after another 4 weeks when treated with 40 mg/d *2862* Mean decrease of 30% observed in 6 patients with heterozygous familial hypercholesterolemia following treatment with 40 mg/d for 8 weeks *2702* In 6 patients with heterozygous familial hypercholesterolemia treatment with pravstatin for 12 weeks caused mean decrease of 27% *1725* Significant reduction from mean of 343 mg/dL to 246 mg/dL in 9 patients with familial hypercholesterolemia treated with 40 mg daily for 16 weeks *1930* In 6 patients with IDDM mean concentration significantly decreased from 157 mg/dL to 93 mg/dL with treatment for 1 year *2247*

LDL-Cholesterol:HDL-Cholesterol Ratio
Serum No Effect Physiological In 10 patients with recent pancreatic transplants (6 with kidney transplants also) treatment with pravastatin (mean 11.7 ± 0.8 mg/d) initiated 250 ± 53 days after the transplant and continued for an average of 143 ± 18 days caused a nonsignificant decrease from 3.0 ± 0.3 to 2.4 ± 0.3 *100*

LDL-Triglycerides *Serum Decrease Physiological* In 7 patients with familial hypercholesterolemia treatment with 40 mg/d for 4 weeks caused significant reduction from mean baseline of 0.45 ± 0.08 mg/dL to 0.30 ± 0.03 mmol/L *6208*

Leukocytes *Blood Decrease Physiological* In 91 patients with type 2 diabetes mellitus treatment pravastatin caused nonsignificant change from mean baseline of 6545 ± 185 /μL to 5294 ± 349 /μL after 4 weeks and 6550 ± 206 /μL after 12 weeks *5961*

Lipoprotein Lp(a) *Serum Decrease Physiological* In 75 patients with coronary artery disease treatment with up to 40 mg/d for 3 years caused an insignificant change from mean baseline of 32.0 ± 2.81 mg/dL to 28.9 ± 0.85 mg/dL after 3 years *835*
Serum Increase Physiological In 7 hyperlipidemic men treatment with 40 mg/d for 48 weeks caused a 9% increase from mean baseline of 15.6 mg/dL *1450*
Serum No Effect Physiological In 24 hypercholesterolemic patients treatment with up to 40 mg/d for 18 weeks had no effect on log concentration of 2.5 ± 9.1 U/L *3599* In 14 hypercholesterolemic patients treated over 2 years no significant change in concentration observed *1858* In 16 patients with primary hypercholesterolemia treatment with 10 mg/d for 8 weeks caused nonsinificant reduction from mean baseline of 44.6 ± 46.7 mg/dL to 41.6 ± 41.3 mg/dL *988* In 79 patients treated for 12 weeks nonsignificant reduction to 11.99 mg/dL observed from mean baseline of 12.04 mg/dL and nonsignificant increase to 12.33 mg/dL observed after 48 weeks treatment *2779* In 51 patients with hypercholesterolemia treatment with 10 mg/d for at least 3 months caused no significant change from mean baseline of 23.1 ± 18.0 mg/dL *6286*

Luteinizing Hormone *Plasma Decrease Physiological* Significant reduction from mean baseline of 8.8 IU/L to 5.1 IU/L in 12 hypercholesterolemic men treated with 40 mg/d for 24 months *1859*
Plasma No Effect Physiological In 12 hypercholesterolemic patients treatment with 40 mg/d for 6 months caused nonsignificant change from 34.8 ± 3.3 mIU/mL to 35.0 ± 4.7 mIU/mL and in 22 hypercholesterolemic men from 4.5 ± 0.6 mIU/mL to 4.1 ± 0.7 mIU/mL *1451*

Methylsterols *Serum Decrease Physiological* In 7 patients with familial hypercholesterolemia treatment with 40 mg/d for 4 weeks caused significant decrease from mean of 0.42 mmol/mol cholesterol to 0.30 mmol/mol cholesterol *6208*

Methylsterols, Esterified *Serum Decrease Physiological* In 7 patients with familial hypercholesterolemia treatment with 40 mg/d caused slight decrease from mean baseline of o.2 mmol/mol cholesterol to 0.1 mmol/mol cholesterol after 4 weeks *6208*

Methylsterols, Free *Serum Decrease Physiological* In 7 patients with familial hypercholesterolemia treatment with 40 mg/d caused significant reduction from mean 1.1 mmol/mol cholesterol to 0.35 mmol/mol cholesterol after 1 week with increase from nadir to 0.75 mmol/mol cholesterol after 2 weeks and 0.8 mmol/mol cholesterol after 4 weeks *6208*

Mevalonate *Urine Decrease Physiological* Administration of 10 mg on two occasions within 3 days to 9 healthy men caused a significant decrease from 2.32 ± 0.65 μmol/d to 1.47 ± 0.49 μmol/d in 105 healthy women *2620*

Neutral Steroids *Feces Decrease Physiological* In 7 patients with familial hypercholesterolemia treatment with 40 mg/d for 4 weeks caused nonsignificant decrease from mean of 12.3 ± 1.1 mg/d/kg to 10.5 ± 1.2 mg/d/kg *6208*

Partial Thromboplastin Time
Plasma No Effect Physiological In 51 patients with hypercholesterolemia treatment with 10 mg/d for at least 3 months caused nonsignificant change from mean baseline of 32.5 ± 5.7 s to 32.7 ± 6.1 s *6286*

Phospholipids *Bile Decrease Physiological* Concentration reduced to about 60% of basal concentration in patients with biliary fistula following a single oral dose of 80 mg *4175*
Serum Decrease Physiological Slight reduction in 33 patients with primary hypercholesterolemia when treated with doses of from 5 to 40 mg daily in 33 patients with primary hypercholesterolemia when treated for 4 weeks. Effect significantly increased when cholestyramine also given *4492*

Plasmin-α_2-Plasmin Inhibitor Complex
Plasma Increase Physiological In 51 patients with hypercholesterolemia treatment with 10 mg/d for at least 3 months caused significant increase from mean baseline of 0.53 ± 0.28 μg/mL to 0.83 ± 0.72 μg/mL *6286*

Plasminogen Activator Inhibitor-1
Plasma Decrease Physiological In 51 patients with hypercholesterolemia treatment with 10 mg/d for at least 3 months caused significant reduction from mean baseline of 69.6 ± 68.9 ng/mL to 30.4 ± 31.6 ng/mL *6286*

Platelets *Blood Decrease Physiological* In 91 patients with type 2 diabetes mellitus treatment pravastatin caused significant change from mean baseline of 25.8 ± 0.8 x 10^4/μL to 24.2 ± 1.3 x 10^4/μL after 4 weeks and 24.9 ± 0.8 x 10^4/μL (non-significant) after 12 weeks *5961*

Potassium *Serum No Effect Physiological* In 91 patients with type 2 diabetes mellitus treatment pravastatin caused non-significant change from mean baseline of 4.4 ± 0.05 mmol/L to 4.4 ± 0.04 mmol/L after 4 weeks and 5.0 ± 0.58 mmol/L after 12 weeks *5961*

Progesterone *Plasma Decrease Physiological* In 12 hypercholesterolemic women treatment with 40 mg/d for 6 months caused nonsignificant reduction from mean baseline of 0.19 ± 0.03 ng/dL to 0.17 ± 0.03 ng/dL and in 22 hypercholesterolemic men from 0.32 ± 0.04 ng/dL to 0.26 ± 0.02 ng/dL *1451*

Protein *Serum No Effect Physiological* In 12 patients with type II hyperproteinemia mean value of 74 ± 4 g/L not significantly changed to 70 ± 3 g/L following treatment with 5-19 mg/d for an average of 13.9 weeks *6083* In 91 patients with type 2 diabetes mellitus treatment pravastatin caused non-significant change from mean baseline of 72 ± 0.7 g/L to 71 ± 0.16 g/L after 4 weeks and 72 ± 0.9 g/L after 12 weeks *5961*

Prothrombin Time *Plasma No Effect Physiological* In 51 patients with hypercholesterolemia treatment with 10 mg/d for at least 3 months caused nonsignificant change from mean baseline of 12.0 ± 0.7 s to 12.1 ± 0.6 s *6286*

Renin Activity *Plasma Increase Physiological* In 35 hypercholesterolemic patients treatment with up to 80 mg/d for 12 months caused increase from mean baseline of 2.72 ± 0.24 ng/mL/h to 6.17 ± 3.45 ng/mL/h *1451*

Sex-Hormone Binding Globulin
Serum No Effect Physiological In a group of patients with heterozygous familial hypercholesterolemia treatment for 12 weeks had no significant effect on concentration *2912*

Sitosterol *Serum Increase Physiological* In 7 patients with familial hypercholesterolemia treatment with 40 mg/d caused increase from mean baseline of 146 ± 18 100 x mmol/mol cholesterol by 10 +/ 6, 9 ± 5 and 19 ± 6 100 x mmol/mol cholesterol respectively after 1, 2 and 4 weeks *6209*

Sodium *Serum No Effect Physiological* In 91 patients with type 2 diabetes mellitus treatment pravastatin caused non-significant change from mean baseline of 139.7 ± 0.3 mmol/L to 141.2 ± 0.5 mmol/L after 4 weeks and 140.7 ± 0.4 mmol/L after 12 weeks *5961*

Sperm Count *Semen Decrease Physiological* In 10 men treatment for 6 months with 40 mg/d caused significant reduction with return towards baseline after another 6 months *1451*

Squalene *Serum Decrease Physiological* In 7 patients with familial hypercholesterolemia treatment with 40 mg/d for 4 weeks caused insignificant decrease from 15 ± 4 x 10^2 mmol/L during treatment period to 12 ± x 10^2 mmol/L with return to pretreatment concentrations after 4 weeks without drug *6208*
Serum No Effect Physiological In 7 patients with familial hypercholesterolemia treatment with 40 mg/d for 4 weeks caused no significant change from mean baseline of 15 ± 4 100 x mmol/mol cholesterol *6209*

Steroids *Feces Decrease Physiological* In 7 patients with familial hypercholesterolemia treatment with 40 mg/d for 4 weeks caused significant decrease from mean of 19.4 ± 2.0 mg/d/kg to 15.2 ± 1.5 mg/d/kg *6208*

Testosterone *Serum Decrease Physiological* In 22 hypercholesterolemic men treatment with up to 80 mg/d caused reduction of concentration from mean baseline of 504 ng/dL to 460 ng/dL: reduction observed in 72% *1451* Significant reduction from mean baseline concentration of 4.9 μg/L to 4.2 μg/L in 12 hypercholesterolemic men after treatment with 40 mg/d for 24 months *1859*
Serum Increase Physiological In 12 hypercholesterolemic women treatment with 40 mg/d for 6 months caused increase from mean baseline of 16.3 ± 2.0 ng/dL to 18.8 ± 2.0 ng/dL *1451*
Serum No Effect Physiological In a group of patients with heterozygous familial hypercholesterolemia treatment for 12 weeks had no significant effect *2912*

Testosterone, Free *Serum Decrease Physiological* In 22 hypercholesterolemic men treatment with 40 mg/d for 6 months caused decrease from 17.2 ± 0.8 pg/mL to 15.6 ± 1.0 pg/mL and from 0.5 ± 0.1 pg/mL to 0.4 ± 0.1 pg/mL in 12 women *1451*

Thrombin/Antithrombin III Complex
Plasma Decrease Physiological Mean concentration in 51 patients with hypercholesterolemia treated with 10 mg/d for at least 3 months 8.45 ± 9.20 ng/mL significantly reduced to 2.85 ± 1.81 ng/mL *6286*

Thrombomodulin *Plasma Decrease Physiological* In 51 patients with hypercholesterolemia treatment with 10 mg/d for at least 3 months caused significant reduction from mean baseline of 4.44 ± 2.02 ng/mL to 2.23 ± 0.63 ng/mL *6286*

Tissue Plasminogen Activator
Plasma No Effect Physiological In 51 patients with hypercholesterolemia treatment with 10 mg/d for at least 3 months caused nonsignificant change from mean baseline of 12.1 ± 7.80 ng/mL to 12.3 ± 6.40 ng/mL *6286*

Triglyceride:LDL-Cholesterol Ratio
Serum Decrease Physiological In a group of hypertriglyceridemic patients treatment with 10 mg/d for 4 weeks caused an decrease in ratio to 1.13, with 20 mg/d causing an decrease to 0.92 and 40 mg/d an decrease to 0.98 *5796*

Triglycerides *Serum Decrease Physiological* In 30 patients with familial defective apolipoprotein B-100 treatment with 40 mg/d for 8 weeks caused a significant change from mean baseline of 1.37 mmol/L to 1.16 mmol/L *2445* In 16 patients with type II hyperproteinemia mean concentration of 251 mg/dL pretreatment significantly reduced to 182 mg/dL following treatment with 10 - 15 mg/d for an average of 10.2 weeks *6083* In 58 patients with types IIa or IIb primary hypercholesterolemia treatment with up to 40 mg/d for 12 weeks caused decrease of mean concentration from 168 mg/dL to 148 mg/dL *245* In 90 individuals aged 64 - 90 y with primary (type II) hypercholesterolemia treatment with up to 40 mg/d caused significant change (-16.7%) from mean baseline of 144.1 ± 41.5 mg/dL to 121.8 ± 39.1 mg/dL after 16 weeks *5266* In 79 patients treatment caused significant decrease from mean baseline of 124 mg/dL to 105 mg/dL after 12 weeks and 99 mg/dL after 48 weeks *2779* In 82 patients with primary hypercholesterolemia treatment with 40 mg/d for 16 weeks caused 20% reduction from mean baseline of 1.64 mmol/L to 1.31 mmol/L *5140* Mean reductions of up to 23.9% observed in 150 patients with primary hypercholesterolemia treated with

Pravastatin *(continued)*

Triglycerides *(continued)*

doses from 5 mg/d to 40 mg/d for 8 weeks *2974* In 75 patients with coronary artery disease treatment with up to 40 mg/d for 3 years caused an insignificant change from mean baseline of 160.2 ± 6.6 mg/dL to 154.5 ± 5.0 mg/dL after 3 years *835* In 450 patients with coronary atherosclerosis treatment with pravastatin caused significant change from baseline of 1.77 mmol/L to 1.65 mmol/L after 2 months, 1.60 mmol/L after 12 months and 1.46 mmol/L after 24 months *2987* In 137 diabetic patients with hypercholesterolemia treatment for 12 weeks caused 29 mg/dL decrease from mean baseline of 173 mg/dL and in 51 nondiabetic patients caused reduction of 17 mg/dL from baseline of 136 mg/dL *3080* In 63-69 patients with hypercholesterolemia treatment for 12 weeks caused significant decrease from mean baseline of 1.79 ± 0.10 mmol/L to 1.53 ± 0.08 mmol/L (14.2%) *6463* Treatment of 13 patients with primary moderate hypercholesterolemia for 6 weeks with 40 mg daily caused mean reduction of 19% *4491* In a group of hypertriglyceridemic patients treatment with 10 mg/d for 4 weeks caused significant 22% decrease, with 20 mg/d causing 25% decrease and 40 mg/d a 35% decrease *5796* In 51 patients with hypercholesterolemia treatment with 10 mg/d for at least 3 months was associated with reduction from mean baseline of 199 ± 178 mg/dL to 164 ± 158 mg/dL *6286* Treatment of 33 hypercholesterolemic patients for 4 weeks with 10, 20 or 40 mg daily caused mean decrease of 6-9% *4491* In 39 patients with hypercholesterolemia treatment with 40 mg/d caused decrease of 17.8% after 2 weeks, 18.9% after 4 weeks and 14.4% after 8 weeks *1271* In 7 hyperlipidemic men treatment with 40 mg/d for 48 weeks caused a 16.4% decrease from mean baseline of 136 mg/dL to 114 mg/dL *1450* In 9014 patients with a history of myocardial infarction or hospitalization for unstable angina treated with 40 mg/d 12% with triglyceride concentrations < 133 mg/dL, 12% with triglycerides between 133 and 230 mg/dL, and 14% with concentrations ≥231 mg/dL died compared with 16%, 15% and 18% with same concentrations in control group *5994* In 7 patients with familial hypercholesterolemia treatment with 40 mg/d caused insignificant reduction of 0.30 ± 0.27 mmol/L from mean baseline of 1.56 ± 0.37 mmol/L after 1 week, 0.68 ± 0.32 mmol/L after 2 weeks and by 0.49 ± 0.25 mmol/L after 4 weeks *6209* Treatment of 10 normocholesterolemic patients with gallstone disease with 40 mg daily for 3 weeks caused mean reduction of 14% *4491* In 7 patients with failial hypercholesterolemia treatment with 40 mg/d for 4 weeks was associated with nonsignificant reduction from mean 1.56 ± 0.37 mmol/L to 1.08 ± 0.17 mmol/L *6208* In the Cholesterol and Recurrent Events Trial of 4,159 patients treatment with 40 mg/d for 5.0 years caused mean decrease of 14% and the West of Scotland Trial of 6,595 patients treatment with 40 mg/d for 4.9 years caused mean decrease of 14% *3115* In one study of 77 hypercholesteroleic patients treatment with 20 mg/d for 16 weeks caused a 9% reduction in concentration *4534* Significant reduction from mean of 146 mg/dL to 127 mg/dL in 9 patients with familial hypercholesterolemia treated with 40 mg daily for 16 weeks *1930* In 16 patients with primary hypercholesterolemia treatment with 10 mg/d for 8 weeks caused nonsignificant decrease from mean baseline of 131.9 ± 59.7 mg/dL to 122.4 ± 49.3 mg/dL *988* In patients with nephrotic syndrome treatment with 20 mg pravastatin caused a decreasing trend in concentration *4440* In 10 patients with recent pancreatic transplants (6 with kidney transplants also) treatment with pravastatin (mean 11.7 ± 0.8 mg/d) initiated 250 ± 53 days after the transplant and continued for an average of 143 ± 18 days caused a nonsignificant decrease from 221 ± 37 mg/dL to 176 ± 32 mg/dL *100* Mean reduction of 15% in 10 patients with gallstone disease treated with 40 mg daily for 3 weeks *4904* Reduction by mean of 6 to 9% in 33 patients with primary hypercholesterolemia when treated with doses of from 5 to 40 mg daily for 4 weeks. Slight increase above baseline observed when cholestyramine coadministered *4492* In hypercholesterolemic patients treatment with 20 mg/d for 8-16 weeks caused 14% reduction in nonelderly and 15% reduction in elderly: with 40 mg/d reductions were 15% and 23% respectively. Treatment for 48 weeks caused 14% reduction in nonelderly and 13% in elderly *3945* In healthy normocholesterolemic individuals with 10 days treatment with 20 mg/day mean decrease of 9% observed, with 24% decrease with 40 mg/day and 26% decrease with 80 mg/day *4493* Consistent non-dose-dependent finding in patients with either familial or nonfamilial hypercholesterolemia *3924* Slight decrease observed with treatment over 12 weeks with 40 mg/d *372*

Serum No Effect Physiological No significant effect observed in 20 patients with types IIa and IIb hyperlipidemias treated with 10-20 mg/d for 8 to 16 weeks *2716* In 24 hypercholesterolemic patients treatment with up to 40 mg/d for 18 weeks caused nonsignificant change from mean baseline of 1.8 ± 0.2 mmol/L *3599* In 10 patients with heterozygous familial hypercholesterolemia with 40 mg/d for 6 months had no significant effect on concentration *2002* In 20 patients with type IIa hypercholesterolemia treatment with 40 mg/d for 4 weeks caused mean 2.7% increase from mean baseline of 150 ± 124 mg/dL *4033* In 18 patients with primary hypercholesterolemia treatment with up to 40 mg/d for 8 weeks caused insignificant decrease from mean baseline of 1.50 ± 0.15 mmol/L to 1.38 ± 0.13 mmol/L (8%) *2862* In 23 patients with dietary-resistant hypercholesterolemia treatment for one year had no significant effect *1452* In 82 patients with primary hypercholesterolemia treatment caused reduction but same effect observed when treated with placebo *5140* No significant change observed in 30 patients with type IIa or IIb hyperlipoproteinemia treated with up to 40 mg daily for 24 weeks *5302*

Ubiquinone *Serum Decrease Physiological* Treatment of 6 patients with heterozygous familial hypercholesterolemia for 12 weeks caused mean decrease of 29% *1725*

Ubiquinone Q_{10} *Serum Decrease Physiological* Treatment of 6 patients with heterozygous familial hypercholesterolemia for 12 weeks caused mean decrease of 29% *1725*

Urea Nitrogen *Serum No Effect Physiological* In 91 patients with type 2 diabetes mellitus treatment pravastatin caused nonsignificant change from mean baseline of 16.6 ± 0.5 mg/dL to 16.2 ± 0.7 mg/dL after 4 weeks and 17.6 ± 0.8 mg/dL after 12 weeks *5961*

Uric Acid *Serum No Effect Physiological* In 91 patients with type 2 diabetes mellitus treatment pravastatin caused nonsignificant change from mean baseline of 5.4 ± 0.2 mg/dL to 4.9 ± 0.3 mg/dL after 4 weeks and 5.0 ± 0.2 mg/dL after 12 weeks *5961*

Viscosity *Plasma Decrease Physiological* In 16 patients with type II hyperproteinemia mean viscosity of 1.39 mPa/s significantly reduced to 1.36 mPa/s following treatment with 10-15 mg/d for an average of 10.2 weeks *6083*

Vitamin D_3 *Serum Increase Physiological* Significant increase from mean baseline concentration of 36 pg/mL to 41 pg/mL in 12 hypercholesterolemic men treated with 40 mg/d for 24 months *1859*

VLDL-Cholesterol *Serum Decrease Physiological* Concentration reduced over 12 weeks with treatment with 40 mg/d *372* In 18 patients with primary hypercholesterolemia treatment with 20 mg/d for 4 weeks caused nonsignificant decrease (18%) from mean baseline of 0.56 ± 0.07 mmol/L to 0.46 ± 0.05 mmol/L but significant decrease (27%) to 0.41 ± 0.04 mmol/L after another 4 weeks treatment with 40 mg/d *2862* Insignificant reduction from mean of 31.0 mg/dL to 19.7 mg/dL in 9 patients with familial hypercholesterolemia treated with 40 mg daily for 16 weeks *1930* In 16 patients with primary hypercholesterolemia treatment with 10 mg/d for 8 weeks caused significant reduction from mean baseline of 30.1 ± 17.4 mg/dL to 22.4 ± 11.5 mg/dL *988* In 63-69 patients with hypercholesterolemia treatment for 12 weeks caused significant decrease from mean baseline of 0.63 ± 0.05 mmol/L to 0.49 mmol/L (21.9%) *6463* Reduced concentration by 31% in 10 patients with primary moderate hypercholesterolemia compared with placebo *6220* Mean decrease of 14% in 10 patients with gallstone disease treated with 40 mg daily for 3 weeks *4904* In 7 patients with familial hypercholesterolemia treatment with 40 mg/d for 4 weeks was associated with reduction from mean of 0.48 ± 0.19 mmol/L to 0.29 ± 0.08 mmol/L *6208*

Serum No Effect Physiological In 24 hypercholesterolemic patients treatment with up to 40 mg/d for 18 weeks caused nonsignificant decrease from 0.9 ± 0.1 mmol/L to 0.8 ± 0.1 mmol/L *3599*

VLDL-Triglycerides *Serum Decrease Physiological* Mean decrease of 28% in 10 patients with gallstone disease treated with 40 mg daily for 3 weeks *4904* In 16 patients with primary hypercholesterolemia treatment with 10 mg/d for 8 weeks caused nonsignificant decrease from mean baseline of 89.0 ±

51.0 mg/dL to 84.6 ± 43.0 mg/dL *988* In 7 patients with familial hypercholesterolemia treatment with 40 mg/d for 4 weeks caused nonsignificant decrease from mean of 0.76 ± 0.30 mmol/L to 0.50 ± 0.16 mmol/L *6208*

Serum No Effect Physiological In 18 patients with primary hypercholesterolemia treatment with up to 40 mg/d for 4 weeks caused nonsignificant reduction from mean baseline of 0.92 ± 0.16 mmol/L to 0.87 ± 0.09 mmol/L (5%) *2862* In 24 hypercholesterolemic patients treatment with up to 40 mg/d for 18 weeks caused nonsignificant decrease from mean baseline of 1.1 ± 0.2 mmol/L to 1.2 ± 0.2 mmol/L *3599*

Volume *Semen Decrease Physiological* In 10 hypercholesterolemic men treatment with 40 mg/d for 6 months caused significant decrease although values returned to baseline after another 6 months *1451*

von Willebrand Factor *Plasma No Effect Physiological* In 51 patients with hypercholesterolemia treatment with 10 mg/d for 3 months caused nonsignificant reduction from mean baseline of 123 ± 26% to 117 ± 23% *6286*

Warfarin *Plasma No Effect Physiological* Administration of pravastatin together with warfarin to 10 healthy men for 6 days caused no effect on the bioavailability of either compound *728*

Prazepam

Benzodiazepine *Urine Positive Analytical* At concentrations of 0.2 μg/mL or greater produces positive result with Syva EMIT II assay *1785*

Catecholamines *Plasma No Effect Analytical* No effect on HPLC method of Koller for dopamine, epinephrine and norepinephrine *3230*

Praziquantel

Alanine Aminotransferase *Serum Increase Physiological* Mild to moderate increases that are transient and reversible observed relatively infrequently *1384*

Albendazole *Serum Increase Physiological* 40 mg/kg praziquantel increased mean plasma concentration of albendazole and its AUC by about 10% in healthy people *5635*

Aspartate Aminotransferase *Serum Increase Physiological* Relatively rare reversible transient increases observed *1384*

Prazosin

Alanine Aminotransferase *Serum Increase Physiological* In fewer than 1% of treated patients liver function test abnormalities noted *4649*

Aldosterone *Plasma No Effect Physiological* No significant change with monotherapy for 12 mo in 15 patients *5919*

Alkaline Phosphatase *Serum Increase Physiological* In fewer than 1% of treated patients liver function test abnormalities noted *4649*

Serum No Effect Physiological No significant effect in 60 hypertensive patients treated with up to 8 mg daily for 20 weeks *5813*

Allopurinol *Serum No Effect Physiological* Coadministration of prazosin with allopurinol had no apparent adverse drug interaction in limited clinical experience *4649*

Amylase *Serum Increase Physiological* In fewer than 1% of treated patients pancreatitis noted but not unequivocally linked to administration of prazosin *4649*

Apolipoprotein A-I *Serum Decrease Physiological* Significant reduction observed in 12 mildly hypertensive patients treated with up to 20 mg daily for 12 weeks *5902*

Serum No Effect Analytical At a concentration of 130 μmol/L no significant effect observed on automated immunoturbidimetric method on Baxter Paramax analyzer *3005*

Serum No Effect Physiological No significant change observed in 10 hypertensive patients treated with up to 2.0 mg/d for up to 20 weeks *3823* Increase by 1 mg/dL in 16 patients given 1 to 3 mg daily for 8 weeks *4213* No change in 8 men with mild to moderate hypertension treated with up to 20 mg daily for 12 weeks *5931*

Apolipoprotein B *Serum Decrease Physiological* Significant reduction in 12 mildly hypertensive patients treated with up to 20 mg daily for 12 weeks. Effect greater than on apolipoprotein A-I so that ratio of A-I to B increased by 35% *5902* Mean reduction from 98 mg/dL to 75 mg/dL in 8 men with mild to moderate hypertension treated with up to 20 mg daily for 12 weeks *5931*

Serum No Effect Analytical At a concentration of 130 μmol/L no significant effect observed on automated immunoturbidimetric method on Baxter Paramax analyzer *3005*

Serum No Effect Physiological Decrease by -8 mg/dL in 16 patients given 1 to 3 mg daily for 8 weeks *4213* No significant effect in 15 hypertensives given 4 mg/d for 10 weeks *1840* No significant change observed in 10 hypertensives treated with up to 2.0 mg/d for up to 20 weeks *3823*

Apolipoprotein C-II *Serum No Effect Physiological* No change in 16 patients given 1 to 3 mg daily for 8 weeks *4213* No significant effect observed in 10 hypertensives treated with up to 2.0 mg/d for up to 20 weeks *3823*

Apolipoprotein C-III *Serum No Effect Physiological* No change in 16 patients given 1 to 3 mg daily for 8 weeks *4213* No significant change observed in 10 hypertensives treated with up to 2.0 mg/d for up to 20 weeks *3823*

Aspartate Aminotransferase *Serum Increase Physiological* In fewer than 1% of treated patients liver function test abnormalities noted *4649*

Serum No Effect Physiological No significant effect in 60 hypertensive patients treated with up to 8 mg daily for 20 weeks *5813*

Atrial Natriuretic Peptide *Plasma Decrease Physiological* Significant suppression observed in elderly patients with mild essential hypertension both at rest and during exercise *3224*

Bilirubin *Serum Increase Physiological* In fewer than 1% of treated patients liver function test abnormalities noted *4649*

Chlordiazepoxide *Serum No Effect Physiological* Coadministration of prazosin with chlordiazepoxide had no apparent adverse drug interaction in limited clinical experience *4649*

Chlorpropamide *Serum No Effect Physiological* Coadministration of prazosin with chlorpropamide had no apparent adverse drug interaction in limited clinical experience *4649*

Cholesterol *Serum Decrease Physiological* In 15 hypertensive patients given 4 mg/d for 10 weeks with mean reduction from 202 to 188 mg/dL *1840* In 37 patients with hypertension treatment for 6 months caused mean reduction of 0.4 mmol/L (9%) from pretreatment value *3609* Significantly decreased concentration observed with administration of alpha$_1$-inhibitors such as prazosin over 8 weeks *3730* From 5 to 12% in several studies involving 25 to 50 patients for up to 6 mo *141* Significant reduction observed in 10 hypertensives treated with up to 2.0 mg/d for up to 20 weeks from mean baseline concentration of 213 mg/dL to 196 mg/dL *3823* In 186 hypertensive patients treated with up to mg/d for 8 weeks mean concentration decreased by 9.3 mg/dL (0.24 mmol/L) *3841* Slight reduction from mean of 223 mg/dL to 215 mg/dL in 12 mildly hypertensive patients treated with up to 20 mg daily for 12 weeks *5902* Increase by 9% in 23 healthy hypertensives treated for 8 weeks *3522*

Serum No Effect Physiological No significant change with monotherapy for 12 mo in 15 patients *5919* In clinical trials there was generally no effect of prazosin on the lipid profile *4649* In 22 mild/moderate male hypertensives treated for 8 weeks versus controls. Effect not significant though slight decrease *2781* No significant change in 8 men with mild to moderate hypertension treated with up to 20 mg daily for 12 weeks *5931* Decrease by 12 mg/dL in 16 patients given 1 to 3 mg daily for 8 weeks *4213* Insignificant reduction by mean of 5 mg/dL in 185 patients treated with up to 20 mg daily for up to 5 months *5041* In 16 hypertensive patients given 2 mg daily for 3 mo *3737* Effect observed with doses as low as 1 to 3 mg/d *5274* No significant effect in 20 hypertensive patients treated with up to 20 mg daily for 4 weeks *1808*

Colchicine *Serum No Effect Physiological* Coadministration of prazosin with colchicine had no apparent adverse drug interaction in limited clinical experience *4649*

Creatinine *Serum No Effect Physiological* No significant effect in 60 hypertensive patients treated with up to 8 mg daily for 20 weeks *5813*

Prazosin *(continued)*

Cyclosporine *Blood No Effect Analytical* At a concentration of 3 mg/L had no significant effect on Syva EMIT method *495*

Diazepam *Serum No Effect Physiological* Coadministration of prazosin with diazepam had no apparent adverse drug interaction in limited clinical experience *4649*

Digitalis-like Immunoreactivity
Serum No Effect Physiological Coadministration of prazosin with digitalis had no apparent adverse drug interaction in limited clinical experience *4649*

Digoxin *Serum Increase Physiological* Significant increase when prazosin co-administered with digoxin but mechanism not determined *1131*
Serum No Effect Physiological Coadministration of prazosin with digoxin had no apparent adverse drug interaction in limited clinical experience *4649*

Drugs of Abuse Screen *Urine No Effect Analytical* No effect at concentration of 100 µg/mL on EZ-SCREEN procedure for cannabinoids and cocaine *1739*

Fatty Acids (FFA), Free *Serum Decrease Physiological* In 10 hypertensives treatment with up to 2.0 mg/d for up to 20 weeks caused mean from mean baseline of 0.67 mEq/L to 0.48 mEq/L *3823* In 10 hypertensives treatment with up to 2.0 mg/d for up to 20 weeks caused decrease from mean baseline of 0.67 mEq/L to 0.48 mEq/L *3823*
Serum Increase Physiological With 2 mg in 12 hypertensives (6 with normal and 6 with abnormal glucose tolerance) *366*
Serum No Effect Physiological No effect of treatment with up to 20 mg daily for 12 weeks in 12 mildly hypertensive patients *5902*

Gastrin *Serum No Effect Physiological* With 2 mg in 12 hypertensives (6 with normal and 6 with abnormal glucose tolerance) *366*

Glucose *Serum Increase Physiological* With 2 mg in 12 hypertensives (6 with normal and 6 with abnormal glucose tolerance) *366*
Serum No Effect Physiological No effect of treatment with up to 20 mg daily for 12 weeks in 12 mildly hypertensive patients *5902*

Glucose Tolerance *Serum Increase Physiological* Decreased glucose response to intravenous glucose tolerance test associated with decreased early insulin response mediated by increased circulating catecholamines *3608*
Serum No Effect Physiological No significant effect observed in 10 hypertensives treated with up to 2.0 mg/d for up to 20 weeks *3823*

γ-Glutamyltransferase *Serum Increase Physiological* In fewer than 1% of treated patients liver function test abnormalities noted *4649*

HDL_2-Cholesterol *Serum No Effect Physiological* No significant change in 8 men with mild to moderate hypertension treated with up to 20 mg daily for 12 weeks *5931*

HDL_3-Cholesterol *Serum Increase Physiological* Mean increase from 24 mg/dL to 26 mg/dL in 8 men with mild to moderate hypertension treated with up to 20 mg daily for 12 weeks *5931*

HDL-Cholesterol *Serum Increase Physiological* In 10 hypertensive patients treatment with up to 2.0 mg/d for up to 20 weeks caused increase from mean baseline of 46 mg/dL to 48 mg/dL *3823* Mean increase from 36 to 40.5 mg/dL in 15 hypertensives given 4 mg/d for weeks *1840* Significantly increased concentration observed with administration of $alpha_1$-inhibitors such as prazosin over 8 weeks *3730* Significant increase from mean of 38 mg/dL to 46 mg/dL in 12 mildly hypertensive patients treated with up to 20 mg daily for 12 weeks *5902* After 6 mg/d for 12 mo average increase of 17% in 15 patients *5919* Increased concentration observed with administration of $alpha_1$-inhibitors such as prazosin *3730* Effect observed with doses as low as 1 to 3 mg/d *5274*
Serum No Effect Physiological In 22 mild/moderate male hypertensives treated for 8 weeks versus controls insignificant reduction noted *2781* In clinical trials there was generally no effect of prazosin on the lipid profile *4649* No change in 16 patients given 1 to 3 mg daily for 8 weeks *4213* No significant effect in 20 hypertensive patients treated with up to 20 mg daily for 4 weeks *1808* No significant change in 8 men with mild to moderate hypertension treated with up to 20 mg daily for 12 weeks *5931* In 23 healthy hypertensives treated for 8 weeks *3522* In 16 hypertensive patients given 2 mg daily for 3 mo *3737* In several studies involving 25 to 50 patients for up to 6 mo *141* Insignificant reduction in 184 patients treated with up to 20 mg daily for up to 5 months *5041*

Hemoglobin *Blood No Effect Physiological* No significant effect in 60 hypertensive patients treated with up to 8 mg daily for 20 weeks *5813*

Hemoglobin A_{1c} *Blood No Effect Physiological* No significant effect observed in 10 hypertensives treated with up to 2.0 mg/d for 20 weeks *3823*

Histamine *Plasma No Effect Analytical* Although 50% inhibition of radio-enzyme assay at 17 µg/mL unlikely to be of clinical significance since therapeutic concentration 0.001 - 0.019 µg/mL *2492*

Indomethacin *Serum No Effect Physiological* Coadministration of prazosin with indomethacin had no apparent adverse drug interaction in limited clinical experience *4649*

Insulin *Plasma Decrease Physiological* Ambient concentrations lower at all times of day studied in 12 mildly hypertensive patients treated with up to 20 mg daily for 12 weeks *5902*
Plasma Increase Physiological With 2 mg in 12 hypertensives (6 with normal and 6 with abnormal glucose tolerance) *366*
Plasma No Effect Physiological Coadministration of prazosin with insulin had no apparent adverse drug interaction in limited clinical experience *4649*

Lactate *Plasma No Effect Physiological* No effect of treatment with up to 20 mg daily in 12 mildly hypertensive patients *5902*

LDL-Cholesterol *Serum Decrease Physiological* Decreased concentration observed with administration of $alpha_1$-inhibitors such as prazosin *3730* Reduction from mean of 133 mg/dL to 120 mg/dL in 8 men with mild to moderate hypertension treated for 12 weeks with up to 20 mg daily *5931* Mean reduction from 130 mg/dL to 125 mg/dL in 12 mildly hypertensive patients treated with up to 20 mg/day for 12 weeks *5902* Significant reduction by mean of 8 mg/dL in 177 patients treated with up to 20 mg daily for up to 5 months *5041*
Serum No Effect Physiological In clinical trials there was generally no effect of prazosin on the lipid profile *4649* No significant effect in 20 hypertensive patients treated with up to 20 mg daily for 4 weeks *1808* In 16 hypertensive patients given 2 mg daily for 3 mo *3737*

LDL-Triglycerides *Serum Decrease Physiological* Mean decrease from 19 mg/dL to 16 mg/dL in 12 mildly hypertensive patients treated with up to 20 mg daily for 12 weeks *5902*

Leukocytes *Blood Decrease Physiological* Mean reduction of 300 /µL in 60 patients with hypertension treated for 20 weeks with up to 8 mg daily *5813*

Lipase *Serum Increase Physiological* In fewer than 1% of treated patients pancreatitis noted but not unequivocally linked to administration of prazosin *4649*

Lipoprotein Lipase *Serum Increase Physiological* Mean increase from 28.4 to 37.7 µmol/L per minute given 4 mg/d for 10 weeks *1840*

Normetanephrine *Urine Increase Physiological* In 5 patients given 12 to 24 mg/d prazosin for 10 to 12 days average increase of 42% in the excretion of the urinary metabolite of norepinephrine *4649*

Phenformin *Serum No Effect Physiological* Coadministration of prazosin with phenformin had no apparent adverse drug interaction in limited clinical experience *4649*

Phenobarbital *Serum No Effect Physiological* Coadministration of prazosin with phenobarbital had no apparent adverse drug interaction in limited clinical experience *4649*

Phenylbutazone *Serum No Effect Physiological* Coadministration of prazosin with phenylbutazone had no apparent adverse drug interaction in limited clinical experience *4649*

Platelet Aggregation *Blood Decrease Physiological* High value in essential hypertension in response to ADP normalized with treatment *2809*

Blood *No Effect* *Physiological* No significant effect on aggregation in response to epinephrine, collagen and adenosine diphosphate observed in 18 hypertensives following treatment with 2-8 mg daily for 7 days although basal aggregation significantly higher in hyper- than normotensives *4396*

Potassium *Serum* *No Effect* *Physiological* No significant effect in 60 hypertensive patients treated with up to 8 mg daily for 20 weeks *5813*

Probenecid *Serum* *No Effect* *Physiological* Coadministration of prazosin with probenecid had no apparent adverse drug interaction in limited clinical experience *4649*

Procainamide *Serum* *No Effect* *Physiological* Coadministration of prazosin with procainamide had no apparent adverse drug interaction in limited clinical experience *4649*

Prolactin *Plasma* *No Effect* *Physiological* With 2 mg in 12 hypertensives (6 with normal and 6 with abnormal glucose tolerance) *366*

Propoxyphene *Serum* *No Effect* *Physiological* Coadministration of prazosin with propoxyphene had no apparent adverse drug interaction in limited clinical experience *4649*

Propranolol *Serum* *No Effect* *Physiological* Coadministration of prazosin with propranolol had no apparent adverse drug interaction in limited clinical experience *4649*

Renin Activity *Plasma* *No Effect* *Physiological* No significant change with monotherapy for 12 mo in 15 patients *5919*

Salicylate *Serum* *No Effect* *Physiological* Coadministration of prazosin with aspirin had no apparent adverse drug interaction in limited clinical experience *4649*

Sodium *Serum* *No Effect* *Physiological* No significant effect in 60 hypertensive patients treated with up to 8 mg daily for 20 weeks *5813*

β-Thromboglobulin *Plasma* *Decrease* *Physiological* 30% higher value in essential hypertensives, normalized with treatment *2809*

Plasma *No Effect* *Physiological* No significant change observed in 18 hypertensives treated with 2-8 mg/d for 7 days although median basal concentration 250% higher in hypertensives than normotensives *4396*

Thyroid Stimulating Hormone

Serum *Increase* *Physiological* In 19 hypertensives treated for 12 weeks caused change from 3.63 μU/mL to 4.83 μU/mL *697*

Thyroxine (T4) *Serum* *Increase* *Physiological* In 19 hypertensives treated for 12 weeks caused change from 10.03 μg/dL to 10.85 μg/dL *697*

Tolazamide *Serum* *No Effect* *Physiological* Coadministration of prazosin with tolazamide had no apparent adverse drug interaction in limited clinical experience *4649*

Tolbutamide *Serum* *No Effect* *Physiological* Coadministration of prazosin with tolbutamide had no apparent adverse drug interaction in limited clinical experience *4649*

Triglycerides *Serum* *Decrease* *Physiological* From 10 to 22% in several studies involving 25 to 50 patients for up to 6 mo *141* Effect observed with doses as low as 1 to 3 mg/d *5274* Mean decrease from 156 mg/dL to 144 mg/dL with treatment with up to 20 mg daily for 12 weeks in 12 mildly hypertensive patients *5902* Decrease by 20 mg/dL in 16 patients given 1 to 3 mg daily for 8 weeks *4213* Decrease by 16% in 23 healthy hypertensives treated for 8 weeks *3522* Significantly decreased concentration observed with administration of alpha$_1$-inhibitors such as prazosin over 8 weeks *3730* In 22 mild/moderate hypertensives treated for 8 weeks versus controls (average effect 9.5%) *2781*

Serum *Increase* *Physiological* Marked mean increase of 30 mg/dL in 185 patients treated with up to 20 mg daily for up to 5 months *5041*

Serum *No Effect* *Physiological* No significant effect in 15 hypertensives given 4 mg/d for 10 weeks *1840* No significant change observed in 10 hypertensives treated with up to 2.0 mg/d for up to 20 weeks *3823* In 16 hypertensive patients given 2 mg daily for 3 mo *3737* In clinical trials there was generally no effect of prazosin on the lipid profile *4649* No significant change with monotherapy for 12 mo in 15 patients *5919* No significant effect observed in patients receiving prazosin *4989* No significant change in 8 men with mild to moderate hypertension treated with up to 20 mg daily for 12 weeks *5931*

Uric Acid *Serum* *No Effect* *Physiological* In 23 healthy hypertensives treated for 8 weeks *3522*

Vanillylmandelic Acid *Urine* *Increase* *Physiological* In 5 patients given 12 to 24 mg/d prazosin for 10 to 12 days average increase of 17% in the excretion of urinary VMA *4649*

Verapamil *Serum* *No Effect* *Physiological* Although pharmacokinetics of prazosin were markedly affected by coadministration of verapamil, verapamil pharmacokinetics were not affected *5411* In 8 healthy volunteers coadministration of 1 mg prazosin and 160 mg verapamil had no effect on kinetics of verapamil *4545*

VLDL-Cholesterol *Serum* *Decrease* *Physiological* Increase by 10% in 23 healthy hypertensives treated for 8 weeks *3522* Mean reduction from 38 mg/dL to 27 mg/dL in 12 mildly hypertensive patients treated with up to 20 mg daily for 12 weeks *5902*

Serum *No Effect* *Physiological* No significant effect in 20 hypertensive patients treated with up to 20 mg daily for 4 weeks *1808* In 16 hypertensive patients given 2 mg daily for 3 mo *3737*

VLDL-Triglycerides *Serum* *Decrease* *Physiological* Mean decrease from 110 mg/dL to 101 mg/dL in 12 mildly hypertensive patients treated with up to 20 mg daily for 12 weeks *5902*

Prednisolone

Absorbance at 450 nm *Amniotic Fluid* *Decrease* *Analytical* Time-dependent reduction in absorbance of bilirubin when added *in vitro4061*

α$_1$-Acid Glycoprotein *Serum* *Decrease* *Physiological* Treatment of 88 patients with Crohn's disease with up to 30 mg/d for 10 weeks caused significant reduction from mean baseline of 1.3 ± 0.6 g/L to 1.2 ± 0.4 g/L after 8 weeks *5161*

Serum *No Effect* *Physiological* In 12 healthy volunteers ingestion of 20 mg caused nonsignificant change from mean baseline of 0.74 g/L to 0.77 g/L after 7 hours *853* In 12 healthy volunteers treatment with 20 mg/d for 3 days had no significant effect on the plasma concentration *853*

Albumin *Serum* *Increase* *Physiological* In 25 patients with nephrotic syndrome treatment for 8 weeks initially daily then on alternate days with up to 40 mg/d caused increase from mean baseline of 19.5 g/L to 39.6 g/L *4236* In 12 healthy volunteers administration of 20 mg/d for 3 days caused statistically significant increase (p = 0.004) after 7 hours *853* In 12 healthy volunteers ingestion of 20 mg caused significant change from mean baseline of 40.2 g/L to 42.1 g/L after 7 hours *853*

Alkaline Phosphatase *Serum* *Decrease* *Physiological* In 14 patients at a mean dose of 40 mg/d mean activity 141 U/L significantly less than 164 U/L at mean dose of 7 mg/d compared with reference range of 69 - 245 U/L *3729* Decrease from mean baseline of 2.68 μkat/L to 2.33 μkat/L in 12 healthy volunteers after inhaling 5 mg/d, to 2.24 μkat/L after inhaling either 10 or 20 mg/d *2928*

Alkaline Phosphatase, Bone Isoenzyme

Serum *Decrease* *Physiological* In 14 patients at a mean dose of 40 mg/d mean activity of 84 U/L measured by precipitation with wheatgerm lectin nonsignificantly less than 98 U/L at mean dose of 7 mg/d compared with reference range of 17 - 128 U/L *3729*

α-Amino-Nitrogen *Plasma* *Increase* *Physiological* After 4 d of oral therapy *3787*

Amino-terminal Propeptide of Type III Procollagen

Serum *Decrease* *Physiological* In 36 patients with early rheumatoid arthritis mean concentration 0.789 ± 0.282 U/mL changed significantly to an average of 0.590 ± 0.217 U/mL during treatment for 24 months with prednisolone *5473*

Amylase *Serum* *Increase* *Physiological* May rarely cause pancreatitis *51* Pancreatitis may occur as an adverse reaction *3977*

Androstenedione *Plasma* *Decrease* *Physiological* In 12 healthy volunteers reduction from mean baseline of 6.1 nmol/L to 5.7 nmol/L when 5 mg/d inhaled, to 4.8 nmol/L when 10 mg/d inhaled and to 3.7 nmol/L when 20 mg/d inhaled *2928*

Angiotensin-converting Enzyme

Serum *Decrease* *Physiological* Mean concentration of 23.3 ± 9.8 mU/mL in 12 patients with MCTD decreased to 13.5 ± 2.7 mU/mL after treatment for 1 to 4 months with 40 mg/d prednisolone *4472*

Prednisolone *(continued)*

Angiotensin-converting Enzyme *(continued)*
Serum No Effect Analytical After 96 h incubation *in vitro* at high doses produced marked reduction: unlikely to be factor *in vivo5119*
Serum No Effect Physiological 75 mg drug orally had no effect in 10 patients with sarcoidosis on diurnal variation or enzyme activity *6014* In 8 patients with sarcoidosis no significant difference in concentration observed after prednisolone *6014*

α_1-Antichymotrypsin *Serum Increase Physiological* In 12 healthy volunteers ingestion of 20 mg caused significant change from mean baseline of 0.53 g/L to 0.56 g/L after 7 hours *853* In 12 healthy volunteers administration of 20 mg/d for 3 days caused significant increase from mean baseline of 0.53 g/L (p = 0.038) at 7 hours to 0.56 g/L at 72 hours *853*

α_1-Antitrypsin *Serum No Effect Physiological* In 12 healthy volunteers administration of 20 mg/d for 3 days caused no significant effect on concentration *853* In 12 healthy volunteers ingestion of 20 mg caused nonsignificant change from mean baseline of 1.18 g/L to 1.19 g/L after 7 hours *853*

Apolipoprotein A *Serum Increase Physiological* Significant increase from mean baseline of 1.61 g/L to 1.99 g/L in 25 children with nephrotic syndrome given up to 40 mg/d initially daily then on alternate days for a total of 8 weeks *4236*

Apolipoprotein B *Serum Decrease Physiological* Significant decrease from mean baseline of 3.41 g/L to 1.68 g/L in 25 children with nephrotic syndrome treated for 4 weeks with up to 40 mg/d then for another 4 weeks with the same dose on alternate days *4236*

Bicarbonate *Serum Increase Physiological* Hypochloremic alkalosis may occur *51*

Calcium *Urine Increase Physiological* Effect of all corticosteroids *51*

Chloride *Serum Decrease Physiological* Hypochloremic alkalosis may occur *51*

Cholesterol *Serum Decrease Physiological* In 25 children with nephrotic syndrome treatment with up to 40 mg/d initially daily then on alternate days caused decrease from mean baseline of 13.65 mmol/L to 6.16 mmol/L after 8 weeks *4236*
Serum Increase Physiological Rose from 4.81 to 6.58 mmol/L in women receiving drug for mean of 3.1 y *2917*
Serum No Effect Analytical At concentration of 8 mg/L had no effect on method using catalase-Hantzsch reaction *5704* At concentration of 8 mg/L had no effect on CHOD-PAP method *5704*
Serum No Effect Physiological In men receiving drug for mean of 3.1 y *2917*
Urine Decrease Physiological Significant decrease from mean pretreatment of 22.2 µmol/d to 7.0 µmol/d in 25 children with nephrotic syndrome treated with up to 40 mg/d for 4 weeks then with the same dose on alternate days for another 4 weeks *4236*

Cholinesterase *Serum No Effect Analytical* No effect observed at concentration of 1 µg/mL with butyrylthiocholine method on Kodak Ektachem® *2504*

Color *Feces Increase Analytical* Black color reported with ingestion of prednisolone *3388*

Cortisol *Plasma Decrease Physiological* Treatment of 88 patients with Crohn's disease with up to 30 mg/d for 10 weeks caused significant reduction from mean baseline of 13.5 µg/dL to 3.0 µg/dL after 8 weeks *5161* Slight increase in concentration with 5 mg/d but decrease to 310 nmol/L with 10 mg/d and to 210 nmol/L with 20 mg/d when drug inhaled by 12 healthy individuals *2928*
Plasma Increase Analytical At concentration of 0.16 mg/L (usual serum concentration up to 0.8 mg/L) caused 51.2% cross reactivity with method on Baxter Stratus *5705* High and equal cross reactivity with RIA and competitive protein binding *1803* Prednisolone caused a significant cross-reactivity of 60.9% with method on Bayer Technicon Immuno 1® *419*

Cortisol, Free *Urine No Effect Analytical* No significant interference observed with HPLC method of Turpeinen et al *6105*

C-Reactive Protein *Serum Decrease Physiological* In 12 healthy volunteers ingestion of 20 mg caused significant change from mean baseline of 1.5 mg/L to 1.0 mg/L after 7 hours *853* Treatment of 88 patients with Crohn's disease with up to 30 mg/d for 10 weeks caused significant reduction from mean baseline of 23 ± 29 mg/L to 15 ± 20 mg/L after 8 weeks *5161*
Urine Decrease Physiological In 10 patients with rheumatoid arthritis with mean age 63 ± 12 y and duration of disease of 4.4 ± 5.8 y mean concentration after 2 - 4 weeks treatment of 6 ± 5 mg/L significantly different from 71 ± 61 mg/L before treatment *5825*

Creatinine *Serum No Effect Analytical* At concentration of 200 mg/L had no effect on Jaffe-Fading-Fraction method *5704* At concentration of 0.23 mg/L had no effect on creatinine iminohydrolase method *5704* At concentration of 200 mg/L had no effect on Jaffe-Fuller's earth method *5704*
Urine No Effect Physiological In 10 patients with rheumatoid arthritis with mean age 63 ± 12 y and duration of disease of 4.4 ± 5.8 y mean excretion after 2 - 4 weeks treatment of 8.69 ± 2.58 mmol/d not significantly different from 8.51 ± 2.33 mmol/d before treatment *5825*

Cyclosporine *Blood Increase Physiological* Coadministration of prednisolone with cyclosporine resulted in a 15% increase of the area under the concentration-time curve and increase of half-life from 2.9 h to 4.3 h *859*
Blood No Effect Analytical At a concentration of 12 mg/L had no effect on Syva EMIT method *495*
Serum Increase Physiological Increased concentrations reported when drugs coadministered *1384* Coadministration of prednisolone with cyclosporine resulted in a 15% increase of the area under the concentration-time curve and increase of half-life from 2.9 h to 4.3 h *859*
Serum No Effect Analytical No interference observed with Incstar RIA procedure *2930*

Cytidine Deaminase *Serum Increase Physiological* In 18 patients with early rheumatoid arthritis mean concentration 14.65 ± 3.73 U/mL changed significantly to an average of 19.22 ± 7.24 U/mL during treatment for 24 months with prednisolone *5473*

Dehydroepiandrosterone Sulfate
Plasma Decrease Physiological Reduction from mean baseline of 3.9 nmol/L to 2.6 nmol/L after inhalation of 5 mg/d in 12 healthy volunteers, to 2.8 nmol/L when 10 mg/d inhaled and to 2.2 nmol/L when 20 mg/d inhaled *2928*

Diclofenac *Serum No Effect Physiological* Coadministration of prednisolone with diclofenac did not significantly affect the peak concentration or AUC of diclofenac *1025*

Digitoxin *Serum No Effect Analytical* At concentrations up to 1.4 mg/L recovery affected by less than 10% with method on Baxter Stratus *5705*

Digoxin *Serum Increase Analytical* At 50 ng/mL equals 0.5 ng/mL by RIA *6638* At normal concentrations in serum if no preincubation *4688*
Serum No Effect Analytical Cross reactivity of less than 10% observed with method on Baxter Stratus *5705* At concentrations up to 50 µg/mL no significant effect observed with method on Ciba Corning ACS:180 *1412*

Eosinophils *Blood Decrease Physiological* In one 77-year old female patient with bullous pemphigoid treatment with 1 mg/kg body weight for 1 week followed by dose tapered by 0.1 mg/kg each week caused significant reduction from initial concentration of about 2300 /µL to close to 0 /µL after one day of treatment *6578*

Erythrocyte Sedimentation Rate
Blood Decrease Physiological In 10 patients with rheumatoid arthritis with mean age 63 ± 12 y and duration of disease of 4.4 ± 5.8 y mean rate after 2 - 4 weeks treatment of 32 ± 17 mm/h significantly different from 62 ± 28 mm/h before treatment *5825* Treatment of 88 patients with Crohn's disease with up to 30 mg/d for 10 weeks caused significant reduction from mean baseline of 25 ± 21 mm/h to 17 ± 14 mm/h after 8 weeks *5161*

Fractional Excretion of Magnesium
Urine Increase Physiological In 8 renal transplant patients receiving azathioprine and prednisolone mean fractional excretion of 18.0 % significantly greater than 3.5 % in 10 healthy individuals *106*

Glucagon *Plasma Increase Physiological* After 4 d fasting level increased 24 pg/mL *3787*
Plasma No Effect Physiological Intravenous injection failed to modify concentration *3787*

Glucocorticoid Receptors
Monocytes Decrease Physiological In 7 of 8 women patients with dermatomyositis/polymyositis treatment with prednisolone (initial doses 40 to 60 mg/d) concentration significantly decreased *5940*

Glucose *Serum Increase Physiological* Treatment of 88 patients with Crohn's disease with up to 30 mg/d for 10 weeks caused significant increase from mean baseline of 83 mg/dL to 97 mg/dL after 8 weeks *5161* After 4 d of oral therapy After i.v. 6 mg/dL at 150 minutes to 15 at 4 h *3787*
Serum No Effect Analytical At concentration of 25 mg/L had no effect on GOD/POD-PAP method *5704*

Glucose Tolerance *Serum Decrease Physiological* Metabolic effect *51* Decreased carbohydrate tolerance may occur as an adverse reaction *3977*

Glycosaminoglycan *Serum No Effect Physiological* In 36 patients with early rheumatoid arthritis mean concentration 26.66 ± 7.71 µg/mL changed nonsignificantly to an average of 27.22 ± 6.52 µg/mL during treatment for 24 months with prednisolone *5473*

Haptoglobin *Serum No Effect Physiological* In 12 healthy volunteers treatment with 20 mg/d for 3 days caused no significant effect on mean concentration *853* In 12 healthy volunteers ingestion of 20 mg caused nonsignificant change from mean baseline of 1.07 g/L to 1.02 g/L after 7 hours *853*

HDL-Cholesterol *Serum Decrease Physiological* Fell from 1.99 to 1.10 mmol/L in women receiving drug for mean of 3.1 y *2917*
Serum No Effect Physiological In men receiving drug for mean of 3.1 y *2917*

Histamine *Plasma No Effect Analytical* No significant inhibition of radio-enzyme assay even at concentrations much greater than physiological *2492*

Hyaluronan *Serum Decrease Physiological* In 35 patients with early rheumatoid arthritis mean concentration 86.67 ± 1.86 ng/mL changed significantly to an average of 65.96 ± 1.95 ng/mL during treatment for 24 months with prednisolone *5473*

Hydroxyproline *Urine Decrease Physiological* Reductions observed in 12 healthy volunteers who inhaled 5, 10 or 20 mg/d but greatest reduction observed with 10 mg/d *2928*

Hypoxanthine *Serum Decrease Physiological* In 7 patients treated with up to 60 mg/d mean concentration reduced to 0.20 ± 0.04 µg/mL not significantly less than 0.23 ± 0.11 µg/mL in 5 healthy controls *2626*
Urine Decrease Physiological In 7 patients treated with up to 60 mg/d mean concentration significantly reduced to 9.9 ± 5.2 mg/d from 18.4 ± 3.7 mg/d in 5 healthy controls *2626*

Immunoglobulin G *Serum Decrease Physiological* In 12 patients with cystic fibrosis receiving prednisolone mean concentration decreased from baseline of 17.8 ± 1.5 g/L to 12.3 ± 1.5 g/L after 12 weeks treatment *2300*

Insulin *Plasma Increase Physiological* In 7 children with Crohn's disease treatment with up to 2 mg/kg/d for 4 weeks caused significant increase in median from 11.0 mUL to 14.0 mU/L *6005* After 4 d of oral therapy *3787*
Plasma No Effect Physiological Intravenous injection failed to modify concentration *3787*

Insulin-like Growth Factor-I *Serum Increase Physiological* In 16 children with Crohn's disease treatment with up to 2 mg/kg/d for 4 weeks caused significant increase in median from 0.65 U/mL to 1.06 U/mL *6005*

Insulin-like Growth Factor Binding Protein-1
Serum Decrease Physiological In 8 children with Crohn's disease treatment with up to 2 mg/kg/d for 4 weeks caused significant decrease in median from 62.6 µg/L to 35.2 µg/L *6005*

Interleukin-1α *Serum Decrease Physiological* In 12 patients with cystic fibrosis receiving prednisolone mean concentration decreased from baseline of 561 ± 141 pg/mL to 356 ± 100 pg/mL after 14 days of treatment and 311 ± 91.4 pg/mL after 12 weeks treatment *2300*

Ionized Magnesium
Red Blood Cells Decrease Physiological In 8 renal transplant patients receiving azathioprine and prednisolone mean concentration of 2.30 mmol/L significantly lower than 2.56 mmol/L in 10 healthy individuals *106*
Serum Decrease Physiological In 8 renal transplant patients receiving azathioprine and prednisolone mean concentration of 0.48 mmol/L significantly lower than 0.58 mmol/L in 10 healthy individuals *106*

Isoniazid *Serum Decrease Physiological* 25-40% reduction observed in group of patients when prednisolone coadministered possibly due to enhanced hepatic metabolism or renal excretion *5272*

Keratan Sulfate *Serum No Effect Physiological* In 36 patients with early rheumatoid arthritis mean concentration 629 ± 181 ng/mL changed nonsignificantly to an average of 640 ± 184 ng/mL during treatment for 24 months with prednisolone *5473*

Lecithin:Cholesterol Acyltransferase
Serum Increase Physiological Significant increase from mean pretreatment concentration of 64 nmol/mL/h to 94 nmol/mL/h in 25 children with nephrotic syndrome treated with up to 40 mg daily for 4 weeks then with the same dose on alternate days for another 4 weeks *4236*

Leukocytes *Blood Decrease Physiological* Leukopenia *3810*
Blood Increase Physiological Leukocytosis observed occasionally *3810*

Lipase *Serum Increase Physiological* Pancreatitis may occur as an adverse reaction *3977*

Magnesium *Serum Decrease Physiological* In 8 renal transplant patients receiving azathioprine and prednisolone mean concentration of 0.62 mmol/L significantly lower than 0.86 mmol/L in 10 healthy individuals *106*
Urine No Effect Physiological In 13 renal transplant patients receiving azathioprine and prednisolone mean excretion of 3.8 mmol/d not significantly different from 4.4 mmol/d in 10 healthy individuals *106*

Mycophenolic Acid *Serum No Effect Analytical* No significant interference observed with HPLC method of Shipkova et al *5526*

Mycophenolic Acid Glucuronide
Serum No Effect Analytical No significant interference observed with HPLC method of Shipkova et al *5526*

Myelin Basic Protein *Serum Decrease Physiological* In one 77-year old female patient with bullous pemphigoid treatment with 1 mg/kg body weight for 1 week followed by dose tapered by 0.1 mg/kg each week caused significant reduction from initial concentration of about 600 ng/mL to about 30 ng/mL after 10 days treatment and 20 ng/mL after 17 days treatment *6578*

Nitrate *Urine Decrease Physiological* In 10 patients with rheumatoid arthritis with mean age 63 ± 12 y and duration of disease of 4.4 ± 5.8 y mean baseline excretion of 223 ± 126 µmol/mmol creatinine significantly reduced to 162 ± 83 µmol/mmol creatinine after 2 - 4 weeks of treatment although excretion remained increased compared with rhat in 18 age and sex comparable controls *5825*

Nitroblue Tetrazolium Test *Blood No Effect Physiological* No effect observed in uremic patients *6528*

Nitrogen *Urine Increase Physiological* Negative nitrogen balance due to protein catabolism *51*

Nitrogen Balance *Patient Negative Physiological* Negative nitrogen balance due to protein catabolism may occur as an adverse reaction *3977*

N-terminal Telopeptide of Type I Collagen
Serum Decrease Physiological In 9 patients with early rheumatoid arthritis mean concentration 50.12 ± 24.26 nmol/mmol changed nonsignificantly to an average of 42.83 ± 24.83 nmol/mmol during treatment for 24 months with prednisolone *5473*

Occult Blood *Feces Increase Physiological* Peptic ulcer with possible subsequent perforation and hemorrhage may occur as an adverse reaction *3977* May activate peptic ulcer with hemorrhage *51*

Osteocalcin *Serum Decrease Physiological* Reduction from mean baseline of 3.4 µg/L to 2.9 µg/L when 5 mg/d inhaled by 12 healthy volunteers, to 2.7 µg/L when 10 mg/d inhaled and to 2.2 µg/L when 20 mg/d inhaled *2928* Reduction from mean baseline of 3.4 µ.g/L to 2.9 µg/L when 5 mg/d inhaled by 12 healthy volunteers, to 2.7 µg/L when 10 mg/d

Prednisolone *(continued)*

Osteocalcin *(continued)*
inhaled and to 2.2 µg/L when 20 mg/d inhaled *2928* In 24 patients with early rheumatoid arthritis mean concentration 23.11 ± 7.51 ng/mL changed significantly to an average of 17.15 ± 5.56 ng/mL during treatment for 24 months with prednisolone *5473* In 14 patients at a mean dose of 40 mg/d mean concentration 13.2 µg/L significantly less than 28.5 µg/L at mean dose of 7 mg/d compared with reference range of 5.2 - 55.9 µg/L *3729*

p-Aminophenol *Urine No Effect Analytical* With addition of drugs at a concentration of 100 mg/L and of related compounds at 50 mg/L no significant effect observed on colorimetric method of van Bocxlaer on Cobas Mira analyzer which involves reacting free p-aminophenol with resorcinol in the presence of magnesium ions to form an indophenol dye measured at 550 nm *6163*

pH *Blood Increase Physiological* Hypokalemic alkalosis may occur as an adverse reaction *3977*

Phenylalanine *Plasma No Effect Analytical* No interference observed with rapid quantitative whole blood method of Campbell et al using phenylalanine dehydrogenase *867*

Potassium *Serum Decrease Physiological* Potassium loss may occur as an adverse reaction *3977* Slight mineralocorticoid effect *128*
Urine Increase Physiological Slight mineralocorticoid effect *128*

Prealbumin *Serum Increase Physiological* Administration of 20 mg/d for 3 days caused significant increase (p = 0.041) after 7 hours *853* In 12 healthy volunteers ingestion of 20 mg caused significant change from mean baseline of 291 mg/L to 296 mg/L after 7 hours *853*

Pro-Matrix Metalloproteinase 1
Serum Decrease Physiological In 17 patients with early rheumatoid arthritis mean concentration 29.67 ± 2.01 ng/mL changed significantly to an average of 24.05 ± 2.10 ng/mL during treatment for 24 months with prednisolone *5473*

Pro-Matrix Metalloproteinase 3
Serum Increase Physiological In 35 patients with early rheumatoid arthritis mean concentration 58.56 ± 2.18 ng/mL changed significantly to an average of 90.02 ± 1.67 ng/mL during treatment for 24 months with prednisolone *5473*

Protein *Cerebrospinal Fluid No Effect Analytical* No significant effect when added in vitro to concentration of 10.0 mg/dL when measured by Kodak Ektachem® method *3654*
Urine Decrease Physiological In 25 children with nephrotic syndrome treatement with 40 mg/d initially daily then on alternate days over 8 weeks caused decrease from mean baseline of 4.74 g/d to 0.76 g/d *4236*

Protein Electrophoresis *Serum No Effect Analytical* At concentration of 7.2 mg/L had no effect on automated Olympus-Hite method except for slight displacement of fractions *5704*

Sodium *Serum Increase Physiological* Very slight mineralocorticoid effect *128*

Soluble Interleukin-2 Receptor
Serum Decrease Physiological In 12 patients with cystic fibrosis receiving prednisolone mean concentration decreased from baseline of 412 ± 91.2 IU/mL to 212 ± 32.6 IU/mL after 14 days of treatment and 234 ± 28.2 IU/mL after 12 weeks treatment *2300*

Tacrolimus *Blood No Effect Analytical* No interference observed with radioreceptor method of Murthy et al *4191*

Theophylline *Serum No Effect Physiological* No documented significant interaction with theophylline reported *6117* No clinically significant effect on theophylline concentration observed when drugs coadministered *5999*

Thromboxane *Plasma No Effect Physiological* No effect of up to 100 µmol/L on formation during blood clotting *4817*

Triglycerides *Serum Decrease Physiological* In 25 children with nephrotic syndrome treatment with 40 mg/d initially daily then on alternate days caused decrease from mean baseline of 3.06 mmol/L to 1.29 mmol/L after 8 weeks *4236*
Serum Increase Physiological Rose from 0.91 to 1.84 mmol/L in women receiving drug for mean of 3.1 y *2917*
Serum No Effect Analytical At concentration of 230 mg/L had no effect on GPO-PAP method *5704*
Serum No Effect Physiological In men receiving drug for mean of 3.1 y *2917*

Uric Acid *Serum Decrease Physiological* In 14 patients treated with up to 60 mg/d mean concentration 3.8 ± 0.9 mg/dL compared with 5.5 ± 0.9 mg/dL in 10 healthy controls *2626*
Serum No Effect Analytical At concentration of 200 mg/L had no effect on Kageyama-Hantzsch method *5704* At concentration of 25 mg/L had no effect on uricase-PAP method *5704* At concentration of 200 mg/L had no effect on catalase-AIDH method *5704*
Urine Increase Physiological In 14 patients treated with up to 60 mg/d nonsignificant increase to 391 ± 139 mg/d from 361 ± 146 mg/d in 10 healthy controls *2626*

Xanthine *Serum No Effect Physiological* In 7 patients treated with up to 60 mg/d no difference in mean concentration of 0.11 ± 0.04 µg/L compared with 5 controls *2626*
Urine Decrease Physiological In 7 patients treated with up to 60 mg/d significant reduction to 12.6 ± 6.4 mg/d compared with 20.8 ± 4.8 mg/d in 5 healthy controls *2626*

Prednisone

Acetylsalicylic Acid *Serum Decrease Physiological* Plasma concentration lower and renal excretion augmented when drugs are coadministered probably through an effect on metabolism *4062* In one case report of a child receiving chronic salicylate therapy coadministration of 15 mg/day prednisone caused reduction of serum concentration by 67% *3247*

Acid Phosphatase *Serum No Effect Physiological* Treatment of 10 euthyroid patients with Graves' disease with prednisone for 12 weeks had no significant effect on enzyme activity *4804*

Adenosine Monophosphate *Urine No Effect Physiological* In 6 patients who needed high-dose corticosteroid therapy concentration changed nonsignificantly from mean baseline of 395 ± 135 nmol/mmol creatinine to 407 ± 124 nmol/mmol creatinine after 15 days treatment with 29.1 mg/d *3625*

Aggregation Index *Red Blood Cells Decrease Physiological* In 29 children with nephrotic syndrome treatment with prednisone for 3 weeks caused mean basal aggregation index of 23.8 ± 5.3 to decrease significantly to 18.2 ± 3.3 (18.3 ± 3.2 in steroid-sensitive and 17.5 ± 4.0 in steroid-resistant) *175*

Albumin *Serum Decrease Physiological* Fell within 3 d in adult hospitalized patients given 40-50 mg/d orally. Concentration paralleled that of zinc *6398*
Serum Increase Physiological In 11 patients with HIV-associated nephropathy treatment with 60 mg/d prednisone for 2 to 11 weeks caused an average increase in serum albumin concentration from mean baseline of 24.4 ± 3.6 g/L to 29.3 ± 2.6 g/L *5623*

Alkaline Phosphatase *Serum Decrease Physiological* Augmented response in cirrhotics when drug added to therapeutic regime *1004* In 10 euthyroid patients with Graves' disease treatment with prednisone for 12 weeks caused decrease in mean activity from 1.15 ± 0.33 µkat/L to 0.83 ± 0.22 µkat/L at 4 weeks and 0.88 ± 0.40 µkat/L at 12 weeks *4804* In 6 patients who needed high-dose corticosteroid therapy concentration changed nonsignificantly from mean baseline of 88.1 ± 30 U/L to 71 ± 30.4 U/L after 15 days treatment with 29.1 mg/d *3625*
Serum No Effect Physiological In 8 patients with autoimmune disorders treatment with prednisone decreasing from 1.0 to 0.1 mg/kg body weight/d for 4 months caused no significant change from mean baseline of 141 ± 27 U/L to 139 ± 16 U/L after one month, 128 ± 17 U/L after 2 months and 114 ± 15 U/L after 4 months *1118* No consistent change noted in 14 hospitalized adult patients when given 40-50 mg/d *6398* No significant effect of treatment with 10-25 mg/day in 23 patients requiring long-term glucocorticoid therapy *4896*

Amino-terminal Propeptide of Type III Procollagen
Serum Decrease Physiological In 8 patients with autoimmune disorders treatment with prednisone decreasing from 1.0 to 0.1 mg/kg body weight/d for 4 months caused significant decrease from mean baseline of 2.2 ± 0.3 ng/mL to 1.6 ± 0.3 ng/mL after one month, 1.5 ± 0.2 ng/mL after 2 months but rose to baseline value of 1.8 ± 0.2 ng/mL after 4 months *1118*

Serum *No Effect* *Physiological* In 8 patients with autoimmune disorders treatment with prednisone decreasing from 1.0 to 0.1 mg/kg body weight/d for 4 months caused significant decrease from mean baseline of 2.2 ± 0.3 ng/mL to 1.6 ± 0.3 ng/mL after one month, 1.5 ± 0.2 ng/mL after 2 months but rose to baseline value of 1.8 ± 0.2 ng/mL after 4 months *1118*

Amylase *Serum* *Increase* *Physiological* May cause pancreatitis *2754*

Angiotensin-converting Enzyme
Serum *Decrease* *Physiological* Marked reduction after 1 week in patients in whom initial value was high, no effect in others *5077*
Serum *No Effect* *Analytical* No effect on colorimetric method of Boomsma and Schalekamp *4703*

Antithrombin III *Plasma* *Increase* *Physiological* In 29 children with nephrotic syndrome treatment with prednisone for 3 weeks caused mean basal concentration of 81 ± 21% to increase significantly to 120 ± 26% (126 ± 21% in steroid-sensitive and 98 ± 33% in steroid-resistant) *175*

α_1-Antitrypsin *Serum* *Increase* *Physiological* In 29 children with nephrotic syndrome treatment with prednisone for 3 weeks caused mean basal concentration of 1.7 ± 0.9 g/L to increase nonsignificantly to 1.9 ± 0.7 g/L (2.1 ± 0.6 g/L in steroid-sensitive and 1.3 ± 0.5 g/L in steroid-resistant) *175*

Apolipoprotein A-I *Serum* *No Effect* *Physiological* No change noted after 1 mo but ratio of HDL-Cholecterol to apo A-I increased, apparent in 48 h *6667*

Apolipoprotein A-II *Serum* *No Effect* *Physiological* No change noted after 1 mo *6667*

Apolipoprotein E *Serum* *No Effect* *Physiological* No change noted after 1 mo *6667*

Aspartate Aminotransferase
Serum *Decrease* *Physiological* Augmented response in cirrhotics when drug added to therapeutic regime *1004*

Bicarbonate *Serum* *Increase* *Physiological* May cause hypokalemic alkalosis *2754*

Bilirubin *Serum* *Decrease* *Physiological* Augmented response in cirrhotics when drug added to therapeutic regime *1004*

BSP Retention *Serum* *Decrease* *Physiological* Augmented response in cirrhotics when drug added to therapeutic regime *1004*

Calcium *Serum* *Decrease* *Physiological* If elevation due to sarcoidosis or vitamin D *128*
Serum *Increase* *Physiological* Significant increase in patients requiring long-term glucocorticoid therapy during the first 2 months of treatment with 10-25 mg/day but concentration fell to normal after this time *4896*
Serum *No Effect* *Physiological* Although given for 1 to 50 mo *6467* In 6 patients who needed high-dose corticosteroid therapy concentration changed nonsignificantly from mean baseline of 2.37 ± 0.12 mmol/L to 2.37 ± 0.09 mmol/L after 15 days treatment with 29.1 mg/d *3625*
Urine *No Effect* *Physiological* No significant effect in 23 patients requiring long-term glucocorticoid therapy when they received 10-25 mg/day for 12 months *4896* In 6 patients who needed high-dose corticosteroid therapy concentration changed nonsignificantly from mean baseline of 0.45 ± 0.25 mmol/mmol creatinine to 0.47 ± 0.01 mmol/mmol creatinine after 15 days treatment with 29.1 mg/d *3625*

Cholesterol *Serum* *Increase* *Physiological* Augmented response in cirrhotics when drug added to therapeutic regime *1004* 17% increase in group of men and women during 1 mo *6667* Significant reduction of mean concentration to 213 mg/dL in 35 women with SLE or rheumatoid arthritis treated with mean dose of 10.8 mg/d for 3 months compared with mean concentration of 205 mg/dL in 44 control untreated women with rheumatoid arthritis *6318*

Cholinesterase *Serum* *No Effect* *Analytical* No effect observed at concentration of 0.1 µg/mL with butyrylthiocholine method on Kodak Ektachem® *2504*

Chondrex *Serum* *No Effect* *Analytical* Concentrations up to 1 g/L had no significant effect on sandwich-type ELISA procedure of Harvey et al *2491*

Cortisol *Plasma* *Increase* *Analytical* At concentration of 0.16 mg/L (usual serum concentration up to 0.05 mg/L) 10.0% cross reactivity observed with method on Baxter Stratus *5705* High and equal cross reactivity with RIA and competitive protein binding *1803*
Plasma *No Effect* *Analytical* Prednisone caused an insignificant cross-reactivity of 3.2% with method on Bayer Technicon Immuno 1® *419*

Cortisol, Free *Urine* *No Effect* *Analytical* No significant interference observed with HPLC method of Turpeinen et al *6105*

C-Peptide *Plasma* *Increase* *Physiological* Significant and progressive increase with short-term treatment *4477*

C-Reactive Protein *Serum* *Decrease* *Physiological* In 15 patients with polyarthralgia rheumatica treated with 12.5 mg/d showed decrease from mean baseline of 6.6 ± 4.5 mg/dL to 0.5 ± 0.5 mg/dL after 1 month and 0.7 ± 0.5 mg/dL after 6 months *5207*

Creatine Kinase *Serum* *Decrease* *Physiological* Low activities below normal range, observed in several patients some of whom were receiving other drugs but not observed in all patients *2610*

Creatinine *Serum* *Decrease* *Physiological* In 17 patients with HIV-associated nephropathy treatment with 60 mg/d prednisone for 2 to 11 weeks caused decrease in serum creatinine concentration from mean baseline of 717 ± 103 µmol/L to 262 ± 31 µmol/L *5623*
Serum *Increase* *Physiological* In 9 patients with Graves' disease treatment with 60 mg/d for 2 weeks caused significant increase in mean concentration from baseline of 68 ± 4 µmol/L to 76 ± 4 µmol/L *6162*
Serum *No Effect* *Analytical* No effect observed at concentrations up to 2.5 mg/L with Jaffe method used on a Technicon SMAC® *6162*
Urine *Decrease* *Physiological* Excretion less than anticipated in comparison with controls *2712*
Urine *Increase* *Physiological* In 9 patients with Graves' disease treatment with 60 mg/d for 2 weeks caused significant increase from mean baseline of 510 ± 40 µmol/h to 570 ± 40 µmol/h *6162* Increase from mean of 190 mg/24 h to 261 mg/24 h in 67 boys with Duchenne's muscular dystrophy treated for 6 months with either 0.75 mg/kg/day or 1.5 mg/kg/day *3951*

Creatinine Clearance *Urine* *Decrease* *Physiological* In comparison with controls probably due to decreased muscle mass in drug treated patients in relation to total body weight *2712*
Urine *Increase* *Physiological* In 9 patients with Graves' disease mean clearance increased from 111± 5 mL/min/1.73 sq m to 120 mL/min/1.73 sq m after 2 weeks treatment with 60 mg/d *6162*

C-terminal Telopeptide of Type I Collagen
Serum *No Effect* *Physiological* In 8 patients with autoimmune disorders treatment with prednisone decreasing from 1.0 to 0.1 mg/kg body weight/d for 4 months caused no significant change from mean baseline of 2.8 ± 0.2 ng/mL to 2.7 ± 0.4 ng/mL after one month, 3.0 ± 0.4 ng/mL after 2 months and 2.4 ± 0.3 ng/mL sfter 4 months *1118*

Cyclosporine *Blood* *No Effect* *Analytical* At a concentration of 12 mg/L had no effect on Syva EMIT method *495*
Serum *Increase* *Physiological* Increased concentrations reported when drugs coadministered *1384*

Digitoxin *Serum* *No Effect* *Analytical* Recovery affected by less than 10% at concentration of 1.4 mg/L with method on Baxter Stratus *5705*

Digoxin *Serum* *Increase* *Analytical* At 50 ng/mL equals 0.2 ng/mL by RIA *6638* At normal concentrations in serum if no preincubation *4688*

1,25-Dihydroxy Vitamin D *Serum* *No Effect* *Physiological* No significant effect in 23 patients requiring long-term glucocorticoid therapy when they received 10-25 mg/day for 12 months *4896*

1,25-Dihydroxy Vitamin D_3 *Serum* *Decrease* *Physiological* In children being treated for renal disease: dose dependent *985*

24,25-Dihydroxy Vitamin D *Serum* *No Effect* *Physiological* No significant effect in 23 patients requiring long-term glucocorticoid therapy when they received 10-25 mg/day for 12 months *4896*

Prednisone *(continued)*

Effective Renal Plasma Flow
Patient Increase Physiological In 9 patients with Graves' disease treatment with 60 mg/d for 2 weeks caused significant increase from mean baseline of 465 ± 25 mL/min/1.73 sq m to 490 mL/min/1.73 sq m *6162*

Eosinophils *Blood Decrease Physiological* Striking decrease in absolute count with 2 weeks therapy *5532*

Erythrocyte Sedimentation Rate
Blood Decrease Physiological In 15 patients with polyarthralgia rheumatica treated with 12.5 mg/d showed decrease from mean baseline of 82 ± 31 mm/h to 13 ± 9 mm/h after 1 month and 17 ± 13 mm/h after 6 months *5207* Augmented response in cirrhotics when drug added to therapeutic regime *1004*

Factor VIII Antigen *Plasma Decrease Physiological* In 29 children with nephrotic syndrome treatment with prednisone for 3 weeks caused mean basal concentration of 231 ± 68% to decrease significantly to 165 ± 59% (157 ± 53% in steroid-sensitive and 196 ± 72% in steroid-resistant) *175*

Factor VIII Coagulant *Plasma Decrease Physiological* In 29 children with nephrotic syndrome treatment with prednisone for 3 weeks caused mean basal concentration of 267 ± 77% to decrease significantly to 194 ± 77% (189 ± 77% in steroid-sensitive and 214 ± 78% in steroid-resistant) *175*

Factor XII *Plasma Increase Physiological* In 29 children with nephrotic syndrome treatment with prednisone for 3 weeks caused mean basal concentration of 45 ± 20% to increase significantly to 104 ± 36% (114 ± 25% in steroid-sensitive and 67 ± 49% in steroid-resistant) *175*

Fibrin Degradation Products *Urine Decrease Physiological* In 2 - 3 d in 2/3 patients with proliferative glomerulonephritis *1053*

Fibrinogen *Plasma Decrease Physiological* In 29 children with nephrotic syndrome treatment with prednisone for 3 weeks caused mean basal concentration of 5.9 ± 1.8 g/L to decrease significantly to 2.5 ± 0.7 g/L (2.5 ± 0.8 g/L in steroid-sensitive and 2.4 ± 0.7 g/L in steroid-resistant) *175*

Filtration Fraction *Urine No Effect Physiological* In 9 patients with Graves' disease treatment with 60 mg/d for 2 weeks caused nonsignificant change from mean baseline of 0.20 ± 0.0 to 0.21 *6162*

Filtration Index *Blood No Effect Physiological* In 29 children with nephrotic syndrome treatment with prednisone for 3 weeks caused mean basal filtration index of 12.0 ± 7.2 to increase nonsignificantly to 13.0 ± 4.9 (12.9 ± 4.0 in steroid-sensitive and 13.7 ± 8.5 in steroid-resistant) *175*

Follicle Stimulating Hormone
Plasma Decrease Physiological In 23 male patients with rheumatoid arthritis taking prednisone mean concentration of 241 ± 160 µg/L not significantly less than 343 ± 212 µg/L in 12 patients with rheumatoid arthritis not taking prednisone *3808*
Plasma No Effect Physiological No apparent effect, unlike that on testosterone, in 67 year old males with chronic pulmonary disease taking drug for at least 1 mo *3707*

γ-Globulin *Serum Decrease Physiological* Augmented response in cirrhotics when drug added to therapeutic regime *1004*

Glomerular Filtration Rate *Urine Increase Physiological* In 9 patients with Graves' disease treatment with 60 mg/d for 2 weeks caused significant increase from mean baseline of 93 ± 4 mL/min/1.73 sqm to 102 ± 5 mL/min/1.73 sq m *6162*

Glucose *Serum Increase Physiological* Fasting concentration progressively and significantly increased with short-term treatment *4477* Glucocorticoid effect *4174*
Urine Decrease Analytical Low results observed with Clinistix® , Diastix® *1826*
Urine No Effect Analytical No effect observed with Tes-Tape® *1826*

Glucose Tolerance *Serum Decrease Physiological* Endocrine action *2754* Moderate reduction in tolerance in response to oral glucose *4477*

Growth Hormone *Plasma Decrease Physiological* In prepubertal children with acute lymphoblastic leukemia receiving chemotherapy administration of 40 mg/m²/d prednisone was associated with a GH concentration of 2 ng/mL whereas the concentration after prednisone was 13 ng/mL *679*

HDL-Cholesterol *Serum Increase Physiological* 68% average effect in both men and women *6667* Mean concentration of 57 mg/dL in 35 women with SLE or rheumatoid arthritis treated with mean dose of 10.8 mg/dL for 3 months compared with mean concentration of 54 mg/dL in 44 untreated women with rheumatoid arthritis *6318*

25-Hydroxy Vitamin D *Serum No Effect Physiological* No significant change in 23 patients requiring long-term glucocorticoid therapy when they received 10-25 mg/day for 12 months *4896*

Hydroxyproline *Urine Decrease Physiological* In 23 patients requiring long-term glucocorticoid therapy receiving 10-25 mg/day concentration fell significantly during first 2 months and continued to fall thereafter *4896*
Urine No Effect Physiological In 6 patients who needed high-dose corticosteroid therapy concentration changed non-significantly from mean baseline of 1.75 ± 0.8 mmol/mmol creatinine to 2.05 ± 0.98 mmol/mmol creatinine after 15 days treatment with 29.1 mg/d *3625* Urinary hydroxyproline/creatinine ratio remained unchanged in 10 euthyroid patients with Graves' disease treated with prednisone for 12 weeks *4804*

Immunoglobulin G *Serum No Effect Physiological* Shortens half life but increased synthesis (no net change) *2331*

Insulin *Plasma Increase Physiological* Progressive and significant increase with short-term treatment *4477*

6-Keto-Prostaglandin $F_{1\alpha}$ *Plasma No Effect Physiological* No significant change with up to 25 mg drug for up to 14 d: no effect on production during clotting *4817*

LDL-Cholesterol *Serum Decrease Physiological* Mean concentration of 120 mg/dL in 35 women with SLE or rheumatoid arthritis treated with mean dose of 10.8 mg daily for 3 months compared with mean concentration of 128 mg/dL in 44 untreated control women *6318*
Serum No Effect Physiological Insignificant increase (11%) in both men and women after 1 mo *6667*

Leukocytes *Blood Decrease Analytical* Low count by Coulter S, ?due to fragile cells *3677*
Blood Increase Physiological Significant effect with increase of 6,000 /µL by second week *5532* Augmented response in cirrhotics when drug added to therapeutic regime *1004* Observed in 2 of 676 cases, no obvious cause *663*

Luteinizing Hormone *Plasma Decrease Physiological* In 23 male patients with rheumatoid arthritis taking prednisone mean concentration of 36 ± 21 µg/L not significantly less than 53 ± 34 µg/L in 12 patients with rheumatoid arthritis not taking prednisone *3808*
Plasma No Effect Physiological No apparent effect, unlike that on testosterone, in 67 year old males with chronic pulmonary disease taking drug for at least 1 mo *3707*

Lymphocyte B-Cells *Blood Decrease Physiological* Reduced but not to same extent as T-lymphocytes *5532*

Lymphocyte T-Cells *Blood Decrease Physiological* Proportional greatest reduction with steroids *5532*

Lymphocytes *Blood Decrease Physiological* Maximal change in third week of therapy due to redistribution of cells out of circulation *5532*

α_2-Macroglobulin *Serum Decrease Physiological* In 29 children with nephrotic syndrome treatment with prednisone for 3 weeks caused mean basal concentration of 9.6 ± 3.4 g/L to decrease nonsignificantly to 6.5 ± 2.2 g/L (6.0 ± 1.7 g/L in steroid-sensitive and 8.2 ± 3.4 g/L in steroid-resistant) *175*
Serum No Effect Physiological No consistent change noted in 14 hospitalized adult patients when given 40-50 mg/d *6398*

Monocytes *Blood Increase Physiological* Changes parallel those of neutrophils *5532*

Mycophenolic Acid *Serum No Effect Analytical* No significant interference observed with HPLC method of Shipkova et al *5526*

Mycophenolic Acid Glucuronide
Serum No Effect Analytical No significant interference observed with HPLC method of Shipkova et al *5526*

Neutrophils *Blood Increase Physiological* Maximum reached in second week of therapy, thereafter falls *5532*

Nitrogen Balance *Patient Negative Physiological* Due to protein catabolism *2754*

Occult Blood *Feces Increase Physiological* May cause hemorrhage and ulceration of gastrointestinal tract *929*

2',5'-Oligoadenylate Synthetase
Neutrophils *Decrease* *Physiological* In healthy volunteers following a single intramuscular injection of interferon *6519*

Osteocalcin *Serum* *Decrease* *Physiological* In 10 euthyroid patients with Graves' disease treatment for 12 weeks caused decrease of mean from 3.0 ± 2.1 µg/L to 1.7 ± 1.1 µg/L after 4 weeks and 2.4 ± 1.9 µg/L after 12 weeks *4804* In 8 patients with autoimmune disorders treatment with prednisone decreasing from 1.0 to 0.1 mg/kg body weight/d for 4 months caused significant decrease from mean baseline of 5.3 ± 0.4 ng/mL to 2.9 ± 0.4 ng/mL after one month but returned to baseline levels of treatment of 4.7 ± 0.4 ng/mL after 2 months and 4.1 ± 0.3 ng/mL after 4 months *1118* Concentration reduced during chronic glucocorticoid treatment, but also observed with short term treatment. Nocturnal rise of osteocalcin inhibited *4287*
Serum *No Effect* *Physiological* In 8 patients with autoimmune disorders treatment with prednisone decreasing from 1.0 to 0.1 mg/kg body weight/d for 4 months caused significant decrease from mean baseline of 5.3 ± 0.4 ng/mL to 2.9 ± 0.4 ng/mL after one month but returned to baseline levels of treatment of 4.7 ± 0.4 ng/mL after 2 months and 4.1 ± 0.3 ng/mL *1118*

Parathyroid Hormone *Plasma* *Decrease* *Physiological* Serum intact-PTH concentration seemed to decrease slightly in 10 euthyroid patients with Graves' disease when treated for 12 weeks *4804*
Plasma *Increase* *Physiological* Significant effect although calcium normal *6467*
Plasma *No Effect* *Physiological* No significant effect in 23 patients requiring long-term glucocorticoid therapy who received 10-25 mg/day for 12 months *4896* In 6 patients who needed high-dose corticosteroid therapy concentration changed nonsignificantly from mean baseline of 40.9 ± 17 pmol/L to 42.8 ± 16 pmol/L after 15 days treatment with 29.1 mg/d *3625*

Phosphate *Serum* *No Effect* *Physiological* In 6 patients who needed high-dose corticosteroid therapy concentration changed nonsignificantly from mean baseline of 1.16 ± 0.12 mmol/L to 1.19 ± 0.16 mmol/L after 15 days treatment with 29.1 mg/d *3625*

Platelets *Blood* *Decrease* *Physiological* Immunologic response occurring in months *2385* In 29 children with nephrotic syndrome treatment with prednisone for 3 weeks caused mean basal concentration of 524 ± 172 10^9/L to decrease significantly to 440 ± 142 10^9/L (425 ± 143 10^9/L in steroid-sensitive and 498 ± 138 10^9/L in steroid-resistant) *175*

Potassium *Serum* *Decrease* *Physiological* Slight mineralocorticoid effect only *128*
Urine *Increase* *Physiological* Slight mineralocorticoid effect only *128*

Prealbumin *Serum* *Increase* *Physiological* Occurs with decreased thyroxine binding globulin *102*

Protein *Cerebrospinal Fluid* *No Effect* *Analytical* No significant effect when added in vitro to concentration of 10.0 mg/dL when measured by Kodak Ektachem® method *3654*
Serum *Increase* *Physiological* In 29 children with nephrotic syndrome treatment with prednisone for 3 weeks caused mean basal concentration of 43.9 ± 4.7 g/L to increase significantly to 55.8 ± 6.9 g/L (58.7 ± 2.9 g/L in steroid-sensitive and 44.7 ± 6.7 g/L in steroid-resistant) *175*
Serum *No Effect* *Physiological* In prepubertal children with acute lymphoblastic leukemia receiving chemotherapy administration of 40 mg/m²/d prednisone was associated with no change in protein concentration from mean of 67.0 ± 2.6 g/L to 66.3 ± 2.0 g/L *679*
Urine *Decrease* *Physiological* In 13 patients with HIV-associated nephropathy treatment with 60 mg/d prednisone for 2 to 11 weeks caused an average decrease in urine protein excretion from mean baseline of 9.1 ± 1.8 g/d to 3.2 ± 0.6 g/d *5623*

Protein C *Plasma* *Increase* *Physiological* In 29 children with nephrotic syndrome treatment with prednisone for 3 weeks caused mean basal concentration of 153 ± 46% to increase significantly to 247 ± 70% (232 ± 64% in steroid-sensitive and 288 ± 77% in steroid-resistant) *175*

Protein S *Plasma* *Increase* *Physiological* In 29 children with nephrotic syndrôme treatment with prednisone for 3 weeks caused mean basal concentration of 117 ± 29% to increase significantly to 139 ± 22% (143 ± 21% in steroid-sensitive and 115 ± 21% in steroid-resistant) *175*

Protein S, Free *Plasma* *Increase* *Physiological* In 29 children with nephrotic syndrome treatment with prednisone for 3 weeks caused mean basal concentration of 91 ± 33% to increase nonsignificantly to 128 ± 41% (136 ± 38% in steroid-sensitive and 82 ± 31% in steroid-resistant) *175*

Sodium *Serum* *Increase* *Physiological* Slight effect only *128*

Soluble CD4+ *Serum* *Decrease* *Physiological* In 15 patients with polyarthralgia rheumatica treated with 12.5 mg/d showed significant change from mean baseline of 10.1 ± 13.0 U/mL to 5.7 ± 7.3 U/mL after 6 months although no real change up to 3 months *5207*
Serum *No Effect* *Physiological* In 15 patients with polyarthralgia rheumatica treated with 12.5 mg/d showed nonsignificant change from mean baseline of 10.1 ± 13.0 U/mL to 10.6 ± 13.5 U/mL after 1 month *5207*

Soluble CD8+ *Serum* *Decrease* *Physiological* In 15 patients with polyarthralgia rheumatica treated with 12.5 mg/d showed change from mean baseline of 410 ± 153 U/mL to 400 ± 142 U/mL after 1 month and 343 ± 154 U/mL after 6 months although no real change up to 3 months *5207*

Soluble Interleukin-2 Receptor
Serum *Decrease* *Physiological* In 26 patients with chronic hepatitis B infection treatment orally for 4 weeks caused reduction from mean of 673.6 ± 52.9 U/mL to 584.8 ± 39.4 U/mL *3528* In 15 patients with polyarthralgia rheumatica treated with 12.5 mg/d showed decrease from mean baseline of 819 ± 421 U/mL to 464 ± 259 U/mL after 1 month and 470 ± 374 U/mL after 6 months *5207*

T3 Binding Capacity *Serum* *Decrease* *Physiological* Lowered with 1-2 mg/kg/d for 2-4 weeks in 10 children *5606*

Testosterone *Serum* *Decrease* *Physiological* In 23 male patients with rheumatoid arthritis taking prednisone mean concentration of 3.56 ± 1.59 ng/mL significantly less than 4.32 ± 1.07 ng/mL in 70 healthy male controls *3808* Reduced by more than 50% in 14 of 16 men aged 67 y with chronic pulmonary disease taking drug for at least 1 mo. Testosterone concentration inversely related to dose of drug. Serum protein binding unaffected. Effect probably due to suppression of secretion of gonadotropin releasing hormone by hypothalamus *3707*

Theophylline *Serum* *Increase* *Analytical* At concentration of 40 mg/L produced positive bias of 2.30 mg/L at theophylline concentration of 20 mg/L with method used with Syntex Accµ Level *1122*
Serum *No Effect* *Analytical* At concentration of 40 mg/L produced no interference with methods used with Kodak DT-60, Abbott TDx, Abbott Vision with both whole blood and serum, 3M Diagnostics TheoFAST and Ames Seralyzer *1122*
Serum *No Effect* *Physiological* No clinically significant effect on theophylline concentration observed when drugs coadministered *5999* No documented significant interaction with theophylline reported *6117*

Thromboxane *Plasma* *No Effect* *Physiological* No significant change with up to 25 mg drug for up to 14 d: no effect on production during clotting *4817*

Thyroid Stimulating Hormone
Serum *Increase* *Physiological* Basal value increased two fold in 10 children given 1-2 mg/kg/h for 2-4 weeks but TSH response to TRH unchanged *5606*

Thyroxine Binding Globulin
Serum *Decrease* *Physiological* Decreases concentration of thyroxine binding globulin, increases thyroxine binding prealbumin *5869*

Thyroxine (T4) *Serum* *No Effect* *Physiological* Insignificant change in 10 children treated for 2-4 weeks *5606*

Tri-iodothyronine, Reverse (rT3)
Serum *Decrease* *Physiological* Significant effect in 10 children given 1-2 mg/kg/h for 2-4 weeks *5606*
Serum *Increase* *Physiological* Considerable rise with 1-2 mg/kg/d for 2-4 weeks in 10 children *5606*

Tri-iodothyronine (T3) *Serum* *Decrease* *Physiological* Significant effect in 10 children given 1-2 mg/kg/h for 2-4 weeks *5606* Significant decrease with 1-2 mg/kg/d for 2-4 weeks in 10 children *5606*

Prednisone *(continued)*

Triglycerides *Serum Increase Physiological* In all 6 women slight effect in 1 mo *6667* Mean concentration of 173 mg/dL in 35 women with SLE or rheumatoid arthritis treated with mean dose of 10.8 mg daily for 3 months compared with mean concentration of 129 mg/dL in 44 untreated women controls *6318*

Serum No Effect Physiological No effect in men during 1 mo *6667*

TSH response to TRH *Serum No Effect Physiological* No significant effect with 1-2 mg/kg/d for 2-4 weeks in 10 children *5606*

Urea Nitrogen *Serum Decrease Physiological* 3.7% of 81 cases with low serum urea nitrogen concentrations associated with prednisone administration *3680*

Uric Acid *Serum Increase Physiological* Promotes nucleic acid catabolism *5869*

Viscosity *Blood Decrease Physiological* In 29 children with nephrotic syndrome treatment with prednisone for 3 weeks caused mean viscosity of 10.7 ± 1.6 mPa/s at shear rate 3.2 /s, 6.2 ± 0.7 mPa/s at shear rate 20.4 /s and 4.4 ± 0.5 mPa/s at shear rate of 128 /s to significantly decrease to 8.8 ± 0.9 mPa/s, 5.4 ± 0.4 mPa/s and 3.9 ± 0.3 mPa/s respectively with increase from 21.1 ± 1.8 mPa/s to 24.0 ± 3.8 mPa/s at shear rate of 0.20 /s and decrease from 19.3 ± 2.6 mPa/s to 18.7 ± 2.2 mPa/s at shear rate of 0.51 /s. Effects comparable in steroid-sensitive and steroid-resistant groups *175*

Plasma Decrease Physiological In 29 children with nephrotic syndrome treatment with prednisone for 3 weeks caused mean basal viscosity of 1.35 ± 0.15 mPa/s to decrease significantly to 1.20 ± 0.08 mPa/s (1.21 ± 0.7 mPa/s in steroid-sensitive and 1.15 ± 0.09 mPa/s in steroid-resistant) *175*

Zinc *Serum Decrease Physiological* Within 3 d average fell from 12.6 µmol/L to 11.1 µmol/L in 14 adult hospitalized patients given 40-50 mg daily; level rose to above normal then reverted normal in 2 weeks *6398*

Urine No Effect Physiological No consistent change noted in 14 hospitalized adult patients when given 40-50 mg/d *6398*

Prenalterol

Renin Activity *Plasma No Effect Physiological* Not significantly different from control state in 23 patients with stage III heart disease over 1 mo under controlled conditions *6361*

Prilocaine

Erythrocytes *Blood Decrease Physiological* Hemolysis with doses greater than 400 mg *128*

Hematocrit *Blood Decrease Physiological* Hemolysis with doses greater than 400 mg *128*

Hemoglobin *Blood Decrease Physiological* Hemolysis with doses greater than 400 mg *128*

Methemoglobin *Blood Increase Physiological* o-toluidine produced as metabolite causes hemolysis *1163*

Primaquine

Bilirubin *Serum Increase Physiological* May cause hemolysis with G-6-PD deficiency *402*

Color *Urine Increase Analytical* Rusty yellow or brown color *606*

Erythrocytes *Blood Decrease Physiological* Hemolytic anemia in G-6-PD deficient persons *1212*

Glutathione, Reduced
Red Blood Cells Decrease Physiological Associated with hemolysis and G-6-PD deficiency *5310*

Granulocytes *Blood Decrease Physiological* Agranulocytosis occasionally reported *1384*

Haptoglobin *Serum Decrease Physiological* May cause hemolytic anemia *3810*

Heinz Body Formation *Blood Positive Physiological* May occur in early stages of hemolysis *536*

Hematocrit *Blood Decrease Physiological* Hemolytic anemia in G-6-PD deficient persons *1212*

Hemoglobin *Blood Decrease Physiological* Hemolytic anemia in G-6-PD deficient persons *1212* Hemolysis in glucose-6-phosphate dehydrogenase deficiency or methemoglobin reductase deficiency may be caused by drug *2873*

Leukocytes *Blood Decrease Physiological* Agranulocytosis/Leukopenia *3810*

Methemoglobin *Blood Increase Physiological* May cause hemolysis in G-6-PD deficiency *128*

Primidone

Amino-4-Imidazole-5-Carboxamide Ribotide
Urine Increase Physiological If megaloblastic anemia occurs *5054*

Amino Acids *Urine Increase Analytical* Unusual orange spot with ninhydrin migrating in all TLC systems close to threonine *2605*

Barbiturate *Serum Increase Physiological* Phenobarbital is major metabolite *2009*

Serum No Effect Analytical No significant interference observed at a concentration of 100 µg/mL (0.46 mmol/L) with method on Du Pont aca *1511*

Bilirubin *Serum No Effect Physiological* Insignificant displacement from protein in neonates *6314*

Carbamazepine *Serum Decrease Physiological* Simultaneous administration causes marked reduction of plasma carbamazepine concentration *282* Drugs that induce CYP 3A4 enhance metabolism of carbamazepine producing clinically meaningful effect *1039* Typically reduction of concentrations when drugs coadministered due to hepatic enzyme induction but may be slight increase *1384* Decreases plasma concentration through hepatic enzyme induction *3118*

Serum No Effect Analytical At a concentration of 200 µg/mL had no significant cross-reactivity with carbamazepine at a concentration of 4.0 µg/mL when measured by method on Bayer Technicon Immuno 1® system *417* Cross reactivity of about 0.05% observed with method on Baxter Stratus *5705* No cross-reactivity observed with method on Du Pont aca *1513*

Chloride *Serum Decrease Analytical* At 10 times therapeutic concentration caused statistically significant decrease with method used on Technicon SRA-2000 *4348*

Clonazepam *Serum Decrease Physiological* Slight and clinically unimportant reduction due to enhanced hepatic metabolism *6501* Stimulates hepatic metabolism to reduce plasma concentration *1384*

Crystals *Urine Increase Physiological* In acute poisoning case crystals may occur due to primidone *329*

Cyclosporine *Blood Decrease Physiological* Coadministration with cyclosporine reported in one patient to decrease trough cyclosporine concentrations probably through induction of CYP enzymes in liver with dramatic increase in concentration after primidone withdrawn *859*

Serum Decrease Physiological Reported effect presumably as result of induction of hepatic microsomal enzymes *1069* Coadministration with cyclosporine reported in one patient to decrease trough cyclosporine concentrations probably through induction of CYP enzymes in liver with dramatic increase in concentration after primidone withdrawn *859* In one renal transplant patient during treatment concentration was 210 µg/L but increased to 1080 µg/L within 12 days of discontinuing treatment *3188* In one renal transplant patient coadministration of primidone caused a reduction in concentration of cyclosporine *6595*

Eosinophils *Blood Increase Physiological* May be allergic type of response *654*

Erythrocytes *Blood Decrease Physiological* Megaloblastic anemia secondary to disturbance in folic acid metabolism *4932*

Ethosuximide *Serum Decrease Physiological* Reported to decrease plasma concentration *1384*

Serum No Effect Analytical Insignificant cross-reactivity observed with method used on Du Pont aca *1523*

Felbamate *Serum No Effect Analytical* No significant interference observed with GLC method of Rifai et al even though it is co-extracted *4958*

Folate *Cerebrospinal Fluid Decrease Physiological* Occurs in many long-treated epileptics *4931* Low folate in from 27 to 91% of treated epileptics in different studies *3383*

Red Blood Cells Decrease Physiological Low serum folate in from 27 to 91% of treated epileptics in different studies *3383* Impaired deconjugation of polyglutamates in gut *1647*
Serum Decrease Physiological Low serum folate in from 27 to 91% of treated epileptics in different studies *3383* May cause megaloblastic anemia (impairs absorption) *5054*
Test Conditions No Effect Analytical No effect on *L. casei* or *S. fecalis4014*

Glucaric Acid *Urine Increase Physiological* Dose-dependent effect but less potent than carbamazepine *4623* More potent inducer of hepatic enzymes than phenobarbital *3430*

Glucose *Serum No Effect Analytical* At concentration of 2.4 mg/L had no effect on Kodak Ektachem® method *5704*
Serum No Effect Physiological No significant effect observed in epileptic patients receiving primidone *4077*

Griseofulvin *Serum Decrease Physiological* Decreases systemic absorption from gastrointestinal tract *1384*

Hematocrit *Blood Decrease Physiological* Megaloblastic anemia secondary to disturbance in folic acid metabolism *4932*

Hemoglobin *Blood Decrease Physiological* Megaloblastic anemia secondary to disturbance in folic acid metabolism *4932*

Histamine *Plasma No Effect Analytical* Improbable inhibition of radio-enzyme assay at physiological concentrations *2492*

Indomethacin *Serum No Effect Analytical* No effect on HPLC method of Roberts and Smith *4978*

Lactate *Plasma No Effect Physiological* No significant effect observed in epileptic patients receiving primidone *4077*

Lamotrigine *Serum Decrease Physiological* Coadministration of primidone with lamotrigine caused a significant approximately 40% reduction in the plasma concentration of lamotrigine *2160*

LE Cells *Blood Positive Physiological* Less frequent than with many anticonvulsants *654*

Leucine Aminopeptidase Isoenzymes
Serum Increase Physiological Increased slower running components *5155*

Leukocytes *Blood Decrease Physiological* Pancytopenia (AMA Blood dyscrasias) *4017*

MCV *Blood Increase Physiological* Megaloblastic anemia secondary to disturbance in folic acid metabolism *4932*

Mexiletine *Serum Decrease Physiological* Hepatic enzyme induction may decrease elimination half-life by 50% *3281*

Mycophenolic Acid *Serum No Effect Analytical* No significant interference observed with HPLC method of Shipkova et al *5526*

Mycophenolic Acid Glucuronide
Serum No Effect Analytical No significant interference observed with HPLC method of Shipkova et al *5526*

Neutrophils *Blood Decrease Physiological* Occasional case of agranulocytosis reported *6264*

N-Formiminoglutamic Acid *Urine Increase Physiological* If megaloblastic anemia occurs *5054*

Phenobarbital *Serum Increase Physiological* Metabolic conversion *in vivo5093*
Serum No Effect Analytical No interference observed at a concentration of 250 µmol/L with Sung and Neely modification of Syva EMIT procedure *148* At maximum physiological or pharmacological concentrations no cross-reactivity observed with phenobarbital method on Bayer Technicon Immuno 1® *427* Cross-reactivity of less than 1.3% observed with method on Baxter Stratus *5705* No significant cross-reactivity observed with method on Du Pont aca *1537* At concentration of 500 µg/mL (2291 µmol/L) has no effect on method on Du Pont Dimension *1582*

Phenylalanine *Plasma No Effect Analytical* No interference observed with rapid quantitative whole blood method of Campbell et al using phenylalanine dehydrogenase *867*

Phenytoin *Serum No Effect Analytical* No effect at concentration of 500 µg/mL (2290 µmol/L) on method on Du Pont Dimension *1583* No significant interference observed at a concentration of 500 µg/mL (2.29 mmol/L) with method on Du Pont aca *1538* At a concentration of 20 µg/mL no cross-reactivity observed with phenytoin at a concentration of 10 µg/mL when measured by the method on Bayer Technicon Immuno 1® *428*

Phosphate *Serum Decrease Analytical* At 10 times therapeutic concentration caused statistically significant decrease with method on Technicon SRA-2000 *4348*

Platelets *Blood Decrease Physiological* Pancytopenia (AMA Blood dyscrasias) *4017*

Potassium *Serum No Effect Analytical* At concentration of 10 mg/L had no effect on measurement by ISE with predilution *5704*

Protein *Serum Increase Analytical* At 10 times therapeutic concentration caused statistically significant increase with method used on Technicon SRA-2000 *4348*

Prothrombin Time *Plasma Decrease Physiological* May shorten action of anticoagulants *2753*

Pyruvate *Plasma No Effect Physiological* No significant effect observed in epileptic patients receiving primidone *4077*

SDZ PSC 833 *Blood No Effect Analytical* At a concentration of 10.1 mg/L had no effect on HPLC method of Scott et al when used to measure PSC (with CsD as internal standard) at a concentration of 5 mg/L *5418*

Sodium *Serum No Effect Analytical* At concentration of 10 mg/L had no effect on measurement by ISE with predilution *5704*

T3-Uptake *Serum No Effect Physiological* In 5 epileptic patients treated on average for 6 mo *3568*

Tacrolimus *Blood No Effect Analytical* No significant effect observed at a concentration of 16 mg/L with MEIA method on Abbott IMx analyzer *1871*
Serum No Effect Analytical At a concentration of 16 mg/L had no significant effect on ELISA method *6329*

Testosterone *Serum No Effect Physiological* Usual effect but may be slight increase *2836*

Testosterone, Free *Serum Decrease Physiological* Observed effect *2836*

Thyroid Stimulating Hormone
Serum No Effect Physiological In 5 epileptic patients treated on average for 6 mo *3568*

Thyroxine (T4) *Serum Decrease Physiological* Associated with enzyme induction *6412*
Serum No Effect Physiological In 5 epileptic patients treated on average for 6 mo *3568*

Thyroxine (T4) Index, Free *Serum Decrease Physiological* Associated with enzyme induction *6412*
Serum No Effect Physiological In 5 epileptic patients treated on average for 6 mo *3568*

Thyroxine (T4) (Murphy-Pattee)
Serum No Effect Physiological In 5 epileptic patients treated on average for 6 mo *3568*

Tri-iodothyronine, Reverse (rT3)
Serum No Effect Physiological In 5 epileptic patients treated on average for 6 mo *3568*

Tri-iodothyronine (T3) *Serum No Effect Physiological* In 5 epileptic patients treated on average for 6 mo *3568* Associated with enzyme induction *6412*

Urea Nitrogen *Serum No Effect Analytical* At concentration of 2.4 mg/L had no effect on Kodak Ektachem® method *5704*

Valproic Acid *Serum Decrease Physiological* By increasing the expression of hepatic enzymes, especially those that increase the amount of glucuronosyl transferases, may increase the clearance of valproate twofold *17* Through induction of hepatic enzymes may increase the plasma clearance of valproate *15*
Serum No Effect Analytical No significant interference observed at a concentration of 1000 µ.g/mL (4582 µmol/L) with method on Du Pont aca *1560* No significant interference observed at a concentration of 1000 µg/mL (4582 µmol/L) with method on Du Pont aca *1560* At concentrations up to 1000 µg/mL had no significant cross-reactivity in valproic acid method on Bayer Technicon Immuno 1® *437*

Prinomide

C-Reactive Protein *Serum Decrease Physiological* In 88 patients with rheumatoid arthritis treated for up to 20 weeks caused reduction from mean increased baseline to almost normal *1083*

Prinomide *(continued)*

Erythrocyte Sedimentation Rate
Blood Decrease Physiological In 88 patients with rheumatoid arthritis treatment for up to 20 weeks caused decrease (median decreasing from 37 to 34 mm/h) but with decrease in 75th percentile from 50 to 40 mm/h and in 25th percentile from 31 to 18 mm/h *1083*

Interleukin-6 *Serum No Effect Physiological* In 88 patients with rheumatoid arthritis treatment with prinomide for up to 20 weeks had no significant effect on concentration *1083*

Pristinamycin

Cyclosporine *Serum Increase Physiological* Drug is known to inhibit cytochrome P-450 thereby inhibiting cyclosporine metabolism *1069*

Pristinomycin

Cyclosporine *Blood Increase Physiological* Coadministration of pristinomycin with cyclosporine caused a 65% increase in the blood cyclosporine concentration in bone marrow transplant recipients *859*
Serum Increase Physiological Coadministration of pristinomycin with cyclosporine caused a 65% increase in the blood cyclosporine concentration in bone marrow transplant recipients *859*

Probenecid

Acetaminophen *Serum Increase Physiological* Probenecid increases the mean plasma elimination half-life of the drug with an increase in its plasma concentration *3960* In 10 healthy volunteers coadministration of probenecid with acetaminophen caused maximal concentration to increase significantly to mean 23.5 µg/mL from mean baseline of 18.2 µg/mL due to uncompetitive inhibition of glucuronidation in the liver *3017*
Urine Decrease Physiological In a group of healthy volunteers pretreatment with probenecid caused a significant decrease in acetaminophen clearance from 6.23 to 3.42 mL/min/kg and urinary excretion of acetaminophen sulfate and acetaminophen glucuronide decreased from 243 to 193 mg and from 348 to 74.5 mg respectively *3017*

Acyclovir *Serum Increase Physiological* Coadministration of probenecid with intraveous acyclovir increases mean half-life and area under concentration curve with corresponding reduction of urinary excretion and renal clearance of acyclovir *2151*

Adenosine Diphosphate
Red Blood Cells No Effect Physiological No effect in 5 volunteers 2 h after 2 g probenecid *6584*

Adenosine Monophosphate *Plasma Increase Physiological* In 8 healthy young men. Probable effect on carrier mediated process to clear plasma cyclic AMP *2206*
Red Blood Cells No Effect Physiological No effect in 5 volunteers 2 h after 2 g probenecid *6584*
Urine No Effect Physiological In 8 healthy young men *2206*

Adenosine Triphosphate
Red Blood Cells No Effect Physiological No effect in 5 volunteers 2 h after 2 g probenecid *6584*

Alanine Aminotransferase *Serum Increase Physiological* Hepatotoxic effect (centrolobular necrosis) *3810* Probenecid has been reported to cause hepatic necrosis *3960*
Serum No Effect Analytical No effect at therapeutic concentration on Boehringer Mannheim Reflotron method *3231* No effect up to 1000 mg/L on Boehringer Mannheim Reflotron method but above this concentration inhibition of enzyme activity although of no clinical significance since normal therapeutic concentrations 100-200 mg/L *5706*

Albumin *Serum No Effect Analytical* At concentration of 1300 mg/L had no effect on BCG method *5704*

Alkaline Phosphatase *Serum Increase Physiological* Probenecid has been reported to cause hepatic necrosis *3960* Hepatotoxic effect (centrolobular necrosis) *3810*

Aminohippurate *Serum Increase Physiological* Renal transport decreased and plasma concentration increased *1384*

Aminosalicylic Acid *Serum Increase Physiological* Increases by 2-4 fold (inhibits renal excretion) *2452* Concentration increased probably as result of inhibition of renal excretion *897*

Ampicillin *Serum Increase Physiological* Administration of probenecid with ampicillin has been associated with increased blood concentrations of ampicillin with possible toxicity *6563*

Amylase *Serum No Effect Analytical* No effect of concentrations up to 1000 mg/L on method on Boehringer Mannheim Reflotron *5706*

Amylase, Pancreatic Isoenzyme
Serum No Effect Analytical No significant effect observed at a concentration of 1000 mg/L with method on Boehringer Mannheim Reflotron *3647*

Aspartate Aminotransferase *Serum Increase Physiological* Hepatotoxic effect (centrolobular necrosis) *3810* Probenecid has been reported to cause hepatic necrosis *3960*
Serum No Effect Analytical No effect at therapeutic concentration on Boehringer Mannheim Reflotron method *3231* No effect at 1000 mg/L on Boehringer Mannheim Reflotron method *5706*

Benzylpenicillin *Serum Increase Physiological* Drug inhibits tubular excretion of penicillin in a dose-related manner *4462*

Bicarbonate *Serum No Effect Analytical* At concentration of 1300 mg/L had no effect on method using phenolphthalein *5704*

Bile *Urine Increase Physiological* Possible hepatotoxicity *3810*

Bilirubin *Serum Increase Physiological* Hepatotoxic effect (centrolobular necrosis) *3810* Probenecid has been reported to cause hepatic necrosis *3960*
Serum No Effect Analytical At concentration of 1000 mg/L no effect on method on Boehringer Mannheim Reflotron system *5706* At concentration of 1300 mg/L had no effect on Jendrassik and Grof method *5704*

Blood *Urine Increase Physiological* Reported to cause hematuria with formation of uric acid stones in gouty patients unless urine alkalinized with a liberal fluid intake *3960*

BSP Retention *Serum Increase Physiological* Hepatotoxic effect (centrolobular necrosis) *6515*

Calcium *Serum No Effect Analytical* At concentration of 1300 mg/L had no effect on cresolphthalein method *5704*

Calculi *Urine Increase Physiological* May occur if little fluid drunk or little excreted *211*

Captopril *Serum Increase Physiological* Slight increase observed in healthy volunteers when drugs coadministered *5578*

Carbenicillin *Serum Increase Physiological* Concentration may be increased and prolonged when probenecid coadministered *4647*

Carprofen *Serum Increase Physiological* Significant decrease in clearance previously reported. In this article demonstration of reduced clearance of both carprofen enantiomers and their glucuronides and conversion of enantiomers to glucuronides *5734*

Catecholamines *Plasma No Effect Analytical* No effect on HPLC method of Koller for dopamine, epinephrine, and norepinephrine *3230*

Cefaclor *Serum Increase Physiological* Administration of probenecid prior to cefaclor increased serum concentration of cefaclor and delayed its urinary excretion *765* Renal excretion reduced when probenecid coadministered *1627*

Cefadroxil *Serum Increase Physiological* Pretreatment with 500 mg probenecid caused increased an increased half-life and peak serum concentration while reducing systemic clearance *765*

Cefamandole *Serum Increase Physiological* Coadministration increased cefamandole concentration although cefamandole given intramuscularly. Clearance reduced from 229 to 57 mL/min/sq m with similar changes after different therapeutic regimes *765*

Cefazedone *Serum Increase Physiological* Following a single intravenous dose of cefazedone of 1000 mg elimination rate of cefazodone decreased with decreased volume of distribution and delayed recovery in urine *765*

Cefazolin *Serum Increase Physiological* Probenecid may decrease renal tubular secretion of cephalosporins when used concurrently, resulting in increased and more prolonged cephalosporin blood concentrations *5637* With prior probenecid administration plasma concentration of cefazolin increased after intramuscular injection. Following a single oral dose of probenecid 2 g cefazolin intravenously resulted in a significant decrease in the cefazolin elimination rate and sustained serum concentrations over the subsequent 24 hours *765*

Cefdinir *Serum Increase Physiological* Concomitant administration of probenecid with cefdinir inhibits its renal excretion resulting in an approximate doubling of its area under the curve and a 54% increase in its peak plasma concentration *4528*

Cefmenoxime *Serum Increase Physiological* Coadministration reduced clearance without a change in the volume of distribution of cefmenoxime *765*

Cefmetazole *Serum Increase Physiological* Pretreatment with probenecid resulted in decreased elimination rate, increased area under the curve and delayed urinary recovery of cefmetazole *765*

Cefonicid *Serum Increase Physiological* Probenecid given 1000 mg orally with 500 mg cefonicid intramuscularly caused increased plasma concentration, reduced elimination rate and decreased clearance *765*

Cefoperazone *Serum No Effect Physiological* Concomitant administration had no effect on concentration *893*

Ceforanide *Serum No Effect Physiological* Coadministration of 1000 mg probenecid did not affect elimination rate, area under the curve, clearance and maximum plasma concentration *765*

Cefotaxime *Serum Increase Physiological* Reduced clearance of cefotaxime and its metabolites observed with administration of probenecid *765*

Cefoxitin *Serum Increase Physiological* Serum half-life and urinary recovery of cefoxitin prolonged with prior administration of probenecid. Area under the concentration curve increased *765*

Cefpodoxime *Serum Increase Physiological* Administration of probenecid inhibited excretion of cefpodoxime, resulting in an approximate 31% increase in its AUC and 20% increase in peak concentration *4684*

Cefruoxime *Serum Increase Physiological* At therapeutic plasma concentration of cefruoxime coadministration of probenecid caused almost complete blockage of tubular excretion of cefruoxime *6231*

Cefsulodin *Serum No Effect Physiological* Concomitant administration had no effect on concentration *893*

Ceftazidime *Serum No Effect Physiological* Concomitant administration had no effect on concentration *893* Pharmacokinetics and serum concentrations not affected by oral administration of probenecid *765*

Ceftizoxime *Serum No Effect Physiological* Elimination rate and volume of distribution not affected in 6 volunteers when probenecid 500 mg orally 7 and 1 h before 1000 mg ceftizoxime but when 1000 mg probenecid given orally with an intramuscular injection of 1000 mg ceftizoxime elimination rate reduced and increase in the area under the curve noted *765*

Ceftriaxone *Serum No Effect Physiological* Concomitant administration had no effect on concentration *893* Prior administration of probenecid had no effect on plasma concentration of ceftriaxone *765*

Cefuroxime *Serum Increase Physiological* Coadministration of probenecid with cefuroxime increases the latter's area under the serum concentration versus time curve by 50%: The peak serum concentration of cefuroxime after a 1.5 g single dose increases to 14.8 µg/mL when taken with probenecid compared with 12.2 µg/mL in the absence of probenecid *2153* Probenecid before and after a single intramuscular injection of cefuroxime caused a 30% higher maximum plasma concentration, a 20% reduction in the volume of distribution and a 32% decrease in the elimination rate when compared with administration of cefuroxime alone *765*

Cephalexin *Serum Increase Physiological* Following oral administration of probenecid rate of clearance of cefalexin reduced and clinically relevant serum cefalexin concentrations prolonged. Urinary recovery of cefalexin does not appear to be reduced but may be delayed *765* Reduces renal clearance *2452*

Cephaloridine *Serum Increase Physiological* Reduces renal clearance *2452*

Cephalothin *Serum Increase Physiological* Reduces renal clearance *2452* Coadministration of oral probenecid and intravenous cefalothin caused impaired clearance of cefalothin and delayed recovery of cefalothin in the urine. Prolonged therapeutic concentration of cefalothin observed *765*

Cephradine *Serum Increase Physiological* Coadministration of probenecid with cefradine caused increase in cefradine concentration and delayed urinary recovery of the antibiotic *765*

Chloride *Serum No Effect Analytical* At concentration of 1300 mg/L had no effect on mercurimetric method *5704*

Chlorpropamide *Serum Increase Physiological* Renal tubular secretion inhibited when probenecid coadministered *4636* Drugs that are highly protein-bound compete with chlorpropamide for binding sites and may potentiate hypoglycemic action of sulfonylurea *4644*

Cholesterol *Serum No Effect Analytical* At concentration of 1300 mg/L had no effect on Liebermann-Burchard method *5704* At concentration of 1000 mg/L no effect on method on Boehringer Mannheim Reflotron system *5706* At concentration of 280 mg/L had no effect on CHOD-PAP method *5704* At concentration of 260 mg/L had no effect on CHOD-Iodide method *5704* No effect at therapeutic concentration on Boehringer Mannheim Reflotron method *3231* At concentration of 260 mg/L had no effect on catalase-AIDH method *5704* At concentration of 260 mg/L had no effect on method using catalase-Hantzsch reaction *5704*

Ciprofloxacin *Serum Increase Physiological* Concurrent administration of ciprofloxacin with probenecid results in decreased renal tubular secretion of ciprofloxacin and an increase in its plasma concentration *416*

Clofibrate *Serum Increase Physiological* probenecid can inhibit the hepatic conjugation of clofibrate with glucuronide and reducing its renal clearance increasing its plasma concentration. Probenecid may also displace clofibrate from its protein-binding sites *3668*

Cortisol *Plasma No Effect Analytical* At concentration of 1000 mg/L marginally increase observed on CEDIA method (worst case 111% recovery) *1097*

Creatinine *Serum No Effect Analytical* At concentration of 1300 mg/L had no effect on Technicon AutoAnalyzer® Jaffe method *5704* At concentration of 200 mg/L had no effect on Jaffe-Fading-Fraction method *5704* At concentration of 1,000 mg/L had no effect on kinetic Jaffe method on BKA-2 *5704* At concentration of 200 mg/L had no effect on Jaffe-Fuller's earth method *5704*

Creatinine Clearance *Urine Decrease Physiological* When coadministered with digoxin probenecid caused significant reduction of 22%, either due to a reduction of GFR by probenecid or inhibition of the secretory component of creatinine elimination. Nevertheless digoxin clearance appeared to be unaffected *2527*

Dapsone *Serum Increase Physiological* 50% increase after 4 h, inhibits excretion *2452* In one study dapsone concentrations increased by about 50% at 4 hours and 25% at 8 hours when drugs coadministered probably due to probenecid inhibition of dapsone excretion *2243* Increased plasma concentration *886*

Digoxin *Serum No Effect Physiological* No effect observed on plasma, renal, or biliary clearance of digoxin, nor on elimination half-life or its volume of distribution *2527*

1,25-Dihydroxy Vitamin D_3 *Serum No Effect Physiological* In 8 healthy young men *2206*

Diphylline *Serum Increase Physiological* In one study substantial increase in dyphylline concentrations when drugs coadministered probably through inhibition of renal excretion *3854*

Erythrocytes *Blood Decrease Physiological* Hemolytic anemia (sensitivity dependent) *1212*
Urine Increase Physiological ?Due to sensitivity, or toxicity *637*

Estradiol *Urine Decrease Physiological* Tubular excretion may be blocked *54*

Estriol *Urine Decrease Physiological* Tubular excretion may be blocked *54*

Probenecid *(continued)*

Estrone *Urine Decrease Physiological* Tubular excretion may be blocked *54*

Furosemide *Serum Increase Physiological* Coadministration of probenecid with furosemide caused significant increase in concentration from 1.79 ± 0.65 μg/L to 2.77 ± 1.71 μg/L *6281* Coadministration of probenecid reduces active tubular secretion of furosemide. Plasma clearance fell from 155 to 85 mL/min and plasma half-life increased from 36 to 61 minutes *2693*

Furosemide Acylglucuronide
Serum Increase Physiological Coadministration of probenecid with furosemide caused significant increase in concentration from 0.09 ± 0.06 μg/L to 0.18 ± 0.12 μg/L *6281*

Gabapentin *Serum No Effect Physiological* Probenecid had no effect on the pharmacokinetics of gabapentin *4526*

Ganciclovir *Serum Increase Physiological* At an oral dose of 1000 mg ganciclovir every 8 h mean steady-state AUC of ganciclovir increased 53 ± 91% in the presence of probenecid 500 mg every 6 h. Renal clearance of ganciclovir decreased 22 ± 20% *5018* Increased plasma concentration *886*

Glucose *Serum Decrease Physiological* Reported effect *192*
Serum No Effect Analytical At concentration of 40 mg/L had no effect on Kodak Ektachem® method *5704* No effect at therapeutic concentration on Boehringer Mannheim Reflotron method *3231* At concentration of 1000 mg/L no effect on method on Boehringer Mannheim Reflotron system *5706* At concentration of 200 mg/L had no effect on hexokinase/G-6-PDH method *5704*
Urine Increase Analytical May cause false positive result with Ames Clinitest tablet procedure *4034*
Urine No Effect Analytical Has no effect on Ames Keto-Diastix, Diastix, Multistix and Clinistix procedures *4034* No effect on glucose oxidase methods *2452*

γ-Glutamyltransferase *Serum Increase Physiological* Probenecid has been reported to cause hepatic necrosis *3960*
Serum No Effect Analytical No effect at therapeutic concentration on Boehringer Mannheim Reflotron method *3231* At concentration of 1000 mg/L no effect on method on Boehringer Mannheim Reflotron system *5706*

Guanosine Diphosphate
Red Blood Cells No Effect Physiological No effect in 5 volunteers 2 h after 2 g probenecid *6584*

Guanosine Triphosphate
Red Blood Cells No Effect Physiological No effect in 5 volunteers 2 h after 2 g probenecid *6584*

HDL-Cholesterol *Serum No Effect Analytical* At a concentration up to 1000 mg/L had no significant effect on Reflotron method for whole blood cholesterol *6352*

Hematocrit *Blood Decrease Physiological* Probenecid has been reported to cause both hemolytic and aplastic anemias *3960* Hemolytic anemia (sensitivity dependent) *1212*

Hemoglobin *Blood Decrease Physiological* Probenecid has been reported to cause both hemolytic and aplastic anemias *3960* Hemolytic anemia (sensitivity dependent) *1212*
Urine Increase Physiological Actual bleeding caused by drug *1714*

Histamine *Plasma No Effect Analytical* Minimal inhibition of radio-enzyme assay at 100 μg/mL but therapeutic concentration 35.3 - 149 μg/mL *2492*

Homovanillic Acid
Cerebrospinal Fluid Increase Physiological Approximately 6 fold at 9 h, 9 fold at 18 h *2249*

4-Hydroxy-3-Methoxy-Phenylglycol
Cerebrospinal Fluid Increase Physiological 60% increase on average if 100 mg/kg over 18 h *2249*

4-Hydroxy-3-Methoxy-Phenylglycol Sulfate
Cerebrospinal Fluid Increase Physiological Small but not significant increase after 9 h *2249*

25-Hydroxy Vitamin D_3 *Serum No Effect Physiological* In 8 healthy young men *2206*

5-Hydroxyindoleacetic Acid
Cerebrospinal Fluid Increase Physiological Approximately 4 fold at 9 h, 5 fold at 18 h *2249*

Hypoxanthine *Red Blood Cells No Effect Physiological* No effect observed in 5 volunteers 2 h after administration of 2 g probenecid *6584*
Serum Decrease Physiological Occurs as result of rapid decrease of plasma uric acid due to uricosuric action of drug *6584* Within 2 hours of ingestion of 2 grams significant reduction occurred in 5 healthy individuals *6582*
Urine No Effect Physiological No significant effect observed although uric acid excretion markedly increased as result of uricosuric action of drug *6584*

Indomethacin *Serum Increase Physiological* Inhibits renal tubular secretion *2452* Probenecid increases the mean plasma elimination half-life of the drug with an increase in its plasma concentration *3960* When indomethacin is given to patients receiving probenecid plasma concentration of indomethacin is likely to be increased *3980* Renal tubular secretion of indomethacin inhibited by probenecid when administered concurrently *5593* Observed effect with coadministration of drugs *1384*

Inosine Monophosphate
Red Blood Cells No Effect Physiological No effect observed in 5 volunteers 2 h after 2 g probenecid *6584*

Iodomethamate *Serum Increase Physiological* Renal transport decreased and plasma concentration increased *1384*

Ketoprofen *Serum Increase Physiological* Probenecid increases the mean plasma elimination half-life of the drug with an increase in its plasma concentration *3960* In 6 healthy volunteers concurrent administration of probenecid with ketoprofen caused inhibition of hepatic metabolism of ketoprofen *6133* Probenecid increases the concentration of both free and bound ketoprofen by reducing the plasma ketoprofen concentration to about one third *6564*

Ketorolac *Serum No Effect Physiological* Coadministration of probenecid with ketorolac caused decreased clearance of ketorolac and significant increase in the ketorolac plasma concentration with AUC increasing from 5.4 to 17.8 μg/h/mL *5035*

17-Ketosteroids *Plasma Increase Physiological* Renal transport decreased and plasma concentration increased *1384*
Urine Decrease Physiological Decrease of up to 50% reported *1967*

Lactate *Plasma No Effect Analytical* At concentration of 200 mg/L had no effect on enzyme method *5704*

Latamoxef *Serum No Effect Physiological* Elimination rate, volume of distribution and clearance not affected by prior administration of probenecid *765*

Leukocytes *Blood Decrease Physiological* Occasional aplastic anemia seen *2753* Probenecid has been reported to cause leukopenia *3960*

Levofloxacin *Serum Increase Physiological* No significant effect observed of probenecid on the rate and extent of levofloxacin absorption but AUC and half-life of levofloxacin increased by 27 - 38% and 30% respectively *3916* Concurrent administration of probenecid with levofloxacin increased AUC and and half-life of levofloxacin by 27-38% and 30% respectively *3916*
Serum No Effect Physiological The AUC of levofloxacin was increased 27 - 38% in healthy volunteers but not enough to require alteration of dosage *4448*

Lomerfloxacin *Serum Increase Physiological* Probenecid slows the renal elimination with a 63% increase in the AUC and 4% in the maximum concentration in one study of 6 individuals *2068*

Loracarbef *Serum Increase Physiological* Coadministration of probenecid with loracarbef caused an 80% increase in the AUC for lorcarbef *1701*

Lorazepam *Serum Increase Physiological* Probenecid increases the mean plasma elimination half-life of the drug with an increase in its plasma concentration *3960*

Meclofenamate *Serum Increase Physiological* Probenecid increases the mean plasma elimination half-life of the drug with an increase in its plasma concentration *3960*

Methemoglobin *Blood Increase Physiological* May cause hemolysis with G-6-PD deficiency *6015*

Methotrexate *Serum Increase Physiological* Probenecid has been reported to increase plasma concentration in both animals and humans *3960* Administration of probenecid with methotrexate been demonstrated to increase its elimination half-life and an increase in its AUC *3909* Marked increase in serum concentration observed when drugs coadministered probably due to inhibition of tubular secretion of methotrexate *70*

Moxalactam *Serum No Effect Physiological* Concomitant administration had no effect on concentration *893*

Nalidixic Acid *Serum No Effect Physiological* In one patient very high concentration of nalidixic acid observed probably due to reduced renal excretion when drugs coadministered *1243*

Naproxen *Serum Increase Physiological* Exact mechanism not established but presumed to be related to reduced renal excretion and hepatic metabolism *5156* Probenecid increases the mean plasma elimination half-life of the drug with an increase in its plasma concentration *3960* Plasma concentration and half-life increased *1384*

Norfloxacin *Serum Increase Physiological* Coadministration of probenecid with norfloxacin reported to reduce urinary excretion of norfloxacin *3987* Reduced urinary excretion of norfloxacin has been reported with concomitant administration of probenecid, leading to increased serum concentration *4981*
Urine Decrease Physiological Coadministration of probenecid with norfloxacin reported to reduce urinary excretion of norfloxacin *3987* Reduced urinary excretion of norfloxacin has been reported with concomitant administration of probenecid, leading to increased serum concentration *4981*

Oxypurinol *Serum No Effect Physiological* In 5 healthy men coadministration of probenecid with allopurinol had no significant effect on plasma concentration *6581*
Urine Increase Physiological Coadministration of probenecid with allopurinol in 5 healthy men caused significant increase in ratio of excretion of oxypurinol to creatinine from 0.72 ± 0.11 to 1.17 ± 0.07 *6581*

p-Aminohippurate *Serum Increase Physiological* Renal transport decreased and plasma concentration increased *1384*

PAH Clearance *Urine Decrease Physiological* Renal clearance impaired *3906*

Pantothenic Acid *Serum Increase Physiological* Renal clearance decreased and plasma concentration increased *1384*

Parathyroid Hormone *Plasma No Effect Physiological* In 8 healthy young men *2206*

Penicillin *Serum Increase Physiological* Probenecid increases the plasma concentration of penicillin and other β-lactams *3960* Inhibits renal transport and increases plasma concentration *1384*

Phenolsulfonphthalein *Serum Increase Physiological* Renal transport decreased and plasma concentration increased *1384*

Phenprocoumon *Plasma Increase Physiological* 500 mg q.i.d. for 7 days in 17 healthy volunteers caused mean decrease of area under curve from 295 µg/h/mL to 157 µg/h/mL and a reduction in the fraction of the dose excreted by the kidneys. Effects probably due to inhibition of glucuronidation *4095*

Phenylalanine *Cerebrospinal Fluid No Effect Physiological* No effect on concentration observed *3903*

Phosphate *Serum No Effect Analytical* At concentration of 1300 mg/L had no effect on phosphomolybdate method *5704*

Platelets *Blood Decrease Physiological* Occasional aplastic anemia seen *2753*

Potassium *Serum No Effect Analytical* At concentration of 400 mg/L had no effect on measurement by ISE without predilution *5704* At concentration of 1300 mg/L had no effect on measurement by ISE with predilution *5704*

Pramipexole *Serum No Effect Physiological* Coadministration of pramipexole with probenecid had no effect on the pharmacokinetics of pramipexole *4680*

Prazosin *Serum No Effect Physiological* Coadministration of prazosin with probenecid had no apparent adverse drug interaction in limited clinical experience *4649*

Procainamide *Serum No Effect Physiological* Coadministration in 6 healthy volunteers had no significant effect on renal clearance or other parameters *3374*

Protein *Serum Decrease Physiological* Probenecid has been reported to cause nephrotic syndrome *3960*
Serum No Effect Analytical At concentration of 1300 mg/L had no effect on biuret method with blank correction *5704*
Urine Increase Physiological Nephrotoxic effect *2451 6515* Probenecid has been reported to cause nephrotic syndrome *3960*

Protein Electrophoresis *Serum No Effect Analytical* At concentration of 400 mg/L had no effect on automated Olympus-Hite method *5704*

Prothrombin Time *Plasma Increase Physiological* Probably displaces anticoagulant from binding protein *2452*

PSP Excretion *Urine Decrease Physiological* Inhibits renal transport of PSP *6515*

Rifampin *Serum Increase Physiological* When rifampin is taken with probenecid the rifampin concentration may increase due to reduced hepatic metabolism *2652* Inconsistent effect when when two drugs coadministered probably due to effect on hepatic uptake. Serum concentration increased by 86% *3110* Probenecid increases the mean plasma elimination half-life of the drug with an increase in its plasma concentration *3960*

Sodium *Serum No Effect Analytical* At concentration of 1300 mg/L had no effect on measurement by ISE with predilution *5704* At concentration of 400 mg/L had no effect on measurement by ISE without predilution *5704*

Sparfloxacin *Serum No Effect Physiological* Probenecid has no effect on the pharmacokinetics of sparfloxacin *4943*

Sugar *Urine Increase Analytical* False positive with Benedict's or Clinitest® *5869* Reducing substances with Benedict's, Clinitest® *882*

Sulfide *Serum No Effect Physiological* Probenecid, when coadministered with sulindac, increases insignificantly the plasma sulfide concentration *3960*

Sulfinpyrazone *Serum Increase Physiological* Inhibits renal tubular secretion *2452* Effect due to inhibition of tubular excretion of sulfinpyrazone and its major metabolite when drugs coadministered *4603*

Sulfobromophthalein *Serum Increase Physiological* Renal transport decreased and plasma concentration increased *1384*

Sulfonamides *Serum Increase Physiological* Decreases renal transport and increases plasma concentration, mainly of inactive conjugates *1384*

Sulfonamides, Conjugated *Serum Increase Physiological* Probenecid increases significantly the plasma concentration of conjugated sulfonamides *3960*

Sulfonamides, Free *Serum Increase Physiological* Probenecid increases insignificantly the plasma concentration of free sulfonamides *3960*

Sulfone *Serum Increase Physiological* Probenecid, when coadministered with sulindac, increases insignificantly the plasma sulfide concentration but significantly increased those of sulindac and sulfone *3960*

Sulfonylureas *Serum Increase Physiological* Inhibits renal transport and increases plasma concentration *1384*

Sulindac *Serum Increase Physiological* Probenecid, when coadministered with sulindac, increases insignificantly the plasma sulfide concentration but significantly increased those of sulindac and sulfone *3960*

Tenoxicam *Serum Increase Physiological* In 6 healthy volunteers co-treatment with 2 g/d probenecid for 4 days caused significant increase of maximum plasma concentration from 2.8 µg/mL to 3.5 µg/mL after a single oral dose of 20 mg tenoxicam *1294*

Theophylline *Serum Increase Analytical* Probenecid has been reported to increase concentration when measured by the Schack and Waxler technique *3960*

Thyroxine (T4), Free *Serum Increase Analytical* Increase observed when FT4 concentration measured by Boehringer Mannheim Enzymun procedure *2617*

Ticarcillin *Serum Increase Physiological* In patients receiving probenecid with ticarcillin renal tubular excretion of ticarcillin impaired resulting in prolonged half-life of ticarcillin *5661*

Tolbutamide *Serum No Effect Physiological* Probably has no effect on plasma concentration *2452*

Triglycerides *Serum No Effect Analytical* At concentration of 1300 mg/L had no effect on lipase/esterase method *5704* No effect at 1000 mg/L on Boehringer Mannheim Reflotron method *5706* No effect at therapeutic concentration on Boehringer Mannheim Reflotron method *3231*

Probenecid *(continued)*

Urea Nitrogen *Serum Increase Physiological* Possible nephrotoxicity *2451*
Serum No Effect Analytical No effect at therapeutic concentration on Boehringer Mannheim Reflotron method *3231* At concentration of 1300 mg/L had no effect on diacetylmonoxime method *5704* No effect at 1000 mg/L on Boehringer Mannheim Reflotron method *5706* At concentration of 40 mg/L had no effect on Kodak Ektachem® method *5704*

Uric Acid *Serum Decrease Physiological* Uricosuric action *2378* Within 2 hours of ingestion of 2 grams significant decrease of uric acid occurred in 5 healthy individuals *6582*
Serum No Effect Analytical No effect at therapeutic concentration on Boehringer Mannheim Reflotron method *3231* At concentration of 1300 mg/L had no effect on phosphotungstate reduction method *5704* No effect at 570 mg/L on uricase method on Ames Seralyzer *5706* At concentration of 570 mg/L had no effect on Seralyzer method *5704* At concentration of 280 mg/L had no effect on Kageyama-Hantzsch method *5704* No effect at 1000 mg/L on Boehringer Mannheim Reflotron method *5706* At concentration of 200 mg/L had no effect on catalase-AIDH method *5704*
Urine Decrease Physiological Small doses depress secretion *2242*
Urine Increase Physiological Uricosuric action *2378* Reported to cause hematuria with formation of uric acid stones in gouty patients unless urine alkalinized with a liberal fluid intake *3960* Ratio of urinary uric acid to creatinine increased within 2 hours of ingestion of 2 grams of drug in 5 healthy individuals *6582*

Xanthine *Serum Decrease Physiological* Occurs as result of rapid decrease of plasma concentration of uric acid due to uricosuric action of drug *6584* Within 2 hours of ingestion of 2 grams significant reduction occurred in 5 healthy individuals *6582*
Urine No Effect Physiological No significant effect observed in association with decreased serum concentration and increased urinary excretion of uric acid *6584*

Zalcitabine *Serum Increase Physiological* When single doses of zalcitabine 1.5 mg and probenecid 500 mg at 8 and 2 hours before and 4 hours after zalcitabine were administered to 12 HIV-positive patients, mean renal clearance of zalcitabine decreased from 310 mL/min to 180 mL/min and AUC increased from 59 ng.h/mL to 91 ng.h/mL *5023*

Zidovudine *Serum Increase Physiological* Increased plasma concentration *886* Coadministration of probenecid with zidovudine may increase the concentration of zidovudine by inhibiting glucuronidation and/or reducing its renal excretion *2163* Inhibits both hepatic glucuronidation and renal excretion and thus reduces total body clearance by up to 65% *6590*

Probucol

Aldolase *Serum Decrease Physiological* Mechanism obscure *1235*

Apolipoprotein A-I *Serum Decrease Physiological* In 14 hypercholesterolemic men treatment with probucol produced significant reduction in concentration *496* In 22 patients with hyperlipoproteinemia type II treatment with 1000 mg/d for 12 weeks caused significant reduction from mean baseline of 128.8 ± 21.8 mg/dL to 98.1 ± 19.6 mg/dL *2688* In 50 diabetics given 500 mg/d for 16 weeks and reduction greatest in highest cholesterol and triglyceride patients *2506* Decreased synthesis. Expression of apo E. Activation of cholesterol ester transfer protein *264*
Serum Increase Physiological In 62 hypercholesterolemic patients treatment with up to 1000 mg/d probucol and up to 400 mg/d bezafibrate caused change from mean baseline of 100 ± 2.0 mg/dL to 110 ± 20.6 mg/dL (significant) at 3 months, 111 ± 2.3 mg/dL at 6 months (nonsignificant) and 106 ± 2.1 mg/dL at 12 months (nonsignificant) *5196*

Apolipoprotein A-II *Serum Decrease Physiological* In 22 patients with hyperlipoproteinemia type II mean concentration significantly decreased from baseline of 35.6 ± 6.4 mg/dL to 30.3 ± 6.1 mg/dL with treatment with 1000 mg/d for 12 weeks *2688*
Serum Increase Physiological In 62 hypercholesterolemic patients treatment with up to 1000 mg/d probucol and up to 400 mg/d bezafibrate caused change from mean baseline of 30.4 ± 0.6 mg/dL to 38.0 ± 0.6 mg/dL (significant) at 3 months, 38.8 ± 0.7 mg/dL at 6 months (significant) and 37.7 ± 0.7 mg/dL at 12 months (significant) *5196*
Serum No Effect Physiological No significant change observed in 14 hypercholesterolemic men treated with drug *496*

Apolipoprotein B *Serum Decrease Physiological* In 22 patients with hyperlipoproteinemia type II mean baseline concentration of 157.7 ± 30.4 mg/dL significantly reduced to 121.2 ± 23.6 mg/dL with treatment with 1000 mg/d for 12 weeks *2688* Decrease from mean concentration of 203 mg/dL to 162 mg/dL in 81 patients with hypercholesterolemia treated with 1 g/day for 12 weeks *4704*
Serum No Effect Physiological In 22 patients with hyperlipoproteinemia type II treatment with 1000 mg/d for 12 weeks caused nonsignificant reduction from mean baseline of 8.8 ± 7.3 mg/dL to 6.7 ± 6.6 mg/dL *2688* In 62 hypercholesterolemic patients treatment with up to 1000 mg/d probucol and up to 400 mg/d bezafibrate caused change from mean baseline of 107 ± 1.6 mg/dL to 103 ± 1.7 mg/dL (nonsignificant) at 3 months, 105 ± 1.9 mg/dL at 6 months (nonsignificant) and 99.5 ± 1.8 mg/dL at 12 months (nonsignificant) *5196* No significant effect observed in 14 hypercholesterolemic men treated with drug *496*

Apolipoprotein C-II *Serum Decrease Physiological* In 50 diabetics given 500 mg/d for 16 weeks and reduction greatest in highest cholesterol and triglyceride patients *2506* In 22 patients with hyperlipoproteinemia type II treatment with 1000 mg/d for 12 weeks caused significant reduction from mean baseline of 5.9 ± 1.7 mg/dL to 4.9 ± 1.7 mg/dL *2688*
Serum No Effect Physiological In 22 patients with hyperlipoproteinemia type II treatment with 1000 mg/d for 12 weeks caused nonsignificant reduction from mean baseline of 1.5 ± 1.3 mg/dL to 1.4 ± 1.0 mg/dL *2688* In 62 hypercholesterolemic patients treatment with up to 1000 mg/d probucol and up to 400 mg/d bezafibrate caused change from mean baseline of 4.4 ± 0.1 mg/dL to 4.3 ± 0.1 mg/dL (nonsignificant) at 3 months, 4.4 ± 0.1 mg/dL at 6 months (nonsignificant) and 4.1 ± 0.1 mg/dL at 12 months (nonsignificant) *5196*

Apolipoprotein C-III *Serum Decrease Physiological* In 62 hypercholesterolemic patients treatment with up to 1000 mg/d probucol and up to 400 mg/d bezafibrate caused change from mean baseline of 10.6 ± 0.2 mg/dL to 8.4 ± 0.2 mg/dL (significant) at 3 months, 8.2 ± 0.3 mg/dL at 6 months (significant) and 8.0 ± 0.2 mg/dL at 12 months (significant) *5196* In 22 patients with hyperlipoproteinemia type II treatment with 1000 mg/d for 12 weeks caused significant decrease from mean baseline of 14.2 ± 4.8 mg/dL to 11.0 ± 4.9 mg/dL *2688*

Apolipoprotein E *Serum Decrease Physiological* In 62 hypercholesterolemic patients treatment with up to 1000 mg/d probucol and up to 400 mg/d bezafibrate caused change from mean baseline of 6.9 ± 0.1 mg/dL to 6.2 ± 0.1 mg/dL (significant) at 3 months, 6.3 ± 0.1 mg/dL at 6 months (significant) and 5.7 ± 0.1 mg/dL at 12 months (significant) *5196*
Serum No Effect Physiological In 22 patients with hyperlipoproteinemia type II treatment with 1000 mg/d for 12 weeks caused nonsignificant change from mean baseline of 6.6 ± 1.5 mg/dL to 7.1 ± 1.9 mg/dL *2688*

Bicarbonate *Serum Increase Physiological* Mechanism obscure (effect slight) *1235*

Calcium *Serum Decrease Physiological* Mechanism obscure (effect slight) *1235*

Cholesterol *Serum Decrease Physiological* 14 hypercholesterolemic men treatment with probucol produced significant reduction in concentration *496* In patients with familial hypercholesterolemia with apolipoprotein E_4 reduction from mean of 327 mg/dL to 237 mg/dL after 3 months treatment with 1 g/d and from 303 mg/dL to 262 mg/dL with the same treatment in those without apolipoprotein E_4 *1765* Reduction from mean concentration of 323 mg/dL to 285 mg/dL in 81 patients with hypercholesterolemia treated with 1 g/day for 12 weeks *4704* In 22 patients with hyperlipoproteinemia type II treatment with 1000 mg/d for 12 weeks caused significant decrease from mean baseline of 291.6 ± 37.9 mg/dL to 234.5 ± 41.1 mg/dL *2688* In 50 diabetics given 500 mg/d for 16 weeks and reduction greatest in highest cholesterol and triglyceride patients *2506* In 97 patients with hypercholesterolemia treatment with 1.0 g/d for 12 weeks caused a mean decrease of 10% *3982* In 29 patients with familial hypercholesterolemia already treated with cholestyramine addition of 1000 mg probucol daily caused further decrease of 15% *5376* In 62 hypercholesterolemic patients treatment with up to 1000 mg/d probucol and up to 400 mg/d bezafibrate caused change from mean baseline of 5.77 ± 0.09 mmol/L to 5.50 ± 0.08 mmol/L (significant) at 3 months, 5.47 ± 0.08 mmol/L at 6 months (significant) and 5.26 ± 0.08 mmol/L at 12 months (significant) *5196* Lowered by more than 20 mg/dL in most patients *1235*

Serum No Effect Physiological In 2 patients with NIDDM treatment of probucol combined with pravastatin for 4-5 months had no effect on concentration *2808*

Cholesterol Ester Transfer Protein
Serum Increase Physiological In 22 patients with hyperlipoproteinemia type II treatment with 1000 mg/d for 12 weeks caused significant increase in activity from mean baseline of 126.6 ± 50.6 units to 172.8 ± 40.2 units *2688*

Cholesterol:HDL-Cholesterol Ratio
Serum Increase Physiological In 97 patients with hypercholesterolemia treatment with 1.0 g/d for 12 weeks caused a mean increase of 23% *3982*

Creatine Kinase *Serum Increase Physiological* About 2% patients have demonstrated increased activity on one or more occasions *3982*

Creatine Kinase MM-Isoenzyme
Serum Increase Physiological About 2% patients have demonstrated increased activity on one or more occasions, attributable to the CK-MM fraction *3982*

Cyclosporine *Blood Decrease Physiological* 28% decrease observed in area under the concentration-time curve 0 to 11 hours after administration of probucol to 6 heart transplant patients with increase in cyclosporine clearance of 60% with increase in cyclosporine concentration once probucol withdrawn from therapeutic regime *859*

Serum Decrease Physiological 28% decrease observed in area under the concentration-time curve 0 to 11 hours after administration of probucol to 6 heart transplant patients with increase in cyclosporine clearance of 60% with increase in cyclosporine concentration once probucol withdrawn from therapeutic regime *859*

Eosinophils *Blood Increase Physiological* Hypersensitivity response (less than 10%) *1235*

Growth Hormone *Plasma Decrease Physiological* Mechanism obscure *1235*

HDL_2-Apolipoprotein A-I *Serum Decrease Physiological* In 22 patients with hyperlipoproteinemia type II treatment with 1000 mg/d for 12 weeks caused significant reduction from mean baseline of 22.5 ± 12.9 mg/dL to 12.6 ± 5.8 mg/dL *2688* Mean reduction of 47.0% observed with 12 weeks treatment *2689*

HDL_2-Cholesterol *Serum Decrease Physiological* Mean reduction of 43.0% observed with 12 weeks treatment *2689* In 22 patients with hyperlipoproteinemia type II treatment with 1000 mg/d for 12 weeks caused significant decrease from mean baseline of 17.3 ± 8.9 mg/dL to 10.1 ± 4.1 mg/dL *2688*

Serum No Effect Physiological In 62 hypercholesterolemic patients treatment with up to 1000 mg/d probucol and up to 400 mg/d bezafibrate caused change from mean baseline of 0.52 ± 0.016 mg/dL to 0.56 ± 0.017 mg/dL (nonsignificant) at 3 months, 0.55 ± 0.019 mg/dL at 6 months (nonsignificant) and 0.56 ± 0.018 mg/dL at 12 months (nonsignificant) *5196*

HDL_2-Phospholipids *Serum Decrease Physiological* In 22 patients with hyperlipoproteinemia type II treatment with 1000 mg/d for 12 weeks caused significant decrease from mean baseline of 26.9 ± 12.4 mg/dL to 16.0 ± 6.6 mg/dL *2688*

HDL_2-Triglycerides *Serum Decrease Physiological* In 22 patients with hyperlipoproteinemia type II treatment with 1000 mg/d for 12 weeks caused significant decrease to 3.2 ± 1.5 mg/dL from mean baseline of 5.1 ± 2.4 mg/dL *2688* Mean reduction of 43.6% observed with 12 weeks treatment *2689*

HDL_3-Apolipoprotein A-I *Serum Decrease Physiological* In 22 patients with hyperlipoproteinemia type II treatment with 1000 mg/d for 12 weeks caused significant reduction from mean baseline of 62.6 ± 18.8 mg/dL to 49.4 ± 17.5 mg/dL *2688* Mean reduction of 19.2% observed with 12 weeks treatment *2689*

HDL_3-Cholesterol *Serum Decrease Physiological* In 22 patients with hyperlipoproteinemia type II treatment with 1000 mg/d for 12 weeks caused significant reduction from mean baseline of 21.6 ± 5.1 mg/dL to 17.2 ± 6.0 mg/dL *2688* Mean reduction of 18.0% observed with 12 weeks treatment *2689*

Serum No Effect Physiological In 62 hypercholesterolemic patients treatment with up to 1000 mg/d probucol and up to 400 mg/d bezafibrate caused change from mean baseline of 0.49 ± 0.010 mg/dL to 0.53 ± 0.011 mg/dL (nonsignificant) at 3 months, 0.54 ± 0.012 mg/dL at 6 months (nonsignificant) and 0.50 ± 0.011 mg/dL at 12 months (nonsignificant) *5196*

HDL_3-Phospholipids *Serum Decrease Physiological* In 22 patients with hyperlipoproteinemia type II treatment with 1000 mg/d for 12 weeks caused significant reduction from mean baseline of 51.0 ± 11.8 mg/dL to 40.5 ± 9.6 mg/dL *2688*

HDL_3-Triglycerides *Serum No Effect Physiological* In 22 patients with hyperlipoproteinemia treatment with 1000 mg/d for 12 weeks caused nonsignificant reducton from mean baseline of 6.0 ± 2.4 mg/dL to 5.3 ± 1.9 mg/dL *2688*

HDL-Cholesterol *Serum Decrease Physiological* In 97 patients with hypercholesterolemia treatment with 1.0 g/d for 12 weeks caused a mean decrease of 23% *3982* Reduction from mean concentration of 45 mg/dL to 33 mg/dL in 81 patients with hypercholesterolemia treated with 1 g/day for 12 weeks *4704* In 2 NIDDM patients treated with a combination of probucol and pravastatin HDL-cholesterol concentration decreased markedly 4-5 mo after combination treatment started: in one it decreased from 48 mg/dL to 14 mg/dL and in the other from 34 mg/dL to 17 mg/dL *2808* When probucol administered with clofibrate reduction of HDL-cholesterol concentration may be enhanced *3668* Marked reduction may occur due to decreased synthesis of HDL apolipoproteins *5586* Added treatment with 1000 mg probucol daily of 29 patients with familial hypercholesterolemia already receiving cholestyramine caused further reduction of 26% *5376* When used alone probucol may decrease the HDL-cholesterol concentration, with the effect exaggerated when gemfibrozil, clofibrate or bezafibrate is coadministered *3668* Reduction from mean concentration of 42 mg/dL to 33 mg/dL in patients with familial hypercholesterolemia and with apolipoprotein E_4 with treatment for 3 months with 1 g/d and from 51 mg/dL to 42 mg/dL in those patients without apolipoprotein E_4 *1765* In 22 individuals with hyperlipoproteinemia type II treatment with 1000 mg/d for 12 weeks caused significant reduction from mean baseline of 50.0 ± 13.0 mg/dL to 32.2 ± 7.8 mg/dL *2688* Decreased synthesis of apo A-I. Expression of apo E. Activation of cholesterol ester transfer protein *264* Significant reduction observed in 14 hypercholesterolemic men in response to treatment *496* In 50 diabetics given 500 mg/d for 16 weeks and reduction greatest in highest cholesterol and triglyceride patients *2506*

Serum No Effect Physiological In 62 hypercholesterolemic patients treatment with up to 1000 mg/d probucol and up to 400 mg/d bezafibrate caused change from mean baseline of 0.99 ± 0.021 mg/dL to 1.00 ± 0.021 mg/dL (nonsignificant) at 3 months, 1.08 ± 0.024 mg/dL at 6 months (nonsignificant) and 1.05 ± 0.022 mg/dL at 12 months (nonsignificant) *5196*

HDL-Phospholipids *Serum Increase Physiological* In 62 hypercholesterolemic patients treatment with up to 1000 mg/d probucol and up to 400 mg/d bezafibrate caused change from mean baseline of 1.03 ± 0.021 mg/dL to 1.13 ± 0.022 mg/dL (significant) at 3 months, 1.18 ± 0.024 mg/dL at 6 months (significant) and 1.12 ± 0.023 mg/dL at 12 months (nonsignificant) *5196*

HDL-Triglycerides *Serum Decrease Physiological* In 62 hypercholesterolemic patients treatment with up to 1000 mg/d probucol and up to 400 mg/d bezafibrate caused change from mean baseline of 0.21 ± 0.005 mg/dL to 0.18 ± 0.005 mg/dL (significant) at 3 months, 0.19 ± 0.006 mg/dL at 6 months (significant) and 0.19 ± 0.005 mg/dL at 12 months (significant) *5196*

Hepatic Triglyceride Lipase *Serum No Effect Physiological* No significant effect of treatment for 12 weeks observed *2689*

IDL-Apolipoprotein B *Serum Decrease Physiological* Mean reduction of 23.8% observed with 12 weeks treatment *2689*

IDL-Cholesterol *Serum Decrease Physiological* In 22 patients with hyperlipoproteinemia type II treatment with 1000 mg/d for 12 weeks caused significant decrease from mean baseline of 15.4 ± 8.1 mg/dL to 12.6 ± 7.2 mg/dL *2688* Mean reduction of 26.7% observed with 12 weeks treatment *2689*

Probucol *(continued)*

IDL-Phospholipids *Serum No Effect Physiological* In 22 patients with hyperlpoproteinemia type II treatment with 1000 mg/d for 12 weeks caused nonsignificant reduction from mean baseline of 13.6 ± 4.9 mg/dL to 12.0 ± 5.8 mg/dL *2688*

IDL-Triglycerides *Serum No Effect Physiological* In 22 patients with hyperlipoproteinemia treatment with 1000 mg/d for 12 weeks caused nonsignificant reduction from mean baseline of 14.4 ± 5.5 mg/dL to 13.2 ± 8.2 mg/dL *2688*

LDL_1-Apolipoprotein B *Serum Decrease Physiological* Mean reduction of 23.2% observed with 12 weeks treatment *2689* In 22 patients with hyperlipoproteinemia type II treatment with 1000 mg/d for 12 weeks caused significant reduction from mean baseline of 58.7 ± 25.8 mg/dL to 44.5 ± 18.9 mg/dL *2688*

LDL_1-Cholesterol *Serum Decrease Physiological* In 22 patients with hyperlipoproteinemia type II treatment with 1000 mg/d for 12 weeks caused significant reduction from mean baseline of 117.2 ± 47.4 mg/dL to 84.7 ± 43.3 mg/dL *2688* Mean reduction of 27.8% observed with 12 weeks treatment *2689*

LDL_1-Phospholipids *Serum Decrease Physiological* In 22 patients with hyperlipoproteinemia type II treatment with 1000 mg/d for 12 weeks caused significant reduction from mean baseline of 86.1 ± 35.4 mg/dL to 69.8 ± 30.5 mg/dL *2688*

LDL_1-Triglycerides *Serum No Effect Physiological* In 22 patients with hyperlipoproteinemia type II treatment with 1000 mg/d for 12 weeks caused nonsignificant reduction from 22.5 ± 7.4 mg/dL to 21.2 ± 5.6 mg/dL *2688*

LDL_2-Apolipoprotein B *Serum No Effect Physiological* In 22 patients with hyperlipoproteinemia type II treatment with 1000 mg/d for 12 weeks caused nonsignificant increase to 17.5 ± 9.4 mg/dL from mean baseline of 20.4 ± 8.7 mg/dL *2688* No significant effect observed with 12 weeks treatment *2689*

LDL_2-Cholesterol *Serum No Effect Physiological* No significant change observed with 12 weeks treatment *2689* In 22 patients with hyperlipoproteinemia type II treatment with 1000 mg/d for 12 weeks caused nonsignificant increase from mean baseline of 33.0 ± 17.2 mg/dL to 36.1 ± 12.5 mg/dL *2688*

LDL_2-Phospholipids *Serum No Effect Physiological* In 22 patients with hyperlipoproteinemia type II treatment with 1000 mg/d for 12 weeks caused nonsignificant increase from mean baseline of 21.0 ± 10.1 mg/dL to 23.9 ± 8.0 mg/dL *2688*

LDL_2-Triglycerides *Serum No Effect Physiological* In 22 patients with hyperlipoproteinemia type II treatment with 1000 mg/d for 12 weeks caused nonsignificant increase from mean baseline of 5.5 ± 3.6 mg/dL to 6.7 ± 3.2 mg/dL *2688*

LDL-Cholesterol *Serum Decrease Physiological* In patients with familial hypercholesterolemia with apolipoprotein E_4 reduction from mean concentration of 251 mg/dL to 178 mg/dL with treatment with 1 g/d for 3 months and from 225 mg/dL to 191 mg/dL in those without apolipoprotein E_4 *1765* In 29 patients with familial hypercholesterolemia already receiving cholestyramine additional treatment with 1000 mg probucol daily caused further decrease of 17% *5376* 14 hypercholesterolemic men showed significant reduction with treatment *496* Reduction from mean concentration of 251 mg/dL to 227 mg/dL in 81 patients with hypercholesterolemia treated with 1 g/day for 12 weeks *4704* In 97 patients with hypercholesterolemia treatment with 1.0 g/d for 12 weeks caused a mean decrease of 8% *3982*

Serum No Effect Physiological In 62 hypercholesterolemic patients treatment with up to 1000 mg/d probucol and up to 400 mg/d bezafibrate caused change from mean baseline of 4.15 ± 0.076 mg/dL to 4.04 ± 0.079 mg/dL (nonsignificant) at 3 months, 4.12 ± 0.088 mg/dL at 6 months (nonsignificant) and 3.94 ± 0.083 mg/dL at 12 months (nonsignificant) *5196*

LDL-Cholesterol:HDL-Cholesterol Ratio
Serum Increase Physiological In 97 patients with hypercholesterolemia treatment with 1.0 g/d for 12 weeks caused a mean increase of 26% *3982*

LDL-Phospholipids *Serum No Effect Physiological* In 62 hypercholesterolemic patients treatment with up to 1000 mg/d probucol and up to 400 mg/d bezafibrate caused change from mean baseline of 1.34 ± 0.027 mg/dL to 1.39 ± 0.028 mg/dL (nonsignificant) at 3 months, 1.39 ± 0.032 mg/dL at 6 months (nonsignificant) and 1.30 ± 0.030 mg/dL at 12 months (nonsignificant) *5196*

LDL-Triglycerides *Serum No Effect Physiological* In 62 hypercholesterolemic patients treatment with up to 1000 mg/d probucol and up to 400 mg/d bezafibrate caused change from mean baseline of 0.50 ± 0.020 mg/dL to 0.52 ± 0.021 mg/dL (nonsignificant) at 3 months, 0.57 ± 0.023 mg/dL at 6 months (nonsignificant) and 0.55 ± 0.022 mg/dL at 12 months (nonsignificant) *5196*

Lecithin:Cholesterol Acyltransferase
Serum Decrease Physiological In 62 hypercholesterolemic patients treatment with up to 1000 mg/d probucol and up to 400 mg/d bezafibrate caused change from mean baseline of 97.0 ± 1.6 nmol/mL/h to 84.1 ± 1.6 nmol/mL/h (significant) at 3 months, 75.7 ± 1.8 nmol/mL/h at 6 months (significant) and 75.7 ± 1.7 nmol/mL/h at 12 months (significant) *5196*

Serum No Effect Physiological In 22 patients with hyperlipoproteinemia type II treatment with 1000 mg/d for 12 weeks caused nonsignificant change from mean baseline of 92.8 ± 19.1 nmol/mL/h to 94.0 ± 21.2 nmol/mL/h *2688*

Lipoprotein Lipase *Serum Decrease Physiological* Treatment for 12 weeks caused decrease from mean of 2.53 ± 0.71 µmol free fatty acids/mL/h to 1.71 ± 0.71 µmol free fatty acids/mL/h *2689*

Lipoprotein Lp(a) *Serum Decrease Physiological* In 62 hypercholesterolemic patients treatment with up to 1000 mg/d probucol and up to 400 mg/d bezafibrate caused change from mean baseline of 29 ± 1 mg/dL to 30 ± 1 mg/dL (nonsignificant) at 3 months, 27 ± 1 mg/dL at 6 months (significant) and 25 ± 1 mg/dL at 12 months (significant) *5196*

Phospholipids *Serum No Effect Physiological* In 62 hypercholesterolemic patients treatment with up to 1000 mg/d probucol and up to 400 mg/d bezafibrate caused change from mean baseline of 2.73 ± 0.03 mmol/L to 2.80 ± 0.03 mmol/L (nonsignificant) at 3 months, 2.82 ± 0.04 mmol/L at 6 months (nonsignificant) and 2.72 ± 0.03 mmol/L at 12 months (nonsignificant) *5196*

Platelet Aggregation *Blood Decrease Physiological* Epinephrine-induced aggregation decreased in 14 hypercholesterolemic men treated with drug *496*

Platelets *Blood Decrease Physiological* Some reduction observed in 29 patients with familial hypercholesterolemia already receiving cholestyramine when 1000 mg daily of probucol added to regime *5376*

Pravastatin *Serum No Effect Physiological* Coadministration with pravastatin caused no significant effect on bioavailability of pravastatin *728*

Triglycerides *Serum Decrease Physiological* In patients with familial hypercholesterolemia reduction from mean concentration of 170 mg/dL to 133 mg/dL in those with apolipoprotein E_4 when treated with 1 g/d for 3 months but increase from 135 mg/dL to 143 mg/dL in patients without apo E_4 *1765* In 62 hypercholesterolemic patients treatment with up to 1000 mg/d probucol and up to 400 mg/d bezafibrate caused change from mean baseline of 1.49 ± 0.05 mmol/L to 1.13 ± 0.05 mmol/L (significant) at 3 months, 1.21 ± 0.06 mmol/L at 6 months (significant) and 1.15 ± 0.05 mmol/L at 12 months (significant) *5196* In 50 diabetics given 500 mg/d for 16 weeks and reduction greatest in highest cholesterol and triglyceride patients *2506*

Serum No Effect Physiological No significant change in 81 patients with hypercholesterolemia treated with 1 g/day for 12 weeks *4704* In 2 patients with NIDDM treatment with a combination of probucol and pravastatin for 4-5 months had no effect on concentration *2808* In 22 patients with hyperlipoproteinemia type II mean concentration not significantly reduced from baseline of 172.4 ± 65.8 mg/dL to 156.8 ± 67.3 mg/dL when treated with 1000 mg/d for 12 weeks *2688* In 97 patients with hypercholesterolemia treatment with 1.0 g/d for 12 weeks caused a mean increase of 1% *3982*

Uric Acid *Serum Increase Physiological* Effect noted in women only *1235*

VLDL-Apolipoprotein B *Serum No Effect Physiological* No significant effect of 12 weeks treatment observed *2689*

VLDL-Cholesterol *Serum Decrease Physiological* In 62 hypercholesterolemic patients treatment with up to 1000 mg/d probucol and up to 400 mg/d bezafibrate caused change from mean baseline of 0.59 ± 0.026 mg/dL to 0.43 ± 0.027 mg/dL (significant) at 3 months, 0.37 ± 0.030 mg/dL at 6 months (significant) and 0.46 ± 0.028 mg/dL at 12 months (significant)

5196 In 97 patients with hypercholesterolemia treatment with 1.0 g/d for 12 weeks caused a mean decrease of 13% *3982* In 22 patients with hyperlipoproteinemia type II treatment with 1000 mg/d for 12 weeks caused significant reduction from mean baseline of 19.5 ± 13.9 mg/dL to 14.2 ± 10.1 mg/dL *2688* In patients with familial hypercholesterolemia with apolipoprotein E_4 reduction from mean concentration of 34 mg/dL to 26 mg/dL with 3 months treatment with 1 g/d whereas in patients without apo E_4 increase from 27 mg/dL to 29 mg/dL with same treatment *1765*
Serum *No Effect* *Physiological* No significant effect observed with treatment for 12 weeks *2689*

VLDL-Phospholipids *Serum* *Decrease* *Physiological* In 22 patients with hyperlipoproteinemia type II treatment with 1000 mg/d for 12 weeks caused significant reduction from mean baseline of 26.5 ± 15.8 mg/dL to 19.0 ± 11.8 mg/dL *2688* In 62 hypercholesterolemic patients treatment with up to 1000 mg/d probucol and up to 400 mg/d bezafibrate caused change from mean baseline of 0.35 ± 0.018 mg/dL to 0.26 ± 0.019 mg/dL (significant) at 3 months, 0.25 ± 0.021 mg/dL at 6 months (significant) and 0.30 ± 0.020 mg/dL at 12 months (significant) *5196*

VLDL-Triglycerides *Serum* *Decrease* *Physiological* In 62 hypercholesterolemic patients treatment with up to 1000 mg/d probucol and up to 400 mg/d bezafibrate caused change from mean baseline of 0.81 ± 0.038 mg/dL to 0.51 ± 0.040 mg/dL (significant) at 3 months, 0.56 ± 0.044 mg/dL at 6 months (significant) and 0.55 ± 0.042 mg/dL at 12 months (significant) *5196*
Serum *No Effect* *Physiological* No significant effect observed with treatment for 12 weeks *2689* In 22 patients with hyperlipoproteinemia type II treatment with 1000 mg/d for 12 weeks caused nonsignificant reduction from mean baseline of 78.1 ± 47.5 mg/dL to 62.9 ± 41.6 mg/dL *2688*

Procainamide

Acetaminophen *Serum* *No Effect* *Analytical* No interference observed at a concentration of 2000 µg/mL (736 µmol/L) with method on Du Pont aca *1506*

Alanine Aminotransferase *Serum* *Increase* *Physiological* Hepatotoxic effect *3810*

Albumin *Serum* *No Effect* *Analytical* At concentration of 50 mg/L had no effect on BCG method *5704* No effect on Technicon SMA 12/60 method at 35 mg/dL *4390*

Alkaline Phosphatase *Serum* *Increase* *Physiological* Reversible hepatic toxicity reported *1714*
Serum *No Effect* *Analytical* No effect on Technicon SMA 12/60 method at 35 mg/dL *4390*

Aminobenzoic Acid *Urine* *Increase* *Physiological* Up to 10% excreted as this *2242*

Anti-Histone Antibodies *Serum* *Positive* *Physiological* Antibodies to histone induced by drug *4755*

Antinuclear Antibodies *Serum* *Increase* *Physiological* Reported to occur in 50% patients *5869* 50-80% patients have antibodies after 3 to 6 mo *3183*

Aspartate Aminotransferase *Serum* *Increase* *Physiological* Hepatotoxic effect *3810*
Serum *No Effect* *Analytical* No effect on Technicon SMA 12/60 method at 35 mg/dL *4390*

Basophils *Blood* *Decrease* *Physiological* Occasional severe reduction noted *2591*

Benzoylecgonine *Urine* *No Effect* *Analytical* Negative result obtained at a concentration of 1000 µg/mL (4.25 mmol/L) with method on Du Pont aca *1558*

Bicarbonate *Serum* *No Effect* *Analytical* At concentration of 50 mg/L had no effect on method using phenolphthalein *5704*

Bile *Urine* *Increase* *Physiological* Hepatotoxic effect *3810*

Bilirubin *Serum* *Increase* *Physiological* Reversible hepatic toxicity reported *2451* In 3% of all patients receiving drug, but in 14% of patients with direct Coombs' test *3183*
Serum *No Effect* *Analytical* No effect on Technicon SMA 12/60 method at 35 mg/dL *4390* At concentration of 350 mg/L had no effect on Kodak Ektachem® method *5704* At concentration of 50 mg/L had no effect on Jendrassik and Grof method *5704*

Bilirubin, Indirect *Serum* *Increase* *Physiological* In 3% of all patients receiving drug, but in 14% of patients with direct Coombs' test *3183*

BSP Retention *Serum* *Increase* *Physiological* Reported case of hepatic toxicity *2451*

Calcium *Serum* *No Effect* *Analytical* At concentration of 50 mg/L had no effect on cresolphthalein method *5704* No effect on Technicon SMA 12/60 method at 35 mg/dL *4390*

Chloride *Serum* *No Effect* *Analytical* At concentration of 50 mg/L had no effect on mercurimetric method *5704*

Cholesterol *Serum* *No Effect* *Analytical* No effect on Technicon SMA 12/60 method at 35 mg/dL *4390*

Cholinesterase *Serum* *Decrease* *Analytical* At activity of 4.5 kU/L procainamide at a concentration of 10 mg/dL decreases activity by 0.47 kU/L when measured by butyrylthiocholine method on Kodak Ektachem® *2504* Reduction of 0.40 U/mL at a concentration of 5 µg/mL, 0.67 U/mL at 10 µg/mL, 1.25 U/mL at 20 µg/mL, 2.70 U/mL at 40 µg/mL with method on Du Pont aca *3271*
Serum *Decrease* *Physiological* At therapeutic concentration *in vitro* inhibition of enzyme by 15 to 30% *3019* Reduction of 0.16 U/mL at a concentration of 5 µg/mL, 0.60 U/mL at 10 µg/mL, 0.96 U/mL at 20 µg/mL, 3.30 U/mL at 40 µg/mL with method on Du Pont Dimension *3271*

Coombs' Test *Blood* *Positive* *Physiological* Mechanism obscure *2453*

Coombs' Test, Direct *Blood* *Positive* *Physiological* Doubled incidence in individuals receiving drug compared with control with production of red cell autoantibody *3183*

Creatine Kinase Isoenzymes *Serum* *No Effect* *Analytical* No interference observed at a concentration of 25 mg/L (106.2 µmol/L) with CK-MB method on Du Pont aca *1519*

Creatinine *Serum* *No Effect* *Analytical* At concentration of 50 mg/L had no effect on Technicon AutoAnalyzer® Jaffe method *5704* No effect on Technicon SMA 12/60 method at 35 mg/dL *4390*

Digoxin *Serum* *No Effect* *Physiological* No significant effect when drug coadministered *3449* No significant effect observed *1384*

Drugs of Abuse Screen *Urine* *No Effect* *Analytical* No effect at concentration of 100 µg/mL on EZ-SCREEN procedure for cannabinoids and cocaine *1739*

Eosinophils *Blood* *Decrease* *Physiological* Occasional severe reduction noted *2591*
Blood *Increase* *Physiological* Evidence of allergic response to drug *5395*

Erythrocyte Sedimentation Rate
Blood *Increase* *Physiological* Associated with SLE-like syndrome *1475*

Erythrocytes *Blood* *Decrease* *Physiological* May cause hemolytic anemia *4265* Pancytopenia may occur with/without lupus-like syndrome *5395* Agranulocytosis, bone marrow depression, neutropenia, hypoplastic anemia and thrombocytopenia have been reported in patients receiving procainamide at a rate of approximately 0.5% *4530*

Glucose *Serum* *No Effect* *Analytical* No effect on Technicon SMA 12/60 method at 35 mg/dL *4390* No effect of concentrations up to 11.4 mg/L on method on Kodak Ektachem® *5706*

Granulocytes *Blood* *Decrease* *Physiological* Agranulocytosis, bone marrow depression, neutropenia, hypoplastic anemia and thrombocytopenia have been reported in patients receiving procainamide at a rate of approximately 0.5% *4530* Agranulocytosis observed in 2.6% of patients versus 0.07% of controls *3098* Agranulocytosis occasionally observed as manifestation of hypersensitivity *1384*

Haptoglobin *Serum* *Decrease* *Physiological* In 3% of all patients receiving drug, but in 14% of patients with direct Coombs' test *3183*

Hematocrit *Blood* *Decrease* *Physiological* Observed with SLE-like syndrome, hemolytic anemia *1475* Agranulocytosis, bone marrow depression, neutropenia, hypoplastic anemia and thrombocytopenia have been reported in patients receiving procainamide at a rate of approximately 0.5% *4530*

Hemoglobin *Blood* *Decrease* *Physiological* Agranulocytosis, bone marrow depression, neutropenia, hypoplastic anemia and thrombocytopenia have been reported in patients receiving

Procainamide *(continued)*

Hemoglobin *(continued)*
procainamide at a rate of approximately 0.5% *4530* Significant reduction in one patient 31 days after start of treatment *5514* Observed with SLE-like syndrome, hemolytic anemia *1475*

Histamine *Plasma No Effect Analytical* Possible inhibition of radio-enzyme assay since 50% inhibition at 36 µg/mL and therapeutic concentration 4 - 30 µg/mL *2492*

Isoniazid *Serum Increase Physiological* Concomitant administration of procainamide slightly prolongs half-life of isoniazid but probably not to an extent that has clinical significance: due to effect on acetylation *5357*

Lactate Dehydrogenase *Serum No Effect Analytical* No effect on Technicon SMA 12/60 method at 35 mg/dL *4390*

Latex Fixation *Serum Positive Physiological* Associated with drug induced lupus *1466*

LE Cells *Blood Positive Physiological* Reported effect *3360* 10-20% patients eventually develop drug-induced lupus syndrome *3183*

Leukocytes *Blood Decrease Physiological* Significant association observed with therapy with sustained release form of drug at normal therapeutic concentration of drug *1724* Agranulocytosis *5934* Reduction observed in one patient 31 days after first receiving drug *5514* Pancytopenia may occur with/without lupus-like syndrome *5395*

Lidocaine *Serum No Effect Analytical* No significant interference observed at a concentration of 100 µg/mL (425 µmol/L) with method on Du Pont aca *1534* At a concentration of 1250 mg/L (normal therapeutic concentration up to 10 mg/L) had less than 10% effect on method on Baxter Stratus *5705*

Lithium *Serum Decrease Analytical* May cause negative bias when lithium measured by an ion-specific electrode *3590*
Serum Increase Analytical May cause positive bias at high concentrations when lithium measured by an ion-specific electrode *3590*

Lymphocytotoxic Antibodies *Serum Positive Physiological* 50-80% patients have antibodies after 3 to 6 mo *3183*

Midazolam *Serum No Effect Analytical* On GC-ECD method of Ha et al *2387*

N-Acetylprocainamide *Serum No Effect Analytical* No significant interference at a concentration of 100 µg/mL (425 µmol/L) with method on Du Pont aca *1536*

Neutrophils *Blood Decrease Physiological* Occasional case of agranulocytosis reported *6264* Agranulocytosis, bone marrow depression, neutropenia, hypoplastic anemia and thrombocytopenia have been reported in patients receiving procainamide at a rate of approximately 0.5% *4530* Occasional severe reduction noted *2591* Marked reduction in one patient 31 days after start of treatment *5514*

Phenylalanine *Plasma No Effect Analytical* No interference observed with rapid quantitative whole blood method of Campbell et al using phenylalanine dehydrogenase *867*

Phosphate *Serum No Effect Analytical* At concentration of 50 mg/L had no effect on phosphomolybdate method *5704* No effect on Technicon SMA 12/60 method at 35 mg/dL *4390*

Platelets *Blood Decrease Physiological* Effect observed in one patient with sustained release form of drug, also associated with decreased marrow megakaryocytes *5514* Pancytopenia may occur with/without lupus-like syndrome *5395* Agranulocytosis, bone marrow depression, neutropenia, hypoplastic anemia and thrombocytopenia have been reported in patients receiving procainamide at a rate of approximately 0.5% *4530*

Potassium *Serum Increase Analytical* At concentrations above 8 mg/L (normal therapeutic concentration 10 mg/L) raised concentration as measured by ISE with predilution *5704*

Prazosin *Serum No Effect Physiological* Coadministration of prazosin with procainamide had no apparent adverse drug interaction in limited clinical experience *4649*

Protein *Serum No Effect Analytical* No effect on Technicon SMA 12/60 method at 35 mg/dL *4390* At concentration of 50 mg/L had no effect on biuret method with blank correction *5704*

Quinidine *Serum No Effect Analytical* Procainamide at a concentration of 100 µg/mL had no significant cross-reactivity with quinidine at a concentration of 2.0 µg/mL in method on Bayer Technicon Immuno 1® *431* No significant interference observed at a concentration of 100 µg/mL (425 µmol/L) with method on Du Pont aca *1543* At concentrations greater than 1000 mg/L causes 30% increase in concentration as measured by method on Baxter Stratus but physiological concentrations are up to 10 mg/L only *5705*

Reticulocytes *Blood Increase Physiological* In 3% of all patients receiving drug, but in 14% of patients with direct Coombs' test *3183*

SDZ PSC 833 *Blood No Effect Analytical* At a concentration of 8.9 mg/L had no effect on HPLC method of Scott et al when used to measure PSC (with CsD as internal standard) at a concentration of 5 mg/L *5418*

Sodium *Serum No Effect Analytical* At concentration of 50 mg/L had no effect on measurement by ISE with predilution *5704*

Tacrolimus *Blood No Effect Analytical* No interference observed with radioreceptor assay of Murthy et al *4191* No significant effect observed at concentrations of 10 and 16 mg/L respectively for procainamide and NAPA with MEIA method on Abbott IMx analyzer *1871*
Serum No Effect Analytical At a concentration of 15 mg/L of procainamide and N-acetylprocainamide had no significant effect on ELISA method *6329*

Triglycerides *Serum No Effect Analytical* At concentration of 50 mg/L had no effect on lipase/esterase method *5704*

Urea Nitrogen *Serum No Effect Analytical* At concentration of 50 mg/L had no effect on diacetylmonoxime method *5704* At concentration of 11.4 mg/L had no effect on Kodak Ektachem® method *5704*

Uric Acid *Serum No Effect Analytical* No effect on Technicon SMA 12/60 method at 35 mg/dL *4390* At concentration of 50 mg/L had no effect on phosphotungstate reduction method *5704*

Procaine

Alanine Aminotransferase *Serum No Effect Analytical* No effect at 2 mg/L on Boehringer Mannheim Reflotron method *5706* No effect at therapeutic concentration on Boehringer Mannheim Reflotron method *3231*

Albumin *Serum No Effect Analytical* At concentration of 2 mg/L had no effect on BCG method *5704*

Amylase *Serum No Effect Analytical* No effect of concentrations up to 2 mg/L on method on Boehringer Mannheim Reflotron *5706*

Amylase, Pancreatic Isoenzyme
Serum No Effect Analytical No significant effect observed at a toxic concentration of 10 mg/L with method on Boehringer Mannheim Reflotron *3647*

Aspartate Aminotransferase *Serum No Effect Analytical* No effect at therapeutic concentration on Boehringer Mannheim Reflotron method *3231* No effect at 2 mg/L on Boehringer Mannheim Reflotron method *5706*

Bicarbonate *Serum No Effect Analytical* At concentration of 2 mg/L had no effect on method using phenolphthalein *5704*

Bilirubin *Serum No Effect Analytical* At concentration of 2 mg/L no effect on method on Boehringer Mannheim Reflotron system *5706* No effect at 1.0 mg/L on Ames Seralyzer method *5706* At concentration of 2 mg/L had no effect on Jendrassik and Grof method *5704*

Calcium *Serum No Effect Analytical* At concentration of 2 mg/L had no effect on cresolphthalein method *5704*

Cannabinoids *Urine No Effect Analytical* No effect on Roche Abuscreen method *5006*

Chloride *Serum No Effect Analytical* At concentration of 2 mg/L had no effect on mercurimetric method *5704*

Cholesterol *Serum No Effect Analytical* No effect at 1.0 mg/L on Ames Seralyzer method *5706* At concentration of 2 mg/L had no effect on Liebermann-Burchard method *5704* No effect at therapeutic concentration on Boehringer Mannheim Reflotron method *3231* At concentration of 2 mg/L no effect on method on Boehringer Mannheim Reflotron system *5706*

Cocaethylene *Urine No Effect Analytical* No interference observed with TLC method of Bailey *328*

Cortisol *Plasma No Effect Analytical* At concentration of 10 mg/L no significant effect observed on CEDIA method (worst case 97.4% recovery) *1097*

Creatine Kinase *Serum No Effect Analytical* No effect at 1.0 mg/L on method on Ames Seralyzer *5706*

Creatinine *Serum No Effect Analytical* At concentration of 2 mg/L had no effect on Technicon AutoAnalyzer® Jaffe method *5704* No effect at 1.0 mg/L on method on Ames Seralyzer *5706*

Drugs of Abuse Screen *Urine No Effect Analytical* No effect at concentration of 100 µg/mL on EZ-SCREEN procedure for cannabinoids and cocaine *1739*

Glucose *Serum No Effect Analytical* At concentration of 40 mg/L had no effect on hexokinase/G-6-PDH method *5704* No effect at therapeutic concentration on Boehringer Mannheim Reflotron method *3231* No effect at 1.0 mg/L on glucose oxidase method on Ames Seralyzer *5706* At concentration of 2 mg/L no effect on method on Boehringer Mannheim Reflotron system *5706*

γ-Glutamyltransferase *Serum No Effect Analytical* At concentration of 2 mg/L no effect on method on Boehringer Mannheim Reflotron system *5706* No effect at therapeutic concentration on Boehringer Mannheim Reflotron method *3231*

HDL-Cholesterol *Serum No Effect Analytical* At a concentration up to 2 mg/L had no significant effect on Reflotron method for whole blood cholesterol *6352*

Histamine *Plasma No Effect Analytical* Possible inhibition at physiological concentration of 12 - 42.7 µg/mL since 50% inhibition of assay observed at concentration of 34 µg/mL *2492*

Lactate *Plasma No Effect Analytical* At concentration of 40 mg/L had no effect on enzymatic method *5704*

Lactate Dehydrogenase *Serum No Effect Analytical* No effect at 1.0 mg/L on method on Ames Seralyzer *5706*

N-Acetylprocainamide *Serum No Effect Analytical* No significant interference observed at a concentration of 100 µg/mL (423 µmol/L) with method on Du Pont aca *1536*

Phosphate *Serum No Effect Analytical* At concentration of 2 mg/L had no effect on phosphomolybdate method *5704*

Porphobilinogen *Urine Increase Analytical* Interferes with Ehrlich's aldehyde reaction *6515*

Potassium *Serum No Effect Analytical* At concentration of 2 mg/L had no effect on measurement by ISE with predilution *5704*

Procainamide *Serum No Effect Analytical* No significant interference observed at a concentration of 100 µg/mL (423 µmol/L) with method on Du Pont aca *1542*

Protein *Cerebrospinal Fluid Increase Analytical* Interferes with Folin-Ciocalteu reagent *2024*
Serum No Effect Analytical At concentration of 2 mg/L had no effect on biuret method with blank correction *5704*

Sodium *Serum No Effect Analytical* At concentration of 2 mg/L had no effect on measurement by ISE with predilution *5704*

Sulfa as Sulfanilamide *Serum Increase Analytical* Metabolized to PABA which interferes with assay procedure *2242*

Triglycerides *Serum No Effect Analytical* At concentration of 2 mg/L had no effect on lipase/esterase method *5704* No effect at 2 mg/L on Boehringer Mannheim Reflotron method *5706* No effect at therapeutic concentration on Boehringer Mannheim Reflotron method *3231*

Urea Nitrogen *Serum No Effect Analytical* No effect at 1.0 mg/L on method on Ames Seralyzer *5706* No effect at therapeutic concentration on Boehringer Mannheim Reflotron method *3231* No effect at 2 mg/L on Boehringer Mannheim Reflotron method *5706* At concentration of 2 mg/L had no effect on diacetylmonoxime method *5704*

Uric Acid *Serum No Effect Analytical* No effect at 2 mg/L on Boehringer Mannheim Reflotron method *5706* At concentration of 2 mg/L had no effect on phosphotungstate reduction method *5704* No effect at therapeutic concentration on Boehringer Mannheim Reflotron method *3231*

Urobilinogen *Urine Increase Analytical* Interferes with Ehrlich's aldehyde reaction *6515*

Procarbazine

Bilirubin *Serum Increase Physiological* Reported effect. ?mechanism *2451*

Color *Feces Increase Analytical* Black color reported with ingestion of procarbazine *3388*

Eosinophils *Blood Increase Physiological* Administration of procabazine has been associated with eosinophilia *5029*

Erythrocytes *Blood Decrease Physiological* Anemia and bone marrow depression *128*

Heinz Body Formation *Blood Positive Physiological* May occur with hemolysis *2754*

Hematocrit *Blood Decrease Physiological* Administration of procabazine has been associated frequently with anemia *5029*

Hemoglobin *Blood Decrease Physiological* May cause hemolysis *1384* Administration of procabazine has been associated frequently with anemia *5029*

Homocysteine *Plasma Increase Physiological* As a vitamin B_6 antagonist causes increased concentration *6123*

Leukocytes *Blood Decrease Physiological* Administration of procabazine has been associated frequently with leukopenia *5029* Leukopenia and bone marrow depression *128* May be dose limiting adverse event but may be delayed for several weeks *1384*

Occult Blood *Feces Increase Physiological* Melena and gastrointestinal tract bleeding *128*

Platelets *Blood Decrease Physiological* Usually dose limiting adverse effect but may be delayed for several weeks *1384* Thrombocytopenia and bone marrow depression *128*

Prochlorperazine

Alanine Aminotransferase *Serum Increase Physiological* May produce cholestatic jaundice, and rare cases of fatty changes in the liver of patients who have died while receiving the drug *5638* Cholestatic effect *128*

Albumin *Serum No Effect Analytical* At concentration of 1 mg/L had no effect on BCG method *5704*

Alkaline Phosphatase *Serum Increase Physiological* May produce cholestatic jaundice, and rare cases of fatty changes in the liver of patients who have died while receiving the drug *5638* Cholestatic effect *128*

Aspartate Aminotransferase *Serum Increase Physiological* May produce cholestatic jaundice, and rare cases of fatty changes in the liver of patients who have died while receiving the drug *5638* Cholestatic effect *128*

Bicarbonate *Serum No Effect Analytical* At concentration of 1 mg/L had no effect on method using phenolphthalein *5704*

Bile *Urine Increase Physiological* Cholestatic effect *128*

Bilirubin *Serum Increase Physiological* May produce cholestatic jaundice, and rare cases of fatty changes in the liver of patients who have died while receiving the drug *5638* Cholestatic effect *128*
Serum No Effect Analytical At concentration of 1 mg/L had no effect on Jendrassik and Grof method *5704*

BSP Retention *Serum Increase Physiological* Cholestatic effect *128*

Calcium *Serum No Effect Analytical* At concentration of 1 mg/L had no effect on cresolphthalein method *5704*

Catecholamines *Urine Increase Physiological* Increased metabolism, decreased organ uptake of norepinephrine *6515*

Chloride *Serum No Effect Analytical* At concentration of 1 mg/L had no effect on mercurimetric method *5704*

Cholesterol *Serum Increase Physiological* Cholestatic effect *128*
Serum No Effect Analytical At concentration of 1 mg/L had no effect on CHOD-PAP method *5704*

Creatinine *Serum No Effect Analytical* At concentration of 1 mg/L had no effect on Technicon AutoAnalyzer® Jaffe method *5704*

Dopamine *Urine Increase Physiological* Up to 79% increase after 30 mg in controls *2616*

Epinephrine *Urine No Effect Physiological* No significant effect with up to 30 mg in controls *2616*

Prochlorperazine *(continued)*

Glucose *Serum* *No Effect* *Analytical* At concentration of 1 mg/L had no effect on GOD/POD-PAP method *5704*

γ-Glutamyltransferase *Serum* *Increase* *Physiological* May produce cholestatic jaundice, and rare cases of fatty changes in the liver of patients who have died while receiving the drug *5638*

Granulocytes *Blood* *Decrease* *Physiological* Leukemia and agranulocytosis may occur in patients while receiving the drug *5638*

Histamine *Plasma* *No Effect* *Analytical* Improbable inhibition of radio-enzyme assay at physiological concentrations *2492*

17-Hydroxycorticosteroids *Urine* *Decrease* *Analytical* Abnormal yellow-pink color, blank not adequate *882*

Leukocytes *Blood* *Decrease* *Physiological* Leukemia and agranulocytosis may occur in patients while receiving the drug *5638* Agranulocytosis due to interference in development *133*

Lysergic Acid Diethylamide *Urine* *Increase* *Analytical* Minimum concentration that caused a positive result with EMIT method to measure LSD 10 mg/L *4968*

Metanephrines, Total *Urine* *Increase* *Physiological* Increased metabolism, decreased organ uptake of norepinephrine *6515*

Neutrophils *Blood* *Decrease* *Physiological* Occasional case of agranulocytosis reported *6264*

Norepinephrine *Urine* *No Effect* *Physiological* No significant effect with up to 30 mg in controls *2616*

Phenylketones *Urine* *Positive* *Analytical* Light purple with $FeCl_3$, also with Phenistix® *1195* May produce false positive test for phenylketonuria *5638*

Phenytoin *Serum* *Increase* *Physiological* Reported impairment of metabolism *3340*

Phosphate *Serum* *No Effect* *Analytical* At concentration of 1 mg/L had no effect on phosphomolybdate method *5704*

Potassium *Serum* *No Effect* *Analytical* At concentration of 1 mg/L had no effect on flame-photometric method *5704*

Prolactin *Plasma* *Increase* *Physiological* Increase may be observed especially in response to chronic treatment *5638* Typical dose-related response to i.m. administered drug due to antidopaminergic actions *3402*

Propranolol *Serum* *Increase* *Physiological* When drugs are coadministered the plasma concentrations of both are increased *5638*

Protein *Serum* *No Effect* *Analytical* At concentration of 1 mg/L had no effect on biuret method with blank correction *5704*

Prothrombin Time *Plasma* *Increase* *Physiological* Associated with impaired excretion of bile salts *128*

Sodium *Serum* *No Effect* *Analytical* At concentration of 1 mg/L had no effect on flame-photometric method *5704*

Triglycerides *Serum* *No Effect* *Analytical* At concentration of 1 mg/L had no effect on lipase/esterase method *5704*

Urea Nitrogen *Serum* *No Effect* *Analytical* At concentration of 1 mg/L had no effect on diacetylmonoxime method *5704*

Uric Acid *Serum* *No Effect* *Analytical* At concentration of 1 mg/L had no effect on phosphotungstate reduction method *5704*

Urobilinogen *Feces* *Decrease* *Physiological* Pale stools associated with cholestasis *128*
Urine *Decrease* *Physiological* Cholestatic effect *128*

Vanillylmandelic Acid *Urine* *Increase* *Physiological* Increased metabolism, decreased organ uptake of norepinephrine *6515*
Urine *No Effect* *Physiological* No significant effect with up to 30 mg in controls *2616*

Procyclidine

Amylase *Serum* *Increase* *Physiological* May cause acute parotitis (theoretical effect) *2754*

Proflavine

Chromosomes *Test Conditions* *Abnormal* *Physiological* Clastogenic in human hela cultures *5484*

Progabide

Alanine Aminotransferase *Serum* *Increase* *Physiological* Several fold increase in one patient necessitating stopping treatment *5349*

Aspartate Aminotransferase *Serum* *Increase* *Physiological* Several fold increase in one patient necessitating stopping treatment *5349*

Carbamazepine *Serum* *Decrease* *Physiological* Significant reduction in concentration observed in 27 patients after first dose which persisted for 3 months but that of epoxide of drug increased. Effect probably due to displacement of carbamazepine from protein and inhibition of metabolism of epoxide *2299*

Phenobarbital *Serum* *Increase* *Physiological* Increased concentration in patients who had a therapeutic response *5349*

Phenytoin *Serum* *Increase* *Physiological* Increased concentration in patients who had a therapeutic response *5349*

Progesterone

Alanine Aminotransferase *Serum* *Increase* *Physiological* Progesterone with estrogens may affect hepatic function tests *5685* Hepatotoxicity *3810*

Albumin *Serum* *Increase* *Physiological* Not observed with combined therapy *1223*

Alkaline Phosphatase *Serum* *Increase* *Physiological* Progesterone with estrogens may affect hepatic function tests *5685* Hepatotoxicity *3810*

Alkaline Phosphatase, Bone Isoenzyme
Serum *No Effect* *Analytical* At a concentration of 250 mg/L had no effect on Tandem-MP Ostase method *777*

Amino Acids *Plasma* *Decrease* *Physiological* Specific amino acids affected in men *1154* Given i.m. to men decreases free and total *1155*

α-Amino-Nitrogen *Plasma* *Decrease* *Physiological* Catabolic effect *1155*
Urine *No Effect* *Physiological* Almost no effect in normal males *5992*

Aspartate Aminotransferase
Serum *Decrease* *Physiological* Observed in healthy individuals when only treatment *1654*
Serum *Increase* *Physiological* Hepatotoxicity *3810* Progesterone with estrogens may affect hepatic function tests *5685*

Bile *Urine* *Increase* *Physiological* Hepatotoxicity *3810*

Bilirubin *Serum* *Increase* *Physiological* Progesterone with estrogens may affect hepatic function tests *5685* Hepatotoxicity also transient familial increase *3810*

BSP Retention *Serum* *Increase* *Physiological* Hepatic toxicity occasional occurrence *4135*

Calcium *Serum* *Increase* *Physiological* Probable effect with remission of metastases *3810*

Catecholamines *Plasma* *No Effect* *Physiological* No significant change in 7 postclimacteric women following single oral dose of 200 mg *5947*

Ceruloplasmin *Serum* *No Effect* *Physiological* No effect reported over several months *5869*

Cholesterol *Serum* *Decrease* *Physiological* Slight effect when only treatment *1654*

Copper *Serum* *No Effect* *Physiological* No effect reported over several months *5869*

Cortisol *Plasma* *No Effect* *Analytical* Progesterone caused an insignificant cross-reactivity of 0.3% with method on Bayer Technicon Immuno 1® *419*

11-Dehydro-thromboxane B_2 *Saliva* *No Effect* *Analytical* Cross-reactivity at maximum concentration In women with polycystic ovaries of 26,300 pmol/L < 0.100% *5937*

Digitoxin *Serum* *No Effect* *Analytical* At concentration of 0.01 mg/L caused no cross reactivity with method on Baxter Stratus *5705*

Digoxin *Serum No Effect Analytical* Cross reactivity of less than 10% observed with method on Baxter Stratus *5705*

Estradiol *Plasma No Effect Analytical* No significant cross-reactivity observed at concentrations up to 300 ng/mL with method on Abbott IMx *334* At a concentration of 100,000 ng/mL had less than 0.01% cross-reactivity with method on Bayer Technicon Immuno 1® *422*

17β-Estradiol *Saliva No Effect Analytical* Cross-reactivity at maximum concentration In natural cycle of 736 pmol/L 0.100% *5937*

Estrone *Urine Increase Physiological* Not significant change however *1654*

Factor VII *Plasma Increase Physiological* Progesterone with estrogens may increase prothrombin factors *5685*

Factor VIII *Plasma Increase Physiological* Progesterone with estrogens may increase prothrombin factors *5685*

Factor IX *Plasma Increase Physiological* Progesterone with estrogens may increase prothrombin factors *5685*

Factor X *Plasma Increase Physiological* Progesterone with estrogens may increase prothrombin factors *5685*

γ-Globulin *Serum Decrease Physiological* Observed in healthy women when only treatment *1654*
Serum Increase Physiological Not observed with combined therapy *1223*

Glucaric Acid *Urine Increase Physiological* Reported induction of hepatic enzymes *2782*

Glucose *Serum Decrease Physiological* Slight insignificant effect (contrast with estrogens) *1654*

17-Hydroxycorticosteroids *Urine Decrease Physiological* Exact mechanism not known *55*

16-α-Hydroxyprogesterone *Plasma Increase Analytical* Up to 25% cross reactivity *38*

6-Keto-Prostaglandin $F_{1\alpha}$ *Urine Decrease Physiological* Significant decrease in 7 postclimacteric women following single oral dose of 200 mg *5947*

Luteinizing Hormone *Plasma Decrease Physiological* Suppresses LH peak *5424*

Magnesium *Serum Increase Physiological* Significantly higher than in controls *1222*

Pregnanediol *Urine Decrease Physiological* Significant decrease with treatment (from 3.5 to 2.0 mg/24 h) *1654*

Progesterone *Plasma Increase Analytical* Cross-reactivity of 5% observed with method on Abbott IMx *1908* 11 - 24% cross reactivity RIA procedure of Cameron *858*
Plasma Increase Physiological Significant increase observed in 7 postclimacteric women following single oral dose of 200 mg *5947*

Prostaglandins *Urine Decrease Physiological* Following single oral dose of 200 mg in 7 postclimacteric women significantly increased excretion observed *5947*

Protein *Serum Increase Physiological* Metabolic effect *1223*

Sodium *Serum Increase Physiological* May cause sodium retention *3669*
Urine Increase Physiological May occur with high doses *4014*

Sulfobromophthalein *Serum Increase Physiological* Progesterone with estrogens may increase BSP retention *5685*

Testosterone *Serum No Effect Analytical* No detectable cross-reactivity observed with in testosterone method on Bayer Technicon Immuno 1® *433*

Thyroxine Binding Globulin *Serum Increase Physiological* Increased synthesis *6515*

Transferrin *Serum No Effect Physiological* No significant effect after 6-9 mo *5869*

Progestogens

δ-Aminolevulinic Acid *Urine Increase Physiological* May precipitate attack of acute porphyria *1687*

Corticosteroid-Binding Globulin
Serum No Effect Physiological No effect with progestogen-only pill *815*

Cortisol *Plasma No Effect Physiological* No effect with progestogen-only pill *815*

Cortisol, Protein Bound *Plasma No Effect Physiological* No effect with progestogen-only pill *815*

Leucine Aminopeptidase *Serum No Effect Physiological* No effect observed *2465*

Nitroblue Tetrazolium Test *Blood No Effect Physiological* When administered alone no effect observed *252*

Porphyrin, Total *Urine Increase Physiological* May precipitate attack of acute porphyria *1687*

Proguanil

Erythrocytes *Urine Increase Physiological* Actual bleeding may be caused by drug *1714*

Hemoglobin *Urine Increase Physiological* Actual bleeding caused by drug *1714*

Promazine

Alanine Aminotransferase *Serum Increase Physiological* May cause cholestatic (hepatocanalicular) jaundice *402*

Alkaline Phosphatase *Serum Increase Physiological* May cause cholestatic (hepatocanalicular) jaundice *402*

Aspartate Aminotransferase *Serum Increase Physiological* May cause cholestatic (hepatocanalicular) jaundice *402*

Bile *Urine Increase Physiological* May cause cholestasis *3810*

Bilirubin *Serum Increase Physiological* May cause cholestatic (hepatocanalicular) jaundice *402*

BSP Retention *Serum Increase Physiological* May cause cholestasis *3810*

Catecholamines *Plasma No Effect Analytical* No effect on HPLC method of Koller for dopamine, epinephrine, and norepinephrine *3230*

Cholesterol *Serum Increase Physiological* May cause cholestatic (hepatocanalicular) jaundice *402*

17-Hydroxycorticosteroids *Urine Decrease Physiological* Acts on hypothalamus to decrease ACTH secretion *661*

5-Hydroxyindoleacetic Acid *Urine Decrease Analytical* Interferes with method of Goldenberg *2219*

^{131}I Uptake *Serum Decrease Physiological* Sparine® contains tetraiodofluorescein *4360*

Leukocytes *Blood Decrease Physiological* Agranulocytosis *1869*

Neutrophils *Blood Decrease Physiological* Occasional case of agranulocytosis reported *6264*

p-Aminophenol *Urine No Effect Analytical* With addition of drugs at a concentration of 100 mg/L and of related compounds at 50 mg/L no significant effect observed on colorimetric method of van Bocxlaer on Cobas Mira analyzer which involves reacting free p-aminophenol with resorcinol in the presence of magnesium ions to form an indophenol dye measured at 550 nm *6163*

Platelets *Blood Decrease Physiological* May rarely cause bone marrow aplasia *2385*

Prolactin *Plasma Increase Physiological* Marked effect in male and female psychiatric patients treated for up to 4 weeks *6098*
Plasma No Effect Physiological No significant change in response to 25 mg i.m *2352*

Protein *Urine Increase Analytical* Affects turbidity tests for up to 3 d *116*
Urine Increase Physiological Affects turbidity tests for up to 3 d *116*

Prothrombin Time *Plasma Increase Physiological* Associated with failure of excretion of bile salts *2803*

Urobilinogen *Feces Decrease Physiological* Pale stools as result of cholestasis *2803*
Urine Decrease Physiological Cholestatic effect *2803*

Promethazine

Alanine Aminotransferase *Serum Increase Physiological* May cause cholestasis *3810*

Promethazine *(continued)*

Alanine Aminotransferase *(continued)*
Serum No Effect Analytical At acute overdose concentration (20 mg/dL) on Technicon SMAC® method *6266*

Albumin *Serum No Effect Analytical* At concentration of 200 mg/L had no effect on BCG method *5704* At acute overdose concentration (20 mg/dL) on Technicon SMAC® method *6266*

Alkaline Phosphatase *Serum Increase Physiological* May cause cholestasis *3810*
Serum No Effect Analytical At acute overdose concentration (20 mg/dL) on Technicon SMAC® method *6266*

Amphetamine/Methamphetamine *Urine Positive Analytical* False positive result observed in some patients taking promethazine with/without chlorprothixene when measured by Syva EMIT II procedure *5634*

Aspartate Aminotransferase *Serum Increase Physiological* May cause cholestasis *3810*
Serum No Effect Analytical At acute overdose concentration (20 mg/dL) on Technicon SMAC® method *6266*

Bicarbonate *Serum No Effect Analytical* At concentration of 200 mg/L had no effect on method using phenolphthalein *5704*

Bile *Urine Increase Physiological* May cause cholestasis *3810*

Bilirubin *Serum Increase Physiological* May cause cholestasis *3810*
Serum No Effect Analytical At concentration of 200 mg/L had no effect on Jendrassik and Grof method *5704* At acute overdose concentration (20 mg/dL) on Technicon SMAC® method *6266*

BSP Retention *Serum Increase Physiological* May cause cholestasis *3810*

Calcium *Serum No Effect Analytical* At concentration of 200 mg/L had no effect on cresolphthalein method *5704* At acute overdose concentration (20 mg/dL) on Technicon SMAC® method *6266*

Cannabinoids *Urine No Effect Analytical* No effect observed at a concentration of 125 µg/mL (0.44 mmol/L) on method on Du Pont aca *1557* No effect on Roche Abuscreen method *5006*

Catecholamines *Plasma Increase Physiological* Increased metabolism, decreased organ uptake of norepinephrine *899*
Plasma No Effect Analytical No effect on HPLC method of Koller for dopamine, epinephrine, and norepinephrine *3230*

Chloride *Serum No Effect Analytical* At concentration of 1 mg/L had no effect on mercurimetric method *5704*

Cholesterol *Serum No Effect Analytical* At concentration of 200 mg/L had no effect on Liebermann-Burchard method *5704* At concentration of 1 mg/L had no effect on CHOD-PAP method *5704* At acute overdose concentration (20 mg/dL) on Technicon SMAC® method *6266*

Creatine Kinase *Serum Increase Physiological* In one individual injected intramuscularly with 1 mL fluid activity increased from mean baseline of 61 U/L to 70 U/L after 12 h and 173 U/L after 24 h *309*
Serum No Effect Analytical At acute overdose concentration (20 mg/dL) on Technicon SMAC® method *6266*

Creatinine *Serum No Effect Analytical* At concentration of 200 mg/L had no effect on Technicon AutoAnalyzer® Jaffe method *5704* At acute overdose concentration (20 mg/dL) on Technicon SMAC® method *6266*

Cyclosporine *Blood No Effect Analytical* At a concentration of 100 mg/L had no effect on Syva EMIT method *495*

Ethosuximide *Serum No Effect Analytical* Insignificant cross-reactivity observed with method on Du Pont aca *1523*

Glucose *Serum Decrease Physiological* If given i.v. or i.m *1334*
Serum No Effect Analytical At concentration of 1 mg/L had no effect on GOD/POD-PAP method *5704* At acute overdose concentration (20 mg/dL) on Technicon SMAC® method *6266*

Glucose Tolerance *Serum Decrease Physiological* An increase in blood glucose has been reported in patients receiving promethazine *6565*

Granulocytes *Blood Decrease Physiological* One case of agranulocytosis has been reported in patients receiving promethazine *6565*

Histamine *Cerebrospinal Fluid Increase Physiological* Mean concentration increased to about 1.8 pmol/L from mean baseline of about 0.6 pmol/L in 8 patients about one hour after they were given 0.08 mg/kg orally *5724*
Plasma No Effect Analytical Improbable inhibition of radioenzyme assay at physiological concentration of about 0.02 although 50% inhibition at 36 µg/mL *2492*

17-Hydroxycorticosteroids *Urine Decrease Analytical* Interference with Porter-Silber reaction *5869*

5-Hydroxyindoleacetic Acid *Urine No Effect Analytical* No effect observed with FPIA method on Abbott TDx *695*

^{131}I Uptake *Serum Decrease Physiological* Phenergan®, Mepergan® contain tetraiodofluorescein *4360*

Iron *Serum No Effect Analytical* At acute overdose concentration (20 mg/dL) on Technicon SMAC® method *6266* At concentration of 200 mg/L had no effect on Ferrozine method *5704*

Lactate Dehydrogenase *Serum No Effect Analytical* At acute overdose concentration (20 mg/dL) on Technicon SMAC® method *6266*

Leukocytes *Blood Decrease Physiological* Agranulocytosis/Leukopenia *6044* Rarely leukopenia has been reported in patients receiving promethazine *6565*

Methadone *Urine No Effect Analytical* Insignificant cross-reactivity of 0.6% observed with Roche Abuscreen ONTRAK method *3279*

Methylhistamine *Cerebrospinal Fluid Increase Physiological* Mean concentration of 1.92 pmol/L observed in 4 of 8 patients about one hour after they were given 0.08 mg/kg *5724*

Midazolam *Serum No Effect Analytical* On GC-ECD method of Ha et al *2387*

Neutrophils *Blood Decrease Physiological* Occasional case of agranulocytosis reported *6264*

p-Aminophenol *Urine No Effect Analytical* With addition of drugs at a concentration of 100 mg/L and of related compounds at 50 mg/L no significant effect observed on colorimetric method of van Bocxlaer on Cobas Mira analyzer which involves reacting free p-aminophenol with resorcinol in the presence of magnesium ions to form an indophenol dye measured at 550 nm *6163*

Phosphate *Serum Decrease Analytical* Turbidity produced, PO_4 concentration decreased in method of Fiske *1688*
Serum No Effect Analytical At concentration of 200 mg/L had no effect on phosphomolybdate method *5704* At acute overdose concentration (20 mg/dL) on Technicon SMAC® method *6266*

Platelets *Blood Decrease Physiological* Rarely thrombocytopenia has been reported in patients receiving promethazine *6565*

Potassium *Serum No Effect Analytical* At concentration of 1 mg/L had no effect on flame-photometric method *5704*

Pregnancy Tests *Serum Negative Analytical* May produce false positive or false negative reaction with immunological pregnancy tests *6565*
Serum Positive Analytical May produce false positive or false negative reaction with immunological pregnancy tests *6565*

Prolactin *Plasma No Effect Analytical* No significant response to 25 mg i.m *2352*

Protein *Serum No Effect Analytical* At acute overdose concentration (20 mg/dL) on Technicon SMAC® method *6266* At concentration of 200 mg/L had no effect on biuret method with blank correction *5704*

Sodium *Serum No Effect Analytical* At concentration of 1 mg/L had no effect on flame-photometric method *5704*

Tricyclic Antidepressants *Urine Increase Analytical* Large proportion of false positive results with Abbott ADx due to promethazine *4535*

Tricyclic Antidepressants Screen
Serum No Effect Analytical No significant effect observed at a concentration of 500 ng/mL (1.76 µmol/L) with method on Du Pont aca *1550*

Triglycerides *Serum No Effect Analytical* At acute overdose concentration (20 mg/dL) on Technicon SMAC® method

6266 At concentration of 200 mg/L had no effect on lipase/esterase method *5704*

Urea Nitrogen *Serum No Effect Analytical* At concentration of 200 mg/L had no effect on diacetylmonoxime method *5704* At acute overdose concentration (20 mg/dL) on Technicon SMAC® method *6266*

Uric Acid *Serum No Effect Analytical* At acute overdose concentration (20 mg/dL) on Technicon SMAC® method *6266* At concentration of 200 mg/L had no effect on phosphotungstate reduction method *5704*

Propafenone

Alanine Aminotransferase *Serum Increase Physiological* Cholestasis observed in 0.2% patients and hepatitis in 0.03% *3204* Activity increased to 402 U/L in one 85-year old woman treated with 450 mg/d for 30 days when she developed cholestatic hepatitis *3509* Rare effect observed *1384*

Alkaline Phosphatase *Serum Increase Physiological* Activity increased to 1054 U/L in one 85-year old woman who had been treated with 450 mg/d for 30 days and who developed cholestatic hepatitis *838* Cholestasis observed in 0.2% patients and hepatitis in 0.03% *3204*

Amitriptyline *Serum Increase Physiological* When coadministered, by inhibiting cytochrome P450 2D6, may increase the concentration of amitriptyline *6645*

Antinuclear Antibodies *Serum Increase Physiological* Positive ANA titer has been observed as a consequence of propafenone administration in 0.7% patients *3204*

Aspartate Aminotransferase *Serum Increase Physiological* Activity increased to 241 U/L in one 85-year old woman who developed cholestatic hepatitis following ingestion of 450 mg/d for 30 days *838* Cholestasis observed in 0.2% patients and hepatitis in 0.03% *3204* Rare effect observed *1384*

Bilirubin *Serum Increase Physiological* In one 85-year old woman who had received 450 mg/d for 30 days concentration increased to 4.6 mg/dL when cholestatic hepatitis developed *838*

Bilirubin, Direct *Serum Increase Physiological* In one 85-year old woman receiving 450 mg/d for 30 days concentration increased to 3.2 mg/dL die to cholestatic hepatitis *838*

Bleeding Time *Patient Increase Physiological* Increased bleeding time observed as a consequence of propafenone administration in some patients *3204*

Creatinine *Serum Increase Physiological* Kidney failure has been observed as a consequence of propafenone administration in some patients *3204*

Digoxin *Serum Increase Physiological* Coadministration with digoxin may increase the digoxin concentration *2161* Concentration increased in healthy individuals and patients partly due to reduction of nonrenal clearance *4316* Variable response observed but with most concentrations being increased when 900 mg/d propafenone administered. Literature cites 37% increase, 83% increase, mean 37% increase, 13.8% increase and 59% increase but also no statistically significant change *559* Dose related increases in plasma digoxin concentration observed with treatment ranging from about 35% at a propafenone dose of 450 mg/d to 85% at 900 mg/d *3204* Reported effect *2600* 37% increase when drugs coadministered due to decreased renal clearance *472*

Eosinophils *Blood Increase Physiological* In one 85-year old woman treatment with 450 mg/d for 30 days was associated with an increase to 20% of a total leukocyte count of 7200 /µL *838*

Erythrocyte Sedimentation Rate *Blood Increase Physiological* In one 85-year old woman treated with 450 mg/d for 30 days cholestatic hepatitis developed with increased ESR of 32 mm/h *838*

Glucose *Serum Increase Physiological* Hyperglycemia observed as a consequence of propafenone administration in some patients *3204*

γ-Glutamyltransferase *Serum Increase Physiological* Activity increased to 1140 U/L in one 85-year old woman who developed cholestatic hepatitis after ingestion of 450 mg/d for 30 days *838*

Granulocytes *Blood Decrease Physiological* Rare effect observed *1384* In U.S. clinical trials one case of agranulocytosis reported after 8 weeks of treatment *3204*

Hematocrit *Blood Decrease Physiological* Anemia observed as a consequence of propafenone administration *3204*

Hemoglobin *Blood Decrease Physiological* Anemia observed as a consequence of propafenone administration in some patients *3204*

Leukocytes *Blood Decrease Physiological* Decreased from mean of 6800 to 5900 /µL in 45 patients treated over 1 y *2429* Leukopenia observed as a consequence of propafenone administration in some patients *3204*
Blood No Effect Physiological In one 85-year old woman treatment with 450 mg/d for 30 days was associated with cholestatic hepatitis and concentration of 7200 /µL *838*

Metoprolol *Serum Increase Physiological* Reported effect *2600* Coadministration of propafenone with metoprolol reduced its plasma clearance by up to 80% and increased its plasma concentration by 2-5 times compared with controls *6293* Concomitant administration of propafenone with metoprolol resulted in a substantial increase in the metoprolol concentration and its elimination half-life *3204*

Neutrophils *Blood Decrease Physiological* Rare neutropenia observed *1384*

Platelets *Blood Decrease Physiological* Thrombocytopenia and purpura observed as a consequence of propafenone administration in some patients *3204*

Propranolol *Serum Increase Physiological* Reported effect *2600* Increased concentrations observed *1384* Concomitant administration of propafenone with propranolol resulted in a substantial increase in the propranolol concentration *3204*

Prothrombin Time *Plasma Increase Physiological* Concomitant administration of propafenone with warfarin in 8 healthy volunteers resulted in a 39% increase in the warfarin concentration with a 25% increase in the prothrombin time *3204*

Sodium *Serum Decrease Physiological* Hyponatremia with inappropriate ADH secretion observed as a consequence of propafenone administration in some patients *3204* Rare hyponatremia observed *1384*

Theophylline *Serum Increase Physiological* Increases serum theophylline concentration by about 40% due to decreased theophylline clearance *6117* Decreases theophylline clearance and also has pharmacologic interaction and increases serum theophylline concentration by about 40% *3125* Decreases theophylline clearance and increases theophylline concentration by about 40% *5999*

Urea Nitrogen *Serum Increase Physiological* Kidney failure has been observed as a consequence of propafenone administration in some patients *3204*

Warfarin *Plasma Increase Physiological* Possibly due to impairment of hepatic metabolism of warfarin. No displacement of warfarin from plasma proteins *3062* Observed effect with coadministration *1384* Concomitant administration of propafenone with warfarin in 8 healthy volunteers resulted in a 39% increase in the warfarin concentration with a 25% increase in the prothrombin time *3204* Reported effect *2600*

Propanidid

Basophils *Blood Decrease Physiological* Marked fall within 3 minutes of i.v. injection *3648*

Histamine *Plasma Increase Physiological* Immediate rise after i.v. injection without anaphylaxis *3648*

Hydrochloric Acid *Gastric Fluid Increase Physiological* Stimulation paralleled plasma histamine concentration *3648*

Propantheline

Acetaminophen *Serum Decrease Physiological* Delayed absorption with delayed gastric emptying *6403*

Bicarbonate *Serum Increase Analytical* Significant effect on method on Kodak Ektachem® but no effect on method on Beckman Astra® 8 *3233*

Propantheline *(continued)*

Bromide *Serum Increase Physiological* Theoretical possibility if bromide salt is administered since it contains 17.8% bromide *5116*

Cefpodoxime *Serum Decrease Physiological* Administration of propantheline delayed peak plasma concentration but did not affect the AUC *4684*

Chloride *Serum Increase Analytical* Substantial increase with method on Kodak Ektachem® and minor effect on method on Beckman Astra® 8 *3233*

Chlorothiazide *Serum Increase Physiological* Absorption window increased with absorption window or dissolution *6403*

Digoxin *Serum Increase Physiological* Increased absorption with augmented dissolution *6403* With tablets of low bioavailability due to reduction of bowel motility *4631* Concentration increased especially with slowly dissolving preparations due to decreased gastrointestinal motility *3772* By decreasing gut motility may increase digoxin absorption thus coadministration with digoxin may increase the digoxin concentration *2161*

Ethanol *Serum Decrease Physiological* Reduced rate of absorption with delayed gastric emptying *6403*

Glucose *Serum Decrease Physiological* In 4 patients with insulin dependent diabetes mellitus mean decrease of 96 mg/dL with same dose of insulin following oral administration of 45 mg *1273*

Growth Hormone *Plasma Decrease Physiological* In 4 patients with insulin dependent diabetes mellitus decrease from mean of 56 ng/mL to 12 ng/mL after treatment with 45 mg orally. Sleep related plasma peaks reduced *1273*

Hydrochlorothiazide *Serum Increase Physiological* Delayed but increased absorption with delayed gastric emptying *6403*

Lithium *Serum Decrease Physiological* Delayed absorption with delayed gastric emptying *6403*

Nitrofurantoin *Serum Increase Physiological* By reducing gastrointestinal motility bioavailability increased with increased absorption and increased serum concentration *2882*

Ranitidine *Serum Increase Physiological* Significantly reduced time to peak concentration but area under curve increased *3146* May delay absorption from gastrointestinal tract and increase peak serum concentration and bioavailability *1384*

β-Propiolactone

Alkaline Phosphatase *Serum Decrease Physiological* Increase by 8 U/L when plasma from BPL treated blood compared with plasma in 25 specimens *351*

Aspartate Aminotransferase
Serum No Effect Physiological But inhibition when drug added to plasma negated by increase from hemolysis *351*

Bicarbonate *Serum Decrease Physiological* Increase by 14 mmol/L when plasma from BPL treated blood compared with plasma in 25 specimens *351*

Bilirubin *Serum Decrease Physiological* Increase by 1 µmol/L when plasma from BPL treated blood compared with plasma in 25 specimens *351*

Calcium *Serum Increase Physiological* Increase by 0.1 mmol/L when plasma from BPL treated blood compared with plasma in 25 specimens *351*

Chloride *Serum Decrease Physiological* Increase by 10 mmol/L when plasma from BPL treated blood compared with plasma in 25 specimens *351*

Hemoglobin *Plasma Increase Physiological* When plasma from BPL treated blood compared with plasma in 25 specimens *351*

Lactate Dehydrogenase *Serum Increase Physiological* Increase by 75 U/L when plasma from BPL treated blood compared with plasma in 25 specimens *351*

Neopterin *Urine No Effect Analytical* No effect observed on radioimmunoassay method using Henning Berlin kit reagents *5491*

Potassium *Serum Increase Physiological* Significant effect by 0.7 mmol/L when plasma from BPL treated blood compared with plasma in 25 specimens *351*

Protein *Serum Increase Physiological* Increase by 3.5 g/L when plasma from BPL treated blood compared with plasma in 25 specimens *351*

Sodium *Serum Increase Physiological* Significant effect by 7 mmol/L when plasma from BPL treated blood compared with plasma in 25 specimens *351*

Propofol

Bicyclo-Prostaglandin E_2 *Plasma Increase Physiological* In 8 volunteers mean concentration increased after injection of mean dose of 3.1 mg/kg from baseline of 123 ± 44 pg/mL to 159 ± 41 pg/mL after 1 minute and 170 ± 51 pg/mL after 5 minutes *4713*

Remifentanil *Serum No Effect Physiological* Remifentanil clearance is not altered when propofol coadministered *2165*

Propoxyphene

Acetaminophen *Serum No Effect Analytical* No interference observed at a concentration of 2160 µg/mL (588 µmol/L) with method on Du Pont aca *1506*

Alanine Aminotransferase *Serum Increase Physiological* Cholestatic effect *3177*
Serum No Effect Analytical At acute overdose concentration (2.5 mg/dL) on Technicon SMAC® method *6266*

Albumin *Serum No Effect Analytical* At acute overdose concentration (2.5 mg/dL) on Technicon SMAC® method *6266* At concentration of 25 mg/L had no effect on BCG method *5704*

Alkaline Phosphatase *Serum Increase Physiological* In 3 patients within 10 d of start of drug treatment *1909* Hepatotoxic response observed in 2 patients *3477* Hepatic toxicity (cholestatic hepatitis) *3177*
Serum No Effect Analytical At acute overdose concentration (2.5 mg/dL) on Technicon SMAC® method *6266*

Alprazolam *Serum Decrease Physiological* Concomitant administration of propoxyphene with alprazolam caused a decrease in the maximum concentration of alprazolam of 6%, decreased its plasma clearance by 36% and increased its half-life by 58% *4685*

Amitriptyline *Serum Increase Analytical* May cause false positive reaction with HPLC methods for amitriptyline *3590*

Amphetamine *Urine No Effect Analytical* Negative result observed with method on Du Pont aca at a concentration of 1000 µg/L (2.94 mmol/L) *1554*

Aspartate Aminotransferase *Serum Increase Physiological* In 3 patients within 10 d of start of drug treatment *1909* Hepatotoxic response observed in 2 patients *3477* Cholestatic effect *3177*
Serum No Effect Analytical At acute overdose concentration (2.5 mg/dL) on Technicon SMAC® method *6266*

Barbiturate *Serum No Effect Analytical* No significant interference observed at a concentration of 100 µg/mL (0.30 mmol/L) with method on Du Pont aca *1511*
Urine No Effect Analytical Negative result obtained at a concentration of 1000 µg/mL (2.94 mmol/L) with method on Du Pont aca *1555*

Benzodiazepine *Urine No Effect Analytical* Negative result observed at a concentration of 1000 µg/mL (2.94 mmol/L) with method on Du Pont aca *1556*

Benzodiazepine Screen *Serum No Effect Analytical* No significant effect observed at a concentration of 100 µg/mL (0.30 mmol/L) with method on Du Pont aca *1512*

Benzoylecgonine *Urine No Effect Analytical* Negative result obtained at a concentration of 500 µg/mL (1.47 mmol/L) with method on Du Pont aca *1558* No significant interference observed at a concentration of 900 µmol/L with Sung and Neely modification of Syva EMIT procedure *148*

Bile *Urine Increase Physiological* Cholestatic effect *3177*

Bilirubin *Serum Increase Physiological* In 3 patients within 10 d of start of drug treatment *1909* Hepatotoxic response observed in 2 patients *3477* Cholestatic effect *3177*
Serum No Effect Analytical At acute overdose concentration (2.5 mg/dL) on Technicon SMAC® method *6266* At concentration of 25 mg/L had no effect on Jendrassik and Grof method *5704*

BSP Retention *Serum Increase Physiological* Cholestatic effect *3177*

Calcium *Serum No Effect Analytical* At acute overdose concentration (2.5 mg/dL) on Technicon SMAC® method *6266* At concentration of 25 mg/L had no effect on cresolphthalein method *5704*

Cannabinoids *Urine No Effect Analytical* No effect of dextropropoxyphene on Roche Abuscreen method *5006* No effect on Roche Abuscreen method *5006* No effect observed at a concentration of 100 µg/mL (0.29 mmol/L) on method on Du Pont aca *1557*

Carbamazepine *Serum Increase Physiological* Inhibits metabolism and increases concentration with possible clinical toxicity *3118* Due to effect on hepatic metabolism *1384* Addition of 195 mg propoxyphene to carbamazepine regime on which 6 patients had been stabilized caused mean increase of carbamazepine concentration by 66% *2439* Drugs that inhibit CYP 3A4 inhibit metabolism of carbamazepine producing clinically meaningful effect *1039* Inhibits metabolism of carbamazepine thereby may cause toxic effects *1384* Concomitant administration with carbamazepine causes marked increase of plasma carbamazepine concentration resulting in toxicity in some cases *282*

Carbon Dioxide Partial Pressure
Blood Increase Physiological Large doses may produce respiratory depression *2242*

Cholesterol *Serum No Effect Analytical* At concentration of 25 mg/L had no effect on Liebermann-Burchard method *5704* At acute overdose concentration (2.5 mg/dL) on Technicon SMAC® method *6266*

Cocaethylene *Urine No Effect Analytical* No interference observed with TLC method of Bailey *328*

Creatine Kinase *Serum No Effect Analytical* At acute overdose concentration (2.5 mg/dL) on Technicon SMAC® method *6266*

Creatinine *Serum No Effect Analytical* At concentration of 25 mg/L had no effect on Technicon AutoAnalyzer® Jaffe method *5704* At acute overdose concentration (2.5 mg/dL) on Technicon SMAC® method *6266*

Doxepin *Serum Increase Physiological* In one patient coadministration of propoxyphene caused marked increase in plasma doxepin concentration probably due to inhibition of hepatic metabolism *36*

Drugs of Abuse Screen *Urine No Effect Analytical* No effect at concentration of 100 µg/mL on EZ-SCREEN procedure for cannabinoids and cocaine *1739*

Glucose *Serum Decrease Physiological* Hypoglycemia allegedly occurred in one case *6440*
Serum No Effect Analytical At acute overdose concentration (2.5 mg/dL) on Technicon SMAC® method *6266* At concentration of 1.8 mg/L had no effect on Kodak Ektachem® method *5704*
Urine Decrease Analytical Low with Clinistix® , Diastix® *1826*
Urine No Effect Analytical No effect on TesTape® *1826*

γ-Glutamyltransferase *Serum Increase Physiological* Hepatotoxic response observed in 2 patients *3477*

11-Hydroxycorticosteroids *Urine Decrease Physiological* Slight effect only (probably physiological action) *1184*

17-Hydroxycorticosteroids *Urine Decrease Physiological* Probable action on hypothalamic pituitary. ACTH secretion *1184*

^{131}I Uptake *Serum Decrease Physiological* Darvon® contains tetraiodofluorescein *4360*

Iron *Serum No Effect Analytical* At acute overdose concentration (2.5 mg/dL) on Technicon SMAC® method *6266* At concentration of 25 mg/L had no effect on Ferrozine method *5704*

17-Ketosteroids *Urine Decrease Physiological* Probable action on hypothalamic pituitary. ACTH secretion *1184*

Lactate Dehydrogenase *Serum Increase Physiological* Cholestatic effect *3177*
Serum No Effect Analytical At acute overdose concentration (2.5 mg/dL) on Technicon SMAC® method *6266*

Methadone *Urine No Effect Analytical* Insignificant cross-reactivity of 0.2% observed with d-propoxyphene and Roche Abuscreen ONTRAK method *3279*

Metoprolol *Serum Increase Physiological* Significant increase observed with coadministration of both drugs due to inhibition of hepatic metabolism *3686*

Morphine *Urine No Effect Analytical* No significant interference observed at a concentration of 900 µmol/L with Sung and Neely modification of Syva EMIT procedure *148* Insignificant cross reactivity with EMIT procedure for opiates. Insignificant cross reactivity with hemagglutination inhibition. Insignificant cross reactivity with RIA procedures *4163*

5'-Nucleotidase *Serum Increase Physiological* Due to cholestasis *2911*

Opiates *Urine No Effect Analytical* No effect observed at a concentration of 1000 µg/mL (2.94 mmol/L) on method on Du Pont aca *1559*

Phenobarbital *Serum Increase Physiological* Concomitant administration increases phenobarbital concentration slightly probably through inhibition of hepatic metabolizing enzymes *2439*

Phenylalanine *Plasma No Effect Analytical* No inteference observed with rapid quantitative whole blood method of Campbell et al using phenylalanine dehydrogenase *867*

Phenytoin *Serum Increase Physiological* Reported impairment of metabolism, increased plasma concentration *3340*

Phosphate *Serum No Effect Analytical* At acute overdose concentration (2.5 mg/dL) on Technicon SMAC® method *6266* At concentration of 25 mg/L had no effect on phosphomolybdate method *5704*

Platelet Aggregation *Blood Decrease Physiological* Observed *in vitro*, may cause gastrointestinal bleeding etc *915*

Potassium *Serum No Effect Analytical* At concentration of 5 mg/L had no effect on measurement by ISE with predilution *5704*

Prazosin *Serum No Effect Physiological* Coadministration of prazosin with propoxyphene had no apparent adverse drug interaction in limited clinical experience *4649*

Propoxyphene *Serum Increase Physiological* 0.2 mg/L after 200 mg orally, 0.3 mg/L after 50 mg i.v *3868*

Propranolol *Serum Increase Physiological* Significant increase in propranolol concentration observed when drugs coadministered due to reduced hepatic metabolism *3686*

Protein *Serum No Effect Analytical* At concentration of 25 mg/L had no effect on biuret method with blank correction *5704* At acute overdose concentration (2.5 mg/dL) on Technicon SMAC® method *6266*

Sodium *Serum No Effect Analytical* At concentration of 5 mg/L had no effect on measurement by ISE with predilution *5704*

Tricyclic Antidepressants Screen
Serum No Effect Analytical No significant effect observed at a concentration of 500 µg/mL (1.47 mmol/L) with method on Du Pont aca *1550*

Triglycerides *Serum No Effect Analytical* At acute overdose concentration (2.5 mg/dL) on Technicon SMAC® method *6266* At concentration of 25 mg/L had no effect on lipase/esterase method *5704*

Urea Nitrogen *Serum No Effect Analytical* At concentration of 25 mg/L had no effect on diacetylmonoxime method *5704* At concentration of 1.8 mg/L had no effect on Kodak Ektachem® method *5704* At acute overdose concentration (2.5 mg/dL) on Technicon SMAC® method *6266*

Uric Acid *Serum No Effect Analytical* At concentration of 25 mg/L had no effect on phosphotungstate reduction method *5704* At acute overdose concentration (2.5 mg/dL) on Technicon SMAC® method *6266*

Propranolol

Adenosine Monophosphate
Plasma Decrease Physiological Substantially lower in patients receiving drug than in those receiving either pindolol or metoprolol *6511*
Platelets Decrease Physiological Significantly less than in patients receiving either pindolol or metoprolol *6511*

Adenosine Triphosphate
Red Blood Cells Decrease Physiological Significant effect, also inhibits glucose utilization by 60% *4594*

Propranolol *(continued)*

Alanine Aminotransferase *Serum Increase Physiological* Plasma activity may be increased when propranolol administered *6558* Low incidence drug induced increase *4014*

Albumin *Serum No Effect Analytical* No effect at 0.1 mg/dL on Technicon SMA 12/60 method *4390* At concentration of 0.2 mg/L had no effect on BCG method *5704*

Aldosterone *Plasma No Effect Physiological* No effect observed in resting state in 12 moderately hypertensive men treated with up to 160 mg/day for 8 weeks *5861*
Urine Decrease Physiological Change less than with renin *801*

Alkaline Phosphatase *Serum Increase Physiological* Low incidence drug induced increase *4014* Plasma activity may be increased when propranolol administered *6558*
Serum No Effect Analytical No effect at 0.1 mg/dL on Technicon SMA 12/60 method *4390*

Alprazolam *Serum No Effect Physiological* 240 mg daily had no effect on alprazolam clearance *4355*

Angiotensin-I *Plasma No Effect Physiological* Concentration not significantly affected by administration of 120 mg daily in 6 healthy male volunteers *473*

Angiotensin-II *Plasma No Effect Physiological* No effect in 6 healthy male volunteers given 120 mg drug *473*

Angiotensin-converting Enzyme
Serum Decrease Physiological Almost complete inhibition of activity 2 hours after administration of 120 mg drug in 6 healthy male volunteers, with 60% inhibition after 24 hours *473*

Antipyrine *Serum Increase Physiological* Plasma concentration increased with coadministration of propranolol *6558*

Apolipoprotein A-I *Serum No Effect Physiological* No change observed in 11 patients *4100* Decrease by -3 mg/dL in 8 patients given 30 to 60 mg daily for 8 weeks *4213*

Apolipoprotein B *Serum No Effect Physiological* No change observed in 11 patients *4100* Increase by 5 mg/dL in 8 patients given 30 to 60 mg daily for 8 weeks *4213*

Apolipoprotein C-II *Serum No Effect Physiological* Increase by 2 mg/dL in 8 patients given 30 to 60 mg daily for 8 weeks *4213*

Apolipoprotein C-III *Serum Increase Physiological* Increase by 4 mg/dL in 8 patients given 30 to 60 mg daily for 8 weeks *4213*

Apolipoprotein E *Serum No Effect Physiological* Increase by 2 mg/dL in 11 patients given 30 to 60 mg daily for 8 weeks *4213*

Aspartate Aminotransferase *Serum Increase Physiological* Occasionally seen, probably not due to hepatotoxicity *4174* Plasma activity may be increased when propranolol administered *6558*
Serum No Effect Analytical No effect at 0.1 mg/dL on Technicon SMA 12/60 method *4390*

Benazepril *Serum No Effect Physiological* No clinically important pharmacokinetic interactions observed when drugs coadministered *1033*

Bicarbonate *Serum No Effect Analytical* At concentration of 0.2 mg/L had no effect on method using phenolphthalein *5704*

Bilirubin *Serum Increase Analytical* 4-hydroxypropranolol metabolite increases bilirubin concentration when measured with diazo reaction. Metabolite present as sulfate or glucuronide *93*
Serum No Effect Analytical No effect at 0.1 mg/dL on Technicon SMA 12/60 method *4390* No effect at concentration of 2 mg/L on method on Kodak Ektachem® systems *5706* At concentration of 0.2 mg/L had no effect on Jendrassik and Grof method *5704*

Bilirubin, Conjugated *Serum No Effect Analytical* No effect at concentration of 2 mg/L on method on Kodak Ektachem® systems *5706*

Bilirubin, Unconjugated *Serum No Effect Analytical* No effect at concentration of 2 mg/L on method on Kodak Ektachem® *5706*

Bleeding Time *Patient Increase Physiological* Greater than 200% increase observed in 3 of 5 volunteers over 4 day ingestion *1617*

Calcium *Serum Increase Physiological* Increase by 0.34 mg/dL in approximately 120 patients with essential hypertension treated for 1 y *6248*
Serum No Effect Analytical No effect at 0.1 mg/dL on Technicon SMA 12/60 method *4390* At concentration of 0.2 mg/L had no effect on cresolphthalein method *5704*
Serum No Effect Physiological In 340 patients given drug for 10 weeks to reduce diastolic BP to less than 90 mm Hg *6247* No significant effect in 12 healthy volunteers over 24 hours following single dose of 160 mg *3452*
Urine No Effect Physiological No significant effect in 12 healthy volunteers over 24 hours following single oral dose of 160 mg *3452*

Chloride *Serum No Effect Analytical* At concentration of 0.2 mg/L had no effect on mercurimetric method *5704*
Serum No Effect Physiological No significant effect in 12 healthy volunteers over 24 hours following single dose of 160 mg *3452*
Urine No Effect Physiological No significant effect in 12 healthy volunteers over 24 hours following single oral dose of 160 mg *3452*

Chlorpromazine *Serum Increase Physiological* Coadministration of drugs caused significant increase in chlorpromazine concentration due to inhibition of metabolism *4588* Concomitant administration increases the concentrations of both drugs *5659* Plasma concentrations of both drugs increased when they are coadministered *6558*

Cholesterol *Serum Increase Physiological* Mean increase from 213 to 222 mg/dL in 16 hypertensives given 80 mg daily for up to 12 mo *3737* Increase by 9 mg/dL in approximately 120 patients with essential hypertension treated for 1 y *6248*
Serum No Effect Analytical At concentration of 0.2 mg/L had no effect on CHOD-PAP method *5704* No effect at 0.1 mg/dL on Technicon SMA 12/60 method *4390*
Serum No Effect Physiological Insignificant change after 6 mo treatment in 16 hypertensives *1293* In 23 hypertensive men given up to 160 mg/d for 8 weeks *3521* In 23 hypertensive men aged 47-55 y treated for 8 weeks *2547* No significant effect in about 20 hypertensives receiving 160 mg/day for 2 years *1899* In 22 mild/moderate hypertensive males treated for 8 weeks: insignificant increase noted *2781* In 50 volunteers given 160 mg daily for 3 mo *3574* Increase by 2 mg/dL in 8 patients given 30 to 60 mg daily for 8 weeks *4213* In 53 hypertensives given 80 mg twice daily for 3 mo *1292* In 340 patients given drug for 10 weeks to reduce diastolic BP to less than 90 mm Hg *6247* General effect observed in multiple studies *142* Range from -2 to 9% change but mostly no change in many studies *141* Increase by 1.0-1.5 mmol/L in 20 hypertensive diabetic patients *6544* In 20 hypertensive diabetic patients *6544*

Cholinesterase *Serum No Effect Analytical* No effect observed at concentration of 5 µg/dL with butyrylthiocholine method on Kodak Ektachem® *2504*

Chromogranin-A *Plasma No Effect Physiological* Inpatients with uni- or bilateral adrenalectomy concentration unaffected by propranolol treatment *5930*

C-Peptide *Urine No Effect Physiological* In 14 hypertensives with type 2 diabetes treated for 3 weeks, with or without added hydrochlorothiazide *1476*

Creatine Kinase *Serum Increase Physiological* In 4 of 27 patients with essential hypertension, effect mainly in MM isoenzyme: effect not very marked *5275*

Creatine Kinase Isoenzymes *Serum No Effect Analytical* No interference observed at a concentration of 200 mg/L (771 µmol/L) with CK-MB method on Du Pont aca *1519*

Creatinine *Serum No Effect Analytical* At concentration of 0.2 mg/L had no effect on Technicon AutoAnalyzer® method *5704* At 100 mg/L on reversed phase liquid chromatographic procedure of Zhiri et al *6656* No effect at 0.1 mg/dL on Technicon SMA 12/60 method *4390* At concentration of 0.16 mg/L had no effect on creatinine iminohydrolase method *5704*
Serum No Effect Physiological No significant effect in 12 healthy volunteers over 24 hours following single dose of 160 mg *3452* In approximately 120 patients with essential hypertension treated for 1 y *6248* In 340 patients given drug for 10 weeks to reduce diastolic BP to less than 90 mm Hg *6247* No significant effect on renal function in 15 patients with essential hypertension over 1 mo *6376*

Urine No Effect Physiological No significant effect in 12 healthy volunteers over 24 hours following single oral dose of 160 mg *3452*

Diazepam *Serum Increase Physiological* 240 mg daily reduced clearance by about 16% *4355*

Serum No Effect Physiological 160 mg daily increased area under diazepam concentration curve by about 20% *2517*

2,3-Diphosphoglycerate

Red Blood Cells Decrease Physiological Shifts hemoglobin-O_2 dissociation curve to right *4594*

Disopyramide *Serum No Effect Physiological* When drugs coadministered no significant effect observed on the pharmacokinetics of either drug *2069*

Doxazosin *Serum No Effect Physiological* Coadministration with doxazosin had no effect on its pharmacokinetics *4642*

Effective Renal Plasma Flow

Patient Decrease Physiological May occur with decreased cardiac output *5688*

Epinephrine *Plasma Increase Physiological* Decreased clearance by 80% in hypertensives and similar effect in normals *6658*

Plasma No Effect Physiological In 20 patients with hypertension following head injury treatment with a single dose of 160 mg caused nonsignificant increase from mean baseline of 768 ± 57 pg/mL to 856 ± 134 pg/mL after 2 h and 831 ± 123 pg/mL after 4 h *3480*

Fatty Acids (FFA), Free *Serum Decrease Physiological* Especially during and after exercise *112* But not significant in hyperthyroid patients given 40 mg every 6 h in 6 patients *540* Marked effect in 53 hypertensives given 80 mg twice daily for 3 mo *1292* Slight effect with pharmacological doses *2346* Significant reduction of basal concentration after 3 mo treatment in 16 hypertensives, but close to normal after 6 mo *1293*

Serum No Effect Physiological In 5 hyperthyroid patients given 10 mg every 8 h for 4 d *540*

Flecainide *Serum Increase Physiological* Small increases in plasma concentration are observed (20%) when propranolol coadministered with flecainide *3702*

Fluvastatin *Serum No Effect Physiological* Administration of propranolol with fluvastatin to patients with hypercholesterolemia had no effect on the metabolism and excretion of fluvastatin *5232*

Glimepiride *Serum Increase Physiological* When propranolol at a dose of 40 mg t.i.d. coadministered with glimepiride peak concentration, AUC and half-life of glimepiride increased by 23%, 22% and 15% respectively *2639*

Glomerular Filtration Rate *Urine Decrease Physiological* 13% decrease on average in hypertensives *2804*

Glucagon *Plasma Decrease Physiological* In 18 patients with mild essential hypertension treated with chlorothiazide concomitantly over 4 weeks *1734* Slight effect with pharmacological doses *2346*

Plasma Increase Physiological Glucagon release reduced in normal subjects, but marked increase observed in cirrhotics following intravenous administration of 10 mg drug *5555*

Plasma No Effect Physiological In hyperthyroid patients given 40 mg every 6 h in 6 patients *540* In 5 hyperthyroid patients given 10 mg every 8 h for 4 d *540* No change in basal concentration or after glucose in 16 hypertensives *1293*

Glucose *Serum Decrease Physiological* Has slight effect like that of prolonging insulin *5869* Rare cases due to inhibition of glycogenolysis in nondiabetics *4369* 6 episodes of hypoglycemia observed in 5 nondiabetic patients on chronic hemodialysis, due to β-adrenergic blockage *2283* In one patient with hepatic cirrhosis and severe hyperandrogenemia administration of 60 mg propranolol per day caused reducton of plasma glucose concentration to 1.1 mmol/L *3911*

Serum Increase Physiological Overt diabetes developed or after glucose challenge in 40 hypertensives *4089* Slight effect with pharmacological doses *2346* Increase by 2 mg/dL in 340 patients given drug for 10 weeks to reduce diastolic BP to less than 90 mm Hg *6247* In 14 hypertensive men with type 2 diabetes when treated for 3 weeks, marked increase when propranolol coadministered *1476* To extent of diabetic coma in 2 diabetics when propranolol given with hydrochlorothiazide: exact mechanism not known *4223* Increase by 8 mg/dL in approximately 120 patients with essential hypertension treated for 1 y *6248* Mean increase from 101 to 108 mg/dL after 16 weeks treatment in approximately 120 hypertensives *3837* Increase by 1.0-1.5 mmol/L in 20 hypertensive diabetic patients *6544*

Serum No Effect Analytical At concentration of 80 mg/L had no effect on GOD/POD-PAP method *5704* No effect at 0.1 mg/dL on Technicon SMA 12/60 method *4390*

Serum No Effect Physiological In 18 patients with mild essential hypertension treated with chlorothiazide concomitantly over 4 weeks *93* No significant effect in 6 healthy volunteers following single oral dose of 40 mg *4064* After 12 mo treatment of 53 previously untreated hypertensives *507* Insignificantly reduced after 3 or 6 mo treatment in 16 nondiabetic hypertensives, but lower after glucose ingestion *1293* No effect on short term administration *2676* In 5 hyperthyroid patients given 10 mg every 8 h for 4 d *540* No effect observed with i.v. infusion *5186*

Glucose Tolerance *Serum Decrease Physiological* Raised concentration during later part of i.v. glucose tolerance test *2346* Overt diabetes developed or after glucose challenge in 40 hypertensives *4089*

Glycerol *Serum Decrease Physiological* In hyperthyroid patients given 40 mg every 6 h in 6 patients *540*

Serum No Effect Physiological In 5 hyperthyroid patients given 10 mg every 8 h for 4 d *540*

Granulocytes *Blood Decrease Physiological* Agranulocytosis observed in 8.2% of patients taking drug compared with 2.3% of control patients (stratified relative risk estimate 4.3) *3098*

Growth Hormone *Plasma Increase Physiological* One out of six produce response *593* Marked increase observed in 11 hypertensives also treated with diuretics. Also caused marked effect in 3 of 4 acromegalics *1819*

Plasma No Effect Physiological No effect unless with epinephrine then sharp increase *3833* No effect on concentration at 3 or 6 mo treatment *1293* No significant effect on baseline concentration in either controls or hyperthyroid patients or in growth hormone response between the 2 groups in response to oral glucose tolerance test *3372*

Haloperidol *Serum No Effect Physiological* Minimal interaction observed when drugs coadministered *2315*

HDL-Cholesterol *Serum Decrease Physiological* From no change to 29% reduction in several studies *141* Mean decrease from 49 to 45 mg/dL in approximately 120 hypertensives after 16 weeks therapy *3837* Marked effect in 53 hypertensives given 80 mg twice daily for 3 mo *1292* Decrease by -3 mg/dL in 8 patients given 30 to 60 mg daily for 8 weeks *4213* Reduction observed in mild to moderate hypertensives following treatment with 80 mg t.i.d. Rise noted in cholesterol/HDL ratio *4232* Decrease from 30-32% in about 20 hypertensives treated with 160 mg/day for 2 years *1899* From 42 to 36 mg/dL in 15 hypertriglyceridemic hypertensives after 12 weeks *552* Significant decrease observed in both normocholesterolemic and hypercholesterolemic hypertensive patients treated with 160 mg/d for 6 months: but percentage change less in hypercholesterolemics than in normocholesterolemics *1900* Primarily observed effect with nonselective β-blockers is reduction of HDL-cholesterol *3730* Mean decrease from 53 to 48 mg/dL in 16 hypertensives given 80 mg daily for up to 12 mo *3737* Increase by 13% in 23 hypertensive men aged 47-55 y treated for 8 weeks *2547* Approximately 10% decrease noted in 22 mild or moderate hypertensives treated for 8 weeks: inverse relationship to dose given *2781* Increase by 13% in 23 hypertensive men given up to 160 mg/d for 8 weeks *3521*

Serum No Effect Physiological General effect observed in multiple studies *142* In 17 patients with hypertension followed for 3 mo *1614* In 50 volunteers given 160 mg daily for 3 mo *3574*

HDL-Triglycerides *Serum Increase Physiological* From 21 to 32 mg/dL in 15 hypertriglyceridemic hypertensives after 12 weeks *552*

Hematocrit *Blood Decrease Physiological* Associated with altered morphology of red cells *4594*

Hemoglobin A_{1c} *Blood Increase Physiological* In 14 hypertensive men with type 2 diabetes when treated for 3 weeks, marked increase when propranolol coadministered *1476*

Histamine *Plasma No Effect Analytical* Improbable inhibition of radio-enzyme assay at therapeutic concentrations *2492*

Hydrochloric Acid *Gastric Fluid Decrease Physiological* Affects basal and histamine stimulated *2097*

Propranolol *(continued)*

Hydroxyproline *Urine Decrease Physiological* In hyperthyroid patients possible effect due to membrane-stabilizing property of drug *539*

^{131}I Uptake *Serum No Effect Physiological* No effect in euthyroid patients *573*

Insulin *Plasma Decrease Physiological* Significantly less in nondiabetic treated hypertensives than in diabetic- treated patients *4089*
Plasma No Effect Physiological After 12 mo treatment of 53 previously untreated hypertensives *507* In 5 hyperthyroid patients given 10 mg every 8 h for 4 d *540* No change in basal concentrations or after glucose in 16 hypertensives *1293* No significant effect although drug affects glucose concentration *2346* In 20 hypertensive diabetic patients *6544* In 18 patients with mild essential hypertension treated with chlorothiazide concomitantly over 4 weeks *1734*

Insulin Tolerance *Plasma Increase Physiological* Decreases glucose rebound at end of test *5501*

Ketones *Serum Decrease Physiological* In hyperthyroid patients given 40 mg every 6 h in 6 patients *540*
Serum No Effect Physiological In 5 hyperthyroid patients given 10 mg every 8 h for 4 d *540*

17-Ketosteroids *Urine No Effect Analytical* No effect observed on concentration when measured by Zimmermann method *4421*

Lactate Dehydrogenase *Serum Increase Physiological* Plasma activity may be increased when propranolol administered *6558*
Serum No Effect Analytical No effect at 0.1 mg/dL on Technicon SMA 12/60 method *4390*

LDL-Cholesterol *Serum Decrease Physiological* Appreciable decrease (130 to 111 mg/dL) after treatment for 12 weeks in 15 hypertriglyceridemic hypertensives *552*
Serum Increase Physiological Mean increase from 126 to 134 mg/dL in 16 hypertensives given 80 mg daily for up to 12 mo *3737*
Serum No Effect Physiological In 17 patients with hypertension followed for 3 mo *1614* In several studies *141* Or slight reduction in 53 hypertensives given 80 mg twice daily for 3 mo *1292* No significant effect in about 20 hypertensives receiving 160 mg/day for 2 years *1899* In 50 volunteers given 160 mg daily for 3 mo *3574* General effect observed in multiple studies *142*

LDL-Triglycerides *Serum No Effect Physiological* No change in 15 hypertriglyceridemic hypertensives after 12 weeks *552*

Lecithin:Cholesterol Acyltransferase
Serum Decrease Physiological In vitro reduction of activity to 54.6 ± 25.7% of control observed at concentration of 0.5 µmol/L *5316*

Lidocaine *Serum Increase Physiological* Plasma concentration increased when propranolol coadministered *6558* Clearance reduced by more than 20% probably associated with inhibition of hepatic microsomal metabolizing enzymes *414*
Serum No Effect Analytical No significant interference observed at a concentration of 100 µg/mL (386 µmol/L) with method on Du Pont aca *1534* At a concentration of 1250 mg/L (normal therapeutic concentration up to 0.3 mg/L) had less than 10% effect on method on Baxter Stratus *5705*

Lipase *Serum No Effect Analytical* No effect of concentrations up to 10 mg/L on method on Kodak Ektachem® *5706*

Lisinopril *Serum No Effect Physiological* Coadministration of lisinopril with propranolol appears to have no effect on the pharmacokinetics of either drug *3990*

Lorazepam *Serum No Effect Physiological* 240 mg daily had no effect on plasma concentration or clearance *4355*

Lovastatin *Serum No Effect Physiological* Coadministration of single doses of lovastatin and propranolol had no effect on the pharmacokinetics of either drug *3982*

Magnesium *Serum No Effect Physiological* No significant effect in 12 healthy volunteers over 24 hours following single dose of 160 mg *3452*
Urine No Effect Physiological No significant effect in 12 healthy volunteers over 24 hours following single oral dose of 160 mg *3452*

Melatonin *Urine Decrease Physiological* Nonsignificant reduction in 10 hypertensive patients treated with mean dose of 305 mg/day for 4 weeks *724*

Metformin *Serum No Effect Physiological* In a single dose study during which propranolol and metformin were coadministered propranolol appeared to have no effect on the pharmacokinetics of metformin *726*

Midazolam *Serum No Effect Analytical* On GC-ECD method of Ha et al *2387*

N-Acetylprocainamide *Serum No Effect Analytical* No significant interference observed at a concentration of 100 µg/mL (386 µmol/L) with method on Du Pont aca *1536*

Nefazodone *Serum No Effect Physiological* In 18 healthy male volunteers (15 phenotyped as P450IID6 extensive metabolizers) coadministration of nefazodone 200 mg b.i.d. with 40 mg b.i.d. propranolol for 5.5 days had no effect on the concentration of nefazodone *729*

Neutrophils *Blood Decrease Physiological* Occasional case of agranulocytosis reported *6264*

Nifedipine *Serum Increase Physiological* Oral administration increased concentration of nifedipine by about 50% even when nifedipine was administered intravenously with reduction of liver blood flow *3181*

Nisoldipine *Serum Increase Physiological* Coadministration caused increase in area under curve of 30% and peak plasma concentration of 57% *3542*
Serum No Effect Physiological Administration of propranolol with nisoldipine caused a variable and insignificant change in the AUC of nisoldipine *6650*

Norepinephrine *Plasma Increase Physiological* Decreased clearance by 20% in hypertensives and similar effect in normals *6658* In 20 patients with hypertension following head injury treatment with a single dose of 160 mg caused non-significant increase from mean baseline of 1020 ± 158 pg/mL to 1178 ± 173 pg/mL after 2 h and 1164 ± 215 pg/mL after 4 h *3480*

Oxygen Partial Pressure *Blood No Effect Physiological* In 20 patients with hypertension following head injury a single dose of 160 mg caused nonsignificant change of arterial pO_2 from mean baseline of 86 ± 7 mm Hg to 86 ± 5 mm Hg after 2 h and 84 ± 5 mm Hg after 4 h *3480*

Parathyroid Hormone *Plasma No Effect Physiological* In hyperthyroid patients possible effect due to membrane-stabilizing property of drug *539*

Phenylalanine *Plasma No Effect Analytical* No interference observed with rapid quantitative whole blood method of Campbell et al using phenylalanine dehydrogenase *867*

Phosphate *Serum No Effect Analytical* At concentration of 0.2 mg/L had no effect on phosphomolybdate method *5704* No effect at 0.1 mg/dL on Technicon SMA 12/60 method *4390*
Serum No Effect Physiological No significant effect in 12 healthy volunteers over 24 hours following single dose of 160 mg *3452*
Urine No Effect Physiological No significant effect in 12 healthy volunteers over 24 hours following single oral dose of 160 mg *3452*

Platelet Aggregation *Blood Decrease Physiological* Lower threshold in patients receiving 80 mg b.i.d. than in those receiving either pindolol or metoprolol *6511*
Blood No Effect Physiological No effect on ADP induced aggregation. In healthy volunteers after single dose or after 1 week treatment *6260*

Platelets *Blood Decrease Physiological* Purpura probably reflects allergic response *2476*
Blood Increase Physiological Significant increase in healthy volunteers after single dose or after 1 week treatment *6260* Significantly higher in patients receiving this drug than in those receiving metoprolol, also higher in those receiving pindolol but not significantly so *6511*

Potassium *Serum Increase Physiological* Increases of 0.3 to 0.5 mmol/L when doses of 160 to 640 mg/d given, although never to value above 4.5 mmol/L *4739* Moderate increase observed in several trials due to redistribution from intracellular to extracellular compartments, not due to retention in body *3685* Approximately 5% increase in both men and women with treatment for 3 y *4149* Pronounced and prolonged increase in patients who had acute myocardial infarction *4324*

Increase by 0.2 mmol/L in 340 patients given drug for 10 weeks to reduce diastolic BP to less than 90 mm Hg *6247* Increases observed of 0.3, 0.2 and 0.3 mmol/L at 2, 3 and 4 hours respectively following single oral dose of 40 mg in 6 healthy volunteers *4064* Slight increase at 24 hours, but not before, in 12 healthy volunteers following single dose of 160 mg *3452* Increase by 0.17 mmol/L in approximately 120 patients with essential hypertension treated for 1 y *6248* In 15 patients with essential hypertension when treated for 1 mo *6376* In healthy individuals given 160 mg propranolol daily for 8 weeks postmaximal exercise potassium increased from 4.81 mmol/L to 5.05 mmol/L, significantly greater than in placebo control group *1890* Usual effect if aldosterone decreased *801*

Serum No Effect Analytical At concentration of 0.2 mg/L had no effect on flame-photometric method *5704* No effect up to 10 mg/L on method on Ames Seralyzer but at higher concentrations apparently lower potassium concentration *5706*

Serum No Effect Physiological No effect observed in 12 moderately hypertensive men treated with up to 160 mg/day for 8 weeks *5861* After 12 mo treatment of 53 previously untreated hypertensives *507*

Urine No Effect Physiological No significant effect in 12 healthy volunteers over 24 hours following single oral dose of 160 mg *3452*

Prazosin *Serum No Effect Physiological* Coadministration of prazosin with propranolol had no apparent adverse drug interaction in limited clinical experience *4649*

Prealbumin *Serum Increase Physiological* In euthyroid patients due to inhibition of peripheral deiodination of thyroxine and on binding protein metabolism *1939*

Procainamide *Serum Increase Analytical* Propranolol may enhance the fluorescence of procainamide and NAPA since it has native fluorescence close to to the procainamide and NAPA wavelengths *4530*

Serum No Effect Analytical No significant interference observed at a concentration of 100 µg/mL (386 µmol/L) with method on Du Pont aca *1542*

Prochlorperazine *Serum Increase Physiological* When drugs are coadministered the plasma concentrations of both are increased *5638*

Propafenone *Serum No Effect Physiological* Concomitant administration of propafenone with propranolol resulted in a substantial increase in the propranolol concentration but no effect on the concentration of propafenone *3204*

Protein *Serum No Effect Analytical* No effect at 0.1 mg/dL on Technicon SMA 12/60 method *4390* At concentration of 0.2 mg/L had no effect on biuret method with blank correction *5704*

Quinidine *Serum Increase Physiological* Coadministration of propranolol with quinidine usually does not affect quinidine pharmacokinetics, but in some cases the peak concentration of quinidine may be increased, and the volume of its distribution is decreased *5996*

Serum No Effect Analytical No significant interference observed at a concentration of 100 µg/mL (386 µmol/L) with method on Du Pont aca *1543* Propranolol at a concentration of 100 µg/mL had no significant cross-reactivity with quinidine at a concentration of 2.0 µg/mL in method on Bayer Technicon Immuno 1® *431* Concentrations greater than 1000 mg/L cause 30% increase with method on Baxter Stratus but physiological concentrations up to 0.3 mg/L only *5705*

Serum No Effect Physiological Coadministration of propranolol with quinidine usually does not affect quinidine pharmacokinetics, but in some cases the peak concentration of quinidine may be increased, and the volume of its distribution is decreased *5996*

Renal Blood Flow *Patient Decrease Physiological* 13% decrease if continued orally or after i.v. injection *2804*

Patient No Effect Physiological In 9 cirrhotic patients 80 mg propranolol caused an insignificant reduction from 454.1 ± 77.3 mL/min to 413.9 ± 60.3 mL/min *5772*

Renin Activity *Plasma Decrease Physiological* Significant effect over 5 weeks in 10 patients with essential hypertension with mean plasma concentration of drug about 244 ng/mL *1836* Observed in all patients, maximum if high initially *801* Reduction from mean of 1.40 ng/mL/h to 0.56 ng/mL/h in 12 moderately hypertensive men treated with up to 160 mg/day for 8 weeks *5861*

Plasma No Effect Physiological No significant effect in 6 healthy male volunteers given 120 mg drug *473*

SDZ PSC 833 *Blood No Effect Analytical* At a concentration of 128 µg/L had no effect on HPLC method of Scott et al when used to measure PSC (with CsD as internal standard) at a concentration of 5 mg/L *5418*

Sodium *Serum No Effect Analytical* At concentration of 0.2 mg/L had no effect on flame-photometric method *5704*

Serum No Effect Physiological No significant effect in 12 healthy volunteers over 24 hours following single dose of 160 mg *3452*

Urine Decrease Physiological Impaired in normals and patients *4014*

Urine No Effect Physiological No significant effect in 12 healthy volunteers over 24 hours following single oral dose of 160 mg *3452*

Sumatriptan *Serum No Effect Physiological* Pretreatment with 160 mg/d propranolol for 7 days had no effect on the pharmacokinetics of a single oral 300 mg dose of sumatriptan *2158*

T3-Uptake *Serum Increase Physiological* Significant increase from mean baseline of 1.06 arbitrary units to 1.13 arbitrary units after 1 week and 1.24 arbitrary units after 3 weeks when 8 healthy young normotensive men were treated with 160 mg/d *3076*

Serum No Effect Physiological No significant effect in 11 hyperthyroid patients treated with 80 mg daily for 7 days *4610*

Theophylline *Serum Increase Physiological* Theophylline clearance reduced when theophylline coadministered with propranolol *6558* Decreases theophylline clearance by inhibiting cytochrome P450 1A2 and also has pharmacologic interaction and increases serum theophylline concentration by 100% *3125* Decreases theophylline clearance by inhibiting cytochrome P450 1A2, increasing theophylline concentration by about 100% *5999* Up to 100% increase in serum theophylline concentration due to decreased theophylline clearance caused by inhibition of cytochrome P450 1A2 *6117* Clearance markedly reduced in healthy individuals given drug orally 40 mg/6 h, possibly due to a metabolite binding to cytochrome P-450 *1116* Dose-dependent increase in theophylline concentration due to inhibition of hepatic microsomal enzymes; effect most marked in smokers *1116*

Thioridazine *Serum Increase Physiological* Coadministration of drugs caused 3-4 fold increase in plasma concentration of thioridazine due to inhibition of metabolism *2315*

Thyroid Stimulating Hormone

Serum Increase Physiological In 8 healthy normotensive men treatment with 160 mg daily caused significant increase from mean baseline of 1.91 mU/L to 2.44 mU/L after 1 week but with fall to 1.68 mU/L after 3 weeks treatment *3076*

Serum No Effect Physiological In 15 euthyroid hypertensives treated for 30 d given 80 to 480 mg/d *3291* In euthyroid patients treatment with propranolol had no effect on TSH concentration *2412* No significant effect in euthyroid patients *1939* Basal concentration unaffected by treatment *1269* In 10 healthy volunteers treated for 2 weeks *4895* In 8 healthy volunteers given 80 mg b.i.d. and followed serially, in spite of reduction of free T4 *6458*

Thyroxine Binding Globulin

Serum Decrease Physiological In 8 healthy volunteers given 80 mg b.i.d. and followed serially, fell by average of 1.2 mg/L *6458* Circulating concentration decreased with treatment *1269* In euthyroid patients due to peripheral inhibition of peripheral deiodination of thyroxine and on binding protein metabolism *1939*

Thyroxine (T4) *Serum Increase Physiological* In euthyroid patients treatment with propranolol caused slight increase in concentration *2412* In 12 hyperthyroid patients given 160 mg/d for 2 weeks due to effect on peripheral metabolism *2485* In 6 patients on large daily doses of drug (480 ± 155 mg) without clinical evidence of hyperthyroidism, due to drug-induced blockage of iodothyronine deiodination *1125* Slight tendency in 10 healthy volunteers treated for 2 weeks *4895* Nonsignificant increase observed in 8 healthy normotensive young men from mean baseline concentration of 91 nmol/L to 101 nmol/L after treatment for 1 week with 160 mg/d and to 103 nmol/L after 3 weeks treatment *3076* Increase by 16% in 15 euthyroid hypertensives treated for 30 d given 80 to 480 mg/d *3291*

Serum No Effect Physiological No effect observed in 11 hyperthyroid patients treated with 80 mg daily for 7 days *4610* No effect observed with treatment *1269*

Propranolol *(continued)*

Thyroxine (T4), Free *Serum Increase Physiological* Increase from mean baseline concentration of 16.5 pmol/L to 20.2 pmol/L (nonsignificant) after treatment for 1 week and to 20.1 pmol/L (significant) after 3 weeks treatment with 160 mg/d in 8 healthy young normotensive men *3076* In 6 patients on large daily doses of drug (480 ± 155 mg) without clinical evidence of hyperthyroidism, due to drug-induced blockade of iodothyronine deiodination *1125* Increase by 18% in 15 euthyroid hypertensives treated for 30 d given 80 to 480 mg/d *3291* Concentration increased during treatment or unaffected *1269* In 8 healthy volunteers given 80 mg b.i.d. and followed serially, increased by average of 3.3 pmol/L *6458* In euthyroid patients due to peripheral inhibition of peripheral deiodination of thyroxine and on binding protein metabolism *1939* Treatment of euthyroid patients with propranolol caused slight increase in concentration *2412*

Thyroxine (T4) Index, Free *Serum Increase Physiological* Increase from mean baseline of 104 arbitrary units to 120 arbitrary units (nonsignificant) after treatment for 1 week with 160 mg/d and to 126 arbitrary units (significant) after 3 weeks treatment in 8 healthy young normotensive men *3076*
Serum No Effect Physiological In hyperthyroid patients given 40 mg every 6 h in 6 patients *540* In 5 hyperthyroid patients given 10 mg every 8 h for 4 d *540*

Tirofiban *Serum No Effect Physiological* Coadministration had no significant effect on plasma clearance of tirofiban *3957*

Tri-iodothyronine, Free (fT3)
Serum Decrease Physiological In euthyroid patients treatment with propranolol caused concentration to decrease to low or low-normal level *2412* Effect most obvious in patients with hypothyroidism or in hypothyroid patients receiving thyroxine with only small change in euthyroid patients. Propranolol inhibits 5'-deiodination so T3 production is decreased *2412* In 8 healthy volunteers given 80 mg b.i.d. and followed serially, fell by average of 1.2 pmol/L *6458* Slight effect in euthyroid patients due to peripheral inhibition of peripheral deiodination of thyroxine and on binding protein metabolism *1939* Effect observed during treatment (reduction typically of the order of 15%) *1269*
Serum No Effect Physiological In 15 euthyroid hypertensives treated for 30 d given 80 to 480 mg/d *3291*

Tri-iodothyronine, Reverse (rT3)
Serum Increase Physiological Effect most marked in hypothyroid patients including those receiving thyroxine. Propranolol inhibits 5'-deiodination causing decreased production rate of T3 but that of rT3 remains unchanged *2412* Marked increase observed with treatment *1269* In 10 healthy volunteers treated for 2 weeks *4895* Increase from mean baseline concentration of 0.43 nmol/L to 0.55 nmol/L at 1 week and significant increase to 0.58 nmol/L after 3 weeks treatment with 160 mg/d in 8 healthy young normotensive men *3076* increase from mean of 0,83 nmol/L to 0.96 nmol/L in 11 hyperthyroid patients treated with 80 mg daily for 7 days *4610* In 6 patients on large daily doses of drug (155 mg) without clinical evidence of hyperthyroidism, due to drug-induced blockage of iodothyronine deiodination *1125* In euthyroid patients treatment with propranolol caused increase in rT3 concentration *2412* In euthyroid patients due to peripheral inhibition of peripheral deiodination of thyroxine and on binding protein metabolism *1939*

Tri-iodothyronine, Reverse (rT3), Free
Serum Increase Physiological Effect most marked in hypothyroid patients including those receiving thyroxine. 5'-deiodination inhibited so T3 production rate reduced although that of rT3 unchanged. Metabolic clearance rate of rT3 reduced *2412* In 8 healthy volunteers given 80 mg b.i.d. and followed serially increased by average of 0.16 nmol/L *6458*

Tri-iodothyronine (T3) *Serum Decrease Physiological* In 12 hyperthyroid patients given 160 mg/d for 2 weeks due to effect on peripheral metabolism *2485* Thyroxine may result in a lower tri-iodothyronine concentration than expected when coadministered with propranolol *6558* Change most obvious in hypothyroid patients or in hypothyroid patients receiving thyroxine with only small change in euthyroid patients. 5'-deiodination inhibited so production rate of T3 reduced. Conversion of T4 to T3 reduced *2412* Reduction from mean of 5.6 nmol/L to mean of 4.7 nmol/L in 11 patients with hyperthyroidism given 80 mg/day for 7 days. Effect probably due to inhibition of 5'-deiodinase enzyme *4610* In hyperthyroid patients possible effect due to membrane-stabilizing property of drug *539* Nonsignificant decrease from mean baseline concentration of 2.2 nmol/L to 2.1 nmol/L after 1 week and 2.0 nmol/L after 3 weeks treatment with 160 mg/d in 8 healthy young normotensive men *3076* In hyperthyroid patients given 40 mg every 6 h in 6 patients *540* In 10 healthy volunteers treated for 2 weeks *4895* In thyrotoxic patients due to effect of drug on peripheral conversion of thyroxine to tri-iodothyronine *1939* In euthyroid patients treatment with propranolol cuased concentration to decrease to low or low-normal concentration *2412*
Serum No Effect Physiological In 5 hyperthyroid patients given 10 mg every 8 h for 4 d *540* In 6 patients on large daily doses of drug (480 ± 155 mg) without clinical evidence of hyperthyroidism, due to drug-induced blockage of iodothyronine deiodination *1125* In 15 euthyroid hypertensives treated for 30 d given 80 to 480 mg/d *3291* No effect observed with treatment *1269*

Trifluoperazine *Serum Increase Physiological* Concomitant administration of propranolol with trifluoperazine increases the plasma concentration of both drugs *5656*

Triglycerides *Serum Increase Physiological* In 20 hypertensive diabetic patients *6544* Increase by 24% in 23 hypertensive men aged 47-55 y treated for 8 weeks *2547* Increase by 24% in 23 hypertensive men given up to 160 mg/d for 8 weeks *3521* Increase by 42 mg/dL in approximately 120 patients with essential hypertension treated for 1 y *6248* From 256 to 369 mg/dL after 12 weeks treatment in 15 hypertriglyceridemic- hypertensive subjects *552* Increase from 33-43% in about 20 hypertensives treated with 160 mg/day for 2 years *1899* Marked increase after 6 mo treatment in 16 patients *1293* Increase by 15 mg/dL in 8 patients given 30 to 60 mg daily for 8 weeks *4213* Mean increase from 151 to 197 mg/dL after 16 weeks treatment in approximately 120 hypertensives *3837* From no change to 65% increase in many studies *141* Mean increase from 146 to 211 mg/dL in 16 hypertensives given 80 mg daily for up to 12 mo *3737* Marked effect in 53 hypertensives given 80 mg twice daily for 3 mo *1292* Primarily observed effect with nonselective β-blockers is increase of triglyceride concentration *3730* Increase by 25 mg/dL in 340 patients given drug for 10 weeks to reduce diastolic BP to less than 90 mm Hg *6247* In both normocholesterolemic and hypercholesterolemic hypertensives administration of 160 mg/d for 6 months caused significant increase but percentage effect less marked in hypercholesterolemics than in normocholesterolemics *1900*
Serum No Effect Analytical At concentration of 92 mg/L had no effect on GPO-PAP method *5704* At concentration of 0.2 mg/L had no effect on lipase/esterase method *5704*
Serum No Effect Physiological General effect observed in multiple studies *142* After 12 mo treatment of 53 previously untreated hypertensives *507* In 22 mild/moderate hypertensive males treated for 8 weeks: insignificant increase noted *2781*

TSH response to TRH *Serum No Effect Physiological* Typically no change observed with treatment *1269*

Urea Nitrogen *Serum Increase Physiological* Increase by 1.1 mg/dL in 340 patients given drug for 10 weeks to reduce diastolic BP to less than 90 mm Hg *6247* Slight but significant in 20 hypertensive diabetic patients *6544* May occur secondary to decreased ERPF *5688* Approximately 10% increase in women without significant change in men when treated over 3 y *4149* Plasma concentration may be increased when propranolol administered *6558*
Serum No Effect Analytical At concentration of 0.2 mg/L had no effect on diacetylmonoxime method *5704*
Serum No Effect Physiological In approximately 120 patients with essential hypertension treated for 1 y *6248* No significant effect on renal function in 15 patients with essential hypertension over 1 mo *6376* No significant effect in 12 healthy volunteers over 24 hours following single dose of 160 mg *3452*
Urine No Effect Physiological No significant effect in 12 healthy volunteers over 24 hours following single oral dose of 160 mg *3452*

Uric Acid *Serum Increase Physiological* Increase by 10% in 23 hypertensive men given up to 160 mg/d for 8 weeks *3521* Approximately 10% increase in both men and women with treatment for 3 y *4149* In 15 patients with essential hypertension when treated for 1 mo *6376* But only by 0.1 mg/dL in approximately 120 patients with essential hypertension treated for 1 y *6248* Mean increase from 6.1 to 6.6 mg/dL in approximately 120 hypertensives after 16 weeks therapy *3837* Increase by 10% in 23 hypertensive men aged 47-55 y treated for 8 weeks *2547*

Serum No Effect Analytical At 100 mg/L on reversed phase liquid chromatographic procedure of Zhiri et al *6656* At concentration of 0.2 mg/L had no effect on phosphotungstate reduction method *5704* At concentration of 80 mg/L had no effect on uricase-PAP method *5704* No effect at 0.1 mg/dL on Technicon SMA 12/60 method *4390*

Serum No Effect Physiological No significant effect in 12 healthy volunteers over 24 hours following single dose of 160 mg *3452* In 340 patients given drug for 10 weeks to reduce diastolic BP to less than 90 mm Hg *6247* After 12 mo treatment of 53 previously untreated hypertensives *507*

Urine No Effect Physiological No significant effect in 12 healthy volunteers over 24 hours following single oral dose of 160 mg *3452*

Verapamil *Serum Decrease Physiological* During concomitant treatment verapamil area under the curve was reduced by 32% and its maximum plasma concentration reduced by 33% *5411*

Serum No Effect Physiological No effect observed on plasma concentration when drugs coadministered *6358*

VLDL-Cholesterol *Serum Increase Physiological* Significant increase from 58 to 80 mg/dL after 12 weeks in 15 hypertriglyceridemic hypertensives *552* Mean increase from 34 to 41 mg/dL in 16 hypertensives given 80 mg daily for up to 12 mo *3737* In several studies *141*

Serum No Effect Physiological In 23 hypertensive men given up to 160 mg/d for 8 weeks *3521* In 17 patients with hypertension followed for 3 mo *1614* General effect observed in multiple studies *142* In several studies *141*

VLDL-Triglycerides *Serum Increase Physiological* Significant increase from 184 mg/dL to 308 mg/dL after 12 weeks in 15 hypertriglyceridemic hypertensives *552* Significant effect in 53 hypertensives given 80 mg twice daily for 3 mo *1292*

Volume *Plasma Decrease Physiological* Decreased by approximately 8% usually. ?mechanism *5949*

Plasma No Effect Physiological No significant change observed *2804*

Urine No Effect Physiological No significant effect in 12 healthy volunteers over 24 hours following single dose of 160 mg *3452*

Zinc *Serum No Effect Physiological* No significant effect in 12 healthy volunteers over 24 hours following single dose of 160 mg *3452*

Urine No Effect Physiological No significant effect in 12 healthy volunteers over 24 hours following single oral dose of 160 mg *3452*

Propylhexedrine

Drugs of Abuse Screen *Urine Increase Analytical* False positive result with Abbott ADx method for amphetamine/methamphetamine *4279*

Propyliodone

Thyroxine (T4) *Serum Increase Analytical* At very high concentrations only *572*

Propylphenazone

p-Aminophenol *Urine No Effect Analytical* With addition of drugs at a concentration of 100 mg/L and of related compounds at 50 mg/L no significant effect observed on colorimetric method of van Bocxlaer on Cobas Mira analyzer which involves reacting free p-aminophenol with resorcinol in the presence of magnesium ions to form an indophenol dye measured at 550 nm *6163*

Propylthiouracil

Alanine Aminotransferase *Serum Increase Physiological* In one 24 year old woman who developed fulminant hepatic failure with lymphocyte sensitization *4030* In 15 of 54 patients with hyperthyroidism treatment for 2 months caused significant increase with peaks ranging from 0.65 to 3.85 µkat/L but changed towards normal during a further 3 months of treatment *3558* Hepatotoxic effect (centrolobular necrosis) *3810* Single case of chronic active hepatitis reported. 2 others with bridging necrosis. Recovery with drug withdrawal *3725*

Alkaline Phosphatase *Serum Increase Physiological* Temporary effect associated with drug administration regressed with cessation *4537* In one 24 year old woman who developed fulminant hepatic failure with lymphocyte sensitization *4030* Drug induced liver damage: either acute or chronic active hepatitis *6394* Hepatotoxic effect (centrolobular necrosis) *3810* In 15 of 54 patients with hyperthyroidism treated with propylthiouracil for 2 months ALT activity increased and mean alkaline phosphatase activity increased nonsignificantly from 2.04 ± 0.12 µkat/L to 2.17 ± 0.23 µkat/L compared with reduction to 1.99 ± 0.14 µkat/L in 39 patients in whom ALT activity did not increase *3558*

Amylase *Serum Decrease Physiological* Reported effect *402*

Antinuclear Antibodies *Serum Increase Physiological* Observed in 10 of 53 treated cases without adequate criteria for diagnosis of SLE *6504*

Serum No Effect Physiological Incidence no different from controls *944*

Aspartate Aminotransferase *Serum Increase Physiological* In one 24 year old woman who developed fulminant hepatic failure with lymphocyte sensitization *4030* Hepatotoxic effect (centrolobular necrosis) *3810* Drug induced liver damage: either acute or chronic active hepatitis *6394* Temporary effect associated with drug administration, regressed with cessation of treatment *4537* Single case of chronic active hepatitis reported. 2 others with bridging necrosis. Recovery with drug withdrawal *3725*

Bile *Urine Increase Physiological* Hepatotoxic effect (centrolobular necrosis) *3810*

Bilirubin *Serum Increase Physiological* Drug induced liver damage: either acute or chronic active hepatitis *6394* Temporary effect associated with drug administration regressed with cessation *4537* In one 24 year old woman who developed fulminant hepatic failure with lymphocyte sensitization *4030* Rare case of hepatotoxicity reported *2451*

Serum No Effect Analytical At concentration of 170 mg/L had no effect on Jendrassik and Grof method *5704*

Bilirubin, Direct *Serum Increase Physiological* In one 24 y old woman who developed fulminant hepatic failure with lymphocyte sensitization *4030* Temporary effect associated with drug administration regressed with cessation of treatment *4537*

BSP Retention *Serum Increase Physiological* Hepatotoxic effect (centrolobular necrosis) *3810*

Calcium *Serum No Effect Analytical* At concentration of 170 mg/L had no effect on cresolphthalein method *5704*

Cholinesterase *Serum No Effect Analytical* No effect observed at concentration of 10 µg/mL with butyrylthiocholine method on Kodak Ektachem® *2504*

Cortisol *Plasma No Effect Analytical* At a concentration of 100 mg/L had no significant effect on Enzymun method *1097*

Erythrocytes *Blood Decrease Physiological* Occasional immunologically associated anemia *6504* Occasional case of aplastic anemia reported *6264*

Urine Increase Physiological In one 24 y old woman who developed fulminant hepatic failure with lymphocyte sensitization *4030*

Fatty Acids (FFA), Free *Serum Decrease Physiological* Marked effect in 5 hyperthyroid individuals given 10 mg every 8 h for 4 d *540*

Fructosamine *Serum No Effect Analytical* No interference observed at any concentration tested with Roche method on Cobas Fara *5152* No effect observed when added to a concentration of 1.0 mmol/L on Cobas-Bio with Roche reagents *5153*

γ-Globulin *Serum Increase Physiological* Possibly related to production of nonspecific drug-stimulated polyclonal antibodies *6504*

Glucagon *Plasma No Effect Physiological* In 5 hyperthyroid individuals given 10 mg every 8 h for 4 d *540*

Propylthiouracil *(continued)*

Glucose *Serum* *Increase* *Analytical* At 1 mmol/L affects Technicon SMA 12/60 method *5576*
Serum *No Effect* *Analytical* No effect at 10 mmol/L on glucokinase based assay of Scott *5414*
Serum *No Effect* *Physiological* In 5 hyperthyroid individuals given 10 mg every 8 h for 4 d *540*

Glycerol *Serum* *Decrease* *Physiological* Marked effect in 5 hyperthyroid individuals given 10 mg every 8 h for 4 d *540*

Glycocholic Acid *Serum* *Increase* *Physiological* In one 24 y old woman who developed fulminant hepatic failure with lymphocyte sensitization *4030*

Hematocrit *Blood* *Decrease* *Physiological* Occasional immunologically associated anemia *6504*

Hemoglobin *Blood* *Decrease* *Physiological* Occasional immunologically associated anemia *6504*

Hydroxyproline *Urine* *No Effect* *Physiological* In hyperthyroid patients and normal controls *539*

^{131}I Uptake *Serum* *Decrease* *Physiological* Effect lasts up to 8 d *2451*
Serum *No Effect* *Physiological* No effect reported *3669*

Insulin *Plasma* *No Effect* *Physiological* In 5 hyperthyroid individuals given 10 mg every 8 h for 4 d *540*

Interleukin-6 *Serum* *Decrease* *Physiological* In 16 patients with Graves' disease mean concentration of 23 pg/mL changed significantly to 3 pg/mL and in 9 patients with toxic modular goiter mean concentration of 26.5 pg/mL changed significantly to 10.0 pg/mL after 6 weeks treatment with 300 mg/d for 6 weeks *934*

Ketones *Serum* *Decrease* *Physiological* Marked effect in 5 hyperthyroid individuals given 10 mg every 8 h for 4 d *540*

Lactate Dehydrogenase *Serum* *Increase* *Physiological* Temporary effect associated with drug administration regressed with cessation *4537* In one 24 year old woman who developed fulminant hepatic failure with lymphocyte sensitization *4030*

LE Cells *Blood* *Positive* *Physiological* May produce LE-like syndrome *5869*

Leukocytes *Blood* *Decrease* *Physiological* In one 24 year old woman who developed fulminant hepatic failure with lymphocyte sensitization *4030* Occasional case of aplastic anemia reported *6264* Agranulocytosis (incidence 1 in 200) *1101*

Lymphocytes *Blood* *Increase* *Physiological* In one 24 year old woman who developed fulminant hepatic failure with lymphocyte sensitization *4030*

Monocytes *Blood* *Increase* *Physiological* In one 24 y old woman who developed fulminant hepatic failure with lymphocyte sensitization *4030*

Neutrophils *Blood* *Decrease* *Physiological* Reported in about 4% of treated individuals *6504* Occasional case of agranulocytosis reported *6264* Occasional reported case of drug-induced neutropenia *241*

Occult Blood *Feces* *Increase* *Physiological* In one 24 year old woman who developed fulminant hepatic failure with lymphocyte sensitization *4030*

Parathyroid Hormone *Plasma* *No Effect* *Physiological* In hyperthyroid patients and normal controls *539*

Phosphate *Serum* *No Effect* *Analytical* At concentration of 170 mg/L had no effect on phosphomolybdate method *5704*

Platelets *Blood* *Decrease* *Physiological* Occasional case of aplastic anemia reported *6264* Associated with platelet associated IgG *6504* In one 24 year old woman who developed fulminant hepatic failure with lymphocyte sensitization *4030*

Propylthiouracil *Serum* *Increase* *Analytical* Reacts with 2,6-DQC (procedure of Ratliff) *4872*

Protein *Serum* *No Effect* *Analytical* At concentration of 170 mg/L had no effect on biuret method with blank correction *5704*

Prothrombin Time *Plasma* *Increase* *Physiological* Deficiency of prothrombin and proconvertin *128* In one 24 year old woman who developed fulminant hepatic failure with lymphocyte sensitization *4030* Observed occasionally in absence of abnormal liver function *6504*

T3-Uptake *Serum* *Decrease* *Physiological* Action of drug *2451*
Serum *No Effect* *Analytical* 97% recovery when added at a concentration of 1.0 mg/dL (59 nmol/L) with method on Du Pont aca *1545* At concentration of 1000 µg/dL (58.7 µmol/L) has no effect on method on Du Pont Dimension *1586*

Thyroxine Binding Globulin *Serum* *No Effect* *Physiological* In 15 of 54 patients with hyperthyroidism treatment for 2 months caused increased ALT activity and nonsignificant decrease of TBG from 242 ± 16.7 nmol/L to 233 ± 28.3 nmol/L and in 39 with normal ALT activity nonsignificant increase of TBG to 247 ± 21.9 nmol/L *3558*

Thyroxine (T4) *Serum* *Decrease* *Physiological* Inhibits synthesis, stops iodination of tyrosine *2451* In 16 patients with Graves' disease mean concentration of 274.9 ± 46 nmol/L decreased to 110.5 ± 39 nmol/L and in 9 patients with toxic modular goiter mean concentration of 230.6 ± 67 nmol/L decreased to 89.8 ± 30 nmol/L after 6 weeks treatment with 300 mg/d for 6 weeks *934*
Serum *Increase* *Analytical* 105% recovery when added at a concentration of 1.0 mg/dL (59 nmol/L) and measured by method on Du Pont aca *1546* *1588*
Serum *Increase* *Physiological* In one 24 year old woman who developed fulminant hepatic failure with lymphocyte sensitization *4030* In 15 of 54 patients with hyperthyroidism treated for 2 months mean concentration increased to 270 ± 12.9 nmol/L from mean baseline of 239 ± 9.01 nmol/L whereas concentration did not change in 39 in whom ALT activity remained normal *3558*
Serum *No Effect* *Analytical* Cross-reactivity of less than 0.05% observed with EIA method on Bio-Rad RADIAS analyzer *4819* Cross-reactivity of less than 0.1% observed with method on Baxter Stratus *5705* At concentration of 1000 µg/dL (5.87 µmol/L) has no effect on method on Du Pont Dimension *1587*

Thyroxine (T4), Free *Serum* *Increase* *Physiological* In 15 of 54 patients with hyperthyroidism who developed increased ALT activity after 2 months treatment mean free thyroxine concentration increased to 91.4 ± 11.6 pmol/L from mean baseline of 81.1 ± 6.44 pmol/L. In 39 patients with normal ALT activity concentration decreased nonsignificantly to 77.2 ± 7.72 pmol/L *3558*
Serum *No Effect* *Analytical* 6-N-propyl-2-thiouracil at a concentration of 5.0 µg/dL had no cross-reactivity FT4 in method on Bayer Technicon Immuno 1® *424*

Thyroxine (T4) Index, Free *Serum* *No Effect* *Physiological* In 5 hyperthyroid individuals given 10 mg every 8 h for 4 d *540*

Tri-iodothyronine, Free (fT3) *Serum* *No Effect* *Analytical* At a concentration of 5.0 x 10^{-5} g/L cross-reactivity of less than 0.1% with free triiodothyronine method on Bayer Technicon Immuno 1® system *425*

Tri-iodothyronine (T3) *Serum* *Decrease* *Physiological* In 16 patients with Graves' disease mean concentration of 7.83 ± 2.9 nmol/L decreased to 2.59 ± 1.1 nmol/L and in 9 patients with toxic modular goiter mean concentration of 6.60 ± 2.4 nmol/L decreased to 2.32 ± 0.9 nmol/L after 6 weeks treatment with 300 mg/d for 6 weeks *934* In hyperthyroid patients and normal controls *539* Significant reduction in 5 hyperthyroid individuals given 10 mg every 8 h for 4 d *540* Associated with decreased plasma concentration *2412*
Serum *Increase* *Physiological* In 15 of 54 patients treated for 2 months ALT activity increased from mean baseline of 6.23 ± 0.35 nmol/L to 7.22 ± 0.72 nmol/L but in 39 in whom activity remained normal concentration decreased slightly to 5.85 ± 0.39 nmol/L *3558*
Serum *No Effect* *Analytical* No cross-reactivity observed with method on Baxter Stratus *5705*

Tumor Necrosis Factor-α *Serum* *No Effect* *Physiological* In 16 patients with Graves' disease mean concentration of 20 pg/mL changed nonsignificantly to 20 pg/mL and in 9 patients with toxic modular goiter mean concentration of 5.0 pg/mL changed nonsignificantly to 5.0 pg/mL after 6 weeks treatment with 300 mg/d for 6 weeks *934*

Urea Nitrogen *Serum* *Increase* *Physiological* Anaphylactic nephritis reported *128*
Serum *No Effect* *Analytical* At concentration of 170 mg/L had no effect on diacetylmonoxime method *5704*

Uric Acid *Serum* *Increase* *Analytical* At concentrations above 150 mg/L raised concentration as measured by phosphotungstate reduction method *5704* At 1 mmol/L affects Technicon SMA 12/60, Henry methods *5576*

Proscillaridin

Digoxin *Serum Increase Analytical* Reported to affect RIA methods *6638*

ProSobee®

Amino Acids *Urine Increase Analytical* Reddish-pink spot with DL-methionine with ninhydrin on thin-layer chromatography *2109*

Methionine *Urine Increase Physiological* Contained in large amount in infant formula *2859*

Prostacyclin

D-Dimer *Plasma Increase Physiological* In 5 patients with chronic renal failure undergoing hemodialysis using 5 ng/kg body weight/min prostacyclin mean arterial concentration of 636 ± 119 ng/mL at baseline changed significantly overall to 735 ± 117 ng/mL after 10 min, 959 ± 255 ng/mL after 60 min, 5450 ± 1444 ng/mL after 120 min and 7722 ± 2359 ng/mL after 180 min *4337*

Fibrinogen *Plasma No Effect Physiological* In 5 patients with chronic renal failure undergoing hemodialysis using 5 ng/kg body weight/min prostacyclin mean arterial concentration of 336 ± 43 mg/dL at baseline changed insignificantly to 365 ± 55 mg/dL after 180 min *4337*

Fibrinopeptide A *Plasma No Effect Physiological* No significant effect observed in 14 post-myocardial infarction patients compared with 13 controls following infusion of 5 ng/kg/min for 72 hours *6002*

6-Keto-Prostaglandin $F_{1\alpha}$ *Plasma Increase Physiological* With 72 hour infusion of 5 ng/kg/min in 14 patients wiyh unstable angina concentration increased from mean baseline concentration < 20 pg/mL to 605 pg/mL during infusion *6002*

Plasmin-Plasmin Inhibitor Complex
Plasma Increase Physiological In 5 patients with chronic renal failure undergoing hemodialysis using 5 ng/kg body weight/min prostacyclin mean arterial concentration of 361 ± 20 ng/mL at baseline changed significantly overall to 365 ± 39 ng/mL after 10 min, 463 ± 59 ng/mL after 60 min, 624 ± 106 ng/mL after 120 min and 1472 ± 369 ng/mL after 180 min *4337*

Platelet Aggregation *Blood Decrease Physiological* In 14 patients with post-myocardial infarction infusion of 5 ng/kg/min for 72 hours caused approximately 50% reduction during the infusion with return to baseline on discontinuation of infusion *6002*

Platelet Factor 4 *Plasma No Effect Physiological* No significant effect observed in 14 post-myocardial patients compared with 13 controls following infusion of 5 ng/kg/min for 72 hours *6002*

Thrombin/Antithrombin III Complex
Plasma Increase Physiological In 5 patients with chronic renal failure undergoing hemodialysis using 5 ng/kg body weight/min prostacyclin mean arterial concentration of 2.5 ± 0.3 ng/mL at baseline changed significantly overall to 2.6 ± 0.3 ng/mL after 10 min, 28.7 ± 8 ng/mL after 60 min, 142 ± 36 ng/mL after 120 min and 126.8 ± 46.1 ng/mL after 180 min *4337*

β-Thromboglobulin *Plasma No Effect Physiological* No significant effect observed in 14 post-myocardial patients compared with 13 controls following infusion of 5 ng/kg/min for 72 hours *6002*

Thromboxane B_2 *Plasma No Effect Physiological* No significant effect observed in 14 post-myocardial patients compared with 13 controls following infusion of 5 ng/kg/min for 72 hours *6002*

Protamine

Aminopeptidase M *Plasma No Effect Physiological* No inhibitory effect observed with concentration up to 100 µg/mL *5938*

Angiotensin-converting Enzyme
Serum No Effect Physiological No inhibitory effect observed on angiotensin I converting enzyme (kininase II) at concentration up to 100 µg/mL *5938*

Antithrombin III *Plasma No Effect Analytical* No interference observed at a concentration of 0.25 mg/mL with method on Du Pont aca *1510* At concentration of 250 mg/L had no effect on Do Pont aca method *5704*

Carboxypeptidase N *Serum Decrease Physiological* Inhibition of hydrolysis of furylacrylolyl(FA)-Ala-Lys by enzyme observed. Also inhibited hydrolysis of bradykinin and C_3a8 *5938*

Endopeptidase 24,11 *Serum No Effect Physiological* No inhibitory effect observed on activity of endopeptidase 24.11 (enkephalinase) at concentration up to 100 µg/mL *5938*

Fibrinogen *Plasma No Effect Analytical* At concentration of 250 mg/L had no effect on Du Pont aca method *5704*

Heparin *Plasma Decrease Analytical* With method on Du Pont aca concentration reduced although not to the extent of full neutralization *917*

Histamine *Plasma No Effect Analytical* No inhibition of radio-enzyme assay at therapeutic concentrations *2492*

Lipase *Serum Decrease Physiological* Inhibition occurs whether specimen heparinized or not *5057*

Lipids *Serum Increase Physiological* Mechanism not established *2242*

Lipoprotein Lipase *Serum Decrease Physiological* Inhibition occurs whether heparinized or not *5057*

Malondialdehyde *Serum Increase Analytical* Addition of 1 - 3 U/mL to each of 5 specimens produced no effect on measured MDA (0.90 ± 0.23 µmol/L without protamine versus 0.94 ± 0.16 and 0.85 ± 0.24 µmol/L for 1 and 3 U/mL, respectively) *388*
Serum Increase Physiological In 4 patients who underwent femoropopliteal bypass surgery mean concentration increased between 15 and 60 min after reperfusion of the extremity from 1.07 ± 0.1 µmol/L to 1.54 ± 0.18 µmol/L *388*

Midazolam *Serum No Effect Analytical* On GC-ECD method of Ha et al *2387*

Plasminogen *Plasma No Effect Analytical* At concentration of 250 mg/L had no effect on Du Pont aca method *5704* At concentration of 0.25 g/L observed to have no effect on method on Du Pont aca *1540*

Potassium *Serum No Effect Analytical* At concentration of 10 mg/L had no effect on measurement by ISE with predilution *5704*

Sodium *Serum No Effect Analytical* At concentration of 10 mg/L had no effect on measurement by ISE with predilution *5704*

Thromboplastin Generation *Blood Decrease Physiological* Possesses anticoagulant action *2242*

Protein Hydrolysate

Alkaline Phosphatase *Serum Increase Physiological* Transient effect with hyperalimentation in infants *6060*

Aspartate Aminotransferase
Serum No Effect Physiological No effect with hyperalimentation in infants *6060*

Bilirubin *Serum Increase Physiological* Hyperalimentation i.v. infants may cause cholestasis *6060*

Bilirubin, Direct *Serum Increase Physiological* Hyperalimentation i.v. in infants may cause cholestasis *6060*

Protionamide

Alanine Aminotransferase *Serum Increase Physiological* Reported to affect liver function *4265*

Alkaline Phosphatase *Serum Increase Physiological* Temporary side effect *4014*

Aspartate Aminotransferase *Serum Increase Physiological* Reported to affect liver function *4265*

Bilirubin *Serum Increase Physiological* Temporary side effect *4014*

Leukocytes *Blood Decrease Physiological* Single case reported *4014*

Protriptyline

Alanine Aminotransferase *Serum* *Increase* *Physiological* Transient reversible cholestasis *128*

Alkaline Phosphatase *Serum* *Increase* *Physiological* Transient reversible cholestasis *128*

Aspartate Aminotransferase *Serum* *Increase* *Physiological* Transient reversible cholestasis *128*

Bile *Urine* *Increase* *Physiological* Transient reversible cholestasis *128*

Bilirubin *Serum* *Increase* *Physiological* Transient reversible cholestasis *128*

Carbamazepine *Serum* *No Effect* *Analytical* Cross reactivity of 0.17% observed with method on Baxter Stratus *5705*

Eosinophils *Blood* *Increase* *Physiological* Rare allergic response *2753*

Glucose *Serum* *Decrease* *Physiological* Reported effect *2753*
Serum *Increase* *Physiological* Reported effect *2753*

Leukocytes *Blood* *Decrease* *Physiological* Transient agranulocytosis or leukopenia *128*

Platelets *Blood* *Decrease* *Physiological* Rare allergic response *2753*

Pseudoephedrine

Amino Acids *Urine* *Increase* *Analytical* Red spot with ninhydrin on thin-layer chromatography when combined with triprolidine in Actifed® *2109*

Amphetamine *Urine* *No Effect* *Analytical* Cross-reactivity of less than 1% observed with Roche Abuscreen method when adapted for use with Roche Cobas Mira analyzer *5120*

Amphetamine/Methamphetamine
Serum *No Effect* *Analytical* At a concentration of 3000 mg/mL caused no detectable cross-reactivity with methods on Abbott AxSYM and TDx *6404*

Cetirizine *Serum* *No Effect* *Physiological* No clinically significant effect observed *4661*

Cholinesterase *Serum* *No Effect* *Analytical* No effect observed at concentration of 3 mg/dL with butyrylthiocholine method on Kodak Ektachem® *2504*

Drugs of Abuse Screen *Urine* *No Effect* *Analytical* No effect at concentration of 100 µg/mL on EZ-SCREEN procedure for cannabinoids and cocaine *1739*

Epinephrine *Plasma* *Increase* *Physiological* In one patient with pheochromocytoma before removal of the tumor after two doses mean concentration increased from 34.8 pg/mL to 72.4 pg/mL but in two others no significant effect observed *2250*
Plasma *No Effect* *Physiological* In 8 normal subjects administration of two doses of Demazin caused nonsignificant change from 17 ± 3 pg/mL to 19 ± 7 pg/mL *2250*

Fexofenadine *Serum* *No Effect* *Physiological* Coadministration of drugs has no effect on the pharmacokinetics of each other *2637*

Methamphetamine *Urine* *No Effect* *Analytical* Less than 0.5% cross-reactivity with Hycor accuPINCH method *162* Less than 1% cross-reactivity with Roche Abuscreen Online assay as performed on Roche Cobas Mira *6347*

Norepinephrine *Plasma* *Increase* *Physiological* In 2 of 3 patients with pheochromocytoma before removal of the tumor administration of two doses of Demazin caused increases from 1067 pg/mL to 3200 pg/mL and 1605 pg/mL to 2842 pg/mL whereas no significant effect was observed in the third *2250*
Plasma *No Effect* *Physiological* In 8 normal subjects administration of two doses of Demazin caused nonsignificant change from 115 ± 12 pg/mL to 108 ± 10 pg/mL *2250*

Theophylline *Serum* *Increase* *Analytical* At concentration of 40 mg/L produced positive bias of 3.65 mg/L at theophylline concentration of 20 mg/L when measured by 3M TheoFAST analyzer *1122*
Serum *No Effect* *Analytical* At concentration of 40 mg/L produced no interference with methods used on Kodak DT60, Abbott TDx, Abbott Vision with either whole blood or serum, 3M Diagnostics TheoFAST or Ames Seralyzer *1122*

Psyllium

Apolipoprotein A-I *Serum* *Increase* *Physiological* In 37 hypercholesterolemic patients treated with high fat diet and 10.2 g/d psyllium mean concentration not significantly from 145.2 ± 5.6 mg/dL to 144.5 ± 6.9 mg/dL and in 81 given low fat diet and 10.2 g/d increased from mean baseline of 147.2 mg/dL to 155.7 ± 5.3 mg/dL *5757*

Apolipoprotein B *Serum* *Decrease* *Physiological* In 37 hypercholesterolemic patients treatment with 10.2 g/d and high fat diet for 8 weeks caused decrease from mean baseline of 136.0 ± 5.1 mg/dL to 127 ± 7.1 mg/dL and in 81 given 10.2 g/d and low fat diet decreased from 130.5 mg/dL to 122.2 ± 3.4 mg/dL *5757*

Cholesterol *Serum* *Decrease* *Physiological* In 37 hypercholesterolemic patients treated with 10.2 g/d psyllium and high fat diet for 8 weeks mean concentration decreased from 6.8 ± 0.1 mmol/L to 6.4 ± 0.2 mmol/L: in 81 patients receiving 10.2 g/d and low fat diet for 8 weeks mean concentration decreased from 6.5 ± 0.1 mmol/L to 6.2 ± 0.1 mmol/L *5757* In 42 patients with hyperlipidemia mean concentration decreased by 6.4% after treatment for 2 weeks (from 6.76 ± 0.12 mmol/L to 6.33 ± 0.12 mmol/L) *6524*

Glucose *Serum* *Decrease* *Physiological* In 18 noninsulin-dependent diabetic patients maximum glucose increase following meals reduced by 14% at breakfast and 20% at dinner relative to placebo *4551*

HDL-Cholesterol *Serum* *Decrease* *Physiological* In 42 patients with hyperlipidemia mean concentration decreased significantly after treatment for 2 weeks from 1.14 ± 0.05 mmol/L to 1.10 ± 0.05 mmol/L) *6524*
Serum *No Effect* *Physiological* In 37 hypercholesterolemic patients treated with 10.2 g/d and high fat diet for 8 weeks mean concentration unchanged at 1.1 ± 0.1 mmol/L and in 81 given low fat diet with 10.2 g/d mean concentration was unchanged at 1.2 ± 0.0 mmol/L *5757*

Insulin *Plasma* *Decrease* *Physiological* Postprandial increase in 18 noninsulin-dependent diabetic patients reduced by 12% relative to placebo after breakfast *4551*

LDL-Cholesterol *Serum* *Decrease* *Physiological* In 37 hypercholesterolemic patients given 10.2 g/d and high fat diet for 8 weeks mean concentration decreased from 4.70 ± 0.1 mmol/L to 4.4 ± 0.1 mmol/L and in 81 given 10.2 g/d and low fat diet concentration decreased from 4.5 ± 0.1 mmol/L to 4.2 ± 0.1 mmol/L *5757* In 42 patients with hyperlipidemia mean concentration decreased by 7.8% after treatment for 2 weeks (from 4.73 ± 0.12 mmol/L to 4.36 ± 0.11 mmol/L) *6524*

Triglycerides *Serum* *Decrease* *Physiological* In 37 hypercholesterolemic patients treated with high fat diet and 10.2 g/d psyllium for 8 weeks mean concentration decreased from 2.3 ± 0.3 mmol/L to 2.1 ± 0.2 mmol/L and in 81 treated with low fat diet and 10.2 g/d psyllium mean concentration was unchanged at 1.7 ± 0.1 mmol/L *5757*
Serum *No Effect* *Physiological* In 42 patients with hyperlipidemia mean concentration changed insignificantly after treatment for 2 weeks *6524*

Puromycin

Chromosomes *Test Conditions* *Abnormal* *Physiological* Clastogenic in human cells *5484*

Protein *Urine* *Increase* *Physiological* May cause nephrotoxicity *5377*

Urea Nitrogen *Serum* *Increase* *Physiological* May cause nephrotoxicity *5377*

Pyrantel

Aspartate Aminotransferase *Serum* *Increase* *Physiological* Transient increases reported *4140* *1384*

Fibrinogen *Plasma* *No Effect* *Analytical* On potassium mercuric thiocyanate procedure of Roberts *4986*

Pyrazinamide

Acetone *Urine* *Increase* *Analytical* Produces a pink-brown color with Acetest® *3468*

Alanine Aminotransferase *Serum Increase Physiological* May produces a dose-related hepatotoxicity which may occur at any time during treatment *3468* In 72 patients with tuberculosis all receiving isoniazid and rifampin and, in addition, pyrazinamide in 72.2%, ethambutol in 80% and streptomycin in 16.7% drug-induced hepatitis observed with AST activity reaching mean of 330.2 ± 425.5 U/L *5577* Low toxicity with daily doses of 20 to 30 mg/kg body weight but overall incidence of hepatitis of 0.3% *1074* Hepatotoxic in 1 to 5% patients (previously reported to be toxic in as many as 25%) *6197* Hepatic toxicity reported (viral-hepatitis like) *5360*

Albumin *Serum Decrease Physiological* Hepatotoxicity (viral-hepatitis like) *128*

Alkaline Phosphatase *Serum Increase Physiological* Hepatotoxic effect (viral-hepatitis like) *3810* May produces a dose-related hepatotoxicity which may occur at any time during treatment *3468* Hepatotoxic in 1 to 5% patients (previously reported to be toxic in as many as 25%) *6197*

Aspartate Aminotransferase *Serum Increase Physiological* In 72 patients with tuberculosis all receiving isoniazid and rifampin and, in addition, pyrazinamide in 72.2%, ethambutol in 80% and streptomycin in 16.7% drug-induced hepatitis observed with AST activity reaching mean of 428.4 ± 666.0 U/L *5577* Low toxicity with daily doses of 20 to 30 mg/kg body weight but overall incidence of hepatitis of 0.3% *1074* May produces a dose-related hepatotoxicity which may occur at any time during treatment *3468* Hepatic toxicity reported (viral-hepatitis like) *5360* Hepatotoxic in 1 to 5% patients (previously reported to be toxic in as many as 25%) *6197*

Bile *Urine Increase Physiological* Hepatotoxic effect (viral-hepatitis like) *3810*

Bilirubin *Serum Increase Physiological* May produces a dose-related hepatotoxicity which may occur at any time during treatment *3468* Hepatotoxic in 1 to 5% patients (previously reported to be toxic in as many as 25%) *6197* In 72 patients with tuberculosis all receiving isoniazid and rifampin and, in addition, pyrazinamide in 72.2%, ethambutol in 80% and streptomycin in 16.7% drug-induced hepatitis observed with bilirubin concentration reaching mean of 5.34 ± 4.68 mg/dL *5577* Hepatic toxicity (approximately 3 %) (dose related) *5360*

BSP Retention *Serum Increase Physiological* Hepatic toxicity (approximately 4%) (dose related) *5360*

Fibrinogen *Plasma Increase Physiological* Reported effect *128*

γ-Globulin *Serum Decrease Physiological* Reported effect (viral-hepatitis like) *128*

Hematocrit *Blood Decrease Physiological* Rare anemia reported *4014* Sideroblastic anemia with erythroid hyperplasia and vacuolation of erythrocytes has been reported as a rare side effect *3468*

Hemoglobin *Blood Decrease Physiological* Sideroblastic anemia with erythroid hyperplasia and vacuolation of erythrocytes has been reported as a rare side effect *3468* Rare anemia reported *4014*

Histamine *Plasma No Effect Analytical* No inhibition of radio-enzyme assay at therapeutic concentration *2492*

Hypoxanthine *Serum Decrease Physiological* Within 2 hours of ingestion of 3 grams by 5 healthy individuals significant reduction occurred *6582*

Iron *Serum Decrease Analytical* At peak concentration in serum negative measurement of 100 to 500 µg/dL with Ferrochem II instrument *4489*
Serum Decrease Physiological Negative concentration of -317.19 µmol/L observed with Ferrochem II method at a concentration of 600 µg/mL and -185.55 µmol/L at a Rifater concentration of 240 µg/mL of pyrazinamide versus 9.91 µmol/L in control *5217*
Serum Increase Physiological Sideroblastic anemia with erythroid hyperplasia and vacuolation of erythrocytes with increased serum iron concentration has been reported as a rare side effect *3468*
Serum No Effect Analytical At a concentration of 600 µg/mL (240 µg/mL in Rifater) caused insignificant change in concentration to 11.55 µg/mL by atomic absorption versus 11.40 µmol/L in controls *5217*

Ketones *Urine Increase Analytical* Produces a pink-brown color with Ketostix® *3468* Pink-brown with Ketostix® , Acetest® and Rothera"s test *199*

17-Ketosteroids *Urine Decrease Physiological* Temperature decreased excretion reported *2242*

Oxypurinol *Serum No Effect Physiological* In 5 healthy men coadministration of pyrazinamide with allopurinol had no significant effect on plasma concentration of oxypurinol *6581*
Urine Decrease Physiological Ratio of excretion of oxypurinol to creatinine decreased from 0.98 ± 0.24 to 0.45 ± 0.13 when pyrazinamide coadministered with allopurinol *6581*

Platelets *Blood Decrease Physiological* Thrombocytopenia has been reported as a rare side effect *3468* Thrombocytopenia reported to occur *2385*

Protein *Serum Decrease Physiological* Part of hepatotoxicity (viral-hepatitis like) *2242*

Prothrombin Time *Plasma Increase Physiological* Reduces concentration of prothrombin *128*

Uric Acid *Serum Increase Physiological* Inhibits tubular secretion of urate *5781* Decreases tubular secretion, may result in clinical manifestations of gout *6197* Significant increase in 5 healthy individuals within 2 hours of ingesting 3 grams of drug *6582*
Urine Decrease Physiological Increased tubular reabsorption of urate *5360*

Xanthine *Serum No Effect Physiological* No significant change occurred in 5 healthy individuals within 2 hours of ingesting 3 grams of drug *6582*

Pyrazinoic Acid

Erythrocytes *Blood Decrease Physiological* Sideroblastic type of anemia may occur *536*

Uric Acid *Urine Decrease Physiological* Inhibition of renal tubular secretion *485*

Pyrazinoylguanidine

Aldosterone *Plasma Decrease Physiological* In 12 mild to moderate hypertensives treatment with 1200 mg/d for 4 weeks caused mean concentration to decrease from 12.4 µg/d to 10.7 µg/d *954*

Chloride *Serum No Effect Physiological* In 12 mild to moderate hypertensives treatment with 1200 mg/d for 4 weeks had no significant effect on serum concentration *954*

Cholesterol *Serum No Effect Physiological* In 12 mild to moderate hypertensives treatment with 1200 mg/d for 4 weeks caused decrease from mean baseline of 243 mg/dL to 232 mg/dL *954*

HDL-Cholesterol *Serum No Effect Physiological* In 12 mild to moderate hypertensives treatment with 1200 mg/d for 4 weeks caused insignificant reduction from mean baseline of 47 mg/dL to 45 mg/dL *954*

LDL-Cholesterol *Serum Decrease Physiological* In 12 mild to moderate hypertensives treatment with 1200 mg/d for 4 weeks caused a decrease from mean of 166 mg/dL to 155 mg/dL, but the extent of drug inhibition depends on the initial predrug concentrations of cholesterol and LDL: the higher the greater the PZG-reduction *954*

Potassium *Serum No Effect Physiological* In 12 mild to moderate hypertensives treatment with 1200 mg/d for 4 weeks had no significant effect on concentration *954*

Renin Activity *Plasma Decrease Physiological* In 12 mild to moderate hypertensives treatment with 1200 mg/d for 4 weeks caused decrease of mean from 1.0 µg/mL/h to 0.8 µg/L/h (20%) *954*

Sodium *Serum No Effect Physiological* In 12 mild to moderate hypertnsives treatment with 1200 mg/d for 4 weeks had no significant effect on concentration *954*
Urine Increase Physiological In 12 mild to moderate hypertensives treatment with 1200 mg/d for 4 weeks caused significant increase from mean baseline of 135 mmol/d to 160 mmol/d *954*

Pyrazolones

Erythrocytes *Blood Decrease Physiological* Aplastic/hemolytic anemia *3810*

Pyrazolones *(continued)*

Erythrocytes *(continued)*
Urine *Increase* *Physiological* May cause actual bleeding *1714*

Hematocrit *Blood* *Decrease* *Physiological* Aplastic/hemolytic anemia *3810*

Hemoglobin *Blood* *Decrease* *Physiological* Aplastic/hemolytic anemia *3810*
Urine *Increase* *Physiological* Actual bleeding caused by drug *1714*

Leukocytes *Blood* *Decrease* *Physiological* Aplastic/hemolytic anemia (may be agranulocytosis) *3810*

Neutrophils *Blood* *Decrease* *Physiological* Myelotoxic effect of drugs *4014*

Occult Blood *Feces* *Increase* *Physiological* May cause gastrointestinal tract bleeding *3810*

Platelets *Blood* *Decrease* *Physiological* Thrombocytopenia *3810*

Protein *Urine* *Increase* *Physiological* Nephrotoxic effect *2024* *1714*

Sugar *Urine* *Increase* *Analytical* Interferes with copper reducing methods *1714*

Urea Nitrogen *Serum* *Increase* *Physiological* May cause nephrotoxicity *2024*

Pyridamole

Alanine Aminotransferase *Serum* *No Effect* *Analytical* No effect at 100 mg/L on Boehringer Mannheim Reflotron method *5706* No effect at therapeutic concentration on Boehringer Mannheim Reflotron method *3231*

Amylase *Serum* *No Effect* *Analytical* No effect of concentrations up to 20 mg/L on method on Boehringer Mannheim Reflotron *5706*

Amylase, Pancreatic Isoenzyme
Serum *No Effect* *Analytical* No significant effect observed at a toxic concentration of 20 mg/L with method on Boehringer Mannheim Reflotron *3647*

Aspartate Aminotransferase *Serum* *No Effect* *Analytical* No effect at 100 mg/L on Boehringer Mannheim Reflotron method *5706* No effect at therapeutic concentration on Boehringer Mannheim Reflotron method *3231*

Bilirubin *Serum* *No Effect* *Analytical* At concentration of 100 mg/L no effect on method on Boehringer Mannheim Reflotron system *5706*

Cholesterol *Serum* *No Effect* *Analytical* No effect at therapeutic concentration on Boehringer Mannheim Reflotron method *3231* At concentration of 100 mg/L no effect on method on Boehringer Mannheim Reflotron system *5706*

Glucose *Serum* *No Effect* *Analytical* No effect at therapeutic concentration on Boehringer Mannheim Reflotron method *3231* At concentration of 100 mg/L no effect on method on Boehringer Mannheim Reflotron system *5706*

γ-Glutamyltransferase *Serum* *No Effect* *Analytical* At concentration of 100 mg/L no effect on method on Boehringer Mannheim Reflotron system *5706* No effect at therapeutic concentration on Boehringer Mannheim Reflotron method *3231*

Triglycerides *Serum* *No Effect* *Analytical* No effect at 100 mg/L on Boehringer Mannheim Reflotron method *5706* No effect at therapeutic concentration on Boehringer Mannheim Reflotron method *3231*

Urea Nitrogen *Serum* *No Effect* *Analytical* No effect at therapeutic concentration on Boehringer Mannheim Reflotron method *3231* No effect at 100 mg/L on Boehringer Mannheim Reflotron method *5706*

Uric Acid *Serum* *No Effect* *Analytical* No effect at therapeutic concentration on Boehringer Mannheim Reflotron method *3231* No effect at 100 mg/L on Boehringer Mannheim Reflotron method *5706*

Pyridinol Carbamate

Isocitrate Dehydrogenase *Serum* *Increase* *Physiological* Noticeable effect, cause not discussed *4224*

Valproic Acid *Serum* *Decrease* *Physiological* By increasing the expression of hepatic enzymes, especially those that increase the amount of glucuronosyl transferases, may increase the clearance of valproate twofold *17*

Pyridoglutethimide

Aldosterone *Plasma* *No Effect* *Physiological* In 10 postmenopausal women with breast cancer treatment with up to 2400 mg/d for 2 weeks had no significant effect on concentration *1486*

Androstenedione *Plasma* *Decrease* *Physiological* In10 postmenopausal women with breast cancer treatment with doses up to 2400 mg/d for 2 weeks caused significant reduction *1486*

Cortisol *Plasma* *No Effect* *Physiological* In 10 postmenopausal women with breast cancer treatment with doses as high as 2400 mg/d for 2 weeks had no significant effect on concentration *1486*

Dehydroepiandrosterone *Plasma* *Decrease* *Physiological* In 10 postmenopausal women with breast cancer treatment with doses up to 2400 mg/d for 2 weeks caused significant reduction *1486*

Dehydroepiandrosterone Sulfate
Plasma *Decrease* *Physiological* In 10 postmenopausal women treatment with doses from 400 mg/d to 2400 mg/d for 2 weeks showed dose-related decrease *1486*

Estradiol *Plasma* *Decrease* *Physiological* In 9 postmenopausal women with breast cancer with treatment with 400 mg/d for 2 weeks concentration reduced from mean baseline of 21 pmol/L to 13 pmol/L, with 800 mg/d for 2 weeks to 13 pmol/L, with 1600 mg/d for 2 weeks to 12 pmol/L and with 2400 mg/d for 2 weeks to 12 pmol/L *1486*

Estrone *Plasma* *Decrease* *Physiological* In 9 postmenopausal women with breast cancer treatment for 2 weeks with pyridoglutethimide caused reduction from mean baseline of 58 ± 14 pmol/L so that with 400 mg/d concentration was reduced to less than 30 pmol/L in 7 patients, with 800 mg/d in 8 patients, with 1600 mg/d in 6 of 7 patients and with 2400 mg/d in 5 of 6 patients *1486*

Follicle Stimulating Hormone
Plasma *No Effect* *Physiological* In 9 postmenopausal women with breast cancer no significant effect observed with treatment with up to 2400 mg/d for 2 weeks *1486*

17-Hydroxyprogesterone *Plasma* *Increase* *Physiological* In 10 postmenopausal women treated with doses from 400 mg/d to 2400 mg/d for 2 weeks dose-related increase in 17α-hydroxyprogesterone concentration observed *1486*

Luteinizing Hormone *Plasma* *No Effect* *Physiological* In 9 postmenopausal women with breast cancer treatment with up to 2400 mg/d for 2 weeks had no significant effect *1486*

Prolactin *Plasma* *No Effect* *Physiological* In 10 postmenopausal women with breast cancer treatment with up to 2400 mg/d for 2 weeks had no significant effect on concentration *1486*

Sex-Hormone Binding Globulin
Serum *No Effect* *Physiological* In 10 postmenopausal women treatment with up to 2400 mg/d for 2 weeks had no significant effect on concentration *1486*

Testosterone *Serum* *Decrease* *Physiological* In 10 postmenopausal women with breast cancer treatment with doses up to 2400 mg/d for 2 weeks caused significant reduction *1486*

Thyroid Stimulating Hormone
Serum *No Effect* *Physiological* In 10 postmenopausal women with breast cancer treatment with up to 2400 mg/d for 2 weeks had no significant effect on concentration *1486*

Pyridostigmine

Bicarbonate *Serum* *Increase* *Analytical* Significant effect on method on Kodak Ektachem® with bromide salt without comparable effect on Beckman Astra® 8 *3233*

Bromide *Serum Increase Physiological* Observed in one woman with myasthenia gravis who received 150 mg pyridostigmine bromide orally every three hours and 180 mg of sustained release compound at bedtime with serum concentration of bromide of 5 mmol/L observed at time patient was confused *5116* Theoretical possibility if bromide salt is administered since it contains 30.6% bromide *5116*

Chloride *Serum Increase Analytical* Significantly greater effect on method on Kodak Ektachem® with bromide salt than on Beckman Astra® 8, although this method also affected *3233*

Cholinesterase *Serum Decrease Physiological* Direct action of drug *1883*

Growth Hormone *Plasma Increase Physiological* In 30 healthy individuals after administration of 120 mg pyridostigmine 26 increased their growth hormone concentration with peaks between 90 and 120 minutes. The mean response in men was 4.82 ± 1.89 mU/L and 19.45 ± 3.63 mU/L in women (difference between men and women highly significant) *3673*

Pyridyltetrazole

Cholesterol *Serum Decrease Physiological* Effect greater than with nicotinic acid *4602*

Fatty Acids (FFA), Free *Serum Decrease Physiological* Reduction of up to 200 Eq/L, then rebound increase *4602*

Pyrimethamine

Alanine Aminotransferase *Serum Increase Physiological* Biopsy-proven granulomatous hepatitis due to sulfadoxine moiety of drug reported in two individuals receiving drug prophylactically possibly due to sulfonamide hypersensitivity *3445*

Alkaline Phosphatase *Serum Increase Physiological* Biopsy-proven granulomatous hepatitis due to sulfadoxine moiety of drug reported in two individuals receiving drug prophylactically possibly due to sulfonamide hypersensitivity *3445*

Amino-4-Imidazole-5-Carboxamide Ribotide
Urine Increase Physiological If megaloblastic anemia occurs *6541*

Aspartate Aminotransferase *Serum Increase Physiological* Biopsy-proven granulomatous hepatitis due to sulfadoxine moiety of drug reported in two individuals receiving drug prophylactically possibly due to sulfonamide hypersensitivity *3445*

Blood *Urine Increase Physiological* At doses used to treat toxoplasmosis may produce hematuria *2173*

Eosinophils *Blood Increase Physiological* Biopsy-proven granulomatous hepatitis due to sulfadoxine moiety of drug reported in two individuals receiving drug prophylactically possibly due to sulfonamide hypersensitivity *3445*

Erythrocytes *Blood Decrease Physiological* Megaloblastic anemia *6541*

Folate *Red Blood Cells Decrease Physiological* Inhibits dihydrofolate reductase *3383*
Serum Decrease Physiological Inhibits folate reductase, causes megaloblastic anemia *5054* Inhibits dihydrofolate reductase *3383*

Hematocrit *Blood Decrease Physiological* Megaloblastic anemia *6541* At doses used to treat toxoplasmosis may produce megaloblastic anemia *2173*

Hemoglobin *Blood Decrease Physiological* At doses used to treat toxoplasmosis may produce megaloblastic anemia *2173* Megaloblastic anemia *6541*

Histamine *Plasma No Effect Analytical* 50% inhibition of radio-enzyme assay at 10 times therapeutic concentration *2492*

Leukocytes *Blood Decrease Physiological* May occur with severe megaloblastic anemia *6541* At doses used to treat toxoplasmosis may produce leukopenia *2173*

MCV *Blood Increase Physiological* At doses used to treat toxoplasmosis may produce megaloblastic anemia *2173* Megaloblastic anemia *6541*

Neutrophils *Blood Decrease Physiological* Occasional case of agranulocytosis reported *6264*

N-Formiminoglutamic Acid *Urine Increase Physiological* If megaloblastic anemia occurs *6541*

Phenylalanine *Plasma Increase Physiological* Hyperphenylalaninemia has been reported as a rare complication of treatment *2173* *2174*

Platelets *Blood Decrease Physiological* At doses used to treat toxoplasmosis may produce thrombocytopenia *2173* May occur with severe megaloblastic anemia *6541*

Quinine *Serum Increase Physiological* May displace from plasma protein binding *2452*

Pyrithioxine

Acetylcholine Receptor Antibodies
Serum Increase Physiological With dose of 400-600 mg/d; associated with development of immune complex nephritis and other penicillamine-like toxic reactions *2881*

Platelets *Blood Decrease Physiological* With dose of 400-600 mg/d: associated with development of immune complex nephritis and other penicillamine-like toxic reactions *2881*

Protein *Urine Increase Physiological* With dose of 400-600 mg/d: associated with development of immune complex nephritis and other penicillamine-like toxic reactions *2881*

Pyritinol

Alanine Aminotransferase *Serum No Effect Analytical* No effect at 20 mg/L on Boehringer Mannheim Reflotron method *5706* No effect at therapeutic concentration on Boehringer Mannheim Reflotron method *3231*

Amylase *Serum No Effect Analytical* Concentrations up to 20 mg/L had no effect on method on Boehringer Mannheim Reflotron system *5706*

Amylase, Pancreatic Isoenzyme
Serum No Effect Analytical No significant effect observed at a toxic concentration of 20 mg/L with method on Boehringer Mannheim Reflotron *3647*

Aspartate Aminotransferase *Serum No Effect Analytical* No effect at therapeutic concentration on Boehringer Mannheim Reflotron method *3231* No effect at 20 mg/L on Boehringer Mannheim Reflotron method *5706*

Bilirubin *Serum No Effect Analytical* At concentration of 20 mg/L no effect on method on Boehringer Mannheim Reflotron system *5706*

Cholesterol *Serum No Effect Analytical* At concentration of 20 mg/L no effect on method on Boehringer Mannheim Reflotron systems *5706* No effect at therapeutic concentration on Boehringer Mannheim Reflotron method *3231*

Glucose *Serum No Effect Analytical* At concentration of 20 mg/L no effect on method on Boehringer Mannheim Reflotron system *5706* No effect at therapeutic concentration on Boehringer Mannheim Reflotron method *3231*

γ-Glutamyltransferase *Serum No Effect Analytical* At concentration of 20 mg/L no effect on method on Boehringer Mannheim Reflotron system *5706* No effect at therapeutic concentration on Boehringer Mannheim Reflotron method *3231*

HDL-Cholesterol *Serum No Effect Analytical* At a concentration up to 20 mg/L had no significant effect on Reflotron method for whole blood cholesterol *6352*

Triglycerides *Serum No Effect Analytical* No effect at 20 mg/L on Boehringer Mannheim Reflotron method *5706* No effect at therapeutic concentration on Boehringer Mannheim Reflotron method *3231*

Urea Nitrogen *Serum No Effect Analytical* No effect at 20 mg/L on Boehringer Mannheim Reflotron method *5706* No effect at therapeutic concentration on Boehringer Mannheim Reflotron method *3231*

Uric Acid *Serum No Effect Analytical* No effect at 20 mg/L on Boehringer Mannheim Reflotron method *5706* No effect at therapeutic concentration on Boehringer Mannheim Reflotron method *3231*

Pyrogallol

Color *Urine Increase Analytical* Brown to black, darkens on standing *3810*

Pyrvinium

Color *Feces Increase Physiological* Stains feces bright red *1384*

Quazepam

Alanine Aminotransferase *Serum Increase Physiological* Increased activity observed in less than 1% of 234 treated patients *6322*

Albumin *Serum Decrease Physiological* Decreased concentration observed in less than 1% of 234 treated patients *6322*

Alkaline Phosphatase *Serum Increase Physiological* Increased activity observed in less than 1% of 234 treated patients *6322*

Aspartate Aminotransferase *Serum Increase Physiological* Increased activity observed in 1.3% of 234 treated patients *6322*

Bilirubin *Serum Increase Physiological* Increased concentration observed in less than 1% of 234 treated patients *6322*

Creatinine *Serum Increase Physiological* Increased concentration observed in less than 1% of 234 treated patients *6322*

Eosinophils *Blood Increase Physiological* Increased eosinophil count observed in 1.5% of 234 treated patients *6322*

Epithelial Cells *Urine Increase Physiological* Increased excretion observed in 2.5% of 234 treated patients *6322*

Hematocrit *Blood Decrease Physiological* Reduced hematocrit observed in 1.5% of 234 treated patients *6322*

Hemoglobin *Blood Decrease Physiological* Reduced hemoglobin observed in 1.4% of 234 treated patients *6322*

Leukocytes *Blood Decrease Physiological* Abnormal count observed in less than 1% of 234 treated patients *6322*
Urine Increase Physiological Increased excretion observed in 2.6% of 234 treated patients *6322*

Lymphocytes *Blood Decrease Physiological* Reduced lymphocyte count observed in 1.3% of 234 treated patients *6322*
Blood Increase Physiological Increased lymphocyte count observed in 1.6% of 234 treated patients *6322*

Monocytes *Blood Increase Physiological* Increased monocyte count observed in 1.1% of 234 treated patients *6322*

Platelets *Blood Decrease Physiological* Abnormal count observed in less than 1% of 234 treated patients *6322*

Protein *Serum Decrease Physiological* Decreased concentration observed in less than 1% of 234 treated patients *6322*

Urea Nitrogen *Serum Increase Physiological* Increased concentration observed in less than 1% of 234 treated patients *6322*

Quinacrine

Alanine Aminotransferase *Serum Increase Physiological* Hepatitis reported (centrolobular necrosis) *128*

Alkaline Phosphatase *Serum Increase Physiological* Hepatotoxic effect *3810*

Aspartate Aminotransferase *Serum Increase Physiological* Hepatitis reported (centrolobular necrosis) *128*

Bile *Urine Increase Physiological* Hepatotoxic effect *3810*

Bilirubin *Serum Increase Physiological* Hemolysis may occur with G-6-PD deficiency *402* Hepatotoxic effect *3810*

Bilirubin, Direct *Serum Increase Physiological* Hemolysis may occur with G-6-PD deficiency *2024*

BSP Retention *Serum Increase Physiological* Hepatotoxic effect *3810*

Color *Urine Increase Analytical* Deep yellow color on acidification *2242* Produces yellow coloration *684*

Diagnex Blue Excretion *Urine Increase Analytical* Release of dye from resin *2025*

Erythrocytes *Blood Decrease Physiological* Occasional case of aplastic anemia reported *6264* May cause hemolysis with G-6-PD deficiency *402* May produce aplastic anemia *3810*

Hematocrit *Blood Decrease Physiological* May cause hemolysis with G-6-PD deficiency *402*

Hemoglobin *Blood Decrease Physiological* May cause hemolysis with G-6-PD deficiency *402*

Icteric Index *Serum Increase Physiological* Hemolysis may occur with G-6-PD deficiency *2024*

Leukocytes *Blood Decrease Physiological* Leukopenia/agranulocytosis/aplastic anemia *4013* Occasional case of aplastic anemia reported *6264*

Methemoglobin *Blood Increase Physiological* May cause hemolysis with G-6-PD deficiency *6015*

Platelets *Blood Decrease Physiological* Occasional case of aplastic anemia reported *6264* Thrombocytopenia or aplastic anemia may occur *3810*

Spermidine Oxidase *Serum No Effect Analytical* At concentration of 0.2 mmol/L had no effect on method of Tabor and Kellogg *1884*

Quinapril

Alanine Aminotransferase *Serum Increase Physiological* Abnormal liver function tests occured with treatment in less than 1% of 4787 patients *4516*

Albumin *Serum No Effect Physiological* In 17 patients with essential hypertension treatment with up to 40 mg/d quinapril caused caused no significant change in concentration after 12 weeks *4810*
Urine Decrease Physiological In 17 patients with essential hypertension treatment with up to 40 mg/d quinapril caused decrease in albumin excretion rate from mean baseline of 55 µg/min to 33 µg/min after 12 weeks *4810* In 17 patients with mild to moderate essential hypertension treatment with up to 40 mg daily for 12 weeks caused mean excretion to decrease from 55 to 33 µg/min *4810* In 99 patients with mild to moderate essential hypertension treated with up to 40 mg/d for 12 weeks mean excretion reduced from baseline of 21.6 ± 28.7 mg/d to 14.2 ± 15.5 mg/d *3414*

Alkaline Phosphatase *Serum Increase Physiological* Abnormal liver function tests occured with treatment in less than 1% of 4787 patients *4516*

Amylase *Serum Increase Physiological* Pancreatitis occured with treatment in less than 1% of 4787 patients *4516*

Angiotensin-converting Enzyme
Serum Decrease Physiological Even after single oral dose of 0.625 mg marked reduction of ACE observed at 30 minutes in volunteers with almost complete inhibition at 1 hour with larger doses with approximately 50% inhibition continuing for 24 hours with doses from 2.5 to 80 mg *1936*

Aspartate Aminotransferase *Serum Increase Physiological* Abnormal liver function tests occured with treatment in less than 1% of 4787 patients *4516*

Bilirubin *Serum Increase Physiological* Abnormal liver function tests occured with treatment in less than 1% of 4787 patients *4516*

C_1-Esterase Inhibitor *Serum Decrease Physiological* In 22 patients treated with quinapril who developed angioedema mean concentration of 0.312 ± 0.06 g/L significantly less than 0.342 ± 0.05 g/L in 48 who did not develop angioedema *5550*

Calcium *Serum No Effect Physiological* In 17 patients with essential hypertension treatment with up to 40 mg/d quinapril caused insignificant increase in calcium concentration from mean baseline of 0.3 mg/dL after 12 weeks *4810* Treatment of 8 patients with mild to moderate essential hypertension with 5-10 mg/d for 12 weeks caused nonsignificant change from mean baseline of 9.6 ± 0.3 mg/dL to 9.7 ± 0.2 mg/dL *4464*
Urine Decrease Physiological In 17 hypertensive patients with mild to moderate renal impairment treatment with up to 40 mg/d for 12 weeks caused significant decrease from 219 mg/d to 188 mg/d *4810* In 17 patients with essential hypertension treatment with up to 40 mg/d quinapril caused decrease in calcium excretion from mean baseline of 219 mg/d to 188 mg/d after 12 weeks *4810*

Carboxypeptidase N *Serum Decrease Physiological* In 22 patients treated with quinapril who developed angioedema mean activity 7.23 ± 1.06 nmol/mL/min less than 8.02 ± 1.62 nmol/mL/min in 48 who did not develop angioedema *5550*

Chloride *Serum No Effect Physiological* Treatment of 8 patients with mild to moderate essential hypertension with 5-10 mg/d for 12 weeks caused nonsignificant change from mean baseline of 103.4 ± 1.0 mmol/L to 103.4 ± 2.7 mmol/L *4464*

Cholesterol *Serum No Effect Physiological* No significant change observed in 16 hypertensive patients treated with up to 80 mg daily for 12 weeks *3255*

Complement C_4 *Serum No Effect Physiological* In 22 patients treated with quinapril who developed angioedema mean concentration of 0.358 ± 0.151 g/L not significantly less than 0.382 ± 0.106 g/L in 48 who did not develop angioedema *5550*

Complement CH50 *Serum No Effect Physiological* In 22 patients treated with quinapril who developed angioedema mean activity 235.0 ± 54.4 units not significantly less than 248.3 ± 79.8 units in 48 who did not develop angioedema *5550*

Creatinine *Serum Increase Physiological* Acute renal failure or worsening renal failure occured with treatment in less than 1% of 4787 patients *4516*

Serum No Effect Physiological Treatment of 8 patients with mild to moderate essential hypertension with 5-10 mg/d for 12 weeks caused nonsignificant change from mean baseline of 0.8 ± 0.2 mg/dL to 0.8 ± 0.2 mg/dL *4464*

Urine Decrease Physiological In 99 patients with mild to moderate essential hypertension treated with up to 40 mg/d for 12 weeks mean concentration reduced nonsignificantly from baseline of 95.5 ± 17.5 µmol/L to 94.7 ± 16.7 µmol/L *3414*

Creatinine Clearance *Urine No Effect Physiological* In 99 patients with mild to moderate essential hypertension treated with up to 40 mg/d for 12 weeks mean excretion reduced nonsignificantly from baseline of 1.5 ± 0.5 mL/s to 1.5 ± 0.4 mL/s *3414* In 9 patients with moderate renal impairment treatment with up to 40 mg/d caused nonsignificant increase from mean baseline of 47.4 ± 2.6 mL/min to 47.0 ± 2.6 mL/min and in 13 with chronic renal failure from 21.2 ± 0.9 mL/min to 22.5 mL/min *4050*

Digoxin *Serum No Effect Physiological* Coadministration of quinapril with digoxin did not affect its pharmacokinetics *4516*

Endothelin *Plasma No Effect Physiological* In 12 patients with congestive cardiac failure treatment with up to 40 mg/d for 16 weeks caused nonsignificant change from mean baseline of 11.9 ± 2.9 pg/mL to 12.3 ± 3.4 pg/mL *6064*

Epinephrine *Plasma No Effect Physiological* Insignificant decrease from mean concentration of 47.0 ng/L to 44.8 ng/L in 10 healthy men treated with 40 mg daily for 4 weeks *2371*

Glomerular Filtration Rate *Urine Increase Physiological* Treatment of 8 patients with mild to moderate essential hypertension with 5-10 mg/d for 12 weeks caused significant increase from mean baseline of 43.4 ± 6.4 mL/min/1.73 m^2 to 53.5 ± 4.6 mL/min/1.73 m^2*4464*

Glucose *Serum Decrease Physiological* Incidence of 0.7% observed in French Pharmacovigilance database *4106*

γ-Glutamyltransferase *Serum Increase Physiological* Abnormal liver function tests occured with treatment in less than 1% of 4787 patients *4516*

Granulocytes *Blood Decrease Physiological* Agranulocytosis occured with treatment in less than 1% of 4787 patients *4516*

HDL-Cholesterol *Serum No Effect Physiological* No significant change observed in 16 hypertensive patients treated with up to 80 mg daily for 12 weeks *3255*

Hematocrit *Blood Decrease Physiological* Hemolytic anemia occured with treatment in less than 1% of 4787 patients *4516*

Hemoglobin *Blood Decrease Physiological* Hemolytic anemia occured with treatment in less than 1% of 4847 patients *4516*

Hydrochlorothiazide *Serum No Effect Physiological* Coadministration of quinapril with hydrochlorothiazide did not affect its pharmacokinetics *4516*

LDL-Cholesterol *Serum No Effect Physiological* No significant change observed in 16 hypertensive patients treated with up to 80 mg daily for 12 weeks *3255*

Lipase *Serum Increase Physiological* Pancreatitis occured with treatment in less than 1% of 4787 patients *4516*

Lithium *Serum Increase Physiological* Coadministration of lithium with ACE inhibitors may cause an increase in lithium concentration and even lithium toxicity *4516*

Norepinephrine *Plasma No Effect Physiological* Insignificant increase from mean concentration of 201.5 ng/L to 220.1 ng/L in 10 healthy men treated with 40 mg daily for 4 weeks *2371*

Platelets No Effect Physiological Insignificant reduction from mean of 55.6 to 51.6 pg/mg platelet weight in 10 healthy men treated with 40 mg daily for 4 weeks *2371*

Occult Blood *Feces Increase Physiological* Gastrointestinal hemorrhage occured with treatment in less than 1% of 4787 patients *4516*

Phosphate *Serum No Effect Physiological* Treatment of 8 patients with mild to moderate essential hypertension with 5-10 mg/d for 12 weeks caused nonsignificant change from mean baseline of 3.3 ± 0.3 mg/dL to 3.1 ± 0.5 mg/dL *4464*

Platelet Aggregation *Blood No Effect Physiological* No significant change in epinephrine, collagen or ADP induced aggregation observed in 10 healthy men treated with 40 mg daily for 4 weeks *2371* No significant effect on aggregation induced by epinephrine, collagen and adenosine diphosphate in 10 white men with mild to moderate hypertension treated with 40 mg daily for 4 weeks *2371*

Platelet Distribution Width *Blood No Effect Physiological* No significant effect observed in 10 white men with mild to moderate hypertension treated with 40 mg/d for 4 weeks *2371* No significant effect observed in 10 healthy men treated with 40 mg daily for 4 weeks *2371*

Platelet Factor 4 *Plasma No Effect Physiological* Insignificant increase from mean of 14.0 µg/L to 17.4 µg/L in 10 healthy white men with mild to moderate hypertenson treated with 40 mg daily for 4 weeks *2371* Insignificant increase from mean of 14.0 µg/L to 17.4 µg/L in 10 healthy men treated with 40 mg daily for 4 weeks *2371*

Platelets *Blood Decrease Physiological* Thrombocytopenia occured with treatment in less than 1% of 4787 patients *4516*

Blood No Effect Physiological No significant effect observed in 10 healthy men treated with 40 mg daily for 4 weeks *2371* No significant effect observed in 10 white men with mild to moderate hypertension treated with 40 mg/d for 4 weeks *2371*

Potassium *Serum Increase Physiological* Hyperkalemia occured with treatment in less than 1% of 4787 patients *4516* Treatment of 8 patients with mild to moderate essential hypertension with 5-10 mg/d for 12 weeks caused significant change from mean baseline of 4.0 ± 0.2 mmol/L to 4.2 ± 0.2 mmol/L *4464*

Protein *Urine Decrease Physiological* In 9 patients with moderate renal failure treated with up to 40 mg/d mean excretion decreased from 1199.4 ± 163.5 mg/d to 628.4 ± 163.5 mg/d and in 13 with chronic renal failure from 1750.8 ± 147.5 mg/d to 1232.2 ± 147.5 mg/d *4050*

Prothrombin Time *Plasma No Effect Physiological* Coadministration of quinapril with a single dose of warfarin had no significant effect on prothrombin time *4516*

Renal Plasma Flow *Patient Increase Physiological* Treatment of 8 patients with mild to moderate essential hypertension with 5-10 mg/d for 12 weeks caused significant increase from mean baseline of 203.9 ± 33.3 mL/min/1.73 m^2 to 245.4 ± 36.7 mL/min/1.73 m^2*4464*

Sodium *Serum No Effect Physiological* Treatment of 8 patients with mild to moderate essential hypertension with 5-10 mg/d for 12 weeks caused nonsignificant change from mean baseline of 141.2 ± 1.0 mmol/L to 140.7 ± 2.5 mmol/L *4464*

Tetracycline *Serum Decrease Physiological* Coadministration of tetracycline with quinapril caused a decrease in absorption of 28 to 37%, possibly due to the high magnesiu concentration in accupril tablets *4516*

β-Thromboglobulin *Plasma No Effect Physiological* Insignificant increase from mean of 43.7 µg/L to 49.6 µg/L in 10 healthy men with mild to moderate hypertension treated with 40 mg daily for 4 weeks *2371* Insignificant increase from mean of 43.7 µg/L to 49.6 µg/L in 10 healthy men treated with 40 mg daily for 4 weeks *2371*

Triglycerides *Serum No Effect Physiological* No significant change observed in 16 hypertensive patients treated with up to 80 mg daily for 12 weeks *3255*

Urea Nitrogen *Serum Increase Physiological* In 10 patients with moderate renal impairment treatment with up to 8.4 ± 0.8 mmol/L to 12.9 ± 0.8 mol/L but in 15 with chronic renal failure essentially unchanged from 26.7 ± 0.9 mmol/L to

Quinapril *(continued)*

Urea Nitrogen *(continued)*
28.4 ± 0.9 mmol/L *4050* Acute renal failure or worsening renal failure occured with treatment in less than 1% of 4787 patients *4516*
Serum No Effect Physiological Treatment of 8 patients with mild to moderate essential hypertension with 5-10 mg/d for 12 weeks caused nonsignificant increase from mean baseline of 14.1 ± 3.2 mg/dL to 15.7 ± 2.7 mg/dL *4464*

Uric Acid *Serum No Effect Physiological* Treatment of 8 patients with mild to moderate essential hypertension with 5-10 mg/d for 12 weeks caused nonsignificant change from mean baseline of 5.4 ± 1.2 mg/dL to 5.8 ± 1.2 mg/dL *4464*

Quinethazone

Alanine Aminotransferase *Serum Increase Physiological* May cause cholestatic jaundice *3810*

Alkaline Phosphatase *Serum Increase Physiological* May cause cholestatic jaundice *3810*

Aspartate Aminotransferase *Serum Increase Physiological* May cause cholestatic jaundice *3810*

Bile *Urine Increase Physiological* May cause cholestatic jaundice *3810*

Bilirubin *Serum Increase Physiological* May cause cholestatic jaundice *4555*

BSP Retention *Serum Increase Physiological* May cause cholestatic jaundice *3810*

Eosinophils *Blood Increase Physiological* Isolated case report *4014*

Erythrocytes *Blood Decrease Physiological* Theoretical bone marrow depression *2754*

Glucose *Serum Increase Physiological* May precipitate latent diabetes or aggravate exist *3810*
Urine Increase Physiological Occurs as consequence of hyperglycemia *3810*

Glucose Tolerance *Serum Decrease Physiological* Similar effect to thiazides *2754*

LE Cells *Blood Positive Physiological* Theoretical possibility of this type of drug *2754*

Leukocytes *Blood Decrease Physiological* Theoretical bone marrow depression *2754*

Platelets *Blood Decrease Physiological* Theoretical bone marrow depression *2754*

Potassium *Serum Decrease Physiological* Diuretic action *4014*
Urine Increase Physiological Relatively small increase *2754*

Sodium *Serum Decrease Physiological* Diuretic action with sodium depletion *3810*
Urine Increase Physiological Intended effect, high Na/K ratio *2754*

Sugar *Urine Increase Analytical* False positive with Benedict's reagent *3810*

Urea Nitrogen *Serum Increase Physiological* Observed effect (?due to dehydration) *4014*

Uric Acid *Serum Increase Physiological* Increased up to 4 mg/dL, inhibits tubular secretion *711*

Quingestanol

Cholesterol *Serum No Effect Physiological* No significant effect with 300 µg/d 6 mo *2193*

Lipoprotein Electrophoresis *Serum No Effect Physiological* No significant effect with 300 µg/d for 6 mo *2193*

Monoglyceride Lipase *Serum No Effect Physiological* No significant effect with 300 µg/d for 6 mo *2193*

Polymorphic Epithelial Mucin
Serum No Effect Physiological In women with breast cancer diagnostic (test) accuracy for breast cancer 39.4% by ACS BR, 50.3% by Centocor CA 15-3, 40.4% by Enzymun-Test CA 15-3 and 40.4% by IMx CA 15-3 respectively *645*

Postheparin Lipase *Plasma No Effect Physiological* No significant effect with 300 µg/d 6 mo *2193*

Triglyceride Lipase *Serum No Effect Physiological* No significant effect with 300 µg/d for 6 mo *2193*

Triglycerides *Serum Decrease Physiological* May be slight effect with 300 µg/d *2193*
Serum No Effect Physiological At 300 µg/d usually no effect *2193*

Quinidine

Acetaminophen *Serum No Effect Analytical* No interference observed at a concentration of 2000 µg/mL (616 µmol/L) with method on Du Pont aca *1506*

Alanine Aminotransferase *Serum Increase Physiological* Isolated case of hepatic toxicity (granulomatous hepatitis) *1354* In single case of severe quinidine hypersensitivity *1350* A few cases of hepatotoxicity, including granulomatous hepatitis, have occurred with quinidine administration *5996* Hypersensitivity reaction reported in one patient *5601*
Serum No Effect Analytical No effect at therapeutic concentration on Boehringer Mannheim Reflotron method *3231* No effect at 60 mg/L on Boehringer Mannheim Reflotron method *5706* At acute overdose concentration (20 mg/dL) Technicon SMAC® method *6266*

Albumin *Serum Decrease Physiological* In single case of severe quinidine hypersensitivity *1350*
Serum No Effect Analytical At acute overdose concentration (20 mg/dL) Technicon SMAC® method *6266* At concentration of 210 mg/L had no effect on BCG method *5704* At 26 mg/dL no effect on Technicon SMA 12/60 method *4390*
Serum No Effect Physiological Hypersensitivity observed in 32 of 487 patients who had received drug *2077*

Aldolase *Serum Increase Physiological* If given intramuscularly, possibly due to increase in intracellular calcium *5395*

Alkaline Phosphatase *Serum Increase Physiological* Hypersensitivity observed in 32 of 487 patients who had received drug *2077* A few cases of hepatotoxicity, including granulomatous hepatitis, have occurred with quinidine administration *5996* In single case of severe quinidine hypersensitivity *1350* Isolated case of reversible granulomatous hepatitis from quinidine hypersensitivity and granuloma induction within 3 d of quinidine readministration *690* May cause mild hepatic impairment in few patients *4185*
Serum No Effect Analytical At acute overdose concentration (20 mg/dL) Technicon SMAC® method *6266* At 26 mg/dL no effect on Technicon SMA 12/60 method *4390*

Amitriptyline *Serum Increase Physiological* When coadministered, by inhibiting cytochrome P450 2D6, may increase the concentration of amitriptyline *6645*

Amylase *Serum No Effect Analytical* Concentrations up to 60 mg/L had no effect on method on Boehringer Mannheim Reflotron system *5706*

Amylase, Pancreatic Isoenzyme
Serum No Effect Analytical No significant effect observed at a toxic concentration of 60 mg/L with method on Boehringer Mannheim Reflotron *3647*

Anisindione *Plasma Increase Physiological* Potentiates action *2452*

Anti-DNA Antibodies *Serum Increase Physiological* Observed in several patients with drug induced rheumatic syndromes *1080*

Anti-ds DNA Antibodies *Serum No Effect Physiological* Reported in 5 cases of an SLE-like syndrome induced by the drug *3437*

Anti-Histone Antibodies *Serum No Effect Physiological* Reported in 5 cases of an SLE-like syndrome induced by the drug *3437*

Anti-Ribonuclear Protein Antibodies
Serum No Effect Physiological Reported in 5 cases of an SLE-like syndrome induced by the drug *3437*

Anti-Scl-70 Antibodies *Serum No Effect Physiological* Reported in 5 cases of an SLE-like syndrome induced by the drug *3437*

Anti-Sjögren's Syndrome A Antibodies (SSA[Ro#)
Serum No Effect Physiological Reported in 5 cases of an SLE-like syndrome induced by the drug *3437*

Anti-Sjögren's Syndrome B Antibodies (SSB[La#])
Serum No Effect Physiological Reported in 5 cases of an SLE-like syndrome induced by the drug *3437*

Anti-Smith Antibodies *Serum No Effect Physiological* Reported in 5 cases of an SLE-like syndrome induced by the drug *3437*

Antinuclear Antibodies *Serum Increase Physiological* Reported in 5 cases of an SLE-like syndrome induced by the drug *3437*

Antipyrine *Serum No Effect Physiological* No significant effect observed on plasma concentration, apparent oral clearance or half-life when quinidine given as pretreatment prior to administration of antipyrine in 6 healthy men *676*

Aspartate Aminotransferase *Serum Increase Physiological* Hypersensitivity observed in 32 of 487 patients who had received drug *2077* Hypersensitivity reaction reported in one patient *5601* In single case of severe quinidine hypersensitivity *1350* A few cases of hepatotoxicity, including granulomatous hepatitis, have occurred with quinidine administration *5996* May cause mild hepatic impairment in few patients *4185*
Serum No Effect Analytical At 26 mg/dL no effect on Technicon SMA 12/60 method *4390* At acute overdose concentration (20 mg/dL) Technicon SMAC® method *6266* No effect at 60 mg/L on Boehringer Mannheim Reflotron method *5706* No effect at therapeutic concentration on Boehringer Mannheim Reflotron method *3231*

Bicarbonate *Serum No Effect Analytical* At concentration of 210 mg/L had no effect on method using phenolphthalein *5704*

Bilirubin *Serum Increase Physiological* Causes hemolytic anemia *3895* Hypersensitivity observed in 32 of 487 patients who had received drug *2077*
Serum No Effect Analytical At concentration of 60 mg/L had no effect on method on Boehringer Mannheim Reflotron system *5706* At 26 mg/dL no effect on Technicon SMA 12/60 method *4390* At concentration of 210 mg/L had no effect on Jendrassik and Grof method *5704* No effect at 5 mg/L on Ames Seralyzer method *5706* At acute overdose concentration (20 mg/dL) Technicon SMAC® method *6266*

Bilirubin, Direct *Serum Increase Physiological* Causes hemolytic anemia *3895*

Calcium *Serum No Effect Analytical* At acute overdose concentration (20 mg/dL) Technicon SMAC® method *6266* At 26 mg/dL no effect on Technicon SMA 12/60 method *4390* At concentration of 210 mg/L had no effect on cresolphthalein method *5704*

Catecholamines *Urine No Effect Analytical* If Hathaway procedure used *2452*

Chloride *Serum No Effect Analytical* At concentration of 210 mg/L had no effect on mercurimetric method *5704*

Cholesterol *Serum No Effect Analytical* At concentration of 210 mg/L had no effect on Liebermann-Burchard method *5704* No effect at 5 mg/L on Ames Seralyzer method *5706* No effect at therapeutic concentration on Boehringer Mannheim Reflotron method *3231* At acute overdose concentration (20 mg/dL) Technicon SMAC® method *6266* At concentration of 60 mg/L no effect on method on Boehringer Mannheim Reflotron system *5706* At 26 mg/dL no effect on Technicon SMA 12/60 method *4390*

Cocaethylene *Urine No Effect Analytical* No interference observed with TLC method of Bailey *328*

Codeine *Cerebrospinal Fluid Decrease Physiological* In 8 patients given 200 mg quinidine with 125 mg codeine median concentration 2 h later 308 nmol/L compared with 387 nmol/L when codeine given alone *5571*

Coombs' Test *Blood Positive Physiological* Immunological response to drug (γ antibody) *2453*

Coombs' Test, Direct *Blood Positive Physiological* Associated with hemolytic anemia *2452* Occasional hemolytic anemia and hypersensitivity observed in 32 of 487 patients who had received drug *2077*

Cortisol *Plasma No Effect Analytical* At a concentration of 60 mg/L no significant effect on CEDIA or Enzymun methods *1097*

Creatine Kinase *Serum Increase Physiological* If given intramuscularly, possibly due to increase in intracellular calcium *5395*
Serum No Effect Analytical No effect at 5 mg/L on method on Ames Seralyzer *5706* At acute overdose concentration (20 mg/dL) Technicon SMAC® method *6266*

Creatine Kinase Isoenzymes *Serum No Effect Analytical* No interference observed at a concentration of 8 mg/L (24.7 μmol/L) with CK-MB method on Du Pont aca *1519*

Creatinine *Serum No Effect Analytical* At 26 mg/dL no effect on Technicon SMA 12/60 method *4390* No interference observed with liquid chromatographic method of Paroni *4540* At concentration of 210 mg/L had no effect on Technicon AutoAnalyzer® Jaffe method *5704* No effect at 5 mg/L on Ames Seralyzer method *5706* At acute overdose concentration (20 mg/dL) Technicon SMAC® method *6266*

Diagnex Blue Excretion *Urine Increase Analytical* Release of dye from resin *2025*

Digitoxin *Serum Increase Physiological* Quinidine slows the elimination of digitoxin but effect appears to be less than with digoxin *5996* Effect less marked than with digoxin but still significant *1384*

Digoxin *Bile Decrease Physiological* In 5 patients concomitant administration of quinidine reduced biliary clearance by an average of 42%. Note nonrenal clearance of digoxin is about 30% of total clearance *180*
Serum Increase Physiological Volume of distribution and nonrenal clearance increased, half-time of elimination greatly increased but total clearance and renal clearance greatly decreased *558* Observed in 7 of 9 patients with mean concentration changing from 1.43 to 2.61 nmol/L, probably due to displacement of quinidine from binding sites in tissues and reduced renal clearance *3775* Quinidine slows the elimination of digoxin and also reduces its apparent volume of distribution *5996* When coadministered with quinidine: so effect of 0.2 mg with quinidine was comparable to that of 0.4 mg without *471* 2.5 fold increase with more than 50% decrease in renal clearance *1457* Absorption rate constant increased, with decreased lag time and peak time. Systemic availability of digoxin increased from 68% to 79%, but no effect on biotransformation *4582* 20 to 330% increase after 3 d of quinidine in 17 patients *1214* Approximate 2-fold increase due to decreased total body clearance but renal clearance negligible and not affected by chronic renal failure *1834* Clearance reduced by coadministration of quinidine: effect further augmented by addition of spironolactone to regime *1833* Coadministration with digoxin may increase the digoxin concentration *2161*

Diltiazem *Serum No Effect Physiological* Quinidine has no effect on the pharmacokinetics of diltiazem *5996*

Disopyramide *Serum Increase Physiological* When concurrent quinidine given: effect small but significant: no significant change in elimination half-life *332* When drugs coadministered slight increase in plasma disopyramide concentration observed together with a slight decrease in the plasma quinidine concentration *2069*

Donepezil *Serum Increase Physiological* Quinidine inhibits CYP450 2D6 inhibiting donepezil metabolism in vitro although in vivo inhibition has not yet been demostrated *0*

Erythrocyte Sedimentation Rate
Blood Increase Physiological Reported in 5 cases of an SLE-like syndrome induced by the drug *3437*

Erythrocytes *Blood Decrease Physiological* Immune mediated hemolytic anemia associated with high titers of IgG antibodies *5395* Occasional hemolytic anemia and hypersensitivity observed in 32 of 487 patients who had received drug *2077* Hemolytic anemia (sensitivity dependent) G-6-PD deficiency *6181*

Felodipine *Serum No Effect Physiological* Quinidine has no effect on the plasma nifedipine concentration as quinidine has no effect on the P450IIIA4 enzyme metabolizing system *5996*

Flecainide *Serum No Effect Physiological* Quinidine has no effect on the pharmacokinetics of flecainide *5996*

Glucose *Serum No Effect Analytical* At concentration of 60 mg/L has no effect on method on Boehringer Mannheim Reflotron system *5706* No effect at therapeutic concentration on Boehringer Mannheim Reflotron method *3231* At acute overdose concentration (20 mg/dL) on Technicon SMAC® method *6266* At concentration of 5.6 mg/L had no effect on Kodak Ektachem® method *5704* No effect at 5 mg/L on glucose

Quinidine *(continued)*

Glucose *(continued)*
oxidase method on Ames Seralyzer *5706* At 26 mg/dL no effect on Technicon SMA 12/60 method *4390*

γ-Glutamyltransferase *Serum Increase Physiological* A few cases of hepatotoxicity, including granulomatous hepatitis, have occurred with quinidine administration *5996* Isolated case of reversible granulomatous hepatitis from quinidine hypersensitivity and granuloma induction within 3 d of quinidine readministration *690* Hypersensitivity reaction reported in one patient *5601*
Serum No Effect Analytical No effect at therapeutic concentration on Boehringer Mannheim Reflotron method *3231* At concentration of 60 mg/L no effect on method on Boehringer Mannheim Reflotron system *5706*

Granulocytes *Blood Decrease Physiological* Occasionally observed *1384* A few cases of agranulocytosis have occurred with quinidine administration *5996*
Blood No Effect Physiological Although agranulocytosis observed in 1.5% patients versus 0.6% controls no evidence of association of drug with agranulocytosis reported *3098*

Haloperidol *Serum Increase Physiological* Quinidine increases plasma haloperidol concentration when quinidine coadministered *5996*

Haptoglobin *Serum Decrease Physiological* Causes hemolytic anemia *3895*

HDL-Cholesterol *Serum No Effect Analytical* At a concentration up to 60 mg/L had no significant effect on Reflotron method for whole blood cholesterol *6352*

Hematocrit *Blood Decrease Physiological* Hemolytic anemia (sensitivity dependent) G-6-PD deficiency *6181* Nonsignificant increased risk of aplastic anemia in patients taking drug *3098*

Hemoglobin *Blood Decrease Physiological* Nonsignificant increased risk of aplastic anemia in patients taking drug *3098* Hemolytic anemia (sensitivity dependent) G-6-PD deficiency *6181*

Histamine *Plasma No Effect Analytical* Although 50% inhibition of radio-enzyme assay at 32 μg/mL unlikely to be of clinical significance since therapeutic concentration 2-6 μg/mL *2492*

17-Hydroxycorticosteroids *Urine Increase Analytical* Metabolite interferes with Zimmermann reaction *2025*

^{131}I Uptake *Serum Decrease Physiological* Lilly product contains tetraiodofluorescein *4360*

Indinavir *Serum No Effect Physiological* Administration of a single dose of indinavir (400 mg) with quinidine sulfate (200 mg) resulted in a 10 ± 26% increase in indinavir AUC *3966*

Iron *Serum No Effect Analytical* At concentration of 200 mg/L had no effect on Ferrozine method *5704* At acute overdose concentration (20 mg/dL) Technicon SMAC® method *6266*

17-Ketosteroids *Urine Increase Analytical* Metabolite interferes with Zimmermann reaction *1714*

Lactate Dehydrogenase *Serum Increase Physiological* May cause mild hepatic impairment in few patients *4185* Isolated case of reversible granulomatous hepatitis from quinidine hypersensitivity and granuloma induction within 3 d of quinidine readministration *690* In single case of severe quinidine hypersensitivity *1350* If given intramuscularly, possibly due to increase in intracellular calcium *5395*
Serum No Effect Analytical At acute overdose concentration (20 mg/dL) Technicon SMAC® method *6266* At 26 mg/dL no effect on Technicon SMA 12/60 method *4390* No effect at 5 mg/L on method on Ames Seralyzer *5706*

Leucine Aminopeptidase *Serum Increase Physiological* Isolated case of hepatic toxicity (granulomatous hepatitis) *1354*

Leukocytes *Blood Decrease Physiological* Agranulocytosis after 8 weeks of drug treatment *1682* Nonsignificant increase in risk of aplastic anemia in patients taking drug *3098* Agranulocytosis/Leukopenia *3810*
Blood Increase Physiological Marked leukocytosis in 2 patients in association with quinidine fever, normalized after drug discontinued *450*

Lidocaine *Serum No Effect Analytical* At a concentration of 1250 mg/L (normal therapeutic concentration 2 - 5 mg/L) had less than 10% effect on method on Baxter Stratus *5705* No significant interference observed at a concentration of 100 μg/mL (308 μmol/L) with method on Du Pont aca *1534*

Lithium *Serum Decrease Analytical* May cause negative bias when lithium measured colorimetrically *3590* May cause negative bias when lithium measured by an ion-specific electrode *3590*
Serum Increase Analytical May cause positive bias at high concentrations when lithium measured by an ion-specific electrode *3590*

Mephenytoin *Serum No Effect Physiological* Quinidine has no effect on the pharmacokinetics of mephenytoin *5996*

Methemoglobin *Blood Increase Physiological* May cause hemolysis in G-6-PD deficiency *6015*

Metoprolol *Serum Increase Physiological* Mean increase of 85% observed in patients receiving 50 mg quinidine compared with controls due to reduced metabolism *3483*
Serum No Effect Physiological Quinidine has no effect on the pharmacokinetics of metoprolol *5996*

Midazolam *Serum No Effect Analytical* On GC-ECD method of Ha et al *2387*

Morphine *Cerebrospinal Fluid Decrease Physiological* In 8 patients given 200 mg quinidine with 125 mg codeine median concentration 2 h later 0.23 nmol/L compared with 3.63 nmol/L when codeine given alone *5571*

Mycophenolic Acid *Serum No Effect Analytical* No significant interference observed with HPLC method of Shipkova et al *5526*

Mycophenolic Acid Glucuronide
Serum No Effect Analytical No significant interference observed with HPLC method of Shipkova et al *5526*

N-Acetylprocainamide *Serum No Effect Analytical* No significant interference observed at a concentration of 100 μg/mL (308 μmol/L) with method on Du Pont aca *1536*

Neutrophils *Blood Decrease Physiological* Occasional agranulocytosis reported *5395*

Nicardipine *Serum No Effect Physiological* Had no effect on plasma protein binding in vitro and presumed to have no effect on nicardipine concentration in vivo *5016* Quinidine has no effect on the plasma nicardipine concentration as quinidine has no effect on the P450IIIA4 enzyme metabolizing system *5996*

Nifedipine *Serum Increase Physiological* Quinidine increases plasma nifedipine concentration by slowing its metabolism *5996*

Nimodipine *Serum No Effect Physiological* Quinidine has no effect on the plasma nimodipine concentration as quinidine has no effect on the P450IIIA4 enzyme metabolizing system *5996*

Nisoldipine *Serum Decrease Physiological* Administration of quinidine 648 mg twice daily with nisoldipine caused a 26% reduction of the AUC of nisoldipine but had no effect on its peak concentration *6650*

Phenindione *Plasma Increase Physiological* Potentiates action *2452*

Phenylalanine *Plasma No Effect Analytical* No interference observed with rapid quantitative whole blood method of Campbell et al using phenylalanine dehydrogenase *867*

Phosphate *Serum No Effect Analytical* At 26 mg/dL no effect on Technicon SMA 12/60 method *4390* At concentration of 210 mg/L had no effect on phosphomolybdate method *5704* At acute overdose concentration (20 mg/dL) Technicon SMAC® method *6266*

Platelet Aggregation *Blood Decrease Physiological* At concentrations of 1 to 1.5 mmol/L marked inhibition of aggregation due to adenosine diphosphate, epinephrine, collagen and arachidonate observed *999*
Blood No Effect Physiological No significant effect observed at physiological concentrations of quinidine (10 μmol/L) in response to adenosine diphosphate, collagen, arachidonate, and ristocetin but variable response to epinephrine ranging from 9 to 80% aggregation in healthy people *999* No effect observed at quinidine concentrations of 1 to 1.5 mmol/L in response to ristocetin *999*

Platelets *Blood Decrease Physiological* Allergic reaction/pancytopenia/purpura *6181* Isolated case of reversible granulomatous hepatitis from quinidine hypersensitivity and granuloma induction within 3 d of quinidine readministration

690 Several cases of platelet-associated IgG and thrombocytopenia *3102* Nonsignificant increase in risk of aplastic anemia in patients taking drug *3098*

Potassium *Serum No Effect Analytical* At concentration of 210 mg/L had no effect on ISE measurement without predilution *5704*

Pramipexole *Serum Increase Physiological* Coadministration of quinidine with pramipexole presumed to decrease the oral clearance of pramipexole by about 20% *4680*

Procainamide *Serum Increase Physiological* Quinidine increases plasma procainamide concentration by competing for pathways of renal clearance *5996*
Serum No Effect Analytical No significant interference observed at a concentration of 100 µg/mL (308 µmol/L) with method on Du Pont aca *1542*

Propafenone *Serum Increase Physiological* Small doses of quinidine inhibit the metabolism of propafenone *1384*
Serum No Effect Physiological Quinidine has no effect on the pharmacokinetics of propafenone *5996*

Propranolol *Serum No Effect Physiological* Quinidine has no effect on the pharmacokinetics of propranolol *5996*

Protein *Serum No Effect Analytical* At concentration of 210 mg/L had no effect on biuret method with blank correction *5704* At acute overdose concentration (20 mg/dL) Technicon SMAC® method *6266* At 26 mg/dL no effect on Technicon SMA 12/60 method *4390*

Prothrombin Time *Plasma Increase Physiological* Probable interaction with warfarin when drugs coadministered *2625* Quinidine potentiates the anticoagulatory action of warfarin *5996* Addition of quinidine to regime of patients who were receiving warfarin caused prolongation of prothrombin time but effect not observed in all patients. Decreases prothrombin formation in the liver *3209* If administration with indandiones, coumarin *2452*
Plasma No Effect Physiological Hypersensitivity observed in 32 of 487 patients who had received drug *4856* No effect observed in volunteers *5501*

Quinidine *Cerebrospinal Fluid Increase Physiological* In 9 patients given 200 mg quinidine median concentration 4 h later 11 nmol/L *5571*
Serum Increase Physiological In 9 patients given 200 mg quinidine median concentration 4 h later 735 nmol/L *5571*

Quinidine, Free *Cerebrospinal Fluid Increase Physiological* In 9 patients given 200 mg quinidine median concentration 4 h later 10.3 nmol/L *5571*
Serum Increase Physiological In 9 patients given 200 mg quinidine median concentration 4 h later 115 nmol/L *5571*

Quinine *Serum No Effect Physiological* Quinidine has no effect on the pharmacokinetics of quinine *5996*

Reticulocytes *Blood Increase Physiological* Occasional hemolytic anemia and hypersensitivity observed in 32 of 487 patients who had received drug *2077*

SDZ PSC 833 *Blood No Effect Analytical* At a concentration of 4.7 mg/L had no effect on HPLC method of Scott et al when used to measure PSC (with CsD as internal standard) at a concentration of 5 mg/L *5418*

Sodium *Serum No Effect Analytical* At concentration of 210 mg/L had no effect on ISE measurement with predilution *5704*

Tacrolimus *Blood No Effect Analytical* No significant effect observed at a concentration of 4 mg/L with MEIA method on Abbott IMx analyzer *1871*
Serum No Effect Analytical At a concentration of 4 mg/L had no significant effect on ELISA method *6329*

Timolol *Serum No Effect Physiological* Quinidine has no effect on the pharmacokinetics of timolol *5996*

Tocainide *Serum No Effect Physiological* Quinidine has no effect on the pharmacokinetics of tiocainide *5996*

Tramadol *Serum Increase Physiological* Coadministration of quinidine with tramadol caused a significant decrease in the metabolism of tramadol because it is metabolized to M1 by the CYP2D6 P-450 isoenzyme which is inhibited by quinidine *3918*

Tricyclic Antidepressants *Serum Increase Physiological* Interacts pharmacokinetically to inhibit metabolism of tricyclic antidepressants *3590*

Triglycerides *Serum No Effect Analytical* At concentration of 210 mg/L had no effect on lipase/esterase method *5704* At acute overdose concentration (20 mg/dL) Technicon SMAC® method *6266* No effect at therapeutic concentration on Boehringer Mannheim Reflotron method *3231* No effect at 60 mg/L on Boehringer Mannheim Reflotron method *5706*

Urea Nitrogen *Serum No Effect Analytical* At concentration of 5.6 mg/L had no effect on Kodak Ektachem® method *5704* At acute overdose concentration (20 mg/dL) Technicon SMAC® method *6266* No effect at therapeutic concentration on Boehringer Mannheim Reflotron method *3231* At concentration of 210 mg/L had no effect on diacetylmonoxime method *5704* No effect at 5 mg/L on method on Ames Seralyzer *5706* No effect at 60 mg/L on Boehringer Mannheim Reflotron method *5706*

Uric Acid *Serum No Effect Analytical* No effect at 60 mg/L on method on Boehringer Mannheim Reflotron *5706* At 26 mg/dL no effect on Technicon SMA 12/60 method *4390* No effect at therapeutic concentration on Boehringer Mannheim Reflotron method *3231* At concentration of 210 mg/L had no effect on phosphotungstate reduction method *5704* At acute overdose concentration (20 mg/dL) Technicon SMAC® method *6266*

Warfarin *Plasma Increase Physiological* Potentiates action *2452*

Quinine

Alanine Aminotransferase *Serum No Effect Analytical* At acute overdose concentration (1.5 mg/dL) on Technicon SMAC® method *6266*

Albumin *Serum No Effect Analytical* At acute overdose concentration (1.5 mg/dL) on Technicon SMAC® method *6266* At concentration of 30 mg/L had no effect on BCG method *5704*

Alkaline Phosphatase *Serum No Effect Analytical* At acute overdose concentration (1.5 mg/dL) on Technicon SMAC® method *6266*

Aspartate Aminotransferase *Serum No Effect Analytical* At acute overdose concentration (1.5 mg/dL) on Technicon SMAC® method *6266*

Astemizole *Serum Increase Physiological* Concomitant administration of quinine with astemizole causes increased astemizole and desmethylastemizole concentrations *2901*

Bicarbonate *Serum No Effect Analytical* At concentration of 30 mg/L had no effect on method using phenolphthalein *5704*

Bilirubin *Serum Increase Physiological* May cause hemolytic anemia *3895*
Serum No Effect Analytical At acute overdose concentration (1.5 mg/dL) on Technicon SMAC® method *6266* At concentration of 30 mg/L had no effect on Jendrassik and Grof method *5704*

Bilirubin, Direct *Serum Increase Physiological* May cause hemolytic anemia *3895*

Bromide *Serum Increase Physiological* Theoretical possibility if hydrobromide salt is administered since it contains 17% bromide *5116*

Calcium *Serum No Effect Analytical* At acute overdose concentration (1.5 mg/dL) on Technicon SMAC® method *6266* At concentration of 30 mg/L had no effect on cresolphthalein method *5704*

Cannabinoids *Urine No Effect Analytical* No effect on Roche Abuscreen method *5006*

Chloride *Serum No Effect Analytical* At concentration of 30 mg/L had no effect on mercurimetric method *5704*

Cholesterol *Serum No Effect Analytical* At acute overdose concentration (1.5 mg/dL) on Technicon SMAC® method *6266* At concentration of 30 mg/L had no effect on Liebermann-Burchard method *5704*

Chromosomes *Test Conditions No Effect Physiological* No effect observed on human leucocytes at concentrations 1/6-3 times normal *1790*

Cocaethylene *Urine No Effect Analytical* No interference observed with TLC method of Bailey *328*

Color *Urine Increase Analytical* Brown color *1714*

Coombs' Test *Blood Positive Physiological* Immunological response to drug *2453*

Quinine *(continued)*

Coombs' Test, Direct *Blood Positive Physiological* Associated with hemolytic anemia *2452*

Creatine Kinase *Serum No Effect Analytical* At acute overdose concentration (1.5 mg/dL) on Technicon SMAC® method *6266*

Creatinine *Serum No Effect Analytical* At concentration of 30 mg/L had no effect on Technicon AutoAnalyzer® Jaffe method *5704* At acute overdose concentration (1.5 mg/dL) on Technicon SMAC® method *6266*

Diagnex Blue Excretion *Urine Increase Analytical* Release of dye from resin *4012*

Digitoxin *Serum Increase Physiological* Increased concentrations observed with concomitant administration of digitoxin and quinine *1384*

Digoxin *Serum Increase Physiological* Total body clearance reduced with increase of renal elimination half-life. Urine excretion increased *6336* Interaction may produce 50% increase in concentration *827* Stepwise increase with increasing quinine dose due to impairment of extrarenal digoxin clearance *4583*

Drugs of Abuse Screen *Urine No Effect Analytical* No effect at concentration of 100 µg/mL on EZ-SCREEN procedure for cannabinoids and cocaine *1739*

Erythrocyte Sedimentation Rate
Blood Decrease Physiological At therapeutic concentration, maximum at 200 minutes with 2 mg/dL *4977*

Erythrocytes *Blood Decrease Physiological* Hemolytic anemia (sensitivity dependent) G-6-PD deficiency *461*

Glucose *Serum Decrease Physiological* Intravenous drug reduced concentration from 88 to 68 mg/dL in normal volunteers *6426*
Serum No Effect Analytical At acute overdose concentration (1.5 mg/dL) on Technicon SMAC® method *6266*

Haptoglobin *Serum Decrease Physiological* May cause hemolytic anemia *3895*

Hematocrit *Blood Decrease Physiological* Hemolytic anemia (sensitivity dependent) G-6-PD deficiency *461*

Hemoglobin *Blood Decrease Physiological* Hemolytic anemia (sensitivity dependent) G-6-PD deficiency *461*
Urine Increase Physiological Possible contributing factor *128*

Histamine *Plasma No Effect Analytical* 50% inhibition of radio-enzyme assay at about 4 times therapeutic concentration *2492*

17-Hydroxycorticosteroids *Urine Increase Analytical* Reddy method affected, not Porter-Silber method *5869*
Urine No Effect Analytical No effect on modified Porter-Silber reaction *2452*

Insulin *Plasma Increase Physiological* Intravenous drug in normal volunteers increased concentration from 8.9 to 17.1 mU/L *6426*

Iron *Serum No Effect Analytical* At acute overdose concentration (1.5 mg/dL) on Technicon SMAC® method *6266* At concentration of 15 mg/L had no effect on Ferrozine method *5704*

Lactate Dehydrogenase *Serum No Effect Analytical* At acute overdose concentration (1.5 mg/dL) on Technicon SMAC® method *6266*

Leukocytes *Blood Decrease Physiological* Leukopenia (AMA Blood dyscrasias) *4017*
Blood Increase Physiological Primary increase, especially of lymphocytes (splenic contractions) *2242*

Methemalbumin *Serum Increase Physiological* If given concurrently with pamaquine *2242*

Methemoglobin *Blood Increase Physiological* May cause hemolysis in G-6-PD deficiency *6015*

Neutrophils *Blood Decrease Physiological* Occasional case of agranulocytosis reported *6264*

p-Aminophenol *Urine No Effect Analytical* With addition of drugs at a concentration of 100 mg/L and of related compounds at 50 mg/L no significant effect observed on colorimetric method of van Bocxlaer on Cobas Mira analyzer which involves reacting free p-aminophenol with resorcinol in the presence of magnesium ions to form an indophenol dye measured at 550 nm *6163*

Phosphate *Serum No Effect Analytical* At acute overdose concentration (1.5 mg/dL) on Technicon SMAC® method *6266* At concentration of 30 mg/L had no effect on phosphomolybdate method *5704*

Platelets *Blood Decrease Physiological* Several cases of immune thrombocytopenia reported *4139* Quinine dependent antibody caused platelet lysis *1044* Immunological mechanism *1170*

Potassium *Serum No Effect Analytical* At concentration of 30 mg/L had no effect on measurement by ISE with predilution *5704*

Pramipexole *Serum Increase Physiological* Coadministration of quinine with pramipexole presumed to decrease the oral clearance of pramipexole by about 20% *4680*

Protein *Serum No Effect Analytical* At concentration of 30 mg/L had no effect on biuret method with blank correction *5704* At acute overdose concentration (1.5 mg/dL) on Technicon SMAC® method *6266*
Urine Increase Physiological May rarely cause renal damage *2242*

Prothrombin Time *Plasma Increase Physiological* Depresses prothrombin formation in liver *1405*

Quinidine *Serum No Effect Analytical* No significant interference observed at a concentration of 20 µg/mL (61.6 µmol/L) with method on Du Pont aca *1543* At concentrations greater than 1000 mg/L concentration as measured by Baxter Stratus increased by 30% but physiological concentration only up to 7 mg/L *5705* Quinine at a concentration of 20 µg/mL had no significant cross-reactivity with quinidine at a concentration of 2.0 µg/mL in method on Bayer Technicon Immuno 1® *431*
Serum No Effect Physiological Quinine has no effect on the pharmacokinetics of quinidine *5996*

Riluzole *Serum No Effect Physiological* No effect on riluzole binding observed *4941*

Sodium *Serum No Effect Analytical* At concentration of 30 mg/L had no effect on measurement by ISE with predilution *5704*

Triglycerides *Serum No Effect Analytical* At concentration of 30 mg/L had no effect on lipase/esterase method *5704* At acute overdose concentration (1.5 mg/dL) on Technicon SMAC® method *6266*

Urea Nitrogen *Serum Increase Physiological* May cause renal damage (rare) *2242*
Serum No Effect Analytical At concentration of 30 mg/L had no effect on diacetylmonoxime method *5704* At acute overdose concentration (1.5 mg/dL) on Technicon SMAC® method *6266*

Uric Acid *Serum No Effect Analytical* At concentration of 30 mg/L had no effect on phosphotungstate reduction method *5704* At acute overdose concentration (1.5 mg/dL) on Technicon SMAC® method *6266*

Quinocide

Erythrocytes *Blood Decrease Physiological* May cause hemolysis with G-6-PD deficiency *3094*

Hematocrit *Blood Decrease Physiological* May cause hemolysis with G-6-PD deficiency *3094*

Hemoglobin *Blood Decrease Physiological* May cause hemolytic anemia *3094*

Quinolones

Alanine Aminotransferase *Serum Increase Physiological* Transient increases in activity noted in 2-3% treated patients *2704*

Aspartate Aminotransferase *Serum Increase Physiological* Transient increases noted in 2-3% treated patients *2704*

Crystals *Urine Increase Physiological* When large doses given and urine alkaline crystalluria may occur but without renal toxicity *2704*

Cyclosporine A *Blood No Effect Physiological* No interaction between caffeine and ofloxacin reported: unknown whether ofloxacin has this specific effect *3914*

Eosinophils *Blood Increase Physiological* Transient eosinophilia noted in 0.2-2% patients treated with drugs *2704*

Hemoglobin *Urine Increase Physiological* Rare cases of hematuria reported following treatment with acute interstitial nephritis and acute renal failure *2704*

Leukocytes *Blood Decrease Physiological* Transient mild leukopenia noted in 0.2-3% treated patients *2704*

Warfarin *Plasma Increase Physiological* Some quinolones reported to enhance the effect of warfarin reported: unknown whether ofloxacin has this specific effect *3914*

R-568

Calcium *Urine Increase Physiological* In 8 postmenopausal women with mild primary hyperparathyroidism receiving 160 mg/d R-568 median excretion increased from about 260 mg/g creatinine to 630 mg/g creatinine after 4 hours and 390 mg/g creatinine after 8 hours *5556*

ionized Calcium *Serum Decrease Physiological* In 8 postmenopausal women with mild primary hyperparathyroidism receiving 160 mg/d R-568 median concentration decreased from almost 1.35 mmol/L to 1.295 mmol/L after 4 hours and 1.31 mmol/L after 8 hours *5556*

Parathyroid Hormone *Plasma Decrease Physiological* In 20 postmenopausal women with mild primary hyperparathyroidism receiving either 20, 80 or 160 mg/d R-568 median concentration decreased by 26% from 77 ± 11 pg/mL to 57 ± 10 pg/mL 2 h after the 20 mg dose, by 42% from 79 ± 22 pg/mL to 46 ± 7 pg/mL after the 80 mg dose and by 51% from 65 ± 12 pg/mL to 32 ± 10 pg/mL after the 160 mg dose, but no significant effect observed after 4 and 10 mg doses *5556*

Radioactive Compounds

Erythrocytes *Blood Decrease Physiological* Aplastic anemia *3810*

Leukocytes *Blood Decrease Physiological* May cause marrow depression *3810*

Prothrombin Time *Plasma Increase Physiological* Also exaggerated response to anticoagulants *2242*

Uric Acid *Serum Increase Physiological* May occur with tissue destruction *467*

Radioactive Iodine

Apolipoprotein A-I *Serum No Effect Physiological* In 28 hyperthyroid patients treatment with RAI caused mean concentration to change not significantly to 2.24 ± 0.49 g/L from baseline of 2.07 ± 0.42 g/L *3322*

Apolipoprotein B *Serum Increase Physiological* In 28 hyperthyroid patients treatment with RAI caused mean concentration to increase to 0.97 ± 0.28 g/L significantly different from baseline of 0.66 ± 0.23 g/L *3322*

Apolipoprotein Lp(a) *Serum Increase Physiological* In 28 hyperthyroid patients treatment with RAI caused mean concentration to increase to 119 IU/L significantly different from baseline of 81 IU/L *3322*

Cholesterol *Serum Increase Physiological* In 28 hyperthyroid patients treatment with RAI caused mean concentration to increase to 5.45 ± 1.63 mmol/L significantly different from baseline of 4.07 ± 0.80 mmol/L *3322*

HDL-Cholesterol *Serum No Effect Physiological* In 28 hyperthyroid patients treatment with RAI caused mean concentration to change not significantly to 0.97 ± 0.24 mmol/L from baseline of 1.05 ± 0.33 mmol/L *3322*

LDL-Cholesterol *Serum Increase Physiological* In 28 hyperthyroid patients treatment with RAI caused mean concentration to increase to 3.81 ± 1.65 mmol/L significantly different from baseline of 2.47 ± 0.77 mmol/L *3322*

Leukocytes *Blood Increase Physiological* Incidence of acute leukemia higher *128*

Thyroxine (T4) Index, Free *Serum Decrease Physiological* In 28 hyperthyroid patients treatment with RAI caused mean index to decrease to 112 ± 30 significantly different from baseline of 302 ± 80 *3322*

Triglycerides *Serum Increase Physiological* In 28 hyperthyroid patients treatment with RAI caused mean concentration to increase to 1.56 ± 0.70 mmol/L significantly different from baseline of 1.18 ± 0.44 mmol/L *3322*

Radiographic Agents

Alanine Aminopeptidase *Urine Increase Physiological* In 10 control individuals administration of digital subtraction angiography caused mean increase from baseline of 1.62 U/mmol creatinine to 1.93 U/mmol creatinine with other changes to 3.69, 1.72 and 1.53 U/mmol creatinine on days 2, 3 and 4 respectively *2784* Marked increase within 1 d when used for arteriography: effect persisted for many days: effect less when used for urography *5455*

Albumin *Urine Increase Physiological* Mean increase from 34 mg/d to 1873 mg/d in 37 patients day following arteriography *4284*

Alkaline Phosphatase *Urine Increase Physiological* May occur after i.v. pyelography or aortography *135*

Amylase *Pancreatic Fluid No Effect Analytical* No effect of Gastrografin® *1152*
Serum Increase Physiological Cholangiography may cause transient increase *2452*

Appearance *Urine Abnormal Physiological* Cloudy, in acid urine *684*

Aspartate Aminotransferase *Urine Increase Physiological* Transient increase if injected in renal artery *5935*

Bilirubin *Serum Increase Physiological* Competition for excretion through bile canaliculi *189*

BSP Retention *Serum Increase Physiological* Compete for excretory mechanism *834*

Casts *Urine Increase Physiological* Nephrotoxic manifestation *1009*

Catalase *Urine Increase Physiological* Transient increase with slight renal damage if injected into renal artery *5935*

Catecholamines *Urine Decrease Physiological* Competes for excretion after i.v. pyelography *1444*

Creatine Kinase *Urine Increase Physiological* Transient increase if injected into renal artery *5935*

Creatinine *Serum Increase Physiological* Frequency of renal impairment following CT brain scan with infusion 2.1% compared with 1.3% in control group *1157* Occasional effect following aortography *116* Incidence of clinically-important contrast-induced renal failure in diabetic patients with preexisting renal insufficiency was 8.8% compared with 1.6% for controls. No clinically important acute renal failure in nondiabetics with normal renal function *4512* In normal people 2%: in patients with renal dysfunction 30% subclinical damage following non-renal angiography *1364*
Serum No Effect Physiological No significant change observed when agents given for either urography or arteriography *5455*

Crystals *Urine Increase Physiological* Diatrizoate may produce crystals in acid urine *684*

β-Endorphin *Cerebrospinal Fluid Increase Analytical* Artifactual increase observed when radiographic contrast media injected into cerebral ventricles due to interference of radiographic agent with antigen-antibody binding and quenching of γ radiation emitted by iodinated peptide ligands *1435*

Erythrocytes *Urine Increase Physiological* Nephrotoxic manifestation *1009*

Glomerular Filtration Rate *Urine Decrease Physiological* If concentrated solutions used for aortography *116*

Glucose *Urine Decrease Analytical* Hypaque Meglumine may cause reduced reactivity and false negative reaction with Ames Clinitest tablet procedure *4034*
Urine No Effect Analytical Hypaque Meglumine has no effect on Ames Keto-Diastix, Diastix, Multistix and Clinistix procedures *4034*

γ-Glutamyltransferase *Urine Increase Physiological* In 10 control individuals administration of digital subtraction angiography excretion increased from mean baseline of 3.56 U/mmol creatinine to 3.77 U/mmol creatinine with subsequent changes to 5.96, 3.32 and 3.10 U/mmol on days 2, 3 and 4 respectively *2784*

Radiographic Agents *(continued)*

Hematocrit *Blood Decrease Physiological* Transient fall following rapid i.v. injection *927*

Histamine *Plasma Increase Physiological* Observed in some patients if administered i.v *694*

Immunoglobulin G *Urine Increase Physiological* Mean increase from 6.1 mg/d to 206.3 mg/d in 37 patients day following arteriography *4284*

Lactate Dehydrogenase *Urine Increase Physiological* Transient increase if injected into renal artery *5935*

Leucine Aminopeptidase *Urine Increase Physiological* Facilitates permeation of enzyme into tubules *4826*

Lipase *Pancreatic Fluid No Effect Analytical* No effect of Gastrografin® *1152*

Lysozyme *Urine Increase Physiological* Marked increase within 1 d when used for arteriography: effect persisted for many days: effect less when used for urography *5455*
Urine No Effect Physiological No change from 3.3 mg/d to 3.3 mg/d in 37 patients day following arteriography *4284*

β_2-Microglobulin *Urine No Effect Physiological* Mean increase from 2.9 mg/d to 5.4 mg/d in 37 patients day following arteriography *4284*

Myoglobin *Serum No Effect Analytical* No significant effect of iodine-containing contrast media with iodine concentrations up to 24 g/L on nephelometric method of Behringwerke *1360* Addition of Omnipaque to a final iodine concentration of 24 g/L had no effect on Behring Turbiquant method *1359*

N-Acetyl-Glucosaminidase *Urine Increase Physiological* Marked increase within 1 d when used for arteriography: effect persisted for many days: effect less when used for urography *5455* In 10 control patients given digital subtraction angiography mean excretion increased from baseline of 7.0 U/mmol creatinine to 7.8 U/mmol creatinine with increases to 10.4, 7.8 and 8.0 U/mmol creatinine on days 2, 3 and 4 respectively *2784*

PAH Clearance *Urine Decrease Physiological* If concentrated solutions used for aortography *116*
Urine No Effect Physiological No effect of arteriography *4284*

Partial Thromboplastin Time
Plasma Increase Physiological ?Transient inactivation of coagulation factors *2452*

Phosphate Clearance *Urine Decrease Physiological* Mean decrease from 12.9 mL/min/1.73 m^2 to 7.1 mL/min/1.73 m^2 day following arteriography in 37 patients *4284*

Protein *Cerebrospinal Fluid Increase Analytical* Causes turbidity if sulfosalicylic acid procedure used *5869* Bias of 1000 mg/dL or more with Isovue-M and 20-30 mg/dL with Omnipaque with method on Kodak Ektachem® systems *2519*
Serum Increase Analytical May produce interfering turbidity *3810*
Urine Increase Analytical Affects biuret part of Doetsch procedure *1458* Affects turbidimetric methods for some days *5869* May cause false positive with Sulfosalicylic Acid and Exton's reagent tests *4034* Affects sulfosalicylic, heat and acetic acid tests *3044* Turbidity if acid procedures used *2787*
Urine Increase Physiological May occur following aortography *116* Mean increase from 129 mg/d to 2760 mg/d in 37 patients day following arteriography *4284* Observed in small number of patients receiving agents for arteriography *5455*
Urine No Effect Analytical On Combistix® , Urostix, Albustix etc *3044* Have no effect on protein test area on Ames Multistix and other reagent test strips *4034*

Protein Electrophoresis *Serum Positive Analytical* Produce uninterpretable pattern *6515*

Prothrombin Time *Plasma Increase Physiological* ?Transient inactivation of coagulation factors *2452*

PSP Excretion *Urine Increase Physiological* Affect renal excretion *2024*

Specific Gravity *Urine Increase Analytical* Presence of high molecular weight substance *5869* *2787* Increase observed when specific gravity measured by either T.S. meter (refractometer) or urinometr (hydrometer) *4034*
Urine No Effect Analytical No effect observed when measured by Ames Multistix and other reagent strip tests *4034*

Sugar *Urine Increase Analytical* Green-black reaction with reducing procedures *882*

Thyroid Stimulating Hormone
Serum Increase Physiological Observed after administration of iodine-containing radiographic contrast agents *1269* Substantial increase 3 d after oral cholecystography *3422*

Thyroxine (T4) *Serum Increase Analytical* Orabilix and Dionosil® affect at 1 mg *5402*
Serum Increase Physiological In first few days following oral cholecystographic agents *3422*
Serum No Effect Analytical Most agents in low concentration *5402*

Thyroxine (T4), Free *Serum Increase Physiological* Observed after administration of iodine-containing contrast agents, probably due to inhibition of 5'-monodeiodoination of T4: effect observed 3-4 days after administration and disappears after 14 days *1269*

Transferrin *Urine Increase Physiological* Mean increase from 2.8 mg/d to 147.1 mg/d in 37 patients day following arteriography *4284*

Tri-iodothyronine, Free (fT3)
Serum Decrease Physiological Observed after administration of iodine-containing contrast agents *1269*

Tri-iodothyronine, Reverse (rT3)
Serum Increase Physiological Marked increase observed after administration of iodine-containing contrast agents, probably largely due to inhibition of 5'-monodeiodoination of reverse T3: effect maximal 3-4 days after administration and disappears within 14 days *1269* In first few days following oral cholecystographic agents *3422*

Tri-iodothyronine (T3) *Serum Decrease Physiological* In first few days following oral cholecystographic agents *3422* Associated with decreased plasma concentration *2412*

Trypsin *Feces Decrease Analytical* Inhibition of esterase by Gastrografin® *1152*

TSH response to TRH *Serum Increase Physiological* Observed after administration of iodine-containing contrast agents *1269*

Urea Nitrogen *Serum Increase Physiological* May produce azotemia or renal failure *128*

Uric Acid *Serum Decrease Physiological* Interferes with reabsorption *4847*

Uric Acid Clearance *Urine No Effect Physiological* No effect of arteriography *4284*

Urobilinogen *Urine Increase Analytical* Turbidity in acid solutions *882*

Vanillylmandelic Acid *Urine Decrease Physiological* Competes for excretion after i.v. pyelography *1444*

Raloxifene

Albumin *Serum Decrease Physiological* Small decreases in concentration observed with treatment *1696*

Alkaline Phosphatase, Bone Isoenzyme
Serum Decrease Physiological In approximately 150 postmenopausal women receiving 60 mg/d raloxifene median activity decreased by 23.1% over a period of 24 months *1371*

Apolipoprotein A-I *Serum Increase Physiological* Increased concentration observed with treatment *1696*
Serum No Effect Physiological In 390 healthy postmenopausal women randomized to treatment with 60 mg/d or 120 mg/d raloxifene or 0.625 mg/d conjugated equine estrogen and 2.5 mg/d medroxyprogesterone acetate caused insignificant changes of 2 ± 2% increase with 60 mg/d raloxifene and 5 ± 1% with 120 mg/d at 6 months *6332*

Apolipoprotein B *Serum Decrease Physiological* Decreased concentration observed with treatment *1696* In 390 healthy postmenopausal women randomized to treatment with 60 mg/d or 120 mg/d raloxifene or 0.625 mg/d conjugated equine estrogen and 2.5 mg/d medroxyprogesterone acetate caused insignificant changes of 9 ± 2% decrease with 60 mg/d raloxifene and 9 ± 1% with 120 mg/d at 6 months *6332*

Apolipoprotein Lp(a) *Serum Decrease Physiological* Decreased concentration observed with treatment *1696*

Calcium *Serum Decrease Physiological* Small decreases in concentration observed with treatment *1696*

Cholesterol *Serum Decrease Physiological* In approximately 150 postmenopausal women receiving either 30, 60 or 150 mg/d raloxifene median concentration decreased by approximately 3%, 5% and 9% respectively over a period of 3 months with little further change being observed over the next 21 months *1371* Reduces concentration by 6 to 11% *1696*

Corticosteroid-Binding Globulin *Serum Increase Physiological* Moderately increases concentration and bound hormones with treatment *1696*

Digoxin *Serum No Effect Physiological* Has no effect on the pharmacokinetics of digoxin *1696*

Fibrinogen *Plasma Decrease Physiological* In 390 healthy postmenopausal women randomized to treatment with 60 mg/d or 120 mg/d raloxifene or 0.625 mg/d conjugated equine estrogen and 2.5 mg/d medroxyprogesterone acetate caused significant changes of 12 ± 11% decrease with 60 mg/d raloxifene and 14 ± 4% with 120 mg/d at 6 months *6332* Decreased concentration observed with treatment *1696*

Fibrinopeptide A *Plasma No Effect Physiological* In 390 healthy postmenopausal women randomized to treatment with 60 mg/d or 120 mg/d raloxifene or 0.625 mg/d conjugated equine estrogen and 2.5 mg/d medroxyprogesterone acetate caused insignificant changes of 9 ± 3% increase with 60 mg/d raloxifene and 9 ± 6% with 120 mg/d at 6 months *6332*

HDL_2-Cholesterol *Serum Increase Physiological* In 390 healthy postmenopausal women randomized to treatment with 60 mg/d or 120 mg/d raloxifene or 0.625 mg/d conjugated equine estrogen and 2.5 mg/d medroxyprogesterone acetate caused significant changes of 15 ± 6% increase with 60 mg/d raloxifene and 17 ± 7% with 120 mg/d at 6 months *6332*

HDL-Cholesterol *Serum Decrease Physiological* In approximately 150 postmenopausal women receiving either 30, 60 or 150 mg/d raloxifene median concentration decreased nonsignificantly by approximately 3%, 4% and 5% respectively over a period of 24 months *1371*
Serum No Effect Physiological Has no significant effect on concentration *1696* In 390 healthy postmenopausal women randomized to treatment with 60 mg/d or 120 mg/d raloxifene or 0.625 mg/d conjugated equine estrogen and 2.5 mg/d medroxyprogesterone acetate caused insignificant changes of 1 ± 2% increase with 60 mg/d raloxifene and 4 ± 1% with 120 mg/d at 6 months *6332*

LDL-Cholesterol *Serum Decrease Physiological* In 390 healthy postmenopausal women randomized to treatment with 60 mg/d or 120 mg/d raloxifene or 0.625 mg/d conjugated equine estrogen and 2.5 mg/d medroxyprogesterone acetate caused median decrease of 11 ± 2% decrease with both doses of raloxifene at both 3 and 6 months *6332* Reduces concentration by 6 to 11% *1696* In approximately 150 postmenopausal women receiving either 30, 60 or 150 mg/d raloxifene median concentration decreased by approximately 5%, 8% and 13% respectively over a period of 3 months with little further change being observed over the next 21 months *1371*

Lipoprotein Lp(a) *Serum Decrease Physiological* In 390 healthy postmenopausal women randomized to treatment with 60 mg/d or 120 mg/d raloxifene or 0.625 mg/d conjugated equine estrogen and 2.5 mg/d medroxyprogesterone acetate caused significant changes of 4 ± 2% decrease with 60 mg/d raloxifene and 4 ± 3% with 120 mg/d at 6 months *6332*

Osteocalcin *Serum Decrease Physiological* In approximately 150 postmenopausal women receiving 60 mg/d raloxifene median concentration decreased from 24.6 ± 0.4 µg/L by 15.0% over a period of 24 months *1371*

Phosphate *Serum Decrease Physiological* Small decreases in concentration observed with treatment *1696*

Plasminogen Activator Inhibitor-1 *Plasma No Effect Physiological* In 390 healthy postmenopausal women randomized to treatment with 60 mg/d or 120 mg/d raloxifene or 0.625 mg/d conjugated equine estrogen and 2.5 mg/d medroxyprogesterone acetate caused insignificant changes of 2 ± 3% decrease with 60 mg/d raloxifene and 2 ± 4% with 120 mg/d at 6 months *6332*

Platelets *Blood Decrease Physiological* Small decreases in concentration observed with treatment *1696*

Protein *Serum Decrease Physiological* Small decreases in concentration observed with treatment *1696*

Prothrombin Fragment 1.2 *Plasma No Effect Physiological* In 390 healthy postmenopausal women randomized to treatment with 60 mg/d or 120 mg/d raloxifene or 0.625 mg/d conjugated equine estrogen and 2.5 mg/d medroxyprogesterone acetate caused insignificant changes of 2 ± 2% decrease with 60 mg/d raloxifene and 1± 3% with 120 mg/d at 6 months *6332*

Prothrombin Time *Plasma Decrease Physiological* Reported to cause a 10% decrease in prothrombin time in patients receiving warfarin when coadministered with warfarin *1696*

Sex-Hormone Binding Globulin *Serum Increase Physiological* Moderately increases concentration and bound hormones with treatment *1696*

Thyroxine Binding Globulin *Serum Increase Physiological* Moderately increases concentration and bound hormones with treatment *1696*

Thyroxine (T4) *Serum Increase Physiological* Moderately increases concentration and bound hormones with treatment *1696*

Triglycerides *Serum No Effect Physiological* Has no significant effect on concentration *1696* In 390 healthy postmenopausal women randomized to treatment with 60 mg/d or 120 mg/d raloxifene or 0.625 mg/d conjugated equine estrogen and 2.5 mg/d medroxyprogesterone acetate caused insignificant changes of 4 ± 2% decrease with 60 mg/d raloxifene and 0 ± 4% with 120 mg/d at 6 months *6332* In approximately 150 postmenopausal women receiving either 30, 60 or 150 mg/d raloxifene median concentration decreased nonsignificantly by approximately 0%, 3% and 1% respectively over a period of 24 months *1371*

Type I Collagen Cross-linked C-telopeptide *Urine Decrease Physiological* In approximately 150 postmenopausal women receiving 60 mg/d raloxifene median excretion decreased from 292.5 ± 6.5 µg/mmol creatinine by 34.0% over a period of 24 months *1371*

Ramipril

Alanine Aminopeptidase *Urine No Effect Physiological* In 11 patients with congestive heart failure mean excretion unchanged following administration of 5 mg/d for 2 weeks *2542*

Alanine Aminotransferase *Serum Increase Physiological* Rarely clinically important change noted with treatment *2638*

Albumin *Urine Decrease Physiological* In 11 patients with congestive heart failure treatment with 5 mg/d ramipril for 2 weeks caused significant decrease from mean baseline of 23.8 ± 27.4 mg/d to 12.4 ± 12.7 mg/d on day 15 *2542*

Aldosterone *Plasma Decrease Physiological* In response to 10 mg and 20 mg on successive days in 9 patients with severe chronic congestive heart failure *1180* In 111 patients with mild or moderate congestive heart failure treatment for 12 weeks caused significant reduction from mean baseline of 387 ± 317 pmol/L to 274 ± 165 pmol/L *5551*

Alkaline Phosphatase *Serum Increase Physiological* Rarely clinically important change noted with treatment *2638*

Angiotensin-II *Plasma Decrease Physiological* In response to 10 mg and 20 mg on successive days in 9 patients with severe chronic congestive heart failure *1180* In 111 patients with mild or moderate congestive heart failure treatment for 12 weeks caused significant reduction from mean baseline of 14.4 ± 18.5 pmo/L to 11.7 ± 15.5 pmol/L *5551*

Angiotensin-converting Enzyme *Serum Decrease Physiological* Almost 100% inhibition after 2 hours in 10 patients with essential hypertension following 10 mg orally *6212* In 111 patients with mild or moderate congestive heart failure treatment for 12 weeks caused significant reduction from mean baseline of 1.45 ± 0.53 µkat/L to 0.41 ± 0.38 µkat/L *5551* In response to 10 mg and 20 mg on successive days in 9 patients with severe chronic congestive heart failure *1180*

Antidiuretic Hormone *Plasma No Effect Physiological* In response to 10 mg and 20 mg on successive days in 9 patients with severe chronic congestive heart failure *1180*

Aspartate Aminotransferase *Serum Increase Physiological* Rarely clinically important change noted with treatment *2638*

Ramipril *(continued)*

Atrial Natriuretic Peptide *Plasma Decrease Physiological* In 111 patients with mild or moderate congestive heart failure treatment for 12 weeks caused significant reduction from mean baseline of 241 ± 138 pg/mL to 204 ± 123 pg/mL *5551*

Bilirubin *Serum Increase Physiological* Rarely clinically important change noted with treatment *2638*

Catecholamines *Plasma No Effect Physiological* In response to 10 mg and 20 mg on successive days in 9 patients with severe chronic congestive heart failure *1180*

Cholesterol *Serum Decrease Physiological* Slight reduction observed in 21 hypertensive noninsulin dependent diabetics given mean dose of 5 mg/d for 12 weeks although effect might be partly due to associated weight loss *2896*

Cortisol *Plasma No Effect Physiological* In response to 10 mg and 20 mg on successive days in 9 patients with severe chronic congestive heart failure *1180*

C-Peptide *Plasma No Effect Physiological* No significant effect observed in 21 noninsulin dependent hypertensive diabetics given mean dose of 5 mg/d for 12 weeks *2896*

Creatinine *Serum Increase Physiological* In response to 10 mg and 20 mg on successive days in 9 patients with severe chronic congestive heart failure *1180* Increases in serum creatinine concentration occurred in 1.2% of 651 patients in controlled clinical trials when ramipril give alone and in 1.5% when a diuretic coadministered *2638* In some patients with congestive cardiac failure treatment with ACE inhibitors may be associated with oliguria and/or progressive azotemia and rarely with acute renal failure. May also be observed in hypertensives with unilateral or bilateral renal artery stenosis *2638*

Creatinine Clearance *Urine Increase Physiological* In 11 patients with congestive heart failure treatment with 5 mg/d for 2 weeks caused significant increase from mean baseline of 78.8 ± 38.3 mL/min to 91.7 ± 36.4 mL/min *2542*

Digoxin *Serum No Effect Physiological* When ramipril coadministered with digoxin no effect observed on its concentration *2638*

Effective Renal Plasma Flow
Patient No Effect Physiological In 7 patients with essential hypertension treatment with 10 mg daily for 2 to 4 weeks had insignificant increase on average *118*

Eosinophils *Blood Increase Physiological* Scattered clinically important change noted with treatment *2638*

Erythrocytes *Blood Decrease Physiological* Pancytopenia,hemolytic anemia and thrombocytopenia may occur as complications *2638*

Furosemide *Serum No Effect Physiological* When ramipril coadministered with furosemide no effect observed on the action of either drug *2638*

Glucose *Serum Decrease Physiological* Slight but significant reduction from mean baseline concentration of 8.5 mmol/L to 8.0 mmol/L in 21 hypertensive patients with noninsulin dependent diabetes mellitus treated with 5 mg/d for 12 weeks *2896* Incidence of 1.6% observed in French Pharmacovigilance database *4106*
Serum Increase Physiological Rarely clinically important change noted with treatment *2638*

γ-Glutamyltransferase *Urine No Effect Physiological* In 11 patients with congestive heart failure treatment with 5 mg/d for 2 weeks had no significant effect on excretion *2542*

HDL-Cholesterol *Serum Increase Physiological* Slight increase observed in 21 hypertensive noninsulin dependent diabetics given mean dose of 5 mg/d for 12 weeks although effect might be partly due to associated weight loss *2896*

Hematocrit *Blood Decrease Physiological* In a clinical trial of 561 patients a decrease of 5% occurred rarely (in 0.4% patients receiving ramipril alone and in 1.5% in patients in whom a diuretic was coadministered) *2638*

Hemoglobin *Blood Decrease Physiological* In a clinical trial of 561 patients a decrease of 5 g/dL occurred rarely (in 0.4% patients receiving ramipril alone and in 1.5% in patients in whom a diuretic was coadministered) *2638*

Hemoglobin A_{1c} *Blood Decrease Physiological* Slight but significant reduction from mean baseline of 10.0% to 9.7% in 21 hypertensive noninsulin dependent diabetics given mean dose of 5 mg/d for 12 weeks *2896*

Indomethacin *Serum No Effect Physiological* When ramipril coadministered with indomethacin no effect observed on the action of either drug *2638*

Lactate Dehydrogenase *Urine Decrease Physiological* In 11 patients with congestive heart failure treatment with 5 mg/d for 2 weeks caused significant decrease from mean baseline of 12.8 ± 9.0 U/d to 4.7 ± 3.7 U/d on day 15 *2542*

Leukocytes *Blood Decrease Physiological* Pancytopenia, hemolytic anemia and thrombocytopenia may occur as complications *2638*

Lithium *Serum Increase Physiological* When ramipril coadministered with lithium the lithium concentration was typically increased *2638*

Norepinephrine *Plasma Decrease Physiological* In 111 patients with mild or moderate congestive heart failure treatment for 12 weeks caused significant reduction from mean baseline of 2.69 ± 1.52 nmol/L to 2.48 ± 0.98 pmol/L *5551*

Phenprocoumon *Plasma No Effect Physiological* When ramipril coadministered with phenprocoumon no effect observed on the anticoagulant effect of phenprocoumon *2638*

Platelets *Blood Decrease Physiological* Pancytopenia,hemolytic anemia and thrombocytopenia may occur as complications *2638*

Potassium *Serum Increase Physiological* In clinical trials serum potassium concentrations above 5.7 mmol/L were observed in about 1% patients *2638* In response to 10 mg and 20 mg on successive days in 9 patients with severe chronic congestive heart failure *1180* Ramipril decreases aldosterone secretion and may increase plasma concentration of potassium *2638*
Urine Decrease Physiological In response to 10 mg and 20 mg on successive days in 9 patients with severe chronic congestive heart failure *1180*

Prolidase *Serum No Effect Analytical* Slight inhibitory effect in vitro but at much higher concentrations than therapeutic *4197*

Propranolol *Serum No Effect Physiological* When ramipril coadministered with propranolol no adverse effects observed on dynamic parameters *2638*

Protein *Urine Increase Physiological* Scattered clinically important change noted with treatment *2638*

Renin Activity *Plasma Increase Physiological* In response to 10 mg and 20 mg on successive days in 9 patients with severe chronic congestive heart failure *1180* Increase from mean baseline concentration of about 12 μU/mL to 40 μU/mL at 2 hours and 45 μU/mL at 3 hours in 10 patients with essential hypertension following single oral dose of 10 mg *6212*

Simvastatin *Serum No Effect Physiological* When ramipril coadministered with simvastatin no effect observed on the action of either drug *2638*

Sodium *Serum Decrease Physiological* Rarely clinically important change noted with treatment *2638*
Serum Increase Physiological In response to 10 mg and 20 mg on successive days in 9 patients with severe chronic congestive heart failure *1180*
Urine Decrease Physiological In response to 10 mg and 20 mg on successive days in 9 patients with severe chronic congestive heart failure *1180*

Urea Nitrogen *Serum Increase Physiological* Increases in serum urea nitrogen concentration occurred in 0.5% of 651 patients in controlled clinical trials when ramipril give alone and in 3% when a diuretic coadministered *2638* In some patients with congestive cardiac failure treatment with ACE inhibitors may be associated with oliguria and/or progressive azotemia and rarely with acute renal failure. May also be observed in hypertensive with unilateral or bilateral renal artery stenosis *2638*

Uric Acid *Serum Increase Physiological* Rarely clinically important change noted with treatment *2638*

Warfarin *Plasma No Effect Physiological* When ramipril coadministered with warfarin no effect observed on the anticoagulant effect of warfarin *2638*

Ramixotidine

Estradiol *Plasma No Effect Physiological* No significant effect on estradiol-17β concentration of treatment with 750 mg/day for 2 weeks in healthy male volunteers *1092*

Gastrin *Serum No Effect Physiological* No significant effect observed in healthy male volunteers treated with 750 mg/day for 2 weeks *1092*

Prolactin *Plasma No Effect Physiological* No significant effect of treatment with 750 mg/day for 2 weeks in healthy male volunteers *1092*

Testosterone *Serum No Effect Physiological* No significant effect of treatment with 750 mg/day for 2 weeks in healthy male volunteers *1092*

Ranitidine

Acetylsalicylic Acid *Serum No Effect Physiological* Pretreatment with 300 mg daily for 7 days did not affect area under the curve or elimination half-life *4062*

Alanine Aminotransferase *Serum Increase Physiological* In normal volunteers activities increased to at least twice the pretreatment levels in 6 of 12 patients receiving 100 mg q.i.d. intravenously for 7 days and in 4 of 24 patients receiving 50 mg q.i.d. intravenously for 5 days. There have been occasional reports of hepatitis, hepatocellular or hepatocanalicular or mixed, with or without jaundice *2169*

Aldosterone *Plasma Decrease Physiological* Significant reduction in plasma aldosterone in both recumbent overnight concentration and after 2 h ambulation with 3-day oral course *5219*

Plasma No Effect Analytical No effect of up to 5 µg/mL on method of Sancho and Haber *5219*

Plasma No Effect Physiological No effect observed with ranitidine administration *2169* Bolus injections have no effect on basal secretion *3872*

Alendronate *Serum Increase Physiological* Intravenous administration of ranitidine doubled the bioavailability of alendronate *3976*

Alkaline Phosphatase *Serum Increase Physiological* There have been occasional reports of hepatitis, hepatocellular or hepatocanalicular or mixed, with or without jaundice *2169*

Amoxicillin *Serum Decrease Physiological* Slight but significant reduction in 10 healthy volunteers when 3 doses of 150 mg given with 1000 mg amoxicillin (concentration reduced from 11.4 mg/L to 10.0 mg/L) *1386*

Amphetamine *Urine No Effect Analytical* No false positive results obtained with Abbott TDx amphetamine/methamphetamine II assay in urine specimens containing 7-271 mg/L drug *4728*

Urine Positive Analytical At concentration of 200 mg/L (amount that would be expected to be achieved therapeutically) false positive with Syva® EMIT monoclonal assay although negative with polyclonal assay procedure *2339* At concentrations greater than 91 mg/L positive reaction occurred with Syva d.a.u. EMIT amphetamine/methamphetamine assay. Note all false positives occurred with first or second voiding after ingestion. No false positives observed in same specimens with polyclonal assay *4728*

Aspartate Aminotransferase *Serum Increase Physiological* There have been occasional reports of hepatitis, hepatocellular or hepatocanalicular or mixed, with or without jaundice *2169*

Atenolol *Serum No Effect Physiological* Minimal effect of coadministration on atenolol pharmacokinetics *3146*

Azelastine *Serum No Effect Physiological* Coadministration of ranitidine (150 mg b.i.d.) with azelastine had no significant effect on the concentration of azelastine *6320*

Basal Acid Output *Gastric Fluid Decrease Physiological* Ranitidine inhibits both daytime and nocturnal basal acid secretion and that after stimulation by food, betazole and pentagastrin *2169*

Bilirubin *Serum Increase Physiological* There have been occasional reports of hepatitis, hepatocellular or hepatocanalicular or mixed, with or without jaundice *2169*

Bilirubin, Conjugated *Serum No Effect Analytical* No effect at concentration of 0.2 mg/L on method on Kodak Ektachem® *5706*

Bilirubin, Unconjugated *Serum No Effect Analytical* No effect at concentration of 0.2 mg/L on method on Kodak Ektachem® *5706*

Carbamazepine *Serum No Effect Physiological* Has no effect on carbamazepine kinetics *3119*

^{14}Carbon *Breath Increase Physiological* In 26 patients with H. pylori infection receiving 150 mg ranitidine twice daily radioactive ^{14}C in exhaled carbon dioxide significantly increased compared with controls *5812*

Cefaclor *Serum No Effect Physiological* When coadministered with cefaclor reported to have no effect on its rate or extent of absorption *1627*

Cefpodoxime *Serum Decrease Physiological* Administration of H_2-blockers reduced peak plasma concentration by 42% and the extent of absorption by 32% *4684*

Cephalexin *Serum Decrease Physiological* Reduction from mean of 29.9 mg/L to 24.1 mg/L in 10 healthy volunteers given 3 doses of 150 mg concomitantly with 1000 mg cephalexin *1386*

Chlormethiazole *Serum Increase Physiological* At least in one patient prolongation of elimination half-life *3146*

Cholesterol *Serum No Effect Physiological* In 25 patients pretreatment concentration 171 mg/dL, changed insignificantly to 175 mg/dL over 5 weeks with treatment *5986*

Cholinesterase (True) *Serum Decrease Physiological* Inhibited by therapeutic doses *3146*

Cifenline *Serum No Effect Physiological* No significant effect observed in 12 healthy volunteers when 160 mg cifenline given in combination with 150 mg ranitidine twice daily *3836*

Cisapride *Serum No Effect Physiological* Coadministration of ranitidine with cisapride had no effect on the peak concentration or AUC of cisapride *2903*

Cocaethylene *Urine No Effect Analytical* No interference observed with TLC method of Bailey *328*

Corticotropin *Plasma Increase Physiological* In 9 healthy male volunteers treatment with 300 mg/d for 14 days caused significant increase of concentration at 8:00 h of 38.0 ± 34.2 pg/mL to 50.4 ± 39.3 pg/mL after treatment but concentration at 20:00 h unchanged from mean baseline of 9.4 ± 5.3 pg/mL *4096*

Cortisol *Plasma Decrease Physiological* Compared to control state after 3 d 150 mg/12 h cortisol level significantly lower at rest and after 30 minutes ambulation *5219*

Plasma Increase Physiological In 9 healthy male volunteers administration of 300 mg/d for 14 days caused no change of concentration of 20.2 mg/dL at 8:00 a.m. but significant increase from baseline concentration of 3.9 mg/dL at 20:00 h to 5.9 mg/dL after treatment *4096*

Plasma No Effect Physiological No effect observed with ranitidine administration *2169* No effect with i.v. bolus of much as 300 mg *1368*

Cortisol, Free *Urine Decrease Physiological* In 9 healthy male volunteers given 300 mg/d for 14 days mean concentration decreased from 337.5 ± 15.4 mg/d to 21.7 ± 10.9 mg/d *4096*

Creatinine *Serum Increase Physiological* There have been occasional reports of hypersensitivity reactions including increases in plasma creatinine concentration *2169*

Serum No Effect Physiological No effect reported although other drugs with same overall action blocks tubular secretion of creatinine *5697*

Cyclosporine *Blood No Effect Analytical* At a concentration of 200 mg/L had no effect on Syva EMIT method *495*

Serum Increase Physiological Ranitidine reported to increase risk of nephrotoxicity although mechanism not discussed *1069*

Serum No Effect Physiological Coadministration of ranitidine with cyclosporine had no effect on cyclosporine concentration *6596* Trough serum concentration, area under curve and clearance not signicantly different before or during treatment in 2 renal transplant patients *2908*

Diazepam *Serum Decrease Physiological* May reduce absorption from gastrointestinal tract and reduce plasma concentration by 25% *1384*

Serum No Effect Physiological Steady-state plasma concentration, clearance and elimination half-life not affected *3146*

Ranitidine *(continued)*

Didanosine *Serum No Effect Physiological* No significant effect observed on the concentration of either drug when two drugs coadministered *730*

Diltiazem *Serum Increase Physiological* Coadministration of ranitidine with diltiazem to 6 healthy volunteers caused a nonsignificant increase in peak diltiazem concentration and its AUC *2643* Administration of diltiazem concurrently with ranitidine resulted in a nonsignificant increase in the diltiazem concentration and area under the curve after one week *4937*
Serum No Effect Physiological Administration of a single dose of 60 mg diltiazem concomitantly with ranitidine to 6 healthy volunteers caused a nonsignificant increase in diltiazem concentration *1911* No significant effect observed when two drugs coadministered *6505*

Doxepin *Serum No Effect Physiological* No effect observed on plasma concentrations when drugs coadministered *5880*

Doxycycline *Serum No Effect Physiological* No significant effect on peak plasma concentration in 10 healthy volunteers given 3 doses of 150 mg and 200 mg doxycycline concomitantly *1383*

Drugs of Abuse Screen *Urine Increase Analytical* With EMIT d.a.u. assay in 8 individuals taking up to 300 mg/day 5 urine specimens observed to produce a positive test: all positive tests were obtained on specimens obtained within 9 hours of subject having ingested a dose of the drug *3099*

Enoxacin *Serum Decrease Physiological* Coadministration of ranitidine with enoxacin reduces the bioavailability of enoxacin by 60% *4940*

Eosinophils *Blood Increase Physiological* There have been occasional reports of hypersensitivity reactions including eosinophilia *2169* Isolated case reported within 1 mo of treatment being started, reverted to normal 2 weeks after drug stopped. Probable hypersensitive or idiosyncratic reaction *5516*

Estradiol *Plasma No Effect Physiological* No effect observed with ranitidine administration *2169* After 4 weeks or 6 mo treatment (300 mg and 150 mg daily respectively) in male patients with duodenal ulcer *1134*

Estriol *Plasma No Effect Physiological* No effect observed with ranitidine administration *2169*

Estrone *Plasma No Effect Physiological* No effect observed with ranitidine administration *2169*

Ethanol *Serum Increase Physiological* In 8 healthy men treatment with 300 mg/d for 1 week caused mean peak concentration and area under curve to increase by 34% (from 6.86 ± 0.86 to 9.08 ± 0.61 mmol/L) and 41% (from 8.41 ± 1.34 to 11.49 mmol/L/h) respectively when 0.3 mg/kg body weight alcohol ingested *1436*
Serum No Effect Physiological Ingestion of ranitidine for several days prior to alcohol was not associated with any change in the integrated postprandial blood alcohol concentration *1947* No effect on peak concentration or area under the curve with pretreatment with drug *5437* Peak plasma concentration and area under curve unaffected *3146*

Fluvastatin *Serum Increase Physiological* Administration of ranitidine with fluvastatin was associated with a 70% increase in the maximum fluvastatin concentration and 24 - 33% increase in its AUC and 18 - 23% decrease in plasma clearance *5232*

Follicle Stimulating Hormone
Plasma No Effect Physiological After 4 weeks or 6 mo treatment (300 mg and 150 mg daily respectively) in male patients with duodenal ulcer *1134* No effect with i.v. bolus of much as 300 mg *1368* With up to 450 mg/d in 20 males with chronic duodenal ulcer *4874* No significant effect observed in 20 men treated daily with ranitidine for 12 months *6626* No effect observed with ranitidine administration *2169*

Gastrin *Serum No Effect Physiological* No effect reported in spite of long term treatment *2736*

Glimepiride *Serum No Effect Physiological* When ranitidine at a dose of 150 mg b.i.d. coadministered with a single oral dose of 4 mg glimepiride no effect on absorption and disposition of glimepiride noted *2639*

Glipizide *Serum Increase Physiological* Concentration increased and hypoglycemic effect enhanced when drugs coadministered due to inhibition of hepatic metabolism of glipizide *3723*

Glyburide *Serum No Effect Physiological* No effect observed in healthy volunteers when drugs coadministered *3311*

Granulocytes *Blood Decrease Physiological* Marked reduction in one elderly woman following 2 weeks of treatment with 300 mg/ daily: normalized when treatment stopped *710*

Growth Hormone *Plasma No Effect Physiological* No effect observed with ranitidine administration *2169* No effect with i.v. bolus of much as 300 mg *1368*

HDL_2-Cholesterol *Serum No Effect Physiological* In 8 ulcer patients given 300 mg/d for 1 mo *6490*

HDL_3-Cholesterol *Serum No Effect Physiological* In 8 ulcer patients given 300 mg/d for 1 mo *6490*

HDL-Cholesterol *Serum No Effect Physiological* In 8 ulcer patients given 300 mg/d for 1 mo *6490* In 25 patients pretreatment 40 mg/dL, after 38 mg/dL over 5 weeks *5986*

Histamine *Plasma No Effect Analytical* Improbable inhibition of radio-enzyme assay at physiological concentration of 0.24 - 0.63 µg/mL although 50% inhibition at 17 µg/mL *2492*

Hydrochloric Acid *Gastric Fluid Decrease Physiological* Reduced to 10% of normal in healthy volunteers *5695*

17-Hydroxycorticosteroids *Urine Increase Physiological* In 9 healthy male volunteers administration of 300 mg/d for 14 days caused nonsignificant increase from mean of 12.1 ± 5.4 mg/d to 15.7 ± 2.4 mg/d *4096*

6-β-Hydroxycortisol *Urine No Effect Physiological* In 9 healthy male volunteers administration of 300 mg/d for 14 days caused change in excretion from 0.464 ± 0.097 mg/d to 0.542 ± 0.129 mg/d although change not significant *4096*

5-Hydroxytryptamine *Blood Decrease Physiological* Significant reduction in one man with carcinoid syndrome with immediate cessation of flushing during drug administration *4320*

Ibuprofen *Serum No Effect Physiological* Cimetidine has been shown to have no effect on ibuprofen concentrations *3200* Coadministration of ranitidine with ibuprofen had no effect on the ibuprofen serum concentration *3913*

itraconazole *Serum Decrease Physiological* Decreased oral bioavailability *886*

Ketoconazole *Serum Decrease Physiological* Decreased oral bioavailability *886* Probable effect when drugs coadministered *1384*

Ketone Body Ratio *Serum No Effect Analytical* When added at a concentration of 50 mg/L had no significant effect on AKBR method of Uno et al *6131*

Leukocytes *Blood Decrease Physiological* Significant reduction in one patient previously given 150 mg drug twice daily for 3 weeks: Problem recurred when cimetidine given to replace ranitidine *3607* Isolated case reported within 1 mo of treatment being started, reverted to normal 2 weeks after drug stopped. Probable hypersensitive or idiosyncratic reaction *5516* Marked reduction in one elderly woman following 2 weeks of treatment with 300 mg/ daily: normalized when treatment stopped *710*

Lidocaine *Serum No Effect Physiological* Insignificant effect on drug kinetics when co-administered *3146*

Lorazepam *Serum No Effect Physiological* Not affected: normally conjugated in liver *3146*

Luteinizing Hormone *Plasma No Effect Physiological* No effect with i.v. bolus of much as 300 mg *1368* With up to 450 mg/d in 20 males with chronic duodenal ulcer *4874* After 4 weeks or 6 mo treatment (300 mg and 150 mg daily respectively) in male patients with duodenal ulcer *1134* No significant effect observed in 20 men treated with ranitidine daily for 12 months *6339* No effect observed with ranitidine administration *2169*

Metoprolol *Serum Increase Physiological* Significantly increased area under curve and peak plasma concentration *3146* In one study of healthy volunteers coadministration of ranitidine with metoprolol increased metoprolol concentration significantly *5733*

Serum No Effect Physiological No effect of daily administration of 300 mg on pharmacokinetics of metoprolol (200 mg daily) in 12 volunteers over 8 days *6054*

Mexiletine *Serum No Effect Physiological* No effect of coadministration on distribution or elimination of drug, nor its overall kinetics or excretion of its metabolites *733*

Midazolam *Serum Increase Physiological* Bioavailability significantly increased *3146*
Serum No Effect Physiological Unlike cimetidine, because it does not inhibit cytochrome P450 3A4, has no effect on plasma clearance of midazolam when drugs coadministered. Coadministration caused a nonsignificant increase in concentration from 57 to 62 ng/mL *5037*

Moricizine *Serum No Effect Physiological* Concomitant administration of ranitidine with moricizine has no effect on its pharmacokinetics or plasma concentration *1062*

Neutrophils *Blood Decrease Physiological* Marked reduction in one patient previously given 150 mg twice daily for 3 weeks: problem recurred when ranitidine replaced with cimetidine *3607* Isolated case reported within 1 mo of treatment being started, reverted to normal 2 weeks after drug stopped. Probable hypersensitive or idiosyncratic reaction *5516*

Nifedipine *Serum Increase Physiological* Significant increase in area under the curve when coadministered probably related to increase in gastric pH *49* Coadministration of ranitidine with nifedipine caused a small nonsignificant increase in peak plasma nifedipine concentration probably mediated by inhibition of hepatic cytochrome P450 *4652* 25% in mean plasma concentration and area under curve *3146*
Serum No Effect Physiological In 18 healthy men mean peak concentration increased insignificantly to 39 ± 27 µg/L from 33 ± 14 µg/L with placebo when ranitidine coadministered with nifedipine. Area under curve increased insignificantly to 111 ± 45 µg/L/h compared with 105 ± 40 µg/L with placebo *3127* Peak plasma concentration and AUC of nifedipine may cause small and nonsignificant increase following administration of cimetidine, possibly mediated by inhibition of cytochrome P-450 *415* In 12 subjects given 300 mg daily together with up to 60 mg nifedipine daily for 1 week no effect observed on either nifedipine pharmacokinetics or pharmacodynamic response *5397*

Nisoldipine *Serum Decrease Physiological* Administration of ranitidine 150 mg twice daily with nisoldipine caused an insignificant 15 - 20% decrease in the AUC of nisoldipine *6650*

Nitrendipine *Serum Decrease Physiological* Clearance reduced with coadministration and plasma concentration increased although no alteration of systolic time intervals observed *3151*

Occult Blood *Feces No Effect Analytical* No effect on Hemoquant method *6172*

Oxaprozin *Serum Increase Physiological* Coadministration of ranitidine with oxaprozin caused a 20% decrease in its total body clearance *2065*

Pepsin *Gastric Material No Effect Physiological* Ranitidine has little or no effect on concentration *2169*

pH *Gastric Material Increase Physiological* Mean pH increased to 4.3 with single daily dose of 150 mg in 15 outpatients and to 6.5 with evening and morning doses of 150 mg in 12 outpatients compared with pH of 2.16 in 15 placebo treated controls *1607* pH 5 reached approximately 1 h after 50 mg *4253*
Urine Increase Physiological Mean increase of 0.4 in healthy volunteers *5697*

Phenytoin *Serum Increase Physiological* Mean concentration increased from 36.1 µmol/L to 39.3 µmol/L after coadministration *3146* Increased serum concentration *886*
Serum No Effect Physiological No significant effect observed on drug metabolism *6368*

Piroxicam *Serum No Effect Physiological* In 15 healthy individuals no effect observed on droxicam kinetics when 300 mg ranitidine given twice daily for 6 weeks coadministered with 20 mg droxicam (maximum concentration 1.14 to 1.86 µg/mL reached after mean of 7.5 ± 2.1 h) *390*

Potassium *Serum No Effect Physiological* No effect of 3-d of 150 mg/12 h *5219*
Urine No Effect Physiological No effect of 3-d of 150 mg/12 h *5219*

Pramipexole *Serum Increase Physiological* Coadministration of ranitidine with pramipexole presumed to decrease the oral clearance of pramipexole by about 20% *4680*

Procainamide *Serum Increase Physiological* Significantly increased area under curve and reduced renal clearance *3146* Renal clearance reduced without change in half-life. Increased area under curve for both procainamide and NAPA. Also slightly reduced gastrointestinal absorption: probably blocks tubular secretion of drug *5695* Concomitant administration of ranitidine with procainamide caused increase in plasma procainamide concentration due to reduction of tubular secretion and possible reduced absorption from gastrointestinal tract. N-acetylprocainamide also affected *5697*
Serum No Effect Physiological No effect on serum concentration or steady-state pharmacokinetics *5053*

Progesterone *Plasma No Effect Physiological* After 4 weeks or 6 mo treatment (300 mg and 150 mg daily respectively) in male patients with duodenal ulcer *1134*

Prolactin *Plasma Decrease Physiological* Compared with control state after 3 d 150 mg/12 h lower during ambulation and at rest *5219*
Plasma Increase Physiological Small transient dose-related increases have been observed after bolus intravenous injections of 100 mg or more *2169* No effect up to 100 mg i.v., but mean increase of 1.3 ng/mL in 5 subjects *1368* Significant increase in basal value *4609*
Plasma No Effect Physiological No significant effect during treatment *4253* No effect is usually observed at recommended oral or intravenous doses *2169* No difference in TRH-stimulated concentration compared with control in 10 ulcer patients or in prestimulation concentration *2612* No significant effect observed in 20 men treated with ranitidine daily for 12 months *6339*

Propranolol *Serum No Effect Physiological* No significant effect on plasma concentration, area under curve or elimination half-life *3146* In 12 volunteers treated with 300 mg daily no effect observed on concentration time profile of propranolol *1467*

Protein *Urine Increase Analytical* False positive tests may occur with Multistix® *2169*
Urine No Effect Analytical False positive tests may occur with Multistix® but no effect on methods using sulfosalicylic acid *2169*

Prothrombin Time *Plasma Decrease Physiological* In patients receiving both ranitidine and warfarin both increased and decreased prothrombin times reported *2169*
Plasma Increase Physiological In patients receiving both ranitidine and warfarin both increased and decreased prothrombin times reported *2169*
Plasma No Effect Physiological In patients receiving both ranitidine up to 400 mg/d and warfarin no interaction occurred, and had no effect on warfarin clearance *2169*

Quinidine *Serum Increase Physiological* By mechanisms not understood concentration of quinidine increased when ranitidine coadministered *5996*

Renin Activity *Plasma No Effect Physiological* No effect of 3-d of 150 mg/12 h *5219*

Sodium *Serum No Effect Physiological* No effect of 3-d of 150 mg/12 h *5219*
Urine No Effect Physiological No effect of 3-d of 150 mg/12 h *5219*

Sperm Count *Semen No Effect Physiological* No significant effect observed in 20 men treated with ranitidine daily for 12 months *6339* No effect observed with ranitidine administration *2169* With up to 450 mg/d in 20 males with chronic duodenal ulcer *4874*

Sperm Morphology *Semen No Effect Physiological* No significant effect observed in 20 men treated with ranitidine daily for 12 months *6339* No effect observed with ranitidine administration *2169* With up to 450 mg/d in 20 males with chronic duodenal ulcer *4874*

Sperm Motility *Semen No Effect Physiological* No significant effect observed in 20 men treated with ranitidine daily for 12 months *6339* No effect observed with ranitidine administration *2169*

Tacrolimus *Serum No Effect Analytical* In HPLC/MS method of Christians et al no significant interference observed with measurement of FK 506 *1010*

Ranitidine *(continued)*

Testosterone *Serum No Effect Physiological* No significant effect observed in 20 men treated with ranitidine daily for 12 months *6339* With up to 450 mg/d in 20 males with chronic duodenal ulcer *4874* After 4 weeks or 6 mo treatment (300 mg and 150 mg daily respectively) in male patients with duodenal ulcer *1134*

Theophylline *Serum Increase Physiological* Reduced clearance when ranitidine added to therapeutic regime with theophylline. Toxicity occurred in some cases but serum theophylline concentration returned to normal when ranitidine withdrawn *5135* Similar effect to cimetidine in reducing plasma clearance *3146*

Serum No Effect Physiological No significant effect on ranitidine pharmacokinetics *4767* No clinically significant effect on theophylline concentration observed when drugs coadministered *5999* No effect observed in 15 patients with chronic obstructive airway disease when 300 mg given daily for one week *627* In 17 patients with COPD given theophylline for 42 days coadministration of cimetidine caused nonsignificant change in mean $AUC_{0\text{-}12}$ from 113.95 mg/h/L to 119.05 mg/h/L and mean maximum concentration from 9.5 mg/L to 9.9 mg/L *316* No documented significant interaction with theophylline reported *6117*

Thyroid Stimulating Hormone
Serum No Effect Physiological After 4 weeks or 6 mo treatment (300 mg and 150 mg daily respectively) in male patients with duodenal ulcer *1134* No effect with i.v. bolus of much as 300 mg *1368* No effect of treatment on values *4609* In 10 peptic ulcer patients no effect of 150 mg twice daily for 28 d *2612* No effect observed with ranitidine administration *2169*

Thyroxine Binding Globulin *Serum No Effect Physiological* No difference in thyroid hormone binding protein in 10 ulcer patients after 150 mg twice daily for 28 d *2612*

Thyroxine (T4) *Serum Decrease Physiological* Small reduction noted in 10 ulcer patients after 150 mg twice daily for 28 d ratio: total T4/total T3 fell *2612* Slight reduction after 4 weeks of 300 mg daily, but returned to normal after 6 mo of 150 mg daily in men with duodenal ulcers *1134*

Thyroxine (T4), Free *Serum Decrease Physiological* Similar small effect noted as for total hormone concentration: ratio fT4/fT3 fell significantly *2612*

Tirofiban *Serum No Effect Physiological* Coadministration had no significant effect on plasma clearance of tirofiban *3957*

Tolbutamide *Serum No Effect Physiological* No significant effect observed on tolbutamide kinetics observed in healthy volunteers *922*

Tri-iodothyronine, Free (fT3) *Serum Increase Physiological* Similar small effect noted as for total hormone concentration *2612*

Tri-iodothyronine (T3) *Serum Increase Physiological* Small increase noted in ulcer patients after 150 mg twice daily for 28 d *2612*

Serum No Effect Physiological No effect of treatment on values *4609* After 4 weeks or 6 mo treatment (300 mg and 150 mg daily respectively) in male patients with duodenal ulcer *1134*

Triglycerides *Serum No Effect Physiological* In 25 patients pretreatment concentration 121 mg/dL, after treatment 137 mg/dL over 5 weeks *5986*

TSH response to TRH *Serum Decrease Physiological* In response to i.v. drug: may cause decrease of basal concentration in hypothyroidism *3146*

Valproic Acid *Serum No Effect Physiological* Coadministration with valproic acid did not affect its clearance *17* In a study involving the coadministration of ranitidine with valproate resulted in no significant effect on the trough plasma concentrations of valproate *15*

Vitamin B_{12} *Serum Decrease Physiological* Significant decreased absorption of protein bound compound *3146*

Volume *Gastric Fluid Decrease Physiological* Significant inhibition following treatment *4253* Reduced to 10% of normal in healthy volunteers *5695* Significant reduction to mean of 11.3 mL in 12 outpatients given evening and morning doses of 150 mg from mean of 19.9 mL in placebo treated controls but no significant reduction in 15 outpatients given single morning dose of 150 mg *1607*

Warfarin *Plasma No Effect Physiological* No effect on plasma concentration or prothrombin time during coadministration *3146*

Zolpidem *Serum No Effect Physiological* Coadministration of ranitidine with zolpidem had no effect on the pharmacokinetics or pharmacodynamics of zolpidem *2062*

Rapamycin

Mycophenolic Acid *Serum No Effect Analytical* No significant interference observed with HPLC method of Shipkova et al *5526*

Mycophenolic Acid Glucuronide
Serum No Effect Analytical No significant interference observed with HPLC method of Shipkova et al *5526*

Tacrolimus *Serum No Effect Analytical* In HPLC/MS method of Christians et al no significant interference observed with measurement of FK 506 *1010*

Triglycerides *Serum Increase Physiological* Administration of sirolimus (rapomycin) to 9 renal transplant patients was associated with rise in serum triglyceride concentration to 11.7 to 42 mmol/L 2 to 4 months after renal transplantation *700*

Rauwolfia

Catecholamines *Urine Increase Physiological* Release of stored norepinephrine *3669*

Hydrochloric Acid *Gastric Fluid Increase Physiological* Stimulates gastric secretion *3669*

4-Hydroxy-3-Methoxy-Phenylglycol
Urine Increase Physiological Release of stored norepinephrine *3669*

17-Hydroxycorticosteroids *Urine Decrease Physiological* Probably due to depressed central synthesis *55*

5-Hydroxyindoleacetic Acid *Urine Increase Physiological* Result of release of 5-HT from brain, tissues *2242*

Sodium *Serum Increase Physiological* May cause electrolyte retention or edema *3810*

Vanillylmandelic Acid *Urine Increase Physiological* Release of stored norepinephrine *3669*

Razoxane

Leukocytes *Blood Decrease Physiological* Leukopenia is principal toxic effect *1384*

Remifentanil

Histamine *Plasma No Effect Physiological* No increase in concentration of histamine observed in patients or healthy volunteers after administration in doses up to 30 µg/kg over 60 seconds *2165*

Remoxipride

Prolactin *Plasma Increase Physiological* Area under curve increased progressively with dose in 8 elderly psychiatric patients with doses increased from 50 mg/d to 200 mg t.i.d. over 2 weeks *6436*

Renacidin

Magnesium *Serum Increase Physiological* One case reported of child who developed severe hypermagnesemia *6483*

Reserpine

Albumin *Serum No Effect Analytical* No effect at 0.02 mg/dL on Technicon SMA 12/60 method *4390*

Alkaline Phosphatase *Serum No Effect Analytical* No effect at 0.02 mg/dL on Technicon SMA 12/60 method *4390*

Amphetamine *Serum Decrease Physiological* Gastrointestinal acidifying agents lower absorption of amphetamines including dextroamphetamine *5641*

Aspartate Aminotransferase *Serum No Effect Analytical* No effect at 0.02 mg/dL on Technicon SMA 12/60 method *4390*

Bilirubin *Serum Increase Analytical* At concentrations above 61 mg/L raised concentration as measured by Jendrassik and Grof method *5704*
Serum No Effect Analytical No effect at 0.02 mg/dL on Technicon SMA 12/60 method *4390*

Calcium *Serum No Effect Analytical* No effect at 0.02 mg/dL on Technicon SMA 12/60 method *4390* At concentration of 61 mg/L had no effect on cresolphthalein method *5704*

Catecholamines *Plasma Decrease Physiological* Observed normal response to therapy *4014*
Urine Decrease Physiological Decreased norepinephrine synthesis *1175*
Urine Increase Physiological Release of stored norepinephrine *3669*

Cholesterol *Serum No Effect Analytical* No effect at 0.02 mg/dL on Technicon SMA 12/60 method *4390*
Serum No Effect Physiological No significant change in small number of patients treated for up to 2.5 mo *142*

Creatinine *Serum No Effect Analytical* No effect at 0.02 mg/dL on Technicon SMA 12/60 method *4390*
Urine Increase Analytical No effect at 0.02 mg/dL on Technicon SMA 12/60 method *4390*

Epinephrine *Urine No Effect Physiological* Not affected (unlike norepinephrine) *4471*

Fatty Acids (FFA), Free *Serum Increase Physiological* 78% increase after 2.5 mg injected i.m *2675*

Glucose *Serum Increase Physiological* Hyperglycemia may follow administration *3806*
Serum No Effect Analytical No effect at 0.02 mg/dL on Technicon SMA 12/60 method *4390*
Urine Increase Physiological Occurs as consequence of hyperglycemia *3806*

Guaiacols Spot Test *Urine Positive Analytical* False reaction with screening test of Rogers *5061*

Homovanillic Acid *Urine Increase Physiological* Maximum during second day of treatment *6465*

Hydrochloric Acid *Gastric Fluid Increase Physiological* Excess secretion may activate peptic ulcers *2242*

4-Hydroxy-3-Methoxy-Phenylglycol
Urine Decrease Physiological Long term administration produces decrease *660*
Urine Increase Physiological Release of stored norepinephrine *3669*

17-Hydroxycorticosteroids *Urine Decrease Analytical* Interference with Porter-Silber reaction *5869*
Urine Decrease Physiological Probably due to depressed central synthesis *55*

5-Hydroxyindoleacetic Acid *Urine Increase Physiological* Release of 5-HT from brain and tissues *4012*
Urine No Effect Analytical No effect observed with FPIA method on Abbott TDx *695*

5-Hydroxytryptamine *Plasma Decrease Physiological* Observed normal response to therapy *4014*

Lactate Dehydrogenase *Serum No Effect Analytical* No effect at 0.02 mg/dL on Technicon SMA 12/60 method *4390*

LE Cells *Blood Positive Physiological* SLE may occur, usually normalizes when stopped *5102*

Norepinephrine *Urine Decrease Physiological* Contributes to fall of total catecholamines *4471*

Occult Blood *Feces Increase Physiological* May activate peptic ulcers and cause bleeding *6487*

Pepsin *Gastric Material Increase Physiological* Greatly augments secretion *929*

Phenytoin *Serum Decrease Physiological* Coadministration with phenytoin may decrease plasma phenytoin concentration *4522* When reserpine ingested with fosphenytoin concentration of phenytoin may be decreased *4519*

Phosphate *Serum No Effect Analytical* At concentration of 61 mg/L had no effect on phosphomolybdate method *5704* No effect at 0.02 mg/dL on Technicon SMA 12/60 method *4390*

Platelets *Blood Decrease Physiological* Thrombocytopenia with purpura may occur *4017*

Prolactin *Plasma Increase Physiological* Marked effect in male and female hypertensives treated for up to 6 weeks *6098* Dose-related at doses greater than 0.25 mg/d *697*

Protein *Serum No Effect Analytical* No effect at 0.02 mg/dL on Technicon SMA 12/60 method *4390* At concentration of 61 mg/L had no effect on biuret method with blank correction *5704*

Prothrombin Time *Plasma Decrease Physiological* Short term treatment blocks action of anticoagulant *2242*
Plasma Increase Physiological Long term treatment markedly enhances anticoagulant *2242*

Quinidine *Serum No Effect Analytical* No significant interference observed at a concentration of 100 µg/mL (164 µmol/L) with method on Du Pont aca *1543*

Thyroxine (T4) *Serum Decrease Physiological* Increased metabolism by hepatic microsomes *5869*

Triglycerides *Serum No Effect Physiological* No significant change in small number of patients treated for up to 2.5 mo *142*

Tyramine Test *Patient Decrease Physiological* Inhibits responsiveness (produces false negative) *2213*

Urea Nitrogen *Serum No Effect Analytical* At concentration of 61 mg/L had no effect on diacetylmonoxime method *5704*

Uric Acid *Serum No Effect Analytical* At concentration of 61 mg/L had no effect on phosphotungstate reduction method *5704* No effect at 0.02 mg/dL on Technicon SMA 12/60 method *4390*

Vanillylmandelic Acid *Urine Decrease Physiological* Depletion of catecholamine stores *4012*
Urine Increase Physiological Release of stored norepinephrine *3669*
Urine No Effect Analytical No effect on Gitlow method *2452*

Residronate

N-terminal Telopeptide of Type I Collagen
Serum Decrease Physiological Treatment of 3 patients with Paget's disease with 30 mg/d for 8 weeks caused mean concentrations to decrease from about 350, 370 and 580 nmol BCE/L to 200, 100 and 100 nmol BCE/L respectively with continuation at approximately the same rate for another 17 weeks *1054*
Urine Decrease Physiological Treatment of 3 patients with Paget's disease with 30 mg/d for 8 weeks caused mean concentrations to decrease from about 3100, 2700 and 1700 nmol BCE/mmol creatinine to 1900, 400 and 500 nmol BCE/mmol creatinine respectively with continuation at approximately the same rate for another 17 weeks *1054*

Reteplase

Fibrinogen *Plasma Decrease Physiological* Causes a reduction in plasma fibrinogen concentration *629*

Ribavirin

Creatinine *Serum No Effect Analytical* No effect noted on liquid chromatographic method of Paroni et al *4540*

Theophylline *Serum No Effect Physiological* No effect on clearance noted in either adults or children *1945*

Rifabutin

Alanine Aminotransferase *Serum Increase Physiological* In 566 treated patients increased activity occurred in 9% compared with 11% in 580 placebo treated controls *4681*

Alkaline Phosphatase *Serum Increase Physiological* In 566 treated patients increased activity occurred in < 1% compared with 3% in 580 placebo treated controls *4681*

Aspartate Aminotransferase *Serum Increase Physiological* In 566 treated patients increased activity occurred in 7% compared with 12% in 580 placebo treated controls *4681*

Rifabutin *(continued)*

Barbiturate *Serum Decrease Physiological* Rifabutin induces liver activity reducing the effects of many drugs including barbiturates *4681*

Chloramphenicol *Serum Decrease Physiological* Rifabutin induces liver activity reducing the effects of many drugs including chloramphenicol *4681*

Clofibrate *Serum Decrease Physiological* Rifabutin induces liver activity reducing the effects of many drugs including clofibrate *4681*

Color *Feces Increase Physiological* May be brown-orange due to drug and some of its metabolites *4681*
Saliva Increase Physiological May be brown-orange due to drug and some of its metabolites *4681*
Sputum Increase Physiological May be brown-orange due to drug and some of its metabolites *4681*
Sweat Increase Physiological May be brown-orange due to drug and some of its metabolites *4681*
Urine Increase Physiological May be brown-orange due to drug and some of its metabolites *4681*

Corticosteroids *Plasma Decrease Physiological* Increased metabolism, loss of efficacy *886*

Cyclosporine *Serum Decrease Physiological* In one renal transplant case, effect on cyclosporine clearance appeared to be delayed and of less magnitude than that of rifampin *6207*

Cyclosporine A *Blood Decrease Physiological* Rifabutin induces liver activity reducing the activity of many drugs including cyclosporine *4681*

Dapsone *Serum Decrease Physiological* Rifabutin induces liver activity reducing the activity of many drugs including dapsone *4681*

Diazepam *Serum Decrease Physiological* Rifabutin induces liver activity reducing the effects of many drugs including diazepam *4681*

Didanosine *Serum No Effect Physiological* No significant effect observed on the concentration of either drug when two drugs coadministered *730*

Digoxin *Serum Decrease Physiological* Rifabutin induces liver activity reducing the activity of many drugs including cardiac glycosides *4681*

Disopyramide *Serum Decrease Physiological* Rifabutin induces liver activity reducing the effects of many drugs including disopyramide *4681*

Eosinophils *Blood Increase Physiological* In 566 treated patients increased concentration occurred in 1% compared with 1% in 580 placebo treated controls *4681*

γ-Glutamyltransferase *Serum No Effect Physiological* No significant change in activity noted in 8 normal subjects given 300 mg daily for 7 days *4622*

Hematocrit *Blood Decrease Physiological* In 566 treated patients decreased value occurred in 6% compared with 7% in 580 placebo treated controls *4681*

Hemoglobin *Blood Decrease Physiological* In 566 treated patients decreased concentration occurred in 6% compared with 7% in 580 placebo treated controls *4681*

17-Hydroxycorticosteroids *Urine No Effect Physiological* No significant effect in 8 normal subjects treated with 300 mg daily for 7 days *4622*

6-β-Hydroxycortisol *Urine Increase Physiological* Increased excretion noted in 8 volunteers given 300 mg daily for 7 days *4622*

Indinavir *Serum Decrease Physiological* Administration of indinavir 800 mg every 8 hours with rifabutin 300 mg/d for 10 days resulted in a 32 ± 19% decrease in indinavir AUC and a 204 ± 142% decrease in rifabutin AUC *3966* Causes a 32% decrease in area under the concentration curve when rifabutin coadministered *1891*

itraconazole *Serum Decrease Physiological* Itraconazole and its major metabolite hydroxyitraconazole inhibit the cytochrome P450 3A enzyme system thereby affecting the metabolism of drugs by this system: rifabutin postulated to reduce the concentration of itraconazole *2905* Increased metabolism, loss of efficacy *886*

Ketoconazole *Serum Decrease Physiological* Increased metabolism, loss of efficacy *886* Rifabutin induces liver activity reducing the effects of many drugs including ketoconazole *4681*

Leukocytes *Blood Decrease Physiological* In 566 treated patients decreased concentration occurred in 17% compared with 16% in 580 placebo treated controls *4681*

Methadone *Serum Decrease Physiological* Rifabutin induces liver activity reducing the activity of many drugs including methadone *4681* Increased metabolism, loss of efficacy *886*
Serum No Effect Physiological In 24 methadone maintained former injecting drug users infected with the HIV virus coadministration of 300 mg/d rifabutin for 15 days had no significant effect on methadone peak plasma concentration, time to peak plasma concentration, area under the plasma concentration-time curve systemic clearance or renal clearance *767*
Urine No Effect Physiological In 24 methadone maintained former injecting drug users infected with the HIV virus coadministration of 300 mg/d rifabutin for 15 days had no significant effect on methadone peak plasma concentration, time to peak plasma concentration, area under the plasma concentration-time curve systemic clearance or renal clearance *767*

Mexiletine *Serum Decrease Physiological* Rifabutin induces liver activity reducing the effects of many drugs including mexiletine *4681*

Nelfinavir *Serum Decrease Physiological* Causes a 32% decrease in area under the concentration curve when rifabutin coadministered *1891* Coadministration of rifabutin with nelfinavir caused a decrease of 32% in the plasma AUC of nelfinavir *66*

Neutrophils *Blood Decrease Physiological* In 566 treated patients decreased concentration occurred in 25% compared with 20% in 580 placebo treated controls *4681*

Phenytoin *Serum Decrease Physiological* Increased metabolism, loss of efficacy *886*

Platelets *Blood Decrease Physiological* In 566 treated patients decreased concentration occurred in 5% compared with 4% in 580 placebo treated controls *4681*

Prothrombin Time *Plasma Decrease Physiological* In patients receiving warfarin increased metabolism of warfarin, loss of efficacy *886*

Quinidine *Serum Decrease Physiological* Rifabutin induces liver activity reducing the activity of many drugs including quinidine *4681*

Saquinavir *Serum Decrease Physiological* Decreases the area under the concentration curve by 40% when rifabutin coadministered *1891* Coadministration of saquinavir 600 mg t.i.d. with rifabutin to 12 HIV patients produced approximately 40% decrease of AUC when saquinavir was given alone *5024* Increased metabolism, loss of efficacy *886*

Tacrolimus *Serum Decrease Physiological* By inducing cytochrome P-450 IIIA enzyme systems may stimulate the metabolism of tacrolimus *1987*

Theophylline *Serum Decrease Physiological* Rifabutin induces liver activity reducing the effects of many drugs including theophylline *4681*
Serum No Effect Physiological Coadministration to 12 adult male volunteers of rifabutin 300 mg/d with 5 mg/kg theophylline caused a signifcant reduction in area under concentration-time curve from 136 ± 48 μg.h/mL to 128 ± 45 μg.h/mL but serum concentration nonsignificantly reduced from 11.0 ± 1.2 μg/mL to 10.3 ± 0.8 μg/mL *2123* No clinically significant effect on theophylline concentration observed when drugs coadministered *5999* No documented significant interaction with theophylline reported *6117*

Verapamil *Serum Decrease Physiological* Rifabutin induces liver activity reducing the effects of many drugs including verapamil *4681*

Zidovudine *Serum Decrease Physiological* In 10 healthy adult volunteers and 8 HIV positive patients steady state plasma concentrations and AUC of zidovudine were reduced by 48% and 32% respectively *4681*

Rifampin

Acenocoumarol *Plasma Decrease Physiological* Decreased serum concentration due to hepatic enzyme induction *44*

Acetaminophen *Urine Increase Physiological* Significantly greater proportion excreted as glucuronide in response to coadministration of drug *621*

Alanine Aminotransferase *Serum Decrease Analytical* At 5 times upper limit of therapeutic range on method on Technicon SMAC® *3525*

Serum Increase Physiological Observed in one patient receiving drug who developed porphyria cutanea tarda *4038* Rarely hepatitis or a shock-like syndrome with hepatic involvement and abnormal liver function tests may occur *1037* Transient increases observed with rifampin treatment *2652* Minimal abnormalities of liver function are common: severe liver damage in about 0.6% patients *6197* In 72 patients with tuberculosis all receiving isoniazid and rifampin and, in addition, pyrazinamide in 72.2%, ethambutol in 80% and streptomycin in 16.7% drug-induced hepatitis observed with AST activity reaching mean of 330.2 ± 425.5 U/L *5577* Hepatic toxicity occurs in up to 7% patients *2549* In 61% of 18 children receiving drug in combination with isoniazid *3598*

Serum No Effect Analytical At 5 times upper limit of therapeutic range on method on Abbott-VP, Du Pont aca, Roche Cobas-Bio, and KDA *3525*

Albumin *Serum No Effect Analytical* At 5 times upper limit of therapeutic range on methods on Technicon SMAC® , Kodak Ektachem® , Hitachi® 705 and KDA *3525*

Alkaline Phosphatase *Serum Increase Physiological* Minimal abnormalities of liver function are common: severe liver damage in about 0.6% patients *6197* Can be serious but reversible liver damage *4689* Rarely hepatitis or a shock-like syndrome with hepatic involvement and abnormal liver function tests may occur *1037* Transient increases observed with rifampin treatment *2652* Observed in one patient receiving drug who developed porphyria cutanea tarda *4038*

Serum No Effect Analytical At 5 times upper limit of therapeutic range on methods on Technicon SMAC® , Roche Cobas-Bio, Abbott-VP, Du Pont aca, Hitachi® 705 and KDA *3525* On method involving hydrolysis of p-nitrophenyl phosphate *352*

Amylase *Serum No Effect Analytical* At 5 times upper limit of therapeutic range on methods on Du Pont aca, Roche Cobas-Bio and Kodak Ektachem® *3525*

Aspartate Aminotransferase *Serum Decrease Analytical* At 3.5 mg/L and above decreased activity when methods using absorbance at 340 nm used, since drug absorbs at this wavelength *352*

Serum Increase Physiological Hepatic toxicity occurs in up to 7% patients *2549* Minimal abnormalities of liver function are common: severe liver damage in about 0.6% patients *6197* In 72 patients with tuberculosis all receiving isoniazid and rifampin and, in addition, pyrazinamide in 72.2%, ethambutol in 80% and streptomycin in 16.7% drug-induced hepatitis observed with AST activity reaching mean of 428.4 ± 666.0 U/L *5577* Transient increases observed with rifampin treatment *2652* In 83% of 18 children receiving drug in combination with isoniazid *3598* Rarely hepatitis or a shock-like syndrome with hepatic involvement and abnormal liver function tests may occur *1037*

Serum No Effect Analytical At 5 times upper limit of therapeutic range on methods on Technicon SMAC® , Roche Cobas-Bio, Abbott-VP, Du Pont aca, Hitachi® 705 and KDA *3525*

Barbiturate *Serum Decrease Physiological* Because of its hepatic enzyme inducing capability reduces drug concentration *2652*

Bile Acids *Serum Increase Physiological* Significant increase possibly due to blocking uptake by plasma membrane of hepatocytes *2007* Marked changes may occur when given alone or in combination with isoniazid in the absence of other abnormal liver function tests, possibly due to inhibition of uptake of bile acids into hepatocytes *498*

Bilirubin *Serum Increase Analytical* At 5 times upper limit of therapeutic concentration on methods on Kodak Ektachem® and Roche Cobas-Bio *3525* Due to yellow coloration of drug *4708* Marked effect when measured by bilirubinometer *352*

Serum Increase Physiological Inhibits hepatic excretion *43* Significant increase in all subjects after single dose of 900 mg *2007* Observed in one patient receiving drug who developed porphyria cutanea tarda *4038* Minimal abnormalities of liver function are common: severe liver damage in about 0.6% patients *6197* Rarely hepatitis or a shock-like syndrome with hepatic involvement and abnormal liver function tests may occur *1037* In 72 patients with tuberculosis all receiving isoniazid and rifampin and, in addition, pyrazinamide in 72.2%, ethambutol in 80% and streptomycin in 16.7% drug-induced hepatitis observed with bilirubin concentration reaching mean of 5.34 ± 4.68 mg/dL *5577*

Serum No Effect Analytical No effect at concentration of 14 mg/L on method on Kodak Ektachem® *5706* No significant effect observed at a concentration of 500 μg/dL (6.1 μmol/L) with method on Du Pont aca *1548* At 5 times upper limit of therapeutic concentration on methods on Technicon SMAC® , Du Pont aca, Hitachi® 705 and KDA *3525* Minimal effect on Jendrassik/Grof methods, although some effect at drug concentration of 15 mg/L *352* No effect up to 35 mg/L on Ames Seralyzer method but at higher concentrations increased apparent bilirubin concentration; possibly of clinical significance *5706*

Serum No Effect Physiological Probably no significant displacement from protein in neonates *6314*

Bilirubin, Conjugated *Serum No Effect Analytical* No effect at concentration of 12 mg/L on method on Kodak Ektachem® *5706* At concentration of 500 μg/dL (6.1 μmol/L) had no effect on method on Du Pont aca *1517*

Bilirubin, Direct *Serum Increase Physiological* Transient effect *2000*

Bilirubin, Unconjugated *Serum Increase Analytical* At concentrations above 1 mg/L increases measurement as determined by method on Kodak Ektachem® : probably of clinical significance since therapeutic concentration is 4-16 mg/L *5706*

Blood *Urine Increase Physiological* Rarely hemoglobinuria or hematuria have occurred with rifampin treatment, probably as a hypersensitivity reaction *2652* Rarely hematuria has been observed *1037*

BSP Retention *Serum Increase Physiological* Inhibits hepatic excretion (probably) *2855* Initial increase of serum concentration due to reduced excretion in bile *44*

Calcitonin *Plasma No Effect Physiological* No change observed in 8 healthy men taking drug for 2 weeks *738*

Calcium *Serum No Effect Analytical* At 5 times upper limit of therapeutic range on method on Technicon SMAC® , Abbott-VP, Du Pont aca, Kodak Ektachem® , Hitachi® 705 and KDA *3525*

Capillary Fragility *Patient Increase Physiological* Reported in patient with macroglobulinemia *1763*

Carbamazepine *Serum Decrease Physiological* Drugs that induce CYP 3A4 enhance metabolism of carbamazepine producing clinically meaningful effect *1039*

Carvedilol *Serum Decrease Physiological* In 8 healthy individuals coadministration of 600 mg/d rifampin for 12 days with carvedilol decreased the AUC and maximum concentration of carvedilol by about 70% *5639*

Casts *Urine Increase Physiological* Rare reported side effect *2549*

Chenodeoxycholic Acid *Serum Increase Physiological* Significant increase possibly due to blocking uptake by plasma membrane of hepatocytes *2007*

Chloramphenicol *Serum Decrease Physiological* Metabolism of chloramphenicol probably stimulated *4792* Because of its hepatic enzyme inducing capability reduces drug concentration *2652* Due to hepatic enzyme induction *1384*

Serum No Effect Analytical No effect at 100 mg/L on coupled enzymatic method *4122*

Cholesterol *Serum Decrease Analytical* At 5 times upper limit of therapeutic concentration on method on Roche Cobas-Bio *3525*

Serum No Effect Analytical No effect of concentrations up to 100 mg/L on method on Kodak Ektachem® *5706* At 5 times upper limit of therapeutic concentration on methods on Technicon SMAC® , Abbott-VP, Du Pont aca, Kodak Ektachem® , Hitachi® 705 and KDA *3525* No effect at 300 mg/L on Ames Seralyzer method *5706*

Rifampin *(continued)*

Cholic Acid *Serum Increase Physiological* Significant increase possibly due to blocking uptake by plasma membrane of hepatocytes *2007*

Ciprofloxacin *Serum No Effect Physiological* Pharmacokinetics unaltered by coadministration *2704* Coadministration of rifampin with ciprofloxacin had no effect on ciprofloxacin pharmacokinetics *657*

Clindamycin *Serum Positive Analytical* Interfere with bioassays *3858*

Clofibrate *Serum Decrease Physiological* Rifampin induces hepatic microsomal enzymes increasing the metabolism of clofibrate and reducing its plasma concentration *3668* Because of its hepatic enzyme inducing capability reduces drug concentration *2652* Hepatic metabolism enhanced with reduction of plasma concentration by 40% in 5 healthy volunteers when drugs coadministered *2732*

Colistin *Serum Positive Analytical* Interferes with bioassays *3858*

Color *Feces Increase Analytical* Orange-red color due to drug and metabolites *51*
Feces Increase Physiological May be colored red-orange by rifampin and its metabolites *1037*
Saliva Increase Physiological May be colored red-orange by rifampin and its metabolites *1037*
Sputum Increase Physiological May be colored red-orange by rifampin and its metabolites *1037*
Sweat Increase Physiological May be colored red-orange by rifampin and its metabolites *1037*
Tears Increase Physiological May be colored red-orange by rifampin and its metabolites *1037*
Urine Increase Analytical Red-orange due to drug and metabolites *2579* Causes orange-pink color in saliva, tears, urine, sweat *6197*
Urine Increase Physiological May be colored red-orange by rifampin and its metabolites *1037*

Coombs' Test, Direct *Blood Positive Physiological* Weak response in 8% patients *4748*

Coombs' Test, Indirect *Blood Positive Physiological* Positive response in 33% patients after 3 mo *4748*

Corticosteroids *Plasma Decrease Physiological* Decreased serum concentration due to hepatic enzyme induction *44* Increased metabolism, loss of efficacy *886*

Cortisol *Plasma Decrease Physiological* In critically ill patients relative hypoadrenalism observed with rifampin therapy because of its effect of increasing the metabolism of cortisol *3381*

Cortisone *Plasma Decrease Physiological* Metabolism enhanced with reduction of circulating drug concentration: cortisol production rate increased *2985*

C-Peptide *Plasma Increase Physiological* Increased rate of secretion after oral administration of 100 g glucose *5925*

Creatine Kinase *Serum No Effect Analytical* At 5 times upper limit of therapeutic range on methods on Technicon SMAC® , Abbott-VP, Du Pont aca, Roche Cobas-Bio, and Hitachi® 705 *3525* No effect at 300 mg/L on method·on Ames Seralyzer *5706*

Creatinine *Serum No Effect Analytical* No effect up to 40 mg/L on method on Ames Seralyzer but at higher concentrations clinically insignificantly increased creatinine concentration *5706* No effect of concentrations up to 15 mg/L on single slide method on Kodak Ektachem® *5706* No effect of concentrations up to 100 mg/L on 2-slide method on Kodak Ektachem® *5706*

Cyclosporine *Blood Decrease Physiological* Coadministration of rifampin with cyclosporine caused a sharp reduction of cyclosporine concentration within 2 days of its administration with further decrease over the first 10 days of its administration. The cyclosporine concentration:dose ratio typically stabilizes at 25 to 50% (or more) of the baseline value. The effect is due to inhibition of CYP enzymes in the liver *859* In 6 healthy men while normal clearance 0.30 L/h/kg, volume distribution at steady state 1.68 L/kg and bioavailability 27% coadministration of rifampin caused increase of clearance to 0.42 L/h/kg, increase of volume of distribution to 1.35 L/kg and decreased bioavailability to 10% *2524* Induces cytochrome P-450 hepatic enzymes thereby increasing clearance of cyclosporine *6166*
Serum Decrease Physiological May decrease cyclosporine concentration by inducing hepatic cytochrome P-450 III A which metabolizes cyclosporine *5236* Although normal clearance of cyclosporine 0.55 L/h/kg,and volume of distribution at steady state1.68 L/kg, and bioavailability 33% coadministration of rifampin changed these values to 0.79 L/h/kg, 1.35 L/kg and 9% respectively *2524* Coadministration of rifampin with cyclosporine caused a sharp reduction of cyclosporine concentration within 2 days of its administration with further decrease over the first 10 days of its administration. The cyclosporine concentration:dose ratio typically stabilizes at 25 to 50% (or more) of the baseline value. The effect is due to inhibition of CYP enzymes in the liver *859* Cyclosporine bioavailability reduced by 20% when rifampin coadministered, possibly by decreasing cyclosporine absorption and/or inducing intestinal P-450 enzyme metabolism *657* Marked decreases in concentration observed when rifampin coadministered with cyclosporine probably due to hepatic enzyme induction *6595* Clearance enhanced when drugs coadministered *1384* Marked reduction of concentration due to hepatic enzyme induction *1075* Clearance increased with concomitant treatment with rifampin, a potent hepatic enzyme inducer *6207* Concentration reduced when drugs coadministered but exact mechanism not yet established *3403*

Cyclosporine A *Blood Decrease Physiological* Coadministration with cyclosporine A decreases its concentration *5240*

Dapsone *Serum Decrease Physiological* Because of its hepatic enzyme inducing capability reduces drug concentration *2652* Rifampin lowers dapsone concentration 7- to 10-fold by increasing its plasma clearance *2873* Decreased serum concentrations observed when rifampin coadministered: mean half-life of dapsone reduced by 63% and mean trough dapsone concentration decreased by 23% *4708* Increased plasma clearance, but interaction may not be clinically significant *44*

Deoxycholic Acid *Serum Increase Physiological* Significant increase possibly due to blocking uptake by plasma membrane of hepatocytes *2007*

Dexamethasone *Serum Decrease Physiological* May enhance metabolic clearance resulting in decreased plasma concentrations and lessened physiologic effects *3969*
Serum Increase Physiological Coadministration with dexamethasone led to more rapid clearance of dexamethasone due to enhanced hepatic enzyne activity possibly leading to an increase in the false positive rate with the dexamethasone suppression test for the diagnosis of Cushing's syndrome *6538*

Diazepam *Serum Decrease Physiological* Concentration reduced due to stimulated hepatic metabolism: half-life reduced from 58 to 14 hours *4354* Because of its hepatic enzyme inducing capability reduces drug concentration *2652* After administration of 1200 mg rifampin a mean 300% increase in mean oral clearance of diazepam observed *657*

Digitoxin *Serum Decrease Physiological* Decreased serum concentration due to hepatic enzyme induction *44* Coadministration of drugs caused reduction of half-life of digitoxin presumably through induction of hepatic microsomal enzymes *6665* May be reduced to subtherapeutic concentration by induction of mixed function oxidases *4631*

Digoxin *Serum Decrease Physiological* Observed in patients receiving antituberculous treatment in addition to drug for cardiac irregularity *828* Decreased serum concentration due to hepatic enzyme induction *44* Due to induction of detoxifying enzymes *6197* Effect probably due to induction of hepatic microsomal enzymes although biliary secretion might also be increased *2052*

1,25-Dihydroxy Vitamin D_3 *Serum No Effect Physiological* No change observed in 8 healthy men taking drug for 2 weeks *738*

Diltiazem *Serum Decrease Physiological* Coadministration decreases diltiazem concentration through induction of diltiazem metabolism *657*

Disopyramide *Serum Decrease Physiological* Coadministration of rifampin with disopyramide reduces concentration by 50% with reduction of half-life by the same amount *657* Plasma disopyramide concentrations reduced by about 50% in 12 patients with tuberculosis when rifampin coadministered. Effect due to stimulated hepatic metabolism *73* Because of its hepatic enzyme inducing capability reduces drug concentration *2652*

Enalapril *Serum No Effect Physiological* With coadministration of rifampin with enalapril its AUC not affected but that of enalaprilat (its active metabolite) decreased by 9% *657*

Eosinophils *Blood Decrease Physiological* Eosinophilia may occur with hypersensitivity reaction *1037*
Blood Increase Physiological Allergic reaction *2549* Isolated case of eosinophilia attributable to drug only *4171* Eosinophilia in one patient clearly linked to drug only since declined once drug withdrawn *3476*

Erythrocytes *Blood Decrease Physiological* Possible antibody-mediated immune reaction *6197* Hemolytic anemia has been observed *1037*
Urine Increase Physiological Rare reported side effect *2549*

Erythromycin *Serum Increase Analytical* Interferes with bioassays *3858*

Fleroxacin *Serum No Effect Physiological* Coadministration of fleroxacin after 5 days pretreatment with rifampin had no effect on peak fleroxacin concentration, time to its maximum concentration, or its renal clearance *5378*

Fluconazole *Serum Decrease Physiological* Rifampin pretreatment caused 22% decrease in mean fluconazole half-life and 23% decrease in mean AUC *657* Increased metabolism, loss of efficacy *886* Rifampin accelerates the metabolism of fluconazole, whose dose should be increased if rifampin is coadministered. After 600 mg/d rifampin administered to 8 healthy men for 15 days ingestion of a single oral 200 mg dose of fluconazole caused a reduction of 23 ± 9% of its AUC with a significant reduction of its half-life *4645*

Fludrocortisone *Serum Decrease Physiological* Decreased concentration observed when drugs coadministered due increased metabolic clearance of fludrocortisone because of induction of hepatic enzymes *221*

Fluvastatin *Serum Decrease Physiological* Administration of fluvastatin to patients pretreated with rifampin resulted in a 59% decrease in the fluvastatin concentration, 51% reduction in its AUC and 95% increase in its plasma clearance *5232*

Folate *Serum Decrease Analytical* Therapeutic concentrations of rifampin may inhibit standard microbiological methods for maeasuring serum vitamin B_{12} and folate *2652* Rifampin at therapeutic concentrations may inhibit standard assays *1037*

Glucaric Acid *Urine Increase Physiological* Manifestation of hepatic enzyme induction *44*

Glucose *Serum Increase Analytical* At 5 times upper limit of therapeutic concentration on method on Du Pont aca *3525*
Serum Increase Physiological Early phase hyperglycemia after oral administration of 100 g glucose *5925*
Serum No Effect Analytical At concentration of 150 mg/L had no effect on hexokinase/G-6-PDH method *5704* At 5 times upper limit of therapeutic concentration on methods on Technicon SMAC® , Abbott-VP, Roche Cobas-Bio, Kodak Ektachem® , Hitachi® 705 and KDA *3525* No effect up to 18 mg/L on glucose oxidase method on Ames Seralyzer but above this concentration apparent reduction of glucose concentration of probable clinical significance *5706*

γ-Glutamyltransferase *Serum Increase Physiological* Slight but statistically significant increase in 8 normal subjects given 600 mg daily for 7 days *4622*
Serum No Effect Analytical On method using hydrolysis of γ-glutamyl p-nitroanilide with absorbance of product at 410 nm *352* At 5 times upper limit of therapeutic range on methods on Technicon SMAC® , Abbott-VP, and Hitachi® 705 *3525*

Glyburide *Serum Decrease Physiological* Coadministration caused significant reduction with dramatic rise (5 to 6-fold) on cessation of administration of rifampin *5925*

Haloperidol *Serum Decrease Physiological* In individuals taking rifampin as well as mean haloperidol concentration reduced by 50%, with shortening of haloperidol half-life *657*

Hematocrit *Blood Decrease Physiological* Hemolytic anemia has occurred with rifampin treatment *2652*

Hemoglobin *Blood Decrease Physiological* Observed effect *2794* Hemolytic anemia has occurred with rifampin treatment *2652* Rarely acute hemolytic anemia occurs associated with circulating drug dependent antibodies in high titer *2135* Hemolytic anemia has been observed *1037*
Urine Increase Physiological Rarely hemoglobinuria has been observed *1037* Rarely hemoglobinuria or hematuria have occurred with rifampin treatment, probably as a hypersensitivity reaction *2652*

Hexobarbital *Serum Decrease Physiological* Concentration reduced when drugs coadministered due to stimulated hepatic metabolism *6664*

Histamine *Plasma No Effect Analytical* Minimal inhibition of radio-enzyme assay at 4 times therapeutic concentration *2492*

Hydrocortisone *Serum Decrease Physiological* Metabolism enhanced with reduction of circulating drug concentration: cortisol production rate increased *2985*

25-Hydroxy Vitamin D_3 *Serum Decrease Physiological* Secondary to induction of hepatic microsomal enzymes: decrease of 70% with short course in 8 healthy men *738*

17-Hydroxycorticosteroids *Urine No Effect Physiological* No significant effect of treatment with 600 mg daily for 7 days in 8 normal subjects *4622*

6-β-Hydroxycortisol *Urine Increase Physiological* Marked increase reflecting hepatic enzyme induction *621* In 14 healthy male volunteers administration of 600 mg/d for 7 days caused significant increase n excretion from mean baseline of 160.8 ± 41.4 μg/4 h to 544.8 ± 120.7 μg/4 h *5378* Mean excretion increased by 498% in patients receiving rifampin *2016* Markedly increased excretion in 8 normal subjects given 600 mg daily for 7 days *4622*

Indinavir *Serum Decrease Physiological* Increased metabolism, loss of efficacy *886* Causes a 92% decrease in area under the concentration curve when rifampin coadministered *1891*

Indocyanine Green *Serum Increase Physiological* Delayed elimination following i.v. injection *4014*

Insulin *Plasma Increase Physiological* Increased rate of secretion after oral administration of 100 g glucose *5925*

Iron *Serum Increase Analytical* Slight increase in apparent iron concentration at therapeutic concentration by method on Ferrochem II instrument *4489*
Serum No Effect Analytical At 5 times upper limit of therapeutic range on Ferrozine method on Technicon SMAC® *3525* No significant effect observed at a concentration of 70 μg/mL with method on Ferrochem II (mean with rifampin 10.03 μmol/L versus 9.91 μmol/L in controls) and 11.62 μmol/L by atomic absorption versus control of 11.40 μmol/L *5217*

itraconazole *Serum Decrease Physiological* Increased metabolism, loss of efficacy *886* Itraconazole and its major metabolite hydroxyitraconazole inhibit the cytochrome P450 3A enzyme system thereby affecting the metabolism of drugs by this system: rifampin reduces the concentration of itraconazole *2905*
Serum Increase Physiological Coadministration of rifampin with Itraconazole inhibits its metabolism thereby increasing the plasma concentration of itraconazole *2905*

Ketoconazole *Serum Decrease Physiological* Increased metabolism of ketoconazole and decreased serum concentration of rifampin *886* When rifampin is taken with ketoconazole both the rifampin and ketoconazole concentrations may decrease due to augmented hepatic metabolism *2652* In patients taking rifampin with ketoconazole significant reduction of plasma concentration of ketoconazole and area under the concentration curve *657* Plasma concentration reduced by about 33% with concomitant administration *696*

Lactate *Plasma No Effect Analytical* At concentration of 150 mg/L had no effect on enzymatic method *5704*

Lactate Dehydrogenase *Serum Increase Analytical* At 5 times upper limit of therapeutic range on method on KDA *3525*
Serum No Effect Analytical At 5 times upper limit of therapeutic range on method on Technicon SMAC® , Abbott-VP, Roche Cobas-Bio and Hitachi® 705 *3525* No effect up to 60 mg/L on method on Ames Seralyzer but at higher concentrations nonclinically significant inhibition of enzyme activity *5706*

Leukocytes *Blood Decrease Physiological* Transient leukopenia has occurred with rifampin treatment *2652* Toxic or allergic response (usually transient) *4708* Transient leukopenia has been observed *1037*

Lipase *Serum No Effect Analytical* No effect of concentrations up to 14 mg/L on method on Kodak Ektachem® *5706*

Lorcainide *Serum Decrease Physiological* In one patient coadministration of rifampin with lorcainide caused a need to increase the lorcainide dosage threefold to reach therapeutic plasma concentrations. Effect due to stimulated hepatic metab-

Rifampin *(continued)*

Lorcainide *(continued)*
olism *3853* In one patient coadministration of rifampin necessitated increase in dose of lorcainide to maintain plasma concentration and to suppress arrhythmia *657*

Methadone *Serum Decrease Physiological* Decreased serum concentration due to hepatic enzyme induction *44* Because of its hepatic enzyme inducing capability reduces drug concentration *2652* Hepatic metabolism of methadone increased as evidenced in one study of 30 patients on methadone when rifampin coadministered *3283* Increased metabolism, loss of efficacy *886*
Urine Increase Physiological Hepatic metabolism of methadone increased as evidenced in one study of 30 patients on methadone when rifampin coadministered. Decreased plasma concentration of methadone associated with increased urinary excretion *3283*

Metoprolol *Serum Decrease Physiological* Coadministration of rifampin with metoprolol requires increase of metoprolol dose to maintain effect *657* Bioavailability markedly reduced with concomitant administration due to enhanced hepatic metabolism *486*

Metronidazole *Serum Increase Analytical* Interferes with bioassays *3858*

Mexiletine *Serum Decrease Physiological* Hepatic enzyme induction may reduce elimination half-life by 50% *3281* Because of its hepatic enzyme inducing capability reduces drug concentration *2652* In 8 healthy volunteers administration of 600 mg rifampin daily for 10 days caused reduction of area under curve by 38% and reduced elimination half-life from 8.5 to 5.0 hours following single oral dose of 400 mg mexiletine compared with control *4596*

Midazolam *Serum No Effect Physiological* Administration of itraconazole caused the AUC of midazolam to increase insignificantly by 2.3% *317*

Morphine *Serum Decrease Physiological* Decreased serum concentration due to hepatic enzyme induction *44*

Nelfinavir *Serum Decrease Physiological* Coadministration of rifampin with nelfinavir caused a 82% increase in the plasma AUC of nelfinavir *66* Causes a 82% decrease in area under the concentration curve when rifampin coadministered *1891*

Neutrophils *Blood Decrease Physiological* Occasional case of agranulocytosis reported *6264* Neutropenia may occur *5373*

Nifedipine *Serum Decrease Physiological* In one patient coadministration caused dramatic decrease in plasma concentration *657* In 6 healthy volunteers coadministration of nifedipine with rifampin caused induction of cytochrome P450 3A4 with reduction of area under the curve from 38.1 ± 4.8 ng.h/mL to 26.7 ± 12.0 ng.h/mL *2685*

Nitrazepam *Serum Decrease Physiological* After administration of 600 mg/d rifampin clearance of 5 mg nitrazepam increased by 83% *657*

Novobiocin *Serum Decrease Physiological* Coadministration of rifampin with novobiocin caused its half-life to be reduced from 5.85 h to 2.66 h *657*

Parathyroid Hormone *Plasma No Effect Physiological* No change observed in 8 healthy men taking drug for 2 weeks *738*

Pefloxacin *Serum Decrease Physiological* Coadministration of rifampin with pefloxacin caused plasma concentration of pefloxacin to decrease from 4.26 ± 1.57 mg/L to 2.70 ± 1.00 mg/L, and area under concentration-time curve and elimination half-life also decreased *657*

Phenobarbital *Serum Decrease Physiological* Because of its hepatic enzyme inducing capability reduces drug concentration *2652*

Phenylalanine *Plasma No Effect Analytical* No interference observed with rapid quantitative whole blood method of Campbell et al using phenylalanine dehydrogenase *867*

Phenytoin *Serum Decrease Physiological* Possibly capable of reducing concentration when drugs coadministered *1384* Increased metabolism, loss of efficacy *886* Metabolism stimulated by rifampin with dose increase required to maintain effect *657*

Phosphate *Serum Increase Analytical* At 5 times upper limit of therapeutic concentration on methods on Du Pont aca and Hitachi® 705 *3525*
Serum No Effect Analytical At 5 times upper limit of therapeutic concentration on methods on Technicon SMAC® and KDA *3525*

Piroxicam *Serum No Effect Physiological* Coadministration of rifampin with piroxicam had no effect on its mean plasma concentration, time to peak plasma concentration, half-life or piroxicam AUC *657*

Platelets *Blood Decrease Physiological* Isolated case of severe reduction in platelet count after one dose in patient receiving treatment 4 mo previously *2397* Possible antibody-mediated immune reaction *6197* Occurs with antibody production *1763* Thrombocytopenia has been observed especially when rifampin coadministered with ethambutol *1037* Rare event but may occur when high doses are given twice weekly but this report cited one case occurring within 4 days of start of low dose treatment and the other occurred following a prolonged interruption of therapy *3472* Rare thrombocytopenia reported: rapid fall after dose given *2135* Several cases of immune mediated thrombocytopenia reported *4139* Thrombocytopenia, transient and reversible, has occurred primarily with high dose intermittent therapy but also has been observed after interruption of rifampin treatment *2652*

Polymyxin *Serum Increase Analytical* Interferes with bioassays *3858*

Prednisolone *Serum Decrease Physiological* Significant increase in systemic clearance and plasma concentration and area under curve due to induction of liver enzymes *3866*

Progestins *Serum Decrease Physiological* Because of its hepatic enzyme inducing capability reduces drug concentration *2652*

Prolactin *Plasma Decrease Physiological* For at least 12 h in normals *1356*

Propafenone *Serum Decrease Physiological* A single case report indicated that coadministration of rifampin with propafenone caused reduction of plasma propafenone and loss of rhythm control *657*

Propranolol *Serum Decrease Physiological* Amount of propranolol administered may need to be increased with coadministration of rifampin *657* Clearance greatly increased when drugs coadministered *6558* Concomitant administration of rifampin caused marked reduction of propranolol concentration due to enhanced hepatic metabolism *5466*

Protein *Serum Decrease Physiological* Due to impaired hepatic metabolism *4708*
Serum Increase Analytical At 5 times upper limit of therapeutic concentration on methods on biuret method on Kodak Ektachem® *3525*
Serum No Effect Analytical No effect of concentrations up to 100 mg/L on method on Kodak Ektachem® *5706* At 5 times upper limit of therapeutic concentration on methods on Technicon SMAC® , Abbott-VP, Hitachi® 705 and KDA *3525*
Urine Increase Physiological Attributed to drug in 2 cases *4014*

Prothrombin Time *Plasma Decrease Physiological* Due to induction of enzymes metabolizing warfarin when coadministered *6197* When coadministered with warfarin increases its metabolic clearance *2625* Occurs in some patients, especially if on anticoagulants *2282* Significantly decreased INR in patients receiving warfarin *886*
Plasma Increase Physiological May prolong action of anticoagulants *2753*

Quinidine *Serum Decrease Physiological* Reduction in peak concentration reported in one patient *44* Hepatic elimination of quinidine accelerated when rifampin coadministered because of increased production of cytochrome P450IIIA4 *5996* Coadministration reduces concentration of quinidine because of stimulated hepatic metabolism: associated with 6-fold reduction in elimination half-life in one study of 8 healthy volunteers *6112* Observed in patients receiving antituberculous treatment in addition to drug for cardiac irregularity *828* Because of its hepatic enzyme inducing capability reduces drug concentration *2652*
Serum Increase Physiological Concentration of metabolites increased with probable maintenance of therapeutic effects *827*

Quinine *Serum Decrease Physiological* In 9 healthy individuals mean maximum concentration of 4.6 ± 1.0 mg/L following a single oral dose of 600 mg quinine sulfate reduced to 2.2 ± 1.1 mg/L when volunteers pretreated with rifampin *6346*

Ritonavir *Serum Decrease Physiological* Decreases area under the concentration curve by 35% when fluoxetine coadministered *1891* Increased metabolism, loss of efficacy *886*

Saquinavir *Serum Decrease Physiological* Increased metabolism, loss of efficacy *886* Coadministration of saquinavir 600 mg t.i.d. with rifampin 600 mg q.d. to 12 healthy volunteers produced approximately 50% decrease of AUC and maximum concentration compared when saquinavir was given alone *5024* Decreases the area under the concentration curve by 80% when rifampin coadministered *1891*

Sildenafil *Serum Decrease Physiological* Theoretical effect: drug likely to decrease area under concentration curve of sildenafil due to induction of CYP3A4 *4657*

Sulfobromophthalein *Serum Increase Physiological* Transient increases in BSP retention observed with rifampin treatment *2652* False positive BSP test may be observed so test should be performed prior to the morning dose of rifampin to avoid false results *1037*

Tacrolimus *Serum Decrease Physiological* By inducing cytochrome P-450 IIIA enzyme systems may stimulate the metabolism of tacrolimus *1987*

Temazepam *Serum No Effect Physiological* Pharmacokinetics of a single dose of 10 mg not affected by coadministration of rifampin *657*

Terbinafine *Serum Decrease Physiological* Rifampin increased the clearance of terbinafine by 100%, a CyP450 enzyme inducer *5231*

Testosterone *Serum Increase Physiological* Probably due to increase in microsomal activity and increased biosynthesis *2836*

Tetracycline *Serum Increase Analytical* Interferes with bioassays *3858*

Theophylline *Serum Decrease Physiological* Reduced area under concentration curve and increased metabolic clearance and volume of distribution *4769* Coadministration reduced theophylline half-life from 9.6 h to 5.5 h but when diltiazem also added half-life increased to 6.2 h *657* Up to 40% decrease in serum theophylline concentration due to increased theophylline clearance caused by increasing cytochrome P450 1A2 and 3A3 activity *6117* Increases theophylline clearance by inhibiting cytochrome P450 1A2 and 3A3 activity and decreases serum theophylline concentration by 20 to 40% *3125* Significantly increased mean oral clearance of drug with elimination rate constant increased by mean of 25% *5843* 25% reduction in area under curve when coadministered and reduction of half-life from 7.0 to 4.8 h *6130* Increases theophylline clearance by increasing cytochrome P450 1A2 and 3A3 activity, decreasing theophylline concentration by 20 - 40% *5999* Because of its hepatic enzyme inducing capability reduces drug concentration *2652* Clearance increased by more than 25% when drugs coadministered *677*
Serum No Effect Physiological No effect observed on half-life *1384* Coadministration to 12 adult male volunteers of rifampin 300 mg/d with 5 mg/kg theophylline caused a significant reduction in area under concentration-time curve from 140 ± 37 µg.h/mL to 100 ± 24 µg.h/mL but serum concentration nonsignificantly reduced from 10.9 ± 1.3 µg/mL to 10.6.± 1.1 µg/mL *2123*

Thyroid Stimulating Hormone
Serum Increase Physiological In one patient with primary hypothyroidism receiving constant replacement dose of L-thyroxine: tri-iodothyronine clearance retarded *2835*

Thyroxine (T4) *Serum Decrease Physiological* In one patient with primary hypothyroidism receiving constant replacement dose of L-thyroxine: tri-iodothyronine clearance retarded *2835*

Tocainide *Serum Decrease Physiological* Following a single oral dose of 600 mg tocainide when rifampin being coadministered reduction of tocainide half-life from 13.2 h to 9.4 h (34%) *657*

Tolbutamide *Serum Decrease Physiological* Concentration reduced due to stimulation of hepatic microsomal enzymes *6664* Decreased serum concentration due to hepatic enzyme induction *44*

Tri-iodothyronine (T3) *Serum Increase Physiological* In one patient with primary hypothyroidism receiving constant replacement dose of L-thyroxine: tri-iodothyronine clearance retarded *2835*

Tricyclic Antidepressants *Serum Decrease Physiological* Interacts pharmacokinetically to induce metabolism of tricyclic antidepressants *3590*

Triglycerides *Serum Decrease Analytical* At 5 times upper limit of therapeutic concentration on method on KDA *3525*
Serum No Effect Analytical At 5 times upper limit of therapeutic concentration on method on Technicon SMAC® , Abbott-VP, Kodak Ektachem® and Hitachi® 705 *3525*

Trimethoprim *Serum Increase Analytical* Interferes with bioassays *3858*

Urea Nitrogen *Serum Increase Physiological* Rarely increased concentration has been observed and even more rarely renal insufficiency or acute renal failure has occurred. These are probably hypersensitivity reactions *1037* Increased concentration has occurred with rifampin treatment *2652* Temporary renal failure reported *1484*
Serum No Effect Analytical At 5 times upper limit of therapeutic range on method on echnicon SMAC® , Abbott-VP, Roche Cobas-Bio, Kodak Ektachem® , Hitachi® 705 and KDA *3525* No effect at 300 mg/L on method on Ames Seralyzer *5706*

Uric Acid *Serum Increase Analytical* Substantial increase at upper limit of therapeutic range on methods on KDA and Hitachi® 705 *3525*
Serum Increase Physiological Increased concentration has occurred with rifampin treatment *2652* Rarely increased concentration has been observed This is probably a hypersensitivity reaction *1037* Temporary renal failure reported *1484*
Serum No Effect Analytical At 5 times upper limit of therapeutic range on methods on Technicon SMAC® , Abbott-VP, Du Pont aca, Kodak Ektachem® and Roche Cobas-Bio *3525*

Valproic Acid *Serum Decrease Physiological* In a study involving the administration of a single dose of valproate (7 mg/kg) 36 hours after 5 nights of daily dosing with 600 mg rifampin revealed a 40% increase in the oral clearance of valproate *15* Administration of a single dose of valproate (7 mg/kg: 36 h after 5 nights of daily dosing with rifampin (600 mg) revealed a 40% increase in the oral clearance of valproate *17*

Vancomycin *Serum No Effect Analytical* No significant interference observed at a concentration of 500 µg/mL (608 µmol/L) with method on Du Pont aca *1561*

Verapamil *Serum Decrease Physiological* Because of its hepatic enzyme inducing capability reduces drug concentration *2652* Hepatic enzyme induction causes reduction of concentration *1384* Coadministration of rifampin with verapamil may markedly reduce the bioavailability of verapamil *3470* Coadministration reduced verapamil bioavailability *657* Rifampin may reduce bioavailability of verapamil *1037* Coadministration may markedly reduce verapamil concentration but mechanism not specified *3201* When drugs coadministered rifampin may markedly reduce bioavailability of verapamil *2063* Marked reduction observed in four individuals following single oral dose of 40 mg: effect due to induction of hepatic metabolism *4835*

Vitamin B_{12} *Serum Decrease Analytical* Rifampin at therapeutic concentrations may inhibit standard assays *1037* Therapeutic concentrations of rifampin may inhibit standard microbiological methods for maeasuring serum vitamin B_{12} and folate *2652*

Warfarin *Plasma Decrease Physiological* Catabolism of drug increased due to induction of hepatic microsomal enzymes *5073* Decreased serum concentration due to hepatic enzyme induction *44*

Zidovudine *Serum Decrease Physiological* Increased metabolism, loss of efficacy *886*
Serum Increase Physiological Coadministration of rifampin (600 mg) with zidovudine (200 mg) decreased the plasma AUC of zidovudine by 48 ± 34% *2163*
Serum No Effect Analytical No effect on liquid chromatographic method of Hedaya and Sawchuk *2525*

Riluzole

Alanine Aminotransferase *Serum Increase Physiological* In 13 of 77 patients with amyotrophic lateral sclerosis treatment with 100 mg/d riluzole caused reversible increase of activity (to over 3 times upper limit of normal in 6 compared with 3 in

Riluzole *(continued)*

Alanine Aminotransferase *(continued)*
placebo group) *489* Experience in about 800 patients with amyotrophic lateral sclerosis shows that about 50% patients develop increased enzyme activity: 8% have increased activity more than 3 times ULN, and about 2% have activity more than 5 times ULN: maximum increases usually occur within 3 months of the start of treatment and were usually transient when less than 5 times ULN *4941*

Alkaline Phosphatase *Serum* *Increase* *Physiological* Infrequently increased activity observed with treatment *4941*

Aspartate Aminotransferase *Serum* *Increase* *Physiological* Infrequently increased activity observed with treatment *4941* In 77 patients with amyotrophic lateral sclerosis treatment with 100 mg/d caused reversible increased activity in 11 patients compared with increase in 3 in placebo group *489*

Calcium *Serum* *Increase* *Physiological* Rare hypercalcemia observed with treatment *4941*

Cholesterol *Serum* *Increase* *Physiological* Rare hypercholesterolemia observed with treatment *4941*

Coombs' Test, Direct *Blood* *Positive* *Physiological* Infrequently positive direct Coomb's test observed with treatment *4941*

γ-Globulin *Serum* *Increase* *Physiological* Infrequently increased concentration observed with treatment *4941*

Glucose *Serum* *Increase* *Physiological* Infrequent diabetes mellitus observed with treatment *4941*

γ-Glutamyltransferase *Serum* *Increase* *Physiological* Infrequently increased activity observed with treatment *4941*

Hematocrit *Blood* *Decrease* *Physiological* Infrequent anemia observed with treatment *4941*

Hemoglobin *Blood* *Decrease* *Physiological* Infrequent anemia observed with treatment *4941*

Lactate Dehydrogenase *Serum* *Increase* *Physiological* Rarely increased activity observed with treatment *4941*

Leukocytes *Blood* *Decrease* *Physiological* Infrequent leukopenia observed with treatment *4941*
Blood *Increase* *Physiological* Infrequent leukocytosis observed with treatment *4941*

Neutrophils *Blood* *Decrease* *Physiological* Rare neutropenia observed with treatment *4941* In about 400 patients with amyotrophic lateral sclerosis there were three cases of marked neutropenia *4941*

Occult Blood *Feces* *Increase* *Physiological* Rare hematemesis or melena observed with treatment *4941*

Potassium *Serum* *Decrease* *Physiological* Infrequent hypokalemia observed with treatment *4941*

Sodium *Serum* *Decrease* *Physiological* Infrequent hyponatremia observed with treatment *4941*

Uric Acid *Serum* *Increase* *Physiological* Infrequent gout observed with treatment *4941*

Warfarin *Plasma* *No Effect* *Physiological* Riluzole had no effect on warfarin binding *4941*

Rimeterol

Aldosterone *Plasma* *No Effect* *Physiological* No significant change in 4 healthy men given therapeutic i.v. dose *4690*

Calcium *Serum* *Decrease* *Physiological* Dose related significant change in 4 healthy men given therapeutic i.v. dose *4690*

Corticosteroids *Plasma* *Decrease* *Physiological* Dose related significant change in 4 healthy men given therapeutic i.v. dose *4690*

Glucose *Serum* *Increase* *Physiological* Dose related significant change in 4 healthy men given therapeutic i.v. dose *4690*

β-Hydroxybutyrate *Serum* *No Effect* *Physiological* No significant change in 4 healthy men given therapeutic i.v. dose *4690*

Insulin *Plasma* *Increase* *Physiological* Dose related significant change in 4 healthy men given therapeutic i.v. dose *4690*

Ketones *Serum* *Increase* *Physiological* Dose related significant change in 4 healthy men given therapeutic i.v. dose *4690*

Lactate *Plasma* *Increase* *Physiological* Dose related significant change in 4 healthy men given therapeutic i.v. dose *4690*

Magnesium *Serum* *Decrease* *Physiological* Dose related significant change in 4 healthy men given therapeutic i.v. dose *4690*

Phosphate *Serum* *Decrease* *Physiological* Dose related significant change in 4 healthy men given therapeutic i.v. dose *4690*

Potassium *Serum* *Decrease* *Physiological* Dose related significant change in 4 healthy men given therapeutic i.v. dose *4690*

Renin Activity *Plasma* *Increase* *Physiological* Dose related significant change in 4 healthy men given therapeutic i.v. dose *4690*

Rioprostil

Gastric Inhibitory Polypeptide
Plasma *Decrease* *Physiological* Doses up to 600 µg/day delayed and reduced the normal 3-hour postprandial release in 9 healthy male volunteers *1380*

Gastrin *Serum* *No Effect* *Physiological* Doses up to 600 µg/day did not modify normal postglucose release in 9 healthy male volunteers *1380* Both basal gastrin and postprandial gastrin concentrations unaffected in normal healthy volunteers when treated with 600 µg for 4 weeks *3242*

Glucose *Serum* *No Effect* *Physiological* Neither basal nor postprandial glucose concentrations significantly modified in 9 healthy male volunteers *1380*

Hydrochloric Acid *Gastric Fluid* *No Effect* *Physiological* Treatment of healthy male volunteers with 600 µg/day for 4 weeks had no effect *3242*

Pancreatic Polypeptide *Plasma* *No Effect* *Physiological* Treatment with 600 µg/day for 4 weeks in healthy male volunteers caused no effect *3242*

Risperidone

Alanine Aminotransferase *Serum* *Increase* *Physiological* Infrequent increased enzyme activity observed with administration of risperidone, with rare hepatic failure, cholestatic hepatitis, cholecystitis, cholelithiasis or hepatocellular damage *2904*

Alkaline Phosphatase *Serum* *Increase* *Physiological* Rare hepatic failure, cholestatic hepatitis, cholecystitis, cholelithiasis or hepatocellular damage observed with risperidone treatment *2904*

Aspartate Aminotransferase *Serum* *Increase* *Physiological* Infrequent increased enzyme activity observed with administration of risperidone, with rare hepatic failure, cholestatic hepatitis, cholecystitis, cholelithiasis or hepatocellular damage *2904*

Blood *Urine* *Increase* *Physiological* Infrequent hematuria observed with administration of risperidone *2904*

Clara Cell Protein *Serum* *No Effect* *Physiological* In 10 schizophrenics treated with risperidone mean concentration of 22.0 ± 3.9 ng/mL not significantly different from that in 14 untreated schizophrenics in whom the mean concentration was 19.3 ± 5.2 ng/mL *3732*

Creatine Kinase *Serum* *Increase* *Physiological* In 11 acutely psychotic patients treatment with olanzapine and haloperidol (2 - 8 determinations per patient) was associated with 15 marked elevations (in 10.0% of the patients) *3947* Infrequent increase in enzyme activity observed with administration of risperidone *2904*

Creatinine *Serum* *Increase* *Physiological* Rare renal insufficiency observed with administration of risperidone *2904*

Glucose *Serum* *Increase* *Physiological* Infrequent diabetes mellitus observed with administration of risperidone *2904*

Hematocrit *Blood* *Decrease* *Physiological* Infrequent hypochromic anemia and rare hypochromic anemia observed with risperidone treatment *2904*

Hemoglobin *Blood* *Decrease* *Physiological* Infrequent hypochromic anemia and rare hypochromic anemia observed with risperidone treatment *2904*

Interleukin-1 Receptor Antagonist
Serum No Effect Physiological In 10 schizophrenics treated with risperidone mean concentration of 0.29 ± 0.18 U/mL not significantly different from that in 14 untreated schizophrenics in whom the mean concentration was 0.29 ± 0.18 U/mL *3732*

Iron *Serum Decrease Physiological* Rare decrease in serum iron concentration observed with administration of risperidone *2904*

Leukocytes *Blood Decrease Physiological* Rare leukocytosis or leukopenia observed with risperidone treatment *2904*
Blood Increase Physiological Rare leukocytosis or leukopenia observed with risperidone treatment *2904*

Phosphate *Serum Increase Physiological* Rare hyperphosphatemia observed with administration of risperidone *2904*

Platelets *Blood Decrease Physiological* Rare thrombocytopenia observed with risperidone treatment *2904*

Potassium *Serum Decrease Physiological* Rare hypokalemia observed with administration of risperidone *2904*

Prolactin *Plasma Increase Physiological* As with other drugs antagonizing dopamine D_2 receptors concentration increased and persists during chronic administration *2904*

Protein *Serum Decrease Physiological* Rare hypoproteinemia observed with administration of risperidone *2904*

Sodium *Serum Decrease Physiological* Infrequent hyponatremia observed with administration of risperidone *2904*

Soluble $CD8^+$ *Serum No Effect Physiological* In 10 schizophrenics treated with risperidone mean concentration of 430 ± 131 U/mL not significantly different from that in 14 untreated schizophrenics in whom the mean concentration was 82 ± 82 U/mL *3732*

Soluble Interleukin-2 Receptor
Serum Increase Physiological In 10 schizophrenics treated with risperidone mean concentration of 131 ± 112 U/mL significantly higher than that in 14 untreated schizophrenics in whom the mean concentration was 82 ± 82 U/mL *3732*

β-Thrombomodulin *Plasma Increase Physiological* Rare hepatic failure, cholestatic hepatitis, cholecystitis, cholelithiasis or hepatocellular damage observed with risperidone treatment *2904*

Triglycerides *Serum Increase Physiological* Rare hypertriglyceridemia observed with administration of risperidone *2904*

Urea Nitrogen *Serum Increase Physiological* Rare renal insufficiency observed with administration of risperidone *2904*

Uric Acid *Serum Decrease Physiological* Rare hypoglycemia observed with administration of risperidone *2904*
Serum Increase Physiological Rare hyperuricemia observed with administration of risperidone *2904*

Ritanserin

Prolactin *Plasma Decrease Physiological* Marked decrease observed in patients with functional and puerperal hyperprolactinemia *1788*
Plasma No Effect Physiological No significant effect observed in normoprolactinemic patients and in those with prolactin-secreting pituitary adenomas *1788*

Ritodrine

Adenosine Monophosphate *Plasma Increase Physiological* Intravenous infusion of ritrodine may increase plasma concentration of cyclic AMP *281*

Drugs of Abuse Screen *Urine Increase Analytical* False positive result obtained for amphetamine/methamphetamine assay using Abbott ADx. Concentration of about 83 mg/L produces ADx concentration of 0.50 mg/L for amphetamine/methamphetamine *4279*

Fatty Acids (FFA), Free *Serum Increase Physiological* Intravenous infusion of ritrodine may increase plasma concentration of FFA *281*

Glucose *Serum Increase Physiological* Moderate effect when given intravenously for premature labor *1400* Intravenous administration may increase plasma insulin and glucose concentrations *281*
Urine Increase Physiological Intravenous infusion of ritrodine may cause glycosuria in association with increased blood glucose concentration *281*

Insulin *Plasma Increase Physiological* Intravenous administration may increase plasma insulin and glucose concentrations *281*

Lactate *Plasma Increase Physiological* Moderate effect when given intravenously for premature labor *1400* Intravenous infusion of ritrodine may cause lactic acidosis *281*

pH *Blood Decrease Physiological* Intravenous infusion of ritrodine may cause lactic acidosis *281*

Potassium *Serum Decrease Physiological* Intravenous administration may decrease plasma potassium concentration but this is usually transient and returns to normal within 24 h *281*

Pyruvate *Plasma No Effect Physiological* Little effect noted in patients given drug intravenously for premature labor, with consequent increase in lactate/pyruvate ratio *1400*

Ritonavir

Alanine Aminotransferase *Serum Increase Physiological* Increased activity observed in in fewer than 10% treated patients, but occurring at least twice as often as in control individuals *1891* In one study of advanced patients 6.1% of those receiving ritonavir had an activity above 215 U/L different from 2.6% in those receiving placebo *23*

Albumin *Serum No Effect Physiological* In one study of advanced patients 0.2% of those receiving ritonavir had a concentration below 2.0 g/dL not different from 0.6% in those receiving placebo *23*

Alfentanil *Serum Increase Physiological* Ritonavir has a high affinity for several cytochrome P450 isoforms inhibiting the metabolism of other drugs. In HIV-infected patients coadministration of ritonavir greatly increased (more than 3 times) the AUC of alfentanil *23*

Alkaline Phosphatase *Serum No Effect Physiological* In one study of advanced patients 1.4% of those receiving ritonavir had an activity above 550 U/L not different from 1.7% in those receiving placebo *23*

Alprazolam *Serum Increase Physiological* Increased plasma concentration *886*

Amitriptyline *Serum Increase Physiological* Ritonavir has a high affinity for several cytochrome P450 isoforms inhibiting the metabolism of other drugs. In HIV-infected patients coadministration of ritonavir moderately increased (1.5 to 3 times) the AUC of amitriptyline *23*

Amlodipine *Serum Increase Physiological* Ritonavir has a high affinity for several cytochrome P450 isoforms inhibiting the metabolism of other drugs. In HIV-infected patients coadministration of ritonavir greatly increased (more than 3 times) the AUC of amlodipine *23*

Aspartate Aminotransferase *Serum Increase Physiological* Increased activity observed in in fewer than 10% treated patients, but occurring at least twice as often as in control individuals *1891*
Serum No Effect Physiological In one study of advanced patients 3.8% of those receiving ritonavir had an activity above 180 U/L not different from 4.3% in those receiving placebo *23*

Astemizole *Serum Increase Physiological* Decreased metabolism resulting in cardiac toxicity or arrhythmia *886*

Atovaquone *Serum Decrease Physiological* Ritonavir has a high affinity for several cytochrome P450 isoforms inhibiting the metabolism of other drugs. In HIV-infected patients coadministration of ritonavir caused a possible decrease of the AUC of atovaquone *23*

Bilirubin *Serum No Effect Physiological* In one study of advanced patients 1.2% of those receiving ritonavir had a concentration above 3.6 mg/dL not different from 0.2% in those receiving placebo *23*

Bromocriptine *Serum Increase Physiological* Ritonavir has a high affinity for several cytochrome P450 isoforms inhibiting the metabolism of other drugs. In HIV-infected patients coadministration of ritonavir greatly increased (more than 3 times) the AUC of bromocriptine *23*

Ritonavir *(continued)*

Calcium *Serum No Effect Physiological* In one study of advanced patients 1.2% of those receiving ritonavir had a concentration below 6.9 mEq/L not different from 0.9% in those receiving placebo *23*

Carbamazepine *Serum Increase Physiological* Ritonavir has a high affinity for several cytochrome P450 isoforms inhibiting the metabolism of other drugs. In HIV-infected patients coadministration of ritonavir greatly increased (more than 3 times) the AUC of carbamazepine *23*

CD4+ Lymphocytes *Blood Increase Physiological* In 84 HIV-positive patients treatment with up to 600 mg/12 h caused increase of up to 130 cells/µL after 3 weeks *1234*

Chlorpromazine *Serum Increase Physiological* Ritonavir has a high affinity for several cytochrome P450 isoforms inhibiting the metabolism of other drugs. In HIV-infected patients coadministration of ritonavir moderately increased (1.5 to 3 times) the AUC of chlorpromazine *23*

Cisapride *Serum Increase Physiological* Decreased metabolism resulting in cardiac toxicity or arrhythmia *886*

Clarithromycin *Serum Increase Physiological* Ritonavir has a high affinity for several cytochrome P450 isoforms inhibiting the metabolism of other drugs. In HIV-infected patients coadministration of ritonavir moderately increased (1.5 to 3 times) the AUC of clarithromycin *23* Increased plasma concentration *886* Increases the area under the concentration curve by 77% when ritonavir coadministered *1891*

Clofibrate *Serum Decrease Physiological* Ritonavir has a high affinity for several cytochrome P450 isoforms inhibiting the metabolism of other drugs. In HIV-infected patients coadministration of ritonavir caused a possible decrease of the AUC of clofibrate *23*

Clomipramine *Serum Increase Physiological* Ritonavir has a high affinity for several cytochrome P450 isoforms inhibiting the metabolism of other drugs. In HIV-infected patients coadministration of ritonavir moderately increased (1.5 to 3 times) the AUC of clomipramine *23*

Clonazepam *Serum Increase Physiological* Ritonavir has a high affinity for several cytochrome P450 isoforms inhibiting the metabolism of other drugs. In HIV-infected patients coadministration of ritonavir moderately increased (1.5 to 3 times) the AUC of clonazepam *23*

Codeine *Serum Decrease Physiological* Ritonavir has a high affinity for several cytochrome P450 isoforms inhibiting the metabolism of other drugs. In HIV-infected patients coadministration of ritonavir possibly decreased the AUC of codeine *23*

Creatine Kinase *Serum Increase Physiological* In one study of advanced patients 8.6% of those receiving ritonavir had an activity above 1000 U/L different from 4.5% in those receiving placebo *23*

Creatinine *Serum No Effect Physiological* In one study of advanced patients 0.2% of those receiving ritonavir had a concentration above 3.6 mg/dL not different from 0.2% in those receiving placebo *23*

Cyclophosphamide *Serum Decrease Physiological.* Ritonavir has a high affinity for several cytochrome P450 isoforms inhibiting the metabolism of other drugs. In HIV-infected patients coadministration of ritonavir moderately decreased (1.5 to 3 times) the AUC of cyclophosphamide *23*
Serum Increase Physiological Ritonavir has a high affinity for several cytochrome P450 isoforms inhibiting the metabolism of other drugs. In HIV-infected patients coadministration of ritonavir moderately increased (1.5 to 3 times) the AUC of cyclophosphamide *23*

Cyclosporine A *Blood Increase Physiological* Ritonavir has a high affinity for several cytochrome P450 isoforms inhibiting the metabolism of other drugs. In HIV-infected patients coadministration of ritonavir greatly increased (more than 3 times) the AUC of cyclosporine *23*

Desipramine *Serum Increase Physiological* Ritonavir has a high affinity for several cytochrome P450 isoforms inhibiting the metabolism of other drugs. In HIV-infected patients coadministration of ritonavir moderately increased (1.5 to 3 times) the AUC of desipramine *23* Increases the area under the concentration curve by 145% when ritonavir coadministered *1891* Increased plasma concentration *886*

Dexamethasone *Serum Increase Physiological* Ritonavir has a high affinity for several cytochrome P450 isoforms inhibiting the metabolism of other drugs. In HIV-infected patients coadministration of ritonavir greatly increased (more than 3 times) the AUC of dexamethasone *23*

Dexfenfluramine *Serum Increase Physiological* Ritonavir has a high affinity for several cytochrome P450 isoforms inhibiting the metabolism of other drugs. In HIV-infected patients coadministration of ritonavir moderately increased (1.5 to 3 times) the AUC of dexfenfluramine *23*

Diazepam *Serum Increase Physiological* Increased plasma concentration *886*

Diclofenac *Serum Decrease Physiological* Ritonavir has a high affinity for several cytochrome P450 isoforms inhibiting the metabolism of other drugs. In HIV-infected patients coadministration of ritonavir caused a moderate decrease or increase (1.5 to 3 times) of the AUC of diclofenac *23*
Serum Increase Physiological Ritonavir has a high affinity for several cytochrome P450 isoforms inhibiting the metabolism of other drugs. In HIV-infected patients coadministration of ritonavir caused a moderate decrease or increase (1.5 to 3 times) of the AUC of diclofenac *23*

Didanosine *Serum Decrease Physiological* Decreases the area under the concentration curve by 13% when ritonavir coadministered *1891* Ritonavir has a high affinity for several cytochrome P450 isoforms affecting the metabolism of other drugs. The mean decrease in AUC was 13% *23*

Diltiazem *Serum Increase Physiological* Ritonavir has a high affinity for several cytochrome P450 isoforms inhibiting the metabolism of other drugs. In HIV-infected patients coadministration of ritonavir greatly increased (more than 3 times) the AUC of diltiazem *23*

Diphenoxylate *Serum Decrease Physiological* Ritonavir has a high affinity for several cytochrome P450 isoforms inhibiting the metabolism of other drugs. In HIV-infected patients coadministration of ritonavir caused a possible decrease of the AUC of diphenoxylate *23*

Disopyramide *Serum Increase Physiological* Ritonavir has a high affinity for several cytochrome P450 isoforms inhibiting the metabolism of other drugs. In HIV-infected patients coadministration of ritonavir moderately increased (1.5 to 3 times) the AUC of disopyramide *23*

Doxazosin *Serum Increase Physiological* Ritonavir has a high affinity for several cytochrome P450 isoforms inhibiting the metabolism of other drugs. In HIV-infected patients coadministration of ritonavir caused a possible increase of the AUC of doxazosin *23*

Doxepin *Serum Increase Physiological* Ritonavir has a high affinity for several cytochrome P450 isoforms inhibiting the metabolism of other drugs. In HIV-infected patients coadministration of ritonavir caused a possible increase of the AUC of doxepin *23*

Dronabinol *Serum Increase Physiological* Ritonavir has a high affinity for several cytochrome P450 isoforms inhibiting the metabolism of other drugs. In HIV-infected patients coadministration of ritonavir moderately increased (1.5 to 3 times) the AUC of dronabinol *23*

Eosinophils *Blood No Effect Physiological* In one study of advanced patients 1.8% of those receiving ritonavir had a concentration above 1.0 x 10^9/L not different from 2.6% in those receiving placebo *23*

Erythrocytes *Blood No Effect Physiological* In one study of advanced patients 14.9% of those receiving ritonavir had a concentration below 3 million /µL not different from 19.7% in those receiving placebo *23*

Erythromycin *Serum Increase Physiological* Ritonavir has a high affinity for several cytochrome P450 isoforms inhibiting the metabolism of other drugs. In HIV-infected patients coadministration of ritonavir greatly increased (more than 3 times) the AUC of erythromycin *23* Increased plasma concentration *886*

Ethinyl Estradiol *Serum Decrease Physiological* Decreases the area under the concentration curve by 40% when ritonavir coadministered *1891* Ritonavir has a high affinity for several cytochrome P450 isoforms affecting the metabolism of other drugs. The mean decrease in AUC of ethinyl estradiol from oral contraceptives was 40% with concomitant administration of ritanavir 500 mg q.i.d *23*

Ethosuximide *Serum Increase Physiological* Ritonavir has a high affinity for several cytochrome P450 isoforms inhibiting the metabolism of other drugs. In HIV-infected patients coadministration of ritonavir moderately increased (1.5 to 3 times) the AUC of ethosuximide *23*

Etoposide *Serum Increase Physiological* Ritonavir has a high affinity for several cytochrome P450 isoforms inhibiting the metabolism of other drugs. In HIV-infected patients coadministration of ritonavir moderately increased (1.5 to 3 times) the AUC of etoposide *23*

Felbamate *Serum Increase Physiological* Ritonavir has a high affinity for several cytochrome P450 isoforms inhibiting the metabolism of other drugs. In HIV-infected patients coadministration of ritonavir greatly increased (more than 3 times) the AUC of felodipine *23*

Felodipine *Serum Increase Physiological* Ritonavir has a high affinity for several cytochrome P450 isoforms affecting the metabolism of other drugs. Significant increase in AUC observed *23*

Fentanyl *Serum Increase Physiological* Ritonavir has a high affinity for several cytochrome P450 isoforms inhibiting the metabolism of other drugs. In HIV-infected patients coadministration of ritonavir greatly increased (more than 3 times) the AUC of fentanyl *23*

Fluoxetine *Serum Increase Physiological* Ritonavir has a high affinity for several cytochrome P450 isoforms inhibiting the metabolism of other drugs. In HIV-infected patients coadministration of ritonavir moderately increased (1.5 to 3 times) the AUC of fluoxetine *23*

Flurbiprofen *Serum Increase Physiological* Ritonavir has a high affinity for several cytochrome P450 isoforms inhibiting the metabolism of other drugs. In HIV-infected patients coadministration of ritonavir caused a moderate decrease or increase (1.5 to 3 times) of the AUC of flurbiprofen *23*

Fluvastatin *Serum Increase Physiological* Ritonavir has a high affinity for several cytochrome P450 isoforms inhibiting the metabolism of other drugs. In HIV-infected patients coadministration of ritonavir greatly increased (more than 3 times) the AUC of fluvastatin *23*

Glimepiride *Serum Decrease Physiological* Ritonavir has a high affinity for several cytochrome P450 isoforms inhibiting the metabolism of other drugs. In HIV-infected patients coadministration of ritonavir moderately decreased (1.5 to 3 times) the AUC of glimepiride *23*
Serum Increase Physiological Ritonavir has a high affinity for several cytochrome P450 isoforms inhibiting the metabolism of other drugs. In HIV-infected patients coadministration of ritonavir moderately increased (1.5 to 3 times) the AUC of glimepiride *23*

Glipizide *Serum Decrease Physiological* Ritonavir has a high affinity for several cytochrome P450 isoforms inhibiting the metabolism of other drugs. In HIV-infected patients coadministration of ritonavir moderately decreased (1.5 to 3 times) the AUC of glipizide *23*
Serum Increase Physiological Ritonavir has a high affinity for several cytochrome P450 isoforms inhibiting the metabolism of other drugs. In HIV-infected patients coadministration of ritonavir moderately increased (1.5 to 3 times) the AUC of glipizide *23*

Glucose *Serum Increase Physiological* Increased concentration observed in in fewer than 10% treated patients, but occurring at least twice as often as in control individuals *1891*
Serum No Effect Physiological In one study of advanced patients 0.4% of those receiving ritonavir had hyperglycemia above 250 mg/dL not significantly different from 1.1% in those receiving placebo *23*

γ-Glutamyltransferase *Serum Increase Physiological* In one study of advanced patients 14.7% of those receiving ritonavir had an activity above 300 U/L different from 6.7% in those receiving placebo *23*

Glyburide *Serum Increase Physiological* Ritonavir has a high affinity for several cytochrome P450 isoforms inhibiting the metabolism of other drugs. In HIV-infected patients coadministration of ritonavir moderately increased (1.5 to 3 times) the AUC of glyburide *23*

Haloperidol *Serum Increase Physiological* Ritonavir has a high affinity for several cytochrome P450 isoforms inhibiting the metabolism of other drugs. In HIV-infected patients coadministration of ritonavir moderately increased (1.5 to 3 times) the AUC of haloperidol *23*

Hematocrit *Blood No Effect Physiological* In one study of advanced patients 11.7% of those receiving ritonavir had a concentration below 30% not different from 16.0% in those receiving placebo *23*

Hemoglobin *Blood No Effect Physiological* In one study of advanced patients 2.9% of those receiving ritonavir had a concentration below 80 g/L not different from 2.4% in those receiving placebo *23*

HIV-1 RNA *Serum Decrease Physiological* In 84 HIV-positive patients treatment with up to 600 mg/12 h caused decrease of about 1.0 log copies/mL between after one week *1234*

HIV p24 Antigen *Serum Decrease Physiological* In 84 HIV-positive patients treatment with up to 600 mg/12 h caused decrease of between 75 and 100% after one week *1234*

Hydrocodone *Serum Increase Physiological* Ritonavir has a high affinity for several cytochrome P450 isoforms inhibiting the metabolism of other drugs. In HIV-infected patients coadministration of ritonavir moderately increased (1.5 to 3 times) the AUC of hydrocodone *23*

Hydromorphone *Serum Decrease Physiological* Ritonavir has a high affinity for several cytochrome P450 isoforms inhibiting the metabolism of other drugs. In HIV-infected patients coadministration of ritonavir possibly decreased the AUC of hydromorphone *23*

Ibuprofen *Serum Decrease Physiological* Ritonavir has a high affinity for several cytochrome P450 isoforms inhibiting the metabolism of other drugs. In HIV-infected patients coadministration of ritonavir caused a moderate decrease or increase (1.5 to 3 times) of the AUC of ibuprofen *23*
Serum Increase Physiological Ritonavir has a high affinity for several cytochrome P450 isoforms inhibiting the metabolism of other drugs. In HIV-infected patients coadministration of ritonavir caused a moderate decrease or increase (1.5 to 3 times) of the AUC of ibuprofen *23*

Ifosfamide *Serum Increase Physiological* Ritonavir has a high affinity for several cytochrome P450 isoforms inhibiting the metabolism of other drugs. In HIV-infected patients coadministration of ritonavir moderately increased (1.5 to 3 times) the AUC of ifosfamide *23*

Imipramine *Serum Increase Physiological* Ritonavir has a high affinity for several cytochrome P450 isoforms inhibiting the metabolism of other drugs. In HIV-infected patients coadministration of ritonavir moderately increased (1.5 to 3 times) the AUC of imipramine *23*

Indinavir *Serum Increase Physiological* Ritonavir has a high affinity for several cytochrome P450 isoforms inhibiting the metabolism of other drugs. In HIV-infected patients coadministration of ritonavir greatly increased (more than 3 times) the AUC of indinavir *23*

Indomethacin *Serum Decrease Physiological* Ritonavir has a high affinity for several cytochrome P450 isoforms inhibiting the metabolism of other drugs. In HIV-infected patients coadministration of ritonavir caused a moderate decrease or increase (1.5 to 3 times) of the AUC of indomethacin *23*
Serum Increase Physiological Ritonavir has a high affinity for several cytochrome P450 isoforms inhibiting the metabolism of other drugs. In HIV-infected patients coadministration of ritonavir caused a moderate decrease or increase (1.5 to 3.0 times) of the AUC of indomethacin *23*

Isradipine *Serum Increase Physiological* Ritonavir has a high affinity for several cytochrome P450 isoforms inhibiting the metabolism of other drugs. In HIV-infected patients coadministration of ritonavir greatly increased (more than 3 times) the AUC of isradipine *23*

itraconazole *Serum Increase Physiological* Increased plasma concentration observed *886* Ritonavir has a high affinity for several cytochrome P450 isoforms inhibiting the metabolism of other drugs. In HIV-infected patients coadministration of ritonavir greatly increased (more than 3 times) the AUC of itraconazole *23*

Ritonavir *(continued)*

Ketoconazole *Serum Increase Physiological* Ritonavir has a high affinity for several cytochrome P450 isoforms inhibiting the metabolism of other drugs. In HIV-infected patients coadministration of ritonavir greatly increased (more than 3 times) the AUC of ketoconazole *23* Increased plasma concentration observed *886*

Ketoprofen *Serum Decrease Physiological* Ritonavir has a high affinity for several cytochrome P450 isoforms inhibiting the metabolism of other drugs. In HIV-infected patients coadministration of ritonavir caused a possible decrease of the AUC of ketoprofen *23*

Ketorolac *Serum Decrease Physiological* Ritonavir has a high affinity for several cytochrome P450 isoforms inhibiting the metabolism of other drugs. In HIV-infected patients coadministration of ritonavir caused a possible decrease of the AUC of ketorlac *23*

Lactate Dehydrogenase *Serum No Effect Physiological* In one study of advanced patients 1.0% of those receiving ritonavir had an activity above 1170 U/L not different from 0.2% in those receiving placebo *23*

Lamotrigine *Serum Decrease Physiological* Ritonavir has a high affinity for several cytochrome P450 isoforms inhibiting the metabolism of other drugs. In HIV-infected patients coadministration of ritonavir caused a possible decrease of the AUC of lamotrigine *23*

Lansoprazole *Serum Decrease Physiological* Ritonavir has a high affinity for several cytochrome P450 isoforms inhibiting the metabolism of other drugs. In HIV-infected patients coadministration of ritonavir moderately decreased (1.5 to 3 times) the AUC of lansoprazole *23*

Serum Increase Physiological Ritonavir has a high affinity for several cytochrome P450 isoforms inhibiting the metabolism of other drugs. In HIV-infected patients coadministration of ritonavir moderately increased (1.5 to 3 times) the AUC of lansoprazole *23*

Leukocytes *Blood Decrease Physiological* In one study of advanced patients 25.1% of those receiving ritonavir had a concentration below 2500 /µL different from 51.4% in those receiving placebo *23*

Blood No Effect Physiological In one study of advanced patients 1.8% of those receiving ritonavir had a concentration above 25,000 /µL not different from 0.7% in those receiving placebo *23*

Lidocaine *Serum Increase Physiological* Ritonavir has a high affinity for several cytochrome P450 isoforms inhibiting the metabolism of other drugs. In HIV-infected patients coadministration of ritonavir greatly increased (more than 3 times) the AUC of lidocaine *23*

Loperamide *Serum Decrease Physiological* Ritonavir has a high affinity for several cytochrome P450 isoforms inhibiting the metabolism of other drugs. In HIV-infected patients coadministration of ritonavir caused a possible decrease of the AUC of loperamide *23*

Loratadine *Serum Increase Physiological* Ritonavir has a high affinity for several cytochrome P450 isoforms inhibiting the metabolism of other drugs. In HIV-infected patients coadministration of ritonavir greatly increased (more than 3 times) the AUC of loratadine *23*

Lorazepam *Serum Decrease Physiological* Ritonavir has a high affinity for several cytochrome P450 isoforms inhibiting the metabolism of other drugs. In HIV-infected patients coadministration of ritonavir caused a possible decrease of the AUC of lorazepam *23*

Losartan *Serum Decrease Physiological* Ritonavir has a high affinity for several cytochrome P450 isoforms inhibiting the metabolism of other drugs. In HIV-infected patients coadministration of ritonavir moderately decreased (1.5 to 3 times) the AUC of losartan *23*

Serum Increase Physiological Ritonavir has a high affinity for several cytochrome P450 isoforms inhibiting the metabolism of other drugs. In HIV-infected patients coadministration of ritonavir moderately increased (1.5 to 3 times) the AUC of losartan *23*

Lovastatin *Serum Increase Physiological* Ritonavir has a high affinity for several cytochrome P450 isoforms inhibiting the metabolism of other drugs. In HIV-infected patients coadministration of ritonavir greatly increased (more than 3 times) the AUC of lovastatin *23*

Magnesium *Serum No Effect Physiological* In one study of advanced patients 0.4% of those receiving ritonavir had a concentration below 1.0 mEq/L not different from 0.4% in those receiving placebo *23*

Maprotiline *Serum Increase Physiological* Ritonavir has a high affinity for several cytochrome P450 isoforms inhibiting the metabolism of other drugs. In HIV-infected patients coadministration of ritonavir moderately increased (1.5 to 3 times) the AUC of maprotiline *23*

Methadone *Serum Increase Physiological* Ritonavir has a high affinity for several cytochrome P450 isoforms inhibiting the metabolism of other drugs. In HIV-infected patients coadministration of ritonavir greatly increased (more than 3 times) the AUC of methadone *23*

Methamphetamine *Serum Increase Physiological* Ritonavir has a high affinity for several cytochrome P450 isoforms inhibiting the metabolism of other drugs. In HIV-infected patients coadministration of ritonavir moderately increased (1.5 to 3 times) the AUC of methamphetamine *23*

Metoprolol *Serum Increase Physiological* Ritonavir has a high affinity for several cytochrome P450 isoforms inhibiting the metabolism of other drugs. In HIV-infected patients coadministration of ritonavir moderately increased (1.5 to 3 times) the AUC of metoprolol *23*

Mexiletine *Serum Increase Physiological* Ritonavir has a high affinity for several cytochrome P450 isoforms inhibiting the metabolism of other drugs. In HIV-infected patients coadministration of ritonavir moderately increased (1.5 to 3 times) the AUC of mexiletine *23*

Miconazole *Serum Increase Physiological* Ritonavir has a high affinity for several cytochrome P450 isoforms inhibiting the metabolism of other drugs. In HIV-infected patients coadministration of ritonavir greatly increased (more than 3 times) the AUC of miconazole *23*

Morphine *Serum Decrease Physiological* Ritonavir has a high affinity for several cytochrome P450 isoforms inhibiting the metabolism of other drugs. In HIV-infected patients coadministration of ritonavir possibly decreased the AUC of morphine *23*

Naproxen *Serum Decrease Physiological* Ritonavir has a high affinity for several cytochrome P450 isoforms inhibiting the metabolism of other drugs. In HIV-infected patients coadministration of ritonavir caused a possible decrease of the AUC of naproxen *23*

Nefazodone *Serum Increase Physiological* Ritonavir has a high affinity for several cytochrome P450 isoforms inhibiting the metabolism of other drugs. In HIV-infected patients coadministration of ritonavir greatly increased (more than 3 times) the AUC of nefazodone *23*

Nelfinavir *Serum Increase Physiological* Causes a 152% increase in area under the concentration curve when ritonavir coadministered *1891* Coadministration of ritonavir with nelfinavir caused a 152% increase in AUC of nelfinavir *66*

Neutrophils *Blood No Effect Physiological* In one study of advanced patients 4.0% of those receiving ritonavir had a concentration below or equal to 0.5 x 10^9/L not different from 6.9% in those receiving placebo *23* In one study of advanced patients 1.8% of those receiving ritonavir had a concentration above 20 x 10^9/L not different from 0.9% in those receiving placebo *23*

Nicardipine *Serum Increase Physiological* Ritonavir has a high affinity for several cytochrome P450 isoforms inhibiting the metabolism of other drugs. In HIV-infected patients coadministration of ritonavir greatly increased (more than 3 times) the AUC of nicardipine *23*

Nifedipine *Serum Increase Physiological* Ritonavir has a high affinity for several cytochrome P450 isoforms inhibiting the metabolism of other drugs. In HIV-infected patients coadministration of ritonavir greatly increased (more than 3 times) the AUC of nifedipine *23*

Nimodipine *Serum Increase Physiological* Ritonavir has a high affinity for several cytochrome P450 isoforms inhibiting the metabolism of other drugs. In HIV-infected patients coadministration of ritonavir greatly increased (more than 3 times) the AUC of nimodipine *23*

Nisoldipine *Serum Increase Physiological* Ritonavir has a high affinity for several cytochrome P450 isoforms inhibiting the metabolism of other drugs. In HIV-infected patients coadministration of ritonavir greatly increased (more than 3 times) the AUC of nisoldipine *23*

Nitrendipine *Serum Increase Physiological* Ritonavir has a high affinity for several cytochrome P450 isoforms inhibiting the metabolism of other drugs. In HIV-infected patients coadministration of ritonavir greatly increased (more than 3 times) the AUC of nitrendipine *23*

Nortriptyline *Serum Increase Physiological* Ritonavir has a high affinity for several cytochrome P450 isoforms inhibiting the metabolism of other drugs. In HIV-infected patients coadministration of ritonavir moderately increased (1.5 to 3 times) the AUC of nortriptyline *23*

Omeprazole *Serum Decrease Physiological* Ritonavir has a high affinity for several cytochrome P450 isoforms inhibiting the metabolism of other drugs. In HIV-infected patients coadministration of ritonavir moderately decreased (1.5 to 3 times) the AUC of omeprazole *23*

Serum Increase Physiological Ritonavir has a high affinity for several cytochrome P450 isoforms inhibiting the metabolism of other drugs. In HIV-infected patients coadministration of ritonavir moderately increased (1.5 to 3 times) the AUC of omeprazole *23*

Ondansetron *Serum Increase Physiological* Ritonavir has a high affinity for several cytochrome P450 isoforms inhibiting the metabolism of other drugs. In HIV-infected patients coadministration of ritonavir moderately increased (1.5 to 3 times) the AUC of ondanestron *23*

Oxazepam *Serum Decrease Physiological* Ritonavir has a high affinity for several cytochrome P450 isoforms inhibiting the metabolism of other drugs. In HIV-infected patients coadministration of ritonavir caused a possible decrease of the AUC of oxazepam *23*

Oxycodone *Serum Increase Physiological* Ritonavir has a high affinity for several cytochrome P450 isoforms inhibiting the metabolism of other drugs. In HIV-infected patients coadministration of ritonavir moderately increased (1.5 to 3 times) the AUC of oxycodone *23*

Paclitaxel *Serum Increase Physiological* Ritonavir has a high affinity for several cytochrome P450 isoforms inhibiting the metabolism of other drugs. In HIV-infected patients coadministration of ritonavir moderately increased (1.5 to 3 times) the AUC of paclitaxel *23*

Paroxetine *Serum Increase Physiological* Ritonavir has a high affinity for several cytochrome P450 isoforms inhibiting the metabolism of other drugs. In HIV-infected patients coadministration of ritonavir moderately increased (1.5 to 3 times) the AUC of paroxetine *23*

Penbutolol *Serum Increase Physiological* Ritonavir has a high affinity for several cytochrome P450 isoforms inhibiting the metabolism of other drugs. In HIV-infected patients coadministration of ritonavir moderately increased (1.5 to 3 times) the AUC of penbutolol *23*

Perphenazine *Serum Increase Physiological* Ritonavir has a high affinity for several cytochrome P450 isoforms inhibiting the metabolism of other drugs. In HIV-infected patients coadministration of ritonavir moderately increased (1.5 to 3 times) the AUC of perphenazine *23*

Phenytoin *Serum Increase Physiological* Ritonavir has a high affinity for several cytochrome P450 isoforms inhibiting the metabolism of other drugs. In HIV-infected patients coadministration of ritonavir moderately increased (1.5 to 3 times) the AUC of phenytoin *23*

Pindolol *Serum Increase Physiological* Ritonavir has a high affinity for several cytochrome P450 isoforms inhibiting the metabolism of other drugs. In HIV-infected patients coadministration of ritonavir moderately increased (1.5 to 3 times) the AUC of pindolol *23*

Platelets *Blood No Effect Physiological* In one study of advanced patients 0.4% of those receiving ritonavir had a concentration below 20 x 10^9/L not different from 0.6% in those receiving placebo *23*

Potassium *Serum No Effect Physiological* In one study of advanced patients 0.4% of those receiving ritonavir had a concentration above 6.0 mmol/L not different from 0.2% in those receiving placebo *23* In one study of advanced patients 2.0% of those receiving ritonavir had a concentration below 3.0 mmol/L not different from 1.1% in those receiving placebo *23*

Pravastatin *Serum Increase Physiological* Ritonavir has a high affinity for several cytochrome P450 isoforms inhibiting the metabolism of other drugs. In HIV-infected patients coadministration of ritonavir moderately increased (1.5 to 3 times) the AUC of pravastatin *23*

Prazosin *Serum Increase Physiological* Ritonavir has a high affinity for several cytochrome P450 isoforms inhibiting the metabolism of other drugs. In HIV-infected patients coadministration of ritonavir caused a possible increase of the AUC of prazosin *23*

Prednisone *Serum Increase Physiological* Ritonavir has a high affinity for several cytochrome P450 isoforms affecting the metabolism of other drugs. Moderate increase in AUC observed *23*

Prochlorperazine *Serum Decrease Physiological* Ritonavir has a high affinity for several cytochrome P450 isoforms inhibiting the metabolism of other drugs. In HIV-infected patients coadministration of ritonavir moderately decreased (1.5 to 3 times) the AUC of prochlorperazine *23*

Serum Increase Physiological Ritonavir has a high affinity for several cytochrome P450 isoforms inhibiting the metabolism of other drugs. In HIV-infected patients coadministration of ritonavir caused a possible increase of the AUC of prochlorperazine *23*

Proguanil *Serum Decrease Physiological* Ritonavir has a high affinity for several cytochrome P450 isoforms inhibiting the metabolism of other drugs. In HIV-infected patients coadministration of ritonavir moderately decreased (1.5 to 3 times) the AUC of proguanil *23*

Serum Increase Physiological Ritonavir has a high affinity for several cytochrome P450 isoforms inhibiting the metabolism of other drugs. In HIV-infected patients coadministration of ritonavir moderately increased (1.5 to 3 times) the AUC of proguanil *23*

Promethazine *Serum Decrease Physiological* Ritonavir has a high affinity for several cytochrome P450 isoforms inhibiting the metabolism of other drugs. In HIV-infected patients coadministration of ritonavir moderately decreased (1.5 to 3 times) the AUC of promethazine *23*

Serum Increase Physiological Ritonavir has a high affinity for several cytochrome P450 isoforms inhibiting the metabolism of other drugs. In HIV-infected patients coadministration of ritonavir caused a possible increase of the AUC of promethazine *23*

Propofol *Serum Decrease Physiological* Ritonavir has a high affinity for several cytochrome P450 isoforms inhibiting the metabolism of other drugs. In HIV-infected patients coadministration of ritonavir caused a possible decrease of the AUC of propofol *23*

Propranolol *Serum Decrease Physiological* Ritonavir has a high affinity for several cytochrome P450 isoforms inhibiting the metabolism of other drugs. In HIV-infected patients coadministration of ritonavir moderately decreased (1.5 to 3 times) the AUC of propranolol *23*

Serum Increase Physiological Ritonavir has a high affinity for several cytochrome P450 isoforms inhibiting the metabolism of other drugs. In HIV-infected patients coadministration of ritonavir moderately increased (1.5 to 3 times) the AUC of propranolol *23*

Prothrombin Time *Plasma No Effect Physiological* In one study of advanced patients 1.0% of those receiving ritonavir had a concentration above 1.5 upper limit of normal not different from 1.3% in those receiving placebo *23*

Quinine *Serum Increase Physiological* Ritonavir has a high affinity for several cytochrome P450 isoforms inhibiting the metabolism of other drugs. In HIV-infected patients coadministration of ritonavir greatly increased (more than 3 times) the AUC of quinine *23*

Rifabutin *Serum Increase Physiological* Increases the area under the concentration curve by 350% when ritonavir coadministered *1891* Increased plasma concentration

Ritonavir *(continued)*

Rifabutin *(continued)*
observed *886* When ritonavir coadministered with rifabutin mean minimum and maximum concentrations and AUC of rifabutin increased by approximately 6-, 2.5- and 4-fold respectively *920*

Risperidone *Serum Increase Physiological* Ritonavir has a high affinity for several cytochrome P450 isoforms inhibiting the metabolism of other drugs. In HIV-infected patients coadministration of ritonavir moderately increased (1.5 to 3 times) the AUC of risperidone *23*

Saquinavir *Serum Increase Physiological* Coadministration of ritonavir 400 or 600 mg b.i.d. with saquinavir produced greater than 20-fold increase in steady-state dose-normalized saquinavir concentrations in healthy individuals *5024* Increases the area under the concentration curve by more than 2000% when ritonavir coadministered *1891* Coadministration of ritonavir with saquinavir caused 50-fold and 22-fold increases of the AUC and peak plasma concentration of saquinavir *2744* Ritonavir has a high affinity for several cytochrome P450 isoforms affecting the metabolism of other drugs. The metabolism of sequiavir was extensively inhibited when ritonavir 400 - 600 mg b.i.d. was coadministered resulting in a 20-fold increase in steady state dose-normalized concentrations in healthy individuals *23*

Sertraline *Serum Increase Physiological* Ritonavir has a high affinity for several cytochrome P450 isoforms inhibiting the metabolism of other drugs. In HIV-infected patients coadministration of ritonavir greatly increased (more than 3 times) the AUC of sertraline *23*

Simvastatin *Serum Increase Physiological* Ritonavir has a high affinity for several cytochrome P450 isoforms inhibiting the metabolism of other drugs. In HIV-infected patients coadministration of ritonavir greatly increased (more than 3 times) the AUC of simvastatin *23*

Tacrolimus *Serum Increase Physiological* Ritonavir has a high affinity for several cytochrome P450 isoforms inhibiting the metabolism of other drugs. In HIV-infected patients coadministration of ritonavir greatly increased (more than 3 times) the AUC of tacrolimus *23*

Tamoxifen *Serum Increase Physiological* Ritonavir has a high affinity for several cytochrome P450 isoforms inhibiting the metabolism of other drugs. In HIV-infected patients coadministration of ritonavir greatly increased (more than 3 times) the AUC of tamoxifen *23*

Temazepam *Serum Decrease Physiological* Ritonavir has a high affinity for several cytochrome P450 isoforms inhibiting the metabolism of other drugs. In HIV-infected patients coadministration of ritonavir caused a possible decrease of the AUC of temazepam *23*

Terazosin *Serum Increase Physiological* Ritonavir has a high affinity for several cytochrome P450 isoforms inhibiting the metabolism of other drugs. In HIV-infected patients coadministration of ritonavir caused a possible increase of the AUC of terazosin *23*

Terfenadine *Serum Increase Physiological* Decreased metabolism resulting in cardiac toxicity or arrhythmia *886*

Theophylline *Serum Decrease Physiological* Ritonavir has a high affinity for several cytochrome P450 isoforms affecting the metabolism of other drugs. The metabolism of theophylline was extensively affected when ritonavir was coadministered resulting in a 43% decrease in theophylline concentrations in healthy individuals *23* Decreases the area under the concentration curve by 43% when ritonavir coadministered *1891*

Thioridazine *Serum Increase Physiological* Ritonavir has a high affinity for several cytochrome P450 isoforms inhibiting the metabolism of other drugs. In HIV-infected patients coadministration of ritonavir moderately increased (1.5 to 3 times) the AUC of thioridazine *23*

Timolol *Serum Increase Physiological* Ritonavir has a high affinity for several cytochrome P450 isoforms inhibiting the metabolism of other drugs. In HIV-infected patients coadministration of ritonavir moderately increased (1.5 to 3 times) the AUC of timolol *23*

Tocainide *Serum Increase Physiological* Ritonavir has a high affinity for several cytochrome P450 isoforms inhibiting the metabolism of other drugs. In HIV-infected patients coadministration of ritonavir caused a possible increase of the AUC of tocainide *23*

Tolbutamide *Serum Decrease Physiological* Ritonavir has a high affinity for several cytochrome P450 isoforms inhibiting the metabolism of other drugs. In HIV-infected patients coadministration of ritonavir moderately decreased (1.5 to 3 times) the AUC of tolbutamide *23*
Serum Increase Physiological Ritonavir has a high affinity for several cytochrome P450 isoforms inhibiting the metabolism of other drugs. In HIV-infected patients coadministration of ritonavir moderately increased (1.5 to 3 times) the AUC of tolbutamide *23*

Tramadol *Serum Increase Physiological* Ritonavir has a high affinity for several cytochrome P450 isoforms inhibiting the metabolism of other drugs. In HIV-infected patients coadministration of ritonavir moderately increased (1.5 to 3 times) the AUC of tramadol *23*

Trazodone *Serum Increase Physiological* Ritonavir has a high affinity for several cytochrome P450 isoforms inhibiting the metabolism of other drugs. In HIV-infected patients coadministration of ritonavir moderately increased (1.5 to 3 times) the AUC of trazodone *23*

Triglycerides *Serum Increase Physiological* In one study of advanced patients 7.9% of those receiving ritonavir had a fasting concentration above 1500 mg/dL significantly different from 0.4% in those receiving placebo *23*

Trimethoprim *Serum Increase Physiological* Increases the area under the concentration curve by 20% when ritonavir coadministered *1891*

Trimipramine *Serum Increase Physiological* Ritonavir has a high affinity for several cytochrome P450 isoforms inhibiting the metabolism of other drugs. In HIV-infected patients coadministration of ritonavir moderately increased (1.5 to 3 times) the AUC of trimipramine *23*

Uric Acid *Serum Increase Physiological* In one study of advanced patients 3.6% of those receiving ritonavir had a concentration above 12 mg/dL different from 0.2% in those receiving placebo *23*

Valproic Acid *Serum Decrease Physiological* Ritonavir has a high affinity for several cytochrome P450 isoforms inhibiting the metabolism of other drugs. In HIV-infected patients coadministration of ritonavir caused a possible decrease of the AUC of valproic acid *23*

Venlafaxine *Serum Increase Physiological* Ritonavir has a high affinity for several cytochrome P450 isoforms inhibiting the metabolism of other drugs. In HIV-infected patients coadministration of ritonavir moderately increased (1.5 to 3 times) the AUC of venlafaxine *23*

Verapamil *Serum Increase Physiological* Ritonavir has a high affinity for several cytochrome P450 isoforms inhibiting the metabolism of other drugs. In HIV-infected patients coadministration of ritonavir greatly increased (more than 3 times) the AUC of verapamil *23*

Vinblastine *Serum Increase Physiological* Ritonavir has a high affinity for several cytochrome P450 isoforms inhibiting the metabolism of other drugs. In HIV-infected patients coadministration of ritonavir moderately increased (1.5 to 3 times) the AUC of vinblastine *23*

Vincristine *Serum Increase Physiological* Ritonavir has a high affinity for several cytochrome P450 isoforms inhibiting the metabolism of other drugs. In HIV-infected patients coadministration of ritonavir moderately increased (1.5 to 3 times) the AUC of vincristine *23*

Warfarin *Serum Decrease Physiological* Ritonavir has a high affinity for several cytochrome P450 isoforms inhibiting the metabolism of other drugs. In HIV-infected patients coadministration of ritonavir moderately decreased (1.5 to 3 times) the AUC of S-warfarin *23*
Serum Increase Physiological Ritonavir has a high affinity for several cytochrome P450 isoforms inhibiting the metabolism of other drugs. In HIV-infected patients coadministration of ritonavir moderately increased (1.5 to 3 times) the AUC of R-warfarin or S-warfarin *23*

Zidovudine *Serum Decrease Physiological* Decreases the area under the concentration curve by 25% when ritonavir coadministered *1891*

Ro 4-2137

Urea Nitrogen *Serum* *Increase* *Physiological* Slight increase up to 70 mg/dL in some patients *3121*

Ro 16-0521

Cholesterol *Serum* *No Effect* *Physiological* Although compound inhibits gastrointestinal absorption in man appears not to affect serum concentration *3114*

Ro 42-5892

Angiotensin-I *Plasma* *Decrease* *Physiological* In 14 healthy indviduals ingestion of 600 mg orally caused significant reduction from mean baseline of 6.48 ± 0.79 pmol/L to 2.00 ± 0.39 pmol/L after 30 minutes and to 3.40 ± 1.03 pmol/L after 30 minutes with 1200 mg *856*
Plasma *Increase* *Physiological* In 14 healthy individuals ingestion of 100 mg caused nonsignificant increase attfer 30 minutes to 10.04 ± 2.18 pmol/L from baseline of 6.48 ± 0.79 pmol/L *856*

Angiotensin-II *Plasma* *Decrease* *Physiological* In 14 healthy individuals ingestion of 100 mg caused reduction from mean baseline of 3.67 ± 0.99 pmol/L to 2.99 ± 0.54 pmol/L after 30 minutes, to 1.81 ± 0.36 pmol/L (significant) with 600 mg after 30 minutes and to 2.38 ± 0.43 pmol/L after 30 minutes with 1200 mg *856* Decrease by 80-90% 10 minutes after intravenous dose and by 30-40% after single oral dose in 9 men with essential hypertension remaining low for 8 h after oral dose but returning to baseline 4 h after low intravenous dose and 6 h after high i.v. dose *6178*

Renin Activity *Plasma* *Decrease* *Physiological* Activity fell to undetectably low values in 10 minutes after either single intravenous or oral dose in 9 men with uncomplicated essential hypertension *6178* In 14 healthy volunteers administration of intravenous drug (0.001 mg/kg to 1 mg/kg) caused maximal suppression in dose-dependent manner at end of infusion. After oral ingestion of up to 1200 mg mean concentration decreased from baseline of 0.82 ± 0.12 ng Ang-I/mL/h to 0.66 ± 0.12 ng Ang-I/mL/h after 100 mg, 0.32 ± 0.08 ng Ang-I/mL/h after 600 mg and 0.39 ± 0.15 ng Ang-I/mL/h after 1200 mg *856* In 6 healthy individuals intravenous administration administration of up to 320 mg or oral administration of 800 mg caused dose-dependent decrease lasting for more than 12 h. Almost maximal decrease of activity observed after 10 mg intravenous dose whereas greater than 50% reduction observed after 100 mg and 90% inhibition after higher doses *3182*

Renin Concentration *Plasma* *Increase* *Physiological* In 14 healthy indviduals ingestion of 100 mg caused increase in active renin concentration after 30 minutes from mean baseline of 22.3 ± 3.4 pg/mL to 23.0 ± 5.7 pg/mL with 100 mg drug, to 25.7 ± 4.4 pg/mL (significant) with 600 mg and to 42.2 ± 8.5 pg/mL (significant) with 1200 mg *856*

Rolitetracycline

Glucose *Serum* *No Effect* *Analytical* At concentration of 4 mg/L had no effect on GOD/POD-PAP method *5704*

Protein *Urine* *Increase* *Physiological* May cause nephropathy *4265*

Tacrolimus *Serum* *No Effect* *Analytical* In HPLC/MS method of Christians et al no significant interference observed with measurement of FK 506 *1010*

Triglycerides *Serum* *No Effect* *Analytical* At concentration of 4 mg/L had no effect on GPO-PAP method *5704*

Urea Nitrogen *Serum* *Increase* *Physiological* May cause nephropathy *4265*

Uric Acid *Serum* *No Effect* *Analytical* At concentration of 4 mg/L had no effect on uricase-PAP method *5704*

Ropinirol

Dopamine *Plasma* *No Effect* *Physiological* No effect of acute administration of 1 mg observed in 8 healthy men *1320*

Epinephrine *Plasma* *No Effect* *Physiological* No effect of acute administration of 1 mg observed in 8 healthy men *1320*

Norepinephrine *Plasma* *No Effect* *Physiological* No effect of acute administration of 1 mg observed in 8 healthy men *1320*

Prolactin *Plasma* *Decrease* *Physiological* Dose related reduction observed in 8 healthy men with effect lasting longer with the higher doses *1320*

Rotenone

Glucose *Serum* *Decrease* *Physiological* Severe hypoglycemia reported with poisoning *2183*

Roxatidine

Theophylline *Serum* *No Effect* *Physiological* No effect observed on pharmacokinetics after infusion of aminophylline when compared with placebo situation in 9 healthy volunteers *6606*

Roxithromycin

Carbamazepine *Serum* *No Effect* *Physiological* Has no effect on metabolism of carbamazepine *3118* No effect on pharmacokinetics when added to stable therapeutic regime *5187*

Cyclosporine *Blood* *Increase* *Physiological* Coadministration of roxithromycin with cyclosporine caused a nonsignificant small increase in the blood cyclosporine concentration *859*
Serum *Increase* *Physiological* Coadministration of roxithromycin with cyclosporine caused a nonsignificant small increase in the blood cyclosporine concentration *859*

Theophylline *Serum* *No Effect* *Physiological* No documented significant interaction with theophylline reported *6117* Little effect on pharmacokinetics when added to stable therapeutic regime *5187* No clinically significant effect on theophylline concentration observed when drugs coadministered *5999*

Rubella Virus Vaccine

Platelets *Blood* *Decrease* *Physiological* Self limiting, occurring within 10 d or purpura *392*

Saccharated Iron Oxide

Albumin *Serum* *No Effect* *Physiological* In 9 individuals given 40 mg/d i.v. daily for up to 42 d *4388*

Calcium *Serum* *No Effect* *Physiological* In 9 individuals given 40 mg/d i.v. daily for up to 42 d *4388*

Creatinine *Serum* *No Effect* *Physiological* In 9 individuals given 40 mg/d i.v. daily for up to 42 d *4388*

Hematocrit *Blood* *Increase* *Physiological* In 9 individuals given 40 mg/d i.v. daily for up to 42 d *4388*

Hemoglobin *Blood* *Increase* *Physiological* In 9 individuals given 40 mg/d i.v. daily for up to 42 d *4388*

Phosphate *Serum* *Decrease* *Physiological* Stepwise significant reduction with 40 mg i.v. daily for up to 42 d *4388*
Urine *No Effect* *Physiological* In 9 individuals given 40 mg/d i.v. daily for up to 42 d *4388*

Potassium *Serum* *No Effect* *Physiological* In 9 individuals given 40 mg/d i.v. for up to 42 d *4388*

Safflower Oil

HDL-Cholesterol *Serum* *Decrease* *Physiological* Nonsignificant reduction observed in 11 mildly hypercholesterolemic men fed 14 g/d for 6 weeks *7*

LDL-Cholesterol *Serum* *Decrease* *Physiological* Mean decrease of 0.18 mmol/L in 11 mildly hypercholesterolemic men fed 14 g/d for 6 weeks *7*

Triglycerides *Serum* *No Effect* *Physiological* In 11 mildly hypercholesterolemic men supplement with 14 g/d had no effect at 6 weeks *7*

Sagamicin

Amikacin *Serum No Effect Analytical* No interference observed with method on Abbott TDx *3858*

Gentamicin *Serum Increase Analytical* Interferes with method on Abbott TDx *3858*

Kanamycin *Serum No Effect Analytical* No interference observed with method on Abbott TDx *3858*

Neomycin *Serum No Effect Analytical* No interference observed with method on Abbott TDx *3858*

Netilmicin *Serum Increase Analytical* Interferes with method on Abbott TDx *3858*

Streptomycin *Serum No Effect Analytical* No interference observed with method on Abbott TDx *3858*

Tobramycin *Serum No Effect Analytical* No interference observed with method on Abbott TDx *3858*

Vancomycin *Serum No Effect Analytical* No interference observed with method on Abbott TDx *3858*

Salicylamide

Histamine *Plasma No Effect Analytical* Insignificant inhibition of radio-enzyme assay at concentrations 2-5 times physiological *2492*

Phenylalanine *Plasma No Effect Analytical* No interference observed with rapid quantitative whole blood method of Campbell et al using phenylalanine dehydrogenase *867*

Salicylate *Serum No Effect Analytical* At a concentration of 30 mg/dL has no significant effect on method on Kodak Ektachem® systems *2519*

Salicylate

Acetaminophen *Serum Increase Analytical* Increases results with unmodified Glynn and Kendal technique *318*
Serum No Effect Analytical No interference of salicylic acid at a concentration of 4000 µg/mL (2896 µmol/L) with method on Du Pont aca *1506* At 200 and 500 mg/L had no effect on HPLC method *5775*

Acid Phosphatase *Serum No Effect Analytical* At concentration of 100 mg/dL (7.2 mmol/L) had no effect on method on Du Pont Dimension *1562*

Alanine Aminopeptidase *Urine Decrease Physiological* When 0.5 g given orally to 20 healthy adult volunteers and urine studied over next 3 h *2984*

Alanine Aminotransferase *Serum No Effect Analytical* No effect at 1000 mg/L on method on Ames Seralyzer *5706* No effect of concentrations up to 350 mg/L on method on Kodak Ektachem® *5706* No effect at concentration of 100 mg/dL (7.24 mmol/L) on method on Du Pont Dimension *1563*

Albumin *Serum No Effect Analytical* At concentration of 600 mg/L had no effect on BCG method *5704* No interference observed at a concentration of 271 mg/L (1.94 mmol/L) with method on Du Pont aca *1507* At concentration of 100 mg/dL (7.2 mmol/L) had no effect on method on Du Pont Dimension *1564* No significant effect even at 1 g/L on BCG method *4335* At concentration of 1000 mg/L had no effect on method on Kodak Ektachem® *5706*

Alkaline Phosphatase *Serum No Effect Analytical* At concentration of 100 mg/dL (7.2 mmol/L) had no effect on method on Du Pont Dimension *1565*

Ammonia *Plasma No Effect Analytical* No effect at concentration of 100 mg/dL (7.2 mmol/L) on method on Du Pont Dimension *1566*

Amphetamine *Urine Decrease Analytical* In specimens to which salicylate added to a concentration of 1000 ng/mL 40% negative interference observed with Syva EMIT II method *6291*

Amylase *Serum No Effect Analytical* No effect at concentration of 1000 mg/L on method on Kodak Ektachem® *5706* At concentration of 100 mg/dL (7.2 mmol/L) had no effect on method on Du Pont Dimension *1567*

Aspartate Aminotransferase *Serum Increase Physiological* Concentration related effect in 9 of 17 patients with acute rheumatic fever also given phenoxymethyl penicillin: in patients with low albumin effect most marked *2138*
Serum No Effect Analytical No effect at concentration of 100 mg/dL (7.24 mmol/L) on method on Du Pont Dimension *1568* No effect of concentrations up to 350 mg/L on method on Kodak Ektachem® *5706*

Barbiturate *Urine No Effect Analytical* At salicylate concentrations up to 330 mg/dL no significant interference observed with Syva EMIT II method on Hitchi 704 *6291*

Benzoylecgonine *Urine No Effect Analytical* No significant interference observed at a concentration of 724 µmol/L with Sung and Neely modification of Syva EMIT procedure *148*

Bicarbonate *Serum Increase Analytical* At concentration of 20 mmol/L increase in concentration of 76% as measured by Kodak Ektachem® 700 *2828*
Serum No Effect Analytical At concentration of 500 mg/L had no effect on method using phenolphthalein *5704*

Bilirubin *Serum Increase Physiological* Clinically significant displacement from protein in neonates *6314*
Serum No Effect Analytical No significant interference observed from salicylic acid at a concentration of 100 mg/dL (7 mmol/L) with method on Du Pont aca *1548* At concentration of 500 mg/L had no effect on Jendrassik and Grof method *5704* No effect at 200 mg/L on Ames Seralyzer method *5706* At concentration of 350 mg/L had no effect on Kodak Ektachem® method *5704* No effect at concentration of 100 mg/dL (7.24 mmol/L) on method on Du Pont Dimension *1589*
Urine No Effect Analytical No effect on bilirubin test area of Ames Multistix, other Ames reagent strip tests and Ictotest reagent tablets *4034*

Bilirubin, Conjugated *Serum No Effect Analytical* No effect at concentration of 1000 mg/L on method on Kodak Ektachem® *5706* Salicylic acid at a concentration of 100 mg/dL (7 mmol/L) had no effect on method on Du Pont aca *1517*

Bilirubin, Direct *Serum No Effect Analytical* At concentration of 100 mg/dL (7.24 mmol/L) had no effect on method on Du Pont Dimension *1574*

Bilirubin, Unconjugated *Serum No Effect Analytical* No effect at concentration of 1000 mg/L on method on Kodak Ektachem® *5706*

Calcium *Serum No Effect Analytical* No effect of concentrations up to 1000 mg/L with method on Kodak Ektachem® *5706* At concentration of 500 mg/L had no effect on cresolphthalein method *5704* No effect at concentration of 100 mg/dL (7.2 mmol/L) on method on Du Pont Dimension *1569*

Chloramphenicol *Serum No Effect Analytical* No effect at 100 mg/L on coupled enzymatic method *4122*

Chloride *Serum Increase Analytical* When chloride measured by the Roche Cobas Integra method with 1 mmol/L salicylate producing an apparent chloride concentration of 5.3 mmol/L. Interference observed with both indirect and modified direct methods, but interference with the indirect method was greater *5048*
Serum No Effect Analytical Although interference observed with both indirect and modified direct methods with Roche Cobas Integra methods, no interference observed at the same concentration with the methods on the J&J Vitros, Beckman CX3 δ and Hitachi 717 analyzers which use both direct and indirect ISE procedures *5048* No effect of concentrations up to 350 mg/L on method on Kodak Ektachem® *5706* At concentration of 500 mg/L had no effect on mercurimetric method *5704*

Chlorpropamide *Serum Increase Physiological* Drugs that are highly protein-bound compete with chlorpropamide for binding sites and may potentiate hypoglycemic action of sulfonylurea *4644*

Cholesterol *Serum No Effect Analytical* No effect at 200 mg/L on Ames Seralyzer method *5706* No effect of concentrations up to 1000 mg/L on method on Kodak Ektachem® *5706* At concentration of 500 mg/L had no effect on Liebermann-Burchard method *5704* At concentration of 100 mg/dL (7.2 mmol/L) had no effect on method on Du Pont Dimension *1570* At concentration of 500 mg/L had no effect on method using catalase-Hantzsch reaction *5704*

Cocaine *Urine Decrease Analytical* At salicylate concentrations of up to 300 ng/mL 37% negative interference observed with Syva EMIT II method *6291*

Color *Feces Increase Analytical* Pink to red black due to gastrointestinal bleeding *1957*

C-Reactive Protein *Serum* *No Effect* *Analytical* No interference observed at a concentration up to 80 mg/dL (5.76 μmol/L) with method on Du Pont aca *1518* At concentration of 800 mg/L (5.76 μmol/L) had no effect on method on Du Pont aca *5403*

Creatine Kinase *Serum* *No Effect* *Analytical* No effect of concentrations up to 350 mg/L on method on Kodak Ektachem® *5706*

Creatine Kinase Isoenzymes *Serum* *No Effect* *Analytical* No interference observed at a concentration of 800 mg/L (5.8 μmol/L) with CK-MB method on Du Pont aca *1519* At concentration of 100 mg/dL (7.2 mmol/L) had no effect on method for measuring CK-MB isoenzyme on Du Pont Dimension *1571*

Creatinine *Serum* *No Effect* *Analytical* No effect of concentrations up to 1000 mg/L on 2-slide method on Kodak Ektachem® *5706* At concentration of 150 mg/L had no effect on creatinine iminohydrolase method *5704* At concentration of 500 mg/L had no effect on Technicon AutoAnalyzer® Jaffe method *5704* No effect at concentration of 100 mg/dL (7.2 mmol/L) on method on Du Pont Dimension *1572* No effect at 200 mg/L on method on Ames Seralyzer *5706*

Cyclosporine *Blood* *No Effect* *Analytical* At a concentration of 500 mg/L had no effect on Syva EMIT method *495*

Digoxin *Serum* *No Effect* *Analytical* At concentration of 1.00 mg/mL (145 mmol/L) had no effect on method on Du Pont Dimension *1573*

Estrogens *Urine* *Decrease* *Analytical* Competes for enzyme used for hydrolysis *55*

Ferric Chloride Test *Urine* *Positive* *Analytical* May produce stable purple color *684*

Fibrin Degradation Products *Plasma* *No Effect* *Analytical* No interference observed at concentrations up to 800 mg/dL (57.9 mmol/L) with method on Du Pont aca *1525*

Glucose *Serum* *Decrease* *Analytical* At concentrations up to 6.30 mmol/L caused significant reduction of up to 0.28 mmol/L with whole blood glucose measurement by Miles Ames Glucostix *5904* At concentrations up to 6.30 mmol/L caused nonsignificant reduction of up to 0.09 mmol/L in whole blood glucose concentration as measured by Medisense Satellite G analyzer *5904*

Serum *Decrease* *Physiological* In noninsulin-dependent diabetics blood glucose concentration decreased by inhibition of prostaglandin E synthesis and may enhance effect of oral hypoglcemics, eg chlorpropamide, by displacing them from their protein binding sites *1384*

Serum *Increase* *Analytical* At concentrations up to 6.30 mmol/L caused nonsignificant increase of up to 0.14 mmol/L in whole blood glucose concentration as measured by Medisense Exatech analyzer *5904*

Serum *No Effect* *Analytical* At concentrations up to 350 mg/L had no significant effect on whole blood measurement on One Touch II meter *3137* No effect of concentrations up to 1000 mg/L on method on Kodak Ektachem® *5706* At concentration of 100 mg/dL (7.24 mmol/L) has no effect on method on Du Pont Dimension *1575* No effect at 3000 mg/L on hexokinase method on Ames Seralyzer *5706* At concentration of 133 mg/L had no effect on Kodak Ektachem® method *5704* At concentrations up to 500 mg/L no effect on method on Fuji Drichem 1000 *5706* At concentrations up to 6.30 mmol/L had no significant effect on whole blood glucose concentration as measured by Boehringer Mannheim BM 1-44 analyzer *5904* No effect of salicylic acid at 2.5 mmol/L on glucokinase based assay of Scott *5414*

Urine *No Effect* *Analytical* At concentration of 5,000 mg/L had no effect on Diabur-test *5704*

γ-Glutamyltransferase *Serum* *No Effect* *Analytical* No effect of concentrations up to 350 mg/L on method on Kodak Ektachem® *5706* At concentration of 100 mg/dL (7.24 mmol/L) has no effect on method on Du Pont Dimension *1579*

Urine *Decrease* *Physiological* When 0.5 g given orally to 20 healthy adult volunteers and urine studied over next 3 h *2984*

HDL-Cholesterol *Serum* *No Effect* *Analytical* No effect at concentration of 100 mg/dL (7.24 mmol/L) on method on Du Pont Dimension *1576* No effect of concentrations up to 350 mg/L on method on Kodak Ektachem® *5706*

17-Hydroxycorticosteroids *Urine* *Decrease* *Analytical* Inhibits β-glucuronidase during hydrolysis *55*

Iron *Serum* *No Effect* *Analytical* No effect at concentration of 100 mg/dL (7.24 mmol/L) on method on Du Pont Dimension *1577*

Iron-Binding Capacity, Total *Serum* *No Effect* *Analytical* No effect at concentration of 100 mg/dL (7.24 mmol/L) on method on Du Pont Dimension *1590*

Ketones *Urine* *No Effect* *Analytical* No effect observed with Ames Multistix and other reagent strip tests and with Ames Acetest reagent tablets *4034*

Ketorolac *Serum* *Increase* *Physiological* With salicylate administration the binding of ketorolac to plasma proteins was reduced from 99.2% to 97.5%, representing a potential twofold increase in unbound ketorolac concentration *5035*

Lactate Dehydrogenase *Serum* *No Effect* *Analytical* At concentration of 100 mg/dL (7.24 mmol/L) has no effect on method on Du Pont Dimension *1578* No effect of concentrations up to 350 mg/L on method on Kodak Ektachem® *5706* No effect at 200 mg/L on method on Ames Seralyzer *5706*

Leucine Aminopeptidase *Urine* *Decrease* *Physiological* When 0.5 g given orally to 20 healthy adult volunteers and urine studied over next 3 h *2984*

Leukocytes *Urine* *No Effect* *Analytical* At concentration of 1,000 mg/L had no effect on Cytur-Test *5704*

Lipase *Serum* *No Effect* *Analytical* At concentration of 100 mg/dL (7.24 mmol/L) has no effect on method on Du Pont Dimension *1580*

Magnesium *Gastric Material* *Decrease* *Physiological* When 0.5 g given orally to 20 healthy adult volunteers and urine studied over next 3 h *2984*

Serum *No Effect* *Analytical* No effect at concentration of 100 mg/dl (7.24 mmol/L) on method on Du Pont Dimension *1581*

Morphine *Urine* *No Effect* *Analytical* No significant interference observed at a concentration of 724 μmol/L with Sung and Neely modification of Syva EMIT procedure *148*

Mycophenolic Acid *Serum* *No Effect* *Analytical* No significant interference observed with HPLC method of Shipkova et al *5526*

Mycophenolic Acid Glucuronide

Serum *No Effect* *Analytical* No significant interference observed with HPLC method of Shipkova et al *5526*

N-Acetyl-Glucosaminidase *Urine* *No Effect* *Analytical* No interference observed with color development of test pad of Boehriger Mannheim dipstick at concentrations up to 2 g/L *3767*

Opiates *Urine* *Decrease* *Analytical* At concentration of salicylate up to 330 mg/dL 59% negative interference observed with Syva EMIT II method on Hitachi 704 analyzer *6291*

Phenobarbital *Serum* *No Effect* *Analytical* No significant interference observed at a concentration of 7200 μmol/L with Sung and Neely modification of Syva EMIT method *148*

Phenytoin *Serum* *Increase* *Physiological* When salicylates ingested with fosphenytoin concentration of phenytoin may be increased *4519*

Serum *No Effect* *Analytical* No effect at concentration of 100 mg/dL (7.24 mmol/L) on method on Du Pont Dimension *1583*

Phenytoin, Free *Serum* *Increase* *Physiological* Causes increase in free fraction when drugs coadministered *6350*

Phosphate *Serum* *No Effect* *Analytical* At concentration of 100 mg/dL (7.24 mmol/L) has no effect on method on Du Pont Dimension *1584* At concentration of 500 mg/L had no effect on phosphomolybdate method *5704* No effect of concentrations up to 350 mg/L on method on Kodak Ektachem® *5706*

Piroxicam *Serum* *Decrease* *Physiological* When salicylates coadministered plasma levels of piroxicam depressed to 80% of their prior concentrations *4646*

Potassium *Serum* *No Effect* *Analytical* At concentration of 30,000 mg/L had no effect on measurement by ISE with predilution *5704* At concentration of 350 mg/L had no effect on measurement by ISE on Kodak Ektachem® *5704* At salicylic acid concentration of 400 mg/L nonsignificant interference of -0.7% observed with method on Abbott Vision *681* No effect up to 500 mg/L on method on Ames Seralyzer but at higher concentrations apparently reduced potassium concentration *5706*

Protein *Cerebrospinal Fluid* *No Effect* *Analytical* At 100 mg/dL on TCA dye method of Pesce *4625*

Salicylate *(continued)*

Protein *(continued)*
Serum *No Effect* *Analytical* At concentration of 100 mg/dL (7.24 mmol/L) had negligible effect on method on Du Pont Dimension *1591* At concentration of 500 mg/L had no effect on biuret method with blank correction *5704* No effect of concentrations up to 1000 mg/L on method on Kodak Ektachem® *5706*
Urine *No Effect* *Analytical* At 100 mg/dL on TCA dye method of Pesce *4625*

SDZ PSC 833 *Blood* *No Effect* *Analytical* At a concentration of 330 mg/L had no effect on HPLC method of Scott et al when used to measure PSC (with CsD as internal standard) at a concentration of 5 mg/L *5418*

Sodium *Serum* *No Effect* *Analytical* No interference observed at concentration of 500 mg/L with Technicon Chromolyte method *969* At concentration of 30,000 mg/L had no effect on measurement by ISE with predilution *5704*

Sucrose *Serum* *No Effect* *Analytical* Using automated procedure involving sucrose phosphorylase, phosphoglutamase and glucose-6-phosphatase of Vinet et al no significant interference observed at a concentration of 20 mmol/L *6267*
Urine *No Effect* *Analytical* Using automated procedure involving sucrose phosphorylase, phosphoglutamase and glucose-6-phosphatase of Vinet et al no significant interference observed at a concentration of 20 mmol/L *6267*

T3-Uptake *Serum* *No Effect* *Analytical* No significant effect observed with salicylic acid at a concentration of 30 mg/dL (2.17 mmol/L) with method on Du Pont aca *1545* At concentration of 100 mg/dL (7.24 mmol/L) has no effect on method on Du Pont Dimension *1586*

Tacrolimus *Blood* *No Effect* *Analytical* No significant effect observed at a concentration of 500 mg/L with MEIA method on Abbott IMx analyzer *1871*
Serum *No Effect* *Analytical* At a concentration of 500 mg/L had no significant effect on ELISA method *6329*

Theophylline *Serum* *Increase* *Analytical* Increment of +6 µmol/L with theophylline concentration of 28 µmol/L and salicylate concentration of 460 µmol/L to +23 µmol/L at same theophylline concentration but at salicylate concentration of 7300 µmol/L on Kodak Ektachem® DTSC method *302* Concentrations above 150 mg/L increase result as determined by method on Kodak Ektachem® : this effect is clinically important since therapeutic range exceeds concentration at which increased effect was observed *5706*
Serum *No Effect* *Analytical* Insignificant positive interference at concentration of 5.2 mmol/L on method on Kodak Ektachem® *6100* At concentration of 100 mg/dL (7.24 mmol/L) had no effect on method on Du Pont Dimension *1585*
Serum *No Effect* *Physiological* In 8 elderly smokers with normal renal function concomitant administration of 650 mg acetylsalicylic acid when the individuals were taking theophylline had no effect on its concentration *1217*

Thyroxine (T4) *Serum* *Decrease* *Physiological* Binding of thyroxine to thyroxine-binding prealbumin inhibited by salicylates *277* Due to competition for transport proteins *6412* Concentration decreased by inhibition of binding to TBG *2412*
Serum *No Effect* *Analytical* Cross-reactivity of less than 0.05% observed with EIA method on Bio-Rad RADIAS analyzer *4819* No significant effect observed from salicylic acid at a concentration of 30 mg/dL (2.17 mmol/L) with method on Du Pont aca *1546* *1588* At concentration of 100 mg/dL (7.24 mmol/L) has no effect on method on Du Pont Dimension *1587*

Thyroxine (T4), Free *Serum* *No Effect* *Analytical* At concentrations up to 400 mg/L had no effect on method on Baxter Stratus *5705*
Serum *No Effect* *Physiological* Binding of thyroxine to thyroxine-binding prealbumin inhibited by salicylates but measurement of free thyroxine enables accurate assessment of thyroid function to be determined *277*

Tri-iodothyronine, Free (fT3) *Serum* *Increase* *Analytical* Assay on Ciba Corning ACS:180 affected by high concentrations of salicylate because of displacement of T3 from serum binding proteins, as with equilibrium dialysis methods *2054*

Tri-iodothyronine (T3) *Serum* *Decrease* *Physiological* Due to competition for transport proteins *6412* Inhibits binding of T3 to TBG *2412*

Triglycerides *Serum* *No Effect* *Analytical* At concentration of 500 mg/L had no effect on lipase/esterase method *5704* At concentration of 100 mg/dL (7.24 mmol/L) has no effect on method on Du Pont Dimension *1592* No effect of concentrations up to 1000 mg/L on method on Kodak Ektachem® *5706* At concentration of 594 mg/L had no effect on GPO-PAP method *5704*

Urea Nitrogen *Serum* *No Effect* *Analytical* At concentration of 500 mg/L had no effect on diacetylmonoxime method *5704* At concentration of 300 mg/L had no effect on Ames Seralyzer method *5704* At concentration of 133 mg/L had no effect on Kodak Ektachem® method *5704* No effect at 100 mg/L on method on Ames Seralyzer *5706* No effect at concentration of 100 mg/dL (7.2 mmol/L) on method on Du Pont Dimension *1593*

Uric Acid *Serum* *Decrease* *Physiological* Large doses have uricosuric effect *1384*
Serum *Increase* *Physiological* Analgesic doses usually cause uric acid retention in contrast to uricosuric effect of large doses *1384*
Serum *No Effect* *Analytical* No effect at concentration of 100 mg/dL (7.24 mmol/L) on method on Du Pont Dimension *1594* No effect observed with salicylic acid at a concentration of 30 mg/dL (2.2 mmol/L) on method on Du Pont aca *1552* No effect on Tripyridyl-s-triazine method of Morin *4117* At concentration of 300 mg/L had no effect on Ames Seralyzer method *5704* No effect at 300 mg/L on uricase method on Ames Seralyzer *5706* No effect of concentrations up to 1000 mg/L on method on Kodak Ektachem® *5706* At concentration of 967 mg/L had no effect on uricase-PAP method *5704* At concentration of 500 mg/L had no effect on phosphotungstate reduction method *5704* At concentration of 300 mg/L had no effect on uricase method on Du Pont aca *5704*
Urine *Decrease* *Physiological* Usual analgesic doses cause uric acid retention in contrast to uricosuric effect of large doses *1384*
Urine *Increase* *Physiological* Large doses have uricosuric effect *1384*

Valproic Acid, Free *Serum* *Increase* *Physiological* Causes increase in free fraction when drugs coadministered *6350* May displace valproic acid from protein binding sites to such an extent as to produce toxicity from free valproic acid *1384*

Zidovudine *Serum* *No Effect* *Analytical* No effect on liquid chromatographic method of Hedaya and Sawchuk *2525*

Salicylic Acid

Apolipoprotein A-I *Serum* *No Effect* *Analytical* At a concentration of 3.6 mmol/L no significant effect observed on automated immunoturbidimetric method on Baxter Paramax analyzer *3005*

Apolipoprotein B *Serum* *No Effect* *Analytical* At a concentration of 3.6 mmol/L no significant effect observed on automated immunoturbidimetric method on Baxter Paramax analyzer *3005*

Glycated Hemoglobin *Blood* *No Effect* *Analytical* At a concentration of 400 mg/L had an insignificant - 2.0% interference with method on Abbott Vision *1885*

p-Aminophenol *Urine* *No Effect* *Analytical* With addition of drugs at a concentration of 100 mg/L and of related compounds at 50 mg/L no significant effect observed on colorimetric method of van Bocxlaer on Cobas Mira analyzer which involves reacting free p-aminophenol with resorcinol in the presence of magnesium ions to form an indophenol dye measured at 550 nm *6163*

Salmeterol

Eosinophil Cationic Protein *Serum* *No Effect* *Physiological* In 20 asthmatic patients treated with salmeterol 50 µg twice daily for two weeks caused insignificant change from mean baseline of 12.8 ± 2.8 µg/L to 15.0 ± 3.2 µg/L *3364*

Soluble Interleukin-2 Receptor
Serum *No Effect* *Physiological* In 20 asthmatic patients treated with salmeterol 50 µg twice daily for two weeks caused insignificant change from mean baseline of 505.9 ± 52.1 U/mL to 512.2 ± 44.0 U/mL *3364*

Tryptase *Serum No Effect Physiological* In 20 asthmatic patients treated with salmeterol 50 µg twice daily for two weeks caused insignificant change from mean baseline of 1.34 ± 0.01 U/L to 1.35 ± 0.01 U/L *3364*

Salol

Color *Urine Increase Analytical* Dark color on standing *3810*

Salsalate

Albumin *Serum Decrease Physiological* Associated with minimal change nephrotic syndrome in one patient *6158*

Creatinine *Serum Increase Physiological* Associated with minimal change nephrotic syndrome in one patient *6158*

Protein *Urine Increase Physiological* Associated with minimal change nephrotic syndrome in one patient *6158*

Thyroid Stimulating Hormone
Serum No Effect Physiological In 16 individuals treated with a mean dose of 2609 mg/d for at least 3 weeks 1.9 ± 0.3 mU/L not significantly greater than 1.5 ± 0.2 mU/L in 22 controls *585*

Thyroxine (T4) *Serum Decrease Physiological* Salicylate-containing drugs compete for binding with plasma proteins - may cause depressed thyroxine concentration *940* In 16 individuals ingesting mean dose of 2609 mg/d for at least 3 weeks mean concentration decreased significantly to 57 ± 4 nmol/L compared with 94 ± 4 nmol/L in 22 controls *585*
Serum Increase Physiological Salicylate competes with thyroid hormones for binding to plasma proteins although thyroid function is unaffected *3700*

Thyroxine (T4) Index, Free *Serum Decrease Physiological* In 16 individuals treated with mean dose of 2609 mg/d for at least 3 weeks mean FTI 54 ± 5 significantly less than 93 ± 4 in 22 controls *585*

Tri-iodothyronine (T3) *Serum Decrease Physiological* In 16 individuals treated with mean dose of 2609 mg/d for at least 3 weeks mean concentration of 1.4 ± 0.1 nmol/L significantly less than 2.0 ± 0.1 nmol/L in 22 controls *585*

Uric Acid *Serum Increase Physiological* Salicylates antagonize the uricosuric acid of drugs used to treat gout *3700*
Urine Decrease Physiological Salicylates antagonize the uricosuric acid of drugs used to treat gout *3700*

Santonin

Color *Feces Increase Analytical* Deep yellow with 65-70 mg *3810*
Urine Increase Analytical Bright yellow (NaOH causes color to change to pink, scarlet) *3810*

Sugar *Urine Increase Analytical* False positive with Benedict's reagent *4053*

Saquinavir

Alanine Aminotransferase *Serum Increase Physiological* Increased activity observed in in fewer than 10% treated patients, but occurring at least twice as often as in control individuals *1891*
Serum No Effect Physiological Administration of saquinavir to 327 patients in NV14256 study had caused an increase in ALT activity in 2% patients *5024*

Amylase *Serum No Effect Physiological* Administration of saquinavir to 327 patients in NV14256 study had caused an increase in amylase activity in 1% patients *5024*

Aspartate Aminotransferase *Serum Increase Physiological* Increased activity observed in in fewer than 10% treated patients, but occurring at least twice as often as in control individuals *1891*
Serum No Effect Physiological Administration of saquinavir to 327 patients in NV14256 study had caused an increase in AST activity in 2% patients *5024*

Bilirubin *Serum Increase Physiological* Increased concentration observed in in fewer than 10% treated patients, but occurring at least twice as often as in control individuals *1891*
Serum No Effect Physiological Administration of saquinavir to 327 patients in NV14256 study had caused an increase in bilirubin concentration in less than 1% patients *5024*

Calcium *Serum No Effect Physiological* Administration of saquinavir to 327 patients in NV14256 study had caused a decrease in calcium concentration in less than 1% patients *5024*

Creatine Kinase *Serum No Effect Physiological* Administration of saquinavir to 327 patients in NV14256 study had caused an increase in creatine kinase activity in less than 1% patients *5024*

Glucose *Serum Decrease Physiological* Administration of saquinavir to 327 patients in NV14256 study had caused a decrease in glucose concentration in 5% patients *5024*
Serum Increase Physiological Increased concentration observed in in fewer than 10% treated patients, but occurring at least twice as often as in control individuals *1891*
Serum No Effect Physiological Administration of saquinavir to 327 patients in NV14256 study had caused an increase in glucose concentration in 1% patients *5024*

Hematocrit *Blood Decrease Physiological* Administration of saquinavir has been associated with anemia, microhemorrhages, pancytopenia, splenomegaly and thrombocytopenia *5024*

Hemoglobin *Blood Decrease Physiological* Administration of saquinavir has been associated with anemia, microhemorrhages, pancytopenia, splenomegaly and thrombocytopenia *5024*

Ketoconazole *Serum No Effect Physiological* The area under the concentration curve unaffected when saquinavir coadministered *1891* Coadministration of saquinavir 600 mg t.i.d. with ketoconazole 200 mg q.d. to 12 healthy volunteers had no significant effect on ketoconazole pharmacokinetics *5024*

Nelfinavir *Serum Increase Physiological* Coadministration of saquinavir with nelfinavir caused a 18% increase in AUC of nelfinavir *66* Causes a 18% increase in area under the concentration curve when saquinavir coadministered *1891*

Occult Blood *Feces Increase Physiological* Administration of saquinavir has been associated with melena, blood-stained feces and gastrointestinal hemorrhage *5024*

Platelets *Blood Decrease Physiological* Administration of saquinavir has been associated with anemia, microhemorrhages, pancytopenia, splenomegaly and thrombocytopenia *5024*

Potassium *Serum No Effect Physiological* Administration of saquinavir to 327 patients in NV14256 study had caused an increase in potassium concentration in less than 1% patients and a decrease in 2% *5024*

Sodium *Serum No Effect Physiological* Administration of saquinavir to 327 patients in NV14256 study had caused an decrease in sodium concentration in less than 1% patients *5024*

Zalcitabine *Serum No Effect Physiological* The area under the concentration curve unaffected when saquinavir coadministered *1891* Coadministration of zalcitabine and zidovudine with saquinavir had no effect on the absorptions, metabolisms or excretions of any of the drugs in adults *5024*

Zidovudine *Serum No Effect Physiological* Coadministration of zalcitabine and zidovudine with saquinavir had no effect on the absorptions, metabolisms or excretions of any of the drugs in adults *5024*

Sargramostim

Alanine Aminotransferase *Serum Increase Physiological* In 13% of 53 patients receiving allogeneic bone marrow transplants increased enzyme activity reported as complication of drug administration *2816*

Albumin *Serum Decrease Physiological* In 27% of 53 patients receiving allogeneic bone marrow transplants hypoalbuminemia reported as complication of drug administration *2816*

Alkaline Phosphatase *Serum Increase Physiological* In 13% of 53 patients receiving allogeneic bone marrow transplants increased enzyme activity reported as complication of drug administration *2816*

Sargramostim *(continued)*

Bilirubin *Serum Increase Physiological* In 30% of 53 patients receiving allogeneic bone marrow transplants hyperbilirubinemia reported as complication of drug administration *2816*

Blood *Feces Increase Physiological* In 11% of 53 patients receiving allogeneic bone marrow transplants gastrointestinal hemorrhage reported as complication of drug administration *2816*

Urine Increase Physiological In 9% of 53 patients receiving allogeneic bone marrow transplants hematuria reported as complication of drug administration *2816*

Calcium *Serum Decrease Physiological* In 27% of 53 patients receiving allogeneic bone marrow transplants hypocalcemia reported as complication of drug administration *2816*

Cholesterol *Serum Increase Physiological* In 17% of 53 patients receiving allogeneic bone marrow transplants increased plasma concentration reported as complication of drug administration *2816*

Creatinine *Serum Increase Physiological* In 15% of 53 patients receiving allogeneic bone marrow transplants increased plasma creatinine concentration reported as complication of drug administration *2816*

Glucose *Serum Increase Physiological* In 41% of 53 patients receiving allogeneic bone marrow transplants hyperglycemia reported as complication of drug administration *2816*

Leukocytes *Blood Decrease Physiological* In 17% of 53 patients receiving allogeneic bone marrow transplants leukopenia reported as complication of drug administration *2816*

Magnesium *Serum Decrease Physiological* In 15% of 53 patients receiving allogeneic bone marrow transplants decreased plasma magnesium concentration reported as complication of drug administration *2816*

Platelets *Blood Decrease Physiological* In 19% of 53 patients receiving allogeneic bone marrow transplants thrombocytopenia reported as complication of drug administration *2816*

Urea Nitrogen *Serum Increase Physiological* In 27% of 53 patients receiving allogeneic bone marrow transplants increased plasma concentration reported as complication of drug administration *2816*

SC-16102

Bicarbonate *Urine Increase Physiological* Minor increase observed within 2 h *2952*

Chloride *Urine Increase Physiological* Duration of diuretic action short *2952*

Creatinine Clearance *Urine No Effect Physiological* No effect noted during study *2952*

Leukocytes *Blood Increase Physiological* Mechanism not explained *2952*

Potassium *Serum Decrease Physiological* Duration of diuretic action short *2952*

Urine Increase Physiological Duration of diuretic action short *2952*

Sodium *Urine Increase Physiological* Duration of diuretic action short *2952*

Uric Acid *Urine Increase Physiological* Minor increased clearance noted *2952*

Volume *Urine Increase Physiological* Duration of diuretic action short *2952*

Scopolamine

Bromide *Serum Increase Physiological* Theoretical possibility if hydrobromide salt is administered since it contains 28.8% bromide *5116*

Chromosomes *Test Conditions Abnormal Physiological* Clastogenic in human cells *5484*

Creatinine *Serum No Effect Analytical* Scopolamine bromide at a concentration of 20 mg/L had no effect on creatinine iminohydrolase method *5704* Scopolamine bromide at a concentration of 20 mg/L had no effect on kinetic Jaffe method on BKA-2 *5704*

Glucose *Serum No Effect Analytical* Scopolamine bromide at a concentration of 20 mg/L had no effect on GOD/POD-PAP method *5704*

Midazolam *Serum No Effect Analytical* On GC-ECD method of Ha et al *2387*

Triglycerides *Serum No Effect Analytical* Scopolamine bromide at a concentration of 20 mg/L had no effect on GPO-PAP method *5704*

Uric Acid *Serum No Effect Analytical* Scopolamine bromide at a concentration of 20 mg/L had no effect on uricase-PAP method *5704*

Seclazone

Uric Acid *Serum Decrease Physiological* Marked antigout response *2888*

Urine Increase Physiological Uricosuric action *2888*

Secobarbital

Acenocoumarol *Plasma Decrease Physiological* Coadministration of secobarbital with acenocoumarol probably reduces its plasma concentration and decreases its anticoagulant effect *1708*

Acetaminophen *Serum No Effect Analytical* No interference observed at a concentration of 2000 µg/mL (696 µmol/L) with method on Du Pont aca *1506*

Alanine Aminotransferase *Serum No Effect Analytical* At acute overdose concentration (20 mg/dL) on Technicon SMAC® method *6266*

Albumin *Serum No Effect Analytical* At acute overdose concentration (20 mg/dL) on Technicon SMAC® method *6266* At concentration of 200 mg/L had no effect on BCG method *5704*

Alkaline Phosphatase *Serum No Effect Analytical* At acute overdose concentration (20 mg/dL) on Technicon SMAC® method *6266*

Amphetamine *Urine No Effect Analytical* Negative result observed with method on Du Pont aca at a concentration of 1000 µg/L (4.20 mmol/L) *1554*

Aspartate Aminotransferase *Serum No Effect Analytical* At acute overdose concentration (20 mg/dL) on Technicon SMAC® method *6266*

Benzodiazepine *Urine No Effect Analytical* Negative result obtained with method on Du Pont aca at a concentration of 1000 µg/mL (4.20 mmol/L) *1556*

Benzodiazepine Screen *Serum No Effect Analytical* No significant effect observed at a concentration of 100 µg/mL (0.38 mmol/L) with method on Du Pont aca *1512*

Benzoylecgonine *Urine No Effect Analytical* No significant interference observed at a concentration of 384 µmol/L with Sung and Neely modification of Syva EMIT procedure *148* Negative result at a concentration of 1000 µg/mL (4.20 mmol/L) with method on Du Pont aca *1558*

Bicarbonate *Serum No Effect Analytical* At concentration of 100 mg/L had no effect on method using phenolphthalein *5704*

Bilirubin *Serum No Effect Analytical* At concentration of 200 mg/L had no effect on Jendrassik and Grof method *5704* At acute overdose concentration (20 mg/dL) on Technicon SMAC® method *6266*

Calcium *Serum No Effect Analytical* At acute overdose concentration (20 mg/dL) on Technicon SMAC® method *6266* At concentration of 200 mg/L had no effect on cresolphthalein method *5704*

Cannabinoids *Urine No Effect Analytical* No effect on Roche Abuscreen method *5006* No effect observed at a concentration of 1000 µg/mL (4.20 mmol/L) on method on Du Pont aca *1557*

Carbamazepine *Serum No Effect Analytical* No cross-reactivity observed with method on Du Pont aca *1513*

Chloride *Serum No Effect Analytical* At concentration of 100 mg/L had no effect on mercurimetric method *5704*

Cholesterol *Serum No Effect Analytical* At concentration of 200 mg/L had no effect on Liebermann-Burchard method *5704* At acute overdose concentration (20 mg/dL) on Technicon

SMAC® method *6266* At concentration of 1 mg/L had no effect on CHOD-PAP method *5704*

Creatine Kinase *Serum No Effect Analytical* At acute overdose concentration (20 mg/dL) on Technicon SMAC® method *6266*

Creatinine *Serum No Effect Analytical* At acute overdose concentration (20 mg/dL) on Technicon SMAC® method *6266* At concentration of 200 mg/L had no effect on Technicon AutoAnalyzer® Jaffe method *5704*

Dicumarol *Plasma Decrease Physiological* Coadministration of secobarbital with dicumarol probably reduces its plasma concentration and decreases its anticoagulant effect *1708*

Doxycycline *Serum Decrease Physiological* Coadministration of secobarbital with doxycycline shortens its half-life for as long as 2 weeks after barbiturate therapy is discontinued *1708*

Drugs of Abuse Screen *Urine No Effect Analytical* No effect at concentration of 100 µg/mL on EZ-SCREEN procedure for cannabinoids and cocaine *1739*

Estradiol *Plasma Decrease Physiological* Coadministration of secobarbital with estradiol probably reduces its concentration by increasing its metabolism as has been reported for phenobarbital *1708*

Ethosuximide *Serum No Effect Analytical* Insignificant cross-reactivity with method on Du Pont aca *1523*

Glucose *Serum No Effect Analytical* At concentration of 1 mg/L had no effect on GOD/POD-PAP method *5704* At acute overdose concentration (20 mg/dL) on Technicon SMAC® method *6266*

Urine Decrease Analytical Low with Clinistix®, Diastix® *1826*

Urine No Effect Analytical No effect observed with Tes-Tape® *1826*

Griseofulvin *Serum Decrease Physiological* Coadministration of secobarbital with griseofulvin probably reduces its absorption and decreases its plasma concentration *1708*

^{131}I Uptake *Serum Decrease Physiological* Seconal™, tuinal contain tetraiodofluorescein *4360*

Iron *Serum No Effect Analytical* At acute overdose concentration (20 mg/dL) on Technicon SMAC® method *6266* At concentration of 200 mg/L had no effect on Ferrozine method *5704*

17-Ketosteroids *Urine Increase Analytical* Metabolite interferes with Zimmermann reaction *1714*

Lactate Dehydrogenase *Serum No Effect Analytical* At acute overdose concentration (20 mg/dL) on Technicon SMAC® method *6266*

Morphine *Urine No Effect Analytical* No significant interference observed at a concentration of 384 µmol/L with Sung and Neely modification of Syva EMIT procedure *148*

Opiates *Urine No Effect Analytical* No effect observed at a concentration of 1000 µg/mL (4.20 mmol/L) on method on Du Pont aca *1559*

Phenobarbital *Serum Increase Analytical* Significant interference observed at a concentration of 100 µmol/L with Sung and Neely modification of Syva EMIT procedure *148*

Serum No Effect Analytical No significant cross-reactivity observed with method on Du Pont aca *1537* Cross-reactivity of less than 1.3% only observed with method on Baxter Stratus *5705* At concentration of 500 µg/mL (1921 µmol/L) has no effect on method on Du Pont Dimension *1582*

Phenprocoumon *Plasma Decrease Physiological* Coadministration of secobarbital with phenprocoumon probably reduces its plasma concentration and decreases its anticoagulant effect *1708*

Phenylalanine *Plasma No Effect Analytical* No interference observed with rapid quantitative whole blood method of Campbell et al using phenylalanine dehydrogenase *867*

Phenytoin *Serum Decrease Physiological* Coadministration of secobarbital with phenytoin probably decreases its concentration or have no effect on it as has been reported for phenobarbital *1708*

Serum No Effect Analytical No significant interference observed at a concentration of 500 µg/mL (1.92 mmol/L) with method on Du Pont aca *1538* No effect at concentration of 500 µg/mL (2100 µmol/L) on method on Du Pont Dimension *1583*

Phosphate *Serum No Effect Analytical* At concentration of 200 mg/L had no effect on phosphomolybdate method *5704* At acute overdose concentration (20 mg/dL) on Technicon SMAC® method *6266*

Potassium *Serum No Effect Analytical* At concentration of 100 mg/L had no effect on measurement by ISE with predilution *5704* At concentration of 1 mg/L had no effect on flame-photometric method *5704*

Primidone *Serum No Effect Analytical* At concentrations above 1250 mg/L causes 25% increase in concentration as measured by method on Baxter Stratus but physiological concentration only up to 5 mg/L *5705* No significant cross-reactivity with method on Du Pont aca *1541*

Protein *Serum No Effect Analytical* At acute overdose concentration (20 mg/dL) on Technicon SMAC® method *6266* At concentration of 200 mg/L had no effect on biuret method with blank correction *5704*

Prothrombin Time *Plasma Decrease Physiological* Coadministration of secobarbital with dicumarol probably reduces its plasma concentration and decreases its anticoagulant effect *1708* Increase in plasma clearance of warfarin *4431* Induces metabolism of administered coumarins *4998* With 0.1 g/d in 10 patients receiving warfarin due to hepatic microsomal enzyme induction *6118*

Secobarbital *Serum Increase Physiological* 600 mg orally produces concentration of 4.8 mg/L *3868*

Sodium *Serum No Effect Analytical* At concentration of 100 mg/L had no effect on measurement by ISE with predilution *5704* At concentration of 1 mg/L had no effect on flame-photometric method *5704*

Tricyclic Antidepressants Screen
Serum No Effect Analytical No significant effect observed at a concentration of 500 µg/mL (1.92 mmol/L) with method on Du Pont aca *1550*

Triglycerides *Serum No Effect Analytical* At concentration of 100 mg/L had no effect on lipase/esterase method *5704* At acute overdose concentration (20 mg/dL) on Technicon SMAC® method *6266*

Urea Nitrogen *Serum No Effect Analytical* At acute overdose concentration (20 mg/dL) on Technicon SMAC® method *6266* At concentration of 200 mg/L had no effect on diacetylmonoxime method *5704*

Uric Acid *Serum No Effect Analytical* At acute overdose concentration (20 mg/dL) on Technicon SMAC® method *6266* At concentration of 200 mg/L had no effect on phosphotungstate reduction method *5704*

Warfarin *Plasma Decrease Physiological* Coadministration of secobarbital with warfarin probably reduces its plasma concentration and decreases its anticoagulant effect *1708*

Secretin

Ammonia *Urine Decrease Physiological* Reduced formation with increased alkalinization *4370*

Amylase *Pancreatic Fluid Increase Physiological* Normal above 14.9 U/kg/80 minutes *746*

Bicarbonate *Bile No Effect Physiological* In normals, increased in cirrhotics *624*

Pancreatic Fluid Increase Physiological Normal above 90 mEq/L *746*

Urine Increase Physiological When i.v. infusion given *4370*

Bile Acids *Bile Decrease Physiological* Slight in normals, marked in cirrhotics *624*

Calcium *Serum Increase Physiological* Increased by 0.6 mEq/L in normals, ?cause *720*

Chloride *Bile Increase Physiological* Slight in normals, marked decrease in cirrhotics *624*

Cholecystokinin *Plasma No Effect Analytical* No significant cross reactivity with RIA procedure of Harvey *2490*

Estradiol *Plasma No Effect Physiological* No significant effect observed in 8 healthy normally cycling women with infusion of 2.0 CU/kg/h during either follicular or luteal phase or at midcycle *2682* Intravenous infusions of up to 2.0 CU/kg/h had no effect on concentration in 6 healthy women *2683*

Gastrin *Serum Decrease Physiological* Basal secretion after injection in normals *2446*

Secretin *(continued)*

Glucagon *Plasma No Effect Physiological* No effect observed if injected i.v *4419*

Glucose *Serum Increase Physiological* Intravenous infusion causes increase *2909*
Serum No Effect Physiological No change after 1 unit/kg i.v *4419*

Hydrochloric Acid *Gastric Fluid Decrease Physiological* Pancreatic secretion also at peak *3240*
Pancreatic Fluid Decrease Physiological Reciprocal relationship to bicarbonate *542*

Insulin *Plasma Increase Physiological* Only from 3 to 6 minutes after i.v. injection *4419* More than 2 fold increased with 15 U pulse *3523*

Lipase *Serum Increase Physiological* May cause spasm of sphincter of Oddi *6377*

Pepsin *Gastric Material Increase Physiological* Rises to 2.5 times basal, falls in 30 minutes *2751*

Prolactin *Plasma Decrease Physiological* At steady-state concentrations at 30 and 60 min dose-related and significant decrease observed in 6 women following intravenous infusion (control: 350 mIU/L; 290 with 0.5, 259 with 1.0 and 222 with 2.0 CU/kg/h respectively) *2683* 2.0 CU/kg/h infusion in 8 healthy normally cycling women caused significant reduction after 30 and 60 minutes during the follicular and luteal phases but nonsignificant reduction at midcycle *2682*

Secretin *Plasma Increase Physiological* Steady-state concentration significantly increased at 30 min following intravenous infusion of 0.5 CU/kg/h *2683*

Sodium *Urine Increase Physiological* Interferes with reabsorption, exchange for H^+ *4370*

Somatostatin *Plasma Increase Physiological* At steady state at 30 and 60 minutes during infusion of 2.0 CU/kg/h in 8 healthy and normally cycling women significant increase observed during luteal phase and at midcycle but no effect observed in follicular phase *2682*
Plasma No Effect Physiological Intravenous infusions of up to 2.0 CU/kg/h had no effect on concentration in 6 healthy women *2683*

Titratable Acidity *Urine Decrease Physiological* Reduced formation with increased alkalinization *4370*

Vasoactive Intestinal Polypeptide
Plasma No Effect Physiological No significant effect observed in 8 healthy normally cycling women infused with 2.0 CU/kg/h during either follicular or luteal phase or at midcycle *2682* Graded intravenous infusions up to 2.0 CU/kg/h had no effect on concentration in 6 healthy women *2683*

Volume *Bile Increase Physiological* Slight effect in normals, marked in cirrhotics *593*
Pancreatic Fluid Increase Physiological Normal response over 3.2 mL/kg/80 minutes *746*

Selective Serotonin-reuptake Inhibitors

Tricyclic Antidepressants *Serum Increase Physiological* Interacts pharmacokinetically to inhibit metabolism of tricyclic antidepressants *3590*

Selegiline

Dihydroxyphenylacetic Acid
Plasma Decrease Physiological From mean of 730 to 370 ng/mL in 12 depressed or Alzheimer's disease patients given 60 mg drug daily for at least 3 weeks *2887*

Dihydroxyphenylalanine *Plasma No Effect Physiological* In 12 depressed or Alzheimer's disease patients given 60 mg drug daily for at least 3 weeks *1680*

3,4-Dihydroxyphenylglycol *Plasma Decrease Physiological* From mean of 820 to 240 ng/mL in 12 depressed or Alzheimer's disease patients given 60 mg drug daily for at least 3 weeks *1680*

Epinephrine *Plasma No Effect Physiological* In 12 depressed or Alzheimer's disease patients given 60 mg drug daily for at least 3 weeks *1680*

Glucose *Serum Decrease Physiological* In one 70 year old man with Parkinson's disease treated with 10 mg/d for 3 weeks marked hypoglycemia (down to 22 mg/dL) induced with concentration remaining low for 1 week after drug discontinued *5127*

Homovanillic Acid
Cerebrospinal Fluid Decrease Physiological In 43 patients with depression or Alzheimer's disease chronically treated with drug *4965*

5-Hydroxyindoleacetic Acid
Cerebrospinal Fluid Decrease Physiological In 43 patients with depression or Alzheimer's disease chronically treated with drug *4965*

Monoamine Oxidase-B *Platelets Decrease Physiological* In 16 healthy individuals 79.6 ± 15.1% inhibition observed after 0.5 mg selegiline intravenously and in 8 of the volunteers 84.9 ± 11.9% and 95.6 ± 4.5% inhibition observed *2541*

Norepinephrine *Plasma No Effect Physiological* In 12 depressed or Alzheimer's disease patients given 60 mg drug daily for at least 3 weeks *1680*

Occult Blood *Feces Increase Physiological* Gastrointestinal bleeding as a result of exacerbation of preexisting ulcer disease observed as an adverse reaction *5689*

Pramipexole *Serum No Effect Physiological* Coadministration of pramipexole with selegiline did not affect the pharmacokinetics of pramipexole *4680*

Semustine

Alanine Aminotransferase *Serum Increase Physiological* Abnormal hepatic function reported as an adverse effect *1384*

Aspartate Aminotransferase *Serum Increase Physiological* Hepatotoxicity observed as an adverse effect *1384*

Creatinine *Serum Increase Physiological* Delayed nephrotoxicity including renal failure reported frequenly particularly in children with nephrotoxicity apparently related to the total cumulative dose *1384*

Leukocytes *Blood Decrease Physiological* Dose-limiting toxicity is myelosuppression with delayed leukopenia with nadir of white cell count occurring 6 weeks after administration *1384*

Platelets *Blood Decrease Physiological* Dose-limiting toxicity is myelosuppression with nadir of platelet counts occurring after about 4 weeks *1384*

Urea Nitrogen *Serum Increase Physiological* Delayed nephrotoxicity including renal failure has been reported frequently particularly in children *1384*

Sertraline

Amitriptyline *Serum Increase Physiological* When coadministered, by inhibiting cytochrome P450 2D6, may increase the concentration of amitriptyline *6645*

Antipyrine *Serum Decrease Physiological* Coadministration of sertaline (200 mg/d for 21 days) caused a statistically significant 5% reduction in antipyrine half-life reflecting a significant change in hepatic metabolism *4660*

Atenolol *Serum No Effect Physiological* Coadministration of sertaline with atenolol had no significant effect on its pharmacological effects *4660*

Carbamazepine *Serum No Effect Physiological* Coadministration of sertaline 50 - 200 mg/d for 21 days with carbamazepine caused no significant effect on plasma concentration of carbamazepine although carbamazepine metabolized by cytochrome P450 3A4 *4660*

Diazepam *Serum Increase Physiological* Coadministration of sertaline 50 - 200 mg/d for 21 days with diazepam caused 32% decrease in diazepam clearance relative to baseline compared to 19% decrease with placebo *4660*

Digoxin *Serum No Effect Physiological* Coadministration of sertaline for 17 days in healthy volunteers with digoxin had no significant effect on serum digoxin concentration or its renal clearance *4660*

Flecainide *Serum No Effect Physiological* Coadministration of sertaline postulated to cause increase in flecainide concentration because of its potential to inhibit cytochrome P450 2D6 *4660*

Lithium *Serum No Effect Physiological* Coadministration of two doses of sertaline with lithium to normal volunteers had no effect on lithium concentration *4660*

Lysergic Acid Diethylamide *Urine Increase Analytical* Minimum concentration that caused a positive result with EMIT method to measure LSD 0.2 mg/L *4968*

Propafenone *Serum No Effect Physiological* Coadministration of sertaline postulated to cause increase in propafenone concentration because of its potential to inhibit cytochrome P450 2D6 *4660*

Prothrombin Time *Plasma Increase Physiological* Mean increase of 8% in prothrombin time when sertaline (50 - 200 mg/d) coadministered with warfarin (0.75 mg/kg) for 21 days compared with 1% increase with placebo poosibly due to displacement of warfarin from protein *4660*

Sodium *Serum Decrease Physiological* Several cases of hyponatremia reported, reversible with discontinuation of sertaline treatment *4660*

Terfenadine *Serum No Effect Physiological* Coadministration of sertaline 50 - 200 mg/d for 21 days with terfenadine caused no significant effect on plasma concentration of terfenadine although terfenadine metabolized by cytochrome P450 3A4 *4660*

Tolbutamide *Serum Increase Physiological* Coadministration of sertaline at a concentration of 200 mg/d for several days caused a 16% statistically significant decrease in tolbutamide clearance due to altered metabolism of the drug *4660*

Tricyclic Antidepressants *Serum Increase Physiological* Interacts pharmacokinetically to inhibit metabolism of tricyclic antidepressants *3590*

Uric Acid *Serum Decrease Physiological* At recommended dose had mild uricosuric effect of about 7% although clinical significance unknown *4660*

Sevoflurane

Albumin *Urine Increase Physiological* When given for 4 hours caused statistically significant transient injury to glomeruli *1669*

Creatinine *Serum Increase Physiological* When given for 4 hours caused statistically significant transient injury to glomeruli *1669*

Fluoride *Serum Increase Physiological* In 8 patients given sevoflurane anesthesia mean concentration increased to a peak of 55.8 ± 3.4 μmol/L 1 hour after anesthesia *2599* In 40 children undergoing mean 2.7 ± 1.6 hours of anesthesia with sevoflurane mean peak concentration 3 h after anesthesia 15.8 ± 4.6 μmol/L *3543* When given for 2 hours caused statistically significant increase in concentration maximal at the end of anesthesia: peak concentration 62 ± 15 μmol/L, average concentration 39 ± 6 μmol/L: after 8 h peak concentration increased to 106 ± 20 μmol/L and average concentration increased to 74 ± 13 μmol/L *1669*

Glucose *Urine Increase Physiological* When given for 4 hours caused statistically significant transient injury to glomeruli and proximal tubules *1669*

Glutathione S-Transferase *Urine Increase Physiological* When given for 4 hours caused statistically significant transient injury to glomeruli and proximal tubules *1669*

Sibutramine

Alanine Aminotransferase *Serum Increase Physiological* Increased activity reported in 1.6% of treated obese patients compared with 0.8% of control patients *3203*

Alkaline Phosphatase *Serum Increase Physiological* Increased activity reported in 1.6% of treated obese patients compared with 0.8% of control patients *3203*

Aspartate Aminotransferase *Serum Increase Physiological* Increased activity reported in 1.6% of treated obese patients compared with 0.8% of control patients *3203*

Bilirubin *Serum Increase Physiological* Increased concentration reported in 1.6% of treated obese patients compared with 0.8% of control patients *3203*

γ-Glutamyltransferase *Serum Increase Physiological* Increased activity reported in 1.6% of treated obese patients compared with 0.8% of control patients *3203*

Lactate Dehydrogenase *Serum Increase Physiological* Increased activity reported in 1.6% of treated obese patients compared with 0.8% of control patients *3203*

Sildenafil

Alanine Aminotransferase *Serum Increase Physiological* Abnormal liver function tests observed in some patients when sildenafil administered *4657*

Alkaline Phosphatase *Serum Increase Physiological* Abnormal liver function tests observed in some patients when sildenafil administered *4657*

Amlodipine *Serum No Effect Physiological* No interaction observed when amlodipine and sildenafil (100 mg) coadministered to hypertensive patients *4657*

Aspartate Aminotransferase *Serum Increase Physiological* Abnormal liver function tests observed in some patients when sildenafil administered *4657*

Bleeding Time *Patient No Effect Physiological* No effect observed on bleeding time when sildenafil coadministered with 150 mg aspirin *4657*

Glucose *Serum Decrease Physiological* Hypoglycemic reaction observed in some patients when sildenafil administered *4657*
Serum Increase Physiological Unstable diabetes or hyperglycemia observed in some patients when sildenafil administered *4657*

Hematocrit *Blood Decrease Physiological* Anemia observed in some patients when sildenafil administered *4657*

Hemoglobin *Blood Decrease Physiological* Anemia observed in some patients when sildenafil administered *4657*

Leukocytes *Blood Decrease Physiological* Leukopenia observed in some patients when sildenafil administered *4657*

Occult Blood *Feces Increase Physiological* Rectal hemorrhage observed in some patients when sildenafil administered *4657*

Sodium *Serum Increase Physiological* Hypernatremia observed in some patients when sildenafil administered *4657*

Tolbutamide *Serum No Effect Physiological* No interaction observed when sildenafil coadministered with 250 mg tolbutamide which is metabolized by CYP2C9 *4657*

Uric Acid *Serum Increase Physiological* Gout observed in some patients when sildenafil administered *4657*

Warfarin *Plasma No Effect Physiological* No interaction observed when sildenafil coadministered with 40 mg warfarin which is metabolized by CYP2C9 *4657*

Silver

Chloride *Serum Decrease Physiological* Observed after silver nitrate antisepsis *4014*

^{131}I Uptake *Serum No Effect Physiological* No effect reported *3107*

Occult Blood *Feces Increase Physiological* May cause hemorrhagic gastroenteritis *2242*

pH *Blood Increase Physiological* Observed after silver nitrate antisepsis *4014*

Protein *Urine Increase Physiological* May cause nephrotoxicity *5377*

Silver *Serum Increase Physiological* In burned patients treated with silver sulfadiazine cream plasma concentration may be as high as 50 μg/L within 6 h of treatment and can reach a maximum of 310 μg/L *6335*
Urine Increase Physiological In burned patients treated with silver sulfadiazine cream silver is detectable in urine after one day and may reach a maximum of 400 μg/d *6335*

Sodium *Serum Decrease Physiological* Observed after silver nitrate antisepsis *4014*

T3-Uptake *Serum No Effect Physiological* No effect on resin procedures *3107*

Urea Nitrogen *Serum Increase Physiological* May cause nephrotoxicity *5377*

Simethicone

Prothrombin Time *Plasma Decrease Physiological* Impairs absorption of oral anticoagulant *2452*

Simvastatin

Alanine Aminotransferase *Serum Decrease Physiological* In various clinical trials persistent increases above 3 times the upper limit of normal was observed with treatment with 10, 20, 40, and 60 mg/d. The incidences were 0.2%, 0.2%, 0.6% and 2.3% respectively *4534*

Serum Increase Physiological Simvastatin caused increases of activity to above 3 times the upper limit of normal in 1% of patients in clinical trials *3998* Increase to less than 200% of baseline observed in 3 of 12 patients with type III hyperlipoproteinemia when treated with 80 mg simvastatin daily for 6 weeks *5856* In one obese woman treatment for 3 months was followed on one occasion by increase to 419 U/L (normal range 10-38 U/L) *589* In 10 of 15 patients with hyperlipoproteinemia treated with up to 40 mg q.p.m. for 12 weeks increased above normal range but in most activity decreased without adjustment of dosage *6621* Increase above 3 times upper limit of normal observed in 2.7% of cases *619* Increase to less than 200% of baseline observed in 3 of 12 patients with type III hyperlipoprtoeinemia when treated with 80 mg simvastatin daily for 6 weeks *5856*

Serum No Effect Physiological No significant effect observed in 8 patients with moderate grade familial hypercholesterolemia treated with 10 mg daily for 8 weeks *6155*

Aldolase *Serum Increase Physiological* In one man taking simvastatin 20 mg/d for 3 months was associated with polymyositis and an increase of activity to 24.2 U/L *2128*

Alkaline Phosphatase *Serum No Effect Physiological* No significant effect observed in 8 patients with moderate grade familial hypercholesterolemia treated with 10 mg daily for 8 weeks *6155*

Amylase *Serum Increase Physiological* Simvastatin has caused pancreatitis in a small number of patients *3998*

α_2-Antiplasmin *Plasma No Effect Physiological* In 12 men and 17 women with familial hypercholesterolemia treatment with up to 20 mg/d for 14 weeks changed mean concentration nonsignificantly from 86.0% to 86.0% in the men and from 89.0% to 86.5% in the women *2933*

Antipyrine *Serum No Effect Physiological* When simvastatin coadministered with antipyrine no effect on pharmacokinetics of antipyrine observed *3998* Simvastatin had no effect on pharmacokinetics of antipyrine *3998*

Antithrombin III *Plasma No Effect Physiological* In 12 men and 17 women with familial hypercholesterolemia treatment with up to 20 mg/d for 14 weeks changed mean concentration nonsignificantly from 112% to 118% in the men and from 118% to 107% in the women *2933*

Apolipoprotein A *Serum No Effect Physiological* No significant effect observed in 27 hypercholesterolemic patients when treated with 40 mg daily for 3 months *3889*

Apolipoprotein A-I *Serum Increase Physiological* In 14 patients with familial hypercholesterolemia treatment with up to 40 mg/d for 4 months caused increase from mean baseline of 117 mg/dL to 146 mg/dL *1209* Mean increase of 17% in 10 patients with primary hypercholesterolemia treated with up to 40 mg daily for 24 weeks *921* In 23 patients with hypercholesterolemia and nephrotic syndrome treatment with up to 40 mg/d for 24 weeks caused nonsignificant increase from mean baseline of 129 mg/dL to 144 mg/dL *6007* In 36 patients with hypercholesterolemia mean baseline concentration of 1322 mg/L on placebo nonsignificantly increased to 1373 mg/L (3.9%) when treated with 40 mg/d simvastatin for 12 weeks *5605* In 28 patients with type II hyperlipoproteinemia treatment with up to 10 mg/d for 12 weeks caused significant change from mean baseline of 145.7 ± 22.7 mg/dL to 152.6 ± 25.3 mg/dL *2692*

Serum No Effect Physiological Treatment with up to 40 mg/d for 3 months of 10 patients with primary renal disease and nephrotic syndrome and in 8 with diabetic nephropathy and nephrotic syndrome caused no significant changes from mean baselines of 181 ± 10 mg/dL and 168 ± 15 mg/dL respectively to 175 ± 16 mg/dL and 176 ± 13 mg/dL *6343* No significant change observed in 8 patients with moderate grade familial hypercholesterolemia treated for 8 weeks with 10 mg daily *6155* No effect of treatment with up to 5 mg/day for 8 months in 29 patients with moderate to severe hypercholesterolemia *5194* No significant effect observed in 10 hypercholesterolemic patients on continuous ambulatory peritoneal dialysis treated with up to 40 mg/d for 24 weeks *3848* In 8 patients with moderate familial hypercholesterolemia treatment with 10 mg/d for 8 weeks caused nonsignificant change from mean baseline of 134 ± 11 mg/dL to 137 ± 13 mg/dL *4920* In 13 patients with primary hypercholesterolemia treatment for 24 weeks with 10-40 mg/d caused insignificant change from 138 ± 17 mg/dL to 140 ± 9 mg/dL and in 10 patients with NIDDM from 135 ± 19 mg/dL to 137 ± 13 mg/dL *4019* In 48 hypercholesterolemic NIDDM patients treatment for 1 month caused +1% change from mean baseline of 135 mg/dL and in 35 nondiabetic patients mean change of +2% from mean baseline of 131 mg/dL *3082* Nonsignificant increase from mean baseline concentration of 1802 mg/L to 1918 mg/L in 12 patients with type III hyperlipoproteinemia treated with 80 mg daily for 6 weeks *5856* In 24 hypercholesterolemic patients treatment with up to 40 mg/d for 18 weeks caused nonsignificant decrease from mean baseline of 135.2 ± 5.9 mg/dL to 128.4 ± 4.1 mg/dL *3599* In 16 patients with type IIa hyperlipidemia treatment with 20 mg/d for 3 months caused no significant change from mean baseline of 149 ± 23 mg/dL to 147 ± 26 mg/dL and in 10 patients with type IIb hyperlipidemia from 144 ± 22 mg/dL to 149 ± 27 mg/dL *1805* In 23 elderly hypercholesterolemic patients treatment with up to 40 mg/d caused nonsignificant change from mean baseline of 164.5 ± 22.0 g/L to 167.8 ± 16.4 g/L after one month, 175.8 ± 17.1 g/L (significant) after 1 year and 176.7 ± 20.5 g/L after 2 years *5150* Insignificant increase in 12 individuals with primary hypercholesterolemia when treated with up to 40 mg daily for 12 weeks *5385* No change observed in 19 patients with heterozygous familial hypercholesterolemia when treated with up to 40 mg/d for 16 weeks *1393* Treatment of 27 patients with primary hypercholesterolemia with 20 mg/day for up to 10 weeks had no effect on concentration *371*

Apolipoprotein A-I:Apolipoprotein A-II Ratio
Serum Increase Physiological In 8 patients with moderate familial hypercholesterolemia treatment with 10 mg/d for 8 weeks caused increase of 12% from mean baseline of 2.5 ± 0.4 to 2.8 ± 0.5 *4920*

Apolipoprotein A-I:Apolipoprotein B Ratio
Serum Increase Physiological In 10 hypercholesterolemic patients on continuous ambulatory peritoneal dialysis treatment with up to 40 mg/d caused significant increase from mean baseline of 0.82 to 1.07 at 6 weeks, 1.19 at 12 weeks, 1.20 at 18 weeks and 1.22 at 24 weeks *3848*

Apolipoprotein A-II *Serum Decrease Physiological* In 8 patients with moderate familial hypercholesterolemia treatment with 10 mg/d for 8 weeks caused 9% reduction from mean baseline of 54 ± 8 mg/dL to 49 ± 6 mg/dL *4920*

Serum Increase Physiological In 24 hypercholesterolemic patients treatment with up to 40 mg/d for 18 weeks caused significant increase from mean baseline of 34.8 ± 1.9 mg/dL to 39.8 ± 1.5 mg/dL *3599* Mean increase of 25% in 10 patients with primary hypercholesterolemia when treated with up to 40 mg daily for 24 weeks *921*

Serum No Effect Physiological In 28 patients with type II hyperlipoproteinemia treatment with up to 10 mg/d for 12 weeks caused nonsignificant change from mean baseline of 38.8 ± 7.3 mg/dL to 37.6 ± 6.2 mg/dL *2692* No significant effect observed in 10 hypercholesterolemic patients on continuous ambulatory peritoneal dialysis treated with up to 40 mg/d for 24 weeks *3848* Nonsignificant increase from mean baseline of 561 mg/L to 637 mg/L in 12 patients with type III hyperlipoproteinemia treated with 80 mg daily for 6 weeks *5856* Treatment of 27 patients with primary hypercholesterolemia for 4 weeks had no effect but slight reduction at 6 weeks and again no effect at 10 weeks *371* No effect of 8 months treatment with up to 5 mg/day in 29 patients with moderate to severe hypercholesterolemia *5194*

Apolipoprotein A-IV *Serum No Effect Physiological* No significant change observed in 10 hypercholesterolemic patients on continuous ambulatory peritoneal dialysis treated with up to 40 mg/d for 24 weeks *3848*

Apolipoprotein B *Serum Decrease Physiological* In 11 hypercholesterolemic patients on continuous ambulatory peritoneal dialysis treatment with up to 40 mg/d caused significant reduction from mean baseline of 136 mg/dL to 107 mg/dL at 6 weeks, 102 mg/dL at 12 weeks and 90 mg/dL at 24 weeks *3848* In 28 patients with type II hyperlipoproteinemia treatment with up to 10 mg/d for 12 weeks caused significant change from mean baseline of 150.4 ± 21.3 mg/dL to 110.0 ± 20.6 mg/dL *2692* In 16 patients with type IIa hyperlipidemia treatment with 20 mg/d for 3 months caused marked decrease from mean baseline of 166 ± 24 mg/dL to 125 ± 23 mg/dL and in 10 with type IIb hyperlipidemia from 173 ± 19 mg/dL to 136 ± 18 mg/dL *1805* In 8 patients with moderate familial hypercholesterolemia treatment with 10 mg/d for 8 weeks caused 18% reduction from mean baseline of 124 ± 11 mg/dL to 101 ± 14 mg/dL *4920* In one study of 45 hypercholesterolemic patients treatment with 10 mg/d for 16 weeks caused a 30% reduction in concentration *4534* In 48 hypercholesterolemic NIDDM patients treatment for 1 month caused -18% change from mean baseline of 118 mg/dL and in 35 nondiabetic patients mean change of -26% from mean baseline of 129 mg/dL *3082* Reduction from mean concentration of 203 mg/dL to 137 mg/dL in 82 patients with hypercholesterolemia treated with 20 mg daily for 12 weeks and to 116 mg/dL in 80 patients treated with 40 mg daily for 12 weeks *4704* Significant effect observed in 27 hypercholesterolemic patients treated with 40 mg daily for 4 weeks *3889* Decrease from mean of 133 mg/dL to mean of 104 mg/dL (21%) in 29 patients with moderate to severe hypercholesterolemia treated for 4 months with 2.5 mg/day, and 23% after another 4 months treatment with 5 mg/day *5194* Mean decrease from 2.21 to 1.57 g/L (29%) in 11 patients with familial hypercholesterolemia and from 1.53 to 1.09 g/L (29%) in 10 cases with polygenic hypercholesterolemia after 24 weeks of treatment with up to 40 mg/day *4091* 38% reduction in 12 individuals with primary hypercholesterolemia treated with up to 40 mg daily for 12 weeks *5385* Treatment with up to 40 mg/d for 3 months of 10 patients with primary renal disease and nephrotic syndrome and in 8 with diabetic nephropathy and nephrotic syndrome caused significant changes from mean baselines of 182 ± 13 mg/dL and 172 ± 13 mg/dL respectively to 125 ± 11 mg/dL and 93 ± 14 mg/dL *6343* In 19 patients with heterozygous familial hypercholesterolemia treated with up to 40 mg/d for 16 weeks concentration decreased from 243 mg/dL to 162 mg/dL *1393* Mean reduction of 19% in 10 patients with primary hypercholesterolemia when treated with up to 40 mg daily for 24 weeks *921* In 8 patients with hypercholesterolemia treatment with up to 40 mg daily for 24 weeks caused reduction from mean concentration of 1.45 g/L to 1.00 g/L *5628* Significant reduction of 33% after 4 weeks and 31% reduction after 8 weeks treatment with 10 mg daily in 8 patients with moderate grade familial hypercholesterolemia *6155* In 23 elderly hypercholesterolemic patients treatment with up to 40 mg/d caused significant reduction from mean baseline of 177.8 ± 30.5 g/L to 131.1 ± 27.0 g/L after 1 month, 120.0 ± 25.7 g/L after 12 months and 142.5 ± 38.4 g/L after 24 months *5150* In 36 patients with hypercholesterolemia treated with 40 mg/d for 12 weeks mean concentration significantly decreased from 1581 mg/L on placebo to 1087 mg/L (31.2%) *5605* Significant reduction by 19-33% in 10 patients with type II hyperlipoproteinemia treated with 20 or 40 mg daily for 3 years *1238* Treatment of 14 patients with familial hypercholesterolemia with up to 40 mg/d for 4 months caused decrease from mean baseline of 218 mg/dL to 153 mg/dL *1209* Significant reduction from mean baseline of 1285 mg/L to 669 mg/L in 12 patients with type III hyperlipoproteinemia treated with 80 mg daily for 6 weeks *5856* In 10 patients with NIDDM treatment with 10-40 mg/d for 24 wk caused significant decrease from mean 210 ± 55 mg/dL to 140 ± 40 mg/dL (33%) and in 13 patients with primary hypercholesterolemia from 214 ± 54 mg/dL to 161 ± 36 mg/dL (25% reduction) *4019* In 24 hypercholesterolemic patients treatment with up to 40 mg/d for 18 weeks caused significant decrease from mean baseline of 156.5 ± 4.1 mg/dL to 102.6 ± 4.2 mg/dL *3599* Treatment of 27 patients with primary hypercholesterolemia with 20 mg/day for 4 weeks caused 28% reduction, with 31% reduction at 6 weeks and 34% reduction at 10 weeks *371*

Serum Increase Physiological Slight increase of 5-13% observed in 10 patients with type II hyperlipoproteinemia treated with 20 or 40 mg daily for 3 years *1238*

Apolipoprotein B-100 *Serum Decrease Physiological* In 23 patients with hypercholesterolemia and nephrotic syndrome mean concentration decreased from mean baseline of 156 mg/dL by 31% after treatment with up to 40 mg/d for 24 weeks *6007*

Apolipoprotein B:Apolipoprotein A-I Ratio

Serum Decrease Physiological In 48 hypercholesterolemic NIDDM patients treatment for 1 month caused -18% change from mean baseline of 0.9 and in 35 nondiabetic patients mean change of -24% from mean baseline of 1.0 *3082* In 8 patients with moderate familial hypercholesterolemia treatment with 10 mg/d for 8 weeks caused decrease of 19% from mean baseline of 0.93 ± 0.1 to 0.75 ± 0.1 *4920*

Apolipoprotein C-II *Serum Decrease Physiological* In 28 patients with type II hyperlipoproteinemia treatment with up to 10 mg/d for 12 weeks caused significant change from mean baseline of 5.4 ± 1.9 mg/dL to 4.4 ± 1.4 mg/dL *2692* Mean decrease of 26.6% in 10 patients with primary hypercholesterolemia when treated with up to 40 mg daily for 24 weeks *921*

Serum No Effect Physiological Nonsignificant reduction from mean baseline of 8.1 mg/dL to 6.1 mg/dL in 10 hypercholesterolemic patients on continuous ambulatory peritoneal dialysis treated with up to 40 mg/d for 24 weeks *3848* In 14 patients with familial hypercholesterolemia treatment with up to 40 mg/d for 4 months caused insignificant decrease from mean baseline of 3.3 mg/dL to 3.1 mg/dL *1209* In 8 patients with moderate familial hypercholesterolemia treatment with 10 mg/d for 8 weeks caused nonsignificant reduction from mean baseline of 4.0 ± 0.3 mg/dL to 3.7 ± 0.4 mg/dL *4920*

Apolipoprotein C-III *Serum Decrease Physiological* Mean reduction of 30.1% in 10 patients with primary hypercholesterolemia when treated with up to 40 mg daily for 24 weeks *921* In 8 patients with moderate familial hypercholesterolemia treatment with 10 mg/d for 8 weeks caused 12% reduction from mean baseline of 15.5 ± 2.8 mg/dL to 13.7 ± 1.4 mg/dL *4920* Treatment of 27 patients with primary hypercholesterolemia with 20 mg/day caused 19% reduction at 6 weeks although no significant change at 10 weeks *371* In 28 patients with type II hyperlipoproteinemia treatment with up to 10 mg/d for 12 weeks caused significant change from mean baseline of 14.7 ± 4.9 mg/dL to 12.8 ± 3.8 mg/dL *2692* Treatment of 14 patients with familial hypercholesterolemia with up to 40 mg/d for 4 months caused insignificant reduction from mean baseline of 8.8 mg/dL to 8.0 mg/dL *1209*

Apolipoprotein E *Serum Decrease Physiological* Treatment of 14 patients with familial hypercholesterolemia with up to 40 mg/d for 4 months caused decrease from mean baseline of 8.4 mg/dL to 6.9 mg/dL *1209* Mean decrease of 35.0% in 10 patients with primary hypercholesterolemia when treated with up to 40 mg daily for 24 weeks *921* In 28 patients with type II hyperlipoproteinemia treatment with up to 10 mg/d for 12 weeks caused significant change from mean baseline of 8.1 ± 1.8 mg/dL to 6.0 ± 1.5 mg/dL *2692* Significant reduction from mean baseline concentration of 175 mg/L to 110 mg/L in 12 patients with type III hyperlipoproteinemia treated with 80 mg daily for 6 weeks *5856* Treatment of 27 patients with primary hypercholesterolemia with 20 mg/day caused 20% reduction after 4 and 6 weeks but no effect observed at 10 weeks *371* In 48 hypercholesterolemic NIDDM patients treatment for 1 month caused -13% change from mean baseline of 6.7 mg/dL and in 35 nondiabetic patients mean change of -27% from mean baseline of 7.9 mg/dL *3082* In 8 patients with moderate familial hypercholesterolemia treatment with 10 mg/d for 8 weeks caused reduction from mean baseline of 7.1 ± 0.9 mg/dL to 6.2 ± 0.9 mg/dL *4920* Significant reduction observed after 24 weeks treatment in hyperlipidemic patients and in those in whom hypercholesterolemia followed CAPD *3848* In 10 hypercholesterolemic patients on continuous ambulatory peritoneal dialysis treatment with up to 40 mg/d caused significant decrease from mean baseline of 7.4 mg/dL to 2.7 mg/dL at 24 weeks *3848*

Ascorbic Acid *Serum No Effect Physiological* In 25 patients with familial hypercholesterolemia treatment changed concentration from mean baseline of 49.29 ± 11.24 μmol/L to 43.72 ± 26.63 μmol/L after 4 weeks, 55.36 ± 19.99 μmol/L after 8 weeks and 54.28 ± 15.27 μmol/L after 14 weeks. In 21 patients without familial hypercholesterolemia corresponding values were 53.83 ± 17.37 μmol/L, 49.17 ± 21.12 μmol/L, 53.03 ± 17.77 μmol/L and 65.81 ± 16.47 μmol/L respectively *2770*

Simvastatin *(continued)*

Aspartate Aminotransferase
Serum Decrease Physiological In various clinical trials persistent increases above 3 times the upper limit of normal was observed with treatment with 10, 20, 40, and 60 mg/d. The incidences were 0.2%, 0.2%, 0.6% and 2.3% respectively *4534*
Serum Increase Physiological In one obese woman after treatment for 3 months on one occasion associated with muscle pain and weakness in her legs activity increased to 2070 U/L (normal range 7-35 U/L) *589* Increase of more than 3 times upper limit of normal occurred in 1.4% cases *619* Persistent increases of more than three times the upper limit of normal observed in 1% of patients receiving drug *3998*
Serum No Effect Physiological No significant effect observed in 8 patients with moderate grade familial hypercholesterolemia treated with 10 mg daily for 8 weeks *6155* No significant adverse effect observed in 27 hypercholesterolemic patients treated with 40 mg/d for 3 months *3889*

Cholesterol *Neutrophils Decrease Physiological* In 12 hypercholesterolemic patients treatment with simvastatin for 6 weeks caused a significant decrease from mean baseline of 4.19 fmol/cell to 3.52 fmol/cell *1289*
Serum Decrease Physiological Significant reduction by 19-34% in 10 patients with hyperlipoproteinemia treated with 20 or 40 mg daily for 3 years *1238* In 48 hypercholesterolemic patients treated for 4 weeks with simvastatin mean concentration decreased by 34%. After 1-3 years treatment mean reduction was 26-29% *4090* In 13 hypercholesterolemic patients treatment with up to 20 mg/d caused significant decrease from mean baseline of 315.6 ± 34.1 mg/dL to 268.4 ± 21.3 mg/dL after 4 weeks, 239.7 ± 24.6 mg/dL after 8 weeks and 231.4 ± 15.6 mg/dL after 24 weeks *1253* In 8 patients with primary moderate hypercholesterolemia treatment with 10 mg/d for 8 weeks caused significant decrease from mean baseline of 259 ± 18 mg/dl to 214 ± 22 mg/dL (17%) *4920* In 23 elderly hypercholesterolemic individuals treatment with up to 40 mg/d caused significant decrease from mean baseline of 299.4 ± 36.4 mg/dL to 223.4 ± 38.3 mg/dL after 1 month, to 211.9 ± 28.3 mg/dL after 12 months and 225.4 ± 40.5 mg/dL after 24 months *5150* Decrease of 18% (from mean of 263 mg/dL to 216 mg/dL) in 29 patients with moderate to severe hypercholesterolemia given 2.5 mg/day for 4 months, and decrease of 17% at 8 months after 5 mg/day for second 4 months *5194* In 10 patients with NIDDM following treatment with 10-40 mg/d for 24 weeks significant reduction from mean baseline of 332 ± 91 mg/dL to 221 ± 50 mg/dL (34%) and in 13 patients with primary hypercholesterolemia from 419 ± 76 mg/dL to 291 45 g/dL (30%) *4019* In one study of 45 hypercholesterolemic patients treatment with 10 mg/d for 16 weeks caused a 24% reduction in concentration *4534* In 10 patients with primary hypercholesterolemia treatment with up to 40 mg daily for 24 weeks caused mean reduction of 30% *921* Mean 35% reduction observed in 8 patients with heterozygous familial hypercholesterolemia treated with 80 mg/d for 8-22 weeks *4786* In 120 patients with heterozygous familial hypercholesterolemia treatment with 40 mg daily for 12 weeks caused mean reduction of 33% *1312* Treatment of 6 patients with familial hypercholesterolemia with 80 mg/d for 24 months caused decrease from mean baseline of 442 mg/dL to 324 mg/dL. When combined with cholestyramine in 8 patients decrease from mean baseline of 424 mg/dL to 262 mg/dL *1209* In 19 patients with heterozygous familial hypercholesterolemia treatment with up to 40 mg/d for 16 weeks caused decrease from mean baseline of 447 mg/dL to 299 mg/dL *1393* In 12 hypercholesterolemic patients treatment with simvastatin for 6 weeks caused a significant decrease from mean baseline of 8.95 mmol/L to 6.55 mmol/L *1289* In 16 patients with type IIa hyperlipidemia treatment with 20 mg/d for 3 months caused significant decrease fro mean baseline of 8.76 ± 1.25 mmol/L to 6.31 ± 1.02 mmol/L and in 10 with type IIb hyperlipidemia from 7.59 ± 0.85 mmol/L to 5.99 ± 0.65 mmol/L *1805* In four patients with familial hypercholesterolemia treated with diet and simvastatin for at least 3 months (with two also receiving cholestyramine) concentrations decreased from 10.9 to 7.8 mmol/L, 9.2 to 8.7 mmol/L, 15.6 to 8.0 mmol/L and 12.9 to 8.0 mmol/L respectively *6405* In 58 postmenopausal women with fasting serum cholesterol concentrations greater than 250 mg/dL treatment with 10 mg simvastatin for 8 weeks caused significant change from mean baseline of 307 ± 43 mg/dL to 227 ± 33 mg/dL *1239* In 7 mildly hypercholesterolemic patients mean concentration of 7.5 mmol/L fell significantly to 5.3 mmol/L after 10 weeks treatment with 20 mg/d *2059* In 28 patients with type II hyperlipoproteinemia treatment with up to 10 mg/d for 12 weeks caused significant change from mean baseline of 307.7 ± 48.3 mg/dL to 225.1 ± 35.7 mg/dL *2692* In patients with nephrotic syndrome treatment with simvastatin caused a 33% decrease in concentration *4440* In 25 patients with familial hypercholesterolemia treatment reduced concentration from mean baseline of 8.78 ± 1.66 mmol/L to 7.31 ± 1.41 mol/L after 4 weeks, 6.92 ± 1.43 mmol/L after 8 weeks and 7.16 ± 1.21 mmol/L after 14 weeks. In 21 patients without familial hypercholesterolemia corresponding values were 7.97 ± 1.41 mmol/L, 6.73 ± 1.08 mmol/L, 6.21 ± 1.25 mmol/L and 5.99 ± 1.04 mmol/L respectively *2770* Reduction from mean concentration of 323 mg/dL to 240 mg/dL in 82 patients with hypercholesterolemia treated with 20 mg daily for 12 weeks and to 216 mg/dL in 80 patients treated with 40 mg daily for 12 weeks *4704* Simvastatin administered in doses of 20 mg/d, 40 mg/d, 80 mg/d and 160 mg/d to about 27 hypercholesterolemic patients at each level caused reductions of 17%, 24%, 25% and 28% respectively *3998* Significant decrease from mean concentration of 326 mg/dL to 239 mg/dL in 83 patients taking 20 mg/day and from 317 mg/dL to 215 mg/dL in 82 patients taking 40 mg daily *3035* 30% reduction in 12 individuals with primary hypercholesterolemia treated with up to 40 mg daily for 12 weeks *5385* Mean decrease from 10.51 to 6.71 mmol/L (36%) in 11 patients with familial hypercholesterolemia and from 6.55 to 4.54 mmol/L (31%) in 10 patients with polygenic hypercholesterolemia after 24 weeks treatment with up to 40 mg/day *4091* In 10 patients with type II hyperlipidemia mean concentration decreased significantly from 351 ± 46 mg/dL to 252 ± 39 mg/dL after 6 months treatment *5585* In the Scandinavian Simvastatin Survival Study of 4,444 patients treatment with 20 or 40 mg/d for 5.4 years caused mean decrease of 25% *3115* In 12 patients with stable angina pectoris and mild to moderate hypercholesterolemia treatment with 10 mg b.i.d. caused significant reduction from mean baseline of 267 ± 22 mg/dL to 209 ± 24 mg/dL after 1 month and 210 ± 32 mg/dL after 3 months *1307* In 36 patients with hypercholesterolemia mean concentration decreased significantly to 5.60 mmol/L from baseline of 8.16 mmol/L (31.7%) after treatment with 40 mg/d for 12 weeks *5605* In 12 patients with type II hyperproteinemia mean concentration of 260 mg/dL pretreatment significantly reduced to 207 mg/dL following treatment with 5 - 10 mg/d for an average of 13.9 weeks *6083* In 8 patients with hypercholesterolemia treatment with up to 40 mg daily for 24 weeks caused reduction of mean cholesterol concentration from 9.3 mmol/L to 6.4 mmol/L *5628* In 48 hypercholesterolemic NIDDM patients treatment for 1 month caused 19% reduction from mean baseline of 261 mg/dL and in 35 nondiabetic patients mean reduction of 24% from mean baseline of 278 mg/dL *3082* In 12 patients with type III hyperlipoproteinemia 80 mg daily for 6 weeks caused reduction from mean baseline of 12.3 mmol/L to 5.3 mmol/L (54%) *5856* In 12 elderly noninsulin-dependent diabetics treatment with 30 mg/d for 3 weeks caused decrease from mean baseline concentration of 7.9 mmol/L to 5.3 mmol/L *4500* In 12 men and 17 women with familial hypercholesterolemia treatment with up to 20 mg/d for 14 weeks reduced mean concentration from 9.55 mmol/L to 7.00 mmol/L in the men and from 9.50 mmol/L to 7.40 mmol/L in the women *2933* Mean reduction of 36-51% observed in 12 patients with familial dysβlipoproteinemia (type III hyperlipoproteinemia) when treated with 40 mg/d for 66 weeks *5855* Mean reduction of 36-51% observed in 12 patients with familial dysbetalipoproteinemia (type III hyperlipoproteinemia) when treated with 40 mg/d for 66 weeks *5855* In 24 patients with familial and nonfamilial hypercholesterolemia treatment with up to 40 mg/d for 30 months caused mean decrease of 30% *6003* In 23 patients with hypercholesterolemia and nephrotic syndrome mean decrease of 30% when treated with 10 mg/d for 4 weeks. By 24 weeks after further treatment with up to 40 mg/d total concentration had decreased by 33% *6007* In a population of patients with primary hypercholesterolemia treatment for 12 weeks caused a 31.7% reduction in concentration *4349* Mean reduction of 27 % in 76 patients with primary hypercholesterolemia treated with mean dose of 17.3 mg daily for 12 weeks *6031* Reduction of 27% observed after 4 weeks and 26% after 8 weeks treatment with 10 mg daily in 8 patients with moderate grade familial

hypercholesterolemia *6155* Treatment with up to 40 mg/d for 3 months of 10 patients with primary renal disease and nephrotic syndrome and in 8 with diabetic nephropathy and nephrotic syndrome caused significant changes from mean baselines of 395 ± 20 mg/dL and 381 ± 26 mg/dL respectively to 272 ± 15 mg/dL and 219 ± 28 mg/dL *6343* In 44 patients with primary hypercholesterolemia treatment with upto 40 mg/d and cholestyramine 4 g/d for 30 weeks caused significant reduction from mean baseline of 11.0 ± 1.9 mmol/L by 19 ± 10% after 6 weeks, 24 ± 9% after 12 weeks, 29 ± 10% after 18 weeks and 32 ± 13% after 30 weeks *5564* Reduction to mean of 7.2 mmol/L from mean of 11.1 mmol/L in 15 patients with hyperlipoproteinemia type II treated with up to 40 mg q.p.m. for 12 weeks *6621* In 27 patients with primary hypercholesterolemia treatment with 20 mg/day caused reduction of 26% after 4 weeks, 26% after 6 weeks and 35% at 10 weeks *371* Significant reduction observed after 24 weeks treatment in patients with hypercholesterolemia following CAPD *3848* In 11 hypercholesterolemic patients on continuous ambulatory peritoneal dialysis treatment with up to 40 mg/d caused significant decrease from mean baseline concentration of 310 mg/dL to 222 mg/dL at 6 weeks and to 201 mg/dL at 12 weeks *3848* Significant effect observed in 27 hypercholesterolemic patients treated with 40 mg daily at 4 weeks *3889* In 24 patients with hypercholesterolemia treatment with up to 40 mg/d for 18 weeks caused significant decrease from mean baseline of 8.6 ± 0.3 mmol/L to 5.8 ± 0.2 mmol/L *3599* In 20 hypercholesterolemic men treatment with 20 mg/d for 4 weeks caused significant reduction from mean baseline of 7.4 mmol/L to 5.5 mmol/L *3352*

Cholesterol Ester Transfer Protein
Serum Decrease Physiological In 28 patients with type II hyperlipoproteinemia treatment with up to 10 mg/d for 12 weeks caused significant change from mean baseline of 121.1 ± 31.4 units to 82.4 ± 27.2 units *2692*

Cholesterol:HDL-Cholesterol Ratio
Serum Decrease Physiological Simvastatin administered in doses of 20 mg/d, 40 mg/d, 80 mg/d and 160 mg/d to about 27 hypercholesterolemic patients at each level caused decreases of 22%, 29%, 30% and 36% respectively *3998* In 48 hypercholesterolemic NIDDM patients treatment for 1 month caused -21% change from mean baseline of 5.3 and in 35 nondiabetic patients mean change of -27% from mean baseline of 6.1 *3082*

Coenzyme Q_{10} *Serum Decrease Physiological* In 25 patients with familial hypercholesterolemia treatment changed concentration significantly from mean baseline of 1519 ± 503 nmol/L to 1134 ± 444 nmol/L after 4 weeks, 1203 ± 489 nmol/L after 8 weeks and 1131 ± 419 nmol/L after 14 weeks. In 21 patients without familial hypercholesterolemia corresponding values were 1409 ± 347 nmol/L, 1212 ± 450 nmol/L, 1058 ± 281 nmol/L and 1043 ± 373 nmol/L respectively *2770*

Cortisol *Plasma No Effect Physiological* No significant difference in 8 patients with heterozygous familial hypercholesterolemia before and after treatment with 80 mg/d for 8-22 weeks *4786*

Cortisol, Free *Urine No Effect Physiological* No significant difference between baseline concentrations in 8 patients with heterozygous familial hypercholesterolemia before and after treatment with 80 mg/d for 8-22 weeks *4786*

Creatine Kinase *Serum Increase Physiological* When simvastatin administered about 5% patients had increases of CK activity of 3 or more times normal on one or more occasions *3998* In one obese female patient marked rhabdomyolysis observed with total CK activity of 26010 U/L *589* Simvastatin caused rare cases of rhabdomyolysis with acute renal failure secondary to myoglobinuria *3998* In 3 of 19 patients with heterozygous familial hypercholesterolemia treatment with up to 40 mg/d for 16 weeks was associated with increases of up to 320 U/L on one occasion in each *1393* In one man taking simvastatin 20 mg/d for 3 months was associated with polymyositis and an increase of CK activity to 503 U/L compared with normal of < 170 U/L *2128*
Serum No Effect Physiological No significant effect observed in 8 patients with moderate grade familial hypercholesterolemia treated with 10 mg daily for 8 weeks *6155* No significant adverse effect observed in 27 hypercholesterolemic patients treated with 40 mg/d for 3 months *3889*

Creatine Kinase Isoenzymes *Serum Increase Physiological* In one obese women after administration of drug for 3 months increased activity to 26010 U/L observed, all of which was CK-MM (137 times the upper limit of normal) *589*

Creatinine Clearance *Urine No Effect Physiological* In 18 normolipidemic patients treated with 20 mg/d for 17 days mean clearance changed nonsignificantly from mean baseline of 135.35 ± 21.75 mL/min to 136.52 ± 25.59 mL/min *2725*

D-Dimer *Plasma Decrease Physiological* In 17 women with familial hypercholesterolemia treatment with up to 20 mg/d for 14 weeks changed mean concentration significantly from 12.0 µg/L to 8.85 µg/L *2933*
Plasma No Effect Physiological In 12 men with familial hypercholesterolemia treatment with up to 20 mg/d for 14 weeks changed mean concentration nonsignificantly from 3.90 µg/L to 4.85 µg/L *2933*

Digoxin *Serum Decrease Physiological* Simvastatin concomitantly administered with digoxin caused a slight increase (less than 0.3 ng/mL) in the mean plasma digoxin concentration *3998*
Serum Increase Physiological When simvastatin coadministered with digoxin caused slight (less than 0.3 ng/mL) increase in mean plasma concentration *3998*

Fatty Acids (FFA), Free *Serum Decrease Physiological* In 12 elderly noninsulin-dependent diabetics treatment with 30 mg/d for 3 weeks caused decrease from mean baseline concentration of 1106 mmol/L to 818 mmol/L *4500*

Fibrinogen *Plasma Decrease Physiological* In 13 hypercholesterolemic patients treatment with up to 20 mg/d caused decrease from mean baseline of 3.82 ± 0.70 g/L to 3.71 ± 0.65 g/L after 4 weeks, 3.48 ± 0.59 g/L after 8 weeks and 3.34 ± 0.56 g/L after 24 weeks *1253* In 12 patients with type II hyperproteinemia mean concentration of 313 mg/dL not significantly reduced to 302 mg/dL following treatment with 5 - 10 mg/d for an average of 13.9 weeks *6083*
Plasma Increase Physiological In 12 men with familial hypercholesterolemia treatment with up to 20 mg/d for 14 weeks changed mean concentration significantly from 2.75 g/L to 2.99 g/L in the men *2933*
Plasma No Effect Physiological No significant effect observed in 27 hypercholesterolemic patients treated with 40 mg/d for 3 months *3889* In 17 women with familial hypercholesterolemia treatment with up to 20 mg/d for 14 weeks changed mean concentration nonsignificantly from 3.31 g/L to 3.37 g/L in the women *2933*

Glucose *Serum Decrease Physiological* In 12 elderly noninsulin-dependent diabetics treatment with 30 mg/d for 3 weeks caused decrease from mean baseline concentration of 7.4 mmol/L to 6.6 mmol/L *4500*
Serum No Effect Physiological In 10 patients with NIDDM and 13 patients with primary hypercholesterolemia treatment with up to 40 mg/d for 24 weeks had no significant effect *4019*

Glyburide *Serum Increase Physiological* In 16 healthy individuals coadministration of 20 mg simvastatin in single dose caused 19% increase and in multiple doses caused 31% increase in maximum glyburide concentration relative to placebo-treated controls *227*

HDL_2-Apolipoprotein A-I *Serum Increase Physiological* In 19 patients with heterozygous familial hypercholesterolemia treatment with up to 40 mg/d for 16 weeks caused increase from mean baseline of 21 mg/dL to 26 mg/dL *1393*

HDL_2-Cholesterol *Serum Increase Physiological* Mean increase of 38.9% in 10 patients with primary hypercholesterolemia when treated with up to 40 mg daily for 24 weeks *921*
Serum No Effect Physiological No change observed in 19 patients with heterozygous familial hypercholesterolemia treated with up to 40 mg/d for 16 weeks *1393* Treatment with up to 40 mg/d for 3 months of 10 patients with primary renal disease and nephrotic syndrome and in 8 with diabetic nephropathy and nephrotic syndrome caused nonsignificant changes from mean baselines of 12 ± 2 mg/dL and 11 ± 2 mg/dL respectively to 11 ± 2 mg/dL and 12 ± 2 mg/dL *6343* In 28 patients with type II hyperlipoproteinemia treatment with up to 10 mg/d for 12 weeks caused nonsignificant change from mean baseline of 21.3 ± 7.0 mg/dL to 23.6 ± 9.4 mg/dL *2692*

HDL_2-Lipoprotein *Serum Increase Physiological* In 7 mildly hypercholesterolemic individuals treatment with 20 mg/d for 10 weeks caused significant increase in HDL_2-lipoprotein from mean baseline of 39 mg/dL to 63 mg/dL *2059*

Simvastatin *(continued)*

HDL_2-Triglycerides *Serum No Effect Physiological* In 28 patients with type II hyperlipoproteinemia treatment with up to 10 mg/d for 12 weeks caused nonsignificant change from mean baseline of 4.1 ± 2.6 mg/dL to 4.1 ± 2.0 mg/dL *2692*

HDL_{2b}-Cholesterol *Serum Increase Physiological* In 22 hypercholesterolemic patients treatment with doses of 10 mg/d for 6 weeks caused significant mean increase of 30% *2948*

HDL_3-Apolipoprotein A-I *Serum Increase Physiological* In 19 patients with heterozygous familial hypercholesterolemia treatment with up to 40 mg/d for 16 weeks caused increase from mean baseline of 62 mg/dL to 70 mg/dL *1393*

HDL_3-Cholesterol *Serum Increase Physiological* Mean increase of 15.8% in 10 patients with primary hypercholesterolemia when treated with up to 40 mg daily for 24 weeks *921*

Serum No Effect Physiological Treatment with up to 40 mg/d for 3 months of 10 patients with primary renal disease and nephrotic syndrome and in 8 with diabetic nephropathy and nephrotic syndrome caused nonsignificant changes from mean baselines of 42 ± 4 mg/dL and 42 ± 5 mg/dL respectively to 44 ± 4 mg/dL and 35 ± 4 mg/dL *6343* In 28 patients with type II hyperlipoproteinemia treatment with up to 10 mg/d for 12 weeks caused nonsignificant change from mean baseline of 23.9 ± 8.0 mg/dL to 24.1 ± 4.5 mg/dL *2692* Insignificant change from baseline of 32 mg/dL to 31 mg/dL observed in 19 patients with heterozygous familial hypercholesterolemia treated with up to 40 mg/d for 16 weeks *1393*

HDL_3-Lipoprotein *Serum No Effect Physiological* In 7 mildly hypercholesterolemic individuals treatment with 20 mg/d for 10 weeks caused nonsignificant increase of HDL_3 lipoprotein from mean baseline of 249 mg/dL to 262 mg/dL *2059*

HDL_3-Triglycerides *Serum No Effect Physiological* In 28 patients with type II hyperlipoproteinemia treatment with up to 10 mg/d for 12 weeks caused nonsignificant change from mean baseline of 4.1 ± 1.9 mg/dL to 4.3 ± 1.8 mg/dL *2692*

HDL_{3a}-Cholesterol *Serum Increase Physiological* In 22 hypercholesterolemic patients treatment with 10 mg/d for 6 weeks caused a significant increase (12%) in concentration *2948*

HDL-Apolipoprotein A-I *Serum No Effect Physiological* No significant change from mean baseline concentration of 112 mg/dL in 5 hypercholesterolemic patients on CAPD treated with up to 40 mg/d for 24 weeks *3848*

HDL-Apolipoprotein E *Serum Decrease Physiological* Significant reduction from mean baseline concentration of 5.6 mg/dL to 1.6 mg/dL in 5 hypercholesterolemic patients on CAPD treated with up to 40 mg/d for 24 weeks *3848*

HDL-Cholesterol *Serum Decrease Physiological* In 28 patients with type II hyperlipoproteinemia treatment with up to 10 mg/d for 12 weeks caused significant change from mean baseline of 50.8 ± 9.1 mg/dL to 53.9 ± 12.3 mg/dL *2692* In one study of 45 hypercholesterolemic patients treatment with 10 mg/d for 16 weeks caused a 7% increase in concentration *4534* In 12 patients with type II hyperproteinemia mean concentration of 52 mg/dL pretreatment nonsignificantly reduced to 49 mg/dL following treatment with 5 - 10 mg/d for an average of 13.9 weeks *6083*

Serum Increase Physiological Significant increase, by 24%, in 10 patients with primary hypercholesterolemia when treated with up to 40 mg daily for 24 weeks *921* In a population of patients with primary hypercholesterolemia treatment for 12 weeks caused significant 13.3% increase in concentration *4349* In 44 patients with primary hypercholesterolemia treatment with upto 40 mg/d and cholestyramine 4 g/d for 30 weeks caused significant increase from mean baseline of 1.1 ± 0.3 mmol/L by 11 ± 13% after 6 weeks, 9 ± 12% after 12 weeks, 13 ± 14% after 18 weeks and 10 ± 15% after 30 weeks *5564* Treatment of 24 patients with familial and nonfamilial hypercholesterolemia with up to 40 mg/d for 30 months caused mean increase of 11% *6003* In the Scandinavian Simvastatin Survival Study of 4,444 patients treatment with 20 or 40 mg/d for 5.4 years caused mean increase of 8% *3115* Increase to 50 mg/dL from 45 mg/dL in 82 patients with hypercholesterolemia treated with 20 mg daily for 12 weeks and in 80 treated with 40 mg daily for 12 weeks *4704* In 25 patients with familial hypercholesterolemia treatment increased concentration from mean baseline of 1.15 ± 0.34 mmol/L to 1.25 ± 0.32 mmol/L after 4 weeks, 1.22 ± 0.32 mmol/L after 8 weeks and 1.26 ± 0.38 mmol/L after 14 weeks. In 21 patients without familial hypercholesterolemia corresponding values were 1.38 ± 0.39 mmol/L, 1.50 ± 0.34 mmol/L, 1.47 ± 0.36 mmol/L and 1.48 ± 0.35 mmol/L respectively *2770* In 12 hypercholesterolemic patients treatment with simvastatin for 6 weeks caused a nonsignificant increase from mean baseline of 1.20 mmol/L to 1.38 mmol/L *1289* Simvastatin administered in doses of 20 mg/d, 40 mg/d, 80 mg/d and 160 mg/d to about 27 hypercholesterolemic patients at each level caused increases of 7%, 9%, 11% and 12% respectively *3998* Mean 9% increase in 8 patients with heterozygous familial hypercholesterolemia treated with 80 mg/d for 8-22 weeks *4786* In 48 patients with hypercholesterolemia treatment with simvastatin for up to 3 years caused 10-14% increase in concentration *4090* Mean increase of 9% in 76 patients with primary hypercholesterolemia treated with mean dose of 17.3 mg daily for 12 weeks *6031* In 6 patients with familial hypercholesterolemia 80 mg/d for 24 months caused increase from mean baseline of 45 mg/dL to 49 mg/dL. When combined with cholestyramine in 8 patients mean concentration increased from 41 mg/dL to 51 mg/dL after 24 months *1209* In 15 patients with hyperlipoproteinemia type II after 12 weeks treatment with up to 40 mg q.p.m. nonsignificant increase of 9% observed *6621* Treatment of 14 patients with familial hypercholesterolemia with 10 mg/d for 4 weeks caused increase to mean of 46 mg/dL from 43 mg/dL, with 20 mg/d caused increase to 47 mg/dL and with 40 mg/d for 8 weeks caused increase to mean of 47 mg/dL *1209* Mean increase of 7% observed in 120 patients with familial heterozygous hypercholesterolemia treated with 40 mg daily for 12 weeks *1312* Significant effect observed in most of 27 patients with hypercholesterolemia when treated with 40 mg/d for 3 months *3889* Increase occurred in 12 individuals with primary hypercholesterolemia when treated with up to 40 mg daily for 12 weeks but not significant *5385* In 19 patients with heterozygous familial hypercholesterolemia treatment with up to 40 mg/d for 16 weeks caused increase from mean baseline of 51 mg/dL to 57 mg/dL *1393* Mean concentration increased in patients with both familial and polygenic hypercholesterolemia treated with up to 40 mg daily for 24 weeks, with both HDL_2 and HDL_3 fractions affected *4091* In 10 patients with type IIb hyperlipidemia treatment with 20 mg/d for 3 months caused increase from mean baseline of 1.07 ± 0.20 mmol/L to 1.23 ± 0.15 mmol/L *1805* In 36 patients with hypercholesterolemia mean concentration increased from 1.30 mmol/L to 1.44 mmol/L (11.2%) after treatment with 40 mg/d simvastatin for 12 weeks *5605* Significant increase from mean of 48 mg/dL to 52 mg/dL after 8 months treatment with up to 5 mg/day in 29 patients with moderate to severe hypercholesterolemia *5194* In 48 hypercholesterolemic NIDDM patients treatment for 1 month caused 4% change from mean baseline of 52 mg/dL and in 35 nondiabetic patients mean change of 10% from mean baseline of 49 mg/dL *3082*

Serum No Effect Physiological Nonsignificant increase from mean baseline of 38.5 mg/dL to 44.0 mg/dL in 5 hypercholesterolemic patients on CAPD treated with up to 40 mg/d for 24 weeks *3848* In 12 men and 17 women with familial hypercholesterolemia treatment with up to 20 mg/d for 14 weeks changed mean concentration nonsignificantly from 1.25 mmol/L to 1.14 mmol/L in the men and from 1.45 mmol/L to 1.36 mmol/L in the women *2933* Nonsignificant increase from mean baseline of 0.89 mmol/L to 0.96 mmol/L in 12 patients with type III hyperlipoproteinemia treated with 80 mg daily for 6 weeks *5856* Treatment with up to 40 mg/d for 3 months of 10 patients with primary renal disease and nephrotic syndrome and in 8 with diabetic nephropathy and nephrotic syndrome caused nonsignificant changes from mean baselines of 53 ± 5 mg/dL and 55 ± 6 mg/dL respectively to 54 ± 7 mg/dL and 48 ± 4 mg/dL *6343* In 7 mildly hypercholesterolemic individuals treatment with 20 mg/d for 10 weeks caused nonsignificant increase from mean baseline of 1.29 mmol/L to 1.30 mmol/L *2059* In 58 postmenopausal women with fasting serum cholesterol concentrations greater than 250 mg/dL treatment with 10 mg simvastatin for 8 weeks caused nonsignificant change from mean baseline of 64 ± 17 mg/dL to 68 ± 17 mg/dL *1239* No significant change observed in 11 hypercholesterolemic patients on continuous ambulatory peritoneal dialysis receiving up to 40 mg/d for 24 weeks *3848* In 12 patients with stable angina pectoris and mild to moderate hypercholesterolemia treatment with 10 mg b.i.d. caused no significant change from mean baseline of 49 ± 17 mg/dL to 55 ± 14 mg/dL after 1 month and 52 ± 11 mg/dL after 3 months *1307* In 23 patients with hypercholesterolemia and nephrotic syndrome mean concentration not significantly changed by treatment with up to 40 mg/d for 24 weeks *6007* In 10 patients with NIDDM treatment for 24 weeks with up to 40 mg/d caused insignificant increase from 45 ± 10 mg/dL to 47 ± 9 mg/dL and in 13 patients with primary hypercholesterolemia no change from baseline of 48 ± 7 mg/dL observed *4019* In 24 patients with hypercholesterolemia treatment with up to 40 mg/d for 18 months caused nonsignificant increase from mean baseline of 1.1 ± 0.1 mmol/L to 1.2 ± 0.1 mmol/L *3599* In 23 elderly hypercholesterolemic patients treatment with up to 40 mg/d caused no significant change from mean baseline of 50.2 ± 12.0 mg/dL to 53.6 ± 12.3 mg/dL after 1 month, 50.3 ± 9.1 mg/dL after 12 months and 51.0 ± 11.7 mg/dL after 24 months *5150* Insignificant increase from mean concentration of 45 mg/dL to 48 mg/dL in 83 patients taking 20 mg daily and from 44 mg/dL to 49 mg/dL in those taking 40 mg daily *3035* In 16 patients with type IIa hyperlipidemia treatment with 20 mg/d for 3 months caused no significant change from mean baseline of 1.39 ± 0.29 mmol/L to 1.41 ± 0.30 mmol/L *1805* Insignificant increase from mean concentration of 0.9 mmol/L to 1.0 mmol/L in 8 patients with hypercholesterolemia treated with up to 40 mg daily for 24 weeks *5628* Insignificant change of -3 to +6% in 10 patients with type II hyperlipoproteinemia treated with 20 or 40 mg daily for 3 years *1238* In 8 patients with moderate familial hypercholesterolemia treatment with 10 mg/d for 8 weeks caused nonsignificant increase of 2% from mean baseline of 43 ± 8 mg/dL to 44 ± 8 mg/dL *4920* In 20 hypercholesterolemic men treatment with 20 mg/d for 4 weeks caused nonsignificant change from mean baseline of 1.26 mmol/L to 1.36 mmol/L *3352* No change observed after 4 weeks and 4% reduction after 8 weeks treatment with 10 mg daily in 8 patients with moderate grade familial hypercholesterolemia *6155* Treatment of 27 patients with primary hypercholesterolemia with 20 mg/day over 10 weeks had no effect on concentration *371* No significant change observed in 11 patients with hypercholesterolemia treated with 10-40 mg/d for 12 weeks *4216*

HDL-Phospholipids *Serum No Effect Physiological* Treatment of 27 patients with primary hypercholesterolemia with 20 mg/day for 10 weeks had no significant effect on concentration *371* Treatment with up to 40 mg/d for 3 months of 10 patients with primary renal disease and nephrotic syndrome and in 8 with diabetic nephropathy and nephrotic syndrome caused nonsignificant changes from mean baselines of 108 ± 10 mg/dL and 108 ± 11 mg/dL respectively to 114 ± 14 mg/dL and 109 ± 7 mg/dL *6343*

HDL-Triglycerides *Serum Decrease Physiological* Treatment of 8 patients with diabetic nephropathy and nephrotic syndrome with up to 40 mg/d for 3 months caused significant change from mean baseline of 40 ± 6 mg/dL to 24 ± 3 mg/dL *6343*

Serum No Effect Physiological Treatment with up to 40 mg/d for 3 months of 10 patients with primary renal disease and nephrotic syndrome caused nonsignificant change from mean baseline of 21 ± 3 mg/dL to 26 ± 3 mg/dL *6343* Nonsignificant increase from mean baseline of 17.0 mg/dL to 20.0 mg/dL in 5 hypercholesterolemic patients on CAPD with up to 40 mg/d for 24 weeks *3848*

Hematocrit *Blood Decrease Physiological* In 12 patients with stable angina pectoris and mild to moderate hypercholesterolemia treatment with 10 mg b.i.d. caused no significant change from mean baseline of 45 ± 4% to 43 ± 4% after 1 month but significant reduction to 43 ± 4% after 3 months *1307*

Hemoglobin A_{1c} *Blood No Effect Physiological* In 10 patients with NIDDM treatment with 10-40 mg/d for 24 weeks had no effect on concentration (8%) *4019*

Hepatic Triglyceride Lipase *Serum No Effect Physiological* No significant effect of treatment with up to 5 mg/day for 8 months in 29 patients with moderate to severe hypercholesterolemia *5194*

HMG-CoA Reductase

White Blood Cells Increase Physiological Activity unchanged in 21 hypercholesterolemic patients after 4 weeks treatment with 40 mg/d for 4 weeks but 87% increase after 3 months *3889*

17-Hydroxycorticosteroids *Urine No Effect Physiological* No significant difference observed in 8 patients with heterozygous familial hypercholesterolemia before and after treatment with 80 mg/d for 8-22 weeks *4786* In 18 normolipidemic patients treatment with 20 mg/d for 17 days caused nonsignificant change from mean baseline of 8.75 ± 2.65 mg/d to 8.64 ± 2.8 mg/d *2725*

6-β-Hydroxycortisol *Urine Increase Physiological* In 18 normolipidemic patients treated with 20 mg/d for 17 days mean excretion increased significantly from baseline of 293.2 ± 67.4 µg/d to 358.6 ± 135.9 µg/d *2725*

IDL-Cholesterol *Serum Decrease Physiological* In 28 patients with type II hyperlipoproteinemia treatment with up to 10 mg/d for 12 weeks caused significant change from mean baseline of 15.5 ± 8.2 mg/dL to 9.8 ± 4.7 mg/dL *2692*

IDL-Triglycerides *Serum Decrease Physiological* In 28 patients with type II hyperlipoproteinemia treatment with up to 10 mg/d for 12 weeks caused significant change from mean baseline of 15.7 ± 10.9 mg/dL to 10.8 ± 4.5 mg/dL *2692*

17-Ketosteroids *Urine No Effect Physiological* No significant difference between baseline concentrations in 8 patients with heterozygous familial hypercholesterolemia before and after treatment with 80 mg/d for 8-22 weeks *4786*

Lactate Dehydrogenase *Serum Increase Physiological* In one man taking simvastatin 20 mg/d for 3 months was associated with polymyositis and an increase of activity to 518 U/L compared with upper limit of normal of < 150 U/L *2128*

LDL_1-Apolipoprotein B *Serum Decrease Physiological* Significant reduction from mean baseline concentration of 22.9 mg/dL to 13.6 mg/dL in 5 hypercholesterolemic patients on CAPD treated with up to 40 mg/d for 24 weeks *3848*

LDL_1-Apolipoprotein E *Serum No Effect Physiological* Nonsignificant reduction from mean baseline concentration of 0.9 mg/dL to 0.5 mg/dL in 5 hypercholesterolemic patients on CAPD treated with up to 40 mg/d for 24 weeks *3848*

LDL_1-Cholesterol *Serum Decrease Physiological* Significant reduction from mean baseline of 52.9 mg/dL to 30.1 mg/dL in 5 hypercholesterolemic patients on CAPD receiving up to 40 mg/d for 24 weeks *3848* In 28 patients with type II hyperlipoproteinemia treatment with up to 10 mg/d for 12 weeks caused significant change from mean baseline of 135.0 ± 54.4 mg/dL to 88.4 ± 28.1 mg/dL *2692*

LDL_1-Lipoprotein *Serum Decrease Physiological* In 7 mildly hypercholesterolemic patients treatment with 20 mg/d for 10 weeks caused significant decrease from mean baseline of 58 mg lipoprotein/dL to 40 mg lipoprotein/dL *2059*

LDL_1-Triglycerides *Serum Decrease Physiological* In 28 patients with type II hyperlipoproteinemia treatment with up to 10 mg/d for 12 weeks caused significant change from mean baseline of 19.2 ± 7.6 mg/dL to 12.9 ± 3.8 mg/dL *2692*

Serum No Effect Physiological Nonsignificant reduction from mean baseline concentration of 66.9 mg/dL to 50.2 mg/dL in 5 hypercholesterolemic patients on CAPD treated with up to 40 mg/d for 24 weeks *3848*

LDL_2-Apolipoprotein B *Serum Decrease Physiological* Significant reduction from mean baseline of 113 mg/dL to 73 mg/dL observed in 5 hypercholesterolemic patients on CAPD treated with up to 40 mg/d for 24 weeks *3848*

LDL_2-Apolipoprotein E *Serum No Effect Physiological* Nonsignificant reduction from mean baseline of 1.3 mg/dL to 0.8 mg/dL observed in 5 hypercholesterolemic patients on CAPD treated with up to 40 mg/d for 24 weeks *3848*

LDL_2-Cholesterol *Serum Decrease Physiological* Significant reduction from mean baseline concentration of 182.3 mg/dL to 106.8 mg/dL in 5 hypercholesterolemic patients on CAPD treated with up to 40 mg/d for 24 weeks *3848* In 28 patients with type II hyperlipoproteinemia treatment with up to 10 mg/d for 12 weeks caused significant change from mean baseline of 32.5 ± 15.1 mg/dL to 25.9 ± 14.0 mg/dL *2692*

LDL_2-Lipoprotein *Serum Decrease Physiological* In 7 mildly hypercholesterolemic individuals treatment with 20 mg/d for 10 weeks caused significant reduction from mean baseline of 218 mg lipoprotein/dL to 133 mg lipoprotein/dL *2059*

LDL_2-Triglycerides *Serum Decrease Physiological* Nonsignificant reduction from mean baseline concentration of 138 mg/dL to 81 mg/dL in 5 hypercholesterolemic patients on

Simvastatin *(continued)*

LDL$_2$-Triglycerides *(continued)*
CAPD treated with up to 40 mg/d for 24 weeks *3848* In 28 patients with type II hyperlipoproteinemia treatment with up to 10 mg/d for 12 weeks caused nonsignificant change from mean baseline of 4.1 ± 2.7 mg/dL to 3.4 ± 1.5 mg/dL *2692*

LDL$_3$-Lipoprotein *Serum Decrease Physiological* In 7 mildly hypercholesterolemic patients treatment with 20 mg/d for 10 weeks caused nonsignificant decrease from mean baseline of 103 mg lipoprotein/dL to 72 mg lipoprotein/dL *2059*

LDL-Apolipoprotein B *Serum Decrease Physiological* In 19 patients with heterozygous familial hypercholesterolemia treatment with up to 40 mg/d for 16 weeks caused decrease from mean baseline of 144 mg/dL to 91 mg/dL *1393*

LDL-Cholesterol *Serum Decrease Physiological* Mean reduction of 32% following treatment with 10-40 mg/d for 12 weeks in 11 patients with hypercholesterolemia *4216* In 23 patients with hypercholesterolemia and nephrotic syndrome treatment with 10 mg/d for 4 weeks caused significant 30% decrease. After further treatment with up to 40 mg/d for a total of 24 weeks mean concentration decreased by a total of 33% *6007* Reduction from mean concentration of 251 mg/dL to 168 mg/dL in 82 patients with hypercholesterolemia treated with 20 mg daily for 12 weeks and to 142 mg/dL in 80 patients treated with 40 mg daily for 12 weeks *4704* Treatment with 20 mg/day of 27 patients with primary hypercholesterolemia caused 29% reduction at 4 weeks, 30% reduction at 6 weeks and 46% reduction at 10 weeks *371* Simvastatin administered in doses of 20 mg/d, 40 mg/d, 80 mg/d and 160 mg/d to about 27 hypercholesterolemic patients at each level caused reductions of 24%, 33%, 33% and 40% respectively *3998* Treatment of 12 elderly noninsulin-dependent diabetics with 30 mg/d for 3 weeks caused decrease from mean baseline concentration of 7.2 mmol/L to 4.3 mmol/L *4500* Mean decrease from 8.87 to 5.05 mmol/L (43%) in 11 patients with familial hypercholesterolemia and from 4.97 to 3.12 mmol/L (37%) in 10 patients with polygenic hypercholesterolemia after 24 weeks treatment with up to 40 mg/day *4091* In the Scandinavian Simvastatin Survival Study of 4,444 patients treatment with 20 or 40 mg/d for 5.4 years caused mean decrease of 35% *3115* 36% reduction after 4 weeks and 35% reduction after 8 weeks treatment with 10 mg daily in 8 patients with moderate grade familial hypercholesterolemia *6155* Mean 45% reduction in 8 patients with heterozygous familial hypercholesterolemia treated with 80 mg/d for 8-22 weeks *4786* In 7 mildly hypercholesterolemic individuals treatment with 20 mg/d for 10 weeks caused significant decrease from mean baseline of 5.29 mmol/L to 3.25 mmol/L *2059* Treatment with up to 40 mg/d for 3 months of 10 patients with primary renal disease and nephrotic syndrome and in 8 with diabetic nephropathy and nephrotic syndrome caused significant changes from mean baselines of 278 ± 21 mg/dL and 253 ± 30 mg/dL respectively to 179 ± 15 mg/dL and 116 ± 22 mg/dL *6343* Mean reduction of 34 % in 76 patients with primary hypercholesterolemia treated with mean dose of 17.3 mg daily for 12 weeks *6031* In 8 patients with moderate familial hypercholesterolemia treatment with 10 mg/d for 8 weeks caused significant decrease from mean baseline of 182 ± 9 mg/dL to 144 ± 21 mg/dL (21%) *4920* In 7 mildly hypercholesterolemic individuals treatment with 20 mg/d for 10 weeks mean concentration of LDL lipoprotein decreased significantly from mean baseline of 379 mg/dL to 245 mg/dL *2059* In a population of patients with primary hypercholesterolemia treatment for 12 weeks caused 41.0% reduction in concentration *4349* In 48 patients with hypercholesterolemia treatment for 4 weeks caused mean 42% reduction *4090* In 48 hypercholesterolemic NIDDM patients treatment for 1 month caused 28% reduction from mean baseline of 178 mg/dL and in 35 nondiabetic patients mean reduction of 34% from mean baseline of 197 mg/dL *3082* In 23 elderly hypercholesterolemic patients treatment with up to 40 mg/d caused significant decrease from mean baseline of 210.3 ± 30.0 mg/dL to 141.7 ± 32.0 mg/dL after 1 month, 129.0 ± 21.3 mg/dL after 12 months and 140.5 ± 34.0 mg/dL after 24 months *5150* In 24 patients with familial and nonfamilial hypercholesterolemia treatment with up to 40 mg/d for 30 months caused mean decrease of 40% *6003* Decrease on average by 24% (from mean of 180 mg/dL to mean of 136 mg/dL) in 29 patients with moderate to severe hypercholesterolemia treated with 2.5 mg/day for 4 months, and 24% after another 4 months with 5 mg/day *5194* In 19 patients with heterozygous familial hypercholesterolemia treatment with up to 40 mg/d for 16 weeks caused decrease from mean of 273 mg/dL to 159 mg/dL *1393* In 20 hypercholesterolemic men treatment with 20 mg/d for 4 weeks caused significant reduction from mean baseline of 4.6 mmol/L to 3.0 mmol/L *3352* In 16 patients with type IIa hyperlipidemia treatment with 20 mg/d for 3 months caused significant decrease from mean baseline of 6.90 ± 1.15 mmol/L to 4.44 ± 0.91 mmol/L and in 10 with type IIb hyperlipidemia from mean baseline of 5.12 ± 0.91 mmol/L to 3.65 ± 0.66 mmol/L *1805* In 10 Patients with NIDDM treatment with 10-40 mg/d for 24 weeks caused significant reduction from 258 ± 85 mg/dL to 154 ± 62 mg/dL (40%) and in 13 patients with primary hypercholesterolemia from 350 ± 79 mg/dL to 218 ± 43 mg/dL (38%) *4019* Treatment of 120 patients with heterozygous familial hypercholesterolemia with 40 mg daily for 12 weeks caused mean reduction of 38% *1312* 37% reduction in 12 individuals with primary hypercholesterolemia treated with up to 40 mg daily for 12 weeks *5385* In 22 patients with hypercholesterolemia treated with doses of 10 mg/d for 6 weeks caused significant 31% reduction of concentration *2948* In one study of 45 hypercholesterolemic patients treatment with 10 mg/d for 16 weeks caused a 30% reduction in concentration *4534* In 36 patients with hypercholesterolemia treated with 40 mg/d simvastatin for 12 weeks calculated mean concentration decreased from baseline on placebo of 5.53 mmol/L to 2.99 mmol/L (45.9%) *5605* In a group of hypertriglyceridemic patients treatment with 10 mg/d for 4 weeks caused significant 27% decrease *5796* In patients with nephrotic syndrome treatment with simvastatin caused a 31% decrease in concentration *4440* In 12 patients with stable angina pectoris and mild to moderate hypercholesterolemia treatment with 10 mg b.i.d. caused a significant change from mean baseline of 81 ± 20 mg/dL to 125 ± 19 mg/dL after 1 month and 127 ± 26 mg/dL after 3 months *1307* Treatment of 12 patients with type III hyperlipoproteinemia for 6 weeks with 80 mg daily caused reduction from mean baseline of 3.1 mmol/L to 1.8 mmol/L *5856* In 24 hypercholesterolemic patients treatment with up to 40 mg/d for 18 weeks caused significant decrease from mean baseline of 6.5 ± 0.3 mmol/L to 4.1 ± 0.2 mmol/L *3599* In two patients with familial hypercholesterolemia treated with diet and simvastatin for at least 3 months (with one also receiving cholestyramine) concentrations decreased from 8.5 to 5.4 mmol/L and 7.5 to 6.3 mmol/L respectively *6405* In 44 patients with primary hypercholesterolemia treatment with upto 40 mg/d and cholestyramine 4 g/d for 30 weeks caused significant reduction from mean baseline of 9.0 ± 2.0 mmol/L by 22 ± 11% after 6 weeks, 30 ± 10% after 12 weeks, 35 ± 11% after 18 weeks and 38 ± 14% after 30 weeks *5564* Significant reduction by 26-44% in 10 patients with type II hyperlipoproteinemia treated with 20 or 40 mg daily for 3 years *1238* After 12 weeks on up to 40 mg q.p.m. 15 patients with hyperlipoproteinemia type II had mean reduction of 40% *6621* In 6 patients with familial hypercholesterolemia treatment with 80 mg/d for 24 months caused decrease from mean baseline of 363 mg/dL to 247 mg/dL. When combined with cholestyramine decrease from baseline of 356 mg/dL to 188 mg/dL observed *1209* In 8 patients with hypercholesterolemia treatment with up to 40 mg daily caused reduction from mean concentration of 7.5 mmol/L to 4.7 mmol/L *5628* In 14 patients with familial hypercholesterolemia 10 mg/d for 4 weeks caused decrease from mean baseline of 359 mg/dL to 312 mg/dL, with 20 mg/d for 4 weeks to 277 mg/dL and with 40 mg/d for 8 weeks reduced mean concentration to 244 mg/dL *1209* In 25 patients with familial hypercholesterolemia treatment reduced concentration from mean baseline of 7.09 ± 1.59 mmol/L to 5.22 ± 1.44 mmol/L after 4 weeks, 5.07 ± 1.46 mmol/L after 8 weeks and 5.12 ± 1.29 mmol/L after 14 weeks. In 21 patients without familial hypercholesterolemia corresponding values were 6.01 ± 1.15 mmol/L, 4.46 ± 1.06 mmol/L, 4.17 ± 1.22 mmol/L and 3.88 ± 1.08 mmol/L respectively *2770* In 11 hypercholesterolemic patients on continuous ambulatory peritoneal dialysis treatment with up to 40 mg/d caused significant decrease from mean baseline of 224 mg/dL to 142 mg/dL at 6 weeks and 130 mg/dL at 24 weeks *3848* Treatment of 10 patients with primary hypercholesterolemia with up to 40 mg daily caused mean reduction of 40% *921* Significant decrease in mean concentration from 249 mg/dL to 165 mg/dL in 83 patients taking 20 mg daily and from 242 mg/dL to 143 mg/dL in those taking 40 mg daily *3035* Significant effect observed at 4 weeks in 27 patients with hypercholesterolemia when treated with 40 mg daily *3889* In 12 men and 17 women with familial hypercholesterolemia treatment with up to 20 mg/d for 14 weeks reduced mean concentration from 7.54 mmol/L to 4.81 mmol/L in the men and from 7.34 mmol/L to 6.11 mmol/L in the women *2933* In 58 postmenopausal women with fasting serum cholesterol concentrations greater than 250 mg/dL treatment with 10 mg simvastatin for 8 weeks caused significant change from mean baseline of 211 ± 40 mg/dL to 154 ± 29 mg/dL *1239* Significant reduction observed after 24 weeks treatment in patients with hypercholesterolemia following CAPD *3848* Significant reduction observed in 12 patients with familial dysβlipoproteinemia (type III hyperlipoproteinemia) when treated with 40 mg/d for 66 weeks *5855*

LDL-Cholesterol:HDL-Cholesterol Ratio
Serum Decrease Physiological In 8 patients with moderate familial hypercholesterolemia treatment with 10 mg/d for 8 weeks caused 21% reduction from mean baseline of 7.1 ± 0.9 to 6.2 ± 0.9 *4920* Simvastatin administered in doses of 20 mg/d, 40 mg/d, 80 mg/d and 160 mg/d to about 27 hypercholesterolemic patients at each level caused decreases of 27%, 37%, 36% and 46% respectively *3998* In a population of patients with primary hypercholesterolemia treatment for 12 weeks caused significant reduction of 46.7% *4349*

LDL-Phospholipids *Serum Decrease Physiological* Treatment with up to 40 mg/d for 3 months of 10 patients with primary renal disease and nephrotic syndrome and in 8 with diabetic nephropathy and nephrotic syndrome caused significant changes from mean baselines of 188 ± 14 mg/dL and 177 ± 15 mg/dL respectively to 116 ± 12 mg/dL and 108 ± 28 mg/dL *6343* In 27 patients with primary hypercholesterolemia treatment with 20 mg/day caused reduction of 34% at 4 weeks, 29% at 6 weeks and 43% at 10 weeks *371*

LDL-Triglycerides *Serum Decrease Physiological* Treatment with up to 40 mg/d for 3 months of 10 patients with primary renal disease and nephrotic syndrome and in 8 with diabetic nephropathy and nephrotic syndrome caused significant changes from mean baselines of 76 ± 9 mg/dL and 76 ± 10 mg/dL respectively to 54 ± 6 mg/dL and 37 ± 5 mg/dL *6343* In 48 patients with hypercholesterolemia treatment for up to 3 years caused decrease of 10-27% *4090*

Lecithin:Cholesterol Acyltransferase
Serum Increase Physiological In 19 patients with heterozygous familial hypercholesterolemia with up to 40 mg/d for 16 weeks caused increase from mean of 3.60 fractional esterification rate %/h to 4.84 fractional esterification rate %/h *1393*
Serum No Effect Physiological No significant effect in 29 patients with moderate to severe hypercholesterolemia when treated with up to 5 mg/day for 8 months *5194*

Lipase *Serum Increase Physiological* Simvastatin has caused pancreatitis in a small number of patients *3998*

Lipoprotein B Cholesterol *Serum Decrease Physiological* In 27 patients with primary hypercholesterolemia treatment with 20 mg/day caused 27% reduction at 4 weeks, 26% reduction at 6 weeks and 45% reduction at 10 weeks *371*

Lipoprotein B Phospholipids
Serum Decrease Physiological Treatment of 27 patients with primary hypercholesterolemia with 20 mg/day caused 30% reduction at 4 weeks, 20% reduction at 6 weeks and 45% reduction at 10 weeks *371*

Lipoprotein Lipase *Serum No Effect Physiological* No significant effect of 8 months treatment with up to 5 mg/day in 29 patients with moderate to severe hypercholesterolemia *5194*

Lipoprotein Lp(a) *Serum Increase Physiological* In 23 elderly hypercholesterolemic patients treatment with up to 40 mg/d caused increase from mean baseline of 190.5 mg/L to 220.0 mg/L (significant) after 1 month, 195 mg/L after 12 months and 203 mg/L after 24 months *5150* In 28 patients with type II hyperlipoproteinemia treatment with up to 10 mg/d for 12 weeks caused nonsignificant change from mean baseline of 24.0 ± 30.0 mg/dL to 30.3 ± 23.5 mg/dL *2692*
Serum No Effect Physiological Treatment with up to 40 mg/d for 3 months of 10 patients with primary renal disease and nephrotic syndrome and in 8 with diabetic nephropathy and nephrotic syndrome caused significant changes from mean baselines of 57 ± 21 mg/dL and 50 ± 14 mg/dL respectively to 59 ± 20 mg/dL and 53 ± 16 mg/dL *6343* In 58 postmenopausal women with fasting serum cholesterol concentrations greater than 250 mg/dL treatment with 10 mg simvastatin for 8 weeks caused nonsignificant change from mean baseline of 34.9 ± 39.2 mg/dL to 33.7 ± 37.6 mg/dL *1239* Insignificant decrease from mean concentration of 317 U/L to 307 U/L in 8 patients with hypercholesterolemia treated with up to 40 mg daily for 24 weeks *5628* In 24 hypercholesterolemic patients treatment with up to 40 mg/d for 18 weeks caused no change in log concentration of 2.3 ± 0.3 U/L *3599* No significant effect observed in 27 hypercholesterolemic patients when treated with 40 mg/d for 3 months *3889* In 36 patients with hypercholesterolemia treatment with 40 mg/d simvastatin caused nonsignificant increase from baseline on placebo of 359 mg/L to 464 mg/L. However, in patients with high Lp(a) concentration simvastatin administration may further increase it *5605* In 16 patients with type IIa hyperlipidemia treatment with 20 mg/d for 3 months caused nonsignificant change from mean baseline of 23.7 ± 23.5 mg/dL to 23.2 ± 23.7 mg/dL and in 10 with type IIb hyperlipidemia from 29.1 ± 36.2 mg/dL to 33.8 ± 47.8 mg/dL *1805* Nonsignificant reduction from mean baseline of 39 mg/dL to 36 mg/dL in 10 hypercholesterolemic patients on continuous ambulatory peritoneal dialysis treated with up to 40 mg/d for 24 weeks *3848*

Mevalonate *Urine Decrease Physiological* Reduction from mean excretion of 3.80 μmol/d to 2.75 μmol/d following treatment with 80 mg/d for 8-22 weeks in 8 patients with heterozygous familial hypercholesterolemia *4786*

Myoglobin *Serum Increase Physiological* In one obese women treated for 3 months muscle pain and leg weakness developed on one occasion with concentration of 5580 μg/L (normal range 10-90 μg/L) *589*
Urine Increase Physiological In one patient after 3 months treatment muscle pain and leg weakness developed on one occasion with myoglobin detectable in her urine *589* Simvastatin caused rare cases of rhabdomyolysis with acute renal failure secondary to myoglobinuria *3998*

Myosin *Serum Increase Physiological* In one woman after 3 months treatment with muscle pain and leg weakness developing on one occasion serum myosin concentration was 10,078 μU/L (normal range 10-400 μU/L) *589*

NADPH Oxidase *Neutrophils No Effect Physiological* In 12 hypercholesterolemic patients treatment with simvastatin for 6 weeks caused a nonsignificant change in maximum rate from mean baseline of 45.6 nmol/10^7 cells/min to 44.4 nmol/10^7 cells/min with a nonsignificant change from 62.1 s to 58.5 s in lag phase *1289*

Phospholipids *Serum Decrease Physiological* Treatment with up to 40 mg/d for 3 months of 10 patients with primary renal disease and nephrotic syndrome and in 8 with diabetic nephropathy and nephrotic syndrome caused significant changes from mean baselines of 366 ± 13 mg/dL and 369 ± 20 mg/dL respectively to 279 ± 7 mg/dL and 230 ± 17 mg/dL *6343* In 27 patients with primary hypercholesterolemia treatment with 20 mg/day for 4 weeks caused 21% reduction, with 17% reduction at 6 weeks and 20% reduction at 10 weeks *371*

Plasmin-α_2-Plasmin Inhibitor Complex
Plasma Increase Physiological In 12 men with familial hypercholesterolemia treatment with up to 20 mg/d for 14 weeks changed mean concentration significantly from 0.21 mg/L to 0.39 mg/L *2933*
Plasma No Effect Physiological In 17 women with familial hypercholesterolemia treatment with up to 20 mg/d for 14 weeks changed mean concentration nonsignificantly from 0.39 mg/L to 0.46 mg/L *2933*

Plasminogen Activator Inhibitor-1 Activity
Plasma No Effect Physiological In 12 men and 17 women with familial hypercholesterolemia treatment with up to 20 mg/d for 14 weeks changed mean concentration nonsignificantly from 29.6 IU/L to 33.5 IU/L in the men and from 35.3 IU/L to 39.0 IU/L in the women *2933*

Propranolol *Serum Decrease Physiological* When simvastatin coadministered with propranolol significant decrease in mean plasma concentration observed although AUC unaffected *3998*

Prothrombin Time *Plasma Increase Physiological* At a dose of 20 - 40 mg/d simvastatin concomitantly administered with coumarin modestly potentiated the prothrombin time increasing the INR from 1.7 to 1.8 and 2.6 to 3.4 in studies of healthy volunteers and hypercholesterolemic patients respectively *3998*

Simvastatin *(continued)*

Retinol *Serum No Effect Physiological* In 25 patients with familial hypercholesterolemia treatment changed concentration insignificantly from mean baseline of 2.69 ± 0.63 μmol/L to 2.63 ± 0.74 μmol/L after 4 weeks, 2.60 ± 0.75 μmol/L after 8 weeks and 2.67 ± 0.70 μmol/L after 14 weeks. In 21 patients without familial hypercholesterolemia corresponding values were 2.98 ± 0.83 μmol/L, 3.03 ± 1.08 μmol/L, 2.98 ± 1.02 μmol/L and 3.05 ± 1.05 μmol/L respectively *2770*

Thrombin/Antithrombin III Complex
Plasma No Effect Physiological In 12 men and 17 women with familial hypercholesterolemia treatment with up to 20 mg/d for 14 weeks changed mean concentration nonsignificantly from 1.50 μg/L to 1.46 μg/L in the men and from 1.65 μg/L to 1.52 μg/L in the women *2933*

Thrombin/Antithrombin III Complex:Plasmin/α_2-antiplasmin Complex Ratio *Plasma Decrease Physiological* In 12 men with familial hypercholesterolemia treatment with up to 20 mg/d for 14 weeks changed the mean ratio significantly from 6.11 to 5.04 *2933*
Plasma No Effect Physiological In 17 women with familial hypercholesterolemia treatment with up to 20 mg/d for 14 weeks changed mean ratio nonsignificantly from 4.39 to 4.23 *2933*

Thromboxane B_2 *Urine Decrease Physiological* In 10 patients with type II hyperlipidemia mean excretion decreased significantly from 76 ± 38 ng/h to 48 ± 15 ng/h after 6 months treatment *5585*

Tirofiban *Serum No Effect Physiological* Coadministration had no significant effect on plasma clearance of tirofiban *3957*

Tissue Plasminogen Activator Antigen
Plasma No Effect Physiological In 12 men and 17 women with familial hypercholesterolemia treatment with up to 20 mg/d for 14 weeks changed mean concentration nonsignificantly from 9.95 ng/mL to 10.7 ng/mL in the men and from 7.75 ng/mL to 9.21 ng/mL in the women *2933*

α-Tocopherol *Serum Decrease Physiological* In 25 patients with familial hypercholesterolemia treatment reduced concentration from mean baseline of 43.0 ± 6.2 μmol/L to 37.9 ± 7.2 μmol/L after 4 weeks, 37.6 ± 6.4 μmol/L after 8 weeks and 38.4 ± 6.4 μmol/L after 14 weeks. In 21 patients without familial hypercholesterolemia corresponding values were 47.7 ± 11.7 μmol/L, 43.2 ± 20.5 μmol/L, 41.2 ± 14.9 μmol/L and 40.1 ± 13.3 μmol/L respectively *2770*

Tolbutamide *Serum Decrease Physiological* In 16 healthy individuals coadministration of 20 mg simvastatin in either single or multiple doses caused 7% decrease of maximum tolbutamide concentration *227*

Triglyceride:LDL-Cholesterol Ratio
Serum Decrease Physiological In a group of hypertriglyceridemic patients treatment with 10 mg/d for 4 weeks caused significant decrease in ratio to 1.0 *5796*

Triglycerides *Serum Decrease Physiological* 14% reduction in 12 individuals with primary hypercholesterolemia treated with up to 40 mg daily for 12 weeks *5385* In 12 patients with familial dysβlipoproteinemia (type III hyperlipoproteinemia) mean reduction of 32-55% observed after treatment with 40 mg/d for 66 weeks *5855* Treatment of 14 patients with familial hypercholesterolemia with 10 mg/d for 4 wk caused decrease from mean baseline of 147 mg/dL to 121 mg/dL, with 20 mg/d for 4 wk concentration maintained at 121 mg/dL and with 40 mg/d for 8 wk reduced to 120 mg/dL *1209* In 10 hypercholesterolemic patients on continuous ambulatory peritoneal dialysis receiving up to 40 mg/d slight decrease from mean baseline of 263 mg/dL to 203 mg/dL at 12 weeks and 195 mg/dL at 24 weeks but no significant change observed at 6 and 12 wk *3848* In 12 patients with type III hyperlipoproteinemia treatment with 80 mg daily for 6 weeks caused reduction from mean baseline of 8.8 mmol/L to 3.6 mmol/L (48%) *5856* Mean reduction from 173 mg/dL to 136 mg/dL after 8 months treatment with up to 5 mg/day in 29 patients with moderate to severe hypercholesterolemia *5194* In 12 patients with familial dysbetalipoproteinemia (type III hyperlipoproteinemia) mean reduction of 32-55% observed after treatment with 40 mg/d for 66 weeks *5855* In 24 patients with familial and nonfamilial hypercholesterolemia treatment with up to 40 mg/d for 30 months caused mean decrease of 25% *6003* In 23 elderly hypercholesterolemic patients treatment with up to 40 mg/d caused reduction from mean baseline of 184.7 ± 72.9 mg/dL to 166.5 ± 62.6 mg/dL (significant) after 1 month, 157.6 ± 54.4 mg/dL (significant) after 12 months and 19.3 ± 59.3 mg/dL (nonsignificant) after 24 months *5150* Significant decrease from mean concentration of 164 mg/dL to 128 mg/dL in 83 patients taking 20 mg/day and from 155 mg/dL to 118 mg/dL in 82 patients taking 40 mg daily *3035* In 23 patients with hypercholesterolemia and nephrotic syndrome treatment with up to 40 mg/d for 24 weeks caused mean decrease of 25% from mean baseline of 2.8 mmol/L *6007* Mean reduction of 7% in 76 patients with primary hypercholesterolemia treated with mean dose of 17.3 mg/day for 12 weeks *6031* In 12 patients with type III hyperlipoproteinemia treatment with 80 mg daily for 6 weeks caused mean reduction from mean baseline of 8.8 mmol/L to 3.6 mmol/L (48%) *5856* In 6 patients with familial hypercholesterolemia treatment with 80 mg/d for 24 months caused increase from baseline of 166 mg/dL to 139 mg/dL and when combined with cholestyramine in 8 patients caused decrease from 132 mg/dL to 114 mg/dL after 24 months *1209* In the Scandinavian Simvastatin Survival Study of 4,444 patients treatment with 20 or 40 mg/d for 5.4 years caused mean decrease of 15% *3115* In 8 patients with moderate familial hypercholesterolemia treatment with 10 mg/d for 8 weeks caused significant decrease from mean baseline of 161 ± 46 mg/dL to 127 ± 28 mg/dL (28%) *4920* Nonsignificant reduction of 19% observed in 10 patients with primary hypercholesterolemia when treated with up to 40 mg daily for 24 weeks *921* In 36 patients with hypercholesterolemia treatment with 40 mg/d simvastatin for 12 weeks caused decrease from mean concentration on placebo of 2.00 mmol/L to 1.58 mmol/L (21.0%) *5605* In 19 patients with heterozygous familial hypercholesterolemia treatment with up to 40 mg/d for 16 weeks caused decrease from mean baseline of 155 mg/dL to 110 mg/dL *1393* Treatment of 120 patients with heterozygous familial hypercholesterolemia with 40 mg daily for 12 weeks caused mean decrease of 19% *1312* In 27 patients with primary hypercholesterolemia treatment with 20 mg/day caused 17% reduction at 4 weeks and 13% reduction at 6 weeks but no significant change at 10 weeks *371* Reduction from mean concentration of 158 mg/dL to 120 mg/dL in 82 patients with hypercholesterolemia treated with 20 mg daily for 12 weeks and to 121 mg/dL in 80 patients treated with 40 mg daily for 12 weeks *4704* Moderate decrease of 2-23% in 10 patients with type II hyperlipoproteinemia treated with 20 or 40 mg daily for 3 years *1238* In 48 patients with hypercholesterolemia treatment for up to 3 years caused mean 15-27% reduction *4090* In 12 patients with type II hyperproteinemia mean concentration of 209 mg/dL pretreatment significantly reduced to 159 mg/dL following treatment with 5 - 10 mg/d for an average of 13.9 weeks *6083* In 44 patients with primary hypercholesterolemia treatment with upto 40 mg/d and cholestyramine 4 g/d for 30 weeks caused significant reduction from mean baseline of 2.4 ± 1.3 mmol/L by 13 ± 26% after 6 weeks, 15 ± 19% after 12 weeks, 23 ± 21% after 18 weeks and 25 ± 22% after 30 weeks *5564* Significant effect observed in most of 27 patients with hypercholesterolemia treated with 40 mg daily for 3 months *3889* Treatment of 12 elderly noninsulin-dependent diabetics with 30 mg/d for 3 weeks caused decrease from mean baseline concentration of 2.9 mmol/L to 2.1 mmol/L *4500* In 48 hypercholesterolemic NIDDM patients treatment for 1 month caused 7% reduction from mean baseline of 158 mg/dL and in 35 nondiabetic patients mean reduction of 7% from mean baseline of 162 mg/dL *3082* In 15 patients with hyperlipoproteinemia treated with up to 40 mg q.p.m. for 12 weeks mean reduction of 20% observed *6621* In 58 postmenopausal women with fasting serum cholesterol concentrations greater than 250 mg/dL treatment with 10 mg simvastatin for 8 weeks caused significant change from mean baseline of 160 ± 75 mg/dL to 125 ± 48 mg/dL *1239* In a group of hypertriglyceridemic patients treatment with 10 mg/d for 4 weeks caused significant 26% decrease *5796* Treatment for 12 weeks of a population of patients with primary hypercholesterolemia caused nonsignificant reduction in concentration *4349* In one study of 45 hypercholesterolemic patients treatment with 10 mg/d for 16 weeks caused a 15% reduction in concentration *4534* 3% reduction after 4 weeks and 16% reduction after 8 weeks treatment with 10 mg daily in 8 patients with moderate grade familial hypercholesterolemia *6155* Simvastatin administered in doses of 20 mg/d, 40 mg/d, 80 mg/d and 160 mg/d to about 27 hypercholesterolemic patients at each level caused decreases of 10%, 10%, 19%

and 19% respectively *3998* In 12 hypercholesterolemic patients treatment with simvastatin for 6 weeks caused a nonsignificant decrease from mean baseline of 2.18 mmol/L to 1.86 mmol/L *1289* In 7 mildly hypercholesterolemic individuals treatment with 20 mg/d for 10 weeks caused nonsignificant reduction from mean baseline of 1.89 mmol/L to 1.50 mmol/L *2059* Treatment with up to 40 mg/d for 3 months of 10 patients with primary renal disease and nephrotic syndrome and in 8 with diabetic nephropathy and nephrotic syndrome caused nonsignificant changes from mean baselines of 286 ± 60 mg/dL and 414 ± 58 mg/dL respectively to 226 ± 30 mg/dL and 314 ± 6 mg/dL *6343* In 28 patients with type II hyperlipoproteinemia treatment with up to 10 mg/d for 12 weeks caused significant change from mean baseline of 137.1 ± 55.9 mg/dL to 107.7 ± 38.8 mg/dL *2692*

Serum Increase Physiological In 10 patients with type IIb hyperlipidemia treatment with 20 mg/d for 3 months caused increase from mean baseline of 3.08 ± 1.09 mmol/L to 3.84 ± 3.29 mmol/L *1805*

Serum No Effect Physiological In 24 patients with hypercholesterolemia treatment with up to 40 mg/d for 18 weeks caused nonsigificant change from mean baseline of 1.7 ± 0.2 mmol/L to 1.5 ± 0.2 mmol/L *3599* In 12 men and 17 women with familial hypercholesterolemia treatment with up to 20 mg/d for 14 weeks changed mean concentration nonsignificantly from 1.51 mmol/L to 1.55 mmol/L in the men and from 1.26 mmol/L to 1.15 mmol/L in the women *2933* In 20 hypercholesterolemic men treatment with 20 mg/d for 4 weeks caused nonsignificant change from mean baseline of 2.61 mmol/L to 2.27 mmol/L *3352* Insignificant reduction from mean concentration of 1.8 mmol/L to 1.6 mmol/L in 8 patients with hypercholesterolemia treated with up to 40 mg daily for 24 weeks *5628* In 10 patients with NIDDM treatment with up to 40 mg/d for 24 weeks caused nonsignificant reduction from 148 ± 27 mg/dL to 146 ± 31 mg/dL and in 13 patients with primary hypercholesterolemia from 105 ± 41 mg/dL to 96 ± 29 mg/dL *4019* In 12 patients with stable angina pectoris and mild to moderate hypercholesterolemia treatment with 10 mg b.i.d. caused no significant change from mean baseline of 140 ± 51 mg/dL to 136 ± 57 mg/dL after 1 month and 139 ± 53 mg/dL after 3 months *1307* No significant effect observed in 11 patients with hypercholesterolemia treated with 10-40 mg/d for 12 weeks *4216* In 16 patients with type IIa hyperlipidemia treatment with 20 mg/d for 3 months caused no significant change from mean baseline of 1.03 ± 0.29 mmol/L to 1.02 ± 0.51 mmol/L *1805* Mean 1% decrease observed in 8 patients with heterozygous familial hypercholesterolemia treated with 80 mg/d for 8-22 weeks *4786*

Ubiquinone *Muscle Increase Physiological* In 20 hypercholesterolemic men treatment with 20 mg/d for 4 weeks caused significant change from mean baseline of 0.060 mg/g to 0.088 mg/g *3352*

Serum Decrease Physiological In 20 hypercholesterolemic men treatment with 20 mg/d for 4 weeks caused significant reduction from mean baseline of 1.86 mg/L to 1.28 mg/L *3352*

Ubiquinone Q_{10} *Serum Decrease Physiological* Treatment with 20 mg daily caused reduction from mean baseline concentration of 0.82 μg/mL to 0.67 μg/mL in 83 patients and treatment with 40 mg daily caused reduction from baseline of 0.83 μg/mL to 0.62 μg/mL in 82 patients, close to normolipemic level *3035*

Viscosity *Blood No Effect Physiological* No significant effect observed in 27 hypercholesterolemic patients treated with 40 mg/d for 3 months *3889*

Plasma No Effect Physiological In 12 patients with type II hyperproteinemia mean concentration of 1.30 mPa/s not significantly changed to 1.32 mPa/s at following treatment with 5 - 10 mg/d for an average of 13.9 weeks *6083* In 12 patients with stable angina pectoris and mild to moderate hypercholesterolemia treatment with 10 mg b.i.d. caused no significant change from mean baseline of 2.1 ± 0.6 cP to 1.9 ± 0.5 cP after 1 month and 1.8 ± 0.6 cP after 3 months *1307*

Viscosity 50^{-5} *Blood No Effect Physiological* In 12 patients with stable angina pectoris and mild to moderate hypercholesterolemia treatment with 10 mg b.i.d. caused no significant change from mean baseline of 4.9 ± 0.7 cP to 5.2 ± 0.9 cP after 1 month and 5.3 ± 0.6 cP after 3 months *1307*

Viscosity 199^{-5} *Blood No Effect Physiological* In 12 patients with stable angina pectoris and mild to moderate hypercholesterolemia treatment with 10 mg b.i.d. caused no significant change from mean baseline of 5.7 ± 0.9 cP to 6.0 ± 1.2 cP after 1 month and 5.9 ± 0.7 cP after 3 months *1307*

VLDL-Apolipoprotein B *Serum Decrease Physiological* Nonsignificant reduction from mean of 40 mg/dL to 28 mg/dL in 19 patients with heterozygous familial hypercholesterolemia treated with up to 40 mg/d for 16 weeks *1393* In 5 hypercholesterolemic patients on CAPD treatment with up to 40 mg/d for 24 weeks caused significant decrease from mean baseline of 15.3 mg/dL to 5.8 mg/dL *3848*

VLDL-Apolipoprotein E *Serum No Effect Physiological* Nonsignificant reduction from mean baseline of 0.7 mg/dL to 0.3 mg/dL in 5 patients with hypercholesterolemia on CAPD treated with up to 40 mg/d for 24 weeks *3848*

VLDL-Cholesterol *Serum Decrease Physiological* Significant reduction from mean baseline of 48.3 mg/dL to 19.8 mg/dL in 5 hypercholesterolemic patients on CAPD treated with up to 40 mg/d for 24 weeks *3848* Significant effect observed in most of 27 hypercholesterolemic patients treated with 40 mg daily for 3 months *3889* In 24 hypercholesterolemic patients treatment with up to 40 mg/d for 18 weeks caused signifcant decrease from mean baseline of 0.9 ± 0.1 mmol/L to 0.6 mmol/L *3599* In 28 patients with type II hyperlipoproteinemia treatment with up to 10 mg/d for 12 weeks caused significant change from mean baseline of 15.9 ± 15.0 mg/dL to 9.9 ± 5.8 mg/dL *2692* In 12 patients with type III hyperlipoproteinemia treatment with 80 mg daily for 6 weeks caused reduction from mean baseline concentration of 8.3 mmol/L to 2.5 mmol/L *5856* Significant reduction observed in 12 patients with familial dysβlipoproteinemia (type III hyperlipoproteinemia) when treated with 40 mg/d for 66 weeks *5855* Treatment with 20 mg/day of 27 patients with primary hypercholesterolemia caused reduction of 36% at 4 weeks, 34% at 6 weeks and 37% at 10 weeks *371* In 24 patients with familial and nonfamilial hypercholesterolemia treatment with up to 40 mg/d for 30 months caused mean decrease of 26% *6003* In 23 patients with hypercholesterolemia and nephrotic syndrome treatment with up to 40 mg/d for 24 weeks caused significant 48% reduction from mean baseline of 1.7 mmol/L *6007* Treatment with up to 40 mg/d for 3 months of 10 patients with primary renal disease and nephrotic syndrome and in 8 with diabetic nephropathy and nephrotic syndrome caused significant changes from mean baselines of 64 ± 16 mg/dL and 74 ± 18 mg/dL respectively to 39 ± 7 mg/dL and 55 ± 14 mg/dL *6343* Nonsignificant reduction of 19% in 10 patients with primary hypercholesterolemia when treated with up to 40 mg daily for 24 weeks *921* In 19 patients with heterozygous familial hypercholesterolemia treatment with up to 40 mg/d for 16 weeks caused decrease from mean 75 mg/dL to 50 mg/dL *1393* In 7 mildly hypercholesterolemic individuals treatment with 20 mg/d for 10 weeks caused nonsignificant decrease from mean baseline of 0.90 mmol/L to 0.74 mmol/L *2059*

Serum No Effect Physiological No significant effect of treatment with up to 40 mg daily for 12 weeks in 12 individuals with primary hypercholesterolemia *5385* No change observed in 8 patients with heterozygous familial hypercholesterolemia treated with 80 mg/d for 8-22 weeks *4786*

VLDL-Phospholipids *Serum Decrease Physiological* Treatment with up to 40 mg/d for 3 months of 10 patients with primary renal disease and nephrotic syndrome and in 8 with diabetic nephropathy and nephrotic syndrome caused significant changes from mean baselines of 70 ± 15 mg/dL and 84 ± 10 mg/dL respectively to 48 ± 8 mg/dL and 54 ± 8 mg/dL *6343*

VLDL-Triglycerides *Serum Decrease Physiological* Treatment with up to 40 mg/d for 3 months of 10 patients with primary renal disease and nephrotic syndrome and in 8 with diabetic nephropathy and nephrotic syndrome caused nonsignificant changes from mean baselines of 187 ± 56 mg/dL and 313 ± 63 mg/dL respectively to 146 ± 28 mg/dL and 245 ± 53 mg/dL *6343* In 28 patients with type II hyperlipoproteinemia treatment with up to 10 mg/d for 12 weeks caused significant change from mean baseline of 54.5 ± 33.3 mg/dL to 43.7 ± 24.8 mg/dL *2692*

Serum No Effect Physiological No significant change observed in 5 hypercholesterolemic patients on CAPD treated with up to 40 mg/d for 24 weeks *3848* In 24 hypercholesterolemic patients treatment with up to 24 mg/d for 18 months caused nonsignificant decrease from mean baseline of 1.1 ± 0.2 mmol/L to 1.0 ± 0.2 mmol/L *3599*

Sinorphan

Aldosterone *Plasma Decrease Physiological* Significant decrease observed with nadir 1 hour after peak for enkephalinase in 11 patients with cirrhosis and ascites following a single oral dose of 100 mg. Effect of 30 mg significant but less marked *1632* Significant decrease observed with nadir 1 hour after peak for enkephalinase in 11 patients with cirrhosis and ascites following a single oral dose of 100 mg. Effect of 30 mg significant but less marked *1632*

Atrial Natriuretic Peptide *Plasma Increase Physiological* Increase of 1.8 times basal concentration observed in 11 patients with cirrhosis and ascites 60 minutes following single oral dose of 100 mg. Effect of 30 mg significant but less marked *1632* Increase of 1.8 times basal concentration observed in 11 patients with cirrhosis and ascites 60 minutes following single oral dose of 100 mg. Effect of 30 mg significant but less marked *1632*

Creatinine Clearance *Urine No Effect Physiological* No significant change observed in 11 patients with cirrhosis and ascites following a single oral dose of 100 mg *1632*

Enkephalinase *Serum Decrease Physiological* At a dose of 100 mg in 11 patients with cirrhosis and ascites inhibition of 70% of enkephalinase activity observed 60 minutes after ingestion *1632*

Guanosine Monophosphate *Plasma Increase Physiological* Increase of 1.5 times basal concentration observed in 11 patients with cirrhosis with ascites at 60 minutes following a single oral dose of 100 mg. Effect of 30 mg significant but less marked *1632*
Urine Increase Physiological Increase observed over 6 hours in 11 patients with cirrhosis and ascites following a single oral dose of 100 mg *1632*

Renin Activity *Plasma No Effect Physiological* Mean activity unaffected in 11 patients with cirrhosis and ascites following a single oral dose of 100 mg *1632*

Sodium *Urine Increase Physiological* Transient increase observed over 2 hours following oral ingestion of 100 mg by 11 patients with cirrhosis with ascites *1632*

Sisomicin

Alanine Aminopeptidase *Urine Increase Physiological* Approximately 8 fold increase in 23 patients given therapeutic amounts of drug for 2 weeks *4283*

Amikacin *Serum No Effect Analytical* No interference observed with method on Abbott TDx *3858* No interference observed at a concentration of 100 µg/mL (223 µmol/L) with method on Du Pont aca *1508*

Creatinine *Serum Increase Physiological* 38% increase in elderly patients with average initial creatinine clearance of 66 mL/min *1971*

Gentamicin *Serum Increase Analytical* Cross-reactivity of 5.3% observed with competitive immunoassay developed for PB Diagnostics OPUS analyzer *5486* Significant cross-reactivity observed with method used on Du Pont aca *1526* Interferes with method on Abbott TDx *3858* Specimens containing sisomicin showed 45.2% cross-reactivity when gentamicin measured by method on Bayer Technicon Immuno 1® system, invalidating the use of the method for such specimens *426*

Glucose *Urine No Effect Analytical* On TesTape® at physiological concentration. On Diastix® at physiological concentration. On Clinitest® at physiological concentration *4538*

Immunoglobulin Light Chains
Urine Increase Physiological Seen in all patients given drug in therapeutic amounts for 2 weeks *4283*

Kanamycin *Serum No Effect Analytical* No interference observed with method on Abbott TDx *3858*

Lysozyme *Urine No Effect Physiological* No significant effect seen in 23 patients given therapeutic amounts for 2 weeks *4283*

β_2-Microglobulin *Serum No Effect Physiological* In 23 patients given drug for 2 weeks in therapeutic amounts *4283*
Urine Increase Physiological Increased up to 2 times in 23 patients given therapeutic amounts for 2 weeks *4283*

N-Acetyl-Glucosaminidase *Urine No Effect Physiological* No significant effect seen in 23 patients given therapeutic amounts for 2 weeks *4283*

Neomycin *Serum No Effect Analytical* No interference observed with method on Abbott TDx *3858*

Netilmicin *Serum Increase Analytical* Interferes with method on Abbott TDx *3858*

Retinol-binding Protein *Serum No Effect Physiological* In 23 patients given drug for 2 weeks in therapeutic amounts *4283*
Urine No Effect Physiological No significant effect seen in 23 patients given therapeutic amounts for 2 weeks *4283*

Streptomycin *Serum No Effect Analytical* No interference observed with method on Abbott TDx *3858*

Tobramycin *Serum No Effect Analytical* No interference observed with method on Abbott TDx *3858* No detectable cross-reactivity observed with tobramycin method on Bayer Technicon Immuno 1® *435* No significant effect observed at concentrations less than 100 µ.g/mL (223 µ.mol/L) with method on Du Pont aca *1547* No significant effect observed at concentrations less than 100 µg/mL (223 µmol/L) with method on Du Pont aca *1547*

Transferrin *Urine No Effect Physiological* No significant change in 23 patients given therapeutic amounts of drug for 2 weeks *4283*

Vancomycin *Serum No Effect Analytical* No interference observed with method on Abbott TDx *3858*

Sitosterols

Cholesterol *Serum Decrease Physiological* Inhibits absorption of endogenous and exogenous compound *2226*

β-Lipoprotein *Serum Decrease Physiological* Therapeutic intent *2754*

Triglycerides *Serum No Effect Physiological* No effect observed *3486*

SKF-101468

Catecholamines *Plasma No Effect Analytical* Interference observed with 500 µg/L when HPLC with electrochemical detection method of Meineke et al used, but no effect observed at 100 µg/L and therapeutic concentration normally about 50 µg/L *3938*

SKF-12185

17-Hydroxycorticosteroids *Urine Decrease Physiological* Direct effect on adrenal steroidogenesis *55*

Smallpox Vaccine

Platelets *Blood Decrease Physiological* May occasionally cause thrombocytopenic purpura *3810*

Sodium Bicarbonate

Acetylsalicylic Acid *Serum Increase Physiological* Absorption is faster from preparations containing sodium bicarbonate: maximum concentration is also increased in both fasting and nonfasting individuals *4062*

Ammonia *Plasma No Effect Analytical* No effect at concentration of 3,360 mg/L on method on Kodak Ektachem® *5706*

Amphetamine *Serum Increase Physiological* Gastrointestinal alkalinizing agents increase absorption of amphetamines including dextroamphetamine *5641*

Chloride *Serum No Effect Analytical* No effect of concentrations up to 40 mmol/L with method on Kodak Ektachem® *5706*

Creatinine *Serum No Effect Analytical* No effect of concentrations up to 3360 mg/L on 2-slide method on Kodak Ektachem® *5706* No effect of concentrations up to 40 mmol/L on single slide method on Kodak Ektachem® *5706*

Drugs of Abuse Screen *Urine No Effect Analytical* At concentration of 250 g/L on Syva® EMIT, Roche RIA and TDx methods except for 18% increase for amphetamine by RIA, 8% for barbiturate by EMIT and 14% by RIA, and 6% decrease for opiates by EMIT and increase of 60% by RIA and 14% decrease for phencyclidine by Abbott TDx *6349*

Ephedrine *Serum Increase Physiological* Through alkalinization of urine ionization of ephedrine reduced and tubular reabsorption increased *6460*

Hemoglobin *Blood No Effect Analytical* No effect of concentrations up to 15 mmol/L on method on Kodak Ektachem® *5706*

Lithium *Serum Decrease Physiological* Effect probably related to increased urinary excretion possibly associated with increased sodium since excretion of lithium correlates well with intake of sodium *6017*

Lithium Clearance *Urine Increase Physiological* A single dose of the compound effectively increases lithium clearance *4399*

Mecamylamine *Serum Increase Physiological* Alkalinizes urine and increases renal tubular reabsorption of mecamylamine when coadministered *105*

Mexiletine *Serum Increase Physiological* Alkalinization of urine causes increase in half-life of drug and reduction in renal clearance. Normal renal clearance in acid urine 40-50% of total clearance but with urine of typical pH renal elimination may be reduced to 10% of total *4596*

Naproxen *Serum Increase Physiological* Theoretical possibility as rate of absorption is increased *1384*

pH *Blood Increase Physiological* Affects acid-base balance *in vivo3810*
Urine Increase Physiological Used to alkalinize urine *128*

Potassium *Serum Decrease Physiological* Causes potassium to shift into cells *128*

Protein *Urine Increase Analytical* False positive with Labstix® due to high pH *2451*

Pseudoephedrine *Serum Increase Physiological* Alkalinization of urine reduces ionization of pseudoephedrine with resulting increased tubular reabsorption and reduced urinary excretion *3326*

Quinidine *Serum Increase Physiological* Alkalinizes urine, increases reabsorption *2452* By alkalinization of urine proportion of nonionized quinidine increased with consequent increase in tubular reabsorption *4060* Drugs that alkalinize the urine reduce the renal elimination of quinidine *5996*

Quinine *Serum Increase Physiological* Alkalinization of urine reduces excretion of quinine since more is unionized and reabsorbed in renal tubules *2388*

Sodium *Serum Increase Physiological* May cause sodium retention *128*

Tolfenamic Acid *Serum No Effect Physiological* No significant effect observed on absorption or on plasma concentration *4259*

Urobilinogen *Urine Increase Physiological* Increased clearance when urine alkaline *4060*

Sodium Bromide

Amylase *Serum No Effect Analytical* No interference observed at a concentration of 4.5 mg/dL (0.44 mol/L) with method on Du Pont aca *1509*

Bicarbonate *Serum Increase Analytical* Significant effect on method on Kodak Ektachem® but no effect on method on Beckman Astra® 8 *3233*

Chloride *Serum Increase Analytical* Significant effect on method on Kodak Ektachem® and with lesser effect on method on Beckman Astra® 8 *3233* As measured by Technicon C_{800} instrument in one patient receiving bromide therapy *4947*
Serum No Effect Analytical On Beckman Astra® 8 and Corning/EEL 920 chloride meter: chloride meter produced results with 5 mmol/L bromide *4947*

Cholesterol *Serum No Effect Analytical* No interference reported at concentration of 11 mg/dL (1.07 mmol/L) with method on Du Pont aca *1516*

Cortisol *Plasma No Effect Physiological* No effect in 10 men, 10 women receiving 1 mg/kg/d during 8 weeks or 2 full menstrual cycles *5246*

Estradiol *Plasma No Effect Physiological* No effect in 10 men, 10 women receiving 1 mg/kg/d during 8 weeks or 2 full menstrual cycles *5246*

Follicle Stimulating Hormone
Plasma No Effect Physiological No effect in 10 men, 10 women receiving 1 mg/kg/d during 8 weeks or 2 full menstrual cycles *5246*

immunoglobulin A *Serum No Effect Analytical* Insignificant effect on method on Du Pont aca at a concentration of 11 mg/dL (1.07 mmol/L) *1528*

Immunoglobulin G *Serum No Effect Analytical* No significant interference observed at a concentration of 15 mg/dL (1.46 mmol/L) with method on Du Pont aca *1529*

Immunoglobulin M *Serum No Effect Analytical* No significant interference observed at a concentration of 11 mg/dL (1.07 mmol/L) with method on Du Pont aca *1530*

Luteinizing Hormone *Plasma No Effect Physiological* No effect in 10 men, 10 women receiving 1 mg/kg/d during 8 weeks or 2 full menstrual cycles *5246*

Progesterone *Plasma No Effect Physiological* No effect in 10 men, 10 women receiving 1 mg/kg/d during 8 weeks or 2 full menstrual cycles *5246*

Prolactin *Plasma No Effect Physiological* No effect in 10 men, 10 women receiving 1 mg/kg/d during 8 weeks or 2 full menstrual cycles *5246*

Testosterone *Serum No Effect Physiological* No effect in 10 men, 10 women receiving 1 mg/kg/d during 8 weeks or 2 full menstrual cycles *5246*

Thyroid Stimulating Hormone
Serum No Effect Physiological No effect in 10 men, 10 women receiving 1 mg/kg/d during 8 weeks or 2 full menstrual cycles *5246*

Thyroxine Binding Globulin *Serum No Effect Physiological* No effect in 10 men, 10 women receiving 1 mg/kg/d during 8 weeks or 2 full menstrual cycles *5246*

Thyroxine (T4) *Serum No Effect Physiological* No effect in 10 men, 10 women receiving 1 mg/kg/d during 8 weeks or 2 full menstrual cycles *5246*

Thyroxine (T4), Free *Serum No Effect Physiological* No effect in 10 men, 10 women receiving 1 mg/kg/d during 8 weeks or 2 full menstrual cycles *5246*

Tri-iodothyronine (T3) *Serum No Effect Physiological* No effect in 10 men, 10 women receiving 1 mg/kg/d during 8 weeks or 2 full menstrual cycles *5246*

Sodium Chenodeoxycholate

Creatinine *Serum No Effect Analytical* No interference observed with method on Technicon SMAC® II, two kinetic picrate and two enzymatic methods on IL Monarch *369*

Sodium Cholate

Creatinine *Serum No Effect Analytical* No inteference observed with method on Technicon SMAC® II, two kinetic picrate and two enzymatic methods on IL Monarch *369*

Sodium Cromoglycate

Alkaline Phosphatase *Serum No Effect Physiological* In 13 children treated with 30 µg/d for 2 months by inhalation caused nonsignificant reduction from mean baseline of 262.64 ± 112.56 U/L to 240.73 ± 126.15 U/L *3817*

Alkaline Phosphatase, Bone Isoenzyme
Serum No Effect Physiological In 13 children treatment with 30 µg/d for 2 months caused nonsignificant decrease from mean baseline of 206.64 ± 88.41 U/L to 174.91 ± 136.11 U/L *3817*

Osteocalcin *Serum No Effect Physiological* In 13 children treatment with 30 µg/d for 2 months by inhalation caused nonsignificant increase from mean baseline of 16.12 ± 4.20 µg/L to 17.95 ± 4.64 µg/L *3817*

Sodium Cromoglycate *(continued)*

Parathyroid Hormone *Plasma No Effect Physiological* In 13 children treatment by inhalation with 30 µg/d for 2 months caused nonsignificant reduction from mean baseline of 21.64 ± 6.39 µ.g/L to 19.36 ± 6.00 µ.g/L *3817*

Type I Collagen Teleopeptide
Serum No Effect Physiological In 13 children treated with 30 µg/d for 2 months by inhalation nonsignificant decrease from mean baseline of 11.79 ± 3.72 µg/L to 11.08 ± 3.06 µg/L observed *3817*

Sodium Enibomal

Platelets *Blood Decrease Physiological* Immunologically induced thrombocytopenic purpura *3051*

Sodium Iodate

Bilirubin *Serum Increase Physiological* Clinically significant effect with displacement from protein possible in neonate *6314*

Sodium Ipodate

Tri-iodothyronine (T3) *Serum Decrease Physiological* Concentration fell from 4.90 nmol/L to 0.30 nmol/L in 7 Graves' hyperthyroid patients with four days treatment with 500 mg daily *502*

Sodium Lauryl Sulfate

Lipid Glycerol *Serum Decrease Analytical* Inhibits phospholipase C with method of Horney *4437*

Protein *Test Conditions No Effect Analytical* Lowry procedure when referenced with chemical only used *2936*

Sodium Phosphate ^{32}P

Erythrocytes *Blood Decrease Physiological* Anemia if excess used *128*

Leukocytes *Blood Decrease Physiological* Leukopenia if excess used *128*

Platelets *Blood Decrease Physiological* Thrombocytopenia if excess used *128*

Sodium Phytate

Calcium *Serum Decrease Physiological* Decreased gastrointestinal tract absorption *128*
Urine Decrease Physiological Decreased gastrointestinal tract absorption *1714*

Sodium Salicylate

Glucose *Serum No Effect Analytical* Sodium salicylate at a concentration of 1,000 mg/L had no effect on GOD/POD-PAP method *5704*

Phenytoin *Serum Decrease Analytical* Sodium salicylate at concentrations above 85 µg/mL caused a decrease of at least 10% in phenytoin concentrations as measured by the method on Bayer Technicon Immuno 1® *428*

Thyroxine (T4), Free *Serum No Effect Analytical* Toxic concentration of sodium salcylate caused change of less than 0.01 ng/dL with method on Technicon Immuno-1® *1296* Sodium salicylate at a concentration of 45,000 µg/dL had no cross-reactivity with FT4 in method on Bayer Technicon Immuno 1® *424*

Tri-iodothyronine (T3) *Serum No Effect Analytical* No cross-reactivity observed from sodium salicylate with method on Baxter Stratus *5705*

Uric Acid *Serum No Effect Analytical* Sodium salicylate at a concentration of 10 mg/dL had no effect on method of Klein *3173*

Sodium Sulfate

Ammonia *Feces Increase Physiological* Modest rise observed *65*

Calcium *Serum Decrease Physiological* If given i.v. may cause hypocalcemia *128*
Urine Increase Physiological Promotes excretion *2242*

Magnesium *Serum Decrease Physiological* May be excreted combined with sulfate *128*

pH *Feces No Effect Physiological* No effect observed *65*

Potassium *Serum Decrease Physiological* May be excreted combined with sulfate *5509*

Sodium *Serum Increase Physiological* If given i.v. may cause fluid retention and coma *5509*

Sodium Taurocholate

Gentamicin *Serum No Effect Analytical* No difference between plate-diffusion and tube dilution *2092*

Somatostatin

Albumin *Serum Increase Physiological* In 12 healthy adults injection of 0.1 mg somatostatin analog caused significant change from baseline of 45.4 ± 0.9 g/L to 46.9 ± 1.1 g/L 60 min later *6211*

Amylase *Serum Decrease Physiological* In 8 patients with acute pancreatitis infusion of 3.5 µg/kg/48 h caused mean decrease of 48% at 24 hours *182*

Catecholamines *Plasma No Effect Physiological* Infusion of somatostatin had no effect on catecholamine concentration *5930*

Elastase 1 *Serum Decrease Physiological* Mean decrease of 63% observed at 48 hours in 8 patients with acute pancreatitis following intravenous infusion of 3.5 µg/kg/ 48 h *182*

Fatty Acids (FFA), Free *Serum Increase Physiological* In 6 healthy individuals infusion of 250 µg/h for 4 hours caused an increase from a mean baseline of about 570 µmol/L to 670 µmol/L after 60 minutes, 1200 µmol/L after 120 minutes and 1300 µmol/L after 180 minutes *3389*

Glucose *Serum Decrease Physiological* In 6 healthy individuals infusion of 250 µg/h for 4 hours caused a mean decrease of 20% after 120 minutes although concentration subsequently increased to above baseline *3389*
Serum Increase Physiological In 6 healthy individuals infusion of 250 µg/h for 4 hours caused caused decrease of up to 20% at 120 minutes but a subsequent increase by about 6% after 4 hours *3389*

17-Hydroxyprogesterone *Plasma Increase Physiological* In 12 healthy adults injection of 0.1 mg somatostatin analog caused nonsignificant change from baseline of 4.5 ± 0.3 nmol/L to 5.1 ± 0.5 nmol/L 60 min later *6211*

Lipase *Serum Decrease Physiological* Infusion of 3.5 µg/kg/48 h in 8 patients with acute pancreatitis caused mean decrease of 63% at 24 hours *182*

Sex-Hormone Binding Globulin
Serum Increase Physiological In 12 healthy adults injection of 0.1 mg somatostatin analog caused significant change from baseline of 41.9 ± 4.7 nmol/L to 43.6 ± 4.7 nmol/L 60 min later *6211*

Sodium *Serum Decrease Physiological* Water intoxication observed in 2 patients given drug i.v., although creatinine remained constant *2416*

Somatostatin *Plasma Increase Physiological* During infusion in 8 patients with acute severe pancreatitis prompt increase of plasma activity observed after beginning of infusion with a slower increase between 6 and 36 h, and a rapid increase at 48 h *182*

Testosterone, Free *Serum No Effect Physiological* In 12 healthy adults injection of 0.1 mg somatostatin analog caused nonsignificant change from baseline of 231.3 ± 36.2 pmol/L to 238.7 ± 22.9 pmol/L 60 min later *6211*

Thyroid Stimulating Hormone
Serum Decrease Physiological In hypothyroid and euthyroid patients and reduced response to TRH: drug is inhibitor of TSH release *6412*

Thyroxine (T4) *Serum* *Decrease* *Physiological* With infusion probable inhibition of TSH release *6412*

Tri-iodothyronine, Free (fT3)
Serum *Decrease* *Physiological* With infusion probable inhibition of TSH release *6412*

Tri-iodothyronine (T3) *Serum* *Decrease* *Physiological* With infusion probable inhibition of TSH release *6412*

Trypsinogen *Serum* *Decrease* *Physiological* Infusion of 3.5 μg/kg/48 h in 8 patients with acute pancreatitis caused mean decrease of 77% at 48 hours *182*

Somatostatin 14

Insulin-like Growth Factor Binding Protein-1
Serum *Increase* *Physiological* In 5 healthy volunteers infusion of 500 μg/h caused concentration to increase slowly from 6.3 ± 6.2 μg/L to 36.1 ± 14.8 μg/L reaching a maximum after 7 hours *4439*

Somatotropin

Amylase *Serum* *Increase* *Physiological* Administration of recombinant growth hormone has been reported to cause pancreatitis rarely *2082*

Calcium *Serum* *No Effect* *Physiological* Administration of recombinant growth hormone to adults with inadequate secretion of endogenous growth hormone or chronic renal insufficiency resulted in slightly increased serum phosphate concentration but no significant effect on the serum calcium concentration *2082*

Cholesterol *Serum* *Decrease* *Physiological* Administration of recombinant growth hormone to normal adults resulted in decreased serum cholesterol concentration *2082*

Fatty Acids (FFA), Free *Serum* *Increase* *Physiological* Acute administration of pituitary derived human growth hormone to normal adults resulted in lipid mobilization with FFA concentration increasing in plasma within 2 hours of hormone administration *2082*

Glucose *Serum* *No Effect* *Physiological* Administration to normal adults, patients with chronic renal insufficiency, and patients who lacked adequate secretion of endogenous growth hormone results in increases in mean fasting and postprandial insulin concentrations, but serum glucose and blood hemoglobin A_{1c} concentrations remain within normal limits *2082*

Glucose Tolerance *Serum* *Decrease* *Physiological* Administration may decrease glucose tolerance in children *2082*

Hemoglobin A_{1c} *Blood* *No Effect* *Physiological* Administration to normal adults, patients with chronic renal insufficiency, and patients who lacked adequate secretion of endogenous growth hormone results in increases in mean fasting and postprandial insulin concentrations, but serum glucose and blood hemoglobin A_{1c} concentrations remain within normal limits *2082*

Hydroxyproline *Urine* *Increase* *Physiological* Administration of recombinant growth hormone stimulates synthesis of chondroitin sulfate and collagen as well as the urinary excretion of hydroxyproline *2082*

Insulin *Plasma* *Increase* *Physiological* Administration to normal adults, patients with chronic renal insufficiency, and patients who lacked adequate secretion of endogenous growth hormone results in increases in mean fasting and postprandial insulin concentrations *2082*

Lipase *Serum* *Increase* *Physiological* Administration of recombinant growth hormone has been reported to cause pancreatitis rarely *2082*

Phosphate *Serum* *Increase* *Physiological* Administration of recombinant growth hormone to adults with inadequate secretion of endogenous growth hormone or chronic renal insufficiency resulted in slightly increased serum phosphate concentration due to metabolic activity associated with bone growth as well as increased tubular reabsorption of phosphate by the kidney *2082*

Phosphate Reabsorption *Urine* *Increase* *Physiological* Administration of recombinant growth hormone to adults with inadequate secretion of endogenous growth hormone or chronic renal insufficiency resulted in slightly increased serum phosphate concentration due to metabolic activity associated with bone growth as well as increased tubular reabsorption of phosphate by the kidney *2082*

Potassium *Serum* *Increase* *Physiological* Administration of recombinant growth hormone to adults with inadequate secretion of endogenous growth hormone or chronic renal insufficiency resulted in potassium retention from cellular growth *2082*

Sodium *Serum* *Increase* *Physiological* Administration of recombinant growth hormone to adults with inadequate secretion of endogenous growth hormone or chronic renal insufficiency resulted in sodium retention *2082*

Thyroxine (T4) *Serum* *Decrease* *Physiological* Or no change associated with accelerated conversion *6412*

Tri-iodothyronine (T3) *Serum* *Increase* *Physiological* Or no change associated with accelerated conversion *6412*

Somatrem

Alkaline Phosphatase *Serum* *Increase* *Physiological* Activity may increase with administration of recombinant growth hormone *2083*

Calcium *Serum* *No Effect* *Physiological* Administration of recombinant growth hormone to adults with inadequate secretion of endogenous growth hormone or chronic renal insufficiency resulted in slightly increased serum phosphate concentration but no significant effect on the serum calcium concentration *2083*

Cholesterol *Serum* *Decrease* *Physiological* Administration of recombinant growth hormone to normal adults resulted in decreased serum cholesterol concentration *2083*

Fatty Acids (FFA), Free *Serum* *Increase* *Physiological* Acute administration of pituitary derived human growth hormone to normal adults resulted in lipid mobilization with FFA concentration increasing in plasma within 2 hours of hormone administration *2083*

Glucose *Serum* *Increase* *Physiological* In children with growth hormone deficiency fasting hypoglycemia is improved with treatment with somatrem *2083*
Serum *No Effect* *Physiological* Somatrem may increase mean fasting and postprandial insulin concentration in normal adults and patients who lack adequate secretion of endogenous growth hormone, although plasma glucose and blood hemoglobin A_{1c} concentrations are unaffected *2083*

Glucose Tolerance *Serum* *Decrease* *Physiological* Somatrem may decrease glucose tolerance in growth hormone deficient children *2083*

Hemoglobin A_{1c} *Blood* *No Effect* *Physiological* Somatrem may increase mean fasting and postprandial insulin concentration in normal adults and patients who lack adequate secretion of endogenous growth hormone, although plasma glucose and blood hemoglobin A_{1c} concentrations are unaffected *2083*

Hydroxyproline *Urine* *Increase* *Physiological* Administration of recombinant growth hormone stimulates synthesis of chondroitin sulfate and collagen as well as the urinary excretion of hydroxyproline *2083*

Insulin *Plasma* *Increase* *Physiological* Somatrem may increase mean fasting and postprandial insulin concentration in normal adults and patients who lack adequate secretion of endogenous growth hormone *2083*

Insulin-like Growth Factor-I *Serum* *Increase* *Physiological* Concentrations are low in growth hormone-deficient children and adolescents but increase with treatment with somatrem *2083*

Parathyroid Hormone *Plasma* *Increase* *Physiological* Concentration may increase with administration of recombinant growth hormone *2083*

Phosphate *Serum* *Increase* *Physiological* Administration of recombinant growth hormone to adults with inadequate secretion of endogenous growth hormone or chronic renal insufficiency resulted in slightly increased serum phosphate concentration due to metabolic activity associated with bone growth as well as increased tubular reabsorption of phosphate by the kidney *2083*

Somatrem *(continued)*

Phosphate Reabsorption *Urine Increase Physiological* Administration of recombinant growth hormone to adults with inadequate secretion of endogenous growth hormone or chronic renal insufficiency resulted in slightly increased serum phosphate concentration due to metabolic activity associated with bone growth as well as increased tubular reabsorption of phosphate by the kidney *2083*

Potassium *Serum Increase Physiological* Administration of recombinant growth hormone to adults with inadequate secretion of endogenous growth hormone or chronic renal insufficiency resulted in potassium retention from cellular growth *2083*

Sodium *Serum Increase Physiological* Administration of recombinant growth hormone to adults with inadequate secretion of endogenous growth hormone or chronic renal insufficiency resulted in sodium retention *2083*

Urea Nitrogen *Serum Decrease Physiological* Linear growth in children is facilitated in part by growth hormone stimulation of protein synthesis: this is reflected in nitrogen retention with treatment with somatrem *2083*

Urine Decrease Physiological Linear growth in children is facilitated in part by growth hormone stimulation of protein synthesis: this is reflected in nitrogen retention with treatment with somatrem *2083*

Somatropin

Alkaline Phosphatase *Serum Increase Physiological* In children with growth hormone deficiency administration of somatotropin increases serum alkaline phosphatase activity in association with stimulated growth *1698*

Amylase *Serum Increase Physiological* In growth hormone deficient patients administration of somatotropin may rarely cause pancreatitis *1698*

Blood *Urine Increase Physiological* Administration of somatropin reported to cause hematuria infrequently *4675*

Calcium *Serum No Effect Physiological* In children with growth hormone deficiency administration of somatotropin has no significant effect on serum calcium concentration *1698* Administration of somatropin causes no significant effect on the plasma calcium concentration *4675*

Urine No Effect Physiological Administration of somatropin causes no significant effect on the plasma calcium concentration but may increase urinary excretion *4675*

Fatty Acids *Serum Increase Physiological* In growth hormone deficient patients administration of somatropin may mobilize lipids and increase plasma fatty acid concentrations *4675*

Fatty Acids (FFA), Free *Serum Decrease Physiological* In children with growth hormone deficiency administration of somatotropin may cause lipid mobilization and increased plasma fatty acids *1698*

Glucose *Serum Increase Physiological* In healthy adults administration of somatotropin occasionally caused hyperglycemia and glycosuria *1698* In children with hypopituitarism who have fasting hypoglycemia administration of somatropin may restore concentration to normal. Hyperglycemia reported in some treated patients *4675*

Urine Increase Physiological In healthy adults administration of somatotropin occasionally caused hyperglycemia and glycosuria *1698*

Glucose Tolerance *Serum Decrease Physiological* In children with growth hormone deficiency administration of somatotropin may cause impaired glucose tolerance *1698* Large doses of human growth hormone may impair glucose tolerance *4675*

Insulin-like Growth Factor-I *Serum Increase Physiological* In children with growth hormone deficiency administration of somatotropin increases IGF-I concentration *1698*

Lipase *Serum Increase Physiological* In growth hormone deficient patients administration of somatotropin may rarely cause pancreatitis *1698*

Nitrogen *Urine Decrease Physiological* Nitrogen retention with decreased urinary excretion of nitrogen and decreased plasma concentration of urea nitrogen occurs following introduction of somatotropin treatment *4675* In children with growth hormone deficiency administration of somatotropin causes nitrogen retention and decreased urinary nitrogen *1698*

Nitrogen Balance *Patient Increase Physiological* Nitrogen retention with decreased urinary excretion of nitrogen and decreased plasma concentration occurs following introduction of somatotropin treatment *4675*

Phosphate *Serum Increase Physiological* In children with growth hormone deficiency administration of somatotropin may cause phosphate retention and increased serum concentration *1698* Administration of somatropin causes phosphate retention and increase in the plasma phosphate concentration *4675*

Thyroxine (T4) *Serum Decrease Physiological* Administration of somatropin reported to cause hypothyroidism infrequently *4675* In children with growth hormone deficiency administration of somatotropin may precipitate hypothyroidism *1698*

Urea Nitrogen *Serum Decrease Physiological* In children with growth hormone deficiency administration of somatotropin causes nitrogen retention and decreased serum and urinary nitrogen *1698* Nitrogen retention with decreased urinary excretion of nitrogen and decreased plasma concentration of urea nitrogen occurs following introduction of somatotropin treatment *4675*

Sorbitol

Alanine Aminotransferase *Serum No Effect Physiological* Increase by 0.3-0.8 mg/dL after i.v. infusion *1920*

Ammonia *Feces Increase Physiological* Modest rise observed *65*

Aspartate Aminotransferase
Serum No Effect Physiological Increase by 0.3-0.8 mg/dL after i.v. infusion *1920*

Bilirubin *Serum Increase Physiological* Increase by 0.3-0.8 mg/dL after i.v. infusion *1920*

Estrogens *Urine No Effect Analytical* On fluorometric procedure at concentration of 1 g/dL *6543*

Glucose *Serum No Effect Analytical* On glucose oxidase procedure at 1 g/dL. On p-HBAH procedure of Lever at 1 g/dL. On alkaline ferricyanide procedure at 1 g/dL. On o-toluidine procedure at 1 g/dL *3531*

Lactate *Plasma Increase Physiological* In response to i.v. infusion *1920*

pH *Feces No Effect Physiological* No effect observed *65*

Pyruvate *Plasma Decrease Physiological* In response to i.v. infusion (effect slight) *1920*

Theophylline *Serum No Effect Physiological* No documented significant interaction with theophylline reported, even with purgative doses *6117* No clinically significant effect on theophylline concentration observed when sorbitol, even at purgative dose level, coadministered *5999*

Uric Acid *Serum No Effect Physiological* Increase by 0.3-0.8 mg/dL after i.v. infusion *1920*

Sorbose

Protein *Test Conditions Increase Analytical* Interferes with Folin-Ciocalteu method of Lowry *6104*

Sorivudine

5-Fluorouracil *Serum Increase Physiological* Administration of sorivudine with 5-fluorouracil causes inhibition of dihydropyridimine dehydrogenase which is responsible for more than 80% of the metabolism of 5-FU leading to a significant increase in its plasma AUC *3909*

Leukocytes *Blood Decrease Physiological* Administration of toxic amounts of sorivudine associated with bloody diarrhea and marked decreases in blood white cell and platelet counts *3909*

Occult Blood *Feces Increase Physiological* Administration of toxic amounts of sorivudine associated with bloody diarrhea and marked decreases in blood white cell and platelet counts *3909*

Platelets *Blood Decrease Physiological* Administration of toxic amounts of sorivudine associated with bloody diarrhea and marked decreases in blood white cell and platelet counts *3909*

Sotalol

Cholesterol *Serum Increase Physiological* Increased from mean of 5.49 mmol/L to 6.37 mmol/L at 12 mo in group of essential hypertensives *3506* Significant increase of 16% reported from one long term study (12 mo) *3499*
Serum No Effect Physiological General effect in 2 studies but overall progressive deterioration in lipid profile *142*

Fatty Acids (FFA), Free *Serum Decrease Physiological* At 1, 3, 6 and 12 mo in group of essential hypertensives given drug orally for 12 mo *3506*

HDL-Cholesterol *Serum Decrease Physiological* Primarily observed effect with nonselective β-blockers is decrease of HDL-cholesterol concentration *3730* Significant average decrease of 28% reported from one 12 mo study *3499* Marked reduction and ratio of HDL-cholesterol to total cholesterol in essential hypertensives after 12 mo *3506* No change in one study: general effect in 2 studies but overall progressive deterioration in lipid profile *142*

LDL-Cholesterol *Serum Increase Physiological* No change or up to 30%: general effect in 2 studies but overall progressive deterioration in lipid profile *142* Significant increase of 32% reported from one 12 mo study *3499*

Metanephrine *Urine Increase Analytical* In urine with a concentration of less than 5.5 µmol/d to sotalol added to a concentration of 200 mg/L concentration measured as 32.2 µmol/d at 350 nm and 17.2 µmol/d at 360 nm with Pisano method *5299*

Metanephrines, Total *Urine Increase Analytical* Cause shift in absorbance peak with Pisano method (may be large enough to double apparent concentration) *5299*

T3-Uptake *Serum No Effect Physiological* No significant effect in 10 hyperthyroid patients treated with 80 mg daily for 7 days *4610*

Thyroxine (T4) *Serum No Effect Physiological* No effect observed in 10 hyperthyroid patients treated with 80 mg daily for 7 days *4610*

Tri-iodothyronine, Reverse (rT3)
Serum No Effect Physiological No effect observed in 10 hyperthyroid patients treated with 80 mg daily for 7 days *4610*

Tri-iodothyronine (T3) *Serum No Effect Physiological* No effect observed in 10 hyperthyroid patients treated with 80 mg daily for 7 days *4610*

Triglycerides *Serum Decrease Physiological* Primarily observed effect with nonselective β-blockers is increase of triglyceride concentration *3730*
Serum Increase Physiological Simultaneous increase with other lipid changes; change from 1.14 to 1.89 mmol/L over 12 mo *3506* Significant increase of 66% reported from one long-term study (12 mo) *3499*
Serum No Effect Physiological General effect in 2 studies but overall progressive deterioration in lipid profile *142*

VLDL-Cholesterol *Serum No Effect Physiological* No change in one study: general effect in 2 studies but overall progressive deterioration in lipid profile *142*

Sparfloxacin

Alanine Aminotransferase *Serum Increase Physiological* In phase 3 trials in the United States increased activity observed in 2.0% patients *4943*

Aspartate Aminotransferase *Serum Increase Physiological* In phase 3 trials in the United States increased activity observed in 2.3% patients *4943*

Caffeine *Serum No Effect Physiological* Since sparfloxacin has no effect on the pharmacokinetics of theophylline it is unlikely to have any effect on the plasma concentration of caffeine *4943*

Digoxin *Serum No Effect Physiological* Sparfloxacin has no effect on the pharmacokinetics of digoxin *4943*

Leukocytes *Blood Increase Physiological* In phase 3 trials in the United States increased concentration observed in 1.1% patients *4943*

Theophylline *Serum No Effect Physiological* Sparfloxacin has no effect on the pharmacokinetics of theophylline *4943*

Warfarin *Plasma No Effect Physiological* Sparfloxacin has no effect on the anticoagulant effect of warfarin *4943*

Spartene

Digoxin *Serum No Effect Physiological* 0.8 g/d had no effect on serum concentration *471*

Spectinomycin

Alanine Aminotransferase *Serum Increase Physiological* Mechanism not discussed *196*

Alkaline Phosphatase *Serum Increase Physiological* Mechanism not discussed *196*

Creatinine *Serum No Effect Analytical* No effect of concentrations up to 15 mg/L on single slide method on Kodak Ektachem® *5706*

Creatinine Clearance *Urine Decrease Physiological* Mechanism not discussed *196*

Hematocrit *Blood Decrease Physiological* Mechanism not discussed *196*

Hemoglobin *Blood Decrease Physiological* Mechanism not discussed *196*

Histamine *Plasma No Effect Analytical* No inhibition of radio-enzyme assay at about therapeutic concentration *2492*

Urea Nitrogen *Serum Increase Physiological* Mechanism not discussed *196*

Volume *Urine Decrease Physiological* Mechanism not discussed *196*

Spiramycin

Creatinine *Serum No Effect Physiological* No significant effect observed in 6 male heart transplant patients given 3 MIU b.d. for 10 days as outpatients after stable cyclosporine concentration achieved *2361*

Cyclosporine *Serum No Effect Physiological* No significant change observed during coadministration, probably since it does not form a stable complex with cytochrome P_{450} so that inhibition of cyclosporine metabolism is less likely than with other macrolide antibiotics *6595* Coadministration had no effect at either 1 day nor at 2 weeks on area under curve, maximum plasma concentration or time to reach maximum concentration *6236* Unlike erythromycin appears to have no effect on plasma concentration of cyclosporine in renal transplant patients *3116* No significant effect in 6 male heart transplant patients given 3 MIU b.d. as outpatients for 10 days after stable cyclosporine concentrations achieved *2361*

Spirapril

Digoxin *Serum No Effect Physiological* No significant effect observed on serum concentration of digoxin when spirapril coadministered in 15 healthy volunteers. Also no effect observed on area under the curve, peak digoxin concentration, time to peak, or urinary excretion or on renal clearance *2955*

Spirogermanium

Alanine Aminotransferase *Serum Increase Physiological* Transient increases observed *1384*

Aspartate Aminotransferase *Serum Increase Physiological* Transient increases observed *1384*

Creatinine *Serum Increase Physiological* Renal toxicity is uncommon *1384*

Urea Nitrogen *Serum Increase Physiological* Renal toxicity is uncommon *1384*

Spironolactone

Aldosterone *Plasma Increase Physiological* Observed with chronic administration of drug *4739* In 5 normal subjects given 300 mg daily for 7 d *4037* Marked increase in supine concentration on constant diet *1879* Mean increase of 386 pg/mL in 3 men given drug 100 mg b.i.d. for 1 week *6303*
Urine Increase Physiological Significant increase observed in 6 volunteers given 300 mg daily for 3 days *1813*

Angiotensin-II *Plasma Increase Physiological* Change varies with renin activity *4037*

Antidiuretic Hormone *Urine No Effect Physiological* No significant effect observed in 6 volunteers given 300 mg/day for 3 days *1813*

Antipyrine *Serum Decrease Physiological* Spironolactone is a weak hepatic enzyme inducing agent stimulating metabolism of antipyrine *2756*

Calcium *Serum Increase Physiological* Nonsignificant increase observed in 9 patients treated with an average dose of 144 mg/d for 1 year *4809*
Urine Decrease Physiological Significant reduction observed in 9 patients treated with mean dose of 144 mg/d for 1 year when expressed as urinary calcium to creatinine ratio and as fractional excretion *4809*
Urine Increase Physiological Probably artifact as tablets each contain 40 mg calcium *4772*

Chloride *Urine Increase Physiological* Diuretic action *2242*

Cholesterol *Serum Decrease Physiological* Increase by 24 mg/dL in 11 men simultaneously with starting diet to reduce cholesterol *145*
Serum Increase Physiological Maximum average increase of 4% in 3 studies *143*
Serum No Effect Analytical At concentration of 20 mg/L had no effect on CHOD-PAP method *5704* At concentration of 20 mg/L had no effect on Liebermann-Burchard method *5704* At concentration of 20 mg/L had no effect on catalase-AIDH method *5704* At concentration of 20 mg/L had no effect on method using catalase-Hantzsch reaction *5704* At concentration of 20 mg/L had no effect on CHOD-Iodide method *5704*
Serum No Effect Physiological Nonsignificant increase from mean baseline of 5.58 mmol/L to 5.78 mmol/L in 9 patients treated with mean dose of 144 mg/d for 1 year *4809* No significant change in 17 subjects treated with drug for less than 1 y *2336*

Cholinesterase *Serum No Effect Analytical* No effect observed at concentration of 0.5 µg/mL with butyrylthiocholine method on Kodak Ektachem® *2504*

Corticosteroids *Plasma Increase Analytical* Marked effect on fluorometric procedure *2452*

Corticosterone *Plasma No Effect Physiological* In 5 normal subjects given 300 mg daily for 7 d *4037*

Cortisol *Plasma Increase Analytical* Fluorometric methods may be affected *3688*
Plasma No Effect Analytical At concentration of 4.0 mg/L causes no cross reactivity with method on Baxter Stratus *5705*
Plasma No Effect Physiological In 5 normal subjects given 300 mg daily for 7 d *4037*

Cortisol, Free *Urine No Effect Analytical* No significant interference observed with HPLC method of Turpeinen et al *6105*

Creatinine *Serum No Effect Analytical* At concentration of 50 mg/L had no effect on kinetic Jaffe method on BKA-2 *5704* At concentration of 20 mg/L had no effect on Jaffe-Fuller's earth method *5704* At concentration of 20 mg/L had no effect on Jaffe-Fading-Fraction method *5704* At concentration of 1 mg/L had no effect on creatinine iminohydrolase method *5704*

Creatinine Clearance *Urine No Effect Physiological* No significant effect observed in 6 volunteers given 300 mg/day for 3 days *1813*

Deoxycorticosterone *Plasma Increase Physiological* In 5 normal subjects given 300 mg daily for 7 d *4037*

Digitoxin *Serum No Effect Analytical* Recovery affected by less than 10% at concentration of 1.4 mg/L with method on Baxter Stratus *5705*
Serum No Effect Physiological May depress level but not to subtherapeutic value due to induction of mixed function oxidases *4631*

Digoxin *Serum Increase Analytical* Cross-reactivity possibly with metabolites with antibodies observed with several radioimmunoassay kits *6009* At normal concentrations in serum if no preincubation *4688* At 250 ng/mL equals 1.4 ng/mL by RIA *6638*
Serum Increase Physiological Increased concentration when given with spironolactone than when given alone *6303* Significant effect as measured by 8 different methods, especially in patients with hepatic or renal disease *4123* Clearance reduced by coadministration of spironolactone: effect more marked when quinidine also administered: renal tubular secretion of digoxin inhibited *1833* In 6 healthy individuals 0.5 to 1 mg digoxin given orally for 6 days but on seventh day when 0.7 times oral dose given intravenously with 200 mg spironolactone mean plasma clearance with spironolactone 224 mL/min compared with 255 mL/min and reduced renal clearance by an average of 13% without affecting biliary clearance *2526* Drug-induced decrease in renal clearance observed *6009*
Serum No Effect Analytical Cross reactivity of less than 10% observed with method on Baxter Stratus *5705* Spironolactone had no detectable cross-reactivity with method on Bayer Technicon Immuno 1® *421* No significant effect observed at a concentration of 30 µg/mL with method on Ciba Corning ACS:180 *1412*

Eosinophils *Blood Increase Physiological* Relative lymphocytosis and 15% eosinophilia observed in a single patient during period of agranulocytosis *5846*

Estradiol *Plasma No Effect Physiological* No significant effect in males for 2 weeks *4597*
Urine Increase Physiological In males for 2 weeks from 2.6 to 3.5 µg/24 h *4597*

Estriol *Plasma No Effect Physiological* No significant effect in males for 2 weeks *4597*
Urine Increase Physiological In males for 2 weeks from 8.1 to 11.8 µg/24 h *4597*

Estrone *Plasma No Effect Physiological* No significant effect in males for 2 weeks *4597*
Urine No Effect Physiological No significant effect in men *4597*

Felodipine *Serum No Effect Physiological* No significant effect observed on either felodipine or spironolactone concentrations when drugs coadministered *266*

Glucaric Acid *Urine Increase Physiological* Weak hepatic microsomal enzyme inducer *5969*

Glucose *Serum No Effect Analytical* At concentration of 8 mg/L had no effect on Kodak Ektachem® method *5704* At concentration of 1 mg/L had no effect on GOD/POD-PAP method *5704*
Serum No Effect Physiological In 15 patients with primary hypertension treated with 100 mg daily for 1 y *1789*

Glucose Tolerance *Serum Decrease Physiological* Transient effect in 15 primary hypertension patients at 6 mo after 100 mg drug daily *1789*

Granulocytes *Blood Decrease Physiological* A few cases of agranulocytosis have been reported in association with treatment *2061* Complete agranulocytosis observed in a single patient *5846*
Blood No Effect Physiological No significant association between use and agranulocytosis *3098*

Growth Hormone *Plasma No Effect Physiological* In 15 patients with primary hypertension treated with 100 mg daily for 1 y *1789*

HDL-Cholesterol *Serum Decrease Physiological* Average fell from 1.5 to 1.1 mmol/L at 6 mo, and to 1.0 mmol/L in 15 patient with primary hypertension given 100 mg/d *1789*
Serum No Effect Physiological Nonsignificant increase from mean baseline of 1.08 mmol/L to 1.19 mmol/L in 9 patients treated with mean dose of 144 mg/d for 1 year *4809* No significant change in 3 studies *143* No significant change in 17 subjects treated with drug for less than 1 y *2336*

Hematocrit *Blood Increase Physiological* When compared with results when patients treated with warfarin alone: augmented effect when spironolactone coadministered probably due to hemoconcentration due to diuresis *4428*

Histamine *Plasma No Effect Analytical* Improbable inhibition of radio-enzyme assay at therapeutic concentrations *2492*

17-Hydroxycorticosteroids *Urine Increase Analytical* Metabolite interferes with Porter-Silber reaction *5869*

18-Hydroxycorticosterone *Plasma Increase Physiological* In 5 normal subjects given 300 mg daily for 7 d *4037*

18-Hydroxydeoxycorticosterone
Plasma No Effect Physiological In 5 normal subjects given 300 mg daily for 7 d *4037*

Insulin *Plasma Increase Physiological* Average rose from 16 to 29 mU/L in 15 primary hypertension patients at 6 mo after 100 mg drug daily *1789*

Kallikrein *Urine Decrease Physiological* In healthy premenopausal women normal rise in luteal phase abolished by spironolactone administration *88*

17-Ketogenic Steroids *Urine Increase Analytical* Metabolite interferes with Zimmermann reaction *5869*

17-Ketosteroids *Urine Decrease Physiological* Decreased in 5 of 7 men over 2 weeks *4597*
Urine Increase Analytical Metabolite interferes with Zimmermann reaction *5869*

LDL-Cholesterol *Serum Increase Physiological* Maximum average increase of 5% in 3 studies *143*
Serum No Effect Physiological No significant change in 17 subjects treated with drug for less than 1 y *2336*

Leukocytes *Blood Decrease Physiological* Documented single case after 5 weeks of 100 mg/d when no other treatment given in 70 year old woman. Probable immunoallergic mechanism *5846*

Lithium *Serum Increase Physiological* Concentration increased when spironolactone (100 mg/day) coadministered but mechanism not established *2122*

Lithium Clearance *Urine No Effect Physiological* A single dose of the drug has no effect on lithium clearance *4399*

Luteinizing Hormone *Plasma Increase Physiological* In males for 2 weeks *4597*

Lymphocytes *Blood Increase Physiological* Relative lymphocytosis and 15% eosinophilia observed in a single patient during period of agranulocytosis *5846*

Magnesium *Red Blood Cells No Effect Physiological* In 9 patients treated with mean dose of 144 mg/d for 1 year concentration remained unchanged at 0.04 pmol/100 cells *4809*
Serum No Effect Physiological 100 mg did not increase serum concentration *5169* In 9 patients treated with mean dose of 144 mg/d for 1 year mean concentration changed insignificantly from 0.84 mmol/L to 0.83 mmol/L *4809*
Urine No Effect Physiological In 9 patients treated with mean dose of 144 mg/d for 1 year excretion decreased insignificantly from mean of 127 mmol/d to 123 mmol/d *4809* 100 mg/d for 6 mo had sparing properties but may be related to aldosterone status *5169*

Neutrophils *Blood Decrease Physiological* Occasional case of agranulocytosis reported *6412*

Occult Blood *Feces Increase Physiological* A few cases of gastric bleeding have been reported in association with treatment *2061*

pH *Blood Decrease Physiological* May cause mild acidosis *2754*

Platelets *Blood Decrease Physiological* Immunologically induced thrombocytopenia *3051*

Potassium *Red Blood Cells No Effect Physiological* In 9 patients treated with mean dose of 144 mg/d for 1 year concentration increased insignificantly from 0.79 pmol/100 cells to 0.85 pmol/100 cells *4809*
Serum Decrease Physiological Diuretic action (not marked) *5869*
Serum Increase Physiological Mean increase of 0.4 mmol/L in 3 men given drug for 1 week *6303* In 9 patients treated with mean dose of 144 mg/d for 1 year concentration increased from mean baseline of 4.0 mmol/L to 4.6 mmol/L *4809* Increase from mean of 4.2 mmol/L to 4.7 mmol/L in 6 volunteers given 300 mg/d for 3 days *1813* Binds to cytoplasmic hormone receptor on pericapillary side of distal tubular cells, blunting normal response to aldosterone *4739* Inhibits Na/K exchange in renal tubules *2242* Increase by 0.4 mmol/L after 7 d in 5 volunteers *4037*
Serum No Effect Analytical At concentration of 80 mg/L had no effect on measurement by ISE without predilution *5704*
Serum No Effect Physiological In 15 patients with primary hypertension treated with 100 mg daily for 1 y *1789*
Urine No Effect Physiological No significant change in 5 volunteers over 7 d *4037* In 9 patients treated with mean dose of 144 mg/d for 1 year mean concentration increased insignificantly from 76 mmol/d to 79 mmol/d *4809*

Propoxyphene *Serum Increase Physiological* Spironolactone probably inhibits metabolism of propoxyphene increasing serum concentration *3560*

Prostaglandin $F_{2\alpha}$ *Urine No Effect Physiological* No effect observed in 6 volunteers given 300 mg daily for 3 days *1813*

Prostaglandins *Urine No Effect Physiological* No effect observed in 6 volunteers given 300 mg daily for 3 days *1813*

Protein Electrophoresis *Serum No Effect Analytical* At concentration of 80 mg/L had no effect on automated Olympus-Hite method *5704*

Prothrombin Time *Plasma Decrease Physiological* When compared with results when patients treated with warfarin alone: augmented effect when spironolactone coadministered probably due to hemoconcentration due to diuresis *4428*

Renin Activity *Plasma Increase Physiological* Significant increase observed in 6 volunteers given 300 mg daily for 3 days *1813* Usual response observed *1076* Marked increase in supine activity on constant diet *1879* 9.5 fold increase after 5 d in 5 volunteers *4037*

Sodium *Serum Decrease Physiological* Reduction by 4 mmol/L after 5 d in 5 volunteers *4037* Aldosterone antagonism with consequent diuresis *3810*
Serum No Effect Analytical At concentration of 80 mg/L had no effect on measurement by ISE without predilution *5704*
Serum No Effect Physiological Slight effect observed in 6 volunteers given 300 mg daily for 3 days *1813*
Urine Increase Physiological Diuretic action *2242* Marked natriuresis with start of treatment *4037*

Tacrolimus *Serum No Effect Analytical* In HPLC/MS method of Christians et al no significant interference observed with measurement of FK 506 *1010*

Testosterone *Serum Decrease Physiological* In males for 2 weeks from 729 ng/mL to 634 ng/mL *4597* Inhibits biosynthesis in the testis *1499* Also displaces DHT from its cytosolic receptors *2836*

Thyroid Stimulating Hormone
Serum No Effect Physiological Increased response to TRH with action upon hypophyseal T3 receptors *6412*

Triglycerides *Serum Decrease Physiological* Increase by 58 mg/dL in 11 men simultaneously with starting diet to reduce cholesterol *145* Average fell from 2.4 to 2.0 mmol/L in 15 primary hypertension patients at 6 mo after 100 mg drug daily *1789*
Serum Increase Physiological Nonsignificant increase from mean baseline of 1.24 mmol/L to 1.53 mmol/L in 9 patients treated with mean dose of 144 mg/d for 1 year *4809* Maximum average increase of 19% in 3 studies *143*
Serum No Effect Analytical At concentration of 1.3 mg/L had no effect on GPO-PAP method *5704*
Serum No Effect Physiological No significant change in 17 subjects treated with drug for less than 1 y *2336* No significant effect observed in patients receiving spironolactone *4989*

Urea Nitrogen *Serum Increase Physiological* Especially if increased at start of therapy *2754*
Serum No Effect Analytical At concentration of 8 mg/L had no effect on Kodak Ektachem® method *5704*

Uric Acid *Serum Decrease Physiological* Average fell from 380 to 342 mmol/L in 15 primary hypertension patients at 6 mo after 100 mg drug daily *1789*
Serum Increase Physiological Decreased urate clearance *3810*
Serum No Effect Analytical At concentration of 20 mg/L had no effect on Kageyama-Hantzsch method *5704* At concentration of 20 mg/L had no effect on catalase-AIDH method *5704* At concentration of 1 mg/L had no effect on uricase-PAP method *5704*
Serum No Effect Physiological No effect observed *2452*

VLDL-Cholesterol *Serum No Effect Physiological* No significant change in 3 studies *143* No significant change in 17 subjects treated with drug for less than 1 y *2336*

VLDL-Triglycerides *Serum No Effect Physiological* No significant change in 17 subjects treated with drug for less than 1 y *2336*

Spironolactone *(continued)*

Volume *Plasma Decrease Physiological* Dehydration observed in 3.4% *2313*

Warfarin *Plasma No Effect Physiological* No consistent change in concentration when spironolactone coadministered *4428*

Stanozolol

Alanine Aminotransferase *Serum Increase Physiological* May cause intrahepatic cholestasis *1174* Cholestatic jaundice may occur with rarely hepatic necrosis and death occurring *5261*

Alkaline Phosphatase *Serum Increase Physiological* Cholestatic jaundice may occur with rarely hepatic necrosis and death occurring *5261* May cause intrahepatic cholestasis *2754*

Serum No Effect Physiological No significant effect observed in 11 healthy men given 6 mg daily for 6 weeks *6012*

Apolipoprotein A-I *Serum Decrease Physiological* In 11 healthy men mean decrease from 124 mg/dL to 74 mg/dL when treated with 6 mg daily for 6 weeks *6012* Increase by 41% in 10 normolipidemic postmenopausal osteoporotic women treated for 6 weeks *5914* Oral administration to men and postmenopausal women caused a significant reduction of 58% in concentration primarily due to a reduction in its synthesis and increased catabolism *5499*

Apolipoprotein A-II *Serum Decrease Physiological* Increase by 24% in 10 normolipidemic postmenopausal osteoporotic women treated for 6 weeks *5914* Oral administration to men and postmenopausal women caused a significant reduction of 31% in concentration primarily due to reduction in synthesis and increased catabolism *5499*

Apolipoprotein B *Serum Increase Physiological* In 11 healthy men given 6 mg daily for 6 weeks mean change from 89 mg/dL to 120 mg/dL *6012*

Serum No Effect Physiological Insignificant increase with 6 weeks treatment reverted to normal by 5 weeks after treatment stopped *91*

Apolipoprotein D *Serum Decrease Physiological* Increase by 23% with 6 weeks treatment reverted to normal by 5 weeks after treatment stopped *394* By 23% with 6 week's treatement: reverted to normal by 5 weeks after treatment stopped *91*

Aspartate Aminotransferase *Serum Increase Physiological* May cause intrahepatic cholestasis *1174* Cholestatic jaundice may occur with rarely hepatic necrosis and death occurring *5261*

Bilirubin *Serum Increase Physiological* Cholestatic jaundice may occur with rarely hepatic necrosis and death occurring *5261* May cause intrahepatic cholestasis *2242*

Serum No Effect Physiological No significant effect observed in 11 healthy men given 6 mg daily for 6 weeks *6012*

BSP Retention *Serum Increase Physiological* Due to intrahepatic cholestasis *1174*

Cholesterol *Serum No Effect Physiological* In 10 normolipidemic postmenopausal osteoporotic women treated for 6 weeks *5914* No significant effect of 6 mg daily in 11 healthy men treated for 6 weeks *6012* Oral administration to men and postmenopausal women had no significant effect on concentration *5499*

Follicle Stimulating Hormone

Plasma Decrease Physiological In 11 healthy men significant reduction first observed after 1 week when given 6 mg daily *6012* From 2.7 to 1.8 U/L after 1 week in 9 healthy men given 10 mg/d for 14 d *5607*

β-Glucuronidase *Serum Increase Physiological* Metabolic effect *368*

γ-Glutamyltransferase *Serum Increase Physiological* Cholestatic jaundice may occur with rarely hepatic necrosis and death occurring *5261*

Haptoglobin *Serum Increase Physiological* Metabolic effect *368*

HDL_2-Cholesterol *Serum Decrease Physiological* In 11 healthy men mean decrease from 0.36 mmol/L to 0.08 mmol/L when treated with 6 mg daily for 6 weeks *6012* Increase by 85% in 10 normolipidemic postmenopausal osteoporotic women treated for 6 weeks *5914*

HDL_3-Cholesterol *Serum Decrease Physiological* Increase by 35% in 10 normolipidemic postmenopausal osteoporotic women treated for 6 weeks *5914* In 11 healthy men mean decrease from 0.80 mmol/L to 0.62 mmol/L when treated with 6 mg daily for 6 weeks *6012*

HDL-Cholesterol *Serum Decrease Physiological* Increase by 53% in 10 normolipidemic postmenopausal osteoporotic women treated for 6 weeks *5914* In 11 healthy men mean decrease from 1.16 mmol/L to 0.70 mmol/L when treated with 6 mg daily for 6 weeks *6012* Oral administration to men and postmenopausal women decreased concentration by 50% *5499*

Hemoglobin *Blood Increase Physiological* Effective in some patients with aplastic anemia *2753*

25-Hydroxy Vitamin D_3 *Serum Decrease Physiological* From 64 to 54.5 nmol/L after 1 week in 9 healthy men given 10 mg/d for 14 d *5607*

LDL-Cholesterol *Serum Increase Physiological* In 11 healthy men mean increase from 2.87 mmol/L to 3.70 mmol/L after 6 weeks treatment with 6 mg daily *6012* Increase by 21% in 10 normolipidemic postmenopausal osteoporotic women treated for 6 weeks *5914* Oral administration to men and postmenopausal women increased concentration by 13% *5499*

Lecithin:Cholesterol Acyltransferase

Serum Decrease Physiological Increase by 30% with 6 weeks treatment: reverted to normal by 5 weeks after treatment stopped *91*

Lipase, Hepatic *Serum Increase Physiological* Oral administration to men and postmenopausal women increased concentration more than three-fold *5499*

Lipoprotein Lipase *Serum No Effect Physiological* Oral administration to men and postmenopausal women had no significant effect on concentration *5499*

Lipoprotein Lp(a) *Serum Decrease Physiological* By average of 65% with 6 weeks treatment reverted to normal by 5 weeks after treatment stopped *91*

Luteinizing Hormone *Plasma Decrease Physiological* From 6.5 to 4.5 IU/L after 1 week in 9 healthy men given 10 mg/d for 14 d *5607* Significant change in 11 healthy men given 6 mg daily for 6 weeks, first observed after 1 week *6012*

Osteocalcin *Serum Increase Physiological* Treatment of healthy adult volunteers causes marked increase of 80-90% by decreasing plasma clearance of osteocalcin and increasing osteoblastic activity *5948*

Plasminogen *Plasma Increase Physiological* Metabolic effect *368*

Prothrombin Time *Plasma Increase Physiological* Anabolic steroids may increase sensitivity to anticoagulants thereby prolonging the prothrombin time *5261*

Sex-Hormone Binding Globulin

Serum Decrease Physiological From 20.7 to 12.2 nmol/L after 1 week in 9 healthy men given 10 mg/d for 14 d *5607* Mean reduction of almost 50% in normal individuals with drug administration for 3 days with less marked responses in patients with partial androgen insensitivity *5582*

Sialic Acid *Serum Increase Physiological* Metabolic effect *368*

Sperm Count *Semen Decrease Physiological* Stanozolol may be associated with oligospermia in men *5261*

Sulfobromophthalein *Serum Increase Physiological* Cholestatic jaundice may occur with rarely hepatic necrosis and death occurring. BSP retention may occur *5261*

T3-Uptake *Serum Increase Physiological* Anabolic steroids may decrease concentration of TBG, thereby decreasing total T4 concentration, and increased resin uptake of T3 and T4 *5261*

Testosterone *Serum Decrease Physiological* Decrease by 55% (from 22.1 to 10.6 nmol/L) after 1 week in 9 healthy men given 10 mg/d for 14 d *5607* In 11 healthy male volunteers mean concentration decreased from 22.5 mmol/L to 11.1 mmol/L after 6 weeks treatment with 6 mg daily *6012*

Testosterone, Free *Serum Decrease Physiological* From 398 to 226 pmol/L after 1 week in 9 healthy men given 10 mg/d for 14 d *5607*

Thyroid Stimulating Hormone
Serum No Effect Physiological 1.95 mU/L before treatment, 2.31 after 2 weeks in 9 healthy men given 10 mg/d for 14 d *5607*

Thyroxine Binding Globulin
Serum Decrease Physiological Anabolic steroids may decrease concentration of TBG *5261* From 22.5 to 17.0 mg/L after 1 week in 9 healthy men given 10 mg/d for 14 d *5607*

Thyroxine (T4) *Serum Decrease Physiological* Anabolic steroids may decrease concentration of TBG, thereby decreasing total T4 concentration *5261* From 106.2 to 90.4 nmol/L after 1 week in 9 healthy men given 10 mg/d for 14 d *5607*

Thyroxine (T4), Free *Serum No Effect Physiological* 18.5 pmol/L before treatment, 19.0 pmol/L after 2 weeks in 9 healthy men given 10 mg/ day for 14 d *5607* Anabolic steroids may decrease concentration of TBG, thereby decreasing total T4 concentration, but has no effect on free thyroxine concentration *5261*

Tri-iodothyronine (T3) *Serum Decrease Physiological* From 2.21 to 1.52 nmol/L after 1 week in 9 healthy men given 10 mg/d for 14 d *5607*

Triglycerides *Serum Decrease Physiological* In 11 healthy men mean decrease from 1.50 mmol/L to 1.25 mmol/L when treated with 6 mg daily for 6 weeks *6012*
Serum No Effect Physiological In 10 normolipidemic postmenopausal osteoporotic women treated for 6 weeks *5914* Oral administration to men and postmenopausal women had no significant effect on concentration *5499*

Vitamin D Binding Globulin *Serum Decrease Physiological* From 270 to 230 mg/L after 1 week in 9 healthy men given 10 mg/d for 14 d *5607*

Statins

Cholesterol *Serum Decrease Physiological* In 39 patients with combined hyperlipidemia treatment with either pravastatin 20 mg/d or simvastatin 10 mg/d for 2 years caused significant reduction of 24.5% *1718*

Cholesterol:HDL-Cholesterol Ratio
Serum Decrease Physiological In 39 patients with combined hyperlipidemia treatment with either pravastatin 20 mg/d or simvastatin 10 mg/d for 2 years caused significant decrease from 8.62 pretreatment to 6.08 *1718*

HDL-Cholesterol *Serum Increase Physiological* In 39 patients with combined hyperlipidemia treatment with either pravastatin 20 mg/d or simvastatin 10 mg/d for 2 years caused significant increase of 15.0% *1718*

LDL-Cholesterol *Serum Decrease Physiological* In 39 patients with combined hyperlipidemia treatment with either pravastatin 20 mg/d or simvastatin 10 mg/d for 2 years caused significant reduction of 30.5% *1718*

LDL-Cholesterol:HDL-Cholesterol Ratio
Serum Decrease Physiological In 39 patients with combined hyperlipidemia treatment with either pravastatin 20 mg/d or simvastatin for 2 years caused significant decrease from 5.30 pretreatment to 3.28 *1718*

Triglycerides *Serum Decrease Physiological* In 39 patients with combined hyperlipidemia treatment with either pravastatin 20 mg/d or simvastatin 10 mg/d for 2 years caused significant reduction of 9.2% *1718*

Stavudine

Alanine Aminotransferase *Serum Increase Physiological* In 412 HIV-infected patients treatment with 40 mg b.i.d. for a median of 79 weeks caused an increase to above 5.0 times the upper limit of normal in 11 patients *731*

Aspartate Aminotransferase *Serum Increase Physiological* In 412 HIV-infected patients treatment with 40 mg b.i.d. for a median of 79 weeks caused an increase to above 5.0 times the upper limit of normal in 13 patients *731*

Bilirubin *Serum Increase Physiological* In 412 HIV-infected patients treatment with 40 mg b.i.d. for a median of 79 weeks caused an increase to above 1.4 times the upper limit of normal in 14 patients *731* In 412 HIV-infected patients treatment with 40 mg b.i.d. for a median of 79 weeks caused an increase to above 5.0 times the upper limit of normal in 2 patients *731*

Hemoglobin *Blood No Effect Physiological* In 412 HIV-infected patients treatment with 40 mg b.i.d. for a median of 79 weeks caused no decreases to below 80 g/L *731*

Indinavir *Serum No Effect Physiological* Causes no significant effect on area under the concentration curve when stavudine coadministered *1891* Administration of indinavir 800 mg every 8 hours with stavudine 40 mg every 12 hours for 1 week resulted in no change in indinavir AUC and a 25 ± 26% increase in stavudine AUC *3966*

Nelfinavir *Serum No Effect Physiological* Coadministration of stavudine with nelfinavir had no effect on the pharmacokinetics of either drug *66*

Neutrophils *Blood Decrease Physiological* In 412 HIV-infected patients treatment with 40 mg b.i.d. for a median of 79 weeks caused an decrease to below 750 /µL in 5 patients *731*

Platelets *Blood Decrease Physiological* In 412 HIV-infected patients treatment with 40 mg b.i.d. for a median of 79 weeks caused an decrease to below 50,000 /µL in 3 patients *731*

Stearylamine

Lipid Glycerol *Serum Increase Analytical* Possible effect in method of Horney *4437*

Steroids

Aggregation Index *Red Blood Cells Decrease Physiological* In 25 children with steroid-sensitive nephrotic syndrome mean aggregation index of 18.2 ± 3.3 following 3 weeks of steroid treatment significantly different from pretreatment index of 23.8 ± 5.3 *175*

Antithrombin III *Plasma Increase Physiological* In 25 children with nephrotic syndrome who were steroid sensitive mean concentration increased to 126 ± 21% from 80 ± 21% pretreatment *175*

Factor VIII Antigen *Plasma Decrease Physiological* In 25 children with nephrotic syndrome who were steroid sensitive mean concentration decreased to 189 ± 77% from 276 ± 80% pretreatment *175*

Factor VIII Coagulant *Plasma Decrease Physiological* In 25 children with nephrotic syndrome who were steroid sensitive mean concentration decreased to 189 ± 77% from 276 ± 80% pretreatment *175*

Factor XII *Plasma Increase Physiological* In 25 children with nephrotic syndrome who were steroid sensitive mean concentration increased to 114 ± 25% from 48 ± 20% pretreatment *175*

Fibrinogen *Plasma Decrease Physiological* In 25 children with nephrotic syndrome who were steroid sensitive mean concentration decreased to 2.5 ± 0.8 g/L from 6 ± 2 g/L pretreatment *175*

Filtration Index *Blood Increase Physiological* In 25 children with steroid-sensitive nephrotic syndrome mean filtration index of 12.0 ± 7.2 not significantly increased to 13.0 ± 4.9 after 3 weeks of steroid treatment *175*

α_2-Macroglobulin *Serum Decrease Physiological* In 25 children with nephrotic syndrome who were steroid sensitive mean concentration decreased to 6.0 ± 1.7 g/L from 9.9 ± 3.6 g/L pretreatment *175*

Platelets *Blood Increase Physiological* In 25 children with nephrotic syndrome who were steroid sensitive mean concentration increased to 509 ± 129 /µL from 425 ± 143 /µL pretreatment *175*

Protein *Serum Increase Physiological* In 25 children with nephrotic syndrome who were steroid sensitive mean concentration increased to 59.7 ± 2.9 g/L from 43.8 ± 4.9 g/L pretreatment *175*

Protein C *Plasma Increase Physiological* In 25 children with nephrotic syndrome who were steroid sensitive mean concentration increased to 232 ± 64% from 154 ± 43% pretreatment *175*

Steroids *(continued)*

Protein S *Plasma Increase Physiological* In 25 children with nephrotic syndrome who were steroid sensitive mean concentration increased to 143 ± 21% from 118 ± 28% pretreatment *175*

Protein S, Free *Plasma Increase Physiological* In 25 children with nephrotic syndrome who were steroid sensitive mean concentration increased to 136 ± 38% from 86 ± 31% pretreatment *175* In 25 children with nephrotic syndrome who were steroid sensitive mean concentration increased to 2.1 ± 0.6 g/L from 1.6 ± 0.7 g/L pretreatment *175*

Relative Viscosity *Blood Decrease Physiological* In 25 children with steroid-sensitive nephrotic syndrome mean relative viscosity of 20.4 ± 3.1 mPa/s reduced to 16.1 ± 2.7 mPa/s at shear rate 0.20 s^{-1} and 15.6 ± 1.5 mPa/s versus pretreatment value of 14.5 ± 1.9 mPa/s at shear rate 0.51 s]sup,-1] after treatment for 3 weeks with steroids *175*

Blood Increase Physiological In 25 children with steroid-sensitive nephrotic syndrome mean relative viscosity of 7.4 ± 0.5 mPa/s at shear rate 3.2 s^{-1} increased to 7.9 ± 0.9 mPa/s pretreatment, 4.7 ± 0.5 mPa/s versus 4.7 ± 0.3 mPa/s at shear rate 20.4 s^{-1}, 3.2 ± 0.3 mPa/s at shear rate 128 s^{-1} versus 3.3 ± 0.2 mPa/s after treatment for 3 weeks with steroids *175*

Viscosity *Blood Decrease Physiological* In 29 children with nephrotic syndrome mean viscosity of 18.7 ± 2.2 mPa/s significantly different from pretreatment value of 19.3 ± 2.6 mPa/s at shear rate 0.51 s^{-1} and 8.8 ± 0.9 mPa/s versus pretreatment value of 10.7 ± 1.6 mPa/s at shear rate 3.2 s]sup,-1], 5.4 ± 0.4 mPa/s at shear rate 20.4 s^{-1} versus 6.2 ± 0.7 mPa/s pretreatment and 3.9 ± 0.3 mPa/s versus 4.4 ± 0.5 mPa/s at shear rate 128 s^{-1} after treatment for 3 weeks with steroids *175*

Blood Increase Physiological In 25 children with nephrotic syndrome who were steroid-sensitive mean viscosity of 24.0 ± 3.8 mPa/s significantly different from pretreatment value of 21.1 ± 3.8 mPa/s at shear rate 0.20 s^{-1} after treatment for 3 weeks with steroids *175*

Plasma Decrease Physiological In 25 children with nephrotic syndrome who were steroid sensitive mean viscosity decreased to 1.20 ± 0.08 mPa/s from 1.35 ± 0.15 mPa/s pretreatment *175*

Stibophen

Alanine Aminotransferase *Serum Increase Physiological* Hepatitis reported *128*

Aspartate Aminotransferase *Serum Increase Physiological* Hepatitis reported *128*

Bilirubin *Serum Increase Physiological* Produces hemolytic anemia *3895*

Bilirubin, Direct *Serum Increase Physiological* Produces hemolytic anemia *3895*

Coombs' Test, Direct *Blood Positive Physiological* Produces hemolytic anemia *3895*

Erythrocytes *Blood Decrease Physiological* Produces hemolytic anemia *3895*

Haptoglobin *Serum Decrease Physiological* Produces hemolytic anemia *3895*

Hematocrit *Blood Decrease Physiological* May produce hemolytic anemia *3895*

Hemoglobin *Blood Decrease Physiological* May produce hemolytic anemia *3895*

Platelets *Blood Decrease Physiological* Immunological mechanism (often with purpura) *1170*

Protein *Urine Increase Physiological* Renal irritation reported *128*

Vanillylmandelic Acid *Urine Increase Analytical* At neutral or alkaline pH affects Gitlow procedure *6506*

Streptokinase

Alanine Aminotransferase *Serum Increase Physiological* Transient increases may occur as a result of treatment but clinical significance is unknown *278* Substantial but not as marked as GGT *5350*

Alkaline Phosphatase *Serum Increase Physiological* Substantial not as marked as GGT *5350* Transient dysfunction of liver, returning to normal when treatment discontinued *5204*

α_2-Antiplasmin *Plasma Decrease Physiological* Effect more marked than after t-PA after myocardial infarction *1384*

α_1-Antitrypsin *Serum Increase Physiological* Significant effect after infusion in infarct patients *2257*

Aspartate Aminotransferase *Serum Increase Physiological* Substantial effect not as marked as GGT *5350* Transient increases may occur as a result of treatment but clinical significance is unknown *278* Transient dysfunction of liver, returning to normal when treatment discontinued *5204* Earlier peak of CK-MB observed in patients on thrombolytic therapy due to reperfusion of ischemic myocardium *2232*

Bilirubin *Serum No Effect Physiological* Transient dysfunction of liver, returning to normal when treatment discontinued *5204*

Bilirubin, Direct *Serum No Effect Physiological* Although transient dysfunction of liver observed, which reverts to normal when treatment stopped *5204*

Bleeding Time *Patient Increase Physiological* Dissolves blood clots *3810*

BSP Retention *Serum Increase Physiological* Possible acute hypoxic or toxic liver damage *5350*

Cholesterol *Serum Decrease Physiological* In 31 patients who received streptokinase 1.5-15 hours after onset of chest pain mean decrease of 0.4 mmol/L observed, with the magnitude of the decrease correlated with the pre-streptokinase concentration *1978*

Cholinesterase *Serum Decrease Physiological* Possible acute hypoxic or toxic liver damage *5350*

Creatine Kinase *Serum Increase Physiological* Earlier peak of CK-MB observed in patients on thrombolytic therapy due to reperfusion of ischemic myocardium *2232*

Serum No Effect Physiological Although marked effect on liver *5350*

Creatine Kinase Isoenzymes *Serum Increase Physiological* Earlier peak of CK-MB observed in patients on thrombolytic therapy due to reperfusion of ischemic myocardium *2232*

Creatinine *Serum Increase Physiological* Nephrotoxic effect (with tubular damage) *3810*

D-Dimer *Plasma Increase Physiological* In 23 patients with acute myocardial infarction treatment with streptokinase 1.5 x 10^6 units for 60 min was associated with increase from mean baseline of 450 µg/L on admission to 1350 µg/L after lysis and peak of 2250 µg/L *2088*

Doxazosin *Serum No Effect Physiological* Coadministration with doxazosin had no effect on its pharmacokinetics *4642*

Eosinophils *Blood Increase Physiological* Allergic response *3810*

Erythrocytes *Urine Increase Physiological* Severe internal bleeding may occur with hematuria as a result of treatment *278*

Euglobulin Lysis Time *Blood Decrease Physiological* Significant effect in patients with myocardial infarct *2257*

Factor V *Plasma Decrease Physiological* Effect more marked than with t-PA after myocardial infarction *1384*

Fibrin Degradation Products
Plasma Increase Physiological Effect more marked than with t-PA following myocardial infarction *1384*

Fibrin Degradation Products (D-Dimer)
Plasma Increase Physiological Intravenous administration into coronary arteries for indications other than myocardial infarction caused marked increase in time, usually normalizing within 12 - 24 h which also caused prolongation of clotting times *278*

Fibrinogen *Plasma Decrease Physiological* Intravenous administration into coronary arteries for myocardial infarction caused marked decrease in concentration, usually normalizing within 12 - 24 h *278* Effect more marked than t-PA after myocardial infarction *1384* Significant effect in infarct patients *2257* In patients receiving streptokinase therapy mean concentration reduced compared with healthy controls when measured by ACL, biuret, Fibrin-timer and Chromo-timer methods *2921*

Plasma Increase Analytical When measured immunonephelometrically using Behring Nephelometer analyzer fibrinogen concentrations increased due to presence of FDP *2921*

Fibrinolytic Time *Plasma Increase Physiological* Significant effect if given parenterally *658*

Fibronectin *Plasma Increase Physiological* In patients with acute myocardial infarction who had received intracoronary streptokinase significantly higher concentration observed than in those who had not received such treatment *1640*

Glutamate Dehydrogenase *Serum Increase Physiological* Disproportionate increase but not as marked as GGT *5350*

γ-Glutamyltransferase *Serum Increase Physiological* Occurring in approximately 25% increase by four times *5350* Transient dysfunction of liver, returning to normal when treatment discontinued *5204*

Hematocrit *Blood Decrease Physiological* Decreased by more than 15% in 23 of 147 patients in one study *3649*

Hemoglobin *Blood Decrease Physiological* Decreased by more than 5 g/dL in 23 of 147 patients in one study *3649*
Urine Increase Physiological Severe internal bleeding may occur with hematuria as a result of treatment *278*

Lactate Dehydrogenase *Serum Increase Physiological* Earlier peak of CK-MB observed in patients on thrombolytic therapy due to reperfusion of ischemic myocardium *2232*
Serum No Effect Physiological Although marked effect on liver *5350*

Lactate Dehydrogenase Isoenzymes
Serum Increase Analytical Broadening of band between LD-3 and LD-4 and absent LD-5. Complex formed between LD-3 and IgA. Unusual band disappeared *6161*

Leucine Aminopeptidase *Urine Increase Physiological* Activates peptidases by plasminogen *4826*

Leukocytes *Blood Increase Physiological* Due to eosinophilia *3810*

α_2-Macroglobulin *Serum Decrease Physiological* Significant effect remained low for 2 weeks after infusion *2257*

Myoglobin *Serum Increase Physiological* Earlier peak of CK-MB observed in patients on thrombolytic therapy due to reperfusion of ischemic myocardium *2232*

Occult Blood *Feces Increase Physiological* Severe internal bleeding may occur as a result of treatment *278*

Partial Thromboplastin Time
Plasma Increase Physiological Intravenous administration into coronary arteries for myocardial infarction caused marked increase in time, usually normalizing within 12 - 24 h *278*

Plasmin *Plasma Increase Physiological* Stimulates conversion of plasminogen to plasmin by forming an activator complex *5162*

Plasminogen *Plasma Decrease Physiological* Effect more marked than with t-PA after myocardial infarction *1384* Intravenous administration into coronary arteries for myocardial infarction caused marked decrease in concentration, usually normalizing within 12 - 24 h *278* Effect observed after myocardial infarction *2257*

Plasminogen Activator Inhibitor-1
Plasma Increase Physiological In 23 patients with acute myocardial infarction treatment with streptokinase 1.5 x 10^6 units for 60 min was associated with increase from mean baseline of 53 μg/L on admission to 70 μg/L after lysis and peak of 140 μg/L *2088*

Plasminogen Activator Inhibitor-1 Antigen
Plasma Increase Physiological In 27 patients treated with 1.5 million units over 60 minutes concentration increased significantly over baseline peaking about 3 hours after stopping of therapy and returned to normal on day 2 *2087*

Protein *Urine Increase Physiological* Renal damage reported *3810*

Prothrombin Time *Plasma Increase Physiological* Intravenous administration into coronary arteries for myocardial infarction caused marked increase in time, usually normalizing within 12 - 24 h *278*

Thrombin Time *Blood Increase Physiological* Intravenous administration into coronary arteries for myocardial infarction caused marked increase in time, usually normalizing within 12 - 24 h *278* Reflects extent of fibrinogen breakdown *5507*

β-Thromboglobulin *Plasma Increase Physiological* In 24 patients with AMI mean concentration on admission (3.5 ± 1.5 h after onset of symptoms) 105 ± 27 IU/mL increased to 191 ± 58 IU/mL at 3 h after administration of 1.5 million IU in 1 h. In patients without streptokinase concentration did not change significantly over the same time period *5210*
Plasma No Effect Physiological In 24 patients with AMI mean concentration on admission (3.5 ± 1.5 h after onset of symptoms) 105 ± 27 IU/mL increased to 191 ± 58 IU/mL at 3 h after administration of 1.5 million IU in 1 h but thereafter decreased on third day to 130 IU/mL not significantly different 125 IU/mL in untreated patients with continuing absence of significant differences on days 5 and 7 *5210*

Tissue Plasminogen Activator-1
Plasma No Effect Physiological In 23 patients with acute myocardial infarction treatment with streptokinase 1.5 x 10^6 units for 60 min was associated with increase from mean baseline of 17 μg/L on admission to 20 μg/L after lysis and peak of 19 μg/L *2088*

Troponin I *Serum No Effect Analytical* At concentrations up to 1.0 g/L had no significant effect on Abbott ELISA method for cardiac troponin I *6010*

Urea Nitrogen *Serum Increase Physiological* Renal tubular damage in one case *1009*

Streptomycin

Acetaminophen *Serum No Effect Analytical* No effect at therapeutic concentration on method using o-cresol *949*

Alanine Aminotransferase *Serum Increase Physiological* In 72 patients with tuberculosis all receiving isoniazid and rifampin and, in addition, pyrazinamide in 72.2%, ethambutol in 80% and streptomycin in 16.7% drug-induced hepatitis observed with AST activity reaching mean of 330.2 ± 425.5 U/L *5577*

Alkaline Phosphatase *Urine Increase Physiological* Due to nephrotoxic effect of drug *4826*

Amikacin *Serum No Effect Analytical* No interference observed at a concentration of 500 μg/mL (860 μmol/L) with method on Du Pont aca *1508* No interference observed with method on Abbott TDx *3858* Error of less than 5% observed when streptomycin added at a concentration of 100 mg/L to a specimen containing 15 mg/L amikacin and measured on Baxter Stratus *5705*

Aspartate Aminotransferase *Serum Increase Physiological* In 72 patients with tuberculosis all receiving isoniazid and rifampin and, in addition, pyrazinamide in 72.2%, ethambutol in 80% and streptomycin in 16.7% drug-induced hepatitis observed with AST activity reaching mean of 428.4 ± 666.0 U/L *5577*

Bilirubin *Serum Increase Physiological* May cause hemolytic anemia *3810* In 72 patients with tuberculosis all receiving isoniazid and rifampin and, in addition, pyrazinamide in 72.2%, ethambutol in 80% and streptomycin in 16.7% drug-induced hepatitis observed with bilirubin concentration reaching mean of 5.34 ± 4.68 mg/dL *5577*
Serum No Effect Analytical At concentration of 58 mg/L had no effect on Jendrassik and Grof method *5704*
Serum No Effect Physiological Clinically insignificant displacement from protein in neonates *6314*

Bilirubin, Conjugated *Serum No Effect Analytical* At concentration of 7.2 μg/mL (12.3 μmol/L) had no effect on method on Du Pont aca *1517*

Calcium *Serum No Effect Analytical* At concentration of 58 mg/L had no effect on cresolphthalein method *5704*

Casts *Urine Increase Physiological* Cylindruria may develop *2242*

Chloramphenicol *Serum No Effect Analytical* No effect at 100 mg/L on coupled enzymatic method *4122*

Chromosomes *Test Conditions No Effect Physiological* Not clastogenic in human cells *5484*

Coombs' Test *Blood Positive Physiological* Mechanism obscure *2453*

Creatine Kinase Isoenzymes *Serum No Effect Analytical* No interference observed at a concentration of 40 mg/L (68.8 μmol/L) with CK-MB method on Du Pont aca *1519*

Streptomycin *(continued)*

Creatinine *Serum Increase Physiological* Nephrotoxicity may occur in 2% *4691* Occasional nephrotoxicity, although less than with other aminoglycosides *6197* Nephrotoxicity occurs rarely *4655*
Serum No Effect Analytical No effect of concentrations up to 15 mg/L on single slide method on Kodak Ektachem® *5706*

Eosinophils *Blood Increase Physiological* Hematopoietic reaction (occurs in 50% cases) *128* Commonly found in patients treated with streptomycin *4655*

Erythrocytes *Blood Decrease Physiological* Occasional case of aplastic anemia reported *2135* Aplastic/hemolytic anemia (sensitivity dependent) *3810*

Gentamicin *Serum No Effect Analytical* No interference observed with method on Abbott TDx *3858* Has cross-reactivity of less than 0.1% with method on Baxter Stratus *5705* No interference observed at concentrations up to 500 µg/mL (860 µmol/L) with method on Du Pont aca *1526*

Glucose *Urine No Effect Analytical* No effect on glucose oxidase methods *2452* Has no effect on Ames Keto-Diastix, Diastix, Multistix, Clinistix and Clinitest procedures *4034* No effect at up to 1 mg/mL on any glucose concentration as measured by Clinitest®, Diastix®, and TesTape® *3710*

Granulocytes *Blood Decrease Physiological* Rare agranulocytosis reported *2135*

Haptoglobin *Serum Decrease Physiological* May cause hemolytic anemia *3810*

Hematocrit *Blood Decrease Physiological* Hemolytic anemia (sensitivity dependent) *1212* Hemolytic anemia or pancytopenia less frequently found in patients treated with streptomycin than eosinophilia *4655*

Hemoglobin *Blood Decrease Physiological* Hemolytic anemia (sensitivity dependent) *1212* Hemolytic anemia or pancytopenia less frequently found in patients treated with streptomycin than eosinophilia *4655*

Histamine *Plasma No Effect Analytical* No inhibition of radio-enzyme assay at 3 times therapeutic concentration *2492*

Kanamycin *Serum No Effect Analytical* No interference observed with method on Abbott TDx *3858*

LE Cells *Blood Positive Physiological* May produce LE-like syndrome *5869*

Leucine Aminopeptidase *Urine Increase Physiological* Facilitates permeation of enzyme into tubules *4826*

Leukocytes *Blood Decrease Physiological* Less frequently found in patients treated with streptomycin than eosinophilia *4655* Occasional case of aplastic anemia reported *2135* Agranulocytosis/Leukopenia/neutropenia *3810*

Midazolam *Serum No Effect Analytical* On GC-ECD method of Ha et al *2387*

Neomycin *Serum No Effect Analytical* No interference observed with method on Abbott TDx *3858*

Netilmicin *Serum No Effect Analytical* No interference observed with method on Abbott TDx *3858*

Neutrophils *Blood Decrease Physiological* Occasional case of agranulocytosis reported *6264*

Nonprotein Nitrogen *Serum Increase Physiological* Nephrotoxicity may occur in 2% *4691*

Phenylalanine *Plasma No Effect Analytical* No interference observed with rapid quantitative whole blood method of Campbell et al using phenylalanine dehydrogenase *867*

Phosphate *Serum No Effect Analytical* At concentration of 58 mg/L had no effect on phosphomolybdate method *5704*

Platelets *Blood Decrease Physiological* Pancytopenia/thrombocytopenia *1212* Occasional case of aplastic anemia reported *2135* Less frequently found in patients treated with streptomycin than eosinophilia *4655*

Potassium *Serum No Effect Analytical* At concentration of 400 mg/L had no effect on measurement by ISE with predilution *5704*

Protein *Cerebrospinal Fluid Increase Analytical* Reacts as phenol if Folin-Ciocalteu reaction used *5869*
Serum No Effect Analytical At concentration of 58 mg/L had no effect on biuret method with blank correction *5704*
Urine Increase Analytical Reacts as phenol if Folin-Ciocalteu reaction used *5869*
Urine Increase Physiological Occasional nephrotoxicity, although less than with other aminoglycosides *6197* May cause nephrotoxicity *2242*

Prothrombin Time *Plasma Increase Physiological* May decrease vitamin K synthesis by gut bacteria *2452*

Sodium *Serum No Effect Analytical* At concentration of 400 mg/L had no effect on measurement by ISE with predilution *5704*

Sugar *Urine Increase Analytical* Acts as reducing agent affects Benedict's, Galatest procedures *6515* False positive with copper reduction procedures *5869*

Tobramycin *Serum No Effect Analytical* No detectable cross-reactivity observed with tobramycin method on Bayer Technicon Immuno 1® *435* At a concentration of 1250 mg/L increased concentration by 15% when measured by method on Baxter Stratus but therapeutic concentration only up to 20 mg/L *5705* No significant effect on method on Du Pont aca at concentrations less than 1000 µg/mL (1.72 mmol/L) *1547* No interference observed with method on Abbott TDx *3858*

Urea Nitrogen *Serum Decrease Analytical* Inhibits Berthelot reaction *5869*
Serum Increase Physiological Nephrotoxicity occurs rarely *4655* Occasional nephrotoxicity, although less than with other aminoglycosides *6197* Nephrotoxicity may occur in 2% *4691*
Serum No Effect Analytical At concentration of 1450 mg/L had no effect on urease/Berthelot method *5704* At concentration of 58 mg/L had no effect on diacetylmonoxime method *5704*

Uric Acid *Serum No Effect Analytical* At concentration of 58 mg/L had no effect on phosphotungstate reduction method *5704*

Vancomycin *Serum No Effect Analytical* No interference observed with method on Abbott TDx *3858*

Zidovudine *Serum No Effect Analytical* No effect on liquid chromatographic method of Hedaya and Sawchuk *2525*

Streptonigrin

Chromosomes *Test Conditions Abnormal Physiological* Clastogenic in human cells *in vitro* for up to 1 mo *5484*

Streptozocin

Acetoacetate *Serum Increase Physiological* Temporary effect following infusion *4190*

Alanine Aminotransferase *Serum Increase Physiological* Abnormal liver function is common and hepatotoxicity may occasionally be severe *1384*

Albumin *Serum Decrease Physiological* May occasionally cause hepatotoxicity with decreased plasma concentration *4686*

Amino Acids *Urine Increase Physiological* Renal dysfunction occurs in 28-73% patients with both glomerular and tubular toxicity with renal tubular acidosis occurring *1384*

Aspartate Aminotransferase *Serum Increase Physiological* May occasionally cause hepatotoxicity *4686* Abnormal lver function is common with hepatotoxicity occasionally severe *1384*

Bicarbonate *Serum Decrease Physiological* Associated with low potassium and polyuria *4190*

Calcium *Serum Decrease Physiological* To normal in few cases of following administration *3426*

Creatinine *Serum Increase Physiological* Renal dysfunction is major dose-limiting toxicity and occurs in 28-73% of patients *1384*

Fatty Acids (FFA), Free *Serum Decrease Physiological* Mechanism not established yet *4190*

Gastrin *Serum Decrease Physiological* Gastric hypersecretion reduced *4190*

Glucose *Urine Increase Physiological* Occurs as a manifestation of renal damage with both glomeruli and tubules affected: glucosuria is associated with renal tubular acidosis *1384* Rarely exceeds 25 mg/dL *4190*

Glucose Tolerance *Serum Decrease Physiological* Mild to moderate, generally reversible, abnormalities of glucose tolerance have been observed with treatment *4686*

Hematocrit *Blood Decrease Physiological* May occasionally cause mild hematological toxicity, although fatal toxicity with substantial reductions in platelet and leukocyte concentrations have been reported *4686*

5-Hydroxyindoleacetic Acid *Urine Decrease Physiological* If carcinoid treated *1826*

Insulin *Plasma Increase Physiological* ?due to release from damaged beta cells *4190*

Ketones *Urine Increase Physiological* Observed in association with renal tubular acidosis occurring subsequent to glomerular and tubular damage *1384*

Lactate *Plasma Increase Physiological* Temporary effect following infusion *4190*

Lactate Dehydrogenase *Serum Increase Physiological* May occasionally cause hepatotoxicity with increased enzyme activity *4686*

Leukocytes *Blood Decrease Physiological* May occasionally cause mild hematological toxicity, although fatal toxicity with substantial reductions in platelet and leukocyte concentrations have been reported *4686*

Platelets *Blood Decrease Physiological* May occasionally cause mild hematological toxicity, although fatal toxicity with substantial reductions in platelet and leukocyte concentrations have been reported *4686*

Potassium *Serum Decrease Physiological* Associated with polyuria *4190*
Urine Increase Physiological In spite of low serum concentration *4190*

Pyruvate *Plasma Increase Physiological* Temporary effect following infusion *4190*

Volume *Urine Increase Physiological* Noted ten days after infusion (with polydipsia) *4190*

Strychnine

Albumin *Serum No Effect Analytical* At concentration of 12 mg/L had no effect on BCG method *5704*

Bicarbonate *Serum No Effect Analytical* At concentration of 12 mg/L had no effect on method using phenolphthalein *5704*

Bilirubin *Serum No Effect Analytical* At concentration of 12 mg/L had no effect on Jendrassik and Grof method *5704*

Calcium *Serum No Effect Analytical* At concentration of 12 mg/L had no effect on cresolphthalein method *5704*

Chloride *Serum No Effect Analytical* At concentration of 12 mg/L had no effect on mercurimetric method *5704*

Cholesterol *Serum No Effect Analytical* At concentration of 12 mg/L had no effect on Liebermann-Burchard method *5704*

Creatinine *Serum No Effect Analytical* At concentration of 12 mg/L had no effect on Technicon AutoAnalyzer® Jaffe method *5704*

Leukocytes *Blood Increase Physiological* Probably due to release of epinephrine from adrenal *2183*

Phosphate *Serum No Effect Analytical* At concentration of 12 mg/L had no effect on phosphomolybdate method *5704*

Potassium *Serum No Effect Analytical* At concentration of 12 mg/L had no effect on measurement by ISE with predilution *5704*

Protein *Serum No Effect Analytical* At concentration of 12 mg/L had no effect on biuret method with blank correction *5704*

Sodium *Serum No Effect Analytical* At concentration of 12 mg/L had no effect on measurement by ISE with predilution *5704*

Triglycerides *Serum No Effect Analytical* At concentration of 12 mg/L had no effect on lipase/esterase method *5704*

Urea Nitrogen *Serum No Effect Analytical* At concentration of 12 mg/L had no effect on diacetylmonoxime method *5704*

Uric Acid *Serum No Effect Analytical* At concentration of 12 mg/L had no effect on phosphotungstate reduction method *5704*

SU-9055

Aldosterone *Urine Decrease Physiological* May inhibit aldosterone production *4605*

Succimer

Salicylate *Serum No Effect Analytical* At a concentration of 1.2 mg/dL has no significant effect on method on Kodak Ektachem® systems *2519*

Succinimide

δ-Aminolevulinic Acid *Urine Increase Physiological* May precipitate acute porphyria *2210*

Coproporphyrin *Feces Increase Physiological* May precipitate acute porphyria *2210*
Urine Increase Physiological May precipitate acute porphyria *2210*

Phenytoin *Serum Increase Physiological* Coadministration of succinimides with phenytoin may increase plasma phenytoin concentration *4522* When succinimides ingested with fosphenytoin concentration of phenytoin may be increased *4519*

Porphobilinogen *Urine Increase Physiological* May precipitate acute porphyria *2210*

Porphyrin, Total *Urine Increase Physiological* May precipitate attack of acute porphyria *1687*

Protoporphyrin *Feces Increase Physiological* May precipitate acute porphyria *2210*

Pyridoxal Phosphate *Serum Decrease Physiological* Increase by 20% at 4 weeks, 60% at 12 weeks *4910*

Succinylcholine

Creatine Kinase *Serum Increase Physiological* Significant if given with anesthesia (effect of injection) *2823* Marked effect on CK if administered during anesthesia *4692* Occurs if given with halothane *6092*

Histamine *Plasma Increase Physiological* Observed with injection for anesthesia *3648*
Plasma No Effect Analytical No significant effect at physiological concentrations on radio-enzyme assay *2492*

ionized Calcium *Serum Increase Physiological* Rise not marked following i.v. administration *1756*

Midazolam *Serum No Effect Analytical* On GC-ECD method of Ha et al *2387*

Myoglobin *Serum Increase Physiological* Occasional result of i.v. injection in children *5164*
Urine Increase Physiological Occasional result of i.v. injection in children *5164*

Potassium *Serum Increase Physiological* Due to increased chemosensitivity of muscle membrane due to development of receptor sites in extrajunctional areas *2344* If injected i.v *5869* Caused transient hyperkalemia in patients undergoing general anesthesia *4739*

Succinylsulfathiazole

Prothrombin Time *Plasma Increase Physiological* May cause vitamin K deficiency *128*

Sucralfate

Acetaminophen *Serum No Effect Physiological* No effect observed on absorption when drugs are coadministered *3873*

Acetylsalicylic Acid *Serum No Effect Analytical* Coadministration had no effect on salicylate pharmacokinetics *4062*
Serum No Effect Physiological No effect observed on absorption when aspirin coadministered with sucralfate *3873*

Sucralfate *(continued)*

Aluminum *Serum Increase Physiological* Total dose of 4 g/day for 21 days increased mean concentration in 25 healthy individuals from about 2 µg/L to more than 5 µg/L. Effect due to gastrointestinal absorption of aluminum from drug. Concentration declined rapidly once sucralfate stopped *104* Serum concentration in uremic patients comparable to that when patients receive aluminum hydroxide *3527*
Urine Increase Physiological Mean excretion increased from less than 5 µg daily to more than 30 µg in 25 healthy individuals given 4 g daily for 21 days. Excretion did not revert to normal for up to 10 days after drug administration stopped *104*

Aminophylline *Serum Decrease Physiological* Absorption and bioavailability of a single dose substantially reduced when drugs are coadministered *3873*

Amitriptyline *Serum Decrease Physiological* Absorption and bioavailability of a single dose of amitriptyline reduced when drugs coadministered *3873*

Azithromycin *Serum Decrease Physiological* Decreased oral availability *886*

Calcium *Serum No Effect Physiological* No effect in uremic patients or when previous aluminum hydroxide regime replaced *3527*

Ceftizoxime *Serum Decrease Physiological* May reduce the extent of absorption (bioavailability) of a single dose of the drug *2642*

Chlorpropamide *Serum Decrease Physiological* Slight reduction in area under curve observed when two drugs coadministered *3526*

Cimetidine *Serum Decrease Physiological* May reduce the extent of absorption (bioavailability) of a single dose of the drug *2642* Insignificant delay in absorption of cimetidine observed when drugs are coadministered *3873*

Ciprofloxacin *Serum Decrease Physiological* Decreased oral availability *886* May reduce the extent of absorption (bioavailability) of a single dose of the drug *2642* Absorption from gastrointestinal tract reduced probably through formation of nonabsorbable chelates *2704* Concurrent administration of ciprofloxacin with sucralfate may substantially interfere with the absorption of ciprofloxacin and plasma and urine concentrations less than desired *416* Absorption and bioavailability of single dose substantially reduced when drugs are coadministered *3873*
Urine Decrease Physiological Concurrent administration of ciprofloxacin with sucralfate may substantially interfere with the absorption of ciprofloxacin and plasma and urine concentrations less than desired *416*

Diazepam *Serum No Effect Physiological* No significant effect on absorption observed when drugs are coadministered *3873*

Diclofenac *Serum No Effect Physiological* Area under concentration curve not significantly different in healthy volunteers with or without sucralfate *6129*

Digoxin *Serum Decrease Physiological* May reduce the extent of absorption (bioavailability) of a single dose of the drug *2642* Absorption and bioavailability of a single dose substantially reduced when drugs are coadministered although bioavailability of digoxin not affected if given 2 hours before sucralfate *3873*

Doxycycline *Serum Decrease Physiological* Significantly decreased oral availability *886*

Erythromycin *Serum No Effect Physiological* No significant effect observed on absorption when drugs are coadministered *3873*

Ethinyl Estradiol *Serum No Effect Physiological* No significant effect observed on absorption when drugs are coadministered *3873*

Ibuprofen *Serum No Effect Physiological* No signifcant effect observed on absorption when drugs are coadministered *3873*

Imipramine *Serum No Effect Physiological* No significant effect observed on absorption when drugs are coadministered *3873*

Indinavir *Serum Decrease Physiological* Decreased oral availability *886*

Indomethacin *Serum No Effect Physiological* No significant effect observed on absorption when drugs are coadministered *3873*

Isoniazid *Serum Decrease Physiological* Decreased oral availability *886*

Ketoconazole *Serum Decrease Physiological* May reduce the extent of absorption (bioavailability) of a single dose of the drug *2642* Decreased oral availability *886*

Ketoprofen *Serum No Effect Physiological* No significant effect observed on absorption when drugs are coadministered *3873*

Lansoprazole *Serum Decrease Physiological* When sucralfate (1 g) administered concomitantly with a single oral dose of 30 mg lansoprazole its absorption was delayed and its bioavailability wa reduced by 17% *5946*

Lomerfloxacin *Serum Decrease Physiological* Forms complex with lomerfloxacin interfering with its bioavailability with reduction of lomerfloxacin by about 30% when sucralfate administered 2 hours previously *2068*

Nalidixic Acid *Urine Decrease Physiological* May interfere with the absorption of nalidixic acid resulting in lower urine concentrations than desired *5255*

Naproxen *Serum No Effect Physiological* No significant effect observed on absorption when drugs are coadministered *3873*

Norfloxacin *Serum Decrease Physiological* Absorption from gastrointestinal tract reduced probably through formation of nonabsorbable chelates *2704* Gastrointestinal absorption reduced *1384* Multivitamins, or other products containing iron or zinc, may interfere with the absorption of norfloxacin resulting in lower plasma and urine concentrations *4981* Absorption and bioavailability of a single dose substantially reduced when drugs are coadministered *3873* Administration of sucralfate within two hours of norfloxacin administration reported to reduce gastrointestinal absorption of norfloxacin with reduction of plasma and urinary concentrations *3987* Decreased oral availability *886*
Urine Decrease Physiological Multivitamins, or other products containing iron or zinc, may interfere with the absorption of norfloxacin resulting in lower plasma and urine concentrations *4981* Administration of sucralfate within two hours of norfloxacin administration reported to reduce gastrointestinal absorption of norfloxacin with reduction of plasma and urinary concentrations *3987*

Ofloxacin *Serum Decrease Physiological* Quinolines form chelates with alkaline earth and transition metal cations resulting in reduced absorption *3914* May reduce the extent of absorption (bioavailability) of a single dose of the drug *2642*

Omeprazole *Serum Decrease Physiological* When sucralfate (1 g) administered concomitantly with a single oral dose of 20 mg omeprazole its absorption was delayed and its bioavailability wa reduced by 16% *5946*

Phenytoin *Serum Decrease Physiological* Coadministration with phenytoin may decrease plasma phenytoin concentration *4522* May reduce the extent of absorption (bioavailability) of a single dose of the drug *2642* Absorption and bioavailability of a single dose of phenytoin substantially reduced when drugs are coadministered although bioavailability of phenytoin not affected if given 2 hours before sucralfate *3873*

Phosphate *Serum Decrease Physiological* Rare side effect reported *3873* Comparable effect to that of aluminum hydroxide in patients with uremia *3527*

Piroxicam *Serum No Effect Physiological* Area under concentration curve not significantly different in healthy volunteers with or without sucralfate *6129*

Prednisone *Serum No Effect Physiological* No significant effect observed on absorption when drugs are coadministered *3873*

Propranolol *Serum No Effect Physiological* No significant effect observed on absorption when drugs are coadministered *3873*

Prothrombin Time *Plasma Decrease Physiological* May reduce the extent of absorption (bioavailability) of a single dose of warfarin, thereby causing subtherapeutic prothrombin times *2642*
Plasma No Effect Physiological Although reported to reduce the absorption of warfarin, two studies have shown no effect on plasma warfarin concentrations and prothrombin times *2642*

Quinidine *Serum Decrease Physiological* May reduce the extent of absorption (bioavailability) of a single dose of the drug *2642*
Serum No Effect Physiological No significant effect observed on absorption when drugs are coadministered *3873*

Ranitidine *Serum Decrease Physiological* Insignificant delay in absorption of ranitidine observed when drugs are coadministered *3873* May reduce the extent of absorption (bioavailability) of a single dose of the drug *2642*

Sparfloxacin *Serum No Effect Physiological* Sucralfate forms chelation complex with sparfloxacin and must be given either 2 hours before or after sparfloxacin to avoid reducing its bioavailability *4943*

Tetracycline *Serum Decrease Physiological* Absorption and bioavailability of a single dose substantially reduced when drugs coadministered although bioavailability of tetracycline not affected if given 2 hours before sucralfate *3873* May reduce the extent of absorption (bioavailability) of a single dose of the drug *2642*

Theophylline *Serum Decrease Physiological* May reduce the extent of absorption (bioavailability) of a single dose of the drug *2642* Absorption and bioavailability of a single dose substantially reduced when drugs coadministered *3873* Decreases absorption of theophylline *3125*
Serum No Effect Physiological No clinically significant effect on theophylline concentration observed when drugs coadministered *5999* No documented significant interaction with theophylline reported *6117*

Tirofiban *Serum No Effect Physiological* Coadministration had no significant effect on plasma clearance of tirofiban *3957*

Trovafloxacin *Serum Decrease Physiological* Coadministration significantly reduces the absorption of trovafloxacin *4663*

Warfarin *Plasma No Effect Physiological* Although reported to reduce the absorption of warfarin, two studies have shown no effect on plasma warfarin concentrations and prothrombin times *2642* No significant effect observed on absorption when drugs are coadministered *3873*

Sufotidine

Gastrin *Serum Increase Physiological* Median integrated plasma gastrin concentration increased from 416 pmol/h/L to 927 pmol/h/L in 7 patients with duodenal ulcer given 1200 mg/d *5618*

Hydrochloric Acid *Gastric Fluid Decrease Physiological* Median integrated 24 hour intragastric acidity decreased by 95% in 7 patients with duodenal ulcer from 1000 mmol/h/L to 51 mmol/h/L when treated with 1200 mg/d *5618*

Sulbactam

Creatinine *Serum Increase Analytical* When specimens drawn from an intravenous line containing sulbactam and measured by Jaffe procedure concentration 96 µmol/L as measured on Boehringer Mannheim Hitachi 736 and 159 µmol/L as measured on Beckman Synchron CX3 compared with 53 µmol/L obtained by enzymatic method on Kodak Ektachem® *1186*

Sulfacarbamide

Glucose *Urine No Effect Analytical* At concentration of 1600 mg/L had no effect on Diabur-test *5704*

Sulfacetamide

Bilirubin *Serum Increase Physiological* May cause hemolysis in G-6-PD deficiency *402*

Erythrocytes *Blood Decrease Physiological* May cause hemolysis with G-6-PD deficiency *3094*

Haptoglobin *Serum Decrease Physiological* May cause hemolysis if G-6-PD deficiency *402*

Hematocrit *Blood Decrease Physiological* May cause hemolysis if G-6-PD deficiency *402*

Hemoglobin *Blood Decrease Physiological* May cause hemolysis if G-6-PD deficiency *402*

Methemoglobin *Blood Increase Physiological* May cause hemolysis if G-6-PD deficiency *6015*

Sulfachlorpyridazine

Alanine Aminotransferase *Serum Increase Physiological* Occasional hepatitis-like reaction *2754*

Amylase *Serum Increase Physiological* Occasional cause of pancreatitis *2754*

Bilirubin *Serum Increase Physiological* Occasional hepatitis-like reaction *2754*

Creatinine *Serum No Effect Analytical* No effect of concentrations up to 15 mg/L on single slide method on Kodak Ektachem® *5706*

Erythrocytes *Blood Decrease Physiological* May be aplastic or hemolytic anemia *2754*

LE Cells *Blood Positive Physiological* Observed occasionally *2754*

Leukocytes *Blood Decrease Physiological* Leukopenia, aplastic anemia may occur *2754*

Methemoglobin *Blood Increase Physiological* Due to hemolysis *2754*

Platelets *Blood Decrease Physiological* Purpura/thrombocytopenia *2754*

Prothrombin Time *Plasma Increase Physiological* Due to decreased prothrombin *2754*

Sulfa as Sulfanilamide *Serum Increase Physiological* After 4 g rises to 22 mg/dL at 3 h *2754*

Sulfadiazine

Alanine Aminotransferase *Serum Increase Physiological* May cause cholestasis with cholangiolitis *3171*

Albumin *Serum No Effect Analytical* At concentration of 1500 mg/L had no effect on BCG method *5704*

Alkaline Phosphatase *Serum Increase Physiological* May cause intrahepatic cholestasis *2377*

Aspartate Aminotransferase *Serum Increase Physiological* May cause cholestasis with cholangiolitis *3171*

Bicarbonate *Serum No Effect Analytical* At concentration of 1500 mg/L had no effect on method using phenolphthalein *5704*

Bilirubin *Serum Increase Physiological* May cause intrahepatic cholestasis *2377* Displacement from protein in neonates *6314*
Serum No Effect Analytical At concentration of 1500 mg/L had no effect on Jendrassik and Grof method *5704* At concentration of 150 mg/L had no effect on Kodak Ektachem® method *5704*

Calcium *Serum No Effect Analytical* At concentration of 1500 mg/L had no effect on cresolphthalein method *5704*

Chloride *Serum No Effect Analytical* At concentration of 1500 mg/L had no effect on mercurimetric method *5704*

Cholesterol *Serum Increase Physiological* May cause intrahepatic cholestasis *2377*
Serum No Effect Analytical At concentration of 1500 mg/L had no effect on Liebermann-Burchard method *5704*

Creatinine *Serum No Effect Analytical* At concentration of 1500 mg/L had no effect on Technicon AutoAnalyzer® Jaffe method *5704* No effect of concentrations up to 15 mg/L on single slide method on Kodak Ektachem® *5706*

Crystals *Urine Increase Physiological* Observed in the urine of four patients with AIDS and toxoplasmic encephalitis: reversible with rehydration and urine alkalinization *4092* Low solubility in acid urine *4691*

Erythrocytes *Blood Decrease Physiological* May cause hemolytic anemia *3810*
Urine Increase Physiological Associated with crystalluria and oliguria *4691*

Glucose *Serum No Effect Analytical* No effect on glucose oxidase method of Boehringer *5480*

Sulfadiazine *(continued)*

Haptoglobin *Serum Decrease Physiological* May cause hemolytic anemia *3810*

Hematocrit *Blood Decrease Physiological* May cause hemolytic anemia *3810*

Hemoglobin *Blood Decrease Physiological* May cause hemolytic anemia *3810*
Urine Increase Physiological Associated with crystalluria and hematuria *4691*

^{131}I Uptake *Serum Decrease Physiological* Dulcet contains tetraiodofluorescein *4360*

Leukocytes *Blood Decrease Physiological* Agranulocytosis/Leukopenia *3810*

Phosphate *Serum No Effect Analytical* At concentration of 1500 mg/L had no effect on phosphomolybdate method *5704*

Potassium *Serum No Effect Analytical* At concentration of 1500 mg/L had no effect on measurement by ISE with predilution *5704*

Protein *Cerebrospinal Fluid Increase Analytical* Reacts as if phenol with Folin-Ciocalteu procedure *6681*
Cerebrospinal Fluid No Effect Analytical At 100 mg/dL on TCA dye method of Pesce *4625*
Serum No Effect Analytical At concentration of 1500 mg/L had no effect on biuret method with blank correction *5704*
Urine Increase Physiological Due to crystalluria and hematuria *4691*
Urine No Effect Analytical At 100 mg/dL on TCA dye method of Pesce *4625*

Sodium *Serum No Effect Analytical* At concentration of 1500 mg/L had no effect on measurement by ISE with predilution *5704*

Tolbutamide *Serum No Effect Physiological* Appears to have no effect on plasma concentration *2452*

Triglycerides *Serum No Effect Analytical* At concentration of 1500 mg/L had no effect on lipase/esterase method *5704*

Urea Nitrogen *Serum No Effect Analytical* No effect on Berthelot procedure *3033* At concentration of 80 mg/L had no effect on urease/Berthelot method *5704* At concentration of 1500 mg/L had no effect on diacetylmonoxime method *5704*

Uric Acid *Serum No Effect Analytical* At concentration of 1500 mg/L had no effect on phosphotungstate reduction method *5704*

Urobilinogen *Urine Increase Analytical* May produce greenish color with Ehrlich's reagent *703* Gives greenish-yellow color with Ehrlich's reagent *409*

Volume *Urine Decrease Physiological* Associated with crystalluria and hematuria *4691*

Sulfadimethoxine

Alanine Aminotransferase *Serum Increase Physiological* Reversible hypersensitive cholestatic response *3070*

Alkaline Phosphatase *Serum Increase Physiological* Granulomatous reaction in liver *1762*

Aspartate Aminotransferase *Serum Increase Physiological* Granulomatous reaction in liver *1762*

Bile *Urine Increase Physiological* Granulomatous reaction in liver *1762*

Bilirubin *Serum Increase Physiological* Granulomatous reaction in liver *1762*
Urine Increase Physiological Granulomatous reaction in liver *1762*

Bilirubin, Direct *Serum Increase Physiological* Granulomatous reaction in liver *1762*

BSP Retention *Serum Increase Physiological* Reversible cholestasis *1762*

LE Cells *Blood Positive Physiological* Implicated as activator of SLE *1608*

Platelets *Blood Decrease Physiological* Aplastic anemia/thrombocytopenia with sulfonamides *3810*

Tolbutamide *Serum No Effect Physiological* Appears to have no effect on plasma concentration *2452*

Urobilinogen *Feces Decrease Physiological* Pale stools with reversible cholestasis *1762*
Urine Decrease Physiological Occurs with reversible cholestasis *1762*

Sulfadimidine

Cyclosporine *Blood Decrease Physiological* Intravenous administration with cyclosporine caused the concentration of cyclosporine to become unmeasureable within 7 days although in one study cyclosporine concentration normalized after oral sulfadimidine was substituted for intravenous *859*
Serum Decrease Physiological When given intravenously with or without trimethoprim decreases concentration but mechanism not discussed *1069* In patients in whom trimethoprim was administered with sulfadimidine cyclosporine concentration decreased but mechanism not known: effect has been attributed to sulfadimidine *6595* Reduction when given i.v.; not seen if given orally: mechanism not clear *6288* Intravenous administration with cyclosporine caused the concentration of cyclosporine to become unmeasureable within 7 days although in one study cyclosporine concentration normalized after oral sulfadimidine was substituted for intravenous *859*

Platelets *Blood Decrease Physiological* Immunologically-induced thrombocytopenic purpura *3051*

Sulfadoxine

Bilirubin *Serum Increase Physiological* Isolated cases reported when given with pyrimethamine for treatment of malaria *4413*

Neutrophils *Blood Decrease Physiological* Isolated cases reported when given with pyrimethamine for treatment of malaria *4413*

Sulfaguanidine

Albumin *Serum No Effect Analytical* At concentration of 500 mg/L had no effect on BCG method *5704*

Bicarbonate *Serum No Effect Analytical* At concentration of 500 mg/L had no effect on method using phenolphthalein *5704*

Bilirubin *Serum No Effect Analytical* At concentration of 500 mg/L had no effect on Jendrassik and Grof method *5704*

Calcium *Serum No Effect Analytical* At concentration of 500 mg/L had no effect on cresolphthalein method *5704*

Chloride *Serum No Effect Analytical* At concentration of 500 mg/L had no effect on mercurimetric method *5704*

Cholesterol *Serum No Effect Analytical* At concentration of 500 mg/L had no effect on Liebermann-Burchard method *5704*

Creatinine *Serum No Effect Analytical* At concentration of 500 mg/L had no effect on Technicon AutoAnalyzer® Jaffe method *5704*

Cyclosporine *Blood Decrease Physiological* Intravenous administration with cyclosporine caused the concentration of cyclosporine to become unmeasureable within 7 days although in one study cyclosporine concentration normalized after oral sulfadimidine was substituted for intravenous *859*

Glucose *Serum No Effect Analytical* No effect on Boehringer GOD-PERID glucose oxidase method *5480*

Phosphate *Serum No Effect Analytical* At concentration of 500 mg/L had no effect on phosphomolybdate method *5704*

Potassium *Serum No Effect Analytical* At concentration of 500 mg/L had no effect on measurement by ISE with predilution *5704*

Protein *Cerebrospinal Fluid Increase Analytical* Reacts as if phenol with Folin-Ciocalteu procedure *6681*
Serum No Effect Analytical At concentration of 500 mg/L had no effect on biuret method with blank correction *5704*

Sodium *Serum No Effect Analytical* At concentration of 500 mg/L had no effect on measurement by ISE with predilution *5704*

Triglycerides *Serum No Effect Analytical* At concentration of 500 mg/L had no effect on lipase/esterase method *5704*

Urea Nitrogen *Serum No Effect Analytical* At concentration of 500 mg/L had no effect on diacetylmonoxime method *5704*

Uric Acid *Serum No Effect Analytical* At concentration of 500 mg/L had no effect on phosphotungstate reduction method *5704*

Sulfamerazine

Crystals *Urine Increase Physiological* Presence of drug *128*

17-Hydroxycorticosteroids *Urine Increase Analytical* Alleged effect on method of Reddy *2451*

Protein *Cerebrospinal Fluid Increase Analytical* Reacts as if phenol with Folin-Ciocalteu procedure *6681*

Sulfamethizole

Alanine Aminotransferase *Serum Increase Physiological* Reversible cholestasis *3211*

Alkaline Phosphatase *Serum Increase Physiological* Reversible cholestasis *3211*

Amylase *Serum Increase Physiological* Case of pancreatitis reported *385*

Aspartate Aminotransferase *Serum Increase Physiological* Reversible cholestasis *3211*

Bile *Urine Increase Physiological* Reversible cholestasis *3211*

Bilirubin *Serum Increase Physiological* May cause cholestatic jaundice *3211*

BSP Retention *Serum Increase Physiological* Reversible cholestasis *3211*

Erythrocytes *Blood Decrease Physiological* Hemolytic anemia/aplastic anemia *4780*

Glucose *Serum No Effect Analytical* No effect on glucose oxidase method of Boehringer *5480*

Haptoglobin *Serum Decrease Physiological* May cause hemolytic anemia *4780*

Hematocrit *Blood Decrease Physiological* Hemolytic anemia *4780*

Hemoglobin *Blood Decrease Physiological* Hemolytic anemia *4780*

Leukocytes *Blood Decrease Physiological* Agranulocytosis *4780*

Methemoglobin *Blood Increase Physiological* May cause hemolytic anemia *4780*

Platelets *Blood Decrease Physiological* Agranulocytosis/aplastic anemia/thrombocytopenia *4780*

Prothrombin Time *Plasma Increase Physiological* Reaction may occur with all sulfonamides *2754*

Sulfhemoglobin *Blood Increase Physiological* May occur with hemolytic anemia *4780*

Urobilinogen *Feces Decrease Physiological* Pale stools with reversible cholestasis *3211*

Urine Decrease Physiological Occurs with reversible cholestasis *3211*

Urine Increase Analytical Yellow color with Ehrlich's (extracted into $CHCl_3$) *3892*

Sulfamethoxazole

Alanine Aminotransferase *Serum Increase Physiological* When given with trimethoprim, fever and malaise: successful response to treatment *3206* Cholestatic jaundice may occur *3211* Occasional case of cholestasis with or without hepatic necrosis *5804* Hepatitis or hepatocellular necrosis associated with drug administration observed in some treated patients *5021*

Serum No Effect Analytical No effect at therapeutic concentration on Boehringer Mannheim Reflotron method *3231* No effect up to 100 mg/L on Boehringer Mannheim Reflotron method but above this concentration inhibition of enzyme activity although of no clinical significance since normal therapeutic concentration 2.5-60 mg/L *5706*

Albumin *Urine No Effect Analytical* At concentration of 600 mg/dL had no significant effect on Boehringer Mannheim Tinaquant method *2799*

Alkaline Phosphatase *Serum Increase Physiological* Cholestatic jaundice may occur *3211* Occasional case of cholestasis with or without hepatic necrosis *5804* Hepatitis or hepatocellular necrosis associated with drug administration observed in some treated patients *5021* When given with trimethoprim, fever and malaise: successful response to treatment *3206*

α-Amino-Nitrogen *Plasma Increase Analytical* Measured in naphthoquinone method of Frame *4953*

Amylase *Serum Increase Physiological* Isolated case of drug-induced pancreatitis. Patient had been sensitized previously by treatment with a different sulfonamide *704* Pancreatitis associated with drug administration observed in some treated patients *5021*

Serum No Effect Analytical At concentration of 600 mg/L had no effect on method on Boehringer Mannheim Reflotron system *5706*

Amylase, Pancreatic Isoenzyme

Serum No Effect Analytical No significant effect observed at a toxic concentration of 600 mg/L with method on Boehringer Mannheim Reflotron *3647*

Anion Gap *Serum No Effect Physiological* In 105 patients with various infections 80 were treated with trimethoprim 320 mg/d and sulfamethoxazole 1600 mg/d. No significant change observed in anion gap *82*

Aspartate Aminotransferase *Serum Increase Physiological* Hepatitis or hepatocellular necrosis associated with drug administration observed in some treated patients *5021* Cholestatic jaundice may occur *3211* Occasional case of cholestasis with or without hepatic necrosis *5804*

Serum No Effect Analytical No effect at 600 mg/L on Boehringer Mannheim Reflotron method *5706* No effect at therapeutic concentration on Boehringer Mannheim Reflotron method *3231*

Bicarbonate *Serum No Effect Physiological* In 105 patients with various infections 80 were treated with trimethoprim 320 mg/d and sulfamethoxazole 1600 mg/d. No significant change observed in bicarbonate concentration *82*

Bile *Urine Increase Physiological* Reversible cholestasis *3810*

Bilirubin *Serum Increase Physiological* Occasional case of cholestasis with or without hepatic necrosis *5804* Displacement from protein in neonates *6314* Reversible cholestasis or hemolytic anemia *3810* Hepatitis or hepatocellular necrosis associated with drug administration observed in some treated patients *5021*

Serum No Effect Analytical No effect at 250 mg/L on Ames Seralyzer method *5706* At concentration of 600 mg/L no effect on method on Boehringer Mannheim Reflotron system *5706* At concentration of 60 mg/L had no effect on Kodak Ektachem® method *5704*

BSP Retention *Serum Increase Physiological* Reversible cholestasis *3810*

Chloride *Serum No Effect Physiological* In 105 patients with various infections 80 were treated with trimethoprim 320 mg/d and sulfamethoxazole 1600 mg/d. No significant change observed in chloride concentration *82*

Cholesterol *Serum No Effect Analytical* At concentration of 600 mg/L no effect on method on Boehringer Mannheim Reflotron system *5706* No effect at therapeutic concentration on Boehringer Mannheim Reflotron method *3231* No effect at 250 mg/L on Ames Seralyzer method *5706*

Cholinesterase *Serum No Effect Analytical* No effect observed at concentration of 350 μg/mL with butyrylthiocholine method on Kodak Ektachem® *2504*

Clindamycin *Serum Positive Analytical* Interferes with bioassays *3858*

Colistin *Serum Positive Analytical* Interferes with bioassays *3858*

Color *Urine Increase Analytical* Brown color observed *1714*

Cortisol *Plasma No Effect Analytical* At a concentration of 600 mg/L no significant effect observed on CEDIA or Enzymun methods *1097*

Creatine Kinase *Serum Decrease Analytical* At high doses only 80% recovery observed with whole blood method on Boehringer Mannheim Reflotron *2714*

Sulfamethoxazole *(continued)*

Creatine Kinase *(continued)*
Serum No Effect Analytical No effect at 250 mg/L on method on Ames Seralyzer *5706*

Creatinine *Serum Increase Analytical* At concentrations above 200 mg/L raised concentration as measured by kinetic Jaffe method *5704*
Serum Increase Physiological In 105 patients with various infections 80 were treated with trimethoprim 320 mg/d and sulfamethoxazole 1600 mg/d. Serum urea nitrogen increased nonsignificantly from 102.5 ± 49.5 μmol/L to 126.1 ± 70.7 μmol/L 4.6 ± 2.2 days after treatment started *82* Increased concentration associated with drug administration observed in some treated patients, with occasional toxic nephrosis with oliguria and anuria *5021*
Serum No Effect Analytical At concentration of 200 mg/L had no effect on Technicon AutoAnalyzer® Jaffe method *5704* No effect at 250 mg/L on method on Ames Seralyzer *5706* No effect on alkaline picrate (Jaffe) procedure *505* No effect of concentrations up to 15 mg/L on single slide method on Kodak Ektachem® *5706*
Serum No Effect Physiological Insignificant reduction in 5 volunteers after 7 d *5136*

Creatinine Clearance *Urine Decrease Physiological* When given with trimethoprim, fever and malaise: successful response to treatment *3206*

Crystals *Urine Increase Physiological* Low solubility in acid urine *4691*

Cyclosporine *Blood No Effect Analytical* At a concentration of 400 mg/L had no effect on Syva EMIT method *495*
Serum Decrease Physiological When admistered with trimethoprim reported to decrease concentration of cyclosporine *1384*
Serum Increase Physiological Reversible deterioration in renal function with effect on tubular function and nephrotoxicity *6288*

D-Lactate *Urine Decrease Physiological* In one patient receiving trimethoprim-sulfamethoxazole on admission to hospital D-lactate concentration 21.9 mmol/L compared with reference interval of 0 - 0.25 mmol/L *1137*

Doxazosin *Serum No Effect Physiological* Coadministration with doxazosin had no effect on its pharmacokinetics *4642*

Eosinophils *Blood Decrease Physiological* Agranulocytosis observed associated with drug administration observed in some treated patients *5021*
Blood Increase Physiological Allergic response *3211* When given with trimethoprim, fever and malaise: successful response to treatment *3206* Eosinophilia associated with drug administration observed in some treated patients *5021*

Erythrocyte Sedimentation Rate
Blood Increase Physiological When given with trimethoprim fever and malaise; successful response to treatment *3206*

Erythrocytes *Blood Decrease Physiological* May cause hemolytic anemia *3211*
Urine Increase Physiological May cause hematuria with crystalluria *4691*

Erythromycin *Serum Increase Analytical* Interferes with bioassays *3858*

Glucose *Serum Decrease Physiological* Hypoglycemia associated with drug administration observed rarely in treated patients *5021*
Serum No Effect Analytical At concentration of 320 mg/L had no effect on hexokinase/G-6-PDH method *5704* At concentration of 600 mg/L no effect on method on Boehringer Mannheim Reflotron system *5706* No effect at 250 mg/L on glucose oxidase method on Ames Seralyzer *5706* No effect at therapeutic concentration on Boehringer Mannheim Reflotron method *3231*
Urine No Effect Analytical At concentration of 1300 mg/L had no effect on Diabur-test *5704*

γ-Glutamyltransferase *Serum Increase Physiological* Hepatitis or hepatocellular necrosis associated with drug administration observed in some treated patients *5021*
Serum No Effect Analytical At concentrations up to 600 mg/L no effect on method on Boehringer Mannheim Reflotron system but at concentrations above this reduced enzyme activity observed but therapeutic range is 2.5 to 60 mg/L *5706* No effect at therapeutic concentration on Boehringer Mannheim Reflotron method *3231*

Haptoglobin *Serum Decrease Physiological* May cause hemolytic anemia *3211*

HDL-Cholesterol *Serum No Effect Analytical* At a concentration up to 600 mg/L had no significant effect on Reflotron method for whole blood cholesterol *6352*

Hematocrit *Blood Decrease Physiological* Aplastic or hemolytic anemia probably associated with drug administration observed in some treated patients *5021* May cause hemolytic anemia *3211*

Hemoglobin *Blood Decrease Physiological* Aplastic or hemolytic anemia probably associated with drug administration observed in some treated patients *5021* May cause hemolytic anemia *3211*
Urine Increase Physiological May cause hematuria with oliguria *4691*

Indinavir *Serum No Effect Physiological* Administration of indinavir 400 mg every 6 hours with trimethoprim/sulfamethoxazole (one double strength tablet every 12 hours) for 1 week resulted in no change in indinavir AUC, a 19 ± 31% increase in trimethoprim AUC and no change in sulfamethoxazole AUC *3966*

Lactate *Plasma No Effect Analytical* At concentration of 320 mg/L had no effect on enzymatic method *5704*

Lactate Dehydrogenase *Serum Increase Physiological* May cause hemolytic anemia *3211* Hepatitis or hepatocellular necrosis associated with drug administration observed in some treated patients *5021*
Serum No Effect Analytical No effect at 250 mg/L on method on Ames Seralyzer *5706*

Lamivudine *Serum Increase Physiological* Coadministration of trimethoprim/sulfamethoxazole (TMP 160 mg/SMX 800 mg) once daily for 5 days with 300 mg lamivudine caused a significant 44 ± 23% increase in the AUC of lamivudine and a decrease of 30 ± 36% in its renal clearance, although the pharmacokinetic properties of trimethoprim and sulfamethoxazole were not affected *2174*

Leukocytes *Blood Decrease Physiological* Toxic reaction to drug *3211* Leukopenia probably associated with drug administration observed in some treated patients *5021*
Blood Increase Physiological When given with trimethoprim, fever and malaise: successful response to treatment *3206*

Lipase *Serum Increase Physiological* Pancreatitis associated with drug administration observed in some treated patients *5021*

Methemoglobin *Blood Decrease Physiological* Methemoglobinemia probably associated with drug administration observed in some treated patients *5021*

Metronidazole *Serum Increase Analytical* Interferes with bioassays *3858*

Mycophenolate *Serum No Effect Physiological* Coadministration of single doses of mycophenolate mofentil (1.5 g) with trimethoprim/sulfamethoxazole in 12 healthy male volunteers no effect on the bioavailability of mycophenolate was observed *5017*

N-Acetyl-Glucosaminidase *Urine No Effect Analytical* At concentration of 600 mg/dL had no significant effect on Boehringer Mannheim CPR method *3174*

Neutrophils *Blood Decrease Physiological* Neutropenia associated with drug administration observed in some treated patients *5021*

PAH Clearance *Urine Decrease Analytical* Although accurate measurements possible in urine without extraction, drug in blood component reacts like PAH producing falsely low clearance. Effect can be avoided by extracting plasma or serum with isoamyl acetate *4781*

pH *Blood Decrease Physiological* In one patient receiving trimethoprim-sulfamethoxazole on admission to hospital D-lactate concentration 21.9 mmol/L compared with reference interval of 0 - 0.25 mmol/L and blood pH 7.37 reflecting mild lactate acidosis *1137*

Phenylalanine *Plasma No Effect Analytical* No interference observed with rapd quantitative whole blood method of Campbell et al using phenylalanine dehydrogenase *867*

Phenytoin, Free *Serum Increase Physiological* In vitro studies showed significant effect at albumin concentrations of 25 and 32 g/L but at 47 g/L displacement is only significant at higher concentrations of antibiotic. Effect predictable in vivo *1242*

Platelets *Blood Decrease Physiological* Thrombocytopenia *3211* Thrombocytopenia probably associated with drug administration observed in some treated patients *5021*

Polymyxin *Serum Increase Analytical* Interferes with bioassays *3858*

Porphyrin, Total *Urine Increase Analytical* May cause false positive with fluorescent methods *1714*

Potassium *Serum Increase Physiological* In a woman with transplanted lungs a potassium concentration of 6.8 mmol/L was observed with high dose treatment with trimethoprim-sulfamethoxazole for Pneumocystis carnii pneumonia. She was concomitantly receiving enalapril. Combination of ACE inhibition and potassium-sparing diuretics (trimethoprim has an amiloride-like effect on the distal nephron) is known to cause hyperkalemia *800* Hyperkalemia observed in 20 - 53% patients with AIDS with high dose treatment with trimethoprim-sulfamethoxazole for Pneumocystis carnii pneumonia. Trimethoprim has an amiloride-like effect on the distal nephron which is probably responsible for the hyperkalemia *3930* In patients with AIDS high dose trimethoprim-sulfamethoxazole has been associated with hyperkalemia, attributable to trimethoprim acting like the potassium sparing diuretic amiloride with a reduction in potassium excretion *4601* In 105 patients with various infections 80 were treated with trimethoprim 320 mg/d and sulfamethoxazole 1600 mg/d. Serum potassium increased by 1.21 mmol/L from 3.89 ± 0.46 mmol/L to 5.1 ± 0.56 mmol/L 4.6 ± 2.2 days after treatment started *82*
Urine Decrease Physiological In patients with AIDS high dose trimethoprim-sulfamethoxazole has been associated with hyperkalemia, attributable to trimethoprim acting like the potassium sparing diuretic amiloride with a reduction in potassium excretion *4601*

Prostate-specific Antigen, Free *Serum No Effect Analytical* Trimethoprim/sulfamethoxazole at a concentration of 9.7 mg/L had no significant effect on the Hybritech Tandem® -R free PSA immunoassay *4286*

Protein *Urine Increase Analytical* May interfere with sulfosalicylic acid methods *1714*
Urine Increase Physiological May cause hematuria with crystalluria *4691*

Prothrombin Time *Plasma Increase Physiological* Displaces warfarin from its binding sites on albumin *6036* Hypoprothrombinemia probably associated with drug administration observed in some treated patients *5021* Possibly due to drug-induced vitamin K deficiency *3211*

PSP Excretion *Urine Decrease Physiological* More common effect *1714*
Urine Increase Physiological Possible large dose effect *1714*

Sodium *Serum No Effect Physiological* In 105 patients with various infections 80 were treated with trimethoprim 320 mg/d and sulfamethoxazole 1600 mg/d. No significant change observed in sodium concentration *82*

Sugar *Urine Increase Analytical* May cause positive reaction with fluorescent methods *1714*

Tacrolimus *Serum No Effect Analytical* In HPLC/MS method of Christians et al no significant interference observed with measurement of FK 506 *1010*

Tetracycline *Serum Increase Analytical* Interferes with bioassays *3858*

Triglycerides *Serum No Effect Analytical* No effect at therapeutic concentration on Boehringer Mannheim Reflotron method *3231* No effect at 600 mg/L on Boehringer Mannheim Reflotron method *5706*

Trimethoprim *Serum No Effect Analytical* No interference observed with bioassay *3858*

Urea Nitrogen *Serum Increase Physiological* In 105 patients with various infections 80 were treated with trimethoprim 320 mg/d and sulfamethoxazole 1600 mg/d. Serum urea nitrogen increased nonsignificantly from 7.92 ± 5.7 mmol/L to 9.2 ± 5.8 mmol/L 4.6 ± 2.2 days after treatment started *82*
Serum No Effect Analytical No effect at therapeutic concentration on Boehringer Mannheim Reflotron method *3231* No effect at 250 mg/L on method on Ames Seralyzer *5706* No effect at 600 mg/L on Boehringer Mannheim Reflotron method *5706*

Uric Acid *Serum Decrease Physiological* Presumed uricosuric effect *6612*
Serum No Effect Analytical No effect at therapeutic concentration on Boehringer Mannheim Reflotron method *3231* No effect at 600 mg/L on Boehringer Mannheim Reflotron method *5706*
Urine Increase Physiological Presumed uricosuric effect *6612*

Urobilinogen *Feces Decrease Physiological* Pale stools with reversible cholestasis *3810*
Urine Decrease Physiological Occurs with reversible cholestasis *3810*
Urine Increase Analytical May react with Ehrlich's reagent to produce false color *139*

Vancomycin *Serum No Effect Analytical* No significant interference observed at a concentration of 600 µg/mL (2369 µmol/L) with method on Du Pont aca *1561*

Volume *Urine Increase Physiological* Diuresis associated with drug administration observed rarely in treated patients *5021*

Zidovudine *Serum No Effect Analytical* No effect on liquid chromatographic method of Hedaya and Sawchuk *2525*

Sulfamethoxydiazine

Cholesterol *Serum No Effect Analytical* At concentration of 231 mg/L had no effect on CHOD-PAP method *5704* At concentration of 231 mg/L had no effect on method using catalase-Hantzsch reaction *5704* At concentration of 231 mg/L had no effect on Liebermann-Burchard method *5704* At concentration of 231 mg/L had no effect on catalase-AIDH method *5704*

Creatinine *Serum No Effect Analytical* At concentration of 500 mg/L had no effect on kinetic Jaffe method on BKA-2 *5704* At concentration of 200 mg/L had no effect on Technicon AutoAnalyzer® Jaffe method *5704* At concentration of 200 mg/L had no effect on Jaffe-Fading-Fraction method *5704* At concentration of 200 mg/L had no effect on Jaffe-Fuller's earth method *5704*

Glucose *Serum No Effect Analytical* At concentration of 20 mg/L had no effect on Kodak Ektachem® method *5704* No effect of concentrations up to 20 mg/L on method on Kodak Ektachem® *5706*

Potassium *Serum No Effect Analytical* At concentration of 200 mg/L had no effect on measurement by ISE with predilution *5704* At concentration of 200 mg/L had no effect on measurement by ISE without predilution *5704*

Protein Electrophoresis *Serum No Effect Analytical* At concentration of 200 mg/L had no effect on automated Olympus-Hite method *5704*

Sodium *Serum No Effect Analytical* At concentration of 200 mg/L had no effect on measurement by ISE with predilution *5704* At concentration of 200 mg/L had no effect on measurement by ISE without predilution *5704*

Urea Nitrogen *Serum No Effect Analytical* At concentration of 20 mg/L had no effect on Kodak Ektachem® method *5704*

Uric Acid *Serum No Effect Analytical* At concentration of 300 mg/L had no effect on catalase-AIDH method *5704* At concentration of 230 mg/L had no effect on Kageyama-Hantzsch method *5704*

Sulfamethoxypyridazine

Creatinine *Serum No Effect Analytical* At concentration of 70 mg/L had no effect on creatinine iminohydrolase method *5704* No effect of concentrations up to 15 mg/L on single slide method on Kodak Ektachem® *5706*

Glucose *Serum No Effect Analytical* At concentration of 70 mg/L had no effect on GOD/POD-PAP method *5704*

Triglycerides *Serum No Effect Analytical* At concentration of 70 mg/L had no effect on GPO-PAP method *5704*

Uric Acid *Serum No Effect Analytical* At concentration of 70 mg/L had no effect on uricase-PAP method *5704*

Sulfamethoxypyridine

Alanine Aminotransferase *Serum Increase Physiological* Reversible cholestasis *3810*

Alkaline Phosphatase *Serum Increase Physiological* Reversible cholestasis *3810*

Aspartate Aminotransferase *Serum Increase Physiological* Reversible cholestasis *3810*

Bile *Urine Increase Physiological* Reversible cholestasis *3810*

Bilirubin *Serum Increase Physiological* May cause hemolysis with G-6-PD deficiency *402*

BSP Retention *Serum Increase Physiological* Reversible cholestasis *3810*

Eosinophils *Blood Increase Physiological* Observed with hypersensitivity hepatitis *3238*

Erythrocytes *Blood Decrease Physiological* Anemia (AMA Blood dyscrasias) *4017*

Haptoglobin *Serum Decrease Physiological* May cause hemolytic anemia *4017*

Hematocrit *Blood Decrease Physiological* Hemolytic/aplastic anemia *3810*

Hemoglobin *Blood Decrease Physiological* Hemolytic/aplastic anemia *3810*

Lactate Dehydrogenase *Serum Increase Physiological* May occur with preponderance of LD-5 *3238*

LE Cells *Blood Positive Physiological* Implicated as activator of SLE *1608*

Leukocytes *Blood Decrease Physiological* Leukopenia (AMA Blood dyscrasias) *4017*

Methemoglobin *Blood Increase Physiological* May cause hemolytic anemia *4017*

Ornithine Carbamoyltransferase
Serum Increase Physiological Reversible cholestasis may occur *3237*

Platelets *Blood Decrease Physiological* Thrombocytopenia may occur after days to weeks *4017*

Urobilinogen *Feces Decrease Physiological* May cause reversible cholestasis *3810*
Urine Decrease Physiological Occurs with reversible cholestasis *3810*

Sulfanilamide

Alanine Aminotransferase *Serum Increase Physiological* May cause reversible cholestasis *3669*

Albumin *Serum No Effect Analytical* At concentration of 1,000 mg/L had no effect on BCG method *5704*

Alkaline Phosphatase *Serum Increase Physiological* May cause reversible cholestasis *3669*

Amikacin *Serum No Effect Analytical* No interference observed at a concentration of 500 µg/mL (2903 µmol/L) with method on Du Pont aca *1508*

Aspartate Aminotransferase *Serum Increase Physiological* May cause reversible cholestasis *3669*

Bicarbonate *Serum No Effect Analytical* At concentration of 1,000 mg/L had no effect on method using phenolphthalein *5704*

Bilirubin *Serum Increase Physiological* May cause hemolysis with G-6-PD deficiency *402*
Serum No Effect Analytical At concentration of 1,000 mg/L had no effect on Jendrassik and Grof method *5704* At concentration of 103 mg/L had no effect on Kodak Ektachem® method *5704*

Calcium *Serum No Effect Analytical* At concentration of 1,000 mg/L had no effect on cresolphthalein method *5704*

Chloride *Serum No Effect Analytical* At concentration of 1,000 mg/L had no effect on mercurimetric method *5704*

Cholesterol *Serum No Effect Analytical* At concentration of 1,000 mg/L had no effect on Liebermann-Burchard method *5704*

Creatinine *Serum No Effect Analytical* At concentration of 1,000 mg/L had no effect on Technicon AutoAnalyzer® Jaffe method *5704*

Erythrocytes *Blood Decrease Physiological* May cause hemolytic anemia *402*

Gentamicin *Serum No Effect Analytical* No interference observed at concentrations up to 500 µg/mL (2905 µmol/L) with method on Du Pont aca *1526*

Glucose *Serum No Effect Analytical* At concentration of 300 mg/L had no effect on Ames Seralyzer method *5704* No effect at 300 mg/L on glucose oxidase method on Ames Seralyzer *5706*

Haptoglobin *Serum Decrease Physiological* May cause hemolytic anemia *402*

Heinz Body Formation *Blood Positive Physiological* May occur in early stages of hemolysis *536*

Hematocrit *Blood Decrease Physiological* May cause hemolytic anemia *402*

Hemoglobin *Blood Decrease Physiological* Hemolysis and Heinz body formation may be exaggerated in individuals with a glucose-6-phosphate dehydrogenase deficiency or methemoglobin reductase deficiency, or hemoglobin M, often dose-related response *2873* May cause hemolytic anemia *402*

Methemoglobin *Blood Increase Physiological* May cause hemolytic anemia *4017*

Moxalactam *Serum Increase Analytical* Cannot be assayed by HPLC method used at Mayo Clinic in presence of sulfanilamide *3858*

Phosphate *Serum No Effect Analytical* At concentration of 1,000 mg/L had no effect on phosphomolybdate method *5704*

Potassium *Serum No Effect Analytical* At concentration of 1,000 mg/L had no effect on measurement by ISE with predilution *5704*

Protein *Cerebrospinal Fluid Increase Analytical* Reacts as if phenol with Folin-Ciocalteu method *6681*
Serum No Effect Analytical At concentration of 1,000 mg/L had no effect on biuret method with blank correction *5704*

Sodium *Serum No Effect Analytical* At concentration of 1,000 mg/L had no effect on measurement by ISE with predilution *5704*

Sugar *Urine Increase Analytical* False positive with Benedict's reagent *2559*

Tobramycin *Serum No Effect Analytical* No significant effect observed on method on Du Pont aca at concentrations less than 1000 µg/mL (5.81 mmol/L) *1547*

Triglycerides *Serum No Effect Analytical* At concentration of 1,000 mg/L had no effect on lipase/esterase method *5704*

Urea Nitrogen *Serum No Effect Analytical* At concentration of 1,000 mg/L had no effect on diacetylmonoxime method *5704*

Uric Acid *Serum Increase Analytical* At concentrations above 250 mg/L raised concentration as measured by Ames Seralyzer method *5704*
Serum No Effect Analytical At concentration of 1,000 mg/L had no effect on phosphotungstate reduction method *5704*

Urobilinogen *Urine Increase Analytical* Gives greenish-yellow color with Ehrlich's reagent *409*

Sulfaphenazole

Glucose *Serum Decrease Physiological* Reported effect *3810*

Phenytoin *Serum Increase Physiological* Reported impairment of metabolism *3340*

Tolbutamide *Serum Increase Physiological* Displaces from protein, inhibits carboxylation *2452* Half-life increased from 9.5 to 28.6 hours in 2 healthy volunteers probably due to inhibition of microsomal mixed function oxidase *4740*

Sulfapyridine

Alanine Aminotransferase *Serum Increase Physiological* May cause reversible cholestasis *3669*

Alkaline Phosphatase *Serum Increase Physiological* May cause reversible cholestasis *3669*

Aspartate Aminotransferase *Serum Increase Physiological* May cause reversible cholestasis *3669*

Bilirubin *Serum Increase Physiological* May cause hemolysis with G-6-PD deficiency *402* Displacement from protein in neonates *6314*
Serum No Effect Analytical No effect at concentration of 40 mg/L on method on Kodak Ektachem® *5706*

Bilirubin, Conjugated *Serum Increase Analytical* Increased value obtained with method on Kodak Ektachem® at concentrations above 10 mg/L. Clinical significance of this has not been established *5706*
Serum No Effect Analytical At concentrations up to 100 µg/mL had no effect on method on Kodak Ektachem® 400 *1942*

Bilirubin, Unconjugated *Serum No Effect Analytical* At concentrations up to 100 µg/mL had no effect on method on Kodak Ektachem® 400 *1942* No effect at concentration of 40 mg/L on method on Kodak Ektachem® *5706*

Erythrocytes *Blood Decrease Physiological* May cause hemolytic anemia *402*

Haptoglobin *Serum Decrease Physiological* May cause hemolytic anemia *402*

Hematocrit *Blood Decrease Physiological* May cause hemolytic anemia *402*

Hemoglobin *Blood Decrease Physiological* May cause hemolytic anemia *402*

Leukoagglutinins *Serum Positive Physiological* Reported observation *1240*

Lipase *Serum No Effect Analytical* No effect of concentrations up to 230 mg/L on method on Kodak Ektachem® *5706*

Methemoglobin *Blood Increase Physiological* May cause hemolytic anemia *4017*

Protein *Serum No Effect Analytical* At concentration of 80 mg/L had no effect on biuret method with blank correction *5704*

Urobilinogen *Urine Increase Analytical* Yields greenish color with Ehrlich's reagent *703*

Sulfarthrol

Platelets *Blood Increase Physiological* Mechanism of action unknown *1823*

Sulfasalazine

Alanine Aminotransferase *Serum Increase Physiological* Rare hepatotoxicity reported associated with noncaseating granuloma or focal inflammation with or without necrosis *1855* Occasional case of drug-induced toxic hepatitis *2365*

Alkaline Phosphatase *Serum Increase Physiological* In 2 cases with drug induced hepatotoxicity of hypersensitivity type of reaction: reversed on drug withdrawal *5624* In 14 female patients with rheumatoid arthritis treatment for 24 weeks caused a significant increase in activity *6011* As part of systemic hypersensitivity reaction in woman with inflammatory bowel disease *5723* Rare hepatotoxicity reported associated with noncaseating granuloma or focal inflammation with or without necrosis *1855* Occasional case of drug-induced toxic hepatitis *2365*

Alkaline Phosphatase, Bone Isoenzyme
Serum Increase Physiological In female patients with rheumatoid arthritis treatment caused significant increase from week 0 to week to 24 weeks *6011*

Anti-DNA Antibodies *Serum Increase Physiological* Antinative or double stranded DNA positive in a single patient with drug-induced lupus erythematosus *1056*

Antinuclear Antibodies *Serum Increase Physiological* ANA test positive and homogenous in a single patient with drug-induced lupus erythematosus *1056*

Aspartate Aminotransferase *Serum Increase Physiological* Hepatotoxic hypersensitivity reaction like sulfonamide hypersensitivity *3651* Rare hepatotoxicity reported associated with noncaseating granuloma or focal inflammation with or without necrosis *1855* Occasional case of drug-induced toxic hepatitis *2365* As part of systemic hypersensitivity reaction in woman with inflammatory bowel disease *5723* In 2 cases with drug induced hepatotoxicity of hypersensitivity type of reaction: reversed on drug withdrawal *5624*

Bilirubin *Serum Increase Physiological* Occasional case of drug-induced toxic hepatitis *2365* Theoretical displacement from protein in neonates although not observed in practice *6314* Hepatotoxic hypersensitivity reaction like sulfonamide hypersensitivity *3651* In 2 cases with drug induced hepatotoxicity of hypersensitivity type of reaction: reversed on drug withdrawal *5624* As part of systemic hypersensitivity reaction in woman with inflammatory bowel disease *5723*
Serum No Effect Analytical No effect at concentration of 38 mg/L on method on Kodak Ektachem® *5706* At therapeutic concentrations that had positive effect on conjugated bilirubin and negative effect on unconjugated bilirubin, had no effect on total as measured by Kodak Ektachem® 400 *1942*
Serum No Effect Physiological Characteristically associated with rare cases of hepatotoxicity *1855*

Bilirubin, Conjugated *Serum Increase Analytical* Conjugated concentration may be higher than total concentration as measured in Kodak Ektachem® 400 analyzer (same effect on Ektachem® 700 analyzer but algorithm prevented reporting of information) due to drug's strong absorbance at 400 nm *1941* At concentrations above 2 mg/L increases measurement as determined by method on Kodak Ektachem® : of clinical importance since normal therapeutic concentration is 20-40 mg/L *5706* At therapeutic concentrations (5-100 µg/mL) increased concentration as measured on Kodak Ektachem® 400 in a linear and dose related manner *1942*

Bilirubin, Direct *Serum Increase Physiological* Occasional case of drug-induced toxic hepatitis *2365*

Bilirubin, Unconjugated *Serum Decrease Analytical* Concentration reduced as measured by Kodak Ektachem® 400 to negative value at therapeutic concentrations of drug *1942* Decreases value as measured by Kodak Ektachem® at concentrations above 2 mg/L: of clinical significance since therapeutic concentration is 20-40 mg/L *5706*

Blood *Urine Increase Physiological* Toxic nephrosis, nephritis or nephrotic syndrome with hematuria, crystaluria or proteinuria reported with administration of sulfasalazine in fewer than 1 per thousand treated patients *4665*

Cholinesterase *Serum No Effect Analytical* No effect observed at concentration of 40 µg/mL with butyrylthiocholine method on Kodak Ektachem® *2504*

Chondrex *Serum No Effect Analytical* Concentrations up to 1 g/L had no significant effect on sandwich-type ELISA procedure of Harvey et al *2491*

Color *Urine Increase Analytical* Orange-yellow color observed following ingestion of sulfasalazine *3388*

C-Reactive Protein *Serum Decrease Physiological* Significant effect observed in about 300 patients with active rheumatoid arthritis treated for 3-6 months but with continued reduction for up to 60 months *5587* In 35 patients with juvenile chronic arthritis treated with 50 mg/kg/d for 24 weeks mean concentration decreased by 0.45 mg/L compared with 0.01 mg/L in 34 placebo treated controls *6196*

Creatinine *Serum Increase Analytical* At concentrations above 500 mg/L (normal therapeutic concentration 70 mg/L) raised concentration as measured by kinetic Jaffe method on BKA-2 *5704*
Serum Increase Physiological Toxic nephrosis, nephritis or nephrotic syndrome reported with administration of sulfasalazine in fewer than 1 per thousand treated patients *4665*

Crystals *Urine Increase Physiological* Toxic nephrosis, nephritis or nephrotic syndrome with hematuria, crystaluria or proteinuria reported with administration of sulfasalazine in fewer than 1 per thousand treated patients *4665*

Deoxypyridinoline *Urine Increase Analytical* Increased concentration observed due to overlapping peak when measured by HPLC *4587*

Digoxin *Serum Decrease Physiological* Reduces bioavailability in gastrointestinal tract *4631* Coadministration causes reduction in serum concentration but mechanism for this not established *2986* Absorption may be reduced when drugs given together *1384* Reduced absorption has been reported with concomitant administration of sulfasalazine *4665* By decreasing intestinal digoxin absorption may decrease the digoxin concentration *2161*

Eosinophils *Blood Increase Physiological* Characteristically associated with rare cases of hepatotoxicity *1855* Hepatotoxic hypersensitivity reaction like sulfonamide hyper-

Sulfasalazine *(continued)*

Eosinophils *(continued)*
sensitivity *3651* Observed in 11% of 18 patients treated with drug who had rheumatoid arthritis *5617* As part of systemic hypersensitivity reaction in woman with inflammatory bowel disease *5723*

Erythrocyte Sedimentation Rate
Blood Decrease Physiological In 35 patients with rheumatoid arthritis treatment with 1000 mg/d sulfasalazine and 400 mg/d hydroxychloroquine caused significant reduction from mean baseline of 45 ± 27 mm/h to 36 ± 29 mm/h after 9 mo and 16 ± 12 mm/h after 24 h *4361* Significant reduction observed with 3-6 months treatment in about 300 patients with active rheumatoid arthritis with continued reduction observed for up to 60 months *5587* In 35 patients with juvenile chronic arthritis treated with 50 mg/kg/d for 24 weeks mean rate decreased by 0.74 mm/h compared with 0.04 mm/h in 34 placebo treated controls *6196*

Erythrocytes *Blood Decrease Physiological* Pancytopenia reported plus reductions of individual series of cells *4814*

Folate *Red Blood Cells Decrease Physiological* Inversely correlated with drug dosage in 45 outpatients taking drug orally for ulcerative colitis *3642* Due to malabsorption with prolonged use *5055* Folate absorption from gastrointestinal tract may be inhibited to a minor degree: may lead to megaloblastic anemia if severe nutritional deficiency or celiac disease *3383*
Serum Decrease Physiological Reduced absorption has been reported with concomitant administration of sulfasalazine *4665* Due to malabsorption with prolonged use *5055* Folate deficiency is common in patients treated with sulfasalazine *1384* Folate absorption from gastrointestinal tract may be inhibited to a minor degree: may lead to megaloblastic anemia if severe nutritional deficiency or celiac disease *3383*
Serum No Effect Physiological No significant difference from controls in 45 outpatients taking drug orally for ulcerative colitis *3642*

γ-Glutamyltransferase *Serum Increase Physiological* Occasional case of drug-induced toxic hepatitis *2365* Rare hepatotoxicity reported associated with noncaseating granuloma or focal inflammation with or without necrosis *1855*

Granulocytes *Blood Decrease Physiological* Aplastic anemia or granulocytosis reported with administration of sulfasalazine in fewer than 1 per thousand treated patients *4665* Rare cases of agranulocytosis and other blood dyscrasias reported *1384*

HDL_3-Lipoprotein A-I *Serum Decrease Physiological* In37 patients with rheumatoid arthritis treatment with parenteral gold for 37 weeks caused mean rate to decrease from 50 ± 36 mm/h to 25 ± 17 mm/h *3999*

Hematocrit *Blood Decrease Physiological* Infrequent hemolytic anemia reported with administration of sulfasalazine *4665*

Hemoglobin *Blood Decrease Physiological* Either immune or nonimmune hemolytic anemia may occur *1384* Hemolysis quite common, but frank hemolytic anemia rare *4814* Infrequent hemolytic anemia reported with administration of sulfasalazine *4665*

Histamine *Plasma No Effect Analytical* Slight inhibition of radio-enzyme assay at twice therapeutic concentration *2492*

5-Hydroxyindoleacetic Acid *Urine Increase Analytical* In patients in whom sulfasalazine administered it coeluted at the same time with 5-HIAA when measured by liquid chromatographic method of Richards and Titheradge, although interference could be eliminated by alteration of pH of phosphate moiety of mobile phase *1150*

immunoglobulin A *Serum Decrease Physiological* In 35 patients with juvenile chronic arthritis treated with 50 mg/kg/d for 24 weeks mean concentration decreased significantly by 0.70 g/L compared with increase of 0.16 g/L in 34 placebo treated controls *6196* Reported reversible or permanent deficiency induced by sulfasalazine *2426*

Immunoglobulin G *Serum Decrease Physiological* In 35 patients with juvenile chronic arthritis treated with 50 mg/kg/d for 24 weeks mean concentration decreased significantly by 2.85 g/L compared with 0.10 g/L in 34 placebo treated controls *6196*

Immunoglobulin M *Serum Decrease Physiological* In 35 patients with juvenile chronic arthritis treated with 50 mg/kg/d for 24 weeks mean concentration decreased significantly by 0.50 g/L compared with increase of 0.09 g/L in 34 placebo treated controls *6196*

Lactate Dehydrogenase *Serum Increase Physiological* Rare hepatotoxicity reported associated with noncaseating granuloma or focal inflammation with or without necrosis *1855* In 2 cases with drug induced hepatotoxicity of hypersensitivity type of reaction: reversed on drug withdrawal *5624*

Leukocytes *Blood Decrease Physiological* Leukopenia reported with administration of sulfasalazine in fewer than 1 per thousand treated patients *4665* Pancytopenia reported plus reductions of individual series of cells *4814*
Blood Increase Physiological Characteristically associated with rare cases of hepatotoxicity *1855* Hepatotoxic hypersensitivity reaction like sulfonamide hypersensitivity *3651*

Lipase *Serum No Effect Analytical* No effect of concentrations up to 230 mg/L on method on Kodak Ektachem® *5706*

MCV *Blood Decrease Physiological* Megaloblastic anemia reported with administration of sulfasalazine in fewer than 1 per thousand treated patients *4665*

Methemoglobin *Blood Decrease Physiological* Methemoglobinemia reported with administration of sulfasalazine in fewer than 1 per thousand treated patients *4665*

Neutrophils *Blood Decrease Physiological* Neutropenia reported with administration of sulfasalazine in fewer than 1 per thousand treated patients *4665* Hemolysis quite common, but frank hemolytic anemia rare *4814* Rare cases of neutropenia reported *241*

Platelets *Blood Decrease Physiological* Pancytopenia reported plus reductions of individual series of cells *4814* Thrombocytopenia reported with administration of sulfasalazine in fewer than 1 per thousand treated patients *4665* Several cases of immune-mediated thrombocytopenia reported *4139*

Potassium *Serum Decrease Analytical* At concentrations above 1,000 mg/L (normal therapeutic concentration 70 mg/L) lowered concentration as measured by ISE without predilution *5704*

Protein *Semen No Effect Analytical* No effect when Du Pont aca turbidimetric method is used with 100 fold dilution of sperm *4116*
Serum Decrease Analytical Spuriously low values with biuret methods on Du Pont aca related to overblanking *4116*
Serum Increase Analytical When measured on a Beckman Synchron CX7 analyzer concentration of a specimen from a man taking 3 g sulfasalazine daily was 25 g/L compared with 43 g/L on a Kodak Ektachem® 700 and BMC-Hitachi 747-100 analyzer. Discrepancy probably related to polychromatics used to blank the biuret reaction in the CX7 analyzer *4155* At steady-state concentrations (2-5 mg/dL, 50-130 µmol/L) decrease results as determined by method on Du Pont aca by 20-40%. At serum concentrations below 0.1 mg/dL (25 µmol/L) no effect observed *1549*
Serum No Effect Analytical At concentration of 50 mg/L had no effect on biuret method with blank correction *5704*
Urine Increase Physiological Toxic nephrosis, nephritis or nephrotic syndrome with hematuria, crystaluria or proteinuria reported with administration of sulfasalazine in fewer than 1 per thousand treated patients *4665*

Protein Electrophoresis *Serum No Effect Analytical* At concentration of 1600 mg/L had no effect on automated Olympus-Hite method except for slight displacement of fractions *5704*

Prothrombin Time *Plasma Decrease Physiological* Hypoprothrombinemia reported with administration of sulfasalazine in fewer than 1 per thousand treated patients *4665*

Pyridinoline *Urine Increase Analytical* In patients with rheumatoid arthritis concentration increased when measured by HPLC procedure due to presence of overlapping peak *4587*

Sodium *Serum No Effect Analytical* At concentration of 1600 mg/L had no effect on measurement by ISE without predilution *5704*

Soluble Interleukin-2 Receptor
Serum Decrease Physiological In37 patients with rheumatoid arthritis treatment with sulfasalazine for 37 weeks caused mean concentration to decrease from 1031 ± 724 U/mL to 851 ± 432 U/mL *3999*

Sperm Count *Semen Decrease Physiological* Reversible oligospermia reported in one third of male patients with administration of sulfasalazine *4665* Often with abnormal sperm in high proportion of men: effect reversible *1499* Reversible oligospermia and infertility described *1384*

Urea Nitrogen *Serum Increase Physiological* Toxic nephrosis, nephritis or nephrotic syndrome reported with administration of sulfasalazine in fewer than 1 per thousand treated patients *4665*

Sulfathiazole

Ammonia *Plasma No Effect Analytical* No effect at concentration of 60 mg/L on method on Kodak Ektachem® *5706* At concentration of 60 mg/L had no effect on Kodak Ektachem® method *5704*

Aspartate Aminotransferase *Serum Increase Analytical* At 1 mmol/L affects Technicon SMA 12/60 method *5576*

Bilirubin *Serum No Effect Analytical* At concentration of 255 mg/L had no effect on Jendrassik and Grof method *5704* At concentration of 60 mg/L had no effect on Kodak Ektachem® method *5704*

Bilirubin, Conjugated *Serum No Effect Analytical* No effect at concentration of 60 mg/L on method on Kodak Ektachem® *5706*

Bilirubin, Unconjugated *Serum No Effect Analytical* No effect at concentration of 60 mg/L on method on Kodak Ektachem® *5706*

Calcium *Serum No Effect Analytical* At concentration of 255 mg/L had no effect on cresolphthalein method *5704*

Chloride *Serum No Effect Analytical* No effect of concentrations up to 60 mg/L on method on Kodak Ektachem® *5706*

Cholesterol *Serum No Effect Analytical* No effect of concentrations up to 60 mg/L on method on Kodak Ektachem® *5706*

Creatinine *Serum No Effect Analytical* No effect of concentrations up to 60 mg/L on single slide method on Kodak Ektachem® *5706* At concentration of 60 mg/L had no effect on Kodak Ektachem® method *5704* No effect of concentrations up to 60 mg/L on 2-slide method on Kodak Ektachem® *5706*

Glucose *Serum No Effect Analytical* At concentration of 50 mg/L had no effect on Kodak Ektachem® method *5704*

HDL-Cholesterol *Serum No Effect Analytical* No effect of concentrations up to 60 mg/L on method on Kodak Ektachem® *5706*

Hemoglobin *Blood No Effect Analytical* No effect of concentrations up to 60 mg/L on method on Kodak Ektachem® *5706*

Histamine *Plasma No Effect Analytical* No effect observed at therapeutic concentrations on radio-enzyme assay *2492*

Lipase *Serum No Effect Analytical* No effect of concentrations up to 60 mg/L on method on Kodak Ektachem® *5706*

Phosphate *Serum No Effect Analytical* At concentration of 255 mg/L had no effect on phosphomolybdate method *5704*

Protein *Serum No Effect Analytical* At concentration of 255 mg/L had no effect on biuret method with blank correction *5704*

Sugar *Urine Increase Analytical* Yellow-orange with Benedict's reagent *882*

Triglycerides *Serum No Effect Analytical* No effect of concentrations up to 60 mg/L on method on Kodak Ektachem® *5706*

Urea Nitrogen *Serum No Effect Analytical* At concentration of 255 mg/L had no effect on diacetylmonoxime method *5704* At concentration of 50 mg/L had no effect on Kodak Ektachem® method *5704*

Uric Acid *Serum No Effect Analytical* No effect of concentrations up to 1000 mg/L on method on Kodak Ektachem® *5706*

Urobilinogen *Urine Increase Analytical* Yields greenish color with Ehrlichs reagent *703*

Sulfhydryl Compounds

Alkaline Phosphatase *Serum Decrease Analytical* Inhibit enzyme activity in laboratory methods *6026*

Sulfinpyrazone

Aminohippurate *Serum Increase Physiological* Decreases renal transport and increases plasma concentration *1384*

Bilirubin *Serum Increase Physiological* Jaundice reported in cases with overdose *2754*

Cyclosporine *Serum Decrease Analytical* One case reported in whom cyclosporine concentration increased threefold when sulfinpyrazone discontinued. Presumed to be due to effect on analytical method *1069*

Erythrocytes *Blood Decrease Physiological* Rare blood dyscrasia *128*

p-Aminohippurate *Serum Increase Physiological* Decreases renal transport and increases plasma concentration *1384*

PAH Clearance *Urine Decrease Physiological* Inhibits tubular transport *128*

Phenolsulfonphthalein *Serum Increase Physiological* Inhibits renal tubular transport and increases plasma concentration *1384*

Phenprocoumon *Plasma No Effect Physiological* No effect on plasma concentration *4427*

Platelet Aggregation *Blood Decrease Physiological* Inhibits collagen induced aggregation *5112*

Prothrombin Time *Plasma Increase Physiological* May prolong action of anticoagulants *2753* When warfarin coadministered prolongs prothrombin time through stereoselective inhibition of clearance of S isomer *2625* When free warfarin concentration increased due to displacement from protein *4427* Drug may potentiate the action of coumarin-type anticoagulants when coadministered *1022*

PSP Excretion *Urine Decrease Physiological* Competition for excretion *1622*

Salicylate *Serum Increase Physiological* Inhibits renal tubular transport and increases plasma concentration *1384*

Sulfadiazine *Serum Increase Physiological* Displaces from protein binding *2452*

Sulfisoxazole *Serum Increase Physiological* Displaces from protein binding *2452*

Theophylline *Serum Decrease Physiological* Increases theophylline clearance by increasing demethylation and hydroxylation. By decreasing renal clearance of theophylline decreases its concentration by 20% *3125* Up to 20% decrease in serum theophylline concentration due to increased theophylline clearance caused by increased demethylation and hydroxylation and decreased renal clearance of theophylline *6117* Increases theophylline clearance by increasing hydroxylation and demethylation and decreases renal clearance of theophylline, decreasing theophylline concentration by about 20% *5999*

Uric Acid *Serum Decrease Physiological* Uricosuric action *2378* Drug has potent uricosuric effect *1022*
Urine Increase Physiological Drug has potent uricosuric effect *1022* Uricosuric action *2378*

Warfarin *Plasma Increase Physiological* Increased concentration due to displacement from protein *4427*

Sulfisoxazole

Alanine Aminotransferase *Serum Increase Physiological* May cause cholestasis *3211* Hepatitis or hepatocellular necrosis associated with drug administration observed in some treated patients *5022*

Albumin *Serum No Effect Analytical* No significant effect on BCG method at 500 mg/L *4335*

Alkaline Phosphatase *Serum Increase Physiological* Reversible cholestasis *3810* Hepatitis or hepatocellular necrosis associated with drug administration observed in some treated patients *5022*

Amylase *Serum Increase Physiological* May cause pancreatitis occasionally *2754*

Sulfisoxazole *(continued)*

Aspartate Aminotransferase *Serum Increase Physiological* Reversible cholestasis *3810* Hepatitis or hepatocellular necrosis associated with drug administration observed in some treated patients *5022*

Bile *Urine Increase Physiological* May cause reversible cholestasis *3810*

Bilirubin *Serum Decrease Physiological* In newborn combined with penicillin has effect *5869*
Serum Increase Physiological Hepatitis or hepatocellular necrosis associated with drug administration observed in some treated patients *5022* Displacement from protein in neonates *6314* May cause cholestatic jaundice or hemolysis *3211*
Serum No Effect Analytical At concentration of 60 mg/L had no effect on Kodak Ektachem® method *5704*

Bilirubin, Conjugated *Serum No Effect Analytical* No effect at concentration of 60 mg/L on method on Kodak Ektachem® *5706*

Bilirubin, Unconjugated *Serum No Effect Analytical* No effect at concentration of 60 mg/L on method on Kodak Ektachem® *5706*

Blood *Urine Increase Physiological* Hematuria associated with drug administration observed in some treated patients *5022*

BSP Retention *Serum Increase Physiological* May cause cholestasis *3211*

Creatinine *Serum Increase Physiological* Increased concentration associated with drug administration observed in some treated patients *5022*
Serum No Effect Analytical No effect of concentrations up to 15 mg/L on single slide method on Kodak Ektachem® *5706*

Crystals *Urine Increase Physiological* Crystaluria associated with drug administration observed in some treated patients *5022* May occur particularly in acidic urine *6455*

Diagnex Blue Excretion *Urine Increase Physiological* Displacement of diagnex blue from resin *6515*

Eosinophils *Blood Increase Physiological* Eosinophilia associated with drug administration observed in some treated patients *5022* Allergic response *3211*

Erythrocytes *Blood Decrease Physiological* Agranulocytosis/aplastic anemia *4780* As result of bone marrow depression or hemolysis (in patients with glucose-6-phosphate dehydrogenase deficiency) *6455*

Fibrinogen *Plasma Decrease Physiological* Decreased concentration associated with drug administration observed in some treated patients *5022*

Folate *Serum Decrease Analytical* Affects standard autoclave method *2965*

Glucose *Serum Decrease Physiological* Hypoglycemia associated with drug administration observed rarely in treated patients *5022*
Serum No Effect Analytical No effect on Boehringer GOD-PERID glucose oxidase method *5480*

γ-Glutamyltransferase *Serum Increase Physiological* Hepatitis or hepatocellular necrosis associated with drug administration observed in some treated patients *5022*

Granulocytes *Blood Decrease Physiological* Agranulocytosis associated with drug administration observed in some treated patients *5022*

Haptoglobin *Serum Decrease Physiological* May cause hemolytic anemia *3211*

Hematocrit *Blood Decrease Physiological* Aplastic or hemolytic anemia associated with drug administration observed in some treated patients *5022* Agranulocytosis/aplastic anemia *4780*

Hemoglobin *Blood Decrease Physiological* Aplastic or hemolytic anemia associated with drug administration observed in some treated patients *5022* Agranulocytosis/aplastic anemia *4780*

Lactate Dehydrogenase *Serum Increase Physiological* May cause hemolytic anemia *3211* Hepatitis or hepatocellular necrosis associated with drug administration observed in some treated patients *5022*

LE Cells *Blood Positive Physiological* May cause LE phenomenon (rare) *2754*

Leukocytes *Blood Decrease Physiological* Agranulocytosis/aplastic anemia *4780* Leukopenia associated with drug administration observed in some treated patients *5022*

Lipase *Serum Increase Physiological* Rare effect on pancreas, salivary glands *4014*

Methemoglobin *Blood Increase Physiological* May cause hemolytic anemia *5008* Sulfhemoglobinemia associated with drug administration observed in some treated patients *5022*

Methotrexate *Serum Increase Physiological* Displaces from plasma protein binding *2452*

Occult Blood *Feces Increase Physiological* Gastrointestinal hemorrhage or melena associated with drug administration observed in some treated patients *5022*

Phenytoin *Serum Increase Physiological* Displaces from protein *in vitro2452*

Platelets *Blood Decrease Physiological* Agranulocytosis/aplastic anemia (after days) *4780* Isolated case of platelet-associated IgG and thrombocytopenia *3102*

Potassium *Serum No Effect Analytical* At concentration of 80,000 mg/L had no effect on measurement by ISE with predilution *5704*

Protein *Cerebrospinal Fluid Increase Analytical* Causes turbidity if sulfosalicylic acid used *5869*
Cerebrospinal Fluid No Effect Analytical At 100 mg/dL on TCA dye method of Pesce *4625*
Urine Increase Analytical Causes turbidity if sulfosalicylic acid used *5869* May produce turbidity with acid methods *703* False positive with Exton's reagent. No effect with acetic acid and heat methods *684* May cause false positive with Sulfosalicylic Acid and Exton's reagent tests *4034*
Urine No Effect Analytical At 100 mg/dL on TCA dye method of Pesce *4625* No effect on Albustix *703* No effect observed with protein test areas on Ames Multistix and other reagent strip tests *4034*

Prothrombin *Plasma Decrease Physiological* Decreased concentration associated with drug administration observed in some treated patients *5022*

Prothrombin Time *Plasma Increase Physiological* Occurs with failure of excretion of bile salts *1405*

Sodium *Serum No Effect Analytical* At concentration of 80,000 mg/L had no effect on measurement by ISE with predilution *5704*

Sulfhemoglobin *Blood Increase Physiological* Sulfhemoglobinemia associated with drug administration observed in some treated patients *5022*

Tolbutamide *Serum Increase Physiological* Displaces from protein *2452*

Urea Nitrogen *Serum Increase Physiological* Increased concentration associated with drug administration observed in some treated patients *5022*

Urobilinogen *Feces Decrease Physiological* Pale stools with reversible cholestasis *3211*
Urine Decrease Physiological With reversible cholestasis *3211*
Urine Increase Analytical Reacts with Urobilistix® *2452*

Volume *Urine Increase Physiological* Diuresis associated with drug administration observed rarely in treated patients *5022*

Sulfobromophthalein

Acetone *Urine Increase Analytical* Development of color at alkaline pH (Rothera test) *6515*

Alkaline Phosphatase *Serum Increase Analytical* If final color developed in alkaline solution *882*

Bilirubin *Serum No Effect Analytical* At a concentration of 150 µg/mL had no significant effect on method on Kodak Ektachem® systems *2519*

Calcium *Serum Increase Analytical* Affects methylthymol method of Gindler/King *2126* May interfere with colorimetric procedures *4012*

Color *Feces Increase Analytical* Alkaline stools may appear bloody *882*
Urine Increase Analytical Red in alkaline urine *5619*

Creatine *Serum Increase Analytical* Presence of interfering color *3810*

Creatinine *Serum Increase Analytical* Presence of interfering color *3810*
Serum No Effect Analytical No interference observed at a concentration of 10 mg/L althoughndetected by HPLC method of Rosano et al because it elutes at 18.0 minutes compared with 8.9 minutes for creatinine *5083* No interference observed at a concentration of 10 mg/L although detected by HPLC method of Rosano et al because it elutes at 18.0 minutes compared with 8.9 minutes for creatinine *5083*

^{131}I Uptake *Serum No Effect Physiological* No effect on uptake reported *3669*

Ketones *Urine Increase Analytical* Produces purple color with alkaline nitroprusside *882* False positive color react with BiliLabstix® in acid urine *2452*

Occult Blood *Feces No Effect Analytical* No effect on tests for occult blood *882*

Protein *Serum Increase Analytical* Color augmentation with alkaline biuret *879*

PSP Excretion *Urine Increase Analytical* Development of color at alkaline pH *6515*

Urobilinogen *Urine Increase Analytical* Color development with Ehrlich's aldehyde reagent *6515*
Urine Increase Physiological Presence of BSP in urine and liver disease *1714*

Vanillylmandelic Acid *Urine Increase Analytical* Occurs unless completely extracted *140*

Sulfomethane

δ-Aminolevulinic Acid *Urine Increase Physiological* May provoke attack of porphyria *2210*

Color *Urine Increase Analytical* Red-brown (may provoke porphyria) *3810*

Coproporphyrin *Blood Increase Physiological* May provoke attack of porphyria *2210*
Feces Increase Physiological May provoke attack of porphyria *2210*
Urine Increase Physiological May provoke attack of porphyria *2210*

Methemoglobin *Blood Increase Physiological* May cause hemolytic anemia *4017*

Porphobilinogen *Urine Increase Physiological* May provoke attack of porphyria *2210*

Porphyrin, Total *Urine Increase Physiological* Stimulates formation of ALA-synthetase *2242*

Protoporphyrin *Blood Increase Physiological* May provoke attack of porphyria *2210*
Feces Increase Physiological May provoke attack of porphyria *2210*

Uroporphyrin *Urine Increase Physiological* May provoke attack of porphyria *2210*

Sulfonamides

Chlorpropamide *Serum Increase Physiological* Drugs that are highly protein-bound compete with chlorpropamide for binding sites and may potentiate hypoglycemic action of sulfonylurea *4644*

Color *Feces Increase Analytical* Black color reported following ingestion of sulfonamides *3388*

Glucose *Urine Increase Analytical* May interfere with Ames 2-drop Clinitest method at concentrations below 0.5 g/dL *4034*
Urine No Effect Analytical Have no effect on Ames Keto-Diastix, Diastix, Multistix and Clinistix methods *4034*

Phenytoin *Serum Increase Physiological* Coadministration of sulfonamides with phenytoin may increase plasma phenytoin concentration *4522* When sulfonamides ingested with fosphenytoin concentration of phenytoin may be increased *4519* Some sulfonamides cause increase in concentration when drugs coadministered through enzyme inhibition *6350* Significant increase in concentrations when drugs coadministered *1384*

Uric Acid *Serum No Effect Analytical* No effect up to 150 mg/L on uricase method on Ames Seralyzer but at higher concentrations disproportionately increased concentrations observed *5706*

Urobilinogen *Urine Increase Analytical* May react with urobilinogen test area of Ames Multistix and other reagent strips *4034*
Urine No Effect Analytical No effect observed with Watson semi-quantitative test if blank is used *4034*

Sulfones

Alanine Aminotransferase *Serum Increase Physiological* May affect liver function *3810*

Alkaline Phosphatase *Serum Increase Physiological* May affect liver function *3810*

Aspartate Aminotransferase *Serum Increase Physiological* May affect liver function *3810*

Bile *Urine Increase Physiological* May affect liver function *3810*

Bilirubin *Serum Increase Physiological* May cause hemolysis with G-6-PD deficiency *402*

BSP Retention *Serum Increase Physiological* May affect liver function *3810*

Erythrocytes *Blood Decrease Physiological* Hemolysis may occur with G-6-PD deficiency *3810*
Urine Increase Physiological May have nephrotoxic effect *3810*

Glutathione, Reduced
Red Blood Cells Decrease Physiological Falls sharply preceding hemolysis *3094*

Haptoglobin *Serum Decrease Physiological* May cause hemolytic anemia *402*

Heinz Body Formation *Blood Positive Physiological* Reported effect in first few days *2242*

Hematocrit *Blood Decrease Physiological* May cause hemolysis *128*

Hemoglobin *Blood Decrease Physiological* May cause hemolysis *128*
Plasma Increase Physiological May occur with hemolysis *4013*
Urine Increase Physiological May have nephrotoxic effect *1714*

Leukocytes *Blood Decrease Physiological* Agranulocytosis/Leukopenia *128*

Methemoglobin *Blood. Increase Physiological* Hemolysis may occur with G-6-PD deficiency *128*

Protein *Urine Increase Physiological* May have nephrotoxic effect *1714*

Reticulocytes *Blood Increase Physiological* Occurs during recovery phase *3094*

Sulfonylureas

Acetaldehyde *Blood Increase Physiological* Mechanism not yet elucidated *2242*

Alanine Aminotransferase *Serum Increase Physiological* Moderate elevation with cholangiolitis *5310*

Alkaline Phosphatase *Serum Increase Physiological* Elevation with cholangiolitis *5310*

Aspartate Aminotransferase *Serum Increase Physiological* Moderate elevation with cholangiolitis *5310*

Bilirubin *Serum Increase Physiological* In some cases probably attributable to drug *4014*

Cholesterol *Serum No Effect Physiological* In 72 insulin treated patients with NIDDM mean concentration 6.2 ± 1.4 mmol/L not significantly different from 6.3 ± 1.4 mmol/L in 20 diet treated patients *2532* Usual effect reported *492*

Coombs' Test *Blood Positive Physiological* May cause immune hemolytic anemia *575*

Creatinine *Serum Decrease Physiological* In 57 sulfonylurea treated patients with NIDDM mean concentration of 75 ± 14 µmol/L not significantly less than 92 ± 25 µmol/L in 20 diet treated patients *2532*

Sulfonylureas *(continued)*

Eosinophils *Blood Increase Physiological* May occur in association with cholangiolitis *5310*

Erythrocytes *Blood Decrease Physiological* Occasional case of aplastic anemia reported *6264* Pancytopenia *3810*

Glucose *Serum Decrease Physiological* Incidence of 11.3% observed in French Pharmacovigilance database *4106* May cause severe hypoglycemia *4014*
Serum Increase Physiological In 57 sulfonylurea treated patients with NIDDM mean concentration 9.2 ± 3.1 mmol/L compared with 6.5 ± 1.9 mmol/L in diet treated patients *2532*

Glycated Hemoglobin *Blood Increase Physiological* In 57 sulfonylurea treated NIDDM patients mean concentration of 8.2 ± 1.7 % significantly higher than 6.6 ± 1.2 % in 20 diet treated patients *2532*

HDL-Cholesterol *Serum No Effect Physiological* In 57 sulfonylurea treated patients with NIDDM mean concentration of 6.5 ± 1.4 mmol/L not significantly different from 6.3 ± 1.4 mmol/L in 20 diet treated patients *2532*

^{131}I Uptake *Serum Decrease Physiological* Due to impaired synthesis of thyroxine *3107*

Leukocytes *Blood Decrease Physiological* Occasional case of aplastic anemia reported *6264* Pancytopenia/agranulocytosis *3810*

Lipoprotein Lp(a) *Serum No Effect Physiological* In 57 sulfonylurea treated patients with NIDDM mean concentration of 173 U/L not significantly different from 190 U/L in 20 diet treated controls *2532*

Phenytoin, Free *Serum Increase Physiological* Cause increase in free fraction when drugs coadministered *6350*

Platelets *Blood Decrease Physiological* Occasional case of aplastic anemia reported *6264* Pancytopenia *3810*

Sodium *Serum Decrease Physiological* Potentiates vasopressin, causes water retention *1864*

T3-Uptake *Serum Increase Physiological* Resin uptake increase due to impaired synthesis of T4 *3107*
Serum No Effect Physiological Probably no effect in most patients *2452*

Thyroxine (T4) *Serum Decrease Physiological* Due to competition for transport proteins *6412* Sulfonylurea derivatives inhibit T4 binding to TBG *2412* Due to impaired synthesis *3107*

Tri-iodothyronine (T3) *Serum Decrease Physiological* Sulfonylurea derivatives nihibit binding of T3 to TBG *2412*

Triglycerides *Serum Decrease Physiological* Effect reported for some compounds *492*
Serum No Effect Physiological In 57 sulfonylurea treated patients with NIDDM mean concentration of 1.82 mmol/L not significantly different from 1.93 mmol/L in 20 diet patients *2532*

Urea Nitrogen *Serum Increase Analytical* Theoretical effect of ureide group on diacetyl method *882*

Sulforidazine

Bilirubin *Serum No Effect Analytical* At concentration of 200 mg/L had no effect on Jendrassik and Grof method *5704*

Calcium *Serum No Effect Analytical* At concentration of 200 mg/L had no effect on cresolphthalein method *5704*

Cholesterol *Serum No Effect Analytical* At concentration of 200 mg/L had no effect on Liebermann-Burchard method *5704*

Creatinine *Serum No Effect Analytical* At concentration of 200 mg/L had no effect on Technicon AutoAnalyzer® Jaffe method *5704*

Iron *Serum No Effect Analytical* At concentration of 200 mg/L had no effect on Ferrozine method *5704*

Phosphate *Serum No Effect Analytical* At concentration of 200 mg/L had no effect on phosphomolybdate method *5704*

Protein *Serum No Effect Analytical* At concentration of 200 mg/L had no effect on biuret method with blank correction *5704*

Triglycerides *Serum No Effect Analytical* At concentration of 200 mg/L had no effect on lipase/esterase method *5704*

Urea Nitrogen *Serum No Effect Analytical* At concentration of 200 mg/L had no effect on diacetylmonoxime method *5704*

Uric Acid *Serum No Effect Analytical* At concentration of 200 mg/L had no effect on phosphotungstate reduction method *5704*

Sulfoxone

Bilirubin *Serum Increase Physiological* May cause hemolysis in G-6-PD deficiency *402*

Erythrocytes *Blood Decrease Physiological* May cause hemolytic anemia *402*

Haptoglobin *Serum Decrease Physiological* May cause hemolytic anemia *402*

Hematocrit *Blood Decrease Physiological* May cause hemolytic anemia *402*

Hemoglobin *Blood Decrease Physiological* May cause hemolytic anemia *402*

Methemoglobin *Blood Increase Physiological* May cause hemolysis in G-6-PD deficiency *6015*

Sulindac

Alanine Aminotransferase *Serum Increase Physiological* Sulindac administration may cause hypersensitivity reactions or cholestatichepatitis. Borderline increases of liver function tests may occur in as many as 15% of patients receiving the drug. Increases above 3 times the upper limit of normal may occur in less than 1% patients *3963* Incidence of acute liver injury of 148.1 per 100,000 treated patients with reported in United Kingdom. Liver damage among all cases primarily hepatocellular in some and primarily cholestatic in others *5049* Isolated case of cholestatic jaundice 12 d after therapy started *3901*

Aldosterone *Plasma No Effect Physiological* In 10 furosemide treated patients with well controlled congestive heart failure given 400 mg/d for 2 d *1749*

Alkaline Phosphatase *Serum Increase Physiological* Isolated case of cholestatic jaundice 12 d after therapy started *3901* Sulindac administration may cause hypersensitivity reactions or cholestatichepatitis. Borderline increases of liver function tests may occur in as many as 15% of patients receiving the drug *3963*

Amylase *Serum Increase Physiological* Sulindac administration has been reported to cause pancreatitis *3963*

Aspartate Aminotransferase *Serum Increase Physiological* Sulindac administration may cause hypersensitivity reactions or cholestatichepatitis. Borderline increases of liver function tests may occur in as many as 15% of patients receiving the drug. Increases above 3 times the upper limit of normal may occur in less than 1% patients *3963* Incidence of acute liver injury of 148.1 per 100,000 treated patients with reported in United Kingdom. Liver damage among all cases primarily hepatocellular in some and primarily cholestatic in others *5049* Isolated case of cholestatic jaundice 12 d after therapy started *3901*

Bilirubin *Serum Increase Physiological* Isolated case of cholestatic jaundice 12 d after therapy started *3901* Sulindac administration has been reported to cause pancreatitis *3963* Sulindac administration may cause hypersensitivity reactions or cholestatichepatitis. Borderline increases of liver function tests may occur in as many as 15% of patients receiving the drug *3963*

Bleeding Time *Patient Increase Physiological* Like aspirin increases bleeding time: effect transient and not detectable 24 hours after discontinuation of drug *1384*

Blood *Urine Increase Physiological* Sulindac administration may cause hematuria in less than 1% of treated patients. Long-term sulindac administration has been reported to cause acute interstitial nephritis with hematuria, proteinuria and occasionally nephrotic syndrome *3963*

Chloride *Urine No Effect Physiological* In 10 furosemide treated patients with well controlled congestive heart failure given 400 mg/d for 2 d *1749*

Chondrex *Serum No Effect Analytical* Concentrations up to 5 g/L had no significant effect on sandwich-type ELISA procedure of Harvey et al *2491*

Color *Urine Increase Physiological* Sulindac administration may cause abnormal color *3963*

Creatinine *Serum Increase Physiological* Sulindac administration may cause renal impairment including renal failure in less than 1% of treated patients *3963*
Serum No Effect Physiological No significant change in patients with chronic glomerular disease *1018*

Creatinine Clearance *Urine Decrease Physiological* Small but significant effect with treatment for 9 d in 9 patients with stable renal insufficiency *4070*
Urine No Effect Physiological No significant change in patients with chronic glomerular disease *1018* When given for 14 d to patients with rheumatoid arthritis and heart failure. Marked effect *5889*

Crystals *Urine Increase Physiological* Sulindac administration may cause crystalluria in less than 1% of treated patients *3963*

Cyclosporine *Serum Increase Physiological* More than 2-fold increase observed in one 47-year old renal transplant patient together with < 0.5 mg/dL increase in plasma creatinine conentration. After sulindac discontinued plasma cyclosporine and creatinine concentrations reverted to normal *6596* More than 2-fold increase observed in one renal transplant recipient when sulindac given as 300 mg/day, but associated with increase in serum creatinine concentration of < 0.5 mg/dL within 1 to 2 days of sulindac therapy *5453*

2,3-Dinor-6-Keto-Prostaglandin $F_{1\alpha}$
Urine Decrease Physiological Effect observed in mildly hypertensive patients after 7 days treatment after two weeks without antihypertensive therapy *4065*

2,3-Dinor-Thromboxane B_2 *Urine Decrease Physiological* Reduced excretion observed in mildly hypertensive patients after 7 days treatment following two weeks without antihypertensive medication *4065*

Effective Renal Plasma Flow
Patient No Effect Physiological In 9 individuals with stable renal insufficiency when treated for 9 d *4070*

Fractional Excretion of Potassium
Urine Decrease Physiological In individuals treated with 200 mg twice times daily caused 10% reduction, 11.5% in elderly and 12.5% in elderly with renal insufficiency *4189*

Fractional Excretion of Sodium
Urine Decrease Physiological In individuals treated with 200 mg twice times daily caused 0.6% reduction, 0.9% in elderly and 1.4% in elderly with renal insufficiency *4189*

Glucose *Serum Increase Physiological* Sulindac administration has been possibly associated with hyperglycemia *3963*

γ-Glutamyltransferase *Serum Increase Physiological* Sulindac administration may cause hypersensitivity reactions or cholestatichepatitis. Borderline increases of liver function tests may occur in as many as 15% of patients receiving the drug *3963* Isolated case of cholestatic jaundice 12 d after therapy started *3901*

Granulocytes *Blood Decrease Physiological* Sulindac administration may cause agranulocytosis in less than 1% of treated patients *3963*

Hematocrit *Blood Decrease Physiological* Sulindac administration may cause aplastic or hemolytic anemia in less than 1% of treated patients *3963*

Hemoglobin *Blood Decrease Physiological* Sulindac administration may cause aplastic or hemolytic anemia in less than 1% of treated patients *3963*

6-Keto-Prostaglandin $F_{1\alpha}$ *Urine Decrease Physiological* Effect observed in mildly hypertensive patients after 7 days treatment following 2 weeks without antihypertensive medication *4065*
Urine No Effect Physiological No significant change in patients with chronic glomerular disease *1018*

Lactate Dehydrogenase *Serum Increase Physiological* Observed with other laboratory evidence of hepatitis in 1 child *3072*

Leukocytes *Blood Decrease Physiological* Sulindac administration may cause leukopenia in less than 1% of treated patients *3963*

Lipase *Serum Increase Physiological* Sulindac administration has been reported to cause pancreatitis *3963*

Lithium *Serum No Effect Physiological* Sulindac administration appears to have no effect on plasma lithium concentration *4399* 300 mg/d did not significantly affect plasma concentration in several studies *4831*

Lithium Clearance *Urine No Effect Physiological* No significant effect observed in one study involving a patient population with a mean age of 59 years *4831*

Neutrophils *Blood Decrease Physiological* Sulindac administration may cause neutropenia in less than 1% of treated patients *3963*

Occult Blood *Feces Increase Physiological* Sulindac administration may cause peptic ulceration and gastrointestinal bleeding. Occurs in less than 1% of treated patients *3963*

PAH Clearance *Urine No Effect Physiological* No significant change in patients with chronic glomerular disease *1018*

Platelet Aggregation *Blood Decrease Physiological* Like aspirin inhibits platelet aggregation but effect transient and not detectable 24 hours after discontinuation of drug *1384*

Platelets *Blood Decrease Physiological* After 3 d of 400 mg/d in one patient reversible but mechanism not understood. No other effects on bone marrow noted *3039* Sulindac administration may cause thrombocytopenia in less than 1% of treated patients *3963*

Potassium *Serum Increase Physiological* Sulindac administration may cause hyperkalemia in less than 1% of treated patients *3963*

Prostaglandin $F_{2\alpha}$ *Urine Decrease Physiological* When given for 14 d to patients with rheumatoid arthritis and heart failure. Marked effect *5889*
Urine No Effect Physiological In 10 furosemide treated patients with well controlled congestive heart failure *1749*

Prostaglandins *Urine Decrease Physiological* When given for 14 d to patients with rheumatoid arthritis and heart failure. Marked effect *5889* In 11 normal volunteers contrary to concept of sparing renal but inhibiting systemic prostaglandins *698*
Urine No Effect Physiological No significant change in patients with chronic glomerular disease *1018*

Protein *Serum Decrease Physiological* Long-term sulindac administration has been reported to cause occasionally nephrotic syndrome *3963*
Urine Increase Physiological Long-term sulindac administration has been reported to cause acute interstitial nephritis with hematuria, proteinuria and occasionally nephrotic syndrome *3963*

Prothrombin Time *Plasma Increase Physiological* Sulindac administration with coumadin and other oral anticoagulants may cause increased prothrombin time *3963*

Renal Blood Flow *Patient Decrease Physiological* Long-term sulindac administration has been occasionally associated in patients with prerenal and renal conditions with a form of renal toxicity that leads to reduced renal blood flow or blood volume. In such patients a dose dependent reduction in prostaglandin formation occurs with overt renal decompensation *3963*

Renin Activity *Plasma Decrease Physiological* When given for 14 d to patients with rheumatoid arthritis and heart failure. Marked effect *5889*
Plasma No Effect Physiological No significant change in patients with chronic glomerular disease *1018* In 10 furosemide treated patients with well controlled congestive heart failure given 400 mg/d for 2 d *1749* In 9 individuals with stable renal insufficiency when treated for 9 d *4070*

Sodium *Urine No Effect Physiological* In 9 individuals with stable renal insufficiency when treated for 9 d *4070* In 10 furosemide treated patients with well controlled congestive heart failure given 400 mg/d for 2 d *1749*

Thromboxane B_2 *Plasma Decrease Physiological* 85% reduction in patients with chronic glomerular disease *1018*
Urine Decrease Physiological In 11 normal volunteers contrary to concept of sparing renal but inhibiting systemic prostaglandins *1214*
Urine No Effect Physiological No significant effect observed in mildly hypertensive patients after 7 days treatment following two weeks without antihypertensive medication *4065*

Thyroid Stimulating Hormone
Serum No Effect Physiological In 12 individuals treated with a mean dose of 383 mg/d for at least 3 weeks mean concentration of 1.4 ± 0.2 mU/L not significantly different from 1.5 ± 0.2 mU/L in 22 controls *585*

Sulindac *(continued)*

Thyroxine (T4) *Serum No Effect Physiological* In 12 individuals treated with a mean dose of 383 mg/d for at least 3 weeks mean concentration of 93 ± 4 nmol/L not significantly different from 94 ± 4 nmol/L in 22 controls *585*

Thyroxine (T4) Index, Free *Serum No Effect Physiological* In 12 individuals treated with a mean dose of 383 mg/d for at least 3 weeks mean FTI 85 ± 4 not significantly different from 93 ± 4 in 22 controls *585*

Tolbutamide *Serum No Effect Physiological* No significant effect noted on plasma concentration *5166*

Tri-iodothyronine (T3) *Serum No Effect Physiological* In 12 individuals treated with a mean dose of 383 mg/d for at least 3 weeks mean concentration of 1.8 ± 0.1 nmol/L not significantly different from 2.0 ± 0.1 nmol/L in 22 controls *585*

Urea Nitrogen *Serum Increase Physiological* Sulindac administration may cause renal impairment including renal failure in less than 1% of treated patients *3963*

Volume *Blood Decrease Physiological* Long-term sulindac administration has been occasionally associated in patients with prerenal and renal conditions with a form of renal toxicity that leads to reduced renal blood flow or blood volume. In such patients a dose dependent reduction in prostaglandin formation occurs with overt renal decompensation *3963*
Urine No Effect Physiological In 10 furosemide treated patients with well controlled congestive heart failure given 400 mg/d for 2 d *1749* In 9 individuals with stable renal insufficiency when treated for 9 d *4070*

Sulodexide

Albumin *Urine Decrease Physiological* In 7 type-I diabetics with microalbuminuria and 7 with macroalbuminuria treatment with 60 mg/d for 10 days then 50 mg for 21 days caused significant change from median baseline of 298 mg/d to 181 mg/d after 10 days and 46 after the additional 21 days *4752*

Cholesterol *Serum No Effect Physiological* In 7 type-I diabetics with microalbuminuria and 7 with macroalbuminuria treatment with 60 mg/d for 10 days then 50 mg for 21 days caused no significant change from mean baseline of 185 ± 19 mg/dL to 186 ± 8 mg/dL *4752*

Creatinine *Serum No Effect Physiological* In 7 type-I diabetics with microalbuminuria and 7 with macroalbuminuria treatment with 60 mg/d for 10 days then 50 mg for 21 days caused no significant change from mean baseline of 1.2 ± 0.2 mg/dL to 1.0 ± 0.5 mg/dL *4752*

Creatinine Clearance *Urine No Effect Physiological* In 7 type-I diabetics with microalbuminuria and 7 with macroalbuminuria treatment with 60 mg/d for 10 days then 50 mg for 21 days caused no significant change from mean baseline of 94.5 ± 21.3 mL/min to 88.7 ± 15.6 mL/min *4752*

Fibrinogen *Plasma No Effect Physiological* In 7 type-I diabetics with microalbuminuria and 7 with macroalbuminuria treatment with 60 mg/d for 10 days then 50 mg for 21 days caused no significant change from mean baseline of 264 ± 54 mg/dL to 248 ± 48 mg/dL *4752*

Glycated Hemoglobin *Blood No Effect Physiological* In 7 type-I diabetics with microalbuminuria and 7 with macroalbuminuria treatment with 60 mg/d for 10 days then 50 mg for 21 days caused no significant change from mean baseline of 6.9 ± 0.4% to 7.1 ± 0.2% *4752*

HDL-Cholesterol *Serum No Effect Physiological* In 7 type-I diabetics with microalbuminuria and 7 with macroalbuminuria treatment with 60 mg/d for 10 days then 50 mg for 21 days caused no significant change from mean baseline of 44 ± 4 mg/dL to 42 ± 5 mg/dL *4752*

Hematocrit *Blood No Effect Physiological* In 7 type-I diabetics with microalbuminuria and 7 with macroalbuminuria treatment with 60 mg/d for 10 days then 50 mg for 21 days caused no significant change from mean baseline of 43.0 ± 0.4% to 42.7 ± 0.5% *4752*

Partial Thromboplastin Time
Plasma No Effect Physiological In 7 type-I diabetics with microalbuminuria and 7 with macroalbuminuria treatment with 60 mg/d for 10 days then 50 mg for 21 days caused no significant change from mean baseline of 1.06 ± 0.13 to 1.07 ± 0.09 *4752*

Triglycerides *Serum No Effect Physiological* In 7 type-I diabetics with microalbuminuria and 7 with macroalbuminuria treatment with 60 mg/d for 10 days then 50 mg for 21 days caused no significant change from mean baseline of 87 ± 5 mg/dL to 86 ± 3 mg/dL *4752*

Sulpiride

Cholesterol *Serum Decrease Analytical* At 15 mg/dL affects conventional methods when added to serum *2877*

Estradiol *Plasma No Effect Physiological* In 11 healthy women between 6 and 9 weeks of pregnancy given 150 mg daily for 2 weeks *6602*

Glucose *Serum Decrease Analytical* At 15 mg/dL with conventional methods when added to serum *2877*

Histamine *Plasma No Effect Analytical* Although 50% inhibition of radio-enzyme assay occurs at 14 μg/mL no clinical effects likely since physiological concentration 0.18 - 0.32 μg/mL *2492*

Metanephrine *Urine No Effect Analytical* At 2 mg/L on HPLC method *557*

Normetanephrine *Urine No Effect Analytical* At 2 mg/L on HPLC method *557*

p-Aminophenol *Urine No Effect Analytical* With addition of drugs at a concentration of 100 mg/L and of related compounds at 50 mg/L no significant effect observed on colorimetric method of van Bocxlaer on Cobas Mira analyzer which involves reacting free p-aminophenol with resorcinol in the presence of magnesium ions to form an indophenol dye measured at 550 nm *6163*

Placental Lactogen *Plasma No Effect Physiological* In 11 healthy women between 6 and 9 weeks of pregnancy given 150 mg daily for 2 weeks *6602*

Progesterone *Plasma No Effect Physiological* In 11 healthy women between 6 and 9 weeks of pregnancy given 150 mg daily for 2 weeks *6602*

Prolactin *Plasma Increase Physiological* After 1 and 2 weeks in 11 healthy women between 6 and 9 weeks of pregnancy given 150 mg daily for 2 weeks *6602* General effect observed *2836*

Testosterone *Serum No Effect Physiological* General effect observed *2836* In 11 healthy women between 6 and 9 weeks of pregnancy given 150 mg daily for 2 weeks *6602*

Sulthiame

Carbonic Anhydrase
Red Blood Cells Decrease Physiological Metabolic action of drug *2306*

Crystals *Urine Increase Physiological* In poisoning identified as pure drug *4014*

Leukocytes *Blood Decrease Physiological* Leukopenia/also increases half life of diphenylhydantoin *2242*

Occult Blood *Feces Increase Physiological* One case reported with poisoning *4014*

Phenytoin *Serum Increase Physiological* Concomitant administration of sulthiame probably inhibits hepatic metabolism of diphenylhydantoin *2441* Increase from 10 to 20 μg/mL (at dose of 200-800 mg/d) *3339* Probably acts on liver enzymes *4951*

Sultopride

Cortisol *Plasma No Effect Physiological* When given 300-600 mg/d for 5 weeks in 5 schizophrenic women *4080*

Estradiol *Plasma No Effect Physiological* When given 300-600 mg/d for 5 weeks in 5 schizophrenic women *4080*

Follicle Stimulating Hormone
Plasma No Effect Physiological When given 300 - 600 mg/d for 5 weeks in 5 schizophrenic women *4080*

Growth Hormone *Plasma Decrease Physiological* After 1 week, but normal after 3-5 weeks *4080*

Insulin *Plasma No Effect Physiological* When given 300-600 mg/d for 5 weeks in 5 schizophrenic women *4080*

Luteinizing Hormone *Plasma No Effect Physiological* When given 300 - 600 mg/d for 5 weeks in 5 schizophrenic women *4080*

Prolactin *Plasma Increase Physiological* After 1 d, maximum at 1 week increase throughout treatment, probably by blocking pituitary dopamine receptors *4080*

Thyroid Stimulating Hormone
Serum No Effect Physiological When given 300-600 mg/d for 5 weeks in 5 schizophrenic women *4080*

Sumatriptan

Alanine Aminotransferase *Serum Increase Physiological* Infrequent disturbances of liver function tests with drug administration *2158*

Aspartate Aminotransferase *Serum Increase Physiological* Infrequent disturbances of liver function tests with drug administration *2158*

Corticotropin *Plasma Decrease Physiological* In 22 healthy men administration of 100 and 200 mg orally caused reduction in trough concentration of 18% and 25% respectively over 4 hours. 5 hour postprandial peaks were reduced by 21% and 20% respectively. No effect observed after 11 h *1738*

Cortisol *Plasma Decrease Physiological* In 22 healthy men administration of 50, 100 and 200 mg orally caused reduction in trough concentration of 15%, 14% and 24% respectively over 4 hours. 5 hour postprandial peaks were reduced by 16% and 15% respectively. No effect observed after 11 h *1738*

Glucose *Serum Decrease Physiological* Rare decreases in concentration reported with drug administration *2158*
Serum Increase Physiological Rare increases in concentration reported with drug administration *2158*

Hematocrit *Blood Decrease Physiological* Rare anemia reported with drug administration *2158*

Hemoglobin *Blood Decrease Physiological* Rare anemia reported with drug administration *2158*

Occult Blood *Feces Increase Physiological* Rare gastrointestinal bleeding, hematemesis and melena reported with drug administration *2158*

Thyroid Stimulating Hormone
Serum Increase Physiological Rare increases in concentration reported with drug administration *2158*

Thyroxine (T4) *Serum Decrease Physiological* Rare hypothyroidism reported with drug administration *2158*

Suprofen

Creatinine *Serum Increase Physiological* Case reported of a man with nonoliguric acute renal failure following two doses of drug *4570* Occasional renal failure observed but mechanism not known *39*

Creatinine Clearance *Urine Decrease Physiological* Case reported of a man with nonoligouric acute renal failure following two doses of drug *4570*

Erythrocytes *Urine Increase Physiological* Reported in a man who developed nonoliguric acute renal failure following two doses of drug *4570* Occasional renal failure observed but mechanism not known *39*

Hemoglobin *Urine Increase Physiological* Occasional renal failure observed but mechanism not known *39*

Protein *Urine Increase Physiological* Occasional renal failure observed but mechanism not known *39*

Urea Nitrogen *Serum Increase Physiological* Occasional renal failure observed but mechanism not known *39*

Suramin

Alanine Aminotransferase *Serum Decrease Analytical* At a concentration of 300 mg/L caused a decrease in activity of about 20 U/L with method on Kodak Ektachem® 700 analyzer *2324*

Albumin *Urine Increase Physiological* May cause albuminuria *1384*

Amylase *Serum Increase Analytical* At concentrations of 300 mg/L and 500 mg/L caused an almost 50% increase in activity with method on Kodak Ektachem® 700 analyzer *2324*

Aspartate Aminotransferase *Serum Decrease Analytical* At a concentration of 300 mg/L caused a decrease in activity of about 20 U/L with method on Kodak Ektachem® 700 analyzer *2324*

Calcium *Serum Decrease Analytical* At a concentration of 300 mg/L caused a 10% decrease in concentration with method on Kodak Ektachem® 700 analyzer *2324*

Casts *Urine Increase Physiological* Cylindruria reported *128* May cause increased excretion of casts as a side effect *1384*

Cortisol *Plasma Decrease Physiological* In critically ill patients relative hypoadrenalism observed with suramin therapy because of its interfering effect on corticotropin action *3381*

Creatinine *Serum Increase Physiological* May occasionally cause nephritis or renal failure *1384*

Erythrocytes *Blood Decrease Physiological* Hemolytic anemia reported *128*
Urine Increase Physiological May cause actual bleeding *1714*

Factor II *Plasma No Effect Physiological* In 11 patients treated for 2 weeks mean activity 99% compared with 50 to 150% in healthy controls *2720*

Factor V *Plasma No Effect Physiological* In 14 patients treated with suramin for 2 weeks mean activity 62 ± 8% compared with 50 to 150% in healthy controls although inhibition observed in vitro *2720*

Factor VII *Plasma No Effect Physiological* In 11 patients treated with suramin for 2 weeks mean activity 84 ± 23% compared with 50 to 150% in healthy controls *2720*

Factor VIII *Plasma No Effect Physiological* In 11 patients treated with suramin for 2 weeks mean activity 143 ± 43% compared with 50 to 150% in healthy controls although inhibition observed in vitro *2720*

Factor IX *Plasma No Effect Physiological* In 11 patients treated with suramin for 2 weeks mean activity 124 ± 20% compared with 50 to 150% in healthy controls although inhibition observed in vitro *2720*

Factor X *Plasma No Effect Physiological* In 11 patients treated with suramin for 2 weeks mean activity 87 ± 14% compared with 50 to 150% in healthy controls although inhibition observed in vitro *2720*

Factor XI *Plasma No Effect Physiological* In 11 patients treated with suramin for 2 weeks mean activity 71 ± 22% compared with 50 to 150% in healthy controls although inhibition observed in vitro *2720*

Factor XII *Plasma No Effect Physiological* In 11 patients treated with suramin for 2 weeks mean activty 75 ± 27% compared with 50 to 150% in healthy controls although inhibition observed in vitro *2720*

Granulocytes *Blood Decrease Physiological* May cause agranulocytosis as a rare adverse effect *1384*

Hematocrit *Blood Decrease Physiological* Hemolytic anemia reported *128*

Hemoglobin *Blood Decrease Physiological* May occasionally cause hemolytic anemia *1384* Hemolytic anemia reported *128*
Urine Increase Physiological Actual bleeding caused by drug *2024* May cause hematuria as side effect *1384*

Lactate Dehydrogenase *Serum Decrease Analytical* At a concentration of 300 mg/L caused a slight decrease in activity with method on Kodak Ektachem® 700 analyzer *2324*

Leukocytes *Blood Decrease Physiological* Agranulocytosis reported *128*

Lipase *Serum No Effect Analytical* At a concentration of 500 mg/L caused no significant effect on activity with method on Kodak Ektachem® 700 analyzer *2324*

Partial Thromboplastin Time
Plasma No Effect Physiological In 14 patients treated with suramin for 2 weeks mean time 37.7 ± 3.5 seconds compared with reference interval of 25.8 to 38.6 seconds *2720*

Protein *Urine Increase Physiological* Nephrotoxic effect *1714* Usual effect during treatment of acute stage *128*

Suramin *(continued)*

Prothrombin Time *Plasma Increase Physiological* In 14 patients after treatment for 2 weeks mean time increased to 18.0 ± 1.3 seconds compared with reference interval of 10.5 to 13.2 seconds *2720*

Thrombin Time *Blood Increase Physiological* In 14 patients treated with suramin for 2 weeks mean time 42 ± 11 seconds compared with reference interval of 25 to 35 seconds *2720*

Urea Nitrogen *Serum Increase Physiological* May occasionally cause nephritis and renal failure *1384*

Synephrine

Catecholamines *Plasma No Effect Analytical* No effect on HPLC method of Koller for dopamine, epinephrine, and norepinephrine *3230*

Syrosingopine

Catecholamines *Urine Increase Physiological* Release of stored norepinephrine *3669*

Hydrochloric Acid *Gastric Fluid Increase Physiological* Excessive amounts may be released *3669*

4-Hydroxy-3-Methoxy-Phenylglycol
Urine Increase Physiological Release of stored norepinephrine *3669*

Platelets *Blood Decrease Physiological* Purpura due to thrombocytopenia may occur *51*

Vanillylmandelic Acid *Urine Increase Physiological* Release of stored norepinephrine *3669*

Tacrine

Acetylcholine *Cerebrospinal Fluid Increase Physiological* In 15 patients with Alzheimer's disease treated with 75 - 150 mg/d tacrine for 9 weeks concentration increased *4342*

Alanine Aminotransferase *Serum Increase Physiological* In almost half the 15 patients with Alzheimer's disease treated with 75 - 150 mg/d tacrine for 9 weeks activity increased *4342* Occasional reversible dose-dependent increase not associated with significant hepatic pathology *5862* In one of 8000 patients in clinical trials bilirubin concentration increased to 5.3 times upper limit of normal and aminotransferase activities more than 20 times the upper limit of normal. In a 35 week study 258 of 479 patients had ALT activities above the upper limit of normal (38% above 2 times ULN, 29% above 3 times ULN, and 6% above 10 times ULN) *4521*

Aspartate Aminotransferase *Serum Increase Physiological* In almost half the 15 patients with Alzheimer's disease treated with 75 - 150 mg/d tacrine for 9 weeks activity increased *4342* Occasional reversible dose-dependent increase not associated with significant hepatic pathology *5862* In one of 8000 patients in clinical trials bilirubin concentration increased to 5.3 times upper limit of normal and aminotransferase activities more than 20 times the upper limit of normal. In a 35 week study 258 of 479 patients had ALT activities above the upper limit of normal (38% above 2 times ULN, 29% above 3 times ULN, and 6% above 10 times ULN) *4521*

Bilirubin *Serum Increase Physiological* In one of 8000 patients in clinical trials bilirubin concentration increased to 5.3 times upper limit of normal and aminotransferase activities more than 20 times the upper limit of normal *4521*

Diazepam *Serum No Effect Physiological* Coadministration of tacrine with diazepam had no major effect on its pharmacokinetics *4521*

Digoxin *Serum No Effect Physiological* Coadministration of tacrine with digoxin had no major effect on its pharmacokinetics *4521*

Glucose *Serum Increase Physiological* Administration of tacrine was associated infrequently with diabetes *4521*
Urine Increase Physiological Administration of tacrine was associated infrequently with diabetes *4521*

Hematocrit *Blood Decrease Physiological* Administration of tacrine was associated infrequently with anemia and rarely with hemolysis or pancytopenia *4521*

Hemoglobin *Blood Decrease Physiological* Administration of tacrine was associated infrequently with anemia and rarely with hemolysis or pancytopenia *4521*

Homovanillic Acid
Cerebrospinal Fluid Increase Physiological In 15 patients with Alzheimer's disease treated with 75 - 150 mg/d tacrine for 9 weeks concentration increased *4342*

5-Hydroxyindoleacetic Acid
Cerebrospinal Fluid Increase Physiological In 15 patients with Alzheimer's disease treated with 75 - 150 mg/d tacrine for 9 weeks concentration increased *4342*

Leukocytes *Blood Decrease Physiological* Administration of tacrine was associated rarely with leukopenia and rarely with pancytopenia *4521*

Neutrophils *Blood Decrease Physiological* Absolute count of less than 500 cells/μL observed in 4 patients, and 6 had counts of less than 1500 cells/μL in association with increased ALT activities in clinical trials with 8000 patients *4521*

Occult Blood *Feces Increase Physiological* Administration of tacrine was associated infrequently with gastrointestinal bleeding *4521*

Platelets *Blood Decrease Physiological* Administration of tacrine was associated rarely with thrombocytopenia and rarely with pancytopenia *4521*

Prothrombin Time *Plasma No Effect Physiological* Coadministration of tacrine with warfarin had no major effect on its anticoagulant activity *4521*

Theophylline *Serum Increase Physiological* Coadministration of tacrine with theophylline increased theophylline elimination half-life and average plasma theophylline concentration by approximately two-fold *4521* Decreases theophylline clearance by inhibiting cytochrome P450 1A2 and increases renal clearance, increasing theophylline concentration by about 90% *5999* Decreases theophylline clearance by inhibiting cytochrome P450 1A2 and increases renal clearance of theophylline and increases serum theophylline concentration by 90% *3125* Up to 90% increase in serum theophylline concentration due to decreased theophylline clearance caused by inhibition of cytochrome P450 1A2 and increased renal clearance of theophylline *6117*

Thyroxine (T4) *Serum Decrease Physiological* Administration of tacrine was associated rarely with hyperthyroidism or hypothyroidism *4521*
Serum Increase Physiological Administration of tacrine was associated rarely with hyperthyroidism or hypothyroidism *4521*

Tacrolimus

Alanine Aminotransferase *Serum Increase Physiological* Cholangitis and cholestatic jaundice observed in patients receiving tacrolimus *1987*

Alkaline Phosphatase *Serum Increase Physiological* Cholangitis and cholestatic jaundice observed in patients receiving tacrolimus *1987*

Apolipoprotein A-I *Serum No Effect Physiological* In 27 post-renal transplant patients at least one year after surgery with cholesterol concentrations greater than 240 mg/dL treatment with tacrolimus for 6 months had no significant effect on the plasma apolipoprotein A-I concentration *3884*

Apolipoprotein B *Serum Decrease Physiological* In 27 post-renal transplant patients at least one year after surgery with cholesterol concentrations greater than 240 mg/dL treatment with tacrolimus for 6 months caused a 36 mg/dL (23%) reduction in concentration *3884*

Aspartate Aminotransferase *Serum Increase Physiological* Cholangitis and cholestatic jaundice observed in patients receiving tacrolimus *1987*

Bilirubin *Serum Increase Physiological* Cholangitis and cholestatic jaundice observed in patients receiving tacrolimus *1987* In two post-transplant patients administration of tacrolimus caused microangiopathic hemolytic anemia to develop with bilirubin concentration increasing to 22 μmol/L in one *3715*

Calcium *Serum Decrease Physiological* Hypocalcemia observed in patients receiving tacrolimus *1987*

Cholesterol *Serum Decrease Physiological* Unexpectedly low concentrations observed in 36 renal transplant recipients *5776* In 27 post-renal transplant patients at least one year after surgery with cholesterol concentrations greater than 240 mg/dL treatment with tacrolimus for 6 months caused a 55 mg/dL (16%) reduction in concentration *3884*

Creatinine *Serum Increase Physiological* In 263 patients mean concentration increased from baseline of 1.0 ± 0.4 mg/dL (88 ± 35 μmol/L) to 1.5 ± 0.5 mg/dL (133 ± 44 μmol/L) 1 year after liver transplant with FK 506 used as immunosuppressant *6000* Nephrotoxicity noted in 40% and 33% of liver transplantation patients receiving tacrolimus in US and European randomized trials *1987* In 283 adult patients who received orthoptic liver transplants and immunosuppression with FK 506 serum creatinine invariably increased in the perioperative period. 76% of the patients had a serum creatinine greater than 2.0 mg/dL at 7 days postoperatively *3875* Following initial rise in first week of treatment in 20 liver transplant patients serum creatinine tended to show slight decrease over next 3 weeks although concentration remained above pretreatment concentration *3874* In two post-transplant patients administration of tacrolimus caused microangiopathic hemolytic anemia to develop with creatinine concentration increasing to 242 μmol/L in one and 121 μmol/L in the other *3715*

Cyclosporine *Blood Increase Physiological* Cyclosporine metabolism reportedly inhibited by tacrolimus in two studies which theoretically would result in an increased cyclosporine concentration *859*
Serum Increase Physiological Cyclosporine metabolism reportedly inhibited by tacrolimus in two studies which theoretically would result in an increased cyclosporine concentration *859*

Effective Renal Plasma Flow
Patient Decrease Physiological In 116 recently liver-transplanted patients mean decrease of 7% observed *5958*

Glomerular Filtration Rate *Urine Decrease Physiological* In 263 patients mean concentration increased from baseline of 85.5 ± 27.8 mL/min to 59.2 ± 21.5 mL/min 1 year after liver transplant with FK 506 used as immunosuppressant *6000*
Urine No Effect Physiological In 116 recently liver-transplanted patients no change observed *5958*

Glucose *Serum Increase Physiological* Observed in 47% and 29% in patients receiving tacrolimus in US and European clinical trials *1987* In 263 patients hyperglycemia observed in 45 (18%) 1 year after liver transplant with FK 506 used as immunosuppressant *6000*
Serum No Effect Physiological In 27 post-renal transplant patients at least one year after surgery with cholesterol concentrations greater than 240 mg/dL treatment with tacrolimus for 6 months caused no significant effect on plasma concentration *3884*

Haptoglobin *Serum Decrease Physiological* In two post-transplant patients administration of tacrolimus caused microangiopathic hemolytic anemia to develop with haptoglobin concentration decreasing to less than 65 mg/L in one and less than 60 mg/L in the other *3715*

HDL-Cholesterol *Serum No Effect Physiological* In 27 post-renal transplant patients at least one year after surgery with cholesterol concentrations greater than 240 mg/dL treatment with tacrolimus for 6 months had no significant effect on the plasma HDL-cholesterol concentration *3884*

Hematocrit *Blood Decrease Physiological* Hypochromic anemia observed in 47% and 4% patients receiving tacrolimus in US and European clinical trials respectively *1987*

Hemoglobin *Blood Decrease Physiological* Hypochromic anemia observed in 47% and 4% patients receiving tacrolimus in US and European clinical trials respectively *1987* In two post-transplant patients administration of tacrolimus caused microangiopathic hemolytic anemia to develop with hemoglobin decreasing to 7.1 g/dL in both *3715*

Hemoglobin A_{1c} *Blood No Effect Physiological* In 27 post-renal transplant patients at least one year after surgery with cholesterol concentrations greater than 240 mg/dL treatment with tacrolimus for 6 months caused no significant effect on blood concentration *3884*

Lactate Dehydrogenase *Serum Increase Physiological* In two post-transplant patients administration of tacrolimus caused microangiopathic hemolytic anemia to develop with LD activity increasing to 2,034 U/L in one *3715*

LDL-Cholesterol *Serum Decrease Physiological* In 27 post-renal transplant patients at least one year after surgery with cholesterol concentrations greater than 240 mg/dL treatment with tacrolimus for 6 months caused a 48 mg/dL (25%) reduction in concentration *3884*

Leukocytes *Blood Decrease Physiological* Leukopenia observed in patients receiving tacrolimus *1987*
Blood Increase Physiological Leukocytosis observed in 32% and 8% patients receiving tacrolimus in US and European clinical trials respectively *1987*
Blood No Effect Physiological In two post-transplant patients administration of tacrolimus caused microangiopathic hemolytic anemia to develop but with leukocyte count remaining at 186 x 10^9L in one *3715*

Lipids *Serum Increase Physiological* Hyperlipemia observed in patients receiving tacrolimus *1987*

Magnesium *Serum Decrease Physiological* In 283 adult patients who received orthoptic liver transplants and immunosuppression with FK 506 serum magnesium concentration decreased in 26% after 7 days, 40% after 14 days, 52% after 28 days, 55% after 60 days and thereafter the number of patients with hypomagnesemia decreased to 17% after 450 days *3875*
Serum Increase Physiological Observed in 48% and 15% patients receiving tacrolimus in US and European clinical trials *1987*

Mycophenolic Acid *Serum No Effect Analytical* No significant interference observed with HPLC method of Shipkova et al *5526*

Mycophenolic Acid Glucuronide
Serum No Effect Analytical No significant interference observed with HPLC method of Shipkova et al *5526*

Occult Blood *Feces Increase Physiological* Gastrointestinal hemorrhage observed in patients receiving tacrolimus *1987*

pH *Blood Decrease Physiological* Acidosis observed in patients receiving tacrolimus *1987*
Blood Increase Physiological Alkalosis observed in patients receiving tacrolimus *1987*

Phosphate *Serum Decrease Physiological* Hypophosphatemia observed in patients receiving tacrolimus *1987*
Serum Increase Physiological Hyperphosphatemia observed in patients receiving tacrolimus *1987*

Platelets *Blood Decrease Physiological* Thrombocytopenia observed in 24% and 10% patients receiving tacrolimus in US and European clinical trials respectively *1987* In two post-transplant patients administration of tacrolimus caused microangiopathic hemolytic anemia to develop with platelet count decreasing to 36 x 10^9L in one and 40 x 10^9/L in the other *3715*

Potassium *Serum Decrease Physiological* Observed in 29% and 11% in patients receiving tacrolimus in US and European clinical trials respectively *1987*
Serum Increase Physiological Mild to severe hyperkalemia noted in 44% and 10% of liver transplantation patients receiving tacrolimus in US and European randomized trials *1987* In 263 patients hyperkalemia observed in 45 (17%) 1 year after liver transplant with FK 506 used as immunosuppressant *6000* Observed in many post liver transplant patients when treated with FK-506 but associated in all cases with low or low normal plasma renin and aldosterone concentrations *3874*

Protein *Serum Decrease Physiological* Hypoproteinemia observed in patients receiving tacrolimus *1987*
Urine Increase Physiological In 6 patients treated with FK-506 2 showed evidence of glomerular damage and 4 showed evidence of both glomerular and tubular damage *2728*

Prothrombin Time *Plasma Decrease Physiological* Prothrombin time observed to be decreased in patients receiving tacrolimus *1987*

Reticulocytes *Blood Increase Physiological* In two post-transplant patients administration of tacrolimus caused microangiopathic hemolytic anemia to develop with reticulocyte count increasing to 186 x 10^9L in one and 145 x 10^9 in the other *3715*

Tacrolimus *(continued)*

Schizocytes *Blood Decrease Physiological* In two post-transplant patients administration of tacrolimus caused microangiopathic hemolytic anemia to develop with numerous schizocytes appearing in both *3715*

Sodium *Serum Decrease Physiological* Hyponatremia observed in patients receiving tacrolimus *1987*

Triglycerides *Serum Decrease Physiological* In 27 post-renal transplant patients at least one year after surgery with cholesterol concentrations greater than 240 mg/dL treatment with tacrolimus for 6 months caused a nonsignificant decrease in the plasma triglyceride concentration *3884*

Urea Nitrogen *Serum Increase Physiological* In two post-transplant patients administration of tacrolimus caused microangiopathic hemolytic anemia to develop with urea nitogen concentration increasing to 16 mmol/L in one *3715* Nephrotoxicity noted in 40% and 33% of liver transplantation patients receiving tacrolimus in US and European randomized trials *1987*

Uric Acid *Serum Increase Physiological* Observed in patients receiving tacrolimus *1987* Hyperuricemia observed in patients receiving tacrolimus *1987*
Serum No Effect Physiological Minimal effect observed in 36 renal transplant recipients *5776*

VLDL-Cholesterol *Serum No Effect Physiological* In 27 post-renal transplant patients at least one year after surgery with cholesterol concentrations greater than 240 mg/dL treatment with tacrolimus for 6 months had no significant effect on the plasma VLDL-cholesterol concentration *3884*

Volume *Urine Decrease Physiological* Nephrotoxicity noted in 40% and 33% of liver transplantation patients receiving tacrolimus in US and European randomized trials *1987*

Talbutal

Barbiturate *Urine Increase Analytical* At a concentration of 2.0 µg/mL (8.9 µmol/L) with method on Du Pont aca *1555*

Talinolol

Lecithin:Cholesterol Acyltransferase
Serum No Effect Physiological At in vitro concentration of 0.5 µmol/L nonsignificant reduction of activity to 97.9 ± 4.0% observed *5316*

Tamoxifen

α_1-Acid Glycoprotein *Serum Decrease Physiological* Significant change due to mild estrogenic effect of drug in breast cancer patients *5114*

Alkaline Phosphatase *Serum Decrease Physiological* In 67 postmenopausal women with breast cancer treatment for 12 months caused reduction from baseline of 79 ± 18 U/L to 62 U/L (21%) *3663* Observed in nonresponders with breast cancer *1847* In 18 women treated for at least 5 years significant reduction in concentration observed *4319*

Alkaline Phosphatase, Bone Isoenzyme
Serum Increase Physiological In 18 women with breast cancer treatment for 5 years was associated with nonsignificant increase *4319*

Amylase *Serum Increase Physiological* In a 58 y-old women with a history of familial hypertriglyceridemia 3 months after mastectomy for adenocarcinoma of the breast and treatment with 20 mg/d tamoxifen serum amylase activity was increased to 83 U/L. With withdrawal of tamoxifen, and administration of gemfibrozil for 3 weeks, amylase activity decreased to 37 U/L *3028*

Androstenedione *Plasma Decrease Physiological* In 32 postmenopausal women with advanced breast cancer mean concentration decreased from 1.57 nmol/L to 1.51 nmol/L (3.9%) after 3 to 12 months treatment *3643*

δ_4-Androstenedione *Plasma No Effect Physiological* In 42 postmenopausal women with biopsy diagnosed breast estrogen receptor positive cancer mean concentration of 1.90 ± 0.18 ng/mL changed nonsignificantly to 1.89 ± 0.20 ng/mL after 6 months treatment with tamoxifen *3258*

Antithrombin III *Plasma Decrease Physiological* Lowered functional activity in 42% treated patients *1732*

α_1-Antitrypsin *Serum Increase Physiological* When 10 mg given twice daily to 30 Z homozygous α_1-antitrypsin-deficient subjects for 30 d although change slight *6420* Significant change due to mild estrogenic effect of drug in breast cancer patients *5114*

Aspartate Aminotransferase *Serum Increase Physiological* Isolated case of drug induced cholestasis in one patient *594* Increased activity above 100 U/L in North America and more than 1.25 times the upper limit of normal in Eastern Europe and Scandinavia has been reported with frequencies of 2%, 15% and 17% in North America, Eastern Europe and Scandinavia respectively *5329*

Bilirubin *Serum Increase Physiological* Increased activity above 2.0 mg/dL in North America and more than 1.25 times the upper limit of normal in Eastern Europe and Scandinavia has been reported with frequencies of 2%, < 1% and 1.5% in North America, Eastern Europe and Scandinavia respectively *5329* Isolated case of drug induced cholestasis in one patient *594*

CA549 *Serum No Effect Analytical* No statistically significant effect observed over a concentration range of 0.4 to 5 mg/L with BRESMARQ assay *958* No effect observed with concentrations up to 5 mg/L with immunoradiometric BRESMARQ procedure *958*

Calcium *Serum Decrease Physiological* In 18 women with breast cancer treatment for at least 5 years was associated with significant reduction *4319*
Serum Increase Physiological In patients with previous hypercalcemia and in patients with metastatic bone disease. Probable overall incidence less than 0.1% *4561* Especially in people with pre-existing hypercalcemia and with widespread skeletal metastases *2530* Life-threatening hypercalcemia observed in a single case following treatment *3423* In 2 patients in whom calcium rose to above 18.0 mg/dL: reverted to normal once drug withdrawn *3397*

Ceruloplasmin *Serum Increase Physiological* Significant change due to mild estrogenic effect of drug in breast cancer patients *5114*

Cholesterol *Serum Decrease Physiological* Concentration in women with stage I and II breast cancer taking tamoxifen fell by more than 10 mg/dL in 73% patients whereas fell by 10 mg/dL in only 35% control women not taking tamoxifen: fall of more than 40 mg/dL observed in 40% tamoxifen patients *5314* Effect on increased concentration in breast cancer patients *5114* In 25 healthy postmenopausal women treatment with 20 mg/d for 2 months caused a significant change from mean value with placebo of 212 ± 31 mg/dL to 185 ± 31 mg/dL *2359* Significant reduction observed in 140 postmenopausal women treated by surgery with/without radiation for breast cancer when treated for 3 months with 20 mg tamoxifen daily: effect persisted at 6 and 12 months *3664* After 4 - 8 weeks treatment with 20 mg/d in a group of low risk women with breast cancer mean 32 mg/dL (15%) decrease from baseline of 205 ± 24 mg/dL observed and 54 mg/dL (19%) decrease from mean baseline of 282 ± 38 mg/dL in women with high risk *1447* In 24 women with breast cancer treatment with 20 mg/d caused mean 17% decrease *1447* Concentration reduced by tamoxifen which may also inhibit atherogenesis by directly affecting the metabolism of low-density lipoproteins in the arteries *4450*
Serum Increase Physiological In one woman previously treated by segmental mastectomy for breast cancer and subsequently with radiation therapy and tamoxifen four years after treatment begun serum cholesterol concentration increased to 750 mg/dL greater than it had been on all previous 6-monthly follow-ups. Change of treatment to gemfibrozil caused the concentration to decrease to 279 mg/dL within 3 weeks *3028* In a 58 y-old women with a history of familial hypertriglyceridemia 3 months after mastectomy for adenocarcinoma of the breast and treatment with 20 mg/d tamoxifen serum cholesterol concentration was 750 mg/dL. With withdrawal of tamoxifen, and administration of gemfibrozil for 3 weeks, cholesterol concentration decreased to 279 mg/dL *3028* Insignificant increase from mean of 193 mg/dL to 204 mg/dL in 8 postmenopausal women treated with 20 mg daily for 3 months *324*
Serum No Effect Physiological In 8 postmenopausal women treatment with 20 mg/d for 3 months had no significant effect on concentration with baseline concentration 193 ± 23 mg/dL

and posttreatment concentration 204 ± 14 mg/dL *324* In 16 normolipidemic patients with breast cancer treated with tamoxifen for 2 months mean cholesterol concentration remained unchanged over 2 months *2742* In 6 women with breast cancer treatment for 1 month caused nonsignificant change from mean baseline of 5.12 ± 1.16 mmol/L to 4.58 ± 1.42 mmol/L and to 4.86 ± 1.11 mmol/L after 3 months *5511*

Cholesterol, Esterified *Serum Increase Physiological* Insignificant increase from mean of 127 mg/dL to 145 mg/dL in 8 postmenopausal women treated with 20 mg/day for 3 months *324*

Cholesterol, Free *Serum Decrease Physiological* In 8 postmenopausal women treatment with 20 mg/d for 3 months caused significant decrease from mean baseline of 66.5 ± 6.5 mg/dL to 59.6 ± 4.6 mg/dL *324*

Corticosteroid-Binding Globulin
Serum Increase Physiological False positive results for dexamethasone suppression test may be observed due to increased corticosteroid binding globulin concentration in the circulation *6538*

Cyclosporine *Serum Increase Physiological* Reported effect although no details discussed *1069*

Dehydroepiandrosterone *Plasma Decrease Physiological* In 32 postmenopausal women with advanced breast cancer mean concentration decreased from 8.46 nmol/L to 7.22 nmol/L (14.6%) after 3 to 12 months treatment *3643*

Dehydroepiandrosterone Sulfate
Plasma Decrease Physiological In 32 postmenopausal women with advanced breast cancer mean concentration decreased from 2.11 µmol/L to 1.99 µmol/L (6.0%) after 3 to 12 months treatment *3643*
Plasma No Effect Physiological In 42 postmenopausal women with biopsy diagnosed breast estrogen receptor positive cancer mean concentration of 2.72 ± 0.24 µmol/L changed nonsignificantly to 2.86 ± 0.27 µmol/L after 6 months treatment with tamoxifen *3258*

Desdimethyl-tamoxifen *Plasma Increase Physiological* In 32 postmenopausal women with advanced breast cancer mean concentration at steady state 32.9 ng/mL *3643*

Desmethyl-4-hydroxytamoxifen
Plasma Increase Physiological In 32 postmenopausal women with advanced breast cancer mean concentration at steady state 21.6 ng/mL *3643*

Desmethyltamoxifen *Plasma Increase Physiological* In 32 postmenopausal women with advanced breast cancer mean concentration at steady state 218.5 ng/mL *3643*

Dexamethasone Suppression
Patient Abnormal Physiological False positive results for dexamethasone suppression test may be observed due to increased corticosteroid binding globulin concentration in the circulation *6538*

1,25-Dihydroxy Vitamin D *Serum No Effect Physiological* In 34 postmenopausal women with breast cancer treatment for 2 years caused nonsignificant increase from mean baseline of 88 ± 27 pmol/L to 100 ± 35 pmol/L *3663*

Erythrocyte Sedimentation Rate
Blood Decrease Physiological Observed in nonresponders with breast cancer *1847*

Estradiol *Plasma Decrease Physiological* In 32 postmenopausal women with advanced breast cancer mean concentration decreased from 18.9 pmol/L to 16.6 pmol/L (12.1%) after 3 to 12 months treatment *3643*
Plasma Increase Physiological Effect on estradiol-17β concentration observed with treatment in men with oligozoospermia *1229* When 20 mg/day given to 6 premenopausal women with uterine fibromyomata for at least 3 months concentration increased in association with lengthened luteal phase *3681* 2 to 8 fold increase in 6 healthy volunteers given 20 mg/d for 5 to 10 d. In postmenopausal breast cancer women who did not respond to drug *2530* Increase during treatment from mean of 0.044 nmol/L to 0.084 nmol/L in 13 men with idiopathic oligozoospermia *2431* In 8 premenopausal women with stage I or II breast cancer concentration increased 1- to 3-fold up to 72 months after mastectomy *2982*
Plasma No Effect Physiological In 42 postmenopausal women with biopsy diagnosed breast estrogen receptor positive cancer mean concentration of 0.05 ± 0.005 nmol/L changed nonsignificantly to 0.08 ± 0.01 nmol/L after 6 months treatment with tamoxifen *3258*
Urine Increase Physiological In 32 postmenopausal women with advanced breast cancer mean excretion increased from 0.93 nmol/d to 1.09 nmol/d (16.9%) after 3 to 12 months treatment *3643*

17β-Estradiol *Plasma Increase Physiological* In 25 healthy postmenopausal women treatment with 20 mg/d for 2 months caused a nonsignificant change from mean value with placebo of 22 ± 28 pg/mL to 35 ± 76 pg/mL *2359*

Estriol *Urine Increase Physiological* In 32 postmenopausal women with advanced breast cancer mean excretion increased from 8.61 nmol/d to 9.85 nmol/d (16.9%) after 3 to 12 months treatment *3643*

Estrogens *Urine Increase Physiological* In 32 postmenopausal women with advanced breast cancer mean excretion increased from 33.9 nmol/d to 35.8 nmol/d (5.8%) after 3 to 12 months treatment *3643*

Estrone *Plasma Decrease Physiological* In 32 postmenopausal women with advanced breast cancer mean concentration decreased from 74.4 pmol/L to 70.9 pmol/L (6.9%) after 3 to 12 months treatment *3643*
Plasma Increase Physiological In 8 premenopausal women with stage I or II breast cancer treatment for up to 72 mo after mastectomy caused 1- to 3-fold increase in concentration *2982*
Urine Increase Physiological In 32 postmenopausal women with advanced breast cancer mean excretion increased from 5.79 nmol/d to 6.72 nmol/d (16.0%) after 3 to 12 months treatment *3643*

Estrone Glucuronide *Urine Increase Physiological* When 20 mg/day given for at least 3 months to 6 premenopausal women with uterine fibromyomata concentration increased in conjunction with lengthened luteal phase *3681*

Estrone Sulfate *Plasma Increase Physiological* In 32 postmenopausal women with advanced breast cancer mean concentration increased from 424.5 pmol/L to 501.7 pmol/L (18.2%) after 3 to 12 months treatment *3643*

Follicle Stimulating Hormone
Plasma Decrease Physiological In 42 postmenopausal women with biopsy diagnosed breast estrogen receptor positive cancer mean concentration of 47.55 ± 3.18 IU/L decreased significantly to 31.92 ± 1.86 IU/L after 6 months treatment with tamoxifen *3258* In postmenopausal women with breast cancer treated for 2 weeks *2530* In 32 postmenopausal women with advanced breast cancer mean concentration decreased from 61.7 IU/L to 33.6 IU/L (45.5%) after 3 to 12 months treatment *3643*
Plasma Increase Physiological Effect observed with treatment in men with oligozoospermia *1229* Significant increase during luteal phase from mean of 2.0 U/L to 8.0 U/L in 6 premenopausal women with uterine fibromyomata treated with 20 mg/day for at least 3 months *3681* Increase of mean from 4.97 U/L to 7.66 U/L during treatment of 13 men with idiopathic oligozoospermia *2431*
Plasma No Effect Physiological After oral administration of 20 mg/d for 5 or 10 d to 6 healthy women during follicular phase of menstrual cycle. In 10 anovulatory women given up to 40 mg/d for 5 d *2530* In 8 premenopausal women with stage I or II breast cancer treatment for up to 72 months after mastectomy maintained concentration within normal range *2982*

Haptoglobin *Serum Decrease Physiological* Significant change due to mild estrogenic effect of drug in breast cancer patients *5114*

HDL_2-Cholesterol *Serum Increase Physiological* In 8 postmenopausal women treatment with 20 mg/d for 3 months caused nonsignificant increase from mean baseline of 9.7 ± 3.6 mg/dL to 14.4 ± 13.3 mg/dL *324* Insignificant increase from mean of 100 mg/L to 140 mg/L in 8 postmenopausal women treated with 20 mg daily for 3 months *324*

HDL_2-Cholesterol, Esterified *Serum Increase Physiological* Insignificant increase from mean of 60 mg/L to 90 mg/L in 8 women treated with 20 mg daily for 3 months *324*

HDL_2-Cholesterol, Free *Serum No Effect Physiological* No effect of treatment for 3 months with 20 mg daily in 8 postmenopausal women *324*

HDL_2-Lecithin *Serum Decrease Physiological* Nonsignificant reduction from mean of 189 µmol/L to 184 µmol/L in 8 postmenopausal women treated with 20 mg daily for 3 months *324*

Tamoxifen *(continued)*

HDL_2-Lysolecithin *Serum Decrease Physiological* Nonsignificant decrease from mean of 28 µmol/L to 26 µmol/L in 8 postmenopausal women treated with 20 mg daily for 3 months *324*

HDL_2-Phosphatidylethanolamine *Serum Decrease Physiological* Nonsignificant reduction from mean of 39 µmol/L 37 µmol/L in 8 postmenopausal women treated with 20 mg daily for 3 months *324*

HDL_2-Phosphoinositol *Serum Decrease Physiological* Significant reduction from mean of 37 µmol/L to 27 µmol/L in 8 postmenopausal women treated with 20 mg daily for 3 months *324*

HDL_2-Sphingomyelin *Serum Decrease Physiological* Nonsignificant decrease from mean of 48 µmol/L to 41 µmol/L in 8 postmenopausal women treated with 20 mg daily for 3 months *324*

HDL_2-Triglycerides *Serum Increase Physiological* Insignificant increase from mean of 40 mg/L to 50 mg/L in 8 postmenopausal women treated with 20 mg daily for 3 months *324*

HDL_3-Cholesterol *Serum No Effect Physiological* No change from mean baseline concentration of 350 mg/L in 8 postmenopausal women treated with 20 mg daily for 3 months *324*

HDL_3-Cholesterol, Esterified *Serum No Effect Physiological* No change from mean baseline concentration of 260 mg/L in 8 postmenopausal women treated with 20 mg daily for 3 months *324*

HDL_3-Cholesterol, Free *Serum No Effect Physiological* No change from mean baseline of 90 mg/L in 8 postmenopausal women treated with 20 mg daily for 3 months *324*

HDL_3-Lecithin *Serum Increase Physiological* Nonsignificant increase from mean of 619 µmol/L to 641 µmol/L in 8 postmenopausal women treated with 20 mg daily for 3 months *324*

HDL_3-Lysolecithin *Serum Decrease Physiological* Significant reduction from mean of 117 µmol/L to 92 µmol/L in 8 postmenopausal women treated with 20 mg daily for 3 months *324*

HDL_3-Phosphatidylethanolamine *Serum Decrease Physiological* Nonsignificant reduction from mean of 56 µmol/L to 49 µmol/L in 8 postmenopausal women treated with 20 mg daily for 3 months *324*

HDL_3-Phosphoinositol *Serum Increase Physiological* Nonsignificant increase from mean of 44 µmol/L to 46 µmol/L in 8 postmenopausal women treated with 20 mg daily for 3 months *324*

HDL_3-Sphingomyelin *Serum Decrease Physiological* Nonsignificant reduction from mean of 90 µmol/L to 80 µmol/L in 8 postmenopausal women treated with 20 mg daily for 3 months *324*

HDL_3-Triglycerides *Serum Increase Physiological* Insignificant increase from mean of 160 mg/L to 190 mg/L in 8 postmenopausal women treated with 20 mg daily for 3 months *324*

HDL-Cholesterol *Serum Decrease Physiological* In one woman previously treated by segmental mastectomy for breast cancer and subsequently with radiation therapy and tamoxifen four years after treatment begun serum HDL-cholesterol concentration decreased to 20 mg/dL lower than it had been on all previous 6-monthly follow-ups. Change of treatment to gemfibrozil caused the concentration to increase to 37 mg/dL within 3 weeks *3028* In a 58 y-old women with a history of familial hypertriglyceridemia 3 months after mastectomy for adenocarcinoma of the breast and treatment with 20 mg/d tamoxifen serum HDL-cholesterol concentration was 20 mg/dL. With withdrawal of tamoxifen, and administration of gemfibrozil for 3 weeks, HDL-cholesterol concentration increased to 37 mg/dL *3028* Small but significant decrease observed in 140 postmenopausal women with prior breast cancer treated by surgery with/without radiation when given 20 mg/d tamoxifen *3664*
Serum No Effect Physiological In 25 healthy postmenopausal women treatment with 20 mg/d for 2 months caused a nonsignificant change from mean value with placebo of 58 ± 18 mg/dL to 56 ± 16 mg/dL *2359* In 6 women with breast cancer treatment with tamoxifen caused nonsignificant change from mean baseline of 1.18 ± 0.30 mmol/L to 1.16 ± 0.29 mmol/L after 1 month and 1.15 ± 0.29 mmol/L after 3 months *5511* In 20 women with breast cancer treatment with 20 mg/d for 4 - 8 weeks caused nonsignificant change to 57 ± 8 mg/dL from mean baseline of 55 ± 13 mg/dL *1447*

Hemoglobin *Blood Decrease Physiological* In a small proportion of patients with associated reductions of platelet and white cell counts *2530*

Hepatic Triglyceride Lipase *Serum Decrease Physiological* In 16 normolipidemic patients with breast cancer treated with tamoxifen for 2 months mean activity decreased significantly from 0.252 µmol/mL/min to 0.202 µmol/mL/min *2742*

11β-Hydroxyandrostenedione *Plasma Increase Physiological* During treatment of 13 men with idiopathic oligozoospermia increase of mean concentration from 10.1 nmol/L to 13.9 nmol/L *2431*

2-Hydroxyestradiol *Urine Decrease Physiological* In 32 postmenopausal women with advanced breast cancer mean excretion decreased from 1.51 nmol/d to 1.46 nmol/d (3.0%) after 3 to 12 months treatment *3643*

2-Hydroxyestrone *Urine Decrease Physiological* In 32 postmenopausal women with advanced breast cancer mean excretion decreased from 5.59 nmol/d to 4.01 nmol/d (28.4%) after 3 to 12 months treatment *3643*

4-Hydroxyestrone *Urine Decrease Physiological* In 32 postmenopausal women with advanced breast cancer mean excretion decreased from 0.61 nmol/d to 0.56 nmol/d (9.4%) after 3 to 12 months treatment *3643*

16α-Hydroxyestrone *Urine Increase Physiological* In 32 postmenopausal women with advanced breast cancer mean excretion increased from 2.70 nmol/d to 3.10 nmol/d (14.8%) after 3 to 12 months treatment *3643*

16β-Hydroxyestrone *Urine Increase Physiological* In 32 postmenopausal women with advanced breast cancer mean excretion increased from 1.54 nmol/d to 1.81 nmol/d (17.6%) after 3 to 12 months treatment *3643*

17-Hydroxyprogesterone *Plasma Increase Physiological* Increase of 17α-hydroxyprogesterone concentration from mean of 3.47 nmol/L to 5.79 nmol/L during treatment in 13 men with idiopathic oligozoospermia *2431*
Plasma No Effect Physiological In 42 postmenopausal women with biopsy diagnosed breast estrogen receptor positive cancer mean concentration of 1.55 ± 0.13 nmol/L changed nonsignificantly to 1.95 ± 0.24 nmol/L after 6 months treatment with tamoxifen *3258*

4-Hydroxytamoxifen *Serum Increase Physiological* In 32 postmenopausal women with advanced breast cancer mean concentration at steady state 2.5 ng/mL *3643*

Insulin-like Growth Factor-I *Serum Decrease Physiological* In about 10 healthy postmenopausal women treatment with 20 mg/d caused significant decrease from mean baseline of 19.19 ± 1.70 nmol/L to 13.50 ± 2.30 nmol/L after 4 weeks, 13.75 ± 2.19 nmol/L after 8 weeks and 14.19 ± 2.24 nmol/L after 12 weeks *5512*
Serum Increase Physiological In 24 out of 27 postmenopausal women treated with 20 or 30 mg/d mean concentration of 14.8 nmol/L before treatment decreased to 10.2 nmol/L during treatment *3566*

Insulin-like Growth Factor Binding Protein-3 *Serum No Effect Physiological* In about 10 healthy postmenopausal women treatment with 20 mg/d caused nonsignificant change from mean baseline of 3.62 ± 0.16 mg/mL to 3.86 ± 0.28 mg/mL after 4 weeks, 3.72 ± 0.23 mg/mL after 8 weeks and 3.50 ± 0.16 mg/mL after 12 weeks *5512*

16-Keto-Estradiol *Urine Increase Physiological* In 32 postmenopausal women with advanced breast cancer mean excretion increased from 1.28 nmol/d to 1.70 nmol/d (32.8%) after 3 to 12 months treatment *3643*

LDL-Cholesterol *Serum Decrease Physiological* From 5.11 to 4.10 mmol/L accountable for much of total change *5114* Significant reduction observed in 140 postmenopausal women who had had breast cancer treated by surgery with/without radiation after 3 months treatment with 20 mg/d for 3 months: effect persisted at 6 and 12 months *3664* Observed in one elderly woman treated for breast cancer. Possibly due to reduction of activities of postheparin plasma lipoprotein lipase and hepatic triglyceride lipase *781* In 8 postmenopausal women treatment with 20 mg/d for 3 months caused concentration to decrease (estrogenic effect) *324* In a group of women with low risk breast cancer treatment with 20 mg/d for 4 - 8 weeks caused significant 33 mg/dL (26%) decrease from mean baseline of 126 ± 26 mg/dL and 63 mg/dL (32%) reduction from mean baseline of 200 ± 35 mg/dL in high risk group *1447* In 25 healthy postmenopausal women treatment with 20 mg/d for 2 months caused a significant change from mean value with placebo of 134 ± 29 mg/dL to 108 ± 32 mg/dL *2359* Significant reduction from mean of 1220 mg/L to 1150 mg/L in 8 postmenopausal women treated with 20 mg daily for 3 months *324* In 6 womenwith breast cancer treatment with tamoxifen caused significant reduction in calculated LDL-cholesterol concentration from mean baseline of 3.18 ± 0.91 mmol/L to 2.61 ± 0.80 mmol/L after 1 month and 2.79 ± 0.52 mmol/L after 3 months *5511* Concentration reduced by tamoxifen which may also inhibit atherogenesis by directly affecting the metabolism of low-density lipoproteins in the arteries *4450*

LDL-Cholesterol, Esterified *Serum No Effect Physiological* No significant change observed in 8 postmenopausal women treated with 20 mg daily for 3 months *324*

LDL-Cholesterol, Free *Serum Decrease Physiological* Significant reduction from mean of 380 mg/L to 300 mg/L in 8 postmenopausal women treated with 20 mg daily for 3 months *324*

LDL-Cholesterol:HDL-Cholesterol Ratio
Serum Decrease Physiological Significant mean 33% reduction observed in 24 women (both pre- and postmenoausal) with breast cancer treated with 20 mg/d *1447*

LDL-Lecithin *Serum Increase Physiological* Nonsignificant increase from mean of 770 µmol/L to 777 µmol/L in 8 postmenopausal women treated with 20 mg daily for 3 months *324*

LDL-Lysolecithin *Serum Decrease Physiological* Nosignificant reduction from mean of 43 µmol/L to 38 µmol/L in 8 postmenopausal women treated with 20 mg daily for 3 months *324*

LDL-Phosphatidylethanolamine
Serum Increase Physiological Nonsignificant increase from mean of 45 µmol/L to 48 µmol/L in 8 postmenopausal women treated with 20 mg daily for 3 months *324*

LDL-Phosphoinositol *Serum Increase Physiological* Nonsignificant increase from mean of 45 µmol/L to 48 µmol/L in 8 postmenopausal women treated with 20 mg daily for 3 months *324*

LDL-Sphingomyelin *Serum Decrease Physiological* Nosignificant reduction from mean of 274 µmol/L to 260 µmol/L in 8 postmenopausal women treated for 3 months with 20 mg daily *324*

LDL-Triglycerides *Serum Increase Physiological* Nonsignificant increase from mean of 490 mg/L to 540 mg/L in 8 postmenopausal women treated with 20 mg daily for 3 months *324* From 0.46 to 0.56 mmol/L accountable for much of total change *5114*

Lecithin *Serum Increase Physiological* Insignificant increase from mean of 1.99 mmol/L to 2.13 mmol/L in 8 postmenopausal women treated with 20 mg daily for 3 months *324*
Serum No Effect Physiological In 8 postmenopausal women treatment with 20 mg/d for 3 months had no significant effect on plasma concentration *324*

Leukocytes *Blood Decrease Physiological* Moderate leukopenia reported with tamoxifen administration but usually not enough to require cessation of treatment *4450* In up to 20% of treated patients *2530*

Lipoprotein Lp(a) *Serum Decrease Physiological* In 6 women with breast cancer treatment for 1 month caused significant decrease from mean baseline of 12.3 ± 9.5 mg/dL to 7.5 ± 6.9 mg/dL *5511* In about 10 healthy postmenopausal women treatment with 20 mg/d caused decrease from mean baseline of 8.9 ± 1.4 mg/dL to 6.4 ± 1.8 mg/dL after 4 weeks (nonsignificant), 5.8 ± 1.8 mg/dL after 8 weeks (nonsignificant) and 5.5 ± 1.8 mg/dL (significant) after 12 weeks *5512*

Luteinizing Hormone *Plasma Decrease Physiological* In 32 postmenopausal women with advanced breast cancer mean concentration decreased from 31.8 IU/L to 16.5 IU/L (48.1%) after 3 to 12 months treatment *3643* In 42 postmenopausal women with biopsy diagnosed breast estrogen receptor positive cancer mean concentration of 20.27 ± 1.83 IU/L decreased significantly to 12.97 ± 1.35 IU/L after 6 months treatment with tamoxifen *3258* In postmenopausal women with breast cancer treated for 2 weeks *2530*
Plasma Increase Physiological During treatment of 13 men with idiopathic oligozoospermia increase of mean from 6.75 U/L to 11.3 U/L *2431* Effect observed following treatment in men with oligozoospermia *1229* In 10 anovulatory women given up to 40 mg/d for 5 d *2530*
Plasma No Effect Physiological After oral administration of 20 mg/d for 5 or 10 d to 6 healthy women during follicular phase of menstrual cycle *2530* In 8 premenopausal women treatment of stage I or II breast cancer for up to 72 mo after mastectomy had no effect on concentration *2982*

Lysolecithin *Serum Decrease Physiological* Insignificant reduction from mean of 177 µmol/L to 158 µmol/L in 8 postmenopausal women treated with 20 mg daily for 3 months *324*

Metabolite Y *Plasma Increase Physiological* In 32 postmenopausal women with advanced breast cancer mean concentration at steady state 25.8 ng/mL *3643*

2-Methoxyestrone *Urine Decrease Physiological* In 32 postmenopausal women with advanced breast cancer mean excretion decreased from 1.94 nmol/d to 1.41 nmol/d (27.4%) after 3 to 12 months treatment *3643*

Osteocalcin *Serum Decrease Physiological* In 35 postmenopausal women with breast cancer treatment for 2 years caused significant reduction from mean baseline of 2244 ± 928 pmol/L to 972 ± 669 pmol/L (52 ± 27% reduction) *3663*
Serum Increase Physiological In 18 women with breast cancer treated for at least 5 years significant increase in concentration observed *4319*

Parathyroid Hormone *Plasma Increase Physiological* Significant increase observed in 18 women with breast cancer treated for at least 5 years *4319*
Plasma No Effect Physiological In 35 postmenopausal women with breast cancer treatment for 2 years caused nonsignificant increase from mean baseline of 2.2 ± 0.7 pmol/L to 2.6 ± 0.8 pmol/L *3663*

Phosphatidylethanolamine *Serum Increase Physiological* Insignificant increase from mean of 147 µmol/L to 156 µmol/L in 8 postmenopausal women treated with 20 mg daily for 3 months *324*

Phosphoinositol *Serum Decrease Physiological* In 8 postmenopausal women treatment with 20 mg/d for 3 months caused tendency for plasma phosphoinositol concentration to decrease *324*
Serum Increase Physiological Insignificant increase from mean of 116 µmol/L to 124 µmol/L in 8 postmenopausal women treated with 20 mg daily for 3 months *324*

Platelets *Blood Decrease Physiological* In up to 20% of treated patients given 400 mg/d for 2 d *2530* Moderate thrombocytopenia reported with tamoxifen administration but usually not enough to require cessation of treatment *4450*

Postheparin Lipoprotein Lipase
Plasma Decrease Physiological In 16 normolipidemic patients with breast cancer treated with tamoxifen for 2 months mean concentration decreased significantly from 0.409 µmol/mL to 0.377 µmol/mL *2742*
Plasma Increase Physiological In 16 normolipidemic patients with breast cancer treated with tamoxifen for 2 months mean mass increased significantly from 207 ng/mL to 271 ng/mL *2742*

Pregnanediol *Urine Increase Physiological* When 20 mg/day given for at least 3 months to 6 women with uterine fibromyomata concentration increased in conjunction with lengthened luteal phase *3681*

Progesterone *Plasma Increase Physiological* When 20 mg/day given to 6 premenopausal women with uterine fibromyomata for at least 3 months concentration increased in association with lengthened luteal phase *3681* Effect observed with treatment in men with oligozoospermia *1229* In 8 premenopausal women with stage I or II breast cancer treated for up to 72 mo after mastectomy concentration increased 1- to 3-fold *2982*
Plasma No Effect Physiological After oral administration of 20 mg/d for 5 or 10 d to 6 healthy women during follicular phase of menstrual cycle *2530*

Tamoxifen *(continued)*

17α-Progesterone *Plasma Increase Physiological* Effect observed with treatment in men with oligozoospermia *1229*

Prolactin *Plasma Decrease Physiological* In 42 postmenopausal women with biopsy diagnosed breast estrogen receptor positive cancer mean concentration of 502.75 ± 82.00 mIU/L changed significantly to 290.20 ± 86.80 mIU/L after 6 months treatment with tamoxifen *3258* Significant effect in 6 healthy volunteers given 20 mg/d for 5 to 10 d *2530* In 8 premenopausal women with stage I or II breast cancer for 72 mo after mastectomy mean concentration decreased 30-40% *2982*

Plasma No Effect Physiological No effect observed with treatment in men with oligozoospermia *1229* No consistent change, but with concentrations fluctuating wildly, in 13 men with idiopathic oligozoospermia during treatment *2431*

Prothrombin Time *Plasma Increase Physiological* Observed in some patients when warfarin coadministered with tamoxifen: probably due to displacement of warfarin from protein binding sites *1384* May cause increased prothrombin time when coadministered with coumadin-type anticoagulants *6648* Probable interaction with warfarin when drugs coadministered *2625*

Sex-Hormone Binding Globulin

Serum Increase Physiological Observed effect with treatment *324* Mean increase from 1.3 ng/dL to 2.8 ng/dL in 8 postmenopausal women treated with 20 mg tamoxifen daily for 3 months *324* In 8 postmenopausal women treatment with 20 mg/d for 3 months had significant estrogenic effect on liver so that plasma concentration increased *324* During treatment increase from mean of 48.6 nmol/L to 62.8 nmol/L in 13 men with idiopathic oligozoospermia *2431* In 42 postmenopausal women with biopsy diagnosed breast estrogen receptor positive cancer mean concentration of 68.49 ± 4.80 nmol/L changed significantly to 126.22 ± 8.69 nmol/L after 6 months treatment with tamoxifen *3258* In 32 postmenopausal women with advanced breast cancer mean concentration increased from 49.0 nmol/L to 81.0 nmol/L (65.2%) after 3 to 12 months treatment *3643*

Serum No Effect Physiological In 8 premenopausal women with stage I or II breast cancer mean concentration unaffected for 72 mo after mastectomy *2982* No effect observed in men with oligozoospermia in response to treatment *1229*

Sperm Count *Semen Increase Physiological* Significant increase in sperm density, motility, and morphology in men with oligozoospermia in response to treatment *1229* Increased in oligozoospermic men if FSH concentration low or normal *1499*

Semen No Effect Physiological No significant change during treatment of 20 men with idiopathic oligozoospermia *2431*

Sperm Motility *Semen Increase Physiological* 3 months treatment of 20 men with idiopathic oligozoospermia caused significant enhancement *2431*

Sphingomyelin *Serum Increase Physiological* Insignificant increase from mean of 424 µmol/L to 453 µmol/L in 8 postmenopausal women treated with 20 mg daily for 3 months *324*

T3-Uptake *Serum Increase Physiological* In 14 postmenopausal women treated with 20 mg tamoxifen daily for 3 months mean concentration 142.43 ± 6.82 ng/dL significantly higher than 119.93 ± 3.48 ng/dL in 14 postmenopausal women treated with placebo for s months *3761*

Tamoxifen *Serum Increase Physiological* In 32 postmenopausal women with advanced breast cancer mean concentration at steady state 125.3 ng/mL *3643* In 25 healthy postmenopausal women treatment with 20 mg/d for 2 months caused a mean serum soncentration of 154 ± 140 ng/mL compared to not detectable amounts in placebo treated patients *2359*

Testosterone *Serum Decrease Physiological* In 32 postmenopausal women with advanced breast cancer mean concentration decreased from 1.09 nmol/L to 0.96 nmol/L (11.9%) after 3 to 12 months treatment *3643*

Serum Increase Physiological Increase from mean of 14.7 nmol/L to 28.4 nmol/L during treatment of 13 men with idiopathic oligozoospermia *2431* Effect observed with treatment in men with oligozoospermia *1229*

Serum No Effect Physiological In 42 postmenopausal women with biopsy diagnosed breast estrogen receptor positive cancer mean concentration of 1.28 ± 0.09 nmol/L changed nonsignificantly to 1.32 ± 0.10 nmol/L after 6 months treatment with tamoxifen *3258*

Testosterone, Free *Serum Decrease Physiological* In 42 postmenopausal women with biopsy diagnosed breast estrogen receptor positive cancer mean concentration of 6.48 ± 0.55 pmol/L changed significantly to 4.58 ± 0.65 pmol/L after 6 months treatment with tamoxifen *3258*

Thyroid Stimulating Hormone

Serum Increase Physiological In 14 postmenopausal women treated with 20 mg tamoxifen daily for 3 months mean concentration 2.28 ± 0.36 µIU/mL not significantly higher than 1.84 ± 0.22 µIU/mL in 14 postmenopausal women treated with placebo for s months *3761*

Thyroxine Binding Globulin *Serum Increase Physiological* Nonsignificant increase from mean of 36.0 nmol/L to 45.0 nmol/L in 8 postmenopausal women treated with 20 mg daily for 3 months *324* Raised in all 6 patients with breast cancer studied *2248* In 14 postmenopausal women treated with 20 mg tamoxifen daily for 3 months mean concentration 26.94 ± 1.81 µg/L not significantly higher than 20.94 ± 0.71 µg/L in 14 postmenopausal women treated with placebo for s months *3761*

Thyroxine (T4) *Serum Increase Physiological* In 10 of 50 postmenopausal patients with breast cancer. Also rose in other patients with start of treatment. Effect not observed in normal volunteers *2248* May cause increased concentration, probably due to increases in TBG, as observed in a few patients in postmarketing studies *6648* In 14 postmenopausal women treated with 20 mg tamoxifen daily for 3 months mean concentration 8.39 ± 0.46 µg/dL not significantly higher than 7.34 ± 0.42 µg/dL in 14 postmenopausal women treated with placebo for s months *3761*

Thyroxine (T4), Free *Serum Increase Physiological* Observed in one patient with persistently high thyroxine of 50 postmenopausal patients with breast cancer *2248*

Thyroxine (T4) Index, Free *Serum No Effect Physiological* In 14 postmenopausal women treated with 20 mg tamoxifen daily for 3 months mean concentration 0.059 ± 0.003 ng/ng not significantly higher than 0.062 ± 0.004 ng/ng in 14 postmenopausal women treated with placebo for s months *3761*

Transforming Growth Factor-β2

Serum Increase Physiological In 10 of 20 patients with metastatic breast cancer and 7 patients with primary breast cancer without evident metastases who responded to treatment significantly increased concentrations observed after 4 weeks of treatment *3244*

Serum No Effect Physiological In 7 of 20 patients with metastatic breast cancer and 7 patients with primary breast cancer without evident metastases who did not respond to treatment no change in concentrations observed after 4 weeks of treatment *3244*

Tri-iodothyronine (T3) *Serum Increase Physiological* In 2 of 10 postmenopausal patients with breast cancer with increased thyroxine concentration *2248*

Triglycerides *Serum Increase Physiological* Insignificant increase from mean of 137 mg/dL to 157 mg/dL in 8 postmenopausal women treated with 20 mg daily for 3 months *324* Up to 2.8 g/dL observed in one elderly woman treated for breast cancer. Possibly due to reduction of activities of postheparin plasma lipoprotein lipase and hepatic triglyceride lipase *781* In 16 normolipidemic patients with breast cancer treated with tamoxifen for 2 months mean triglyceride concentration increased significantly from 134 mg/dL to 182 mg/dL with concentration at 12 months similar *2742* In one woman previously treated by segmental mastectomy for breast cancer and subsequently with radiation therapy and tamoxifen four years after treatment begun serum triglyceride concentration increased to 4420 mg/dL when it had been less than 770 mg/dL on all previous 6-monthly follow-ups. Change of treatment to gemfibrozil caused the concentration to decrease to 218 mg/dL within 3 weeks *3028* In a 58 y-old women with a history of familial hypertriglyceridemia 3 months after mastectomy for adenocarcinoma of the breast and treatment with 20 mg/d tamoxifen serum triglyceride concentration was 795 mg/dL which increased over 4 y to 4420 mg/dL. With withdrawal of tamoxifen, and administration of gemfibrozil for 3 weeks, triglyceride concentration decreased to 218 mg/dL *3028*

On slightly higher concentration in breast cancer patients *5114* Concentration increased in 140 postmenopausal women with prior breast cancer treated by surgery with/without radiation when given 20 mg/d tamoxifen *3664*

Serum No Effect Physiological In 8 postmenopausal women treatment with 20 mg/d for 3 months had no significant effect on concentration with pretreatment concentration 137 ± 59 mg/dL changing to 157 ± 110 mg/dL after treatment *324* In 6 women with breast cancer treatment caused nonsignificant change from mean baseline of 1.66 ± 1.06 mmol/L to 1.76 ± 1.41 mmol/L after 1 month and 2.00 ± 2.31 mmol/L after 3 months *5511* In 25 healthy postmenopausal women treatment with 20 mg/d for 2 months caused a nonsignificant change from mean value with placebo of 103 ± 71 mg/dL to 106 ± 64 mg/dL *2359*

VLDL-Cholesterol *Serum Decrease Physiological* Nonsignificant decrease from mean of 230 mg/L to 210 mg/L in 8 postmenopausal women treated with 20 mg daily for 3 months *324*

Serum Increase Physiological Up to 241 mg/dL observed in one elderly woman treated for breast cancer. Possibly due to reduction of activities of postheparin plasma lipoprotein lipase and hepatic triglyceride lipase *781*

VLDL-Cholesterol, Esterified

Serum No Effect Physiological No significant change in 8 postmenopausal women treated for 3 months with 20 mg daily *324*

VLDL-Cholesterol, Free *Serum Decrease Physiological* Nonsignificant decrease from mean of 110 mg/L to 90 mg/L in 8 postmenopausal women treated with 20 mg daily for 3 months *324*

VLDL-Lecithin *Serum Increase Physiological* Nonsignificant increase from mean of 236 µmol/L to 325 µmol/L in 8 postmenopausal women treated with 20 mg daily for 3 months *324*

VLDL-Lysolecithin *Serum Increase Physiological* Nonsignificant increase from mean of 14 µmol/L to 18 µmol/L in 8 postmenopausal women treated with 20 mg daily for 3 months *324*

VLDL-Phosphatidylethanolamine

Serum Increase Physiological Nonsignificant increase from mean of 33 µmol/L to 38 µmol/L in 8 postmenopausal women treated with 20 mg daily for 3 months *324*

VLDL-Phosphoinositol *Serum Decrease Physiological* Nonsignificant reduction from mean of 26 µmol/L to 25 µmol/L in 8 postmenopausal women treated with 20 mg daily for 3 months *324*

VLDL-Sphingomyelin *Serum No Effect Physiological* No change from mean baseline concentration of 480 µmol/L in 8 postmenopausal women treated with 20 mg daily for 3 months *324*

VLDL-Triglycerides *Serum Increase Physiological* Nonsignificant increase from mean of 743 mg/L to 967 mg/L in 8 postmenopausal women treated with 20 mg daily for 3 months *324*

Volume *Semen No Effect Physiological* No significant change observed during treatment in 20 men with idiopathic oligozoospermia *2431*

Taurocholate

Lipase *Serum Increase Analytical* Sodium salts prevent inactivation of enzyme *6027*

TCDD

Thymosin-α_1 *Serum Decrease Physiological* In individuals exposed to 2,3,7,8-tetrachlorodibenzo-p-dioxin (977 ng/L versus 1149 ng/L in unexposed controls) with some correlation with duration of exposure *5790*

Temazepam

Benzodiazepine *Urine Positive Analytical* At concentrations of 0.2 µg/mL or greater produces positive result with Syva EMIT II assay *1785* Detectable limit 0.06 µg/mL with improved EMIT assay with Syva ETS system compared with 0.2 µg/mL with former d.a.u. assay *3370*

Drugs of Abuse Screen *Urine Increase Analytical* Cross-reactivity observed of 57.9% with Syva EMIT II, 73.7% with Abbott AD_x, 36.8% with Syva EMIT II and 52.6% with Abbott AD_x in different laboratories 10 hours after dosing *4699* Following ingestion of 15 mg and testing by Syva EMIT II and Abbott ADx over 24 hours positive results observed in 37 - 74% subjects *4698*

Remifentanil *Serum No Effect Physiological* Remifentanil clearance is not altered when temazepam coadministered *2165*

Tirofiban *Serum No Effect Physiological* Coadministration had no significant effect on plasma clearance of tirofiban *3957*

Temocillin

Prothrombin Time *Plasma No Effect Physiological* 4 g intravenously 12 hourly had no effect in 8 weeks *4341*

Tenidap

Digoxin *Serum No Effect Physiological* Coadministration of tenidap sodium with digoxin to healthy young men caused no significant change in plasma digoxin concentration although it took 0.5 h longer to reach the peak concentration *1404*

Phenytoin *Serum No Effect Physiological* In 12 healthy young men tenidap sodium 120 mg/d increased the percentage of unbound phenytoin in plasma by approximately 25% but did not significantly affect the area under the concentration-time curve (0.48 h) or maximum concentration *610*

Phenytoin, Free *Serum Increase Physiological* In 12 healthy young men tenidap sodium 120 mg/d increased the percentage of unbound phenytoin in plasma by approximately 25% but did not significantly affect the area under the concentration-time curve (0.48 h) or maximum concentration *610*

Tolbutamide *Serum No Effect Physiological* Administration to 12 healthy young men of tenidap sodium 120 mg/d for 22 days with intravenous administration of 1000 mg tolbutamide intravenously had no effect on clearance or plasma protein binding of tolbutamide *6481*

Tenoxicam

Bleeding Time *Patient. No Effect Physiological* In 8 healthy volunteers administration of 20 mg/d for 14 days had no effect *1676*

Factor II *Plasma No Effect Physiological* In 8 healthy volunteers administration of 20 mg/d for 14 days had no effect on factor II activity *1676*

Factor V *Plasma No Effect Physiological* In 8 healthy volunteers administration of 20 mg/d for 14 days had no effect on factor V activity *1676*

Factor VII *Plasma No Effect Physiological* In 8 healthy volunteers administration of 20 mg/d for 14 days had no effect on factor VII activity *1676*

Factor IX *Plasma No Effect Physiological* In 8 healthy volunteers administration of 20 mg/d for 14 days had no effect on factor IX activity *1676*

Factor X *Plasma No Effect Physiological* In 8 healthy volunteers administration of 20 mg/d for 14 days had no effect *1676*

Partial Thromboplastin Time

Plasma No Effect Physiological In 8 healthy volunteers administration of 20 mg/d for 14 days had no effect *1676*

Prothrombin Time *Plasma No Effect Physiological* In 8 healthy volunteers administration of 20 mg/d for 14 days had no effect *1676*

Thrombin Time *Blood No Effect Physiological* In 8 volunteers treatment with 20 mg/d for 14 days had no effect *1676*

Warfarin *Plasma No Effect Physiological* In 8 volunteers receiving 20 mg/d for 14 days no effect observed on plasma warfarin concentration or on prothrombin time *1676*

Teprotide

Angiotensin-converting Enzyme
Serum Decrease Physiological 43% inhibition reported with method using benzyloxycarbonyl-phenylalanyl- histidyl-leucine as substrate *5409*

Bradykinin *Serum Increase Physiological* Transient effect with i.v. or subcutaneous drug in one renal transplant patient *6205*

Terazosin

Albumin *Serum Decrease Physiological* Small but statistically significant decrease observed in controlled clinical trials, probably related to hemodilution *21*
Serum No Effect Physiological In 9 patients with essential hypertension treated with terazosin for 6 months baseline value of 43 ± 2 g/L not significantly changed to 43 ± 3 g/L *2237*

Apolipoprotein A-I *Serum No Effect Physiological* No significant effect in 64 mildly hypertensive patients treated with up to 10 mg daily for 10 weeks *3691*

Apolipoprotein B *Serum No Effect Physiological* no significant effect in 64 mildly hypertensive patients treated with up to 10 mg daily for 10 weeks *3691*

Captopril *Serum No Effect Physiological* In 6 individuals coadministration of terazosin with captopril had no significant effect on the concentration of captopril *21*

Cholesterol *Serum Decrease Physiological* Increase by 5.4 mg/dL with up to 20 mg daily over 4 weeks in patients with moderate hypertension *1348* Statistically significant reduction in 65 patients with mild hypertension when treated with up to 10 mg daily for 10 weeks *3691* Significant reduction observed with treatment of hypertensive Blacks *3692* In 34 hypertensive patients with impaired glucose tolerance significant reduction observed with 6 months treatment *5522*
Serum No Effect Physiological In 9 patients with essential hypertension treated with terazosin for 6 months baseline value of 5.4 ± 0.9 mmol/L not significantly changed to 5.3 ± 1.0 mmol/L *2237*

Creatinine *Serum Decrease Physiological* In 9 patients with essential hypertension treated with terazosin for 6 months baseline value of 70 ± 17 µmol/L significantly changed to 56 ± 13 µmol/L *2237*

Fibrinogen *Plasma No Effect Physiological* In 9 patients with essential hypertension treated with terazosin for 6 months baseline value of 2.19 ± 0.78 g/L not significantly changed to 2.11 ± 0.48 g/L *2237*

Filtration Rate *Red Blood Cells Increase Physiological* In 9 patients with essential hypertension treated with terazosin for 6 months baseline value of 65 ± 10 µL/s significantly changed to 75 ± 12 µL/s *2237*

Fructosamine *Serum Decrease Physiological* In 34 hypertensive patients with impaired glucose tolerance significant reduction observed with 6 months treatment *5522*

Glucose *Serum No Effect Physiological* In 9 patients with essential hypertension treated with terazosin for 6 months baseline value of 5.6 ± 0.5 mmol/L not significantly changed to 5.4 ± 0.7 mmol/L *2237* In 53 hypertensive patients treatment for 6 months had no significant effect on concentration *5522*

Glucose Tolerance *Serum Increase Physiological* In 34 hypertensive patients with impaired glucose tolerance treatment for 6 months reduced degree of glucose intolerance *5522*

HDL-Cholesterol *Serum Increase Physiological* Significantly increased concentration observed with administration of alpha$_1$-inhibitors such as terazosin over 8 weeks *3730*
Serum No Effect Physiological In 9 patients with essential hypertension treated with terazosin for 6 months baseline value of 1.3 ± 0.3 mmol/L not significantly changed to 1.4 ± 0.3 mmol/L *2237* No significant effect in 65 patients with mild hypertension treated with up to 10 mg daily for 10 weeks *3691* No significant effect with up to 20 mg daily over 4 weeks in patients with moderate hypertension *1348*

Hematocrit *Blood Decrease Physiological* Small but statistically significant decrease observed in controlled clinical trials, probably related to hemodilution *21*
Blood No Effect Physiological In 9 patients with essential hypertension treated with terazosin for 6 months baseline value of 0.42 ± 0.06 not significantly changed to 0.41 ± 0.05 *2237*

Hemoglobin *Blood Decrease Physiological* Small but statistically significant decrease observed in controlled clinical trials, probably related to hemodilution *21*

Hemoglobin A$_{1c}$ *Blood Decrease Physiological* In 34 hypertensive patients with impaired glucose tolerance treatment for 6 months significant reduction of mean concentration observed *5522*

LDL-Cholesterol *Serum Decrease Physiological* Significantly decreased concentration observed with administration of alpha$_1$-inhibitors such as terazosin in short and long term studies *3730*

Leukocytes *Blood Decrease Physiological* Small but statistically significant decrease observed in controlled clinical trials, probably related to hemodilution *21*

Prostate-specific Antigen, Free *Serum No Effect Analytical* Terazosin hydrochloride at a concentration of 1.45 g/L had no significant effect on the Hybritech Tandem® -R free PSA immunoassay *4286*

Protein *Serum Decrease Physiological* Small but statistically significant decrease observed in controlled clinical trials, probably related to hemodilution *21*

Triglycerides *Serum Decrease Physiological* Significant reduction in 65 mildly hypertensive patients treated with up to 10 mg daily for 10 weeks *3691* Significant reduction observed with treatment of hypertensive Blacks *3692* In 9 patients with essential hypertension treated with terazosin for 6 months baseline value of 1.7 ± 1.3 mmol/L not significantly changed to 1.2 ± 0.7 mmol/L *2237* In 34 hypertensive patients with impaired glucose tolerance treatment for 6 months caused significant reduction *5522*
Serum No Effect Physiological No significant effect with up to 20 mg daily over 4 weeks in patients with moderate hypertension *1348*

Viscosity *Blood Decrease Physiological* In 9 patients with essential hypertension treated with terazosin for 6 months significant reduction observed over shear rate from 22.5 to 450 /s *2237*
Plasma No Effect Physiological In 9 patients with essential hypertension treated with terazosin for 6 months no significant change over shear rate from 2.25 to 450 /s *2237*

VLDL + LDL-Cholesterol *Serum Decrease Physiological* Decrease by 6.1 mg/dL with up to 20 mg daily over 4 weeks in patients with moderate hypertension *1348* Statistically significant reduction in 65 mildly hypertensive patients treated with up to 10 mg daily for 10 weeks *3691*

VLDL-Cholesterol *Serum Decrease Physiological* Significantly decreased concentration observed with administration of alpha$_1$-inhibitors such as terazosin in short and long term studies *3730*

Terbinafine

Alanine Aminotransferase *Serum Increase Physiological* Rare cases of hepatobiliary dysfunction including cholestatic hepatitis have been reported *5231*

Alkaline Phosphatase *Serum Increase Physiological* Rare cases of hepatobiliary dysfunction including cholestatic hepatitis have been reported *5231*

Antipyrine *Serum No Effect Physiological* Terbinafine has no effect on the clearance of antipyrine *5231*

Aspartate Aminotransferase *Serum Increase Physiological* Rare cases of hepatobiliary dysfunction including cholestatic hepatitis have been reported *5231*

Bilirubin *Serum Increase Physiological* Rare cases of hepatobiliary dysfunction including cholestatic hepatitis have been reported *5231*

Caffeine *Serum Increase Physiological* Terbinafine decreased the clearance of intravenously administered caffeine by 19% *5231*

Cyclosporine A *Blood Decrease Physiological* Terbinafine increased the clearance of cyclosporine by 15% *5231*

γ-Glutamyltransferase *Serum Increase Physiological* Rare cases of hepatobiliary dysfunction including cholestatic hepatitis have been reported *5231*

Lymphocytes *Blood Decrease Physiological* Transient decreases in absolute lymphocyte count have been reported (8 of 465 patients) in clinical trials *5231*

Neutrophils *Blood Decrease Physiological* Isolated decreases in neutrophil count have been reported in clinical trials *5231*

Terfenadine *Serum No Effect Physiological* Terbinafine has no effect on the clearance of terfenadine *5231*

Warfarin *Plasma No Effect Physiological* Terbinafine has no effect on the clearance of warfarin *5231*

Terbutaline

Alanine *Plasma No Effect Physiological* No significant effect observed in either 6 insulin-infused initially euglycemic IDDM patients or 6 healthy nondiabetic individuals after either 5.0 mg orally or 0.25 mg subcutaneously *6446*

Alanine Aminotransferase *Serum Increase Physiological* Rare reports of increased liver enzyme activities and of hypersensitivity vasculitis *2641* Rare reports of increased activity of liver enzymes and hypersensitivity vasculitis *1024*

Albumin *Serum No Effect Physiological* In 6 normal men treated with therapeutic amounts for 2 weeks *5319*

Aspartate Aminotransferase *Serum Increase Physiological* Rare reports of increased liver enzyme activities and of hypersensitivity vasculitis *2641* Rare reports of increased activity of liver enzymes and hypersensitivity vasculitis *1024*

Cholesterol *Serum No Effect Physiological* No significant effect observed after 2 weeks in 15 subjects *2705*

Cortisol *Plasma No Effect Physiological* In 6 healthy nondiabetic individuals administration of either 2.5 or 5.0 mg orally or 0.25 mg subcutaneously no significant effect observed. In diabetics no significant effect observed *6446*

C-Peptide *Plasma Increase Physiological* In 6 healthy nondiabetic individuals significant increase observed after administration of 0.25 mg subcutaneously *6446*

Epinephrine *Plasma No Effect Physiological* In 6 normal men treated with therapeutic amounts for 2 weeks *5319* In 6 healthy nondiabetic individuals oral administration of 2.5 or 5.0 mg or 0.25 mg subcutaneously had no significant effect. In diabetics no significant effect observed *6446*

Fatty Acids (FFA), Free *Serum Increase Physiological* Nonsignificant increase observed in 6 nondiabetic healthy individuals after 5.0 mg orally or 0.25 mg subcutaneously. Increase more marked in diabetics *6446*

Serum No Effect Physiological In 6 normal men treated with therapeutic amounts for 2 weeks *5319*

Gastrin *Serum Increase Physiological* Subcutaneous or oral drug increased concentration in normal subjects and in patients with Zollinger-Ellison syndrome and in vagotomized individuals *6004*

Glucagon *Plasma No Effect Physiological* In 6 healthy nondiabetic individuals administration of either 2.5 or 5.0 mg orally or 0.25 mg subcutaneously had no significant effect. No effect observed in diabetics *6446*

Glucose *Serum Decrease Physiological* With overdosage varying degrees of hyperglycemia and rise in insulin levels may occur followed by rebound hypoglycemia *2641*

Serum Increase Physiological Observed following infusion of 0.25 mg or 5 mg 3 times/d on first day of treatment *479* With overdosage varying degrees of hyperglycemia and rise in insulin levels may occur followed by rebound hypoglycemia *2641* In 6 healthy nondiabetics administration of 2.5 mg orally caused significant increase from mean baseline of 5.4 ± 0.2 mmol/L to a peak of 5.8 ± 0.2 mmol/L and from 5.6 ± 0.3 mmol/L to 6.3 ± 0.3 mmol/L at 60 minutes after 5.0 mg orally. Increase from 5.3 ± 0.3 mmol/L to 6.0 ± 0.3 mmol/L observed after subcutaneous administration of 0.25 mg although none of the increases were significant. In diabetics substantial dose-related increases observed *6446* Large doses of intravenous terbutaline have been shown to aggravate preexisting diabetes mellitus and ketoacidosis *1024*

Serum No Effect Physiological In 6 normal men treated with therapeutic amounts for 2 weeks *5319*

Growth Hormone *Plasma No Effect Physiological* Administration of 2,5 or 5.0 mg orally or 0.25 mg subcutaneously to 6 healthy nondiabetic individuals had no significant effect on concentration. In diabetics no significant effect observed *6446*

HDL-Cholesterol *Serum Increase Physiological* 10% increase with 2 weeks treatment in 15 subjects *2705*

Hydrochloric Acid *Gastric Fluid Decrease Physiological* Reduces mean concentration in response to a variety of challenges in spite of an increase in serum gastrin concentration *6004*

β-Hydroxybutyrate *Serum Increase Physiological* In 6 healthy individuals nonsignificant increase observed after 5.0 mg orally or 0.25 mg subcutaneously. Effect more marked in diabetics *6446*

Insulin *Plasma Increase Physiological* Observed following infusion of 0.25 mg or 5 mg 3 times/d on first day of treatment *479* With overdosage varying degrees of hyperglycemia and rise in insulin levels may occur followed by rebound hypoglycemia *2641* In 6 healthy nondiabetics administration of either 2.5 or 5.0 mg orally or 0.25 mg subcutaneously caused significant increase up to 120 pmol/L from baseline of about 40 pmol/L *6446*

Plasma No Effect Physiological In 6 normal men treated with therapeutic amounts for 2 weeks *5319*

Ketones *Serum Increase Physiological* Large doses of intravenous terbutaline have been shown to aggravate preexisting diabetes mellitus and ketoacidosis *1024*

Lactate *Plasma Increase Physiological* In 6 healthy nondiabetic individuals insignificant dose-related increase observed. In diabetics dose-related significant increase observed *6446*

LDL-Cholesterol *Serum No Effect Physiological* No significant effect observed after 2 weeks in 15 subjects *2705*

Norepinephrine *Plasma Increase Physiological* In 6 healthy nondiabetics administration of 0.25 mg subcutaneously caused significant increase from mean baseline of about 1.4 nmol/L to peak of about 2.5 nmol/L. In diabetics same effect observed *6446*

Plasma No Effect Physiological In 6 normal men treated with therapeutic amounts for 2 weeks *5319*

Pancreatic Polypeptide *Plasma No Effect Physiological* In 6 healthy nondiabetic individuals administration of 2.5 or 5.0 mg orally or 0.25 mg subcutaneously had no significant effect on concentration. In diabetics no significant effect observed *6446*

Potassium *Serum Decrease Physiological* Observed following infusion of 0.25 mg or 5 mg 3 times/d on first day of treatment *479* With overdosage hypokalemia may occur in the early stages *2641*

Serum Increase Physiological Due to β_2-adrenergic mediated uptake of potassium in skeletal muscle and other tissues (decrease of about 0.8 mmol/L) *2977*

Serum No Effect Physiological In 6 normal men treated with therapeutic amounts for 2 weeks *5319* No reduction after oral treatment for 13 d *479*

Prealbumin *Serum No Effect Physiological* In 6 normal men treated with therapeutic amounts for 2 weeks *5319*

Protein *Serum No Effect Physiological* In 6 normal men treated with therapeutic amounts for 2 weeks *5319*

Theophylline *Serum Decrease Physiological* 0.075 mg 3 times per day caused average reduction of serum concentration from 13.8 to 10.8 µg/mL when sustained release drug given *1236* Administration of 2.5 mg t.d.s. to 6 adult asthmatic patients together with 200-400 mg b.d. sustained release theophylline decreased serum trough concentration from 8.1 to 7.3 µg/mL although peak concentration and timing unaffected. Clearance increased *2038*

Serum Increase Analytical At concentration of 4 mg/L produced positive bias of 2.90 mg/L at theophylline concentration of 20.0 mg/L when serum analyzed by Abbott Vision system and bias of 5.05 mg/L when measured by 3M Diagnostics TheoFAST method *1122*

Serum No Effect Analytical At concentration of 4 mg/L produced no interference with methods used with Kodak DT60, Abbott TDx, Abbott Vision when whole blood analyzed, Syntex AccµLevel, and Ames Seralyzer *1122*

Serum No Effect Physiological No clinically significant effect on theophylline concentration observed when systemic terbutaline coadministered *5999* No documented significant interaction with theophylline reported *6117*

Thyroid Stimulating Hormone
Serum No Effect Physiological In 6 normal men treated with therapeutic amounts for 2 weeks *5319*

Terbutaline *(continued)*

Thyroxine Binding Globulin *Serum No Effect Physiological* In 6 normal men treated with therapeutic amounts for 2 weeks *5319*

Thyroxine (T4) *Serum Decrease Physiological* From 7.2 to 6.7 µg/dL on average in 6 normal men after 2 weeks treatment *5319* In 6 normal men after 15 mg/d for 2 weeks with non-significant change from 6.7 to 7.2 mg/dL *5319*

Thyroxine (T4), Free *Serum No Effect Physiological* In 6 normal men treated with therapeutic amounts for 2 weeks *5319*

Tri-iodothyronine, Free (fT3) *Serum No Effect Physiological* In 6 normal men treated with therapeutic amounts for 2 weeks *5319*

Tri-iodothyronine, Reverse (rT3) *Serum No Effect Physiological* In 6 normal men treated with therapeutic amounts for 2 weeks *5319*

Tri-iodothyronine (T3) *Serum Increase Physiological* In 6 normal men after 15 mg/d for 2 weeks with average of 160 ng/dL versus 136 ng/dL in controls *5319*

Triglycerides *Serum No Effect Physiological* No significant effect observed after 2 weeks in 15 subjects *2705*

Terfenadine

Carbamazepine *Serum Increase Physiological* Drugs that inhibit CYP 3A4 inhibit metabolism of carbamazepine producing clinically meaningful effect *1039*

Clarithromycin *Serum No Effect Physiological* Coadministration of clarithromycin with terfenadine had no significant effect on the concentration of clarithromycin *11*

Histamine *Plasma No Effect Analytical* Improbable inhibition of radio-enzyme assay at physiological concentrations *2492*

Terbinafine *Serum Increase Physiological* Terfenadine decreased the clearance of terbinafine by 16% *5231*

Theophylline *Serum No Effect Physiological* No documented significant interaction with theophylline reported *6117* No clinically significant effect on theophylline concentration observed when drugs coadministered *5999*

Zafirlukast *Serum Decrease Physiological* In 16 healthy men coadministration of zafirlukast (320 mg/d) with terfenadine (120 mg/d) caused a significant decrease of 66% in the mean plasma concentration and 54% decrease in the area under the time/concentration curve of zafirlukast *6641*

Terguride

6-β-Hydroxycortisol *Urine No Effect Physiological* Excretion remained constant at mean of 0.29 mg/d before and during treatment with doses from 0.50 mg daily for 1 week to 1.50 mg daily for 1 week in 10 healthy volunteers *3277*

Prolactin *Plasma Decrease Physiological* Slight lowering effect observed in men during first two hours after 0.05 mg intravenously. With oral administration clear cut dose dependent depression of plasma concentration both in morning and two hours after drug *3277*

Terodiline

Thrombotest *Plasma No Effect Physiological* No effect observed in 23 healthy young volunteers given 50 mg daily for 2 weeks concomitantly with warfarin *2663*

Warfarin *Plasma No Effect Physiological* No effect observed in 23 healthy young volunteers given 50 mg/day over two weeks *2663*

Tertatolol

Albumin *Urine No Effect Physiological* In 8 patients with essential hypertension treatment with a mean dose of 4.1 mg/d for 3 months caused nonsignificant change from mean baseline of 20 ± 8 µg/min to 19 ± 9 µg/min over 24 hours and during clearances from 25 ± 7 µg/min to 23 ± 9 µg/min *4945*

Aldosterone *Plasma No Effect Physiological* In 8 patients with essential hypertension treatment with a mean dose of 4.1 mg/d for 3 months caused nonsignificant change from mean baseline of 13.9 ± 2.7 ng/dL to 13.0 ± 2.6 ng/dL *4945*

Apolipoprotein A-I *Serum Increase Physiological* In 39 hypertensives treatment with 5 mg/d for 9 months caused 6% increase from mean baseline of 1.48 ± 0.05 g/L to 1.59 ± 0.08 g/L *1423*

Apolipoprotein A-I:Apolipoprotein B Ratio *Serum Decrease Physiological* In 39 hypertensives treatment with 5 mg/d for 9 months 7% reduction from mean baseline of 1.38 ± 0.15 to 1.29 ± 0.08 *1423*

Apolipoprotein A-II *Serum Increase Physiological* In 39 hypertensive patients treatment with 5 mg/d for 9 months caused significant increase of 24% from mean baseline of 0.37 ± 0.02 g/L to 0.46 g/L *1423*

Apolipoprotein B *Serum Increase Physiological* In 39 hypertensives treatment with 5 mg/d for 9 months caused significant 13% increase from mean baseline of 1.13 ± 0.06 g/L to 1.28 ± 0.07 g/L *1423*

Calcium *Serum No Effect Physiological* No significant effect in 12 healthy volunteers over 24 hours following single dose of 5 mg *3452*
Urine No Effect Physiological No significant effect in 12 healthy volunteers over 24 hours following single oral dose of 5 mg *3452*

Chloride *Serum No Effect Physiological* No significant effect in 12 healthy volunteers over 24 hours following single dose of 5 mg *3452*
Urine No Effect Physiological No significant effect in 12 healthy volunteers over 24 hours following single oral dose of 5 mg *3452*

Cholesterol *Serum No Effect Physiological* In 39 patients with mid to moderate hypertension treatment with 5 mg/d for 9 months caused nonsignificant change from mean baseline of 6.48 ± 0.32 mmol/L to 6.36 ± 0.32 mmol/L *1423*

Creatinine *Serum No Effect Physiological* No significant effect in 12 healthy volunteers over 24 hours following single dose of 5 mg *3452*
Urine No Effect Physiological No significant effect in 12 healthy volunteers over 24 hours following single oral dose of 5 mg *3452*

Effective Renal Plasma Flow *Patient No Effect Physiological* In 8 patients with essential hypertension treatment with a mean dose of 4.1 mg/d for 3 months caused nonsignificant change from mean baseline of 425 ± 31 mL/min/1.73 sq m to 444 ± 43 mL/min/1.73 sq m *4945*

Epinephrine *Plasma No Effect Physiological* In 20 patients with hypertension following head injury treatment with a single dose of 5 mg caused nonsignificant increase from mean baseline of 697 ± 86 pg/mL to 761 ± 138 pg/mL after 2 h and 926 ± 120 pg/mL after 4 h *3480*

Filtration Fraction *Urine No Effect Physiological* In 8 patients with essential hypertension treatment with a mean dose of 4.1 mg/d for 3 months caused nonsignificant change from mean baseline of 0.25 ± 0.02 to 0.23 ± 0.01 *4945*

Glomerular Filtration Rate *Urine No Effect Physiological* In 8 patients with essential hypertension treatment with a mean dose of 4.1 mg/d for 3 months caused nonsignificant change from mean baseline of 104 ± 6 mL/min/1.73 sq m to 101 ± 6 mL/min/1.73 sq m *4945*

HDL-Cholesterol *Serum No Effect Physiological* In 39 hypertensives mean concentration of 1.07 ± 0.05 mmol/L not significantly reduced to 1.04 ± 0.07 mmol/L after treatment with 5 mg/d for 9 months *1423*

Inulin Clearance *Urine No Effect Physiological* No significant change observed in 14 patients given 5 mg daily for 2 months *3801*

Kallikrein *Urine No Effect Physiological* In 8 patients with essential hypertension treatment with a mean dose of 4.1 mg/d for 3 months caused nonsignificant change from mean baseline of 8.0 ± 1.9 nkat/d to 7.2 ± 2.0 nkat/d and during clearance from 15.9 ± 3.7 pkat/min to 13.5 ± 3.7 pkat/min *4945*

LDL-Cholesterol *Serum No Effect Physiological* In 39 hypertensive individuals treatment with 5 mg/d for 9 months caused nonsignificant reduction from mean baseline of 4.69 ± 0.29 mmol/L to 4.38 ± 0.27 mmol/L *1423*

Magnesium *Serum No Effect Physiological* No significant effect in 12 healthy volunteers over 24 hours following single dose of 5 mg *3452*
Urine No Effect Physiological No significant effect in 12 healthy volunteers over 24 hours following single oral dose of 5 mg *3452*

Norepinephrine *Plasma Increase Physiological* In 20 patients with hypertension following head injury a single dose of 5 mg caused significant increase from mean baseline of 1189 ± 202 pg/mL to 1377 ± 232 pg/mL after 2 h and 1431 ± 189 pg/mL after 4 h *3480*

Oxygen Partial Pressure *Blood Increase Physiological* In 20 patients with hypertension following head injury admnistation of 5 mg caused nonsignificant increase of arterial pO_2 from mean baseline of 92 ± 8 mm Hg to 97 ± 6 mm Hg after 2 h and 100 ± 10 mm Hg after 4 h *3480*

PAH Clearance *Urine No Effect Physiological* No significant change observed in 14 patients given 5 mg daily for 2 months *3801*

Phosphate *Serum Increase Physiological* Significant effect in 12 healthy volunteers at 24 hours following single dose of 5 mg but effect slight and not clinically significant. No apparent change earlier *3452*
Urine No Effect Physiological No significant effect in 12 healthy volunteers over 24 hours following single oral dose of 5 mg *3452*

Potassium *Serum Increase Physiological* In 8 patients with essential hypertension treatment with a mean dose of 4.1 mg/d for 3 months caused significant change from mean baseline of 3.6 ± 0.1 mmol/L to 3.8 ± 0.1 mmol/L *4945*
Serum No Effect Physiological No significant effect in 12 healthy volunteers over 24 hours following single dose of 5 mg *3452*
Urine No Effect Physiological In 8 patients with essential hypertension treatment with a mean dose of 4.1 mg/d for 3 months caused nonsignificant change from mean baseline of 59 ± 7 mmol/d to 47 ± 8 mmol/d *4945* No significant effect in 12 healthy volunteers over 24 hours following single oral dose of 5 mg *3452*

Renin Activity *Plasma Decrease Physiological* In 8 patients with essential hypertension treatment with a mean dose of 4.1 mg/d for 3 months caused significant change from mean baseline of 2.98 ± 0.86 ng/mL/h to 0.69 ± 0.19 ng/mL/h *4945*

Sodium *Serum No Effect Physiological* No significant effect in 12 healthy volunteers over 24 hours following single dose of 5 mg *3452* In 8 patients with essential hypertension treatment with a mean dose of 4.1 mg/d for 3 months caused nonsignificant change from mean baseline of 140 ± 1 mmol/L to 141 ± 1 mmol/L *4945*
Urine No Effect Physiological No significant effect in 12 healthy volunteers over 24 hours following single oral dose of 5 mg *3452* In 8 patients with essential hypertension treatment with a mean dose of 4.1 mg/d for 3 months caused nonsignificant change from mean baseline of 123 ± 12 mmol/d to 108 ± 14 mmol/d *4945*

Triglycerides *Serum No Effect Physiological* In 39 hypertensive patients treatment with 5 mg/d for 9 months caused nonsignificant change from mean baseline of 2.16 ± 0.28 mmol/L to 2.19 ± 0.17 mmol/L *1423*

Urea *Urine No Effect Physiological* In 8 patients with essential hypertension treatment with a mean dose of 4.1 mg/d for 3 months caused nonsignificant change from mean baseline of 358 ± 17 mmol/d to 377 ± 29 mmol/d *4945*

Urea Nitrogen *Serum Increase Physiological* Significant effect in 12 healthy volunteers at 24 hours following single dose of 5 mg, although no increase observed earlier *3452*
Urine No Effect Physiological No significant effect in 12 healthy volunteers over 24 hours following single oral dose of 5 mg *3452*

Uric Acid *Serum No Effect Physiological* No effect in 12 healthy volunteers over 24 hours following single dose of 5 mg *3452*
Urine No Effect Physiological No significant effect in 12 healthy volunteers over 24 hours following single oral dose of 5 mg *3452*

VLDL-Cholesterol *Serum No Effect Physiological* In 39 hypertensives treatment with 5 mg/d for 9 months caused nonsignificant increase from mean baseline of 0.86 ± 0.12 mmol/L to 0.88 ± 0.09 mmol/L *1423*

Volume *Urine No Effect Physiological* No significant effect in 12 healthy volunteers over 24 hours following single oral dose of 5 mg *3452*

Zinc *Serum No Effect Physiological* No significant effect in 12 healthy volunteers over 24 hours following single dose of 5 mg, although slight reduction observed at 6 hours *3452*
Urine No Effect Physiological No significant effect in 12 healthy volunteers over 24 hours following single oral dose of 5 mg *3452*

Testolactone

Androstenedione *Serum Increase Analytical* Produces marked cross-reactivity with Sanofi DSL coated tube RIA procedure *1193*

Calcium *Serum Increase Physiological* Probable effect during remission of metastases *128*

Estradiol *Plasma No Effect Analytical* Produces no cross-reactivity with Intermedico DPC Coat-a-Count RIA procedure *1193*

17-Ketosteroids *Urine Increase Physiological* Reported effect *2451*

Testosterone *Serum Increase Analytical* Produces marked cross-reactivity with Medicorp ImmuChem double antibody RIA procedure *1193*

Tetrabenazine

Homovanillic Acid
Cerebrospinal Fluid Increase Physiological Significant effect in chorea after oral administration *3908*

5-Hydroxyindoleacetic Acid
Cerebrospinal Fluid No Effect Physiological No significant effect in Huntington's chorea *3908*

Tetracaine

Protein *Cerebrospinal Fluid Increase Analytical* Interferes with Folin-Ciocalteu reagent *2024*

Sulfa as Sulfanilamide *Serum Increase Analytical* Yields diazotization reaction *409*

Tetrachloroethylene

Protein *Urine Increase Physiological* May cause nephrotoxicity *5377*

Urea Nitrogen *Serum Increase Physiological* May cause nephrotoxicity *5377*

Tetrachlorothyronine

Thyroxine (T4) *Serum Decrease Physiological* Displaces thyroxine from thyroxine binding globulin *5869*

Tetracosactrin

Adenosine Monophosphate *Plasma Increase Physiological* Increase from baseline value of 18.2 nmol/L to maximum of 24.2 nmol/L in 21 normal volunteers following i.v. injection of 0.25 mg. Increase began 5 minutes after injection and persisted for 60 minutes *1950*

Alanine *Plasma Increase Physiological* In healthy volunteers given 1 mg intramuscularly for up to 60 h *2962*

Aldolase *Serum Increase Physiological* Probably due to muscle damage at injection site *463*

Corticosteroids *Plasma Increase Physiological* Therapeutic intent has prolonged action *3091*

Cortisol *Plasma Increase Physiological* Rise of 21 µg/dL in 6 h after i.m. injections *463* 3 fold increase in healthy vol-

Tetracosactrin *(continued)*

Cortisol *(continued)*
unteers given 1 mg intramuscularly for up to 60 h *2962* Rise in concentration parallels increase in concentration of cyclic AMP *1950*

Fatty Acids (FFA), Free *Serum No Effect Physiological* In healthy volunteers given 1 mg intramuscularly for up to 60 h *2962*

Glucose *Serum Increase Physiological* From 5.2 to 7.2 mmol/L healthy volunteers given 1 mg intramuscularly for up to 60 h *2962*

Glycerol *Serum No Effect Physiological* In healthy volunteers given 1 mg intramuscularly for up to 60 h *2962*

Growth Hormone *Plasma Increase Physiological* Associated with change in cortisol concentration *463*

Hematocrit *Blood Decrease Physiological* Maximum effect observed after 24 h *463*

Insulin *Plasma Increase Physiological* From 5.2 to 13.1 mU/L healthy volunteers given 1 mg intramuscularly for up to 60 h *2962*

Ketones *Serum No Effect Physiological* In healthy volunteers given 1 mg intramuscularly for up to 60 h *2962*

Lactate *Plasma Increase Physiological* In healthy volunteers given 1 mg intramuscularly for up to 60 h *2962*

Leukocytes *Blood Increase Physiological* Increase (mainly NPL) of 7,000 seen in 1 d *4996*

Pyruvate *Plasma Increase Physiological* In healthy volunteers given 1 mg intramuscularly for up to 60 h *2962*

Tetracycline

Acetaminophen *Serum Decrease Analytical* Slight reduction of up to 18% at just above upper therapeutic concentration on method using o-cresol reaction *949*

Alanine Aminotransferase *Serum Increase Physiological* Hepatotoxic especially in pregnant women *4691*
Serum No Effect Analytical At 5 times upper limit of therapeutic range on methods on Technicon SMAC® , Abbott-VP, Roche Cobas-Bio, Du Pont aca, and KDA *3525*

Albumin *Serum No Effect Analytical* At concentration of 300 mg/L had no effect on BCG method *5704* At 5 times upper limit of therapeutic range on methods on Technicon SMAC® , Kodak Ektachem® , Hitachi® 705 and KDA *3525*

Alkaline Phosphatase *Serum Increase Physiological* May occur with cholestasis *2451* 2 cases of drug-associated fatty liver of pregnancy *6408*
Serum No Effect Analytical At 5 times upper limit of therapeutic range on methods on Technicon SMAC® , Abbott-VP, Roche Cobas-Bio, Du Pont aca, Hitachi® 705 and KDA *3525*

Amikacin *Serum No Effect Analytical* Error of less than 5% observed when tetracycline added at a concentration of 100 mg/L to a specimen containing 15 mg/L amikacin and measured on Baxter Stratus *5705* No interference observed at a concentration of 1000 µg/mL (2250 µmol/L) with method on Du Pont aca *1508*

Amino Acids *Urine Increase Physiological* Nephrotoxic effect with degraded tetracycline *2024*

Ammonia *Plasma Decrease Physiological* Reduces production by gut bacteria *2452*
Plasma Increase Physiological If given i.v. in large doses *2451*

Amylase *Serum Increase Physiological* Toxic effect especially in pregnant women *2451*
Serum No Effect Analytical At 5 times upper limit of therapeutic range on methods on Du Pont aca, Roche Cobas-Bio and Kodak Ektachem® *3525*

Antithrombin III *Plasma No Effect Analytical* At concentration of 1,000 mg/L had no effect on Du Pont aca method *5704*

Ascorbic Acid *White Blood Cells Decrease Physiological* Other antibiotics also have effect *5964*

Aspartate Aminotransferase *Serum Increase Physiological* 2 cases of drug-associated fatty liver of pregnancy *6408* Hepatotoxic especially in pregnant women *4691*
Serum No Effect Analytical At 5 times upper limit of therapeutic range on methods on Technicon SMAC® , Abbott-VP, Roche Cobas-Bio, Du Pont aca, Hitachi® 705 and KDA *3525*

Bence-Jones Protein *Urine Positive Physiological* Nephrotoxic effect with degraded tetracycline *1714*

Bicarbonate *Serum Decrease Physiological* May cause acidosis with nephrotoxicity *128*
Serum No Effect Analytical At concentration of 4 mg/L had no effect on method using phenolphthalein *5704*

Bilirubin *Serum Increase Physiological* 2 cases of drug-associated fatty liver of pregnancy *6408* Hepatic injury may occur especially if given i.v *563*
Serum No Effect Analytical At 5 times upper limit of therapeutic range on methods on Technicon SMAC® , Roche Cobas-Bio, Du Pont aca, Kodak Ektachem® , Hitachi® 705 and KDA *3525* At concentration of 300 mg/L had no effect on Jendrassik and Grof method *5704* At concentration of 10 mg/L had no effect on Kodak Ektachem® method *5704*

Bilirubin, Conjugated *Serum No Effect Analytical* No effect at concentration of 30 mg/L on method on Kodak Ektachem® *5706* At concentration of 3.6 µg/mL (8.1 µmol/L) had no effect on method on Du Pont aca *1517*

Bilirubin, Direct *Serum Increase Physiological* 2 cases of drug-associated fatty liver of pregnancy *6408* Cholestatic effect *1485*

Bilirubin, Unconjugated *Serum No Effect Analytical* No effect at concentration of 30 mg/L on method on Kodak Ektachem® *5706*

BSP Retention *Serum Increase Physiological* Cholestatic especially in pregnant women *4691*

Calcium *Serum Decrease Physiological* Observed in pregnant women *4014*
Serum No Effect Analytical At concentration of 300 mg/L had no effect on cresolphthalein method *5704* At 5 times upper limit of therapeutic range on methods on Technicon SMAC® , Abbott-VP, Du Pont aca, Kodak Ektachem® , Hitachi® 705 and KDA *3525*

Cannabinoids *Urine No Effect Analytical* No effect on Roche Abuscreen method *5006*

Catecholamines *Plasma Increase Analytical* Interferes with fluorometric techniques *189*
Urine Increase Analytical Produces interfering fluorescence *2999*

Chloramphenicol *Serum No Effect Analytical* No effect at 100 mg/L on coupled enzymatic method *4122*

Chloride *Serum No Effect Analytical* At concentration of 300 mg/L had no effect on mercurimetric method *5704*

Cholesterol *Serum Decrease Physiological* Hepatotoxicity may occur *4691*
Serum Increase Analytical At concentrations above 50 mg/L (normal therapeutic concentration 8 mg/L) raised concentration as measured by CHOD-Iodide method *5704*
Serum No Effect Analytical At concentration of 200 mg/L had no effect on method using catalase-Hantzsch reaction *5704* At 5 times upper limit of therapeutic range on methods on Technicon SMAC® , Abbott-VP, Roche Cobas-Bio, Kodak Ektachem® , Hitachi® 705 and KDA *3525* At concentration of 200 mg/L had no effect on CHOD-PAP method *5704* At concentration of 300 mg/L had no effect on Liebermann-Burchard method *5704* At concentration of 200 mg/L had no effect on catalase-AIDH method *5704*
Serum No Effect Physiological No effect seen even when administered orally *2452*

Chromosomes *Test Conditions No Effect Physiological* Not clastogenic in human cells *5484*

Clindamycin *Serum Positive Analytical* Interfere with bioassays *3858*

Clotting Time *Blood Increase Physiological* Delayed coagulation reported *3810*

Colistin *Serum Positive Analytical* Interfere with bioassays *3858*

Color *Feces Increase Analytical* Red if glucosamine potentiated syrup form *3810*
Urine Increase Analytical Greenish blue *3810*

Coombs' Test *Blood Positive Physiological* Mechanism obscure *2453*

Creatine Kinase *Serum No Effect Analytical* At 5 times upper limit of therapeutic range on methods on Technicon SMAC® , Abbott-VP, Roche Cobas-Bio, Du Pont aca and Hitachi® 705 *3525*

Creatinine *Serum Increase Physiological* Nephrotoxicity may cause Fanconi like syndrome *4691*
Serum No Effect Analytical No effect of concentrations up to 15 mg/L on single slide method on Kodak Ektachem® *5706* No effect of concentrations up to 15 mg/L on 2-slide method on Kodak Ektachem® *5706* At concentration of 60 mg/L had no effect on creatinine iminohydrolase method *5704* At concentration of 200 mg/L had no effect on Jaffe-Fading-Fraction method *5704* At 5 times upper limit of therapeutic range on methods on Technicon SMAC® , Abbott-VP, Du Pont aca, Roche Cobas-Bio, Kodak Ektachem® , Hitachi® 705 and KDA *3525* At concentration of 200 mg/L had no effect on Jaffe-Fuller's earth method *5704* At concentration of 40 mg/L had no effect on kinetic Jaffe method on BKA-2 *5704* At concentration of 300 mg/L had no effect on Technicon AutoAnalyzer® Jaffe method *5704*

Drugs of Abuse Screen *Urine No Effect Analytical* No effect at concentration of 100 µg/mL on EZ-SCREEN procedure for cannabinoids and cocaine *1739*

Eosinophils *Blood Increase Physiological* Allergic response *2484* Eosinophilia reported as a side effect *3461*

Erythrocytes *Blood Decrease Physiological* May cause hemolytic anemia *3810*

Erythromycin *Serum Increase Analytical* Interferes with bioassays *3858*

Folate *Serum Decrease Analytical* Inhibits growth of *L. casei5869*
Serum Decrease Physiological Isolated case of impaired absorption *2965*
Serum No Effect Analytical Allegedly no effect on autoclave method *2965*

Gentamicin *Serum Increase Analytical* At concentrations up to 750 mg/L caused 25% increase with method on Baxter Stratus but not clinically relevant since clinical concentrations only up to 30 mg/L *5705*
Serum No Effect Analytical No interference observed at concentrations up to 500 µg/mL (1125 µmol/L) with method on Du Pont aca *1526*

Glucose *Serum Decrease Analytical* Ascorbic acid in preparation may affect glucose oxidase procedure *882* At concentrations above 20 mg/L (normal therapeutic concentration 8 mg/L) lowered concentration as measured by GOD/POD-PAP method *5704*
Serum Increase Analytical Mg for mg (approximately) effect with MBTH procedure of Neeley *4241* Slight effect on hexokinase, o-toluidine methods *4240*
Serum No Effect Analytical At concentration of 20 mg/L had no effect on Kodak Ektachem® method *5704* At concentration of 500 mg/L had no effect on Ames Seralyzer method *5704* No effect on glucose oxidase method *4240* No effect at 1000 mg/L on hexokinase method on Ames Seralyzer *5706* No significant effect at 1 g/L on glucokinase based assay of Scott *5414* No effect at 500 mg/L on glucose oxidase method on Ames Seralyzer *5706* At 5 times upper limit of therapeutic range on methods on Technicon SMAC® , Abbott-VP, Du Pont aca, Roche Cobas-Bio, Kodak Ektachem® , Hitachi® 705 and KDA *3525*
Urine Decrease Analytical Prevents oxidation of chromogen in glucose oxidase methods *4012* False negative dipstick test if buffered with ascorbic acid *1828*
Urine Increase Physiological Degraded material may cause Fanconi-like syndrome *4014* Degraded drug may cause Fanconi like syndrome *4691*

γ-Glutamyltransferase *Serum No Effect Analytical* At 5 times upper limit of therapeutic range on methods on Technicon SMAC® , Abbott-VP and Hitachi® 705 *3525*

Hematocrit *Blood Decrease Physiological* Hemolytic anemia reported as a side effect *3461* May cause hemolytic anemia *3810*

Hemoglobin *Blood Decrease Physiological* May cause hemolytic anemia *3810* Hemolytic anemia reported as a side effect *3461*
Urine Decrease Analytical In large amounts if buffered with ascorbate *882*

Histidine *Urine Increase Physiological* Unexplained mechanism *2242*

^{131}I Uptake *Serum Decrease Physiological* Panmycin® contains tetraiodofluorescein *4360*
Serum No Effect Physiological No effect with 2 g/d for 11 d *882*

Iron *Serum No Effect Analytical* At 5 times upper limit of therapeutic range on Ferrozine method on Technicon SMAC® *3525*

Lactate Dehydrogenase *Serum Increase Physiological* 2 cases of drug-associated fatty liver of pregnancy *6408*
Serum No Effect Analytical At 5 times upper limit of therapeutic range on methods on Technicon SMAC® , Abbott-VP, Roche Cobas-Bio, Hitachi® 705 and KDA *3525*

LE Cells *Blood Positive Physiological* May produce LE-like syndrome *5869*

Leukocytes *Blood Decrease Physiological* Leukopenia (AMA Blood dyscrasias) *4017*
Blood Increase Physiological Leukocytosis with atypical lymphocytes *2242*
Urine Decrease Analytical High concentrations may cause false negative results with leukocyte test area on Ames Multistix and other reagent strip tests *4034*

Lipase *Serum No Effect Analytical* No effect of concentrations up to 30 mg/L on method on Kodak Ektachem® *5706*

Methotrexate *Serum Decrease Physiological* Concomitant administration of tetracycline may decrease absorption of methotrexate *2818*

Metronidazole *Serum Increase Analytical* Interfere with bioassays *3858*

Neutrophils *Blood Decrease Physiological* Neutropenia may occur occasionally *2754* Neutropenia reported as a side effect *3461*

N-Formiminoglutamic Acid *Urine Increase Physiological* Isolated case of folic acid deficiency reported *2965*

Nitrogen *Urine Increase Physiological* Due to antianabolic effect *128*

Nonprotein Nitrogen *Serum Increase Physiological* Due to nephrotoxicity or antianabolic effect *3810*

Occult Blood *Feces Increase Physiological* May occur with hematemesis and melena *1485*

p-Aminophenol *Urine No Effect Analytical* With addition of drugs at a concentration of 100 mg/L and of related compounds at 50 mg/L no significant effect observed on colorimetric method of van Bocxlaer on Cobas Mira analyzer which involves reacting free p-aminophenol with resorcinol in the presence of magnesium ions to form an indophenol dye measured at 550 nm *6163*

Partial Thromboplastin Time
Plasma Decrease Physiological Tetracyclines reported to partially counteract the anticoagulant action of sodium heparin *6557*

pH *Blood Decrease Physiological* May cause acidosis with renal impairment *3669*

Phenylalanine *Plasma No Effect Analytical* No interference observed with rapid quantitative whole blood method of Campbell et al using phenylalanine dehydrogenase *867*

Phosphate *Serum Decrease Physiological* May occur with Fanconi syndrome *128*
Serum Increase Physiological May occur with nephrotoxicity *3810*
Serum No Effect Analytical At concentration of 300 mg/L had no effect on phosphomolybdate method *5704* At 5 times upper limit of therapeutic range on methods on Technicon SMAC® , Du Pont aca, Hitachi® 705 and KDA *3525*
Urine Increase Physiological Degraded material may cause Fanconi syndrome *4014*

Plasminogen *Plasma No Effect Analytical* At concentration of 1,000 mg/L had no effect on Du Pont aca method *5704*

Platelets *Blood Decrease Physiological* Thrombocytopenia reported as a side effect *3461* Thrombocytopenia/pancytopenia *3810*

Polymyxin *Serum Increase Analytical* Interfere with bioassays *3858*

Porphyrin, Total *Urine Increase Analytical* Interfering fluorescence *2025*

Tetracycline *(continued)*

Potassium *Serum Decrease Physiological* Fanconi like syndrome may occur with degraded compound *2451*
Serum Increase Physiological Occurs with azotemia *128*
Serum No Effect Analytical At concentration of 4 mg/L had no effect on flame-photometric method *5704* At concentration of 20,000 mg/L had no effect on measurement by ISE with predilution *5704* At concentration of 400 mg/L had no effect on measurement by ISE without predilution *5704*

Protein *Cerebrospinal Fluid Increase Analytical* Reacts as if phenol with Folin-Ciocalteu procedure *6681* At concentration of 3 mg/L on SDS/Coomassie Blue method of Huang caused a positive interference of 3% when compared against Du Pont aca method *2745*
Serum No Effect Analytical At 5 times upper limit of therapeutic range on methods on Technicon SMAC® , Abbott-VP, Kodak Ektachem® , Hitachi® 705 and KDA *3525*
Urine Increase Physiological Nephrotoxic effect with degraded tetracycline *2024*

Protein Electrophoresis *Serum No Effect Analytical* At concentration of 400 mg/L had no effect on automated Olympus-Hite method *5704*

Prothrombin Time *Plasma Decrease Physiological* Reported to depress prothrombin time so dose of anticoagulants may need to be reduced *3461* May partially counteract action of heparin *2753*
Plasma Increase Physiological Associated with cholestasis, and reduced activity *1485*

Sex-Hormone Binding Globulin
Serum No Effect Physiological No effect reported *2836* In 9 men with acne given compound for 3 d *4811*

Sodium *Serum Increase Physiological* May cause hypernatremia with renal impairment *3669*
Serum No Effect Analytical At concentration of 20,000 mg/L had no effect on measurement by ISE with predilution *5704* At concentration of 4 mg/L had no effect on flame-photometric method *5704* At concentration of 400 mg/L had no effect on measurement by ISE without predilution *5704*
Urine Increase Physiological Natriuretic and diuretic effects of drug *754*

Sugar *Urine Increase Analytical* False positive with Benedict's and Clinitest® *2451* False positive copper reduction procedure *5869*

T3-Uptake *Serum No Effect Physiological* No effect with 2 g/d for 11 d *882*

Testosterone *Serum Decrease Physiological* Fell from 21 to 17 nmol/L in 9 men after 3 d treatment: mechanism not established *4811* By about 10-20% *2836*
Serum No Effect Analytical No effect given at 100 µg/mL on radioimmunoassay *4811*

Testosterone, Free *Serum Decrease Physiological* By about 10-20% *2836*

Theophylline *Serum No Effect Analytical* At concentration of 10 mg/L produced no interference with methods used on Kodak DT60, Abbott TDx, Abbott Vision with both whole blood and serum, 3M Diagnostics TheoFAST, Syntex AccµLevel and Ames Seralyzer *1122*
Serum No Effect Physiological No effect observed on half-life *1384* No documented significant interaction with theophylline reported *6117* No clinically significant effect on theophylline concentration observed when drugs coadministered *5999*

Threonine *Urine Increase Physiological* Unexplained mechanism *2242*

Thromboplastin Generation *Blood Decrease Physiological* Impaired rate of regeneration observed *2242*

Tobramycin *Serum No Effect Analytical* At a concentration of 1250 mg/L increased concentration by 15% when measured by method on Baxter Stratus but therapeutic concentration only 4 to 8 mg/L *5705* No significant effect observed with concentrations up to 1000 µg/mL (2.25 mmol/L) with method on Du Pont aca *1547*

Triglycerides *Serum No Effect Analytical* At 5 times upper limit of therapeutic range on methods on Technicon SMAC® , Abbott-VP, Kodak Ektachem® , Hitachi® 705 and KDA *3525* At concentration of 300 mg/L had no effect on lipase/esterase method *5704* At concentration of 60 mg/L had no effect on GPO-PAP method *5704*

Trimethoprim *Serum Increase Analytical* Interfere with bioassays *3858*

Tryptophan *Urine Increase Physiological* Unexplained mechanism *2242*

Urea Nitrogen *Serum Increase Analytical* At concentrations above 40 mg/L (normal therapeutic concentration 8 mg/L) raised concentration as measured by Kodak Ektachem® method *5704*
Serum Increase Physiological Dose related increase in concentration reported *3461* Anti-anabolic action, amino acids degraded to urea *754* May be dose related renal toxicity *2754*
Serum No Effect Analytical At concentration of 300 mg/L had no effect on diacetylmonoxime method *5704* No effect at 100 mg/L on method on Ames Seralyzer *5706* At 5 times upper limit of therapeutic range on methods on Technicon SMAC® , Abbott-VP, Roche Cobas-Bio, Kodak Ektachem® , Hitachi® 705 and KDA *3525*

Uric Acid *Serum Decrease Analytical* At concentrations above 150 mg/L (normal therapeutic concentration 8 mg/L) lowered concentration as measured by Kageyama-Hantzsch method *5704*
Serum Increase Analytical At concentrations above 30 mg/L (normal therapeutic concentration 8 mg/L) raised concentration as measured by phosphotungstate reduction method *5704*
Serum No Effect Analytical At concentration of 100 mg/L had no effect on Ames Seralyzer method *5704* No effect at 100 mg/L on uricase method on Ames Seralyzer *5706* At concentration of 200 mg/L had no effect on catalase-AIDH method *5704* At 5 times upper limit of therapeutic range on methods on Technicon SMAC® , Abbott-VP, Du Pont aca, Roche Cobas-Bio, Kodak Ektachem® , Hitachi® 705 and KDA *3525*

Urobilinogen *Feces Decrease Physiological* Reduces flora in gastrointestinal tract *2451*
Urine Decrease Physiological Reduces flora in gastrointestinal tract *2451*
Urine Increase Analytical Yellow color extracted into $CHCl_3$ (Ehrlich's procedure) *3892*

Volume *Urine Increase Physiological* May have diuretic or nephrotoxic action *754*

Tetragastrin

Glucagon *Plasma No Effect Physiological* No effect observed if given i.v *4419*

Glucose *Serum No Effect Physiological* No change after 4 µg/kg i.v *4419*

Hydrochloric Acid *Gastric Fluid Increase Physiological* Effect similar to pentagastrin *2443*

Insulin *Plasma Increase Physiological* Slight rise but not significant *4419*

Tetrahydrolipstatin

Atenolol *Serum No Effect Physiological* In 8 healthy male volunteers administration of 100 mg atenolol with or without tetrahydrolipstatin 50 mg three times daily concentration atenolol increased nonsignificantly from mean 578 ± 116 ng/mL without tetrahydrolipstatin to 636 ± 236 ng/mL with tetrahydrolipstatin *6374*

Captopril *Serum No Effect Physiological* In 8 healthy male volunteers administration of 50 mg captopril with or without tetrahydrolipstatin 50 mg three times daily concentration captopril decreased nonsignificantly from mean 374 ± 132 ng/mL without tetrahydrolipstatin to 358 ± 40 ng/mL with tetrahydrolipstatin *6374*

Furosemide *Serum Decrease Physiological* In 8 healthy male volunteers administration of 100 mg atenolol with or without tetrahydrolipstatin 50 mg three times daily concentration furosemide decreased nonsignificantly from mean 369 ± 89 ng/mL without tetrahydrolipstatin to 235 ± 89 ng/mL with tetrahydrolipstatin *6374*

Nifedipine *Serum No Effect Physiological* In 8 healthy male volunteers administration of 20 mg nifedipine with or without tetrahydrolipstatin 50 mg three times daily concentration nifedipine decreased nonsignificantly from mean 67.1 ± 24.5 ng/mL without tetrahydrolipstatin to 63.8 ± 31.7 ng/mL with tetrahydrolipstatin *6374*

Tetraiodoacetic Acid

Thyroxine (T4) *Serum Increase Analytical* 105% recovery when added at a concentration of 2.5 μg/dL (16.9 nmol/L) and measured by method on Du Pont aca *1546*

Tetraiodofluorescein

^{131}I Uptake *Serum Decrease Physiological* Iodine derivative is a constituent of capsules of many pharmaceuticals *4360*

Thyroxine (T4) *Serum No Effect Physiological* No effect observed *6280*

Urobilin *Urine Increase Analytical* Pink color with mauve fluorescence *2559*

Tetraiodophthalein

BSP Retention *Serum Increase Physiological* Competitive uptake and excretion of dye *2855*

Precipitable Iodine *Serum Increase Analytical* Iodine contamination *2024*

Thalidomide

CD4+ Lymphocytes *Blood No Effect Physiological* In 20 adults with HIV-infection treatment with thalidomide for 4 weeks had no significant effect on count *2870*

CD8+ Lymphocytes *Blood No Effect Physiological* In 20 adults with HIV-infection treatment with thalidomide for 4 weeks had no significant effect on count *2870*

Creatinine *Serum No Effect Analytical* No effect at therapeutic concentrations on Jaffe procedure on Beckman Astra® and Technicon SMAC® *1181*

Soluble Tumor Necrosis Factor Receptor-II *Serum Increase Physiological* In 20 adults with HIV-infection prior to treatment for aphthous ulcers mean concentration of 3.8 ng/mL, significantly greater than 2.1 ± 0.7 ng/mL in healthy controls, increased by 1.5 ng/mL after 2 weeks treatment with thalidomide and by 0.5 ng/mL after 4 weeks treatment *2870*

Tumor Necrosis Factor-α *Serum Increase Physiological* In 20 adults with HIV-infection prior to treatment for aphthous ulcers mean concentration of 37.0 pg/mL, significantly greater than 9.5 ± 5.7 pg/mL in healthy controls, increased by 12.2 pg/mL after 2 weeks treatment with thalidomide and by 4.0 pg/mL after 4 weeks treatment *2870*

Thallium

Alanine Aminotransferase *Serum Increase Physiological* Due to hepatic necrosis *2183*

Casts *Urine Increase Physiological* Damage to renal tubular epithelium *2183*

Cells *Urine Increase Physiological* Damage to renal tubular epithelium *2183*

Occult Blood *Feces Increase Physiological* Due to ingestion of toxic dose *2183*

Protein *Urine Increase Physiological* Damage to renal tubular epithelium *2183*

Urea Nitrogen *Serum Increase Physiological* May cause nephrotoxicity *5377*

Thebaine

Opiates *Urine Positive Analytical* Cross-reactivity of over 50% observed with Roche Abuscreen Online procedure as adapted to Roche Cobas Fara II analyzer *5547* Significant cross-reactivity observed with Roche Abuscreen method adapted for use with Olympus AU 5121 and 5131 analyzers *214*

Thenalidine

Leukocytes *Blood Decrease Physiological* Leukopenia (AMA Blood dyscrasias) *4017*

Neutrophils *Blood Decrease Physiological* Occasional case of drug-induced neutropenia *241*

Theobromine

Acetaminophen *Serum No Effect Analytical* At 10 mg/L had no effect on HPLC method *5775*

Albumin *Serum No Effect Analytical* At concentration of 2,000 mg/L had no effect on BCG method *5704*

Bicarbonate *Serum No Effect Analytical* At concentration of 2,000 mg/L had no effect on method using phenolphthalein *5704*

Bilirubin *Serum No Effect Analytical* At concentration of 2,000 mg/L had no effect on Jendrassik and Grof method *5704*

Calcium *Serum No Effect Analytical* At concentration of 2,000 mg/L had no effect on cresolphthalein method *5704*

Catecholamines *Plasma No Effect Analytical* No effect on HPLC method of Koller for dopamine, epinephrine, and norepinephrine *3230*

Chloride *Serum No Effect Analytical* At concentration of 2,000 mg/L had no effect on mercurimetric method *5704*

Cholesterol *Serum No Effect Analytical* At concentration of 2,000 mg/L had no effect on Liebermann-Burchard method *5704*

Chromosomes *Test Conditions Abnormal Physiological* Clastogenic in human cells *5484*

Creatinine *Serum No Effect Analytical* At concentration of 2,000 mg/L had no effect on Technicon AutoAnalyzer® method *5704*

p-Aminophenol *Urine No Effect Analytical* With addition of drugs at a concentration of 100 mg/L and of related compounds at 50 mg/L no significant effect observed on colorimetric method of van Bocxlaer on Cobas Mira analyzer which involves reacting free p-aminophenol with resorcinol in the presence of magnesium ions to form an indophenol dye measured at 550 nm *6163*

Phenylalanine *Plasma No Effect Analytical* No interference observed with rapid quantitative whole blood method of Campbell et al using phenylalanine dehydrogenase *867*

Phosphate *Serum No Effect Analytical* At concentration of 2,000 mg/L had no effect on phosphomolybdate method *5704*

Protein *Serum No Effect Analytical* At concentration of 2,000 mg/L had no effect on biuret method with blank correction *5704*

Theophylline *Serum Increase Analytical* At 200 mg/L produced positive bias of 5.25 mg/L at concentration of 20.0 mg/L with Abbott Vision with serum, "interfering substance" when whole blood used with Abbott Vision, unreadable test strip with Ames Seralyzer and 5.60 mg/L with 3M TheoFAST *1122*
Serum No Effect Analytical No effect of concentrations up to 20 mg/L on method on Kodak Ektachem® *5706* Cross-reactivity of 0.6% observed with method on Baxter Stratus *5705* At concentration of 200 mg/L produced no interference with methods on Kodak DT60, Abbott TDx and Syntex AccμLevel *1122* No significant effect observed on method on Kodak Ektachem® systems *2519* No significant interference observed at a concentration of 10 μg/mL (56 μmol/L) with method on Du Pont aca *1544* No effect at concentration of 10 μg/mL (56 μmol/L) on method on Du Pont Dimension *1585*

Triglycerides *Serum No Effect Analytical* At concentration of 2,000 mg/L had no effect on lipase/esterase method *5704*

Urea Nitrogen *Serum No Effect Analytical* At concentration of 2,000 mg/L had no effect on diacetylmonoxime method *5704*

Uric Acid *Serum No Effect Analytical* At concentration of 2,000 mg/L had no effect on phosphotungstate reduction method *5704*

Theophylline

Acetaminophen *Serum No Effect Analytical* At 20 mg/L had no effect on HPLC method *5775* No interference observed at a concentration of 2000 μg/mL (1110 μmol/L) with method on Du Pont aca *1506*

Acid Phosphatase *Serum No Effect Analytical* At concentration of 100 μg/mL (555 μmol/L) had no effect on method on Du Pont Dimension *1562*

Theophylline *(continued)*

Adenosine *Serum Decrease Physiological* Theophylline blocks adenosine receptors requiring higher doses of adenosine to achieve desired effect *3125* Coadministration with adenosine antagonizes its effects *1985*

Adenosine Monophosphate *Plasma Increase Physiological* Insignificant increase from mean of 14.3 nmol/L to 18.1 nmol/L in 8 patients with renal transplants treated with 8 mg/kg/day for 8 weeks *340*

Urine No Effect Physiological No significant change observed in 8 postrenal transplant patients treated with 8 mg/kg/day for 8 weeks *340* In normals given 400 mg b.i.d. for 5 d *3920*

Alanine Aminotransferase *Serum No Effect Analytical* At 5 times upper limit of therapeutic range on methods on Technicon SMAC® , Abbott-VP, Du Pont aca, Roche Cobas-Bio and KDA *3525* No effect at concentration of 100 µg/mL (555 µmol/L) on method on Du Pont Dimension *1563* No effect at 200 mg/L on Boehringer Mannheim Reflotron method *5706* No effect at therapeutic concentration on Boehringer Mannheim Reflotron method *3231*

Albumin *Serum No Effect Analytical* At concentration of 100 µg/mL (555 µmol/L) had no effect on method on Du Pont Dimension *1564* At 5 times upper limit of therapeutic range on methods on Technicon SMAC® , Kodak Ektachem® , Hitachi® 705 and KDA *3525* At concentration of 2,000 mg/L had no effect on BCG method *5704*

Alkaline Phosphatase *Serum Decrease Analytical* At 5 times upper limit of therapeutic range on methods on Technicon SMAC® , KDA, Roche Cobas-Bio and Hitachi® 705 *3525* Approximately 10% reduction in activity at drug concentration of 2 mg/dL *6266*

Serum No Effect Analytical No effect at concentration of 20 mg/L on method on Kodak Ektachem® *5706* At concentration of 100 µg/mL (555 µmol/L) had no effect on method on Du Pont Dimension *1565* At 5 times upper limit of therapeutic range on methods on Abbott-VP and Du Pont aca *3525*

Ammonia *Plasma No Effect Analytical* No effect at concentration of 100 µg/mL (555 µmol/L) on method on Du Pont Dimension *1566*

Amylase *Serum No Effect Analytical* At 5 times upper limit of therapeutic range on Du Pont aca, Roche Cobas-Bio and Kodak Ektachem® *3525* At concentration of 100 µg/mL (555 µmol/L) had no effect on method on Du Pont Dimension *1567* Concentrations up to 200 mg/L had no effect on method on Boehringer Mannheim Reflotron system *5706*

Amylase, Pancreatic Isoenzyme

Serum No Effect Analytical No significant effect observed at a toxic concentration of 100 mg/L with method on Boehringer Mannheim Reflotron *3647*

Aspartate Aminotransferase *Serum No Effect Analytical* No effect at concentration of 100 µg/mL (555 µmol/L) on method on Du Pont Dimension *1568* At 5 times upper limit of therapeutic range on methods on Technicon SMAC® , Abbott-VP, Du Pont aca, Roche Cobas-Bio, Hitachi® 705 and KDA *3525* No effect at therapeutic concentration on Boehringer Mannheim Reflotron method *3231* No effect at 200 mg/L on Boehringer Mannheim Reflotron method *5706*

Barbiturate *Serum Increase Analytical* In certain gas-chromatographic procedures may produce falsely high values *1338*

Bicarbonate *Serum No Effect Analytical* At concentration of 2,000 mg/L had no effect on method using phenolphthalein method *5704*

Bilirubin *Serum Decrease Analytical* Causes depression of color formation *3810*

Serum No Effect Analytical No significant effect observed at a concentration of 40 µg/dL (2.2 µmol/L) with method on Du Pont aca *1548* At concentration of 2,000 mg/L had no effect on Jendrassik and Grof method *5704* No effect at 12 mg/L on Ames Seralyzer method *5706* At concentration of 200 mg/L no effect on method on Boehringer Mannheim Reflotron system *5706* No effect at concentration of 100 µg/mL (555 µmol/L) on method on Du Pont Dimension *1589* At 5 times upper limit of therapeutic range on methods on Technicon SMAC® , Roche Cobas-Bio, Du Pont aca, Kodak Ektachem® , Hitachi® 705 and KDA *3525*

Bilirubin, Conjugated *Serum No Effect Analytical* No effect at concentration of 100 mg/L on method on Kodak Ektachem® *5706* At concentration of 40 µg/dL (2.2 µmol/L) had no effect on method on Du Pont aca *1517*

Bilirubin, Direct *Serum No Effect Analytical* At concentration of 100 µg/mL (555 µmol/L) had no effect on method on Du Pont Dimension *1574*

Bilirubin, Unconjugated *Serum No Effect Analytical* No effect at concentration of 100 mg/L on method on Kodak Ektachem® *5706*

Caffeine *Serum Increase Physiological* In patients receiving theophylline mean concentration of caffeine correlated with theophylline concentration: at mean concentration of 7.2 mg/L mean caffeine concentration 0.76 mg/L, at 16.4 mg/L mean caffeine concentration 0.82 mg/L, at 17.2 mg/Lmean caffeine concentration 0.81 mg/L and at mean theophylline concentration of 34.7 mg/L mean caffeine concentration 3.58 ± 3.1 mg/L *5722*

Calcium *Serum Decrease Physiological* Observed in a single case of massive overdose (theophylline concentration 117 mg/L) who had extensive tissue damage and seizures *1759*

Serum Increase Physiological In overdose with theophylline toxicity hypercalcemia was observed *3125* 11 of 60 patients with theophylline toxicity but reverted to normal when drug withdrawn. Also in normals with 400 mg b.i.d. for 5 d *3920* Manifestation of theophylline toxicity *5999*

Serum No Effect Analytical At 5 times upper limit of therapeutic range on methods on Technicon SMAC® , Abbott-VP, Du Pont aca, Kodak Ektachem® , Hitachi® 705 and KDA *3525* At concentration of 120 mg/L had no effect on cresolphthalein method *5704* No effect at 100 µg/mL (555 µmol/L) on method on Du Pont Dimension *1569*

Serum No Effect Physiological No effect in response to i.v. infusion *6631*

Urine No Effect Physiological In normals given 400 mg b.i.d. for 5 d *3920*

Calcium, Ultrafiltratable *Serum Increase Physiological* Apparent log dose response correlation with drug concentration in individuals with toxicity *3920*

Carbamazepine *Serum Decrease Physiological* Drugs that induce CYP 3A4 enhance metabolism of carbamazepine producing clinically meaningful effect *1039*

Carbon Dioxide Partial Pressure

Blood Decrease Physiological Mean decrease of 9% after 2 months treatment with 10 mg/kg body weight/day in 60 patients with chronic pulmonary disease *4177*

Catecholamines *Plasma No Effect Analytical* No effect on HPLC method of Koller for dopamine, epinephrine, and norepinephrine *3230*

Urine Increase Physiological Normal response even when given orally *288*

Cetirizine *Serum Increase Physiological* Small decrease in clearance of cetirizine observed with a single 400 mg dose of theophylline *4661*

Chloride *Serum No Effect Analytical* At concentration of 2,000 mg/L had no effect on mercurimetric method *5704*

Cholesterol *Serum Increase Physiological* At serum concentrations of 10 - 20 µg/mL a moderate increase of serum total cholesterol from a mean of 140 mg/dL to 160 mg/dL occurred as a result of its pharmacological effects *3125*

Serum No Effect Analytical At concentration of 100 µg/mL (555 µmol/L) had no effect on method on Du Pont Dimension *1570* At concentration of 200 mg/L no effect on method on Boehringer Mannheim Reflotron system *5706* No effect at therapeutic concentration on Boehringer Mannheim Reflotron method *3231* At 5 times upper limit of therapeutic range on methods on Technicon SMAC® , Abbott-VP, Roche Cobas-Bio, Kodak Ektachem® , Hitachi® 705 and KDA *3525* No effect at 12 mg/L on Ames Seralyzer method *5706* At concentration of 20 mg/L had no effect on CHOD-PAP method *5704* At concentration of 2,000 mg/L had no effect on Liebermann-Burchard method *5704*

Cholinesterase *Serum No Effect Analytical* No effect observed at a concentration of 100 µg/mL with method on Du Pont Dimension *3271* No effect observed at concentration of 25 mg/dL with butyrylthiocholine method on Kodak Ektachem® *2504* Insignificant reduction of 0.01 U/mL at a concentration of 100 µg/mL with method on Du Pont aca *3271*

Chromosomes *Test Conditions Abnormal Physiological* Clastogenic in human cells *5484*

Color *Feces Increase Analytical* Black color reported following ingestion of theophylline *3388*

Cortisol *Plasma No Effect Analytical* At concentration of 100 mg/L no significant effect observed on CEDIA method (88.5% recovery with one specimen and 100.1% with a second) or on Enzymun method *1097*

Plasma No Effect Physiological No effect on hepatic metabolism so concentration unaffected *2985* No effect in response to i.v. infusion of aminophylline *923* In 7 patients with chronic obstructive pulmonary disease niether of two different treatment regimes had an effect on either the plasma concentration or circadian variation *2125*

Cortisol, Free *Urine Increase Physiological* At serum concentrations of 10 - 20 µg/mL a moderate increase of urinary free cortisol from a mean of 44 µg/d to 63 µg/d occurred as a result of its pharmacological effects *3125*

C-Reactive Protein *Serum No Effect Analytical* No interference observed at concentrations up to 50 µg/mL (278 µmol/L) with method on Du Pont aca *1518* At concentration of 500 mg/L (278 µmol/L) had no effect on method on Du Pont aca *5403*

Creatine Kinase *Serum Increase Physiological* In overdose with theophylline toxicity rhabdomyolysis was observed with increased serum creatine kinase activity and myoglobin concentration *3125* Massive increase to over 1 million U/L in a single case with serum concentration of theophylline of 117 mg/L probably due to extensive tissue damage and seizures *1759* Manifestation of theophylline toxicity *5999*

Serum No Effect Analytical No effect at 12 mg/L on method on Ames Seralyzer *5706* At 5 times upper limit of therapeutic range on methods on Technicon SMAC® , Abbott-VP, Roche Cobas-Bio, Du Pont aca and Hitachi® 705 *3525*

Creatine Kinase Isoenzymes *Serum No Effect Analytical* No interference observed at a concentration of 40 mg/L (222 µmol/L) with CK-MB method on Du Pont aca *1519* At concentration of 100 µg/mL (555 µmol/L) had no effect on method for measuring CK-MB isoenzyme on Du Pont Dimension *1571*

Creatinine *Serum No Effect Analytical* No effect of concentrations up to 100 mg/L on 2-slide method on Kodak Ektachem® *5706* At 5 times upper limit of therapeutic range on methods on Technicon SMAC® , Abbott-VP, Du Pont aca, Roche Cobas-Bio, Kodak Ektachem® , Hitachi® 705 and KDA *3525* No effect of concentrations up to 20 mg/L on single slide method on Kodak Ektachem® *5706* At concentration of 2,000 mg/L had no effect on Technicon AutoAnalyzer® Jaffe method *5704* At 1.0 g/L on reversed phase liquid chromatographic procedure of Zhiri et al *6656* No effect at 12 mg/L on method on Ames Seralyzer *5706* No interference observed at a concentration of 2 mg/L although detected by HPLC method of Rosano et al because it elutes at 10.0 minutes compared with 8.9 minutes for creatinine *5083* No effect at concentration of 100 µg/mL (555 µmol/L) on method on Du Pont Dimension *1572*

Urine No Effect Physiological No significant effect of treatment for 7 days in 8 healthy normals, 8 patients with chronic obstructive pulmonary disease and 8 patients with stable asthma *6382*

Creatinine Clearance *Urine No Effect Physiological* No significant effect observed in 8 patients with renal transplants treated with 8 mg/kg/day for 8 weeks *340*

Cyclosporine *Blood No Effect Analytical* At a concentration of 250 mg/L had no effect on Syva EMIT method *495*

Dexamethasone *Serum No Effect Physiological* Coadministration appeared to have no effect on plasma concentration or clearance *748* No effect on hepatic metabolism so concentration unaffected *2985*

Epinephrine *Urine No Effect Physiological* In 8 patients receiving 450-750 mg/d for at least 2 months excretion remained within normal range *4478*

Erythromycin *Serum Decrease Physiological* Up to 35% decrease in serum erythromycin concentration observed at the same time as theophylline concentration increased *6117* Coadministration of theophylline with erythromycin decreases erythromycin concentration by about 35% *5999*

Serum Increase Physiological Erythromycin metabolite decreases theophylline clearance by inhibiting cytochrome P450 3A3 and increases serum theophylline concentration by 35%. At the same time the clearance of erythromycin is also decreased by 35% *3125*

Serum No Effect Physiological No effect on area under curve although appeared to be increased elimination *2603*

Erythropoietin *Serum Decrease Physiological* Reduction from mean of 60 U/L to 9 U/L in 8 renal transplant recipients with erythrocytosis following 8 weeks treatment (8 mg/kg/day) and from 6.9 U/L to 4.7 U/L in 5 normal controls with similar treatment *340*

Serum Increase Physiological In 8 premature infants with a mean birth weight of 1546 g treated with up to 4 mg/kg/d mean concentration 25 mU/mL at 4 weeks and 22.1 mU/mL at 5 weeks compared with a control group of 11 infants with a mean birth weight of 1629 g in whom mean concentration was 10.3 mU/mL at 4 weeks and 8.6 mU/mL at 5 weeks at comparable degrees of anemia *2239*

Fatty Acids (FFA), Free *Serum Increase Physiological* Rapid pronounced and prolonged rise associated with aminophylline to produce therapeutic concentration of theophylline *923* At serum concentrations of 10 - 20 µg/mL a moderate increase of serum FFA from a mean of 451 µeq/dL to 800 µeq/dL as a result of its pharmacological effects *3125* 123% increase after 4 d of treatment in 10 healthy volunteers *6334*

Felbamate *Serum No Effect Analytical* No significant interference observed with GLC method of Rifai et al even though it is co-extracted *4958*

Ferritin *Serum Increase Physiological* Increase from mean baseline of 27 µg/L to 271 µg/L following 8 weeks treatment of 8 mg/kg/day in 8 patients with renal transplants (iron coadministered in some patients) *340*

Fibrin Degradation Products *Plasma No Effect Analytical* No interference observed at concentrations up to 50 µg/mL (278 µmol/L) with method on Du Pont aca *1525*

Glucagon *Plasma No Effect Physiological* No effect in response to i.v. infusion of aminophylline *923*

Glucose *Serum Decrease Physiological* Hypoglycemia observed in 98% patients in a study of 157 patients with acute overdose and in 18% of 92 patients with chronic overdoses *5999*

Serum Increase Physiological Follows overdose, but decreased glucose tolerance also observed in infants and others *5761* In a study of acute overdose hyperglycemia was observed in 98% of patients and in one study of chronic toxicity hyperglycemia occurred in 18% patients *3125* At serum concentrations of 10 - 20 µg/mL a moderate increase of serum glucose from a mean of 88 mg/dL to 98 mg/dL occurred as a result of its pharmacological effects *3125* Effect small in response to i.v. infusion of aminophylline *923*

Serum No Effect Analytical At concentration of 23 mg/L had no effect on Kodak Ektachem® method *5704* At concentration of 100 µg/mL (555 µmol/L) has no effect on method on Du Pont Dimension *1575* No effect at 12 mg/L on glucose oxidase method on Ames Seralyzer *5706* At concentration of 20 mg/L had no effect on GOD/POD-PAP method *5704* No effect at therapeutic concentration on Boehringer Mannheim Reflotron method *3231* At concentration of 200 mg/L no effect on method on Boehringer Mannheim Reflotron system *5706* At 5 times upper limit of therapeutic range on methods on Technicon SMAC® , Abbott-VP, Du Pont aca, Roche Cobas-Bio, Kodak Ektachem® , Hitachi® 705 and KDA *3525*

Urine Increase Physiological Follows overdose, but decreased glucose tolerance also observed in infants and others *5761*

γ-Glutamyltransferase *Serum No Effect Analytical* At 5 times upper limit of therapeutic range on methods on Technicon SMAC® , Abbott-VP,and Hitachi® 705 *3525* No effect at therapeutic concentration on Boehringer Mannheim Reflotron method *3231* At concentration of 200 mg/L no effect on method on Boehringer Mannheim Reflotron system *5706* At concentration of 100 µg/mL (555 µmol/L) has no effect on method on Du Pont Dimension *1579*

Glycated Hemoglobin *Blood No Effect Analytical* At a concentration of 80 mg/L had an insignificant 0.0% interference with method on Abbott Vision *1885*

Growth Hormone *Plasma No Effect Physiological* No effect in response to i.v. infusion of aminophylline *923*

HDL-Cholesterol *Serum Increase Physiological* At serum concentrations of 10 - 20 µg/mL a moderate increase of serum HDL-cholesterol from a mean of 36 mg/dL to 50 mg/dL occurred as a result of its pharmacological effects *3125*

Theophylline *(continued)*

HDL-Cholesterol *(continued)*
Serum No Effect Analytical No effect at concentration of 100 µg/mL (555 µmol/L) on method on Du Pont Dimension *1576* At a concentration up to 200 mg/L had no significant effect on Reflotron method for whole blood cholesterol *6352*

HDL-Cholesterol:LDL-Cholesterol Ratio
Serum Increase Physiological At serum concentrations of 10 - 20 µg/mL a moderate increase of serum HDL-cholesterol from a mean of 0.5 to 0.7 occurred as a result of its pharmacological effects *3125*

Hematocrit *Blood Decrease Physiological* Reduction from mean of 0.58 to 0.46 in 8 renal transplant recipients following 8 weeks treatment (8 mg/kg/day) and from 0.43 to 0.39 in 5 healthy controls after similar treatment *340*

Histamine *Plasma No Effect Analytical* Improbable inhibition of radio-enzyme assay at therapeutic concentrations *2492*

Indomethacin *Serum No Effect Analytical* No effect on HPLC method of Roberts and Smith *4978*

Insulin *Plasma No Effect Physiological* No effect in response to i.v. infusion of aminophylline *923*

Iron *Serum No Effect Analytical* No interference observed with method on Kodak Ektachem® *2792* No effect at concentration of 100 µg/mL (555 µmol/L) on method on Du Pont Dimension *1577* At 5 times upper limit of therapeutic range on Ferrozine method on Technicon SMAC® *3525*

Iron-Binding Capacity, Total *Serum No Effect Analytical* No effect at concentration of 100 µg/mL (555 µmol/L) on method on Du Pont Dimension *1590*

Lactate Dehydrogenase *Serum Decrease Analytical* Effect small and can be ignored at therapeutic concentration *6266*
Serum No Effect Analytical At 5 times upper limit of therapeutic range on methods on Technicon SMAC® , Abbott-VP, Roche Cobas-Bio, Hitachi® 705 and KDA *3525* No effect at 12 mg/L on method on Ames Seralyzer *5706* At concentration of 100 µg/mL (555 µmol/L) has no effect on method on Du Pont Dimension *1578*

Leukocytes *Blood Increase Physiological* Manifestation of theophylline toxicity *5999* In overdose with theophylline toxicity leukocytosis was observed *3125*

Levofloxacin *Serum No Effect Physiological* Concurrent administration of levofloxacin with theophylline had no effect on levofloxacin absorption and disposition *3916* No significant effect observed of theophylline on absorption and disposition of levofloxacin observed in 14 healthy volunteers *3916*

Lipase *Serum No Effect Analytical* At concentration of 100 µg/mL (555 µmol/L) has no effect on method on Du Pont Dimension *1580*

Lithium *Serum Decrease Physiological* Theophylline increases renal lithium clearance and decreases serum lithium concentration requiring an increase in dose of about 60% *3125* Decrease in serum lithium concentration observed requiring an increase on average of 60% in lithium dose to achieve same effect *6117* Lithium clearance enhanced by coadministration of theophylline with increased amounts of lithium recovered from urine *1119* Coadministration of theophylline with lithium increases lithium clearance and substantially decreases lithium concentration, requiring an increase in dose of about 60% *5999*
Serum Increase Physiological Increase concentration by reducing renal elimination *3590*

Lithium Clearance *Urine Increase Physiological* Theophylline increases renal lithium clearance and decreases serum lithium concentration requiring an increase in dose of about 60% *3125*

Magnesium *Serum Decrease Physiological* In overdose with theophylline toxicity hypomagnesemia observed as complication *3125* Manifestation of theophylline toxicity *5999*
Serum Increase Physiological In single case of massive overdose (theophylline concentration 117 mg/L) as result of seizures and massive tissue destruction. Normal finding with overdose is hypomagnesemia *1759*
Serum No Effect Analytical No effect at concentration of 100 µg/mL (555 µmol/L) on method on Du Pont Dimension *1581*
Serum No Effect Physiological No effect in response to i.v. infusion *6631*

3-Methylhistidine *Urine Increase Physiological* Treatment for 7 days with theophylline caused increase from mean baseline of 176 µmol/d to 206 µmol/d in patients with chronic obstructive pulmonary disease and from 190 µmol/d to 216 µmol/d in patients with stable asthma but little increase in normals *6382*

Mibefradil *Serum No Effect Physiological* Theophylline coadministration had no significant effect on pharmacokinetics of mibefradil *5009*

Mycophenolic Acid *Serum No Effect Analytical* No significant interference observed with HPLC method of Shipkova et al *5526*

Mycophenolic Acid Glucuronide
Serum No Effect Analytical No significant interference observed with HPLC method of Shipkova et al *5526*

Myoglobin *Serum Increase Physiological* Manifestation of theophylline toxicity *5999* In overdose with theophylline toxicity rhabdomyolysis was observed with increased serum creatine kinase activity and myoglobin concentration *3125*

N-Acetyl-Glucosaminidase *Urine No Effect Analytical* At 3 mg/L had no effect on 2 colorimetric analytical methods *2254*

Norepinephrine *Urine No Effect Physiological* In 8 patients receiving 450-750 mg/d for at least 2 months excretion remained within normal limits *4478*

Occult Blood *Feces Increase Physiological* In large doses may cause gastric hemorrhage *2754*

Oxygen Partial Pressure *Blood Increase Physiological* Mean increase of 9% in 60 patients with chronic pulmonary disease following 2 months therapy (10 mg/kg/day) *4177*

p-Aminophenol *Urine No Effect Analytical* With addition of drugs at a concentration of 100 mg/L and of related compounds at 50 mg/L no significant effect observed on colorimetric method of van Bocxlaer on Cobas Mira analyzer which involves reacting free p-aminophenol with resorcinol in the presence of magnesium ions to form an indophenol dye measured at 550 nm *6163*

Parathyroid Hormone *Plasma No Effect Physiological* In patients with drug toxicity *3920*

Penciclovir *Serum No Effect Physiological* No significant effect on pharmacokinetics of penciclovir observed following single-dose administatration of 500 mg famciclovir after pretreatment with multiple doses of theophylline *5646*

pH *Blood Decrease Physiological* In single case of massive overdose (theophylline concentration 117 mg/L) pH of 6.88 observed in contrast to more usual respiratory alkalosis or less common metabolic acidosis observed with theophylline overdose *1759*
Urine No Effect Physiological In healthy volunteers given drug intravenously *2603*

Phenylalanine *Plasma No Effect Analytical* No interference observed with rapid quantitative whole blood method of Campbell et al using phenylalanine dehydrogenase *867*

Phenytoin *Serum Decrease Physiological* Decrease in serum phenytoin concentration of about 40% observed due to decreased absorption *6117* Induces microsomal enzyme activity, decreasing phenytoin concentration by about 40% *5999* Mean value decreased by 21% when theophylline coadministered; rebound when drug discontinued *5968* Theophylline increases phenytoin clearance by induction of microsomal enzyme activity and decreases serum phenytoin concentration by about 40% *3125*
Serum No Effect Analytical No effect at concentration of 100 µg/mL (555 µmol/L) on method on Du Pont Dimension *1583*

Phosphate *Serum Decrease Physiological* Response to i.v. infusion, returned to baseline in 4 h *6631* In overdose with theophylline toxicity hypophosphatemia observed as complication *3125* Manifestation of theophylline toxicity *5999*
Serum Increase Physiological In single case of massive overdose (theophylline concentration 117 mg/L) probably as result of massive tissue damage and seizures as hypophosphatemia more typical finding with overdose *1759*
Serum No Effect Analytical At 5 times upper limit of therapeutic range on methods on Technicon SMAC® , Du Pont aca, Hitachi® 705 and KDA *3525* At concentration of 100 µg/mL (555 µmol/L) has no effect on method on Du Pont Dimension *1584* At concentration of 2,000 mg/L had no effect on phosphomolybdate method *5704*

Urine *No Effect* *Physiological* In normals given 400 mg b.i.d. for 5 d *3920*

Potassium *Serum* *Decrease* *Physiological* In two studies of acute overdose hypokalemia was observed in 79% and 85% of patients and in two studies of chronic toxicity hypokalemia occurred in 44% and 43% patients *3125* Hypokalemia observed in 85% and 79% patients in two studies of patients with acute overdose and 44% and 43% in two studies of patients with chronic overdoses *5999* Response to i.v. infusion, returned to baseline in 4 h *6631*

Serum *Increase* *Physiological* In single case of massive overdose (theophylline concentration 117 mg/L) concentration of 6.2 mmol/L observed probably resulting from massive tissue damage and seizures since hypokalemia more typical of theophlline overdose *1759*

Serum *No Effect* *Analytical* At concentration of 80 mg/L nonsignificant interference of -0.3% observed with method on Abbott Vision *681* No effect up to 60 mg/L on method on Ames Seralyzer but at higher concentrations apparently reduced potassium concentration although of no clinical significance *5706* At concentration of 20 mg/L had no effect on flame-photometric method *5704* At concentration of 1,000 mg/L had no effect on measurement by ISE with predilution *5704*

Protein *Serum* *No Effect* *Analytical* At 5 times upper limit of therapeutic range on methods on Technicon SMAC® , Abbott-VP, Kodak Ektachem® , Hitachi® 705 and KDA *3525* At concentration of 100 µg/mL (555 µmol/L) had negligible effect on method on Du Pont Dimension *1591* At concentration of 2,000 mg/L had no effect on biuret method with blank correction *5704*

Urine *Increase* *Physiological* When high doses sodium glycinate salt given *3810*

Pyridoxal *Serum* *No Effect* *Physiological* No effect observed in healthy men *6115*

Pyridoxal Kinase *Red Blood Cells* *Increase* *Physiological* Nearly twofold increase in apparently healthy men from mean of 24.2 nmol to 46.9 nmol pyridoxal phosphate per gram hemoglobin per hour *6115*

Pyridoxal Phosphate

Red Blood Cells *Decrease* *Physiological* Significant decrease from pretreatment values in apparently healthy men *6115*

Serum *Decrease* *Physiological* Significant reduction in concentration in apparently healthy young men. Effect due to noncompetitive inhibition of erythrocyte pyridoxal kinase *6115*

Pyridoxine Phosphate Oxidase

Red Blood Cells *No Effect* *Physiological* No effect observed in apparently healthy men *6115*

Red Cell Mass *Blood* *Decrease* *Physiological* Decrease from mean of 3197 mL to 2273 mL in 8 patients with renal transplants following treatment with 8 mg/kg/day for 8 weeks *340*

SDZ PSC 833 *Blood* *No Effect* *Analytical* At a concentration of 24.07 mg/L had no effect on HPLC method of Scott et al when used to measure PSC (with CsD as internal standard) at a concentration of 5 mg/L *5418*

Sodium *Serum* *Decrease* *Physiological* Significant effect 8 h after i.v. infusion *6631*

Serum *No Effect* *Analytical* At concentration of 20 mg/L had no effect on flame-photometric method *5704* At concentration of 1,000 mg/L had no effect on measurement by ISE with predilution *5704*

Somatostatin *Plasma* *Decrease* *Analytical* Interferes with binding in radioimmunoassays with 3 different antisera *5588*

Plasma *Increase* *Analytical* With a variety of different antibodies for RIA measurement inhibits tracer binding at concentrations normally achieved therapeutically *5588*

T3-Uptake *Serum* *No Effect* *Analytical* No significant effect observed at a concentration of 100 µg/mL (555 µmol/L) with method on Du Pont aca *1545* At concentration of 100 µg/mL (555 µmol/L) has no effect on method on Du Pont Dimension *1586*

Tacrolimus *Blood* *No Effect* *Analytical* No interference observed with radiorecptor assay of Murthy et al *4191* No significant effect observed at a concentration of 20 mg/L with MEIA method on Abbott IMx analyzer *1871*

Serum *No Effect* *Analytical* At concentration of 20 mg/L had no significant effect on ELISA method *6329*

Thyroid Stimulating Hormone

Serum *No Effect* *Physiological* Increased response to TRH: due to increased intracellular ATP which exerts action on TRH *6412*

Thyroxine (T4) *Serum* *No Effect* *Analytical* No significant effect observed at a concentration of 100 µg/mL (555 µmol/L) with method on Du Pont aca *1588* At concentration of 100 µg/mL (555 µmol/L) has no effect on method on Du Pont Dimension *1587* No significant effect observed at a concentration of 100 µg/mL (555 µmol/L) with method on Du Pont aca *1546*

Tri-iodothyronine (T3) *Serum* *Decrease* *Physiological* At serum concentrations of 10 - 20 µg/mL a transient moderate decrease of serum tri-iodothyronine occurred from a mean of 144 ng/dL before treatment to 131 ng/dL one week after treatment started and 142 ng/dL after 4 weeks of treatment as a result of its pharmacological effects *3125*

Triglycerides *Serum* *No Effect* *Analytical* At 5 times upper limit of therapeutic range on methods on Technicon SMAC® , Abbott-VP, Kodak Ektachem® , Hitachi® 705 and KDA *3525* No effect at therapeutic concentration on Boehringer Mannheim Reflotron method *3231* No effect at 200 mg/L on Boehringer Mannheim Reflotron method *5706* At concentration of 100 µg/mL (555 µmol/L) has no effect on method on Du Pont Dimension *1592* At concentration of 2,000 mg/L had no effect on lipase/esterase method *5704*

Trovafloxacin *Serum* *No Effect* *Physiological* No significant interaction observed *4663*

Urea Nitrogen *Serum* *No Effect* *Analytical* No effect at concentration of 100 µg/mL (555 µmol/L) on method on Du Pont Dimension *1593* No effect at 200 mg/L on Boehringer Mannheim Reflotron method *5706* No effect at therapeutic concentration on Boehringer Mannheim Reflotron method *3231* At concentration of 23 mg/L had no effect on Kodak Ektachem® method *5704* At concentration of 2,000 mg/L had no effect on diacetylmonoxime method *5704* No effect at 12 mg/L on method on Ames Seralyzer *5706* At 5 times upper limit of therapeutic range on methods on echnicon SMAC® , Abbott-VP, Roche Cobas-Bio, Kodak Ektachem® , Hitachi® 705 and KDA *3525*

Urine *No Effect* *Physiological* Nonsignificant reduction observed in 8 healthy volunteers treated for 7 days but nonsignificant increase observed after 7 days in both patients with chronic obstructive pulmonary disease and stable asthma *6382*

Uric Acid *Serum* *Increase* *Analytical* Reduction of phosphotungstate by metabolites *3669*

Serum *Increase* *Physiological* At serum concentrations of 10 - 20 µg/mL a moderate increase of serum uric acid from a mean of 4 mg/dL to 6 mg/dL occurred as a result of its pharmacological effects *3125* Significant effect dose related and unrelated to reduced clearance. Slight inhibitory effect on hypoxanthine guanine phosphoribosyl transferase *4120* Increased concentration observed due to augmented purine catabolism *6579*

Serum *No Effect* *Analytical* No effect at therapeutic concentration on Boehringer Mannheim Reflotron method *3231* No effect at 200 mg/L on Boehringer Mannheim Reflotron method *5706* At 5 times upper limit of therapeutic range on methods on Technicon SMAC® , Abbott-VP, Du Pont aca, Roche Cobas-Bio, Kodak Ektachem® , Hitachi® 705 and KDA *3525* At 1.0 g/L on reversed phase liquid chromatographic procedure of Zhiri et al *6656* No effect at concentration of 100 µg/mL (555 µmol/L) on method on Du Pont Dimension *1594* At concentration of 2,000 mg/L had no effect on phosphotungstate reduction method *5704*

Urine *Increase* *Analytical* Reduction of phosphotungstate by metabolites *880*

Volume *Urine* *Increase* *Physiological* 4.7 mL/min versus 1.9 mL/min in 11 healthy subjects when given drug intravenously *2603*

Xanthurenic Acid *Urine* *Increase* *Physiological* Substantial increase in response to tryptophan load test after 4 weeks treatment with theophylline, but test normalized after 1 week of pyridoxine supplementation *6115*

Zafirlukast *Serum* *Decrease* *Physiological* In 13 asthmatic patients coadministration of zafirlukast (80 mg/d) at steady state with erythromycin (6 mg/kg) for 5 days to steady state caused a significant decrease of 30% in the mean plasma concentration of zafirlukast due to a decrease in its bioavailability *6641*

Thiabendazole

Alanine Aminotransferase *Serum Increase Physiological* May occasionally cause hypersensitivity-mediated idiosyncratic cholestatic reaction *1384* Has been reported to cause jaundice, cholestasis and parenchymal liver damage *3984*

Aldolase *Serum Increase Physiological* Probably of muscle origin although taken orally *4014*

Alkaline Phosphatase *Serum Increase Physiological* One case of drug-induced cholestasis reported *4925* Rare cholestasis *2911* Has been reported to cause jaundice, cholestasis and parenchymal liver damage *3984* May occasionally cause a hypersensitivity-mediated idiosyncratic cholestatic reaction *1384*

Aspartate Aminotransferase *Serum Increase Physiological* May rarely cause a transient increase in activity. Has been reported to cause jaundice, cholestasis and parenchymal liver damage *3984* One case of drug-induced cholestasis reported *4925* May occasionally cause hypersensitivity-mediated idiosyncratic cholestatic reaction *1384*

Bilirubin *Serum Increase Physiological* One case of drug-induced cholestasis reported *4925* Has been reported to cause jaundice, cholestasis and parenchymal liver damage *3984* May occasionally cause cholestasis probably due to a hypersensitivity-mediated idiosyncratic reaction *1384*

Blood *Urine Increase Physiological* Has been reported to cause hematuria *3984*

BSP Retention *Serum Increase Physiological* Rare cholestasis *3984*

Cholesterol *Serum Increase Physiological* Cholestatic effect *3984*

Crystals *Urine Increase Physiological* May occasionally cause crystalluria *1384* Low solubility of drug, especially at neutral pH *3984*

Glucose *Serum Decrease Physiological* Asymptomatic lowering observed *128*
Serum Increase Physiological Rare case of hyperglycemia reported *2451* May occasionally cause hyperglycemia *1384* Has been reported to cause hyperglycemia *3984*

γ-Glutamyltransferase *Serum Increase Physiological* Has been reported to cause jaundice, cholestasis and parenchymal liver damage *3984*

Hemoglobin *Urine Increase Physiological* May occasionally cause hematuria *1384*

Leukocytes *Blood Decrease Physiological* Has been reported to cause transient leukopenia or agranulocytosis *3984* May occasionally cause transient leukopenia *1384*

Myoglobin *Urine No Effect Physiological* Not observed although serum aldolase increased *4014*

5'-Nucleotidase *Serum Increase Physiological* Rare cholestasis *2911*

Odor *Urine Increase Physiological* Odor similar to that after ingestion of asparagine *3984*

Platelets *Blood Decrease Physiological* Thrombocytopenia *3984*

Protein *Urine Increase Physiological* May cause nephrotoxicity *2451*

Theophylline *Serum Increase Physiological* Decreases theophylline clearance and increases serum theophylline concentration by 190% *3125* Up to 190% increase in serum theophylline concentration due to decreased theophylline clearance *6117* May cause increase in concentration through competing for metabolic sites in the liver *3984* Decreases theophylline clearance, increasing theophylline concentration by about 190% *5999* May interfere with metabolism and increase plasma drug concentration *1384*

Urobilinogen *Feces Decrease Physiological* Pale stools, cholestatic effect *3984*
Urine Decrease Physiological Cholestatic effect *3984*

Thiacetazone

Alanine Aminotransferase *Serum Increase Physiological* May cause hepatitis *2135* May cause cholestatic (hepatocanalicular) jaundice *402*

Alkaline Phosphatase *Serum Increase Physiological* May cause cholestatic (hepatocanalicular) jaundice *402*

Aspartate Aminotransferase *Serum Increase Physiological* May cause hepatitis *2135* May cause cholestatic (hepatocanalicular) jaundice *402*

Bile *Urine Increase Physiological* May cause cholestasis *402*

Bilirubin *Serum Increase Physiological* May cause cholestatic (hepatocanalicular) jaundice *402*

BSP Retention *Serum Increase Physiological* May cause cholestasis *402*

Cholesterol *Serum Increase Physiological* May cause cholestatic (hepatocanalicular) jaundice *402*

Erythrocytes *Blood Decrease Physiological* Rare Stevens-Johnson syndrome induced *4014*

Hemoglobin *Blood Decrease Physiological* May cause hemolytic anemia; may fall without frank anemia *2135*

Leukocytes *Blood Decrease Physiological* Drug related agranulocytosis (rare) *4014*

Neutrophils *Blood Decrease Physiological* May cause agranulocytosis *2135*

Urobilinogen *Feces Decrease Physiological* Pale stools, occurs with cholestasis *402*
Urine Decrease Physiological May cause cholestasis *402*

Thiamine

Albumin *Urine No Effect Analytical* Using a fluorimetric assay with Albumin Blue 580 on a Cobas Fara centrifugal analyzer for the detection of microalbuminuria no significant interference was detected at a concentration of 3.0 mg/L *3117*

Creatinine *Serum No Effect Analytical* At 500 mg/L on reversed phase liquid chromatographic procedure of Zhiri et al *6656*

Lymphocytes *Blood Decrease Physiological* Significant effect with megadose supplementation *2245*

Neutrophils *Blood No Effect Physiological* No effect with megadose supplementation *2245*

Uric Acid *Serum No Effect Analytical* At 500 mg/L on reversed phase liquid chromatographic procedure of Zhiri et al *6656*

Thiamylal

Protein *Test Conditions Increase Analytical* Reacts with Folin-Ciocalteu method of Lowry *1102*

T3-Uptake *Serum No Effect Physiological* No effect on test *882*

Thiazides

Adenosine Monophosphate
Plasma Decrease Physiological Administration of thazide diuretics with sodium restriction improves gastrointestinal absorption of calcium and reduce urine calcium excretion in glucocorticoid-treated patients and decrease cyclic AMP and iPTH *6526*

Alanine Aminotransferase *Serum Increase Physiological* May cause cholestasis *3810*

Alkaline Phosphatase *Serum Increase Physiological* Cholestatic hepatitis reported *2242*

Ammonia *Plasma Increase Physiological* Associated with potassium depletion and alkalosis *2025*

Amphetamine *Serum Increase Physiological* Urinary alkalinizing agents, including some thiazides, increase the nonionized part of the amphetamine molecule, thereby decreasing urinary excretion *5641*

Amylase *Serum Increase Physiological* May increase up to 200% in a week *1136*

Aspartate Aminotransferase *Serum Increase Physiological* May cause cholestasis *3810*

Bicarbonate *Serum Increase Physiological* Over 60% have value over 30 mEq/L in long term *455*

Bilirubin *Serum Increase Physiological* Cholestatic hepatitis reported to occur *2242*

Bromide *Urine Increase Physiological* In cases of bromide intoxication *2242*

BSP Retention *Serum Increase Physiological* Reduced plasma volume and hepatic blood flow *2451*

Calcium *Serum Increase Physiological* May increase up to 0.25 mEq/L *4555*
Urine Decrease Physiological Observed effect associated with increased bone density and improved calcium balance *3359* Administration of thazide diuretics with sodium restriction improves gastrointestinal absorption of calcium and reduce urine calcium excretion in glucocorticoid-treated patients and decrease cyclic AMP and iPTH *6526* By up to 50% (appear to have extra-renal effect) *4555*

Chloride *Serum Decrease Physiological* Diuretic action (impaired tubular reabsorption) *3810*
Urine Increase Physiological Diuretic action *2242*

Cholesterol *Serum Decrease Physiological* Mean 9 mg/dL decrease observed in 1021 patients in MRFIT study treated for 6 years *167*
Serum Increase Physiological In 310 hypertensives treatment with thiazides for one year caused significant 14.3 ± 2.9 mg/dL increase in concentration *1721* Mean 5% increase observed after 1 year in 302 patients in NHLB study *167* Infrequent cholestatic effect *2803*

Citrate *Urine Decrease Physiological* By up to 30% *4555*

Cortisol *Urine Decrease Physiological* ?Changed secretion or renal handling *1672*

Creatine *Urine Decrease Physiological* Clearance tests decreased by 10-20% *4013*

Creatinine *Serum Increase Physiological* Nephrotoxic effect with large doses *3669*
Urine Decrease Physiological Clearance tests decreased by 10-20% *4013*

Creatinine Clearance *Urine Decrease Physiological* May cause decrease by up to 20% *4013*

1,25-Dihydroxy Vitamin D *Serum Decrease Physiological* In 25 postmenopausal women mean concentration 60.8 ± 16.2 pmol/L less than 77.0 ± 18.7 pmol/L in postmenopausal non-users in the winter/spring *1287*

Erythrocytes *Blood Decrease Physiological* Rare hypersensitive depression of bone marrow *3810*
Urine Increase Physiological May cause actual bleeding *1714*

Glomerular Filtration Rate *Urine Decrease Physiological* Especially if administered i.v *2242*

Glucose *Serum Increase Physiological* Decreased glucose tolerance *129* In 310 hypertensives treatment with thiazides for one year caused significant 10.3 ± 4.7 mg/dL increase in concentration *1721*
Urine Increase Physiological May occur especially in prediabetics *705*

Glucose Tolerance *Serum Decrease Physiological* Diabetogenic-like action of drug *4555*

HDL-Cholesterol *Serum Decrease Physiological* Mean 1 mg/dL decrease observed in 1021 patients in MRFIT study treated for 6 years *167*
Serum No Effect Physiological In short term studies administration of thiazides had no significant effect on concentration within a year *3730*

Hemoglobin *Urine Increase Physiological* Actual bleeding caused by the drug *1714*

Histamine Test *Patient Decrease Physiological* False negative due to hypotensive effect of drug *2451*

^{131}I Uptake *Serum No Effect Physiological* No effect observed in most patients *2452*

LDL-Cholesterol *Serum Increase Physiological* Mean 10% increase observed in 302 patients in NHLB study treated for 1 year *167* In short term studies administration of thiazides increased concentration of LDL-cholesterol by 6 to 10% within a year *3730*

LE Cells *Blood Positive Physiological* SLE may occur, usually normalizes when stopped *5102*

Leukocytes *Blood Decrease Physiological* Reported to cause agranulocytopenia *4555*

Lithium *Serum Increase Physiological* Long-term administration decreases renal clearance with corresponding increase in plasma concentration *5678* Increase reabsorption of lithium in the proximal tube *3590*

Lithium Clearance *Urine No Effect Physiological* A single dose of the drug has no effect on lithium clearance *4399*

Magnesium *Serum Decrease Physiological* Consequence of diuresis *2858*
Urine Increase Physiological Increase of 33% reported *5633*

Methotrexate *Serum Increase Physiological* Effect probably due to reduced renal excretion but mechanism not conclusively established *4438*

5'-Nucleotidase *Serum Increase Physiological* Due to cholestasis *2911*

Osteocalcin *Serum Decrease Physiological* In 10 postmenopausal women mean concentration in summer/fall 2.89 ± 0.82 µg/L versus 3.65 ± 1.02 µg/L in non-users and 2.54 ± 0.80 µg/L versus 3.47 ± 1.07 µg/L in non-users in winter/spring *1287*

Parathyroid Hormone *Plasma Decrease Physiological* In 25 postmenopausal thiazide users mean concentration of 26.2 ± 7.6 ng/L less than 31.0 ± 11.7 ng/mL in postmenopausal non-users in the winter/spring *1287*

Parathyroid Hormone, Intact
Plasma Decrease Physiological Administration of thazide diuretics with sodium restriction improves gastrointestinal absorption of calcium and reduce urine calcium excretion in glucocorticoid-treated patients and decrease cyclic AMP and iPTH *6526*

Phentolamine Test *Patient Decrease Physiological* False negative due to hypotensive effect of drug *2451*

Platelets *Blood Decrease Physiological* Reported to cause thrombocytopenia *4555*

Potassium *Serum Decrease Physiological* Administration of thazide diuretics may aggravate glucocorticoid-induced hypokalemia *6526* In 310 hypertensives treatment with thiazides for one year caused significant 0.08 ± 0.04 mmol/L decrease in concentration *1721* Consequence of diuresis *2242*
Urine Increase Physiological Diuretic action *2242*

Prothrombin Time *Plasma Increase Physiological* Associated with failure of excretion of bile salts *2803*

PSP Excretion *Urine Decrease Physiological* Competition for excretion by tubules *1622*

Quinidine *Serum Increase Physiological* Alkalinize urine, increase reabsorption *2452*

Sildenafil *Serum No Effect Physiological* CYP2D6 inhibitors such as thiazides and related diuretics did not affect the pharmacokinetics of sildenafil *4657*

Sodium *Serum Decrease Physiological* Diuretic action with sodium depletion *129*
Urine Increase Physiological Diuretic action *2242*

Sugar *Urine Increase Analytical* Interferes with Benedict's reagent *1714*

T3-Uptake *Serum Decrease Physiological* Slight effect observed only *3933*

Triglycerides *Serum Increase Physiological* Mean 17 mg/dL increase observed in 1021 patients in MRFIT study treated for 6 years *167* In short term studies administration of thiazides increased concentration of triglycerides by 15 to 20% within a year *3730* Concentration increased in patients receiving thiazides *4989*

Tyramine Test *Patient Decrease Physiological* May attenuate response to tyramine *1733*

Urea Nitrogen *Serum Increase Physiological* Nephrotoxic effect in large doses *1714*

Uric Acid *Serum Increase Physiological* Decreased renal excretion *2024*
Urine Decrease Physiological Decreased renal excretion (18% in long term) *455*

Uric Acid Clearance *Urine Decrease Physiological* Decreased renal clearance *4014*

Urobilinogen *Feces Decrease Physiological* May cause cholestasis with pale stools *2803*
Urine Decrease Physiological Cholestatic effect *2803*

Volume *Plasma Decrease Physiological* Due to diuretic action *2242*

Thiazolidine

Amino Acids *Urine Increase Analytical* Positive reaction observed with ninhydrin in paper chromatography, paper electrophoresis and ion-exchange chromatography *4761*

Sugar *Urine Increase Analytical* Reacts positively with Clinitest *4761*

Thiazolsulfone

Bilirubin *Serum Increase Physiological* Hemolytic anemia *3810*

Color *Urine Increase Analytical* Red, pink, purple, orange and rust color *2024*

Erythrocytes *Blood Decrease Physiological* May cause hemolytic anemia *3810*

Haptoglobin *Serum Decrease Physiological* Hemolytic anemia *3810*

Hematocrit *Blood Decrease Physiological* May cause hemolytic anemia *3810*

Hemoglobin *Blood Decrease Physiological* May cause hemolytic anemia *3810*

Methemoglobin *Blood Increase Physiological* Hemolytic anemia *3810*

Thiethylperazine

Alanine Aminotransferase *Serum Increase Physiological* Occasional cases of cholestatic jaundice and hepatotoxicity described *5133* Few cases of cholestasis reported *2754*

Alkaline Phosphatase *Serum Increase Physiological* Occasional cases of cholestatic jaundice and hepatotoxicity described *5133*

Aspartate Aminotransferase *Serum Increase Physiological* Occasional cases of cholestatic jaundice and hepatotoxicity described *5133* Few cases of cholestasis reported *2754*

Bilirubin *Serum Increase Physiological* Few cases of cholestasis reported *2754* Occasional cases of cholestatic jaundice and hepatotoxicity described *5133*

γ-Glutamyltransferase *Serum Increase Physiological* Occasional cases of cholestatic jaundice and hepatotoxicity described *5133*

Prolactin *Plasma Increase Physiological* Significant response to drug given i.m. or orally *2352*

Thiocarlide

Alanine Aminotransferase *Serum Increase Physiological* Reported effect in 4% subjects *4014*

Bilirubin *Serum Increase Physiological* Rare observation *4014*

Glucose *Serum Decrease Physiological* Hypoglycemic reactions observed *4014*

Leukocytes *Blood Decrease Physiological* Associated with relative lymphocytosis and monocytosis *4014*

Thiocolchicine

Eosinophils *Blood Increase Physiological* May cause eosinophilia *3535*

Erythrocytes *Blood Decrease Physiological* May cause anemia (rare) *3535*

Lymphocytes *Blood Increase Physiological* May cause real increase *3535*

Neutrophils *Blood Decrease Physiological* May be reduced although lymphocytes increased *3535*

Platelets *Blood Decrease Physiological* May cause thrombocytopenia occasionally *3535*

Thiocyanate

Alanine Aminotransferase *Serum Increase Physiological* May cause hepatic necrosis *2242*

Aspartate Aminotransferase *Serum Increase Physiological* May cause hepatic necrosis *2242*

Erythrocytes *Blood Decrease Physiological* Several cases of aplastic anemia reported *6264* May cause anemia *3810*

^{131}I Uptake *Serum No Effect Physiological* Does not affect uptake by thyroid *3669*

ionized Calcium *Serum No Effect Analytical* No effect observed with concentrations of thiocyanate likely to be found in smokers with AVL and Nova ion-selective electrodes *4898*

Ionized Magnesium *Serum Decrease Analytical* Significant reduction observed with increasing concentrations of thiocyanate likely to be found in smokers with Nova ion-selective electrode: extent related to baseline magnesium concentration *4898*
Serum No Effect Analytical No effect observed with concentrations of thiocyanate likely to be found in smokers with AVL ion-selective electrode *4898*

Leukocytes *Blood Decrease Physiological* Several cases of aplastic anemia reported *6264*

Platelets *Blood Decrease Physiological* Several cases of aplastic anemia reported *6264*

Protein *Urine Increase Physiological* May cause nephrosis *2242*

Urea Nitrogen *Serum Increase Physiological* May cause nephrosis *2242*

Thioglycolate

Leukocytes *Blood Decrease Physiological* Reported effect *4017*

Thioguanine

Alanine Aminotransferase *Serum Increase Physiological* Liver enzymes and other liver function tests are occasionally abnormal *2180* May cause cholestasis *3810*

Alkaline Phosphatase *Serum Increase Physiological* Liver enzymes and other liver function tests are occasionally abnormal *2180* Transient increase in 3 of 29 patients with polycythemia rubra vera *4055* May cause cholestasis *3810*

Aspartate Aminotransferase *Serum Increase Physiological* Liver enzymes and other liver function tests are occasionally abnormal *2180* Transient increase in 3 of 29 patients with polycythemia rubra vera *4055* May cause cholestasis *3810*

Bile *Urine Increase Physiological* May cause cholestasis *3810*

Bilirubin *Serum Increase Physiological* Liver enzymes and other liver function tests are occasionally abnormal *2180* May cause cholestasis *3810*

BSP Retention *Serum Increase Physiological* May cause cholestasis *3810*

Chromosomes *Test Conditions Abnormal Physiological* Clastogenic in human cells *5484*

Hematocrit *Blood Decrease Physiological* In 29 patients with polycythemia rubra vera; effect usually apparent in 2 weeks *4055*

Hemoglobin *Blood Decrease Physiological* In 29 patients with polycythemia rubra vera; effect usually apparent in 2 weeks *4055*

Leukocytes *Blood Decrease Physiological* May cause marrow depression *822* In 29 patients with polycythemia rubra vera; effect usually apparent in 2 weeks *4055* Observed in 7 patients with chronic granulocytic leukemia *5745*

Neutrophils *Blood Decrease Physiological* Observed in 7 patients with chronic granulocytic leukemia *5745*

Platelets *Blood Decrease Physiological* Immunologically induced thrombocytopenia *822* In 29 patients with polycythemia rubra vera; effect usually apparent in 2 weeks *4055* Observed in 7 patients with chronic granulocytic leukemia *5745*

Protein *Test Conditions Increase Analytical* Reacts in Folin-Ciocalteu method of Lowry *2566*

Uric Acid *Serum Increase Physiological* Rapid destruction of tissues due to nucleic acid catabolism *2242*
Urine Increase Physiological Due to augmented tissue catabolism *2242*

Thioneine

Uric Acid *Serum Increase Analytical* Affects phosphotungstate reduction methods *5868*

Thiopental

Alanine Aminotransferase *Serum Increase Physiological* 1 case out of 24 3-5 d after anesthesia, more longer period after anesthesia pyrexia and jaundice in one case after repeated anesthesia *615*
Serum No Effect Analytical At acute overdose concentration (20 mg/dL) on Technicon SMAC® method *6266*

Albumin *Serum No Effect Analytical* At concentration of 200 mg/L had no effect on BCG method *5704* At acute overdose concentration (20 mg/dL) on Technicon SMAC® method *6266*

Alkaline Phosphatase *Serum Increase Physiological* 1 case out of 24 3-5 d after anesthesia, more longer period after anesthesia pyrexia and jaundice in one case after reported anesthesia *615*
Serum No Effect Analytical At acute overdose concentration (20 mg/dL) on Technicon SMAC® method *6266*

Aspartate Aminotransferase *Serum Increase Physiological* 1 case out of 24 3-5 d after anesthesia, more longer period after anesthesia pyrexia and jaundice in one case after repeated anesthesia *615*
Serum No Effect Analytical At acute overdose concentration (20 mg/dL) on Technicon SMAC® method *6266*

Basophils *Blood Decrease Physiological* Significant fall within 3 minutes of i.v. injection *3648*

Bicarbonate *Serum No Effect Analytical* At concentration of 70 mg/L had no effect on method using phenolphthalein method *5704*

Bicyclo-Prostaglandin E_2 *Plasma Increase Physiological* In 8 volunteers mean concentration increased after injection of mean dose of 6.0 mg/kg from baseline of 86 ± 34 pg/mL to 111 ± 33 pg/mL after 1 minute and 113 ± 24 pg/mL after 5 minutes *4713*

Bilirubin *Serum Increase Physiological* 1 case out of 24 3-5 d after anesthesia, more longer period after anesthesia *615*
Serum No Effect Analytical At acute overdose concentration (20 mg/dL) on Technicon SMAC® method *6266* At concentration of 200 mg/L had no effect on Jendrassik and Grof method *5704*

Calcium *Serum No Effect Analytical* At concentration of 200 mg/L had no effect on cresolphthalein method *5704* At acute overdose concentration (20 mg/dL) on Technicon SMAC® method *6266*

Chloride *Serum No Effect Analytical* At concentration of 200 mg/L had no effect on mercurimetric method *5704*

Cholesterol *Serum No Effect Analytical* At acute overdose concentration (20 mg/dL) on Technicon SMAC® method *6266* At concentration of 200 mg/L had no effect on Liebermann-Burchard method *5704*

Creatine Kinase *Serum No Effect Analytical* At acute overdose concentration (20 mg/dL) on Technicon SMAC® method *6266*

Creatinine *Serum No Effect Analytical* At acute overdose concentration (20 mg/dL) on Technicon SMAC® method *6266* At concentration of 200 mg/L had no effect on Technicon AutoAnalyzer® Jaffe method *5704*

Glucaric Acid *Urine Increase Physiological* Enhanced excretion with anesthesia *3*

Glucose *Serum No Effect Analytical* At acute overdose concentration (20 mg/dL) on Technicon SMAC® method *6266*
Serum No Effect Physiological No effect except during surgery which causes increase *1620*

γ-Glutamyltransferase *Serum Increase Physiological* 1 case out of 24 3-5 d after anesthesia, more with longer period after anesthesia *615*

Guaiacols Spot Test *Urine Positive Analytical* False reaction with screening test of Rogers *5061*

Histamine *Plasma Increase Physiological* Normal response even up by 350% at 5 minutes *3648*
Plasma No Effect Analytical No inhibition of radio-enzyme assay observed at physiological concentration *2492*

Hydrochloric Acid *Gastric Fluid Increase Physiological* Stimulation of secretion parallels plasma histamine *3648*

Iron *Serum No Effect Analytical* At acute overdose concentration (20 mg/dL) on Technicon SMAC® method *6266* At concentration of 200 mg/L had no effect on Ferrozine method *5704*

Lactate Dehydrogenase *Serum Increase Physiological* Pyrexia and jaundice in one case after repeated anesthesia *615*
Serum No Effect Analytical At acute overdose concentration (20 mg/dL) on Technicon SMAC® method *6266*

Midazolam *Serum No Effect Analytical* On GC-ECD method of Ha et al *2387*

Phosphate *Serum No Effect Analytical* At concentration of 200 mg/L had no effect on phosphomolybdate method *5704* At acute overdose concentration (20 mg/dL) on Technicon SMAC® method *6266*

Protein *Serum No Effect Analytical* At concentration of 200 mg/L had no effect on biuret method with blank correction *5704* At acute overdose concentration (20 mg/dL) on Technicon SMAC® method *6266*

Remifentanil *Serum No Effect Physiological* Remifentanil clearance is not altered when thiopental coadministered *2165*

T3-Uptake *Serum No Effect Physiological* No effect on test *882*

Triglycerides *Serum No Effect Analytical* At concentration of 200 mg/L had no effect on lipase/esterase method *5704* At acute overdose concentration (20 mg/dL) on Technicon SMAC® method *6266*

Urea Nitrogen *Serum No Effect Analytical* At acute overdose concentration (20 mg/dL) on Technicon SMAC® method *6266* At concentration of 200 mg/L had no effect on diacetylmonoxime method *5704*

Uric Acid *Serum No Effect Analytical* At concentration of 200 mg/L had no effect on phosphotungstate reduction method *5704* At acute overdose concentration (20 mg/dL) on Technicon SMAC® method *6266*

Thioproline

Sugar *Urine Increase Analytical* Reacts positively with Clinitest *4761*

Thiopronine

Acetylcholine Receptor Antibodies
Serum No Effect Physiological No occurrence of myasthenia gravis or other autoimmune syndromes reported *2881*

Leukocytes *Blood No Effect Physiological* Toxicity similar to penicillamine and other sulfhydryl drugs *2881*

Platelets *Blood Decrease Physiological* Toxicity similar to penicillamine and other sulfhydryl drugs *2881*

Protein *Urine Increase Physiological* Toxicity similar to penicillamine and other sulfhydryl drugs *2881*

Thiopropazate

Homovanillic Acid
Cerebrospinal Fluid No Effect Physiological No significant effect in Huntington's chorea *3908*

5-Hydroxyindoleacetic Acid
Cerebrospinal Fluid No Effect Physiological No significant effect in Huntington's chorea *3908*

Leukocytes *Blood Decrease Physiological* Rare leukopenia *128*

Thioridazine

Alanine Aminotransferase *Serum Increase Physiological* Hepatotoxicity *3025* Administration of thioridazine causes occasional jaundice or biliary stasis *5233*

Thioridazine *(continued)*

Albumin *Urine No Effect Analytical* Using a fluorimetric assay with Albumin Blue 580 on a Cobas Fara centrifugal analyzer for the detection of microalbuminuria no significant interference was detected at a concentration of 10 mg/L *3117*

Alkaline Phosphatase *Serum Increase Physiological* Hypersensitivity reaction *3025* Administration of thioridazine causes occasional jaundice or biliary stasis *5233*

Amitriptyline *Serum No Effect Analytical* Cross-reactivity less than 5% with Abbott TDx procedure *2487*

Amphetamine *Urine No Effect Analytical* No false positive results observed in 12 assays using Syva EMIT amphatamine method with either monoclonal or polyclonal antibodies *1160*

Aspartate Aminotransferase *Serum Increase Physiological* Hepatotoxicity *3025* Administration of thioridazine causes occasional jaundice or biliary stasis *5233*

Bile *Urine Increase Physiological* Hepatotoxicity *3025*

Bilirubin *Serum Decrease Physiological* ?Due to effect on bilirubin metabolism *2670*
Serum Increase Physiological Hepatotoxicity (questionable) *3025* Administration of thioridazine causes occasional jaundice or biliary stasis *5233*

BSP Retention *Serum Increase Physiological* Hepatotoxicity *3025*

Carbamazepine *Serum No Effect Physiological* No significant effect observed with either 100 mg or 200 mg thioridazine in 8 epileptic patients *5748*

Carbamazepine-10,11-Epoxide
Serum No Effect Physiological No significant effect observed in 8 epileptic patients following ingestion of either 100 mg or 200 mg daily *5748*

Eosinophils *Blood Increase Physiological* Administration of thioridazine causes mild transient increase in concentration *5233*

Erythrocytes *Blood Decrease Physiological* Occasionally seen with phenothiazines *2754*

γ-Glutamyltransferase *Serum Increase Physiological* Administration of thioridazine causes occasional jaundice or biliary stasis *5233*

Gonadotropin, Pituitary *Urine Decrease Physiological* Total gonadotrophic activity reduced *5957*

Granulocytes *Blood Decrease Physiological* Agranulocytosis with hepatitis observed in one patient with progression to hepatic encephalopathy *1384* Administration of thioridazine causes mild transient decrease in concentration with occasional agranulocytosis *5233*

Growth Hormone *Plasma No Effect Physiological* No significant difference in patients receiving drug on continuing basis versus controls *6491*

Hematocrit *Blood Decrease Physiological* Significant decrease reported *2670* Administration of thioridazine causes mild transient decrease in value with anemia or aplastic anemia *5233*

Hemoglobin *Blood Decrease Physiological* Significant effect reported *2670*

Histamine *Plasma No Effect Analytical* Although 50% inhibition of radio-enzyme assay at 39 μg/mL no effect likely to occur clinically since physiological concentration 0.05 - 2.0 μg/mL *2492*

Imipramine *Serum No Effect Analytical* Cross-reactivity of less than 5% observed with Abbott TDx procedure *2473*

Leukocytes *Blood Decrease Physiological* Administration of thioridazine causes mild transient decrease in concentration *5233* Agranulocytosis due to inhibition of development *4714*

Luteinizing Hormone *Plasma Decrease Physiological* Significantly less in 42 male schizophrenics than when they ingested other neuroleptic agents *772*

Lysergic Acid Diethylamide *Urine Increase Analytical* Minimum concentration that caused a positive result with EMIT method to measure LSD 2 mg/L *4968*

Neutrophils *Blood Decrease Physiological* Occasional case of agranulocytosis reported *6264* Administration of thioridazine reported to cause neutropenia infrequently *5233*

Nortriptyline *Serum No Effect Analytical* Cross-reactivity less than 5% with Abbott TDx procedure *2487*

p-Aminophenol *Urine No Effect Analytical* With addition of drugs at a concentration of 100 mg/L and of related compounds at 50 mg/L no significant effect observed on colorimetric method of van Bocxlaer on Cobas Mira analyzer which involves reacting free p-aminophenol with resorcinol in the presence of magnesium ions to form an indophenol dye measured at 550 nm *6163*

Peptides, Low-molecular Weight
Urine Decrease Physiological In one schizophrenic patient treatment with 150 mg/d for 5 weeks caused significant reduction from 116.5 μmol/d to 22.3 μmol/d *4901*

Phenytoin *Serum Increase Physiological* Significant increase in 15% patients with combined therapy, reduction in 7%. No change in others *5245* Two cases reported of increased plasma concentration due to competition for metabolism by cytochrome P-450 *6263*

Pindolol *Serum Increase Physiological* When drugs coadministered plasma pindolol concentration may be increased *5244* Administration of thioridazine with pindolol observed to cause higher than expected pindolol concentration *5233*

Platelets *Blood Decrease Physiological* Occasionally seen with phenothiazines *2754* Administration of thioridazine causes mild transient decrease in concentration *5233*

Pregnancy Tests *Urine Positive Analytical* With Prognosticon and other tests *2452*

Prolactin *Plasma Increase Physiological* Significant response to drug given orally (50 mg) *2352* Administration of thioridazine observed to cause hyperprolactinemia *5233* Significant increase within 45 minutes of ingestion of 50 mg orally and 8 to 19 times baseline at 2 h. Functions as potent dopamine antagonist in the tuberoinfundibular system. Effect dose related *5179*

Testosterone *Serum Decrease Physiological* Slight effect in patients on long-term treatment *2836* Significantly less in 42 male schizophrenics than when they ingested other neuroleptic agents *772*

Tricyclic Antidepressants *Serum Increase Analytical* May cause false positive reaction in immunoassays for tricyclic antidepressants *3590*

Tricyclic Antidepressants Screen
Serum Positive Analytical Cross-reactivity observed and may give positive result with method on Du Pont aca *1550*

Thiosemicarbazones

Alanine Aminotransferase *Serum Increase Physiological* May affect liver function *3810*

Alkaline Phosphatase *Serum Increase Physiological* May affect liver function *3810*

Aspartate Aminotransferase *Serum Increase Physiological* May affect liver function *3810*

Bile *Urine Increase Physiological* May affect liver function *3810*

Bilirubin *Serum Increase Physiological* May affect liver function *3810*

BSP Retention *Serum Increase Physiological* May affect liver function *3810*

Erythrocytes *Blood Decrease Physiological* Hydrazone complex formed with pyridoxal PO_4*5054*

Hematocrit *Blood Decrease Physiological* Large dose effect *2242*

Hemoglobin *Blood Decrease Physiological* Large dose effect *2242*

Leukocytes *Blood Decrease Physiological* Leukopenia/agranulocytosis in 0.5% *2242*

Protein *Urine Increase Physiological* Nephrotoxic effect *1714 2024*

Thiotepa

Cholinesterase *Serum Decrease Physiological* Mild depressive effects reported *2452*

Color *Feces Increase Analytical* Black color reported following ingestion of thiotepa *3388*

Erythrocytes *Blood Decrease Physiological* 10 of 25 patients given drug intravesically had at least one incident of acute myelosuppression; 5 of 29 patients had chronic myelosuppression *2674* May cause bone marrow depression *128* Hematopoietic toxicity can occur following overdose *2820*

Hematocrit *Blood Decrease Physiological* May be rapid decrease *4014*

Hemoglobin *Blood Decrease Physiological* May be rapid decrease *4014* 10 of 25 patients given drug intravesically had at least one incident of acute myelosuppression; 5 of 29 patients had chronic myelosuppression *2674*

Leukocytes *Blood Decrease Physiological* Hematopoietic toxicity can occur following overdose *2820* May cause bone marrow depression *128* 10 of 25 patients given drug intravesically had at least one incident of acute myelosuppression; 5 of 29 patients had chronic myelosuppression *2674*

Occult Blood *Feces Increase Physiological* May be ulceration of gastrointestinal tract *4014*

Platelets *Blood Decrease Physiological* Hematopoietic toxicity can occur following overdose *2820* May cause bone marrow depression *128* 10 of 25 patients given drug intravesically had at least one incident of acute myelosuppression; 5 of 25 patients had chronic myelosuppression *2674*

Sperm Count *Semen Decrease Physiological* Impaired spermatogenesis may occur *1384*

Uric Acid *Serum Increase Physiological* Due to cell destruction, may cause nephropathy *2754*

Thiothixene

Alanine Aminotransferase *Serum Increase Physiological* Transient increases in activity have been infrequently observed in some patients *4650* Hepatotoxic effect (reversible cholestasis) *3810*

Alkaline Phosphatase *Serum Increase Physiological* Hepatotoxic effect (reversible cholestasis) *1714* Transient increases in activity have been infrequently observed in some patients *4650*

Aspartate Aminotransferase *Serum Increase Physiological* Hepatotoxic effect (reversible cholestasis) *3810* Transient increases in activity have been infrequently observed in some patients *4650*

Bile *Urine Increase Physiological* Hepatotoxic effect (reversible cholestasis) *3810*

Bilirubin *Serum Increase Physiological* Hepatotoxic effect (reversible cholestasis) *3810*
Serum No Effect Physiological No cases of jaundice attributable to thiothixene have been reported *4650*

BSP Retention *Serum Increase Physiological* Hepatotoxic effect (reversible cholestasis) *3810*

Eosinophils *Blood Increase Physiological* Reported with other phenothiazines *2754*

Erythrocytes *Blood Decrease Physiological* Reported with other phenothiazines *2754*

Glucose *Serum Decrease Physiological* Observed with some phenothiazines *2753* Both hypoglycemia and hyperglycemia have been attributed occasionally to thiothixene administration *4650*
Serum Increase Physiological Both hypoglycemia and hyperglycemia have been attributed occasionally to thiothixene administration *4650* Observed with some phenothiazines *2753*
Urine Increase Physiological Both hypoglycemia and hyperglycemia have been attributed occasionally to thiothixene administration *4650* Observed with some phenothiazines *2753*

Leukocytes *Blood Decrease Physiological* Both leukopenia and leukocytosis have been attributed occasionally to thiothixene administration *4650* Transitory leukopenia *3810*
Blood Increase Physiological Both leukopenia and leukocytosis have been attributed occasionally to thiothixene administration *4650* Transient leukocytosis may occur *2753*

Platelets *Blood Decrease Physiological* Reported with other phenothiazines *2754*

Pregnancy Tests *Urine Positive Analytical* Falsely positive tests have been attributed to phenothiazines *4650* Observed with some phenothiazines *2753*

Prolactin *Plasma Increase Physiological* Typical dose-related response to i.m. administered drug due to antidopaminergic action *3402*

Prothrombin Time *Plasma Decrease Physiological* Rarely reported side effect *128*

Vanillylmandelic Acid *Urine No Effect Physiological* No effect on short term administration *2676*

Thiouracil

Alanine Aminotransferase *Serum Increase Physiological* May cause cholestasis with cholangiolitis *3171*

Alkaline Phosphatase *Serum Increase Physiological* May cause intrahepatic cholestasis *2377*

Aspartate Aminotransferase *Serum Increase Physiological* May cause cholestasis with cholangiolitis *3171*

Bilirubin *Serum Increase Physiological* May cause intrahepatic cholestasis *2377*

Cholesterol *Serum Decrease Analytical* At 13 mg/dL decreased by 30-40 mg/dL *882*
Serum Increase Analytical Interferes with Zlatkis-Zak reaction *5869*
Serum Increase Physiological May cause intrahepatic cholestasis *2377*

Glucose *Serum Decrease Physiological* Reported effect *192*

Histamine *Plasma No Effect Analytical* No inhibition of radio-enzyme assay at therapeutic concentrations *2492*

Leukocytes *Blood Decrease Physiological* Agranulocytosis (in about 1% cases) *6071*

Platelets *Blood Decrease Physiological* Thrombocytopenia *4309*

Thiourea

Histamine *Plasma No Effect Analytical* No inhibition of radio-enzyme assay at therapeutic concentrations *2492*

Propylthiouracil *Serum Increase Analytical* Reacts with 2,6-DQC (procedure of Ratliff) *4872*

Protein *Test Conditions Increase Analytical* Reacts with Folin-Ciocalteu method of Lowry *1102*

Thiouric Acid

Uric Acid *Serum Increase Analytical* 6-thiouric acid (metabolite of 6-mercaptopurine) reported to produce positive interference with uricase methods *1552*

Thiproline

Amino Acids *Urine Increase Analytical* Positive reaction observed with ninhydrin in paper chromatography, paper electrophoresis and ion-exchange chromatography *4761*

Thorium Dioxide

Alanine Aminotransferase *Serum Increase Physiological* Increased about 10% after injection *5270*

Albumin *Serum Decrease Physiological* May produce severe liver damage with years *5270*

Aldolase *Serum Increase Physiological* Time related liver damage (eventual tumor) *5270*

Alkaline Phosphatase *Serum Increase Physiological* Very common (related to time since injection) *5270*

Aspartate Aminotransferase *Serum Increase Physiological* Increased in about 15% after injection *5270*

Bilirubin *Serum Increase Physiological* Time related liver damage *5270*

Bilirubin, Direct *Serum Increase Physiological* Time related liver damage *5270*

BSP Retention *Serum Increase Physiological* May induce liver damage in half cases *5270*

Thorium Dioxide *(continued)*

Chromosomes *Test Conditions Abnormal Physiological* Clastogenic in human cells *5484*

α_2-Globulin *Serum Increase Physiological* May produce severe liver damage after years *5270*

β-Globulin *Serum Increase Physiological* May produce severe liver damage after years *5270*

γ-Globulin *Serum Increase Physiological* May produce severe liver damage after years *5270*

Leucine Aminopeptidase *Serum Increase Physiological* Common finding (related to time since injection) *5270*

Thrombolytic Therapy

Creatine Kinase MB-Isoenzyme *Serum Increase Analytical* Specimens from patients receiving thrombolytic therapy may yield falsely high results when CK-MB measured by method on Bayer Technicon Immuno 1® system *420*

Endothelin *Plasma Decrease Physiological* In patients with AMI significant decrease from mean baseline of 7.5 ng/L observed with thrombolytic therapy with normal activity recurring after about 20 weeks with return occurring earlier in patients with early reperfusion *3459*

Thymopentin

$CD4^+$:$CD8^+$ Lymphocyte Ratio
Blood No Effect Physiological In 3 children with rheumatoid arthritis receiving treatment with 1 mg/kg intraarticularly once weekly for 10 weeks mean ratio decreased significantly from the third week onwards, due to an increase in the concentration of $CD8^+$ cells *5865*

$CD4^+$ Lymphocytes *Blood No Effect Physiological* In 25 patients with rheumatoid arthritis receiving treatment with 50 mg i.v. 3 times weekly for 3 weeks mean concentration changed insignificantly *5865*

$CD8^+$ Lymphocytes *Blood No Effect Physiological* In 25 patients with rheumatoid arthritis receiving treatment with 50 mg i.v. 3 times weekly for 3 weeks mean concentration changed insignificantly *5865*

Erythrocyte Sedimentation Rate
Blood Decrease Physiological In 3 children with rheumatoid arthritis receiving treatment with 1 mg/kg intraarticularly once weekly for 10 weeks mean rate changed significantly from 100 to 70 mm/h during the first 6 weeks and more slowly thereafter *5865*

Hemoglobin *Blood Increase Physiological* In 3 children with rheumatoid arthritis receiving treatment with 1 mg/kg intraarticularly once weekly for 10 weeks mean concentration changed significantly from 8.5 to 11.0 g/dL *5865*

immunoglobulin A *Serum Decrease Physiological* In 20 patients with rheumatoid arthritis receiving treatment with 50 mg i.v. every second day for 1 month mean concentration changed significantly *5865*

Immunoglobulin M *Serum Decrease Physiological* In 20 patients with rheumatoid arthritis receiving treatment with 50 mg i.v. every second day for 1 month mean concentration changed significantly *5865*

Leukocytes *Blood Decrease Physiological* In 748 patients with rheumatoid arthritis receiving treatment with 50 mg i.v. every other day for 4 - 6 weeks mean concentration decreased significantly from 8461 ± 567 /μL to 6680 ± 364 μL *5865*
Blood No Effect Physiological In 3 children with rheumatoid arthritis receiving treatment with 1 mg/kg intraarticularly once weekly for 10 weeks mean concentration changed insignificantly *5865*

Thyroid

Basal Metabolic Rate *Patient Increase Physiological* Metabolic effect of hormone *3669*

Cholesterol *Serum Decrease Physiological* Physiological effect *2451*

Glucose *Serum Increase Physiological* Metabolic action of hormone *1009*

Hydroxyproline *Urine Increase Physiological* Due to catabolic action *6111*

^{131}I Uptake *Serum Decrease Physiological* Consequence of treatment *2451*

Protein *Serum Increase Physiological* Physiological effect exerts anabolic effect *1095*

Prothrombin Time *Plasma Increase Physiological* Prolongs action of anticoagulants *3810*

T3-Uptake *Serum Increase Physiological* Consequence of treatment *2451*

Thyroxine (T4) *Serum Increase Physiological* Increased available thyroxine *3669*

Thyronine

Protein *Cerebrospinal Fluid Increase Analytical* 1.0 mg reacts as if 2.9 mg in Folin-Ciocalteu procedure *882*

Thyrotropin Releasing Hormone

Cortisol *Plasma No Effect Physiological* No effect in normal subjects after i.v. administration *163*

Epinephrine *Plasma Increase Physiological* Mean increase of 28% in 2nd to 4th minute after i.v. injection regardless of whether patient was initially hypo- or hyperthyroid *4871*

Fatty Acids (FFA), Free *Serum No Effect Physiological* After single dose of 1.0 mg synthetic TRH *6453*

Follicle Stimulating Hormone
Plasma No Effect Physiological No effect in normal subjects after i.v. administration *163*

Glucose *Serum No Effect Physiological* After single dose of 1.0 mg synthetic TRH *6453*

Growth Hormone *Plasma No Effect Physiological* No effect in normal subjects after i.v. administration *163*

Insulin *Plasma No Effect Physiological* After single dose of 1.0 mg synthetic TRH *6453*

Interleukin-1β *Serum Increase Physiological* In 8 healthy volunteers and 8 women with galactorrhea standard TRH test caused nonsignificant increase in mean concentration from baseline of 38.1 ± 2.9 fmol/mL to peak concentration of 43.3 ± 2.3 fmol/mL *3234*

Interleukin-2 *Serum Increase Physiological* In 8 healthy volunteers and 8 women with galactorrhea standard TRH test caused significant increase in mean concentration from baseline of 45.6 ± 7.8 fmol/mL to peak concentration of 79.9 ± 16.4 fmol/mL *3234*

Interleukin-6 *Serum Decrease Physiological* In 8 healthy volunteers and 8 women with galactorrhea standard TRH test caused nonsignificant decrease in mean concentration from baseline of 7.9 ± 0.6 fmol/mL to peak concentration of 8.4 ± 0.6 fmol/mL *3234*

Luteinizing Hormone *Plasma No Effect Physiological* No effect in normal subjects *163* No effect seen with 1 mg i.v. in normals *6443*

Norepinephrine *Plasma Increase Physiological* Mean increase of 21% in 2nd to 4th minute after i.v. injection regardless of whether patient was initially hypo- or hyperthyroid *4871*

Prolactin *Plasma Increase Physiological* Response within 5 minutes to i.v. injection *2866* In 8 healthy volunteers and 8 women with galactorrhea standard TRH test caused significant increase in mean concentration from baseline of 15.3 ± 2.3 ng/mL to peak concentration of 46.4 ± 8.8 ng/mL *3234* Maximum effect 15-30 minutes after i.v *2382*

Thyroid Stimulating Hormone
Serum Increase Physiological Threefold increase in 30 minutes *163* In 8 healthy volunteers and 8 women with galactorrhea standard TRH test caused significant increase in mean concentration from baseline of 2.0 ± 0.3 uIU/mL to peak concentration of 12.3 ± 2.2 uIU/mL *3234* Dose related when given i.v.-effect 20 mg orally *1779*

Thyroxine (T4) *Serum Increase Physiological* In 8 healthy volunteers and 8 women with galactorrhea standard TRH test caused significant increase in mean concentration from baseline of 7.9 ± 0.4 pg/dL to peak concentration of 9.6 ± 0.5 pg/dL *3234* But no change in % free T4 (variable response) *2672*

Tri-iodothyronine (T3) *Serum Increase Physiological* In 8 healthy volunteers and 8 women with galactorrhea standard TRH test caused significant increase in mean concentration from baseline of 178.0 ± 16.4 ng/dL to peak concentration of 248.7 ± 21.1 ng/dL *3234* But no change in percent free T3 *2672*

Thyroxine

LDL-Receptor Activity *Tissue Increase Physiological* Increased activity observed with thyroxine administration *3730*

Prothrombin Time *Plasma Increase Physiological* When coadministered with warfarin increases metabolism of coagulation factors *2625*

Thyroglobulin *Serum Decrease Physiological* With 0.1 mg/day for 3 months in 49 patients with solitary thyroid nodules in 18 in whom nodule decreased by more than 50% concentration decreased from mean of 425 µg/L to 61 µg/L whereas in nonresponders mean concentration did not change significantly *4119*

Thyroid Stimulating Hormone
Serum Decrease Physiological Marked decrease from about 1.30 mU/L to about 0.06 mU/L in 49 patients with solitary thyroid nodules treated with 0.1 mg/day for 3 months regardless of whether they responded to treatment or not *4119*

Thyroxine (T4) *Serum Increase Physiological* In both responders and nonresponders mean concentration increased in patients with solitary thyroid nodules with treatment with 0.1 mg/day for 3 months from about 120 nmol/L to about 155 nmol/L *4119*

Thyroxine (T4), Free *Serum Increase Physiological* Increase from about 15 pmol/L to about 22 pmol/L in 49 patients with solitary thyroid nodules treated with 0.1 mg/day for 3 months regardless of whether they responded to treatment or not *4119*

Tri-iodothyronine, Free (fT3) *Serum Increase Physiological* In 49 patients with solitary thyroid nodules increase from mean of 5.08 to 5.80 pmol/L in responders and from 5.23 to 6.42 pmol/L in nonresponders in response to 0.1 mg/day for 3 months *4119*
Serum No Effect Analytical At a concentration of 5.0 x 10^{-5} g/L cross-reactivity of less than 0.1% with free triiodothyronine method on Bayer Technicon Immuno 1® system *425* No significant cross-reactivity observed with either D- or L-thyroxine with method on Organon Teknika AuraFlex random access immunoassay analyzer *885*

Tri-iodothyronine, Reverse (rT3)
Serum Increase Physiological Increase from mean of 0.32 to 0.45 nmol/L in responders and from 0.29 to 0.50 nmol/L in nonresponders in 49 patients with solitary thyroid nodules treated with 0.1 mg/day for 3 months *4119*

Tri-iodothyronine (T3) *Serum No Effect Analytical* Cross-reactivity of only 0.08% observed in triiodothyronine method on Bayer Technicon Immuno 1® *436* No significant interference observed from L-thyroxine with method on Organon Teknika AuraFlex random access immunoassay analyzer *2120*
Serum No Effect Physiological In very preterm infants treatment with up to 10 mg/kg body weight for 6 weeks had no effect on plasma tri-iodothyronine concentration *6199* Insignificant increase in both responders and nonresponders with solitary thyroid nodules with treatment with 0.1 mg/day for 3 months *4119*

TSH response to TRH *Serum Decrease Physiological* Baseline concentration of 1.5 mIU/L and maximum of 14.0 mIU/L at 30 min in control state but when treated with thyroxine basal concentration of 0.09 mIU/L and 0.8 mIU/L at 30 min after TRH *1743*

Tiadenol

Cholesterol *Serum Decrease Physiological* Observed in different forms of hyperlipoproteinemia due to reduction of liver lipoprotein secretion but long-term results are not very satisfactory *5586*

Triglycerides *Serum Decrease Physiological* Effective in various forms of hyperlipoproteinemia due to reduction of lipoprotein secretion but long-term effects not very satisfactory *5586*

Tiapamil

Digoxin *Serum Increase Physiological* When coadministered with digoxin increased its area under the concentration curve, its half-life and steady state plasma concentration (59%) *5345* Significant increase in concentration when coadministered with tiapamil *3524*

Tiapride

Albumin *Urine No Effect Analytical* Using a fluorimetric assay with Albumin Blue 580 on a Cobas Fara centrifugal analyzer for the detection of microalbuminuria no significant interference was detected at a concentration of 22 mg/L *3117*

Tiaprofenic Acid

Creatinine *Serum No Effect Analytical* No effect observed with liquid chromatographic method of Paroni et al *4540*

Uric Acid *Serum Decrease Physiological* Interference with transport of uric acid from intra- to extra cellular fluid *3696* In 10 healthy subjects given 300 mg b.i.d *3697*
Urine Increase Physiological Impedes reabsorption in renal tubules thereby increasing clearance *3696* In 10 healthy subjects given 300 mg b.i.d., but effect occurs early so no increased excretion may be observed later *3697*

Tibolone

Androstenedione *Plasma No Effect Physiological* In 11 healthy postmenopausal women administration of 2.5 mg/d for 3 months had no significant effect on plasma concentration which remained within the reference range *839*

Apolipoprotein A *Serum No Effect Physiological* In 11 healthy postmenopausal women administration of 2.5 mg/d for 3 months caused an insignificant change from mean baseline concentration of 247.6 ± 18.9 mg/dL to 208.2 ± 19.0 mg/dL *839*

Apolipoprotein A:Apolipoprotein B Ratio
Serum No Effect Physiological In 11 healthy postmenopausal women administration of 2.5 mg/d for 3 months caused an insignificant change from mean baseline ratio of 3.59 ± 0.76 to 2.91 ± 0.37 *839*

Apolipoprotein B *Serum No Effect Physiological* In 11 healthy postmenopausal women administration of 2.5 mg/d for 3 months caused an insignificant change from mean baseline concentration of 78.9 ± 9.3 mg/dL to 79.4 ± 9.9 mg/dL *839*

Cholesterol *Serum Decrease Physiological* In 39 postmenopausal women treatment with 2.5 mg/d for 6 months caused significant reduction from mean baseline of 6.55 ± 0.15 mmol/L to 5.75 ± 0.17 mmol/L *1800*
Serum No Effect Physiological In 11 healthy postmenopausal women administration of 2.5 mg/d for 3 months caused an insignificant change from mean baseline concentration of 4.62 ± 0.34 mmol/L to 4.28 ± 0.32 mmol/L *839*

C-Peptide *Plasma No Effect Physiological* In 11 healthy postmenopausal women administration of 2.5 mg/d for 3 months caused an insignificant change from mean baseline concentration of 287.6 ± 33.3 pmol/L to 258.7 ± 17.9 pmol/L *839*

C-terminal Telopeptides of Type I Collagen Degradation Products *Serum Decrease Physiological* In 180 healthy postmenopausal women at least 10 years postmenopause those receiving either 1.25 mg/d or 2.5 mg/d showed approximately 50% decrease in concentration after 3 months treatment which was sustained with continuing treatment *1008*
Urine Decrease Physiological In 180 healthy postmenopausal women at least 10 years postmenopause those receiving either 1.25 mg/d or 2.5 mg/d showed approximately 65% decrease in concentration after 3 months treatment which was sustained with continuing treatment *1008*

Dehydroepiandrosterone Sulfate
Plasma No Effect Physiological In 11 healthy postmenopausal women administration of 2.5 mg/d for 3 months had no significant effect on plasma concentration which remained within the reference range *839*

Tibolone *(continued)*

Estradiol *Plasma No Effect Physiological* In 11 healthy postmenopausal women administration of 2.5 mg/d for 3 months had no significant effect on plasma concentration which remained within the reference range *839*

Glucose *Serum Decrease Physiological* In 11 healthy postmenopausal women administration of 2.5 mg/d for 3 months caused a significant change in fasting blood glucose from mean baseline concentration of 4.49 ± 0.18 mmol/L to 4.16 ± 0.19 mmol/L *839*

Glucose Tolerance *Serum No Effect Physiological* In 11 healthy postmenopausal women administration of 2.5 mg/d for 3 months caused no significant change on oral glucose tolerance *839*

HDL_2-Cholesterol *Serum Decrease Physiological* In 39 postmenopausal women treatment with 2.5 mg/d for 6 months caused significant reduction from mean baseline of 0.42 ± 0.03 mmol/L to 0.27 ± 0.02 mmol/L *1800*

HDL_3-Cholesterol *Serum Decrease Physiological* In 39 postmenopausal women treatment with 2.5 mg/d for 6 months caused significant reduction from mean baseline of 1.19 ± 0.04 mmol/L to 1.07 ± 0.04 mmol/L *1800*

HDL-Cholesterol *Serum Decrease Physiological* In 39 postmenopausal women treatment with 2.5 mg/d for 6 months caused significant reduction from mean baseline of 1.65 ± 0.06 mmol/L to 1.36 ± 0.19 mmol/L *1800*

Serum No Effect Physiological In 11 healthy postmenopausal women administration of 2.5 mg/d for 3 months caused an insignificant change from mean baseline concentration of 1.18 ± 0.1 mmol/L to 1.11 ± 0.1 mmol/L *839*

HDL-Cholesterol:Cholesterol Ratio
Serum No Effect Physiological In 11 healthy postmenopausal women administration of 2.5 mg/d for 3 months caused an insignificant change from mean baseline ratio of 0.27 ± 0.04 to 0.28 ± 0.04 *839*

Insulin *Plasma No Effect Physiological* In 11 healthy postmenopausal women administration of 2.5 mg/d for 3 months caused an insignificant change from mean baseline concentration of 58.9 ± 10.7 pmol/L to 56.6 ± 7.3 pmol/L *839*

Insulin-like Growth Factor-I *Serum No Effect Physiological* Treatment of 30 normal healthy post-menopausal women with 2.5 mg/d caused an insignificant decrease in concentration from mean baseline of 173 ± 37 ng/mL to 163 ± 37 ng/mL after 36 months *2707*

Insulin-like Growth Factor Binding Protein-3
Serum No Effect Physiological Treatment of 30 normal healthy post-menopausal women with 2.5 mg/d caused an insignificant change in concentration from mean baseline of 4.18 ± 0.79 mg/L to 4.27 ± 0.88 mg/L after 36 months *2707*

LDL-Cholesterol *Serum Decrease Physiological* In 39 postmenopausal women treatment with 2.5 mg/d for 6 months caused nonsignificant reduction from mean baseline of 4.32 ± 0.15 mmol/L to 4.00 ± 0.19 mmol/L *1800*

Lipoprotein Lp(a) *Serum Decrease Physiological* In 39 postmenopausal women treatment with 2.5 mg/d for 6 months caused significant reduction from mean baseline of 245 mg/L to 152 mg/L (39%) *1800*

Progesterone *Plasma No Effect Physiological* In 11 healthy postmenopausal women administration of 2.5 mg/d for 3 months had no significant effect on plasma concentration which remained within the reference range *839*

Testosterone *Serum No Effect Physiological* In 11 healthy postmenopausal women administration of 2.5 mg/d for 3 months had no significant effect on plasma concentration which remained within the reference range *839*

Triglycerides *Serum Decrease Physiological* In 11 healthy postmenopausal women administration of 2.5 mg/d for 3 months caused a significant change (27 ± 5%) from mean baseline concentration of 0.9 ± 0.07 mmol/L to 0.65 ± 0.06 mmol/L *839* In 39 postmenopausal women treatment with 2.5 mg/d for 6 months caused significant reduction from mean baseline of 1.46 ± 0.14 mmol/L to 1.15 ± 0.10 mmol/L *1800*

VLDL-Cholesterol *Serum Decrease Physiological* In 39 postmenopausal women treatment with 2.5 mg/d for 6 months caused significant reduction from mean baseline of 0.58 ± 0.06 mmol/L to 0.38 ± 0.04 mmol/L *1800*

Ticarcillin

Alanine Aminotransferase *Serum Increase Physiological* Activity may be increased in some patients receiving ticarcillin with clavulanate, but rarely transient hepatitis and cholestatic jaundice may occur as with other penicillins and some cephalosporins *5661* As with other semi-synthetic penicillins increased activity has been observed with treatment *5660*

Alkaline Phosphatase *Serum Increase Physiological* Activity may be increased in some patients receiving ticarcillin with clavulanate, but rarely transient hepatitis and cholestatic jaundice may occur as with other penicillins and some cephalosporins *5661*

Amikacin *Serum No Effect Analytical* No interference observed at a concentration of 500 µg/mL (1301 µmol/L) with method on Du Pont aca *1508*

Aspartate Aminotransferase *Serum Increase Physiological* As with other semi-synthetic penicillins increased activity has been observed with treatment *5660* Activity may be increased in some patients receiving ticarcillin with clavulanate, but rarely transient hepatitis and cholestatic jaundice may occur as with other penicillins and some cephalosporins *5661*

Bilirubin *Serum Increase Physiological* Concentration may be increased in some patients receiving ticarcillin with clavulanate, but rarely transient hepatitis and cholestatic jaundice may occur as with other penicillins and some cephalosporins *5661*

Bleeding Time *Patient Increase Physiological* At high concentrations platelet aggregation may be inhibited and cause prolonged bleeding *1384* Bleeding time may be increased in some patients receiving ticarcillin with clavulanate *5661*

Clotting Time *Blood Increase Physiological* Bleeding manifestations have occurred in some patients receiving β-lactam antibiotics associated with abnormalities of coagulation tests such as clotting time, platelet aggregation and prothrombin time *5661*

Creatinine *Serum Increase Physiological* Concentration may be increased in some patients receiving ticarcillin with clavulanate *5661*

Serum No Effect Analytical No effect of concentrations up to 15 mg/L on single slide method on Kodak Ektachem® *5706*

Cyclosporine *Serum Increase Physiological* Observed effect and confirmed through rechallenge although mechanism not described *1069*

Eosinophils *Blood Increase Physiological* As with other penicillins eosinophilia has been observed with treatment *5660* Eosinophilia may occur in some patients receiving ticarcillin with clavulanate *5661*

Glucose *Urine Increase Analytical* Falsely elevated values with Clinitest® *3446*

Urine No Effect Analytical Concentrations measured accurately with Diastix® and TesTape® *3446*

Hematocrit *Blood Decrease Physiological* Anemia may occur in some patients receiving ticarcillin with clavulanate *5661* As with other penicillins anemia has been observed with treatment *5660*

Hemoglobin *Blood Decrease Physiological* As with other penicillins anemia has been observed with treatment *5660* Anemia may occur in some patients receiving ticarcillin with clavulanate *5661*

Lactate Dehydrogenase *Serum Increase Physiological* Activity may be increased in some patients receiving ticarcillin with clavulanate, but rarely transient hepatitis and cholestatic jaundice may occur as with other penicillins and some cephalosporins *5661*

Leukocytes *Blood Decrease Physiological* As with other penicillins leukopenia has been observed with treatment *5660* Leukopenia may occur in some patients receiving ticarcillin with clavulanate *5661*

Neutrophils *Blood Decrease Physiological* As with other penicillins neutropenia has been observed with treatment *5660* Neutropenia may occur in some patients receiving ticarcillin with clavulanate *5661*

Platelet Aggregation *Blood Decrease Physiological* At high concentrations binds to adenosine diphosphate receptors and prevents normal platelet aggregation *1384* Bleeding manifestations have occurred in some patients receiving β-lactam antibiotics associated with abnormalities of coagulation tests such as clotting time, platelet aggregation and prothrombin time *5661*

Platelets *Blood Decrease Physiological* As with other penicillins thrombocytopenia has been observed with treatment *5660* Thrombocytopenia may occur in some patients receiving ticarcillin with clavulanate *5661*

Potassium *Serum Decrease Physiological* Rare cases of hypokalemia reported *5661* Large doses given intravenously may cause hypokalemia due to the large amount of nonreabsorbable anion in the distal renal tubules *1384*

Protein *Urine Increase Analytical* In patients receiving ticarcillin false increase observed with sulfosalicylic acid and boiling test, acetic acid test, biuret reaction and nitric acid test *5661*

Urine No Effect Analytical In patients receiving ticarcillin no false reaction observed with bromphenol blue (Multi-Stix) reagent strip test *5661*

Prothrombin Time *Plasma Increase Physiological* Bleeding manifestations have occurred in some patients receiving β-lactam antibiotics associated with abnormalities of coagulation tests such as clotting time, platelet aggregation and prothrombin time *5661*

Sodium *Serum Increase Physiological* Concentration may be increased in some patients receiving ticarcillin with clavulanate *5661*

Urea Nitrogen *Serum Increase Physiological* Concentration may be increased in some patients receiving ticarcillin with clavulanate *5661*

Uric Acid *Serum Decrease Physiological* Concentration may be decreased in some patients receiving ticarcillin with clavulanate *5661*

Ticlopidine

Alanine Aminotransferase *Serum Increase Physiological* Activity increased to 140 U/L in one 92-year old man who developed cholestasis after treatment with 500 mg/d for 3 months *2334* Abnormal liver function reported in 1.0% of 2048 patients treated with ticlopidine in comparison with 0% of 530 pattients treated with placebo *5034* Abnormal liver function occasionally observed. Rare cholestasis or hepatitis reported *1384*

Alkaline Phosphatase *Serum Increase Physiological* Hepatitis, hepatocellular jaundice, cholestatic jaundice or hepatic necrosis reported rarely in some patients treated with ticlopidine *5034* Activity increased to 577 U/L in one 92-year old man after treatment with 500 mg/d for 3 months occurring as part of unusual cholestatic reaction *2334*

Antipyrine *Serum Increase Physiological* Ticlopidine treatment has been reported to cause a 30% increase in the plasma half-life of antipyrine *5034*

Aspartate Aminotransferase *Serum Increase Physiological* Activity increased to 236 U/L in one 92 year old man who developed cholestasis after treatment with 500 mg/d for 3 months *2334* Abnormal liver function reported in 1.0% of 2048 patients treated with ticlopidine in comparison with 0% of 530 patients treated with placebo *5034* Occasional abnormal liver function tests observed. Rare cholestasis or hepatitis reported *1384*

Bilirubin *Serum Increase Physiological* Rarely reported side effect, possibly in association with cholestasis *1384* Hepatitis, hepatocellular jaundice, cholestatic jaundice or hepatic necrosis reported rarely in some patients treated with ticlopidine *5034* In one 92-year old man who had received 500 mg/d for 3 months concentration increased to 22.1 mg/dL as part of cholestatic picture *2334*

Bilirubin, Direct *Serum Increase Physiological* In one 92-year old man treated with 500 mg/d for 3 months mean concentration increased to 17.5 mg/dL as part of cholestatic reaction *2334*

Bleeding Time *Patient Increase Physiological* When combined with warfarin has potential for increasing risk of warfarin-associated bleeding *2625* May prolong bleeding time *1384* Ticlopidine treatment prolongs template bleeding time *5034*

Blood *Urine Increase Physiological* Hematuria reported in some patients treated with ticlopidine *5034*

Cholesterol *Serum Increase Physiological* In stroke patients mean baseline concentration already increased at 6.3 mmol/L but further increase noted at one month with concentration stabilizing by month 4. Mean increase of 9 ± 20% observed *2500* Ticlopidine treatment causes increased plasma cholesterol concentrations by 8 to 10% within one month of commencement of treatment and remain increased *5034*

Creatinine *Serum Increase Physiological* Renal failure or nephrotic syndrome reported rarely in some patients treated with ticlopidine *5034*

Cyclosporine *Blood Decrease Physiological* Coadministration of ticlopidine with cyclosporine caused a decrease in cyclosporine concentration from 136 ± 44 µg/L to 72 ± 20 µ g/L despite a 10% reduction in its dose possibly due to inhibition of the microsomal drug hydroxylating enzymes in the liver *859*

Serum Decrease Physiological May decrease cyclosporine concentration by inducing hepatic cytochrome P-450 III A which metabolizes cyclosporine *5236* Coadministration of ticlopidine with cyclosporine caused a decrease in cyclosporine concentration from 136 ± 44 µg/L to 72 ± 20 µ g/L despite a 10% reduction in its dose possibly due to inhibition of the microsomal drug hydroxylating enzymes in the liver *859*

Digoxin *Serum Decrease Physiological* Ticlopidine administration with digoxin has been reported to cause a 15% decrease in the plasma concentration of digoxin *5034*

Eosinophils *Blood Increase Physiological* Eosinophilia reported in some patients treated with ticlopidine *5034*

Erythrocytes *Blood Decrease Physiological* Observed occasionally with pancytopenia *1384*

Urine Increase Physiological Microscopic hematuria occurred in small number of patients receiving drug as follow-up to stroke *2500*

Fibrinogen *Plasma Decrease Physiological* Decrease observed with treatment *3186*

Granulocytes *Blood Decrease Physiological* Agranulocytosis, pancytopenia and aplastic anemia have been occasionally reported *5034* Observed with agranulocytosis or pancytopenia as rare side effect *1384*

Hematocrit *Blood Decrease Physiological* Hemolytic or aplastic anemia reported rarely in some patients treated with ticlopidine *5034*

Hemoglobin *Blood Decrease Physiological* Hemolytic or aplastic anemia reported rarely in some patients treated with ticlopidine *5034* Agranulocytosis, pancytopenia and aplastic anemia have been occasionally reported *5034*

LDL-Cholesterol *Serum Increase Physiological* Observed effect *1384*

Leukocytes *Blood Decrease Physiological* Decrease observed with treatment *3186* Severe neutropenia developed in 13 of 1529 patients receiving drug between 1 and 3 months of start of treatment but all episodes resolved within 3 weeks of treatment being stopped. Mild to moderate neutropenia occurred in 22 patients *2500* Most serious side-effect observed either as leukopenia, agranulocytosis or pancytopenia *1384*

Neutrophils *Blood Decrease Physiological* Neutopenia with neutrophil count less than 1200 cells/µL occurred in 50 of 2048 stroke patients (2.4%) stroke patients who received ticlopidine in clinical trials. Neutropenia of less than 450 cells/µL occurred in 17 patients (0.8%), but count returned to normal in 1 to 3 weeks when drug discontinued *5034* Severe neutropenia occurred in 13 of 1529 patients treated as follow-up to stroke. In all cases occurred within 1 to 3 months of start of therapy and resolved within 3 weeks of treatment being stopped. Mild to moderate neutropenia seen in 22 patients *2500*

Occult Blood *Feces Increase Physiological* Ticlopidine treatment prolongs template bleeding time and may cause gastrointestinal bleeding *5034*

Phenytoin *Serum Increase Physiological* Several cases reported in which ticlopidine administration with phenytoin in normal volunteers was associated with increased plasma phenytoin concentration *5034*

Ticlopidine *(continued)*

Platelet Aggregation *Blood Decrease Physiological* Inhibits ADP-induced aggregation but has variable effect on epinephrine induced aggregation and aggregation by thrombin, platelet-activating factor, arachidonic acid and collagen *1384*

Platelet-associated IgG *Blood Increase Physiological* Concentration of 1270 ng per 10^7 cells observed in one 67-year old man with thrombocytopenia who had received 200 mg drug daily for 4 years (compared with normal of 9 to 25 ng per 10^7 cells) just after withdrawal of drug but normal seven weeks later *5928*

Platelets *Blood Decrease Physiological* Occasional pancytopenia observed *1384* Thrombocytopenia may occur with or without neutopenia. Rarely immune thrombocytopenia and thrombotic thrombocytopenic purpura have been reported *5034* Single case reported of a 67-year old man who had received 200 mg daily for 4 years. Platelet count was 32000/µL on admission. Concentration unaffected by reduction of dose but reverted to close to normal after several weeks when drug withdrawn *5928*

Blood Increase Physiological Thrombocytosis reported in some patients treated with ticlopidine *5034*

Protein *Urine Increase Physiological* Renal failure or nephrotic syndrome reported rarely in some patients treated with ticlopidine *5034*

Reticulocytes *Blood Decrease Physiological* Reticulocytosis with hemolytic anemia reported rarely in some patients treated with ticlopidine *5034*

Sodium *Serum Decrease Physiological* Hyponatremia reported rarely in some patients treated with ticlopidine *5034*

Theophylline *Serum Increase Physiological* Ticlopidine administration with theophylline in normal volunteers has been reported to cause a significant increase in the theophylline elimination half-life from 8.6 to 12.2 hours and a comparable reduction in total plasma clearance of theophylline *5034* Up to 60% increase in serum theophylline concentration due to decreased theophylline clearance *6117* Decreases theophylline clearance and increases serum theophylline concentration by 60% *3125* Decreases theophylline clearance, increasing theophylline concentration by about 60% *5999*

Triglycerides *Serum Increase Physiological* Ticlopidine treatment causes increased plasma cholesterol and triglyceride concentrations *5034*

Urea Nitrogen *Serum Increase Physiological* Renal failure or nephrotic syndrome reported rarely in some patients treated with ticlopidine *5034*

VLDL-Cholesterol *Serum Increase Physiological* Observed consequence of treatment *1384*

Tilidine

p-Aminophenol *Urine No Effect Analytical* With addition of drugs at a concentration of 100 mg/L and of related compounds at 50 mg/L no significant effect observed on colorimetric method of van Bocxlaer on Cobas Mira analyzer which involves reacting free p-aminophenol with resorcinol in the presence of magnesium ions to form an indophenol dye measured at 550 nm *6163*

Tiludronate

Digoxin *Serum No Effect Physiological* Pharmacokinetics of digoxin not significantly affected when tiludronate coadministered *5258*

Timegadine

α_1-Acid Glycoprotein *Serum No Effect Physiological* In 23 patients with rheumatoid arthritis given 250 to 750 mg/d for 48 weeks *3864*

Albumin *Serum No Effect Physiological* In 23 patients with rheumatoid arthritis given 250 to 750 mg/d for 48 weeks *3864*

Creatinine *Serum No Effect Physiological* In 23 patients with rheumatoid arthritis given 250 to 750 mg/d for 48 weeks *3864*

Erythrocyte Sedimentation Rate
Blood No Effect Physiological In 23 patients with rheumatoid arthritis given 250 to 750 mg/d for 48 weeks *3864*

Erythrocytes *Blood No Effect Physiological* In 23 patients with rheumatoid arthritis given 250 to 750 mg/d for 48 weeks *3864*

Urine No Effect Physiological In 23 patients with rheumatoid arthritis given 250 to 750 mg/d for 48 weeks *3864*

Glucose *Urine No Effect Physiological* In 23 patients with rheumatoid arthritis given 250 to 750 mg/d for 48 weeks *3864*

Hemoglobin *Blood No Effect Physiological* In 23 patients with rheumatoid arthritis given 250 to 750 mg/d for 48 weeks *3864*

immunoglobulin A *Serum Decrease Physiological* But not significantly in 23 patients with rheumatoid arthritis given 250 to 750 mg/d for 48 weeks *3864*

Immunoglobulin G *Serum Decrease Physiological* But not significantly in 23 patients with rheumatoid arthritis given 250 to 750 mg/d for 48 weeks *3864*

Immunoglobulin M *Serum Decrease Physiological* But not significantly in 23 patients with rheumatoid arthritis given 250 to 750 mg/d for 48 weeks *3864*

Leukocytes *Blood No Effect Physiological* In 23 patients with rheumatoid arthritis given 250 to 750 mg/d for 48 weeks *3864*

Platelets *Blood No Effect Physiological* In 23 patients with rheumatoid arthritis given 250 to 750 mg/d for 48 weeks *3864*

Protein *Urine No Effect Physiological* In 23 patients with rheumatoid arthritis given 250 to 750 mg/d for 48 weeks *3864*

Rheumatoid Factor *Serum No Effect Physiological* In 23 patients with rheumatoid arthritis given 250 to 750 mg/d for 48 weeks *3864*

Thyroxine (T4) *Serum No Effect Physiological* In 23 patients with rheumatoid arthritis given 250 to 750 mg/d for 48 weeks *3864*

Timolol

Alanine Aminotransferase *Serum Increase Physiological* Timolol may cause hepatomegaly and abnormal liver function tests *3995* Administration of timolol has been associated with increases in liver function tests *3961*

Albumin *Serum Decrease Physiological* Significant decrease from mean baseline concentration of 637 µmol/L to 602 µmol/L at 4 hours and reversion to baseline concentration in 5 patients with hyperthyroidism treated for one week *3077*

Serum No Effect Analytical At concentration of 0.01 mg/L had no effect on BCG method *5704*

Alkaline Phosphatase *Serum Increase Physiological* Timolol may cause hepatomegaly and abnormal liver function tests *3995* Administration of timolol has been associated with increases in liver function tests *3961*

Aspartate Aminotransferase *Serum Increase Physiological* Timolol may cause hepatomegaly and abnormal liver function tests *3995* Administration of timolol has been associated with increases in liver function tests *3961*

Bicarbonate *Serum No Effect Analytical* At concentration of 0.01 mg/L had no effect on method using phenolphthalein *5704*

Bilirubin *Serum Increase Physiological* Timolol may cause hepatomegaly and abnormal liver function tests *3995* Administration of timolol has been associated with increases in liver function tests *3961*

Serum No Effect Analytical At concentration of 0.01 mg/L had no effect on Jendrassik and Grof method *5704*

Calcium *Serum No Effect Analytical* At concentration of 0.01 mg/L had no effect on cresolphthalein method *5704*

Chloride *Serum No Effect Analytical* At concentration of 0.01 mg/L had no effect on mercurimetric method *5704*

Cholesterol *Serum No Effect Analytical* At concentration of 0.01 mg/L had no effect on CHOD-PAP method *5704*

Serum No Effect Physiological In 15 patients treated for 1 mo *6450*

Creatinine *Serum Increase Physiological* Timolol may cause renal failure, renal dysfunction or interstitial nephritis *3995*

Serum No Effect Analytical At concentration of 0.01 mg/L had no effect on Technicon AutoAnalyzer® Jaffe method *5704*

Fatty Acids (FFA), Free *Serum No Effect Physiological* In 5 hyperthyroid patients given 10 mg every 8 h for 4 d *540*

Glucagon *Plasma No Effect Physiological* In 5 hyperthyroid patients given 10 mg every 8 h for 4 d *540*

Glucose *Serum Decrease Physiological* Timolol has been reported to both increase and decrease the plasma glucose concentration *3961*

Serum Increase Physiological Timolol may cause hyperglycemia and glycosuria *3995* Timolol has been reported to both increase and decrease the plasma glucose concentration *3961*

Serum No Effect Analytical At concentration of 0.01 mg/L had no effect on GOD/POD-PAP method *5704*

Serum No Effect Physiological In 5 hyperthyroid patients given 10 mg every 8 h for 4 d *540*

Urine Increase Physiological Timolol may cause hyperglycemia and glycosuria *3995*

Glycerol *Serum No Effect Physiological* In 5 hyperthyroid patients given 10 mg every 8 h for 4 d *540*

Gonadotropin-releasing Hormone

Plasma Decrease Physiological Timolol may cause rarely leukopenia, agranulocytosis, thrombocytopenia, aplastic or hemolytic anemia *3995*

HDL-Cholesterol *Serum Decrease Physiological* Administration of timolol has been associated with creases in concentration *3961* Primarily observed effect with nonselective β-blockers is decrease of HDL-cholesterol concentration *3730* Topical application of timolol to the eye caused significant decrease in concentration *1089*

Hematocrit *Blood Decrease Physiological* Administration of timolol has been associated with slight decreases in value *3961* Timolol may cause rarely leukopenia, agranulocytosis, thrombocytopenia, aplastic or hemolytic anemia *3995*

Hemoglobin *Blood Decrease Physiological* Timolol may cause rarely leukopenia, agranulocytosis, thrombocytopenia, aplastic or hemolytic anemia *3995* Administration of timolol has been associated with slight decreases in concentration *3961*

Histamine *Plasma No Effect Analytical* Improbable inhibition of radio-enzyme assay at therapeutic concentrations *2492*

Hydroxyproline *Urine No Effect Physiological* No effect in hyperthyroid patients *539*

Insulin *Plasma No Effect Physiological* In 5 hyperthyroid patients given 10 mg every 8 h for 4 d *540*

Ketones *Serum No Effect Physiological* In 5 hyperthyroid patients given 10 mg every 8 h for 4 d *540*

Leukocytes *Blood Decrease Physiological* Timolol may cause rarely leukopenia, agranulocytosis, thrombocytopenia, aplastic or hemolytic anemia *3995*

Parathyroid Hormone *Plasma No Effect Physiological* No effect in hyperthyroid patients *539*

Phosphate *Serum Increase Physiological* In 5 patients with hyperthyroidism increase from mean baseline value of 1.04 mmol/L to 1.32 mmol/L at 4 hours and 1.11 mmol/L after one week *3077*

Serum No Effect Analytical At concentration of 0.01 mg/L had no effect on phosphomolybdate method *5704*

Platelets *Blood Decrease Physiological* Timolol may cause rarely leukopenia, agranulocytosis, thrombocytopenia, aplastic or hemolytic anemia *3995*

Potassium *Serum Increase Physiological* Pronounced and prolonged increase in patients who had acute myocardial infarction *4324* Administration of timolol has been associated with slight increases in concentration *3961* Has rarely caused hyperkalemia *1384* Slight increase in patients treated with moderate doses of drug *4739*

Serum No Effect Analytical At concentration of 0.01 mg/L had no effect on flame-photometric method *5704*

Protein *Serum No Effect Analytical* At concentration of 0.01 mg/L had no effect on biuret method with blank correction *5704*

Sodium *Serum No Effect Analytical* At concentration of 0.01 mg/L had no effect on flame-photometric method *5704*

Thyroxine (T4) Index, Free *Serum No Effect Physiological* In 5 hyperthyroid patients given 10 mg every 8 h for 4 d *540*

Tri-iodothyronine (T3) *Serum No Effect Physiological* No effect in hyperthyroid patients *539* In 5 hyperthyroid patients given 10 mg every 8 h for 4 d *540*

Triglycerides *Serum Increase Physiological* Significant increase observed when timolol applied to the eye *1089* Administration of timolol has been associated with slight increases in concentration *3961* Primarily observed effect with nonselective β-blockers is increase of triglyceride concentration *3730*

Serum No Effect Analytical At concentration of 0.01 mg/L had no effect on lipase/esterase method *5704*

Serum No Effect Physiological In 15 patients treated for 1 mo *6450*

Urea Nitrogen *Serum Increase Physiological* Administration of timolol has been associated with slight increases in concentration *3961* Timolol may cause renal failure, renal dysfunction or interstitial nephritis *3995*

Serum No Effect Analytical At concentration of 0.01 mg/L had no effect on diacetylmonoxime method *5704*

Uric Acid *Serum Increase Physiological* Administration of timolol has been associated with slight increases in concentration *3961* Timolol may cause hyperuricemia *3995*

Serum No Effect Analytical At concentration of 0.01 mg/L had no effect on phosphotungstate reduction method *5704*

Tissue-type Plasminogen Activator

Aminoterminal Propeptide of Type III Collagen

Serum Increase Physiological In 41 patients given rt-PA significant increase observed at 3 and 6 hours after administration compared with those given placebo *2729*

C-terminal Propeptide of Type I Procollagen

Serum No Effect Physiological In 41 patients given rt-PA no significant difference observed at any time after administration compared with those given placebo *2729*

D-Dimer *Plasma Increase Physiological* In 17 patients with acute myocardial infarction treatment with rt-PA 10 mg in a bolus over 2 min, then 50 mg during first hour and 20 mg in each of second and third hours was associated with increase from mean baseline of 500 µg/L on admission to 1800 µg/L after lysis and peak of 2600 µg/L *2088*

Lactate Dehydrogenase Isoenzymes

Serum Decrease Physiological In 319 patients with myocardial infarctions treatment within 3 h of onset of symptoms caused mean reduction of LD-1 activity by 32% from 13.3 µkat/L to 9.0 µkat/L versus placebo *4966*

Plasminogen Activator Inhibitor-1

Plasma Increase Physiological In 17 patients with acute myocardial infarction treatment with rt-PA 10 mg in a bolus over 2 min, then 50 mg during first hour and 20 mg in each of second and third hours was associated with increase from mean baseline of 50 µg/L on admission to 75 µg/L after lysis and peak of 130 µg/L *2088*

Plasminogen Activator Inhibitor-1 Antigen

Plasma Increase Physiological In 10 patients with suspected myocardial infarction treatment with recombinant tissue-type plasminogen activator 100 mg over 3 hours caused significant increase peaking 3 hours after end of thrombolytic therapy and returned to normal by day 2 *2087*

Tobramycin

Alanine Aminotransferase *Serum Increase Physiological* Reported change possibly related to tobramycin administration *1703*

Urine No Effect Physiological No significant effect in 15 volunteers up to 24 hours after receiving 1 mg/kg intravenously *1730*

Alkaline Phosphatase *Urine No Effect Physiological* No significant effect in 15 volunteers up to 24 hours after receiving 1 mg/kg intravenously *1730*

Amikacin *Serum Increase Analytical* 2.3% cross-reactivity observed with method on Abbott TDx *3858* At a concentration of 200 mg/L causes error of 25% when added to a specimen containing 15 mg/L amikacin and measured on a Baxter Stratus analyzer *5705*

Tobramycin *(continued)*

Amikacin *(continued)*
Serum No Effect Analytical No interference observed at a concentration of 100 µg/mL (214 µmol/L) with method on Du Pont aca *1508*

Antithrombin III *Plasma No Effect Analytical* At concentration of 15 mg/L had no effect on Du Pont aca method *5704*

Aspartate Aminotransferase *Serum Increase Physiological* Reported change possibly related to tobramycin administration *1703*
Urine No Effect Physiological No significant effect in 15 volunteers up to 24 hours after receiving 1 mg/kg intravenously *1730*

Bilirubin *Serum Increase Physiological* Reported change possibly related to tobramycin administration *1703*
Serum No Effect Analytical At concentration of 5 mg/L had no effect on Kodak Ektachem® method *5704*
Serum No Effect Physiological Clinically insignificant displacement from protein in neonates *6314*

Bilirubin, Conjugated *Serum No Effect Analytical* No effect at concentration of 5 mg/L on method on Kodak Ektachem® *5706*

Bilirubin, Unconjugated *Serum No Effect Analytical* No effect at concentration of 5 mg/L on method on Kodak Ektachem® *5706*

Calcium *Serum Decrease Physiological* Reported change possibly related to tobramycin administration *1703*

Casts *Urine Increase Physiological* At dose of 4.5 mg/kg/d for 12 d in 90 patients nephrotoxicity observed in up to 39%, reversible in most *1067* Manifestation of drug induced nephrotoxicity but tend to decrease as serum creatinine begins to climb *5325*

Chloramphenicol *Serum No Effect Analytical* No effect at 100 mg/L on coupled enzymatic method *4122*

Creatine Kinase Isoenzymes *Serum No Effect Analytical* No interference observed at a concentration of 20 mg/L (42,8 µmol/L) with CK-MB method on Du Pont aca *1519* No interference observed at a concentration of 20 mg/L (42.8 µmol/L) with CK-MB method on Du Pont aca *1519*

Creatinine *Serum Increase Physiological* Reported change, most often in patients with a history of renal impairment who are treated for longer periods or with higher doses than those recommended *1703* In 4 of 59 patients whose drug concentrations were monitored *2050* In 12% of patients with sepsis. Mean increase of only 0.1 mg/dL in all patients studied *5615* 18.4% incidence of nephrotoxicity in 49 patients given drug with creatinine concentration measured by McHenry method versus 16.7% in 48 patients given drug and creatinine measured by Sawchuk/Zaske method *3850* At dose of 4.5 mg/kg/d for 12 d in 90 patients nephrotoxicity observed in up to 39%, reversible in most *1067* 12% incidence of nephrotoxicity but unrelated to initial renal function or prior use of aminoglycosides, drug concentration, amount given duration of treatment or concurrent treatment with other drugs *5325*
Serum No Effect Analytical At therapeutic concentration had no effect on method on Kodak Ektachem® 700 *586* No interference observed at a concentration of 10 mg/L with HPLC method of Rosano et al *5083* No effect of concentrations up to 15 mg/L on single slide method on Kodak Ektachem® *5706*

Cylinders *Urine Increase Physiological* Reported change, most often in patients with a history of renal impairment who are treated for longer periods or with higher doses than those recommended *1703*

Eosinophils *Blood Increase Physiological* Reported change possibly related to tobramycin administration *1703*

Gentamicin *Serum No Effect Analytical* Has cross-reactivity of less than 0.1% with method on Baxter Stratus *5705* Specimens containing tobramycin showed no cross-reactivity when gentamicin measured by method on Bayer Technicon Immuno 1® system *426* No interference observed at concentrations up to 500 µg/mL (1069 µmol/L) with method on Du Pont aca *1526* No interference observed with method on Abbott TDx *3858*

Glucose *Urine No Effect Analytical* No effect at up to 250 µg/mL on any glucose concentration as measured by Clinitest® , Diastix® or TesTape® *3710*

γ-Glutamyltransferase *Urine No Effect Physiological* No significant effect in 15 volunteers up to 24 hours after receiving 1 mg/kg intravenously *1730*

Granulocytes *Blood Decrease Physiological* Reported change possibly related to tobramycin administration *1703*

Hematocrit *Blood Decrease Physiological* Reported change possibly related to tobramycin administration *1703*

Hemoglobin *Blood Decrease Physiological* Reported change possibly related to tobramycin administration *1703*
Urine Increase Physiological At dose of 4.5 mg/kg/d for 12 d in 90 patients nephrotoxicity observed in up to 39%, reversible in most *1067*

Histamine *Plasma No Effect Analytical* No inhibition of radio-enzyme assay at 10 times therapeutic concentration *2492*

Kanamycin *Serum Increase Analytical* Interferes with method on Abbott TDx *3858*

Lactate Dehydrogenase *Serum Increase Physiological* Reported change possibly related to tobramycin administration *1703*
Urine No Effect Physiological No significant effect in 15 volunteers up to 24 hours after receiving 1 mg/kg intravenously *1730*

Leucine Aminopeptidase *Urine No Effect Physiological* No significant effect in 15 volunteers up to 24 hours after receiving 1 mg/kg intravenously *1730*

Leukocytes *Blood Decrease Physiological* Reported change possibly related to tobramycin administration *1703*
Blood Increase Physiological Reported change possibly related to tobramycin administration *1703*

Magnesium *Serum Decrease Physiological* Reported change possibly related to tobramycin administration *1703*
Serum No Effect Analytical No effect at therapeutic concentration on method on Kodak Ektachem® 700 *586*

β_2-Microglobulin *Urine Increase Physiological* Manifestation of drug induced nephrotoxicity but tend to decrease as serum creatinine begins to climb *5325*
Urine No Effect Physiological Up to i.v. dose of 2 mg/kg does not affect renal excretion *6282*

Mycophenolic Acid *Serum No Effect Analytical* No significant interference observed with HPLC method of Shipkova et al *5526*

Mycophenolic Acid Glucuronide
Serum No Effect Analytical No significant interference observed with HPLC method of Shipkova et al *5526*

Neomycin *Serum No Effect Analytical* No interference observed with method on Abbott TDx *3858*

Netilmicin *Serum No Effect Analytical* No interference observed with method on Abbott TDx *3858*

Nonprotein Nitrogen *Serum Increase Physiological* Reported change, most often in patients with a history of renal impairment who are treated for longer periods or with higher doses than those recommended *1703*

Phenylalanine *Plasma No Effect Analytical* No interference observed with rapid quantitative whole blood method of Campbell et al using phenylalanine dehydrogenase *867*

Plasminogen *Plasma No Effect Analytical* At concentration of 15 mg/L had no effect on Du Pont aca method *5704*

Platelets *Blood Decrease Physiological* Reported change possibly related to tobramycin administration *1703*

Potassium *Serum Decrease Physiological* Reported change possibly related to tobramycin administration *1703*

Protein *Cerebrospinal Fluid No Effect Analytical* No significant effect when added in vitro to concentration of 100 mg/dL when measured by Kodak Ektachem® slide method *3654*
Urine Increase Physiological Manifestation of drug induced nephrotoxicity but tend to decrease as serum creatinine begins to climb *5325* At dose of 4.5 mg/kg/d for 12 d in 90 patients nephrotoxicity observed in up to 39%, reversible in most *1067* Reported change, most often in patients with a history of renal impairment who are treated for longer periods or with higher doses than those recommended *1703*

SDZ PSC 833 *Blood No Effect Analytical* At a concentration of 7.3 mg/L had no effect on HPLC method of Scott et al when used to measure PSC (with CsD as internal standard) at a concentration of 5 mg/L *5418*

Sodium *Serum Decrease Physiological* Reported change possibly related to tobramycin administration *1703*

Streptomycin *Serum No Effect Analytical* No interference observed with method on Abbott TDx *3858*

Tacrolimus *Blood No Effect Analytical* No significant effect observed at a concentration of 10 mg/L with MEIA method on Abbott IMx analyzer *1871*
Serum No Effect Analytical At concentration of 10 mg/L had no significant rffect on ELISA method *6329*

Theophylline *Serum No Effect Analytical* No effect at 20 mg/L on method on Ames Seralyzer *5706*

Thyroxine (T4) *Serum No Effect Physiological* When given i.v. with cloxacillin to 13 patients *1602*

Tri-iodothyronine, Reverse (rT3)
Serum No Effect Physiological When given i.v. with cloxacillin to 13 patients *1602*

Tri-iodothyronine (T3) *Serum No Effect Physiological* When given i.v. with cloxacillin to 13 patients *1602*

Urea Nitrogen *Serum Increase Physiological* Reported change, most often in patients with a history of renal impairment who are treated for longer periods or with higher doses than those recommended *1703*

Vancomycin *Serum No Effect Analytical* No significant interference observed at a concentration of 100 µg/mL (214 µmol/L) with method on Du Pont aca *1561* No interference observed with method on Abbott TDx *3858*
Serum No Effect Physiological No significant effect observed on pharmacokinetics when drugs coadministered *4169*

Tocainide

Alanine Aminotransferase *Serum Increase Physiological* Abnormal liver function tests observed, particularly with the early stages of treatment. Hepatitis and jaundice have been reported in some patients *268* Occasional abnormality reported associated with reversible hepatitis *3281*

Alkaline Phosphatase *Serum Increase Physiological* Abnormal liver function tests observed, particularly with the early stages of treatment. Hepatitis and jaundice have been reported in some patients *268*

Antinuclear Antibodies *Serum Increase Physiological* Rare finding in fewer than 0.2% patients *3281*

Aspartate Aminotransferase *Serum Increase Physiological* Abnormal liver function tests observed, particularly with the early stages of treatment. Hepatitis and jaundice have been reported in some patients *268* Occasional abnormality reported associated with reversible hepatitis *3281*

Bilirubin *Serum Increase Physiological* Abnormal liver function tests observed, particularly with the early stages of treatment. Hepatitis and jaundice have been reported in some patients *268*

Cimetidine *Serum No Effect Physiological* No clinically significant interaction observed *268*

Digoxin *Serum No Effect Physiological* No clinically significant interaction observed *268*

Erythrocytes *Blood Decrease Physiological* Blood dyscrasias occur in fewer than 0.2% patients *3281*

γ-Glutamyltransferase *Serum Increase Physiological* Abnormal liver function tests observed, particularly with the early stages of treatment. Hepatitis and jaundice have been reported in some patients *268*

Granulocytes *Blood Decrease Physiological* Occasionally observed in patients treated with drug *1384*

Hemoglobin *Blood Decrease Physiological* Occasional hypoplastic or hemolytic anemia observed in patients treated with drug *1384*

LE Cells *Blood Positive Physiological* Rare finding in fewer than 0.2% patients *3281*

Leukocytes *Blood Decrease Physiological* Blood dyscrasias occur in fewer than 0.2% patients *3281* Leukopenia occasionally observed in patients treated with drug *1384*

Lidocaine *Serum No Effect Analytical* At a concentration of 1250 mg/L (normal therapeutic concentration up to 10 mg/L) had less than 10% effect on method on Baxter Stratus *5705*

Neutrophils *Blood Decrease Physiological* Estimated incidence of 0.18% *5043* Blood dyscrasias occur in fewer than 0.2% patients *3281*

Platelets *Blood Decrease Physiological* Occasional thrombocytopenia observed in patients treated with drug *1384* Blood dyscrasias occur in fewer than 0.2% patients *3281*

Theophylline *Serum No Effect Physiological* No documented significant interaction with theophylline reported *6117* No clinically significant effect on theophylline concentration observed when drugs coadministered *5999*

Warfarin *Plasma No Effect Physiological* No clinically significant interaction observed *268*

Tolazamide

Alanine Aminotransferase *Serum Increase Physiological* Cholestatic effect *3810*
Serum No Effect Analytical No effect at 500 mg/L on method on Ames Seralyzer *5706*

Alkaline Phosphatase *Serum Increase Physiological* Intrahepatic cholestatic jaundice *139*

Aspartate Aminotransferase *Serum Increase Physiological* Cholestasis may occur *3810*

Bile *Urine Increase Physiological* Cholestatic effect *3810*

Bilirubin *Serum Increase Physiological* Cholestatic jaundice *3810*

BSP Retention *Serum Increase Physiological* Cholestasis may occur *3810*

Creatinine *Serum No Effect Analytical* Insignificant effect on manual Jaffe procedure or on automated methods on Technicon SMAC® , Beckman Astra® , Du Pont aca or Roche Cobas-Bio at 5 times therapeutic concentration *4976*

Erythrocytes *Blood Decrease Physiological* May cause hemolytic anemia *2242*

γ-Globulin *Serum Increase Physiological* Transient increases reported *4014*

Glucose *Serum Decrease Analytical* Inhibits oxidation chromogen with Boehringer glucose oxidase method *5480* At concentrations above 10 mg/L lowered concentration as measured by GOD-PERID method *5704*
Serum Decrease Physiological Sulfonylurea derivative stimulates insulin secretion *5481*
Serum No Effect Analytical No effect on hexokinase, o-toluidine methods *4240* If guiacum or phenolaminophenazone with glucose oxidase *5480* No effect at 5000 mg/L on hexokinase method on Ames Seralyzer *5706* At concentration of 200 mg/L had no effect on GOD/POD-PAP method *5704*

Insulin *Plasma Decrease Physiological* Return to normal usually if high initially *492*
Plasma Increase Physiological Usual effect observed *492*

Leukocytes *Blood Decrease Physiological* Leukopenia/agranulocytosis *2242*

5'-Nucleotidase *Serum Increase Physiological* Due to cholestasis *2911*

Osmolality *Urine Decrease Physiological* Normal diuretic response *4136*

Platelets *Blood Decrease Physiological* Thrombocytopenia/pancytopenia *2242*

Prazosin *Serum No Effect Physiological* Coadministration of prazosin with tolazamide had no apparent adverse drug interaction in limited clinical experience *4649*

Prothrombin Time *Plasma Increase Physiological* Occurs with failure to excrete bile salts *3810*

Urobilinogen *Feces Decrease Physiological* Pale stools with cholestasis *3810*
Urine Decrease Physiological Cholestatic effect *3810*

Volume *Urine Increase Physiological* Normal diuretic response *4136*

Water Clearance, Free *Urine Increase Physiological* Normal diuretic response *4136*

Tolazoline

Alanine Aminotransferase *Serum Increase Physiological* Hepatitis may occur as an adverse event but frequency not known *1036*

Tolazoline *(continued)*

Alkaline Phosphatase *Serum Increase Physiological* Hepatitis may occur as an adverse event but frequency not known *1036*

Aspartate Aminotransferase *Serum Increase Physiological* Hepatitis may occur as an adverse event but frequency not known *1036*

Bilirubin *Serum Increase Physiological* Hepatitis may occur as an adverse event but frequency not known *1036*

Blood *Urine Increase Physiological* Hematuria may occur as an adverse event but frequency not known *1036*

Erythrocytes *Blood Decrease Physiological* Pancytopenia (AMA Blood dyscrasias) *4017*

Histamine *Plasma No Effect Analytical* Although 50% inhibition of radio-enzyme assay at 46 µg/mL unlikely to be of clinical significance since therapeutic concentration 7-8 µg/mL *2492*

Hydrochloric Acid *Gastric Fluid Increase Physiological* Also enhances histamine stimulation *2242*

Leukocytes *Blood Decrease Physiological* Pancytopenia (AMA Blood dyscrasias) *4017* Leukopenia may occur as adverse event but frequency not known *1036*

Occult Blood *Feces Increase Physiological* Gastrointestinal hemorrhage may occur as adverse event but frequency not known *1036* Gastrointestinal distension and hemorrhage observed as a side effect of treatment *1384*

Pepsin *Gastric Material Increase Physiological* Also enhances histamine stimulation *2242*

Platelets *Blood Decrease Physiological* Thrombocytopenia may occur as adverse event but frequency not known *1036* Pancytopenia (AMA Blood dyscrasias) *4017* Thrombocytopnia is relatively common as a side effect *1384*

Tolbutamide

Alanine Aminotransferase *Serum Increase Physiological* May cause cytotoxic liver damage or cholestasis *402*

Albumin *Serum No Effect Analytical* At concentration of 220 mg/L had no effect on Kodak Ektachem® method *5706* At concentration of 100 mg/L had no effect on BCG method *5704*

Alkaline Phosphatase *Serum Increase Physiological* May cause intrahepatic cholestatic syndrome *402* Bone isoenzyme activity increased: inversely influenced by serum 25-hydroxyvitamin D concentration *5810*

δ-Aminolevulinic Acid *Urine Increase Physiological* May precipitate porphyria attack *2210*

Aspartate Aminotransferase *Serum Increase Analytical* At 1 mmol/L affects Technicon SMA 12/60 method *5576*
Serum Increase Physiological May cause cytotoxic liver damage or cholestasis *402*

Bicarbonate *Serum No Effect Analytical* At concentration of 100 mg/L had no effect on method using phenolphthalein *5704*

Bile *Urine Increase Physiological* Cholestatic jaundice reported *2451*

Bilirubin *Serum Increase Physiological* Cholestatic jaundice reported *2451*
Serum No Effect Analytical At concentration of 270 mg/L had no effect on Jendrassik and Grof method *5704*

BSP Retention *Serum Increase Physiological* May cause cytotoxic liver damage or cholestasis *402*

Calcium *Serum No Effect Analytical* At concentration of 270 mg/L had no effect on cresolphthalein method *5704*
Serum No Effect Physiological Slight, but not significant reduction, associated with increased bone organic matrix turnover *5810*

Chloride *Serum No Effect Analytical* No effect of concentrations up to 220 mg/L on method on Kodak Ektachem® *5706* At concentration of 100 mg/L had no effect on mercurimetric method *5704*

Cholesterol *Serum Decrease Physiological* Inhibits hepatic synthesis (?also absorption) *1381*
Serum No Effect Analytical At concentration of 480 mg/L had no effect on Liebermann-Burchard method *5704* At concentration of 480 mg/L had no effect on CHOD-PAP method *5704* At concentration of 480 mg/L had no effect on method using catalase-Hantzsch reaction *5704* At concentration of 480 mg/L had no effect on CHOD-Iodide method *5704* At concentration of 480 mg/L had no effect on catalase-AIDH method *5704*

Cholinesterase *Serum No Effect Analytical* No effect observed at concentration of 100 mg/dL with butyrylthiocholine method on Kodak Ektachem® *2504*

Coombs' Test, Direct *Blood Positive Physiological* Probably due to autoantibody complex on RBC surface *575* Not definitive proof, hemolytic anemia *2452*

Coproporphyrin *Blood Increase Physiological* May precipitate cutaneous porphyria *2210*
Feces Increase Physiological May precipitate cutaneous porphyria *2210*
Urine Increase Physiological May precipitate porphyria attack *2210*

Creatinine *Serum No Effect Analytical* At concentration of 400 mg/L had no effect on Jaffe-Fading-Fraction method *5704* No effect of concentrations up to 220 mg/L on single slide method on Kodak Ektachem® *5706* No effect at concentrations up to 220 mg/L on 2-slide method on Kodak Ektachem® *5706* No interference observed at a concentration of 3 mg/L with HPLC method of Rosano et al Tolbutamide elutes at 14.4 minutes compared with 8.9 minutes for creatinine *5083* No interference noted with liquid chromatographic method of Paroni et al *4540* At concentration of 400 mg/L had no effect on Jaffe-Fuller's earth method *5704* No significant effect on manual Jaffe procedure or on automated methods on Technicon SMAC® , Beckman Astra® , Roche Cobas-Bio or Du Pont aca at 5 times therapeutic concentration *4976* At concentration of 500 mg/L had no effect on creatinine iminohydrolase method *5704* At concentration of 500 mg/L had no effect on kinetic Jaffe method on BKA-2 *5704* At concentration of 100 mg/L had no effect on Technicon AutoAnalyzer® Jaffe method *5704*

Erythrocytes *Blood Decrease Physiological* Agranulocytosis/aplastic anemia *132*

Fatty Acids (FFA), Free *Serum Increase Physiological* Slight initial rise then fall to 25% at 90 minutes *2511*

Fluvastatin *Serum No Effect Physiological* In 16 healthy individuals coadministration of tolbutamide with fluvastatin had no significant effect on the latter's concentration *227*

Gastrin *Serum Decrease Physiological* After 5 minutes of i.v. infusion in patients with atrophic gastritis, duodenal ulcer, diabetes mellitus and healthy volunteers significant decrease. Reduction from mean of 84 pg/mL to 73 pg/mL at 30 min and 62 pg/mL at 60 min after 1 g orally in normals *993*

Glucagon *Plasma No Effect Physiological* No effect i.v. if given slowly or rapidly *4590*

Glucose *Serum Decrease Analytical* At concentrations above 500 mg/L (normal therapeutic concentration 110 mg/L) lowered concentration as measured by GOD-PERID method *5704*
Serum Decrease Physiological Significant reduction in normal volunteers to mean of 57 mg/dL 120 minutes after oral ingestion of 1 g *993* Incidence of 11.1% observed in French Pharmacovigilance database *4106* Therapeutic intent (promotes insulin secretion) *1897*
Serum Increase Analytical False increase (little effect at normal concentration) with glucose oxidase procedure *5481*
Serum No Effect Analytical No effect on glucose oxidase, o-toluidine, hexokinase procedures *4240* At concentration of 1,000 mg/L had no effect on GOD/POD-PAP method *5704* No effect at 5000 mg/L on hexokinase method on Ames Seralyzer *5706* No effect at 10 mmol/L on glucokinase based assay of Scott *5414* At concentration of 220 mg/L had no effect on Kodak Ektachem® method *5704* No effect on Boehringer GOD-PERID method *5480*

Glycated Hemoglobin *Blood No Effect Analytical* At a concentration of 1000 mg/L had an insignificant - 7.3% interference with method on Abbott Vision *1885*

Glycerol *Serum Decrease Physiological* Response similar to that of free fatty acids *2511*

Hematocrit *Blood Decrease Physiological* Agranulocytosis/aplastic anemia *132*

Hemoglobin *Blood Decrease Physiological* Agranulocytosis/aplastic anemia *132*
Blood No Effect Analytical No effect of concentrations up to 220 mg/L on method on Kodak Ektachem® *5706*

Histamine *Plasma No Effect Analytical* Improbable inhibition of radio-enzyme assay at therapeutic concentrations *2492*

25-Hydroxy Vitamin D_3 *Serum Decrease Physiological* Associated with turnover of bone organic matrix *5810*

Hydroxyproline *Urine Increase Physiological* Associated with turnover of bone organic matrix *5810*

^{131}I Uptake *Serum Decrease Physiological* Uncommon reported effect *3669*

Insulin *Plasma Decrease Physiological* Effect observed in some patients *492*
Plasma Increase Physiological Marked rise associated with hypoglycemia *1897* Significant increase in normal volunteers after 1 g orally with peak value of mean of 12 µU/mL at 30 minutes *993* Slight effect maximum in 15 minutes *501*

Ketorolac *Serum No Effect Physiological* At therapeutic concentrations had no effect on ketorolac-protein binding *5035*

Leukocytes *Blood Decrease Physiological* Agranulocytosis/aplastic anemia *967*

Neutrophils *Blood Decrease Physiological* Occasional case of drug-induced neutropenia *241* Occasionally observed *4014* Occasional case of agranulocytosis reported *6264*

5'-Nucleotidase *Serum Increase Physiological* Due to cholestasis *2911*

Phenprocoumon *Plasma No Effect Physiological* No effect noted with coadministration on half-life or plasma concentration *2538*

Phenylalanine *Plasma No Effect Analytical* No interference observed with rapid quantitative whole blood method of Campbell et al using phenylalanine dehydrogenase *867*

Phenytoin *Serum Increase Physiological* When tolbutamide ingested with fosphenytoin concentration of phenytoin may be increased *4519* Coadministration with phenytoin may increase plasma phenytoin concentration *4522*

Phosphate *Serum No Effect Analytical* At concentration of 270 mg/L had no effect on phosphomolybdate method *5704*

Platelets *Blood Decrease Physiological* Agranulocytosis/aplastic anemia *967*

Porphobilinogen *Urine Increase Physiological* May precipitate porphyria attack *2210*

Potassium *Serum No Effect Analytical* At concentration of 400 mg/L had no effect on measurement by ISE without predilution *5704* At concentration of 100 mg/L had no effect on flame-photometric method *5704* At concentration of 2,000 mg/L had no effect on measurement by ISE with predilution *5704*

Prazosin *Serum No Effect Physiological* Coadministration of prazosin with tolbutamide had no apparent adverse drug interaction in limited clinical experience *4649*

Protein *Cerebrospinal Fluid Increase Analytical* Causes turbidity if sulfosalicylic acid used *5869*
Serum No Effect Analytical At concentration of 270 mg/L had no effect on biuret method with blank correction *5704*
Urine Increase Analytical Affects heat and acetic acid test *3044* May cause false positive with Sulfosalicylic Acid and Exton's reagent tests *4034* Causes turbidity if sulfosalicylic acid used *5415*
Urine No Effect Analytical No effect on Albustix *703* Has no effect on protein test areas on Ames Multistix reagent test strips and other reagent strip tests *4034*

Protein Electrophoresis *Serum No Effect Analytical* At concentration of 400 mg/L had no effect on automated Olympus-Hite method *5704*

Prothrombin Time *Plasma Decrease Physiological* Stimulates metabolism of anticoagulants *2452*
Plasma Increase Physiological Occurs with failure to excrete bile salts *1405*

Protoporphyrin *Blood Increase Physiological* May precipitate cutaneous porphyria *2210*
Feces Increase Physiological May precipitate cutaneous porphyria *2210*

Sildenafil *Serum No Effect Physiological* CYP2C9 inhibitors such as tolbutamide did not affect the pharmacokinetics of sildenafil *4657*

Simvastatin *Serum No Effect Physiological* In 16 healthy individuals coadministration of tolbutamide with simvastatin had no significant effect on the latter's concentration *227*

Sodium *Serum No Effect Analytical* At concentration of 2,000 mg/L had no effect on measurement by ISE with predilution *5704* At concentration of 100 mg/L had no effect on flame-photometric method *5704* At concentration of 400 mg/L had no effect on measurement by ISE without predilution *5704*

Somatostatin *Plasma Increase Physiological* Intravenous bolus injection increased concentration in biphasic manner in both healthy individuals and in patients with impaired glucose tolerance *5430*

T3-Uptake *Serum Increase Physiological* Increase by 5-10% with 1 g i.v *882*

Thyroxine (T4) *Serum Decrease Physiological* Displaces from thyroxine binding globulin *5869*

Triglycerides *Serum No Effect Analytical* At concentration of 100 mg/L had no effect on lipase/esterase method *5704* At concentration of 540 mg/L had no effect on GPO-PAP method *5704*

Urea Nitrogen *Serum No Effect Analytical* At concentration of 270 mg/L had no effect on diacetylmonoxime method *5704* At concentration of 220 mg/L had no effect on Kodak Ektachem® method *5704*

Uric Acid *Serum No Effect Analytical* At concentration of 260 mg/L had no effect on Kageyama-Hantzsch method *5704* At concentration of 500 mg/L had no effect on uricase-PAP method *5704* At concentration of 270 mg/L had no effect on phosphotungstate reduction method *5704* At concentration of 400 mg/L had no effect on catalase-AIDH method *5704*

Urobilinogen *Feces Decrease Physiological* Pale stools with cholestasis may occur *2803*
Urine Decrease Physiological Possible cholestatic effect *2803*

Uroporphyrin *Urine Increase Physiological* May precipitate porphyria attack *2210*

Tolcapone

Alanine Aminotransferase *Serum Increase Physiological* Tolcapone administration has been associated with severe liver damage *5011*

Alkaline Phosphatase *Serum Increase Physiological* Tolcapone administration has been associated with severe liver damage *5011*

Aspartate Aminotransferase *Serum Increase Physiological* Tolcapone administration has been associated with severe liver damage *5011*

Bilirubin *Serum Increase Physiological* Tolcapone administration has been associated with severe liver damage *5011*

Blood *Urine Increase Physiological* May cause hematuria in 4% of patients with doses of 100 mg and 5% with doses of 200 mgcompared with 2% with placebo *5011*

Catechol-O-Methyltransferase
Red Blood Cells Decrease Physiological Causes reversible inhibition of erythrocyte COMT. With a 200 mg dose of tolcapone maximum inhibitory activity of COMT is on average greater than 80% *5011*

Catecholamines *Plasma No Effect Physiological* Tolcapone had no significant effect on the effect of ephedrine on the hemodynamics of catecholamines *5011*

Cholesterol *Serum Increase Physiological* Tolcapone administration is associated with infrequent hypercholesterolemia *5011*

Color *Urine Increase Physiological* Tolcapone caused abnormal color in 2% of 290 patients receiving 100 mg and in 7% of 298 patients receiving 200 mg compared with 1% in 298 placebo-treated controls *5011*

Creatine Kinase *Serum Increase Physiological* Tolcapone administration has been associated with severe rhabdomyolysis *5011*

Desipramine *Serum No Effect Physiological* Tolcapone had no significant effect on pharmacokinetics of desipramine *5011*

Tolcapone *(continued)*

3,4-Dihydroxyphenylalanine
Plasma Increase Physiological When administered with levodopa tolcapone increases the bioavailability of levodopa twofold by decreasing its clearance, although plasma concentration may be unaffected *5011*

Glucose *Serum Increase Physiological* Tolcapone administration is associated with infrequent diabetes mellitus *5011*

Hematocrit *Blood Decrease Physiological* Tolcapone administration is associated with infrequent anemia *5011*

Hemoglobin *Blood Decrease Physiological* Tolcapone administration is associated with infrequent anemia *5011*

Leukocytes *Blood Increase Physiological* Tolcapone administration is associated with rare leukemia *5011*

3-Methoxy-4-hydroxyl-phenylalanine
Plasma Decrease Physiological When administered with levodopa or carbidopa tolcapone causes a dose-dependent decrease 3-OMD *5011*

Occult Blood *Feces Increase Physiological* Tolcapone administration is associated with infrequent gastrointestinal hemorrhage *5011*

Platelets *Blood Decrease Physiological* Tolcapone administration is associated with rare thrombocytopenia *5011*

Tolbutamide *Serum No Effect Physiological* Tolcapone had no significant effect on pharmacokinetics of tolbutamide *5011*

Tolfenamic Acid

Histamine *Plasma No Effect Analytical* Insignificant inhibition of radio-enzyme assay at concentrations up to 50 times physiological *2492*

Tolmetin

Alanine Aminotransferase *Serum Increase Physiological* In fewer than 1% of recipients tolmetin administration has been reported to produce hepatitis or liver function test abnormalities *3917*
Serum No Effect Physiological Observed in single case of 49 y old man who had taken drug as needed for arthritis for 1 y *5759*

Alkaline Phosphatase *Serum Increase Physiological* Observed in single case of 49 y old man who had taken drug as needed for arthritis for 1 y *5759* In fewer than 1% of recipients tolmetin administration has been reported to produce hepatitis or liver function test abnormalities *3917*

Aspartate Aminotransferase *Serum Increase Physiological* In fewer than 1% of recipients tolmetin administration has been reported to produce hepatitis or liver function test abnormalities *3917*

Bilirubin *Serum Increase Physiological* In fewer than 1% of recipients tolmetin administration has been reported to produce hepatitis or liver function test abnormalities *3917* Observed in single case of 49 y old man who had taken drug as needed for arthritis for 1 y *5759*
Urine Increase Physiological Observed in single case of 49 y old man who had taken drug as needed for arthritis for 1 y *5759*

Bleeding Time *Patient Increase Physiological* Like aspirin prolongs bleeding time *1384*

Blood *Urine Increase Physiological* In fewer than 1% of recipients tolmetin administration has been reported to produce hematuria *3917*

Chondrex *Serum No Effect Analytical* Concentrations up to 10 g/L had no significant effect on sandwich-type ELISA procedure of Harvey et al *2491*

Coombs' Test, Direct *Blood Positive Physiological* Strongly positive: Observed in single case of 49 y old man who had taken drug as needed for arthritis for 1 y *5759*

Drugs of Abuse Screen *Urine Increase Analytical* False positive results obtained with Syva EMIT assays for barbiturates, benzodiazepines, THC, opiates, PCP, benzoylecgonine, methaqualone, and amphetamines *4783*

Erythrocytes *Blood Decrease Physiological* In 2% of patients in trials for treatment of juvenile rheumatoid arthritis *386*

γ-Glutamyltransferase *Serum Increase Physiological* Observed in single case of 49 y old man who had taken drug as needed for arthritis for 1 y *5759*

Granulocytes *Blood Decrease Physiological* In fewer than 1% of recipients tolmetin administration has been reported to produce granulocytopenia or agranulocytosis *3917*

Haptoglobin *Serum Decrease Physiological* Observed in single case of 49 y old man who had taken drug as needed for arthritis for 1 y *5759*

Hematocrit *Blood Decrease Physiological* In more than 1% of recipients tolmetin administration has been reported to produce small and transient decreases in hemoglobin and hematocrit not associated with gastrointestinal bleeding *3917* Observed in single case of 49 y old man who had taken drug as needed for arthritis for 1 y *5759*

Hemoglobin *Blood Decrease Physiological* In more than 1% of recipients tolmetin administration has been reported to produce small and transient decreases in hemoglobin and hematocrit not associated with gastrointestinal bleeding *3917*

Lactate Dehydrogenase *Serum Increase Physiological* Observed in single case of 49 y old man who had taken drug as needed for arthritis for 1 y *5759*

Occult Blood *Feces Increase Physiological* In fewer than 1% of recipients tolmetin administration has been reported to produce gastrointestinal bleeding with/without evidence of peptic ulcer *3917*

Partial Thromboplastin Time
Plasma Increase Physiological In 1% of patients in trials for treatment of juvenile rheumatoid arthritis *386*

Platelet Aggregation *Blood No Effect Physiological* Unlike aspirin has minimal effect on platelet aggregation *1384*

Platelets *Blood Decrease Physiological* In fewer than 1% of recipients tolmetin administration has been reported to produce thrombocytopenia *3917*

Protein *Urine Increase Analytical* With acid precipitation procedures causes pseudoproteinuria *1384* Tolmetin administration has been reported to yield metabolites that give positive tests for proteinuria which rely on acid precipitation as their endpoint (e.g. sulfosalicylic acid) *3917* May cause false positive with sulfosalicylic acid and Exton's reagent tests *4034*
Urine Increase Physiological In 1% of patients in trials for treatment of juvenile rheumatoid arthritis *386* In fewer than 1% of recipients tolmetin administration has been reported to produce proteinuria *3917*
Urine No Effect Analytical Tolmetin administration has been reported to yield metabolites that give positive tests for proteinuria which rely on acid precipitation as their endpoint (e.g. sulfosalicylic acid), but not on those that use dye-binding properties (e.g. Albustix® or Uristix®) *3917* Tolmetin sodium has no effect on protein test area of Ames Multistix and other reagent strips *4034*

Prothrombin Time *Plasma Increase Physiological* Tolmetin administration has been reported to increase prothrombin time and cause bleeding in some individuals receiving warfarin *3917*
Plasma No Effect Physiological Tolmetin administration had no effect on prothrombin time in individuals receiving warfarin *3917*

Reticulocytes *Blood Increase Physiological* Observed in single case of 49 y old man who had taken drug as needed for arthritis for 1 y *5759*

Urea Nitrogen *Serum Increase Physiological* In more than 1% of recipients tolmetin administration has been reported to increase the plasma urea nitrogen concentration *3917*

Urobilinogen *Urine Increase Physiological* Observed in single case of 49 y old man who had taken drug as needed for arthritis for 1 y *5759*

Tolonium

Color *Urine Increase Analytical* Green and blue color *1714*

Erythrocytes *Blood Decrease Physiological* May cause hemolysis with G-6-PD deficiency *536*

Heinz Body Formation *Blood Positive Physiological* May cause hemolysis with G-6-PD deficiency *536*

Hematocrit *Blood Decrease Physiological* May cause hemolysis with G-6-PD deficiency *536*

Hemoglobin *Blood Decrease Physiological* May cause hemolysis with G-6-PD deficiency *536*

Toloxatone

Amitriptyline *Serum No Effect Physiological* In 17 patients treated for major depressive illness when 600 mg/d toloxatone added to regime of 125 mg/d amitriptyline for 2 weeks small increase of amitriptyline/nortriptyline ratio from 0.68 to 0.78 but plasma concentration of amitriptyline not significantly affected *6202*

Urine No Effect Physiological In 17 depressed patients coadministration of toloxatone 600 mg/d to a regime of 125 mg/d amitriptyline for 2 weeks had no significant effect on excretion *6202*

Tolrestat

Albumin *Urine Decrease Physiological* In 20 patients with diabetic nephropathy treatment with 200 mg/d caused significant decrease from mean baseline of 219 ± 32.5 µg/min to 196 ± 28.5 µg/min at 2 mo, 172.6 ± 25.5 µg/min at 4 mo, and 158.6 ± 19.3 µg/min at 6 mo *4548*

Creatinine *Serum No Effect Physiological* In 20 patients with diabetic nephropathy treatment with 200 mg/d had no effect over 6 months *4548*

Glomerular Filtration Rate *Urine Decrease Physiological* During treatment of 20 patients with diabetic nephropathy with 200 mg/d GFR decreased from basal value of 158 ± 14 mL/min/1.73 sq m to 142 ± 13.7 mL/min/sq m at 2 mo, 128 ± 12.4 mL/min/1.73 sq m at 4 mo and 123.7 ± 13.0 mL/min/1.73 sq m at 6 mo *4548*

Renal Plasma Flow *Patient No Effect Physiological* In 20 patients with diabetic nephropathy treatment with 200 mg/d for 6 months had no effect on plasma flow *4548*

Topotecan

Alanine Aminotransferase *Serum Increase Physiological* Transient increases observed in 5% of 452 patients with greater increases occurring in < 1% *5648*

Aspartate Aminotransferase *Serum Increase Physiological* Transient increases observed in 5% of 452 patients with greater increases occurring in < 1% *5648*

Bilirubin *Serum Increase Physiological* Grade 3/4 increases observed in < 3% of 452 patients *5648*

Hematocrit *Blood Decrease Physiological* Anemia with hemoglobin of less than 8 g/dL observed in 40% of patients and in 16% of all courses of treatment, with nadir occurring with median of 15 days of treatment *5648*

Leukocytes *Blood Decrease Physiological* Leukopenia with WBC of less than 3000 cells/µL observed in 98% of 452 patients and in 77% of 2375 courses of treatment, and count of less than 1000 cells/µL occurred in 32% patients and in 11 courses *5648*

Neutrophils *Blood Decrease Physiological* Neutropenia is the dose-limiting toxicity of topotecan. Counts of less than 500/µL observed in 40% of all courses of treatment, with nadir occurring with median of 11 days of treatment *5648*

Platelets *Blood Decrease Physiological* Counts of less than 25,000/µL observed in 26% of patients and in 9% of all courses of treatment, with nadir occurring with median of 15 days of treatment *5648*

Toremifene

Alanine Aminotransferase *Serum Decrease Physiological* Activity decreased in healthy postmenopausal volunteers at doses above 220 mg *3165*

Alkaline Phosphatase *Serum Decrease Physiological* Activity decreased in healthy postmenopausal volunteers at doses above 220 mg *3165*

Serum Increase Physiological Increased activity above 200 U/L in North America and more than 1.25 times the upper limit of normal in Eastern Europe and Scandinavia has been reported with frequencies of 19%, 10% and 8% in North America, Eastern Europe and Scandinavia respectively *5329*

Aspartate Aminotransferase

Serum Decrease Physiological Activity decreased in healthy postmenopausal volunteers at doses above 220 mg *3165*

Serum Increase Physiological Increased activity above 100 U/L in North America and more than 1.25 times the upper limit of normal in Eastern Europe and Scandinavia has been reported with frequencies of 5%, 19% and 15% in North America, Eastern Europe and Scandinavia respectively *5329*

Bilirubin *Serum Increase Physiological* Increased activity above 2.0 mg/dL in North America and more than 1.25 times the upper limit of normal in Eastern Europe and Scandinavia has been reported with frequencies of 1.5%, 1% and 1% in North America, Eastern Europe and Scandinavia respectively *5329*

Calcium *Serum Increase Physiological* Hypercalcemia and tumor flare have been reported in patients with breast cancer during the first weeks of treatment. In one study the incidence was 3% *5329*

Estradiol *Plasma Decrease Physiological* In 15 postmenopausal women with breast cancer treatment with 60 mg/d continuously mean concentration changed nonsignificantly from mean baseline of 600 pmol/L to 130 pmol/Land in 15 given 300 mg/d for 12 weeks caused nonsignificant change from mean baseline of 420 pmol/L to 100 pmol/L *5905*

Follicle Stimulating Hormone

Plasma Decrease Physiological Reduction observed in healthy postmenopausal volunteers *3165*

immunoglobulin A *Serum Decrease Physiological* Significant decrease observed with treatment of women with breast cancer *4474*

Immunoglobulin G *Serum Decrease Physiological* Significant reduction observed in women undergoing treatment for breast cancer *4474*

Immunoglobulin M *Serum Decrease Physiological* Significant reduction observed in women undergoing treatment for breast cancer *4474*

Leukocytes *Blood Decrease Physiological* Apparent causal relationship in some patients receiving toremifene treatment *5329*

Blood Increase Physiological Concentration increased in healthy postmenopausal volunteers at doses above 220 mg *3165*

Luteinizing Hormone *Plasma Decrease Physiological* Concentration reduced in healthy postmenopausal volunteers *3165*

Platelets *Blood Decrease Physiological* Apparent causal relationship in some patients receiving toremifene treatment *5329*

Prolactin *Plasma Decrease Physiological* In 15 postmenopausal women with breast cancer treatment with 60 mg/d continuously mean concentration changed significantly from mean baseline of 398 ± 62 mU/L to 192 ± 40 mU/mL and in 15 given 300 mg/d for 12 weeks caused significant change from mean baseline to 178 ± 36 mU/L *5905*

Prothrombin Time *Plasma Increase Physiological* Observed interaction with warfarin leading to prolonged prothrombin time *5329*

Sex-Hormone Binding Globulin

Serum Increase Physiological Concentration increased in healthy postmenopausal volunteers *3165* In 15 postmenopausal women with breast cancer treatment with 60 mg/d continuously mean concentration changed significantly from mean baseline of 60 nmol/L to 90 nmol/L and in 15 given 300 mg/d for 12 weeks caused significant change from mean baseline of 75 nmol/L to 95 nmol/L *5905*

Torsemide

Calcium *Urine Increase Physiological* Similar effects to that of furosemide *1456*

Torsemide *(continued)*

Carvedilol *Serum No Effect Physiological* In 12 healthy individuals coadministration of drugs (5 mg/d torsemide and 25 mg/d carvedilol) for 5 days had no clinically relevant effect on pharmacokinetics of either compound *5639*

Chloride *Urine Increase Physiological* Similar effects to that of furosemide *1456*

Creatinine Clearance *Urine Increase Physiological* Similar effects to that of furosemide *1456*

Magnesium *Urine Increase Physiological* Similar effects to that of furosemide *1456*

Potassium *Urine Increase Physiological* Similar effects to that of furosemide *1456*

Sodium *Urine Increase Physiological* Similar effects to that of furosemide *1456*

Volume *Urine Increase Physiological* Similar effects to that of furosemide *1456*

Tosylate Bretylium

Catecholamines *Urine Decrease Physiological* Inhibits release of norepinephrine *6277*

Prothrombin Time *Plasma Increase Physiological* Enhances anticoagulant activity *2242*

Tramadol

Alanine Aminotransferase *Serum Increase Physiological* Administration of tramadol reported to cause hepatitis in some patients *3918*

Albumin *Urine No Effect Analytical* Using a fluorimetric assay with Albumin Blue 580 on a Cobas Fara centrifugal analyzer for the detection of microalbuminuria no significant interference was detected at a concentration of 20 mg/L *3117*

Alkaline Phosphatase *Serum Increase Physiological* Administration of tramadol reported to cause hepatitis in some patients *3918*

Aspartate Aminotransferase *Serum Increase Physiological* Administration of tramadol reported to cause hepatitis in some patients *3918*

Bilirubin *Serum Increase Physiological* Administration of tramadol reported to cause hepatitis in some patients *3918*

Creatinine *Serum Increase Physiological* Administration of tramadol reported to cause increases in serum creatinine concentration *3918*

Digoxin *Serum Increase Physiological* Administration of tramadol reported to cause digoxin toxicity in some patients *3918*

Hemoglobin *Blood Decrease Physiological* Administration of tramadol reported to cause decreases in hemoglobin concentration *3918*

Occult Blood *Feces Increase Physiological* Administration of tramadol reported to cause gastrointestinal bleeding in some patients *3918*

Protein *Urine Increase Physiological* Administration of tramadol reported to cause proteinuria in some patients *3918*

Prothrombin Time *Plasma Increase Physiological* Administration of tramadol reported to alter warfarin effect in some patients with actual increase of prothrombin time *3918*

Trandolapril

Alanine Aminotransferase *Serum Increase Physiological* Increased ALT activity concentration observed in fewer than 1.0% patients treated with trandolapril *3202*

Angiotensin-converting Enzyme
Serum Decrease Physiological Activity begins to decrease within 30 minutes of administration with maximum decrease at 2 to 4 hours. Same effect observed with any dose from 0.125 mg to 32.0 mg *4552*

Bilirubin *Serum Increase Physiological* Increased serum bilirubin concentration observed in 0.2% patients *3202*

Chloride *Urine No Effect Physiological* No significant change in excretion in 24 hours following doses up to 32.0 mg *4552*

Creatinine *Serum Increase Physiological* Increased serum creatinine concentration observed in 1.1% patients treated with trandolapril alone and in 7.3% patients treated with tranolapril and a diuretic *3202*

Digoxin *Serum No Effect Physiological* Trandolapril did not affect the plasma concentration (pre-dose and 2 h post-dose) of oral digoxin 0.25 mg *3202*

Furosemide *Serum No Effect Physiological* Coadministration of furosemide with trandolapril led to a 25% increase in the renal clearance of trandoprilat but had no effect on the pharmacokinetics of furosemide *3202*

Glomerular Filtration Rate *Urine No Effect Physiological* In 23 hypertensive patients treated with 2 mg/d for 3 weeks mean flow 76.29 ± 6.18 mL/min not significantly different from 73.79 ± 6.11 mL/min in placebo-treated patients *4790*

Leukocytes *Blood Decrease Physiological* Leukopenia observed in fewer than 1.0% patients treated with trandolapril *3202*

Neutrophils *Blood Decrease Physiological* Neutropenia observed in fewer than 1.0% patients treated with trandolapril *3202*

Potassium *Serum Increase Physiological* In clinical trials with trandolapril hyperkalemia with plasma potassium above 6.0 mmol/L occurred in about 0.4% hypertensive patients. In most cases these were isolated situations and resolved with continued therapy *3202*
Urine No Effect Physiological No significant change in excretion in 24 hours following doses up to 32.0 mg *4552*

Renal Plasma Flow *Patient No Effect Physiological* In 23 hypertensive patients treated with 2 mg/d for 3 weeks mean flow 338.24 ± 29.65 mL/min not significantly different from 309.16 ± 29.41 mL/min in placebo-treated patients *4790*

Sodium *Urine No Effect Physiological* No significant change in 24 h following doses up to 32.0 mg *4552*

Urea Nitrogen *Serum Increase Physiological* Increased serum urea nitrogen concentration observed in 0.6% patients treated with trandolapril alone and in 1.4% patients treated with tranolapril and a diuretic *3202*

Warfarin *Plasma No Effect Physiological* Administration of trandolapril with warfarin had no significant on either the warfarin concentration or plasma prothrombin time *3202*

Tranexamic Acid

Antiplasmin *Plasma Increase Physiological* In 15 patients who had received 20 mg/kg body weight total dose mean concentration of 128 ± 5 ng/mL significantly higher than control of 115 ± 3 ng/mL on the morning of the day after operation *599*

D-Dimer *Plasma Decrease Physiological* In 15 patients who had received 20 mg/kg body weight total dose mean concentration of 613 ± 84 ng/mL significantly less than control of 1412 ± 266 ng/mL on the morning of the day after operation *599*

Hematocrit *Blood No Effect Physiological* In 15 patients who had received 20 mg/kg body weight total dose mean of 34.0 ± 0.7% not significantly higher than control of 32.1 ± 0.9% on the morning of the day after operation *599*

Histamine *Plasma No Effect Analytical* No inhibition of radio-enzyme assay at therapeutic concentrations *2492*

Plasminogen Activator Inhibitor-1
Plasma No Effect Physiological In 15 patients who had received 20 mg/kg body weight total dose mean concentration of 129.7 ± 24.8 ng/mL not significantly higher than control of 105.2 ± 18.0 ng/mL on the morning of the day after operation *599*

Platelet Aggregation *Blood No Effect Physiological* In 15 patients who had received 20 mg/kg body weight total dose mean ADP-induced platelet aggregation of 89.0 ± 1.2% not significantly higher than control of 87.1 ± 1.4% on the morning of the day after operation *599*

Tissue Plasminogen Activator
Plasma *No Effect* *Physiological* In 15 patients who had received 20 mg/kg body weight total dose mean concentration of 10.6 ± 0.9 ng/mL not significantly higher than control of 9.3 ± 1.2 ng/mL on the morning of the day after operation *599*

Tranquilizers

17-Hydroxycorticosteroids *Urine* *Increase* *Analytical* Some artifactually increase value *467*

17-Ketosteroids *Urine* *Increase* *Analytical* Some artifactually increase value *467*

Tranylcypromine

Alanine Aminotransferase *Serum* *Increase* *Physiological* May affect liver function (?hypersensitivity) *3810*

Alkaline Phosphatase *Serum* *Increase* *Physiological* May affect liver function (?hypersensitivity) *3810*

α-Amino-Nitrogen *Plasma* *Increase* *Physiological* Majority of amino acids increased *1276*

Amphetamine/Methamphetamine
Serum *No Effect* *Analytical* At a concentration of 100000 ng/mL caused no detectable cross-reactivity with methods on Abbott AxSYM and TDx *6404*

Aspartate Aminotransferase *Serum* *Increase* *Physiological* May affect liver function (?hypersensitivity) *3810*

Aspartic Acid *Plasma* *Decrease* *Physiological* Observed effect in normal individuals *1276*

Bile *Urine* *Increase* *Physiological* May affect liver function (?hypersensitivity) *3810*

Bilirubin *Serum* *Increase* *Physiological* May affect liver function (?hypersensitivity) *3810*

BSP Retention *Serum* *Increase* *Physiological* Hepatotoxic/cholestatic syndromes *2242*

Carbamazepine *Serum* *No Effect* *Physiological* No apparent effect observed on plasma concentration of either drug with coadministration *3118*

Citrulline *Plasma* *Decrease* *Physiological* Observed effect in normal individuals *1276*

Dihydroxyphenylacetic Acid
Plasma *Decrease* *Physiological* From mean of 710 to 63 ng/L in 6 patients with depression or Alzheimer's disease treated with up to 40 mg daily for at least 3 weeks *1680*

Dihydroxyphenylalanine *Plasma* *No Effect* *Physiological* In 6 patients with depression or Alzheimer's disease treated with up to 40 mg daily for at least 3 weeks *1680*

3,4-Dihydroxyphenylglycol *Plasma* *Decrease* *Physiological* From mean of 850 to 210 ng/L in 6 patients with depression or Alzheimer's disease treated with up to 40 mg daily for at least 3 weeks *1680*

Epinephrine *Plasma* *No Effect* *Physiological* In 6 patients with depression or Alzheimer's disease treated with up to 40 mg daily for at least 3 weeks *1680*

Granulocytes *Blood* *Decrease* *Physiological* Agranulocytosis reported as side effect of administration *5653*

Hematocrit *Blood* *Decrease* *Physiological* Anemia reported as side effect of administration *5653*

Hemoglobin *Blood* *Decrease* *Physiological* Anemia reported as side effect of administration *5653*

^{131}I Uptake *Serum* *Decrease* *Physiological* Parnate contains tetraiodofluorescein *4360*

Leukocytes *Blood* *Decrease* *Physiological* Theoretical effect of this type of drug *128* Leukopenia reported as side effect of administration *5653*

Norepinephrine *Plasma* *No Effect* *Physiological* In 6 patients with depression or Alzheimer's disease treated with up to 40 mg daily for at least 3 weeks *1680*

Ornithine *Plasma* *No Effect* *Physiological* No effect observed *1276*

Platelets *Blood* *Decrease* *Physiological* Thrombocytopenia reported as side effect of administration *5653*

Proline *Plasma* *No Effect* *Physiological* No effect observed *1276*

Protein *Cerebrospinal Fluid* *No Effect* *Analytical* No significant effect when added in vitro to concentration of 6.0 mg/dL when measured by Kodak Ektachem® method *3654*

Taurine *Plasma* *Decrease* *Physiological* Observed effect in normal individuals *1276*

Trastuzumab

Alanine Aminotransferase *Serum* *Increase* *Physiological* Hepatic failure and/or hepatitis reported in at least 1 of 958 treated patients *2079*

Alkaline Phosphatase *Serum* *Increase* *Physiological* Hepatic failure and/or hepatitis reported in at least 1 of 958 treated patients *2079*

Amylase *Serum* *Increase* *Physiological* Pancreatitis reported in at least 1 of 958 treated patients *2079*

Aspartate Aminotransferase *Serum* *Increase* *Physiological* Hepatic failure and/or hepatitis reported in at least 1 of 958 treated patients *2079*

Bilirubin *Serum* *Increase* *Physiological* Hepatic failure and/or hepatitis reported in at least 1 of 958 treated patients *2079*

Blood *Urine* *Increase* *Physiological* Hematuria reported in at least 1 of 958 treated patients *2079*

Calcium *Serum* *Increase* *Physiological* Hypercalcemia reported in at least 1 of 958 treated patients *2079*

Erythrocytes *Blood* *Decrease* *Physiological* Pancytopenia reported in at least 1 of 958 treated patients *2079*

Glucose *Serum* *Decrease* *Physiological* Hypoglycemia reported in at least 1 of 958 treated patients *2079*

Hematocrit *Blood* *Decrease* *Physiological* Anemia reported in 4 of 352 patients when administered by itself, 14 of 91 patients when administered with pacitaxel and in 36 of 143 patients when administered with anthracycline and cyclophosphamide *2079*

Hemoglobin *Blood* *Decrease* *Physiological* Anemia reported in 4 of 352 patients when administered by itself, 14 of 91 patients when administered with pacitaxel and in 36 of 143 patients when administered with anthracycline and cyclophosphamide *2079*

Leukocytes *Blood* *Decrease* *Physiological* Leukopenia reported in 8 of 352 patients when administered by itself, 10 of 91 patients when administered with pacitaxel and in 11 of 143 patients when administered with anthracycline and cyclophosphamide *2079*

Lipase *Serum* *Increase* *Physiological* Pancreatitis reported in at least 1 of 958 treated patients *2079*

Lymphocytes *Blood* *Decrease* *Physiological* Pancytopenia reported in at least 1 of 958 treated patients *2079*

Magnesium *Serum* *Decrease* *Physiological* Hypomagnesemia reported in at least 1 of 958 treated patients *2079*

Occult Blood *Feces* *Increase* *Physiological* Hematemesis and esophageal ulcers reported in at least 1 of 958 treated patients *2079*

Platelets *Blood* *Decrease* *Physiological* Pancytopenia reported in at least 1 of 958 treated patients *2079*

Sodium *Serum* *Decrease* *Physiological* Hyponatremia reported in at least 1 of 958 treated patients *2079*

Thyroxine (T4) *Serum* *Decrease* *Physiological* Hypoythroidism reported in at least 1 of 958 treated patients *2079*

Trazodone

Albumin *Serum* *Decrease* *Physiological* Significant decrease from mean baseline concentration of 4.5 g/L to 4.3 g/L in 36 patients with depression treated for 6 weeks *4615*
Urine *No Effect* *Analytical* Using a fluorimetric assay with Albumin Blue 580 on a Cobas Fara centrifugal analyzer for the detection of microalbuminuria no significant interference was detected at a concentration of 4 mg/L *3117*

Calcium *Serum* *Decrease* *Physiological* Significant decrease from mean baseline concentration of 9.7 mg/dL to 9.5 mg/dL in 36 patients with depression treated for 6 weeks *4615*

Trazodone *(continued)*

Cholesterol *Serum Decrease Physiological* Significant decrease from mean baseline concentration of 205 mg/dL to 191 mg/dL in 36 patients with depression treated for 6 weeks *4615*

Digoxin *Serum Increase Physiological* Increased concentration reported when drugs coadministered *220* Observed to increase plasma concentration *1384*

Drugs of Abuse Screen *Urine No Effect Analytical* No effect at concentration of 100 µg/mL on EZ-SCREEN procedure for cannabinoids and cocaine *1739*

Erythrocytes *Blood Decrease Physiological* Decrease from mean baseline concentration of 4.78 million/µL to 4.54 million /µL in 36 patients treated for 6 weeks *4615*

Glucose *Serum No Effect Analytical* At concentration of 50 mg/L had no effect on GOD/POD-PAP method *5704*

Hematocrit *Blood Decrease Physiological* Significant decrease observed in 36 patients from mean of 43.0% to 40.9% following treatment for 6 weeks *4615*

Hemoglobin *Blood Decrease Physiological* Significant decrease from mean baseline of 14.4 g/L to 13.8 g/L in 36 patients with depression treated for 6 weeks *4615*

Leukocytes *Blood Decrease Physiological* Occasional low counts observed but not usually of clinical significance *220*

Lysergic Acid Diethylamide *Urine Increase Analytical* Minimum concentration that caused a positive result with EMIT method to measure LSD 15 mg/L *4968*

Neutrophils *Blood Decrease Physiological* Occasional low counts observed but not usually of clinical significance *220*

p-Aminophenol *Urine No Effect Analytical* With addition of drugs at a concentration of 100 mg/L and of related compounds at 50 mg/L no significant effect observed on colorimetric method of van Bocxlaer on Cobas Mira analyzer which involves reacting free p-aminophenol with resorcinol in the presence of magnesium ions to form an indophenol dye measured at 550 nm *6163*

Phenytoin *Serum Increase Physiological* Increased concentration reported when drugs coadministered *220* Possibly capable of increasing plasma concentration when drugs coadministered *1384* When trazodone ingested with fosphenytoin concentration of phenytoin may be increased *4519* Coadministration with phenytoin may increase plasma phenytoin concentration *4522*

Prothrombin Time *Plasma Decrease Physiological* Both increased and decreased prothrombin times reported in warfarinized patients patients taking trazodone *220*
Plasma Increase Physiological Both increased and decreased prothrombin times reported in warfarinized patients patients taking trazodone *220*

Triglycerides *Serum No Effect Analytical* At concentration of 50 mg/L had no effect on GPO-PAP method *5704*

Uric Acid *Serum No Effect Analytical* At concentration of 50 mg/L had no effect on uricase-PAP method *5704*

Tretinoin

Alanine Aminotransferase *Serum Increase Physiological* Up to 60% of treated patients develop abnormal liver function tests during treatment *5038*

Alkaline Phosphatase *Serum Increase Physiological* Up to 60% of treated patients develop abnormal liver function tests during treatment *5038*

Amylase *Serum Increase Physiological* Isolated cases of pancreatitis observed in treated patients *5038*

Aspartate Aminotransferase *Serum Increase Physiological* Up to 60% of treated patients develop abnormal liver function tests during treatment *5038*

Basophils *Blood Increase Physiological* Isolated cases reported in treated patients *5038*

Bilirubin *Serum Increase Physiological* Up to 60% of treated patients develop abnormal liver function tests during treatment *5038*

Calcium *Serum Increase Physiological* Isolated cases observed in treated patients *5038*

Cholesterol *Serum Increase Physiological* Up to 60% of treated patients develop hypercholesterolemia or hypertriglyceridemia, which was reversible at the end of the treatment *5038*

Creatinine *Serum Increase Physiological* Renal insufficiency observed in 11% of treated patients *5038*

Histamine *Plasma Increase Physiological* Isolated cases reported in treated patients *5038*

Leukocytes *Blood Increase Physiological* About 40% of treated patients develop rapidly evolving leukocytosis *5038*

Lipase *Serum Increase Physiological* Isolated cases of pancreatitis observed in treated patients *5038*

Occult Blood *Feces Increase Physiological* 34% of treated patients develop gastrointestinal hemorrhage *5038*

Triglycerides *Serum Increase Physiological* Up to 60% of treated pattients develop hypercholesterolemia or hypertriglyceridemia, which was reversible at the end of treatment *5038*

Urea Nitrogen *Serum Increase Physiological* Renal insufficiency observed in 11% of treated patients *5038*

Triacetyloleandomycin

Ergotamine *Urine Increase Physiological* Triacetyloleandomycin inhibits the metabolism of ergotamine *3657*

Triamcinolone

Amino Acids *Urine Increase Analytical* Purple spot with ninhydrin on thin-layer chromatography when combined with neomycin and nystatin in Kenacomb *2109*
Urine Increase Physiological Negative nitrogen balance with protein catabolism *2754*

Amylase *Serum Increase Physiological* May occasionally cause pancreatitis *2754*

Calcium *Urine Increase Physiological* Typical action of all corticosteroids *2754*

Color *Feces Increase Analytical* Black color reported following ingestion of triamcinolone *3388*

Cortisol *Plasma Decrease Physiological* Marked decrease in 2 children given injections of compound with suppression of hypothalamic-pituitary axis *1199*
Plasma No Effect Analytical Reactivity of less than 1% possible with RIA *1803* At concentration of 4.0 mg/L caused no cross reactivity with method on Baxter Stratus *5705*

Glucose *Serum Increase Physiological* Glucocorticoid effect *4174*
Urine Increase Physiological Consequence of hyperglycemia *4174*

Glucose Tolerance *Serum Decrease Physiological* Latent diabetes manifestation, endocrine effect *2754*

Nitrogen Balance *Patient Negative Physiological* Due to protein catabolism *2754*

Occult Blood *Feces Increase Physiological* May activate peptic ulcer or cause perforation *2754*

pH *Blood Increase Physiological* May cause hypokalemic alkalosis *2754*

Potassium *Urine Increase Physiological* Only in exceedingly large doses *128*

Sodium *Urine Increase Physiological* Mild diuresis with sodium loss in first few days *128*

Tacrolimus *Serum No Effect Analytical* In HPLC/MS method of Christians et al no significant interference observed with measurement of FK 506 *1010*

Volume *Plasma Increase Physiological* May cause sodium and fluid retention *2754*

Triamterene

Aldosterone *Plasma Increase Physiological* Mean increase of 125 pg/mL in 3 men given drug 50 mg tid for 1 week *6303*
Urine Increase Physiological Significant increase observed in 6 volunteers given 200 mg daily for 3 days *1813*

Amantadine *Serum Decrease Physiological* In one patient dyazide (triamterene/hydrochlorothiazide) reported to cause increased amantadine concentration but not known which component of drug was responsible *1600*

Amino-4-Imidazole-5-Carboxamide Ribotide
Urine Increase Physiological If megaloblastic anemia occurs *6370*

Ammonia *Urine No Effect Physiological* Does not cause excessive excretion *2754*

Antidiuretic Hormone *Urine No Effect Physiological* No significant effect in 6 volunteers given 200 mg/day for 3 days *1813*

Bicarbonate *Serum Decrease Physiological* Nephrotoxic effect *1714*

Calcium *Serum No Effect Physiological* No significant effect observed *6309*
Urine Increase Physiological Impairs reabsorption *4555*

Carbon Dioxide Partial Pressure
Blood No Effect Physiological No effect in normals (decreased in diabetics) *6308*

Catecholamines *Urine Decrease Analytical* When measured with Bio-Rad laboratories catecholamines column test procedure, fluorescence of drug interferes with high blank production *400*

Chloride *Serum Decrease Physiological* Diuretic action with impaired tubular reabsorption *1009*
Serum Increase Physiological Nephrotoxic and azotemic effect *3810*
Urine Increase Physiological Diuretic action *2242*

Cholinesterase *Serum No Effect Analytical* No effect observed at concentration of 6 mg/dL with butyrylthiocholine method on Kodak Ektachem® *2504*

Color *Urine Increase Analytical* Green, blue with blue fluorescence *1714*

Creatinine *Serum Increase Physiological* Nephrotoxic effect (causes reduced GFR) *3810*

Creatinine Clearance *Urine Decrease Physiological* Probably reduced renal blood flow *6309*
Urine No Effect Physiological No significant effect observed in 6 volunteers given 200 mg daily for 3 days *1813*

Crystals *Urine Increase Physiological* Either free or as part on conglomerations and also in large round brown bodies; common at pH < 6.0 *1786*

Cyclosporine *Blood No Effect Analytical* at a concentration of 2.8 mg/L had no effect on Syva EMIT method *495*

Diagnex Blue Excretion *Urine Increase Analytical* Increased dye release from resin *2024*

Digoxin *Serum Increase Analytical* At 500 ng/mL equals 0.3 ng/mL by RIA *6638*
Serum Increase Physiological Higher concentration when given in association with triamterene than when given alone *6303*

Eosinophils *Blood Increase Physiological* Allergic response *2484*

Erythrocytes *Blood Decrease Physiological* May cause megaloblastic anemia (folic acid antagonist) *6370*
Blood No Effect Physiological No significant difference observed in elderly chronic triamterene users and in those not taking the drug *3830*

Folate *Serum Decrease Physiological* Inhibits dihydrofolate reductase *6370* Identified as folate antagonist *5055*
Serum No Effect Physiological No significant difference observed in elderly people between those taking drug and those not doing so *3830* No significant difference observed in elderly people between those taking drug chronically and those not doing so *3830*

Glomerular Filtration Rate *Urine Decrease Physiological* Causes reduced glomerular filtration rate *1009*

Glucose *Serum Increase Physiological* Triamterene may cause increased concentration *5642* Effect less common than with thiazides *3308*
Serum No Effect Physiological In normals but increased in diabetics *6308*

Glucose Tolerance *Serum Decrease Physiological* Increase up to 250 mg/dL seen in normals even *6308*

Hematocrit *Blood Decrease Physiological* May cause megaloblastic anemia (folic acid antagonist) *6370*
Blood No Effect Physiological Usually no effect in normals *6308*

Hemoglobin *Blood Decrease Physiological* May cause megaloblastic anemia (folic acid antagonist) *6370*
Blood No Effect Physiological No significant difference between elderly people taking drug and those not taking drug *3830*

Histamine *Plasma No Effect Analytical* Improbable inhibition of radio-enzyme assay at therapeutic concentrations *2492*

Leukocytes *Blood Increase Physiological* Due to eosinophilia *3810*

Lithium *Serum Increase Physiological* Reported in 2 cases taking lithium: drug also given with hydrochlorothiazide: due to reduced clearance of lithium *3934*

Magnesium *Serum Increase Physiological* Slight increased effect observed in normals *6309*
Urine Increase Physiological Increased clearance observed *6309*
Urine No Effect Physiological Spared renal excretion with 37.5 mg/d *5169*

MCV *Blood Increase Physiological* Megaloblastic anemia *6370*
Blood No Effect Physiological No significant difference observed in elderly people between those taking drug and those not taking it *3830*

N-Formiminoglutamic Acid *Urine Increase Physiological* If megaloblastic anemia occurs *6370*

Nitrogen Balance *Patient Increase Physiological* Triamterene may cause mild nitrogen retention *5642*

pH *Blood No Effect Physiological* No effect in normals when given 100 mg b.i.d *6308*
Urine Increase Physiological Slight alkalinization (mechanism not known) *2242*

Phosphate *Serum No Effect Physiological* No significant effect observed *6309*

Potassium *Serum Decrease Physiological* Diuretic action *5869*
Serum Increase Physiological Increase from mean of 4.2 mmol/L to 4.4 mmol/L in 6 volunteers given 200 mg/day for 3 days *1813* Mean increase of 0.3 mmol/L in 3 men given drug for 1 week *6303* Potassium sparing action (affects Na/K exchange) *3810* Triamterene tends to conserve potassium rather than promoting its excretion like many other diuretics, and in rare cases may cause hyperkalemia *5642*

Pramipexole *Serum Increase Physiological* Coadministration of triamterene with pramipexole presumed to decrease the oral clearance of pramipexole by about 20% *4680*

Prostaglandin $F_{2\alpha}$ *Urine Increase Physiological* Increase of 192% in 6 volunteers given 200 mg daily for 3 days *1813*

Prostaglandins *Urine Increase Physiological* Increase of 474% observed in 6 volunteers given 200 mg daily for 3 days *1813*

Quinidine *Serum Increase Analytical* Triamterene may interfere with the fluorometric measurement of quinidine *5642*

Renin Activity *Plasma Increase Physiological* Significant increase observed in 6 volunteers given 200 mg daily for 3 days *1813*

Sodium *Serum Decrease Physiological* Diuretic action *3810*
Serum No Effect Physiological No effect of 200 mg/day for 3 days in 6 volunteers *1813*
Urine Increase Physiological Diuretic action (increased clearance) *2242* Reduces availability of potassium within distal tubular cells for secretion into distal lumen *4739*

Titratable Acidity *Urine No Effect Physiological* Does not cause excessive excretion *2754*

Triglycerides *Serum No Effect Physiological* No significant effect observed in patients receiving triamterene *4989*

Urea Nitrogen *Serum Increase Physiological* Nephrotoxic effect (with excessive diuresis) *2127*

Uric Acid *Serum Increase Physiological* Triamterene may cause increased concentration especially in persons predisposed to gouty arthritis *5642* Significant effect in about 17% cases *2451*
Serum No Effect Physiological Unless predisposition to gouty arthritis *2754*
Urine Increase Physiological Slight uricosuric action *2024*

Triamterene *(continued)*

Uric Acid Clearance *Urine Decrease Physiological* Reduced in proportion to creatinine clearance *6309*

Zinc *Urine Increase Physiological* Increase by 18% in 9 patients with hypertension for 2 weeks *6418*
Urine No Effect Physiological No effect observed *4484*

Triaziquone

Chromosomes *Test Conditions Abnormal Physiological* Clastogenic in human cells *5484*

Triazolam

Albumin *Urine Increase Physiological* Administration reported to increase excretion in 1.1% of 380 treated patients *4677*
Urine No Effect Analytical Using a fluorimetric assay with Albumin Blue 580 on a Cobas Fara centrifugal analyzer for the detection of microalbuminuria no significant interference was detected at a concentration of 0.4 mg/L *3117*

Alkaline Phosphatase *Serum Increase Physiological* Administration reported to increase activity in 2.2% of 380 treated patients *4677*

Aspartate Aminotransferase *Serum Increase Physiological* Administration reported to increase activity in 5.3% of 380 treated patients *4677*

Basophils *Blood Decrease Physiological* Administration reported to decrease concentration in 1.7% of 380 treated patients *4677*
Blood Increase Physiological Administration reported to increase concentration in 2.1% of 380 treated patients *4677*

Benzodiazepine *Urine Positive Analytical* Detectable limit 0.08 µg/mL with improved EMIT assay with Syva ETS system compared with 0.5 µg/mL with former d.a.u. assay *3370* At concentrations of 0.5 µg/mL or greater produces positive result with Syva EMIT II assay *1785*

Benzodiazepine Screen *Serum Increase Analytical* Cross-reacts in method on Du Pont aca *1512*

Bilirubin *Serum Increase Physiological* Administration reported to increase concentration in 1.5% of 380 treated patients *4677*

Cortisol *Urine Decrease Physiological* Observed in 9 poor sleepers given 0.5 mg/d for 3 weeks: overnight urinary cortisol measured. Immediate rebound increase on withdrawal *45*

Creatinine *Serum Decrease Physiological* Administration reported to decrease concentration in 2.4% of 380 treated patients *4677*
Serum Increase Physiological Administration reported to increase concentration in 1.9% of 380 treated patients *4677*

Eosinophils *Blood Decrease Physiological* Administration reported to decrease concentration in 10.2% of 380 treated patients *4677*
Blood Increase Physiological Administration reported to increase concentration in 3.2% of 380 treated patients *4677*

Erythrocytes *Urine Increase Physiological* Administration reported to increase excretion in 2.9% of 380 treated patients *4677*

Leukocytes *Blood Decrease Physiological* Administration reported to decrease concentration in 1.7% of 380 treated patients *4677*
Blood Increase Physiological Administration reported to increase concentration in 2.1% of 380 treated patients *4677*
Urine Increase Physiological Administration reported to increase excretion in 11.7% of 380 treated patients *4677*

Lymphocytes *Blood Decrease Physiological* Administration reported to decrease concentration in 2.3% of 380 treated patients *4677*
Blood Increase Physiological Administration reported to increase concentration in 4.0% of 380 treated patients *4677*

Midazolam *Serum No Effect Analytical* On GC-ECD method of Ha et al *2387*

Monocytes *Blood Decrease Physiological* Administration reported to decrease concentration in 3.6% of 380 treated patients *4677*

Neutrophils *Blood Decrease Physiological* Administration reported to decrease concentration in 1.5% of 380 treated patients *4677*
Blood Increase Physiological Administration reported to increase concentration in 1.5% of 380 treated patients *4677*

Tribromethanol

Albumin *Serum No Effect Analytical* At concentration of 90 mg/L had no effect on BCG method *5704*

Bicarbonate *Serum No Effect Analytical* At concentration of 90 mg/L had no effect on method using phenolphthalein *5704*

Bilirubin *Serum No Effect Analytical* At concentration of 90 mg/L had no effect on Jendrassik and Grof method *5704*

Calcium *Serum No Effect Analytical* At concentration of 90 mg/L had no effect on cresolphthalein method *5704*

Chloride *Serum No Effect Analytical* At concentration of 90 mg/L had no effect on mercurimetric method *5704*

Cholesterol *Serum No Effect Analytical* At concentration of 90 mg/L had no effect on Liebermann-Burchard method *5704*

Creatinine *Serum No Effect Analytical* At concentration of 90 mg/L had no effect on Technicon AutoAnalyzer® Jaffe method *5704*

Phosphate *Serum No Effect Analytical* At concentration of 90 mg/L had no effect on phosphomolybdate method *5704*

Protein *Serum No Effect Analytical* At concentration of 90 mg/L had no effect on biuret method with blank correction *5704*

Triglycerides *Serum No Effect Analytical* At concentration of 90 mg/L had no effect on lipase/esterase method *5704*

Urea Nitrogen *Serum No Effect Analytical* At concentration of 90 mg/L had no effect on diacetylmonoxime method *5704*

Uric Acid *Serum No Effect Analytical* At concentration of 90 mg/L had no effect on phosphotungstate reduction method *5704*

Trichlormethiazide

Alanine Aminotransferase *Serum Increase Physiological* May rarely cause cholestasis *2754*

Albumin *Serum No Effect Physiological* In 9 patients with essential hypertension treated with trichlormethiazide for 6 months baseline value of 42 ± 2 g/L not significantly changed to 42 ± 4 g/L *2237*

Alkaline Phosphatase *Serum Increase Physiological* May rarely cause cholestasis *2754*

Amylase *Serum Increase Physiological* May occasionally cause pancreatitis *2754*

Apolipoprotein A-I *Serum No Effect Physiological* Decrease by -5 mg/dL in 15 patients given 4 mg daily for 3 mo but note marked difference between responders and nonresponder populations *4213*

Apolipoprotein B *Serum No Effect Physiological* Increase by 1 mg/dL in 15 patients given 4 mg daily for 3 mo but note marked difference between responders and nonresponder populations *4213*

Apolipoprotein C-II *Serum No Effect Physiological* Increase by 2 mg/dL in 15 patients given 4 mg daily for 3 mo but note marked difference between responders and nonresponder populations *4213*

Apolipoprotein C-III *Serum Increase Physiological* Increase by 6 mg/dL in 15 patients given 4 mg daily for 3 mo but note marked difference between responders and nonresponder populations *4213*

Apolipoprotein E *Serum No Effect Physiological* Increase by 1 mg/dL in 15 patients given 4 mg daily for 3 mo but note marked difference between responders and nonresponder populations *4213*

Aspartate Aminotransferase *Serum Increase Physiological* May rarely cause cholestasis *2754*

Bilirubin *Serum Increase Physiological* May rarely cause cholestasis *2754*

Calcium *Serum Increase Physiological* Impaired excretion *5869*
Urine Decrease Physiological Impaired excretion *5869*

Cholesterol *Serum No Effect Physiological* Decrease by -17 mg/dL in 15 patients given 4 mg daily for 3 mo but note marked difference between responders and nonresponder populations *4213* In 9 patients with essential hypertension treated with trichlormethiazide for 6 months baseline value of 5.2 ± 0.1 mmol/L not significantly changed to 5.2 ± 0.7 mmol/L *2237*

Creatinine *Serum Decrease Physiological* In 9 patients with essential hypertension treated with trichlormethiazide for 6 months baseline value of 86 ± 22 µmol/L significantly changed to 71 ± 18 µmol/L *2237*

Erythrocytes *Blood Decrease Physiological* May cause bone marrow depression *2754*

Fatty Acids (FFA), Free *Serum Increase Physiological* Significant increase in fasting state (0.37 vs 0.31 mEq/L) and 60 minutes (0.33 vs 0.26 mEq/L) after 75 g glucose orally *4213*

Fibrinogen *Plasma No Effect Physiological* In 9 patients with essential hypertension treated with trichlormethiazide for 6 months baseline value of 2.20 ± 0.46 g/L not significantly changed to 2.28 ± 0.40 g/L *2237*

Filtration Rate *Red Blood Cells No Effect Physiological* In 9 patients with essential hypertension treated with trichlormethiazide for 6 months baseline value of 62 ± 11 µL/s not significantly changed to 64 ± 13 µL/s *2237*

Glucose *Serum Increase Physiological* Diabetogenic like action of drug: affects glucose tolerance test *5869* At 30 and 60 minutes in 6 patients given orally 75 g glucose values versus controls were 158 and 170 versus 136 and 156 mg/dL respectively *4213*

Serum No Effect Physiological In 9 patients with essential hypertension treated with trichlormethiazide for 6 months baseline value of 5.7 ± 0.4 mmol/L not significantly changed to 5.6 ± 0.3 mmol/L *2237*

Urine Increase Physiological Diabetogenic-like action of drug *5869*

HDL-Cholesterol *Serum Decrease Physiological* Decrease by -11 mg/dL in 15 patients given 4 mg daily for 3 mo but note marked difference between responders and nonresponder populations *4213*

Serum No Effect Physiological In 9 patients with essential hypertension treated with trichlormethiazide for 6 months baseline value of 1.3 ± 0.7 mmol/L not significantly changed to 1.4 ± 0.7 mmol/L *2237*

Hematocrit *Blood No Effect Physiological* In 9 patients with essential hypertension treated with trichlormethiazide for 6 months baseline value of 0.42 ± 0.04 not significantly changed to 0.41 ± 0.02 *2237*

Insulin *Plasma Increase Physiological* Significant increase versus controls in 6 patients given 75 g glucose orally at 30 minutes (79 vs 54 µU/mL) and 60 minutes (99 vs 76 µU/mL) *4213*

Leukocytes *Blood Decrease Physiological* May cause bone marrow depression *2754*

Magnesium *Red Blood Cells Decrease Physiological* Significant reduction in 14 patients with mild hypertension treated with 4 mg/d with or without a potassium sparing diuretic *3162*

Oxacillin *Serum Increase Analytical* Cannot be assayed in presence of trichlormethiazide by HPLC method used at Mayo Clinic *3858*

Platelets *Blood Decrease Physiological* May occur with/without purpura, bone marrow depression *2754*

Postheparin Lipase *Plasma Decrease Physiological* Significant effect during 3 mo drug administration (2.3 vs 3.3 µmol free fatty acid/mL/h respectively) *4213*

Potassium *Red Blood Cells No Effect Physiological* No effect of treatment with 4 mg/d in 14 patients with mild hypertension with or without a potassium sparing diuretic *3162*

Serum Decrease Physiological Diuretic action *5869*

Sodium *Red Blood Cells No Effect Physiological* No effect of 4 mg/d in 14 patients with mild hypertension with or without a potassium sparing diuretic *3162*

Urine Increase Physiological Therapeutic intent : diuretic action *2754*

Triglycerides *Serum Decrease Physiological* In 9 patients with essential hypertension treated with trichlormethiazide for 6 months baseline value of 2.3 ± 2.5 mmol/L not significantly changed to 1.5 ± 0.9 mmol/L *2237*

Serum Increase Physiological Increase by 44 mg/dL in 15 patients given 4 mg daily for 3 mo but note marked difference between responders and nonresponder populations *4213*

Uric Acid *Serum Increase Physiological* Inhibition of tubular secretion of urate *2378*

Viscosity *Blood No Effect Physiological* In 9 patients with essential hypertension treated with trichlormethiazide for 6 months no significant change over shear rate from 2.25 to 450 /s *2237*

Plasma No Effect Physiological In 9 patients with essential hypertension treated with trichlormethiazide for 6 months no significant change over shear rate from 2.25 to 450 /s *2237*

Trichloroethylene

Alanine Aminotransferase *Serum Increase Physiological* Potentially hepatotoxic *128*

Aspartate Aminotransferase *Serum Increase Physiological* Potentially hepatotoxic *128*

Bilirubin *Serum Increase Physiological* Potentially hepatotoxic *128*

β_2-Microglobulin *Urine No Effect Physiological* No significant increase in workers exposed to 15 parts per million compared with controls *4210*

Protein *Urine Increase Physiological* In workers probably exposed to 15 parts per million in air slightly higher excretion than in controls although not significantly increased *4210*

Tricine

Protein *Test Conditions Decrease Analytical* Lowry procedure, non linear absorption *2936*

Tricyclic Antidepressants

Sildenafil *Serum No Effect Physiological* CYP2D6 inhibitors such as tricyclic antidepressants did not affect the pharmacokinetics of sildenafil *4657*

Tridodecylmethylammonium Heparin

Potassium *Serum No Effect Analytical* No effect when serum passed through catheters containing this heparin salt when measured by methods on Beckman Astra® 8, Kodak Ektachem® 700, Baxter Paramax, American Monitor Parallel, flame photometry, Abbott Spectrum, du Pont Dimension and IL Monarch *3208*

Sodium *Serum No Effect Analytical* No effect seen when serum passed through catheters containing this heparin salt when measured by methods on Beckman Astra® , Kodak Ektachem® 700, Baxter Paramax, American Monitor Parallel, flame-photometry, Abbott Spectrum, IL Monarch and du Pont Dimension *3208*

Trientine

Copper *Urine Increase Physiological* In selected patients with Wilson's disease previously treated with penicillamine for one year after a single dose of 1.2 g excretion increased from baseline of 19 µg/6 h to 234 µg/6 h. In 8 previously untreated patients treatment with 1.2 g caused significant increase in excretion from 71 µg/6 h to 1326 µg/6 h *3994*

Copper, Free *Serum Decrease Physiological* In patients with Wilson's disease adequate treatment results in a concentration less than 10 µg/dL *3994*

Hematocrit *Blood Decrease Physiological* In 4 patients with primary biliary cirrhosis treatment with trientine was associated with hypochromic microcytic anemia *3994*

Hemoglobin *Blood Decrease Physiological* In 4 patients with primary biliary cirrhosis treatment with trientine was associated with hypochromic microcytic anemia *3994*

Occult Blood *Feces Increase Physiological* In 4 patients with primary biliary cirrhosis treatment with trientine was associated with acute gastritis and melena *3994*

Triethanolamine

Potassium *Serum No Effect Analytical* At concentration of 200 mg/L had no effect on measurement by ISE with predilution *5704*

Sodium *Serum No Effect Analytical* At concentration of 200 mg/L had no effect on measurement by ISE with predilution *5704*

Triethylenemelamine

Alanine Aminotransferase *Serum Increase Physiological* Hepatotoxicity with prolonged treatment and large doses *128*

Aspartate Aminotransferase *Serum Increase Physiological* Hepatotoxicity (prolonged treatment, large dose) *128*

Bilirubin *Serum Increase Physiological* May cause hemolytic anemia *3895*

Cholinesterase *Serum Decrease Physiological* Observed *in vitro*, probable effect *in vivo6684*

Chromosomes *Test Conditions Abnormal Physiological* Clastogenic in human cells *5484*

Coombs' Test, Direct *Blood Positive Physiological* May cause hemolytic anemia *3895*

Crystals *Urine Increase Physiological* Due to crystalization out of drug *2754*

Erythrocytes *Blood Decrease Physiological* May cause bone marrow depression *128* May cause hemolytic anemia *3810*
Urine Increase Physiological Due to nephrotoxicity *2754*

Hemoglobin *Blood Decrease Physiological* May cause hemolytic anemia *3810*
Urine Increase Physiological Due to nephrotoxicity *2754*

Leukocytes *Blood Decrease Physiological* May cause bone marrow depression *128*

Platelets *Blood Decrease Physiological* May cause bone marrow depression *128*

Protein *Urine Increase Physiological* Due to nephrotoxicity *2754*

Urea Nitrogen *Serum Increase Physiological* Nephrotoxicity with nitrogen retention *2754*

Triflocin

Ammonia *Urine Increase Physiological* Inhibits carbonic anhydrase *67*

Potassium *Urine Increase Physiological* Diuretic action *67*

Sodium *Urine Increase Physiological* Diuretic action *67*

Titratable Acidity *Urine Increase Physiological* Inhibits carbonic anhydrase *67*

Trifluoperazine

Alanine Aminotransferase *Serum Increase Physiological* Cholestatic effect *2803* Jaundice of the cholestatic type of hepatitis or liver damage has been reported to occur in patients receiving trifluoperazine *5656*

Albumin *Serum No Effect Analytical* At concentration of 1 mg/L had no effect on BCG method *5704*

Alkaline Phosphatase *Serum Decrease Physiological* Not very marked *358*
Serum Increase Physiological Jaundice of the cholestatic type of hepatitis or liver damage has been reported to occur in patients receiving trifluoperazine *5656* Cholestatic effect *2803*

Amphetamine *Urine No Effect Analytical* No false positive results observed in 1 assay using Syva EMIT amphatamine method with either monoclonal or polyclonal antibodies *1160*

Aspartate Aminotransferase
Serum Decrease Physiological Noticeable effect *358*
Serum Increase Physiological Jaundice of the cholestatic type of hepatitis or liver damage has been reported to occur in patients receiving trifluoperazine *5656* Cholestatic effect *2803*

Bicarbonate *Serum No Effect Analytical* At concentration of 1 mg/L had no effect on method using phenolphthalein *5704*

Bilirubin *Serum Increase Physiological* Jaundice of the cholestatic type of hepatitis or liver damage has been reported to occur in patients receiving trifluoperazine *5656* Cholestatic effect *2803*
Serum No Effect Analytical At concentration of 1 mg/L had no effect on Jendrassik and Grof method *5704*

BSP Retention *Serum Increase Physiological* Cholestatic effect *2803*

Calcium *Serum No Effect Analytical* At concentration of 1 mg/L had no effect on cresolphthalein method *5704*

Cannabinoids *Urine No Effect Analytical* No effect on Roche Abuscreen method *5006*

Chloride *Serum No Effect Analytical* At concentration of 1 mg/L had no effect on mercurimetric method *5704*

Cholesterol *Serum Increase Physiological* Increase of up to 35 mg/dL reported *4909*
Serum No Effect Analytical At concentration of 1 mg/L had no effect on Liebermann-Burchard method *5704*

Creatinine *Serum No Effect Analytical* At concentration of 1 mg/L had no effect on Technicon AutoAnalyzer® method *5704*

Eosinophils *Blood Increase Physiological* Administration of trifluoperazine reported to cause various blood dyscrasias including pancytopenia and eosinophilia *5656*

Erythrocytes *Blood Decrease Physiological* Pancytopenia (AMA Blood dyscrasias) *4017* Administration of trifluoperazine reported to cause various blood dyscrasias including pancytopenia *5656*

Glucose *Serum Decrease Physiological* Administration of trifluoperazine reported to cause hypoglycemia *5656*
Serum Increase Physiological Administration of trifluoperazine reported to cause hyperglycemia *5656*
Serum No Effect Analytical At concentration of 1 mg/L had no effect on GOD/POD-PAP method *5704*
Urine Increase Physiological Administration of trifluoperazine reported to cause glycosuria *5656*

γ-Glutamyltransferase *Serum Increase Physiological* Jaundice of the cholestatic type of hepatitis or liver damage has been reported to occur in patients receiving trifluoperazine *5656*

Granulocytes *Blood Decrease Physiological* Decreased values noted (not marked) *358* Administration of trifluoperazine reported to cause various blood dyscrasias including pancytopenia and granulocytopenia *5656*

Hematocrit *Blood Decrease Physiological* Administration of trifluoperazine reported to cause various blood dyscrasias including pancytopenia and hemolytic or aplastic anemia *5656*

Hemoglobin *Blood Decrease Physiological* Administration of trifluoperazine reported to cause various blood dyscrasias including pancytopenia and hemolytic or aplastic anemia *5656*

Leukocytes *Blood Decrease Physiological* Administration of trifluoperazine reported to cause various blood dyscrasias including pancytopenia and leukopenia *5656* Pancytopenia (AMA Blood dyscrasias) *4014* Transient leukopenia reported occasionally *1384*

Phenylketones *Urine Positive Analytical* Administration of trifluoperazine may produce false positive test for phenylketonuria *5656*

Phosphate *Serum No Effect Analytical* At concentration of 1 mg/L had no effect on phosphomolybdate method *5704*

Platelets *Blood Decrease Physiological* Administration of trifluoperazine reported to cause various blood dyscrasias including pancytopenia and thrombocytopenic purpura *5656* Pancytopenia (AMA Blood dyscrasias) *4017*

Potassium *Serum No Effect Analytical* At concentration of 1 mg/L had no effect on flame-photometric method *5704*

Pregnancy Tests *Urine Positive Analytical* Administration of trifluoperazine reported to cause false positive pregnancy tests *5656*

Prolactin *Plasma Increase Physiological* Hyperprolactinemia has been reported to occur in patients receiving trifluoperazine, but the significance of this is unknown *5656* Typical response to i.m. administered drug: effect dose related *3402*

Propranolol *Serum Increase Physiological* Concomitant administration of propranolol with trifluoperazine increases the plasma concentration of both drugs *5656*

Protein *Cerebrospinal Fluid Increase Physiological* Administration of trifluoperazine reported to alter cerebrospinal fluid proteins *5656*
Serum No Effect Analytical At concentration of 1 mg/L had no effect on biuret method with blank correction *5704*
Urine Increase Analytical In 2 patients receiving up to 30 mg daily on Ponceau S dye method in comparison with sulfosalicylic acid and trichloracetic acid methods *6611*

Prothrombin Time *Plasma Increase Physiological* Associated with failure of excretion of bile salts *2803*

Sodium *Serum No Effect Analytical* At concentration of 1 mg/L had no effect on flame-photometric method *5704*

Triglycerides *Serum No Effect Analytical* At concentration of 1 mg/L had no effect on lipase/esterase method *5704*

Urea Nitrogen *Serum No Effect Analytical* At concentration of 1 mg/L had no effect on diacetylmonoxime method *5704*

Uric Acid *Serum No Effect Analytical* At concentration of 1 mg/L had no effect on phosphotungstate reduction method *5704*

Urobilinogen *Feces Decrease Physiological* Pale stools with cholestasis *2803*
Urine Decrease Physiological Cholestatic effect *2803*

Trifluperidol

Alanine Aminotransferase *Serum Increase Physiological* Hepatocellular changes observed *2242*

Bilirubin *Serum Increase Physiological* Elevated in chronic and acute hepatitis *1714*

Catecholamines *Plasma No Effect Analytical* No effect on HPLC method of Koller for dopamine, epinephrine, and norepinephrine *3230*

Cholesterol *Serum Decrease Physiological* Inhibits biosynthesis in liver *2242*

Desmosterol *Serum Increase Physiological* Further metabolism inhibited so accumulates *2242*

Eosinophils *Blood Increase Physiological* Allergic response *3810*

Leukocytes *Blood Decrease Physiological* Rare leukopenia/agranulocytosis *2242*
Blood Increase Physiological Due to eosinophilia *3810*

Triflupromazine

Bilirubin *Serum Increase Physiological* Liver dysfunction exceptionally rare *128*

Leukocytes *Blood Decrease Physiological* Agranulocytosis due to inhibition of development *4714*

Triflusal

Albumin *Urine Decrease Physiological* In 9 normotensive insulin-dependent diabetics with urinary albumin excretion between 30 and 103 µg/min 5 days of treatment with 900 mg/d albumin excretion reduced from 59 µg/min to 33 µg/min *1760*

Filtration Fraction *Urine Decrease Physiological* In 9 normotensive insulin-dependent diabetic patients mean reduced from 0.24 to 0.20 with treatment with 900 mg/d for 5 days *1760*

Glucose *Serum No Effect Physiological* In 9 normotensive insulin-dependent diabetics treatment with 900 mg/d for 5 days caused insignificant change from mean of 10.3 mmol/L to 10.1 mmol/L *1760*

6-Keto-Prostaglandin $F_{1\alpha}$ *Plasma No Effect Physiological* No significant change from mean baseline of 22 pg/mL in 9 normotensive insulin-dependent diabetic patients treated with 900 mg/day for 5 days. Final mean concentration 17 pg/mL *1760*
Urine No Effect Physiological No significant effect in 9 normotensive insulin-dependent diabetics treated with 900 mg/d for 5 days *1760*

Potassium *Urine No Effect Physiological* No significant effect observed in 9 normotensive insulin-dependent diabetics treated with 900 mg/d for 5 days *1760*

Prostaglandin E_2 *Urine No Effect Physiological* No significant effect observed in 9 normotensive insulin-dependent diabetics treated with 900 mg/d for 5 days *1760*

Renal Plasma Flow *Patient Increase Physiological* In 9 normotensive insulin-dependent diabetics treatment with 900 mg/d for 5 days caused increase from mean of 648 mL/min/1.73 sq m to 722 mL/min/1.73 sq m *1760*

Renin Activity *Plasma No Effect Physiological* No significant change observed in 9 insulin-dependent normotensive diabetics treated with 900 mg/d for 5 days *1760*

Sodium *Urine No Effect Physiological* No significant change observed in 9 normotensive insulin-dependent diabetics treated with 900 mg/d for 5 days *1760*

Thromboxane B_2 *Plasma Decrease Physiological* In 9 normotensive insulin-dependent diabetics treated with 900 mg/d for significant decrease from mean concentration of 130 pg/mL to 52 pg/mL *1760*
Urine Decrease Physiological Significant reduction in excretion from mean of 523 pg/min to 312 pg/min in 9 insulin-dependent normotensive dependent diabetics treated with 900 mg/d for 5 days *1760*

Volume *Urine No Effect Physiological* No significant effect observed in 9 normotensive insulin-dependent diabetics treated with 900 mg/d for 5 days *1760*

Trihexyphenidyl

Volume *Urine Decrease Physiological* Retention due to parasympatholytic effect *2754*

Triiodothyronine

Adenosine Monophosphate *Plasma Increase Physiological* In 23 euthyroid asthmatic children treatment for 30 days caused significant increase compared with pretest concentrations and in controls *3126*
Sputum Increase Physiological In 23 euthyroid children with asthma treatment for 30 days caused significant increase in concentration *3126*

Angiotensin-converting Enzyme
Serum Increase Physiological In 7 normal women aged 18-27 y given 25 µg/d three times daily for 14 d. Effect observed on endothelium-associated proteins but not on hepatically synthesized proteins *2294*

Antithrombin III *Plasma No Effect Physiological* In 7 normal women aged 18-27 y given 25 µg/d three times daily for 14 d. Effect observed on endothelium-associated proteins but not on hepatically synthesized proteins *2294*

α_1-Antitrypsin *Serum No Effect Physiological* In 7 normal women aged 18-27 y given 25 µg/d three times daily for 14 d. Effect observed on endothelium-associated proteins but not on hepatically synthesized proteins *2294*

Ceruloplasmin *Serum No Effect Physiological* In 7 normal women aged 18-27 y given 25 µg/d three times daily for 14 d. Effect observed on endothelium-associated proteins but not on hepatically synthesized proteins *2294*

Cholesterol *Serum Decrease Physiological* Physiological consequence of hormone *5869*

2,3-Diphosphoglycerate Mutase
Blood No Effect Physiological No effect on amount of 2,3-DPG produced *6057*

Factor VIII Antigen *Plasma Increase Physiological* In 7 normal women aged 18-27 y given 25 µg/d three times daily for 14 d. Effect observed on endothelium-associated proteins but not on hepatically synthesized proteins *2294*

Fibronectin *Plasma Increase Physiological* In 7 normal women aged 18-27 y given 25 µg three times daily for 14 d. Effect observed on endothelium-associated proteins but not on hepatically synthesized proteins *2294*

Haptoglobin *Serum No Effect Physiological* In 7 normal women aged 18-27 y given 25 µg/d three times daily for 14 d. Effect observed on endothelium-associated proteins but not on hepatically synthesized proteins *2294*

^{131}I Uptake *Serum Decrease Physiological* Marked decrease in obese with 150 µg/d *702*

Triiodothyronine *(continued)*

Prealbumin *Serum* *No Effect* *Physiological* In 7 normal women aged 18-27 y given 25 µg/d three times daily for 14 d. Effect observed on endothelium-associated proteins but not on hepatically synthesized proteins *2294*

T3-Uptake *Serum* *No Effect* *Analytical* D-tri-iodothyronine at concentration of 1.5 µg/dL (23.1 nmol/L) 99% recovery observed with method on Du Pont aca *1545* 99% recovery observed when L-tri-iodothyronine added at a concentration of 1.5 µg/dL (23.1 nmol/L) with method on Du Pont aca *1545*
Serum *No Effect* *Physiological* No significant effect with 150 µg/d in obese *702*

Thyroid Stimulating Hormone
Serum *Decrease* *Physiological* Effect marked in euthyroid, hypothyroid subjects *6139*

Thyroxine Binding Globulin *Serum* *No Effect* *Analytical* On radioimmunoassay procedure of Van Herle *6188*
Serum *No Effect* *Physiological* In 7 normal women aged 18-27 y given 25 µg/d three times daily for 14 d. Effect observed on endothelium-associated proteins but not on hepatically synthesized proteins *2294*

Thyroxine (T4) *Serum* *Decrease* *Physiological* Marked decrease in obese with 150 µg/d *702* In 7 normal women aged 18-27 y given 25 µg/d three times daily for 14 d. Effect observed on endothelium-associated proteins but not on hepatically synthesized proteins *2294* Diminished synthesis *5869*
Serum *Increase* *Analytical* 112% recovery when D-tri-iodothyronine at concentration of 1.5 µg/dL (23.1 nmol/L) added when measured by method on Du Pont aca *1588* 111% recovery when L-tri-iodothyronine added at concentration of 1.5 lmu]g/dL (23.1 nmol/L) and measured by method on Du Pont aca *1588* 111% recovery when L-tri-iodothyronine added at concentration of 1.5 µg/dL (23.1 nmol/L) and measured by method on Du Pont aca *1546* 112% recovery when D-tri-iodothyronine at concentration of 1.5 µg/dL (23.1 nmol/L) added when measured by method on Du Pont aca *1546*
Serum *No Effect* *Analytical* Caused less than 2.4% cross-reactivity with EIA method on Bio-Rad RADIAS analyzer *4819* No significant cross-reactivity observed in T4 method on Bayer Technicon Immuno 1® *434* Cross-reactivity of 1.9% observed with method on Baxter Stratus *5705*

Thyroxine (T4), Free *Serum* *Increase* *Analytical* Has cross-reactivity of 3.9% with method on Baxter Stratus *5705*
Serum *No Effect* *Analytical* At toxic concentration of D-tri-iodothyronine change of less than 0.01 ng/dL observed with method on Technicon Immuno-1 *1296* L-triiodothyronine at a concentration of 5.0 µg/dL had no cross-reactivity FT4 in method on Bayer Technicon Immuno 1® *424* Toxic concentration of L-tri-iodothyronine caused change of less than 0.01 ng/dL with method on Technicon Immuno-1 *1296*

Tissue Plasminogen Activator Antigen
Plasma *Increase* *Physiological* In 7 normal women aged 18-27 y given 25 µg/d three times daily for 14 d. Effect observed on endothelium-associated proteins but not on hepatically synthesized proteins *2294*

Transferrin *Serum* *No Effect* *Physiological* In 7 normal women aged 18-27 y given 25 µg/d three times daily for 14 d. Effect observed on endothelium-associated proteins but not on hepatically synthesized proteins *2294*

Tri-iodothyronine (T3) *Serum* *Increase* *Physiological* Cross-reactivity of 100% observed from D-tri-iodothyronine with method on Behring Opus immunoassay system *4964* Marked increase in obese with 150 µg/d *702*
Serum *No Effect* *Physiological* In 7 normal women aged 18-27 y given 25 µg/d three times daily for 14 d. Effect observed on endothelium-associated proteins but not on hepatically synthesized proteins *2294*

Tyrosine *Plasma* *Increase* *Physiological* Slight increase in obese with 150 µg/d *702*

Trilostane

Cortisol *Plasma* *Decrease* *Physiological* In critically ill patients relative hypoadrenalism observed with trilostane therapy because of its effect on cortisol synthesis *3381*

Trimazosin

Cholesterol *Serum* *No Effect* *Physiological* In 2 studies with 13 and 48 subjects treated for 2.5 to 12 mo *142*

HDL-Cholesterol *Serum* *No Effect* *Physiological* In 2 studies with 13 and 48 subjects treated for 2.5 to 12 mo *142*

Renin Activity *Plasma* *No Effect* *Physiological* No significant change observed *1353*

Sodium *Urine* *No Effect* *Physiological* No significant effect noted *1353*

Triglycerides *Serum* *No Effect* *Physiological* In 2 studies with 13 and 48 subjects treated for 2.5 to 12 mo *142*

Trimeprazine

Alanine Aminotransferase *Serum* *Increase* *Physiological* May cause cholestasis *128*

Amphetamine/Methamphetamine
Urine *No Effect* *Analytical* No false positive results observed in 35 urines from 34 patients taking drug when measured by Syva EMIT II procedure *5634*

Aspartate Aminotransferase *Serum* *Increase* *Physiological* May cause cholestasis *128*

Bile *Urine* *Increase* *Physiological* May cause cholestasis *128*

Bilirubin *Serum* *Increase* *Physiological* May cause cholestasis *128*

Granulocytes *Blood* *Decrease* *Physiological* Absence reported in one case *680*

Leukocytes *Blood* *Decrease* *Physiological* May cause leukopenia or agranulocytosis *128*

Neutrophils *Blood* *Decrease* *Physiological* Occasional case of agranulocytosis reported *6264*

Trimethadione

Alanine Aminotransferase *Serum* *Increase* *Physiological* May cause hepatotoxicity with necrosis *3810*

Alkaline Phosphatase *Serum* *Increase* *Physiological* Hepatotoxicity with centrolobular necrosis *3810*

Antinuclear Antibodies *Serum* *Increase* *Physiological* Related to number of drugs, higher in women *6411*

Aspartate Aminotransferase *Serum* *Increase* *Physiological* May cause hepatotoxicity with necrosis *3810*

Bicarbonate *Serum* *Decrease* *Physiological* Converted to dimethadione *in vivo* with same effects *6518*

Bile *Urine* *Increase* *Physiological* May cause hepatotoxicity with necrosis *3810*

Bilirubin *Serum* *Increase* *Physiological* Hepatotoxicity with centrolobular necrosis *3810*

BSP Retention *Serum* *Increase* *Physiological* Hepatotoxicity with centrolobular necrosis *3810*

Calcium *Serum* *Decrease* *Physiological* Theoretical effect of type of drug *2403*

Casts *Urine* *Increase* *Physiological* May have nephrotoxic effect *3810*

Cholesterol *Serum* *Increase* *Physiological* May affect liver function (hepatitis) *3810*

Erythrocytes *Blood* *Decrease* *Physiological* Aplastic anemia *4017*
Urine *Increase* *Physiological* Hematuria may occur especially in children *3669*

Felbamate *Serum* *No Effect* *Analytical* No significant interference observed with GLC method of Rifai et al *4958*

Folate *Test Conditions* *No Effect* *Analytical* No effect on *L. casei* or *S. fecalis4014*

Granulocytes *Blood* *Decrease* *Physiological* Occasionally observed in association with bone marrow depression *1384*

Hematocrit *Blood* *Decrease* *Physiological* Aplastic anemia *4995*

Hemoglobin *Blood* *Decrease* *Physiological* Aplastic anemia *4995*
Urine *Increase* *Physiological* Hematuria may occur especially in children *3669*

25-Hydroxy Vitamin D_3 *Serum Decrease Physiological* Theoretical effect of type of drug *2403*

LE Cells *Blood Positive Physiological* Rare immune response observed *2010*

Leukocytes *Blood Decrease Physiological* Aplastic anemia *4995*

Neutrophils *Blood Decrease Physiological* Moderate neutropenia quite common *2242* Occasional agranulocytosis reported *6264*

Occult Blood *Feces Increase Physiological* Gastrointestinal bleeding reported (may affect many organs) *1714*

pH *Blood Decrease Physiological* Converted to dimethadione *in vivo* with same effects *6518*

Platelets *Blood Decrease Physiological* Aplastic anemia may occur rarely *4995*

Protein *Serum Decrease Physiological* Reversible effect due to urinary loss *3669*
Urine Increase Physiological May have nephrotoxic effect *2585 2451*

Urea Nitrogen *Serum Increase Physiological* Nephropathy reported *128*

Trimethaphan

Chromogranin-A *Plasma Decrease Physiological* Selective disruption of sympathetic outflow caused decrease of basal concentration by 25% *5930*

Histamine *Plasma Increase Physiological* Observed with injection associated with anesthesia *3648*

Trimethobenzamide

Amphetamine *Urine Positive Analytical* In an RIA method for amphetamine/methamphetamine positive reaction observed not seen with GC-MS but false positive results also obtained with Abbott FPIA and Syva EMIT methods *2975*

Bilirubin *Serum Increase Physiological* Rare cases of jaundice reported *2754* Jaundice reported as a complication of treatment *4984*

Trimethoprim

Alanine Aminotransferase *Serum Increase Physiological* Increased activity reported with administration *5036*
Serum No Effect Analytical No effect at 18 mg/L on Boehringer Mannheim Reflotron method *5706* No effect at therapeutic concentration on Boehringer Mannheim Reflotron method *3231*

Albumin *Serum Decrease Physiological* In 7 patients with HIV infection treatment with trimethoprim-sulfamethoxazole caused nonsignificant mean decrease of 0.6 g/L at time of peak hyperkalemia from mean baseline of 29.8 ± 1.3 g/L *2309*
Urine No Effect Analytical At concentration of 20 mg/dL no significant effect observed on Boehringer Mannheim Tina-quant method *2799*

Alkaline Phosphatase *Serum Increase Physiological* Transient increase in the absence of abnormal liver function tests in two patients when drug combined with sulfamethoxazole *1402*

Amylase *Serum No Effect Analytical* Concentrations up to 18 mg/L had no effect on method on Boehringer Mannheim Reflotron system *5706*

Amylase, Pancreatic Isoenzyme
Serum No Effect Analytical No significant effect observed at a toxic concentration of 20 mg/L with method on Boehringer Mannheim Reflotron *3647*

Anion Gap *Serum No Effect Physiological* In 105 patients with various infections 80 were treated with trimethoprim 320 mg/d and sulfamethoxazole 1600 mg/d. No significant change observed in anion gap *82*

Aspartate Aminotransferase *Serum Increase Physiological* Increased activity reported with administration *5036*
Serum No Effect Analytical No effect at 18 mg/L on Boehringer Mannheim Reflotron method *5706* No effect at therapeutic concentration on Boehringer Mannheim Reflotron method *3231*

Bicarbonate *Serum Decrease Physiological* In 25 patients with HIV infection treatment with trimethoprim-sulfamethoxazole mean concentration decreased by 0.6 mol/L from mean baseline of 22.9 ± 0.6 mmol/L at time of peak hyperkalemia *2309*
Serum No Effect Physiological In 105 patients with various infections 80 were treated with trimethoprim 320 mg/d and sulfamethoxazole 1600 mg/d. No significant change observed in bicarbonate concentration *82*

Bilirubin *Serum Increase Physiological* Increased activity reported with administration *5036*
Serum No Effect Analytical At concentration of 18 mg/L no effect on method on Boehringer Mannheim Reflotron system *5706* No effect at 50 mg/L on Ames Seralyzer method *5706*
Serum No Effect Physiological No clinically significant displacement from protein likely at pharmacological concentrations in neonates *6314*

Cephalothin *Serum Increase Analytical* Cannot be assayed by HPLC method used at Mayo Clinic in presence of trimethoprim *3858*

Chloramphenicol *Serum No Effect Analytical* No effect at 100 mg/L on coupled enzymatic method *4122*

Chloride *Serum Decrease Physiological* In 25 patients with HIV infection when treated with trimethoprim-sulfamethoxazole at time of peak hyperkalemia mean concentration decreased by 3.2 mmol/L from mean baseline of 101 ± 0.7 mmol/L *2309*
Serum No Effect Physiological In 105 patients with various infections 80 were treated with trimethoprim 320 mg/d and sulfamethoxazole 1600 mg/d. No significant change observed in chloride concentration *82*

Chlorpropamide *Serum Increase Physiological* May potentiate action by effects on metabolism *1070*

Cholesterol *Serum No Effect Analytical* No effect at 50 mg/L on Ames Seralyzer method *5706* At concentration of 18 mg/L no effect on method on Boehringer Mannheim Reflotron system *5706* No effect at therapeutic concentration on Boehringer Mannheim Reflotron method *3231*
Serum No Effect Physiological In 7 patients with HIV infection treated with trimethoprim-sulfamethoxazole mean concentration increased insignificantly by 0.1 mmol/L at time of peak hyperkalemia from mean baseline of 3.42 ± 0.5 mmol/L *2309*

Cholinesterase *Serum No Effect Analytical* No effect observed at concentration of 25 µg/mL with butyrylthiocholine method on Kodak Ektachem® *2504*

Clindamycin *Serum Positive Analytical* Interferes with bioassays *3858*

Colistin *Serum Positive Analytical* Interferes with bioassays *3858*

Cortisol *Plasma No Effect Analytical* At a concentration of 20 mg/L no significant effect observed on CEDIA or Enzymun methods *1097*

Creatine Kinase *Serum Increase Physiological* In 13 patients with HIV infection treatment with trimethoprim-sulfamethoxazole caused nonsignificant mean increase of 838 nmol/s/L at time of peak hyperkalemia from mean baseline of 1040 ± 277 nmol/s/L *2309*
Serum No Effect Analytical No effect at 50 mg/L on method on Ames Seralyzer *5706*

Creatinine *Serum Increase Analytical* May interfere with methods to measure methotrexate when Jaffe alkaline picrate reaction used, causing serum concentrations in normal range to be overestimated by about 10% *2162*
Serum Increase Physiological In 25 patients with HIV infection concentration increased by mean 28.3 µmol/L from baseline of 84.8 ± 6.4 µmol/L when treated with trimethoprim-sulfamethoxazole at time of peak hyperkalemia *2309* Increased concentration may occur as a complication of treatment *2162* In 105 patients with various infections 80 were treated with trimethoprim 320 mg/d and sulfamethoxazole 1600 mg/d. Serum urea nitrogen increased nonsignificantly from 102.5 ± 49.5 µmol/L to 126.1 ± 70.7 µmol/L 4.6 ± 2.2 days after treatment started *82* Due to co-trimoxazole component, but effect is slight *5136* In elderly increased by more than 50% and by 20% in young males. Tubular secretion affected *3059*

Trimethoprim *(continued)*

Creatinine *(continued)*
Increase by 0.2 mg/dL in 21 patients when given with sulfamethoxazole; also when given by itself; probably due to competitive inhibition of tubular secretion mechanism *505*
Serum No Effect Analytical At concentration of 5 mg/L had no effect on Technicon AutoAnalyzer® Jaffe method *5704* No effect at 50 mg/L on method on Ames Seralyzer *5706* At concentration of 5 mg/L had no effect on kinetic Jaffe method *5704* On Jaffe reaction with alkaline picrate *505*

Crystals *Urine Increase Physiological* May occur with high doses especially if severe renal insufficiency *1070*

Cyclosporine *Blood No Effect Analytical* At a concentration of 20 mg/L had no effect on Syva EMIT method *495*
Serum Decrease Physiological Marked reduction when drug given with sulfadimidine i.v. due to effect on hepatic metabolism *1075*
Serum Increase Physiological Reversible deterioration of renal function with effect on tubular function and nephrotoxicity *6288*

Dapsone *Serum Increase Physiological* When coadministered with dapsone (100 mg/d) trimethoprim (3 mg/kg/q6 h) on day 7 dapsone concentration averaged 2.1 ± 1.0 µg/mL compared with 1.5 ± 0.5 µg/mL when dapsone given alone and trimethoprim concentration averaged 18.4 ± 5.2 µg/mL compared with 12.4 ± 4.5 µg/mL when given alone *2873* Increased concentration observed when drugs coadministered in patients with AIDS *1384*

Digoxin *Serum Increase Physiological* Tubular secretion reduced with increase in serum concentration as a consequence *4634*

D-Lactate *Urine Decrease Physiological* In one patient receiving trimethoprim-sulfamethoxazole on admission to hospital D-lactate concentration 21.9 mmol/L compared with reference interval of 0 - 0.25 mmol/L *1137*

EDTA Clearance *Urine No Effect Physiological* True glomerular filtration rate not affected by drug *3059*

Erythrocyte Sedimentation Rate
Blood Decrease Physiological With sulfa caused marked decrease in rheumatoids *3015*

Erythrocytes *Blood Decrease Physiological* Folic acid antagonist. ?megaloblastic anemia *6370* Isolated case when drug given alone, but clear evidence of pancytopenia. Megaloblastic anemia may occur with prolonged use *5489*

Erythromycin *Serum Increase Analytical* Interferes with bioassays *3858*

Folate *Red Blood Cells Decrease Physiological* Reported association with megaloblastic anemia by inhibiting dihydrofolate reductase although other reports dispute drug as cause of megaloblastic anemia *3383*
Serum Decrease Physiological Reported association with megaloblastic anemia by inhibiting dihydrofolate reductase although other reports dispute drug as cause of megaloblastic anemia *3383* Usually prescribed with sulfa drugs: no hematological abnormality observed *4691*

Glucose *Serum No Effect Analytical* No effect at therapeutic concentration on Boehringer Mannheim Reflotron method *3231* No effect at 50 mg/L on glucose oxidase method on Ames Seralyzer *5706* At concentration of 18 mg/L no effect on method on Boehringer Mannheim Reflotron system *5706*
Urine No Effect Analytical At concentration of 500 mg/L had no effect on Diabur-test *5704*

γ-Glutamyltransferase *Serum No Effect Analytical* No effect at therapeutic concentration on Boehringer Mannheim Reflotron method *3231* At concentration of 18 mg/L no effect on method on Boehringer Mannheim Reflotron system *5706*

HDL-Cholesterol *Serum No Effect Analytical* At a concentration up to 18 mg/L had no significant effect on Reflotron method for whole blood cholesterol *6352*

Hematocrit *Blood Decrease Physiological* Megaloblastic anemia reported with administration *5036* Megaloblastic anemia may occur as a complication of treatment *2162* Folic acid antagonist ?megaloblastic anemia *6370*

Hemoglobin *Blood Decrease Physiological* Megaloblastic anemia reported with administration *5036* Megaloblastic anemia may occur as a complication of treatment *2162* Folic acid antagonist. ?megaloblastic anemia *6370* Isolated case when drug given alone, but clear evidence of pancytopenia. Megaloblastic anemia may occur with prolonged use *5489*
Blood No Effect Physiological In 25 patients with HIV infection treatment with trimethoprim-sulfamethoxazole caused non-significant increase of 0.17 mmol/L at time of peak hyperkalemia from mean baseline of 6.96 ± 0.25 mmol/L *2309*

Histamine *Plasma No Effect Analytical* Minimal inhibition of radio-enzyme assay at more than 10 times therapeutic concentration *2492*

Indinavir *Serum No Effect Physiological* Administration of indinavir 400 mg every 6 hours with trimethoprim/sulfamethoxazole (one double strength tablet every 12 hours) for 1 week resulted in no change in indinavir AUC, a 19 ± 31% increase in trimethoprim AUC and no change in sulfamethoxazole AUC *3966*

Lactate Dehydrogenase *Serum No Effect Analytical* No effect at 50 mg/L on method on Ames Seralyzer *5706*
Serum No Effect Physiological In 6 patients with HIV infection treatment with trimethoprim-sulfamethoxazole caused non-significant increase of activity by 158 nmol/s/L at time of peak hyperkalemia from mean baseline of 7560 ± 1100 nmol/s/L *2309*

Lamivudine *Serum Increase Physiological* Coadministration of trimethoprim/sulfamethoxazole (TMP 160 mg/SMX 800 mg) once daily for 5 days with 300 mg lamivudine caused a significant 44 ± 23% increase in the AUC of lamivudine and a decrease of 30 ± 36% in its renal clearance, although the pharmacokinetic properties of trimethoprim and sulfamethoxazole were not affected *2174*

Leukocytes *Blood Decrease Physiological* Leukopenia reported with administration *5036* Isolated case when drug given alone, but clear evidence of pancytopenia. Megaloblastic anemia may occur with prolonged use *5489* Leukopenia may occur as a complication of treatment *2162*

MCV *Blood Increase Physiological* Megaloblastic anemia may occur as a complication of treatment *2162* Occurs with megaloblastic anemia *6370*

Methemoglobin *Blood Decrease Physiological* Methemoglobinemia may occur as a complication of treatment *2162* Methemoglobinemia reported with administration *5036*

Methotrexate *Serum Increase Analytical* May interfere with competitive binding protein binding techniques when a bacterial dihydrofolate reductase is used as the binding protein *2162*
Serum No Effect Analytical Does not interfere when RIA is used to measure methotrexate *2162* No significant interference observed at a concentration of 100 µmol/L with method on Du Pont aca *1535*

Metronidazole *Serum Increase Analytical* Interferes with bioassays *3858*

Mycophenolate *Serum No Effect Physiological* Coadministration of single doses of mycophenolate mofentil (1.5 g) with trimethoprim/sulfamethoxazole in 12 healthy male volunteers no effect on the bioavailability of mycophenolate was observed *5017*

N-Acetyl-Glucosaminidase *Urine No Effect Analytical* At concentration of 20 mg/dL had no significant effect on Boehringer Mannheim CPR method *3174*

N-Acetylprocainamide *Serum Increase Physiological* Concentration increased because of decreased renal clearance *1384*

Neutrophils *Blood Decrease Physiological* Occasional cases of neutropenia reported *241* Observed at least once in 57% of 49 children given trimethoprim-sulfamethoxazole over 10 day treatment period *1829* Neutropenia reported with administration *5036* Neutropenia may occur as a complication of treatment *2162*

5'-Nucleotidase *Serum Increase Physiological* Transient increase in the absence of abnormal liver function tests in two patients when drug combined with sulfamethoxazole *1402*

pH *Blood Decrease Physiological* In one patient receiving trimethoprim-sulfamethoxazole on admission to hospital D-lactate concentration 21.9 mmol/L compared with reference interval of 0 - 0.25 mmol/L and blood pH 7.37 reflecting mild lactate acidosis *1137*

Blood *No Effect* *Physiological* In 13 patients with HIV infection treatment with trimethoprim-sulfamethoxazole caused non-significant decrease of 0.01 at time of peak hyperkalemia from mean baseline of 7.48 ± 0.01 *2309*

Phenylalanine *Plasma* *No Effect* *Analytical* No interference observed with rapid quantitative whole blood method of Campbell et al using phenylalanine dehydrogenase *867*

Phenytoin *Serum* *Increase* *Physiological* May potentiate action by effects on metabolism *1070* Significant increase in concentration when drugs coadministered *1384* Coadministration of trimethoprim with phenytoin caused considerable increase in the half-life of phenytoin due to inhibition of its hepatic metabolism *2440* May inhibit the hepatic metabolism of phenytoin. At clinical dose of trimethoprim increased the phenytoin half-life by 51% and decreased the phenytoin metabolic clearance rate by 30% *2162*

Phenytoin, Free *Serum* *Increase* *Physiological* In vivo, in presence of bactrim, concentration of free phenytoin increased from calculated value of 2.7-9.6 μmol/L to 3.1-11.5 μmol/L in 5 patients treated with both phenytoin and bactrim *1242*

Platelets *Blood* *Decrease* *Physiological* Thrombocytopenia may occur as a complication of treatment *2162* Thrombocytopenia reported with administration *5036* Isolated case when drug given alone, but clear evidence of pancytopenia. Megaloblastic anemia may occur with prolonged use *5489* Most common serious toxic effect *4894*

Polymyxin *Serum* *Increase* *Analytical* Interferes with bioassays *3858*

Potassium *Serum* *Decrease* *Physiological* Hypokalemia may occur as a complication of treatment *2162*

Serum *Increase* *Physiological* Hyperkalemia observed in 20 - 53% patients with AIDS with high dose treatment with trimethoprim-sulfamethoxazole for Pneumocystis carnii pneumonia. Trimethoprim has an amiloride-like effect on the distal nephron which is probably responsible for the hyperkalemia *3930* In 30 patients with AIDS treatment with 20 mg/kg/d increased mean serum potassium by 0.6 mmol/L *6222* In 105 patients with various infections 80 were treated with trimethoprim 320 mg/d and sulfamethoxazole 1600 mg/d. Serum potassium increased by 1.21 mmol/L from 3.89 ± 0.46 mmol/L to 5.1 ± 0.56 mmol/L 4.6 ± 2.2 days after treatment started *82* In 25 patients with HIV infection taking high dose trimethoprim-sulfamethoxazole had significant increase by mean 1.1 mmol/L from mean baseline of 4.1 ± 0.1 mmol/L 9.8 ± 0.5 days after starting treatment with progressive increase with continuing treatment and decline after cessation *2309* In a woman with transplanted lungs a potassium concentration of 6.8 mmol/L was observed with high dose treatment with trimethoprim-sulfamethoxazole for Pneumocystis carnii pneumonia. She was concomitantly receiving enalapril. Combination of ACE inhibition and potassium-sparing diuretics (trimethoprim has an amiloride-like effect on the distal nephron) is known to cause hyperkalemia *800* In patients with AIDS high dose trimethoprim-sulfamethoxazole has been associated with hyperkalemia, attributable to trimethoprim acting like the potassium sparing diuretic amiloride with a reduction in potassium excretion *4601*

Urine *Decrease* *Physiological* In patients with AIDS high dose trimethoprim-sulfamethoxazole has been associated with hyperkalemia, attributable to trimethoprim acting like the potassium sparing diuretic amiloride with a reduction in potassium excretion *4601*

Procainamide *Serum* *Increase* *Physiological* Decreased mean clearance of procainamide by 45% and clearance of N-acetylprocainamide by 26% with increase of area under curve of both compounds from 0 to 12 hours after dosing increased by 39% and 27% respectively *6273* Administration of trimethoprim with procainamide led to plasma procainamide concentrations greater than those with procainamide alone *4530* Increases concentration and its major metabolite by decreasing renal clearance *1384* Increased area under curve of procainamide by 63% and of NAPA by 52% with decreases of renal clearances by 47% and 13% respectively, with 39% increase in urinary recovery of NAPA in 8 healthy men given both trimethoprim and procainamide *3256*

Prostate-specific Antigen, Free *Serum* *No Effect* *Analytical* Trimethoprim/sulfamethoxazole at a concentration of 9.7 mg/L had no significant effect on the Hybritech Tandem® -R free PSA immunoassay *4286*

Prothrombin Time *Plasma* *Increase* *Physiological* In patients receiving warfarin increased INR observed *886* When given with warfarin and sulfamethoxazole causes stereoselective inhibition of clearance of S isomer of warfarin *2625*

Sodium *Serum* *Decrease* *Physiological* Impairs free water clearance: effect noted when combined with diuretic *1645* Hyponatremia may occur as a complication of treatment *2162* In 25 patients with HIV infection mean concentration decreased by 4.0 mmol/L at time of peak hyperkalemia from mean baseline of 137 ± 0.7 mmol/L when treated with trimethoprim-sulfamethoxazole *2309*

Serum *No Effect* *Physiological* In 105 patients with various infections 80 were treated with trimethoprim 320 mg/d and sulfamethoxazole 1600 mg/d. No significant change observed in sodium concentration *82*

Urine *Increase* *Physiological* Impairs free water clearance: effect noted when combined with diuretic *1645*

Tacrolimus *Serum* *No Effect* *Analytical* In HPLC/MS method of Christians et al no significant interference observed with measurement of FK 506 *1010*

Tetracycline *Serum* *Increase* *Analytical* Interferes with bioassays *3858*

Tolbutamide *Serum* *Increase* *Physiological* May potentiate action by effects on metabolism *1070*

Triglycerides *Serum* *No Effect* *Analytical* No effect at therapeutic concentration on Boehringer Mannheim Reflotron method *3231* No effect at 18 mg/L on Boehringer Mannheim Reflotron method *5706*

Urea Nitrogen *Serum* *Increase* *Physiological* Increased concentration may occur as a complication of treatment *2162* In 105 patients with various infections 80 were treated with trimethoprim 320 mg/d and sulfamethoxazole 1600 mg/d. Serum urea nitrogen increased nonsignificantly from 7.92 ± 5.7 mmol/L to 9.2 ± 5.8 mmol/L 4.6 ± 2.2 days after treatment started *82* In 25 patients with HIV infection treatment with high doses caused mild increase from 4.3 ± 0.5 mmol/L to 6.4 ± 0.7 mmol/L 7 to 10 days after start of treatment *2309*

Serum *No Effect* *Analytical* No effect at 18 mg/L on Boehringer Mannheim Reflotron method *5706* No effect at 50 mg/L on method on Ames Seralyzer *5706* No effect at therapeutic concentration on Boehringer Mannheim Reflotron method *3231*

Uric Acid *Serum* *No Effect* *Analytical* No effect at therapeutic concentration on Boehringer Mannheim Reflotron method *3231* No effect at 18 mg/L on Boehringer Mannheim Reflotron method *5706*

Vancomycin *Serum* *No Effect* *Analytical* No significant interference observed at a concentration of 25 μg/mL (86 μmol/L) with method on Du Pont aca *1561*

Warfarin *Plasma* *Increase* *Physiological* May potentiate action by effects on metabolism *1070*

Zidovudine *Serum* *No Effect* *Analytical* No effect on liquid chromatographic method of Hedaya and Sawchuk *2525*

Trimetozine

Glucose *Urine* *Increase* *Analytical* False positive with glucose oxidase (Combistix®) reported *1047*

Urine *Increase* *Physiological* Hyperglycemia reported in one patient *2452*

Sugar *Urine* *Increase* *Analytical* Interferes with Benedict's reagent *1714*

Trimetrexate

Alanine Aminotransferase *Serum* *Increase* *Physiological* Transient effect in small proportion of patients although reverted to normal with continued treatment *107* Activity greater than 5 times the upper limit of normal observed in 12 (11.0%) of 109 patients treated with trimetrexate and leucovorin *6138* Transient increases commonly observed *1384*

Alkaline Phosphatase *Serum* *Increase* *Physiological* Activity greater than 5 times the upper limit of normal observed in 5 (4.6%) of 109 patients treated with trimetrexate and leucovorin *6138*

Aspartate Aminotransferase *Serum* *Increase* *Physiological* Transient effect in small proportion of patients although

Trimetrexate *(continued)*

Aspartate Aminotransferase *(continued)*
reverted to normal with continued treatment *107* Activity greater than 5 times the upper limit of normal observed in 15 (13.8%) of 109 patients treated with trimetrexate and leucovorin *6138* Transient increases commonly observed *1384*

Bilirubin *Serum Increase Physiological* Transient effect in small proportion of patients although reverted to normal with continued treatment *107* Concentration greater than 2.5 times the upper limit of normal observed in 2 (1.8%) of 109 patients treated with trimetrexate and leucovorin *6138*

Calcium *Serum Decrease Physiological* Hypocalcemia observed in 2 (1.8%) of 109 patients treated with trimetrexate and leucovorin *6138*

Creatinine *Serum Increase Physiological* Concentration greater than 3 times the upper limit of normal observed in 1 (0.9%) of 109 patients treated with trimetrexate and leucovorin *6138* Nephrotoxicity reported in some patients following treatment, possibly associated with prior reduced renal function *2631*

Creatinine Clearance *Urine Decrease Physiological* Nephrotoxicity reported in some patients following treatment, possibly associated with prior reduced renal function *2631*

Hemoglobin *Blood Decrease Physiological* Anemia occurs occasionally *1384* Anemia with hemoglobin less than 8 g/dL observed in 8 (7.5%) of 109 patients treated with trimetrexate and leucovorin *6138*

Leukocytes *Blood Decrease Physiological* Myelosuppression is dose-limiting toxicity but with thrombocytopenia in excess of neutropenia *1384*

Neutrophils *Blood Decrease Physiological* Neutropenia in from 6 to 30% patients given different regimes *107* Neutropenia of less than 1000 cells/µL observed in 33 (30.3%) of 109 patients treated with trimetrexate and leucovorin *6138*

Platelets *Blood Decrease Physiological* Thrombocytopenia of less than 75,000 cells/µL observed in 11 (10.1%) of 109 patients treated with trimetrexate and leucovorin *6138* Myelosuppression is dose-limiting toxicity with thrombocytopenia in excess of neutropenia *1384*

Sodium *Serum Decrease Physiological* Hyponatremia observed in 5 (4.6%) of 109 patients treated with trimetrexate and leucovorin *6138*

Urea Nitrogen *Serum Increase Physiological* Nephrotoxicity reported in some patients following treatment, possibly associated with prior reduced renal function *2631*

Uric Acid *Serum Increase Physiological* Nephrotoxicity reported in some patients following treatment, possibly associated with prior reduced renal function *2631*

Trimipramine

Alanine Aminotransferase *Serum Increase Physiological* Altered liver function with jaundice, simulating obstructive, may occur with treatment *6571*

Albumin *Urine No Effect Analytical* Using a fluorimetric assay with Albumin Blue 580 on a Cobas Fara centrifugal analyzer for the detection of microalbuminuria no significant interference was detected at a concentration of 20 mg/L *3117*

Alkaline Phosphatase *Serum Increase Physiological* Altered liver function with jaundice, simulating obstructive, may occur with treatment *6571*

Aspartate Aminotransferase *Serum Increase Physiological* Altered liver function with jaundice, simulating obstructive, may occur with treatment *6571*

Bilirubin *Serum Increase Physiological* Altered liver function with jaundice, simulating obstructive, may occur with treatment *6571*

Cortisol *Plasma Decrease Physiological* After a single oral dose of 75 mg mean decrease of cortisol concentration observed at 3 hours from baseline of 117 to 43 µg/L in 8 healthy volunteers *6442* Marked decrease of nocturnal concentration in 3 men after 200 mg drug. Delayed early morning rise also noted *5792*

Eosinophils *Blood Increase Physiological* Bone marrow depression may occur with eosinophilia *6571*

Follicle Stimulating Hormone
Plasma No Effect Physiological Nocturnal secretion not affected in 3 men given single dose of 200 mg *5792*

Glucose *Serum Decrease Physiological* Hypoglycemia or hyperglycemia may occur with treatment *6571*
Serum Increase Physiological Hyperglycemia or hypoglycemia may occur with treatment *6571*

Granulocytes *Blood Decrease Physiological* Bone marrow depression may occur with agranulocytosis *6571*

Growth Hormone *Plasma No Effect Physiological* Nocturnal secretion not affected by dose of 200 mg *5792* No significant effect on concentration in 8 volunteers 3 hours after single oral dose of 75 mg *6442*

Luteinizing Hormone *Plasma No Effect Physiological* Nocturnal secretion in 3 men not affected by administration of 200 mg drug *5792*

Platelets *Blood Decrease Physiological* Bone marrow depression may occur with thrombocytopenia and purpura *6571*

Prolactin *Plasma Increase Physiological* Nocturnal concentration increased in 3 men following 200 mg drug but concentration reverted to normal with withdrawal *5792* After single oral dose of 75 mg mean increase observed at 3 hours in 8 healthy volunteers was to 16.3 µg/L from baseline of 6 µg/L *6442*

Testosterone *Serum No Effect Physiological* Nocturnal secretion not affected by administration of 200 mg *5792*

Trinitrotoluene

Color *Urine Increase Analytical* Red brown due to hemoglobin *3810*

Erythrocytes *Blood Decrease Physiological* May cause hemolysis *4017* May cause hemolysis with G-6-PD deficiency *2349*
Urine Increase Physiological May cause hemolysis *3810*

Hematocrit *Blood Decrease Physiological* May cause hemolysis *4017*

Hemoglobin *Blood Decrease Physiological* May cause hemolysis with G-6-PD deficiency *2349*
Urine Increase Physiological May cause hemolysis *3810*

Methemoglobin *Blood Increase Physiological* Associated with hemolysis *4017*

Sulfhemoglobin *Blood Increase Physiological* Associated with methemoglobinemia and hemolysis *4017*

Trioxsalen

Alanine Aminotransferase *Serum Increase Physiological* May affect liver function *3810*

Alkaline Phosphatase *Serum Increase Physiological* May affect liver function *3810*

Aspartate Aminotransferase *Serum Increase Physiological* May affect liver function *3810*

Bile *Urine Increase Physiological* May affect liver function *3810*

Bilirubin *Serum Increase Physiological* May affect liver function *3810*

BSP Retention *Serum Increase Physiological* May affect liver function *3810*

Histamine *Plasma No Effect Analytical* Improbable inhibition of radio-enzyme assay at therapeutic concentrations *2492*

Tripamide

Glucose *Serum No Effect Physiological* No effect in hypertensives with or without diabetes *1115*

Glucose Tolerance *Serum No Effect Physiological* No effect in hypertensives with or without diabetes *1115*

Insulin *Plasma No Effect Physiological* No effect in hypertensives with or without diabetes *1115*

Tripelennamine

Alanine Aminotransferase *Serum No Effect Analytical* At acute overdose concentration (20 mg/dL) on Technicon SMAC® methods *6266*

Albumin *Serum No Effect Analytical* At acute overdose concentration (20 mg/dL) on Technicon SMAC® methods *6266* At concentration of 200 mg/L had no effect on BCG method *5704*

Alkaline Phosphatase *Serum No Effect Analytical* At acute overdose concentration (20 mg/dL) on Technicon SMAC® methods *6266*

Aspartate Aminotransferase *Serum No Effect Analytical* At acute overdose concentration (20 mg/dL) on Technicon SMAC® methods *6266*

Bilirubin *Serum No Effect Analytical* At concentration of 200 mg/L had no effect on Jendrassik and Grof method *5704* At acute overdose concentration (20 mg/dL) on Technicon SMAC® methods *6266*

Calcium *Serum No Effect Analytical* At acute overdose concentration (20 mg/dL) on Technicon SMAC® methods *6266* At concentration of 200 mg/L had no effect on cresolphthalein method *5704*

Cholesterol *Serum No Effect Analytical* At acute overdose concentration (20 mg/dL) on Technicon SMAC® methods *6266* At concentration of 200 mg/L had no effect on Liebermann-Burchard method *5704*

Creatine Kinase *Serum No Effect Analytical* At acute overdose concentration (20 mg/dL) on Technicon SMAC® methods *6266*

Creatinine *Serum No Effect Analytical* At acute overdose concentration (20 mg/dL) on Technicon SMAC® methods *6266* At concentration of 200 mg/L had no effect on Technicon AutoAnalyzer® Jaffe method *5704*

Erythrocytes *Blood Decrease Physiological* Hemolytic anemia may occur as adverse reaction *1041* Hemolytic anemia *4014*

Glucose *Serum Decrease Physiological* Reported effect *192*
Serum No Effect Analytical At acute overdose concentration (20 mg/dL) on Technicon SMAC® method *6266*

Granulocytes *Blood Decrease Physiological* Agranulocytosis or aplastic anemia may occur as adverse reaction *1041*

Haptoglobin *Serum Decrease Physiological* Hemolytic anemia *1212*

Hematocrit *Blood Decrease Physiological* Hemolytic anemia *1212*

Hemoglobin *Blood Decrease Physiological* Hemolytic anemia *1212* Hemolytic or aplastic anemia may occur as adverse reaction *1041*

Iron *Serum No Effect Analytical* At concentration of 200 mg/L had no effect on Ferrozine method *5704* At acute overdose concentration (20 mg/dL) on Technicon SMAC® methods *6266*

Lactate Dehydrogenase *Serum No Effect Analytical* At acute overdose concentration (20 mg/dL) on Technicon SMAC® methods *6266*

Leukocytes *Blood Decrease Physiological* Agranulocytosis/Leukopenia (rare) *6044* May occur as adverse reaction *1041*

p-Aminophenol *Urine No Effect Analytical* With addition of drugs at a concentration of 100 mg/L and of related compounds at 50 mg/L no significant effect observed on colorimetric method of van Bocxlaer on Cobas Mira analyzer which involves reacting free p-aminophenol with resorcinol in the presence of magnesium ions to form an indophenol dye measured at 550 nm *6163*

Phosphate *Serum No Effect Analytical* At acute overdose concentration (20 mg/dL) on Technicon SMAC® methods *6266* At concentration of 200 mg/L had no effect on phosphomolybdate method *5704*

Platelets *Blood Decrease Physiological* Selective thrombocytopenia or aplastic anemia *2385* Thrombocytopenia or aplastic anemia may occur as adverse reaction *1041*

Protein *Serum No Effect Analytical* At concentration of 200 mg/L had no effect on biuret method with blank correction *5704* At acute overdose concentration (20 mg/dL) on Technicon SMAC® methods *6266*

Triglycerides *Serum No Effect Analytical* At concentration of 200 mg/L had no effect on lipase/esterase method *5704* At acute overdose concentration (20 mg/dL) on Technicon SMAC® methods *6266*

Urea Nitrogen *Serum No Effect Analytical* At acute overdose concentration (20 mg/dL) on Technicon SMAC® methods *6266* At concentration of 200 mg/L had no effect on diacetylmonoxime method *5704*

Uric Acid *Serum No Effect Analytical* At acute overdose concentration (20 mg/dL) on Technicon SMAC® methods *6266* At concentration of 200 mg/L had no effect on phosphotungstate reduction method *5704*

Triple Bromides

Bicarbonate *Serum Increase Analytical* Significant effect on method on Kodak Ektachem® , whereas no effect on method on Beckman Astra® 8 *3233*

Chloride *Serum Increase Analytical* Significant effect on method on Kodak Ektachem® , with minor effect on Beckman Astra® 8 *3233*

Triprolidine

Amino Acids *Urine Increase Analytical* Red spot with ninhydrin on thin-layer chromatography when combined with pseudoephedrine in Actifed® *2109*

Tris (2-Butoxyethyl) Phosphate (TBEP)

Lidocaine *Serum Decrease Analytical* By up to 17% at 12.7 µmol/L when used as plasticizer in evacuated blood tubes *1401*

Quinidine *Serum Decrease Analytical* By up to 32% at 4.4 µmol/L when used as plasticizer in evaluated blood tubes *1401*

Trisodium Phosphonoformate

Hepatitis B Virus DNA *Serum Decrease Physiological* In 8 male patients with chronic persistent or chronic active hepatitis concentration fell with treatment with continuous infusion of 0.15 mg/kg/min for 7 days or 180 mg/kg/day for 3 days over 2 weeks. Mean reduction from 533 pg/40 µL to 401 pg/40 µL *330*

Troglitazone

Acetaminophen *Serum No Effect Physiological* Coadministration of acetaminophen with troglitazone had no significant effect on the concentration of either drug *4532*

Alanine Aminotransferase *Serum Increase Physiological* During troglitazone treatment of 2510 type II diabetics during North American clinical trials typically for 6 months increased ALT activity (more than 3 times the upper limit of normal) observed in 48 (1.9%) compared with 0.6% of placebo treated controls *6362* In 2510 patients receiving troglitazone 20 were withdrawn from treatment because of liver function test abnormalities. Two were shown to have idiosyncratic drug reactions *4532*

Alkaline Phosphatase *Serum Increase Physiological* In 2510 patients receiving troglitazone 20 were withdrawn from treatment because of liver function test abnormalities. Two were shown to have idiosyncratic drug reactions *4532*

Apolipoprotein B *Serum No Effect Physiological* Following treatment with troglitazone no change in concentration observed although increases observed in total cholesterol and LDL-cholesterol concentrations *4532*

Aspartate Aminotransferase *Serum Increase Physiological* In 2510 patients receiving troglitazone 20 were withdrawn from treatment because of liver function test abnormalities. Two were shown to have idiosyncratic drug reactions *4532*

Troglitazone *(continued)*

Cholesterol *Serum Increase Physiological* In 350 patients with poorly controlled non-insulin dependent diabetes mellitus despite treatment with at least 30 units of insulin daily, treatment with insulin and 200 mg/d troglitazone for 26 weeks caused an increase of the cholesterol concentration from 217 ± 38 mg/dL to 224 ± 45 mg/dL: treatment with 600 mg/d caused an increase from 208 ± 40 mg/dL to 220 ± 52 mg/dL *5404* Following treatment with troglitazone concentration increases *4532*

Cholesterol:HDL-Cholesterol Ratio
Serum No Effect Physiological Following treatment with troglitazone no change in ratio observed *4532*

Creatine Kinase *Serum Increase Physiological* Following treatment with troglitazone some patients observed to have increased activity in postintroduction reports *4532*

Digoxin *Serum No Effect Physiological* In 12 healthy individuals treatment with 400 mg/d troglitazone together with digoxin 0.25 mg/d digoxin caused nonsignificant change in maximum plasma concentration , AUC, and total urinary excretion of digoxin (146 mL/min to 154 mL/min) *3637*

Ethinyl Estradiol *Serum Decrease Physiological* In women taking oral contraceptives containing ethinyl estradiol and norethindrone coadministration of troglitazone caused reduction of approximately 30% in the concentration of both steroids *4532*

Glucagon *Plasma Decrease Physiological* In 12 obese individuals treated with 400 mg/d for 12 weeks mean concentration changed nonsignificantly from 144 ± 52 ng/L to 132 ± 64 ng/L *4314*

Glucose *Serum Decrease Physiological* In 12 obese individuals treated with 400 mg/d for 12 weeks mean concentration changed significantly from 99 ± 4 mg/dL to 95 ± 4 mg/dL *4314* In 350 patients with poorly controlled non-insulin dependent diabetes mellitus despite treatment with at least 30 units of insulin daily, treatment with insulin and 200 mg/d troglitazone for 26 weeks caused a reduction of glucose concentration of 35 mg/dL: treatment with 600 mg/d caused reduction of 49 mg/dL, whereas treatment with placebo caused an increase of 0.8 mg/dL *5404* During troglitazone treatment of 14 type II diabetics for 3 months blood glucose concentration decreased by 4.8 mmol/L (25%) *2827* In patients receiving troglitazone together with insulin potential for hypoglycemia observed although no effect observed when troglitazone given by itself *4532*

Glucose Tolerance *Serum Increase Physiological* In 12 obese individuals treated with 400 mg/d for 12 weeks mean 2 hour concentration changed significantly from 146 ± 25 mg/dL to 126 ± 17 mg/dL and plasma insulin incremental area under the concentration curve by 40% *4314*

γ-Glutamyltransferase *Serum Increase Physiological* In 2510 patients receiving troglitazone 20 were withdrawn from treatment because of liver function test abnormalities. Two were shown to have idiosyncratic drug reactions *4532*

Glyburide *Serum No Effect Physiological* Coadministration of glyburide with troglitazone had no significant effect on the pharmacokinetics of either drug but may further decrease plasma glucose concentration *4532*

Glycated Hemoglobin *Blood Decrease Physiological* In 350 patients with poorly controlled non-insulin dependent diabetes mellitus despite treatment with at least 30 units of insulin daily, treatment with insulin and 200 mg/d troglitazone for 26 weeks caused a reduction of glycated hemoglobin of 0.8%: treatment with 600 mg/d caused reduction of 1.4%, whereas treatment with placebo caused an decrease of 0.1 *5404*
Blood No Effect Physiological During troglitazone treatment of 15 type II diabetics for 3 months no significant effect observed on glycated hemoglobin concentration *2827*

HDL-Cholesterol *Serum Increase Physiological* Following treatment with troglitazone concentration increases *4532* In 350 patients with poorly controlled non-insulin dependent diabetes mellitus despite treatment with at least 30 units of insulin daily, treatment with insulin and 200 mg/d troglitazone for 26 weeks caused an increase of the HDL-cholesterol concentration from 39 ± 9 mg/dL to 41 ± 10 mg/dL: treatment with 600 mg/d caused an increase from 38 ± 9 mg/dL to 41 ± 11 mg/dL *5404*
Serum No Effect Physiological In 12 obese individuals treated with 400 mg/d for 12 weeks mean concentration changed nonsignificantly from 35 ± 7 mg/dL to 36 ± 7 mg/dL *4314*

HDL-Cholesterol:LDL-Cholesterol Ratio
Serum No Effect Physiological Following treatment with troglitazone no change in ratio observed *4532*

Hemoglobin *Blood Decrease Physiological* In 2510 patients receiving troglitazone hemoglobin decreased by 3 to 4% compared with 1 to 2% in controls, possibly due to increased plasma volume *4532* Following treatment with troglitazone hemoglobin concentration declined by 3 - 4% compared with 1 - 2% in placebo-treated controls during first 4 - 8 weeks of treatment *4532*

Insulin *Plasma Decrease Physiological* In 12 obese individuals treated with 400 mg/d for 12 weeks mean concentration changed significantly from 18 ± 8 μU/mL to 10 ± 4 μU/mL *4314*

LDL-Cholesterol *Serum Increase Physiological* Following treatment with troglitazone concentration increases *4532* In 350 patients with poorly controlled non-insulin dependent diabetes mellitus despite treatment with at least 30 units of insulin daily, treatment with insulin and 200 mg/d troglitazone for 26 weeks caused an increase of the LDL-cholesterol concentration from 135 ± 34 mg/dL to 144 ± 38 mg/dL: treatment with 600 mg/d caused an increase from 125 ± 34 mg/dL to 220 ± 52 mg/dL *5404*
Serum No Effect Physiological In 12 obese individuals treated with 400 mg/d for 12 weeks mean concentration changed nonsignificantly from 113 ± 35 mg/dL to 121 ± 39 mg/dL *4314*

Leukocytes *Blood Decrease Physiological* In 2510 patients receiving troglitazone leukocyte count decreased slightly within the first 4 to 8 weeks of treatment, then stabilized and remained stable for 2 years with continued treatment. Effect might be due to dilutional effect of increased plasma volume *4532*

Norethindrone *Serum Decrease Physiological* In women taking oral contraceptives containing ethinyl estradiol and norethindrone coadministration of troglitazone caused reduction of approximately 30% in the concentration of both steroids *4532*

Prothrombin Time *Plasma No Effect Physiological* Coadministration of troglitazone with warfarin had no significant effect on the plasma prothrombin time *4532*

Terfenadine *Serum Decrease Physiological* Coadministration of terfenadine with troglitazone decreases plasma concentration of terfenadine and its metabolites by 50 to 70% *4532*

Triglycerides *Serum Decrease Physiological* In 350 patients with poorly controlled non-insulin dependent diabetes mellitus despite treatment with at least 30 units of insulin daily, treatment with insulin and 200 mg/d troglitazone for 26 weeks caused an decrease of the triglyceride concentration from 222 ± 112 mg/dL to 209 ± 141 mg/dL: treatment with 600 mg/d caused an decrease from 239 ± 175 mg/dL to 203 ± 150 mg/dL *5404*
Serum No Effect Physiological In 12 obese individuals treated with 400 mg/d for 12 weeks mean concentration changed nonsignificantly from 146 ± 63 mg/dL to 145 ± 62 mg/dL *4314*

Trolamine

ionized Calcium *Serum Decrease Analytical* At concentrations more than 0.1 mmol/L on calcium specific electrode *820* By up to 12% if added to standards *3361*

Troleandomycin

Alanine Aminotransferase *Serum Increase Physiological* In 30% individuals treated with 1 g/d for 3-4 weeks. Jaundice typically occurs after 2 weeks mixed in type with both cholestasis and mild hepatocytic necrosis *4627* In 6 healthy male volunteers activity 78 U/L after 2 g troleandomycin per day for 10 days compared with 30 U/L after placebo *6146*

Alkaline Phosphatase *Serum Increase Physiological* In 6 healthy male volunteers mean activity 191 U/L after 2 g/d for 10 days compared with 170 U/L after placebo *6146*

Aspartate Aminotransferase *Serum Increase Physiological* In 30% individuals treated with 1 g/d for 3-4 weeks. Jaundice typically occurs after 2 weeks mixed in type with both cholestasis and mild hepatocytic necrosis *4627* Mean activity increased to 61 U/L compared with 26 U/L in control period in 6 healthy male volunteers given 2 g troleandomycin per day for 10 days *6146*

Bilirubin *Serum Increase Physiological* Mean concentration 17 μmol/L in 6 healthy male volunteers after 2 g/d troleandomycin for 10 days compared with 13.2 μmol/L after placebo *6146* In 4% individuals treated with 1 g/d for 3-4 weeks. Jaundice typically occurs after 2 weeks mixed in type with both cholestasis and mild hepatocytic necrosis *4627*

BSP Retention *Serum Increase Physiological* In 50% individuals treated with 1 g/d for 3-4 weeks. Jaundice typically occurs after 2 weeks mixed in type with both cholestasis and mild hepatocytic necrosis *4627*

Carbamazepine *Serum Increase Physiological* Forms complexes with cytochrome P-450 and increases plasma concentration of carbamazepine resulting in toxicity *3118* Inhibits hepatic drug metabolism *1384* Due to effect on hepatic metabolism *1384* Concentration increased as result of impaired hepatic metabolism *1493* Drugs that inhibit CYP 3A4 inhibit metabolism of carbamazepine producing clinically meaningful effect *1039*

Cisapride *Serum Increase Physiological* By inhibiting cytochrome P450 3A4 inhibits metabolism of cisapride and increases its plasma concentration *2903*

Cortisol *Plasma No Effect Physiological* Nonsignificant reduction from mean baseline of 428 nmol/L to 372 nmol/L in 6 healthy male volunteers given 2 g/d for 10 days *6146*

Cortisol, Free *Urine Decrease Physiological* Nonsignificant reduction from mean baseline of 159 nmol/d to 104 nmol/d in 6 healthy male volunteers given 2 g/d for 10 days *6146*

Creatinine *Serum No Effect Analytical* At 200 mg/L on reversed phase liquid chromatographic method of Zhiri et al *6656*

Cyclosporine *Serum Increase Physiological* Inhibits hepatic metabolism and increases plasma concentration *1384*

Dehydroepiandrosterone Sulfate
Plasma No Effect Physiological Nonsignificant increase from mean baseline of 10.6 μmol/L to 11.3 μmol/L in 6 healthy male volunteers given 2 g/d for 10 days *6146*

Digoxin *Serum Increase Physiological* When given orally alters gastrointestinal tract flora and prevents inactivation of digoxin *1384*

Disopyramide *Serum Increase Physiological* Inhibits hepatic metabolism *1384*

Estradiol *Plasma Increase Physiological* Significant increase from mean baseline of 110 pmol/L to 143 pmol/L in 6 healthy male volunteers given 2 g/d for 10 days *6146*

Follicle Stimulating Hormone
Plasma No Effect Physiological Nonsignificant increase from mean baseline of 1.66 IU/L to 1.75 IU/L in 6 healthy male volunteers given 2 g/d for 10 days *6146*

γ-Glutamyltransferase *Serum Increase Physiological* Mean activity 32 U/L after 2 g/d for 10 days in 6 healthy male volunteers compared with 15 U/L after placebo *6146*

6-β-Hydroxycortisol *Urine Decrease Physiological* Significant reduction from mean baseline of 472 nmol/d to 301 nmol/d in 6 healthy male volunteers given 2 g/d for 10 days *6146*
Urine Increase Physiological Increased excretion due to hepatic enzyme induction observed in healthy volunteers *6146*

Luteinizing Hormone *Plasma Increase Physiological* Nonsignificant increase from mean baseline of 1.84 IU/L to 2.30 IU/L in 6 healthy male volunteers given 2 g/d for 10 days *6146*

Methylprednisolone *Serum Increase Physiological* Clearance reduced in asthmatic patients when drugs coadministered *1384*

Testosterone, Free *Serum Increase Physiological* Significant increase from mean baseline of 93 pmol/L to 106 pmol/L in 6 healthy male volunteers given 2 g/d for 10 days *6146*

Theophylline *Serum Increase Physiological* Dose-dependent 33 - 100% increase in serum theophylline concentration due to decreased theophylline clearance caused by inhibition of cytochrome P450 3A3 by an erythromycin metabolite *6117* Reduction of about 50% in clearance from plasma probably associated with impaired hepatic metabolism *6386* Troleandomycin metabolite decreases theophylline clearance by inhibiting cytochrome P450 3A3 and increases serum theophylline concentration by 33 to 100% depending on the dose *3125* Metabolite decreases theophylline clearance by inhibiting cytochrome P450 3A3, increasing theophylline concentration by about 33 - 100% depending on troleandomycin dose *5999* Has a steroid-sparing action and also prolongs half-life of theophylline by reducing its clearance *1384*

Thyroid Stimulating Hormone
Serum Decrease Physiological Decreased concentration observed in some healthy volunteers *6146* In 6 healthy male volunteers 2 g troleandomycin per day for 10 days caused decrease from mean of 1.82 mU/L to 1.52 mU/L *6146*

Thyroxine (T4) *Serum No Effect Physiological* In 6 healthy male volunteers 2 g/d for 10 days caused nonsignificant increase from mean of 104 nmol/L to 113 nmol/L *6146*

Thyroxine (T4), Free *Serum No Effect Physiological* Nonsignificant increase from mean of 19.0 pmol/L to 21.4 pmol/L in 6 healthy male volunteers given 2 g/d for 10 days *6146*

Tri-iodothyronine, Free (fT3)
Serum No Effect Physiological Nonsignificant increase from mean baseline of 6.95 pmol/L to 7.40 pmol/L in 6 healthy male volunteers given 2 g/d for 10 days *6146*

Tri-iodothyronine, Reverse (rT3)
Serum No Effect Physiological No change from baseline concentration of 0.45 nmol/L in 6 healthy male volunteers given 2 g/d for 10 days *6146*

Triazolam *Serum Increase Physiological* Inhibits hepatic metabolism *1384*

Uric Acid *Serum No Effect Analytical* At 200 mg/L on reversed phase liquid chromatographic procedure of Zhiri et al *6656*

Warfarin *Plasma Increase Physiological* Inhibits hepatic metabolism and prolongs prothrombin time *1384*

Tromethamine

Amino Acids *Urine Increase Analytical* Peak observed near to or on tyrosine when short-column postcolumn derivitization used with HPLC method. Results likely to be similar regardless whether o-phthaldehyde or ninhydrin used as detection system *714*

Ammonia *Plasma Decrease Analytical* Indophenol color formation (Berthelot reaction) inhibition *4368*

Bicarbonate *Serum Increase Physiological* Correction of respiratory acidosis *4993*

Carbon Dioxide Partial Pressure
Blood Decrease Physiological Correction of respiratory acidosis *4993*

Creatinine *Serum Decrease Analytical* With single-slide method on Kodak Ektachem® systems approximately 50% decrease in results observed *2519*

Dopamine *Plasma Increase Analytical* Markedly increased concentration when progressively increasingly diluted with tris and radio enzymatic method used for quantitation *1188*

Epinephrine *Plasma Increase Analytical* Markedly increased concentration when progressively increasingly diluted with tris and radio enzymatic method used for quantitation *1188*

Glucose *Serum Decrease Physiological* Hypoglycemia especially if i.v., also transient if oral *4993*

ionized Calcium *Serum Decrease Analytical* At concentrations greater than 0.1 mmol/L on calcium specific electrode *820*

Norepinephrine *Plasma Increase Analytical* Markedly increased concentration when progressively increasingly diluted with tris and radio enzymatic method used for quantitation *1188*

Orthophosphate *Test Conditions Decrease Analytical* Total inhibition at 0.1 mol/L on method of Horder *2713*

pH *Blood Increase Physiological* Can correct metabolic or hypercapnic acidosis *4993*

Potassium *Serum Increase Physiological* Reported effect *4993*

Protein *Test Conditions Decrease Analytical* Lowry procedure, non linear absorption *2936*

Tropicamide

Histamine *Plasma No Effect Analytical* No effect at physiological concentration on radio-enzyme assay *2492*

Tropine

Creatinine *Serum No Effect Analytical* No interference observed with liquid chromatographic method of Paroni *4540*

Tropococaine

Benzoylecgonine *Urine Positive Analytical* Cross-reactivity of 1.5% observed with Serex CoMA EIA method *4084*

Trovafloxacin

Alanine Aminotransferase *Serum Increase Physiological* Increased activity probably attributable to trovafloxacin observed in fewer than 1% of treated patients. Activity greater than 9% of upper limit of normal in patients with chronic bacterial prostatitis *4663*

Albumin *Serum Decrease Physiological* Decreased concentration probably attributable to trovafloxacin observed in fewer than 1% of treated patients *4663*

Alkaline Phosphatase *Serum Increase Physiological* Increased activity probably attributable to trovafloxacin observed in fewer than 1% of treated patients *4663*

Aspartate Aminotransferase *Serum Increase Physiological* Increased activity probably attributable to trovafloxacin observed in fewer than 1% of treated patients. Activity greater than 3 times upper limit of normal in 9% of patients with chronic bacterial prostatitis but declined with cessation of treatment *4663*

Bicarbonate *Serum Decrease Physiological* Decreased concentration probably attributable to trovafloxacin observed in fewer than 1% of treated patients *4663*

Cimetidine *Serum No Effect Physiological* No significant interaction observed *4663*

Creatinine *Serum Increase Physiological* Increased concentration probably attributable to trovafloxacin observed in fewer than 1% of treated patients *4663*

Cyclosporine A *Blood No Effect Physiological* No significant interaction observed *4663*

Digoxin *Serum No Effect Physiological* No significant interaction observed *4663*

Eosinophils *Blood Increase Physiological* Eosinophilia probably attributable to trovafloxacin observed in fewer than 1% of treated patients *4663*

Hematocrit *Blood Decrease Physiological* Anemia probably attributable to trovafloxacin observed in fewer than 1% of treated patients *4663*

Hemoglobin *Blood Decrease Physiological* Anemia probably attributable to trovafloxacin observed in fewer than 1% of treated patients *4663*

Heparin *Plasma No Effect Physiological* No significant interaction observed *4663*

Leukocytes *Blood Decrease Physiological* Increased and decreased counts probably attributable to trovafloxacin observed in fewer than 1% of treated patients *4663*

Blood Increase Physiological Increased and decreased counts probably attributable to trovafloxacin observed in fewer than 1% of treated patients *4663*

Occult Blood *Feces Increase Physiological* Melena observed in fewer than 1% of treated patients *4663*

Platelets *Blood Decrease Physiological* Thrombocytopenia probably attributable to trovafloxacin observed in fewer than 1% of treated patients *4663*

Protein *Serum Decrease Physiological* Decreased concentration probably attributable to trovafloxacin observed in fewer than 1% of treated patients *4663*

Sodium *Serum Decrease Physiological* Decreased concentration probably attributable to trovafloxacin observed in fewer than 1% of treated patients *4663*

Theophylline *Serum No Effect Physiological* No significant interaction observed *4663*

Urea Nitrogen *Serum Increase Physiological* Increased concentration probably attributable to trovafloxacin observed in fewer than 1% of treated patients *4663*

Trypan Blue

Glucose *Serum Decrease Analytical* Affects glucose oxidase method of Boehringer *5480*

Tryparsamide

Alanine Aminotransferase *Serum Increase Physiological* May cause liver damage *128*

Aspartate Aminotransferase *Serum Increase Physiological* May cause liver damage *128*

Tubocurarine

Cholinesterase *Test Conditions Decrease Analytical* Inhibitory effect observed *4821*

Creatine Kinase *Serum Increase Physiological* Due to i.m. injections or histamine release *1079*

γ-Globulin *Serum Increase Physiological* Positive correlation between sensitivity and concentration *5841*

Histamine *Plasma Increase Physiological* Observed with administration for anesthesia *3648*

Plasma No Effect Analytical Improbable effect on radio-enzyme assay method although 50% inhibition produced at 19 μg/mL since physiological concentration 0.7 - 1.1 μg/mL *2492*

pH *Blood Decrease Physiological* Large dose effect with prolonged recovery *3669*

Blood Increase Physiological Respiratory alkalosis with low doses *3669*

Tumor Necrosis Factor

Corticotropin *Plasma Increase Physiological* In 9 patients with inoperable cancer treatment with 125 - 275 μg/sq m intravenously caused significant increase from mean baseline of 18.5 pmol/L to peak of 78.2 pmol/L *4317*

Cortisol *Plasma Increase Physiological* In 9 patients with inoperable cancer intravenous administration of 125 - 275 μg/sq m caused significant increase from mean baseline of 464 nmol/L to a peak of 993 nmol/L *4317*

Urine Increase Physiological In 9 patients with inoperable cancer intravenous injection of 125 to 275 μg/sq m caused significant increase from mean baseline of 51 nmol/d on a control day to 318 nmol/d on the day of administration *4317*

Growth Hormone *Plasma Increase Physiological* In 9 patients with inoperable cancer intravenous administration of 125 - 275 μg/sq m caused significant increase from mean baseline of 6.3 μg/L to a peak of 11.3 lmu]g/L *4317*

Prolactin *Plasma Increase Physiological* In 9 patients with inoperable cancer intravenous administration of 125 - 275 μg/sq m caused significant increase from mean baseline of 6.5 μg/L to a peak of 19.3 μg/L *4317*

Sperm Motility *Semen Decrease Physiological* At concentrations of 500 U/mL and above significant reduction of progressive and total motility after 4 and 21 hours of incubation when compared with controls *1681*

Typhoid Vaccine

α_1-Antitrypsin *Serum Increase Physiological* May be considerable rise after single injection *3314*

Nitroblue Tetrazolium Test *Blood Increase Physiological* False positive after typhoid/paratyphoid vaccination *4276*

Tyropanoic Acid

Thyroid Stimulating Hormone *Serum Increase Physiological* Intrahypophyseal conversion of T4 to T3 involved *6412*

Thyroxine (T4) *Serum Increase Physiological* Impaired conversion of T4 to T3 *6412*

Tri-iodothyronine (T3) *Serum Decrease Physiological* Impaired conversion of T4 to T3 *6412*

Tyrothricin

Bilirubin *Serum Increase Physiological* Hemolysis even when applied topically *128*

Erythrocytes *Blood Decrease Physiological* Hemolysis even when applied topically *128*

Hematocrit *Blood Decrease Physiological* May cause hemolysis even if applied topically *128*

Hemoglobin *Blood Decrease Physiological* May cause hemolysis even if applied topically *128*

Ulinastatin

Ketone Body Ratio *Serum No Effect Analytical* When added at a concentration of 2500 kU/L had no significant effect on AKBR method of Uno et al *6131*

Unfractionated Heparin

Alanine Aminotransferase *Serum No Effect Physiological* In 24 patients with chronic renal failure undergoing hemodialysis mean activity changed nonsignificantly from baseline of 7.11 ± 5.08 U/L to 7.66 ± 4.62 U/L after 6 months *3302*

Apolipoprotein A-I *Serum No Effect Physiological* In 24 patients with chronic renal failure undergoing hemodialysis mean concentration changed nonsignificantly from baseline of 115.7 ± 33.4 mg/dL to 121.9 ± 34.3 mg/dL after 6 months *3302*

Apolipoprotein A-IV *Serum No Effect Physiological* In 24 patients with chronic renal failure undergoing hemodialysis mean concentration changed nonsignificantly from baseline of 27.0 ± 11.9 mg/dL to 31.1 ± 7.5 mg/dL after 6 months *3302*

Apolipoprotein B *Serum Decrease Physiological* In 24 patients with chronic renal failure undergoing hemodialysis mean concentration changed nonsignificantly from baseline of 99.6 ± 40.2 mg/dL to 89.9 ± 30.4 mg/dL after 6 months *3302*

Aspartate Aminotransferase *Serum No Effect Physiological* In 24 patients with chronic renal failure undergoing hemodialysis mean activity changed nonsignificantly from baseline of 6.81 ± 3.52 U/L to 6.83 ± 2.99 U/L after 6 months *3302*

Cholesterol *Serum No Effect Physiological* In 24 patients with chronic renal failure undergoing hemodialysis mean concentration changed nonsignificantly from baseline of 159.1 ± 44.0 mg/dL to 154.4 ± 41.9 mg/dL after 6 months *3302*

Creatinine *Serum No Effect Physiological* In 24 patients with chronic renal failure undergoing hemodialysis mean concentration changed nonsignificantly from baseline of 10.49 ± 2.10 mg/dL to 10.61 ± 2.24 mg/dL after 6 months *3302*

D-Dimer *Plasma No Effect Physiological* In 5 patients with chronic renal failure undergoing hemodialysis using 750 - 1000 IU/h unfractionated heparin mean arterial concentration of 694 ± 142 ng/mL at baseline changed insignificantly to 714 ± 119 ng/mL after 10 min, 820 ± 194 ng/mL after 60 min, 745 ± 121 ng/mL after 120 min and 744 ± 153 ng/mL after 180 min *4337*

Fibrinogen *Plasma No Effect Physiological* In 5 patients with chronic renal failure undergoing hemodialysis using 750 - 1000 IU/h unfractionated heparin mean arterial concentration of 390 ± 36 mg/dL at baseline changed insignificantly to 418 ± 39 mg/dL after 180 min *4337*

γ-Glutamyltransferase *Serum No Effect Physiological* In 24 patients with chronic renal failure undergoing hemodialysis mean activity changed nonsignificantly from baseline of 11.79 ± 5.55 U/L to 14.56 ± 8.09 U/L after 6 months *3302*

HDL-Cholesterol *Serum No Effect Physiological* In 24 patients with chronic renal failure undergoing hemodialysis mean concentration changed nonsignificantly from baseline of 31.0 ± 13.0 mg/dL to 37.7 ± 17.5 mg/dL after 6 months *3302*

Heptest *Plasma Increase Physiological* Increase in clotting time observed with peak of 53 s after 60 mg subcutaneously after 1 hour *2709*

LDL-Cholesterol *Serum No Effect Physiological* In 24 patients with chronic renal failure undergoing hemodialysis mean concentration changed nonsignificantly from baseline of 94.1 ± 38.0 mg/dL to 89.9 ± 32.3 mg/dL after 6 months *3302*

Leukocytes *Blood No Effect Physiological* In 24 patients with chronic renal failure undergoing hemodialysis mean concentration changed nonsignificantly from baseline of 7880 ± 2320 /µL to 7650 ± 2260 /µL after 6 months *3302*

Lipoprotein Lp(a) *Serum No Effect Physiological* In 24 patients with chronic renal failure undergoing hemodialysis mean concentration changed nonsignificantly from baseline of 23.2 ± 33.2 mg/dL to 21.3 ± 27.0 mg/dL after 6 months *3302*

Plasmin-Plasmin Inhibitor Complex *Plasma Increase Physiological* In 5 patients with chronic renal failure undergoing hemodialysis using 750 - 1000 IU/h unfractionated heparin mean arterial concentration of 432 ± 62 ng/mL at baseline changed significantly overall to 373 ± 77 ng/mL after 10 min, 507 ± 113 ng/mL after 60 min, 517 ± 66 ng/mL after 120 min and 627 ± 100 ng/mL after 180 min *4337*

Protein *Serum No Effect Physiological* In 24 patients with chronic renal failure undergoing hemodialysis mean concentration changed nonsignificantly from baseline of 63.9 ± 7.7 g/L to 66.2 ± 5.3 g/L after 6 months *3302*

Thrombin/Antithrombin III Complex *Plasma No Effect Physiological* In 5 patients with chronic renal failure undergoing hemodialysis using 750 - 1000 IU/h unfractionated heparin mean arterial concentration of 3.6 ± 1.2 ng/mL at baseline changed insignificantly to 2.1 ± 0.1 ng/mL after 10 min, 2.8 ± 0.4 ng/mL after 60 min, 2.7 ± 0.5 ng/mL after 120 min and 3.5 ± 1.2 ng/mL after 180 min *4337*

Tissue Factor Pathway Inhibitor *Plasma Increase Physiological* Increase in concentration observed with peak of 170 ng/mL after 60 mg subcutaneously after 1 hour *2709*

Triglycerides *Serum Decrease Physiological* In 24 patients with chronic renal failure undergoing hemodialysis mean concentration changed nonsignificantly from baseline of 148.9 ± 94.3 mg/dL to 121.4 ± 88.8 mg/dL after 6 months *3302*

Urea *Serum No Effect Physiological* In 24 patients with chronic renal failure undergoing hemodialysis mean concentration changed nonsignificantly from baseline of 149.2 ± 38.7 mg/dL to 134.8 ± 39.6 mg/dL after 6 months *3302*

Uracil Mustard

Alanine Aminotransferase *Serum Increase Physiological* May affect liver function *3810*

Alkaline Phosphatase *Serum Increase Physiological* May affect liver function *3810*

Aspartate Aminotransferase *Serum Increase Physiological* May affect liver function *3810*

Bile *Urine Increase Physiological* May affect liver function *3810*

Bilirubin *Serum Increase Physiological* May affect liver function *3810*

BSP Retention *Serum Increase Physiological* May affect liver function *3810*

Erythrocytes *Blood Decrease Physiological* May cause bone marrow depression *128*

Leukocytes *Blood Decrease Physiological* May cause bone marrow depression *128*

Platelets *Blood Decrease Physiological* May cause bone marrow depression *128*

Urapidil

Aldosterone *Plasma Increase Physiological* Nonsignificant increase observed in 7 hypertensives treated with 60 or 90 mg/d for 12 days *2621*

Urapidil *(continued)*

Aldosterone *(continued)*
Plasma *No Effect* *Physiological* No significant effect observed in 7 patients with moderate essential hypertension treated with up to 90 mg/d for 12 days *2621*

Atrial Natriuretic Peptide *Plasma* *Decrease* *Physiological* Significant reduction of 26% observed in 7 patients with moderate essential hypertension treated with 60 or 90 mg/d for 12 days *2621* Significant reduction of 26% observed in 7 hypertensive patients treated with 60 or 90 mg/d for 12 days *2621*

Calcium *Serum* *No Effect* *Physiological* No effect observed in 7 hypertensives treated with 60 or 90 mg/d for 12 days *2621*

Catecholamines *Plasma* *No Effect* *Physiological* No significant effect observed in 7 patients with moderate essential hypertension treated with up to 90 mg/d for 12 days *2621*

Creatinine *Serum* *No Effect* *Physiological* No change observed in 7 hypertensive hospitalized patients treated with 60 or 90 mg/d for 12 days *2621*

Epinephrine *Plasma* *Increase* *Physiological* Nonsignificant increase observed in 7 hypertensive hospitalized patients treated with 60 or 90 mg/d for 12 days *2621*

Fibrinogen *Plasma* *Decrease* *Physiological* In 17 patients with essential hypertension treatment with 60 mg twice daily for 12 weeks caused 24% reduction in concentration *2398*

Filtration Fraction *Urine* *Decrease* *Physiological* Nonsignificant reduction of less than 10% observed in 7 hypertensives treated with 60 or 90 mg/d for 12 days *2621*

Glomerular Filtration Rate *Urine* *Increase* *Physiological* Nonsignificant increase of less than 10% observed in 7 hospitalized hypertensives treated with 60 or 90 mg/d for 12 days *2621*
Urine *No Effect* *Physiological* No significant change observed in 7 patients with moderate essential hypertension treated with up to 90 mg/d for 12 days *2621*

Glucose *Serum* *No Effect* *Physiological* In 17 patients with essential hypertension treatment with 60 mg twice daily for 12 weeks had no significant effect on concentration *2398*

Glucose Tolerance *Serum* *No Effect* *Physiological* In 17 patients with essential hypertension treatment with 60 mg twice daily for 12 weeks had no significant effect on OGTT *2398*

HDL-Cholesterol *Serum* *No Effect* *Physiological* In 17 patients with essential hypertension treatment with 60 mg twice daily for 12 weeks caused nonsignificant reduction of 5% *2398*

HDL-Triglycerides *Serum* *No Effect* *Physiological* In 17 patients with essential hypertension treatment with 60 mg twice daily for 12 weeks caused nonsignificant reduction of 5% *2398*

Hematocrit *Blood* *No Effect* *Physiological* In 17 patients with essential hypertension treatment with 60 mg twice daily for 12 weeks had no significant effect on value *2398*

Hemoglobin *Blood* *No Effect* *Physiological* In 17 patients with essential hypertension treatment with 60 mg twice daily for 12 weeks had no significant effect on concentration *2398*

Hemoglobin A_{1c} *Blood* *No Effect* *Physiological* In 17 patients with essential hypertension treatment with 60 mg twice daily for 12 weeks had no significant effect on concentration *2398*

Insulin *Plasma* *No Effect* *Physiological* In 17 patients with essential hypertension treatment with 60 mg twice daily for 12 weeks had no significant effect on concentration *2398*

LDL-Cholesterol *Serum* *No Effect* *Physiological* No significant effect observed in 78 hypertensive patients treated with up to 180 mg/d for 8 weeks *1441*

Norepinephrine *Plasma* *Increase* *Physiological* Nonsignificant increase observed in 7 hypertensive patients treated with 60 or 90 mg/d for 12 days *2621*

Plasminogen Activator Inhibitor Activity
Plasma *Decrease* *Physiological* In 17 patients with essential hypertension treatment with 60 mg twice daily for 12 weeks caused nonsignificant 4% reduction in concentration *2398*

Potassium *Serum* *No Effect* *Physiological* No significant effect observed in 78 hypertensive patients treated with up to 180 mg/d for 8 weeks *1441* No effect observed in 7 hypertensive patients treated with 60 or 90 mg/d for 12 days *2621*

Protein *Serum* *No Effect* *Physiological* Nonsignificant reduction of 0.3 g/dL observed in 7 hypertensive patients treated with 60 or 90 mg/d for 12 days in comparison with controls *2621*

Renal Blood Flow *Patient* *Increase* *Physiological* In 7 hospitalized patients with moderate essential hypertension treatment with up to 90 mg/d for 12 days caused mean increase of about 10% *2621*

Renin Activity *Plasma* *Decrease* *Physiological* Nonsignificant reduction observed in 7 hypertensives treated with 60 or 90 mg/d for 12 days *2621*
Plasma *No Effect* *Physiological* No significant effect observed in 7 patients with moderate essential hypertension treated with up to 90 mg/d for 12 days *2621*

Sodium *Serum* *No Effect* *Physiological* No significant change observed in 7 hypertensive patients treated with 60 or 90 mg/d for 12 days *2621*
Urine *Decrease* *Physiological* Nonsignificant reduction from 187 uEq/min/sq m to 166 uEq/min/sq m observed in 7 hypertensive patients treated with 60 or 90 mg/d for 12 days *2621* Nonsignificant reduction from 187 µEq/min/sq m to 166 µEq/min/sq m observed in 7 hypertensive patients treated with 60 or 90 mg/d for 12 days *2621*

Triglycerides *Serum* *Decrease* *Physiological* In 17 patients with essential hypertension treatment with 60 mg twice daily for 12 weeks caused nonsignificant 13% reduction in concentration *2398*

Urea Nitrogen *Serum* *Decrease* *Physiological* Nonsignificant reduction from 15.5 mg/dL to 15.2 mg/dL observed in 7 hypertensives treated with 60 or 90 mg/d for 12 days *2621*

Uric Acid *Serum* *Decrease* *Physiological* Nonsignificant reduction from 6.2 mg/dL to 5.7 mg/dL observed in 7 hypertensive patients treated with 60 or 90 mg/d for 12 days *2621*
Serum *No Effect* *Physiological* In 17 patients with essential hypertension treatment with 60 mg twice daily for 12 weeks had no significant effect on concentration *2398* No significant effect observed in 78 hypertensive patients treated with up to 180 mg/d for 8 weeks *1441*

VLDL-Triglycerides *Serum* *Decrease* *Physiological* In 17 patients with essential hypertension treatment with 60 mg twice daily for 12 weeks caused nonsignificant 22% reduction in concentration *2398*

Urate Oxidase

Uric Acid *Serum* *Decrease* *Physiological* In one patient with stage C chronic lymphatic leukemia treatment with fludarabine 25 mg/m^2 caused significant increase to 1761 µmol/L but treatment with urate oxidase 100 U/kg/d intravenously for five consecutive days caused reduction to 29 µmol/L by second day. Similar results observed in two other patients *3447*

Urethan

Alanine Aminotransferase *Serum* *Increase* *Physiological* May cause liver damage and necrosis *128*

Aspartate Aminotransferase *Serum* *Increase* *Physiological* May cause liver damage and necrosis *128*

Bilirubin *Serum* *Increase* *Physiological* Hepatotoxicity with centrolobular necrosis *128*

Erythrocytes *Blood* *Decrease* *Physiological* Bone marrow aplasia/pancytopenia *3810*

Hematocrit *Blood* *Decrease* *Physiological* May occur with bone marrow depression *4014*

Hemoglobin *Blood* *Decrease* *Physiological* May occur with bone marrow depression *4014*

Leukocytes *Blood* *Decrease* *Physiological* Bone marrow aplasia/pancytopenia *128*

Platelets *Blood* *Decrease* *Physiological* Bone marrow aplasia/pancytopenia *128*

Urokinase

Blood *Urine* *Increase* *Physiological* Complication observed as a result of internal bleeding *10*

D-Dimer *Plasma* *Increase* *Physiological* In 17 patients with acute myocardial infarction treatment with urokinase 2 x 10^6 units for 15 min was associated with increase from mean baseline of 225 µg/L on admission to 1425 µg/L after lysis and peak of 2200 µg/L *2088*

Fibrinolytic Time *Plasma* *Increase* *Physiological* Significant effect if given parenterally *658*

Occult Blood *Feces* *Increase* *Physiological* Complication observed as a result of internal bleeding *10*

Oxygen Partial Pressure *Blood* *Increase* *Physiological* In patients with pulmonary embolism *5507*

Plasmin *Plasma* *Increase* *Physiological* Acts directly in converting plasminogen to plasmin *5162*

Plasminogen Activator Inhibitor-1
Plasma *Increase* *Physiological* In 17 patients with acute myocardial infarction treatment with urokinase 2 x 10^6 units for 15 min was associated with increase from mean baseline of 65 µg/L on admission to 45 µg/L after lysis and peak of 140 µg/L *2088*

Plasminogen Activator Inhibitor-1 Antigen
Plasma *Increase* *Physiological* In 18 patients with suspected myocardial infarction treatment with 2 million units over 10 minutes caused significant increase peaking 3 hours after end of infusion and returning to normal by day 2 *2087*

Thrombin Time *Blood* *Increase* *Physiological* In patients with pulmonary embolism *5507*

Tissue Plasminogen Activator-1
Plasma *No Effect* *Physiological* In 17 patients with acute myocardial infarction treatment with urokinase 2 x 10^6 units for 15 min was associated with increase from mean baseline of 16 µg/L on admission to 14 µg/L after lysis and peak of 17 µg/L *2088*

Troponin I *Serum* *No Effect* *Analytical* At concentrations up to 1.0 g/L had no significant effect on Abbott ELISA method for cardiac troponin I *6010*

Ursodiol

Alanine Aminotransferase *Serum* *Decrease* *Physiological* Administration has been shown to decrease activity in liver disease *1020* Treatment of 13 patients with chronic active hepatitis with 450 mg/d caused reduction of mean activity from 213 U/L after 12 weeks although on withdrawal of treatment activity increased to 152 U/L after 4 weeks *5067* Significant reduction from mean baseline activity of 2.69 times upper limit of normal to 1.16 times upper limit of normal in over 70 patients with primary biliary cirrhosis treated with up to 15 mg/kg/d for 2 years *4763* In 30 patients with chronic hepatitis treatment with 600 mg/d caused significant decrease from mean baseline of 200 ± 98 U/L to 169 ± 115 U/L after 3 months, 165 ± 100 U/L after 6 months and 163 ± 116 U/L after 12 months, with decrease greater in patients with cirrhosis than in others *465* Mean reduction of 33% observed in 12 patients with chronic hepatitis treated with 600 mg/d for 2 months *4724*
Serum *Increase* *Physiological* Hypersensitivity related increase reported rarely *1384*

Albumin *Serum* *Decrease* *Physiological* In 51 patients with primary sclerosing cholangitis treatment with 13 - 15 mg/kg caused a significant decrease from mean baseline concentration of 39 ± 4 g/L at baseline to 39 ± 6 g/L after 12 months and 37 ± 7 g/L after 2 y *3593*
Serum *Increase* *Physiological* Moderately significant increase from mean baseline concentration of 38.9 g/L in over 70 patients with primary biliary cirrhosis to 39.8 g/L treated with up to 15 mg/kg/d for 2 years *4763*
Serum *No Effect* *Physiological* No significant change observed in 13 patients with chronic active hepatitis treated with 450 mg/d for 12 weeks *5067*

Alkaline Phosphatase *Serum* *Decrease* *Physiological* In comparison with placebo significant reduction in activity observed with treatment *300* In 51 patients with primary sclerosing cholangitis treatment with 13 - 15 mg/kg caused a significant decrease from mean baseline concentration of 1102 ± 762 U/L at baseline to 592 ± 462 U/L after 12 months and 655 ± 481 U/L after 2 y *3593* In 13 patients with chronic active hepatitis treatment with 450 mg/d for 12 weeks caused decrease from mean baseline of 274 U/L to 174 U/L although 4 weeks after treatment stopped activity had increased to 215 U/L *5067* Significant reduction from mean baseline activity of 5.68 times upper limit of normal to 2.04 times upper limit of normal in over 70 patients with primary biliary cirrhosis treated with up to 15 mg/kg/d for 2 years *4763* In 23 patients with primary biliary cirrhosis treatment with 12 - 15 mg/kg/d for 2 years caused significant change of - 649 ± 128 U/L from mean baseline *4026*
Serum *Increase* *Physiological* Hypersensitivity-related increase reported rarely *1384*

Antimitochondrial Antibodies
Serum *Decrease* *Physiological* Significant reduction from mean baseline titer of 1:1800 to 1:730 in over 70 patients with primary biliary cirrhosis treated with up to 15 mg/kg/d for 2 years *4763*

Aspartate Aminotransferase
Serum *Decrease* *Physiological* In 51 patients with primary sclerosing cholangitis treatment with 13 - 15 mg/kg caused a significant decrease from mean baseline concentration of 120 ± 78 U/L at baseline to 70 ± 71 U/L after 12 months and 68 ± 47 U/L after 2 y *3593* Administration has been shown to decrease activity in liver disease *1020* In comparison with placebo significant reduction in activity observed with treatment *300* In 13 patients with chronic active hepatitis treatment with 450 mg/d caused reduction from mean baseline of 139 U/L to 67 U/L after 12 weeks although activity increased after treatment stopped *5067* Mean reduction of 35% observed in 12 patients with chronic hepatitis given 600 mg/d for 2 months *4724* In 30 patients with chronic hepatitis treated with 600 mg/d activity decreased from mean baseline of 128 ± 54 U/L to 90 ± 48 U/L after 3 months, 89 ± 48 U/L after 6 months and 88 ± 48 U/L after 12 months, with decrease greater in patients with cirrhosis than in others *465* Significant reduction from mean baseline activity of 2.44 times upper limit of normal to 1.14 times upper limit of normal in over 70 patients with primary biliary cirrhosis treated for 2 years with up to 15 mg/kg/d *4763*
Serum *Increase* *Physiological* Hypersensitivity related increase reported rarely without hepatic damage occurring *1384*

Bile Acids *Serum* *Increase* *Physiological* In 29 patients with primary biliary cirrhosis mean concentration increased from 30.5 µmol/L to 52.7 µmol/L after treatment with 750 - 1000 mg/d for 6 to 12 months *5827*

Bilirubin *Serum* *Decrease* *Physiological* In 13 patients with chronic active hepatitis treatment with 450 mg/d caused significant 21% reduction *5067* Significant reduction from mean baseline concentration of 23.2 µmol/L to 12.3 µmol/L in over 70 patients with primary biliary cirrhosis treated with up to 15 mg/kg/d for 2 years *4763* In 13 patients with chronic active hepatitis treatment with 450 mg/d caused significant 21% reduction from mean baseline after 12 weeks *5067* In 51 patients with primary sclerosing cholangitis treatment with 13 - 15 mg/kg caused a decrease from mean baseline concentration of 1.6 ± 1.6 mg/dL at baseline to 1.3 ± 1.4 mg/dL after 12 months and 1.5 ± 2.1 mg/dL after 2 y *3593* In comparison with placebo significant improvement in concentration observed with treatment *300*
Serum *No Effect* *Physiological* In 23 patients with primary biliary cirrhosis treatment with 12 - 15 mg/kg/d for 2 years caused nonsignificant change of - 1.4 ± 4.5 µmol/L from mean baseline *4026*

Campesterol *Serum* *Increase* *Physiological* In 23 patients with primary biliary cirrhosis treatment with 12 - 15 mg/kg/d for 2 years caused nonsignificant change of + 37 ± 49 x 10 mmol/mol cholesterol from mean baseline of 530 ± 76 x 10 mmol/mol cholesterol *4026*

Cholestanol *Serum* *Decrease* *Physiological* In 23 patients with primary biliary cirrhosis treatment with 12 - 15 mg/kg/d for 2 years caused nonsignificant change of - 15 ± 10 x 10 mmol/mol cholesterol from mean baseline of 412 ± 50 x 10 mmol/mol cholesterol *4026*

δ^8-Cholestanol *Serum* *Increase* *Physiological* In 23 patients with primary biliary cirrhosis treatment with 12 - 15 mg/kg/d for 2 years caused significant change of + 2.4 ± 1.0 x 10 mmol/mol cholesterol from mean baseline of 8.2 ± 1.0 x 10 mmol/mol cholesterol *4026*

Cholesterol *Serum* *Decrease* *Physiological* Significant reduction from mean baseline concentration of 7.3 mmol/L to 6.2 mmol/L in over 70 patients with primary biliary cirrhosis

Ursodiol *(continued)*

Cholesterol *(continued)*
treated with up to 15 mg/kg/d for 2 years *4763* In 88 patients with primary biliary cirrhosis treatment caused decrease from mean baseline of 288.3 ± 121.7 mg/dL by -58.0 ± 76.5 mg/dL after 12 months and by -82.0 ± 55.3 mg/dL after 24 months *342* In 23 patients with primary biliary cirrhosis treatment with 12 - 15 mg/kg/d for 2 years caused significant change of - 0.90 ± 0.39 mmol/L from mean baseline of 6.47 ± 0.98 mmol/L *4026*
Serum No Effect Physiological No significant effect with 600 mg daily in patients with endogenous hypertriglyceridemia *905*

Cholesterol, Esterified *Serum Decrease Physiological* In 23 patients with primary biliary cirrhosis treatment with 12 - 15 mg/kg/d for 2 years caused significant change of - 0.57 ± 0.25 mmol/L from mean baseline of 4.47 ± 0.31 mmol/L *4026*

Cholesterol, Free *Serum Decrease Physiological* In 23 patients with primary biliary cirrhosis treatment with 12 - 15 mg/kg/d for 2 years caused nonsignificant change of - 0.33 ± 0.16 mmol/L from mean baseline of 2.01 ± 0.17 mmol/L *4026*

Cholinesterase *Serum No Effect Analytical* No effect observed at concentration of 15 µg/mL with butyrylthiocholine method on Kodak Ektachem® *2504*

Creatinine *Serum Increase Physiological* Treatment reported to increase concentration in 1.3% patients after 24 months *300*

Cyclosporine A *Blood Increase Physiological* In 7 liver transplant patients 600 mg ursodiol coadministration with cyclosporine A had no significant effect on absorption of cyclosporine A with AUC unchanged from 5486 ng/h/mL to 5011 ng/h/mL and maximum concentration 871 ng/mL compared with 832 ng/mL *3706*

Desmosterol *Serum Increase Physiological* In 23 patients with primary biliary cirrhosis treatment with 12 - 15 mg/kg/d for 2 years caused significant change of + 6 ± 3 x 10 mmol/mol cholesterol from mean baseline of 56 ± 3 x 10 mmol/mol cholesterol *4026*

Erythrocytes *Blood No Effect Physiological* No significant change observed in count in 13 patients with chronic active hepatitis treated with 450 mg/d for 12 weeks *5067*

γ-Globulin *Serum Decrease Physiological* Significant reduction from mean baseline concentration of 18.2 g/L to 15.9 g/L in over 70 patients with primary biliary cirrhosis treated with up to 15 mg/kg/d for 2 years *4763*
Serum No Effect Physiological No significant change observed in 13 patients with chronic active hepatitis treated with 450 mg/d for 12 weeks *5067*

Glucose *Serum Increase Physiological* Treatment reported to increase concentration in 1.2% patients after 12 months and 1.3% patients after 24 months *300*

γ-Glutamyltransferase *Serum Decrease Physiological* Significant reduction from mean baseline activity of 13.0 times upper limit of normal to 3.5 times upper limit of normal in over 70 patients with primary biliary cirrhosis treated with up to 15 mg/kg/d for 2 years *4763* In 13 patients with chronic active hepatitis treatment with 450 mg/d for 12 weeks caused decrease from mean baseline of 92 U/L to 48 U/L after 12 weeks although 4 weeks after treatment stopped activity had risen to 68 U/L *5067* Mean reduction of 41% observed in 12 patients with chronic hepatitis treated with 600 mg/d for 2 months *4724* In 30 patients with chronic hepatitis treatment with 600 mg/d caused significant decrease from mean baseline of 73 ± 54 U/L to 41 ± 25 U/L after 3 months, 39 ± 25 U/L after 6 months and 37 ± 22 U/L after 12 months, with decrease greater in patients with cirrhosis than in others *465*

HDL-Cholesterol *Serum Decrease Physiological* In 23 patients with primary biliary cirrhosis treatment with 12 - 15 mg/kg/d for 2 years caused significant change of - 0.29 ± 0.09 mmol/L from mean baseline of 1.68 ± 0.15 mmol/L *4026*
Serum No Effect Physiological In 8 normolipemic patients receiving 1,000 mg drug daily *3510* In more than 40 patients with primary biliary cirrhosis treatment for 12 months caused nonsignificant reducton of 2.67 ± 22.0 mg/dL from mean baseline of 63.1 ± 23.6 mg/dL and reduction of 2.41 ± 24.5 mg/dL after 24 months *342* No significant effect with 600 mg daily in patients with endogenous hypertriglyceridemia *905* In 88 patients with primary biliary cirrhosis treatment caused insignificant change from mean baseline of 63.1 ± 23.6 mg/dL by -2.67 ± 22.0 mg/dL after 12 months and by -2.41 ± 24.5 mg/dL after 24 months *342*

HDL-Cholesterol, Esterified *Serum Decrease Physiological* In 23 patients with primary biliary cirrhosis treatment with 12 - 15 mg/kg/d for 2 years caused significant change of - 0.16 ± 0.07 mmol/L from mean baseline of 1.21 ± 0.10 mmol/L *4026*

HDL-Cholesterol, Free *Serum Decrease Physiological* In 23 patients with primary biliary cirrhosis treatment with 12 - 15 mg/kg/d for 2 years caused significant change of - 0.13 ± 0.04 mmol/L from mean baseline of 0.47 ± 0.06 mmol/L *4026*

HDL-Phospholipids *Serum Decrease Physiological* In 23 patients with primary biliary cirrhosis treatment with 12 - 15 mg/kg/d for 2 years caused significant change of - 0.44 ± 0.08 mmol/L from mean baseline of 1.78 ± 0.14 mmol/L *4026*

HDL-Triglycerides *Serum Decrease Physiological* In 23 patients with primary biliary cirrhosis treatment with 12 - 15 mg/kg/d for 2 years caused nonsignificant change of - 0.03 ± 0.02 mmol/L from mean baseline of 0.21 ± 0.02 mmol/L *4026*
Serum No Effect Physiological In 8 normolipemic patients receiving 1,000 mg drug daily *3510*

Hematocrit *Blood No Effect Physiological* No significant change observed in 13 patients with chronic active hepatitis treated with 450 mg/d for 12 weeks *5067*

Hemoglobin *Blood No Effect Physiological* No significant change observed in 13 patients with chronic active hepatitis treated with 450 mg/d for 12 weeks *5067*

IDL-Cholesterol *Serum Increase Physiological* In 23 patients with primary biliary cirrhosis treatment with 12 - 15 mg/kg/d for 2 years caused significant change of + 0.06 ± 0.03 mmol/L from mean baseline of 0.19 ± 0.04 mmol/L *4026*

IDL-Cholesterol, Esterified *Serum Increase Physiological* In 23 patients with primary biliary cirrhosis treatment with 12 - 15 mg/kg/d for 2 years caused nonsignificant change of + 0.04 ± 0.02 mmol/L from mean baseline of 0.12 ± 0.03 mmol/L *4026*

IDL-Cholesterol, Free *Serum Increase Physiological* In 23 patients with primary biliary cirrhosis treatment with 12 - 15 mg/kg/d for 2 years caused significant change of + 0.01 ± 0.01 mmol/L from mean baseline of 0.07 ± 0.01 mmol/L *4026*

IDL-Phospholipids *Serum Increase Physiological* In 23 patients with primary biliary cirrhosis treatment with 12 - 15 mg/kg/d for 2 years caused nonsignificant change of + 0.01 ± 0.01 mmol/L from mean baseline of 0.09 ± 0.02 mmol/L *4026*

IDL-Triglycerides *Serum Increase Physiological* In 23 patients with primary biliary cirrhosis treatment with 12 - 15 mg/kg/d for 2 years caused significant change of + 0.03 ± 0.01 mmol/L from mean baseline of 0.08 ± 0.01 mmol/L *4026*

immunoglobulin A *Serum Decrease Physiological* Significant reduction from mean baseline concentration of 1.14 times upper limit of normal to 1.01 times upper limit of normal in over 70 patients with primary biliary cirrhosis treated with up to 15 mg/kg/d for 2 years *4763*

Immunoglobulin G *Serum Decrease Physiological* Significant reduction from mean baseline concentration of 1.21 times upper limit of normal to 1.10 times upper limit of normal in over 70 patients with primary biliary cirrhosis treated with up to 15 mg/kg/d for 2 years *4763*

Immunoglobulin M *Serum Decrease Physiological* Significant reduction from mean baseline concentration of 2.54 times upper limit of normal to 1.65 times upper limit of normal in over 70 patients with primary biliary cirrhosis treated with up to 15 mg/kg/d for 2 years *4763* In comparison with placebo significant improvement in concentration observed with treatment *300*

Lathosterol *Serum Increase Physiological* In 23 patients with primary biliary cirrhosis treatment with 12 - 15 mg/kg/d for 2 years caused significant change of + 12 ± 7 x 10 mmol/mol cholesterol from mean baseline of 85 ± 8 x 10 mmol/mol cholesterol *4026*

LDL-Cholesterol *Serum Decrease Physiological* In 30 healthy individuals treatment with 15 mg/kg/d caused mean reduction from 4.3 mmol/L to 3.9 mmol/L and with 30 mg/kg/d from 4.7 mmol/L to 3.7 mmol/L *181* In 23 patients with primary biliary cirrhosis treatment with 12 - 15 mg/kg/d for 2 years caused nonsignificant change of - 0.44 ± 0.28 mmol/L from mean baseline of 3.58 ± 0.28 mmol/L *4026*

Serum *No Effect* *Physiological* In 8 normolipemic patients receiving 1,000 mg drug daily *3510*

LDL-Cholesterol, Esterified *Serum* *Decrease* *Physiological* In 23 patients with primary biliary cirrhosis treatment with 12 - 15 mg/kg/d for 2 years caused nonsignificant change of - 0.28 ± 0.19 mmol/L from mean baseline of 2.43 ± 0.21 mmol/L *4026*

LDL-Cholesterol, Free *Serum* *Decrease* *Physiological* In 23 patients with primary biliary cirrhosis treatment with 12 - 15 mg/kg/d for 2 years caused nonsignificant change of - 0.16 ± 0.11 mmol/L from mean baseline of 1.15 ± 0.11 mmol/L *4026*

LDL-Phospholipids *Serum* *Decrease* *Physiological* In 23 patients with primary biliary cirrhosis treatment with 12 - 15 mg/kg/d for 2 years caused nonsignificant change of - 0.18 ± 0.16 mmol/L from mean baseline of 1.27 ± 0.20 mmol/L *4026*

LDL-Triglycerides *Serum* *Decrease* *Physiological* In 23 patients with primary biliary cirrhosis treatment with 12 - 15 mg/kg/d for 2 years caused nonsignificant change of - 0.01 ± 0.02 mmol/L from mean baseline of 0.29 ± 0.03 mmol/L *4026*

Serum *No Effect* *Physiological* In 8 normolipemic patients receiving 1,000 mg drug daily *3510*

Leukocytes *Blood* *Decrease* *Physiological* Treatment reported to decrease concentration in 2.6% patients after 24 months *300*

Blood *No Effect* *Physiological* No significant change observed in 13 patients with chronic active hepatitis treated with 450 mg/d for 12 weeks *5067*

Phospholipids *Serum* *Decrease* *Physiological* In 23 patients with primary biliary cirrhosis treatment with 12 - 15 mg/kg/d for 2 years caused significant change of - 0.93 ± 0.27 mmol/L from mean baseline of 3.93 ± 0.27 mmol/L *4026*

Platelets *Blood* *No Effect* *Physiological* No significant change observed in 13 patients with chronic active hepatitis treated with 450 mg/d for 12 weeks *5067*

Protein *Serum* *No Effect* *Physiological* No significant change observed in 13 patients with chronic active hepatitis treated with 450 mg/d for 12 weeks *5067*

Prothrombin Time *Plasma* *No Effect* *Physiological* Nonsignificant increase from mean baseline of 95.9% to 97.0% in over 70 patients with primary biliary cirrhosis treated with up to 15 mg/kg/d for 2 years *4763*

Sitosterol *Serum* *Decrease* *Physiological* In 23 patients with primary biliary cirrhosis treatment with 12 - 15 mg/kg/d for 2 years caused nonsignificant change of - 26 ± 52 x 10 mmol/mol cholesterol from mean baseline of 414 ± 70 x 10 mmol/mol cholesterol *4026*

Squalene *Serum* *Increase* *Physiological* In 23 patients with primary biliary cirrhosis treatment with 12 - 15 mg/kg/d for 2 years caused nonsignificant change of + 2.0 ± 2.3 x 10 mmol/mol cholesterol from mean baseline of 30.2 ± 2.8 x 10 mmol/mol cholesterol *4026*

Triglycerides *Serum* *Decrease* *Physiological* In 23 patients with primary biliary cirrhosis treatment with 12 - 15 mg/kg/d for 2 years caused nonsignificant change of - 0.12 ± 0.06 mmol/L from mean baseline of 1.18 ± 0.11 mmol/L *4026*

Serum *No Effect* *Physiological* In 8 normolipemic patients receiving 1,000 mg drug daily *3510* In 88 patients with primary biliary cirrhosis treatment caused insignificant change from mean baseline of 102.0 ± 50.4 mg/dL by +3.76 ± 55.4 mg/dL after 12 months and by +13.62 ± 58.0 mg/dL after 24 months *342* No significant effect with 600 mg daily in patients with endogenous hypertriglyceridemia *905*

Ursodeoxycholic Acid *Serum* *Increase* *Physiological* In 21 patients treated with 600 mg/d caused significant increase from mean baseline of 0.9 ± 0.2 μmol/L to 25.6 ± 2.8 μmol/L after 3 months, 24.6 ± 3.7 μmol/L after 6 months and 19.5 ± 2.2 μmol/L after 12 months *465*

VLDL-Cholesterol *Serum* *Decrease* *Physiological* In 23 patients with primary biliary cirrhosis treatment with 12 - 15 mg/kg/d for 2 years caused significant change of - 0.11 ± 0.04 mmol/L from mean baseline of 0.40 ± 0.06 mmol/L *4026*

Serum *No Effect* *Physiological* In 8 normolipemic patients receiving 1,000 mg drug daily *3510*

VLDL-Cholesterol, Esterified

Serum *Decrease* *Physiological* In 23 patients with primary biliary cirrhosis treatment with 12 - 15 mg/kg/d for 2 years caused significant change of - 0.08 ± 0.03 mmol/L from mean baseline of 0.24 ± 0.09 mmol/L *4026*

VLDL-Cholesterol, Free *Serum* *Decrease* *Physiological* In 23 patients with primary biliary cirrhosis treatment with 12 - 15 mg/kg/d for 2 years caused significant change of - 0.04 ± 0.02 mmol/L from mean baseline of 0.17 ± 0.02 mmol/L *4026*

VLDL-Phospholipids *Serum* *Decrease* *Physiological* In 23 patients with primary biliary cirrhosis treatment with 12 - 15 mg/kg/d for 2 years caused significant change of - 0.05 ± 0.02 mmol/L from mean baseline of 0.23 ± 0.04 mmol/L *4026*

VLDL-Triglycerides *Serum* *Decrease* *Physiological* In 23 patients with primary biliary cirrhosis treatment with 12 - 15 mg/kg/d for 2 years caused nonsignificant change of - 0.05 ± 0.03 mmol/L from mean baseline of 0.49 ± 0.03 mmol/L *4026*

Serum *No Effect* *Physiological* In 8 normolipemic patients receiving 1,000 mg drug daily *3510*

Valaciclovir

Digoxin *Serum* *No Effect* *Physiological* Coadministration of valaciclovir with digoxin had no effect on the pharmacokinetics of either drug *5725*

Valproic Acid

Acetaminophen *Serum* *No Effect* *Analytical* No interference observed at a concentration of 2000 μg/mL (1386 μmol/L) with method on Du Pont aca *1506*

Serum *No Effect* *Physiological* Coadministration of valproate with acetaminophen had no effect on the phamacokinetic parameters of acetaminophen in 3 epileptic patients *15*

Acetoacetate *Serum* *Decrease* *Physiological* In 10 children with epilepsy receiving long-term treatment with valproic acid mean concentration 19.7 ± 4.04 μmol/L significantly different compared with 108.9 ± 28.6 μmol/L in 12 healthy age and sex-matched controls *3941*

α_1-Acid Glycoprotein *Serum* *No Effect* *Physiological* Mean concentration in 35 epileptic patients receiving 18.7 mg/kg/d 0.6 g/L not significantly different from 0.58 g/L in normal controls *5944*

Acylcarnitine *Serum* *Decrease* *Physiological* In 10 children with epilepsy receiving long-term treatment with valproic acid mean concentration 7.63 ± 1.35 μmol/L significantly different compared with 10.1 ± 0.96 μmol/L in 12 healthy age and sex-matched controls *3941*

Serum *Increase* *Physiological* Significant increase in patients treated with valproic acid compared with controls *5052*

Urine *Decrease* *Physiological* In 10 children with epilepsy receiving long-term treatment with valproic acid mean excretion 72.6 ± 18.0 μmol/d significantly different compared with 136.4 ± 47.7 μmol/d in 12 healthy age and sex-matched controls *3941*

Alanine *Plasma* *Increase* *Physiological* Incidence of high concentration higher in children given valproic acid alone or when combined with other antiepileptic drugs than when other drugs only given *2807* In normal humans, oral or intravenous administration enhances concentration *1143* When 1 g given orally to fasting individuals *6101*

Alanine Aminotransferase *Serum* *Increase* *Physiological* Rise in about 15 to 30% cases transient and usually maximal to 10 to 12 weeks after beginning treatment *774* Increased activity observed in 2.0% of 50 patients when treated with low dose valproic acid *6323* Administration of valproic acid associated with frequent minor increases in activity that appear to be dose related *15* Fatal case reported in child also given phenytoin *2665* Acute hepatic centrilobular necrosis with severe fatty change in small number of patients *6348* Observed in 4 of 25 patients treated with drug: reversible with reduction of dose or withdrawal of drug *6476* In 1 of 9 patients with epilepsy poorly controlled *5878* Dose related increase in 44% of treated patients *1494* Administration of valproate has been associated with frequent minor increases in activity *16* Transient increase in 44% of patients without change of dosage *2914*

Serum *No Effect* *Physiological* In chronically treated patients with monotherapy only, but increases when combined with other antiepileptics *2405* In 93 epileptic patients treated with valproic acid mean activity of 13.2 ± 14.1 U/L not significantly increased compared with 13.5 ± 5.5 U/L in healthy controls *6234*

Valproic Acid *(continued)*

Albumin *Serum Decrease Physiological* Reduced to below 35 g/L in 4 of 9 patients *5878* Observed in 4 of 25 patients treated with drug: reversible with reduction of dose or withdrawal of drug *6476*

Alkaline Phosphatase *Serum Increase Physiological* In 1 of 9 patients with epilepsy poorly controlled *5878* Acute hepatic centrilobular necrosis with severe fatty change in small number of patients *6348* Reported in children with coadministration only *2914*

Aluminum *Serum Increase Physiological* Reported in one woman on chronic hemodialysis *4272*

γ-Aminobutyric Acid *Plasma Increase Physiological* Increased concentration observed by third day in 10 normal subjects given 1600 mg/day sodium valproate *3336*

δ-Aminolevulinic Acid *Serum Increase Physiological* Mean increase to 130 nmol/L from 99 nmol/L in controls *2246*

Amitriptyline *Serum Increase Physiological* Coadministration of valproate (1000 mg/d) with a single oral dose of amitriptyline (50 mg) caused a 21% decrease in plasma clearance of amitriptyline and a 34% decrease in the net clearance of nortriptyline *15* Coadministration of valproic acid with amitriptyline caused a 21% decrease in plasma clearance of amitriptyline and of 34% in the clearance of nortriptyline *17*

Ammonia *Plasma Increase Physiological* Nondose dependent effect in some patients with both normal and abnormal liver function *2045* About half of patients comedicated with phenobarbital had increase; especially noted when concentrations high *2406* Incidence of 19% in 75 epileptic children when treated with drug alone and 20% when treated with valproic acid and other antiepileptic drugs *2807* In the absence of clinical hepatic dysfunction, hyperammonemia occurs as a reversible side effect *1143* Probably due to inhibition of enzymes involved in glycine clearance in liver analogous to ketotic hyperglycinemias *2878* Associated with inhibition of carbamyl phosphate synthetase I and interference with mitochondrial glycine transport *1146* Some patients with epilepsy receiving valproic acid reported to have hyperamonnemia occurring even in the absence of abnormal liver function tests *15* In 29 of 55 patients receiving drug versus none in control population on other anticonvulsants; values especially high when phenytoin also taken *4182* Administration of valproate has been associated with hyperammonemia *16* Occasional hyperammonemia when given alone, more frequent when given with phenytoin when effect also more marked *3795*

Plasma No Effect Physiological In patients on monotherapy but increases seen with coadministration of other antiepileptics *2406* No striking abnormality when given to epileptics *6233*

Amylase *Serum Increase Physiological* Administration of valproic acid associated with occasional increased activity but fatalities have been reported *15* In 1 of 100 epileptic children when given alone or combined with other anticonvulsants *1147* Almost 20% patients had mild increase *346* Increase observed in two patients with pancreatitis following valproic acid ingestion. Activity returned to normal with withdrawal of drug. About 20 cases of this adverse reaction previously reported *3653* Associated with dysphagia and epigastric discomfort in one adult patient who subsequently died *4184* Reported in one woman on chronic hemodialysis *4272* Apparently drug related case of acute pancreatitis *5281* Administration of valproate has been associated with acute pancreatitis *16*

Androgen Index, Free (FAI) *Plasma Increase Physiological* Insignificant increase to mean of 108 in 7 male epileptic patients treated for mean of 5.4 years compared with 87 in healthy control subjects *2840* In 21 epileptic patients treated with sodium valproate for a median of 10.7 years median index in follicular and luteal phases significantly higher than in controls *4178*

Androstenedione *Plasma No Effect Physiological* In 6 women with PCOS treatment with sodium valproate 1200 mg/d for 5 days caused mean concentration to change nonsignificantly from mean of 15.9 ± 2.2 nmol/L to 15.3 ± 1.6 nmol/L *4753*

δ_4-Androstenedione *Plasma Increase Physiological* In 21 epileptic patients treated with sodium valproate for a median of 10.7 years median concentration in follicular and luteal phases significantly higher than in controls *4178*

Anti-DNA Antibodies *Serum Increase Physiological* Observed in two patients who developed systemic lupus erythematosus and in whom other probable causes were excluded *600*

Anti-ds DNA Antibodies *Serum Increase Physiological* Significant titer observed in one patient who developed systemic lupus erythematosus and in whom other probable causes had been excluded *600*

Anti-Histone Antibodies *Serum Positive Physiological* Observed in one patient who had taken valproic acid and who developed systemic lupus erythematosus in the absence of probable other causes *600*

Antinuclear Antibodies *Serum Increase Physiological* Observed in two patients who developed systemic lupus erythematosus and had received valproic acid and in whom other probable causes had been excluded *600*

Apolipoprotein A-I *Serum No Effect Physiological* In 16 epileptic children treated with valproate for a mean of 1.34 years mean concentration of 155.79 ± 71.01 mg/dL not significantly different from 111.65 ± 59.75 mg/dL in 57 healthy control children *5727*

Apolipoprotein B *Serum No Effect Physiological* In 16 epileptic children treated with valproate for a mean of 1.34 years mean concentration of 74.43 ± 33.89 mg/dL not significantly different from 75.15 ± 39.67 mg/dL in 57 healthy control children *5727*

Aspartate Aminotransferase *Serum Increase Physiological* Administration of valproate has been associated with frequent minor increases in activity *16* Administration of valproic acid associated with frequent minor increases in activity that appear to be dose related *15* Transient increase in 44% of patients without change of dosage *2914* In 4 of 9 patients with epilepsy poorly controlled *5878* Acute hepatic centrilobular necrosis with severe fatty change in small number of patients *6348* In 93 epileptic patients treated with valproic acid mean activity of 27.8 ± 22.2 U/L significantly increased compared with 15.1 ± 5.6 U/L in 42 healthy controls *6234* Observed in 4 of 25 patients treated with drug: reversible with reduction of dose or withdrawal of drug *6476* In 44% of 100 epileptic children when given alone or combined with other anticonvulsants *1147* Fatal case reported in child also given phenytoin *2665* Observed in 3% of 109 patients: reports of fatalities in some studies *2915* Dose related increase in 44% of treated patients *1494* Rise in about 15 to 30% cases transient and usually maximal to 10 to 12 weeks after beginning treatment *774* Slight increase in 20% patients on chronic monotherapy: enzyme activity linearly and directly correlated with drug concentration *2405*

Aspirin Esterase *Serum Increase Physiological* Significant increase from mean of 186 μg/mL/h in controls to 300 μg/mL/h in epileptics receiving valproic acid only *4807* Substantially higher activity in treated epileptics than in controls *4806*

Barbiturate *Serum Decrease Physiological* Phenobarbital administration with valproic acid reported to accelerate metabolism of phenobarbital *22*

Bilirubin *Serum Decrease Physiological* Mean reduction of 2.1 μmol/L versus controls in 22 epileptic patients treated for several years *2267*

Serum Increase Physiological Administration of valproic acid associated with occasional increased concentration and other abnormal liver function tests *15* Administration of valproate has been associated with occasional increase in bilirubin concentration and other abnormal liver function tests *16* Acute hepatic centrilobular necrosis with severe fatty change in small number of patients *6348*

Biotin *Serum Decrease Physiological* Dose related effect in long term treated epileptics compared with controls effect not as marked as with other anticonvulsants *3275*

Bleeding Time *Patient Increase Physiological* In 23% of 30 epileptic children with epilepsy treated with valproic acid bleeding time prolonged *3286* In 3 of 9 patients with poorly controlled epilepsy *5878*

Carbamazepine *Serum Decrease Physiological* Valproate administration with carbamazepine to epileptic patients caused a 17% decrease of carbamazepine and a 45% increase of carbamazepine-10,11-epoxide concentrations *15* In 25 epileptic patients receiving both valproic acid and carbamazepine withdrawal of valproic acid for 4 weeks caused increase of carbamazepine concentration by 10% compared with baseline *1619*

Displaces carbamazepine from protein increasing free carbamazepine fraction which is then available for metabolism and concentration of total carbamazepine in plasma is reduced *3118* Coadministration to epileptic patients of valproic acid with carbamazepine caused a decrease of 17% in the concentration of carbamazepine and increased by 45% the concentration of carbamazepine-10,11-epoxide did not affect its clearance *17* Slight or no effect in 25 patients studied for 5 to 9 mo *6452*

Serum Increase Physiological Reported increase when valproic acid co-administered *207* Concurrent administration causes increase in carbamazepine concentration *4846* May increase concentration as inhibits metabolism *3118*

Serum No Effect Analytical At a concentration of 1000 µg/mL had no significant cross-reactivity with carbamazepine at a concentration of 4.0 µg/mL when measured by method on Bayer Technicon Immuno 1® system *417*

Serum No Effect Physiological Coadministration of valproic acid with carbamazepine had no significant on the total carbamazepine concentration *4846* No significant change in 12 epileptics when valproic acid coadministered *4846* May be no effect on plasma concentration because concentration increased through inhibition of metabolism but free component increased and subsequently metabolised thereby reducing plasma concentration *3118* No significant effect on area under curve in patients with steady state valproate concentration although did prolong its elimination half life by 12% *3721*

Carbamazepine-10,11-Epoxide

Serum Increase Physiological Total plasma carbamazepine concentration may be unchanged but concentration of epoxide metabolite may be increased due to inhibition of epoxide hydrolase *3118* Drugs that inhibit CYP 3A4 inhibit metabolism of carbamazepine producing clinically meaningful effect *1039* Simultaneous administration of valproic acid with carbamazepine causes increased ratio of plasma carbamazepine-trans-10,11-epoxide to carbamazepine concentration *282* Effect on carbamazepine concentration may be variable depending on whether displacement from protein binding sites or inhibition of metabolism predominates but effect on carbamazepine epoxide remains constant *1384* In 14 children coadministration of valproic acid and carbamazepine caused increase of epoxide metabolite up to 13 µg/mL although concentrations of carbamazepine were within normal range *4838* Significant increase from mean of 1.2 µg/mL to 3.8 µg/mL in 12 epileptic patients when valproic acid coadministered *4846* Valproate administration with carbamazepine to epileptic patients caused a 17% decrease of carbamazepine and a 45% increase of carbamazepine-10,11-epoxide concentrations *15* Coadministration to epileptic patients of valproic acid with carbamazepine caused a decrease of 17% in the concentration of carbamazepine and increased by 45% the concentration of carbamazepine-10,11-epoxide did not affect its clearance *17* Mean decrease of 24% observed in 25 epileptic patients receiving both valproic acid and carbamazepine 4 weeks after withdrawal of valproic acid *1619*

Carbamazepine-10,11-Epoxide, Free

Serum Increase Physiological Significant increase from mean of 0.5 µg/mL to 1.4 µg/mL in 12 patients with epilepsy when valproic acid coadministered *4846* Mean decrease from 0.33 µmol/L at baseline to 0.24 µmol/L 3 weeks after withdrawal of valproic acid in 25 epileptic patients receiving both drugs *1619* Significant increase from mean of 0.5 µ.g/mL to 1.4 µg/mL in 12 patients with epilepsy when valproic acid coadministered *4846*

Carbamazepine, Free *Serum Decrease Physiological* In 25 epileptic patients withdrawal of valproic acid for 4 weeks caused mean increase of 16% compared with baseline *1619*

Serum Increase Physiological Displaces carbamazepine from plasma proteins thereby increasing plasma concentration of free drug but free drug is available for metabolism *3118*

Serum No Effect Physiological No significant effect in 12 epileptics when valproic acid coadministered *4846* Coadministration of valproic acid with carbamazepine had no significant effect on the free carbamazepine concentration *4846*

Carnitine *Serum Decrease Physiological* In 10 children with epilepsy receiving long-term treatment with valproic acid mean concentration 33.5 ± 4.45 µmol/L significantly different compared with 43.6 ± 1.63 µmol/L in 12 healthy age and sex-matched controls *3941* In 53 epileptic children treated with valproic acid mean concentration of total carnitine of 35.6 ± 11.7 nmol/mL significantly reduced compared with 57.8 ± 15.4 nmol/mL in 32 healthy control children *2757* Decreased concentration observed in serum and liver following drug administration *1143* Lower concentrations observed in diabetic patients and in patients taking valproic acid *3879* Reversibly reduced, inversely related to drug dose and plasma ammonia concentration *4386* Significant reduction observed with either polytherapy or monotherapy *4423* Administration of valproate has been associated with a decreased carnitine concentration, although the clinical relevance is undetermined *16*

Serum No Effect Physiological Mean concentration 55.7 ± 12.4 mmol/L in 45 valproate treated epileptics not significantly different from 57.6 ± 12.1 mmol/L in 45 age-matched controls *2622*

Urine Decrease Physiological In 10 children with epilepsy receiving long-term treatment with valproic acid mean excretion 116.8 ± 29.9 µmol/d significantly different compared with 290.4 ± 92.9 µmol/d in 12 healthy age and sex-matched controls *3941*

Carnitine, Free *Serum Decrease Physiological* Reduction observed in 76.5% of adult patients treated with drug compared with a decrease in only 21.5% treated with other anticonvulsants *5052* In 10 children with epilepsy receiving long-term treatment with valproic acid mean concentration 25.9 ± 3.72 µmol/L significantly different compared with 33.5 ± 1.81 µmol/L in 12 healthy age and sex-matched controls *3941*

Serum No Effect Physiological Mean concentration 42.7 ± 9.9 mmol/L in 45 valproate treated epileptics not significantly different from 44.4 ± 9.9 mmol/L in 45 age-matched controls *2622* In 53 epileptic children mean concentration in those treated with valproic acid of 27.8 ± 10.9 nmol/L not significantly different from 42.5 ± 14.1 nmol/mL in 32 healthy control children *2757*

Urine Decrease Physiological In 10 children with epilepsy receiving long-term treatment with valproic acid mean excretion 44.3 ± 12.6 µmol/d significantly different compared with 154.0 ± 56.2 µmol/d in 12 healthy age and sex-matched controls *3941*

Cholesterol *Serum Decrease Physiological* Significantly reduced concentration observed in chronically treated epileptics compared with age and sex matched controls *843*

Serum No Effect Physiological In 16 epileptic children treated with valproate for a mean of 1.34 years mean concentration of 165.79 ± 42.15 mg/dL not significantly different from 155.10 ± 35.66 mg/dL in 57 healthy control children *5727*

Cholesterol:HDL-Cholesterol Ratio

Serum No Effect Physiological In 16 epileptic children treated with carbamazepine for a mean of 1.34 years mean ratio of 3.91 ± 1.19 not significantly different from 3.83 ± 10.3 in 57 healthy control children *5727*

Cholinesterase *Serum Increase Physiological* Significant increase in controls from 4.77 U/L in controls to 7.01 U/L in epileptics treated with valproic acid only *4807*

Cholinesterase (True) *Serum Increase Physiological* Substantially higher activity in treated epileptics than in controls *4806*

Clonazepam *Serum No Effect Physiological* No definite effect in 25 patients studied for 5 to 9 mo *6452*

Clozapine *Serum Increase Physiological* In one patient in whom the drugs were coadministered minor increase observed in clozapine metabolites *938*

Serum No Effect Physiological Coadministration of valproic acid with clozapine had no effect on its metabolism *17* Coadministration of valproate with clozapine to 11 psychotic patients had no effect on the phamacokinetic parameters of clozapine *15*

Complement, Total *Serum Decrease Physiological* Low concentrations observed in two patients who developed systemic lupus erythematosus following treatment with valproic acid and other probable causes had been excluded *600*

Copper *Serum Decrease Physiological* Reduction from mean of 93.0 µg/dL to 71.3 µg/dL in 13 patients being treated for epilepsy *4710*

Serum Increase Physiological In 29 epileptic patients treated for 1 month significant increase to 93.7 ± 25.4 µg/dL compared with 74.7 ± 9.4 µg/dL in 30 healthy controls *3344*

Serum No Effect Physiological In 19 epileptic children receiving valproic acid mean concentration of 1.22 ± 0.30 µg/mL not significantly different from 1.28 ± 0.369 µg/mL in 20 healthy control children *3331*

Valproic Acid *(continued)*

Corticotropin *Plasma Decrease Physiological* In 6 adult women with Nelson's syndrome administration of 1 g valproic acid caused mean decrease of 37 ± 10% in the plasma ACTH concentration *3956*
Plasma No Effect Physiological In patients with Addison's and Cushing's diseases *137* Normal concentration in maternal and umbilical cord blood in one pregnant woman *2505*

Cortisol *Plasma No Effect Physiological* Normal concentrations in maternal and umbilical cord blood in one pregnant woman *2505*

Cortisol, Free *Urine No Effect Analytical* No significant interference observed with HPLC method of Turpeinen et al *6105*

C-Peptide *Plasma No Effect Physiological* No change observed in 10 normal subjects and in 1 with somatostatinoma treated with 1600 mg/day for 6 days *3336*

Creatinine *Serum Decrease Physiological* Administration of valproic acid associated with occasional reduction of serum creatinine concentration but significance not understood *15*
Serum No Effect Analytical At 1.0 g/L on reversed phase liquid chromatographic procedure of Zhiri et al *6656* At concentration of 100 mg/L had no effect on creatinine iminohydrolase method *5704*

Cyclosporine *Blood No Effect Analytical* At a concentration of 500 mg/L had no effect on Syva EMIT method *495*
Serum Increase Physiological Effect occurs as result of hepatic cytochrome P-450 induction *1069*
Serum No Effect Physiological No significant effect observed when valproic acid coadministered with cyclosporine *6595*

Dehydroepiandrosterone Sulfate
Plasma Decrease Physiological In 21 epileptic patients treated with sodium valproate for a median of 10.7 years median index in follicular and luteal phases not significantly lower than in controls *4178*
Plasma Increase Physiological Insignificant mean increase to 9.8 µmol/L in 7 male epileptic patients treated for mean of 5.4 years compared with 8.0 µmol/L in healthy control subjects *2840*
Plasma No Effect Physiological In 6 women with PCOS treatment with sodium valproate 1200 mg/d for 5 days caused mean concentration to change nonsignificantly from mean of 6.7 ± 0.8 nmol/L to 6.4 ± 0.6 nmol/L *4753*

Diazepam *Serum Increase Physiological* In one study of 6 healthy volunteers coadministration of valproic acid caused significant increase in serum concentration probably due to inhibition of hepatic metabolism. Diazepam also displaced from plasma protein binding sites *1408* Valproate administration (1500 mg/d) with diazepam (10 mg/d) to epileptic patients caused a 90% increase of free diazepam, by displacing it from its plasma albumin-binding sites, and a 25% decrease of plasma clearance of diazepam *15*

Diazepam, Free *Serum Increase Physiological* Coadministration of valproic acid (1500 mg/d) increased the free fraction of diazepam (10 mg) by 90% in 6 healthy volunteers *17* Valproate administration (1500 mg/d) with diazepam (10 mg/d) to epileptic patients caused a 90% increase of free diazepam, by displacing it from its plasma albumin-binding sites, and a 25% decrease of plasma clearance of diazepam *15*

Eosinophils *Blood Increase Physiological* Administration of valproic acid associated with occasional eosinophilia *15* Administration of valproate has been associated with eosinophilia *16*

Estradiol *Plasma Decrease Physiological* In 21 epileptic patients treated with sodium valproate for a median of 10.7 years median concentration in follicular phase significantly lower than median in 20 age-matched controls *4178* In 6 women with PCOS treatment with sodium valproate 1200 mg/d for 5 days caused mean concentration to change nonsignificantly from mean of 214 ± 60 pmol/L to 184 ± 64 pmol/L *4753*
Plasma Increase Physiological Mean increase to 0.25 nmol/L in 7 male epileptic patients treated for mean of 5.4 years compared with 0.15 nmol/L in healthy control subjects *2840* In 21 epileptic patients treated with sodium valproate for a median of 10.7 years median concentration in luteal phase significantly higher than median in 20 age-matched controls *4178*

Ethinyl Estradiol *Serum No Effect Physiological* Coadministration of valproate (400 mg/d) with ethinylestradiol (50 µg/d) and 250 µg/d levonorgestrel to 6 pregnant women for 2 months had no effect on the phamacokinetic parameters of either steroid *15*

Ethosuximide *Serum Increase Physiological* Administration of a single 500 mg dose of ethosuximide with valproic acid (8 to 1600 mg/d) to 6 healthy volunteers was associated with a 25% increase in elimination half life *17* Reported increase when valproic acid co-administered *207* Valproate (800 to 1600 mg/d) coadministration with a single dose of ethosuximide (500 mg) to 6 healthy volunteers caused a 25% increase in elimination half-life of ethosuximide and a 15% decrease in its total clearance *15*
Serum No Effect Physiological No definite effect in 25 patients studied for 5 to 9 mo *6452*

Factor VIII Complex *Plasma Decrease Physiological* A reduction of concentration was observed in 33% of 30 epileptic children *3286*

Fatty Acids (FFA), Free *Serum Increase Analytical* With colorimetric method of Duncombe (overestimation by about 40% at plasma concentration) *86*
Serum No Effect Physiological In 10 children with epilepsy receiving long-term treatment with valproic acid mean concentration 835.5 ± 93.2 µmol/L not significantly different compared with 832.5 ± 64.4 µmol/L in 12 healthy age and sex-matched controls *3941*

Felbamate *Serum No Effect Analytical* No significant interference observed with GLC method of Rifai et al *4958*
Serum No Effect Physiological Addition of valproic acid to felbamate regime had no significant effect on steady state felbamate concentration *6323* With coadministration no significant effect observed on the concentration of felbamate at steady-state *6324*

Fibrinogen *Plasma Decrease Physiological* Reduced to 0.9 to 1.6 g/L in 9 patients with epilepsy poorly controlled *5878* In 30 children with epilepsy treatment with valproate was associated with a reduction in the plasma fibrinogen concentration *3286* Administration of valproate has been associated with hypofibrinogenemia *16* Some patients with epilepsy receiving valproic acid reported to have low plasma fibrinogen concentrations *15* Reported to reduce plasma concentration *3694* In one 6-year old patient receiving valproate 500 mg/d plasma fibrinogen concentration less than 50 mg/dL on two occasions *709*

Follicle Stimulating Hormone
Plasma Decrease Physiological Marked reduction of mean to 2.4 U/L in 7 male epileptic patients treated for mean of 5.4 years compared with mean of 6.2 U/L in healthy control subjects *2840*
Plasma No Effect Physiological In 21 epileptic patients treated with sodium valproate for a median of 10.7 years median concentration of 8.0 mIU/mL in follicular phase and 5.7 mIU/mL in luteal phase not markedly different from medians of 8.1 and 9.4 mIU/mL in 20 age-matched controls *4178* In 6 women with PCOS treatment with sodium valproate 1200 mg/d for 5 days caused mean concentration to change nonsignificantly from mean of 4.3 ± 0.5 IU/L to 5.0 ± 0.8 IU/L *4753*

Glucaric Acid *Urine Increase Physiological* Slightly higher but not statistically significant *4623* Selective induction of hepatic metabolizing enzymes *1329*

Glucose *Serum Decrease Physiological* In 10 children with epilepsy receiving long-term treatment with valproic acid mean concentration 4.94 ± 0.22 mmol/L not significantly different compared with 5.41 ± 0.27 mmol/L in 12 healthy age and sex-matched controls *3941* Reduced concentration observed in 1 patient with somatostatinoma during treatment with 1600 mg/day for 6 days but no effect observed in normal subjects *3336*
Serum Increase Physiological Administration of valproic acid associated with fatal outcome in one patient with with preexisting nonketotic hyperglycemia *15*
Serum No Effect Analytical At concentration of 100 mg/L had no effect on GOD/POD-PAP method *5704*
Serum No Effect Physiological No significant effect observed in epileptic patients receiving valproic acid *4077*

Glutamine *Plasma No Effect Physiological* No striking abnormality when given to epileptics *6233*

γ-Glutamyltransferase *Serum Increase Physiological* Transient increase in 44% of patients without change of dosage *2914*
Serum No Effect Physiological In 35 epileptic patients receiving 18.7 mg/kg/d mean activity increased by less than 10 U/L compared with controls *5944* In spite of induction of some hepatic enzymes *1329*

Glutathione Peroxidase *Serum Increase Physiological* In 19 epileptic children receiving valproic acid mean activity of 0.73 ± 0.0996 U/mL significantly different from 0.624 ± 0.08 U/mL in 20 healthy control children *3331*

Glutathione Reductase
Red Blood Cells Decrease Physiological Reduction from mean of 35.4 U/g hemoglobin to 30.1 U/g hemoglobin in 13 epileptic patients, secondary to depletion of selenium which is cofactor for enzyme *4710*

Glycerol *Serum Increase Physiological* When 1 g given orally to fasting individuals *6101*

Glycine *Plasma Increase Physiological* Incidence of high concentration greater in children treated with valproic acid alone or when combined with other antiepileptic drugs than when other drugs only given *2807* Associated with inhibition of carbamyl phosphate synthetase I and interference *1146* Administration of valproate has been associated with hyperglycinemia in a patient with preexistent nonketotic hyperglycinemia *16* Probably due to inhibition of enzymes involved in glycine clearance in liver analogous to ketotic hyperglycinemias *2878*
Plasma No Effect Physiological No striking abnormality when given to epileptics *6233*

Growth Hormone *Plasma Decrease Physiological* Release of hormone in epileptics treated with sodium valproate less than when other antiepileptics used *1164*

HDL-Cholesterol *Serum No Effect Physiological* In 16 epileptic children treated with valproate for a mean of 1.34 years mean concentration of 43.50 ± 4.78 mg/dL not significantly different from 41.31 ± 4.91 mg/dL in 57 healthy control children *5727*

HDL-Cholesterol:LDL-Cholesterol Ratio
Serum No Effect Physiological In 16 epileptic children treated with valproate for a mean of 1.34 years mean ratio of 2.60 ± 1.12 not significantly different from 2.29 ± 1.04 in 57 healthy control children *5727*

Hemoglobin *Blood Increase Physiological* Administration of valproate has been associated with anemia which may be macrocytic with or without folate deficiency, bone marrow depression, and acute intermittent porphyria *16*

3-Hydroxybutyrate *Serum Decrease Physiological* In 10 children with epilepsy receiving long-term treatment with valproic acid mean concentration 58.6 ± 4.09 μmol/L significantly different compared with 265.6 ± 39.6 μmol/L in 12 healthy age and sex-matched controls *3941* 78% reduction when 1 g given orally to fasting individuals *6101*

β-Hydroxybutyrate *Serum Decrease Physiological* Ketogenesis inhibited. Ketone concentration in plasma reduced after oral or intravenous drug administration *1143*

6-β-Hydroxycortisol *Urine No Effect Physiological* No significant effect on excretion when administered alone to 8 healthy male subjects *3721*

Immunoglobulins *Serum Decrease Physiological* Deficiency occurred in 29% of 41 epileptic patients on anticonvulsant therapy. Users of drug in general had lower concentrations than in controls *2983*

Indomethacin *Serum No Effect Analytical* No effect on HPLC method of Roberts and Smith *4978*

Ketones *Serum Decrease Physiological* 60% reduction when 1 g given orally to fasting individuals *6101*
Urine Increase Analytical Valproate partially eliminated in urine as a keto-metabolite which may lead to misinterpretations of urine ketone tests *15* Single drug eliminated as ketones may give false positive test *774* Valproate is partially eliminated in the urine as a keto-metabolite which may lead to a false interpretation of the urine ketone test *16*

Lactate *Plasma Decrease Physiological* Significant reduction in lactate concentration and in lactate:pyruvate ratio in epileptic patients receiving valproic acid *4077* In normal humans, after oral or intravenous administration, concentration initially increases, then declines *1143*
Plasma Increase Physiological When 1 g given orally to fasting individuals *6101* Dose related effect in long term treated epileptics compared with controls: effect not as marked as with other anticonvulsants *3275*

Lactate Dehydrogenase *Serum Increase Physiological* Acute hepatic centrilobular necrosis with severe fatty change in small number of patients *6348* In 2 of 9 patients with epilepsy poorly controlled *5878* Administration of valproate has been associated with frequent minor increases in activity *16* Administration of valproic acid associated with frequent minor increases in activity that appear to be dose related *15*

Lamotrigine *Serum Increase Physiological* Administration of lamotrigine with valproic acid caused an increase of 165% in the lamotogrine half life *17* Coadministration of valproic acid with lamotrigine caused a significant increase (approximately 2-fold) in the plasma concentration of lamotrigine *2160* In 10 healthy volunteers the elimination half-life of lamotrigine increased from 26 to 70 hours (165% increase) with valproate coadministration *15*

LDL-Cholesterol *Serum Decrease Physiological* Significantly reduced concentration observed in chronically treated epileptics compared with age and sex matched controls *843*
Serum No Effect Physiological In 16 epileptic children treated with valproate for a mean of 1.34 years mean concentration of 111.46 ± 45.50 mg/dL not significantly different from 92.85 ± 38.65 mg/dL in 57 healthy control children *5727*

Leukocytes *Blood Decrease Physiological* Administration of valproate has been associated with leukopenia *16* In 27% of 100 epileptic children when given alone or combined with other anticonvulsants *1147*

Levonorgestrel *Serum No Effect Physiological* Coadministration of valproate (400 mg/d) with ethinylestradiol (50 μg/d) and 250 μg/d levonorgestrel to 6 pregnant women for 2 months had no effect on the phamacokinetic parameters of either steroid *15*

Lipase *Serum Increase Physiological* Administration of valproate has been associated with acute pancreatitis *16* Administration of valproic acid associated with occasional increased activity but fatalities have been reported *15* Three cases reported in whom activity increased substantially but which reverted to normal when drug treatment stopped *3653*
Serum No Effect Analytical No effect observed on Kodak Ektachem® slide method when 500 mg/L added to a serum pool *3653*

Lithium *Serum No Effect Physiological* Coadministration of valproic acid with lithium had no effect on its steady state kinetics *17* Coadministration of valproate (1000 mg/d) with 900 mg/d lithium carbonate to 16 normal male volunteers had no effect on the steady state kinetics of lithium *15*

Long-chain Fatty Acid Carnitine Esters
Serum No Effect Physiological In 53 epileptic children treated with valproic acid caused nonsignificant reduction to 2.4 ± 0.7 nmol/mL compared with 3.1 ± 2.5 nmol/mL in 32 healthy control children *2757*

Lorazepam *Serum No Effect Physiological* Coadministration of valproate (1000 mg/d) with 2 mg/d lorazepam to 9 normal male volunteers caused a 17% decrease in the plasma clearance of lorazepam *15* Treatment of 16 healthy male volunteers with 500 mg/12 h valproic acid in addition to 1 mg/12 h lorazepam for 12 days caused significant increase in mean plasma concentration of lorazepam from 24.9 ± 5.2 ng/mL to 26.8 ± 5.7 ng/mL *5211*

Luteinizing Hormone *Plasma Decrease Physiological* Reduction to mean of 4.5 IU/L in 7 male epileptic patients treated for mean of 5.4 years compared with mean of 8.0 IU/L in healthy control subjects *2840* In 60 healthy postmenopausal women administration of valproic acid at doses from 300 to 1,200 mg orally caused 14 - 20% decrease in concentration. 1,200 mg significantly decreased concentration in 30 premenstrual women during the luteal phase of their menstrual cycle *4754*
Plasma Increase Physiological In 21 epileptic patients treated with sodium valproate for a median of 10.7 years median concentration of 9.6 mIU/mL in follicular phase and 19.3 mIU/mL in luteal phase higher than medians of 7.4 and 9.4 mIU/mL in 20 age-matched controls *4178*
Plasma No Effect Physiological In 6 women with PCOS treatment with sodium valproate 1200 mg/d for 5 days caused mean concentration to change nonsignificantly from mean of

Valproic Acid *(continued)*

Luteinizing Hormone *(continued)*
9.1 ± 0.6 IU/L to 9.0 ± 0.8 IU/L *4753* In 50 healthy postmenopausal women who had been on estrogen replacement therapy administration of valproic acid at doses from 300 to 1,200 mg orally had no significant effect on concentration *4754* In 9 women during late follicular phase of two successive menstrual cycles given 400 mg every 8 h on the 2 days preceding their second session and 400 mg at 9:00 a.m. on the day of the session no significant difference observed in pulse amplitude or relative pulse amplitude between first and second menstrual cycle (with and without drug). Similarly no effect observed in individuals ingesting sodium valproate chronically *3362*

Luteinizing Hormone:Follicle Stimulating Hormone Ratio
Plasma Increase Physiological In 21 epileptic patients treated with sodium valproate for a median of 10.7 years median ratio of 3.2 in luteal phase significantly different from median of 1.0 in 20 age-matched controls *4178*
Plasma No Effect Physiological In 21 epileptic patients treated with sodium valproate for a median of 10.7 years median ratio of 1.5 in follicular phase not markedly different from median of 0.9 in 20 age-matched controls *4178*

Lymphocytes *Blood Increase Physiological* Administration of valproic acid associated with relative lymphocytosis *15* Administration of valproate has been associated with relative lymphocytosis *16*

Macrocytes *Blood Increase Physiological* Administration of valproate has been associated with macrocytosis *16*

Magnesium *Serum No Effect Physiological* In 19 epileptic children receiving valproic acid mean concentration of 24.62 ± 6.94 μg/mL not significantly different from 21.32 ± 5.21 μg/mL in 20 healthy control children *3331*

Manganese *Serum No Effect Physiological* In 19 epileptic children receiving valproic acid mean concentration of 50.09 ± 22.29 ng/mL not significantly different from 46.29 ± 15.56 ng/mL in 20 healthy control children *3331*

Mephobarbital *Serum Increase Physiological* May increase plasma concentration of mephobarbital by shortening decreasing its metabolism *5254*

Nortriptyline *Serum Increase Physiological* Coadministration of valproate (1000 mg/d) with a single oral dose of amitriptyline (50 mg) caused a 21% decrease in plasma clearance of amitriptyline and a 34% decrease in the net clearance of nortriptyline *15*

Organic Acids *Urine Increase Physiological* Dose related effect in long term treated epileptics compared with controls. Effect not as marked as with other anticonvulsants *3275*

Ornithine *Plasma No Effect Physiological* No striking abnormality when given to epileptics *6233*

Phenobarbital *Serum Increase Physiological* Coadministration of valproic acid with phenobarbital causes an increase in plasma phenobarbital concentration *1706* Nonsignificant reduction of 15% observed in 3 epileptic patients receiving both drugs 4 weeks after withdrawal of valproic acid *1619* Reported increase when valproic acid coadministered *207* Causes increased concentration. Acidifies urine enhances reabsorption of phenobarbital with an increase in its half life leading to a 10 - 40% increase in its concentration after 24 - 26 days *6350* In patients taking primidone *774* Coadministration has been observed to increase plasma concentration by as much as 25-68% and phenobarbital dose must be adjusted accordingly *1384* Coadministration of valproate with phenobarbital may increase the phenobarbital concentration by impairment of non-renal clearance *16* In 4 patients decreased conversion to hydroxyphenyl-phenobarbital *784* Valproate (700 mg/d for 14 days) coadministration with phenobarbital to 6 healthy volunteers caused a 50% increase in half-life of phenobarbital and a 30% decrease in its total clearance. The fraction of phenobarbital excreted unchanged increased by 50% in the presence of valproate *15* Higher concentration obtained, especially in children, with increase of its biological half-life and decrease in its metabolic clearance *1143* Coadministration of valproic acid (500 mg/d for 14 days) caused a 50% increase in half-life and 30% decrease in plasma clearance of phenobarbital (60 mg single dose) *17* Several studies have shown that valproic acid inhibits hepatic metabolism of phenobarbital *6452* Increased half-life, relaxed plasma clearance, and other effects suggesting inhibition of metabolism *4553*
Serum No Effect Analytical No interference observed at a concentration of 5000 μmol/L with Sung and Neely modification of Syva EMIT procedure *148*

Phenytoin *Serum Decrease Physiological* During first several weeks of therapy concentration may decrease by about 30%. Interaction between valproic acid and phenytoin is complex since valproic acid displaces phenytoin from plasma albumin but also inhibits biotransformation of phenytoin *1384* Bound concentration falls, although free concentration unchanged *4097* Proportion of free concentration increased from 9.1% to 15.8% as serum concentration fell from 19.7 to 15.3 μg/mL *1966* Clearance markedly increased when phenytoin given i.v *1968* When valproic acid ingested with fosphenytoin concentration of phenytoin may be decreased or increased *4519* Coadministration of valproic acid (1200 mg/d) with 250 mg phenytoin in 7 healthy volunteers caused a 60% increase in the free fraction of phenytoin and 30% increase in plasma clearance of phenytoin *17* Coadministration of valproate with phenytoin has been associated with both increased and decreased total plasma phenytoin concentration *16* In one study of epileptic patients coadministration of valproic acid caused reduction of about 30% in plasma diphenylhydantoin concentration probably as result of stimulated hepatic metabolism although concentration returned to normal after several weeks *375* Due to displacement from protein and reduction in total serum concentration but free concentration unchanged *5262* Displaces from protein-binding sites and inhibited metabolism in some patients *783* Valproate displaces phenytoin from its plasma albumin-binding sites and inhibits its hepatic metabolism. Valproate (1200 mg/d) coadministration with phenytoin (250 mg) to 7 healthy volunteers caused a 60% increase in the free fraction of phenytoin and a 30% increase in the total plasma clearance of phenytoin *15* Due to displacement from albumin in 25 patients studied for 5 to 9 mo *6452*
Serum Increase Physiological Coadministration of valproate with phenytoin has been associated with both increased and decreased total plasma phenytoin concentration *16* Displaces from its plasma-protein binding sites and inhibits its oxidative metabolism *1143* When valproic acid ingested with fosphenytoin concentration of phenytoin may be decreased or increased *4519* Caused increased concentration which led to hepatic damage *4488*
Serum No Effect Analytical No significant interference observed at a concentration of 1000 μg/mL (6.93 mmol/L) with method on Du Pont aca *1538* No effect at concentration of 1000 μg/mL (6930 μmol/L) on method on Du Pont Dimension *1583*
Serum No Effect Physiological No significant effect observed in 25 epileptic patients receiving both valproic acid and phenytoin 4 weeks after withdrawal of valproic acid *1619*

Phenytoin, Free *Serum Increase Physiological* Valproate displaces phenytoin from its plasma albumin-binding sites and inhibits its hepatic metabolism. Valproate (1200 mg/d) coadministration with phenytoin (250 mg) to 7 healthy volunteers caused a 60% increase in the free fraction of phenytoin and a 30% increase in the total plasma clearance of phenytoin. The clearance and apparent volume of distribution of free phenytoin was reduced by 25% *15* Coadministration of valproate with phenytoin has been associated with an increased free phenytoin concentration in proportion to protein-bound phenytoin *16* Significant reduction from 0.11 μmol/L at baseline to 0.07 μmol/L after 2 weeks of withdrawal of valproic acid in 25 epileptic patients *1619*
Serum No Effect Physiological In spite of displacement of diphenylhydantoin from albumin and effect on metabolism concentration of free diphenylhydantoin unaffected *1384*

Platelet Aggregation *Blood Decrease Physiological* Some patients with epilepsy receiving valproic acid reported to have inhibition of secondary phase of platelet aggregation *15*

Platelets *Blood Decrease Physiological* In 30 epileptic children treatment with valproic acid was associated with a reduction in platelet concentration *3286* Platelet-bound antibody found in 4 of 31 patients and serum antiplatelet antibody found in 1 patient *5228* Reported to cause thrombocytopenia *3694* In 1 of 100 epileptic children when given alone or combined with other anticonvulsants *1147* 34 of 126 patients with epilepsy (27%) receiving approximately 50 mg valproic acid/kg/d on average had at least one platelet count of less than 75,000 /μL, with count normalizing with discontinuation of treatment *15*

In 4 of 9 patients with epilepsy poorly controlled *5878* Administration of valproate has been associated with thrombocytopenia and inhibition of the secondary phase of platelet aggregation *16*

Potassium *Serum No Effect Analytical* No effect of concentrations up to 1730 mg/L on method on Kodak Ektachem® *5706*

Primidone *Serum Increase Physiological* Coadministration of valproate with primidone which is metabolized to phenobarbital which may increase the phenobarbital concentration by impairment of non-renal clearance *16* In patients taking primidone *774*

Progesterone *Plasma Decrease Physiological* In 21 epileptic patients treated with sodium valproate for a median of 10.7 years median concentration in luteal phase significantly lower in 63.6% than 12.7 nmol/L *4178*
Plasma Increase Physiological Insignificant mean increase to 1.10 nmol/L in 7 male epileptic patients treated for mean of 5.4 years compared with 1.01 nmol/L in healthy control subjects *2840*
Plasma No Effect Physiological In 21 epileptic patients treated with sodium valproate for a median of 10.7 years median concentration in follicular phase not significantly different from that in controls *4178*

Prolactin *Plasma Decrease Physiological* Significant effect in women 30-180 minutes after 400 mg orally *3943* Significant effect in both normal women and in hyperprolactinemic women *3943* Insignificant reduction to mean of 8.6 µg/L in 7 male epileptic patients treated for mean of 5.4 years compared with 9.5 µg/L in healthy control subjects *2840*
Plasma No Effect Physiological In 6 women with PCOS treatment with sodium valproate 1200 mg/d for 5 days caused mean concentration to change nonsignificantly from mean of 203 ± 81 mU/L to 205 ± 68 mU/L *4753* In 21 epileptic patients treated with sodium valproate for a median of 10.7 years median concentration of 16.8 ng/mL in follicular phase and 16.8 ng/mL in luteal phase not markedly different from medians of 15.1 and 14.2 ng/mL in 20 age-matched controls *4178*

Propionic Acid *Serum Increase Physiological* Associated with inhibition of carbamyl phosphate synthetase I and interference with mitochondrial glycine transport *1146*

Protein *Serum Decrease Analytical* At 10 times therapeutic concentration caused statistically significant decrease with method used on Technicon SRA-2000 *4348*

Prothrombin Time *Plasma Increase Physiological* Associated with other effects on coagulation *774* In 3 of 9 volunteers with epilepsy poorly controlled *5878* Observed in 4 of 25 patients treated with drug: reversible with reduction of dose or withdrawal of drug *6476*

Pyruvate *Plasma Increase Physiological* When 1 g given orally to fasting individuals *6101* In normal humans, concentration initially increases, then declines *1143*

Ristocetin Cofactor Activity
Plasma Decrease Physiological Decrease observed in 66% of 30 epileptic children treated with valproic acid *3286*

SDZ PSC 833 *Blood No Effect Analytical* At a concentration of 105 mg/L had no effect on HPLC method of Scott et al when used to measure PSC (with CsD as internal standard) at a concentration of 5 mg/L *5418*

Secobarbital *Serum Increase Physiological* Coadministration of valproic acid with secobarbital probably causes an increase in plasma secobarbital concentration as has been reported for phenobarbital *1708*

Selenium *Serum Decrease Physiological* Mean reduction from 15.9 µg/dL to 11.1 µg/dL in 13 epileptic patients *4710*
Serum No Effect Physiological In 18 epileptic children receiving valproic acid mean concentration of 122.61 ± 26.66 ng/mL not significantly different from 110.72 ± 25.41 ng/mL in 20 healthy control children *3331*

Serine *Plasma Increase Physiological* High concentration more common in epileptic children given valproic acid alone or combined with other antiepileptic drugs than when other antiepileptic drugs only given *2807*

Sex-Hormone Binding Globulin
Serum Decrease Physiological Insignificant reduction to mean of 24.2 nmol/L in 7 male epileptic patients treated for mean of 5.4 years compared with mean of 27.2 nmol/L in healthy control subjects *2840*
Serum Increase Physiological In 6 women with PCOS treatment with sodium valproate 1200 mg/d for 5 days caused mean concentration to change nonsignificantly from mean of 32 ± 6.3 nmol/L to 32 ± 5.6 nmol/L *4753*

Short-chain Fatty Acid Carnitine Esters
Serum No Effect Physiological In 53 epileptic children treated with valproic acid mean concentration of 8.6 ± 4.0 nmol/mL not significantly less than 15.4 ± 9.1 nmol/mL in 32 healthy control children *2757*

Sodium *Serum Decrease Physiological* Administration of valproate has been associated with hyponatremia and inappropriate ADH secretion *16*
Serum Increase Analytical At 10 times therapeutic concentration caused statistically significant increase with method used on Technicon SRA-2000 *4348*
Serum Increase Physiological Administration of valproic acid associated with occasional hyponatremia and inappropriate ADH secretion *15*

Somatostatin *Plasma Decrease Physiological* 40% reduction observed in 10 normal subjects and 63% reduction observed in 1 patient with somatostatinoma after 6 days of treatment with 1600 mg/day sodium valproate *3336*

Superoxide Dismutase
Red Blood Cells Decrease Physiological Reduction from mean of 2527 U/g hemoglobin to 2288 U/g hemoglobin in 13 epileptic patients associated with reduction in concentration of trace element cofactors *4710*
Serum No Effect Physiological In 19 epileptic children receiving valproic acid mean activity of copper:zinc superoxide dismutase of 0.682 ± 0.307 U/mL not significantly different from 0.681 ± 0.298 U/mL in 20 healthy control children *3331*

T3-Uptake *Serum No Effect Physiological* In 10 epileptic patients treated average of 8 mo *3568* In 23 epileptic patients treated with valproic acid mean uptake ratio of 0.85 ± 0.1 not significantly decreased compared with 0.91 ± 0.1 in 32 healthy controls *6234*

Tacrolimus *Blood No Effect Analytical* No significant effect observed at a concentration of 75 mg/L with MEIA method on Abbott IMx analyzer *1871* No interference observed with radioreceptor assay of Murthy et al *4191*
Serum No Effect Analytical At a concentration of 75 mg/L had no significant effect on ELISA method *6329*

Taurine *Plasma Increase Physiological* Concentration higher in patients with primary generalized seizure disorder receiving valproate than other drugs *2241*

Testosterone *Serum Increase Physiological* In 21 epileptic patients treated with sodium valproate for a median of 10.7 years median concentration in follicular and luteal phases significantly higher than in controls *4178* In 6 women with PCOS treatment with sodium valproate 1200 mg/d for 5 days caused mean concentration to increase from mean of 5.6 ± 1.0 nmol/L to 9.1 ± 2.0 nmol/L *4753*
Serum No Effect Physiological Mean concentration of 23 nmol/L in 7 male epileptic patients treated for mean of 5.4 years, same as in healthy control subjects *2840* Usual effect although slight increase may occur *2836*

Testosterone, Free *Serum Decrease Physiological* Observed effect *2836*
Serum No Effect Physiological Mean concentration of 91 pmol/L in 7 male epileptic patients treated for mean of 5.4 years, same as in healthy control subjects *2840*

Thyroid Stimulating Hormone
Serum Increase Physiological Insignificant mean increase to 2.1 mU/L in 7 male epileptic patients treated for mean of 5.4 years compared with 1.4 mU/L in healthy control subjects *2840* In 11 patients with chronic epilepsy treated with valproic acid mean concentration 2.9 ± 1.8 mU/L significantly increased compared with 1.7 ± 0.8 mU/L in 28 healthy controls *2839*
Serum No Effect Physiological In 10 epileptic patients treated average of 8 mo *3568*

Thyroxine (T4) *Serum Decrease Physiological* Insignificant mean reduction to 85 nmol/L in 7 male epileptic patients treated for mean of 5.4 years compared with mean of 93 nmol/L in healthy control subjects *2840*
Serum No Effect Physiological In 10 epileptic patients treated average of 8 mo *3568* In 23 epileptic patients treated with valproic acid mean concentration of 90 ± 19 nmol/L not significantly different from 99 ± 19 nmol/L in 32 healthy con-

Valproic Acid *(continued)*

Thyroxine (T4) *(continued)*
trols *6234* In 11 patients with chronic epilepsy treatment with valproic acid long term mean concentration 90.0 ± 16.2 nmol/L not significantly different from 91.6 ± 12.9 nmol/L in 28 healthy controls *2839*

Thyroxine (T4), Free *Serum Increase Physiological* Mean increased to 18.4 pmol/L in 7 male epileptic patients treated for mean of 5.4 years compared with mean of 16.5 pmol/L in healthy controls *2840* In 11 chronic epileptic patients treatment with long term valproic acid caused significant increase to 19.0 ± 3.0 pmol/L compared with 16.3 ± 2.4 pmol/L in 28 healthy controls *2839*

Thyroxine (T4) Index, Free *Serum No Effect Physiological* In 23 epileptic patients treated with valproic acid mean concentration of 106.8 ± 12.9 nmol/L not different from 106.8 ± 15.4 nmol/L in 32 healthy controls *6234* In 10 epileptic patients treated average of 8 mo *3568*

Tri-iodothyronine, Reverse (rT3)
Serum No Effect Physiological In 10 epileptic patients treated average of 8 mo *3568*

Tri-iodothyronine (T3) *Serum Increase Physiological* In 11 chronic epileptics treated with long term valproic acid mean concentration 1.9 ± 0.3 nmol/L slightly higher when compared with 1.7 ± 0.2 nmol/L in 28 healthy controls *2839* Insignificant increase to mean of 1.8 nmol/L in 7 male epileptic patients treated for mean of 5.4 years compared with 1.7 nmol/L in healthy control subjects *2840*
Serum No Effect Physiological In 10 epileptic patients treated average of 8 mo *3568*

Triglycerides *Serum No Effect Analytical* At concentration of 1010 mg/L had no effect on GPO-PAP method *5704*
Serum No Effect Physiological In 16 epileptic children treated with valproate for a mean of 1.34 years mean concentration of 82.50 ± 36.67 mg/dL not significantly different from 98.22 ± 38.83 mg/dL in 57 healthy control children *5727*

Uric Acid *Serum No Effect Analytical* At 1.0 g/L on reversed phase liquid chromatographic procedure of Zhiri et al *6656* At concentration of 100 mg/L had no effect on uricase-PAP method *5704*

VLDL-Cholesterol *Serum No Effect Physiological* In 16 epileptic children treated with valproate for a mean of 1.34 years mean concentration of 15.15 ± 4.78 mg/dL not significantly different from 21.69 ± 19.06 mg/dL in 57 healthy control children *5727*

von Willebrand Factor *Plasma Decrease Physiological* Decrease observed in 83% of 30 treated epileptic children *3286*

Zidovudine *Serum Increase Physiological* Coadministration of valproic acid (750 - 1500 mg/d) with 300 mg zidovudine in 6 patients with AIDS caused a 38% decrease in plasma clearance of zidovudine *17* In 6 HIV-positive volunteers coadministration of 250 - 500 mg/8 h daily with zidovudine (100 mg/8 h) for 4 d increased the plasma zidovudine AUC by 79 ± 61% *2163* In HIV-positive patients the clearance of zidovudine (300 mg/d) decreased by 38% after administration of valproate (750 to 1500 mg/d) coadministration without affecting zidovudine half-life *15*
Serum No Effect Physiological Coadministration of valproic acid with acetaminophen had no effect on any of its pharmacokinetic parameters *17*

Zidovudine Glucuronide *Serum Decrease Physiological* In 6 HIV-positive volunteers coadministration of 250 - 500 mg/8 h daily with zidovudine (100 mg/8 h) for 4 d increased the plasma zidovudine AUC by 79 ± 61% but decreased its glucuronide AUC by 22 ± 10% *2163*
Urine Decrease Physiological In 6 HIV-positive volunteers coadministration of 250 - 500 mg/8 h daily with zidovudine (100 mg/8 h) for 4 d increased the plasma zidovudine AUC by 79 ± 61% but decreased its glucuronide AUC by 22 ± 10%. The GZDV/zidovudine urinary excretion ratio declined by 58 ± 12% *2163*

Zinc *Serum Decrease Physiological* Reduction from mean of 670.0 µg/dL to 432.7 µg/dL in patients being treated for epilepsy *4710*
Serum No Effect Physiological In 29 epileptic patients treated for 1 month insignificant reduction to 73.4 ± 11.7 µg/dL compared with 78.4 ± 12.8 µg/dL in 30 controls *3344* In 19 epileptic children receiving valproic acid mean concentration of 3.706 ± 0.77 µg/mL not significantly different from 3.44 ± 1.09 µg/mL in 20 healthy control children *3331*

Valsartan

Alanine Aminotransferase *Serum Increase Physiological* In controlled clinical trials increases of greater than 150% were occasionally observed *1042*

Amlodipine *Serum No Effect Physiological* In controlled clinical trials no pharmacologic interaction observed *1042*

Aspartate Aminotransferase *Serum Increase Physiological* In controlled clinical trials increases of greater than 150% were occasionally observed *1042*

Atenolol *Serum No Effect Physiological* In controlled clinical trials no pharmacologic interaction observed *1042*

Cimetidine *Serum No Effect Physiological* In controlled clinical trials no pharmacologic interaction observed *1042*

Creatinine *Serum Increase Physiological* In controlled clinical trials minor increases were observed in 0.8% drug treated patients compared with 0.6% in placebo-treated patients *1042*

Digoxin *Serum No Effect Physiological* In controlled clinical trials no pharmacologic interaction observed *1042*

Furosemide *Serum No Effect Physiological* In controlled clinical trials no pharmacologic interaction observed *1042*

Glibenclamide *Serum No Effect Physiological* In controlled clinical trials no pharmacologic interaction observed *1042*

Hematocrit *Blood Decrease Physiological* In controlled clinical trials greater than 20% decreases were observed in 0.8% drug treated patients compared with 0.1% in placebo-treated patients *1042*

Hemoglobin *Blood Decrease Physiological* In controlled clinical trials greater than 20% decreases were observed in 0.4% drug treated patients compared with 0.1% in placebo-treated patients *1042*

Hydrochlorothiazide *Serum No Effect Physiological* In controlled clinical trials no pharmacologic interaction observed *1042*

Indomethacin *Serum No Effect Physiological* In controlled clinical trials no pharmacologic interaction observed *1042*

Leukocytes *Blood Decrease Physiological* In controlled clinical trials neutropenia was observed in 1.9% drug treated patients compared with 0.8% in placebo-treated patients *1042*

Potassium *Serum Increase Physiological* In controlled clinical trials increases greater than 20% were observed in 4.4% drug treated patients compared with 2.9% in placebo-treated patients *1042*

Vancomycin

Amikacin *Serum No Effect Analytical* Error of less than 5% observed when vancomycin added at a concentration on 100 mg/L to a specimen containing 15 mg/L amikacin and measured on Baxter Stratus *5705* No interference observed with method on Abbott TDx *3858*

Bilirubin *Serum No Effect Physiological* Clinically significant displacement from protein in neonates *6314*

Casts *Urine Increase Physiological* Occasional evidence of mild nephrotoxicity *2571*

Chloramphenicol *Serum No Effect Analytical* No effect at 100 mg/L on coupled enzymatic method *4122*

Clindamycin *Serum Positive Analytical* Interferes with bioassays *3858*

Colistin *Serum Positive Analytical* Interferes with bioassays *3858*

Creatinine *Serum Increase Physiological* Occasional renal damage (usually reversible) *198* Occasional evidence of mild nephrotoxicity *2571* Nephrotoxicity in 5% of 60 patients given drug alone but much higher incidence when given with aminoglycosides *4364* In 5 to 20% of cases co-treatment with gentamicin increases risk of nephrotoxicity *5170* Rarely renal failure may occur, mainly in patients given large doses of drug. Rare cases of interstitial nephritis have been reported *1710*

Serum *No Effect* *Analytical* At therapeutic concentration had no effect on method on Kodak Ektachem® 700 *586* No interference observed at a concentration of 1 mg/L with HPLC method of Rosano et al *5083* No effect of concentrations up to 15 mg/L on single slide method on Kodak Ektachem® *5706* No effect at therapeutic concentrations on Jaffe procedure on Beckman Astra® and Technicon SMAC® *1181*

Creatinine Clearance *Urine* *Decrease* *Physiological* Occasional renal damage (usually reversible) *198*

Cyclosporine *Blood* *No Effect* *Analytical* At a concentration of 630 mg/L had no effect on Syva EMIT method *495*
Blood *No Effect* *Physiological* Coadministration with cyclosporine appeared to have no significant effect on its concentration *859*
Serum *No Effect* *Physiological* Coadministration with cyclosporine appeared to have no significant effect on its concentration *859*

Eosinophils *Blood* *Increase* *Physiological* Occasional hypersensitivity reaction noted *2571* Allergic response *2484*

Erythromycin *Serum* *Increase* *Analytical* Interferes with bioassays *3858*

Gentamicin *Serum* *No Effect* *Analytical* Has cross-reactivity of less than 0.1% with method on Baxter Stratus *5705* No interference observed with method on Abbott TDx *3858*

Granulocytes *Blood* *Decrease* *Physiological* Reversible agranulocytosis has been rarely attributed to drug administration *1710*

Hemoglobin *Urine* *Increase* *Physiological* Occasional evidence of mild nephrotoxicity *2571*

Iron *Serum* *No Effect* *Analytical* No interference observed with method on Kodak Ektachem® *2792*

Kanamycin *Serum* *No Effect* *Analytical* No interference observed with method on Abbott TDx *3858*

Lactate *Plasma* *No Effect* *Analytical* No effect at final concentration of 50 µg/mL with method on Kodak Ektachem® *2793*

Leukocytes *Blood* *Decrease* *Physiological* Favorable response of antibiotic-associated colitis to drug *5974*
Blood *Increase* *Physiological* Due to eosinophilia *3810*

Magnesium *Serum* *No Effect* *Analytical* No effect at therapeutic concentration on method on Kodak Ektachem® 700 *586*

Metronidazole *Serum* *Increase* *Analytical* Interferes with bioassays *3858*

Mycophenolic Acid *Serum* *No Effect* *Analytical* No significant interference observed with HPLC method of Shipkova et al *5526*

Mycophenolic Acid Glucuronide
Serum *No Effect* *Analytical* No significant interference observed with HPLC method of Shipkova et al *5526*

Neomycin *Serum* *No Effect* *Analytical* No interference observed with method on Abbott TDx *3858*

Netilmicin *Serum* *No Effect* *Analytical* No interference observed with method on Abbott TDx *3858*

Neutrophils *Blood* *Decrease* *Physiological* Observed in one patient with renal failure after 3 g drug *58* Reversible neutropenia, usually starting one or more weeks after start of therapy, or after a total dose of 25 g, has been reported for several dozen patients. Neutropenia stops when drug is stopped *1710* Occasional reversible side effect *2571*

Phenylalanine *Plasma* *No Effect* *Analytical* No interference observed with rapid quantitative whole blood method of Campbell et al using phenylalanine dehydrogenase *867*

Platelets *Blood* *Decrease* *Physiological* Reversible thrombocytopenia has been reported rarely *1710*

Polymyxin *Serum* *Increase* *Analytical* Interferes with bioassays *3858*

Protein *Cerebrospinal Fluid* *Increase* *Analytical* 100 mg/L solution gave color corresponding to 130 mg/L protein when measured with Kodak Ektachem® method, but effect uncertain clinically since drug does not readily diffuse across normal meninges although does diffuse across inflamed meninges *3654*
Cerebrospinal Fluid *No Effect* *Analytical* No effect observed at final concentration of 5 µg/mL with method on Kodak Ektachem® *2791* At concentration of 40 mg/L on SDS/Coomassie Blue method of Huang *2745*

Urine *Increase* *Physiological* Occasional evidence of mild nephrotoxicity *2571* May cause nephrotoxicity *5377*

SDZ PSC 833 *Blood* *No Effect* *Analytical* At a concentration of 36 mg/L had no effect on HPLC method of Scott et al when used to measure PSC (with CsD as internal standard) at a concentration of 5 mg/L *5418*

Streptomycin *Serum* *No Effect* *Analytical* No interference observed with method on Abbott TDx *3858*

Tacrolimus *Blood* *No Effect* *Analytical* No significant effect observed at a concentration of 50 mg/L with MEIA method on Abbott IMx analyzer *1871*
Serum *Increase* *Analytical* In HPLC/MS method of Christians et al interference observed with measurement of metabolites of FK 506 because of similar retention time *1010*
Serum *No Effect* *Analytical* At concentration of 50 mg/L had no significant effect on ELISA method *6329*

Tetracycline *Serum* *Increase* *Analytical* Interferes with bioassays *3858*

Tobramycin *Serum* *Increase* *Analytical* At a concentration of 1250 mg/L increases concentration by 15% when measured by method on Baxter Stratus but therapeutic concentration up to 30 mg/L only *5705*
Serum *No Effect* *Analytical* No interference observed with method on Abbott TDx *3858*
Serum *No Effect* *Physiological* No significant effect observed on pharmacokinetics when drugs coadministered *4169*

Trimethoprim *Serum* *Increase* *Analytical* Interferes with bioassays *3858*

Urea Nitrogen *Serum* *Increase* *Physiological* Nephrotoxicity in 5% of 60 patients given drug alone but much higher incidence when given with aminoglycosides *4364* Nephrotoxic effect (may even be fatal) *2024* Occasional evidence of mild nephrotoxicity *2571* Rarely renal failure may occur, mainly in patients given large doses of drug. Rare cases of interstitial nephritis have been reported *1710*

Vasopressin

Aldolase *Serum* *Increase* *Physiological* Rhabdomyolysis observed in 2 patients following intravenous drug administration *61*

Aldosterone *Plasma* *No Effect* *Physiological* In 7 healthy individuals infusion of either 0.5 or 2 ng/kg/min had no significant effect *911*
Urine *No Effect* *Physiological* If not overhydrated no effect *2244*

Aspartate Aminotransferase *Serum* *Increase* *Physiological* Rhabdomyolysis observed in 2 patients following intravenous drug administration *61*

Atrial Natriuretic Peptide *Plasma* *Increase* *Physiological* In 7 normal individuals sequential 20-min infusions at 0.5 and 2 ng/kg/min caused significant increase at the end of both the first and second infusion periods *911*

Corticosteroids *Plasma* *Increase* *Physiological* Significant effect 30-45 minutes after i.v. in normals *5778*

Corticotropin *Plasma* *Increase* *Physiological* Small but significant effect after i.v. in normals *5778*

Cortisol *Plasma* *Increase* *Physiological* May be rise of up to 6 µg/dL or more *6085*

Creatine Kinase *Serum* *Increase* *Physiological* Rhabdomyolysis observed in 2 patients following intravenous drug administration *61*

Creatinine *Serum* *Increase* *Physiological* Progressive deterioration in renal function observed in one patient given drug i.v *61*

Epinephrine *Plasma* *No Effect* *Physiological* In 7 healthy individuals infusion of either 0.5 or 2 ng/kg/min for 20 min had no significant effect on concentration *911*

Growth Hormone *Plasma* *Increase* *Physiological* Observed effect in normals *593*

Lactate Dehydrogenase *Serum* *Increase* *Physiological* Rhabdomyolysis observed in 2 patients following intravenous drug administration *61*

Leucine Aminopeptidase *Urine* *Increase* *Physiological* Activates peptidases by release of plasminogen *4826*

Vasopressin *(continued)*

Myoglobin *Urine Increase Physiological* Rhabdomyolysis observed in 2 patients following intravenous drug administration *61*

Norepinephrine *Plasma No Effect Physiological* In 7 healthy individuals 20-min infusion of either 0.5 or 2 ng/kg/min had no significant effect on concentration *911*

Renin Activity *Plasma Decrease Physiological* In 7 healthy individuals infusion of sequential infusions of 0.5 and 2 ng/kg/min caused significant decrease at the end of the infusion *911*

Plasma No Effect Physiological No demonstrable effect if not overhydrated *2244*

Sodium *Serum Decrease Physiological* May occur with water retention *128*

Urea Nitrogen *Serum Increase Physiological* Progressive deterioration in renal function observed in one patient given drug *61*

Volume *Urine Decrease Physiological* Therapeutic intent *128*

Vecuronium

Bromide *Serum Increase Physiological* Theoretical possibility if bromide salt is administered since it contains 25% bromide *5116*

Histamine *Plasma No Effect Analytical* Although 50% inhibition of radio-enzyme assay at 5.8 µg/mL unlikely to be of clinical significance since physiological concentration 0.09 - 0.2 µg/mL *2492*

Plasma No Effect Physiological Apparently no effect on concentration with doses up to 0.2 mg/kg in group of 10 patients *871*

Ketone Body Ratio *Serum No Effect Analytical* When added at a concentration of 40 mg/L had no significant effect on AKBR method of Uno et al *6131*

Venlafaxine

Abnormal Erythrocytes *Blood Increase Physiological* Rarely abnormal erythrocytes associated with administration of venlafaxine *6555*

Alanine Aminotransferase *Serum Increase Physiological* Hepatitis and jaundice have been infrequently associated with administration of venlafaxine *6555*

Albumin *Urine Increase Physiological* Albuminuria frequently observed *6555*

Alkaline Phosphatase *Serum Increase Physiological* Hepatitis and jaundice have been infrequently associated with administration of venlafaxine *6555*

Aspartate Aminotransferase *Serum Increase Physiological* Hepatitis and jaundice have been infrequently associated with administration of venlafaxine *6555*

Basophils *Blood Increase Physiological* Rare basophilia associated with administration of venlafaxine *6555*

Bilirubin *Serum Increase Physiological* Hepatitis and jaundice have been infrequently associated with administration of venlafaxine *6555*

Blood *Urine Increase Physiological* Hematuria frequently observed *6555*

Cholesterol *Serum Increase Physiological* Increased plasma cholesterol concentration infrequently associated with administration of venlafaxine *6555*

Creatinine *Serum Increase Physiological* Increased plasma creatinine concentration infrequently associated with administration of venlafaxine *6555* Uremia rarely observed *6555*

Crystals *Urine Increase Physiological* Calcium crystalluria frequently observed *6555*

Desmethyldiazepam *Serum No Effect Physiological* When a single 10 mg dose of diazepam was administered to 18 healthy men no effect observed on steady state pharmacokinetics of diazepam or desmethyldiazepam when venlafaxine administered 50 mg every 8 hours *6555*

Diazepam *Serum No Effect Physiological* When a single 10 mg dose of diazepam was administered to 18 healthy men no effect observed on steady state pharmacokinetics of diazepam or desmethyldiazepam when venlafaxine administered 50 mg every 8 hours *6555*

Eosinophils *Blood Increase Physiological* Rare eosinophilia associated with administration of venlafaxine *6555*

Glucose *Serum Decrease Physiological* Hypoglycemia infrequently associated with administration of venlafaxine *6555*

Serum Increase Physiological Increased plasma glucose concentration infrequently associated with administration of venlafaxine *6555*

Urine Increase Physiological Increased plasma glucose concentration with glycosuria infrequently associated with administration of venlafaxine *6555*

Hematocrit *Blood Decrease Physiological* Infrequent anemia associated with administration of venlafaxine *6555*

Hemoglobin *Blood Decrease Physiological* Infrequent anemia associated with administration of venlafaxine *6555*

Leukocytes *Blood Decrease Physiological* Infrequent leukopenia associated with administration of venlafaxine *6555*

Blood Increase Physiological Infrequent leukocytosis associated with administration of venlafaxine *6555*

Lipids *Serum Increase Physiological* Hyperlipidemia infrequently associated with administration of venlafaxine *6555*

Lymphocytes *Blood Increase Physiological* Infrequent lymphocytosis associated with administration of venlafaxine *6555*

Occult Blood *Feces Increase Physiological* Rectal hemorrhage has been infrequently associated with administration of venlafaxine *6555*

Phosphate *Serum Decrease Physiological* Hypophosphatemia rarely associated with administration of venlafaxine *6555*

Serum Increase Physiological Hyperphosphatemia rarely associated with administration of venlafaxine *6555*

Platelets *Blood Increase Physiological* Infrequent thrombocythemia associated with administration of venlafaxine *6555*

Potassium *Serum Decrease Physiological* Hypokalemia infrequently associated with administration of venlafaxine *6555*

Serum Increase Physiological Hyperkalemia rarely associated with administration of venlafaxine *6555*

Protein *Serum Decrease Physiological* Hypoproteinemia rarely associated with administration of venlafaxine *6555*

Sodium *Serum Decrease Physiological* Hyponatremia rarely associated with administration of venlafaxine *6555*

Thyroxine (T4) *Serum Decrease Physiological* Rare hypothyroidism associated with administration of venlafaxine *6555*

Serum Increase Physiological Rare hyperthyroidism associated with administration of venlafaxine *6555*

Urea Nitrogen *Serum Increase Physiological* Increased concentration rarely associated with administration of venlafaxine: uremia rarely observed *6555*

Uric Acid *Serum Increase Physiological* Hyperuricemia infrequently associated with administration of venlafaxine *6555*

Venoms

Protein *Urine Increase Physiological* May cause nephrotoxicity *5377*

Urea Nitrogen *Serum Increase Physiological* May cause nephrotoxicity *5377*

Veralipride

Luteinizing Hormone *Plasma No Effect Physiological* 200 mg daily for 30 days in 15 postmenopausal women caused significant reduction of plasma concentration *1870*

Prolactin *Plasma Increase Physiological* Significant increase in 15 postmenopausal women treated with 200 mg/day for 30 days *1870*

Verapamil

Adriamycin *Serum Increase Physiological* In 5 patients with small cell lung cancer coadministration with verapamil caused increased peak plasma concentration, terminal half-life and volume of distribution at steady state but plasma clearance reduced *3111*

Alanine Aminotransferase *Serum Increase Physiological* Increased activity has been reported with treatment *2063* Observed in a single case, reverted to normal as soon as drug withdrawn *4225* Increased enzyme activity, sometimes transient, and even decreasing during continuing treatment have been observed, but several cases of hepatocellular damage have also been reported *3201* Increased aminotransferase activity with/without concomitant increases in alkaline phosphatase and bilirubin have been reported. Increases may be transient and subside even with continued treatment. Hepatocellular injury related to treatment may occur *3470*

Serum No Effect Physiological In 437 patients with essential hypertension treatment with verapamil SR 240 mg/d for 6 months caused nonsignificant reduction from mean baseline of 22 ± 10 U/L to 21 ± 8 U/L *3559*

Albumin *Urine Increase Physiological* Nonsignificant increase from mean baseline of 78 µg/mg creatinine to 83 µg/mg after 10 weeks, 193 µg/mg after 20 weeks and 251 µg/mg in 18 hypertensive diabetic patients *1849*

Aldosterone *Plasma Decrease Physiological* Significant effect in 15 patients with uncomplicated essential hypertension *1362*

Plasma Increase Physiological In 15 hypertensive patients with mild to chronic renal failure when treated with verapamil SR 240 mg/d for 4 weeks mean concentration of 882.1 ± 349.5 pmol/L significantly greater than 740.7 ± 302.4 pmol/L when treated with placebo *5372* Concentration initially lower in hypertensives and increased gradually up to fourth month. Exact mechanism still to be elucidated *6676*

Plasma No Effect Physiological No significant effect in 9 patients with normal renin hypertension when receiving either low or high sodium diet *2759* No significant change in 8 healthy women treated with 240 mg/day for 7 days *6392* No change compared with placebo in 11 patients treated with up to 360 mg daily for 6 weeks *5710* No significant effect observed in 15 patients with essential hypertension treated with 480 mg slow release preparation daily for 2 months *3068*

Alkaline Phosphatase *Serum Increase Physiological* In hypertensive patients activity increased, largely from bone *5589* Increased enzyme activity, sometimes transient, and even decreasing during continuing treatment have been observed, but several cases of hepatocellular damage have also been reported *3201* Increased activity has been reported with treatment *2063* Increased aminotransferase activity with/without concomitant increases in alkaline phosphatase and bilirubin have been reported. Increases may be transient and subside even with continued treatment. Hepatocellular injury related to treatment may occur *3470*

Serum No Effect Physiological In 10 patients with recent AMI treated with 360 mg/d verapamil for 6 months mean activity of 218 U/L not significantly different from 200 U/L in 9 placebo-treated AMI patients *636*

Angiotensin-II *Plasma Increase Physiological* In 15 hypertensive patients with mild to severe chronic renal failure when treated with verapamil 240 mg/d for 4 weeks mean concentration 14.3 ± 3.8 ng/L significantly greater than 12.9 ± 4.7 ng/L when treated with placebo *5372*

Plasma No Effect Physiological In 15 patients with uncomplicated essential hypertension *1362* No significant effect in 8 healthy women treated with 240 mg daily for 7 days *6392* No significant effect observed in 15 patients with essential hypertension treated with 480 mg slow release preparation daily for 2 months *3068* No change compared with placebo in 11 patients treated with up to 360 mg daily for 6 weeks *5710*

Antidiuretic Hormone *Plasma No Effect Physiological* No change compared with placebo in 11 patients treated with up to 360 mg daily *5710*

Antipyrine *Serum Increase Physiological* Decreased clearance observed with coadministration of verapamil *5151* Administration of 80 mg t.i.d. caused significant increase in plasma concentration probably due to inhibition of hepatic metabolism *411*

Aspartate Aminotransferase *Serum Increase Physiological* Observed in a single case, reverted to normal as soon as drug withdrawn *4225* Increased aminotransferase activity with/without concomitant increases in alkaline phosphatase and bilirubin have been reported. Increases may be transient and subside even with continued treatment. Hepatocellular injury related to treatment may occur *3470* Increased enzyme activity, sometimes transient, and even decreasing during continuing treatment have been observed, but several cases of hepatocellular damage have also been reported *3201* Increased activity has been reported with treatment *2063*

Serum No Effect Physiological In 437 patients with essential hypertension treatment with verapamil SR 240 mg/d for 6 months caused no change from mean baseline of 21 ± 9 U/L *3559*

Atenolol *Serum Increase Physiological* A decrease in atenolol clearance has been reported when the drug is coadministered with verapamil *3470* Moderate increases in plasma concentration and area under curve observed with coadministration: effect due to enhanced gastrointestinal absorption and reduced renal clearance *3896*

Serum No Effect Physiological Coadministration had no significant effect on plasma atenolol concentration *3087* In 10 patients with coronary artery disease receiving long term maintenance treatment with atenolol and verapamil mean atenolol concentration and area under the curve were not affected compared with atenolol treatment alone *5411*

Atrial Natriuretic Peptide *Plasma Increase Physiological* Both in young and elderly hypertensives treatment with 360 mg daily for 4 weeks caused increase to mean of 66.4 pg/mL in young hypertensives and 78.8 pg/mL in elderly hypertensives after 30 minutes in supine position *6164* In elderly hypertensives treatment with 240 mg orally daily for 4 months significantly increased concentration. Increase in adult hypertensives not significant *216* In elderly hypertensives treatment with 240 mg orally daily for 4 months significantly increased concentration. Increase in adult hypertensives not significant *216*

Plasma No Effect Physiological No significant effect in 9 patients with normal renin hypertension when receiving either low or high sodium diet *2759*

Bilirubin *Serum Increase Physiological* Observed in a single case, reverted to normal as soon as drug withdrawn *4225* Increased enzyme activity, sometimes transient, and even decreasing during continuing treatment have been observed, but several cases of hepatocellular damage have also been reported *3201* Increased aminotransferase activity with/without concomitant increases in alkaline phosphatase and bilirubin have been reported. Increases may be transient and subside even with continued treatment. Hepatocellular injury related to treatment may occur *3470*

Bilirubin, Direct *Serum Increase Physiological* Observed in a single case reverted to normal as soon as drug withdrawn *4225*

Buspirone *Serum Increase Physiological* In 9 healthy volunteers coadministration of verapamil with buspirone caused increase of AUC of buspirone by 3.4-fold with a 3.4-fold increase in peak plasma concentration *3376*

Calcium *Serum No Effect Physiological* No significant effect in 9 patients with normal renin hypertension when receiving either low or high sodium diet *2759* In 10 patients with recent AMI treatment with 360 mg/d for 6 months had no different effect from treatment with placebo *636*

Urine No Effect Physiological No significant effect in 9 patients with normal renin hypertension when receiving either low or high sodium diet *2759*

Carbamazepine *Serum Increase Physiological* Drugs that inhibit CYP 3A4 inhibit metabolism of carbamazepine producing clinically meaningful effect *1039* Concentration increased during coadministration probably due to inhibition of hepatic oxidative metabolism *3119* Concomitant administration of calcium channel blockers with carbamazepine causes marked increase of plasma carbamazepine concentration resulting in toxicity in some cases *282* The pharmacokinetic interaction betwen verapamil and carbamazepine may increase the plasma carbamazepine concentration *3470* When drugs coadministered serum carbamazepine concentration may be increased *2063* Coadministration may increase carbamazepine concentration

Verapamil *(continued)*

Carbamazepine *(continued)*
but mechanism not specified *3201* Addition of 120 mg/day verapamil to 6 patients receiving carbamazepine as chronic anticonvulsant therapy caused decrease in carbamazepine clearance of about 40% with reduction of metabolites *3722* Inhibits metabolism and potentiates neurotoxicity of carbamazepine *1384* 2 cases of increased concentration observed when verapamil coadministered with carbamazepine. In another study carbamazepine concentrations rose 46% when 120 mg carbamazepine administered three times daily for 7 days *5411*

Carbamazepine-10,11-Epoxide
Serum No Effect Physiological No change in concentration observed when verapamil coadministered with carbamazepine even though carbamazepine concentration markedly increased *5411*

Cholesterol *Serum Decrease Physiological* In 12 patients when angina or hypertension treated for 6 weeks. Where change occurred it was of the order of 10% *6328* In 52 newly diagnosed hypertensives treatment with 240 mg/d for 6 weeks caused significant mean reduction of 0.26 mmol/L *378* In 437 patients with essential hypertension treatment with verapamil SR 240 mg/d for 6 months caused significant reduction from mean baseline of 5.77 ± 1.08 mmol/L to 5.35 ± 0.88 mmol/L *3559*
Serum No Effect Physiological In 64 patients in post-myocardial infarction comparison against placebo *5852*

Cortisol *Plasma No Effect Physiological* With 80 mg 3-4/d orally no significant effect on resting concentration or after ACTH stimulation in mild hypertensives *6676*

Creatinine *Serum No Effect Physiological* In 142 hypertensives treatment with 240 mg/d for 6 weeks had no significant effect on concentration *378* No effect in 8 healthy women of treatment with 240 mg daily for 7 days *6392* No significant effect in 9 patients with normal renin hypertension when given either low or sodium diet *2759*
Urine No Effect Physiological No significant effect in 9 patients with normal renin hypertension when receiving either low or high sodium diet *2759*

Creatinine Clearance *Urine No Effect Physiological* In 142 hypertensives treatment with 240 mg/d for 6 weeks had no significant effect on clearance *378* No significant effect in 9 patients with normal renin hypertension when receiving either low or high sodium diet *2759*

Cyclosporine *Blood Increase Physiological* Coadministration with cyclosporine reported to increase trough cyclosporine concentrations probably due to inhibtion of CYP enzymes in liver. This allows reduction of cyclosporine dosage by 33 to 50% *859*
Serum Increase Physiological Concentration increased in 12 cardiac transplant patients and 14 renal transplant recipients when drug coadministered for treatment of hypertension or arrhythmia: associated with renal deterioration in heart patients but not in renal patients *6596* Coadministration may increase cyclosporine concentration but mechanism not specified *3201* After 1 week of concurrent therapy in 5 patients concentration increased up to 4 times *6220* Coadministration of verapamil to renal transplant recipients caused significant increase *6058* Increased concentration reported when drugs coadministered *1384* 45% increase in area under curve in 11 verapamil-treated patients with renal transplants. Maximum concentration, steady-state concentration and trough levels of both cyclosporine and metabolite 17 also increased *6058* May increase cyclosporine concentration by inhibiting hepatic cytochrome P-450 III A which metabolizes cyclosporine *5236* Coadministration with cyclosporine reported to increase trough cyclosporine concentrations probably due to inhibtion of CYP enzymes in liver. This allows reduction of cyclosporine dosage by 33 to 50% *859* Coadministration of verapamil with cyclosporine was associated with increased cyclosporine concentration due to reduction of cyclosporine clearance due to inhibition of hepatic microsomal drug metabolism. Effect dose related *5411*

Cyclosporine A *Blood Increase Physiological* When drugs coadministered serum cyclosporine A concentration may be increased *2063* Coadministration with cyclosporine A increases its concentration *5240* Coadministration of verapamil with cyclosporine may increase its concentration *3470*

Digitoxin *Serum Increase Physiological* Slight increase observed with coadministration *1384* Concentration increased by up to 35% when two drugs coadministered *3318* In 10 patients receiving concurrent verapamil (240 mg/d) and digitoxin plasma digitoxin concentrations increased 27% after 2-3 weeks due to decreased clearance of digitoxin *5345*

Digoxin *Serum Increase Physiological* When drugs coadministered chronically serum digoxin concentration may be increased by 50% to 75% during the first week of therapy *2063* Total body clearance reduced after single dose from mean of 4.68 mL/min/kg to 3.29 mL/min/kg and increased plasma half-life from 32.5 to 41.3 h. Increase in plasma concentration of from 35 to 75% reported due to decreased renal and extrarenal clearance *4584* With chronic administration of verapamil with digoxin plasma digoxin concentration may be increased by 50 to 75%. The effect is magnified in patients with hepatic cirrhosis *3470* Coadministration with digoxin may increase the digoxin concentration *2161* In patients in whom verapamil coadministered with digoxin digoxin's area under the concentration curve, its half-life and plasma concentration were increased. Steady state plasma concentrations increased by 77%, 61%, 53%, 155% and 60% respectively in 5 different studies *5345* Average increase from 0.96 to 1.63 ng/mL in 41 patients when given 240 mg/d *3175* Marked increase observed in patients undergoing hemodialysis and taking digoxin *4916* An increase of 50% to 70% has been observed in the plasma digoxin concentration when the drug was coadministered chronically with verapamil. The effect was exaggerated in patients with hepatic cirrhosis *3201*

1,25-Dihydroxy Vitamin D_3 *Serum No Effect Physiological* No significant effect in 9 patients with normal renin hypertension when receiving either low or high sodium diet *2759*

Doxorubicin *Serum Increase Physiological* Prior administration of verapamil to 5 patients with cancer caused decrease in average clearance of doxorubicin of 33% with increase in half-life from 23.6 to 32.5 hours probably due to inhibition of hepatic metabolism of doxorubicin *3111* In patients in whom verapamil was coadministered with doxorubicin mean doxorubicin area under the concentration curve doubled (not significant) and its clearance decreased by 32%. Nevertheless because patients also received other drugs verapamil may not have been responsible for all effects *5345*

Epinephrine *Plasma Decrease Physiological* Significant effect in 15 patients with uncomplicated essential hypertension *1362*

Filtration Fraction *Urine No Effect Physiological* In 15 hypertensive patients with mild to severe chronic renal failure mean fraction 23.6 ± 10.9% when treated with 240 mg/d verapamil SR for 4 weeks compared with 22.3 ± 10.0% when treated with placebo *5372*

Flecainide *Serum No Effect Physiological* Area under the flecainide curve and half-life of flecainide unaffected by coadministration *5345*

Glomerular Filtration Rate *Urine No Effect Physiological* In 15 patients with hypertension and mild to severe chronic renal failure mean of 27.3 ± 17.8 mL/min when treated with verapamil SR 240 mg/d for 4 weeks not significantly different from 25.8 ± 16.9 mL/min when treated with placebo *5372* No change compared with placebo in 11 patients treated with up to 360 mg daily for 6 weeks *5710* No significant effect observed in 15 patients with essential hypertension treated with 480 mg slow release preparation daily for 2 months *3068*

Glucagon *Plasma Decrease Physiological* Significant change during tolerance test when drug and glucose coadministered *1837*
Plasma No Effect Physiological No effect observed even in individuals fasted for 36 h when infused at rate of 5 mg/h or 3 h *166*

Glucose *Serum Decrease Physiological* In 437 patients with essential hypertension treatment with verapamil SR 240 mg/d for 6 months caused significant reduction from mean baseline of 5.4 ± 0.8 mmol/L to 5.2 ± 0.6 mmol/L *3559* Incidence of 1.0% observed in French Pharmacovigilance database *4106* When infused i.v. at rate of 5 mg/h for 3 h in prolonged fasted individuals but not in overnight fasted subjects *166*
Serum No Effect Physiological In 18 hypertensive diabetic patients treatment for up to 30 weeks had no significant effect on concentration *1849*

Glucose Tolerance *Serum Decrease Physiological* Significant impairment when glucose and drug co-administered *1837*

Serum No Effect Physiological No significant effect observed in diabetics with hypertension *1140*

HDL-Cholesterol *Serum Decrease Physiological* In 12 patients with angina or hypertension treated for 6 weeks. Where change occurred it was of the order of 10% *6328*
Serum Increase Physiological In 437 patients with essential hypertension treatment with verapamil SR 240 mg/d for 6 months caused significant increase from mean baseline of 1.16 ± 0.31 mmol/L to 1.27 ± 0.28 mmol/L *3559* In 52 newly diagnosed hypertensives treatment with 240 mg/d for 6 weeks caused nonsignificant mean increase of 0.12 mmol/L *378*
Serum No Effect Physiological In 64 patients in post-myocardial infarction comparison against placebo *5852*

Hemoglobin A_{1c} *Blood Decrease Physiological* In 77 hypertensive diabetics treatment with 240 mg/d for 6 weeks caused nonsignificant mean reduction of 0.01% *378*
Blood No Effect Physiological Treatment of 18 hypertensive diabetic patients for 30 weeks had no significant effect on concentration *1849* No significant effect observed in diabetics with hypertension *1140*

Histamine *Plasma No Effect Analytical* Although 50% inhibition of radio-enzyme assay at 32 µg/mL unlikely to be of clinical significance since therapeutic concentration 0.031 - 0.134 µg/mL *2492*

Homovanillic Acid
Cerebrospinal Fluid Increase Physiological In 7 chronically ill schizophrenic patients when administered for 5 weeks *4694*
Plasma Increase Physiological In 7 chronically ill schizophrenic patients when administered for 5 weeks *4694*

4-Hydroxy-3-Methoxy-Phenylglycol
Urine Decrease Physiological In 7 chronically ill schizophrenic patients when administered for 5 weeks *4694*

Insulin *Plasma Increase Physiological* Significant change during tolerance test when drug and glucose coadministered *1837*
Plasma No Effect Physiological No effect observed even in individuals fasted for 36 h when infused at rate of 5 mg/h for 3 h *166*

ionized Calcium *Serum No Effect Physiological* No significant effect in 9 patients with normal renin hypertension when receiving either low or high sodium diet but baseline value when receiving high sodium diet significantly less than when receiving low sodium *2759*

Lactate Dehydrogenase *Serum Increase Physiological* Observed in a single case, reverted to normal as soon as drug withdrawn *4225*

LDL-Cholesterol *Serum Decrease Physiological* In 437 patients with essential hypertension treatment with verapamil SR 240 mg/d for 6 months caused significant reduction from mean baseline of 3.70 ± 1.08 mmol/L to 3.39 ± 0.96 mmol/L *3559* In 52 newly diagnosed hypertensives treatment with 240 mg/d for 6 weeks caused nonsignificant mean decrease of 0.16 mmol/L *378*
Serum No Effect Physiological In 64 patients in postmyocardial infarction in comparison against placebo *5852*

Lithium *Serum Decrease Physiological* Verapamil has been shown to reduce the concentration of plasma lithium concentration under steady state conditions *3201* The pharmacokinetic interaction betwen verapamil and lithium may cause a reduction in the plasma lithium concentration *3470*
Serum Increase Physiological Possible effect of verapamil in inducing lithium toxicity but patients also receiving drugs that might have contributed to toxicity *5345*

Lysergic Acid Diethylamide *Urine Increase Analytical* Minimum concentration that caused a positive result with EMIT method to measure LSD 5 mg/L *4968*

Methadone *Urine Increase Analytical* False positive results observed with metabolites of verapamil when methadone measured by Diagnostics Reagents kit *3561*

Metoprolol *Serum Increase Physiological* When drugs coadministered clearance of metoprolol decreased *2063* Chronic coadministration increased area under concentration curve of metoprolol from mean of 1107 mg/h/mL to 1467 mg/h/mL in patients with stable coronary disease *3087* A decrease in metoprolol clearance has been observed when it was coadministered with verapamil *3201* A decrease in metoprolol clearance has been reported when the drug is coadministered with verapamil *3470* In 9 patients with coronary artery disease coadministration of verapamil and metoprolol in different amounts for one week per phase caused increase in maximum concentration and area under the curve by 41% and 33% respectively *5411*

Midazolam *Serum Increase Physiological* By inhibiting cytochrome P450 3A4 may reduce plasma clearance of midazolam when drugs coadministered. Half-life of midazolam increased from 5 to 7 hours *5037*
Serum No Effect Analytical On GC-ECD method of Ha et al *2387*

Norepinephrine *Plasma Increase Physiological* Insignificant change in 15 patients with uncomplicated essential hypertension *1362*
Plasma No Effect Physiological No significant effect observed in 15 patients treated with 480 mg slow release compound daily for 2 months (mean concentration 0.88 nmol/L versus 1.33 nmol/L with placebo) *3068* In 15 hypertensive patients with mild to severe chronic renal failure treatment with verapamil 240 mg/d for 4 weeks associated with mean concentration of 420 ± 104 ng/L not significantly different from 426 ± 173 ng/L when treated with placebo *5372*

Osmolality *Serum No Effect Physiological* No significant effect in 9 patients with normal renin hypertension given either low or high sodium diet *2759*
Urine Decrease Physiological Significant reduction in 9 patients with normal renin hypertension when receiving either low or high sodium diet associated with reduced clearance *2759*

Osteocalcin *Serum No Effect Physiological* No significant difference observed between 10 patients who had had a recent myocardial infarct treated with 360 mg/d for 6 months compared with 9 treated with placebo (8.2 µg/L versus 8.0 µg/L) *636*

Parathyroid Hormone *Plasma Increase Physiological* In hypertensive patients concentration increased 10% after 2 months treatment *5589*
Plasma No Effect Physiological In 10 patients with recent AMI treated with 360 mg/d for 6 months had no different effect from placebo in 9 placebo-treated patients *636* In 14 premenopausal women given 240 mg sustained release verapamil parathyroid concentration changed nonsignificantly from mean baseline of about 15.5 ng/L to 15.0 ng/L and no change observed over 28 days *6372* No significant effect in 9 patients with normal renin hypertension when receiving either low or high sodium diet *2759*

Phenytoin *Serum Increase Physiological* Reported increase as with other anticonvulsants when verapamil coadministered with phenytoin *5411*

Phosphate *Serum No Effect Physiological* In 10 patients with recent AMI treatment with 360 mg/d had no significantly different effect from placebo in 9 other patients *636*

Platelet Aggregation *Blood No Effect Physiological* No significant alteration in threshold values for epinephrine-induced aggregation at doses of 40 mg t.i.d. or 80 mg t.i.d. in 12 healthy volunteers *6510* No significant change in threshold for ADP-induced aggregation with either 40 mg t.i.d. or 80 mg t.i.d. in 12 healthy volunteers *6510*

Platelet Factor 4 *Plasma Decrease Physiological* Mean reduction of about 1 ng/mL in 12 healthy volunteers given 40 mg t.i.d. but reduction with 80 mg t.i.d. not significant *6510*

Potassium *Serum No Effect Physiological* In 437 patients with essential hypertension treatment with verapamil SR 240 mg/d for 6 months caused no change from mean baseline of 4.2 ± 0.4 mmol/L *3559*
Urine No Effect Physiological No significant effect in 8 healthy women treated with 240 mg daily for 7 days *6392*

Pramipexole *Serum Increase Physiological* Coadministration of verapamil with pramipexole presumed to decrease the oral clearance of pramipexole by about 20% *4680*

Prazosin *Serum Increase Physiological* Concomitant administration caused increase from mean of 5.2 ng/mL when prazosin given alone to 9.6 ng/mL with verapamil also in 8 normotensive volunteers: effect probably due to reduced first-pass clearance but possible pharmacodynamic interaction also

Verapamil *(continued)*

Prazosin *(continued)*
4545 In 8 normotensive volunteers concurrent treatment with 160 mg verapamil and 1 mg prazosin caused maximum concentration of prazosin to increase by 86% and area under its concentration curve to increase by 62% although its half-life was not affected. Similar effects were seen in hypertensive patients *5411*

Prolactin *Plasma Increase Physiological* In 449 male outpatients receiving verapamil the mean prolactin concentration was 267 ± 205 mU/L significantly greater than mean of 203 ± 118 mU/L in 166 controls *5075* In 7 chronically ill schizophrenic patients when administered for 5 weeks *4694*

Propranolol *Serum Increase Physiological* In 6 patients receiving propranolol 80 mg twice daily and verapamil 120 mg three times daily for several weeks mean total propranolol maximum plasma concentration and area under the concentration curve increased by 94% and 66% respectively. With single doses of each drug in healthy volunteers propranolol area under the curve and maximum plasma concentration increased by 57% and 79% respectively. Mean area under the curve for D-propranolol increased by 58% and for L-propranolol by 46% in one study *5411* When drugs coadministered clearance of propranolol decreased *2063* Moderate but significant increase of plasma concentration and area under concentration curve when compounds coadministered *3897*

Protein Kinase C *Lymphocytes Decrease Physiological* In 9 healthy male volunteers administration of up to 360 mg/d mean concentration decreased significantly from baseline of 5.07 ± 0.76 pmol/µg protein/min to 3.50 ± 0.20 pmol/µg protein/min after 1 week and 3.14 ± 0.27 pmol/µg protein/min after 2 weeks *1385*

Quinidine *Serum Increase Physiological* Hepatic clearance of quinidine is significantly reduced during coadministration of verapamil *5996* Concentration increased in one patient receiving concomitant verapamil and quinidine. Following verapamil quinidine half-life increased by 83% and clearance was reduced by 51%. In another study in 6 healthy volunteers oral clearance of quinidine reduced by about 33% and half-life increased by about 30-35% *5345* Clearance of quinidine reduced with coadministration *1384* Concomitant administration may increase quinidine concentration *1384* Pretreatment with up to 360 mg verapamil daily caused reduction of quinidine clearance from 17 L/h to 11 L/h and significantly increased elimination half-life *1666* In 6 volunteers administration of verapamil immediately prior to quinidine caused increase in serum concentration with prolongation of half-life from 6.9 to 9.0 hours. Quinidine clearance reduced. Metabolism of quinidine to 3-hydroxyquinidine reduced *1666*

Renal Blood Flow *Patient Decrease Physiological* Mean 9% reduction observed in 15 patients with essential hypertension treated with 480 mg slow release preparation daily for 2 months *3068*
Patient Increase Physiological In 15 patients with hypertension and mild to severe chronic renal failure administration of sustained release verapamil 240 mg/d for 4 weeks caused significant increase to 511 ± 196 mL/min compared with 471 ± 195 mL/min when treated with placebo *5372*
Patient No Effect Physiological No change compared with placebo in 11 patients treated with up to 360 mg daily for 6 weeks *5710*

Renin Activity *Plasma No Effect Physiological* No significant effect in 9 patients with normal renin hypertension when receiving either low or high sodium diet *2759* Insignificant increase from mean of 1.1 ng/mL/h to 1.4 ng/mL/h in 8 healthy women treated with 240 mg/day for 7 days *6392* In 15 hypertensive patients with mild to severe chronic renal failure when treated with verapamil SR 240 mg/d for 4 weeks mean concentration 1.13 ± 0.53 ng/L/s compared with 1.11 ± 0.59 ng/L/s when treated with placebo *5372* No significant effect observed in 15 patients with essential hypertension treated with 480 mg slow release preparation daily for 2 months *3068* In 15 patients with uncomplicated essential hypertension *1362*

Sodium *Red Blood Cells Increase Physiological* When given with digoxin increased concentration more than with controls with digoxin only *4581*
Red Blood Cells No Effect Physiological No effect when drug given alone *4581*
Serum No Effect Physiological No significant effect in 9 patients with normal renin hypertension when receiving either low or high sodium diet *2759* In 437 patients with essential hypertension treatment with verapamil SR 240 mg/d for 6 months caused nonsignificant reduction from mean baseline of 141 ± 5 mmol/L to 140 ± 3 mmol/L *3559*
Urine Increase Physiological Marked enhancement in 15 patients with uncomplicated essential hypertension *1362*
Urine No Effect Physiological No significant effect in 9 patients with normal renin hypertension when on low sodium diet but significant increase when receiving high sodium diet *2759* Insignificant increase in 8 healthy women treated with 240 mg daily for 7 days *6392*

Tacrolimus *Serum Increase Physiological* By inhibiting cytochrome P-450 IIIA enzyme systems may inhibit the metabolism of tacrolimus *1987*

Terazosin *Serum Increase Physiological* In a study of 24 individuals coadministration of verapamil with terazosin caused a 11% increase in the terazosin AUC after the first dose of verapamil and a 24% increase after 3 weeks together with a 25% increase in maximum concentration and 32% increase in minimum concentration *21*

Testosterone *Serum Decrease Physiological* In 15 male outpatients receiving verapamil the mean testosterone concentration was 6.16 ± 2.52 nmol/L significantly lower than mean of 9.42 ± 3.92 nmol/L in 9 patients in whom verapamil had been discontinued *5075*

Theophylline *Serum Increase Physiological* In healthy nonsmokers concomitant administration of verapamil with theophylline caused decrease in theophylline clearance by 14 to 22.5%. In another study of healthy nonsmokers nonsignificant decrease of theophylline clearance of 11.5% observed after 80 mg verapamil given orally every 8 hours *5345* Significant increase observed in 7 healthy volunteers given 360 mg verapamil daily for 7 days when 5 mg theophylline given i.v. Theophylline clearance reduced from mean of 45.2 mL/h/kg to 36.1 mL/h/kg and terminal half-life increased from 6.8 to 8.23 h *4290* Decreases theophylline clearance by inhibiting hydroxylation and demethylation, increasing theophylline concentration by about 20% *5999* When drugs coadministered serum cyclosporine A concentration may be increased *2063* Decreases theophylline clearance by inhibiting hydroxylation and demethylation and increases serum theophylline concentration by 20% *3125* Coadministration of verapamil in one patient caused marked increase in theophylline concentration probably as result of inhibition of hepatic metabolism *819* Up to 20% increase in serum theophylline concentration due to decreased theophylline clearance caused by inhibition of hydroxylation and demethylation *6117*

β-Thromboglobulin *Plasma Decrease Physiological* Mean decrease of about 16 ng/mL in 12 healthy volunteers when given low-dose (40 mg t.i.d) therapy but reduction not significant when given 80 mg t.i.d *6510*

Triglycerides *Serum Decrease Physiological* In 437 patients with essential hypertension treatment with verapamil SR 240 mg/d for 6 months caused significant decrease from mean baseline of 1.76 ± 0.87 mmol/L to 1.61 ± 0.75 mmol/L *3559* In 52 newly diagnosed hypertensives treatment with 240 mg/d for 6 weeks caused significant mean decrease of 0.32 mmol/L *378*
Serum No Effect Physiological In 64 patients in post-myocardial infarction comparison against placebo *5852* No significant effect observed in patients receiving verapamil *4989* In 12 patients when angina or hypertension treated for 6 weeks. Where change occurred it was of the order of 10% *6328*

Urea *Serum No Effect Physiological* In 437 patients with essential hypertension treatment with verapamil SR for 6 months caused nonsignificant reduction from mean baseline of 13.6 ± 3.9 mmol/L to 13.2 ± 3.6 mmol/L *3559*

Urea Nitrogen *Serum No Effect Physiological* In 142 hypertensives treatment with 240 mg/d for 6 weeks had no significant effect on concentration *378*

Uric Acid *Serum Decrease Physiological* In 437 patients with essential hypertension treatment with verapamil SR for 6 months caused significant reduction from mean baseline of 303 ± 83 µmol/L to 285 ± 59 µmol/L *3559* In 15 hypertensive patients with mild to moderate severe chronic renal failure treatment with 240 mg/d for 4 weeks caused significant reduction in concentration *5372*

Urine Increase Physiological In 15 hypertensive patients with mild to moderate chronic renal failure treatment with 240 mg/d sustained release verapamil for 4 weeks caused significant increase *5372*

Valproic Acid *Serum Increase Physiological* Reported increased concentration, as with other anticonvulsants, when verapamil coadministered with valproic acid *5411*

VLDL-Triglycerides *Serum No Effect Physiological* In 12 patients with angina or hypertension treated for 6 weeks. Where change occurred it was of the order of 10% *6328*

Volume *Plasma Increase Physiological* Due to decreased arterial and venous resistance in 15 patients with uncomplicated essential hypertension *1362*

Vidarabine

Alanine Aminotransferase *Serum Increase Physiological* No change of greater than 5-fold observed in 6 patients with AIDS treated with drug intravenously daily for 10-42 days *5184*

Alkaline Phosphatase *Serum Increase Physiological* Increase of greater than 2.6 times observed in 1 of 6 patients with AIDS treated with drug intravenously for 10-42 days *5184*

Aspartate Aminotransferase *Serum Increase Physiological* Occasional increase observed with treatment *1384*
Serum No Effect Physiological No change of greater than 5-fold observed in 6 patients with AIDS treated with intravenous drug daily for 10-42 days *5184*

Bilirubin *Serum Increase Physiological* Occasional increases observed with treatment *1384*

Calcium *Serum No Effect Physiological* No significant change observed in 6 patients with AIDS treated with drug intravenously for 10-42 days *5184*

Creatinine *Serum No Effect Physiological* No effect observed in 6 patients with AIDS treated with drug intravenously for 10-42 days *5184*

Glucose *Serum Increase Physiological* Observed in one patient with AIDS treated with drug intravenously for 10-42 days *5184*

Hematocrit *Blood Decrease Physiological* Occasional reduction observed *1384*

Hemoglobin *Blood Decrease Physiological* Occasional effect observed *1384* Observed decrease below 79 g/L in 4 of 6 patients with AIDS treated with drug intravenously for 10-42 days *5184*

Histamine *Plasma No Effect Analytical* No effect on radioenzyme assay at therapeutic concentrations *2492*

Leukocytes *Blood Decrease Physiological* Occasional leukopenia reported with therapy *1384* Occasional reduction observed with treatment *1384*

Neutrophils *Blood Decrease Physiological* Reduced below 5000/μL in 1 of 6 patients with AIDS treated with drug intravenously for 10-42 days *5184* Reduced below 5000 /μL in 1 of 6 patients with AIDS treated with drug intravenously for 10-42 days *5184*

Phosphate *Serum Decrease Physiological* Hypophosphatemia observed in 1 of 6 patients with AIDS treated with drug intravenously for 10-42 days *5184*

Platelets *Blood Decrease Physiological* Occasional thrombocytopenia reported with treatment *1384*

Potassium *Serum Decrease Physiological* Observed in 2 of 6 patients with AIDS treated with drug intravenously for 10-42 days *5184*

Protein *Urine Increase Physiological* Observed in 1 of 6 patients with AIDS treated with drug intravenously for 10-42 days *5184*

Sodium *Serum Decrease Physiological* Hyponatremia observed in 1 of 6 patients with AIDS treated with drug intravenously for 10-42 days *5184*

Zidovudine *Serum No Effect Analytical* No effect on liquid chromatographic method of Hedaya and Sawchuk *2525*

Vigabatrin

Alanine Aminotransferase *Serum Decrease Analytical* In 36 patients with epilepsy steep reduction in ALT activity observed in 75% from baseline of 17.1 ± 1.76 U/L to 6.11 ± 0.81 U/L after initiation of 2000 mg/d vigabatrin due to function as competitive cosubstrate for ALT *2767*
Serum Decrease Physiological In 3 individuals treated with vigabatrin caused profound decreases of serum ALT activity to less than 1 U/L due to inhibition of GABA-transaminase *5168* In 12 children aged 2 to 17 years with epilepsy treatment caused a decrease of 31% to 100% from initial normal ALT activity *6464*

Amino Acids *Urine Increase Analytical* False positive reaction observed since compound reacts with ninhydrin, yielding several reactive bands with high-voltage electrophoresis of urine: also affects thin-layer chromatographic methods *4873*

γ-Aminobutyric Acid
Cerebrospinal Fluid Increase Physiological In 4 patients with succinic semialdehyde dehydrogenase deficiency treatment with 40 - 100 mg/kg/d vigabatrin for 1 month to 1 year caused increase of 143% to 229% *2106*

Aspartate Aminotransferase *Serum No Effect Analytical* In patients with epilepsy has no effect, unlike that on ALT, since it does not function as a competitive cosubstrate *2767*

Carbamazepine *Serum Decrease Physiological* Coadministration caused delay in absorption of carbamazepine and reduction of its plasma concentration. Area under concentration curve reduced by 17% *101*

Cortisol, Free *Urine No Effect Analytical* No significant interference observed with HPLC method of Turpeinen et al *6105*

4-Hydroxybutyrate
Cerebrospinal Fluid Decrease Physiological In 4 patients with succinic semialdehyde dehydrogenase deficiency treatment with 40 - 100 mg/kg/d vigabatrin for 1 month to 1 year caused decrease of 26% to 47% *2106*

Phenytoin *Serum Decrease Physiological* Coadministration of vigabatrin with phenytoin caused delayed absorption of phenytoin and reduced its plasma concentration. Area under the concentration curve reduced by 21% *101*

Pyroglutamic Acid *Urine Increase Physiological* Increased excretion observed in patients with intractable convulsions treated with this compound, presumably due to inhibition of 4-aminobutyrate aminotransferase *4873*
Urine Positive Physiological Observed during metabolic screening for organic acidurias in two patients taking vigabatrin although not found in all such patients *651*

Vinyl-γ-Aminobutyric Acid *Urine Positive Physiological* Ingestion of drug causes presence of ninhydrin-reacting (bright purple) compound by both high voltage electrophoresis and paper chromatography which eluted with ethanolamine on an amino acid analyzer *5519*

Viloxazine

Carbamazepine *Serum Increase Physiological* Increases plasma carbamazepine concentration with possible toxicity *3118*

Metanephrine *Urine No Effect Analytical* No influence on liquid chromatographic measurement as drug elutes at different time *557*

Normetanephrine *Urine Increase Analytical* Substantial effect on liquid chromatographic measurement as drug elutes at same time *557*

Theophylline *Serum Increase Physiological* Significant increase in plasma concentration, and area under the curve and decreased its body clearance. Effect probably due to interference with biotransformation although exact mechanism not known *4600*

Vinblastine

CA549 *Serum No Effect Analytical* No statistically significant effect observed over a concentration range of 0.1 to 1.3

Vinblastine *(continued)*

CA549 *(continued)*
mg/L with BRESMARQ assay *958* No interference observed at concentrations from 0.1 - 1.3 mg/L with immunoradiometric BRESMARQ procedure *958*

Carcinoembryonic Antigen *Serum No Effect Analytical* At a concentration of up to 1384 µg/mL caused less than 10% error in the concentration of CEA as measured by the method on Bayer Technicon Immuno 1® *418*

Erythrocytes *Blood Decrease Physiological* Anemia (secondary to leukopenia) *128* Anemia is uncommon adverse effect of treatment *1384*

Granulocytes *Blood Decrease Physiological* Leukopenia (granulocytopenia), the most common side effect, is usually the dose limiting side effect *1711*

Hematocrit *Blood Decrease Physiological* Anemia may occur as a side effect *1711*

Hemoglobin *Blood Decrease Physiological* Anemia may occur as a side effect *1711* Anemia is uncommon side effect *1384*

Histamine *Plasma No Effect Analytical* Apparently no inhibition of radio-enzyme assay at concentrations approximating steady-state therapeutic concentration *2492*

Leukocytes *Blood Decrease Physiological* Dose-limiting leukopenia is most common toxic effect with nadir occurring within 5-10 days but with recovery within 7-10 days *1384* Leukopenia *128* Leukopenia (granulocytopenia), the most common side effect, is usually the dose limiting side effect *1711*

Methotrexate *Serum No Effect Analytical* No significant interference at a concentration of 50 µmol/L with method on Du Pont aca *1535*

Occult Blood *Feces Increase Physiological* Hemorrhagic enterocolitis or bleeding from an old peptic ulcer may be associated with rectal bleeding *1711*

Phenytoin *Serum Decrease Physiological* Capable of reducing plasma concentration when drugs are coadministered *1384*

Platelets *Blood Decrease Physiological* Thrombocytopenia is uncommon adverse effect *1384* Thrombocytopenia may occur as a side effect as a result of bone marrow suppression *1711* May cause bone marrow depression *128*

Reticulocytes *Blood Decrease Physiological* Absence from peripheral blood observed *2242*

Uric Acid *Serum Decrease Physiological* Of theoretical value in acute gout *2222*

Vincristine

Carcinoembryonic Antigen *Serum No Effect Analytical* At a concentration of 1384 µg/mL caused less than 10% error in the concentration of CEA as measured by the method on Bayer Technicon Immuno 1® *418*

Erythrocytes *Blood No Effect Physiological* No effect observed on erythrocytes although mild leukopenia may develop as result of action on bone marrow *1384*

Hematocrit *Blood Decrease Physiological* Anemia reported in some individuals receiving vincristine but rare *1704*

Hemoglobin *Blood Decrease Physiological* Anemia reported in some individuals receiving vincristine but rare *1704*

Leukocytes *Blood Decrease Physiological* Usually reversible leukopenia *128* Reported change in some individuals, particularly when previous therapy or the disease itself has reduced bone marrow function *1704*

Methotrexate *Serum No Effect Analytical* No significant interference observed at a concentration of 50 µmol/L with method on Du Pont aca *1535*

Osmolality *Urine Increase Physiological* May produce clinically impaired water excretion *1343*

Phenytoin *Serum Decrease Physiological* When phenytoin coadministered with vincristine concentration of phenytoin reported to be reduced *1704*

Platelets *Blood Decrease Physiological* Reported change in some individuals, particularly when previous therapy or the disease itself has reduced bone marrow function *1704* May cause bone marrow depression *2242*

Blood No Effect Physiological No effect observed on platelets although effect on bone marrow may cause leukopenia *1384*

Protein *Cerebrospinal Fluid No Effect Analytical* No significant effect when added in vitro to concentration of 0.04 mg/dL when measured by Kodak Ektachem® method *3654*

Sodium *Serum Decrease Physiological* Drug has been reported to promote release of antidiuretic hormone which has rarely caused hyponatremia *1384* May be inappropriate ADH secretion *2754* Rare syndrome of inappropiate ADH hormone secretion reported with vincristine administration including hyponatremia and increased urinary sodium secretion *1704*

Urine Increase Physiological Rare syndrome of inappropiate ADH hormone secretion reported with vincristine administration including hyponatremia and increased urinary sodium secretion *1704* May be inappropriate ADH secretion *2754*

Uric Acid *Serum Increase Physiological* Increased nucleic acid catabolism *5869*

Vindesine

Leukocytes *Blood Decrease Physiological* Myelosuppression is dose-limiting toxicity but with neutropenia predominating over thrombocytopenia *1384*

Platelets *Blood Decrease Physiological* Myelosuppression is dose-limiting toxicity but with neutropenia predominating over thrombocytopenia *1384*

Vinorelbine

Aspartate Aminotransferase *Serum Increase Physiological* In a study of 346 patients receiving vinorelbine 67% had an increased enzyme activity *2178*

Bilirubin *Serum Increase Physiological* In a study of 351 patients receiving vinorelbine 13% had an increased bilirubin concentration *2178*

Granulocytes *Blood Decrease Physiological* Granulocytopenia may be dose-limiting side effect. In a study of 365 patients receiving vinorelbine 90% had a cell count of less than 2000 cells/µL and 36% had a count of less than 500 cells/µL *2178*

Hemoglobin *Blood Decrease Physiological* n a study of 365 treated patients 5% had a hemoglobin concentration of less than 11 g/dL and 9% had a concentration of less than 8 g/dL *2178*

Leukocytes *Blood Decrease Physiological* Granulocytopenia may be dose-limiting side effect. In a study of 365 treated patients 92% had a white cell count of less than 4000 cells/µL and 15% had a count of less than 1000 cells/µL *2178*

Platelets *Blood Decrease Physiological* Thrombocytopenia may be dose-limiting side effect. In a study of 365 treated patients 5% had a platelet cell count of less than 100,000 cells/µL and 1% had a count of less than 50,000 cells/µL *2178*

Vinpocetine

Imipramine *Serum No Effect Physiological* No apparent effect of 30 mg vinpocetine daily when 75 mg imipramine given daily to 18 healthy volunteers although large interindividual variation observed *2628*

Oxazepam *Serum No Effect Physiological* In 16 healthy individuals 10 mg three times daily of vinpocetine together with 10 mg oxazepam three times daily caused area under oxazepam concentration curve of 4716 ± 2296 ng/mL/h compared with 4737 ± 2448 ng/mL/h in the absence of vinpocetine *5836*

Viomycin

Bicarbonate *Serum Increase Physiological* Altered electrolyte balance *2024*

Calcium *Serum Decrease Physiological* May cause tetany with electrolyte imbalance *128*

Urine Increase Physiological Promotes urinary loss *2024*

Casts *Urine Increase Physiological* Nephrotoxicity with cylindruria *128*

Chloride *Urine Increase Physiological* Promotes urinary loss *128*

Cholesterol *Serum Increase Analytical* Interferes with Zlatkis-Zak reaction *5869*

Creatinine *Serum Increase Physiological* Nephrotoxic may cause nitrogen retention *3810*

Creatinine Clearance *Urine Decrease Physiological* Occasional renal damage observed *198*

Eosinophils *Blood Increase Physiological* Allergic response *2484*

Erythrocytes *Urine Increase Physiological* May cause actual bleeding *2024*

Hemoglobin *Urine Increase Physiological* Actual bleeding caused by drug *2024*

Leukocytes *Blood Increase Physiological* Due to eosinophilia *3810*

Potassium *Serum Decrease Physiological* May occur with nephrotoxicity *3810*
Urine Increase Physiological Promotes urinary loss *128*

Protein *Urine Increase Physiological* May have nephrotoxic effect *2024*

Urea Nitrogen *Serum Increase Physiological* Frequent complication *2242*

Vitamin B Complex

Catecholamines *Plasma Increase Analytical* May be interference with fluorescence *2451*

Cholesterol *Serum No Effect Analytical* At concentration of 12.9 mg/L had no effect on catalase-AIDH method *5704* At concentration of 12.9 mg/L had no effect on Liebermann-Burchard method *5704* At concentration of 12.9 mg/L had no effect on CHOD-Iodide method *5704* At concentration of 12.9 mg/L had no effect on method using catalase-Hantzsch reaction *5704* At concentration of 12.9 mg/L had no effect on CHOD-PAP method *5704*

Creatinine *Serum No Effect Analytical* At concentration of 12.9 mg/L had no effect on Jaffe-Fuller's earth method *5704* At concentration of 800 mg/L had no effect on kinetic Jaffe method on BKA-2 *5704* At concentration of 12.9 mg/L had no effect on Jaffe-Fading-Fraction method *5704*

Diagnex Blue Excretion *Urine Increase Analytical* Release of dye from resin *2025*

Glucose *Serum No Effect Analytical* No effect of concentrations up to 2.3 mg/L on method on Kodak Ektachem® *5706* At concentration of 2.3 mg/L had no effect on Kodak Ektachem® method *5704*

Iron *Serum No Effect Analytical* At concentration of 1.4 mg/L had no effect on Ferrozine method *5704*

Potassium *Serum No Effect Analytical* At concentration of 23.3 mg/L had no effect on measurement by ISE without predilution *5704*

Protein Electrophoresis *Serum No Effect Analytical* At concentration of 23.3 mg/L had no effect on automated Olympus-Hite method *5704*

Sodium *Serum No Effect Analytical* At concentration of 23.3 mg/L had no effect on measurement by ISE without predilution *5704*

Urea Nitrogen *Serum No Effect Analytical* At concentration of 23.3 mg/L had no effect on Kodak Ektachem® method *5704*

Uric Acid *Serum No Effect Analytical* At concentration of 32 mg/L had no effect on Kageyama-Hantzsch method *5704* At concentration of 12.9 mg/L had no effect on catalase-AIDH method *5704*

Vitamin D

Alkaline Phosphatase *Serum Decrease Physiological* Reported effect with excess vitamin D ingestion *3679*
Serum Increase Physiological May be affected in some cases *1648*

Alkaline Phosphatase, Bone Isoenzyme
Serum No Effect Analytical At a concentration of 20 mg/L had no effect on Tandem-MP Ostase method *777*

Bilirubin *Serum No Effect Analytical* No significant effect observed at a concentration of 300 μg/dL (10.5 μmol/L) with method on Du Pont aca *1548*

Calcium *Feces Decrease Physiological* Due to excessive absorption *1647*
Serum Increase Physiological In one study of 40 patients with nonmalignant causes of hypercalcemia and low intact PTH concentrations 3 were due to excess vitamin D therapy in non-chronic renal failure *3774* Effect of increased gastrointestinal tract absorption *6515*
Serum No Effect Physiological In 15 vitamin D treated hypoparathyroid patients mean concentration of 2.25 mmol/L not significantly significantly different from mean of 2.36 mmol/L in 12 normal individuals *4127*
Urine Increase Physiological In 146 men and 167 women aged more than 65 years treatment with 500 mg calcium and 700 IU vitamin D_3 (cholecalciferol) per day for 3 years caused a significant change of 35 ± 51 mg/g creatinine from mean baseline of 98 ± 50 mg/g creatinine in the men and of 67 ± 64 mg/g creatinine from mean baseline 113 ± 64 mg/g creatinine in the women *1288* Associated with hypercalcemia *1714*

Calculi *Urine Increase Physiological* High incidence in people with self medication *5971*

Cholesterol *Serum Increase Analytical* Interferes with Zlatkis-Zak reaction *5869*
Serum Increase Physiological In men by 25 mg/dL in ages 35-54 y old *1221*

Creatinine *Serum Increase Physiological* Manifestation of hypervitaminosis D *128*

1,25-Dihydroxy Vitamin D *Serum Increase Physiological* In 15 vitamin D treated hypoparathyroid patients mean concentration of 206 pmol/L significantly greater than mean of 80 pmol/L in 12 normal individuals *4127* In elderly patients with very low serum 25-hydroxyvitamin D concentrations administration of 1000 U/d for 40 weeks caused increase from mean baseline of 89 pmol/L to 105 pmol/L *5718*
Serum No Effect Physiological In 146 men and 167 women aged more than 65 years treatment with 500 mg calcium and 700 IU vitamin D_3 (cholecalciferol) per day for 3 years caused a nonsignificant change of -6.3 ± 11.0 pg/mL from mean baseline of 33.6 ± 7.0 pg/mL in the men and of -5.8 ± 9.5 pg/mL from mean baseline 36.5 ± 7.3 pg/mL in the women *1288*

1,25-Dihydroxy Vitamin D_3 *Serum Increase Physiological* In elderly patients with very low serum 25-hydroxyvitamin D concentrations administration of 1000 U/d for 40 weeks caused increase from mean baseline of 89 pmol/L to 105 pmol/L *5718*

25-Hydroxy Vitamin D *Serum Increase Physiological* In patients with Cushing's syndrome large doses of vitamin D (25,000 to 50,000 IU three times per week) requires several weeks to achieve equilibrium levels, and may lead to prolonged toxic concentrations *6526* In 146 men and 167 women aged more than 65 years treatment with 500 mg calcium and 700 IU vitamin D_3 (cholecalciferol) per day for 3 years caused a significant increase of 11.8 ± 11.6 ng/mL from mean baseline of 33.0 ± 16.3 ng/mL in the men and of 16.1 ± 14.3 ng/mL from mean baseline 28.7 ± 13.3 ng/mL in the women *1288*

Hydroxyproline *Urine Increase Physiological* In vitamin-sensitive rickets *6111*

ionized Calcium *Serum Increase Physiological* In 146 men and 167 women aged more than 65 years treatment with 500 mg calcium and 700 IU vitamin D_3 (cholecalciferol) per day for 3 years caused a significant increase of 0.1 ± 0.2 mg/dL from mean baseline of 5.0 ± 0.2 mg/dL in the men and of 0.1 ± 0.1 mg/dL (nonsignificant) from mean baseline 5.1 ± 0.2 mg/dL in the women *1288*
Serum No Effect Physiological No effect observed in elderly patients with very low serum 25-hydroxyvitamin D concentrations when given 1000 U/day for 40 weeks *5718*

Magnesium *Serum No Effect Physiological* In 15 vitamin D treated hypoparathyroid patients mean concentration of 0.82 mmol/L not significantly significantly different from mean of 0.84 mmol/L in 12 normal individuals *4127*

Nonprotein Nitrogen *Serum Increase Physiological* Manifestation of hypervitaminosis D *3810*

Vitamin D *(continued)*

Osteocalcin *Serum Decrease Physiological* In 146 men and 167 women aged more than 65 years treatment with 500 mg calcium and 700 IU vitamin D_3 (cholecalciferol) per day for 3 years caused a significant change of -0.5 ± 1.4 ng/mL from mean baseline of 5.3 ± 1.3 ng/mL in the men and of -0.9 ± 1.9 ng/mL from mean baseline 6.9 ± 1.3 ng/mL in the women *1288*

Parathyroid Hormone *Plasma Decrease Physiological* In one study of 40 patients with low intact PTH concentration and hypercalcemia not due to malignant disease 3 had increased concentration due to excess vitamin D therapy but without chronic renal failure *3774* Concentration decreased from mean of 32 ng/L to 27 ng/L in elderly patients with very low serum 25-hydroxyvitamin D concentrations when given 1000 U/d for 40 weeks *5718* In 146 men and 167 women aged more than 65 years treatment with 500 mg calcium and 700 IU vitamin D_3 (cholecalciferol) per day for 3 years caused a significant change of -7.0 ± 12.9 pg/mL from mean baseline of 38.0 ± 19.1 pg/mL in the men and of -5.5 ± 13.2 pg/mL from mean baseline 37.4 ± 15.3 pg/mL in the women *1288* In 15 vitamin D treated hypoparathyroid patients mean concentration of PTH(1-84) of 8.1 pg/mL significantly less than mean of 45.1 pg/mL in 12 normal individuals *4127*

Phosphate *Feces Decrease Physiological* Due to excessive absorption *1647*

Serum Increase Physiological Effect of increased gastrointestinal tract and renal absorption *6515*

Serum No Effect Physiological In 15 vitamin D treated hypoparathyroid patients mean concentration of 1.25 mmol/L not significantly significantly different from mean of 1.24 mmol/L in 12 normal individuals *4127*

Urine Increase Physiological May be normal in many cases *6327*

Protein *Urine Increase Physiological* Nephrotoxic effect with hypercalcemia *1714*

Urea Nitrogen *Serum Increase Physiological* Manifestation of hypervitaminosis D *128*

Vitamin D_2

1,25-Dihydroxy Vitamin D *Serum Increase Physiological* In 46 elderly women with radiological evidence of vertebral osteoporosis treatment with 500 - 1000 IU/d caused nonsignificant change from mean baseline of 62.6 ± 4.3 pmol/L to 61.2 ± 5.7 pmol/L after 3 months and 60.3 ± 5.7 pmol/L after 6 months *1935*

25-Hydroxy Vitamin D *Serum Increase Physiological* In 46 elderly women with radiological evidence of vertebral osteoporosis treatment with 500 - 1000 IU/d caused significant change from mean baseline of 35.9 ± 5.0 nmol/L to 58.8 ± 5.4 nmol/L after 3 months and 60.7 ± 4.6 nmol/L after 6 months *1935*

Parathyroid Hormone *Plasma No Effect Physiological* In 46 elderly women with radiological evidence of vertebral osteoporosis treatment with 500 - 1000 IU/d caused nonsignificant change from mean baseline of 2.58 ± 0.24 pmol/L to 2.56 ± 0.26 pmol/L after 3 months and 2.39 ± 0.25 pmol/L after 6 months *1935*

Vitamin D_3

Alkaline Phosphatase, Bone Isoenzyme

Serum Decrease Physiological In 17 healthy postmenopausal women treatment with 300 IU/d vitamin D_3 caused a significant change in activity from mean baseline of 93.3 ± 10.4 U/L to 82.7 ± 9.6 U/L at 6 months and 85.7 ± 9.1 U/L at 12 months *2535*

Serum No Effect Analytical At a concentration of 1 g/L had no effect on EIA method of Gomez et al *2234*

Calcium *Serum Increase Physiological* Increase to low normal range in elderly institutionalized patients with initially low concentrations when treated with 5 mg i.m. at monthly intervals for 3 months but no effect observed in those with initially normal calcium concentrations *2362*

C-terminal Telopeptide of Type I Collagen

Serum No Effect Physiological In 17 healthy postmenopausal women treatment with 300 IU/d vitamin D_3 caused an insignificant change in concentration from mean baseline of 3.34 ± 0.19 µg/L to 3.56 ± 0.15 µg/L at 6 months and 3.26 ± 0.13 µg/L at 12 months *2535*

1,25-Dihydroxy Vitamin D_3 *Serum Increase Physiological* In 16 elderly individuals with low serum calcium concentrations 5 mg i.m. at monthly intervals for 3 months caused increase from mean of 22.9 ng/L to 32.6 ng/L but effect not observed in individuals with normal serum calcium concentrations *2362*

25-Hydroxy Vitamin D_2 *Serum Increase Physiological* In 40 elderly institutionalized patients with initially low 25-(OH)D_2 concentrations 3 i.m. injections over 3 months caused increase from about 4.5 µg/L to 26 µg/L *2362*

Osteocalcin *Serum Increase Physiological* Transient significant increase from mean of 10.6 µg/L to 14.1 µg/L in elderly patients with initially low serum calcium concentrations, but not in others, when treated with 5 mg i.m. monthly for 3 months *2362*

Serum No Effect Physiological In 17 healthy postmenopausal women treatment with 300 IU/d vitamin D_3 caused an insignificant change in concentration from mean baseline of 3.34 ± 0.62 ng/mL to 3.79 ± 0.64 ng/mL at 6 months and 4.07 ± 0.62 ng/mL at 12 months *2535*

Vitamin K

Bilirubin *Serum Increase Physiological* Large doses in neonates or G-6-PD deficiency *402*

Calcium *Urine Decrease Physiological* In patients with a mean calcium:creatinine ratio of more than 0.5 significant mean decrease of 0.2 observed when treated with vitamin K for 1 month *2937* Excretion reduced, especially in fast calcium losers, in postmenopausal women treated with 1 mg/day for 2 weeks *3196*

Urine Increase Physiological In patients with a mean calcium:creatinine ratio of less than 0.2 mean increase of 0.06 observed when treated with vitamin K for 1 month *2937*

Erythrocytes *Blood Decrease Physiological* Vitamins K_3 and K_4 only, especially with G-6-PD deficiency *3453*

Hematocrit *Blood Decrease Physiological* Vitamins K_3 and K_4 only, especially with G-6-PD deficiency *3453*

Hemoglobin *Blood Decrease Physiological* Vitamins K_3 and K_4 only, especially with G-6-PD deficiency *3453*

Urine Increase Physiological Effect of treatment of hemorrhagic states in children *128*

17-Hydroxycorticosteroids *Urine Increase Analytical* Alleged *in vitro* interference with Reddy method *2451*

Hydroxyproline *Urine Decrease Physiological* Reduced excretion in parallel with reduced calcium excretion in postmenopausal women treated with 1 mg daily for 2 weeks *3196*

Leukocytes *Blood Decrease Physiological* Pancytopenia reported after vitamins K_3 and K_4*4014*

Osteocalcin *Serum Increase Physiological* Treatment with 1 mg/day for 2 weeks increased serum immunoreactive osteocalcin in postmenopausal women although no effect was observed in premenopausal women *3196*

Platelets *Blood Decrease Physiological* Pancytopenia reported after vitamins K_3 and K_4*4014*

Porphyrin, Total *Urine Increase Physiological* Reported side effect *4014*

Protein *Urine Increase Physiological* Reported side effect *4014*

Prothrombin Time *Plasma Decrease Physiological* Therapeutic intent, affects action of warfarin *3810*

Urobilinogen *Urine Increase Physiological* Hemolytic anemia in G-6-PD deficiency *2242*

Vitamin K Antagonists

γ-Carboxyglutamic Acid, Free
Plasma Decrease Physiological In 12 patients taking vitamin K antagonists mean concentration of 76 ± 33 pmol/mL significantly lower than that in 19 healthy men and women aged between 35 and 65 years in whom mean concentration was 146 ± 34 pmol/mL *2447*

Vitamin Preparations

Albumin *Serum No Effect Analytical* No effect at expected concentration with Technicon SMA 12/60 procedure *4391*

Alkaline Phosphatase *Serum No Effect Analytical* No effect at expected concentration with Technicon SMA 12/60 procedure *4391*

Aspartate Aminotransferase *Serum No Effect Analytical* No effect at expected concentration with Technicon SMA 12/60 procedure *4391*

Calcium *Serum No Effect Analytical* No effect at expected concentration with Technicon SMA 12/60 procedure *4391*

Cholesterol *Serum No Effect Analytical* No effect at expected concentration with Technicon SMA 12/60 procedure *4391*

Ciprofloxacin *Serum Decrease Physiological* Following ingestion of ciproloxacin with one tablet of Centrum Forte peak serum concentration reduced by 1.4 mg/L and area under curve reduced by 5.4 mg/Lh due to oxidation of ferrous to ferric iron and binding of ferric iron by ciprofloxacin *3038*

Creatinine *Serum No Effect Analytical* No effect at expected concentration with Technicon SMA 12/60 procedure *4391*

Glucose *Serum No Effect Analytical* No effect at expected concentration with Technicon SMA 12/60 procedure *4391*
Urine Decrease Analytical Low measurements with Clinistix® and Diastix® *1826*
Urine No Effect Analytical No effect observed with Tes-Tape® *1826*

^{131}I Uptake *Serum Decrease Physiological* If preparations contain iodine *3669* Daylets contain tetraiodofluorescein *4360*

Lactate Dehydrogenase *Serum No Effect Analytical* No effect at expected concentration with Technicon SMA 12/60 procedure *4391*

Norfloxacin *Serum Decrease Physiological* Multivitamins, or other products containing iron or zinc, may interfere with the absorption of norfloxacin resulting in lower plasma and urine concentrations *4981*
Urine Decrease Physiological Multivitamins, or other products containing iron or zinc, may interfere with the absorption of norfloxacin resulting in lower plasma and urine concentrations *4981*

Phosphate *Serum No Effect Analytical* No effect at expected concentration with Technicon SMA 12/60 procedure *4391*

Protein *Serum No Effect Analytical* No effect at expected concentration with Technicon SMA 12/60 procedure *4391*

Urea Nitrogen *Serum No Effect Analytical* No effect at expected concentration with Technicon SMA 12/60 procedure *4391*

Uric Acid *Serum No Effect Analytical* No effect at expected concentration with Technicon SMA 12/60 procedure *4391*

Voglibose

1,5-Anhydroglucitol *Serum Decrease Physiological* In 25 patients with NIDDM treated with 0.2 mg voglibose three times daily for 1 week 1,5-anhydroglucitol concentration decreased from a mean of 4.8 ± 1.2 µg/mL to 6.7 ± 1.8 µg/mL *6610*

Glucose *Serum Decrease Physiological* In 25 patients with NIDDM treated with 0.2 mg voglibose three times daily for 1 week glucose concentration decreased from a mean of 7.2 ± 2.0 mmol/L to 6.1 ± 0.9 mmol/L *6610*

Hemoglobin A_{1c} *Blood No Effect Physiological* In 25 patients with NIDDM treated with 0.2 mg voglibose three times daily for 1 week hemoglobin A_{1c} concentration changed insignificantly from a mean of 8.9 ± 1.9% to 8.8 ± 1.8% *6610*

Warfarin

Alanine Aminotransferase *Serum Increase Physiological* Rare cases of intrahepatic cholestasis in patients with previous history of hypersensitivity reported *4899*
Serum No Effect Analytical No effect at 10 mg/L on method on Ames Seralyzer *5706*

Albumin *Serum No Effect Analytical* No interference observed at a concentration of 1.3 mg/L (4.2 µmol/L) with method on Du Pont aca *1507* At concentration of 100 mg/L had no effect on BCG method *5704*

Alkaline Phosphatase *Serum Increase Physiological* Rare cases of intrahepatic cholestasis in patients with previous history of hypersensitivity reported *4899*

Antithrombin III *Plasma No Effect Physiological* In 12 patients with cardioembolic stroke treatment caused nonsignificant change from mean baseline of 97 ± 11% to 93 ± 11% *6587*

Aspartate Aminotransferase *Serum Increase Physiological* Rare cases of intrahepatic cholestasis in patients with previous history of hypersensitivity reported *4899*

Bicarbonate *Serum No Effect Analytical* At concentration of 100 mg/L had no effect on method using phenolphthalein *5704*

Bilirubin *Serum No Effect Analytical* At concentration of 100 mg/L had no effect on Jendrassik and Grof method *5704*

Bleeding Time *Patient Increase Physiological* May be prolonged *2183*

Calcium *Serum No Effect Analytical* At concentration of 100 mg/L had no effect on cresolphthalein method *5704*

Chloride *Serum No Effect Analytical* At concentration of 100 mg/L had no effect on mercurimetric method *5704*

Cholesterol *Serum No Effect Analytical* At concentration of 100 mg/L had no effect on Liebermann-Burchard method *5704* At concentration of 1.5 mg/L had no effect on CHOD-PAP method *5704*
Serum No Effect Physiological In 12 men treatment with up to 2.5 mg/d for 8 weeks caused no significant change from mean baseline of 5.93 mmol/L *2678*

Clotting Time *Blood Increase Physiological* May be prolonged *2183*

Color *Feces Increase Analytical* Black color reported following ingestion of warfarin *3388*
Urine Increase Analytical Orange-yellow color observed following ingestion of warfarin *3388*

Creatinine *Serum No Effect Analytical* At concentration of 100 mg/L had no effect on Technicon AutoAnalyzer® Jaffe method *5704* No interference noted with liquid chromatographic method of Paroni et al *4540*
Serum No Effect Physiological No effect on renal function noted with continuing administration *3954*

Cyclosporine *Serum Increase Physiological* Poorly documented effect reported *1069*

D-Dimer *Plasma Decrease Physiological* In 39 patients with congestive cardiac failure treatment with warfarin sufficient to maintain an INR of 1.5 to 3.0 for 3 months caused a significant decrease in concentration from mean baseline of 622 ± 427 ng/mL to 358 ± 229 ng/mL after 1 month, 370 ± 361 ng/mL after 2 months and 382 ± 291 ng/mL after 3 months *2884* In 12 patients with cardioembolic stroke treatment caused significant reduction from mean baseline of 669 ± 751 ng/mL to 183 ± 124 ng/mL *6587* In 31 patients with chronic atrial fibrillation initial median concentration of 158 ng/mL (interquartile range 3.0 - 4.7 ng/mL) significantly changed to 50 ng/mL (interquartile range 50 - 60 ng/mL) after treatment with warfarin for 2 months, below median concentration of 76 ng/mL (interquartile range 53 - 103 ng/mL) in 158 controls with sinus rhythm *2130*

Erythrocytes *Urine Increase Physiological* Excessive doses may cause hematuria *1492*

Factor II *Plasma Decrease Physiological* Therapeutic action *2754*

Factor VII *Plasma Decrease Physiological* Therapeutic action *2754* At the beginning of warfarin therapy factor VII concentration decreases rapidly *2014*

Warfarin *(continued)*

Factor VII Activity *Plasma Decrease Physiological* In 12 men treatment with 1.25 mg/d for 4 weeks caused 5.3% reduction to 107 U/dL from mean baseline of 113 U/dL and treatment with 2.5 mg/d for another 4 weeks caused 18.8% reduction to 91 U/dL, but returned to normal within 4 weeks of cessation of treatment *2678*

Factor VII Antigen *Plasma Decrease Physiological* In 74 cardiovascular patients on long-term warfarin therapy mean concentration of 1.18 ng/mL (range 0.29 - 4.17) compared with age and sex-matched control concentrations of 2.69 ± 0.78 ng/mL *5191*

Factor VII Coagulant *Plasma Decrease Physiological* In 74 cardiovascular patients on long-term warfarin therapy mean concentration of 48.2% (range 23.3 - 96.0) compared with age and sex-matched control concentrations of 120 ± 25% *5191*

Factor IX *Plasma Decrease Physiological* Therapeutic action *2754*

Factor X *Plasma Decrease Physiological* Therapeutic action *2754* In 12 patients treatment with 1.25 mg/d for 4 weeks caused significant decrease from mean baseline of 106 U/dL to 102 U/dL and to 89 U/dL after treatment with 2.5 mg/d for another 4 weeks *2678* In 74 cardiovascular patients on long-term warfarin therapy mean concentration of 42.8% (range 9.8 - 75.4) compared with commercially available standard human plasma of 100% *5191* 3 - 9 days after the initiation of warfarin therapy factor X concentration decreases *2014*

Famotidine *Serum No Effect Physiological* Peak plasma concentration, time to peak concentration, and area under plasma concentration curve unaffected during maintenance therapy with warfarin compared with values obtained with famotidine alone in 8 healthy male volunteers *1316*

Fibrinogen *Plasma No Effect Physiological* In 31 patients with chronic atrial fibrillation initial median concentration of 3.78 g/L (interquartile range 3.0 - 4.7 g/L) not significantly changed to 3.50 g/L (interquartile range 2.95 - 4.70 g/L) after treatment with warfarin for 2 months *2130*

Fibrinopeptide A *Plasma Decrease Physiological* In 12 patients with cardioembolic stroke mean concentration non-significantly reduced from mean baseline of 11.4 ± 13.6 ng/mL to 4.1 ± 2.3 ng/mL *6587*

Glucose *Serum No Effect Analytical* At concentration of 1.5 mg/L had no effect on GOD/POD-PAP method *5704* No effect at 100 mg/L on hexokinase method on Ames Seralyzer *5706*

γ-Glutamyltransferase *Serum Increase Physiological* Rare cases of intrahepatic cholestasis in patients with previous history *4899*

Glycated Hemoglobin *Blood No Effect Analytical* At a concentration of 100 mg/L had an insignificant - 1.9% interference with method on Abbott Vision *1885*

Hemoglobin *Blood No Effect Physiological* In 12 men treatment with 1.25 mg/d for 4 weeks and then 2.5 mg/d for 4 weeks had no significant effect on concentration *2678*
Urine Increase Physiological Due to overdosage in some cases *2183*
Urine No Effect Physiological No association observed in over 1000 men aged 60 years and older between warfarin ingestion and dipstick hematuria *732*

Histamine *Plasma No Effect Analytical* No inhibition of radio-enzyme assay at therapeutic concentrations *2492*

^{131}I Uptake *Serum Decrease Physiological* Panwarfin® contains tetraiodofluorescein *4360*

Ketorolac *Serum No Effect Physiological* At therapeutic concentrations had no effect on ketorolac-protein binding *5035*

Levofloxacin *Serum No Effect Physiological* Concurrent administration of levofloxacin with warfarin had no effect on levofloxacin absorption and disposition *3916*

MCV *Blood Decrease Physiological* May be secondary microcytic hypochromic anemia *2183*

Neutrophils *Blood Decrease Physiological* May cause neutropenia *4265*

Nicardipine *Serum No Effect Physiological* Had no effect on plasma protein binding in vitro and presumed to have no effect on nicardipine concentration in vivo *5016*

Nisoldipine *Serum No Effect Physiological* No significant interaction observed between nisoldipine and warfarin *6650*

Occult Blood *Feces Increase Physiological* May cause intramural hemorrhage even if no ulcer *5864*

Phenyramidol *Plasma Increase Physiological* Impairs metabolism *4426*

Phenytoin *Serum No Effect Physiological* With concurrent therapy typically had no effect *5966*

Phosphate *Serum No Effect Analytical* At concentration of 100 mg/L had no effect on phosphomolybdate method *5704*

Plasmin-α_2-Plasmin Inhibitor Complex
Plasma Decrease Physiological In 12 patients with cardioembolic stroke treatment caused significant reduction from mean baseline of 1.9 ± 1.6 μg/mL to 0.8 ± 0.3 μg/mL *6587*

Platelet Aggregation *Blood Decrease Physiological* If caused by ADP, thrombin, collagen, epinephrine *941*

Potassium *Serum No Effect Analytical* At concentration of 1.5 mg/L had no effect on flame-photometric method *5704* At concentration of 100 mg/L had no effect on measurement by ISE with predilution *5704* At concentration of 100 mg/L non-significant interference of -0.8% observed with method on Abbott Vision *681*

Pravastatin *Serum No Effect Physiological* Administration of pravastatin together with warfarin to 10 healthy men for 6 days caused no effect on the bioavailability of either compound *728*

Protein *Serum No Effect Analytical* At concentration of 100 mg/L had no effect on biuret method with blank correction *5704*

Protein C *Plasma Decrease Physiological* In 74 cardiovascular patients on long-term warfarin therapy mean concentration of 49.0% (range 16.9 - 86.7) compared with commercially available standard human plasma of 100% *5191* At the beginning of warfarin therapy protein C concentration decreases rapidly *2014*

Protein C Activity *Plasma Decrease Physiological* In patients with cardioembolic stroke mean activity decreased significantly from baseline of 120 ± 39% to 39 ± 26% *6587*

Protein C Antigen *Plasma Decrease Physiological* In 12 patients with cardioembolic stroke treatment caused significant reduction from mean baseline of 130 ± 46% to 73 ± 17% *6587*

Protein S *Plasma Decrease Physiological* Although concentration in 12 men not reduced when they were treated with 1.25 mg/d for 4 weeks it was reduced by 14.7% when they were treated with 2.5 mg/d for 4 weeks *2678* Normal mean concentration of 16.34 mg/L but in 47 plasma specimens from patients receiving warfarin mean concentration 8.2 mg/L (SD 2.33 mg/L) *673*

Protein S, Free *Plasma Decrease Physiological* In 12 men treatment with 1.25 mg/d for 4 weeks caused 34.9% reduction after 4 weeks and with 2.5 mg/d 29.8% reduction after 4 weeks *2678*

Prothrombin *Plasma Decrease Physiological* 3 - 9 days after the initiation of warfarin therapy prothrombin concentration decreases *2014*

Prothrombin Fragment 1.2 *Plasma Decrease Physiological* Mean concentration of prothrombin fragment 1.2 in platelet-poor plasma from 5 patients stably anticoagulated with warfarin of 0.20 ± 0.04 nmol/L slightly reduced compared with that in 268 healthy individuals less than 44 years of age 0.51 nmol/L with 95% reference interval of 0.21 - 2.78 nmol/L *2307* In 12 men treatment with 1.25 mg/d for 4 weeks caused decrease of mean concentration from 1.60 mmol/L to 1.27 mmol/L. When treated with 2.5 mg/d for 4 weeks concentration decreased to about 1.05 mmol/L *2678* In 39 patients with congestive cardiac failure treatment with warfarin sufficient to maintain an INR of 1.5 to 3.0 for 3 months caused a significant decrease in concentration from mean baseline of 1.7 ± 1.2 mol/L to 0.6 ± 0.5 mol/L after 1 month, 0.8 ± 1.8 mol/L after 2 months and 0.6 ± 0.5 mol/L after 3 months *2884*

Prothrombin Time *Plasma Decrease Physiological* In 12 men treatment with 1.25 mg/d for 4 weeks caused nonsignificant change from mean baseline of 107% but treatment with 2.5 mg/d for 4 weeks caused significant reduction to 81%. Trough prothrombin time values were 70% and 35% respectively with 1.25 mg and 2.5 mg respectively *2678*
Plasma Increase Physiological In 8 healthy male volunteers administration of 4.0 mg warfarin daily caused increase of mean from 12.22 seconds to 16.98 seconds *1316* Therapeutic intent (inhibits prothrombin formation) *2242*

Plasma *No Effect* *Physiological* Coadministration of losartan with warfarin had no significant effect on the prothrombin time *1596*

Riluzole *Serum* *No Effect* *Physiological* No effect on riluzole binding observed *4941*

Sildenafil *Serum* *No Effect* *Physiological* CYP2C9 inhibitors such as warfarin did not affect the pharmacokinetics of sildenafil *4657*

Sodium *Serum* *No Effect* *Analytical* At concentration of 1.5 mg/L had no effect on flame-photometric method *5704* At concentration of 100 mg/L had no effect on measurement by ISE with predilution *5704*

T3-Uptake *Serum* *No Effect* *Physiological* No effect at dose of 5 mg/d *882*

Thrombin/Antithrombin III Complex
Plasma *Decrease* *Physiological* In 39 patients with congestive cardiac failure treatment with warfarin sufficient to maintain an INR of 1.5 to 3.0 for 3 months caused a significant decrease in concentration from mean baseline of 3.0 ± 2.8 ng/mL to 1.8 ± 1.1 ng/mL after 1 month, 2.2 ± 2.2 ng/mL after 2 months and 1.7 ± 1.0 ng/mL after 3 months *2884* In 12 patients with cardioembolic stroke treatment caused nonsignificant reduction from mean baseline of 12.2 ± 15.6 ng/mL to 2.8 ± 1.5 ng/mL *6587*

Tocainide *Serum* *No Effect* *Physiological* No clinically significant interaction observed *268*

Tolbutamide *Serum* *No Effect* *Physiological* No effect apparent on plasma concentration or metabolism *5595*

Triglycerides *Serum* *Increase* *Physiological* In 12 men treatment with up to 2.5 mg/d for 8 weeks caused slight increase from mean baseline of 1.62 mmol/L at baseline to 1.83 mmol/L *2678*
Serum *No Effect* *Analytical* At concentration of 100 mg/L had no effect on lipase/esterase method *5704*

Trovafloxacin *Serum* *No Effect* *Physiological* No significant interaction observed *4663*

Urea Nitrogen *Serum* *No Effect* *Analytical* At concentration of 100 mg/L had no effect on diacetylmonoxime method *5704*
Serum *No Effect* *Physiological* No effect on renal function noted with continuing administration *3954*

Uric Acid *Serum* *Increase* *Physiological* Noted in men at all levels of renal function without alteration of renal clearance of uric acid, possibly related to increased production: effect up to 25% *3954*
Serum *No Effect* *Analytical* At concentration of 100 mg/L had no effect on phosphotungstate reduction method *5704* At concentration of 26 mg/L had no effect on Kageyama-Hantzsch method *5704*
Serum *No Effect* *Physiological* No change observed in 40 patients before and after treatment in contrast to prior reports *6312*

von Willebrand Factor *Plasma* *No Effect* *Physiological* In 31 patients with chronic atrial fibrillation initial median concentration of 152 IU/dL (interquartile range 108 - 198 IU/dL) not significantly changed to 169 IU/dL (interquartile range 118 - 227 IU/dL) after treatment with warfarin for 2 months *2130*

Warfarin Metabolites

Factor II *Plasma* *Decrease* *Physiological* Slight effect with some compounds only *3552*

Factor VII *Plasma* *Decrease* *Physiological* Usually marked effect all compounds *3552*

Factor IX *Plasma* *Decrease* *Physiological* Usually marked effect all compounds *3552*

Factor X *Plasma* *Decrease* *Physiological* Usually marked effect all compounds *3552*

WEB 2086

Alanine Aminotransferase *Serum* *No Effect* *Physiological* No effect observed in 12 healthy men given 300 mg daily for 7 days *52*

Alkaline Phosphatase *Serum* *No Effect* *Physiological* No effect observed in 12 healthy men given 300 mg daily for 7 days *52*

Aspartate Aminotransferase
Serum *No Effect* *Physiological* No effect observed in 12 healthy men given 300 mg daily for 7 days *52*

Bilirubin *Serum* *No Effect* *Physiological* No effect observed in 12 healthy men given 300 mg daily for 7 days *52*
Urine *No Effect* *Physiological* No significant effect observed in 12 healthy men given 300 mg daily for 7 days *52*

Bleeding Time *Patient* *No Effect* *Physiological* No significant effect observed in 12 healthy men given 300 mg daily for 7 days *52*

Calcium *Serum* *No Effect* *Physiological* No effect observed in 12 healthy men given 300 mg daily for 7 days *52*

Chloride *Serum* *No Effect* *Physiological* No effect observed in 12 healthy men given 300 mg daily for 7 days *52*

Cholesterol *Serum* *No Effect* *Physiological* No effect observed in 12 healthy men given 300 mg daily for 7 days *52*

Creatinine *Serum* *No Effect* *Physiological* No effect observed in 12 healthy men given 300 mg daily for 7 days *52*

Erythrocyte Sedimentation Rate
Blood *No Effect* *Physiological* No significant effect observed in 12 healthy men given 300 mg daily for 7 days *52*

Erythrocytes *Blood* *No Effect* *Physiological* No significant effect observed in 12 healthy men given 300 mg daily for 7 days *52*
Urine *No Effect* *Physiological* No significant effect observed in 12 healthy men given 300 mg daily for 7 days *52*

Fatty Acids (FFA), Free *Serum* *No Effect* *Physiological* No effect observed in 12 healthy men given 300 mg daily for 7 days *52*

Fibrinogen *Plasma* *No Effect* *Physiological* No significant effect observed in 12 healthy men given 300 mg daily for 7 days *52*

Glucose *Serum* *No Effect* *Physiological* No effect observed in 12 healthy men given 300 mg daily for 7 days *52*
Urine *No Effect* *Physiological* No significant effect observed in 12 healthy men given 300 mg daily for 7 days *52*

γ-Glutamyltransferase *Serum* *No Effect* *Physiological* No effect observed in 12 healthy men given 300 mg daily for 7 days *52*

Hematocrit *Blood* *No Effect* *Physiological* No effect observed with 300 mg/day for 7 days in 12 healthy men *52*

Hemoglobin *Blood* *No Effect* *Physiological* No significant effect in 12 healthy men given 300 mg daily for 7 days *52*

Ketones *Urine* *No Effect* *Physiological* No significant effect observed in 12 healthy men given 300 mg daily for 7 days *52*

Lactate *Plasma* *No Effect* *Physiological* No effect observed in 12 healthy men given 300 mg daily for 7 days *52*

Lactate Dehydrogenase *Serum* *No Effect* *Physiological* No effect observed in 12 healthy men given 300 mg daily for 7 days *52*

Leukocytes *Blood* *No Effect* *Physiological* No significant effect observed in 12 healthy men given 300 mg daily for 7 days; no effect on differential count observed *52*

Lipase *Serum* *No Effect* *Physiological* No effect observed in 12 healthy men given 300 mg daily for 7 days *52*

MCHC *Blood* *No Effect* *Physiological* No significant effect observed in 12 healthy men given 300 mg daily for 7 days *52*

MCV *Blood* *No Effect* *Physiological* No significant effect observed in 12 healthy men given 300 mg daily for 7 days *52*

Microscopy *Urine* *No Effect* *Physiological* No effect observed in 12 healthy men given 300 mg daily for 7 days *52*

Nitrate *Urine* *No Effect* *Physiological* No significant effect observed in 12 healthy men given 300 mg daily for 7 days *52*

Partial Thromboplastin Time
Plasma *No Effect* *Physiological* No significant effect observed in 12 healthy men given 300 mg daily for 7 days *52*

pH *Urine* *No Effect* *Physiological* No significant effect observed in 12 healthy men given 300 mg daily for 7 days *52*

Phosphate *Serum* *No Effect* *Physiological* No effect observed in 12 healthy men given 300 mg daily for 7 days *52*

Platelets *Blood* *No Effect* *Physiological* No effect observed in 12 healthy men given 300 mg daily for 7 days *52*

Potassium *Serum* *No Effect* *Physiological* No effect observed in 12 healthy men given 300 mg daily for 7 days *52*

WEB 2086 *(continued)*

Protein *Serum No Effect Physiological* No effect observed in 12 healthy men given 300 mg daily for 7 days *52*
Urine No Effect Physiological No significant effect observed in 12 healthy men given 300 mg daily for 7 days *52*

Protein Electrophoresis *Serum No Effect Physiological* No effect observed in 12 healthy men given 300 mg daily for 7 days *52*

Reticulocytes *Blood No Effect Physiological* No significant effect observed in 12 healthy men given 300 mg daily for 7 days *52*

Sodium *Serum No Effect Physiological* No effect observed in 12 healthy men given 300 mg daily for 7 days *52*

Specific Gravity *Urine No Effect Physiological* No significant effect observed in 12 healthy men given 300 mg daily for 7 days *52*

Thrombin Time *Blood No Effect Physiological* No significant effect in 12 healthy men given 300 mg daily for 7 days *52*

Thromboplastin Time *Plasma No Effect Physiological* No significant effect observed in 12 healthy men given 300 mg daily for 7 days *52*

Thyroid Stimulating Hormone
Serum No Effect Physiological No effect observed in 12 healthy men given 300 mg daily for 7 days *52*

Thyroxine (T4) *Serum No Effect Physiological* No effect observed in 12 healthy men given 300 mg daily for 7 days *52*

Tri-iodothyronine (T3) *Serum No Effect Physiological* No effect observed in 12 healthy men given 300 mg daily for 7 days *52*

Triglycerides *Serum No Effect Physiological* No effect observed in 12 healthy men given 300 mg daily for 7 days *52*

Urea Nitrogen *Serum No Effect Physiological* No effect observed in 12 healthy men given 300 mg daily for 7 days *52*

Uric Acid *Serum No Effect Physiological* No effect observed in 12 healthy men given 300 mg daily for 7 days *52*

Urobilinogen *Urine No Effect Physiological* No significant effect observed in 12 healthy men given 300 mg daily for 7 days *52*

Xamoterol

Aldosterone *Plasma No Effect Physiological* In 12 patients with moderate heart failure 0.2 mg/kg intravenously caused nonsignificant increase to 282 pmol/L after 2 h (from mean placebo concentration of 249 pmol/L) to 26 pmol/L after 5 h *665*

Angiotensin-II *Plasma No Effect Physiological* In 12 patients with moderate heart failure 0.2 mg/kg intravenously caused nonsignificant change from placebo of 39 pmol/L to 38 pmol/L after 2 h and from 42 pmol/L with placebo and 54 pmol/L with xamoterol after 5 h *665*

Creatinine Clearance *Urine No Effect Physiological* In 12 patients with moderate heart failure 0.2 mg/kg intravenously caused nonsignificant change from baseline of 90.7 ± 4.5 mL/min to 91.0 ± 4.5 mL/min after 5 hours *665*

Filtration Fraction *Urine No Effect Physiological* In 12 patients with moderate heart failure 0.2 mg/kg intravenously caused nonsignificant change from mean baseline of 0.29 ± 0.03 to 0.28 ± 0.02 *665*

Glomerular Filtration Rate *Urine No Effect Physiological* In 12 patients with moderate heart failure administration of 0.2 mg/kg caused nonsignificant increase from mean baseline of 70 ± 2 mL/min to 71 ± 2 mL/min after 5 hours *665*

Lithium Clearance *Urine No Effect Physiological* In 12 patients with moderate heart failure 0.2 mg/kg intravenously caused nonsignificant reduction from baseline of 16.4 ± 2.9 mL/min to 13.9 ± 2.7 mL/min after 5 hours *665*

Potassium Clearance *Urine No Effect Physiological* In 12 patients with moderate heart failure 0.2 mg/kg intravenously caused nonsignificant reduction from mean baseline of 11.0 ± 2.0 mL/min to 7.9 ± 1.4 mL/min *665*

Renal Plasma Flow *Patient No Effect Physiological* In 12 patients with moderate heart failure intravenous infusion of 0.2 mg/kg caused nonsignificant change from mean baseline of 244 ± 9 mL/min to 252 ± 10 mL/min after 5 hours *665*

Sodium Clearance *Urine Decrease Physiological* In 12 patients with moderate heart failure 0.2 mg/kg intravenously caused significant reduction from baseline of 0.59 ± 0.13 mL/min to 0.32 ± 0.12 mL/min after 5 hours *665*

Uric Acid Clearance *Urine No Effect Physiological* In 12 patients with moderate heart failure 0.2 mg/kg intravenously caused nonsignificant change from baseline of 5.8 ± 1.9 mL/min to 5.4 ± 1.9 mL/min *665*

Volume *Urine Decrease Physiological* In 12 patients with moderate heart failure after 0.2 mg/kg intravenously flow rate decreased from 5.1 ± 1.5 mL/min after 2 h to 3.3 ± 1.5 mL/min after 5 h *665*

Xipamide

Aldosterone *Plasma Increase Physiological* In 6 healthy volunteers treatment for 16 weeks with 20 mg/d caused significant increase to 1.00 (range 0.59-1.58) nmol/L from 0.27 (0.15-0.60) nmol/L in placebo treatment period *3572* In 6 healthy men mean increase from 0.27 nmol/L to 1.00 nmol/L when treated with 20 mg daily for 16 weeks when compared with placebo period *3575*
Urine Increase Physiological Mean increase of 24 h excretion from 29 nmol to 69 nmol in 6 healthy men treated with 20 mg daily for 16 weeks *3575* In 6 healthy volunteers treated with 20 mg/d for 16 weeks caused significantly increased excretion to 69 (range 61-114) nmol/d from 29 (range 19-69) nmol/d during placebo period *3572*

Atrial Natriuretic Peptide *Plasma Decrease Physiological* In 6 healthy men 20 mg daily for 16 weeks caused reduction of mean concentration from 9.0 pmol/L to 4.7 pmol/L *3575* In 6 healthy volunteers treatment with 20 mg/d for 16 weeks caused significant decrease to 4.7 (range 2.7-7.3) pmol/L compared with 9.0 (4.6-11.3) pmol/L during placebo treatment period *3572*

Creatinine *Serum No Effect Physiological* No significant change in 12 healthy men treated with 20 mg daily for 16 weeks *3575*

Erythrocytes *Blood Increase Physiological* In 6 healthy men 20 mg daily for 16 weeks caused mean increase from 4.94 million /μL to 5.14 million /μL *3575*

Hematocrit *Blood Increase Physiological* In 6 healthy men 20 mg daily for 16 weeks caused mean increase from 0.45 to 0.47 *3575*

Hemoglobin *Blood Increase Physiological* In 6 healthy men 20 mg daily for 16 weeks caused mean increase from 9.2 mmol/L to 9.6 mmol/L *3575*

Kallikrein *Urine Increase Physiological* In 6 healthy volunteers treatment with 20 mg/d for 16 weeks caused significant increase to 1.25 (range 0.34-2.56) U/d from 0.43 (0.07-1.00) U/d in placebo period *3572* Mean increase from 0.43 U/24 h to 1.25 U/24 h in 6 healthy men treated with 20 mg daily for 16 weeks *3575*

Leukocytes *Blood No Effect Physiological* No significant effect observed in 12 healthy men treated with 20 mg daily for 16 weeks *3575*

Potassium *Serum Decrease Physiological* Reduction from mean of 4.30 mmol/L to 3.79 mmol/L in 6 healthy men treated with 20 mg daily for 16 weeks *3575*
Urine No Effect Physiological In 12 healthy volunteers treatment with 20 mg/d for 16 weeks caused no significant change from mean baseline of 85 ± 7 mmol/d *3572*

Renin Activity *Plasma Increase Physiological* Increase from mean of 0.29 nmol/L/h to 2.02 nmol/L/h in 6 healthy men treated with 20 mg daily for 16 weeks *3575* In 6 healthy volunteers treatment with 20 mg/d for 16 weeks caused significant increase to mean of 2.02 (range 1.28-2.84) nmol/L/h compared with 0.29 (range 0.15-0.44) nmol/L/h in placebo treatment period *3572*

Sodium *Serum Decrease Physiological* Reduction by 1 mmol/L in 6 healthy men treated with 20 mg daily for 16 weeks *3575*
Urine No Effect Physiological In 12 healthy volunteers treatment with 20 mg/d for 16 weeks caused no significant change from mean baseline of 171 ± 18 mmol/d *3572*

Xylometazoline

Histamine *Plasma No Effect Analytical* Improbable inhibition of radio-enzyme assay at therapeutic concentrations *2492*

Yohimbine

Antidiuretic Hormone
Cerebrospinal Fluid No Effect Physiological No effect observed on arginine vasopressin concentration following administration to 7 normal young men *4626*
Plasma No Effect Physiological No significant effect in 7 young normal men following administration *4626*

Norepinephrine *Cerebrospinal Fluid Increase Physiological* Significant increase observed in 7 young normal men following administration *4626*
Plasma Increase Physiological Significant increase in 7 normal young men following administration *4626*

Zabicipril

Glomerular Filtration Rate *Urine No Effect Physiological* In 16 healthy men (both old and young) no significant change observed over 4 hours with doses ranging up to 2.5 mg *4203*

Renal Plasma Flow *Patient Increase Physiological* After dose of 2.5 mg mean flow increased from baseline of 540 ± 17 mL/min to 653 ± 33 mL/min after 4 hours in 8 healthy young men and from 355 ± 22 mL/min to 415 ± 48 mL/min in 8 healthy old men but no significant effect at lesser concentrations and over less time in either population *4203*

Zacopride

Aldosterone *Plasma Increase Physiological* In 28 healthy mean administration of a single oral dose of 400 µg caused a significant increase of plasma aldosterone concentration from 289 ± 62 pmol/L to 453 ± 105 pmol/L over the next 3 hours *3488* In 8 healthy volunteers pretreated with dexamethasone administration of 400 µg zacopride caused a significant increase of 172 ± 60% (compared with 37 ± 25% in placebo treated controls) *3487*

Corticotropin *Plasma No Effect Physiological* In 28 healthy mean administration of a single oral dose of 400 µg had no effect on plasma ACTH concentration over the next 3 hours *3488* In healthy volunteers pretreated with dexamethasone which caused suppression of corticotropin concentration subsequent administration of zacopride had no effect on concentration *3487*

Cortisol *Plasma No Effect Physiological* In 8 healthy volunteers pretreatment with dexamethasone caused significant reduction of concentration but subsequent administration of zacopride had no effect on already reduced concentration *3487* In 28 healthy mean administration of a single oral dose of 400 µg had no effect on plasma cortisol concentration over the next 3 hours *3488*

Potassium *Serum No Effect Physiological* In 8 healthy volunteers pretreatment with dexamethasone prior to aministration of zacopride had no effect on plasma concentration *3487*

Zafirlukast

Alanine Aminotransferase *Serum No Effect Physiological* In 4058 patients taking zafirlukast significant increase observed in 1.5% patients compared with 1.1% in 2032 individuals receiving placebo *6641* In several clinical trials frequency of increases to above twice the upper limit of normal similar in drug-treated and placebo-treated groups *845*

Ethinyl Estradiol *Serum No Effect Physiological* In 39 healthy women taking oral contraceptives coadministration of zafirlukast (80 mg/d) had no significant effect on the ethinyl estradiol concentration *6641*

Prothrombin Time *Plasma Increase Physiological* Coadministration of zafirlukast and warfarin to healthy male volunteers caused a significant increase in prothrombin time unless warfarin dose modified *6641*

Theophylline *Serum No Effect Physiological* In 13 asthmatic patients coadministration of zafirlukast (80 mg/d) at steady state with erythromycin (6 mg/kg) for 5 days to steady state caused no significant effect on the plasma theophylline concentration *6641*

Warfarin *Plasma Increase Physiological* Coadministration of zafirlukast 160 mg/d to 16 healthy male volunteers with a single 25 mg dose of warfarin-S caused a 63% mean increase in the area under the concentration/time curve and half-life of 36% probably due to inhibition of the cytochrome P450 2C9 isoenzyme *6641*

Zalcitabine

Alanine Aminotransferase *Serum Increase Physiological* Zalcitabine reported to cause increased activity in 5.7% of 615 treated patients in one trial when administered with zidovudine *5023* Zalcitabine reported to cause rare cases of potentially fatal lactic acidosis in the absence of hypoxemia and severe hepatomegaly with steatosis, and rare cases of hepatic failure related to underlying hepatitis B *5023*

Albumin *Urine Increase Physiological* Zalcitabine reported to cause albuminuria in some patients *5023*

Alkaline Phosphatase *Serum Increase Physiological* Zalcitabine reported to cause rare cases of potentially fatal lactic acidosis in the absence of hypoxemia and severe hepatomegaly with steatosis, and rare cases of hepatic failure related to underlying hepatitis B *5023*

Amylase *Serum Increase Physiological* Zalcitabine reported to cause pancreatitis in up to 1.1% cases when administered alone or with zidovudine: increased amylase activity observed in 1.6% patients with zalcitabine monotherapy. Amylase activity increased above 5 times the upper limit of normal in 5.1% of 237 patients treated with zalcitabine monotherapy, and 1.5% of 615 patients treated with combined therapy with zidovudine *5023*

Aspartate Aminotransferase *Serum Increase Physiological* Zalcitabine reported to cause rare cases of potentially fatal lactic acidosis in the absence of hypoxemia and severe hepatomegaly with steatosis, and rare cases of hepatic failure related to underlying hepatitis B *5023*

Bicarbonate *Serum Decrease Physiological* Zalcitabine reported to cause decreased concentration *5023*

Bilirubin *Serum Increase Physiological* Zalcitabine reported to cause increased concentration in 0.8% of 237 treated patients in one trial when administered alone *5023*

Calcium *Serum Decrease Physiological* Zalcitabine reported to cause hypocalcemia *5023*
Serum Increase Physiological Zalcitabine reported to cause hypercalcemia *5023*

CD4+ Lymphocytes *Blood Increase Physiological* During Phase I trials treatment of adults with advanced HIV-1 infection caused transient increases of CD4 count *2623*

Creatine Kinase *Serum Increase Physiological* Zalcitabine reported to cause increased activity in 0.8% of 237 treated patients in one trial when administered alone *5023*

Eosinophils *Blood Increase Physiological* Zalcitabine reported to cause eosinophilia in 2.5% of 237 treated patients in one trial when administered alone *5023*

Glucose *Serum Decrease Physiological* Zalcitabine reported to cause hypoglycemia *5023*
Serum Increase Physiological Zalcitabine reported to cause hyperglycemia in 2.0% of 615 treated patients in one trial when administered with zidovudine, but in none of 237 patients treated with zalcitabine alone *5023*
Serum No Effect Physiological Zalcitabine reported to cause hyperglycemia in 2.0% of 615 treated patients in one trial when administered with zidovudine, but in none of 237 patients treated with zalcitabine alone *5023*
Urine Increase Physiological Zalcitabine reported to cause increased concentration *5023*

γ-Glutamyltransferase *Serum Increase Physiological* Zalcitabine reported to cause rare cases of potentially fatal lactic acidosis in the absence of hypoxemia and severe hepatomegaly with steatosis, and rare cases of hepatic failure related to underlying hepatitis B *5023*

Zalcitabine *(continued)*

Hematocrit *Blood Decrease Physiological* Zalcitabine reported to cause anemia in 8.4% of 237 treated patients in one trial when administered alone *5023*

Hemoglobin *Blood Decrease Physiological* Zalcitabine reported to cause anemia in 8.4% of 237 treated patients in one trial when administered alone *5023*

HIV p24 Antigen *Serum Decrease Physiological* Concentration reduced in adults with HIV-1 infection during Phase I trials *2623*

Leukocytes *Blood Decrease Physiological* Zalcitabine reported to cause leukopenia in 13.1% of 237 treated patients in one trial when administered alone *5023*

Lipase *Serum Increase Physiological* Zalcitabine reported to cause pancreatitis in up to 1.1% cases when administered alone or with zidovudine *5023* Zalcitabine reported to cause increased activity in 1.0% of 615 treated patients in one trial when administered with zidovudine *5023*

Lipids *Serum Increase Physiological* Zalcitabine reported to cause hyperlipemia *5023*

Loperamide *Serum No Effect Physiological* Coadministration of loperamide and single doses of zalcitabine 1.5 mg to 12 HIV-positive patients had no significant effect on pharmacokinetics of either drug *5023*

Magnesium *Serum Decrease Physiological* Zalcitabine reported to cause hypomagnesemia *5023*

Neutrophils *Blood Increase Physiological* Zalcitabine reported to cause neutropenia in 16.9% of 237 treated patients in one trial when administered alone *5023*

Nonprotein Nitrogen *Serum Increase Physiological* Zalcitabine reported to cause increased nonprotein nitrogen concentration *5023*

Occult Blood *Feces Increase Physiological* Zalcitabine reported to cause abdominal bleeding and rectal bleeding *5023*

Phosphate *Serum Decrease Physiological* Zalcitabine reported to cause hypophosphatemia *5023*

Platelets *Blood Increase Physiological* Zalcitabine reported to cause thrombocytopenia in 16.9% of 237 treated patients in one trial when administered alone *5023*

Potassium *Serum Decrease Physiological* Zalcitabine reported to cause hypokalemia *5023*
Serum Increase Physiological Zalcitabine reported to cause hyperkalemia *5023*

Saquinavir *Serum No Effect Physiological* Coadministration of zalcitabine and zidovudine with saquinavir had no effect on the absorptions, metabolisms or excretions of any of the drugs in adults *5024*

Sodium *Serum Decrease Physiological* Zalcitabine reported to cause hyponatremia *5023*
Serum Increase Physiological Zalcitabine reported to cause hypernatremia *5023*

Triglycerides *Serum Increase Physiological* Zalcitabine reported to cause increased concentration *5023*

Urea Nitrogen *Serum Increase Physiological* Zalcitabine reported to cause increased blood urea nitrogen concentration and abnormal renal function (including renal failure) in some patients *5023*

Uric Acid *Serum Increase Physiological* Zalcitabine reported to cause gout *5023*

Zidovudine *Serum No Effect Physiological* When single doses of zalcitabine 1.5 mg and zidovudine 200 mg were coadministered to 12 HIV-positive patients no significant pharmacokinetic interaction observed *5023*

Zanamivir

Erythrocytes *Blood No Effect Physiological* Administration to 417 individuals with influenza-virus infection showed no drug-related effects on blood counts *2518*

Leukocytes *Blood No Effect Physiological* Administration to 417 individuals with influenza-virus infection showed no drug-related effects on blood counts *2518*

Platelets *Blood No Effect Physiological* Administration to 417 individuals with influenza-virus infection showed no drug-related effects on blood counts *2518*

Zidovudine

Alanine Aminotransferase *Serum Increase Physiological* In 402 HIV-infected patients treatment with 200 mg t.i.d. for a median of 53 weeks caused an increase to above 5.0 times the upper limit of normal in 11 patients *731* In 619 patients treatment with 200 mg q8 h 3.6% demonstrated increased activity *5023* In studies of several thousand patients with HIV infection treated with zidovudine alone for 24 weeks ALT activity greater than 5.0 ULN observed in 3.6% *2174* Increase observed in one patient 6 days after treatment discontinued with predominantly cholestatic pattern of liver function abnormalities *1606* In 276 children with AIDS treatment with zidovudine for a median of 19 months 18% had serum alanine aminotransferase activity exceeding 10 times the upper limit of normal *1736* At recommended dose in ACTG 1168/117 and 116A trials of almost 500 adult patients caused ALT activity of more than 5 times ULN in 6 and 6% patients respectively, and of greater than 10 times ULN in 7% of 281 children *730*

Albumin *Serum No Effect Physiological* In 14 patients with HIV-1 infection pretreatment concentration decreased by 1.5% after 3 - 30 months treatment *2137*

Alkaline Phosphatase *Serum Increase Physiological* At recommended dose in ACTG 1168/117 and 116A trials of almost 500 adult patients caused alkaline phosphatase activity of more than 5 times ULN in 1 and 1% patients respectively, and of greater than 2 times ULN in 10% of 281 children *730* Increase observed in one patient 6 days after treatment discontinued with cholestatic liver function abnormalities *1606*

Amylase *Serum Decrease Physiological* In studies of several thousand patients with HIV infection treated with zidovudine alone for 24 weeks amylase activities above 2.0 ULN observed in 1.5% patients *2174*
Serum Increase Physiological At recommended dose in ACTG 1168/117 and 116A trials of almost 500 adult patients caused amylase activity of more than 1.4 times ULN in 12 and 5% patients respectively, and of greater than 3.1 ULN in 7% children *730* In 402 HIV-infected patients treatment with 200 mg t.i.d. for a median of 53 weeks caused an increase to above 1.4 times the upper limit of normal in 13 patients *731* In 276 children with AIDS treatment with zidovudine for a median of 19 months 30% had serum amylase activity exceeding 3 times the upper limit of normal *1736* In 619 patients treatment with 200 mg q8 h 1.0% demonstrated increased activity *5023*

Anti-p24 Antibody *Serum No Effect Physiological* No effect in either patients with AIDS or ARC given 250 mg every 4 hours for one month or in control patients *947*

Aspartate Aminotransferase *Serum Increase Physiological* Increase observed in one patient 6 days after treatment discontinued with cholestatic pattern of liver function abnormalities *1606* In 619 patients treatment with 200 mg q8 h 2.9% demonstrated increased activity *5023* At recommended dose in ACTG 1168/117 and 116A trials of almost 500 adult patients caused AST activity of more than 5 times ULN in 4 and 6% patients respectively, and in 16% of 281 children *730* In studies of several thousand patients with HIV infection treated with zidovudine alone for 24 weeks AST activity greater than 5.0 ULN observed in 1.8% *2174* In 402 HIV-infected patients treatment with 200 mg t.i.d. for a median of 53 weeks caused an increase to above 5.0 times the upper limit of normal in 10 patients *731*

Atovaquone *Serum No Effect Physiological* In 14 HIV-positive volunteers coadministration of 750 mg/12 h atovaquone daily with steady state zidovudine conditions (200 mg/8 h) had no effect on atovaquone pharmacokinetics *2163*

Bilirubin *Serum Increase Physiological* In studies of several thousand patients with HIV infection treated with zidovudine alone for 24 weeks bilirubin concentration greater than 2.5 ULN observed in 1.5% *2174* In patients with asymptomatic HIV infection mild drug-associated increases have been reported rarely *2163* At recommended dose in ACTG 1168/117 and 116A trials in almost 500 adult patients caused an increase in bilirubin concentration to more than 2.6 times ULN in 1 and 1% patients respectively, and in 4% of 281 children *730* In 619 patients treatment with 200 mg q8 h 0.5% demonstrated increased concentration *5023* Increase observed in one patient 6 days after treatment discontinued with predominantly cholestatic pattern of liver function abnormalities *1606* In 276 children with AIDS treatment with zidovudine for a median of 19 months 10% had serum total bilirubin concentration exceeding 2.6 times the upper limit of normal *1736* In 402 HIV-infected patients treatment with 200 mg t.i.d. for a median of 53 weeks caused an increase to above 5.0 times the upper limit of normal in 2 patients *731*

CD4⁺ Lymphocytes *Blood Increase Physiological* In 79 patients with AIDS or ARC treatment for 8-12 weeks caused significant mean increase of 20 cells /µL *2871* In 14 patients with HIV-1 infection pretreatment concentration 275 x 10^6/L increased by 32% after 3 - 14 months treatment and 16% after 14 - 30 months treatment *2137* Sustained rise observed in patients with AIDS treated for 12 weeks. Count increased from mean of 321/µL to 412/µL in those receiving 300 mg/day but decreased from 316/µL to 296/µL (not significant) in those receiving 600 mg/day. No change with 1500 mg/d *1094* Significant increase observed in one patient with AIDS and nephropathy following treatment with 800 mg zidovudine daily for 7 weeks *3373* Sustained rise observed in patients with AIDS treated for 12 weeks. Count increased from mean of 321 /µL to 412 /µL in those receiving 300 mg/day but decreased from 316 /µL to 296 /µL (not significant) in those receiving 600 mg/day. No change with 1500 mg/d *1094* Transient effect observed in patients with AIDS, but count fell often to baseline after 16 to 20 weeks therapy *6590* In a study of 366 previously untreated patients with HIV infection treated with zidovudine alone for 24 weeks mean CD4 count increased from 352 cells/µL by up to 30 cells/µL *2174*

Blood No Effect Physiological In 20 men with HIV-1 p_{24} antigenemia treatment with 1 g daily for 92 weeks after stabilization caused insignificant change in CD4+ count form 0.4 /nL to 0.45 /nL *4160*

CD8⁺ Lymphocytes *Blood Increase Physiological* Significant increase observed in a single patient with AIDS and nephrotic syndrome treated with 800 mg zidovudine daily for 7 weeks *3373*

Creatine Kinase *Serum Increase Physiological* Mitochondrial myopathy observed as a toxic side effect in some patients positive for HIV *1220* In 619 patients treatment with 200 mg q8 h 5.8% demonstrated increased activity *5023* Prolonged treatment of patients with HIV-infection can cause a myopathy characterized by inhibition of mitochondrial DNA replication which may be difficult to distinguish from the myopathy caused by HIV-1 itself *2623* At recommended dose in ACTG 152 trial of 281patients caused creatine kinase activity of more than 5.1 times ULN in 8% patients. Increased creatine kinase activity also observed in adults in association with rhabdomyolysis *730*

Creatinine *Serum Decrease Physiological* In one patient with AIDS and nephrotic syndrome treatment with 800 mg daily caused reduction of serum creatinine to 195 µmol/L after 2 weeks and to 133 µmol/L after another 5 weeks from an initial concentration of 345 µmol/L *3373*

Erythrocytes *Blood Decrease Physiological* Prolonged treatment may cause anemia although incidence less since doses reduced *2623* Pancytopenia observed in two patients with rheumatoid arthritis treated with 100 mg daily, with effects occurring within 3 and 8 weeks of start of treatment *2935*

Erythropoietin *Serum Increase Physiological* At time of first required transfusion in patients with AIDS treated with drug, suggesting that anemia is due to red cell hypoplasia or aplasia *6317*

Ganciclovir *Serum Decrease Physiological* At an oral dose of 1000 mg ganciclovir every 8 h mean steady-state AUC of ganciclovir decreased 17 ± 25% in the presence of zidovudine 100 mg every 4 h *5018*

Glucose *Serum Increase Physiological* In 619 patients treatment with 200 mg q8 h 0.8% demonstrated increased concentration *5023*

γ-Glutamyltransferase *Serum Increase Physiological* In 619 patients treatment with 200 mg q8 h 0.5% demonstrated increased activity *5023* Increase in one patient within 7 days following treatment with 200 mg every 4 hours with predominantly cholestatic pattern of laboratory abnormalities *1606*

Granulocytes *Blood Decrease Physiological* Occurred in 47% of zidovudine treated versus 10% of placebo treated patients: occurence correlated inversely with the number of CD4 lymphocytes and granulocytes at start of treatment *1384* In patients with AIDS receiving 1500 mg drug daily mean decrease of 13, 22 and 25% respectively at 4, 8 and 12 weeks, whereas no change observed at these times in patients receiving either 300 or 600 mg daily *1094* In asymptomatic patients treated with 500 mg/d granulocytopenia of > 750 cells/µL observed in 1.8% patients, in patients with early HIV disease treated with 1200 mg/d incidence of 4% observed, in advanced patients with CD4 counts above 200 cells/µL treated with 1500 mg/d incidence 10% and in patients with ≤200 cells/µL treated with 600 or 1500 mg/d incidence of granulocytopenia 37% and 47% respectively *2163* At recommended dose in ACTG 1168/117 and 116A trials of almost 500 adult patients caused granulocyte concentrations of less than 750/µL in 19 and 15% patients respectively, and 27% in 281 children *730*

Hematocrit *Blood Decrease Physiological* Coadministration with ganciclovir, dapsone, flucytosine, vincristine, vinblastine, adriamycin or interferon-α increases the risk of toxicity in some patients with advanced HIV disease *2163* In 619 patients treatment with 200 mg q8 h 1.8% demonstrated anemia *5023*

Hemoglobin *Blood Decrease Physiological* Decrease to below 90 g/L observed in 2.4% of 125 patients with AIDS without neutropenia and in 4.8% in those with neutropenia also when treated with up to 1200 mg daily. When hematotoxic drugs also given anemia and neutropenia observed in 2.4% patients *2124* Prolonged treatment may cause anemia although frequency of this problem has been lessened since doses have been reduced *2623* In 276 children with AIDS treatment with zidovudine for a median of 19 months 26% had hemoglobin concentration of less than 7.5 g/dL *1736* Profound effect observed in one male homosexual with AIDS unlikely related to other factors *1913* In 402 HIV-infected patients treatment with 200 mg t.i.d. for a median of 53 weeks caused an decrease to below 80 g/L in 3 patients *731* In studies of several thousand patients with HIV infection treated with zidovudine alone for 24 weeks anemia with hemoglobin concentration of less than 8.0 g/dL observed in 1.8% *2174* 25% reduction observed in 45% zidovudine treated patients but only in 14% of placebo recipients: occurence correlated inversely with number of CD4 lymphocytes and granulocytes at start of treatment *1384* Anemia developed in 6 of 15 patients treated with drug requiring transfusion (Hemoglobin less than 100 g/L) at mean of 6 weeks after starting treatment *6317* Effect observed in patients with AIDS treated with doses of 300, 600 and 1500 mg daily but most marked in those receiving 600 mg or 1500 mg. Mean decreases at 12 weeks of 4 g/L with 300 mg, 12 g/L with 600 mg and 18 g/L with 1500 mg/day *1094* In 619 patients treatment with 200 mg q8 h 1.8% demonstrated anemia *5023* At recommended dose in ACTG 1168/117 and 116A trials of almost 500 adult patients caused hemoglobin concentrations of less than 80 g/L in 8 and 5% patients respectively, and hemoglobin of less than 75 g/L in 10% of 281 children *730* In patients with advanced HIV disease treated with zidovudine anemia occurs due to impaired erythrocyte maturation as evidenced by macrocytosis *2163* Coadministration with ganciclovir, dapsone, flucytosine, vincristine, vinblastine, adriamycin or interferon-α increases the risk of toxicity in some patients with advanced HIV disease *2163*

HIV-1 RNA *Serum Decrease Physiological* In a study of 366 previously untreated patients with HIV infection treated with 300 mg lamivudine b.i.d alone for 24 weeks mean HIV RNA decreased by about 0.4 copies/mL with a greater response when coadministered with lamivudine *2174*

HIV Core Antigen *Serum Decrease Physiological* Decreased from average of 111 pg/mL to 46 pg/mL after 4 weeks treatment with 250 mg every 4 hours in 32 patients with AIDS or ARC *947*

HIV p24 Antibody *Serum No Effect Physiological* No significant change observed in 89 patients with AIDS or ARC treated for 8-12 weeks *2871*

HIV p24 Antigen *Serum Decrease Physiological* In 12 patients with AIDS or ARC receiving up to 1500 mg/day for up to 72 weeks but concentration rose in 2 patients with discontinuance of treatment *4887* Good correlation observed with serum β_2-microglobulin concentration during initial response to zidovudine treatment in patients with asymptomatic HIV infection *4161* In 90 patients with AIDS or ARC treatment for 8-12 weeks caused mean decrease of 63 ng/mL *2871* Reduction observed in patients with AIDS of comparable magnitude regardless of whether treated with 300 mg or 600 mg daily *1094* Sustained reduction is typical response to treatment with zidovudine although disease progression may continue *4160*

Zidovudine *(continued)*

4-Hydroxy-3-Methoxy-Phenylglycol
Cerebrospinal Fluid No Effect Physiological In 14 patients with HIV-1 infection median pretreatment concentration 6.4 ng/mL compared with reference interval of 6.0 - 16 ng/mL ncreased by 10% after 3 - 14 months treatment and decreased by 12% after 14 - 30 months treatment *2137*

5-Hydroxyindoleacetic Acid
Cerebrospinal Fluid No Effect Physiological In 14 patients with HIV-1 infection median pretreatment concentration 20 ng/mL compared with reference interval of 13 - 42 ng/mL decreased by 2.2% after 3 - 14 months treatment and increased by 4.7% after 14 - 30 months *2137*

IgG Index *Cerebrospinal Fluid No Effect Physiological* In 14 patients with HIV-1 infection pretreatment concentration increased above upper limit of 0.7 decreased by 7.2% after 3 - 14 months treatment and increased by 3.6% after 14 - 30 months treatment *2137*

Indinavir *Serum Increase Physiological* Causes a 13% increase in area under the concentration curve when zidovudine coadministered *1891* Administration of indinavir 1000 mg every 8 hours with zidovudine 200 mg every 8 hours for 1 week resulted in a 13 ± 48% increase in indinavir AUC *3966*
Serum No Effect Physiological Administration of indinavir 800 mg every 8 hours with zidovudine 200 mg every 8 hours in combination with lamivudine 150 mg twice daily for 1 week resulted in no change in indinavir AUC a 36% increase in zidovudine AUC and a 6% decrease in lamivudine AUC *3966*

Lamivudine *Serum Decrease Physiological* Administration of indinavir 800 mg every 8 hours with zidovudine 200 mg every 8 hours in combination with lamivudine 150 mg twice daily for 1 week resulted in no change in indinavir AUC a 36% increase in zidovudine AUC and a 6% decrease in lamivudine AUC *3966*

Leukocytes *Blood Decrease Physiological* Pancytopenia observed in two patients with rheumatoid arthritis treated with 100 mg daily. Effect occurred after 3 weeks in one patient and 8 weeks in the other *2935* In patients with HIV-1 infection who had received prolonged treatment leukopenia frequently observed *2623* Profound effect observed in one male homosexual with AIDS unlikely related to other factors *1913* Decrease of neutrophils to below 1000/ µL observed in 21.2% of 125 patients with AIDS treated with up to 1200 mg without hematotoxic drugs daily and 12.0% when hematotoxic drugs also given *2124* At recommended dose in ACTG 1168/117 and 116A trials of almost 500 adult patients caused leukocyte concentrations of less than 2000/µL in 26 and 32% patients respectively, but less than 1% in 281 children *730* Coadministration with ganciclovir, dapsone, flucytosine, vincristine, vinblastine, adriamycin or interferon-α increases the risk of toxicity in some patients with advanced HIV disease *2163*

MCV *Blood Increase Physiological* Effect observed in patients with AIDS beginning in 2 weeks of start of treatment with doses from 300 mg to 1500 mg daily: effect sustained for 24 weeks *1094* In patients with advanced HIV disease treated with zidovudine anemia occurs due to impaired erythrocyte maturation as evidenced by macrocytosis *2163* Marked effect in patients with AIDS being treated with drug and not developing anemia *6317* In 100 patients with macrocytosis (MCV greater than 110 fL) 47 had AIDS of whom 44 were treated with zidovudine *5664*

Methadone *Serum No Effect Physiological* In 9 HIV-positive volunteers coadministration of a 30 to 90 mg methadone daily with steady state zidovudine conditions (200 mg/4 h) had no effect on methadone kinetics over 14 days *2163* Although methadone appears to increase concentration when drugs coadministered in drug-using patients with HIV infection zidovudine appears to have no effect on methadone concentration *5393*

β_2-Microglobulin *Serum Decrease Physiological* In 34 individuals with mild symptomatic HIV infection treatment for 4 weeks caused significant reduction from mean baseline of 3.01 mg/L to 2.69 mg/L and reached its lowest concentration at 8 weeks, but returned to pretreatment values at approximately 24 weeks after treatment stopped *397* In 18 initially asymptomatic HIV-1 p_{24} antigenemic patients treated with zidovudine and followed for 2.5 years median serum concentration decreased from 2.5 mg/L to 2.3 mg/L after 12 weeks *4161* Significant mean reduction of 59 nmol/L in 90 patients with AIDS or ARC treated for 8-12 weeks *2871*

Nelfinavir *Serum No Effect Physiological* Has no significant effect on area under the concentration curve when zidovudine coadministered *1891*

Neopterin *Cerebrospinal Fluid Decrease Physiological* In 14 patients with HIV-1 infection median pretreatment concentration 15.2 nmol/L compared with reference interval of < 4.2 nmol/L decreased by 45% after 3 - 14 months treatment and 39% after 14 - 30 months treatment *2137*
Serum Decrease Physiological In 14 patients with HIV-1 infection median pretreatment concentration 19.0 nmol/L compared with reference interval of < 8.4 nmol/L decreased by 32% after 3 - 14 months treatment and 22% after 14 - 30 months treatment *2137* In 34 individuals with mild symptomatic HIV infection mean concentration decreased from 15.76 nmol/L before treatment to 12.73 nmol/L after 4 weeks treatment, with lowest concentration observed at 8 weeks, but subsequently the mean value of plasma neopterin increased but remained below pretreatment concentration for more than one year *397* Significant mean reduction of 5 nmol/L in 89 patients with AIDS or ARC treated for 8-12 weeks *2871*

Neutrophils *Blood Decrease Physiological* In studies of several thousand patients with HIV infection treated with zidovudine alone for 24 weeks neutrophil counts of less than 750 /µL observed in 5.4% *2174* In 619 patients treatment with 200 mg q8 h 1.9% demonstrated neutropenia *5023* In 125 patients with AIDS treatment with up to 1200 mg daily without other drugs decrease to below 1000 /µL observed in 21.2% patients and when given with hematoxic drugs observed in 12.0% patients *2124* In 276 children with AIDS treatment with zidovudine for a median of 19 months 74% had absolute neutrophil count of less than 500 cells/µL *1736* In 402 HIV-infected patients treatment with 200 mg t.i.d. for a median of 53 weeks caused an decrease to below 750 /µL in 9 patients *731*

Phenytoin *Serum No Effect Physiological* In 12 HIV-positive volunteers coadministration of a single 300 mg dose of phenytoin with steady state zidovudine conditions (200 mg/4 h) had no effect on phenytoin kinetics *2163*

Platelets *Blood Decrease Physiological* In 402 HIV-infected patients treatment with 200 mg t.i.d. for a median of 53 weeks caused an decrease to below 50,000 /µL in 3 patients *731* Profound effect observed in one male homosexual with AIDS unlikely related to other factors *1913* In studies of several thousand patients with HIV infection treated with zidovudine alone for 24 weeks platelet counts of less than 50,000 /µL observed in 1.3% *2174* In patients with advanced HIV disease 12% of patients receiving zidovudine had thrombocytopenia with a > 50% decrease from baseline count compared with 5% of those receiving placebo *2163* In 619 patients treatment with 200 mg q8 h 1.1% demonstrated thrombocytopenia *5023* Pancytopenia observed in two patients with rheumatoid arthritis treated with 100 mg daily. Effect observed in one patient after 3 weeks in one patient and 8 weeks in the other *2935* At recommended dose in ACTG 1168/117 and 116A trials of about 500 adult patients caused platelet concentrations of less than 50,000/µL in 4 and 3% patients respectively, and 7% in 281 children *730*
Blood Increase Physiological Observed in some patients with thrombocytopenia induced by AIDS but may be reduced late in the course of zidovudine therapy *6590* In patients with AIDS began to rise within 1 week of start of treatment and rose into normal range within 2 weeks in 6 of 7 patients studied *2801* In patients with HIV disease successful treatment was associated with significantly increased concentration *2163*

Protein *Urine No Effect Physiological* No change observed in proteinuria in a patient with AIDS and proteinuria when treated with 800 mg daily for up to 7 months although serum creatinine significantly reduced *3373*

Reticulocytes *Blood Decrease Physiological* Earliest peripheral blood indicator of drug toxicity in patients with AIDS treated with drug *6317*

Ritonavir *Serum No Effect Physiological* Has no effect on the area under the concentration curve when zidovudine coadministered *1891*

Saquinavir *Serum No Effect Physiological* No effect observed on the area under the concentration curve when zidovudine coadministered *1891* Coadministration of zalcitabine and zidovudine with saquinavir had no effect on the absorptions, metabolisms or excretions of any of the drugs in adults *5024*

Thymidine Kinase *Serum Increase Physiological* Significant increase in patients with AIDS and predictive association with development of bone marrow toxicity described *4580*

Tryptophan *Cerebrospinal Fluid Increase Physiological* In 14 patients with HIV-1 infection median pretreatment concentration 224 ng/mL significantly less than reference interval of 371 - 513 ng/mL increased by median of 40% after 3 - 14 months treatment and 41% after 14 - 30 months treatment *2137*

Plasma Increase Physiological In 14 patients with HIV-1 infection median pretreatment blood tryptophan concentration 6.0 µg/mL at lower limit of reference interval of 6.0 - 11 µg/mL increased by 23% 3 - 14 months treatment and 33% after 14 - 30 months treatment *2137*

Uric Acid *Serum Increase Physiological* At recommended dose in ACTG 1168/117 and 116A trials caused increased uric acid concentration to more than 12 mg/dL in 1 and 1% patients respectively, and to above 3.5 times ULN in less than 1% of 281 children *730*

Zalcitabine *Serum No Effect Analytical* At a concentration of 30 mg/L had less than 0.01% cross-reactivity with solid phase extraction and RIA method of Roberts et al *4990*

Serum No Effect Physiological When single doses of zalcitabine 1.5 mg and zidovudine 200 mg were coadministered to 12 HIV-positive patients no significant pharmacokinetic interaction observed *5023*

Zileuton

Alanine Aminotransferase *Serum Increase Physiological* In placebo-controlled clinical trials the frequency of increased ALT activity more than 3 times the upper limit of normal was 1.9% in drug-treated patients versus 0.2% in placebo treated patients *29*

Digoxin *Serum No Effect Physiological* Drug-drug interactions in healthy individuals have shown no significant interaction *29*

Ethinyl Estradiol *Serum No Effect Physiological* Although ethinyl estradiol is metabolized by the P450 3A4 isoenzyme no significant interaction observed in healthy volunteers *29*

Leukocytes *Blood Decrease Physiological* In placebo-controlled clinical trials the frequency of decreased leukocyte counts below 2800 /µL was 1.0% in 1678 drug treated patients versus 0.6% in placebo treated patients *29*

Naproxen *Serum No Effect Physiological* Drug-drug interactions in healthy individuals have shown no significant interaction *29*

Phenytoin *Serum No Effect Physiological* Drug-drug interactions in healthy individuals have shown no significant interaction *29*

Prednisone *Serum No Effect Physiological* Although prednisone is metabolized by the P450 3A4 isoenzyme no significant interaction observed in healthy volunteers *29*

Propranolol *Serum Increase Physiological* In 16 healthy male volunteers coadministration of zileuton 600 mg every 6 h for 5 d and a single 80 mg dose of propranolol caused a 62% decrease in propranolol clearance and an increase of 52% in propranolol C_{max} and of 104% in the AUC *29*

Prothrombin Time *Plasma Increase Physiological* In 30 healthy male volunteers coadministration of zileuton 600 mg every 6 h and a fixed dose of warfarin caused a 15% decrease in R-warfarin clearance and a significant increase in the prothrombin time *29*

Sulfasalazine *Serum No Effect Physiological* Drug-drug interactions in healthy individuals have shown no significant interaction *29*

Terfenadine *Serum Increase Physiological* In 16 healthy volunteers coadministration of zileuton 600 mg every 6 h for 7 d with 60 mg terfenadine every 12 h caused a 22% decrease in terfenadine clearance and an increase of 35% terfenadine C_{max} and a statistically significant increase in the AUC *29*

Theophylline *Serum Increase Physiological* In 16 healthy volunteers coadministration of zileuton 800 mg every 12 h and theophylline 200 mg every 6 hours for 5 days caused a 50% decrease in steady state clearance of theophyllinewith an approximate doubling of the AUC and an increase of theophylline C_{max} of 73% *29*

Warfarin *Plasma Increase Physiological* In 30 healthy male volunteers coadministration of zileuton 600 mg every 6 h and a fixed dose of warfarin caused a 15% decrease in R-warfarin clearance and an increase of the AUC of 22%. The pharmacokinetics of S-warfarin were not affected *29*

Zimeldine

Alanine Aminotransferase *Serum Increase Physiological* Reported in 2 patients in association with headaches, possibly due to fall in blood concentration of 5-hydroxytryptamine *5694* 7 of 14 patients treated for more than 1 week demonstrated toxic syndrome. ?immunological mechanism or related to high initial dose *3406* In several of 147 patients although 16 had initially high values *6307* In 64% of 21 inpatients with endogenous depression given 225 mg daily for 4 weeks *3419*

Alkaline Phosphatase *Serum Increase Physiological* 7 of 14 patients treated for more than 1 week demonstrated toxic syndrome. ?immunological mechanism or related to high initial dose *3406* In 45% of 21 inpatients with endogenous depression given 225 mg daily for 4 weeks *3419* In several of 147 patients although 16 had initially high values *6307*

Aspartate Aminotransferase *Serum Increase Physiological* 7 of 14 patients treated for more than 1 week demonstrated toxic syndrome. ?immunological mechanism or related to high initial dose *3406* In 64% of 21 inpatients with endogenous depression given 225 mg daily for 4 weeks *3419* Reported in 2 patients in association with headaches, possibly due to fall in blood concentration of 5-hydroxytryptamine *5694* In several of 147 patients although 16 had initially high values *6307*

Bilirubin *Serum No Effect Physiological* In 1 study involving 147 patients no significant change seen *6307*

Cortisol *Plasma No Effect Physiological* In group of depressed patients *846*

Creatinine *Serum Increase Physiological* Observed in 23 of approximately 147 patients *3419*

Erythrocyte Sedimentation Rate

Blood No Effect Physiological In 1 study involving 147 patients no significant change seen *6307*

Erythrocytes *Blood No Effect Physiological* In 1 study involving 147 patients no significant change seen *6307*

Urine Increase Physiological 3 of 14 patients treated for more than 1 week presented mild abnormality *3406*

γ-Glutamyltransferase *Serum Increase Physiological* Reported in 2 patients in association with headaches, possibly due to fall in blood concentration of 5-hydroxytryptamine *5694*

Homovanillic Acid

Cerebrospinal Fluid Increase Physiological Insignificant effect in 43 chronically treated patients with depression or Alzheimer's disease *4965*

5-Hydroxyindoleacetic Acid

Cerebrospinal Fluid Decrease Physiological Significant effect in 43 chronically treated patients with depression or Alzheimer's disease *4965*

Leukocytes *Blood Decrease Physiological* 7 of 14 patients treated for more than 1 week demonstrated toxic syndrome. ?immunological mechanism or related to high initial dose *3406*

Blood No Effect Physiological In 1 study involving 147 patients no significant change seen *6307*

Luteinizing Hormone *Plasma No Effect Physiological* In group of depressed patients *846*

Platelets *Blood Decrease Physiological* 7 of 14 patients treated for more than 1 week demonstrated toxic syndrome. ?immunological mechanism or related to high initial dose *3406*

Blood No Effect Physiological In 1 study involving 147 patients no significant change seen *6307*

Prolactin *Plasma Increase Physiological* Response only after chronic pretreatment in group of depressed patients *846*

Protein *Urine Increase Physiological* 3 of 14 patients treated for more than 1 week preserved mild abnormality *3406*

Zinc Sulfate

Norfloxacin *Urine Decrease Physiological* When zinc sulfate coingested with 400 mg norfloxacin urinary excretion reduced by 56% over next 24 hours due to interference with absorption *865*

Potassium *Serum No Effect Analytical* Negligible effect at a concentration of 20 μmol/L on spectrophotometric enzymatic method of Berry et al *523*

Sodium *Serum No Effect Analytical* Negligible effect at a concentration of 20 μmol/L on spectrophotometric enzymatic method of Berry et al *523*

Zirconium Salts

γ-Globulin *Serum Increase Physiological* Observed with zirconium granulomas *4508*

Zolmitriptan

Alanine Aminotransferase *Serum Increase Physiological* Administration of zolmitriptan reported to cause infrequent abnormalities of liver function tests *6653*

Alkaline Phosphatase *Serum Increase Physiological* Administration of zolmitriptan reported to cause infrequent abnormalities of liver function tests *6653*

Amylase *Serum Increase Physiological* Administration of zolmitriptan reported to cause pancreatitis rarely *6653*

Aspartate Aminotransferase *Serum Increase Physiological* Administration of zolmitriptan reported to cause infrequent abnormalities of liver function tests *6653*

Bilirubin *Serum Increase Physiological* Administration of zolmitriptan reported to cause infrequent abnormalities of liver function tests *6653*

Eosinophils *Blood Increase Physiological* Administration of zolmitriptan reported to cause rare eosinophilia *6653*

Glucose *Serum Increase Physiological* Administration of zolmitriptan reported to cause rare hyperglycemia *6653*

Leukocytes *Blood Decrease Physiological* Administration of zolmitriptan reported to cause rare leukopenia *6653*

Lipase *Serum Increase Physiological* Administration of zolmitriptan reported to cause pancreatitis rarely *6653*

Occult Blood *Feces Increase Physiological* Administration of zolmitriptan reported to cause gastritis, hematemesis and melena rarely *6653*

Platelets *Blood Decrease Physiological* Administration of zolmitriptan reported to cause rare thrombocytopenia *6653*

Zolodex

Prostate-specific Antigen *Serum No Effect Analytical* Zolodex at a concentration of up to 7.2 μg/mL caused less than 0.1% cross-reactivity with method on PSA method on Bayer Technicon Immuno 1® *430*

Zolpidem

Alanine Aminotransferase *Serum Increase Physiological* Infrequent increased activity observed with treatment *2062*

Alkaline Phosphatase *Serum Increase Physiological* Rarely increased activity observed with treatment *2062*

Aspartate Aminotransferase *Serum Increase Physiological* Rarely increased activity observed with treatment *2062*

Bilirubin *Serum Increase Physiological* Rarely increased concentration observed with treatment *2062*

Cholesterol *Serum Increase Physiological* Rarely increased concentration observed with treatment *2062*

Digoxin *Serum No Effect Physiological* Coadministration of zolpidem with digoxin had no effect on digoxin kinetics *2062*

Drugs of Abuse Screen *Urine No Effect Analytical* No cross-reactivity observed or its metabolites with Syva EMIT II and Abbott AD urine drug screen procedures up to 24 hours after ingestion of zolpidem *4699* Following ingestion of 10 mg and testing by Syva EMIT II and Abbott ADx over 24 hours no significant effect observed on methods *4698*

Erythrocyte Sedimentation Rate *Blood Increase Physiological* Rare increase observed with treatment *2062*

Glucose *Serum Increase Physiological* Infrequently increased concentration observed with treatment *2062*

Hematocrit *Blood Decrease Physiological* Rare anemia observed with treatment *2062*

Hemoglobin *Blood Decrease Physiological* Rare anemia observed with treatment *2062*

Imipramine *Serum Decrease Physiological* Coadministration of zolpidem with imipramine caused a 20% decrease in the maximum concentration of imipramine *2062*

Leukocytes *Blood Decrease Physiological* Rare anemia observed with treatment *2062*

Occult Blood *Feces Increase Physiological* Rare gastritis, hemorrhoids or rectal hemorrhage observed with treatment *2062*

Prothrombin Time *Plasma No Effect Physiological* Coadministration of zolpidem with warfarin had no effect on the plasma prothrombin time *2062*

Urea Nitrogen *Serum Increase Physiological* Rarely increased concentration observed with treatment *2062*

Uric Acid *Serum Increase Physiological* Rarely increased concentration observed with treatment *2062*

Zomepirac

Cannabinoids *Urine No Effect Analytical* No effect on Roche Abuscreen method *5006*

Coombs' Test, Direct *Blood Positive Physiological* Case reported of immune hemolysis *5381*

Hemoglobin *Blood Decrease Physiological* Case reported of immune hemolysis *5381*

Zonisamide

immunoglobulin A *Serum No Effect Physiological* No significant effect observed in 19 patients with refractory epilepsy receiving multiple antiepileptic drugs given mean dose of 389 mg daily for mean of 863 days *1983*

Immunoglobulin G *Serum No Effect Physiological* No effect observed in 19 patients with refractory epilepsy receiving multiple antiepileptic drugs treated with mean dose of 389 mg daily for mean of 863 days *1983*

Immunoglobulin M *Serum No Effect Physiological* No significant effect observed in 19 patients with refractory epilepsy receiving multiple antiepileptic drugs treated with mean dose of 389 mg daily for mean duration of 863 days *1983*

Phenytoin *Serum No Effect Physiological* No significant effect on phenytoin concentration observed when zonisamide coadministered with phenytoin *5952*

Valproic Acid *Serum No Effect Physiological* No significant effect on valproic acid concentration observed when zonisamide coadministered with sodium valproate *5952*

Zopiclone

Cortisol, Free *Urine No Effect Analytical* No significant interference observed with HPLC method of Turpeinen et al *6105*

p-Aminophenol *Urine No Effect Analytical* With addition of drugs at a concentration of 100 mg/L and of related compounds at 50 mg/L no significant effect observed on colorimetric method of van Bocxlaer on Cobas Mira analyzer which involves reacting free p-aminophenol with resorcinol in the presence of magnesium ions to form an indophenol dye measured at 550 nm *6163*

Zotepine

Prolactin *Plasma Increase Physiological* In 24 schizophrenic inpatients treatment with up to 200 mg/d for 4 weeks caused significant from mean baseline of 10.0 ± 8.2 ng/mL to 21.6 ± 17.5 ng/mL with progressive increases observed after each of the four weeks. Significant correlation with zotepine concentration observed *4459*

Zoxazolamine

Alanine Aminotransferase *Serum Increase Physiological* May produce viral-hepatitis like syndrome *3171*

Aspartate Aminotransferase *Serum Increase Physiological* May produce viral-hepatitis like syndrome *3171*

Bilirubin *Serum Increase Physiological* May produce viral-hepatitis like syndrome *3171*

Protein *Urine Increase Physiological* May have nephrotoxic effect *2451*

Zuclopenthixol

Peptides, Low-molecular Weight
Urine Decrease Physiological In one schizophrenic patient treatment with depot 400 mg every 14 days over 5 weeks caused significant reduction from 57.6 µmol/d to 18.6 µmol/d *4901*

4 REFERENCES

1 Aadland E, Odegaard OR, Roseth A et al. Free protein S deficiency in patients with Crohn's disease. *Scand J Gastroenterol*, 29, 333-335 (1994)

2 Aanderud S, Myking OL, Strandjord RE. The influence of carbamazepine on thyroid hormones and thyroxine binding globulin in hypothyroid patients substituted with thyroxine. *Clin Endocrinol*, 15, 247-252 (1981)

3 Aarts EM. D-glucaric acid excretion as a test for hepatic enzyme induction. *Lancet*, 1, 859 (1971)

4 Aarts EM. Drug-induced stimulation of the glucuronic acid system. *PhD Thesis, Nijmegen, The Netherlands* (1968)

5 Aaser E, Gullestad L, Tollofsrud S, et al. Effect of bolus injection versus continuous infusion of furosemide on diuresis and neurohormonal activation in patients with severe congestive heart failure. *Scand J Clin Lab Invest*, 57, 361-368 (1997)

6 Abassi ZA, Klein H, Golomb E et al. Urinary endothelin: a possible biological marker of renal damage. *Am J Hypertens*, 6, 1046-1054 (1993)

7 Abbey M, Clifton P, Kessin M et al. Effect of fish oil on lipoproteins, lecithin:cholesterol acyltransferase, and lipid transfer protein activity in humans. *Arterioscler Thromb*, 10, 85-94 (1990)

8 Abbiati G, Arrigoni M, Frignani S et al. Effect of salmon calcitonin on deoxypyridinoline (Dpyr) urinary excretion in healthy volunteers. *Calcif Tissue Int*, 55, 346-348 (1994)

9 Abboix M, Frati ME, Laporte J-R. The potentiation of acenocoumarol anticoagulant effect by amiodarone. *Br J Clin Pharmacol*, 18, 355-360 (1984)

10 Abbott Laboratories. Manufacturer's literature on Abbokinase® . North Chicago, IL 60064 (1994)

11 Abbott Laboratories. Manufacturer's literature on Biaxin® . North Chicago, IL 60064 (1996)

12 Abbott Laboratories. Manufacturer's literature on Calcijex® . North Chicago, IL 60064 (1995)

13 Abbott Laboratories. Manufacturer's literature on Cartrol® . North Chicago, IL 60064 (1997)

14 Abbott Laboratories. Manufacturer's literature on Cylert® . North Chicago, IL 60064 (1996)

15 Abbott Laboratories. Manufacturer's literature on Depacon™. North Chicago, IL 60064 (1997)

16 Abbott Laboratories. Manufacturer's literature on Depakene® . North Chicago, IL 60064 (1997)

17 Abbott Laboratories. Manufacturer's literature on Depakote® . North Chicago, IL 60064 (1996)

18 Abbott Laboratories. Manufacturer's literature on Desoxyn® . North Chicago, IL 60064 (1997)

19 Abbott Laboratories. Manufacturer's literature on Enduron® . North Chicago, IL 60064 (1997)

20 Abbott Laboratories. Manufacturer's literature on Ery-Tab® . North Chicago, IL 60064 (1997)

21 Abbott Laboratories. Manufacturer's literature on Hytrin® . North Chicago, IL 60064 (1995)

22 Abbott Laboratories. Manufacturer's literature on Nembutal® . North Chicago, IL 60064 (1992)

23 Abbott Laboratories. Manufacturer's literature on Norvir™. North Chicago, IL60064 (1996)

24 Abbott Laboratories. Manufacturer's literature on Oretic® . North Chicago, IL 60064 (1997)

25 Abbott Laboratories. Manufacturer's literature on Phenurone® . North Chicago, IL 60064 (1997)

26 Abbott Laboratories. Manufacturer's literature on Placidyl® . North Chicago, IL 60064 (1997)

27 Abbott Laboratories. Manufacturer's literature on Prosom™. North Chicago, IL 60064 (1997)

28 Abbott Laboratories. Manufacturer's literature on Tranxene® . North Chicago, IL 60064 (1997)

29 Abbott Laboratories. Manufacturer's literature on Zyflo™. North Chicago, IL (1996)

30 Abbruzzese A, Swanson J. Jaundice after therapy with chlordiazepoxide hydrochloride. *N Engl J Med*, 273, 321 (1965)

31 Abdalla HI, Hart DM, Beastall GH. Reduced serum free thyroxine concentration in postmenopausal women receiving oestrogen treatment. *Br Med J*, 288, 754-755 (1984)

32 Abe A, Yamashita S, Noma A. Sensitive, direct colorimetric assay for copper in serum. *Clin Chem*, 35, 552-554 (1989)

33 Abelson JL, Glitz D, Cameron OG et al. Endocrine, cardiovascular, and behavioral response to clonidine in patients with panic disorder. *Biol Psychiat*, 32, 8-25 (1992)

34 Abernethy DR, Divoll M, Ochs R et al. Increased metabolic clearance of acetaminophen with oral contraceptive use. *Obstet Gynecol*, 60, 338-341 (1982)

35 Abernethy DR, Greenblatt DJ, Divoll M et al. Impairment of diazepam metabolism by low-dose estrogen-containing oral contraceptive steroids. *N Engl J Med*, 306, 791-792 (1982)

36 Abernethy DR, Greenblatt DJ, Steel K et al. Impairment of hepatic drug oxidation by propoxyphene. *Ann Intern Med*, 97, 223-224 (1982)

37 Abraham AS, Meshulam Z, Rosenmann D et al. Influence of chronic diuretic therapy on serum, lymphocyte and erythrocyte potassium, magnesium and calcium concentrations. *Cardiology*, 75, 17-23 (1988)

38 Abraham GE, Samojlik E, Kyle FW et al. Radioimmunoassay of plasma 16α-hydroxyprogesterone. *Anal Lett*, 6, 675 (1973)

39 Abreo K, Labarre J. Suprofen, acute renal failure, and hematuria. *Ann Intern Med*, 105, 799 (1986)

40 Acien P, Shaw RW, Irvine L et al. CA 125 levels in endometriosis patients before, during and after treatment with danazol or LHRH agonists. *Eur J Obstet Gynecol Reprod Biol*, 32, 241-246 (1989)

41 Ackermann H, Steva E, Blackwood J et al. A dry chemistry multilayer immunoassay test for valproic acid. *Clin Chem*, 36, 1038 (1990)

42 Acland JD. The interpretation of the serum protein bound iodine: a review. *J Clin Pathol*, 24, 187 (1971)

43 Acocella G, Billing BH. Effect of drugs on the hepatic transport of bilirubin. In. *Therapeutic Agents and the Liver. N McIntyre, S Sherlock, eds*, Oxford, Blackwell (1965)

44 Acocella G, Conti R. Interaction of rifampicin with other drugs. *Tubercle*, 61, 171-177 (1980)

45 Adam K, Oswald I, Shapiro C. Effects of loprazolam and triazolam on sleep and overnight urinary cortisol. *Psychopharmacology*, 82, 389-394 (1984)

46 Adams EC. Differentiation of myoglobin and hemoglobin in biological fluids. *Ann Clin Lab Sci*, 1, 208 (1971)

47 Adams JS, Diz MM, Sharma OP. Effective reduction in the serum 1,25-dihydroxyvitamin D and calcium concentration in sarcoidosis-associated hypercalcemia with short-course chloroquine therapy. *Ann Intern Med*, 111, 437-438 (1989)

48 Adams JS, Sharma OP, Diz MM et al. Ketoconazole decreases the serum 1,25-dihydroxyvitamin D and calcium concentration in sarcoidosis-associated hypercalcemia. *J Clin Endocrinol Metab*, 70, 1090-1095 (1990)

49 Adams LJ, Antonow DR, McClain CJ et al. Effect of ranitidine on bioavailability of nifedipine. *Gastroenterology*, 90, 1320 (1986)

50 Adams PW, Godsland I, Melrose J et al. The influence of oral contraceptive formulation on carbohydrate and lipid metabolism. *J Pharmacother*, 3, 54-63 (1980)

51 Adams RG, Harrison JF, Scott P. The development of cadmium induced proteinuria, impaired renal function and osteomalacia. *Q J Med*, 38, 425 (1969)

52 Adamus WS, Heuer H, Meade CJ et al. Safety, tolerability, and pharmacologic activity of multiple doses of the new platelet activating factor antagonist WEB 2086 in human subjects. *Clin Pharmacol Ther*, 45, 270-276 (1989)

53 Adebayo GI, Coker HAB, Fagbure F. Renal effects of nifedipine in healthy normotensive volunteers. Effects of dose, formulation, duration of treatment, and chlorothiazide coadministration. *Fundam Clin Pharmacol*, 2, 541-549 (1988)

54 Adlercreutz H. Drug interference in urinary estrogen determination. *Proc V International Symposium on Quality Control in Clinical Chemistry*, Geneva, Switzerland (1973)

55 Adlercreutz H. Drug interference in urinary steroid hormone assay. *First European Congress of Clinical Chemistry*, Munich (1974)

56 Adlercreutz H, Soininen K, Harkonen M. Oral contraceptives and serum amylase. *Br Med J*, 3, 529 (1972)

57 Adnitt PI. Hypoglycemic action of monoamine oxidase inhibitors (MAOI's). *Diabetes*, 17, 628 (1968)

58 Adrouny A, Meguerditchian S, Koo CH et al. Agranulocytosis related to vancomycin therapy. *Am J Med*, 81, 1059-1061 (1986)

59 Adu D, Turney J, Michael J et al. Hyperkalaemia in cyclosporin treated renal allograft recipients. *Lancet*, 2, 370-372 (1983)

60 Adverse Drug Reactions Advisory Committee. Mianserin: a possible cause of neutropenia and agranulocytosis. *Med J Aust*, 2, 673-674 (1980)

61 Affarah HB, Mars RL, Someren A et al. Myoglobinuria and acute renal failure associated with intravenous vasopressin infusion. *South Med J*, 77, 918-921 (1984)

62 Aggeler PM, O'Reilly RA, Leong L. Potentiation of anticoagulant effect of warfarin by phenylbutazone. *N Engl J Med*, 276, 496 (1967)

63 Agnelli G, Del Favero A, Parise P et al. Cephalosporins-induced hypoprothrombinemia: is the N-methyl-thiotetrazole side chain the culprit?. *Antimicrob Agent Chemother*, 29, 1108-1109 (1986)

64 Agnelli G, Piovella F, Buoncristiani P, et al. Enoxaprin plus compression stockings compared with compression stockings alone in the prevention of venous thromboembolism after elective neurosurgery. *N Engl J Med*, 339, 80-85 (1998)

65 Agostini L, Down PF, Murison J et al. Faecal ammonia and pH during lactulose administration in man. *Gut*, 13, 859 (1972)

66 Agouron Pharmaceuticals, Inc. Manufacturer's literature on Viracept. La Jolla, CA (1997)

67 Agus ZS, Goldberg M. Renal mechanisms of the natriuretic and antiphosphaturic effects of triflocin - a new diuretic. *J Lab Clin Med*, 76, 280 (1970)

68 AH Robins. Manufacturer's literature on Dopram® . AH Robins, Richmond VA

69 Ahearn MJ, Hicks JE, Andriole VT. Neutropenia during high dose intravenous oxacillin therapy. *Yale J Biol Med*, 49, 351-360 (1976)

70 Aherne GW, Piall E, Marks V et al. Prolongation and enhancement of methotrexate concentrations by probenecid. *Br Med J*, 1, 1097-1099 (1978)

71 Ahmad S. Nifedipine-phenytoin interaction. *J Am Coll Cardiol*, 2, 1581-1582 (1984)

72 Ahmed AR, Moy R. Azathioprine. *Int J Dermatol*, 20, 461-467 (1981)

73 Aitio ML. The effect of enzyme induction on the metabolism of disopyramide in man. *Br J Clin Pharmacol*, 11, 279 (1981)

74 Aitken JM, Hart DM, Smith DA. The effect of long-term mestranol administration on calcium and phosphorus homeostasis in oophorectomized women. *Clin Sci*, 41, 233 (1971)

75 Aitken RG, Northall H, York GA. High serum concentrations of paraquat increase apparent creatinine concentrations. *Ann Clin Biochem*, 31, 198-199 (1994)

76 Aitken RG, Robinson CS. The effect of lithium on thyroid function. *Proc ACB Natl Meet*, 52 (1989)

77 Aizawa T, Suzuki S, Asawa T et al. Dipyridamole reduces urinary albumin excretion in diabetic patients with normo- or microalbuminuria. *Clin Nephrol*, 33, 130-135 (1990)

78 Ajdukiewicz AB, Grainger J, Scheuer PJ et al. Jaundice due to iprindole. *Gut*, 12, 705 (1971)

79 Ajel LA. Positive diphenhydramine interference in the Emit-d.a.u. assay. *Clin Chem*, 31, 340-341 (1985)

80 Akalin S. Effects of ketoconazole in hirsute women. *Acta Endocrinol*, 124, 19-22 (1991)

81 Akpolat T, Ozdemir O, Arik N et al. Effect of desmopressin (DDAVP) on protein C and protein C inhibitors in uremia. *Nephron*, 64, 232-234 (1993)

82 Alappan R, Perazella MA, Buller GK. Hyperkalemia in hospitalized patients treated with trimethoprim-sulfamethoazole. *Ann Intern Med*, 124, 316-320 (1996)

83 Alarcon-Segovia D, Fishbein E, Alcala H. Isoniazid acetylation rate and development of antinuclear antibodies upon isoniazid treatment. *Arth Rheum*, 14, 748 (1971)

84 Alarcon-Segovia D, Wakim KG, Worthington JW et al. Clinical and experimental studies on the hydralazine syndrome. *Medicine*, 46, 1 (1967)

85 Alaupovic P, Hodis HN, Knight-Gibson C et al. Effects of lovastatin on ApoA- and ApoB-containing lipoproteins: families in a subpopulation of patients participating in the monitored atherosclerosis regression study (MARS). *Arterioscler Thromb*, 14, 1906-1914 (1994)

86 Albani F, Riva R, Perucca E et al. Interference of valproic acid in the colorimetric determination of free fatty acids in plasma. *Clin Chem*, 28, 1398 (1982)

87 Albani F, Theodore WH, Washington P et al. Effect of felbamate on plasma levels of carbamazepine and its metabolites. *Epilepsia*, 32, 130-132 (1991)

88 Albano JDM, Campbell SK, Farrer A et al. Gender differences in urinary kallikrein excretion in man: variation throughout the menstrual cycle. *Clin Sci*, 86, 227-231 (1994)

89 Albayrak D, Islek I, Kalayci AG, et al. Acute immune thrombocytopenic purpura: a comparative study of very high oral doses of methylprednisolone and intravenously administered immune globulin. *J Pediatr*, 125, 1004-1007 (1994)

90 Albers JJ, Grundy SM, Cleary PA et al. National cooperative gallstone study: the effect of chenodeoxycholic acid on lipoproteins and apolipoproteins. *Gastroenterology*, 82, 638-646 (1982)

91 Albers JJ, Taggart HM, Appelbaum-Bowden D et al. Reduction of lecithin cholesterol acyltransferase, apolipoprotein D and the Lp(a) lipoprotein with the anabolic steroid stanozolol. *Biochim Biophys Acta*, 795, 293-296 (1984)

92 Albert M, Stansell MJ. Vascular symptomatic relief during administration of ethylchlorophenoxyisobutyrate, clofibrate. *Metabolism*, 18, 635 (1969)

93 AL-Damluji S, Meek JH. Interference of a propranolol metabolite with serum bilirubin estimation in chronic renal failure. *Br Med J*, 2, 1414 (1980)

94 Alen M, Rahkila P, Reinila M et al. Androgenic-anabolic steroid effects on serum thyroid, pituitary and steroid hormones in athletes. *Am J Sports Med*, 15, 357-361 (1987)

95 Alestig K, Eilard T, Norrby R et al. Ceftazidime in clinical practice. *J Antimicrob Chemother*, 12, Suppl A, 111-114 (1983)

96 Alestig K, Trollfors B, Andersson R et al. Ceftazidine and renal function. *J Antimicrob Chemother*, 13, 177-181 (1984)

97 Alexander DP, Russo ME, Fohrman DE et al. Nafcillin-induced platelet dysfunction and bleeding. *Antimicrob Agent Chemother*, 23, 59-62 (1983)

98 Alexander MR, Louie SG, Guernsey BG. Isoniazid-associated hepatitis. *Clin Pharm*, 1, 148-153 (1982)

99 Alexieva-Figusch J, Blankenstein MA, Hop WCJ et al. Treatment of metastatic breast cancer patients with different doses of megesterol acetate: dose relations, metabolic and endocrine effects. *Eur J Cancer Clin Oncol*, 20, 33-40 (1981)

100 Al'Halawani MH, Larsen JL, Miller S, et al. Pravastatin reduces serum cholesterol and low density lipoprotein concentrations following pancreas transplantation. *Transplantation*, 58, 1204-1209 (1994)

101 Al-Hassan MI, Bawazir SA, Al-Khamis KI et al. The interaction potential of vigabatrin with phenytoin and carbamazepine. *Int J Pharmaceutics*, 93, 7-12 (1993)

102 AL-Hujaj M, Schonthal H. Hyperuricemia and levodopa. *N Engl J Med*, 285, 859 (1971)

103 Allain CC, Poon LS, Chan CSG et al. Enzymatic determination of total serum cholesterol. *Clin Chem*, 20, 470 (1974)

104 Allain P, Mauras Y, Krari N et al. Plasma and urine aluminium concentration in healthy subjects after administration of sucralfate. *Br J Clin Pharmacol*, 29, 391-395 (1990)

105 Allanby KD, Trounce JR. Excretion of mecamylamine after intravenous and oral administration. *Br Med J*, 2, 1219-1221 (1957)

106 Allegra A, Corica F, Ientile R, et al. Plasma (total and ionized), erythrocyte and platelet magnesium levels in renal transplant recipients during cyclosporine and/or azathioprine treatment. *Magnesium Res*, 11, 11-18 (1998)

107 Allegra CJ, Chabner BA, Tuazon CU et al. Trimetrexate for the treatment of pneumocystis carinii pneumonia in patients with the acquired immunodeficiency syndrome. *N Engl J Med*, 317, 978-985 (1987)

108 Allen JK, Fraser IS. Cholesterol, high density lipoprotein and danazol. *J Clin Endocrinol Metab*, 53, 149-152 (1981)

109 Allen LC, Kadljevic L, Romaschin AD. An enzymatic method for oxalate automated with the Cobas Fara centrifugal analyzer. *Clin Chem*, 35, 2098-2100 (1989)

110 Allen LC, Michalko K, Coons C. More on cephalosporin interference with creatinine determinations. *Clin Chem*, 28, 555-556 (1982)

111 Allergan, Inc. Manufacturer's literature on Gris-PEG® . Irvine, CA 92623 (1995)

112 Allison SP, Chamberlain MJ, Miller JE et al. Effects of propranolol on blood sugar, insulin and free fatty acids. *Diabetologia*, 5, 339 (1969)

113 Allolio B, Dorr H, Stuttman R et al. Effect of a single bolus of etomidate upon 8 major corticosteroid hormones and plasma ACTH. *Clin Endocrinol*, 22, 281-286 (1985)

114 Allon M, Pasque CB, Rodriguez M. Acute effects of captopril and ibuprofen on proteinuria in patients with nephrosis. *J Lab Clin Med*, 116, 462-468 (1990)

115 Almen T. A steering device for selective angiography and some vascular and enzymatic reactions observed. *Acta Radiol*, Suppl 260, 1 (1966)

116 Almen T. Toxicity of radio contrast agents. *International Encyclopedia of Pharmacology and Therapeutics*, New York, Pergamon Press, 2, 19 (1971)

117 Almond PS, Gillingham KJ, Sibley R et al. Renal transplant function after ten years of cyclosporine. *Transplantation*, 53, 316-323 (1992)

118 Al-Nahhas AM, Nimmon CC, Britton KE et al. The effect of ramipril. A new angiotensin-converting enzyme inhibitor on cortical nephron flow and effective renal plasma flow in patients with essential hypertension. *Nephron*, 54, 47-52 (1990)

119 Aloia JF, Vaswani A, Yeh JK et al. Biochemical short-term changes produced by hormonal replacement therapy. *J Endocrinol Invest*, 14, 927-934 (1991)

120 Alora BD, Estrada FA, Lansang SL. Parenteral sodium epicillin in acute infections. *Curr Ther Res*, 14, 358 (1972)

121 Al-Refaie FN, De Silva CE, Wonke B et al. Changes in transferrin saturation after treatment with the oral iron chelator deferiprone in patients with iron overload. *J Clin Pathol*, 48, 110-114 (1995)

122 Altamirano A, Bondani A. Adverse reactions to furazolidone and other drugs: a comparative review. *Scand J Gastroenterol*, 24, Suppl 169, 70-80 (1989)

123 Altemus M, Swedo SE, Leonard HL et al. Changes in cerebrospinal fluid neurochemistry during treatment of obsessive-compulsive disorder with clomipramine. *Arch Gen Psychiat*, 51, 794-803 (1994)

124 Altmeyer P, Buhles N, Holzel C et al. Influence of topical corticosteroids on hormones in urine and plasma. *Arz Forsch Drug Res*, 36, 993-996 (1986)

125 Alvarsson M, Grill V. Impact of nicotinic acid treatment on insulin secretion and insulin sensitivity in low and high insulin responders. *Scand J Clin Lab Invest*, 56, 563-570 (1996)

126 Alvir JMJ, Lieberman JA, Safferman AZ et al. Clozapine-induced agranulocytosis: incidence and risk factors in the United States. *N Engl J Med*, 329, 162-167 (1993)

127 Alza Pharmaceuticals. Manufacturer's literature on Ethyol® . Palo Alto, CA 94303 (1996)

128 AMA Council on Drugs. *AMA Drug Evaluations*, Chicago IL, American Medical Association (1973)

129 AMA Council on Drugs. *New Drugs*, Chicago IL, American Medical Association (1967)

130 AMA Council on Drugs. A copper-chelating agent: penicillamine (cuprimine®). *J Am Med Ass*, 189, 847 (1964)

131 AMA Council on Drugs. A new antibiotic - lincomycin. *J Am Med Ass*, 194, 545 (1965)

132 AMA Council on Drugs. Registry on adverse reactions. Chicago IL, American Medical Association (1964)

133 AMA Council on Drugs. Registry on adverse reactions, tabulation of reports - panel on hematology. Chicago IL, American Medical Association (1964)

134 Amador E. Automated urinary glucose analyses. *Am J Clin Pathol*, 59, 735 (1973)

135 Amador E, Wacker WEC. Enzymes in genitourinary disease. In. *Diagnostic Enzymology. EL Coodley (ed)*, Philadelphia PA, Lea and Febiger (1970)

136 Ambre JJ, Fischer LJ. Effect of coadministration of aluminum and magnesium hydroxides on absorption of anticoagulants in man. *Clin Pharmacol Ther*, 14, 231-237 (1973)

137 Ambrosi B, Bochicchio D, Riva E et al. Effects of sodium valproate administration on plasma ACTH levels in patients with ACTH hypersecretion. *J Endocrinol Invest*, 6, 305-306 (1983)

138 Amdisen A, Andersen CJ. Lithium treatment and thyroid function. a survey of 237 patients in long-term lithium treatment. *Pharmacopsychiatry*, 15, 149-155 (1982)

139 American Hospital Formulary Service. American hospital formulary service. Washington DC, American Society of Hospital Pharmacists

140 Amery A, Conway J. A critical review of diagnostic tests for pheochromocytoma. *Am Heart J*, 73, 129 (1967)

141 Ames RP. The effect of antihypertensive drugs on serum lipids and lipoproteins. i Diuretics. *Drugs*, 32, 260-278 (1986)

142 Ames RP. The effects of antihypertensive drugs on serum lipids and lipoproteins. II Nondiuretic drugs. *Drugs*, 32, 335-357 (1986)

143 Ames RP. The influence of nonβ-blocking drugs on the lipid profile: are diuretics outclassed as initial therapy for hypertension?. *Am Heart J*, 114, 998-1006 (1987)

144 Ames RP, Kiyasu JY. Alpha$_1$- adrenoreceptor blockade with doxazosin in hypertension: effects on blood pressure and lipoproteins. *J Clin Pharmacol*, 28, 123-127 (1989)

145 Ames RP, Peacock PB. Serum cholesterol during treatment of hypertension with diuretic drugs. *Arch Intern Med*, 144, 710-714 (1984)

146 Amgen Inc. Manufacturer's literature on Epogen® . Thousand Oaks, CA 91320 (1994)

147 Amgen Inc. Manufacturer's literature on Neupogen. Thousand Oaks, CA (1995)

148 Ammann H, Vinet B. Accuracy, precision, and interferences of three modified EMIT procedures for determining serum phenobarbital, urine morphine, and urine cocaine metabolites with a Cobas-Fara. *Clin Chem*, 37, 2139-2141 (1991)

149 Amsterdam JD, Maislin G. Effect of erythromycin on tricyclic antidepressant metabolism. *J Clin Psychopharmacol*, 11, 203-206 (1991)

150 Amsterdam JD, Maislin G, Skolnick B et al. Multiple hormone responses to clonidine administration in depressed patients and volunteers. *Biol Psychiat*, 26, 265-278 (1989)

151 Anast CS. The unreliability of the titan yellow method for the determination of magnesium. *Clin Chem*, 9, 544 (1963)

152 Anastasiou-Nanam, Koutras DA, Levis G et al. The correlation of serum amiodarone levels with abnormalities in the metabolism of thyroxine. *J Endocrinol Invest*, 7, 405-407 (1984)

153 Anastassiades E, Lane DA, Ireland H et al. A low molecular weight heparin ('fragmin') for routine hemodialysis; a crossover trial comparing three dose regimens with a standard regimen of commercial unfractionated heparin. *Clin Nephrol*, 32, 290-296 (1989)

154 Anastassiadis PA, Common RH. Some aspects of the reliability of chemical analyses. *Anal Biochem*, 22, 409 (1968)

155 Ancill RJ. Ulcerogenic action of azapropazone. *Br Med J*, 1, 1469-1470 (1977)

156 Andersen AN, Schioler V, Hertz J et al. Effect of metoclopramide induced hyperprolactinaemia on the gonadotrophic response to oestradiol and LRH. *Acta Endocrinol*, 100, 1-9 (1982)

157 Andersen P, Smith P, Seljeflot I et al. Effects of gemfibrozil on lipids and haemostasis after myocardial infarction. *Thromb Haemostas*, 63, 174-177 (1990)

158 Andersen PH, Richelsen B, Bak J et al. Influence of short-term dexfenfluramine therapy on glucose and lipid metabolism in obese non-diabetic patients. *Acta Endocrinol*, 128, 251-258 (1993)

159 Anderson BN, Henrikson IR. Jaundice and eosinophilia associated with amitriptyline. *J Clin Psychiat*, 39, 730-731 (1978)

160 Anderson CJ, Kaufman PL, Sturm RJ et al. Toxicity of combined therapy with carbonic anhydrase inhibitors and aspirin. *Am J Ophthalmol*, 86, 516-519 (1978)

161 Anderson D, Cremase M, Forte E et al. False negative results for benzoylecgonine in urine using GC/MS analysis due to fluconazole. *Clin Chem*, 39, 1233-1234 (1993)

162 Anderson G, Colletti A, Dino J et al. Evaluation of a methamphetamine screening kit. *Clin Chem*, 37, 999 (1991)

163 Anderson MS, Bowers CY, Kastin AJ et al. Synthetic thyrotropin-releasing hormone: a potent stimulator of thyrotropin secretion in man. *N Engl J Med*, 285, 1279 (1971)

164 Anderson OO, Persson I. Carbohydrate metabolism during treatment with chlorthalidone and ethacrynic acid. *Br Med J*, 2, 798 (1968)

165 Andersson B, Zimmermann ME, Hedner T et al. Haemodynamic, metabolic and endocrine effects of short-term dexfenfluramine treatment in young, obese women. *Eur J Clin Pharmacol* (1991)

166 Andersson DEH, Rojdmark S. Blood glucose lowering effect of verapamil in fasted man. *Horm Metab Res*, 16, Suppl 1, 160-163 (1984)

167 Andersson OK, Gubrandsson T, Jamerson K. Metabolic adverse effects of thiazide diuretics: the importance of normokalemia. *J Intern Med*, 229, Suppl 2, 89-96 (1991)

168 Andersson S, Carlson LA, Oro L et al. Effect of nicotinic acid on gastric secretion of acid in human subjects and in dogs. *Scand J Gastroenterol*, 6, 693 (1971)

169 Andersson T. Omeprazole drug interaction studies. *Clin Pharmacokinet*, 21, 195-212 (1991)

170 Andersson T, Andren K, Cederberg C et al. Effect of omeprazole and cimetidine on plasma diazepam levels. *Eur J Clin Pharmacol*, 39, 51-54 (1990)

171 Andersson T, Cederberg C, Edvardsson G et al. Effect of omeprazole treatment on diazepam plasma levels in slow versus normal rapid metabolizers of omeprazole. *Clin Pharmacol Ther*, 47, 79-85 (1990)

172 Andersson T, Lagerstrom PO, Unge P. A study of the interaction between omeprazole and phenytoin in epileptic patients. *Ther Drug Monit*, 12, 329-333 (1990)

173 Andersson T, Lundborg P, Regardh CG. Lack of effect of omeprazole treatment on steady-state plasma levels of metoprolol. *Eur J Clin Pharmacol*, 40, 61-65 (1991)

174 Anderton JL, Kincaid-Smith P. Diuretics: II clinical considerations. *Drugs*, 1, 141 (1971)

175 Andre E, Voisin P, Andre JL, et al. Hemorheological and hemostatic parameters in children with nephrotic syndrome undergoing steroid therapy. *Nephron*, 68, 184-191 (1994)

176 Andrejak M, Hary L, Andrejak M-TH et al. Diltiazem increases steady state digoxin serum levels in patients with cardiac disease. *J Clin Pharmacol*, 27, 967-970 (1987)

177 Andreone P, Cursaro C, Gramenzi A et al. Indomethacin enhances serum 2',5'-oligoadenylate synthetase in patients with hepatitis B and C virus chronic active hepatitis. *J Hepatol*, 21, 984-988 (1994)

178 Andress DL, Norris KC, Coburn JW et al. Intravenous calcitriol in the treatment of refractory osteitis fibrosa of chronic renal failure. *N Engl J Med*, 321, 274-279 (1989)

179 Aneckstein AG, Weingold AB. Chlorothiazide-induced hepatic coma in pregnancy. *Am J Obstet Gynecol*, 95, 136 (1966)

180 Angelin B, Arvidsson A, Hedman A et al. Quinidine reduces biliary clearance of digoxin in man. *Eur J Clin Invest*, 17, 262-265 (1987)

181 Angelin B, Eusufzai S. Effects of ursodeoxycholic acid on plasma lipids. *Scand J Gastroenterol*, 29, 24-26 (1994)

182 Annibale B, Ribaldi S, Anania MC et al. Somatostatin infused during acute pancreatitis retains its biological activity. *Pancreas*, 4, 674-679 (1989)

183 Anonymous. *Med Lett*, 13, 101 (1971)

184 Anonymous. Aluminum nicotinate reduces level of serum cholesterol. *J Am Med Ass*, 209, 353 (1969)

185 Anonymous. Amicar® and hyperfibrinolysis. *Med Lett*, 9, 10 (1967)

186 Anonymous. Antithrombotic therapy. *Otsuka Pharmaceutical Co. Ltd.*, Japan

187 Anonymous. Clindamycin. *Med Lett*, 15, 25 (1973)

188 Anonymous. Diazoxide: a review of its pharmacological properties and therapeutic use in hypertensive crisis. *Drugs*, 2, 78 (1971)
189 Anonymous. Drugs and other factors affecting laboratory tests. *Med Lett*, 13, 82 (1971)
190 Anonymous. Drugs for parasitic infections. *Med Lett*, 11, 21 (1969)
191 Anonymous. Etoposide (VP 15-213: Vepesid). *Med Lett*, 26, 48-49 (1984)
192 Anonymous. 52 factors that can affect blood glucose levels. *Clin Toxicol*, 4, 297 (1971)
193 Anonymous. False positive and false negative reactions with various tests for glycosuria. Ames Company, Elkhart IN
194 Anonymous. False positive and false negative reactions with various tests for proteinuria. Ames Company, Elkhart IN
195 Anonymous. FDA approved new drug literature - sodium dicloxacillin monohydrate. *Drug Intell Clin Pharm*, 2, 251 (1968)
196 Anonymous. FDA drug efficacy study implementation. *Drug Therapy*, 1, 81 (1971)
197 Anonymous. Glibenclamide: a review. *Drugs*, 1, 116 (1971)
198 Anonymous. Handbook of antimicrobial therapy. *Med Lett*, 14, 1 (1972)
199 Anonymous. Interference of drugs with chemical diagnostic tests. *Drug Ther Bull*, 10, 69 (1972)
200 Anonymous. Intravenous feeding with amino acids and fats. *Drug Ther Bull*, 10, 49 (1972)
201 Anonymous. Mafenide acetate cream: a review. *Drugs*, 1, 461 (1971)
202 Anonymous. Methotrexate in the treatment of psoriasis. *Med Lett*, 14, 41 (1972)
203 Anonymous. Microstix and other office tests for detection of urinary tract infection. *Med Lett*, 16, 13 (1974)
204 Anonymous. Minocycline (minocin®). *Med Lett*, 14, 9 (1972)
205 Anonymous. Penicillamine nephropathy. *Br Med J*, 1, 761-762 (1981)
206 Anonymous. Sodium dextrothyroxine (Choloxin®). *Med Lett*, 9, 103 (1967)
207 Anonymous. Sodium valproate reassessed. *Drug Ther Bull*, 19, 93-95 (1981)
208 Anonymous. Today's drugs: diazoxide. *Br Med J*, 4, 417 (1972)
209 Anonymous. Today's drugs: drugs for rheumatoid disorders. *Br Med J*, 1, 545 (1964)
210 Anonymous. Today's drugs: treatment of trigeminal neuralgia. *Br Med J*, 2, 583 (1972)
211 Anonymous. Use of probenecid in antimicrobial therapy. *Med Lett*, 13, 85 (1971)
212 Anonymous. Venoglobulin® -I. Alpha Therapeutic Corporation, Los Angeles, CA (1988)
213 Antcliff AC, Beevers DG, Hamilton M et al. The use of amiloride hydrochloride in the correction of hypokalaemic alkalosis induced by diuretics. *Postgrad Med J*, 47, 644 (1971)
214 Antonian E, McNally AJ, Ng CF et al. An Abuscreen Online immunoassay for opiates in urine on the Olympus AU 5121 and 5131 automated analyzers. *Clin Chem*, 37, 1000 (1991)
215 Antoniazzi F, Radetti G, Zamboni G et al. Effects of 1,25-dihydroxyvitamin D_3 and growth hormone therapy on serum osteocalcin levels in children with growth hormone deficiency. *Bone Miner*, 21, 151-156 (1993)
216 Antonicelli R, Tomassini PF, Galletti P et al. Age-related antihypertensive and haemodynamic effects of verapamil SR: clinical results and effects on atrial natriuretic peptide. *Eur J Clin Pharmacol*, 39, Suppl 1, S29-S33 (1990)
217 Antonsen S, Qvist N, Wanscher M. Aspects of preanalytical variation of lactoferrin and elastase/alpha$_1$-protease inhibitor complexes. *Scand J Clin Lab Invest*, 53, 263-274 (1993)
218 Anumonye A, Reading HW, Knight F et al. Uric acid metabolism in manic-depressive illness and during lithium therapy. *Lancet*, 1, 1290 (1968)
219 Apothecon. Manufacturer's literature on Amikin® . Princeton, NJ 08543 (1993)
220 Apothecon. Manufacturer's literature on Desyrel® . Princeton, NJ 08543 (1993)
221 Apothecon. Manufacturer's literature on Florinef® . Princeton, NJ 08543 (1991)
222 Apothecon. Manufacturer's literature on Fungizone® . Princeton, NJ 08543 (1993)
223 Apothecon. Manufacturer's literature on Nydrazid® . Princeton. NJ 08543 (1990)
224 Apothecon. Manufacturer's literature on Prolixin® . Princeton. NJ 08543 (1996)
225 Appel GB. A decade of penicillin related acute interstitial nephritis - more questions than answers. *Clin Nephrol*, 13, 151-154 (1980)
226 Appel GB, D'Agati V, Bergman M et al. Nephrotic syndrome and immune complex glomerulonephritis associated with chlorpropamide therapy. *Am J Med*, 74, 337-342 (1983)
227 Appel S, Rufenacht T, Kalafsky G, et al. Lack of interaction between fluvastatin and oral hypoglycemic agents in healthy subjects and in patients with non-insulin-dependent diabetes mellitus. *Am J Cardiol*, 76, 29A-32A (1995)
228 Appelboom TM, Flowers FP. Acyclovir. *South Med J*, 76, 905-909 (1983)
229 Apperloo AJ, de Zeeuw D, Sluiter HE et al. Differential effects of enalapril and atenolol on proteinuria and renal haemodynamics in non-diabetic renal disease. *Br Med J*, 303 (1991)
230 Aquaron R. Protein-bound iodine and hormonal iodine after ioxitalamic acid. *Clin Chim Acta*, 41, 175 (1972)
231 Arabshahi L, Gotze A, Hui R et al. Abuscreen Online immunoassay for the detection of benzodiazepines in urine on the Cobas Mira. *Clin Chem*, 37, 995 (1991)
232 Arad Y, Ramakrishnan R, Ginsberg HN. Lovastatin therapy reduces low density lipoprotein apoB levels in subjects with combined hyperlipidemia by reducing the production of apoB-containing lipoproteins: implications for the pathophysiology of apoB production. *J Lipid Res*, 31, 567-582 (1990)
233 Aramaki T, Okumura H, Ichikawa T. Studies on aspirin induced hepatic injury. *Jpn J Pharmacol*, 22, 118 (1972)
234 Arana GW, Epstein S, Molloy M et al. Carbamazepine-induced reduction of plasma alprazolam concentrations; a clinical case report. *J Clin Psychiat*, 49, 448-449 (1988)
235 Arana GW, Goff DC, Friedman H et al. Does carbamazepine-induced reduction of plasma haloperidol levels worsen psychotic symptoms?. *Am J Psychiat*, 143, 650-651 (1986)
236 Aranow RB, Hudson JI, Pope HG JR et al. Elevated plasma levels after addition of fluoxetine. *Am J Psychiat*, 146, 911-913 (1989)
237 Arcieri G, Griffith E, Gruenwaldt G. Ciprofloxacin: an update on clinical experience. *Am J Med*, 82, Suppl 4A, 381-386 (1987)
238 Arem R, Patsch W. Lipoprotein and apolipoprotein levels in subclinical hypothyroidism. Effect of levothyroxine therapy. *Arch Intern Med*, 150, 2097-2100 (1990)
239 Arias IM. Effects of plant acid (icterogenin) and certain anabolic steroids on hepatic metabolism of bilirubin and BSP. *Ann NY Acad Sci*, 104, 1014 (1963)
240 Armstrong P, Rae PWH, Gray WM et al. Nitrous oxide and formiminoglutamic acid: excretion in surgical patients and anaesthetists. *Br J Anaes*, 66, 163-169 (1991)
241 Arneborn P, Palmblad J. Drug-induced neutropenia - a survey for Stockholm 1973-1978. *Acta Med Scand*, 212, 289-292 (1982)
242 Arnesen E, Huseby N-E, Brenn T et al. The Tromso heart study: distribution of, and determinants for, γ-glutamyltransferase in a free-living population. *Scand J Clin Lab Invest*, 46, 63-70 (1986)
243 Arneson GA. Phenothiazine derivatives and glucose metabolism. *J Neuropsychiat*, 5, 181 (1964)

244 Arnon R, Sehayek E, Eisenberg S. Disparate effects of a triglyceride lowering diet and of bezafibrate on the HDL system: a study in patients with hypertriglyceridemia and low HDL-cholesterol levels. *Eur J Clin Invest*, 23, 492-498 (1993)

245 Arntz H-R, Bonner G, Kikis D et al. Efficacy of pravastatin and bezafibrate in primary hypercholesterolaemia. *Dtsch Med Wschr*, 116, 7-12 (1991)

246 Aro A, KyllastinenM, Kostiainen E et al. No effect on serum lipids by moderate and high doses of vitamin C in elderly subjects with low plasma ascorbic acid levels. *Ann Nutr Metab*, 32, 133-137 (1988)

247 Aro J, Haapiainen R, Sane T et al. Effects of orchiectomy and polyestradiol phosphate therapy on serum lipoprotein lipids and glucose tolerance in prostatic cancer patients. *Eur Urol*, 17, 229-235 (1990)

248 Aron NB. Phenoxybenzamine-induced hyponatremia simulating the syndrome of inappropriate antidiuretic hormone secretion. *Ann Intern Med*, 107, 119 (1987)

249 Aronoff GR, Brier RA, Sloan RS et al. Interactions of ceftazidime and tobramycin in patients with normal and impaired renal function. *Antimicrob Agent Chemother*, 34, 1139-1142 (1990)

250 Aronow WS, Harding PR, Khursheed M et al. Effect of halofenate on serum uric acid. *Clin Pharmacol Ther*, 14, 371 (1973)

251 Arranto AJ, Sotaniemi EA. Morphologic alterations in patients with α-melthyldopa-induced liver damage after short- and long-term exposure. *Scand J Gastroenterol*, 16, 853-863 (1981)

252 Arrowsmith D, Morin RJ. Oral contraceptives and the N.B.T. test. *Lancet*, 1, 148 (1973)

253 Arsura E, Lichstein E, Guadagnino V et al. Methemoglobin levels produced by organic nitrates in patients with coronary artery disease. *J Clin Pharmacol*, 24, 160-164 (1984)

254 Arthur JB, Ashby DWR, Bremer C et al. Trial of clofibrate in the treatment of ischaemic heart disease. *Br Med J*, 4, 767 (1971)

255 Arthur S, Greenberg A. Hyperkalemia associated with intravenous labetalol therapy for acute hypertension in renal transplant recipients. *Clin Nephrol*, 33, 269-271 (1990)

256 Arze RS, Ramos JM, Rashid HU et al. Amenorrhoea, galactorrhoea, and hyperprolactinaemia induced by methyldopa. *Br Med J*, 283, 194 (1981)

257 Asberg M, Bertilsson L, Tuck D et al. Indoleamine metabolites in the cerebrospinal fluid of depressed patients before and during treatment. *Clin Pharmacol Ther*, 14, 277 (1973)

258 Asfeldt VH. Plasma corticosteroids in normal individuals. *Scand J Clin Lab Invest*, 28, 61 (1971)

259 Ashraf M, Scotchel PL, Krall JM et al. Cisplatin-induced hypomagnesemia and peripheral neuropathy. *Gynecol Oncol*, 16, 309-318 (1983)

260 Ashraf N, Locksley R, Arieff AI. Thiazide-induced hyponatremia associated with death or neurologic damage in outpatients. *Am J Med*, 70, 1163-1168 (1981)

261 Ashton A, Alexander DP, DeBellis C et al. Leukocyturia in cyclosporine-treated renal allograft recipients. *Am J Clin Pathol*, 89, 113-117 (1988)

262 Ashwell K, Hopton MR, Harrop JS. Serum free thyroxine concentrations in subjects with high circulating levels of thyroxine-binding globulin. *Ann Clin Biochem*, 20, 285-288 (1983)

263 Assadi FK, Chow-Tung E. Renal handling of beta$_2$-microglobulin in neonates treated with gentamicin. *Nephron*, 49, 114-118 (1988)

264 Assmann G. Drugs affecting HDL-cholesterol. *Cardiology*, 78, 236-242 (1991)

265 Astles R, Petros WP, Peters WP et al. Artifactual hypoglycemia with hematopoietic cytokines. *Clin Chem*, 41, S202 (1995)

266 Astra Merck Inc. Manufacturer's literature on Plendil® . Wayne, PA 19087 (1995)

267 Astra Merck Inc. Manufacturer's literature on Prilosec® . Wayne, PA 19087 (1995)

268 Astra Merck Inc. Manufacturer's literature on Tonocard® . Wayne, PA 19087 (1995)

269 Astra Pharmaceuticals, L.P.. Manufacturer's literature on Atacand® . Wayne, PA 19087 (1998)

270 Astra USA, Inc. Manufacturer's literature on Amikacin Sulfate. Westborough, MA 01581 (1995)

271 Astra USA, Inc. Manufacturer's literature on Aredia® . Westborough, MA 01581 (1996)

272 Astra USA, Inc. Manufacturer's literature on Dalgan® . Westborough, MA 01581 (1994)

273 Astra USA, Inc. Manufacturer's literature on Doxorubicin. Westborough, MA 01581 (1996)

274 Astra USA, Inc. Manufacturer's literature on Duranest® . Westborough, MA 01581 (1993)

275 Astra USA, Inc. Manufacturer's literature on Etoposide. Westborough, MA 01581 (1995)

276 Astra USA, Inc. Manufacturer's literature on Foscavir® . Westborough, MA 01581 (1997)

277 Astra USA, Inc. Manufacturer's literature on Levothyroxine. Westborough, MA 01581 (1995)

278 Astra USA, Inc. Manufacturer's literature on Streptase® . Westborough, MA 01581 (1994)

279 Astra USA, Inc. Manufacturer's literature on Toprol-XL® . Westborough, MA 01581 (1996)

280 Astra USA, Inc. Manufacturer's literature on Xylocaine. Westborough, MA 01581 (1992)

281 Astra USA, Inc. Manufacturer's literature on Yutopar® . Westborough, MA 01581 (1995)

282 Athena Neurosciences, Inc. Manufacturer's literature on Atretol® . South San Francisco, CA 94080 (1995)

283 Athena Neurosciences, Inc. Manufacturer's literature on Permax® . South San Francisco, CA 94080 (1995)

284 Atkinson K, Biggs J, Dodds A et al. Cyclosporine-associated hepatotoxicity after allogeneic marrow transplantation in man: differentiation from other causes of post-transplant liver disease. *Transplant Proc*, 15, Suppl 1, 2761-2767 (1983)

285 Atkinson K, Biggs JC, Hayes J et al. Cyclosporin A associated nephrotoxicity in the first 100 days after allogeneic bone marrow transplantation: three distinct syndromes. *Br J Haematol*, 54, 59-67 (1983)

286 Atkinson RL. Endocrine and metabolic effects of opiate antagonists. *J Clin Psychiat*, 45, 20-24 (1984)

287 Atlas SA, Case DB, Yu ZY et al. Hormonal and metabolic effects of angiotensin converting enzyme inhibitors: possible differences between enalapril and captopril. *Am J Med*, 77, Suppl 2A, 13-17 (1984)

288 Atuk NO, Blaydes MC, Westervelt FB Jr et al. Effect of aminophylline on urinary excretion of epinephrine and norepinephrine in man. *Circulation*, 35, 745 (1967)

289 Aubertin E, Sudre J. Purpura thrombocytopenique hemorrhagique due a l'esidrex. *J Med Bordeaux*, 141, 1735 (1964)

290 Auerbach M, Witt D, Toler W et al. Clinical use of the total dose intravenous infusion of iron dextran. *J Lab Clin Med*, 111, 566-570 (1988)

291 Auld WHR, Murdoch WR. Clinical trial of mefruside, a new diuretic. *Br Med J*, 4, 786 (1971)

292 Aurell M, Delin K, Herlitz H. Captopril in treatment-resistant essential and renal hypertension. *Scand J Urol Nephrol*, 16, 243-249 (1982)

293 Aurell M, Vikgren P. Plasma renin activity in supine muscular exercise. *J Appl Physiol*, 31, 839 (1971)

294 Avall-Lundqvist E, Economidou-Karaoglou A, Sjovall K et al. Serum alkaline DNase activity in normal or nonhospitalized individuals. *Clin Chim Acta*, 185, 35-44 (1989)

295 Avellone G, Di Garbo V, Cordova R et al. Effect of gemfibrozil treatment on fibrinolysis system in patients with hypertriglyceridemia. *Curr Ther Res*, 52, 338-348 (1992)

296 Avellone G, Di Garbo V, Cordova R et al. Fibrnolytic effect of gemfibrozil versus placebo administration in response to venous occlusion. *Fibrinolysis*, 7, 416-421 (1993)

297 Averna MR, Barbagallo CM, Pata G et al. Effects of two different administration regimens of gemfibrozil on plasma lipids, lipoproteins and apoproteins. *Curr Ther Res*, 49, 47-53 (1991)

298 Avila JL, Convit J. Heterogeneity of acid phosphatase activity in human polymorphonuclear leukocytes. *Clin Chim Acta*, 44, 21 (1973)

299 Aviles A, Herrera J, Ramos E et al. Hepatic injury during doxorubicin therapy. *Arch Pathol Lab Med*, 108, 912-913 (1984)

300 Axcan Pharma U.S. Inc. Manufacturer's literature on Urso®. Minneapolis, MN 55247 (1998)

301 Ayd FJ. Amitriptyline reappraisal after six years experience. *Dis Nerv Sys*, 26, 719 (1965)

302 Ayers GJ, Baldwin AJ, Fowler AM et al. Theophylline assay on Kodak Ektachem® DTSC: performance and interference by structurally-related compounds and salicylate. *Ann Clin Biochem*, 26, 268-273 (1989)

303 Aylward M, Maddock J. Plasma tryptophan levels in depression. *Lancet*, 1, 936 (1973)

304 Aymard B, Aymard JP, Netter P et al. Cytopenies sanguines associees a la prise de cimetidine. *Therapie*, 39, 545-553 (1984)

305 Aynsley-Green A, Alberti KGM. Serum insulin or plasma insulin?. *Lancet*, 1, 318 (1972)

306 Azizi F. Environmental iodine intake affects the response to methimazole in patients with diffuse toxic goiter. *J Clin Endocrinol Metab*, 61, 374-377 (1985)

307 Azizi F, Vagenakis AG, Portnay GI et al. Thyroxine transport and metabolism in methadone and heroin addicts. *Ann Intern Med*, 80, 194 (1974)

308 Azrolan N, Brown CD, Thomas L et al. Cyclosporin A has divergent effects on plasma LDL cholesterol (LDL-C) and lipoprotein (a) [Lp(a)] levels in renal transplant recipients. *Arterioscler Thromb*, 14, 1393-1398 (1994)

309 Azzam Z, Krivoy N, Alroy G et al. Serum creatine kinase levels after a single intramuscular injection - dependence on injection volume. *Ann Clin Biochem*, 31, 193-194 (1994)

310 Baba T, Boku A, Ishizaki T et al. Renal effects of nicardipine in patients with mild-to-moderate essential hypertension. *Am Heart J*, 111, 552-557 (1986)

311 Baba T, Kodama T, Ishizaki T. Effect of chronic treatment with enalapril on glucose tolerance and serum insulin in non-insulin-resistant Japanese patients with essential hypertension. *Eur J Clin Pharmacol*, 45, 23-27 (1993)

312 Baba T, Murabayashi S, Tomiyama T et al. Comparison of the renal effects of dilevalol and carteolol in patients with mild to moderate hypertension. *Eur J Clin Pharmacol*, 38, 305-307 (1990)

313 Bachmann H. Propranolol versus chlorthalidone - a prospective therapeutic trial in children with chronic hypertension. *Helv Paediat Acta*, 39, 55-61 (1984)

314 Bachmann K, Nunlee M, Martin M et al. Changes in the steady-state pharmacokinetics of theophylline during treatment with dirithromycin. *J Clin Pharmacol*, 30, 1001-1005 (1990)

315 Bachmann K, Schwartz JI, Forney R JR et al. The effect of erythromycin on the disposition kinetics of warfarin. *Pharmacologist*, 28, 171-176 (1984)

316 Bachmann KA, Sullivan TJ, Jauregui L et al. Drug interactions of H_2-receptor antagonists. *Scand J Gastroenterol*, 29, 14-19 (1994)

317 Backman JT, Kivistö KT, Olkkola KT, Neuvonen PJ. The area under the plasma concentration-time curve for oral midazolam is 400-fold larger during treatment with itraconazole than with rifampicin. *Eur J Clin Pharmacol*, 54, 53-58 (1998)

318 Badcock NR, Penna AC, Everett DS et al. Aspirin metabolites causing misinterpretation of paracetamol results. *Ann Clin Biochem*, 21, 527-530 (1984)

319 Badrick TC, Campbell B. Effects of intravenous infusion of ascorbate on common clinical chemistry tests. *Clin Chem*, 38, 2160 (1992)

320 Baer DM, Jones RN, Mullooly JP et al. Protocol for the study of drug interferences in laboratory tests: cefotaxime interference in 24 clinical tests. *Clin Chem*, 29, 1736-1740 (1983)

321 Bagdade JD, Buchanan WF, Pollare T, Lithell H. Effects of hydrochlorothiazide and captopril on lipoprotein lipid composition in patients with essential hypertension. *Eur J Clin Pharmacol*, 49, 355-359 (1996)

322 Bagdade JD, Porte D Jr, Bierman EL. Steroid-induced lipemia: a complication of high-dosage corticosteroid therapy. *Arch Intern Med*, 125, 129 (1970)

323 Bagdade JD, Subbaiah PV. Effects of estropipate treatment on plasma lipids and lipoprotein lipid composition in postmenopausal women. *J Clin Endocrinol Metab*, 72, 283-286 (1991)

324 Bagdade JD, Wolter J, Subbaiah PV et al. Effects of tamoxifen treatment on plasma lipids and lipoprotein lipid composition. *J Clin Endocrinol Metab*, 70, 1132-1135 (1990)

325 Bagnoud M-A, Reymond J-Ph. Interference of metamizole (dipyrone) on the determination of creatinine with the Kodak dry chemistry slide: comparison with the enzymatic method from Boehringer. *Eur J Clin Chem Clin Biochem*, 31, 753-757 (1993)

326 Bailey CC, Geary CG, Israels MCG et al. Cytosine arabinoside in the treatment of acute myeloblastic leukemia. *Lancet*, 1, 1268 (1971)

327 Bailey DG, Freeman DJ, Melendez LJ et al. Quinidine interaction with nifedipine and felodipine: pharmacokinetic and pharmacodynamic evaluation. *Clin Pharmacol Ther*, 53, 354-359 (1993)

328 Bailey DN. Thin-layer chromatographic detection of cocaethylene in human urine. *Am J Clin Pathol*, 101, 342-345 (1994)

329 Bailey DN, Jatlow PI. Chemical analysis of massive crystalluria following primidone overdose. *Am J Clin Pathol*, 58, 583 (1972)

330 Bain FG, Daniels HM, Chanas A et al. Foscarnet therapy in chronic hepatitis B virus E antigen carriers. *J Med Virol*, 29, 152-155 (1989)

331 Baitsch G, Walter N. Comparative hypolipidemic potency of beclofibrate, gemfibrozil, and various forms of diet. In: Kostner GM, Sirtori CR (eds). *Beclofibrate, a New Lipoprotein Regulator. GM Kostner, CR Sirtori (eds)*, Toronto ONT, Hogrefe and Huber, 83-87 (1990)

332 Baker B, Gammill J, Massengill J et al. Concurrent use of quinidine and disopyramide: evaluation of serum concentrations and electrocardiographic effects. *Am Heart J*, 105, 12-15 (1983)

333 Baker DA, Salvatore W, Milch PO. Effect of low-dose oral contraceptives on natural killer cell activity. *Contraception*, 39, 119-124 (1989)

334 Baker HN, Massei MK, Ramp SK et al. Development of a fully automated immunoassay for estradiol on the Abbott IMx automated immunoassay system. *Clin Chem*, 37, 1037 (1991)

335 Baker N, Huebotter RJ. Immobilizing and hyperglycemic effects of benzyl alcohol. *Life Sci*, 10, 1193 (1971)

336 Baker Norton Pharmaceuticals, Inc. Manufacturer's literature on Elmiron®. Miami, FL 33137 (1996)

337 Baker Norton Pharmaceuticals, Inc. Manufacturer's literature on Proglycem®. Miami, FL 33137 (1995)

338 Bakker-Arkema RG, Best J, Fayyad R, et al. A brief review paper of the efficacy and safety of atorvastatin in early clinical trials. *Atherosclerosis*, 131, 17-23 (1997)

339 Bakris GL. Effects of diltiazem or lisinopril on massive proteinuria associated with diabetes mellitus. *Ann Intern Med*, 112, 707-708 (1990)

340 Bakris GL, Sauter ER, Hussey JL et al. Effects of theophylline on erythropoietin production in normal subjects and in patients with erythrocytosis after renal transplantation. *N Engl J Med*, 323, 86-90 (1990)

341 Bakris GL, Weber RR, Nelson K et al. Comparison of the effects of dopamine and fenoldopam, a selective dopamine-1 agonist, on parathyroid hormone release in man. *Mineral Elect Metab*, 14, 343-346 (1988)

342 Balan V, Dickson ER, Jorgensen RA et al. Effect of ursodeoxycholic acid on serum lipids of patients with primary biliary cirrhosis. *Mayo Clin Proc*, 69, 923-929 (1994)

343 Balazs M, Kovach G. Chronic aggressive hepatitis after methyldopa treatment: case report with electron microscopy study. *Hepatogastroenterology*, 28, 199-202 (1981)

344 Baldessarini RJ, Frankenburg FR. Clozapine: a novel antipsychotic agent. *N Engl J Med*, 324, 726-754 (1991)

345 Baldwin DS, Levine BB, McCluskey RT et al. Renal failure and interstitial nephritis due to penicillin and methicillin. *N Engl J Med*, 279, 1245 (1968)

346 Bale JF Jr, Gay PE, Madsen JA. Monitoring of serum amylase levels during valproic acid therapy. *Ann Neurol*, 11, 217-218 (1982)

347 Bale Oenick MD, Hilborn D, Danielson S et al. Thin-film enzyme immunoassay for the measurement of phenytoin in human serum. *Clin Chem*, 37, 1035 (1991)

348 Balestrieri A, Benassi P, Cassano GB et al. Clinical comparative evaluation of maprotiline, a new antidepressant drug. *Int Pharmacopsychiat*, 6, 236 (1971)

349 Balfour JA, McTavish D, Heel RC. Fenofibrate: a review of its pharmacodynamic and pharmacokinetic properties and its use in dyslipidaemia. *Drugs*, 40, 260-290 (1990)

350 Ball JH, Kaminsky NI, Hardman JG et al. Effect of catecholamines and adrenergic-blocking agents on plasma and urinary cyclic nucleotides in man. *J Clin Invest*, 51, 2124 (1972)

351 Ball MJ, Griffiths D. Effect on chemical analyses of β-propiolactone treatment of whole blood and plasma. *Lancet*, 1, 1160-1161 (1985)

352 Ball MJ, Paul J, Kay JDS. Analytical interference by rifampicin with tests of liver function.. *Ann Clin Biochem*, 24, Suppl S1, 75-77 (1987)

353 Ballantyne CM, Podet EJ, Patsch WP et al. Effects of cyclosporine therapy on plasma lipoprotein levels. *J Am Med Ass*, 262, 53-56 (1989)

354 Balschun D, Burchardt U, Klagge M et al. Infradian rhythms of alanine aminopeptidase excretion during gentamicin therapy. *Eur J Clin Chem Clin Biochem*, 29, 783-786 (1991)

355 Balzano S, Cappa M, Migliari R et al. The effect of flutamide on basal and ACTH-stimulated plasma levels of adrenal androgens in patients with advanced prostatic cancer. *J Endocrinol Invest*, 11, 693-696 (1988)

356 Banerji A, Shriner S. Development of phenytoin II (monoclonal) assay for the Abbott AxSYM immunoassay analyzer. *Clin Chem*, 41, S121 (1995)

357 Bang NU. Acquired abnormalities of platelet function. *N Engl J Med*, 324, 1672 (1991)

358 Bankier RG. A comparison of fluspirilene and trifluoperazine in the treatment of acute schizophrenic psychosis. *J Clin Pharmacol*, 13, 44 (1973)

359 Bansal OP. Agranulocytosis during unitheben therapy. *Ind Practitioner*, 18, 616 (1965)

360 Bantle JP, Boudreau RJ, Ferris TF. Suppression of plasma renin activity by cyclosporine. *Am J Med*, 83, 59-64 (1987)

361 Bar RS, Wilson HE, Mazzaferri EL. Hypomagnesemic hypocalcemia secondary to renal magnesium wasting. *Ann Intern Med*, 82, 646-649 (1975)

362 Barbarino A, De Marinis L, Folli G et al. Corticotropin-releasing hormone inhibition of gonadotropin secretion during the menstrual cycle. *Metabolism*, 38, 504-506 (1989)

363 Barbhaiya RH, Shukla UA, Greene DS. Lack of interaction between nefazodone and cimetidine: a steady state pharmacokinetic study in humans. *Br J Clin Pharmacol*, 40, 161-165 (1995)

364 Barbhaiya RH, Shukla UA, Greene DS, et al. Coadministration of nefazodone and benzodiazepines: II A pharmacokinetic interaction study with triazolam. *J Clin Psychopharmacol*, 15, 320-326 (1995)

365 Barbhaiya RH, Shukla UA, Greene DS, et al. Investigation of pharmacokinetic and pharmacodynamic interactions after coadministration of nefazodone and haloperidol. *J Clin Psychopharmacol*, 16, 26-34 (1996)

366 Barbieri C, Caldara R, Ferrari C et al. Metabolic effect of prazosin. *Clin Pharmacol Ther*, 27, 313-316 (1980)

367 Barbieri C, Ferrari C, Caldara R et al. Endocrine and metabolic effects of labetalol in man. *J Cardiovasc Pharmacol*, 3, 986-991 (1981)

368 Barbosa J, Seal US, Doe RP. Effects of anabolic steroids on haptoglobin, orosomucoid, plasminogen, fibrinogen, transferrin, ceruloplasmin. *J Clin Endocrinol Metab*, 33, 388 (1971)

369 Barbour HM. Four methods compared for determining plasma creatinine with the Monarch centrifugal analyzer. *Clin Chem*, 37, 474 (1991)

370 Barbour HM, Pritchard JL, Blundell G et al. Does cefixime interfere in creatinine assays?. *Proc ACB Natl Meet*, 117 (1991)

371 Bard J-M, Luc G, Douste-Blazy P et al. Effect of simvastatin on plasma lipids, apolipoproteins and lipoprotein particles in patients with primary hypercholesterolaemia. *Eur J Clin Pharmacol*, 37, 545-550 (1989)

372 Bard J-M, Parra HJ, Douste-Blazy P et al. Effect of pravastatin, an HMG CoA reductase inhibitor, and cholestyramine, a bile acid sequestrant, on lipoprotein particles defined by their apolipoprotein composition. *Metabolism*, 39, 269-273 (1990)

373 Bardana EJ Jr, Gabourel JD, Davies GH et al. Effects of phenytoin on man's immunity: evaluation of changes in serum immunoglobulins, complement and antinuclear antibody. *Am J Med*, 74, 289-296 (1984)

374 Bardin CW, Ross GT, Lipsett MB. Site of action of clomiphene citrate in man: a study of the pituitary-Leydig cell axis. *J Clin Endocrinol Metab*, 27, 1558 (1967)

375 Bardy A, Hari A, Lehtovaara R et al. Valproate may lower serum phenytoin. *Lancet*, 2, 1297-1298 (1976)

376 Barkia A, Steinmetz A, Brayana C et al. Low-dose oral contraceptive lower plasma levels of Lp AI, Lp B, Lp CIII, Lp E. *Clin Chem*, 36, 953 (1990)

377 Barlow DH, Beastall GH, Abdalla HI et al. Effect of long-term hormone replacement on plasma prolactin concentrations in women after oophorectomy. *Br Med J*, 23, 589-591 (1985)

378 Barnes C, Hamilton PG, Lebel M. Effects of monotherapy with sustained-release verapamil on blood pressure, lipid levels, renal function, diabetic control, and patient well-being in patients with mild to moderate hypertension. *Curr Ther Res*, 54, 127-141 (1993)

379 Barnes DB, Pierce GF, Lichtl D et al. Effects of dextran on five biuret-based procedures for total protein in serum. *Clin Chem*, 31, 2018-2019 (1985)

380 Barnes PC, Leonard JHC. Hypokalemic myopathy and myoglobinuria due to carbenoxolone sodium. *Postgrad Med J*, 47, 813 (1971)

381 Barnes RB, Rosenfield RL, Burstein S et al. Pituitary-ovarian responses to nafarelin testing in the polycystic ovary syndrome. *N Engl J Med*, 320, 559-565 (1989)

382 Barness LA. Safety considerations with high ascorbic acid dosage. *Ann NY Acad Sci*, 258, 523-528 (1975)

383 Baron JM. Chlordiazepoxide (librium®) and thyroid function tests. *Br Med J*, 1, 699 (1967)

384 Barreca T, Picciotto A, Franceschini R et al. Long term therapy with recombinant interferon alpha 2b in patients with chronic hepatitis C: effects on thyroid function and autoantibodies. *J Biol Reg Homeostat Agents*, 7, 58-62 (1994)

385 Barrett PV, Thier SO. Meningitis and pancreatitis associated with sulfamethizole. *N Engl J Med*, 268, 36 (1963)

386 Barron KS, Person DA, Brewer EJ. The toxicity of nonsteroidal anti-inflammatory drugs in juvenile rheumatoid arthritis. *J Rheumatol*, 9, 149-155 (1982)

387 Bartalena L, Grasso L, Brogioni S et al. Serum interleukin-6 in amiodarone-induced thyrotoxicosis. *J Clin Endocrinol Metab*, 78, 423-427 (1994)

388 Bartels C, Horpacsy G, Horsch S. Modification of malondialdehyde concentration by administration of protamine sulfate. *Clin Chem*, 41, 1544 (1995)

389 Barthelmebs M, Mbou P, Stephan D et al. Renal dopamine excretion in healthy volunteers after oral ingestion of L-Dopa. *Fundam Clin Pharmacol*, 7, 11-16 (1993)

390 Bartlett A, Costa A, Martinez L et al. The effect of antacid and ranitidine on doxicam pharmacokinetics. *J Clin Pharmacol*, 32, 1115-1119 (1992)

391 Barton CH, Pahl M, Vaziri ND et al. Renal magnesium wasting associated with amphotericin B therapy. *Am J Med*, 77, 471-474 (1984)

392 Bartos HR. Thrombocytopenia associated with rubella vaccination. *NY State J Med*, 72, 499 (1972)

393 Bartter FC, Elea CS, Halberg F. A map of blood and urinary changes related to circadian variations in adrenal cortical function in normal subject. *Ann NY Acad Sci*, 98, 969 (1962)

394 Barzel US. The role of bone in acid base metabolism. In:. *Osteoporosis, US Barzel (ed)*, New York NY, Grune and Stratton (1970)

395 Basaran MM, Barlan IB, Tukenmez F et al. Effect of interferon-α therapy on serum IgE, IL-4, and sCD23 levels in childhood asthma. *Clin Chem*, 32, 215-220 (1995)

396 Bascoul J, Goze C, Domergue N et al. Serum level of 7α-hydroxycholesterol in hypercholesterolemic patients treated with cholestyramine. *Biochim Biophys Acta Lipids Lipid Metab*, 1044, 357-360 (1990)

397 Bass HZ, Hardy WD, Mitsuyasu RT et al. The effect of zidovudine treatment on serum neopterin and β-microglobulin levels in mildly symptomatic, HIV type 1 seropositive indiviuals. *J Acq Immune Defic Syndromes*, 5, 215-221 (1992)

398 Bassol S, Barraza-Vazquez A, Nava MP, Recio R. Effects of oral buserelin on urinary LH secretion in male infants. *Contraception*, 55, 311-314 (1997)

399 Batch J, Ma A, Bird D, et al. The effects of ingestion time of gliclazide in relationship to meals on plasma glucose, insulin and C-peptide levels. *Eur J Clin Pharmacol*, 38, 465-467 (1990)

400 Bateh RP, Bowie LJ. Triamterene interferes in urinary catecholamine analyses. *Clin Chem*, 29, 1325-1326 (1983)

401 Bates MC, Warren SG, Grubb S et al. Effectiveness of low-dose lovastatin in lowering serum cholesterol: experience with 56 patients. *Arch Intern Med*, 150, 1947-1950 (1990)

402 Batsakis JG, Briere RO. *Interpretive Enzymology*, Springfield, IL, CC Thomas (1967)

403 Batsakis JG, Preston JA, Briere Rogiesen PC. Iatrogenic aberrations of serum enzyme activity. *Clin Biochem*, 2, 125 (1968)

404 Battistini B, D'Orleans-Juste P, Sirois P. Endothelins: circulating plasma levels and presence in other biologic fluids. *Lab Invest*, 68, 600-628 (1993)

405 Batty KT, Davis TME, Ilett KF et al. The effect of ciprofloxacin on theophylline pharmacokinetics in healthy subjects. *Br J Clin Pharmacol*, 39, 305-311 (1995)

406 Bauch M, Ester A, Kimura B et al. Atrial natriuretic peptide as a marker for doxorubicin-induced cardiotoxic effects. *Cancer*, 69, 1492-1497 (1992)

407 Bauer D, Gaertner HJ. Wirkungen der neuroleptika auf die leberfunktion, das blutbildende system, den blutdruck und die temperature regulation. *Pharmacopsychiatry*, 16, 23-29 (1983)

408 Bauer JD, Ackermann PG, Toro G. Bray's Clinical Laboratory Methods. 6th edition. St Louis, MO, CV Mosby (1962)

409 Bauer JD, Ackermann PG, Toro G. Bray's Clinical Laboratory Methods. 7th edition. St Louis, MO, CV Mosby (1968)

410 Bauer LA, Edwards WAD, Randolph FP et al. Cimetidine-induced decrease in lidocaine metabolism. *Am Heart J*, 108, 413-415 (1984)

411 Bauer LA, Stenwall M, Horn JR et al. Changes in antipyrine and indocyanine green kinetics during nifedipine, verapamil and diltiazem therapy. *Clin Pharmacol Ther*, 40, 239-242 (1986)

412 Baulieu E-E. RU-486 as an antiprogesterone steroid; from receptor to contrgestion and beyond. *J Am Med Ass*, 262, 1808-1814 (1989)

413 Bautista J, Huster M. Syva EMIT 2000 theophylline assay. *Clin Chem*, 37, 998-999 (1991)

414 Bax NDS, Tucker GT, Lennard MS et al. The impairment of lidocaine clearance by propranolol -- major contribution from enzyme inhibition. *Br J Clin Pharmacol*, 19, 597-603 (1985)

415 Bayer Corporation. Manufacturer's literature on Adalat® CC. West Haven, CT (1997)

416 Bayer Corporation. Manufacturer's literature on Cipro® . West Haven, CT (1997)

417 Bayer Corporation, Business Group Diagnostics. Manufacturer's literature on Technicon Immuno 1® System Carbamazepine. Tarrytown, NY 10591, February (1997)

418 Bayer Corporation, Business Group Diagnostics. Manufacturer's literature on Technicon Immuno 1® System Carcinoembryonic antigen. Tarrytown, NY 10591, November (1996)

419 Bayer Corporation, Business Group Diagnostics. Manufacturer's literature on Technicon Immuno 1® System Cortisol. Tarrytown, NY 10591, November (1995)

420 Bayer Corporation, Business Group Diagnostics. Manufacturer's literature on Technicon Immuno 1® System Creatine Kinase-MB. Tarrytown, NY 10591, July (1996)

421 Bayer Corporation, Business Group Diagnostics. Manufacturer's literature on Technicon Immuno 1® System Digoxin. Tarrytown, NY 10591, September (1995)

422 Bayer Corporation, Business Group Diagnostics. Manufacturer's literature on Technicon Immuno 1® System Estradiol. Tarrytown, NY 10591, September (1995)

423 Bayer Corporation, Business Group Diagnostics. Manufacturer's literature on Technicon Immuno 1® System Folate. Tarrytown, NY 10591, November (1996)

424 Bayer Corporation, Business Group Diagnostics. Manufacturer's literature on Technicon Immuno 1® System Free Thyroxine (FT4). Tarrytown, NY 10591, July (1996)

425 Bayer Corporation, Business Group Diagnostics. Manufacturer's literature on Technicon Immuno 1® System Free Triiodothyronine (FT3). Tarrytown, NY 10591, December (1996)

426 Bayer Corporation, Business Group Diagnostics. Manufacturer's literature on Technicon Immuno 1® System Gentamicin. Tarrytown, NY 10591, September (1995)

427 Bayer Corporation, Business Group Diagnostics. Manufacturer's literature on Technicon Immuno 1® System Phenobarbital. Tarrytown, NY 10591, September (1995)

428 Bayer Corporation, Business Group Diagnostics. Manufacturer's literature on Technicon Immuno 1® System Phenytoin. Tarrytown, NY 10591, September (1995)

429 Bayer Corporation, Business Group Diagnostics. Manufacturer's literature on Technicon Immuno 1® System Progesterone. Tarrytown, NY 10591, April (1996)

430 Bayer Corporation, Business Group Diagnostics. Manufacturer's literature on Technicon Immuno 1® System Prostate Specific Antigen. Tarrytown, NY 10591, November (1996)

431 Bayer Corporation, Business Group Diagnostics. Manufacturer's literature on Technicon Immuno 1® System Quinidine. Tarrytown, NY 10591, February (1997)

432 Bayer Corporation, Business Group Diagnostics. Manufacturer's literature on Technicon Immuno 1® System RBC Folate. Tarrytown, NY 10591, March (1996)

433 Bayer Corporation, Business Group Diagnostics. Manufacturer's literature on Technicon Immuno 1® System Testosterone. Tarrytown, NY 10591, December (1996)

434 Bayer Corporation, Business Group Diagnostics. Manufacturer's literature on Technicon Immuno 1® System Thyroxine (T4). Tarrytown, NY 10591, September (1995)

435 Bayer Corporation, Business Group Diagnostics. Manufacturer's literature on Technicon Immuno 1® System Tobramycin. Tarrytown, NY 10591, September (1995)

436 Bayer Corporation, Business Group Diagnostics. Manufacturer's literature on Technicon Immuno 1® System Triiodothyronine (T3). Tarrytown, NY 10591, July (1996)

437 Bayer Corporation, Business Group Diagnostics. Manufacturer's literature on Technicon Immuno 1® System Valproic Acid. Tarrytown, NY 10591, February (1997)

438 Bayer Corporation, Business Group Diagnostics. Manufacturer's literature on Technicon Immuno 1® System Vancomycin. Tarrytown, NY 10591, February (1997)

439 Bayer Corporation, Business Group Diagnostics. Manufacturer's literature on Technicon Immuno 1® System Vitamin B_{12}. Tarrytown, NY 10591, November (1996)

440 Bayly GR, Bartlett WA, Jones AF. A non-isotopic method for estimating 11β hydroxysteroid dehydrogenase activity in vivo. *Ann Clin Biochem*, 34, 521-526 (1997)

441 Beastall GH, Cowan RA, Gray JMB et al. Hormone binding globulins and anticonvulsant therapy. *Scott Med J*, 30, 101-105 (1985)

442 Beaugrand M, Gavillon C, Ferrier J-P. High levels of endoplasmic reticulum antibody titer in a case of α-methyldopa-induced chronic active hepatitis. *Gastroenterol Clin Biol*, 4, 219-221 (1980)

443 Beck RP, Fawcett DM, Morcos F. Thyroid function studies in different phases of the menstrual cycle and in women receiving norethindrone. *Am J Obstet Gynecol*, 112, 369 (1972)

444 Beck RP, Morcos F, Fawcett D et al. Adrenocortical function studies during the normal menstrual cycle and in women receiving norethindrone. *Am J Obstet Gynecol*, 112, 364 (1972)

445 Becker CE, Gorden P, Robbins J. Hepatitis from methimazole during adrenal steroid therapy for malignant exophthalmos. *J Am Med Ass*, 206, 1787 (1968)

446 Beckerhoff R, Vetter W, Armbruster H et al. Plasma-aldosterone during oral contraceptive therapy. *Lancet*, 1, 1218 (1973)

447 Beckett GJ, Foster GR, Hussey AJ et al. Plasma glutathione S-transferase and F protein are more sensitive than alanine aminotransferase as markers of paracetamol (acetaminophen)-induced liver damage. *Clin Chem*, 35, 2186-2189 (1989)

448 Beckett GJ, Kellett HA, Gow SM et al. Raised plasma glutathione-S-transferase values in hyperthyroidism and in hypothyroid patients receiving thyroxine replacement: evidence for hepatic damage. *Br Med J*, 291, 427-431 (1985)

449 Beck-Peccoz P, Medri G, Piscitelli G et al. Treatment of inappropriate secretion of thyrotropin with somatostatin analog SMS 201-995. *Horm Res*, 29, 121-123 (1988)

450 Bedell SA, Kang JL. Leukocytosis and left shift associated with quinidine fever. *Am J Med*, 77, 345-346 (1984)

451 Beeley L, Kendall MJ. Effect of aspirin on renal clearance of I-diatrizoate. *Br Med J*, 1, 707 (1971)

452 Beer NA, Jakubowicz DJ, Beer RM et al. Effects of nitrendipine on glucose tolerance and serum insulin and dehydroepiandrosterone sulfate levels in insulin-resistant obese and hypertensive men. *J Clin Endocrinol Metab*, 76, 178-183 (1993)

453 Beerman B, Ericsson JLE, Hellstrom K et al. Transient cholestasis during treatment with ajmaline and chronic xanthomatous cholestasis. *Acta Med Scand*, 190, 241 (1971)

454 Beevers DG, Blackwood RA, Garnham S et al. Comparison of lisinopril versus atenolol for mild to moderate essential hypertension. *Am J Cardiol*, 67, 59-62 (1991)

455 Beevers DG, Hamilton M, Harpur JE. The long-term treatment of hypertension with thiazide diuretics. *Postgrad Med J*, 47, 639 (1971)

456 Begg EJ, Chinwah PM, Webb C et al. Enhanced metabolism of mexiletine after phenytoin administration. *Br J Clin Pharmacol*, 14, 219-223 (1982)

457 Beierle FA, Bailey L. Cyclosporine metabolism impeded/blocked by co-administration of phenobarbital. *Clin Chem*, 35, 1160 (1989)

458 Beil FU, Schrameyer-Wernecke A, Beisiegel U et al. Lovastatin versus bezafibrate: efficacy, tolerability, and effect on urinary mevalonate. *Cardiology*, 77, Suppl 4, 22-32 (1990)

459 Belgorosky A, Chahin S, Rivarola MA. Elevation of serum luteinizing hormone levels during hydrocortisone treatment in infant girls with 21-hydroxylase deficiency. *Acta Paediat*, 85, 1172-1175 (1996)

460 Belisle S, Patry M, Tetreault L. Cimetidine and plasma levels of gonadotropins, prolactin and gonadal steroids in women. *Can Med Ass J*, 127, 29-32 (1982)

461 Belkin GA. Cocktail purpura: an unusual case of quinine sensitivity. *Ann Intern Med*, 66, 583 (1967)

462 Bell GD, Whitney B, Dowling RH. Gallstone dissolution in man using chenodeoxycholic acid. *Lancet*, 2, 1213 (1972)

463 Bell R, Jones J. Cortisol, growth hormone response, and pain following tetracosactrin depot and ACTH gel. *S Afr Med J*, 46, 1305 (1972)

464 Bellamy WE Jr, Mauck HP Jr, Hennigar GR et al. Jaundice associated with the administration of sodium p-aminosalicylic acid: review of the literature. *Ann Intern Med*, 44, 764 (1956)

465 Bellantani S, Podda M, Tiribelli C et al. Ursodiol in the long-term treatment of chronic hepatitis: a double-blind multicenter clinical trial. *J Hepatol*, 19, 459-464 (1993)

466 Bellinger JF, Buist NRM. Rapid column-chromatographic measurement of orotic acid. *Clin Chem*, 17, 1132 (1971)

467 Bellon EM. Haemolytic anemia due to nalidixic acid. *Lancet*, 2, 691 (1965)

468 Belmaker RH, Zohar J, Klein E. Are the effects of carbamazepine on blood levels of haloperidol clinically relevant? In:. *International Clinical Psychopharmacology. H Emrich, W Schiwy, T Silverstone (eds)*, London, Clinical Neuroscience Publishers, 5, (Suppl 1), 67-72 (1990)

469 Belmaker RH, Zohar J, Klein E. Are the effects of carbamazepine on blood levels of haloperidol clinically relevant? In:. *International Clinical Psychopharmacology. H Emrich, W Schiwy, T Silverstone (eds)*, London, Clinical Neuroscience Publishers London, 5, (Suppl 1), 67-72 (1990)

470 Belz GG, Aust PE, Munkes R. Digoxin plasma concentrations and nifedipine. *Lancet*, 1, 844-845 (1981)

471 Belz GG, Doering W, Aust PE et al. Quinidine-digoxin interaction: cardiac efficacy of elevated serum digoxin concentration. *Clin Pharmacol Ther*, 31, 548-554 (1982)

472 Belz GG, Doering W, Munkes R et al. Interaction between digoxin and calcium antagonists and antiarrhythmic drugs. *Clin Pharmacol Ther*, 33, 410-417 (1983)

473 Belz GG, Essig J, Kleinbloesem CH et al. Interactions between cilazapril and propranolol in man: plasma drug concentrations, hormone and enzyme responses, haemodynamics, agonist dose-effect curves and baroreceptor reflex. *Br J Clin Pharmacol*, 26, 547-556 (1988)

474 Belz GG, Wistuba S, Matthews JH. Digoxin and bepridil: pharmacokinetic and pharmacodynamic interactions. *Clin Pharmacol Ther*, 39, 65-71 (1986)

475 Bender W, LA France N, Walker WG. Mechanism of deterioration in renal function in patients with renovascular hypertension treated with enalapril. *Hypertension*, 6, Suppl 1, 193-197 (1984)

476 Bendvold E, Gottlieb C, Svanborg K et al. The effect of naproxen on the concentration of prostaglandins in human seminal fluid. *Fertil Steril*, 43, 922 (1985)

477 Beneke M, Wingender W, Horstmann R et al. Neuroendocrine effects of ipsapirone on the hypothalamic-pituitary adrenal axis: CRF, ACTH and cortisol in healthy volunteers. *Eur J Clin Pharmacol*, 42, 163-169 (1992)

478 Ben-Ezer D, Shany S, Conforty A et al. Oral administration of 24,25$(OH)_2$ D_3 suppresses the the serum parathyroid hormone levels of dialysis patients. *Nephron*, 58, 283-287 (1991)

479 Bengtsson B. Plasma concentration and side effects of terbutaline. *Eur J Respir Dis*, 65, Suppl 134, 231-235 (1984)

480 Bengzon A, Hippius H, Kanig K. Some changes in the serum during treatment with psychotropic drugs. *J Nerv Ment Dis*, 143, 369 (1966)

481 Benigni A, Gregorini G, Frusca T et al. Effect of low dose aspirin on fetal and maternal generation of thromboxane by platelets in women at risk for pregnancy-induced hypertension. *N Engl J Med*, 321, 357-362 (1989)

482 Benjamin SB, Ishak KG, Zimmerman HJ et al. Phenylbutazone liver injury: a clinical pathologic survey of 23 cases and review of the literature. *Hepatology*, 1, 255-263 (1981)

483 Benke A, Gogolak G, Stumpf C et al. Althesin and hydroxydione: comparative laboratory and clinical investigations. *Postgrad Med*, 48, Suppl 2, 120 (1972)

484 Bennett JR. Myopathy from ε-aminocaproic acid: a second case. *Postgrad Med J*, 48, 440 (1972)

485 Bennett JS, Bond J, Singer I et al. Hypouricemia in Hodgkin's disease. *Ann Intern Med*, 76, 751 (1972)

486 Bennett PN, John VA, Whitmarsh VB. Effects of rifampin on metoprolol and antipyrine kinetics. *Br J Clin Pharmacol*, 13, 387-391 (1982)

487 Bennett RM, Mohla C. A solid-phase radioimmunoassay for the measurement of lactoferrin in human plasma: variations with age, sex and disease. *J Lab Clin Med*, 88, 156-166 (1976)

488 Bensaid J, Aldigier J-C, Gualde N. Systemic lupus erythematosus syndrome induced by pindolol. *Br Med J*, 2, 1603-1604 (1979)

489 Bensimon G, Lacomblez L, Meininger V et al. A controlled trial of riluzole in amyotrophic lateral sclerosis. *N Engl J Med*, 330, 585-591 (1994)

490 Benzie IFF, Strain JJ. The effect of ascorbic acid on the measurement of total cholesterol and triglycerides: possible artefactual lowering in individuals with high plasma concentration of ascorbic acid. *Clin Chim Acta*, 239, 185-190 (1995)

491 Berardi RR, Hyneck ML, Cohen IA. Effect of cimetidine on serum uric acid concentration. *Clin Pharm*, 3, 56-59 (1984)

492 Berchtold P, Bjorntorp P, Gustafson A et al. Glucose tolerance, plasma insulin and lipids in diabetic subjects before and after treatment. *Eur J Clin Pharmacol*, 4, 22 (1971)

493 Berchtold P, Dahlquist A, Gustafson A et al. Effects of a biguanide (metformin) on vitamin B_{12} and folic acid absorption and intestinal enzyme activities. *Scand J Gastroenterol*, 6, 751 (1971)

494 Berendes E, Mölhoff T, van Aken H, et al. Efects of dopexamine on creatinine clearance, systemic inflammation, and splanchnic oxygenation in patients undergoing coronary artery bypass grafting. *Anesth Analg*, 84, 950-957 (1997)

495 Beresini MH, Davalian D, Alexander S et al. Evaluation of EMIT cyclosporine assay for use with whole blood. *Clin Chem*, 39, 2235-2241 (1993)

496 Berg A, Baumstark MW, Frey I et al. Clinical and therapeutic use of probucol. *Eur J Clin Pharmacol*, 40, Suppl 1, S81-S84 (1991)

497 Berg B. Ascorbate interference in the estimation of urinary glucose by test strips. *J Clin Chem Clin Biochem*, 24, 89-96 (1986)

498 Berg JD, Pandov HI, Sammons HG. Serum total bile acid levels in patients receiving rifampicin and isoniazid. *Ann Clin Biochem*, 21, 218-222 (1984)

499 Berg MJ, Fischer LJ, Rivey MP et al. Phenytoin and folic acid interaction: a preliminary report. *Ther Drug Monit*, 5, 389-394 (1983)

500 Berger M, Potter DE. Pitfall in diagnosis of viral hepatitis in haemodialysis unit. *Lancet*, 2, 95-96 (1977)

501 Berger W, Goschke H, Moppert J et al. Insulin concentrations in portal venous and peripheral venous blood in man following administration of glucose. *Horm Metab Res*, 5, 4 (1973)

502 Berghout A, Wiersinga WM, Brummelkamp WH. Sodium ipodate in the preparation of Graves' hyperthyroid patients for thyroidectomy. *Horm Res*, 31, 256-260 (1989)

503 Bergink EW, Holma P, Pyorala T. Effect of oral contraceptive combinations containing levonorgestrel or desogestrel on serum proteins and androgen binding. *Scand J Clin Lab Invest*, 41, 663-668 (1981)

504 Bergink EW, Kloosterboer HJ, Lund L et al. Effects of levonorgestrel and desogestrel in low-dose oral contraceptive combinations on serum lipids, apolipoproteins A-I and B and glycosylated proteins. *Contraception*, 30, 61-72 (1984)

505 Berglund F, Killander J, Pompeius R. Effect of trimethoprim-sulfamethoxazole on the renal excretion of creatinine in man. *J Urol*, 114, 802-808 (1975)

506 Berglund G. Diuretics in long-term treatment of hypertension: a comparison to β-blockers. *J Cardiovasc Pharmacol*, 6, S256-S259 (1984)

507 Berglund G, Andersson O, Larsson O et al. Antihypertensive effect and side effects of bendroflumethiazide and propranolol. *Acta Med Scand*, 199, 499-506 (1976)

508 Bergman A, Andreen M, Blomback M. Plasma substitution with 3% Dextran-60 in orthopaedic surgery: influence on plasma colloid osmotic pressure, coagulation parameters, immunoglobulins and other plasma constituents. *Acta Anaesthesiol Scand*, 34, 21-29 (1990)

509 Bergman D, Futterweit W, Segal R et al. Increased oestradiol in diazepam related gynecomastia. *Lancet*, 2, 1225-1226 (1981)

510 Berkman K, Tozun N, Taga Y et al. The effect of chronic guanfacine administration on high plasma vasopressin levels in essential hypertension. *Int J Clin Pharmacol Ther Toxicol*, 28, 67-71 (1990)

511 Berkowitz D. Clinical experiences with halofenate, a new hypolipemic and hypouricemic agent. *Circulation*, 46, 251-256 (1977)

512 Berkowitz D. Long-term treatment of hyperlipidemic patients with clofibrate. *J Am Med Ass*, 218, 1002 (1971)

513 Berkowitz D, Spitzer JJ, Likoff WP. Practical significance of serum triglycerides and radioactive fat tolerance: their relation to current therapy. *Am J Cardiol*, 10, 198 (1962)

514 Berlin I, Deray G, Maistre G et al. Cicletanine does not affect plasma atrial natriuretic peptide concentration in healthy subjects. *Eur J Clin Pharmacol*, 39, 593-594 (1991)

515 Berliner AD, Lackner H. Hemorrhagic diathesis after prolonged infusion of low molecular weight Dextran. *Am J Med Sci*, 263, 397 (1972)

516 Bernard GR, Wheeler AP, Russell JA, et al. The effects of ibuprofen on the physiology and survival of patients with sepsis. *N Engl J Med*, 336, 912-918 (1997)

517 Bernasconi S, Orlandini G, Reali N et al. Effect of GnRH on blood polyamines and LH levels in normal and obese children. *Horm Metab Res*, 20, 648-651 (1988)

518 Berneis K, Vosmeer S, Keller U. Effects of glucocorticoids and of growth hormone on serum leptin concentrations. *Eur J Endocrinol*, 135, 663-665 (1996)

519 Bernstein DE, Jeffers L, Erhardtsen E, et al. Recombinant factor VIIa corrects prothrombin time in cirrhotic patients: a preliminary study. *Gastroenterology*, 113, 1930-1937 (1997)

520 Bernstein V, Peretz DI. Lidoflazine - a new drug in the treatment of angina pectoris. *Curr Ther Res*, 14, 483 (1972)

521 Berrettini WH, Garrick NA, Nurnberger JI Jr et al. Intravenous physostigmine increases cerebrospinal fluid neuropeptide-Y. *Biol Psychiat*, 26, 623-630 (1989)

522 Berry JN. Acute myeloblastic leukemia in a benzedrine addict. *South Med J*, 59, 1169 (1966)

523 Berry MN, Mazzachi RD, Peake MJ. Enzymatic spectrophotometric determination of sodium and potassium ions in serum or urine: a simple and satisfactory alternative to the use of flame photometry or ion-selective electrodes. *J Int Fed Clin Chem*, 3, 18-23 (1991)

524 Bershad S, Rubinstein A, Paterniti JR et al. Changes in plasma lipids and lipoproteins during isotretinoin therapy for acne. *N Engl J Med*, 313, 981-985 (1985)

525 Berthelot P, Billing BH. Effect of bunamiodyl on hepatic uptake of sulfobromophthalein in the rat. *Am J Physiol*, 211, 395 (1966)

526 Berthold H, Del Pozo E. Antidiuretic effect of sandostatin (SMS 201-995) in healthy volunteers. *Acta Endocrinol*, 120, 708-714 (1989)

527 Bertino JS Jr, Kozak AJ, Reese RE et al. Hypoprothrombinemia associated with cefamandole: use in a rural teaching hospital. *Arch Intern Med*, 146, 1125-1128 (1986)

528 Bertoli A, Fusco A, Magnani A , et al. Efficacy of low-dose GnRH analogue (Buserelin) in the treatment of hirsutism. *Exp Clin Endocrinol*, 103, 15-20 (1995)

529 Bertorini TE, Palmieri GMA, Griffin JA et al. Effect of dantrolene in Duchenne muscular dystrophy. *Muscle Nerv*, 14, 503-507 (1991)

530 Besa EC, Gorshein D, Gardner FH. Blood volume change in normal and various anemic states in man after androgen administration. *Ann Intern Med*, 76, 869 (1972)

531 Besana C, Zocchi MR, Storti M et al. Effects of short-term lithium treatment on peripheral blood lymphocytes and granulocytes in healthy volunteers. *Ric Clin Lab*, 13, 373-379 (1983)

532 Besser GM, Butler PW, Landon J, Rees L. Influence of amphetamines on plasma corticosteroid and growth hormone levels in man. *Br Med J*, 4, 528 (1969)

533 Bessman AN, Chandrasekar S. Effect of pentylenetetrazol (metrazol) on blood cholesterol concentration in man. *J Am Geriatr Soc*, 17, 25 (1969)

534 Best PJM, Berger PB, Miller VM, Lerman A. The effect of estrogen replacement therapy on plasma hitric oxide and endothelin-1 levels in postmenopausal women. *Ann Intern Med*, 128, 285-288 (1998)

535 Bettoli V, Tosti A, Capobianco C et al. Creatine kinase values during isotretinoin treatment. *Dermatologica*, 180, 54-55 (1990)

536 Beutler E. Drug-induced anemia. *Fed Proc*, 31, 141 (1972)

537 Bevilacqua M, Bettica P, Milani M, et al. Effect of fluvastatin on lipids and fibrinolysis in coronary disease. *Am J Cardiol*, 79, 84-87 (1997)

538 Beyeler C, reichen J, Thomann SR, et al. Quantitative liver function in patients with rheumatoid arthritis treated with low-dose methotrexate: a longitudinal study. *Br J Rheumatol*, 36, 338-344 (1997)

539 Beylot M, Borson F, David L et al. Reduction by propranolol of urinary hydroxyproline excretion in human hyperthyroidism: a β-receptor blockade or a membrane stabilizing mechanism. *Metabolism*, 33, 124-128 (1984)

540 Beylot M, Riou JP, Borson F et al. Reduction of increased levels of blood glycerol and ketone bodies by propranolol in human hyperthyroidism: role of the fall of triiodothyronine levels. *Metabolism*, 33, 1080-1083 (1984)

541 Bhatnagar D, Durrington PN, Mackness MI et al. Effects of treatment of hypertriglyceridemia with gemfibrozil on serum lipoproteins and the transfer of cholesteryl ester from high density lipoproteins to low density lipoproteins. *Atherosclerosis*, 92, 49-57 (1992)

542 B'Hend P, Hadorn B, Haldemann B et al. Stimulation of pancreatic secretion in man by secretin snuff. *Lancet*, 1, 509 (1973)

543 Bhutta ZA, Mansoorali N, Hussain R. Plasma cytokines in paedriatric typhoidal salmonellosis: correlation with clinical course and outcomes. *J Infect*, 35, 253-256 (1997)

544 Biaggioni I, Onrot J, Hollister AS et al. Cardiovascular effects of adenosine infusion in man and their modulation by dipyridamole. *Life Sci*, 39, 2229-2236 (1986)

545 Bianchi S, Bigazzi R, Baldari G et al. Microalbuminuria in patients with essential hypertension: effects of several antihypertensive drugs. *Am J Med*, 93, 525-528 (1992)

546 Bichet DG, Razi M, Arthus M-F et al. Epinephrine and DDAVP® administration in patients with congenital nephrogenic diabetes insipidus. Evidence for a pre-cyclic AMP V_2 receptor defective mechanism. *Kidney Int*, 36, 859-866 (1989)

547 Bick RL, Thompson WB. Fibrinolytic activity: changes induced with oral contraceptives. *Obstet Gynecol*, 39, 213 (1972)

548 Bidlingmaier A, Hammermaier A, Nagyivanyi P et al. Gastrointestinal blood loss induced by three different non-steroidal anti-inflammatory drugs. *Arz Forsch Drug Res*, 45, 491-493 (1995)

549 Bieck PR, Firkusny L, Schick C et al. Monoamine oxidase inhibition by phenelzine and brofaromine in healthy volunteers. *Clin Pharmacol Ther*, 45, 260-269 (1989)

550 Bieger R, Dejonge H, Loeliger EA. Influence of nitrazepam on oral anticoagulation with phenprocoumon. *Clin Pharmacol Ther*, 13, 361 (1972)

551 Bielmann P, Leduc G, Gutkowska J et al. Effects of ketanserin on lipids, lipoproteins, and plasma atrial natriuretic factor in patients with essential hypertension. *J Clin Pharmacol*, 30, 438-443 (1990)

552 Bielmann P, Leduc G, Jequier J-C et al. Changes in the lipoprotein composition after chronic administration of metoprolol and propranolol in hypertriglyceridemic - hypertensive subjects. *Curr Ther Res*, 30, 956-967 (1981)

553 Bielmann P, Leduc G, Thibault G et al. Effects of chlorthalidone and metoprolol alone or in combination (logotron) on blood pressure, lipids, lipoproteins and circulating plasma ANF levels in essential hypertension, 5232

554 Biemond I, Crobach LFSJ, Jansen JBMJ et al. Effect of intermittent administration of omeprazole on serum pepsinogens in duodenal ulcer patients and healthy volunteers. *Br J Clin Pharmacol*, 29, 465-472 (1990)

555 Bierenbaum ML, Reichstein RP, Watkins TR et al. Effects of canola oil on serum lipids in humans. *J Am Coll Nutr*, 10, 228-233 (1991)

556 Biesma DH, van de Wiel A, Beguin Y et al. Erythropoietic activity and iron metabolism in autologous blood donors during recombinant human erythropoietin therapy. *Eur J Clin Invest*, 24, 426-432 (1994)

557 Bieva C, Ladmirant IH, Scheirs I et al. Administered viloxazine interferes in liquid-chromatographic assay of normetanephrines. *Clin Chem*, 33, 1677-1678 (1987)

558 Bigger JT Jr. The quinidine digoxin interaction. *Mod Concept Cardiovasc Dis*, 51, 73-78 (1982)

559 Bigot M-C, Debruyne D, Bonnefoy L et al. Serum digoxin levels related to plasma propafenone levels during concomitant treatment. *J Clin Pharmacol*, 31, 521-626 (1991)

560 Bijvoet OLM. Natriuretic effect of calcitonin in man. *N Engl J Med*, 284, 681 (1971)

561 Bikle DD, Gee E, Halloran B et al. Free 1,25-dihydroxyvitamin D levels in serum from normal subjects, pregnant subjects, and subjects with liver disease. *J Clin Invest*, 74, 1966-1971 (1984)

562 Bilezikian JP. Management of acute hypercalcemia. *N Engl J Med*, 326, 1196-1203 (1992)

563 Billing BH, Black M. The action of drugs on bilirubin metabolism in man. *Ann NY Acad Sci*, 179, 403 (1971)

564 Billing BH, Maggiore Q, Cartter MA. Hepatic transport of bilirubin. *Ann NY Acad Sci*, 111, 319 (1963)

565 Billing BH, Maggiore QS, Goulis G. Action of cholecystographic contrast media and novobiocin on hepatic transport of bilirubin. In:. *Biliary System, W Taylor (ed)*, Oxford, Blackwell (1965)

566 Bimmermann A, Boerschmann C, Schwartzkopff W, et al. Effective therapeutic measures for reducing lipoprotein (A) in patients with dyslipidemia. Lipoprotein (A) reduction with sustained release bezafibrate. *Curr Ther Res*, 49, 635-643 (1991)

567 Bindoli A, Rigobello MP, Cavallini L et al. Decrease of serum malondialdehyde in patients treated with chlorpromazine. *Clin Chim Acta*, 169, 329-332 (1987)

568 Bing RF, Russell GI, Swales JD et al. Indapamide and bendrofluazide: a comparison in the management of essential hypertension. *Br J Clin Pharmacol*, 12, 883-886 (1981)

569 Bing RF, Russell GI, Thurston H et al. Hydralazine in hypertension: is there a safe dose?. *Br Med J*, 2, 353-354 (1980)

570 Biochemex Laboratories. Diagnostic interferences. Materials affecting the diagnostic specificity of laboratory tests. Biochemex Laboratories Inc, Elmont, NY

571 Biollaz J, Munafo A, Buclin T et al. Whole-blood pharmacokinetics and metabolic effects of the topical carbonic anhydrase inhibitor dorzolamide. *Eur J Clin Pharmacol*, 47, 453-460 (1995)

572 Bio-Science Handbook. Specialized Diagnostic Laboratory Tests. *9th Edition*, Bio-Science Laboratories, Van Nuys, CA (1971)

573 Biran S, Tal E. Effect of β-blocking drug propranolol on ^{131}I utilization in euthyroid patients. *J Clin Pharmacol*, 12, 105 (1972)

574 Birch CA. Jaundice due to phenobarbital. *Lancet*, 1, 478 (1936)

575 Bird GW, Eeles GH, Litchfield JA et al. Haemolytic anaemia associated with antibodies to tolbutamide and phenacetin. *Br Med J*, 1, 718 (1972)

576 Bird GWG, McEvoy MW, Wingham J. Acute haemolytic anaemia due to IgM penicillin antibody in a 3 year old child: a sequel to oral penicillin. *J Clin Pathol*, 28, 321-323 (1975)

577 Bird HA, Le Gallez P, Dixon JS et al. A clinical and biochemical assessment of a nonthiol ACE inhibitor (Pentopril; CGS-13945) in active rheumatoid arthritis. *J Rheumatol*, 17, 603-608 (1990)

578 Birke G, Diczfalusy E, Plantin LO. Assessment of the functional capacity of the adrenal cortex: II clinical application of the ACTH test. *J Clin Endocrinol Metab*, 20, 593 (1960)

579 Birkeland KI, Mowinckel P, Furuseth K et al. Long-term randomized placebo-controlled double-blind therapeutic comparison of glipizide and glyburide. *Diabetes Care*, 17, 45-49 (1994)

580 Birnbaum D, Karmeli F, Tefera M. The effect of diazepam on human gastric secretion. *Gut*, 12, 616 (1971)

581 Birnbaum D, Levy M. Diuretics and adverse gastrointestinal reaction. *Digestion*, 4, 362 (1971)

582 Birnie GG, Fitzsimons CP, Czarnecki D et al. Hepatic metabolic function in patients receiving long-term methotrexate therapy: comparison with topically treated psoriatics, patient controls and cirrhotics. *Hepatogastroenterology*, 32, 163-167 (1985)

583 Bisgaard H, Nielsen MD, Andersen B et al. Adrenal function in children with bronchial asthma treated with beclomethasone dipropionate or budesonide. *J Allerg Clin Immunol*, 81, 1088-1095 (1988)

584 Bishell GP, Lewis H, Rooke RA et al. Interference by Parvolex with chloride estimation by the Ag/AgCl method. *Ann Clin Biochem*, 31, 181-183 (1994)

585 Bishnoi A, Carlson HE, Gruber BL et al. Effects of commonly prescribed nonsteroidal anti-inflammatory drugs on thyroid hormone measurements. *Am J Med*, 96, 235-238 (1994)

586 Bissell MG, Hussain S, Sanghavi P et al. A user evaluation of four Kodak Ektachem® slide assays. *Clin Chem*, 34, 964-965 (1988)

587 Bisset LR, Rothen M, Joller-Jemelka HI, et al. Change in circulating levels of the chemokines macrophage inflammatory proteins 1α and 1β, RANTES, monocytic chemotactic protein-1 and interleukin-16 following treatment of severely immunodeficient HIV-infected individuals with indinavir. *AIDS*, 11, 485-491 (1997)

588 Bissonnette F, Lussier-Cacan S, Fugre P, Bırubı S. Metabolic effect of two hormonal preparations in postmenopausal women. *Maturitas*, 27, 275-284 (1997)

589 Bizzaro N, Bagolin E, Milani L et al. Massive rhabdomyolysis and simvastatin. *Clin Chem*, 38, 1504 (1992)

590 Bjorck S, Svalander C, Westberg G. Hydralazine-associated glomerulonephritis. *Acta Med Scand*, 218, 261-269 (1985)

591 Blachley JD, Hill JB. Renal and electrolyte disturbances associated with cisplatin. *Ann Intern Med*, 95, 628-632 (1981)

592 Black JA, Henderson MH. Activation and inhibition of human erythrocyte pyruvate kinase by organic phosphates, amino acids, peptides. *Biochim Biophys Acta*, 284, 115 (1972)

593 Blackard WG. Control of growth hormone secretion in man. *Postgrad Med J*, 49, Suppl, 122 (1973)

594 Blackburn AM, Amiel SA, Millis RR et al. Tamoxifen and liver damage. *Br Med J*, 289, 288 (1984)

595 Blackshear JL, Davidman M, Stillman MT. Identification of risk for renal insufficiency from nonsteroidal anti-inflammatory drugs. *Arch Intern Med*, 143, 1130-1134 (1983)

596 Blackwell CP, Harding SM. The clinical pharmacology of ondansetron. *Eur J Cancer Clin Oncol*, 25, Suppl 1, S21-S24 (1989)

597 Blank DW, Joffe RT. Effect of carbamazepine on thyroid hormone measurement in vitro. *Clin Chim Acta*, 143, 173-176 (1984)

598 Blaschke TF, Elin RJ, Berk PD et al. Effects of induced fever on sulfobromophthalein kinetics in man. *Ann Intern Med*, 78, 221 (1973)

599 Blauhut B, Harringer W, Bettelheim P et al. Comparison of the effects of aprontin and tranexamic acid on blood loss and related variables after cardiopulmonary bypass. *J Thorac Cardiovasc Surg*, 108, 1083-1091 (1994)

600 Bleck P, Smith MC. Possible induction of systemic lupus erythematosus by valproate. *Epilepsia*, 31, 343-345 (1990)

601 Bleyer WA. The clinical pharmacology of methotrexate: new application of an old drug. *Cancer*, 41, 36-51 (1978)

602 Blickstein I, Hagay Z, Goldschmidt R et al. Nifedipine may cause falsely increased spectrophotometric values of urinary vanillylmandelic acid. *Clin Chem*, 39, 365-366 (1993)

603 Bliss BP, Kirk CJC, Newall RG. The effect of fenfluramine on glucose tolerance, insulin, lipid and lipoprotein levels in patients. *Postgrad Med J*, 48, 409 (1972)

604 Bloch A. More on infantile methemoglobinemia due to benzocaine suppository. *J Pediatr*, 67, 509 (1965)

605 Bloch-Michel H, Kyriaco C, Juvin E. Notre experience de l'indomethacine dans les rheumatismes inflammatoires. *Therapie*, 22, 45 (1967)

606 Block LH, Lamy PP. These drugs discolor the feces or urine. *Am Prof Pharm*, 34, 27 (1968)

607 Blohme I, Idstrom J-P, Andersson T. A study of the interaction between omeprazole and cyclosporine in renal transplant patients. *Br J Clin Pharmacol*, 35, 156-160 (1993)

608 Bloomquist JN, Laddu A, Engler R. Adverse effects of acebutolol in chronic stable angina: drug-induced positive antinuclear antibody. *J Cardiovasc Pharmacol*, 6, 735-738 (1984)

609 Blöchl-Daum B, Pehamberger H, Kurz C, et al. Effects of cisplatin on urinary thromboxane B_2 excretion. *Clin Pharmacol Ther*, 58, 418-424 (1995)

610 Blum RA, Schentag JJ, Gardner MJ, Wilner KD. The effect of tenidap sodium on the disposition and plasma protein binding of phenytoin in healthy male volunteers. *Br J Clin Pharmacol*, 39, 35S-38S (1995)

611 Blum RH, Carter SK. Adriamycin® . a new anticancer drug with significant clinical activity. *Ann Intern Med*, 80, 249 (1974)

612 Blumenkrantz N, Sboe-Hansen G. New method for quantitative determination of uronic acids. *Anal Biochem*, 54, 484 (1973)

613 Blumsohn A, Naylor KE, Assiri AMA et al. Different responses of biochemical markers of bone reabsorption to biphosphonate therapy in Paget disease. *Clin Chem*, 41, 1592-1598 (1995)

614 Blunden RW, Lloyd JV, Rudzki Z et al. Changes in serum ferritin levels after intravenous iron. *Ann Clin Biochem*, 18, 215-217 (1981)

615 Blunnie WP, Zacharias M, Dundee JW et al. Liver enzyme studies with continuous intravenous anesthesia. *Anesthesia*, 36, 152-156 (1981)

616 Blyden GT, Greenblatt DJ, Scavone JM. Metronidazole impairs clearance of phenytoin but not alprazolam or lorazepam. *Clin Pharmacol Ther*, 39, 181 (1986)

617 Boardman PL, Hart FD. Side effects of indomethacin. *Ann Rheum Dis*, 26, 127 (1967)

618 Bocchetta A, Bernardi F, Pedditzi M et al. Thyroid abnormalities during lithium treatment. *Acta Psychiat Scand*, 83, 193-198 (1991)

619 Boccuzzi SJ, Bocanegra TS, Walker JF et al. Long-term safety and efficacy profile of simvastatin. *Am J Cardiol*, 68, 1127-1131 (1991)

620 Bock KD, Merguet P, Brandt T et al. Experimental studies with clonidine hydrochloride in normotensive and hypertensive subjects. In:. *Catapres® in Hypertension. ME Conolly (ed)*, London, Butterworth (1970)

621 Bock KW, Wiltfang J, Blume R et al. Paracetamol as test drug to determine glucuronide formation in man. Effects of inducers and of smoking. *Eur J Clin Pharmacol*, 31, 677-683 (1987)

622 Bockner V, Roman W. Oral contraceptives and thyroid status. *Lancet*, 1, 163 (1967)

623 Bodansky O. Methemoglobinemia and methemoglobin-producing compounds. *Pharmacol Rev*, 3, 144 (1951)

624 Bode C, Zelder O, Goeball H et al. Choleresis induced by secretin: distinctly increased response in cirrhotics. *Scand J Gastroenterol*, 7, 697 (1972)

625 Bodenham A, Hoskins R, Carlyle AK et al. The effect of the inotropic agents dopamine, dobutamine and dopexamine on the evening rise of TSH. *Proc ACB Natl Meet*, 52 (1989)

626 Body JJ, Delmas PD. Urinary pyridinium cross-links as markers of bone resorption in tumor-associated hypercalcemia. *J Clin Endocrinol Metab*, 74, 471-475 (1992)

627 Boehning W. Effect of cimetidine and ranitidine on plasma theophylline in patients with chronic obstructive airways disease treated with theophylline and corticosteroids. *Eur J Clin Pharmacol*, 38, 43-45 (1990)

628 Boehringer K, Weidmann P, Mordasini R et al. Menopause-dependent plasma lipoprotein alterations in diuretic treated women. *Ann Intern Med*, 97, 206-209 (1982)

629 Boehringer Mannhein Corp, Therapeutics Division. Manufacturer's literature on Retavase™. Gaithersburg, MD 20878 (1996)

630 Boeijinga JJ, Boerstra EE, Ris P, et al. Interaction between paracetamol and coumarin anticoagulants. *Lancet*, 1, 506 (1982)

631 Boekenoogen SJ, Sholiton LJ, Werk EE Jr et al. Prednisolone disposition and protein binding in oral contraceptive users. *J Clin Endocrinol Metab*, 56, 702-709 (1983)

632 Boer P, van Rijn HJM, Koomans HA et al. Urinary oxalate excretion during intravenous infusion of diuretics in man. *Biochim Clin*, 13, Suppl 1, 229 (1989)

633 Boer WH, Koomans HA, Dorhout Mess EJ. Acute effects of thiazides, with and without carbonic anhydrase inhibiting activity, on lithium and free water clearance in man. *Clin Sci*, 76, 539-545 (1989)

634 Boers M, Dijkmans BAC, Breedveld FC, et al. No effect of misoprostol on renal function of rheumatoid patients treated with diclofenac. *Br J Rheumatol*, 30, 56-59 (1991)

635 Boesgaard S, Hagen C, Andersen AN et al. Effect of fenoldopam, a dopamine D-1 receptor agonist, on pituitary, gonadal and thyroid hormone secretion. *Clin Endocrinol*, 30, 231-239 (1989)

636 Boesgaard S, Hyldstrup L, Feldstedt M. Changes in calcium homeostasis and bone formation in patients recovering from acute myocardial infarction: effect of verapamil treatment. *Eur J Clin Pharmacol*, 41, 521-523 (1991)

637 Boger WP, Strickland SC. Gout. *Lancet*, 1, 420 (1954)

638 Boguneiwicz M, Jaffe HS, Izu A et al. Recombinant γ interferon in treatment with atopic dermatitis and elevated IgE levels. *Am J Med*, 88, 365-370 (1990)

639 Bohler J, Becker A, Reetze-Bonorden P et al. Effect of antihypertensive drugs on glomerular hyperfiltration and renal haemodynamics: comparison of captopril with nifedipine, metoprolol and celiprolol. *Eur J Clin Pharmacol*, 44, Suppl 1, S57-S61 (1993)

640 Boidin MP, Stuurman A, Erdmann W. Ascorbic acid prevents cimetidine-induced decrease of serum hydrocortisone concentrations. *Pharm Weekbl (Sci)*, 12, 151-153 (1990)

641 Bolognese RJ, Corson SL, Touchstone JC. Factors affecting the yield of urinary estriol. *Obstet Gynecol*, 39, 683 (1972)

642 Bolton CH, Jackson L, Roberts CJC et al. Enzyme induction and serum and lipoprotein lipids: a study of glutethimide in normal subjects. *Clin Sci*, 58, 419-421 (1980)

643 Boman G. Mechanism of the inhibitory effect of PAS granules on the absorption of rifampicin: absorption of rifampicin by an excipient, bentonite. *Eur J Clin Pharmacol*, 8, 293 (1975)

644 Bon GB, Soldan S, Cazzolato G et al. Efficacy and tolerability of bezafibrate slow-release formulation vs fenofibrate in the treatment of patients with type IIb hyperlipoproteinemia. *Curr Ther Res*, 47, 735-742 (1990)

645 Bon GG, von Mensdorff-Pouilly S, Kenemans P, et al. Clinical and technical evaluation of ACS™ BR serum assay of MUCI gene-derived glycoprotein in breast cancer, and comparison with CA 15-3 assays. *Clin Chem*, 43, 585-593 (1997)

646 Bonaa KH, Bjerve KS, Straume B et al. Effects of eicosapentaenoic and docosahexaenoic acids on blood pressure in hypertension: a population-based intervention trial from the Tromso study. *N Engl J Med*, 322, 795-801 (1990)

647 Bond PA, Jenner FA, Lee CR et al. The effect of lithium salts on the urinary excretion of α-oxoglutarate in man. *Br J Pharmacol*, 46, 116 (1972)

648 Bond WS. Toxic reactions and side effects of glucocorticoids in man. *Am J Hosp Pharm*, 34, 479-485 (1977)

649 Bondar RJL, Mead DC. Evaluation of glucose-6-phosphate dehydrogenase from leuconostoc mesenteroides in the hexokinase method. *Clin Chem*, 20, 586 (1974)

650 Bonde J, Bdtker S, Angelo HR et al. Atenolol inhibits the elimination of disopyramide. *Eur J Clin Pharmacol*, 28, 41-43 (1985)

651 Bonham JR, Rattenbury JM, Meeks A et al. Pyroglutamicaciduria from vigabatrin. *Lancet*, 1, 1452-1453 (1989)

652 Bonnet G. A multicenter study of doxazosin in the treatment of essential hypertension in France. *Am Heart J*, 121, II Suppl, 335-340 (1991)

653 Bonneterre J, Nguyen M, Hecquet B et al. Dyslipemie induite par l'aminoglutethimide. *Bull Cancer*, 72, 99-103 (1985)

654 Booker HE. Primidone toxicity. In:. *Antiepileptic Drugs, DM Woodbury, JK Penry, RP Schmidt (eds)*, New York NY, Raven Press (1972)

655 Booth JB, Todd GB. Subclinical scurvy - hypovitaminosis C. *Geriatrics*, 27, 130 (1972)

656 Booth RJ, Bullock JY, Wilson JD. Antinuclear antibodies in patients on acebutolol. *Br J Clin Pharmacol*, 9, 515-517 (1980)

657 Borcherding SM, Baciewicz AM, Self TH. Update on rifampin drug interactions. *Arch Intern Med*, 152, 711-716 (1992)

658 Bordia A, Bansal HC. Essential oil of garlic in prevention of atherosclerosis. *Lancet*, 2, 1491 (1973)

659 Borowski GD, Garofano CD, Rose LI et al. Effect of long-term amiodarone therapy on thyroid hormone levels and thyroid function. *Am J Med*, 78, 443-450 (1985)

660 Borud O, Gjessing LR. Excretion of vanylglycol in human urine under dietary control, and during treatment with antibiotics, disulfiram. *Scand J Clin Lab Invest*, 25, 251 (1970)

661 Borushek S, Gold JJ. Commonly used medications that interfere with routine endocrine laboratory procedures. *Clin Chem*, 10, 41 (1964)

662 Borusiak P, Korn-Merker E, Holert N, Boenigk H-E. Hyponatremia induced by oxcarbazine in children. *Epilep Res*, 30, 241-246 (1998)

663 Boston Collaborative Drug Surveillance Program. Acute adverse reactions to prednisone in relation to dosage. *Clin Pharmacol Ther*, 13, 694 (1972)

664 Botana MA, Castillo L, Pesquera C et al. Lack of effect of octreotide on parathyroid levels and urinary excretion of epidermal growth factor. *Horm Metab Res*, 25, 37-39 (1993)

665 Botker HE, Jensen HK, Krusell LR et al. Renal effects of xamoterol in patients with moderate heart failure. *Cardiovasc Drug Ther*, 7, 111-116 (1993)

666 Bottiger LE, Westerholm B. Oral contraceptives and thromboembolic disease. *Acta Med Scand*, 190, 455 (1971)

667 Bouchard P, Sai P, Reach G et al. Diabetes mellitus following pentamidine-induced hypoglycemia in humans. *Diabetes*, 31, 40-45 (1982)

668 Bouillon R, Vanderschueren D, Van Herck E et al. Homologous radioimmunoassay of human osteocalcin. *Clin Chem*, 38, 2055-2060 (1992)

669 Bouloux P-M, Rees LH, Clement-Jones V et al. Erroneous diagnosis of phaeochromocytoma in hypertensive patient on labetalol. *J Roy Soc Med*, 78, 588-589 (1985)

670 Bouloux P-MG, Perrett D. Interference of labetalol metabolites in the determination of plasma catecholamines by HPLC with electrochemical determination. *Clin Chim Acta*, 150, 111-117 (1985)

671 Bönner G, Schmieder R, Chrosch R, Weidinger G. Effect of bunazosin and atenolol on glucose metabolism in obese, nondiabetic patients with primary hypertension. *Cardiovasc Drug Ther*, 11, 21-26 (1997)

672 Bourbigot B, Guiserix J, Airiau J et al. Nicardipine increases cyclosporine blood levels. *Lancet*, 1, 1447 (1986)

673 Bovill EG, Landesman MM, Busch SA et al. Studies on the measurement of protein S in plasma. *Clin Chem*, 37, 1708-1714 (1991)

674 Bowersox JC, Andersen CA. Acute effects of intravenous lipid emulsion infusion on plasma fibronectin. *Nutr Res*, 9, 867-871 (1989)

675 Bowes WA Jr, Katta LR, Droegemueller W et al. Triphasic randomized clinical trial: comparison of effects on carbohydrate metabolism. *Am J Obstet Gynecol*, 161, 1402-1407 (1989)

676 Bowles SK, Cardozo L, Edwards DJ. Quinidine does not alter antipyrine metabolism. *J Clin Pharmacol*, 30, 267-271 (1990)

677 Boyce EG, Dukes GE, Rollins DE et al. The effect of rifampin on theophylline kinetics. *Clin Pharmacol Ther*, 37, 183 (1985)

678 Boyer TD, Rouff SL. Acetaminophen-induced hepatic necrosis and renal failure. *J Am Med Ass*, 218, 440 (1971)

679 Bozzola M, Locatelli F, Gambarana B, et al. Effect of corticosteroid therapy on growth hormone secretion. *Horm Res*, 36, 183-186 (1991)

680 Brachman PS, Mccreary TW, Florence R. Agranulocytosis induced by trimeprazine. *N Engl J Med*, 260, 378 (1959)

681 Brackett J, Durley B, Janczak R et al. Centrifugal ion-selective electrode system for potassium in whole blood. *Clin Chem*, 36, 2126-2130 (1990)

682 Bradford RH, Shear CL, Chremos AN et al. Expanded clinical evaluation of lovastatin (EXCEL) study results. I. Efficacy in modifying plasma lipoproteins and adverse event profile in 8245 patients with moderate hypercholesterolemia. *Arch Intern Med*, 151, 43-49 (1991)

683 Bradford RH, Shear CL, Chremos AN et al. Expanded clinical evaluation of lovastatin (EXCEL) study results: two-year efficacy and safety follow-up. *Am J Cardiol*, 74, 667-673 (1994)

684 Bradley GM, Benson ES. Examination of the urine. In:. *Todd-Sanford Clinical Diagnosis by Laboratory Methods, I Davidsohn, JB Henry (eds)*, Philadelphia PA, WB Saunders (1974)

685 Braeman J. PHA response and cytotoxic drugs. *Lancet*, 2, 818 (1972)

686 Brahen LS, Capone TJ, Capone DM. Naltrexone: lack of effect on hepatic enzymes. *J Clin Pharmacol*, 28, 64-70 (1988)

687 Brainerd H. Current Diagnosis and Treatment -1970. Los Altos CA, Lange Medical Publishers (1970)

688 Brambilla F, Belloi L, Perna G et al. Plasma interleukin-1 beta concentrations in panic disorder. *Psychiat Res*, 54, 135-142 (1994)

689 Bramble MG, Record CO. Drug-induced gastrointestinal disease. *Drugs*, 15, 451-463 (1978)

690 Bramlet DA, Posalaky Z, Olson R. Granulomatous hepatitis as a manifestation of quinidine hypersensitivity. *Arch Intern Med*, 140, 395-397 (1980)

691 Brandle E, Gottwald E, Melzer H et al. Influence of oral contraceptive agents on kidney function and protein metabolism. *Eur J Clin Pharmacol*, 43, 643-646 (1992)

692 Brans YW, Shaffer SG, Bell EF et al. Antipyrine interferes with chemical determination of bromide with simultaneous estimation of total body water and extracellular water. *Clin Chem*, 35, 1367-1370 (1989)

693 Branum E, Cummins L, Bartilson M et al. Effect of two anticoagulants on leukocyte yield and function, and on lysosomal enzyme activity. *Clin Chem*, 34, 110-113 (1988)

694 Brasch RC, Rockoff SC, Kuhn C et al. Contrast media as histamine liberators. *Invest Radiol*, 6, 510 (1971)

695 Brashear J, Zeitvogel C, Jackson J et al. Fluorescent polarization immunoassay of urinary 5-hydroxy-3-indoleacetic acid. *Clin Chem*, 35, 355-359 (1989)

696 Brass C, Galgiani JN, Blaschke TF et al. Disposition of ketoconazole, an oral antifungal, in humans. *Antimicrob Agent Chemother*, 21, 151-158 (1982)

697 Brass EP. Effects of antihypertensive drugs on endocrine function. *Drugs*, 27, 447-458 (1984)

698 Brater DC, Anderson S, Baird B et al. Effects of ibuprofen, naproxen, and sulindac on prostaglandins in men. *Kidney Int*, 27, 66-73 (1985)

699 Brater DC, Brown-Cartwright D, Anderson SA. Effect of high dose etodolac on renal function. *Clin Pharmacol Ther*, 42, 283-289 (1987)

700 Brattström C, Wilczek H, Tydın G, et al. Hyperlipidemia in renal transplant recipients treated with sirolimus (rapamycin). *Transplantation*, 65, 1272-1274 (1998)

701 Braunsteiner H, Herbst M, Sandhofer F. Long-term therapy of adult cases of primary hypertriglyceridaemia with clofibrate. *Germ Med*, 13, 65 (1968)

702 Bray GA, Melvin KEW, Chopra IJ. Effect of tri-iodothyronine on some metabolic responses of obese patients. *Am J Clin Nutr*, 26, 715 (1973)

703 Bray WE. Clinical Laboratory Methods. *5th edition*, St Louis, MO, CV Mosby (1957)

704 Brazer SR, Medoff JR. Sulfonamide-induced pancreatitis. *Pancreas*, 3, 583-586 (1988)

705 Breckenridge A, Welborn TA, Dollery CT et al. Glucose tolerance in hypertensive patients on long-term diuretic therapy. *Lancet*, 1, 61 (1967)

706 Breithaupt K, Belz GG, Spielmanns DG et al. Antihypertensive treatment with cilazapril: resting and exercise blood pressure, hormones and enzymes. *Arz Forsch Drug Res*, 40, 136-141 (1990)

707 Breland BD, Hicks GS Jr. Hepatitis and hemolytic anemia associated with methyldopa therapy. *Drug Intell Clin Pharm*, 16, 489 (1982)

708 Bremer HA, Rotmans N, Brommer EJP et al. Effect of low-dose aspirin during pregnancy on fibrinolytic variables before and after parturition. *Am J Obstet Gynecol*, 172, 986-991 (1995)

709 Breningstall GN, Cich JA. Pseudo valproate-induced hypofibrinogenemia. *Pediatr Neurol*, 14, 345 (1996)

710 Brenner LO. Agranulocytosis and ranitidine. *Ann Intern Med*, 104, 896 (1986)

711 Brest AN, Heider C, Mehbod H. Drug control of diuretic-induced hyperuricemia. *J Am Med Ass*, 195, 42 (1966)

712 Brewer EJ, Giannini EH, Baum J et al. Aspirin and fenoprofen (nalfon®) in the treatment of juvenile rheumatoid arthritis. *J Rheumatol*, 9, 123-128 (1982)

713 Brewer NS, Hellinger WC. The monolactams. *Mayo Clin Proc*, 66, 1152-1157 (1991)

714 Brewster MA, Starrett W. Therapeutic agents affecting amino acid chromatograms. *Clin Chem*, 35, 1999-2000 (1989)

715 Brezin JH, Katz SM, Schwartz AB et al. Reversible renal failure and nephrotic syndrome associated with non-steroidal anti-inflammatory drugs. *N Engl J Med*, 301, 1271-1273 (1979)

716 Brichard S, Ketelslegers JM, Lambert AE. Renal function, glycemic control and peridopril in diabetic patients. *Clin Exp Hypertens*, 11, Suppl 2, 545-554 (1989)

717 Brickman AS, Carlson HE, Deftos LJ. Prolactin and calcitonin responses to parathyroid hormone infusion in hypoparathyroid, pseudohypoparathyroid and normal subjects. *J Clin Endocrinol Metab*, 53, 661-664 (1981)

718 Brickman AS, Coburn JW, Koppel M et al. Effect of hydrochlorothiazide on calcium metabolism. *J Clin Invest*, 50, 13 (1971)

719 Brickman AS, Coburn JW, Massry SG et al. Biologic actions of 1,25-dihydroxycholecalciferol in man. *Clin Res*, 21, 250 (1973)

720 Brickman AS, Isenberg JI. Secretin increases serum calcium in man. *Clin Res*, 20, 236 (1972)

721 Brigden ML, Edgell D, McPherson M et al. High incidence of significant urinary ascorbic acid concentrations in a west coast population -- implications for routine urinalysis. *Clin Chem*, 38, 426-431 (1992)

722 Briggs M, Briggs M. Endocrine effects on serum vitamin B_{12}. *Lancet*, 2, 1037 (1972)

723 Briggs MH, Briggs M. Anti-estrogenic effects of progestogens in normal women. *Life Sci*, 11, 949 (1972)

724 Brismar K, Hylander B, Eliasson K et al. Melatonin secretion related to side-effects of β-blockers from the central nervous system. *Acta Med Scand*, 223, 525-530 (1988)

725 Bristol-Myers Squibb Company. Manufacturer's literature on Avapro® . Princeton, NJ 08543 (1997)

726 Bristol-Myers Squibb Company. Manufacturer's literature on Glucophage® . Princeton, NJ (1998)

727 Bristol-Myers Squibb Company. Manufacturer's literature on Maxipime® . Princeton, NJ 08543 (1997)

728 Bristol-Myers Squibb Company. Manufacturer's literature on Pravachol® . Princeton. NJ (1997)

729 Bristol-Myers Squibb Company. Manufacturer's literature on Serzone® . Princeton, NJ 08543 (1996)

730 Bristol-Myers Squibb Company. Manufacturer's literature on Videx® . Princeton, NJ 08543 (1997)

731 Bristol-Myers Squibb Company. Manufacturer's literature on Zerit® . Princeton, NJ 08543 (1996)

732 Britton JP, Dowell AC, Whelan P. Dipstick haematuria: its association with smoking and nonsteroidal anti-inflammatory drugs. *J Roy Soc Med*, 83, 149-151 (1990)

733 Brockmeyer NH, Breithaupt H, Ferdinand W et al. Kinetics of oral and intravenous mexiletine: lack of effect on cimetidine and ranitidine. *Eur J Clin Pharmacol*, 36, 375-378 (1989)

734 Brockmeyer NH, Kreuzfelder E, Chalabi N et al. The immunomodulatory potency of cimetidine in healthy volunteers. *Int J Clin Pharmacol Ther Toxicol*, 27, 458-462 (1989)

735 Brod J, Horbach L, Just H et al. Acute effects of clonidine on central and peripheral haemodynamics and plasma renin activity. *Eur J Clin Pharmacol*, 4, 107 (1972)

736 Brodie A. Aromatase and its inhibitors - an overview. *J Steroid Biochem Mol Biol*, 40, 255-261 (1991)

737 Brodie MJ, Boobis AR, Hillyard CJ et al. Effect of isoniazid on vitamin D metabolism and hepatic monooxygenase activity. *Clin Pharmacol Ther*, 30, 363-367 (1981)

738 Brodie MJ, Boobis PR, Dollery CT et al. Rifampicin and vitamin D metabolism. *Clin Pharmacol Ther*, 27, 810-814 (1980)

739 Brodie MJ, MacPhee GJ. Carbamazepine neurotoxicity precipitated by diltiazem. *Br Med J*, 292, 1170-1171 (1986)

740 Broekhuysen J, Deger F, Douchamps J et al. Effect of oxametacin on endogenous uric acid clearance rate in healthy volunteers. *Eur J Clin Pharmacol*, 24, 671-673 (1983)

741 Brogden RN, Speight TM, Avery GS. Levodopa: a review of its pharmacological properties and therapeutic uses. *Drugs*, 2, 262 (1971)

742 Brohee D, Piro P, Kennes B et al. In vitro effects of flunarizine on human lymphocytes. *Cytobios*, 45, 139-146 (1986)

743 Brohult A, Brohult J, Brohult S. Effects of alkoxyglycerols on the serum ornithine carbamoyl transferase in connection with radiation treatment. *Experientia*, 28, 146 (1972)

744 Brompton Hospital/Medical Research Council Collaboration. Long-term study of disodium cromoglycate in treatment of severe extrinsic or intrinsic bronchial asthma in adults. *Br Med J*, 4, 383 (1972)

745 Brook I. Leukopenia and agranulocytopenia after oxacillin therapy. *South Med J*, 70, 565-566 (1977)

746 Brooks FP. Testing pancreatic function. *N Engl J Med*, 286, 300 (1972)

747 Brooks PM, Cossum PA, Boyd GW. Rebound rise in renin concentrations after cessation of salicylates. *N Engl J Med*, 303, 562-564 (1980)

748 Brooks SM, Sholiton LJ, Werk EE Jr et al. The effects of ephedrine and theophylline on dexamethasone metabolism in bronchial asthma. *J Clin Pharmacol*, 17, 308-318 (1977)

749 Brooks SM, Werk EE, Ackerman SJ et al. Adverse effects of phenobarbital on corticosteroid metabolism in patients with bronchial asthma. *N Engl J Med*, 286, 1125-1128 (1972)

750 Brosen K, Hansen JG, Nielsen KK, et al. Inhibition by paroxetine of desipramine metabolism in extensive but not in poor metabolizers of sparteine. *Eur J Clin Pharmacol*, 44, 349-355 (1993)

751 Broulik PD, Stepan JJ, Soucek K et al. Alterations in human serum alkaline phosphatase and its bone isoenzyme by chronic administration of lithium. *Clin Chim Acta*, 140, 151-155 (1984)

752 Bröijersın A, Eriksson M, Angelin B, Hjemdahl P. Gemfibrozil enhances platelet activity in patients with combined hyperlipoproteinemia. *Arterioscler Thromb*, 15, 121-127 (1995)

753 Brown BA, Griffiths DE, Girard W, et al. Relationship of adverse events to serum drug levels in patients receiving high-dose azithromycin for mycobacterial lung disease. *Clin Infect Dis*, 24, 958-964 (1997)

754 Brown CB. Tetracycline and renal function. *Br Med*, 4, 428 (1971)

755 Brown CD, Azrolan N, Thomas L et al. Reduction of lipoprotein(a) following treatment with lovastatin in patients with unremitting nephrotic syndrome. *Am J Kid Dis*, 26, 170-177 (1995)

756 Brown CH III, Bradshaw MW, Natelson EA et al. Defective platelet function following the administration of penicillin compounds. *Blood*, 47, 949-956 (1976)

757 Brown CL, Backhouse CI, Grippat JC et al. The effect of perindopril and hydrochlorothiazide alone and in combination on blood pressure and on the renin-angiotensin system in hypertensive subjects. *Eur J Clin Pharmacol*, 39, 327-332 (1990)

758 Brown CR, Forrest WH Jr, Hayden J et al. Respiratory effects of hydromorphone in man. *Clin Pharmacol Ther*, 14, 331 (1973)

759 Brown CS, Wells BG, Cold JA et al. Possible influence of carbamazepine on plasma imipramine concentrations in children with attention deficit hyperactivity disorder. *J Clin Psychopharmacol*, 10, 359-362 (1990)

760 Brown DD, Juhl RP. Decreased bioavailability of digoxin due to antacids and kaolin-pectin. *N Engl J Med*, 295, 1034-1037 (1976)

761 Brown DD, Juhl RP, Warner SL. Decreased bioavailability of digoxin due to hypocholesterolemic interventions. *Circulation*, 58, 164-172 (1978)

762 Brown DD, Schmid J, Long RA et al. A steady-state evaluation of the effects of propantheline bromide and cholestyramine on the the bioavailability of digoxin when administered as tablets or capsules. *J Clin Pharmacol*, 25, 360-364 (1985)

763 Brown DW, Keller TA, Crumlish J et al. Carbamazepine-induced increases in total serum cholesterol: clinical and theoretical implications. *J Clin Psychopharmacol*, 12, 431-437 (1992)

764 Brown GM, Garfinkel PE, Warsh JJ et al. Effect of carbidopa on prolactin, growth hormone and cortisol secretion in man. *J Clin Endocrinol Metab*, 43, 236-239 (1976)

765 Brown GR. Cephalosporin-probenecid drug interactions. *Clin Pharmacokinet*, 24, 289-300 (1993)

766 Brown JH, Murphy BG, Douglas AF, et al. Influence of immunosuppressive therapy on lipoprotein(a) and other lipoproteins following renal transplantation. *Nephron*, 75, 277-282 (1997)

767 Brown LS, Sawyer RC, Li R, et al. Lack of a pharmacologic interaction between rifabutin and methadone in HIV-infected former injecting drug users. *Drug Alcohol Dep*, 43, 71-77 (1996)

768 Brown PJE, Lesna M, Hamlyn AN et al. Primary biliary cirrhosis after long-term practolol administration. *Br Med J*, 2, 1591 (1978)

769 Brown RD, Billman GE, Kem DC et al. The effect of metoclopramide and dopamine on plasma aldosterone concentrations in normal man and rhesus monkeys (Macaca Mulatta): a new model to study dopamine control of aldosterone secretion. *J Clin Endocrinol Metab*, 55, 828-832 (1982)

770 Brown RR. Aminoaciduria resulting from cycloleucine administration in man. *Science*, 157, 432 (1967)

771 Brown S, Miller WG. Determination of magnesium in serum by the Technicon SMAC with a calmagite method with blank correction. *Clin Chem*, 36, 1990-1991 (1990)

772 Brown WA, Laughren TP, Williams B. Differential effects of neuroleptic agents on the pituitary gonadal axis in men. *Arch Gen Psychiat*, 38, 1270-1272 (1981)

773 Brown WV, Dujovne CA, Farquhar JW et al. Effects of fenofibrate on plasma lipids. double-blind, multicenter study in patients with type IIa or type IIb hyperlipidemia. *Arterioscler Thromb*, 6, 670-678 (1986)

774 Browne TR. Valproic acid. *N Engl J Med*, 302, 661-666 (1980)

775 Browning RH, Donnerberg RL. Capreomycin experiences in patient acceptance and toxicity. *Ann NY Acad Sci*, 135, 1057 (1966)

776 Broxson EH Jr, Stork LC, Allen RH et al. Changes in plasma methionine and total homocysteine levels in patients receiving methotrexate infusions. *Cancer Res*, 49, 5879-5883 (1989)

777 Broyles DL, Nielsen RG, Bussett EM, et al. Analytical and clinical performance characteristics of Tandem-MP Ostase, a new immunoassay for serum bone alkaline phosphatase. *Clin Chem*, 44, 2139-2147 (1998)

778 Brtel T, Billing B, Dahlqvist R. Felodipine reduces the absorption of theophylline in man. *Eur J Clin Pharmacol*, 36, 481-485 (1989)

779 Bruckner FE, Randle AP. The use of indomethacin in rheumatoid arthritis. *Ann Phys Med*, 8, 100 (1965)

780 Bruckner HW, Creasey WA. The administration of 5-fluorouracil by mouth. *Cancer*, 33, 14-18 (1974)

781 Brun LD, Gagne C, Rousseau C et al. Severe lipemia induced by tamoxifen. *Cancer*, 57, 2123-2126 (1986)

782 Brune GG, Pflughaupt KW. Effects of L-dopa treatment on indole metabolism in Parkinson's disease. *Experientia*, 27, 516 (1971)

783 Bruni J, Lee CS, Perchalski RJ et al. Interactions of valproic acid with phenytoin. *Neurology*, 30, 1233-1236 (1980)

784 Bruni J, Wilder BJ, Perchalski RJ et al. Valproic acid and plasma levels of phenobarbital. *Neurology*, 30, 94-97 (1980)

785 Brunkhorst R, Wrenger E, Koch KM. Low-dose prednisolone/chloramphenicol therapy in patients with severe membranous glomerulonephritis. *Clin Investig*, 72, 277-282 (1994)

786 Brunkhorst R, Wrenger E, Kuhn K et al. Effects of a captopril-therapy on sodium- and water-excretion in patients with liver cirrhosis and ascites. *Klin Wschr*, 67, 774-783 (1989)

787 Brussaard HE, Gevers Leuven JA, Kluft C, et al. Effect of 17β-estradiol on plasma lipids and LDL oxidation in postmenopausal women with type II diabetes mellitus. *Areterioscler Vasc Biol*, 17, 324-330 (1997)

788 Brutigam C, Wevers RA, Jansen RJT, et al. Biochemical hallmarks of tyrosine hydroxylase deficiency. *Clin Chem*, 44, 1897-1904 (1998)

789 Bruton J, Li TK, Smith GD. Comparison of results by 4 different procedures for determination of 17-hydroxycorticosteroids. *Clin Chem*, 19, 748 (1973)

790 Bryant JM, Yu TF, Berger L et al. Hyperuricemia induced by the administration of chlorthalidone and other sulfonamide diuretics. *Am J Med*, 33, 408 (1962)

791 Bryskov J, Freund L, Rasmussen SN et al. A placebo-controlled, double-blind, randomized trial of cyclosporine therapy in active chronic Crohn's disease. *N Engl J Med*, 321, 845-850 (1989)

792 Buchanan GR, Holtkamp CA, Johnson A. Reduced serum haptoglobin values in hemophiliacs receiving monoclonally purified factor VIII concentrates. *Am J Hematol*, 33, 234-237 (1990)

793 Buchanan RA. Ethosuximide toxicity. In:. *Antiepileptic Drugs, DM Woodbury, JK Penry, RP Schmidt (eds)*, New York NY, Raven Press (1972)

794 Bucht G, Wahlin A. Renal concentrating capacity in long-term lithium treatment and after withdrawal of lithium. *Acta Med Scand*, 207, 309-314 (1980)

795 Buckley JE, Clark VL, Meyer TJ et al. Hypomagnesemia after cisplatin combination chemotherapy. *Arch Intern Med*, 144, 2347-2348 (1984)

796 Buckman MT, Kaminsky N, Conway M et al. Water-load - a new test for prolactin suppression. *Clin Res*, 21, 486 (1973)

797 Buckman MT, Peake GT. Estrogen potentiation of phenothiazine-induced prolactin secretion in man. *J Clin Endocrinol Metab*, 37, 977 (1973)

798 Budaj A, Herbaczynska-Cedro K, Kokot F, Ceremuzynski L. Effect of early captopril treatment on blood adrenaline levels in acute myocardial infarction (the substudy of ISIS-4). *Am J Cardiol*, 81, 335-339 (1998)

799 Bueno J, Amiguet JA, Carasusan J et al. Bisoprolol vs chlorthalidone: a randomized, double-blind , comparative study in arterial hypertension. *J Cardiovasc Pharmacol*, 16, Suppl 5, S189-S192 (1990)

800 Bugge JF. Severe hyperkalemia induced by trimethoprim in combination with an angiotensin-converting enzyme inhibitor in a patient with transplanted lungs. *J Intern Med*, 240, 249-252 (1996)

801 Buhler FR, Laragh JH, Baer L et al. Propranolol inhibition of renin secretion. *N Engl J Med*, 287, 1209 (1972)

802 Bulbrook RD, Hayward JL. Excretion of urinary 17-hydroxycorticosteroids and 11-deoxy-17-oxosteroids by women. *Lancet*, 2, 1033 (1969)

803 Bull J, MacKinnon J. Phenylbutazone and anticoagulant control. *Practitioner*, 215, 767-769 (1975)

804 Bunney WE Jr, Goodwin FK, Davis JM et al. A behavioral-biochemical study of lithium treatment. *Am J Psychiat*, 125, 499 (1968)

805 Burack DA, Griffith BP, Thompson ME et al. Hyperuricemia and gout among heart transplant recipients receiving cyclosporine. *Am J Med*, 92, 141-146 (1992)

806 Burch PG, Migeon CJ. Systemic absorption of topical steroids. *Arch Ophthalmol*, 79, 174 (1968)

807 Burch RE, Parker M, Luby RJ et al. Oral contraceptives and trace metals. *Clin Res*, 20, 774 (1972)

808 Burckart GJ, Venkataramanan R, Starzy TE et al. Cyclosporine clearance in children following organ transplantation. *J Clin Pharmacol*, 24, 412 (1984)

809 Burdick L, Panigo F, Pini C. Effects of etozolin on lipid metabolism in hypertensive patients. *Curr Ther Res*, 43, 997-1001 (1988)

810 Burger A, Dinichert D, Nicod P et al. Effect of amiodarone on serum tri-iodothyronine, reverse tri-iodothyronine, thyroxine and thyrotropin: a drug influencing peripheral metabolism of thyroid hormones. *J Clin Invest*, 58, 255-259 (1976)

811 Burgess E, Cutler RE, Blair AD. Cimetidine pharmacokinetics in hemodialysis patients and inhibition of creatinine secretion in healthy subjects. *Clin Pharmacol Ther*, 27, 247 (1980)

812 Burgess JL, Birchall R. Nephrotoxicity of amphotericin B, with emphasis on changes in tubular function. *Am J Med*, 53, 77 (1972)

813 Burgunder JM, Varriale A, Lauterburg BH. Effect of N-acetylcysteine on plasma cystine and glutathione following paracetamol administration. *Eur J Clin Pharmacol*, 36, 127-131 (1989)

814 Buris L, Varga M. Change of alcohol dehydrogenase activity in sera after alcoholism treatment. *Eur J Clin Chem Clin Biochem*, 30, 203-204 (1992)

815 Burke CW. The effect of oral contraceptives on cortisol metabolism. *J Clin Pathol*, 3, suppl, 11 (1969)

816 Burkman RT, Robinson JC, Kruzson-Moran D et al. Lipid and lipoprotein changes associated with oral contraceptive use: a randomized clinical trial. *Obstet Gynecol*, 71, 33-38 (1988)

817 Burkman RT, Zacur HA, Kimball AW et al. Oral contraceptives and lipids and lipoproteins; Part 1; Variations in mean levels by oral contraceptive type. *Contraception*, 40, 553-561 (1989)

818 Burland WL. Fenfluramine and haemolytic anaemia. *Br Med J*, 1, 419 (1973)

819 Burnakis TG, Seldon M, Dzalplicki AD. Increased serum theophylline concentrations secondary to oral verapamil. *Clin Pharmacol Ther*, 3, 458-461 (1983)

820 Burr RG. A source of error with the calcium-specific ion electrode. solvent effects in aqueous solution. *Clin Chim Acta*, 43, 311 (1973)

821 Burrell CD. Fatal marrow aplasia after treatment with carbimazole. *Br Med J*, 1, 1456 (1956)

822 Burroughs Wellcome Co. Treatment of neoplastic diseases - manufacturer's brochure. Tuckahoe, NY (1971)

823 Burrow GN, Burke WR, Himmelhoch JM et al. Effect of lithium on thyroid function. *J Clin Endocrinol Metab*, 32, 647 (1971)

824 Burry HC, Dieppe PA. Apparent reduction of endogenous creatinine clearance by salicylate treatment. *Br Med J*, 2, 16-17 (1976)

825 Burstein S, Klaiber EL. Phenobarbital-induced increase in 6-β-hydroxycortisol excretion: clue to its significance in human urine. *J Clin Endocrinol Metab*, 25, 293 (1965)

826 Buscaglia AJ, Cowden FE, Brill H. Pulmonary infiltrates associated with naproxen. *J Am Med Ass*, 25, 65-66 (1984)

827 Bussey HI. Update on the influence of quinidine and other agents on digitalis glycosides. *Am Heart J*, 107, 143-146 (1984)

828 Bussey HI, Farringer J, Merritt GJ. Influence of rifampin on quinidine and digoxin. *Arch Intern Med*, 144, 1021-1023 (1984)

829 Bussien JP, d'Amore TF, Perret L et al. Single and repeated dosing of the converting enzyme inhibitor perindopril to normal subjects. *Clin Pharmacol Ther*, 39, 554-558 (1986)

830 Butler KM, Husson RN, Balis FM et al. Dideoxyinosine in children with symptomatic human immunodeficiency virus infection. *N Engl J Med*, 324, 137-144 (1991)

831 Butler WT, Bennett JE, Hill GJ II et al. Electrocardiographic and electrolyte abnormalities caused by amphotericin B in dog and man. *Proc Soc Exp Biol Med*, 116, 857 (1964)

832 Butler WT, Rossen RD. Effect of corticosteroids on immunity in man. *J Clin Invest*, 52, 2629 (1973)

833 Buttery JE, Boord S, Ludvigsen N. Ascorbate interference in the urinary screen for acetaminophen. *Clin Chem*, 34, 769 (1988)

834 Buttner H. Question and answer section. *Germ Med*, 13, 247 (1968)

835 Byington RP, Furberg CD, Crouse III JR, et al. Pravastatin, lipids, and atherosclerosis in the carotid arteries (PLAC-II). *Am J Cardiol*, 76, 54C-59C (1995)

836 Byrd RB, Horn BR, Griggs GA et al. Isoniazid chemoprophylaxis: association with detection and incidence of liver toxicity. *Arch Intern Med*, 137, 1130-1133 (1977)

837 Cacoub P, Deray G, Baumelou A et al. Disopyramide-induced hypoglycemia: case report and review of the literature. *Fundam Clin Pharmacol*, 3, 527-535 (1989)

838 Cadeddu G, Lipponi G, Gasparrini PM et al. Cholestatic hepatitis due to propafenone therapy: a case report. *Curr Ther Res*, 50, 442-447 (1991)

839 Cagnacci A, Mallus E, Tuveri F, et al. Effect of tibolone on glucose and lipid metabolism in postmenopausal women. *J Clin Endocrinol Metab*, 82, 251-253 (1997)

840 Cain MD, Walters WA, Catt KJ. Effects of oral contraceptive therapy on the renin-angiotensin system. *J Clin Endocrinol Metab*, 33, 671 (1971)

841 Cairo MS. Adverse reactions of L-asparaginase. *Am J Pediat Hematol Oncol*, 4, 335-339 (1982)

842 Calandre EP, Porta BS, Garcia de la Calzada D. The effect of chronic phenytoin treatment on serum lipid profile in adult epileptic patients. *Epilepsia*, 33, 154-157 (1992)

843 Calandre EP, Rodriguez-Lopez C, Blazquez A et al. Serum lipids, lipoproteins and apolipoproteins A and B in epileptic patients treated with valproic acid, carbamazepine or phenobarbital. *Acta Neurol Scand*, 83, 250-253 (1991)

844 Caldara R, Cambielli M, Masci E et al. Effect of loperamide and naloxone on gastric acid secretion in healthy man. *Gut*, 22, 720-723 (1981)

845 Calhoun WJ. Summary of clinical trials with zafirlukast. *Am J Resp Crit Care Med*, 157, 5238-5246 (1998)

846 Calil HM, Lesieur P, Gold PW et al. Hormonal responses to zimeldine and desipramine in depressed patients. *Psychiat Res*, 13, 231-242 (1984)

847 Callaghan JT, Tsuru M, Holtzman JL et al. Effect of cholestyramine and colestipol on the absorption of phenytoin. *Eur J Clin Pharmacol*, 24, 675-678 (1983)

848 Callis L, Vila A, Nieto J et al. Effect of cyclosporin A on proteinuria in patients with Alport's syndrome. *Pediatr Nephrol*, 6, 140-144 (1992)

849 Callister TQ, Raggi P, Cooil B, et al. Effect of HMG-CoA reductase inhibitors on coronary artery disease as assessed by electron-beam computed tomography. *N Engl J Med*, 339, 1972-1978 (1998)

850 Calne DB, Karoum F, Ruthven CRJ. The metabolism of orally administered L-dopa in Parkinsonism. *Br J Pharmacol*, 37, 57 (1969)

851 Calo L, Cantaro S, Favaro S et al. Urinary excretion of prostanoids during treatment with enalapril compared with captopril. *Curr Ther Res*, 49, 376-382 (1991)

852 Cals MJ, Bailly M. Interference of Drugs in Enzymology. In:. *Reference Values In Human Chemistry, G Siest (ed)*, Basel, Karger, 292 (1973)

853 Calvin J, Pountain GD, Hazelman BL. Effect of short-term corticosteroid administration on the concentration of serum proteins. *Ann Clin Biochem*, 32, 213-215 (1995)

854 Cam JM, Luck VA, Eastwood JB et al. The effect of aluminum hydroxide orally on calcium, phosphorus and aluminum metabolism in normal subjects. *Clin Sci Mol Med*, 51, 407-414 (1976)

855 Camara PD, Audette L, Velletri K et al. False-positive immunoassay results for urine benzodiazepine in patients receiving oxaprozin (Daypro). *Clin Chem*, 41, 115-116 (1995)

856 Camenzind E, Nussberger J, Juillerat L et al. Effect of the renin response during renin inhibition: oral Ro 42-5892 in normal humans. *J Cardiovasc Pharmacol*, 18, 299-307 (1991)

857 Cameron A, Eisen AA, Niranjan LM. Aplastic anemia due to phenylbutazone. *Postgrad Med J*, 42, 49 (1966)

858 Cameron EHD, Scarisbrick JJ. Radioimmunoassay of plasma progesterone. *Clin Chem*, 19, 1403 (1973)

859 Campana C, Regazzi MB, Buggia I, Molinaro M. Clinically significant drug interactions with cyclosporin. *Clin Pharmacokinet*, 30, 141-179 (1996)

860 Campbell CA, Peet M, Ward NI. Vanadium and other trace elements in patients taking lithium. *Biol Psychiat*, 24, 775-761 (1988)

861 Campbell DJ, Mendelsohn FAO, Adam WR et al. Is aldosterone secretion under dopaminergic control?. *Circ Res*, 49, 1217-1227 (1981)

862 Campbell MA, Plachetka JR, Jackson JE et al. Cimetidine decreases theophylline clearance. *Ann Intern Med*, 95, 68-69 (1981)

863 Campbell NRC, Hasinoff BB. Iron supplements: a common cause of drug interactions. *Br J Clin Pharmacol*, 31, 251-255 (1991)

864 Campbell NRC, Hasinoff BB, Stalts H et al. Ferrous sulfate reduces thyroxine efficacy in patients with hypothyroidism. *Ann Intern Med*, 117, 1010-1013 (1992)

865 Campbell NRC, Kara M, Hasinoff BB et al. Norfloxacin interaction with antacids and minerals. *Br J Clin Pharmacol*, 33, 115-116 (1992)

866 Campbell NRG, Wickert WA, Shumak SL. Frusemide causes acute increases in lipid concentrations. *Br J Clin Pharmacol*, 36, 607-609 (1993)

867 Campbell RS, Hollifield RD, Varsani H et al. Development of an enzyme-mediated assay for phenylalanine in blood spots. *Ann Clin Biochem*, 31, 140-146 (1994)

868 Campos H, Wilson PW, Jimenez D et al. Differences in apolipoproteins and low-density lipoprotein subfractions in postmenopausal women on and off estrogen therapy: results from the Framingham Offspring study. *Metabolism*, 39, 1033-1038 (1990)

869 Campos H, Wilson PWF, Jimenez D et al. Differences in apolipoproteins and low-density lipoprotein subfractions in postmenopausal women on and off estrogen therapy: results from the Framingham Offspring study. *Metabolism*, 39, 1033-1038 (1990)

870 Canadian Multicentre Transplant Study Group. A randomized clinical trial of cyclosporine in cadaveric renal transplantation. *N Engl J Med*, 309, 809-815 (1983)

871 Cannon JE, Fahey MR, Moss J et al. Large doses of vecuronium and plasma histamine concentrations. *Can J Anaes*, 35, 350-353 (1988)

872 Cano A, Parrilla JJ, Abad L. Effect of exogenous and endogenous gonadotropin-releasing hormone on prolactin secretion in perimenopausal women. *Gynecol Obstet Invest*, 26, 308-312 (1988)

873 Canoso RT, De Oliveira RM. Chlorpromazine-induced anticardiolipin antibodies and lupus anticoagulant: Absence of thrombosis. *Am J Hematol*, 27, 272-275 (1988)

874 Cantatore FP, Carrozzo M, Magil DM et al. The action of anabolic steroids in increasing serum 1,25$(OH)_2D_3$ and Gla protein in osteoporotic females. *Clin Trials J*, 25, 65-71 (1988)

875 Cantwell BMJ, Pooley J, Harris AL. False-positive ketonuria during ifosfamide and mesna therapy. *Eur J Cancer Clin Oncol*, 22, 229-230 (1986)

876 Capewell S, Freestone S, Critchley JAJH et al. Gross reduction in felodipine bioavailability in patients taking anticonvulsants. *Br J Clin Pharmacol*, 24, 243-244 (1987)

877 Capizzi RL, Bertino JR, Handschumacher RE. L-asparaginase. *Ann Rev Med*, 21, 433 (1970)

878 Capurso A. Drugs affecting triglycerides. *Cardiology*, 78, 218-225 (1991)

879 Caraway WT. Chemical and diagnostic specificity of laboratory tests. *Am J Clin Pathol*, 37, 445 (1962)

880 Caraway WT. Non-urate chromogens in body fluids. *Clin Chem*, 15, 720 (1969)

881 Caraway WT. Sources of error in clinical chemistry. *Stand Meth Clin Chem*, 5, 19 (1965)

882 Caraway WT, Kammeyer CW. Chemical interference by drugs and other substances with clinical laboratory test procedures. *Clin Chim Acta*, 41, 395 (1972)

883 Carballo-Dieguez A, Sahs J, Goetz R. The effect of methadone on immunological parameters among HIV-positive and HIV-negative drug users. *Am J Drug Alcohol Abuse*, 20, 317-329 (1994)

884 Carbo M, Segura J, de la Torre R et al. Effect of quinolones on caffeine disposition. *Clin Pharmacol Ther*, 45, 234-240 (1989)

885 Cardinaels C, Rijntjes J. FT3 assay for the Auraflex immunoassay system. *Clin Chem*, 41, S45 (1995)

886 Carey DL, Day RO, Bowden FJ. Managing HIV: Quick reference; drug interactions. Common drug interactions in HIV medicine. *Med J Aust*, 164, 605-606 (1996)

887 Carey HM. Principles of oral contraceptives: 2. Side effects of oral contraceptives. *Med J Aust*, 2, 1242 (1971)

888 Carloss HW, Tavassoli M, Mcmillan R. Cimetidine-induced granulocytopenia. *Ann Intern Med*, 93, 57-58 (1980)

889 Carlsen JE, Jensen HE, Rehling M et al. Long term haemodynamic effects of pinacidil and hydralazine in arterial hypertension. *Drugs*, 36, Suppl 7, 55-63 (1988)

890 Carlsen JE, Kober L, Torp-Pedersen C et al. Relationship between dose of bendrofluazide, antihypertensive effect, and adverse biochemical effects. *Br Med J*, 300, 975-978 (1990)

891 Carlson HE, Brickman AS, Bottazzo GF. Prolactin deficiency in pseudohypoparathyroidism. *N Engl J Med*, 296, 140-144 (1977)

892 Carlstrom K, Doberl A, Rannevik G. Peripheral androgen levels in danazol-treated premenopausal women. *Fertil Steril*, 39, 499-504 (1983)

893 Carmine AA, Brogden RN, Heel RC et al. Moxalactam (latamoxef) a review of its antibacterial activity, pharmacokinetic properties and therapeutic use. *Drugs*, 26, 279-333 (1983)

894 Carney SL, Gillies A, Heller RF et al. Effects of pindolol, or a pindolol/clopamide combination preparation, on plasma lipid levels in essential hypertension. *Med J Aust*, 150, 646-652 (1989)

895 Caroldi S, de Paris P, Zotti S et al. Effects of disulfiram on serum dopamine-β-hydroxylase and blood carbon disulphide concentrations in alcoholics. *J Appl Toxicol*, 14, 77-80 (1994)

896 Carpentiere G, Marino S, Castello F. Furosemide and theophylline. *Ann Intern Med*, 103, 957 (1985)

897 Carr DT, Karlson AG, Bridge EV. Concentration of PAS and tuberculostatic potency of serum after administration of PAS with and without Benemid® . *Proc Staff Meet Mayo Clin*, 27, 209-215 (1952)

898 Carr RE, Humphreys SM, Frayn KN. Catecholamine interference with enzymatic determination of nonesterified fatty acids in two commercially available test kits. *Clin Chem*, 41, 455-457 (1995)

899 Carruthers M, Taggart P, Conway N et al. Validity of plasma catecholamine estimations. *Lancet*, 2, 62 (1970)

900 Carstairs KC, Breckenridge A, Dollery CT. Incidence of a positive direct Coombs' test in patients on α-methyldopa. *Lancet*, 2, 133 (1966)

901 Carter BL, Small RE, Mandel MD et al. Phenytoin-induced hyperglycemia. *Am J Hosp Pharm*, 38, 1508-1512 (1981)

902 Carter DC, Dozois RR, Kirkpatrick JR. Insulin infusion test of gastric acid secretion. *Br Med J*, 2, 202 (1972)

903 Carter SA. Potentiation of the effect of orally administered anticoagulants by phenyramidol hydrochloride. *N Engl J Med*, 273, 423 (1965)

904 Cartier J-L, Leclerc P, Pouliot M, et al. Toxic levels of acetaminophen produce a major positive interference on Glucometer Elite and Accu-chek Advantage glucose meters. *Clin Chem*, 44, 893-895 (1998)

905 Carulli N, Ponz de Leon M, Podda M , et al. Chenodeoxycholic acid and ursodeoxycholic acid effects in endogenous hypertriglyceridemias: a controlled double-blind trial. *J Clin Pharmacol*, 21, 436-442 (1981)

906 Casagrande P, Valvo E, Bedogna V et al. Antihypertensive therapy with ketanserin: effects on central and renal hemodynamics, and microalbuminuria. *Int J Clin Pharmacol Ther Toxicol*, 28, 79-83 (1990)

907 Casale TB, Macher AM, Fauci AS. Complete hematologic and hepatic recovery in a patient with chloramphenicol hepatitis-pancytopenia syndrome. *J Pediatr*, 101, 1025-1027 (1982)

908 Casaneuva FF, Burguera B, Muruais C et al. Acute administration of corticoids: a new and peculiar stimulus of growth hormone secretion in man. *J Clin Endocrinol Metab*, 70, 234-237 (1990)

909 Casaretto ME, Bates M, Brenner C et al. Abuscreen Online immunoassay for the detection of phencyclidine (PCP) in urine on the Cobas Mira. *Clin Chem*, 37, 996 (1991)

910 Cascinu S, Ficaeelli R, Safi MAA, et al. A phase I study of paclitaxel and 5-fluorouracil in advanced gastric cancer. *Eur J Cancer*, 33, 1699-1702 (1997)

911 Cases Amenos A, Munoz I, Jimenez W et al. Arginine vasopressin infusion increases plasma levels of atrial natriuretic factor in humans. *Horm Metab Res*, 24, 127-129 (1992)

912 Cashin-Hemphill L, Spencer CA, Nicoloff JT et al. Alterations in serum thyroid hormonal indices with colestipol-niacin therapy. *Ann Intern Med*, 107, 324-329 (1987)

913 Casi MT, Dunovic S, Maric S. Acute phase proteins in children with urinary tract infections. *Clin Biochem Rev*, 14, 210 (1993)

914 Cassia L, Tonolo G, Glorioso N et al. Atrial natriuretic factor release during transient myocardial ischemia: a placebo-controlled study in man. *Am J Noninvas Cardiol*, 7, 325-332 (1993)

915 Casteels-Van Daele M. Gastrointestinal bleeding: a possible association with ibuprofen. *Lancet*, 1, 1021 (1972)

916 Castellani WJ. Mercurochrome interference with the Abbott TDx. *Clin Chem*, 38, 1190-1191 (1992)

917 Castellani WJ, Hodges ED, Bode AP. Effect of protamine sulfate on the aca heparin assay. *Clin Chem*, 37, 1119 (1991)

918 Castillo-Ferrando J, Garcia M, Carmona J. Digoxin levels and diazepam. *Lancet*, 2, 368 (1980)

919 Castleden CM, Richens A. Chronic phenytoin therapy and carbohydrate tolerance. *Lancet*, 2, 966 (1973)

920 Cat A III, Cavanaugh J, Shi H, et al. The effect of multiple doses of ritonavir on the pharmacokinetics of rifabutin. *Clin Pharmacol Ther*, 63, 414-421 (1998)

921 Catalano M, Aronica A, Carzaniga G et al. Simvastatin and the apolipoprotein profile in primary hypercholesterolemia. *Curr Ther Res*, 48, 85-90 (1990)

922 Cate EW, Rogers JF, Powell JR. Inhibition of tolbutamide elimination by cimetidine but not ranitidine. *J Clin Pharmacol*, 26, 372-377 (1986)

923 Cathcart-Rake WF, Kyner JL, Azarnoff DL. Metabolic responses to plasma concentrations of theophylline. *Clin Pharmacol Ther*, 26, 89-95 (1979)

924 Cathro DM, Saez JM, Bertrand J. The effect of clomiphene on the plasma androgens of prepubertal and pubertal boys. *J Endocrinol*, 50, 387 (1971)

925 Catlin DH, Poland RE, Gorelick DA et al. Intravenous infusion of β-endorphin increases serum prolactin, but not growth hormone or cortisol, in depressed subjects and withdrawing methadone addicts. *J Clin Endocrinol Metab*, 50, 1021-1025 (1980)

926 Cattaneo AG, Caviezel F, Pozza G. Pharmacological interaction between tolbutamide and acetylsalicylic acid: study on insulin secretion in man. *Int J Clin Pharmacol Ther Toxicol*, 28, 229-234 (1990)

927 Cattell WR. Excretory pathways for contrast media. *Invest Radiol*, 6, 473 (1971)

928 Cattin L, Da Col PG, Feruglio FS et al. Efficacy of ciprofibrate in primary type II and type IV hyperlipidemia: the Itialian Multicenter study. *Clin Ther*, 12, 482-488 (1990)

929 Caulin C. Les troubles digestifs d'origine medicamenteuse. *Presse Med*, 79, 2117 (1971)

930 Cavallo-Perin P, Estivi P, Boine L et al. Benfluorex and blood glucose control in non insulin-dependent diabetic patients. *J Endocrinol Invest*, 14, 109-113 (1991)

931 Caviet NL, Klaassen CHL. Trombocytopenie veroorzaakt door alprenolol. *Ned Tijdschr Geneeskd*, 123, 18-20 (1979)

932 Cazzola M, Brancaccio V, De Giglio C et al. Flomoxef, a new oxacephem antibiotic, does not cause hemostatic defects. *Int J Clin Pharmacol Ther Toxicol*, 11, 148-152 (1993)

933 Cedeno J, Mendoza SG, Velazquez E et al. Effects of ketoconazole on plasma sex hormones, lipids, lipoproteins, and apolipoproteins, and apolipoproteins in hyperandrogenic women. *Metabolism*, 39, 511-517 (1990)

934 Celik I, Akalin S, Erbas T. Serum levels of interleukin 6 and tumor necrosis factor-α in hyperthyroid patients before and after propylthiouracil treatment. *Eur J Endocrinol*, 132, 668-672 (1995)

935 Centeon. Manufacturer's literature on Bioclate™. King of Prussia, PA 19406 (1997)

936 Centeon. Manufacturer's literature on Gammar® -P I.V.. King of Prussia, PA 19406 (1996)

937 Centeon. Manufacturer's literature on Helixate® . King of Prussia, PA 19406 (1997)

938 Centorrino F, Baldessarini RJ, Kando J et al. Serum concentrations of clozapine and its major metabolites: effects of cotreatment with fluoxetine or valproate. *Am J Psychiat*, 151, 123-125 (1994)

939 Central Pharmaceuticals, Inc. Manufacturer's literature on Guaimax-D® . Seymour, IN 47274 (1997)

940 Central Pharmaceuticals, Inc. Manufacturer's literature on Mono-Gesic® Tablets. Seymour, IN 47274 (1997)

941 Cepelak V, Roubal Z, Cepelakova H. Aggregation of blood platelets and its inhibition by coumarin derivatives. *Blood*, 39, 588 (1972)

942 Cersosimo RJ, Lee -M. Creatine kinase elevation associated with 5-fluorouracil and levamisole therapy for carcinoma of the colon. *Cancer*, 77, 1250-1253 (1996)

943 Cervera H, Jara LJ, Pizarro S et al. Danazol for systemic lupus erythematosus with refractory autoimmune thrombocytopenia or Evans' syndrome. *J Rheumatol*, 22, 1867-1871 (1995)

944 Cetina JA, Fishbein EA, Alarcon-Segovia D. Antinuclear antibodies and propylthiouracil therapy. *J Am Med Ass*, 220, 1012 (1972)

945 Cetkovsky P, Koza V, Cepelak V et al. Haemostasis in patients with acute myeloid leukemia treated with intermediate dose of cytosine arabinoside and mitoxantrone: the influence of chemotherapy, infection and remission status on haemostasis. *Fibrinolysis*, 9, 165-169 (1995)

946 Chaffman M, Brogden RN, Heel RC et al. Auranofin: a preliminary review of its pharmacological properties and therapeutic use in rheumatoid arthritis. *Drugs*, 27, 378-424 (1984)

947 Chaisson RE, Leuther MD, Allain J-P et al. Effect of zidovudine on serum human immunodeficiency virus core antigen levels. *Arch Intern Med*, 148, 2151-2153 (1988)

948 Chakrabarti R, Fearnley GR, Evans JF. Effects of clofibrate on fibrinolysis, platelet stickiness, plasma fibrinogen and serum cholesterol. *Lancet*, 2, 1007 (1968)

949 Chakrabarty AK. Interference by antibiotics in plasma paracetamol determination. *Ann Clin Biochem*, 16, 217 (1979)

950 Challis TW, Reid LC, Hinton JW. Study of some factors which influence the level of serum amylase in dogs and humans. *Gastroenterology*, 33, 818 (1957)

951 Chalmers A, Thompson D, Stein HE et al. Systemic lupus erythematosus during penicillamine therapy for rheumatoid arthritis. *Ann Intern Med*, 97, 659-663 (1982)

952 Chalmers DM, Brown RC, Miller MG et al. The influence of long-term cimetidine as an adjuvant to pancreatic enzyme therapy in cystic fibrosis. *Acta Paediat Scand*, 74, 114-117 (1985)

953 Chamberlain JS, Hill DM, Shenkin A. Hypercholesterolaemia and HMG-CoA reductase inhibition: response determination by apolipoprotein and lipase gene variants. *Proc ACB Natl Meet*, 51 (1995)

954 Chambers CE, Vesell ES, Helm C et al. Pyrazinoylguanidine: antihypertensive, hypocholesterolemic, and renin effects. *J Clin Pharmacol*, 32, 1128-1134 (1992)

955 Chambers LA, Donovan LM, Kruskall MS. Ceftazidime-induced hemolysis in a patient with drug-dependent antibodies reactive by immune complex and drug absorption mechanisms. *Am J Clin Pathol*, 95, 393-396 (1991)

956 Champion MC, Sullivan SN, Bloom SR et al. The effects of naloxone and morphine on postprandial gastrointestinal hormone secretion. *Am J Gastroenterol*, 77, 617-620 (1982)

957 Chan AC, Sack K. Danazol therapy in autoimmune hemolytic anemia associated with systemic lupus erythematosus. *J Rheumatol*, 18, 280-282 (1991)

958 Chan DW, Beveridge RA, Bhargava A et al. Breast cancer marker CA549: a multicenter study. *Am J Clin Pathol*, 101, 465-470 (1994)

959 Chan JCN, Cockram CS, Tomlinson B et al. Metabolic and hemodynamic effects of metformin and glibenclamide in normotensive NIDDM patients. *Diabetes Care*, 16, 1035-1038 (1993)

960 Chan JCN, Tomlinson B, Yeung VTF et al. The effects of enalapril and nifedipine on carbohydrate and lipid metabolism in NIDDM. *Diabetes Care*, 17, 859-862 (1994)

961 Chan PCK, Robinson JD, Yeung WC et al. Lovastatin in glomerulonephritis patients with hyperlipidaemia and heavy proteinuria. *Nephrol Dial Transplant*, 7, 93-99 (1992)

962 Chan TM, Cheng IKP, Tam SCF. Hyperlipidemia after renal transplantation: treatment with gemfibrozil. *Nephron*, 67, 317-321 (1994)

963 Chan V, Besser GM, Landon J. Effects of oestrogens on urinary thyroxine excretion. *Br Med J*, 4, 699 (1972)

964 Chandler B, Lavin PT. Efficacy and tolerability of enalapril and its effect on serum lipids in patients with mild uncomplicated essential hypertension. *Curr Ther Res*, 43, 1143-1149 (1988)

965 Chang TW. Cold urticaria and photosensitivity due to griseofulvin. *J Am Med Ass*, 193, 848 (1965)

966 Chanu B, Rouffy J, Noseda G et al. Comparative study of the effects of pindolol and atenolol on blood lipids. *Curr Ther Res*, 49, 588-595 (1991)

967 Chapman I, Cheung WH. Pancytopenia associated with tolbutamide therapy. *J Am Med Ass*, 186, 595 (1963)

968 Chapman JR, Griffiths D, Harding NGL et al. Reversibility of cyclosporine nephrotoxicity after three months treatment. *Lancet*, 2, 128-129 (1985)

969 Chapoteau E, Gebauer CR, Chimenti MZ et al. Principles and performance of the Technicon Chromolyte sodium method. Accuracy, interferences and multisite imprecision studies. *Clin Chem*, 36, 1065 (1990)

970 Charache S, Terrin ML, Moore RD et al. Effect of hydroxyurea on the frequency of painful crises in sickle cell anemia. *N Engl J Med*, 332, 1317-1322 (1995)

971 Charest L, Comtois R, Beauregard H et al. Growth hormone rebound after cessation of SMS 201-995 treatment in acromegaly. *Can J Neurol Sci*, 16, 442-445 (1989)

972 Charles BG, Renshaw PJ, Kay JJ et al. Effect of metoclopramide on the bioavailability of long-acting propranolol. *Br J Clin Pharmacol*, 11, 517 (1981)

973 Charles MA, Danforth E Jr. Nonketoacidotic hyperglycemia and coma during intravenous diazoxide therapy in uremia. *Diabetes*, 20, 501 (1971)

974 Charles S, Ketelslegers J-M, Buysschaert M et al. Hyperglycaemic effect of nifedipine. *Br Med J*, 283, 19-20 (1981)

975 Chazan R, Droszcz W, Bobilewicz D et al. Changes in plasma high density lipoproteins (HDL) levels after salbutamol. *Int J Clin Pharmacol Ther Toxicol*, 23, 427-429 (1985)

976 Chee HD, Bronsveld W, Lips PTAM et al. Adrenocortical suppression in multiply injured patients: a complication of etomidate treatment. *Br Med J*, 288, 485 (1984)

977 Chen JH, Ottolengi P, Distenfeld A. Oxyphenbutazone-induced sialadenitis. *J Am Med Ass*, 238, 1399 (1977)

978 Chen JJS, Berlin FS, Margolis S. Effect of large dose progesterone on plasma levels of lipids, lipoproteins and apolipoproteins in males. *J Endocrinol Invest*, 9, 281-285 (1986)

979 Chen MF, Boyce HW Jr, Hsu JM. Effect of ascorbic acid on plasma alcohol clearance. *J Am Coll Nutr*, 9, 185-189 (1990)

980 Chen S-S, Shen M-R, Chen T-J et al. Effects of antiepileptic drugs on sperm motility of normal controls and epileptic patients with long-term therapy. *Epilepsia*, 33, 149-153 (1992)

981 Cheng M, Reyes G. Serum myosin as a biochemical indicator for myocardial injury during intravenous inotropic drug therapy. *Abstracts, 5th APCCB, Kobe* (1991)

982 Cheng MH, Wang C-I. Changes in serum cholesterol levels in patients with cystic fibrosis before and after intravenous antibiotics. *Clin Chem*, 37, 923 (1991)

983 Cheng SH, White A. Effect of orally administered neomycin on the absorption of penicillin V. *N Engl J Med*, 267, 1296-1297 (1962)

984 Chesney RW. Drug-induced hypokalemia. *Am J Dis Child*, 130, 1055-1056 (1976)

985 Chesney RW, Hamstr AJ, Mazees RB et al. Reduction of serum 1,25-dihydroxy vitamin D in children receiving glucocorticoids. *Lancet*, 2, 1123-1125 (1978)

986 Chesnut CH III, Bell NH, Clark GS, et al. Hormone replacement therapy in postmenopausal women: urinary N-telopeptide of type I collagen monitors therapeutic effect and predicts response of bone mineral density. *Am J Med*, 102, 29-37 (1997)

987 Chetty M, Miller R, Moodley SV. Smoking and body weight influence the clearance of chlorpromazine. *Eur J Clin Pharmacol*, 46, 523-526 (1994)

988 Cheung MC, Austin MA, Moulin P et al. Effects of pravastatin on apolipoprotein-specific high density lipoprotein subpopulations and low density lipoprotein subclass phenotypes in patients with primary hypercholesterolemia. *Atherosclerosis*, 102, 107-119 (1993)

989 Cheung M-K, Williams M, Haden B et al. Evaluation of Synchron CX lactate reagent on the Synchron CX4/5. *Clin Chem*, 37, 976 (1991)

990 Chey WD, Kochman ML, Traber PG, et al. Possible nizatidine-induced subfulminant hepatic failure. *J Clin Gastroenterol*, 20, 164-167 (1995)

991 Chiariello M, Volpe M, Rengo F et al. Effect of furosemide on plasma concentration and β-blockade by propranolol. *Clin Pharmacol Ther*, 26, 433-436 (1979)

992 Chiasson J-L, Nathan DM, Josse RG, et al. The effect of acarbose on insulin sensitivity in subjects with impaired glucose tolerance. *Diabetes Care*, 19, 1190-1193

993 Chiba T, Okimura Y, Kodama H et al. Tolbutamide inhibits gastrin release in man. *Horm Metab Res*, 20, 641-644 (1988)

994 Childs PA, Rodin I, Martin NJ , et al. Effect of fluoxetine on melatonin in patients with seasonal affective disorder and matched controls. *Br J Psychiat*, 166, 196-198 (1995)

995 Chinitz JL, Kim KE, Onesti G et al. Pathophysiology and prevention of Dextran-40-induced anuria. *J Lab Clin Med*, 77, 76 (1971)

996 Chiodera P, Coiro V, Zanardi G et al. Effect of metoclopramide on serum GH levels in normal women. *Horm Metab Res*, 14, 103-104 (1982)

997 Chiron Therapeutics. Manufacturer's literature on Proleukin® . Emeryville, CA 94606 (1994)

998 Cho C, Flynn RJ. Hepatic enzyme induction by antiepileptic drugs. *Lab Med*, 21, 823-826 (1990)

999 Chong BH, Kaplin IJ. Effect of quinidine on platelets. *Haemostasis*, 20, 106-111 (1990)

1000 Chow CC, Lai KN, Leung JCK et al. Serum soluble interleukin 2 receptor in hyperthyroid Graves' disease and effect of carbimazole therapy. *Clin Endocrinol*, 33, 317-321 (1990)

1001 Chow CC, Lee S, Wing YK et al. Thyroid abnormalities associated with long term lithium therapy in Hong Kong: a controlled study. *Clin Biochem Rev*, 14, 254 (1993)

1002 Christensen CK, Morgensen CE, Hanberg Sorensen F. Renal function and cimetidine. urinary albumin and $beta_2$ - microglobulin excretion and creatinine clearance during cimetidine treatment. *Scand J Gastroenterol*, 16, 129-134 (1981)

1003 Christensen CK, Pedersen OL, Mikkelsen E. Renal effects of acute calcium blockade with nifedipine in hypertensive patients receiving β-adrenoceptor blocking drugs. *Clin Pharmacol Ther*, 32, 572-576 (1982)

1004 Christensen E, Schlichting P, Fauerholdt L et al. Changes of laboratory variables with time in cirrhosis: prognostic and therapeutic significance. *Hepatology*, 5, 843-853 (1985)

1005 Christensen LK, Skovsted L. Inhibition of drug metabolism by chloramphenicol. *Lancet*, 2, 1397-1399 (1969)

1006 Christensen P, Gram LF, Lolk A et al. The cortisol suppressing effect of dexamethasone and oxazepam in depressed patients; significance of spontaneous levels and interindividual distribution. *J Affect Disord*, 13, 273-278 (1987)

1007 Christenson RH, Gregory LC, Duh S-H et al. Hemoglobin based blood substitutes: interference with routine chemical tests. *Clin Chem*, 39, 1129 (1993)

1008 Christgau S, Rosenquist C, Alexandersen P, et al. Clinical evaluation of the serum CrossLaps™ One Step ELISA, a new assay measuring the serum concentration of bone-derived degradation products of type I collagen C-telopeptides. *Clin Chem*, 44, 2290-2300 (1998)

1009 Christian DG. Drug interference with laboratory blood chemistry determinations. *Am J Clin Pathol*, 54, 118 (1970)

1010 Christians U, Braun F, Schmidt M et al. Specific and sensitive measurement of Fk506 and its metabolites in blood and urine of liver-graft recipients. *Clin Chem*, 38, 2025-2032 (1992)

1011 Christiansen C, Rodbro P, Tjellsen L. Serum alkaline phosphatase during hormone treatment in early postmenopausal women. *Acta Med Scand*, 216, 11-17 (1984)

1012 Christiansen J, Dam M. Influence of phenobarbital and diphenylhydantoin on plasma carbamazepine levels in patients with epilepsy. *Acta Neurol Scand*, 49, 543-546 (1973)

1013 Chrysant SG, Dunn M, Marples D et al. Severe reversible azotemia from captopril therapy: report of three cases and review of the literature. *Arch Intern Med*, 143, 437-441 (1983)

1014 Chrysant SG, Luu TM. Effects of amiloride on arterial pressure and renal function. *J Clin Pharmacol*, 20, 332-337 (1980)

1015 Chu J-Y, O'Connor DM, Schmidt RR et al. The mechanism of oxacillin-induced neutropenia. *J Pediatr*, 90, 668 (1977)

1016 Chung EK. Digitalis intoxication. *Postgrad Med J*, 48, 163 (1972)

1017 Chyatte SB, Basmajian JV. Dantrolene sodium: long-term effects in severe spasticity. *Arch Phys Med Rehabil*, 54, 311 (1973)

1018 Ciabattoni G, Cinotti GA, Pierucci A et al. Effects of sulindac and ibuprofen in patients with chronic glomerular disease. evidence for the dependence of renal function on prostacyclin. *N Engl J Med*, 310, 279-283 (1984)

1019 Cianci P, Reitz RE, Werner HV et al. Role of free fatty acids in growth hormone regulation during fasting. *Ann Intern Med*, 76, 857 (1972)

1020 Ciba-Geigy Corporation. Manufacturer's literature on Actigall® . Summit, NJ 07901 (1996)

1021 Ciba-Geigy Corporation. Manufacturer's literature on Anafranil® . Summit, NJ 07901 (1996)

1022 Ciba-Geigy Corporation. Manufacturer's literature on Anturane® . Summit, NJ 07901 (1996)

1023 Ciba-Geigy Corporation. Manufacturer's literature on Apresoline® . Summit, NJ 07901 (1995)

1024 Ciba-Geigy Corporation. Manufacturer's literature on Brethine® . Summit, NJ 07901 (1995)

1025 Ciba-Geigy Corporation. Manufacturer's literature on Cataflam® and Voltaren® . Summit, NJ 07901 (1996)

1026 Ciba-Geigy Corporation. Manufacturer's literature on Cytadren® . Summit, NJ 07901 (1996)

1027 Ciba-Geigy Corporation. Manufacturer's literature on Desferal® . Summit, NJ 07901 (1994)

1028 Ciba-Geigy Corporation. Manufacturer's literature on Esidrix® . Summit, NJ 07901 (1996)

1029 Ciba-Geigy Corporation. Manufacturer's literature on Ismelin® . Summit, NJ 07901 (1996)

1030 Ciba-Geigy Corporation. Manufacturer's literature on Lamprene® . Summit, NJ 07901 (1995)

1031 Ciba-Geigy Corporation. Manufacturer's literature on Lioresal® . Summit, NJ 07901 (1996)

1032 Ciba-Geigy Corporation. Manufacturer's literature on Lopressor® . Summit, NJ 07901 (1996)

1033 Ciba-Geigy Corporation. Manufacturer's literature on Lotensin® . Summit, NJ 07901 (1995)

1034 Ciba-Geigy Corporation. Manufacturer's literature on Ludiomil® . Summit, NJ 07901 (1996)

1035 Ciba-Geigy Corporation. Manufacturer's literature on Metopirone® . Summit, NJ 07901 (1996)

1036 Ciba-Geigy Corporation. Manufacturer's literature on Priscoline® . Summit, NJ 07901 (1989)

1037 Ciba-Geigy Corporation. Manufacturer's literature on Rimactane® . Summit, NJ 07901 (1992)

1038 Ciba-Geigy Corporation. Manufacturer's literature on Ritalin® . Summit, NJ 07901 (1996)

1039 Ciba-Geigy Corporation. Manufacturer's literature on Tegretol® . Summit, NJ 07901 (1996)

1040 Ciba-Geigy Corporation. Manufacturer's literature on Tofranil® . Summit, NJ 07901 (1994)

1041 Ciba-Geigy Corporation. Manufacturer's literature on Tripelennamine® . Summit, NJ 07901 (1996)

1042 CibaGeneva Pharmaceuticals, Ciba-Geigy Corporation. Manufacturer's literature on Diovan™. Summit, NJ 07901 (1996)

1043 Ciccarelli E, Grottoli S, Razzore P, wt al. Hexarelin, a synthetic growth hormone releasing peptide, stimulates prolactin secretion in acromegalic but not in hyperprolactinaemic patients. *Clin Endocrinol*, 44, 67-71 (1996)

1044 Cimo PL. Documenting suspected drug-induced thrombocytopenia. *Arch Intern Med*, 143, 1117-1118 (1983)

1045 Ciotta L, Marletta E, Cianci A et al. Clinical and endocrine effects of finasteride, a 5α-reductase inhibitor, in women with idiopathic hirsutism. *Fertil Steril*, 64, 299-306 (1995)

1046 Claas FHJ, Van Der Meer JWM, Langerak J. Immunological effect of co-trimoxazole on platelets. *Br Med J*, 2, 898-899 (1979)

1047 Claghorn JL, Kinrose-Wright J, McIsaac WM. False positive urine glucose test in two patients receiving trioxazine. *J New Drugs*, 6, 153 (1966)

1048 Claiborne RA, Dutt AK. Isoniazid-induced pure red cell aplasia. *Am Rev Resp Dis*, 131, 947-949 (1985)

1049 Clark DW, Goldberg LI. Guancydine: a new antihypertensive agent. *Ann Intern Med*, 76, 579 (1972)

1050 Clark PMS, Clark JDA, Wheatley T. Urine discoloration after acetaminophen overdose. *Clin Chem*, 32, 1777-1778 (1986)

1051 Clark PMS, Kricka LJ. Interference by diazepam in the determination of 5-hydroxyindoleacetic acid. *Ann Clin Biochem*, 14, 233-234 (1977)

1052 Clarke RJ, Mayo G, Price P et al. Suppression of thromboxane A_2 but not of systemic prostacyclin by controlled release aspirin. *N Engl J Med*, 325, 1137-1141 (1991)

1053 Clarkson AR, MacDonald MK, Cash JD et al. Modification by drugs of urinary fibrin/fibrinogen degradation products in glomerulonephritis. *Br Med J*, 3, 255 (1972)

1054 Clemens JD, Herrick MV, Singer FR, Eyre DR. Evidence that serum NTx (collagen-type I N-telopeptides) can act as an immunochemical marker of bone resorption. *Clin Chem*, 43, 2058-2063 (1997)

1055 Clemente C, Russo F, Caruso MG et al. Ceruloplasmin serum level in post-menopausal women treated with oral estrogens administered at different times. *Horm Metab Res*, 24, 191-193 (1992)

1056 Clementz GL, Dolin BJ. Sulfasalazine-induced lupus erythematosus. *Am J Med*, 84, 535-538 (1988)

1057 Clemenzia G, Russo G, Gentile V et al. Remarks on the behaviour of certain enzymurias in subjects treated with pipemidic acid. *Minerva Med*, 77, 621-626 (1986)

1058 Clerson P, Carre A, Berthet P et al. Glucose tolerance parameters in nondiabetic hypertensive patients treated with cicletanine. *Arch Mal Coeur*, 82, Special Issue 4, 139-143 (1989)

1059 Clifford NJ, Weil J. Cortisol metabolism in persons occupationally exposed to DDT. *Arch Environ Health*, 24, 145 (1972)

1060 Clifton G, McMahon G, Ryan J et al. The effects of enoximone on renal function in patients with congestive heart failure. *Clin Pharmacol Ther*, 45, 85-91 (1989)

1061 Closa AS, Lambert C, du Souich P. Lack of effect of cimetidine on furosemide kinetics and dynamics in patients with hepatic cirrhosis. *Int J Clin Pharmacol Ther Toxicol*, 31, 461-466 (1993)

1062 Clyne CA, Estes NAM III, Wang PJ. Moricizine. *N Engl J Med*, 327, 255-260 (1992)

1063 Coates JE, LeGatt DF. Lack of interference by therapeutic concentrations of Inocor® (amrinone lactate) in the TDx assay for digoxin. *Clin Chem*, 34, 1004-1005 (1988)

1064 Cobb MM, Teitelbaum HS, Breslow JL. Lovastatin efficacy in reducing low-density lipoprotein cholesterol levels on high- vs low-fat diets. *J Am Med Ass*, 265, 997-1001 (1991)

1065 Cobb MN, Deai J, Brown LS Jr, et al. The effect of fluconazole on the clinical pharmacokinetics of methadone. *Clin Pharmacol Ther*, 63, 655-662 (1998)

1066 Coblyn JS, Weinblatt M, Holdsworth D et al. Gold induced thrombocytopenia: a clinical and immunogenetic study of twenty- three patients. *Ann Intern Med*, 95, 178-181 (1981)

1067 Coca A, Blade J, Martinez A et al. Tobramycin nephrotoxicity: a prospective clinical study. *Postgrad Med J*, 55, 791-796 (1979)

1068 Coccheri S, Biagi G, Legnani C et al. Acute effects of defibrotide, an experimental antithrombotic agent, on fibrinolysis and blood prostanoids in man. *Eur J Clin Pharmacol*, 35, 151-156 (1988)

1069 Cockburn ITR, Krupp P. An appraisal of drug interactions with Sandimmune. *Transplant Proc*, 21, 3845-3850 (1989)

1070 Cockerill FR III, Edson RS. Trimethoprim-sulfamethoxazole. *Mayo Clin Proc*, 58, 147-153 (1983)

1071 Cockerill FR III, Edson RS. Trimethoprim-sulfamethoxazole. *Mayo Clin Proc*, 62, 921-929 (1987)

1072 Cody RJ Jr, Calabrese LH, Clough JD. Development of antinuclear antibodies during acebutolol therapy. *Clin Pharmacol Ther*, 25, 800-805 (1979)

1073 Coffey VJ. Myxoedema during cyclophosphamide therapy. *Br Med J*, 4, 682 (1971)

1074 Cohen CD, Sayed AR, Kirsch RE. Hepatic complications of antituberculosis therapy revisited. *S Afr Med J*, 63, 960-963 (1983)

1075 Cohen DJ, Loertscher R, Rubin MF et al. Cyclosporine: a new immunosuppressive agent for organ transplantation. *Ann Intern Med*, 101, 667-682 (1984)

1076 Cohen EL, Grim CE, Conn JW et al. Accurate and rapid measurement of plasma renin activity by radioimmunoassay. *J Lab Clin Med*, 77, 1025 (1971)

1077 Cohen HN, Beastall GH, Ratcliffe WA et al. Effects on human thyroid function of sulphonamide and trimethoprim combination drugs. *Br Med J*, 281, 646-647 (1980)

1078 Cohen IA, Johnson CE, Berardi RR et al. Cimetidine-theophylline interaction: effects of age and cimetidine dose. *Ther Drug Monit*, 7, 426-434 (1985)

1079 Cohen LC. CPK tests - effect of intramuscular injection in myocardial infarction. *J Am Med Ass*, 219, 625 (1972)

1080 Cohen MG, Kevat S, Prowse MV et al. Two distinct quinidine-induced rheumatic syndromes. *Ann Intern Med*, 108, 369-371 (1988)

1081 Cohen MM, Debas HT, Holubitsky IB et al. Caffeine and pentagastrin stimulation of human gastric secretion. *Gastroenterology*, 61, 440 (1971)

1082 Cohen MS, Washton HE, Barranco SF. Multicenter clinical trial of cefoperazone sodium in the United States. *Am J Med*, 77. Suppl 1b, 35-41 (1984)

1083 Cohick CB, Furst DE, Quagliata S et al. Analysis of elevated serum interleukin-6 levels in rheumatoid arthritis: correlation with erythrocyte sedimentation rate or C-reactive protein. *J Lab Clin Med*, 123, 721-727 (1994)

1084 Coiro V, Passeri M, Volpi R et al. Different effects of aging on the opioid mechanisms controlling gonadotropin and cortisol secretion in man. *Horm Res*, 32, 119-123 (1989)

1085 Col DI G, Cevaro G, Lombardo F et al. L'indapamide nei traitment dell ipertensione arteriosa essenziale dell anziano: influenza sui metabolismo glico-lipidico. *Boll Soc Ital Cardiol*, 26, 1527-1530 (1981)

1086 Colantonio D, Casale R, Desiati P et al. Short-term effects of atenolol and nifedipine on atrial natriuretic peptide, plasma renin activity, and plasma aldosterone in patients with essential hypertension. *J Clin Pharmacol*, 31, 238-242 (1991)

1087 Cold JA, ZumBrunnen TL, Simpson MA, et al. Increased lithium serum and red blood cell concentrations during ketorolac coadministration. *J Clin Psychopharmacol*, 18, 33-37 (1998)

1088 Cole RM, Raghavan D, Caterson I et al. Danazol treatment of advanced prostate cancer: clinical and hormonal effects. *Prostate*, 9, 15-20 (1986)

1089 Coleman AL, Diehl DL, Jampel HD et al. Topical timolol decreases plasma high-density lipoprotein cholesterol level. *Arch Ophthalmol*, 108, 1260-1263 (1990)

1090 Coley TP, Kunches LM, Saunders CA et al. Once-daily administration of 2',3'-dideoxyinosine (ddi) in patients with the acquired immunodeficiency syndrome or AIDS-related complex. *N Engl J Med*, 322, 1340-1345 (1990)

1091 Colin JN, Farinotti R, Fredj G et al. Kinetics of allopurinol after chronic oral administration: interaction with benzbromarone. *Eur J Clin Pharmacol*, 31, 53-58 (1986)

1092 Colle M, Ruedas E, Cazenave J et al. Plasma prolactin, sex steroids and gastrin in human volunteers treated for 2 weeks with therapeutic doses of cimetidine or the new histamine H_2-receptor antagonist ramixotidine (CM 57755A). *Eur J Clin Pharmacol*, 35, 529-534 (1988)

1093 Collen MJ. Cimetidine-associated thrombocytopenia and leukopenia. *West J Med*, 132, 257-258 (1980)

1094 Collier AC, Bozzette S, Coombs RW et al. A pilot study of low-dose zidovudine in human immunodeficiency virus infection. *N Engl J Med*, 323, 1015-1021 (1990)

1095 Collins RD. Illustrated Manual of Laboratory Diagnosis. Philadelphia PA, JB Lippincott (1968)

1096 Collinson PO, Kind PRN, Slavin B et al. False diagnosis of phaeochromocytoma in patients on sinemet® . *Lancet*, 1, 14 (1984)

1097 Collinsworth W. Personal communication. Boehringer Mannheim, Indianapolis IN

1098 Collste P, Seideman P, Borg K-O et al. Influence of pentobarbital on effect and plasma levels of alprenolol and 4-hydroxyalprenolol. *Clin Pharmacol Ther*, 25, 423-427 (1979)

1099 Colt EWD, Kimbrell D, Fieve RR. Renal impairment, hypercalcaemia, and lithium therapy. *Am J Psychiat*, 138, 106-108 (1981)

1100 Colucci R, Glue P, Holt B, et al. Effect of felbamate on the pharmacokinetics of lamotrigine. *J Clin Pharmacol*, 36, 634-638 (1996)

1101 Colwell AR Jr, Sando DE, Lang SJ. Propylthiouracil-induced agranulocytosis, toxic hepatitis, and death. *J Am Med Ass*, 148, 639 (1952)

1102 Combs AB, Giri SN, Peoples SA. A new method for analysis of phenylthiourea in biological fluids. *Anal Biochem*, 44, 570 (1971)

1103 Cominacini L, Garbin U, Bossello O et al. Effect of gemfibrozil on the composition of very-low-density lipoproteins: Interrelationships with low-density lipoprotein cholesterol levels. *Curr Ther Res*, 46, 1045-1058 (1989)

1104 Commentz J, Willig R. No effect of ethinylestradiol treatment on melatonin secretion in healthy pubertal girls. *Exp Clin Endocrinol*, 103, 52-57 (1995)

1105 Comoy E, Bohoun C. Isohomovanillic acid determination in human urine. *Clin Chim Acta*, 35, 369 (1971)

1106 Cone EJ, Darwin WD, Dickerson SL et al. Evaluation of the Abuscreen ONTRAK assay for cocaine metabolites. *Clin Chem News*, July, 40 (1991)

1107 Conget JI, Halperin I, Ferrer J et al. Evaluation of clinical and hormonal effects in hirsute women treated with ketoconazole (1994)

1108 Conn JW. Hypertension, the potassium ion and impaired carbohydrate tolerance. *N Engl J Med*, 273, 1135 (1965)

1109 Connell JMC, Rapeport WG, Beastall GH et al. Changes in circulating androgens during short term carbamazepine therapy. *Br J Clin Pharmacol*, 17, 347-351 (1984)

1110 Connell JMC, Rapeport WG, Gordon S et al. Changes in circulating thyroid hormones during short-term hepatic enzyme induction with carbamazepine. *Eur J Clin Pharmacol*, 26, 453-456 (1984)

1111 Conner CS. Etomidate and adrenal suppression. *Drug Intell Clin Pharm*, 18, 393-394 (1984)

1112 Conney AH, Spark RS, Robinson SH et al. Drug metabolism and therapeutics. *N Engl J Med*, 280, 653 (1969)

1113 Connolly P, Comeau L, Lino K et al. An automated chemiluminescence immunoassay for progesterone. *Clin Chem*, 39, 1259 (1993)

1114 Conrad KA, Byers JM III, Finley PR et al. Lidocaine elimination: effects of metoprolol and of propranolol. *Clin Pharmacol Ther*, 33, 133-138 (1983)

1115 Conrad KA, Fagan TC, Lee SM et al. Effects of tripamide on glucose tolerance in patients with hypertension. *Clin Pharmacol Ther*, 40, 476-479 (1986)

1116 Conrad KA, Nyman DW. Effects of metropolol and propranolol on theophylline elimination. *Clin Pharmacol Ther*, 28, 463-467 (1980)

1117 Conrad ME, Knochel JP, Crosby WH. Novobiocin jaundice: demonstration of a hemolytic state. *Antibiot Med*, 7, 382 (1960)

1118 Conti A, Sartorio A, Ferrero S, et al. Modifications of biochemical markers of bone and collagen turnover during corticosteroid therapy. *J Endocrinol Invest*, 19, 127-130 (1996)

1119 Cook BL, Smith RE, Perry PJ et al. Theophylline-lithium interaction. *J Clin Psychiat*, 46, 278-279 (1985)

1120 Cook FJ, Chandler DW, Snyder DK. Effect of busiprone on urinary catecholamine assays. *N Engl J Med*, 332, 401 (1995)

1121 Cook J, Daneman D, Spino M et al. Angiotensin converting enzyme inhibitor therapy to decrease microalbuminuria in normotensive children with insulin-dependent diabetes mellitus. *J Pediatr*, 117, 39-45 (1990)

1122 Cook JD, Platoff GE, Koch TR et al. Accuracy and precision of methods for theophylline measurement in physicians' offices. *Clin Chem*, 36, 780-783 (1990)

1123 Coon WW, Willis PW III. Some aspects of the pharmacology of oral anticoagulants. *Clin Pharmacol Ther*, 11, 312 (1970)

1124 Cooper CM, Foster GR, Cooper AE et al. Serum F-protein concentration following halothane or isoflurane anaesthesia. *Clin Chim Acta*, 202, 73-82 (1991)

1125 Cooper DS, Daniels GH, Ladenson PW et al. Hyperthyroxinemia in patients treated with high-dose propranolol. *Am J Med*, 73, 867-871 (1982)

1126 Cooper DS, Gelenberg AJ, Wojcik JC et al. The effect of amoxapine and imipramine on serum prolactin levels. *Arch Intern Med*, 141, 1023-1025 (1981)

1127 Cooperberg AA, Eidlow S. Haemolytic anemia, jaundice and diabetes mellitus following chlorpromazine therapy. *Can Med Ass J*, 75, 746 (1956)

1128 Coore JR, Patel S, Selby C et al. The effect of frusemide therapy on urinary microalbumin excretion. *Proc ACB Natl Meet*, 118 (1993)

1129 Copeland JG, Channick JM, Gittes RF. Complications of a "Mayo enema". *Calif Med*, 116, 65 (1972)

1130 Copur MS, Tasdemir I, Turgan C et al. Effects of nitrendipine on blood pressure and blood cyclosporin A level in patients with post-transplant hypertension. *Nephron*, 52, 227-230 (1989)

1131 Copur S, Tokgozoglu L, Oto A et al. Effects of oral prazosin on total plasma digoxin levels. *Fundam Clin Pharmacol*, 2, 13-17 (1988)

1132 Corder CN, Goldberg MR, Alaupovic PA et al. Lipid and apolipoprotein levels during therapy with pinacidil combined with hydrochlorothiazide. *Eur J Clin Pharmacol*, 42, 65-70 (1992)

1133 Corder CN, Kloer HU, Price MD. CI-924 effects on plasma lipids in patients with type II and type IV hyperlipoproteinemias. *Eur J Clin Pharmacol*, 37, 477-481 (1989)

1134 Corinaldesi R, Pasquali R, Paternico A et al. Effects of short- and long-term administrations of famotidine and ranitidine on some pituitary, sexual and thyroid hormones. *Drugs Exp Clin Res*, 13, 647-654 (1987)

1135 Corn TH, Hale AS, Thompson C et al. A comparison of the growth hormone responses to clonidine and apomorphine in the same patient with endogenous depression. *Br J Psychiat*, 144, 636-639 (1984)

1136 Cornish AL, McClellan JT, Johnston DH. Effects of chlorothiazide on the pancreas. *N Engl J Med*, 265, 673 (1961)

1137 Coronado BE, Opal SM, Yoburn DC. Antibiotic-induced D-lactic acidosis. *Ann Intern Med*, 122, 839-842 (1995)

1138 Corrado ML, Struble WE, Chennekatu P et al. Norfloxacin: review of safety studies. *Am J Med*, 82, Suppl 6b, 22-26 (1987)

1139 Corsi CM, Nafziger AN, Pieper JA et al. Lack of effect of atenolol and nadolol on the metabolism of theophylline. *Br J Clin Pharmacol*, 29, 265-268 (1990)

1140 Cortassa G, Odetti P, Borgoglio A et al. Effects of antihypertensive therapy with verapamil and insulin secretion in type II diabetics. *Curr Ther Res*, 49, 843-853 (1991)

1141 Cortelazzo S, Finazzi G, Ruggeri M et al. Hydroxyurea for patients with essential thrombocythemia and a high risk of thrombosis. *N Engl J Med*, 332, 1132-1136 (1995)

1142 Corvetta A, Luchetti MM, Pomponio G et al. Interleukin-2, soluble interleukin-2 receptor and tumor necrosis factor in sera from patients with rheumatoid arthritis. *Res Clin Lab*, 20, 275-281 (1990)

1143 Cotariu D, Zaidman JL. Valproic acid and the liver. *Clin Chem*, 34, 890-897 (1988)

1144 Coty W, Kauffman L, Johnson F et al. Development of a CEDIA digoxin assay and application to the Hitachi 717. *Clin Chem*, 37, 993 (1991)

1145 Couet W, Istin B, Ingrand I et al. Effect of ponsinomycin on single-dose kinetics and metabolism of carbamazepine. *Ther Drug Monit*, 12, 144-149 (1990)

1146 Coulter DL, Allen RJ. Secondary hyperammonaemia: a possible mechanism for valproate encephalopathy. *Lancet*, 1, 1310-1311 (1980)

1147 Coulter DL, Wu H, Allen RJ. Valproic acid therapy in childhood epilepsy. *J Am Med Ass*, 244, 785-788 (1980)

1148 Coursin DB. Discussion of paper. *Ann NY Acad Sci*, 80, 894 (1959)

1149 Cowan RE, Wright JT. Dapsone and severe hypoalbuminaemia in dermatitis herpetiformis. *Br J Dermatol*, 104, 201-204 (1981)

1150 Coward S, Boa FG, Sherwood RA. Sulfasalazine interference with HPLC assay of 5-hydroxyindole-3-acetic acid. *Clin Chem*, 41, 765-766 (1995)

1151 Cowden EA, Ratcliffe WA, Beastall GH et al. Laboratory assessment of prolactin status. *Ann Clin Biochem*, 16, 113-121 (1979)

1152 Cowen AE, McGeary HM, Campbell CB. Interference by gastrografin® with a spectrophotometric trypsin assay. *Gut*, 13, 395 (1972)

1153 Cox J, Staedter M, Blackwood J et al. Dry chemistry multilayer immunoassay test for carbamazepine. *Clin Chem*, 36, 1036 (1990)

1154 Craft IL, Peters TJ. Quantitative changes in plasma amino acids induced by oral contraceptives. *Clin Sci*, 41, 301 (1971)

1155 Craft IL, Wise I. Plasma amino acids and oral contraceptives. *Lancet*, 2, 1138 (1969)

1156 Craig WA, Kunin CM. Trimethoprim-sulfamethoxazole: pharmacodynamic effect of urinary pH and impaired renal function. *Ann Intern Med*, 78, 491 (1973)

1157 Cramer BC, Parfrey PS, Hutchinson TA et al. Renal function following infusion of radiologic contrast material: a prospective controlled study. *Arch Intern Med*, 145, 87-89 (1985)

1158 Crammer JL, Elkes A. Agranulocytosis after desipramine. *Lancet*, 1, 105 (1967)

1159 Crandell WB, Pappas SG, MacDonald A. Nephrotoxicity associated with methoxyflurane anesthesia. *Anesthesiology*, 27, 591 (1966)

1160 Crane T, Dawson CM, Tickner TR. False-positive results from the Syva EMIT d.a.u. monoclonal amphetamine assay as a result of antipsychotic drug therapy. *Clin Chem*, 39, 549 (1993)

1161 Crave J-C, Fimbel S, Lejeune H, et al. Effects of diet and metformin administration on sex hormone binding globulin, androgens, and insulin in hirsute and obese women. *J Clin Endocrinol Metab*, 80, 2057-2062 (1995)

1162 Crawford GA, Gallery EDM, Gyory AZ. Removal of interference by antihypertensive drugs in the spectrophotometric assay of metanephrines. *Clin Chim Acta*, 169, 117-120 (1987)

1163 Crawford OB. Methemoglobin in man following the use of prilocaine. *Acta Anaesthesiol Scand*, 16, Suppl, 183 (1965)

1164 Crawford PM, Belchetz P, Davis C et al. Growth hormone response to diazepam, clonidine and glucagon in patients with epilepsy. *Epilepsy Res*, 3, 63-69 (1989)

1165 Crawford WA, Franks HM, Hensley VR et al. The effect of disodium cromoglycate on human performance, alone and in combination with ethanol. *Med J Aust*, 1, 997-999 (1976)

1166 Crawhall JC. Proteinuria in D-penicillamine-treated rheumatoid arthritis. *J Rheumatol*, 8, Suppl 7, 161-163 (1981)

1167 Cremata VY Jr, Koe BK. Clinical-pharmacological evaluation of p-chlorophenylalanine: new serotonin-depleting agent. *Clin Pharmacol Ther*, 7, 768 (1966)

1168 Crespi HG. Topical corticosteroid therapy for children: alclometasone dipropionate cream 0.05%. *Clin Ther*, 8, 203-210 (1986)

1169 Crobach LFSJ, Jansen JBMJ, Lamers CBHW. Effect of intermittent weekend therapy with omeprazole on basal and bombesin- and pentagastrin-stimulated gastric acid and serum gastrin. *Scand J Gastroenterol*, 23, 407-412 (1988)

1170 Croft JD, Swisher SN, Gilliland BC et al. Coombs' - test positivity induced by drugs. *Ann Intern Med*, 68, 176 (1968)

1171 Crofton PM. Positive and negative interference in the benzethonium chloride method for urine protein. *Ann Clin Biochem*, 26, 104-105 (1989)

1172 Crooij MJ, de Nooyer CCA, Rao BR et al. Termination of early pregnancy by the 3β-hydroxysteroid dehydrogenase inhibitor epostane. *N Engl J Med*, 319, 813-817 (1988)

1173 Crook D, Gardner R, Worthington M et al. Zoladex versus danazol in the treatment of pelvic endometriosis: effects on plasma lipid risk factors. *Horm Res*, Suppl 1, 157-160 (1989)

1174 Cross FC, Canada AT Jr, Davis NM. Effects of certain drugs on the results of some common laboratory diagnostic procedures. *Am J Hosp Pharm*, 23, 235 (1966)

1175 Crout JR. Catecholamines in urine. *Stand Meth Clin Chem*, 3, 62 (1961)

1176 Crowell EB Jr, Clatanoff DV, Kiekhofer W. The effect of oral contraceptives on factor VIII levels. *J Lab Clin Med*, 77, 551 (1971)

1177 Crowley MF, Rosser A. Oestrogen determination in pregnancy urine using enzymatic hydrolysis of oestrogen conjugates. *Clin Chim Acta*, 49, 115 (1973)

1178 Crowley VEF, Olukoga AO, Stewart MF et al. Ciprofibrate: a cause of low HDL cholesterol?. *Proc ACB Natl Meet*, 137-138 (1995)

1179 Croxatto HB, Diaz S, Robertson DN et al. Clinical chemistry in women with levonorgestrel implants (Norplant ™) or a TCU 200 IUD. *Contraception*, 27, 281-288 (1983)

1180 Crozier IG, Ikram H, Nicholls MG et al. Acute hemodynamic, hormonal and electrolyte effects of ramipril in severe congestive heart failure. *Am J Cardiol*, 59, 155D-163D (1987)

1181 Cruickshank AM, Ballantyne FC, Shenkin A. Negative interference in a kinetic Jaffe method for serum creatinine determination. *Ann Clin Biochem*, 25, 112-113 (1988)

1182 Crumpacker CS. Ganciclovir. *N Engl J Med*, 335, 721-729 (1996)

1183 Crussell-Porter LL, Rindone JP, Ford MA et al. Low-dose fluconazole therapy potentiates the hypoprothrombinemic response of warfarin sodium. *Arch Intern Med*, 153, 102-04 (1993)

1184 Cryer PE, Sode J. Drug interference with measurement of adrenal hormones in urine: analgesics and tranquilizer-sedatives. *Ann Intern Med*, 75, 697 (1971)

1185 Csako G. False-positive results for ketone with the drug mesna and other free sulfhydryl compounds. *Clin Chem*, 33, 289-292 (1987)

1186 Csako G, Costello R, Pucino F. Positive interference with the Jaffe reaction by sulbactam. *Clin Chem*, 39, 1144-1145 (1993)

1187 Cubeddu LX, Hoffmann IS, Fuenmayor NT et al. Efficacy of Ondanesetron (GR 38032F) and the role of serotonin in cisplatin-induced nausea and vomiting. *N Engl J Med*, 322, 810-816 (1990)

1188 Cuche J-L, Seiz F, Ruget G et al. Dilution of plasma with tris buffer increases measured catecholamines in plasma. *Clin Chem*, 33, 408-411 (1987)

1189 Cuche L-L, Brochier P, Klioua N et al. Conjugated catecholamines in human plasma: where are they coming from?. *J Lab Clin Med*, 116, 681-686 (1990)

1190 Cucuianu M, Bornuz F, Macavei I. Effect of L-asparaginase therapy upon serum pseudocholinesterase and ceruloplasmin levels in patients. *Clin Chim Acta*, 38, 97 (1972)

1191 Cullen SI, Catalano PM. Griseofulvin-warfarin antagonism. *J Am Med Ass*, 199, 582 (1967)

1192 Cumming FJ, Briggs MH. Changes in plasma vitamin A in lactating and nonlactating oral contraceptive users. *Br J Obstet Gynaecol*, 90, 73-77 (1983)

1193 Cummings EA, Salisbury SR, Givner ML, Rittmaster RS. Testolactone-associated high androgen levels, a pharmacologic effect or laboratory artifact?. *J Clin Endocrinol Metab*, 83, 784-787 (1998)

1194 Cummings JN. Migraine - a biochemical disorder?. *Fourth Symposium of the Migraine Trust, London* (1970)

1195 Cunningham GC. Phenylketonuria testing - its role in pediatrics and public health. *Crit Rev Clin Lab Sci*, 2, 45 (1971)

1196 Cunningham GR, Hirshkowitz M. Inhibition of steroid 5α-reductase with finasteride: sleep-related erections, potency, and libido in healthy men. *J Clin Endocrinol Metab*, 80, 1934-1940 (1995)

1197 Cunningham JJ, Mearkle PL, Brown RG. Vitamin C: an aldolase reductase inhibitor that normalizes erythrocyte sorbitol in insulin-dependent diabetes mellitus. *J Am Coll Nutr*, 13, 344-350 (1994)

1198 Cunningham SK, Loughlin T, Culliton M et al. The relationship between sex steroids and sex hormone-binding globulin in plasma in physiological and pathological conditions.. *Ann Clin Biochem*, 22, 489-497 (1985)

1199 Curtis JA, Cormode E, Laski B et al. Endocrine complications of topical and intralesional corticosteroid therapy. *Arch Dis Child*, 57, 204-207 (1982)

1200 Cuschieri A. Activation of the kinin-forming system during therapy with cyclophosphamide. *Clin Chem*, 20, 19 (1974)

1201 Cushman P Jr. Plasma testosterone in narcotic addiction. *Am J Med*, 55, 452 (1973)

1202 Cushman P Jr, Grieco MH. Hyperimmunoglobulinemia associated with narcotic addiction: effects of methadone maintenance treatment. *Am J Med*, 54, 320 (1973)

1203 Custro N, Scafidi V, Costanza G et al. Effect of long-term treatment with therapeutic doses of domperidone on circulating thyroid-stimulating hormone levels in euthyroid patients. *Curr Ther Res*, 44, 287-291 (1988)

1204 Cuthbert MF. Adverse reactions to nonsteroidal antirheumatic drugs. *Curr Med Res Opin*, 2, 600-610 (1974)

1205 Cwikiel M, Persson SU, Larsson H et al. Changes of blood viscosity in patients treated with 5-fluorouracil - a link to cardiotoxicity. *Acta Oncol*, 34, 83-85 (1995)

1206 Czejka MJ, Schuller J, Jager W et al. Influence of different doses of interferon-α-2b on the blood plasma levels of 5-fluorouracil. *Eur J Drug Metab Pharmacokinet*, 18, 247-250 (1993)

1207 Czekalski S, Widecka K, Gozdzik J et al. Atrial natriuretic peptide and cyclic guanosine monophosphate plasma concentrations in patients with thyrotoxicosis and atrial fibrillation. Effect of short-term methimazole therapy. *J Endocrinol Invest*, 17, 341-346 (1994)

1208 Czerwinski AW, Czerwinski AB, Whitsett TI et al. Effects of a single, large, intravenous injection of dexamethasone. *Clin Pharmacol Ther*, 13, 638 (1972)

1209 Da Col PG, Cattin L, Valenti M et al. Efficacy of simvastatin plus cholestyramine in the two-year treatment of heterozygous hypercholesterolemia. *Curr Ther Res*, 48, 798-808 (1990)

1210 Daae LNW, Juell A. A new and more ascorbic acid resistant dipstick test for the detection of glucosuria has been introduced. *Scand J Clin Lab Invest*, 45, 289 (1985)

1211 Daae LNW, Juell A. Rapid diagnostic tests for glucosuria are still influenced by ascorbic acid. *Scand J Clin Lab Invest*, 43, 747-749 (1983)

1212 Dacie JV. The Haemolytic Anaemias part IV. New York NY, Grune and Stratton (1967)

1213 Dahl JR. Diphenylhydantoin toxic psychosis with associated hyperglycemia. *Calif Med*, 107, 345 (1967)

1214 Dahlquist R, Ejvinsson G, Schenck-Gustafsson K. Effect of quinidine on plasma concentration and renal clearance of digoxin: a clinically important drug interaction. *Br J Clin Pharmacol*, 9, 413-418 (1980)

1215 Dahlqvist R, Steiner E, Koike Y et al. Induction of theophylline metabolism by pentobarbital. *Ther Drug Monit*, 11, 408-410 (1989)

1216 Daidoh H, Morita H, Mune T et al. Responses of plasma adrenocortical steroids to low dose ACTH in normal subjects. *Clin Endocrinol*, 43, 311-315 (1995)

1217 Daigneault EA, Hamdy RC, Ferslew KE et al. Investigation of the influence of acetylsalicylic acid on the steady state of long-term therapy with theophylline in elderly male patients with normal renal function. *J Clin Pharmacol*, 34, 86-90 (1994)

1218 Dal Canton A, Fuiano G, Conte G et al. Mechanism of increased plasma urea after diuretic therapy in uraemic patients. *Clin Sci*, 68, 255-261 (1985)

1219 Dal Negro R, Pomari C, Turco P. Famotidine and theophylline pharmacokinetics: an unexpected cimetidine-like interaction in patients with chronic obstructive pulmonary disease. *Clin Pharmacokinet*, 24, 255-258 (1993)

1220 Dalakas M, Illa I. Mitochondrial myopathy caused by long-term zidovudine therapy. *N Engl J Med*, 323, 994 (1990)

1221 Dalderup LM. Ischaemic heart disease and vitamin D. *Lancet*, 2, 92 (1973)

1222 Dale E, Simpson G. Serum magnesium levels of women taking an oral or long-term injectable progestational contraceptive. *Obstet Gynecol*, 39, 115 (1972)

1223 Dale E, Spivey SH. Serum proteins of women utilizing combination oral or long-acting injectable progestational contraceptives. *Contraception*, 4, 241 (1971)

1224 Dale J, Landmark KH, Myhre E. The effects of nifedipine, a calcium antagonist, on platelet function. *Am Heart J*, 105, 103-105 (1983)

1225 Dallongeville J, Fruchart JC, Pfister P et al. Effect of fluvastatin on plasma apolipoprotein-B-containing particles, including lipoprotein(a). *J Intern Med*, 236, 95-101 (1994)

1226 Dallos V, Heathfield K, Stone P et al. The comparative value of amantadine and levodopa. *Postgrad Med J*, 48, 354 (1972)

1227 Dalrymple RW, Stearns FM. Diflunisal interference with determination of salicylate by the Trinder, Abbott TDx, and du Pont aca methods. *Clin Chem*, 32, 230 (1986)

1228 Dalton MJ, Powell JR, Messenheimer JA Jr. The influence of cimetidine on single dose carbamazepine pharmacokinetics. *Epilepsia*, 26, 127-130 (1985)

1229 Damber J-E, Abramsson L, Duchek M. Tamoxifen treatment of idiopathic oligozoospermia; Effect on hCG-induced testicular steroidogenesis and semen variables. *Scand J Urol Nephrol*, 23, 241-246 (1989)

1230 Dana-Haeri J, Oxley J, Richens A. Reduction of free testosterone by antiepileptic drugs. *Br Med J*, 284, 85-86 (1982)

1231 Dandona D, Junglee D, Katrak A. Increased serum pancreatic enzymes after treatment with methylprednisolone: possible evidence of subclinical pancreatitis. *Br Med J*, 291, 24 (1985)

1232 Daniel D, Dappen G, Winterkorn R et al. Development of the Kodak Ektachem clinical chemistry slides for ethanol. *Clin Chem*, 36, 1197 (1990)

1233 Daniels AL, Everson GJ. Influence of acetylsalicylic acid (aspirin) on urinary excretion of ascorbic acid. *Proc Soc Exp Biol Med*, 35, 20 (1936)

1234 Danner SA, Carr A, Leonard JM et al. A short-term study of the safety, pharmacokinetics, and efficacy of ritonavir, an inhibitor of HIV-1 protease. *N Engl J Med*, 333, 1528-1533 (1995)

1235 Danowski TS, Vester JW, Sunder JH et al. Endocrine and metabolic indices during administration of a lipophilic bis-phenol, probucol. *Clin Pharmacol Ther*, 12, 929 (1971)

1236 Danziger Y, Garty M, Volwitz B et al. Reduction of serum theophylline levels by terbutaline in children with asthma. *Clin Pharmacol Ther*, 37, 469-471 (1985)

1237 Danzinger RG, Hofmann AF, Schoenfield LJ et al. Dissolution of cholesterol gallstones by chenodeoxycholic acid. *N Engl J Med*, 286, 1 (1972)

1238 Darioli R, Bovet P, Brunner H-R et al. Effectiveness, tolerance and safety of three-year simvastatin therapy in primary hypercholesterolemia. *Schweiz Med Wschr*, 120, 85-89 (1990)

1239 Darling GM, Harris SSJohns JA, McCloud PI, Davis SR. Estrogen and progestin compared with simvastatin for hypercholesterolemia in postmenopausal women. *N Engl J Med*, 337, 595-601 (1997)

1240 Das KM, Eastwood MA, Mcmanus JPA et al. Adverse reactions during salicylasulfapyridine therapy and the relation with drug metabolism and acetylator. *N Engl J Med*, 289, 491 (1973)

1241 Dasgupta A, Dennen DA, Dean R. Effect of serum albumin on in vitro displacement of valproic acid by ceftriaxone and nafcillin. *Clin Chem*, 36, 825-826 (1990)

1242 Dasgupta A, Dennen DA, Dean R et al. Displacement of phenytoin from serum protein carriers by antibiotics: studies with ceftriaxone, nafcillin, and sulfamethoxazole. *Clin Chem*, 37, 98-100 (1991)

1243 Dash H, Mills J. Severe metabolic acidosis associated with nalidixic acid overdose. *Ann Intern Med*, 84, 570-571 (1976)

1244 Dash RJ, Ahmad J, Sethi BK et al. Failure of long-term cyproheptadine therapy in lowering growth hormone levels in acromegaly. *Clin Endocrinol*, 30, 639-644 (1989)

1245 Data JL, Wilkinson GR, Nies AS. Interaction of quinidine with anticonvulsant drugs. *N Engl J Med*, 294, 699-702 (1976)

1246 Datey KK, Deshmukh SN, Dalvi CP et al. Hepatocellular damage with ethacrynic acid. *Br Med J*, 3, 152 (1967)

1247 Datta P. Oxaprozin and 5-(p-hydroxyphenyl)-5-phenylhydantoin interference in phenytoin immunoassays. *Clin Chem*, 43, 1468-1469 (1997)

1248 Daudon M, Estıpa L, Viard JP , et al. Urinary stones in HIV-positive positive patients treated with indinavir. *Lancet*, 349, 1294 (1997)

1249 Daugaard G, Abildgaard U, Holstein-Rathlou H-E et al. Renal tubular function in patients treated with high-dose cisplatin. *Clin Pharmacol Ther*, 44, 164-172 (1988)

1250 D'Auria L, Cordiali Fei P, Pietravalle M, et al. The serum levels of sE-selectin are increased in patients with bullous pemphigoid or pemphigus vulgaris. Correlation with the number of skin lesions and recovery after corticosteroid therapy. *Br J Dermatol*, 137, 59-64 (1997)

1251 Davenport A, Davison AM, Newton KE et al. Urinary aluminium excretion following renal transplantation and the effect of pulse steroid therapy. *Ann Clin Biochem*, 27, 25-32 (1990)

1252 Davenport HW. Physiology of the Digestive Tract. Chicago IL, Year Book Medical Publishers (1961)

1253 Davi G, Averna MR, Catalano I et al. Plasma fibrinogen levels in hypercholesterolemia: effects of simvastatin therapy. *Curr Ther Res*, 50, 79-83 (1991)

1254 David J. Hyperglucagonaemia and treatment with danazol for systemic lupus erythematosus. *Br Med J*, 291, 1170-1171 (1985)

1255 Davidsohn I, Wells BB. Clinical Diagnosis by Laboratory Methods. *13th edition*, Philadelphia PA, WB Saunders (1962)

1256 Davidson BJ, Rea CD, Valenzuela GJ. Atrial natriuretic peptide, plasma renin activity, and aldosterone in women on estrogen therapy and with premenstrual syndrome. *Fertil Steril*, 50, 743-746 (1988)

1257 Davidson DF. Urinary catecholamines assay by HPLC: in vitro interference by some drugs. *Ann Clin Biochem*, 25, 583-584 (1988)

1258 Davidson DGD, Eastham WN. Acute liver necrosis following overdose of paracetamol. *Br Med J*, 2, 497 (1966)

1259 Davidson M, Davis BM, Bastiaens L et al. Growth hormone response to edrophonium in patients with Alzheimer's disease and normal control subjects. *Am J Psychiat*, 145, 1007-1009 (1988)

1260 Davidson MB, Bernstein JM. Effect of nicotinic acid on growth hormone induced glucose intolerance and lipolysis. *Clin Res*, 20, 237 (1972)

1261 Davidson MB, Holzman GB. Role of growth hormone in the alteration of carbohydrate metabolism induced by oral contraceptive agents. *J Clin Endocrinol Metab*, 36, 246 (1973)

1262 Davidson MH, Nawrocki JW, Weiss SR, et al. Effectiveness of atorvastatin for reducing low-density lipoprotein cholesterol to National Cholesterol Education Program Treat ment goals, 347-348 (1997)

1263 Davidson W, Barbour HM. Determination of urinary magnesium using the Magon dye method on the Monarch centrifugal analyzer. *Ann Clin Biochem*, 27, 595-596 (1990)

1264 Davie MWJ, Worsfold M, Sharp CA et al. Anomalous rise of serum osteocalcin following desferrioxamine treatment in aluminum intoxication. *Nephron*, 65, 245-248 (1993)

1265 Davie SJ, Gould BJ, Yudkin JS. Artifactual increase in electrophoretic measurement of glycated haemoglobin caused by vitamin C. *Proc ACB Natl Meet*, 40 (1990)

1266 Davie SJ, Gould BJ, Yudkin JS. The effect of vitamin C on glycation of proteins in vivo. *Proc ACB Natl Meet*, 40 (1990)

1267 Davie SJ, Gould BJ, Yudkin JS. The effect of vitamin C on glycosylation of proteins. *Diabetes*, 41, 167-173 (1992)

1268 Davies DL, Lant AF, Millard NR et al. Some aspects of the clinical pharmacology of bumetanide, a new potent oral diuretic. *Br J Pharmacol*, 47, 618 (1973)

1269 Davies PH, Franklyn JA. The effects of drugs on tests of thyroid function. *Eur J Clin Pharmacol*, 40, 439-451 (1991)

1270 Davies RO, Gomez HJ, Irvin JD et al. An overview of the clinical pharmacology of enalapril. *Br J Clin Pharmacol*, 18, Suppl 2, 215s-229s (1984)

1271 Davignon J, Roederer G, Montigny M et al. Comparative efficacy and safety of pravastatin, nicotinic acid and the two combined in patients with hypercholesterolemia. *Am J Cardiol*, 73, 339-345 (1994)

1272 Davila R, Manero E, Zumarraga M et al. Plasma homovanillic acid as a predictor of response to neuroleptics. *Arch Gen Psychiat*, 45, 564-567 (1988)

1273 Davis B, Davis K. Effect of propantheline on growth hormone and blood glucose levels. *Lancet*, 1, 1382 (1986)

1274 Davis GL, Balart LA, Schiff ER et al. Treatment of chronic hepatitis C with recombinant interferon alfa. A multicenter randomized, controlled trial. *N Engl J Med*, 321, 1501-1506 (1989)

1275 Davis GL, Esteban-Mur R, Rustgi V, et al. Interferon alfa-2b alone or with ribavirin for the treatment of relapse of chronic hepatitis C. *N Engl J Med*, 339, 1493-1499 (1998)

1276 Davis JM, Spaide JK, Heimwich HE. Effects of tranylcypromine and L-cysteine on plasma amino acids in controls and schizophrenic patients. *Am J Clin Nutr*, 25, 302 (1972)

1277 Davis M, Eddleston ALWF, Williams R. Hypersensitivity and jaundice due to azathioprine. *Postgrad Med J*, 56, 274-275 (1980)

1278 Davis P. Undesirable effects of gold salts. *J Rheumatol*, 6, Suppl 5, 18-24 (1979)

1279 Davis PJ. Factors affecting the determination of the serum protein-bound iodine. *Am J Med*, 40, 918 (1966)

1280 Davis PJ, Hsu TH, Bianchine J et al. Effects of a new hypolipidemic agent, MK-185, on serum thyroxine binding globulin (TBG). *J Clin Endocrinol Metab*, 34, 200 (1972)

1281 Davis RB. Metabolic studies in carcinoid syndrome: observations on use of α-methyldopa, isonicotinic acid hydrazide. *Metabolism*, 10, 1035 (1961)

1282 Davis RL, Berman W Jr, Wernly JA et al. Warfarin-nafcillin interaction. *J Pediatr*, 118, 300-303 (1991)

1283 Davis RL, Kelly HW, Quenzer RW et al. Effect of norfloxacin on theophylline metabolism. *Antimicrob Agent Chemother*, 33, 212-214 (1989)

1284 Davoren PM, Kelly W, Gries FA, et al. Long-term effects of a sustained-release preparation of acipimox on dyslipidemia and glucose metabolism in noninsulin-dependent diabetes mellitus. *Metabolism*, 47, 250-256 (1998)

1285 Dawood MY, Obasiolu CW, Ramos J, Khan-Dawood FS. Clinical, endocrine, and metabolic effects of two doses of gestrinone in treatment of pelvic endometriosis. *Am J Obstet Gynecol*, 176, 387-394 (1997)

1286 Dawood MY, Ramos J, Khan-Dawood FS. Depot leuprolide acetate versus danazol for treatment of pelvic endometriosis: changes in vertebral bone mass and serum estradiol and calcitonin. *Fertil Steril*, 63, 1177-1183 (1995)

1287 Dawson-Hughes B, Harris S. Thiazides and seasonal bone change in healthy postmenopausal women. *Bone Miner*, 21, 41-51 (1993)

1288 Dawson-Hughes B, Harris SS, Krall EA, Dallal GE. Effect of calcium and vitamin D supplementation on bone density in men and women 65 years of age or older. *N Engl J Med*, 337, 670-676 (1997)

1289 Day AP, Bellavia S, Jones OTG, Stansbie D. Effect of simvastatin therapy on cell membrane cholesterol content and membrane function as assessed by polymorphonuclear cell NADPH oxidase activity. *Ann Clin Biochem*, 34, 269-275 (1997)

1290 Day AP, Feher MD, Chopra R et al. The effect of bezafibrate on serum alkaline phosphatase isoenzyme activities both fasting and after an oral fat load. *Proc ACB Natl Meet*, 120 (1992)

1291 Day HJ, Holmsen H. Laboratory tests of platelet function. *Ann Clin Lab Sci*, 2, 63 (1972)

1292 Day JL, Metcalfe J, Simpson CN. Adrenergic mechanisms in control of plasma lipid concentrations. *Br Med J*, 284, 1145-1148 (1982)

1293 Day JL, Simpson N, Metcalfe J et al. Metabolic consequences of atenolol and propranolol in treatment of essential hypertension. *Br Med J*, 1, 77-80 (1979)

1294 Day RO, Geisslinger G, Paull P et al. Neither cimetidine nor probenecid affect the pharmacokinetics of tenoxicam in normal volunteers. *Br J Clin Pharmacol*, 37, 79-81 (1994)

1295 Day RO, Paull PD, Lam S et al. The effect of concurrent aspirin upon plasma concentrations of tenoxicam. *Br J Clin Pharmacol*, 26, 455-462 (1988)

1296 Dayal S, Schwarzberg M. Technicon free thyroxine assay: a fully automated direct immunoassay for the determination of free thyroxine in human serum. *Clin Chem*, 37, 1032 (1991)

1297 Dayan AD, Lewis PD. Idoxuridine and jaundice. *Lancet*, 2, 1073 (1970)

1298 Daymond TJ. Cholecystography and renal failure. *Lancet*, 2, 549 (1971)

1299 D'Costa DF, Basu SK, Gunasekera NP et al. ACE inhibitors and diuretics causing hypokalemia. *Br J Clin Pract*, 44, 26-27 (1990)

1300 De Backer G. Multicentre study of the efficacy and tolerance of acebutolol versus atenolol in the long term treatment of mild arterial hypertension. *Drugs*, 36, Suppl 2, 51-56 (1988)

1301 De Bellis MD, Geracioti TD Jr, Altemus M et al. Cerebrospinal fluid monoamine metabolites in fluoxetine-treated patients with major depression and in healthy volunteers. *Biol Psychiat*, 33, 636-641 (1993)

1302 de Boer A, Kluft C, Kasper FJ et al. Interaction study between nifedipine and recombinant tissue-type plasminogen activator in healthy subjects. *Br J Clin Pharmacol*, 36, 99-104 (1993)

1303 de Bruin TWA, van Barlingen H, van Linde-Sibenius Trip M et al. Lipoprotein(a) and apolipoprotein B plasma concentrations in hypothyroid, euthyroid, and hyperthyroid subjects. *J Clin Endocrinol Metab*, 76, 121-126 (1993)

1304 De Cesaris R, Rainieri G, Chiarappa R et al. Interaktionen einiger Calcium-antagonisten mit der Wirksamkeit von Digitalis. *Biol Med*, 6, 169-177 (1984)

1305 De Cesaris R, Ranieri G, Filitti V et al. Effects of atenolol and enalapril on kidney function in hypertensive diabetic patients. *J Cardiovasc Pharmacol*, 22, 208-214 (1993)

1306 De Cesaris R, Ranieri G, Filitti V et al. Glucose and lipid metabolism in essential hypertension: effects of diuretics and ACE-inhibitors. *Cardiology*, 83, 165-172 (1993)

1307 de Divitiis M, Rubba P, Di Somma S, et al. Effects of short-term reduction in serum cholesterol with simvastatin in patients with stable angina pectoris and mild to moderate hypercholesterolemia. *Am J Cardiol*, 78, 763-768 (1996)

1308 de Gislain C, Dumas M, d'Athis P et al. Evolution de la creatininemie lors d'injections repetees de cisplatine. Influence des associations medicamenteuses. *Therapie*, 45, 423-427 (1990)

1309 de Graaf J, Swinkels DW, Demacker PNM et al. Differences in the low density lipoprotein subfraction profile between oral contraceptive users and controls. *J Clin Endocrinol Metab*, 76, 197-202 (1993)

1310 De Gramont A, Rioux E, Drolet Y et al. Erythrocyte mean corpuscular volume during cytotoxic therapy and the risk of secondary leukemia. *Cancer*, 55, 493-495 (1985)

1311 De Haan RM, Schellenberg D, Vanden Bosch WD. Clindamycin palmitate in healthy men: general tolerance and effect on stools. *Curr Ther Res*, 14, 81 (1972)

1312 De Kniff P, Stalenhoef AFH, Mol MJTM et al. Influence of apo E polymorphism on the response to simvastatin treatment of patients with heterozygous familial hypercholesterolemia. *Atherosclerosis*, 83, 89-97 (1990)

1313 De Lange WE, Visser JWE, Doorenbos H. Hormonal influences on the concentration of tyrosine in blood. *Clin Chim Acta*, 42, 21 (1972)

1314 De Leacy EA, Brown NN, Clague AE. Nitromethane interferes in assay of creatinine by the Jaffe reaction. *Clin Chem*, 35, 1772-1774 (1989)

1315 De Leacy EA, McLeay CD, Eadie MJ et al. Effects of subjects' sex, and intake of tobacco, alcohol and oral contraceptives on plasma phenytoin levels. *Br J Clin Pharmacol*, 8, 33-36 (1979)

1316 De Lepeleire I, van Hecken A, Verbesselt R et al. Lack of interaction between famotidine and warfarin. *Int J Clin Pharmacol Res*, 10, 167-171 (1990)

1317 de Maat MPM, Knipscheer HC, Kastelein JJP, Kluft C. Modulation of plasma fibrinogen levels by ciprofibrate and gemfibrozil in primary hyperlipidaemia. *Thromb Haemostas*, 77, 75-79 (1997)

1318 De Marinis L, Mancini A, Calabaro F et al. Evaluation of dopaminergic tone in postmenopausal women: effects of piribedil on anterior pituitary hormones. *Horm Metab Res*, 23, 30-34 (1991)

1319 de May C, Brendel E, Enterling D. Carvedilol increases the systemic bioavailability of oral digoxin. *Br J Clin Pharmacol*, 29, 486-490 (1990)

1320 de May C, Enterling D, Meineke I et al. Effects of the novel D_2-dopaminergic agonist ropinirol on supine resting and stimulated circulatory and neuroendocrine variables in healthy volunteers. *Arz Forsch Drug Res*, 40, 7-13 (1990)

1321 De Pinho RA, Goldberg CS, Lefkowitch JH. Azathioprine and the liver. Evidence favoring idiosyncratic, mixed cholestatic- hepatocellular injury in humans. *Gastroenterology*, 86, 162-165 (1984)

1322 De Ritis L. Un caso di neutropenia da chlorothiazide. *Arcisped S Anna Ferrera*, 16, 985 (1963)

1323 De Schepper PJ, Imperato-McGinley J, Van Hecken A et al. Hormonal effects, tolerability, and preliminary kinetics in men of MK-906, a 5α-reductase inhibitor. *Steroids*, 56, 469-471 (1991)

1324 De Virgilio R, Zampieri A, De Lazzari M et al. Intravenous administration of clodronate in normocalcemic patients with tumoral bone metastases: effect on serum parathormone and biochemical markers of bone turnover. *Curr Ther Res*, 49, 182-186 (1991)

1325 de Vries RJM, Dunselman PHJM, Sung UGCK, et al. Effects of lacidipine on peak oxygen consumption, neurohormones and invasive haemodynamics in patients with mild to moderate chronic failure. *Heart*, 75, 159-164 (1996)

1326 de Vries RJM, Querı M, Lok DJA, et al. Comparison of effects on peak oxygen consumption, quality of life, and neurohormones of felodipine and enalapril in patients with congestive heart failure. *Am J Cardiol*, 76, 1253-1258 (1995)

1327 De Wit R, Bakker PJM, Reiss P et al. Temporary increase in serum β_2-microglobulin during treatment with interferon-α for AIDS-associated Kaposi's sarcoma. *AIDS*, 4, 459-462 (1990)

1328 De Wit R, Raasveld MHM, Ten Berghe RJM et al. Interleukin-6 concentrations in the serum of patients with AIDS-associated kaposi's sarcoma during treatment with interferon-α. *J Intern Med*, 229, 539-542 (1991)

1329 De Wolff FA, Peters ACB, Van Kempen GMJ. Valproate induces urinary D-glucaric acid excretion. *Lancet*, 1, 843 (1981)

1330 de Zeeuw D, Gansevoort RT, Dullaart RPF et al. Angiotensin II antagonism improves the lipoprotein profile in patients with nephrotic syndrome. *J Hypertens*, 13, Suppl 1, S53-S58 (1995)

1331 Deadman NM. Evaluation of chromogens suitable for occult blood in faeces. *Clin Chim Acta*, 35, 273 (1971)

1332 Dean RP, Talbert RL. Bleeding associated with concurrent warfarin and metronidazole therapy. *Drug Intell Clin Pharm*, 14, 864-866 (1980)

1333 Deary G, Maistre G, Le Hoang P et al. Effect of cyclosporine on atrial natriuretic factor in patients with uveitis. *N Engl J Med*, 332, 336 (1990)

1334 Deblasi S. Azione del fargan sulla glicemia e sulla curva glicemia de carico nell'uomo e nel cane. *Minerva Anesthesiol*, 19, 66 (1953)

1335 Debruyne D, Commeau Ph, Grollier G et al. Nicardipine does not significantly affect serum digoxin concentrations at the steady state of patients with congestive heart failure. *Int J Clin Pharmacol Res*, 9, 15-19 (1989)

1336 Decensi A, Torrisi R, Marroni P et al. Effect of the nonsteroidal antiandrogen nilutamide on adrenal androgen secretion. *Prostate*, 24, 17-23 (1994)

1337 Dechend R, Hauck S, Eichhorn J et al. Effects of low-molecular weight and high-molecular weight heparin on the intrinsic and extrinsic endogenous fibrinolytic system. *Fibrinolysis*, 8, 71-74 (1994)

1338 Dechtiaruk W, Crawford R, Frye R. Theophylline interference in phenobarbital quantitation. *Clin Chem*, 25, 2055 (1979)

1339 Declerck PJ, Boden G, Degreef H et al. Influence of oral intake of retinoids on the human plasma fibrinolytic system. *Fibrinolysis*, 7, 347-351 (1993)

1340 Deenamode MJMJ, Sherwood RA, Sherman DIN et al. Amylase and lipase activity following paracetamol overdose. *Proc ACB Natl Meet*, 153 (1995)

1341 Deeny M, Farish E, Tillman J et al. Changes in the bone and liver isoenzymes of alkaline phosphatase in postmenopausal women being treated with norethisterone. *Clin Chim Acta*, 171, 103-108 (1988)

1342 Defelice EA, Mehta DJ, Cahn MM et al. Evaluation of safety, serum levels and urinary excretion of hetacillin in normal volunteers. *Toxicol Appl Pharmacol*, 11, 20 (1967)

1343 Defronzo RA, Braine H, Calvin OM et al. Water intoxication in man after cyclophosphamide therapy. *Ann Intern Med*, 78, 861 (1973)

1344 Defronzo RA, Colvin OM, Braine H et al. Cyclophosphamide - induced hyponatremia. *Clin Res*, 20, 891 (1972)

1345 Defronzo RA, Goodman AM, Multicenter Metformin Study Group. Efficacy of metformin in patients with non-insulin-dependent diabetes mellitus. *N Engl J Med*, 333, 541-549 (1995)

1346 Deftos LJ, Parthemore J, Roos B. Effect of gastrin on calcitonin (CT) secretion in man. *Clin Res*, 21, 489 (1973)

1347 Degaute JP, Leeman M, Reuse C et al. Acute and chronic effects of lisinopril on renal and sytematic hemodynamics in hypertension. *Cardiovasc Drug Ther*, 6, 489-494 (1992)

1348 Deger G. Effect of terazosin on serum lipids. *Am J Med*, 80, Suppl 5B, 82-85 (1986)

1349 Degli Uberti EC, Trasforini G, Margutti A et al. Stimulation of growth hormone and corticotropin release by angiotensin II in man. *Metabolism*, 39, 1063-1067 (1990)

1350 Deglin JM, Poll K. Quinidine-induced fever and hepatic dysfunction. *Drug Intell Clin Pharm*, 14, 216-217 (1980)

1351 Degnbol B, Dorph S, Marner T. The effect of different diuretics on elevated blood pressure and serum potassium. *Acta Med Scand*, 193, 407 (1973)

1352 Degroot LJ, Hoye K. Dexamthasone suppression of serum T3 and T4. *J Clin Endocrinol Metab*, 42, 976-978 (1976)

1353 Deguia D, Mendlowitz M, Vlachakis ND et al. CP-19,106 - a new oral antihypertensive agent. *Clin Res*, 20, 862 (1972)

1354 Deisseroth A, Morganroth J, Winokru S. Quinidine-induced liver disease. *Ann Intern Med*, 77, 595 (1972)

1355 Del Arbol LR, Moreira V, Moreno A et al. Bridging hepatic necrosis associated with cimetidine. *Am J Gastroenterol*, 74, 267-269 (1980)

1356 Del Pozo E, Brun Del RER, Varga L et al. The inhibition of prolactin secretion in man by CB-154 (2-Br-α-ergocryptine). *J Clin Endocrinol Metab*, 35, 768 (1972)

1357 Del Rio G, Velardo A, Zizzo G et al. Sex differences in catecholamine response to clonidine. *Int J Obesity*, 17, 465-469 (1993)

1358 Delage JM, Lehner-Netsch G, Brisson J. The classical and alternate pathways of complement in oral contraceptive users. *Contraception*, 36, 627-632 (1987)

1359 Delanghe J, Chapelle J-P, El Allaf M et al. Quantitative turbidimetric assay for determining myoglobin evaluated. *Ann Clin Biochem*, 28, 474-479 (1991)

1360 Delanghe JR, Chapelle J-P, Vanderschueren SC. Quantitative nephelometric assay for determining myoglobin evaluated. *Clin Chem*, 36, 1675-1678 (1990)

1361 Delbeke FT, Debackere M. The influence of diuretics on the excretion and metabolism of doping agents – I. Mephentermine. *J Pharmacol Biomed Anal*, 3, 141-148 (1985)

1362 Deleeuw PW, Birkenhager WH. Effects of verapamil in hypertensive patients. *Acta Med Scand*, 215, Suppl 681, 125-128 (1984)

1363 Delfs TM, Baars S, Fook C et al. Sex steroids do not alter melatonin secretion in the human. *Hum Reprod*, 9, 49-54 (1994)

1364 D'Elia JA, Gleason RE, Alday M. Nephrotoxicity from angiographic contrast material: a prospective study. *Am J Med*, 72, 719-725 (1982)

1365 Delitala G, Devilla L, Arata L. Opiate receptors and anterior pituitary hormone secretion in man. *Acta Endocrinol*, 97, 150-156 (1981)

1366 Delitala G, Devilla L, Lotti G. Domperidone, an extracerebral inhibitor of dopamine receptors, stimulates thyrotropin and prolactin release in man. *J Clin Endocrinol Metab*, 50, 1127-1130 (1980)

1367 Delitala G, Devilla L, Lotti G. TSH and prolactin stimulation by the decarboxylase inhibitor benserazide in primary hypothyroidism. *Clin Endocrinol*, 12, 313-316 (1980)

1368 Delitala G, Devilla L, Pende A et al. Effects of the H_2-receptor antagonist ranitidine on anterior hormone secretion in men. *Eur J Clin Pharmacol*, 22, 207-211 (1982)

1369 Della JE, Maxson WS, Breen JL. Methoxyflurane hepatitis: two cases following obstetric analgesia. *Int J Gynaecol Obstet*, 21, 89-93 (1983)

1370 Dellaportas DI, Shorvon SD, Galbraith AW et al. Chronic toxicity in epileptic patients receiving single drug treatment. *Br Med J*, 285, 409-410 (1982)

1371 Delmas PD, Bjarnason NH, Mitlak BH, et al. Effects of raloxifene on bone mineral density, serum cholesterol concentrations, and uterine endometrium in postmenopausal women. *N Engl J Med*, 337, 1641-1647 (1997)

1372 Delmas PD, Demiaux B, Malaval L et al. Osteocalcin (bone gla-protein): a new biological marker for the study of skeletal pathology. *Presse Med*, 15, 643-646 (1986)

1373 Delpre G, Grinblat J, Kadish U et al. Immunological studies in a case of hepatitis following methyldopa administration. *Am J Med Sci*, 277, 207-213 (1979)

1374 Delrio FG, Park Y, Herzlich B, Drob D. Case report: diclofenac-induced rhabdomyolysis. *Am J Med Sci*, 312, 95-97 (1996)

1375 Delva NJ, Matthews DR, Cowen PJ. Brain serotonin (5-HT) neuroendocrine function in patients taking cholesterol-lowering drugs. *Biol Psychiat*, 39, 100-106 (1996)

1376 Demarie BK, Bakris GL. Effects of different calcium antagonists on proteinuria associated with diabetes mellitus. *Ann Intern Med*, 113, 987-988 (1990)

1377 Demers LM, Melby JC, Wilson TE et al. The effects of CGS 16949A, an aromatase inhibitor on adrenal mineralocorticoid biosynthesis. *J Clin Endocrinol Metab*, 70, 1162-1166 (1990)

1378 Demetriou JA, Austin FG. A rapid competitive protein-binding assay for plasma progesterone. *Clin Chim Acta*, 33, 21 (1971)

1379 Demke DM. Drug interaction between thyroxine and lovastatin. *N Engl J Med*, 321, 1341-1342 (1989)

1380 Demol P, Wingender W. Effects of rioprostil on the postprandial glucose, GIP, insulin and gastrin levels in volunteers. *Scand J Gastroenterol*, 164, Suppl 24, 112-117 (1989)

1381 Dempsey ME. The effect of hypoglycemic agents on cholesterol biosynthesis. *Adv Exp Med Biol*, 4, 511 (1968)

1382 Dennis PM, Ericksen CM. Interference of metronidazole (flagyl®) with serum aspartate aminotransferase (AST) assays. *Med J Aust*, 2, 343-344 (1980)

1383 Denny A, Adams J, Miller TC. Oxacillin and the liver. *Ann Intern Med*, 90, 277 (1979)

1384 Department of Drugs, Division of Drugs and Toxicology. Drug Evaluations Annual 1991. Chicago IL, American Medical Association (1991)

1385 DePetrillo PB, Abernethy DR, Wainer IW et al. Verapamil decreases lymphocyte protein kinase C activity in humans. *Clin Pharmacol Ther*, 55, 44-49 (1994)

1386 Deppermann K-M, Lode H, Hoffken G et al. Influence of ranitidine, pirenzepine, and aluminum magnesium hydroxide on the bioavailability of various antibiotics, including amoxicillin, cephalexin, doxycycline, and amoxicillin-clavulanic acid. *Antimicrob Agent Chemother*, 33, 1901-1907 (1989)

1387 Depre M, Friedman B, Tanaka W et al. Biochemical activity, pharmacokinetics, and tolerability of MK-866, a leukotriene biosynthesis inhibitor, in humans. *Clin Pharmacol Ther*, 53, 602-607 (1993)

1388 Dequeker J, Mardjuardi A. Treatment of rheumatoid arthritis with flurbiprofen: a comparison with enteric - coated aspirin. *Curr Med Res Opin*, 7, 418-428 (1981)

1389 Deray G, Khayat D, Jacquiaud C et al. Renal effects of S10036 in man. *Cancer Chemother Pharmacol*, 26, 467-468 (1990)

1390 Deringer PM, Maniatis A. Chlorpheniramine-induced bone marrow suppression. *Lancet*, 1, 432 (1976)

1391 Derkx FHM, Stuenkel C, Schalekamp MPA et al. Immunoreactive renin, prorenin, and enzymatically active renin in plasma during pregnancy and in women taking oral contraceptives. *J Clin Endocrinol Metab*, 63, 1008-1015 (1986)

1392 Desager JP, Harvengt C, Bianchetti G et al. The effect of cimetidine on the pharmacokinetics of single oral doses of alfuzosin. *Int J Clin Pharmacol Ther Toxicol*, 31, 568-571 (1993)

1393 Desager JP, Horsmans Y, Harvengt C. Lecithin:cholesterol acyltransferase activity in familial hypercholesterolemia treated with simvastatin and simvastatin plus low-dose colestipol. *J Clin Pharmacol*, 31, 537-542 (1991)

1394 Desager JP, Hulhoven R, Harvengt C et al. Effect of cimetidine on the pharmacodynamics, pharmacokinetics and biotransformation of a single oral dose of alpidem. *Int J Clin Pharmacol Ther Toxicol*, 28, 498-503 (1990)

1395 Desai TK, Maliakkal J, Kinzie JL et al. Taurine deficiency after intensive chemotherapy and/or radiation. *Am J Clin Nutr*, 55, 708-711 (1992)

1396 Desborough JP, Griffin RA, Moore CM et al. Growth hormone secretion in response to surgery: effects of cholinergic blockade and octreotide. *Horm Metab Res*, 25, 640-643 (1993)

1397 Desborough JP, Hall GM, Hart GR et al. Midazolam modifies pancreatic and anterior pituitary hormone secretion during upper abdominal surgery. *Br J Anaes*, 67, 390-396 (1991)

1398 Dessypris EN, Redline S, Harris JW et al. Diphenylhydantoin-induced pure red cell aplasia. *Blood*, 65, 789-794 (1985)

1399 Deuber HJ, Schulz W. Reduced lipid concentrations during four years of dialysis with low molecular weight heparin. *Kidney Int*, 40, 496-500 (1991)

1400 Devilla L, Pende A, Morgano A et al. Morphine-induced TSH release in normal and hypothyroid subjects. *Neuroendocrinology*, 40, 303-308 (1985)

1401 Devine JE. Drug-protein binding interferences caused by the plasticizer TBEP. *Clin Biochem*, 17, 345-347 (1984)

1402 Devito GA Jr. Transient elevation of alkaline phosphatase possibly related to trimethoprim- sulfamethoxazole therapy. *J Pediatr*, 100, 998-999 (1982)

1403 Devlin RD, Retallack RW, Fenton AJ et al. Long-term elevation of 1,25-dihydroxyvitamin D after short-term intravenous administration of pamidronate (aminohydroxypropylidene bisphosphonate, APD) in Paget's disease of bone. *J Bone Miner Res*, 9, 81-85 (1994)

1404 Dewland PM, Grimwood VC, Rapeport WG et al. Effect of tenidap sodium on digoxin pharmacokinetics in healthy young men. *Br J Clin Pharmacol*, 39, 43S-46S (1995)

1405 Deykin D. Warfarin therapy. *N Engl J Med*, 283, 801 (1970)

1406 Deykin D, Janson P, McMahon L. Ethanol potentiation of aspirin - induced prolongation of the bleeding time. *N Engl J Med*, 306, 852-854 (1982)

1407 Dezube BJ, Pardee AB, Chapman B et al. Pentoxifyline decreases tumor necrosis factor expression and serum triglycerides in people with AIDS. *J Acq Immune Defic Syndromes*, 6, 787-794 (1993)

1408 Dhillion S, Richens A. Valproic acid and diazepam interaction in vivo. *Br J Clin Pharmacol*, 13, 553-560 (1982)

1409 Dhondt JL, Farriaux JP, Millot F et al. Hyperphenylalaninemia during high-dose methotrexate therapy. *Arch Fr Pediat*, 48, 249-251 (1991)

1410 Di Bisceglie AM, Martin P, Kassianides C et al. Recombinant interferon alpha therapy for chronic hepatitis C: a randomized, double-blind, placebo-controlled trial. *N Engl J Med*, 321, 1506-1510 (1989)

1411 Di Leo A, Ferrari L, Bajetta E et al. Biological and clinical evaluation of lanreotide (BIM 23014), a somatostatin analogue, in the treatment of advanced breast cancer. *Breast Cancer Res Treat*, 34, 237-244 (1993)

1412 Di Minno G, Mancini M. Drugs affecting plasma fibrinogen levels. *Cardiovasc Drug Ther*, 6, 25-27 (1992)

1413 Di Pasquale P, Valdes L, Albano V, et al. Early captopril treatment reduces plasma endothelin concentrations in the acute and subacute phases of myocardial infarction: a pilot study. *J Cardiovasc Pharmacol*, 29, 1-7 (1997)

1414 Di Sant-Agnese PA. Personal communication (1972)

1415 Di Veroli C. The effects of nitrendipine on glycemia, uricemia, lipids, and body mass index during long-term antihypertensive treatment. *Curr Ther Res*, 50, 449-453 (1991)

1416 Diagnostic Systems Laboratories. Manufacturer's Product Insert on Active androstanediol glucuronide. Webster, TX

1417 Diamond JR, Cheung JY, Fang LST. Nifedipine-induced renal dysfunction. alterations in renal hemodynamics. *Am J Med*, 77, 905-909 (1984)

1418 Diamond T, Vine J, Smart R et al. Thyrotoxic bone disease in women: a potentially reversible disorder. *Ann Intern Med*, 120, 8-11 (1994)

1419 Diaz S, Croxatto HB, Pavez M. Clinical chemistry in women treated with six levonorgestrel covered rods or with a copper IUD. *Contraception*, 31, 321-330 (1985)

1420 DiBanco R, Shabetal R, Kostuk W et al. A comparison of oral milrinone, digoxin, and their combination in the treatment of patients with chronic heart failure. *N Engl J Med*, 320, 677-683 (1989)

1421 Dickes R, Schenker V, Deutsch C. Serial liver function and blood studies in patients receiving chlorpromazine. *N Engl J Med*, 256, 1 (1957)

1422 Dickinson DS, Bailey WC, Hirschowitz BI et al. Risk factors for isoniazid (INH)-induced liver dysfunction. *J Clin Gastroenterol*, 3, 271-279 (1981)

1423 Diehm C, Jacobsen O, Amendt K. The effects of tertatolol on lipid profile. *Cardiology*, 83, Suppl 1, 32-40 (1993)

1424 Diem K. Scientific Tables. *6th edition*, Basel, Documenta Geigy (1962)

1425 Dietrichson O. Chronic active hepatitis: aetiological considerations based on clinical and serological studies. *Scand J Gastroenterol*, 10, 617-624 (1975)

1426 Diffet B, Piers LS, Soares MJ, O'Dea K. The effect of oral contraceptive agents on the basal metabolic rate of young women. *Br J Nutr*, 77, 853-862 (1997)

1427 Digiesi V, Cantini F, Bisi G et al. Mechanism of action of coenzyme Q10 in essential hypertension. *Curr Ther Res*, 51, 668-672 (1992)

1428 Dijkmans BAC, Van Rijthoven AWAM, Goei The HS et al. Effect of cyclosporine on serum creatinine in patients with rheumatoid arthritis. *Eur J Clin Pharmacol*, 31, 541-545 (1987)

1429 Dillon HC Jr, Bridges RA, Null WA et al. Erythropoietic changes associated with chloramphenicol therapy. *Ala J Med Sci*, 1, 368 (1964)

1430 Dimeski G, Cheung K, Ormiston B. Interference from bicarbonate reagent in magnesium measurements on the BM/Hitachi 747. *Clin Chem*, 40, 851-852 (1994)

1431 Dimmitt DC. Pharmacokinetics of cardizem and propranolol when administered alone and in combination. *Pharmaceut Res*, 4, S82 (1987)

1432 Dimsdale JE, Hartley LH, Ruskin J et al. Effect of beta blockade on plasma catecholamine levels during psychological and exercise stress. *Am J Cardiol*, 54, 182-185 (1984)

1433 Dinscoy HP, Saelinger DA. Haloperidol-induced chronic cholestatic liver disease. *Gastroenterology*, 83, 694-700 (1982)

1434 Dinsmore WW, O'Hara MD, Callender ME. Postanesthetic carbimazole jaundice. *N Engl J Med*, 309, 438 (1983)

1435 Dionne RA, Mueller GP, Young RF et al. Contrast medium causes the apparent increase in β-endorphin levels in human cerebrospinal fluid following brain stimulation. *Pain*, 20, 313-321 (1984)

1436 DiPadova C, Roine R, Frezza M et al. Effects of ranitidine on blood alcohol levels after ethanol ingestion. *J Am Med Ass*, 267, 83-86 (1992)

1437 Dippe S, Jones R. Marijuana, glucose and insulin. *Clin Res*, 20, 237 (1972)

1438 Dista Products and Eli Lilly and Company. Manufacturer's literature on Keflex® . Indianapolis, IN 46285 (1995)

1439 Dista Products and Eli Lilly and Company. Manufacturer's literature on Nalfon® . Indianapolis, IN 46285 (1995)

1440 Dista Products Company. Manufacturer's literature on Prozac® . Indianapolis, IN (1997)

1441 Distler A, Haerlin R, Hilgenstock G et al. Clinical aspects of antihypertensive therapy with urapidil. Comparison with hydrochlorothiazide. *Drugs*, 40, Suppl 4, 21-27 (1990)

1442 Ditschuneit HH, Flechtner-Mors M, Dolderer M et al. Endocrine and metabolic effects of dexfenfluramine in patients with android obesity. *Horm Metab Res*, 25, 573-578 (1993)

1443 Diver MJ, Hipkin LJ. Changes in serum testosterone following two different treatments for hirsutism. *Proc ACB Natl Meet*, 124 (1995)

1444 Division of Clinical Biochemistry. Special Tests Instruction Booklet. *Institute of Medical and Veterinary Sciences, Adelaide, South Australia*

1445 Djurica SN, Plecas V, Milojevic Z et al. Direct effects of cytostatic therapy on the functional state of the thyroid gland and TBG in serum of patients. *Exp Clin Endocrinol*, 96, 57-63 (1990)

1446 Djurup R, Chiabrando C, Jorres A et al. Rapid direct enzyme immunoassay of 11-keto-thromboxane B_2 in urine, validated by immunoaffinity/gas chromatography-mass spectrometry. *Clin Chem*, 39, 2470-2477 (1993)

1447 Dnistrian AM, Schwartz MK, Greenberg EJ et al. Effect of tamoxifen on serum cholesterol and lipoproteins during chemohormonal therapy. *Clin Chim Acta*, 223, 43-52 (1993)

1448 Doar JWH, Wynn V. Serum lipid levels during oral contraceptive and glucocorticoid administration. *J Clin Pathol*, 55 (1969)

1449 Dobkin AB, Levy AA. Blood serum fluoride levels with methoxyflurane anesthesia. *Can J Anaes*, 20, 81 (1973)

1450 Dobs AS, Prasad M, Goldberg A, et al. Changes in serum lipoprotein(a) in hyperlipidemic subjects undergoing long-term treatment with lipid-lowering drugs. *Cardiovasc Drug Ther*, 9, 677-684

1451 Dobs AS, Sarma PS, Schteingart D. Long-term endocrine function in hypercholesterolemic patients treated with pravastatin, a new 3-hydroxy-3-methylglutaryl coenzyme A reductase inhibitor. *Metabolism*, 42, 1146-1152 (1993)

1452 Dobs AS, Sarma PS, Wilder L. Lipid-lowering diets in patients taking pravastatin, a new HMG-CoA reductase inhibitor: Compliance and adequacy. *Am J Clin Nutr*, 54, 696-700 (1991)

1453 Dobson HM, Muir MM, Hume R. The effect of ascorbic acid on the seasonal variations in serum cholesterol levels. *Scott Med J*, 29, 176-182 (1984)

1454 Dockens RC, Greene DS, Barbhaiya RH. Assessment of pharmacokinetic and pharmacodynamic drug interactions between nefazodone and digoxin in healthy male volunteers. *J Clin Pharmacol*, 36, 160-167 (1996)

1455 Dodds WN, Davidson RJL. Thrombocytopenia due to slow release oxprenolol. *Lancet*, 2, 683 (1978)

1456 Dodion L, Ambroes Y, Lamaire N. A comparison of the pharmacokinetics and diuretic effects of two loop diuretics, torasemide and furosemide, in normal volunteers. *Eur J Clin Pharmacol*, 31, Suppl, 21-27 (1986)

1457 Doering W. Quinidine-digoxin interaction. *N Engl J Med*, 301, 400-404 (1979)

1458 Doetsch K, Gadsden RH. Determination of total urinary protein, combining Lowry sensitivity and biuret specificity. *Clin Chem*, 19, 1170 (1973)

1459 Dogan P, Dogan M, Klockenkamper R. Determination of trace elements in blood serum of patients with Behcet's disease by total reflection X-ray fluorescence analysis. *Clin Chem*, 39, 1037-1041 (1993)

1460 Dollery CT. Methyldopa in hypertension. *Am Heart J*, 65, 139 (1963)

1461 Dollery CT, Duncan H, Schumer B. Hyperuricaemia related to treatment of hypertension. *Br Med J*, 2, 832 (1960)

1462 Dona G, Arditi M, Frontespezi S. Evaluation of the absorption of iron-protein-succinylate in different gastric and duodenal biochemical conditions. *Curr Ther Res*, 44, 348-352 (1988)

1463 Donadio C, Tramonti G, Giordani R et al. Effects on renal hemodynamics and tubular function of the contrast medium iohexol in renal patients. *Renal Fail*, 12, 141-146 (1990)

1464 Donaldson GWK, Graham JG. Aplastic anaemia following the administration of tegretol® . *Br J Clin Pract*, 19, 699 (1965)

1465 Donker JM. Nephrotoxicity of angiotensin converting enzyme inhibition. *Kidney Int*, 31, Suppl 20, S132-S137 (1987)

1466 Donlan CJ Jr, Forker AD. Cardiac tamponade in procainamide induced lupus erythematosus. *Chest*, 61, 685 (1972)

1467 Donn KH, Powell JR, Rogers JF et al. The influence of H_2-receptor antagonists on steady-state concentrations of propranolol and 4-hydroxypropranolol. *J Clin Pharmacol*, 24, 500-508 (1984)

1468 Donnachie EM, Seccombe DW, Urquhart NI et al. Indocyanine green interference in the Kodak Ektachem® determination of total bilirubin. *Clin Chem*, 35, 899-900 (1989)

1469 Dooley MA, Cush JJ, Lipsky PE et al. The effects of nonsteroidal antiinflammatory drug therapy in early rheumatoid arthritis on serum levels of soluble interleukin-2 receptor, CD4, and CD8. *J Rheumatol*, 20, 1857- 1862 (1993)

1470 Doppelbauer A, Zeitlhofer J, Obergottsberger S et al. The significance of laboratory findings in patients on long term antiepileptic therapy. *Dtsch Med Wschr*, 116, 41-47 (1991)

1471 D'Orazio P, Parker B. Interference by the oxidizable pharmaceuticals acetaminophen and dopamine at electrochemical sensors for blood glucose. *Clin Chem*, 41, S156 (1995)

1472 Dorchy H, Duchateau J, Bosson D et al. Transfer from purified porcine insulins to semisynthetic human insulins decreases insulin antibodies and circulating immune complexes in diabetic children and adolescents. A two-year follow-up. *Diabete Metab*, 15, 107-110 (1989)

1473 Dordoni B, Willson RA, Thompson RPH et al. Reduction of absorption of paracetamol by activated charcoal and cholestyramine: a possible therapeutic measure. *Br Med J*, 3, 86-87 (1973)

1474 Dorea JG, Costa THM, Marques AO. Effects of contraceptives on mother's serum and milk zinc. *J Nutr Biochem*, 4, 86-91 (1993)

1475 Dorfmann H, Kahn MF, De Seze S. Iatrogenic lupus: current status of the question. *Nouv Presse Med*, 1, 2907 (1972)

1476 Dornhorst A, Powell SH, Pensky J. Aggravation by propranolol of hyperglycemic effect of hydrochlorothiazide in type II diabetics without alteration of insulin secretion. *Lancet*, 1, 123-126 (1985)

1477 Dorsky DI, Crumpacker CS. Drugs five years later: acyclovir. *Ann Intern Med*, 107, 859-874 (1987)

1478 Dorwart WV. Metronidazole interference in hexokinase glucose determinations. *Clin Chem*, 29, 995 (1983)

1479 Doss M, Nawrocki P, Schmidt A et al. The influence of diet, glycine and alcohol on porphyrinuria in chronic hepatic porphyria. *Germ Med*, 1, 85 (1971)

1480 Douglass JF. Atherosclerosis. In. *Annual Reports in Medicinal Chemistry 1970, CK Cain (ed)*, New York NY, Academic Press (1971)

1481 Douste-Blazy P, Montastruc JL, Bonnet B et al. Influence of amiodarone on plasma and urine digoxin concentrations. *Lancet*, 1, 905 (1984)

1482 Doutremepuich C, Paillet D, De Seze O et al. Bleeding time after administration of acetyl salicylic acid at different dosages in healthy volunteers. *Ann Pharm Fr*, 46, 35-39 (1988)

1483 Douwes FR. Clinical value of NBT test. *N Engl J Med*, 287, 822 (1972)

1484 Dow Chemical Company. Manufacturer's literature. Indianapolis, IN (1971)

1485 Dowling HF, Lepper MH. Hepatic reactions to tetracycline. *J Am Med Ass*, 188, 307 (1964)

1486 Dowsett M, MacNeill F, Mehta A et al. Endocrine, pharmacokinetic and clinical studies of the aromatase inhibitor 3-ethyl-3-(4-pyridyl)piperidine-2,6-dione ('pyridoglutethimide') in postmenopausal breast cancer patients. *Br J Cancer*, 64, 887-894 (1991)

1487 Dowsett M, Mehta A, King N et al. An endocrine and pharmacokinetic study of four oral doses of formestane in postmenopausal breast cancer patients. *Eur J Cancer*, 28, 415-420 (1992)

1488 Dowsett M, Murray RML, Pitt P et al. Biochemical basis for the antagonism between aminoglutethimide and danazol in the endocrine treatment of breast cancer. *Ann Clin Biochem*, 23, 277-284 (1986)

1489 Doyle DR, McCurley TL, Sergent JS. Fatal polymyositis in D-penicillamine-treated rheumatoid arthritis. *Ann Intern Med*, 98, 327-330 (1983)

1490 Draeger KE, Wernicke-Panten K, Lomp H-J, et al. Long-term treatment of type 2 diabetic patients with the new oral antidiabetic agent Glimepiride (Amaryl®): a double-blind comparison with glibenclamide. *Horm Metab Res*, 28, 419-425 (1996)

1491 Drake S, Massie JD, Postlethwaite AE et al. Pamidronate sodium and calcitonin-resistant Paget's disease. Immediate response in a patient. *Arch Intern Med*, 149, 401-403 (1989)

1492 Drash A, Wolff FW. Drug therapy in leucine-sensitive hypoglycemia. *Metabolism*, 13, 487 (1964)

1493 Dravet C, Mesdjian E, Cenraud B et al. Interaction between carbamazepine and triacetyloleandomycin. *Lancet*, 2, 810-811 (1977)

1494 Dreifuss FE, Langer DH. Hepatic considerations in the use of antiepileptic drugs. *Epilepsia*, 28, Suppl 2, S23-S29 (1987)

1495 Drew SI, Carter BM, Nathanson DS et al. Levamisole-associated neutropenia and autoimmune granulocytoxins. *Ann Rheum Dis*, 39, 59-63 (1980)

1496 Drexler H, Kurz S, Jeserich M, et al. Effect of chronic angiotensin-converting enzyme inhibition on endothelial function in patients with chronic heart failure. *Am J Cardiol*, 76, 13E-18E (1995)

1497 Drici M-D, Candito M, Ferrari E et al. Clinical and biological evaluation of dilevalol vasodilating properties in mild to moderate hypertension. *Int J Clin Pharmacol Ther Toxicol*, 29, 361-365 (1991)

1498 Dries DJ, Walenga JM, Hoppensteadt D, Fareed J. Molecular markers of hemostatic activation and inflammation following major injury: effect of therapy with IFN-γ. *J Interferon Cytokine Res*, 18, 327-335 (1998)

1499 Drife JO. The effects of drugs on sperm. *Drugs*, 53, 610-622 (1987)

1500 Drinka PJ, Nolten WE. Effects of iodinated glycerol on thyroid function studies in elderly nursing home residents. *J Am Geriatr Soc*, 36, 911-913 (1988)

1501 Driskell JA, Geders JM, Urban MC. Vitamin B_6 status of young men, women, and women using oral contraceptives. *J Lab Clin Med*, 87, 813-821 (1976)

1502 Druml W, Polzleitner D, Laggner AN et al. Dextran-40, acute renal failure, and elevated plasma oncotic pressure. *N Engl J Med*, 318, 252-253 (1988)

1503 Drummond K, Levy-Marchal C, Laborde K et al. Enalapril does not alter renal function in normotensive, normoalbuminuric, hyperfiltering Type 1 (insulin-dependent) diabetic children. *Diabetologia*, 32, 255-260 (1989)

1504 Drummond KN, Michael AF. Specificity of the inhibition of tubular phosphate reabsorption by certain amino acids. *Nature*, 201, 1333 (1964)

1505 Drutz DJ, Fan JH, Tai TY et al. Hypokalemic rhabdomyolysis and myoglobinuria following amphotericin B therapy. *J Am Med Ass*, 211, 824 (1970)

1506 Du Pont aca package insert for acetaminophen. Du Pont, Wilmington DE (10/84)

1507 Du Pont aca package insert for albumin. Du Pont, Wilmington DE (5/83)

1508 Du Pont aca package insert for amikacin. Du Pont, Wilmington DE (8/86)

1509 Du Pont aca package insert for amylase. Du Pont, Wilmington DE (9/84)

1510 Du Pont aca package insert for antithrombin III. Du Pont, Wilmington DE (11/85)

1511 Du Pont aca package insert for barbiturates screen. Du Pont, Wilmington DE (11/87)

1512 Du Pont aca package insert for benzodiazepines screen. Du Pont, Wilmington DE (11/87)

1513 Du Pont aca package insert for carbamazepine. Du Pont, Wilmington DE (5/83)

1514 Du Pont aca package insert for carbon dioxide. Du Pont, Wilmington DE (5/83)

1515 Du Pont aca package insert for cerebrospinal fluid protein. Du Pont, Wilmington DE (5/83)

1516 Du Pont aca package insert for cholesterol. Du Pont, Wilmington DE (3/86)

1517 Du Pont aca package insert for conjugated bilirubin. Du Pont, Wilmington DE (10/89)

1518 Du Pont aca package insert for C-reactive protein. Du Pont, Wilmington DE (11/86)

1519 Du Pont aca package insert for creatine kinase isoenzymes. Du Pont, Wilmington DE (1/86)

1520 Du Pont aca package insert for creatinine. Du Pont, Wilmington DE (1/86)

1521 Du Pont aca package insert for digitoxin. Du Pont, Wilmington DE (7/89)

1522 Du Pont aca package insert for digoxin. Du Pont, Wilmington DE (8/86)

1523 Du Pont aca package insert for ethosuximide. Du Pont, Wilmington DE (5/83)

1524 Du Pont aca package insert for fibrinogen. Du Pont, Wilmington DE (6/87)

1525 Du Pont aca package insert for fibrinogen degradation products. Du Pont, Wilmington DE (12/87)

1526 Du Pont aca package insert for gentamicin. Du Pont, Wilmington DE (4/86)

1527 Du Pont aca package insert for glucose. Du Pont, Wilmington DE (10/83)

1528 Du Pont aca package insert for immunoglobulin A. Du Pont, Wilmington DE (5/83)

1529 Du Pont aca package insert for immunoglobulin G. Du Pont, Wilmington DE (5/83)

1530 Du Pont aca package insert for immunoglobulin M. Du Pont, Wilmington DE (5/83)

1531 Du Pont aca package insert for lactic acid. Du Pont, Wilmington DE (6/83)

1532 Du Pont aca package insert for γ-glutamyl transferase. Du Pont, Wilmington DE (5/83)

1533 Du Pont aca package insert for γ-glutamyltransferase. Du Pont, Wilmington DE (5/83)

1534 Du Pont aca package insert for lidocaine. Du Pont, Wilmington DE (10/83)

1535 Du Pont aca package insert for methotrexate. Du Pont, Wilmington DE (1/89)

1536 Du Pont aca package insert for N-acetylprocainamide. Du Pont, Wilmington DE (10/83)

1537 Du Pont aca package insert for phenobarbital. Du Pont, Wilmington DE (6/83)

1538 Du Pont aca package insert for phenytoin. Du Pont, Wilmington DE (9/84)

1539 Du Pont aca package insert for phosphorus. Du Pont, Wilmington DE (6/83)

1540 Du Pont aca package insert for plasminogen. Du Pont, Wilmington DE (6/83)

1541 Du Pont aca package insert for primidone. Du Pont, Wilmington DE (6/83)

1542 Du Pont aca package insert for procainamide. Du Pont, Wilmington DE (1/84)

1543 Du Pont aca package insert for quinidine. Du Pont, Wilmington DE (6/84)

1544 Du Pont aca package insert for theophylline. Du Pont, Wilmington DE (3/87)

1545 Du Pont aca package insert for thyronine uptake. Du Pont, Wilmington DE (7/90)

1546 Du Pont aca package insert for thyroxine. Du Pont, Wilmington DE (7/90)

1547 Du Pont aca package insert for tobramycin. Du Pont, Wilmington DE (12/85)

1548 Du Pont aca package insert for total bilirubin. Du Pont, Wilmington DE (3/87)

1549 Du Pont aca package insert for total protein. Du Pont, Wilmington DE (5/83)

1550 Du Pont aca package insert for tricyclic antidepressants screen. Du Pont, Wilmington DE (3/87)

1551 Du Pont aca package insert for triglyceride. Du Pont, Wilmington DE (10/84)

1552 Du Pont aca package insert for uric acid. Du Pont, Wilmington DE (3/87)

1553 Du Pont aca package insert for urinary protein. Du Pont, Wilmington DE (6/86)

1554 Du Pont aca package insert for urine amphetamines screen. Du Pont, Wilmington DE (9/87)

1555 Du Pont aca package insert for urine barbiturates screen. Du Pont, Wilmington DE (9/87)

1556 Du Pont aca package insert for urine benzodiazepines screen. Du Pont, Wilmington DE (12/87)

1557 Du Pont aca package insert for urine cannabinoids screen. Du Pont, Wilmington DE (1/88)

1558 Du Pont aca package insert for urine cocaine metabolite screen. Du Pont, Wilmington DE (6/87)

1559 Du Pont aca package insert for urine opiates screen. Du Pont, Wilmington DE (6/87)

1560 Du Pont aca package insert for valproic acid. Du Pont, Wilmington DE (7/90)

1561 Du Pont aca package insert for vancomycin. Du Pont, Wilmington DE (7/90)

1562 Du Pont Dimension package insert for acid phosphatase. Du Pont, Wilmington DE (12/89)

1563 Du Pont Dimension package insert for alanine aminotransferase. Du Pont, Wilmington DE (9/89)

1564 Du Pont Dimension package insert for albumin. Du Pont, Wilmington DE (7/1/88)

1565 Du Pont Dimension package insert for alkaline phosphatase. Du Pont, Wilmington DE (5/1/89)

1566 Du Pont Dimension package insert for ammonia. Du Pont, Wilmington DE (9/1/88)

1567 Du Pont Dimension package insert for amylase. Du Pont, Wilmington DE (7/1/88)

1568 Du Pont Dimension package insert for aspartate aminotransferase. Du Pont, Wilmington DE (7/89)

1569 Du Pont Dimension package insert for calcium. Du Pont, Wilmington DE (12/15/87)

1570 Du Pont Dimension package insert for cholesterol. Du Pont, Wilmington DE (9/1/88)

1571 Du Pont Dimension package insert for creatine kinase. Du Pont, Wilmington DE (10/1/88)

1572 Du Pont Dimension package insert for creatinine. Du Pont, Wilmington DE (12/15/87)

1573 Du Pont Dimension package insert for digoxin. Du Pont, Wilmington DE (6/87)

1574 Du Pont Dimension package insert for direct bilirubin. Du Pont, Wilmington DE (9/1/88)

1575 Du Pont Dimension package insert for glucose. Du Pont, Wilmington DE (12/15/87)

1576 Du Pont Dimension package insert for high density lipoprotein cholesterol. Du Pont, Wilmington DE (9/15/88)

1577 Du Pont Dimension package insert for iron. Du Pont, Wilmington DE (7/20/88)

1578 Du Pont Dimension package insert for lactate dehydrogenase. Du Pont, Wilmington DE (7/1/88)

1579 Du Pont Dimension package insert for γ-glutamyltransferase. Du Pont, Wilmington DE (7/1/88)

1580 Du Pont Dimension package insert for lipase. Du Pont, Wilmington DE (5/1/88)

1581 Du Pont Dimension package insert for magnesium. Du Pont, Wilmington DE (5/30/88)

1582 Du Pont Dimension package insert for phenobarbital. Du Pont, Wilmington DE (12/15/86)

1583 Du Pont Dimension package insert for phenytoin. Du Pont, Wilmington DE (7/20/88)

1584 Du Pont Dimension package insert for phosphorus. Du Pont, Wilmington DE (5/1/88)

1585 Du Pont Dimension package insert for theophylline. Du Pont, Wilmington DE (10/1/88)

1586 Du Pont Dimension package insert for thyronine uptake. Du Pont, Wilmington DE (12/31/87)

1587 Du Pont Dimension package insert for thyroxine. Du Pont, Wilmington DE (12/31/87)

1588 Du Pont Dimension package insert for thyroxine. Du Pont, Wilmington DE (7/90)

1589 Du Pont Dimension package insert for total bilirubin. Du Pont, Wilmington DE (8/15/88)

1590 Du Pont Dimension package insert for total iron binding capacity. Du Pont, Wilmington DE (10/1/88)

1591 Du Pont Dimension package insert for total protein. Du Pont, Wilmington DE (10/15/88)

1592 Du Pont Dimension package insert for triglyceride. Du Pont, Wilmington DE (10/15/88)

1593 Du Pont Dimension package insert for urea nitrogen. Du Pont, Wilmington DE (5/30/88)

1594 Du Pont Dimension package insert for uric acid. Du Pont, Wilmington DE (5/30/88)

1595 Du Pont Pharma. Manufacturer's literature on Coumadin® . Wilmington, DE 19805 (1995)

1596 Du Pont Pharma. Manufacturer's literature on Cozaar® . Wilmington, DE (1996)

1597 Du Pont Pharma. Manufacturer's literature on Hespan® . Wilmington, DE 19805 (1996)

1598 Du Pont Pharma. Manufacturer's literature on Pentaspan® . Wilmington, DE 19805 (1995)

1599 Du Pont Pharma. Manufacturer's literature on Revia™. Wilmington, DE 19805 (1995)

1600 Du Pont Pharma. Manufacturer's literature on Symmetrel® . Wilmington, DE 19805 (1996)

1601 Du Souich P, Caille G, Larochelle P. Enhancement of nadolol elimination by activated charcoal and antibiotics. *Clin Pharmacol Ther*, 33, 585-590 (1983)

1602 Du Souich P, Pisson C, Pedneault L et al. Effect of aminoglycosides on the disposition of thyroid hormones and thyroglobulin. *Clin Pharmacol Ther*, 38, 686-691 (1985)

1603 Duane WC. Effects of lovastatin in humans on biliary lipid composition and secretion as a function of dosage and treatment interval. *J Pharm Exp Ther*, 270, 841-845 (1994)

1604 Duarte PA, Chow CC, Simmons F et al. Fatal hepatitis associated with ketoconazole therapy. *Arch Intern Med*, 144, 1069-1070 (1984)

1605 Dubick MA, Summary JJ, Greene JY et al. In vitro and in vivo effects of hypertonic saline/dextran-70 on protein determinations in serum or plasma. *Clin Chem*, 37, 1801-1802 (1991)

1606 Dubin G, Braffman MN. Zidovudine-induced hepatotoxicity. *Ann Intern Med*, 110, 85-86 (1989)

1607 Dubin SA, Silverstein PI, Wakefield ML et al. Comparison of the effects of oral famotidine and ranitidine on gastric volume and pH. *Anesth Analg*, 69, 680-683 (1989)

1608 Dubois EL. Current status of the LE cell test. *Semin Arth Rheum*, 1, 97 (1971)

1609 Dubois EL, Tallman E, Wonka RA. Chlorpromazine - induced systemic lupus erythematosus. *J Am Med Ass*, 221, 595 (1972)

1610 Ducharme MP, Slaughter RL, Warbasse LH, et al. Itraconazole and hydroxyitraconazole serum concentrations are reduced more than tenfold by phenytoin. *Clin Pharmacol Ther*, 58, 617-624 (1995)

1611 Duchin KL, Waclawski AP, Tu JI et al. Pharmacokinetics, safety, and pharmacologic effects of fosinopril sodium, an angiotensin-converting enzyme inhibitor in healthy subjects. *J Clin Pharmacol*, 31, 58-64 (1991)

1612 Duckworth WC, Solomon SS, Kitabachi AE. Effect of chronic sulfonylurea therapy on plasma insulin and proinsulin levels. *J Clin Endocrinol Metab*, 35, 585 (1972)

1613 Duhring JL, Mckean HE, Greene JW Jr. Diurnal variation of estriol excretion in human pregnancy. *Am J Obstet Gynecol*, 115, 875 (1973)

1614 Dujovne CA, Decoursey S, Krehbiel P et al. Serum lipids in normo - and hyperlipidemics after methyldopa and propranolol. *Clin Pharmacol Ther*, 36, 157-162 (1984)

1615 Dulbecco A, Albenga C, Borretta G et al. Effect of acipimox on plasma glucose levels in patients with non-insulin-dependent diabetes mellitus. *Curr Ther Res*, 46, 478-483 (1989)

1616 Duma RJ. Summary of comparative clinical studies of ceftizoxime and cefamandole, cefazolin and tobramycin. *J Antimicrob Chemother*, 10, Suppl C, 303-309 (1982)

1617 Duncan A, Tracy RP, Vliestra RL. Influence of propranolol on platelet function. *Clin Chem*, 26, 1039 (1980)

1618 Duncan DA. Colistin toxicity: neuromuscular and renal manifestations. *Minn Med*, 56, 31 (1973)

1619 Duncan JS, Patsalos PN, Shorvon SD. Effects of discontinuation of phenytoin, carbamazepine, and valproate on concomitant antiepileptic medication. *Epilepsia*, 32, 101-115 (1991)

1620 Dundee JW. Effect of thiopentone on blood sugar and glucose tolerance. *Br J Pharmacol*, 11, 458 (1956)

1621 Dundee JW, Fee JPH, Moore J et al. Changes in serum enzyme levels following ketamine infusions. *Anesthesia*, 35, 12-16 (1980)

1622 Dunea G, Freedman P. Phenolsulfonphthalein excretion test. *J Am Med Ass*, 204, 621 (1968)

1623 Dunselmann PHJM, Scaf AMJ, Kuntze KI et al. Digoxin-felodipine interaction in patients with congestive heart failure. *Eur J Clin Pharmacol*, 35, 461-465 (1988)

1624 Dupont AG. Effects of carvedilol on renal function. *Eur J Clin Pharmacol*, 38, S96-S100 (1990)

1625 Duprez D, Baele G, De Buyzere M et al. Comparison of the fibrinolytic response to desmopressin acetate (DDAVP) infusion versus venous occlusion in patients with coronary artery disease. *Eur Heart J*, 12, 800-802 (1991)

1626 Dura Pharmaceuticals. Manufacturer's literature on Capastat® . San Diego, CA 92121 (1995)

1627 Dura Pharmaceuticals. Manufacturer's literature on Ceclor® . San Diego, CA 92121 (1996)

1628 Dura Pharmaceuticals. Manufacturer's literature on Tornalate® . San Diego, CA 92121 (1995)

1629 Duraj FF, Backman L, Dati F et al. Monitoring low-molecular weight serum proteins in cyclosporine A-treated bone marrow transplant recipients. *Transplant Proc*, 22, 203-204 (1990)

1630 Durham SR, Bignell AHC, Wise R. Interference of cefoxitin in the creatinine estimation and its clinical relevance. *J Clin Pathol*, 32, 1148-1151 (1979)

1631 Durst RY, Pipek R, Levy Y. Hyponatremia caused by omeprazole treatment. *Am J Med*, 97, 400-401 (1994)

1632 Dussaule J-C, Grange J-D, Wolf J-P et al. Effect of sinorphan, an enkephalinase inhibitor, on plasma atrial natriuretic factor and sodium urinary excretion in cirrhotic patients with ascites. *J Clin Endocrinol Metab*, 72, 653-659 (1991)

1633 Dusterdieck G, McElwee G. Estimation of angiotensin II concentration in human plasma by radioimmunoassay. *Eur J Clin Invest*, 2, 32 (1971)

1634 Dutt MK, Moody P, Northfield TC. Effect of cimetidine on renal function in man. *Br J Clin Pharmacol*, 12, 47-50 (1981)

1635 Duttera MJ. Personal communication

1636 Duttera MJ, Carolla RL, Callelli JF et al. Hematuria and crystalluria after high-dose 6-mercaptopurine administration. *N Engl J Med*, 287, 292 (1972)

1637 Dutton J, Copeland LG, Playfer JR et al. Measuring L-dopa in plasma and urine to monitor therapy of elderly patients with Parkinson disease treated with L-dopa and a dopa decarboxylase inhibitor. *Clin Chem*, 39, 629-634 (1993)

1638 Duvernoy WFC. Positive phentolamine test in hypertension induced by a nasal decongestant. *N Engl J Med*, 280, 877 (1969)

1639 Dvorak K, Blazkova E. Acute thrombocytopenic purpura after phenylbutazone. *Vnitr Lek*, 11, 1000 (1965)

1640 Dyck RF, Orchard RC, Senger DL. The response of plasma fibronectin to acute myocardial infarction in humans. *Clin Invest Med*, 13, 107-110 (1990)

1641 Dyck WP, Hightower NC, Janowitz HD. Effect of acetazolamide on human pancreatic secretion. *Gastroenterology*, 62, 547 (1972)

1642 Dymling J-F, Jeppsson S, Rannevik G. Effect of danazol on thyroid function in post menopausal women. *Acta Obstet Gynecol Scand*, Suppl 123, 137-139 (1984)

1643 Earl RA, Timmins PW, Markin RS. Ampicillin interference in the fluorometric measurement of phenylalanine. *Clin Chem*, 36, 1115 (1990)

1644 East C, Bilheimer DW, Grundy SM. Combination drug therapy for familial combined hyperlipidemia. *Ann Intern Med*, 108, 25-32 (1988)

1645 Eastell R, Edmonds CJ. Hyponatraemia associated with trimethoprim and a diuretic. *Br Med J*, 289, 1658-1659 (1984)

1646 Eastep SJ, Benson PJ, Preese LM et al. Factitiously high sodium activities on the Ektachem® 400 owing to interferences by high γ-globulin concentrations. *Clin Chem*, 35, 333-334 (1989)

1647 Eastham RD. Biochemical Values in Clinical Medicine. *4th edition*, Baltimore MD, Williams and Wilkins (1971)

1648 Eastham RD. Laboratory Guide to Clinical Diagnosis. Baltimore MD, Williams and Wilkins (1970)

1649 Easton JD. Potential hazards of hydantoin use. *Ann Intern Med*, 77, 998 (1972)

1650 Eastwood MA, Brydon WG, Anderson DMW. The effects of dietary gum tragacanth in man. *Toxicol Lett*, 21, 73-81 (1984)

1651 Ebeling T, Turtola H, Voutilainen E et al. Comparison between lovastatin and cholestyramine in the treatment of moderate to severe primary hypercholesterolaemia. *Ann Med*, 24, 121-127 (1992)

1652 Eckert B, Hartmann M, Blaut H et al. Electrochemical immunoassay for FT4 using the random-access analyzer Elecsys. *Clin Chem*, 41, S60 (1995)

1653 Eckert B, von Bulow S, Cully M et al. Electro-chemiluminescent immunoassays for free T3 and total T3 using the random-access analyzer Elecsys. *Clin Chem*, 41, S52 (1995)

1654 Eckstein P, Whitby M, Fotherby K et al. Clinical and laboratory findings in a trial of norgestrel, a low-dose progestogen. *Br Med J*, 3, 195 (1972)

1655 Edelman J, Davis P, Owen ET. Prevalence of eosinophilia during gold therapy for rheumatoid arthritis. *J Rheumatol*, 10, 121-123 (1983)

1656 Edelman J, Donnelly R, Graham DN et al. Liver dysfunction associated with gold therapy for rheumatoid arthritis. *J Rheumatol*, 10, 510-511 (1983)

1657 Edelman S, Witztum JL. Hyperkalemia during treatment with HMG-CoA reductase inhibitor. *N Engl J Med*, 320, 1219-1220 (1989)

1658 Editorial. *Geneesk Ned T*, 109, 2046 (1965)

1659 Editorial. Hemolytic anemia caused by penicillin. *N Engl J Med*, 274, 222 (1966)

1660 Edmondson RPS, Thomas R, Hilton PJ et al. Leukocyte electrolytes in cardiac and noncardiac patients receiving diuretics. *Lancet*, 1, 12 (1974)

1661 Edner M, Jogestrand T. Oral salbutamol decreases serum digoxin concentration. *Eur J Clin Pharmacol*, 38, 195-197 (1990)

1662 Edner M, Jogestrand T, Dahlqvist R. Effect of salbutamol on digoxin pharmacokinetics. *Eur J Clin Pharmacol*, 42, 197-201 (1992)

1663 Edner M, Ponikowski P, Jogestrand T. The effect of digoxin on the serum potassium concentration. *Scand J Clin Lab Invest*, 53, 187-189 (1993)

1664 Edwards BD, Bhatnagar D, Mackness MI et al. Effect of low-dose cyclosporin on plasma lipoproteins and markers of cholestasis in patients with psoriasis. *Q J Med*, 88, 109-113 (1995)

1665 Edwards C, Monkman S, Cholerton S et al. Lack of effect of co-trimoxazole on the pharmacokinetics and pharmacodynamics of nifedipine. *Br J Clin Pharmacol*, 30, 889-891 (1990)

1666 Edwards DJ, Lavoie R, Beckmann H et al. The effect of co-administration of verapamil on the pharmacokinetics and metabolism of quinidine. *Clin Pharmacol Ther*, 41, 68-73 (1987)

1667 Edwards MS, Curtis JR. Decreased anticoagulant tolerance with oxymetholone. *Lancet*, 2, 221 (1971)

1668 Egeland GM, Kuller LH, Matthews KA et al. Hormone replacement therapy and lipoprotein changes during early menopause. *Obstet Gynecol*, 76, 776-782 (1990)

1669 Eger EI II, Gong D, Koblin DD, et al. Dose-related biochemical markers of renal injury after sevoflurane versus desflurane anesthesia in volunteers. *Anesth Analg*, 85, 1154-1163 (1997)

1670 Egilmez A, Dobkin AB. Enflurane (ethrane® , compound 347) in man. *Anesthesia*, 27, 171 (1972)

1671 Ehmer B, van der Does R, Rudorf J. Influence of carvedilol on blood glucose and glycohaemoglobin A_1 in non-insulin-dependent diabetics. *Drugs*, 36, Suppl 6, 136-140 (1988)

1672 Ehrlich EN. Reciprocal variations in urinary cortisol and aldosterone in response to increased salt intake in humans. *J Clin Endocrinol Metab*, 26, 1160 (1966)

1673 Ehrmann DA, Cavaghan MK, Imperial J, et al. Effects of metformin on insulin secretion, insulin action, and ovarian steroidogenesis in women with polycystic ovary syndrome. *J Clin Endocrinol Metab*, 82, 524-530 (1997)

1674 Eichhorn EJ, McGhie I, Bedotto JB et al. Effects of bucindolol on neurohormonal activation in congestive heart failure. *Am J Cardiol*, 67, 67-73 (1991)

1675 Eichhorn JH, Hedley-Whyte J, Steinman TI et al. Renal failure following enflurane anesthesia. *Anesthesiology*, 45, 557-560 (1976)

1676 Eichler H-G, Jung M, Kyrle PA et al. Absence of interaction between tenoxicam and warfarin. *Eur J Clin Pharmacol*, 42, 227-229 (1992)

1677 Eimer M, Carter BL. Elevated serum carbamazepine concentrations following diltiazem initiation. *Drug Intell Clin Pharm*, 21, 340-342 (1987)

1678 Einhorn N. Acute leukemia after chemotherapy (melphalan). *Cancer*, 41, 444-447 (1978)

1679 Eisenbery AB, Mathew R, Kiechle FL. Mannitol interference in an automated serum phosphate assay. *Clin Chem*, 33, 2308-2309 (1987)

1680 Eisenhofer G, Goldstein DS, Stull R et al. Simultaneous liquid-chromatographic determination of 3,4-dihydroxyphenylglycol, catecholamines, and 3,4-dihydroxyphenylalanine in plasma, and their responses to inhibition of monoamine oxidase. *Clin Chem*, 32, 2030-2033 (1986)

1681 Eisermann J, Register KB, Strickler RC et al. The effect of tumor necrosis factor on human sperm motility in vitro. *J Androl*, 10, 270-274 (1989)

1682 Eisner EV, Carr RM, MacKinney AA. Quinidine-induced agranulocytosis. *J Am Med Ass*, 238, 884-886 (1977)

1683 Eisner EV, Shahidi NT. Immune thrombocytopenia due to a drug metabolite. *N Engl J Med*, 287, 376 (1972)

1684 El Bashir B, Rostom A, Wright J. Nutrition and IGF-I in patients with cancer cachexia. *Proc ACB Natl Meet*, 50 (1993)

1685 El Matri A, Larabi MS, Kechrid C et al. Fatal bone marrow suppression associated with captopril. *Br Med J*, 283, 277-278 (1981)

1686 El weshi A, Thieblimont C, Cottin V, et al. Cisplatin-induced hyponatremia and renal sodium wasting. *Acta Oncol*, 34 (1995)

1687 Elder GH, Gray CH, Nicholson DC. The porphyrias: a review. *J Clin Pathol*, 25, 1013 (1972)

1688 El-Dorry HFA, Medina H, Bacila M. Interference of phenothiazine compounds in the colorimetric determination of inorganic phosphate. *Anal Biochem*, 47, 329 (1972)

1689 Eldridge JC, Strandhoy J, Buckalew VM Jr. Endocrinologic effects of antihypertensive therapy with guanabenz or hydrochlorothiazide. *J Cardiovasc Pharmacol*, 6, Suppl 5, S776-S780 (1984)

1690 El-Ghobarey AF, Capell HA. Levamisole-induced thrombocytopenia. *Br Med J*, 2, 555-556 (1977)

1691 Eli Lilly and Company. Manufacturer's literature on Axid® . Indianapolis, IN 46285 (1995)

1692 Eli Lilly and Company. Manufacturer's literature on Ceclor® . Indianapolis, IN 46285 (1996)

1693 Eli Lilly and Company. Manufacturer's literature on Cefurox® . Indianapolis, IN 46285 (1995)

1694 Eli Lilly and Company. Manufacturer's literature on Diethylstilbestrol. Indianapolis, IN 46285 (1994)

1695 Eli Lilly and Company. Manufacturer's literature on Dymelor® , Loridine, Keflin® , glucagon. Indianapolis, IN 46285

1696 Eli Lilly and Company. Manufacturer's literature on Evista® . Indianapolis, IN 46285 (1997)

1697 Eli Lilly and Company. Manufacturer's literature on Gemzar® . Indianapolis, IN 46285 (1996)

1698 Eli Lilly and Company. Manufacturer's literature on Humatrope® . Indianapolis, IN 46285 (1996)

1699 Eli Lilly and Company. Manufacturer's literature on Keftab® . Indianapolis, IN 46285 (1996)

1700 Eli Lilly and Company. Manufacturer's literature on Kefzol® . Indianapolis, IN 46285 (1995)

1701 Eli Lilly and Company. Manufacturer's literature on Lorabid® . Indianapolis, IN 46285 (1996)

1702 Eli Lilly and Company. Manufacturer's literature on Mandol® . Indianapolis, IN 46285 (1996)

1703 Eli Lilly and Company. Manufacturer's literature on Nebcin® . Indianapolis, IN 46285 (1996)

1704 Eli Lilly and Company. Manufacturer's literature on Oncovin® . Indianapolis, IN 46285 (1995)

1705 Eli Lilly and Company. Manufacturer's literature on Papaverine. Indianapolis, IN 46285 (1990)

1706 Eli Lilly and Company. Manufacturer's literature on Phenobarbital. Indianapolis, IN 46285 (1991)

1707 Eli Lilly and Company. Manufacturer's literature on Reopro™. Indianapolis, IN 46285 (1997)

1708 Eli Lilly and Company. Manufacturer's literature on Seconal® . Indianapolis, IN 46285 (1995)

1709 Eli Lilly and Company. Manufacturer's literature on Tazidime® . Indianapolis, IN 46285 (1996)

1710 Eli Lilly and Company. Manufacturer's literature on Vancocin® . Indianapolis, IN 46285 (1995)

1711 Eli Lilly and Company. Manufacturer's literature on Velban® . Indianapolis, IN 46285 (1995)

1712 Elias AN, Gwinup G. Effects of some clinically encountered drugs on steroid synthesis and degradation. *Metabolism*, 29, 582-595 (1986)

1713 Eliasson K, Lins L-E, Rossner S. Serum lipoprotein changes during atenolol treatment of essential hypertension. *Eur J Clin Pharmacol*, 20, 335-338 (1981)

1714 Elking MP, Kabat HF. Drug induced modifications of laboratory test values. *Am J Hosp Pharm*, 25, 485 (1968)

1715 Elkington SG. Hepatic injury caused by L-α-methyldopa. *Circulation*, 40, 589 (1969)

1716 Elkins BN, Worsinger NG. Evaluation of theophylline slides for the Kodak Ektachem® 700. *Clin Chem*, 34, 1190 (1988)

1717 Ellekilde G, Holm J, Hemmingsen L et al. Impact of inhibition of angiotensin-converting enzyme on urinary excretion of proteins in chronic heart failure. *Clin Chem*, 38, 1377-1378 (1992)

1718 Ellen RLB, McPherson R. Long-term efficacy and safety of fenofibrate and a statin in the treatment of combined hyperlipidemia. *Am J Cardiol*, 81 (4A), 60B-65B (1998)

1719 Elling H, Kiilerich, Sabro J et al. Influence of a nonsteroid antirheumatic drug on serum and urinary zinc in healthy volunteers. *Scand J Rheumatol*, 9, 161-163 (1980)

1720 Elliott HC Jr, Murdaugh HV Jr. Effects of acetylsalicylic acid on excretion of endogenous metabolites by man. *Proc Soc Exp Biol Med*, 109, 333 (1962)

1721 Elliott WJ. Glucose and cholesterol elevations during thiazide therapy: intention-to-treat versus actual on-therapy experience. *Am J Med*, 99, 261-269 (1995)

1722 Ellis CN, Fradin MS, Messana JM et al. Cyclosporine for plaque-type psoriasis: results of a multidose, double-blind trial. *N Engl J Med*, 324, 277-284 (1991)

1723 Ellis NF, MacGillivray MH, Voorhess ML. Effect of clonidine on plasma cortisol concentrations. *Clin Pharmacol Ther*, 39, 660-663 (1986)

1724 Ellrodt AG, Murata GH, Riedinger MS et al. Severe neutropenia associated with sustained - release procainamide. *Ann Intern Med*, 100, 197-201 (1984)

1725 Elmberger PG, Kalen A, Lund E et al. Effects of pravastatin and cholestyramine on products of the mevalonate pathway in familial hypercholesterolemia. *J Lipid Res*, 32, 935-940 (1991)

1726 El-Sayed YM, Al-Meshal MA, Al-Angary AA et al. Effects of oral administration of colestipol and cholestyramine on the pharmacokinetics of ketoprofen administered intramuscularly in man. *Int J Pharmacol*, 109, 107-113 (1994)

1727 El-Yousef MK, Manier DH. Tricyclic antidepressants and phenothiazines. *J Am Med Ass*, 229, 1419 (1974)

1728 Emancipator K, Rehak NN, Kroll MH. Different types of bromide interferences on chloride ion specific electrodes. *Abstracts*, ACLPS meeting (1989)

1729 Emanuele R, Robuschi G, Tagliaferri A et al. Iodothyronine and thyrotropin concentrations after iodoamide administration for angiographic studies. *Ric Clin Lab*, 12, 589-594 (1982)

1730 Emanuelli G, Anfossi G, Calcamuggi G et al. Urinary enzyme release following aminoglycoside administration in single low dose. *Enzyme*, 39, 119-122 (1988)

1731 Emtage LA, George J, Boughton BJ et al. Hemostatic changes during hormone manipulation in advanced prostate cancer: a comparison of DES 3 mg/day and goserelin 3.6 mg/month. *Eur J Cancer*, 26, 315-319 (1990)

1732 Enck RE, Rios CN. Tamoxifen treatment of metastatic breast cancer and antithrombin III levels. *Cancer*, 1984, 2607-2609 (1984)

1733 Engelman K, Horwitz D, Ambrose IM. Further evaluation of the tyramine test for pheochromocytoma. *N Engl J Med*, 278, 705 (1968)

1734 England JDF. β-adrenoreceptor-blocking drugs once daily in essential hypertension: a comparison of propranolol, pindolol and atenolol. *Aust NZ J Med*, 11, 35-40 (1981)

1735 England JM, Coles M. Effect of co-trimoxazole on phenylalanine metabolism in man. *Lancet*, 2, 1341 (1972)

1736 Englund JA, Baker CJ, Raskino C, et al. zidovudine, didanosine, or both as the initial treatment for symptomatic HIV-infected children. *N Engl J Med*, 336, 1704-1712 (1997)

1737 Enright H, Coyle M, O'Connell LG. C-reactive protein concentrations pre- and post-transfusion. *Clin Lab Haematol*, 12, 25-29 (1990)

1738 Entwisle SJ, Fowler PA, Thomas M et al. The effects of oral sumatriptan, a 5-HT1 receptor agonist, on circulating ACTH and cortisol concentrations in man. *Br J Clin Pharmacol*, 39, 389-395 (1995)

1739 Environmental Diagnostics Manufacturer's Literature. EZ-SCREEN: Cannabinoid/Cocaine, Performance characteristics. Burlington, NC (1989)

1740 Eraz J, Hauknecht R. Diminished urinary estriol due to mandelamine® administration during pregnancy. *Am J Obstet Gynecol*, 104, 924 (1969)

1741 Erbil MK, Ozcan N, Ozbay T et al. Effect of captopril on serum lipids, lipoproteins and apolipoproteins in patients with hypertension. *Clin Chem*, 37, 927 (1991)

1742 Erden F, Hacisalihoglu A, Kocer Z et al. Effects of vitamin C intake on whole blood plasma, leucocyte and urine ascorbic acid and urine oxalic acid levels. *Acta Vitaminol Enzymol*, 7, 123-130 (1985)

1743 Erfurth EM, Hedner P. Delayed suppression of TSH secretion during thyroxine administration. *Horm Metab Res*, 21, 161-163 (1989)

1744 Eri LM, Haug E, Tveter KJ. Effects on the endocrine system of long-term treatment with the luteinizing hormone-releasing hormone agonist leuprolide in patients with benign prostatic hyperplasia. *Scand J Clin Lab Invest*, 56, 319-325 (1996)

1745 Eri LM, Haug E, Tveter KJ. Effects on the endocrine system of long-term treatment with the non-steroidal anti-androgen Casodex in patients with benign prostatic hyperplasia. *Br J Urol*, 75, 335-340 (1995)

1746 Eri LM, Urdal P. Effects of the nonsteroidal antiandrogen Casodex on lipoproteins, fibrinogen and plasminogen activator inhibitor in patients with benign prostatic hyperplasia. *Eur Urol*, 27, 274-279 (1995)

1747 Eriksson BI, Wille-Jorgensen P, Klebo P, et al. A comparison of recombinant hirudin with a low molecular weight heparin to prevent thromboembolic complications after total hip replacement. *N Engl J Med*, 337, 1329-1335 (1997)

1748 Eriksson I, Berggren L. Effect of repeated doses of benzodiazepines on arterial blood gases and transcutaneous pO_2. *Acta Anaesthesiol Scand*, 31, 357-361 (1987)

1749 Eriksson L-O, Beermann B, Kallner M. Renal function and tubular transport effect of sulindac and naproxen in chronic heart failure. *Clin Pharmacol Ther*, 42, 646-654 (1987)

1750 Eriksson L-O, Wahlin-Boll E, Liedholm H et al. Influence of chronic diflunisal treatment on the plasma levels, metabolism and excretion of indomethacin. *Eur J Clin Pharmacol*, 37, 7-15 (1989)

1751 Erle G, Basso M, Federspil G et al. Effect of chlorpromazine on blood glucose and plasma insulin in man. *Eur J Clin Pharmacol*, 11, 15-18 (1977)

1752 Erlemeier H-H, Kupper W, Bleifield W. Acute haemodynamic and neurohumoral effects of intravenous nisoldipine in patients with severe cogestive heart failure. *Eur J Clin Pharmacol*, 38, 11-15 (1990)

1753 Ernaelsteen D, Williams R. Jaundice due to nitrofurantoin. *Gastroenterology*, 41, 590 (1961)

1754 Ernst E, Bergmann H. Influence of cilazapril on blood rheology in healthy subjects: a pilot study. *Am J Med*, 87, Suppl B, 70S-71S (1989)

1755 Ernst JA, Sy ER. Effect of azlocillin on uric acid levels in serum. *Antimicrob Agent Chemother*, 24, 609-610 (1983)

1756 Eryasa Y, Chang PM, Pittinger CB. Serum ionic calcium changes in man following succinylcholine administration. *Fed Proc*, 29, 548 (1970)

1757 Eschbach JW, Adamson JW. Improvement in the anemia of chronic renal failure with fluoxymesterone. *Ann Intern Med*, 78, 527 (1973)

1758 Escolar G, Cases A, Monteagudo J et al. Uremic plasma after infusion of desmopressin (DDAVP®) improves the interaction of normal platelets with vessel subendothelium. *J Lab Clin Med*, 114, 36-42 (1989)

1759 Eshleman SHS, Shaw LM. Massive theophylline overdose with atypical metabolic abnormalities. *Clin Chem*, 36, 398-399 (1990)

1760 Esmatjes E, Conget JI, Gaya J et al. Effects of thromboxane synthesis inhibitor flusinal on renal hemodynamics in microalbuminuric diabetic patients. *Diabetes Care*, 13, 1114-1117 (1990)

1761 Esmatjes E, Ricart MJ, Ferrer JP et al. Cyclosporine's effect on insulin secretion in patients with kidney transplants. *Transplantation*, 52, 500-503 (1991)

1762 Espiritu CR, Kim TS, Levine RA. Granulomatous hepatitis associated with sulfadimethoxine hypersensitivity. *J Am Med Ass*, 202, 985 (1967)

1763 Esposito R, Vitali D. Rifampicin and thrombocytopenia. *Lancet*, 2, 491 (1971)

1764 Etchason JA, Miller TD, Squires RW et al. Niacin-induced hepatitis: a potential side effect with low-dose time-release niacin. *Mayo Clin Proc*, 66, 23-28 (1991)

1765 Eto M, Sato T, Watanabe K et al. Effects of probucol on plasma lipids and lipoproteins in familial hypercholesterolemic patients with and without apolipoprotein E_4. *Atherosclerosis*, 84, 49-53 (1990)

1766 Ette EI, Brown-Awala EA, Essien EE. Chloroquine elimination in humans: effect of low-dose cimetidine. *J Clin Pharmacol*, 27, 813-816 (1987)

1767 Evans DJ, Taylor DM, Zetterstorm O, et al. A comparison of low-dose inhaled budesonide plus theophylline and high-dose inhaled budesonide for moderate asthma. *N Engl J Med*, 337, 1412-1418 (1997)

1768 Evans JR, Shankel SW, Cutler RE. Low osmolar contrast agents and nephrotoxicity. *Ann Intern Med*, 107, 116 (1987)

1769 Evans RA. Hypercalcaemia: what does it signify?. *Drugs*, 31, 64-74 (1986)

1770 Evans RL, Nelson MV, Melethil S et al. Evaluation of the interaction of lithium and aprazolam. *J Clin Psychopharmacol*, 10, 355-359 (1990)

1771 Ewen LM, Griffiths J. γ-Glutamyl transpeptidase: elevated activities in certain neurologic diseases. *Am J Clin Pathol*, 59, 2-9 (1973)

1772 Eykyn S. Use and control of cephalosporins. *J Clin Pathol*, 24, 419 (1971)

1773 Eyssen H, Evrard E, Vanderhaeghe H. Cholesterol lowering effects of N-methylated neomycin and basic antibiotics. *J Lab Clin Med*, 68, 753 (1966)

1774 Ezzat S, Ren S-G, Braunstein GD et al. Octreotide stimulates insulin-like growth factor binding protein-1 (IGFBP-1) levels in acromegaly. *J Clin Endocrinol Metab*, 73, 441 (1991)

1775 Faas FM, Norman J, Carter WJ. Cefoxitin interference with urinary 17-hydroxycorticosteroid determination. *Clin Chem*, 29, 1311-1313 (1983)

1776 Faber OK, Beck-Nielsen H, Binder C et al. Acute actions of sulfonylurea drugs during long-term treatment of NIDDM. *Diabetes Care*, 13, Suppl 3, 26-31 (1990)

1777 Fabre J, Wintsch J, Peter-Contesse R et al. Effects of bopindolol: on renal function. *J Cardiovasc Pharmacol*, 8, Suppl 6, 545-550 (1986)

1778 Fagerberg B, Berglund A, Holme E et al. Metabolic effects of controlled-release metoprolol in hypertensive men with impaired or diabetic glucose tolerance: a comparison with atenolol. *J Intern Med*, 227, 37-43 (1990)

1779 Faglia G, Beck-Peccoz P, Ambrosi B et al. The effects of a synthetic thyrotropin releasing hormone (TRH) in normal and endocrinopathic subjects. *Acta Endocrinol*, 71, 209 (1972)

1780 Faguer de Moustier B, Paoli V. The influence of nicardipine in type 2 diabetic patients with slight hypertension. *J Cardiovasc Pharmacol*, 16, Suppl 2, S26-S33 (1990)

1781 Fahmy K, Khairy M, Allam G et al. Effect of depo-medroxyprogesterone acetate on coagulation factors and serum lipids in Egyptian women. *Contraception*, 44, 431-444 (1991)

1782 Fahraeus L, Larsson-Cohn U, Ljungberg S et al. Plasma lipoproteins during and after danazol treatment. *Acta Obstet Gynecol Scand*, 63, Suppl 123, 133-135 (1984)

1783 Fahraeus L, Larsson-Cohn V, Wallentin L. Lipoproteins during oral and cutaneous administration of oestradiol-17β to menopausal women. *Acta Endocrinol*, 101, 597-602 (1982)

1784 Fahraeus L, Sydsjo A, Wallentin L. Lipoprotein changes during treatment of pelvic endometriosis with medroxyprogesterone acetate. *Fertil Steril*, 45, 503-506 (1986)

1785 Fairchild L, Bartlett C, Myers D et al. Emit II benzodiazepine, a two-reagent assay for detection of benzodiazpine in urine on high volume analyzers. *Clin Chem*, 37, 999 (1991)

1786 Fairley KF, Birch DF, Haines I. Abnormal urinary sediment in patients on triamterene. *Lancet*, 1, 421-422 (1983)

1787 Fakeye O, Balogh S. Effect of NORPLANT contraceptive use on hemoglobin, packed cell volume and menstrual bleeding patterns. *Contraception*, 39, 265-274 (1989)

1788 Falaschi P, Rosa M, Rocco A et al. Effect of ritanserin, specific 5HT-2 antagonist, on PRL secretion in normal subjects and in different hyperprolactinemic conditions. *Clin Endocrinol*, 34, 449-453 (1991)

1789 Falch DK, Schreiner A. The effect of spironolactone on lipid, glucose and uric acid levels in blood during long-term administration to hypertensives. *Acta Med Scand*, 213, 27-30 (1983)

1790 Falek A, Jordan RB, King BJ et al. Human chromosomes and opiates. *Arch Gen Psychiat*, 27, 511 (1972)

1791 Falkner B, Canessa M, Anzalone D. Effect of angiotensin converting enzyme inhibitor (Lisinopril) on insulin sensitivity and sodium transport in mild hypertension. *Am J Hypertens*, 8, 454-460 (1995)

1792 Fallon JA, Tall AR, Janis MG et al. Oxacillin-induced granulocytopenia. *Acta Haematol*, 59, 167-170 (1978)

1793 Faloon WW. Metabolic effects of nonabsorbable antibacterial agents. *Am J Clin Nutr*, 23, 645 (1970)

1794 Falsetti L, Zanagnolo V, Galbignani E. Cabergoline treatment in hyperprolactinaemic women. *J Obstet Gynecol*, 11, 68-71 (1991)

1795 Fann WE, Davis JM, Janowsky DS et al. Chlorpromazine: effects of antacids on its gastrointestinal absorption. *J Clin Pharmacol*, 13, 388-390 (1973)

1796 Faraj JH. Hyperosmolality due to antacid treatment. *Anesthesia*, 44, 911-912 (1989)

1797 Farci P, Mandas A, Coiana A et al. Treatment of chronic hepatitis D with interferon alfa-2a. *N Engl J Med*, 330, 88-94 (1994)

1798 Farid NR, Johnson RJ, Low WT. Hemolytic reaction to mefenamic acid. *Lancet*, 2, 382 (1971)

1799 Farid Z, Smith JH, Bassily S et al. Hepatotoxicity after treatment of schistosomiasis with hycanthone. *Br Med J*, 2, 88 (1972)

1800 Farish E, Barnes JF, Rolton HA et al. Effects of tibolone on lipoprotein(a) and HDL subfractions. *Maturitas*, 20, 215-219 (1995)

1801 Farish E, Fletcher CD, Hart DM et al. The effects of hormone implants on serum lipoproteins and steroid hormones in bilaterally oophorectomized women. *Acta Endocrinol*, 106, 116-120 (1984)

1802 Farkkila AM, Iivanainen MV, Farkilla MA. Disturbance of the water and electrolyte balance during high-dose interferon treatment. *J Interferon Res*, 10, 221-227 (1990)

1803 Farmer RW, Pierce CE. Plasma cortisol determination: radioimmunoassay and competitive protein binding compared. *Clin Chem*, 20, 411 (1974)

1804 Farmos Diagnostica Product Insert. SHBG IRMA: Immunoradiometric assay for sex hormone binding globulin. Farmos Diagnostica, Orion Corporation, Oulunsalo, Finland (1991)

1805 Farnier M, Bonnefous F, Debbas N et al. Comparative efficacy and safety of micronized fenofibrate and simvastatin in patients with primary type IIa or IIb hyperlipidemia. *Arch Intern Med*, 154, 441-449 (1994)

1806 Farrell G, Lin R, Schoeman M et al. Interferon alfa-2b for chronic active hepatitis C: interim results of an Australian trial. *J Hepatol*, 11, Suppl 1, S157 (1990)

1807 Farringer JA, Green JA, O'Rourke RA et al. Nifedipine-induced alterations in serum quinidine concentrations. *Am Heart J*, 108, 1570-1572 (1984)

1808 Farry JP, Fischl SJ, Tighe MJ et al. Effects of prazosin and labetalol on blood pressure control and blood lipid levels in patients with mild-to-moderate essential hypertension. *Am J Med*, 86, Suppl 1b, 41-44 (1989)

1809 Fass RJ, Saslaw S. Clindamycin: clinical and laboratory evaluation of parenteral therapy. *Am J Med Sci*, 263, 368 (1972)

1810 Fattovich G, Betterle C, Brollo L et al. Autoantibodies during α-interferon therapy for chronic hepatitis B. *J Med Virol*, 34, 132-135 (1991)

1811 Fauler J, Thon A, Tsikas D et al. Enhanced synthesis of cysteinyl leukotrienes in juvenile rheumatoid arthritis. *Arth Rheum*, 37, 93-97 (1994)

1812 Faulkner A, Peake MJ. Bicarbonate interference with Hitachi chloride electrodes. *Ann Clin Biochem*, 28, 107-108 (1991)

1813 Favre L, Glasson P, Riondel A et al. Interaction of diuretics and non-steroidal anti-inflammatory drugs in man. *Clin Sci*, 64, 407-415 (1983)

1814 Favreau M, Tannenbaum H, Lough J. Hepatic toxicity associated with gold therapy. *Ann Intern Med*, 87, 717-719 (1977)

1815 Fawcett J, Kravitz HM. The long term management of bipolar disorders with lithium, carbamazepine, and antidepressants. *J Clin Psychiat*, 46, 58-60 (1985)

1816 Faynor SM, Espina V. Fluoxetine inhibition of imipramine metabolism. *Clin Chem*, 35, 1180 (1989)

1817 Feagan BG, Rochon J, Fedorak RN et al. Methotrexate for the treatment of Crohn's disease. *N Engl J Med*, 332, 292-297 (1995)

1818 Fee JPH, Black GW, Dundee JW et al. A prospective study of liver enzyme and other changes following repeat administration of halothane and enflurane. *Br J Anaes*, 51, 1133-1140 (1979)

1819 Feely J. β-adrenoceptor-blocking drugs, growth hormone and acromegaly. *Postgrad Med J*, 56, 236-237 (1980)

1820 Feely J. Enhanced sulphonylurea-induced hypoglycaemia with cimetidine. *Br J Clin Pharmacol*, 16, 607p (1983)

1821 Feely J, Wilkinson GR, Wood AJJ. Reduction of liver blood flow and propranolol metabolism by cimetidine. *N Engl J Med*, 304, 692-695 (1981)

1822 Feely J, Wood AJJ. Effects of cimetidine on the elimination and actions of ethanol. *J Am Med Ass*, 247, 2819-2821 (1982)

1823 Feiks FK. Uber eine weitere indikation zu parenteraler schwefeltherapie. *Wien Med Wschr*, 117, 899 (1967)

1824 Feld R, Roberts P. Measurement of β-hydroxybutyrate (BHB) in urine on the Hitachi 705. *Clin Chem*, 37, 947 (1991)

1825 Feldman JM, Kelley WN, Lebovitz HE. Inhibition of glucose oxidase paper tests by reducing metabolites. *Diabetes*, 19, 337 (1970)

1826 Feldman JM, Lebovitz FL. Tests for glucosuria. An analysis of factors that cause misleading results. *Diabetes*, 22, 115 (1973)

1827 Feldman JM, Lebovitz HE. Endocrine and metabolic effects of glibenclamide. *Diabetes*, 20, 745 (1971)

1828 Feldman JM, Lebovitz HE. Levodopa and tests for urinary glucose. *N Engl J Med*, 283, 1053 (1970)

1829 Feldman S, Doolittle M, Lott L et al. Similar hematologic changes in children receiving trimethoprim-sulfamethoxazole or amoxicillin for otitis media. *J Pediatr*, 106, 995-1000 (1985)

1830 Feldmann U, Gaus W, Kretschmer F-J et al. Analgesic use, agranulocytosis, and aplastic anemia. *J Am Med Ass*, 257, 2590-2591 (1987)

1831 Fellman JH, Joyce JR, Strandholm JJ. Analysis in human plasma of 3-methoxytyrosine: a metabolite of dopa. *Clin Chim Acta*, 32, 313 (1971)

1832 Fenech FF, Bannister WH, Grech JL. Hepatitis with biliverdinaemia in association with indomethacin therapy. *Br Med J*, 3, 155 (1967)

1833 Fenster PE, Hager WD, Goodman MM. Digoxin-quinidine-spironolactone interaction. *Clin Pharmacol Ther*, 36, 70-73 (1984)

1834 Fenster PE, Hager WD, Perrier D et al. Digoxin-quinidine interaction in patients with chronic renal failure. *Circulation*, 66, 1277-1280 (1982)

1835 Ferguson RM, Sutherland DER, Simmons RL et al. Ketoconazole, cyclosporine metabolism and renal transplantation. *Lancet*, 2, 882-883 (1982)

1836 Ferlinz J, Easthope JL, Hughes D et al. Right ventricular performance in essential hypertension after β-blockade. *Br Heart J*, 46, 23-29 (1981)

1837 Ferlito S, Modica L, Romano F et al. Effects of verapamil on glucose, insulin and glucagon levels after oral glucose load in normal and diabetic subjects. *Panminerva Med*, 24, 221-226 (1982)

1838 Fermo I, de Vecchi E, Vigano S et al. Total plasma homocysteine: influence of some common physiological variables. *Amino Acids*, 5, 17-21 (1993)

1839 Fernandez AA, Jacobs SL. Porphyrins, porphobilinogen and aminolevulinic acid in urine. *Stand Meth Clin Chem*, 6, 57 (1970)

1840 Ferrara LA, Marotta T, Rubba P et al. Effects of α-adrenergic and β-adrenergic receptor blockade on lipid metabolism. *Am J Med*, 80, 104-108 (1986)

1841 Ferrara LA, Soro S, Fasano ML. Effects of nitrendipine on glucose and lipid serum concentrations. *Curr Ther Res*, 37, 614-618 (1985)

1842 Ferrari C, Frezzati S, Romussi M et al. Effects of short term clofibrate administration on glucose tolerance and insulin secretion in patients with chemical diabetes or hypertriglyceridemia. *Metabolism*, 26, 129-139 (1977)

1843 Ferrari C, Mattel A, Melis GB et al. Cabergoline; long-acting oral treatment of hyperprolactinemic disorders. *J Clin Endocrinol Metab*, 68, 1201-1206 (1989)

1844 Ferrari C, Paracchi A, Romano C et al. Long-lasting lowering of serum growth hormone and prolactin levels by single and repetitive cabergoline administration in dopamine-responsive acromegalic patients. *Clin Endocrinol*, 29, 467-476 (1988)

1845 Ferrari C, Testori G, Scanni A et al. Reduction of serum alkaline phosphatase and γ-Glutamyl transpeptidase activities by short-term clofibrate. *N Engl J Med*, 295, 449 (1976)

1846 Ferrari L, Zilembo N, Bajetta E et al. Effect of 4-hydroxyandrostenedione doses on serum insulin-like growth factor I levels in advanced breast cancer. *Breast Cancer Res Treat*, 30, 127-132 (1994)

1847 Ferrazzi E, Cartei G, De Besi P et al. Tamoxifen in disseminated breast cancer. *Tumori*, 63, 463-468 (1977)

1848 Ferre C, Panadero AM, Castineiras MJ et al. Interference by cyclosporine assessed. *Clin Chem*, 32, 1590-1591 (1986)

1849 Ferrier C, Ferrari P, Weidmann P et al. Antihypertensive therapy with Ca^{2+}: antagonist verapamil and/or ACE inhibitor enalapril in NIDDM patients. *Diabetes Care*, 14, 911-914 (1991)

1850 Ferrier CP, Kurtz A, Lehner P et al. Stimulation of renin secretion by potassium-channel activation with cromakalim. *Eur J Clin Pharmacol*, 36, 443-447 (1989)

1851 Ferris TF, Gorden P. Effect of angiotensin and norepinephrine upon urate clearance in man. *Am J Med*, 44, 359 (1968)

1852 Fessel WJ. Hyperuricemia in health and disease. *Semin Arth Rheum*, 1, 275 (1972)

1853 Festen HPM, Thijs JC, Lamers CBHW et al. Effect of oral omeprazole on serum gastrin and serum pepsinogen levels. *Gastroenterology*, 87, 1030-1034 (1984)

1854 Few JD, Cashmore GC. Plasma cortisone in man: its determination, physiological variation, and significance. *Ann Clin Biochem*, 17, 227-232 (1980)

1855 Fich A, Schwartz J, Braverman D et al. Sulfasalazine hepatotoxicity. *Am J Gastroenterol*, 79, 401-402 (1984)

1856 Fichman MP, Vorherr H, Kleeman CR et al. Diuretic - induced hyponatremia. *Ann Intern Med*, 75, 853 (1971)

1857 Fields WS, Hass WK (eds). Aspirin, platelets and stroke: background for a clinical trial. St Louis, MO, Green (1971)

1858 Fieseler H-G, Armstrong VW, Wieland E et al. Serum Lp(a) concentrations are unaffected by treatment with the HMG-CoA reductase inhibitor pravastatin: results of a 2-year investigation. *Clin Chim Acta*, 204, 292-300 (1991)

1859 Fieseler HG, Wieland E, Thiery J et al. Long term treatment with the HMG-CoA reductase inhibitor pravastatin has no major effect on steroid and pituitary gland hormone concentrations in hypercholesterolemic patients. *Diag Lab*, 27, Suppl, 132 (1991)

1860 Fiet J, Villette J-M, Galons H et al. The application of a new highly-sensitive radioimmunoassay for plasma 21-deoxycortisol to the detection of steroid-21-hydroxylase deficiency. *Ann Clin Biochem*, 31, 56-64 (1994)

1861 Figg WD, Thibault A, Surtor AO et al. Hypothyroidism associated with aminoglutethimide in patients with prostate cancer. *Arch Intern Med*, 154, 1023-1025 (1994)

1862 Figge HL, Figge J. The effects of amiodarone on thyroid hormone function: a review of the physiology and clinical manifestations. *J Clin Pharmacol*, 30, 588-595 (1990)

1863 Findling JW, Backstrom D, Rawsthorne L et al. Indomethacin-induced hyperkalemia in three patients with gouty arthritis. *J Am Med Ass*, 244, 1127-1128 (1980)

1864 Fine D, Shedrovilzky H. Hyponatremia due to chlorpropamide, a syndrome resembling inappropriate secretion of antidiuretic hormone. *Ann Intern Med*, 72, 83 (1970)

1865 Fingerhut B. A non-mercurimetric automated method for serum chloride. *Clin Chim Acta*, 41, 247 (1972)

1866 Finkelstein JS, Klibanski A, Schaefer EH et al. Parathyroid hormone for the prevention of bone loss induced by estrogen deficiency. *N Engl J Med*, 331, 1618-1623 (1994)

1867 Finlay GD, Whitsett TL, Cucinell EA et al. Augmentation of sodium and potassium excretion, glomerular filtration rate and renal plasma flow by levodopa. *N Engl J Med*, 284, 865 (1971)

1868 Fiore CE, Malatino LS, Kanis JA. Effects of cimetidine on parathyroid metabolism. *Lancet*, 1, 501 (1981)

1869 Fiore JM, Noonan FM. Agranulocytosis due to mepazine (phenothiazine). *N Engl J Med*, 260, 375 (1959)

1870 Fioretti P, Cagnacci A, Paoletti AM et al. Effects of the antidopaminergic drug veralipride on LH and PRL secretion in postmenopausal women. *J Endocrinol Invest*, 12, 295-301 (1989)

1871 Firdaous I, Hassoun A, Otte JB et al. HPLC-microparticle enzyme immunoassay specific for tacrolimus in whole blood of hepatic and renal transplant patients. *Clin Chem*, 41, 1292-1296 (1995)

1872 Firkin FC, Mariani AF. Agranulocytosis due to dapsone. *Med J Aust*, 2, 247-251 (1977)

1873 Fisch IR, Freedman SH. Oral contraceptives and the red blood cell. *Clin Pharmacol Ther*, 14, 245 (1973)

1874 Fischer HW, Hoak JC. Mimicry of acute cholecystitis by erythromycin estolate reactions: Report of two cases. *Am J Med Sci*, 247, 283 (1964)

1875 Fischer J, Verbruggen B, Wessels H et al. Interference of coumarin therapy with the "Heptest" owing to declining prothrombin concentrations. *Clin Chem*, 35, 483-486 (1989)

1876 Fischereder M, Jaffe JP. Thrombocytopenia following acute acetaminophen overdose. *Am J Hematol*, 45, 258-259 (1994)

1877 Fisher B, Keenan AM, Garra BS et al. Interleukin-2 induces profound reversible cholestasis: a detailed analysis in treated cancer patients. *J Clin Oncol*, 7, 1852-1862 (1989)

1878 Fisher CE, Woo J, Horton R. Effect of spironolactone on aldosterone and renin in normal man and in primary aldosteronism. *Clin Res*, 20, 217 (1972)

1879 Fisher CE, Woo J, Horton R. Effects of spironolactone on aldosterone and renin in man. *Abstracts IV Int Congr Endocrinol, Washington DC*, 111 (1972)

1880 Fishman WH. Pindolol: a new β-adrenoceptor antagonist with partial agonist activity. *N Engl J Med*, 308, 940-944 (1983)

1881 Fitzgerald PH, Pickering AF, Ferguson DD. Depressed lymphocyte response to PHA in long-term users of oral contraceptives. *Lancet*, 1, 615 (1973)

1882 Fizazi K, Cojean I, Pignon J-P, et al. Normal serum neuron specific enolase (NSE) value after the first cycle of chemotherapy. *Cancer*, 82, 1049-1055 (1998)

1883 Flacke W. Drug therapy: treatment of myasthenia gravis. *N Engl J Med*, 288, 27 (1973)

1884 Flayeh KA. Spermidine oxidase activity in serum of normal and schizophrenic subjects. *Clin Chem*, 34, 401-403 (1988)

1885 Flechtner M, Ramp J, England B et al. Affinity binding assay of glycohemoglobin by two-dimensional electrophoresis referenced to hemoglobin A_{1c}. *Clin Chem*, 38, 2372-2379 (1992)

1886 Fleischer N, Brown H, Graham DY et al. Chronic laxative-induced hyperaldosteronism and hypokalemia simulating Bartter's syndrome. *Ann Intern Med*, 70, 791 (1969)

1887 Fleisher WR. Enzymatic methods for lactic and pyruvic acids. *Stand Meth Clin Chem*, 6, 245 (1970)

1888 Fletcher CD, Farish E, Dagen MM et al. Short-term changes in lipoproteins and apoproteins during cyclical oestrogen-progestogen replacement therapy. *Maturitas*, 14, 33-42 (1991)

1889 Fletcher CD, Farish E, Leggate J et al. Prevention of bone loss by hormone replacement therapy is probably not due to stimulation of calcitonin secretion. *Acta Endocrinol*, 124, 353-356 (1991)

1890 Fletcher GF, Fletcher BJ, Sweeney ME. Effects of exercise testing, training and beta blockade on serum potassium in normal subjects. *Am J Cardiol*, 65, 1242-1245 (1990)

1891 Flexner C. HIV-protease inhibitors. *N Engl J Med*, 338, 1281-1292 (1998)

1892 Flink EB. Hypomagnesemia in the patient receiving digitalis. *Arch Intern Med*, 145, 625 (1985)

1893 Flordal PA, Sahlin S. Use of desmopressin to prevent bleeding complications in patients treated with aspirin. *Br J Surg*, 80, 723-724 (1993)

1894 Flordal PA, Svensson J, Ljungstrom K-G. Effects of desmopressin and dextran on coagulation and fibrinolysis in healthy volunteers. *Thromb Res*, 62, 355-364 (1991)

1895 Florent C, Cogoni C, Joubert M et al. Effect of two-week treatment with enpostil (35 µg twice a day) on 24-hour serum gastrin levels. *Dig Dis Sci*, 35, 1352-1357 (1990)

1896 Florijn KW, Derkx FHM, Visser W et al. Plasma immunoreactive endothelin-1 in pregnant women with and without pre-eclampsia. *J Cardiovasc Pharmacol*, 17, Suppl 7, S446-S448 (1991)

1897 Floyd JC Jr, Fajans SS, Knopf RF et al. Plasma insulin in hyperinsulinism: comparative effects of tolbutamide, leucine and glucose. *J Clin Endocrinol Metab*, 24, 747 (1964)

1898 Flynn A, Pories WJ, Strain WH et al. Rapid serum-zinc depletion associated with corticosteroid therapy. *Lancet*, 2, 1169 (1971)

1899 Fogari R, Zoppi A, Pasotti C et al. Plasma lipids during chronic antihypertensive therapy with different β-blockers. *J Cardiovasc Pharmacol*, 14, Suppl 7, S28-S32 (1988)

1900 Fogari R, Zoppi A, Tettamanti F et al. β-blocker effects on plasma lipids in antihypertensive therapy: importance of the duration of treatment and the lipid status before treatment. *J Cardiovasc Pharmacol*, 16, Suppl 5, S76-S80 (1990)

1901 Fogari R, Zoppi A, Tettamanti F et al. The effect of celiprolol on the blood lipid profile in hypertensive patients with high cholesterol levels. *Cardiovasc Drug Ther*, 4, Suppl 6, 1287-1290 (1990)

1902 Foley RJ, Hamner RW, Weinman EJ. Serum potassium concentrations in cyclosporine and azathioprine-treated renal transplant patients. *Nephron*, 40, 280-285 (1985)

1903 Folsom AR, Qamhieh HT, Flack JM et al. Plasma fibrinogen: levels and correlates in young adults. *Am J Epidemiol*, 138, 1023-1036 (1993)

1904 Fong HJ, Cohen AH. Ibuprofen-induced acute renal failure with acute tubular necrosis. *Am J Nephrol*, 2, 28-31 (1982)

1905 Foo Y, Konecny P. Hyperamylasaemia in asymptomatic HIV patients. *Ann Clin Biochem*, 34, 259-262 (1997)

1906 Foo Y, Rosalki SB. Carbohydrate deficient transferrin measurement. *Ann Clin Biochem*, 35, 345-350 (1998)

1907 Ford HC, Johnson LA. Ascorbic acid interferes with an automated urinary iodide determination based on the ceric-arsenious acid reaction. *Clin Chem*, 37, 759 (1991)

1908 Ford K, Caplan DE, Tobias DD et al. Automated direct immunoassay of progesterone on the Abbott IMx analyzer. *Clin Chem*, 36, 1099 (1990)

1909 Ford MJ, Kellett RJ, Busuttil A et al. Dextropropoxyphene and jaundice. *Br Med J*, 2, 674 (1977)

1910 Forest Pharmaceuticals. Manufacturer's literature on Flumadine® . St. Louis, MO 63045 (1995)

1911 Forest Pharmaceuticals. Manufacturer's literature on Tiazac™. St. Louis, MO 63045 (1996)

1912 Forest Pharmaceuticals, Inc. Manufacturer's literature on Monurol™. St. Louis, MO 63045 (1997)

1913 Forester G. Profound cytopenia secondary to azidothymidine. *N Engl J Med*, 317, 772 (1987)

1914 Forman MB, Uderman H, Jackson EK et al. Effects of indomethacin on systemic and coronary hemodynamics in patients with coronary artery disease. *Am Heart J*, 110, 311-318 (1985)

1915 Forman SD, Bissette G, Yao J et al. Cerebrospinal fluid corticotropin-releasing factor increases following haloperidol withdrawal in chronic schizophrenia. *Schiz Res*, 12, 43-51 (1994)

1916 Formisano R, Falaschi P, Cerbo R et al. Nimodipine in migraine: clinical efficacy and endocrinological effects. *Eur J Clin Pharmacol*, 41, 69-71 (1991)

1917 Forrest FM, Forrest IS, Serra MT. Modification of chlorpromazine metabolism by some other drugs frequently administered to psychiatric patients. *Biol Psychiat*, 2, 53-58 (1970)

1918 Forshaw J. Muscle paresis and hypokalaemia after treatment with duogastrone. *Br Med J*, 2, 674 (1969)

1919 Forslund T, Franzen P, Backman R. Comparison of fosinopril and hydrochlorothiazide in patients with mild to moderate hypertension. *J Intern Med*, 230, 511-517 (1991)

1920 Forster H. Safety of xylitol. *N Engl J Med*, 286, 790 (1972)

1921 Forster HW. Hepatitis from hydralazine. *N Engl J Med*, 302, 1362 (1980)

1922 Fortman CS, Witte DL. Serum 5'-nucleotidase in patients receiving antiepileptic drugs. *Am J Clin Pathol*, 84, 197-201 (1985)

1923 Foss OP, Jensen K. The effect of captopril and metoprolol as monotherapy or combined with bendroflumethiazide on blood lipids. *J Intern Med*, 227, 119-123 (1990)

1924 Foster PN, Swan CHJ. Dapsone and fatal hypoalbuminemia. *Lancet*, 2, 806 (1981)

1925 Fouad FM, EL-Tobgi S, Tarazi RC et al. Captopril in congestive heart failure resistant to other vasodilators. *Eur Heart J*, 5, 47-54 (1984)

1926 Fouad FM, Tarazi RC, Bravo EL et al. Hemodynamic and antihypertensive effects of the new oral angiotensin-converting enzyme inhibitor MK-421 (enalapril). *Hypertension*, 6, 167-174 (1984)

1927 Foucan L, Bourhis V, Bangou J, et al. A randomized trial of captopril for microalbumunuria in normotensive adults with sickle cell anemia. *Am J Med*, 104, 339-342 (1998)

1928 Foulds G, Hilligos DM, Henry EB et al. The effects of an antacid or cimetidine on the serum concentrations of azithromycin. *J Clin Pharmacol*, 31, 164-167 (1991)

1929 Franceschini G, Lovati MR, Manzoni C et al. Effect of gemfibrozil treatment in hypercholesterolemia on low density lipoprotein (LDL) subclass distribution and LDL-cell interaction. *Atherosclerosis*, 114, 61-71 (1995)

1930 Franceschini G, Sirtori M, Vaccarino V et al. Plasma lipoprotein changes after treatment with pravastatin and gemfibrozil in patients with familial hypercholesterolemia. *J Lab Clin Med*, 114, 250-259 (1989)

1931 Franceschini G, Werba JP, D'Acquarica AL et al. Microsomal enzyme inducers raise plasma high-density lipoprotein cholesterol levels in healthy control subjects but not in patients with primary hypoalphalipoproteinemia. *Clin Pharmacol Ther*, 57, 434-440 (1995)

1932 Franceschini R, Cataldi A, Barreca T et al. Plasma β-endorphin, ACTH and cortisol secretion in man after nasal spray administration of calcitonin. *Eur J Clin Pharmacol*, 37, 341-343 (1989)

1933 Franceschini R, Corsini G, Cataldi A et al. Lack of variation of plasma β-endorphin after clodronate infusion in patients with increased bone resorption. *Curr Ther Res*, 54, 214-220 (1993)

1934 Francis KL, Jenis EH, Jensen GE et al. Gold-associated nephropathy. *Arch Pathol Lab Med*, 108, 234-238 (1984)

1935 Francis RM. Is there a differential response to alfacalcidiol and vitamin D in the treatment of osteoporosis. *Calcif Tissue Int*, 60, 111-114 (1997)

1936 Frank GJ, Knapp LE, Olson SC et al. Overview of quinapril, a new ACE inhibitor. *J Cardiovasc Pharmacol*, 15, Suppl 2, S14-S23 (1990)

1937 Franken N, Lenz H, Maier J et al. Sensitive, fully mechanized TSH enzyme immunoassay using streptavidin/biotin technology. *Clin Chem*, 37, 1035 (1991)

1938 Franklyn JA, Davis JR, Gammage MD et al. Amiodarone and thyroid hormone action. *Clin Endocrinol*, 22, 257-264 (1985)

1939 Franklyn JA, Wilkins MR, Wilkinson R et al. The effect of propranolol on circulating thyroid hormone measurements in thyrotoxic and euthyroid subjects. *Acta Endocrinol*, 108, 351-355 (1985)

1940 Franks RD, Dubovsky SL, Lifshitz M et al. Long-term lithium carbonate therapy causes hyperparathyroidism. *Arch Gen Psychiat*, 39, 1074-1077 (1982)

1941 Franquemont DW, Sutphen JL, Herold DA et al. Characterization of sulfasalazine's interference in the measurement of conjugated bilirubin by the Ektachem® slide method. *Clin Chem*, 35, 1760-1762 (1989)

1942 Franquemont DW, Sutphen JL, Herold DA et al. Clinically important interference of sulfasalazine in the measurement of conjugated bilirubin by the Ektachem® slide method. *Clin Chem*, 35, 1158 (1989)

1943 Franssen AMHW, Kauer FM, Chadha DR et al. Endometriosis; treatment with gonadotropin-releasing hormone agonist Buserelin. *Fertil Steril*, 51, 401-408 (1989)

1944 Franzen F, Eysell K. Biologically Active Amines Found in Man. New York NY, Pergamon Press (1969)

1945 Fraschini F, Scaglione F, Maierna G et al. Ribavirin influence on theophylline plasma levels in adult and children. *Int J Clin Pharmacol Ther Toxicol*, 26, 30-32 (1988)

1946 Frascino JA. Effect of inorganic fluoride on the renal concentrating mechanism. *J Lab Clin Med*, 79, 192 (1972)

1947 Fraser AG, Rosalki SB, Pounder RE. Effects of H_2-receptor antagonists on blood alcohol levels. *J Am Med Ass*, 267, 2469 (1992)

1948 Fraser DG, Ludden TM, Evens RP et al. Displacement of phenytoin from plasma binding sites by salicylate. *Clin Pharmacol Ther*, 27, 165-169 (1980)

1949 Fraser PM, Doll R, Langman MJS et al. Clinical trial of a new carbenoxolone analogue (BX24), zinc sulfate and vitamin A in treatment of gastric ulcer. *Gut*, 13, 459 (1972)

1950 Fraser WD, Gray CE, O'Reilly D St J. The plasma cAMP response to tetracosactrin (Synacthen). *Proc ACB Natl Meet*, 51 (1989)

1951 Frassinelli-Gundersen EP, Margen S, Brown JR. Iron stores in users of oral contraceptive agents. *Am J Clin Nutr*, 41, 703-712 (1985)

1952 Frayn KN, Adnitt PI, Turner P. The hypoglycaemic action of metformin. *Postgrad Med J*, 47, 777 (1971)

1953 Freaney R, McBrinn Y, McKenna M. Secondary hyperparathyroidism in elderly people: combined effect of renal insufficiency and vitamin D deficiency. *Am J Clin Nutr*, 58, 187-191 (1993)

1954 Freche JP, Decolin D, Siest JP et al. Variation chez l'homme de l'excretion du 6-β-hydroxycortisol urinaire apres administration d'un nouveau derive de l'isoquinoleine, PK-11195 (52028 RP). *Therapie*, 44, 327-330 (1989)

1955 Freedman SH, Anderson NE. Spirometry and oral contraceptives. *Am J Obstet Gynecol*, 116, 682 (1973)

1956 Freeman DJ, Laupacis A, Keown PA et al. Evaluation of cyclosporine-phenytoin interaction with observations on cyclosporine metabolites. *Br J Clin Pharmacol*, 18, 887-893 (1984)

1957 Freeman JA, Beeler MF. *Laboratory Medicine: Clinical Microscopy*, Philadelphia PA, Lea and Febiger (1974)

1958 Freeman RB, Maher JF, Schreiner GE et al. Renal tubular necrosis due to nephrotoxicity of organic mercurial diuretics. *Ann Intern Med*, 57, 34 (1962)

1959 Fregly MJ, McCarthy JS. Effect of diuretics on renal iodide excretion by humans. *Toxicol Appl Pharmacol*, 25, 289 (1973)

1960 Frenkel EP, McCall MS, Sheehan RG. Cerebrospinal fluid folate, and vitamin B_{12} in anticonvulsant induced megaloblastosis. *J Lab Clin Med*, 81, 105 (1973)

1961 Frick J, Aulitzky W, Kalla NR. Clinical microdose study of gossypol: effect on sperm motility and renal function. *Contraception*, 37, 153-162 (1988)

1962 Frick MH, Elo O, Haapa K et al. Helsinki heart study: primary - prevention trial with gemfibrozil in middle - aged men with dyslipidemia. *N Engl J Med*, 317, 1237-1245 (1987)

1963 Friedman AC, Lautin EM. Cis-platinum (III) diamine dichloride: another cause of bilateral small kidneys. *Urology*, 16, 584-586 (1980)

1964 Friedman E, Shadel M, Halkin H et al. Thiazide-induced hyponatremia: Reproducibility by single dose rechallenge and an analysis of pathogenesis. *Ann Intern Med*, 110, 24-30 (1989)

1965 Friedman GD, Siegelaub AB, Seltzer CC et al. Smoking habits and the leukocyte count. *Arch Environ Health*, 26, 137 (1973)

1966 Friel PN, Leal KW, Wilensky AJ. Valproic acid-phenytoin interaction. *Ther Drug Monit*, 1, 243-248 (1979)

1967 Friend DG. Uricosuric drugs. *Practitioner*, 200, 153 (1968)

1968 Frigo GM, Lecchini S, Gatti G et al. Modification of phenytoin clearance by valproic acid in normal subjects. *Br J Clin Pharmacol*, 8, 553-556 (1979)

1969 Friis T, Pedersen LR. Serum lipids in hyper- and hypothyroidism before and after treatment. *Clin Chim Acta*, 162, 155-163 (1987)

1970 Friman G, Nystrom-Rosander C, Jonsell G et al. Agranulocytosis associated with malaria prophylaxis with maloprim. *Br Med J*, 286, 1244-1245 (1983)

1971 Frimodt-Moller N, Maigaard S, Madsen PO. Comparative nephrotoxicity among aminoglycosides and β-lactam antibiotics. *Infection*, 6, 283-289 (1980)

1972 Frings CS, Queen C, Foster LB. Improved colorimetric method for assay of amphetamines in urine. *Clin Chem*, 17, 1016 (1971)

1973 Frishman WH. Carvedilol. *N Engl J Med*, 339, 1759-1765 (1998)

1974 Fritschka E, Gotzen R, Kittler R et al. Effect of metoprolol on 24 hour urinary excretion of adrenal steroids and kallikrein in patients with essential hypertension. *Br J Pharmacol*, 81, 245-253 (1984)

1975 Frohlich ED, Dustan HP, Page IH. Some clinical effects of guanoxan. *Clin Pharmacol Ther*, 7, 599 (1966)

1976 Frolich C, Wilson TW, Carr K et al. Urinary prostaglandins: release from the kidney by angiotensin in dog and man. *Clin Res*, 21, 687 (1973)

1977 Fröhlich M, Schunkert H, Hense H-W, et al. Effects of hormone replacement therapies on fibrinogen and plasma viscosity in postmenopausal women. *Br J Haematol*, 100, 577-581 (1998)

1978 Fry IDR, Chua TP, Frankel RJ. Fall in serum cholesterol concentration after streptokinase therapy for acute myocardial infarction. *Proc ACB Natl Meet*, 119 (1992)

1979 Fry J, Southgate HJ, Taylor C et al. Foscarnet induced hypocalcaemia in patients with acquired immunodeficiency syndrome: an inappropriate PTH response. *Proc ACB Natl Meet*, 76 (1993)

1980 Frystyk J, Skjaerback C, Alexander N, et al. Lanreotide reduces serum free and total insulin-like growth factor-I after angioplasty. *Circulation*, 94, 2465-2471 (1996)

1981 Fuentes A, Goldkrand JW. Angiotensin-converting enzyme activity in hypertensive subjects after magnesium sulfate therapy. *Am J Obstet Gynecol*, 156, 1375-1379 (1987)

1982 Fujimoto VY, Downey D, Monroe SE, et al. Dose-related suppression of serum luteinizing hormone in women by a potent new gonadotropin-releasing antagonist (Ganirelix) administered by intranasal spray. *Fertil Steril*, 67, 469-473 (1997)

1983 Fujimoto Y, Ikoma R, Shimizu T et al. Effect of zonisamide on serum immunoglobulins. *Arz Forsch Drug Res*, 40, 855-858 (1990)

1984 Fujino Y, Nishimura M, Nishimura S, et al. Prolonged administration of isoflurane to patients with severe renal dysfunction. *Anesth Analg*, 86, 440-441 (1998)

1985 Fujisawa USA, Inc. Manufacturer's literature on Adenocard® IV and Adenoscan® . Deerfield, IL 60015 (1995)

1986 Fujisawa USA, Inc. Manufacturer's literature on Cefizox® . Deerfield, IL 60015 (1995)

1987 Fujisawa USA, Inc. Manufacturer's literature on Prograf® . Deerfield, IL 60015 (1997)

1988 Fujita J, Nakamura H, Takigawa K et al. Serial measurements of plasma elastase alpha$_1$-proteinase inhibitor complexes in patients receiving cancer chemotherapy. *Chest*, 104, 522-526 (1993)

1989 Fujita T, Chan JCM, Bartter FC. Effects of oral furosemide and salt loading on parathyroid function in normal subjects. *Nephron*, 38, 109-114 (1984)

1990 Fukagawa M, Okazaki R, Takano K et al. Regression of parathyroid hyperplasia by calcitriol-pulse therapy in patients on long-term dialysis. *N Engl J Med*, 323, 421 (1990)

1991 Furst DE, Anderson W. Differential effects of diclofenac and aspirin on serum glutamic oxaloacetic transaminase elevations in patients with rheumatoid arthritis and osteoarthritis. *Arth Rheum*, 36, 804-810 (1993)

1992 Furst P, Guanieri G, Hultman E. The effect of the administration of L-tryptophan on synthesis of urea and gluconeogenesis in man. *Scand J Clin Lab Invest*, 27, 183 (1971)

1993 Fuse H, Sakamoto M, Ohta S et al. Effect of pentoxifylline on sperm motion. *Arch Androl*, 31, 9-15 (1993)

1994 Fushimi R, Suehisa E, Matsui M et al. Effect of ethamsylate, anti-haemorrhagic drug, in peroxidase-coupled enzymatic assay of serum creatinine. *Clin Biochem Rev*, 14, 363 (1993)

1995 Fuss M, Bergmann P, Bergans A et al. Correction of low circulating levels of 1,25-dihydroxyvitamin D by 25-hydroxyvitamin D during reversal of hypomagnesaemia. *Clin Endocrinol*, 31, 31-38 (1989)

1996 Fyhrquist F, Karppinen K, Honkanen T et al. High serum erythropoietin levels are normalized during treatment of congestive heart failure with enalapril. *J Intern Med*, 226, 257-260 (1989)

1997 Fyles J, Byrne D, Chambers D et al. Multilayer slide enzyme immunoassay for the measurement of carbamazepine in human serum. *Clin Chem*, 41, S57 (1995)

1998 Gabor EP. Hemolytic anemia as adverse reaction to salicylazosulfapyridine. *N Engl J Med*, 289, 1372 (1973)

1999 Gabriel R. Ethambutol and a false-positive screening test for phaeochromocytoma. *Br Med J*, 3, 332 (1972)

2000 Gabriel R. Rifampicin jaundice. *Br Med J*, 3, 182 (1971)

2001 Gabriel R, Caldwell J, Hartley RB. Acute tubular necrosis, caused by therapeutic doses of paracetamol?. *Clin Nephrol*, 18, 269-271 (1982)

2002 Gaddi A, Arca M, Ciarrocchi A et al. Pravastatin in heterozygous familial hypercholesterolemia: low density lipoprotein (LDL) cholesterol-lowering effect and LDL receptor activity on skin fibroblasts. *Metabolism*, 40, 1074-1078 (1991)

2003 Gailani S, Holland JF, Glick A. Effects of boxidine on human serum sterols and neoplasms. *Clin Pharmacol Ther*, 13, 91 (1972)

2004 Gainer JV, Morrow JD, Loveland A, et al. Effect of bradykinin-receptor blockade on the response to angiotensin-converting-enzyme inhibitor in normotensive and hypertensive subjects. *N Engl J Med*, 339, 1285-1292 (1998)

2005 Gal I, Parkinson C, Craft I. Effect of oral contraceptives on human plasma vitamin A levels. *Br Med J*, 2, 436 (1971)

2006 Galbraith RA, Michnovicz JJ. The effects of cimetidine on the oxidative metabolism of estradiol. *N Engl J Med*, 321, 269-274 (1989)

2007 Galeazzi R, Lorenzini I, Orlandi F. Rifampicin-induced elevation of serum bile acids in man. *Dig Dis Sci*, 25, 108-112 (1980)

2008 Galeone F, Giacomelli A, Rossi A et al. Effect of famotidine on serum immunoreactive parathyroid hormone in chronic hemodialysis patients. *Curr Ther Res*, 44, 355-358 (1988)

2009 Gallagher B, Baumel IP. Primidone: biotransformation. In:. *Antiepileptic Drugs, DM Woodbury, JK Penry, RP Schmidt (eds)*, New York NY, Raven Press (1972)

2010 Gallagher BB. Trimethadione and other oxagolidinediones: toxicity. In:. *Antiepileptic Drugs, DM Woodbury, JK Penry, RP Schmidt (eds)*, New York NY, Raven Press (1972)

2011 Gallagher JC, Goldgar D. Treatment of postmenopausal osteoporosis with high doses of synthetic calcitriol: a randomized controlled study. *Ann Intern Med*, 113, 649-655 (1990)

2012 Gallant DM, Bishop MP. Quide vs mellaril® in chronic schizophrenic patients. *Curr Ther Res*, 14, 10 (1972)

2013 Galler M, Folkert VW, Schlondorff D. Reversible acute renal insufficiency and hyperkalemia following indomethacin therapy. *J Am Med Ass*, 246, 154-155 (1981)

2014 Gallerani M, Manfredini R, Moratelli S. Non-hemorrhagic adverse reactions of oral anticoagulant therapy. *Int J Cardiol*, 49, 1-7 (1995)

2015 Galletti F, Strazzullo P, Gagliardi R et al. Metabolic effects of long-term therapy with muzolimine and chlorthalidone in hypertension. *Eur J Clin Pharmacol*, 33, 515-517 (1987)

2016 Galteau MM, Ghribi S, Siest JP et al. 6β-hydroxycortisol urinary excretion as a noninvasive test for drug induction or inhibition exploration. *Ann Clin Biol*, 50, 525 (1992)

2017 Gambardella S, Frontoni S, Lala A et al. Regression of microalbuminuria in type II diabetic, hypertensive patients after long-term indapamide treatment. *Am Heart J*, 122, 1232-1238 (1991)

2018 Gambini G, Rossi S, Valori C. Absence of effects of ketanserin on renal prostacyclin and thromboxane A2 in essential hypertension. *Eur Heart J*, 12, 550-553 (1991)

2019 Gandini R, Cunietti E, Pappalepore V et al. Effects of intravenous high doses of ketoprofen on blood clotting, bleeding time and platelet aggregation. *J Intern Med Res*, 11, 243-246 (1983)

2020 Gangji D, Juvent M, Niset G et al. Study of the influence of nifedipine on the pharmacokinetics and pharmacodynamics of propranolol, metoprolol and atenolol. *Br J Clin Pharmacol*, 17, 29s-35s (1984)

2021 Ganguli PC, Hunter WM. Radioimmunoassay of gastrin in human plasma. *J Physiol*, 220, 499 (1972)

2022 Ganguli R, Yang Z, Shurin G et al. Serum interleukin-6 concentration in schizophrenia: elevation associated with duration of illness. *Psychiat Res*, 51, 1-10 (1994)

2023 Gao Y, Shimizu M, Yamada S, et al. The effects of chemotherapy including cisplatin on vitamin D metabolism. *Endocrine J*, 40, 737-742 (1993)

2024 Garb S. Clinical Guide to Undesirable Drug Interactions and Drug Interferences. New York NY, Springer Publishing Co (1971)

2025 Garb S. Laboratory Tests in Common Use. *4th edition*, New York NY, Springer Publishing Co (1966)

2026 Garcia M, Miller M, Moses AM. Chlorpropamide-induced water retention in patients with diabetes mellitus. *Ann Intern Med*, 75, 549 (1971)

2027 Garcia-Borreguero D, Jacobsen FM, Nurphy DL et al. Hormonal responses to the administration of m-chlorophenylpiperazine in patients with seasonal affective disorder and controls. *Biol Psychiat*, 37, 740-749 (1995)

2028 Garcia-Buey L, Garcia-Monzon C, Garcia-Sanchez A et al. Treatment of chronic NANB viral hepatitis with recombinant interferon alfa-2b. Preliminary clinical and immunological results. *J Hepatol*, 11, Suppl 1, S158 (1990)

2029 Garden JM, Freinkel RK. Systemic absorption of topical steroids. metabolic effects as an index of mild hypercortisolism. *Arch Dermatol*, 122, 1007-1010 (1986)

2030 Gardner DF, Centor RM, Utiger RD. Effects of low dose oral iodide supplementation on thyroid function in normal men. *Clin Endocrinol*, 28, 283-288 (1988)

2031 Gardner DF, Utiger RD, Schwartz SL et al. Effects of oral erythrosine (2', 4', 5', 7'-tetraiodofluorescein) on thyroid function in normal men. *Toxicol Appl Pharmacol*, 91, 299-304 (1987)

2032 Garg A, Grundy SM. Cholestyramine therapy for dyslipidemia in non-insulin-dependent diabetes mellitus. *Ann Intern Med*, 121, 416-422 (1994)

2033 Garg A, Grundy SM. Nicotinic acid as therapy for dyslipidemia in non-insulin-dependent diabetes mellitus. *J Am Med Ass*, 264, 723-726 (1990)

2034 Garibotto G, Gurreri G, Robaudo C et al. Erythropoietin treatment and amino acid metabolism in hemodialysis patients. *Nephron*, 65, 533-536 (1993)

2035 Garnero P, Sornay-Rendu E, Delmas PD. Decreased bone turnover in oral contraceptive users. *Bone*, 16, 499-503 (1995)

2036 Garnett ES, Cohen H, Nahmias C et al. The roles of carbohydrate, renin and aldosterone in sodium retention during and after total starvation. *Metabolism*, 22, 867 (1973)

2037 Garrettson LK, Perel JM, Dayton PG. Methylphenidate interaction with both anticonvulsants and ethyl biscoumacetate: a new action of methylphenidate. *J Am Med Ass*, 207, 2053 (1969)

2038 Garty M, Paul-Keslin L, Ilfeld DN et al. Increased theophylline clearance in asthmatic patients due to terbutaline. *Eur J Clin Pharmacol*, 36, 25-28 (1989)

2039 Garvey MJ, Hollon SD, DeRubeis RJ. Changes in urinary MHPG during treatment of depression with imipramine. *Biol Psychiat*, 34, 562-564 (1993)

2040 Garvey MJ, Noel M. Is carbamazepine associated with NAG elevations suggestive of renal disease?. *Brain Dev*, 17, 222-224 (1995)

2041 Gary NE, Dodelson R, Eisinger RP. Indomethacin-associated acute renal failure. *Am J Med*, 69, 135-136 (1980)

2042 Garza-Flores J, De la Cruz DL, Valles de Bourges V et al. Long-term effects of depot-medroxyprogesterone acetate on lipoprotein metabolism. *Contraception*, 44, 61-71 (1991)

2043 Gascon N, Otal C, Martinez-Bru C et al. Dipyrone interference on several common biochemical tests. *Clin Chem*, 39, 1033-1038 (1993)

2044 Gascon-Roche N, Mora-Brugues J, Rodriguez-Espinosa J et al. In vitro effect of dipyrone on several peroxidase labelled immunoassays. *Eur J Clin Chem Clin Biochem*, 33, 221-224 (1995)

2045 Gaskins JD, Holt RJ, Postelnick M. Nondosage-dependent valproic acid induced hyperammonemia and coma. *Clin Pharm*, 3, 313-316 (1984)

2046 Gaspard UJ. Metabolic effects of oral contraceptives. *Am J Obstet Gynecol*, 157, 1029-1041 (1987)

2047 Gaspard UJ, Buret J, Gillain D et al. Serum lipid and lipoprotein changes induced by new oral contraceptives containing ethinylestradiol plus levonorgestrel or desogestrel. *Contraception*, 81, 395-408 (1985)

2048 Gate Pharmaceuticals. Manufacturer's literature on Moban® . Sellersville, PA 18960 (1996)

2049 Gate Pharmaceuticals. Manufacturer's literature on Orap® . Sellersville, PA 18960 (1996)

2050 Gatell JM, San Miguel JG, Zamora L et al. Comparison of the nephrotoxicity and auditory toxicity of tobramycin and amikacin. *Antimicrob Agent Chemother*, 23, 897-901 (1983)

2051 Gaudreault P, Temple AR, Lovejoy FH Jr. The relative severity of acute versus chronic salicylate poisoning in children: a clinical comparison. *Pediatrics*, 70, 566-569 (1982)

2052 Gault H, Longerich L, Dawe M et al. Digoxin-rifampin interaction. *Clin Pharmacol Ther*, 35, 750-754 (1984)

2053 Gaumann DM, Tassonyi E, Rivest RW et al. Cardiovascular and endocrine effects of clonidine premedication in neurosurgical patients. *Can J Anaes*, 38, 837-843 (1991)

2054 Gaumond B, Lindsey K, Sanborn K et al. An automated chemiluminescence immunoassay test for free triiodothyronine. *Clin Chem*, 41, S57 (1995)

2055 Gaunt R, Steinetz BG, Chart JJ. Pharmacologic alteration of steroid hormone functions. *Clin Pharmacol Ther*, 9, 657 (1968)

2056 Gaut ZN, Pocelinko R, Solomon HM et al. Oral glucose tolerance, plasma insulin, and uric acid excretion in man during chronic administration. *Metabolism*, 20, 1031 (1971)

2057 Gavish D, Breslow JL. Lipoprotein(a) reduction by N-acetylcysteine. *Lancet*, 337, 203-204 (1991)

2058 Gavras I, Graff LG, Rose BD et al. Fatal pancytopenia associated with the use of captopril. *Ann Intern Med*, 94, 58-59 (1981)

2059 Gaw A, Packard CJ, Murray EF et al. Effects of simvastatin on apoB metabolism and LDL subfraction distribution. *Arterioscler Thromb*, 13, 170-189 (1993)

2060 Gawaz MP, Ward RA. Effects of hemodialysis on platelet-derived thrombospondin. *Kidney Int*, 40, 257-265 (1991)

2061 G.D. Searle & Co. Manufacturer's literature on Aldactone® . Chicago. IL 60680 (1992)

2062 G.D. Searle & Co. Manufacturer's literature on Ambien® . Chicago. IL 60680 (1996)

2063 G.D. Searle & Co. Manufacturer's literature on Calan® . Chicago, IL 60680 (1995)

2064 G.D. Searle & Co. Manufacturer's literature on Cytotec® . Chicago, IL 60680 (1995)

2065 G.D. Searle & Co. Manufacturer's literature on Daypro® . Chicago, IL 60680 (1996)

2066 G.D. Searle & Co. Manufacturer's literature on Flagyl® . Chicago, IL 60680 (1995)

2067 G.D. Searle & Co. Manufacturer's literature on Kerlone® . Chicago, IL 60680 (1995)

2068 G.D. Searle & Co. Manufacturer's literature on Maxaquin® . Chicago, IL 60680 (1995)

2069 G.D. Searle & Co. Manufacturer's literature on Norpace® . Chicago, IL 60680 (1996)

2070 G.D. Searle & Co. Manufacturer's literature on Synarel® . Chicago, IL 60680 (1995)

2071 Geaney DP, Carver JG, Aronson JK et al. Interaction of azapropazone with phenytoin. *Br Med J*, 284, 1373 (1982)

2072 Geffner DL, Sladek J, Hershman JM. Pharmacokinetics and clinical effects of atenolol in therapy of hyperthyroidism. *Drugs Exp Clin Res*, 16, 167-173 (1990)

2073 Gehr TWB, Sica DA, Grasela DM et al. Fosinopril pharmacokinetics and pharmacodynamics in chronic ambulatory peritoneal dialysis patients. *Eur J Clin Pharmacol*, 41, 165-169 (1991)

2074 Geissler AH, Turnlund JR, Cohen RD. Effect of chlorthalidone on zinc levels, testosterone and sexual function in man. *Drug Nutr Interact*, 4, 275-283 (1986)

2075 Gelander L, Lindstedt G, Selstam G et al. Effects of acute intravenous injection of two growth hormone-releasing hormones (GHRH 1-40 and 1-29) on serum growth hormone and other pituitary hormones in short children with pulsatile growth hormone secretion. *Horm Res*, 31, 213-220 (1989)

2076 Gelfand MD. Ischemic colitis associated with a depot synthetic progestogen. *Am J Dig Dis*, 17, 275 (1972)

2077 Geltner D, Chajek T, Rubinger D et al. Quinidine hypersensitivity and liver involvement. *Gastroenterology*, 70, 650-652 (1976)

2078 Genant HK, Lucas J, Weiss S, et al. Low dose esterified estrogen therapy: Effects on bone, plasma estradiol concentrations, endometrium, and lipid levels. *Arch Intern Med*, 157, 2609-2615 (1997)

2079 Genentech Biotechnology. Manufacturer's Literature on Herceptin® . South San Francisco, CA (1998)

2080 Genentech, Inc. Manufacturer's literature on Actimmune® . South San Francisco, CA 94080 (1995)

2081 Genentech, Inc. Manufacturer's literature on Activase® . South San Francisco, CA 94080 (1995)

2082 Genentech, Inc. Manufacturer's literature on Nutropin® . South San Francisco, CA 94080 (1995)

2083 Genentech, Inc. Manufacturer's literature on Protropin® . South San Francisco, CA 94080 (1995)

2084 Geneve J, Le Dinh T, Brouard A et al. Changes in indocyanine green kinetics after the administration of enalapril to healthy subjects. *Br J Clin Pharmacol*, 30, 297-300 (1990)

2085 Gennari C, Agnusdei D, Nardi P et al. Estrogen preserves a normal intestinal responsiveness to 1,25-dihydroxyvitamin D_3 in oophorectomized women. *J Clin Endocrinol Metab*, 71, 1288-1293 (1990)

2086 Genser N, Fink FM, Mair J et al. Plasma concentrations of CKMB mass and troponin T in children receiving anthracycline chemotherapy. *Clin Chem*, 39, 1170 (1993)

2087 Genser N, Lechleitner P, Maier J et al. PAI-1 increase after thrombolytic therapy in patients with suspected myocardial infarction. *Clin Chem*, 39, 1129 (1993)

2088 Genser N, Lechleitner P, Maier J, et al. Rebound increase of plasminogen activator inhibitor type I after cessation of thrombolytic treatment for acute myocardial infarction is independent of type of plasminogen activator used. *Clin Chem*, 44, 209-214 (1998)

2089 Gentry LO, Wood BA, Natelson EA. Effects of apalcillin on platelet function in normal volunteers. *Antimicrob Agent Chemother*, 27, 683-684 (1985)

2090 Genzyme Corporation. Manufacturer's literature on Ceredase® . Cambridge, MA 02139 (1995)

2091 George MS, Rosenstein D, Rubinow DR et al. CSF magnesium in affective disorder: lack of correlation with clinical course of treatment. *Psychiat Res*, 51, 139-146 (1994)

2092 George RH. Gentamicin assay in jaundice. *Lancet*, 1, 838 (1973)

2093 Gerber A, Weidmann P, Saner R et al. Increased serum high density lipoprotein cholesterol in hypertensive men treated with the potent vasodilator caprazidil. *Metabolism*, 33, 342-346 (1984)

2094 Gerber N, Lynn R, Oates J. Acute intoxication with 5,5-diphenylhydantoin (dilantin®) associated with impairment of biotransformation. *Ann Intern Med*, 77, 765 (1972)

2095 Gertig H, Nowaczyk W, Gniadek M. Effect of aldrin, dieldrin and lindane on lactic acid dehydrogenase and cholinesterase activity. *Diss Pharmaceut Pharmacol*, 22, 253 (1970)

2096 Getaz EP, Beckley S, Fitzpatrick J et al. Cisplatin-induced hemolysis. *N Engl J Med*, 302, 334-335 (1980)

2097 Geumei A, Issa I, EL-Gendi M et al. Inhibitory effect of β-adrenergic-blocking agent propranolol on histamine-stimulated gastric acid secretion in man. *Am J Dig Dis*, 17, 55 (1972)

2098 Gevers Leuven JA, Dersjant-Roorda MC, Helmerhorst FM et al. Effects of oral contraceptives on lipid metabolism. *Am J Obstet Gynecol*, 163, Suppl II, 1410-1413 (1990)

2099 Gevers Leuven JA, Dersjant-Roorda MC, Helmerhorst FM et al. Estrogenic effect of gestodene- or desogestrel-containing oral contraceptives on lipoprotein metabolism. *Am J Obstet Gynecol*, 263, 358-362 (1990)

2100 Ghanem MH, Fahmi MH, Abdel Malek AT. Eosinopenic effect of antiserotonin (methysergide). *Alexandria Med J*, 11, 400 (1965)

2101 Ghose K, Taylor A. Hypercupricaemia induced by antiepileptic drugs. *Hum Toxicol*, 3, 519-529 (1983)

2102 Giansiracusa DF, Blumberg S, Kantrowitz FG. Aseptic meningitis associated with ibuprofen. *Arch Intern Med*, 140, 1553 (1980)

2103 Gianturco SH, Bradley WA, Nozaki S et al. Effects of lovastatin on the levels, structure, and atherogeneity of VLDL in patients with moderate hypertriglyceridemia. *Arterioscler Thromb*, 13, 472-481 (1993)

2104 Giaufre E, Bruguerolle B, Morisson-Lacombe G et al. Influence of midazolam on the plasma concentrations of mepivacaine after lumbar epidural injection in children. *Eur J Clin Pharmacol*, 38, 91-92 (1990)

2105 Gibb DM, Dunger D, Levin M et al. Absence of effect of dipyridamole on renal and platelet function in diabetes mellitus. *Arch Dis Child*, 65, 93-98 (1990)

2106 Gibson KM, Jakobs C, Ogier H et al. Vigabatrin therapy in six patients with succinic semialdehyde dehydrogenase deficiency. *J Inher Metab Dis*, 18, 143-146 (1995)

2107 Gidal BE, Anderson GD, Seaton TL et al. Evaluation of the effect of fluoxetine on the formation of carbamazepine epoxide. *Ther Drug Monit*, 15, 405-409 (1993)

2108 Gifford RW Jr. Catapres® (ST 155) in the management of hypertension. In:. *Catapres® in Hypertension. ME Conolly (ed)*, London, Butterworth (1970)

2109 Giguere R, Auray-Blais C, Draper P et al. Diet and medications giving positive ninhydrin reactions in TLC in a newborn urinary screening program. *Clin Biochem*, 13, 103-105 (1980)

2110 Gil-Ad I, Bar-Yoseph J, Smadja Y et al. Effect of clonidine on plasma β-endorphin, cortisol and growth hormone secretion in opiate-addicted subjects. *Isr J Med Sci*, 21, 601-604 (1985)

2111 Gil-Ad I, Leibowitch N, Josefsberg Z et al. Effect of oral clonidine, insulin-induced hypoglycemia and exercise on plasma GHRH levels in short-stature children. *Acta Endocrinol*, 122, 89-95 (1990)

2112 Gilbert EF, Dasilva AQ, Queen DM. Intrahepatic cholestasis with fatal termination following norethandrolone therapy. *J Am Med Ass*, 185, 538 (1963)

2113 Gilbertson C, Jones DR. Haemolytic anaemia with nalidixic acid. *Br Med J*, 4, 493 (1972)

2114 Gilead Sciences. Manufacturer's literature on Vistide® . Foster City, CA 94404 (1996)

2115 Gilhus NE, Lea T. Carbamazepine: Effect on IgG subclass in epileptic patients. *Epilepsia*, 29, 317-320 (1988)

2116 Gilhus NE, Strandjord RE, Aarli JA. The effect of carbamazepine on serum immunoglobulin concentrations. *Acta Neurol Scand*, 66, 172-179 (1982)

2117 Gill JS, Beevers DG. Bucindol: effects on blood pressure, airways resistance and serum creatine phosphokinase. *Eur J Clin Pharmacol*, 27, 265-268 (1984)

2118 Gill MJ, Ratliff DA, Harding LK. Hypoglycemic coma, jaundice, and pure RBC aplasia following chlorpropamide therapy. *Arch Intern Med*, 140, 714-715 (1980)

2119 Gill TS, Hopkins KJ, Bottomley J et al. Cimetidine-nicoumalone interaction in man: stereochemical considerations. *Br J Clin Pharmacol*, 27, 469-474 (1989)

2120 Gilligan E, Lequin R. T3 assay for the Auraflex immunoassay system. *Clin Chem*, 41, S38 (1995)

2121 Gillman MA, Katzeff I, Vermaak WJH et al. Hormonal response to analgesic nitrous oxide in man. *Horm Metab Res*, 20, 751-754 (1988)

2122 Gillman MA, Lichtigfeld FJ. Synergism of spironolactone and lithium in mania. *Br Med J*, 292, 661-662 (1986)

2123 Gillum JG, Sesler JM, Bruzzese VL, et al. Induction of theophylline clearance by rifampin and rifabutin in healthy male volunteers. *Antimicrob Agent Chemother*, 40, 1866-1869 (1996)

2124 Gimenez S, Bagheri H, Marchou B et al. Bilan d'un suivi de pharmacovigilance de la zidovudine. *Therapie*, 45, 407-409 (1990)

2125 Gimeno F, Steenhuis EJ, Jonkman JHG. Effect of theophylline on cortisol plasma concentrations in patients with chronic pulmonary disease. *Int J Clin Pharmacol Ther Toxicol*, 28, 139-143 (1990)

2126 Ginder EM, King JD. Rapid colorimetric determination of calcium in biologic fluids with methylthymol blue. *Am J Clin Pathol*, 58, 376 (1972)

2127 Ginsberg DJ, Saad A, Gabuzda GJ. Metabolic studies with the diuretic triamterene in patients with cirrhosis and ascites. *N Engl J Med*, 271, 1229 (1964)

2128 Giordano N, Senesi M, Mattii G, et al. Polymyositis associated with simvastatin. *Lancet*, 349, 1600-1601 (1997)

2129 Giorgi PL, Oggiano N, Biraghi M et al. Effect of high doses of inhaled flunisolde on hypothalamic-pituitary-adrenal axis function in children with asthma. *Curr Ther Res*, 49, 778-783 (1991)

2130 Gip GYH, Lowe GDO, Rumley A et al. Increased markers of thrombogenesis in chronic atrial fibrillation: effects of warfarin treatment. *Br Heart J*, 73, 527-533 (1995)

2131 Gips CH, Reitsema A. Influence of nonprotein nitrogen substances on the indophenol reaction. *Clin Chim Acta*, 33, 257 (1971)

2132 Girbes ARJ, van Velhuisen DJ, Smit AJ et al. Renal and neurohumoral effects of ibopamine and metoclopramide in normal man. *Br J Clin Pharmacol*, 31, 701-704 (1991)

2133 Girbes ARL. Clinical studies with new dopamine agonists. *Doctoral thesis, University of Groningen* (1991)

2134 Giri S, Thompson PD, Taxel P, et al. Oral estrogen improves serum lipids, homocysteine and fibrinolysis in elderly men. *Atherosclerosis*, 137, 359-366 (1998)

2135 Girling DJ. Adverse effects of antituberculosis drugs. *Drugs*, 23, 56-74 (1982)

2136 Giroud M, Fabre JL, Brun JM et al. Diphenylhydantoin effects on thyroid function. *Therapie*, 40, 119-122 (1985)

2137 Gisslen M, Larsson M, Norkrans G et al. Tryptophan concentrations increase in cerebrospinal fluid and blood after zidovudine treatment in patients with HIV type 1 infection. *AIDS*, 10, 947-951 (1994)

2138 Gitlin N. Salicylate hepatotoxicity: the potential role of hypoalbuminemia. *J Clin Gastroenterol*, 2, 281-285 (1980)

2139 Gitsch E, Spona J. Serum estradiol and LH during normal and induced menstrual cycles. *Endocrinol Exp*, 7, 53 (1973)

2140 Giugliano D, Torella R, Caciapuoti F et al. Impairment of insulin secretion in man by nifedipine. *Eur J Clin Pharmacol*, 18, 395-398 (1980)

2141 Giuntoli F, Galeone F, Gabbani S et al. Nitrendipine does not impair long-term glucose control in hypertensive noninsulin-dependent diabetic patients. *Clin Ther*, 13, 216-223 (1991)

2142 Giustina A, Bussi AR, Licini M et al. Acute effects of hydrocortisone on circulating growth hormone levels in patients with acromegaly. *Horm Res*, 37, 213-216 (1992)

2143 Givers Leuven JA, Dersjant-Roorda MC, Helmerhorst RM et al. Estrogenic effects of gestodene- or desogestrel-containing oral contraceptives on lipoprotein levels. *Am J Obstet Gynecol*, 163, 358-362 (1990)

2144 Gjone E, Blomhoff JP, Ritland S et al. Laxative-induced chronic liver disease. *Scand J Gastroenterol*, 7, 395 (1972)

2145 Gjone E, Stave R. Liver disease associated with a non-constipating iron preparation. *Lancet*, 1, 421 (1973)

2146 Glass AR. Ketoconazole-induced stimulation of gonadotropin output in men: basis for a potential test of gonadotropin reserve.. *J Clin Endocrinol Metab*, 63, 1121-1125 (1986)

2147 Glass AR, Cerletty JM, Elliott W et al. Ketoconazole reduces elevated serum levels of 1,25-dihydroxyvitamin D in hypercalcemic sarcoidoss. *J Endocrinol Invest*, 13, 407-413 (1990)

2148 Glass AR, Eil C. Ketoconazole-induced reduction in serum 1, 25-dihydroxyvitamin D. *J Clin Endocrinol Metab*, 63, 766-769 (1986)

2149 Glass AR, Eil C. Ketoconazole-induced reduction in serum 1,25-dihydroxyvitamin D and total serum calcium in hypercalcemic patients. *J Clin Endocrinol Metab*, 66, 934-938 (1988)

2150 Glass D, Evans JI, Daly JR. Sleep associated growth hormone (GH) release and the effect of corticotropin injections. *Clin Sci*, 43, 5p (1972)

2151 Glaxo Wellcome Co. Manufacturer's literature on Zovirax® . Research Triangle Park, NC 27709 (1996)

2152 Glaxo Wellcome Co. Manufacturer's literature on Zyloprim. Research Triangle Park, NC 27709 (1996)

2153 Glaxo Wellcome, Inc. Manufacturer's literature on Ceftin® . Research Triangle Park, NC 27709 (1997)

2154 Glaxo Wellcome Inc. Manufacturer's literature on Ceptaz® . Research Triangle Park, NC 27709 (1996)

2155 Glaxo Wellcome Inc. Manufacturer's literature on Digibind® . Research Triangle Park, NC 27709 (1994)

2156 Glaxo Wellcome Inc. Manufacturer's literature on Flolan® . Research Triangle Park, NC 27709 (1996)

2157 Glaxo Wellcome Inc. Manufacturer's literature on Fortaz® . Research Triangle Park, NC 27709 (1996)

2158 Glaxo Wellcome Inc. Manufacturer's literature on Imitrex® . Research Triangle Park, NC 27709 (1997)

2159 Glaxo Wellcome Inc. Manufacturer's literature on Imuran® . Research Triangle Park, NC 27709 (1996)

2160 Glaxo Wellcome, Inc. Manufacturer's literature on Lamictal® . Research Triangle Park, NC 27709 (1997)

2161 Glaxo Wellcome Inc. Manufacturer's literature on Lanoxin® . Research Triangle Park, NC 27709 (1996)

2162 Glaxo Wellcome Inc. Manufacturer's literature on Proloprim® . Research Triangle Park, NC 27709 (1996)

2163 Glaxo Wellcome, Inc. Manufacturer's literature on Retrovir® . Research Triangle Park, NC 27709 (1996)

2164 Glaxo Wellcome Inc. Manufacturer's literature on Trandate® . Research Triangle Park, NC 27709 (1995)

2165 Glaxo Wellcome, Inc. Manufacturer's literature on Ultiva™. Research Triangle Park, NC 27709 (1996)

2166 Glaxo Wellcome Inc. Manufacturer's literature on Vasoxyl® . Research Triangle Park, NC 27709 (1996)

2167 Glaxo Wellcome Inc. Manufacturer's literature on Ventolin® . Research Triangle Park, NC 27709 (1996)

2168 Glaxo Wellcome Inc. Manufacturer's literature on Wellbutrin® . Research Triangle Park, NC 27709 (1996)

2169 Glaxo Wellcome Inc. Manufacturer's literature on Zantac® . Research Triangle Park, NC 27709 (1996)

2170 Glaxo Wellcome Inc. Manufacturer's literature on Zinacef® . Research Triangle Park, NC 27709 (1996)

2171 Glaxo Wellcome Inc. Manufacturer's literature on Zyban™. Research Triangle Park, NC (1997)

2172 Glaxo Wellcome Oncology/HIV. Manufacturer's literature on Alkeran® . Research Triangle Park, NC 27709 (1996)

2173 Glaxo Wellcome Oncology/HIV. Manufacturer's literature on Daraprim® . Research Triangle Park, NC 27709 (1994)

2174 Glaxo Wellcome Oncology/HIV. Manufacturer's literature on Epivir® . Research Triangle Park, NC 27709 (1996)

2175 Glaxo Wellcome Oncology/HIV. Manufacturer's literature on Leukeran® . Research Triangle Park, NC 27709 (1996)

2176 Glaxo Wellcome Oncology/HIV. Manufacturer's literature on Mepron® . Research Triangle Park, NC 27709 (1996)

2177 Glaxo Wellcome Oncology/HIV. Manufacturer's literature on Myleran® . Research Triangle Park, NC 27709 (1996)

2178 Glaxo Wellcome Oncology/HIV. Manufacturer's literature on Navelbine® . Research Triangle Park, NC 27709 (1996)

2179 Glaxo Wellcome Oncology/HIV. Manufacturer's literature on Purinethol® . Research Triangle Park, NC 27709 (1996)

2180 Glaxo Wellcome Oncology/HIV. Manufacturer's literature on Thioguanine. Research Triangle Park, NC 27709 (1996)

2181 Glaxo Wellcome Oncology/HIV. Manufacturer's literature on Zofran® . Research Triangle Park, NC 27709 (1996)

2182 Glazko AJ. Antiepileptic drugs: biotransformation, metabolism, and serum half-life. *Epilepsia*, 16, 367-391 (1975)

2183 Gleason MN, Gosslein RE, Hodge HC. Clinical Toxicology of Commercial Products. Baltimore, MD, Williams and Wilkins (1957)

2184 Gleeson JM, Dukes CS, Elstad NL et al. Effects of estrogen/progestin agents on plasma retinoids and chylomicron remnant metabolism. *Contraception*, 35, 69-78 (1987)

2185 Gleiter CH, Schreeb KH, Goldbach S, et al. Fenoterol increases erythropoietin concentrations during tocolysis. *Br J Clin Pharmacol*, 45, 157-159 (1998)

2186 Glick JH. Deficiencies of Sigma Diagnostics urinary oxalate method in the presence of ascorbate. *Clin Chem*, 33, 419-420 (1987)

2187 Gloggler A, Bulla M, Furst P. Effect of low dose supplementation of L-carnitine on lipid metabolism in hemodialyzed children. *Kidney Int*, 36, Suppl 27, S147-S151 (1989)

2188 Glorieux FH, Bishop NJ, Plotkin H, et al. Cyclic administration of pamidronate in children with severe osteogenesis imperfecta. *N Engl J Med*, 339, 947-952 (1998)

2189 Glovinsky D, Kalogeras KT, Kirch DG et al. Cerebrospinal fluid oxytocin concentration in schizophrenic patients does not differ from control subjects and is not changed by neuroleptic medication. *Schiz Res*, 11, 273-276 (1994)

2190 Gluck Z, Baumgartner G, Weidmann P et al. Increased ratio between serum β- and α-lipoproteins during diuretic therapy: an adverse effect?. *Clin Sci Mol Med*, 55, 325s-328s (1978)

2191 Gluck Z, Weidmann P, Mordasini R et al. Einfluss einer diuretic-therapie auf die serumlipoproteine: ein unerwunschter effect. *Schweiz Med Wschr*, 109, 104-108 (1979)

2192 Glueck CJ. Effects of oxandrolone on plasma triglycerides and postheparin lipolytic activity. *Metabolism*, 20, 691 (1971)

2193 Glueck CJ, Ford S Jr, Steiner P et al. Effects of a progestational oral contraceptive on lipids and lipases. *Am J Obstet Gynecol*, 116, 689 (1973)

2194 Glueck CJ, Glueck HI, Hamer T et al. Beta blockers, Lp(a), hypertension, and reduced basal fibrinolytic actity. *Am J Med Sci*, 307, 317-324 (1994)

2195 Gluszko P, Undas A, Amenta S et al. Administration of γ interferon in human subjects decreases plasminogen activation and fibrinolysis without influencing C_1 inhibitor. *J Lab Clin Med*, 123, 232-240 (1994)

2196 Glynn KP, Cafaro AF, Fowler CW et al. False elevations of serum glutamic-oxaloacetic transaminase due to para-aminosalicylic acid. *Ann Intern Med*, 72, 525 (1970)

2197 Gochman N. Personal communication (1972)

2198 Godeau B, Zini J-M, Schaeffer A et al. High-dose methylprednisolone is an alternative treatment for adults with autoimmune thrombocytopenic purpura refractory to intravenous immunoglobulins and oral corticosteroids. *Am J Hematol*, 48, 282-284 (1995)

2199 Godfrey NF, Peter A, Simon TM et al. IV N-acetylcysteine treatment of hematologic reactions to chrysotherapy. *J Rheumatol*, 9, 519-526 (1982)

2200 Godsall JW, Baron R, Insogna KL. Vitamin D metabolism and bone histomorphometry in a patient with antacid- induced osteomalacia. *Am J Med*, 77, 747-750 (1984)

2201 Godsland IF, Crook D, Simpson R et al. The effects of different formulations of oral-contraceptive agents on lipid and carbohydrate metabolism. *N Engl J Med*, 323, 1375-1381 (1990)

2202 Godsland IF, Crook D, Wynn V. Coronary heart disease risk markers in users of low-dose oral contraceptives. *J Reprod Med Obstet Gynecol*, 36, Suppl, 226-237 (1991)

2203 Goedel-Meinen L, Schmidt G, Wirtzfeld A et al. The influence of amiodarone on the function of the thyroid gland. *Z Kardiol*, 73, 399-404 (1984)

2204 Goerdt C, Keith M, Bloomfield Rubins H. Effects of phenytoin on plasma high-density lipoprotein cholesterol levels in men with low levels of high-density lipoprotein cholesterol. *J Clin Pharmacol*, 35, 767-775 (1995)

2205 Goff DC, Midha KK, Brotman AW et al. Elevations of plasma concentrations of haloperidol after the addition of fluoxetine. *Am J Psychiat*, 148, 790-792 (1991)

2206 Gogel E, Halloran BP, Strewler GJ. Probenecid inhibits the secretion of nephrogenous adenosine-3'-5'-monophosphate in normal man. *J Clin Endocrinol Metab*, 57, 689-693 (1983)

2207 Golan A, Bukovsky I, Winraub Z et al. The effect of chorionic gonadotropic-releasing hormone analog (D-Trp-6) treatment on elevated and normal serum prolactin levels. *Fertil Steril*, 51, 532-534 (1989)

2208 Gold EJ, Mertelsmann RH, Itri LM et al. Phase I clinical trial of 13-cis-retinoic acid in myelodysplastic syndromes. *Cancer Treat Rep*, 67, 981-986 (1983)

2209 Gold GL, Fritz RD. Hyperuricemia associated with the treatment of acute leukemia. *Ann Intern Med*, 47, 428 (1957)

2210 Goldberg A. Porphyrins and porphyrias In:. *Recent Advances in Haematology, A Goldberg, McBrain, (eds)*, New York NY, Churchill-Livingstone (1971)

2211 Goldberg IJ, Brown LK, Rayfield EJ. Disopyramide (Norpace®)-induced hypoglycemia. *Am J Med*, 69, 463-466 (1980)

2212 Goldberg IJL, Lawton K, Redding JR et al. Effect of penicillamine on blood levels and urinary excretion of gold. *Ann Clin Biochem*, 20, 220 (1983)

2213 Goldberg LI. Monoamine oxidase inhibitors: adverse reactions and possible mechanisms. *J Am Med Ass*, 190, 456 (1964)

2214 Goldberg MA, Brugnara C, Dover GJ et al. Treatment of sickle cell anemia with hydroxyurea and erythropoietin. *N Engl J Med*, 323, 366-372 (1990)

2215 Goldberg R, La Belle P, Zupkis R et al. Comparison of the effects of lovastatin and gemfibrozil on lipids and glucose control in non-insulin-dependent diabetes mellitus. *Am J Cardiol*, 66, 16B-21B (1990)

2216 Goldberg RB, Roth D. A preliminary report of the safety and efficacy of fluvastatin for hypercholesterolemia in renal transplant patients receiving cyclosporine. *Am J Cardiol*, 76, 107A-109A (1995)

2217 Golden NH, Pepper GM, Sacker I et al. The effects of a dopamine antagonist on luteinizing hormone and prolactin release in women with anorexia nervosa and in normal controls. *J Adolesc Health*, 13, 155-160 (1992)

2218 Golden RL, Hsiao J, Lane E et al. The effects of intravenous clomipramine on neurohormones in normal subjects. *J Clin Endocrinol Metab*, 68, 632-637 (1989)

2219 Goldenberg H. Specific photometric determination of 5-hydroxyindoleacetic acid in urine. *Clin Chem*, 13, 697 (1967)

2220 Goldenberg H. Specific photometric determination of 5-hydroxyindoleacetic acid in urine. *Clin Chem*, 19, 38 (1973)

2221 Goldenberg LF, Olivari MT, Levine TB et al. Effect of dobutamine on plasma potassium in congestive heart failure secondary to idiopathic or ischemic cardiomyopathy. *Am J Cardiol*, 63, 843-846 (1989)

2222 Goldfinger SE. Drug therapy - treatment of gout. *N Engl J Med*, 285, 1303 (1971)

2223 Goldhaber SZ, Hennekens CH, Spark RF et al. Plasma renin substrate, renin activity and aldosterone levels in a sample of oral contraceptive users from a community survey. *Am Heart J*, 107, 119-122 (1984)

2224 Goldman AI, Steele BW, Schnaper HW et al. Serum lipoprotein levels during chlorthalidone therapy. *J Am Med Ass*, 244, 1691-1695 (1980)

2225 Goldman JA, Eckerling B. Effect of a progestogen oral contraceptive compound on carbohydrate metabolism. *Isr J Med Sci*, 8, 1724 (1972)

2226 Goldsmith GA. Therapy of hypercholesterolemia. *Am J Dig Dis*, 9, 651 (1964)

2227 Goldsmith NF, Goldsmith JR. Epidemiological aspects of magnesium and calcium metabolism. *Arch Environ Health*, 12, 607 (1966)

2228 Goldstein G. Sarcoid reaction associated with phenylbutazone hypersensitivity. *Ann Intern Med*, 59, 97 (1963)

2229 Goldstein P, Sundaram S, Manimekalai S. Maternal serum α-Fetoprotein: effect of bacterial infection. *Clin Chem*, 38, 1022 (1992)

2230 Goldstein P, Sundaram S, Manimekalai S et al. Effect of drug ingestion on maternal serum α-Fetoprotein. *Clin Chem*, 37, 934 (1991)

2231 Goldzieher JW, Kleber JW, Moses LE et al. A cross-sectional study of plasma FSH and LH levels in women. *Contraception*, 2, 225 (1970)

2232 Golf SW, Temme H, Kempf DK et al. Systemic short-term fibrinolysis with high dose streptokinase in acute myocardial infarction: time course of biochemical parameters. *J Clin Chem Clin Biochem*, 22, 723-729 (1984)

2233 Golland IM, Vaughan-Williams CA, Shalet SM et al. Influence of danazol and goserelin on insulin and glucagon in non-obese women with endometriosis. *Acta Endocrinol*, 123, 405-410 (1990)

2234 Gomez B Jr, Ardakani S, Ju J et al. Monoclonal antibody assay for measuring bone-specific alkaline phosphatase activity in serum. *Clin Chem*, 41, 1560-1566 (1995)

2235 Gomez J-L, Dupont A, Cusan L et al. Incidence of liver toxicity associated with the use of flutamide in prostate cancer patients. *Am J Med*, 92, 465-470 (1992)

2236 Gomez-Rubio M, Porres JC, Castillo I et al. Prolonged treatment (18 months) of chronic hepatitis C with recombinant α-interferon in comparison with a control group. *J Hepatol*, 11, Suppl 1, S63-S67 (1990)

2237 Gomi T, Ikeda T, Ikegami F. Beneficial effect of α-blocker on hemorheology in patients with essential hypertension. *Am J Hypertens*, 10, 886-892 (1997)

2238 Gonano F, Pirisi M, Soardo G et al. Changes in lipid metabolism by treatment with interferon alpha in patients with chronic viral liver disease. *Clin Biochem Rev*, 14, 225 (1993)

2239 Gonzalez MT, Sherwood JB, Brion LP et al. Erythropoietin levels during theophylline treatment in premature infants. *J Pediatr*, 124, 128- 130 (1994)

2240 Goodale RM. Clinical Interpretation of Laboratory Tests. *5th edition*, Philadelphia PA, Davis (1964)

2241 Goodman HO, Shihabi Z, Oles KS. Antiepileptic drugs and plasma and platelet taurine in epilepsy. *Epilepsia*, 30, 201-207 (1989)

2242 Goodman LS, Gilman A. The Pharmacological Basis of Therapeutics. *4th edition*, New York NY, MacMillan and Co (1970)

2243 Goodwin CS, Sparell G. Inhibition of dapsone excretion by probenecid. *Lancet*, 2, 884-885 (1969)

2244 Goodwin FJ, Ledingham JG, Laragh JH. The effects of prolonged administration of vasopressin and oxytocin on renin, aldosterone and sodium balance. *Clin Sci*, 39, 641 (1970)

2245 Goodwin JS, Garry PJ. Relationship between megadose vitamin supplementation and immunological function in a healthy elderly population. *Clin Exp Immunol*, 51, 647-653 (1983)

2246 Gorchein A, Webber R, Burnett D et al. Effect of anticonvulsant drugs on serum δ-aminolevulinic acid levels in non-porphyric subjects. *Br J Clin Pharmacol*, 24, 847-848 (1987)

2247 Gordon B, Chang S, Kavanagh M et al. The effects of lipid lowering on diabetic retinopathy. *Am J Ophthalmol*, 112, 385-391 (1991)

2248 Gordon D, Beastall GH, McArdle CS et al. The effect of tamoxifen therapy on thyroid function tests. *Cancer*, 58, 1422-1425 (1986)

2249 Gordon EK, Oliver J, Goodwin FK et al. Effect of probenecid on free 3-methoxy-4-hydroxyphenylethylene glycol (MHPG) and its sulfate in human CSF. *Neuropharmacology*, 12, 391 (1973)

2250 Gordon RD, Ballantine DM, Bachmann AW. Effects of repeated doses of pseudoephedrine on blood pressure and plasma catecholamines in normal subjects and in patients with phaeochromocytoma. *Clin Exp Pharmacol Physiol*, 19, 287-290 (1992)

2251 Gordon RD, Pawsey CGK, O'Halloran MW et al. Use of home blood pressure measurement to compare the efficacy of two diuretics. *Med J Aust*, 2, 565 (1971)

2252 Gordon T. Factors associated with serum alkaline phosphatase level. *Arch Pathol Lab Med*, 117, 187-190 (1993)

2253 Goren MP, Pratt CB. False-positive ketone tests: a bedside measure of urinary mesna. *Cancer Chemother Pharmacol*, 25, 371-372 (1990)

2254 Goren MP, Wright PK, Osborne S. Two automated procedures for N-acetyl-β-glucosaminidase determination evaluated for detection of drug-induced tubular nephrotoxicity. *Clin Chem*, 32, 2052-2055 (1986)

2255 Goren MP, Wright RK, Horowitz ME et al. Cancer chemotherapy induced tubular nephrotoxicity evaluated by immunochemical determination of urinary adenosine binding protein. *Am J Clin Pathol*, 86, 780-783 (1986)

2256 Gormley GJ, Stoner E, Rittmaster RS et al. Effects of Finasteride (MK-906), a 5α-reductase inhibitor on circulating androgens in male volunteers. *J Clin Endocrinol Metab*, 70, 1136-1141 (1990)

2257 Gormsen J. Biochemical evaluation of standard treatment with streptokinase in acute myocardial infarction. *Acta Med Scand*, 191, 77 (1972)

2258 Gorski J, Holm G, Krotkiewski M. Effect of isoproterenol on the plasma C-peptide and insulin levels in humans. *Horm Res*, 31, 175-179 (1989)

2259 Gosling P, Andrews D, Chesner I. Non-steroidal anti-inflammatory drugs reduce albumin excretion in normal subjects. *Proc ACB Natl Meet*, 88 (1990)

2260 Gosling R, Kerry RJ, Owen G. Creatine phosphokinase activity during lithium treatment. *Br Med J*, 3, 327 (1972)

2261 Gosney K, Adachi-Kirkland J, Schiller HS. Evaluation of lidocaine interference in the Kodak Ektachem® 700 analyzer single slide method for creatinine. *Clin Chem*, 33, 2311 (1987)

2262 Goss H, Dickhaus DW. Increased bishydroxycoumarin requirements in patients receiving phenobarbital. *N Engl J Med*, 273, 1094 (1965)

2263 Goto F, Tamachi H, Hata Y et al. Effects of nifedipine slow-release tablets on blood pressure and serum lipid metabolism in patients with essential hypertension. *Curr Ther Res*, 48, 638-650 (1990)

2264 Goto Y, Tamachi H, Fusegawa Y et al. Effects of carvediol on serum lipids in patients with essential hypertension. *J Cardiovasc Pharmacol*, 18, Suppl 4, S45-S50 (1991)

2265 Goto Y, Tamachi H, Hata Y et al. Effects of nifedipine slow-release on blood pressure and serum lipid metabolism in patients with essential hypertension. *Curr Ther Res*, 48, 638-650 (1990)

2266 Gottlieb NL, Buchoff HS, Vidal AF et al. The course of severe gold associated granulocytopenia. *Clin Res*, 30, 659a (1982)

2267 Gough H, Goggin T, Crowley M et al. Serum bilirubin levels with antiepileptic drugs. *Epilepsia*, 30, 597-602 (1989)

2268 Gougoux A, Michaud G, Vinay P. The uricosuric action of benziodarone in man and dog. *Clin Res*, 18, 747 (1970)

2269 Goursot G, Deriaz H, Dufieux P et al. Haemodynamics, plasma histamine and osmolality during aortic arteriography. *Ann Fr Anesth Reanim*, 3, 90-93 (1984)

2270 Gouyette A, Pico JL, Dro JP et al. Pharmacocinetique et metabolisme du VP-16 et du cisplatine admistres a fortes doses avec autogreffe de moelle. *Bull Cancer*, 73, 406 (1986)

2271 Gow IF, Flapan AD, Morris M et al. A lack of effect of captopril on platelet aggregation in patients with congestive cardiac failure. *Eur J Clin Pharmacol*, 41, 47-49 (1991)

2272 Gow JA, Ebbeling L, Gerrard JM. The effect of regular and enteric-coated aspirin on bleeding time, thromboxane, and prostacyclin. *Prostaglandins Leukot Essent Fatty Acids*, 49, 515-520 (1993)

2273 Gow SM, Caldwell G, Toft AD et al. Different hepatic responses to thyroxine replacement in spontaneous and ^{125}I-induced primary hypothyroidism. *Clin Endocrinol*, 30, 505-512 (1989)

2274 Goyot C, Debray Q, Hug R et al. Basal plasma level evaluation of three anterior pituitary hormones during acute or chronic treatment with tricyclic antidepressants. *Encephale*, 11, 45-51 (1985)

2275 Grace E, Emans SJ, Drum DE. Hematologic abnormalities in adolescents who take oral contraceptive pills. *J Pediatr*, 101, 771-774 (1982)

2276 Gradon JD, Fricchione L, Sepkowitz D. Severe hypomagnesemia associated with pentamidine therapy. *Rev Infect Dis*, 13, 511-512 (1991)

2277 Graef V, Staudinger H. Studies on specificity of the fluorometric determination of plasma 11-hydroxycorticoids. *Z Klin Chem Klin Biochem*, 8, 368 (1970)

2278 Graf M, Tarlov A. Agranulocytosis with monohistiocytosis associated with ampicillin therapy. *Ann Intern Med*, 69, 91 (1968)

2279 Graft DF, Chesney PJ. Use of ticarcillin following carbenicillin-associated hepatotoxicity. *J Pediatr*, 100, 497-499 (1982)

2280 Graham GG, Champion GD, Day RO et al. Patterns of plasma concentrations and urinary excretion of salicylate in rheumatoid arthritis. *Clin Pharmacol Ther*, 22, 410-420 (1977)

2281 Graham P, Naidoo D. False-positive Ketostix® in a diabetic on antihypertensive therapy. *Clin Chem*, 33, 1490 (1987)

2282 Graisely B, Emery JP, Hugues FC et al. Rifampicine et ictere observations chez l'homme. *Therapie*, 26, 655 (1971)

2283 Grajower MM, Walter L, Albin J. Hypoglycemia in chronic hemodialysis patients: association with propranolol use. *Nephron*, 26, 126-129 (1980)

2284 Gralnick HR, McGinniss M, Elton W et al. Hemolytic anemia associated with cephalothin. *J Am Med Ass*, 217, 1193 (1971)

2285 Gralnick HR, Wright LD Jr, McGinniss MH. Coombs' positive reactions associated with sodium cephalothin therapy. *J Am Med Ass*, 199, 725 (1967)

2286 Gram J, Bollerslev J, Nielsen HK et al. Increased serum concentrations of type I procollagen C-terminal propeptide and osteocalcin during a short course of calcitriol administration to adult male volunteers. *Acta Endocrinol*, 125, 609-613 (1991)

2287 Gram J, Jespersen J, Dooijewaard G et al. The effect of gliclazide on plasma urokinase-related fibrinolysis. The results from an exploratory study. *Fibrinolysis*, 8, 60-62 (1994)

2288 Gram LF, Hansen MGJ, Sindrup SH et al. Citalopram: interaction studies with levomepromazine, imipramine, and lithium. *Ther Drug Monit*, 15, 18-24 (1993)

2289 Gran JT, Husby G, Thorsby E. HLA DR antigens and gold toxicity. *Ann Rheum Dis*, 42, 63-66 (1983)

2290 Granberg PO, Wahlin A. The effect of methoxyflurane (penthrane®) on the renal function with special reference to tubular rejection. *Acta Anaesthesiol Scand*, 16, 216 (1972)

2291 Grandjean P, Nielsen GD, Jorgensen PJ et al. Reference intervals for trace elements in blood: significance of risk factors. *Scand J Clin Lab Invest*, 52, 321-337 (1992)

2292 Granerus G, Wetterqvist H, White T. Histamine metabolism in healthy subjects before and during treatment with aminoguanidine. *Scand J Clin Lab Invest*, 22, Suppl 104, 39 (1968)

2293 Granerus G, Wetterqvist H, White T. Urinary excretion of histamine, methylhistamine and methylimadazoleacetic acids in man. *Scand J Clin Lab Invest*, 22, Suppl 104, 59 (1968)

2294 Graninger W, Pirich KR, Speiser W et al. Effect of thyroid hormones on plasma protein concentrations in man. *J Clin Endocrinol Metab*, 63, 407-411 (1986)

2295 Grant C, Routh JI, Lawton W, Witte DL. The effects of therapy for mild hypertension on circulating dopamine-β-hydroxylase. *Clin Chim Acta*, 69, 333-340 (1976)

2296 Grau JJ, Estape J, Daniels M et al. Cisplatin and plasma iron levels. *Ann Intern Med*, 103, 158-159 (1985)

2297 Graves GR, Kennedy TG, Weick RF et al. The effect of nalmefene on pulsatile secretion of luteinizing hormone and prolactin in men. *Hum Reprod*, 8, 1598-1603 (1993)

2298 Graves J, Kenamond TG, Whittier FC. Acute effects of nifedipine on renal electrolyte excretion in normal and hypertensive subjects. *Am J Med Sci*, 31, 114-118 (1988)

2299 Graves NM, Fuerst RH, Cloyd JC et al. Progabide-induced changes in carbamazepine metabolism. *Epilepsia*, 29, 775-780 (1988)

2300 Greally P, Hussain MJ, Vergani D et al. Interleukin-1α, soluble interleukin-2 receptor, and IgG concentrations in cystic fibrosis treated with prednisolone. *Arch Dis Child*, 71, 35-39 (1994)

2301 Green AJE, Halloran SP, Mould GP et al. Cephalosporin interference with creatinine determination. *Proc ACB Natl Meet*, 72 (1990)

2302 Green AJE, Halloran SP, Mould GP et al. Interference by newer cephalosporins in current methods for measuring creatinine. *Clin Chem*, 36, 2139-2140 (1990)

2303 Green D, Davies RO, Holmes GI et al. Effects of diflunisal on platelet function and fecal blood loss. *Clin Pharmacol Ther*, 30, 378-384 (1981)

2304 Green D, Ts'ao C-H, Cerullo L et al. Clinical and laboratory investigations of the effects of ε-aminocaproic acid on hemostasis. *J Lab Clin Med*, 105, 321-327 (1985)

2305 Green JA, Clementi WA, Porter C et al. Nifedipine-quinidine interaction. *Clin Pharmacol Ther*, 2, 461-465 (1983)

2306 Green JR, Kupferberg HJ. Sulfonamides and derivatives: sulthiame. In:. *Antiepileptic Drugs, DM Woodbury, JK Penry, RP Schmidt (eds)*, New York NY, Raven Press (1972)

2307 Greenberg CS, Hursting MJ, Macik BG et al. Evaluation of preanalytical variables associated with measurement of prothrombin fragment 1.2. *Clin Chem*, 40, 1962-1969 (1994)

2308 Greenberg GR, Feagan BG, Martin F et al. Oral budesonide for active Crohn's disease. *N Engl J Med*, 331, 836-841 (1994)

2309 Greenberg S, Reiser IW, Chou S-Y et al. Trimethoprim-sulfamethoxazole induces reversible hyperkalemia. *Ann Intern Med*, 119, 291-295 (1993)

2310 Greenberg SR. More on levodopa - implications for adrenal function. *N Engl J Med*, 286, 375 (1972)

2311 Greenblatt DJ, Duhme DW, Allen MD et al. Clinical toxicity of furosemide in hospitalized patients. *Am Heart J*, 94, 6-13 (1977)

2312 Greenblatt DJ, Duhme DW, Koch-Weser J. Pain and CPK elevation after intramuscular digoxin. *N Engl J Med*, 288, 689 (1973)

2313 Greenblatt DJ, Koch-Weser J. Adverse reactions to spironolactone. *J Am Med Ass*, 225, 39 (1973)

2314 Greenblatt DJ, Preskorn SH, Cotreau MM. Fluoxetine impairs clearance of alprazolam but not of clonazepam. *Clin Pharmacol Ther*, 52, 479-486 (1992)

2315 Greendyke RM, Kanter DR. Plasma propranolol levels and their effect on plasma thioridazine and haloperidol concentrations. *J Clin Psychopharmacol*, 7, 178-182 (1987)

2316 Greene DS, Salazar DE, Dockens RC, et al. Coadministration of nefazodone and benzodiazepines: III A pharmacokinetic interaction study with alprazolam. *J Clin Psychopharmacol*, 15, 399-408 (1995)

2317 Greene DS, Salazar DE, Dockens RC, et al. Coadministration of nefazodone and benzodiazepines: IV A pharmacokinetic interaction study with lorazepam. *J Clin Psychopharmacol*, 15, 399-408 (1995)

2318 Greene HL, Graham EL, Werner JA et al. Toxic and therapeutic effects of amiodarone in the treatment of cardiac arrhythmias. *J Am Coll Cardiol*, 2, 1114-1128 (1983)

2319 Greene ML, Fujimoto WY, Seegmiller JE. Urinary xanthine stones, a rare complication of allopurinol therapy. *N Engl J Med*, 280, 426 (1969)

2320 Greenlaw R, Pryor J, Winnacker J et al. Osteomalacia (OM) from anticonvulsant drugs (ACV): therapeutic implications. *Clin Res*, 20, 56 (1972)

2321 Greenstein AJ, Kaynan A, Singer A et al. A comparative study of pentazocine and meperidine on the biliary passage pressure. *Am J Gastroenterol*, 58, 47 (1972)

2322 Greenstein R, Nogeire C, Ohnuma T et al. Management of asparaginase induced hemorrhagic pancreatitis complicated by pseudocyst. *Cancer*, 43, 718-722 (1979)

2323 Gregorio F, Ambrosi F, Manfrinin S, et al. Metformin, plasma glucose and free fatty acids in type II diabetic out-patients: results of a clinical study. *Diabet Res Clin Pract*, 37, 21-33 (1997)

2324 Gregory LC, Eisenberger M, Sinibaldi V et al. Suramin interferes with measurements of total calcium and serum amylase by the Kodak Ektachem 700 analyzer and may inhibit liver enzyme activity. *Clin Chem*, 38, 2552-2553 (1992)

2325 Grennan DM, Ferry DG, Ashworth ME et al. The aspirin-ibuprofen interaction in rheumatoid arthritis. *Br J Clin Pharmacol*, 8, 497-503 (1979)

2326 Gresser U, Kamilli I, Kronawitter U et al. Uricosuric effect of different doses of irtemazole in normouricaemia subjects. *Eur J Clin Pharmacol*, 38, 489-491 (1990)

2327 Gretzer I, Rossner S. Long-term effects of pindolol on serum lipoproteins in hypertensive patients. *Acta Med Scand*, 219, 367-370 (1986)

2328 Griffin B, Farish E, Walsh D et al. Response of plasma low density lipoprotein subfractions to oestrogen replacement therapy following surgical menopause. *Clin Endocrinol*, 39, 463-468 (1993)

2329 Griffiths ID, Richardson J. Lupus-type illness associated with labetalol. *Br Med J*, 2, 496 (1979)

2330 Griffiths J, Linklater H. A radioisotope method for catechol-O-methyl transferase in blood. *Clin Chim Acta*, 39, 383 (1972)

2331 Griggs RC, Condemi JJ, Vaughan JH. Effect of therapeutic dosage of prednisone on human immunoglobulin G metabolism. *J Allerg Clin Immunol*, 49, 267 (1972)

2332 Grigoriou O, Papoulias I, Vitoratos N, et al. Effects of nasal administration of calcitonin in oophorectomized women: 2-year controlled double-blind study. *Maturitas*, 28, 147-151 (1997)

2333 Grimbert S, Pessayre D, Degott C, Benhamou J-P. Acute hepatitis induced by HMG-CoA reductase inhibitor, lovastatin. *Dig Dis Sci*, 39, 2032-2033 (1994)

2334 Grimm IS, Litynski JJ. Severe cholestasis associated with ticlopidine. *Am J Gerontol*, 89, 279-280 (1994)

2335 Grimm RH Jr, Flack JM, Grandits GA, et al. Long-term effects on plasma lipids of diet and drugs to treat hypertension. *J Am Med Ass*, 275, 1549-1556 (1996)

2336 Grimm RH Jr, Leon AS, Hunninghake DB et al. Diuretics and plasma lipids: effects of thiazides and spironolactone. In:. *Lipoproteins and Coronary Atherosclerosis. Noseda et al (eds)*, Amsterdam, Elsevier Biomedical Press, 371-376 (1982)

2337 Grimm RH Jr., Leon AS, Hunninghake DB et al. Effect of thiazide diuretics on plasma lipids and lipoproteins in mildly hypertensive patients. *Ann Intern Med*, 94, 7-11 (1981)

2338 Grino JM, Sabate I, Castelao AM et al. Influence of diltiazem on cyclosporine clearance. *Lancet*, 1, 1387 (1986)

2339 Gristead GF. Ranitidine and high concentrations of phenylpropanolamine cross react in the EMIT monoclonal amphetamine/methamphetamine assay. *Clin Chem*, 35, 1998-1999 (1989)

2340 Grob PJ, Herold GE. Immunological abnormalities and hydantoins. *Br Med J*, 2, 561 (1972)

2341 Grob U, Honcamp M, Daume E, et al. Hormonal oral contraceptives, urinary porphyrin excretion and porphyrias. *Horm Metab Res*, 27, 379-383 (1995)

2342 Groel JT, Tadros SS, Dreslinski GR et al. Long-term antihypertensive therapy with captopril. *Hypertension*, 5, Suppl 3, 145-151 (1983)

2343 Grol M, Stock W, Ebert C. Fully automated steroid determination on the immuno-analyzer ES 300: development and performance of a new direct highly sensitive enzyme immunoassay for serum estradiol. *Clin Chem*, 37, 1027-1028 (1991)

2344 Gronert GA, Theye RA. Pathophysiology of hyperkalemia induced by succinylcholine. *Anesthesiology*, 43, 89-99 (1975)

2345 Gronhagen-Riska C, Hellstrom P-E, Froseth B. Predisposing factors in hepatitis induced by isoniazid-rifampin treatment of tuberculosis. *Am Rev Resp Dis*, 118, 461-466 (1978)

2346 Groop L, Totterman KJ, Harno K et al. Influence of β-blocking drugs on glucose metabolism in hypertensive, non- diabetic patients. *Acta Med Scand*, 213, 9-14 (1983)

2347 Groop P-H, Groop LC, Totterman KJ et al. The effect of dexamethasone on the enteroinsular axis. *Scand J Clin Lab Invest*, 47, 491-495 (1987)

2348 Gross L. Oxyphenbutazone-induced parotitis. *Ann Intern Med*, 70, 1229 (1969)

2349 Grossbard L, Marks PA. Enzymes in hematologic disease. In:. *Diagnostic Enzymology. EL Coodley (ed)*, Philadelphia PA, Lea and Febiger (1970)

2350 Grossman RM, Delaney RJ, Brinton EA et al. Hypertriglyceridemia in patients with psoriasis treated with cyclosporine. *J Am Acad Dermatol*, 25, 648-651 (1991)

2351 Grotsch H, Hajdu P. Interference by the new antibiotic cefipirome and other cephalosporins in clinical laboratory tests, with special regard to the Jaffe reaction. *J Clin Chem Clin Biochem*, 25, 49-52 (1987)

2352 Gruen PH, Sachar EJ, Langer G et al. Prolactin responses to neuroleptics in normal and schizophrenic subjects. *Arch Gen Psychiat*, 35, 108-116 (1978)

2353 Grunding E, Birnbaumer E, Kollner U et al. Influence of drugs on aminotransferase activity in human blood serum and cerebrospinal fluid. *Lab*, 4, 323 (1977)

2354 Gruneberger S, Dreyer M, Kangah R et al. Reduction of plasma lipid concentration by lovastatin: results of a clinical study in patients with primary hypercholesterolemia. *Dtsch Med Wschr*, 114, 1734-1739 (1989)

2355 Guagnellini E, Bertolini G, Cappelletti M et al. Thrombin inhibitors in women on oral contraceptives. *Acta Haematol*, 65, 205-210 (1981)

2356 Guanabens N, Pares A, Navasa M et al. Cyclosporin A increases the biochemical markers of bone remodeling in primary biliary cirrhosis. *J Hepatol*, 21, 24-28 (1994)

2357 Guemei A, Issa I, El-Gindi M et al. β-adrenergic receptors and gastric acid secretion. *Surgery*, 66, 663-668 (1969)

2358 Guerra M. Toxicity of indomethacin: Report of a case of acute pancreatitis. *J Am Med Ass*, 200, 552 (1967)

2359 Guetta V, Lush RM, Figg WD, et al. Effects of the antiestrogen Tamoxifen on low-density lipoprotein concentrations and oxidation in postmenopausal women. *Am J Cardiol*, 76, 1072-1073 (1995)

2360 Gugler R, Jensen JC. Interaction between cimetidine and metronidazole. *N Engl J Med*, 309, 1518-1519 (1983)

2361 Guillemain R, Billaud E, Dreyfus G et al. The effects of spiramycin on plasma cyclosporin A concentrations in heart transplant patients. *Eur J Clin Pharmacol*, 36, 97-98 (1989)

2362 Guillemant S, Guillemant J, Feteanu D et al. Effect of vitamin D_3 administration on serum 25-hydroxyvitamin D_3, 1,25-dihydroxyvitamin D_3 and osteocalcin in vitamin D-deficient elderly people. *J Steroid Biochem*, 33, 1155-1159 (1989)

2363 Guliana JM, Guillausseau PJ, Caron J et al. Effects of short-term subcutaneous administration of SMS 201-995 on calcitonin plasma levels in patients suffering from medullary thyroid carcinoma. *Horm Metab Res*, 21, 584-586 (1989)

2364 Gulick RM, Mellors JW, Havlir D, et al. Treatment with indinavir, zidovudine, and lamivudine in adults with human immunodeficiency virus infection and prior antiretroviral therapy. *N Engl J Med*, 337, 734-739 (1997)

2365 Gulley RM, Mirza A, Kelly CE. Hepatotoxicity of salicylazosulfapyridine. *Am J Gastroenterol*, 72, 561-564 (1979)

2366 Gumaste VV, Sereny G, Dave P et al. Serum lipase levels in chronic alcoholics. *J Clin Gastroenterol*, 13, 407-410 (1991)

2367 Gundersen K, Demissianos HV. The effects of 5-methylpyrazole-3-carboxylic acid (V-19425) and nicotinic acid (NA) on free fatty acids (FFA). *Adv Exp Med Biol*, 4, 213 (1968)

2368 Gunneberg A, Gillett MG, Goldie DJ. A high serum concentration of azlocillin affects routine biochemical analyses. *Ann Clin Biochem*, 30, 329-330 (1993)

2369 Gunstone RF, Wing AJ, Shani HGP et al. Clinical experience with metolazone in fiftytwo African patients: synergy with frusemide. *Postgrad Med J*, 47, 789 (1971)

2370 Gupta KK. Guanethidine and glucose tolerance in diabetics. *Br Med J*, 3, 679 (1968)

2371 Gupta RK, Kjeldsen SE, Motley E et al. Platelet function during antihypertensive treatment with quinapril, a novel angiotensin converting enzyme inhibitor. *J Cardiovasc Pharmacol*, 17, 13-19 (1991)

2372 Gupta RN, Price D, Keane PM. Modified Pisano method for estimating urinary metanephrines. *Clin Chem*, 19, 611 (1973)

2373 Gupta SK, Bakran A, Johnson RWG et al. Cyclosporin-erythromycin interaction in renal transplant patients. *Br J Clin Pharmacol*, 27, 475-481 (1989)

2374 Gustafson A, Bjorntorp P, Fahlen M. Metformin administration in hyperlipidemic states. *Acta Med Scand*, 190, 491 (1971)

2375 Gustavsson S, Adami H-O, Loof L et al. Rapid healing of duodenal ulcers with omeprazole: double-blind dose comparative trial. *Lancet*, 2, 124-125 (1983)

2376 Gutigliano G, Vadruccio F. Serum β_2-microglobulin as a possible early indicator of glomerular filtration impairment in subjects receiving long-term lithium treatment. *Eur Psychiat*, 9, 201-203 (1994)

2377 Gutman AB. Drug reactions characterized by cholestasis associated with intrahepatic biliary tract obstruction. *Am J Med*, 23, 841 (1957)

2378 Gutman AB. Uricosuric drugs, with special reference to probenecid and sulfinpyrazone. *Adv Pharmacol*, 4, 91 (1966)

2379 Gutteridge DH, Retallack RW, Ward LC, et al. Clinical, biochemical, hematologic, and radiographic responses in Paget's disease following intravenous pamidronate disodium: a 2-year study. *Bone*, 19, 387-394 (1996)

2380 Guttormsen AB, Ueland PM, Lonning PE, et al. Kinetics of plasma total homocysteine in patients receiving high-dose methotrexate therapy. *Clin Chem*, 44, 1987-1989 (1998)

2381 Guven H, Tuncok Y, Guneri S et al. Age-related digoxin-alprazolam interaction. *Clin Pharmacol Ther*, 54, 42-44 (1993)

2382 Guyda HJ, Friesen HG. Serum prolactin levels in humans from birth to adult life. *Pediatr Res*, 7, 534 (1973)

2383 Gylling H, Vanhanen H, Miettinen TA. Effects of ketoconazole on cholesterol precursors and low density lipoprotein kinetics in hypercholesterolemia. *J Lipid Res*, 34, 39-67 (1993)

2384 Gylling H, Vanhanen H, Miettinen TA. Hypolipidemic effect and mechanisms of ketoconazole without and with cholestyramine in familial hypercholesterolemia. *Metabolism*, 40, 35-41 (1991)

2385 Gynn TN, Messmore HL, Friedman IA. Drug induced thrombocytopenia. *Med Clin North Am*, 56, 65 (1972)

2386 Gyorke ZS, Sulyok E, Guignard J-P. Ammonium chloride metabolic acidosis and the activity of renin-angiotensin-aldosterone system in children. *Eur J Pediatr*, 150, 547-549 (1991)

2387 Ha HR, Funk B, Maitre PO et al. Midazolam in plasma from hospitalized patients as measured by gas-liquid chromatography with electron-capture detection. *Clin Chem*, 34, 676-679 (1988)

2388 Haag HB, Larson PS, Schwartz JJ. The effect of urinary pH on the elimination of quinine in man. *J Pharmacol*, 79, 136-139 (1943)

2389 Haalboom JRE, Deenstra M, Struyvenberg A. Hypokalemia induced by inhalation of fenoterol. *Lancet*, 1, 1125-1127 (1985)

2390 Haalboom JRE, Struyvenberg A. The mechanism underlying chlorthalidone-induced hypokalaemia: effects of sodium restriction, potassium supplementation, spironolactone and triamterene. *Neth J Med*, 25, 184-192 (1982)

2391 Haas HG, Dambacher MA, Guncaga J et al. Renal effects of calcitonin and parathyroid extract in man. *J Clin Invest*, 50, 2689 (1971)

2392 Haavaldsen R, Ingraldsen P. Biological effects of lithium salts. *Lancet*, 1, 1390 (1973)

2393 Habbal ZM, Touma EH. Positive interference from homocystinuria urine in a Spot test for molybdenum cofactor deficiency. *Clin Chem*, 41, 1056 - 1057 (1995)

2394 Habersetzer F, Larrey D, Babany G et al. Clotiazepam-induced acute hepatitis. *J Hepatol*, 9, 256-259 (1989)

2395 Hadden JW, Metzner RJ. Pseudoketosis and hyperacetaldehydemia in paraldehyde acidosis. *Am J Med*, 47, 642 (1969)

2396 Haden HT. Thyroid function tests: physiologic basis and clinical interpretation. *Postgrad Med*, 40, 129 (1966)

2397 Hadfield JW. Rifampicin-induced thrombocytopenia. *Postgrad Med J*, 56, 59-60 (1980)

2398 Haenni A, Lithell H. Uradipil treatment decreases plasma fibrinogen concentration in essential hypertension. *Metabolism*, 45, 1221-1229 (1996)

2399 Haffner SM, Knapp JA, Stern MP et al. Coffee consumption, diet, and lipids. *Am J Epidemiol*, 122, 1-12 (1985)

2400 Hagnevik K, Gordon E, Lins LE et al. Glycerol-induced hemolysis with hemoglobinuria and acute renal failure. *Lancet*, 1, 75 (1974)

2401 Hahn E. Dimenhydrinate interferes with radioimmunoassay of theophylline. *Clin Chem*, 26, 1759-1760 (1980)

2402 Hahn TJ, Haddad JG, Hendin BA. Effect of chronic anticonvulsant therapy on serum 25 OH vitamin D levels. *Clin Res*, 20, 238 (1972)

2403 Hahn TJ, Hendin BA, Scharp CR et al. Effect of chronic anticonvulsant therapy on serum 25-hydroxycalciferol levels in adults. *N Engl J Med*, 287, 900 (1972)

2404 Hahn TJ, Hendin BA, Scharp CR et al. Serum 25-hydroxycalciferol levels and bone mass in children in chronic anticonvulsant therapy. *N Engl J Med*, 292, 550-554 (1975)

2405 Haidukewych D, John G. Chronic valproic acid and coantileptic drug therapy and incidence of increases in serum liver enzymes. *Ther Drug Monit*, 8, 407-410 (1986)

2406 Haidukewych D, John G, Zielinski JJ et al. Chronic valproic acid therapy and incidence of increases in venous plasma ammonia. *Ther Drug Monit*, 7, 290-294 (1985)

2407 Haidukewych D, Rodin EA. Effect of phenothiazines on serum antiepileptic drug concentrations in psychiatric patients with seizure disorder. *Ther Drug Monit*, 7, 401-404 (1985)

2408 Hailer S, Pogarell O, Keller C, Wolfram G. Effect of fluvastatin or bezafibrate on the distribution of high density lipoprotein subpopulations in patients with familial hypercholesterolemia. *Arz Forsch Drug Res*, 46, 879-883 (1996)

2409 Hainer JW, Terry JG, Connell JM et al. Effect of the acyl-CoA:cholesterol acyltransferase inhibitor DuP 128 on cholesterol absorption and serum cholesterol in humans. *Clin Pharmacol Ther*, 56, 65-74 (1994)

2410 Hajos P, Berlin I, Intody Z et al. The effect of oral contraceptives on serum lipids, γ-glutamyltranspeptidase, and excretion of D-glucaric acid. *Int J Clin Pharmacol Ther Toxicol*, 19, 117-123 (1981)

2411 Hall CD, Dafni U, Simpson D, et al. Failure of cytarabine in progressive multifocal leukoencephalopathy associated with human immunodeficiency virus infection. *N Engl J Med*, 338, 1345-1351 (1998)

2412 Hall R. The clinical and technical background to the use of free hormone measurements in thyroid disease. Amersham UK, Kodak Clinical Diagnostics (1992)

2413 Halla JT, Cassidy J, Hardin JG. Sequential gold and penicillamine therapy in rheumatoid arthritis: comparative study of effectiveness and toxicity and review of literature. *Am J Med*, 72, 423-426 (1982)

2414 Haller J. A review of the long term effects of hormonal contraceptives. *Contraception*, 1, 233 (1970)

2415 Halliday A, Jawetz E. Sodium nitrofurantoin administered intravenously. *N Engl J Med*, 266, 427 (1962)

2416 Halma C, Jansen JBMJ, Janssens AR et al. Life-threatening water intoxication during somatostatin therapy. *Ann Intern Med*, 107, 518-520 (1987)

2417 Halmi KA, Noyes RJC, Millard SA. Effect of lithium on plasma cortisol and adrenal response to adrenocorticotropin in man. *Clin Pharmacol Ther*, 13, 699 (1972)

2418 Halsted JA, Hackley BM, Smith JC. Plasma zinc and copper in pregnancy and after oral contraceptives. *Lancet*, 2, 278 (1968)

2419 Hamada Y, Odagaki Y, Sakakibara F et al. Effects of an aldolase reductase inhibitor on erythrocyte fructose 3-phosphate and sorbitol 3-phosphate levels in diabetic patients. *Life Sci*, 57, 23-29 (1995)

2420 Hamalainen E, Korpela JT, Adlercreutz H. Effect of oxytetracycline administration on intestinal metabolism of oestrogens and on plasma sex hormones in healthy men. *Gut*, 28, 439-445 (1987)

2421 Hamer A, Peter T, Mandel WJ et al. The potentiation of warfarin anticoagulation by amiodarone. *Circulation*, 65, 1025-1029 (1982)

2422 Hamet P, Kuchel O, Genest J. Effect of upright posture and isoproterenol infusion on cyclic adenosine monophosphate excretion. *J Clin Endocrinol Metab*, 36, 218 (1973)

2423 Hamilton CR, Bliss JM, Horwich A. The late effects of cis-platinum on renal function. *Eur J Cancer Clin Oncol*, 25, 185-189 (1989)

2424 Hamilton DV, Saunders J. Carbimazole-induced agranulocytosis in two sisters. *Curr Med Res Opin*, 4, 607-608 (1977)

2425 Hamman BL, Martin MM. Separation of six urinary 17-ketosteroids by two-dimensional thin-layer chromatography: control values. *J Clin Endocrinol Metab*, 24, 1195 (1964)

2426 Hammarstrom L, Smith CIE. Captopril-induced IgA deficiency. *Lancet*, 337, 436 (1991)

2427 Hammerman C, Zaia W, Wu H-H. Severe hyponatremia with indomethacin - a more serious toxicity than previously realized?. *Dev Pharmacol Ther*, 8, 260-267 (1985)

2428 Hammerstein J, Daume E, Simon A, et al. Influence of gestodene and desogestrel of low-dose oral contraceptives on the pharmacokinetics of ethinyl estradiol (EE_2), on serum CBG and on urinary cortisol and 6β-hydroxycortisol. *Contraception*, 47, 263-281 (1993)

2429 Hammill SC, Sorenson PB, Wood DL et al. Propafenone for the treatment of refractory complex ventricular ectopic activity. *Mayo Clin Proc*, 61, 98-103 (1986)

2430 Hammond WP IV, Price TH, Souza LM et al. Treatment of cyclic neutropenia with granulocyte colony-stimulating factor. *N Engl J Med*, 320, 1306-1311 (1989)

2431 Hampl R, Heresova J, Lachman M et al. Hormonal changes in tamoxifen treated men with idiopathic oligozoospermia. *Exp Clin Endocrinol*, 92, 211-216 (1988)

2432 Hanefeld M, Fischer S, Schulze J et al. Therapeutic potentials of acarbose as first line drug in NIDDM insufficiently treated with diet alone. *Diabetes Care*, 14, 732-737 (1991)

2433 Hanger DP, Jevons S, Shaw JTB. Fluconazole and testosterone: In vivo and in vitro studies. *Antimicrob Agent Chemother*, 32, 646-648 (1988)

2434 Hanger FM, Gutman AB. Post-arsphenamine jaundice. *J Am Med Ass*, 115, 263 (1940)

2435 Haning RV Jr, Carlson IH, Cortes J et al. Danazol and its principal metabolites interfere with binding of testosterone, cortisol and thyroxine by plasma proteins. *Clin Chem*, 28, 696-698 (1982)

2436 Hannon R, Blumsohn A, Naylor K, Eastell R. Response of bone markers of bone turnover to hormone replacement therapy: impact of biological variability. *J Bone Miner Res*, 13, 1124-1133 (1998)

2437 Hannuksela M, Kesaniemi YA, Savolainen MJ. Evaluation of plasma cholesteryl ester transfer protein (CETP) activity as a marker of alcoholism. *Alcohol Alcoholism*, 27, 557-562 (1992)

2438 Hansell JR. Effect of therapeutic digoxin antibodies on digoxin assays. *Arch Pathol Lab Med*, 113, 1259-1262 (1989)

2439 Hansen BS, Dam M, Brandt J et al. Influence of dextropropoxyphene on steady state serum levels and protein binding of three anti-epileptic drugs in man. *Acta Neurol Scand*, 61, 357-367 (1980)

2440 Hansen JM, Kampmann JM, Siersbaek-Nielsen K et al. The effect of different sulfonamides on phenytoin metabolism in man. *Acta Med Scand*, 624, Suppl, 106-110 (1979)

2441 Hansen JM, Kristensen M, Skovsted L. Sulthiame (Ospolot) as inhibitor of diphenylhydantoin metabolism. *Epilepsia*, 9, 17-22 (1968)

2442 Hansen JM, Siersboek-Nielsen K, Skovsted L. Carbamazepine-induced acceleration of diphenylhydantoin and warfarin metabolism in man. *Clin Pharmacol Ther*, 12, 539-543 (1971)

2443 Hansen OH, Madsen P. The effect of tetragastrin on gastric acid secretion. *Scand J Gastroenterol*, 7, 171 (1972)

2444 Hansen PR, Hovgaard D. Disparate effects of interleukin-3 on serum lipoprotein(a), and low- and high-density lipoprotein cholesterol levels. *Am J Cardiol*, 75, 296-297 (1995)

2445 Hansen PS, Meinertz H, Gerdes LU, et al. Treatment of patients with familial defective apolipoprotein B-100 with pravastatin and gemfibrozil. *Clin Investig*, 22, 1065-1070 (1994)

2446 Hansky J, Soveny C, Korman MG. The effect of glucagon on serum gastrin, I. studies in normal subjects. *Gut*, 14, 457 (1973)

2447 Hanss M, Coppere B, Gineyts E et al. Increased plasma free γ-carboxyglutamic acid levels during deep vein thrombosis and intravascular disseminated coagulation. *Thromb Res*, 73, 185-192 (1994)

2448 Hanss M, Trzeciak MC, Ninet J et al. Decreased plasma fibrin degradation products during hormonal stimulation for in vitro fertilisation. *Fibrinolysis*, 7, 341-346 (1993)

2449 Hanssen LE, Schrumpf E, Jacobsen MB et al. Extended experience with recombinant α-2b interferon with or without hepatic artery embolization in the treatment of midgut carcinoid tumors. A preliminary report. *Acta Oncol*, 30, 523-527 (1991)

2450 Hansson P, Hedstrom S-A, Hultberg B et al. Fusidic acid interferes in enzymatic determination of bile acids. *Clin Chim Acta*, 125, 241-243 (1982)

2451 Hansten PD. Drug Interactions. Philadelphia PA, Lea and Febiger (1971)

2452 Hansten PD. Drug Interactions. *2nd edition*, Philadelphia PA, Lea and Febiger (1973)

2453 Hansten PD. Drugs in the production of direct Coombs' test positivity. *Am J Hosp Pharm*, 28, 629 (1971)

2454 Hansten PD, Hayton WL. Effects of antacids and ascorbic acid on serum salicylate concentration. *J Clin Pharmacol*, 24, 326-331 (1980)

2455 Hantman DA, Donaldson CL, Hulley SB. Abnormal urinary sediment during therapy with synthetic sodium calcitonin. *J Clin Endocrinol Metab*, 33, 564 (1971)

2456 Haragsim L, Dalal R, Bagga H, Bastani B. Ketorlac-induced acute renal failure and hyperkalemia: report of three cases. *Am J Kid Dis*, 24, 578-580 (1994)

2457 Haran N, Gurwicz S, Gallati H et al. Effect of 1α-hydroxyvitamin D_3 treatment on production of tumor necrosis factor-α by peripheral blood mononuclear cells and on serum concentrations of soluble tumor necrosis factor receptors in hemodialysis patients. *Nephron*, 66, 262-266 (1994)

2458 Harding S, Munro AJ. Frusemide and renal enzyme excretion. *Br Med J*, 2, 1431 (1978)

2459 Hardy BG, Schentag JJ. Lack of effect of cimetidine on the metabolism of quinidine: effect on renal clearance. *Int J Clin Pharmacol Ther Toxicol*, 26, 388-391 (1988)

2460 Hardy BG, Zador IT, Golden L et al. Effect of cimetidine on the pharmacokinetics and pharmacodynamics of quinidine. *Am J Cardiol*, 52, 172-175 (1983)

2461 Hare DL, Hicks BH. Thrombocytopenia due to oxprenolol. *Med J Aust*, 2, 259 (1979)

2462 Hare TA, Beasley BL, Chambers RA et al. Dopa and amino acid levels in plasma and cerebrospinal fluid of patients with Parkinson's disease. *Clin Chim Acta*, 45, 273 (1973)

2463 Harenberg J, Stehle G, Dempfle CE et al. Influence of the low molecular weight heparin CY 216 on blood coagulation and lipases. *Arztl Lab*, 35, 73-79 (1989)

2464 Hargreaves KM, Schmidt EA, Mueller GP et al. Dexamethasone alters plasma levels of β-endorphin and postoperative pain. *Clin Pharmacol Ther*, 42, 601-607 (1987)

2465 Hargreaves T. Oral contraceptives and liver function. *J Clin Pathol*, 1 (1969)

2466 Hargreaves T, Lathe GH. Drugs affecting biliary secretion. In:. *Therapeutic Agents and the Liver. N McIntyre, S Sherlock (eds)*, Oxford, Blackwell (1965)

2467 Hargreaves T, Lathe GH. Inhibitory aspects of bile secretion. *Nature*, 200, 1172 (1963)

2468 Harjai KJ, Licata AA. Effects of amiodarone on thyroid function. *Ann Intern Med*, 126, 6-73 (1997)

2469 Harju E, Pakarinen A. The effect of iron treatment on serum ferritin concentrations and bone marrow stainable iron in iron deficient outpatients with gastritis, gastric ulcer and duodenal ulcer. *J Intern Med Res*, 12, 56-58 (1984)

2470 Harmse DP. Clinical experience with doxazosin in general medical practice in the Netherlands. *Am Heart J*, 121, II Suppl, 341-345 (1991)

2471 Harney J, Glasberg MR. Myopathy and hypersensitivity to phenytoin. *Neurology*, 33, 790-791 (1983)

2472 Harno K, Valimaki M, Verho M. Effects of a new diuretic piretanide on glucose tolerance, insulin secretion and ^{125}i-insulin binding. *Eur J Clin Pharmacol*, 27, 697-700 (1985)

2473 Harrington CA, Adamczyk M, Johnson D et al. Development of a TDx assay for the analysis of imipramine and desipramine in patient plasma or serum. *Clin Chem*, 37, 1006 (1991)

2474 Harrington JM. Risk of mercurial poisoning in laboratories using volumetric gas analysis. *Lancet*, 1, 86 (1974)

2475 Harrington WL Sr, Kolodny L, Horstman LL, et al. Danazol for paroxysmal nocturnal hemoglobinuria. *Am J Hematol*, 54, 149-154 (1997)

2476 Harris A. Long term treatment of paroxysmal cardiac arrhythmias with propranolol. *Am J Cardiol*, 18, 431 (1966)

2477 Harris AB, Hartley J, Moor A. Reduced ascorbic acid excretion and oral contraceptives. *Lancet*, 2, 201 (1973)

2478 Harris J, Jessop JD, Chaput DE et al. Further experience with azathioprine in rheumatoid arthritis. *Br Med J*, 4, 463 (1971)

2479 Harris L, Mckenna WJ, Rowland E et al. Side effects of long-term amiodarone therapy. *Circulation*, 67, 45-51 (1983)

2480 Harris WS, Dujovne CA, von Bergmann K et al. Effects of the ACAT inhibitor CL 277082 on cholesterol metabolism in humans. *Clin Pharmacol Ther*, 48, 189-194 (1990)

2481 Harris WS, Rayford A. LCAT inhibitors interfere with the enzymatic determination of cholesterol and triglycerides. *Lipids*, 25, 341-343 (1990)

2482 Harrison RJ. Vitamin B_{12} levels in erythrocytes in hypochromic anaemia. *J Clin Pathol*, 24, 698 (1971)

2483 Harrison SP. Naproxen interference with the ion-selective electrode in the RA-1000. *Clin Chem*, 33, 421 (1987)

2484 Harrison TR. Principles of Internal Medicine. *6th edition. M Wintrobe (ed)*, New York NY, McGraw-Hill (1970)

2485 Harrower ADB, Fyffe JA, Horn DB et al. Thyroxine and triodothyronine levels in hyperthyroid patients during treatment with propranolol. *Clin Endocrinol*, 7, 41-44 (1977)

2486 Hartshorn EA. Drug interactions. *Drug Intell Clin Pharm*, 2, 174 (1968)

2487 Hartter D, Adamczyk M, Roberts B et al. Development of TDx assays for the analysis of amitriptyline and nortriptyline in patient serum/plasma. *Clin Chem*, 37, 1006 (1991)

2488 Haruta T, Kuroki S, Okura K et al. Clinical studies of aspoxicillin in pediatrics. *Jpn J Antibiot*, 38, 1898-1904 (1985)

2489 Harvengt C, Desager JP, Gaspard U et al. Changes in lipoprotein composition in women receiving two low-dose oral contraceptives containing ethinylestradiol and gonane progestins. *Contraception*, 37, 565-575 (1988)

2490 Harvey RF, Dowsett L, Hartog M et al. A radioimmunoassay for cholecystokinin-pancreozymin. *Lancet*, 2, 826 (1973)

2491 Harvey S, Weisman M, O'Dell J, et al. Chondrex: a new marker of joint disease. *Clin Chem*, 44, 509-516 (1998)

2492 Harvima RJ, Harvima RT, Kajander EO et al. Effect of drugs on histamine radio-enzyme assay. *Clin Chim Acta*, 180, 231-240 (1989)

2493 Hashimoto R, Ozaki N, Ohta T et al. Total biopterin levels of plasma in patients with depression. *Neuropsychobiology*, 17, 176-177 (1987)

2494 Hashimoto S, Miwa M, Akasofu K et al. Changes in serum proteins of post-menopausal women. *Maturitas*, 13, 23-33 (1991)

2495 Hashimoto T, Sato T, Kawai K et al. Effect of growth-hormone-releasing factor (GRF) on prolactin and thyrotropin release in patients with pituitary dwarfism. *Abstracts*, 5th APCCB, Kobe (1991)

2496 Hasibeder H, Staab HJ, Seibel K et al. Clinical pharmacology of the hypocholesterolemic agent K 12.148 (lifibrol) in healthy volunteers. *Eur J Clin Pharmacol*, 40, Suppl 1, S91-S94 (1991)

2497 Haskell CM, Canellos GP, Leventhal BG et al. L-asparaginase therapeutic and toxic effects in patients with neoplastic disease. *N Engl J Med*, 281, 1028 (1969)

2498 Haskovec L, Rysanek K. Excretion of 3-methoxy-4-hydroxymandelic acid and 5-hydroxyindoleacetic acid in depressed patients. *J Psychiat Res*, 5, 213 (1967)

2499 Hasling C, Charles P, Mosekilde L. Etidronate sodium for treating hypercalcaemia of malignancy: a double blind, placebo-controlled study. *Eur J Clin Invest*, 16, 433-437 (1986)

2500 Hass WK, Easton JD, Adams HP Jr et al. A randomized trial comparing ticlopidine hydrochloride with aspirin for the prevention of stroke in high-risk patients. *N Engl J Med*, 321, 501-507 (1989)

2501 Hassager C, Podenphant J, Riis BJ et al. Changes in soft tissue body composition and plasma lipid metabolism during nadrolone decanoate therapy in postmenopausal osteoporotic women. *Metabolism*, 38, 238-242 (1989)

2502 Hassan J, Feighery C, Bresnihan B et al. Serum IgA and IgG subclasses during treatment for acute respiratory exacerbation in cystic fibrosis: analysis of patients colonised with mucoid or non-mucoid strains of pseudomonas aeruginosa. *Immunol Invest*, 23, 1-13 (1994)

2503 Hassan M, Oberg G, Bjorkholm M et al. Influence of prophylactic anticonvulsant therapy on high-dose busulphan kinetics. *Cancer Chemother Pharmacol*, 33, 181-186 (1993)

2504 Hasselberg S, Bodman V, Kane M et al. A Kodak Ektachem thin-film assay for serum cholinesterase using potassium hexacyanoferrate (III) as color indicator. *Diag Lab*, 27, 100 (1991)

2505 Hatjis CG, Rose JC, Pippitt C et al. Effect of treatment with sodium valproate on plasma adrenocorticotropic hormone and cortisol concentrations in pregnancy. *Am J Obstet Gynecol*, 152, 315-316 (1985)

2506 Hattori M, Tsuda K, Taminato T et al. Effect of probucol on serum lipids and apoproteins in patients with noninsulin- dependent diabetes mellitus. *Curr Ther Res*, 42, 967-973 (1987)

2507 Hauf-Zachariou U, Widmann L, Zulsdorf B et al. A double-blind comparison of the effects of carvedilol and captopril on serum lipid concentrations in patients with mild to moderate essential hypertension and dyslipidaemia. *Eur J Clin Pharmacol*, 45, 95-100 (1993)

2508 Hauger-Klevene JH, Reader C, Mayer E et al. A comparative study of endralazine and captopril in essential hypertension: effect on renal levels, pulmonary function studies and lipid profile. *Int J Clin Pharmacol Res*, 6, 275-281 (1986)

2509 Haughton MA, Mason RS. Immunonephelometric assay of vitamin-D binding protein. *Clin Chem*, 38, 1796-1801 (1992)

2510 Haukamaa M, Gummerus M. Decrease of serum oestriol during intravenous hexoprenaline or salbutamol treatment. *Br J Obstet Gynaecol*, 89, 917-920 (1982)

2511 Haupt E, Koberich W, Beyer J et al. Pharmacodynamic aspects of tolbutamide, glibenclamide, glibonuride, and glisoxepide. *Diabetologia*, 7, 449 (1971)

2512 Hauser A, Quigley ML, Driever CW et al. More on false-positive 'Hemoccult® ' reaction with cimetidine. *N Engl J Med*, 304, 847-848 (1981)

2513 Hautanen A, Manttari M, Manninen V et al. Gemfibrozil treatment i associated with elevated adrenal androgen, androstanediol glucuronide and cortisol levels in dyslipidemic men. *J Steroid Biochem Mol Biol*, 51, 307-313 (1994)

2514 Havel RJ, Hunninghake DB, Illingworth DR et al. Lovastatin (mevinolin) in the treatment of heterozygous familial hypercholesterolemia. *Ann Intern Med*, 107, 609-615 (1987)

2515 Havel RJ, Segel N, Balasse EO. Effect of 5-methylpyrazole-3-carboxylic acid (MPCA) on fat mobilization, ketogenesis and glucose metabolism. *Adv Exp Med Biol*, 4, 105 (1968)

2516 Hawkins RC. Furosemide interference in newer free thyroxine assays. *Clin Chem*, 44, 2550-2551 (1998)

2517 Hawksworth G, Betts T, Crowe A et al. Diazepam/β-adrenoceptor antagonist interactions. *Br J Clin Pharmacol*, 17, 69s-76s (1984)

2518 Hayden FG, Osterhaus ADME, Treanor JJ, et al. Efficacy and safety of the neuraminidase inhibitor zanamivir in the treatment of influenza virus infections. *N Engl J Med*, 337, 874-880 (1997)

2519 Haynes DC. Summary of interference testing data for Kodak Ektachem Clinical Chemistry systems, Personal Communication (1994)

2520 Haznedaroglu IC, Tokgozoglu L, Caglar M et al. The effect of chronic angiotensin converting enzyme inhibition on circulating prolactin in systemic hypertension. *Horm Metab Res*, 26, 491-493 (1994)

2521 Healey LA, Harrison M, Decker JL. Uricosuric effect of chlorprothixene. *N Engl J Med*, 272, 526 (1965)

2522 Heaney RP, Whedon GD. Impairment of hepatic bromosulfophthalein clearance by two 17-substituted testosterones. *J Lab Clin Med*, 52, 169 (1955)

2523 Heaton KW, Pomare EW. Effect of bran on blood lipids and calcium. *Lancet*, 1, 49 (1974)

2524 Hebert MF, Roberts JP, Prueksaritanont T et al. Bioavailability of cyclosporine with concomitant rifampin administration is markedly less than predicted by hepatic enzyme induction. *Clin Pharmacol Ther*, 52, 453-457 (1992)

2525 Hedaya MA, Sawchuk RJ. A sensitive liquid-chromatographic method for determination of 3'-azido-3'-deoxythymidine (AZT) in plasma and urine. *Clin Chem*, 34, 1565-1568 (1988)

2526 Hedman A, Angelin B, Arvidsson A et al. Digoxin-interactions in man: spironolactone reduces renal but not biliary digoxin clearance. *Eur J Clin Pharmacol*, 42, 481-485 (1992)

2527 Hedman A, Angelin B, Arvidsson A et al. No effect of probenecid on the renal and biliary clearance of digoxin in man. *Br J Clin Pharmacol*, 32, 63-67 (1991)

2528 Hedner T, Samuelsson O, Lindholm L. Effects of antihypertensive therapy on glucose tolerance: focus on calcium antagonists. *J Intern Med*, 229, Suppl 2, 101-111 (1991)

2529 Hedrick R, Williams F, Morin R et al. Carbamazepine-erythromycin interaction leading to carbamazepine in four epileptic children. *Ther Drug Monit*, 5, 405-407 (1983)

2530 Heel RC, Brogden RN, Speight TM et al. Tamoxifen: a review of its pharmacological and therapeutic use in the treatment of breast cancer. *Drugs*, 16, 1-24 (1978)

2531 Heering P, Grabensee B. Influence of cyclosporin A on renal tubular function after kidney transplantation. *Nephron*, 59, 66-70 (1991)

2532 Heesen BJ, Wolffenbuttel BHR, Leurs PB et al. Lipoprotein (a) levels in relation to diabetic complications in patients with non-insulin-dependent diabetes. *Eur J Clin Invest*, 23, 580-584 (1993)

2533 Heeter C, McMillan KD. Creatinine, PAP adaptation on the Beckman Synchron CX5 system avoids interference from three cephalosporin drugs. *Clin Chem*, 37, 933 (1991)

2534 Heidemann PH, Stubbe P, Beck W. Transient secondary hypothyroidism and thyroxine binding globulin deficiency in leukemic children during polychemotherapy: an effect of L-asparaginase. *Eur J Pediatr*, 136, 291-295 (1981)

2535 Heikkinen A-M, Parviainen M, Niskanen L, et al. Biochemical bone markers and bone mineral density during postmenopausal hormone replacement therapy with and without vitamin D_3: a prospective, controlled, randomized study. *J Clin Endocrinol Metab*, 82, 2476-2482 (1997)

2536 Heikkinen J, Maentausta O, Ylostalo P et al. Serum bile acid levels in intrahepatic cholestasis of pregnancy during treatment with phenobarbital or cholestyramine. *Eur J Obstet Gynecol Reprod Biol*, 14, 153-162 (1982)

2537 Heikkinen J, Ylostalo P, Maentausta O et al. Serum bile acids during biphasic contraceptive treatment with ethinyl estradiol and norgestrel. *Contraception*, 25, 89-95 (1982)

2538 Heine P, Kewitz H, Wiegboldt K-A. The influence of hypoglycaemic sulfonylureas on elimination and efficacy of phenprocoumon following a single oral dose in diabetic patients. *Eur J Clin Pharmacol*, 10, 31-36 (1976)

2539 Heinegard D, Tiderstrom G. Determination of serum creatinine by a direct colorimetric method. *Clin Chim Acta*, 43, 305 (1973)

2540 Heinicke RM, Van Der Wal L, Yokoyama M. Effect of bromelain (ananase) on human platelet aggregation. *Experientia*, 28, 844 (1972)

2541 Heinonen EH, Antilla MI, Nyman LM, et al. Inhibition of platelet monoamine oxidase type B by selegiline. *J Clin Pharmacol*, 37, 597-601 (1997)

2542 Heintz B, Verho M, Brockmeier D et al. Influence of ramipril on renal function in patients with chronic congestive heart failure. *J Cardiovasc Pharmacol*, 18, Suppl 2, S174-S179 (1991)

2543 Heinze E, Fussganger R, Teller WM. Influence of calcium on insulin secretion in newborns. *Pediatr Res*, 7, 100 (1973)

2544 Helander A, Carlsson S. Use of leukocyte aldehyde dehydrogenase acyivity to monitor inhibitory effect of disulfiram treatment. *Alcohol Clin Exp Res*, 14, 48-52 (1990)

2545 Helander A, Vabö E, Levin K, Borg S. Intra- and inter-individual variability of carbohydrate-deficient transferrin, γ-glutamyltransferase, and mean corpuscular volume in teetotalers. *Clin Chem*, 44, 2120-2125 (1998)

2546 Helfgott SM, Sandberg-Cook J, Zakim D et al. Diclofenac-associated hepatotoxicity. *J Am Med Ass*, 264, 2660-2662 (1990)

2547 Helgeland A. The impact on serum lipids of combinations of diuretics and β-blockers and of β- blockers alone. *J Cardiovasc Pharmacol*, 6, S474-S476 (1984)

2548 Hellstrom PE, Repo UK. Capreomycin, ethambutol, and rifampicin in apparently incurable pulmonary tuberculosis. *Scand J Resp Dis*, 69 Suppl, 1 (1969)

2549 Hellstrom PE, Repo UK, Mattson K. New drugs in tuberculosis. *Drugs*, 1, 349 (1971)

2550 Henauer SA, Hollister LE. Cimetidine interaction with imipramine and nortriptyline. *Clin Pharmacol Ther*, 35, 183-187 (1984)

2551 Hendel J, Nyfors A. Impact of methotrexate therapy on the folate status of psoriatic patients. *Clin Exp Dermatol*, 10, 30-33 (1985)

2552 Henderson MJ, Dear PRF. Role of the clinical biochemistry laboratory in the management of very low birth weight infants. *Ann Clin Biochem*, 30, 341-354 (1993)

2553 Hene RJ, Koomans HA, Boer P et al. Effect of captopril in Bartter's syndrome. *Nephron*, 35, 275 (1983)

2554 Henkin Y, Oberman A, Hurst DC et al. Niacin revisited: clinical observations on an important but underutilized drug. *Am J Med*, 91, 239-246 (1991)

2555 Henning RJ, Becker H, Vincent J-L et al. Use of methylprednisolone in patients following acute myocardial infarction. *Chest*, 79, 186-194 (1981)

2556 Henrich WL. Nephrotoxicity of nonsteroidal anti-inflammatory agents. *Am J Kid Dis*, 11, 478-484 (1983)

2557 Henry DA, Lowe JM, Donnelly T. Jaundice during cyproheptadine treatment. *Br Med J*, 1, 753 (1978)

2558 Henry JA. Overdose and safety with fluvoxamine. *Int J Clin Psychopharmacol*, 6, Suppl 3, 41-47 (1991)

2559 Henry RJ. Clinical Chemistry: Principles and Technics. New York NY, Harper and Row Hoeber Division (1964)

2560 Henry RL, Washnock MA, Taylor GW. Mistabron effects on platelets and blood coagulation. *J Intern Med Res*, 12, 277-280 (1984)

2561 Henry RR, Gumbiner B, Ditzler T et al. Intensive conventional insulin therapy for type II diabetes: metabolic effects during a 6-mo outpatient trial. *Diabetes Care*, 16, 21-31 (1993)

2562 Henzl MR, Corson SL, Moghissi K et al. Administration of nasal nafarelin as compared with oral danazol for endometriosis: a multicenter double-blind comparative trial. *N Engl J Med*, 318, 485-489 (1988)

2563 Heptner G, Dkomschke S, Domschke W. Comparison of CA 72-4 with CA 19-9 and carcinoembryonic antigen in the serodiagnostics of gastrointestinal malignancies. *Scand J Gastroenterol*, 24, 745-750 (1989)

2564 Herbeth B, Bangrel A, Dalo B et al. Influence of oral contraceptives of differing dosages on α_1-antitrypsin, γ-glutamyltransferase and alkaline phosphatase. *Clin Chim Acta*, 112, 293-299 (1981)

2565 Herchberg S, Galan P, Soustre Y et al. Effects of iron supplementation on serum ferritin and other hematological indices of iron status in menstruating women. *Ann Nutr Metab*, 29, 232-238 (1985)

2566 Herd JK. Interference of hexosamines in the Lowry reaction. *Anal Biochem*, 44, 404 (1971)

2567 Herlitz J, Hjalmarson A, Waagstein F. Early use of metoprolol and serum potassium in suspected acute myocardial infarction. *Int J Cardiol*, 22, 169-175 (1989)

2568 Herlong HF, Reid PR, Boitnott JK et al. Aprindine hepatitis. *Ann Intern Med*, 89, 359-361 (1978)

2569 Hermann LS, Karlsson JE, Sjostrand A et al. Prospective comparative study in NIDDM patients of metformin and glibenclamide with special reference to lipid profiles. *Eur J Clin Pharmacol*, 41, 263-265 (1991)

2570 Hermann LS, Kjellstrom T, Nilsson-Ehle P. Effects of metformin and glibenclamide alone and in combinations on serum lipids and lipoproteins in patients with non-insulin-dependent diabetes mellitus. *Diabete Metab*, 17, 174-179 (1991)

2571 Hermans PE, Wilhelm MP. Vancomycin. *Mayo Clin Proc*, 62, 901-905 (1987)

2572 Hernandez Hernandez R, Carvajal AR, Guerrero Pajuelo J et al. The effect of doxazosin on platelet aggregation in normotensive subjects and patients with hypertension: an in vitro study. *Am Heart J*, 121, II Suppl, 389-394 (1991)

2573 Herold DA, Reed AE. Interference by endogenous glycerol in an enzymatic assay of phosphatidylglycerol in amniotic fluid. *Clin Chem*, 34, 560-563 (1988)

2574 Heroz AG, Levesque LA, Drislane FW et al. Phenytoin-induced elevation of serum estradiol and reproductive dysfunction in men with epilepsy. *Epilepsia*, 32, 550-553 (1991)

2575 Herreman F. Iatrogenic pathology in cardiology. *Nouv Presse Med*, 1, 413 (1972)

2576 Herrmann JM, Zieseniss E, Freischutz G. Betablockertherapie der hypertonie und koronaren herzkrankheit. *Munch Medizin Wschr*, 42, 735-740 (1988)

2577 Hersh AD, Kelly JG, Laher MS, et al. Effect of hydrochlorothiazide on the pharmacokinetics of enalapril in hypertensive patients with varying renal function. *J Cardiovasc Pharmacol*, 27, 7-11 (1996)

2578 Hersh EM, Wong VG, Henderson ES. Hepatotoxic effect of methotrexate. *Cancer*, 19, 600 (1966)

2579 Herxheimer A. Rifampicin. *Drug Ther Bull*, 8, 11 (1970)

2580 Herzig RH, Wolff SN, Lazarus HM et al. High-dose cytosine arabinoside therapy for refractory leukemia. *Blood*, 62, 361-369 (1983)

2581 Herzog AG, Levesque LA, Drislane FW et al. Phenytoin-induced elevation of serum estradiol and reproductive dysfunction in men with epilepsy. *Epilepsia*, 32, 550-553 (1991)

2582 Heshmati HM, Turpin G, Touitou Y et al. Lack of effect in vivo of clofibrate on adrenal steroid secretion. *Eur J Clin Pharmacol*, 36, 87-89 (1989)

2583 Hess JW, MacDonald RP. Serum creatine phosphokinase activity: a new diagnostic aid in myocardial and skeletal muscle disease. *J Mich Med Soc*, 62, 1095 (1963)

2584 Hewlett JS, Bodey GP, Coltman CA et al. Intermittent guanazole therapy in adult acute leukemia. *Clin Pharmacol Ther*, 14, 271 (1973)

2585 Heymann W. Nephrotic syndrome after use of trimethadione and paramethadione in petit mal. *J Am Med Ass*, 202, 893 (1967)

2586 Heymann W, Grupe WE. Increase in proteinuria due to steroid medication in chronic renal disease. *J Pediatr*, 74, 356 (1969)

2587 Hibbard DM, Peters JR, Hunninghake DB. Effects of cholestyramine and colestipol on the plasma concentrations of propranolol. *Br J Clin Pharmacol*, 18, 337-342 (1984)

2588 Hichens M, Hogans AF. Radioimmunoassay for dexamethasone in plasma. *Clin Chem*, 20, 266 (1974)

2589 Hickman PE, Mather P, Boyne P. Variation among instruments in interference by cephalosporin in the Jaffe reaction for creatinine. *Clin Chem*, 34, 215-216 (1988)

2590 Hicks JM, Soldin SJ, Iosefsohn M. Determination of serum and plasma iron using Kodak slides for pediatric patients. *Clin Chem*, 37, 967 (1991)

2591 Hickson B, Davidson RJL, Walker W. Agranulocytosis caused by procainamide. *Scott Med J*, 17, 165 (1972)

2592 Hida M, Aiba Y, Sawamura S, et al. Inhibition of the accumulation of uremic toxins in the blood and their precursors in the feces after oral administration of Lebenin® , a lactic acid bacteria preparation, to uremic patients undergoing hemodialysis. *Nephron*, 74, 349-355 (1996)

2593 Hiemke C, Weigmann H, Hartter S et al. Elevated levels of clozapine in serum after addition of fluvoxamine. *J Clin Psychopharmacol*, 14, 279-281 (1994)

2594 Higaki J, Ogihara T, Kumahara Y. Effects of frusemide and captopril on the relationship between biologically and immunologically active renin in human plasma. *Clin Sci*, 75, 669-672 (1988)

2595 Higaki J, Ogihara T, Nakamura M et al. Effects of carvedilol on plasma hormonal and biochemical factors and renal function in Japanese patients with essential hypertension. *Drugs*, 36, Suppl 6, 64-68 (1988)

2596 Higashi A, Ikeda T, Matsukura M et al. Serum zinc and vitamin E concentrations in handicapped children treated with anticonvulsants. *Dev Pharmacol Ther*, 5, 109-113 (1982)

2597 Higbee MD, Wood JS, Mead RA. Procainamide, cimetidine interaction: a potential toxic interaction in the elderly. *J Am Geriatr Soc*, 32, 162-164 (1984)

2598 Higgens CS, Scott JT. The uricosuric action of azapropazone: dose response and comparison with probenecid. *Br J Clin Pharmacol*, 18, 439-443 (1984)

2599 Higuchi H, Sumikura H, Sumita S et al. Renal function in patients with high serum fluoride concentrations after prolonged sevoflurane anesthesia. *Anesthesiology*, 83, 449-458 (1995)

2600 HIll JTY, Duff HJ, Burgess ED. Clinical pharmacokinetics of propafenone. *Clin Pharmacokinet*, 21, 1-10 (1991)

2601 Hilborn DA, Bale Oenick M, Danielson S et al. Thin-film enzyme immunoassay for the measurement of phenobarbital in human serum. *Clin Chem*, 37, 1034-1035 (1991)

2602 Hilbrands LB, Demacker PNM, Hoitsma AJ et al. The effects of cyclosporine and prednisone on serum lipid and (apo)lipoprotein levels in renal transplant recipients. *J Am Soc Nephrol*, 5, 2073-2081 (1995)

2603 Hildebrandt R, Moller H, Gundert-Remy U. Influence of theophylline on the renal clearance of erythromycin. *Int J Clin Pharmacol Ther Toxicol*, 25, 601-604 (1987)

2604 Hiles BW. Hyperglycemia and glycosuria following chlorpromazine therapy. *J Am Med Ass*, 162, 1651 (1956)

2605 Hill A, Casey R, Zaleski WA. Difficulties and pitfalls in the interpretation of screening tests for the detection of inborn errors of metabolism. *Clin Chim Acta*, 72, 1-15 (1976)

2606 Hill JM, Roberts J, Loeb E et al. L-asparaginase therapy for leukemia and other malignant neoplasms. *J Am Med Ass*, 202, 882 (1967)

2607 Hill NS, Antman EM, Green LH et al. Intravenous nitroglycerin: a review of pharmacology, indications, therapeutic effects and complications. *Chest*, 79, 69-76 (1981)

2608 Hill RP, Hindle EJ, Howey JEA et al. Recommendations for adopting standard conditions and analytical procedures in the measurement of serum fructosamine concentration. *Ann Clin Biochem*, 27, 413-424 (1990)

2609 Hillmer T, Frerichs H, Creutzfeldt W et al. Kolenhydrat- und fettstoffwechselveranderungen wahrend der behandlung mit einem ovulations = hemmer (eugynon). *Verh 3 Kongress D Dtsch Diabetesgesellschaft, Gottingen* (1968)

2610 Hinderks GJ, Frohlich J. Low serum creatine kinase values associated with administration of steroids. *Clin Chem*, 25, 2050-2051 (1979)

2611 Hindmarsh PC, Pringle PJ, Stanhope R, Brook CGD. The effect of a continuous infusion of a somatostatin analogue (octreotide) for two years on growth hormone secretion and height prediction in tall children. *Clin Endocrinol*, 42, 509-515 (1995)

2612 Hine KR, Harrop JS, Hopton MR et al. The effects of ranitidine on pituitary-thyroid function. *Br J Clin Pharmacol*, 18, 608-611 (1984)

2613 Hinks LJ, Clayton BE, Lloyd RS. Zinc and copper concentrations in leukocytes and erythrocytes in healthy adults and the effect of oral contraceptives. *J Clin Pathol*, 36, 1016-1021 (1983)

2614 Hinman AR, Wolinsky E. Nephrotoxicity associated with the use of cephaloridine. *J Am Med Ass*, 200, 724 (1967)

2615 Hinshaw JR, Hobler KE, Borja AR. Pentazocine: a potent, nonaddicting analgesic. *Am J Med Sci*, 251, 57 (1966)

2616 Hinterberger H, Wilcken DE. The effect of prolonged glucagon infusions on the urinary excretion of catecholamines. *Clin Chim Acta*, 52, 153 (1974)

2617 Hintze G, Briehl E, Jaworek D et al. Evaluation of a new enzyme immunoassay system for free thyroxine (Enzymun-test FT4). *J Clin Chem Clin Biochem*, 28, 427-433 (1990)

2618 Hirakata H, Onoyama K, Iseki K et al. Worsening of anemia induced by long-term use of captopril in hemodialysis patients. *Am J Nephrol*, 4, 355-360 (1984)

2619 Hiramatsu K, Yamagishi F, Kubota T et al. Acute effects of the calcium antagonist, nifedipine, on blood pressure, pulse rate and renin-aldosterone-angiotensin system in patients with essential hypertension. *Am Heart J*, 104, 1346-1350 (1982)

2620 Hiramatsu M, Hayashi A, Hidaka H, et al. Enzyme immunoassay of urinary mevalonic acid and its clinical application. *Clin Chem*, 44, 2152-2157 (1998)

2621 Hirata Y, Hayakawa H, Suzuki E et al. Renal and endocrine effects of urapidil in patients with essential hypertension. *Curr Ther Res*, 49, 961-968 (1991)

2622 Hirose S, Mitsudome A, Yasumoto S, et al. Valproate therapy does not deplete carnitine levels in otherwise healthy children. *Pediatrics*, 101, 1-5 (1998)

2623 Hirsch MS, D'Aqula RT. Drug therapy: therapy for human immunodeficiency virus infection. *N Engl J Med*, 328, 1686-1695 (1993)

2624 Hirschel B. Amodiaquine and hepatitis. *Lancet*, 1, 467 (1986)

2625 Hirsh J. Oral anticoagulant drugs. *N Engl J Med*, 324, 1865-1875 (1991)

2626 Hisatome I, Ishiko R, Sasaki N et al. Effect of prednisolone on urate and oxypurine excretion. *Horm Metab Res*, 23, 513-514 (1991)

2627 Hitz J, Steinmetz J, Henny J et al. Effets de l'aldatense sur les examens de laboratoire. comparaison avec la population de reference. *Ann Biol Clin*, 42, 289-293 (1984)

2628 Hitzenberger G, Schmid R, Braun W et al. Vinpocetine therapy does not change imipramine pharmacokinetics in man. *Int J Clin Pharmacol Ther Toxicol*, 28, 99-104 (1990)

2629 Hjelm M, De Verdier CH. Biochemical effects of aromatic amines. 1. methaemoglobinaemia, haemolysis and Heinz-body formation. *Biochem Pharmacol*, 14, 1119 (1965)

2630 Ho AD, Klotzbucher A, Gross A et al. Induction of intracellular and plasma 2',5'-oligoadenylate synthetase by pentostatin. *Leukemia*, 6, 209-214 (1992)

2631 Ho DHW, Covington WP, Legha SS et al. Clinical pharmacology of trimetrexate. *Clin Pharmacol Ther*, 42, 351-356 (1987)

2632 Ho KY, Weissberger AJ. Secretory patterns of growth hormone according to sex and age. *Horm Res*, 33, 7-11 (1990)

2633 Ho KY, Weissberger AJ, Marbach P et al. Therapeutic efficacy of the somatostatin analog SMS 201-995 (Octreotide) in acromegaly. *Ann Intern Med*, 112, 173-181 (1990)

2634 Hobbs CJ, Plymate SR, Rosen CJ et al. Testosterone administration increases insulin-like growth factor-I levels in normal men. *J Clin Endocrinol Metab*, 77, 776-779 (1993)

2635 Hodsman AB, Fraher LI. Biochemical responses to sequential human parathyroid hormone (1-38) and calcitonin in osteoporotic patients. *Bone Miner*, 9, 137-152 (1990)

2636 Hodsman GP, Brown JJ, Cumming AMM et al. Enalapril in the treatment of hypertension with renal artery stenosis. *Br Med J*, 287, 1413-1417 (1983)

2637 Hoechst Marion Roussel. Manufacturer's literature on Allegra™. Kansas City, MO 64134 (1996)

2638 Hoechst Marion Roussel. Manufacturer's literature on Altace® . Kansas City, MO 64134 (1995)

2639 Hoechst Marion Roussel. Manufacturer's literature on Amaryl® . Kansas City, MO 64134 (1995)

2640 Hoechst Marion Roussel. Manufacturer's literature on Bentyl® . Kansas City, MO 64134 (1995)

2641 Hoechst Marion Roussel. Manufacturer's literature on Bricanyl® . Kansas City, MO 64134 (1992)

2642 Hoechst Marion Roussel. Manufacturer's literature on Carafate® . Kansas City, MO 64134 (1995)

2643 Hoechst Marion Roussel. Manufacturer's literature on Cardizem® . Kansas City, Mo 64134 (1996)

2644 Hoechst Marion Roussel. Manufacturer's literature on Claforan® . Kansas City, MO 64134 (1995)

2645 Hoechst Marion Roussel. Manufacturer's literature on Clomid® . Kansas City, MO 64134 (1995)

2646 Hoechst Marion Roussel. Manufacturer's literature on Diaβeta® . Kansas City, MO 64134 (1995)

2647 Hoechst Marion Roussel. Manufacturer's literature on Lasix® . Kansas City, MO 64134 (1994)

2648 Hoechst Marion Roussel. Manufacturer's literature on Nilandron™. Kansas City, MO 64134 (1996)

2649 Hoechst Marion Roussel. Manufacturer's literature on Nitro-Bid® . Kansas City, MO 64134 (1995)

2650 Hoechst Marion Roussel. Manufacturer's literature on Norpramin® . Kansas City, MO 64134 (1996)

2651 Hoechst Marion Roussel. Manufacturer's literature on Pentasa® . Kansas City, MO 64134 (1995)

2652 Hoechst Marion Roussel. Manufacturer's literature on Rifadin® . Kansas City, MO 64134 (1995)

2653 Hoechst Marion Roussel. Manufacturer's literature on Seldane® . Kansas City, MO 64134 (1995)

2654 Hoechst Marion Roussel. Manufacturer's literature on Trental® . Kansas City, MO 64134 (1995)

2655 Hoeck HC, Laurberg G, Laurberg P. Hypercalcaemic crisis after excessive topical use of a vitamin D derivative. *J Intern Med*, 235, 281-282 (1994)

2656 Hoeg JM, Schaefer EJ, Romano CA et al. Neomycin and plasma lipoproteins in type II hyperlipoproteinemia. *Clin Pharmacol Ther*, 36, 555-565 (1984)

2657 Hoekenga MT, Bunde CA, Cho YW et al. Double blind multicenter evaluation of a new antianginal drug: perhexiline maleate. *Clin Pharmacol Ther*, 13, 140 (1972)

2658 Hoffer A. Niacin Therapy in Psychiatry. Springfield IL, CC Thomas (1962)

2659 Hoffman RS. Evaluation of coagulation factor abnormalities in long-acting anticoagulant overdose. *Clin Toxicol*, 26, 233-248 (1988)

2660 Hoffman WH, DiPiro JT, Tackett RL et al. Relationship of plasma clonidine to growth hormone concentrations in children and adolescents. *J Clin Pharmacol*, 29, 538-542 (1989)

2661 Hofmann GE, Rao CV, Brown MJ et al. Epidermal growth factor in urine of nonpregnant women and pregnant women throughout pregnancy and at delivery. *J Clin Endocrinol Metab*, 66, 119-123 (1988)

2662 Hoge SK, Biederman J. Liver function tests during treatment with desipramine in children and adolescents. *J Clin Psychopharmacol*, 7, 87-89 (1987)

2663 Hoglund P, Paulsen O, Bogentoft S. No effect of terodiline on anticoagulation effect of warfarin and steady-state plasma levels of warfarin enantiomers in healthy volunteers. *Ther Drug Monit*, 11, 667-673 (1989)

2664 Hoikka V, Alhava EM, Karjalainen P et al. Carbamazepine and bone mineral metabolism. *Acta Neurol Scand*, 68, 77-80 (1984)

2665 Hojer B, Rane A. Fatal hepatic failure in a child treated with phenytoin and valproic acid. *Dev Med Child Neurol*, 24, 846-849 (1982)

2666 Hokfelt B, Hedeland H, Dymling JF. The influence of Catapres® on catecholamines, renin and aldosterone in man. In:. *Catapres® in Hypertension. ME Conolly (ed)*, London, Butterworth (1970)

2667 Hokin DB. Blank correction for metronidazole interference with continuous flow measurement of aspartate aminotransferase. *Clin Chem*, 29, 406-407 (1983)

2668 Holazo AA, Choma N, Brown SY et al. Effect of cimetidine on the disposition of rimantadine in healthy subjects. *Antimicrob Agent Chemother*, 33, 820-823 (1989)

2669 Holdaas H, Hartmann A, Stenstrom J et al. Effect of fluvastatin for safety lowering atherogenic lipids in renal transplant patients receiving cyclosporine. *Am J Cardiol*, 76, 102A-106A (1995)

2670 Holden JMC, Itil TM. Laboratory changes with chlordiazepoxide and thioridazine, alone and combined. *Can J Psychiat*, 14, 299 (1969)

2671 Holdstock DJ. Gastrointestinal bleeding: a possible association with ibuprofen. *Lancet*, 1, 541 (1972)

2672 Hollander CS, Mitsuma T, Shenkman L et al. Thyrotropin-releasing hormone: evidence for thyroid response to intravenous injection in man. *Science*, 175, 209 (1972)

2673 Hollenbeck CB, Johnston P, Varasteh BB et al. Effects of metformin on glucose, insulin and lipid metabolism in patients with mild hypertriglyceridemia and non-insulin dependent diabetes mellitus by glucose intolerance test criteria. *Diabete Metabol*, 17, 483-489 (1991)

2674 Hollister D Jr, Coleman M. Hematologic effects of intravesicular Thiotepa therapy for bladder carcinoma. *J Am Med Ass*, 244, 2065-2067 (1980)

2675 Hollister LE. Prediction of therapeutic uses of psychotherapeutic drugs from experiences with normal volunteers. *Clin Pharmacol Ther*, 13, 803 (1972)

2676 Hollister LE. Some human pharmacological studies of three psychotropic drugs: thiothixene, molindone, and W-18677. *J Clin Pharmacol*, 8, 95 (1968)

2677 Hollister LE. Status report on clinical pharmacology of marijuana. *Ann NY Acad Sci*, 191, 132 (1972)

2678 Holm J, Berntorp E, Carlsson R et al. Low-dose warfarin decreases coagulability without affecting prothrombin complex activity. *J Intern Med*, 234, 303-308 (1993)

2679 Holmberg L, Boman G. Pulmonary reactions to nitrofurantoin. *Eur J Respir Dis*, 62, 180-189 (1981)

2680 Holmberg L, Boman G, Bottiger LE. Adverse reactions to nitrofurantoin: analysis of 921 reports. *Am J Med*, 69, 733-738 (1980)

2681 Holmes TH, Morgan BA, Woolf CR. The effect of disodium cromoglycate on plasma 17-hydroxycorticoid concentration during exercise. *Am Rev Resp Dis*, 106, 610 (1972)

2682 Holst N, Jenssen TG, Burhol PG et al. Prolactin response to secretin during the spontaneous menstrual cycle in women. *Gynecol Obstet Invest*, 31, 37-41 (1991)

2683 Holst N, Jenssen TG, Burhol PG et al. The effects of secretin on prolactin, estradiol, vasoactive intestinal polypeptide, and somatostatin levels in women. *Acta Endocrinol*, 122, 313-318 (1990)

2684 Holt RJ. Neuroleptic drug-induced changes in platelet levels. *J Clin Psychopharmacol*, 4, 130-132 (1984)

2685 Holtbecker N, Fromm MF, Kroemer HK, et al. The nifedipine-rifampin interaction: evidence for induction of gut wall metabolism. *Drug Metab Dispos*, 24, 1121-1123 (1996)

2686 Homayouni H, Gross PA, Setia U et al. Leukopenia due to penicillin and cephalosporin homologues. *Arch Intern Med*, 139, 827-828 (1979)

2687 Homi J, Konchigeri HN, Eckenhoff JE et al. A new anesthetic agent - Forane® : preliminary observations in man. *Anesth Analg*, 51, 439 (1972)

2688 Homma Y, Kobayashi T, Yamaguchi H et al. Decrease of plasma large, light LDL (LDL1), HDL_2 and HDL_3 levels with concomitant increase of cholesterylester transfer protein (CETP) activity by probucol in type II hyperlipoproteinemia. *Artery*, 20, 1-18 (1993)

2689 Homma Y, Moriguchi EH, Sakane H et al. Effects of probucol on plasma lipoprotein subfractions and activities of lipoprotein lipase and hepatic triglyceride lipase. *Atherosclerosis*, 88, 175-181 (1991)

2690 Homma Y, Ohshima K, Yamaguchi H et al. Effects of eicosapentaenoic acid on plasma lipoprotein subfractions and activities of lecithin:cholesterol acyltransferase and lipid transfer protein. *Atherosclerosis*, 91, 145-153 (1991)

2691 Homma Y, Ozawa H, Kobayashi T et al. Effects of bezafibrate therapy on subfractions of plasma low-density lipoprotein and high-density lipoprotein, and on activities of lecithin:cholesterol acyltransferase and cholesteryl ester transfer protein in patients with hyperlipoproteinemia. *Atherosclerosis*, 106, 191-201 (1994)

2692 Homma Y, Ozawa H, Kobayashi T et al. Effects of simvastatin on plasma lipoprotein subfractions, cholesterol esterification rate, and cholesteryl transfer protein in type II hyperlipoproteinemia. *Atherosclerosis*, 114, 223-234 (1995)

2693 Honari J, Blair AD, Cutler RE. Effects of probenecid on furosemide kinetics and natriuresis in man. *Clin Pharmacol Ther*, 22, 395 (1977)

2694 Honer WG, Thompson C, Lightman SC et al. No effect of naloxone on plasma oxytocin in normal men. *Psychoneuroendocrinology*, 11, 245-248 (1986)

2695 Honet JC. False positive urinary test for 5-HIAA due to methocarbomal and mephenesin carbamate. *N Engl J Med*, 261, 188 (1959)

2696 Hong CY, Huang JJ, Wu P. The inhibitory effect of gossypol on human sperm motility: relationship with time, temperature and concentration. *Hum Toxicol*, 8, 49-51 (1989)

2697 Hong MK, Romm PA, Reagan KA et al. Effects of estrogen replacement therapy on serum lipid values and angiographically defined coronary artery disease in postmenopausal women. *Am J Cardiol*, 69, 176-178 (1992)

2698 Honger PE, Rossing N. Albumin metabolism and oral contraception. *Clin Sci*, 36, 41 (1969)

2699 Honig PK, Wortham DC, Hull R et al. Itraconazole affects single-dose terfenadine pharmacokinetics and cardiac repolarization pharmacodynamics. *J Clin Pharmacol*, 33, 1201-1206 (1993)

2700 Honig PK, Wortham DC, Zamani K et al. Terfendine-ketoconazole interaction. *J Am Med Ass*, 269, 1513-1518 (1993)

2701 Hood JW, Toth WN. Jaundice caused by phenazopyridine hydrochloride. *J Am Med Ass*, 198, 1366 (1966)

2702 Hoogerbrugge-Vd Linden, De Rooy FWM, Jansen H et al. Effects of pravastatin on biliary lipid composition and bile acid synthesis in familial hypercholesterolemia. *Gut*, 31, 348-350 (1990)

2703 Hoogwerf BJ, Grund VR, Hunninghake DB. Effect of cimetidine on plasma lipids and lipoproteins. *Clin Pharmacol Ther*, 36, 217-220 (1984)

2704 Hooper DC, Wolfson JS. Fluoroquinolone antimicrobial agents. *N Engl J Med*, 324, 384-394 (1991)

2705 Hooper PL, Woo W, Visconti L et al. Terbutaline raises high-density-lipoprotein-cholesterol levels. *N Engl J Med*, 305, 1455-1457 (1981)

2706 Hooper WD, Franklin ME, Glue P, et al. Effect of felbamate on valproic acid disposition in healthy volunteers: inhibition of β-oxidation. *Epilepsia*, 37, 91-07 (1996)

2707 Hopkins KD, Parker JR, Lehmann ED, et al. Insulin-like growth factor (IGF)-I levels in postmenopausal women receiving tibolone. *Horm Metab Res*, 27, 387-388 (1995)

2708 Hoppensteadt DA, Kahn S, Fareed J. Factor X values as a means to assess the extent of oral anticoagulation in patients receiving antithrombin drugs. *Clin Chem*, 43, 1786-1788 (1997)

2709 Hoppensteadt DA, Walenga JM, Fasanella A et al. TFPI antigen levels in normal human volunteers after intravenous and subcutaneous administration of unfractionated heparin and a low molecular weight heparin. *Thromb Res*, 77, 175-185 (1995)

2710 Hoppichler F, Sandholzer C, Moncayo R et al. Thyroid hormone (fT4) reduces lipoprotein(a) plasma levels. *Atherosclerosis*, 115, 65-71 (1995)

2711 Hoppin EC, Greenberg BR, Walter RM. Agranulocytosis secondary to pentazocine therapy. *Arch Intern Med*, 138, 533-534 (1978)

2712 Horber FF, Scheidegger J, Frey FJ. Overestimation of renal function in glucocorticosteroid treated patients. *Eur J Clin Pharmacol*, 28, 537-541 (1985)

2713 Horder M. Colorimetric determination of orthophosphate in the assay of inorganic pyrophosphatase activity. *Anal Biochem*, 49, 37 (1972)

2714 Horder M, Jorgensen PJ, Hafkenscheid JCM et al. Creatine kinase determination: a European evaluation of the creatine kinase determination in serum, plasma and whole blood with the Reflotron system. *Eur J Clin Chem Clin Biochem*, 29, 691-696 (1991)

2715 Horie Y, Udagawa M, Hirayama C. Clinical usefulness of cimetidine for the treatment of acute intermittent porphyria - a preliminary report. *Clin Chim Acta*, 167, 267-271 (1987)

2716 Horiuchi I, Ohya T, Tazuma S et al. Effects of pravastatin (CS-154) on biliary lipid metabolism in patients with hyperlipidemia. *Metabolism*, 40, 226-230 (1991)

2717 Horn K, Casineiras MJ, Ortola J et al. The determination of thyroxine and thyroxine uptake with new homogeneous enzyme immunoassays using Boehringer-Mannheim/Hitachi analysis systems. *Eur J Clin Chem Clin Biochem*, 29, 697-703 (1991)

2718 Horn M. Coadministration of itraconazole with hypolipidemic agents may induce rhabdomyolysis in healthy individuals. *Arch Dermatol*, 132, 1254 (1996)

2719 Horne CHW, Mallinson AC, Ferguson J et al. Effect of estrogen and progestogen on serum levels of α_2-macroglobulin, transferrin and IgG. *J Clin Pathol*, 24, 464 (1971)

2720 Horne MK III, Wilson OJ, Cooper M et al. The effect of suramin on laboratory tests of coagulation. *Thromb Haemostas*, 67, 434-439 (1992)

2721 Hornych A, Boisson J, Gaschard JC. Decreased prostaglandin synthesis in patients with essential hypertension: stimulating effect of cicletanine. *Arch Mal Coeur*, 82, Special Issue 4, 85-90 (1989)

2722 Horowitz J, Keynan A, Ben-Ishay D. A syndrome of inappropriate ADH secretion induced by cyclothiazide. *J Clin Pharmacol*, 12, 337 (1972)

2723 Horowitz S, Patwardhan R, Marcus E. Hepatotoxic reactions associated with carbamazepine therapy. *Epilepsia*, 29, 149-154 (1988)

2724 Horsmans Y, Desager JP, Harvengt C. Effects of gemfibrozil on the activities of plasma lipolytic enzymes in normolipidemic subjects. *Clin Chim Acta*, 218, 223-228 (1993)

2725 Horsmans Y, Desager JP, Van den Berge V et al. Effects of simvastatin and pravastatin on 6β-hydroxycortisol excretion, a potential marker of cytochrome P-450 3A. *Pharmacol Res*, 28, 243-248 (1993)

2726 Horus Therapeutics. Manufacturer's literature on Thalitone® . Rochester, NY 14623 (1994)

2727 Horwitz CA, Garmezy L, Lyon F et al. A comparative study of five immunologic pregnancy tests. *Am J Clin Pathol*, 58, 305 (1972)

2728 Hossein-Nia M, Devlin JJ, Tredger JM et al. Excretion of urinary proteins as a marker of drug-induced renal damage. *Proc ACB Natl Meet*, 122 (1991)

2729 Host NB, Stoltenberg MB, Jensen LT et al. Effect on collagen metabolism of thrombolytic therapy with tissue-plasminogen activator. A randomized, placebo-controlled study. *Eur J Clin Invest*, 25, 15-18 (1995)

2730 Hotta N, Koh N, Sakakibara F, et al. Effect of acarbose on blood glucose profiles and plasma 1,5-anhydro-D-glucitol in type 2 diabetes poorly controlled by sulfonylurea therapy. *Biomed Pharmacother*, 50, 297-302 (1996)

2731 Houdent C, Noblet C, Vandoren C et al. Cibenzoline-induced hypoglycaemia in the elderly. *Rev Med Interne*, 12, 143-145 (1991)

2732 Houin G, Tillement JP. Clofibrate and enzymatic induction in man. *Int J Clin Pharmacol Biopharm*, 16, 150-154 (1978)

2733 Houston MC, Olafsson L, Burger MC. Effects of nifedipine (GTIS) and atenolol monotherapy on serum lipids, blood pressure, heart rate, and weight gain in mild to moderate hypertension. *Angiology*, 42, 681-690 (1991)

2734 Hoverstad T, Carlstedt-Duke B, Lingaas E et al. Influence of ampicillin, clindamycin and metronidazole on faecal excretion of short-chain fatty acids in healthy subjects.. *Scand J Gastroenterol*, 21, 621-626 (1986)

2735 Howard G, Blair M, Fotherby K et al. Some metabolic effects of long-term use of the injectable contraceptive norethisterone oenanthate. *Lancet*, 1, 423-425 (1982)

2736 Howard JM, Chremos AN, Collen MJ et al. Famotidine, a new potent, long-acting histamine H_2-receptor antagonist: comparison with cimetidine and ranitidine in the treatment of Zollinger-Ellison syndrome. *Gastroenterology*, 88, 1026-1033 (1985)

2737 Howard KM, Roelli AP, Worth HGJ. Some effects of combined contraceptive therapy on cortisol measurements. *Ann Clin Biochem*, 24, Suppl S1, 191-192 (1987)

2738 Howard RP, Brusco OJ, Furman RH. Effect of cholestyramine administration on serum lipids and on nitrogen balance in familial hypercholesterolemia. *J Lab Clin Med*, 68, 12 (1966)

2739 Howes CA, Pullar T, Sourindhrin I et al. Reduced steady-state plasma concentrations of chlorpromazine and indomethacin in patients receiving cimetidine. *Eur J Clin Pharmacol*, 24, 99-102 (1983)

2740 Howitz PF. The effect of apurin (allopurinol) on liver function and serum iron. *Dan Med Bull*, 17, 203 (1970)

2741 Howrie DL, Gartner JC Jr. Gold-induced hepatotoxicity: case report and review of the literature. *J Rheumatol*, 9, 727-729 (1982)

2742 Hozumi, Y, Kawano M, Saito T, Miyata M. Effect of tamoxifen on serum lipid metabolism. *J Clin Endocrinol Metab*, 83, 1633-1635 (1998)

2743 Hsieh K-H, Chou C-C, Huang S-F. Interleukin 2 therapy in severe atopic dermatitis. *J Clin Immunol*, 11, 22-28 (1991)

2744 Hsu A, Granneman R, Cao G, et al. Pharmacokinetic interactions between two human immunodeficiency virus protease inhibitors, ritonavir and saquinavir. *Clin Pharmacol Ther*, 63, 453-464 (1998)

2745 Huang CM. Development and evaluation of an automated dye-binding assay for protein in cerebrospinal fluid. *Clin Chem*, 34, 980-983 (1988)

2746 Huang CM, Elin RJ, Ruddel M et al. Changes in laboratory results for cancer patients treated with interleukin-2. *Clin Chem*, 36, 431-434 (1990)

2747 Huang CM, Kroll MH, Ruddel M et al. An enzymatic method for 5-fluorocytosine. *Clin Chem*, 34, 59-62 (1988)

2748 Huang SM, Chan SH, Wu TJ, Chow NH. Effect of thyroid hormone on urinary excretion of epidermal growth factor. *Eur Surg Res*, 29, 222-238 (1997)

2749 Huang S-M, Weintraub HS, Marriott TB et al. Etintidine-propranolol interaction study in humans. *J Pharm Biopharm*, 15, 557-567 (1987)

2750 Hubbuch A, Lang FS, Stockmann W. Multicentre evaluation of a sensitive urinary albumin method in 8 laboratories. *Clin Chem*, 37, 962 (1991)

2751 Hubel KA. Secretin: a long progress note. *Gastroenterology*, 62, 318 (1972)

2752 Hucker RS, Smith GT, Minty PSB. Evaluation of enzymic assay for paracetamol: clinical and forensic experiences. *J Pharmacol Biomed Anal*, 2, 549-554 (1984)

2753 Huff B, Brogeler E, Felknor L et al (eds). Physicians' Desk Reference. Supplement B. Oradell NJ, Medical Economics (1973)

2754 Huff B, Brogeler E, Felknor L, Muller T (eds). Physicians' Desk Reference. *26th edition*, Oradell NJ, Medical Economics (1972)

2755 Huffman DH, Azarnoff DL, Shoeman DW et al. The interaction between halofenate and propranolol. *Clin Pharmacol Ther*, 19, 807-812 (1976)

2756 Huffman DH, Shoeman DW, Pentikainen P et al. The effect of spironolactone on antipyrine metabolism in man. *Pharmacology*, 10, 338-344 (1973)

2757 Hug G, McGraw CA, Bates SR et al. Reduction of serum carnitine concentrations during anticonvulsant therapy with phenobarbital, valproic acid, phenytoin, and carbamazepine in children. *J Pediatr*, 119, 799-802 (1991)

2758 Hughes GS, Francom SF, Spillers CR et al. The effect of ketoconazole and transdermal estradiol on serum sex steroid hormone levels. *Eur J Clin Pharmacol*, 38, 555-560 (1990)

2759 Hughes GS Jr, Cowart TD, Oexmann MJ et al. Verapamil-induced natriuretic and diuretic effects: dependency on sodium intake. *Clin Pharmacol Ther*, 44, 400-407 (1988)

2760 Hughes JA, Sudell W. Hemolytic anemia associated with naproxen. *Arth Rheum*, 26, 1054 (1983)

2761 Hughes JM, Gallagher DL, Olson JE. Plasma free thyroxine concentrations in patients receiving levothyroxine for thyroid suppression. *Surgery*, 106, 951-955 (1989)

2762 Hughes W, Seamonds B, Cohen S et al. The relation of serum ionized calcium to the alkaline tide. *Clin Res*, 20, 733 (1972)

2763 Hugues JN, Perret G, Sebaoun J et al. Effects of cimetidine on thyroid hormones. *Clin Endocrinol*, 17, 297-302 (1982)

2764 Huguley CM Jr. Agranulocytosis induced by dipyrone, a hazardous antipyretic and analgesic. *J Am Med Ass*, 189, 938 (1964)

2765 Hui R, Trube A, Lissner D et al. Interactions between 1,25-dihydroxyvitamin D_3 and vitamin D_2: effects of pharmacologic doses in normal individuals. *Clin Pharmacol Ther*, 42, 641-645 (1988)

2766 Huis in't Veld LG. Drug Information Service Note no 6. *IFCC Committee on Standards*

2767 Huisman J. The influence of vigabatrin on ALAT-activity measurements. *Clin Chem*, 39, 1142 (1993)

2768 Huisman JW. Interference by diflunisal with the FETI method for serum thyroxine. *Ann Clin Biochem*, 23, 223-224 (1986)

2769 Hulthen UL, Van Brummelen P, Amann FW et al. Antihypertensive efficacy of the new long-acting β-blocker bopindolol as related to age. *J Cardiovasc Pharmacol*, 5, 426-429 (1983)

2770 Human JA, Ubbink JB, Jerling JJ, et al. The effect of simvastatin on the plasma antioxidant concentrations in patients with hypercholesterolemia. *Clin Chim Acta*, 263, 67-77 (1997)

2771 Humble MW, Eykyn SJ, Phillips I. Staphylococcal bacteremia, fusidic acid, and jaundice. *Br Med J*, 1, 1495-1498 (1980)

2772 Hume R, Johnstone JMS, Weyers E. Interaction of ascorbic acid and warfarin. *J Am Med Ass*, 219, 1479 (1972)

2773 Hummer M, Kurz M, Kurzthaler I, et al. Hepatotoxicity of clozapine. *J Clin Psychopharmacol*, 17, 314-317 (1997)

2774 Humpel M, Tauber U, Kuhnz W et al. Comparison of serum ethinyl estradiol, sex hormone-binding globulin, corticoid-binding globulin and cortisol levels in women using two low-dose combined oral contraceptives. *Horm Res*, 33, 35-39 (1990)

2775 Humphries JE, Siragy H. Significant hyponatremia following DDAVP administration in a healthy adult. *Am J Hematol*, 44, 12-15 (1993)

2776 Humphries JE, Wheby MS, VandenBerg SR. Fluoxetine and the bleeding time. *Arch Pathol Lab Med*, 114, 727-728 (1990)

2777 Hunninghake D, Goldberg A, Insull W et al. Pravastatin: a tissue-selective once-daily HMG-CoA reductase inhibitor in the treatment of primary hypercholesterolemia. *J Am Coll Cardiol*, 11, 8A (1988)

2778 Hunninghake DB, King S, La Croix K. The effect of cholestyramine and colestipol on the absorption of hydrochlorothiazide. *Int J Clin Pharmacol Ther Toxicol*, 20, 151-154 (1982)

2779 Hunninghake DB, Stein EA, Mellies MJ. Effects of one year of treatment with pravastatin, an HMG-CoA reductase inhibitor, on lipoprotein A. *J Clin Pharmacol*, 33, 574-580 (1993)

2780 Hunter E, Raik E, Gordon S et al. Incidence of positive Coombs' test, LE cells and antinuclear factor in patients on α-methyldopa (Aldomet®). *Med J Aust*, 2, 810 (1971)

2781 Hunter Hypertension Group. Changes in serum lipid levels during antihypertensive therapy. *Med J Aust*, 140, 522-524 (1984)

2782 Hunter J, Maxwell JD, Carrella M et al. Urinary D-glucaric acid excretion as a test for hepatic enzyme induction in man. *Lancet*, 1, 572 (1971)

2783 Hunter J, Maxwell JD, Stewart DA et al. Altered calcium metabolism in epileptic children on anticonvulsants. *Br Med J*, 4, 202 (1971)

2784 Hunter JV, Kind PRN. Nonionic iodinated contrast media: potential renal damage assessed with enzymuria. *Radiology*, 183, 101-104 (1992)

2785 Huraib S, Al-Momen AK, Gader AMA et al. Effect of recombinant human erythropoietin (rHuEpo) on the hemostatic system in chronic hemodialysis patients. *Clin Nephrol*, 36, 252-257 (1991)

2786 Hursting MJ, Raisys VA, Opheim KE. Drug specific FAB therapy in drug overdose. *Arch Pathol Lab Med*, 111, 693-697 (1987)

2787 Hurt R. The effect of radiographic contrast media on urinalysis. *Am J Med Technol*, 26, 122 (1960)

2788 Hurt RD, Dale LC, Offord KP et al. Serum nicotine and cotinine levels during nicotine-patch therapy. *Clin Pharmacol Ther*, 54, 98-106 (1993)

2789 Hurwitz A, Schlozman DL. Effects of antacids on gastrointestinal absorption of isoniazid in rat and man. *Am Rev Resp Dis*, 109, 41-47 (1974)

2790 Hurwitz A, Vacek JL, Botteron GW et al. Mexiletine effects on theophylline disposition. *Clin Pharmacol Ther*, 50, 299-307 (1991)

2791 Hussain S, Gupta AD, Dean R et al. Performance evaluation and interference study of the Kodak Ektachem slide method for CSF proteins. *Clin Chem*, 36, 1197 (1990)

2792 Hussain S, McLawhon RW, Dasgupta A et al. Performance evaluation and reference range study of the Ektachem slide method for serum iron and total iron binding capacity. *Clin Chem*, 37, 975 (1991)

2793 Hussain S, McLawhon RW, Dean R et al. Performance evaluation and practical consideration of the Kodak Ektachem slide method for lactate. *Clin Chem*, 36, 1197 (1990)

2794 Hussar DA. The new drugs of 1971. *Am J Pharm*, 144, 5 (1972)

2795 Husserl FE. Erythromycin - warfarin interaction. *Arch Intern Med*, 143, 1831-1832 (1983)

2796 Hussey AJ, Howie J, Allan LG et al. Impaired hepatocellular integrity during general anaesthesia, as assessed by measurement of plasma glutathione S-transferase. *Clin Chim Acta*, 161, 19-28 (1986)

2797 Hutchison FN, Perez EA, Gandara DR et al. Renal salt wasting in patients treated with cisplatin. *Ann Intern Med*, 108, 21-25 (1988)

2798 Hutchison JC, Wilkinson WH, Zemlin RD. Long-term experiences with halofenate. *Clin Res*, 21, 469 (1973)

2799 Huubuch A. Results of the multicenter study with Tinaquant albumin in urine. *Wien Klin Wschr*, 103, Suppl 189, 23-29 (1991)

2800 Hwang PLH, Ng CSH, Cheong ST. Effect of oral contraceptives on serum prolactin: longitudinal study in 126 normal premenopausal women. *Clin Endocrinol*, 24, 127-133 (1986)

2801 Hymes KB, Greene JB, Karpatkin S. The effect of azidothymidine on HIV-related thrombocytopenia. *N Engl J Med*, 318, 516-517 (1988)

2802 Hysell JK, Hysell JW, Gray JM. Thrombocytopenic purpura following iopanoic acid ingestion. *J Am Med Ass*, 237, 361-362 (1977)

2803 Iber FL. Cholestasis. *Postgrad Med*, 41, 30 (1967)

2804 Ibsen H, Sederberg-Olsen P. Changes in glomerular filtration rate during long-term treatment with propranolol in patients. *Clin Sci*, 44, 129 (1973)

2805 ICN Pharmaceuticals, Inc. Manufacturer's literature on Android® . Costa Mesa, CA 92626 (1994)

2806 ICN Pharmaceuticals, Inc. Manufacturer's literature on Testred® . Costa Mesa, CA 92626 (1994)

2807 Iinuma K, Hayasaka K, Narisawa K et al. Hyperaminoacidaemia and hyperammonaemia in epileptic children treated with valproic acid. *Eur J Pediatr*, 148, 267-269 (1988)

2808 Ikeda T. Marked decrease in serum HDL cholesterol levels by combined probucol-pravastatin treatment in hypercholesterolemic NIDDM patients. *Diabetes Care*, 16, 849-850 (1993)

2809 Ikeda T, Nonaka Y, Goto A et al. Effects of prazosin on platelet aggregation and plasma β-thromboglobulin in essential hypertension. *Clin Pharmacol Ther*, 37, 601-605 (1985)

2810 Ikeda T, Shibuya Y, Senba U et al. Automated immunoturbidimetric analysis of six plasma apolipoproteins: correlation with radial immunodiffusion assays. *J Clin Lab Anal*, 5, 90-95 (1991)

2811 Ikram H, Maslowski AH, Nicholls MG et al. Haemodynamic and hormonal effects of captopril in primary pulmonary hypertension. *Br Heart J*, 48, 541-545 (1982)

2812 Illingworth DR, Bacon S. Influence of lovastatin plus gemfibrozil on plasma lipids and lipoproteins in patients with heterozygous familial hypercholesterolemia. *Circulation*, 79, 590-596 (1989)

2813 Imaizumi H, Namiki A, Watanabe A et al. Hemolysis and hemoglobinuria following administration of high dose fentanyl. a case report. *Jpn J Anesthesiol*, 35, 639-642 (1986)

2814 Imhof PR, Hushak J, Schumann G et al. Excretion of urinary casts after the administration of diuretics. *Br Med J*, 2, 199 (1972)

2815 Immunex Corporation. Manufacturer's literature on Amicar® . Seattle, WA 98101 (1995)

2816 Immunex Corporation. Manufacturer's literature on Leukine® . Seattle, WA 98101 (1997)

2817 Immunex Corporation. Manufacturer's literature on Levoprome® . Seattle, WA 98101 (1987)

2818 Immunex Corporation. Manufacturer's literature on Methotrexate® . Seattle, WA 98101 (1996)

2819 Immunex Corporation. Manufacturer's literature on Novantrone® . Seattle, WA 98101 (1994)

2820 Immunex Corporation. Manufacturer's literature on Thioplex® . Seattle, WA 98101 (1994)

2821 Imura H, Nakai Y, Matsukura S et al. Effect of intravenous infusion of L-dopa on plasma growth hormone levels in man. *Horm Metab Res*, 5, 41 (1973)

2822 Inman WHW. Study of fatal bone marrow depression with special reference to phenylbutazone and oxyphenbutazone. *Br Med J*, 1, 1500-1505 (1977)

2823 Innes RKR, Stromme JH. Rise in serum creatine phosphokinase associated with agents used in anesthesia. *Br J Anaes*, 45, 185 (1973)

2824 International Union Against Tuberculosis Committee. Efficacy of various durations of isoniazid preventive therapy for tuberculosis: five years of follow-up in the IUAT trial. *Bull WHO*, 60, 555-564 (1982)

2825 Invitti C, De Martin I, Bolla GB et al. Effect of octreotide on catecholamine plasma levels in patients with chromaffin cell tumors. *Horm Res*, 40, 156-160 (1993)

2826 Invitti C, Fatti L, Camboni MG, et al. Effect of chronic treatment with octreotide nasal powder on serum levels of growth hormone, insulin-like growth factor I, insulin-like growth factor binding proteins 1 and 3 in acromegalic patients. *J Endocrinol Invest*, 19, 548-555 (1996)

2827 Inzucchi SE, Maggs DG, Spollett GR, et al. Efficacy and metabolic effects of metformin and troglitazone in type II diabetes mellitus. *N Engl J Med*, 338, 867-872 (1998)

2828 Iosefsohn M, Rifai N, Hyde JE et al. Organic acids and drug interference in the measurement of CO_2 concentrations by the Kodak Ektachem® 700. *Clin Chem*, 35, 1156 (1989)

2829 Iosefsohn M, Rifai N, Myatt L et al. Effect of cyclosporine on serum analytes. *Clin Chem*, 36, 1034 (1990)

2830 Iqbal SJ, Whittaker P, Bourke J et al. Possible interference with calcipotriol on new IDS RIA for 1,25-dihydroxyvitamin D. *Clin Chem*, 42, 112-113 (1996)

2831 Irie M, Tsushima T, Sakuma M. Effect of nicotinic acid administration on plasma hGH, FFA and glucose in obese subjects. *Metabolism*, 19, 972 (1971)

2832 Isaac R, Merceron R, Caillens G et al. Effects of calcitonin on basal and thyrotropin-releasing hormone stimulated prolactin secretion in man. *J Clin Endocrinol Metab*, 50, 1011-1015 (1980)

2833 Isaacsohn JL, Setaro JF, Nicholas C et al. Effects of lovastatin therapy on plasminogen activator inhibitor-1 antigen levels. *Am J Cardiol*, 74, 735-737 (1994)

2834 Ishak KG, Kirchner JP, Dhar JK. Granulomas and cholestatic-hepatocellular injury associated with phenylbutazone: report of two cases. *Am J Dig Dis*, 22, 611-617 (1977)

2835 Isley WL. Effect of rifampin therapy on thyroid function tests in a hypothyroid patient on replacement L-thyroxine. *Ann Intern Med*, 107, 517-518 (1987)

2836 Ismail A, Astley P, Burr WA et al. The role of testosterone measurement in the investigation of androgen disorders. *Ann Clin Biochem*, 23, 113-134 (1986)

2837 Isojarvi JIT. Serum steroid hormones and pituitary function in female epileptic patients during carbamazepine therapy. *Epilepsia*, 31, 438-445 (1990)

2838 Isojarvi JIT, Pakarinen AJ, Myllyla VV. Effects of carbamazepine therapy on serum sex hormone levels in male patients with epilepsy. *Epilepsia*, 29, 781-786 (1988)

2839 Isojarvi JIT, Pakarinen AJ, Myllyla VV. Thyroid function with antiepileptic drugs. *Epilepsia*, 33, 142-148 (1992)

2840 Isojarvi JIT, Pakarinen AJ, Ylipalosaari PJ et al. Serum hormones in male epileptic patients receiving anticonvulsant medication. *Arch Neurol*, 47, 670-676 (1990)

2841 Isojrvi JIT, Pakarinen AJ, Rautio A, et al. Serum sex hormone levels after replacing carbamazepine with oxcarbazepine. *Eur J Clin Pharmacol*, 47, 461-464 (1995)

2842 Isojrvi JIT, Repo M, Pakarinen AJ, et al. Carbamazepine, phenytoin, sex hormones, and sexual function in men with epilepsy. *Epilepsia*, 36, 366-370 (1995)

2843 Israel BC, Blouin RA, McIntyre W et al. Effects of interferon-α monotherapy on hepatic drug metabolism in cancer patients. *Br J Clin Pharmacol*, 36, 229-235 (1993)

2844 Israel R, O'Mara V, Austin B et al. Metoclopramide decreases renal plasma flow. *Clin Pharmacol Ther*, 39, 261-264 (1986)

2845 Itil TM, Stock MJ, Duffy AD et al. Therapeutic trials and EEG investigations with SCH-12,679. *Curr Ther Res*, 14, 136 (1972)

2846 Itoh H. Clinical pharmacology of ibopamine. *Am J Med*, 90, Suppl 5B, 36S-42S (1991)

2847 Itoh S, Ichinoe A, Tsukada Y et al. Hydralazine-induced hepatitis. *Hepatogastroenterology*, 28, 13-16 (1981)

2848 Itoh S, Tanaka K, Kumagae M et al. Effect of subcutaneous injection of a long-acting analogue of somatostatin (SMS 201-995) on plasma thyroid-stimulating hormone in normal human subjects. *Life Sci*, 42, 2691-2699 (1988)

2849 Itoh Y, Okanoue T, Sakamoto S et al. Serum autoantibody against interleukin-1α is unrelated to the etiology or activity of liver disease but can be raised by interferon treatment. *Am J Gastroenterol*, 90, 777-782 (1995)

2850 Itskovitz HD, Flamenbaum W, De Gaetano C et al. Effect of lovastatin on serum lipids in patients with nonfamilial primary hypercholesterolemia. *Clin Ther*, 11, 867-872 (1989)

2851 Iveson TJ, Ryley NG, Kelly PMA et al. Diclofenac associated hepatitis. *J Hepatol*, 10, 85-89 (1990)

2852 Iwahashi K, Miyatake R, Suwaki H et al. The drug-drug interaction effects of haloperidol on plasma carbamazepine levels. *Clin Neuropharmacol*, 18, 233-236 (1995)

2853 Izquierdo JM, Sotorrio P, Rodriguez M et al. Enzymatic determination of sodium in serum in a Cobas Fara analyzer. *Diag Lab*, 27, Suppl, 58 (1991)

2854 Jaatela A, Nikki P, Takki S et al. Effect of dextromoramide, fentanyl, and morphine on the plasma catecholamine levels. *Ann Clin Res*, 3, 107 (1971)

2855 Jablonski P, Owen JA. The clinical chemistry of bromosulfophthalein and other cholephilic dyes. *Adv Clin Chem*, 12, 209 (1969)

2856 Jabotinsky-Rubin K, Durst R, Levitin LA et al. Effects of haloperidol on human plasma magnesium. *J Psychiat Res*, 27, 155-159 (1993)

2857 Jackson B, Johnston CI. Angiotensin converting enzyme during acute and chronic enalapril therapy in essential hypertension. *Clin Exp Pharmacol Physiol*, 11, 355-359 (1984)

2858 Jackson CE, Meier DW. Routine serum magnesium analysis correlation with clinical state in 5,100 patients. *Ann Intern Med*, 69, 743 (1968)

2859 Jackson SH. Problems in screening infants for defects of amino acid metabolism. *Clin Biochem*, 6, 15 (1973)

2860 Jackson SH, Shak K, Debbas NM et al. The interaction between i.v. theophylline and chronic oral dosing with slow release nifedipine in volunteers. *Br J Clin Pharmacol*, 21, 389-392 (1986)

2861 Jackson ST, Rallison ML, Buntin WH et al. Use of oxandrolone for growth stimulation. *Am J Dis Child*, 126, 481 (1973)

2862 Jacob BG, Mohrle W, Richter WO et al. Short- and long term effects of lovasatin and pravastatin alone and in combination with cholestyramine on serum lipids, lipoproteins and apolipoproteins in primary hyercholesterolaemia. *Eur J Clin Pharmacol*, 42, 353-358 (1992)

2863 Jacob RA, Omaye ST, Skala JH et al. Experimental vitamin C depletion and supplementation in young men. Nutrient interactions and dental health effects. *Ann NY Acad Sci*, 498, 333-346 (1987)

2864 Jacob RA, Skala JH, Omaye ST et al. Effect of varying ascorbic acid intakes on copper absorption and ceruloplasmin levels of young men. *J Nutr*, 117, 2109-2115 (1987)

2865 Jacobs JC, Alexander NM. Colorimetry and constant-potential coulometry determinations of transferrin-bound iron, total iron-binding capacity, and total iron in serum containing iron-dextran, with use of sodium dithionite and alumina columns. *Clin Chem*, 36, 1803-1807 (1990)

2866 Jacobs LS, Snyder PJ, Wilber JF et al. Increased serum prolactin after administration of synthetic thyrotropin releasing hormone in man. *J Clin Endocrinol Metab*, 33, 996 (1971)

2867 Jacobs S, Pullan PT, Potter JM et al. Adrenal suppression following extradural steroids. *Anesthesia*, 38, 953-956 (1983)

2868 Jacobs SL, Fernandez AA. Hemoglobin in plasma. *Stand Meth Clin Chem*, 6, 107 (1970)

2869 Jacobson ED, Prior JT, Faloon WW. Malabsorptive syndrome induced by neomycin: morphologic alterations in the jejunal mucosa. *J Lab Clin Med*, 56, 245 (1960)

2870 Jacobson JM, Greenspan JS, Spritzler J, et al. Thalidomide for the treatment of oral aphthous ulcers in patients with human immunodeficiency virus infection. *N Engl J Med*, 336, 1487-1493 (1997)

2871 Jacobson MA, Bacchetti P, Kolokathis A et al. Surrogate markers for survival in patients with AIDS and AIDS related complex treated with zidovudine. *Br Med J*, 302, 73-78 (1991)

2872 Jacobson MA, Gambertoglio JG, Aweeka FT et al. Foscarnet-induced hypocalcemia and effects of foscarnet on calcium metabolism. *J Clin Endocrinol Metab*, 72, 1130-1135 (1991)

2873 Jacobus Pharmaceutical Co., Inc. Manufacturer's literature on Dapsone® . Princeton, NJ 08540 (1996)

2874 Jacobus Pharmaceutical Co., Inc. Manufacturer's literature on Paser® . Princeton, NJ 08540 (1996)

2875 Jacques PF, Hartz SC, McGandy RB et al. Ascorbic acid, HDL, and total plasma cholesterol in the elderly. *J Am Coll Nutr*, 6, 169-174 (1987)

2876 Jacques PF, Sulsky SI, Perrone GA et al. Ascorbic acid and plasma lipids. *Epidemiology*, 5, 19-26 (1994)

2877 Jadin-Starodoubsky A, Delwaide PA, Penders C et al. Psychotropic drug interferences with clinical chemistry determination. In:. *Reference Values in Human Chemistry. G Siest (ed)*, Karger, Basel, 1973, 299

2878 Jaeken J, Casaer P, Corbeel M. Valproate, hyperammonaemia and hyperglycinaemia. *Lancet*, 2, 260 (1980)

2879 Jaffe A, Matzkin H, Gilad S et al. Effect of 5-α-reductase inhibition on sex-hormone-binding globulin in elderly men. *Horm Res*, 41, 215-217 (1994)

2880 Jaffe BM, Behrman HR, Parker CW. Radioimmunoassay measurement of prostaglandins E, A and F in human plasma. *J Clin Invest*, 52, 398 (1973)

2881 Jaffe IA. Adverse effects profile of sulfhydryl compounds in man. *Am J Med*, 80, 471-476 (1986)

2882 Jaffe JM. Effect of propantheline on nitrofurantoin absorption. *J Pharmacol Sci*, 64, 1729-1730 (1975)

2883 Jaffe RM, Kasten B, Young DS et al. False-negative stool occult blood test caused by ingestion of ascorbic acid (vitamin C). *Ann Intern Med*, 83, 824-826 (1975)

2884 Jafri SM, Mammen EF, Masura J, Goldstein S. Effects of warfarin on markers of hypercoagulability in patients with heart failure. *Am Heart J*, 134, 27-36 (1997)

2885 Jaggarao NSV, Sheldon J, Grundy EN et al. The effects of amiodarone on thyroid function. *Postgrad Med J*, 58, 693-696 (1982)

2886 Jahnchen E, Meinertz T, Gilfrich HJ. Interaction of allopurinol with phenprocoumon in man. *Klin Wschr*, 55, 759-761 (1977)

2887 Jaillard J, Sezille G, Scherrereel P et al. Clinical and experimental studies of plasma-lipids modifications induced by alcohol. *Nutr Metab*, 13, 114 (1971)

2888 Jain A, Hoyt H. The early clinical evaluation of W-2354 in gout. *Clin Pharmacol Ther*, 13, 141 (1972)

2889 Jain AK, Ryan JR, McMahon FG. Potentiation of hypoglycemic effect of sulfonylureas by halofenate. *N Engl J Med*, 293, 1283-1286 (1975)

2890 Jakobsen JA, Nossen JO, Jorgensen NP et al. Renal tubular effects of diuretics and X-ray contrast media: a comparative study of equimolar doses in healthy volunteers. *Invest Radiol*, 28, 319-324 (1993)

2891 Jakobsson B, Berg U. Effect of hydrochlorothiazide and indomethacin treatment on renal function in nephrogenic diabetes insipidus. *Acta Paediat*, 83, 522-525 (1994)

2892 Jakubowski AA, Souza L, Kelly F et al. Effects of human granulocyte colony-stimulating factor in a patient with idiopathic neutropenia. *N Engl J Med*, 320, 38-42 (1989)

2893 James C, Prout BJ. Marrow suspension and intravenous cimetidine. *Lancet*, 1, 987 (1978)

2894 James O, Lesna M, Roberts SH et al. Liver damage after paracetamol overdose: comparison of liver function tests, fasting serum bile acids and liver histology. *Lancet*, 2, 579-581 (1975)

2895 James VHT, Mattingly D, Daly JR. Recommended method for the determination of plasma corticosteroids. *Br Med J*, 2, 310 (1971)

2896 Janka HU, Nuber A, Mehnert H. Metabolic effects of ramipril treatment in hypertensive subjects with non-insulin-dependent diabetes mellitus. *Arz Forsch Drug Res*, 40, 432-435 (1990)

2897 Jankowiak ME, Levier RR. Elimination of phosphorus interference in the colorimetric determination of silicon in biological material. *Anal Biochem*, 44, 462 (1971)

2898 Jansen PLM, Froeling PGAM, Schade RWB et al. Intrahepatic cholestasis in hyperthyroidism and the effect of antithyroid and β-blocking drugs. *Neth J Med*, 25, 318-324 (1982)

2899 Janssen Pharmaceutica, Inc. Manufacturer's literature on Alfenta® . Titusville, NJ 08560 (1994)

2900 Janssen Pharmaceutica, Inc. Manufacturer's literature on Ergamisol® . Titusville, NJ 08560 (1995)

2901 Janssen Pharmaceutica, Inc. Manufacturer's literature on Hismanal® . Titusville, NJ 08560 (1996)

2902 Janssen Pharmaceutica, Inc. Manufacturer's literature on Nizoral® . Titusville, NJ 08560 (1995)

2903 Janssen Pharmaceutica, Inc. Manufacturer's literature on Propulsid® . Titusville, NJ 08560 (1996)

2904 Janssen Pharmaceutica, Inc. Manufacturer's literature on Risperdal® . Titusville, NJ 08560 (1996)

2905 Janssen Pharmaceutica, Inc. Manufacturer's literature on Sporonox® . Titusville, NJ 08560 (1997)

2906 Janssen Pharmaceutica, Inc. Manufacturer's literature on Vermox® . Titusville, NJ 08560 (1993)

2907 Jansson J-H, Johansson B, Boman K et al. Effects of doxazosin and atenolol on the fibrinolytic system in patients with hypertension and elevated serum cholesterol. *Eur J Clin Pharmacol*, 40, 321-326 (1991)

2908 Jarowenko MV, Buren CTV, Kramer WG et al. Ranitidine, cimetidine and cyclosporine-treated recipient. *Transplantation*, 42, 311-312 (1986)

2909 Jarrett RJ, Graver HJ, Cohen NM. The effects of infusions of aminoacids, secretin and pancreozymin upon levels of blood sugar and plasma insulin. *Diabetologia*, 5, 421 (1969)

2910 Jarvie DR, Heyworth R, Simpson D. Plasma salicylate analysis: a comparison of colorimetric, HPLC and enzymatic techniques. *Ann Clin Biochem*, 24, 364-373 (1987)

2911 Javitt NB. The cholestatic syndrome - 1971. *Am J Med*, 51, 637 (1971)

2912 Jay RH, Sturley RH, Stirling C et al. Effects of pravastatin and cholestyramine on gonadal and adrenal steroid production in familial hypercholesterolemia. *Br J Clin Pharmacol*, 32, 417-422 (1991)

2913 Jeanjean M, Rousseau M, Harvengt C. Influence of cephalothin therapy on the estimation of 17-keto and 17-ketogenic sterolds. *Arch Int Pharmacol Ther*, 196, Suppl, 302 (1972)

2914 Jeavons PM. Non-dose-related side effects of valproate. *Epilepsia*, 25, Suppl 1, S50-S55 (1984)

2915 Jeavons PM. Sodium valproate and acute hepatic failure. *Dev Med Child Neurol*, 22, 547-548 (1980)

2916 Jefferson JW, Kalin NH. Serum lithium levels and long-term diuretic use. *J Am Med Ass*, 241, 1134-1136 (1979)

2917 Jefferys DB, Lessof MH, Mattock MB. Corticosteroid treatment, serum lipids and coronary artery disease. *Postgrad Med J*, 56, 491-493 (1980)

2918 Jeffrey RF, MacDonald TM, Rutter M et al. The effect of intravenous frusemide on urine dopamine in normal volunteers: studies with indomethacin and carbidopa. *Clin Sci*, 73, 151-157 (1987)

2919 Jelic Z, Majkic-Singh N, Spasic S et al. Effects of analgesic and antirheumatic drugs on the assay of serum enzymes. *J Clin Chem Clin Biochem*, 22, 559-563 (1984)

2920 Jelic-Ivanovic Z, Majkic-Singh N, Spasic S et al. Interference by analgesic and antirheumatic drugs in 25 common laboratory assays. *J Clin Chem Clin Biochem*, 23, 287-292 (1985)

2921 Jelic-Ivanovic Z, Pevcevic N. Fibrinogen determination by five methods in patients receiving streptokinase therapy. *Clin Chem*, 39, 698-699 (1993)

2922 Jelic-Ivanovic Z, Spasic S, Majkk-Singh N et al. Effects of some anti-inflammatory drugs on 12 blood constituents: protocol for the study of in vivo effects of drugs. *Clin Chem*, 31, 1141-1143 (1985)

2923 Jeng KY, Johnson J, Trimpe KL. Development of the AxSYM digoxin assay. *Clin Chem*, 41, S134 (1995)

2924 Jenkins D, Vannucci S, Lingenfelter D et al. CEDIA phenobarbital assay: development and evaluation of performance on the Hitachi 704. *Clin Chem*, 36, 1038 (1990)

2925 Jenkins DAS, Craig K, Cumming AD et al. The acute renal haemodynamic and endocrine response to felodipine in normal man. *Eur J Clin Pharmacol*, 33, 581-585 (1988)

2926 Jenkins RM, Evans DMD. Carbimazole hypersensitivity and liver damage. *Br J Clin Pract*, 35, 415-417 (1981)

2927 Jenner FA. Biochemical studies on the effects of lithium salts. *Biochem Soc Trans*, 1, 88 (1973)

2928 Jennings BH, Andersson K-E, Johansson SA. Assessment of systemic effects of inhaled glucocorticoids: comparison of the effects of inhaled budesonide and oral prednisolone on adrenal function and markers of bone turnover. *Eur J Clin Pharmacol*, 40, 77-82 (1991)

2929 Jensen OB, Mosdal C, Reske-Nielsen E. Hypokalemic myopathy during treatment with diuretics. *Acta Neurol Scand*, 55, 465-482 (1977)

2930 Jensen T, Johanson N, Brudzinski A et al. Specific measurements of cyclosoprin A in kidney, heart, and liver transplant patients by RIA with a monoclonal antibody and ^{125}I tracer. *Clin Chem*, 37, 1019 (1991)

2931 Jensen T, Stender S, Goldstein K et al. Partial normalization by dietary cod liver oil of increased microvascular albumin leakage in patients with insulin-dependent diabetes and albuminuria. *N Engl J Med*, 321, 1572-1577 (1989)

2932 Jepsen LV, Pedersen KH. Changes in zinc and zinc-dependent enzymes in rheumatoid patients during penicillamine treatment. *Scand J Rheumatol*, 13, 282-288 (1984)

2933 Jerling JC, Vorster HH, Oosthuizen W, Vermaak WJH. Effecti of simvastatin, a 3-hydroxy-3-methylglutaryl coenzyme A reductase inhibitor, on the haemostatic balance of familial hypercholesterolemic subjects. *Fibrinolysis*, 11, 91-96 (1997)

2934 Jespersen J, Ingeberg S, Bach E. Antithrombin III and platelets during the normal menstrual cycle and in women receiving oral contraceptives low in oestrogen. *Gynecol Obstet Invest*, 15, 153-162 (1983)

2935 Jeurissen MEC, Boerbooms AMT, Van de Putte LBA. Pancytopenia related to azathioprine in rheumatoid arthritis. *Ann Rheum Dis*, 47, 503-505 (1988)

2936 Ji TH. Interference by detergents, chelating agents and buffers with the Lowry protein determination. *Anal Biochem*, 52, 517 (1973)

2937 Jie K-SG, Gijsbers BLMG, Knapen MHJ et al. Effects of vitamin K and oral anticoagulants on urinary calcium excretion. *Br J Haematol*, 83, 100-104 (1993)

2938 Jilma B, Stohlawetz P, Pernerstorfer T, et al. Glucocorticoids dose-dependently increase plasma levels of granulocyte colony stimulating factor in man. *J Clin Endocrinol Metab*, 83, 1037-1039 (1998)

2939 Joborn C, Ljunghall S, Larsson K et al. Skeletal responsiveness to parathyroid hormone in healthy females: relationship to menopause and oestrogen replacement. *Clin Endocrinol*, 34, 335-339 (1991)

2940 Joffe BI, Haitas B, Edelstein D et al. Clonidine and the hormonal responses to graded exercise in healthy subjects. *Horm Res*, 23, 136-141 (1986)

2941 Joffe RT, Kellner CH, Post RM et al. Lithium increases platelet count. *N Engl J Med*, 311, 674 (1984)

2942 Johannessen SI, Strandjord RE, Munthe-Kass AW. Lack of effect of clonazepam on serum levels of diphenylhydantoin, phenobarbital and carbamazepine. *Acta Neurol Scand*, 55, 506-512 (1977)

2943 Johannson E. Androgen levels in women using Norplant implants. *Contraception*, 34, 157-167 (1986)

2944 Johansson AG, Baylink DJ, Ekenstam E et al. Circulating levels of insulin-like growth factor-I and -II, and IGF-binding protein-3 in inflammation and after parathyroid hormone infusion. *Bone Miner*, 24, 25-31 (1994)

2945 Johansson B, Roos BE. 5-hydroxyindoleacetic and homovanillic acid levels in the cerebrospinal fluid of healthy volunteers and patients. *Life Sci*, 6, 1449 (1967)

2946 Johansson C, Adamsson U, Stierner U et al. Interaction by cholestyramine on the uptake of hydrocortisone in the gastrointestinal tract. *Acta Med Scand*, 204, 509-512 (1978)

2947 Johansson J, Carlson LA. The effects of nicotinic acid treatment on high density lipoprotein particle size subclass levels in hyperlipidaemic subjects. *Atherosclerosis*, 83, 207-216 (1990)

2948 Johansson J, Molgaard J, Olsson AG. Plasma high density lipoprotein particle size alteration by simvastatin treatment in patients with hypercholesterolaemia. *Atherosclerosis*, 91, 175-184 (1991)

2949 Johansson SA. Apparent resistance to oral anticoagulant therapy and influence of hypnotics on some coagulation factors. *Acta Med Scand*, 184, 297 (1968)

2950 John VA, Monk JP, Dorhofer G. Interference of an oxprenolol metabolite with screening tests for 5-hydroxyindole in urine. *Clin Chem*, 29, 743-744 (1983)

2951 Johnson BF. Diazoxide and renal function in man. *Clin Pharmacol Ther*, 12, 815 (1971)

2952 Johnson BF. The diuretic action of an azido pyrimidine in man. *Clin Pharmacol Ther*, 11, 77 (1970)

2953 Johnson BF. The emerging problem of plasma lipid changes during antihypertensive therapy. *J Cardiovasc Pharmacol*, 4, Suppl 2, S213-S221 (1982)

2954 Johnson BF, Errichetti A, Urbach D et al. The effect of once daily minoxidil on blood pressure and plasma lipids.. *J Clin Pharmacol*, 26, 534-538 (1986)

2955 Johnson BF, Wilson J, Johnson J et al. Digoxin pharmacokinetics and spirapril, a new ACE inhibitor. *J Clin Pharmacol*, 31, 527-530 (1991)

2956 Johnson BF, Wilson J, Marwaha R et al. The comparative effects of verapamil and a new dihydropyridine calcium channel blocker on digoxin pharmacokinetics. *Clin Pharmacol Ther*, 42, 66-71 (1987)

2957 Johnson BJ, Romero L, Johnson J et al. Comparative effects of propranolol and prazosin upon serum lipids in thiazide treated hypertensive patients. *Am J Med*, 76, Suppl 2a, 109-112 (1984)

2958 Johnson MR, Lydiard RB, Morton WA et al. Effect of fluvoxamine, imipramine and placebo on catecholamine function in depressed outpatients. *J Psychiat Res*, 27, 161-172 (1993)

2959 Johnson PE, Milne DB, Lykken GI. Effects of age and sex on copper absorption, biological half-life, and status in humans. *Am J Clin Nutr*, 56, 917-925 (1992)

2960 Johnson PJ, McFarlane IG, Williams R. Azathioprine for long-term maintenance of remission in autoimmune hepatitis. *N Engl J Med*, 333, 958-963 (1995)

2961 Johnston BB. Diabetes mellitus in patients on lithium. *Lancet*, 2, 935-936 (1977)

2962 Johnston DG, Gill A, Orskov H et al. Metabolic effects of cortisol in man - studies with somatostatin. *Metabolism*, 31, 312-317 (1982)

2963 Johnston J, McLelland A, O'Reilly DStJ. The relationship between serum cholesterol and serum thyroid hormones in male patients with suspected hypothyroidism. *Ann Clin Biochem*, 30, 256-259 (1993)

2964 Johnston RR, Cromwell TH, Eger EI II et al. The toxicity of fluroxene in animals and man. *Anesthesiology*, 38, 313 (1973)

2965 Jones CC. Megaloblastic anemia associated with long-term tetracycline therapy. *Ann Intern Med*, 78, 910 (1973)

2966 Jones DG, Turnbull MJ, Lenman JAR et al. Effect of amantadine on the urinary excretion of some monoamines and metabolites in normal and Parkinsonian subjects. *J Neurol Sci*, 17, 245 (1972)

2967 Jones DH, King K, Miller AJ et al. A dose-response study of 13-cis-retinoic acid in acne vulgaris. *Br J Dermatol*, 108, 333-343 (1983)

2968 Jones DW, Sands CD. Lack of effect of hydrochlorothiazide on total cholesterol. *Clin Exp Hypertens*, 16, 675-689 (1994)

2969 Jones GW, Ashwood ER. Enzymatic measurement of phosphatidylglycerol in amniotic fluid. *Clin Chem*, 40, 518-525 (1994)

2970 Jones IR, Swai A, Taylor R et al. Lowering of plasma glucose concentrations with bezafibrate in patients with moderately controlled NIDDM. *Diabetes Care*, 13, 855-863 (1990)

2971 Jones Medical Industries, Inc. Manufacturer's literature on Tapazole® . St. Louis, MO 63146 (1996)

2972 Jones MF, Caldwell JR. Acute hemorrhagic pancreatitis associated with administration of chlorthalidone. *N Engl J Med*, 267, 1029 (1962)

2973 Jones PE, Oelbaum MH. Frusemide-induced pancreatitis. *Br Med J*, 1, 133-134 (1975)

2974 Jones PH, Farmer JA, Cressman MD et al. Once-daily pravastatin in patients with primary hypercholesterolemia: a dose-response study. *Clin Cardiol*, 14, 146-151 (1991)

2975 Jones R, Klette K, Kuhlman JJ et al. Trimethobenzamide cross-reacts in imunoassays of amphetamine/methamphetamine. *Clin Chem*, 39, 699-700 (1993)

2976 Jones RJ, Dobrilovic L. Lipoprotein lipid alterations with cholestyramine administration. *J Lab Clin Med*, 75, 953 (1970)

2977 Jonkers R, Van Boxtel CJ, Oosterhuis B. β_2-adrenoreceptor-mediated hypokalaemia and its abolition by oxprenolol. *Clin Pharmacol Ther*, 42, 627-633 (1987)

2978 Jonkman JHG, Nicholson KG, Farrow PR et al. Effects of α-interferon on theophylline pharmacokinetics and metabolism. *Br J Clin Pharmacol*, 27, 795-802 (1989)

2979 Jonkman JM, Van Der Boon WJ, Schoenmaker R et al. Clinical pharmacokinetics of theophylline during cotreatment with cefaclor. *Int J Clin Pharmacol Ther Toxicol*, 24, 88-92 (1986)

2980 Jonsson LE, Lewander T, Gunne LM. Amphetamine psychosis: urinary excretion of catecholamines. *Res Comm Chem Pathol Pharmacol*, 2, 355 (1971)

2981 Joos C, Kewitz H, Reinhold-Kourniati D. Effects of diuretics on plasma lipoproteins in healthy men. *Eur J Clin Pharmacol*, 17, 251-257 (1980)

2982 Jordan VC, Fritz NF, Langan-Fahey S et al. Alteration of endocrine parameters in premenopausal women with breast cancer during long-term adjuvant therapy with tamoxifen as the single agent. *J Natl Cancer Inst*, 83, 1488-1491 (1991)

2983 Joubert PH, Aucamp AK, Potgieter GM et al. Epilepsy and IgA deficiency - the effects of sodium valproate. *S Afr Med J*, 52, 642-644 (1977)

2984 Jovanovic SD, Banic B, Jovanovic E. Influence of salicylates on the activity of AAP, LAP and GGT in urine. *Jugosl Med Biokem*, 2, 188-191 (1983)

2985 Jubiz W, Meikle AW. Alterations of glucocorticoid actions by other drugs and disease states. *Drugs*, 18, 113-121 (1979)

2986 Juhl RP, Summers RW, Guillory JK et al. Effect of sulfasalazine on digoxin bioavailability. *Clin Pharmacol Ther*, 20, 387-394 (1976)

2987 Jukema JW, Bruschke AVG, van Bowen AJ et al. Effects of lipid lowering by pravastatin on progression and regression of coronary artery disease in symptomatic men with normal to moderately elevated serum cholesterol levels: the regression growth evaluation statin study (REGRESS). *Circulation*, 91, 2528-2540 (1995)

2988 Julius S, Pascual AV, Abbrecht PH et al. Effect of β-adrenergic blockage on plasma volume in human subjects. *Proc Soc Exp Biol Med*, 140, 982 (1972)

2989 Julius U, Fritsch H, Fritsch W et al. Impact of hormone replacement therapy on postprandial lipoproteins and lipoprotein (a) in normolipidemic postmenopausal women. *Clin Investig*, 72, 502-507 (1994)

2990 June CH, Thompson CB, Kennedy MS et al. Profound hypomagnesemia and renal magnesium wasting associated with the use of cyclosporine for marrow transplantation. *Transplantation*, 39, 620-624 (1985)

2991 Jung DH, Parekh AC. A new color reaction for cholesterol assay. *Clin Chim Acta*, 35, 73 (1971)

2992 Jung DH, Parekh AC. Urinary inorganic phosphorus determinations. *J Clin Pathol*, 25, 263 (1972)

2993 Jung K, Laube C, Lein M, et al. Kind of sample as preanalytical determinant of matrix metalloproteinases 2 and 9 and tissue inhibitor of metalloproteinase 2 in blood. *Clin Chem*, 44, 1060-1062 (1998)

2994 Jung-Hoffman C, Heidt F, Kuhl H. Effect of two oral contraceptives containing 30 μg ethinylestradiol and 75 μg gestodene or 150 μg desogestrel upon various hormonal parameters. *Contraception*, 38, 593-603 (1988)

2995 Jungst G, Mohr R. Side effects of ofloxacin in clinical trials and in postmarketing surveillance. *Drugs*, 34, suppl 1, 144-149 (1987)

2996 Jurgensen HJ. Comparative effects of pinacidil and nifedipine in the treatment of arterial hypertension. *Drugs*, 36, Suppl 7, 67-69 (1988)

2997 Kaaja R, Valtonen VV. Leucopenia associated with β-lactam antibiotic therapy. *Acta Med Scand*, 216, 531-534 (1984)

2998 Kabasakalian P, Kalliney S, Westcott A. Determination of uric acid in serum with use of uricase and tribromophenol-aminoantipyrine chromogen. *Clin Chem*, 19, 522 (1973)

2999 Kabat HF. Clinical Pharmacy Handbook. Philadelphia PA, Lea and Febiger (1969)

3000 Kaczmarski RS, Mufti GJ. Low-dose filgrastim therapy for chronic neutropenia. *N Engl J Med*, 329, 1280-1281 (1993)

3001 Kader A, ELiu H. Interference of anthracycline derivatives with measurement of proteins with BCA. *Clin Chem*, 43, 2201-2202 (1997)

3002 Kahan Z, Toth I, Vecsernyes M. Low-dose aminoglutethimide therapy without glucocorticoid administration: Clinical and hormonal findings. *Oncology*, 49, 31-34 (1992)

3003 Kahn JB. Oxacillin-induced agranulocytosis. *J Am Med Ass*, 240, 2632 (1978)

3004 Kahn RS, Knott P, Gabriel S et al. Effect of m-chlorophenylpiperazine on plasma homovanillic acid concentrations in healthy subjects. *Biol Psychiat*, 32, 1055-1061 (1992)

3005 Kahn SE, Labbe RF, Pfadenhauer EH et al. Multicenter evaluation of automated immunoturbidimetric aasays for measurement of apolipoproteins A-I and B in serum or plasma. *Clin Chem*, 40, 1722-1729 (1994)

3006 Kahri J, Vuorinen-Markkola H, Tilly-Kiesi M et al. Effect of gemfibrozil on high density lipoprotein subspecies in non-insulin dependent diabetes mellitus. Relations to lipolytic enzymes and to the cholesteryl ester transfer protein activity. *Atherosclerosis*, 102, 79-89 (1993)

3007 Kairisto V, Koskinen P, Mattila K et al. Reference intervals for 24-h urinary normetanephrine, metanephrine, and 3-methoxy-4-hydroxymandelic acid in hypertensive patients. *Clin Chem*, 38, 416-420 (1992)

3008 Kaldor A, Demeczky L, Juvancz P. The effect of disulfiram on the blood catecholamine level in man. *Int Zeitschr Klin Pharmacol Ther Toxicol*, 5, 284 (1971)

3009 Kaldor A, Juvancz P, Demeczky M et al. Enhancement of methyldopa metabolism with barbiturate. *Br Med J*, 3, 518 (1971)

3010 Kalesh DG, Mallikarjuneswara VR, Clemetson CAB. Effect of estrogen-containing oral contraceptives on platelet and plasma ascorbic acid concentrations. *Contraception*, 4, 183 (1971)

3011 Kalff R, Houtkooper MA, Meyer JWA et al. Carbamazepine and serum sodium levels. *Epilepsia*, 25, 390-397 (1984)

3012 Kalkhoff RK. Effects of oral contraceptive agents and sex steroids on carbohydrate metabolism. *Ann Rev Med*, 23, 429 (1972)

3013 Kallenberg CGM, Hoorntje SJ, Smit AJ et al. Antinuclear and antinative DNA antibodies during captopril treatment. *Acta Med Scand*, 211, 297-300 (1982)

3014 Kallio J, Karlsson R, Toppari J, et al. Antenatal dexamethasone treatment decreases plasma catecholamine levels in preterm infants. *Pediatr Res*, 43, 801-807 (1998)

3015 Kalliomaki JL. A therapeutic trial with a combination of trimethoprim-sulfamethoxazole in rheumatoid arthritis. *Curr Ther Res*, 14, 22 (1972)

3016 Kalowski S, Nanra RS, Mathew TH et al. Deterioration in renal function in association with co-trimoxazole therapy. *Lancet*, 1, 394 (1973)

3017 Kamali F. The effect of probenecid on paracetamol metabolism and pharmacokinetics. *Eur J Clin Pharmacol*, 45, 551-553 (1993)

3018 Kamali F, Thomas SHL, Edwards C. The influence of steady-state ciprofloxacin on the pharmacokinetics and pharmacodynamics of a single dose of diazepam in healthy volunteers. *Eur J Clin Pharmacol*, 44, 365-367 (1993)

3019 Kamban JR, Naukam RJ, Sastry BVR. The effect of procainamide on plasma cholinesterase activity. *Can J Anaes*, 34, 579-581 (1987)

3020 Kamerud JO, Schwartz TR, Heinzerling RH. Solid-phase total testosterone RIA. *Clin Chem*, 38, 1094 (1992)

3021 Kamiya Biomedical Company. K-Assay NAG enzyme assay reagent. CA

3022 Kamoun PP, Bardet JI, Di Giulio S et al. Measurements of angiotensin converting enzyme in captopril-treated patients. *Clin Chim Acta*, 118, 333-336 (1982)

3023 Kamper A-L, Nielsen OJ. Effect of enalapril on haemoglobin and serum erythropoietin in patients with chronic nephropathy. *Scand J Clin Lab Invest*, 50, 611-618 (1990)

3024 Kamper A-L, Thomsen HS, Nielsen NL et al. Initial effect of enalapril on kidney function in patients with moderate to severe chronic nephropathy. *Scand J Urol Nephrol*, 24, 69-73 (1990)

3025 Kane FJ Jr, Moore LP. Hepatotoxicity occurring with thioridazine therapy. *South Med J*, 64, 573 (1971)

3026 Kaneko K, Fujimori S, Ishizuka I et al. Effect of ethanol on metabolism of the hypouricemic agents allopurinol and benzbromarone. *Clin Chim Acta*, 193, 181-186 (1990)

3027 Kaneko S. Antiepileptic drug therapy and reproductive consequences: functional and morphologic effects. *Reprod Toxicol*, 5, 179-198 (1991)

3028 Kanel KT, Wolmark N, Thompson PD. Delayed severe hypertriglyceridemia with tamoxifen. *N Engl J Med*, 337, 281 (1997)

3029 Kanno K, Sasaki S, Hirata Y et al. Urinary excretion of aquaporin-2 in patients with diabetes insipidus. *N Engl J Med*, 332, 1540-1545 (1995)

3030 Kanoh T, Jingami H, Uschino H. Aplastic anemia after prolonged treatment with chlorpheniramine. *Lancet*, 1, 546-547 (1977)

3031 Kansal PC, Buse J, Talbert OR et al. The effect of L-dopa on plasma growth hormone, insulin, and thyroxine. *J Clin Endocrinol Metab*, 34, 99 (1972)

3032 Kapil RP, Axelson JE, Mansfield IL et al. Disopyramide pharmacokinetics and metabolism: effect of inducers. *Br J Clin Pharmacol*, 24, 781-791 (1987)

3033 Kaplan A. Urea nitrogen and urinary ammonia. *Stand Meth Clin Chem*, 5, 245 (1965)

3034 Kaplan B, Cardarelli C, Pinnell SR. Levamisole and agranulocytosis. *Cutis*, 24, 429-430 (1979)

3035 Kaplan LA, Fearn JA, Laskarzewski PM et al. Serum ubiquinone Q10 levels: effect of cholesterol-lowering drugs. *Clin Chem*, 36, 963 (1990)

3036 Kaplan NM. Effects of guanabenz on plasma lipid levels in hypertensive patients. *J Cardiovasc Pharmacol*, 6, Suppl 5, S841-S846 (1984)

3037 Kaplan RP, Russell DH, Lowe NJ. Etrinate therapy for psoriasis: clinical responses, remission times, epidermal DNA, and polyamine responses. *J Am Acad Dermatol*, 8, 95-102 (1983)

3038 Kara M, Hasinoff BB, McKay DW et al. Clinical and chemical interactions between iron preparations and ciprofloxacin. *Br J Clin Pharmacol*, 31, 257-261 (1991)

3039 Karachalios GN, Parigorakis JG. Thrombocytopenia and sulindac. *Ann Intern Med*, 104, 128 (1986)

3040 Karawajczyk M, Höglund M, Ericsson J, et al. Administration of G-CSF to healthy subjects: the effects on eosinophil counts and mobilization of eosinophil granule proteins. *Br J Haematol*, 96, 259-265 (1997)

3041 Karege F, Widmer J, Bovier P et al. Platelet serotonin and plasma tryptophan in depressed patients: effect of drug treatment and clinical outcome. *Neuropsychopharmacology*, 10, 207-214 (1994)

3042 Karim A, Nissen C, Azarnoff DL. Clinical pharmacokinetics of disopyramide. *J Pharmacokinet Biopharm*, 10, 465-494 (1982)

3043 Kark RAP, Poskanzer DC, Bullock JD et al. Mercury poisoning and its treatment with N-acetyl-δ-L-penicillamine. *N Engl J Med*, 285, 10 (1971)

3044 Kark RM. Proteinuria II: diagnosis and management. *Hosp Pract*, 6, 59 (1971)

3045 Karkalas Y, Lal H. Jaundice following therapy with imipramine and cyproheptadine. *Clin Toxicol*, 4, 47 (1971)

3046 Karkkainen J, Raisanen M. Nialamide, an MAO inhibitor, increases urinary excretion of endogenously produced bufotenin in man. *Biol Psychiat*, 32, 1042-1048 (1992)

3047 Karlberg BE, Lins LE, Rossner S. Clonidine in mild to moderate hypertension: effects on blood pressure and serum lipoproteins. *J Hypertens*, 3, Suppl, S69-S71 (1985)

3048 Karlson BW, Henning R, Waern AU. Doxazosin and atenolol in mild-to-moderate hypertension. A double-blind 20-week trial with special regard to blood pressure lowering and effects on serum lipoproteins. *Curr Ther Res*, 43, 1003-1009 (1988)

3049 Karlsson R, Eden S, von Schoultz B. Altered growth hormone secretion during oral contraception. *Gynecol Obstet Invest*, 30, 234-238 (1990)

3050 Karon BS, Daly TM, Scott MG. Mechanisms of dopamine and dobutamine interference in biochemical tests that use peroxide and peroxidase to generate chromophore. *Clin Chem*, 44, 155-160 (1998)

3051 Karpatkin S. Drug-induced thrombocytopenia. *Am J Med Sci*, 262, 68 (1971)

3052 Karrenbrock B, Heim J-M, Gerzer R. Effect of molsidomine on ex vivo platelet aggregation and plasma guanosine 3'-5'-cyclic monophosphate levels in healthy volunteers. *Klin Wschr*, 68, 213-217 (1990)

3053 Kasich AM. Clorazepate dipotassium in the treatment of anxiety associated with chronic gastrointestinal disease. *Curr Ther Res*, 15, 83 (1973)

3054 Kasim SE, Bagchi N, Brown TR. Amiodarone-induced changes in lipid metabolism. *Horm Metab Res*, 22, 385-388 (1990)

3055 Kasiske BL, Tortorice KL, Heim-Duhoy KL et al. Lovastatin treatment of hypercholesterolemia in renal transplant recipients. *Transplantation*, 49, 95-100 (1990)

3056 Kassiandes C, Nussenblatt R, Palestine AG et al. Liver injury from cyclosporine A. *Dig Dis Sci*, 35, 693-697 (1990)

3057 Kassianides C, Nussenblatt R, Palestine AG et al. Liver injury from cyclosporine A. *Dig Dis Sci*, 35, 693-697 (1990)

3058 Kaste M, Muuronen A, Nikkila EA. Increase of low serum concentrations of high-density lipoprotein (HDL) cholesterol in TIA-patients treated with phenytoin. *Stroke*, 14, 525-530 (1983)

3059 Kastrup J, Petersen P, Bartram R et al. The effect of trimethoprim on serum creatinine. *Br J Urol*, 57, 265-268 (1985)

3060 Kataoka K, Kanamori N, Oishi M et al. Vitamin E status in pediatric patients receiving antiepileptic drugs. *Dev Pharmacol Ther*, 14, 96-101 (1990)

3061 Kater RMH. Double blind evaluation of analgesic and toxic effects of flufenamic acid and mefenamic acid. *Med J Aust*, 1, 848 (1968)

3062 Kates RE, Yee YG, Kirsten EB. Interaction between warfarin and propafenone in healthy volunteer subjects. *Clin Pharmacol Ther*, 42, 305-311 (1987)

3063 Katila H, Appelberg B, Hurme M et al. Plasma levels of interleukin-1β and interleukin-6 in schizophrenia, other psychoses, and affective disorders. *Schiz Res*, 12, 29-34 (1994)

3064 Kato DB. Dilutional hyponatremia and water intoxication during carbamazepine therapy. *Drug Intell Clin Pharm*, 12, 392-396 (1978)

3065 Katsilambros N, Braaten J, Ferguson BD et al. Muscular syndrome after clofibrate. *N Engl J Med*, 286, 1110 (1972)

3066 Katz WA, Blodgett RC Jr, Pietrusko RG. Proteinuria in gold-treated rheumatoid arthritis. *Ann Intern Med*, 101, 176-179 (1984)

3067 Katzeff HL, Yang M-U, Presta E et al. Calorie restriction and iopanoic acid effects on thyroid hormone metabolism. *Am J Clin Nutr*, 52, 263-266 (1990)

3068 Katzman PL, Henningsen NC, Fagher B et al. Renal and endocrine effects of long-term coverting enzyme inhibition as compared with calcium antagonism in essential hypertension. *J Cardiovasc Pharmacol*, 15, 360-364 (1990)

3069 Katzman PL, Hulthen UL, Hokfelt B. The effect of 8 weeks treatment with the calcium antagonist felodipine on blood pressure, heart rate, working capacity, plasma renin activity, plasma angiotensin II, urinary catecholamines and aldosterone in patients with essential hypertension. *Br J Clin Pharmacol*, 21, 633-640 (1986)

3070 Kaufman F. A rare complication of sulfadimethoxine (madribon) therapy. *Calif Med*, 107, 344 (1967)

3071 Kaukonen K-M, Olkkola KT, Neuvonen PJ. Itraconazole increases plasma concentrations of quinidine. *Clin Pharmacol Ther*, 62, 510-517 (1997)

3072 Kaul A, Reddy JC, Fagman E et al. Hepatitis associated with use of sulindac in a child. *J Pediatr*, 99, 650-651 (1981)

3073 Kauppinen-Makelin R, Bjorses UM, Turpeinen U et al. Interference of iodine-containing contrast materials with assay of urinary 17-ketogenic steroids. *Clin Chem*, 34, 2160-2161 (1988)

3074 Kawakatsu K, Kino T, Yasuba H et al. Effect of Ozagrel (OKY-046), a thromboxane synthetase inhibitor, on theophylline pharmacokinetics in asthmatic patients. *Int J Clin Pharmacol Ther Toxicol*, 28, 158-163 (1990)

3075 Kawamura M, Imanishi M, Matsushima Y et al. A comparison of lisinopril with enalapril by monitoring plasma angiotensin II levels in humans. *Jpn J Pharmacol*, 54, 143-149 (1990)

3076 Kayser L, Perrild H, Feldt-Rasmussen U et al. The thyroid function and size in healthy man during 3 weeks treatment with β-adrenoceptor-antagonists. *Horm Metab Res*, 23, 35-37 (1991)

3077 Kayser L, Perrild H, Fogh-Andersen N et al. Serum phosphate increase during short term β-adrenoceptor blockade in thyrotoxicosis. *Acta Med Scand*, 222, 143-146 (1987)

3078 Kazierad DJ, Martin DE, Blum RA, et al. Effect of fluconazole on the pharmacokinetics of eprosartan and losartan in healthy male volunteers. *Clin Pharmacol Ther*, 62, 417-425 (1997)

3079 Kazmier FJ. A significant interaction between metronidazole and warfarin. *Mayo Clin Proc*, 51, 782-784 (1976)

3080 Kazumi T, Yoshino G, Ishida Y et al. Long-term efficacy and tolerability of pravastatin in hypercholesterolemia in patients with non-insulin-dependent diabetes mellitus. *Diabetes Res Clin Pract*, 27, 61-68 (1995)

3081 Kazumi T, Yoshino G, Matsuba K et al. Effects of bezafibrate on plasma apolipoproteins, lipid concentration, and compositions of lipoproteins in patients with type IV hyperlipoproteinemia. *Curr Ther Res*, 44, 1035-1044 (1988)

3082 Kazumi T, Yoshino G, Ohki A et al. Long-term effects of simvastatin in hypercholesterolemic patients with NIDDM and additional atherosclerotic risk factors. *Horm Metab Res*, 27, 239-243 (1995)

3083 Kazumi T, Yoshino G, Okutani T et al. Plasma lipoprotein and apolipoprotein concentrations and glycemic control during short-term treatment with nifedipine in hypertensive patients with type II diabetes mellitus. *Curr Ther Res*, 46, 951-958 (1989)

3084 Kean WF, Anastassiades TP, Dwosh IL et al. Efficacy and toxicity of D-penicillamine for rheumatoid disease in the elderly. *J Am Geriatr Soc*, 30, 94-100 (1982)

3085 Kean WF, Dwosh IL, Anastassiades TP et al. The toxicity pattern of D-penicillamine therapy: a guide to its use in rheumatoid arthritis. *Arth Rheum*, 23, 158-164 (1980)

3086 Keber I, Lavre J, Suc S et al. The decrease of plasminogen activator inhibitor after normalization of triglycerides during treatment with fibrates. *Fibrinolysis*, 8, 57-59 (1994)

3087 Keech AC, Harper RW, Harrison PM et al. Pharmacokinetic interaction between oral metoprolol and verapamil for angina pectoris. *Am J Cardiol*, 58, 551-552 (1986)

3088 Keefe EB, Reis TC, Berland JE. Hepatotoxicity to both erythromycin estolate and ethylsuccinate. *Dig Dis Sci*, 27, 701-704 (1982)

3089 Keefe EB, Sunderland MC, Gabourel JD. Serum γ-Glutamyl transpeptidase activity in patients receiving chronic phenytoin therapy. *Dig Dis Sci*, 31, 1056-1061 (1986)

3090 Keenan BS, Johnsonbaugh RE, Sode J. Discordant serum growth hormone responses to i.v. and i.m. administration of synthetic 1-24 corticotropin (ACTH). *Clin Res*, 20, 866 (1972)

3091 Keenan J, Thompson JB, Chamberlain MA et al. Prolonged corticotrophic action of a synthetic substituted 1-18 ACTH. *Br Med J*, 3, 742 (1971)

3092 Keilani T, Schlueter WA, Levin ML et al. Improvement of lipid abnormalities associated with proteinuria using fosinopril, an angiotensin-converting enzyme inhibitor. *Ann Intern Med*, 118, 24-254 (1993)

3093 Kelestimur F, Utas C, Ozbakir O, et al. The effects of octreotide in a patient with Nelson's Syndrome. *Postgrad Med J*, 72, 53-54 (1996)

3094 Keller DF. G-6-PD Deficiency. Cleveland OH, CRC Press (1971)

3095 Kelley WN, Goldfinger SE, Hardy HL. Hyperuricemia in chronic beryllium disease. *Ann Intern Med*, 70, 977 (1969)

3096 Kelley WN, Rosenbloom FM, Seegmiller JE. The effects of azathioprine (Imuran®) on purine synthesis in clinical disorders of purine metabolism. *J Clin Invest*, 46, 1518 (1967)

3097 Kellner R, Gervais RH, Pathak D. A pilot study of the short-term antianxiety effects of molindone HCl. *J Clin Pharmacol*, 12, 472 (1972)

3098 Kelly JP, Kaufman DW, Shapiro S. Risks of agranulocytosis and aplastic anemia in relation to the use of cardiovascular drugs: the International agranulocytosis and aplastic anemia study. *Clin Pharmacol Ther*, 49, 330-341 (1991)

3099 Kelly KL. Ranitidine cross-reactivity in the EMIT d.a.u. monoclonal amphetamine/methamphetamine assay. *Clin Chem*, 36, 1391-1392 (1990)

3100 Kelsey WM, Schary JM. Fatal hepatitis probably due to indomethacin. *J Am Med Ass*, 199, 586 (1967)

3101 Kelton JG. Impaired reticuloendothelial function in patients treated with methyldopa. *N Engl J Med*, 313, 596-600 (1985)

3102 Kelton JG, Meltzer D, Moore J et al. Drug-induced thrombocytopenia is associated with increased binding of IgG to platelets both in vivo and in vitro. *Blood*, 58, 524-529 (1981)

3103 Kemmer TP, Malfertheiner P, Buchler M et al. Inhibition of human exocrine pancreatic secretion by the long-acting soamatostatin analogue octreotide (SMS 201-995). *Aliment Phamacol Therap*, 6, 41-50 (1992)

3104 Kemper A, Koalick F, Thiele H et al. Cortisol and β-endorphin response in alcoholics and alcohol abusers following a high naloxone dosage. *Drug Alcohol Dep*, 25, 319-326 (1990)

3105 Kendall MJ, Nutter S, Hawkins CF. Xylose test: effect of aspirin and indomethacin. *Br Med J*, 1, 532 (1971)

3106 Kendall MJ, Quarterman CP, Jack DB et al. Metoprolol pharmacokinetics and the oral contraceptive pill. *Br J Clin Pharmacol*, 14, 120-122 (1982)

3107 Kendall-Taylor P. Hyperthyroidism. *Br Med J*, 2, 337 (1972)

3108 Kennedy P. Liver cross-sensitivity to antipsychotic drugs. *Br J Psychiat*, 143, 312 (1983)

3109 Kent JR, Hill M, Parlow AF et al. Estrogenic supression of the pituitary-gonadal axis and prostatic function. *Clin Pharmacol Ther*, 13, 144 (1972)

3110 Kenwright S, Levi AJ. Impairment of hepatic uptake of rifamycin antibiotics by probenecid and its therapeutic implications. *Lancet*, 2, 1401-1405 (1973)

3111 Kerr DJ, Graham J, Cummings J et al. The effect of verapamil on the pharmacokinetics of adriamycin. *Cancer Chemother Pharmacol*, 18, 239-242 (1986)

3112 Kerry RJ, Ludlow JM, Owen G. Diuretics are dangerous with lithium. *Br Med J*, 281, 371 (1980)

3113 Kes P, Reiner Z. Symptomatic hypomagnesemia associated with gentamicin therapy. *Magnesium Trace Elem*, 9, 54-60 (1990)

3114 Kesaniemi YA, Miettinen TA. Inhibition of cholesterol absorption by neomycin, benzodiazepine derivatives and ketoconazole. *Eur J Clin Pharmacol*, 40, Suppl 1, S65-S67 (1991)

3115 Kesniemi YA. Serum triglycerides and clinical benefit in lipid-lowering trials. *Am J Cardiol*, 81, 70B-73B (1998)

3116 Kessler M, Netter P, Zerrouki M et al. Spiromycin does not increase plasma cyclosporin concentrations in renal transplant patients. *Eur J Clin Pharmacol*, 35, 331-332 (1988)

3117 Kessler MA, Meinitzer A, Petek W, Wolfreis OS. Microalbuminuria and borderline-increased albumin rxcretion determined with a centrifugal analyzer and the Albumin Blue 580 fluorescence assay. *Clin Chem*, 43, 996-1002 (1997)

3118 Ketter TA, Post RM, Worthington K. Principles of clinically important drug interactions with carbamazepine. Part I. *J Clin Psychopharmacol*, 11, 198-203 (1991)

3119 Ketter TA, Post RM, Worthington K. Principles of clinically important drug interactions with carbamazepine. Part II. *J Clin Psychopharmacol*, 11, 306-313 (1991)

3120 Kettlewell M, Nowers A, White R. Effect of digoxin on human red blood cell electrolytes. *Br J Pharmacol*, 44, 165 (1972)

3121 Kew MC, First RG. A trial of Ro 4-2137 in the treatment of hypertension. *Curr Ther Res*, 14, 343 (1972)

3122 Kew MC, Seftel HC, Bloomberg BM. Pregnancy tests and proteinuria. *Lancet*, 1, 902 (1967)

3123 Key LL Jr, Rodriguiz RM, Willi SM et al. Long-term treatment of osteopetrosis with recombinant human interferon γ. *N Engl J Med*, 332, 1594-1599 (1995)

3124 Key Pharmaceuticals, Inc. Manufacturer's literature on Imdur® . Kenilworth, NJ 07033 (1995)

3125 Key Pharmaceuticals, Inc. Manufacturer's literature on Theo-dur® . Kenilworth, NJ 07033 (1995)

3126 Khalek KA, El Kholy M, Rafik M et al. Effect of triiodothyronine on cyclic AMP and pulmonary function tests in bronchial asthma. *J Asthma*, 29, 425-431 (1991)

3127 Khan A, Langley SJ, Mullins FGP et al. The pharmacokinetics and pharmacodynamics of nifedipine at steady state during concomitant administration of cimetidine or high dose ranitidine. *Br J Clin Pharmacol*, 32, 519-522 (1991)

3128 Khanna BK, Gupta VP, Singh MP. Ethambutol-induced hyperuricaemia. *Tubercle*, 65, 195-199 (1984)

3129 Kharasch ED, Thummel KE, Mhyre J et al. Single-dose sulfiram inhibition of chlorzoxazone metabolism: a clinical probe for P450 $2E_1$. *Clin Pharmacol Ther*, 53, 643-650 (1993)

3130 Khoo KC, Mendels J, Rothbart M et al. Influence of phenytoin and phenobarbital on the disposition of a single oral dose of clonazepam. *Clin Pharmacol Ther*, 28, 368-375 (1980)

3131 Khumalo H, Gomo ZAR, Gangaidzo IT, et al. Effect of ascorbic acid administration on serum concentration of transferrin receptors. *Clin Chem*, 44, 1573-1575 (1998)

3132 Kiberd BA. Cyclosporine-induced renal dysfunction in human renal allograft recipients. *Transplantation*, 48, 965-969 (1989)

3133 Kidd JE, Gilchrist NL, Utley RJ et al. Effect of opiate, general anesthesia and surgery on plasma atrial natriuretic peptide levels in man. *Clin Exp Pharmacol Physiol*, 14, 755-760 (1987)

3134 Kieselbach F, Kotanko P. Urinary excretion of N-acetyl-β-D-glucosaminidase in patients after cyclosporin-treated corneal grafting. *Klin Wschr*, 68, 869-871 (1990)

3135 Kihara A. Effect of the calcium antagonist nicardipine hydrochloride on glucose tolerance and insulin secretion. *Am Heart J*, 122, II Suppl, 363-369 (1991)

3136 Kijima Y, Sasauka T, Kanayama M et al. Clofibrate effect on alkaline phosphatase in renal failure. *N Engl J Med*, 297, 113 (1977)

3137 Kilpatrick ES, Rumley AG, Small M. Evaluation of the One Touch II blood glucose meter. *Proc ACB Natl Meet*, 89 (1993)

3138 Kim CJ, Min YK, Ryu WS, et al. Effect of hormone replacement therapy on lipoprotein(a) and lipid levels in postmenopausal women: Influence of various progestogens and duration of therapy. *Arch Intern Med*, 156, 1693-1700 (1996)

3139 Kimura S, Iyama S, Yamaguchi Y, et al. New enzymatic assay with urea amidolyase for determining potassium in serum. *Ann Clin Biochem*, 34, 384-388 (1997)

3140 Kinane K, O'Connor L, Gunzer G. Development of immunoturbidimetric assays for IgG, IgA and IgM on Olympus chemistry analyzers with no sample predilution. *Clin Chem*, 41, S65 (1995)

3141 King A. Positive interference by cephalothin with Zimmermann reaction for 17-ketosteroids. *Clin Chem*, 20, 401 (1974)

3142 King JM, Crouse JR, Terry JG et al. Evaluation of effects of unmodified niacin on fasting and postprandial plasma lipids in normolipidemic men with hypoalphalipoproteinemia. *Am J Med*, 97, 323-331 (1994)

3143 Kingham JGC, Swain P, Swarbrick ET. Dapsone and severe hypoalbuminemia: a report of two cases. *Lancet*, 2, 662-664 (1979)

3144 Kingsley GR, Tager HS. Ion-exchange method for the determination of plasma ammonia nitrogen with the Berthelot reaction. *Stand Meth Clin Chem*, 6, 115 (1970)

3145 Kirberger E. Variable action of MAO inhibiting hydrazines on serotonin metabolism. *Nature*, 197, 1211 (1963)

3146 Kirch W, Hoensch H, Janisch HD. Interactions and non-interactions with ranitidine. *Clin Pharmacokinet*, 8, 493-510 (1984)

3147 Kirch W, Hutt HJ, Heidemann H et al. Drug interactions with nitrendipine. *J Cardiovasc Pharmacol*, 6, S982-S985 (1984)

3148 Kirch W, Janisch JD, Ohnhaus EE et al. Cisapride-cimetidine interaction: enhanced cisapride bioavailability and accelerated cimetidine absorption. *Ther Drug Monit*, 11, 411-414 (1989)

3149 Kirch W, Laskowski M, Ohnhaus EE et al. Effects of felodipine on plasma digoxin levels and haemodynamics in patients with heart failure. *J Intern Med*, 225, 237-239 (1989)

3150 Kirch W, Logemann C, Heidemann H et al. Effect of two different doses of nitrendipine on steady-state plasma digoxin levels and systolic time intervals. *Eur J Clin Pharmacol*, 31, 391-395 (1986)

3151 Kirch W, Nahoui R, Ohnhaus EE. The ranitidine/nitrendipine interaction. *Clin Pharmacol Ther*, 43, 149 (1988)

3152 Kirch W, Schafer-Korting M, Axthelm T et al. Interaction of atenolol with furosemide and calcium and aluminum salts. *Clin Pharmacol Ther*, 30, 429-435 (1981)

3153 Kirch W, Spahn H, Kitteringham NR et al. Interaction between the β-adrenoceptor blockers metoprolol and atenolol with amitriptyline and their effects on oxidative liver metabolism. *Br J Clin Pharmacol*, 17, 65s-68s (1984)

3154 Kirch W, Stenzel J, Dylewicz P et al. Influence of nisoldipine on haemodynamic effects and plasma levels of digoxin. *Br J Clin Pharmacol*, 22, 155-159 (1986)

3155 Kirckmair H, Huber H. Fieberhafte reaktion ('drug fever') unter α-methyldopa. *Wien Klin Wschr*, 77, 699 (1965)

3156 Kirk JM. Probable cefotaxime interference in enzymatic ammonia assay - a cautionary note. *Ann Clin Biochem*, 26, 195-196 (1989)

3157 Kirkwood JM, Ernstoff MS, Davis CA et al. Comparison of intramuscular and intravenous recombinant α_2-interferon in melanoma and other cancers. *Ann Intern Med*, 103, 32-36 (1985)

3158 Kirschbaum BB, Schoolwerth AC. Hyperaluminiumaemia associated with oral citrate and aluminum hydroxide. *Hum Toxicol*, 8, 45-47 (1989)

3159 Kirschner MA, Bardin CW. Androgen production and metabolism in normal and virilized women. *Metabolism*, 21, 667 (1972)

3160 Kirsh MM, Abrams B, Coon W et al. Diphenhydramine (Benadryl®) hydrochloride in the treatment of ammonia intoxication. *Arch Surg*, 91, 466 (1965)

3161 Kisfauldy S, Buki B, Meszaros S. Effect of orally administered amino acids on portal blood ammonia. *Acta Med Hung*, 20, 365 (1964)

3162 Kisters K, Zidek W, Rahn KH. Effects of trichlormethiazide and amiloride on intracellular Mg^{2+}, Na^+ and K^+ concentrations. *Schweiz Med Wschr*, 119, 1837-1839 (1989)

3163 Kistner RW. Present status of oral contraceptives. *Drug Therapy*, 1, 14 (1971)

3164 Kitagawa H, Chang H, Fujita T. Hyperkalemia due to nafamostat mesylate. *N Engl J Med*, 332, 687 (1995)

3165 Kivinen S, Maenpaa J. Effect of toremifene on clinical chemistry, hematology and hormone levels at different doses in healthy postmenopausal women: phase I study. *J Steroid Biochem*, 36, 217-220 (1990)

3166 Kivisto KT, Neuvonen PJ. Enhancement of absorption and effect of glipizide by magnesium hydroxide. *Clin Pharmacol Ther*, 49, 39-43 (1991)

3167 Kivisto KT, Neuvonen PJ. The effect of cholestyramine and activated charcoal on glipizide absorption. *Br J Clin Pharmacol*, 30, 733-736 (1990)

3168 Kiyosawa K, Sodeyama T, Nakano Y et al. Treatment of chronic non-A non-B hepatitis with human interferon beta; a preliminary study. *Antiviral Res*, 12, 151-162 (1989)

3169 Kjellstrom T, Blychert E, Lindgarde F. Felodipine in the treatment of hypertensive type II diabetics: Effect on glucose homeostasis. *J Intern Med*, 229, 233-239 (1991)

3170 Klastersky J, Vanderklen B, Daneau D et al. Carbenicillin and hypokalemia. *Ann Intern Med*, 78, 774 (1973)

3171 Klatskin G. Toxic and drug induced hepatitis. In:. *Diseases of the Liver, 3rd edition. L Schiff (ed)*, Philadelphia PA, JB Lippncott (1969)

3172 Klein AL, Sami MH. Usefulness and safety of cimetidine in patients receiving mexiletine for ventricular arrhythmia. *Am Heart J*, 109, 1281-1286 (1985)

3173 Klein B, Lucas LB. Application of Fe (11)-5-pyridyl benzodiazepin-2-ones to the manual or automated determination of serum uric acid. *Clin Chem*, 19, 67 (1973)

3174 Klein G. Results of the multicenter evaluation of a new method for the determination of β-N-Acetyl-glucosaminidase in urine. *Wien Klin Wschr*, 103, Suppl 189, 30-37 (1991)

3175 Klein HO, Lane R, DI Segni E et al. Verapamil-digoxin interaction. *N Engl J Med*, 303, 160 (1980)

3176 Klein M. Agranulocytosis secondary to chlorthalidone therapy (report of a case). *J Am Med Ass*, 184, 310 (1963)

3177 Klein NC, Magida MG. Propoxyphene (Darvon®) hepatotoxicity. *Am J Dig Dis*, 16, 467 (1971)

3178 Kleinberg DL, Lieberman A, Todd J et al. Pergolide mesylate: a potent day-long inhibitor of prolactin in rhesus monkeys and patients with Parkinson's disease. *J Clin Endocrinol Metab*, 51, 152-154 (1980)

3179 Kleinbloesem CH, Van Brummelen P, Francis RJ et al. Clinical pharmacology of cilazapril. *Am J Med*, 87, Suppl 6b, 45S-49S (1989)

3180 Kleinbloesem CH, Van Brummelen P, Hillers J et al. Interaction between digoxin and nifedipine at steady state in patients with atrial fibrillation. *Ther Drug Monit*, 7, 372-376 (1985)

3181 Kleinbloesem CH, van Brummelen P, Sandberg TWH et al. Pharmacokinetics and haemodynamic interaction between nifedipine and propranolol. *Br J Clin Pharmacol*, 19, 537p (1985)

3182 Kleinbloesem CH, Weber C, Fahrner E et al. Hemodynamics, biochemical effects, and pharmacokinetics of the renin inhibitor remikiren in healthy human subjects. *Clin Pharmacol Ther*, 53, 585-592 (1993)

3183 Kleinman S, Nelson R, Smith L et al. Positive direct antiglobulin tests and immune hemolytic anemia in patients receiving procainamide. *N Engl J Med*, 311, 809-812 (1984)

3184 Kletter G, Parks BR Jr, Bhatnagar A et al. Elevated serum iron levels following administration of cisplatinum. *Oncology*, 45, 421-423 (1988)

3185 Kletter GB, Foster CM, Beitins IZ et al. Acute effects of testosterone infusion and naloxone on luteinizing hormone secretion in normal men. *J Clin Endocrinol Metab*, 75, 1215-1219 (1992)

3186 Klinger B, Ionesco A, Anin S et al. Effect of insulin-like growth factor I on the thyroid axis in patients with Laron-type dwarfism and healthy subjects. *Acta Endocrinol*, 127, 515-519 (1992)

3187 Klingmuller V, Bergmann E, Claassen F. The urinary excretion of alanine aminopeptidase in children: reference values and influence of nephrotropic contrast media. *J Clin Chem Clin Biochem*, 22, 787-789 (1984)

3188 Klintmalm G, Sawe J, Ringden O et al. Cyclosporine plasma levels in renal transplant patients. *Transplantation*, 39, 132-137 (1985)

3189 Klintmalm GBG, Iwatsuki S, Starzl TE. Cyclosporine A hepatotoxicity in 66 renal allograft recipients. *Transplantation*, 32, 488-489 (1981)

3190 Kloosterboer HJ, Van Wayjen RGA, Van Den Ende A. Effects of the oral contraceptive combination 0.150 mg desogestrel + 0.020 mg ethinylestradiol on serum lipids including the HDL subfractions. *Acta Obstet Gynecol Scand*, 66, Suppl 144, 33-36 (1987)

3191 Kloosterboer HJ, Van Wayjen RGA, Van Den Ende A. Effects of three low-dose oral contraceptive combinations on sex-hormone binding globulin, corticosteroid binding globulin and antithrombin III activity in healthy women: Two monophasic desogestrel combinations and 1 triphasic levonorgestrel. *Acta Obstet Gynecol Scand*, 66, Suppl 144, 41-44 (1987)

3192 Klotz MO, Richter H, Meuffels M. Interference by formaldehyde forming drugs in the determination of urinary catecholamines. *Clin Chem*, 10, 372 (1964)

3193 Klotz U, Arvela P, Rosenkranz B. Interaction study of diazepam and procainamide with the new H_2-receptor antagonist famotidine. *Clin Pharmacol Ther*, 37, 205 (1985)

3194 Klotz U, Reimann I. Elevation of steady-state diazepam levels by cimetidine. *Clin Pharmacol Ther*, 30, 513-517 (1981)

3195 Kluge RM, Wilkes R. Reactions to antibiotics. *J Am Med Ass*, 237, 1825 (1977)

3196 Knapen MHJ, Hamulyak K, Vermeer C. The effect of vitamin K supplementation on circulating osteocalcin (bone Gla Protein) and urinary calcium excretion. *Ann Intern Med*, 111, 1001-1005 (1989)

3197 Kniffin JC, Noyes WD, Porter FS. Iron and cholestyramine in erythropoietic protoporphyria. *Clin Res*, 18, 38 (1970)

3198 Knipscheer HC, Nurmohamed MT, van den Ende A et al. Gemfibrozil treatment of the high triglyceride-low high-density lipoprotein cholesterol trait in men with established atherosclerosis. *J Intern Med*, 236, 377-384 (1994)

3199 Knirsch AK, Gralla EJ. Abnormal serum transaminase levels after parenteral ampicillin and carbenicillin administration. *N Engl J Med*, 282, 1081 (1970)

3200 Knoll Pharmaceutical Company. Manufacturer's literature on Ibu® . Mount Olive, NJ 07828 (1995)

3201 Knoll Pharmaceutical Company. Manufacturer's literature on Isoptin® . Mount Olive, NJ 07828 (1992)

3202 Knoll Pharmaceutical Company. Manufacturer's literature on Mavik® . Mount Olive, NJ 07828 (1996)

3203 Knoll Pharmaceutical Company. Manufacturer's literature on Meridia® . Mount Olive, NJ 07828 (1998)

3204 Knoll Pharmaceutical Company. Manufacturer's literature on Rythmol® . Mount Olive, NJ 07828 (1995)

3205 Knopp RH, Ginsberg J, Albers JJ et al. Contrasting effects of unmodified and time-release forms of niacin in lipoproteins in hyperlipidemic subjects: clues to mechanism of action of niacin. *Metabolism*, 34, 642-650 (1985)

3206 Knudsen L, Weismann K. Pustular eruption and damage to internal organs following sulfamethoxazole-trimethoprim. *Ugeskr Laeger*, 139, 1007-1009 (1977)

3207 Knuth UA, Nieschlag E. Effect of different doses of naloxone on serum levels of prolactin and gonadotropins in young male volunteers. *J Endocrinol Invest*, 8, 55-57 (1985)

3208 Koch TR, Cook JD. Benzalkonium interference with test methods for potassium and sodium. *Clin Chem*, 36, 807-808 (1990)

3209 Koch-Weser J. Quinidine-induced hypothrombinemic hemorrhage in patients on chronic warfarin therapy. *Ann Intern Med*, 68, 511-517 (1968)

3210 Koch-Weser J, Sellers EM. Coumarin anticoagulants. *N Engl J Med*, 285, 555 (1971)

3211 Koch-Weser J, Sidel VW, Dexter M et al. Adverse reactions to sulfisoxazole, sulfamethoxazole, and nitrofurantoin. *Arch Intern Med*, 128, 399 (1971)

3212 Kodama J, Katayama S, Tanaka K et al. Effect of captopril on glucose concentration: possible role of augmented postprandial forearm blood flow. *Diabetes Care*, 13, 1109-1111 (1990)

3213 Koenig W, Binner L, Gabrielsen F et al. Catecholamines and the renin-angiotensin-aldosterone system during treatment with felodipine ER or hydrochlorothiazide in essential hypertension. *J Cardiovasc Pharmacol*, 18, 349-353 (1991)

3214 Koenig W, Hehr R, Ditschuneit HH et al. Lovastatin alters blood rheology in primary hyperlipoproteinemia: dependence on lipoprotein(a)?. *J Clin Pharmacol*, 32, 539-545 (1992)

3215 Koenig W, Sund M, Ernst E et al. Effects of felodipine ER and hydrochlorothiazide on blood rheology in essential hypertension - a randomized, double-blind, crossover study. *J Intern Med*, 229, 511-538 (1991)

3216 Koev D, Cvrkalova A-L, Rybka J et al. Improvement of lipoprotein lipid composition in type II diabetic patients with concomitant hyperlipoproteinemia by acipimox treatment. *Diabetes Care*, 16, 1285-1293 (1993)

3217 Koh H, Nambu S, Tsushima M et al. A specific inhibition of insulin secretion by a β_1-selective adrenoceptor blocking drug. *Acta Therapeut*, 9, 325-332 (1983)

3218 Koh KK, Bui MN, Mincemoyer R, Cannon RO III. Effects of hormone therapy on inflammatory cell adhesion molecules in postmenopausal healthy women. *Am J Cardiol*, 80, 1505-1507 (1997)

3219 Koh KK, Mincemover R, Bul MN, et al. Effects of hormone replacement therapy on fibrinolysis in postmenopausal women. *N Engl J Med*, 336, 683-690 (1997)

3220 Kohler M, Harris A. Pharmacokinetics and haematological effects of desmopressin. *Eur J Clin Pharmacol*, 35, 281-285 (1988)

3221 Kohn NN, Myerson RM. Xanthomatous biliary cirrhosis following chlorpromazine. *Am J Med*, 31, 665 (1961)

3222 Kohn RM, Montes M. Hepatic fibrosis following long acting nicotinic acid therapy: a case report. *Am J Med Sci*, 258, 94 (1969)

3223 Kohno M, Takeda T, Ishii M et al. Therapeutic benefits and safety of carvedilol in the treatment of renal hypertension: an open, short term study. *Drugs*, 36, Suppl 6, 129-135 (1988)

3224 Kohno M, Yokokawa K, Yasunari K et al. Acute effects of α- and β-adrenoceptor blockade on plasma atrial natriuretic peptides during exercise in elderly patients with mild hypertension. *Chest*, 99, 847-854 (1991)

3225 Kohvakka A, Salo H, Gordin A et al. Antihypertensive and biochemical effects of different doses of hydrochlorothiazide alone or in combination with triamterene. *Acta Med Scand*, 219, 381-386 (1986)

3226 Koivisto KA, Pelkonen R, Cantell K. Effect of interferon on glucose tolerance and insulin sensitivity. *Diabetes*, 38, 641-647 (1989)

3227 Koizumi J, Haraki T, Yagi K et al. Clinical efficacy of fluvastatin in the long-term treatment of familial hypercholesterolemia. *Am J Cardiol*, 76, 47A-50A (1995)

3228 Kolanowski J, Pizarro MA, Crabbe J. Changes in adrenocortical response to corticotropin (ACTH) administered repeatedly in man. *Abstracts IV Int Congr Endocrinol, Washington DC*, 115 (1972)

3229 Kolb KW, Garnett WR, Small RE et al. Effect of cimetidine on quinidine clearance. *Ther Drug Monit*, 6, 306-312 (1984)

3230 Koller M. Results of 74 substances tested for interference with determination of plasma catecholamines by high-performance liquid chromatography with electrochemical detection. *Clin Chem*, 34, 947-949 (1988)

3231 Koller PU, Tritschler W, Carstensen CA. Systematic drug interference studies on Reflotron. *Clin Chem*, 33, 916 (1987)

3232 Koltringer P, Langsteger W, Lind P et al. Gallopamil und Veranderungen der Adenosin-diphosphat- und Kollagen-induzierten Throbozyten-Aggregation. *Arz Forsch Drug Res*, 41, 786-788 (1991)

3233 Komaiko W, Hussain S, Brecher M et al. Positive interference with Ektachem® chloride and carbon dioxide methods by bromide-containing drugs. *Clin Chem*, 34, 429-430 (1988)

3234 Komorowski J, Stepien H, Pawlikowski M. Increased interleukin-2 levels during standard TRH test in man. *Neuropeptides*, 27, 151-156 (1994)

3235 Koninckx PR, Riittinen L, Seppala M et al. CA-125 and placental protein 14 concentrations in plasma and peritoneal fluid of women with deeply infiltrating pelvic endometriosis. *Fertil Steril*, 57, 523-530 (1992)

3236 Konno M, Nishizawa N, Miyate Y et al. Intraoperative changes in plasma folate and cobalamin levels in patients inhaling nitrous oxide. *Jpn J Anesthesiol*, 34, 1620-1624 (1985)

3237 Konttinen A. Hepatotoxicity of sulfamethoxypyridazine. *Br Med J*, 2, 168 (1972)

3238 Konttinen A, Perasalo J, Eisalo A. Sulfonamide hepatitis. *Acta Med Scand*, 191, 389 (1972)

3239 Konttinen YP. Epsilon-aminocaproic acid in treatment of acute pancreatitis. *Scand J Clin Lab Invest*, 27, 41 (1971)

3240 Konturek S, Gabrys B. Inhibition of gastric secretion of hydrochloric acid by secretin. *Pol Tyg Lek*, 25, 95 (1970)

3241 Konturek SJ, Kwiecien N, Obtulowicz W et al. Effects of nocloprost on gastric functions in man. *Scand J Gastroenterol*, 26, 1145-1151 (1991)

3242 Koop H, Schwarting H, Eckel U et al. Influence of chronic rioprostil treatment on gastric endocrine function. *Scand J Gastroenterol*, 164, Suppl 24, 104-111 (1989)

3243 Koopmans PP, Van Megen T, Thien T et al. The interaction between indomethacin and captopril or enalapril in healthy volunteers. *J Intern Med*, 226, 139-142 (1989)

3244 Kopp A, Jonat W, Schmahl M, Knabbe C. Transforming growth factor β2 (TGF-β2) levels in plasma of patients with metastatic breast cancer treated with tamoxifen. *Cancer Res*, 55, 4512-4515 (1995)

3245 Koppensteiner R, Lang CC, Maclean D et al. Effects of lovastatin on hemorheology in type II hyperlipoproteinemia. *Atherosclerosis*, 83, 53-58 (1990)

3246 Koren G, Hesslein PS, Macleod SM. Digoxin toxicity associated with amiodarone therapy in children. *J Pediatr*, 104, 467-470 (1984)

3247 Koren G, Roifman C, Gelfand E et al. Corticosteroids-salicylate interaction -- a case of juvenile rheumatoid arthritis. *Ther Drug Monit*, 9, 177-179 (1987)

3248 Koren JF, Randall GR, Kincaid RS et al. Phenytoin hypersensitivity reaction: hepatic necrosis. *Drug Intell Clin Pharm*, 14, 252-257 (1980)

3249 Korenman J, Baker B, Waggoner J et al. Long-term remission of chronic hepatitis B after α-interferon therapy. *Ann Intern Med*, 114, 629-634 (1991)

3250 Korman MG, Soveny C, Hansky J. The effect of food on serum gastrin. *Aust NZ J Med*, 1, 299 (1971)

3251 Kornberg A, Kobrin I. IgG antiplatelet antibodies due to carbamazepine. *Acta Haematol*, 68, 68-70 (1970)

3252 Kornfeld JM, Ullmann WW. Penicillin interference with the determination of δ-aminolevulinic acid. *Clin Chim Acta*, 46, 187 (1973)

3253 Kos Pharmaceuticals, Inc.. Manufacturer's literature on Niaspan® . Miami, FL 33131 (1997)

3254 Koskinen P, Kovanen PT, Tuomilehto J et al. Gemfibrozil also corrects dyslipidemia in postmenopausal women and smokers. *Arch Intern Med*, 152, 90-96 (1992)

3255 Koskinen P, Manninen V, Eisalo A. Quinapril and blood lipids. *Br J Clin Pharmacol*, 26, 478-480 (1988)

3256 Kosoglou T, Rocci ML Jr, Vlasses PH. Trimethoprim alters the disposition of procainamide and N-acetylprocainamide. *Clin Pharmacol Ther*, 44, 467-477 (1988)

3257 Kossover MF, Beckham ME, Threefoot SA. Influence of an oral peristaltic stimulant, danthron, on the PSP excretion test. *Am J Med Sci*, 247, 694 (1964)

3258 Kostoglou-Athanassiou I, Ntalles K, Gogas J, et al. Sex hormones in postmenopausal women with breast cancer on tamoxifen. *Horm Res*, 47, 116-120 (1997)

3259 Kosty MP, Hench PK, Tani P et al. Throbocytopenia associated with auranofin therapy: evidence for a gold-dependent immunologic mechanism. *Am J Hematol*, 30, 236-239 (1989)

3260 Koszewski BJ, Hubbard TF. Immunologic agranulocytosis due to mercurial diuretics. *Am J Med*, 20, 958 (1956)

3261 Koumantakis G, Wyndham LE, Gyory AZ. Phenolsulfonphthalein interferes with the measurement of urinary protein in the Du Pont analyzer. *Clin Chem*, 34, 1509-1510 (1988)

3262 Koup JR, Toothaker RD, Posvar E et al. Theophylline dosage adjustment during enoxacin coadministration. *Antimicrob Agent Chemother*, 34, 803-807 (1990)

3263 Kovacs JL, Tuzel I, Aogaichi K et al. False-positive urine protein reaction with cibenzoline, a new antiarrhythmic agent. *J Clin Pharmacol*, 24, 127-128 (1984)

3264 Kovarik JM, Mueller EA, Gaber M et al. Pharmacokinetics of cyclosporine and steady-state aspirin during coadministration. *J Clin Pharmacol*, 33, 513-521 (1993)

3265 Koytchev R, Aiken R-G, Mayer O. Effect of diprafenone on the pharmacokinetics of digoxin. *Eur J Clin Pharmacol*, 50, 97-100 (1996)

3266 Kozlowski BW, Taylor ML, Baer MT et al. Anticonvulsant medication use and circulating levels of total thyroxine, retinol binding protein and vitamin A in children with delayed cognitive development. *Am J Clin Nutr*, 46, 360-368 (1987)

3267 Kracke RR. Relation of drug therapy to neutropenic states. *J Am Med Ass*, 111, 1255 (1938)

3268 Kraiss S, Lenz H, Rotter A et al. Electro-chemiluminescent 3rd generation TSH assay using the random-access analyzer Elecsys. *Clin Chem*, 41, S52 (1995)

3269 Kramer BK, Haussler M, Ress KM et al. Renal effects of the new calcium channel blocking drug isradipine. *Eur J Clin Pharmacol*, 39, 333-335 (1990)

3270 Kramer G, Theisohn M, von Unruh GE et al. Carbamazepine-danazol drug interaction: its mechanism studied by a stable isotope technique. *Ther Drug Monit*, 8, 387-392 (1986)

3271 Kramer S, Watson LL, Lodato DT et al. Assay of pseudocholinesterase on the Dimension clinical chemistry system. *Clin Chem*, 37, 913 (1991)

3272 Krantz JC, Carr CJ. Pharmacologic Principles of Medical Practice. *6th edition*, Baltimore MD, Williams and Wilkins (1965)

3273 Kraupp M, Legenstein E, Linkesch W et al. Influence of recombinant erythropoietin on heme biosynthesis in chronic uremic patients. *Clin Chem*, 36, 974 (1990)

3274 Krause K-H, Berlit P, Bonjour J-P et al. Vitamin status in patients on chronic anticonvulsant therapy. *Int J Vitam Nutr Res*, 52, 375-385 (1982)

3275 Krause K-H, Bonjour J-P, Berlit P et al. Biotin status of epileptics. *Ann NY Acad Sci*, 447, 297-313 (1985)

3276 Krause K-H, Bonjour J-P, Berlit P et al. Effect of long-term treatment with antiepileptic drugs on the vitamin status. *Drug Nutr Interact*, 5, 317-343 (1988)

3277 Krause W, Trager H, Kuhne G et al. Pharmacokinetics and endocrine effects of terguride in healthy subjects. *Eur J Clin Pharmacol*, 38, 609-615 (1990)

3278 Krauss RM, Roys S, Mishell DR Jr et al. Effects of two low-dose oral contraceptives on serum lipids and lipoproteins: differential changes in high-density lipoprotein subclasses. *Am J Obstet Gynecol*, 145, 446-452 (1983)

3279 Kravec CV, Rouse S, Subuhi HS et al. Abuscreen ONTRAK assay for methadone: a rapid latex immunoassay for detection of methadone use. *Clin Chem*, 41, S110 (1995)

3280 Kreeft JH, Langlois S, Ogilvie RI. Comparative trial of indapamide and hydrochlorothiazide in essential hypertension with forearm plethysmography. *J Cardiovasc Pharmacol*, 6, 622-626 (1984)

3281 Kreeger RW, Hammill SC. New antiarrhythmic drugs: tocainide, mexiletine, flecainide, encainide and amiodarone. *Mayo Clin Proc*, 62, 1033-1050 (1987)

3282 Kreek MJ, Dodes L, Kane S et al. Long-term methadone maintenance therapy: effects on liver function. *Ann Intern Med*, 77, 598 (1972)

3283 Kreek MJ, Garfield JW, Gutjahr CL et al. Rifampin-induced methadone withdrawal. *N Engl J Med*, 294, 1104-1106 (1976)

3284 Kreft-Jais C, Billaud EM, Gaudry C et al. Effect of josamycin on plasma cyclosporine levels. *Eur J Clin Pharmacol*, 32, 327-328 (1987)

3285 Kremer JAM, Rolland R, Van der Heijden PFM et al. Return of gonadotropic function in postpartum women during bromocriptine treatment. *Fertil Steril*, 51, 622-627 (1989)

3286 Kreuz W, Linde R, Funk M et al. Valproate therapy induces von Willebrand disease type I. *Epilepsia*, 33, 178-184 (1992)

3287 Kriger HU, Schuler U, Proksch B et al. Investigation of potential interaction of ciprofloxacin with cyclosporine in bone marrow transplant patients. *Antimicrob Agent Chemother*, 34, 1048-1052 (1990)

3288 Kris MT, Dettmer A, Rakette S. Long-term efficacy of beclobrate on plasma lipids and blood glucose. In:. *Beclobrate, a New Lipoprotein Regulator. GM Kostner, CR Sirtori (eds)*, Toronto, Hogrefe and Huber, 45-49 (1990)

3289 Krishnaiah YSR, Satyanarayana S, Visweswaram D. Interaction between tolbutamide and ketoconazole in healthy subjects. *Br J Clin Pharmacol*, 37, 205-207 (1994)

3290 Kristensen BO, Skov J, Peterslund NA. Frusemide-induced increases in serum amylases. *Br Med J*, 281, 978 (1980)

3291 Kristensen BO, Weeke JO. Propranolol-induced increments in total and free serum thyroxine in patients with essential hypertension. *Clin Pharmacol Ther*, 22, 864-867 (1977)

3292 Kristensen M, Hansen JM. Accumulation of chlorpropamide caused by dicumarol. *Acta Med Scand*, 183, 83-86 (1968)

3293 Kristensen ME. Toxic hepatitis induced by disulfiram in a nonalcoholic. *Acta Med Scand*, 209, 335-336 (1981)

3294 Kristinsson A. Fatal reaction to acetazolamide. *Br J Ophthalmol*, 51, 348 (1967)

3295 Kristoff CA, Hayes PE, Barr WH et al. Effect of ibuprofen on lithium plasma and red blood cell concentrations. *Clin Pharm*, 5, 51-55 (1986)

3296 Kroboth FJ, Kroboth PD, Logan T. Phenytoin-theophylline-quinidine interaction. *N Engl J Med*, 308, 725 (1983)

3297 Kroll MH, Hagengruber C, Elin RJ. Effect of dialysis on interference by cefoxitin with determination of creatinine. *Clin Chem*, 30, 1386-1388 (1984)

3298 Kroll MH, Jackson AJ, Elin RJ. Cefoxitin interferes with the 'Clini-skreen' column method for urinary 17-hydroxycorticosteroids. *Clin Chem*, 33, 1219-1222 (1987)

3299 Kroll MH, Koch TR, Drusano GI et al. Lack of interference with creatinine assays by four cephalosporin like antibiotics. *Am J Clin Pathol*, 82, 214-216 (1984)

3300 Kroll MH, Nealon L, Vogel MA et al. How certain drugs interfere negatively with the Jaffe reaction for creatinine. *Clin Chem*, 31, 306-308 (1985)

3301 Kromann NP, Vilhelmsen R, Stahl D. The dapsone syndrome. *Arch Dermatol*, 118, 531-532 (1982)

3302 Kronenberg F, Konig P, Lhotta K et al. Low molecular weight heparin does not necessarily reduce lipids and lipoproteins in hemodialysis patients. *Clin Nephrol*, 43, 399-404 (1995)

3303 Kronvall P, Fahy TA, Isaksson A et al. The clinical relevance of salivary amylase monitoring in bulimia nervosa. *Biol Psychiat*, 32, 156-163 (1992)

3304 Kroon AA, Demacker PNM, Stalenhoef AFH. N-acetylcysteine and serum concentrations of lipoprotein(a). *J Intern Med*, 230, 519-526 (1991)

3305 Kroon C, de Boer A, Hoogkamer JFW et al. Detection of drug interactions with single dose acenocoumarol: a new screening method?. *Int J Clin Pharmacol Ther Toxicol*, 28, 355-360 (1990)

3306 Kruger HU, Schuler U, Zimmermann R et al. Absence of significant interaction of fluconazole with cyclosporin. *J Antimicrob Chemother*, 24, 781-786 (1989)

3307 Krum H, Viskoper RJ, Lacourciere Y , et al. The effect of an endothelin-receptor antagonist, Rosentan, on blood pressure in patients with essential hypertension. *N Engl J Med*, 338, 784-790 (1998)

3308 Krumholz WV, Chipps HI, Merlis S. Clinical effects of trioxazine, with a case report of hyperglycemia as a side effect. *J Clin Pharmacol*, 7, 108 (1967)

3309 Kruse K, Bartels H, Ziegler R et al. Parathyroid function and serum calcitonin in children receiving anticonvulsant drugs. *Eur J Pediatr*, 133, 151-156 (1980)

3310 Kruszynska YT, Greenstone M, Home PD et al. Effect of high dose inhaled beclomethasone dipropionate on carbohydrate and lipid metabolism in normal subjects. *Thorax*, 42, 881-884 (1987)

3311 Kubacka RT, Antal EJ, Juhl RP. The paradoxical effect of cimetidine and ranitidine on glibenclamide pharmacokinetics and pharmacodynamics. *Br J Clin Pharmacol*, 23, 743-751 (1987)

3312 Kubota K, Tamura J, Kurabayashi H et al. Evaluation of increased serum ferritin levels in patients with hyperthyroidism. *Clin Investig*, 72, 26-29 (1993)

3313 Kuchel O, Buu NT, Edwards DJ. Alternative catecholamine pathways after tyrosine hydroxylase inhibition in malignant pheochromocytoma. *J Lab Clin Med*, 115, 449-453 (1990)

3314 Kueppers F, Brackertz D, Czygan PJ. Serum α_1-antitrypsin levels during the ovarian cycle. *Clin Chim Acta*, 39, 131 (1972)

3315 Kuhl H, Jung-Hoffmann C, Fitzner M, et al. Short- and long-term effects on lipid metabolism of oral contraceptives containing 30 μg ethinylestradiol and 150 μg desogestrel or 3-keto-desogestrel. *Horm Res*, 44, 121-125 (1995)

3316 Kuhl H, Marz W, Jung-Hoffman C et al. Effect on lipid metabolism of a biphasic desogestrel-containing oral contraceptive: divergent changes in apolipoprotein B and E and transitory decrease in Lp(a) levels. *Contraception*, 47, 69-83 (1993)

3317 Kuhl H, Marz W, Jung-Hoffman C et al. Time-dependent alterations in lipid metabolism during treatment with low-dose oral contraceptives. *Am J Obstet Gynecol*, 163, 363-369 (1990)

3318 Kuhlmann J. Effects of verapamil, diltiazem, and nifedipine on plasma levels and renal excretion of digitoxin. *Clin Pharmacol Ther*, 38, 667-673 (1986)

3319 Kuhn JM, Basin C, Mollard M et al. Effects of the new somatostatin analogue (BIM 23014) on blood glucose homeostasis in normal men. *Eur J Clin Invest*, 22, 793-799 (1992)

3320 Kuhn J-M, Billebaud T, Navrath H et al. Prevention of the transient adverse effects of a gonadotropin-releasing hormone analogue (buserelin) in metastatic prostatic carcinoma by administration of an antiandrogen (nilutamide). *N Engl J Med*, 321, 413-418 (1989)

3321 Kung AWC, Jones BM, Lai CL. Effects of interferon-γ therapy on thyroid function. T-lymphocyte populations and induction of antibodies. *J Clin Endocrinol Metab*, 71, 1230-1234 (1990)

3322 Kung AWC, Pang RWC, Lauder I et al. Changes in serum lipoprotein(a) and lipids during treatment of hyperthyroidism. *Clin Chem*, 41, 226-231 (1995)

3323 Kuno-Sakai H, Sakai H, Ritzmann SE. Interference of digitoxin with the radioimmunoassay of digoxin. *Lancet*, 2, 326 (1972)

3324 Kuntz E, Liehr H, Pfingst W. Toxische leberschadigung durch athionamid. *Dtsch Med Wschr*, 92, 1718 (1967)

3325 Kuntzman R, Jacobson M, Conney AH. Effect of phenylbutazone on cortisol metabolism in man. *Pharmacologist*, 8, 195 (1966)

3326 Kuntzman RG, Tsai I, Brand L et al. The influence of urinary pH on the plasma half-life of pseudoephedrine in man and dog and a sensitive assay for its determination in human plasma. *Clin Pharmacol Ther*, 12, 62-67 (1971)

3327 Kunz F, Pechlaner C, Tabarelli M et al. Influence of oral contraceptives on coagulation tests in native blood and plasma. *Am J Obstet Gynecol*, 163, 417-420 (1990)

3328 Kuo B, Castell DO. Optimal dosing of omeprazole 40 mg daily: effects on gastric and esophageal pH and serum gastrin in healthy controls. *Am J Gastroenterol*, 91, 1532-1538 (1996)

3329 Kuo PC, Kirshenbaum JM, Gordon J et al. Lovastatin therapy for hypercholesterolemia in cardiac transplant recipients. *Am J Cardiol*, 64, 631-635 (1989)

3330 Kuo PT, Wilson AC, Kostis JB et al. Treatment of type III hyperlipoproteinemia with gemfibrozil to retard progression of coronary heart disease. *Am Heart J*, 116, 85-90 (1988)

3331 Kurekci AE, Alpay F, Tanindi S et al. Plasma trace element, plasma glutathione peroxidase, and superoxide dismutase levels in epileptic children receiving antiepileptic drug therapy. *Epilepsia*, 36, 600-604 (1995)

3332 Kuruvilla A, Peedicayil J, Srikrishna G et al. A study of serum prolactin levels in schizophrenia: a comparison of males and females. *Clin Exp Pharmacol Physiol*, 19, 603-606 (1992)

3333 Kurz D, Roach J, Eyring EJ. Determination of zinc by flameless atomic absorption spectrophotometry. *Anal Biochem*, 53, 586 (1973)

3334 Kurz M. Diamox® und manifestierung von diabetes mellitus. *Wien Med Wschr*, 118, 239 (1968)

3335 Kusaka M, Atarashi K, Matsumoto K et al. Effects of treatment with captopril on exercise tolerance and plasma catecholamines in elderly hypertensives. *J Hypertens*, 7, Suppl 7, S59-S61 (1989)

3336 Kusonoki M, Yamamura T, Ichii S et al. The effects of sodium valproate on plasma somatostatin and insulin in humans. *J Clin Endocrinol Metab*, 67, 1060-1063 (1988)

3337 Kutkaite D, Rudzki Z. Chloral hydrate interferes with estimation of serum vitamin B_{12} by some radioimmunoassay methods. *Clin Chem*, 32, 1983 (1986)

3338 Kutkuhn B, Hollenbeck M, Westhoff A, et al. Renin secretion and captopril stimulation in hypertensive renal transplant recipients. *Urol Int*, 52, 82-86 (1994)

3339 Kutt H. Diphenylhydantoin: interaction with other drugs in man. In:. *Antiepileptic Drugs. DM Woodbury, JK Penry, RP Schmidt (eds)*, New York NY, Raven Press (1972)

3340 Kutt H, Louis S. Anticonvulsant drugs: III clinical pharmacological and therapeutic aspects. *Drugs*, 4, 256 (1972)

3341 Kutti J, Olsson L-B, Lundborg P et al. The peripheral platelet count in response to intravenous infusion of salbutamol. *Acta Med Scand*, 201, 515-517 (1977)

3342 Kutti J, Safai-Kutti S, Sigvaldason A et al. The effect of acetylsalicylic acid in 3 different formulations on in vitro and in vivo platelet function tests. *Scand J Haematol*, 32, 379-384 (1984)

3343 Kuzuya F, Sugino N, Yoshizumi K et al. Clinical investigations in the pharmacology of azosemide (SK-110) in comparison with furosemide in healthy volunteers. *Int J Clin Pharmacol Ther Toxicol*, 22, 291-299 (1984)

3344 Kuzuya T, Hasegawa T, Shimizu K et al. Effect of antiepileptic drugs on serum zinc and copper concentrations in epileptic patients. *Int J Clin Pharmacol Ther Toxicol*, 31, 61-63 (1993)

3345 Kwan D, Bartle WR, Walker SE. Abnormal serum transaminases folloowing therapeutic doses of acetaminophen in the absence of known risk factors. *Dig Dis Sci*, 40, 1951-1955 (1995)

3346 Kwan JT, Foxall PJ, Davidson DG et al. Interaction of cyclosporine and itraconazole. *Lancet*, 2, 282 (1987)

3347 Kwan KC, Brebult GO, Davis RL et al. Effects of concomitant aspirin administration on the pharmacokinetics of indomethacin in man. *J Pharmacokinet Biopharm*, 6, 451-476 (1978)

3348 Kwong NK, Brown BH, Whittacker GE et al. Effects of gastrin 1, secretin and cholecystokinin-pancreozymin on the electrical activity, motor activity. *Scand J Gastroenterol*, 7, 161 (1972)

3349 Kyd PA, De Vooght K, Kerkhoff F, et al. Clinical usefulness of bone alkaline phosphatase in osteoporosis. *Ann Clin Biochem*, 35, 717-725 (1998)

3350 Laake K, Horvel C, Aspoy B et al. Hypomagnesemia during treatment with diuretics. *Curr Ther Res*, 23, 730-733 (1978)

3351 Laake K, Kjeldaas L, Borchgrevink CF. Side effects of piroxicam (Feldene®). *Acta Med Scand*, 215, 81-83 (1984)

3352 Laaksonen R, Jokelainen K, Sahi T et al. Decreases in serum ubiquinone concentrations do not result in reduced levels in muscle tissue during short0term simvastatin treatment in humans. *Clin Pharmacol Ther*, 57, 62-66 (1995)

3353 Laatikainen T, Ruutiainen K, Anttila L et al. Effect of naloxone on plasma insulin, insulin-like growth factor I, and its binding protein 1 in patients with polycystic ovarian disease. *Fertil Steril*, 54, 434-437 (1990)

3354 Labeeunn M, Pozet N, Zech P et al. Magnesuria induced by thiazides and the influence of triamterene. *Fundam Clin Pharmacol*, 1, 225-232 (1987)

3355 Labib M, Marks V. Inadvertent intake of sulphonylurea. *Ann Clin Biochem*, 27, 382-383 (1990)

3356 Labib MH. Lithium, hypercalcaemia and hyperparathyroidism. *Ann Clin Biochem*, 24, Suppl S1, 147-148 (1987)

3357 Lachaal M, Venuto RC. Nephrotoxicity and hyperkalemia in patients with acquired immunodeficiency syndrome treated with pentamidine. *Am J Med*, 87, 260-263 (1989)

3358 Lack SJ, Baldwin DS, Montgomery SA. Lofepramine, desipramine and abnormal tests of liver function: a case report. *Int Clin Psychopharmacol*, 5, 185-190 (1990)

3359 LaCroix AZ, Wienpahl J, White LR et al. Thiazide diuretic agents and the incidence of hip fractures. *N Engl J Med*, 332, 286-290 (1990)

3360 Ladd AT. Procainamide-induced lupus erythematosus. *N Engl J Med*, 267, 1357 (1962)

3361 Ladenson JH, Bowers GN Jr. Free calcium in serum 1. determination with the ion-specific electrode, and factors affecting the results. *Clin Chem*, 19, 565 (1973)

3362 Lado Abeal J, Cabezas Agricola J, Paz Carreira JM et al. Influence of sodium valproate on the late follicular phase pulsatile LH secretion in normal women. *Clin Endocrinol*, 35, 477-483 (1991)

3363 Laforce CF, Miller MF, Chai M. Effect of erythromycin on theophylline clearance in asthmatic children. *J Pediatr*, 99, 153-156 (1981)

3364 Lai CKW, Chan CHS, Ho SS, et al. Inhaled salmeterol and albuterol in asthmatic patients receiving high-dose inhaled corticosteroids. *Chest*, 108, 36-40 (1995)

3365 Lai C-L, Chien R-N, Leung NWY, et al. A one-year trial of lamivudine for chronic hepatitis B. *N Engl J Med*, 339, 61-68 (1998)

3366 Lai KN, Lai FM-M, Li PKT et al. Cyclosporin treatment of IgA nephropathy: a short term controlled trial. *Br Med J*, 295, 1165-1168 (1988)

3367 Laing I, Golland I, Cowen D et al. Androgen interrelationships after treatment with an oral contraceptive containing ethinyl oestradiol and cyproterone acetate in polycystic ovary syndrome. *Proc ACB Natl Meet*, 69 (1992)

3368 Laker MF, Green C, Bhuiyan AKM et al. Isotretinoin and serum lipids: studies on fatty acid, apolipoprotein and intermediary metabolism. *Br J Dermatol*, 117, 203-206 (1987)

3369 Lakhdar AA, Farish E, Dunn FG et al. Amiodarone therapy and glucose tolerance - a prospective trial. *Eur J Clin Pharmacol*, 34, 651-652 (1988)

3370 Lakshmi A, Forni T, Gottwald K. A new and improved EMIT D.A.U. benzodiazepine assay. *Clin Chem*, 37, 998 (1991)

3371 Lal S, Tolis G, McDonald TJ et al. Effect of clonidine on growth hormone and glucagon secretion. *Horm Metab Res*, 13, 648-649 (1981)

3372 Lalau JD, Lourdel C, Sauvanet JP et al. GH secretion in patients with hyperthyroidism; comparison of the effects of long-acting propranolol and betaxolol. *Horm Metab Res*, 20, 67 (1988)

3373 Lam M, Park MJ. HIV-associated nephropathy - beneficial effects of zidovudine therapy. *N Engl J Med*, 323, 1775-1776 (1990)

3374 Lam YWF, Boyd RA, Chin SK et al. Effect of probenecid on the pharmacokinetics and pharmacodynamics of procainamide. *J Clin Pharmacol*, 31, 429-432 (1991)

3375 Lamberg B-A, Tikkanen MJ. Hypercalcaemia due to dihydrotachysterol treatment in patients with hypothyroidism after thyroidectomy. *Br Med J*, 283, 461-462 (1981)

3376 Lamberg TS, Kivistö KT, Neuvonen PJ. Effects of verapamil and diltiazem on the pharmacokinetics and pharmacodynamics of buspirone. *Clin Pharmacol Ther*, 63, 640-645 (1998)

3377 Lamberg-Allardt C, Karkkainen M, Seppanen R et al. Low serum 25-hydroxyvitamin D concentrations and secondary hyperparathyroidism in middle-aged white strict vegetarians. *Am J Clin Nutr*, 58, 684-689 (1993)

3378 Lambert JS, Seidlin M, Reichman RC et al. 2',3'-dideoxyinosine (ddi) in patients with the acquired immunodeficiency syndrome or AIDS-related complex: a phase I trial. *N Engl J Med*, 322, 1333-1340 (1990)

3379 Lamberts SWJ, Del Pozo E. Somatostatin analog treatment of acromegaly: New aspects. *Horm Res*, 29, 115-117 (1988)

3380 Lamberts SWJ, Koper JW, de Jong FH. The endocrine effects of long-term treatment with mifepristone (RU 486). *J Clin Endocrinol Metab*, 73, 187-191 (1991)

3381 Lamberts SWJ, Swanson J, Bruining HA, De Jong FH. Corticosteroid therapy in severe illness. *N Engl J Med*, 337, 1285-1292 (1997)

3382 Lamberts SWJ, Uitterlinden P, Klijn JMG. The effect of the long-acting somatostatin analogue SMS 201-995 on ACTH secretion in Nelson's syndrome and Cushing's disease. *Acta Endocrinol*, 120, 760-766 (1989)

3383 Lambie DG, Johnson RH. Drugs and folate metabolism. *Drugs*, 30, 145-155 (1985)

3384 Lamden MP. Dangers of massive vitamin C intake. *N Engl J Med*, 284, 336 (1971)

3385 Lammers PJ, White L, Ettinger LJ. Cisplatinum-induced renal sodium wasting. *Med Pediatr Oncol*, 12, 343-346 (1984)

3386 Lampe GH, Wauk LZ, Whitendale P et al. Nitrous oxide does not impair hepatic function in young or old surgical patients. *Anesth Analg*, 71, 606-609 (1990)

3387 Lamrani A, Vidon N, Sogni P, et al. Effects of lanreotide, a somatostatin analogue, on postprandial gastric functions and biliopancreatic secretions in humans. *Br J Clin Pharmacol*, 43, 65-70 (1997)

3388 Lance LL, Lacy C, Warren F (eds). Quick Look Drug Book. Hudson OH, Lexi-Comp (1991)

3389 Landau C, Chen Y-DI, Skowronski R et al. Effect of nicotinic acid on plasma glucose concentration in normal individuals. *Horm Metab Res*, 24, 424-428 (1992)

3390 Landay RA, Gonzalez MA, Taylor JC. Effect of phenobarbital on theophylline disposition. *J Allerg Clin Immunol*, 62, 27-29 (1978)

3391 Landesman PW, Lott JA, Zager RA. Mannitol interferes with the du Pont aca method for inorganic phosphorus. *Clin Chem*, 28, 1994-1995 (1982)

3392 Landgraf R, Landgraf-Leurs MMC, Nusser J et al. Effect of somatastatin analogue (SMS 201-995) on cyclosporine levels. *Transplantation*, 44, 725-725 (1987)

3393 Landgren F, Israelsson B, Lindgren A et al. Plasma homocysteine in acute myocardial infarction: homocysteine-lowering effect of folic acid. *J Intern Med*, 237, 381-388 (1995)

3394 Landman D, Sarai A, Sathe SS. Use of pentoxifylline therapy for patients with AIDS-related wasting. *Clin Infect Dis*, 18, 97-99 (1994)

3395 Landon J (1969) cited by Loraine JA, Bell ET. Hormone Assays and their Clinical Application. *3rd edition*, Baltimore MD, Williams and Wilkins (1971)

3396 Landon MJ, Bates D, Kirkley M et al. Effect of anticonvulsant drugs on urinary excretion of γ-glutamyltransferase in women. *Ann Clin Biochem*, 15, 313-315 (1978)

3397 Lane SD, Besa EC, Joseph RR. Tamoxifen and hypercalcemia. *Ann Intern Med*, 91, 414-415 (1979)

3398 Lanes R, Herrera A, Palacios A et al. Decreased secretion of cortisol and ACTH after oral clonidine administration in normal adults. *Metabolism*, 32, 568-570 (1983)

3399 Lang I, Huber K, Capek J et al. Furosemide and increases in liver enzymes. *Ann Intern Med*, 109, 845 (1988)

3400 Lang J, de Villaine JF, Guemei A et al. Absence of pharmacokinetic interaction between perfloxacin and cyclosporin A in patients with renal transplants. *Rev Infect Dis*, 11, Suppl 5, S1094 (1989)

3401 Langelaan DE. Aldomet® interference with melanogen tests. *ACB News Sheet No 125 Sept* (1973)

3402 Langer G, Sachar EJ, Halpern FS et al. The prolactin response to neuroleptic drugs. a test of dopaminergic blockade: neuroendocrine studies in normal men. *J Clin Endocrinol Metab*, 45, 966-1002 (1977)

3403 Langhoff E, Madsen S. Rapid metabolism of cyclosporin and prednisolone in kidney transplant patients receiving tuberculostatic treatment. *Lancet*, 2, 1031 (1983)

3404 Langlands AO, Martin WMC. Jaundice associated with norethisterone acetate treatment of breast cancer. *Lancet*, 1, 584 (1975)

3405 Langlois J. Diamox® et thrombocytopenie. *Arch Ophthalmol*, 26, 701 (1966)

3406 Langlois R, Cournoyer G, De Montigny C et al. High incidence of multisystemic reactions to zimeldine. *Eur J Clin Pharmacol*, 28, 67-71 (1985)

3407 Langman S, Henry DA, Bell GD et al. Cimetidine and ranitidine in duodenal ulcer. *Br Med J*, 281, 473-474 (1980)

3408 Laorden ML, Miralles F, Fuentes T et al. Effect of stress and stress therapy on plasma β-endorphin-like immunoreactivity. *Meth Fund Exp Clin Pharmacol*, 6, 671-674 (1984)

3409 Lapierre G, Stewart RB. Lithium carbonate and leukocytosis. *Am J Hosp Pharm*, 37, 1525-1528 (1980)

3410 Laporte J-R, Capella D, Juan J. Agranulocytosis induced by cinepazide. *Eur J Clin Pharmacol*, 38, 387-388 (1990)

3411 Lapsley M, Singer JM, Hartley JM et al. Long term tubular function in patients treated with ifosfamide. *Proc ACB Natl Meet*, 106-107 (1995)

3412 Lardinois CK, Mazzaferri EL. Cimetidine blocks testosterone synthesis. *Arch Intern Med*, 145, 920-922 (1985)

3413 Larkin JG, McKee PJW, Forrest G et al. Lack of enzyme induction with oxcarbazepine (600 mg daily) in healthy subjects. *Br J Clin Pharmacol*, 31, 65-71 (1991)

3414 Larochelle P. Effect of quinapril on the albumin excretion rate in patients with mild to moderate hypertension. *Am J Hypertens*, 9, 551-559 (1996)

3415 Larochelle P, Cusson JR, du Souich P et al. Renal effects of a nonhypotensive I.V. dose of felodipine. *J Clin Pharmacol*, 33, 732-737 (1993)

3416 Larrey D, Castot A, Pessayre D et al. Amodiaquine-induced hepatitis. *Ann Intern Med*, 104, 801-803 (1986)

3417 Larry D, Henrion J, Heller F et al. Metoprolol-induced hepatitis: rechallenge and drug oxidation phenotyping. *Ann Intern Med*, 108, 67-68 (1988)

3418 Larsen FG, Nielsen-Kudsk F, Jakobsen P et al. Interaction of etrinate with methotrexate pharmacokinetics in psoriatic patients. *J Clin Pharmacol*, 30, 802-807 (1990)

3419 Larsen FW, Hansen CE. Zimeldine versus amitriptyline in endogenous depression. a double-blind study. *Acta Psychiat Scand*, 69, 343-349 (1984)

3420 Larsen J, Fogerson R. Nonsteroidal anti-inflammatory drug interference in TDx assays for abused drugs. *Clin Chem*, 34, 987-988 (1988)

3421 Larsen PR. Inhibition of tri-iodothyronine (T3) binding to thyroxine binding globulin by sodium salicylate. *Metabolism*, 20, 976 (1971)

3422 Larsen PR. Thyroid-pituitary interaction: feedback regulation of thyrotropin secretion by thyroid hormones. *N Engl J Med*, 306, 23-32 (1982)

3423 Larsen W, Fellowes G, Rickman LS. Life-threatening hypercalcemia and tamoxifen. *Am J Med*, 88, 440-442 (1990)

3424 Larsson R, Bodemar G, Kagedal B et al. The effects of cimetidine (Tagamet®) on renal function in patients with renal failure. *Acta Med Scand*, 298, 27-31 (1980)

3425 Larsson-Cohn U. The 2-hour sulfobromophthalein retention test and the transaminase activity during oral contraceptive therapy. *Am J Obstet Gynecol*, 98, 188 (1967)

3426 Laryea EA, Brodrick R, Hidvegi R. Hypercalcemia and streptozotocin. *Ann Intern Med*, 80, 276 (1974)

3427 Laskow DA, Curtis JJ, Luke RG et al. Cyclosporine-induced changes in glomerular filtration rate and urea excretion. *Am J Med*, 88, 497-502 (1990)

3428 Lasser EC, Lang JH. Inhibition of acetylcholinesterase by some organic contrast media. *Invest Radiol*, 1, 237 (1966)

3429 Lassman HB, Hubbard JW, Chen B-L et al. Lack of interaction between cefiprome and alcohol. *Br Soc Antimicrob Chemother*, Suppl A, 47-50 (1992)

3430 Latham AN, Richens A. Pheneturide, a more potent liver enzyme inducer in man than phenobarbitone?. *Br J Pharmacol*, 47, 615 (1973)

3431 Laue L, Lotze ME, Chrousos GP et al. Effect of chronic treatment with the glucocorticoid antagonist RU 486 in man: toxicity, immunological, and hormonal aspects. *J Clin Endocrinol Metab*, 71, 1474-1480 (1990)

3432 Launay C, Fabiani P, Grenet P. Un nouveau cas d'acrodynie avec presence de mercure dans les urines (discussion therapeutique). *Arch Fr Pediat*, 7, 79 (1950)

3433 Laupacis A, Keown PA, Ulan RA et al. Hyperbilirubinaemia and cyclosporin A levels. *Lancet*, 2, 1426 (1981)

3434 Laurell C-B, Rannevik G. A comparison of plasma protein changes induced by danazol, pregnancy, and estrogens. *J Clin Endocrinol Metab*, 49, 719-725 (1979)

3435 Lavan JN. The effect of oral ammonium chloride on the urinary excretion of calcium, magnesium and sodium. *Ir J Med Sci*, 2, 223 (1969)

3436 Laviades C, Mayor G, Diez J et al. Treatment with lisinopril normalizes serum concentrations of procollagen type III amino-terminal peptide in patients with essential hypertension. *Am J Hypertens*, 7, 52-58 (1994)

3437 Lavie CJ, Biundo J, Quinet RJ et al. Systemic lupus erythematosus (SLE) induced by quinidine. *Arch Intern Med*, 145, 446-448 (1985)

3438 Lavigne J-G, Marchand C. Inhibition of the gastrointestinal absorption of p-aminosalicylate (PAS) in rats and humans by diphenhydramine. *Clin Pharmacol Ther*, 14, 404-412 (1973)

3439 Law LK, Cheung CK, Swaminathan R. Possible interference by amiodarone and desethylamiodarone in thyroxine assays. *Clin Chem*, 34, 2154 (1988)

3440 Lawler SD, Lele KP. Chromosomal damage induced by chlorambucil in chronic lymphocytic leukaemia. *Scand J Haematol*, 9, 603 (1972)

3441 Lawrence VA, Loewenstein JE, Eichner ER. Aspirin and folate binding: in vivo and in vitro studies of serum binding and urinary excretion of endogenous folate. *J Lab Clin Med*, 103, 944-948 (1984)

3442 Lawson AA, McArdle T, Ghosh S. Cephradine-associated immune neutropenia. *N Engl J Med*, 312, 651 (1985)

3443 Lawson DH, Lovatt GE, Gurton CS et al. Adverse effects of azathioprine. *Adv Drug React Act Pois Rev*, 3, 161-171 (1984)

3444 Lay WH. Drug-induced haemolytic reactions due to antibodies against the erythrocyte/dipyrone complex. *Vox Sang*, 11, 601 (1966)

3445 Lazar HP, Murphy RL, Phair JP. Fansidar® and hepatic granulomas. *Ann Intern Med*, 102, 722 (1985)

3446 Le Bel M, Paone RP, Lewis GP. Effect of ten new β-lactam antibiotics on urine glucose test methods. *Drug Intell Clin Pharm*, 18, 617-620 (1984)

3447 Leach M, Parsons RM, Reilly JT, Winfield DA. Effect of urate oxidase (uricozyme) in tumor lysis induced urate nephropathy. *Clin Lab Haematol*, 20, 169-172 (1998)

3448 Leaf DA, Connor WE, Illingworth R et al. The hypolipidemic effects of gemfibrozil in type V hyperlipidemia; a double-blind, crossover study. *J Am Med Ass*, 262, 3154-3160 (1989)

3449 Leahey EB Jr, Reiffel JA, Giardina E-GV et al. The effect of quinidine and other oral antiarrhythmic drugs on serum digoxin. *Ann Intern Med*, 92, 605-608 (1980)

3450 Leal T, Dupret P, Hassoun A, Wallemacq PE. Topical application of eosin to burns produces interference in measurement of serum vancomycin by fluorescence polarization immunoassay. *Clin Chem*, 43, 1238-1240 (1997)

3451 Leal-Cerro A, Garcia-Luna PP, Villar J et al. Ketoconazole as an inhibitor of steroid production. *N Engl J Med*, 318, 710-711 (1988)

3452 Leary WP, Reyes AJ, Maharaj B. Effects of atenolol, propranolol, and tertatolol on urinary excretion of water and solutes in healthy subjects. *Curr Ther Res*, 44, 630-640 (1988)

3453 Leavell BS, Thorup OA. *Fundamentals of Clinical Hematology, 3rd edition*, Philadelphia PA, WB Saunders (1971)

3454 Lebacq EG, Tirzmalis A. Metformin and lactic acidosis. *Lancet*, 1, 314 (1972)

3455 Lebel M, Vallee F, St-Laurent M. Influence of lomefloxacin on the pharmacokinetics of theophylline. *Antimicrob Agent Chemother*, 34, 1254-1256 (1990)

3456 Leblanc H, Lombrail P, Marre M et al. Prevalence des anticorps antinucleaires chez les diabetiques hypertendus traites par l'acebutolol. *Presse Med*, 13, 2747-2749 (1984)

3457 Lechin F, van der Dijs B, Benaim M. Benzodiazepines: tolerability in elderly patients. *Psychother Psychosom*, 65, 171-182 (1996)

3458 Lechin F, van der Dijs B, Vitelli-Flores G, et al. Peripheral blood immunological parameters in long-term benzodiazepine users. *Clin Neuropharmacol*, 17, 63-72 (1994)

3459 Lechleitner P, Genser N, Mair J et al. Plasma immunoreactive endothelin in the acute and subacute phases of myocardial infarction in patients undergoing fibrinolysis. *Clin Chem*, 39, 955-959 (1993)

3460 Leden I. Digoxin-hydroxychloroquine interaction?. *Acta Med Scand*, 211, 411-412 (1982)

3461 Lederle Laboratories, Division of American Cyanamid Co. Manufacturer's literature on Achromycin® V. Pearl River, NY 10965 (1997)

3462 Lederle Laboratories, Division of American Cyanamid Co. Manufacturer's literature on Asendin® . Pearl River, NY 10965 (1997)

3463 Lederle Laboratories, Division of American Cyanamid Co. Manufacturer's literature on Declomycin® . Pearl River, NY 07470 (1997)

3464 Lederle Laboratories, Division of American Cyanamid Co. Manufacturer's literature on Loxitane® . Pearl River, NY 10965 (1997)

3465 Lederle Laboratories, Division of American Cyanamid Co. Manufacturer's literature on Minocin® . Pearl River, NY 10965 (1997)

3466 Lederle Laboratories, Division of American Cyanamid Co. Manufacturer's literature on Myambutol® . Pearl River, NY 10965 (1997)

3467 Lederle Laboratories, Division of American Cyanamid Co. Manufacturer's literature on Pipracil® . Pearl River, NY 10965 (1997)

3468 Lederle Laboratories, Division of American Cyanamid Co. Manufacturer's literature on Pyrazinamide. Pearl River, NY 10965 (1997)

3469 Lederle Laboratories, Division of American Cyanamid Co. Manufacturer's literature on Suprax® . Pearl River, NY 10965 (1997)

3470 Lederle Laboratories, Division of American Cyanamid Co. Manufacturer's literature on Verelan® . Pearl River, NY 10965 (1997)

3471 Lederle Laboratories, Division of American Cyanamid Co. Manufacturer's literature on Zebeta® . Pearl River, NY 10965 (1997)

3472 Lee C-H, Lee C-J. Thrombocytopenia - a rare but potentially serious side effect of initial daily and interrupted use of rifampicin. *Chest*, 96, 202-203 (1989)

3473 Lee CR, Pollitt RJ. The effect of lithium salts on the urinary excretion of some dicarboxylic acids. *Biochem Soc Trans*, 1, 108 (1973)

3474 Lee DB, Drinkard JP, Rosen VJ et al. The adult Fanconi syndrome: observations on etiology, morphology, renal function, and mineral metabolism. *Medicine*, 51, 107 (1972)

3475 Lee EJ, Kim KR, Lee HC, et al. Acipimox potentiates growth hormone response to growth-hormone-releasing hormone by decreasing serum free fatty acid levels in hyperthyroidism. *Metabolism*, 44, 1509-1512 (1995)

3476 Lee M, Berger HW. Eosinophilia caused by rifampin. *Chest*, 77, 579 (1980)

3477 Lee TH, Rees PJ. Hepatotoxicity of dextropropoxyphene. *Br Med J*, 2, 296-297 (1977)

3478 Lee T-K, Chen Y-C, Kuo T-L et al. Effect of low dose acetylsalicylic acid upon plasma thromboxane B_2 levels and platelet aggregation in ischemic stroke patients. *Clin Chim Acta*, 184, 323-328 (1989)

3479 Lee-Jones M. Serum transaminases during salicylate therapy. *Br Med J*, 2, 772 (1971)

3480 Leeman M, Naeije R, Degaute J-P et al. Acute central and renal haemodynamic responses to tertatolol and propranolol in patients with arterial hypertension following head injury. *J Hypertens*, 4, 581-587 (1986)

3481 Leeman M, van de Borne P, Collart F et al. Bisoprolol and atenolol in essential hypertension: effects on systemic and renal hemodynamics and on ambulatory blood pressure. *J Cardiovasc Pharmacol*, 22, 785-791 (1993)

3482 Leeman M, Vereerstraeten P, Uytdenhoef M et al. Systemic and renal hemodynamic responses to carvedilol and metoprolol in hypertensive renal transplant patients. *J Cardiovasc Pharmacol*, 22, 706-710 (1993)

3483 Leemann NT, Dayer P, Meyer UA. Single dose quinidine treatment inhibits metoprolol oxidation in extensive metabolizers. *Eur J Clin Pharmacol*, 29, 739-741 (1986)

3484 Lees KR, Hughes DM, McNeill CA et al. Pharmacokinetics of perindopril: therapeutic consequences. *Clin Exp Hypertens*, 11, Suppl 2, 499-506 (1989)

3485 Lees KR, Reid JL. Lisinopril and nifedipine. No acute interaction in normotensives. *Br J Clin Pharmacol*, 25, 307-313 (1988)

3486 Lees RS, Schonfeld G, Myers G et al. The efficacy of sitosterols in the treatment of hypercholesterolemia. *Clin Res*, 20, 409 (1972)

3487 Lefebvre H, Contesse V, Delarue C et al. Effect of the serotonin-4 receptor agonist zacopride on aldosterone secretion from the human adrenal cortex: in vivo and in vitro studies. *J Clin Endocrinol Metab*, 77, 1662-1666 (1993)

3488 Lefebvre H, Contesse V, Delarue C, et al. Lack of effect of the serotonin$_4$ receptor agonist zacopride on ACTH secretion in normal men. *Eur J Clin Pharmacol*, 51, 49-51 (1996)

3489 Lefebvre RA, Bogaert MG, Duprez D. Investigation of possible pharmacokinetic and pharmacodynamic interactions between epanolol and digoxin. *Eur J Clin Pharmacol*, 38, 505-507 (1990)

3490 Lefebvre RA, Flouvat B, Karolac-Tamisier S et al. Influence of lansoprazole treatment on diazepam plasma concentrations. *Clin Pharmacol Ther*, 52, 458-463 (1992)

3491 Lefevre MJP. Incidents et accidents des medications neuroleptiques et psychotropes. *J Med Bordeaux*, 144, 139 (1967)

3492 Leff JA, Busse WW, Pearlman D, et al. Montelukast, a leukotriene receptor antagonist, for the treatment of mild asthma and exercise-induced bronchoconstriction. *N Engl J Med*, 339, 147-152 (1998)

3493 Legg EF, Guy JM. Serum creatinine assays in patients receiving the antibiotic cefpirome (HR 810): a study of three different routine methods compared with a specific HPLC method. *Med Lab Sci*, 49, 248-251 (1992)

3494 Legovini P, De Menis E, Doroldi C et al. Parathormone levels during treatment of acromegaly with octreotide: one-year follow-up. *Clin Ther Res*, 53, 360-366 (1993)

3495 Legro RS, Gentzschein E, Carmina E et al. Alterations in androgen conjugate levels in women and men with alopecia. *Fertil Steril*, 62, 744-750 (1994)

3496 Lehnert H, Schmitz H, Preuss K et al. Effects of nitrendipine on blood pressure, renin-angiotensin-system and atrial natriuretic peptide in hypertensive type I diabetic patients. *Horm Metab Res*, 25, 24-28 (1992)

3497 Lehto P, Kivisto KT, Neuvonen PJ. The effect of ferrous sulfate on the absorption of norfloxacin, ciprofloxacin and ofloxacin. *Br J Clin Pharmacol*, 37, 82-85 (1994)

3498 Lehtonen A. Doxazosin effects on insulin and glucose in hypertensive patients. *Am Heart J*, 121, II Suppl, 1307-1311 (1991)

3499 Lehtonen A. Effect of beta blockers on blood lipid profile. *Am Heart J*, 109, 1192-1196 (1985)

3500 Lehtonen A. Long-term effect of pindolol on plasma lipids, apoproteins A, blood glucose and serum insulin levels. *Int J Clin Pharmacol Ther Toxicol*, 22, 269-272 (1984)

3501 Lehtonen A. The effect of acebutolol on plasma lipids, blood glucose and serum insulin levels. *Acta Med Scand*, 216, 57-60 (1984)

3502 Lehtonen A and the Finnish Multicenter Study Group. Lowered levels of serum insulin, glucose, and cholesterol in hypertensive patients during treatment with doxazosin. *Curr Ther Res*, 47, 278-284 (1990)

3503 Lehtonen A, Gronroos M, Marniemi J et al. Effects of high dose progestin on serum lipids and lipid metabolizing enzymes in patients with endometrial cancer. *Horm Metab Res*, 17, 32-34 (1985)

3504 Lehtonen A, Raiha I, Puumalainen R et al. The effect of the short-term administration of fish oil on serum lipoproteins in old people. *Gerontology*, 35, 311-314 (1990)

3505 Lehtonen A, Tanskanen A, Lehto H et al. The effect of nifedipine on plasma lipids in patients with essential hypertension. *Int J Clin Pharmacol Ther Toxicol*, 24, 357-358 (1986)

3506 Lehtonen A, Viikari J. Long-term effect of sotalol on plasma lipids. *Clin Sci*, 57, 405s-407s (1979)

3507 Lehtonen L, Lankinen KS, Wikberg R et al. Hepatic safety of erythromycin acistrate in 1549 patients with respiratory tract or skin infections. *J Antimicrob Chemother*, 27, 233-242 (1991)

3508 Leibovitz A, Bilchinsky T, Gil I, Habot B. Elevated serum digoxin level associated with coadministered fluoxetine. *Arch Intern Med*, 158, 1152-1153 (1998)

3509 Leinonen E, Lillsunde P, Laukkanen V et al. Effects of carbamazepine on serum antidepressant concentrations in psychiatric patients. *J Clin Psychopharmacol*, 11, 313-318 (1991)

3510 Leiss O, Von Bergmann K. Different effects of chenodeoxycholic acid and ursodeoxycholic acid on serum lipoprotein concentrations in patients with radiolucent gallstones. *Scand J Gastroenterol*, 17, 587-592 (1982)

3511 Lekkerkerker JFF, Liem Ch'ing SZE, Doorenbos H. The influence of chlorthalidone on calcium absorption from the gut in relation to urinary calcium excretion. *Abstracts IV Int Congr Endocrinol, Washington DC*, 239 (1972)

3512 Lemay A, Dewailly SD. Long-term use of the low dose LHRH analogue combined with monthly medroxyprogesterone administration. *Horm Res*, Suppl 1, 141-145 (1989)

3513 Lemberger L, Crabtree R, Callaghan JT. Pergolide, a potent long-acting dopamine receptor agonist. *Clin Pharmacol Ther*, 27, 642-651 (1980)

3514 Lentjes EGWM, Romijn F, Maassen RJ et al. Free cortisol in serum assayed by temperature-controlled ultrafiltration before fluorescence polarization immunoassay. *Clin Chem*, 39, 2518-2521 (1993)

3515 Leon AS, Agre J, McNally C et al. Blood lipid effects of antihypertensive therapy: a double-blind comparison of the effects of methyldopa and propranolol. *J Clin Pharmacol*, 24, 209-217 (1984)

3516 Leonetti G, Bonazzi O, Grazi S et al. Cardiovascular and renal effects of acute administration of a new hypotensive compound, guancydine. *Eur J Clin Pharmacol*, 4, 1 (1971)

3517 Leonhardt W, Hanefeld M, Fischer S et al. Beneficial effects on serum lipids in noninsulin dependent diabetics by acarbose treatment. *Arz Forsch Drug Res*, 41, 735-738 (1991)

3518 Lepage L, Schiele F, Gueguen R et al. Total cholinesterase in plasma: biological variations and reference limits. *Clin Chem*, 31, 545-550 (1985)

3519 Lepage N, Roberts KD, Langlais J. Interference of lysophosphatidylcholine in hormone radioimmunoassays. *Clin Chem*, 39, 865-869 (1993)

3520 Lequin R, Olsen D. Progesterone assay for the Auraflex immunoassay system. *Clin Chem*, 41, S35 (1995)

3521 Leren P, Eide I, Foss OP et al. Antihypertensive drugs and blood lipids: the Oslo study. *J Cardiovasc Pharmacol*, 4, Suppl 2, S222-S224 (1982)

3522 Leren P, Foss PO, Helgeland A et al. Effect of propranolol and prazosin on blood lipids. *Lancet*, II, 4-6 (1980)

3523 Lerner RL, Porte D Jr. Studies of secretin-stimulated insulin responses in man. *J Clin Invest*, 51, 2205 (1972)

3524 Lessem J, Bellinetto A. Interactions between digoxin and the calcium antagonists nicardipine and tiapamil. *Clin Ther*, 5, 592-602 (1983)

3525 Letellier G, Desjarlais F. Analytical interference of drugs in clinical chemistry: 1. Study of twenty drugs on seven different instruments. *Clin Biochem*, 18, 345-351 (1985)

3526 Letendre PW, Carlson JD, Seifert RD et al. Effect of sucralfate on the absorption and pharmacokinetics of chlorpropamide. *J Clin Pharmacol*, 26, 622-625 (1986)

3527 Leung ACT, Henderson IS, Halls DJ et al. Aluminum hydroxide versus sucralfate is a phosphate binder in uraemia. *Br Med J*, 286, 1379-1381 (1983)

3528 Leung NWY, Leung JCK, Tam JS et al. Effects of α-interferon and prednisone on serum-soluble interleukin-2 receptor (sIL-2R) in chronic hepatitis B infection. *Am J Gastroenterol*, 87, 113-117 (1992)

3529 Leuven JAG, van der Mooren MJ, Nuytenhek R. The effect of medrogesterone on plasma lipids and lipoproteins in postmenopausal women using conjugated estrogens: an open randomized comparative study. *Fertil Steril*, 64, 525-531 (1995)

3530 Levenson SA, MacFate RP. Clinical Laboratory Diagnosis. *6th edition*, Philadelphia PA, Lea and Febiger (1961)

3531 Lever M, Powell JC, Killip M, Small CW. A comparison of 4-hydroxybenzoic acid hydrazide (PABAH) with other reagents for the determination of glucose. *J Lab Clin Med*, 82, 649 (1973)

3532 Levesque H, Verdier S, Cailleux N et al. Low molecular weight heparins and hypoaldosteronism. *Br Med J*, 300, 1437-1438 (1990)

3533 Levesque LA, Herzog AG, Seibel MM. The effect of phenytoin and carbamazepine on serum dehydroepiandrosterone sulfate in men and women who have partial seizures with temporal lobe involvement.. *J Clin Endocrinol Metab*, 63, 243-245 (1986)

3534 Levi L. The effect of coffee on the function of the sympatho-adrenomedullary system in man. *Acta Med Scand*, 181, 431 (1967)

3535 Levillain R, Bouaziz I, Cluzan R et al. 15 years of experience with N-desacetylthiocolchicine (thiocolciran) in cancerology. *Therapie*, 27, 77 (1972)

3536 Levin HA, McMillan R, Tavassoll M. Thrombocytopenia associated with gold therapy: observations on the mechanism of platelet destruction. *Am J Med*, 59, 274-280 (1975)

3537 Levin K, Josephson B, Grunewald G. The effect of iodochloro-oxyquinoline and iopanoic acid on the determination of PBI and BEI. *Acta Endocrinol*, 52, 627 (1966)

3538 Levine BD, Yoshimura K, Kobayashi T et al. Dexamethasone in the treatment of acute mountain sickness. *N Engl J Med*, 321, 1707-1713 (1989)

3539 Levine BS, Caplan YH. Isometheptene cross reacts in the amphetamine assay. *Clin Chem*, 33, 1264-1265 (1987)

3540 Levine DN, Collin D, Parker T. Evaluation of the new Roche reagent for measuring triglycerides in serum or plasma. *Clin Chem*, 37, 923 (1991)

3541 Levine M, Jones MW, Sheppard I. Differential effect of cimetidine on serum concentrations of carbamazepine and phenytoin. *Neurology*, 35, 562-565 (1985)

3542 Levine MAH, Ogilvie RI, Leenen FHH. Pharmacokinetic and pharmacodynamic interactions between nisoldipine and propranolol. *Clin Pharmacol Ther*, 43, 39-48 (1988)

3543 Levine MF, Sarner J, Lerman J, et al. Plasma inorganic fluoride concentrations after sevoflurane anesthesia in children. *Anesthesiology*, 84, 348-353 (1996)

3544 Levine RA. Steatorrhea induced by para-aminosalicylic acid. *Ann Intern Med*, 68, 1265 (1968)

3545 Levitt PE, Jones R, Samuell CT. Positive interference by cotrimoxazole in the o-phthaldehyde method for plasma urea. *Proc ACB Natl Meet*, 97 (1991)

3546 Levy M, Eliakim M. Urinary precipitate during cephalothin - cephaloridine treatment. *J Am Med Ass*, 219, 908 (1972)

3547 Levy M, Goodman MW, Van Dyne BJ et al. Granulomatous hepatitis secondary to carbamazepine. *Ann Intern Med*, 95, 64-65 (1981)

3548 Lewandowski R, Sokalski T, Hulanicki A. Influence of aspirin on in vitro direct potentiometry of Cl in serum. *Clin Chem*, 35, 2146 (1989)

3549 Lewin PK. Phenytoin-associated congenital defects with Y-chromosome variant. *Lancet*, 1, 559 (1973)

3550 Lewis IJ, Rosenbloom L. Glandular fever-like syndrome, pulmonary eosinophilia and asthma associated with carbamazepine. *Postgrad Med J*, 58, 100-101 (1982)

3551 Lewis JH, Zimmermann HJ, Ishak KG et al. Enflurane hepatotoxicity: a clinicopathologic study of 24 cases. *Ann Intern Med*, 98, 984-992 (1983)

3552 Lewis RJ, Trager WF, Robinson AJ et al. Warfarin metabolites: the anticoagulant activity and pharmacology of warfarin alcohols. *J Lab Clin Med*, 81, 925 (1973)

3553 Lewis SA, Oswald I, Dunleavy DLF. Chronic fenfluramine administration: some cerebral effects. *Br Med J*, 3, 67 (1971)

3554 Leza MA. Agranulocitosis medicamentossas con plasmacitosis medular e hipery globinemia. *Rev Clin Esp*, 103, 316 (1966)

3555 Liakakos D, Papadopoulos Z, Vlachos P et al. Serum alkaline phosphatase and urinary hydroxyproline values in children receiving phenobarbital with and without vitamin D. *J Pediatr*, 87, 291-296 (1975)

3556 Liakakos D, Valchos P, Anoussakis C. Effect of acetylsalicylic acid (aspirin) on bone collagen. *Clin Chim Acta*, 44, 427 (1973)

3557 Liang E, Hardy J, DeSouza S et al. An enzyme immunoassay for red cell folate using the Bio-Rad Radias system. *Clin Chem*, 41, S74 (1995)

3558 Liaw Y-F, Huang M-J, Fan K-D et al. Hepatic injury during propylthiouracil therapy in patients with hyperthyroidism: a cohort study. *Ann Intern Med*, 118, 424-428 (1993)

3559 Libretti A, Catalano M. Lipid profile during antihypertensive treatment: the SLIP study. *Drugs*, 46, Suppl 2, 16-23 (1993)

3560 Licata AA, Bartter FC. Spironolactone-induced gynecomastia related to allergic reaction to Darvon® compound. *Lancet*, 1, 905 (1976)

3561 Lichtenwalner MR, Mencken T, Tully R, Petosa M. False-positive immunochemical screen for methadone attributable to metabolites of verapamil. *Clin Chem*, 44, 1039-1041 (1998)

3562 Lichtiger B, Rogge K. Spurious serologic test results in patients receiving infusions of intravenous immune γglobulin. *Arch Pathol Lab Med*, 115, 467-469 (1991)

3563 Liddle GW. Tests of pituitary-adrenal supressibility in the diagnosis of Cushing's syndrome. *J Clin Endocrinol Metab*, 20, 1539 (1960)

3564 Lidsky MD, Sharp JT. Jaundice with the use of 4-hydroxypyrazol-(3,4-D)-pyrimidine (4-HPP). *Arth Rheum*, 10, 294 (1967)

3565 Lieberman AN, Kupersmith M, Gopinathan G et al. Bromocriptidine in Parkinson disease: further studies. *Neurology*, 29, 363-369 (1979)

3566 Lien EA, Johannessen DC, Aakvaag A et al. Influence of tamoxifen, aminoglutethimide and goserelin on human plasma IGF-I levels in breast cancer patients. *J Steroid Biochem Mol Biol*, 41, 837-839 (1992)

3567 Lieschke GJ, Burgess AW. Drug therapy: granulocyte colony-stimulating factor and granulocyte-macrophage colony-stimulating factor. *N Engl J Med*, 327, 28-35 (1992)

3568 Liewendahl K, Majuri H, Helenius T. Thyroid function tests in patients on long-term treatment with various anticonvulsant drugs. *Clin Endocrinol*, 8, 185-191 (1978)

3569 Liewendahl K, Tikanoja S, Helenius T et al. Free thyroxine and free tri-iodothyronine as measured by equilibrium dialysis and analog radioimmunoassay in serum of patients taking phenytoin and carbamazepine. *Clin Chem*, 31, 1993-1996 (1985)

3570 Lifton LJ, Kreiser J. False positive stool occult blood tests caused by iron preparations: a controlled study and review of literature. *Gastroenterology*, 83, 860-863 (1982)

3571 Lijnen P, Amery A. Serum lipid changes during α_1- and β_1- adrenergic receptor blockade with doxazosin and atenolol. *Clin Chem*, 36, 968 (1990)

3572 Lijnen P, Fagard R, Staessen J et al. Hormonal effects of the diuretic xipamide in healthy men. *Cardiovasc Drug Ther*, 5, 741-748 (1991)

3573 Lijnen P, Fagard R, Staessen J et al. Humoral and cellular effects of the K^+-channel activator cromakalim in man. *Eur J Clin Pharmacol*, 37, 609-611 (1989)

3574 Lijnen P, Fagard R, Staessen J et al. Serum cholesterol during ketanserin and propranolol administration in hypertensive patients. *J Cardiovasc Pharmacol*, 10, 647-650 (1987)

3575 Lijnen P, Hespel P, Fagard R et al. Plasma atrial natriuretic peptide and the renin-aldosterone system during long-term administration of the diuretic xipamide in man. *Eur J Clin Pharmacol*, 36, 111-117 (1989)

3576 Lillicrap DP, Pinto M, Benford K et al. Heterogeneity of laboratory test results for antiphospholipid antibodies in patients treated with chlorpromazine and other phenothiazines. *Am J Clin Pathol*, 93, 771-775 (1990)

3577 Lilly JR, Hitch DC, Javitt NB. Cimetidine cholestatic jaundice in children. *J Surg Res*, 24, 384-387 (1978)

3578 Lima MC, Ajzen HA, Ribeiro AB et al. Effect of angiotensin II on urinary magnesium, calcium, and sodium excretion. *Am J Med Sci*, 263, 173 (1972)

3579 Limas C, Guiha NH, Freis ED. Treatment of severe resistant hypertension with minoxidil. *Clin Pharmacol Ther*, 13, 145 (1972)

3580 LiMuti C, LaTart D, Mauck J et al. Performance of the Kodak Ektachem clinical chemistry slide (Prot) in the determination of urinary protein. *Clin Chem*, 39, 1135-1136 (1993)

3581 Lin AC, Goldwasser E, Bernard EM et al. Amphotericin B blunts erythropoietin response to anemia. *J Infect Dis*, 161, 348-351 (1990)

3582 Lin H-Y, Rocher LL, McQuillan MA et al. Cyclosporine-induced hyperuricemia and gout. *N Engl J Med*, 321, 287-292 (1989)

3583 Lin MS, Huang CS. Lack of effect of labetalol on platelet aggregation in hypertensive patients. *Int J Clin Pharmacol Ther Toxicol*, 29, 391-393 (1991)

3584 Lin T, Tucci JR. Comparison of provocative tests of growth hormone release. *Clin Res*, 20, 866 (1972)

3585 Lind T, Cederberg C, Olausson M et al. Omeprazole in elderly duodenal ulcer patients: relationship between reduction in gastric acid secretion and fasting plasma gastrin. *Eur J Clin Pharmacol*, 40, 557-560 (1991)

3586 Lindberg U-B, Crona N, Enk L et al. Effects of cyproterone acetate (CPA) on serum lipoproteins when administered alone and in combination with ethinyl estradiol (EE). *Horm Metab Res*, 79, 222-225 (1987)

3587 Lindeberg S, Holm B, Lundborg P et al. The effect of hydralazine on steady-state plasma concentrations of metoprolol in pregnant hypertensive women. *Eur J Clin Pharmacol*, 35, 131-135 (1988)

3588 Lindenbaum J, Maulitz RM, Butler VP Jr. Inhibition of digoxin absorption by neomycin. *Gastroenterology*, 71, 399-404 (1976)

3589 Lindenbaum J, Rund DG, Butler VP Jr et al. Inactivation of digoxin by the gut flora: reversal by antibiotic therapy. *N Engl J Med*, 305, 789-794 (1981)

3590 Linder MW, Keck PE Jr. Standards of laboratory practice: antidepressant drug monitoring. *Clin Chem*, 44, 1073-1084 (1998)

3591 Lindholm J, Schultz-Moller N. Plasma and urinary cortisol in pregnancy and during estrogen-gestagen treatment. *Scand J Clin Lab Invest*, 31, 119 (1973)

3592 Lindhout D, Meinardi H. False-negative pregnancy test in women taking carbamazepine. *Lancet*, 2, 505 (1982)

3593 Lindor KD, Mayo Primary Sclerosing Cholangitis-Ursodeoxycholic Acid Study Group. Ursodiol for primary sclerosing cholangitis. *N Engl J Med*, 336, 691-695 (1997)

3594 Lindquist M, Edwards IR. Endocrine adverse effects of omeprazole. *Br Med J*, 305, 451-452 (1992)

3595 Lindstedt G, Lundberg PA, Tofft M et al. Serum thyrotropin and hypothyroidism during lithium therapy. *Clin Chim Acta*, 48, 127 (1973)

3596 Lindstedt G, Nilsson L-A, Walinder J et al. On the prevalence, diagnosis and management of lithium-induced hypothyroidism in psychiatric patients. *Br J Psychiat*, 130, 452-458 (1977)

3597 Ling BN, Bourke E, Campbell WG Jr et al. Naproxen-induced nephropathy in systemic lupus erythematosus. *Nephron*, 54, 249-255 (1993)

3598 Linna O, Uhari M. Hepatotoxicity of rifampicin and isoniazid in children treated for tuberculosis. *Eur J Pediatr*, 134, 227-229 (1980)

3599 Lintott CJ, Sutherland WHF, Scott RS et al. Treating hypercholesterolaemia with HMG CoA reductase inhibitors: a direct comparison of simvastatin and pravastatin. *Aust NZ J Med*, 23, 381-386 (1993)

3600 Liou H-H, Chiang S-S, Wu S-C et al. Hypokalemic effect of intravenous infusion or nebulization of salbutamol in patients with chronic renal failure: comparative study. *Am J Kid Dis*, 23, 266-271 (1994)

3601 Liou H-H, Huang T-P, Campese VM. Effect of long-term therapy with captopril on proteinuria and renal function in patients with non-insulin-dependent diabetes and with non-diabetic renal diseases. *Nephron*, 69, 41-48 (1995)

3602 Liozon E, Volkov L, Comte L et al. AcSDKP serum concentrations vary during chemotherapy in patients with acute myeloid leukemia. *Br J Haematol*, 89, 917-920 (1995)

3603 Lippi G, Braga V, Adami S, Guidi G. Modification of serum apolipoprotein A-I, apolipoprotein B and lipoprotein(a) levels after bisphosphonates-induced acute phase response. *Clin Chim Acta*, 271, 79-87 (1998)

3604 Lipsett MB, Combs JW, Catt K et al. Problems in contraceptives. *Ann Intern Med*, 74, 251 (1971)

3605 Lissoni P, Ardizzoia A, Perego MS et al. Inhibition of tumor necrosis factor-α secretion by pentoxifylline in advanced cancer patients with abnormally high blood levels of tumor necrosis factor-α. *J Biol Regulators Homeostatic Agents*, 7, 73-75 (1993)

3606 Lissoni P, Barni S, Archili C et al. Endocrine effects of a 24-hour intravenous infusion of interleukin-2 in the immunotherapy of cancer. *Anticancer Res*, 10, 753-757 (1990)

3607 List AF, Beaird DH, Kummet T. Ranitidine-induced granulocytopenia: recurrence with cimetidine administration. *Ann Intern Med*, 108, 566-567 (1988)

3608 Lithell H, Berne C, Waern AU et al. Glucose metabolism during long-term treatment with prazosin. *Diabetes Res*, 2, 297-299 (1985)

3609 Lithell H, Haglund K, Granath F et al. Are effects of antihypertensive treatment on lipoproteins merely "side-effects"?. *Acta Med Scand*, 223, 531-536 (1988)

3610 Lithell H, Weiner L, Selinus I et al. A comparison of the effects of bisoprolol and atenolol on lipoprotein concentrations and blood pressure. *J Cardiovasc Pharmacol*, 8, Suppl, S128-S133 (1986)

3611 Lithell H, Weiner L, Vessby B et al. Effects of small doses of bisoprolol on blood pressure and lipoprotein concentrations in hypertensive patients. *Eur J Clin Pharmacol*, 44, 19-22 (1993)

3612 Littley MD, Gibson S, White A et al. Comparison of the ACTH and cortisol responses to provocative testing with glucagon and insulin hypoglycaemia in normal subjects. *Clin Endocrinol*, 31, 527-533 (1989)

3613 Liu C-S, Wu H-M, Kao S-H, Wei Y-H. Phenytoin-mediated oxidative stress in serum of female epileptics: a possible pathogenesis in the fetal hydantoin syndrome. *Hum Exp Toxicol*, 16, 177-181 (1997)

3614 Liu C-S, Wu H-M, Kao S-H, Wei Y-H. Serum trace elements, glutathione, copper/zinc superoxide dismutase, and lipid peroxidation in epileptic patients with phenytoin or carbamazepine monotherapy. *Clin Neuropharmacol*, 21, 62-64 (1998)

3615 Liu K, Mittelman A, Sproul EE et al. Renal toxicity in man treated with mitomycin-C. *Cancer*, 28, 1314 (1971)

3616 Liu TZ, Oka KH. Spectrophotometric screening method for acetaminophen in serum and plasma. *Clin Chem*, 26, 69-71 (1980)

3617 Liukko P, Erkkola R, Bergink EW. Progestagen-dependent effect on some plasma proteins during oral contraception. *Gynecol Obstet Invest*, 25, 118-122 (1988)

3618 Liukko P, Erokkola R, Pakarinen P et al. Trace elements during 2 years' oral contraception with low-estrogen preparations. *Gynecol Obstet Invest*, 25, 113-117 (1988)

3619 Ljungberg B, Beving H, Egberg N et al. Immediate effects of heparin and LMW heparin on some platelet and endothelial derived factors. *Thromb Res*, 51, 209-217 (1988)

3620 Ljunghall S, Althoff P, Fellstrom B et al. Effects on serum parathyroid hormone of intravenous treatment with alphacalcidol in patients on chronic hemodialysis. *Nephron*, 55, 380-385 (1990)

3621 Ljunghall S, Gardsell P, Johnell O et al. Synthetic human calcitonin in postmenopausal osteoporosis: a placebo-controlled double-blind study. *Calcif Tissue Int*, 49, 17-19 (1991)

3622 Ljutic D, Rumboldt Z. Possible interaction between azithromycin and cyclosporin: a case report. *Nephron*, 70, 130 (1995)

3623 Llerena O, Pearson O. Interference of nalidixic acid in urinary 17-ketosteroid determinations. *N Engl J Med*, 279, 983 (1968)

3624 Lloyd TW. Agranulocytosis associated with paracetamol. *Lancet*, 1, 114 (1961)

3625 Lo Cascio V, Kanis JA, Beneton MNC et al. Acute effects of deflazacort and prednisone on rates of mineralization and bone formation. *Calcif Tissue Int*, 56, 109-112 (1995)

3626 Lo CH, Stelson H. Interference by polysucrose in protein determination by the Lowry method. *Anal Biochem*, 45, 331 (1971)

3627 Lobatto S, Dijkmans BAC, Mattie H et al. Flucloxacillin-associated liver damage. *Neth J Med*, 25, 47-48 (1982)

3628 Lobo RA. Effects of hormonal replacement on lipids and lipoproteins in post menopausal women. *J Clin Endocrinol Metab*, 73, 925-930 (1991)

3629 Loche S, Pintus S, Carta D et al. The effect of atenolol on the growth hormone response to growth hormone-releasing hormone in obese children. *Acta Endocrinol*, 126, 124-127 (1992)

3630 Locker PK, Jungbluth GL, Francom SF et al. Lifibrol: a novel lipid-lowering drug for the therapy of hypercholesterolemia. *Clin Pharmacol Ther*, 57, 73-88 (1995)

3631 Loertscher R, Thiel G, Harder F et al. Persistent elevation of alkaline phosphatase in cyclosporine-treated renal- transplant recipients. *Transplantation*, 36, 115-116 (1983)

3632 Lofaso F, Baud FJ, Halna DU et al. Hypokalemia in massive chloroquine intoxication: two cases. *Presse Med*, 16, 22-24 (1987)

3633 Loga S. Interactions of orphenadrine and phenobarbitone with chlorpromazine: plasma concentrations and effects in man. *Br J Clin Pharmacol*, 2, 197 (1975)

3634 Loga S, Curry S, Lader M. Interaction of chlorpromazine and nortriptyline in patients with schizophrenia. *Clin Pharmacokinet*, 6, 454-462 (1981)

3635 Loh HS, Watters K, Wilson CWM. The effects of aspirin on the metabolic availability of ascorbic acid in humans. *J Clin Pharmacol*, 13, 480 (1973)

3636 Loi C-M, Day JD, Jue SG et al. Dose-dependent inhibition of theophylline metabolism by disulfiram in recovering alcoholics. *Clin Pharmacol Ther*, 45, 476-486 (1989)

3637 Loi C-M, Knowlton PW, Stern R, et al. Effect of troglitazone on steady-state pharmacokinetics of digoxin. *J Clin Pharmacol*, 38, 178-183 (1998)

3638 Loi C-M, Parker BM, Cusack BJ et al. Individual and combined effects of cimetidine and ciprofloxacin on theophylline metabolism in male nonsmokers. *Br J Clin Pharmacol*, 36, 195-200 (1993)

3639 Loi C-M, Rollins E, Dukes GE et al. Effect of cimetidine on verapamil disposition. *Clin Pharmacol Ther*, 37, 654-657 (1985)

3640 Long KP, Marcuson R, Miyashita K et al. Urinary excretion of calcium, dopamine, norepinephrine, and epinephrine in young women following ascorbic acid ingestion. *Nutr Res*, 12, 1051-1063 (1992)

3641 Longo G, Valenti C, Gandini G, et al. Azithromycin-induced intrahepatic cholestasis. *Am J Med*, 102, 217-218 (1997)

3642 Longstreth GF, Green R. Folate status in patients receiving maintenance doses of sulfasalazine. *Arch Intern Med*, 143, 902-904 (1983)

3643 Lonning PE, Johannessen DC, Lien EA et al. Influence of tamoxifen on sex hormones, goadotrophins and sex hormone binding globulin in postmenopausal breast cancer patients. *J Steroid Biochem Mol Biol*, 52, 491-496 (1995)

3644 Looij BJ Jr, Roelfsema F, Van der Heide D et al. The effect of calcitonin on growth hormone secretion in man. *Clin Endocrinol*, 29, 517-527 (1988)

3645 Lopez A, Rene A. Effect of 17 ketosteroids on glucose-6-phosphate dehydrogenase activity on G6PD isoenzymes. *Proc Soc Exp Biol Med*, 142, 258 (1973)

3646 Loraine JA, Bell ET. Hormone Assays and Their Clinical Applications. *3rd edition*, Baltimore MD, Williams and Wilkins (1971)

3647 Lorentz K, Bais R, Bayer PM et al. New method for the determination of pancreatic amylase evaluated. *J Clin Lab Anal*, 5, 410-414 (1991)

3648 Lorenz W, Doenicke A, Meyer R et al. Histamine release in man by propanidid and thiopentone: pharmacological effects and clinical consequences. *Br J Anaes*, 44, 355 (1972)

3649 Loscalzo J, Braunwald E. Tissue plasminogen activator. *N Engl J Med*, 319, 925-931 (1988)

3650 Loschiavo C, Valvo E, Bedogna V et al. Effects of ketanserin administration on lipid metabolism and platelet aggregation in hypertensive patients. *Int J Clin Pharmacol Ther Toxicol*, 28, 455-457 (1990)

3651 Losek JD, Werlin SL. Sulfasalazine hepatotoxicity. *Am J Dis Child*, 135, 1070-1072 (1981)

3652 Lotito CA, Mengel CE. Effect of melphalan in the malignant carcinoid syndrome. *Arch Intern Med*, 124, 36 (1969)

3653 Lott JA, Bond LW, Bobo RC et al. Valproic acid-associated pancreatitis: report of three cases and a brief review. *Clin Chem*, 36, 395-397 (1990)

3654 Lott JA, Warren P. Estimation of reference intervals for total protein in cerebrospinal fluid. *Clin Chem*, 35, 1766-1770 (1989)

3655 Lotti T, Mirone V, Prezioso D et al. Observations on serum hormone fractions in patients with benign prostatic hyperplasia treated with mepartricin. *Curr Ther Res*, 44, 402-409 (1988)

3656 Lotus Biochemical Corporation. Manufacturer's literature on Adapin® . Radford, VA 24143 (1993)

3657 Lotus Biochemical Corporation. Manufacturer's literature on Ergomar® . Radford, VA 24143 (1995)

3658 Lotz J, Hafher G, Röhrich J, et al. False-positive LSD drug screening induced by a mucolytic medication. *Clin Chem*, 44, 1580-1581 (1998)

3659 Loubatieres AL. Confrontation of experimental and clinical pharmacological observations in the field of hypoglycaemic. *Arch Int Pharmacol Ther*, 192, Suppl, 133 (1971)

3660 Loun B, Astles R, Copeland KR et al. Leukocytes magnesium content in leukemia, infection, G-CSF treatment. *Clin Chem*, 41, S222 (1995)

3661 Louria DB, Joselow MM, Browder AA. The human toxicity of certain trace elements. *Ann Intern Med*, 76, 307 (1972)

3662 Love JE, Kelley D, Branch L et al. Effect of dietary n-3 fatty acids (flax seed oil) on plasma lipids, lipoproteins and apolipoproteins in humans. *Clin Chem*, 36, 956 (1990)

3663 Love RR, Mazess RB, Barden HS et al. Effects of tamoxifen on bone mineral density in postmenopausal women with breast cancer. *N Engl J Med*, 326, 852-856 (1992)

3664 Love RR, Newcomb PA, Wiebe DA et al. Effects of tamoxifen therapy on lipid and lipoprotein levels in postmenopausal patients with node-negative breast cancer. *J Natl Cancer Inst*, 82, 1327-1332 (1990)

3665 Loviselli A, Calia MA, Murenu S et al. Circulating soluble IL-2 receptor levels are low in patients with hypothyroid autoimmune thyroiditis. *Horm Metab Res*, 26, 548-551 (1994)

3666 Lowe J, Gray J, Henry DA et al. Adverse reactions to frusemide in hospital patients. *Br Med J*, 2, 360-362 (1979)

3667 Lowenstein FW. Serum magnesium in women during pregnancy, while taking contraceptives, and after menopause. *J Am Coll Nutr*, 6, 313-319 (1987)

3668 Lozada A, Dujovne CA. Drug interactions with fibric acids. *Pharmacol Ther*, 63, 163-176 (1994)

3669 Lubran M. The effects of drugs on laboratory values. *Med Clin North Am*, 53, 211 (1969)

3670 Luby ED, Schwartz D, Rosenbaum H. Lithium carbonate-induced myxedema. *J Am Med Ass*, 218, 1298 (1971)

3671 Luce GG. Biological Rhythms in Psychiatry and Medicine. Washington DC, PHS Publication No 2088 (1970)

3672 Lucena MI, Moreno A, Fernandez MC et al. Digitoxin elimination in healthy subjects taking ampicillin. *Int J Clin Pharmacol Res*, 7, 33-37 (1987)

3673 Lucey JV, O'Keane V, O'Flynn K et al. Gender and age differences in the growth hormone response to pyridostigmine. *Int Clin Psychopharmacol*, 6, 105-109 (1991)

3674 Luciano AA, Hauser KS, Chapler FK et al. Danazol: endocrine consequences in healthy women. *Am J Obstet Gynecol*, 141, 723-727 (1981)

3675 Luder PJ, Siffert B, Witassek F et al. Treatment of hydatid disease with high oral doses of mebendazole. Long-term follow-up of plasma mebendazole levels and drug interactions. *Eur J Clin Pharmacol*, 31, 443-448 (1986)

3676 Ludwig H, Fritz E, Kotzmann H et al. Erythropoietin treatment of anemia associated with multiple myeloma. *N Engl J Med*, 322, 1693-1699 (1990)

3677 Luke RG, Koepke JA, Siegel RR. The effects of immunosuppressive drugs and uremia on automated leukocyte counts. *Am J Clin Pathol*, 56, 503 (1971)

3678 Lukkari E, Juhakoski A, Aranko K, Neuvonen PJ. Itraconazole moderately increases serum concentrations of oxybutynin but does not affect thos of its active metabolite. *Eur J Clin Pharmacol*, 52, 403-406 (1997)

3679 Lum G. Significance of low serum alkaline phosphatase activity in a predominantly adult population. *Clin Chem*, 41, 515-518 (1995)

3680 Lum G, Leal-Khouri S. Significance of low serum urea nitrogen concentrations. *Clin Chem*, 35, 639-640 (1989)

3681 Lumsden MA, West CP, Baird DT. Tamoxifen prolongs luteal phase in premenopausal women but has no effect on the size of uterine fibroids. *Clin Endocrinol*, 31, 335-343 (1989)

3682 Lund C, Qvitzau S, Greulich A et al. Comparison of the effects of extradural clonidine with those of morphine on postoperative pain, stress responses, cardiopulmonary function and motor and sensory block. *Br J Anaes*, 63, 516-519 (1989)

3683 Lund J, Pedersen HE, Olsen PZ et al. Early human studies of a new carbonic anhydrase inhibitor (NSD 3004) with anticonvulsant properties. *Clin Pharmacol Ther*, 12, 902 (1971)

3684 Lundberg B, Nergardh A, Boreus LO. Plasma concentrations of valproate during maintenance therapy in epileptic children. *J Neurol*, 228, 133-141 (1982)

3685 Lundborg P. The effect of adrenergic blockade on potassium concentrations in different conditions. *Acta Med Scand*, 672, Suppl, 121-125 (1983)

3686 Lundborg P, Regard CG. The effect of propoxyphene pretreatment on the disposition of metoprolol and propranolol. *Clin Pharmacol Ther*, 29, 263-264 (1981)

3687 Lupovitch A. Phenothiazine interference and the Porter-Silber reaction. *Clin Chem*, 14, 179 (1968)

3688 Lurie AO. Spironolactone and steroid assay. *Lancet*, 2, 326 (1969)

3689 Lussier-Cacan S, Davignon J, Nestruck AC et al. Influence of a triphasic oral contraceptive preparation on plasma lipids and lipoproteins. *Fertil Steril*, 53, 28-34 (1990)

3690 Lustgarten BP. Catabolic response to lovastatin therapy. *Ann Intern Med*, 109, 171-172 (1988)

3691 Luther RR, Glassman HN, Estep CB et al. The effects of terazosin and methyclothiazide on blood pressure and serum lipids. *Am Heart J*, 117, 842-847 (1989)

3692 Luther RR, Klepper MJ, Maurath CJ et al. Effects of terazosin on serum lipid levels in hypertensive blacks. *J Hum Hypertens*, 4, 154-156 (1990)

3693 Lutz EG. Monocytosis blood dyscrasia and chlorpromazine toxicity. *Int J Neuropsychiat*, 1, 76 (1965)

3694 Lutze G, Breyer J, Zawta B. Useful facts about coagulation: questions and answers. *Useful Facts about Coagulation*, Boehringer Mannheim GmbH, Mannheim (1996)

3695 Luurila H, Kivistö KT, Neuvonen PJ. Effect of itraconazole on the pharmacokinetics and pharmacodynamics of zolpidem. *Eur J Clin Pharmacol*, 54, 163-166 (1998)

3696 Lyfar V, Fernandes L, Thornton E et al. A study of the hypouricaemic effect of tiaprofenic acid. *Ann Clin Biochem*, 25, 595-600 (1988)

3697 Lyfar VJ. A study of the hypouricaemic effect of surgam. *Ann Clin Biochem*, 24, Suppl S1, 32-33 (1987)

3698 Lyons D, Webster J, Fowler G et al. Colestipol at varying dosage intervals in the treatment of moderate hypercholesterolaemia. *Br J Clin Pharmacol*, 37, 59-62 (1994)

3699 Lyons F, Laker MF, Marsden JR et al. Effect of oral 13-cis-retinoic acid on serum lipids. *Br J Dermatol*, 107, 591-595 (1982)

3700 3M Pharmaceuticals. Manufacturer's literature on Disalcid™. St Paul, MN 55133 (1993)

3701 3M Pharmaceuticals. Manufacturer's literature on Norflex™. St Paul, MN 55133 (1993)

3702 3M Pharmaceuticals. Manufacturer's literature on Tambocor™. St Paul, MN 55133 (1994)

3703 3M Riker. Manufacturer's literature on Minitran® . St Paul, MN 55144

3704 Maacks S, Tegtmeyer KF, Wood WG. The influence of blood sampling techniques on plasma concentrations of lactoferrin and elastase-α_1-Pi. *Ann Clin Biochem*, 27, 512-513 (1990)

3705 Maas RD, Venook AP, Linker CA et al. Pentoxifylline and aplastic anemia. *Ann Intern Med*, 107, 427-428 (1987)

3706 Maboundou CW, Paintaud G, Vanlemmens C, et al. A single dose of ursodiol does not affect cyclosporine absorption in liver transplant patients. *Eur J Clin Pharmacol*, 50, 335-337 (1996)

3707 MacAdams MR, White RH, Chipps BE. Reduction of serum testosterone levels during chronic glucocorticoid therapy. *Ann Intern Med*, 104, 648-651 (1986)

3708 Macaulay VM, Begent Rhj, Phillips ME et al. Prophylaxis against hypomagnesemia induced by cis-platinum combination chemotherapy. *Cancer Chemother Pharmacol*, 9, 179-181 (1982)

3709 Macbeth WA, Kass EH, McDermott WV. Treatment of hepatic encephalopathy by alteration of intestinal flora with lactobacillus acidophilus. *Lancet*, 1, 399 (1965)

3710 Maccara ME, Parker WA. In vitro effect of penicillins and aminoglycosides on commonly used tests for glycosuria. *Am J Hosp Pharm*, 38, 1340-1345 (1981)

3711 MacDonald AG, Robinson DS, Sylwester D et al. The effects of phenobarbital, chloral betaine, and glutethimide administration on warfarin plasma levels and hypoprothrombinemic response in man. *Clin Pharmacol Ther*, 10, 80-84 (1969)

3712 MacDonald TM, Jeffrey RF, Lee MR. The renal and haemodynamic effects of a 10 h infusion of glutamyl-L-dopa in normal man. *Br J Clin Pharmacol*, 27, 811-822 (1989)

3713 MacDougall IC, Davies ME, Hutton RD et al. The treatment of renal anemia in CAPD patients with recombinant human erythropoietin. *Nephrol Dial Transplant*, 5, 950-955 (1990)

3714 MacFadyen RJ, Lees KR, Reid JL. Peridopril: a review of its pharmacokinetics and clinical pharmacology. *Drugs*, 39, Suppl 1, 49-63 (1990)

3715 Mach-Pascual S, Samil K, Beris P. Microangiopathic hemolytic anemia complicating FK506 (tacrolimus) therapy. *Am J Hematol*, 52, 310-312 (1996)

3716 Machtey I. Serum uric acid levels following administration of metiazinic acid. *Clin Chim Acta*, 47, 317 (1973)

3717 MacKay EV, Khoo SK. Clinical and laboratory study of a new diuretic agent ('Vectren') in pregnancy. *Med J Aust*, 1, 607 (1969)

3718 MacKinney AA, Booker HE. Diphenylhydantoin effects on human lymphocytes in vitro and in vivo. *Arch Intern Med*, 129, 988 (1972)

3719 Mackintosh W, Jacobs P. Response in serum ferritin and haemoglobin to iron therapy in blood donors. *Am J Hematol*, 27, 17-19 (1988)

3720 MacLeod SM, Sellers EM, Giles HG et al. Interaction of disulfiram with benzodiazepines. *Clin Pharmacol Ther*, 24, 583-589 (1978)

3721 MacPhee GJA, Mitchell JR, Wiseman L et al. Effect of sodium valproate on carbamazepine disposition and psychomotor profile in man. *Br J Clin Pharmacol*, 25, 59-66 (1988)

3722 MacPhee GJA, Thompson GG, McInnes GT et al. Verapamil potentiates carbamazepine neurotoxicity: a clinically important inhibitory interaction. *Lancet*, 1, 700-703 (1986)

3723 MacWalter RS, El Debani AH, Feely J et al. Potentiation by ranitidine of the hypoglycaemic response to glipizide in diabetic patients. *Br J Clin Pharmacol*, 19, 121p-122p (1985)

3724 Maddocks J, Hann S, Hopkins M et al. Effect of methyldopa on creatinine estimation. *Lancet*, 1, 157 (1973)

3725 Maddrey WC, Boitnott JK. Drug-induced chronic liver disease. *Gastroenterology*, 72, 1348-1353 (1977)

3726 Maddrey WC, Boitnott JK. Severe hepatitis from methyldopa. *Gastroenterology*, 68, 351-360 (1975)

3727 Maddux MS, Barriere SL. A review of complications of amphotericin B therapy: recommendations for prevention and management.. *Drug Intell Clin Pharm*, 14, 177-181 (1980)

3728 Madeddu P, Ena P, Dessi-Fulgheri P. Captopril induced proteinuria in hypertensive psoriatic patients. *Nephron*, 44, 358-360 (1986)

3729 Madira W, Igbal SJ, Bourke J et al. Changing dosages of glucocorticoids: effects on total and bone specific alkaline phosphatase compared with bone Gla protein. *Proc ACB Natl Meet*, 64 (1995)

3730 Madu EC, Reddy RC, Madu AN, et al. Review: the effects of antihypertensive agents on serum lipids. *Am J Med Sci*, 312, 76-84 (1996)

3731 Maes M, Bosmans E, Kenis G, De Jong R. In vivo immunomodulatory effects of clozapine in schizophrenia. *Schiz Res*, 26, 221-225 (1997)

3732 Maes M, Bosmans E, Ranjan R, et al. Lower plasma CC16, a natural anti-inflammatory protein, and increased plasma interleukin-1 receptor antagonist in schizophrenia: effects of antipsychotic drugs. *Schiz Res*, 21, 39-50 (1996)

3733 Maes M, Jacobs J-P, Suy E et al. Cortisol, ACTH, prolactin and β-endorphin responses to fenfluramine administration in major-depressed patients. *Neuropsychobiology*, 21, 192-196 (1989)

3734 Maes M, Meltzer HY, Bosmans E et al. Increased plasma concentrations of interleukin-6, soluble interleukin-6 and transferrin receptor in major depression. *J Affect Disord*, 34, 301-309 (1995)

3735 Maesen FPV, Costongs R, Smeets JJ et al. The effect of maximal doses of formoterol and salbutamol from a metered dose inhaler on pulse rates, ECG, and serum potassium concentrations. *Chest*, 99, 1367-1373 (1991)

3736 Maestri E, Manzoni GC, Marchesi G et al. Effect of flunarizine on pituitary secretion by healthy men and in women with migraine. *Eur J Clin Pharmacol*, 32, 525-527 (1987)

3737 Magarian EO, Dietz AJ, Freeman DS et al. Effect of prazosin and β-blocker monotherapy on serum lipids: a crossover, placebo-controlled study. *J Clin Pharmacol*, 27, 756-761 (1987)

3738 Magnusson B, Rodjer S. Alprenolol-induced thrombocytopenia. *Acta Med Scand*, 207, 231-233 (1980)

3739 Maher VMG, Thompson GR. HMG CoA reductase inhibitors as lipid-lowering agents: Five years experience with lovastatin and an appraisal of simvastatin and pravastatin. *Q J Med*, 74, 165-175 (1990)

3740 Maheshwari HG, Butler J, Norman M. Growth hormone binding protein in patients with renal failure. *Acta Endocrinol*, 127, 485-488 (1992)

3741 Maheux P, Facchini F, Jeppsen J et al. Changes in glucose, insulin, lipid, lipoprotein, and apoprotein concentrations and insulin action in doxazosin-treated patients with hypertension. *Am J Hypertens*, 7, 416-424 (1994)

3742 Maj M, Ariano MG, Pirozzi R et al. Platelet monoamine oxidase activity in schizophrenia: relationship to family history of the illness and neuroleptic treatment. *J Psychiat Res*, 18, 131-137 (1984)

3743 Major LF, Goyer PF. Effects of disulfiram and pyridoxine on serum cholesterol. *Ann Intern Med*, 88, 53-56 (1978)

3744 Maki DG, Aughey DR. Comparative study of cefazolin, cefoxitin and ceftizoxine for surgical prophylaxis in colorectal surgery. *Chemotherapy*, 10, Suppl C, 281-287 (1982)

3745 Maki KC, Skorodin MS, Jessen JH, Laghi F. Effects of oral albuterol on serum lipids and carbohydrate metabolism in healthy men. *Metabolism*, 45, 712-717 (1996)

3746 Malacco E, Groothold G, Gnemmi AE et al. An Italian multicenter study on the metabolic effects of indenolol in hypertensive patients with non-insulin-dependent diabetes. *Curr Ther Res*, 49, 1034-1039 (1991)

3747 Malandain H, Cano Y. Interference of glycerol, propylene glycol, and other diols in enzymatic assay of ethylene glycol. *Clin Chem*, 41, S120 (1995)

3748 Malarkey WB, Jacobs LS, Daughaday WH. Levodopa suppression of prolactin in nonpuerperal galactorrhea. *N Engl J Med*, 285, 1160 (1971)

3749 Malatino LS, Glen L, Wilson ESB et al. The effects of low-dose estrogen-progestogen oral contraceptives on blood pressure and the renin-angiotensin system. *Curr Ther Res*, 43, 743-749 (1988)

3750 Maletzky B, Blachly PH. The use of lithium in psychiatry. *Crit Rev Clin Lab Sci*, 2, 279 (1971)

3751 Malherbe C, Burrill KC, Levin SR et al. Effect of diphenylhydantoin on insulin secretion in man. *N Engl J Med*, 286, 339 (1972)

3752 Malini PL, Strocchi E, Ambriosini E. Comparison of the antihypertensive, metabolic and cellular effects of enalapril. *J Hypertens*, 2, Suppl, S101-S105 (1984)

3753 Malinow MR, Duell PB, Hess DL, et al. Reduction of plasma homocyst(e)ine levels by breakfasr cereal fortified with folic acid in patients with coronary heart disease. *N Engl J Med*, 338, 1009-1015 (1998)

3754 Malkonen M, Manninen V, Hirvonen E. Effects of danazol and lynestrenol on serum lipoproteins in endometriosis. *Clin Pharmacol Ther*, 28, 602-604 (1980)

3755 Mallette LE. Successful treatment of Paget's disease of bone with pamidronate. *Arch Intern Med*, 149, 2765-2767 (1989)

3756 Mallette LE, Khouri K, Zengotita H et al. Lithium treatment increases intact and midregion parathyroid hormone concentration and parathyroid volume. *J Clin Endocrinol Metab*, 68, 654-660 (1989)

3757 Mall-Haefeli M, Darragh A, Werner-Zodrow I. Effects of various combined oral contraceptives on sex steroids, gonadotropins and SHBG. *Ir Med J*, 76, 266-272 (1983)

3758 Mallory A, Kern F Jr. Drug-induced pancreatitis: a critical review. *Gastroenterology*, 78, 813-820 (1980)

3759 Malm J, Laurell M, Dahlback B. Changes in the plasma levels of vitamin K-dependent proteins C and S and of C_4b-binding protein during pregnancy and oral contraception. *Br J Haematol*, 68, 437-443 (1988)

3760 Maly J, Schuck O. The influence of benzbromarone and its combination with hydrochlorothiazide on renal excretion of uric acid and electrolytes. *Int J Clin Pharmacol Ther Toxicol*, 28, 443-445 (1990)

3761 Mamby CC, Love RR, Lee KE. Thyroid function test changes with adjuvant tamoxifen therapy in postmenopausal women with breast cancer. *J Clin Oncol*, 13, 854-857 (1995)

3762 Mancini AM, Barontini M, Armando I et al. Effect of bromocriptine on plasma catecholamines in normal subjects and prolactin-secreting tumor patients. *J Endocrinol Invest*, 9, 223-226 (1986)

3763 Maneschi F, Geraci P, Barreca PV et al. Estradiol, progesterone, 17-hydroxyprogesterone, androstenedione and CA 125 in patients with ovarian carcinoma. *Gynecol Endocrinol*, 6, 25-30 (1992)

3764 Maness LJ, Blair DC, Newman N, Coyle TE. Elevation of platelet counts associated with indinavir treatment in human immunodeficiency virus-infected patients. *Clin Infect Dis*, 26, 207-208 (1998)

3765 Manfredi RL, Vessell ES. Inhibition of theophylline metabolism by long-term allopurinol administration. *Clin Pharmacol Ther*, 29, 224-229 (1981)

3766 Manger WM, Steinsland OS, Nahas GG, Wakim KG. Comparison of improved fluorometric methods used to quantitate plasma catecholamines. *Clin Chem*, 15, 1101 (1969)

3767 Mangold D, Traeger U, Feller P. Dipstick for rapid and simple detection of N-Acetylglucosaminidase (NAG) in urine. *Clin Chem*, 37, 911 (1991)

3768 Mann HJ, Schneider JR, Miller JB et al. Cimetidine-associated thrombocytopenia. *Drug Intell Clin Pharm*, 17, 126-128 (1983)

3769 Mannaerts B, Shoham Z, Fauser B, et al. Serum hormone concentrations during treatment with multiple rising doses of recombinant follicle stimulating hormone (Puregon*) in men with hypogonadotropic hypogonadism. *Fertil Steril*, 65, 406-410 (1996)

3770 Mannelli M, Gheri RG, De Feo ML et al. Effects of thyroid replacement therapy on catecholamine plasma levels. *J Endocrinol Invest*, 6, 307-309 (1983)

3771 Manner T, Kanto J, Scheinin H, et al. Meptazinol and pentazocine: plasma catecholamines and other effects in healthy volunteers. *Br J Clin Pharmacol*, 24, 689-697 (1987)

3772 Manninen V, Apajalahti A, Melin J et al. Altered absorption of digoxin in patients given propantheline and metoclopramide. *Lancet*, 1, 398-400 (1973)

3773 Manninen V, Elo MO, Frick MH et al. Lipid alterations and decline in the incidence of coronary heart disease in the Helsinki Heart Study. *J Am Med Ass*, 260, 641-651 (1988)

3774 Manning EMC, Fraser WD. A survey of diagnoses in patients with a low intact parathyroid hormone concentration. *Ann Clin Biochem*, 30, 252-255 (1993)

3775 Manolas EG, Hunt D, Sloman G. Effects of quinidine and disopyramide on serum digoxin concentrations. *Aust NZ J Med*, 10, 426-429 (1980)

3776 Manos J. A long-term study of doxazosin in the treatment of mild or moderate essential hypertension in general medical practice. *Am Heart J*, 121, II Suppl, 346-351 (1991)

3777 Mantarri M, Koskinen P, Manninien V et al. Effect of gemfibrozil on the concentration and composition of serum lipoproteins. *Atherosclerosis*, 81, 11-17 (1990)

3778 Manzato E, Zambon A, Zambon S et al. Serum lipoprotein and apolipoprotein levels during ketanserin or metoprolol administration in hypertensive patients. *Curr Ther Res*, 47, 807-813 (1990)

3779 Maouris P, Dowsett M, Edmonds DK et al. The effect of danazol on pulsatile gonadotropin secretion in women with endometriosis. *Fertil Steril*, 55, 890-894 (1991)

3780 Maouris P, Dowsett M, Rose G et al. The effect of danazol and the LHRH agonist analogue goserelin (Zoladex) on the biological activity of luteinizing hormone in women with endometriosis. *Clin Endocrinol*, 33, 539-546 (1990)

3781 Maqueda IG. Adrenoceptors, endothelial function, and lipid profile: effects of atenolol, doxazosin, and carvedilol. *Coronary Arty Dis*, 5, 909-918 (1994)

3782 Maragno I, Santostasi G, Gaion RM et al. Influence of amiodarone on oral digoxin bioavailability in healthy volunteers. *Int J Clin Pharmacol Res*, 4, 149-153 (1984)

3783 Marangell LB, George MS, Bissette G et al. Carbamazepine increases cerebrospinal fluid thyrotropin-releasing hormone levels in affectively ill patients. *Arch Gen Psychiat*, 51, 625-628 (1994)

3784 Marbet GA, Duckert F, Walter M et al. Interaction study between phenprocoumon and flurbiprofen. *Curr Med Res Opin*, 5, 26-31 (1977)

3785 Marcellin P, Boyer N, Giostra E et al. Recombinant human α-interferon in patients with chronic non-A, non-B hepatitis. A randomized controlled trial from France. *Hepatology*, 13, 393-397 (1991)

3786 Marchetti P, Benzi L, Cerri M et al. Effect of plasma metformin concentrations on serum lipid levels in type II diabetic patients. *Acta Diabetol Lat*, 25, 55-62 (1988)

3787 Marco J, Calle C, Roman D et al. Hyperglucagonism induced by glucocorticoid treatment in man. *N Engl J Med*, 288, 128 (1973)

3788 Marcondes JAM, Luthold WW, Wajchenberg BL et al. Monthly cyproterone acetate in the treatment of hirsute women: clinical and laboratory effects. *Fertil Steril*, 53, 40-44 (1990)

3789 Marcondes JAM, Minnani SL, Luthold WW et al. Treatment of hirsutism in women with flutamide. *Fertil Steril*, 57, 543-547 (1992)

3790 Marcuard SP, Albernaz L, Khaanie PG. Omeprazole therapy causes malabsorption of cyanocobalamin (vitamin B_{12}). *Ann Intern Med*, 120, 211-215 (1994)

3791 Marcus FI. Drug interactions with amiodarone. *Am Heart J*, 106, 924-930 (1983)

3792 Marcus J, Mulvihill FJ. Agranulocytosis and chlorpromazine. *J Clin Psychiat*, 39, 784-786 (1978)

3793 Marek J, Hana V, Krsek M et al. Long-term treatment of acromegaly with the slow-release sommatostatin analogue lanreotide. *Eur J Endocrinol*, 131, 20-26 (1994)

3794 Marena S, Tagliaferro V, Cavallero G et al. Double-blind crossover study of acarbose in type I diabetic patients. *Diabetic Med*, 8, 674-678 (1991)

3795 Marescaux C, Warter JM, Brandt C et al. Adaptation of hepatic ammonia metabolism after chronic valproate administration in epileptics treated with phenytoin. *Eur Neurol*, 24, 191-195 (1985)

3796 Markianos M, Alevizos V, Stefanis C. Plasma sex hormones and urinary biogenic amine metabolites during treatment of male depressed male patients with the monoamine oxidase inhibitor moclobemide. *Neuroendocrinol Lett*, 13, 49-55 (1991)

3797 Markianos M, Sakellariou G, Bistolaki E. Prolactin responses to haloperidol in drug-free and treated schizophrenics. *J Neural Transm Gen Sect*, 83, 37-42 (1991)

3798 Markman M, Rothman R, Reichman B et al. Persistent hypomagnesaemia following cisplatin chemotherapy in patients with ovarian cancer. *J Cancer Res Clin Oncol*, 117, 89-90 (1991)

3799 Marosvari I, Neubauer K. Treatment of neonatal hyperbilirubinemia with flumecinolone, a new enzyme- inducing drug. *Acta Paediat Hung*, 26, 297-302 (1985)

3800 Marotta T, Ferrara LA, Pasanisi F et al. Enhancement of exogenous triglyceride removal following calcium channel blockade. *Artery*, 16, 312-326 (1989)

3801 Marotta T, Lombardi I, Fasano ML et al. β-blockers and renal function: Observations during treatment with tertatolol. *Curr Ther Res*, 43, 1127-1132 (1988)

3802 Marquis J-F, Carruther SG, Spence JD et al. Phenytoin-theophylline interaction. *N Engl J Med*, 307, 1189-1190 (1982)

3803 Mars H, Genuth SM. Potentiation of levodopa stimulation of human growth hormone by systemic decarboxylase inhibition. *Clin Pharmacol Ther*, 14, 390 (1973)

3804 Marsden JR, Trinick TR, Laker MF et al. Effect of isotretinoin on serum lipids and lipoproteins, liver and thyroid function. *Clin Chim Acta*, 143, 243-245 (1984)

3805 Marsh HH. Basic Urine Analysis: Physico-chemical Tests. *Audiovisual Seminar*, Chicago IL, American Society of Clinical Pathologists (1973)

3806 Marshall EF, Tait AC, Todrick A. The effect of reserpine on the blood sugar level in human subjects. *Biochem J*, 69, 41 (1958)

3807 Marshall PW, Williams AJ, Dixon RM, et al. A comparison of the effects of aspirin on bleeding time measured using the Simplate™ method and closure time measured using the PFA-100™, in healthy volunteers. *Br J Clin Pharmacol*, 44, 151-155 (1997)

3808 Martens HF, Sheets PK, Tenover JS et al. Decreased testosterone levels in men with rheumatoid arthritis: effect of low dose prednisone therapy. *J Rheumatol*, 21, 1427-1431 (1994)

3809 Martin CM. Myelography with sodium diatrizoate (Hypaque®). *Calif Med*, 115, 57 (1971)

3810 Martin EW. Hazards of Medication. Philadelphia PA, JB Lippincott (1971)

3811 Martin HE. Clinical studies of magnesium metabolism. *Med Clin North Am*, 36, 1157 (1952)

3812 Martin JH, Gordon M, Wallace R. Methotrexate in psoriasis. precipitation of gout. *Arch Dermatol*, 96, 431 (1967)

3813 Martin JV, Martin PJ, Goldberg DM. Enzyme induction as a possible cause of increased serum triglycerides after oral contraceptives. *Lancet*, 1, 1107-1108 (1976)

3814 Martin P, Tindall H, Rice P et al. Effects of pimobendan (UDCG 115) on renal function in healthy volunteers. *J Intern Med Res*, 20, 267-272 (1992)

3815 Martin WE. Adverse reactions during treatment of Parkinson's disease with levodopa. *J Am Med Ass*, 216, 1979 (1971)

3816 Martina V, Maccario M, Tagliabue M et al. Chronic treatment with pirenzepine decreases growth hormone secretion in insulin-dependent diabetes mellitus. *J Clin Endocrinol Metab*, 68, 392-396 (1989)

3817 Martinati LC, Sette L, Chiocca E et al. Effect of beclomethasone dipropionate nasal aerosol on serum markers of bone metabolism in children with seasonal allergic rhinitis. *Clin Exp Allergy*, 23, 986-991 (1993)

3818 Martinelli R, Pereira LJC, Santos ESC, Rocha H. Clinical effects of intermittent, intravenous cyclophosphamide in severe systemic lupus erythematosus. *Nephron*, 74, 313-317 (1996)

3819 Martinez ME, Del Campo MT, Plaza MA, et al. Pamidronate and biochemical markers of bone turnover. *Scand J Clin Lab Invest*, 57, 581-586 (1997)

3820 Martinez ME, Pastrana P, Snchez-Cabezudo MJ, et al. Effect of clodronate on calcidiol serum levels in women with breast cancer. *Calcif Tissue Int*, 61, 148-150 (1997)

3821 Martinowitz U, Rabinovici J, Goldfarb D et al. Interaction between warfarin sodium and amiodarone. *N Engl J Med*, 304, 671-672 (1981)

3822 Martz W, Schutz HW. Synthetic sweetener cyclamate as a potential source of false-positive amphetamine results in the TDx system. *Clin Chem*, 37, 2016-2017 (1991)

3823 Maruyama H, Saruta T, Itoh H et al. Effect of α-adrenergic blockade on blood pressure, glucose, and lipid metabolism in hypertensive patients with non-insulin-dependent diabetes mellitus. *Am Heart J*, 121, II Suppl, 1302-1305 (1991)

3824 Marx HH. Emphysematous bronchitis. *Germ Med*, 1, 162 (1971)

3825 Masala A, Alagna S, Rovasio PP et al. Suppression of insulin-induced prolactin secretion in man by nomifensine. *Drug Dev Res*, 1, 51-54 (1981)

3826 Mascho G, Alberti D, Janin G, et al. Effect of the angiotensin-converting-enzyme inhibitor benazepril on the progression of chronic renal insufficiency. *N Engl J Med*, 334, 939-945 (1996)

3827 Masel MA. A lupus-like reaction to antituberculosis drugs. *Med J Aust*, 2, 738 (1967)

3828 Masel MA. Erythromycin hepato-sensitivity: a preliminary report of two cases. *Med J Aust*, 1, 560 (1962)

3829 Mason AM. Bleeding massive gastric ulcer on diflunisal (Dolobid®). *Br Med J*, 1, 888 (1979)

3830 Mason JB, Zimmerman J, Otradovec CL et al. Chronic diuretic therapy with moderate doses of triamterene is not associated with folate deficiency. *J Lab Clin Med*, 117, 365-369 (1991)

3831 Mason JW. Drug therapy: Amiodarone. *N Engl J Med*, 316, 455-466 (1987)

3832 Mason NA. Disulfiram-induced hepatitis: Case report and review of the literature. *Dicp Ann Pharmacother*, 23, 872-875 (1989)

3833 Massara F, Camanni F, Molinatti GM. The effect of various adrenergic substances on plasma hGH levels. *Abstracts IV Int Congr Endocrinol, Washington, DC*, 30 (1972)

3834 Massara F, Tangolo D, Godano A et al. Effect of metoclopramide, domperidone, and apomorphine on GH secretion in children and adolescents. *Acta Endocrinol*, 108, 451-455 (1985)

3835 Massarano AA, Brook CGD, Hindmarsh PC. Growth hormone secretion in Turner's syndrome and influence of oxandrolone and ethinyl estradiol. *Arch Dis Child*, 64, 587-592 (1989)

3836 Massarella JW, Defeo TM, Ligouri J et al. The effects of cimetidine and ranitidine on the pharmacokinetics of cifenline. *Br J Clin Pharmacol*, 31, 481-483 (1991)

3837 Massie B, MacCarthy EP, Ramanathan KB et al. Diltiazem and propranolol in mild to moderate essential hypertension as monotherapy or with hydrochlorothiazide. *Ann Intern Med*, 107, 150-157 (1987)

3838 Masters B. Glycerol-blanked triglycerides applications to BM/Hitachi 717, 737, 738 and 747 analyzers. *Clin Chem*, 37, 922 (1991)

3839 Matera MG, De Santis D, Vacca C et al. Quinidine-diltiazem: pharmacokinetic interactions in humans. *Curr Ther Res*, 40, 653-656 (1986)

3840 Matera MG, Di Martino G, De Santis D et al. Acute guanfacine treatment: catecholamines and serotonin in hypertensive patients. *Curr Ther Res*, 46, 919-923 (1989)

3841 Materson BJ, Reda DJ, Cushman WC et al. Single-drug therapy for hypertension in men: a comparison of six antihypertensive agents. *N Engl J Med*, 328, 914-921 (1993)

3842 Matheke ML, Kessler G, Chan K-M. Interference of the chemotherapeutic agent etoposide with the direct phosphotungstic method for uric acid. *Clin Chem*, 33, 2109-2110 (1987)

3843 Mathews JD, Hooper BM, Whittingham S et al. Association of autoantibodies with smoking, cardiovascular morbidity, and death in the Busselton population. *Lancet*, 2, 754 (1973)

3844 Matson AM, Shaw M, Loughnan BA, et al. Pituitary-adrenal, hormonal changes during induced hypotension with labetalol or isoflurane for middle-ear surgery. *Acta Anaesthesiol Scand*, 42, 17-22 (1998)

3845 Matsunaga T, Kojima J, Inoue A et al. Serum hyaluronate levels predict responsiveness to interferonα therapy in patients with chronic hepatitis C. *Clin Chim Acta*, 229, 191-195 (1994)

3846 Matsuoka LY, Wortsman J, Hanifan N et al. Chronic sunscreen use decreases circulating concentration of 25-hydroxyvitamin D. *Arch Dermatol*, 124, 1802-1804 (1988)

3847 Matsuoka M, Otsuka H, Masuda S et al. Changes in the concentrations of vitamin D and its metabolites in the plasma of healthy subjects orally given physiological doses of vitamin D_2 by multivitamin or vitamin D preparations. *J Nutr Sci Vitaminol*, 35, 253-266 (1989)

3848 Matthys E, Schurgers M, Lamberigts G et al. Effect of simvastatin treatment on the dyslipoproteinemia in CAPD patients. *Atherosclerosis*, 86, 183-192 (1991)

3849 Matthysse S, Lipinski J, Shih V. L-dopa and S-adenosylmethionine. *Clin Chim Acta*, 35, 253 (1971)

3850 Matzke GR, Lucarotti RL, Shapiro HS. Controlled comparison of gentamicin and tobramycin nephrotoxicity. *Am J Nephrol*, 3, 11-17 (1983)

3851 Mau Pedersen M, Schmitz A, Bjercegaard Pedersen E et al. Acute and long term renal effects of angiotensin converting enzyme inhibition in normotensive, normoalbuminuric insulin-dependent diabetic patients. *Diabetic Med*, 5, 562-569 (1988)

3852 Maurin N, Fitzner S, Fritz H et al. Influence of recombinant human erythropoietin on hematological and hemostatic parameters with special reference to microhemolysis. *Clin Nephrol*, 43, 196-200 (1995)

3853 Mauro VF, Somani P, Temesy-Armos PN. Drug interaction between lorcainide and rifampicin. *Eur J Clin Pharmacol*, 31, 737-738 (1987)

3854 May DC, Jarboe CH. Effect of probenecid on dyphylline elimination. *Clin Pharmacol Ther*, 33, 822-825 (1983)

3855 May T, Rambeck B. Serum concentrations of valproic acid: influence of dose and comedication. *Ther Drug Monit*, 7, 387-390 (1985)

3856 Mayer J, Eller T, Brauer P et al. Effects of long-term treatment with lovastatin on the clotting system and blood platelets. *Ann Hematol*, 64, 196-201 (1992)

3857 Mayfield D, Brown RG. The clinical laboratory and electroencephalographic effects of lithium. *J Psychiat Res*, 4, 207 (1966)

3858 Mayo Medical Laboratories. Test Catalog. Rochester MN, Mayo Medical Laboratories (1991)

3859 Mays DC, Camisa C, Cheney P et al. Methoxsalen is a potent inhibitor of the metabolism of caffeine in humans. *Clin Pharmacol Ther*, 42, 621-626 (1987)

3860 Mazonson PD, Williams ML, Cantley LK et al. Myxedema coma during long-term amiodarone therapy. *Am J Med*, 77, 751-754 (1984)

3861 Mazza P, Amurri B, Lazzari G, et al. Oral iron chelating therapy: a single center interim report on deferiprone (L1) in thalassemia. *Haematologica*, 83, 496-501 (1998)

3862 Mazzachi BC, Teubner JK, Ryall RL. Factors affecting measurement of urinary oxalate. *Clin Chem*, 30, 1339-1343 (1984)

3863 Mazzola C, Vaccarella A, Serra G et al. The efficacy and safety of doxazosin in the treatment of mild or moderate essential hypertension when dose adjustment is simplified. *Curr Ther Res*, 48, 809-816 (1990)

3864 Mbuyi-Muamba JM, Dequeker J. A comparative trial of timegadine and D-penicillamine in rheumatoid arthritis. *Clin Rheumatol*, 2, 369-374 (1983)

3865 McAllister RA. Inhibition of the cysteine-sulfuric acid reaction for sedoheptulose by ferric iron. *Anal Biochem*, 43, 647 (1971)

3866 McAllister WAC, Thompson PJ, AL-Habet SM et al. Rifampicin reduces effectiveness and bioavailability of prednisolone. *Br Med J*, 286, 923-925 (1983)

3867 McArthur JW, Turnbull BA, Rehrson J, et al. Nalefene enhances LH secretion in a ptoprtion of oligo-amenorrheic athletes. *Acta Endocrinol*, 128, 325-333 (1993)

3868 McBay AJ. Toxicological findings in fatal poisonings. *Clin Chem*, 19, 361 (1973)

3869 McBride WG. Oral contraceptives. *Med J Aust*, 1, 525 (1965)

3870 McCall CE, Steigbigel NH, Finland M. Lincomycin: activity in vitro and absorption and excretion in normal young men. *Am J Med Sci*, 254, 144-155 (1967)

3871 McCance DR, Kennedy L, Sheridan B et al. Ketoconazole as an inhibitor of steroid production. *N Engl J Med*, 318, 710 (1988)

3872 McCarthy DM. Ranitidine or cimetidine. *Ann Intern Med*, 99, 551-553 (1983)

3873 McCarthy DM. Sucralfate. *N Engl J Med*, 325, 1017-1025 (1991)

3874 McCauley J, Fung J, Jain A et al. The effects of FK 506 on renal function after liver transplantation. *Transplant Proc*, 22, Suppl 1, 17-20 (1990)

3875 McCauley J, Fung JJ, Todo S et al. Changes in renal function after liver transplantation under FK 506. *Transplant Proc*, 23, 3143-3145 (1994)

3876 McCloy RF, Baron JH. Intragastric pH and cimetidine, fasting and after food. *Lancet*, 1, 609-610 (1981)

3877 McColl KEL, El Nujumi AM, Dorrian CA et al. Helicobacter pylori and hypergastrinaemia during proton pump inhibitor therapy. *Scand J Gastroenterol*, 27, 93-98 (1992)

3878 McConnell JD, Wilson JD, George FW et al. Finasteride, an inhibitor of 5α-reductase, suppresses prostatic dihydrotestosterone in men with benign prostatic hyperplasia. *J Clin Endocrinol Metab*, 74, 505-508 (1992)

3879 McCormick CP, Shihabi CK, Oles KS et al. Sensitive enzymatic assay for carnitine. *Clin Chem*, 36, 969 (1990)

3880 McCrea JB, Fruncillo RJ, Holland SD et al. Lovastatin does not affect oral glucose tolerance in hypercholesterolemic patients. *J Clin Pharmacol*, 33, 581-585 (1993)

3881 McCrea JB, Lo M-W, Tomasko L, et al. Absence of a pharmacokinetic interaction between losartan and hydrochlorothiazide. *J Clin Pharmacol*, 35, 1200-1206 (1995)

3882 McCreadie RG, Halliday J, MacEwan T, et al. Plasma lipid peroxide and serum vitamin E levels in subjects taking antipsychotic drugs. *J Psychopharmacol*, 10, 295-297 (1996)

3883 McCuistion CH, Lawlis M, Gonzales BB. Human pharmacological studies with griseofulvin. *Arch Dermatol*, 81, 766 (1960)

3884 McCune TR, Thacker LR II, Peters TG, et al. Effects of tacrolimus on hyperlipidemia after successful renal transplantation. *Transplantation*, 65, 87-92 (1998)

3885 McCune WJ, Golbus J, Zeldes W et al. Clinical and immunologic effects of monthly administration of intravenous cyclophosphamide in severe systemic lupus erythematosus. *N Engl J Med*, 318, 1423-1430 (1988)

3886 McDonald EC, Speicher CE. Peliosis hepatitis associated with administration of oxymetholone. *J Am Med Ass*, 240, 243-244 (1978)

3887 McDonald FD. Renal dysfunction with methoxyflurane. *J Am Med Ass*, 217, 79 (1971)

3888 McDonald RK, Weise VK. The effect of certain psychotropic drugs on the urinary excretion of 3-methoxy-4-hydroxymandelic acid in man. *J Pharmacol Exp Ther*, 136, 26 (1962)

3889 McDowell IFW, Smye M, Trinick T et al. Simvastatin in severe hypercholesterolemia: a placebo controlled trial. *Br J Clin Pharmacol*, 31, 340-343 (1991)

3890 McDuffie FC. Bone marrow depression after drug therapy in patients with systemic lupus erythematosus. *Ann Rheum Dis*, 24, 289 (1965)

3891 McElnay JC, Mukhtar HA, D'Arcy PF et al. In vitro experiments on chloroquine and pyrimethamine absorption in the presence of antacid constituents or kaolin. *J Trop Med Hyg*, 85, 153-158 (1982)

3892 McEwen J, Paterson C. Drugs and false-positive screening tests for porphyria. *Br Med J*, 1, 421 (1972)

3893 McFarland KF, Carr AA. Changes in the fasting blood sugar after hydrochlorothiazide and potassium supplementation. *J Clin Pharmacol*, 17, 13-17 (1977)

3894 McFate Smith W, Kulaga SF, Moncloa F et al. Overall tolerance and safety of enalapril. *J Hypertens*, 2, Suppl, S113-S117 (1984)

3895 McGinniss M. Personal communication (1972)

3896 McGourty JC, Silas JH, Solomon SA. Tolerability of combined treatment with verapamil and β-blockers in angina resistant to monotherapy. *Postgrad Med J*, 61, 228-232 (1985)

3897 McGourty JC, Silas JH, Tucker GT et al. The effects of the combined therapy on the pharmacokinetics and pharmacodynamics of verapamil and propranolol in patients with angina pectoris. *Br J Clin Pharmacol*, 25, 349-358 (1988)

3898 McGovern B, Geer VR, Laraia PJ et al. Possible interaction between amiodarone and phenytoin. *Ann Intern Med*, 101, 650-651 (1984)

3899 McGregor RF, Phillips G, Romsdahl MM. Analysis of urinary 5-hydroxyindoleacetic acid by thin layer chromatography: elimination of interference. *Clin Chim Acta*, 40, 59 (1972)

3900 McGuigan JE. A consideration of the adverse effects of cimetidine. *Gastroenterology*, 80, 181-192 (1981)

3901 McIndoe GJ, Menzies KW, Reddy J. Sulindac (Clinoril®) and cholestatic jaundice. *NZ Med J*, 2, 430-431 (1981)

3902 McIntyre PA. Hypokalemia occurring during para-aminosalicylic acid therapy. *Bull Johns Hopkins Hosp*, 92, 210 (1953)

3903 McKean CM. The effects of high phenylalanine concentrations on serotonin and catecholamine metabolism in the human brain. *Brain Res*, 47, 469 (1972)

3904 McKelvie GM, Bayliff CD, Gaska JA et al. Adverse reaction reviews: drug-induced liver diseases: part 3; illustrative cases. *Hosp Pharm*, 17, 562-568 (1982)

3905 McKenney JM, Barnett MD, Wright JT Jr et al. Comparison of gemfibrozil and lovastatin in patients with high low-density lipoprotein and low high-density cholesterol levels. *Arch Intern Med*, 152, 1781-1787 (1992)

3906 McKinney SE, Peck HM, Bochey L et al. Benemid® , p(di-N-propylsulfamyl)-benzoic acid. *J Pharmacol Exp Ther*, 102, 208 (1951)

3907 McLachlan S, Pegg CAS, Atherton MC et al. The effect of carbimazole on thyroid autoantibody synthesis by thyroid lymphocytes. *J Clin Endocrinol Metab*, 60, 1237-1242 (1985)

3908 McLellan DL, Chalmers RJ, Johnson RH. A double-blind trial of tetrabenazine, thiopropazate and placebo in patients with chorea. *Lancet*, 1, 104 (1974)

3909 McLeod HL. Clinically relevant drug-drug interactions in oncology. *Br J Clin Pharmacol*, 45, 539-544 (1998)

3910 McLeroy VJ, Schendel HE. Influence of oral contraceptives on ascorbic acid concentrations in healthy, sexually mature women. *Am J Clin Nutr*, 26, 191 (1973)

3911 McLindon JP, Babbs C, Gordon C et al. Profound hypoglycaemia induced by propranolol in a patient with hepatic cirrhosis and severe hyperandrogenaemia. *Ann Clin Biochem*, 32, 334-336 (1995)

3912 McMillan DC, Simpson JM, Preston T et al. Effect of megesterol acetate on weight loss, body composition and blood screen of gastrointestinal cancer patients. *Clin Nutr*, 13, 85-89 (1994)

3913 McNeil Consumer Products Company. Manufacturer's literature on Motrin® . Fort Washington, PA 19034 (1994)

3914 McNeil Pharmaceutical. Manufacturer's literature on Floxin® . Raritan, NJ 08869 (1994)

3915 McNeil Pharmaceutical. Manufacturer's literature on Haldol® . Raritan, NJ 08869 (1994)

3916 McNeil Pharmaceutical. Manufacturer's literature on Levaquin™. Raritan, NJ 08869 (1996)

3917 McNeil Pharmaceutical. Manufacturer's literature on Tolectin® . Raritan, NJ 08869 (1996)

3918 McNeil Pharmaceutical. Manufacturer's literature on Ultram® . Raritan, NJ 08869 (1996)

3919 McNeil Pharmaceutical. Manufacturer's literature on Vascor® . Raritan, NJ 08869 (1996)

3920 McPherson ML, Prince SR, Atamer ER et al. Theophylline-induced hypercalcemia. *Ann Intern Med*, 105, 52-54 (1986)

3921 McPherson R, Tsoukas C, Baines MG et al. Effects of lovastatin on natural killer cell function and other immunological parameters in man. *J Clin Immunol*, 13, 439-444 (1993)

3922 McPherson RA, Brown KD, Agarwal RP et al. Hydroxyurea interferes negatively with triglyceride measurement by a glycerol oxidase method. *Clin Chem*, 31, 1355-1357 (1985)

3923 McQueen EG. Hormonal steroid contraceptives. IV. adverse reactions and management of the patient. *Drugs*, 2, 138 (1971)

3924 McTavish D, Sorkin EM. Pravastatin: a review of its pharmacological properties and therapeutic potential in hypercholesterolaemia. *Drugs*, 42, 65-89 (1991)

3925 McVeigh GE, Dulie EB, Ravenscroft A et al. Low and conventional dose cyclopenthiazide on glucose and lipid metabolism in mild hypertension. *Br J Clin Pharmacol*, 27, 523-526 (1989)

3926 Mead PB, Gibson M, Schentag JJ et al. Possible alteration of metronidazole metabolism by phenobarbital. *N Engl J Med*, 306, 1490 (1982)

3927 Meatherall RC, Guay DRP, Baxter H. Cephalosporins and urinary protein determination. *Clin Chem*, 31, 165 (1985)

3928 Medeva Pharmaceuticals, Inc. Manufacturer's literature on Mykrox® . Fort Worth, TX 76155 (1996)

3929 Medeva Pharmaceuticals, Inc. Manufacturer's literature on Zaroxolyn® . Fort Worth, TX 76155 (1996)

3930 Medina I, Mills J, Leoung G, et al. Oral therapy for Pneumocystis carnii pneumonia in the acquired immunodeficiency syndrome. A controlled trial of trimethoprim-sulfamethoxazole vs. trimethoprim-dapsone. *N Engl J Med*, 323, 776-782 (1990)

3931 Medline A, Cohen LB, Tobe BA et al. Liver granulomas and allopurinol. *Br Med J*, 1, 1320-1321 (1978)

3932 Meffin PJ, Brooks PM, Bertouch J et al. Diflunisal disposition and hypouricemic response in osteoarthritis. *Clin Pharmacol Ther*, 33, 813-821 (1983)

3933 Mehbod H, Swartz CD, Brest AN. The effect of prolonged thiazide administration on thiazide function. *Arch Intern Med*, 119, 283 (1967)

3934 Mehta BR, Robinson BHB. Lithium toxicity induced by triamterene hydrochlorothiazide. *Postgrad Med J*, 56, 783-784 (1980)

3935 Mehta S. The influence of premedication with diazepam on blood sugar level. *Anesthesia*, 26, 468 (1971)

3936 Meijer P, Kamerling SWA, van de Ham FJ et al. Baseline levels of α_2-antiplasmin-plasmin complex in human plasma. *Fibrinolysis*, 8, 124-125 (1994)

3937 Meikle AW, Cardoso de Sousa JC, Ward JH et al. Reduction of testosterone synthesis after high dose interleukin-2 therapy of metastatic cancer. *J Clin Endocrinol Metab*, 73, 931-935 (1991)

3938 Meineke I, Stuwe E, Henne EM et al. Routine measurement of plasma catecholamines in clinical pharmacology by high-performance liquid chromatography with electrochemical detection. *J Chromatog*, 493, 287-303 (1990)

3939 Mejer LE, Blanchard RC. Fluorometric determination of plasma 11-hydroxycorticosteroids. *Clin Chem*, 19, 710 (1973)

3940 Melby J. Mineralocorticoid assays. *Radioimmunoassay Symposium, Washington, DC* (1974)

3941 melegh B, Pap M, Morava E, et al. Carnitine-dependent changes of metabolic fuel consumption during long-term treatment with valproic acid. *J Pediatr*, 125, 317-321 (1994)

3942 Melikian V, Eddy JD, Paton A. The stimulant effect of drugs on indocyanine green clearance by the liver. *Gut*, 13, 755 (1972)

3943 Melis GB, Paoletti AM, Mais V et al. The effects of the gabaergic drug, sodium valproate, on prolactin secretion in normal and hyperprolactinemic subjects. *J Clin Endocrinol Metab*, 54, 485-489 (1982)

3944 Mellerup ET, Lauritsen B, Dam H et al. Lithium effects on diurnal rhythm of calcium, magnesium, and phosphate metabolism in manic-melancholic disorder. *Acta Psychiat Scand*, 53, 360-370 (1976)

3945 Mellies MJ, DeVault AR, Kassler-Taub K et al. Pravastatin experience in elderly and non-elderly patients. *Atherosclerosis*, 101, 97-110 (1993)

3946 Meltzer HY. Intramuscular chlorpromazine and creatine kinase: acute psychosis or local muscle trauma?. *Science*, 164, 726 (1969)

3947 Meltzer HY, Cola PA, Parsa M. Marked elevations of serum creatine kinase activity associated with antipsychotic drug treatment. *Neuropsychopharmacology*, 15, 395-405 (1996)

3948 Meltzer HY, Fang VS, Tricou BJ et al. Effect of dexamethasone on plasma prolactin and cortisol levels in psychiatric patients. *Am J Psychiat*, 139, 763-768 (1982)

3949 Menard DB, Gisselbrecht C, Marty M et al. Antineoplastic agents and the liver. *Gastroenterology*, 78, 142-164 (1980)

3950 Menczel J, Dreyfuss F. Effect of prednisone on blood coagulation time in patients on dicumarol therapy. *J Lab Clin Med*, 56, 14 (1960)

3951 Mendell JR, Moxley RT, Griggs RC et al. Randomized double-blind six-month trial of prednisone in Duchenne muscular dystrophy. *N Engl J Med*, 320, 1592-1597 (1989)

3952 Mendelson JH, Ellingboe J, Jodson BA et al. Plasma testosterone and luteinizing hormone levels during levo-α-acetylmethadol maintenance and withdrawal. *Clin Pharmacol Ther*, 35, 545-547 (1984)

3953 Menezes S, Rege Vil, Sehgal VN. Dapsone haemolysis in leprosy. *Leprosy India*, 53, 63-69 (1981)

3954 Menon RK, Mikhalidis DP, Bell JL et al. Warfarin administration increases uric acid concentrations in plasma. *Clin Chem*, 32, 1557-1559 (1986)

3955 Menta R, Rossi E, Guariglia A et al. Reversible acute cyclosporin nephrotoxicity induced by colchicine administration. *Nephrol Dial Transplant*, 2, 380-381 (1987)

3956 Mercado-Asis LB, Yanovski JA, Tracer HL, et al. Acute effects of bromcriptine, cyproheptadine, and valproic acid on plasma adrenocorticotropin secretion in Nelson's syndrome. *J Clin Endocrinol Metab*, 82, 514-517 (1997)

3957 Merck & Co.. Manufacturer's literature on Aggrastat® . West Point, PA 19486 (1998)

3958 Merck & Co. Manufacturer's literature on Aldomet® . West Point, PA 19486 (1997)

3959 Merck & Co.. Manufacturer's literature on Basiliximab® . West Point, PA 19486 (1998)

3960 Merck & Co. Manufacturer's literature on Benemid® . West Point, PA 19486 (1988)

3961 Merck & Co. Manufacturer's literature on Blocadren® . West Point, PA 19486 (1985)

3962 Merck & Co. Manufacturer's literature on Chibroxin® . West Point, PA 19486 (1993)

3963 Merck & Co.. Manufacturer's literature on Clinoril® . West Point, PA 19486 (1995)

3964 Merck & Co. Manufacturer's literature on Cosmegen® . West Point, PA 19486 (1995)

3965 Merck & Co. Manufacturer's literature on Cozaar® . West Point, PA 19486 (1996)

3966 Merck & Co. Manufacturer's literature on Crixivan® . West Point, PA 19486 (1996)

3967 Merck & Co. Manufacturer's literature on Cuprimine® . West Point, PA 19486 (1989)

3968 Merck & Co. Manufacturer's literature on Daranide® . West Point, PA 19486 (1994)

3969 Merck & Co. Manufacturer's literature on Decadron® . West Point, PA 19486 (1995)

3970 Merck & Co. Manufacturer's literature on Demser® . West Point, PA 19486 (1985)

3971 Merck & Co. Manufacturer's literature on Diuril® . West Point, PA 19486 (1986)

3972 Merck & Co. Manufacturer's literature on Dolobid® . West Point, PA 19486 (1995)

3973 Merck & Co. Manufacturer's literature on Edecrin® . West Point, PA 19486 (1985)

3974 Merck & Co. Manufacturer's literature on Elspar® . West Point, PA 19486 (1995)

3975 Merck & Co. Manufacturer's literature on Flexeril® . West Point, PA 19486 (1995)

3976 Merck & Co. Manufacturer's literature on Fosamax® . West Point, PA 19486 (1997)

3977 Merck & Co. Manufacturer's literature on Hydeltrasol® . West Point, PA 19486 (1993)

3978 Merck & Co. Manufacturer's literature on Hydrocortone® . West Point, PA 19486 (1995)

3979 Merck & Co. Manufacturer's literature on Hyzaar® . West Point, PA 19486 (1996)

3980 Merck & Co.. Manufacturer's literature on Indocin® . West Point, PA 19486 (1995)

3981 Merck & Co. Manufacturer's literature on Mefoxin® . West Point, PA 19486 (1995)

3982 Merck & Co. Manufacturer's literature on Mevacor® . West Point, PA 19486 (1996)

3983 Merck & Co. Manufacturer's literature on Midamor® . West Point, PA 19486 (1992)

3984 Merck & Co. Manufacturer's literature on Mintezol® . West Point, PA 19486 (1996)

3985 Merck & Co. Manufacturer's literature on Mustargen® . West Point, PA 19486 (1994)

3986 Merck & Co. Manufacturer's literature on Myochrysine® . West Point, PA 19486 (1994)

3987 Merck & Co. Manufacturer's literature on Noroxin® . West Point, PA 19486 (1995)

3988 Merck & Co. Manufacturer's literature on Pepcid® . West Point, PA 19486 (1996)

3989 Merck & Co. Manufacturer's literature on Periactin® . West Point, PA 19486 (1994)

3990 Merck & Co. Manufacturer's literature on Prinivil® . West Point, PA 19486 (1997)

3991 Merck & Co. Manufacturer's literature on Proscar® . West Point, PA 19486 (1996)

3992 Merck & Co. Manufacturer's literature on Singulair® . West Point, PA 19486 (1998)

3993 Merck & Co. Manufacturer's literature on Stromectol® . West Point, PA 19486 (1996)

3994 Merck & Co. Manufacturer's literature on Syprine® . West Point, PA 19486 (1989)

3995 Merck & Co. Manufacturer's literature on Timolide® . West Point, PA 19486 (1995)

3996 Merck & Co. Manufacturer's literature on Vaqta® . West Point, PA 19486 (1996)

3997 Merck & Co. Manufacturer's literature on Vasotec® . West Point, PA 19486 (1995)

3998 Merck & Co. Manufacturer's literature on Zocor® . West Point, PA 19486 (1997)

3999 Merkel PA, Dooley MA, Dawson DV, et al. Interleukin-2 receptor levels in sera of patients with rheumatoid arthritis treated with sulfasalazine, parental gold, or placebo. *J Rheumatol*, 23, 1856-1861 (1996)

4000 Merrell-National Laboratories, Division of Richardson Merrell. Manufacturer's literature on Tenuate. Cincinnati, OH

4001 Merriel SL, Davis A, Smolens B et al. Cephalothin in serious bacterial infection. *Ann Intern Med*, 64, 1 (1966)

4002 Merrit GJ, Hunter BH, Hall WC. Lack of mezlocillin and piperacillin interference in measurement of vancomycin in the Abbott TDx. *Clin Chem*, 33, 2304 (1987)

4003 Merry J. Lithium thyrotoxicosis. *Br Med J*, 2, 765 (1977)

4004 Messana JM, Johnson KJ, Mihatsch MJ. Renal structure and function effects after low dose cyclosporine in psoriasis patients: a preliminary report. *Clin Nephrol*, 43, 150-153 (1995)

4005 Mestman JH, Pocock DS, Kirchner A. Lactic acidosis with recovery in diabetes mellitus on phenformin therapy. *Calif Med*, 111, 181 (1969)

4006 Metcalf MG. Rapid gas chromatographic assay for dehydroepiandrosterone in urine. *Clin Biochem*, 4, 241 (1971)

4007 Metsarinne K, Fyhrquist F, Totterman KJ et al. No effect of short term angiotensin II infusion on plasma renin substrate levels in man. *J Clin Endocrinol Metab*, 68, 386-391 (1989)

4008 Metzler M, Pierre K, Dewberry T. Development of a glycerol blanked triglycerides GPO method for Beckman's Synchron CX 4/5 systems. *Clin Chem*, 36, 959 (1990)

4009 Meulenberg PMM, Hofman JA. The effect of oral contraceptive use and pregnancy on the daily rhythm of cortisol and cortisone. *Clin Chim Acta*, 190, 211-222 (1990)

4010 Meyboom RHB. Thrombocytopenia induced by nalidixic acid. *Br Med J*, 289, 962 (1984)

4011 Meyer FL, Cooper K, Bolick M. Nitrogen and mineral excretion after carbohydrate test meals. *Am J Clin Nutr*, 25, 677 (1972)

4012 Meyers FH, Jawetz E, Goldfien A. Review of Medical Pharmacology. Los Altos CA, Lange (1968)

4013 Meyler L, Herxheimer A (eds). Side Effects of Drugs. The Hague, Excerpta Medica, 5 (1966)

4014 Meyler L, Herxheimer A (eds). Side Effects of Drugs. The Hague, Excerpta Medica, 6 (1968)

4015 MGI Pharma, Inc. Manufacturer's literature on Didronel® . Minnetonka, MN 55343 (1994)

4016 MGI Pharma, Inc. Manufacturer's literature on Salagen® . Minnetonka, MN 55343 (1994)

4017 Miale JB. *Laboratory Medicine: Hematology, 2nd edition*, St Louis MO, CV Mosby (1962)

4018 Miano L, Kolloch R, DE Quattro V. Increased catecholamine excretion after labetalol therapy: a spurious effect of drug metabolites. *Clin Chim Acta*, 95, 211-217 (1979)

4019 Miccoli R, Bertolotto A, Giovannitti MG et al. Simvastatin for lowering cholestertol levels in non-insulin-dependent diabetes mellitus and in primary hypercholesterolemia. *Curr Ther Res*, 51, 66-74 (1992)

4020 Michelet F, Gueguen R, Leroy P et al. Blood and plasma glutathione measured in healthy subjects by HPLC: relation to sex, aging, biological variables, and life habits. *Clin Chem*, 41, 1509-1517 (1995)

4021 Michelson PA. Reversible high dose oxacillin-associated liver injury. *Can J Hosp Pharm*, 34, 83-85 (1981)

4022 Michnovicz JJ, Galbraith RA. Cimetidine inhibits catechol estrogen metabolism in women. *Metabolism*, 40, 170-174 (1991)

4023 Michotte LJ, Wauters M. Clinical test of indomethacin. *Rheumatol Scand*, 10, 273 (1964)

4024 Micossi P, Pontiroli AE, Baron SH et al. Aspirin stimulates insulin and glucagon secretion and increases glucose tolerance in normal and diabetic subjects. *Diabetes*, 27, 1196-1204 (1978)

4025 Mielke CH Jr. Aspirin prolongation of the template bleeding time: influence of venostasis and direction of incision. *Blood*, 60, 1139-1142 (1982)

4026 Miettinen TA, Farkkila M, Vuoristo M, et al. Serum cholestanol, cholesterol precursors, and plant sterols during placebo-controlled treatment of primary biliary cirrhosis with ursodeoxycholic acid or colchicine. *Hepatology*, 21, 1261-1268 (1995)

4027 Miettinen TA, Tarpila S. Serum lipids and cholesterol metabolism during guar gum, plantago ovata and high fibre treatments. *Clin Chim Acta*, 183, 253-262 (1989)

4028 Migeon CJ. Ciba Foundation Colloquia on Endocrinology. London, Churchill, 8 (1954)

4029 Mignault G, Laberque B, Hamel S. Methoxyflurane and nephrotoxicity: a study of renal function in 22 patients anesthetized with methoxyflurane. *Can J Anaes*, 17, 331 (1970)

4030 Mihas AA, Holley P, Koff RS et al. Fulminant hepatitis and lymphocyte sensitization due to propylthiouracil. *Gastroenterology*, 70, 770-774 (1976)

4031 Mikus G, Eichelbaum M, Fischer C et al. Interaction of verapamil and cimetidine: stereochemical aspects of drug metabolism, drug disposition and drug action. *J Pharmacol Exp Ther*, 253, 1042-1048 (1990)

4032 Milanese C, Salmaggi A, La Mantia L et al. Double blind study of intrathecal β-interferon in multiple sclerosis: clinical and laboratory results. *J Neurol Neurosurg Psychiatry*, 53, 554-557 (1990)

4033 Milani M, Cimminello C, Merlo B et al. Effects of fluvastatin and pravastatin on lipid profiles and thromboxane production in type IIa hypercholesterolemia. *Am J Cardiol*, 76, 51A-53A (1995)

4034 Miles Inc. Product Insert for Multistix 10 SG Reagent Strips. Elkhart, IN (2/92)

4035 Miles MV, Tennison MB. Erythromycin effects on multiple-dose carbamazepine kinetics. *Ther Drug Monit*, 11, 47-52 (1988)

4036 Millar AW, Brown PD, Moore J, et al. Results of single and repeat dose studies of the oral metalloproteinase inhibitor marimastat in healthy male volunteers. *Br J Clin Pharmacol*, 45, 21-26 (1998)

4037 Millar JA, Fraser R, Mason P et al. Metabolic effects of high dose amiloride and spironolactone: a comparative study in normal subjects. *Br J Clin Pharmacol*, 18, 369-375 (1984)

4038 Millar JW. Rifampicin-induced porphyria cutanea tarda. *Br J Dis Chest*, 74, 405-408 (1980)

4039 Millar RA. The fluorimetric estimation of epinephrine in peripheral venous plasma during insulin hypoglycemia. *J Pharmacol Exp Ther*, 118, 453 (1956)

4040 Miller A. Reversible hepatotoxicity related to amphotericin B. *Can Med Ass J*, 131, 1245-1247 (1984)

4041 Miller ARO, Addis BJ, Clarke PD. Nitrofurantoin and chronic active hepatitis. *Ann Intern Med*, 97, 452 (1982)

4042 Miller BL, Lin K-M, Djenderedijian A et al. Changes in red blood cell choline and choline-bound lipids with oral lithium. *Experientia*, 46, 454-456 (1990)

4043 Miller DD, Macklin M. Cimetidine-imipramine interaction: a case report. *Am J Psychiat*, 140, 351-352 (1983)

4044 Miller DD, Sawyer JB, Duffy JP. Cimetidine's effect on steady-state serum nortriptyline concentrations. *Drug Intell Clin Pharm*, 17, 904-905 (1983)

4045 Miller HC, McLeod A, Kirby BJ et al. Effect of pentazocine on pulmonary circulation. *Lancet*, 2, 1167 (1972)

4046 Miller KW, Williams DS, Carter SB et al. The effect of Olestra on systemic levels of oral contraceptives. *Clin Pharmacol Ther*, 48, 34-40 (1990)

4047 Miller LC, Kaplan MM. Serum interleukin-2 and tumor necrosis factor-α in primary biliary cirrhosis: decrease by colchicine and relationship to HLA-DR4. *Am J Gastroenterol*, 87, 465-470 (1992)

4048 Miller M. Neuropathy, agranulocytosis and hepatotoxicity following imipramine therapy. *Am J Psychiat*, 120, 185 (1963)

4049 Miller M, Bachorik PS, McCrindle BW et al. Effect of gemfibrozil in men with primary isolated low high-density lipoprotein cholesterol: a randomized, double-blind, placebo-controlled, cross-over study. *Am J Med*, 94, 7-12 (1993)

4050 Miller MA, Texter M, Gmerek A et al. Quinapril hydrochloride effects on renal function in patients with renal dysfunction and hypertension: a drug-withdrawal study. *Cardiovasc Drug Ther*, 8, 271-275 (1994)

4051 Miller MI, Puchner PJ. Effects of finasteride on hematuria associated with benign prostatic hyperplasia: long-term follow-up. *Urology*, 51, 237-240 (1998)

4052 Miller RR, Porter J, Greenblatt DJ. Clinical importance of the interaction of phenytoin and isoniazid: a report from the Boston Collaborative Drug Surveillance Program. *Chest*, 75, 356-358 (1979)

4053 Miller SE. A Textbook of Clinical Pathology. *6th edition*, Baltimore MD, Williams and Wilkins (1960)

4054 Millett B, Sullivan A-M, Morimoto M et al. A third generation immunoassay for tumor necrosis factor-α. *BioTechniques*, 17, 1166-1171 (1994)

4055 Milligan DW, Thein SL, Roberts BE. Secondary treatment of polycythemia rubra vera with 6-thioguanine. *Cancer*, 50, 836-839 (1982)

4056 Milliner DS, Eickholt JT, Bergstralh EJ et al. Results of long-term treatment with orthophosphate and pyridoxine in patients with primary hyperoxaluria. *N Engl J Med*, 331, 1553-1558 (1994)

4057 Mills GA, Walker V, Corina DL. Glyoxal: An artifact from metronidazole and glyoxylic acid in urinary organic acid analysis. *Clin Chem*, 35, 673 (1989)

4058 Mills RM Jr. Severe hypersensitivity reactions associated with allopurinol. *J Am Med Ass*, 216, 799 (1971)

4059 Milman N, Senglov H, Dombernowsky P. Iron status in patients with small cell carcinoma of the lung. Relation to survival. *Br J Cancer*, 64, 895-898 (1991)

4060 Milne MD. Influence of acid-base balance on the efficacy and toxicity of drugs. *Proc Roy Soc Med*, 58, 961-963 (1965)

4061 Milwidsky A, Yagel S, Chaouat M et al. Glucocorticoids directly affect spectrophotometry of bilirubin in amniotic fluid. *Clin Chem*, 30, 677-680 (1984)

4062 Miners JO. Drug interactions involving aspirin (acetylsalicylic acid) and salicylic acid. *Clin Pharmacokinet*, 17, 327-344 (1989)

4063 Mink IB, Courey NG, Moore RH et al. Progestational agents and blood coagulation. IV. changes induced by progestogen alone. *Am J Obstet Gynecol*, 113, 739 (1972)

4064 Minton NA, Baird AR, Henry JA. Modulation of the effects of salbutamol by propranolol and atenolol. *Eur J Clin Pharmacol*, 36, 449-453 (1989)

4065 Minuz P, Barrow SE, Cockcroft JR et al. Effects of non-steroidal anti-inflammatory drugs on prostacyclin and thromboxane biosynthesis in patients with mild essential hypertension. *Br J Clin Pharmacol*, 30, 519-526 (1990)

4066 Minuz P, Lechi C, Arosio E et al. Effect of picotamide on platelet aggregation and on thromboxane A_2 production in vivo. *Thromb Haemostas*, 65, 312-316 (1991)

4067 Mishler JM, Emerson PM. Development of neutrophilia by serially increasing doses of dexamethasone. *Br J Haematol*, 36, 249-257 (1977)

4068 Misiani R, Bellavita P, Fenili D et al. Interferon-alfa2a therapy in cryoglobulinemia associated with hepatitis C virus. *N Engl J Med*, 330, 751-756 (1994)

4069 Missale C, Metra M, Sigala S et al. Inhibition of aldosterone secretion by dopamine, ibopamine, and dihydroergotoxine in patients with congestive heart failure. *J Cardiovasc Pharmacol*, 14, Suppl 8, S72-S76 (1990)

4070 Mistry CD, Lote CJ, Gokal R et al. Effects of sulindac on renal function and prostaglandin synthesis in patients with moderate chronic renal insufficiency. *Clin Sci*, 70, 501-505 (1986)

4071 Mitchell ABS. Duogastrone-induced hypokalemic nephropathy and myopathy with myoglobinuria. *Postgrad Med J*, 47, 807 (1971)

4072 Mitchell P, Smythe G. Hormonal responses to fenfluramine in depressed and control subjects. *J Affect Disord*, 19, 43-51 (1990)

4073 Mitchell RJ. Improved method for specific determination of creatinine in serum and urine. *Clin Chem*, 19, 408 (1973)

4074 Mitchell WD. A comparison of the effect of clofibrate and thyroxine on serum lipids in three hypothyroid subjects. *Clin Chim Acta*, 35, 429 (1971)

4075 Mitchell WD, Murchison LE. The effect of clofibrate on serum and faecal lipids. *Clin Chim Acta*, 36, 153 (1972)

4076 Mitnick PD, Greenberg A, Deoreo PB et al. Effects of two nonsteroidal anti-inflammatory drugs, indomethacin and oxaprozin, on the kidney. *Clin Pharmacol Ther*, 28, 680-689 (1980)

4077 Mitrevski A. Influence of the anticonvulsive drugs on carbohydrate metabolism. *Diag Lab*, 27, Suppl, 84 (1991)

4078 Mitrevski A. Serum γ-glutamyltransferase activity in patients receiving phenobarbitone and carbamazepine. *Biochim Clin*, 13, Suppl 1/8, 262 (1989)

4079 Mitrovic V, Patyna W, v Bruchhausen V et al. Interactions of clonidine and nifedipine in moderately severe hypertensive patients. *J Clin Pharmacol*, 31, 549-555 (1991)

4080 Miyachi Y, Mizuchi A, Hamano H et al. Effects of chronic sultopride treatment on endocrine systems in psychotic women. *Psychopharmacology*, 82, 287-290 (1984)

4081 Miyakawa T, Shionoiri H, Takasaki I et al. The effect of captopril on pharmacokinetics of digoxin in patients with mild congestive heart failure. *J Cardiovasc Pharmacol*, 17, 576-580 (1991)

4082 Mizuta E, Kuno S. Effect of D-penicillamine on pharmacokinetics of levodopa in Parkinson's disease. *Clin Neuropharmacol*, 16, 448-450 (1993)

4083 Moberg E, Hagg E, Asplund K et al. Misleading T3-test values in psychiatric patients treated with orphenadrine. *Acta Med Scand*, 222, 375-379 (1987)

4084 Modh BD, Lenda R, Fitzpatrick J. A simplified, sensitive enzyme immunoassay for detection of the cocaine metabolite benzoylecgonine. *Clin Chem*, 37, 1002 (1991)

4085 Moertel CG, Fleming TR, MacDonald JS et al. Levamisole and fluorouracil for adjuvant therapy of resected colon carcinoma. *N Engl J Med*, 322, 352-358 (1990)

4086 Moezzi B, Fatourechi V, Khozain R et al. The effect of penicillamine on serum digoxin levels. *Jpn Heart J*, 19, 366-375 (1978)

4087 Moghetti P, Castello R, Magnani CM et al. Clinical and hormonal effects of the 5α-reductase inhibitor finasteride in idiopathic hirsutism. *J Clin Endocrinol Metab*, 79, 1115-1121 (1994)

4088 Mogk LG, Cyrlin MN. Blood dyscrasias and carbonic anhydrase inhibitors. *Ophthalmology*, 95, 768-771 (1988)

4089 Mohler H, Bravo EL, Tarazi RC. Glucose intolerance during chronic β-adrenergic blockade in man. *Clin Pharmacol Ther*, 25, 237 (1978)

4090 Molgaard J, Lundh BL, Von Schenck H et al. Long-term efficacy and safety of simvastatin alone and in combination therapy in treatment of hypercholesterolemia. *Atherosclerosis*, 91, Suppl, S21-S28 (1991)

4091 Molgaard J, Von Schenck H, Olsson AG. Effects of simvastatin on plasma lipid, lipoprotein and apolipoprotein concentrations in hypercholesterolaemia. *Eur Heart J*, 9, 541-551 (1988)

4092 Molina J-M, Doco-Lecompte T, Belenfant X et al. Sulfadiazine-induced crystalluria in AIDS patients with toxoplasma encephalitis. *AIDS*, 5, 587-589 (1991)

4093 Moller DE, Moses AC, Jones K et al. Octreotide suppresses both growth hormone (GH) and GH-releasing hormone (GHRH) in acromegaly due to ectopic GHRH secretion. *J Clin Endocrinol Metab*, 68, 499-504 (1989)

4094 Monig H, Baese C, Heidemann HT et al. Effect of oral contraceptive steroids on the pharmacokinetics of phenprocoumon. *Br J Clin Pharmacol*, 30, 115-118 (1990)

4095 Monig H, Bohm M, Ohnhaus EE et al. The effects of frusemide and probenecid on the pharmacokinetics of phenprocoumon. *Eur J Clin Pharmacol*, 39, 261-265 (1990)

4096 Monig H, Hoffmann K, Ohnhaus EE et al. Ranitidine treatment and cortisol metabolism in man. *Eur J Drug Metab Pharmacokinet*, 17, 9-12 (1992)

4097 Monks A, Richens A. Effect of single doses of sodium valproate on serum phenytoin levels and protein binding in epileptic patients. *Clin Pharmacol Ther*, 27, 89-95 (1980)

4098 Monmany J, Domingo P, Gomez JA et al. Effects of long-term treatment with metoprolol and hydrochlorothiazide on plasma lipids and lipoproteins. *J Intern Med*, 228, 323-331 (1990)

4099 Monreal M, Lafoz E, Salvador R et al. Adverse effects of three different forms of heparin therapy: thrombocytopenia, increased transaminases, and hyperkalaemia. *Eur J Clin Pharmacol*, 37, 415-418 (1989)

4100 Montanari G, Gianfranceschi G, Suppa G et al. Plasma lipid and lipoprotein changes in hypertensive patients treated with propranolol and prazosin. In:. *Lipoproteins and Coronary Atherosclerosis. Noseda et al (eds)*, Amsterdam, Elsevier, 389-398 (1982)

4101 Montani E, Picotti GB, Bondiolotti GP et al. Effects of a single oral dose of dihydroergotoxine on plasma catecholamine concentrations and blood pressure in mildly hypertensive patients. *Curr Ther Res*, 43, 577-587 (1988)

4102 Monteleone P, Orazzo C, Natale M et al. Lack of effect of short-term fluoxetine administration on nighttime plasma melatonin levels in healthy subjects. *Biol Psychiat*, 35, 139-142 (1994)

4103 Mooij PNM, Thomas CMG, Doesburg WH, Eskes TKAB. The effects of oral contraceptives and multivitamin supplementation on serum ferritin and hematological parameters. *Int J Clin Pharmacol Ther Toxicol*, 30, 37-62 (1992)

4104 Mooradian AD, Reed RL, Osterweil D et al. Detectable serum levels of tumor necrosis factor alpha may predict early mortality in elderly institutionalized patients. *J Am Geriatr Soc*, 39, 891-894 (1991)

4105 Moore JJ, Sax SM. Elimination of dextran interference in serum protein determinations. *Clin Chem*, 18, 393 (1972)

4106 Moore N, Kreft-Jais C, Haramburu F, et al. Reports of hypoglycemia associated with the use of ACE inhibitors and other drugs: a case/non-case study in the French pharmacovigilance system database. *Br J Clin Pharmacol*, 44, 513-518 (1997)

4107 Mor F, Liebovici L, Cohen O et al. Prospective evaluation of liver function tests in patients treated with aminoglycosides. *Dicp Ann Pharmacother*, 24, 135-137 (1990)

4108 Morady F, Sauve MJ, Malone P et al. Long-term efficacy and toxicity of high-dose amiodarone therapy for ventricular tachycardia or ventricular fibrillation. *Am J Cardiol*, 52, 975-979 (1983)

4109 Morcos F, Crockford PM, Beck RP. The effect of norethindrone with and without estrogen on serum immunoreactive luteinizing hormone secretion. *Am J Obstet Gynecol*, 112, 358 (1972)

4110 Moreira AC, Foss MC, Iazigi N et al. The effect of low-dose naloxone infusion on plasma ACTH and LH in patients with Cushing's and Addison's diseases. *Horm Metab Res*, 20, 230-234 (1988)

4111 Morel D, Bannwarth B, Vincon G et al. Effect of famotidine on renal transplant patients treated with ciclosporine A. *Fundam Clin Pharmacol*, 7, 167-170 (1993)

4112 Moreno M, Murphy C, Goldsmith C. Increase in serum potassium resulting from the administration of hypertonic mannitol or other solutions. *J Lab Clin Med*, 73, 291 (1969)

4113 Morgan DH. Jaundice associated with amitriptyline. *Br J Psychiat*, 115, 105 (1969)

4114 Morgan JP, Bianchine. The uricosuric and thyroxine (T4) displacing effect of MK-185, a new hypolipidemic agent. *Clin Res*, 19, 27 (1971)

4115 Morgan TO. Efficacy of cilazapril compared with hydrochlorothiazide in the treatment of mild-to-moderate essential hypertension. *Am J Med*, 87, Suppl 6B, 37S-41S (1989)

4116 Moriarty AT, Moorehead WR, Ryder KW et al. Sulfasalazine interference in total protein measurements with the du Pont aca. *Clin Chem*, 29, 592-593 (1983)

4117 Morin LG. Determination of serum urate by direct acid Fe^{3+} reduction or by absorbance change (at 293 nm). *Clin Chem*, 20, 51 (1974)

4118 Morishita E, Saito M, Asakura H et al. Increased levels of plasma thrombomodulin in chronic myelogenous leukemia. *Am J Hematol*, 39, 183-187 (1992)

4119 Morita T, Tamai H, Ohshima A et al. Changes in serum thyroid hormone, thyrotropin and thyroglobulin concentrations during thyroxine therapy in patients with solitary thyroid nodules. *J Clin Endocrinol Metab*, 69, 227-230 (1989)

4120 Morita Y, Nishida Y, Kamatani N et al. Theophylline increases serum uric acid levels. *J Allerg Clin Immunol*, 74, 707-712 (1984)

4121 Morley JE, Shafer RB. Thyroid function screening in new psychiatric admissions. *Arch Intern Med*, 142, 591-593 (1982)

4122 Morris HC, Miller J, Campbell RS et al. Development of a rapid enzyme mediated colorimetric assay for chloramphenicol in serum. *Ann Clin Biochem*, 24, Suppl S1, 78-80 (1987)

4123 Morris RG, Frewin DB, Taylor WB et al. The effect of renal and hepatic impairment and of spironolactone on digoxin immunoassays. *Eur J Clin Pharmacol*, 34, 233-239 (1988)

4124 Morris SJ, Kanner R, Chiprut RO et al. Disulfiram hepatitis. *Gastroenterology*, 75, 100-102 (1978)

4125 Morse RM, Valenzuela GA, Greenwald TP et al. Amiodarone-induced liver toxicity. *Ann Intern Med*, 109, 838-839 (1988)

4126 Morselli PL, Marc V, Garattini S et al. Metabolism of exogenous cortisol in humans: influence of phenobarbital treatment on plasma cortisol. *Rev Eur Etudes Clin Biol*, 15, 195 (1970)

4127 Mortensen L, Hyldstrup L, Charles P. Effect of vitamin D treatment in hypoparathyroid patients: q study on calcium, phosphate and magnesium homeostasis. *Eur J Endocrinol*, 136, 52-60 (1997)

4128 Morton MR, Parish RC, Spruill WJ. Lack of theophylline assay interference from pentoxifylline and its metabolites. *Ther Drug Monit*, 11, 347-348 (1989)

4129 Mosekilde L, Melsen F. Anticonvulsant osteomalacia determined by quantitative analysis of bone changes. *Acta Med Scand*, 199, 349-355 (1976)

4130 Moser M. Low-dose diuretic therapy for hypertension. *Clin Ther*, 8, 554-562 (1986)

4131 Moser M, Abraham PA, Bennett WM et al. The effects of benazepril, a new angiotensin-converting enzyme inhibitor, in mild to moderate essential hypertension: a multicenter study. *Clin Pharmacol Ther*, 49, 322-329 (1991)

4132 Moser RH. Bibliographies on diseases of medical progress: reactions to phenothiazine and related drugs. *Clin Pharmacol Ther*, 7, 683 (1966)

4133 Moser RH. Diseases of Medical Progress: A Contemporary Analysis of Illness produced by Drugs. *3rd edition*, Springfield IL, CC Thomas (1964)

4134 Moser RH. Diseases of Medical Progressive: A Study of Iatrogenic Disease. *3rd edition*, Springfield IL, CC Thomas (1969)

4135 Moser RH. Disorders produced by progestational agents. *Clin Pharmacol Ther*, 7, 399 (1966)

4136 Moses AM, Howanitz J et al. Diuretic action of three sulfonylurea drugs. *Ann Intern Med*, 78, 541 (1973)

4137 Moshides JS. Comparison of ascorbic acid interference in HDL-cholesterol estimation by six precipitation methods, with use of a sensitive enzymic cholesterol reagent. *Clin Chem*, 33, 1467-1468 (1987)

4138 Moskovitz R, Devane CL, Harris R et al. Toxic hepatitis and single daily dose imipramine therapy. *J Clin Psychiat*, 43, 165-166 (1982)

4139 Moss RA. Drug-induced immune thrombocytopenia. *Am J Hematol*, 9, 439-446 (1980)

4140 Most H. Treatment of common parasitic infections of man encountered in the United States. *N Engl J Med*, 287, 495 (1972)

4141 Moticello JE, Hilyard K, Nassar R et al. An enzyme-linked no-boil assay for folate using the Stratus family of analyzers. *Clin Chem*, 38, 1101 (1992)

4142 Mouallem R. Comparative efficacy and safety of cephradine and cephalexin in children. *J Intern Med Res*, 4, 265-271 (1976)

4143 Mould GP, Curry SH, Binns TB. Interaction of glutethimide and phenobarbitone with ethanol in man. *J Pharm Pharmacol*, 24, 894-899 (1972)

4144 Mouller KH, Herrmann K. Vertragt sich eine gleichzeitige behandlung mit antikoagulantien und indomethacin?. *Med Welt*, 17, 1553 (1966)

4145 Mountokalakis T, Kallivretakis N, Mayopoulou-Symvoulidou D et al. Enhancement of renal function by a long-acting somatostatin analogue in patients with decompensated cirrhosis. *Nephrol Dial Transplant*, 3, 604-607 (1988)

4146 Mousa SA, Forsythe MS, Bozarth J et al. Effect of single oral dose of aspirin on human platelet function and plasma plasminogen activator inhibitor-1. *Cardiology*, 83, 367-373 (1993)

4147 Moustafa MA. Decreased bioavailability of quinidine sulphate due to interactions with adsorbent antacids and antidiarrheal mixtures. *Int J Pharmacol*, 34, 207 (1987)

4148 Moynot A, Zins B, Nare C et al. One-year treatment of 43 chronic haemodialysis patients, using recombinant human erythropoietin. *Presse Med*, 19, 111-115 (1990)

4149 MRC Working Party on Mild to Moderate Hypertension. Adverse reactions to bendrofluazide and propranolol for the treatment of mild hypertension. *Lancet*, 2, 539-543 (1981)

4150 Mudde AH, Houben AJHM, Nieuwenhuijzen Kruseman AC. Bone metabolism during anti-thyroid drug treatment of endogenous subclinical hyperthyroidism. *Clin Endocrinol*, 41, 421-424 (1994)

4151 Mudge GH. Uricosuric action of cholecystographic agents: a possible factor in nephrotoxicity. *N Engl J Med*, 284, 929 (1971)

4152 Mueller RG, Lang GE. Fluorescent spectra of lysergic acid diethylamine. *Am J Clin Pathol*, 60, 487 (1973)

4153 Muggeo M, Zenti MG, Travia D et al. Serum retinol levels throughout 2 years of cholesterol-lowering therapy. *Metabolism*, 44, 398-403 (1995)

4154 Muir JF, Peiffer G, Richard MO et al. Lack of effect of magnesium-aluminum hydroxide on the absorption of theophylline given as a pH-dependent sustained release preparation. *Eur J Clin Pharmacol*, 44, 85-88 (1993)

4155 Muir S, Turner P, O'Toole V et al. Sulfasalazine interference in total protein measurement on the Beckman CX7. *Clin Chem*, 39, 2028 (1993)

4156 Mulberg E. Syva EMIT 2000 carbamazepine assay. *Clin Chem*, 37, 1005 (1991)

4157 Mulder H, Schop C, Koster JC. Influence of pharmacological doses of calcitonin on serum osteocalcin concentration in patients with Paget's disease of the bone. *Acta Endocrinol*, 120, 721-723 (1989)

4158 Mulder H, Schopman W Jr, Van Der Lely AJ et al. Acute changes in plasma renin activity, plasma aldosterone concentration and plasma electrolyte concentrations following furosemide administration in patients with congestive heart failure - interrelationships and diuretic response. *Horm Metab Res*, 19, 80-83 (1987)

4159 Mulder H, Schopman W Sr, Van der Lely AJ. Extrapancreatic effect of glibenclamide. *Eur J Clin Pharmacol*, 40, 379-381 (1991)

4160 Mulder JW, De Wolf F, Goudsmit J et al. Long-term zidovudine treatment of asymptomatic HIV-1-infected subjects. *Antiviral Res*, 13, 127-138 (1990)

4161 Mulder JW, Krijnen P, Coutinho RA et al. Serum β_2-microglobulin levels in asymptomatic HIV-1-infected subjects during long-term zidovudine treatment. *Genitourin Med*, 67, 188-193 (1991)

4162 Mulder TPJ, Knapen MFCM, van der Mooren MJ, et al. Effects of hormone replacement therapy on plasma glutathione S-transferase A1-! concentrations in healthy postmenopausal women. *Clin Chem*, 44, 666-667 (1998)

4163 Mule SJ, Bastos ML, Jukofsky D. Evaluation of immunoassay methods for detection, in urine, of drugs subject to abuse. *Clin Chem*, 20, 243 (1974)

4164 Muller EO, Schall R, Groenewoud G et al. The effect of benzbromarone on allopurinol/oxypurinol kinetics in patients with gout. *Eur J Clin Pharmacol*, 44, 69-72 (1993)

4165 Muller P, Seitz HK, Simon B et al. Day omeprazole treatment. gastric acid secretion and basal hormone levels in man. *Z Gastroenterol*, 22, 236-240 (1984)

4166 Mullick FG, Ishak KG. Hepatic injury associated with diphenylhydantoin therapy. *Am J Clin Pathol*, 74, 442-452 (1980)

4167 Mullins RE, Hutton PS, Conn RB. Effects of fluosol-DA (artificial blood) on clinical chemistry tests and instruments. *Am J Clin Pathol*, 80, 478-483 (1983)

4168 Mulsant BH, Foglia JP, Sweet RA, et al. The effects of perphenazine on the concentration of nortriptyline and its hydroxymetabolites in older patients. *J Clin Psychopharmacol*, 17, 318-321 (1997)

4169 Munar MY, Elzinga L, Brummett R et al. The effect of tobramycin on the renal handling of vancomycin. *J Clin Pharmacol*, 31, 618-623 (1991)

4170 Mungall IPF, Hague RV. Pancreatitis and the pill. *Postgrad Med J*, 51, 855-857 (1975)

4171 Mungall IPF, Standing VF. Eosinophilia caused by rifampin. *Chest*, 74, 321-322 (1978)

4172 Munion GL, Seaton JF, Harrison TS. HPLC for urinary catecholamines and metanephrines with α-methyldopa. *J Surg Res*, 35, 507-514 (1983)

4173 Munoz JJ, de Salamanca RE, Diaz-Obregon C et al. The effect of clobazam on steady state plasma concentrations of carbamazepine and its metabolites. *Br J Clin Pharmacol*, 29, 763-765 (1990)

4174 Munzenberger P, Emmanuel S. The incidence of drug-diagnostic test interferences in outpatients. *Am J Hosp Pharm*, 28, 789 (1971)

4175 Muraca M, Baggio G, Miconi L et al. Acute effects of HMG-CoA reductase inhibitors on biliary lipids in patients with interrupted enterohepatic circulation. *Eur J Clin Invest*, 21, 204-208 (1991)

4176 Murakami M, Odake K, Matsuda T et al. Effects of anabolic steroids on anticoagulant requirements. *Jpn Circ J*, 29, 243 (1965)

4177 Murciano D, Auclair M-H, Pariente R et al. A randomized, controlled trial of theophylline in patients with severe chronic obstructive pulmonary disease. *N Engl J Med*, 320, 1521-1525 (1989)

4178 Murialdo G, Galimberti CA, Gianelli MV, et al. Effects of valproate, phenobarbital, and carbamazepine on sex steroid setup in women with epilepsy. *Clin Neuropharmacol*, 21, 52-56 (1998)

4179 Muros M, Lopez T, Leon C et al. Analytical interferences from calcium dobesilate in five serum assays. *Clin Chem*, 38, 371 (1993)

4180 Murphy AA, Burkman RT, Cropp CS et al. Effect of low-dose oral contraceptive on gonadotropins, androgens, and sex hormone binding globulin in nonhirsute women. *Fertil Steril*, 53, 35-39 (1990)

4181 Murphy DL, Goodwin FK, Bunney WE. Aldosterone and sodium response to lithium administration in man. *Lancet*, 2, 458 (1969)

4182 Murphy JV, Marquardt K. Asymptomatic hyperammonia in patients receiving valproic acid. *Arch Neurol*, 39, 591-592 (1982)

4183 Murphy MF, Metcalfe P, Grint PCA et al. Cephalosporin-induced immune neutropenia. *Br J Haematol*, 59, 9-14 (1985)

4184 Murphy MJ, Lyon LW, Taylor JW et al. Valproic acid associated pancreatitis in an adult. *Lancet*, 1, 41-42 (1981)

4185 Murphy PJ, Rymer W. Quinidine-induced liver disease. *Ann Intern Med*, 78, 785 (1973)

4186 Murphy R, Swartz R, Watkins PB. Severe acetaminophen toxicity in a patient receiving isoniazid. *Ann Intern Med*, 113, 799-800 (1990)

4187 Murray A, Clinton O, Earl H, et al. Assessment of five serum marker assays in patients with advanced breast cancer treated with medroxyprogesterone acetate. *Eur J Cancer*, 31A, 1605-1610 (1995)

4188 Murray FJ. Outbreak of unexpected reactions among epileptics taking isoniazid. *Am Rev Resp Dis*, 86, 729 (1962)

4189 Murray MD, Lazaridis EN, Brizendine E, et al. The effect of nonsteroidal antiinflammatory drugs on electrolyte homeostasis and blood pressure in young and elderly persons with and without renal insufficiency. *Am J Med Sci*, 314, 80-88 (1997)

4190 Murray-Lyon IM, Cassar J, Coulson R et al. Further studies in streptozotocin therapy for a multiple hormone-producing islet cell carcinoma. *Gut*, 12, 717 (1971)

4191 Murthy JN, Chen Y, Warty VS et al. Radioreceptor assay for quantifying FK-506 immunosuppressant in whole blood. *Clin Chem*, 38, 1307-1310 (1992)

4192 Muscat-Baron JM, Freeman DM. Toxic hepatitis following phenylbutazone therapy. *Br J Clin Pract*, 20, 437 (1966)

4193 Musto P, Matera R, Minervini MM et al. Low serum levels of tumor necrosis factor and interleukin-1β in myelodysplastic syndromes responsive to recombinant erythropoietin. *Haematologica*, 79, 265-268 (1994)

4194 Mutanen M, Mykkanen HM. Effect of ascorbic acid supplementation on selenium bioavailability. *Hum Nutr Clin Nutr*, 39, 221-226 (1985)

4195 Muther RS, Potter DM, Bennett WM. Aspirin-induced depression of glomerular filtration rate in normal humans: role of sodium imbalance. *Ann Intern Med*, 94, 317-321 (1981)

4196 Mutschler E, Spahn H, Kirch W. The interaction between H_2-receptor antagonists and β-adrenoceptor blockers. *Br J Clin Pharmacol*, 17, 51s-57s (1984)

4197 Myara I, Cosson C, Plouin PF et al. Effect of captopril and other inhibitors of angiotensin-converting enzyme on plasma prolidase activity. *Clin Chem*, 34, 172-173 (1988)

4198 Myers ED. The effect of oral dextroamphetamine on plasma cortisol in major depressive disorder. *Biol Psychiat*, 26, 634-636 (1989)

4199 Myers MD, Ross J, Newton L et al. Cyclosporine-associated chronic nephropathy. *N Engl J Med*, 311, 699-705 (1984)

4200 Myren J, Berstad A. Effect of oxyphencyclimine HCl on basic gastric secretion of acid and pepsin in man. *Acta Hepatogastroenterol*, 20, 57 (1973)

4201 Myrup B, Hansen PM, Jensen T et al. Effect of low-dose heparin on urinary excretion in insulin-dependent diabetes mellitus. *Lancet*, 421-422, 345 (1995)

4202 Nademanee K, Piwonka RW, Singh BN et al. Amiodarone and thyroid function. *Prog Cardiovasc Dis*, 31, 427-437 (1989)

4203 Naeije R, Fiasse A, Carlier E et al. Systemic and renal haemodynamic effects of angiotensin converting enzyme inhibition by zabicipril in young and in old normal men. *Eur J Cln Pharmacol*, 44, 35-39 (1993)

4204 Nagahama S, Fujimaki M, Kawabe H et al. Effect of metoclopramide on the secretion of aldosterone and other adrenocortical steroids. *Clin Endocrinol*, 18, 287-293 (1983)

4205 Nagakawa Y, Akedo Y, Kaku S et al. Effect of nicergoline on platelet aggregation, plasma viscosity and erythrocyte deformability in geriatric patients with cerebral infarction. *Arz Forsch Drug Res*, 40, 862-864 (1990)

4206 Naganna B, Rajamma M, Rao KV. On the failure of enzyme paper strips to detect glucose in certain abnormal urines. *Clin Chim Acta*, 17, 219 (1967)

4207 Nagasaka A, Hara I, Imai Y et al. Effect of fusaric acid (a dopamine β-hydroxylase inhibitor) on phaeochromocytoma. *Clin Endocrinol*, 22, 437-444 (1985)

4208 Nagasaki T, Enomoto M, Ito S et al. An enzymatic method for determination of direct bilirubin in serum with bilirubin oxidase. *Clin Chem*, 36, 1072-1073 (1990)

4209 Nagatsu T, Kato T, Kuzuya H et al. Inhibition of human serum dopamine-β-hydroxylase after the oral administration of fusaric acid. *Experientia*, 28, 779 (1972)

4210 Nagaya T, Ishikawa N, Hata H. Urinary total protein and β-2-microglobulin in workers exposed to trichloroethylene. *Environ Res*, 50, 86-92 (1989)

4211 Nagel GA, Wander HE, Blossey HC. Phase II study of aminoglutethimide and medroxyprogesterone acetate in the treatment of patients with advanced breast cancer. *Cancer Res*, 42, Suppl, 3442-3444 (1982)

4212 Nahata MC, Debolt SL, Powell DA. Adverse effects of methicillin, nafcillin, and oxacillin in pediatric patients. *Dev Pharmacol Ther*, 4, 117-123 (1982)

4213 Nakamura H. Effects of antihypertensive drugs on plasma lipids. *Am J Cardiol*, 60, 24E-28E (1987)

4214 Nakamura H, Hirata F, Yasugi T et al. Effects of ketaserin tartrate on serum lipids in patients with essential hypertension. *Drugs*, 36, Suppl 1, 25-34 (1988)

4215 Nakamura T, Matsuzawa Y, Takemura K et al. Combined treatment with chenodeoxycholic acid and pravastatin improves plasma cholestanol levels associated with marked regression of tendon xanthomas in cerebrotendinous xanthomatosis. *Metabolism*, 40, 741-746 (1991)

4216 Nakandakare E, Garcia RC, Rocha JC et al. Effects of simvastatin, bezafibrate and gemfibrozil on the quantity and composition of plasma lipoproteins. *Atherosclerosis*, 85, 211-217 (1990)

4217 Nanji AA. Symptomatic hypercalcaemia precipitated by magnesium therapy. *Postgrad Med J*, 61, 47-48 (1985)

4218 Nanji AA, Mikhael NZ, Stewart DJ. Increase in serum uric acid level associated with cisplatin therapy. *Arch Intern Med*, 145, 2013-2014 (1985)

4219 Nanji AA, Poon R, Hinberg I. Interference by cephalosporins with creatinine measurement by desktop analyzers. *Eur J Clin Pharmacol*, 33, 427-429 (1987)

4220 Nappi JM. Warfarin and phenytoin interaction. *Ann Intern Med*, 90, 852 (1979)

4221 Nappi JM, Dhanani S, Lovejoy JR et al. Severe hypoglycemia associated with disopyramide. *West J Med*, 138, 95-97 (1983)

4222 Narayanan S, Appleton HD. Specificity of accepted procedures for urine creatinine. *Clin Chem*, 18, 270 (1972)

4223 Nardone DA, Bouma DJ. Hyperglycemia and diabetic coma: possible relationship to diuretic-propranolol therapy. *South Med J*, 72, 1607-1608 (1979)

4224 Nash DT. A study on the effects of pyridinol carbamate p-23 on angina pectoris. *J Clin Pharmacol*, 8, 259 (1968)

4225 Nash DT, Feer TD. Hepatic injury possibly induced by verapamil. *J Am Med Ass*, 249, 395-396 (1983)

4226 Nash DT, Schonfeld G, Reeves RL et al. A double blind parallel trial to assess the efficacy of doxazosin, atenolol and placebo in patients with mild to moderate systemic hypertension. *Am J Cardiol*, 59, 87G-90G (1987)

4227 Nash J. Current therapeutics: CCXLII. glymidine. *Practitioner*, 200, 311 (1968)

4228 Nathan DM, Francis TB, Palmer JL. Effect of aspirin on determinations of glycosylated hemoglobin. *Clin Chem*, 29, 466-469 (1983)

4229 Nathan DM, Roussel A, Godine JE. Glyburide or insulin for metabolic control in non-insulin-dependent diabetes mellitus: a randomized double-blind study. *Ann Intern Med*, 108, 334-340 (1988)

4230 Nathan PJ, Norman TR, Burrows GD. Nocturnal plasma melatonin concentrations in healthy volunteers: effect of single doses of d-fenfluramine, paoxetine, and isapirone. *J Pineal Res*, 21, 55-58 (1996)

4231 Nathan RS, Tabrizi MA, Halpern FS et al. Effect of cyproheptadine and atropine on the diurnal prolactin responses to insulin-induced hypoglycemia in normal men. *J Clin Endocrinol Metab*, 51, 90-92 (1980)

4232 Naukkarinen VA. Serum lipid changes in patients with mild to moderate essential hypertension taking nicardipine and propranolol. *Br J Clin Pract*, 42, 509-513 (1988)

4233 Naumann HN. Prevention of pyridium® interference in urinalysis by dithionite reduction or butanol extraction. *Am J Clin Pathol*, 48, 337 (1967)

4234 Navascues I, Gil J, Pascau C et al. Effect of a long-acting somatostatin derivative SMS 201-995 (sandostatin) on glucose homeostasis in type I diabetes mellitus. *Horm Res*, 29, 92-94 (1988)

4235 Navis G, Buter H, de Jong PE, et al. Effect of antiproteinuric treatment on the lipid profile in nondiabetic renal disease. *Contrib Nephrol*, 120, 88-96 (1997)

4236 Nayak SS, Bhaskaranand N, Kamath KS et al. Serum apolipoproteins A and B, lecithin:cholesterol acyl transferase activities and urinary cholesterol levels in nephrotic syndrome patients before and during steroid treatment. *Nephron*, 54, 234-239 (1990)

4237 Nazor SM, Schmidt H. The use of dextranase to remove the interference by dextran in the determination of serum proteins by the biuret procedure. *Z Klin Chem Klin Biochem*, 10, 548 (1973)

4238 Nealon DA, Delaney DW. Validation of a candidate reference method (RIA) for digoxin. *Clin Chem*, 37, 999 (1991)

4239 Neef C, de Voogd-van der Straaten I. An interaction between cytostatic and anticonvulsant drugs. *Clin Pharmacol Ther*, 43, 372-375 (1988)

4240 Neeley WE. Simple automated determination of serum or plasma glucose by a hexokinase/G-6-PD method. *Clin Chem*, 18, 509 (1972)

4241 Neeley WE, Cupas CA. The use of 3-methyl-2-benzothiazolone hydrazone in clinical chemistry. *Clin Biochem*, 6, 246 (1973)

4242 Negrier S, Escuder B, Douillard J-Y, et al. Recombinant human interleukin-2, recombinant human interferon alfa-2a or both in metastatic renal-cell carcinoma. *N Engl J Med*, 338, 1272-1278 (1998)

4243 Neill DW, Carre IJ, McCorry RL et al. A possible source of error in the diagnosis of phaeochromocytoma. *J Clin Pathol*, 14, 415 (1961)

4244 Nelis GF. Nitrofurantoin - induced pancreatitis: report of a case. *Gastroenterology*, 84, 1032-1034 (1983)

4245 Nelson JC, Krueger GG, Wilcox RB et al. Effect of radiocontrast media on the measurement of adrenal steroids in the urine. *J Clin Endocrinol Metab*, 28, 1515 (1968)

4246 Nelson RB. Hepatitis due to carbarsone. *J Am Med Ass*, 160, 764 (1956)

4247 Nemanich JW, Veith RC, Abrass IB et al. Effects of metropolol on rest and exercise cardiac function and plasma catecholamines in chronic congestive heart failure secondary to ischemic or idiopathic cardiomyopathy. *Am J Cardiol*, 66, 843-848 (1990)

4248 Neri A, Zukerman Z, Aygen M et al. The effect of long-term administration of digoxin on plasma androgens and sexual dysfunction. *J Sex Marital Ther*, 13, 58-63 (1987)

4249 Nestel PJ, Hunt D, Wahlqvist ML. Clofibrate raises plasma apoprotein A-I and HDL-cholesterol concentrations. *Atherosclerosis*, 37, 625-629 (1980)

4250 Nestler JE, Barlascini CO, Matt DW et al. Suppression of serum insulin by diazoxide reduces serum testosterone levels in obese women with polycystic ovary syndrome. *J Clin Endocrinol Metab*, 68, 1027-1032 (1989)

4251 Nestler JE, Beer NA, Jakubowicz DJ et al. Effects of insulin reduction with benfluorex on serum dehydroepiandrosterone (DHEA), DHEA sulfate, and blood pressure in hypertensive middle-aged and elderly men. *J Clin Endocrinol Metab*, 80, 700-706 (1995)

4252 Nestler JE, Singh R, Matt DW et al. Suppression of serum insulin level by diazoxide does not alter serum testosterone or sex hormone-binding globulin levels in healthy, nonobese women. *Am J Obstet Gynecol*, 163, 1243-1246 (1990)

4253 Nestler JF, Barlascini CO, Clore JN et al. Dehydroepiandrosterone reduces serum low density lipoprotein levels and body fat but does not alter insulin sensitivity in normal man. *J Clin Endocrinol Metab*, 66, 57-61 (1988)

4254 Nestruck AC, Pande SV, Davignon J. Plasma carnitine and lipid-lowering drugs. *Atherosclerosis*, 55, 353-356 (1985)

4255 Neuvonen P, Gothoni G, Hackman R et al. Interference of iron with the absorption of tetracyclines in man. *Br Med J*, 4, 532-534 (1970)

4256 Neuvonen PJ. The effect of magnesium hydroxide on the oral absorption of ibuprofen, ketoprofen and diclofenac. *Br J Clin Pharmacol*, 31, 263-266 (1991)

4257 Neuvonen PJ, Kannisto H, Hirvisalo EL. Effect of activated charcoal on absorption of tolbutamide and valproate in man. *Eur J Clin Pharmacol*, 24, 243-246 (1983)

4258 Neuvonen PJ, Karkkainen S. Effects of charcoal, sodium bicarbonate, and ammonium chloride on chlorpropamide kinetics. *Clin Pharmacol Ther*, 33, 386-393 (1983)

4259 Neuvonen PJ, Kivisto KT. Effect of magnesium hydroxide on the absorption of tolfenamic and mefenamic acids. *Eur J Clin Pharmacol*, 35, 495-501 (1988)

4260 Neuvonen PJ, Lehtovaara R, Bardy A et al. Antipyretic analgesics in patients on antiepileptic drug therapy. *Eur J Clin Pharmacol*, 15, 263-268 (1979)

4261 Neuvonen PJ, Penttila O. Interaction between doxycycline and barbiturates. *Br Med J*, 1, 535-536 (1974)

4262 Neuvonen PJ, Penttila O, Lehtovaara R et al. Effect of antiepileptic drugs on the elimination of various tetracycline derivatives. *Eur J Pharmacol*, 9, 147-154 (1975)

4263 Neverov NP, Kaysen GA, Tareyeva IE. Effect of lipid-lowering therapy on the progression of renal disease in nondiabetic nephrotic patients. *Contrib Nephrol*, 120, 68-78 (1997)

4264 Nevinny HB, Hall TC. Chemotherapy with hydroxyurea (NSC-32065) in renal cell carcinoma. *J Clin Pharmacol*, 8, 352 (1968)

4265 New Zealand Committee on Adverse Drug Reactions. Three year survey of reactions 1969-1971. *NZ Med J*, 75, 100 (1972)

4266 Newcomb PA, Klein R, Klein BEK et al. Association of dietary and life-style factors with sex hormones in postmenopausal women. *Epidemiology*, 6, 318-321 (1995)

4267 Newman CB, Melmed S, Snyder PJ, et al. Safety and efficacy of long term octreotide therapy of acromegaly: results of a multicenter trial in 103 patients - a clinical research center study. *J Clin Endocrinol Metab*, 80, 2768-2775 (1995)

4268 Newnham HH, Hamblin PS, Long F et al. Effect of oral frusemide on diagnostic indices of thyroid function. *Clin Endocrinol*, 26, 423-431 (1987)

4269 Newton J, Dixon P. Site of action of clomiphene and its use as a test of pituitary function. *J Obstet Gynaecol Br Comm*, 78, 812 (1971)

4270 Newton P, Swinburn WR, Swinson DR. Proteinuria with gold therapy: when should gold be permanently stopped. *Br J Rheumatol*, 22, 11-17 (1983)

4271 Ney GC, Schaul N, Loughlin J et al. Thrombocytopenia in association with adjunctive felbamate use. *Neurology*, 44 (1994)

4272 Ng JYK, Disney APS, Jones TE et al. Acute pancreatitis and sodium valproate. *Med J Aust*, 2, 362 (1982)

4273 Ng RH, Guilmet R, Altaffer M et al. Falsely high results for triglycerides in patients receiving intravenous nitroglycerin. *Clin Chem*, 32, 2098-2099 (1986)

4274 Ng RH, Sparks KM, Chua GT et al. Contrast media interference in the measurement of urine protein by biuret and turbidimetric methods. *Clin Chem*, 36, 1118 (1990)

4275 Ng RH, Sparks KM, Statland BE. Direct measurement of high-density lipoprotein cholesterol by the Reflotron assay with no manual precipitation step. *Clin Chem*, 37, 435-437 (1991)

4276 Ng RP, Chan TK, Todd D. NBT test false-negative and false-positive results. *Lancet*, 1, 1341 (1972)

4277 Nhachi CFB, Murabiwa W, Kasilo OJ et al. Effect of a single oral dose of metrifonate on human plasma cholinesterase levels. *Bull Environ Contam Toxicol*, 47, 641-645 (1991)

4278 Niaudet P, Habib R. Methylprednisolone pulse therapy in the treatment of severe forms of Schönlein-Henoch purpura nephritis. *Pediatr Nephrol*, 12, 238-243 (1998)

4279 Nice A, Maturen A. False-positive urine amphetamine screen with ritodrine. *Clin Chem*, 35, 1542-1543 (1989)

4280 Nicholls A, Snaith ML, Scott JT. Effect of oestrogen therapy on plasma and urinary levels of uric acid. *Br Med J*, 1, 449 (1973)

4281 Nicholls DG, Hampton JR, Mitchell JRA. Cyclical changes in plasma lysolecithin induced by oral contraceptives. *Lancet*, 2, 1428 (1971)

4282 Nicholls MG, Espiner EA, Ikram H et al. Hyponatraemia in congestive heart failure during treatment with captopril. *Br Med J*, 281, 909 (1980)

4283 Nicot G, Merle L, Valette J-P et al. Gentamicin and sisomicin induced renal tubular damage. *Eur J Clin Pharmacol*, 23, 161-166 (1982)

4284 Nicot GS, Mekle LJ, Charmes JP et al. Transient glomerular proteinuria, enzymuria, and nephrotoxic reactions induced by radiocontrast media. *J Am Med Ass*, 252, 2432-2434 (1984)

4285 Nielsen CB, Pedersen EB. Effects of captopril on renal function in healthy uninephrectomized subjects and in healthy control subjects. *J Intern Med*, 235, 359-365 (1994)

4286 Nielsen F, Mikkelsen BB, Nielsen JB, et al. Plasma malondialdehyde as biomarker for oxidative stree: reference interval and effects of life-style factors. *Clin Chem*, 43, 1209-1214 (1997)

4287 Nielsen HK, Charles P, Mosekilde L. The effect of single oral doses of prednisone on the circadian rhythm of serum osteocalcin in normal subjects. *J Clin Endocrinol Metab*, 67, 1025-1030 (1988)

4288 Nielsen MD, Binder C, Starup J. Urinary excretion of different corticosteroid metabolites in oral contraception and pregnancy. *Acta Endocrinol*, 60, 473 (1969)

4289 Nielsen NP, Cesana B, Zizolfi S et al. Therapeutic effects of fengabine, a new GABAergic agent, in depressed outpatients: a double-blind study versus clomipramine. *Acta Psychiat Scand*, 82, 366-371 (1990)

4290 Nielsen-Kudsk JE, Buhl JS, Johannessen AC. Verapamil-induced inhibition of theophylline elimination in healthy humans. *Pharmacol Toxicol*, 66, 101-103 (1990)

4291 Nielsen-Kudsk JE, Mellemkjoer S, Nielsen CB et al. Lack of effect of the vasodilator pinacidil on insulin secretion in healthy humans. *J Clin Pharmacol*, 30, 409-411 (1990)

4292 Niemi TT, Kuitunen AH, Vahtera EM, Rosenberg PH. Haemostatic changes caused by i.v. regional anaesthesia with lignocaine. *Br J Anaes*, 76, 822-828 (1996)

4293 Nightingale J, Nappi JM. Effect of phenytoin on serum disopyramide concentrations. *Clin Pharmacol Ther*, 6, 46-50 (1987)

4294 Nikkila EA, Kaste M, Ehnholm C et al. Increase of serum high-density lipoprotein in phenytoin users. *Br Med J*, 2, 99 (1978)

4295 Nikolaizik WH, Marchant JL, Preece MA, Warner JO. Nocturnal cortisol secretion in healthy adults before and after inhalation of budesonide. *Am J Resp Crit Care Med*, 153, 97-101 (1996)

4296 Nilsson A, Axelsson R. Effects of long-term lithium treatment on thyroid and renal function (serum creatinine and maximal urine osmolality) -- a prospective study in psychiatric patients. *Curr Ther Res*, 46, 85-102 (1989)

4297 Nilsson B, Sodergard R, Damber M-G et al. Free testosterone levels during danazol therapy. *Fertil Steril*, 39, 505-509 (1983)

4298 Nilsson KO, Hokfelt B. Influence of metyrapone on plasma concentrations of testosterone and androsteredione in man. *Acta Endocrinol*, 68, 576 (1971)

4299 Nilsson L, Jones AW. 2,3-butanediol: a potential interfering substance in the assay of ethylene glycol by an enzymatic method. *Clin Chim Acta*, 208, 225-229 (1992)

4300 Niort G, Bulgarelli A, Cassader M et al. Effect of short-term treatment with bezafibrate on plasma fibrinogen, fibrinopeptide A, platelet activation and blood filterability in atherosclerotic hyperfibrinogenemic patients. *Atherosclerosis*, 71, 113-119 (1988)

4301 Niort G, Gambino R, Cassader M et al. Bezafibrate affects lipid, lipo- and apolipoprotein pattern in non-insulin-dependent diabetic patients. *Horm Metab Res*, 25, 372-374 (1993)

4302 Nisbet P. Chlorpropamide-induced hyponatraemia. *Br Med J*, 1, 904 (1977)

4303 Nishida S, Matsuki M, Tsushima K et al. Effects of changes in angiotensin converting enzyme activity on renin release: pretreatment with dexamethasone enhances a plasma renin activity response to captopril in normal subjects. *J Clin Endocrinol Metab*, 72, 547-553 (1991)

4304 Nishide T, Shirai K, Shinomiya M et al. Serum lipid levels in hypertensive patients during captopril treatment. *Clin Ther*, 11, 820-827 (1989)

4305 Nitsch J, Luderitz B. Enhanced elimination of amiodarone by cholestyramine. *Dtsch Med Wschr*, 111, 1241-1244 (1986)

4306 Nix DE, DeVito JM, Whitbread MA et al. Effect of multiple dose oral ciprofloxacillin on the pharmacokinetics of theophylline and indocyanine green. *J Antimicrob Chemother*, 19, 263-269 (1987)

4307 Nixon AL, Long WH, Puopolo PR et al. Bupropion metabolites produce false-positive urine amphetamine results. *Clin Chem*, 41, 955-956 (1995)

4308 Nixon DD. Thrombocytopenia following doxepin treatment. *J Am Med Ass*, 220, 418 (1972)

4309 Nizet A. Antagonistic action of uracil, thiouracil and thiourea on reticulocyte ripening. *Science*, 115, 290 (1952)

4310 Noda K, Umeda F, Nawata H. Effect of acarbose on glucose intolerance in patients with non-insulin-dependent diabetes mellitus. *Diabetes Res Clin Pract*, 37, 129-136 (1997)

4311 Nodine JH, Modi KN, Rhodes M et al. Pharmacodynamics and pharmacokinetics of isosorbide in man. *Clin Pharmacol Ther*, 14, 196 (1973)

4312 Noerpramana NP. Blood-lipid fractions: the side-effects and continuation of Norplant use. *Adv Contracept*, 13, 13-38 (1997)

4313 Noh GW, Lee W, Lee W, Lee K. Effects of intravenous immunoglobulin on plasma interleukin-10 levels in Kawasaki disease. *Immunol Lett*, 63, 19-24 (1998)

4314 Nolan JJ, Ludvik B, Beersden P et al. Improvement in glucose tolerance and insulin resistance in obese subjects treated with troglitazone. *N Engl J Med*, 331, 1188-1193 (1994)

4315 Nolan PE Jr, Marcus FI, Karol MD et al. Effect of phenytoin on the clinical pharmacokinetics of amiodarone. *J Clin Pharmacol*, 30, 1112-1119 (1990)

4316 Nolan PE, Marcus FI, Erstad BL et al. Pharmacokinetic interaction between propafenone and digoxin. *J Am Coll Cardiol*, 11, Suppl, 168a (1988)

4317 Nolten WE, Goldstein D, Lindstrom M et al. Effects of cytokines on the pituitary-adrenal axis in cancer patients. *J Interferon Res*, 13, 349-357 (1993)

4318 Noojin RO, Bradford LG, Osmet LS. Monitoring methotrexate therapy in psoriasis. *Arch Dermatol*, 101, 646 (1970)

4319 Noonan KA, Neal AI, Price CP. Effects of long term administration of tamoxifen on calcium metabolism in women with breast cancer. *Proc ACB Natl Meet*, 77 (1993)

4320 Noppen M, Jacobs A, Van Belle S et al. Inhibitory effects of ranitidine on flushing and serum serotonin concentrations in carcinoid syndrome. *Br Med J*, 296, 682-683 (1988)

4321 Norden CW, Reese R. Oral contraceptives and NBT test. *N Engl J Med*, 287, 254 (1972)

4322 Nordenstrom J, Elvius M, Bagedahl-Strindlund M et al. Biochemical hyperparathyroidism and bone mineral status in patients treated long-term with lithium. *Metabolism*, 43, 1563-1567 (1994)

4323 Nordin BE. The effect of intravenous parathyroid extract on urinary pH, bicarbonate and electrolyte excretion. *Clin Sci*, 19, 311 (1960)

4324 Nordrehaug JE, Johannessen K-A, Von Der Lippe G et al. Effect of timolol on changes in serum potassium concentration during acute myocardial infarction. *Br Heart J*, 53, 388-393 (1985)

4325 Norfleet RG. Green urine. *J Am Med Ass*, 247, 29 (1982)

4326 Norman EJ, Logan D, Terrell P. Falsely high serum B_{12} levels. *Am J Clin Pathol*, 86, 692 (1986)

4327 Norrby SR. Side effects of cephalosporins. *Drugs*, 34, Suppl 2, 105-120 (1987)

4328 Norrby SR, Burman LA, Linderholm H et al. Ceftazidime: pharmacokinetics in patients and effects on the renal function. *J Antimicrob Chemother*, 10, 199-206 (1982)

4329 North JDK. Experience with amiloride - a powerful potassium-sparing diuretic. *S Afr Med J*, 49, Suppl, 9 (1972)

4330 Norton WL, Donnelly RJ. High dose, low frequency parenteral gold administration. *J Rheumatol*, 10, 454-458 (1983)

4331 Nosal T, Kiser WS, Robitaille ML et al. Urinary alkaline phosphatase and lactic dehydrogenase activity in the diagnosis of urologic neoplasms. *Clin Chem*, 12, 542 (1966)

4332 Nosslin B. Bromsulphalein™ retention and jaundice due to unconjugated bilirubin following treatment with male fern extract. *Scand J Clin Lab Invest*, 15, Suppl, 69 (1963)

4333 Notelovitz M, Feldman EB, Gillespy M et al. Lipid and lipoprotein changes in women taking low-dose, triphasic oral contraceptives: a controlled, comparative, 12 month clinical trial. *Am J Obstet Gynecol*, 160, 1269-1280 (1989)

4334 Notelovitz M, Kitchens CS, Coone L et al. Low-dose oral contraceptive usage and coagulation. *Am J Obstet Gynecol*, 141, 71-75 (1981)

4335 Notrica S, Miyada DS, Baysinger V et al. Effects of various medications on values from the HABA and BCG methods for determining albumin. *Clin Chem*, 18, 1537 (1972)

4336 Nourok DS, Glassock RS, Solomon DH. Hypothyroidism following prolonged sodium nitroprusside therapy. *Am J Med Sci*, 248, 129 (1964)

4337 Novacek G, Kapiotis S, Jilma B, et al. Enhanced blood coagulation and enhanced fibrinolysis during hemodialysis with prostacyclin. *Thromb Res*, 88, 283-290 (1997)

4338 Novakova I, Donnelly P, De Witte T et al. Itraconazole and cyclosporin nephrotoxicity. *Lancet*, 2, 920-921 (1987)

4339 Nugent DJ, Bray GL, Counts RB et al. Danazol fails to increase factor VIII or IX levels in a double blind crossover study of patients with hemophilia A or B.. *Br J Haematol*, 64, 493-502 (1986)

4340 Numeroff M, Perlmutter M, Slater S. Falsely elevated values for urinary 17-ketosteroids and 17-hydroxycorticoids. *J Clin Endocrinol Metab*, 19, 1350 (1959)

4341 Nunn B, Baird A, Chamberlain PD. Effect of temocillin and moxalactam on platelet responsiveness and bleeding time in normal volunteers. *Antimicrob Agent Chemother*, 27, 858-862 (1985)

4342 Nyback N, Hassan M, Junthe JJ. Clinical experiences and biochemical findings with tacrine (THA). *Acta Neurol Scand*, 149, Suppl, 36-38 (1993)

4343 Nygard O, Nordrehaug JE, Refsum H, et al. Plasma homocysteine levels and mortality in patients with coronary artery disease. *N Engl J Med*, 337, 230-236 (1997)

4344 Oberg K, Norheim I, Theodorsson E et al. The effects of octreotide on basal and stimulated hormone levels in patients with carcinoid syndrome. *J Clin Endocrinol Metab*, 68, 796-800 (1989)

4345 Obradovic A, Spasic S, Ercegovac D et al. Serum electrolyte levels in long-term antiepileptic therapy. *Biochim Clin*, 13, Suppl 1/8, 335 (1989)

4346 Obradovic D, Spasic S, Golubovic M et al. Serum ceruloplasmin and transferrin values in patients on long-term antiepileptic therapy. *Diag Lab*, 27, Suppl, 157 (1991)

4347 Obradovic D, Spasic S, Golubovic M et al. The effect of long-term antiepileptic therapy on albumin and prealbumin levels. *Diag Lab*, 27, Suppl, 157 (1991)

4348 Obradovic D, Spasic S, Jelic-Ivanovic Z et al. Effects of some antiepileptic drugs on SRA-2000 procedures. *Biochim Clin*, 13, Suppl 1/8, 178 (1989)

4349 O'Brien RC, Simons LA, Clifton P et al. Comparison of simvastatin and cholestyramine in the treatment of primary hypercholesterolemia. *Med J Aust*, 152, 480-483 (1990)

4350 O'Brien RJ, Long MW, Cross FS et al. Hepatotoxicity from isoniazid and rifampin among children treated for tuberculosis. *Pediatrics*, 72, 491-499 (1983)

4351 O'Brien T, Dinneen SF, O'Brien PC et al. Hyperlipidemia in patients with primary and secondary hypothyroidism. *Mayo Clin Proc*, 68, 860-866 (1993)

4352 O'Broin JD, Scott JM, Temperley IJ. A comparison of serum folate estimations using two different methods. *J Clin Pathol*, 26, 80 (1973)

4353 Ochs HR, Greenblatt DJ. Interaction of triazolam with ethanol and isoniazid. *Clin Pharmacol Ther*, 33, 241 (1983)

4354 Ochs HR, Greenblatt DJ, Roberts G-M et al. Diazepam interaction with antituberculosis drugs. *Clin Pharmacol Ther*, 29, 671-678 (1981)

4355 Ochs HR, Greenblatt DJ, Verburg-Ochs B. Propranolol interactions with diazepam, lorazepam, and alprazolam. *Clin Pharmacol Ther*, 36, 451-455 (1984)

4356 Ochs L. Serum protein reagent for use in the Parallel analytical system not susceptible to interference by dextrans. *Clin Chem*, 33, 1953 (1987)

4357 Oclassen Pharmaceuticals, Inc. Manufacturer's literature on Monodox® . San Rafael, CA 94901 (1991)

4358 O'Connor DT, Cervenka JH, Stone RA et al. Dopamine β-hydroxylase immunoreactivity in human cerebrospinal fluid: properties, relationship to central noradrenergic neuronal activity and variation in Parkinson's disease and congenital dopamine β-hydroxylase deficiency. *Clin Sci*, 86, 149-158 (1994)

4359 O'Connor GT, Olmstead EM, Zug K et al. Detection of hepatotoxicity associated with methotrexate therapy for psoriasis. *Arch Dermatol*, 125, 1209-1217 (1989)

4360 Oddie TH, Kossler AW. Tetraiodofluorescein, a contributor to variations in radioiodine uptake. *Am J Hosp Pharm*, 29, 690 (1972)

4361 O'Dell JR, Haire CE, Erikson n, et al. Treatment of rheumatoid arthritis with methotrexate alone, sulfasalazine and hydroxychloroquine, or a combination of all three medications. *N Engl J Med*, 334, 1287-1291 (1996)

4362 O'Dell JR, Haire CE, Palmer W, et al. Treatment of early rheumatoid arthritis with minocycline or placebo. *Arth Rheum*, 40, 842-848 (1997)

4363 Odigne CE, McCulloch AJ, Williams DO et al. A trial of calcium antagonist nisoldipine in hypertensive noninsulin dependent diabetics. *Diabetic Med*, 3, 463-467 (1986)

4364 Odio C, McCracken GH Jr, Nelson JD. Nephrotoxicity associated with vancomycin-aminoglycoside therapy in four children. *J Pediatr*, 105, 491-493 (1984)

4365 Odio CM, Faingezicht I, Paris M et al. The beneficial effects of early dexamethasone administration in infants and children with bacterial meningitis. *N Engl J Med*, 324, 1525-1531 (1991)

4366 Odlind V, Olsson SE. Enhanced metabolism of levonorgestrel during phenytoin treatment in a woman with norplant implants. *Contraception*, 33, 257-261 (1986)

4367 Odman B, Ericsson S, Lindmark M et al. Gemfibrozil in familial combined hyperlipidaemia: effect of added low-dose cholestyramine on plasma and biliary lipids. *Eur J Clin Invest*, 21, 344-349 (1991)

4368 O'Donovan DJ. Inhibition of the indophenol reaction in the spectrophotometric determination of ammonia. *Clin Chim Acta*, 32, 59 (1971)

4369 O'Dwyer WF. Propranolol associated hypoglycaemia in nondiabetics. *J Ir Med Ass*, 73, 173 (1980)

4370 Oetliker O, Hadorn B, Chattas A et al. Secretin induces renal bicarbonate loss in man. *Biol Gastroenterol Belg*, 4, 309 (1971)

4371 Oettgen HF, Stephenson PA, Schwartz MK et al. Toxicity of E coli L-asparaginase in man. *Cancer*, 25, 253 (1970)

4372 Ogata M, Izhushi F. Effects of chlordane on parameters of liver and muscle toxicity in man and experimental animals. *Toxicol Lett*, 56, 327-337 (1991)

4373 Ogawa K, Hatano T, Yamamoto M et al. Hormonal response to acute diuresis - a comparative study of furosemide and azosemide. *Int J Clin Pharmacol Ther Toxicol*, 22, 284-290 (1984)

4374 Ogihara T, Goto Y, Yoshinaga K et al. Dose-effect relationship of carvedilol in essential hypertension: an open study. *Drugs*, 36, Suppl 6, 75-81 (1988)

4375 O'Gorman LP, Borud O, Kham IA et al. The metabolism of L-3,4-dihydroxyphenylalanine in man. *Clin Chim Acta*, 29, 111 (1970)

4376 Ogutman C, Ozben T, Sadan G et al. Morphine increases plasma immunoreactive atrial natriuretic peptide level in humans. *Ann Clin Biochem*, 27, 21-24 (1990)

4377 O'Hare JA, Duggan B, O'Driscoll D et al. Biochemical evidence for osteomalacia with carbamazepine therapy. *Acta Neurol Scand*, 62, 282-286 (1980)

4378 O'Hare JA, Minaker KL, Meneilly GS et al. Effect of insulin on plasma norepinephrine and 3,4-dihydroxyphenylalanine in obese men. *Metabolism*, 38, 322-329 (1989)

4379 Ohashi K, Tateishi T, Sudo T et al. Effects of diltiazem on the pharmacokinetics of nifedipine. *J Cardiovasc Pharmacol*, 15, 96-101 (1990)

4380 Ohashi Y, Nakai H, Ohno Y, et al. Natural course of serum-specific immunoglobulin E and immunoglobulin IgG_4 for a span of eight years in patients with perennial allergic rhinitis. *Laryngoscope*, 107, 382-385 (1997)

4381 Ohashi Y, Nakai H, Okamoto Y, et al. Serum level of interleukin-4 in patients with perennial allergic rhinitis during allergen speficic immunotherapy. *Scand J Immunol*, 43, 680-686 (1996)

4382 Ohashi Y, Nakai Y, Sakamoto H, et al. Serum levels of soluble interleukin-2 receptor in patients with perennial allergic rhinitis before and after immunotherapy. *Ann Allergy*, 77, 203-208 (1996)

4383 Ohman KP, Wiener L, Von Schenck H et al. Antihypertensive and metabolic effects of nifedipine and labetalol alone and in combination in primary hypertension. *Eur J Clin Pharmacol*, 29, 149-154 (1985)

4384 Ohnishi A, Murakami S, Harada M et al. Renal and hormonal responses to repeated treatment with enalapril in non-azotemic cirrhosis with ascites. *J Hepatol*, 20, 223-230 (1994)

4385 Ohsaka A, Saionji K, Igari j. Granulocyte colony-stimulating factor administration increases serum concentrations of soluble selectins. *Br J Haematol*, 100, 66-69 (1998)

4386 Ohtani Y, Endo F, Matsuda I. Carnitine deficiency and hyperammonemia associated with valproic acid therapy. *J Pediatr*, 101, 782-785 (1982)

4387 Ojala J-P, Helve E, Tikkanen MJ. Treatment of combined hyperlipidemia with lovastatin versus gemfibrozil: a comparison study. *Cardiology*, 77, Suppl 4, 39-42 (1990)

4388 Okada M, Imamura K, Iida M et al. Hypophosphatemia induced by intravenous administration of saccharated iron oxide. *Klin Wschr*, 61, 99-102 (1983)

4389 Okada S, Miyai Y, Ichiki K et al. Clinofibrate therapy raises high-density lipoprotein levels and lowers atherogenic index in diabetes mellitus patients. *J Intern Med Res*, 17, 521-525 (1989)

4390 O'Kell RT, Knepper L, Mantzey L et al. Effect of drugs on results of laboratory tests. *Clin Chem*, 18, 1039 (1972)

4391 O'Kell RT, Mantzey L, Knepper L et al. Intravenous vitamins and clinical laboratory tests. *Clin Chem*, 18, 403 (1972)

4392 Oken MM, Hootkin L, Dejager RL. Hepatitis after Konyne® administration. *Am J Dig Dis*, 17, 271 (1972)

4393 Okesina AB, Donaldson D, Lascelles PT. Isoenzymes of alkaline phosphatase in epileptic patients receiving carbamazepine monotherapy. *J Clin Pathol*, 44, 480-482 (1991)

4394 Okesina AB, Donaldson D, Lascelles PT. Serum γ-glutamyltransferase activities in epileptic patients receiving carbamazepine monotherapy. *Ann Clin Biochem*, 28, 307-308 (1991)

4395 Okrucka A, Pechan J, Balazovjech I. The effect of short-term celiprolol therapy on platelet function in essential hypertension. *Cardiology*, 82, 399-404 (1993)

4396 Okrucka A, Pechan J, Mikulecky M. The effect of prazosin therapy on platelet activation in essential hypertension. *Clin Exp Pharmacol Physiol*, 17, 813-819 (1990)

4397 Oksa A, Gajdos M, Fedelesova V et al. Effects of angiotensin-converting enzyme inhibitors on glucose and lipid metabolism in essential hypertension. *J Cardiovasc Pharmacol*, 23, 79-86 (1994)

4398 Okuno T, Shindo M, Arai K et al. 2'-5'-oligoadenylate synthetase activity in peripheral blood mononuclear cells and serum during interferon treatment of chronic non-A, non-B hepatitis. *Gastroenterol Jpn*, 26, 603-610 (1991)

4399 okusa MD, Crystal LJT. Clinical manifestations and management of acute lithium intoxication. *Am J Med*, 97, 383-389 (1994)

4400 Olans RN, Weiner LB. Reversible oxacillin hepatotoxicity. *J Pediatr*, 89, 835-838 (1976)

4401 Olarte MR, Shafer SQ. Levamisole is ineffective in the treatment of amyotrophic lateral sclerosis. *Neurology*, 35, 1063-1066 (1985)

4402 O'Leary TJ, Jones G, Yip A et al. The effects of chloroquine on serum 1,25-dihydroxyvitamin D and calcium metabolism in sarcoidosis. *N Engl J Med*, 315, 727-730 (1986)

4403 O'Leary TJ, Simo IE, Kanigsberg ND et al. Lack of effect of isotretinoin on thyroid function tests. *Clin Chem*, 32, 913-914 (1986)

4404 Oleesky DA, Mir MA. Paradoxical high-density lipoprotein reduction induced by fibrate therapy. *Ann Clin Biochem*, 34, 573-574 (1997)

4405 Olesen KH, Sigurd B, Steiness E et al. Bumetanide, a new potent diuretic. *Acta Med Scand*, 193, 119 (1973)

4406 Oliver MF, Roberts SD, Hayes D. Effect of atromid and ethyl chlorophenoxyisobutyrate on anticoagulant requirements. *Lancet*, 1, 143 (1963)

4407 Oliveros-Palacios MC, Godoy-Godoy N, Colina-Chourio JA. Effects of doxazosin on blood pressure, renin-angiotensin-aldosterone and urinary kallikrein. *Am J Cardiol*, 67, 157-161 (1991)

4408 Olivesi A. Modified elimination of prednisolone in epileptic patients on carbamazepine monotherapy, and in women using low-dose oral contraceptives. *Biomed Pharmacother*, 40, 301-308 (1986)

4409 Olivieri NF. Long-term therapy with deferiprone. *Acta Haematol*, 95, 37-48 (1996)

4410 Olofsson B-O, Nyhlin H, Wester P-O. β-blockade or inhibition of angiotensin converting enzyme does not affect intracellular magnesium or potassium. *Curr Ther Res*, 46, 121-125 (1989)

4411 Olsen KM, Gulliksen M, Christophersen AS. Metabolites of chlorpromazine and brompheniramine may cause false-positive urine amphetamine results with monoclonal EMIT d.a.u. immunoassay. *Clin Chem*, 38, 611-612 (1992)

4412 Olsen NV, Lund J, Jensen PF et al. Dopamine, dobutamine, and dopexamine: a comparison of renal effects in unanesthetized human volunteers. *Anesthesiology*, 79, 685-694 (1993)

4413 Olson VV, Loft S, Christensen KD. Serious reactions during malaria prophylaxis with pyrimethamine sulfadoxine. *Lancet*, 2, 994 (1982)

4414 Olsson R, Broome U, Danielsson A et al. Colchicine treatment of primary sclerosing cholangitis. *Gastroenterology*, 106, 1199-1203 (1995)

4415 Olsson R, Hellner L, Lindstedt G et al. Plasma proteins in patients on long-term antiepileptic treatment. *Clin Chem*, 29, 728-730 (1984)

4416 Olsson R, Tyllstrom J, Zettergren L. Hepatic reactions to cyclofenil. *Gut*, 24, 260-263 (1983)

4417 O'Malley K, Stevenson IH, Crooks J. Impairment of human drug metabolism by oral contraceptive steroids. *Clin Pharmacol Ther*, 13, 552-557 (1972)

4418 Onarato IM, Axelrod JL. Hepatitis from intravenous high-dose oxacillin therapy. *Ann Intern Med*, 89, 497-500 (1978)

4419 Oneda A, Sato M, Yanbe A et al. Plasma glucagon response to blood glucose fall, gastrointestinal hormones and arginine in man. *Tohoku J Exp Med*, 107, 241 (1973)

4420 Ooi TC, Peden NR, Champion MC et al. The effect of cimetidine and ranitidine on serum high density lipoprotein subfractions. *Atherosclerosis*, 57, 159-162 (1985)

4421 Ooiwa H, Shimamoto K, Nakagawa M et al. The interference of acebutolol administration in the measurement of urinary 17-ketosteroid by Zimmermann method. *Endocrinol Jpn*, 35, 485-490 (1988)

4422 Oosterhuis WP, Kramer PA, Poirot MJ et al. Penicillin antibiotic interference of urinary protein determination in the biuret reaction. *Tijdschr Ned Ver Klin Chem*, 14, 198-200 (1989)

4423 Opala G, Winter S, Vance C et al. The effect of valproic acid on plasma carnitine levels. *Am J Dis Child*, 145, 999-1001 (1991)

4424 Orefice G, Troisi E, Selvaggio M et al. Effect of long-term mesoglycan treatment on fibrinogen plasma levels in patients with ischemic cerebrovascular disease. *Curr Ther Res*, 52, 666-670 (1992)

4425 O'Reilly RA. Dynamic interaction between disulfiram and separated enantiomorphs of racemic warfarin. *Clin Pharmacol Ther*, 29, 332-336 (1981)

4426 O'Reilly RA. Interaction of sodium warfarin and disulfiram (Antabuse®) in man. *Ann Intern Med*, 78, 73 (1973)

4427 O'Reilly RA. Phenylbutazone and sulfinpyrazone interaction with oral anticoagulant phenprocoumon. *Arch Intern Med*, 142, 1634-1637 (1982)

4428 O'Reilly RA. Spironolactone and warfarin interaction. *Clin Pharmacol Ther*, 27, 198-201 (1980)

4429 O'Reilly RA. The stereoselective interaction of warfarin and metronidazole in man. *N Engl J Med*, 295, 354-357 (1976)

4430 O'Reilly RA, Motley CH. Racemic warfarin and trimethoprim-sulfamethoxazole interaction in humans. *Ann Intern Med*, 91, 34-36 (1979)

4431 O'Reilly RA, Trager WF, Motley CH et al. Interaction of secobarbital with warfarin pseudoracemates. *Clin Pharmacol Ther*, 28, 187-195 (1980)

4432 Orenstein AA, Yakulis V, Eipe J et al. Immune hemolysis due to hydralazine. *Ann Intern Med*, 86, 450-451 (1977)

4433 Organon Inc. Manufacturer's literature on Durabolin® . West Orange, NJ

4434 Organon Inc. Manufacturer's literature on Remeron® . West Orange, NJ 07062 (1996)

4435 Organon Inc. Manufacturer's literature on Tice® BCG. West Orange, NJ 07062 (1994)

4436 Orme M, Breckenridge A, Brooks RV. Interactions of benzodiazepines with warfarin. *Br Med J*, 3, 611 (1972)

4437 Orney DL. An approach to the measurement of total lipid glycerol in serum. *Clin Chem*, 19, 453 (1973)

4438 Orr LE. Potentiation of myelosuppression from cancer chemotherapy and thiazide diuretics. *Drug Intell Clin Pharm*, 15, 967-970 (1981)

4439 Orskov H, Wolthers T, Grofte T et al. Somatostatin-stimulated insulin-like growth factor binding protein-1 release is abolished by hyperinsulinemia. *J Clin Endocrinol Metab*, 78, 138-140 (1994)

4440 Orth SR, Ritz E. The nephrotic syndrome. *N Engl J Med*, 338, 1202-1211 (1998)

4441 Ortho Biotech Inc.. Manufacturer's literature on Leustatin® . Raritan, NJ 08869 (1995)

4442 Ortho Biotech Inc.. Manufacturer's literature on Micronor® . Raritan, NJ 08869 (1996)

4443 Ortho Biotech Inc.. Manufacturer's literature on Ortho-Est® . Raritan, NJ 08869 (1996)

4444 Ortho Biotech Inc.. Manufacturer's literature on Orthoclone OKT® 3 Sterile Solution. Raritan, NJ 08869 (1995)

4445 Ortho Biotech Inc.. Manufacturer's literature on Procrit® . Raritan, NJ 08869 (1995)

4446 Ortho Biotech Inc.. Manufacturer's literature on Protostat® . Raritan, NJ 08869 (1992)

4447 Ortho Pharmaceutical Corporation. Manufacturer's literature on Grifulvin V®. Raritan, NJ 08869 (1992)

4448 Ortho Pharmaceutical Corporation. Manufacturer's literature on Levaquin™. Raritan, NJ (1997)

4449 Osawa S, Iida S, Yonemitsu H et al. Prostatic acid phosphatase assay with self-indicating substrate 2,6-dichloro-4-acetylphenyl phosphate. *Clin Chem*, 41, 200-203 (1995)

4450 Osborne CK. Tamoxifen in the treatment of breast cancer. *N Engl J Med*, 339, 1609-1618 (1998)

4451 Osborne JC. Hypoprothrombinemia and bleeding due to cefoperazone. *Ann Intern Med*, 102, 721 (1985)

4452 Osei K, Holland G, Falko JM. Indapamide: effect on apoprotein, lipoprotein, and glucoregulation in ambulatory diabetic patients. *Arch Intern Med*, 146, 1973-1977 (1986)

4453 Oshima S, Ogawa H, Mizuno Y, et al. The effects of the angiotensin-converting enzyme inhibitor imidapril on plasma plasminogen activator inhibitor activity in patients with acute myocardial infarction. *Am Heart J*, 134, 961-966 (1997)

4454 Osilesi O et al. Blood pressure and plasma lipids during ascorbic acid supplementation in borderline hypertensive and normotensive adults. *Nutr Res*, 11, 405 (1991)

4455 Osman MA, Patel RB, Schuna A et al. Reduction in oral penicillamine absorption by food, antacid and ferrous sulfate. *Clin Pharmacol Ther*, 33, 465-470 (1983)

4456 Osman MI, Abdalla MI, Toppozada MH et al. Subdermal levonorgestrel implants: serum androgens. *Contracept Deliv Syst*, 4, 127-131 (1983)

4457 Osman MM, Toppozada HK, Ghanem MH et al. The effect of an oral contraceptive on serum lipids. *Contraception*, 5, 105 (1972)

4458 Osmialowska Z, Nartowicz-Skoiewska M, Slominsk JM et al. Effect of nifedipine monotherapy on platelet aggregation in patients with untreated essential hypertension. *Eur J Clin Pharmacol*, 39, 403-404 (1990)

4459 Otani K, Kondo T, Ishida M et al. Prolactin response to zotepine in schizophrenic patients. *Hum Psychopharmacol*, 8, 35-39 (1993)

4460 Otterstad JE, Froeland G, Wasenius Soeyland AK et al. Lipid profile in 100 men with moderate hypertension treated for 1 year with atenolol or hydrochlorothiazide plus amiloride: a double-blind, randomized study. *Scand J Clin Lab Invest*, 52, 83-93 (1992)

4461 Ottosson A-M, Karlberg BE. Nisoldipine - effects on the renin-angiotensin-aldosterone system and catecholamines. Studies in normotensive and hypertensive subjects. *J Intern Med*, 228, 503-509 (1990)

4462 Overbosch D, Van Gulpen C, Hermans J et al. The effect of probenecid on the renal tubular excretion of benzylpenicillin. *Br J Clin Pharmacol*, 25, 51-58 (1988)

4463 Overton CE, Kennedy SH, Egan DE et al. The effect of nafarelin on human plasma adrenocorticotrophic hormone and cortisol concentrations. *Hum Reprod*, 8, 1593-1597 (1993)

4464 Owada A, Nonoguchi H, Terada Y, et al. Effects of quinapril hydrochloride in patients with essential hypertension and renal function. *Clin Exp Hypertens*, 19, 495-502 (1997)

4465 Owen RT. Piroxicam. *Drugs Today*, 16, 115-119 (1980)

4466 Owusu SK. Acute haemolysis complicating co-trimoxazole therapy for typhoid fever in a patient with G-6-PD deficiency. *Lancet*, 2, 819 (1972)

4467 Oyake H, Isono Y, Kudo M. A case of agranulocytosis possibly due to aminobenzyl penicillin. *Iryo*, 22, 676 (1968)

4468 Oyama T, Matsuki A, Kudo T. Effect of ether, thiopentone anesthesia and surgery on plasma thyroid-stimulating hormone concentrations. *Br J Anaes*, 44, 841 (1972)

4469 Oyama T, Matsuki A, Kudo T. Effect of halothane, methoxyflurane anaesthesia and surgery on plasma thyroid-stimulating hormone. *Anesthesia*, 27, 3 (1972)

4470 Oyama T, Matsuki A, Kudo T. Effects of enflurane (Ethrane®) anaesthesia and surgery on carbohydrate and fat metabolism in man. *Anesthesia*, 27, 179 (1972)

4471 Ozawa N, Tokoro T, Hirakawa S et al. Influence of fusaric acid and reserpine on the urinary excretion of catecholamines. *Jpn J Pharmacol*, 22, 113 (1972)

4472 Ozawa T, Ninomiya Y, Honma T et al. Increased serum angiotensin I-converting enzyme activity in patients with mixed connective tissue disease and pulmonary hypertension. *Scand J Rheumatol*, 24, 38-43 (1995)

4473 Ozdemir MA, Sofuoglu S, Tanrikulu G et al. Lithium-induced hematologic changes in patients with bipolar affective disorder. *Biol Psychiat*, 35, 210-213 (1994)

4474 Paavonen T, Aronen H, Pyrhonen S et al. The effect of toremifene therapy on serum immunoglobulin levels in breast cancer. *APMIS*, 99, 849-853 (1991)

4475 Pacifici R, Paris L, Di Carlo S et al. Immunologic aspects of carbamazepine treatment in epileptic patients. *Epilepsia*, 32, 122-127 (1991)

4476 Paciucci PA, Sklarin NT. Mitoxantrone and hepatic toxicity. *Ann Intern Med*, 105, 805-806 (1986)

4477 Pagano G, Bruno A, Cavallo-Perin P et al. Glucose intolerance after short-term administration of corticosteroids in healthy subjects: prednisone, deflazacort, and betamethasone. *Arch Intern Med*, 149, 1098-1101 (1989)

4478 Page K, Massey J. Urine catecholamine excretion in long-term oral theophylline use. *Ann Clin Biochem*, 30, 492-293 (1993)

4479 Page LB, Sidd JJ. Medical management of primary hypertension. *N Engl J Med*, 287, 1018 (1972)

4480 Paine D. Fatal hepatic necrosis associated with aminosalicylic acid: review of literature and report of case. *J Am Med Ass*, 167, 286 (1958)

4481 Pak CYC. Hydrochlorothiazide therapy in nephrolithiasis. *Clin Pharmacol Ther*, 14, 209 (1973)

4482 Pak CYC. Sodium cellulose phosphate: mechanism of action and effect on mineral metabolism. *J Clin Pharmacol*, 13, 15 (1973)

4483 Pak CYC, Delea CS, Bartter FC. Successful treatment of recurrent nephrolithiasis (calcium stones) with cellulose phosphate. *N Engl J Med*, 290, 175 (1974)

4484 Pak CYC, Ruskin B, Diller E. Enhancement of renal excretion of zinc by hydrochlorothiazide. *Clin Chim Acta*, 39, 511 (1972)

4485 Palan PR, Romney SL, Vermund SH et al. Effects of smoking and oral contraception on plasma β-carotene levels in healthy women. *Am J Obstet Gynecol*, 161, 881-885 (1989)

4486 Palazidou E, Skene D, Arendt J et al. The acute and chronic effects of (+) and (-) oxaprotiline upon melatonin secretion in normal subjects. *Psychol Med*, 200, 273-277 (1992)

4487 Palestine AG, Nussenblatt RB, Chan C-C. Side effects of systemic cyclosporine in patients not undergoing transplantation. *Am J Med*, 77, 652-656 (1984)

4488 Palm R, Silseth C, Alvan G. Phenytoin intoxication as the first symptom of fatal liver damage induced by sodium valproate. *Br J Clin Pharmacol*, 17, 597-598 (1984)

4489 Palmer JH, Sapienza TJ, Zink EW. Pyrazinamide interference in the Ferrochem II determination of iron. *Clin Chem*, 34, 1510-1511 (1988)

4490 Palumbo G, Barantani E, Pozzi F et al. Long-term nifedipine treatment and glucose homeostasis in hypertensive patients. *Curr Ther Res*, 43, 171-179 (1988)

4491 Pan HY. Clinical pharmacology of pravastatin, a selective inhibitor of HMG-CoA reductase. *Eur J Clin Pharmacol*, 40, Suppl 1, S15-S18 (1991)

4492 Pan HY, DeVault AR, Swites BJ et al. Pharmacokinetics and pharmacodynamics of pravastatin alone and with cholestyramine in hypercholesterolemia. *Clin Pharmacol Ther*, 48, 201-207 (1990)

4493 Pan HY, Funke PT, Willard DE et al. Pharmacokinetics, pharmacodynamics and safety of pravastatin sodium, a potent inhibitor of HMG-CoA reductase, in healthy volunteers. *Roy Soc Med Int Congress Symp Ser*, 162, 9-22 (1989)

4494 Pandian MR, Morgan CH, Carlton E et al. Modified immunoradiometric assay of parathyroid hormone-related protein: clinical application in the differential diagnosis of hypercalcemia. *Clin Chem*, 38, 282-288 (1992)

4495 Panesar SK, Orr JM, Farrell K et al. The effect of carbamazepine on valproic acid disposition in adult volunteers. *Br J Clin Pharmacol*, 27, 323-328 (1989)

4496 Panidis D, Vavilis D, Rousso D et al. Danazol influences gonadotropin secretion at the hypothalamic level. *Int J Gynaecol Obstet*, 45, 241-246 (1994)

4497 Panidis D, Vavilis D, Rousso D et al. Provocative tests of prolactin before, during and after long-term danazol treatment in patients with endometriosis. *Gynecol Endocrinol*, 6, 19-24 (1992)

4498 Pannall PR, Maas DA. Danazol and thyroid function tests. *Lancet*, 1, 102-103 (1977)

4499 Panz VR, Wing JR, Raal FJ, et al. Improved glucose tolerance after effective lipid-lowering therapy with bezafibrate in a patient with lipoatrophic diabetes mellitus: a putative role for Randle's cycle in its pathogenesis. *Clin Endocrinol*, 46, 365-368 (1997)

4500 Paolisso G, Sgambato S, De Riu S et al. Simvastatin reduces plasma lipid levels and improves insulin action in elderly, non-insulin dependent diabetics. *Eur J Clin Pharmacol*, 40, 27-31 (1991)

4501 Paolisso G, Sgambato S, Passariello N et al. Insulin induces opposite changes in plasma and erythrocyte magnesium concentrations in normal man. *Diabetologia*, 29, 644-647 (1986)

4502 Papademetriou V, Price M, Johnson E et al. Early changes in plasma and urinary potassium in diuretic-treated patients with systemic hypertension. *Am J Cardiol*, 54, 1015-1019 (1984)

4503 Papageorgiou P, Kesarwala HH, Alcid DV et al. Levamisole in chronic pyoderma. *J Clin Lab Immunol*, 8, 121-127 (1982)

4504 Papavasiliou PS, Cotzias GC, Duby SE et al. Levodopa in Parkinsonism: potentiation of central effects with a peripheral inhibitor. *N Engl J Med*, 286, 8 (1972)

4505 Papeschi R, Molina-Negro P, Sourkes Tlerba G. The concentration of homovanillic and 5-hydroxyindoleacetic acids in ventricular and lumbar CSF. *Neurology*, 22, 1151 (1972)

4506 Pappu AS, Illingworth DR. Contrasting effects of lovastatin and cholestyramine on low-density lipoprotein cholesterol and 24-hour urinary mevalonate excretion in patients with heterozygous familial hypercholesterolemia. *J Lab Clin Med*, 114, 554-562 (1989)

4507 Pappu AS, Illingworth DR, Bacon S. Reduction of plasma low-density lipoprotein cholesterol and urinary mevalonic acid by lovastatin in patients with heterozygous hypercholesterolemia. *Metabolism*, 38, 542-549 (1989)

4508 Pardue WO. Severe liver dysfunction during nicotinic acid therapy. *J Am Med Ass*, 175, 137 (1961)

4509 Parent M, St-Laurent M, Lebel M. Safety of fleroxicin coadministered with theophylline to young and elderly volunteers. *Antimicrob Agent Chemother*, 34, 1249-1253 (1990)

4510 Parent X, Hanser AM, Aberer P et al. Interference of high bicarbonate concentration on sodium measurement by ISE. *Clin Biochem Rev*, 14, 195 (1993)

4511 Parfitt AM. Chlorothiazide induced hypercalcemia in juvenile osteoporosis and hyperparathyroidism. *N Engl J Med*, 281, 55 (1969)

4512 Parfrey PS, Griffiths SM, Barrett BJ et al. Contrast material-induced renal failure in patients with diabetes mellitus, renal insufficiency, or both. *N Engl J Med*, 320, 143-149 (1989)

4513 Pariente EA, Bataille C, Bercoff E et al. Acute effects of captopril on systemic and renal hemodynamics and on renal function in cirrhotic patients with ascites. *Gastroenterology*, 88, 1255-1259 (1985)

4514 Pariente EA, Pessayre D, Bentata-Pessayre M et al. Hepatite a l'ajmaline. description de 4 observations et revue de la litterature. *Gastroenterol Clin Biol*, 4, 240-245 (1980)

4515 Parish RC, Gotz VP, Mehta JL. Cimetidine does not increase α_1-acid glycoprotein serum concentrations. *Br J Clin Pharmacol*, 25, 514-517 (1988)

4516 Parke-Davis. Manufacturer's literature on Accupril® . Morris Plains, NJ 07950 (1994)

4517 Parke-Davis. Manufacturer's literature on Benadryl® . Morris Plains, NJ 07950 (1996)

4518 Parke-Davis. Manufacturer's literature on Celontin® . Morris Plains, NJ 07950 (1995)

4519 Parke-Davis. Manufacturer's literature on Cerebyx® . Morris Plains, NJ 07950 (1996)

4520 Parke-Davis. Manufacturer's literature on Chloromycetin® . Morris Plains, NJ 07950 (1994)

4521 Parke-Davis. Manufacturer's literature on Cognex® . Morris Plains, NJ 07950 (1995)

4522 Parke-Davis. Manufacturer's literature on Dilantin® . Morris Plains, NJ 07950 (1995)

4523 Parke-Davis. Manufacturer's literature on Doryx® . Morris Plains, NJ 07950 (1994)

4524 Parke-Davis. Manufacturer's literature on Lopid® . Morris Plains, NJ 07950 (1994)

4525 Parke-Davis. Manufacturer's literature on Nardil® . Morris Plains, NJ 07950 (1995)

4526 Parke-Davis. Manufacturer's literature on Neurontin® . Morris Plains, NJ 07950 (1995)

4527 Parke-Davis. Manufacturer's literature on Nitrostat® . Morris Plains, NJ 07950 (1995)

4528 Parke-Davis. Manufacturer's literature on Omnicef® . Morris Plains, NJ 07950 (1998)

4529 Parke-Davis. Manufacturer's literature on Ponstel® . Morris Plains, NJ 07950 (1995)

4530 Parke-Davis. Manufacturer's literature on Procanbid™. Morris Plains, NJ 07950 (1995)

4531 Parke-Davis. Manufacturer's literature on Pyridium® . Morris Plains, NJ 07950 (1994)

4532 Parke-Davis. Manufacturer's literature on Rezulin™. Morris Plains, NJ 07950 (1998)

4533 Parke-Davis. Manufacturer's literature on Zarontin® . Morris Plains, NJ 07950 (1994)

4534 Parke-Davis, Division of Warner-Lambert Company. Manufacturer's literature on Lipitor™. Morris Plains, NJ 07950 (1997)

4535 Parker KM, Rawlings V, Dunn L. Medical drug screening using the Abbott ADx syatem. *Clin Chem*, 37, 1013 (1991)

4536 Parker WA. Captopril-induced cholestatic jaundice. *Drug Intell Clin Pharm*, 18, 234-235 (1984)

4537 Parker WA. Propylthiouracil-induced hepatotoxicity. *Clin Pharmacol*, 1, 471-474 (1982)

4538 Parker WA, Maccara ME. In vitro effect of new penicillins and aminoglycosides on tests for glycosuria. *Am J Hosp Pharm*, 41, 125-127 (1984)

4539 Parodi FA. Pharmacological and clinical evaluation of the activity and tolerance of new oral antidiabetic compound. *Isr J Med Sci*, 8, 888 (1972)

4540 Paroni R, Arcelloni C, Fermo I et al. Determination of creatinine in serum and urine by a rapid liquid chromatographic method. *Clin Chem*, 36, 830-836 (1990)

4541 Parris WCV, Kambam JR, Naukam RJ et al. Immunoreactive substance P is decreased in saliva of patients with chronic back pain syndromes. *Anesth Analg*, 70, 63-67 (1990)

4542 Parry MF. The tolerance and safety of azlocillin. *J Antimicrob Chemother*, 11, Suppl B, 223-228 (1983)

4543 Parsons WB Jr. Effect of nicotinic acid on serum levels of cholesterol, triglycerides, glucose and uric acid. *Circulation*, Suppl 6, 154 (1968)

4544 Pas AT, Quinn EL. Cholestatic hepatitis following the administration of sodium oxacillin. *J Am Med Ass*, 191, 674 (1965)

4545 Pasanisi F, Elliott HL, Merdith PA et al. Combined α-adrenoceptor antagonism and calcium channel blockade in normal subjects. *Clin Pharmacol Ther*, 36, 716-723 (1984)

4546 Pasic J, Jackson SHD, Johnston A et al. The interaction between chronic oral slow-release theophylline and single-dose intravenous erythromycin. *Xenobiotica*, 17, 493-497 (1987)

4547 Passariello N, Giugliano D, Sgambato S et al. Calcitonin, a diabetogenic hormone. *J Clin Endocrinol Metab*, 53, 318-323 (1981)

4548 Passariello N, Pisano MCA, Sepe J et al. Effect of aldolase reductase inhibitor (tolrestat) on urinary albumin excretion rate and glomerular filtration rate in IDDM subjects with nephropathy. *Diabetes Care*, 16, 789-795 (1993)

4549 Passmore AP, Copeland S, Johnston GD. A comparison of the effects of ibuprofen and indomethacin upon renal haemodynamics and electrolyte excretion in the presence and absence of frusemide. *Br J Clin Pharmacol*, 27, 483-490 (1989)

4550 Pasternack A, Vanttinen T, Solakivi T et al. Normalization of lipoprotein lipase and hepatic lipase by gemfibrozil results in correction of lipoprotein abnormalities in chronic renal failure. *Clin Nephrol*, 27, 163-168 (1987)

4551 Pastors JG, Blaisdell PW, Balm TK et al. Psyllium fiber reduces rise in postprandial glucose and insulin concentrations in patients with non-insulin-dependent diabetes. *Am J Clin Nutr*, 53, 1431-1435 (1991)

4552 Patat A, Surjus A, Le Go A et al. Safety and tolerance of single oral doses of trandolapril (RU 44.570), a new angiotensin converting enzyme inhibitor. *Eur J Clin Pharmacol*, 36, 17-23 (1989)

4553 Patel IH, Levy RH, Cutler RE. Phenobarbital-valproic acid interaction. *Clin Pharmacol Ther*, 27, 515-521 (1980)

4554 Paterson Y, Lawrence EF. Factors affecting creatine phosphokinase levels in normal adult females. *Clin Chim Acta*, 42, 131 (1972)

4555 Pathy MS. The use, action and side effects of diuretics. *Gerontol Clin*, 13, 261 (1971)

4556 Pathy MS, Reynolds AJ. Papaverine and hepatotoxicity. *Postgrad Med J*, 56, 488-490 (1980)

4557 Patoia L, Guerciolini R, Menichetti F et al. Norfloxacin and neutropenia. *Ann Intern Med*, 107, 788-789 (1987)

4558 Paton TW, Walker SE, Leung FY et al. Effect of cimetidine on bioavailability of enteric-coated aspirin tablets. *Clin Pharmacol Ther*, 2, 165-166 (1983)

4559 Patrassi GM, Fallo F, Martinelli S et al. The contact phase of blood coagulation and renin activation in essential hypertension before and after captopril. *Eur Heart J*, 5, 561-567 (1984)

4560 Patsch W, Brown SA, Gotto AM Jr et al. The effect of triphasic oral contraceptives on plasma lipids and lipoproteins. *Am J Obstet Gynecol*, 161, 1396-1401 (1989)

4561 Patterson JS, Furr BJA, Battersby LA. Tamoxifen and hypercalcemia. *Ann Intern Med*, 89, 1013 (1978)

4562 Patterson WP, Khojasteh A. Ifosfamide-induced renal tubular defects. *Cancer*, 63, 649-651 (1989)

4563 Patwardhan RV, Desmond PV, Johnson RF et al. Impaired elimination of caffeine by oral contraceptive steroids. *J Lab Clin Med*, 95, 603-608 (1980)

4564 Pauciullo P, Marotta G, Rubba P et al. Serum lipoproteins, apolipoproteins and very low density lipoprotein subfractions during 6 month fibrate treatment in primary hypertriglyceridemia. *J Intern Med*, 228, 425-430 (1990)

4565 Pauksen K, Elfman L, Ulfgren A-K et al. Serum levels of granulocyte-colony stimulating factor (G-CSF) in bacterial and viral infections, and in atypical pneumonia. *Br J Haematol*, 88, 256-260 (1994)

4566 Pawan GI. Metabolic effects of S992 in man. *Br J Pharmacol*, 41, 416 (1971)

4567 Payne R. Serum uric acid and phenothiazines. *Lancet*, 2, 855 (1969)

4568 Pazmino P. Acute renal failure, skin rash, and eosinophilia associated with aztreonam. *Am J Nephrol*, 8, 68-70 (1988)

4569 Pazmino P. Topical tretinoin for photoaged skin. *J Am Med Ass*, 259, 3271 (1988)

4570 Pazmino PA. Suprofen-induced acute renal failure. *Tex Med*, 83, 32-33 (1987)

4571 Pazmino PA, Pazmino PB. Ketoprofen-induced irreversible renal failure. *Nephron*, 50, 70-71 (1988)

4572 Pazos F, Alvarez JJ, Rubies-Prat J et al. Long term thyroid replacement therapy and levels of lipoprotein(a) and other lipoproteins. *J Clin Endocrinol Metab*, 80, 562-566 (1995)

4573 Pazzucconi F, Mannucci L, Mussoni L et al. Bezafibrate lowers plasma lipids, fibrinogen and platelet aggregability in hypertriglyceridaemia. *Eur J Clin Pharmacol*, 43, 219-223 (1992)

4574 Pearson AJG, Grainger JM, Scheuer PJ et al. Jaundice due to oxyphenisatin. *Lancet*, 1, 994 (1971)

4575 Pearson DWM, Ratcliffe WA, Thomson JA et al. Biochemical and clinical effects of fenclofenac in thyrotoxicosis. *Clin Endocrinol*, 16, 369-373 (1982)

4576 Pearson JR, Binder CI, Neber J. Agranulocytosis following Diamox® therapy. *J Am Med Ass*, 157, 339 (1955)

4577 Peddicord CH, Barnes WA. Ascorbic acid interferogram for cholesterol in the Demand and TDx. *Clin Chem*, 34, 773-774 (1988)

4578 Peden NR, Dow RJ, Isles TE et al. β-Adrenoreceptor blockade and responses of serum lipids to a meal and exercise. *Br Med J*, 288, 1788-1790 (1984)

4579 Pedersen A, Sandström B, van Amelsvoort JMM. The effect of ingestion on blood lipids and gastrointestinal symptoms in healthy females. *Br J Nutr*, 78, 215-222 (1997)

4580 Pedersen C, Ingeberg S, Stubbe T et al. Serum thymidine kinase – a marker of bone marrow toxicity during treatment with zidovudine. *AIDS*, 3, 743-746 (1989)

4581 Pedersen KE, Christiansen BD, Kjaer K et al. Verapamil-induced changes in digoxin kinetics and intraerythrocytic sodium concentrations. *Clin Pharmacol Ther*, 34, 8-13 (1983)

4582 Pedersen KE, Christiansen BD, Klitgaard NA et al. Effect of quinidine on digoxin bioavailability. *Eur J Clin Pharmacol*, 24, 41-47 (1983)

4583 Pedersen KE, Madsen JL, Klitgaard NA et al. Effect of quinine on plasma digoxin concentration and renal digoxin clearance. *Acta Med Scand*, 218, 229-232 (1985)

4584 Pedersen KE, Thayssen P, Klitgaard NA et al. Influence of verapamil on the inotropism and pharmacokinetics of digoxin. *Eur J Clin Pharmacol*, 25, 199-206 (1983)

4585 Pedersen MM, Christensen SE, Sandahl Christiansen J et al. Acute effects of a somatostatin analogue on kidney function in type I diabetic patients. *Diabetic Med*, 7, 304-309 (1990)

4586 Pedersen S, Fuglsang G. Urine cortisol excretion in children with high doses of inhaled corticosteroids: A comparison of budesonide and beclomethasone. *Eur Respir J*, 1, 433-435 (1988)

4587 Peel N, Al-Dehaimi A, Colwell A et al. Sulfasalazine may interfere with HPLC assay of urinary pyridinium crosslinks. *Clin Chem*, 40, 167-168 (1994)

4588 Peet M, Middlemiss DN, Yates RA. Propranolol in schizophrenia II. Clinical and biochemical aspects of combining propranolol with chlorpromazine. *Br J Psychiat*, 139, 112-117 (1981)

4589 Pehan J, Okrucka A. Diltiazem inhibits the spontaneous platelet aggregation in essential hypertension. *Cardiology*, 79, 116-119 (1991)

4590 Pek S, Fajans SS, Floyd JC Jr et al. Failure of sulfonylureas to suppress plasma glucagon in man. *Diabetes*, 21, 216 (1972)

4591 Pelkonen R, Fogelholm R, Nikkila EA. Increase in serum cholesterol during phenytoin treatment. *Br Med J*, 4, 85 (1975)

4592 Pellock JM, Howell J, Kendig EL Jr. Pyridoxine deficiency in children treated with isoniazid. *Chest*, 87, 658-661 (1985)

4593 Penarrubia MJ, Steegman JL, Lavilla E et al. Hypertriglyceridemia may be severe in CML patients treated with interferon-α. *Am J Hematol*, 49, 240-241 (1995)

4594 Pendleton RG, Newman DJ, Sherman SS et al. Effect of propranolol upon the hemoglobin-oxygen dissociation curve. *J Pharmacol Exp Ther*, 180, 647 (1972)

4595 Penney MD, Hampton D. The effect of lithium therapy on arginine vasopressin secretion and thirst in man. *Clin Biochem*, 23, 233-236 (1990)

4596 Pentikainen J, Koivula IH, Hiltunen HA. Effect of rifampicin treatment on the kinetics of mexiletine. *Eur J Clin Pharmacol*, 23, 261-266 (1982)

4597 Pentikainen PJ, Pentikainen LA, Huffman DM et al. The effect of spironolactone on sexual hormones in males. *Clin Res*, 21, 472 (1973)

4598 Pentikainen PJ, Voutilainen E, Aro A et al. Cholesterol lowering effect of metformin in combined hyperlipidemia: placebo controlled double blind trial. *Ann Med*, 22, 307-312 (1990)

4599 Penttila O, Neuvonen PJ, Aho K et al. Interaction between doxycycline and some antiepileptic drugs. *Br Med J*, 2, 470-472 (1974)

4600 Perault MC, Griesemann E, Bouquet S et al. A study of the interaction of viloxazine with theophylline. *Ther Drug Monit*, 11, 520-522 (1989)

4601 Perazella MA, Mahnesmith RL. Trimethoprim-sulfamethoxazole: hyperkalemia is an important complication regardless of dose. *Clin Nephrol*, 46, 187-192 (1996)

4602 Pereira JN, Holland GF, Hochstein F et al. Studies with 5-(3-pyridyl) tetrazole on long acting lipolysis inhibitor. *Adv Exp Med Biol*, 4, 227 (1968)

4603 Perel JM, Dayton PG, Snell M et al. Studies of interactions among drugs in man at the renal level: probenecid and sulfinpyrazone. *Clin Pharmacol Ther*, 10, 834-840 (1969)

4604 Peretz A, Moris M, Willems D et al. Is bone alkaline phosphatase an adequate marker of bone metabolism during acute corticosteroid treatment?. *Clin Chem*, 42, 102-103 (1996)

4605 Perez G, Siegel L, Schreiner GE. Selective hypoaldosteronism with hyperkalemia. *Ann Intern Med*, 76, 757 (1972)

4606 Perkins SL, Ooi DS. Inocor® (amrinone lactate) interferences with TDx digoxin measurement. *Clin Chem*, 33, 1944 (1987)

4607 Perlow MJ, Sassin JF, Boyar R et al. Release of human growth hormone, follicle stimulating hormone, luteinizing hormone. *Dis Nerv Syst*, 33, 804 (1972)

4608 Perrault DJ, Domovitch E. Aminoglutethimide and cholestasis. *Ann Intern Med*, 100, 160 (1984)

4609 Perret G, Hugues JN, Louchahi M et al. Effect of a short-term oral administration of cimetidine and ranitidine on the basal and thyrotropin-releasing hormone-stimulated serum concentrations of prolactin, thyrotropin and thyroid hormones in healthy volunteers.. *Pharmacology*, 32, 101-108 (1986)

4610 Perrild H, Hansen JM, Skovsted L et al. Different effects of propranolol, alprenolol, sotalol, atenolol, and metoprolol on serum T3, and serum rT3 in hyperthyroidism. *Clin Endocrinol*, 18, 139-142 (1983)

4611 Perrild H, Jessen-Jurgensen H, Pedersen F et al. Serum magnesium, calcium, phosphate and PTH following long-term β-blockade in ischaemic disease. *Eur J Clin Pharmacol*, 34, 299-301 (1988)

4612 Perrild H, Madsen SN, Hansen JEM. Irreversible myxoedema after lithium carbonate. *Br Med J*, 1, 1108-1109 (1978)

4613 Perrillo RP, Schiff ER, Davis GL et al. A randomized, controlled trial of interferon alfa-2b alone and after prednisone withdrawal for the treatment of chronic hepatitis B. *N Engl J Med*, 323, 295-301 (1990)

4614 Perry HM Jr, Sakamato A, Tan EM. Relationship of acetylating enzyme to hydralazine toxicity. *J Lab Clin Med*, 70, 1020 (1967)

4615 Perry PJ, Garvey MJ, Dunner DL et al. A report of trazodone-associated laboratory abnormalities. *Ther Drug Monit*, 12, 517-519 (1990)

4616 Perry TL, Hansen S, Hestrin M et al. Exogenous urinary amines of plant origin. *Clin Chim Acta*, 11, 24 (1965)

4617 Perry-Keene DA, Larkins RG, Heyma P et al. The effect of long-term diphenylhydantoin therapy on glucose tolerance and insulin secretion: a controlled trial. *Clin Endocrinol*, 12, 575-580 (1980)

4618 Persson B, Fex G. HDL-increasing effect of cyclofenil. *Acta Med Scand*, 208, 205-207 (1980)

4619 Persson B-E, Ronquist G. Allopurinol treatment results in elevated prostate-specific antigen levels in prostatic fluid and serum of patients with non-bacterial prostatitis. *Eur Urol*, 29, 111-114 (1996)

4620 Peruca E. Reduction of oral bioavailability of lignocaine by induction of first pass metabolism in epileptic patients. *Br J Clin Pharmacol*, 8, 21 (1979)

4621 Perucca E, Garratt A, Hebdige S et al. Water intoxication in epileptic patients receiving carbamazepine. *J Neurol Neurosurg Psychiat*, 41, 713-718 (1978)

4622 Perucca E, Grimaldi R, Frigo GM et al. Comparative effects of rifabutin and rifampicin on hepatic microsomal enzyme activity in normal subjects. *Eur J Clin Pharmacol*, 595-599 (1988)

4623 Perucca E, Hedges A, Makki KA et al. A comparative study of the relative enzyme inducing properties of anticonvulsant drugs in epileptic patients. *Br J Clin Pharmacol*, 18, 401-410 (1984)

4624 Pesavento TE, Jones PA, Julian BA, Curtis JJ. Amlodipine increases cyclosporine levels in hypertensive renal transplant patients: results of a prospective study. *J Am Soc Nephrol*, 7, 831-835 (1996)

4625 Pesce MA, Strande CS. A new micromethod for determination of protein in cerebrospinal fluid and urine. *Clin Chem*, 19, 1265 (1973)

4626 Peskind ER, Veith RC, Dorsa DM et al. Yohimbine increases cerebrospinal fluid and plasma norepinephrine but not arginine vasopressin in humans. *Neuroendocrinology*, 50, 286-291 (1989)

4627 Pessayre D, Larrey D, Funck-Brentano C et al. Drug interactions and hepatitis produced by some macrolide antibiotics. *J Antimicrob Chemother*, 16, Suppl A, 181-194 (1985)

4628 Peters CA, Walsh PC. The effect of nafarelin acetate, a luteinizing hormone-releasing hormone agonist on benign prostatic hyperplasia. *N Engl J Med*, 317, 599-604 (1987)

4629 Peters GR, Metzler CM. The effects of cefmatazole and latamoxef on platelet function in healthy human volunteers. *J Antimicrob Chemother*, 23, Suppl D, 119-123 (1989)

4630 Peters TK. Fluvastatin in severe hypercholesterolemia: analysis of a clinical trial database. *Am J Cardiol*, 76, 71A-75A (1995)

4631 Peters U. Pharmacokinetic review of digitalis glycosides. *Eur Heart J*, 3, Suppl D, 65-78 (1982)

4632 Petersen KC, Silberman H, Berne TV. Hyperkalaemia after cyclosporin therapy. *Lancet*, 1, 1470 (1984)

4633 Petersen KR, Vedel P, Skouby SO et al. Hormonal contraception in women with IDDM. *Diabetes Care*, 18, 800-806 (1995)

4634 Petersen P, Kastrup J, Bartram R et al. Digoxin-trimethoprim interaction. *Acta Med Scand*, 217, 423-427 (1985)

4635 Peterslund NA, Larsen ML, Mygind H. Acyclovir crystalluria. *Scand J Infect Dis*, 20, 225-228 (1988)

4636 Petitpierre B. Behavior of chlorpropamide in renal insufficiency and under the effect of associated drug therapy. *Int J Clin Pharmacol Ther Toxicol*, 6, 120 (1972)

4637 Petraglia A, Scarpitta M, Ansalone D et al. Negligible metabolic effects of long-term oral treatment with a new β_2-agonist: broxaterol. *Int J Clin Pharmacol Res*, 10, 299-304 (1990)

4638 Petraglia F, Bernasconi S, Iughetti L. Naloxone-induced luteinizing hormone secretion in normal, precocious and delayed puberty. *J Clin Endocrinol Metab*, 63, 1112-1116 (1986)

4639 Petrides PE, Beykirch MK, Trapp OM. Anagrelide, a novel platelet lowering option in essential thrombocytopenia: treatment experience in 48 patients in Germany. *Eur J Haematol*, 61, 71-76 (1998)

4640 Pettit WA Jr, Henrich J, Insogna KL et al. Influence of furosemide on parathyroid hormone levels in hyperparathyroidism. *N Engl J Med*, 318, 644-645 (1988)

4641 Petty F, Steinberg J, Kramer GL et al. Desipramine does not alter plasma GABA in patients with major depression. *J Affect Disord*, 29, 53-56 (1993)

4642 Pfizer Inc. Manufacturer's literature on Cardura® . New York, NY 10017 (1997)

4643 Pfizer Inc. Manufacturer's literature on Cefobid® . New York, NY 10017 (1995)

4644 Pfizer Inc. Manufacturer's literature on Diabinase® . New York, NY 10017 (1996)

4645 Pfizer Inc. Manufacturer's literature on Diflucan® . New York, NY 10017 (1996)

4646 Pfizer Inc. Manufacturer's Literature on Feldene® . New York, NY 10017 (1993)

4647 Pfizer Inc. Manufacturer's literature on Geocillin® . New York, NY 10017 (1991)

4648 Pfizer Inc. Manufacturer's literature on Glucotrol XL® . New York, NY 10017 (1995)

4649 Pfizer Inc. Manufacturer's literature on Minipress® . New York, NY 10017 (1990)

4650 Pfizer Inc. Manufacturer's literature on Navane® . New York, NY 10017 (1988)

4651 Pfizer Inc. Manufacturer's literature on Norvasc® . New York, NY 10017 (1996)

4652 Pfizer Inc. Manufacturer's literature on Procardia XL® . New York, NY 10017 (1996)

4653 Pfizer Inc. Manufacturer's literature on Sinequan® . New York, NY 10017 (1996)

4654 Pfizer Inc. Manufacturer's literature on Spectrobid® . New York, NY 10017 (1995)

4655 Pfizer Inc. Manufacturer's literature on Streptomycin. New York, NY 10017 (1995)

4656 Pfizer Inc. Manufacturer's literature on Terramycin® . New York, NY 10017 (1997)

4657 Pfizer Inc. Manufacturer's literature on Viagra® . New York, NY 10017 (1998)

4658 Pfizer Inc. Manufacturer's literature on Vibramycin® . New York, NY 10017 (1993)

4659 Pfizer Inc. Manufacturer's literature on Zithromax® . New York, NY 10017 (1996)

4660 Pfizer Inc. Manufacturer's literature on Zoloft® . New York, NY 10017 (1996)

4661 Pfizer Inc. Manufacturer's literature on Zyrtec® . New York, NY 10017 (1995)

4662 Pfizer U.S. Pharmaceuticals. Manufacturer's literature on Aricept® . New York, NY 10017 (1998)

4663 Pfizer US Pharmaceuticals. Manufacturer's literature on Trovan® . New York, NY 10017 (1998)

4664 Pharmacia & Upjohn Company. Manufacturer's literature on Adriamycin® . Kalamazoo, MI 49001 (1996)

4665 Pharmacia & Upjohn Company. Manufacturer's literature on Azulfidine® . Kalamazoo, MI 49001 (1994)

4666 Pharmacia & Upjohn Company. Manufacturer's literature on Campostar® . Kalamazoo, MI 49001 (1996)

4667 Pharmacia & Upjohn Company. Manufacturer's literature on Caverject® . Kalamazoo, MI 49001 (1995)

4668 Pharmacia & Upjohn Company. Manufacturer's literature on Cleocin® . Kalamazoo, MI 49001 (1996)

4669 Pharmacia & Upjohn Company. Manufacturer's literature on Colestid® . Kalamazoo, MI 49001 (1996)

4670 Pharmacia & Upjohn Company. Manufacturer's literature on Cytosar-U® . Kalamazoo, MI 49001 (1996)

4671 Pharmacia & Upjohn Company. Manufacturer's literature on Depo-Provera® . Kalamazoo, MI 49001 (1996)

4672 Pharmacia & Upjohn Company. Manufacturer's literature on Dipentum® . Kalamazoo, MI 49001 (1994)

4673 Pharmacia & Upjohn Company. Manufacturer's literature on Emcyt® . Kalamazoo, MI 49001 (1994)

4674 Pharmacia & Upjohn Company. Manufacturer's literature on Fragmin® . Kalamazoo, MI 49001 (1996)

4675 Pharmacia & Upjohn Company. Manufacturer's literature on Gentropin™. Kalamazoo, MI 49001 (1996)

4676 Pharmacia & Upjohn Company. Manufacturer's literature on Glynase® . Kalamazoo, MI 49001 (1996)

4677 Pharmacia & Upjohn Company. Manufacturer's literature on Halcion® . Kalamazoo, MI 49001 (1993)

4678 Pharmacia & Upjohn Company. Manufacturer's literature on Halotestin® . Kalamazoo, MI 49001 (1991)

4679 Pharmacia & Upjohn Company. Manufacturer's literature on Idamycin® . Kalamazoo, MI 49001 (1996)

4680 Pharmacia & Upjohn Company. Manufacturer's literature on Mirapex® . Kalamazoo, MI 49001 (1997)

4681 Pharmacia & Upjohn Company. Manufacturer's literature on Mycobutin® . Kalamazoo, MI 49001 (1996)

4682 Pharmacia & Upjohn Company. Manufacturer's literature on Ogen® . Kalamazoo, MI 49001 (1994)

4683 Pharmacia & Upjohn Company. Manufacturer's literature on Provera® . Kalamazoo, MI 49001 (1992)

4684 Pharmacia & Upjohn Company. Manufacturer's literature on Vantin® . Kalamazoo, MI 49001 (1995)

4685 Pharmacia & Upjohn Company. Manufacturer's literature on Xanax® . Kalamazoo, MI 49001 (1996)

4686 Pharmacia & Upjohn Company. Manufacturer's literature on Zanosar® . Kalamazoo, MI 49001 (1994)

4687 Pharmacia & Upjohn Company. Manufacturer's literature on Zinecard® . Kalamazoo, MI 49001 (1994)

4688 Phillips AP. The improvement of specificity in radioimmunoassays. *Clin Chim Acta*, 44, 333 (1973)

4689 Phillips I. Clinical uses and control of rifampicin and clindamycin. *J Clin Pathol*, 24, 410 (1971)

4690 Phillips PJ, Vedig AE, Jones PL et al. Metabolic and cardiovascular side effects of the β_2-adrenoceptor agonists salbutamol and rimiterol. *Br J Clin Pharmacol*, 9, 483-491 (1980)

4691 Philp JR. Untoward effects of antimicrobial drugs: prevention and control. *Postgrad Med*, 50, 193 (1971)

4692 Phornphutkul KS, Anuras S, Koff RS et al. Causes of increased plasma creatine kinase activity after surgery. *Clin Chem*, 20, 340 (1974)

4693 Picard EH. Side effects of metronidazole. *Mayo Clin Proc*, 58, 401 (1983)

4694 Pickar D, Wolkowitz OM, Doran AR et al. Clinical and biochemical effects of verapamil administration to schizophrenic patients. *Arch Gen Psychiat*, 44, 113-118 (1987)

4695 Pickert A, Riedlinger I, Stumvoll M. Interference of cefotiam with total bilirubin measured with the Ektachem analyzer. *Clin Chem*, 38, 599-600 (1992)

4696 Pieniaszek HJ Jr, Davidson AF, Benedek IH. Effect of moricizine on the pharmacokinetics of single-dose theophylline in healthy subjects. *Ther Drug Monit*, 15, 199-203 (1993)

4697 Pierce EH, Chesler DL. Possible association of granulomatous hepatitis with clofibrate therapy. *N Engl J Med*, 299, 314 (1978)

4698 Piergies AA, sainati S, Roth-Schechter B. Lack of cross-reactivity of Ambien (Zolpidem) with drugs in standard urine drug screens. *Arch Pathol Lab Med*, 121, 392-394 (1997)

4699 Piergies AA, SainatiS, Roth-Schechter B. Lack of cross-reactivity of Ambien (Zolpidem) with drugs in standard urine drug screens. *Arch Pathol Lab Med*, 121, 392-394 (1997)

4700 Pieroni RE, Fisher JG. Use of cholestyramine resin in digitoxin toxicity. *J Am Med Ass*, 245, 1939-1940 (1981)

4701 Pierre K, Whitt B, Wolf S. Performance characteristics of Beckman's Synchron CX magnesium reagent on the Synchron CX 4/5 systems. *Clin Chem*, 36, 1067 (1990)

4702 Pierson-Perry JF, Crouse SP, Sistek CG et al. An improved assay for serum lipase on the Du Pont aca discrete clinical analyzer through colipase activation. *Clin Chem*, 37, 910 (1991)

4703 Pietila K, Koivula T. Increase of serum angiotensin-converting enzyme activity after freezing. *Scand J Clin Lab Invest*, 44, 453-455 (1984)

4704 Pietro DA, Alexander S, Mantell G et al. Effects of simvastatin and probucol in hypercholesterolemia (Simvastatin multicenter study group II). *Am J Cardiol*, 63, 682-686 (1989)

4705 Pilewski RM, Scheib ET, Misage JR et al. Technique of controlled drug assay in hypertension. V. comparison of hydrochlorothiazide with a new quinethazone. *Clin Pharmacol Ther*, 12, 843 (1971)

4706 Pillans PI, Cowan P, Whitelaw D. Hyponatraemia and confusion in a patient taking ketoconazole. *Lancet*, 1, 821-822 (1985)

4707 Pillay VK, Gandhi VC, Sharma BK et al. Effect of hydration and furosemide given intravenously on proteinuria. *Arch Intern Med*, 130, 90 (1972)

4708 Pines A, Raafat M, Siddiqui GM. Rifampicin and ethambutol in the treatment of drug resistant and far advanced pulmonary tuberculosis. *J Ir Med Ass*, 63, 82 (1970)

4709 Pintor C, Cella SE, Corda R et al. Clonidine accelerates growth in children with impaired growth hormone secretion. *Lancet*, 1, 1482-1485 (1985)

4710 Pippenger CE, Meng X, Van Lente F et al. Valproate therapy depresses GSH-PX and SOD enzyme activity. A possible mechanism for VPA induced idiosyncratic drug toxicity. *Clin Chem*, 35, 1173 (1989)

4711 Piraud M, Maire I. Interference of amikacin in thin-layer chromatographic screening of urine for oligosaccharidosis. *Clin Chem*, 36, 809 (1990)

4712 Piroso E, Erslev AJ, Caro J. Inappropriate increase in erythropoietin titers during chemotherapy. *Am J Hematol*, 32, 248-254 (1989)

4713 Pirttikangas C-O, Salo M, Riutta A et al. Effects of propofol and Intralipid on immune response and prostaglandin E_2 production. *Anesthesia*, 50, 317-321 (1995)

4714 Pisciotta AV. Agranulocytosis induced by certain phenothiazine derivatives. *J Am Med Ass*, 208, 1862 (1969)

4715 Pitney WR, Oakley CM, Goodwin JF. Therapeutic defibrination with ancrodarvin. *Am Heart J*, 80, 144 (1970)

4716 Pitnick PD, Klein WJ Jr. Piroxicam-induced renal disease. *Arch Intern Med*, 144, 63-64 (1984)

4717 Pitt J. Association between paracetamol and pyroglutamic aciduria. *Clin Chem*, 36, 173-174 (1990)

4718 Piziak VK, Sellman JE, Othmer E. Lithium and hypothyroidism. *J Clin Psychiat*, 39, 709-711 (1978)

4719 Pizzuto J, Aviles A, Ramos E et al. Cytosine arabinoside induced liver damage: histopathologic demonstration. *Med Pediatr Oncol*, 11, 287-290 (1983)

4720 Planas AT, Kranwinkel RN, Soletsky HB et al. Chlorpropamide-induced pure RBC aplasia. *Arch Intern Med*, 140, 707-708 (1980)

4721 Platman SR, Fieve RR. Lithium carbonate and plasma cortisol response in the affective disorders. *Arch Gen Psychiat*, 18, 591 (1968)

4722 Plavinik FL, Rodrigues CIS, Zanella MT et al. Hypokalemia, glucose intolerance, and hyperinsulinemia during diuretic therapy. *Hypertension*, 19, Suppl II, 26-29 (1992)

4723 Plouin P-F, Bertheral J, Chatellier G et al. Short-term effects of octreotide on blood pressure and plasma catecholamines and neuropeptide Y levels in patients with phaeochromocytoma: a placebo-controlled trial. *Clin Endocrinol*, 42, 289-294 (1995)

4724 Podda M, Ghezzi C, Battezzati PM , et al. Effects of ursodeoxycholic acid and taurine on serum liver enzymes and bile acids in chronic hepatitis. *Gastroenterology*, 98, 1044-1050 (1990)

4725 Podolsky S, Pattavina CG, Amaral MA. Effect of marijuana on the glucose-tolerance test. *Ann NY Acad Sci*, 191, 54 (1972)

4726 Poffenbarger PL, Brinkley BR. Colchicine for familial mediterranean fever: possible adverse effects. *N Engl J Med*, 290, 56 (1974)

4727 Poilleux F, Lemercier M. Use of the new antibiotic gentamycin in surgery. *Presse Med*, 75, 1611 (1967)

4728 Poklis A, Hall KV, Still J. Ranitidine interference with the monoclonal EMIT d.a.u. amphetamine/methamphetamine immunoassay. *J Anal Toxicol*, 15, 101-103 (1991)

4729 Polisson RP, Dooley MA, Dawson DV et al. Interleukin-2 receptor levels in the sera of rheumatoid arthritis patients with methotrexate. *Arth Rheum*, 37, 50-56 (1994)

4730 Politi A, Poggio G, Margiotta A. Can amiodarone induce hyperglycaemia and hypertriglyceridaemia?. *Br Med J*, 288, 285 (1984)

4731 Polk RE, Healy DP, Sahai J et al. Effect of ferrous sulfate and multivitamins with zinc on absorption of ciprofloxacin in normal volunteers. *Antimicrob Agent Chemother*, 33, 1841-1844 (1989)

4732 Pollak PT, Sharma AD, Carruthers SG. Creatinine elevation in patients receiving amiodarone correlates with serum amiodarone concentration. *Br J Clin Pharmacol*, 36, 125-127 (1993)

4733 Pollak PT, Sharma AD, Carruthers SG. Elevation of serum total cholesterol and triglyceride levels during amiodarone therapy. *Am J Cardiol*, 62, 562-565 (1988)

4734 Pollak PT, Sharma AD, Carruthers SG. Relation of amiodarone hepatic and pulmonary toxicity to serum drug concentrations and superoxide dismutase activity. *Am J Cardiol*, 65, 1185-1191 (1990)

4735 Pollare T, Lithell H, Berne C. A comparison of the effects of hydrochlorothiazide and captopril on glucose and lipid metabolism in patients with hypertension. *N Engl J Med*, 321, 868-873 (1989)

4736 Pollare T, Lithell H, Morlin C et al. Metabolic effects of diltiazem and atenolol: results from a randomized, double-blind study with parallel groups. *J Hypertens*, 7, 551-559 (1989)

4737 Poller L, Thomson JM, Thomas W. Estrogen/progestogen oral contraception and blood clotting: a long-term follow-up. *Br Med J*, 4, 648 (1971)

4738 Pollock AA, Berger SA, Simberkoff MS et al. Hepatitis associated with high-dose oxacillin therapy. *Arch Intern Med*, 138, 915-917 (1978)

4739 Ponce SP, Jennings AE, Madias NE et al. Drug-induced hyperkalemia. *Medicine*, 64, 357-370 (1985)

4740 Pond SM, Birkett DJ, Wade DN et al. Mechanisms of inhibition of tolbutamide metabolism: phenylbutazone, oxyphenbutazone, sulfaphenazole. *Clin Pharmacol Ther*, 22, 573-579 (1977)

4741 Pond SM, Kretschzmar KM. Effect of phenytoin on meperidine clearance and normeperidine formation. *Clin Pharmacol Ther*, 30, 680-686 (1981)

4742 Ponikowska I. Blood patterns of free fatty acids in healthy subjects and diabetics under insulin, glucose and tolbutamide. *Pol Arch Med Wewn*, 45, 71 (1970)

4743 Pont A, Goldman ES, Sugar AM et al. Ketoconazole-induced increase in estradiol-testosterone ratio. Probable explanation for gynecomastia. *Arch Intern Med*, 145, 1429-1431 (1985)

4744 Pont A, Graybill JR, Craven PC et al. High-dose ketoconazole therapy and adrenal and testicular function in humans. *Arch Intern Med*, 144, 2150-2153 (1984)

4745 Ponte CD, Decker EL. Leukopenia and hepatotoxicity as a possible consequence of chlorpromazine administration. *Drug Intell Clin Pharm*, 76, 562-565 (1976)

4746 Pontiroli AE, Scarpignato C. Effect of bombesin on basal and stimulated secretion of some pituitary hormones in humans. *Horm Res*, 23, 129-135 (1986)

4747 Pool JL. Plasma lipid lowering effect of doxazosin, a new selective $alpha_1$-adrenergic inhibitor for systemic hypertension. *Am J Cardiol*, 59, 46G-50G (1987)

4748 Poole G, Stradling P, Worlledge S. Potentially serious side-effects of high-dose twice-weekly rifampicin. *Postgrad Med J*, 47, 742 (1971)

4749 Poon R, Hinberg I. One-step elimination of interference of free-sulfhydryl-containing drugs with Chemstrip ketone readings. *Clin Chem*, 36, 1527-1528 (1990)

4750 Poon R, Hinberg I, Peterson RG. False-positive urinary ketone tests in patients undergoing N-acetylcysteine treatment. *Clin Chem*, 36, 1111 (1990)

4751 Poon R, Hinberg I, Peterson RG. N-acetylcysteine causes false-positive ketone results with urinary dipsticks. *Clin Chem*, 36, 818-819 (1990)

4752 Poplawska A, Szelachowska M, Topolska J, et al. Effect of glycosaminoglycans on urinary albumin excretion in insulin-dependent diabetic patients with micro- or macroalbuminuria. *Diab Res Clin Pract*, 38, 109-114 (1997)

4753 Popovic V, Spremovic S. The effect of sodium valproate on luteinizing hormone secretion in women with polycystic ovary disease. *J Endocrinol Invest*, 18, 104-108 (1995)

4754 Popovic V, Spremovic-Radjenovic S, Eric-Marinkovic J, Grossman A. Effect of sodium valproate on luteinizing hormone secretion in pre- and postmenopausal women and its modulation by naloxone infusion. *J Clin Endocrinol Metab*, 81, 2520-2524 (1996)

4755 Portanova JP, Rubin RL, Joslin FG. Reactivity of antihistone antibodies induced by procainamide and hydralazine. *Clin Immunol Immunopathol*, 25, 67-79 (1982)

4756 Porter GA. Studies concerning the mechanism of sodium retention associated with carbenoxolone administration. *Gastroenterology*, 62, 795 (1972)

4757 Posner J, Sobel RJ, Glick S. Effect of amiodarone on thyroid hormone economy. *Isr J Med Sci*, 20, 113-117 (1984)

4758 Postlethwaite AE, Bartel AG, Kelley WN. Hyperuricemia due to ethambutol. *N Engl J Med*, 286, 761-762 (1972)

4759 Posvar EL, Sedman AJ. First-in-human studies of synthetic molecules. *Appl Clin Trials*, Oct, 70-74 (1996)

4760 Potter JL. Further observations on ninhydrin reacting compounds in urine. *J Pediatr*, 84, 250 (1974)

4761 Potter JL, Timmons GD, Kofron WG. Interferences by cephalosporin antibiotics in urinary tests for metabolic disorders. *Clin Chem*, 41, 1317-1318 (1995)

4762 Potter JL, Weinberg AG, West R. Ampicillinuria and ampicillin crystalluria. *Pediatrics*, 48, 636 (1971)

4763 Poupon RE, Balkau B, Eschwege E, et al. A multicenter controlled trial of ursodiol for the treament of primary biliary cirrhosis. *N Engl J Med*, 324, 1548-1554 (1991)

4764 Pouw EM, Prummel MF, Oosting H et al. Beclomethasone inhalation decreases serum osteocalcin concentrations. *Br Med J*, 302, 627-628 (1991)

4765 Powell JB, Djuh YY. A comparison of automated methods for glucose analysis in patients with uremia before and after dialysis. *Am J Clin Pathol*, 56, 8 (1971)

4766 Powell JB, Knesel EA, Hoffner PR et al. Effect of clofibrate (atromid S) on T4-by-column measurements. *Am J Clin Pathol*, 59, 764 (1973)

4767 Powell JR, Rogers JF, Wargin WA et al. Inhibition of theophylline clearance by cimetidine but not ranitidine. *Arch Intern Med*, 144, 484-486 (1984)

4768 Powell MG, Hedlin AM, Cerskus I et al. Effects of oral contraceptives on lipoprotein lipids: a prospective study. *Obstet Gynecol*, 63, 764-770 (1984)

4769 Powell-Jackson PR, Jamieson AP, Gray BJ et al. Effect of rifampicin administration on theophylline pharmacokinetics in humans. *Am Rev Resp Dis*, 131, 939-940 (1985)

4770 Powrie JK, Smith GD, Shojaee-Moradie F et al. Mode of action of chloroquine in patients with non-insulin-dependent diabetes mellitus. *Am J Physiol Endocrinol Metab*, 260, E897-E904 (1991)

4771 Prata MM, Nogueira AC, Pinto JR et al. Long-term effect of lovastatin on lipoprotein profile in patients with primary nephrotic syndrome. *Clin Nephrol*, 41, 277-283 (1994)

4772 Prati RC, Alfrey AC, Hull AR. Spironolactone-induced hypercalciuria. *J Lab Clin Med*, 80, 224 (1972)

4773 Pratt CB, Verzosa M. Comparison of crystalline and amorphous asparaginase in treatment of acute leukemia in children. *Clin Pharmacol Ther*, 13, 343 (1972)

4774 Preheim LC, Cuevas TA, Roccaforte JS et al. Ciprofloxacin and antacids. *Lancet*, 2, 48 (1986)

4775 Preiss R, Brovtsyn VK, Perevodchikova NI et al. Effect of methotrexate on the pharmacokinetics and renal excretion of cisplatin. *Eur J Clin Pharmacol*, 34, 139-144 (1988)

4776 Prelevic GM, Wurzburger MI, Balint-Peric L et al. Inhibitory effect of sandostatin on secretion of luteinising hormone and ovarian steroids in polycystic ovary syndrome. *Lancet*, 336, 900-903 (1990)

4777 Prescott LF. Analgesic nephropathy: a reassessment of the role of phenacetin and other analgesics. *Drugs*, 23, 75-149 (1982)

4778 Pressac M, Jardel C, Durand D et al. Interference of bromide in determination of serum chloride. *Clin Chem*, 33, 415-416 (1987)

4779 Pressac M, Morgant G, Farnier MA et al. Enzyme immunoassay of serum erythropoietin in healthy children: reference values. *Ann Clin Biochem*, 28, 345-350 (1991)

4780 Pretty HM, Gosselin G, Colpron G et al. Agranulocytosis: a report of 30 cases. *Can Med Ass J*, 93, 1058 (1965)

4781 Preuss HG, Razavi MH, Slemmer D et al. Colorimetry of p-aminohippurate in the presence of sulfamethoxazole. *Clin Chem*, 34, 422-423 (1988)

4782 Pri D, Blanchet FB, Essig M, et al. Dipyridamole decreases renal phosphate leak and augments serum phosphorus in patients with low renal phosphate threshold. *J Am Soc Nephrol*, 9, 1264-1269 (1998)

4783 Price G, Skogen W. Tolectin (Tolmetin) is a potent interfering substance for the Syva EMIT urine drug screen assays. *Clin Chem*, 36, 1118 (1990)

4784 Price HL. Circulating adrenaline and noradrenaline during diethyl-ether anaesthesia in man. *Clin Sci*, 16, 377 (1957)

4785 Price LH, Nelson JC, Jatlow PI. Effect of desipramine on clinical liver function tests. *Am J Psychiat*, 141, 798-800 (1984)

4786 Prihoda JS, Pappu AS, Smith FE et al. The influence of simvastatin on adrenal corticosteroid production and urinary mevalonate during adrenocorticotropin stimulation in patients with heterozygous familial hypercholesterolemia. *J Clin Endocrinol Metab*, 72, 567-574 (1991)

4787 Primack WA, Gartner LM, McGurk HE et al. Hypernatremia associated with cholestyramine therapy. *J Pediatr*, 90, 1024-1025 (1977)

4788 Prisant LM, Beall SP, Nichoalds GE et al. Biochemical, endocrine, and mineral effects of indapamide in black women. *J Clin Pharmacol*, 30, 121-126 (1990)

4789 Pristautz H, Stradner F. Effect of celiprolol and metoprolol on serum lipids in patients with different types of hyperlipoproteinemia. *Wien Med Wschr*, 136, 443-448 (1986)

4790 Pritchard G, Lyons D, Webster J, et al. Do trandolapril and indomethacin influence renal function and renal functional reserve in hypertensive patients?. *Br J Clin Pharmacol*, 44, 145-149 (1997)

4791 Privitera M, Greden GF, Gardner RW et al. Interference by carbamazepine with the dexamethasone suppression test. *Biol Psychiat*, 17, 611-620 (1982)

4792 Prober CG. Effect of rifampin on chloramphenicol levels. *N Engl J Med*, 312, 788-789 (1985)

4793 Probstfield JL, Lee G, Campion B et al. Colestipol, an investigational bile-acid sequestering agent for lowering serum cholesterol. *Clin Res*, 20, 412 (1972)

4794 Probstfield JL, Lin T-L, Peters J et al. Carotenoids and vitamin A: the effect of hypocholesterolemic agents on serum levels. *Metabolism*, 34, 88-91 (1985)

4795 Probstfield JL, Margitic SE, Byington RP, et al. Results of the primary outcome measure and clinical events from the asymptomatic carotid artery progression study. *Am J Cardiol*, 76, 47C-53C (1995)

4796 Procter & Gamble Pharmaceuticals, Inc.. Manufacturer's literature on Asacol® . Cincinnati, OH 45241 (1996)

4797 Procter & Gamble Pharmaceuticals, Inc.. Manufacturer's literature on Dantrium® . Cincinnati, OH 45241 (1996)

4798 Procter & Gamble Pharmaceuticals, Inc.. Manufacturer's literature on Didronel® . Cincinnati, OH 45241 (1996)

4799 Procter & Gamble Pharmaceuticals, Inc.. Manufacturer's literature on Macrobid® . Cincinnati, OH 45241 (1996)

4800 Procter & Gamble Pharmaceuticals, Inc.. Manufacturer's literature on Macrodantin® . Cincinnati, OH 45241 (1996)

4801 Proctor EA, Barton FL. Polyuric acute renal failure after methoxyflurane and tetracycline. *Br Med J*, 4, 661 (1971)

4802 Proctor SJ, Jackson G, Carey P et al. Improvement of platelet counts in steroid-unresponsive idiopathic immune thrombocytopenic purpura after short-course therapy with recombinant α-2b interferon. *Blood*, 74, 1894-1897 (1989)

4803 Propp RP, Stillman JS. Agranulocytosis and hydroxychloroquine. *N Engl J Med*, 277, 492 (1967)

4804 Prummel MF, Wiersinga WM, Lips P et al. The course of biochemical parameters of bone turnover during treatment with corticosteroids. *J Clin Endocrinol Metab*, 72, 382-386 (1991)

4805 Ptachcinski RJ, Carpenter BJ, Burckart GJ et al. Effect of erythromycin on cyclosporine levels. *N Engl J Med*, 313, 1416-1417 (1985)

4806 Puche E, Garcia de la Serrana H, Mota C et al. Serum aspirin-esterase activity in epileptic patients receiving treatment with phenobarbital, phenytoin, carbamazepine and valproic acid. *Int J Clin Pharmacol Res*, 9, 55-58 (1989)

4807 Puche E, Garcia Morillas M, Garcia de la Serrana H et al. Probable pseudocholinesterase induction by valproic acid, carbamazepine and phenytoin leading to increased serum aspirin-esterase activity in epileptics. *Int J Clin Pharmacol Res*, 9, 309-311 (1989)

4808 Pui C-H, Burghen GA, Bowman WP et al. Risk factors for hyperglycemia in children with leukemia receiving L-asparaginase and prednisone. *J Pediatr*, 99, 46-50 (1981)

4809 Puig JC, Miranda ME, Mateos F et al. Hydrochlorothiazide versus spironolactone: long-term metabolic modifications in patients with essential hypertension. *J Clin Pharmacol*, 31, 455-461 (1991)

4810 Puig JG, Mateos FA, Ramos TH et al. Albumin excretion rate and metabolic modifications in patients with essential hypertension: effects of two angiotensin converting enzyme inhibitors. *Am J Hypertens*, 7, 46-51 (1994)

4811 Pulkkinen MO, Maenpaa J. Decrease in serum testosterone concentration during treatment with tetracycline. *Acta Endocrinol*, 103, 269-272 (1983)

4812 Pulkkinen MO, Willman K. Reduction of maternal estrogen excretion by neomycin. *Am J Obstet Gynecol*, 115, 1153 (1973)

4813 Pulkkinen MO, Willman K. Serum inorganic phosphate during oral contraceptive therapy. *Ann Chir Gynaecol*, 57, 172 (1968)

4814 Pullar T, Capell HA. Sulfasalazine: a 'new' antirheumatic drug. *Br J Rheumatol*, 23, 26-34 (1984)

4815 Puopolo PR, Flood JG. Detection of interference by cyclobenzapine in liquid-chromatographic assays of tricyclic antidepressants. *Clin Chem*, 33, 819-820 (1987)

4816 Puri VN. Increased urinary antidiuretic hormone excretion by imipramine. *Exp Clin Endocrinol*, 88, 112-114 (1986)

4817 Puustinen T, Dahl M-L, Uotila P et al. Glucocorticoids do not decrease thromboxane and prostacyclin levels in human blood. *Prostaglandins Leukot Med*, 15, 409-410 (1984)

4818 Puybasset L, Lacolley P, Laurent S et al. Effects of clonidine on plasma catecholamines and neuropeptide Y in hypertensive patients at rest and during stress. *J Cardiovasc Pharmacol*, 21, 912-919 (1993)

4819 Quarmby V, DeVore K, Breglio S et al. Development of a thyroxine EIA for the Bio-Rad RADIAS system. *Clin Chem*, 39, 1247 (1993)

4820 Quart BD, Gallo DG, Sami MH et al. Drug interaction studies and encainide use in renal and hepatic impairment. *Am J Cardiol*, 58, 104C-113C (1986)

4821 Quastel JH. The action of drugs on enzyme systems. In:. *Enzymes in Health and Disease. DM Greenberg, HA Harper (eds)*, Springfield IL, CC Thomas (1960)

4822 Quattrocchi FP, Robinson JD, Curry RW Jr et al. The effects of ibuprofen on serum digoxin concentrations. *Drug Intell Clin Pharm*, 17, 286-288 (1983)

4823 Quehenberger P, Loner U, Kaplotis S, et al. Increased levels of activated factor VII and decreased plasma protein S activity and circulating thrombomodulin during use of oral contraceptives. *Thromb Haemostas*, 76, 729-734 (1996)

4824 Quintin L, Roudot F, Roux C et al. Effect of clonidine on the circulation and vasoactive hormones after aortic surgery. *Br J Anaes*, 66, 108-115 (1991)

4825 Quottrocchi FP, Robinson JD, Curry RW Jr et al. The effect of ibuprofen on serum digoxin concentrations. *Drug Intell Clin Pharm*, 17, 286-288 (1983)

4826 Raab WP. The diagnostic value of urinary enzyme determinations. *Clin Chem*, 18, 5 (1972)

4827 Raaska K, Neuvonen PJ. Serum concentrations of clozapine and N-desmethylclozapine are unaffected by the potent CYP3A4 inhibitor itraconazole. *Eur J Clin Pharmacol*, 54, 167-170 (1998)

4828 Race TF, Paes IC, Faloon WW. Intestinal malabsorption induced by oral colchicine: comparison with neomycin and cathartic agents. *Am J Med Sci*, 259, 32 (1970)

4829 Radcliff FJ, Wilton NM, Donnelly GL. Clopamide (brinaldix), a new diuretic agent: duration of action and dosage response. *Curr Ther Res*, 10, 103 (1968)

4830 Rado JP, Banos C, Gercsak G et al. Glucose-induced hyperkalemia developing in the upright position in captopril- treated hypertensives. *Res Comm Chem Pathol Pharmacol*, 38, 161-164 (1982)

4831 Ragheb M. The clinical significance of lithium-nonsteroidal anti-inflammatory drug interactions. *J Clin Psychopharmacol*, 10, 350-354 (1990)

4832 Ragheb M, Ban TA, Buchanan D et al. Interaction of indomethacin and ibuprofen with lithium in manic patients under a steady-state lithium level. *J Clin Psychiat*, 41, 397-398 (1980)

4833 Ragni G, De Laurentis L, Bestetti O et al. Gonadal function in male heroin and methadone addicts. *Int J Androl*, 11, 93-100 (1988)

4834 Rahim A, O'Neill PA, Shalet SM. Growth hormone status during long-term hexarelin therapy. *J Clin Endocrinol Metab*, 83, 1644-1649 (1998)

4835 Rahn KH, Mooy J, Bohm R. Reduction of bioavailability of verapamil by rifampin. *N Engl J Med*, 312, 920-921 (1985)

4836 Raine AEG, Carter R, Mann JI et al. Adverse effects of cyclosporin on plasma cholesterol in renal transplant recipients. *Nephrol Dial Transplant*, 3, 458-463 (1988)

4837 Rainsford KD, James C, Hunt RH et al. Effects of misoprostol on the pharmacokinetics of indomethacin in human volunteers. *Clin Pharmacol Ther*, 51, 415-421 (1992)

4838 Rambeck B, Salke-Treumann A, May T et al. Valproic acid-induced carbamazepine-10, 11-epoxide toxicity in children and adolescents. *Eur Neurol*, 30, 79-83 (1990)

4839 Rameis H. On the interaction between phenytoin and digoxin. *Eur J Clin Pharmacol*, 29, 49-53 (1985)

4840 Rameis H, Magometschnigg D, Ganzilnger U. The diltiazem-digoxin interaction. *Clin Pharmacol Ther*, 36, 183-189 (1984)

4841 Ramey JN, Burrow GN, Spaulding SW et al. The effect of aspirin and indomethacin on the TRH response in man. *J Clin Endocrinol Metab*, 43, 107-114 (1976)

4842 Ramey K, Lee K, Patel V et al. Application of p-aminohippuric acid method to the Cobas Mira. *Clin Chem*, 37, 982-983 (1991)

4843 Ramirez G, Narvarte J, Bittle PA et al. Cyclosporine-induced alterations in the hypothalamic hypophyseal gonadal axis in transplant patients. *Nephron*, 58, 27-32 (1991)

4844 Ramond M-J, Novel O, Degott C et al. Hepatite a l'allopurinol. *Gastroenterol Clin Biol*, 6, 138-142 (1982)

4845 Ramsay ID. Carbamazepine-induced jaundice. *Br Med J*, 4, 155 (1967)

4846 Ramsay RE, McManus DQ, Guterman A et al. Carbamazepine metabolites in humans: effect of concurrent anticonvulsant therapy. *Ther Drug Monit*, 12, 235-241 (1990)

4847 Ramsdell CM, Kelley WN. The clinical significance of hypouricemia. *Ann Intern Med*, 78, 239-242 (1973)

4848 Ramsey TA, Mendels J, Stokes JW et al. Lithium carbonate and kidney function: a failure in renal concentrating ability. *J Am Med Ass*, 219, 1446 (1972)

4849 Ranadive GN, Mistry JS, Damodaran K, et al. Rapid, convenient radioimmunoassay of estrone sulfate. *Clin Chem*, 44, 244-249 (1998)

4850 Randall AG, Kent GN, Fisher E et al. Pyridinium crosslink assays in monitoring treatment of Paget's disease of bone with pamidronate. *Clin Biochem Rev*, 14, 352 (1993)

4851 Randall RE Jr, Osheroff RJ, Bakerman S et al. Bismuth nephrotoxicity. *Ann Intern Med*, 77, 481 (1972)

4852 Ranek L, Andreasen PB. Disulfiram hepatotoxicity. *Br Med J*, 2, 94-96 (1977)

4853 Ranganath L, Lewis GA, Nobbs BT et al. Serum lipid changes after conjugated equine oestrogen and cyclical L-norgestrel therapy in postmenopausal women. *Proc ACB Natl Meet*, 113 (1993)

4854 Rannevik G, Doeberl A, Valentin L. Epostane in non-pregnant females: Effects on progesterone, 17α-hydroxyprogesterone, and 17β-estradiol of two dose levels given for one month. *Fertil Steril*, 50, 893-902 (1988)

4855 Rao ML, Clarenbach P, Vahlensieck M et al. Gabapentin augments whole blood serotonin in healthy young men. *J Neural Transm*, 73, 129-134 (1988)

4856 Rao SD, Vakil SK, Calne DB et al. Augmenting the action of levodopa. *Postgrad Med J*, 48, 653 (1972)

4857 Raoof S, Wollschlager C, Khan FA. Ciprofloxacin increases serum levels of theophylline. *Am J Med*, 82, Suppl 4A, 115-118 (1987)

4858 Rapaport MH, Schmidt ME, Risinger R, Manji H. The effects of prolonged lithium exposure on the immune system of normal control subjects: serial soluble interleukin-2 receptor and antithyroid antibody measurements. *Biol Psychiat*, 35, 761-766 (1994)

4859 Raphold HJ, De Bono D, Arnold AER et al. Plasma fibrinopeptide A levels in patients with acute myocardial infarction treated with alteplase: correlation with concomitant heparin, coronary artery patency, and recurrent ischemia. *Circulation*, 85, 928-934 (1992)

4860 Rapoport S, Wing M, Guest GM. Hypoprothrombinemia after salicylate administration in man and rabbits. *Proc Soc Exp Biol Med*, 53, 40 (1943)

4861 Rappelli A, Baldinelli A, Zingaretti O et al. The effects of antihypertensive therapy on renal function. *J Hypertens*, 9, Suppl 3, S37-S40 (1991)

4862 Rappelli A, Dessi-Fulgheri P, Bandiera F et al. Changes in plasma atrial natriuretic peptide levels after a single sublingual dose of nifedipine in hypertensive patients. *Med Sci Res*, 15, 1503-1504 (1987)

4863 Rappelli A, Dessi-Fulgheri P, Bandiera F et al. Increase of plasma atrial natriuretic peptide levels after sublingual administration of nifedipine in essentially hypertensive patients. *Int J Cardiol*, 25, Suppl 1, S25-S28 (1989)

4864 Raptis S, Dollinger HC, Schroder KE et al. Difference in insulin growth hormone and pancreatic enzyme secretion. *N Engl J Med*, 288, 1199 (1973)

4865 Rasanayagam LJ, Lim KL, Beng CG et al. Measurement of urine albumin using bromocresol green. *Clin Chim Acta*, 44, 53 (1973)

4866 Raskind MA, Courtney N, Murbery MM et al. Antipsychotic drugs and plasma vasopressin in normals and acute schizophrenic patients. *Biol Psychiat*, 22, 453-462 (1987)

4867 Rasmussen K, Moller J, Ostergaard K et al. Methylmalonic acid concentrations in serum of normal subjects: biological variability and effect of oral L-isoleucine loads before and after intramuscular administration of cobalamin. *Clin Chem*, 36, 1295-1299 (1990)

4868 Rasmussen L, Oster-Jorgensen E, Qvist N et al. The effects of omeprazole on interdigestive motility and early postprandial levels of gastrin and secretin. *Scand J Gastroenterol*, 27, 119-123 (1992)

4869 Rastogi S, Atkinson JLD, McCarthy JT. Allergic nephropathy associated with ciprofloxacin. *Mayo Clin Proc*, 65, 987-989 (1990)

4870 Rasuli P, McLeish WA, Hammond DI. Anticoagulant effects of contrast materials: in vitro study of iohexol, ioxaglate, and diatrizoate. *Am J Roentgenol*, 152, 309-311 (1989)

4871 Ratge D, Barthels U, Wisser H et al. Nebenwirkungen und verhalten von noradrenalin und adrenalin in plasma beim intravenosen thyroliberin - test bei personen mit normaler und gestorter schilddrusenfunktion. *J Clin Chem Clin Biochem*, 25, 393-400 (1987)

4872 Ratliff CR, Gilliland PF, Hall FF. Serum propylthiouracil: determination by a direct colorimetric procedure. *Clin Chem*, 18, 1373 (1972)

4873 Rattenbury JM, Bonham JR, Allen JC et al. Appearance of Vigabatrin (γ-vinyl-γ-aminobutyric acid, 4-amino-hex-5-enoic acid) in screening tests and analyses for amino acids. *Clin Chem*, 36, 159-160 (1990)

4874 Ratzmann M-L, Rjasanowski I, Bruns W et al. Effects of clofibrate therapy on glucose tolerance, insulin secretion and serum lipids in subjects with hyperlipoproteinemia and impaired glucose tolerance: a follow-up study over a 5 year period.. *Exp Clin Endocrinol*, 82, 216-221 (1983)

4875 Rausch JL, Stahl SM, Hauger RL. Cortisol and growth hormone responses to the 5-HTIA agonist gepirone in depressed patients. *Biol Psychiat*, 28, 73-78 (1990)

4876 Rauscher E, Neumann U, Schaich E et al. Optimized conditions for determining activity concentration of α-amylase in serum, with 1, 4-α-D-4-nitrophenylmaltoheptaoside as substrate. *Clin Chem*, 31, 14-19 (1985)

4877 Raveh D, Arnon R, Israeli A et al. Lovastatin-induced hepatitis. *Isr J Med Sci*, 28, 101-102 (1992)

4878 Ravic M, Johnston A, Turner P et al. A study of the interaction between lornoxicam and warfarin in healthy volunteers. *Hum Exp Toxicol*, 9, 413-414 (1990)

4879 Rawlins MD, Smith SE. Influence of allopurinol on drug metabolism in man. *Br J Pharmacol*, 48, 693-698 (1973)

4880 Ray DC, Aldridge LM, Spens HJ et al. Biological variation and the effect of fasting and halothane anesthesia on plasma glutathione S-transferase concentrations. *Clin Chem*, 41, 668-671 (1995)

4881 Rayfield EJ, Curnow RT, Beisel WR. Acute glucose intolerance during sandfly fever in man: metabolic interrelationships. *Am J Clin Nutr*, 26, 463 (1973)

4882 Realdi G, Diodati G, Bonetti P et al. Recombinant human interferon alfa-2a in community acquired non-A, non-B chronic active hepatitis. Preliminary results of a randomized, controlled trial. *J Hepatol*, 11, Suppl 1, S68-S71 (1990)

4883 Reams G, Lau A, Knaus V et al. The effect of nifedipine GTIS on renal function in hypertensive patients with renal insufficiency. *J Clin Pharmacol*, 31, 468-472 (1991)

4884 Reardon LC, MacPherson DS. Hyperkalemia in outpatients using angiotensin-converting enzyme inhibitors. *Arch Intern Med*, 158, 26-32 (1998)

4885 Rechenberg HK. Phenylbutazone. London, Arnold (1962)

4886 Recker RR, Hassing GS, Lau JR et al. The hyperphosphatemic effect of disodium ethane-1hydroxy-1, 1-diphosphonate (EHDP). *J Lab Clin Med*, 81, 258 (1973)

4887 Reddy MM, McKinley G, England A et al. Effects of azidothymidine (AZT) on p24 antigen levels in patients with AIDS-related complex. *J Clin Lab Anal*, 3, 199-201 (1989)

4888 Redmon JB, Pyzdrowski KL, Robertson RP. No effect of deferoxamine therapy on glucose homeostasis and insulin secretion in individuals with NIDDM and elevated serum ferritin. *Diabetes*, 42, 544-549 (1993)

4889 Redondo FL, Bergon E, Tinture T et al. Urinary enzyme activities in patients treated with gold and other antirheumatic drugs. *Clin Biochem*, 20, 343-347 (1987)

4890 Reed MJ, Gompels MMA, Beranek PA et al. A direct assay for oestrone sulphate and its use to investigate the effect of ampicillin on plasma levels of oestrone sulphate. *Horm Metab Res*, 20, 713-716 (1988)

4891 Reed RG, Guiney WB, Collier SA. Salicylate interference with measurement of acetaminophen. *Clin Chem*, 28, 2178-2179 (1982)

4892 Rees GW, Trull AK, Doyle S. Evaluation of an enzyme-immunometric assay for serum α-glutathione S-transferase. *Ann Clin Biochem*, 32, 575-583 (1995)

4893 Rees LH, Ratcliffe JG, Besser GM et al. Comparison of the redox assay for ACTH with previous assays. *Nature New Biol*, 241, 84 (1973)

4894 Reeves DS. Sulfamethoxazole/trimethoprim: the first two years. *J Clin Pathol*, 24, 430 (1971)

4895 Reeves RA, From GLA, Paul W et al. Nadolol, propranolol and thyroid hormones: evidence for a membrane stabilizing action of propranolol. *Clin Pharmacol Ther*, 37, 157-161 (1985)

4896 Reference Missing. Relates to effects of prednisone on bone measures

4897 Reginster J-YL. Ipriflavone: pharmacological properties and usefulness in postmenopausal osteoporosis. *Bone Miner*, 23, 223-232 (1993)

4898 Rehak NN, Cecco SA, Niemela JE, Elin RJ. Thiocyanate in smokers interferes with the Nova magnesium ion-selective electrode. *Clin Chem*, 43, 1595-1600 (1997)

4899 Rehnqvist N. Intrahepatic jaundice due to warfarin therapy. *Acta Med Scand*, 204, 335-336 (1978)

4900 Reichel H, Deibert B, Geberth S et al. Frusemide therapy and intact parathyroid hormone plasma concentrations in chronic renal insufficiency. *Nephrol Dial Transplant*, 7, 8-15 (1992)

4901 Reichelt KL, Teigland-Gjerstad B. Decreased urinary peptide excretion in schizophrenic patients after neuroleptic treatment. *Psychiat Res*, 58, 171-176 (1995)

4902 Reidenberg MM. Kidney function and drug action. *N Engl J Med*, 313, 816-818 (1985)

4903 Reidenberg MM, Drayer DE, Levy M et al. Polymorphic acetylation of procainamide in man. *Clin Pharmacol Ther*, 17, 722-730 (1975)

4904 Reihner E, Rudling M, Stahlberg D et al. Influence of pravastatin, a specific inhibitor of HMG-CoA reductase, on hepatic metabolism of cholesterol. *N Engl J Med*, 323, 224-228 (1990)

4905 Reilly CS, Bioallaz J, Koshakji RP et al. Enprostil, in contrast to cimetidine, does not inhibit propranolol metabolism. *Clin Pharmacol Ther*, 40, 37-41 (1986)

4906 Reimann IW, Frolich JC. Effects of diclofenac on lithium kinetics. *Clin Pharmacol Ther*, 30, 348-352 (1981)

4907 Reimold EW. The effect of furosemide on hypercalcemia due to dihydrotachysterol. *Metabolism*, 21, 593 (1972)

4908 Reiner M, Cheung HL. Xylose. *Stand Meth Clin Chem*, 5, 257 (1965)

4909 Reinhardt DJ III, Tausig T, Alvarez R. Serum cholesterol elevation with trifluorperazine (Stelazine®) therapy. *Del Med J*, 34, 318 (1962)

4910 Reinken L. The effect of hydantoin and succinimide on vitamin B_6 metabolism. *Clin Chim Acta*, 48, 435 (1973)

4911 Reinken L, Hohenauer L, Ziegler EE. Activity of red cell glutamic oxaloacetic transaminase in epileptic children under antiepileptic treatment. *Clin Chim Acta*, 36, 270 (1972)

4912 Reio L, Wetterberg L. False porphobilinogen reactions in the urine of mental patients. *J Am Med Ass*, 207, 148 (1969)

4913 Reisz G, Pingleton SK, Melethil S et al. The effect of erythromycin on theophylline pharmacokinetics in chronic bronchitis. *Am Rev Resp Dis*, 127, 581-584 (1983)

4914 Remp DG. Uric acid (uricase). *Stand Meth Clin Chem*, 6, 1 (1970)

4915 Renault PF, Schuster CR, Heinrich RI et al. Altered plasma cortisol response in patients on methadone maintenance. *Clin Pharmacol Ther*, 13, 269 (1972)

4916 Rendtorff C, Johannessen AC, Halck S et al. Verapail-digoxin interaction in chronic hemodialysis patients. *Scand J Urol Nephrol*, 24, 137-139 (1990)

4917 Rennie ID, Keen H. Evaluation of clinical methods for detecting proteinuria. *Lancet*, 2, 489 (1967)

4918 Reppas C, Adair CH, Barnett JL et al. High viscosity hydroxypropylmethylcellulose reduces postprandial blood glucose concentrations in NIDDM patients. *Diabetes Res Clin Pract*, 22, 61-69 (1993)

4919 Resta F, Capurso A. Modifications in serum lipids and apolipoproteins induced by gemfibrozil. *Curr Ther Res*, 50, 144-149 (1991)

4920 Resta F, Colacicco AM, Di Tommaso M et al. The effect of low-dose simvastatin on serum lipid, lipoprotein, and apolipoprotein concentrations in primary moderate hypercholesterolemia. *Curr Ther Res*, 54, 508-518 (1993)

4921 Retsas S, Phillips RH, Hanham IWF et al. Agranulocytosis in breast cancer patients treated with levamisole. *Lancet*, 2, 324 (1978)

4922 Reubi FC, Vorbuger C, Butikofer E. A comparison of the short-term and long-term haemodynamic effect of antihypertensive drug therapy. In:. *Catapres® in Hypertension. ME Conolly (ed)*, London, Butterworth (1970)

4923 Reverter JL, Pizarro E, Senti M et al. Relationship between lipoprotein profile and urinary excretion in type II diabetic patients with stable metabolic control. *Diabetes Care*, 17, 189-194 (1994)

4924 Revillion F, Hebbar M, Bonneterre J, Peyrat JP. Plasma c-erbB2 concentrations in relation to chemotherapy in breast cancer patients. *Eur J Cancer*, 32A, 231-234 (1996)

4925 Rex D, Lumeng L, Eble J et al. Intrahepatic cholestasis and sicca complex after thiabendazole. *Gastroenterology*, 85, 718-721 (1983)

4926 Reyes AJ, Leary WP, Van der Byl K et al. Effects of the angiotensin-I converting enzyme inhibitor perindopril on timed urinary excretion of water and solutes in healthy subjects. *Curr Ther Res*, 44, 619-629 (1988)

4927 Reyes E, Lisansky J. Effects of tricyclic antidepressants on platelet monoamine oxidase activity. *Clin Pharmacol Ther*, 35, 531-534 (1984)

4928 Reyes MP, Palutke M, Lerner AM. Granulocytopenia associated with carbenicillin. *Am J Med*, 54, 413 (1973)

4929 Reyniak JV, Wenof M, Aubert JM et al. Incidence of hyperprolactinemia during oral contraceptive therapy. *Obstet Gynecol*, 55, 8-11 (1980)

4930 Reynolds EH. Anticonvulsants, folic acid, and epilepsy. *Lancet*, 1, 1376 (1973)

4931 Reynolds EH, Gallagher BB, Mattson RH et al. Relationship between serum and cerebrospinal fluid folate. *Nature*, 2540, 155 (1972)

4932 Reynolds EH, Milner G, Mathews DM. Anticonvulsant therapy, megaloblastic haemopoiesis and folic acid metabolism. *Q J Med*, 35, 521 (1966)

4933 Reynolds TB, Pelle HC. Effects of a new diuretic amipramidine (MK 870) in patients with cirrhosis and ascites. *Clin Res*, 14, 184 (1966)

4934 Reynolds TB, Peters RL, Yamada S. Chronic active and lupoid hepatitis caused by a laxative, oxyphenisatin. *N Engl J Med*, 285, 813 (1971)

4935 Rhone-Poulenec Rorer Pharmaceuticals Inc. Manufacturer's literature on Calcimar® . Collegeville, PA 19426 (1992)

4936 Rhone-Poulenec Rorer Pharmaceuticals Inc. Manufacturer's literature on DDAVP™. Collegeville, PA 19426 (1996)

4937 Rhone-Poulenec Rorer Pharmaceuticals Inc. Manufacturer's literature on Dilacor® . Collegeville, PA 19426 (1996)

4938 Rhone-Poulenec Rorer Pharmaceuticals Inc. Manufacturer's literature on Lovenox® . Collegeville, PA 19426 (1996)

4939 Rhone-Poulenec Rorer Pharmaceuticals Inc. Manufacturer's literature on Oncaspar® . Collegeville, PA 19426 (1994)

4940 Rhone-Poulenec Rorer Pharmaceuticals Inc. Manufacturer's literature on Penetrex™. Collegeville, PA 19426 (1996)

4941 Rhone-Poulenec Rorer Pharmaceuticals Inc. Manufacturer's literature on Rilutek® . Collegeville, PA 19426 (1996)

4942 Rhone-Poulenec Rorer Pharmaceuticals Inc. Manufacturer's literature on Taxotere® . Collegeville, PA 19426 (1997)

4943 Rhone-Poulenec Rorer Pharmaceuticals Inc. Manufacturer's literature on Zagam® . Collegeville, PA 19426 (1996)

4944 Rhys J, Kadury S, Woodhead JS et al. Fenclofenac and thyroid function tests. *Ann Clin Biochem*, 20, 381-382 (1983)

4945 Ribstein J, Du Cailar G, Brouard R et al. Comparative renal and cardiac effects of tertatolol and enalapril in essential hypertension. *Cardiology*, 83, 57-63 (1993)

4946 Riccardi G, Genovese S, Saldalamacchia G et al. Effects of bezafibrate on insulin secretion and peripheral insulin sensitivity in hyperlipidemic patients with and without diabetes. *Atherosclerosis*, 75, 175-181 (1989)

4947 Ricci N, Toma PM, Pazzi P et al. Bromide can interfere with chloride estimation. *Lancet*, 2, 100 (1982)

4948 Riccio A, del Prato S, de Kreutzenberg SV et al. Glucose and lipid metabolism in non-insulin-dependent diabetes. Effect of metformin. *Diabete Metab*, 17, 180-184 (1991)

4949 Richards DA, Harris DM, Martin LE. Labetalol and urinary catecholamines. *Br Med J*, 1, 685 (1979)

4950 Richards KC, Borgstedt HH. Near fatal reaction to ingestion of the hallucinogenic drug MDA. *J Am Med Ass*, 218, 1826 (1971)

4951 Richens A, Houghton GW. Phenytoin intoxication caused by sulthiame. *Lancet*, 2, 1442 (1973)

4952 Richey JE, Smith RB. Renal failure after methoxyflurane anaesthesia. *Anesthesia*, 27, 9 (1972)

4953 Richterich R. Clinical Chemistry: Theory and Practice. Basel, Karger (1969)

4954 Riddoch D. Gastritis and L-dopa. *Br Med J*, 1, 53 (1972)

4955 Ridolfo AS, Rubin A, Crabtree RE et al. Effects of fenoprofen and aspirin on gastrointestinal microbleeding. *Clin Pharmacol Ther*, 14, 226 (1973)

4956 Riegel W, Horl WH, Heidland A. Long-term effects of nifedipine on carbohydrate and lipid metabolism in hypertensive hemodialyzed patients. *Klin Wochenschr*, 64, 1124-1130 (1986)

4957 Riegelman S, Rowland M, Epstein WL. Griseofulvin-phenobarbital interaction in man. *J Am Med Ass*, 213, 426-431 (1970)

4958 Rifai N, Fuller D, Law T et al. Measurement of felbamate by wide-bore capillary gas chromatography and flame ionization detection. *Clin Chem*, 40, 745-748 (1994)

4959 Rifai N, Iannotti E, DeAngelis K, Law T. Analytical and clinical performance of a homogeneous enzymatic LDL-cholesterol assay compared with the ultracentrifugation-dextran sulfate-Mg^{2+} method. *Clin Chem*, 44, 1242-1250 (1998)

4960 Rigas B, Rosenfeld LE, Barwick KW. Amiodarone hepatotoxicity: a clinicopathologic study of 5 patients. *Ann Intern Med*, 104, 348-351 (1986)

4961 Rigberg LA, Robinson MJ, Espiritu CR. Chlorpropamide - induced granulomas: a probable hypersensitivity reaction in liver and bone marrow. *J Am Med Ass*, 235, 409-410 (1976)

4962 Rigden SPA, Montini G, Morris M et al. Recombinant human erythropoietin therapy in children maintained by hemodialysis. *Pediatr Nephrol*, 4, 618-622 (1990)

4963 Riis B, Christiansen C. Actions of thiazide in vitamin D metabolism a controlled therapeutic trial in normal women early in the menopause. *Metabolism*, 34, 421-424 (1985)

4964 Rines R, Woodring C, Robert T et al. An improved fully automated total T3 assay for Opus immunoassay systems. *Clin Chem*, 41, S38-S39 (1995)

4965 Risby ED, Hsiao JK, Sunderland T et al. The effects of antidepressants on the cerebrospinal fluid homovanillic acid/5-hydroxyindoleacetic acid ratio. *Clin Pharmacol Ther*, 42, 547-554 (1987)

4966 Risenfors M, Hartford M, Dellborg M et al. Effect of early intravenous rt-PA on infarct size estimated from serum enzyme activity: results from the TEAHAT study. *J Intern Med*, 229, 11-18 (1991)

4967 Risler T, Burk M, Peters U et al. On the interaction between digoxin and disopyramide. *Clin Pharmacol Ther*, 34, 176-180 (1983)

4968 Ritter D, Cortese CM, Edwards LC, et al. Interference with testing for lysergic acid diethylamide. *Clin Chem*, 43, 635-637 (1997)

4969 Ritter MA, Gioe TJ, Sieber JM. Systemic effects of polymethylmethacrylate: increased serum levels of γ- glutamyltranspeptidase following arthroplasty. *Acta Orthop Scand*, 55, 411-413 (1984)

4970 Rittmaster RS. Finasteride. *N Engl J Med*, 330, 120-125 (1994)

4971 Rittmaster RS, Stoner E, Thompson DL et al. Effect of MK-906, a specific 5 α-reductase inhibitor, on serum androgens and androgen conjugates in normal men. *J Androl*, 10, 259-262 (1989)

4972 Rittmaster RS, Thompson DL. Effect of leuprolide and dexamethasone on hair growth and hormone levels in hirsute women: the relative importance of the ovary and the adrenal in the pathogenesis of hirsutism. *J Clin Endocrinol Metab*, 70, 1096-1102 (1990)

4973 Riva R, Contin M, Albani F et al. Epileptic children being treated with carbamazepine. *Clin Chem*, 31, 150-151 (1985)

4974 Rivera R, Almonte H, Arreola M et al. The effects of three different regimens of oral contraceptives and three different intrauterine devices on the levels of hemoglobin, serum iron and iron-binding capacity in anemic women. *Contraception*, 27, 311-327 (1983)

4975 Rivera-Calimlim L, Bianchine JR. Effect of L-dopa on plasma free fatty acids and plasma glucose. *Metabolism*, 21, 611 (1972)

4976 Roach NA, Kroll MH, Elin RJ. Interference by sulfonylurea drugs with the Jaffe method for creatinine. *Clin Chim Acta*, 151, 301-307 (1985)

4977 Robbins RC, Harbin JE Jr. The in vitro sensitivity of erythrocyte aggregation to quinine. *Clin Chem*, 17, 31 (1971)

4978 Roberts I, Smith IM. A high performance liquid chromatography method for the analysis of total and free indomethacin in serum. *Ann Clin Biochem*, 24, 167-171 (1987)

4979 Roberts Pharmaceutical Corporation. Manufacturer's literature on Eminase® . Eatontown, NJ 07724 (1997)

4980 Roberts Pharmaceutical Corporation. Manufacturer's literature on Ethmozine® . Eatontown, NJ 07724 (1997)

4981 Roberts Pharmaceutical Corporation. Manufacturer's literature on Noroxin® . Eatontown, NJ 07724 (1989)

4982 Roberts Pharmaceutical Corporation. Manufacturer's literature on Reglan® . Eatontown, NJ 07724 (1997)

4983 Roberts Pharmaceutical Corporation. Manufacturer's literature on Supprelin® . Eatontown, NJ 07724 (1997)

4984 Roberts Pharmaceutical Corporation. Manufacturer's literature on Tigan® . Eatontown, NJ 07724 (1997)

4985 Roberts Pharmaceutical Corporation. Manufacturer's literature on Viokase® . Eatontown, NJ 07724 (1997)

4986 Roberts PS, Regelson W, Kingbury B. Determination of fibrinogen in normal human plasma in the presence and absence of anticoagulants. *J Lab Clin Med*, 82, 822 (1973)

4987 Roberts RK, Desmond PV, Wilkinson GR et al. Disposition of chlordiazepoxide: sex differences and effects of oral contraceptives. *Clin Pharmacol Ther*, 25, 826-831 (1979)

4988 Roberts RK, Grice J, Wood L et al. Cimetidine impairs the elimination of theophylline and antipyrine. *Gastroenterology*, 81, 19-21 (1981)

4989 Roberts WC (ed). The hypertriglyceridemias: risk and management. *Am J Cardiol*, 68, 1A (1991)

4990 Roberts WL, Buckley TJ, Rainey PM et al. Solid-phase extraction combined with radioimmunoassay for measurement of zalcitabine (2',3'-dideoxycytidine) in plasma and serum. *Clin Chem*, 40, 211-215 (1994)

4991 Robertson DM, Mester J, Kellie AE. The measurement of estradiol and progesterone in plasma from normal, infertile and clomiphene treated women. *Acta Endocrinol*, 68, 523 (1971)

4992 Robertson JFR, Nicholson RI, Walker KJ et al. Zoladex in advanced breast cancer. *Horm Res*, 32, Suppl 1, 206-208 (1989)

4993 Robertson NRC. Apnea after THAM administration in the newborn. *Arch Dis Child*, 45, 206 (1970)

4994 Robertson WG, Scurr DS. Prevention of ascorbic acid interference in the measurement of oxalic acid in urine by ion-chromatography. *Clin Chim Acta*, 140, 97-99 (1984)

4995 Robins MM. Aplastic anemia secondary to anticonvulsants. *Am J Dis Child*, 104, 614 (1962)

4996 Robinson AR. Leukocytosis after tetracosactrin. *Br Med J*, 4, 178 (1972)

4997 Robinson DS et al. Interactions of benzodiazepines with warfarin in man. Milan, Italy, Abstracts, Symposium on benzodiazepines (1971)

4998 Robinson DS, Sylvester D. Interaction of commonly prescribed drugs and warfarin. *Ann Intern Med*, 72, 853 (1970)

4999 Robinson J, Birkinshaw G, Dutton J et al. Urinary free PYR and DPYR excretion in the diagnosis and treatment of metabolic bone disease and hypercalcaemia of malignancy. *Proc ACB Natl Meet*, 67-68 (1995)

5000 Robinson JA, Venezio FR, Constanzo-Nordin MR et al. Patients receiving quinolones and cyclosporine after heart transplantation. *J Heart Transplant*, 9, 30-31 (1990)

5001 Robinson RG. Indomethacin in rheumatic disease - a reassessment. *Med J Aust*, 1, 971 (1966)

5002 Robinson RG, Radcliff FJ. The effect of meclofenamic acid on plasma uric acid levels. *Med J Aust*, 1, 1079 (1972)

5003 Robson RA, Begg EJ, Atkinson HC et al. Comparative effects of ciprofloxacin and lomefloxacin on the oxidative metabolism of theophylline. *Br J Clin Pharmacol*, 29, 491-493 (1990)

5004 Robson S, Neuberger J, Alexander G et al. Cyclosporin A nephrotoxicity related to changes in haemoglobin concentration. *Br Med J*, 288, 1417-1418 (1984)

5005 Rocha R, Horstman L, Ahn YS et al. Danazol therapy for cyclic thrombocytopenia. *Am J Hematol*, 36, 140-143 (1991)

5006 Roche Diagnostic Systems. Manufacturer's literature on Abuscreen EIA test kit for cannabinoids. Nutley, NJ 07110 (1987)

5007 Roche Laboratories, Inc. Manufacturer's literature on Dalmane® . Nutley, NJ 07110 (1971)

5008 Roche Laboratories, Inc. Manufacturer's literature on Gantrisin® . Nutley, NJ 07110 (1993)

5009 Roche Laboratories, Inc. Manufacturer's literature on Posicor® . Nutley, NJ 07110 (1997)

5010 Roche Laboratories, Inc. Manufacturer's literature on Rocephin® . Nutley, NJ 07110 (1996)

5011 Roche Laboratories, Inc. Manufacturer's literature on Tasmar® . Nutley, NJ 07110 (1998)

5012 Roche Laboratories, Inc. Manufacturer's literature on Valium® . Nutley, NJ 07110 (1993)

5013 Roche Pharmaceuticals. Manufacturer's literature on Xeloda® . Nutley, NJ 07110 (1998)

5014 Roche Pharmaceuticals, Inc. Manufacturer's literature on Accutane® . Nutley, NJ 07110 (1997)

5015 Roche Pharmaceuticals, Inc. Manufacturer's literature on Ancobon® . Nutley, NJ 07110 (1994)

5016 Roche Pharmaceuticals, Inc. Manufacturer's literature on Cardene® . Nutley, NJ 07110 (1995)

5017 Roche Pharmaceuticals, Inc. Manufacturer's literature on Cellcept® . Nutley, NJ 07110 (1995)

5018 Roche Pharmaceuticals, Inc. Manufacturer's literature on Cytovene® . Nutley, NJ 07110 (1997)

5019 Roche Pharmaceuticals, Inc. Manufacturer's literature on Efudex® . Nutley, NJ 07110 (1995)

5020 Roche Pharmaceuticals, Inc. Manufacturer's literature on FUDR® . Nutley, NJ 07110 (1994)

5021 Roche Pharmaceuticals, Inc. Manufacturer's literature on Gantanol® . Nutley, NJ 07110 (1994)

5022 Roche Pharmaceuticals, Inc. Manufacturer's literature on Gantrisin® . Nutley, NJ 07110 (1993)

5023 Roche Pharmaceuticals, Inc. Manufacturer's literature on Hivid® . Nutley, NJ 07110 (1996)

5024 Roche Pharmaceuticals, Inc. Manufacturer's literature on Invirase® . Nutley, NJ 07110 (1997)

5025 Roche Pharmaceuticals, Inc. Manufacturer's literature on Klonopin® . Nutley, NJ 07110 (1991)

5026 Roche Pharmaceuticals, Inc. Manufacturer's literature on Lariam® . Nutley, NJ 07110 (1994)

5027 Roche Pharmaceuticals, Inc. Manufacturer's literature on Larodopa® . Nutley, NJ 07110 (1991)

5028 Roche Pharmaceuticals, Inc. Manufacturer's literature on Levo-Dromoran® . Nutley, NJ 07110 (1995)

5029 Roche Pharmaceuticals, Inc. Manufacturer's literature on Matulane® . Nutley, NJ 07110 (1996)

5030 Roche Pharmaceuticals, Inc. Manufacturer's literature on Naprosyn® . Nutley, NJ 07110 (1995)

5031 Roche Pharmaceuticals, Inc. Manufacturer's literature on Rocaltrol® . Nutley, NJ 07110 (1996)

5032 Roche Pharmaceuticals, Inc. Manufacturer's literature on Roferon® -A. Nutley, NJ 07110 (1996)

5033 Roche Pharmaceuticals, Inc. Manufacturer's literature on Tegison® . Nutley, NJ 07110 (1994)

5034 Roche Pharmaceuticals, Inc. Manufacturer's literature on Ticlid® . Nutley, NJ 07110 (1995)

5035 Roche Pharmaceuticals, Inc. Manufacturer's literature on Toradol® . Nutley, NJ 07110 (1995)

5036 Roche Pharmaceuticals, Inc. Manufacturer's literature on Trimpex® . Nutley, NJ 07110 (1993)

5037 Roche Pharmaceuticals, Inc. Manufacturer's literature on Versed® . Nutley, NJ 07110 (1997)

5038 Roche Pharmaceuticals, Inc. Manufacturer's literature on Vesanoid® . Nutley, NJ 07110 (1995)

5039 Roche Products, Inc. Manufacturer's literature on Dalmane® . Manati, Puerto Rico 00674 (1988)

5040 Roche Products, Inc. Manufacturer's literature on Librium® . Manati, Puerto Rico 00674 (1993)

5041 Rockhold FW, Goldberg MR, Thompson WL. Beneficial effects of pinacidil on blood lipids: comparisons with prazosin and placebo in patients with hypertension. *J Lab Clin Med*, 114, 646-654 (1989)

5042 Roddis MJ. Paracetamol interference with glucose analysis. *Lancet*, 2, 634-635 (1981)

5043 Roden DM, Woosley RL. Tocainide. *N Engl J Med*, 315, 41-45 (1986)

5044 Rodgers DP, Dover GJ, Noguchi CT et al. Hematologic responses of patients with sickle cell disease to treatment with hyroxyurea. *N Engl J Med*, 322, 1037-1045 (1990)

5045 Rodier M, Ribstein J, Parer-Richard C et al. Renal changes associated with cyclosporine in recent type I diabetes mellitus. *Hypertension*, 18, 334-340 (1991)

5046 Rodin E, Subramanian MG, Gilroy J. Investigation of sex hormones in male epileptic patients. *Epilepsia*, 25, 690-694 (1984)

5047 Rodland O, Aksnes L, Nilsen A et al. Serum levels of vitamin D metabolites in isotretinoin-treated acne patients. *Acta Derm Venereol*, 72, 217-219 (1992)

5048 RodMori L, Waldhuber S. Salicylate interference with the Roche Cobas Integra chloride electrode. *Clin Chem*, 43, 1249-1250 (1997)

5049 Rodriguez LAG, Williams R, Derby LE, et al. Acute liver injury associated with nonsteroidal anti-inflammatory drugs and the role of risk factors. *Arch Intern Med*, 154, 311-316 (1994)

5050 Rodriguez M, Solanki DL, Whang R. Refractory potassium repletion due to cisplatin-induced magnesium depletion. *Arch Intern Med*, 149, 2592-2594 (1989)

5051 Rodriguez V, Bodey GP, McCredie KB et al. Combination 6-mercaptopurine, adriamycin® in refractory adult acute leukemia. *Clin Pharmacol Ther*, 18, 462-466 (1988)

5052 Rodriguez-Segade S, Alonso de la Pena C, Tutor JC et al. Carnitine deficiency associated with anticonvulsant therapy. *Clin Chim Acta*, 181, 175-182 (1989)

5053 Rodvold KA, Paloucek FP, Jung D et al. Interaction of steady state procainamide with H_2 receptor antagonists cimetidine and ranitidine. *Ther Drug Monit*, 9, 378-383 (1987)

5054 Roe DA. Drug-induced deficiency of B vitamins. *NY State J Med*, 71, 2770 (1971)

5055 Roe DA. Drug interference with the assessment of nutritional status. *Clin Lab Med*, 1, 647-664 (1981)

5056 Roe DA. Interactions between drugs and nutrients. *Med Clin North Am*, 63, 985-1007 (1979)

5057 Roe JH, Ticktin HE, Schneider M. Determination and clinical significance of serum lipase. *Enzyme Biol Clin*, 7, 73 (1966)

5058 Roe TF, Podosin RL, Blaskovics ME. Drug interaction -- diazoxide and diphenylhydantoin. *J Pediatr*, 87, 480-484 (1975)

5059 Roenigk HH, Gottlob ME. Estrogen-induced porphyria cutanea tarda - report of 3 cases. *Arch Dermatol*, 102, 260 (1970)

5060 Rofe AM, Pholenz SM, Bais R et al. Inhibitory effect of ascorbic acid in oxalate assays involving oxalate decarboxylase. *Clin Chem*, 31, 1574-1575 (1985)

5061 Rogers LE, Lyon GM Jr, Porter FS. Spot test for vanillylmandelic acid and other guaiacols in urine of patients with neuroblastoma. *Am J Clin Pathol*, 58, 383 (1972)

5062 Rogers SM, Back DJ, Stevenson P et al. Paracetamol interaction with oral contraceptive steroids. *Br J Clin Pharmacol*, 23, 615p (1987)

5063 Rogge MC, Solomon WR, Sedman AJ et al. The theophylline-enoxacin interaction; II. Changes in the disposition of theophylline and its metabolites during intermittent administration of enoxacin. *Clin Pharmacol Ther*, 46, 420-428 (1989)

5064 Roine R, DiPadova C, Frezza M. Effects of omeprazole, cimetidine and ranitidine on blood ethanol concentrations. *Gastroenterology*, 98, A114 (1990)

5065 Roine R, Gentry T, Hernadez-Munoz R et al. Aspirin increases blood alcohol concentration in humans after ingestion of ethanol. *J Am Med Ass*, 264, 2406-2408 (1990)

5066 Rolan PE, Somogyi AA, Drew MJR et al. Phenytoin intoxication during treatment with parenteral miconazole. *Br Med J*, 287, 1760 (1983)

5067 Rolandi E, Franceschini R, Cataldi A, et al. Effects of ursodeoxycholic acid (UDCA) on serum liver damage indices in patients with chronic active hepatitis: A double-blind controlled study. *Eur J Clin Pharmacol*, 40, 473-476 (1991)

5068 Rolandi E, Franceschini R, Marabini A et al. Serum concentrations of PRL, GH, LH, FSH, TSH and cortisol after single administration to man of a new synthetic narcotic analgesic butorphanol. *Eur J Clin Pharmacol*, 26, 563-565 (1984)

5069 Rolland R, van der Heijden PFM. Nafarelin versus danazol in the treatment of endometriosis. *Am J Obstet Gynecol*, 162, 586-588 (1990)

5070 Rollins DE, Jennison TA, Jones G. Investigations of interference by nonsteroidal anti-inflammatory drugs in urine tests for abused drugs. *Clin Chem*, 36, 602-606 (1990)

5071 Rollman O, Loof L. Hepatic toxicity of ketoconazole. *Br J Dermatol*, 108, 376-378 (1983)

5072 Romanelli G, Giustina A, Cimino A et al. Short-term effect of captopril on microalbuminuria induced by exercise in normotensive diabetics. *Br Med J*, 298, 284-288 (1989)

5073 Romankiewicz JA, Ehrman M. Rifampin and warfarin: a drug interaction. *Ann Intern Med*, 82, 224-225 (1975)

5074 Romeo G, Salanitri G, Catonia G. Time-course of anti-Xa effects of calcium heparin and low-molecular-weight heparin given s.c.: insights for thrombosis prevention. *Drugs Exp Clin Res*, 14, 423-427 (1988)

5075 Romeo JH, Dombrowski R, Kwak YS, et al. Hyperprolactinaemia and verapamil: prevalence and potential association with hypogonadism in men. *Clin Endocrinol*, 45, 571-575 (1996)

5076 Romeo R, Boedeker M, Duncan C et al. Comparisons between serum and plasma: analytes measured on the Baxter Paramax. *Clin Chem*, 37, 967 (1991)

5077 Romer FK, Jacobsen F. The influence of prednisone on serum angiotensin-converting enzyme activity in patients with and without sarcoidosis. *Scand J Clin Lab Invest*, 42, 377-382 (1982)

5078 Romero RA, Granadillo VA, Salgado O et al. Desferroxamine B increases urinary lead excretion. *Clin Chem*, 39, 2021-2023 (1993)

5079 Ronchera CL, Hernandez T, Peris JE et al. Pharmacokinetic interaction between high-dose methotrexate and amoxycillin. *Ther Drug Monit*, 15, 375-379 (1993)

5080 Ronnov-Jessen V, Tjernlund A. Hepatotoxicity due to treatment with papaverine: report of four cases. *N Engl J Med*, 281, 1333 (1969)

5081 Roos JC, Boer P, Koomans HA et al. Haemodynamic and hormonal changes during acute and chronic diuretic treatment in essential hypertension. *Eur J Clin Pharmacol*, 19, 107-112 (1981)

5082 Rosalki SB, Tarlow D, Rau D. Plasma γ-Glutamyl transpeptidase elevation in patients receiving enzyme-inducing drugs. *Lancet*, 2, 376 (1971)

5083 Rosano TG, Ambrose RT, Wu AHB et al. Candidate reference method for determining creatinine in serum: method development and interlaboratory validation. *Clin Chem*, 36, 1951-1955 (1990)

5084 Rosano TG, Peaston RT, Bone HG, Borg S. Urinary free deoxypyridinoline by chemiluminascence immunoassay: analytical and clinical evaluation. *Clin Chem*, 44, 2126-2132 (1998)

5085 Rose DP. Aspects of tryptophan metabolism in health and disease: a review. *J Clin Pathol*, 25, 17 (1972)

5086 Rose DP, McGinty F. The influence of adrenocortical hormones and vitamins upon tryptophan metabolism in man. *Clin Sci*, 35, 1 (1968)

5087 Rose DP, Strong R, Adams PW et al. Experimental vitamin B_6 deficiency and the effect of oestrogen-containing oral contraceptives. *Clin Sci*, 42, 465 (1972)

5088 Rose DP, Strong R, Folkhard J et al. Erythrocyte aminotransferase activities in women using oral contraceptives and the effect of vitamin B_6. *Am J Clin Nutr*, 26, 48 (1973)

5089 Rose DP, Toseland PA. Urinary excretion of quinolinic acid and other tryptophan metabolites after deoxypyridoxine. *Metabolism*, 22, 165 (1973)

5090 Rose PG. Paracetamol overdose and liver damage. *Br Med J*, 1, 381 (1969)

5091 Rose S, Hindmarsh JG, Steiger MJ et al. Plasma HVA levels following debrisoquine administration do not reflect cerebral dopamine loss in early Parkinson's disease. *Clin Neuropharmacol*, 17, 260-269 (1994)

5092 Rose S, Price PG. Effect of intramuscular injections on serum creatine phosphokinase. *J Am Med Ass*, 225, 417 (1973)

5093 Rose SW, Smith LD, Penry JK. Blood level determinations of antiepileptic drugs: clinical value and methods. *US Dept HEW, NIH* (1971)

5094 Rosen HN, Moses AC, Garber J, et al. Randomized trial of pamidronate in patients with thyroid cancer: bone density is not reduced by suppressive doses of thyroxine, but is increased by cyclic intravenous pamidronate. *J Clin Endocrinol Metab*, 83, 2324-2330 (1998)

5095 Rosenberry KR, Defusco CJ, Mansmann HC Jr et al. Reduced theophylline half-life induced by carbamazepine therapy. *J Pediatr*, 102, 472-474 (1983)

5096 Rosenblatt JE, Edson RS. Metronidazole. *Mayo Clin Proc*, 58, 154-157 (1983)

5097 Rosenblatt JE, Edson RS. Metronidazole. *Mayo Clin Proc*, 62, 1013-1017 (1987)

5098 Rosenfeld H, Vogelsberg V, Kaufman RA. Development of a stable liquid reagent for ethanol assay on Cobas clinical analyzers. *Clin Chem*, 37, 996 (1991)

5099 Rosenfield RL, Perovic N, Ehrmann DA, Barnes RB. Acute hormonal responses to the gonadotropin releasing hormone agonist leuprolide: dose-response studies and comparison to nafarelin - a Clinical Research Center study. *J Clin Endocrinol Metab*, 81, 3408-3411 (1996)

5100 Rosenheck R, Cramer J, Xu W, et al. A comparison of clozapine and haloperidol in hospitalized patients with refractory schizophrenia. *N Engl J Med*, 337, 809-815 (1997)

5101 Rosenoer VM, Gill GM. Drug interactions in clinical medicine. *Med Clin North Am*, 56, 585 (1972)

5102 Rosenow EC III. The spectrum of drug-induced pulmonary disease. *Ann Intern Med*, 77, 977 (1972)

5103 Rosenquist C, Fledelius C, Christgau S, et al. Serum CrossLaps™ One Step ELISA. First application of monoclonal antibodies for measurement in serum of bone-related degradation products from C-terminal telopeptides of type I collagen. *Clin Chem*, 44, 2281-2289 (1998)

5104 Rosenquist C, Qvist P, Bjarnason N et al. Measurement of a more stable region of osteocalcin in serum by ELISA with two monoclonal antibodies. *Clin Chem*, 41, 1439-1445 (1995)

5105 Rosenthal AF, Tomson MR. Hydrochlorothiazide interference with urinary estriol determination. *Clin Chem*, 18, 471 (1972)

5106 Rosman M, Bertino JR. Azathioprine. *Ann Intern Med*, 79, 694 (1973)

5107 Rosner JM, Conte NF. Evaluation of testicular function by measurement of urinary excretion of testosterone. *J Clin Endocrinol Metab*, 26, 735 (1966)

5108 Ross AR, Sherlock S. A controlled trial of azathioprine in primary biliary cirrhosis. *Gut*, 12, 770 (1971)

5109 Ross DS. Subclinical hyperthyroidism: possible danger of overzealous thyroxine replacement therapy. *Mayo Clin Proc*, 63, 1223-1229 (1988)

5110 Ross RJ, Savadil AP III, Calil HM et al. Effects of desmethylimipramine on plasma norepinephrine, pulse and blood pressure. *Clin Pharmacol Ther*, 33, 429-437 (1983)

5111 Rossi EC, Levin NW. Inhibition of ADP-induced platelet aggregation by furosemide. *J Lab Clin Med*, 81, 140 (1973)

5112 Rossi EC, Levin NW. Inhibition of primary ADP-induced platelet aggregation in normal subjects. *J Clin Invest*, 52, 2457 (1973)

5113 Rossi GP, Semplicini A, Bongiovi S et al. Effect of acute captopril administration on digoxin pharmacokinetics in normal subjects. *Curr Ther Res*, 46, 439-444 (1989)

5114 Rossner S, Wallgren A. Serum lipoproteins and proteins after breast cancer surgery and effects of tamoxifen. *Atherosclerosis*, 52, 339-341 (1984)

5115 Rossner S, Weiner L. Atenolol and metoprolol: comparison of effects on blood pressure and serum lipoproteins and side effects. *Eur J Clin Pharmacol*, 24, 573-577 (1983)

5116 Rothenberg DM, Berns AS, Barkin R et al. Bromide intoxication secondary to pyridostigmine bromide therapy. *J Am Med Ass*, 263, 1121-1122 (1990)

5117 Rothstein E. Warfarin effect enhanced by disulfiram. *J Am Med Ass*, 206, 1574 (1968)

5118 Roti E, Gardini E, Minelli R et al. Methimazole and serum thyroid hormone concentrations in hyperthyroid patients: effects of single and multiple daily doses. *Ann Intern Med*, 111, 181-182 (1989)

5119 Roulston JE, Galloway PJ. In vitro inhibition of angiotensin-converting enzyme by prednisolone and methylprednisolone. *Clin Chem*, 32, 697-698 (1986)

5120 Rouse R, Motter K, McNally A et al. An Abuscreen Online immunoassay for the detection of amphetamine in urine on the Cobas Mira automated analyzer. *Clin Chem*, 37, 995 (1991)

5121 Rousell RH, Budinger MD, Pirofsky B et al. Prospective study on the hepatitis safety of intravenous immunoglobulin, pH 4.25. *Vox Sang*, 60, 65-68 (1991)

5122 Routh JI, Paul WD. Assessment of interference by aspirin with some assays commonly done in the clinical laboratory. *Clin Chem*, 22, 837-842 (1976)

5123 Rouveix B, Coulombel L, Aymard JP et al. Amodiaquine-induced immune granulocytosis. *Br J Haematol*, 71, 7-11 (1989)

5124 Rowe MJ, Dolder MA, Kirby BJ et al. Effect of a nicotinic acid analogue on raised plasma free fatty acids after acute myocardial infarction. *Lancet*, 2, 814 (1973)

5125 Rowinsky EK, Donehower RC. Paclitaxel (Taxol). *N Engl J Med*, 332, 1004-1014 (1995)

5126 Rowland M. Amphetamine blood and urine levels in man. *J Pharmacol Sci*, 58, 508 (1969)

5127 Rowland MJ, Bransome ED Jr, Hendry LB. Hypoglycemia caused by selegiline, an antiParkinsonian drug: can such side effects be predicted?. *J Clin Pharmacol*, 34, 80-85 (1994)

5128 Roxane Laboratories, Inc. Manufacturer's literature on Azathioprine. Columbus, OH 43216 (1995)

5129 Roxane Laboratories, Inc. Manufacturer's literature on DHT™. Columbus, OH 43216 (1994)

5130 Roxane Laboratories, Inc. Manufacturer's literature on lithium carbonate. Columbus, OH 43216 (1994)

5131 Roxane Laboratories, Inc. Manufacturer's literature on Marinol® . Columbus, OH 43216 (1994)

5132 Roxane Laboratories, Inc. Manufacturer's literature on Orlaam® . Columbus, OH 43216 (1995)

5133 Roxane Laboratories, Inc. Manufacturer's literature on Torecan® . Columbus, OH 43216 (1992)

5134 Roxane Laboratories, Inc. Manufacturer's literature on Viramune® . Columbus, OH 43216 (1997)

5135 Roy AK, Cuda MP, Levine RA. Induction of theophylline toxicity and inhibition of clearance rates by ranitidine. *Am J Med*, 85, 525-527 (1988)

5136 Roy MT, First MR, Myre SA et al. Effect of co-trimoxazole and sulfamethoxazole on serum creatinine in normal subjects. *Ther Drug Monit*, 4, 77-79 (1982)

5137 Roy-Byrne P, Fleishaker J, Arnett C et al. Effects of acute and chronic alprazolam treatment on cerebral blood flow, memory, sedation, and plasma catecholamines. *Neuropsychopharmacology*, 8, 161-169 (1993)

5138 Roy-Byrne P, Vittone BJ, Uhde TW. Alprazolam-related hepatotoxicity. *Lancet*, 2, 786-787 (1983)

5139 Rozman B. Clinical experience with leflunomide in rheumatoid arthritis. *J Rheumatol*, 25 Suppl 53, 27-32 (1998)

5140 Rubenfire M, Maciejko JJ, Blevins RD et al. The effect of pravastatin on plasma lipoprotein and apolipoprotein levels in primary hypercholesterolemia. *Arch Intern Med*, 151, 2234-2240 (1991)

5141 Rubin A, Rodda BE, Warrick P et al. Interactions of aspirin with nonsteroidal anti-inflammatory drugs in man. *Arth Rheum*, 16, 635-645 (1973)

5142 Rubinow DR, Post RM, Gold PW et al. Effects of carbamazepine on cerebrospinal fluid somatostatin. *Psychopharmacology*, 85, 210-213 (1985)

5143 Rubins HB, Robins SJ. Effect of reduction of plasma triglycerides with gemfibrozil on high-density-lipoprotein-cholesterol concentrations. *J Intern Med*, 231, 421-426 (1992)

5144 Rubinstein A, Lurie Y, Groskop I et al. Cholesterol-lowering effects of a 10 mg daily dose of lovastatin in patients with initial cholesterol levels 200 to 240 mg/dL (5.18 to 6.21 mmol/L). *Am J Cardiol*, 68, 1123-1126 (1991)

5145 Rubulis A, Rubert M, Faloon WW. Cholesterol lowering fecal bile acid, and sterol changes during neomycin and colchicine. *Am J Clin Nutr*, 23, 1251 (1970)

5146 Rudberg S, Aperia A, Freyschuss U et al. Enalapril reduces microalbuminuria in young normotensive Type I (insulin-dependent) diabetic patients irrespective of its hypotensive effect. *Diabetologia*, 33, 470-476 (1990)

5147 Ruedy J, Davies RO. A comparative clinical trial of guanoxan and guanethidine in essential hypertension. *Clin Pharmacol Ther*, 8, 38 (1967)

5148 Ruffalo RL, Thompson JF, Segal JL. Diazepam-cimetidine drug interaction: a clinically significant effect. *South Med J*, 74, 1075-1078 (1981)

5149 Ruiz Del Arbol L, Moreira V, Moreno A et al. Bridging hepatic necrosis associated with cimetidine. *Am J Gastroenterol*, 74, 267-269 (1980)

5150 Ruiz M-J, Pararas C, Bercher L et al. Simvastatin in the treatment of type II hyperlipoproteinemia in the elderly: a two-year experience. *Curr Ther Res*, 50, 731-739 (1991)

5151 Rumiantsev DO, Piotrovskii VK, Riabokon OS et al. The effect of oral verapamil therapy on antipyrine clearance. *Br J Clin Pharmacol*, 22, 606-609 (1986)

5152 Rumley AG, Paterson JR. Drug interference in the measurement of serum fructosamine. *Ann Clin Biochem*, 27, 384-385 (1990)

5153 Rumley AG, Paterson JR, Dominiczak MH. Drug interference in the serum fructosamine assay. *Proc ACB Natl Meet*, 37 (1989)

5154 Rumpf KW, Barth M, Blech M et al. Bezafibrat-induzierte myolyse und myoglobinurie bei patienten mit eingeschrankter nierenfunktion. *Klin Wschr*, 62, 346-348 (1984)

5155 Rundly AT, Sndell B. Leucine aminopeptidase isoenzyme changes after treatment with anticonvulsant drugs. *Clin Chim Acta*, 44, 377 (1973)

5156 Runkel R, Mroszczak E, Chaplin M et al. Naproxen-probenecid interaction. *Clin Pharmacol Ther*, 24, 706-713 (1978)

5157 Ruokonen A, Kaar K. Effects of desogestrel, levonorgestrel and lynestrenol on serum sex hormone binding globulin, cortisol binding globulin, ceruloplasmin and HDL-cholesterol. *Eur J Obstet Gynecol Reprod Biol*, 20, 13-18 (1985)

5158 Rush JA, Beran RG. Leucopenia as an adverse reaction to carbamazepine therapy. *Med J Aust*, 140, 426-428 (1984)

5159 Russel AS, Sturge RA, Smith MA. Serum transaminases during salicylate therapy. *Br Med J*, 2, 428 (1971)

5160 Russell DW. Low circulating levels of acid-labile hydrazones after oral administration of isonicotinic acid hydrazide. *Clin Chim Acta*, 41, 163 (1972)

5161 Rutgeerts P, Lofberg R, Malchow H et al. A comparison of budesonide with prednisolone for active Crohn's disease. *N Engl J Med*, 331, 842-845 (1994)

5162 Rutkowski DM, Burkle WS. Advances in thrombolytic therapy. *Drug Intell Clin Pharm*, 16, 115-121 (1982)

5163 Rutman JY. Effect of carbamazepine on blood elements. *Ann Neurol*, 3, 373 (1978)

5164 Ryan JF, Kagen LJ, Hyman AI. Myoglobinemia after a single dose of succinylcholine. *N Engl J Med*, 285, 824 (1971)

5165 Ryan JR, Gomez-Perez F, Jain A et al. Metabolic and efficacy studies of MK-270, a new oral hypoglycemic agent. *Clin Pharmacol Ther*, 13, 151 (1972)

5166 Ryan JR, Jain AK, McMahon FG et al. On the question of an interaction between sulindac and tolbutamide in the control of diabetes. *Clin Pharmacol Ther*, 21, 231-233 (1977)

5167 Ryan JR, Maha GE, McMahon FG et al. Effects of a new oral hypoglycemic agent on glucose and insulin after oral glucose loading. *Diabetes*, 20, 734 (1971)

5168 Ryan MF, Young J. Vigabatrin causes profound reduction in serum alanine aminotransferase concentrations in serum. *Proc ACB Natl Meet*, 166-167 (1995)

5169 Ryan MP. Magnesium and potassium-sparing diuretics. *Magnesium*, 5, 282-292 (1986)

5170 Rybak MJ, Albrecht LM, Boike SC et al. Nephrotoxicity of vancomycin, alone and with an aminoglycoside. *J Antimicrob Chemother*, 25, 679-687 (1990)

5171 Rylance HJ, Myhal DR. Taurine excretion and the influence of drugs. *Clin Chim Acta*, 35, 159 (1971)

5172 Rymer W, Greenlaw CW. Hypoprothrombinemia associated with cefamandole. *Drug Intell Clin Pharm*, 14, 780-783 (1980)

5173 Rysanek K, Konig J, Spankova H et al. Influence of hydrocortisone and an allergen on aggregation of thrombocytes with streptokinase. *Blood*, 39, 588 (1972)

5174 Saad MJA, Morais SL, Saad STO. Reduced cortisol secretion in patients with iron deficiency. *Ann Nutr Metab*, 35, 111-115 (1991)

5175 Saag KG, Emkey R, Schnitzer TJ, et al. Alendronate for the prevention and treatment of glucocorticoid induced osteoporosis. *N Engl J Med*, 339, 292-299 (1998)

5176 Saal AK, Werner JA, Greene HL et al. Effect of amiodarone on serum quinidine and procainamide levels. *Am J Cardiol*, 53, 1264-1267 (1984)

5177 Saba P, Galeone F, Giuntoli F et al. Clinical investigation of the hypolipidemic effect of gemfibrozil in hyperlipidemic patients. *Curr Ther Res*, 43, 113-120 (1988)

5178 Sabath LD, Gerstein DA, Finland M. Serum glutamic oxaloacetic transaminase, false elevations during administration of erythromycin. *N Engl J Med*, 279, 1137 (1968)

5179 Sachar EJ, Gruen PH, Karasu TB et al. Thioridazine stimulates prolactin secretion in man. *Arch Gen Psychiat*, 32, 885-886 (1975)

5180 Sachs C, Dobin E, Kindermans C et al. Foscarnet induced functional hypoparathyroidism in AIDS patients is connected with low ionized magnesium: a breakthrough of its electrometric determination. *Proc ACB Natl Meet*, 88 (1994)

5181 Sacks FM, McPherson R, Walsh BW. Effect of postmenopausal estrogen replacement on plasma Lp(a) lipoprotein concentrations. *Arch Intern Med*, 154, 1106-1110 (1994)

5182 Sadayasu T, Nakashima Y, Yashiro A et al. Heparin-releasable platelet factor 4 in patients with coronary artery disease. *Clin Cardiol*, 14, 725-729 (1991)

5183 Saffouri B, Cho JH, Felber N. Chlorpropamide-induced hemolytic anemia. *Postgrad Med J*, 57, 44-45 (1981)

5184 Safrin S, Crumpacker C, Chatis P et al. A controlled trial comparing foscarnet with vidarabine for acyclovir-resistant mucocutaneous herpes simplex in the acquired immunodeficiency syndrome. *N Engl J Med*, 325, 551-555 (1991)

5185 Sahai J, Gallicano K, Garber G et al. Evaluation of the in vivo effect of naproxen on zidovudine pharmacokinetics in patients infected with human immunodeficiency virus. *Clin Pharmacol Ther*, 52, 464-470 (1992)

5186 Sailer S, Sandhofer F, Bolzano K et al. Action of norepinephrine and propranolol on the turnover rate of free fatty acids and the esterification rate. *Adv Exp Med Biol*, 4, 135 (1968)

5187 Saint-Salvi B, Tremblay D, Surjus A et al. A study of the interaction of roxithromycin with theophylline and carbamazepine. *J Antimicrob Chemother*, 20, Suppl B, 121-129 (1987)

5188 Saito I, Kawabe H, Hasegawa C, et al. Effect of L-dopa in young patients with hypertension. *Angiology*, 42, 691-695 (1991)

5189 Sakata H, Kakehashi H, Fujita K et al. Effects of aztreonam on fecal flora and on vitamin K metabolism. *Antimicrob Agent Chemother*, 34, 1045-1047 (1990)

5190 Sakata K, Hoshino T, Yoshida T, et al. Effects of beraprost sodium, a new prostaglandin I_2 analog, on parameters of hemostasis, fibrinolysis and yocardial ischemia in patients with exertional angina. *Cardiovasc Drug Ther*, 9, 601-607 (1995)

5191 Sakata T, Kario K, Matsuo T et al. Suppression of plasma-activated factor VII levels by warfarin therapy. *Arterioscler Thromb*, 15, 241-246 (1995)

5192 Sakemi T, Fujimoto S, Fujimi S et al. Transient renal failure following intravenous methylprednisolone pulse therapy. *Curr Ther Res*, 52, 254-264 (1992)

5193 Saku K, Gartside PS, Hynd BA et al. Mechanism of action of gemfibrozil on lipoprotein metabolism. *J Clin Invest*, 75, 1702-1712 (1985)

5194 Saku K, Sasaki J, Arakawa K. Low-dose effect of simvastatin (MK-733) on serum lipids, lipoproteins, and apolipoproteins in patients with hypercholesterolemia. *Clin Ther*, 11, 247-257 (1989)

5195 Saku K, Ying H, Arakawa K et al. Effects of pinacidil on serum lipid, lipoprotein and apolipoprotein levels in patients with mild to moderate hypertension. *Clin Ther*, 12, 132-138 (1990)

5196 Saku K, Zhang B, Jimi S et al. High-density lipoprotein and apolipoprotein A-I deficiency induced by combination therapy with probucol and bezafibrate. *Eur J Clin Pharmacol*, 48, 209-215 (1995)

5197 Sakuma N, Hasimoto Y, Iwatsuki N. Effects of neostigmine and edrophonium on human erythrocyte acetylcholinesterase activity. *Br J Anaes*, 68, 316-317 (1992)

5198 Salata R, Klein I. Effects of lithium on the endocrine system: a review. *J Lab Clin Med*, 110, 130-136 (1987)

5199 Saleh AAS, Ginsburg KA, Duchon TA et al. Hormonal contraception and platelet function. *Thromb Res*, 78, 363-367 (1995)

5200 Salem P, Khalyl M, Jabboury K et al. Cis-diaminedichlorplatinum (III) 5-day continuous infusion: a new dose schedule with minimal toxicity. *Cancer*, 53, 837-840 (1984)

5201 Salem RB, Breland BD, Mishra SK et al. Effect of cimetidine on phenytoin serum levels. *Epilepsia*, 24, 284-288 (1983)

5202 Salem RR, McIndoe A, Matkin JA et al. The hematologic effects of latamoxef sodium when used as a prophylaxis during surgical treatment. *Surg Gynecol Obstet*, 164, 525-529 (1987)

5203 Salerno DM, Fifield J, Krejci J et al. Encainide-induced hyperglycemia. *Am J Med*, 84, 39-44 (1988)

5204 Sallen MK, Efrusy ME, Kniaz JL et al. Streptokinase-induced hepatic dysfunction. *Am J Gastroenterol*, 78, 523-524 (1983)

5205 Salmela PI, Juustila H, Pyhtinen J et al. Effective clinical response to long term octreotide treatment, with reduced serum concentrations of growth hormone, insulin-like growth factor-I, and the amino-terminal propeptide of type III procollagen in acromegaly. *J Clin Endocrinol Metab*, 70, 1193-1201 (1990)

5206 Salom IL, Silvis SE, Doscherholmen A. Effect of cimetidine on the absorption of vitamin B_{12}. *Scand J Gastroenterol*, 17, 129-131 (1982)

5207 Salvarani C, Boiardi L, Macchioni P et al. Serum soluble CD4 and CD8 levels in polymyalgia rheumatica. *J Rheumatol*, 21, 1865-1869 (1994)

5208 Salvetti A, Abdel-Haq B, Magagna A et al. Indomethacin reduces the antihypertensive action of enalapril. *Clin Exp Hypertens*, 9, 559-567 (1987)

5209 Salvini S, Stampfer MJ, Barbieri RL et al. Effects of age, smoking and vitamins on plasma DHEAS levels: a cross-sectional study in men. *J Clin Endocrinol Metab*, 74, 139-143 (1992)

5210 Salvioni A, Marenzi G, Lauri G et al. β-Thromboglobulin plasma levels in the first week after myocardial infarction: influence of thrombolytic therapy. *Am Heart J*, 128, 472-476 (1994)

5211 Samara EE, Granneman RG, Witt GF, Cavanaugh JH. Effect of valproate on the pharmacokinetics and pharmaxodynamics of lorazeoam. *J Clin Pharmacol*, 37, 442-450 (1997)

5212 Samigun, Mulyono, Santoso B. Lowering of theophylline clearance by isoniazid in slow and rapid acetylators. *Br J Clin Pharmacol*, 29, 570-573 (1990)

5213 Sampson SE, Costello JF, Sampson AP. The effects of inhaled leukotriene B_4 in normal and asthmatic subjects. *Am J Resp Crit Care Med*, 155, 1789-1792 (1997)

5214 Samsioe G. Coagulation and anticoagulation effects of contraceptive steroids. *Am J Obstet Gynecol*, 170, 1523-1527 (1994)

5215 Samuel P, Shalchi OB, Holtzman CM. Reduction of serum cholesterol concentrations by paromomycin in patients with arteriosclerosis. *Proc Soc Exp Biol Med*, 115, 718 (1964)

5216 Samuels MH, Luther M, Henry P et al. Effects of hydrocortisone on pulsatile glycoprotein secretion. *J Clin Endocrinol Metab*, 78, 211-215 (1994)

5217 San Jose ME, Sarandeses A, Alvarez D et al. Determination of iron by the Ferrochem II: interference by tuberculostatics. *Scand J Clin Lab Invest*, 53, 653-658 (1993)

5218 Sanchez RA, Traballi CA, Marco EJ et al. Long-term evaluation of cilazapril in severe hypertension. Assessment of left ventricular and renal function. *Am J Med*, 87, Suppl B, 56S-60S (1989)

5219 Sancho JM, Robles RG, Mancheno E et al. Interference by ranitidine with aldosterone secretion in vivo. *Eur J Clin Pharmacol*, 27, 495-497 (1984)

5220 Sandek CD, Boulter PR, Arky RA. The sodium retention of insulin therapy. *Clin Res*, 20, 883 (1972)

5221 Sander S, Bergan T, Fossberg E. Piperacillin in the treatment of urinary tract infections. *Chemotherapy*, 26, 141-144 (1980)

5222 Sander WE Jr, Johnson JE III, Taggart JG. Adverse reactions to cephalothin and cephapirin. *N Engl J Med*, 290, 424 (1974)

5223 Sanderink G-J, Artur Y, Schiele F et al. Alanine aminopeptidase in serum: biological variations and reference limits. *Clin Chem*, 34, 1422-1426 (1988)

5224 Sanders CV, Greenberg RN, Marier RL. Cefamandole and cefoxitin. *Ann Intern Med*, 103, 70-78 (1985)

5225 Sandhya P, Das UN. Vitamin C therapy for maturity onset diabetes mellitus: relevance to prostaglandin involvement. *IRCS Med Sci: Clin Biochem*, 9, 618 (1981)

5226 Sandler M, Johnson RD, Ruthven CRJ et al. Transamination is a major pathway of L-dopa metabolism following peripheral decarboxylase inhibition. *Nature*, 247, 364 (1974)

5227 Sandler M, Karoum F, Ruthven CR. Metabolism of dopa in Parkinsonism. *N Engl J Med*, 281, 1429 (1969)

5228 Sandler RM, Bevan PC, Roberts GE et al. Interaction between sodium valproate and platelets: a further study. *Br Med J*, 2, 1476 (1979)

5229 Sandoz Pharmaceuticals Corporation. Manufacturer's literature on Clozaril® . East Hanover, NJ 07936 (1996)

5230 Sandoz Pharmaceuticals Corporation. Manufacturer's literature on DynaCirc® . East Hanover, NJ 07936 (1996)

5231 Sandoz Pharmaceuticals Corporation. Manufacturer's literature on Lamisil® . East Hanover, NJ 07936 (1996)

5232 Sandoz Pharmaceuticals Corporation. Manufacturer's literature on Lescol® . East Hanover, NJ 07936 (1996)

5233 Sandoz Pharmaceuticals Corporation. Manufacturer's literature on Mellaril® . East Hanover, NJ 07936 (1995)

5234 Sandoz Pharmaceuticals Corporation. Manufacturer's literature on Mesantoin® . East Hanover, NJ 07936 (1996)

5235 Sandoz Pharmaceuticals Corporation. Manufacturer's literature on Miacalcin® . East Hanover, NJ 07936 (1997)

5236 Sandoz Pharmaceuticals Corporation. Manufacturer's literature on Neoral® . East Hanover, NJ 07936 (1995)

5237 Sandoz Pharmaceuticals Corporation. Manufacturer's literature on Pamelor® . East Hanover, NJ 07936 (1996)
5238 Sandoz Pharmaceuticals Corporation. Manufacturer's literature on Parlodel® . East Hanover, NJ 07936 (1996)
5239 Sandoz Pharmaceuticals Corporation. Manufacturer's literature on Restoril® . East Hanover, NJ 07936 (1996)
5240 Sandoz Pharmaceuticals Corporation. Manufacturer's literature on Sandimmune® . East Hanover, NJ 07936 (1996)
5241 Sandoz Pharmaceuticals Corporation. Manufacturer's literature on Sandostatin® . East Hanover, NJ 07936 (1995)
5242 Sandoz Pharmaceuticals Corporation. Manufacturer's literature on Sansert® . East Hanover, NJ 07936 (1995)
5243 Sandoz Pharmaceuticals Corporation. Manufacturer's literature on Tavist® . East Hanover, NJ 07936 (1994)
5244 Sandoz Pharmaceuticals Corporation. Manufacturer's literature on Visken® . East Hanover, NJ 07936 (1996)
5245 Sands CD, Robinson JD, Salem RB et al. Effect of thioridazine on phenytoin serum concentration: a retrospective study. *Drug Intell Clin Pharm*, 21, 267-272 (1987)
5246 Sangster B, Krajnc EJ, Loeber JG et al. Study of sodium bromide in human volunteers, with special emphasis on the endocrine system. *Hum Toxicol*, 1, 393-402 (1984)
5247 Sanmarti A, Lucas A, Granada ML et al. Effect of clonidine treatment on urinary growth hormone excretion and linear growth in children with short stature. *Horm Res*, 34, 193-196 (1990)
5248 Sanmarti A, Permanyer-Miralda G, Castellanos JM et al. Chronic administration of amiodarone and thyroid function: a follow-up study. *Am Heart J*, 108, 1262-1268 (1984)
5249 Sannour MB, Ibrahim WN, Shaker A. A three-year study of liver function during long-acting progestogen-estrogen administration. *Contraception*, 7, 403 (1973)
5250 Sano T, Hara T, Kawamura T et al. Effects of long-term enalapril treatment on persistent microalbuminuria in well-controlled hypertensive and normotensive NIDDM patients. *Diabetes Care*, 17, 420-424 (1994)
5251 Sanofi Winthrop Pharmaceuticals. Manufacturer's literature on Danocrine® . New York, NY 10016 (1997)
5252 Sanofi Winthrop Pharmaceuticals. Manufacturer's literature on Inocor® . New York, NY 10016 (1997)
5253 Sanofi Winthrop Pharmaceuticals. Manufacturer's literature on Kayexalate® . New York, NY 10016 (1997)
5254 Sanofi Winthrop Pharmaceuticals. Manufacturer's literature on Mebaral® . New York, NY 10016 (1997)
5255 Sanofi Winthrop Pharmaceuticals. Manufacturer's literature on NegGram® . New York, NY 10016 (1997)
5256 Sanofi Winthrop Pharmaceuticals. Manufacturer's literature on Plavix® . New York, NY 10016 (1997)
5257 Sanofi Winthrop Pharmaceuticals. Manufacturer's literature on Primacor® . New York, NY 10016 (1997)
5258 Sanofi Winthrop Pharmaceuticals. Manufacturer's literature on Skelid® . New York, NY 10016 (1996)
5259 Sanofi Winthrop Pharmaceuticals. Manufacturer's literature on Talwin® . New York, NY 10016 (1997)
5260 Sanofi Winthrop Pharmaceuticals. Manufacturer's literature on Trancopal® . New York, NY 10016 (1997)
5261 Sanofi Winthrop Pharmaceuticals. Manufacturer's literature on Winstrol® . New York, NY 10016 (1997)
5262 Sansom LN, Beran RC, Schapel GJ. Interaction between phenytoin and valproate. *Med J Aust*, 2, 212 (1980)
5263 Santen RJ, Demers LM, Lynch J et al. Specificity of low dose fadrozole hydrochloride (CGS 16949A) as an aromatase inhibitor. *J Clin Endocrinol Metab*, 73, 99-106 (1991)
5264 Santen RJ, Leonard JM, Sherins RJ et al. Short and long-term effects of clomiphene citrate on the pituitary-testicular axis. *J Clin Endocrinol Metab*, 33, 970 (1971)
5265 Santen RJ, Lipton A, Kendall J. Successful medical adrenalectomy with aminoglutethimide. *J Am Med Ass*, 230, 1661-1665 (1974)
5266 Santinga JT, Rosman HS, Rubenfire M et al. Efficacy and safety of pravastatin in the long-term treatment of elderly patients with hypercholesterolemia. *Am J Med*, 96, 509-515 (1994)
5267 Santoni J-Ph, Richard C, Pouyollon F et al. Tolerance and safety of perindopril. *Clin Exp Hypertens*, 11, Suppl 2, 605-617 (1989)
5268 Santostasi G, Fantin M, Maragno I et al. Effects of amiodarone on oral and intravenous digoxin kinetics in healthy subjects. *J Cardiovasc Pharmacol*, 9, 385-390 (1987)
5269 Sapira JD, Klaniecki T, Ratkin G. 'Non-pheochromocytoma'. *J Am Med Ass*, 212, 2243 (1970)
5270 Saragoca A, Tavares MH, Barros FB et al. Some clinical and laboratory findings in patients injected with thorium dioxide. *Am J Gastroenterol*, 57, 301 (1972)
5271 Sarai M, Matsunga H. ADH secretion in schizophrenic patients on antipsychotic drugs. *Biol Psychiat*, 26, 576-580 (1989)
5272 Sarma GR, Kailasam S, Nair NGK et al. Effect of prednisone and rifampin on isoniazid metabolism in slow and rapid inactivators of isoniazid. *Antimicrob Agent Chemother*, 18, 661-666 (1980)
5273 Sartori S, Nielsen I, Masotti M et al. Early and late hyperferremia during cisplatin chemotherapy. *J Chemother*, 3, 45-50 (1991)
5274 Saruta T. Studies on the effect of prazosin on blood pressure and serum lipids in japanese hypertensive patients. *Am J Med*, 76, Suppl 2A, 117-120 (1984)
5275 Saruta T, Suzuki H, Kawamura M et al. Serum creatine phosphokinase levels during treatment with β-adrenoreceptor blocking agents. *J Cardiovasc Pharmacol*, 7, 805-808 (1985)
5276 Sasaki H, Naka K, Kishi Y et al. Nicardipine may impair glucose metabolism in hypertensive diabetic patients. *Diabet Res Clin Pract*, 26, 67-75 (1994)
5277 Sasaki J, Arakawa K. Effect of bunitrolol administration on serum lipids, lipoproteins, and apolipoproteins in patients with essential hypertension. *Curr Ther Res*, 40, 903-907 (1986)
5278 Sasaki J, Arakawa K. Effect of captopril on serum lipids, lipoproteins and apolipoproteins in patients with mild essential hypertension. *Curr Ther Res*, 40, 898-902 (1986)
5279 Sasaki J, Ogihara T, Yokoyama M et al. Comparative effects of monatpil, a novel calcium antagonist with α_1-adrenergic-blocking activity, and nitrendipine on lipoprotein and carbohydrate metabolism in patients with hypertension. *Am J Hypertens*, 7, 161S-166S (1994)
5280 Sasaki J, Saku K, Ideishi M et al. Effects of pindolol on serum lipids, apolipoproteins, and lipoproteins in patients with mild to moderate essential hypertension. *Clin Ther*, 11, 219-224 (1989)
5281 Sasaki M, Tonoda S, Aoki Y et al. Pancreatitis due to valproic acid. *Lancet*, 1, 1196 (1980)
5282 Sasaki N, Matsuoka N, Saito Y et al. The effect of nifedipine on serum lipoproteins in hyperlipoproteinemic subjects. *Curr Ther Res*, 43, 317-326 (1988)
5283 Sasaki N, Saito Y, Shinomiya M et al. Effects of pindolol on serum lipoproteins and postheparin lipolytic activities in hypertensive patients. *Clin Ther*, 12, 157-164 (1990)
5284 Sassard J, Geoffroy J, Ferry N et al. Compared effects of isoxicam and indomethacin on the urinary excretion of prostaglandins in degenerative articular disease. *Prostaglandins Leukot Essent Fatty Acids*, 38, 107-111 (1989)

5285 Sassolas G, Khalfallah Y, Chayvialle JA et al. Effects of the somatostatin analog BIM 23014 on the secretion of growth hormone, thyrotropin, and digestive peptides in normal men. *J Clin Endocrinol Metab*, 68, 239-246 (1989)

5286 Sassolas G, Serusclat P, Claustrat B et al. Plasma α-subunit levels during the treatment of pituitary adenomas with the somatostatin analog (SMS 201-995). *Horm Res*, 29, 124-128 (1988)

5287 Sathananthan S, Gershan S. Renal damage due to imipramine. *Lancet*, 1, 833 (1973)

5288 Satoh K, Masuda T, Ikeda Y et al. Hemodynamic changes by recombinant erythropoietin therapy in hemodialyzed patients. *Hypertension*, 15, 262-266 (1990)

5289 Sattler FR, Ko R, Antoniskis D et al. Acetaminophen does not impair clearance of zidovudine. *Ann Intern Med*, 114, 937-940 (1991)

5290 Sattler FR, Waskin H. Pentamidine and fatal hypoglycemia. *Ann Intern Med*, 197, 789-790 (1987)

5291 Sattler FR, Weitekamp MR, Ballard JO. Potential for bleeding with the new β-lactam antibiotics. *Ann Intern Med*, 105, 924-931 (1986)

5292 Saurat J-H, Gumowski SD, Rizzoli R. Topical calcipotriol and hypercalcemia. *Lancet*, 337, 1287 (1991)

5293 Sauter ER, Bakris GL. The effects of enapril on urinary protein excretion in patients with idiopathic membranous nephropathy. *J Clin Pharmacol*, 30, 155-158 (1990)

5294 Sauty A, Pecherstorfer M, Zimmer-Roth I, et al. Interleukin-6 and tumor necrosis factorα levels after bisphosphonates treatment in vitro and in patients with malignancy. *Bone*, 18, 133-139 (1996)

5295 Savaraj N, Troner MB. Aminoglutethimide in the management of metastatic breast cancer. *Med Pediatr Oncol*, 8, 251-263 (1980)

5296 Savege TM, Foley EI, Coultas RJ et al. Ct 1341: some effects in man. *Anesthesia*, 26, 402 (1971)

5297 Saven A, Beutler E. Iron overload after prolonged intramuscular iron therapy. *N Engl J Med*, 321, 331-332 (1989)

5298 Savon JJ, Allen ML, DiMarino AJ Jr et al. Gastrointestinal blood loss with low dose (325 mg) plain and enteric-coated aspirin administration. *Am J Gastroenterol*, 90, 581-585 (1995)

5299 Savory DJ. Interference by sotalol with the Pisano method for urinary metanephrines. *Ann Clin Biochem*, 21, 446 (1984)

5300 Sawers JS, Kellett HA, Brown NS et al. Prolactin response to metoclopramide in hyperthyroidism. *J Clin Endocrinol Metab*, 55, 175-177 (1982)

5301 Sawin CT. Measurement of plasma cortisol in the diagnosis of Cushing's syndrome. *Ann Intern Med*, 68, 624 (1968)

5302 Saxenhofer H, Weidmann P, Riesen WF et al. Therapeutic efficacy of the HMG-CoA-reductase inhibitor pravastatin in hyperlipoproteinemia type II. *Eur J Clin Pharmacol*, 39, 101-105 (1990)

5303 Saxton C, Majid PA, Clough G et al. Effect of ouabain on insulin secretion in man. *Clin Sci*, 42, 57 (1972)

5304 Scalley RD, Roark RD. Oxacillin-induced agranulocytosis. *Drug Intell Clin Pharm*, 11, 420-423 (1977)

5305 Scanlon MF, Rodriguez-Arnao MD, Pourmand M et al. Catecholaminergic interactions in the regulation of thyrotropin (TSH) secretion in man. *J Endocrinol Invest*, 3, 125-129 (1980)

5306 Scanlon MJ, Whorwood CB, Franks S et al. Serum androstanediol glucuronide concentrations in normal and hirsute women and in patients with thyroid dysfunction. *Clin Endocrinol*, 29, 529-538 (1988)

5307 Schade RWB, Demacker PNM, Laar AV'T. Reduction of serum alkaline phosphatase by clofibrate. *Lancet*, 1, 862-863 (1975)

5308 Schadel JM, Rehfeld N. Der einfluss hormonaler kontrazeptiva auf die enzyme aktivitat verschiedenerin blutserum. *Z Med Labor Diagn*, 26, 77-85 (1985)

5309 Schafer-Korting M, Kirch W, Axthelm T et al. Atenolol interaction with aspirin, allopurinol and ampicillin. *Clin Pharmacol Ther*, 33, 283-288 (1983)

5310 Schaffner F. Iatrogenic jaundice. *J Am Med Ass*, 174, 1690 (1960)

5311 Schaffner F, Popper H, Chesrow E. Cholestasis produced by administration of norethandrolone. *Am J Med*, 26, 249 (1959)

5312 Schalhorn A, Wilmanns W, Koczorek CE. The influence of high dose methotrexate therapy on serum iron. *Klin Wschr*, 64, 475-480 (1986)

5313 Schambelan M, Biglieri EG. Deoxycorticosterone production and regulation in man. *J Clin Endocrinol Metab*, 34, 695 (1972)

5314 Schapira DV, Kumar NB, Lyman GH. Serum cholesterol reduction with tamoxifen. *Breast Cancer Res Treat*, 17, 3-7 (1990)

5315 Schatz DL, Palter HC, Russell CS. Effects of oral contraceptives and pregnancy on thyroid function. *Can Med Ass J*, 99, 882 (1968)

5316 Schauer UJW, Schauer I. β-blockers, lecithin:cholesterol acyl transferase activity, and lipoprotein concentrations. *Clin Investig*, 71, 663 (1993)

5317 Schectman G, Kaul S, Mueller RA et al. The effect of interferon on the metabolism of LDLs. *Arterioscler Thromb*, 12, 1053-1062 (1992)

5318 Scheel PJ Jr, Whelton A, Rossiter K et al. Cholestyramine-induced hyperchloremic metabolic acidosis. *J Clin Pharmacol*, 32, 536-538 (1992)

5319 Scheidegger K, O'Connell M, Robbins DC et al. Effects of chronic β-receptor stimulation on sympathetic nervous system avtivity, energy expenditure and thyroid hormones. *J Clin Endocrinol Metab*, 58, 895-903 (1984)

5320 Schein Pharmaceuticals, Inc. Manufacturer's literature on INFeD® . Florham Park, NJ 07932 (1995)

5321 Scheinin M, Erkka KG, Syvalahti EKG, et al. Effects of apomorphine on blood levels of homovanillic acid, growth hormone and prolactin in medicated schizophrenics and healthy control subjects. *Prog Neuropsychopharmacol Biol Psychiat*, 9, 441-449 (1985)

5322 Scheinin M, Koulu M, Laurikainen E, et al. Hypokalemia and other non-bronchial effects of inhaled fenoterol and salbutamol: A placebo-controlled dose-response study in healthy volunteers. *Br J Clin Pharmacol*, 24, 645-653 (1987)

5323 Schenken JR, Grass L. Deferoxamine and autoassay of serum iron. *Clin Toxicol*, 4, 641 (1971)

5324 Schenker JG, Ben-Yoseph Y, Shapira E. Erythrocyte carbonic anhydrase B levels during pregnancy and use of oral contraceptives. *Obstet Gynecol*, 39, 237 (1972)

5325 Schentag JJ, Cerra FB, Plaut ME. Clinical and pharmacokinetic characteristics of aminoglycoside nephrotoxicity in 201 critically ill patients. *Antimicrob Agent Chemother*, 21, 721-726 (1982)

5326 Schering Corporation. Manufacturer's literature on Cedax® . Kenilworth, NJ 07033 (1995)

5327 Schering Corporation. Manufacturer's literature on Claritin® . Kenilworth, NJ 07033 (1997)

5328 Schering Corporation. Manufacturer's literature on Eulexin® . Kenilworth, NJ 07033 (1996)

5329 Schering Corporation. Manufacturer's literature on Fareston® . Kenilworth, NJ 07033 (1997)

5330 Schering Corporation. Manufacturer's literature on Fulvicin® . Kenilworth, NJ 07033 (1992)

5331 Schering Corporation. Manufacturer's literature on Garamycin® . Kenilworth, NJ 07033 (1997)

5332 Schering Corporation. Manufacturer's literature on Hyperstat® . Kenilworth, NJ 07033 (1985)

5333 Schering Corporation. Manufacturer's literature on Intron® A. Kenilworth, NJ 07033 (1997)

5334 Schering Corporation. Manufacturer's literature on Netromycin® . Kenilworth, NJ 07033 (1987)

5335 Schering Corporation. Manufacturer's literature on Normodyne® . Kenilworth, NJ 07033 (1995)

5336 Schering Corporation. Manufacturer's literature on Proventil® . Kenilworth, NJ 07033 (1996)

5337 Schering Corporation. Manufacturer's literature on Solganal® . Kenilworth, NJ 07033 (1984)

5338 Schering Corporation. Manufacturer's literature on Trilafon® . Kenilworth, NJ 07033 (1994)

5339 Schiff E, Peleg E, Goldenberg M et al. The use of aspirin to prevent pregnancy-induced hypertension and lower the ratio thromboxane A_2 to prostacyclin in relatively high risk pregnancies. *N Engl J Med*, 321, 351-356 (1989)

5340 Schifferli J, Leski M, Favre H et al. High-dose intravenous IgG treatment and renal function. *Lancet*, 337, 457-459 (1991)

5341 Schiffl H, Weidmann P, Mordasini R et al. Reversal of diuretic induced increases in serum low density lipoprotein cholesterol by the beta blocker pindolol.. *Metabolism*, 31, 411-415 (1982)

5342 Schifter S, Johannsen L, Bunker C et al. Calcitonin gene-related peptide in small cell lung carcinomas. *Clin Endocrinol*, 39, 59-65 (1993)

5343 Schilsky RL, Barlock A, Ozois RF. Persistent hypomagnesemia following cisplatin therapy for testicular cancer. *Cancer Treat Rep*, 66, 1767-1769 (1982)

5344 Schiodt FV, Rochling FA, Casey DL, Lee Wm. Acetaminophen toxicity in an urban county hospital. *N Engl J Med*, 337, 1112-1117 (1997)

5345 Schlanz KD, Myre SA, Bottorff MB. Pharmacokinetic intercations with calcium channel antagonists (Part I). *Clin Pharmacokinet*, 21, 344-356 (1991)

5346 Schlueter W, Keilani T, Batile DC. Metabolic effects of converting enzyme inhibitors: focus on the reduction of cholesterol and lipoprotein(a) by fosinopril. *Am J Cardiol*, 72, 37H-44H (1993)

5347 Schmid R, Schusdziarra V, Schulte-Frohlinde E at al. Effect of CCK on insulin, glucagon, and pancreatic polypeptide levels in humans. *Pancreas*, 4, 653-661 (1989)

5348 Schmidt D, Flentge C, Place L et al. Development of whole blood phenytoin assay. *Clin Chem*, 36, 1037 (1990)

5349 Schmidt D, Utech K. Progabide for refractory partial epilepsy: a controlled add-on trial. *Neurology*, 36, 217-221 (1986)

5350 Schmidt E, Poliwoda H, Buhl V et al. Observations of enzyme elevations in the serum during streptokinase treatment. *J Clin Pathol*, 25, 650 (1972)

5351 Schmidt GH, Horak DA, Niland JC et al. A randomized controlled trial of prophylactic ganciclovir for cytomegalovirus pulmonary infection in recipients of allogeneic bone marrow transplants. *N Engl J Med*, 324, 1005-1011 (1991)

5352 Schmidt JB, Gebhart W, Kopsa H et al. Does cyclosporine A influence sex hormone level?. *Exp Clin Endocrinol*, 88, 207-211 (1986)

5353 Schmidt P, Zazgornik J, Kopsa H. Hypouricemia after renal transplantation. *N Engl J Med*, 289, 1373 (1973)

5354 Schmitt JK. Indomethacin increases plasma growth hormone levels in man. *Am J Med Sci*, 300, 144-147 (1990)

5355 Schnack C, Prager RJF, Winkler J et al. Effects of 8-week α-glucosidase inhibition on metabolic control, C-peptide secretion, hepatic glucose output, and peripheral insulin sensitivity in poorly controlled type II diabetic patients. *Diabetes Care*, 12, 537-543 (1989)

5356 Schnapp P, Hermann H, Cernak P et al. Nifedipine monotherapy in the hypertensive elderly: a placebo controlled clinical trial. *Curr Med Res Opin*, 10, 407-413 (1987)

5357 Schneck D, Hayes A Jr, Shiroff R et al. Effect of procainamide and isoniazid on each other's acetylation pathway in normal subjects. *Clin Pharmacol Ther*, 21, 116 (1977)

5358 Schneck DW, Callaghan JT, Bergstrom RF et al. Relationship between steady-state plasma nizatidine concentrations and inhibition of basal and stimulated gastric acid secretion. *Clin Pharmacol Ther*, 47, 499-503 (1990)

5359 Schneck DW, Luderer JR, Davis D et al. Effects of nadolol and propranolol on plasma lidocaine clearance. *Clin Pharmacol Ther*, 36, 584-587 (1984)

5360 Schneeweiss J, Poole GW. Hyperuricaemia due to pyrazinamide. *Br Med J*, 2, 830 (1960)

5361 Schneider H, Schmitt Y. Low molecular weight heparin: influence on blood lipids in patients on chronic hemodialysis. *Klin Wschr*, 69, 749-756 (1991)

5362 Schneider J. Effects of metformin on dyslipoproteinemia in non-insulin-dependent diabetes mellitus. *Diabete Metab*, 17, 185-190 (1991)

5363 Schneider J. Serum lipoproteins in hyperlipoproteinemic patients with essential hypertension treated with felodipine for two years. *Curr Ther Res*, 50, 118-126 (1991)

5364 Schneider M, Giardina E-GV. Interference by flexeril® , a tricyclic muscle relaxant, with liquid chromatographic determination of imipramine. *Clin Chem*, 32, 1599 (1986)

5365 Schoch HK. The US Veterans Administration cardiology drug-lipid study: an interim report. *Adv Exp Biol Med*, 4, 405 (1968)

5366 Schoenfeld N, Mamet R. Interference of ofloxacin with determination of urinary porphyrins. *Clin Chem*, 40, 417-419 (1994)

5367 Schoenfield LJ. Sulfobromophthalein transport and metabolism. *Gastroenterology*, 48, 530 (1965)

5368 Schoenfield LJ, Grundy SM, Hofman AF et al. The national cooperative gallstone study viewed by its investigators. *Gastroenterology*, 84, 644-647 (1983)

5369 Schoenfield LJ, Lachin JM et al. Chenodiol (chenodeoxycholic acid) for dissolution of gallstones: the national cooperative gallstone study. a controlled trial of efficacy and safety. *Ann Intern Med*, 95, 257-282 (1981)

5370 Schoenfield LJ, McGill DB, Foulk WT. Studies of BSP metabolism in man, demonstration of a transport maximum for biliary excretion of BSP. *J Clin Invest*, 43, 1424 (1964)

5371 Schoerlin M-P, Mayersohn M, Hoevels B et al. Cimetidine alters the disposition kinetics of the monoamine oxidase-A inhibitor moclobemide. *Clin Pharmacol Ther*, 59, 32-38 (1991)

5372 Schohn DC, Jahn HA, Maareck M et al. Long term effects of sustained release verapamil on the renal and systemic haemodynamic parameters in hypertensive patients with mild to severe chronic renal failure. *Drugs*, 46, Suppl 2, 113-120 (1993)

5373 Schonell M, Dorken E, Grzybowski S. Rifampin. *Can Med Ass J*, 106, 783 (1972)

5374 Schoors DF, Vercruysse I, Musch G et al. Influence of nicardipine on the pharmacokinetics and pharmacodynamics of propranolol in healthy volunteers. *Br J Clin Pharmacol*, 29, 497-501 (1990)

5375 Schou M, Vestergaard P. Lithium and the kidney scare. *Psychosomatics*, 22, 92-94 (1981)

5376 Schouten JA, Danner SA, Hoek FJ et al. Further cholesterol lowering induced by probucol in familial hypercholesterolemia treated with cholestyramine. *Curr Ther Res*, 48, 985-990 (1990)

5377 Schreiner GE, Maher JF. Toxic nephropathy: adverse renal effects caused by drugs and chemicals. *J Am Med Ass*, 191, 849 (1965)

5378 Schrenzel J, Dayer P, Leemann T et al. Influence of rifampin on fleroxacin pharmacokinetics. *Antimicrob Agent Chemother*, 37, 2132-2138 (1993)

5379 Schrier RW, Lieberman R, Ufferman RC. Mechanism of antidiuretic effect of beta adrenergic stimulation. *J Clin Invest*, 51, 97 (1972)

5380 Schrogie JJ, Solomon HM. The hypocholesterolemic effect of phenyramidol. *Clin Pharmacol Ther*, 7, 723 (1966)

5381 Schulenburg BJ, Beck ML, Pierce SR et al. Immune hemolysis associated with zomax. *Transfusion*, 23, 409 (1983)

5382 Schultz AL. Influence of drugs on thyroid ^{131}I uptake and serum chemical protein-bound iodine. *Postgrad Med*, 31, A-34 (1962)

5383 Schultz KL, Badrick TC, Gaffney PT. High oral doses of sodium ascorbate cause significant changes in five common clinical biochemical assays. *Clin Biochem Rev*, 14, 365 (1993)

5384 Schulz H-U, Hartmann M, Steinijans VW et al. Lack of influence of pantoprazole on the disposition kinetics of theophylline in man. *Int J Clin Pharmacol*, 29, 369-375 (1991)

5385 Schulzeck P, Bojanovski M, Jochim A et al. Comparison between simvastatin and bezafibrate in effect on plasma lipoproteins and apolipoproteins in primary hypercholesterolaemia. *Lancet*, 1, 611-612 (1988)

5386 Schumacher HR Jr, Meng Z, Sieck M, et al. Effect of a nonsteroidal antiinflamatory drug on synovial fluid in osteoarthritis. *J Rheumatol*, 23, 1774-1777 (1996)

5387 Schwab M, Ruder H. Hyponatremia and cerebral convulsion due to DDAVP administration in patients with enuresis nocturna or urine concentration testing. *Eur J Pediat*, 156, 668 (1997)

5388 Schwab RS, Poskanzer DC, England AC Jr et al. Amantadine in Parkinson's disease. *J Am Med Ass*, 222, 792 (1972)

5389 Schwab SJ, Hlatky MA, Pieper KS et al. Contrast nephrotoxicity: a randomized control trial of a nonionic and an ionic radiographic contrast agent. *N Engl J Med*, 320, 149-153 (1989)

5390 Schwandt P, Elsasser R, Schmidt C et al. Safety and efficacy of lifibrol upon four-week administration to patients with primary hypercholesterolaemia. *Eur J Clin Pharmacol*, 47, 133-138 (1994)

5391 Schwartz AB, Orquiza CS. The effects of recombinant human erythropoietin on mean corpuscular volume in patients with the anemia of chronic renal failure. *Clin Nephrol*, 43, 256-259 (1995)

5392 Schwartz DE, Schaeffer E, Brewer HB et al. Bioavailability of propranolol following administration of cholestyramine. *Clin Pharmacol Ther*, 31, 268 (1982)

5393 Schwartz EL, et al. Pharmacokinetic interactions of zidovudine and methadone in intravenous drug-using patients with HIV infection. *J AIDS*, 5, 616-626 (1992)

5394 Schwartz FD, Pillay VKG, Kark RM. Ethacrynic acid: its usefulness and untoward effects. *Am Heart J*, 79, 427 (1970)

5395 Schwartz JB, Keefe D, Harrison DC. Adverse effects of antiarrhythmic drugs. *Drugs*, 21, 23-45 (1981)

5396 Schwartz JB, Misliore PJ. Effect of nifedipine on serum digoxin concentration and renal digoxin clearance. *Clin Pharmacol Ther*, 36, 19-24 (1984)

5397 Schwartz JB, Upton RA, Lin ET et al. Effect of cimetidine or ranitidine administration on nifedipine pharmacokinetics and pharmacodynamics. *Clin Pharmacol Ther*, 43, 673-680 (1988)

5398 Schwartz KE, Zaro B, Burton P et al. Reduction of serum lipoproteins in man by the oral administration of a prostaglandin analogue (enprostil). *Atherosclerosis*, 71, 9-16 (1988)

5399 Schwartz KE, Zaro B, Reynolds J et al. Suppression of postprandial glucose, insulin, C-peptide, and glucose-dependent insulinotropic peptide (GIP) in man by oral administration of a prostaglandin analogue (Enprostil). *Horm Metab Res*, 20, 637-640 (1988)

5400 Schwartz MA, Postma E. Metabolism of flurazepam, a benzodiazepine in man and dog. *J Pharm Sci*, 59, 1800 (1970)

5401 Schwartz MK. Interferences in biochemical tests. *Mem Sloan-Kettering Clin Bull*, 1, 11 (1971)

5402 Schwartz MK. Interferences in diagnostic biochemical procedures. *Adv Clin Chem*, 16, 1 (1973)

5403 Schwartz MW, Schifreen RS, Gorman E et al. Development and performance of a fully automated method for assay of C-reactive protein in the aca discrete clinical analyzer. *Clin Chem*, 34, 1646-1649 (1988)

5404 Schwartz S, Raskin P, Fonseca V, et al. Effect of troglitazone in insulin-treated patients with type II diabetes mellitus. *N Engl J Med*, 338, 861-866 (1998)

5405 Schwarz Pharma, Inc. Manufacturer's literature on Univasc® . Milwaukee, WI 53201 (1997)

5406 Schwarz S, Tappeiner G, Hintner H. Hormone binding globulin levels in patients with hereditary angioedema during treatment with danazol. *Clin Endocrinol*, 14, 563-570 (1981)

5407 Schwarze R, Kintzel HW, Hinkel GK. The influence of orotic acid on the serum bilirubin level of mature newborn. *Acta Paediat Scand*, 60, 705 (1971)

5408 Schwarzhoff R, Cody JT. The effects of adultering agents on FPIA analysis of urine for drugs of abuse. *J Anal Toxicol*, 17, 14-17 (1993)

5409 Schweisfurth H, Schioberg-Schiegnitz S. Assay and biochemical characterization of angiotensin-converting enzyme in cerebrospinal fluid. *Enzyme*, 32, 12-19 (1984)

5410 Schweppe K-W, Assman G. Changes of plasma lipids and lipoprotein levels during danazol treatment for endometriosis. *Horm Metab Res*, 16, 593-597 (1984)

5411 Sclanz KD, Myre SA, Bottorff MB. Pharmacokinetic interactions with calcium channel antagonists (Part II). *Clin Pharmacokinet*, 21, 448-460 (1991)

5412 Scnapp P. Acute natriuretic effect of nifedipine in elderly males with essential hypertension. *Int J Clin Pharmacol Ther Toxicol*, 27, 442-444 (1989)

5413 Scobie IN, Maccuish AC, Kesson CM et al. Neutropenia during allopurinol treatment in total therapeutic starvation. *Br Med J*, 1, 1163 (1980)

5414 Scott DA, Goward CR, Scawen MD et al. Colorimetric glucose assay using thermostable glucokinase. *Ann Clin Biochem*, 27, 33-37 (1990)

5415 Scott JT, Hall AP, Grahame R. Allopurinol in treatment of gout. *Br Med J*, 2, 321 (1966)

5416 Scott JT, Higgens CS. Diuretic induced gout: a multifactorial condition. *Ann Rheum Dis*, 51, 259-261 (1992)

5417 Scott JT, Porter IH, Lewis SM et al. Studies of gastrointestinal bleeding caused by corticosteroids, salicylates and other analgesics. *Q J Med*, 30, 167 (1961)

5418 Scott MG, Hock KG, Crimmins DL, Fracasso PM. HPLC method for monitoring SDZ PSC 833 in whole blood. *Clin Chem*, 43, 505-510 (1997)

5419 Scott SM, Rogers C, Backstrom C. Dexamethasone therapy is associated with a rise in urinary epidermal growth factor concentrations in the preterm infant. *Eur J Endocrinol*, 132, 326-330 (1995)

5420 SCS Pharmaceuticals. Manufacturer's literature on Flagyl® . Chicago, IL 60680 (1993)

5421 Seager J. IgA deficiency during treatment of infantile hypothyroidism with thyroxine. *Br Med J*, 288, 1562-1563 (1984)

5422 Sealey JE. Plasma renin activity and plasma prorenin assays. *Clin Chem*, 37, Suppl B, 1811-1819 (1991)

5423 Sebel PS, Verghese C, Makin HIj. Effect on plasma cortisol concentrations of a single induction dose of etomidate on thiopentone. *Lancet*, 2, 625 (1983)

5424 Seddon RJ. Hormonal steroid contraceptives, 1. physiological and pharmacological considerations. *Drugs*, 1, 399 (1971)

5425 Sedlacek SM, Rudolf PM, Kaehny WD. Amoxapine-associated agranulocytosis with thrombocytosis occurring early during recovery. *Am J Med*, 80, 533-536 (1986)

5426 Seed M, Godsland IF, Wynn V et al. The effects of cyproterone acetate and ethinyl oestradiol on carbohydrate metabolism. *Clin Endocrinol*, 21, 689-699 (1984)

5427 Seed M, O'Connor B, Perombelon N et al. The effect of nicotinic acid and acipimox on lipoprotein(a) concentration and turnover. *Atherosclerosis*, 101, 61-68 (1993)

5428 Seeldrayers P, Messina D, Desmedt D et al. CSF levels of neurotransmitters in Alzheimer-type dementia. Effects of ergoloid mesylate. *Acta Neurol Scand*, 71, 411-414 (1985)

5429 Seely EW, LeBoff MS, Brown EM et al. The calcium channel blocker diltiazem lowers serum parathyroid hormone levels in vivo and in vitro. *J Clin Endocrinol Metab*, 68, 1007-1012 (1989)

5430 Segers O, De Vroede M, Michotte Y et al. Basal and tolbutamide-induced plasma somatostatin in healthy subjects and in patients with diabetes and impaired glucose tolerance. *Diabetic Med*, 6, 232-238 (1989)

5431 Segre EJ, Chaplin M, Forchielli E et al. Naproxen-aspirin interactions in man. *Clin Pharmacol Ther*, 15, 374-379 (1974)

5432 Seguchi H, Nakamura H, Aosaki N et al. Effects of carvedilol on serum lipids in hypertensive and normotensive subjects. *Eur J Clin Pharmacol*, 38, S139-S142 (1990)

5433 Seibold JR, Lynch CJ, Medsger JA Jr. Cholestasis associated with D-penicillamine therapy: case report and review of the literature. *Arth Rheum*, 24, 554-556 (1981)

5434 Seidelin R. Cimetidine and renal failure. *Postgrad Med J*, 56, 440-441 (1980)

5435 Seifritz E, Baumann P, Muller MJ, et al. Neuroendocrine effects of a 20-mg citalopram infusion in healthy males: a placebo-controlled evaluation of citalopram as 5-HT function probe. *Neuropsychopharmacology*, 14, 253-263 (1996)

5436 Seitz H, Jaworski ZF. Effect of hydrochlorothiazide on serum and urinary calcium and urinary citrate. *Can Med Ass J*, 90, 414 (1964)

5437 Seitz HK, Bosche J, Czygan P et al. Increased blood ethanol levels following cimetidine but not ranitidine. *Lancet*, 1, 760 (1983)

5438 Sekadde CB, Slaunwhite WR Jr, Aceto T Jr. Rapid radioimmunoassay of triiodothyronine. *Clin Chem*, 19, 1016 (1973)

5439 Selby C. Sex hormone binding globulin: origin, function and clinical significance. *Ann Clin Biochem*, 27, 532-541 (1990)

5440 Sellers EM, Koch-Weser J. Displacement of warfarin from human albumin by diazoxide and ethacrynic, mefenamic and nalidixic acids. *Clin Pharmacol Ther*, 11, 524 (1970)

5441 Sellers EM, Lang M, Koch-Weser J et al. Interaction of chloral hydrate and ethanol in man I. Metabolism. *Clin Pharmacol Ther*, 13, 37-49 (1972)

5442 Selroos O, Edgren J. Lupus-like syndrome associated with pulmonary reaction to nitrofurantoin. *Acta Med Scand*, 197, 125-129 (1975)

5443 Sen S, Mukerjee AB. Hypoglycaemic action of oxytetracycline. *J Ind Med Ass*, 52, 366 (1969)

5444 Sena SF, Syed D, Romeo R et al. Lidocaine metabolite and creatinine measurements in the Ektachem® 700: steps to minimize impact on patient care. *Clin Chem*, 34, 2144-2148 (1988)

5445 Senecal P-E, Kosnett M, Larson S et al. Investigation of an anion gap of minus 88 in a patient taking bromazepam. *Clin Chem*, 36, 1040 (1990)

5446 Sengelov H, Winther K. Effect of felodipine, a new calcium channel antagonist, on platelet function and fibrinolytic activity at rest and after exercise. *Eur J Clin Pharmacol*, 37, 453-457 (1989)

5447 Seo H, Matsui N, Niinomi M et al. Effect of niceritrol on the glucose metabolism in type II diabetes mellitus associated with hyperlipidemia. *Curr Ther Res*, 44, 189-199 (1988)

5448 SEQUUS Pharmaceuticals, Inc. Manufacturer's literature on Doxil® . Menlo Park, CA 94026 (1995)

5449 Series JJ, Caslake MJ, Kilday C et al. Effect of combined therapy with bezafibrate and cholestyramine on low-density lipoprotein metabolism in type IIa hypercholesterolemia. *Metabolism*, 38, 153-158 (1989)

5450 Serlin MJ, Sibeon RG, Mossman S et al. Cimetidine: interactions with oral anticoagulants in man. *Lancet*, 2, 317-319 (1979)

5451 Serono Laboratories, Inc. Manufacturer's literature on Serophene® . Norwell, MA 02061 (1994)

5452 Serri O, Beauregard H, Brazeau P et al. Somatostatin analogue, octreotide, reduces increased glomerular filtration rate and kidney size in insulin-dependent diabetics. *J Am Med Ass*, 265, 888-892 (1991)

5453 Sesin GP, O'Keefe E, Roberto P. Sulindac-induced elevation of serum cyclosporine concentration. *Clin Pharm*, 8, 445 (1989)

5454 Settlage DF, Nakamura RM, Davajan V et al. A quantitative analysis of serum proteins during treatment with oral contraceptive steroids. *Contraception*, 1, 101 (1970)

5455 Severini G, Aliberti LM. Variation of urinary enzymes N-acetyl-β-glucosaminidase, alanine aminopeptidase, and lysozyme in patients receiving radiocontrast agents. *Clin Biochem*, 20, 339-341 (1987)

5456 Seviour PW, Teal TK, Richmond W et al. Chlorpropamide lowers serum and lipoprotein cholesterol in insulin dependent diabetics. *Diabetic Med*, 3, 152-154 (1986)

5457 Seyberth HW. The significance of renal prostaglandins for kidney function in early childhood. *Monatsschr Kinderheilkd*, 135, 178-185 (1987)

5458 Sfogliano L, Benigno R, Bonanno G et al. Effects of long-term administration of the calcium-antagonist nicardipine on kidney function parameters and renin-angiotensin/angiotensin-converting-enzyme/aldosterone system. *Curr Ther Res*, 44, 267-274 (1988)

5459 Sgoutas DS, Abbott KL. Cyclosporine does not interfere in total and high-density lipoprotein cholesterol measurement with use of enzymatic cholesterol assays. *Clin Chem*, 35, 2251-2251 (1989)

5460 Shaaban MM, Elwan SI, Abdalla SA et al. Effect of subdermal contraceptive implants, NORPLANT® , on serum lipids. *Contraception*, 30, 413-419 (1984)

5461 Shaaban MM, Elwan SI, El-Kabsh MY et al. Effect of levonorgestrel contraceptive implants, NORPLANT® , on blood coagulation. *Contraception*, 30, 421-430 (1984)

5462 Shaaban MM, Elwan SI, El-Sharkawy MM et al. Effects of subdermal levonorgestrel contraceptive implants, NORPLANT® , on liver functions. *Contraception*, 30, 407-412 (1984)

5463 Shackleford EJ, Watson FT. Amiodarone-phenytoin interaction. *Drug Intell Clin Pharm*, 21, 921 (1987)

5464 Shaffner F. Diagnosis of drug-induced hepatic damage. *J Am Med Ass*, 191, 466 (1965)

5465 Shah S. Hepatotoxicity due to papaverine hydrochloride. *N Engl J Med*, 282, 1271 (1970)

5466 Shaheen O, Biollaz J, Koshakji R et al. Effect of debrisoquine phenotype on the inducibility of propranolol metabolism. *Clin Pharmacol Ther*, 41, 158 (1987)

5467 Shalev A, Hermesh H, Munitz H. The hypouricemic effect of chlorprothixene. *Clin Pharmacol Ther*, 42, 562-566 (1987)

5468 Shalev O, Mosseri M, Ariel I et al. Methyldopa-induced immune hemolytic anemia and chronic active hepatitis. *Arch Intern Med*, 143, 592-593 (1983)

5469 Shalmi M, Rasmusen H, Amtorp O et al. Effect of chronic oral furosemide administration on the 24-hour cycle of lithium clearance and electrolyte excretion in humans. *Eur J Clin Pharmacol*, 38, 275-280 (1990)

5470 Shamash J, Earl H, Souhami R. Acetazolamide for alkalinisation of urine in patients receiving high-dose methotrexate. *Cancer Chemother Pharmacol*, 28, 150-151 (1991)

5471 Shand DG, Epstein C, Kinberg-Calhoun J et al. The effect of etodolac administration on renal function in patients with arthritis. *J Clin Pharmacol*, 26, 269-274 (1986)

5472 Shapiro ET, Van Cauter E, Tillil H et al. Glyburide enhances the responsiveness of the β-cell to glucose but does not correct the abnormal patterns of insulin secretion in noninsulin-dependent diabetes mellitus. *J Clin Endocrinol Metab*, 69, 571-576 (1989)

5473 Sharif M, Salisbury C, Taylor DJ, Kirwan JR. Changes in biochemical markers of joint tissue metabolism in a randomized controlled trial of glucocorticoid in early rheumatoid arthritis. *Arth Rheum*, 41, 1203-1209 (1998)

5474 Sharifi R, Knoll D, Smith J, Kramolowsky E. Leuprolide acetate (30 mg depot every four months) in the treatment of advanced prostate cancer. *Urology*, 51, 271-276 (1998)

5475 Sharifi R, Lee M, Ojeda L et al. Preliminary report comparing piperacillin and carbenicillin for complicated urinary tract infections. *J Urol*, 128, 755-758 (1982)

5476 Sharma RP, Bissette G, Janicak P et al. Cerebrospinal fluid somatostatin concentrations in schizophrenia and schizoaffective disorder: the effects of antipsychotic treatment. *Schiz Res*, 13, 173-178 (1994)

5477 Sharp AM, Fraser IS, Caterson ID. Further studies on danazol interference in testosterone radioimmunoassays. *Clin Chem*, 29, 141-143 (1983)

5478 Sharp AM, Walters CA, Wong SD et al. IRMA and RIA compared for assessing dexamethasone suppression of corticotropin in plasma. *Clin Chem*, 38, 149 (1992)

5479 Sharp CA, Perks J, Worsfold M et al. Plasma aluminium in a reference population: the effects of antacid consumption and its influence on biochemical indices of bone formation. *Eur J Clin Invest*, 23, 554-560 (1993)

5480 Sharp P. Interference in glucose oxidase-peroxidase blood glucose methods. *Clin Chim Acta*, 40, 115 (1972)

5481 Sharp P, Riley C, Cook JGH et al. Effect of two sulfonylureas on glucose determinations by enzymic methods. *Clin Chim Acta*, 36, 93 (1972)

5482 Shasha SM, Shiller M, Ben Aryeh H et al. Effect of pindolol on blood parathyroid hormone concentration. *Isr J Med Sci*, 17, 1189-1190 (1981)

5483 Shaw DM. Anti-depressant drugs. *Practitioner*, 192, 23 (1964)

5484 Shaw MW. Human chromosome damage by chemical agents. *Ann Rev Med*, 21, 409 (1970)

5485 Shay H, Siplet H. Study of chlorpromazine jaundice: mechanism and prevention. *Gastroenterology*, 32, 571 (1957)

5486 Shea M, D'Eon P, Blackwood J et al. A dry chemistry multilayer immunoassay test for gentamicin. *Clin Chem*, 36, 1045 (1990)

5487 Shea P, Lal R, Kim SS et al. Flecainide and amiodarone interaction. *J Am Coll Cardiol*, 7, 1127-1130 (1986)

5488 Shearer MJ, Bechtold H, Andrassy K et al. Mechanism of cephalosporin-induced hypoprothrombinemia: Relation to cephalosporin side chain, Vitamin K metabolism, and Vitamin K status. *J Clin Pharmacol*, 28, 88-95 (1988)

5489 Sheehan J. Trimethoprim-associated marrow toxicity. *Lancet*, 2, 692 (1981)

5490 Sheehan J, White A. Diuretic-associated hypomagnesaemia. *Br Med J*, 285, 1157-1159 (1982)

5491 Sheldon J, Riches P, Hobbs JR. Neopterin radioimmunoassay results are unaffected by β-propiolactone: safer monitoring of HIV-positive serum samples. *Clin Chem*, 36, 175 (1990)

5492 Sheldon W, Welch RJ, Bonham JR et al. Hypomagnesaemia following treatment of childhood cancer with cisplatinum.. *Ann Clin Biochem*, 24, Suppl S1, 85-86 (1987)

5493 Shelp WD, Bloodworth JMB Jr, Rieselbach RE. Effect of azathioprine on renal histology and function in lupus nephritis. *Arch Intern Med*, 128, 566 (1971)

5494 Shemin D, Elnour M, Amarantes B et al. Oral estrogens decrease bleeding time and improve clinical bleeding in patients with renal failure. *Am J Med*, 89, 436-440 (1990)

5495 Shen M-R, Chiang P-H, Yang R-C et al. Pentoxifylline stimulates human sperm motility both in vitro and after oral therapy. *Br J Clin Pharmacol*, 31, 711-714 (1991)

5496 Shen S, Weir M, Dagher F et al. Effect of cyclosporine on total lymphocyte and T-cell counts in renal transplant recipients. *N Engl J Med*, 314, 447-448 (1986)

5497 Shenkenberg TD, Von Hoff DD. Mitoxantrone: a new anticancer drug with significant clinical activity. *Ann Intern Med*, 105, 67-81 (1986)

5498 Shephard RJ, Killinger D, Fried T. Responses to sustained use of anabolic steroid. *Br J Sport Med*, 11, 170-173 (1977)

5499 Shepherd J. Danazol and plasma lipoprotein metabolism. *Int J Gynaecol Obstet*, 50, Suppl 1, S23-S26 (1995)

5500 Shepherd J, Packard CJ, Stewart JM et al. Apolipoprotein A and B (sf 100-400) metabolism during bezafibrate therapy in hypertriglyceridemic subjects. *J Clin Invest*, 74, 2164-2177 (1984)

5501 Sher SP. Drug enzyme induction and drug interactions: literature tabulation. *Toxicol Appl Pharmacol*, 18, 780 (1971)

5502 Sherlock S. Effects of drugs on the liver. *Ann Clin Biochem*, 7, 75 (1970)

5503 Sherlock S. Halothane hepatitis. *Gut*, 12, 324 (1971)

5504 Sherman HC, Caldwell ML, Adams M. A quantitative comparison of the influence of neutral salts on the activity of pancreatic amylase. *J Am Chem Soc*, 50, 2538 (1928)

5505 Sherman JD, Love DE, Harrington JF. Anemia-positive lupus and rheumatoid factors with methyldopa a report of three cases. *Arch Intern Med*, 120, 321 (1967)

5506 Sherman L, Kim S, Benjamin F et al. Effect of chlorpromazine on serum growth hormone concentration in man. *N Engl J Med*, 284, 72 (1971)

5507 Sherry S. Prospects in antithrombotic therapy. *Am J Cardiol*, 29, 81 (1972)

5508 Sherwin SA, Knost JA, Fein S et al. A multiple dose phase i trial of recombinant leukocyte α-interferon in cancer patients. *J Am Med Ass*, 248, 2461-2466 (1982)

5509 Sherwood LM. Hypernatremia during sodium sulfate therapy. *N Engl J Med*, 277, 314 (1967)

5510 Sherwood RA, Pippard MJ, Peters TJ. Iron homeostasis and the assessment of iron status. *Ann Clin Biochem*, 35, 693-708 (1998)

5511 Shewman DA, Stock JL, Abusamra LC et al. Tamoxifen decreases lipoprotein (a) in patients with breast cancer. *Metabolism*, 43, 531-532 (1994)

5512 Shewmon DA, Stock JL, Rosen CJ et al. Tamoxifen and estrogen lower circulating lipoprotein(a) concentrations in healthy postmenopausal women. *Arterioscler Thromb*, 14, 1586-1593 (1994)

5513 Shi YF, Harris AG, Zhu XF et al. Clinical and biochemical effects of incremental doses of the long-acting somatostatin analogue SMS 201-995 in 10 acromegalic patients. *Clin Endocrinol*, 32, 695-705 (1990)

5514 Shields AF, Berenson JA. Procainamide-associated pancytopenia. *Am J Hematol*, 27, 299-301 (1988)

5515 Shields JE Jr, Praissman M, Berkowitz JM. Plasma gastrin response to oral coffee and calcium carbonate. *Clin Res*, 21, 524 (1973)

5516 Shields LI, Files JA, Doll DC et al. Ranitidine and agranulocytosis. *Ann Intern Med*, 104, 128 (1986)

5517 Shifrine M, Fisher GL. Ceruloplasmin levels in sera from human patients with osteosarcoma. *Cancer*, 38, 244-248 (1976)

5518 Shih VE, Nikiforov V, Carney MM. Acetaminophen metabolite interferes in analysis for amino acids. *Clin Chem*, 31, 148 (1985)

5519 Shih VE, Tenanbaum A. Aminoaciduria due to vinyl-GABA administration. *N Engl J Med*, 323, 1353 (1990)

5520 Shindelman J, Singh H, Hertle V et al. Homogeneous enzyme immunoassay for measurement of human ferritin using recombinant enzyme fragments. *Clin Chem*, 38, 1078-1079 (1992)

5521 Shiohara T, Imanishi K, Sagawa Y et al. Differential effects of cyclosporine and etretinate on serum cytokine levels in patients with psoriasis. *J Am Acad Dermatol*, 27, 568-574 (1992)

5522 Shionoiri H, Gotoh E, Ito T et al. Long-term therapy with terazosin may improve glucose and lipid metabolism in hypertensives. *Am J Med Sci*, 307, Suppl 1, S91-S95 (1994)

5523 Shionoiri H, Iino S, Inoue S. Glucose metabolism during captopril monotherapy and combination therapy in diabetic hypertensive patients: a multiclinic trial. *Clin Exp Hypertens*, 9, 671-674 (1987)

5524 Shionoiri H, Sugimoto K-i, Minamisawa K et al. Glucose and lipid metabolism during long-term treatment with cilazapril in hypertensive patients with or without impaired glucose metabolism. *J Cardiovasc Pharmacol*, 15, 933-938 (1990)

5525 Shionoiri H, Ueda S-i, Gotoh E et al. Glucose and lipid metabolism during long-term lisinopril therapy in hypertensive patients. *J Cardiovasc Pharmacol*, 16, 905-909 (1990)

5526 Shipkova M, Niedmann PD, Armstrong VW, et al. Simultaneous determination of mycophenolic acid and its glucuronide in human plasma using a simple high-performance liqid chromatography procedure. *Clin Chem*, 44, 1481-1488 (1998)

5527 Shirakami A, Hirai Y, Takeichi T et al. Changes in plasma fibronectin levels in thyroid diseases. *Horm Metab Res*, 18, 345-348 (1986)

5528 Shiratori K, Watanabe S-I, Takeuchi T et al. Effect of plaunotol on release of plasma secretin and pancreatic exocrine secretion in humans. *Pancreas*, 4, 323-328 (1989)

5529 Shiratsuki N, Uyama O, Kitada O et al. Effects of hydrocortisone and aminophylline on plasma leukotriene C_4 levels in patients during an asthmatic attack. *Prostaglandins Leukot Essent Fatty Acid*, 40, 285-289 (1990)

5530 Shirley DG, Singer DRJ, Sagnella GA et al. Effect of a single test dose of lithium carbonate on sodium and potassium excretion in man. *Clin Sci*, 81, 59-63 (1991)

5531 Shoenfeld Y, Baruch NB, Livni E et al. Carbamazepine (Tegretol®)-induced thrombocytopenia. *Acta Haematol*, 68, 74 (1982)

5532 Shoenfeld Y, Gurewich Y, Gallant LA et al. Prednisone-induced leukocytosis. *Am J Med*, 71, 773-778 (1981)

5533 Shohat J, Modan M, Rosenfeld JB. Bopindolol: Long-term effects on blood pressure, renal function, plasma renin activity, and plasma aldosterone in mild-to-moderate essential hypertension. *Fundam Clin Pharmacol*, 3, 53-58 (1989)

5534 Shojania AM. Oral contraceptives: effects on folate and vitamin B_{12} metabolism. *Can Med Ass J*, 126, 244-247 (1982)

5535 Shojania AM, Hornady GJ, Barnes PH. The effect of oral contraceptives on folate metabolism. *Am J Obstet Gynecol*, 111, 782 (1971)

5536 Shopsin B. Effects of lithium on thyroid function: a review. *Dis Nerv Sys*, 31, 237 (1970)

5537 Shopsin B, Friedmann R, Gershon S. Lithium and leukocytosis. *Clin Pharmacol Ther*, 12, 923 (1971)

5538 Shotan A, Mehra A, Ostrzega E et al. Plasma cyclic guanosine monophosphate in chronic heart failure: hemodynamic and neurohumoral correlations and response to nitrate therapy. *Clin Pharmacol Ther*, 54, 638-644 (1993)

5539 Shurtleff DB, Hayden PW. The treatment of hydrocephalus with isosorbide, an oral hyperosmotic agent. *J Clin Pharmacol*, 12, 108 (1972)

5540 Shuster F, Napier EA, Henley KS. Serum transaminase activity following morphine, meperidine, and codeine in normals. *Am J Med Sci*, 246, 714 (1963)

5541 Shuster M, Dunn M. Pentamidine and hematuria. *Ann Intern Med*, 105, 146 (1986)

5542 Shusterman NH, Elliott WJ, White WB. Fenoldopam, but not nitroprusside, improves renal function in severely hypertensive patients with impaired renal function. *Am J Med*, 95, 161-168 (1993)

5543 Siebers RWL, Maling TJB, Dineen HJ et al. No interference by amiodarone on albumin estimation by dye-binding methods. *Clin Chem*, 32, 1990 (1986)

5544 Siegel D, Saliba P, Haffner S. Glucose and insulin levels during diuretic therapy in hypertensive men. *Hypertension*, 23, 688-694 (1994)

5545 Siegel SF, Finegold DN, Lanes R et al. ACTH stimulation tests and plasma dehydroepiandrosterone sulfate levels in women with hirsutism. *N Engl J Med*, 323, 849-854 (1990)

5546 Siegert G, Bergmann S, Jaross W. Influence of age, gender and lipoprotein metabolism parameters on the activity of the plasminogen activator inhibitor and the fibrinogen concentration. *Fibrinolysis*, 6, Suppl 3, 47-51 (1992)

5547 Siemon P, Akhabue BE, Hernandez MR et al. An Abuscreen Online immunoassay for opiates in urine on the Cobas Fara II analyzer. *Clin Chem*, 37, 1007 (1991)

5548 Siest G, Bagrel A, Panek E et al. Plasma enzymes - physiological and environmental variations. In:. *Reference Values in Human Chemistry. G Siest (ed)*, Basel, Karger, 28 (1973)

5549 Siff KS, Finkler AE. False-positive barbiturate test in urine owing to phenytoin and 5-(p-hydroxyphenyl)-5-phenylhydantoin. *Clin Chem*, 34, 1359-1360 (1988)

5550 Sigler C, Annis K, Cooper K , et al. Examination of baseline levels of carboxypeptidase N and complement components as potential predictors of angioedema associated with the use of an angiotensin-converting enzyme inhibitor. *Arch Dermatol*, 133, 972-975 (1997)

5551 Sigurdsson A, Amtorp O, Gundersen T et al. Neurohormonal activation in patients with mild or moderately severe congestive heart failure and effects of rampiril. *Br Heart J*, 72, 422-427 (1994)

5552 Silagy CA, McNeil JJ, Donnan GA et al. Adverse effects of low-dose aspirin in a healthy elderly population. *Clin Pharmacol Ther*, 54, 84-89 (1993)

5553 Silber M, Almkvist O, Larsson B et al. The effect of oral contraceptive pills on levels of oxytocin in plasma and on cognitive function. *Contraception*, 36, 641-650 (1987)

5554 Silber M, Larsson B, Uvnas-Moberg K. Oxytocin, somatostatin, insulin and gastrin concentrations vis-a-vis late pregnancy, breast feeding and oral contraceptives. *Acta Obstet Gynecol Scand*, 70, 283-289 (1991)

5555 Silva G, Gomis R, Bosch J et al. Hyperglucagonism and glucagon resistance in cirrhosis. Paradoxical effect of propranolol on plasma glucagon levels. *J Hepatol*, 6, 325-331 (1988)

5556 Silverberg SJ, Bone HG III, Marriott TB, et al. Short-term inhibition of parathyroid hormone secretion by a calcium receptor agonist in patients with primary hyperparathyroidism. *N Engl J Med*, 337, 1506-1510 (1997)

5557 Silverman BA, Rubinstein A. Serum lactate dehydrogenase levels in adults and children with acquired immune deficiency syndrome (AIDS) and AIDS-related complex: possible indicator of B cell lymphoproliferation and disease activity. Effect of intravenous γ-globulin on enzyme levels. *Am J Med*, 78, 728-736 (1985)

5558 Silverman ED, Laxer RM, Greenwald M et al. Intravenous γ globulin therapy in systemic juvenile rheumatoid arthritis. *Arth Rheum*, 33, 1015-1022 (1990)

5559 Silverman G, Braithwaite RA. Benzodiazepines and tricyclic antidepressant plasma levels. *Br Med J*, 3, 18 (1973)

5560 Silverman JL, Wurzel HA. The effect of glyceryl guaiacolate on platelet function and other coagulation factors in vivo. *Am J Clin Pathol*, 51, 35 (1969)

5561 Silverstein MN, Petitt RM, Solberg LA Jr et al. Anagrelide; a new drug for treating thrombocytosis. *N Engl J Med*, 318, 1292-1294 (1988)

5562 Simon G, Peterson S. Pathophysiology of increased urinary N-acetyl-D-glucosaminidase activity in human hypertension: Effect of cilazapril therapy. *Clin Exp Hypertens*, 10, 767-777 (1988)

5563 Simonin R, Roux H, Oliver C et al. Effect of oral administration of 0.500 g L-dopa on the plasmatic level of GH, ACTH, TSH. *Sem Hop Paris*, 49, 617 (1973)

5564 Simons LA. Comparison of atorvastatin alone versus simvastatin ± cholestyramine in the management of severe primary hypercholesterolemia. *Aust NZ J Med*, 28, 327-333 (1998)

5565 Simpson GM, Cooper TB, Braun GA. Further studies on the effects of butyrophenones on cholesterol synthesis in humans. *Curr Ther Res*, 9, 413 (1967)

5566 Simpson GM, Varga V. An investigation of the clinical effect of GPA-1714, a catechol-O-methyl transferase inhibitor. *J Clin Pharmacol*, 12, 417 (1972)

5567 Simpson GR, Dale E. Serum levels of phosphorus, magnesium, and calcium in women utilizing combination oral or long-acting injectable. *Fertil Steril*, 23, 326 (1972)

5568 Simpson RE III, Goldstein DJ, Hjelte GS et al. Acute thrombocytopenia associated with fenoprofen. *N Engl J Med*, 298, 629-630 (1978)

5569 Simpson W. Severe megaloblastic anemia induced by phenytoin sodium. *Oral Surg*, 22, 302 (1966)

5570 Simpson WM Jr. Oral contraceptives and untoward effects coincident with their use: review. *South Med J*, 64, 1184 (1971)

5571 Sindrup SH, Hofmann U, Asmussen J, et al. Impact of quinidine on plasma and cerebrospinal fluid concentrations of codeine and morphine after codeine intake. *Eur J Clin Pharmacol*, 49, 503-509 (1996)

5572 Singer DRJ, Markandu ND, Buckley MG et al. Dietary sodium and inhibition of neutral endopeptidase 24.11 in essential hypertension. *Hypertension*, 18, 798-804 (1991)

5573 Singer DRJ, Markandu ND, Sugden AL et al. A comparison of the acute effects of cicletanine and bendrofluazide on urinary electrolytes and plasma potassium in essential hypertension. *Eur J Clin Pharmacol*, 39, 227-232 (1990)

5574 Singer I, Rotenberg D. Demeclocycline-induced nephrogenic diabetes insipidus. *Ann Intern Med*, 79, 679 (1973)

5575 Singh GB. Clinical significance and experimental studies on amylase. a review. *Ind J Med Sci*, 20, 181 (1966)

5576 Singh HP, Herbert MA, Gault MH. Effect of some drugs on clinical laboratory values as determined by the Technicon® SMA 12/60. *Clin Chem*, 18, 137 (1972)

5577 Singh J, Garg PK, Tandon RK. Hepatotoxicity due to antituberculosis drugs: clinical profile and reintroduction of therapy. *J Clin Gastroenterol*, 22, 211-214 (1996)

5578 Singhvi SM, Duchin KL, Willard DA et al. Renal handling of captopril: effect of probenecid. *Clin Pharmacol Ther*, 32, 182-189 (1982)

5579 Singleton JD, Conyers L. Warfarin and azathioprine: an important drug interaction. *Am J Med*, 92, 217 (1992)

5580 Sinhamahapatra SB, Kirschner MA. Effect of L-dopa on testosterone and luteinizing hormone production. *J Clin Endocrinol Metab*, 34, 756 (1972)

5581 Sinkule JA. Etoposide: a semisynthetic epipodophyllotoxin. *Pharmacotherapy*, 4, 61-73 (1984)

5582 Sinnecker G, Kohler S. Sex hormone-binding globulin response to the anabolic steroid stanozolol: evidence for its suitability as a biological androgen sensitivity test. *J Clin Endocrinol Metab*, 68, 1195-1200 (1989)

5583 Sinofsky FE, Pasquale SA. The effect of fluconazole on circulating ethinyl estradiol levels in women taking oral contraceptives. *Am J Obstet Gynecol*, 178, 300-304 (1998)

5584 Siris SG, Siris ES, Van Kammen DP et al. Effects of dopamine blockade on gonadotropins and testosterone in men. *Am J Psychiat*, 137, 211-214 (1980)

5585 Sirtori CR, Colli S. Influences of lipid-modifying agents on hemostasis. *Cardiovasc Drug Ther*, 7, 817-823 (1993)

5586 Sirtori CR, Manzoni C, Lovati MR. Mechanisms of lipid-lowering agents. *Cardiology*, 78, 226-235 (1991)

5587 Situnayake RD, McConkey B. Clinical and laboratory effects of prolonged therapy with sulfasalazine, gold or penicillamine: the effects of disease duration on treatment response. *J Rheumatol*, 17, 1268-1273 (1990)

5588 Sivitz WI, Chertow BS, Baranetsky NG et al. Theophylline interferes with ligand binding in radioimmunoassays for somatostatin. *J Immunoassay*, 3, 145-154 (1982)

5589 Sjoden G, Rosenquist M, Kriegholm E et al. Verapamil increases serum alkaline phosphatase in hypertensive patients. *J Intern Med*, 228, 339-342 (1990)

5590 Sjogren A, Floren C-H, Nilsson A. Oral administration of magnesium hydroxide to subjects with insulin-dependent diabetes mellitus : effects on magnesium and potassium levels and insulin requirements. *Magnesium*, 7, 117-122 (1988)

5591 Sjostrom R. Absence of effect of para-chlorophenylalanine on 5-hydroxyindoleacetic acid in cerebrospinal fluid in man. *Psychopharmacology*, 27, 393 (1972)

5592 Skeith MD, Healey LA, Cutler RE. Effect of phloridzin on uric acid excretion in man. *Am J Physiol*, 219, 1080 (1970)

5593 Skeith MD, Simkin PA, Healey LA. The renal excretion of indomethacin and its inhibition by probenecid. *Clin Pharmacol Ther*, 9, 89-93 (1968)

5594 Skillen AW, Buamah PK, Cantwell BMJ et al. Urinary protein and enzyme excretion in patients receiving chemotherapy with the cis-platinum analogs carboplatin (CBDCA, JM8) and iproplatin(CHIP, JM9). *Cancer Chemother Pharmacol*, 22, 228-234 (1988)

5595 Skovsted L, Kristensen M, Hansen JM, et al. The effect of different oral anticoagulants on diphenylhydantoin (DPH) and tolbutamide metabolism. *Acta Med Scand*, 199, 513-515 (1976)

5596 Skrede S, Ro JS, Mjolnerod O. Effects of dextrans on the plasma protein changes during the postoperative period. *Clin Chim Acta*, 48, 143 (1973)

5597 Slagboom G, Loeliger EA. Coumarin-associated hepatitis: report of two cases. *Arch Intern Med*, 140, 1028-1029 (1980)

5598 Slanina P, Frech W, Ekstrom L-G et al. Dietary citric acid enhances absorption of aluminum in antacids. *Clin Chem*, 32, 539-541 (1986)

5599 Slattery JT, McRorie TI, Reynolds R et al. Lack of effect of cimetidine on acetaminophen disposition in humans. *Clin Pharmacol Ther*, 46, 591-597 (1989)

5600 Slayton RE, Shnider BI, Elias E et al. New approach to the treatment of hypercalcemia: the effect of short-term treatment with mithramycin. *Clin Pharmacol Ther*, 12, 833 (1971)

5601 Slezak P. Quinidine hepatotoxicity. *Med J Aust*, 1, 139 (1981)

5602 Slowinska-Srzednicka J, Zgliczynski S, Soszynski P et al. Effect of clonidine on β-endorphin, ACTH and cortisol secretion in essential hypertension and obesity. *Eur J Clin Pharmacol*, 35, 115-121 (1988)

5603 Sluiter HE, Huysmans FT, Thien TA et al. Haemodynamic, hormonal, and diuretic effects of felodipine in healthy normotensive volunteers. *Drugs*, 29, Suppl 2, 26-35 (1985)

5604 Slunga L, Asplund K, Johnson O et al. Lipoprotein(a) in a randomly selected 25-64 year old population: the northern Sweden Monica study. *J Clin Epidemiol*, 46, 612-624 (1993)

5605 Slunga L, Johnson O, Dahlen GH. Changes in Lp(a) lipoprotein levels during the treatment of hypercholesterolaemia with simvastatin. *Eur J Clin Pharmacol*, 43, 369-373 (1992)

5606 Sluszkiewicz E. Effect of prednisone therapy on serum levels of thyroxine (T4), triiodothyronine (T3), reverse triiodothyronine (T3), T3-binding capacity, basal TSH level, and TSH response to thyreoliberin (TRH) in children. *Exp Clin Endocrinol*, 85, 191-198 (1985)

5607 Small M, Eastall GH, Semple CG et al. Alteration of hormone levels in normal males given the anabolic steroid stanozolol. *Clin Endocrinol*, 21, 49-55 (1984)

5608 Smalldon KW. Ethanol oxidation by human erythrocytes. *Nature*, 245, 266 (1973)

5609 Smalley DL, Bradley ME. New test for glucose (BM33071) evaluated. *Clin Chem*, 31, 90-92 (1985)

5610 Smellie WSA, Scott R, Couper J et al. The effects of bendrofluazide on proinsulin conversion and insulin secretion. *Proc ACB Natl Meet*, 117 (1993)

5611 Smigan L, Perris C. Cortisol changes in long-term lithium therapy. *Neuropsychobiology*, 11, 219-223 (1984)

5612 Smilkstein MJ, Knapp GL, Kulig KW et al. Efficacy of oral N-acetylcysteine in the treatment of acetaminophen overdose: analysis of the national multicenter study (1976 to 1985). *N Engl J Med*, 319, 1557-1562 (1988)

5613 Smilkstein MJ, Steedle D, Kulig KW et al. Magnesium levels after magnesium-containing cathartics. *Clin Toxicol*, 26, 51-65 (1988)

5614 Smit JW, Wijnne HJ, Schobben F et al. Effects of alcohol and flavastatin on lipid metabolism and hepatic function. *Ann Intern Med*, 122, 678-680 (1995)

5615 Smith CR, Lipsky JJ, Laskin OL et al. Double-blind comparison on the nephrotoxicity and auditory toxicity of gentamicin and tobramycin. *N Engl J Med*, 302, 1106-1109 (1980)

5616 Smith DH, Goldwasser E, Vokes EE. Serum immunoerythropoietin levels in patients with cancer receiving cisplatin-based chemotherapy. *Cancer*, 68, 1101-1105 (1991)

5617 Smith DH, Scott DL, Zaphiropoulos GC. Eosinophilia in D-penicillamine therapy. *Ann Rheum Dis*, 42, 408-410 (1983)

5618 Smith JTL, Pounder RE. Sufotidine 600 mg bd virtually eliminates 24 hour intragastric acidity in duodenal ulcer subjects. *Gut*, 31, 291-293 (1990)

5619 Smith JW (ed.). Manual of Medical Therapeutics. Boston MA, Little Brown Co, 19th edition (1969)

5620 Smith, Kline and French. Manufacturer's literature on Ducon® . Philadelphia, PA

5621 Smith LM, Caslake C, Gunn I. Positive interference by azapropazone (Rheumox) in the measurement of total thyroxine using the Ciba-Corning ACS:180 immunoassay analyser. *Ann Clin Biochem*, 32, 425-425 (1995)

5622 Smith MB, Hiraldo M, Trafton J et al. Performance of an improved AST/IFCC reagent on the Paramax analytical system. *Clin Chem*, 36, 1139 (1990)

5623 Smith MC, Austen JL, Carey JT, et al. Prednisone improves renal function and proteinuria in human immunodeficiency virus-associated nephropathy. *Am J Med*, 101, 41-48 (1996)

5624 Smith MD, Gibson GE, Rowland R. Combined hepatotoxicity and neurotoxicity following sulfosalazine administration. *Aust NZ J Med*, 12, 76-80 (1982)

5625 Smith MJH, Smith PK. The Salicylates: A Critical Bibliographic Reviews. New York NY, Interscience (1966)

5626 Smith PM, Smith EM, Gottlieb NL. Gold distribution in whole blood during chrysotherapy. *J Lab Clin Med*, 82, 930 (1973)

5627 Smith RD, Rodel PV, Mulcahy WS et al. Long-tem renal effects of enalapril therapy in patients with renal insufficiency. *Nephron*, 55, Suppl 1, 49-58 (1990)

5628 Smith SC, Florkowski CM, Lemon M et al. Open study of simvastin action on cholesterol, triglycerides and lipoprotein fractions including Lp(a). *Clin Chem*, 36, 954 (1990)

5629 Smith SR, Kendall HJ, Lobo J et al. Ranitidine and cimetidine drug interactions with single and steady-state nifedipine administration. *Br J Clin Pharmacol*, 23, 311-315 (1987)

5630 Smith SR, Wilkins MR, Jack DB et al. Pharmacokinetic interactions between felodipine and metoprolol. *Eur J Clin Pharmacol*, 31, 575-578 (1987)

5631 Smith WGJ, Dharmasena AD, El Nahas AM et al. Short-term effect of captopril on renal haemodynamics in chronic renal failure. *Nephrol Dial Transplant*, 4, 696-700 (1989)

5632 Smith WM, Feigal DW, Furberg CD et al. Use of diuretics in the treatment of hypertension in the elderly. *Drugs*, 31, Suppl 4, 154-164 (1986)

5633 Smith WO, Kyriakopoulos AA, Hammarstein JF. Magnesium depletion induced by various diuretics. *J Okla State Med Ass*, 55, 248 (1962)

5634 Smith-Kielland A, Olsen KM, Christopherson AS. False-positive results with EMIT II amphetamine/methamphetamine assay in users of common psychotropic drugs. *Clin Chem*, 41, 951-952 (1995)

5635 SmithKline Beecham Pharmaceuticals. Manufacturer's literature on Albenza® . Philadelphia, PA 19101 (1997)

5636 SmithKline Beecham Pharmaceuticals. Manufacturer's literature on Amoxil® . Philadelphia, PA 19101 (1997)

5637 SmithKline Beecham Pharmaceuticals. Manufacturer's literature on Ancef® . Philadelphia, PA 19101 (1997)

5638 SmithKline Beecham Pharmaceuticals. Manufacturer's literature on Compazine® . Philadelphia, PA 19101 (1997)

5639 SmithKline Beecham Pharmaceuticals. Manufacturer's literature on Coreg® . Philadelphia, PA 19101 (1997)

5640 SmithKline Beecham Pharmaceuticals. Manufacturer's literature on Cytomel® . Philadelphia, PA 19101 (1997)

5641 SmithKline Beecham Pharmaceuticals. Manufacturer's literature on Dexedrine® . Philadelphia, PA 19101 (1997)

5642 SmithKline Beecham Pharmaceuticals. Manufacturer's literature on Dyrenium® . Philadelphia, PA 19101 (1997)

5643 SmithKline Beecham Pharmaceuticals. Manufacturer's literature on Eminase® . Philadelphia, PA 19101 (1990)

5644 SmithKline Beecham Pharmaceuticals. Manufacturer's literature on Energix-B® . Philadelphia, PA 19101 (1997)

5645 SmithKline Beecham Pharmaceuticals. Manufacturer's literature on Eskalith® . Philadelphia, PA 19101 (1997)

5646 SmithKline Beecham Pharmaceuticals. Manufacturer's literature on Famvir® . Philadelphia, PA 19101 (1997)

5647 SmithKline Beecham Pharmaceuticals. Manufacturer's literature on Havrix® . Philadelphia, PA 19101 (1997)

5648 SmithKline Beecham Pharmaceuticals. Manufacturer's literature on Hycamtin™. Philadelphia, PA 19101 (1997)

5649 SmithKline Beecham Pharmaceuticals. Manufacturer's literature on Kytril® . Philadelphia, PA 19101 (1997)

5650 SmithKline Beecham Pharmaceuticals. Manufacturer's literature on Menest™. Philadelphia, PA 19101 (1997)

5651 SmithKline Beecham Pharmaceuticals. Manufacturer's literature on Monocid® . Philadelphia, PA 19101 (1997)

5652 SmithKline Beecham Pharmaceuticals. Manufacturer's literature on Nabumetone® . Philadelphia, PA 19101 (1997)

5653 SmithKline Beecham Pharmaceuticals. Manufacturer's literature on Parnate® . Philadelphia, PA 19101 (1997)

5654 SmithKline Beecham Pharmaceuticals. Manufacturer's literature on Paxil® . Philadelphia, PA 19101 (1997)

5655 SmithKline Beecham Pharmaceuticals. Manufacturer's literature on Ridaura® . Philadelphia, PA 19101 (1997)

5656 SmithKline Beecham Pharmaceuticals. Manufacturer's literature on Stelazine® . Philadelphia, PA 19101 (1997)

5657 SmithKline Beecham Pharmaceuticals. Manufacturer's literature on Tagamet® . Philadelphia, PA 19101 (1997)

5658 SmithKline Beecham Pharmaceuticals. Manufacturer's literature on Tazicef® . Philadelphia, PA 19101 (1997)

5659 SmithKline Beecham Pharmaceuticals. Manufacturer's literature on Thorazine® . Philadelphia, PA 19101 (1997)

5660 SmithKline Beecham Pharmaceuticals. Manufacturer's literature on Ticar® . Philadelphia, PA 19101 (1997)

5661 SmithKline Beecham Pharmaceuticals. Manufacturer's literature on Timentin® . Philadelphia, PA 19101 (1997)

5662 SmithKline Beecham Pharmaceuticals. Manufacturer's literature on Urispas® . Philadelphia, PA 19101 (1997)
5663 Snider GB, Gogate SA. Clinical observations following papaverine therapy. *Ohio Med*, 74, 571-573 (1978)
5664 Snower DP, Weil SC. Changing etiology of macrocytosis: zidovudine as a frequent causative factor. *Am J Clin Pathol*, 99, 57-60 (1993)
5665 Snyder S. Fluphenazine jaundice. *Am J Gastroenterol*, 73, 336-340 (1980)
5666 Sobbrio GA, Graata A, D'Arrigo F et al. Treatment of hirsutism related to micropolycystic ovary syndrome (MPCO) with two low-dose oestrogen oral contraceptives: a comparative randomized evaluation. *Acta Eur Fertil*, 21, 139-141 (1990)
5667 Soffer EE, Taylor RJ, Bertram PD et al. Carbamazepine-induced liver injury. *South Med J*, 76, 681-683 (1983)
5668 Sogaard P, Klausen IC, Rungby J, et al. Lipoprotein (a) and oxygen free radicals in survivors of acute myocardial infarction: effects of captopril. *Cardiology*, 87, 18-22 (1996)
5669 Sokoloff B, Michiteru H, Saelhof CC et al. Aging: atherosclerosis and ascorbic acid metabolism. *J Am Geriatr Soc*, 14, 1239 (1966)
5670 Solberg LA Jr, Tefferi A, Oles KJ, et al. The effects of anagrelide on human megakaryocytopoiesis. *Br J Haematol*, 99, 174-180 (1997)
5671 Solinas A, Cossu P, Poddighe P et al. Changes of serum 2',5'-oligoadenylate synthetase activity during interferon treatment of chronic hepatitis C. *Liver*, 13, 253-258 (1993)
5672 Solomon GE, Hilgartner MW, Kutt H. Coagulation defects caused by diphenylhydantoin. *Neurology*, 22, 1165 (1972)
5673 Solomon HM, Abrams WB. Interactions between digitoxin and other drugs in man. *Am Heart J*, 83, 277-280 (1972)
5674 Solomon HM, Barakat MJ, Ashley CJ. Mechanisms of drug interaction. *J Am Med Ass*, 216, 1997 (1971)
5675 Solomon HM, Reich S, Spirt N et al. Interactions between digitoxin and other drugs in vitro and in vivo. *Ann NY Acad Sci*, 179, 362-368 (1971)
5676 Solomon HM, Schrogie JJ. Change in receptor site affinity: a proposed explanation for the potentiating effect of D-thyroxine. *Clin Pharmacol Ther*, 8, 797 (1967)
5677 Solomon HM, Schrogie JJ. Effect of phenyramidol and bishydroxycoumarin on the metabolism of tolbutamide in human subjects. *Metabolism*, 16, 1029-1033 (1967)
5678 Solomon K. Combined use of lithium and diuretics. *South Med J*, 71, 1098-1099 (1978)
5679 SoloPak Laboratories Inc. Manufacturer's literature on Ganite® . Boca Raton, FL 33487 (1996)
5680 SoloPak Laboratories Inc. Manufacturer's literature on Hydralazine. Boca Raton, FL 33487 (1997)
5681 Soloway MS, Chodak G, Vogelzang NJ et al. Zoladex versus orchiectomy in treatment of advanced prostatic cancer: a randomized trial. *Urology*, 37, 46-51 (1991)
5682 Soltero I, Fuenmayor I, Colmenares A et al. Action of indapamide on lipid profiles. *Curr Ther Res*, 46, 163-172 (1989)
5683 Solvay Pharmaceuticals Inc. Manufacturer's literature on Creon® . Marietta, GA 30062 (1994)
5684 Solvay Pharmaceuticals Inc. Manufacturer's literature on Luvox® . Marietta, GA 30062 (1997)
5685 Solvay Pharmaceuticals Inc. Manufacturer's literature on Prometrium® . Marietta, GA 30062 (1998)
5686 SOLVD Investigators. Effect of enalapril on mortality and the development of heart failure in asymptomatic patients with reduced left ventricular ejection fractions. *N Engl J Med*, 327, 685-691 (1992)
5687 Somani P, Temesy-Armos PN, Leighton RF et al. Hyponatremia in patients treated with lorcainide, a new anti-arrhythmic drug. *Am Heart J*, 108, 1443-1448 (1984)
5688 Somani P, Wang RIH. Alpha and beta adrenergic-receptor blocking drugs. *Drug Therapy*, March (1975)
5689 Somerset Pharmaceuticals Inc. Manufacturer's literature on Eldepryl® . Tampa, FL 33607 (1996)
5690 Sommariva D, Branchi A, Tirrito M et al. Differential effects of benfluorex and two fibrate derivatives in serum lipoprotein patterns in hypertriglyceridemic type 2 diabetic patients. *Curr Ther Res*, 40, 859-870 (1986)
5691 Sommer L, Zanger K, Dyong T et al. Seven-day administration of the gonadotropin-releasing hormone antagonist cetrorelix in normal cycling women. *Eur J Endocrinol*, 131, 280-285 (1994)
5692 Sommers DK, Kovarik JM, Meyer EC et al. Effects of diclofenac on isradipine pharmacokinetics and platelet aggregation in volunteers. *Eur J Clin Pharmacol*, 44, 391-393 (1993)
5693 Sommers DK, Schoeman HS. Drug interactions with urate excretion in man. *Eur J Clin Pharmacol*, 32, 499-502 (1987)
5694 Sommerville JM, McLaren EH, Campbell LM et al. Severe headache and disturbed liver function during treatment with zimeldine. *Br Med J*, 285, 1009 (1982)
5695 Somogyi A, Bochner F. Dose and concentration dependent effect of ranitidine on procainamide disposition and renal clearance in man. *Br J Clin Pharmacol*, 18, 175-181 (1984)
5696 Somogyi A, Bochner F, Chen ZR. Lack of effect of paracetamol on the pharmacokinetics and metabolism of codeine in man. *Eur J Clin Pharmacol*, 41, 379-382 (1991)
5697 Somogyi A, McLean A, Heinzow B. Cimetidine-procainamide pharmacokinetic interaction in man: evidence of competition for tubular secretion of basic drugs. *Eur J Clin Pharmacol*, 25, 339-345 (1983)
5698 Somogyi A, Thielscher S, Gugler R. Influence of phenobarbital treatment on cimetidine kinetics. *Eur J Clin Pharmacol*, 19, 343-347 (1981)
5699 Sona M, Fumagalli R, Paoletti R et al. Plasma Lp(a) concentration after oestrogen and progestagen in postmenopausal women. *Lancet*, 337, 612 (1990)
5700 Song S, Chen J-K, He M-L et al. Effect of some oral contraceptives on serum concentrations of sex hormone binding globulin and ceruloplasmin. *Contraception*, 39, 385-399 (1989)
5701 Sonino N. The use of ketoconazole as an inhibitor of steroid production. *N Engl J Med*, 317, 812-818 (1987)
5702 Sonnenblick M, Gottlieb S, Goldstein R et al. Effect of amiodarone on blood lipids. *Cardiology*, 73, 147-150 (1986)
5703 Sonnendecker EWW, Polakow ES. Effects of conjugated equine oestrogens with and without the addition of cyclical medrogestone on hot flushes, liver function, blood pressure and endocrinological indices. *S Afr Med J*, 77, 281-285 (1990)
5704 Sonntag O. Arzneimittel-interferenzen. Stuttgart, Thieme (1985)
5705 Sonntag O. Dry Chemistry Analysis with Carrier-Bound Reagents. Amsterdam, Elsevier (1993)
5706 Sonntag O. Trockenchemie: Analytik mit tragergebundenen Reagenzien. Stuttgart, Thieme (1988)
5707 Sonsalla J, Edmonds D, Flentge C et al. Development of a theophylline II assay for the Abbott Vision system. *Clin Chem*, 36, 1039 (1990)
5708 Sorcini G, Sciarra F, Disilverio F et al. Further studies on plasma androgens and gonadotropins after cyproterone acetate (SH 714). *Folia Endocrinol*, 24, 196 (1971)
5709 Sorensen LB. Suppression of the shunt pathway in primary gout by azathioprine. *Proc Natl Acad Sci USA*, 55, 571 (1966)
5710 Sorensen SS, Thomsen OO, Danielsen H et al. Effect of verapamil on renal plasma flow, glomerular filtration rate and plasma angiotensin II, aldosterone and arginine vasopressin in essential hypertension. *Eur J Clin Pharmacol*, 29, 257-261 (1985)

5711 Sorenson PG, Nissen MH, Groth S et al. β_2-microglobulin excretion: an indicator of long term nephrotoxicity during cis-platinum treatment?. *Cancer Chemother Pharmacol*, 14, 247-249 (1985)

5712 Soreth JT, Dubb JW, Allison NL et al. Effect on the endocrine system of a new dopaminergic agent, ibopamine. *Clin Pharmacol Ther*, 41, 627-632 (1987)

5713 Sorisky A, Watson DC. Positive diphenhydramine interference in the EMIT-ST™ assay for tricyclic antidepressants in serum. *Clin Chem*, 32, 715 (1986)

5714 Soro S, Cocca A, Pasanisi F et al. The effects of nicardipine on sodium and calcium metabolism in hypertensive patients: a chronic study. *J Clin Pharmacol*, 30, 133-137 (1991)

5715 Soro S, Ferrara LA. Effect of lacidipine, a long-acting calcium antagonist, on hypertension and lipids: a 1-year follow-up. *Eur J Clin Pharmacol*, 41, 105-107 (1991)

5716 Sorrell TC, Forbes IJ, Burness FR et al. Depression of immunological function in patients treated with phenytoin sodium (sodium diphenylhydantoin). *Lancet*, 2, 1233 (1971)

5717 Sorva A, Valimaki M, Risteli J et al. Serum ionized calcium, intact PTH and novel markers of bone turnover in bedridden elderly patients. *Eur J Clin Invest*, 24, 806-812 (1994)

5718 Sorva A, Valimaki M, Tilvis R. Effects of vitamin D and calcium supplementation in geriatric patients with low vitamin D status. *Arch Gerontol Geriat*, 12, Suppl 2, 481-484 (1991)

5719 Sorva R, Thtel R, Turpeinen M, et al. Changes in bone markers in children with asthma during inhaled budesonide and nedocromil treatments. *Acta Paediat*, 85, 1176-1180 (1996)

5720 Sorva R, Turpeinen M, Juntunen-Backman K. Effects of inhaled budesonide on serum markers of bone metabolism in children with asthma. *J Allerg Clin Immunol*, 90, 808-815 (1992)

5721 Sotaniemi EA, Hakkarainen HK, Puranen Jalahti RO. Radiologic bone changes and hypocalcemia with anticonvulsant therapy in epilepsy. *Ann Intern Med*, 77, 389 (1972)

5722 Soto J, Sacristan JA, Alsar MJ. Caffeine concentrations in adult patients chronically taking theophylline. *Clin Chem*, 38, 1386-1388 (1992)

5723 Sotolongo RP, Neefe LI, Rudzki C et al. Hypersensitivity reaction to sulfasalazine with severe hepatotoxicity. *Gastroenterology*, 75, 95-99 (1978)

5724 Soujaranta-Ylinen R, Hendolin H, Tuomisto L. The effects of morphine, morphine plus scopolamine, midazolam and promethazine on cerebrospinal fluid histamine concentration and postoperative analgesic consumption. *Agents Actions*, 33, 212-214 (1991)

5725 Soul-Lawton JH, Weatherley BC, Posner J, et al. Lack of interaction between valciclovir, the L-valyl ester of aciclovir, and digoxin. *Br J Clin Pharmacol*, 45, 87-89 (1998)

5726 Souma JA, Green PJ, Coppage AT et al. Changes in thyroid function in pregnancy and with oral contraceptive use. *South Med J*, 74, 684-687 (1981)

5727 Sözuer DT, Atakli D, Dogu O, et al. Serum lipids in epileptic children treated with carbamazepine and valproate. *Eur J Pediatr*, 156, 565-567 (1997)

5728 Souney PF, Mariani G. Effect of various concentrations of flucytosine on the accuracy of serum creatinine determinations. *Am J Hosp Pharm*, 42, 621-622 (1985)

5729 Souney PF, Menard C, Chang JT et al. Effect of cephen antibiotics on creatinine assay. *Am J Hosp Pharm*, 40, 1152 (1983)

5730 Southgate HJ, Townsend J, Barron J. Cherubism: biochemistry and response to treatment with the diphosphonate etidronate. *Proc ACB Natl Meet*, 67 (1995)

5731 Southworth W, Friday KJ, Ruffy R. Possible amiodarone-aprindine interaction. *Am Heart J*, 104, 323 (1982)

5732 Sowers JR, Sharp B, McCallum RW. Effect of domperidone, an extracerebral inhibitor of dopamine receptors, on thyrotropin, prolactin, renin, aldosterone, and 18-hydroxycorticosterone secretion in man. *J Clin Endocrinol Metab*, 54, 869-871 (1982)

5733 Spahn H, Mutschler E, Kirch W et al. Influence of ranitidine on plasma metoprolol and atenolol concentrations. *Br Med J*, 286, 1546-1547 (1983)

5734 Spahn H, Spahn I, Benet LZ. Probenecid-induced changes in the clearance of carprofen enantiomers: a preliminary study. *Clin Pharmacol Ther*, 45, 500-505 (1989)

5735 Spandrio S, Sleiman I, Scalvini T et al. Lipoprotein(a) in thyroid dysfunction before and after treatment. *Horm Metab Res*, 25, 586-589 (1993)

5736 Speed BR, Spelman DW. Sialadenitis and systemic reaction associated with phenylbutazone. *Aust NZ J Med*, 12, 261-264 (1982)

5737 Speight TM, Avery GS. Pancuronium bromide: a review. *Drugs*, 4, 163 (1972)

5738 Speight TM, Avery GS. Pizotifen (BC-105): a review of its pharmacological properties and therapeutic efficacy in vascular headaches. *Drugs*, 3, 159 (1972)

5739 Spellacy WN, Buhi WC, Birk SA et al. Metabolic studies in woman taking norethindrone for 6 months time. *Fertil Steril*, 24, 419 (1973)

5740 Spellacy WN, Buhi WC, Birk SA et al. Studies of ethynodiol diacetate and mestranol on blood glucose and plasma insulin. *Contraception*, 3, 185 (1971)

5741 Spellacy WN, Ellingson AB, Kotlik A et al. Plasma insulin and glucose levels in women using a levonorgestrel-containing triphasic oral contraceptive for 3 months. *Contraception*, 38, 27-35 (1988)

5742 Spellacy WN, McLeod AG, Buhi WC et al. The effect of medroxyprogesterone acetate on carbohydrate metabolism: measurements of glucose, insulin. *Fertil Steril*, 23, 239 (1972)

5743 Spencer H, Kramer L, Osis D et al. Effects of aluminum hydroxide on fluoride and calcium metabolism. *J Environ Pathol Toxicol Oncol*, 6, 33-41 (1985)

5744 Sperber AD, Henkin Y, Zuili. The hypocholesterolemic effect of an antacid containing aluminum hydroxde. *Am J Med*, 91, 597-604 (1991)

5745 Spiers ASD, Galton DAG, Kaur J et al. Thioguanine as primary treatment for chronic granulocytic leukaemia. *Lancet*, 1, 829-832 (1975)

5746 Spigset O, Mjörndal T. The effect of fluvoxamine on serum prolactin and serum sodium concentrations: relation to platelet 5-HT_{2A} receptor status. *J Clin Psychopharmacol*, 17, 292-297 (1997)

5747 Spilker B, Watson BS, Woods JW. Drug interference with measurement of metanephrines in urine. *Ann Clin Lab Sci*, 13, 16-19 (1983)

5748 Spina E, Amendola D'Agostino AM, Ioculano MP et al. No effect of thioridazine on plasma concentrations of carbamazepine and its active metabolite carbamazepine-10,11-epoxide. *Ther Drug Monit*, 12, 511-513 (1990)

5749 Spina E, Avenoso A, Pollicino AM et al. Carbamazepine coadministration with fluoxetine or fluvoxamine. *Ther Drug Monit*, 15, 247-250 (1993)

5750 Spina E, Martines C, Fazio A et al. Effect of phenobarbital on the pharmacokinetics of carbamazepine-10, 11-epoxide, an active metabolite of carbamazepine. *Ther Drug Monit*, 13, 109-112 (1991)

5751 Spina E, Pollicino AM, Avenoso A et al. Effect of fluvoxamine on the pharmacokinetics of imipramine and desipramine in healthy subjects. *Ther Drug Monit*, 15, 243-246 (1993)

5752 Spino M, Sellers EM, Kaplan HL et al. Adverse biochemical and clinical consequences of furosemide administration. *Can Med Ass J*, 118, 1513-1518 (1978)

5753 Spittle CR. Atherosclerosis and vitamin C. *Lancet*, 2, 1280 (1971)

5754 Spitz IM, Bardin CW. Clinical pharmacology of RU 486 - an antiprogestin and antiglucocorticoid. *Contraception*, 48, 403-444 (1993)

5755 Spitz IM, Bardin CW. Drug therapy: mifepristone (RU 486) - a modulator of progestin and glucocorticoid action. *N Engl J Med*, 329, 404-412 (1993)

5756 Spragg J, Weinblatt ME, Coblyn J et al. Effect of cyclosporine on urinary kallikrein excretion in patients with rheumatoid arthritis. *J Lab Clin Med*, 112, 324-332 (1988)

5757 Sprecher DL, Harris BV, Goldberg AC et al. Efficacy of psyllium in reducing serum cholesterol levels in hypercholesterolemic patients on high- or low-fat diets. *Ann Intern Med*, 119, 545-554 (1993)

5758 Spreux-Varoquaux O, Gailledreau J, Vanier B, et al. Initial increase of plasma serotonin: a biological predictor for the antidepressant response to clomipramine. *Biol Psychiat*, 40, 465-473 (1996)

5759 Squires JE, Mintz PD, Clark S. Tolmetin-induced hemolysis. *Transfusion*, 25, 410-413 (1985)

5760 Srauss JS, Rapini RP, Shalita AR et al. Isotretinoin therapy for acne. Results of a multicenter dose response study. *J Am Acad Dermatol*, 10, 490-496 (1984)

5761 Srinivasan G, Singh J, Cattamanchi G et al. Plasma glucose changes in preterm infants during oral theophylline therapy. *J Pediatr*, 103, 473-475 (1983)

5762 Srinivasan SR, Dahlen GH, Jarpa RA et al. Racial (black-white) differences in serum lipoprotein(a) distribution and its relation to parental myocardial infarction in children. *Circulation*, 84, 160-167 (1991)

5763 Sritharan V, Bharadwaj VP, Venkatesan K et al. Dapsone induced hypohaptoglobinemia in lepromatous leprosy patients. *Int J Lepr Other Mycobact Dis*, 49, 307-310 (1981)

5764 Stadtmauer EA, Cassileth PA, Edelstein M et al. Danazol treatment of myelodysplastic syndromes. *Br J Haematol*, 77, 502-509 (1991)

5765 Staessen J, Fiocchi R, Bouillon R et al. Differential responses of plasma aldosterone, cortisol and adrenocorticotropin to two dopamine receptor antagonists. *Meth Fund Exp Clin Pharmacol*, 7, 523-527 (1985)

5766 Stafford BT, Crosby WH. Late onset of gold-induced thrombocytopenia: with a practical note on the injections of dimercaprol. *J Am Med Ass*, 239, 50-51 (1978)

5767 Staib AH, Harder S, Fuhr U et al. Interaction of quinolones with the theophylline metabolism in man: investigations with lomefloxacin and pipemidic acid. *Int J Clin Pharmacol Ther Toxicol*, 27, 289-293 (1989)

5768 Staiger CH, Steger W, Widmann L et al. Double-blind, controlled clinical trial to evaluate the antihypertensive effect of carvedilol in elderly patients with mild to moderate hypertension. *Drugs*, 36, Suppl 6, 169-171 (1988)

5769 Stalla GK, Brockmeier SJ, Renner U et al. Octreotide exerts different effects in vivo and in vitro in Cushing's disease. *Eur J Endocrinol*, 130, 126-131 (1994)

5770 Standefer J, Blackwell W. Enzymatic method for measuring ethylene glycol with a centrifugal analyzer. *Clin Chem*, 37, 1734-1736 (1991)

5771 Stanek B, Renner F, Sedlmayer A et al. Effect of captopril on renin and blood pressure in cirrhosis. *Eur J Clin Pharmacol*, 33, 249-254 (1988)

5772 Stanley AJ, Bouchier IAD, Hayes PC. Acute effect of propranolol and isosorbide-5-mononitrate administration on renal blood flow in cirrhotic patients. *Gut*, 42, 283-287 (!998)

5773 Stanton MF, Lowenstein FW. Serum magnesium in women during pregnancy, while taking oral contraceptives and after menopause. *J Am Coll Nutr*, 6, 313-319 (1987)

5774 Stapleton FB, Nelson B, Vats TS et al. Hypokalemia associated with antibiotic treatment: evidence in children with malignant neoplasms. *Am J Dis Child*, 130, 1104-1108 (1976)

5775 Starkey BJ, Loscombe SM, Smith JM. Paracetamol (acetaminophen) analysis by high performance liquid chromatography: interference studies and comparison with an enzymatic procedure. *Ther Drug Monit*, 8, 78-84 (1986)

5776 Starzl TE, Fung J, Jordan M et al. Kidney transplantation under FK 506. *J Am Med Ass*, 264, 63-67 (1990)

5777 Starzl TE, Putnam CW, Halgrimson CG et al. Cyclophosphamide and whole organ transplantation in human beings. *Surg Gynecol Obstet*, 133, 981 (1971)

5778 Staub JJ, Jenkins JS, Ratcliffe JG et al. Comparison of corticotrophin and corticosteroid response to lysine vasopressin, insulin and pyrogen in man. *Br Med J*, 1, 267 (1973)

5779 Staubli M, Studer H. Amiodarone-treated patients with suppressed TSH test at risk of thyrotoxicosis. *Klin Wschr*, 63, 168-175 (1985)

5780 Steegers-Theunissen RPM, Boers GHJ, Steegers EAP, et al. Effect of sub-50 oral contraceptives on homocysteine metabolism: a preliminary study. *Contraception*, 45, 129-139 (1992)

5781 Steele TH. Control of uric acid excretion. *N Engl J Med*, 284, 1193 (1971)

5782 Steele TH. Dissociation of zinc excretion from other cations in man. *J Lab Clin Med*, 81, 205 (1973)

5783 Steele TH, Oppenheimer S. Factors affecting urate excretion following diuretic administration in man. *Am J Med*, 47, 564 (1969)

5784 Steer PL, Marks MI, Klite PD et al. 5-fluorocytosine: an oral antifungal agent. *Ann Intern Med*, 76, 15 (1972)

5785 Stegeman CA, Dullaart RPF, Meijer S et al. Acute renal effects of somatostatin analogue, octreotide, in insulin-dependent diabetic patients: antagonism by low dose glucagon. *Diab Nutr Metab*, 6, 87-95 (1993)

5786 Stegink LD, Filer LJ Jr, Baker GL. Repeated ingestion of aspartame-sweetened beverage: effect on plasma amino acid concentrations in normal adults. *Metabolism*, 37, 246-251 (1988)

5787 Stegink LD, Filer LJ Jr, Bell EF et al. Effect of repeated ingestion of aspartame-sweetened beverage on plasma amino acid, blood methanol, and blood formate concentrations in normal adults. *Metabolism*, 38, 357-363 (1989)

5788 Stehouwer CDA, Lems WF, Fischer HRA et al. Aggravation of hypoglycemia in insulinoma patients by the long-acting somatostatin analogue octreotide (sandostatin). *Acta Endocrinol*, 121, 34-40 (1989)

5789 Stehr-Green JK, Helmick CG. Pentamidine and renal toxicity. *N Engl J Med*, 313, 694-695 (1985)

5790 Stehr-Green PA, Naylor PH, Hoffman RE. Diminished thymosin-α_1 levels in persons exposed to 2,3,7,8-tetrachlorodibenzo-p-dioxin. *J Toxicol Environ Health*, 28, 285-295 (1989)

5791 Steiger A, Benkert O, Holsboer F. Effects of long-term treatment with the MAO-A inhibitor moclobemide on sleep EEG and nocturnal hormonal secretion in normal men. *Neuropsychobiology*, 30, 101-105 (1994)

5792 Steiger A, Benkert O, Wohrmann S et al. Effects of trimipramine on sleep EEG, penile tumescence and nocturnal hormone secretion. A long-term study in 3 normal controls. *Neuropsychobiology*, 21, 71-75 (1989)

5793 Steiger U, Cotting J, Reichen J. Albendazole treatment of echinococcosis in humans: effects on microsomal metabolism and drug tolerance. *Clin Pharmacol Ther*, 47, 347-353 (1990)

5794 Steimetz A, Bauer K, Jurgensen R et al. Low-dose oral contraceptives lower plasma levels of apolipoprotein E. *Eur J Obstet Gynecol Reprod Biol*, 37, 155-162 (1990)

5795 Steimetz J, Choukaife A, Visvikis S et al. Biological factors affecting concentrations of serum LpA-I lipoprotein particles in serum, and determination of reference limits. *Clin Chem*, 36, 677-679 (1990)

5796 Stein EA, Lane M, Laskarzweski P. Comparison of statins in hypertriglyceridemia. *Am J Cardiol*, 81, 66B-69B (1998)

5797 Stein GH, Matthews K, Bannatyne RE et al. Long-term lipid profiles with isradipine and hydrochlorothiazide treatment in elderly hypertensive patients. *J Cardiovasc Pharmacol*, 15, Suppl, S90-S92 (1990)

5798 Stein HB, Hasan A, Fox IH. Ascorbic acid-induced uricosuria. *Ann Intern Med*, 84, 385-388 (1976)

5799 Stein HD, Keiser HR, Sjoerdsma A. Proline hydroxylase activity in human blood. *Lancet*, 1, 106 (1970)

5800 Stein JH, Rosenson RS. Treatment of severe hypertriglyceridemia lowers plasma viscosity. *Atherosclerosis*, 137, 401-405 (1998)

5801 Stein RS, Howard CL. Clinical assessment of cimetidine myelotoxicity. *South Med J*, 73, 293-297 (1981)

5802 Steinbach G, Pflieger H, Maier V. Falsely increased values for serum creatinine during therapy with cefoxitin. *Clin Chem*, 29, 1700-1701 (1983)

5803 Steinberg WM, King CE, Toskes PP. Malabsorption of protein-bound cobalamin but not unbound cobalamin during cimetidine administration. *Dig Dis Sci*, 25, 188-192 (1980)

5804 Steinbrecher UP, Mishkin S. Sulfamethoxazole-induced hepatic injury. *Dig Dis Sci*, 26, 756-759 (1981)

5805 Steiner J, Cassar J, Mashiter K et al. Effects of methyldopa on prolactin and growth hormone. *Br Med J*, 1, 1186-1188 (1976)

5806 Steingo L, Altona B, Anderson GW et al. Epidemiology of hyperlipidemia and the efficacy of pravastatin therapy. *Curr Ther Res*, 54, 290-299 (1993)

5807 Steinmetz J, Choukaife A, Visvikis S et al. Biological factors affecting concentrations of serum LpAI lipoprotein particles in serum, and determination of reference limits. *Clin Chem*, 36, 677-680 (1990)

5808 Stella L, Crescenti A, Pontiroli AE et al. Enflurane anesthesia affects serum prolactin levels in man. *IRCS Med Sci*, 12, 572 (1984)

5809 Stempel DA, Miller JJ III. Lymphopenia and hepatic toxicity with ibuprofen. *J Pediatr*, 90, 657-658 (1977)

5810 Stepan J, Wilczek H, Justova V et al. Plasma 25-hydroxycholecalciferol in oral sulfonylurea treated diabetes mellitus. *Horm Metab Res*, 14, 98-100 (1982)

5811 Stephensen CB, Alvarez JO, Kohatsu J et al. Vitamin A is excreted in the urine during acute infection. *Am J Clin Nutr*, 60, 388-392 (1994)

5812 Stermer E, Tabak M, Potasman I, et al. Effect of ranitidine on the urea breath test: a controlled trial. *J Clin Gastroenterol*, 25, 323-327 (1997)

5813 Sterndorff B, Johansen P. The antihypertensive effect of pinacidil versus prazosin in mild to moderate hypertensive patients seen in general practice. *Acta Med Scand*, 224, 329-336 (1988)

5814 Sternlieb P, Robinson RM. Stevens-Johnson syndrome plus toxic hepatitis due to ibuprofen. *NY State J Med*, 1239-1243 (1978)

5815 Stevens DA. Miconazole in the treatment of coccidioidomycosis. *Drugs*, 26, 347-354 (1983)

5816 Stevens DA. Miconazole in the treatment of systemic fungal infections. *Am Rev Resp Dis*, 116, 801-806 (1977)

5817 Stevens VC, Goldzieher JW, Vorys N. Effect of mestranol and chlormadinone acetate on urinary excretion of FSH and LH. *Am J Obstet Gynecol*, 102, 95 (1968)

5818 Stevens WC, Eger EL, Joas TA et al. Comparative toxicity of isoflurane, halothane, fluroxene, and diethyl ether in human volunteers. *Can J Anaes*, 20, 357 (1973)

5819 Stevenson HP, Archibold GPR, Johnston P, et al. Misleading serum free thyroxine results during low molecular weight heparin treatment. *Clin Chem*, 44, 1002-1007 (1998)

5820 Stevenson IH, Browning M, Crooks J et al. Changes in human drug metabolism after long-term exposure to hypnotics. *Br Med J*, 4, 322-324 (1972)

5821 Stewart AF, Keating T, Schwartz PE. Magnesium homeostasis following chemotherapy with cisplatin: a prospective study. *Am J Obstet Gynecol*, 153, 660-665 (1985)

5822 Stewart CF, Arbuck CG, Fleming RA et al. Relation of systemic exposure to unbound etoposide and haematologic toxicity. *Clin Pharmacol Ther*, 50, 385-393 (1991)

5823 Stewart GW, Peart WS, Boylston AW. Obstructive jaundice, pancytopenia and hydralazine. *Lancet*, 1, 1207 (1981)

5824 Stewart MJ, Simpson E. Prognosis in paracetamol self-poisoning: the use of plasma paracetamol concentration in a region. *Ann Clin Biochem*, 10, 173 (1973)

5825 Stichtenoth DO, Fauler J, Zeidler H et al. Urinary nitrate excretion in patients with rheumatoid arthritis and reduced by prednisolone. *Ann Rheum Dis*, 54, 820-824 (1995)

5826 Stichtenoth DO, Tsikas D, Gutzki E-M, Frölich JC. Effects of ketoprofen and ibuprofen on platelet aggregation and prostanoid formation in man. *Eur J Clin Pharmacol*, 51, 231-234 (1996)

5827 Stiehl A, Rudolph G, Raedsch R et al, et al. Ursodeoxycholic acid-induced changes of plasma and urinary bile acids in patients with primary biliary cirrhosis. *Hepatology*, 12, 492-497 (1990)

5828 Stjernholm MR, Katz FH. Effects of diphenylhydantoin, phenobarbital and diazepam on the metabolism of methylprednisolone and its sodium succinate. *J Clin Endocrinol Metab*, 41, 887-893 (1975)

5829 Stoa-Birketvedt G, Waldum HL, Vonen B, Florholmen J. Effect of cimetidine on basal and postprandial plasma concentrations of cholecystokinin and gastrin in humans. *Acta Physiol Scand*, 159, 321-325 (1997)

5830 Stocigt JR, Lim C-F, Barlow JW et al. High concentrations of furosemide inhibit serum binding of thyroxine. *J Clin Endocrinol Metab*, 59, 62-66 (1984)

5831 Stoehr GP. The effect of low-dose estrogen-containing oral contraceptives on the pharmacokinetics of triazolam, alprazolam, temazepam and lorazepam. *Drug Intell Clin Pharm*, 18, 495 (1984)

5832 Stoffer SS, Hynes KM, Jiang N et al. The effects of chronic digoxin administration of serum estrogen, serum luteinizing hormone. *Clin Res*, 20, 720 (1972)

5833 Stone MC. Idiopathic hyperglyceridaemia treated with methyltestosterone and methandienone. *Lancet*, 1, 477 (1963)

5834 Stone NN, Clejan SJ. Response of prostate volume, prostate-specific antigen, and testosterone to flutamide in men with benign prostatic hyperplasia. *J Androl*, 12, 376-380 (1991)

5835 Stone SP, Goodwin RM. Dapsone-induced jaundice. *Arch Dermatol*, 114, 947 (1978)

5836 Storm G, OOsterhuis B, Sollie FAE et al. Lack of pharmacokinetic interaction between vinpocetine and oxazepam. *Br J Clin Pharmacol*, 38, 143-146 (1994)

5837 Storm T, Thamsborg G, Steiniche T et al. Effect of intermittent cyclical etridonate therapy on bone mass and fracture rate in women with postmenopausal osteoporosis. *N Engl J Med*, 322, 1265-1271 (1990)

5838 Storm-Mathisen H. Discussion. In:. *Catapres® in Hypertension. ME Conolly (ed)*, London, Butterworth (1970)

5839 Storrow AB, Hernandez AV, Norton JA. Nalmefene and the urine opiate screen. *Clin Chem*, 44, 346-348 (1998)

5840 Stote RM, Smith LH, Wilson DM et al. Hydrochlorothiazide effects on serum calcium and immuno-active parathyroid hormone concentrations. *Ann Intern Med*, 77, 587 (1972)

5841 Stovner J, Theodorsen L, Bjelke E. Sensitivity to dimethyltubocurarine and toxiferine with special reference to serum proteins. *Br J Anaes*, 44, 374 (1972)

5842 Stowell A, Johnsen J, Ripel A et al. Disulfiram-induced acetonemia. *Lancet*, 1, 882-883 (1983)

5843 Straughn AB, Henderson RP, Lieberman PL et al. Effect of rifampin on theophylline disposition. *Ther Drug Monit*, 6, 153-156 (1984)

5844 Straus SE, Dale JK, Tobi M et al. Acyclovir treatment of the chronic fatigue syndrome: lack of efficacy in a placebo-controlled trial. *N Engl J Med*, 319, 1692-1698 (1988)

5845 Stricker BHC, Meyboom RHB, Bleeker PA. Blood disorders associated with pirenzepine. *Br Med J*, 293, 1074 (1986)

5846 Stricker BHC, Oei TT. Agranulocytosis caused by spironolactone. *Br Med J*, 289, 731 (1984)

5847 Strickland D, Sprafka JM, Luepker RV et al. Association of antihypertensive agents and blood lipids in a population-based survey. *Epidemiology*, 5, 96-101 (1994)

5848 Stringer KA, Switzer DF, Abadier R et al. The effect of pirmenol administration on the anti-coagulant activity of warfarin. *J Clin Pharmacol*, 31, 607-610 (1991)

5849 Stringer MD, Steadman CA, Kakkar VV. Gemfibrozil in hyperlipidemic patients with peripheral arterial disease: some undiscovered actions. *Curr Med Res Opin*, 12, 207-214 (1990)

5850 Strom BL, Carson JL, Schinnar R, Shaw M. Is cimetidine associated with neutropenia?. *Am J Med*, 99, 282-290 (1995)

5851 Stromberg A, Wengle B. Chronic active hepatitis induced by nitrofurantoin. *Br Med J*, 2, 174 (1976)

5852 Strunge P, Engby B, Schmidt E et al. Variation of serum lipids in postmyocardial infarction patients treated with verapamil or placebo. *Acta Med Scand*, 215, Supl 681, 53-57 (1984)

5853 Stubbs WA, Delitala G, Besser GM et al. The endocrine and metabolic effects of cimetidine. *Clin Endocrinol*, 18, 167-178 (1983)

5854 Stumvoll M, Nurjhan N, Perriello G et al. Metabolic effects of metformin in non-insulin-dependent diabetes mellitus. *N Engl J Med*, 333, 550-554 (1995)

5855 Stuyt PMJ, Mol MJTM, Stalenhoef AFH. Long-term effects of simvastatin in familial dysbetalipoproteinaemia. *J Intern Med*, 230, 151-155 (1991)

5856 Stuyt PMJ, Mol MJTM, Stalenhoef AFH et al. Simvastatin in the effective reduction of plasma lipoprotein levels in familial dysbetalipoproteinemia (type III hyperlipoproteinemia). *Am J Med*, 88, 42N-45N (1990)

5857 Sudhop T, Lutjohann, Ratman C, et al. Differences in the response of serum lipoproteins to fenofibrate between women and men with primary hypercholesterolemia. *Eur J Clin Pharmacol*, 50, 365-369 (1996)

5858 Suikkari A-M, Tiitinen A, Stenman U-H et al. Oral contraceptives increase insulin-like growth factor binding protein-1 concentration in women with polycystic ovarian disease. *Fertil Steril*, 55, 895-899 (1991)

5859 Suki WN, Dawoud F, Eknoyan G et al. Effects of metolazone on renal function in normal man. *J Clin Pharmacol Exp Ther*, 180, 6 (1972)

5860 Sullivan KM, Small RE, Rock WL et al. Effects of cimetidine or ranitidine on the pharmacokinetics of flurbiprofen. *Clin Pharmacol*, 5, 586-589 (1986)

5861 Sullivan PA, Cervenka J, O'Connor DT et al. Fosinopril, an angiotensin-converting enzyme inhibitor, and propranolol: comparative effects at rest and exercise on blood pressure, hormonal variables, and plasma potassium in essential hypertension. *Cardiovasc Drug Ther*, 3, 57-62 (1989)

5862 Summers WK, Tachiki KH, Kling A. Tacrine in the treatment of Alzheimer's disease. A clinical update and recent pharmacologic studies. *Eur Neurol*, 29, Suppl 3, 28-32 (1989)

5863 Summerskill WHJ, Thorsell F, Feinberg JH et al. Effects of urease inhibition in hyperammonemia: clinical and experimental studies. *Gastroenterology*, 54, 20 (1968)

5864 Sun DCH. Iatrogenic gastrointestinal diseases in the aged. *Geriatrics*, 27, 89 (1972)

5865 Sundal E, Bertelletti D. Thymopentin treatment of rheumatoid arthritis. *Arz Forsch Drug Res*, 44, 1145-1149 (1994)

5866 Sundberg L. Interferences in nickel determinations by atomic absorption spectrometry. *Anal Chem*, 45, 1460 (1973)

5867 Sunderman FW. The chemical measurement of magnesium in biological fluids. *Proficiency Test Service*, 6 (1972)

5868 Sunderman FW. Uric acid in biological fluids. *Proficiency Test Service*, 2, May (1972)

5869 Sunderman FW Jr. Drug interference in clinical biochemistry. *Crit Rev Clin Lab Sci*, 1, 427 (1970)

5870 Sunderman FW Jr. Effects of drugs upon hematological tests. *Ann Clin Lab Sci*, 2, 1 (1972)

5871 Sunderman FW Jr. Measurements of vanilmandelic acid for the diagnosis of pheochromocytoma and neuroblastoma. *Am J Clin Pathol*, 42, 481 (1964)

5872 Sungur C, Akpolat T, Ozdemir O et al. Hematologic profile of dialysis patients receiving α-interferon and erythropoietin concomitantly. *Nephron*, 67, 499 (1994)

5873 Supergen , Inc. Manufacturer's literature on Nipent® . Emeryville, CA 94608 (1994)

5874 Superko HR, Krauss RM, DiRicco C. Effect of fluvastatin on low-density lipoprotein peak particle diameter. *Am J Cardiol*, 80, 78-81 (1997)

5875 Supparatpinyo K, Perriens J, Nelson KE, Sirisanthana T. A controlled trial of itraconazole to prevent relapse of penicillium marnefei infection in patients infected with the human immunodeficiency virus. *N Engl J Med*, 339, 1739-1743 (1998)

5876 Surka MI, DeFesi CR. Normal serum free thyroid hormone concentrations in patients treated with phenytoin or carbamazepine. *J Am Med Ass*, 275, 1495-1498 (1996)

5877 Surtees R, Hyland K. L-3,4-dihydroxyphenylalanine (levodopa) lowers central nervous system S-adenosylmethionine concentrations in humans. *J Neurol Neurosurg Psychiatry*, 53, 569-572 (1990)

5878 Sussman NW, McLain LW Jr. A direct hepatotoxic effect of valproic acid. *J Am Med Ass*, 242, 1173-1174 (1979)

5879 Sutfin T, Balmer K, Bostrom H et al. Stereoselective interaction of omeprazole with warfarin in healthy men. *Ther Drug Monit*, 11, 176-184 (1989)

5880 Sutherland DL, Remillard AJ, Haight KR et al. The influence of cimetidine versus ranitidine on doxepin pharmacokinetics. *Eur J Clin Pharmacol*, 32, 159-164 (1987)

5881 Sutor AH. Thrombocyturia after aspirin. *N Engl J Med*, 288, 794 (1973)

5882 Sutton RAL, Walker VR, Halabe A et al. Chronic hypomagnesemia caused by cisplatin: effect of calcitriol. *J Lab Clin Med*, 117, 40-43 (1991)

5883 Suzuki H, Noguchi K, Nakahata M et al. Effect of iopanoic acid on the pituitary-thyroid axis: time sequence of changes in serum iodothyronines, thyrotropin, and prolactin concentrations and responses to thyroid hormones. *J Clin Endocrinol Metab*, 53, 779-783 (1981)

5884 Suzuki H, Yamazaki N, Suzuki Y et al. Lowering effect of diphenylhydantoin on serum free thyroxine and thyroxine binding globulin (TBG). *Acta Endocrinol*, 105, 477-481 (1984)

5885 Suzuki T, Koizumi J, Moroji T et al. Effects of long-term anticonvulsant therapy on copper, zinc, and magnesium in hair and serum of epileptics. *Biol Psychiat*, 31, 571-581 (1992)

5886 Svedhem A. Toxic hepatitis following ketoconazole treatment. *Scand J Infect Dis*, 16, 123-125 (1984)

5887 Svendsen TL, Kristensen MB, Hansen JM et al. The influence of disulfiram on the half-life and metabolic clearance rate of diphenylhydantoin and tolbutamide in man. *Eur J Clin Pharmacol*, 9, 439-441 (1976)

5888 Svendsen TL, Tango M, Waldorff S et al. Effects of propranolol and pindolol on plasma lignocaine clearance in man. *Br J Clin Pharmacol*, 13, Suppl 2, 223S-226S (1982)

5889 Svendsen UG, Gerstoft J, Hansen TM et al. The renal excretion of prostaglandins and changes in plasma renin during treatment with sulindac or naproxen in patients with rheumatoid arthritis and thiazide treated heart failure. *J Rheumatol*, 11, 779-782 (1984)

5890 Svensson J, Ohlsson C, Jansson J-O, et al. Treatment with the oral growth hormone secretagogue MK-677 increases markers of bone formation and bone resorption in obese young males. *J Bone Miner Res*, 13, 1158-1166 (1998)

5891 Svenstrup B, Herrstedt J, Brunner et al. Sex hormone levels in postmenopausal women with advanced metastatic breast cancer treated with CGS 169 49A. *Eur J Cancer*, 30A, 1254-1258 (1994)

5892 Swaiman KF, Flagler DG. Mercury poisoning with central and peripheral nervous system involvement treated with penicillamine. *Pediatrics*, 48, 639 (1971)

5893 Swainson CP, Walker RJ, Bailey RR. Effects of cilazapril on renal function and hormones in hypertensive patients with renal disease. *Am J Med*, 87, Suppl B, 83S-87S (1989)

5894 Swann AC, Koslow SH, Katz MM et al. Lithium carbonate treatment of mania: cerebrospinal fluid and urinary monoamine metabolites and treatment outcome. *Arch Gen Psychiat*, 44, 345-354 (1987)

5895 Swanson S, Mifflin TE, Boyd JC. Methotrexate interferes with determinations of conjugated bilirubin with the Kodak Ektachem® 400. *Clin Chem*, 32, 863-864 (1986)

5896 Swaroop S, Krant MJ. Rapid estrogen-induced hypercalcemia. *J Am Med Ass*, 223, 913 (1973)

5897 Swart S, O'Malley BP, Vora J et al. The effect of dopaminergic blockade on serum TSH and prolactin levels in thyrotoxicosis. *Acta Endocrinol*, 106, 330-335 (1984)

5898 Swartz SL. Endocrine and vascular responses in hypertensive patients to long-term treatment with diltiazem. *J Cardiovasc Pharmacol*, 9, 391-395 (1987)

5899 Sweeney GD, Saunders SJ, Dowdle E et al. The effects of chloroquine on patients with cutaneous porphyria of the 'symptomatic' type. *Br Med J*, 1, 1281 (1965)

5900 Swidler G. Handbook of Drug Interactions. New York NY, Wiley-Interscience (1971)

5901 Swinkels LMJW, Meulenberg PMM, Ross HA et al. Salivary and plasma free testosterone and androstenedione levels in women using oral contraceptives containing desogestrel or levonorgestrel. *Ann Clin Biochem*, 25, 354-359 (1988)

5902 Swislocki ALM, Hoffman BB, Sheu WH-H et al. Effect of prazosin treatment on carbohydrate and lipoprotein metabolism in patients with hypertension. *Am J Med*, 86, Suppl 1B, 14-18 (1989)

5903 Swislocki ALM, Vestal RE, Reaven GM et al. Acute metabolic effects of clonidine and adenosine in man. *Horm Metab Res*, 25, 90-95 (1993)

5904 Sylvester ECJ, Price CP, Burrin JM. Investigation of the potential for interference with whole blood glucose strips. *Ann Clin Biochem*, 31, 94-96 (1994)

5905 Szamel I, Hindy I, Vineze B et al. Influence of toremifene on the endocrine regulation in breast cancer patients. *Eur J Cancer*, 30A, 154-158 (1994)

5906 Szlavy L, Repa I, Lengyel I et al. Calcium dobesilate (CLS 2210) protects the myocardium in early acute myocardial infarction: a preliminary randomized, double-blind, placebo-controlled study of its effects on biochemical markers. *J Cardiovasc Pharmacol*, 15, 89-95 (1990)

5907 Szollar LG, Meszaros I, Tornoci L et al. Effect of metoprolol and pindolol monotherapy on plasma lipid- and lipoprotein-cholesterol levels (including the HDL subclasses) in mild hypertensive males and females. *J Cardiovasc Pharmacol*, 15, 911-917 (1990)

5908 T Cell Diagnostics. Manufacturer's literature on Assays. Cambridge, MA (1991)

5909 T Cell Sciences. Manufacturer's literature on CELLFREE IL-2R Bead Assay Kit. Cambridge, MA 02139 (1990)

5910 Tabayashi K, Suzuki Y, Nagamine S et al. A clinical trial of allopurinol (zyloric) for myocardial protection. *J Thorac Cardiovasc Surg*, 101, 713-718 (1991)

5911 Tabei K, Furuya H, Asano Y et al. Effect of carteolol on renal function in healthy subjects and patients with hypertension. *Eur J Clin Pharmacol*, 36, 83-86 (1989)

5912 Taga M, Uemura T, Minaguchi H. The effect of hormone replacement therapy in postmenopausal women on urinary C-telopeptide and N-telopeptide of type I collagen, new markers of bone resorption. *J Endocrinol Invest*, 21, 154-159 (1998)

5913 Tagatz GE, McHugh RB. Oral contraceptives, a continuing reappraisal. *Postgrad Med*, 50, 121 (1971)

5914 Taggart HM, Applebaum-Bowden D, Haffner S et al. Reduction in high-density lipoproteins by anabolic steroid (stanozolol) therapy for postmenopausal osteoporosis. *Metabolism*, 31, 1147-1152 (1982)

5915 Taguma Y, Kitamoto Y, Futaki G et al. Effect of captopril on heavy proteinuria in azotemic diabetics. *N Engl J Med*, 313, 1617-1620 (1985)

5916 Tahara Y, Tanaka A, Ikegami H et al. Effects of the calcium antagonist nicardipine on glucose tolerance and secretion of insulin and glucagon in healthy men. *Curr Ther Res*, 43, 106-112 (1988)

5917 Tait RC, Walker ID, Conkie JA et al. Plasminogen levels in healthy volunteers - influence of age, sex, smoking and oral contraceptives. *Thromb Haemostas*, 68, 506-510 (1992)

5918 Takabatake T, Yamamoto Y, Nakamura S et al. Effect of the calcium antagonist nilvadipine on haemodynamics at rest and during cold stimulation in essential hypertension. *Eur J Clin Pharmacol*, 33, 215-219 (1987)

5919 Takabatke T, Ohta H, Maekawa M et al. Effects of long-term prazosin therapy on lipoprotein metabolism in hypertensive patients. *Am J Med*, 76, Suppl 2A, 113-116 (1984)

5920 Takahara K, Kuroiwa A, Matsushima T et al. Effects of nifedipine on platelet function. *Am Heart J*, 109, 4-8 (1985)

5921 Takahashi K, Abu Musa A, Nagata H et al. Serum CA-125 and 17β-estradiol in patients with external endometriosis on danazol. *Gynecol Obstet Invest*, 29, 301-304 (1990)

5922 Takahashi S, Shirahase Y, Watazu Y. The determination of sialic acid with use of N-acetyl-D-mannosamine dehydrogenase. *Abstracts*, 5th APCCB, Kobe (1991)

5923 Takahashi S, Yamamoto T, Moriwaki Y et al. Increased concentrations of serum Lp(a) lipoprotein in patients with primary gout. *Ann Rheum Dis*, 54, 90-93 (1995)

5924 Takamoto S, Onishi T, Morimoto S et al. Serum phosphate, parathyroid hormone and vitamin D metabolites in patients with chronic renal failure: effect of aluminum hydroxide administration. *Nephron*, 40, 286-291 (1985)

5925 Takasu N, Yamada T, Miura H et al. Rifampicin-induced early phase hyperglycemia in humans. *Am Rev Resp Dis*, 125, 23-27 (1982)

5926 Takeda M, Komeyama T, Tsutsu T et al. Changes in urinary excretion of endothelin-1-like immunoreactivity in patients with testicular cancer receiving high-dose cisplatin therapy. *Am J Kid Dis*, 24, 12-16 (1994)

5927 Takeda M, Komeyama T, Tsutsui T et al. Urinary endothelin-1-like immunoreactivity in young male patients with testicular cancer treated by cis-platinum: comparison with other urinary parameters. *Clin Sci*, 86, 703-707 (1994)

5928 Takishita S, Kawazoe N, Yoshida T. Ticlopidine and thrombocytopenia. *N Engl J Med*, 323, 1487 (1990)

5929 Takishita S, Muratani H, Tsuchihashi T et al. Effects of a new calcium channel blocker, nilvadipine, on the renin-angiotensin-aldosterone system in patients with essential hypertension. *Curr Ther Res*, 48, 417-426 (1990)

5930 Takiyyuddin MA, Baron AD, Cervenka JH et al. Suppression of chromogranin-A release from neuroendocrine sources in man: pharmacological studies. *J Clin Endocrinol*, 72, 616-622 (1991)

5931 Takiyyuddin MA, Cervenka JH, Dinh T et al. Selective α-blockade versus angiotensin-converting enzyme inhibition as initial antihypertensive therapy. *Am J Med*, 86, Suppl 1B, 32-35 (1989)

5932 Tal A, Dall L. Didanosine-induced hypertriglyceridemia. *Am J Med*, 95, 247 (1993)

5933 Talbot J, Beeley L. Fusidic acid and jaundice. *Br Med J*, 2, 308 (1980)

5934 Talmers FN, Telmos AJ. Procaine amide hydrochloride (Pronestyl®) induced agranulocytosis. *Mich Med*, 64, 655 (1965)

5935 Talner LB, Rushmer HN, Coel MN. The effect of renal artery injection of contrast material on urinary enzyme excretion. *Invest Radiol*, 7, 311 (1972)

5936 Tamai H, Takaichi Y, Morita T et al. Methimazole-induced agranulocytosis in Japanese patients with Graves' disease. *Clin Endocrinol*, 30, 525-530 (1989)

5937 Tamate K, Charleton M, Gosling JP, et al. Direct colorimetric monoclonal antibody enzyme immunoassay for estradiol-17β in saliva. *Clin Chem*, 43, 1159-1164 (1997)

5938 Tan F, Jackman H, Skidgel RA et al. Protamine inhibits plasma carboxypeptidase N, the inactivator of anaphylatoxins and kinins. *Anesthesiology*, 70, 267-275 (1989)

5939 Tan SY, Shapiro R, Franco R. Indomethacin-induced prostaglandin inhibition with hyperkalemia. *Ann Intern Med*, 90, 783-785 (1979)

5940 Tanaka H, Akama H, Ichikawa Y et al. Glucocorticoid receptors in normal leukocytes: effects of age, gender, season, and plasma cortisol concentrations. *Clin Chem*, 37, 1715-1719 (1991)

5941 Tang M, Gibson D, Sullivan M. Bacteriostatic saline flush interferes with sodium measurement on the Ektachem 700. *Clin Chem*, 39, 2032 (1993)

5942 Tannenberg AM, Wicher KJ, Rose NR. Ampicillin nephropathy. *J Am Med Ass*, 218, 449 (1971)

5943 Tanswell P, Tebbe U, Neuhaus K-L et al. Pharmacokinetics and fibrin specificity of alteplase during accelerated infusions in acute myocardial infarction. *J Am Coll Cardiol*, 19, 1071-1075 (1992)

5944 Tanyalcin T, Kutay F, Soydan I et al. Erythrocyte Na^+, K^+-ATPase activity does not predict therapeutic response to calcium antagonists in essential hypertension. *Clin Chem*, 40, 1532-1536 (1994)

5945 TAP Pharmaceuticals, Inc. Manufacturer's literature on Lupron® . Deerfield, IL 60015 (1996)

5946 TAP Pharmaceuticals, Inc. Manufacturer's literature on Prevacid® . Deerfield, IL 60015 (1996)

5947 Tapanainen J, Kauppila A, Metsa-Ketela T et al. Prostanoids and catecholamines after oral administration of natural progesterone. *Gynecol Endocrinol*, 3, 135-142 (1989)

5948 Tarallo P, Henny J, Fournier B et al. Plasma osteocalcin: biological variations and reference limits. *Scand J Clin Lab Invest*, 50, 649-655 (1990)

5949 Tarazi RC, Frohlich ED, Dustan HP. Plasma volume changes with long-term β-adrenergic blockade. *Am Heart J*, 82, 770 (1971)

5950 Tarssanen L, Huikko M, Rossi M. Amiloride-induced hyponatremia. *Acta Med Scand*, 208, 491-494 (1980)

5951 Tartini R, Kappenberger L, Steinbrunn W et al. Dangerous interaction between amiodarone and quinidine. *Lancet*, 1, 1327-1329 (1982)

5952 Tasaki K, Minami T, Ieiri I et al. Drug interactions of zonisamide with phenytoin and sodium valproate: serum concentrations and protein binding. *Brain Dev*, 17, 182-185 (1995)

5953 Tataranni G, Zavagli G, Farinelli R et al. Usefulness of the assessment of urinary enzymes and microproteins in monitoring ciclosporin nephrotoxicity. *Nephron*, 60, 314-318 (1992)

5954 Tatro DS. Effect of oral contraceptives on plasma minerals and protein. *Hosp Form Manage*, 6, 14 (1971)

5955 Tattersal MHN, Battershy G, Spiers ASD. Antibiotics and hypokalemia. *Lancet*, 1, 630 (1972)

5956 Tauber MT, Tauber JP, Vigoni F et al. Effect of the long-acting somatostatin analogue SMS 201-995 on growth rate and reduction of predicted adult height in ten tall adolescents. *Acta Paediat Scand*, 79, 176-181 (1990)

5957 Taubert HD, Haskins AL, Moszkowski EF. The influence of thioridazine upon urinary gonadotropin excretion. *South Med J*, 59, 1301 (1966)

5958 Tauxe WN, Mochizuki T, McCauley et al. A comparison of the renal effects (ERPF, GFR, and FF) of FK 506 and cyclosporine in patients with liver transplantation. *Transplant Proc*, 23, 3146-3147 (1991)

5959 Tavella M, Corder CN, McConathy W. Effect of gemfibrozil on fatty acids in lipid fractions of plasma from patients with hypertriglyceridemia. *J Clin Pharmacol*, 33, 35-39 (1993)

5960 Taves DR, Fry BW, Freeman RB et al. Toxicity following methoxyflurane anesthesia: fluoride concentration in nephrotoxicity. *J Am Med Ass*, 214, 91 (1970)

5961 Tawara M, Miwa I, Tsuchiya K et al. Clinical efficacy of pravastatin for hyperlipidemia in patients with type 2 diabetes mellitus. *Arz Forsch Drug Res*, 45, 704-708 (1995)

5962 Tawodzera PBP, Bell RMS, Jones JJ. Plasma zinc levels and corticotropin gel. *Lancet*, 1, 1072 (1972)

5963 Taylor DR, Constable J, Sonnekus M et al. Effect of indapamide on serum and red cell cations, with and without magnesium supplementation, in subjects with mild hypertension. *S Afr Med J*, 74, 273-276 (1988)

5964 Taylor G. Vitamin C deficiency. *Lancet*, 2, 1363 (1972)

5965 Taylor HL, Ata HM. Canthaxanthin: a cause of discolored plasma. *Med Lab Prodacol*, Aug, 20-21 (1988)

5966 Taylor JW, Alexander B, Lyon LW. A comparative evaluation of oral anticoagulant phenytoin interactions. *Drug Intell Clin Pharm*, 14, 669-673 (1980)

5967 Taylor JW, Alexander B, Lyon LW. Mathematical analysis of a phenytoin-disulfiram interaction. *Am J Hosp Pharm*, 38, 93-95 (1981)

5968 Taylor JW, Hendeles L, Weinberger M. The interaction of phenytoin and theophylline. *Drug Intell Clin Pharm*, 14, 638 (1980)

5969 Taylor SA, Rawlins MD, Smith SE. Spironolactone - a weak enzyme inducer in man. *J Pharmacokinet Pharmacol*, 24, 578 (1972)

5970 Taylor SH. Efficacy and safety of doxazosin in the treatment of patients with mild or moderate essential hypertension and elevated levels of cholesterol. *Am Heart J*, 121, II Suppl, 362-266 (1991)

5971 Taylor WH. Renal calculi and self-medication with multivitamin preparations containing vitamin D. *Clin Sci*, 42, 515 (1972)

5972 Tazuma S, Ohya T, Mizuno T et al. Effects of fluvastatin on human biliary lipids. *Am J Cardiol*, 76, 110A-113A (1995)

5973 Teasdale PR, Pearce J. Comparative and serial assays of folate metabolism in anticonvulsant treated epileptics. *J Clin Pathol*, 25, 721 (1972)

5974 Tedesco F, Markham R, Gurwith M et al. Oral vancomycin for antibiotic-associated pseudomembranous colitis. *Lancet*, 2, 226-228 (1978)

5975 Tedesco FJ, Mills LR. Diazepam (Valium®) hepatitis. *Dig Dis Sci*, 27, 470-471 (1982)

5976 Teerenhovi L, Heinonen E, Grohn P et al. High frequency of agranulocytosis in breast cancer patients treated with levamisole. *Lancet*, 2, 151-152 (1978)

5977 Telerman-Toppet N, Duret ME, Coers C. Cimetidine interaction with carbamazepine. *Ann Intern Med*, 94, 544 (1981)

5978 Telhag H. Safety and efficacy of piroxicam in the treatment of osteoarthrosis. *Eur J Rheumatol Inflamm*, 1, 352-355 (1978)

5979 Templeton JS. Azapropazone or allopurinol in the treatment of chronic gout and/or hyperuricemia. a preliminary report. *Br J Clin Pract*, 36, 353-358 (1982)

5980 Ten Holt WL, van Iperen CE, Schrijver G, Bartelink AKM. Severe hyponatremia during therapy with fluoxetine. *Arch Intern Med*, 156, 681-682 (1996)

5981 Ten Kate, RW, Tuynman HARE, Festen HPM et al. Effect of high dose omeprazole on gastric pepsin secretion and serum pepsinogen levels in man. *Eur J Clin Pharmacol*, 35, 173-176 (1988)

5982 Teramoto T, Goto Y, Kurokawa K et al. Clinical efficacy of fluvastatin for hyperlipidemia in Japanese patients. *Am J Cardiol*, 76, 33A-36A (1995)

5983 Terent A, Ribacke M, Carlson LA. Long-term effect of pindolol on lipids and lipoproteins in men with newly diagnosed hypertension. *Eur J Clin Pharmacol*, 36, 347-350 (1989)

5984 Terragna A, Spirito L. Porpora trombocitopenic in lattante dopo somministrazione di acido acetilsalicilico alla nutrice. *Minerva Pediatr*, 19, 613 (1967)

5985 Terrell CL, Hermans PE. Antifungal agents used for deep-seated mycotic infections. *Mayo Clin Proc*, 62, 1116-1128 (1987)

5986 Terruzzi V, Minoli G, Tadeo G et al. The influence of cimetidine and ranitidine of the plasma lipid pattern. *Br J Clin Pharmacol*, 19, 846-848 (1985)

5987 Terry SI. Transient dysaesthesiae and persistent leucocytosis after clioquinol therapy. *Br Med J*, 3, 745 (1971)

5988 Terzolo M, Panarelli M, Piovesan A et al. Ketoconazole treatment in Cushing's disease. Effect on the circadian profile of plasma ACTH and cortisol. *J Endocrinol Invest*, 11, 717-721 (1988)

5989 Testa R, Picciotto A, Bardellini E et al. Modifications in the serum concentrations of prolyl hydroxylase in patients with chronic hepatitis B during and after interferon therapy. *J Intern Med Res*, 18, 322-325 (1990)

5990 Testori GP, Frrari C, Lepore R et al. Effect of gemfibrozil treatment on glucose tolerance in hypertriglyceridemic patients with normal or impaired glucose tolerance. *Curr Ther Res*, 47, 390-395 (1990)

5991 Tevaarwerk GJM, Hurst CJ, Uksik P et al. Effect of insulin induced hypoglycemia on the serum concentrations of thyroxine, tri-iodothyronine and reverse tri-iodothyronine. *Can Med Ass J*, 20, 1090-1093 (1979)

5992 Tewksbury DA, Lohrenz FN. Circadian rhythm of human urinary amino acid excretion in fed and fasted states. *Metabolism*, 19, 363 (1970)

5993 The Liposome Company. Manufacturer's literature on Abelcet® . Princeton, NJ 08540 (1996)

5994 The long-term intervention with pravastatin in ischemic disease (LIPID) study group. Prevention of cardiovascular events and death with pravastatin in patients with coronary heart disease and a broad range of inyial cholesterol levels. *N Engl J Med*, 339, 1349-1347 (1998)

5995 The Purdue Frederick Company. Manufacturer's literature on Alferon® N Injection. Norwalk, CT 06850 (1990)

5996 The Purdue Frederick Company. Manufacturer's literature on Cardioquin® . Norwalk, CT 06850 (1995)

5997 The Purdue Frederick Company. Manufacturer's literature on Oxycontin™. Norwalk, CT 06850 (1996)

5998 The Purdue Frederick Company. Manufacturer's literature on Trilisate® . Norwalk, CT 06850 (1995)

5999 The Purdue Frederick Company. Manufacturer's literature on Uniphyl® . Norwalk, CT 06850 (1996)

6000 The US Multicenter FK 506 Liver Study Group. A comparison of tacrolimus (FK 506) and cyclosporine for immunosuppression in liver transplantation. *N Engl J Med*, 331, 1110-1115 (1994)

6001 Thenot A. Hydrochlorothiazide contre pancreas. *Presse Med*, 71, 572 (1963)

6002 Theroux P, Latour J-G, Diodati J et al. Hemodynamic, platelet and clinical responses to prostacyclin in unstable angina pectoris. *Am J Cardiol*, 65, 1084-1089 (1990)

6003 Thiery J, Creuzfeldt C, Creuzfeldt W et al. Effects of long-term treatment with simvastatin on plasma lipids and lipoproteins in patients with primary hypercholesterolemia. *Klin Wschr*, 68, 814-822 (1990)

6004 Thirlby RC, Richardson CT, Chew P et al. Effect of terbutaline, a β-adrenoreceptor agonist, on gastric acid secretion and serum gastrin concentrations in humans. *Gastroenterology*, 95, 913-919 (1988)

6005 Thomas AG, Holly JMP, Taylor F et al. Insulin like growth factor-I, insulin like growth factor binding protein-1, and insulin in childhood Crohn's disease. *Gut*, 34, 944-947 (1993)

6006 Thomas D, Gallus AS, Brooks PM et al. Thrombokinetics in patients with rheumatoid arthritis treated with D-penicillamine. *Ann Rheum Dis*, 43, 402-406 (1984)

6007 Thomas ME, Harris KPG, Ramaswamy C et al. Simvastatin therapy for hypercholesterolemic patients with nephrotic syndrome or significant proteinuria. *Kidney Int*, 44, 1124-1129 (1993)

6008 Thomas MK, Lloyd-Jones DM, Thadhani RI, et al. Hypovitaminosis D in medical inpatients. *N Engl J Med*, 338, 777-783 (1998)

6009 Thomas RW, Maddox RR. The interaction of spironolactone and digoxin: a review and evaluation. *Ther Drug Monit*, 3, 117-120 (1981)

6010 Thome-Kromer B, Michel G. Human cardiotropin I - detectability after myocrdial infarction and severe skeletal muscle damage. *Clin Chem*, 39, 1248 (1993)

6011 Thompson D, Banks R, Beyeler C et al. Alkaline phosphatase (total and bone isoenzyme) in female patients with rheumatoid arthritis. *Proc ACB Natl Meet*, 97 (1993)

6012 Thompson PD, Cullinane EM, Sady SP et al. Contrasting effects of testosterone and stanozolol on serum lipoprotein levels. *J Am Med Ass*, 261, 1165-1168 (1989)

6013 Thompson PD, Gadaleta PA, Yurgalevitch S et al. Effects of exercise and lovastatin on serum creatine kinase activity. *Metabolism*, 40, 1333-1336 (1991)

6014 Thompson PJ, Kemp MW, McAllister WAC et al. Angiotensin-converting enzyme: investigation of diurnal variation, the effect of a large dose of prednisolone, and prednisolone pharmacokinetics in patients with sarcoidosis. *Am Rev Resp Dis*, 134, 1075-1077 (1986)

6015 Thompson RHS, Wootton IDP (eds). Biochemical Disorders in Human Disease. *3rd edition*, New York NY, Academic Press (1971)

6016 Thomsen BS, From A, Jacobsen IA et al. Acute renal failure possibly associated with fenoprofen therapy. *Arth Rheum*, 26, 234-235 (1983)

6017 Thomsen K, Schou M. Renal lithium excretion in man. *Am J Physiol*, 215, 823-827 (1968)

6018 Thomsen O¿, Cortot A, Jewell D, et al. A comparison of budesonide and mesalamine for active Crohn's disease. *N Engl J Med*, 339, 370-374 (1998)

6019 Thomson AH, Thomson GD, Hepburn M et al. A clinically significant interaction between ciprofloxacin and theophylline. *Eur J Clin Pharmacol*, 33, 435-436 (1987)

6020 Thomson DJ, Menkis AG, McKenzie FN. Norfloxacin-cyclosporine interaction. *Transplantation*, 46, 312-313 (1988)

6021 Thornton GHM, Illingworth DG. An evaluation of the benzidine test for occult blood in the feces. *Gastroenterology*, 28, 593 (1955)

6022 Thrift CB. Acute salicylate intoxication: effect on the direct eosinophil count. *Illinois Med J*, 128, 39 (1965)

6023 Thronfeldt C, Cornell RC, Stoughton RB. The effect of alclometasone propionate cream 0.05% on the hypothalamic- pituitary-adrenal axis of normal volunteers. *J Intern Med Res*, 13, 276-280 (1985)

6024 Thurmann P, Odenthal H-J, Rietbrock N. Converting enzyme inhibition in coronary artery disease: a randomized, placebo-controlled trial with benazepril. *J Cardiovasc Pharmacol*, 17, 718-723 (1991)

6025 Tienhaara A, Remes K, Pelliniemi T-T. Alpha interferon raises serum β_2-microglobulin in patients with multiple myeloma. *Br J Haematol*, 77, 335-338 (1991)

6026 Tietz NW (ed). *Fundamentals of Clinical Chemistry*, Philadelphia PA, WB Saunders (1970)

6027 Tietz NW, Repique EV. Proposed standard method for measuring lipase activity in serum by a continuous sampling technique. *Clin Chem*, 19, 1268 (1973)

6028 Tiffany TO, Morton JM, Hall EM et al. Clinical evaluation of kinetic enzymatic fixed time and integral analysis of serum triglycerides. *Clin Chem*, 20, 476 (1974)

6029 Tigelaar RE, Rapport RL II, Inman JK et al. A radioimmunoassay for diphenylhydantoin. *Clin Chim Acta*, 43, 231 (1973)

6030 Tikkanen I, Fyhrquist F, Metsarinne K et al. Plasma atrial natriuretic peptide in cardiac disease and during infusion in healthy volunteers. *Lancet*, 2, 100-101 (1985)

6031 Tikkanen MJ, Bocanegra TS, Walker JF et al. Comparison of low dose simvastatin and gemfibrozil in the treatment of elevated plasma cholesterol. *Am J Med*, 87, Suppl 4A, 47S-53S (1989)

6032 Tikkanen MJ, Nikkila EA, Kuusi T. Effects of oestradiol and levonorgestrel on lipoprotein lipids and postheparin plasma lipase activities in normolipoproteinaemic women. *Acta Endocrinol*, 99, 630-635 (1982)

6033 Tikkanen MJ, Ojala J-P, Helve E. Lovastatin and gemfibrozil in the treatment of type 2a and type 2b hyperlipoprtoeinemia. *Eur J Clin Pharmacol*, 40, Suppl 1, S23-S25 (1991)

6034 Tilkemeier P, Thompson PD. Acute pancreatitis possibly related to enalapril. *N Engl J Med*, 318, 1275-1276 (1988)

6035 Tillman J, Leask JTS, Campbell J et al. Effect of fenoprofen on thyroid function tests. *Clin Chim Acta*, 161, 233-238 (1986)

6036 Tilstone WJ, Gray JMB, Nimmo-Smith RH et al. Interaction between warfarin and sulfamethoxazole. *Postgrad Med J*, 53, 388-390 (1977)

6037 Tilstone WJ, Semple PF, Lawson DH et al. Effects of furosemide on glomerular filtration rate and clearance of practolol, digoxin, cephaloridine, and gentamicin. *Clin Pharmacol Ther*, 22, 389-394 (1977)

6038 Timmer R, Koningsberger JC, Erkelens DW et al. No effect of the long-acting somatostatin analogue octreotide in patients with insulinoma. *Neth J Med*, 38, 199-203 (1991)

6039 Tishler M, Armon S. Nifedipine-induced hypokalemia. *Drug Intell Clin Pharm*, 20, 370-371 (1986)

6040 Tiula E, Neuvonen PJ. Antiepileptic drugs and α_1-acid glycoprotein. *N Engl J Med*, 307, 1148 (1982)

6041 Tjandra-Maga TB, van Hecken A, van Melle P et al. Altered pharmacokinetics of oral flecainide by cimetidine. *Br J Clin Pharmacol*, 22, 108-110 (1986)

6042 Tkach JR. Indomethacin-induced hyperglycemia in psoriatic arthritis. *J Am Acad Dermatol*, 7, 802 (1982)

6043 Tobias JH, Laversuch CV, Wilson N, Robins SP. Neridronate preferentially suppresses the urinary excretion of peptide-bound deoxypyridinoline in postmenopausal women. *Calcif Tissue Int*, 59, 407-409 (1996)

6044 Today's Drugs. Antihistamines, mechanism of action. *Br Med J*, 1, 642 (1962)

6045 Todorovic T, Jelic-Ivanovic Z, Petronijevic A et al. Effect of gentamycin on urinary excretion of some specific proteins. *Diag Lab*, 27, Suppl, 153 (1991)

6046 Tolis G. Long-term management of acromegaly with sandostatin. *Horm Res*, 29, 112-114 (1988)

6047 Tollefson G, Lesar T, Groethe D et al. Alprazolam-related digoxin toxicity. *Am J Psychol*, 141, 1612-1614 (1984)

6048 Tollefson GD, Godes M, Montague-Clouse J et al. Buspirone: effects on prolactin and growth hormone as a function of drug level in generalized anxiety. *J Clin Psychopharmacol*, 9, 132-136 (1989)

6049 Tomecki KJ, Catalano CJ. Dapsone hypersensitivity: the sulfone syndrome revisited. *Arch Dermatol*, 117, 38-39 (1981)

6050 Tomkin GH, Hadden DR, Weaver JA et al. Vitamin B_{12} status of patients on long term metformin therapy. *Br Med J*, 2, 685 (1971)

6051 Tomoda F, Takata M, Izumino K et al. Effects of erythropoietin treatment on thyroid dysfunction in hemodialysis patients with renal anemia. *Nephron*, 66, 307-311 (1994)

6052 Tomokuni K, Ogata M. Direct colorimetric determination of hippuric acid in urine. *Clin Chem*, 18, 349 (1972)

6053 Tomvall P, Walldius G. A comparison between nicotinic acid and acipimox in hypertriglyceridemia - effects on serum lipids, lipoproteins, glucose tolerance and tolerability. *J Intern Med*, 230, 415-421 (1991)

6054 Toon S, Davidson EM, Garstanh FM et al. The racemic metoprolol H_2-antagonist interaction. *Clin Pharmacol Ther*, 43, 283-289 (1988)

6055 Toone BK, Wheeler M, Fenwick PBC. Sex hormone changes in male epileptics. *Clin Endocrinol*, 12, 391-395 (1980)

6056 Torpy DJ, Jackson RV, Grice JE et al. Effect of flumazil on basal and naloxone-stimulated ACTH and cortisol release in humans. *Clin Exp Pharmacol Physiol*, 21, 157-161 (1994)

6057 Torrance JK. Diphosphoglycerate mutase assay: the effect of pyruvate, lactate dehydrogenase and thyroid hormone on the assay. *Clin Chim Acta*, 50, 103 (1974)

6058 Tortorice KL, Heim-Duthoy KL, Awni WM et al. The effects of calcium channel blockers on cyclosporine and its metabolites in renal transplant recipients. *Ther Drug Monit*, 12, 321-328 (1990)

6059 Totani Y, Niinomi M, Takatsuki K et al. Effect of metyrapone pretreatment on adrenocorticotropin secretion induced by corticotropin-releasing hormone in normal subjects and patients with Cushing's disease. *J Clin Endocrinol Metab*, 70, 798-803 (1990)

6060 Touloukian RJ, Downing SE. Cholestasis associated with long-term parenteral hyperalimentation. *Arch Surg*, 106, 58 (1973)

6061 Touminen HP, Svartling NE, Tikkanen IT, Asko-Seljavaara S. The effect of felodipine on endothelin-1 levels, peripheral vasoconstriction and flap survival during microvascular breast reconstruction. *Br J Plast Surg*, 59, 624-631 (1997)

6062 Toupance O, Lavaud S, Canivet E et al. Antihypertensive effect of amlodipine and lack of intereference with cyclosporine metabolism in renal transplant recipients. *Hypertension*, 24, 297-300 (1994)

6063 Tourtellotte WW, Reinglass JL, Newkirk TA. Cerebral dehydration action of glycerol. *Clin Pharmacol Ther*, 13, 159 (1972)

6064 Townend J, Doran J, Jones S et al. Effect of angiotensin converting enzyme inhibition on plasma endothelin in congestive heart failure. *Int J Cardiol*, 43, 299-304 (1994)

6065 Townsend MM, Smith AJ. Factors influencing the urinary excretion of free catecholamines in man. *Clin Sci*, 44, 253 (1973)

6066 Townsend R, Dipette DJ, Evans RR et al. Effects of calcium channel blockade on calcium homeostasis in mild to moderate hypertension. *Am J Med Sci*, 300, 133-137 (1990)

6067 Tozhillin SA, Gonda M, Carbonell G et al. Serum amylases and their inhibitors: 2, clinical and experimental observations - diet and steroid effects. *Am J Gastroenterol*, 77, 26-28 (1982)

6068 Traindl O et al. Cyclosporine A does not cause hyperlipidemia in kidney graft recipients. *Clin Transplant*, 5, 265 (1991)

6069 Trapnell CB, Narang PK, Li R, Lavelle JP. Increased plasma rifabutin levels with concomitant fluconazole therapy in HIV-infected patients. *Ann Intern Med*, 124, 573-576 (1996)

6070 Trapp OM, Beykirch MK, Petrides PE. Anagrelide for treatment of patients with chronic myelogenous leukemia and a high platelet count. *Blood Cells Mol Dis*, 24, 9-13 (1998)

6071 Trasoff A, Wohl MG, Mintz SS. Fatal agranulocytosis with autopsy following the use of thiouracil in a case of thyrotoxicosis. *Am J Med Sci*, 211, 62 (1946)

6072 Travis SF, Sugerman HJ, Ruberg RI et al. Alterations of red-cell glycolytic intermediates and oxygen transport as a consequence of hypophosphatemia. *N Engl J Med*, 285, 763 (1971)

6073 Trollfors B, Alestig K, Carlsten C et al. Unexpected side effects of cefuroxime lysine, new cefuroxine salt. *J Antimicrob Chemother*, 6, 558 (1983)

6074 Trollfors B, Alestig K, Krantz I et al. Quantitative nephrotoxicity of gentamicin in nontoxic doses. *J Infect Dis*, 141, 306-309 (1980)

6075 Troullos E, Hargreaves KM, Dionne RA. Ibuprofen elevates immunoreactive β-endorphin levels in humans during surgical stress. *Clin Pharmacol Ther*, 62, 74-81 (1997)

6076 Trunet PF, Bhatnagar AS, Chaudri HA, Hornberger U. Letrozole (CGS 20267), a new oral aromatase inhibitor for the treatment of advanced breast cancer in postmenopausal patients. *Acta Oncol*, 35, Suppl 5, 15-18 (1996)

6077 Trunet PF, Mueller P, Girard F et al. The effects of fadrozole hydrochloride on aldosterone secretion in healthy male subjects. *J Clin Endocrinol Metab*, 74, 571-576 (1992)

6078 Trybuchowski H. Effect of ampicillin on the urinary output of steroidal hormones in pregnant and nonpregnant women. *Clin Chim Acta*, 45, 9 (1973)

6079 Tryding N, Tufvesson G, Nilsson S. Serum monoamine-oxidase levels during levodopa therapy. *Lancet*, 1, 859 (1971)

6080 Tsao CS, Miyashita K. Effect of large intake of ascorbic acid on the urinary excretion of amino acids and related compounds. *IRCS Med Sci*, 13, 855-856 (1985)

6081 Tsatsakis AM, Psillakis ThK, Tzatzarakis M, et al. Carbamazepine levels in the hair of patients under long-term treatment: a preliminary study. *Clin Chim Acta*, 263, 187-195 (1997)

6082 Tsuchihashi T, Takishita S, Muratani H et al. Effect of single-administration captopril on plasma and urinary vasopressin in normotensive subjects and patients with essential hypertension and primary aldosteronism. *Jpn Circ J*, 53, 1473-1480 (1989)

6083 Tsuda Y, Satoh K, Kitadai M, Takahashi T. Effects of pravastatin sodium and simvastatin on plasma fibrinogen level and blood rheology in type II hyperlipproteinemia. *Atherosclerosis*, 122, 225-233 (1996)

6084 Tsuji H, Murai K, Akagi K et al. Effects of recombinant leukocyte interferon on ribonuclease activities in serum in chronic hepatitis B. *Clin Chem*, 36, 913-916 (1990)

6085 Tucci JR, Espiner EA, Jagger PI et al. Vasopressin in the evaluation of pituitary-adrenal function. *Ann Intern Med*, 69, 191 (1968)

6086 Tucker RM, Haq Y, Denning DW et al. Adverse events associated with itraconazole in 189 patients on chronic therapy. *J Antimicrob Chemother*, 26, 561-566 (1990)

6087 Tucker SC, Lynch JP, Ansell BF Jr. Chlorpropamide - induced agranulocytosis. *J Am Med Ass*, 238, 422 (1977)

6088 Tugwell P, Bennett KJ, Chalmers A et al. Low-dose cyclosporin versus placebo in patients with rheumatoid arthritis. *Lancet*, 335, 1051-1055 (1990)

6089 Tuimala R, Korhonen M, Kortesluoma M. Effects of the oral contraceptive combination 0.150 mg desogestrel + 0.020 mg ethinylestradiol on serum lipids, SHBG, glycosylated proteins and plasma antithrombin III activity in healthy women. *Acta Obstet Gynecol Scand*, 66, Suppl 144, 37-39 (1987)

6090 Tulassay Z, Tulassay T, Szucs L et al. Effects of long acting somatostatin analogue on renal functions. *Horm Metab Res*, 22, 555-556 (1990)

6091 Tulassy Z, Tulassy T, Gupta R et al. Long-acting somatostatin analogue in dumping syndrome. *Br J Surg*, 76, 1294-1295 (1989)

6092 Tummisto T, Airaksinen MM. Increase of creatine kinase activity in serum caused by intermittently administered suxamethonium. *Br J Anaes*, 38, 510 (1966)

6093 Tummon IS, Pepping ME, Binor Z et al. A randomized, prospective comparison of endocrine changes induced with intranasal leuprolide or danazol for treatment of endometriosis. *Fertil Steril*, 51, 390-394 (1989)

6094 Tuncer AM, Hisönmez G, Gumruk F, et al. Serum TNF-α, γ-INF and GM-CSF levels in neutropenic children with acute leukemia treated with short-course, high dose methylprednisolone. *Leuk Res*, 20, 265-269 (1996)

6095 Tunn S, Mollmann H, Barth J et al. Simultaneous measurement of cortisol in serum and saliva after different forms of cortisol administration. *Clin Chem*, 38, 1491-1494 (1992)

6096 Tuppurainen M, Heikkinen A-M, Penttila I et al. Does vitamin D_3 have negative effects on serum levels of lipids? A follow-up study with a sequential combination of estradiol valerate and cyproterone acetate and/or vitamin D_3. *Maturitas*, 22, 55-61 (1995)

6097 Turkington RW. Phenothiazine stimulation test for prolactin reserve: the syndrome of isolated prolactin deficiency. *J Clin Endocrinol Metab*, 34, 246 (1972)

6098 Turkington RW. Prolactin secretion in patients treated with various drugs: phenothiazines, tricyclic antidepressants, reserpine and methyldopa. *Arch Intern Med*, 130, 349-354 (1972)

6099 Turkington VE, Nixon JC, Campbell JS et al. Effect of long-acting steroid contraceptive (medroxyprogesterone acetate) on human female subjects. *Clin Chem*, 17, 667 (1971)

6100 Turkington VE, Robinson VJ. Kodak Ektachem® method for theophylline in serum evaluated. *Clin Chem*, 34, 1512-1513 (1988)

6101 Turnbull DM, Dick DJ, Wilson L et al. Valproate causes metabolic disturbance in normal man. *J Neurol Neurosurg Psychiatry*, 49, 405-410 (1986)

6102 Turnbull MJ, Ballinger BR. Urinary excretion of monoamines and metabolites in patients dependent on and withdrawn from barbiturates. *Psychopharmacology*, 30, 103 (1973)

6103 Turner GA, Ellis RD, Guthrie D et al. Levels of adenosine 3',5' cyclic monophosphate and guanosine 3',5' cyclic guanosine monophosphate in single urine specimens collected from a large population of healthy subjects. *Ann Clin Biochem*, 19, 77-82 (1982)

6104 Turner LV, Manchester KL. Interference of HEPES with the Lowry method. *Science*, 170, 649 (1970)

6105 Turpeinen U, Markkanen H, Vlimki M, Stenman U-H. Determination of urinary free cortisol by HPLC. *Clin Chem*, 43, 1386-1391 (1997)

6106 Turtle JT, Burgess JA, Bauckhan S. The metabolic effects of fenfluramine. *S Afr Med J*, 44, Suppl, 23 (1971)

6107 Tutor JC. Mecanismo de interferecia de la penicilina en la determinacion del acido δ-aminokevulinico urinario. *Laboratorio (Granada)*, 70, 501-508 (1980)

6108 Tutor JC, Fernandez MP, Paz JM. Serum copper concentrations and hepatic enzyme induction during long-term therapy with anticonvulsants. *Clin Chem*, 28, 1367-1370 (1982)

6109 Tutor JC, Paz JM, Ron R et al. Niveles plasmaticas de glutamina y amino-acidos del ciclo de la urea en ninos tratodos con difenilhidantoina y fenobarbital. *Quim Clin*, 4, 115-118 (1985)

6110 Tweeddale MG, Ogilvie RI, Ruedy J. Antihypertensive and biochemical effects of chlorthalidone. *Clin Pharmacol Ther*, 22, 519-527 (1977)

6111 Twek J, Goverde BC. The significance of hydroxyproline assay in urine. The Netherlands, Organon Teknika-Oss (1972)

6112 Twum-Barima Y, Carruthers SG. Quinidine-rifampin interaction. *N Engl J Med*, 304, 1466-1469 (1981)

6113 Tynes BS. The clinical use of amphotericin B. *GP*, 32, 97 (1965)

6114 Tysellje JR. Hepatitis induced by methyldopa (Aldomet®) report of a case and review of the literature. *Am J Dig Dis*, 16, 849 (1971)

6115 Ubbink JB, Delport R, Becker PJ et al. Evidence for a theophylline-induced vitamin B_6 deficiency caused by noncompetitive inhibition of pyridoxal kinase. *J Lab Clin Med*, 113, 15-22 (1989)

6116 Uberti ECD, Trasforini G, Margutti AR et al. Intravenous administration of pentagastrin increases plasma prolactin but not growth hormone in normal women. *Min Endocr*, 7, 249-252 (1982)

6117 UCB Pharma, Inc. Manufacturer's literature on Theophylline. Smyrna (Atlanta), GA 31139 (1996)

6118 Udall JA. Clinical implications of warfarin interactions with five sedatives. *Am J Cardiol*, 35, 67-71 (1975)

6119 Udall JA. Drug interference with warfarin therapy. *Clin Med*, 77, 20 (1970)

6120 Ueda D, Suzuki K, Malyszko J et al. Fibrinolysis and serotonin under cyclosporine A treatment in renal transplant recipients. *Thromb Res*, 76, 97-102 (1994)

6121 Uehara S, Hirayama A. Effects of cilostazol on platelet function. *Arz Forsch Drug Res*, 39, 1531-1534 (1989)

6122 Uehlinger DE, Weidmann P, Gnaedinger MP. Cardiovascular regulation and lipoprotein profile during administration of co-dergocrine in essential hypertension. *Eur J Clin Pharmacol*, 36, 119-125 (1989)

6123 Ueland PM, Refsum H, Stabler SP et al. Total homocysteine in plasma or serum: methods and clinical applications. *Clin Chem*, 39, 1764-1779 (1983)

6124 Uemasu J, Munemura C, Fujihara M et al. Inhibition of endothelin-1 concentration by captopril in patients with essential hypertension. *Clin Nephrol*, 41, 150-152 (1994)

6125 Ueno K, Miyai K, Seki T et al. Interaction between theophylline and mexiletine. *Dicp Ann Pharmacother*, 24, 471-472 (1990)

6126 Ueno T, Tanaka S, Umeda M. Determination of CRP antigen in serum using liposome turbidimetric assay (LTA). *Clin Chem*, 39, 1254 (1993)

6127 Ulick S, Wang JZ, Hanukoglu A et al. The effect of carbenoxalone on the peripheral metabolism of cortisol in human patients. *J Lab Clin Med*, 122, 673-676 (1993)

6128 Unge P, Svedberg L-E, Nordgren A et al. A study of the interaction of omeprazole and warfarin in anticoagulated patients. *Br J Clin Pharmacol*, 34, 509-512 (1992)

6129 Ungethum W. Study on the interaction between sucralfate and diclofenac/piroxicam in healthy volunteers. *Arz Forsch Drug Res*, 41, 797-800 (1991)

6130 Unknown or lost reference

6131 Uno S, Takehiro O, Tabata R et al. Enzymatic method for determining ketone body ratio in arterial blood. *Clin Chem*, 41, 1745-1750 (1995)

6132 Updike SJ, Shults MC, Capelli CC et al. Laboratory evaluation of new reusable blood glucose sensor. *Diabetes Care*, 11, 801-807 (1988)

6133 Upton RA, Williams RL, Buskin JN et al. Effects of probenecid on ketoprofen kinetics. *Clin Pharmacol Ther*, 31, 705-712 (1982)

6134 Urena P, Bererhi L, Houhou S et al. No acute change of serum erythropoietin in response to hypocalcemia or antihypertensive agents in uremic patients. *Nephron*, 70, 197-201 (1995)

6135 Uretsky BF, Generalovich T, Verbalis JG et al. Comparative hemodynamic and hormonal response of enoximone and dobutamine in severe congestive heart failure. *Am J Cardiol*, 58, 110-116 (1986)

6136 Urman B, Pride SM, Yuen BH. Elevated serum testosterone, hirsutism, and virilism associated with combined androgen-estrogen hormone replacement therapy. *Obstet Gynecol*, 77, 595-598 (1991)

6137 U.S. Bioscience, Inc. Manufacturer's literature on Hexalen® . West Conshohocken, PA 19428 (1995)

6138 U.S. Bioscience, Inc. Manufacturer's literature on Neutrexin® . West Conshohocken, PA 19428 (1994)

6139 Utiger RD. In:. *Current Topics in Thyroid Research. C Cassano, M Andreoli (eds)*, New York NY, Academic Press (1965)

6140 Utili R, Boitnott JK, Zimmermann HJ. Dantrolene-associated hepatic injury: incidence and character. *Gastroenterology*, 72, 610-616 (1977)

6141 Utting JE, Whitford JH. Assessment of premedicant drugs using measurements of plasma cortisol. *Br J Anaes*, 44, 43 (1972)

6142 Uygur MC, Arik AI, Altug U, Erol D. Effects of the 5α-reductase inhibitor finasteride on serum levels of gonadal, adrenal, and hypophyseal hormones and its clinical significance: a prospective clinical study. *Steroids*, 63, 208-213 (1998)

6143 Uyttenbroeck W, Korthout M, De Bock R et al. Cimetidine induced pancytopenia. Effect on human CFU-MIX colony formation. *Blut*, 60, 323-327 (1990)

6144 Uza G, Pavel O. Effect of nifedipine on serum inorganic phosphorus and serum magnesium in hypertensive patients. *Magnesium Bull*, 11, 173-176 (1989)

6145 Uzbay IT, Ozcan N, Erbil MK et al. Effect of captopril on serum lipids, lipoproteins, apolipoproteins, and glucose levels in patients with essential hypertension. *Curr Ther Res*, 51, 46-53 (1992)

6146 Uzzan B, Nicolas P, Perret G et al. Effects of troleandomycin and josamycin on thyroid hormone and steroid serum levels, liver function tests and microsomal monooxygenases in healthy volunteers: a double-blind placebo-controlled study. *Fundam Clin Pharmacol*, 5, 513-526 (1991)

6147 Vaag A, Skott P, Damsbo P et al. Effect of the antilipolytic nicotinic acid analogue acipimox on whole-body and skeletal muscle glucose metabolism in patients with non-insulin dependent diabetes mellitus. *J Clin Invest*, 88, 1282-1290 (1991)

6148 Vagenakis AG, Downs P, Braverman LE et al. Control of thyroid hormone secretion in normal subjects receiving iodides. *J Clin Invest*, 52, 528 (1973)

6149 Vague P, Juhan-Vague I, Alessi MC et al. Metformin decreases the high plasminogen activator inhibition capacity, plasma insulin and triglyceride levels in nondiabetic obese subjects. *Thromb Haemostas*, 57, 326-328 (1988)

6150 Vahlquist C, Michaelsson G, Vahlquist A et al. A sequential comparison of etretinate (tigason) and isotretinoin (roaccutane) with special regard to their effects on serum lipoproteins. *Br J Dermatol*, 112, 69-76 (1985)

6151 Valcavi R, Diequez C, Zini M et al. Influence of hyperthyroidism on growth hormone secretion. *Clin Endocrinol*, 38, 515-522 (1993)

6152 Valdiguie P, Lareng L, Dirat MF et al. Action of several anesthetic drugs on serum lactate dehydrogenase. *Pathol Biol*, 20, 131 (1972)

6153 Valensi P, Perret G, Vassy R et al. Effect of nifedipine on thyrotropin, prolactin, and thyroid hormone release in man: a placebo controlled study. *Fundam Clin Pharmacol*, 3, 59-66 (1989)

6154 Valenti G, Denti L, Banchini A et al. Dissociated effect of buserelin on luteinizing hormone (LH) and alpha subunit in men. *J Endocrinol Invest*, 13, 459-467 (1990)

6155 Valerio G, Vigna GB, Vitale E et al. Low-dose simvaststin treatment in patients with moderate-grade familial hypercholesterolemia. *Curr Ther Res*, 48, 701-706 (1990)

6156 Valimaki M, Harno K, Nikkila EA. Serum lipoproteins and indices of glucose tolerance during diuretic therapy. a comparison between hydrochlorothiazide and piretanide. *J Cardiovasc Pharmacol*, 5, 525-530 (1985)

6157 Valimaki M, Nilsson CG, Roine R et al. Comparison between the effects of nafarelin and danazol on serum lipids and lipoproteins in patients with endometriosis. *J Clin Endocrinol Metab*, 69, 1097-1103 (1989)

6158 Valles M, Tovar JL. Salsalate and minimal change nephrotic syndrome. *Ann Intern Med*, 107, 116 (1987)

6159 Valsalan VC, Cooper GL. Carbamazepine intoxication caused by interaction with isoniazid. *Br Med J*, 285, 261-262 (1982)

6160 Valvo E, Casagrande P, Bedogna V et al. Systemic and renal effects of a new angiotensin converting enzyme inhibitor, benazepril, in essential hypertension. *J Hypertens*, 8, 991-995 (1990)

6161 van Acker K, Verbraeken K, Baluwe R. Abnormal patterns of lactate dehydrogenase isoenzymes after streptokinase therapy. *Clin Chem*, 32, 2210 (1986)

6162 van Acker RAC, Prummel MF, Weber JA et al. Effect of prednisone on renal function in man. *Nephron*, 65, 254-259 (1993)

6163 van Bocxlaer JF, Clauwaert KM, Lambert WF, de Leenheer AP. Quantitative colorimetric determination of urinary p-aminophenol with an automated analyzer. *Clin Chem*, 43, 627-634 (1997)

6164 Van Bortel LMAB, Schiffers PMH, Bohm ROB et al. The influence of chronic treatment with verapamil on plasma atrial natriuretic peptide levels in young and elderly hypertensive patients. *Eur J Clin Pharmacol*, 39, Suppl 1, S39-S40 (1990)

6165 van Brummelen P, Buhler FR, Amann FW et al. Effects of a new long-acting β-blocker bopindolol (IT 31-200) on blood pressure, plasma catecholamines, renin and cholesterol in patients with arterial hypertension. *Eur J Clin Pharmacol*, 22, 491-493 (1982)

6166 van Buren D, Wideman CA, Reid M et al. The antagonistic effect of rifampin upon cyclosporine bioavailability. *Transplant Proc*, 16, 1642-1645 (1984)

6167 van Buren M, van Rijn HJM, Koomans HA. Short-term indomethacin administration does not impair excretion of acute potassium load in humans. *Eur J Clin Invest*, 22, 821-826 (1992)

6168 van Dam FE, Overkamp M, Haanen C. The interaction of drugs. *Lancet*, 2, 1027 (1966)

6169 Van de Merwe JP, van Blankenstein M, Wilson JHP. Intrahepatic cholestasis induced by phenylbutazone. *Digestion*, 22, 317-320 (1981)

6170 Van de Walle JGJ, Donckerwolcke RAMG. Association of fever, nasal congestion and rise in serum creatinine with azathioprine. *Pediatr Nephrol*, 4, 67-68 (1990)

6171 van de Walle JGJ, Donckerwolcke RAMG. Association of fever, nasal congestion and rise in serum creatinine with azathioprine. *Pediatr Nephrol*, 4, 67-68 (1990)

6172 Van den Berg JWO, Edixhoven-Bosdijk A, Koole-Lesuis R et al. Faecal haem assay - some practical modifications of the Hemoquant assay for haemoglobin in faeces. *Clin Chim Acta*, 169, 319-322 (1987)

6173 van den Brink HR, van Wijk MJG, Geertzen RGM et al. Influence of corticosteroid pulse therapy on the serum levels of soluble interleukin 2 receptor, interleukin 6 and interleukin 8 in patients with rheumatoid arthritis. *J Rheumatol*, 21, 430-434 (1994)

6174 van den Ende A, Lutjens A, van Wayjen RGA et al. Effects of the oral contraceptive combination 0.150 mg desogestrel plus 0.020 mg ethinylestradiol on carbohydrate metabolism in healthy female volunteers. *Acta Obstet Gynecol Scand*, 66, Suppl 144, 29-32 (1987)

6175 van der Auwera P, Meunier F, Ibrahim S et al. Pharmacodynamic parmeters and toxicity of netilmicin (6 miligrams/kilogram/day) given once daily or in three divided doses to cancer patients with urinary tract infection. *Antimicrob Agent Chemother*, 35, 640-647 (1991)

6176 Van der Auwera P, Meunier F, Ibrahim S et al. Pharmacodynamic parmeters and toxicity of netilmicin (6 miligrams/kilogram/day) given once daily or in three divided doses to cancer patients with urinary tract infection. *Antimicrob Agent Chemother*, 35, 640-647 (1991)

6177 van der Meer JWM, Keuning JJ, Scheijgrond HW et al. The influence of gastric acidity on the bioavailability of ketoconazole. *J Antimicrob Chemother*, 6, 552-554 (1980)

6178 van der Meiracker AH, Admiraal PJJ, Man in't Veld AJ et al. Prolonged blood pressure reduction by orally active renin inhibitor Ro 42-5892 in essential hypertension. *Br Med J*, 301, 205-210 (1990)

6179 van der Vange N, Blankenstein MA, Kloosterboer HJ et al. Effects of seven low-dose combined oral contraceptives on sex hormone binding globulin, corticosteroid binding globulin, total and free testosterone. *Contraception*, 41, 345-352 (1990)

6180 van der Velde CD, Gordon MW. Manic-depressive illness, diabetes mellitus, and lithium carbonate. *Arch Gen Psychiat*, 21, 478 (1969)

6181 van der Weerdt CM. Thrombocytopenia due to quinidine or quinine. *Vox Sang*, 12, 265 (1967)

6182 van Dyk JJ, Falkson HC, van der Merwe AM et al. Unexpected toxicity in patients treated with iphosphamide. *Cancer Res*, 32, 921 (1972)

6183 Van Haelst Pisani C, Kovach JS, Kita H et al. Administration of interleukin-2 (IL-2) results in increased plasma concentrations of IL-5 and eosinophilia in patients with cancer. *Blood*, 78, 1538-1544 (1991)

6184 van Harten J, van Brummelen P, Michiel M et al. Pharmacokinetics and hemodynamic effects of nisoldipine and its interaction with cimetidine. *Clin Pharmacol Ther*, 43, 332-341 (1988)

6185 van Hecken A, de Lepeleire I, Verbesselt R et al. Effect of benazepril, a converting enzyme inhibitor, on plasma levels and activity of acenocoumarol and warfarin. *Int J Clin Pharmacol Res*, 8, 315-319 (1988)

6186 Van Hecken A, Depre M, Schwartz JI et al. Plasma concentrations and effect on testosterone metabolism after single doses of MK-0434, a steroid 5 alpha reductase inhibitor, in healthy subjects. *Eur J Clin Pharmacol*, 46, 123-126 (1994)

6187 van Hecken A, Verbesselt R, Tjandra-Maga TB et al. Pharmacokinetic interaction between indomethacin and diflunisal. *Eur J Clin Pharmacol*, 36, 507-512 (1989)

6188 van Herle AJ, Uller RP, Matthews NL et al. Radioimmunoassay for measurement of thyroglobulin in human serum. *J Clin Invest*, 52, 1320 (1973)

6189 Van Hunsel F, Wauters A, Vandoolaeghe E, et al. Lower total serum protein, albumin, and β- and γ-globulin in major and treatment resistant depression: effects of antidepressant treatments. *Psychiat Res*, 65, 159-169 (1996)

6190 van Leerdam FJM, van der Meulen J, de Vries PMJM et al. The effect of ketoprofen on effective renal plasma flow and glomerular filtration rate in healthy men with and without sodium depletion. *Curr Ther Res*, 48, 676-683 (1990)

6191 van Peenen MJ, Files JB. The effect of medication on laboratory test results. *Am J Clin Pathol*, 52, 666 (1969)

6192 van Praag HM, Leijnse B. The xylose metabolism in depressed patients and its alteration under the influence of antidepressive hydrazines. *Clin Chim Acta*, 11, 13 (1965)

6193 van Riel PLCM, van de Putte LBA, Gribnau FWJ et al. Serum IgA and gold-induced toxic effects in patients with rheumatoid arthritis. *Arch Intern Med*, 144, 1401-1403 (1984)

6194 Van Roon-Djordjevic B, Cerfontain-Van Staalen J. Urinary excretion of histidine metabolites as an indication for folic acid and vitamin B_{12} deficiency. *Clin Chim Acta*, 41, 55 (1972)

6195 van Rooyen RJ, Ziady F. Hypokalemic alkalosis following the abuse of purgatives. Case report. *S Afr Med J*, 46, 998 (1972)

6196 van Rossum MAJ, Fiselier TJW, Franssen MJAM, et al. Sulfasalazine in the treatment of juvenile chronic arthritis: a randomized, double-blind, placebo-controlled multicenter study. *Arth Rheum*, 41, 808-816 (1998)

6197 van Scoy RE, Wilkowske CJ. Antituberculous agents. *Mayo Clin Proc*, 62, 1129-1136 (1987)

6198 Van Stekelenburg GJ, Koorevaar G. Evidence for the existence of mammalian acetoacetate decarboxylase. *Clin Chim Acta*, 39, 191 (1972)

6199 van Wassenaer AG, Kok JH, Endert E et al. Thyroxine administration to infants of less than 30 weeks' gestational age does not increase plasma triiodothyronine concentrations. *Acta Endocrinol*, 129, 139-146 (1993)

6200 van Woert MH, Ambani LM, Levine RJ. Clinical effects of para-chlorophenylalanine in Parkinson's disease. *Dis Nerv Sys*, 33, 777 (1972)

6201 Vandam LD. Analgesic drugs - the mild analgesics. *N Engl J Med*, 286, 20 (1972)

6202 Vandel S, Bertschy G, Perault MC et al. Minor and clinically non-significant interaction between toloxatone and amitriptyline. *Eur J Clin Pharmacol*, 44, 97-99 (1993)

6203 Vandenberghe H, Crosby JE. Evaluation of the DCL and Sigma Ethylalcohol assay on the Hitachi 717. *Proc CliniChem*, 6, 16 (1991)

6204 Vandenburg M, Parfrey P, Wright P et al. Hepatitis associated with captopril treatment. *Br J Clin Pharmacol*, 11, 105-106 (1981)

6205 Vandenburg MJ, Sharman VL, Morton JJ et al. Hormonal and blood pressure changes during converting enzyme inhibition by teprotide. *Postgrad Med J*, 57, 283-288 (1981)

6206 Vandenheuvel WJA, Smith JL, Silber RH. B-(2-methoxyphenoxy)lactic acid, the major urinary metabolite of glyceryl guaiacolate in man. *J Pharm Sci*, 61, 1997 (1972)

6207 Vandevelde C, Chang A, Andrews D et al. Rifampin and ansamycin interactions with cyclosporine after renal transplantation. *Pharmacotherapy*, 11, 88-89 (1991)

6208 Vanhanen H, Kesaniemi YA, Miettinen TA. Pravastatin lowers serum cholesterol, cholesterol-precursor sterols, fecal steroids, and cholesterol absorption in man. *Metabolism*, 41, 588-595 (1992)

6209 Vanhanen H, Miettinen TA. Pravastatin and lovastatin similarly reduce serum cholesterol and its precursor levels in familial hypercholesterolaemia. *Eur J Clin Pharmacol*, 42, 127-130 (1992)

6210 Vanholder R, Patel S, Hsu CH. Effect of uric acid on plasma levels of $1,25(OH)_2$ D in renal failure. *J Am Soc Nephrol*, 4, 1035-1038 (1993)

6211 Vasankari T, Kujala U, Taimela S, et al. Effects of a long acting somatostatin analog on pituitary, adrenal, and testicular function during rest and acute exercise: unexpected stimulation of testosterone secretion. *J Clin Endocrinol Metab*, 80, 3298-3303 (1995)

6212 Vasmant D, Bender N. The renin-angiotensin system and ramipril, a new converting enzyme inhibitor. *J Cardiovasc Pharmacol*, 14, Suppl 4, S46-S52 (1989)

6213 Vathsala A, Verani R, Schoenberg L et al. Proteinuria in cyclosporine-treated renal transplant recipients. *Transplantation*, 49, 35-41 (1990)

6214 Vathsala A, Weinberg RB, Schoenberg L et al. Lipid abnormalities in cyclosporine-prednisone-treated renal transplant recipients. *Transplantation*, 48, 37-43 (1989)

6215 Vaughan-Williams CA, Shalet SM. Glucose tolerance and insulin resistance after danazol treatment. *J Obstet Gynecol*, 9, 229-232 (1989)

6216 Vaz R, Senior B, Morris M et al. Adrenal effects of beclomethasone inhalation therapy in asthmatic children. *J Pediatr*, 100, 660-662 (1982)

6217 Veerman M, Espejo MG, Christopher MA et al. Use of activated charcoal to reduce elevated serum phenobarbital concentration in a neonate. *Clin Toxicol*, 29, 53-58 (1991)

6218 Vega E, Gonzalez D, Ghiringhelli G et al. Acute effect of the intranasal administration of salmon calcitonin in osteoporotic women. *Bone Miner*, 7, 267-273 (1989)

6219 Vega GL, Grundy SM. Lipoprotein responses to treatment with lovastatin, gemfibrozil, and nicotinic acid in normolipidemic patients with hypoalphalipoproteinemia. *Arch Intern Med*, 154, 73-82 (1994)

6220 Vega GL, Krauss RM, Grundy SM. Pravastatin therapy in primary moderate hypercholesterolaemia: Changes in metabolism of apolipoprotein B-containing lipoproteins. *J Intern Med*, 227, 81-94 (1990)

6221 Velazquez EM, Mendoza S, Hamer T et al. Metformin therapy in polycystic ovary syndrome reduces hyperinsulinemia, insulin resistance, hyperandrogenemia, and systolic blood pressure, while facilitating normal menses and pregnancy. *Metabolism*, 43, 647-654 (1994)

6222 Velazquez H, Perazella MA, Wright FS et al. Renal mechanism of trimethoprim-induced hyperkalemia. *Ann Intern Med*, 119, 296-301 (1993)

6223 Veldhuis JD, Lizarralde G, Iranmanesh A. Divergent effects of short term glucocorticoid excess on the gonadotropic and somatotropic axes in normal men. *J Clin Endocrinol Metab*, 74, 96-102 (1992)

6224 Ventura A, Mannarino E, Lupattelli G et al. Efficacy of beclobrate and gemfibrozil in the treatment of hyperlipoproteinemia. In:. *Beclofibrate, a New Lipoprotein Regulator. GM Kostner, CR Sirtori (eds)*, Toronto, Hogrefe and Huber, 57-64 (1990)

6225 Ventura A, Mannarino E, Lupattelli G et al. Efficacy of beclobrate and gemfibrozil in the treatment of hyperlipoproteinemia. In:. *Beclofibrate, a New Lipoprotein Regulator. GM Kostner, CR Sirtori (eds)*, Toronto, Hogrefe and Huber, 57-64 (1990)

6226 Venturini PL, Fasce V, Costantini S et al. Treatment of endometriosis with goserelin depot, a long-acting gonadotropin-releasing hormone agonist analog: endocrine and clinical results. *Fertil Steril*, 54, 1021-1027 (1990)

6227 Verbeelen D, Vanhaelst L, Fuss M et al. Effect of 1, 25-dihydroxyvitamin D_3 and nifedipine on prolactin release in normal man. *J Endocrinol Invest*, 8, 103-106 (1985)

6228 Vercammen M, Goedhuys W, Boeyckens A et al. Iron and total iron-binding capacity in serum of patients receiving iron-dextran: Kodak Ektachem methodologies, spectrophotometry, and atomic-absorption spectrometry compared. *Clin Chem*, 36, 1812-1815 (1990)

6229 Vercruysse I, Massart DL, Dupont AG. Increase in plasma propranolol caused by nicardipine is dependent on the delivery rate of propranolol. *Eur J Clin Pharmacol*, 49, 121-125 (1995)

6230 Veremis SA, Maddux MS, Pollak R et al. Subtherapeutic cyclosporine concentrations during nafcillin therapy. *Transplantation*, 43, 913-915 (1987)

6231 Verhagen CA, Mattie H, Van Strijen E et al. The renal clearance of cefuroxime and ceftazidime and the effect of probenecid on their tubular excretion. *Br J Clin Pharmacol*, 37, 193-197 (1994)

6232 Verho M, Bossaller W, Heinen B. Serum trace element levels in piretanide-treated hypertensives: a double-blind trial against hydrochlorothiazide plus amiloride. *Int J Clin Pharmacol Res*, 7, 5-11 (1987)

6233 Verity CM, Applegarth DA, Farrell K et al. The influence of anticonvulsants on fasting plasma ammonia and amino acid levels. *Clin Biochem*, 16, 344-345 (1983)

6234 Verma NP, Haidukewych D. Differential but infrequent alterations of hepatic enzyme levels and thyroid hormone levels by anticonvulsant drugs. *Arch Neurol*, 51, 381-384 (1994)

6235 Vermorken JB, Pinedo HM. Gastrointestinal toxicity of cis-diaminedichloro-platinum (III). *Neth J Med*, 25, 270-274 (1982)

6236 Vernillet L, Bertault-Peres P, Berland Y et al. Lack of effect of spiramycin on cyclosporin pharmacokinetics. *Br J Clin Pharmacol*, 27, 789-794 (1989)

6237 Verplanke AJW, Herber RFM, de Wit R et al. Comparison of renal function parameters in the assessment of cis-platin induced nephrotoxicity. *Nephron*, 66, 267-272 (1994)

6238 Verschure JCM. Clinical use of measurements of clearance and maximum capacity of the liver. *Acta Med Scand*, 142, 409 (1952)

6239 Verster FDEB, Garoutte J, Ichinosa H et al. Mode of action of diphenylhydantoin. *Fed Proc*, 24, 390 (1965)

6240 Verstraeten L, ledoux MC, Moos B et al. Interference of tienam in colorimetric determination of 5-aminolevulinic acid and porphobilinogen in serum and urine. *Clin Chem*, 38, 2557-2558 (1992)

6241 Verweij WM, Ossenkoppele GJ, Wijermans P. Interference of methotrexate with the determination of the protein content of cerebrospinal fluid.. *Ann Clin Biochem*, 23, 612-613 (1986)

6242 Vessby B, Abelin J, Finnson M et al. Effects of nifedipine treatment on carbohydrate and lipoprotein metabolism. *Curr Ther Res*, 33, 1075-1081 (1983)

6243 Vessell ES. Impairment of drug metabolism by disulfiram in man. *Clin Pharmacol Ther*, 12, 785 (1971)

6244 Vessell ES, Passananti GT, Greene FE. Impairment of drug metabolism in man by allopurinol and nortriptyline. *N Engl J Med*, 283, 1484-1488 (1970)

6245 Vestal RE, Kornhauser DM, Hollifield JW et al. Inhibition of propranolol metabolism by chlorpromazine. *Clin Pharmacol Ther*, 25, 19-24 (1979)

6246 Vestergaard P, Amdisen A, Hansen HE et al. Lithium treatment and kidney function, a survey of 237 patients in long-term treatment. *Acta Psychiat Scand*, 60, 504-520 (1979)

6247 Veterans Administration Cooperative Study Group. Comparison of propranolol and hydrochlorothiazide for the initial treatment of hypertension: i. results of short-term titration with emphasis on racial differences in response.. *J Am Med Ass*, 248, 1996-2003 (1982)

6248 Veterans Administration Cooperative Study Group. Comparison of propranolol and hydrochlorothiazide for the initial treatment of hypertension: III. results of long-term therapy. *J Am Med Ass*, 248, 2004-2011 (1982)

6249 Veterans Administration Cooperative Study Group. Efficacy of nadolol alone and combined with bendroflumethiazide and hydralazine for systemic hypertension. *Am J Cardiol*, 52, 1230-1237 (1983)

6250 Vettor R, Macor C, Rossi E et al. Effect of naltrexone treatment on insulin secretion, insulin action and postprandial thermogenesis in obesity. *Horm Metab Res*, 26, 188-194 (1995)

6251 Veys EM, Mielants H, Verbruggen G et al. Levamisole as basic treatment of rheumatoid arthritis: long term evaluation. *J Rheumatol Dis*, 8, 45-56 (1981)

6252 Vianello F, Dal Santo PL, Plebani M et al. Gastrointestinal hormones and serum group I pepsinogen after intravenous hexaprazol injection in healthy volunteers. *Curr Ther Res*, 46, 505-510 (1989)

6253 Vianello F, Laino G, Dal Santo P et al. Effects of nizatidine on gastric acid and bicarbonate secretion. *Curr Ther Res*, 53, 277-284 (1993)

6254 Viberti G, Mogensen CE, Groop LC et al. Effect of captopril on progression to clinical proteinuria in patients with insulin-dependent diabetes mellitus and microalbuminuria. *J Am Med Ass*, 271, 275-279 (1994)

6255 Vidal-Puig AJ, Munoz-Torres M, Jodar-Gimeno E et al. Ketoconazole therapy: hormonal and clinical effects in no-tumoral hyperandrogenism. *Eur J Clin Endocrinol*, 130, 333-338 (1994)

6256 Vidt DG. Mechanism of action, pharmacokinetics, adverse effects and therapeutic uses of amiloride hydrochloride, a new potassium-sparing diuretic. *Pharmacotherapy*, 1, 179-187 (1981)

6257 Vidt DG, Bravo EL, Fouad FM. Captopril. *N Engl J Med*, 306, 214-219 (1982)

6258 Vigliani EC, Cavagna G, Locatigfoa V. Biological effects of nitroglycol on the metabolism of catecholamines. *Arch Environ Health*, 16, 477 (1968)

6259 Vilaseca MA, Farre C, Ramon F. Phenylalanine determined in plasma with use of phenylalanine dehydrogenase and a centrifugal analyzer. *Clin Chem*, 39, 129-131 (1995)

6260 Vilen L, Kutti J, Freden K et al. The peripheral platelet count and ADP-induced platelet aggregation in response to metoprolol and propranolol as studied in young healthy male volunteers. *Scand J Haematol*, 31, 440-446 (1983)

6261 Villarreal H, Arcila H, Ramirezma S et al. Effect of guancydine on systemic and renal hemodynamics in arterial hypertension. *Clin Pharmacol Ther*, 12, 838 (1971)

6262 Vinceneux P, Canal M, Domart Y et al. Pharmacokinetic and pharmacodynamic interactions between nifedipine and propranolol or betaxolol. *Int J Clin Pharmacol Ther Toxicol*, 24, 153-158 (1986)

6263 Vincent FM. Phenothiazine-induced phenytoin intoxication. *Ann Intern Med*, 93, 56-57 (1980)

6264 Vincent PC. Drug-induced aplastic anemia and agranulocytosis: incidence and mechanisms. *Drugs*, 31, 52-63 (1986)

6265 Vincenti F, Kirkman R, Light S, et al. Interleukin-2-receptor blockade with daclizumab to prevent acute rejection in renal transplantation. *N Engl J Med*, 338, 161-165 (1998)

6266 Vinet B, Letellier G. The in vitro effect of drugs on biochemical parameters determined by a SMAC® system. *Clin Biochem*, 10, 47-51 (1977)

6267 Vinet B, Panzini B, Boucher M, Massicotte J. Automated enzymatic assay for the determination of sucrose in serum and urine and its use as a marker of gastric damage. *Clin Chem*, 44, 2369-2371 (1998)

6268 Vinik AI, Colwell JA, Hyperlipidemia in Diabetes Investigators. Effects of gemfibrozil on triglyceride levels in patients with NIDDM. *Diabetes Care*, 16, 37-44 (1993)

6269 Violi F, Ferro D, Saliola M et al. Effect of oral defibrotide on tissue-plasminogen activator and tissue-plasminogen activator inhibitor balance. *Eur J Clin Pharmacol*, 42, 379-383 (1992)

6270 Vir SC, Love AHG. Zinc and copper nutriture of women taking oral contraceptive agents. *Am J Clin Nutr*, 34, 1479-1483 (1981)

6271 Viswanathan CT, Levy RH. Plasma protein binding interaction between valproic and salicylic acids in rhesus monkeys. *J Pharmacol Sci*, 70, 1279-1281 (1981)

6272 Vivus Inc. Manufacturer's literature on Muse® . Menlo Park, CA 94205 (1997)

6273 Vlasses PH, Kosoglou T, Chase SL et al. Trimethoprim inhibition of the renal clearance of procainamide and N-acetylprocainamide. *Arch Intern Med*, 149, 1350-1353 (1989)

6274 Vogt P, Schorn T, Frei U et al. Ofloxacin in the treatment of urinary tract infection in renal transplant recipients. *Infection*, 16, 175-178 (1988)

6275 Volkert RM, Nadig KB, hannabery J et al. Determination of nifedipine (Dihydropyridine) in human serum or urine using the STC microplate assay. *Clin Chem*, 37, 1048 (1991)

6276 Volpi R, Coiro V, Salvi M et al. Effect of metoclopramide on serum growth hormone levels in cirrhotic men. *J Endocrinol Invest*, 6, 101-105 (1983)

6277 Von Euler US. Pathophysiological aspects of catecholamine production. *Clin Chem*, 18, 1445 (1972)

6278 Voors AW, Srinivasan SR, Hunter SM et al. Smoking, oral contraceptives, and serum lipid and lipoprotein levels in youths. *Prev Med*, 11, 1-12 (1982)

6279 Voskaridou E, Kalotychou V, Loukopoulos D. Clinical and laboratory effects of long-term administration of hydroxyurea to patients with sickle-cell/β-thalassaemia. *Br J Haematol*, 89, 479-484 (1995)

6280 Vought RL, Brown FA, Wolff J. Erythrosine: an adventitious source of iodide. *J Clin Endocrinol Metab*, 34, 747 (1972)

6281 Vree TB, van den Biggelaar-Martea M, Verwey-Van CPWGM. Probenecid inhibits the renal clearance o frusemide and its acyl glucuronide. *Br J Clin Pharmacol*, 39, 692-695 (1995)

6282 Vree TB, Zweens K, Huige PJC et al. Interactions between the renal excretion rates of β_2-microglobulin and tobramycin in man. *Clin Chim Acta*, 138, 49-57 (1984)

6283 Vyden JK, Curnow DH, Beck AB et al. Failure of chlordiazepoxide to influence urinary copper excretion. *Lancet*, 2, 1090 (1972)

6284 Wachter JP, Smeby RR, Free AH. Urinalysis and oral hypoglycemic agents. *Am J Med Technol*, 26, 125 (1960)

6285 Wacker WEC, Parisi AF. Magnesium metabolism. *N Engl J Med*, 278, 712 (1968)

6286 Wada H, Mori Y, Kaneko T et al. Elevated plasma levels of vascular endothelial cell markers in patients with hypercholesterolemia. *Am J Hematol*, 44, 112-116 (1993)

6287 Wade JC, Schimpff SC, Wiernik PH. Antibiotic combination-associated nephrotoxicity in granulocytopenia patients with cancer. *Arch Intern Med*, 141, 1789-1793 (1981)

6288 Wadhwa NF, Schroeder TJ, Pesce AJ et al. Cyclosporine drug interactions: a review. *Ther Drug Monit*, 9, 399-406 (1987)

6289 Waeber B, Nussberger J, Perret L et al. Experience with perindopril in normal volunteers. *Clin Exp Hypertens*, A 11, Suppl 2, 507-519 (1989)

6290 Waeber G, Burnier M, Porchet M et al. Effects of prolonged administration of the angiotensin converting enzyme inhibitor CGS 16617 in normotensive volunteers. *Eur J Clin Pharmacol*, 36, 587-591 (1989)

6291 Wagener RE, Flood K, Valdes R Jr. False negative d.a.u. EMIT results with salicylate-containing urines. *Clin Chem*, 39, 1231 (1993)

6292 Wagener RE, Linder MW, Valdes R Jr. Decreased signal in EMIT assays of drugs of abuse in urine after ingestion of aspirin: potential for false-negative results. *Clin Chem*, 40, 608-612 (1994)

6293 Wagner F, Kalusche D, Trenk D et al. Drug interaction between propafenone and metoprolol. *Br J Clin Pharmacol*, 24, 213-220 (1987)

6294 Wagner ML, Remmel RP, Graves NM et al. Effect of felbamate on carbamazepine and its major metabolites. *Clin Pharmacol Ther*, 53, 536-543 (1993)

6295 Wahl P, Walden C, Knopp R et al. Effect of estrogen/progestin potency on lipid/Lipoprotein cholesterol. *N Engl J Med*, 308, 862-867 (1983)

6296 Wahlbeck K, Rimon R, Fyhrquist F. Elevated angiotensin-converting enzyme (kininase II) in the cerebrospinal fluid of neuroleptic-treated schizophrenic patients. *Schiz Res*, 9, 77-82 (1993)

6297 Wahlberg G, Holmquist L, Walldius G et al. Effects of nicotinic acid on concentrations of serum apolipoproteins B, C-I, C-II, C-III and E in hyperlipidemic patients. *Acta Med Scand*, 224, 319-327 (1988)

6298 Wahlberg G, Walldius G, Olsson AG et al. Effects of nicotinic acid on serum cholesterol concentrations of high density lipoprotein subfractions HDL_2 and HDL_3 in hyperlipoproteinaemia. *J Intern Med*, 228, 151-157 (1990)

6299 Waisbren BA, Evani SV, Ziebert AP. Carbenicillin and bleeding. *J Am Med Ass*, 217, 1243 (1971)

6300 Waite NM, Edwaeds DJ, Arnott WS et al. Effects of ciprofloxacin on testosterone and cortisol concentrations in healthy males. *Antimicrob Agent Chemother*, 33, 1875-1877 (1989)

6301 Walach N, Evans S, Zaidman JL et al. Red blood cell glutathione status in patients with gastrointestinal malignancies treated with 5-fluorouracil. *Clin Chim Acta*, 231, 95-100 (1994)

6302 Waldman FM, Koblin DD, Lampe GH et al. Hematologic effects of nitrous oxide in surgical patients. *Anesth Analg*, 71, 618-624 (1990)

6303 Waldorff S, Hansen PB, Egeblad H et al. Interactions between digoxin and potassium-sparing diuretics. *Clin Pharmacol Ther*, 33, 418-423 (1983)

6304 Waldorff S, Hansen PB, Kjaergard H et al. Amiloride-induced changes in digoxin dynamics and kinetics: abolition of digoxin-induced inotropism with amiloride. *Clin Pharmacol Ther*, 30, 172-176 (1981)

6305 Walenkamp GHIM, Vree TB, Guelen PJM et al. Interaction between the renal excretion rates of β_2-microglobulin and gentamicin in man. *Clin Chim Acta*, 127, 229-238 (1983)

6306 Wales JK, Wolff F. Hematological side effects of diazoxide. *Lancet*, 1, 53 (1967)

6307 Walinder J, Arberg-Wistedt A, Jozwiak H et al. The safety of zimeldine in long-term use in depressive illness. *Acta Psychiat Scand*, 68, Suppl 308, 147-160 (1983)

6308 Walker BR, Capuzzi DM, Alexander F. Hyperkalemia after triamterene in diabetic patients. *J Clin Pharmacol*, 13, 643 (1972)

6309 Walker BR, Hoppe RC, Alexander F. Effect of triamterene on the renal clearance of calcium, magnesium, phosphate and uric acid in man. *Clin Pharmacol Ther*, 13, 245 (1972)

6310 Walker BR, Mackie RM. Serum lipid elevation during isotretinoin therapy for acne in the west of Scotland. *Br J Dermatol*, 122, 531-537 (1990)

6311 Walker FA. Ammonia in fibrin hydrolysates. *N Engl J Med*, 285, 1324 (1971)

6312 Walker FB, Becker DM, Kowal-Neeley B et al. Lack of effect of warfarin on uric acid concentration. *Clin Chem*, 34, 952-954 (1988)

6313 Walker JG. Fatal agranulocytosis complicating treatment with ethacrynic acid. *Ann Intern Med*, 64, 1303 (1966)

6314 Walker PC. Neonatal bilirubin toxicity. a review of kernicterus and the implications of drug-induced bilirubin displacement. *Clin Pharmacokinet*, 13, 26-50 (1987)

6315 Walker PL, Pettit BR, Sandler M. Interference by naproxen in the urinary 5-hydroxyindoleacetic acid assay is due to a metabolite desmethylnaproxen. *Ann Clin Biochem*, 24, 177-181 (1987)

6316 Walker RC, Wright AJ. The quinolones. *Mayo Clin Proc*, 62, 1007-1012 (1987)

6317 Walker RE, Parker RI, Kovacs JA , et al. Anemia and erythropoiesis in patients with acquired immunodeficiency syndrome (AIDS) and Kaposi sarcoma treated with zidovudine. *Ann Intern Med*, 108, 372-376 (1988)

6318 Wallace DJ, Metzger AL, Steher VJ et al. Cholesterol-lowering effect of hydroxychloroquine in patients with rheumatic disease: reversal of deleterious effects of steroids on lipids. *Am J Med*, 89, 322-326 (1990)

6319 Wallace EM, Wu FC et al. Effect of depot medroxyprogesterone acetate and testosterone oenanthate on serum lipoproteins in man. *Contraception*, 41, 63-71 (1990)

6320 Wallace Laboratories. Manufacturer's literature on Astelin® . Cranbury, NJ 08512 (1996)

6321 Wallace Laboratories. Manufacturer's literature on Depen® . Cranbury, NJ 08512 (1992)

6322 Wallace Laboratories. Manufacturer's literature on Doral® . Cranbury, NJ 08512 (1994)

6323 Wallace Laboratories. Manufacturer's literature on Felbatol® . Cranbury, NJ 08512 (1995)

6324 Wallace Laboratories. Manufacturer's literature on Felbatol® . Cranbury, NJ 08512 (1996)

6325 Wallace Laboratories. Manufacturer's literature on Lufyllin® . Cranbury, NJ 08512 (1995)

6326 Wallace SL, Nissen AW. Griseofulvin in acute gout. *N Engl J Med*, 266, 1099 (1962)

6327 Wallach J. *Interpretation of Diagnostic Tests*, Boston MA, Little Brown and Co (1970)

6328 Walldius G. Effect of verapamil on serum lipoproteins in patients with angina pectoris. *Acta Med Scand*, 215, Suppl 681, 43-48 (1984)

6329 Wallemacq PE, Firdaous I, Hassoun A. Improvement and assessment of enzyme-linked immunosorbent assay to detect low FK 506 concentrations in plasma or whole blood within 6 hours. *Clin Chem*, 39, 1045-1049 (1993)

6330 Wallen NH, Larsson PT, Broijersen A et al. Effects of an oral dose of isosorbide nitrate on platelet function and fibrinolysis in healthy volunteers. *Br J Clin Pharmacol*, 35, 143-151 (1993)

6331 Walley TJ, Woods KL, Barnett DB. The effects of intravenous and oral nifedipine on ex vivo platelet function. *Eur J Clin Pharmacol*, 37, 449-452 (1989)

6332 Walsh BW, Kuller LH, Wild RA, et al. Effects of raloxifene on serum lipids and coagulation factors in healthy postmenopausal women. *J Am Med Ass*, 279, 1445-1451 (1998)

6333 Walsh BW, Schiff I, Rosner B et al. Effects of postmenopausal estrogen replacement on the concentrations and metabolism of plasma lipoproteins. *N Engl J Med*, 325, 1196-1204 (1991)

6334 Walstad RA, Myhre KI, Wirum E et al. The influence of sustained release theophylline therapy on free fatty acids in serum. *Acta Pharmacol Toxicol*, 56, 199-203 (1985)

6335 Wan AT, Conyers RAJ, Coombs CJ et al. Determination of silver in blood, urine, and tissues of volunteers and burn patients. *Clin Chem*, 37, 1683-1687 (1991)

6336 Wandell M, Powell JR, Hager WD et al. Effect of quinine on digoxin kinetics. *Clin Pharmacol Ther*, 28, 425-430 (1980)

6337 Wandzilak TR, D'Andre SD, Davis PA et al. Effect of high dose vitamin C on urinary oxalate levels. *J Urol*, 151, 834-837 (1994)

6338 Wang C, Lai CL, Lam KC et al. Effect of cimetidine on gonadal function in man. *Br J Clin Pharmacol*, 13, 791-794 (1982)

6339 Wang C, Wong KL, Lam KC et al. Ranitidine does not affect gonadal function in man. *Br J Clin Pharmacol*, 16, 430-432 (1983)

6340 Wang D-J, Shen D-C, Sheu WH-H et al. Effect of nicardipine treatment on carbohydrate and lipoprotein metabolism in patients with hypertension. *Clin Exp Hypertens*, 15, 557-573 (1993)

6341 Wang Y-S, Hershman JM, Smith V et al. Effect of heparin on free thyroxine as measured by equilibrium dialysis and ultrafiltration. *Clin Chem*, 32, 700 (1986)

6342 Wanka J, Jones LI, Wood PH et al. Indomethacin in rheumatic diseases. *Ann Rheum Dis*, 23, 218 (1964)

6343 Wanner C, Bohler J, Eckardt HG et al. Effects of simvastin on lipoprotein (a) and lipoprotein composition in patients with nephrotic syndrome. *Clin Nephrol*, 41, 138-143 (1994)

6344 Wanner C, Wieland H, Schollmeyer P et al. Beclobrate: pharmacodynamic properties and therapeutic use in hyperlipidemia. *Eur J Clin Pharmacol*, 40, Suppl 1, S85-S89 (1990)

6345 Wanner C, Wieland H, Wackerle B et al. Ketogenic and antiketogenic effects of L-carnitine in hemodialysis patients. *Kidney Int*, 36, Suppl 27, S264-S268 (1989)

6346 Wanwimolruk S, Kang W, Coville PF et al. Marked enhancement by rifampin and lack of effect of isoniazid on the elimination of quinine in man. *Br J Clin Pharmacol*, 40, 87-91 (1995)

6347 Ward C, McNally A, Motter K et al. An Abuscreen Online immunoassay for methamphetamine in urine on the Cobas Mira automated analyzer. *Clin Chem*, 37, 1007 (1991)

6348 Ware S, Millward-Sadler GH. Acute liver disease associated with sodium valproate. *Lancet*, 2, 1110-1113 (1980)

6349 Warner A. Interference of common household chemicals in immunoassay methods for drugs of abuse. *Clin Chem*, 35, 648-651 (1989)

6350 Warner A, Privitera M, Bates D. Standards of laboratory practice: antiepileptic drug monitoring. *Clin Chem*, 44, 1085-1095 (1998)

6351 Warner MD, Peabody CA. Prolactin bioassay before and after treatment with nortriptyline. *Curr Ther Res*, 54, 272-274 (1993)

6352 Warnick GR, Boerma GJM, Assman G et al. Multicenter evaluation of Reflotron direct dry-chemistry assay of high-density lipoprotein cholesterol in venous and fingerstick specimens. *Clin Chem*, 39, 271-277 (1993)

6353 Warrell JP Jr, Israel R, Frisone M et al. Gallium nitrate for acute treatment of cancer-related hypercalcemia: A randomized, double-blind comparison to serotonin. *Ann Intern Med*, 108, 669-674 (1988)

6354 Warrell RP Jr, Isaacs M, Alcock NW et al. Gallium nitrate for treatment of retractory hypercalcemia from parathyroid carcinoma. *Ann Intern Med*, 107, 683-686 (1987)

6355 Warrell RP Jr, Muindi J, Stevens Y-W et al. Induction of profound hypouricemia by a non-sedating thiobarbiturate. *Metabolism*, 38, 550-554 (1989)

6356 Warren K, Hasselberg S, Hilborn D et al. Interference testing on Ektachem clinical chemistry slides (PHYT) for the measurement of phenytoin. *Clin Chem*, 41, S201 (1995)

6357 Warren SE. False-positive urine ketone test with captopril. *N Engl J Med*, 303, 1003-1004 (1980)

6358 Warrington SJ, Holt D, Johnston A et al. Pharmacokinetics and pharmacodynamics of verapamil in combination with atenolol, metoprolol and propranolol. *Br J Clin Pharmacol*, 17, 37s-44s (1984)

6359 Wascher TC, Hermann J, Brezinschek R et al. Serum levels of interleukin-6 and tumour-necrosis-factor-α are not correlated to disease activity in patients with rheumatoid arthritis after treatment with low-dose methotrexate. *Eur J Clin Invest*, 24, 73-75 (1994)

6360 Watanabe J, Sako Y, Umeda F et al. Effects of cilostazol, a phosphodiesterase inhibitor, on urinary excretion of albumin and prostaglandins in non-insulin-dependent diabetic patients. *Diabetes Res Clin Pract*, 22, 53-59 (1993)

6361 Wathen CG, Mackay IG, Glover DR et al. Effect of the partial β-agonist prenalterol on plasma renin activity in patients with left ventricular failure. *Clin Chim Acta*, 162, 97-100 (1987)

6362 Watkins PB, Whitcomb RW. Hepatic dysfunction associated with troglitazone. *N Engl J Med*, 338, 916-917 (1998)

6363 Watschinger B, Watzinger U, Templ H et al. Effect of recombinant human erythropoietin on anterior pituitary function in patients on chronic hemodialysis. *Horm Res*, 36, 22-26 (1991)

6364 Watson CJ. The problem of porphyria - some facts and questions. *N Engl J Med*, 263, 1205 (1960)

6365 Watson PG, Locman RG, Redding VJ. Drug interaction with coumarin derivative anticoagulants. *Br Med J*, 285, 1045-1046 (1982)

6366 Watts GF, Pillay D, Kind PRN. Influence of atenolol on within-subject variation of thyroid function tests. *Ann Clin Biochem*, 27, 599-600 (1990)

6367 Watts NB, Harris ST, Genant HK et al. Intermittent cyclical etidronate treatment of postmenopausal osteoporosis. *N Engl J Med*, 323, 73-79 (1990)

6368 Watts RW, Hetzel DJ, Bochner F et al. Lack of interaction between ranitidine and phenytoin. *Br J Clin Pharmacol*, 15, 499-500 (1983)

6369 Waxman J, Sandow J, Abel P et al. Three-monthly GnRH agonist (buserelin) for prostatic cancer. *Br J Urol*, 65, 43-45 (1990)

6370 Waxman S, Corcino JJ, Herbert V. Drugs, toxins and dietary amino acids affecting vitamin B_{12} or folic acid absorption or utilization. *Am J Med*, 48, 599 (1970)

6371 Way BA, Wilhite TR, Miller R, et al. Vitros digoxin immunoassay evaluated for interference by digoxin-like immunoreactive factors. *Clin Chem*, 44, 1339-1340 (1998)

6372 Wayne AG, Romanski SA, Klee GG et al. Nifedipine, but not verapamil, acutely elevates parathyroid hormone levels in premenopausal women. *Clin Endocrinol*, 42, 9-15 (1995)

6373 Webel ML, Donadio JV Jr. Effects of a large dose of methylprednisolone on renal function. *J Lab Clin Med*, 80, 765 (1972)

6374 Weber C, Tam YK, Schmidtke-Schrezenmeier G, et al. Effect of the lipase inhibitor orlistat on the pharmacokinetics of four different antihypertensive drugs in healthy volunteers. *Eur J Clin Pharmacol*, 51, 87-90 (1996)

6375 Weber JA, van Zanten AP. Interferences in current methods for measurements of creatinine. *Clin Chem*, 37, 695-700 (1991)

6376 Weber MA, Drayer JIM, Kaufman CA. The combined α- and β- adrenergic blocker labetalol and propranolol in the treatment of high blood pressure: similarities and differences. *J Clin Pharmacol*, 24, 103-112 (1984)

6377 Webster PD, Zieve L. Alterations in serum content of pancreatic enzymes. *N Engl J Med*, 267, 654 (1962)

6378 Weeks CE, Conrad GJ, Kvam DC et al. The effect of flecainide acetate, a new antiarrhythmic, on plasma digoxin levels. *J Clin Pharmacol*, 26, 27-31 (1986)

6379 Weetman AP. Effect of the antithyroid drug methimazole on interleukin-1 and interleukin-2 in vitro. *Clin Endocrinol*, 25, 133-142 (1986)

6380 Wegmuller E, Reubi FC. Changes in renal function induced by endralazine, a new antihypertensive drug. *Eur J Clin Pharmacol*, 24, 307-314 (1983)

6381 Wehling M, Muller T, Heim JM et al. Effects of clonidine and dihydralazine on atrial natriuretic factor and cGMP in humans. *J Appl Physiol*, 67, 938-944 (1989)

6382 Wei I, McFadden ER Jr, Hoppel C. Effect of theophylline on urinary excretion of 3-methylhistidine in patients with lung disease. *Metabolism*, 40, 702-706 (1991)

6383 Weidmann P, Bousquet J-C et al. Antihypertensive treatment with bopindolol alone or combined with a diuretic in general practice. *J Cardiovasc Pharmacol*, 8, Suppl 6, 580-587 (1986)

6384 Weidmann P, Gerber A. Effects of treatment with diuretics on serum lipoproteins. *J Cardiovasc Pharmacol*, 6, S260-S268 (1984)

6385 Weinberger I, Rotenberg Z, Fuchs J et al. Amiodarone induced thrombocytopenia. *Arch Intern Med*, 147, 735-736 (1987)

6386 Weinberger M, Hudgel D, Spector S et al. Inhibition of theophylline clearance by troleandomycin. *J Allerg Clin Immunol*, 59, 228-231 (1977)

6387 Weinberger MM, Smith G, Milavetz G et al. Decreased theophylline clearance due to cimetidine. *N Engl J Med*, 304, 672 (1981)

6388 Weinblatt M, Helfgott S, Coblyn J et al. The effects of cyclosporin A on eicosanoid excretion in patients with rheumatoid arthritis. *Arth Rheum*, 34, 481-485 (1991)

6389 Weinstein J. Hypocomplementemia in hydralazine - associated systemic lupus erythematosus. *Am J Med*, 65, 553-556 (1978)

6390 Weinstein L. Antimicrobial agents. In:. *The Pharmacological Basis of Therapeutics. 4th edition. LS Goodman, Gilman (eds)*, New York NY, MacMillan (1970)

6391 Weintraub MS, Eisenberg S, Breslow JL. Lovastatin reduces postprandial lipoprotein levels in hypercholesterolaemic patients with mild hypertriglyceridaemia. *Eur J Clin Invest*, 19, 480-485 (1989)

6392 Weir MR, Klassen DK, Shen SY et al. Acute effects of intravenous cyclosporine on blood pressure, renal hemodynamics, and urine prostaglandin production of healthy humans. *Transplantation*, 49, 41-47 (1990)

6393 Weir RJ, Tree M, Fraser R. Effect of oral contraceptives on blood pressure and on plasma renin, renin substrate and corticosteroids. *J Clin Pathol*, 23, Suppl 3, 49 (1969)

6394 Weiss M, Hassin D, Bank H. Propylthiouracil-induced hepatic damage. *Arch Intern Med*, 140, 1184-1185 (1980)

6395 Weiss P, Bianchine JR. The effect on serum tocopherol levels on drug-induced decrease in serum lipids. *Am J Med Sci*, 258, 275 (1969)

6396 Weiss VC, West DP, Ackerman R et al. Hepatotoxic reactions in a patient treated with etrinate. *Arch Dermatol*, 120, 104-106 (1984)

6397 Weissberger AJ, Ho KKY, Lazarus L. Contrasting effects of oral and transdermal routes of estrogen replacement therapy on 24-hour growth hormone (GH) secretion, insulin-like growth factor I, and GH-binding protein in postmenopausal women. *J Clin Endocrinol Metab*, 72, 374-381 (1991)

6398 Weissman K, Hoyer H. Serum zinc levels during oral glucocorticoid therapy. *J Invest Dermatol*, 86, 715-716 (1986)

6399 Weissman PN, Shenkman L, Gregerman RI. Chlorpropamide hyponatremia. *N Engl J Med*, 284, 65 (1971)

6400 Weisweiler P. Low-dose colestipol plus fenofibrate: effects on plasma lipoproteins, lecithin: cholesterol acyltransferase, and postheparin lipases in familial hypercholesterolemia. *Metabolism*, 38, 271-275 (1989)

6401 Weitekamp MR, Aber RC. Prolonged bleeding times and bleeding diathesis associated with moxalactam administration. *J Am Med Ass*, 249, 69-71 (1983)

6402 Welch S, Wright T, Shuler C. Evaluation of ferritin with a newly formatted assay on the BMC ES 300. *Clin Chem*, 41, S188 (1995)

6403 Welling PG. Interactions affecting drug absorption. *Clin Pharmacokinet*, 9, 404-434 (1984)

6404 Wendland DB, Bishop J, Harrington C et al. Specificity of the amphetamine/methamphetamine assay on the Abbott AxSYM system. *Clin Chem*, 41, S123 (1995)

6405 Wenham PR, Haddad L, Panarelli M, et al. Simplified detection of a mutation causing familial hypercholesterolaemia throughout Britain: evidence for an origin in a common distant ancestor. *Ann Clin Biochem*, 35, 226-235 (1998)

6406 Wenisch C, Myskiw D, Narzt E et al. Serum laminin in Graves' disease. *Eur J Clin Invest*, 25, 425-428 (1995)

6407 Wenisch C, Parschalk B, Burgmann H et al. Decreased serum levels of TGF-β in patients with acute Plasmodium falciparum malaria. *J Clin Immunol*, 15, 69-73 (1995)

6408 Wenk RE, Gebhardt FC, Bhagavan BS et al. Tetracycline-associated fatty liver of pregnancy, including possible pregnancy risk after chronic dermatologic use of tetracycline. *J Reprod Med*, 26, 135-141 (1981)

6409 Wennberg JE, Okum R, Hinman EJ et al. Renal toxicity of oral cholecystographic media. *J Am Med Ass*, 186, 461 (1963)

6410 Wennmalm A, Karwatowska-Prokopczuk E, Wennmalm M. Effect of aminophylline on plasma and urinary catecholamine levels during heavy leg exercise in healthy young men. *Clin Sci*, 76, 255-260 (1989)

6411 Wentz AC, Jones GS, Graeber J. Effect of infused prostaglandin F2α on hormonal levels during early pregnancy. *Am J Obstet Gynecol*, 114, 908 (1972)

6412 Wenzel KW. Pharmacological interference with *in vitro* tests of thyroid function. *Metabolism*, 30, 717-732 (1981)

6413 Werblin TP, Pollack IP, Liss RA. Blood dyscrasias in patients using methazolamide (Neptazane®) for glaucoma. *Ophthalmology*, 87, 350-354 (1980)

6414 Werk EE Jr, Macgee J, Sholiton LJ. Effect of diphenylhydantoin on cortisol metabolism in man. *J Clin Invest*, 43, 1824 (1964)

6415 Werning C, Bayer JM, Fischer N et al. The effect of carbenoxolone sodium on blood pressure. *Germ Med*, 2, 9 (1972)

6416 Wertalik LF, Metz EN, Lobuglio AF et al. Decreased serum B_{12} levels secondary to oral contraceptive agents. *Am J Clin Nutr*, 24, 603 (1971)

6417 Wertmer CA, Cloud H, Ohtake M et al. Effect of long-term administration of anticonvulsants on copper, zinc and ceruloplasmin levels. *Drug Nutr Interact*, 4, 269-270 (1986)

6418 Wester PO. Urinary zinc excretion during treatment with different diuretics. *Acta Med Scand*, 208, 209-212 (1980)

6419 Westerveld HT, Kock LAW, van Rijn HJM et al. 17β-estradiol improves postprandial lipid metabolism in postmenopausal women. *J Clin Endocrinol Metab*, 80, 249-253 (1995)

6420 Wewers MD, Brantly ML, Casolaro MA et al. Effect of tamoxifen as a therapy to augment alpha$_1$-antitrypsin concentrations in Z homozygous alpha$_1$-antitrypsin-deficient subjects. *Am Rev Resp Dis*, 135, 401-402 (1987)

6421 Weykamp CW, Penders TJ, Baadenhuijsen H et al. Vitamin C and glycohemoglobin. *Clin Chem*, 41, 713-716 (1995)

6422 White DJG, Blatchford NR, Cauwenbergh G. Cyclosporine and ketoconazole. *Transplantation*, 37, 214-215 (1984)

6423 White LL. Fatal marrow aplasia during chlorpropamide therapy. *Br Med J*, 1, 691 (1962)

6424 White MC, Kendall-Taylor P. Adrenal hypofunction in patients taking ketoconazole. *Lancet*, 1, 44 (1985)

6425 White MG, Asch MJ. Acid-base effects of topical mafenide acetate in the burned patient. *N Engl J Med*, 284, 1281 (1971)

6426 White NJ, Warrell DJ, Chantavanich P et al. Severe hypoglycemia and hyperinsulinemia in falciparum malaria. *N Engl J Med*, 309, 61-66 (1983)

6427 Whitehead TP, Robinson D, Allaway S et al. Effect of red wine ingestion on the antioxidant capacity of serum. *Clin Chem*, 41, 32-35 (1995)

6428 Whitfield JB, Moss DW, Neale G et al. Changes in γ-Glutamyl transpeptidase activity associated with alterations in drug metabolism in man. *Br Med J*, 1, 316-318 (1973)

6429 Whitfield JB, Pounder RE, Neale G et al. Serum glutamyl transpeptidase activity in liver disease. *Gut*, 13, 702 (1972)

6430 Whiting GFM, McLaran CJ, Bochner F. Severe hyperkalemia with moduretic. *Med J Aust*, 1, 409 (1979)

6431 Whittaker JA, Price Evans DA. Genetic control of phenylbutazone metabolism in man. *Br Med J*, 4, 323-328 (1970)

6432 Whitten CF, Brough AJ. The pathophysiology of acute iron poisoning. *Clin Toxicol*, 4, 585 (1971)

6433 Whitworth JA, Gordon D, Harpley R et al. Acute hormonal and renal effects of oral dilevalol in normal men. *Clin Exp Pharmacol Physiol*, 16, 59-63 (1989)

6434 Wians FH Jr, Norton JT, Wirebaugh SR. False-positive serum tricyclic antidepressant screen with cyproheptadine. *Clin Chem*, 39, 1355-1356 (1993)

6435 Wians FH Jr, Plickert NJ, Heald JI. The modified aca method for serum iron quantification eliminates deferoxamine interference. *Clin Chem*, 34, 1513-1514 (1988)

6436 Widerlov E, Andersson U, Von Bahr C et al. Pharmacokinetics and effects on prolactin of remoxipride in patients with tardive dyskinesia. *Psychopharmacology*, 103, 46-49 (1991)

6437 Widerlov E, Karlman I, Storsater J. Hydralazine-induced neonatal thrombocytopenia. *N Engl J Med*, 303, 1235 (1980)

6438 Widmark P. Safety and efficacy of piroxicam in the treatment of acute gout. *Eur J Rheumatol Inflamm*, 1, 346-355 (1978)

6439 Wiecek A, Fkiser D, Nowicki M, Ritz E. Effect of moxonidine on urinary electrolyte excretion and renal haemodynamics in man. *Eur J Clin Pharmacol*, 48, 203-208 (1995)

6440 Wiederholt IC, Genco M, Foley JM. Recurrent episodes of hypoglycemia induced by propoxyphene. *Neurology*, 17, 703 (1967)

6441 Wiedermann CJ, Vogel W, Tilg H et al. Suppression of thyroid function by interferon-α2 in man. *Nauyn-Schmiedebergs Arch Pharmacol*, 343, 665-668 (1991)

6442 Wiegand M, Berger M. Action of trimipramine on sleep and pituitary hormone secretion. *Drugs*, 38, Suppl 1, 35-42 (1989)

6443 Wiegelmann W, Wildmeister W, Horster FA et al. Radioimmunoassay of hGH, ICSH, and FSH in plasma after i.v. administration of thyrotropin releasing hormone (TRH). *Horm Metab Res*, 4, 482 (1972)

6444 Wiersinga WM, Trip MD, van Beeren MH et al. An increase in plasma cholesterol independent of thyroid function during long-term amiodarone therapy. *Ann Intern Med*, 114, 128-132 (1991)

6445 Wiesener RH, Ludwig J, Lindor KD et al. A controlled trial of cyclosporine in the treatment of primary biliary cirrhosis. *N Engl J Med*, 322, 1419-1424 (1990)

6446 Wiethrop BV, Cryer PE. Glycemic actions of alanine and terbutaline in IDDM. *Diabetes Care*, 16, 1124-1130 (1993)

6447 Wigley RD. Aspirin and the kidney. *NZ Med J*, 74, 301 (1971)

6448 Wijnands WJA, Van Herwaarden CLA, Vree TB. Enoxacin raises plasma theophylline concentrations. *Lancet*, 2, 108-109 (1984)

6449 Wijnja LL, Snijder JA, Nieweg HO. Acetylsalicylic acid as a cause of pancytopenia from bone marrow damage. *Lancet*, 2, 768 (1966)

6450 Wilcox RG. Randomized study of six β-blockers and a thiazide diuretic in essential hypertension. *Br Med J*, 2, 383-385 (1978)

6451 Wilder BJ, Serrano EE, Ramsay RE. Plasma diphenylhydantoin levels after loading and maintenance doses. *Clin Pharmacol Ther*, 14, 797-801 (1973)

6452 Wilder BJ, Willmore LJ, Bruni J et al. Valproic acid: interaction with other anticonvulsant drugs. *Neurology*, 28, 892-896 (1978)

6453 Wildmeister W, Daweke H, Gries FA et al. Influence of synthetic TRH on glucose, free fatty acids and insulin in plasma of healthy persons. *Horm Metab Res*, 4, 368 (1972)

6454 Wiles DH, McCreadie RG, Whitehead A. Pharmacokinetics of haloperidol and fluphenazine decanoates in chronic schizophrenia. *Psychopharmacology*, 101, 274-281 (1990)

6455 Wilhelm MP, Edson RS. Antimicrobial agents in urinary tract infections. *Mayo Clin Proc*, 62, 1025-1031 (1987)

6456 Wilimas JA, Flynn PM, Harris S et al. A randomized study of outpatient treatment with ceftriaxone for selected febrile children with sickle cell disease. *N Engl J Med*, 329, 472-476 (1993)

6457 Wilkes HC, Meade TW, Barzegar S et al. Gemfibrozil reduces plasma prothrombin fragment F1+2 concentration, a marker of coagulability, in patients with coronary heart disease. *Thromb Haemostas*, 67, 503-506 (1992)

6458 Wilkins MR, Franklyn JA, Woods KL et al. Effect of propranolol on thyroid homeostasis of healthy volunteers. *Postgrad Med J*, 61, 391-394 (1985)

6459 Wilkins MR, Lewis HM, West MJ. Captopril reduces the renal response to intravenous atrial natriuretic peptide in normotensives. *J Hum Hypertens*, 1, 47-51 (1987)

6460 Wilkinson GR, Beckett AH. Absorption, metabolism and excretion of the ephedrines in man. *J Pharmacol Exp Ther*, 162, 139-147 (1968)

6461 Wilkinson JH. An Introduction to Diagnostic Enzymology. London, Arnold (1962)

6462 Wilkinson SP, Portmann B, Williams R. Hepatitis from dantrolene sodium. *Gut*, 20, 133-136 (1979)

6463 Wilklund O, Angelin B, Bergman M et al. Pravastatin and gemfibrozil alone and in combination for the treatment of hypercholesterolemia. *Am J Med*, 94, 13-20 (1993)

6464 Williams A, Goldsmith R, Coakley J. Profound suppression of plasma alanine aminotransferase activity in children taking vigabatrin. *Aust NZ J Med*, 23, 65 (1993)

6465 Williams CM. The effect of reserpine on dopamine metabolism in humans. *J Neurochem*, 9, 335 (1962)

6466 Williams G, Lofts F, Fuessl H et al. Treatment with danazol and plasma glucagon concentration. *Br Med J*, 291, 1155-1156 (1985)

6467 Williams GA, Bowser EN, Hargis GK et al. Effect of glucocorticoids on function of the parathyroid glands in man. *Clin Res*, 20, 780 (1972)

6468 Williams GT, Johnson SAN, Dieppe PA et al. Neutropenia during treatment of rheumatoid arthritis. *Ann Rheum Dis*, 37, 366-369 (1978)

6469 Williams L, Carrico J, Georgette C et al. Investigation of possible interference by ibuprofen and naproxen patient samples with EMIT D.A.U. assays for amphetamine, barbiturate, benzodiazepines and cannabinoid. *Clin Chem*, 37, 1009 (1991)

6470 Williams LL, Lopez LM, Thorman AD et al. Plasma lipid profiles and antihypertensive agents: effects of lisinopril, enalapril, nitrendipine, hydralazine, and hydrochlorothiazide. *Drug Intell Clin Pharm*, 22, 546-550 (1988)

6471 Williams M, Young JB, Rosa RM et al. Effect of protein on urinary dopamine excretion. *J Clin Invest*, 78, 1687-1693 (1986)

6472 Williams SJ, Baird-Lambert JA, Farrell GC. Inhibition of theophylline metabolism by interferon. *Lancet*, 2, 939-941 (1987)

6473 Williamson J, Davidson DF, Boag DE. Contamination of a specimen with N-acetyl cysteine infusion: a cause of spurious ketonaemia and hyperglycaemia. *Ann Clin Biochem*, 26, 207 (1989)

6474 Williamson JM, Gibbs WN. Hypoplastic anaemia and hydroflumethiazide. *Scott Med J*, 11, 19 (1966)

6475 Willich SN, Pohjola-Sintonen S, Bhatia SJS et al. Suppression of silent ischemia by metoprolol without alteration of morning increase of platelet aggregability in patients with stable coronary artery disease. *Circulation*, 79, 557-565 (1989)

6476 Willmore LJ, Wilder BJ, Bruni J et al. Effect of valproic acid on hepatic function. *Neurology*, 28, 961-964 (1978)

6477 Willoughby JS, Paton TW, Walker SE et al. The effect of cimetidine on enteric-coated ASA disposition. *Clin Pharmacol Ther*, 33, 268 (1983)

6478 Willoughby MIN, Baird GM, Campbell AM. Levamisole and neutropenia. *Lancet*, 1, 657 (1977)

6479 Wills JH. The measurement and significance of changes in the cholinesterase activities of erythrocytes and plasma in man. *Crit Rev Toxicol*, 1, 153 (1972)

6480 Wilner KD, Gardner MJ. Cimetidine does not alter the clearance or plasma binding of tenidap in healthy male volunteers. *Br J Clin Pharmacol*, 39, 21S-24S (1995)

6481 Wilner KD, Gardner MJ. Tenidap sodium does not alter the clearance or plasma protein binding of tolbutamide in healthy male volunteers. *Br J Clin Pharmacol*, 39, 39S-42S (1995)

6482 Wilner KD, Ziegler MG. Effects of $alpha_1$,-inhibition on renal blood flow and sympathetic nervous activity in systemic hypertension. *Am J Cardiol*, 59, 82G-86G (1987)

6483 Wilson C, Azmy AF, Beattie TJ et al. Hypermagnesemia and progression of renal failure associated with Renacidin® therapy. *Clin Nephrol*, 25, 266-267 (1986)

6484 Wilson CB, Kirkendall WM. The acute effects of mefruside in man: a new diuretic compound. *Pharmacol Exp Ther*, 173, 288 (1970)

6485 Wilson DM, Baldwin RB, Ariagno RL. A randomized placebo-controlled trial of effects of dexamethasone on hypothalamic-pituitary-adrenal axis in preterm infants. *J Pediatr*, 113, 764-768 (1988)

6486 Wilson FA, Dietschy JM. Differential diagnostic approach to clinical problems of malabsorption. *Gastroenterology*, 61, 911 (1971)

6487 Wilson GM. Toxicity of hypotensive drugs. *Practitioner*, 194, 51 (1965)

6488 Wilson IC, Gambill JM, Sandifier MGK Jr. A double blind study comparing imipramine (Tofranil®) with desmethylimipramine (Pertofrane®). *Psychosomatics*, 5, 88 (1964)

6489 Wilson J, Wahbha MMAE, Martin PG et al. The effect of nisoldipine on renal function in the long-term treatment of hypertension in patients with and without renal impairment. *Eur J Clin Pharmacol*, 37, 437-441 (1989)

6490 Wilson JA, Craig IF. Effects of cimetidine and ranitidine on high density lipoprotein cholesterol concentrations. *Br Med J*, 290, 807-808 (1985)

6491 Wilson RG, Hamilton JR, Boyd WD et al. The effect of long term phenothiazine therapy on plasma prolactin. *Br J Psychiat*, 127, 71-74 (1975)

6492 Wilson RG, Singhai VK, Percy Robb I et al. Response of plasma prolactin and growth hormone to insulin hypoglycaemia. *Lancet*, 2, 1283 (1972)

6493 Wilson SP, Kamin DL, Feldman JM. Acetaminophen administration interferes with urinary metanephrine (and catecholamine) determinations. *Clin Chem*, 31, 1093-1094 (1985)

6494 Wilson T, Thong KJ, Howie PW. Decrease in human plasma gravidin levels after medical abortion. *Prostaglandins*, 48, 175-185 (1994)

6495 Wilson TW. Effects of atenolol and enalapril on blood pressure, plasma renin activity and urinary prostanoids. *Clin Invest Med*, 11, 203-208 (1988)

6496 Wilson TW, McCaulay FA, Waslen TA. Effects of aging in responses to furosemide. *Prostaglandins*, 38, 675-689 (1989)

6497 Wilson WL, Bisel HF, Cole D et al. Prolonged low dosage administration of hexamethylmelamine (NC 13875). *Cancer*, 25, 568 (1970)

6498 Wilson WR, Cockeril FR III. Tetracyclines, chloramphenicol, erythromycin and clindamycin. *Mayo Clin Proc*, 62, 906-915 (1987)

6499 Winchester JF, Kellett RJ, Boddy K et al. Metolazone and bendroflumethiazide in hypertension: physiologic and metabolic observations. *Clin Pharmacol Ther*, 28, 611-618 (1980)

6500 Windhorst DB, Nigra T. General clinical toxicology of oral retinoids. *J Am Acad Dermatol*, 6, 675-682 (1982)

6501 Windorfer P. Drug interaction during anticonvulsive therapy. *Int J Clin Pharmacol*, 14, 236 (1976)

6502 Winek CL, Kuhlman JJ Jr, Shanor SP. Detection and interference of some central nervous system stimulants in urine drug screening procedures. *Clin Toxicol*, 17, 337-351 (1980)

6503 Winer N, Kirkendall WM, Canosa FL et al. Placebo-controlled trial of once-a-day isradipine monotherapy in mild to moderately severe hypertension. *J Clin Pharmacol*, 30, 1006-1011 (1990)

6504 Wing SS, Fantus IG. Adverse immunologic effects of antithyroid drugs. *Can Med Ass J*, 136, 121-127 (1987)

6505 Winship LC, McKenney JM, Wright JT et al. The effect of ranitidine and cimetidine on single-dose diltiazem pharmacokinetics. *Pharmacotherapy*, 5, 16-19 (1985)

6506 Winsten S. Collection and preservation of specimens. *Stand Meth Clin Chem*, 5, 1 (1965)

6507 Winston DJ, Murphy W, Young LS et al. Piperacillin therapy for serious bacterial infections. *Am J Med*, 69, 255-261 (1980)

6508 Winter SL, Boyer JL. Hepatic toxicity from large doses of vitamin B_3 (nicotinamide). *N Engl J Med*, 289, 1180 (1973)

6509 Winther K, Bondesen S, Honore Hansen S et al. Lack of effect of 5-aminosalicylic acid on platelet aggregation and fibrinolytic activity in vivo and in vitro. *Eur J Clin Pharmacol*, 33, 419-422 (1987)

6510 Winther K, Jespersen CM, Rydberg B et al. Dose-dependent effects of verapamil and nifedipine on in vivo platelet function in normal volunteers. *Eur J Clin Pharmacol*, 39, 291-293 (1990)

6511 Winther K, Trap-Jensen J. Effects of three β-blockers with different pharmacodynamic properties on platelet aggregation and platelet and plasma cyclic AMP. *Eur J Clin Pharmacol*, 35, 17-20 (1988)

6512 Winthrop Laboratories. Manufacturer's literature on Neggram® . New York, NY

6513 Winthrop Laboratories. Manufacturer's literature on Telepaque. New York, NY

6514 Wintrobe MM. *Clinical Hematology, 6th ed*, Philadelphia PA, Lea and Febiger (1967)

6515 Wirth WA, Thompson RL. The effect of various conditions and substances on the results of laboratory procedures. *Am J Clin Pathol*, 43, 579 (1965)

6516 Wise PH. Clopamide and carbohydrate metabolism. *Med J Aust*, 2, 795 (1969)

6517 Wiseman C, McGregor RF, McCredie KB. Urinary amino acid excretion in acute leukemia. *Cancer*, 38, 219-224 (1976)

6518 Withrow CD, Woodbury DM. Trimethadione and other oxazolidinediones: interactions with other drugs. In:. *Antiepileptic Drugs. DM Woodbury, JK Penry, RP Schmidt (eds)*, New York NY, Raven Press (1972)

6519 Witter FR, Woods AS, Griffin MD et al. Effects of prednisone, aspirin, and acetaminophen on an in vivo biologic response to interferon in humans. *Clin Pharmacol Ther*, 44, 239-243 (1988)

6520 Witzgall HV, Werder K, Weber PC. Mineralocorticoid and prolactin response to the dopamine antagonist metoclopramide in patients with primary aldosteronism. *J Steroid Biochem*, 19, 1671-1676 (1983)

6521 Witzig TE, Kvols LK, Moertel CG et al. Effect of the somatostatin analogue octreotide acetate on hemostasis in humans. *Mayo Clin Proc*, 66, 283-286 (1991)

6522 Wojtukiewicz MZ, Kloczko J, Galar M et al. Decreased plasma protein C levels after high dosage of acetylsalicylic acid. *Thromb Res*, 69, 401-406 (1993)

6523 Wolcott GJ, Hackett TN Jr. Levodopa and tests for ketonuria. *N Engl J Med*, 2183, 1522 (1970)

6524 Wolever TMS, Jenkins DJA, Mueller S et al. Psyllium reduces blood lipids in men and women with hyperlipidemia. *Am J Med Sci*, 307, 269-273 (1994)

6525 Wolff JA, Barshop B, Nyhan WL et al. Effects of ascorbic acid in alkaptonuria: alterations in benzoquinone acetic acid and an ontogenic effect in infancy. *Pediatr Res*, 26, 140-144 (1989)

6526 Wolinsky-Friedland M. Drug-induced metabolic bone disease. *Endocrinol Metab Clin NA*, 24, 395-420 (1995)

6527 Wollheim FA, Lindstrom CG. Liver abnormalities in penicillamine treated rheumatoid arthritis. *Scand J Rheumatol*, , Suppl28, 100-107 (1979)

6528 Wollman MR, David DS, Brennan BL et al. The nitrobluetetrazolium test. *Lancet*, 2, 289 (1972)

6529 Wolpert E, Phillips SF, Summerskill WH. Ammonia production in the human colon: effects of cleansing neomycin and acetohydroxamic acid (AHA). *N Engl J Med*, 283, 159 (1970)

6530 Wolthers T, Grofte T, Flyvbjerg A et al. Dose-dependent stimulation of insulin-like growth factor-binding protein-1 by lanreotide, a somatostatin analog. *J Clin Endocrinol Metab*, 78, 141-144 (1994)

6531 Wong F, Massie D, Hsu P et al. Nifedipine: its effects on renal hemodynamics and sodium homeostasis in well-compensated alcoholic cirrhosis. *J Hepatol*, 21, 64-69 (1994)

6532 Wong LC, Choo YC, MA HK. Use of oral VP 16-213 as primary chemotherapeutic agent in treatment of gestational trophoblastic disease. *Am J Obstet Gynecol*, 15, 924-927 (1984)

6533 Wong L-G, Reilly EB. Effect of acetohexamide on serum creatinine measurement. *Clin Chem*, 28, 1651 (1982)

6534 Wong TC, Palav AB, Kin BJ et al. Changes in serum and urinary electrolytes following intra-amniotic injection of hypertonic saline. *NY State J Med*, 72, 564 (1972)

6535 Wong YY, Ludden TM, Bell RD. Effect of erythromycin on carbamazepine kinetics. *Clin Pharmacol Ther*, 33, 460-464 (1983)

6536 Wongpaitoon V, Mills PR, Russell RI et al. Intrahepatic cholestasis and cutaneous bullae associated with glibenclamide therapy. *Postgrad Med J*, 57, 244-246 (1981)

6537 Wood FC, Cahill GF. Mannose utilization in man. *J Clin Invest*, 42, 1300 (1963)

6538 Wood PJ, Barth JH, Freedman DB, et al. Evidence for the low dose dexamethasone suppression to screen for Cushing's syndrome - recommendations for a protocol for biochemistry laboratories. *Ann Clin Biochem*, 34, 222-229 (1997)

6539 Woodcock BG, Kirsten R, Nelson K et al. A reduction in verapamil concentrations with phenytoin. *N Engl J Med*, 325, 1179 (1991)

6540 Woods JW, Ajzen H. Effect of reserpine and guanethidine on excretion of 3-methoxy-4-hydroxymandelic acid in man. *Proc Soc Exp Biol Med*, 114, 107 (1963)

6541 World Health Organization. Expert Committee on Malaria report. *WHO Tech Rep Ser*, 324, 38 (1966)

6542 Worth D, Harvey J, Brown J et al. The effects of intravenous levodopa on plasma renin activity, renal function, and blood pressure in man. *Eur J Clin Pharmacol*, 35, 137-141 (1988)

6543 Worth HG. The effect of sugars on automated urinary oestrogens estimations in pregnancy. *Clin Chim Acta*, 49, 53 (1973)

6544 Wright AD, Barber SG, Kendall MJ et al. β-adrenoceptor-blocking drugs and blood sugar control in diabetes mellitus. *Br Med J*, 1, 159-161 (1979)

6545 Wright N, Clarkson AR, Brown SS et al. Effects of poisoning on serum enzyme activities. *Br Med J*, 3, 347 (1971)

6546 Wright RA, Flapan AD, Alberti KGMM et al. Effects of captopril therapy on endogenous fibrinolysis in men with recent, uncomplicated myocardial infarction. *J Am Coll Cardiol*, 24, 67-73 (1994)

6547 Wright RA, Perrie AM, Stenhouse F et al. The long-term effects of metoprolol and epanolol on tissue-type plasminogen activator and plasminogen activator inhibitor 1 in patients with ischaemic heart disease. *Eur J Clin Pharmacol*, 46, 279-282 (1994)

6548 Wu M-S, Johnston P, Sheu WH-H et al. Effect of metformin on carbohydrate and lipoprotein metabolism in NIDDM patients. *Diabetes Care*, 13, 1-8 (1990)

6549 Wu YS, Hurt C, Kohne C et al. Determination of urinary/CSF protein using Boehringer Mannheim/Hitachi analyzers. *Clin Chem*, 37, 1063 (1991)

6550 Wyeth-Ayerst Laboratories. Manufacturer's literature on Atromid-S® . Philadelphia, PA 19101 (1997)

6551 Wyeth-Ayerst Laboratories. Manufacturer's literature on Cardene® . Philadelphia, PA 19101 (1997)

6552 Wyeth-Ayerst Laboratories. Manufacturer's literature on Cordarone® . Philadelphia, PA 19101 (1997)

6553 Wyeth-Ayerst Laboratories. Manufacturer's literature on Diucardin® . Philadelphia, PA 19101 (1997)

6554 Wyeth-Ayerst Laboratories. Manufacturer's literature on Duract™. Philadelphia, PA 19101 (1997)

6555 Wyeth-Ayerst Laboratories. Manufacturer's literature on Effexor® . Philadelphia, PA 19101 (1997)

6556 Wyeth-Ayerst Laboratories. Manufacturer's literature on Fluothane® . Philadelphia, PA 19101 (1997)

6557 Wyeth-Ayerst Laboratories. Manufacturer's literature on Heparin. Philadelphia, PA 19101 (1997)

6558 Wyeth-Ayerst Laboratories. Manufacturer's literature on Inderal® LA. Philadelphia, PA 19101 (1990)

6559 Wyeth-Ayerst Laboratories. Manufacturer's literature on Lodine® . Philadelphia, PA 19101 (1996)

6560 Wyeth-Ayerst Laboratories. Manufacturer's literature on Naprelan® . Philadelphia, PA 19101 (1997)

6561 Wyeth-Ayerst Laboratories. Manufacturer's literature on Normiflos® . Philadelphia, PA 19101 (1997)

6562 Wyeth-Ayerst Laboratories. Manufacturer's literature on Norplant® System. Philadelphia, PA 19101 (1997)

6563 Wyeth-Ayerst Laboratories. Manufacturer's literature on Omnipen® . Philadelphia, PA 19101 (1997)

6564 Wyeth-Ayerst Laboratories. Manufacturer's literature on Orudis® and Oruvail® . Philadelphia, PA 19101 (1997)

6565 Wyeth-Ayerst Laboratories. Manufacturer's literature on Phenergan® . Philadelphia, PA 19101 (1997)

6566 Wyeth-Ayerst Laboratories. Manufacturer's literature on Premarin® . Philadelphia, PA 19101 (1997)

6567 Wyeth-Ayerst Laboratories. Manufacturer's literature on Protopam® . Philadelphia, PA 19101 (1997)

6568 Wyeth-Ayerst Laboratories. Manufacturer's literature on Redux™. Philadelphia, PA 19101 (1997)

6569 Wyeth-Ayerst Laboratories. Manufacturer's literature on Sectral® . Philadelphia, PA 19101 (1997)

6570 Wyeth-Ayerst Laboratories. Manufacturer's literature on Serax® . Philadelphia, PA 19101 (1997)

6571 Wyeth-Ayerst Laboratories. Manufacturer's literature on Surmontil® . Philadelphia, PA 19101 (1997)

6572 Wyllie JH, Boulos PB, Lewin MR et al. Plasma gastrin and acid secretion in man following stimulation by food, meat extract and insulin. *Gut*, 13, 887 (1972)

6573 Wyllie JH, Hesselbo T, Black JW. Effects in man of histamine H_2-receptor blockade by burimamide. *Lancet*, 2, 1117 (1972)

6574 Wynn V. Metabolic effects of danazol. *J Intern Med Res*, 5, Suppl 3, 25-35 (1977)

6575 Xanthopoulos B, Koutras DA, Boukis MA et al. The effect of benziodarone on the thyroid hormone levels and the pituitary- thyroid axis. *J Endocrinol Invest*, 9, 337-339 (1986)

6576 Yamada K, Kanba S, Ohnishi K, et al. Changes in symptoms and plasma homovanillic acid with amantadine hydrochloride in chronic schizophrenia. *Biol Psychiat*, 41, 1062-1064 (1997)

6577 Yamada S, Suou T, Kawasaki H. Plasma vitronectin concentrations in patients with chronic hepatitis C treated with interferon alpha. *Clin Chim Acta*, 261, 61-90 (1997)

6578 Yamamoto H, Ninomiya H, Yoshimatsu K, et al. Serum levels of major basic protein in patients with or without eosinophilia: measurement by enzyme linked immunosorbent assay. *Br J Haematol*, 86, 490-495 (1994)

6579 Yamamoto T, Moriwaki Y, Suda M, et al. Theophylline-induced increase in plasma uric acid - purine catabolism increased by theophylline. *Int J Clin Pharmacol Ther Toxicol*, 29, 257-261 (1991)

6580 Yamamoto T, Moriwaki Y, Takahashi S, et al. Effect of allopurinol and benzbromarone on the concentration of uridine in plasma. *Metabolism*, 46, 1473-1475 (1997)

6581 Yamamoto T, Moriwaki Y, Takahashi S, et al. Effects of pyrazinamide, probenecid, and benzbromarone on renal excretion of oxypurinol. *Arch Rheum Dis*, 50, 631-633 (1991)

6582 Yamamoto T, Moriwaki Y, Takahashi S, et al. Renal excretion of purine bases: effects of probenecid, benzbromarone and pyrazinamide. *Nephron*, 48, 116-120 (1988)

6583 Yamamoto T, Takahashi S, Nakaoko M, et al. The effect of phenobarbital on human plasma lipids. *Int J Clin Pharmacol Ther Toxicol*, 27, 463-466 (1989)

6584 Yamamoto T, Takahashi S, Suda M, et al. Effect of probenecid on oxypurines in plasma. *Int J Clin Pharmacol Ther Toxicol*, 27, 510-514 (1989)

6585 Yamashita J-I, Hideshima T, Shirakusa T, Ogawa M. Medroxyprogesterone acetate treatment reduces serum interleukin-6 levels in patients with metastatic breast carcinoma. *Cancer*, 78, 2346-2352 (1996)

6586 Yamashita SK, Ludwig EA, Middleton E , et al. Lack of pharmacokinetic and pharmacodynamic interactions between ketoconazole and prednisolone. *Clin Pharmacol Ther*, 49, 558-570 (1991)

6587 Yamazaki M, Uchiyama S, Maruyama S. Alterations of haemostatic markers in various subtypes and phases of stroke. *Blood Coag Fibrinolysis*, 4, 707-712 (1993)

6588 Yan Y, Davis P. Gold induced marrow suppression: a review of 10 cases. *J Rheumatol*, 17, 47-51 (1990)

6589 Yang C-Y, Gu Z-W, Xie Y-H, et al. Efects of gemfibrozil on very-low-density lipoprotein composition and low-density lipoprotein size in patients with hypertriglyceridemia or combined hyperlipidemia. *Atherosclerosis*, 126, 105-116 (1996)

6590 Yarchoan R, Mitsuya H, Myers CE, et al. Clinical pharmacology of 3'-azido-2',3'-dideoxythymidine (Zidovudine) and related dideoxynucleosides. *N Engl J Med*, 321, 726-738 (1989)

6591 Yasu T, Imanishi M, Kimura G, et al. Short-term increase in prostaglandin I_2 synthesis caused by cicletanine in patients with essential hypertension. *Am J Hypertens*, 8, 944-948 (1995)

6592 Yates VM, Kerr REI. Cimetidine and thrombocytopenia. *Br Med J*, 280, 1453 (1980)

6593 Yatsuhashi H, Inoue O, Inokuchi K, et al. Short and long-term effects of interferon on serum markers of hepatitis C virus replication. *J Gastroenterol Hepatol*, 8, 1-6 (1993)

6594 Yazici H, Pazarli H, Barnes CG, et al. A controlled trial of azathioprine in Behcet's syndrome. *N Engl J Med*, 332, 281-285 (1990)

6595 Yee GC, McGuire TR. Pharmacokinetic drug interactions with cyclosporin (Part I). *Clin Pharmacokinet*, 1, 319-332 (1990)

6596 Yee GC, McGuire TR. Pharmacokinetic drug interactions with cyclosporin (Part II). *Clin Pharmacokinet*, 19, 400-415 (1990)

6597 Yen SSC, Ehara Y, Siler TM. Augmentation of prolactin secretion by estrogen in hypogonadal women. *J Clin Invest*, 53, 652 (1974)

6598 Yen SSC, Tsai CC. The biphasic pattern in the feedback action of ethinyl estradiol on the release of pituitary FSH and LH. *J Clin Endocrinol Metab*, 33, 882 (1971)

6599 Yeung CY, Yu VYH. Phenobarbitone enhancement of bromsulphalein™ clearance in neonatal hyperbilirubinemia. *Pediatrics*, 48, 556 (1971)

6600 Yikorkala O, Nilsson CG, Hirvonen E, et al. Evidence of similar increases in bone turnover during nafarelin and danazol use in women with endometriosis. *Gynecol Endocrinol*, 4, 251-260 (1990)

6601 Yilmaz E, Canberk A, Eroglu L. Nifedipine alters serum theophylline levels in asthmatic patients with hypertension. *Fundam Clin Pharmacol*, 5, 341-345 (1991)

6602 Ylikorkala O, Kivinen S, Ronnberg L, et al. Sulpiride treatment during early human pregnancy: effect on the levels of prolactin, sex steroids, and placental lactogen. *J Clin Endocrinol Metab*, 51, 155-157 (1980)

6603 Yoshida A, Fujita M, Kurosawa N, et al. Effects of diltiazem on plasma level and urinary excretion of digoxin in healthy subjects. *Clin Pharmacol Ther*, 35, 681-685 (1984)

6604 Yoshida K, Kiso Y, Kurihara H , et al. Erythrocyte carbonic anhydrase I concentration in patients receiving thyroxine. *Endocrinol Jpn*, 38, 363-367 (1991)

6605 Yoshimura N, Kodama K, Yoshitake J. Carbohydrate metabolism and insulin release during ether and halothane anesthesia. *Br J Anaes*, 43, 1022 (1971)

6606 Yoshimura N, Takeuchi H, Ogata H, et al. Effects of roxatidine acetate hydrochloride and cimetidine on the pharmacokinetics of theophylline in healthy subjects. *Int J Clin Pharmacol Ther Toxicol*, 27, 308-312 (1989)

6607 Yoshinari M, Yamamoto M, Wakisaka M, et al. Effect of bezafibrate on hypercoagulability assessed by fluorogenic prothrombin time in hyperlipidemic patients with non-insulin-dependent diabetes mellitus. *Thromb Res*, 86, 443-451 (1997)

6608 Yoshino G, Kazumi T, Iwai M, et al. Effects of CS-514 on plasma lipids and lipoprotein composition in hypercholesterolemic subjects. *Atherosclerosis*, 71, 95-101 (1988)

6609 Yoshioka K. Elevation and fluctuation of serum CA 19-9 and SPAN-1 levels after administration of sulfonylurea in a diabetic patient with Lewis(a-,b-) blood phenotype. *Diabetes Care*, 18, 1397-1399 (1995)

6610 Yoshioka K, Azukari K, Yoshida T, Kondo M. Rapid improvement of serum 1,5-anhydroglucitol concentrations after administration of α-glucosidase inhibitor. *Diabetes Care*, 20, 462 (1997)

6611 Yosselson-Superstine S, Sinai Y. Drug interference with urine protein determination. *J Clin Chem Clin Biochem*, 24, 103-106 (1986)

6612 Young DS. *Personal Observation*

6613 Young GP, Bhathal PS, Sullivan JR, et al. Fatal hepatic coma complicating oxymetholone therapy in multiple myeloma. *Aust NZ J Med*, 7, 47-51 (1977)

6614 Young GP, Sullivan J, Hurley T. Hypokalaemia due to gentamicin/cephalexin in leukemia. *Lancet*, 2, 855 (1973)

6615 Young MA, Lettis S, Eastmond R. Concomitant administration of cholestyramine influences the absorption of troglitazone. *Br J Clin Pharmacol*, 45, 37-40 (1998)

6616 Young MM, Jasani C, Smith DA, et al. Some effects of ethinyl oestradiol on calcium and phosphorus metabolism in osteoporosis. *Clin Sci*, 34, 411 (1968)

6617 Young RC, Nachman RL, Horowitz HI. Thrombocytopenia due to digitoxin. *Am J Med*, 41, 605 (1966)

6618 Young RE, Ramsay LE, Murray TS. Barbiturates and serum calcium in the elderly. *Postgrad Med J*, 53, 212-215 (1977)

6619 Young SG, Witztum JL, Carew TE, et al. Colestipol-induced changes in LDL composition and metabolism. II Studies in humans. *J Lipid Res*, 30, 225-238 (1989)

6620 Young SN, Gauthier S, Anderson GM, et al. Tryptophan, 5-hydroxyindoleacetic acid and indoleacetic acid in human cerebrospinal fluid: interrelationships and the influence of age, sex, epilepsy and anticonvulsant drugs. *J Neurol Neurosurg Psychiatry*, 43, 438-445 (1980)

6621 Ytre-Arne K, Nordoy A. Simvastatin and cholestyramine in the long-term treatment of hypercholesterolaemia. *J Intern Med*, 226, 285-290 (1989)

6622 Yu TF, Berger L, Gutman AB. Hypoglycemic and uricosuric properties of acetohexamide and hydroxyhexamide. *Metabolism*, 17, 309 (1968)

6623 Zaccara G, Gangemi PF, Bendoni L, et al. Influence of single and repeated doses of oxcarbazepine on the pharmacokinetic profile of felodipine. *Ther Drug Monit*, 15, 39-42 (1993)

6624 Zaccaria M, Giordano G, Pasquali C, et al. Effects of pirenzepine on plasma insulin, glucagon and pancreatic polypeptide levels in normal man. *Eur J Clin Pharmacol*, 27, 701-705 (1985)

6625 Zacharieva S, Stoeva I, Matrozov P, et al. Serum aldosterone response to metoclopramide in normal subjects and acromegalic patients. *Exp Clin Endocrinol*, 95, 331-338 (1990)

6626 Zager PG, Frey HJ, Gerdes BG. Plasma 18-hydoxycorticosterone during continuous ambulatory peritoneal dialysis. *J Lab Clin Med*, 102, 604-612 (1983)

6627 Zametkin AJ, Hamburger SD. The effect of methylphenidate on urinary catecholamine excretion in hyperactivity: a partial replication. *Biol Psychiat*, 23, 350-356 (1988)

6628 Zametkin AJ, Karoum F, Linnoila M, et al. Stimulants, urinary catecholamines, and indoleamines in hyperactivity. A comparison of methylphenidate and dextroamphetamine. *Arch Gen Psychiat*, 42, 251-255 (1985)

6629 Zanaboni L, Bonfiglioli D, Sommariva D, et al. Increase in lipolysis and decrease in plasma-heparin lipoprotein lipase activity and alpha$_1$ lipoprotein level after aminophylline in man. *Eur J Clin Pharmacol*, 19, 349-351 (1981)

6630 Zannad F, Bray-Desboscs L, El Ghawi R, et al. Effects of lisinopril and hydrochlorothiazide on platelet function and blood rheology in essential hypertension: a randomly allocated double-blind study. *J Hypertens*, 11, 559-564 (1993)

6631 Zantvoort FA, Derkx FHM, Boomsma F, et al. Theophylline and serum electrolytes. *Ann Intern Med*, 104, 134 (1986)

6632 Zarembski PM, Hodgkinson A, Cochran M. Treatment of primary hyperoxaluria with calcium carbimide. *N Engl J Med*, 277, 1000 (1967)

6633 Zarrabi MH, Zucker S, Miller F, et al. Immunologic and coagulation disorders in chlorpromazine-treated patients. *Ann Intern Med*, 91, 194-199 (1979)

6634 Zatz M, Rapaport D, Vainzof M, et al. Effect of mazindol on growth hormone levels in patients with Duchenne muscular dystrophy. *Am J Med Genet*, 31, 821-833 (1988)

6635 Zavagli G, Taddeo U, Bolelli G, et al. Platelet aggregation and evaluation of the ratio thromboxane B$_2$/6-keto-prostaglandin F1α in the plasma of patients on long-term cimetidine treatment. *Prostaglandins Leukot Med*, 19, 241-250 (1985)

6636 Zavaral JH, Haggerty BJ, Winick AG, et al. Efficacy of fluvastatin, a totally synthetic 3-hydroxy-3-methylglutaryl Coenzyme A reductase inhibitor. *Am J Cardiol*, 76, 37A-40A (1995)

6637 Zazgornik J, Schein W, Heimberger K, et al. Potentiation of neurotoxic side effects by coadministartion of imipenem to cyclosporine therapy in kidney transplant recipient - synergism of side effects or drug interaction. *Clin Nephrol*, 26, 265-266 (1986)

6638 Zeegers JJ, Maas AH, Willebrands AF, et al. The radioimmunoassay of plasma digoxin. *Clin Chim Acta*, 44, 109 (1973)

6639 Zelaschi NM, Delucchi GA, Rodriguez JL. High plasma prolactin levels after long-term neuroleptic treatment. *Biol Psychiat*, 39, 900-901 (1996)

6640 Zemba-Palko V, Lacher D. Serum magnesium as affected by drugs. *Clin Chem*, 34, 1913 (1988)

6641 Zeneca Pharmaceuticals. Manufacturer's literature on Accolate® . Wilmington, DE (1997)

6642 Zeneca Pharmaceuticals. Manufacturer's literature on Arimdex® . Wilmington, DE 19850 (1997)

6643 Zeneca Pharmaceuticals. Manufacturer's literature on Casodex® . Wilmington, DE 19850 (1997)

6644 Zeneca Pharmaceuticals. Manufacturer's literature on Cefotan® . Wilmington, DE (1997)

6645 Zeneca Pharmaceuticals. Manufacturer's literature on Elavil® . Wilmington, DE 19850 (1996)

6646 Zeneca Pharmaceuticals. Manufacturer's literature on Kadian™. Wilmington, DE (1997)

6647 Zeneca Pharmaceuticals. Manufacturer's literature on Merrem® . Wilmington, DE (1997)

6648 Zeneca Pharmaceuticals. Manufacturer's literature on Nolvadex® . Wilmington, DE (1997)

6649 Zeneca Pharmaceuticals. Manufacturer's literature on Sorbitrate® . Wilmington, DE (1997)

6650 Zeneca Pharmaceuticals. Manufacturer's literature on Sular® . Wilmington, DE (1996)

6651 Zeneca Pharmaceuticals. Manufacturer's literature on Zestril® . Wilmington, DE (1997)

6652 Zeneca Pharmaceuticals. Manufacturer's literature on Zoladex® . Wilmington, DE (1997)

6653 Zeneca Pharmaceuticals. Manufacturer's literature on Zomig™. Wilmington, DE 19850 (1997)

6654 Zernechel CF. Aminopyrine and agranulocytosis: review and report of six cases. *NC Med J*, 28, 91 (1967)

6655 Zhao S-P, Smelt AHM, Gevers Leuven JA, et al. Changes of lipoprotein profile in familial dysbetalipoproteinemia with gemfibrozil. *Am J Med*, 96, 49-55 (1994)

6656 Zhiri A, Houot O, Wellman-Bednawska M, et al. Simultaneous determination of uric acid and creatinine in plasma by reversed-phase liquid chromatography. *Clin Chem*, 31, 109-112 (1985)

6657 Zhiri A, Wellman-Bednawska M, Siest G. 6β-hydroxycortisol in human urine: diurnal variations and effects of antiepileptic therapy. *Clin Chim Acta*, 157, 267-276 (1986)

6658 Ziegler MG, Chernow B, Woodson LC, et al. The effect of propranolol on catecholamine clearance. *Clin Pharmacol Ther*, 40, 116-119 (1986)

6659 Zielinski JJ, Haidukewych D, Lehata BJ. Carbamazepine-phenytoin interaction: elevation of plasma phenytoin concentrations due to carbamazepine comedication. *Ther Drug Monit*, 7, 51-53 (1985)

6660 Zielinski JJ, Lichten EM, Haidukewych D. Clinically significant danazol-carbamazepine interaction. *Ther Drug Monit*, 9, 24-27 (1987)

6661 Zielinski RM, Lawrence WD. Interferon-α for the hypereosinophilic syndrome. *Ann Intern Med*, 113, 716-718 (1990)

6662 Zietse R, Wenting FJ, Kramer P, et al. Fractional excretion of protein: a marker of the efficacy of cyclosporine A treatment in nephrotic syndrome. *Transplant Proc*, 20, Suppl 4, 280-284 (1988)

6663 Zilembo N, Noerasco C, Bajetta E, et al. Endocrinological and clinical evaluation of exemestane, a new steroidal aromatase inhibitor. *Br J Cancer*, 72, 1007-1012 (1995)

6664 Zilly W, Breimer DD, Richter E. Induction of drug metabolism in man after rifampicin treatment measured by increased hexobarbital and tolbutamide clearance. *Eur J Clin Pharmacol*, 9, 219-227 (1975)

6665 Zilly W, Breimer DD, Richter E. Pharmacokinetic interactions with rifampicin. *Clin Pharmacokinet*, 2, 61-70 (1977)

6666 Zimmermann HJ. Effects of aspirin and acetaminophen on the liver. *Arch Intern Med*, 141, 333-342 (1981)

6667 Zimmermann J, Fainaru M, Eisenberg S. The effects of prednisone therapy on plasma lipoproteins and apolipoproteins: a prospective study. *Metabolism*, 33, 521-526 (1984)

6668 Zinzani PL, Lauria F, Rondelli D, et al. Fludarabine in patients with advanced and/or resistant B-chronic lymphocytic leukemia. *Eur J Haematol*, 51, 93-97 (1993)

6669 Zipes DP, Prystowsky EN, Heger JJ. Amiodarone: electrophysiologic actions, pharmacokinetics and clinical effects. *J Am Coll Cardiol*, 3, 1057-1071 (1984)

6670 Ziporin ZZ, Chambers JS, Taylor RR, et al. The effect of isoniazid administration on the blood ammonia in tuberculous patients. *Am Rev Resp Dis*, 86, 21 (1962)

6671 Zirbes PM, Khaja G, Narahari M. Interference of Rocephin in salicylate determination. *Clin Chem*, 37, 934 (1991)

6672 Zis AP, Haskett RF, Arlav Albala A, et al. Morphine inhibits cortisol and stimulates prolactin secretion in man. *Psychoneuroendocrinology*, 9, 423-427 (1984)

6673 Zis AP, Remick RA, Clark CM, et al. Effect of morphine on cortisol and prolactin secretion in anorexia nervosa and depression. *Clin Endocrinol*, 30, 421-427 (1989)

6674 Zishka MK, Nishimura JS. Effect of glycerol on Lowry and biuret methods of protein determination. *Anal Biochem*, 34, 291 (1970)

6675 Ziun M, Grandinetti G, Camisasca M, et al. A comparison of cholestyramine and diethylaminoethyl-dextran for the treatment of hyperlipidemia and pruritus of primary biliary cirrhosis. *Cur Ther Res Clin Exp*, 49, 622-626 (1991)

6676 Zofkova I. The effect of long-term verapamil treatment on the secretion of cortisol and aldosterone in subjects with normal and high blood pressure. *Exp Clin Endocrinol*, 85, 217-222 (1985)

6677 Zofkova I, Laberg-Allardt C, Kancheva RL, et al. Effect of hypermagnesemia on the adenohypophyseal-gonadal function, parathyroid hormone secretion and some other hormonal indicators. *Horm Metab Res*, 25, 29-33 (1993)

6678 Zofkova I, Scholz G, Starka L. Effect of calcitonin and 1,25$(OH)_2$-vitamin D_3 on the FSH, LH and testosterone secretion at rest and LHRH stimulated secretion. *Horm Metab Res*, 21, 682-685 (1989)

6679 Zohrens G, Armbrust T, Meyer Zum Buschenfelde K-H. Interferon-α_2a increases serum concentration of hyaluronic acid and type III procollagen aminoterminal propeptide in patients with chronic hepatitis B virus infection. *Dig Dis Sci*, 39, 2007-2013 (1994)

6680 Zollner N, Heimstadt P. Effects of a single administration of L-asparaginase on serum lipids. *Nutr Metab*, 13, 344 (1971)

6681 Zondag HA, Van Boetzelaer GL. Determination of protein in cerebrospinal fluid: sources of error in the Lowry method. *Clin Chim Acta*, 5, 155 (1960)

6682 Zsigmond EK, Flynn K. The effect of methotrimeprazine on arterial blood gases in human volunteers. *J Clin Pharmacol*, 28, 1033-1037 (1988)

6683 Zsigmond EK, Flynn K, Shively JG. Effect of hydroxyzine and meperidine on arterial blood gases in patients with chronic obstructive pulmonary disease. *Int J Clin Pharmacol Ther Toxicol*, 31, 124-129 (1993)

6684 Zsigmond EK, Robins G. The effect of a series of anticancer drugs on plasma cholinesterase activity. *Can J Anaes*, 19, 75 (1972)

6685 Zuck TF, Bergin JJ, Perkins RP. Antithrombin III and oestrogen content of oral contraceptives. *Lancet*, 1, 831 (1973)

6686 Zuck TF, Bergin JJ, Raymond JM, et al. Implications of depressed antithrombin III activity associated with oral contraceptives. *Surg Gynecol Obstet*, 133, 609 (1971)

6687 Zucker ML, Budd SE, Dollar LE, et al. Effect of diltiazem and low-dose aspirin on platelet aggregation and ATP release indced by paired agonists. *Thromb Haemostas*, 70, 332-335 (1993)

6688 Zucker P, Daum F, Cohen MI. Aspirin hepatitis. *Am J Dis Child*, 129, 1433-1434 (1975)

6689 Zumkley H, Bertram HP, Preusser P, et al. Renal excretion of magnesium and trace elements during cisplatin treatment. *Clin Nephrol*, 17, 254-257 (1982)

6690 Zusman R, Christensen D, Federman E, et al. Comparison of nifedipine and propranolol used in combination with diuretics for the treatment of hypertension. *Am J Med*, 82, 37-41 (1987)

6691 Zuspan FP, Talledo OE, Chesley LC, et al. Angiotensin and norepinephrine infusions during pregnancy: alterations in plasma epinephrine and norepinephrine. *J Clin Endocrinol Metab*, 33, 929 (1971)

6692 Zweig MH, Jackson A. Ascorbic acid interference in reagent strip reactions for assay of urinary glucose and hemoglobin. *Clin Chem*, 32, 674-677 (1986)

6693 Zweig MH, Nichols HC. Interference with spinal fluid protein results. *Personal Communication*

6694 Zwirska-Korczala K, Kucharzewski M, Buntner B, et al. Serum ferritin, iron and transferrin changes in women with Graves disease before and after methimazole treatment. *Biochim Clin*, 13, Suppl 1/8, 222 (1989)